# Bone and Joint
# IMAGING

## THIRD EDITION

## Donald Resnick, MD

Chief, Musculoskeletal Imaging
Professor of Radiology
University of California, San Diego
San Diego, California

## Mark J. Kransdorf, MD

Chief, Musculoskeletal Imaging
Mayo Clinic
Jacksonville, Florida
Professor of Radiology
Mayo Clinic College of Medicine
Rochester, Minnesota

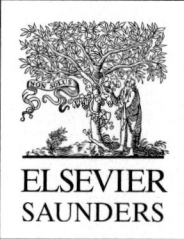

**ELSEVIER**
**SAUNDERS**

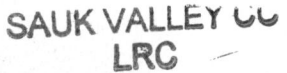

**ELSEVIER**
**SAUNDERS**

The Curtis Center
170 S Independence Mall W 300E
Philadelphia, Pennsylvania 19106

BONE AND JOINT IMAGING                                          ISBN 0-7216-0270-3
**Copyright © 2005, 1996, 1989 by Elsevier Inc.**

---

### NOTICE

Radiology is an ever-changing field. Standard safety precautions must be followed, but as new research and clinical experience broaden our knowledge, changes in treatment and drug therapy may become necessary or appropriate. Readers are advised to check the most current product information provided by the manufacturer of each drug to be administered to verify the recommended dose, the method and duration of administration, and contraindications. It is the responsibility of the treating physician, relying on experience and knowledge of the patient, to determine dosages and the best treatment for each individual patient. Neither the Publisher nor the author assumes any liability for any injury and/or damage to persons or property arising from this publication.

---

**Library of Congress Cataloging-in-Publication Data**

Resnick, Donald.
    Bone and joint imaging/Donald Resnick, Mark J. Kransdorf. – 3rd ed.
        p.; cm.
    Includes bibliographical references and index.
    ISBN 0-7216-0270-3
        1. Bones—Imaging.   2. Joints—Imaging.   3. Bones—Diseases—Diagnosis.
    4. Joints—Diseases—Diagnosis.   I. Kransdorf, Mark J.   II. Title.
        [DNLM: 1. Bone Diseases—diagnosis.   2. Diagnostic Imaging—methods.
    3. Joint Diseases—diagnosis. WE 141 R434b 2005]
    RC930.5.R47 2005
    616.7′10754—dc22                                              2003070436

*Executive Editor:* Allan Ross
*Senior Developmental Editor:* Janice M. Gaillard
*Project Manager:* Linda Lewis Grigg
*Design Manager:* Gene Harris

Printed in USA

Last digit is the print number:  9   8   7   6   5   4   3   2   1

*To our residents and fellows*
*— for their motivation, enthusiasm, and, most important, inspiration*

# CONTRIBUTORS

**Ronald S. Adler, M.D., Ph.D.**
Professor of Radiology, Cornell University Joan and Sanford
I. Weill Medical College and Graduate School of Medical
Sciences; Attending Radiologist, Hospital for Special Surgery,
New York, New York

Diagnostic Ultrasonography

**Wayne H. Akeson, M.D.**
Emeritus Professor of Orthopaedics, University of California,
San Diego, School of Medicine, La Jolla; Chief of
Orthopaedics, Veterans Affairs San Diego Healthcare System,
San Diego, California

Articular Cartilage: Morphology, Physiology, and Function

**Robert Downey Boutin, M.D.**
Executive Musculoskeletal Radiologist, Med-Tel International,
McLean, Virginia

Muscle Disorders

**William Bugbee, M.D.**
Assistant Professor, Department of Orthopaedics,
University of California, San Diego,
School of Medicine, La Jolla, California

Articular Cartilage: Morphology, Physiology, and Function

**Constance R. Chu, M.D.**
Assistant Professor, University of Pittsburgh School of
Medicine; Director, Cartilage Restoration, University of
Pittsburgh Medical Center, Pittsburgh, Pennsylvania

Articular Cartilage: Morphology, Physiology, and Function

**Christine B. Chung, M.D.**
Assistant Professor of Radiology, University of California,
San Diego, School of Medicine, La Jolla; Department of
Radiology, Veterans Affairs San Diego Healthcare System,
San Diego, California

Developmental Dysplasia of the Hip

**James M. Coumas, M.D.**
Musculoskeletal Radiologist, Carolina Hospital Authority,
Charlotte, North Carolina

Interventional Spinal Procedures

**Murray K. Dalinka, M.D.**
Professor of Radiology, Hospital of the University of
Pennsylvania, Philadelphia, Pennsylvania

Radiation Changes

**Jerry R. Dwek, M.D.**
Assistant Clinical Professor, University of California,
San Diego, School of Medicine, La Jolla;
Department of Orthopaedic Surgery,
Veterans Affairs San Diego Healthcare System,
San Diego, California

Developmental Dysplasia of the Hip

**Michael D. Fallon, M.D.\***
Former Assistant Professor of Pathology, University of
Pennsylvania School of Medicine, Philadelphia, Pennsylvania
*deceased

Histogenesis, Anatomy, and Physiology of Bone

**Frieda Feldman, M.D.**
Professor of Radiology, Columbia College of Physicians and
Surgeons; Attending Radiologist, New York Presbyterian
Hospital, New York, New York

Tuberous Sclerosis, Neurofibromatosis, and Fibrous Dysplasia

**Steven R. Garfin, M.D.**
Chairman, Department of Orthopaedic Surgery, University of
California, San Diego, University of California, San Diego,
Medical Center, San Diego, California

Imaging after Spinal Surgery

**Thomas G. Goergen, M.D.**
Associate Clinical Professor, University of California,
San Diego, School of Medicine, La Jolla; Palomar Medical
Center, Escondido, California

Physical Injury: Concepts and Terminology

**Amy Beth Goldman, M.D.**
New York, New York

Heritable Diseases of Connective Tissue, Epiphyseal
Dysplasias, and Related Conditions

**Guerdon D. Greenway, M.D.**
Associate Clinical Professor, Department of Radiology,
University of California, San Diego, School of Medicine,
La Jolla, California; Clinical Associate Professor, Department
of Orthopaedic Surgery, University of Texas Southwestern
Medical Center, Dallas; Attending Physician, Department of
Radiology, Baylor University Medical Center, Dallas, Texas

Tumors and Tumor-like Lesions of Bone: Imaging and
Pathology of Specific Lesions

**W. Bonner Guilford, M.D.**
Musculoskeletal Radiologist, Charlotte Radiology,
Carolina Healthcare System, Charlotte, North Carolina

Interventional Spinal Procedures

**Parviz Haghighi, M.D., F.R.C.P.A.**
Professor of Clinical Pathology, University of California,
San Diego; Staff Pathologist, Veterans Affairs Medical Center,
San Diego, California

Lymphoproliferative and Myeloproliferative Disorders

**Tamara Miner Haygood, M.D., Ph.D.**
Radiology Associates, Corpus Christi, Texas

Radiation Changes

**Thomas E. Herman, M.D.**
Associate Professor, Mallinckrodt Institute of Radiology
and Washington University School of Medicine; Radiologist,
St. Louis Children's Hospital, St. Louis, Missouri

Osteochondrodysplasias, Dysostoses, Chromosomal
Aberrations, Mucopolysaccharidoses, and Mucolipidoses

**Brian A. Howard, M.D., M.B.C.H.B.**
Musculoskeletal Radiologist, Charlotte Radiology,
Carolina Healthcare System, Charlotte, North Carolina

Interventional Spinal Procedures

**Phoebe A. Kaplan, M.D.**
Montreal, Quebec, Canada

Temporomandibular Joint

**Michael Kyriakos, M.D.**
Professor of Surgical Pathology, Washington University
School of Medicine; Senior Pathologist, Barnes Hospital,
St. Louis, Missouri

Tumors and Tumor-like Lesions of Bone: Imaging
and Pathology of Specific Lesions

**Laurence A. Mack, M.D.***
Former Professor of Radiology, Adjunct Professor of
Orthopedics, and Director of Ultrasound, University of
Washington, Seattle, Washington
*deceased

Diagnostic Ultrasonography

**John E. Madewell, M.D.**
Professor of Radiology and Director of Clinical Radiology
Operations, University of Texas M. D. Anderson Cancer
Center, Houston, Texas

Osteonecrosis: Pathogenesis, Diagnostic Techniques,
Specific Situations, and Complications

**Stavros C. Manolagas, M.D., Ph.D.**
Professor of Medicine and Director, Division of
Endocrinology and Metabolism, University of Arkansas for
Medical Sciences, Little Rock, Arkansas

Histogenesis, Anatomy, and Physiology of Bone

**William H. McAlister, M.D.**
Professor of Radiology and Pediatrics, Washington University
School of Medicine and Mallinckrodt Institute of Radiology;
Radiologist-in-Chief, St. Louis Children's Hospital, St. Louis,
Missouri

Osteochondrodysplasias, Dysostoses, Chromosomal
Aberrations, Mucopolysaccharidoses, and Mucolipidoses

**William A. Murphy, Jr., M.D.**
John S. Dunn, Sr., Distinguished Chair and Professor of
Radiology, University of Texas M. D. Anderson Cancer
Center, Houston, Texas

Temporomandibular Joint

**M. B. Ozonoff, M.D.**
Salt Lake City, Utah

Spinal Anomalies and Curvatures

**Mini N. Pathria, M.D.**
Professor of Clinical Radiology, University of California,
San Diego, School of Medicine, La Jolla, California

Imaging after Spinal Surgery; Physical Injury: Spine

**Michael J. Pitt, M.D.**
Professor of Radiology, University of Alabama School of
Medicine; Staff, University Hospital, UAB Children's Hospital
of Alabama, Birmingham, Alabama

Rickets and Osteomalacia

**Jeffrey S. Ross, M.D.**
Head, Radiology Research, and Staff Neuroradiologist,
Cleveland Clinic Foundation, Cleveland, Ohio

Spinal Imaging

**David A. Rubin, M.D.**
Associate Professor of Radiology, Washington University
School of Medicine; Director, Musculoskeletal Section,
Mal&linckrodt Institute of Radiology, St. Louis, Missouri

Magnetic Resonance Imaging: Practical Considerations

**David J. Sartoris, M.D.***
Former Professor of Radiology, University of California,
San Diego; Chief, Quantitative Bone Densitometry,
UCSD Medical Center; Professor of Radiology, Veterans
Affairs Medical Center and Scripps Clinic, Green Hospital,
La Jolla, California
*deceased

Developmental Dysplasia of the Hip

**F. William Scheible, M.D.**
Radiology Consultants of Iowa, Cedar Rapids, Iowa

Diagnostic Ultrasonography

**Robert Schneider, M.D.**
Associate Professor of Radiology, Cornell University Joan
and Sanford I. Weill Medical College and Graduate School of
Medical Sciences; Attending Radiologist, Hospital for Special
Surgery, New York, New York

Radionuclide Techniques

**Carolyn M. Sofka, M.D.**
Associate Professor of Radiology, Cornell University Joan
and Sanford I. Weill Medical College and Graduate School
of Medical Sciences; Assistant Attending Radiologist,
Hospital for Special Surgery, New York, New York

> Diagnostic Ultrasonography

**Donald E. Sweet, M.D.***
Former Clinical Professor of Pathology, Georgetown University
School of Medicine, Washington, D.C.; Clinical Professor
of Pathology, Uniformed Services University of Health
Sciences, Bethesda, Maryland; Chairman, Department of
Orthopedic Pathology, Armed Forces Institute of Pathology,
Washington, D.C.
*deceased

> Osteonecrosis: Pathogenesis, Diagnostic Techniques,
> Specific Situations, and Complications

**Barbara N. Weissman, M.D.**
Professor of Radiology, Harvard Medical School; Vice Chair
for Ambulatory Services, Brigham and Women's Hospital,
Boston, Massachusetts

> Imaging after Surgery in Extraspinal Sites; Imaging of Joint
> Replacement

# PREFACE

Nine years after the publication of the second edition of **Bone and Joint Imaging** and a few years after the publication of the fourth edition of the larger **Diagnosis of Bone and Joint Disorders**, the third edition of **Bone and Joint Imaging** is now ready for dissemination. In common with the first and second editions of this text, the purpose of this book is to present in a logical manner and easy-to-read format the information that we, the authors, believe is essential for those learning musculoskeletal imaging for the first time or for those reviewing the subject one more time. The subject of musculoskeletal imaging is ever changing and constantly growing in scope. Much of this growth relates not to the discovery of new processes or disorders but rather to the development and refinement of advanced imaging methods and techniques. Diagnostic methods now applied routinely to the analysis of musculoskeletal disorders include far more than conventional radiography: CT scanning, MR imaging, ultrasonography, radionuclide studies, and arthrography are among the additional methods that must be mastered by those interpreting images related to bone, joint, and soft tissue disorders. To summarize adequately the many imaging techniques and findings in a text any shorter than this, in our view, would not be appropriate or even possible.

The organization of the text follows that of the previous edition. Basic anatomy and physiology, diagnostic techniques, and postoperative imaging serve as introductory material; this material is then followed by sections dealing with imaging of most of the important diseases that affect the musculoskeletal system. Key images have been selected to illustrate the most important of the imaging findings, and a short but appropriate bibliography is included in each chapter. As before, we have included shortened versions of many chapters written by experts in the field that were part of the larger multivolume textbook. When compared with the second edition, however, there are significant changes in this third edition. Many subjects appear for the first time, countless new and improved illustrations are included, and references are updated. And to do this properly and on time, two editors rather than one have accomplished this task.

Both of us are confident that we have succeeded in condensing the essential material related to musculoskeletal imaging in a manageable textbook. But it is the readers who are the ultimate judge. We are hopeful that whether it is used for consultation on an intermittent basis or read in its entirety, the readers will enjoy the experience and be wiser for it.

Donald Resnick
Mark J. Kransdorf

# ACKNOWLEDGMENTS

We are greatly indebted to a number of individuals without whom this project would not be possible. This includes our many contributing authors, all of whom are highly regarded educators and experts in their respective fields. Their efforts are very much appreciated.

A very special thanks must go to Allan Ross, Executive Editor, and his associates at Elsevier: Janice M. Gaillard, Senior Developmental Editor; Linda Lewis Grigg, Project Manager, Book Production; and Walter Verbitski, Illustration Specialist.

We would also like to acknowledge those individuals whose dedication, commitment, and energy often go unnoticed but who keep the system running smoothly and on time: our administrative assistants Michael Holbrook, Debra Trudell, and Pamela J. Chirico.

# CONTENTS

# Basic Science

# CHAPTER 1

## Histogenesis, Anatomy, and Physiology of Bone

### Donald Resnick, Stavros C. Manolagas, and Michael D. Fallon

## SUMMARY OF KEY FEATURES

Bone is a unique tissue that is constantly undergoing change. It develops through the processes of endochondral and intramembranous ossification and is subsequently modified and refined by the processes of modeling and remodeling to create a structurally and metabolically competent, highly organized architectural marvel. Its cells, including osteoblasts, osteocytes, and osteoclasts, reside in organic matrix, primarily collagen, and inorganic material is deposited in a form that resembles hydroxyapatite. The process of mineralization is complex and incompletely understood.

Bone is essential in maintaining calcium homeostasis, or stabilization of the plasma level of calcium. Its cells are highly responsive to stimuli provided by a number of humoral agents, the most important of which are parathyroid hormone, thyrocalcitonin, and 1,25-dihydroxyvitamin D. Synthesis and resorption of bone, which normally continue in a delicate balance throughout life, are mediated by the action of such humoral agents through processes that include stimulation of osteoblasts to form bone and stimulation of osteoclasts to remove bone.

## INTRODUCTION

Bone is a remarkable tissue. Although its appearance on radiographs might be misinterpreted as indicating inactivity, bone is constantly undergoing change. This occurs not only in the immature skeleton, in which growth and development are readily apparent, but also in the mature skeleton, through the constant and balanced processes of bone formation and resorption. It is when these processes are modified such that one dominates, that a pathologic state may be created. In some instances, the resulting imbalance between bone formation and resorption is easily detectable on the radiograph. In others, a more subtle imbalance exists that may be identified only at the histologic level.

The initial architecture of bone is characterized by an irregular network of collagen, termed woven-fibered bone, which is a temporary material that is either removed to form a marrow cavity or subsequently replaced by a sheetlike arrangement of osseous tissue, termed parallel-fibered, or lamellar, bone. As a connective tissue, bone is highly specialized and differs from other connective tissue by its rigidity and hardness, which relate primarily to the inorganic salts that are deposited in its matrix. These properties are fundamental to a tissue that must maintain the shape of the human body, protect its vital soft tissues, and allow locomotion by transmitting from one region of the body to another the forces generated by the contractions of various muscles. Bone also serves as a reservoir for ions, principally calcium, that are essential to normal fluid regulation; these ions are made available as a response to stimuli produced by a number of hormones, particularly parathyroid hormone, vitamin D, and calcitonin.

## HISTOGENESIS

### Developing Bone

Bone develops by the process of intramembranous bone formation (transformation of condensed mesenchymal tissue), endochondral bone formation (indirect conversion of an intermediate cartilage model), or both. At some locations, such as the bones of the cranial vault (frontal and parietal bones, as well as parts of the occipital and temporal bones), the mandible and maxilla, and the midportion of the clavicle, intramembranous (mesenchymal) ossification is detected; in other locations, such as the bones of the extremities, the vertebral column, the pelvis, and the base of the skull, both endochondral and intramembranous ossification can be identified. The actual processes of bone tissue formation are essentially the same in both intramembranous and endochondral ossification and include the following sequence: (1) osteoblasts differentiate from mesenchymal cells; (2) osteoblasts deposit matrix, which is subsequently mineralized; (3) bone is initially deposited as a network of immature (woven) trabeculae, the primary spongiosa; and (4) the primary spongiosa is replaced by secondary bone, removed to form bone marrow, or converted to primary cortical bone by the filling of spaces between trabeculae.

### Intramembranous Ossification

Intramembranous ossification is initiated by the proliferation of mesenchymal cells about a network of capillaries. At this site, transformation of the mesenchymal cells is accompanied by the appearance of a meshwork of collagen fibers and amorphous ground substance. The primitive cells proliferate, enlarge, and become arranged in groups, transforming into osteoblasts, which are intimately involved in the formation of an eosinophilic matrix within the collagenous tissue. As the osteoid matrix undergoes calcification with the deposition of calcium phosphate, some of the osteoblasts on the surface of the osteoid and woven-fibered bone become entrapped within the substance of the matrix in a space called a lacuna. These cells, now osteocytes, maintain the integrity of the surrounding matrix and are not directly involved in bone formation. Through the continued transformation of mesenchymal cells into osteoblasts, elaboration of an osteoid matrix, and entrapment of osteoblasts within the matrix, the primitive mesenchyme is converted into osseous tissue.

The ultimate characteristics of the tissue depend on its location within the bone: in cancellous areas of the bone, the meshwork of osseous tissue contains intervening vascular connective tissue, representing the embryonic precursor of the bone marrow; in compact areas of the bone, the osseous tissue becomes more condensed and forms cylindric masses containing a central vascular channel, the haversian system. On the external and internal surfaces of the compact bone, fibrovascular layers develop (periosteum and endosteum) and contain cells that remain osteogenic and give bone its ever-changing quality.

### Endochondral Ossification

In endochondral (intracartilaginous) ossification, cartilaginous tissue derived from mesenchyme serves as a template and is replaced with bone (Fig. 1–1). The initial

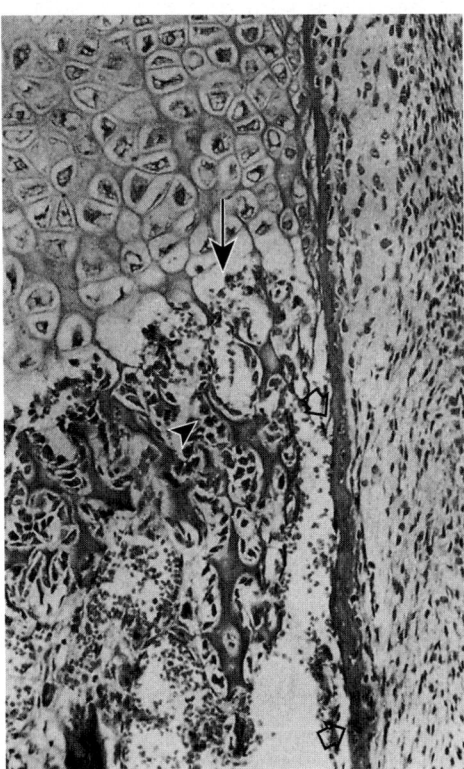

**Figure 1–1.** Endochondral and intramembranous ossification in a tubular bone: radius of a 4½-month-old fetus. The large and confluent cartilage cell lacunae are being penetrated by vascular channels *(solid arrow)*, thereby exposing intervening cores of calcified cartilage matrix. The osteoblasts are depositing osseous tissue on these cartilage matrix cores *(arrowhead)*. Observe the subperiosteal bone formation *(open arrows)*.

sites of bone formation are called centers of ossification. In tubular bones, the primary center of ossification is located in the central portion of the cartilaginous model, whereas later-appearing centers of ossification (secondary centers) are located at the ends of the models within epiphyses and apophyses. Vascular mesenchymal tissue or perichondrium, whose deeper layers contain cells with osteogenic potential, surrounds the cartilaginous model.

The initial changes in the primary center of ossification are hypertrophy of cartilage cells, glycogen accumulation, and reduction of intervening matrix. Subsequently, these cells degenerate, die, and become calcified. Simultaneously, the deeper or subperichondrial cells undergo transformation to osteoblasts, and through a process identical to intramembranous ossification, these osteoblasts produce a subperiosteal collar or cuff of bone that encloses the central portions of the cartilaginous tissue. Periosteal tissue is converted into vascular channels, and the aggressive vascular tissue disrupts the lacunae of the cartilage cells and creates spaces that fill with embryonic bone marrow. Osteoblasts appear and transform the sites of degenerating and dying cartilage cells into foci of ossification by laying down osteoid tissue in the cartilage matrix. Osteoblasts become trapped within the developing bone as osteocytes.

From the center of the tubular bone, ossification proceeds toward the ends of the bone. Similarly, the periosteal collar, which is actively participating in intramembranous ossification, spreads toward the ends of the bone, slightly ahead of the band of endochondral ossification. Through a process of subperiosteal deposition of bone, a cortex becomes evident, grows thicker, and is converted into a system with longitudinally arranged compact bone surrounding vascular channels (haversian system). The front of endochondral ossification that is advancing toward the end of the bone becomes better delineated, and it is this plate that ultimately becomes located between the epiphysis and diaphysis of a tubular bone and forms the growth plate (cartilaginous plate or physis). The plate contains clearly demarcated zones: a resting zone of flattened and immature cells on the epiphyseal aspect of the plate, as well as zones of cell growth and hypertrophy and of transformation, with provisional calcification and ossification on the metaphyseal or diaphyseal aspect of the plate.

The size and shape of the most recently formed portion of the metaphysis of a tubular bone depend on the effects of an encircling fibrochondro-osseous structure, designated the periphysis, that consists of the zone of Ranvier, the ring of La Croix, and the bone bark that they produce (Fig. 1–2). In this setting of progressive ossification of the diaphysis with longitudinal spread toward the ends of the bone, characteristic changes appear within the epiphysis. Epiphyseal invasion by vascular channels is followed by the initiation of endochondral bone formation, which creates secondary centers of ossification. The process is again characterized by cartilage cell hypertrophy and death, followed by calcification.

The epiphyseal ossification center at first develops rapidly, although later the process slows. The epiphyseal cartilage is thus converted to bone, although a layer on its articular aspect persists and is destined to become the

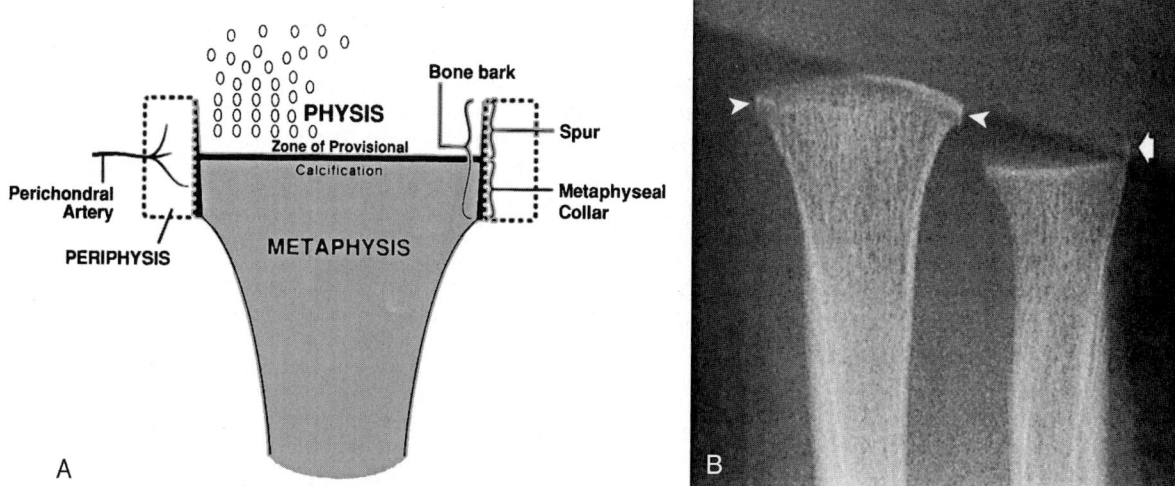

**Figure 1–2.** Endochondral and intramembranous ossification in a tubular bone: periphysis and metaphyseal collar. *A,* In this diagram, observe the periphysis *(dashed boxes)* and metaphyseal collar and spur. The bone bark is indicated. *B,* In the distal portion of the radius of a normal infant, note the straight metaphyseal margins *(white arrowheads)* forming the edges of the metaphyseal collar, in addition to the well-defined bone bark *(white arrow)* at the medial margin of the ulnar physis.

(From Oestreich AE, Ahmad BS: The periphysis and its effect on the metaphysis. I. Definition and normal radiographic pattern. Skeletal Radiol 21:283, 1992.)

articular cartilage of the neighboring joint. With continued maturation of both the epiphysis and the diaphysis, the growth plate is thinned further (Figs. 1–3 and 1–4). The growth plate eventually disappears and thereby allows

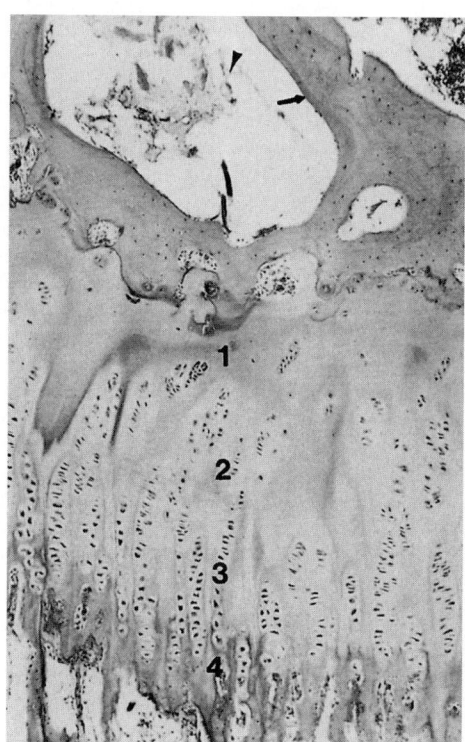

**Figure 1–3.** Cartilaginous growth plate in a 16-year-old patient. Observe the bone *(arrow)* and marrow *(arrowhead)* of the epiphysis. The areas of the growth plate include a zone of resting cartilage (1), proliferating cartilage (2), maturing cartilage (3), and calcifying cartilage (4) (×86).

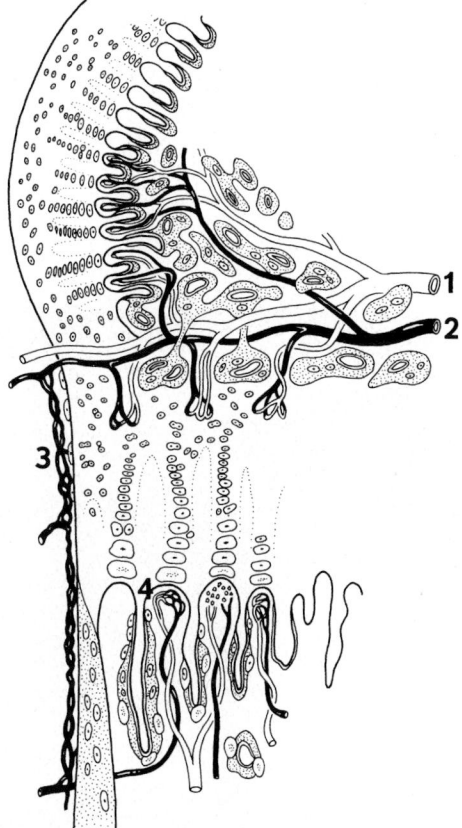

**Figure 1–4.** Cartilage growth plate and adjacent metaphysis and epiphysis. Note the epiphyseal vein (1) and artery (2), the perichondrial vascular ring (3), the terminal loops of the nutrient artery (4) in the metaphysis, and ongoing endochondral ossification in the physis and epiphysis.

(Redrawn from Warwick R, Williams PL [eds]: Gray's Anatomy, 35th Br ed. Philadelphia, WB Saunders, 1973, p 227.)

fusion of the epiphyseal and diaphyseal ossification centers, followed by cessation of endochondral bone formation deep to the articular cartilage of the epiphysis and formation of a subchondral bone plate. Although the growth plate has now ceased to function, a band of horizontally oriented trabeculae may persist and mark the previous location of the plate as a transverse radiopaque fusion line. Abnormalities of endochondral ossification in the physis are well recognized in a number of disorders and are fundamental to the diagnosis of rickets (Fig. 1–5*A*). Transient aberrations of such ossification lead to the development of growth recovery lines (see Fig. 1–5*B*).

## Developing Joint

An articulation eventually appears in the mesenchyme that exists between the developing ends of the bones. In a fibrous joint, the interzonal mesenchyme is modified to form the fibrous tissue that will connect the adjacent bones; in a synchondrosis, it is converted to hyaline cartilage; and in a symphysis, the interzonal mesenchyme is changed to fibrocartilage. In a synovial joint, the central portion of the mesenchyme becomes loosely meshed and is continuous in its periphery with adjacent mesenchyme that is undergoing vascularization (Fig. 1–6). The synovial mesenchyme that is created will later form the synovial membrane, as well as some additional intra-articular structures, whereas the central aspect of the mesenchyme undergoes liquefaction and cavitation and thereby creates the joint space. Condensation of the peripheral mesenchyme leads to joint capsule formation.

## Modeling and Remodeling of Bone

The term *intermediary organization* has been used to describe the control and regulation of coordinated cellular events that occur in the living human skeleton. Intermediary organization is dependent on a number of bone cells, such as osteoblasts and osteoclasts, whose activity is linked. Thus, the processes of bone formation and bone resorption are intertwined.

### Modeling

It is the process of modeling that significantly alters the shape and form of bone. Modeling, or sculpting, of the skeleton is responsive to the mechanical forces placed on it. This process occurs continuously throughout the growth period at varying rates and involves all bone surfaces. Classic examples of the modeling process are (1) drifting of the midshaft of a tubular bone, (2) flaring of the ends of a tubular bone, and (3) enlargement of the cranial vault and modification of cranial curvature. This form of modeling is a prerequisite to the normal development of tubular bones, ribs, and other osseous structures. It is accomplished by resorption, which dominates in one aspect of a bone, and apposition, which dominates in another. In the long tubular bones of the extremity, resorption is more evident on the side of the bone surface that is nearer the body core, and apposition occurs on the opposite surface.

The flaring that is normally evident in the end of a long tubular bone exemplifies bone modeling (Fig. 1–7). As the bone grows in length, the wide metaphyseal

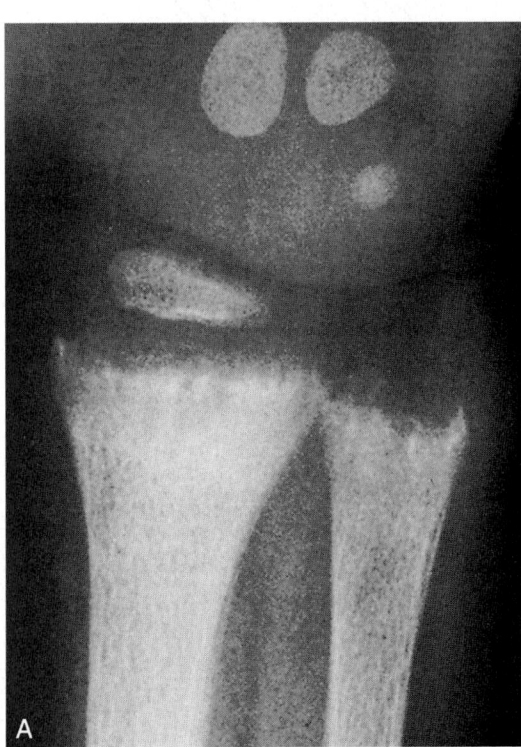
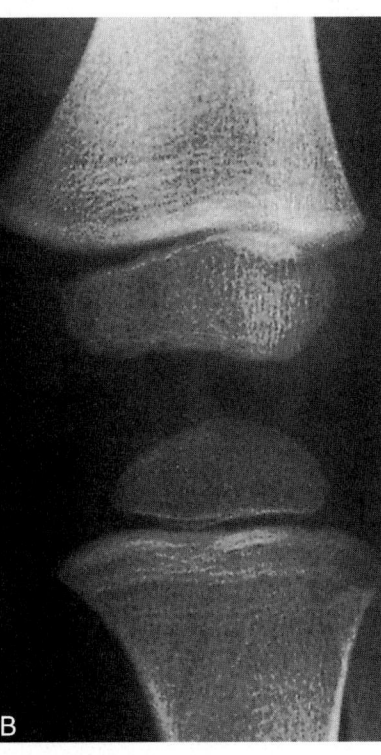

**Figure 1–5.** Abnormalities in endochondral ossification in the growth plate. *A*, Rickets. Widening of the physis and irregularity and enlargement of the metaphysis are among the manifestations of this disease. *B*, Growth recovery lines. Note the multiple wavy, radiodense lines in the metaphyses of the femur and tibia. The configuration of these lines is similar to the shape of the adjacent physis.

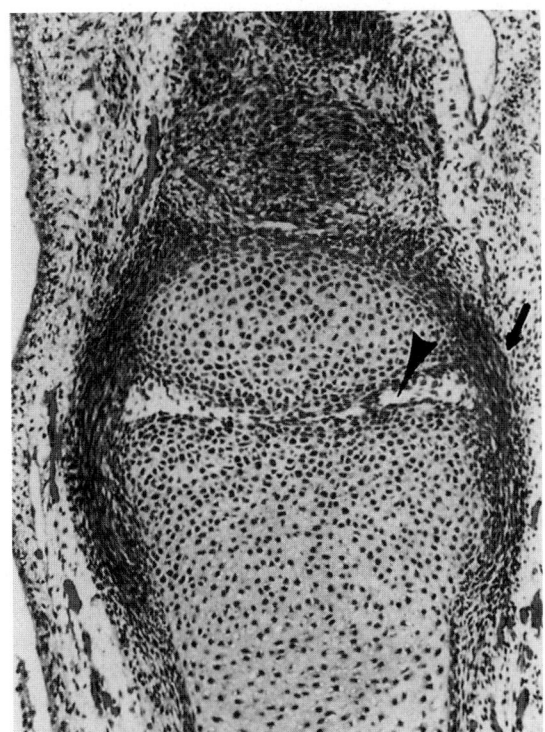

**Figure 1–6.** Development of a synovial joint. Cavitation *(arrowhead)* within the interzone has created the primitive joint cavity. Condensation at the periphery of the joint *(arrow)* will lead to capsule formation (×140).

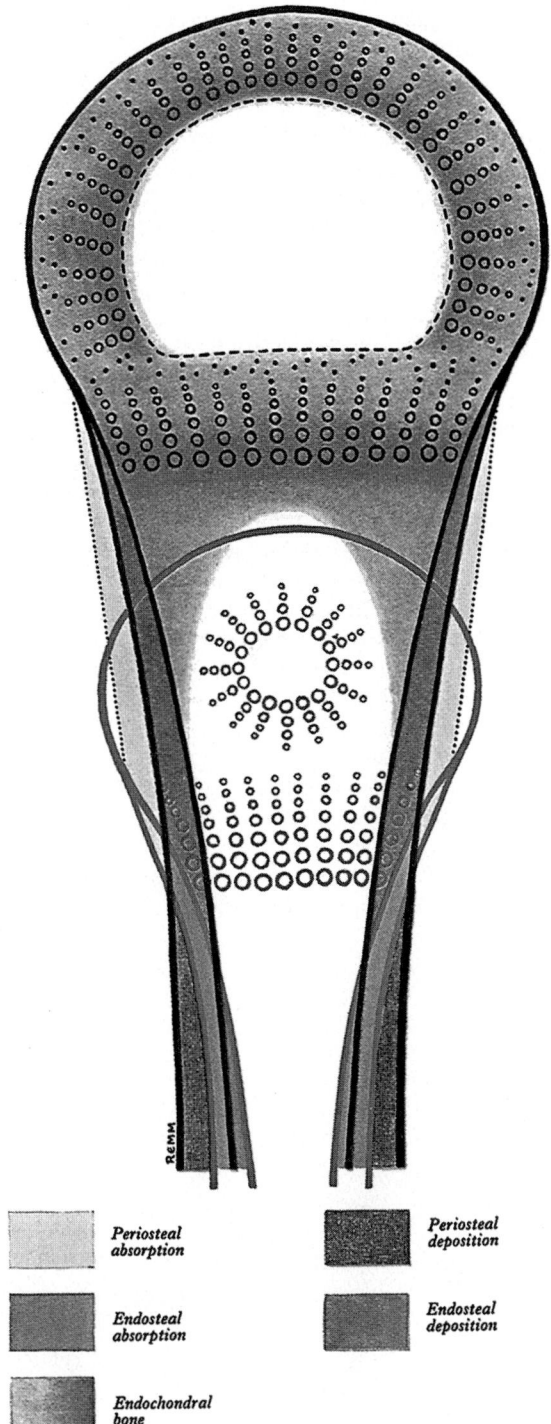

region, a product of the growth plate, is later occupied by a narrow diaphysis, a change that requires close coordination of bone resorption and apposition. Reduction of the metaphysis, with the creation of a metaphyseal funnel, is accomplished by osteoclastic resorption along the periosteal surface, coupled with osteoblastic bone formation in the endosteal surface of the metaphyseal cortex. Subsequently, as the metaphysis migrates shaftward, the marrow cavity is enlarged through the processes of osteoclastic resorption of trabecular bone and endosteal bone resorption, and the overall diameter of the shaft is increased as a result of periosteal bone formation.

## Remodeling

To produce and maintain biomechanically and metabolically competent tissue, transformation of immature, woven-type bone to more compact lamellar bone is required. This process of remodeling is normally most prominent in the young but continues at reduced rates throughout life. The linkage of resorption and formation of bone is very tight; formation follows resorption at the resorption site, not at some other location, and the amount of bone that is formed is almost always nearly equal to the amount that is removed. The remodeling process replaces aged or injured bone tissue with new bone tissue; over time, the repeated strain on skeletal tissue that occurs during ordinary physical activity results in microdamage that, if not repaired, would eventually lead to structural failure.

| | |
|---|---|
| Periosteal absorption | Periosteal deposition |
| Endosteal absorption | Endosteal deposition |
| Endochondral bone | |

**Figure 1–7.** Modeling of bone: growth of a tubular bone. Note the changing shape of the epiphyseal ossification center, the altered organization of the growth plate, and the varying zones of bone deposition and resorption (absorption).
(From Warwick R, Williams PL [eds]: Gray's Anatomy, 35th Br ed. Philadelphia, WB Saunders, 1973, p 230.)

In the endosteal and periosteal surfaces of the cortex, osteoclastic resorption leads to a tube-shaped tunnel designated a resorption canal. Initially, this tunnel is oriented approximately perpendicular to the surface of the bone and corresponds in position to Volkmann's canal. Subsequently, the osteoclasts create longitudinally oriented canals and, by first excavating in one direction and then in the opposite direction, liberate the osteocytes from their lacunae and displace the vascular channels; when these events are followed by osteoblastic apposition, cylinders of bone are formed about linear vascular channels, which is the basic component of the haversian system, or osteon. When viewed longitudinally, the mature cortical remodeling unit consists of a cutting zone lined by osteoclasts (Fig. 1–8).

It must be emphasized that bone remodeling is not confined to the immature skeleton but proceeds throughout life and is modified in accordance with alterations in cellular activities. The processes of resorption and formation predominate on bone surfaces. Although trabecular bone represents only 20% to 25% of the total skeletal volume, it contributes more than 60% of the total surface area; conversely, cortical bone is characterized by a relatively small amount of surface area (Table 1–1). Routine radiography, even when supplemented with magnification techniques, is far more sensitive in detecting changes in cortical bone in the form of subperiosteal or endosteal resorption or intracortical "tunneling" than it is in detecting changes in trabecular bone.

## ANATOMY

### General Structure of Bone

Mature bone consists primarily of an outer shell of compact bone termed the cortex, a looser-appearing meshwork of trabeculae beneath the cortex that represents cancellous or spongy bone, and interconnecting spaces containing myeloid, fatty marrow, or both. Cortical bone is clothed by a periosteal membrane, which contains arterioles and capillaries that pierce the cortex and enter the medullary canal. These vessels, along with larger structures that enter one or more nutrient canals, provide the blood supply to the bone. The periosteum is continuous about the bone, except for a portion that is intra-articular and covered with synovial membrane or cartilage. At sites of attachment to bone, the fibers of tendons and ligaments blend with the periosteum (entheses). The structure of the periosteal membrane varies with a person's age: it is thicker, vascular, active, and loosely attached in infants and children and thinner, inactive, and more firmly adherent in adults. The periosteal membrane in an immature skeleton contains two relatively well-defined layers, an outer fibrous layer and an inner osteogenic layer, whereas that in a mature

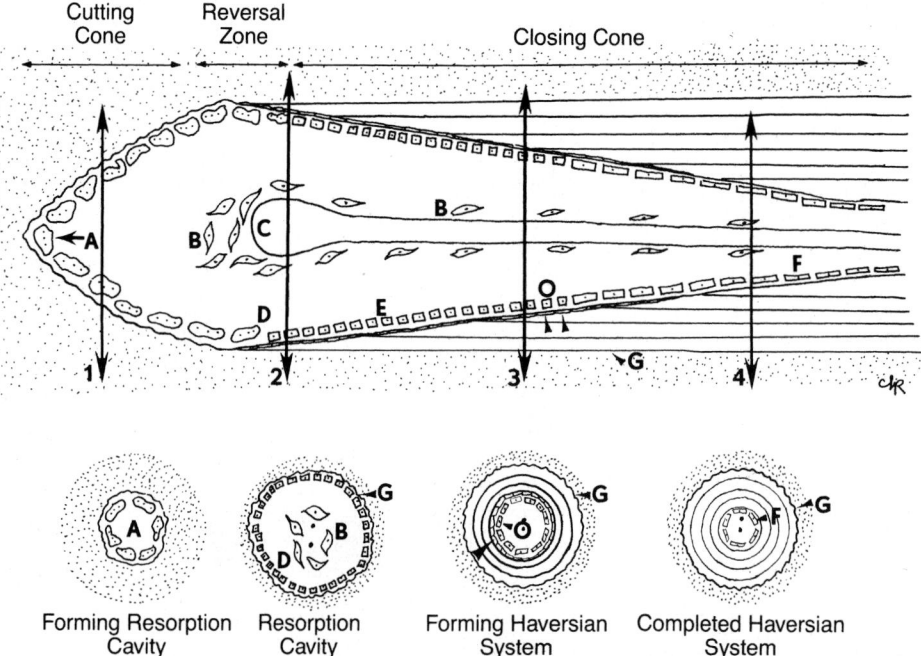

**Figure 1–8.** Remodeling of bone: cortical remodeling unit. *Top,* Diagram shows a longitudinal section through a cortical remodeling unit, with corresponding transverse sections below (1 to 4). A, Multinucleated osteoclasts in Howship's lacunae advancing longitudinally from right to left and radially to enlarge a resorption cavity; B, perivascular spindle-shaped precursor cells; C, capillary loops; D, mononuclear cells lining reversal zones; E, osteoblasts depositing new bone centripetally; F, flattened cells lining the haversian canal of a complete haversian system. *Bottom,* Transverse sections at different stages of development: 1, resorption cavities lined with osteoclasts; 2, completed resorption cavities lined by mononuclear cells, the reversal zone; 3, the forming haversian system, or osteons, lined with osteoblasts that had recently formed three lamellae; 4, the completed haversian system with flattened bone cells lining the canal. Osteoid *(arrowheads)* is present between osteoblast (O) and mineralized bone. G, cement line.

(Redrawn from Parfitt AM: The actions of parathyroid hormone on bone: Relation to bone remodeling and turnover, calcium homeostasis, and metabolic bone disease. Part I of IV parts: Mechanisms of calcium transfer between blood and bone and their cellular basis: Morphological and kinetic approaches to bone turnover. Metabolism 25:809, 1976.)

**Adult Bone Surfaces (Envelopes)**

| Surface | Surface Area ($\times 10^6$ sq mm) |
| --- | --- |
| Cortical surfaces | |
|   Periosteal | 0.5 |
|   Haversian (osteonal) | 3.5 |
|   Corticoendosteal | 0.5 |
| Trabecular surfaces | |
|   Endosteal | 7 |
| Total surfaces | 11.5 |

From Jee WSS: The skeletal tissues. In Weiss L, Lansing L (eds): Histology. Cell and Tissue Biology, 5th ed. New York, Elsevier, 1983, p 221.

skeleton is characterized by a single layer that has resulted from fusion of the fibrous and osteogenic layers. Although a layer that may be identified on the inner surface of the cortex is sometimes called an endosteum to emphasize its similarities with the periosteum, this layer is less well defined than the periosteum and may be involved in significant normal bone formation only in the fetus.

A closer look at the cortex identifies its intricate structure (Fig. 1–9). Spongiosa bone differs in structure from cortical bone. Individual trabeculae in a crosshatched or honeycomb distribution can be identified and divide the marrow space into communicating compartments. The precise distribution, orientation, and size of the individual trabeculae differ from one skeletal site to another, although the trabeculae often appear most numerous and prominent in areas of normal stress, where they align themselves in the direction of physiologic strain.

## Cellular Constituents of Bone

Five types of bone cells are found in skeletal tissue: osteoprogenitor cells, osteoblasts, osteocytes, osteoclasts, and bone-lining cells (Fig. 1–10).

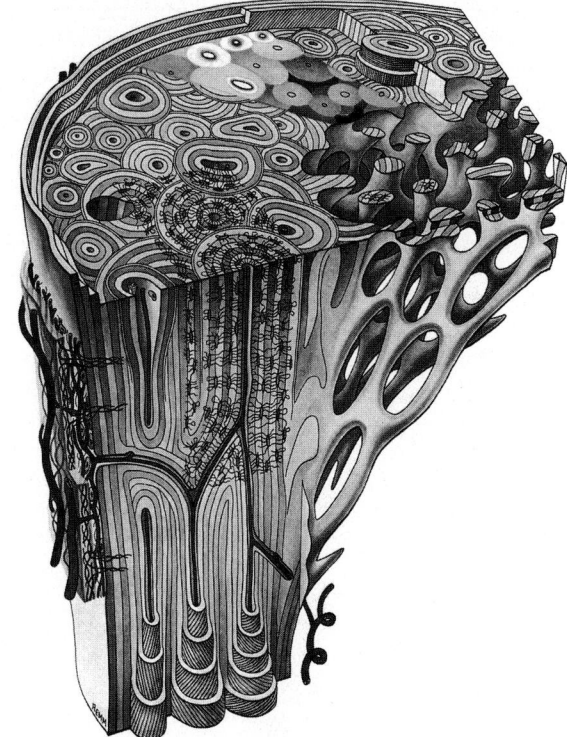

**Figure 1–9.** Features of mature compact and cancellous bone. Note the haversian systems, or osteons, consisting of a central haversian canal surrounded by concentric lamellae of osseous tissue. Osteocytes are identified within lacunae in the lamellae and send out processes through radiating canaliculi. At the bottom of the diagram, note that the orientation of the collagen fibers differs in each lamella.

(From Warwick R, Williams RL [eds]: Gray's Anatomy, 35th Br ed. Philadelphia, WB Saunders, 1973, p 217.)

**Osteoprogenitor Cells.** Undifferentiated stromal cells have the capacity to proliferate by mitotic division and develop into osteoblasts, or bone-forming cells. Osteoclasts are derived from a different source, cells of the hematopoietic system.

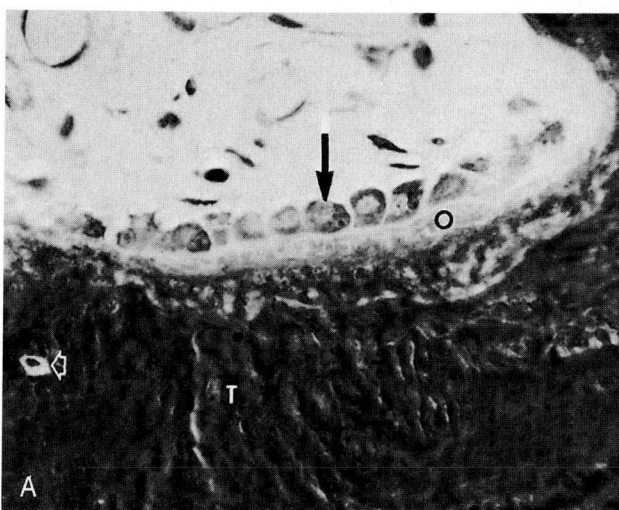
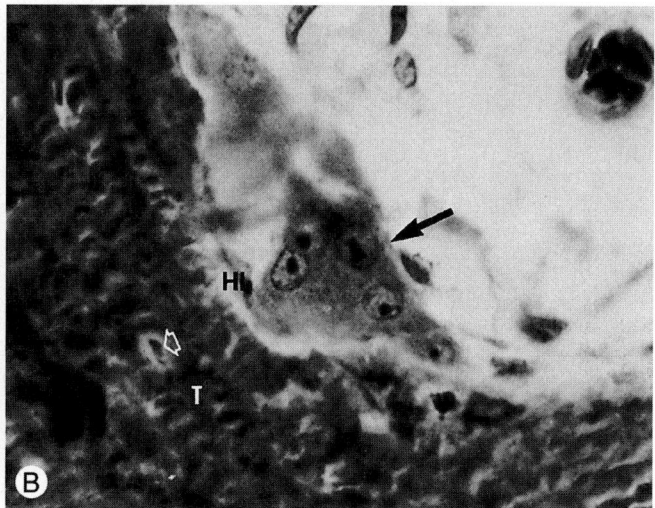

**Figure 1–10.** Cellular constituents of bone: osteoblasts, osteocytes, and osteoclasts. *A*, Prominent osteoblasts *(arrow)* secreting osteoid matrix (O). Note the perinuclear clear zone, which represents the Golgi apparatus. *B*, Multinucleated osteoclast *(arrow)* residing in a resorption bay or Howship's lacuna (HL). Open arrow, osteocyte; T, mineralized trabecular bone (trichrome stain, ×340).

**Osteoblasts.** Osteoblasts are derived from cells that are probably components of the stromal system of bone and marrow. Osteoblasts are intimately involved in the processes of intramembranous and endochondral bone formation. Indeed, any cell that forms bone—whether during growth and modeling, remodeling, or fracture healing—is defined as an osteoblast. The activity of the precursor cells is directly governed by the principle of supply and demand; at times when new bone is required, such as during the healing of a fracture, these cells are called to action in the generation of osteoblasts.

**Osteocytes.** Osteocytes arise from preosteoblasts and osteoblasts. Initially present at the surface of the bone, some, but not all, of the osteoblasts subsequently become entrapped within the osseous tissue as osteocytes. Here, the osteocyte lies in a lacuna. They are unable to divide, so only one cell is present in each lacuna. The osteocyte is concerned with proper maintenance of the bone matrix.

**Osteoclasts.** Another cell, the osteoclast, is a multinucleated cell (2 to 100 nuclei) with a short life span that is intimately related to the process of bone resorption. The origin of the osteoclast has been investigated, and it now appears to be a product of one of the cell lines of the hematopoietic system and is derived from a hematopoietic stem cell (monocyte-phagocyte line).

**Bone-Lining Cells.** The precise nature of the commonly identified flat, elongated cells with spindle-shaped nuclei that line the surface of the bone is not clear, although they are generally believed to be derived from osteoblasts that have become inactive. Lining cells communicate with the syncytium of osteocytes, and although their function is also unknown, it may include maintenance of mineral homeostasis, control of the growth of bone crystals, or the ability to differentiate into other cells, such as osteoblasts.

## Noncellular Constituents of Bone

Water is responsible for about 20% of the wet weight of bone tissue. The major cellular components—osteoblasts, osteocytes, and osteoclasts—account for a very small fraction of the total weight of bone. The other constituents of bone include the remaining organic matrix (collagen and mucopolysaccharides), which accounts for approximately 20% to 30% of osseous tissue by dry weight, and inorganic material, which accounts for approximately 70% to 80% of osseous tissue by dry weight. It is these constituents, in physiologic amounts, that create bone tissue that is both dynamic and uniquely capable of providing the support the body requires.

**Organic Matrix.** The organic matrix of bone, which surrounds the cellular components, is composed primarily of protein, glycoprotein, and polysaccharide. Collagen (type I) is the major constituent (90%) of the organic matrix of bone; the collagen is embedded in a gelatinous mucopolysaccharide material (ground substance). Although mucopolysaccharides represent a minor quantitative part of the structure of osseous tissue, they appear to be very important in the process of bone matrix maturation and mineralization.

**Inorganic Mineral.** The inorganic mineral of bone exists in a crystalline form that resembles hydroxyapatite—$3Ca(PO_4)_2 \bullet Ca(OH)_2$; this mineral is distributed regularly along the length of the collagen fibers and is surrounded by ground substance.

## Bone Marrow

Bone marrow is a soft, pulpy tissue that lies in the spaces between the trabeculae of all bones and even in the larger haversian canals. It is one of the most extensive organs of the human body. Its functions include the provision of a continual supply of red cells, white cells, and platelets to meet the body's demand for oxygenation, immunity, and coagulation. A complex vascular supply relies mainly on a nutrient artery that, in the long tubular bones, pierces the diaphyseal cortex at an angle and extends toward the ends of the tubular bone by running parallel to its long axis. Branches from the nutrient artery enter the endosteal surface of the cortex as capillaries and eventually form primary and collecting sinusoids in an extensive, anastomosing complex among the fat cells of the marrow.

### Marrow Composition

The basic composition of bone marrow consists of mineralized osseous matrix, connective tissue, and a variety of cells. As described previously, the trabeculae in the medullary space represent the osseous component of the bone marrow. The marrow itself occupies the spaces between and around the plates and struts of trabecular (cancellous or spongy) bone, and it is held in place by a network of fine fibrous tissue called a reticulum. The cancellous trabeculae provide architectural support and serve as a mineral depot. The interface between marrow and trabecular bone, the endosteal envelope, is very active metabolically and has a complement of cells, such as osteoblasts and osteoclasts, that are extremely sensitive to metabolic stimuli.

The cells of the marrow consist of all stages of erythrocytic and leukocytic development, as well as fat cells and reticulum cells. Under homeostatic conditions, the production rate of hematopoietic cells precisely equals the destruction rate. The average life span of a human red cell is approximately 120 days, and that of a platelet is 7 to 10 days; the life span of leukocytes is more variable, being relatively short for granulocytes (6 to 12 hours) and long for lymphocytes (months or even years). Fat cells are also a major component of bone marrow. Although smaller than fat cells from extramedullary sites, marrow fat cells are active metabolically and respond to hematopoietic activity by changes in size. During periods of decreased hematopoiesis, the fat cells in bone marrow increase in size and number, whereas during increased hematopoiesis, the fat cells atrophy.

Two forms of bone marrow are encountered, although at any given anatomic site an admixture of the two forms often exists. Red marrow is hematopoietically active marrow and consists of approximately 40% water, 40% fat, and 20% protein; yellow marrow is hematopoietically inactive and consists of approximately 15% water, 80% fat, and 5% protein.

## Marrow Conversion

The amount of red marrow versus yellow marrow at any given time is dependent on the age of the person, the site that is being sampled, and the health of the individual. At birth, red marrow is present throughout the skeleton, but with increasing age, because of the normal conversion process of hematopoietic to fatty marrow, the proportion of hematopoietic marrow decreases. Fatty marrow represents approximately 15% of the total marrow volume in a child but accounts for 60% of this volume by age 80 years. The conversion of red to yellow marrow that occurs during growth and development is predictable and orderly (Fig. 1–11). This replacement commences earlier and is more advanced in the more distal bones of the extremities; further, in each bone, the conversion to yellow marrow proceeds from the distal to the proximal end, although some authors maintain that it commences in the center of the shaft and extends in both directions, but more rapidly in the distal segment. Cartilaginous epiphyses and apophyses lack marrow until they ossify. By the age of 20 to 25 years, marrow conversion is usually complete. At this time, the adult pattern is characterized by the presence of red marrow only in portions of the vertebrae, sternum, ribs, clavicles, scapulae, skull, and innominate bones and in the metaphyses of the femora and humeri. Minor variations in this distribution, however, are encountered.

Although the visualized patterns of signal intensity do not precisely correspond to anatomic sites of red and yellow marrow, magnetic resonance imaging is an effective, albeit indirect, means of determining the cellular characteristics of bone marrow. Composed predominantly of fat, yellow marrow displays the T1 and T2 relaxation patterns of adipose tissue; containing considerable amounts of water and protein, as well as fat, red marrow has T1 and T2 relaxation patterns that differ from those of fatty marrow. Although the major contributor to signal intensity for both types of marrow is fat, on standard T1-weighted spin echo sequences, red marrow demonstrates lower signal intensity than yellow marrow does. Normal age-related conversion of red to yellow marrow in the vertebral bodies and femora is illustrated in Figures 1–12 and 1–13, underscoring the variability of magnetic resonance imaging findings that characterize the normal, orderly process of conversion from hematopoietic to fatty marrow.

When the body's demand for hematopoiesis increases, yellow marrow is reconverted to red marrow. The extent of reconversion depends on the severity and duration of the stimulus, and the process may be initiated or modulated by such factors as temperature, low oxygen tension, hemoglobin blood level, and elevated levels of erythropoietin. The process of reconversion follows that of conversion, but in reverse. Initial changes occur in the

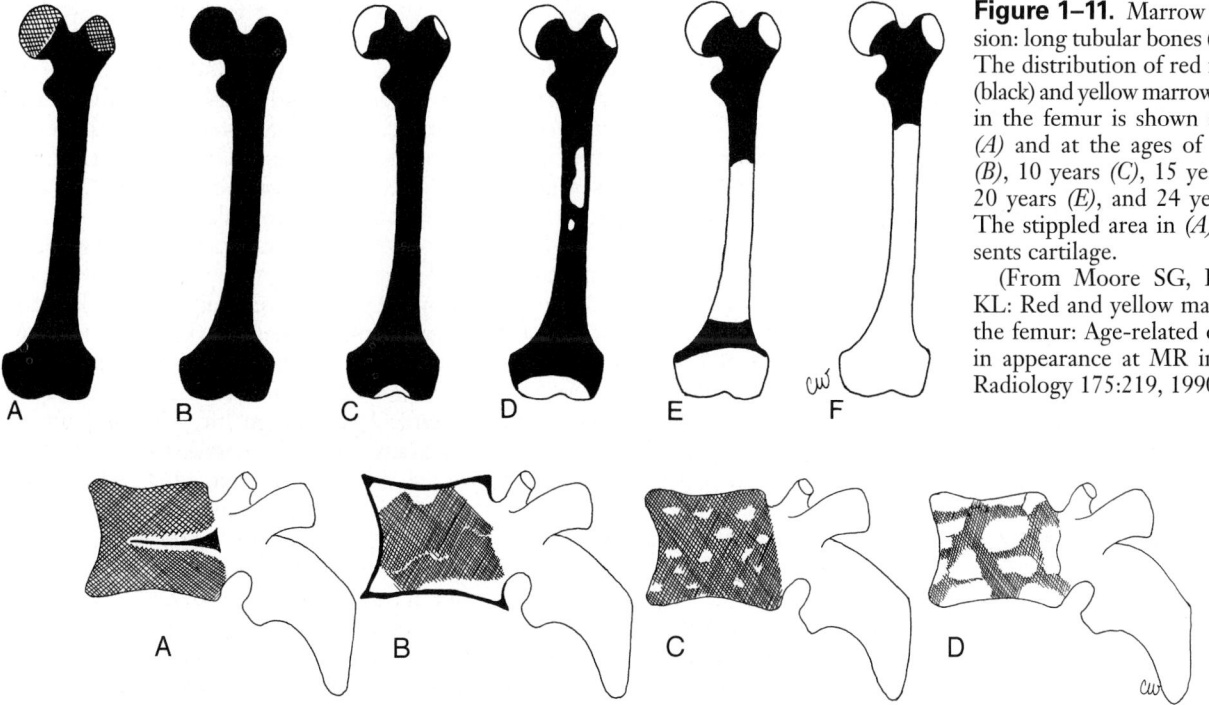

**Figure 1–11.** Marrow conversion: long tubular bones (femur). The distribution of red marrow (black) and yellow marrow (white) in the femur is shown at birth (*A*) and at the ages of 5 years (*B*), 10 years (*C*), 15 years (*D*), 20 years (*E*), and 24 years (*F*). The stippled area in (*A*) represents cartilage.

(From Moore SG, Dawson KL: Red and yellow marrow in the femur: Age-related changes in appearance at MR imaging. Radiology 175:219, 1990.)

**Figure 1–12.** Marrow conversion: vertebral bodies. Appearance on T1-weighted spin echo magnetic resonance images. Four patterns are observed. *A*, Pattern 1 is characterized by the presence of high-signal-intensity fatty marrow confined to linear areas along the basivertebral vein. *B*, Pattern 2 is characterized by bandlike and triangular areas of fatty marrow in a peripheral location. *C*, Pattern 3 is characterized by multiple small regions of high-signal-intensity fatty marrow. *D*, Pattern 4 is characterized by multiple large regions of fatty marrow. Pattern 1 is common in all regions of the spine in the first 2 or 3 decades of life, and patterns 2, 3, and 4 become more dominant after age 30 or 40 years, particularly in the thoracic and lumbar regions.

(From Ricci C, Cova M, Kang YS, et al: Normal age-related patterns of cellular and fatty bone marrow distribution in the axial skeleton: MR imaging study. Radiology 177:83, 1990.)

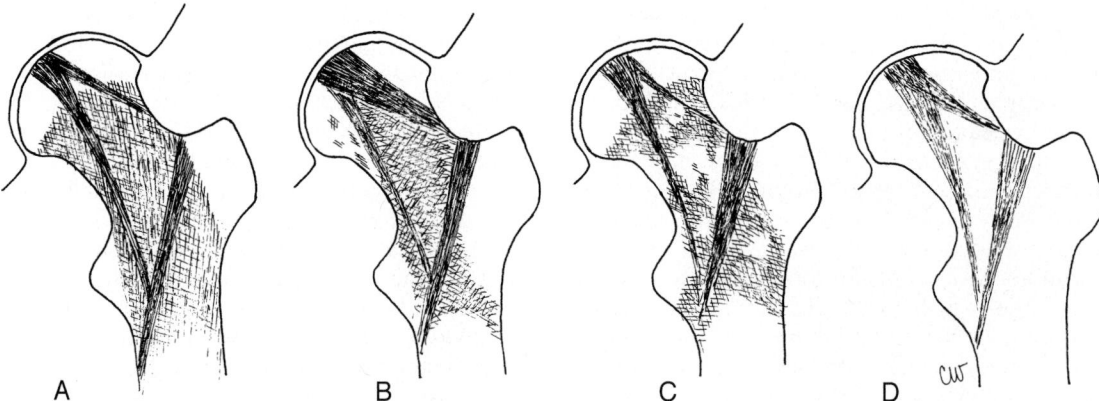

**Figure 1–13.** Marrow conversion: proximal portion of the femur. Appearance on T1-weighted spin echo magnetic resonance images. Four patterns are observed. *A,* Pattern 1 is characterized by high-signal-intensity fatty marrow confined to the capital femoral epiphysis and greater and lesser trochanters. *B,* Pattern 2 resembles pattern 1, with the addition of fatty marrow in the medial portion of the femoral head and in the lateral portion of the intertrochanteric region. *C,* Pattern 3 resembles pattern 1, with the addition of many small, sometimes confluent areas of fatty marrow in the intertrochanteric region. *D,* Pattern 4 is characterized by uniform high-signal-intensity fatty marrow throughout the proximal portion of the femur, with the exception of the regions of the major trabecular groups. Patterns 1 and 2 predominate in the first 3 decades of life, pattern 3 predominates in the fifth and sometimes the fourth decades of life, and pattern 4 predominates after age 50 or 60 years.

(From Ricci C, Cova M, Kang YS, et al: Normal age-related patterns of cellular and fatty bone marrow distribution in the axial skeleton: MR imaging study. Radiology 177:83, 1990.)

axial skeleton and thereafter from a proximal to distal direction in the extremities.

## PHYSIOLOGY

### Mineralization of Bone

At present, no unified concept exists for the mechanism of bone mineralization. The process of biologic calcification, in which hydroxyapatite or some similar material is deposited within an organic matrix, is complex. The ions essential to formation of the crystalline unit in bone are calcium ($Ca^{2+}$) and phosphate ($PO_4^{3-}$). Initial interpretations of the calcification process emphasized precipitation dynamics in which the unique milieu of the organic matrix of bone provided the specific conditions required for the deposition of these ions.

### Calcium Homeostasis

The skeleton contains 99% of the body's calcium and serves as the essential reservoir for the maintenance of stable plasma levels of calcium. Approximately 70% of plasma calcium is believed to be maintained by a continuous exchange of calcium ions between bone tissue and the extracellular fluid; this interchange occurs between the hydroxyapatite crystals of all bone surfaces and proceeds independently of any change in bone volume (i.e., formation and resorption). Hypocalcemia stimulates the release of calcium ions from the bone mineral into the extracellular fluid, and conversely, hypercalcemia promotes an inward flux of calcium ions from the extracellular fluid to the bone mineral. Maintenance of the remaining 30% of plasma calcium may be mediated by the actions of parathyroid hormone and other hormones.

### Bone Resorption and Formation

The processes of resorption and formation occur continuously in normal bone. These processes are prominent in an immature skeleton, in which modeling leads to the major changes in bone size and shape that are required for normal osseous growth and development; in a mature skeleton, these processes are less evident but nonetheless essential for the maintenance of biomechanically competent tissue and calcium homeostasis.

As indicated previously, resorption and apposition dominate on the bone surfaces present in the cortex and spongiosa. Four broad surface areas exist in the skeleton, each of which is functionally distinct (Fig. 1–14). These areas are often referred to as envelopes. The first of these areas, related to the outer surface of the cortex, is the periosteal envelope (or periosteum), which consists of an outer sheath of fibrous connective tissue and an inner, or cambrian, layer of undifferentiated cells. These two distinct histologic layers are not present everywhere; they are absent in intra-articular locations such as the femoral neck, at entheses or sites of tendinous and ligamentous attachments to bone, and about the sesamoid bones. The second of the envelopes, the haversian envelope, lies within the bone cortex and surrounds the individual haversian systems. The corticoendosteal envelope relates to the inner surface of the bone cortex and is therefore the outermost boundary of the medullary bone. It is interrupted at sites where the trabeculae of the medullary cavity are connected to the cortex. This envelope functions primarily as a bone resorptive surface, and it accounts for the general thinning of the cortex that occurs with advancing age in adults. The fourth envelope is the endosteal envelope, which represents the interface of medullary bone and marrow. As indicated previously,

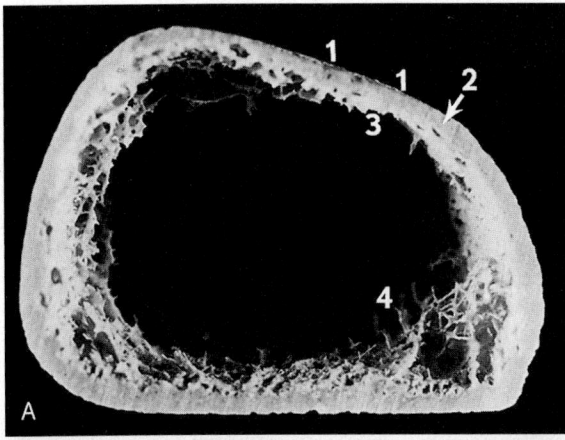

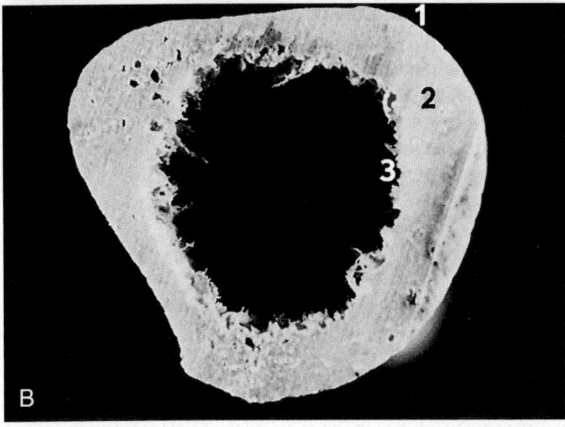

**Figure 1–14.** Bone resorption and formation: available bone envelopes. Transverse sections of the metaphysis *(A)* and diaphysis *(B)* of a tubular bone reveal the osseous envelopes involved in the processes of resorption and apposition. In the cortex, they are the periosteal (1), haversian or osteonal (2), and corticoendosteal (3) envelopes; in the spongiosa, an endosteal or transitional (4) envelope is present.

this envelope is characterized by a very large surface area and is primarily a bone-losing envelope.

Thus, at any particular time, such surfaces may normally be quiescent or, less commonly, actively involved in the synthesis or resorption of bone. Their cellular composition varies according to their functional state. It is the coupling of bone resorption to bone formation that controls the volume of bone that is present at any particular time. It appears likely that the mechanisms responsible for coupling are intrinsic to bone and that an increase in bone resorption must subsequently be coupled to an increase in bone formation if bone volume is to remain unchanged.

## Bone Resorption

Although it has long been held that the osteoclast is the principal cell involved in the degradation of organic bone matrix and in the release of bone mineral, a potential (albeit controversial) role for the osteocyte in removing at least a small amount of perilacunar bone has also been emphasized, and accumulating evidence indicates that mononuclear phagocytes, including peripheral blood monocytes

and tissue macrophages, are involved in bone resorption. Surfaces of bone involved in extensive resorption are sites of accumulation of multinucleated osteoclasts. The finely striated (brush) border of the osteoclast is in contact with the adjacent bone and is in a state of vigorous movement.

Osteoclasts play an active role in the resorption of bone; however, the precise mechanism of the process, including the participation of other cells, is not clear. Osteoclasts appear to be the major cells responsible for the skeletal contribution to regulating the serum concentration of calcium; all the agents that have been shown to increase the serum calcium concentration in vivo have also been shown to increase osteoclastic activity, and the hormones and drugs that lower this concentration have been shown to inhibit osteoclastic activity. Among the substances capable of directly or indirectly stimulating existing osteoclasts, increasing the formation of new osteoclasts, or both are parathyroid hormone, active metabolites of vitamin D, prostaglandin $E_2$, thyroid hormone, heparin, and interleukin-1; among those substances inhibiting resorption are calcitonin, glucocorticoid, diphosphonates, glucagon, phosphate, and carbonic anhydrase inhibitors. Osteoclastic resorption plays a major role in the pathogenesis of a variety of skeletal disorders, including metabolic processes such as osteoporosis, neoplastic and inflammatory conditions accompanied by bone lysis, Paget's disease, and osteopetrosis.

## Bone Formation

The principal cell involved in the formation of bone is the osteoblast. Osteoblasts are derived from mesenchymal osteoprogenitor cells, or preosteoblasts; they are involved in the synthesis of bone matrix and subsequently become either internal osteocytes or inactive bone-lining cells. New bone formation may result from the activation of bone-lining cells, the proliferation and differentiation of preosteoblasts, or both.

The formation of bone occurs in two phases: matrix formation and mineralization. Matrix formation precedes mineralization and occurs at the interface between osteoblasts and existing osteoid; mineralization occurs at the junction of osteoid and newly mineralized bone, a region designated the mineralization front. The layer of unmineralized matrix is termed the osteoid seam. In adults, the usual interval between matrix production and mineralization is 10 days. In certain disease states, such as osteomalacia, the thickness of the osteoid seam is increased.

## Humoral Regulation of Bone Metabolism

Bone metabolism and calcium homeostasis are intimately related to interactions among the skeleton, intestines, and kidneys, and they are involved in the presence of many chemical factors, of which three hormones—parathyroid hormone, calcitonin, and 1,25-dihydroxyvitamin D— are most important.

**Parathyroid Hormone.** An important regulator of skeletal metabolism is parathyroid hormone, the two main functions of which are to stimulate and control the rate of bone remodeling and to influence mechanisms controlling the plasma level of calcium. This hormone is produced by the chief cells of the four parathyroid glands. It has a direct effect on bone (enhancing the mobilization of calcium from the skeleton) and on the kidney (stimulating the absorption of calcium from the glomerular fluid) and has an indirect effect on the intestines (influencing the rate of calcium absorption).

The direct effect of parathyroid hormone on bone (Fig. 1–15) may be either bone resorption or bone formation. An immediate action of parathyroid hormone is to promote the process of osteoclastic resorption, which is fundamental to calcium homeostasis; more prolonged effects of parathyroid hormone are influential on bone remodeling. Thus, at the cellular level, parathyroid hormone influences osteoclasts, osteoblasts, osteocytes, and bone surface cells. A significant increase in the number of osteoclasts and in the ratio of osteoclasts to osteoblasts may occur within hours after administration of the hormone. Osteoblast function is decreased initially; however, subsequent stimulation of osteoblasts results in an increase in bone formation.

**Calcitonin.** Calcitonin is released from the thyroid gland, and secretion of calcitonin is controlled by the circulating levels of calcium. Calcitonin inhibits bone resorption and may lead to significant hypocalcemia and hypophosphatemia. Data also indicate that calcitonin has a stimulatory effect on bone growth in vivo. The importance of calcitonin as a regulator of calcium metabolism in humans, however, is not clear at present.

**Vitamin D.** Vitamin D is one of the most potent humoral factors involved in the regulation of bone metabolism. The biochemistry and mechanisms of action are described in detail in Chapter 42. The general term *vitamin D* refers to both vitamin $D_2$ (ergocalciferol), which originates in plants and is obtained from dietary sources, and vitamin $D_3$ (cholecalciferol), which occurs naturally in the skin. In humans, these two forms of vitamin D have similar potency, so considering them separately has little, if any, clinical significance. The classic biologic role of vitamin D is regulation of intestinal mineral absorption and maintenance of skeletal growth and mineralization. It is now widely accepted that these functions are mediated through the actions of 1,25-dihydroxyvitamin D $(1,25[OH]_2D)$ on the intestine, bone, and kidney.

Additionally, accumulating evidence based on in vitro observations indicates that $1,25(OH)_2D$ has important regulatory effects on blood mononuclear cells and on the immune system. There is also some evidence that $1,25(OH)_2D$ plays a significant role in the intrathymic differentiation of lymphocytes. The clinical relevance of these experimental data regarding the immunoregulatory role of $1,25(OH)_2D$ is not known.

## Metabolic Bone Disorders

### Histologic Techniques

Because differentiation of the two major metabolic bone diseases, osteoporosis and osteomalacia, is based in part on the quantity and quality of bone mineral, the ability to distinguish between calcified and uncalcified bone matrix (osteoid) is critical. The traditional procedures for processing bone require the removal of inorganic matrix to facilitate histologic sectioning; therefore, these procedures prevent subsequent determination of the degree of skeletal mineralization. Because of deficiencies in traditional histologic techniques, additional methods have been used, including qualitative and quantitative microscopic assessment of nondecalcified specimens and the use of in vivo bone markers such as tetracycline. Typically, the iliac crest is used as the biopsy site from which nondecalcified tissue sections are prepared.

In nondecalcified bone sections, osteomalacia is usually characterized by the accumulation of osteoid as a consequence of a defect in the mineralization process. Excess quantities of osteoid, however, may result not only from a decreased rate of mineralization but also from an accelerated rate of bone matrix synthesis. Differentiation between these states is based on a determination of mineralization rates, with tetracycline used as an in vivo bone marker (Table 1–2). Tetracycline fluorescence is evaluated on unstained, nondecalcified tissue sections by ultraviolet light. The first course of tetracycline appears as a discrete fluorescent band within the mineralized bone. The second, more recently administered course of tetracycline is located at the current mineralization front (i.e., mineralized bone–osteoid seam interface). The distance between the two bands represents the amount of new bone synthesized and mineralized over the drug-free interval.

### Normal and Abnormal Histologic Appearance

Normally, the contour of the external cortical margins is smooth. Subperiosteal osteoid deposits, as well as eroded

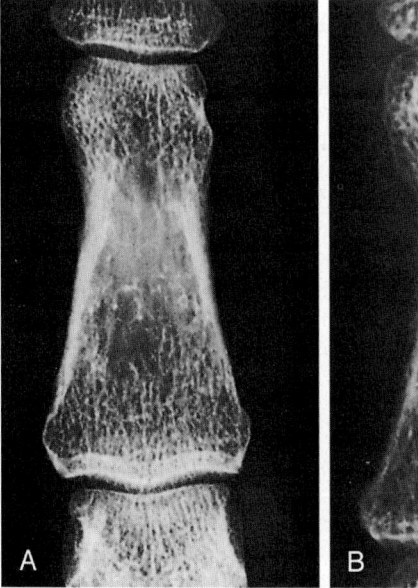
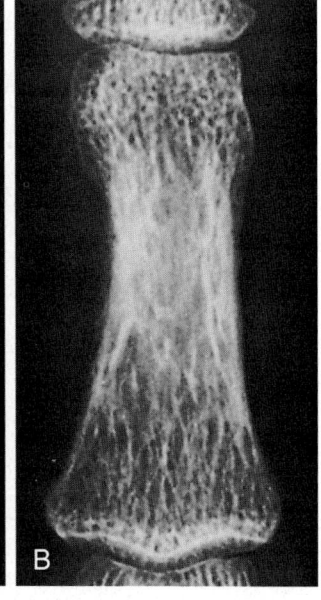

**Figure 1–15.** Osseous effects of parathyroid hormone: hyperparathyroidism. Magnification radiographs of the phalanges in a normal person (*A*) and in a patient with hyperparathyroidism (*B*) reveal the effects of parathyroid hormone on bone. In (*B*), note the osteopenia, indistinct trabeculae, and prominent subperiosteal bone resorption.

**TABLE 1–2**

### Tetracycline-Labeling Regimen for Bone Biopsy

| Day | Regimen |
|---|---|
| 1, 2, 3 | Tetracycline hydrochloride, 250 mg orally four times daily or 500 mg orally twice daily\*† |
| 4–17 | Hiatus (no tetracycline)‡ |
| 18, 19, 20 | Tetracycline hydrochloride, 250 mg orally four times daily or 500 mg orally twice daily† |
| 24 | Bone biopsy§ |

\*Tetracycline is given 1 hour before or 2 hours after meals. A larger dose is used if malabsorption or severe osteomalacia is suspected; up to 3 g/day may be necessary for patients after intestinal bypass.

If the patient has recently received tetracycline hydrochloride, the use of oxytetracycline or demeclocycline in equivalent doses may help distinguish the new tetracycline bone labels from the old because of differences in the fluorescent color produced by the different tetracyclines.

†Avoid all dairy products, antacids, and iron-containing medicines on days 1, 2, 3, 18, 19, and 20.

‡An interval of at least 10 days is required between the two courses of tetracycline.

§Biopsy may be performed several days later, but not sooner.

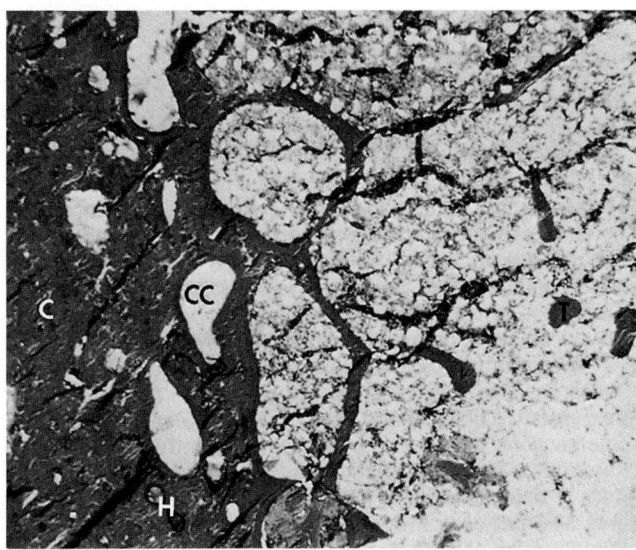

**Figure 1–16.** Cortical bone (C) of an iliac crest biopsy specimen undergoing remodeling. Osteoclasts within cutting cones (CC) resorb endosteal bone, resulting in cortical cancellization (i.e., the formation of cancellous trabecular bone from preexisting cortical bone). A reduction in cortical width ultimately occurs. H, Normal haversian canal before activation (trichrome stain, ×25).

surfaces containing osteoclasts, are normally absent. Subperiosteal bone resorption is evidence of activation of osteoclasts and is seen in states of high bone turnover or accelerated remodeling, such as in hyperparathyroidism.

Loss of cortical bone mass is suggested when cortical thickness is reduced. Activation of osteoclasts leads to increased resorption of bone, thereby enlarging the preexisting vascular canals. Resorption of bone in the longitudinally oriented canals results in the formation of cavities termed cutting cones. The junction between cortical and medullary trabecular bone, which is normally sharply demarcated, is termed the endosteum. Loss of distinction between the cortex and the medullary cavity occurs with increasing cortical porosity as a result of increased cortical osteoclastic resorptive activity, as is seen in severe hyperparathyroidism. Endosteal resorption cavities increase in number and depth until the previously solid cortical bone becomes whittled into what appears to be new, thick trabeculae, a process referred to as cancellization or trabecularization of cortical bone (Fig. 1–16). The total amount and quality of trabecular bone located between the two cortices reflect the weight-bearing properties of the skeleton. Usually, trabecular bone occupies 15% to 25% of the marrow space. A trabecular bone volume below 15% is histologic evidence of osteopenia. Normally, the individual trabeculae are continuous interconnecting or branching bands; atrophic trabeculae appear as struts, bars, or blots (Fig. 1–17), indicating a reduction in mean trabecular plate density.

Decalcified sections taken from the bone core should be examined under polarized light for evidence of woven collagen architecture. Woven bone in a transiliac crest specimen is an abnormal finding in an adult patient and reflects accelerated skeletal turnover. Abnormal patterns of fluorescent label deposition are the hallmark of osteomalacia and represent the morphologic expression of defective mineralization. The amount of tetracycline fluorescence is proportional to the amount of immature amorphous calcium phosphate deposits in the mineralizing foci of the osteoid seam.

The location and extent of bone removal and deposition determine the physical anatomy of the skeleton and the physiologic status of mineral metabolism. Bone remodeling activity is influenced by physical forces, serum levels of endocrine hormones, and nutritional and metabolic factors. Normally, bone resorption and formation are in balance. A net loss of bone tissue may occur from excessive bone resorption, deficient bone formation, or a combination of both processes during the coupling process. Bone diseases resulting from an abnormality of remodeling activity are characterized by failure of the skeleton to provide structural support, generally secondary to a deficiency in skeletal mass. When the bone mass can no longer sustain normal forces, a fracture may ensue and cause pain and deformity. A metabolic bone disease is defined as any generalized disorder of the skeleton, regardless of cause; most metabolic bone diseases result from either an imbalance in remodeling activity or a disorder of matrix mineralization.

Osteopenia refers to a generalized reduction in bone mass that, on radiographic examination, appears as an exaggerated radiolucency of the skeleton. Osteoporosis and osteomalacia are the two major causes of osteopenia. Histologically, osteoporotic diseases may be accompanied by either increased or decreased rates of bone turnover. Osteomalacic syndromes are characterized by histologic evidence of defective mineralization (Table 1–3). High bone turnover diseases (Table 1–4) are characterized by evidence of both increased formation and increased

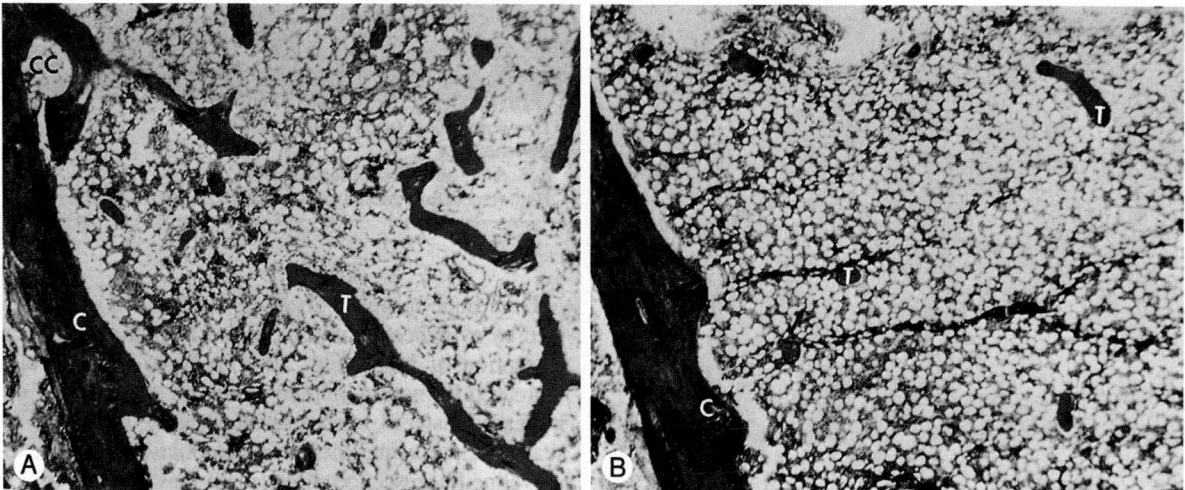

**Figure 1–17.** Normal and abnormal trabecular bone architecture. *A*, Low-power view of an iliac crest biopsy specimen. Cortical thickness is reduced as a result of progressive erosion by cortical cutting cones (CC). Trabecular bone (T), however, exhibits a normal, platelike, connecting architectural pattern (trichrome stain, ×25). *B*, Reduction in trabecular bone (T) volume. Not only is the volume of bone reduced, but the architecture of trabecular bone is also abnormal because of the presence of thin, widely spaced, atrophic rods of bone (trichrome stain, ×25).

---

**TABLE 1–3**

**General Morphologic Classification of Metabolic Bone Diseases**

---

**Osteoporosis**
  High remodeling: active bone turnover
  Low remodeling: inactive bone turnover

**Osteomalacia**
  Low remodeling: pure osteomalacia
  High remodeling: mixed osteomalacia and osteitis fibrosa cystica

resorption of bone. States associated with reduced bone turnover (see Table 1–4) show little evidence of either bone formation or bone resorption. Osteomalacia is usually characterized by excessive quantities of osteoid caused by failure of matrix calcification despite continued matrix synthesis by osteoblasts. Marked increases in the thickness of osteoid seams are characteristic, but osteomalacia may be associated with normal or even reduced quantities of osteoid.

---

**TABLE 1–4**

**Bone Morphology Associated with Specific Metabolic Diseases**

---

**Increased Bone Remodeling Activity (Accelerated Turnover Osteoporosis)**
  Anticonvulsant drug related
  Calcium deficiency states, chronic (secondary hyperparathyroidism)
  Small intestinal disease (early, compensated mineral malabsorption)
  Postgastrectomy (mineral malabsorption)
  Some forms of postmenopausal or senile osteoporosis
  Erythroid hyperplasia
  Hemochromatosis
  Hyperparathyroidism
  Hyperthyroidism
  Osteoporosis of young men
  Mastocytosis

**Decreased Bone Remodeling Activity (Reduced Turnover Osteoporosis)**
  Glucocorticoid associated
  Hepatic disease
    Alcohol related
    Cholestatic
  Hypothyroidism
  Severe systemic disease
  Starvation, malnutrition

  Some forms of postmenopausal or senile osteoporosis
  Total parenteral nutrition (hyperalimentation)

**Osteomalacia (Pure)**
  X-linked hypophosphatemia (vitamin D-resistant rickets)
  Sporadic hypophosphatemia
  Antacid-induced osteomalacia
  Oncogenic osteomalacia
  Primary vitamin D deficiency
  Chronic pancreatitis
  Chronic extrahepatic obstruction
  Metabolic acidosis
  Renal osteodystrophy (aluminium-associated osteomalacia)

**Osteomalacia (Mixed Osteomalacia and Osteitis Fibrosa Cystica)**
  Primary vitamin D deficiency (nutritional, lack of exposure to sunlight)
  Small intestinal disease (vitamin D and calcium malabsorption)
  Postgastrectomy (vitamin D and calcium malabsorption)
  Renal osteodystrophy (mixed)
  Calcium deficiency of children
  Vitamin D-dependent rickets

## FURTHER READING

Aurbach GD, Marx SJ, Spiegel AM: Parathyroid hormone, calcitonin, and the calciferols. In Williams RH (ed): Textbook of Endocrinology, 6th ed. Philadelphia, WB Saunders, 1981, p 922.

Bonucci E: New knowledge on the origin, function and fate of osteoclasts. Clin Orthop 158:252, 1981.

Boskey AL: Current concepts of the physiology and biochemistry of calcification. Clin Orthop 157:225, 1981.

Coccia PF: Cells that resorb bone. N Engl J Med 310:456, 1984.

Feldman RS, Krieger NS, Tashjian AJ: Effects of parathyroid hormone and calcitonin on osteoclast formation in vitro. Endocrinology 107:1137, 1980.

Frost HM: Tetracycline-based histological analysis of bone remodeling. Calcif Tissue Res 3:211, 1969.

Garn SM, Silverman FN, Herzog KP, et al: Lines and bands of increased density: Their implication to growth and development. Med Radiogr Photogr 44:58, 1968.

Holtrop ME, Raisz LG, Simmons HA: The effect of parathyroid hormone, colchicine and calcitonin on the ultrastructure and the activity of osteoclasts in organ culture. J Cell Biol 60:346, 1974.

Jaffe HL: Metabolic, Degenerative, and Inflammatory Diseases of Bones and Joints. Philadelphia, Lea & Febiger, 1972, p 1.

Jee WSS: The skeletal tissues. In Weiss L, Lansing L (eds): Histology: Cell and Tissue Biology, 5th ed. New York, Elsevier Biomedical, 1983.

Kirkpatrick JA Jr: Bone and joint growth—normal and in disease. Clin Rheum Dis 7:671, 1981.

Ledesma-Medina J, Newman B, Oh KS: The skeletal tissues. In Weiss L, Lansing L (eds): Histology: Cell and Tissue Biology, 5th ed. New York, Elsevier Biomedical, 1983.

Levine CD, Schweitzer ME, Ehrlich SM: Pelvic marrow in adults. Skeletal Radiol 23:343, 1994.

McKenna MJ, Frame B: The mast cell and bone. Clin Orthop 200:226, 1985.

Moore SG, Bisset GS III, Siegel MJ, et al: Pediatric musculoskeletal MR imaging. Radiology 179:345, 1991.

Nathan DG: Introduction: Hematologic and hematopoietic diseases. In Wyngaarden JB, Smith LH Jr, Bennett JC (eds): Cecil Textbook of Medicine, 19th ed. Philadelphia, WB Saunders, 1992.

Oestrich AE, Ahmad BS: The periphysis and its effect on the metaphysis. I. Definition and normal radiographic pattern. Skeletal Radiol 21:283, 1992.

Owen M: Lineage of osteogenic cells and their relationship to the stromal system. In Peck WA (ed): Bone and Mineral Research. New York, Elsevier, 1985, p 1.

Posner AS: The mineral of bone. Clin Orthop 200:87, 1985.

Raisz LG: Mechanisms and regulation of bone resorption by osteoclastic cells. In Coe FL, Favus MJ (eds): Disorders of Bone and Mineral Metabolism. New York, Raven Press, 1992, p 287.

Raisz LG, Kream BE: Regulation of bone formation. N Engl J Med 309:29, 1983.

Ricci C, Cova M, Kang YS, et al: Normal age-related patterns of cellular and fatty bone marrow distribution in the axial skeleton: MR imaging study. Radiology 177:83, 1990.

Tatevossian A: Effect of parathyroid extract on blood calcium and osteoclast counts in mice. Calcif Tissue Res 11:251, 1973.

Teitelbaum SL: Osteomalacia and rickets. Clin Endocrinol Metab 9:43, 1980.

VandeBerg BC, Lecouvet FE, Moysan P, et al: MR assessment of red marrow distribution and composition in the proximal femur: Correlation with clinical and laboratory parameters. Skeletal Radiol 26:589, 1997.

VandeBerg BC, Malghem J, Lecouvet FE, et al: Magnetic resonance imaging of the normal bone marrow. Skeletal Radiol 27:471, 1998.

Vogler JB III, Murphy WA: Bone marrow imaging. Radiology 168:679, 1988.

# CHAPTER 2

## Articular Anatomy and Histology

### SUMMARY OF KEY FEATURES

An understanding of the structure of joints is essential to the proper interpretation of radiographs in numerous diseases. Joints can be classified into three types: fibrous, cartilaginous, and synovial. In addition, supporting structures (tendons, aponeuroses, fasciae, and ligaments) influence the manifestation of articular disorders.

### INTRODUCTION

Joints have been classified according to (1) the extent of joint motion and (2) the type of articular histology. The classification of articulations based on the extent of joint motion is as follows:

*Synarthroses:* fixed or rigid joints

*Amphiarthroses:* slightly movable joints

*Diarthroses:* freely movable joints

The classification of joints on the basis of histology emphasizes the type of tissue that characterizes the junctional area (Table 2–1). The following categories are recognized:

*Fibrous articulations:* apposed bony surfaces fastened together by fibrous connective tissue

*Cartilaginous articulations:* apposed bony surfaces initially or eventually connected by cartilaginous tissue

*Synovial articulations:* apposed bony surfaces separated by an articular cavity lined by synovial membrane

This second method of classification can lead to difficulty, because joints that are similar histologically may differ considerably in function and degree of allowable motion; however, it is used in the following discussion.

### FIBROUS ARTICULATIONS

In a fibrous articulation, apposed bony surfaces are fastened together by intervening fibrous tissue. Fibrous articulations can be subdivided into three types: sutures, syndesmoses, and gomphoses.

#### Suture

Limited to the skull, sutures (Fig. 2–1) allow no active motion and exist where broad osseous surfaces are separated only by a zone of connective tissue. Although classically a suture is considered to be a fibrous joint, areas of secondary cartilage formation may be observed during the growth period, and in later life, sutures may undergo bony union or synostosis. Bony obliteration of the sutures is somewhat variable in its time of onset and cranial dis-

| TABLE 2–1 | |
|---|---|
| **Types of Articulations** | |
| **Fibrous** | |
| Suture | Skull |
| Syndesmosis | Distal tibiofibular interosseous membrane |
| | Radioulnar interosseous membrane |
| | Sacroiliac interosseous ligament |
| Gomphosis | Teeth |
| **Cartilaginous** | |
| Symphysis | Symphysis pubis |
| | Intervertebral disc |
| | Manubriosternal joint |
| | Central mandible |
| Synchondrosis | Physeal plate (growth plate) |
| | Neurocentral joint |
| | Spheno-occipital joint |
| **Synovial** | |
| | Large, small joints of extremities |
| | Sacroiliac joint |
| | Apophyseal joint |
| | Costovertebral joint |
| | Sternoclavicular joint |

tribution. This obliteration usually occurs at the bregma and subsequently extends into the sagittal, coronal, and lambdoid sutures, in that order. Despite the normal variations in suture development and closure, their assessment is important in the diagnosis of obstructive hydrocephalus and cranial synostosis. Computed tomography scanning seems to be a superior technique for making this delineation.

#### Syndesmosis

A syndesmosis (Fig. 2–2) is a fibrous joint in which adjacent bony surfaces are united by an interosseous ligament, as in the distal tibiofibular joint, or an interosseous membrane, as at the diaphyses of the radius, ulna, tibia, and fibula. A syndesmosis may demonstrate minor degrees of motion related to stretching of the interosseous ligament or flexibility of the interosseous membrane.

#### Gomphosis

A gomphosis (Fig. 2–3) is a special type of fibrous joint located between the teeth and the maxilla or mandible. At these sites, the articulation resembles a peg that fits into a fossa or socket. The intervening membrane between tooth and bone is termed the periodontal ligament.

### CARTILAGINOUS ARTICULATIONS

There are two types of cartilaginous joints: symphyses and synchondroses.

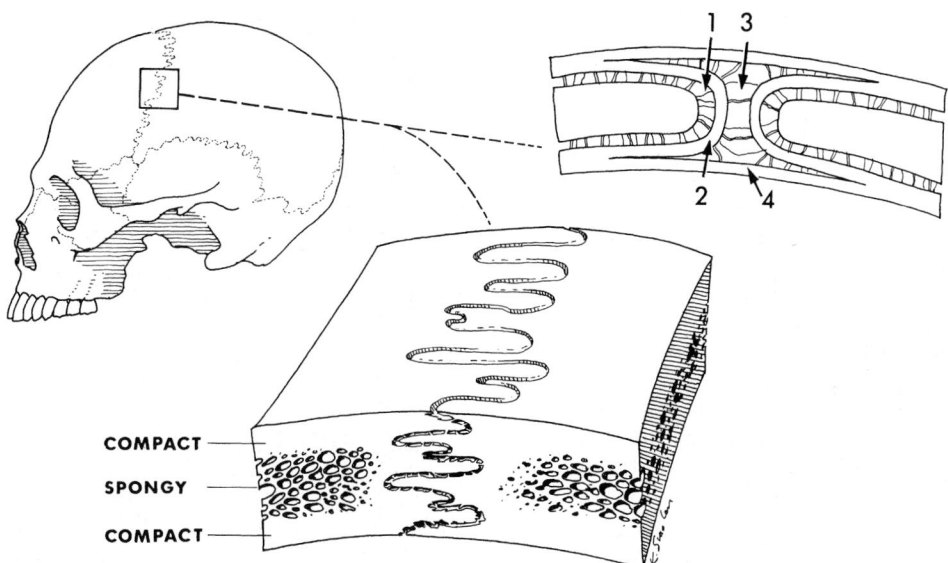

**Figure 2–1.** Fibrous articulation: suture. Schematic drawings indicate the structure of a typical suture in the skull. Note the interdigitations of the osseous surfaces. The specific layers that intervene between the ends of the bones are indicated at the upper right. These include the cambial (1), capsular (2), and middle (3) layers. A uniting (4) layer is also indicated.

(Reproduced in part from Pritchard JJ, Scott JH, Girgis FG: The structure and development of cranial and facial sutures. J Anat 90:73, 1956. Courtesy of Cambridge University Press.)

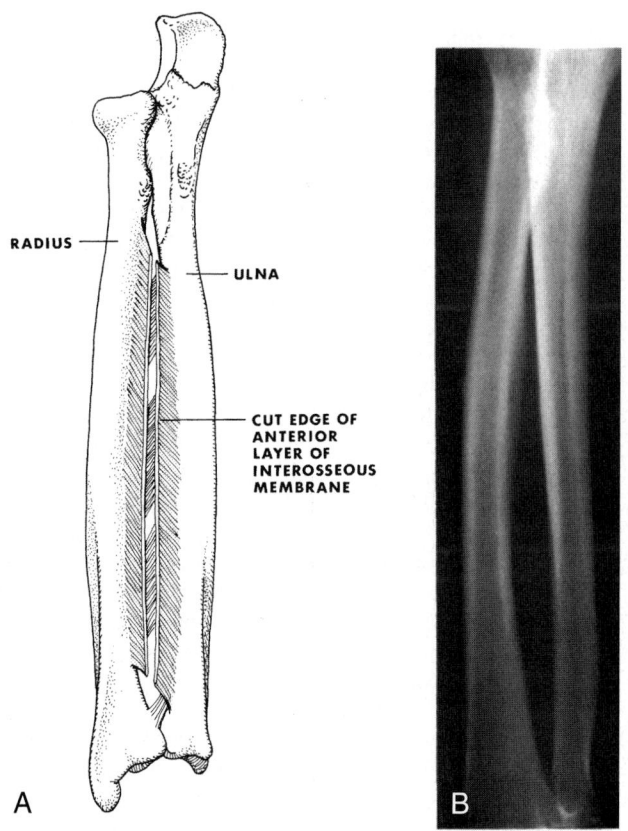

**Figure 2–2.** Fibrous articulation: syndesmosis. *A* and *B*, The interosseous membrane between the medial aspect of the radius and the lateral aspect of the ulna originates approximately 3 cm below the radial tuberosity and extends to the wrist, containing apertures for various interosseous vessels. The radiograph reveals an osseous crest on apposing surfaces of bone.

## Symphysis

In a symphysis (Fig. 2–4), adjacent bony surfaces are connected by a cartilaginous disc, which arises from chondrification of intervening mesenchymal tissue. Eventually, this tissue is composed of fibrocartilaginous or fibrous connective tissue, although a thin layer of hyaline cartilage usually persists, covering the articular surface of the adjacent bone. Symphyses (typified by the symphysis pubis and intervertebral disc) allow a small amount of motion, which occurs through compression or deformation of the intervening connective tissue.

Some symphyses, such as the symphysis pubis and manubriosternal joint, have a small, cleftlike central cavity that contains fluid and may enlarge with advancing age; this cavity may be demonstrable radiographically, owing to the presence of gas (vacuum phenomenon). Symphyses are located within the midsagittal plane of the human body and are permanent structures, unlike synchondroses, which are temporary joints. Infrequently, intra-articular ankylosis or synostosis may obliterate a symphysis, such as occurs at the manubriosternal joint.

## Synchondrosis

Synchondroses (Fig. 2–5) are temporary joints that exist during the growing phase of the skeleton and are composed of hyaline cartilage. Typical synchondroses are the cartilaginous growth plate between the epiphysis and metaphysis of a tubular bone; the neurocentral vertebral articulations; and the unossified cartilage in the chondro-

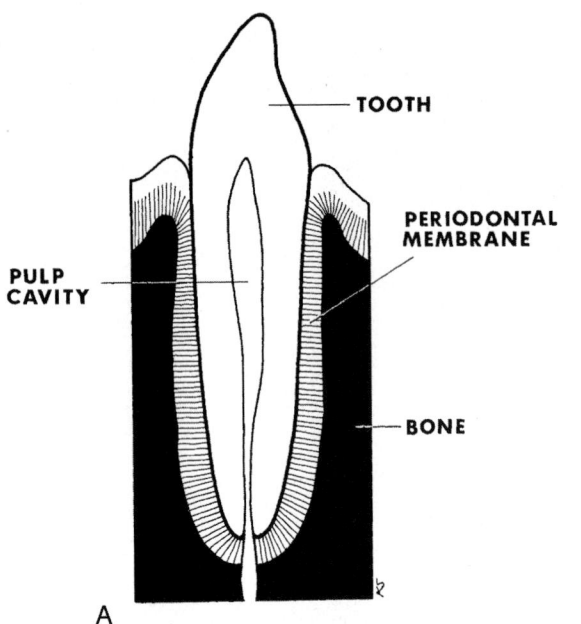

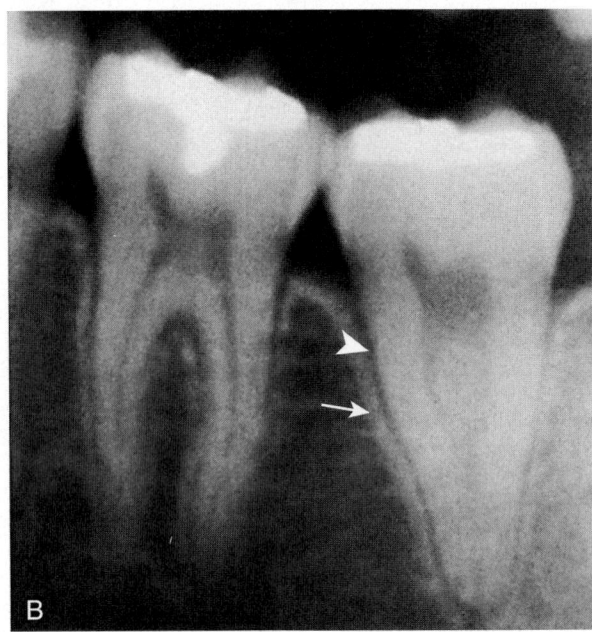

**Figure 2–3.** Fibrous articulation: gomphosis. *A,* Diagrammatic representation of this special type of articulation located between the teeth and the maxilla or mandible. Note the location of the periodontal membrane. *B,* Radiograph reveals the radiolucent periodontal membrane *(arrowhead)* and the radiopaque lamina dura *(arrow)*.

cranium, the spheno-occipital synchondrosis. With skeletal maturation, synchondroses become thinner and are eventually obliterated by bony union or synostosis.

## SYNOVIAL ARTICULATIONS

A synovial joint is a specialized type of joint that is located primarily in the appendicular skeleton (Fig. 2–6). Synovial articulations generally allow unrestricted motion. The structure of a synovial joint differs fundamentally from that of fibrous and cartilaginous joints; osseous surfaces are bound together by a fibrous capsule,

which may be reinforced by accessory ligaments. The inner portion of the articulating surface of the apposing bones is separated by a space, the articular or joint cavity. Articular cartilage covers the ends of both bones; motion between these cartilaginous surfaces is characterized by a low coefficient of friction. The inner aspect of the joint capsule is formed by the synovial membrane, which secretes synovial fluid into the articular cavity. This synovial fluid acts both as a lubricant, encouraging motion, and as a nutritive substance, providing nourishment to the adjacent articular cartilage. In some synovial joints, an intra-articular disc of fibrocartilage partially or completely divides the joint cavity. Additional intra-articular structures, including fat pads and labra, may be noted.

### Articular Cartilage

The articulating surfaces of the bone are covered by a layer of glistening connective tissue, the articular cartilage. Its unique properties include transmission and distribution of high loads, maintenance of contact stresses at acceptably low levels, movement with little friction, and shock absorption. In most synovial joints, the cartilage is hyaline in type. Articular cartilage is devoid of lymphatic vessels, blood vessels, and nerves. A large portion of the cartilage derives its nutrition through diffusion of fluid from the synovial cavity. Small blood vessels pass from the subchondral bone plate into the deepest stratum of cartilage, providing nutrients to this area of articular cartilage. Additionally, a vascular ring is located within the synovial membrane at the periphery of the cartilage.

Articular cartilage is variable in thickness. It may be thicker on one articulating bone than on another. Further,

**Figure 2–4.** Cartilaginous articulation: symphysis (symphysis pubis). Note the central fibrocartilage (FC), with a thin layer of hyaline cartilage (HC) adjacent to the osseous surfaces of the pubis.

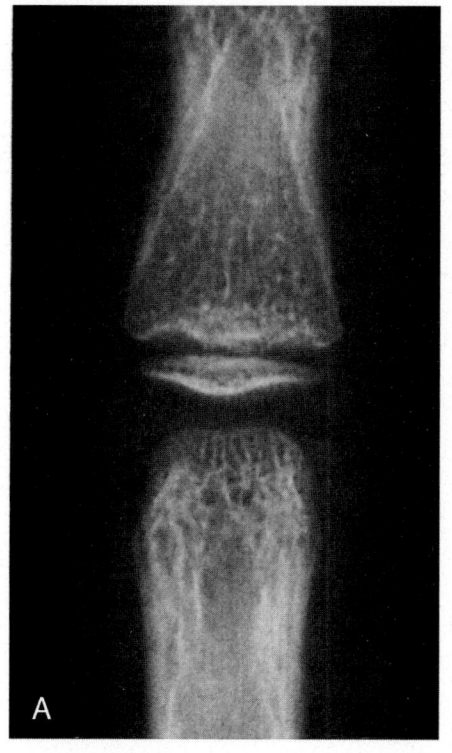

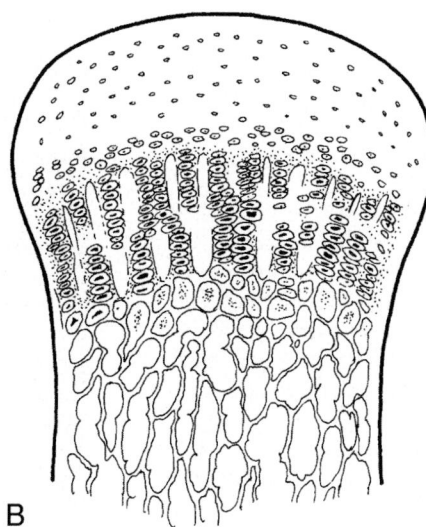

**Figure 2–5.** Cartilaginous articulation: synchondrosis. *A,* Radiograph of the phalanges in a growing child demonstrates a typical epiphysis separated from the metaphysis and diaphysis by the radiolucent growth plate. *B,* Schematic drawing of a growth plate between the cartilaginous epiphysis and the ossified diaphysis of a long bone. Note the transition from hyaline cartilage through various cartilaginous zones, including resting cartilage, cell proliferation, cell hypertrophy, cell calcification, and bone formation.

articular cartilage is not necessarily of uniform thickness over the entire osseous surface. In general, it varies from 1 to 7 mm thick, averaging 2 or 3 mm. Cartilage is thicker (1) in large joints than in small joints; (2) in joints or areas of joints in which there is considerable functional pressure or stress, such as those in the lower extremity; (3) at sites of extensive frictional or shearing force; (4) in poorly fitted articulations (i.e., less congruent joints) compared

with smoothly fitted ones; and (5) in young and middle-aged persons compared with older people.

## Subchondral Bone Plate and Tidemark

The bony or subchondral endplate is a layer of osseous tissue of variable thickness that is located beneath the cartilage. Immediately superficial to the subchondral bone

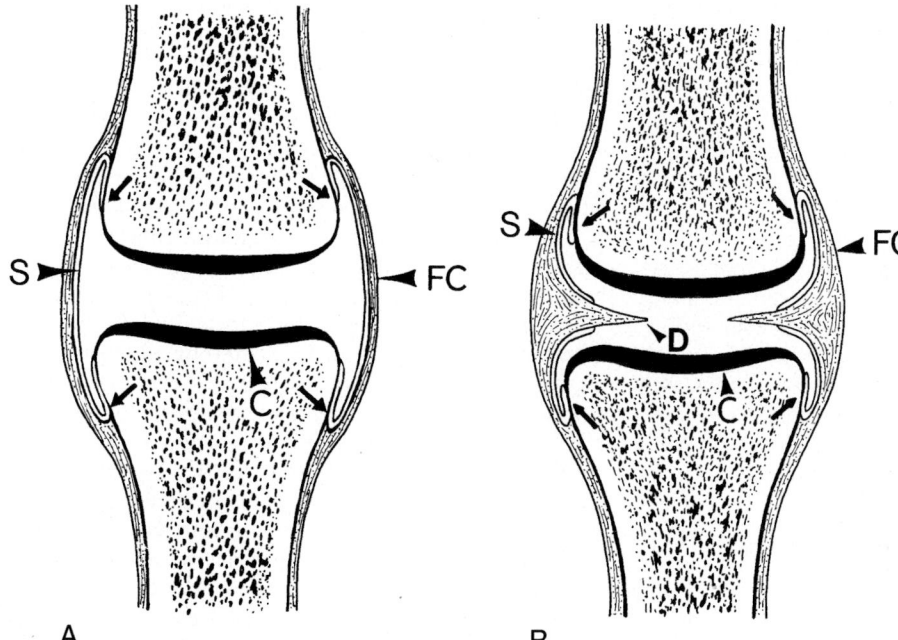

**Figure 2–6.** Synovial articulation: general features. *A,* Typical synovial joint without an intra-articular disc. Diagram of a section through a metacarpophalangeal joint outlines the important structures, including the fibrous capsule (FC), synovial membrane (S), and articular cartilage (C). Note that there are marginal areas of the articulation where synovial membrane abuts on bone without protective cartilage *(arrows). B,* Typical synovial joint containing an articular disc that partially divides the joint cavity. Diagram of a section through the knee joint reveals the fibrous capsule (FC), synovial membrane (S), articular cartilage (C), and articular disc (D). The marginal areas of the joint are indicated by arrows.

plate is the calcified zone of articular cartilage, termed the tidemark. The tidemark serves a mechanical function; it anchors the collagen fibers of the noncalcified portion of cartilage and, in turn, is anchored to the subchondral bone plate. These strong connections resist disruption by shearing force.

## Articular Capsule

The articular capsule is connective tissue that envelops the joint cavity. It is composed of a thick, tough outer layer—the fibrous capsule—and a more delicate, thin inner layer—the synovial membrane.

**Fibrous Capsule.** The fibrous capsule consists of parallel and interlacing bundles of dense white fibrous tissue. At each end of the articulation, the fibrous capsule is firmly adherent to the periosteum of the articulating bones. The site of attachment of the capsule to the periosteum is variable. The fibrous capsule is not of uniform thickness. Ligaments and tendons may attach to it, producing focal areas of increased thickness. Extracapsular accessory ligaments, such as those about the sternoclavicular joint, and intracapsular ligaments, such as the cruciate ligaments of the knee, also may be found. The fibrous capsule is richly supplied with blood and lymphatic vessels and nerves, which may penetrate the capsule and extend down to the synovial membrane.

**Synovial Membrane.** The synovial membrane is a delicate, highly vascular inner membrane of the articular capsule (Fig. 2–7). It lines the nonarticular portion of the synovial joint and any intra-articular ligaments or tendons. The synovial membrane also covers the intracapsular osseous surfaces, which are clothed by periosteum or perichondrium but lack cartilaginous surfaces. These latter areas occur frequently at the peripheral portion of the joint and are termed "marginal" or "bare" areas of the joint.

The synovial membrane demonstrates variable structural characteristics in different segments of the joint. In general, there are two synovial layers: a thin cellular surface layer (intima) and a deeper vascular underlying layer (subintima). The subintimal layer merges on its deep surface with the fibrous capsule. In certain locations, the synovial membrane is attenuated and fails to demonstrate two distinct layers.

The synovial membrane has several functions. First, it is involved in the secretion of a sticky mucoid substance into the synovial fluid. Second, owing to its inherent flexibility, loose synovial folds, villi, and marginal recesses, the synovium facilitates and accommodates the changing shape of the articular cavity that is required for normal joint motion, an ability that is lost in the case of adhesive capsulitis, which is accompanied by a decrease in synovial flexibility. In addition, the synovial membrane aids in the removal of substances from the articular cavity.

## Intra-articular Disc (Meniscus), Labrum, and Fat Pad

A fibrocartilaginous disc, or meniscus, may be found in some joints, such as the knee, wrist, and temporomandibu-

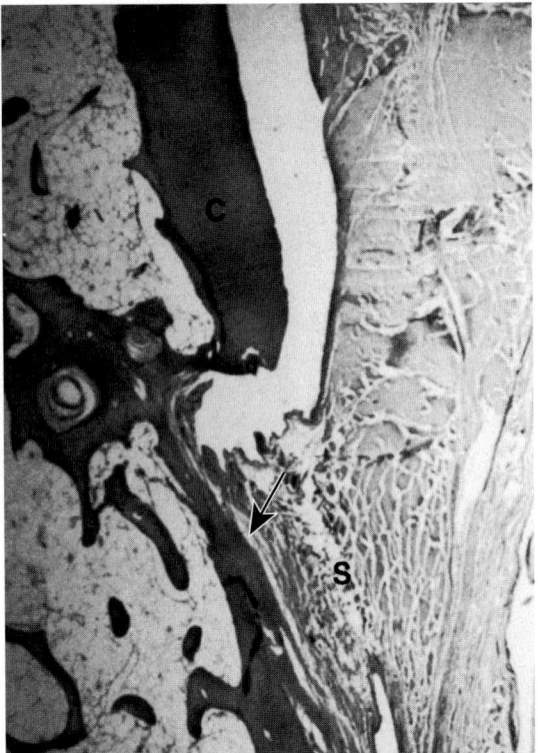

**Figure 2–7.** Synovial articulation: synovial membrane. Low-power (×80) photomicrograph of the chondro-osseous junction about a metacarpophalangeal joint delineates the synovial membrane (S) and articular cartilage (C). The marginal area of the joint where the synovial membrane abuts on bone is well demonstrated (*arrow*).

lar, acromioclavicular, sternoclavicular, and costovertebral joints. The peripheral portion of the disc attaches to the fibrous capsule. Blood vessels and afferent nerves may be noted within this peripheral zone of the disc. Most of the articular disc, however, is avascular. The exact function of intra-articular discs is unknown. Suggested functions include shock absorption, distribution of weight over a large surface, facilitation of various motions (such as rotation) and limitation of others (such as translation), and protection of the articular surface. It has been suggested that intra-articular discs play an important role in the effective lubrication of a joint.

Some joints, such as the hip and glenohumeral articulations, contain circumferential cartilaginous folds termed labra (Fig. 2–8). These lips of cartilage are usually triangular in cross section and are attached to the peripheral portion of an articular surface, thereby acting to enlarge or deepen the joint cavity. They also may help increase contact and congruity of adjacent articular surfaces, particularly at the extremes of joint motion.

Fat pads represent additional structures that may be present within a joint. These structures possess a generous vascular and nerve supply, contain few lymphatic vessels, and are covered by a flattened layer of synovial cells. Fat pads may act as cushions, absorbing forces generated across a joint, thus protecting adjacent bony processes. They also may distribute lubricants in the joint cavity.

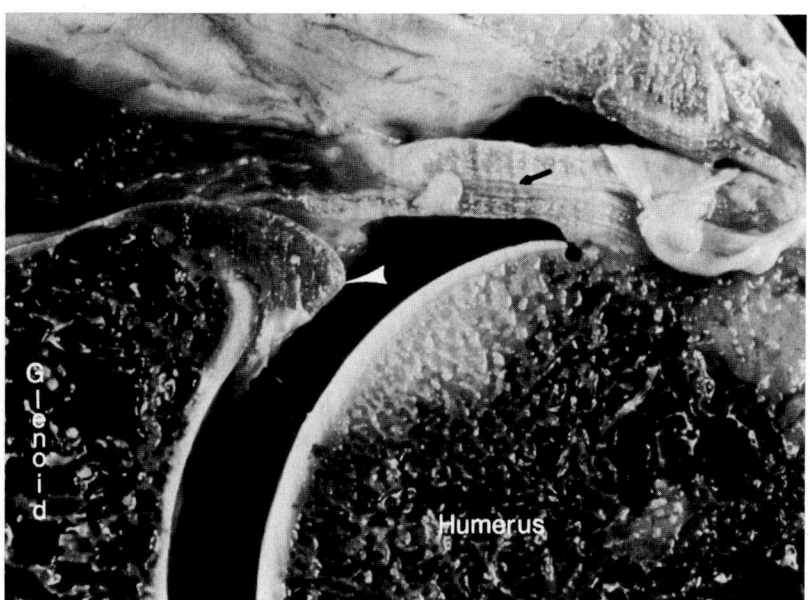

**Figure 2–8.** Synovial articulation: intra-articular labrum. Photograph of a coronal section through the superior aspect of the glenohumeral joint demonstrates a cartilaginous labrum (*arrowhead*) along the superior aspect of the glenoid. Note the adjacent rotator cuff tendons (*arrow*).

## Synovial Fluid

Minute amounts of clear, colorless to pale yellow, highly viscous fluid of slightly alkaline pH are present in healthy joints. The exact composition, viscosity, volume, and color vary somewhat from joint to joint. Particles, cell fragments, and fibrous tissue may also be seen in the synovial fluid as a result of wear and tear of the articular surface. Functions of the synovial fluid are to provide nutrition to the adjacent articular cartilage and disc and lubrication of joint surfaces, which decreases friction and increases joint efficiency.

## Synovial Sheaths and Bursae

Synovial tissue is also found about various tendon sheaths and bursae (Fig. 2–9). This tissue is located at sites where closely apposed structures move in relationship to each other. Tendon sheaths completely or partially cover a portion of the tendon where it passes through fascial slings, osseofibrous tunnels, and ligamentous bands. They function to promote the gliding of tendons and contribute to the nutrition of the intrasheath portion of the tendons.

Bursae represent enclosed, flattened sacs consisting of synovial lining and, in some locations, a thin film of synovial fluid, which provides both lubrication and nourishment for the cells of the synovial membrane. Intervening bursae facilitate motion between apposing tissues. Subcutaneous bursae are found between skin and underlying bony prominences, such as the olecranon and patella; subfascial bursae occur between deep fascia and bone; subtendinous bursae exist where one tendon overlies another tendon; submucosal bursae are located between muscle and bone, tendon, or ligament; interligamentous bursae separate ligaments. When bursae are located near

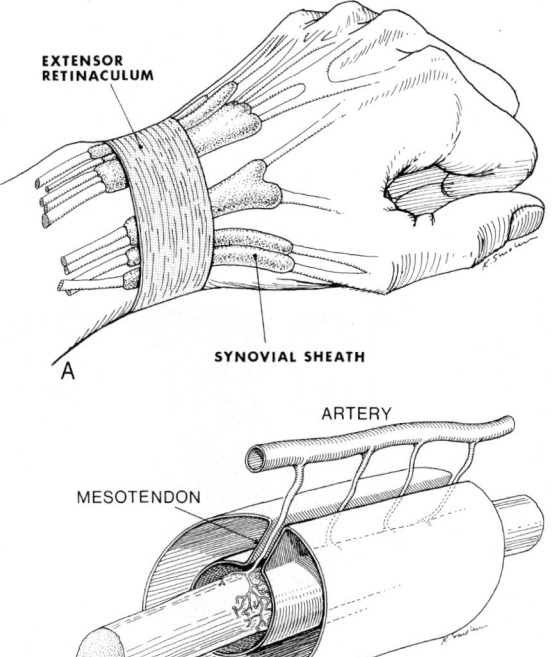

**Figure 2–9.** Tendons and tendon sheaths. *A*, Extensor tendons with surrounding synovial sheaths pass beneath the extensor retinaculum on the dorsum of the wrist. *B*, Drawing of the fine structure of a tendon and tendon sheath reveals an inner coat or visceral layer adjacent to the tendon surface and an outer coat or parietal layer. Note that the invaginated tendon allows apposition of visceral and parietal layers in the form of a mesotendon. This latter structure provides a passageway for adjacent blood vessels.

articulations, the synovial membrane of the bursa may be continuous with that of the joint cavity, producing communicating bursae. This occurs normally about the hip (iliopsoas bursa) and knee (gastrocnemiosemimembranous bursa) and abnormally about the glenohumeral joint (subacromial bursa) owing to defects in the rotator cuff. Distention of communicating bursae may serve to lower intra-articular pressure in cases of joint effusion. At certain sites where skin is subject to pressure and lateral displacement, adventitious bursae may appear, allowing increased freedom of motion. Examples of adventitious bursae include those that may develop over a hallux valgus deformity, those occurring about prominent spinous processes, and bursae located adjacent to exostoses.

## Sesamoid Bones

Sesamoids generally are small ovoid nodules embedded in tendons (Fig. 2–10). They are found in two specific situations in the skeleton.

**Type A.** In type A, the sesamoid is located adjacent to a joint, and its tendon is incorporated into the joint capsule. The sesamoid nodule and adjacent bone form an extension of the articulation. Examples of this type are the patella and the hallucis and pollicis sesamoids.

**Type B.** In type B, the sesamoid is located at sites where tendons are angled about bony surfaces. They are separated from the underlying bone by a synovium-lined bursa. An example of this type of sesamoid is the sesamoid of the peroneus longus.

In both type A and type B situations, the arrangement of the sesamoid nodule and surrounding tissue resembles that of a synovial joint. In the hand, sesamoid nodules adjacent to joints (type A) are present most frequently on the palmar aspect of the metacarpophalangeal joints, particularly the first. In this location, two sesamoids are found in the tendons of the adductor pollicis and flexor pollicis brevis, articulating with facets on the palmar surface of the metacarpal head. Additional sesamoids are most frequent in the second and fifth metacarpophalangeal joints and adjacent to the interphalangeal joint of the thumb. This distribution of sesamoids in the hand is not constant. Sesamoid bones unassociated with synovial joints (type B) are more frequent in the lower extremity than in the upper extremity. In the foot, sesamoids of this type are noted in the tendon of the peroneus longus muscle adjacent to a facet on the tuberosity of the cuboid bone and in the tendon of the tibialis anterior muscle in contact with the medial surface of the medial cuneiform bone.

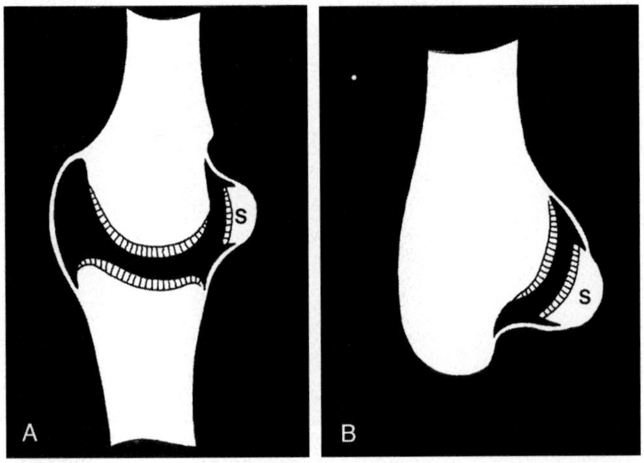

## SUPPORTING STRUCTURES

### Tendons

Tendons represent a portion of a muscle and are of constant length, consisting of collagen fibers that transmit muscle tension to a mobile part of the body. They are flexible cords that can be angulated about bony protuberances, changing the direction of pull of the muscle. Synovial sheaths may surround portions of the tendon. In some locations, such as the flexor tendons about the ankle, fluid is normally observed in these synovial sheaths. The attachment sites of tendons are termed *entheses*.

### Aponeuroses

Aponeuroses consist of several flat layers or sheets of dense collagen fibers associated with the attachment of a muscle. The fasciculi within one layer of an aponeurosis are parallel, and they differ in direction from fasciculi of an adjacent layer.

### Fasciae

*Fascia* is a general term used to describe a focal collection of connective tissue. Superficial fascia consists of a layer of loose areolar tissue of variable thickness beneath the dermis. It is most distinct over the lower abdomen, perineum, and limbs. Deep fascia resembles an aponeurosis, consisting of regularly arranged, compact collagen fibers. Parallel fibers of one layer are angled with respect to the fibers of an adjacent layer. Deep fascia is particularly prominent in the extremities, and in these sites, muscle may arise from the inner aspect of the deep fascia. At sites where deep fascia contacts bone, the fascia fuses with the periosteum. It is well suited to transmit the pull of adjacent musculature. Intermuscular septa extend from deep fascia between groups of muscles, producing functional compartments. These compartments are important with regard to patterns of spread of infection and tumor. Retinacula are transverse thickenings in the deep fascia that are attached to bony protuberances, creating tunnels through which tendons can pass. An example is the dorsal retinaculum of the wrist, under which extend the extensor tendons and their synovial sheaths.

**Figure 2–10.** Sesamoid bones. There are two types of sesamoids: type A *(A)*, in which the sesamoid is located adjacent to an articulation, and type B *(B)*, in which the sesamoid is separated from the underlying bone by a bursa. In both types, the sesamoid is intimately associated with a synovial lining and articular cartilage *(hatched areas)*.

(From Resnick D, Niwayama G, Feingold ML: The sesamoid bones of the hands and feet: Participators in arthritis. Radiology 123:57, 1977.)

## Ligaments

Ligaments represent fibrous bands that unite bones. They do not transmit muscle action directly but are essential in the control of posture and the maintenance of joint stability. Histologically and biomechanically, ligaments resemble tendons, and their sites of osseous attachment (entheses) are similar to those of tendons.

## VASCULAR, LYMPHATIC, AND NERVE SUPPLY

The blood supply of joints arises from periarticular arterial plexuses that pierce the capsule, break up in the synovial membrane, and form a rich and intricate network of capillaries. A circle of vessels (circulus articularis vasculosus) within the synovial membrane is adjacent to the peripheral margin of articular cartilage.

The lymphatics form a plexus in the subintima of the synovial membrane. Efferent vessels pass toward the flexor aspect of the joint and then along blood vessels to regional deep lymph nodes. The nerve supply of movable joints generally arises from the same nerves that supply the adjacent musculature. The fibrous capsule and, to a lesser extent, the synovial membrane are both supplied by nerves.

## FURTHER READING

Barnett CH, Davies DV, MacConaill MA: Snyovial Joints: Their Structure and Mechanics. Springfield, Ill, Charles C Thomas, 1961.

Canoso JJ: Bursae, tendons and ligaments. Clin Rheum Dis 7:189, 1981.

Davies DV: The structure and functions of the synovial membrane. BMJ 1:92, 1950.

Jaffe HL: Metabolic, Degenerative and Inflammatory Diseases of Bones and Joints. Philadelphia, Lea & Febiger, 1972, p 80.

Resnick D, Niwayama G: Entheses and enthesopathy: Anatomical, pathological, and radiological correlation. Radiology 146:1, 1983.

Resnick D, Niwayama G, Feingold ML: The sesamoid bones of the hands and feet: Participators in arthritis. Radiology 123:57, 1977.

Shepherd DET, Seedhom BB: Thickness of human articular cartilage in joints of the lower limb. Ann Rheum Dis 58:27, 1999.

Simkin PA: Friction and lubrication in synovial joints. J Rheumatol 27:567, 2000.

Walmsley R: Joints. In Romanes GJ (ed): Cunningham's Textbook of Anatomy, 11th ed. London, Oxford University Press, 1972, p 207.

Wyke B: The neurology of joints: A review of general principles. Clin Rheum Dis 7:223, 1981.

# CHAPTER 3

## Anatomy of Individual Joints

## SUMMARY OF KEY FEATURES

Anatomic features related to articular and periarticular soft tissue and osseous structures govern the manner in which disease processes become evident on radiographs. This chapter summarizes the basic osseous and soft tissue anatomy of individual joints in the body. The tendinous and ligamentous anatomy is reviewed in greater detail in Chapter 5.

## WRIST

### Osseous Anatomy

The osseous structures about the wrist are the distal portions of the radius and ulna, the proximal and distal rows of carpal bones, and the metacarpals. The distal aspects of the radius and ulna articulate with the proximal row of carpal bones. The articular surface of the radius is divided into an ulnar and a radial portion by a faint central ridge of bone. The ulnar portion articulates with the lunate, and the radial portion articulates with the scaphoid. The medial surface of the distal end of the radius contains the concave ulnar notch, which articulates with the distal end of the ulna. The proximal row of carpal bones consists of the scaphoid, lunate, and triquetrum, as well as the pisiform bone within the tendon of the flexor carpi ulnaris muscle. The distal row of carpal bones contains the trapezium, trapezoid, capitate, and hamate bones. A strong fibrous retinaculum attaches to the palmar surface of the carpus, converting the carpal groove into a carpal tunnel, through which pass the median nerve and flexor tendons.

Ulnar variance relates to the length of the ulna compared with that of the radius. A positive ulnar variance (i.e., ulnar plus) means a relatively long ulna in which the articular surface of the ulna projects distal to that of the radius; this variance is associated with the ulnocarpal abutment, or impaction, syndrome. A negative ulnar variance implies a relatively short ulna and is associated with Kienböck's disease.

When the wrist is in the neutral position without dorsal or palmar flexion, the distal end of the radius articulates with the scaphoid and approximately 50% of the lunate. The degree of radial deviation of the radiocarpal compartment can be measured on a posteroanterior radiograph with the wrist in this neutral attitude. A line is drawn through the longitudinal axis of the second metacarpal at its radial cortex. On a lateral radiograph of a normal wrist in the neutral position without palmar flexion or dorsiflexion, a continuous line can be drawn through the longitudinal axes of the radius, lunate, capitate, and third metacarpal. The alignment of the bones in the wrist joints varies with wrist position (Fig. 3–1).

The complexity of wrist motion has led to differing concepts of functional osseous anatomy. Some regard the wrist as composed of carpal bones arranged in two rows (proximal and distal), with the scaphoid bridging the two. Others describe the joint as a vertical arrangement consisting of three columns. A mobile lateral column contains the scaphoid, trapezium, and trapezoid; osteoarthritis occurs here most frequently. The central column, containing the lunate and capitate, is concerned with flexion and extension and is primarily implicated in most varieties of carpal instability. The medial column is composed of the triquetrum and hamate, and, on the axis of this column, the rotation of the forearm is extended into the wrist. A third concept considers the wrist as a dynamic ring, with a fixed distal half and a mobile proximal half. Distortion or rupture of the mobile segment with respect to the rigid part explains both instability and dislocation.

### Soft Tissue Anatomy

The wrist is not a single joint. Rather, it consists of a series of articulations or compartments (Fig. 3–2).

**Radiocarpal Compartment.** The radiocarpal compartment (Fig. 3–3) is formed proximally by the distal surface of the radius and the triangular fibrocartilage complex and distally by the proximal row of carpal bones exclusive of the pisiform. The triangular fibrocartilage prevents communication of the radiocarpal and inferior radioulnar compartments, whereas a meniscus may attach to the triquetrum, preventing communication of the radiocarpal and pisiform-triquetral compartments. The triangular fibrocartilage, the meniscus, the dorsal and volar radioulnar ligaments, the ulnar collateral ligament, the ulnocarpal ligaments, and (sometimes) the sheath of the extensor carpi ulnaris tendon are the components of the triangular fibrocartilage complex of the wrist and represent important stabilizers about the inferior radioulnar joint (see Chapter 59). Synovial diverticula, or recesses, are common and vary in number and size.

**Inferior Radioulnar Compartment.** The inferior radioulnar compartment (see Fig. 3–2) is an L-shaped joint whose proximal border is the cartilage-covered head of the ulna and ulnar notch of the radius. Its distal limit is the triangular fibrocartilage.

**Midcarpal Compartment.** The midcarpal compartment (see Fig. 3–2) extends between the proximal and distal carpal rows. On the radial aspect of the midcarpal compartment, the trapezium and trapezoid articulate with the distal aspect of the scaphoid. The radial side of this compartment is called the trapezioscaphoid space.

**Pisiform-Triquetral Compartment.** The pisiform-triquetral compartment (Fig. 3–4) exists between the palmar surface of the triquetrum and the dorsal surface of the pisiform. A large proximal synovial recess can be noted.

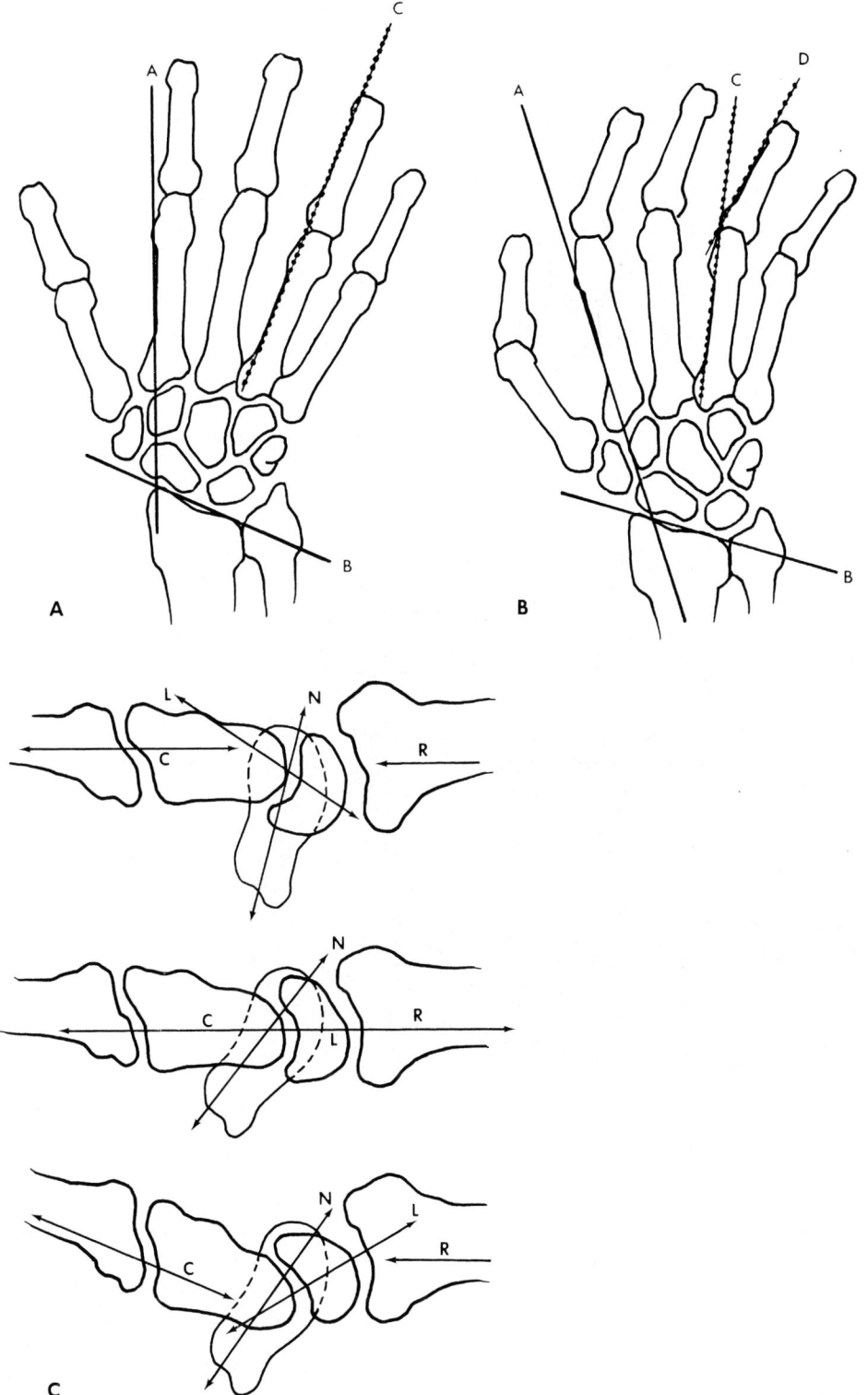

**Figure 3–1.** Hand and wrist: normal and abnormal alignment. *A* and *B*, Frontal projection. The angle of intersection of lines A and B, measuring radial deviation of the radiocarpal compartment, normally averages 112 degrees *(A)* and is increased in rheumatoid arthritis *(B)*. Lines C and D measure ulnar deviation at the metacarpophalangeal joints. *C,* Lateral projection. Line drawings of longitudinal axes of the third metacarpal, navicular (N) or scaphoid, lunate (L), capitate (C), and radius (R) in dorsiflexion instability (upper), in a normal situation (middle), and in palmar flexion instability (lower). When the wrist is normal, a continuous line can be drawn through the longitudinal axes of the capitate, lunate, and radius, and this line intersects a second line through the longitudinal axis of the scaphoid, creating an angle of 30 to 60 degrees. In dorsiflexion instability, the lunate is flexed toward the back of the hand and the scaphoid is displaced vertically. The angle of intersection between the two longitudinal axes is greater than 60 degrees. In palmar flexion instability, the lunate is flexed toward the palm and the angle between the two longitudinal axes is less than 30 degrees.

*(A* and *B,* From Resnick D: Rheumatoid arthritis of the wrist: The compartmental approach. Med Radiogr Photogr 52:50, 1976. *C,* From Linscheid RL, Dobyns JH, Beabout JW, Bryan RS: Traumatic instability of the wrist. Diagnosis, classification, and pathomechanics. J Bone Joint Surg Am 54:1612, 1972.)

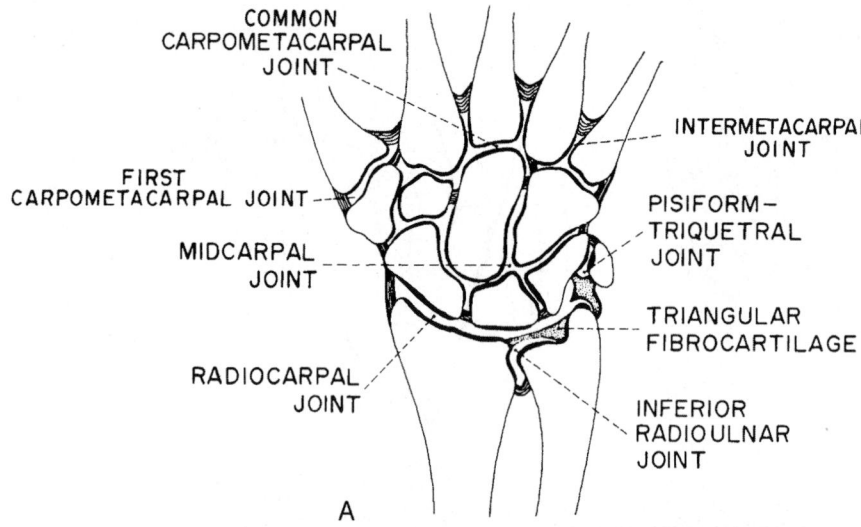

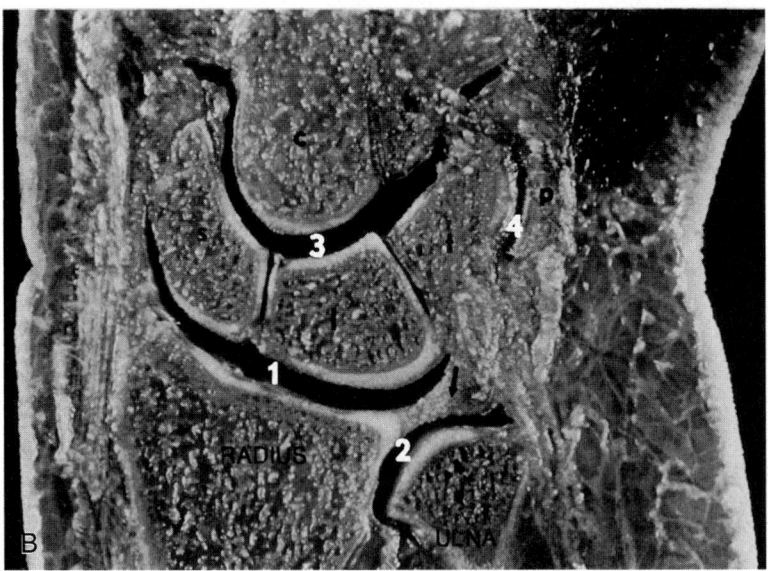

**Figure 3–2.** Articulations of the wrist: general anatomy. The various wrist compartments are depicted on a schematic drawing *(A)* and in a photograph *(B)* of a coronal section. These include the radiocarpal (1), inferior radioulnar (2), midcarpal (3), and pisiform-triquetral (4) compartments. Note the triangular fibrocartilage *(arrow)*. c, capitate; h, hamate; l, lunate; p, pisiform; s, scaphoid; t, triquetrum.

**Common Carpometacarpal Compartment.** This compartment exists between the base of each of the four medial metacarpals and the distal row of carpal bones (see Fig. 3–2). Occasionally, the articulation between the hamate and the fourth and fifth metacarpals is a separate synovial cavity, produced by a ligamentous attachment between the hamate and fourth metacarpal.

**First Carpometacarpal Compartment.** The carpometacarpal compartment of the thumb is a separate saddle-shaped cavity between the trapezium and base of the first metacarpal (see Fig. 3–2).

**Intermetacarpal Compartments.** Three intermetacarpal compartments extend between the bases of the second and third, the third and fourth, and the fourth and fifth metacarpals. These compartments usually communicate with one another and with the common carpometacarpal compartment.

**Communication between Compartments.** Although the wrist compartments are distinct structures, direct communication between compartments has been well documented. Direct communication between the radiocarpal and inferior radioulnar joint has been noted in 7% of the radiocarpal compartment arthrograms of living persons. This communication results from a full-thickness defect of the triangular fibrocartilage, a finding seen more frequently in elderly persons, which relates to cartilaginous degeneration.

Communications have also been demonstrated between the radiocarpal and midcarpal compartments (resulting from a full-thickness defect of the interosseous ligaments that extend between the bones of the proximal carpal row), radiocarpal and pisiform-triquetral compartments, and midcarpal, carpometacarpal, and intermetacarpal compartments. The frequency of these communications is not known. Extensor tendons traverse the dorsum of the wrist, surrounded by synovial sheaths (Fig. 3–5). The attachment

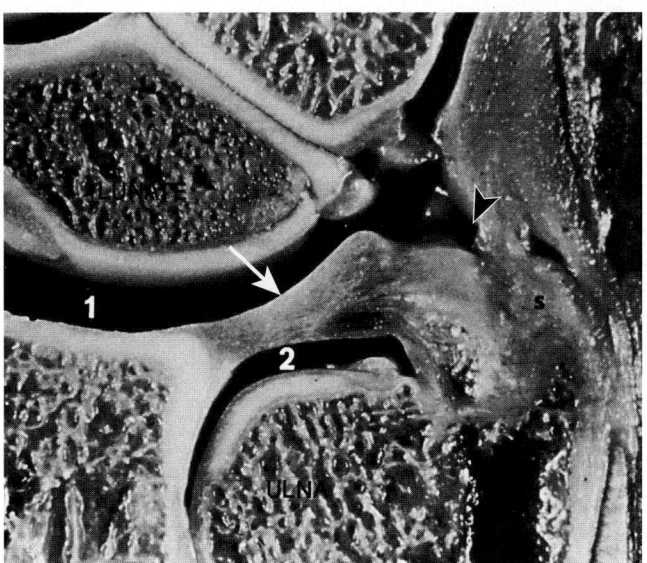

**Figure 3–3.** Articulations of the wrist: specific compartments. Ulnar limit of the radiocarpal compartment (coronal section). Note the extent of this compartment (1), its relationship to the inferior radioulnar compartment (2), the intervening triangular fibrocartilage *(arrow)*, and the prestyloid recess *(arrowhead)*, which is intimate with the ulnar styloid (s).

of the dorsal carpal ligament to the adjacent radius and ulna creates six separate compartments or bundles of tendons. Flexor tendons with surrounding synovial sheaths pass through the carpal tunnel in the palmar aspect of the wrist.

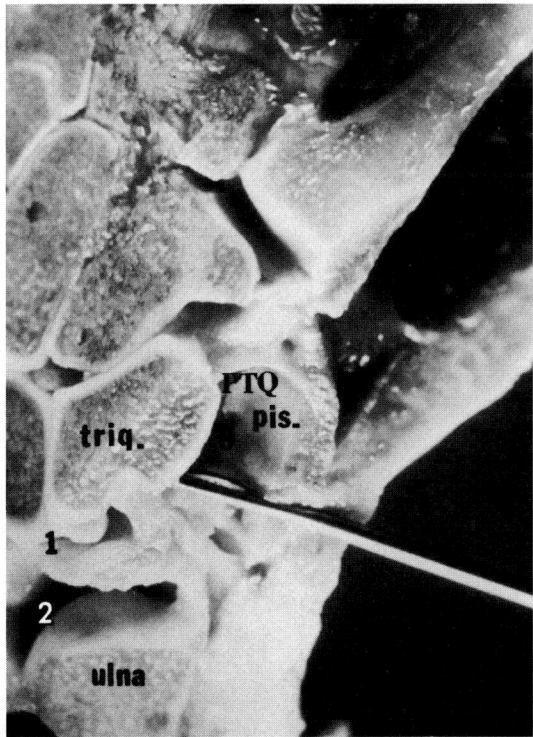

**Figure 3–4.** Articulations of the wrist: specific compartments. Pisiform-triquetral compartment (coronal section). This compartment (PTQ) exists between the triquetrum (triq.) and pisiform (pis.). The radiocarpal (1) and inferior radioulnar (2) compartments are also indicated.

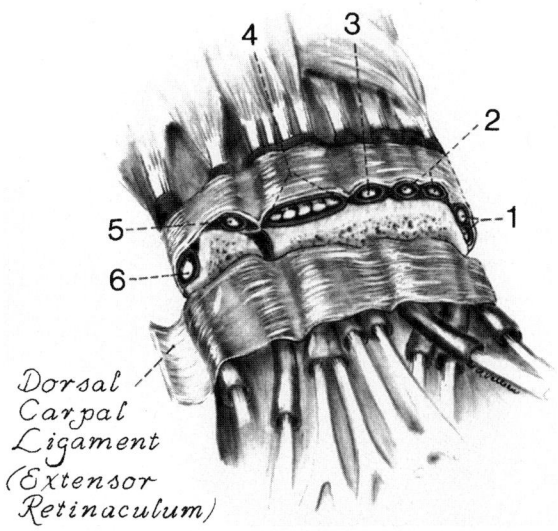

**Figure 3–5.** Extensor tendons and tendon sheaths. Drawing shows the dorsal carpal ligament and extensor tendons surrounded by synovial sheaths traversing the dorsum of the wrist within six separate compartments. These compartments are created by the insular attachment of the dorsal carpal ligament on the posterior and lateral surfaces of the radius and ulna. The extensor carpi ulnaris tendon and its sheath are in the medial compartment (6) and are closely applied to the posterior surface of the ulna.

(From Resnick D: Rheumatoid arthritis of the wrist: The compartmental approach. Med Radiogr Photogr 52:50, 1976.)

Certain tissue planes about the wrist have received attention in the literature. The scaphoid fat pad is a triangular or linear collection of fat between the radial collateral ligament and the synovial sheath of the abductor pollicis longus and extensor pollicis brevis (Fig. 3–6). On radiographs, this fat pad may produce a thin radiolucent line or triangle paralleling the lateral surface of the scaphoid. It is more difficult to discern in children younger than 11 or 12 years. Obliteration, obscuration, or displacement of this fat plane is reported to be common in acute fractures of the scaphoid, the radial styloid process, and the proximal first metacarpal bone.

A second important soft tissue landmark is the fat plane that exists between the pronator quadratus muscle and the tendons of the flexor digitorum profundus (Fig. 3–7). On a lateral radiograph, the fat pad produces a radiolucent region on the volar aspect of the wrist. Displacement, distortion, or obliteration of the pronator quadratus fat pad has been reported in fractures of the distal ends of the radius and ulna, osteomyelitis, and septic arthritis of the wrist.

## METACARPOPHALANGEAL JOINTS

### Osseous Anatomy

At the metacarpophalangeal joints, the metacarpal heads articulate with the proximal phalanges (Fig. 3–8). The medial four metacarpal bones lie side by side; the first

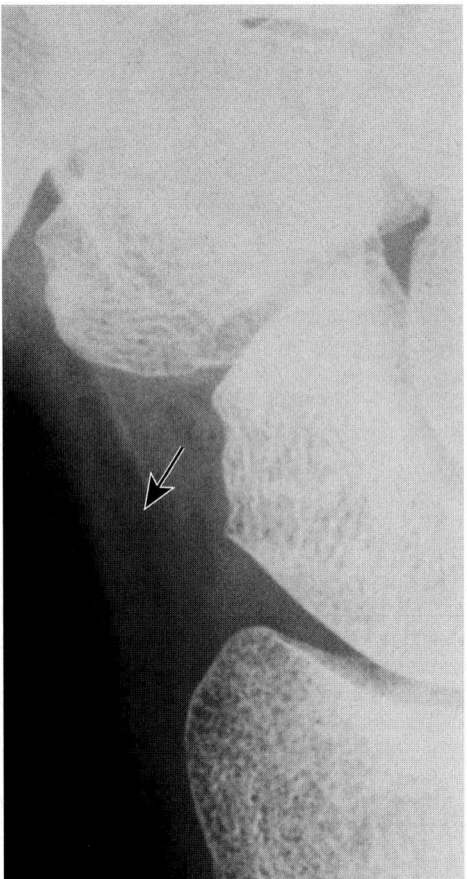

**Figure 3–6.**  Scaphoid fat pad. On a conventional radiograph, the scaphoid fat pad *(arrow)* produces a triangular or linear radiolucent shadow paralleling the lateral surface of the scaphoid.

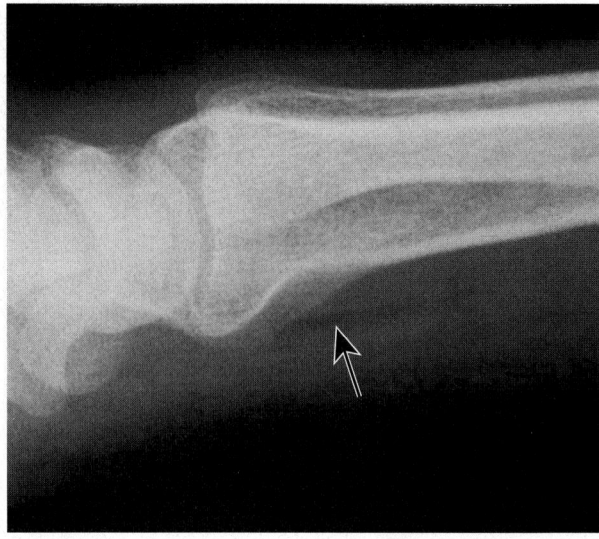

**Figure 3–7.**  Pronator fat pad. In normal situations, a fat plane between the pronator quadratus and tendons of the flexor digitorum profundus creates a radiolucent area *(arrow)* on the volar aspect of the wrist.

metacarpal lies in a more anterior plane and is rotated medially along its long axis through an angle of 90 degrees, allowing the thumb to appose the other four metacarpals during flexion and rotation. Tubercles are found on the heads of all metacarpals; these tubercles occur at the sides of the metacarpal heads where the dorsal surface of the body of the bone extends onto the head. Collateral ligaments attach to the metacarpal tubercles.

### Soft Tissue Anatomy

Each metacarpophalangeal joint has a palmar ligament and two collateral ligaments. The palmar ligament is located on the volar aspect of the articulation and is firmly attached to the base of the proximal phalanx and loosely united to the metacarpal neck. Laterally the palmar ligament blends with the collateral ligaments, and volarly the palmar ligament blends with the deep transverse metacarpal ligaments, which connect the palmar ligaments of the second through fifth metacarpophalangeal joints. The palmar ligament is also grooved for the passage of the flexor tendons, whose fibrous sheaths are attached to the sides of the groove. The collateral ligaments reinforce the fibrous capsule laterally.

## INTERPHALANGEAL JOINTS OF THE HAND

### Osseous Anatomy

At the proximal interphalangeal joints, the head of the proximal phalanx articulates with the base of the adjacent middle phalanx. The articular surface of the phalangeal head is wide (from side to side), with a central groove and ridges on either side for attachment of the collateral ligaments (see Fig. 3–8). The base of the middle phalanx contains a ridge that fits into the groove on the head of the proximal phalanx. At the distal interphalangeal joints, the head of the middle phalanx articulates with the base of the distal phalanx. This phalangeal head, like that of the proximal phalanx, is pulley-like in configuration and conforms to the base of the adjacent phalanx.

### Soft Tissue Anatomy

A fibrous capsule surrounds the articulation, and on its inner aspect, the capsule is covered by synovial membrane, which extends over intracapsular bone not covered by articular cartilage. At the interphalangeal joints, synovial pouches exist proximally on both dorsal and palmar aspects of the articulation. The interphalangeal articulations have a palmar and two collateral ligaments whose anatomy is similar to that of the ligaments about the metacarpophalangeal joints.

## ELBOW

The elbow has three articulations: (1) humeroradial—the area between the capitulum of the humerus and the facet on the radial head; (2) humeroulnar—the area between the trochlea of the humerus and the trochlear notch of the ulna; and (3) superior (proximal) radioulnar—the area between the head of the radius and radial notch of the ulna and the annular ligament.

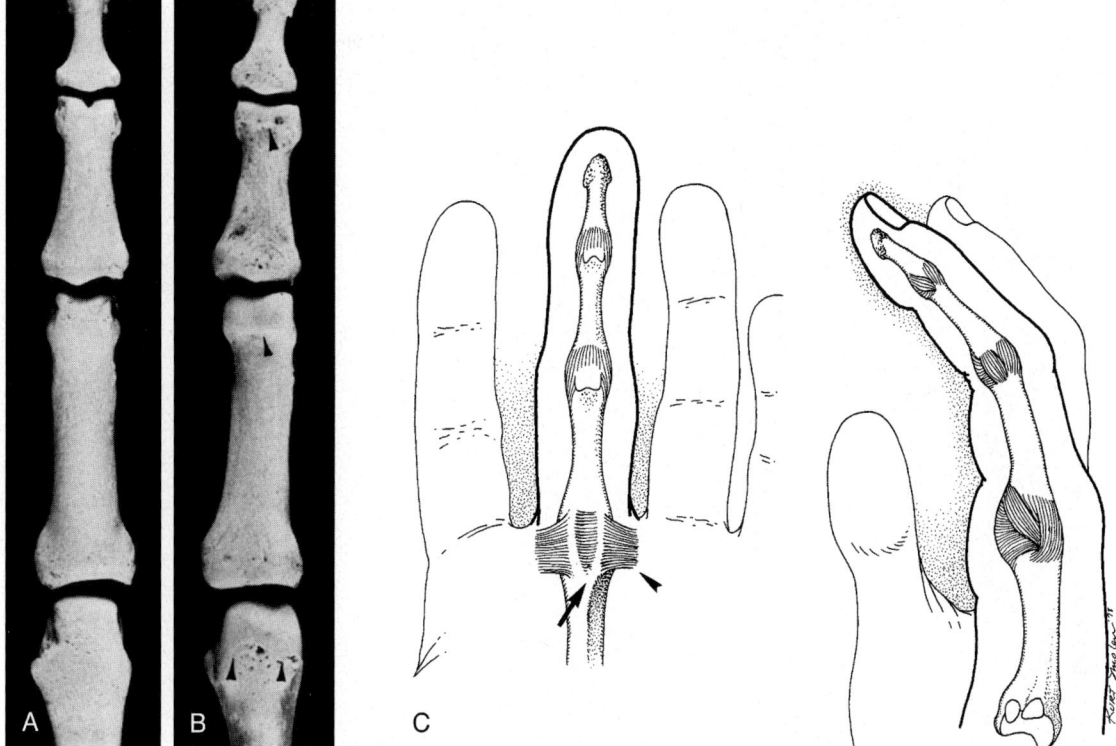

**Figure 3–8.** Metacarpals and phalanges: osseous anatomy. *A* and *B*, Dorsal *(A)* and ventral *(B)* aspects of the third metacarpal and phalanges. Note the more extensive articular surface on the volar aspect of the metacarpal head and phalanges *(arrowheads)*. *C*, Drawings of the palmar and medial aspects of the metacarpophalangeal and interphalangeal joints of the fourth digit reveal the deep transverse metacarpal ligament *(arrowhead)* with its central groove for the flexor tendons *(arrow)* and the capsule of the interphalangeal joints.

## Osseous Anatomy

The proximal end of the ulna contains two processes, the olecranon and the coronoid. The olecranon process is smooth posteriorly at the site of attachment of the triceps tendon. Its anterior surface provides the site of attachment of the capsule of the elbow joint. The coronoid process contains the radial notch, below which is the ulnar tuberosity. The radial head is disc shaped, containing a shallow, cupped articular surface that is intimate with the capitulum of the humerus. The articular circumference of the head is largest medially, where it articulates with the radial notch of the ulna (Fig. 3–9).

The distal aspect of the humerus is a wide, flattened structure. The medial third of its articular surface, termed the trochlea, is intimate with the ulna. Lateral to the trochlea is the capitulum, which articulates with the radius. The sulcus is between the trochlea and the capitulum. A hollow area, termed the olecranon fossa, is found on the posterior surface of the humerus above the trochlea. A smaller fossa, the coronoid fossa, lies above the trochlea on the anterior surface of the humerus, and a radial fossa lies adjacent to it, above the capitulum. When the elbow is fully extended, the tip of the olecranon process is located in the olecranon fossa, and when the elbow is flexed, the coronoid process of the ulna is found in the coronoid fossa and the margin of the radial head is located in the radial fossa (see Fig. 3–9).

## Soft Tissue Anatomy

A fibrous capsule invests the elbow completely. The fibrous capsule is strengthened at the sides of the articulation by the radial and ulnar collateral ligaments. The synovial membrane of the elbow lines the deep surface of the fibrous capsule. It extends from the articular surface of the humerus and contacts the olecranon, radial, and coronoid fossae and the medial surface of the trochlea. A synovial fold projects into the joint between the radius and ulna, partially dividing the articulation into humeroulnar and humeroradial portions.

Several fat pads are located between the fibrous capsule and the synovial membrane (Fig. 3–10). These fat pads, which are extrasynovial but intracapsular, are of radiographic significance. On lateral radiographs, an anterior radiolucent area represents the summation of radial and coronoid fossae fat pads. These fat pads are pressed into their respective fossae by the brachialis muscle during extension of the elbow. A posterior radiolucent region represents the olecranon fossa fat pad. It is pressed into this fossa by the triceps muscle during flexion of the elbow. The anterior fat pad normally assumes a teardrop configuration anterior to the distal end of the humerus on lateral radiographs of the elbow exposed in approximately 90 degrees of joint flexion. The posterior fat pad normally is not visible in radiographs of the elbow exposed in flexion. Any intra-articular process that is associated

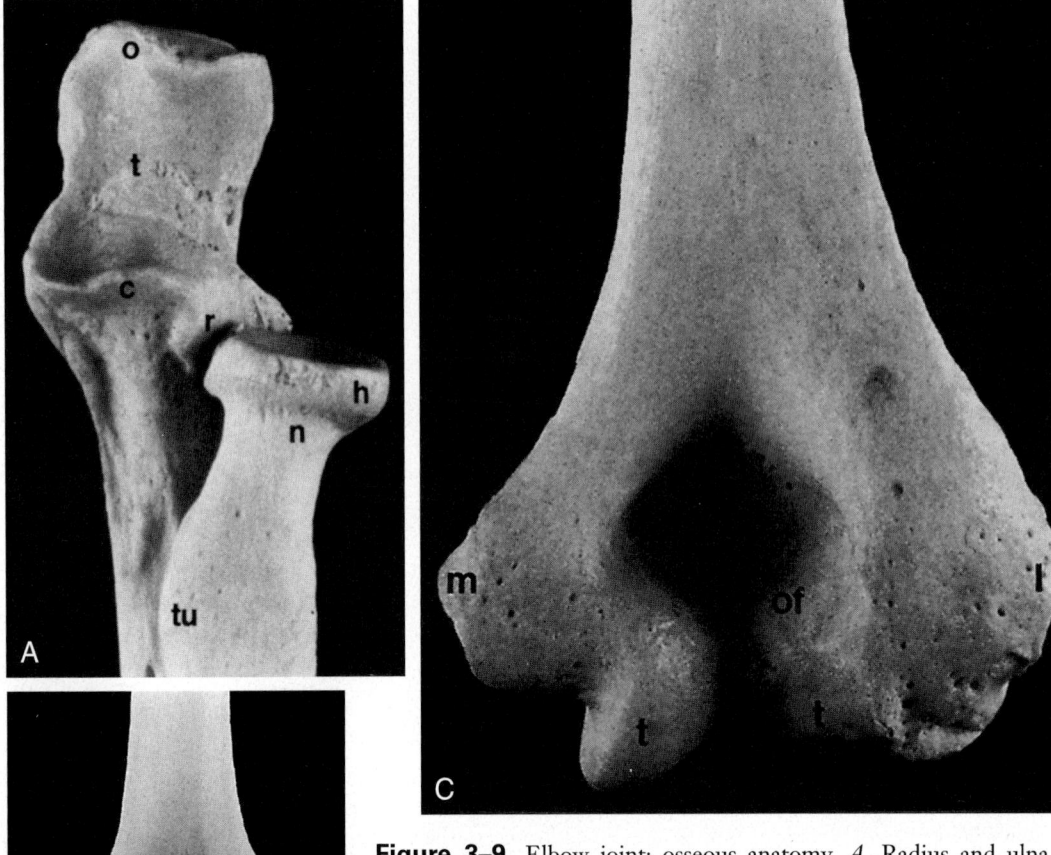

**Figure 3–9.** Elbow joint: osseous anatomy. *A,* Radius and ulna, anterior aspect. Note the olecranon (o), coronoid process (c), trochlear notch (t), radial notch (r), radial head (h), radial neck (n), and radial tuberosity (tu). *B* and *C,* Distal end of the humerus, anterior and posterior aspects. The anterior view *(B)* reveals the trochlea (t), capitulum (c), medial epicondyle (m), lateral epicondyle (l), coronoid fossa (cf), and radial fossa (rf). The posterior view *(C),* oriented in the same fashion, outlines some of the same structures, as well as the olecranon fossa (of).

with a mass or fluid may produce a positive fat pad sign, characterized by elevation and displacement of anterior and posterior fat pads (Fig. 3–11).

## GLENOHUMERAL JOINT

The glenohumeral joint lies between the roughly hemispheric head of the humerus and the shallow cavity of the glenoid region of the scapula. Stability of this articulation is limited for two major reasons: the scapular "socket" is small compared with the size of the adjacent humeral head, so that apposing osseous surfaces provide little inherent stability; and the joint capsule is quite redundant, providing little additional support.

### Osseous Anatomy

The upper end of the humerus consists of the head and the greater and lesser tuberosities (tubercles) (Fig. 3–12). Beneath the head is the anatomic neck of the humerus,

a slightly constricted area that encircles the bone, separating the head from the tuberosities. The anatomic neck is the site of attachment of the capsular ligament of the glenohumeral joint. The greater tuberosity is located on the lateral aspect of the proximal end of the humerus. The tendons of the supraspinatus and infraspinatus muscles insert on its superior portion, whereas the tendon of the teres minor muscle inserts on its posterior aspect. The lesser tuberosity is located on the anterior portion of the proximal humerus, immediately below the anatomic neck. The subscapularis tendon attaches to the medial aspect of this structure, as well as to the humeral neck below the lesser tuberosity. Between the greater and lesser tuberosities is located the intertubercular sulcus or groove (bicipital groove), through which passes the tendon of the long head of the biceps brachii muscle.

The shallow glenoid cavity is located on the lateral margin of the scapula (Fig. 3–13). Although there is variation in the osseous depth of the glenoid region, a fibrocartilaginous labrum encircles and slightly deepens

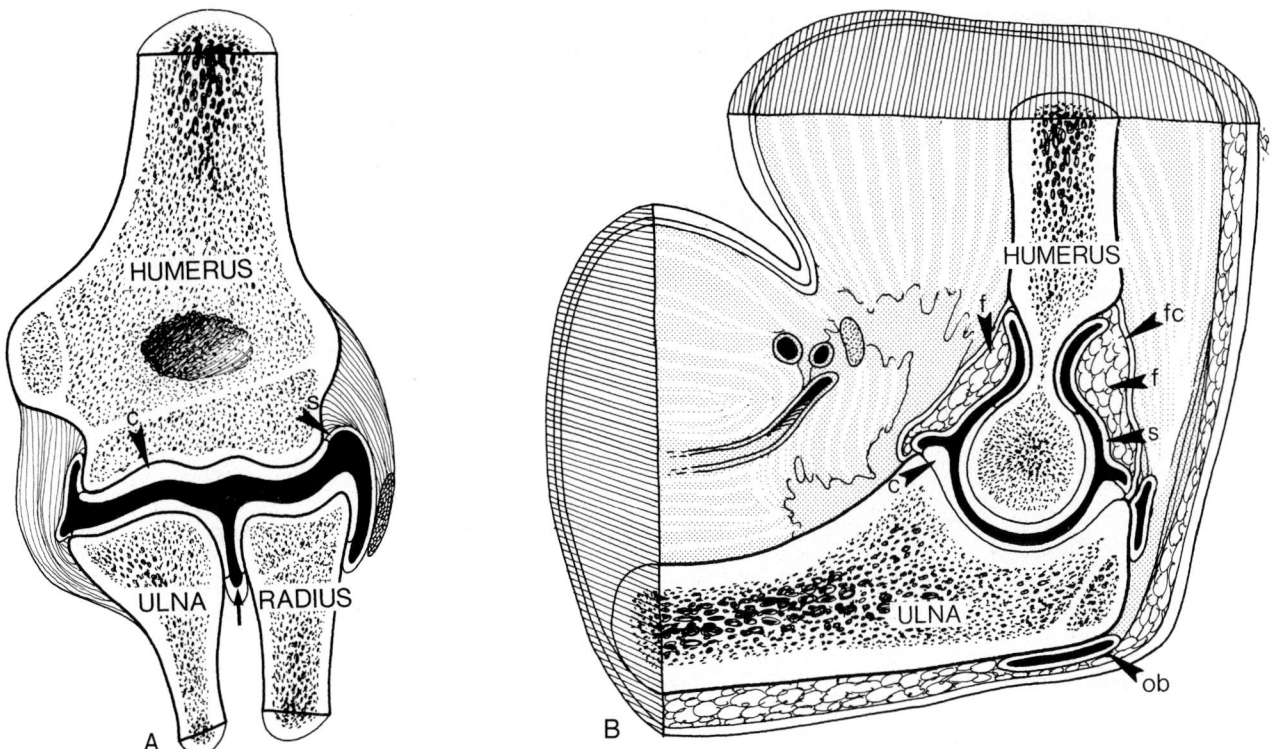

**Figure 3–10.** Elbow joint: normal anatomy. Drawings of coronal *(A)* and sagittal *(B)* sections. Observe the synovium (s), articular cartilage (c), fibrous capsule (fc), anterior and posterior fat pads (f), and olecranon bursa (ob). Note the extension of the elbow joint between the radius and ulna as the superior radioulnar joint *(arrow)*.

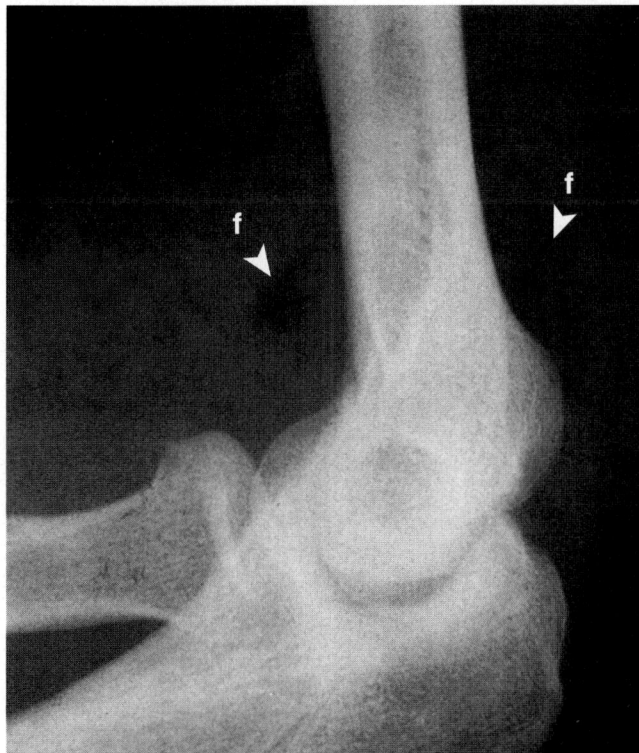

**Figure 3–11.** Elbow joint: abnormal appearance of fat pads. With a joint effusion, both fat pads (f) are elevated. The anterior fat pad assumes a "sail" configuration, whereas the posterior fat pad becomes visible.

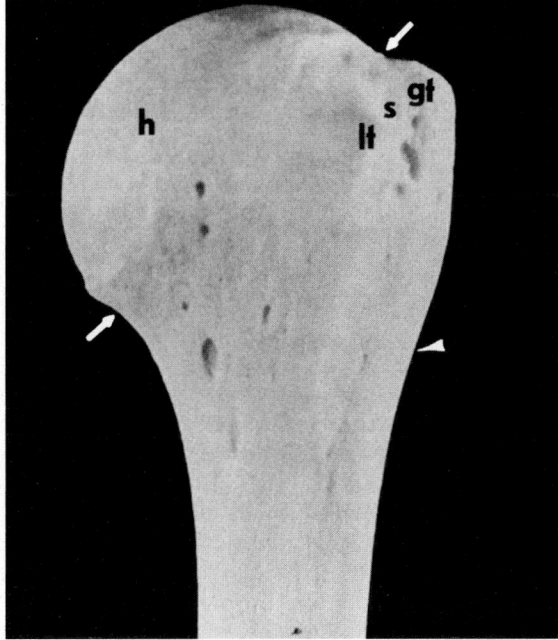

**Figure 3–12.** Proximal end of humerus: osseous anatomy—anterior aspect, external rotation. Observe the articular surface of the humeral head (h), greater tuberosity (gt), lesser tuberosity (lt), intertubercular sulcus (s), anatomic neck *(arrows)*, and surgical neck *(arrowhead)*.

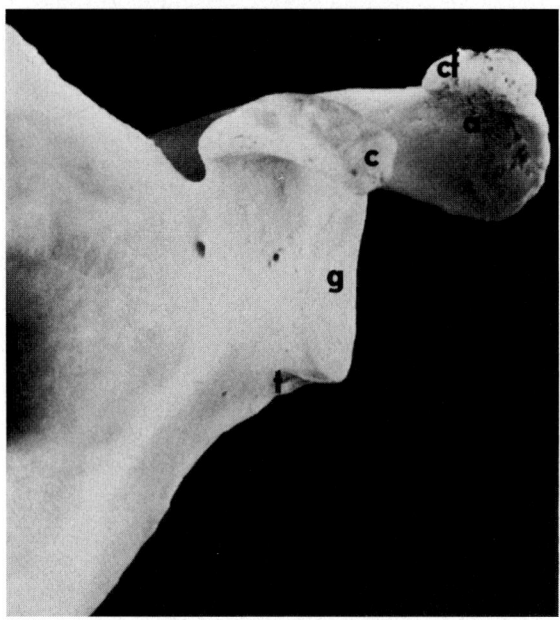

**Figure 3–13.** Scapula: osseous anatomy—anterior (costal) aspect. The scapula is viewed in the position it maintains when an anteroposterior radiograph of the shoulder is obtained. Observe the acromion (a), clavicular facet (cf), coracoid process (c), glenoid cavity (g), and infraglenoid tubercle (t). Note that the glenoid cavity is not seen tangentially.

the glenoid cavity. The glenoid contour may be almost flat or slightly curved, or it may possess a deep, socket-like appearance. A supraglenoid tubercle is located above the glenoid cavity, to which is attached a tendinous portion of the long head of the biceps muscle. Below the cavity is a thickened ridge of bone, the infraglenoid tubercle, which is a site of tendinous attachment for the long head of the triceps muscle.

### Soft Tissue Anatomy

A loose fibrous capsule arises medially from the circumference of the glenoid labrum or, anteriorly, from the neck of the scapula. It inserts distally into the anatomic neck of the humerus and periosteum of the humeral diaphysis. In certain areas, the fibrous capsule is strengthened by its intimate association with surrounding tendons and ligaments. The tendons of the supraspinatus, infraspinatus, teres minor, and subscapularis muscles form a cuff—the rotator cuff—which blends with and reinforces the fibrous capsule. The coracohumeral ligament strengthens the upper part of the capsule and is located (along with the tendon of the long head of the biceps muscle and superior glenohumeral ligament) in a space between the supraspinatus and subscapularis tendon, designated the rotator interval. Anteriorly, the capsule may thicken to form the superior, middle, and inferior glenohumeral ligaments. Portions of the last of these ligaments are referred to collectively as the inferior glenohumeral ligament complex (see Chapter 59).

Several synovium-lined recesses or bursae are present about the glenohumeral joint. The subscapular recess lies

between the subscapularis tendon and the scapula, communicating with the joint via an opening that is usually (but not invariably) located between the superior and middle glenohumeral ligaments. This bursa is readily apparent on shoulder arthrograms as a tongue-shaped collection of contrast material extending medially from the glenohumeral space underneath the coracoid process. The bursa about the infraspinatus tendon is an inconstant bursa that separates the infraspinatus tendon and joint capsule and may communicate with the joint cavity. The subacromial (subdeltoid) bursa lies between the deltoid muscle and joint capsule. It extends underneath the acromion and the coracoacromial ligament and is separated from the articular cavity by the rotator cuff. It does not communicate with the joint unless there has been a perforation of the cuff.

## ACROMIOCLAVICULAR JOINT

The acromioclavicular joint is a synovial articulation between the lateral aspect of the clavicle and the medial aspect of the acromion.

### Osseous Anatomy

The lateral or acromial end of the clavicle articulates with the acromial facet of the scapula and is the site of attachment of the joint capsule of the acromioclavicular joint. The inferior surface of the acromial end of the clavicle possesses a rough osseous ridge, termed the trapezoid line. A conoid tubercle is located at the posterior aspect of the lateral clavicle. The trapezoid line and conoid tubercle are the sites of attachment of the trapezoid and conoid parts of the coracoclavicular ligament. The acromion is a forward protuberance of the lateral aspect of the scapula. The inferior surface of the acromion varies in its slope and configuration, factors that may be important in the pathogenesis of one type of shoulder impingement syndrome and rotator cuff pathology (see Chapter 59).

### Soft Tissue Anatomy

The articular surfaces about the acromioclavicular joint are covered with fibrocartilage. In the central portion of the joint is an articular margin that partially or, more rarely, completely divides the joint cavity. The fibrous capsule surrounds the articular margin and is reinforced on its superior and inferior surfaces. Surrounding ligaments include the acromioclavicular and coracoclavicular ligaments. The former ligament, which is located at the superior portion of the joint, extends between the clavicle and acromion. The coracoclavicular ligament, which attaches to the coracoid process of the scapula and clavicle, is composed of a trapezoid (medial) part and a conoid (lateral) part. The trapezoid and conoid parts of the coracoclavicular ligament may be separated by fat or a bursa.

## STERNOCLAVICULAR JOINT

At the sternoclavicular articulation, the medial end of the clavicle articulates with the clavicular notch of the manubrium sterni and with the cartilage of the first rib (Fig. 3–14).

## Osseous Anatomy

The enlarged medial or sternal end of the clavicle projects above the upper margin of the manubrium. The articular surface is smooth except on its superior portion, where a roughened area allows attachment of an articular disc. The inferior portion of the articular surface is extended to allow articulation with the first costal cartilage. Below each clavicular notch is a rough projection, which receives the first costal cartilage.

## Soft Tissue Anatomy

The articular end of the clavicle is covered with a layer of fibrocartilage that is thicker than the cartilage on the sternum. A flat, circular disc is located between the articulating surfaces of the clavicle and sternum; it divides the joint into two articular cavities. The disc acts as a checkrein against medial displacement of the inner clavicle. Perforations in the disc are frequent in older persons. A fibrous capsule surrounds the joint. The sternoclavicular joint is freely mobile. It participates in movements of the upper extremity, including elevation, depression, protraction, retraction, and circumduction.

## JOINTS OF THE VERTEBRAL BODIES

### Osseous and Soft Tissue Anatomy

Joints separating vertebral bodies are of two types: articulations between vertebral bodies that consist of inter-vertebral discs are symphyses; those between vertebral bodies that consist of anterior and posterior longitudinal ligaments are syndesmoses (Fig. 3–15).

**Intervertebral Discs.** Intervertebral discs separate the vertebral bodies from the axis to the sacrum. The attachments of the discs include the anterior and posterior longitudinal ligaments and the intra-articular ligaments. Discs are thickest in the lumbar region and thinnest in the upper thoracic area. The intervertebral discs between the cervical vertebrae do not extend to the lateral edges of the vertebral bodies (Fig. 3–16). In this area, articular modifications are found on both sides of the intervertebral discs as cleftlike cavities between the superior surface of the uncinate process of one vertebra and the lateral lips of the inferior articulating surface of the vertebra above. These modifications are called the joints of Luschka.

Each disc consists of an inner portion, the nucleus pulposus, surrounded by a peripheral portion, the anulus fibrosus. The nucleus pulposus is soft and gelatinous in young persons, but it is gradually replaced by fibrocartilage with increasing age. The anulus fibrosus encircles the nucleus pulposus and unites the vertebral bodies firmly. The lamellae of the anulus fibrosus are thinner and more closely packed between the nucleus and the dorsal aspect of the intervertebral disc. Anteriorly, the lamellae are stronger and more distinct. The direction in which they are oriented varies with their relative position in the intervertebral disc. More peripherally, the bands of fibers are vertical. At the extreme periphery of the intervertebral disc, the lamellae may become curved, with their convexity facing the periphery of the intervertebral disc.

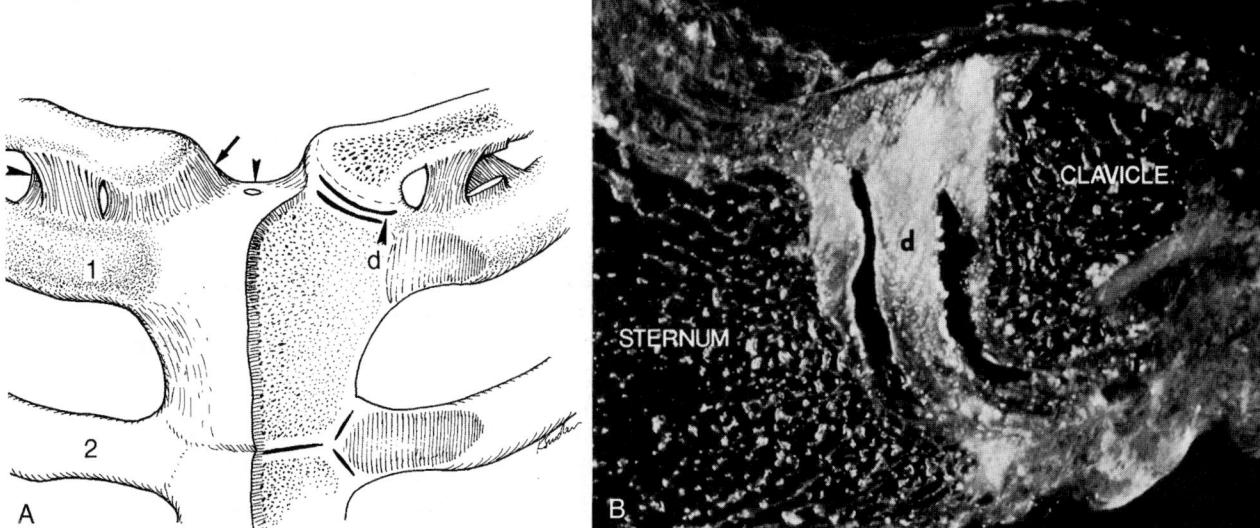

**Figure 3–14.** Sternoclavicular joint: normal anatomy. *A,* Diagram of the anterior aspect of the upper sternum and medial clavicles. On the right-hand side, the superficial bone has been removed, exposing the sternoclavicular, manubriosternal, and second sternocostal joints. Identified structures are the anterior sternoclavicular ligament *(arrow),* costoclavicular ligament *(arrowhead on left),* interclavicular ligament *(arrowhead in center),* and articular disc (d). Note the first (1) and second (2) costal cartilages. *B,* Photographs of a coronal section through the sternoclavicular joint in a cadaver reveal characteristics of the intra-articular disc (d).
(*A,* From Warwick R, Williams P: Gray's Anatomy, 35th Br ed. Philadelphia, WB Saunders, 1973.)

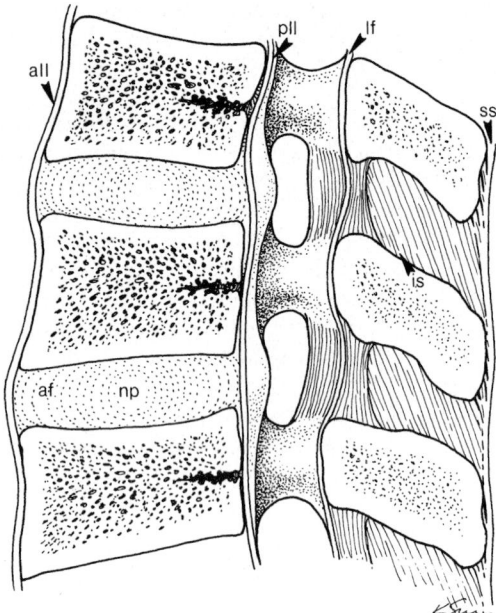

**Figure 3–15.** Vertebral column: normal development and anatomy. Drawing of a sagittal section of an adult spine depicts vertebral bodies separated by intervertebral discs, consisting of the anulus fibrosus (af) and nucleus pulposus (np). The anterior longitudinal ligament (all), posterior longitudinal ligament (pll), ligamentum flavum (lf), and interspinous (is) and supraspinous (ss) ligaments are indicated.

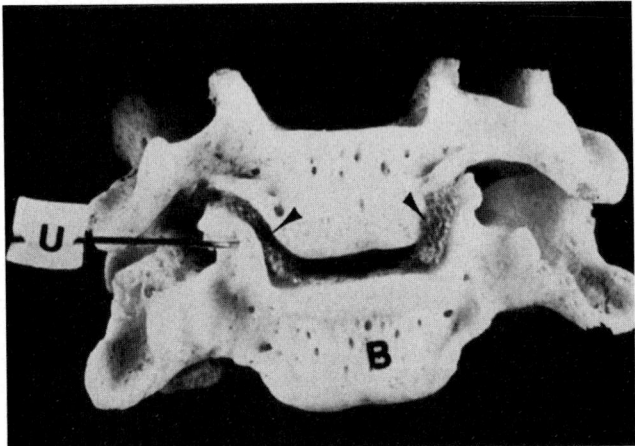

**Figure 3–16.** Cervical spine: joints of Luschka. On a photograph of the anterior aspect of the cervical spine, the joints of Luschka (*arrowheads*) are seen between the superior surface of the uncinate process (U) of one vertebra (B) and the lateral lips of the inferior articulating surface of the vertebra above.

The anulus fibrosus is attached to the adjacent vertebral bodies in two ways. At sites of endochondral ossification, such as the cartilaginous endplates and marginal osseous rims, the attachment consists essentially of fibers that penetrate the cartilaginous endplate and subchondral bony trabeculae. A stronger attachment between anulus fibrosus and vertebral body is apparent at sites of intra-

membranous ossification, such as the anterior vertebral surface. Here, the fibers of the stoutest external lamellar bands, termed Sharpey's fibers, enter the bone at different angles and extend beyond the confines of the intervertebral disc, blending with the periosteum of the vertebral body and longitudinal ligaments.

**Anterior and Posterior Longitudinal Ligaments.** The anterior longitudinal ligament is a strong band of fibers that descends along the anterior surface of the vertebral column. It is relatively narrow in the cervical region and expands in width in the thoracic and lumbar regions; in the latter regions, it covers most of the anterolateral surface of the vertebral bodies and discs. The anterior longitudinal ligament is fixed to the intervertebral discs and vertebral bodies. It is particularly adherent to the articular lip at the edge of each vertebral body but is loosely attached at intermediate levels of the bodies.

The posterior longitudinal ligament extends along the posterior surface of the vertebral bodies and discs from skull to sacrum, within the vertebral canal. Its fibers are attached only to the intervertebral discs and margins of the vertebral bodies, not to the midposterior surface of the bone.

## JOINTS OF THE VERTEBRAL ARCHES

Articulations between vertebral arches consist of synovial joints (between articular processes of vertebrae) and syndesmoses (ligamentum flavum; interspinous, supraspinous, and intertransverse ligaments; and ligamentum nuchae) (Table 3–1).

### Osseous Anatomy

The vertebral arch contains two pedicles and two laminae, the latter joining posteriorly to become the spinous process. The transverse process and two articular facets originate from a mass of bone at the junction of lamina and pedicle. One articular facet passes superiorly and the second one inferiorly, to articulate with a facet from the vertebrae above and below, respectively. The orientation

**TABLE 3–1**

**Articulations of the Spine**

Synovial Joints
  Apophyseal (facet) joints
  Atlas-odontoid process
  Odontoid process–transverse ligament
  Costovertebral joints
    Joints of the heads of the ribs
    Costotransverse joints
  Joints of Luschka*
Symphyses
  Intervertebral discs
Syndesmoses
  Ligamentous connections of vertebral bodies
  Ligamentous connections of vertebral arches

*Resemble synovial joints.

and appearance of the articular processes of the vertebrae vary, depending on the region of the vertebral column. In the cervical spine (C3–C7), the articular processes are large, forming part of a pillar of bone termed the articular mass. In the thoracic spine, the superior articular processes, which face backward, slightly upward, and laterally, appose inferior articular processes that face in the opposite direction (Fig. 3–17). In the lumbar spine, superior processes face medially and posteriorly, whereas inferior processes face laterally and anteriorly (Fig. 3–18). The articulations of the cervical and thoracic portions of the spine are best demonstrated on lateral radiographs, whereas oblique projections are necessary for the lumbar spine. Conventional tomography or computed tomography scanning is frequently required.

The transverse processes of the vertebrae also demonstrate regional differences. In a typical cervical vertebra, the transverse processes have an anterior and a posterior tubercle, connected by a costotransverse lamella. The adjacent foramen transversarium transmits the vertebral artery, veins, and nerves. The transverse processes of the thoracic vertebrae have a tubercle for articulation with the corresponding rib tubercle. Transverse processes in the lumbar spine are flat, and the processes of the third lumbar vertebra may be the longest. In the cervical spine, the spinous processes of the second to fifth vertebrae frequently are bifid. The atlas has no spinous process. In the thoracic spine, spinous processes are long and sloping, whereas in the lumbar spine, these processes are broad and horizontal.

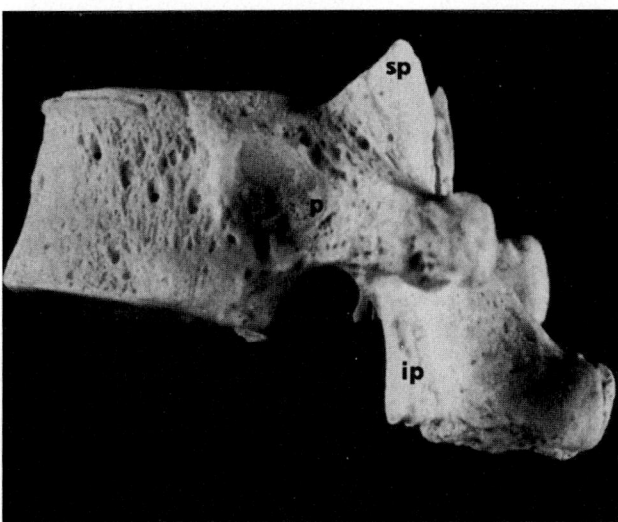

**Figure 3–18.** Articular processes: lumbar spine. Photograph of the lateral aspect of the lumbar vertebrae outlines the superior articular process (sp) and inferior articular process (ip). Also observe the pedicles (p).

## Soft Tissue Anatomy

Synovial joints and syndesmoses exist at the joints of the vertebral arches.

**Articular Processes (Synovial Joints).** The superior articulating process of one vertebra is separated from the inferior articulating process of the vertebra above by a synovial joint, termed the apophyseal joint. This articulation is surrounded by a loose, thin articular capsule, which is attached to the bones of the adjacent articulating processes.

**Ligamentous Articulations (Syndesmoses).** The syndesmoses between the vertebral arches are formed by the paired sets of ligamenta flava, intertransverse ligaments, and interspinous ligaments and by the unpaired supraspinous ligament.

The ligamenta flava connect the laminae of adjacent vertebrae from the second cervical to the lumbosacral levels. The ligamentum flavum, which consists predominantly of yellow elastic fibers extending in a perpendicular fashion, is thin and broad in the cervical region and thicker in the thoracic and lumbar areas. It is the most prominent elastic ligament in the human body; it permits separation of the laminae with flexion of the vertebral column and does not form redundant folds, which might otherwise compromise adjacent nervous tissue when the spine resumes an erect posture. Intertransverse ligaments extend between transverse processes. Their appearance varies at different levels of the spine: in the cervical spine, they are absent or consist of a few irregular, scattered fibers; in the thoracic spine, they are cords of tissue associated with the deep musculature of the back; and in the lumbar spine, they are thin and membranous.

Interspinous ligaments connect adjoining spinous processes, where their attachment extends from the root to the apex of the process. These ligaments, which are located between the ligamentum flavum in front and the

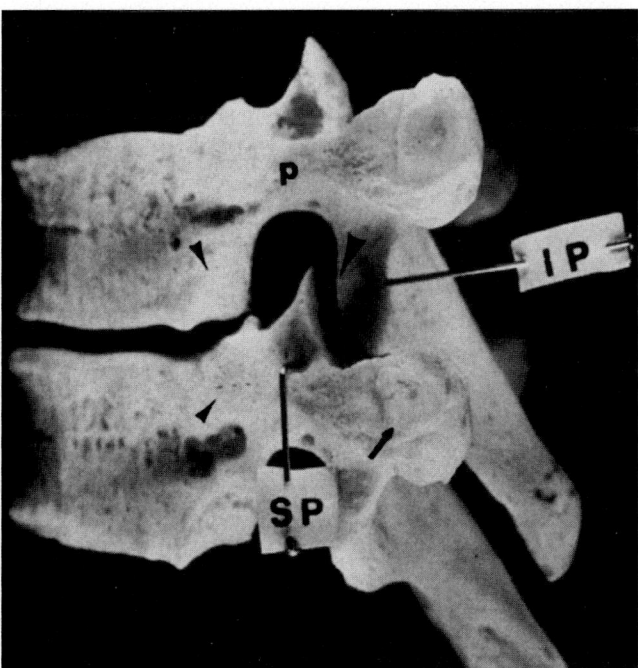

**Figure 3–17.** Articular processes: thoracic spine. Photograph of the lateral aspect of two thoracic vertebrae demonstrates the inferior articular process (ip) and superior articular process (sp), separated by a synovial joint *(large arrowhead)*. Note the pedicle (p), hemifacets for the head of the rib *(small arrowheads)*, and facet for the rib tubercle *(arrow)*.

supraspinous ligament behind, are longest and strongest in the lumbar spine. The supraspinous ligament is broader and thicker in the lumbar spine than in the thoracic spine. In the cervical spine, the supraspinous ligament merges with the triangular ligamentum nuchae, the latter passing from the external occipital protuberance to the seventh cervical vertebra. Ossicles resembling sesamoid bones are common in the ligamentum nuchae.

## ATLANTOAXIAL JOINTS

### Osseous Anatomy

The ringlike first cervical vertebra, the atlas, does not possess a vertebral body or a spinous process (Fig. 3–19). It contains a small anterior arch with a tubercle, a larger posterior arch with a corresponding tubercle, and two bulky lateral masses. The second cervical vertebra, the

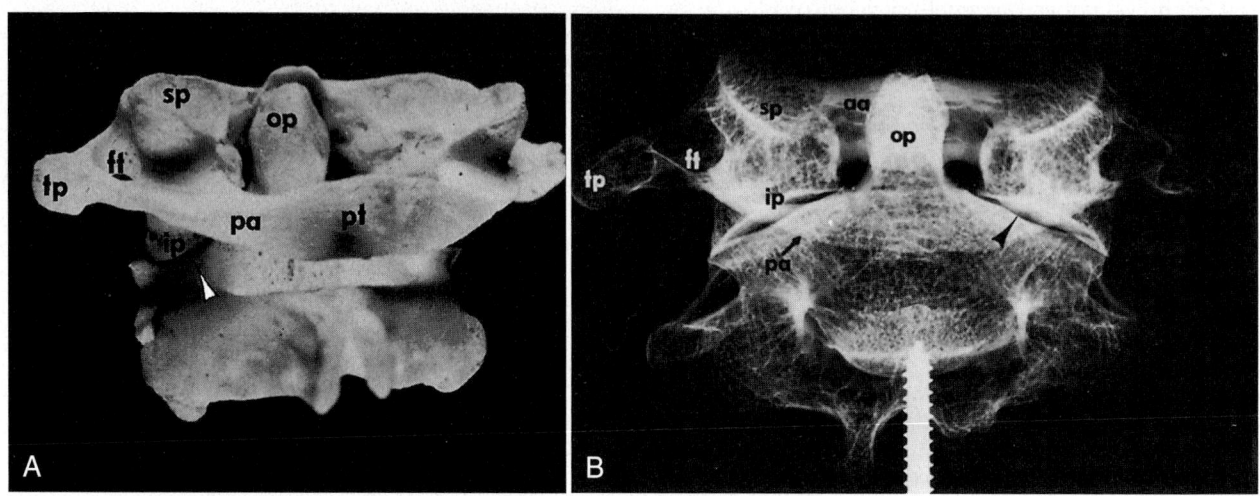

**Figure 3–19.** Atlas and axis: osseous anatomy. *A*, Posterior view. Observe the posterior arch (pa), posterior tubercle (pt), superior articular process (sp), inferior articular process (ip), transverse process (tp), and foramen transversarium (ft) of the atlas, and the odontoid process (op) and superior articular process *(arrowhead)* of the axis. *B*, Frontal radiographs of the atlas and axis with the same structures indicated, as well as the anterior arch (aa).

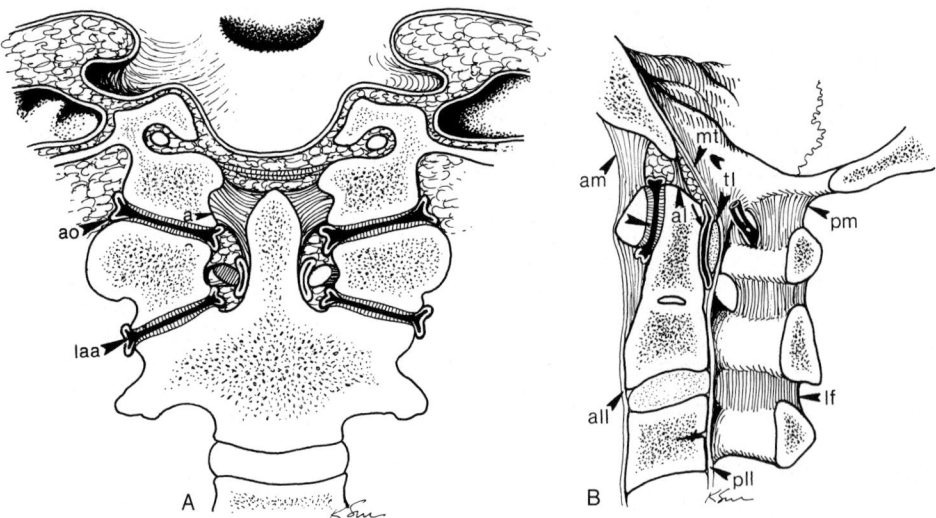

**Figure 3–20.** Atlantoaxial and atlanto-occipital joints. Drawing of coronal *(A)* and sagittal *(B)* sections of the base of the skull and upper cervical spine. Note the lateral atlantoaxial joints (laa), atlanto-occipital synovial joints (ao), anterior median joint *(arrowhead)* between the odontoid process and anterior arch of the atlas, and posterior median joint *(arrow)* between the odontoid process and transverse ligament (tl) of the atlas. Additional structures are the anterior longitudinal ligament (all), posterior longitudinal ligament (pll), membrana tectoria (mt), anterior atlanto-occipital membrane (am), posterior atlanto-occipital membrane (pm), apical ligament of the odontoid process (al), alar ligament (a), and ligamentum flavum (lf).

axis, contains a superior peg of bone, the dens or odontoid process, which possesses a small oval facet for articulation with a facet on the posterior surface of the anterior arch of the atlas. On the posterior surface of the odontoid process is a groove for the transverse ligament of the atlas.

On lateral radiographs of the cervical spine, the normal space between the anterior arch of the atlas and the odontoid process of the axis should be no greater than 2.5 mm in adults. In children, the average distance between the anterior arch of the atlas and the odontoid process is 2 to 2.5 mm in extension and 2 to 3 mm in flexion. This distance should not exceed 4.5 mm in children.

## Soft Tissue Anatomy

Four synovial articulations occur between the atlas and axis: two lateral atlantoaxial joints, one on each side, between the inferior facet of the lateral mass of the atlas and the superior facet of the axis; and two median synovial joints, one between the anterior arch of the atlas and the odontoid process of the axis and the second between the odontoid process and the transverse ligament of the atlas (Fig. 3–20). In addition to these synovial articulations, syndesmoses between the atlas and axis include continuations of the anterior longitudinal ligament anteriorly and the ligamenta flava posteriorly.

## ATLANTO-OCCIPITAL JOINTS

### Osseous Anatomy

The superior surface of each lateral mass of the atlas has a concave, kidney-shaped facet that articulates with the corresponding occipital condyle. This atlantal facet is oriented medially and superiorly. The occipital condyles are oval, located on the anterolateral aspect of the foramen magnum.

### Soft Tissue Anatomy

The atlanto-occipital joints consist of a pair of synovial joints, between the articular facets of the atlas and the condyles of the occiput, and syndesmoses formed by the anterior and posterior atlanto-occipital membranes (see Fig. 3–20). The atlanto-occipital synovial joints are the reciprocally curved superior articular facets separating the lateral masses of the atlas and condyles of the occipital bone. They are surrounded by a fibrous capsule that is particularly thick on its posterior and lateral surfaces but deficient medially. The anterior atlanto-occipital membrane is attached above to the anterior margin of the foramen magnum and below to the anterior arch of the atlas. Its central portion contains fibers continuous with those of the anterior longitudinal ligament. The posterior atlanto-occipital membrane is attached above to the posterior margin of the foramen magnum and below to the posterior arch of the atlas.

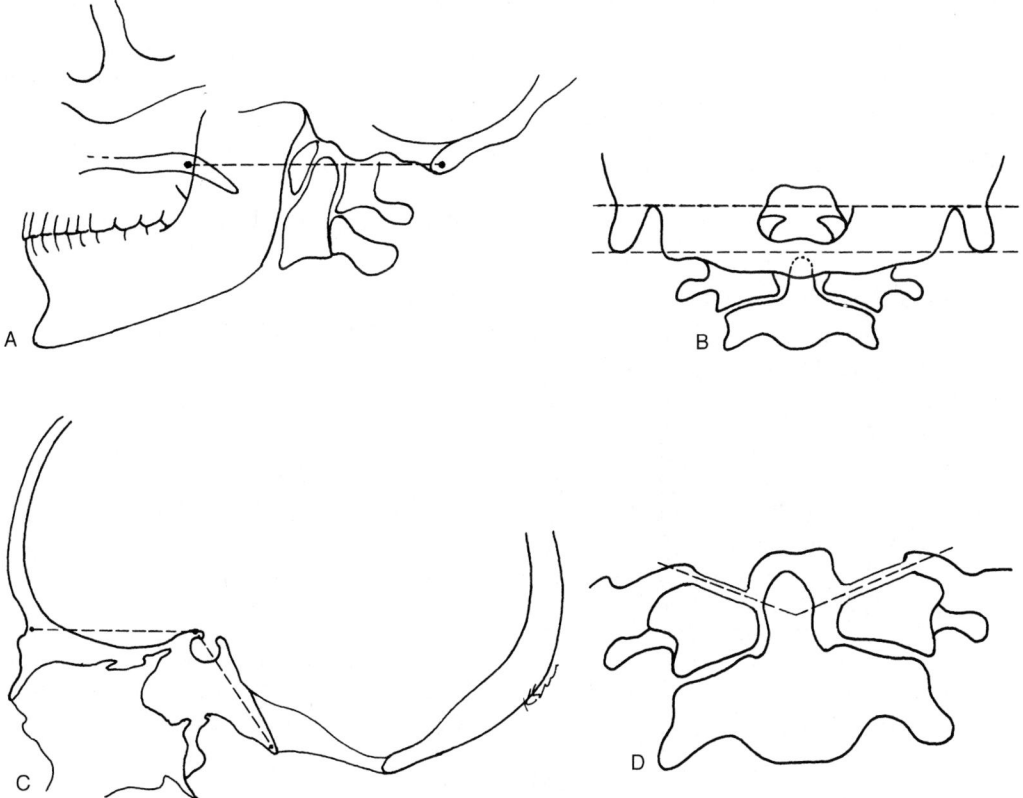

**Figure 3–21.** Cervicobasilar junction: normal osseous relationships. *A,* Chamberlain's line is drawn from the posterior margin of the hard palate to the posterior border of the foramen magnum. The odontoid process normally does not extend more than 5 mm above this line. *B,* The bimastoid line (lower line), connecting the tips of the mastoids, is normally within 2 mm of the odontoid tip. The digastric line (upper line), connecting the digastric muscle fossae, is normally located above the odontoid process. *C,* The basilar angle, which normally exceeds 140 degrees, is formed by the angle of intersection of two lines—one drawn from the nasion to the tuberculum sellae, and the second drawn from the tuberculum sellae to the anterior edge of the foramen magnum. *D,* The atlanto-occipital joint angle, constructed on frontal tomograms by the intersection of two lines drawn along the axes of these articulations, is normally not greater than 150 degrees.

## OSSEOUS RELATIONSHIPS OF CERVICOBASILAR JUNCTION

The osseous relationships at the cervicobasilar junction have received considerable attention. Chamberlain's line can be drawn on a lateral radiograph from the posterior margin of the hard palate to the posterior border of the foramen magnum. In normal situations, the odontoid process should not extend more than 5 mm above this line. A modification of this line, McGregor's line, uses the inferior surface of the occiput rather than the margin of the foramen magnum. In normal persons, the odontoid tip does not extend more than 7 mm above this line. On frontal radiographs, a line connecting the mastoid tips is within 2 mm of the tip of the odontoid, whereas a line connecting the digastric muscle fossae is located at the approximate level of the foramen magnum and above the odontoid process (Fig. 3–21).

The basilar angle is the angle of intersection of two lines—one drawn from the nasion to the tuberculum sellae, and the second drawn from the tuberculum sellae to the anterior edge of the foramen magnum. This angle normally does not exceed 140 degrees. An atlanto-occipital joint angle is constructed on frontal tomograms by drawing a line along this articulation on either side. The angle formed by the intersection of these two lines normally should not exceed 150 degrees.

## SACROILIAC JOINTS

### Osseous Anatomy

The apposing osseous surfaces of the sacrum and the ilium are irregular in character and allow interdigitation of the sacrum and ilium, which contributes to the strength of the joint and to its restricted motion. Irregular osseous pits, which are the sites of attachment of various ligaments, are located posterior to the articular surface.

### Soft Tissue Anatomy

The articulation between articular surfaces of the sacrum and ilium is synovial in type. The articular surface of the sacrum is covered with a thick layer of hyaline cartilage, and the articular surface of the ilium is clothed by a thinner layer of fibrocartilage (Fig. 3–22). This joint has a complete fibrous capsule, which is attached close to the margins of the adjacent surfaces of the sacrum and ilium and is lined with synovial membrane. A thin, broad band of tissue, the ventral sacroiliac ligament, is noted in front of the joint (Fig. 3–23). Posteriorly, a deep, thick interosseous sacroiliac ligament extends above the articular surface to fill the superior cleft between the sacrum and the ilium. Accessory synovial joints are not uncommon between the lateral sacral crest and the posterior or superior iliac spine and ilial tuberosity.

It is important to realize that only the lower one half to two thirds of the space between the sacrum and the ilium represents the synovial joint; the superior aspect of this space is ligamentous. In young adults, the interosseous joint space is 2 to 5 mm, reflecting the combined thickness of sacral and ilial cartilage. Diminution of the joint space is common in persons older than 40 years and increases in frequency thereafter.

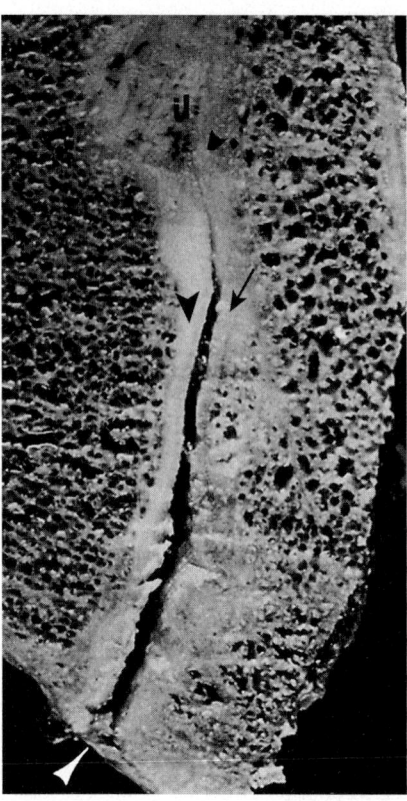

**Figure 3–22.** Sacroiliac joint: coronal section. Photograph reveals the extent of synovial articulation (*large arrowhead*), thick sacral cartilage (*small arrowhead*), and thinner iliac cartilage (*arrow*). Note the interosseous ligament (il) above the synovial joint.

## PELVIC-VERTEBRAL LIGAMENTS

In addition to the iliolumbar ligaments, other important ligaments connecting the pelvis and the vertebral column are the sacrotuberous and sacrospinous ligaments (Fig. 3–24).

## HIP

### Osseous Anatomy

At birth, the acetabulum is cartilaginous, with a triradiate stem extending medially from its deep aspect, producing a Y-shaped physeal plate between ilium, ischium, and pubis. Continued ossification results in eventual fusion of these three bones. The fully developed acetabular cavity is hemispheric in shape and possesses an elevated bony rim (Fig. 3–25). This rim is absent inferiorly, and this defect is termed the acetabular notch. A fibrocartilaginous labrum is attached to the bony rim, deepening the acetabular cavity.

The hemispheric head of the femur extends superiorly, medially, and anteriorly. It is smooth except for a central roughened pit, the fovea, to which is attached the ligament of the head of the femur (i.e., ligamentum teres). The anterior surface of the femoral neck is intracapsular, as the capsular line extends to the intertrochanteric line.

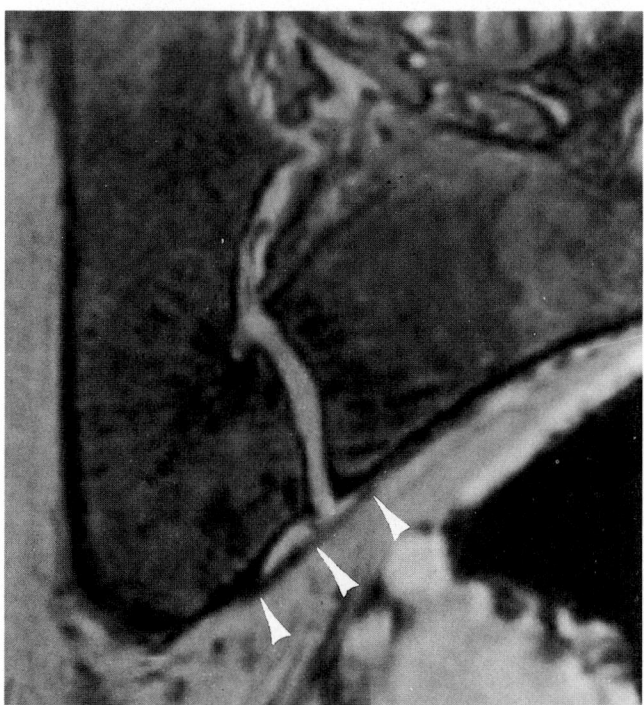

**Figure 3–23.** Ventral sacroiliac ligament. Coronal volumetric SPGR (TR/TE, 60/10; flip angle, 30 degrees) magnetic resonance image reveals the ventral sacroiliac ligament *(arrowheads)* traversing the anteroinferior aspect of the joint.

Radiographic examination of normal osseous structures about the hip has received much attention, and various measurements have been determined. The acetabular angle, iliac angle, and angle of anteversion of the femoral

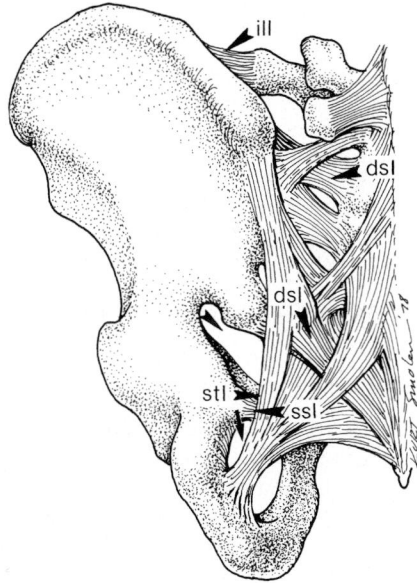

**Figure 3–24.** Pelvic-vertebral ligaments: posterior aspect. Observe the iliolumbar ligament (ill), short and long dorsal sacroiliac ligaments (dsl), sacrotuberous ligament (stl), sacrospinous ligament (ssl), and greater *(arrowhead)* and lesser *(arrow)* sciatic foramina.

(From Warwick R, Williams P: Gray's Anatomy, 35th Br ed. Philadelphia, WB Saunders, 1973.)

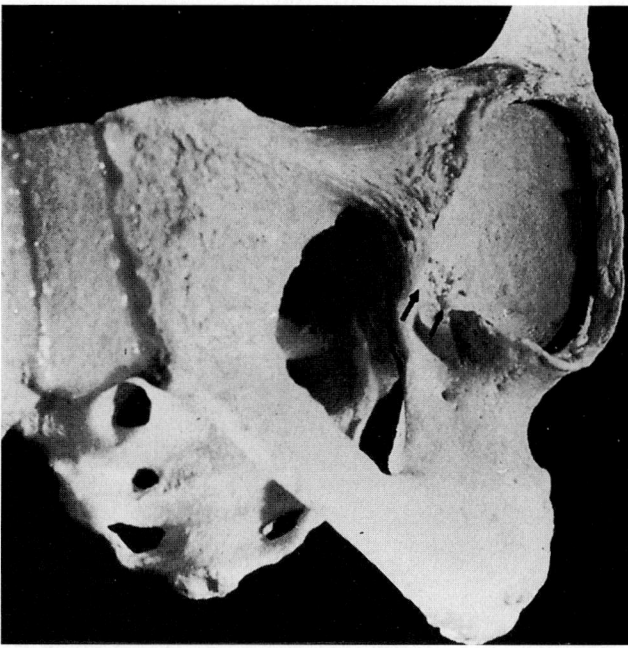

**Figure 3–25.** Acetabular cavity: osseous anatomy (anterior view). A metal marker (black strip) identifies the posterior acetabular rim. This rim is continuous except at the acetabular notch inferiorly *(arrows)*.

(From Armbuster TG, Guerra J Jr, Resnick D, et al: The adult hip: An anatomic study. Part I. The bony landmarks. Radiology 128:1, 1978.)

neck are useful measurements, particularly in the young skeleton. The center-edge (CE) angle of Wiberg is an indication of acetabular depth (Fig. 3–26). It is the angle formed by a perpendicular line through the midportion of the femoral head and a line from the femoral head center to the upper outer acetabular margin. The pelvic radiograph also is useful in outlining certain normal lines and structures (Fig. 3–27). The ilioischial line is formed by that portion of the quadrilateral surface of the ilium that is tangent to the x-ray beam; the iliopubic line is simply the inner margin of the ilium, which forms a continuous line with the inner superior aspect of the pubis. Two columns of bone produce an arch, with the acetabulum located in the concavity of the arch. The ilioischial, or posterior, column is a thick structure that includes a portion of the ilium and extends to the ischial tuberosity. The iliopubic, or anterior, column consists of a portion of ilium and pubis and extends superolaterally to the anterior inferior iliac spine.

The "teardrop" is a U-shaped shadow medial to the hip joint that has been used to detect abnormalities of acetabular depth, thereby establishing a diagnosis of acetabular protrusion (Fig. 3–28). The lateral aspect of the teardrop is the wall of the acetabular fossa, and the medial aspect is the anteroinferior margin of the quadrilateral surface. The configuration of the teardrop varies in normal persons, and it is affected significantly by positioning. Differentiation of normal acetabular depth and acetabular protrusion (protrusio acetabuli) can be accomplished by careful analysis of conventional radiographs in adults. Protrusio acetabuli is diagnosed when the acetabular line projects medial to the ilioischial line by 3 mm or

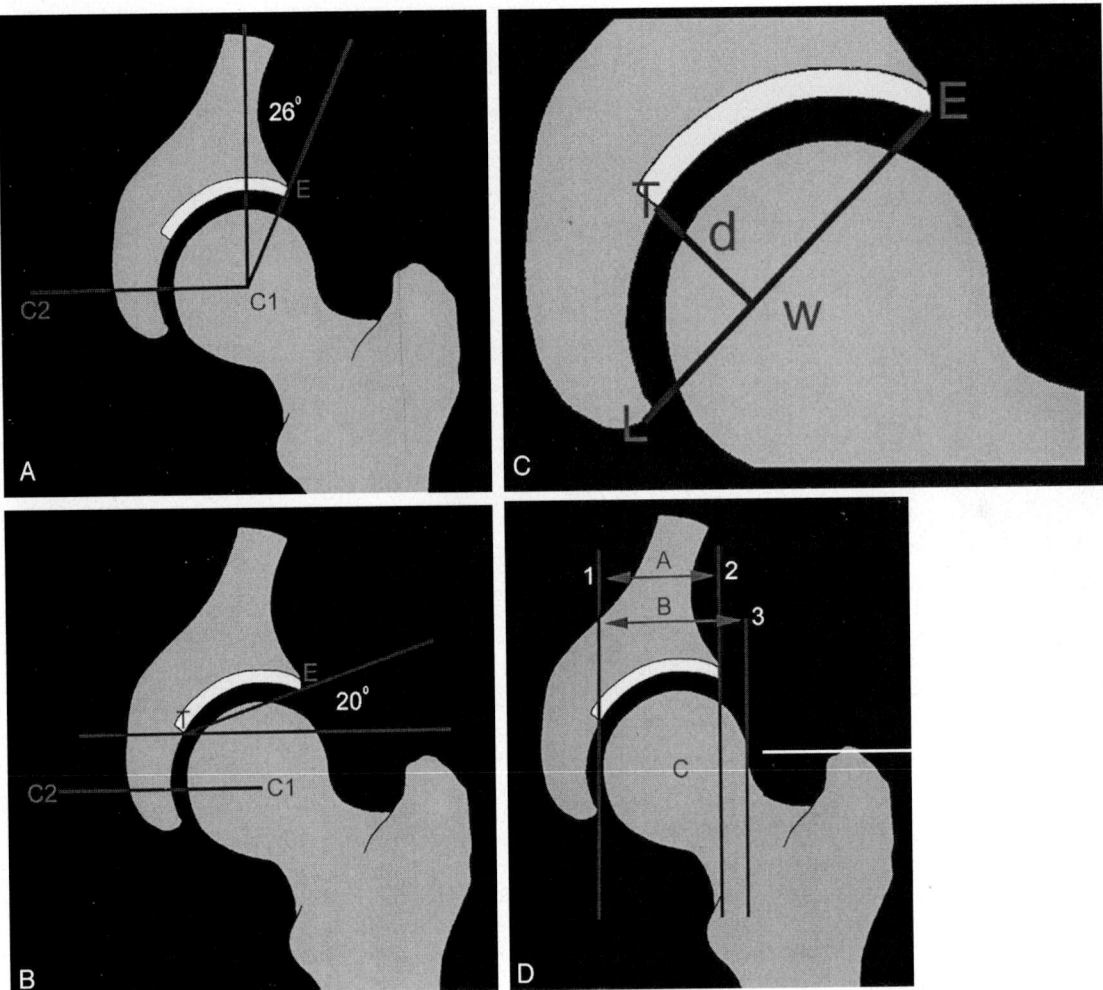

**Figure 3–26.** Hip: radiographic indices. *A,* Center-edge (CE) angle of Wiberg. A horizontal line (C2–C1) is drawn, connecting the center of each femoral head. A perpendicular line is drawn superiorly from the center of the femoral head. The edge (E) of the acetabulum is determined, and a line (C1–E) is constructed. In this case, the value of 26 degrees is considered normal. *B,* "Horizontal toit externe" (HTE) angle of Wiberg. A horizontal line is drawn parallel to the C2–C1 line through the most medial portion of the weight-bearing aspect of the acetabulum (T). A line is then constructed as shown through E. The angle created between the two lines is normally 10 degrees or less. *C,* Acetabular index of depth (d) to width (w). The two lines are constructed as illustrated. The ratio (d/w) × 100 is calculated. This ratio normally measures greater than 38. *D,* Percentage of the femoral head covered by the acetabulum. This represents the relative width of the weight-bearing surface of the acetabulum (A), represented by line 1–2, and that of the femoral head, represented by line 1–3. Normal acetabular coverage is 75% or above when the ratio of 1–2:1–3 is determined.

(Modified from Delaunay S, Dussault RG, Kaplan PA, et al: Radiographic measurements of dysplastic adult hips. Skeletal Radiol 26:75, 1997.)

more in men or by 6 mm or more in women. In children, 1 mm in boys and 3 mm in girls are the corresponding values (Fig. 3–29).

## Soft Tissue Anatomy

The femoral head is covered with articular cartilage, although a small area exists on its surface that is devoid of cartilage, to which attaches the ligament of the head of the femur, or ligamentum teres. A fibrous capsule encircles the joint and much of the femoral neck. The capsule attaches proximally to the acetabulum, labrum, and transverse ligament of the acetabulum. Distally, it surrounds

the femoral neck; in front, it is attached to the trochanteric line at the junction of the femoral neck and shaft; above and below, it is attached to the femoral neck close to the junction with the trochanters; behind, the capsule extends over the medial two-thirds of the neck. Because of these capsular attachments, the physeal plate of the femur is intracapsular, and the physeal plates of the trochanters are extracapsular. The fibers of the fibrous capsule, although oriented longitudinally from pelvis to femur, also consist of a deeply situated circular group of fibers termed the zona orbicularis. The fibrous capsule is strengthened by surrounding ligaments, including the iliofemoral, pubofemoral, and ischiofemoral ligaments. The external surface of the

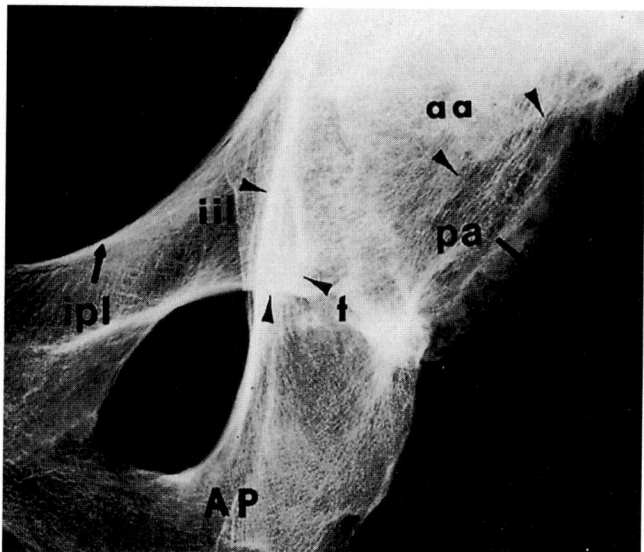

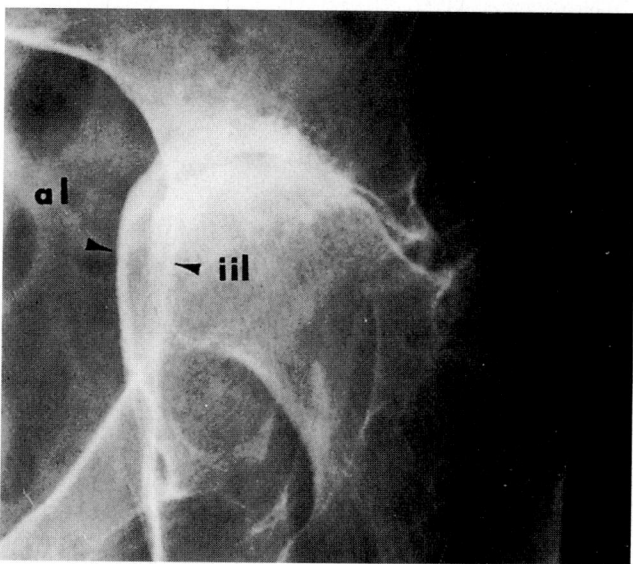

**Figure 3–27.** Normal osseous landmarks of the pelvis: antero-posterior view. The posterior acetabular rim (pa) is more lateral than the anterior acetabular rim (aa). The ilioischial line (iil) is formed by that portion of the quadrilateral surface of the ilium that is tangent to the x-ray beam. The iliopubic line (ipl) is the inner margin of the ilium, which forms a continuous line with the inner superior surface of the pubis. The "teardrop" (t) is labeled.

**Figure 3–29.** Acetabular protrusion. A protrusio acetabuli deformity is present when the acetabular line (al) projects medial to the ilioischial line (iil) by 3 mm or more in men and 6 mm or more in women.

(From Armbuster TG, Guerra J Jr, Resnick D, et al: The adult hip: An anatomic study. Part I. The bony landmarks. Radiology 128:1, 1978.)

capsule is covered by musculature and separated anteriorly from the psoas major and iliacus by a bursa. In this area, the joint may communicate with the subtendinous iliac bursa (iliopsoas bursa) (Fig. 3–30).

A number of periarticular fat planes have been described that can be recognized on radiographs and, when disturbed, may indicate significant intra-articular disease. Four fatty layers can be identified on anteroposterior radiographs (Fig. 3–31): fat plane 1 is medial to the obturator internus muscle; fat plane 2 is medial to the iliopsoas muscle; fat plane 3 is between the gluteus medius

muscle (lateral) and the gluteus minimus muscle (medial); and fat plane 4 has been termed the "capsular" fat plane, although more recent evidence suggests that this fat pad is not related to the joint capsule but lies between the rectus femoris and tensor fasciae latae muscles.

The iliopsoas bursa represents the largest and most important bursa about the hip. It is present in 98% of hips and is located anterior to the joint capsule. It may extend proximally and communicates with the joint space in approximately 15% of normal hips. Extension of hip disease into this bursa has been recognized in a variety of articular diseases. Bursae about the gluteus muscles also may be demonstrated anatomically and radiographically. The bursa deep to the gluteus medius is larger than that deep to the gluteus minimus. Both bursae are intimate with the greater trochanter, and bursitis can lead to pain and soft tissue calcifications in this region.

### KNEE

In this joint, three functional spaces exist: the medial femorotibial space, the lateral femorotibial space, and the patellofemoral space.

### Osseous and Soft Tissue Anatomy

The lower end of the femur contains a medial and lateral condyle, separated posteriorly by an intercondylar fossa, or notch. The medial condyle is larger than the lateral condyle and possesses a superior prominence called the adductor tubercle for attachment of the tendon of the adductor magnus muscle. Below this tubercle is a ridge, the medial epicondyle. The lateral condyle possesses a similar protuberance, the lateral epicondyle. The patella,

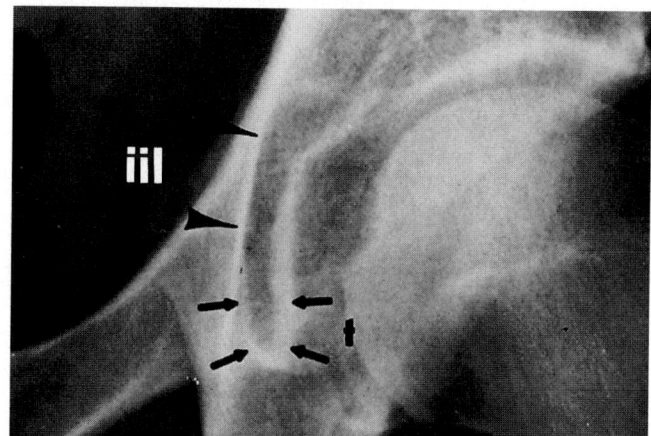

**Figure 3–28.** Teardrop. Frontal radiograph shows the tear-drop (t; *arrows*) and ilioischial line (iil; *arrowheads*). An "open-type" configuration of the teardrop is shown.

(From Armbuster TG, Guerra J Jr, Resnick D, et al: The adult hip: An anatomic study. Part I. The bony landmarks. Radiology 128:1, 1978.)

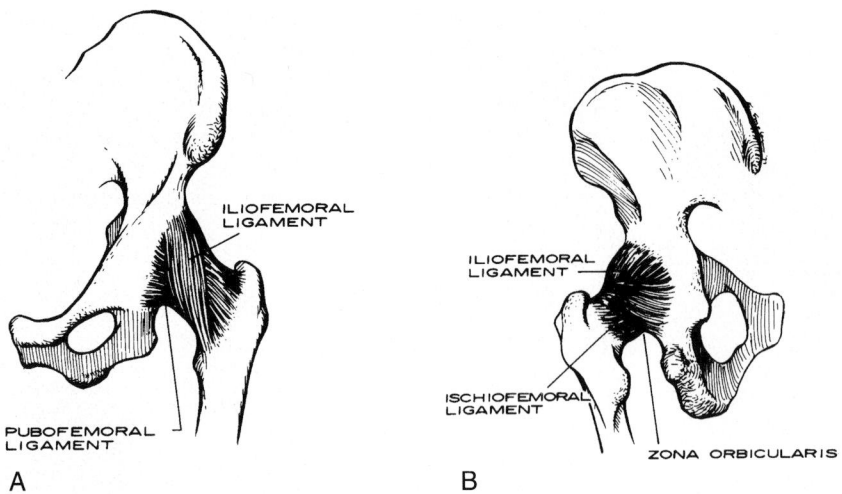

**Figure 3–30.** Normal anatomy. *A,* Capsular ligaments of hip, anterior view. The iliofemoral ligament extends anterior to the pubofemoral ligament. A gap may persist at this crossing, which allows communication between the iliopsoas bursa and the hip joint. *B,* Capsular ligaments of hip, posterior view. The iliofemoral and ischiofemoral ligaments are thick posteriorly and without inherent areas of weakness. The zona orbicularis is created by the crossing of the hip ligaments.

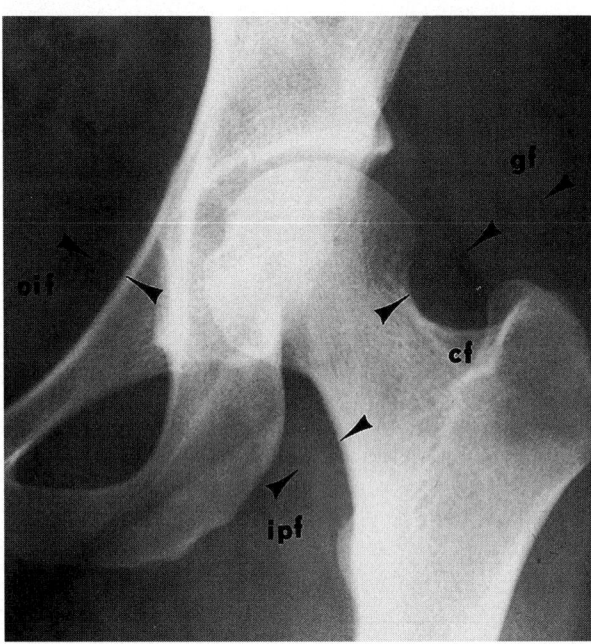

**Figure 3–31.** Periarticular fat planes. The fat planes include fat plane 1 (obturator internus [oif]), fat plane 2 (iliopsoas [ipf]), fat plane 3 (gluteus [gf]), and fat plane 4 ("capsular" [cf]). In each instance, arrowheads indicate the distances from the fat plane to adjacent osseous structures.

(From Guerra J Jr, Armbuster TG, Resnick D, et al: The adult hip: An anatomic study. Part II: The soft-tissue landmarks. Radiology 128:11, 1978.)

the largest sesamoid bone of the body, is embedded within the tendon of the quadriceps femoris. It is oval in outline, with a pointed apex on its inferior surface. The ligamentum patellae (i.e., patellar tendon), a continuation of the quadriceps tendon, is attached to the apex and adjacent bone of the patella.

Articular surfaces of the femur, tibia, and patella are not congruent. The articular surface of the femur comprises the condylar areas and the patellar surface. A shallow groove is present between each condylar surface and the patellar surface. The surface on the lateral femoral condyle appears circular, whereas that on the medial femoral

condyle is large and oval, elongated in an anteroposterior direction. The tibial articular surfaces are the cartilage-clothed condyles, each with a central hollow and peripheral flattened area. The adjacent articular surfaces of the tibia and femur are fitted together more closely by the presence of the medial and lateral menisci. The medial meniscus is nearly semicircular, with a broadened or widened posterior horn. The peripheral aspect of the medial meniscus is attached to the fibrous capsule and tibial collateral ligament. The lateral meniscus, which is of relatively uniform width throughout, resembles a ring. The lateral meniscus is grooved posteriorly by the popliteus tendon and its accompanying tendon sheath. Meniscofemoral ligaments, both anterior and posterior, represent attachments of the posterior horn of the lateral meniscus. A transverse ligament connects the convex anterior portions of both menisci (Fig. 3–32).

The articular surface of the patella is oval and contains an osseous vertical ridge that divides it into a smaller medial area and a larger lateral area. This patellar ridge fits into a corresponding groove on the anterior, or trochlear, surface of the femur. The patellar articulating surface is subdivided further by two poorly defined horizontal ridges of bone into three facets on either side. One additional vertical ridge of bone separates a narrow elongated facet on the medial border of the articular surface. Contact between these various patellar articular facets and the femur varies, depending on the position of the knee.

Trabecular architecture about the knee has been studied, and Blumensaat's line is identified as a condensed linear shadow on the lateral radiograph representing tangential bone in the intercondylar fossa. The location and appearance of Blumensaat's line are extremely sensitive to changes in knee position. In the past, Blumensaat's line was used to provide an indication of the relative position of the patella in lateral projections. Elevation of the distal pole of the patella above this line with the knee flexed 30 degrees was used as an indicator of patella alta (an elevated position of the patella). More recently, other measurements on lateral radiographs have been suggested as more reliable indicators of patellar position (Fig. 3–33). Determination of the ratio of patellar tendon

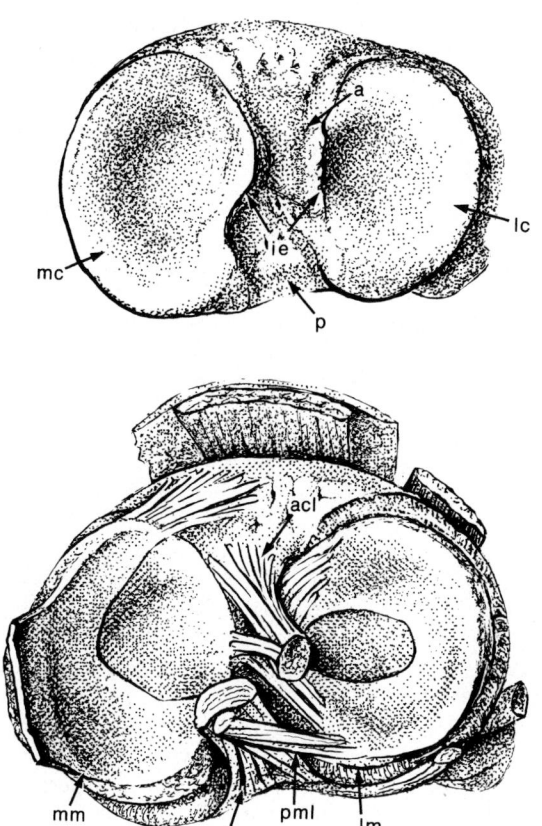

**Figure 3–32.** Meniscal anatomy. Drawings of tibial articular surfaces without (upper) and with (lower) the addition of soft tissue structures. Note the medial condyle (mc), lateral condyle (lc), intercondylar eminences (ie), anterior intercondylar area (a), and posterior intercondylar area (p). Soft tissue structures are the medial meniscus (mm), lateral meniscus (lm), posterior cruciate ligament (pcl), posterior meniscofemoral ligament (pml), and anterior cruciate ligament (acl).

length to greatest diagonal length of the patella has revealed that in the normal situation, both measurements are approximately equal, with a variation of about 20%. A modification of this technique uses the ratio of the distance between the inferior articular surface of the patella and patellar tendon insertion to the length of the articular surface of the patella; a value greater than 2 is considered evidence of patella alta. Another method involves determining the distance between the lower articular surface of the patella and the tibial plateau line. The ratio of this value over the length of the patellar articular surface in normal persons has been reported to be approximately 0.8. The diagnosis of patella alta may have clinical significance, as an abnormally high position of the patella has been recorded in chondromalacia patellae and patellar subluxation or dislocation, whereas a high or low position of the patella has been noted in Osgood-Schlatter disease.

The normal relationships of the anterior surface of the femur and the patella have been studied using axial radiographs (see Fig. 3–33) and computed tomography scanning. In the lateral projection of a mildly flexed knee,

the collapsed suprapatellar pouch creates a sharp vertical radiodense line between an anterior fat pad superior to the patella (anterior suprapatellar fat) and a posterior fat pad in front of the distal supracondylar region of the femur (prefemoral fat pad) (Fig. 3–34). This line is generally less than 5 mm wide but may be between 5 and 10 mm. Shadows of increased thickness suggest the presence of intra-articular fluid.

## TIBIOFIBULAR JOINTS

### Osseous and Soft Tissue Anatomy

Articulations uniting the tibia and the fibula are the proximal (superior) tibiofibular joint (synovial), the crural interosseous membrane (syndesmosis), and the distal tibiofibular joint (syndesmosis). These joints allow limited movement of the fibula with respect to the tibia.

**Proximal Tibiofibular Joint.** The major functions of the proximal tibiofibular joint are dissipating torsional stresses applied at the ankle and providing tensile rather than significant weight-bearing strength. On an anteroposterior radiograph, the medial aspect of the fibular head, which is the actual articulating surface, crosses the lateral border of the tibia. On a lateral radiograph, the fibular head overlies the posterior border of the tibia. Its proper position in this projection can be confirmed by identifying its relationship to the lateral tibial condyle. An important landmark on the lateral knee radiograph for locating the exact position of the fibular head is formed by the posteromedial portion of the lateral tibial condyle. If a line is drawn in an anterior to posterior direction along the lateral tibial spine and continued inferiorly along the posterior aspect of the tibia, this line will identify a groove that separates the midportion of the tibial shaft from the bulk of the bone forming the supporting structure of the lateral tibial condyle posteriorly. The sloping radiodense line observed on the lateral knee radiograph proceeds first posteriorly and inferiorly to form an acute angle posteriorly, which identifies the most posteromedial portion of the lateral tibial condyle. The radiodense line then extends inferiorly and anteriorly from this point in the groove described previously. Knowledge of the exact location of this line greatly assists in the interpretation of lateral knee radiographs in cases of tibiofibular joint dislocation (Fig. 3–35).

**Crural Interosseous Membrane.** The crural interosseous membrane is tightly stretched between the interosseous borders of the tibia and fibula. Its upper limit is just inferior to the proximal tibiofibular joint, and its lower limit contains fibers that blend with those about the distal tibiofibular joint. The oblique fibers in the crural interosseous membrane extend inferiorly and laterally from tibia to fibula. A large oval opening in the superior aspect of the membrane allows passage of the anterior tibial vessels; a smaller distal opening allows passage of the perforating branch of the peroneal artery.

**Distal Tibiofibular Joint.** This fibrous joint consists of a strong interosseous ligament that unites the convex surface of the medial distal fibula and the concave surface of

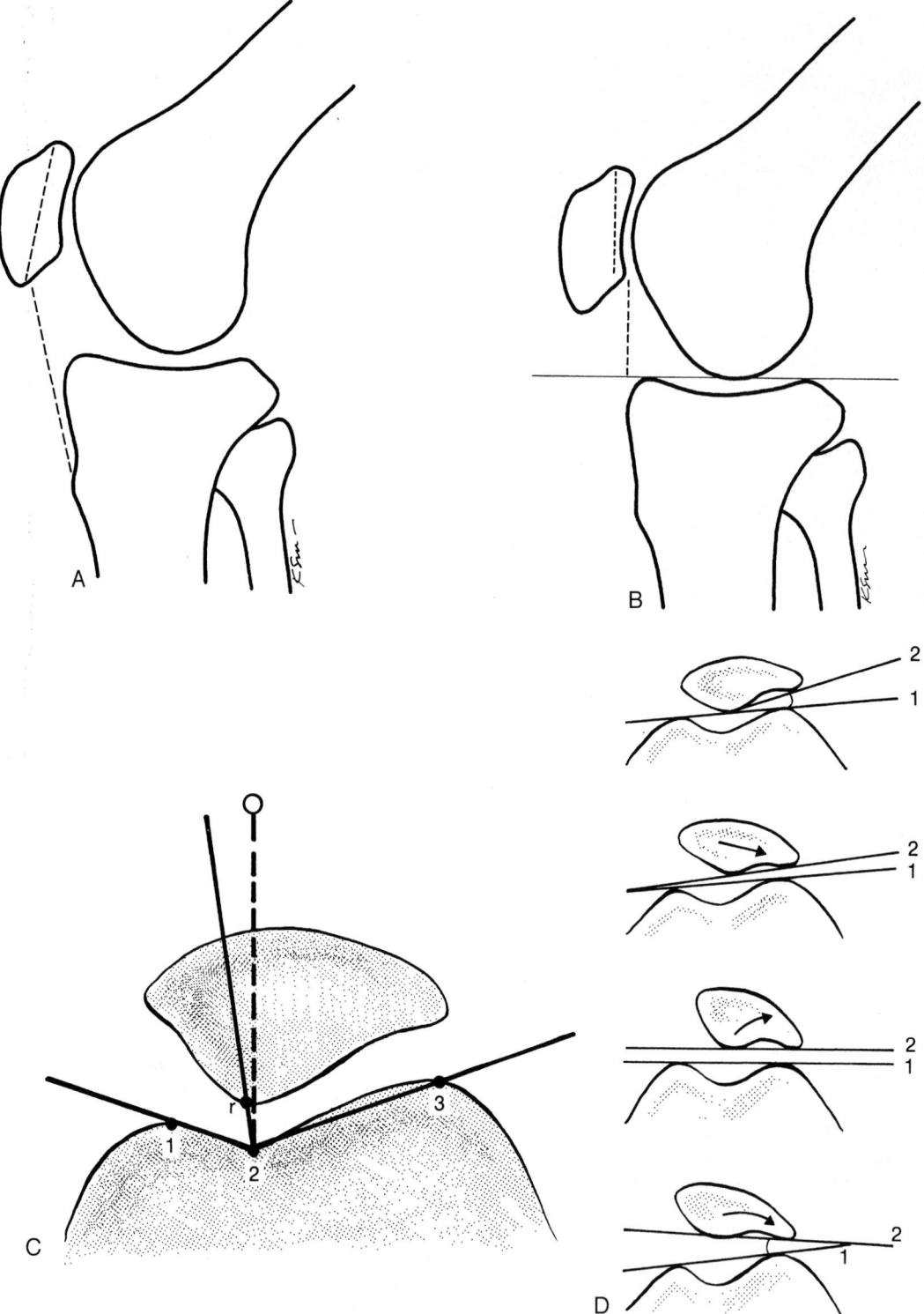

**Figure 3–33.** Patellar position. *A,* The ratio of patellar tendon length to the greatest diagonal length of the patella can be used to diagnose patella alta. *B,* The ratio of the distance between the lower articular surface of the patella and the tibial plateau line to the length of the patellar articular surface has also been used for this purpose. *C,* Merchant and coworkers (J Bone Joint Surg Am 56:1391, 1974) suggested that on an axial radiograph, the line connecting the median ridge of the patella (r) and trochlear depth (2) should fall medial or slightly lateral to a line (O) bisecting angle 1-2-3. Here, the first line lies medial to line O, a normal finding. *D,* Laurin and coworkers proposed other measurements that might be appropriate. The upper two diagrams reveal the normal situation; the lower two diagrams indicate the abnormal situation. On axial radiographs, an angle formed between a line connecting the anterior aspect of the femoral condyles (1) and a second line along the lateral facet of the patella (2) normally opens laterally. In patients with subluxation or abnormal tilting of the patella, these lines are parallel, or the angle of intersection opens medially.

(*D,* From Laurin CA, Levesque HP, Dussault R, et al: The abnormal lateral patellofemoral angle: A diagnostic roentgenographic sign of recurrent patellar subluxation. J Bone Joint Surg Am 60:55, 1978.)

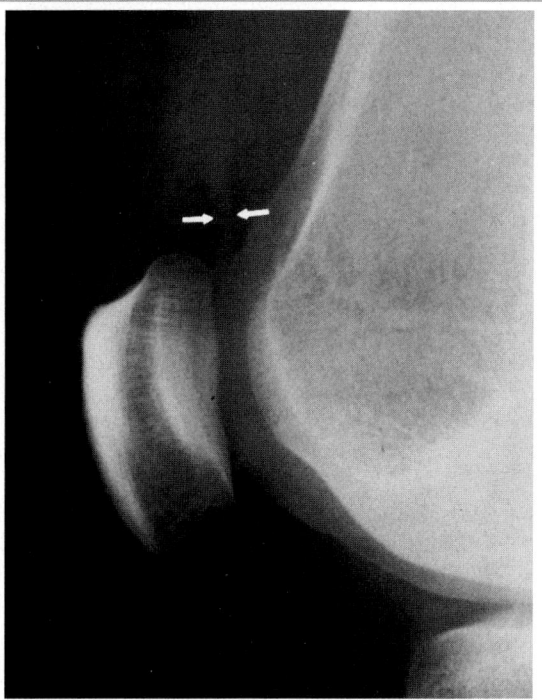

**Figure 3–34.** Diagnosis of a synovial effusion in the knee. In normal situations, the collapsed suprapatellar pouch creates a radiodense area *(arrows)* that is generally less than 5 mm wide but may be between 5 and 10 mm wide.

the adjacent fibular notch of the tibia. Additionally, the anterior and posterior tibiofibular ligaments reinforce this articulation. Below this ligamentous joint, an upward prolongation of the synovial membrane of the ankle (talocrural joint) can extend 3 to 5 mm. This synovial recess may be associated with cartilaginous surfaces on the tibia and fibula.

## ANKLE (TALOCRURAL JOINT)

This synovial articulation exists where the talus relates to the lower ends of the tibia and fibula and to the inferior transverse tibiofibular ligament.

### Osseous Anatomy

The distal end of the tibia contains the medial malleolus and articular surface. The broad malleolus has an articular facet on its lateral surface, which is comma-shaped. On the posterior surface of the distal end of the tibia is a groove, just lateral to the medial malleolus, related to the tendon of the tibialis posterior muscle. The inferior surface of the tibia represents the articular area for the talus. It is smooth and wider anteriorly than posteriorly. The triangular fibular notch is on the lateral side of the tibia. This notch represents the site of attachment of various ligaments that connect the distal portions of the tibia and fibula. The distal end of the fibula contains the

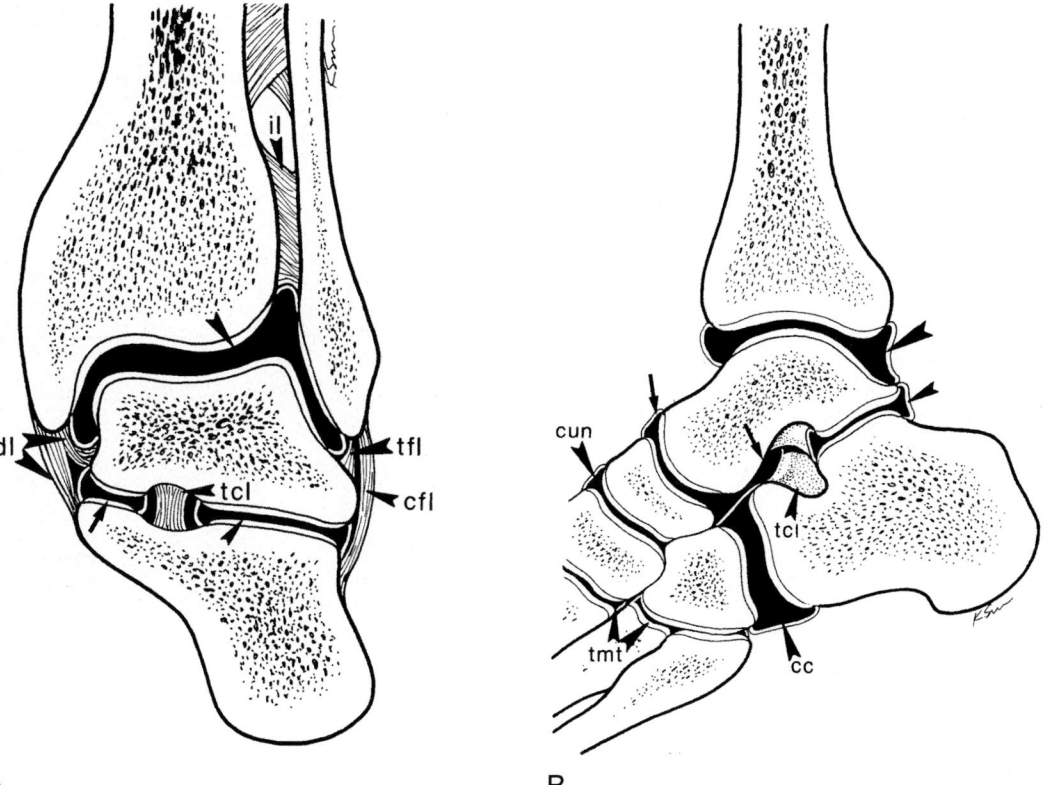

A                                    B

**Figure 3–35.** Ankle joint anatomy. *A,* Drawing of a coronal section through the distal ends of the tibia, fibula, and talus, outlining the ankle joint *(large arrowheads),* interosseous ligament (il) of the tibiofibular syndesmosis, interosseous talocalcaneal ligament (tcl), portions of the deltoid ligament (dl), posterior talofibular ligament (tfl), calcaneofibular ligament (cfl), surrounding tendons, subtalar joint *(small arrowhead),* and talocalcaneonavicular joint *(arrow). B,* Some of the same structures in *(A)* can be identified in a drawing of a sagittal section of the ankle. Additional articulations are the calcaneocuboid (cc), cuneonavicular (cun), and tarsometatarsal (tmt) joints.

lateral malleolus. This structure projects more inferiorly than the medial malleolus and contains a triangular facet on its medial surface for articulation with the talus and an irregular surface above this facet for the interosseous ligament. Posterior to the convex articular facet is a depression, the malleolar fossa.

Assessment of alignment of the ankle on radiographs is important in the post-trauma evaluation of this joint. Small degrees of lateral displacement of the talus on the tibia may result in the rapid development of secondary degenerative arthritis. It has been shown that even 1 mm of lateral displacement of the talus reduces the tibiotalar contact area by 42%. Incomplete ligament tears may result in relatively small amounts of displacement, which may be difficult to detect radiographically.

In adults, the coronal plane of the ankle is oriented in about 15 to 20 degrees of external rotation with reference to the coronal plane of the knee; therefore, the lateral malleolus is slightly posterior to the medial malleolus. To obtain a true anteroposterior film of the tibiotalar articulation, the ankle must be positioned with the medial and lateral malleoli parallel to the tabletop—that is, in about 15 to 20 degrees of internal rotation, or the mortise view. This positioning places the medial articular surface tangent to the x-ray beam, and the short concave line representing the posteromedial surface of the talus falls slightly lateral to the medial articular surface.

The axial relationships of the ankle have been described. The longitudinal axis of the tibia is perpendicular to the horizontal plane of the ankle joint and is continuous with the longitudinal axis of the talus. The tibial angle, the angle formed by the intersection of one line drawn tangentially to the articular surface of the medial malleolus and a second line drawn along the articular surface of the talus, averages 53 degrees (range, 45 to 61 degrees). The fibular angle, drawn in a corresponding way using the lateral malleolus rather than the medial malleolus, averages 52 degrees (range, 45 to 63 degrees).

## Soft Tissue Anatomy

The fibrous capsule is attached superiorly to the medial and lateral malleoli and tibia and inferiorly to the talus. The talar attachment of the capsule is close to the margins of the trochlear surface, except anteriorly, where the attachment to the neck of the talus is located at some distance from the articular margin. The capsule is weak both anteriorly and posteriorly, but it is reinforced medially and laterally by various ligaments. Surrounding ligaments include the deltoid, anterior and posterior talofibular, and calcaneofibular ligaments.

## TENDON SHEATHS AND BURSAE ABOUT THE ANKLE AND CALCANEUS

Tendons with accompanying tendon sheaths are intimate with the ankle joint. Anteriorly, there are sheaths about the tibialis anterior, extensor hallucis longus, extensor digitorum longus, and peroneus tertius tendons. Medially, sheaths are present about the tibialis posterior, flexor digitorum longus, and flexor hallucis longus tendons.

Laterally, the common sheath of the peroneus longus and peroneus brevis tendons is seen.

Important tendons, aponeuroses, and bursae are located about the calcaneus. The plantar aponeurosis contains strong fibers that adhere to the posteroinferior surface of the bone. It has central, medial, and lateral components. The Achilles tendon, which is the thickest and strongest human tendon, attaches to the posterior surface of the calcaneus approximately 2 cm below the upper surface of the bone. The plantaris tendon is located medial to the Achilles tendon. The retrocalcaneal bursa exists between the Achilles tendon and the posterosuperior surface of the calcaneus.

On normal radiographs, the Achilles tendon has a thickness of 4 to 8 mm at the level of the calcaneus or 1 to 2 cm above the top of the calcaneus (Fig. 3–36). A vertical radiolucent area, the retrocalcaneal recess, measures 2 mm or more in length and extends from the posterior aspect of the calcaneus behind the posterior portion of the bone, reflecting fat adjacent to the normal retrocalcaneal bursa (Fig. 3–37). The appearance of the retrocalcaneal recess can be influenced by severe dorsiflexion or plantar flexion of the foot.

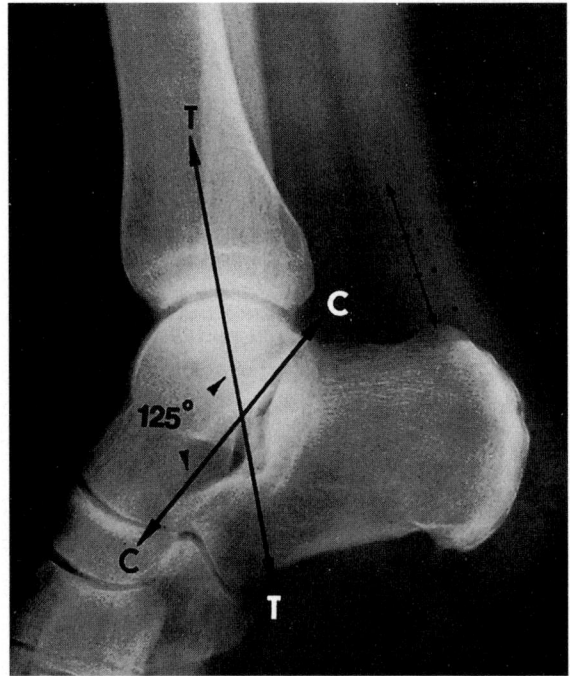

**Figure 3–36.** Achilles tendon: normal radiographic measurements. The thickness of the Achilles tendon is noted at the level of the calcaneus and at 1 and 2 cm above it. The determination of the calcaneal-talar angle guarantees that the radiograph has been taken in a "neutral" position. This angle is formed by the intersection of two lines—one drawn along the longitudinal axis of the tibia (T) and the second drawn along the top of the calcaneus (C). With proper positioning in normal persons, this angle varies from approximately 90 to 140 degrees.

(From Resnick D, Feingold ML, Curd J, et al: Calcaneal abnormalities in articular disorders. Rheumatoid arthritis, ankylosing spondylitis, psoriatic arthritis, and Reiter syndrome. Radiology 125:355, 1977.)

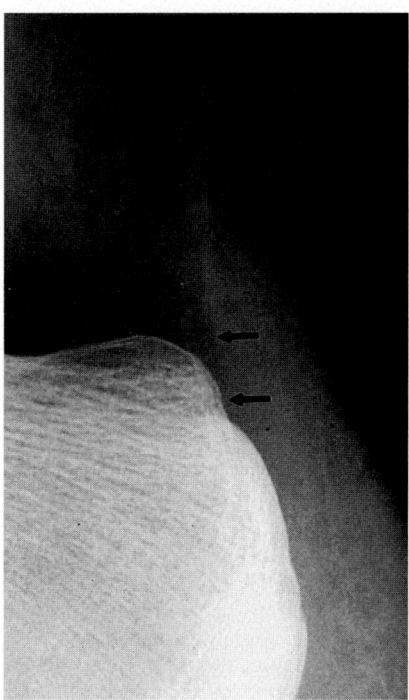

**Figure 3–37.** Retrocalcaneal recess: normal appearance. This recess appears as a triangular radiolucent area between the Achilles tendon and calcaneus. It is normally 2 mm or longer (*between arrows*).

(From Resnick D, Feingold ML, Curd J, et al: Calcaneal abnormalities in articular disorders. Rheumatoid arthritis, ankylosing spondylitis, psoriatic arthritis, and Reiter syndrome. Radiology 125:355, 1977.)

## FURTHER READING

Armbuster TG, Guerra J Jr, Resnick D, et al: The adult hip: An anatomic study. Part I. The bony landmarks. Radiology 128:1, 1978.

Bettinger PC, Linscheid RL, Berger RA, et al: An anatomic study of the stabilizing ligaments of the trapezium and trapeziometacarpal joint. J Hand Surg Am 24:786, 1999.

Cone RO, Szabo R, Resnick D, et al: Computed tomography of the normal soft tissues of the wrist. Invest Radiol 18:546, 1983.

Coventry MB: Anatomy of the intervertebral disc. Clin Orthop 67:9, 1969.

Crockarell JR Jr, Trousdale RT, Guyton JL: The anterior centre-edge angle: A cadaver study. J Bone Joint Surg Br 82:532, 2000.

Curtis DJ, Downey EF Jr, Brower AC, et al: Importance of soft-tissue evaluation in hand and wrist trauma: statistical evaluation. AJR Am J Roentgenol 142:781, 1984.

Danzig LA, Newell JD, Guerra J Jr, et al: Osseous landmarks of the normal knee. Clin Orthop 156:201, 1981.

Delaunay S, Dussault RG, Kaplan PA, et al: Radiographic measurements of dysplastic adult hips. Skeletal Radiol 26:75, 1997.

Grelsamer RP, Meadows S: The modified Insall-Salvati ratio for assessment of patellar height. Clin Orthop 282:170, 1992.

Hall FM: Radiographic diagnosis and accuracy in knee joint effusions. Radiology 115:49, 1975.

Insall J, Salvati E: Patella position in the normal knee joint. Radiology 101:101, 1971.

Jackson H: The diagnosis of minimal atlanto-axial subluxation. Br J Radiol 23:672, 1950.

Jirout J: Patterns of changes in the cervical spine on lateroflexion. Neuroradiology 2:164, 1971.

Kaplan EB: Functional and Surgical Anatomy of the Hand, 2nd ed. Philadelphia, JB Lippincott, 1965, p 114.

Keats TE, Teeslink R, Diamond AE, et al: Normal axial relationships of the major joints. Radiology 87:904, 1966.

Lusted LB, Keats TE: Atlas of Roentgenographic Measurement, 2nd ed. Chicago, Year Book Medical Publishers, 1967, p 122.

MacDonald D: Primary protrusio acetabuli: Report of an affected family. J Bone Joint Surg Br 53:30, 1971.

McGregor M: The significance of certain measurements of the skull in the diagnosis of basilar impression. Br J Radiol 21:171, 1948.

Minns RJ, Hunter JAA: The mechanical and structural characteristics of the tibiofibular interosseous membrane. Acta Orthop Scand 47:236, 1976.

Murphy WA, Siegel MJ: Elbow fat pads with new signs and extended differential diagnosis. Radiology 124:659, 1977.

Paquin JD, Van der Rest M, Marie PJ, et al: Biochemical and morphologic studies of cartilage from the adult human sacroiliac joint. Arthritis Rheum 26:887, 1983.

Reichmann S: Roentgenologic soft tissue appearances in hip disease. Acta Radiol (Diagn) 6:167, 1967.

Resnick D: Arthrography in the evaluation of arthritic disorders of the wrist. Radiology 113:331, 1974.

Resnick D: Inter-relationship between radiocarpal and metacarpophalangeal joint deformities in rheumatoid arthritis. J Can Assoc Radiol 27:29, 1976.

Resnick D: Radiology of the talocalcaneal articulations: Anatomic considerations and arthrography. Radiology 111:581, 1974.

Rothman RH, Marvel JP Jr, Heppenstall RB: Anatomic considerations in the glenohumeral joint. Orthop Clin North Am 6:341, 1975.

Schills JP, Resnick D, Haghighi P, et al: Sternocostal joints: Anatomic, radiographic and pathologic features in adult cadavers. Invest Radiol 24:596, 1989.

Stein MG, Barmeir E, Levin J, et al: The medial acetabular wall: Normal measurements in different population groups. Invest Radiol 17:476, 1982.

Towbin R, Dunbar JS, Towbin J, et al: Teardrop sign: Plain film recognition of ankle effusion. AJR Am J Roentgenol 134:985, 1980.

Vleeming A, Volkers ACW, Snijders CJ, et al: Relation between form and function in the sacroiliac joint. Part II. Biomechanical aspects. Spine 15:133, 1990.

Walmsley R: Joints. In Romanes GJ (ed): Cunningham's Textbook of Anatomy, 11th ed. London, Oxford University Press, 1972, p 214.

Warwick R, Williams PL: Gray's Anatomy, 35th Br ed. Philadelphia, WB Saunders, 1973, p 407.

Weston WJ, Palmer DG: Soft Tissues of the Extremities. New York, Springer-Verlag, 1978, p 61.

Whalen JP, Woodruff CL: The cervical prevertebral fat stripe: A new aid in evaluating the cervical prevertebral soft tissue space. AJR Am J Roentgenol 109:445, 1970.

# CHAPTER 4

## Articular Cartilage: Morphology, Physiology, and Function

Wayne H. Akeson, Constance R. Chu, and William Bugbee

## *SUMMARY OF KEY FEATURES*

Articular cartilage is a highly specialized tissue. The components of the matrix in which the chondrocytes are dispersed, as well as the cells themselves, are important in allowing articular cartilage to fulfill its special functions related to chemistry, synthesis, maturation, and unique interactions. The mechanisms for load carriage, lubrication, and nutrition and their interrelationships are also related to the functional properties of cartilage.

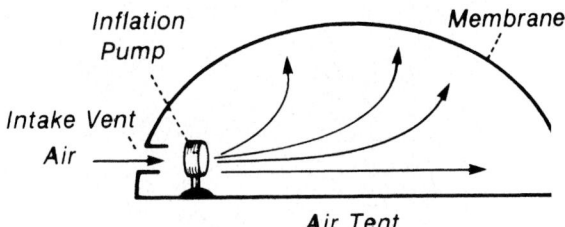

**Figure 4–1.** Air tent–articular cartilage analogy. It is conceptually useful to think of cartilage as a pressurized structure such as an air tent. The system requires a pump, which must be working constantly to maintain inflation of the system because of leaks through the fabric. In the case of cartilage, the surface membrane is the fine collagen fibril network concentrated at the surface. The inflation pump is the proteoglycan molecules, and the inflation medium is an ultrafiltrate of synovial fluid. In cartilage, of course, there is no single intake vent for the inflation medium to enter; rather, the fluid that inflates the tissue enters through the same fabric pores at the surface from which it exits when compressed.

## INTRODUCTION

Articular cartilage is a unique tissue in many respects, but especially with regard to its structural, metabolic, and functional interactions. Articular cartilage possesses unparalleled functional efficiency. Such efficiencies are achieved despite stringent limitations imposed on the tissue, including a lack of blood supply, a tissue thickness that measures only a few millimeters at most, and a limited repair capability.

## OVERVIEW OF CARTILAGE FUNCTION

A useful analogy for the morphology and biochemistry of articular cartilage is the air tent seen in parts of the country as a cover for recreational areas such as swimming pools or tennis courts (Fig. 4–1). The requirements for the tent are a membrane (fabric cover), an inflation medium (air), and an energy source to keep the tent inflated (fan). These elements are interrelated, and a deficiency in any of them results in failure of the system.

Articular cartilage is analogous to the air tent in a number of respects. There is a fabriclike structure at the cartilage surface that consists of fine collagen fibrils packed tightly in a matted pattern; this differs from the structure seen in the deeper layers, where fibers become thicker, the orientation becomes vertical, and the spaces between the fibers increase. The surface "fabric" of cartilage has tiny pores that permit fluid and small molecules access to and egress from the tissue but block the movement of large molecules. The inflation medium in articular cartilage is, of course, fluid, not air. The cartilage fluid is in equilibrium with the synovial fluid, which in turn is essentially an ultrafiltrate of plasma. The fluid in articular cartilage is significantly pressurized. The pump for the

articular cartilage organ is provided by the proteoglycan aggregate molecules. These huge macromolecules are fixed within the articular cartilage fibrillar matrix as a result of their large size and volume. They are too large to move between the fibrils of collagen and much too large to exit through the small pores in the matted, capsulelike surface of the articular cartilage. Internal reactions cause fluid to be pulled into articular cartilage and cause the collagen matrix of the system to expand, creating a swelling pressure within the enclosed cartilage space. The collagen fibers are placed under tension as the fluid pressure rises. In this manner, the cartilage is pressurized and the collagen "fabric" is inflated. The equilibrium state reached is a balance that can be upset by external applied pressure. If the external pressure exceeds the internal pressure, fluid will flow outward until a new equilibrium is reached. This fluid movement is of great interest, as it explains the mechanism of several indispensable elements of the articular cartilage system, such as lubrication, load bearing, and nutrition.

## COLLAGEN
### Morphology of the Collagen Framework

The air tent analogy requires that a pressurized internal medium be constrained from expansion by a membrane. A matted surface layer of collagen fibrils provides this membrane-like function (Fig. 4–2). This model, though not precisely accurate, provides a functional understanding of the concept. Certainly the characteristics of surface fibers differ from those of fibers in deeper layers. The surface collagen fibrils are smaller and more closely packed than are those in the middle and deeper layers. The collagen concentration is greatest at the surface, where the small fibrils are compacted tangentially to the

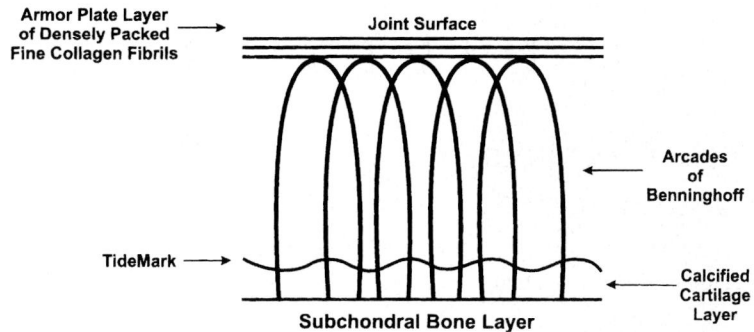

**Figure 4–2.** Schematic diagram of the collagen fibril orientation within articular cartilage. The fibrils are tightly packed near the articular surface in a tangential layer that has been termed the armor plate layer. Fibrils in the deeper layers become progressively larger as they approach the subchondral bone layer. The fibrils also are more widely spaced in the deeper layers of cartilage. The change in orientation from tangential to perpendicular in the deeper layers creates a pattern that has been termed an arcade. The collagen fibrils anchor into the subchondral bone layer after traversing the calcified cartilage, which is demarcated by a change in staining properties termed the tidemark line. The anchoring of these fibrils into bone is analogous to the continuation of ligamentous attachments into bone, termed Sharpey's fibers.

surface. This arrangement creates an effective pore size, which has been calculated to be about 6 nm. The largest molecule that can traverse a pore of this dimension is hemoglobin. Therefore, the surface pores readily admit most of the synovial fluid molecules. Small ions and glucose, for example, easily traverse these pores, but larger molecules such as proteins and hyaluronan (hyaluronic acid) do not enter cartilage in significant amounts under normal conditions.

Collagen fibers in the intermediate layers are no longer oriented principally tangentially to the surface but are directed obliquely or randomly. They are larger than the surface fibrils. The deepest fibrils are the largest in cartilage. They are oriented perpendicular to the joint surface. They perforate the calcified basal layers of cartilage through the tidemark regions and eventually enter the subchondral bone layer, where they are attached firmly, similar to Sharpey's fibers of cortical bone. This anatomic arrangement is the key to the secure structural anchorage of cartilage to the bone that it overlies.

The surface pattern of the collagen framework described has been recognized implicitly for decades by the term *armor plate layer*, referring to the tough, resilient cartilage surface. It has been well demonstrated clinically that loss of the densely packed collagen mat at the surface of cartilage in weight-bearing regions is a prelude to fibrillation, thinning, and ensuing degenerative arthritis. The term *fibrillation* describes the tendency of these fibrils to be split vertically all the way to their subchondral attachment. The villus-like strands so exposed collectively resemble a shag rug.

Routine histologic techniques do not show the collagen fibrils of cartilage well; they tend to be masked by the abundant proteoglycan intertwined within the fibril network. The collagen fibril pattern can be inferred, however, by viewing sections with polarized light, because a fibrillar pattern of preferred orientation will alter the polarized light characteristically (Figs. 4–3 and 4–4).

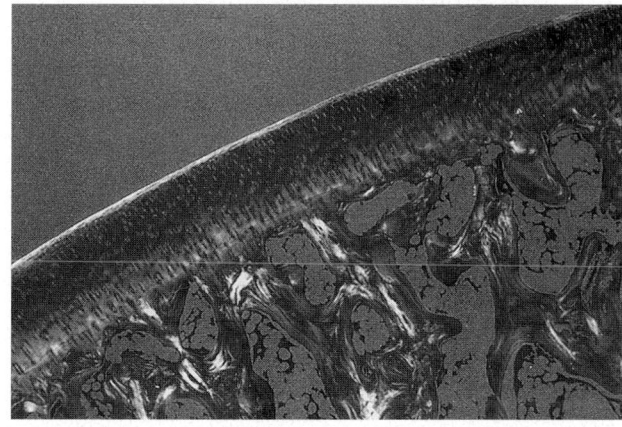

**Figure 4–3.** This photograph of an articular cartilage surface under polarized light shows differences in refractivity of the surface layer compared with deeper layers of articular cartilage. The preferred tangential orientation of the collagen fibrils at the surface creates the refractile difference seen as a bright line (×45). (Compare with Fig. 4–4.)

## Collagen Chemistry

Collagen constitutes 65% to 80% of the mass by dry weight of such specialized connective tissues as tendons, ligaments, skin, joint capsules, and cartilage. It is the only protein with significant tensile force–resisting properties with the exception of elastin, whose functional role is insignificant in comparison. The tensile force–resisting properties of cartilage derive from the precise molecular configuration of the collagen macromolecule. This molecule is one of the largest in the body, forming a rodlike structure. These rods are termed tropocollagen. They are assembled in a three-dimensional array in the extracellular environment, being somehow influenced by environmental stresses and additional biologic factors. The assembly is typically patterned in a quarter stagger, which

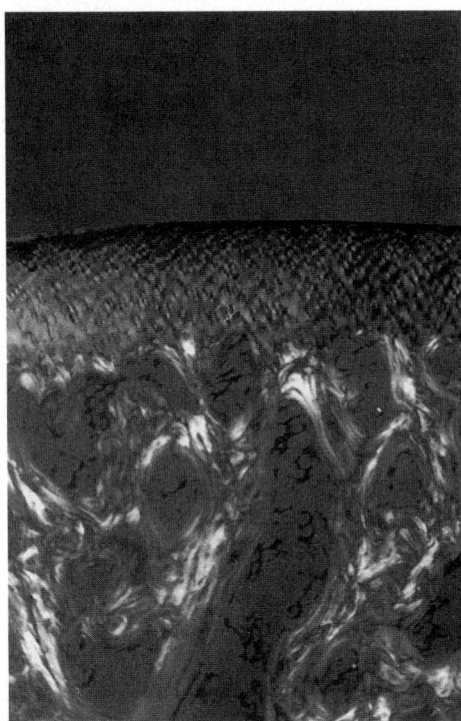

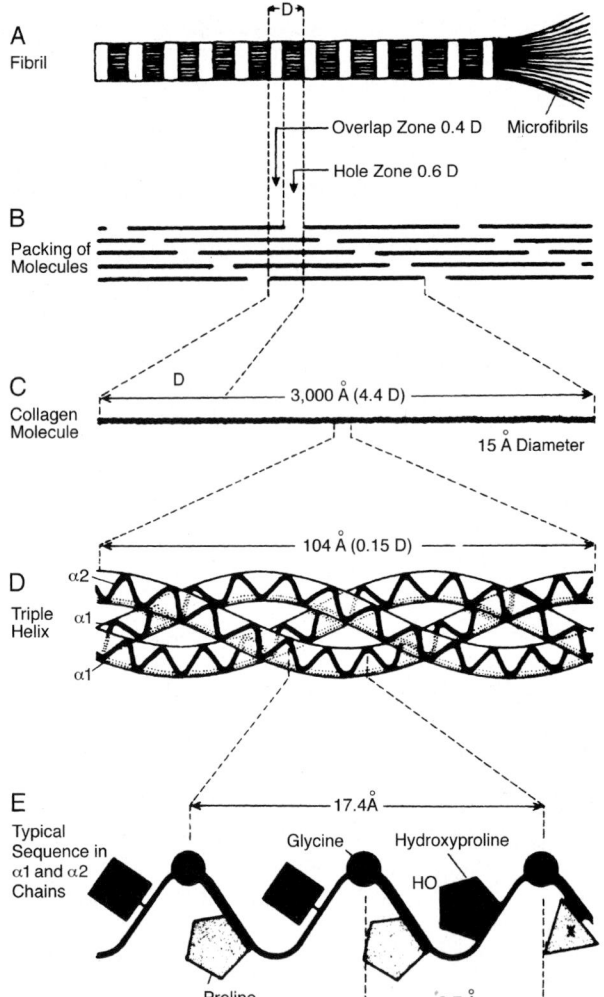

**Figure 4–4.** Articular cartilage surface (same section as in Fig. 4–3) with the polarizing filter rotated 90 degrees, which produces a marked change in the refractile pattern. The surface is now dark rather than bright because of the predominant orientation of the tangential layer of fibrils. The arcade pattern in the deeper layers also can be perceived with the filter in this rotation, in contrast to Figure 4–3. Use of this polarized light technique identifies areas in the tissue where a predominant orientation exists, as opposed to a random pattern of fibrils.

**Figure 4–5.** Relationship of the single-strand protein of the alpha chain to the triple helix, the collagen molecule, and the fully developed fibril. The characteristic feature of the collagen molecule is its rigid and very long, narrow rodlike structure, which is created by the tight winding of three alpha chains into a triple helix termed tropocollagen.

(From Prockop DJ, Kivirikko KI, Tuderman L, Guzman NA: The biosynthesis of collagen and its disorders (first of two parts). N Engl J Med 301:13, 1979.)

is seen on transmission electron micrographs. The individual tropocollagen units are made up of three chains that are synthesized independently intracellularly, in the manner of other proteins (Fig. 4–5). Each chain contains about 1000 amino acids. Most of the chains (called alpha chains) are precisely ordered, with a general sequence of glycine-proline-hydroxyproline, glycine-proline-$x$, or glycine-$x$-proline, in which $x$ is another amino acid. The higher percentages of the amino acids glycine, proline, and hydroxyproline are unique to collagen. Glycine is the smallest amino acid and permits the close packing necessary for the assembly of the three alpha chains into tropocollagen.

The assembly of the three alpha chains into tropocollagen is facilitated by a group of amino acids at the end of each alpha chain called registration peptides. The triple helix plus its registration peptide is larger than the tropocollagen molecule and is called procollagen. Once the assembly of the triple helix is completed, the registration peptides are no longer of utility and are cleaved by an enzyme, procollagen peptidase, as the procollagen passes through the cellular membrane into the extracellular space.

Nineteen different types of collagen have been described in vertebrates. The collagens can be divided into two major classes on the basis of their primary structure and supramolecular assembly: fibril-forming and non–fibril-forming collagens. The fibril-forming collagens include types I, II, III, V, and XI; all these types have a long, central, triple helical domain without any interruptions in the glycine-$x$-$y$ sequence, in which $x$ and $y$ are amino acids. The rest of the collagens belong to the non–fibril-forming class. Although they vary in size, they share the feature of having imperfections in the glycine-$x$-$y$ sequence. Within this class, types IX, XII, and XIV collagens form a subgroup called the fibril-associated collagens with interrupted triple helices (FACIT). They are associated with type I or II collagen fibrils and play a role in the interaction of these fibrils with other matrix components. Although their sizes and primary structures vary, they share several common structural features. Type XVI collagen also appears to be a member of this group. Four collagens have been isolated from articular cartilage: II, VI, IX, and XI (Table 4–1).

## Collagen Crosslinks

Stabilization of collagen occurs extracellularly after assembly into the quarter-stagger arrays that make up filaments, fibrils, and fibers. The stabilization and ultimate tensile strength of the structure are thought to result mainly from the development of intramolecular and intermolecular crosslinks. The former occur between alpha chains of the same tropocollagen molecule; the latter occur between adjacent tropocollagen molecules. The crosslinks result from enzyme-mediated reactions involving mainly lysine and hydroxylysine.

The significance of type II collagen to cartilage is not yet known. The principal differences between this collagen and the more common type I found in fibrous connective tissue are the number of hydroxylysine molecules present and the presence of a small number of cysteine residues (see Table 4–1). The principal crosslinking residues in mature type II collagen fibrils are hydroxylysyl pyridinoline residues. Evidence is being accumulated that type IX collagen, and possibly type XI, makes a critical contribution to the organization and mechanical stability of the type II collagen fibrillar network. Type IX makes up approximately 10% of the collagen protein in fetal mammalian articular cartilage, but the amount decreases to about 1% in adult tissue. It is believed that type IX provides a covalent interface between the surface of type II collagen fibril and the interfibrillar proteoglycan domain. Type IX collagen molecules are heavily crosslinked to type II collagen and also to other type IX collagen molecules, enhancing the mechanical stability of the fibrillar network and serving as a mediator of collagen fiber architecture.

The fundamental process of collagen formation by chondroblasts and chondrocytes seems to be nearly identical to the process of synthesis by fibroblasts and fibrocytes (Fig. 4–6). The collagen turnover in cartilage proceeds at a rate not unlike that seen in connective tissue of the fibrous type. Because significant synthesis occurs in adult cartilage, it is clear that control processes for spatial orientation of the product are crucial.

## PROTEOGLYCANS OF ARTICULAR CARTILAGE

The proteoglycans of articular cartilage serve as the "pump" of the highly pressurized cartilage system. The characteristics of the proteoglycan molecules that permit this crucial function include their very large size and hence their immobility within the collagen fibril meshwork; their densely concentrated, fixed negative charges; and their large number of hydroxyl groups. Collectively, these characteristics serve to attract water and small ions into the cartilage. The sum of this attraction is termed the swelling pressure, which consists of osmotic forces, ionic forces, and Donnan forces.

The original term applied to this group of molecules was *acid mucopolysaccharides*. The more precise chemical term *glycosaminoglycans* has been accepted as preferable. The preferred term for hyaluronic acid is now *hyaluronan*. In most of the glycosaminoglycan molecules, hexosamine alternates with another sugar polymerized in a repeating disaccharide pattern. The predominance of the amine group in this configuration is the reason for the occurrence of *amino* in the term *glycosaminoglycan*. The disaccharide repeating unit for the glycosaminoglycans of articular cartilage is chondroitin 4-sulfate, chondroitin 6-sulfate, hyaluronan, and keratan sulfate (Fig. 4–7). The glycosaminoglycans are covalently bound to core protein in a structure termed aggrecan. The aggrecan structure locates relatively short keratan sulfate side arms preferentially close to the linkage region to hyaluronan.

The ability of proteoglycan to aggregate further by combining with hyaluronan is facilitated and stabilized by small proteins called link proteins. Much attention has been given to the degree of aggregate formation in various tissues and in various pathologic conditions. Clearly, the ability of the proteoglycan molecule to form aggregates of even greater molecular size amplifies its physiologic functional properties as the pump of the system.

In distinction to the covalent linkage of glycosaminoglycans to core protein in proteoglycan subunit, the linkage of proteoglycan subunit to hyaluronan is noncovalent. The linkage is facilitated and strengthened by low-molecular-weight link proteins. Three link proteins have been identified in canine and human articular cartilage. Cartilages from different sources possess differing percentages of aggregation of proteoglycan, but factors controlling this process are not yet fully understood.

## FLUID OF ARTICULAR CARTILAGE

As was noted in the air tent analogy, the inflation medium of articular cartilage is synovial fluid. This is essentially an ultrafiltrate of plasma plus hyaluronan. The hyaluronan molecules are too large to enter cartilage through its surface pores, but most of the remaining ions and molecules of normal synovial fluid, such as water, sodium, potassium, and glucose, are sufficiently small to pass through these pores easily. Movement of fluid into and out of cartilage occurs to some extent by diffusion, but diffusion by itself does not seem adequate to provide for cartilage health. Most of the fluid of articular cartilage is water. The percentage of water in cartilage ranges from more than 60% to nearly 80%. Net flow into and out of cartilage is induced by the normal weight-bearing function of synovial joints. The rate of fluid movement permitted by the small surface pore size and the cartilage microarchitecture, however, is sufficiently slow that cartilage is compressed only partially even after loading for hours. The fluid movement that occurs during the loading process appears to be important for lubrication of the joint surfaces as well as for load carriage. This process provides a fluid film that minimizes cartilage-cartilage contact, thus also minimizing wear.

## NUTRITION

Fluid movement is necessary not only for load carriage and lubrication but also for nutrition of the chondro-

## TABLE 4–1

**Structurally and Genetically Distinct Collagens**

| Type | Tissue Distribution | Molecular Form | Chemical Characterization |
|---|---|---|---|
| Fibrillar collagens | | | |
| I | Bone, tendon, skin, dentin, ligament, uterus, artery | $[\alpha_1 \text{(I)}]_2 \, \alpha_2 \text{(I)}$ | Hybrid composed of two kinds of chains; low in hydroxylysine and glycosylated |
| | Fetal tissues, inflammatory and neoplastic states | $[\alpha_1 \text{(I)}]_3$ | hydroxylysine; small 67-nm banded fibril; increased content of 3- and 4-hydroxyproline and hydroxylysine as compared with the heteropolymer |
| II | Hyaline cartilage, vitreous body | $[\alpha_1 \text{(II)}]_3$ | Relatively high in hydroxylysine and glycosylated hydroxylysine; small 67-nm banded fibril |
| III | Skin, artery, uterus | $[\alpha_1 \text{(III)}]_3$ | High in hydroxyproline and low in hydroxylysine; contains interchain disulfide bonds, associated with type I; small 67-nm banded fibril |
| V | Hamster lung cell culture | $[\alpha_1 \text{(V)}]_3$ | Associated with type I; small fibers; small 67-nm banded fibril; similar to type IV |
| | Skin, bone, fetal membranes | $[\alpha_1 \text{(V)}]_2 \, \alpha_2 \text{(V)}$ | |
| | Synovial membrane, placenta | $\alpha_1 \text{(V)} \, \alpha_2 \text{(V)}$ | |
| | Most interstitial tissues | $\alpha_3 \text{(V)}$ | |
| XI | Hyaline cartilage associated with type II | $\alpha_1 \text{(XI)} \, \alpha_2 \text{(XI)}$ $\alpha_3 \text{(XI)}$ | 67-nm banded fibril |
| FACIT collagens | | | |
| IX | Hyaline cartilage, vitreous humor | $\alpha_1 \text{(IX)} \, \alpha_2 \text{(IX)}$ $\alpha_3 \text{(IX)}$ | Associated with type II; minor cartilage protein; contains attached glycosaminoglycan; NF and FACIT member; FACIT collagen 1 domain |
| XII | Embryonic tendon and skin, periodontal ligament | $[\alpha_1 \text{(XII)}]_3$ | Associated with type I; NF and FACIT member; FACIT collagen 1 domain with similarities to type IX |
| XIV | Fetal tendon and skin | $[\alpha_1 \text{(XIV)}]_3$ | NF and FACIT member; FACIT collagen 1 domain similar to that of type IX |
| XVI | Skin fibroblast, Epidermal keratinocytes | $[\alpha \text{(XVI)}]_3$ | Approximately 65% of molecules composed of repeating glycine-*x*-*y* sequences; 10 separate collagen domains, noncollagen domains contain numerous cystines and often are found in the sequence of cystine-*x*-*y*-cystine, where *x* and *y* are any amino acids |
| XIX | Found in only a few adult tissues: brain, eye, testes | $[\alpha_1 \text{(XIX)}]_3$ | Five triple helix domains flanked by six nonhelical domains |
| Short chain collagens | | | |
| VIII | Descemet's membrane, endothelial cells | $\alpha_1 \text{(VIII)}, \alpha_2 \text{(VIII)},$ $\alpha_1 \text{(X)}$ | NF; small helices linked in tandem |
| X | Growth plate chick embryo chondrocytes, Hypertrophic mineralizing cartilage | $[\alpha_1 \text{(X)}]_3$ | NF; short chain; high in hydroxyproline and hydroxylysine, 25% amino acids high in aromatic residues in noncollagenous regions |
| Basement membrane collagens | | | |
| IV | Basement membranes, including glomerular basement membrane | $[\alpha_1 \text{(IV)}]_2 \, \alpha_2 \text{(IV)}$ Four additional chains $\alpha_3 \text{(IV)}$–$\alpha_6 \text{(IV)}$ are important components of specialized basement membranes | NF; high in hydroxylysine and glycosylated hydroxylysine; may contain large globular regions |
| Multiplexins | | | |
| XV | Broadly expressed in many tissues, but particularly in internal organs | $[\alpha_1 \text{(XV)}]_3$ | Contain multiple triple helix domains with many interruptions |
| XVIII | Broadly expressed in many tissues, but particularly in internal organs | $[\alpha_1 \text{(XVIII)}]_3$ | Contain multiple triple helix domains with many interruptions |

**Structurally and Genetically Distinct Collagens—cont'd**

| Type | Tissue Distribution | Molecular Form | Chemical Characterization |
|---|---|---|---|
| MACITs: collagens with transmembrane domains | | | |
| XIII | A new class of cell adhesion molecule; widely expressed in human tissue, including cartilage and bone | $[\alpha_1 (XIII)]_3$ | Cell surface molecule with multiple extracellular triple helix domains and a transmembrane segment |
| XVII | A new class of cell adhesion molecule; a hemidesmosomal component with extracellular domains connecting with basement membrane | $[\alpha_1 (XVII)]_3$ | Cell surface molecule with multiple extracellular triple helix domains and a transmembrane segment |
| Other collagens | | | |
| VI | Intervertebral disc, skin, vessels | $\alpha_1 (VI)\ \alpha_2 (VI)$ | NF; 100-nm beaded microfibrils; disulfide bonds between tetramers; arginine–glycine–aspartic acid sequences |
| | Most interstitial tissues | $\alpha_1 (VI)$ | |
| VII | Dermoepidermal junction anchoring fibrils produced by keratinocytes | $[\alpha_1 (VII)]_3$ | NF; long chain |

FACIT, fibril-associated collagen with interrupted triple helices; NF, nonfibrillar.

cytes. Cartilage nutrition derives almost entirely from synovial fluid. The pumping action of fluid into and out of cartilage during loading and unloading appears to be a key to this process. Joints that are immobilized suffer relatively quickly in a number of important respects. The metabolic activity of cells appears to be affected, as a loss of proteoglycan and an increase in water content are soon observed. The normal white, glistening appearance of the cartilage changes to a dull bluish color, and the cartilage thickness is reduced. How much of this process is due to nutritional deficiency and how much is due to an upset in the stress-dependent metabolic homeostasis is not yet clear.

## METABOLISM OF ARTICULAR CARTILAGE

It should come as no surprise that articular cartilage—a highly specialized, functionally complex tissue—should be active metabolically. The specialized functional structures of cartilage—the collagen fabric and the proteoglycan pump—require constant maintenance and renewal. By most measures of cellular activity, cartilage cells are nearly as active metabolically as are other cell types from relatively avascular tissue sources.

Chondrocytes use anaerobic pathways for the most part, a choice well suited to the relative isolation of the cells, their lack of cell-to-cell contact, and their remoteness from capillary beds. Proteoglycan aggregation and collagen crosslinking both occur outside the cell. In this respect, the chondrocyte is able to avoid the troublesome problem of exporting and properly locating molecules that are much too large to diffuse through cartilage matrix. As it is, proteoglycan and procollagen are among the largest molecules that mammalian cells are called on to synthesize. Each chain of procollagen has more than

1000 amino acids. Therefore, the messenger RNA is necessarily one of the largest in the cellular protein synthetic apparatus.

## ENZYMES OF ARTICULAR CARTILAGE

The continuation of normal function of articular cartilage depends on the special properties of the constituents of cartilage matrix and the maintenance of their normal concentration within the matrix. If the normal rate of degradation is increased or if synthesis of new matrix is interfered with, the concentration of the various articular cartilage components will change, and this is manifested by a particular disease process. The production, release, and actions of the various enzymes affecting articular cartilage are of primary importance in most articular cartilage diseases. Naturally occurring inhibitors exist in the synovial fluid or serum that can modify the actions of the matrix-degrading enzymes. Most of these inhibitors, however, are relatively large molecules that cannot reach the enzymes in the matrix unless the latter diffuse out of the matrix or until degradation of the matrix causes an increase in its normal impermeability to large molecules. The enzymes active on articular cartilage matrix can be divided into endogenous enzymes peculiar to the cartilage itself and exogenous enzymes arising in the synovium, polymorphonuclear leukocytes, macrophages, or blood serum.

### Endogenous Enzymes

Lysosomes are intracytoplasmic vacuoles enclosed by a lipoprotein membrane; they contain a number of enzymes responsible for digestion of the proteoglycan and collagen molecules of articular cartilage matrix. Chondrocytes may

STAGES ENZYMES

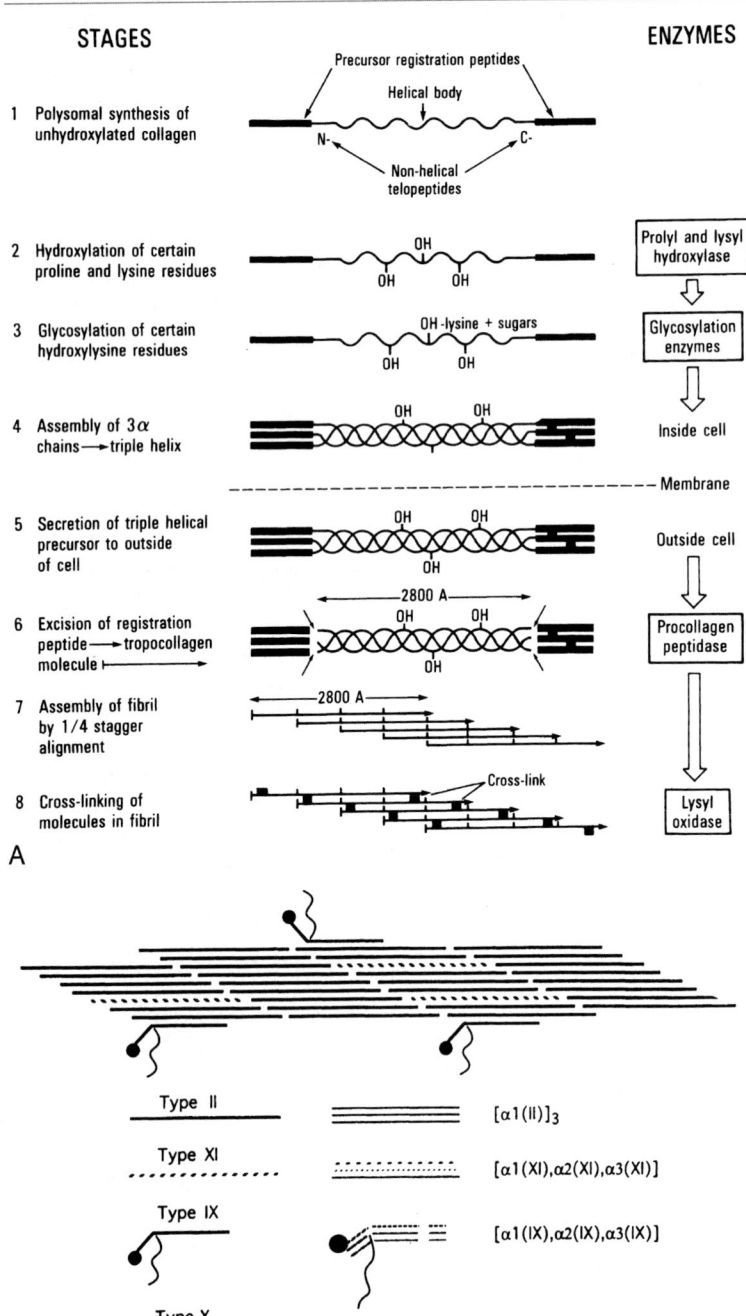

1  Polysomal synthesis of unhydroxylated collagen

Precursor registration peptides
Helical body
N-    C-
Non-helical telopeptides

2  Hydroxylation of certain proline and lysine residues

Prolyl and lysyl hydroxylase

3  Glycosylation of certain hydroxylysine residues

OH -lysine + sugars

Glycosylation enzymes

4  Assembly of 3α chains ⟶ triple helix

Inside cell

——————— Membrane

5  Secretion of triple helical precursor to outside of cell

Outside cell

6  Excision of registration peptide ⟶ tropocollagen molecule

2800 A

Procollagen peptidase

7  Assembly of fibril by 1/4 stagger alignment

2800 A

8  Cross-linking of molecules in fibril

Cross-link

Lysyl oxidase

A

B

Type II        [α1(II)]₃

Type XI        [α1(XI),α2(XI),α3(XI)]

Type IX        [α1(IX),α2(IX),α3(IX)]

Type X         [α1(X)]₃

**Figure 4–6.** Collagen synthesis. *A,* Several enzymatic steps are necessary for the creation of the final collagen molecule and its maturation into a collagen fibril. These enzymatic steps take place partly within the cell and partly outside the cell. Even those steps that occur inside the cell are post-translational; that is, they are not directly under genetic control. However, they are essential for the proper development of the final structure. Defects in many of the steps have been identified in a variety of heritable disorders of connective tissues. The final aggregation of collagen into a structure that becomes crosslinked is essential to produce the requisite tensile stress–resistant properties characteristic of mature connective tissue. *B,* The assembly of tropocollagen II units into fibers and fibrils in cartilage is controlled in part by the minor collagens. Type IX collagen is a surface molecule that binds to type II and to itself. Its side arms interfere with further growth of the fiber by steric interference with the addition of more type II molecules. Type XI collagen is located in the core of the fiber and is also thought to be important in the determination of ultimate fiber size. Type XI is present in largest quantities in small fibers. Type X is found in growth plate cartilage, not in articular cartilage.

(*A,* From Levene CI: Diseases of the collagen molecule. J Clin Pathol Suppl 12:82, 1978.)

be stimulated to release the lysosomal enzymes to the exterior of the cell, where initial degradation of the macromolecules occurs. Subsequently, diffusion of products from the matrix for intracellular digestion in the secondary or digestive lysosomes occurs. In this group of enzymes are the cathepsins, which have maximal activity at acid pH and little or no activity at the neutral pH of the cartilage matrix.

## Exogenous Enzymes

The exogenous enzymes affecting articular cartilage matrix may arise from the synovium of the joint and be secreted into the synovial fluid from lysosomes of lining cells. Enzymes in this category include protease, collagenase, and hyaluronidase. In addition, in pathologic situations, when polymorphonucleocytes and macrophages reach the joint cavity, they may secrete a collagenase, lysozyme, or neutral protease, the last being distinguished from the proteases occurring in the synovial membrane. Collagenases have been implicated in several types of arthritis and have been detected in the synovium in patients with rheumatoid arthritis and nonspecific inflammatory synovial conditions. All synovial tissues have the capacity to produce collagenase; however, it is likely that only in states of chronic proliferative synovitis and inflammation is collagenase produced in sufficient quantities to bring about the destruction of articular tissue. Although type II

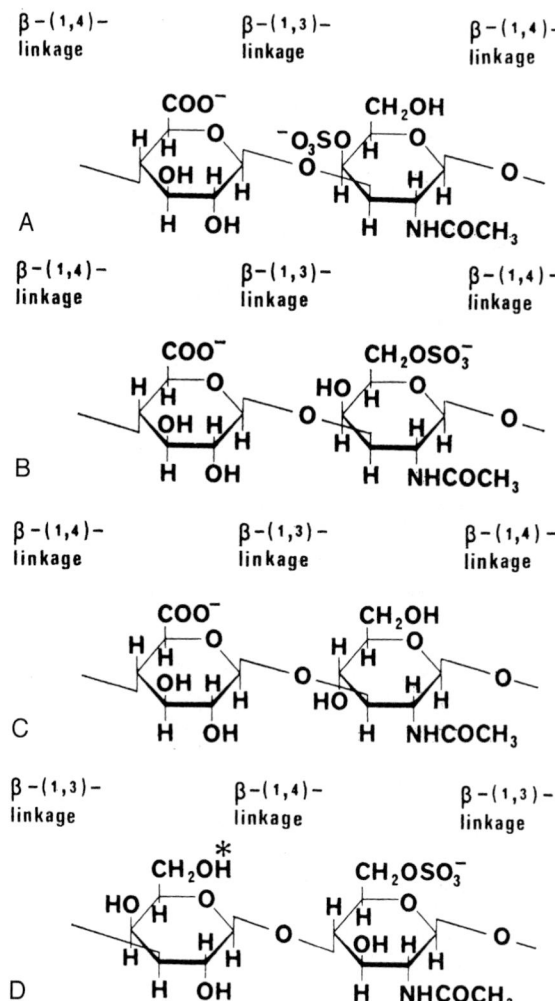

**Figure 4–7.** Disaccharide configuration of the principal glycosaminoglycans of the proteoglycan constituents of articular cartilage. *A,* Molecular configuration of chondroitin 4-sulfate. This differs from chondroitin 6-sulfate *(B)* only in the location of the sulfate group on the hexosamine molecule. Both contain alternating glucuronic acid and galactosamine sugars. *B,* Chondroitin 6-sulfate. *C,* Hyaluronan contains alternating molecules of glucosamine and glucuronic acid but lacks a sulfate group. *D,* Keratan sulfate contains galactose rather than a uronic acid moiety in the disaccharide. The hexosamine is glucosamine, which is sulfated in the C6 position.

collagen is a poorer substrate for collagenase than is interstitial type I collagen, cleavage of the triple helix of collagen can be augmented significantly by raising the temperature above the normal range of 33°C to 36°C. Thus, in an inflamed joint affected by rheumatoid arthritis in which the joint temperature is raised, the rate of cartilage degradation by collagenase would be increased.

## ENZYMES IN ARTICULAR CARTILAGE DISEASE PROCESSES

The avascular nature of adult cartilage has a bearing on its limited capacity to respond to various insults, whether inflammatory, mechanical, or biomechanical. Thus,

although adult joint cartilage has some potential for repair, a given insult usually results in a degenerative lesion mediated by endogenous or exogenous enzymes.

## Osteoarthritis

The cause of articular cartilage destruction in osteoarthritis may be mechanical, but part of the matrix degradation is likely due to enzymatic action. An increase in the activity of enzymes involved in the normal turnover of the matrix may occur, or the degradation may be due to the production and release of special enzymes. The fact that secondary lysosomes are rare in normal articular cartilage but are found readily in the chondrocytes of osteoarthritic cartilage adds weight to this theory. The degradation process is mainly extracellular, but it may be completed within the cell. Several endogenous enzymes have been implicated in osteoarthritis. Although a collagenase capable of splitting the collagen molecule has not been found in normal cartilage, it is present in osteoarthritic human cartilage and is believed to be extralysosomal in origin. It probably is present in minute quantities, and its demonstration indicates prior removal of an inhibitor. Collagenase does occur in the synovial tissue of joints affected by osteoarthritis and has been produced by synovial explants from joints affected by osteoarthritis, but in lesser amounts than in rheumatoid arthritis. In severe osteoarthritis, however, total loss of articular cartilage occurs. Lysozyme also has been implicated in osteoarthritic lesions by the finding of significant elevations of the enzyme in hip and knee joint cartilage affected by osteoarthritis. Various cytokines likewise are important in the development of osteoarthritis.

One additional aspect of the effect of enzymes in the osteoarthritic process is the nature of the matrix synthesis response of chondrocytes to lysosomal enzymes. Although the collagen content of osteoarthritic cartilage does not change, the cartilage synthesizes type I collagen in addition to the usual type II collagen. Thus, the enzymes alter the function of chondrocytes, causing them to synthesize nonspecific collagen molecules, which might lead to weakening of the mechanical structure of the cartilage and its subsequent mechanical destruction.

## Rheumatoid Arthritis

Rheumatoid arthritis is characterized by the destruction of articular cartilage and comprises three interrelated processes: inflammation, synovial proliferation, and tissue destruction. An autoimmune stimulus to the synovial lining cells is involved in this disease and causes inflammation, hyperplasia, and hypertrophy of the cells. The resulting inflammatory rheumatoid tissue, or pannus, growing over and under the articular cartilage is thought to release greatly increased amounts of intracellular lysosomal enzymes, which irreversibly destroy proteoglycan and collagen to produce the erosive focal lesion in the cartilage. Other cellular sources for lysosomal enzyme release are the polymorphonuclear leukocytes and lymphocyte clusters that are present in large numbers in the inflamed synovial cavity and in the synovium, respectively, in rheumatoid arthritis. In addition, the levels of lysozyme in serum and synovial fluid are increased in rheumatoid arthritis and may accompany the loss of cartilage glycosaminoglycans seen in this disease. In contradistinction, in the arthritis of systemic lupus erythematosus, in which usually no cartilage destruction occurs, normal serum lysozyme levels are seen. The fact that continued inflammation hastens cartilage lysis implies that treatment should involve the suppression of inflammation to reduce lysosomal protease accumulation and synovial collagenase production.

## Pyogenic Arthritis

The result of untreated pyogenic arthritis is a severe and rapid destruction of joint cartilage, which invariably evolves into an osteoarthritic process and possibly leads to fibrous or bony ankylosis. The extensive proteoglycan degradation of cartilage is due to the action of several proteinases, which may be derived from neutrophil leukocytes. The leukocytes can release their lysosomal enzymes on encountering bacteria or after the eventual death of the leukocytes. The proteinases incriminated are elastase, cathepsin G, and collagenase, all of which are active at neutral pH. In the body, various inhibitors are secreted into the synovial fluid that can prevent the extracellular activity of the above-mentioned enzymes. It seems logical, however, that in the treatment of septic joints, removal of polymorphonuclear leukocytes by operation or aspiration is essential to minimize cartilage destruction.

## FURTHER READING ———

Arend WP, Dayer JM: Inhibition of the production and effects of interleukin-1 and tumor necrosis factor alpha in rheumatoid arthritis. Arthritis Rheum 38:151, 1995.

Barrett AJ: The possible role of neutrophil proteinases in damage to articular cartilage. Agents Actions 8:11, 1978.

Benninghoff A: Form und Bau der Gelenkknorpel in ihren Beziehungen zur Funktion. Z Anat Entwicklungsgesch 76:43, 1925.

Brandt KD, Doherty M, Lohmander LS: Osteoarthritis. Oxford, Oxford University Press, 1998.

Curtiss PH Jr, Klein L: Destruction of articular cartilage in septic arthritis. J Bone Joint Surg Am 45:797, 1963.

Dingle JT: The role of lysosomal enzymes in skeletal tissues. J Bone Joint Surg Br 55:87, 1973.

Eyre DR, Wu JJ, Woods P: Cartilage-specific collagens: Structural studies. In Kuettner K, et al (eds): Articular Cartilage and Osteoarthritis. New York, Raven Press, 1992, p 119.

Feldmann M, Brennan FM, Maini RN: Role of cytokines in rheumatoid arthritis. Annu Rev Immunol 14:397, 1996.

Glimcher MJ, Krane SM: The organization and structure of bone, and the mechanism of calcification. In Gould BS (ed): Treatise on Collagen. Vol 2, Biology of Collagen. New York, Academic Press, 1968, p 67.

Keller K, Shortkroff S, Sledge CB, et al: Effects of rheumatoid synovial cells on cartilage degradation in vitro. J Orthop Res 8:345, 1990.

Lazarus GS, Daniels JR, Brown RS, et al: Degradation of collagen by a human granulocyte collagenolytic system. J Clin Invest 47:2622, 1968.

Lotke PA: Diffusion in cartilage. In Simon WH (ed): The Human Joint in Health and Disease. Philadelphia, University of Pennsylvania Press, 1978.

Sajdera SW, Hascall VC: Protein-polysaccharide complex from bovine nasal cartilage: A comparison of low and high shear extraction procedures. J Biol Chem 244:77, 1969.

Seyer J, Kang A: Connective tissues of the subendothelium. In Creager M, Dzag V (eds): Vascular Medicine. Boston, Little, Brown, 1996, p 39.

Sternlicht MD, Werb Z: ECM proteinases. In Kreis T, Vale R (eds): Extracellular Matrix, Anchor and Adhesion Proteins, 2nd ed. Oxford, Oxford University Press, 1999, p 505.

Vuorio E, deCrombruggle B: The family of collagen genes. Annu Rev Biochem 59:837, 1990.

Weiss C, Rosenberg L, Helfet AJ: An ultrastructural study of normal young adult human articular cartilage. J Bone Joint Surg Am 50:663, 1968.

Weissmann G: Lysosomal mechanisms of tissue injury in arthritis. Semin Med Beth Israel Hosp 286:141, 1972.

Weissmann G, Spilberg I: Breakdown of cartilage protein polysaccharide by lysosomes. Arthritis Rheum 11:162, 1968.

Ziff M, Gribetz HJ, Lospalluto J: Effect of leukocyte and synovial membrane extracts on cartilage mucoprotein. J Clin Invest 39:405, 1960.

# CHAPTER 5

## Arthrography, Tenography, and Bursography

**TABLE 5–1**

**Indications for Wrist Arthrography**

Evaluation of:
Presence and extent of synovial inflammation
Injuries to the triangular fibrocartilage, interosseous
ligaments, and joint capsule
Soft tissue masses

## SUMMARY OF KEY FEATURES

Although contrast opacification of joint cavities (arthrography), tendon sheaths (tenography), and bursae (bursography) has been used less frequently in recent years, owing to increased reliance on magnetic resonance (MR) imaging, such opacification still has important clinical applications.

Arthrographic procedures generally are simple to perform, and the information they provide may be essential for proper diagnosis and treatment. The technique is used alone or in combination with other technologic methods, such as fluoroscopy, conventional and computed tomography (arthrotomography), and digital radiography. Normal and abnormal arthrographic findings at specific locations in the body are described. Arthrographic abnormalities in patients with joint prostheses are described in Chapter 14.

## INTRODUCTION

Arthrography is applicable in the evaluation of many different joints and can be coupled with fluoroscopy, conventional and computed tomography, digital radiography, and MR imaging. Various radiopaque and radiolucent (air or carbon dioxide) contrast media exist that can be used separately as a single-contrast technique or combined as a double-contrast technique. The administration of epinephrine also increases the quality of arthrograms by reducing simultaneously the egress of contrast material from the joint and the influx of body fluid through the synovial membrane into the joint. Application of stress is a useful technique in the arthrographic evaluation of ligamentous injuries of the ankle, wrist, and first metacarpophalangeal joint.

As performed currently, arthrography is a safe and well-tolerated procedure. Hypersensitivity reaction to iodinated contrast agent is rarely observed.

## WRIST

Several indications exist for wrist arthrography (Table 5–1).

## Technique

Under fluoroscopic control, a needle is introduced into the wrist from a dorsal approach. Most often, the radio-carpal compartment is the site of injection, although other compartments of the wrist may be studied (see later discussion). The needle is guided under the radial lip, entering the radiocarpal compartment between the scaphoid and the radius. Approximately 2 mL of contrast agent is administered. Fluoroscopic monitoring combined with sequential spot filming, videotaping, or digital technique during the injection of contrast material allows more precise delineation of sites of abnormal compartment communication. Selective injection of the midcarpal compartment, rather than the radiocarpal compartment, has been advocated as a superior method for analysis of the scapholunate and lunotriquetral ligaments. Indeed, some authorities recommend sequential injections into the radiocarpal, midcarpal, and inferior radioulnar joints as ideal.

### Normal Wrist Arthrogram

Contrast opacification of the radiocarpal compartment reveals a concave sac with smooth synovial surfaces extending between the distal end of the radius and proximal carpal row (Fig. 5–1). The prestyloid recess appears as a finger-like projection that approaches the ulnar styloid process. Volar radial recesses are located beneath the distal end of the radius. If the midcarpal joint is injected, contrast material normally extends proximally between the scaphoid and lunate and between the lunate and triquetrum to the level of the scapholunate and lunotriquetral interosseous ligaments. It extends distally into the common carpometacarpal and intermetacarpal compartments. If the distal radioulnar joint is injected, contrast material sits like a cap on the articular surface of the ulna. Communication between the radiocarpal compartment and other compartments in the wrist during arthrography may be observed in normal persons. The prevalence of such communication increases in older persons, and it may be seen in as many as 50% of asymptomatic persons.

### Rheumatoid Arthritis

Injection of contrast material into the radiocarpal compartment in patients with rheumatoid arthritis reveals

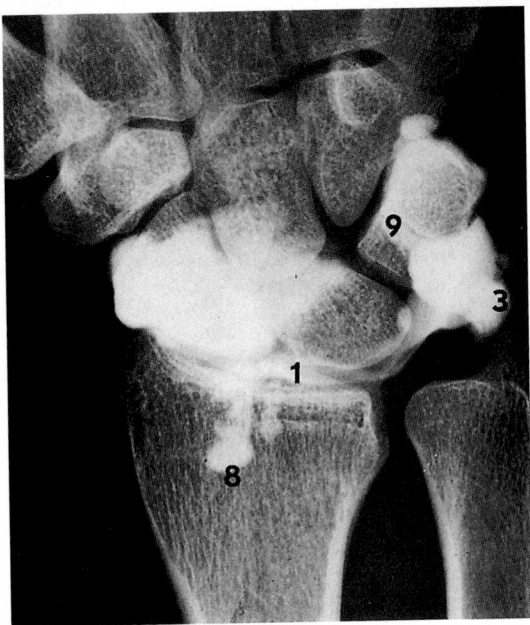

**Figure 5–1.** Wrist arthrography: normal and abnormal arthrograms. Radiocarpal joint injection, frontal view. Observe the contrast-filled radiocarpal compartment (1), which is communicating with the pisiform-triquetral compartment (9). Also note the prestyloid recess (3) and volar radial recesses (8).

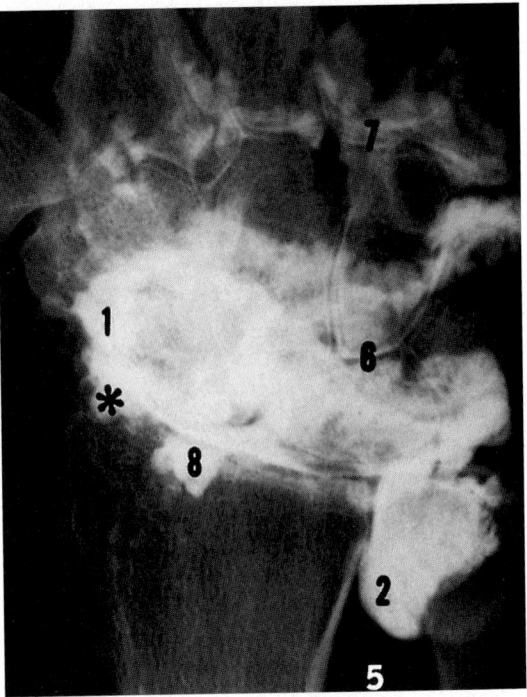

**Figure 5–2.** Wrist arthrography: rheumatoid arthritis. Posteroanterior view after radiocarpal joint arthrography demonstrates severe synovial irregularity or corrugation (*asterisk*); radiocarpal compartment (1) communication with the inferior radioulnar (2), midcarpal (6), and common carpometacarpal (7) compartments; lymphatic filling (5); and prominent volar radial recesses (8).

(From Resnick D: Arthrography in the evaluation of arthritic disorders of the wrist. Radiology 113:331, 1974.)

corrugated irregularity of the contrast material and opacification of lymphatic vessels (Fig. 5–2). These findings are not specific for rheumatoid arthritis but are reliable indicators of synovial inflammation. Communication between the radiocarpal compartment and other compartments of the wrist in rheumatoid arthritis is frequent.

## Trauma

The assessment of injury to the triangular fibrocartilage complex and interosseous carpal ligaments represents the major indication for wrist arthrography today. Arthrographic abnormalities occurring after wrist trauma include compartmental communication, tendon sheath visualization, and mild synovial irregularity. The pattern of compartmental communication depends on the site of trauma. With injuries to the triangular fibrocartilage or ulnar styloid, communication between the radiocarpal and inferior radioulnar compartments is observed (Fig. 5–3). With scaphoid fractures or injuries to the interosseous ligaments between the bones of the proximal carpal row, communication between the radiocarpal and midcarpal compartments is seen (Fig. 5–4). In young persons, compartmental communication may provide presumptive evidence of the site of soft tissue injury when initial radiographs are normal. In older patients, the frequency of such communication in asymptomatic persons limits the value of wrist arthrography.

## Evaluation of Soft Tissue Masses

Although wrist arthrography can provide useful information for the surgeon evaluating a patient with an adjacent soft tissue mass, this assessment is accomplished far better by MR imaging (see Chapters 59 and 71). Such a mass may represent a synovial cyst, a ganglion cyst, or an enlarged tendon sheath.

## ELBOW

Arthrography of the elbow (Table 5–2) is not a commonly performed procedure.

## Technique

Using a lateral approach, the joint is entered between the radial head and capitulum of the humerus. Six to 10 mL of contrast material alone, 0.5 to 1 mL of contrast material plus 6 to 10 mL of air, or 8 to 12 mL of air alone is injected. The injection of contrast material alone is useful for outlining the presence and extent of synovial disorders, capsular integrity, and synovial cysts, whereas the double-contrast study or the single-contrast study with air alone may be superior in demonstrating cartilaginous and osseous defects and free intra-articular bodies.

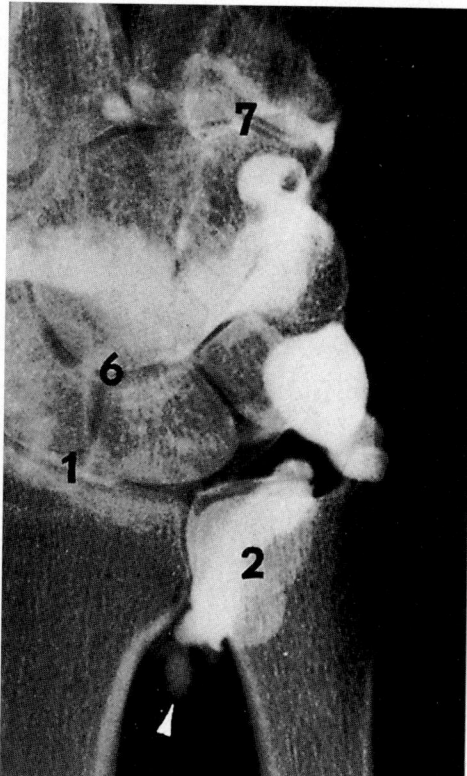

**Figure 5–3.** Wrist arthrography: injury of the triangular fibrocartilage. This young man had pain over the distal end of the ulna after an injury. A radiocarpal joint arthrogram reveals communication between the radiocarpal compartment (1) and inferior radioulnar compartment (2). The midcarpal (6) and common carpometacarpal (7) compartments are also opacified. Small contrast-filled diverticula near the proximal aspect of the inferior radioulnar joint (*arrowhead*) may indicate a capsular tear.

## Normal Elbow Arthrogram

On frontal radiographs, a thin layer of contrast material or air is observed between the humerus, radius, and ulna. A periradial recess is apparent about the proximal portion of the radius, which is indented where the annular ligament surrounds the bone. Proximal extension of contrast material along the anterior surface of the humerus may resemble the ears of a rabbit, the "Bugs Bunny" sign (Fig. 5–5). On a lateral radiograph, the periradial or annular recess again is apparent. In addition, coronoid (anterior) and olecranon (posterior) recesses are seen (see Fig. 5–5). Articular cartilage is of uniform thickness except for a portion of the trochlear notch of the ulna, which lacks cartilage.

### Rheumatoid Arthritis

Synovial inflammation with hypertrophy and villous transformation accounts for an irregular outline of contrast material that may be seen in rheumatoid arthritis (Fig. 5–6). Lymphatic visualization is common, and capsular distention, sacculation, and cystic swelling may be observed.

Nodular filling defects within the contrast-filled elbow joint may represent hypertrophied synovium, as in rheumatoid arthritis, or synovial masses associated with pigmented villonodular synovitis and idiopathic synovial (osteo)chondromatosis (Fig. 5–7).

### Trauma

Opacification of the traumatized elbow joint, particularly after the introduction of air or air and contrast material, may reveal cartilaginous and osseous defects associated with osteochondritis dissecans. Contrast medium may dissect beneath the adjacent osseous fragment or reveal loose or embedded bodies elsewhere in the joint cavity. Computed arthrotomography also may be used (Fig. 5–8).

## SHOULDER

Arthrography of the glenohumeral joint (Table 5–3) is an aid to the diagnosis of rotator cuff tear, adhesive capsulitis, previous dislocation, articular disease, and bicipital tendon abnormalities.

### Technique

Both single-contrast and double-contrast examinations have been advocated for glenohumeral joint arthrography. Conventional and computed arthrotomography may be necessary in certain situations.

**Single-Contrast Examination.** Ten to 15 mL of iodinated contrast material is injected into the glenohumeral joint from an anterior approach. Anteroposterior radiographs are obtained in internal and external rotation, and axillary and tangential bicipital groove radiographs are also obtained. This series of radiographs is repeated after moderate exercise of the shoulder.

| TABLE 5–2 |
| --- |
| **Indications for Elbow Arthrography** |
| Evaluation of:<br>  Presence and extent of synovial inflammation<br>  Intra-articular cartilaginous and osseous bodies<br>  Soft tissue masses<br>  Trauma in children |

| TABLE 5–3 |
| --- |
| **Indications for Glenohumeral Joint Arthrography** |
| Evaluation of:<br>  Rotator cuff tears<br>  Adhesive capsulitis<br>  Bicipital tendon abnormalities<br>  Previous dislocations<br>  Presence and extent of synovial inflammation |

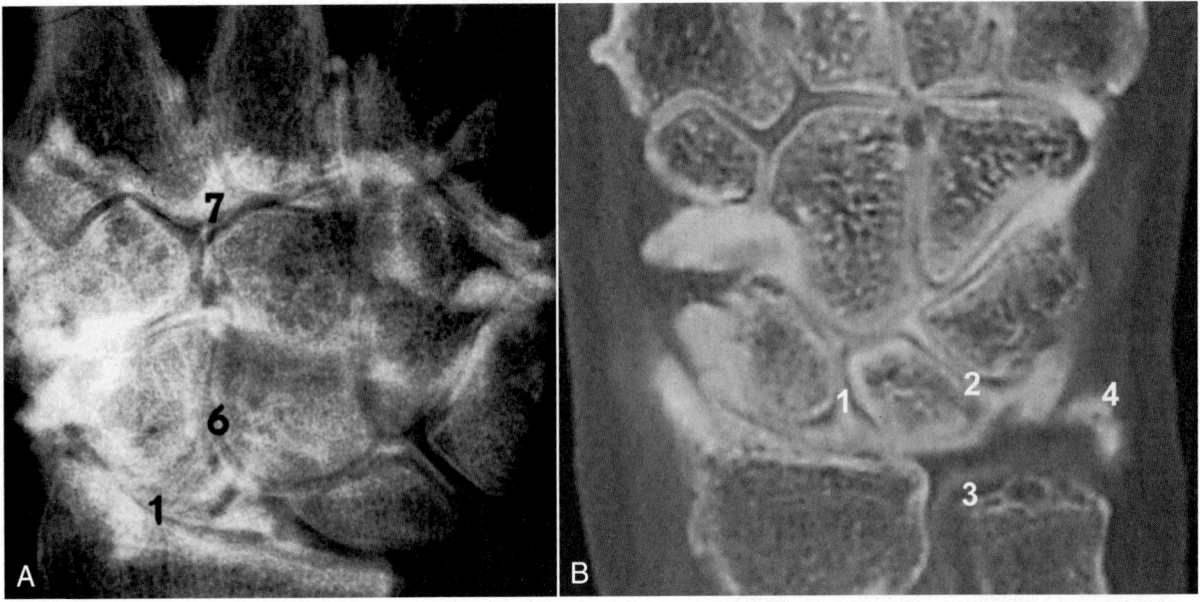

**Figure 5–4.** Wrist arthrography: injuries of the scaphoid and interosseous ligaments of the proximal carpal row. *A*, Scapholunate dissociation with disruption of the scapholunate ligament. After radiocarpal joint arthrography, contrast material has flowed from the radiocarpal compartment (1) into the midcarpal (6) and common carpometacarpal (7) compartments. Contrast material overlies the scapholunate space. *B*, Scapholunate dissociation with disruption of the scapholunate ligament, lunotriquetral ligament, triangular fibrocartilage, and ulnar capsule in a different patient. Computed tomography following radiocarpal joint arthrography shows that contrast material has flowed through the scapholunate ligament (1), lunotriquetral ligament (2), and triangular fibrocartilage (3). Contrast also extends through the ulnar capsule (4).

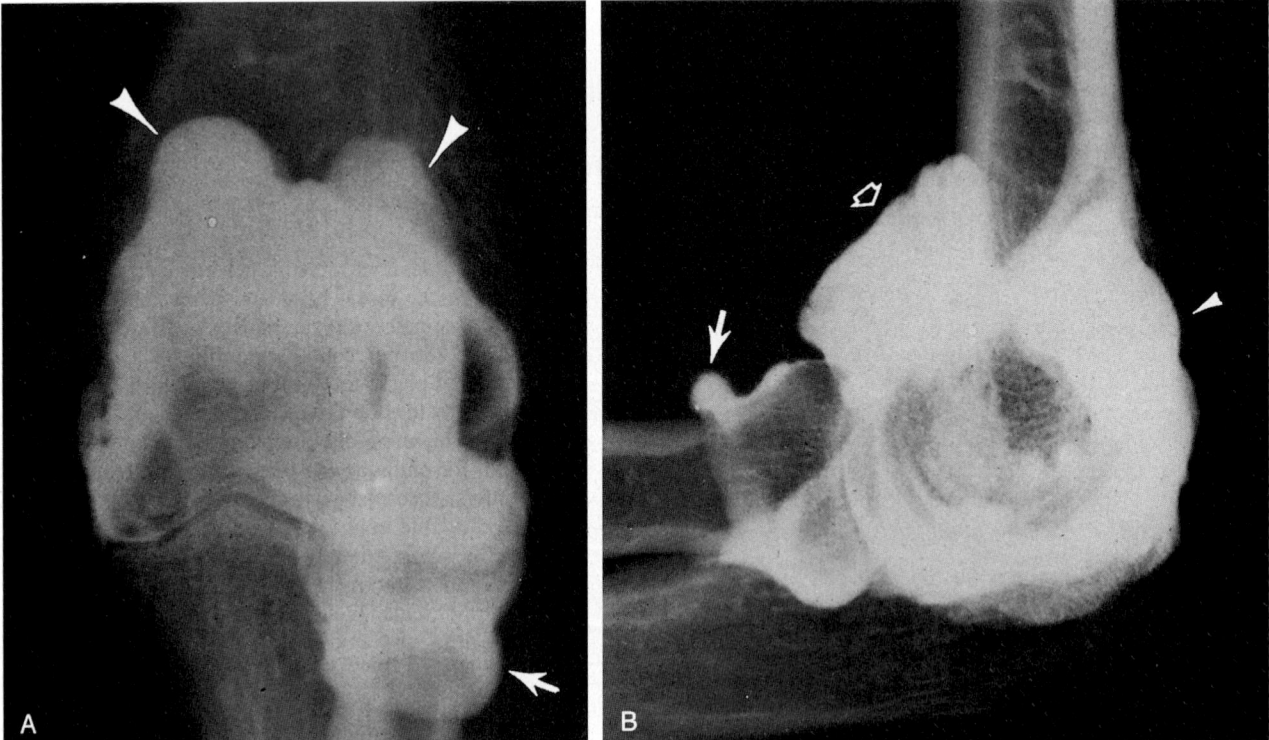

**Figure 5–5.** Elbow arthrography: normal arthrogram. *A*, Anteroposterior radiograph. Observe the thin layer of contrast material between the humerus and ulna; the proximal extension of material in front of the humerus, resembling the ears of a rabbit *(arrowheads)*; and the periradial, or annular, recess *(arrow)*. *B*, Lateral radiograph. Note the periradial, or annular, recess *(arrow)*; the coronoid, or anterior, recess *(open arrow)*; and the olecranon, or posterior, recess *(arrowhead)*.

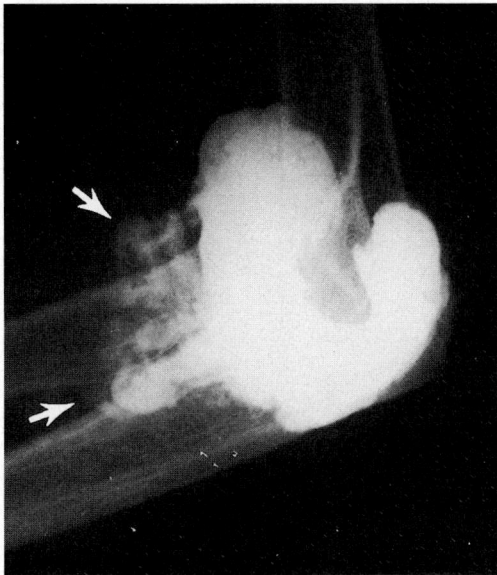

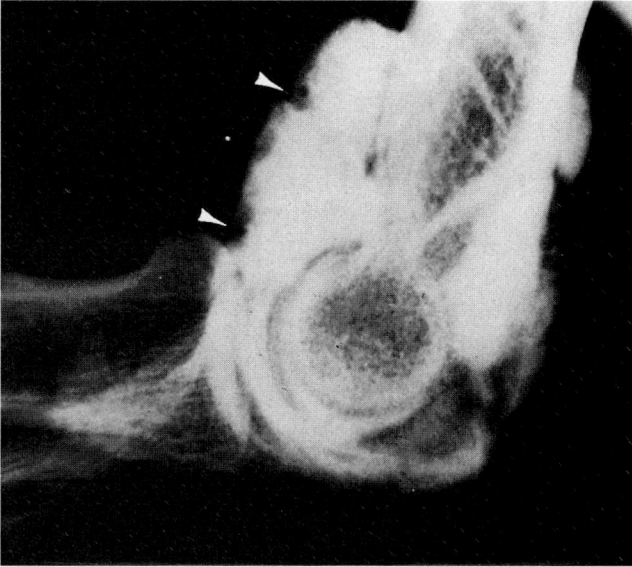

**Figure 5–6.** Elbow arthrography: rheumatoid arthritis. Arthrogram from a 50-year-old man with rheumatoid arthritis and a periarticular mass caused by a synovial cyst. The arthrogram outlines distal cystic dilatation of the articular cavity with irregular synovium *(arrows)*.
(From Ehrlich GE: Antecubital cysts in rheumatoid arthritis—a corollary to popliteal [Baker's] cysts. J Bone Joint Surg Am 54:165, 1972.)

**Figure 5–7.** Elbow arthrography: idiopathic synovial (osteo)-chondromatosis. A lateral view after arthrography delineates irregular nodular filling defects *(arrowheads)* that represent cartilaginous foci resulting from synovial metaplasia.

**Double-Contrast Examination.** Double-contrast shoulder arthrography employs 1 to 4 mL of iodinated contrast agent and 10 to 15 mL of air. The patient then sits upright with a 2.3-kg (5-lb) sandbag in his or her hand. Radiographs in internal and external rotation are obtained with or without a spot film device. The patient returns to the supine position, and internal rotation, external rotation, axillary, and bicipital groove films are made. These radiographs can be repeated after mild exercise of the shoulder. With this technique, the width of the rotator cuff tear and the integrity of cuff tendons can be assessed. In addition, the internal structures of the joint, including the glenoid labrum, are better identified.

### Normal Glenohumeral Joint Arthrogram

Contrast material is identified between the humeral head and the glenoid (Figs. 5–9 and 5–10). On radiographs taken in external rotation, the contrast substance ends abruptly laterally at the anatomic neck of the humerus. In this view, an axillary pouch may be opacified on the undersurface of the humeral head. In internal rotation, a prominent subscapular recess is observed overlying the glenoid and lateral scapular region. The tendon of the long head of the biceps is visible as a radiolucent filling defect within the articular cavity and can be traced for a variable distance within the contrast-filled tendon sheath into the bicipital groove and along the metaphysis of the humerus. In the axillary view, contrast material is identified between the glenoid cavity and humeral head, anterior to the scapula (subscapular recess), and within the bicipital tendon sheath. In this projection, contrast mate-

rial should not overlie the surgical neck of the humerus. The tangential view of the bicipital groove demonstrates an oval filling defect within the contrast-filled sheath, representing the biceps tendon.

### Complete and Incomplete Tears of the Rotator Cuff

Tears in the rotator cuff musculature may involve the entire thickness of the cuff (complete tear) or a portion of the cuff (incomplete or partial tear).

**Complete Tear.** Abnormal communication exists between the glenohumeral joint cavity and the subacromial (subdeltoid) bursa (Fig. 5–11). Contrast material can be identified within the bursa as a large collection superior and lateral to the greater tuberosity and adjacent to the undersurface of the acromion. Using double-contrast shoulder arthrography, the degree of degeneration of the torn rotator cuff can be recognized. Further, the width of the tear itself is identified.

**Incomplete Tear.** A partial tear may involve the deep surface of the rotator cuff, the superficial surface, or the interior substance of the tendon (Fig. 5–12). Tears within the substance of the cuff or involving the superior surface of the cuff are not demonstrated on glenohumeral joint arthrography. Tears on the inferior surface of the rotator cuff can be diagnosed on arthrography as an irregular circular or linear collection of contrast material above the opacified joint cavity.

### Adhesive Capsulitis

Glenohumeral joint arthrography has been used in the diagnosis and treatment of adhesive capsulitis. The main

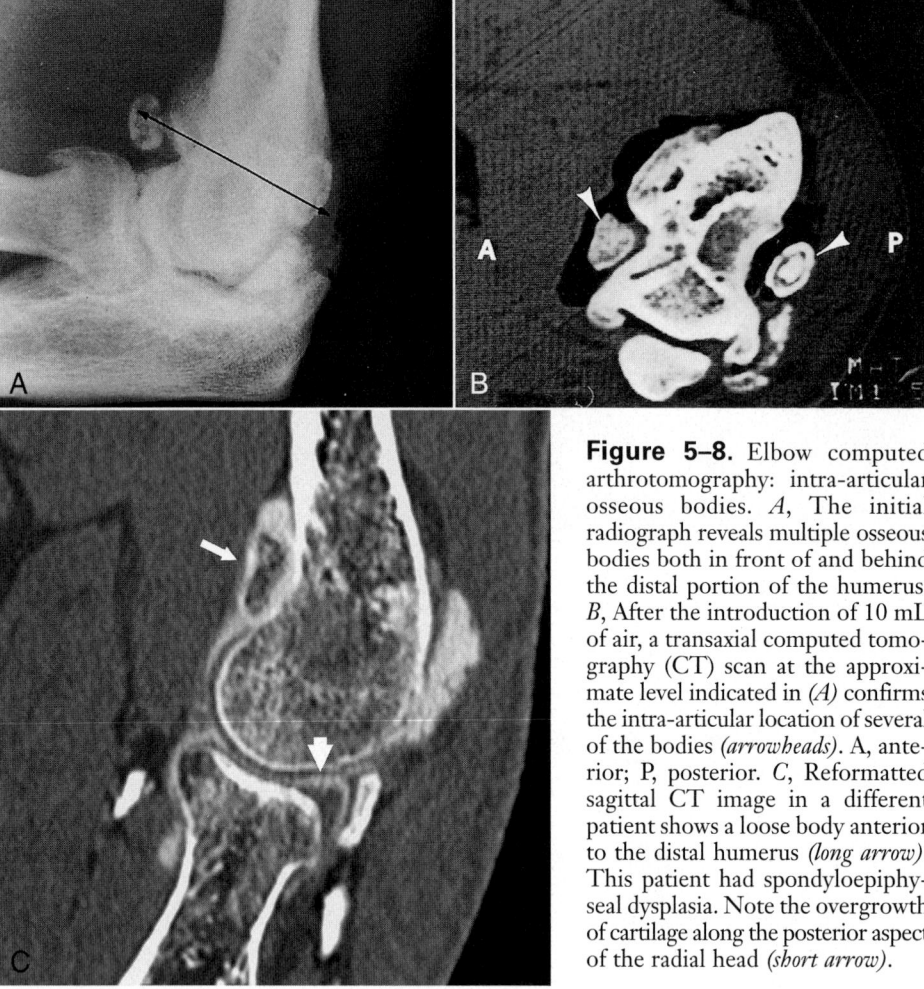

**Figure 5–8.** Elbow computed arthrotomography: intra-articular osseous bodies. *A,* The initial radiograph reveals multiple osseous bodies both in front of and behind the distal portion of the humerus. *B,* After the introduction of 10 mL of air, a transaxial computed tomography (CT) scan at the approximate level indicated in *(A)* confirms the intra-articular location of several of the bodies *(arrowheads).* A, anterior; P, posterior. *C,* Reformatted sagittal CT image in a different patient shows a loose body anterior to the distal humerus *(long arrow).* This patient had spondyloepiphyseal dysplasia. Note the overgrowth of cartilage along the posterior aspect of the radial head *(short arrow).*

arthrographic abnormality in this disorder is a joint of low capacity evidenced by increased resistance to injection and a "tight" feel. Only a small amount of fluid (5 to 8 mL) can be injected successfully. The subscapular and axillary recesses are small or absent, and lymphatic filling may be evident (Fig. 5–13).

Joint distention during arthrography, the "brisement" procedure, may aid in the treatment of this condition. This technique requires slow, intermittent injection of larger and larger volumes of contrast material (mixed with saline solution, corticosteroids, and lidocaine).

## Abnormalities of the Bicipital Tendon

Considering the wide variation in the arthrographic appearance of the bicipital tendon and sheath in normal persons, the radiologist must not rely too heavily on the arthrogram in establishing the existence of a significant abnormality. The arthrographic diagnosis of complete rupture of the bicipital tendon is based on failure to identify the tendon in the opacified sheath. Incomplete tears of the bicipital tendon produce increased width of the tendon and distortion of the synovial sheath. Medial

dislocation of the tendon and sheath from their normal positions in the intertubercular groove can be suspected when the positions of these structures do not change on the internal and external rotation radiographs.

## Abnormalities Occurring after Previous Dislocations

Anterior dislocations of the glenohumeral joint are associated with soft tissue damage. As the dislocating humeral head moves anteriorly, it lifts the articular capsule from the glenoid and neck of the scapula, producing an abnormal recess between the subscapular and axillary recesses. On arthrography, the abnormal recess fills with contrast material, a finding that is more evident on radiographs taken in internal rotation (Fig. 5–14). Additional findings related to anterior dislocation are injuries of cartilage and bone. The Bankart deformity involves an avulsion or compression defect of the anteroinferior rim of the glenoid and may be purely cartilaginous. The arthrogram may outline the cartilaginous abnormalities about the glenoid labrum. A Hill-Sachs compression deformity on the posterolateral aspect of the humeral head also may be detected.

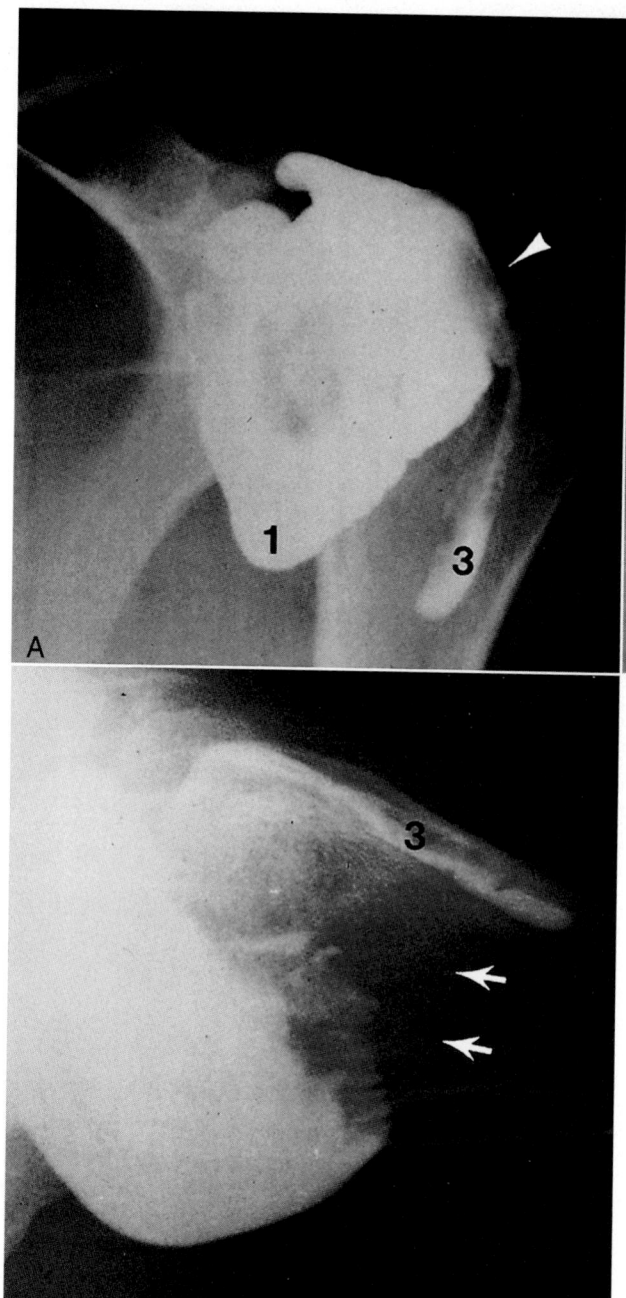

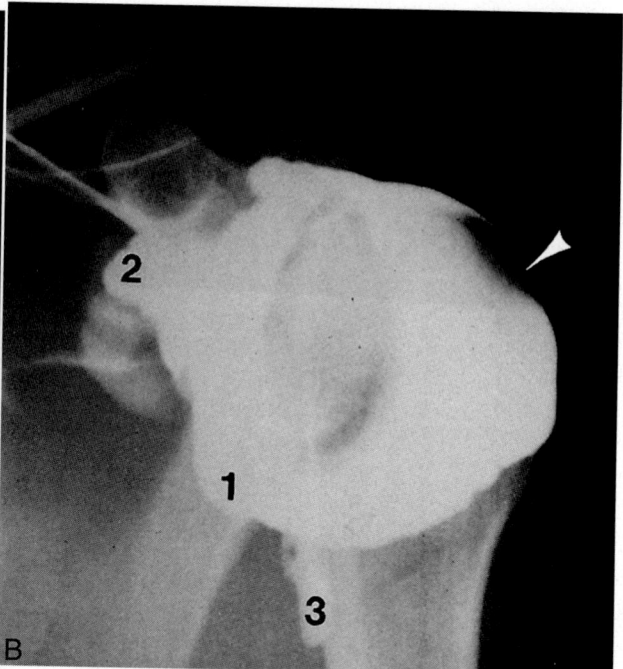

**Figure 5–9.** Glenohumeral joint arthrography: anatomy and normal single-contrast arthrogram. *A,* External rotation. Visualized structures include the axillary pouch (1) and bicipital tendon sheath (3). Note that the subscapular recess is not well seen, and contrast material ends abruptly laterally at the anatomic neck of the humerus *(arrowhead). B,* Internal rotation. Observe the prominent subscapular recess (2), axillary pouch (1), and bicipital tendon sheath (3). The articular cartilage of the humeral head is well seen *(arrowhead).* Minimal extravasation of contrast material has occurred in the axilla near the injection site. *C,* Axillary view. Observe the bicipital tendon (3) and the absence of contrast material over the surgical neck of the humerus *(arrows).*

Conventional and computed arthrotomography has been applied to the diagnosis of abnormalities in the unstable shoulder. Computed arthrotomography is accomplished after the injection of 10 to 15 mL of air with or without 1 mL of radiopaque contrast material. Abnormalities of the glenoid labrum depicted on conventional or computed arthrotomography include fore-shortening or thinning or contrast imbibition along its free margin. the labrum also may be detached completely, along with one or more of the glenohumeral ligaments. An osseous Bankart lesion typically is visualized as an elevation of a small sliver of bone and irregularity of the adjacent glenoid rim. A depression along the posterolateral aspect of the humeral head is indicative of a Hill-Sachs lesion (Fig. 5–15).

## Rheumatoid Arthritis and Other Synovial Disorders

The arthrographic findings of rheumatoid arthritis include a corrugated, enlarged synovial cavity, nodular filling defects, cartilage loss, contrast filling of osseous erosions, lymphatic filling, enlarging axillary lymph nodes, capsulitis with a restricted joint cavity, and rotator cuff tear. In rheumatoid arthritis (and other synovial disorders), synovial cysts about the glenohumeral joint may be documented by arthrography.

Septic arthritis of the glenohumeral joint may lead to synovial irregularity and rupture of the capsule and rotator cuff, with the formation of soft tissue abscesses.

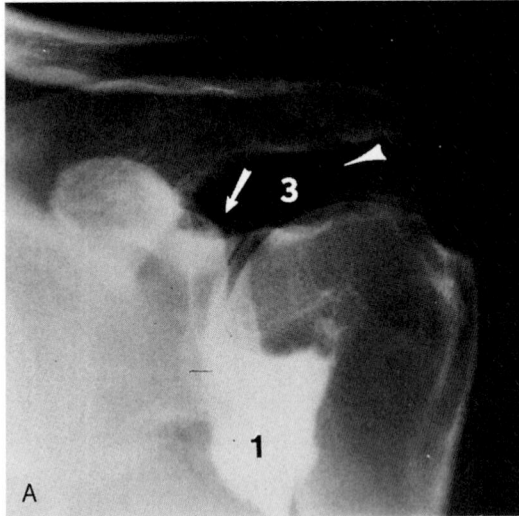

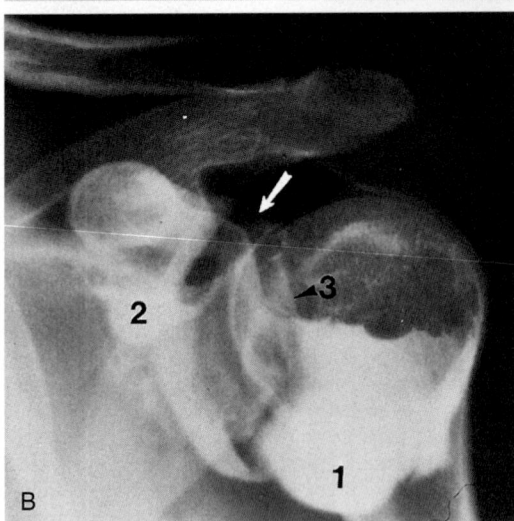

**Figure 5–10.** Glenohumeral joint arthrography: normal double-contrast arthrogram (upright projections). *A,* Normal arthrogram: external rotation. Visualized structures include the axillary pouch (1), bicipital tendon (3), glenoid fibrocartilage *(arrow),* and articular cartilage of the humeral head. The distended articular cavity *(arrowhead)* above the bicipital tendon should not be misinterpreted as filling of the subacromial (subdeltoid) bursa. *B,* Normal arthrogram: internal rotation. Visualized structures include the subscapular recess (2), axillary pouch (1), bicipital tendon (3), glenoid fibrocartilage *(arrow),* and articular cartilage of the humeral head.

## HIP

Hip arthrography may be employed in patients with congenital, traumatic, and articular disorders (Table 5–4).

## Technique

Many techniques exist for puncturing the hip joint. The author uses an anterior approach in performing hip arthrography, with the patient placed supine on the table. In infants and children, an anterolateral subphyseal plate

**TABLE 5–4**

**Indications for Hip Arthrography**

Evaluation of:
Developmental dysplasia of the hip
Septic arthritis and osteomyelitis with epiphyseal separation
Epiphyseal dysplasia and osteonecrosis
Certain synovial disorders
Soft tissue masses
Trauma

site is ideal for contacting the bone. Additional modifications include the supplementation of hip arthrography with conventional tomography or computed tomography (CT) scanning.

## Normal Hip Arthrogram

The normal hip arthrogram in an adult is shown in Figure 5–16.

## Developmental Dysplasia of the Hip

In infants, hip arthrography may be useful in the evaluation of developmental dysplasia of the hip (see Chapter 73).

## Septic Arthritis in Infants

Hip arthrography is useful in the clinical setting of neonatal sepsis and an apparent dislocation of the femoral head.

## Legg-Calvé-Perthes Disease

Hip arthrography may be of benefit in evaluating patients with Legg-Calvé-Perthes disease. This method allows identification of the true position of the cartilaginous head; this information may allow the surgeon to determine which position of the hip will be best during treatment of the condition (Fig. 5–17). MR imaging also can be used in the assessment of hip involvement in Legg-Calvé-Perthes disease.

## Trauma

In patients with dislocations of the femoral head, hip athrography alone or in combination with CT may outline distortion of or defects in the joint capsule, tears of the ligamentum teres, and intra-articular osteocartilaginous bodies. Capsular constriction (adhesive capsulitis) may be seen following injury, although it may be idiopathic. Accurate diagnosis is accomplished with arthrography, during which a low capacity of the joint cavity is demonstrated.

Tears and deformities of the acetabular labrum have been recorded after trauma. Ganglion cyst formation in the labrum also has been identified. Routine radiography may reveal gas-containing soft tissue masses, and during arthrography, contrast material may extend from the joint into the labral tear and ganglion.

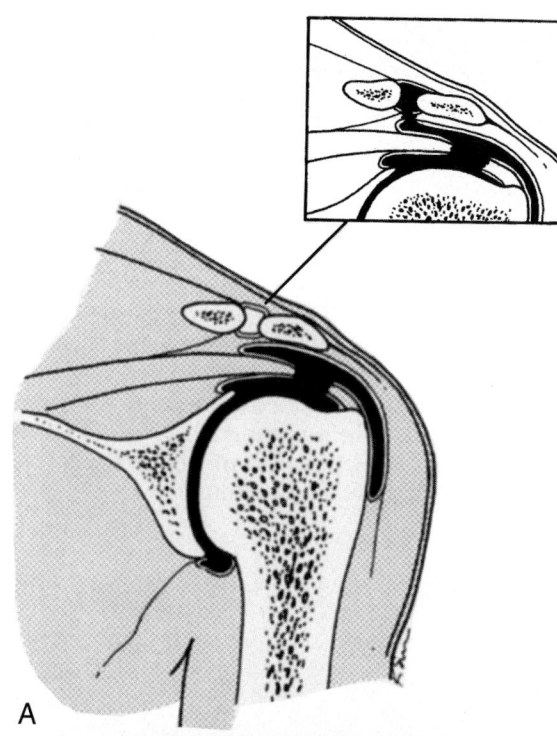

**A**

**Figure 5–11.** Glenohumeral joint arthrography: complete rotator cuff tear. *A,* Arthrographic findings of a complete tear of the rotator cuff. Contrast material extends from the glenohumeral joint through the rotator cuff into the subacromial (subdeltoid) bursa. The inset reveals contrast material extending from the glenohumeral joint through the rotator cuff into the subacromial bursa and from there into the acromioclavicular joint. *B* and *C,* Double-contrast arthrography. The external rotation view *(B)* demonstrates that contrast material has extended from the glenohumeral joint into the subacromial (subdeltoid) bursa *(thin arrows).* The width of the tear of the rotator cuff can be seen *(between heavy arrows).* In another patient with a rotator cuff tear, an axillary view *(C)* reveals a "saddlebag" configuration, with contrast material overlying the surgical neck of the humerus *(arrowheads).*

*(B,* Courtesy of J. Mink, MD, Los Angeles, California.)

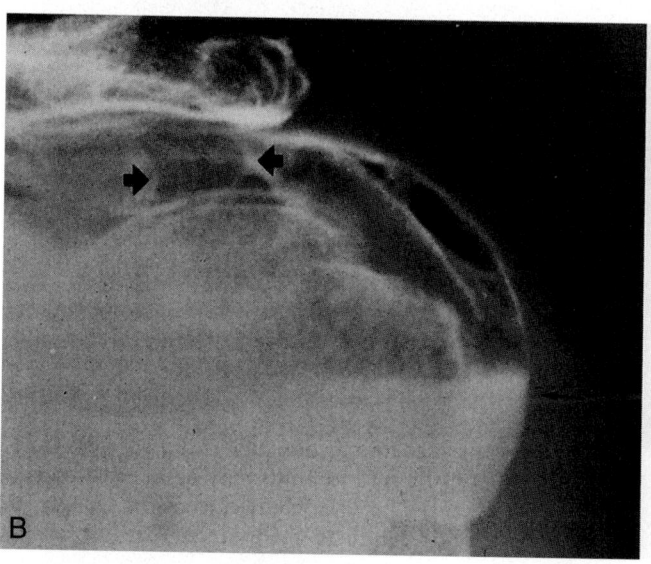

**B**

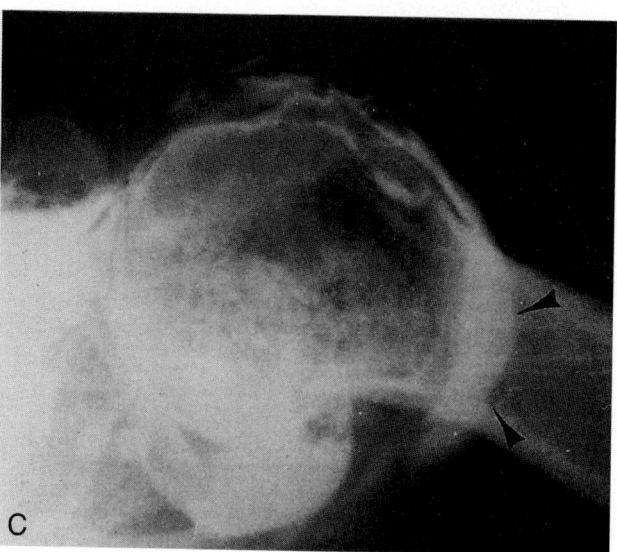

**C**

## Articular Disorders

In idiopathic synovial (osteo)chondromatosis or pigmented villonodular synovitis, the extent of synovial and capsular abnormality can be determined with arthrography (Fig. 5–18). In patients with septic arthritis, hip arthrography provides a technique for aspiration and subsequent culture, as well as a means of evaluating cartilaginous, osseous, and snyovial abnormalities.

## Synovial Cysts

Hip arthrography in rheumatoid arthritis and other synovial disorders reveals the degree of intra-articular alterations and the presence or absence of communicating synovial cysts (Fig. 5–19). Opacification of an enlarged iliopsoas bursa also may be identified. The enlarged iliopsoas bursa may accompany intra-articular diseases such as osteoarthritis, rheumatoid arthritis, pigmented villonodular synovitis, infection, calcium pyrophosphate dihydrate crystal deposition disease, and idiopathic synovial (osteo)chondromatosis, producing a mass in the ilioinguinal region that may stimulate a hernia and cause obstruction of the femoral vein.

## Knee

Although knee arthrography is useful in the assessment of many intra-articular structures (Table 5–5), the current gold standard for the noninvasive assessment of internal derangements of the knee is MR imaging (see Chapter 59).

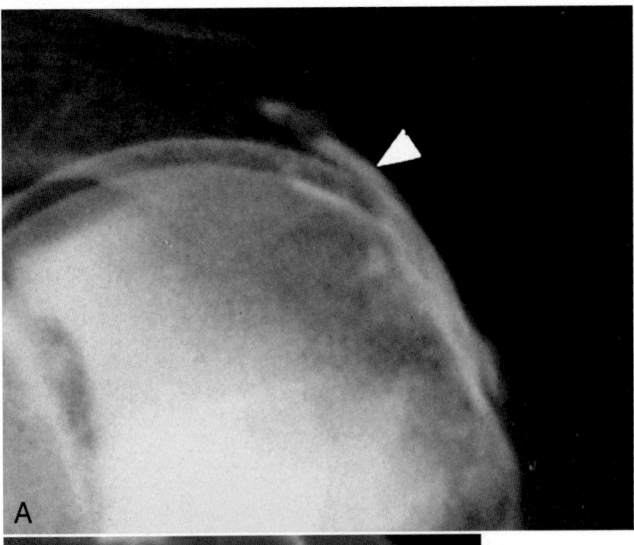

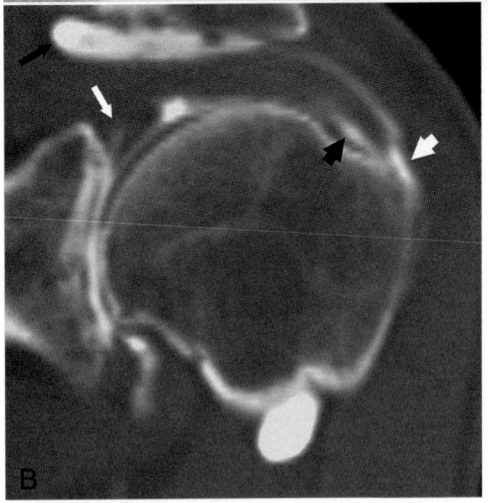

**Figure 5–12.** Glenohumeral joint arthrography. *A,* Incomplete rotator cuff tear. Internal rotation view shows contrast material *(arrowhead)* extending into the undersurface of the rotator cuff in this single-contrast arthrogram. *B,* Reformatted oblique coronal computed tomography image in a different patient shows a thickened supraspinatus tendon with contrast extending into the substance of the tendon *(short black arrow)*, compatible with an incomplete tear. Note contrast extending through the distal supraspinatus at its distal attachment *(short white arrow)*, compatible with a small full-thickness tear. Contrast is seen in the subacromial (subdeltoid) bursa *(long black arrow)*. Note also contrast extending into the superior labrum *(long white arrow)*, compatible with a superior labral tear.

## Technique

After puncture of the joint and aspiration of joint contents, 2 to 5 mL of contrast material and 30 mL of air are injected. The patient then exercises moderately and is placed beneath the fluoroscopic unit. Nine to 18 exposures are made of each meniscus, using slight changes in position and appropriate leg traction. After fluoroscopy, overhead or spot films are taken to evaluate the articular cartilage and cruciate ligaments and to determine whether a popliteal cyst is present. The key to the success of the fluoroscopic technique of knee arthrography is the exam-

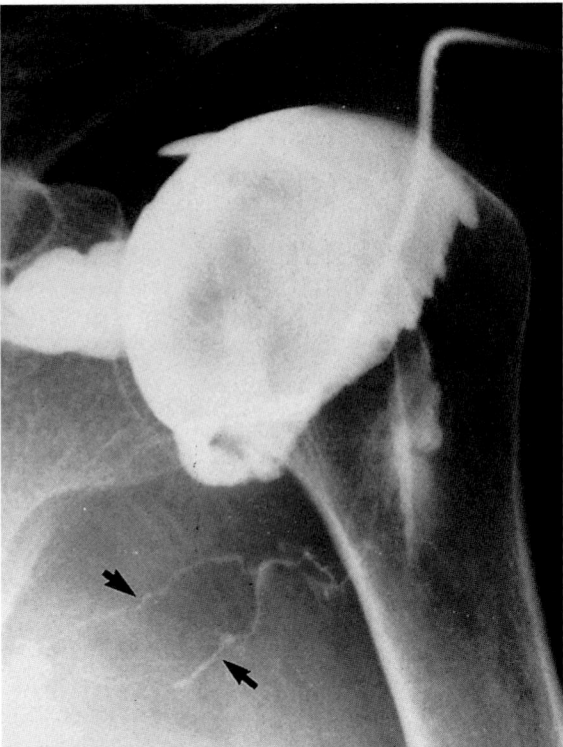

**Figure 5–13.** Glenohumeral joint arthrography: diagnosis of adhesive capsulitis. After the introduction of 10 mL of contrast material, the patient complained of pain, and it was difficult to inject any additional solution. Note the "tight-looking" articulation with a small axillary recess and opacification of the lymphatic channels *(arrows)*.

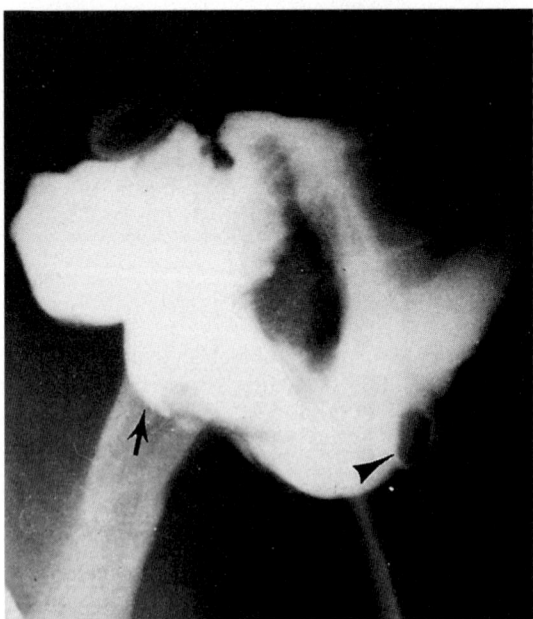

**Figure 5–14.** Glenohumeral joint arthrography. In a patient with previous anterior dislocations of the glenohumeral joint, arthrography demonstrates an abnormal recess *(arrow)* between the axillary pouch and subscapular recess and an intra-articular body *(arrowhead)*.

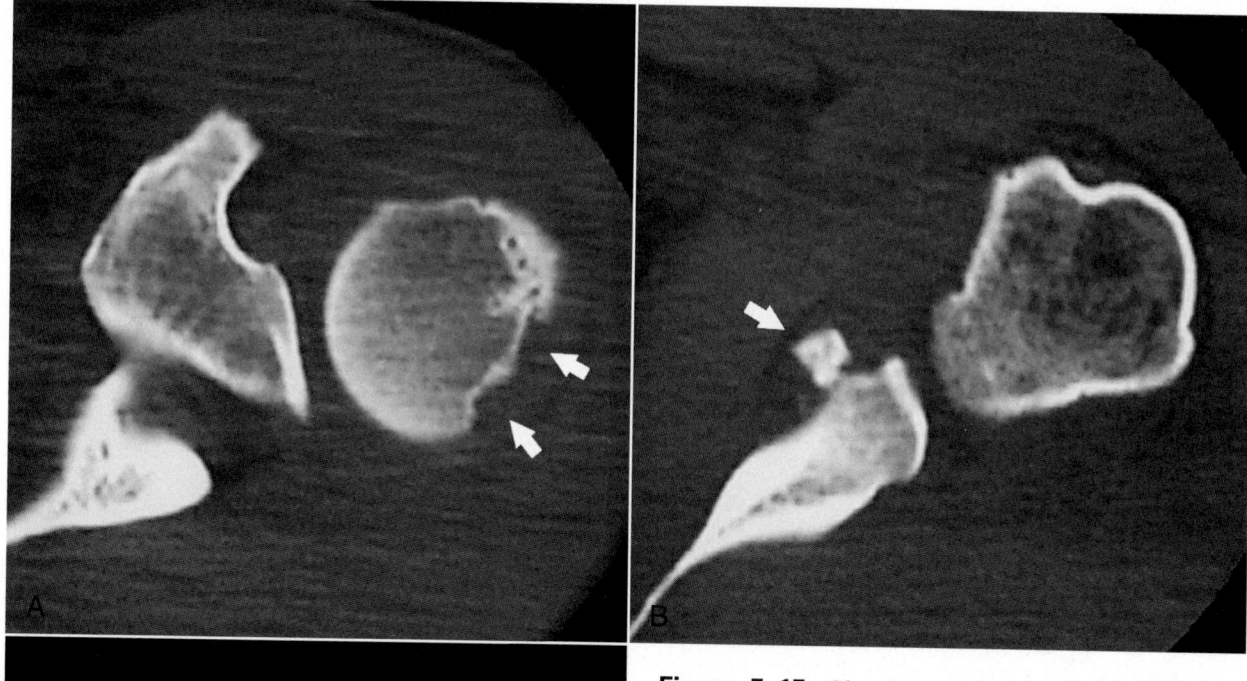

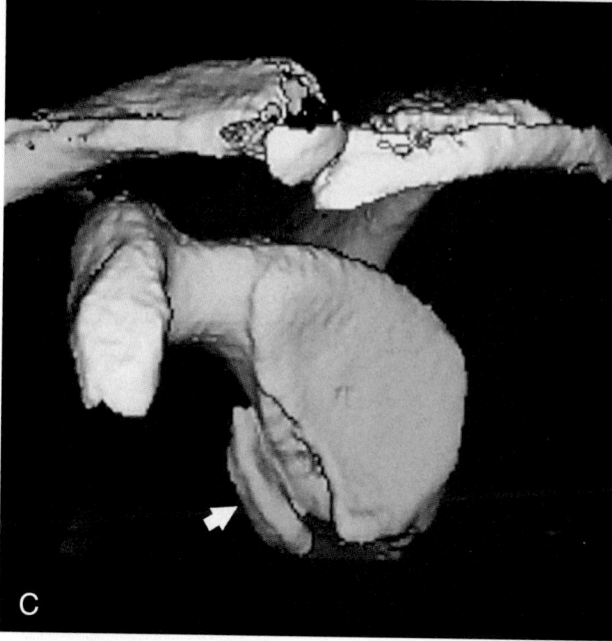

**Figure 5–15.** Glenohumeral joint: glenoid labrum and humeral head abnormalities. *A,* Computed arthrotomography of the glenohumeral joint reveals a Hill-Sachs lesion *(arrows)* in the posterolateral humeral head. *B,* A large osseous fragment is seen adjacent to the anterior inferior aspect of the glenoid labrum *(arrow). C,* Reformatted three-dimensional computed tomography shows the relationship of the osseous Bankart lesion *(arrow)* and the glenoid to better advantage.

---

**TABLE 5-5**

**Indications for Knee Arthrography**

Evaluation of:
  Meniscal tears, cysts, and ossicles
  Discoid menisci
  Postmeniscectomy syndromes
  Ligamentous injuries
  Transchondral fractures
  Chondromalacia patellae
  Degenerative joint disease
  Intra-articular osseous and cartilaginous bodies
  Synovial disorders
  Blount's disease

---

ination of all parts of both menisci. The addition of intra-articular epinephrine (0.2 mL of 1:1000 solution) may enhance meniscal visualization by causing vasoconstriction of synovial vessels, decreasing both the amount of contrast material absorbed from the joint cavity and the amount of intra-articular fluid formed.

## Normal Knee Arthrogram

The medial meniscus is identified as a sharply defined soft tissue triangular shadow (Fig. 5–20). Its posterior horn is usually large, the midportion is somewhat smaller, and the anterior horn is usually the smallest portion. The peripheral surface of the medial meniscus is firmly attached to the medial collateral ligament. A superior recess fre-

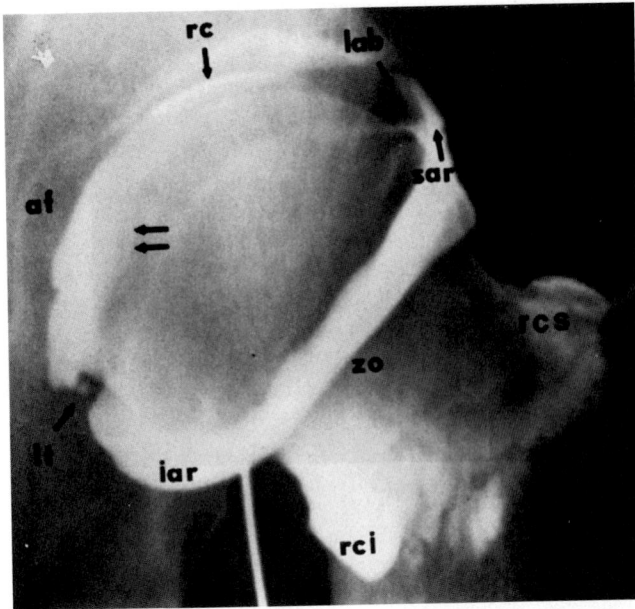

**Figure 5–16.** Hip arthrography: normal arthrogram. The recessus capitis (rc) is a thin, smooth collection of contrast medium between apposing articular surfaces and is interrupted only where the ligamentum teres (*double arrows*) enters the fovea centralis of the femoral head. The ligamentum transversum (It) is seen as a radiolucent defect adjacent to the inferior rim of the acetabulum. The ligamentum teres bridges the acetabular notch and effectively deepens the acetabulum. The inferior articular recess (iar) forms a pouch at the inferior base of the femoral head below the acetabular notch and ligamentum transversum. The superior articular recess (sar) extends cephalad around the acetabular labrum (lab). The acetabular labrum is seen as a triangular radiolucent area adjacent to the superolateral lip of the acetabulum. The zona orbicularis (zo) is a circumferential lucent band around the femoral neck that changes configuration with rotation of the femur. The recessus colli superior (rcs) and recessus colli inferior (rci) are poolings of contrast material located at the apex and base of the intertrochanteric line and are the most caudal extensions of the synovial membrane.

(From Guerra J Jr, Armbuster TC, Resnick D, et al: The adult hip: An anatomic study. Part II: The soft-tissue landmarks. Radiology 128:11, 1978.)

quently is present above the posterior horn of the medial meniscus. The anterior part of the medial meniscus is covered with the base of the infrapatellar fat pad, making evaluation of this region more difficult.

Likewise, the lateral meniscus is projected as a sharply defined triangular radiodense area surrounded by air and contrast material. It changes little in size from its anterior to its posterior horn. Inferior recesses are frequent beneath both the anterior and the posterior horns of the lateral meniscus. The posterior horn of the lateral meniscus is separated from the capsule by the synovial sheath of the popliteus tendon.

## Meniscal Abnormalities

**Meniscal Tear.** Arthrography remains a highly accurate technique for the evaluation of a number of meniscal abnormalities, including tears. A meniscal tear is more frequent on the medial side, involving particularly the posterior horn of the medial meniscus. The lateral meniscal tear most commonly involves the anterior horn.

A vertical concentric tear appears as a vertical radiodense line extending through the meniscus (Fig. 5–21). The inner fragment may be displaced, producing a buckethandle tear, and may lodge in the central portion of the joint. A vertical radial tear along the inner contour of the meniscus produces a contrast-coated inner meniscal margin and a blunted meniscal shadow. Horizontal tears, which are observed more frequently in older persons, produce a radiopaque line of contrast material that extends to the superior or inferior surface (Fig. 5–22).

**Meniscal Cyst.** Meniscal cysts are multiloculated collections of mucinous material that have a predilection for the lateral aspect of the knee. They are associated with meniscal tears and may be opacified because of articular communication (Fig. 5–23).

**Discoid Meniscus.** A discoid meniscus is broad and disclike rather than semilunar in shape. A discoid configuration is seen much more commonly in the lateral meniscus than in the medial meniscus. The pathogenesis of a discoid meniscus is not clear. The usual age of patients at the time of clinical presentation is between 15 and 35 years. These patients commonly have symptoms of a torn cartilage.

Initial plain films in patients with discoid menisci generally are unrewarding. Arthrography reveals the abnormally large and elongated meniscus, frequently extending to the intercondylar notch (Fig. 5–24). An associated meniscal tear frequently is observed.

**Meniscal Ossicle.** Meniscal ossicles represent foci of ossification within the menisci. Patients with meniscal ossicles may be asymptomatic or have local pain and swelling.

Initial films reveal ossification of variable shape in the anterior or posterior portion of either the medial or the lateral meniscus. The most common site is the posterior horn of the medial meniscus. Arthrography confirms the location of the ossification within the meniscus.

Meniscal ossicles may simulate intra-articular osteochondral fragments.

**Meniscectomy.** A total meniscectomy involves the removal of the entire meniscus from its capsular attachment. A partial meniscectomy may involve the removal of the anterior two thirds of the abnormal meniscus; alternatively, only the torn portion of the meniscus may be removed, leaving the remainder of the meniscus intact. Arthrographic evaluation after complete or partial meniscectomy may reveal a retained fragment, a regenerated meniscus, a tear of the opposite meniscus, or additional abnormalities.

The retained posterior horn after incomplete meniscectomy resembles a normal posterior horn, although it may be irregular or contain an obvious tear. After the removal of the inner fragment of a bucket-handle tear, the retained peripheral fragment appears as a truncated shadow with rough, irregular surfaces. With regeneration of the meniscus, a small triangular shadow resembling an equilateral or isosceles triangle is observed. A variety

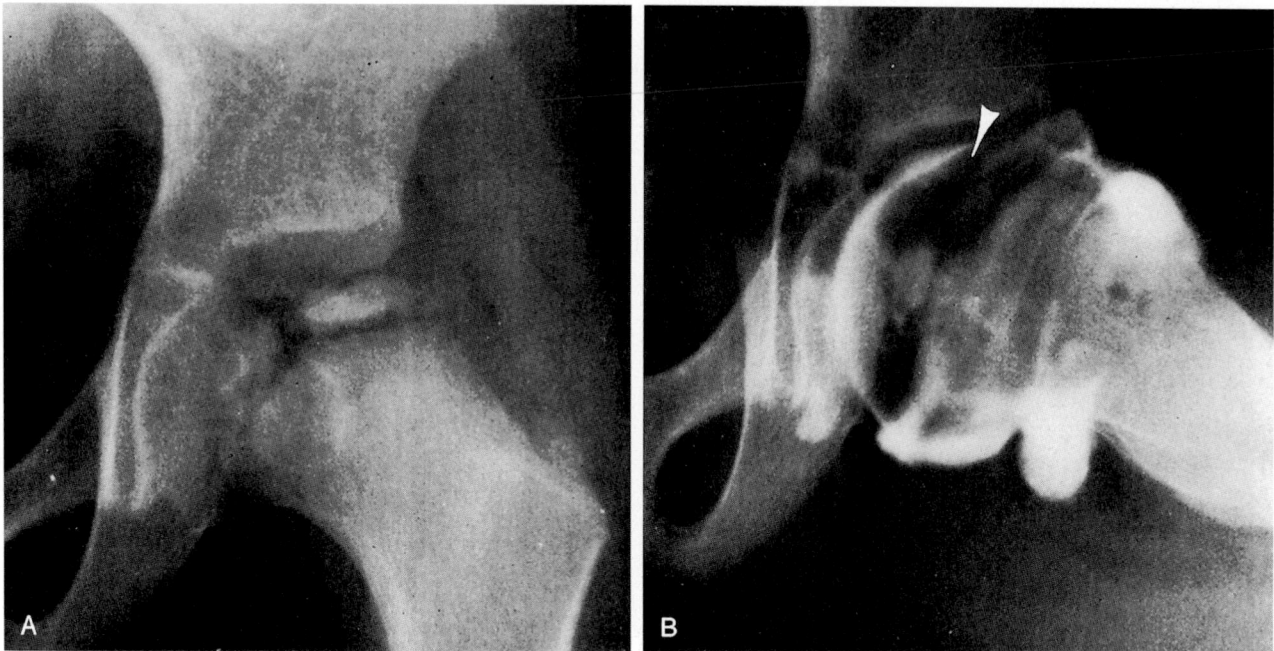

**Figure 5–17.** Hip arthrography: Legg-Calvé-Perthes disease. *A,* On the initial film, epiphyseal fragmentation and metaphyseal irregularity are apparent. *B,* An arthrographic image in hip abduction indicates a relatively smooth radiolucent cartilaginous head *(arrowhead)* that is well covered by the acetabulum.

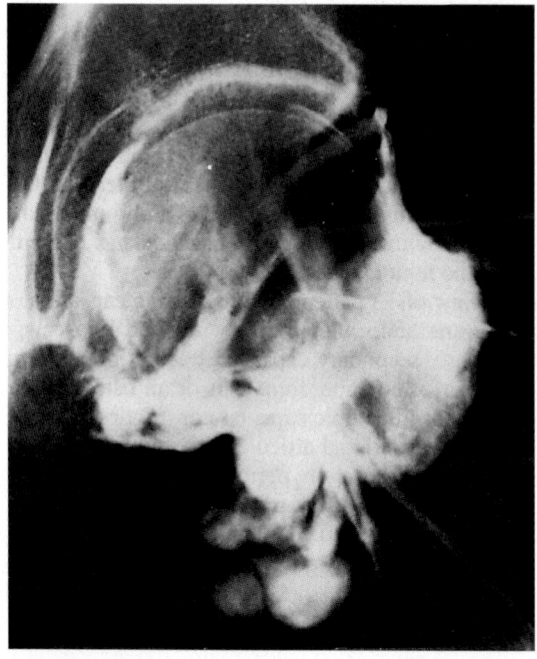

**Figure 5–18.** Hip arthrography: pigmented villonodular synovitis. The initial radiograph of the hip (not shown) in this 57-year-old woman revealed a normal joint space and cystic areas in the femoral head and neck. Aspiration of the joint revealed brown discoloration of the synovial fluid, and arthrography documented an enlarged and irregular joint cavity with small, medial collections, or pools, of contrast material.

(Courtesy of V. Vint, MD, San Diego, California.)

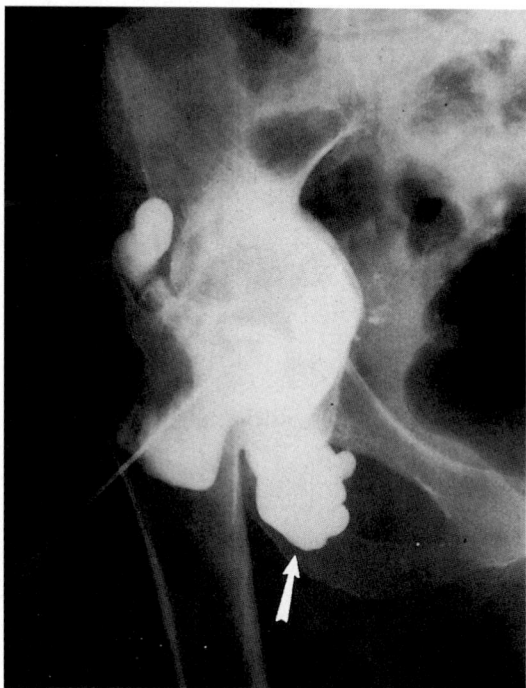

**Figure 5–19.** Hip arthrography: rheumatoid arthritis and synovial cyst formation. In this 65-year-old woman with rheumatoid arthritis and an apparent "femoral" hernia, arthrography indicates that the clinically evident soft tissue mass is related to a synovial cyst *(arrow)*. Observe the sacculation of the articular cavity and a protrusio acetabuli defect.

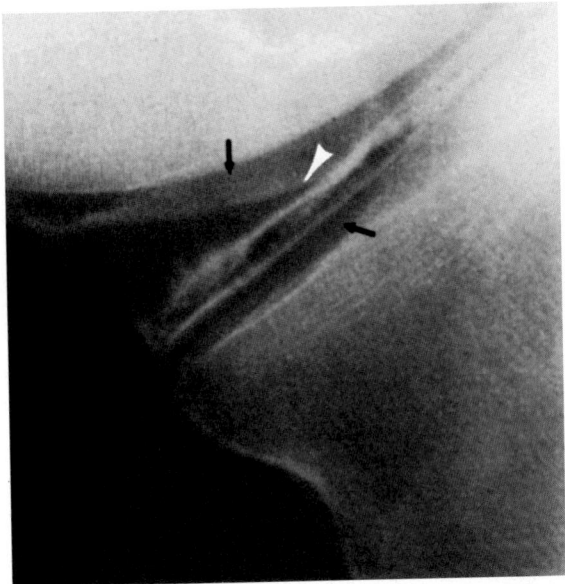

**Figure 5–20.** Knee arthrography: normal arthrography of the posterior horn of the medial meniscus. This segment is relatively large and extends for a considerable distance into the articular cavity (*arrowhead*). The adjacent articular recesses are small. The articular cartilage (*arrows*) is smooth.

of causes exist for postmeniscectomy pain, including ligament injury, loose bodies, and cartilage ulceration.

## Ligamentous Injury

**Collateral Ligament Tears.** Recent tears of the collateral ligaments may be documented by arthrography. Contrast material introduced into the joint space extravasates into the adjacent soft tissues. This finding is more readily apparent on the medial aspect of the knee (Fig. 5–25).

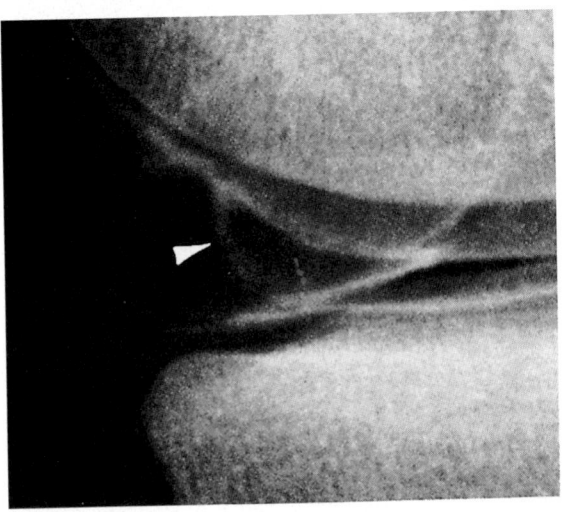

**Figure 5–21.** Knee arthrography: vertical concentric meniscal tear. Observe the contrast- or air-filled linear shadows (*arrowhead*) in the meniscus.

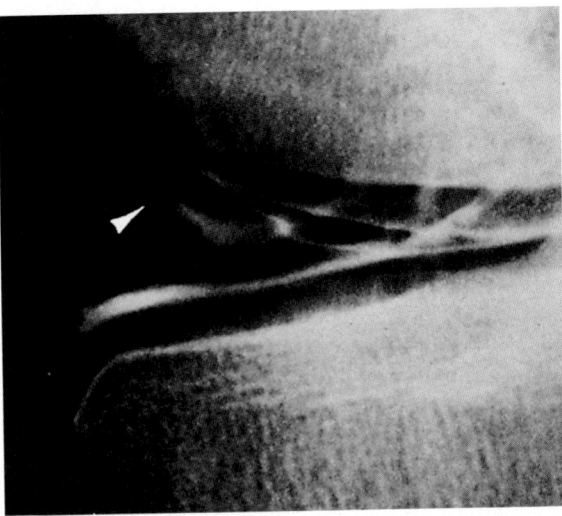

**Figure 5–22.** Knee arthrography: horizontal medial meniscal tear. The tear (*arrowhead*) is filled with contrast material on the arthrogram.

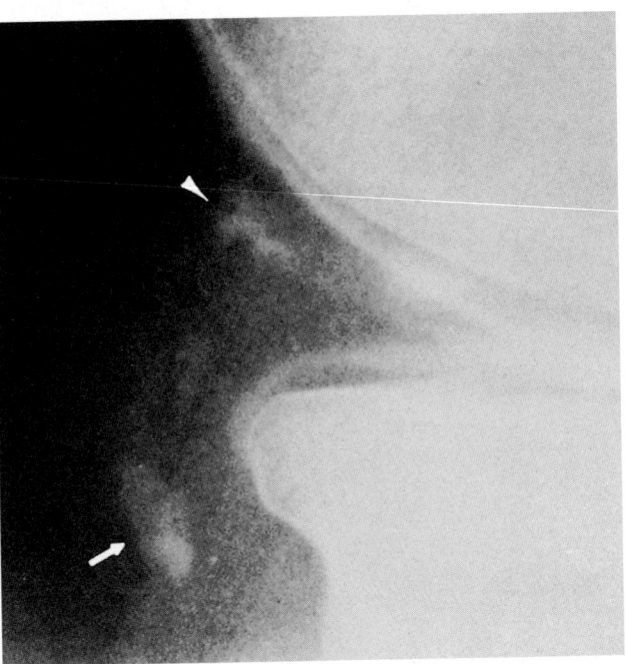

**Figure 5–23.** Knee arthrography: meniscal cyst. A cyst of the medial meniscus is opacified (*arrow*) and is associated with a horizontal tear of the meniscus (*arrowhead*).

**Cruciate Ligament Injuries.** MR imaging is superior to arthrography in the assessment of injuries of the cruciate ligaments (see Chapter 59). The fundamental arthrographic criterion of a normal anterior cruciate ligament is an anterior synovial surface that is "ruler straight" on specialized lateral radiographs. The ligament is considered to be lax but intact if the anterior synovial surface is bowed and concave anteriorly. The arthrographic abnormalities associated with disruption of the anterior cruciate ligament include nonvisualization; a wavy, lumpy, or acutely angulated anterior surface; irregularity of the inferior attachment of the ligament; pooling of the contrast medium in the usual location of the ligament; and

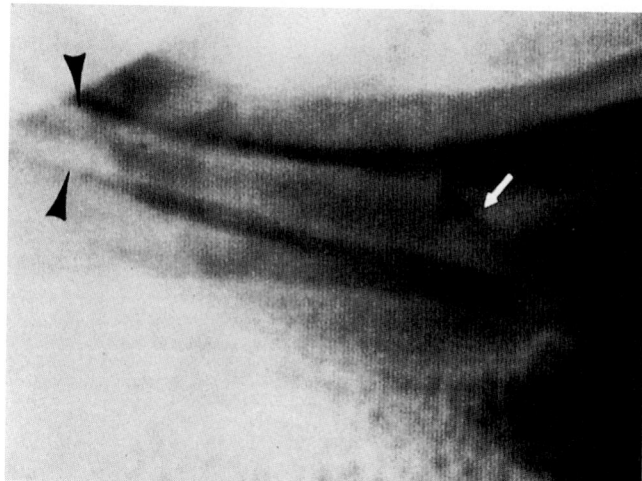

**Figure 5–24.** Knee arthrography: discoid lateral meniscus (slab type) with a tear. Observe that the meniscus extends far into the joint cavity *(arrowheads)*. A vertical tear is evident *(arrow)*.

visualization of the plica synovialis infrapatellaris. It should be emphasized that the abnormal findings frequently are subtle, requiring an examiner with a good deal of experience and knowledge.

## Lesions of Articular Cartilage

Contrast material within the joint cavity allows visualization of portions of articular cartilage. Abnormalities such as osteochondral fracture (osteochondritis dissecans) and chondromalacia may be identified, although they are better studied with MR imaging.

**Osteochondral Fracture (Osteochondritis Dissecans).** Transchondral fractures exist where tangential shearing forces are applied to the articular surface. In the knee, such fractures are most frequent on the lateral surface of the medial femoral condyle. The fracture fragment may consist of cartilage, cartilage and bone, or solely bone. It may remain in situ, with relatively normal overlying cartilage; become depressed, with an indentation of the articular surface; or become detached, existing as a loose body in the articular cavity or as an attached body at a distant synovial site.

Arthrography allows evaluation of the cartilaginous or osseous surface, or both, at the fracture site (Fig. 5–26). Contrast medium may outline a normal, swollen, or depressed cartilaginous surface, or it may dissect beneath the osteochondral fragment. The detection of intra-articular osteochondral bodies accompanying osteochondritis dissecans may require the combination of arthrography and conventional tomography or CT scanning (Fig. 5–27).

**Chondromalacia.** The role of arthrography in the diagnosis of chondromalacia of the patella is not clear. On arthrography, chondromalacia produces absorption or imbibition of contrast material by the patellar cartilage. Nodular elevation, fissuring, or diminution of the cartilaginous surface may be apparent. MR imaging, however, appears to be a superior technique in the evaluation of the articular cartilage.

## Synovial Plicae

Synovial plicae are remnants of synovial tissue that in early development originally divided the joint into three separate compartments; they may be found normally in

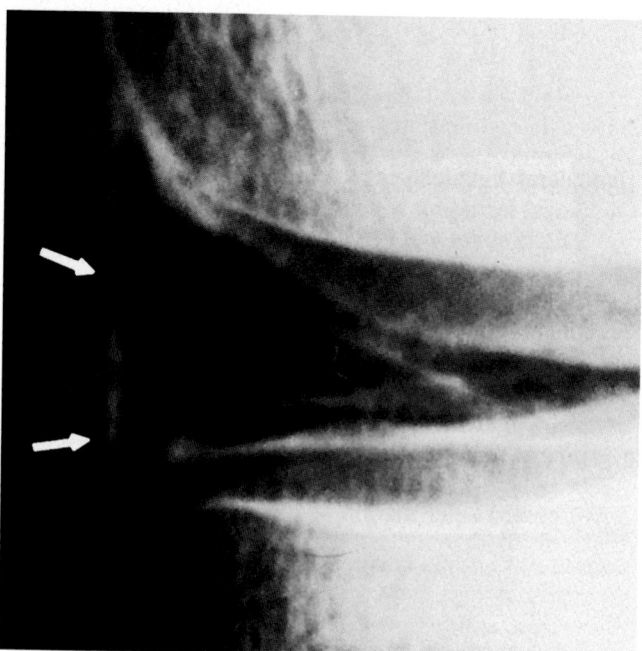

**Figure 5–25.** Knee arthrography: collateral ligament injuries. A tear of the medial collateral ligament allows contrast material to pass from the articular cavity into the soft tissues and outline the outer aspect of the ligament *(arrows)*.

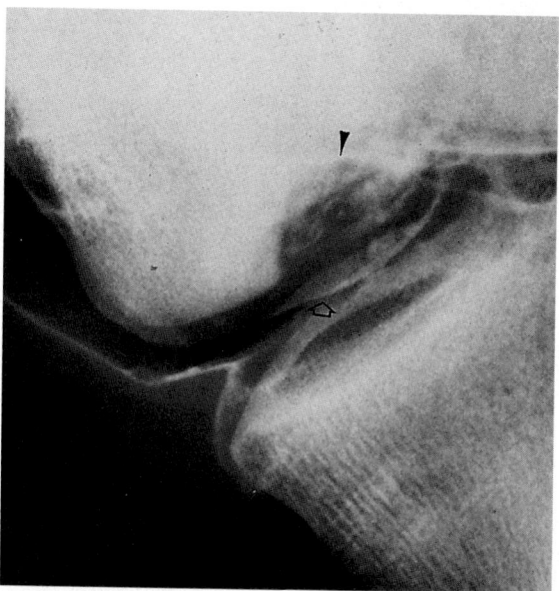

**Figure 5–26.** Knee arthrography: osteochondritis dissecans. Arthrography demonstrates the osseous abnormality *(arrowhead)* and swollen articular cartilage over the lesion *(open arrow)*.

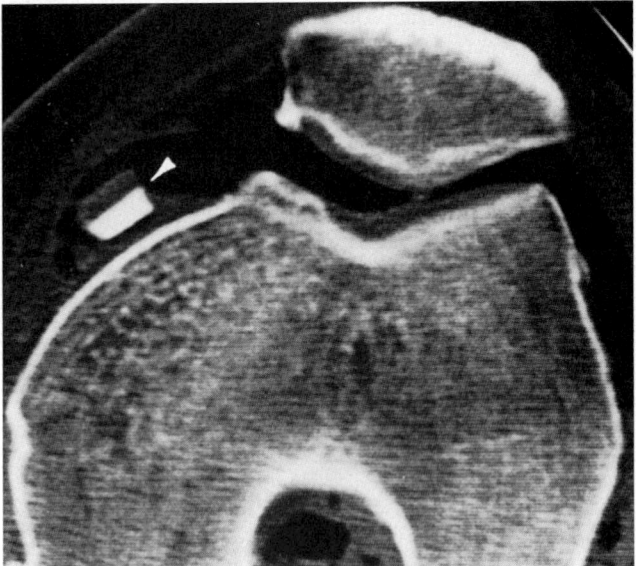

**Figure 5–27.** Knee arthrography: osteochondral fragment. After the introduction of air into the knee joint, a transaxial computed tomography scan reveals the fragment (*arrowhead*), which consists of cartilage and bone, in the medial aspect of the joint.

the adult knee. Usually of no consequence, these structures may become pathologically thickened and lead to significant symptoms. The three plicae encountered most commonly are classified according to the partitions from which they took origin (suprapatellar medial patellar, and infrapatellar). Their identification can be accomplished by arthrography (Figs. 5–28 and 5–29), computed arthrotomography, MR imaging (see Chapter 59), or arthroscopy.

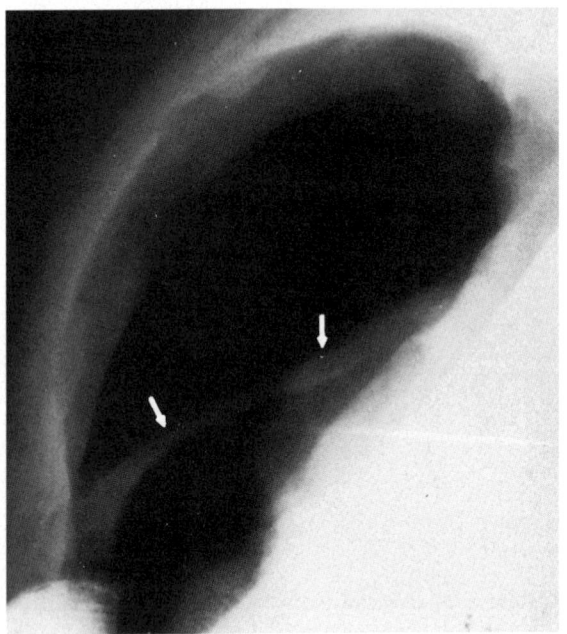

**Figure 5–28.** Knee arthrography: suprapatellar plica (*arrows*).

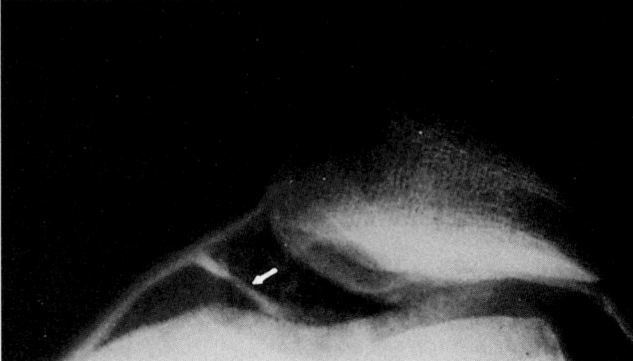

**Figure 5–29.** Knee arthrography: medial patellar plica (*arrow*).

## Articular Disorders (Table 5–6)

**Degenerative Joint Disease.** Contrast examination of the knee in patients with degenerative joint disease delineates abnormalities of the articular cartilage and menisci and the presence of intra-articular osseous bodies and popliteal cysts (Fig. 5–30).

**Rheumatoid Arthritis.** Arthrographic findings in the knee in rheumatoid arthritis include enlargement of the joint cavity or suprapatellar pouch, nodular irregularity or corrugation of the synovial membrane, filling defects within the joint cavity, lymphatic filling, destruction of hyaline cartilage and fibrocartilage, and synovial cyst formation (Fig. 5–31).

**Pigmented Villonodular Synovitis.** The knee arthrogram in diffuse pigmented villonodular synovitis reveals an enlarged synovial cavity, irregular synovial outline with "laking" or pooling of contrast material, and nodular filling defects (Fig. 5–32).

**Idiopathic Synovial (Osteo)Chondromatosis.** Knee arthrography in idiopathic synovial (osteo)chondromatosis reveals an enlarged synovial cavity and multiple small, sharply defined filling defects (Fig. 5–33).

## Synovial Cysts

Synovial cysts about the knee are most frequent in the popliteal region, where communication between the joint and normal posterior bursae can be identified. The bursa involved most commonly is the gastrocnemiosemimembranosus bursa, located posterior to the medial femoral condyle between the tendons of the gastrocnemius and

---

**TABLE 5–6**

**Causes of Multiple Filling Defects on Knee Arthrograms**

Rheumatoid arthritis
Pigmented villonodular synovitis
Idiopathic synovial (osteo)chondromatosis
Hemangioma, angioma
Lipoma arborescens

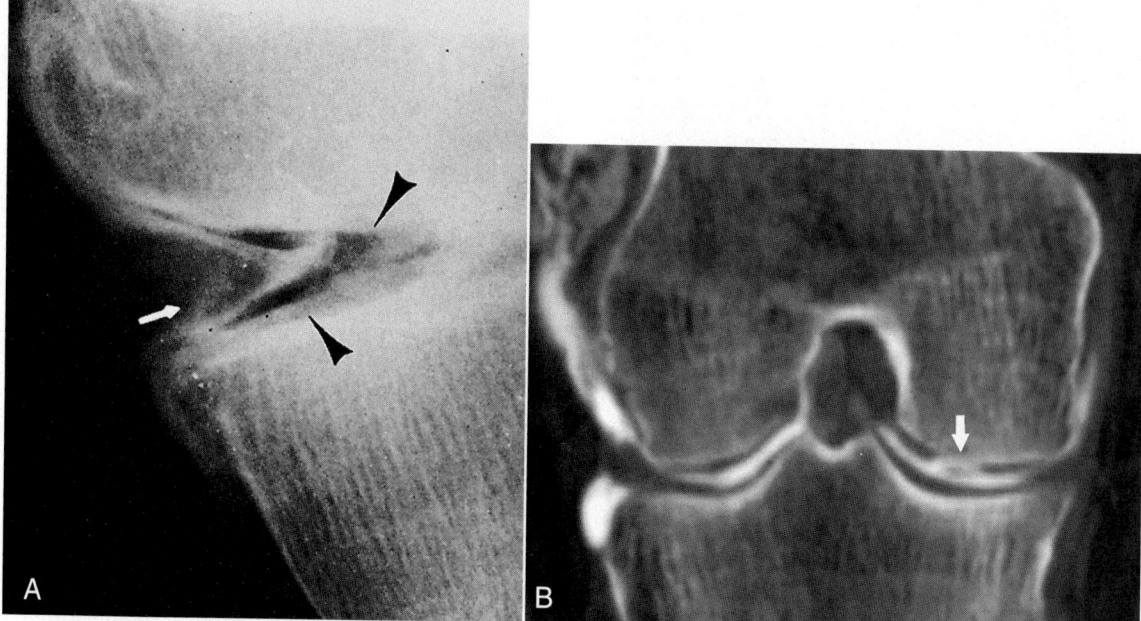

**Figure 5–30.** Knee arthrography: degenerative joint disease. *A*, In the medial compartment, findings include severe denudation of articular cartilage on both the femur and the tibia *(arrowheads)*. The medial meniscus is swollen, with an incomplete vertical tear *(arrow)* and an irregular inner contour. *B*, Reformatted coronal computed tomography image in a different patient after arthrography shows a flap tear of the medial femoral condyle *(arrow)*.

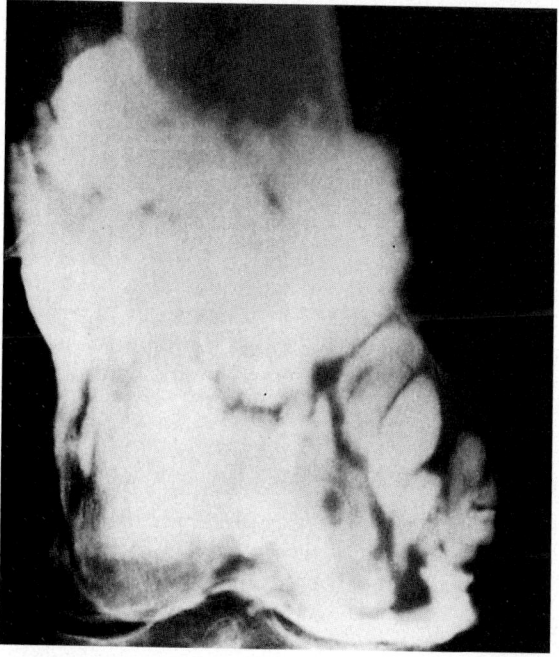

**Figure 5–31.** Knee arthrography: rheumatoid arthritis. Nodular and linear irregularity and pooling of contrast material reflect synovial hypertrophy.

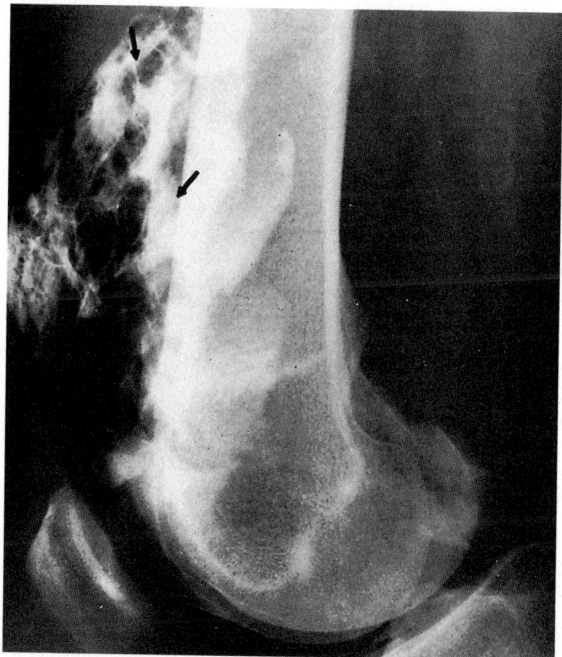

**Figure 5–32.** Knee arthrography: diffuse pigmented villonodular synovitis. Observe the irregular distribution and appearance of contrast material *(arrows)* in the suprapatellar pouch.

(From Dalinka MK, Coren GS, Wershba M: Knee arthroscopy. CRC Crit Rev Radiol Nucl Med 4:1, 1973.)

semimembranosus muscles. Swelling of this posterior bursa is termed a Baker's cyst. Rupture of such a cyst is associated with soft tissue extravasation of fluid contents. Ruptures occurring posteriorly can simulate a compartment syndrome or thrombophlebitis.

Arthrography of the knee is an accurate method of diagnosing synovial cysts, although some investigators

also recommended sonographic or isotopic examination in this clinical situation. MR imaging of such cysts may provide the most detailed information regarding the distribution and extent of the process and the degree of synovial

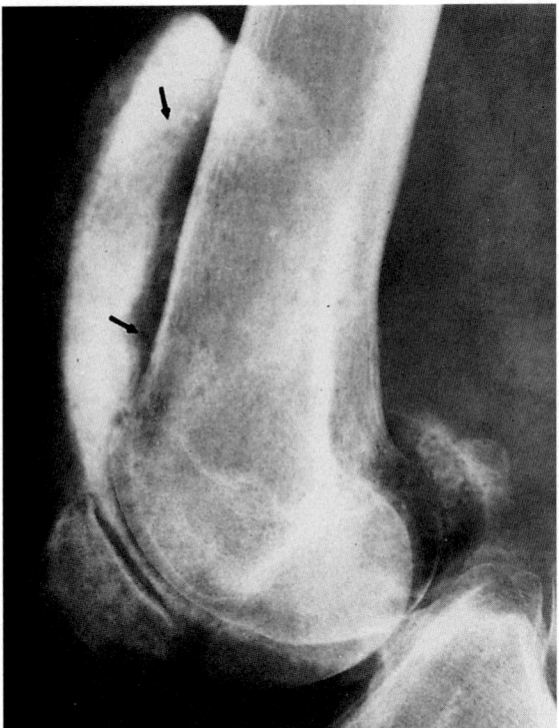

**Figure 5–33.** Knee arthrography: idiopathic synovial (osteo)chondromatosis. Observe the multiple sharply defined filling defects *(arrows)* throughout the articular cavity.
(From Dalinka MK, Coren GS, Wershba M: Knee arthroscopy. CRC Crit Rev Radiol Nucl Med 4:1, 1973.)

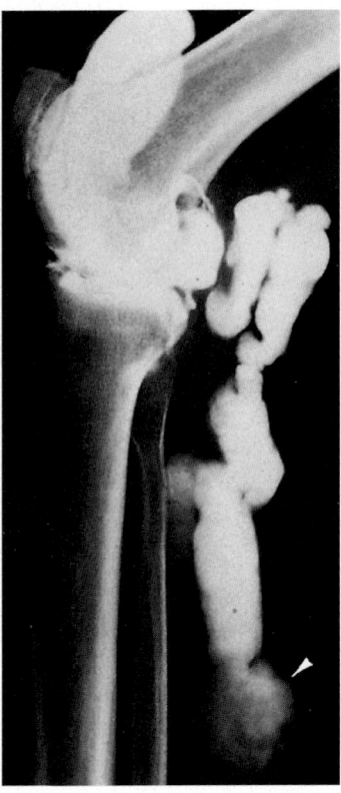

**Figure 5–34.** Knee arthrography: synovial cyst formation in rheumatoid arthritis. A typical large popliteal cyst extending into the calf is filled with contrast material. It is slightly irregular in contour, particularly inferiorly *(arrowhead)*, which may reflect synovial inflammation. No free extravasation into the soft tissues is seen.

inflammation (see Chapter 59). The arthrographic appearance of an abnormal synovial cyst varies. In most instances, a well-defined, lobulated structure filled with air and radiopaque contrast material is revealed. It may have an irregular surface related to hypertrophy of its synovial lining (Fig. 5–34). Alternatively, the entire cyst or a portion of it may rupture, with extravasation of contrast material.

Any inflammatory, degenerative, traumatic, or neoplastic condition that produces a knee effusion can lead to synovial cyst formation. The differential diagnosis of synovial cysts about the knee includes a variety of neoplasms of soft tissue or bone origin, thrombophlebitis and hematomas, varicose veins, aneurysms, and other conditions.

## ANKLE

Arthrography of the ankle is performed for a variety of indications (Table 5–7). Contrast opacification allows identification and delineation of ligamentous injuries and can be combined effectively with routine and stress radiography of the ankle.

### Technique

Ideally, arthrography of the ankle should be performed within a few days of the acute injury, because blood and tissue adhesions about the ligamentous tear may result in false-negative examinations. Six to 10 mL of contrast

agent is injected using an anterior approach. The needle is withdrawn, and radiographs are exposed in anteroposterior, oblique, and lateral projections after mild exercise of the ankle. Stress radiographs also may be obtained.

### Normal Ankle Arthrogram

Under normal circumstances, ankle arthrography results in opacification of the articular cavity without evidence of extra-articular leak, except for filling of the tendon sheath of the flexor hallucis longus or the flexor digitorum longus muscle, or both, in approximately 20% of patients

---

**TABLE 5–7**

**Indications for Ankle Arthrography**

---

Evaluation of:
   Ligamentous injuries
   Transchondral fractures
   Intra-articular osseous and cartilaginous bodies
   Adhesive capsulitis

---

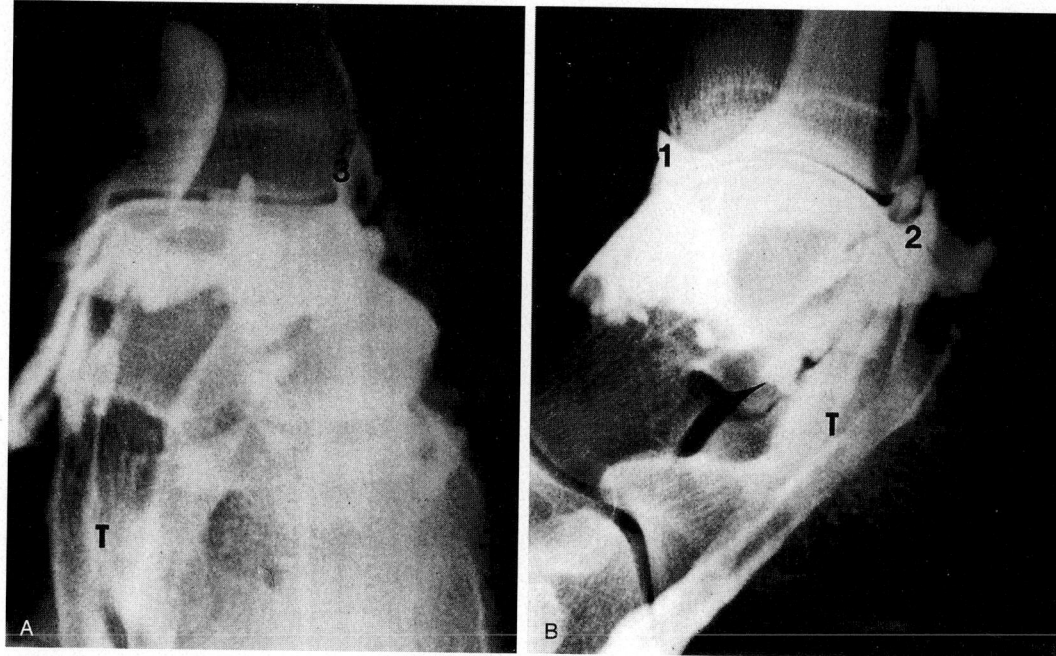

**Figure 5–35.** Knee arthrography: normal arthrogram. Anteroposterior *(A)* and lateral *(B)* views. The tibiotalar joint has been opacified. Note the normal recesses: anterior recess (1), posterior recess (2), and syndesmotic recess (3). Filling of the medial tendon sheaths (T) and posterior subtalar joint *(arrowhead)* is a normal finding.

(Fig. 5–35). The posterior subtalar joint is opacified in approximately 10% of patients.

## Ligamentous Injuries

**Anterior Talofibular Ligament Injury.** The anterior talofibular ligament extends from the anterior surface of the distal portion of the fibula to the talar neck. With tears, contrast material is seen both inferior and lateral to the distal end of the fibula (Fig. 5–36).

**Calcaneofibular Ligament Injury.** The calcaneofibular ligament originates from the posterior aspect of the distal portion of the fibula and inserts on the superior aspect of the calcaneus. When this strong ligament is torn, contrast material fills the peroneal tendon sheaths as the inner aspect of the sheaths is also torn (see Fig. 5–36).

**Distal Anterior Tibiofibular Ligament Injury.** This structure extends from the anterior and lateral aspects of the distal portion of the tibia to the adjacent anterior portion of the distal fibular end. After injury to this ligament, extravasation of contrast material occurs between distal tibia and fibula, beyond the syndesmotic recess.

**Deltoid Ligament Injury.** The deltoid ligament originates from the medial malleolus and extends to the talus and calcaneus. With tears of the deltoid ligament, contrast material extravasates beyond the medial confines of the joint.

Any of these ankle injuries may be associated with abnormalities on plain films, including soft tissue swelling and avulsion fractures at the osseous sites of attachment of the specific ligament. Further, stress radiography may indicate ligament weakening by revealing abnormal widening of the joint. Evidence also indicates a potential role for MR imaging in the identification of sites of ligamentous (and tendinous) injury about the ankle (see Chapter 59).

## Other Traumatic Disorders

**Transchondral Fracture.** Osteochondral fractures (osteochondritis dissecans) of the talar dome are not infrequent. Arthrography in this situation outlines the integrity of the overlying cartilage and the presence of intra-articular cartilaginous bodies.

**Adhesive Capsulitis.** Post-traumatic adhesive capsulitis in the ankle is associated with restricted motion. Arthrography delineates a decrease in the articular capacity, with resistance to injection of contrast material, obliteration of normal anterior and posterior recesses or tibiofibular syndesmosis, opacification of lymphatic vessels, and extravasation of contrast material along the needle track.

## APOPHYSEAL JOINTS

The injection of contrast material, anesthetic agent, corticosteroid preparation, or any combination of the three into the apophyseal joints of the lumbar spine has been advocated in the diagnosis and treatment of the facet syndrome. This syndrome leads to pain, which is exacerbated with rotary motion, in the lower back, thighs, buttocks, and legs and to focal tenderness over the affected joint. The intrinsically curved lumbar apophyseal joints

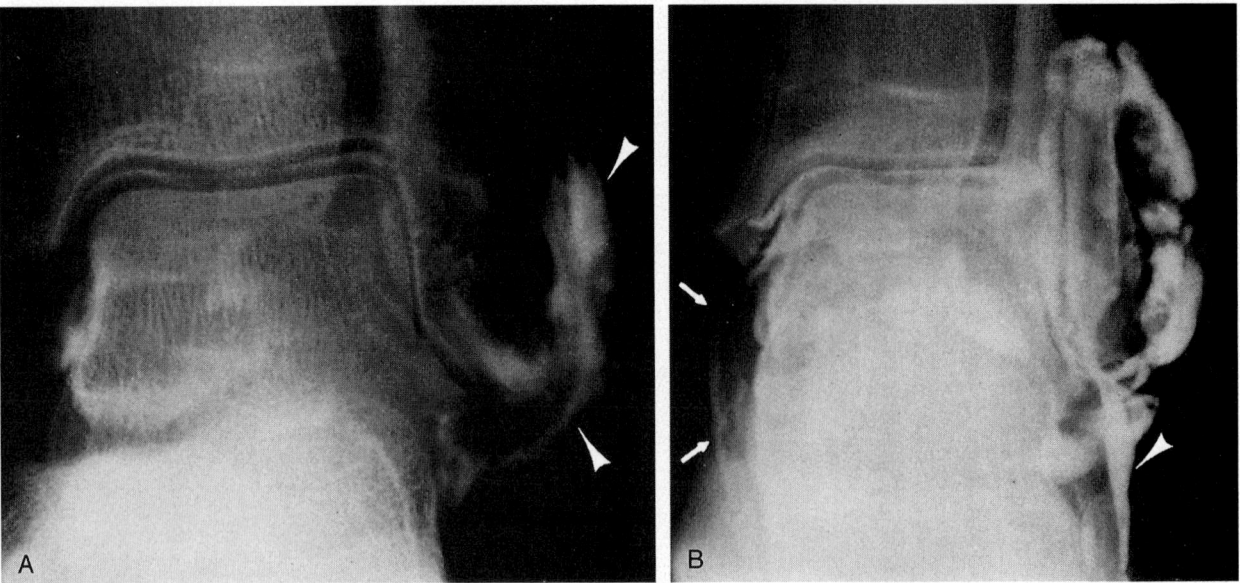

**Figure 5–36.** Ankle arthrography: ligamentous injuries. *A*, Anterior talofibular ligament injury. Contrast material is located inferior and lateral to the tip of the fibula *(arrowheads)*. On a lateral view (not shown), the contrast material would be anterior to the distal portion of the fibula. *B*, Anterior talofibular and calcaneofibular ligament injuries. In addition to extravasation of contrast material lateral to the distal end of the fibula, the peroneal tendon sheaths are visualized *(arrowhead)*. Normal filling of the medial tendon sheaths is noted *(arrows)*.

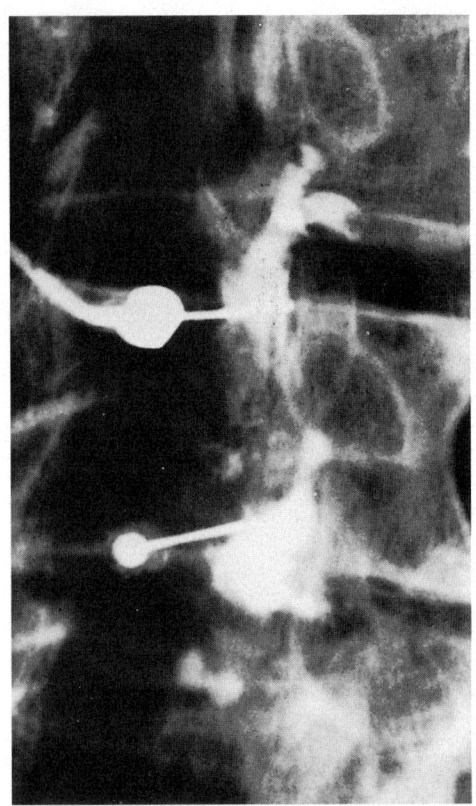

**Figure 5–37.** Arthrography of the lumbar apophyseal joints. Observe the needle placement in two consecutive apophyseal joints. Some extravasation of contrast material is evident at the lower level, whereas in the upper joint, all the contrast agent is within the joint.

are less accessible to direct puncture than are many other articulations of the body; however, the puncture technique is not difficult and can be accomplished with fluoroscopy and, occasionally, CT (Fig. 5–37). Arthrography of the facet joints in the cervical spine has received less attention.

## FURTHER READING

Anderson TM Jr: Arthrography. Radiol Clin North Am 19:215, 1981.

Arndt R-D, Horns JW, Gold RH, et al: Clinical Arthrography. Baltimore, Williams & Wilkins, 1981.

Burk DL Jr, Kanal E, Brunberg JA, et al: 1.5-T surface-coil MRI of the knee. AJR Am J Roentgenol 147:293, 1986.

Burk DL Jr, Karajick D, Kurtz AB, et al: Rotator cuff tears: Prospective comparison of MR imaging with arthrography, sonography, and surgery. AJR Am J Roentgenol 153:87, 1989.

Dalinka MK: Arthrography. New York, Springer-Verlag, 1980.

Destouet JM, Gilula LA, Murphy WA, et al: Lumbar facet joint injection: Indication, technique, clinical correlation, and preliminary results. Radiology 145:321, 1982.

Deutsch AL, Resnick D, Dalinka MK, et al: Synovial plicae of the knee. Radiology 141:627, 1981.

Deutsch AL, Resnick D, Mink JH, et al: Computed and conventional arthrotomography of the glenohumeral joint: Normal anatomy and clinical experience. Radiology 143:603, 1984.

Dory MA: Arthrography of the ankle joint in chronic instability. Skeletal Radiol 15:291, 1986.

El-Khoury GY, Albright JP, Abu Yousef MM, et al: Arthrotomography of the glenoid labrum. Radiology 131:333, 1979.

Freiberger RH, Kaye JJ: Arthrography. New York, Appleton-Century-Crofts, 1979.

Freiberger RH, Pavlov H: Knee arthrography. Radiology 166:489, 1988.

Gilula LA, Reinus WR, Totty WG: Midcarpal wrist arthrography. AJR Am J Roentgenol 146:645, 1986.

Goldman AB, Dines DM, Warren RF: Shoulder Arthrography: Technique, Diagnosis, and Clinical Correlation. Boston, Little, Brown, 1982.

Goldman AB, Ghelman B: The double-contrast shoulder arthrogram: A review of 158 studies. Radiology 127:655, 1978.

Goldman AB, Katz MC, Freiberger RH: Post-traumatic adhesive capsulitis of the ankle: Arthrographic diagnosis. AJR Am J Roentgenol 127:585, 1976.

Hall FM: Arthrography of the discoid lateral meniscus. AJR Am J Roentgenol 128:993, 1977.

Hendrix RW, Lin P-JP, Kane WJ: Simplified aspiration or injection technique for the sacro-iliac joint. J Bone Joint Surg Am 64:1249, 1982.

Herbert TJ, Faithfull RG, McCann DJ, et al: Bilateral arthrography of the wrist. J Hand Surg [Br] 15:233, 1990.

Herman LJ, Beltran L: Pitfalls in MR imaging of the knee. Radiology 167:775, 1988.

Kaye JJ: Knee arthrography today. Radiology 157:265, 1985.

Kaye JJ, Bohne WHO: A radiographic study of the ligamentous anatomy of the ankle. Radiology 125:659, 1977.

Killoran PJ, Marcove RC, Freiberg RH: Shoulder arthrography. AJR Am J Roentgenol 103:658, 1968.

Lequesne M, Becker J, Bard M, et al: Capsular constriction of the hip: Arthrographic and clinical considerations. Skeletal Radiol 6:1, 1981.

Lindgren PG, Willen R: Gastrocnemio-semimembranosus bursa and its relation to the knee joint. I. Anatomy and histology. Acta Radiol Diagn 18:497, 1977.

Middleton WD, Reinus WR, Melson GL, et al: Pitfalls of rotator cuff sonography. AJR Am J Roentgenol 146: 555, 1986.

Mooney V, Robertson J: The facet syndrome. Clin Orthop 115:149, 1976.

Murphy WA, Siegel MJ, Gilula LA: Arthrography in the diagnosis of unexplained chronic hip pain with regional osteopenia. AJR Am J Roentgenol 129:283, 1977.

Newberg AH, Muhn CS, Robbins AH: Complications of arthrography. Radiology 155:605, 1985.

Nicholas JA, Freiberger RH, Killoran PJ: Double contrast arthrography of the knee: Its value in the management of 225 knee derangements. J Bone Joint Surg Am 52:203, 1970.

Olson RW: Arthrography of the ankle: Its use in the evaluation of ankle sprains. Radiology 92:1439, 1969.

Pavlov H, Ghelman B, Warren RF: Double-contrast arthrography of the elbow. Radiology 130:87, 1979.

Pavlov H, Goldman AB: The popliteus bursa: An indicator of subtle pathology. AJR Am J Roentgenol 134:313, 1980.

Pavlov H, Hirschy JC, Torg JS: Computed tomography of the cruciate ligaments. Radiology 132:389, 1979.

Pavlov H, Torg JS: Double contrast arthrographic evaluation of the anterior cruciate ligament. Radiology 126:661, 1978.

Pavlov H, Warren RF, Sherman MF, et al: The accuracy of double-contrast arthrographic evaluation of the anterior cruciate ligament: A retrospective review of one hundred and sixty-three knees with surgical confirmation. J Bone Joint Surg Am 65:175, 1983.

Rafii M, Firooznia H, Golimbu C, et al: CT arthrography of the capsular structures of the shoulder. AJR Am J Roentgenol 146:361, 1986.

Rauschning W: Anatomy and function of the communication between knee joint and popliteal bursae. Ann Rheum Dis 39:354, 1980.

Reicher MA, Bassett LW, Gold RH: High-resolution magnetic resonance imaging of the knee joint: Pathologic correlations. AJR Am J Roentgenol 145:903, 1985.

Resnick D: Rheumatoid arthritis of the wrist: The compartmental approach. Med Radiogr Photogr 52:50, 1976.

Resnick D, André M, Kerr R, et al: Digital arthrography of the wrist: A radiographic and pathologic investigation. AJR Am J Roentgenol 142:1187, 1984.

Ricklin P, Rüttimann A, Del Buono MS: Meniscus Lesions—Practical Problems of Clinical Diagnosis, Arthrography and Therapy. New York, Grune & Stratton, 1971.

Sauser DD, Nelson RC, Lavine MH, et al: Acute injuries of the lateral ligaments of the ankle: Comparison of stress radiography and arthrography. Radiology 148:653, 1983.

Stoker DJ, Renton P, Fulton A: The value of arthrography in the management of internal derangements of the knee: The first 1000 are the worst. Clin Radiol 32:557, 1981.

Stoller DW, Martin C, Cruess JV III, et al: Meniscal tears: Pathologic correlation with MR imaging. Radiology 163: 731, 1987.

Thomas RH, Resnick D, Alazraki NP, et al: Compartmental evaluation of osteoarthritis of the knee: A comparative study of available diagnostic modalities. Radiology 116:585, 1975.

Turner DA, Prodromos CC, Petasnick JP, et al: Acute injury of the ligaments of the knee: Magnetic resonance evaluation. Radiology 154:717, 1985.

Zlatkin MB, Bjorkengren A, Gylys-Morin, V et al: Cross-sectional imaging of the capsular mechanism of the glenohumeral joint. AJR Am J Roentgenol 150:151, 1988.

# CHAPTER 6

## Diagnostic Ultrasonography

Ronald S. Adler, Laurence A. Mack,
F. William Scheible, Carolyn M. Sofka,
and Donald Resnick

## SUMMARY OF KEY FEATURES

Although alternative techniques such as computed tomography (CT) and magnetic resonance (MR) imaging have influenced dramatically the manner in which ultrasonography is used, the benefits of diagnostic ultrasonography—which include lower cost, less time, and less patient discomfort—ensure its place in clinical imaging. Advances in transducer technology and power Doppler techniques have expanded the applicability of ultrasonography to the assessment of many structures, particularly those that are situated superficially. The orthopedic and rheumatologic disorders that can be assessed with ultrasonographic imaging include traumatic, metabolic, degenerative, infectious, and neoplastic processes.

## INTRODUCTION

The ability of ultrasonography to evaluate the musculoskeletal system has increased dramatically with the development of high-frequency linear array real-time transducers, coupled with significant technologic advances that have improved image resolution. This group of devices shares the common characteristics of excellent near-field resolution, electronic focusing, and very high transducer frequency (5 to 15 MHz). These qualities are especially important when imaging tendons and muscles, which are often superficial and whose internal architecture gives rise to a unique appearance on ultrasonography. Further, improvements in color-flow sensitivity allow the demonstration of alterations in blood flow associated with a variety of inflammatory, neoplastic, and traumatic disorders. Although the role of ultrasonography in diagnosing problems related to bones, joints, and soft tissues is somewhat limited compared with that of CT or MR imaging, the technique offers significant information in an increasing number of situations and usually involves less discomfort, risk, cost, and time than alternative radiographic or isotopic procedures. In addition, the real-time nature of this technology enables the performance of provocative maneuvers, as well as visualization during interventional procedures involving the soft tissues.

## CLINICAL USE IN BONE, JOINT, AND SOFT TISSUE DISEASES

### Popliteal Space

The use of ultrasonography to evaluate various swellings in the popliteal space gained early acceptance. Because the fluid-solid distinction was easily accomplished even by early instruments, and because popliteal cysts and popliteal artery aneurysms constitute the majority of masses in this area, sonography has frequently been used to diagnose these lesions.

Popliteal cysts (Baker's cysts) arise in knee joints that have a communication between the knee joint and the gastrocnemiosemimembranosus bursa, as well as an intra-articular abnormality that produces an effusion capable of distending the joint. The gastrocnemiosemimembranosus bursa is situated between the medial head of the gastrocnemius muscle and the semimembranosus muscle more laterally. An anatomic connection between the bursa and the knee joint is present in about 50% of normal persons. Joint effusion can be a response to a number of abnormalities of the knee. As a component in the genesis of popliteal cysts, effusions are most often related to the synovial proliferation of rheumatoid arthritis or to traumatic internal derangements of the knee joint. Indeed, such cysts can develop as a complication of any disorder of the knee that leads to elevation of intra-articular pressure.

Classically, a simple Baker's cyst appears as a focal, hypoechoic, smooth-walled cystic mass located between the tendons of the medial head of the gastrocnemius and semimembranosus muscles. A superior extension, or neck, of the fluid collection that confirms communication with the knee is an important diagnostic feature. Variable amounts of septation, debris, or pannus may be seen within the cyst. Color Doppler sonography may be helpful in differentiating cysts from popliteal artery aneurysms, which are located more centrally within the popliteal fossa. The size threshold for sonographic identification of popliteal cysts is less than 1 cm.

Rupture of a popliteal cyst or hemorrhage into the cyst can lead to a clinical picture that closely mimics deep venous thrombophlebitis. Compression of the popliteal vein by the cyst can also produce physical signs resembling thrombophlebitis. Loss of normal sharp margins along the inferior aspect of the cyst (Fig. 6–1) and superficial fluid spaces with surrounding edema are the most common findings associated with rupture. Such edema may be identified in the medial head of the gastrocnemius muscle, and fluid may track proximally or distally along soft tissue planes; smaller daughter cysts may be evident. However, sonography may fail to detect some ruptured cysts that have completely decompressed.

Ultrasonography may also be helpful in cases in which the synovial membrane herniates through a weakened posterior capsule of the knee joint. This probably occurs

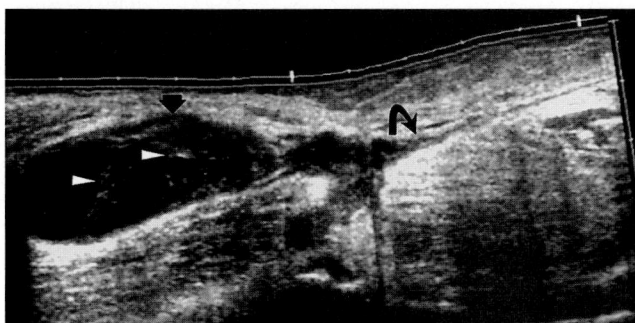

**Figure 6–1.** Synovial (popliteal) cyst with rupture. A longitudinal view of the posterior aspect of the knee shows a popliteal cyst *(straight black arrow)* with internal septations *(arrowheads)* and an irregular inferior tail *(curved arrow)*, the last finding consistent with a recent rupture.

in persons who lack anatomic communication between the joint space and the gastrocnemiosemimembranosus bursa; when rupture occurs, a pseudocapsule forms to contain fluid. Most often, these collections are located between the gastrocnemius and soleus muscles.

Not every swelling in this area is the result of a popliteal cyst, and sonography can conveniently exclude other causes, such as a popliteal artery aneurysm (Fig. 6–2), soft tissue tumor, or abscess. Aneurysms of the popliteal artery are the most common of the peripheral arterial aneurysms. Atheromatous disease is causative in the vast majority of cases, and a significant number of patients have coexisting cardiovascular disease, including an abdominal aortic aneurysm. The lesions are bilateral in

up to 59% of cases, although involvement of only one side may be evident clinically. Popliteal artery aneurysms are commonly associated with thromboembolic complications, including thrombosis, venous occlusion, ulceration, gangrene, and peripheral embolization. The ultrasonographic diagnosis of a popliteal artery aneurysm is relatively straightforward, as long as continuity of the mass with a proximal and a distal vessel can be ascertained. Angiography, the traditional method for diagnosing and evaluating popliteal artery aneurysms, is not necessary. In addition, arteriography has several limitations that are overcome by ultrasonography. For example, thrombus within an aneurysm is easily documented by sonography but is not well seen with arteriography, which opacifies only the patent lumen carrying flowing blood. Thrombus is considered by some clinicians to be an indication for surgery. Clinical diagnosis is not always straightforward, however, such as when pulsation is absent because of a thrombosed aneurysm.

## Knee

The role of ultrasonography in evaluating the knee has been diminished by MR imaging. However, sonography may be helpful in evaluating specific problems. For example, joint fluid, or an effusion, in the knee is easily detected by ultrasonography. Anechoic or hypoechoic fluid is identified in the suprapatellar recess, deep to the quadriceps musculature, and in the medial and lateral joint recesses as well. Intra-articular cartilaginous or osteocartilaginous bodies appear as echogenic foci.

Investigations have centered on the sonographic evaluation of cartilage (Fig. 6–3). In a series of patients with osteoarthritis, ultrasonography was shown to be capable of measuring the thickness of articular cartilage and assess-

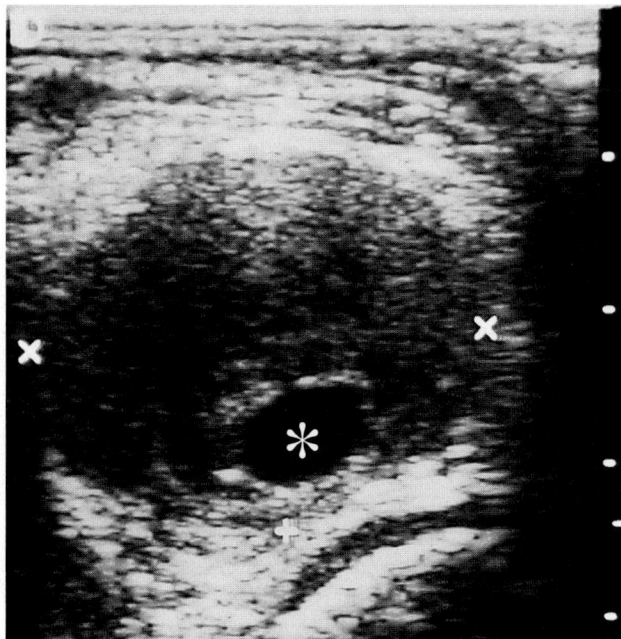

**Figure 6–2.** Popliteal artery aneurysm, presenting as a soft tissue mass. Transaxial image of the popliteal fossa shows a 3-cm popliteal artery aneurysm. Significant thrombus surrounds a residual central lumen *(asterisk).*

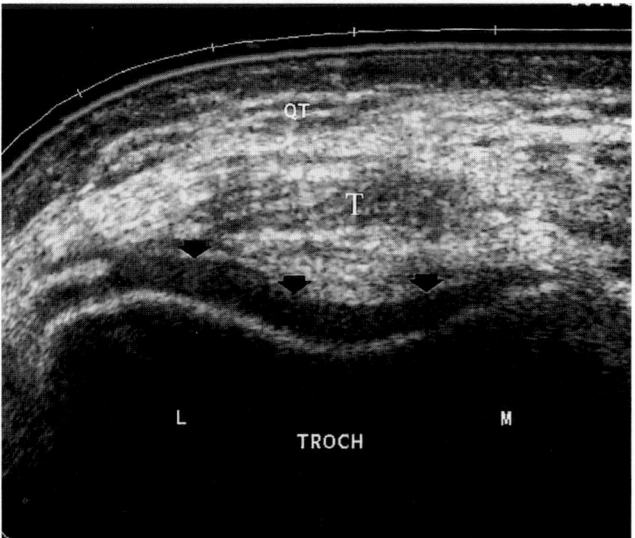

**Figure 6–3.** Articular cartilage. This is a transverse extended field of view of the trochlear cartilage. Note the medial (M) and lateral (L) femoral condyles and the homogeneously hypoechoic articular cartilage of the trochlea (TROCH) *(arrows).* The anterior quadriceps mechanism (QT) and tendon (T) are labeled.

ing its surface characteristics. However, with increasing severity of disease, the sharp interface between cartilage and soft tissue is blurred, making measurement of cartilage thickness more difficult.

Real-time ultrasonography is capable of showing portions of the medial and lateral menisci (Fig. 6–4). The normal meniscus appears as a triangular hyperechoic structure; it is often easier to identify when there is a degree of cartilage loss in the femorotibial compartments and associated peripheral displacement of the meniscus. Meniscal tears are visualized as hypoechoic linear defects within this structure. Vertical concentric tears as small as 2 mm and horizontal tears as small as 4 mm have been seen consistently in vitro. The clinical utility of this technique has not been evaluated systematically, however. Meniscal cysts are a common cause of masses in locations that are atypical for simple popliteal cysts. Such cysts are most common in the lateral meniscus, and the vast majority are associated with tears of the menisci. Because of tightly adherent medial collateral ligaments, medial cysts may lie at some distance from the meniscus, whereas lateral cysts are usually found adjacent to the underlying meniscal lesion. Meniscal cysts are easily identified sonographically as fluid-containing spaces superficial to the menisci and collateral ligaments (Fig. 6–5).

The collateral ligaments of the knee can also be visualized with ultrasonography (Fig. 6–6). In common with other ligaments, these collateral ligaments appear as homogeneous, hyperechoic linear bands of tissue. Disruption of the uniform, compact fibrillar pattern indicates an injury.

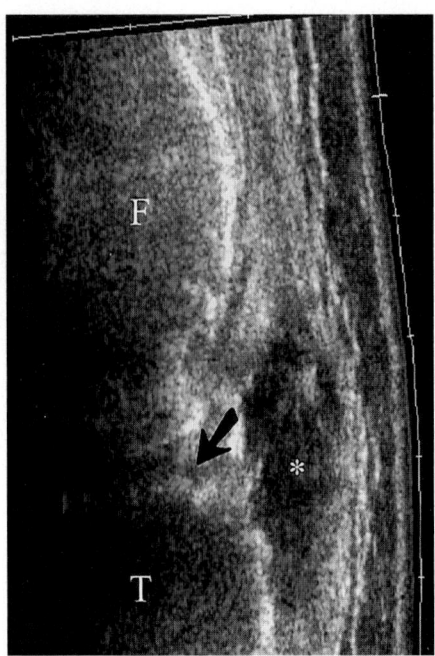

**Figure 6–5.** Meniscal cyst. Longitudinal view of the lateral aspect of the knee demonstrating a horizontal cleavage tear through the lateral meniscus *(arrow)* extending into a meniscal cyst *(asterisk)*. Note the lateral femoral condyle (F) and the lateral tibial plateau (T).

## Patellar Tendon

Jumper's knee, a term describing a group of conditions that commonly cause extra-articular knee pain, is seen in persons whose activities involve frequent, vigorous use of the extensor mechanism of the knee. Athletic activities that include repetitive jumping, running, or kicking are implicated most often. Rather than being the result of a primary inflammatory lesion, jumper's knee is thought to be caused by multiple partial fiber tears of the patellar tendon that lead to degeneration, necrosis, or fibrosis.

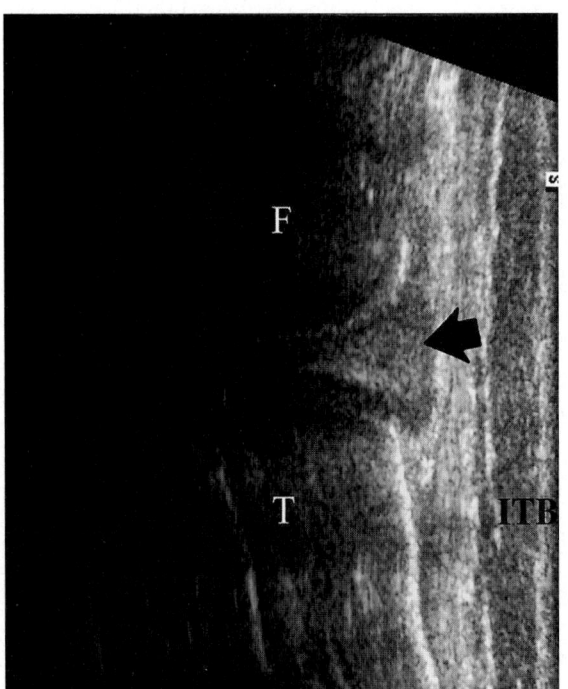

**Figure 6–4.** Menisci of the knee. A longitudinal scan of the lateral meniscus shows the lateral femoral condyle (F) and the lateral tibial plateau (T), as well as the overlying iliotibial band (ITB). The normal lateral meniscus is seen as triangular homogeneously hyperechoic tissue *(black arrow)*.

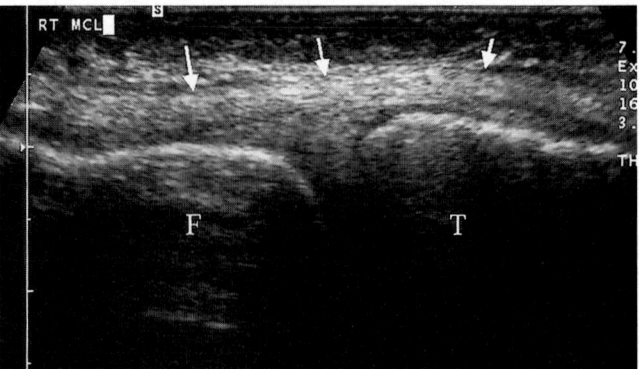

**Figure 6–6.** Collateral ligaments of the knee. A longitudinal image along the medial joint line of the knee demonstrates a normal, homogeneously hyperechoic medial collateral ligament *(arrows)*. Note the medial femoral condyle (F) and the medial tibial plateau (T).

When scanned longitudinally, the normal patellar tendon is visualized as a linear structure of medium echogenicity, approximately 3 to 6 mm thick, located deep to more echogenic subcutaneous fat and the hypoechoic serous pretibial bursa. Deep to the tendon, a second anechoic bursa may be seen. The internal architecture is similar to that of other tendons, with parallel echogenic fibers and homogeneous density (Fig. 6–7). Seventy-seven percent to 90% of abnormalities in patellar tendinosis are visualized at the proximal attachment of the tendon. In early stages of disease, the tendon appears enlarged as a result of edema. If the degenerative process continues, the tendon becomes heterogeneous in its internal architecture, with areas of central hypoechogenicity being the most common sonographic finding, although hyperechoic foci may occasionally be seen.

## Hip

Ultrasonography can be used as a screening procedure to document the presence of intra-articular fluid. In both children and adults, distention of the joint capsule is identified most readily in scans oriented along the long axis of the femoral neck. Ultrasonography can be used to characterize the joint effusion as simple or as containing particulate debris; the latter is suggestive of inflammation, infection, or hemorrhage. Abscess, hematoma, cellulitis, thrombophlebitis, aneurysm, and lymphadenopathy can manifest in nonspecific and overlapping ways. Sonography can often differentiate among these conditions and, if necessary, is a convenient method of guiding percutaneous aspiration or biopsy of possibly abnormal areas. Ultrasonography can also identify fluid collections within the iliopsoas bursa, which are often associated with the synovitis that accompanies many arthritides. In addition, ultrasonography has an important role in the diagnosis of developmental dysplasia of the hip (see Chapter 73).

## Shoulder

Numerous reports using high-resolution linear array realtime ultrasonography have demonstrated that sonography is an alternative means of examining the rotator cuff. Meticulous technique is critical, and examination of the tendons in two orthogonal planes is required whenever possible. Criteria for the diagnosis of rotator cuff tears can be categorized into four groups: (1) nonvisualization of the cuff, (2) localized absence or focal nonvisualization, (3) discontinuity, and (4) focal abnormal echogenicity. No cuff tendon is visualized in patients with large or massive rotator cuff tears.

Joint and bursal effusions commonly accompany large tears and are seen along the biceps tendon and lateral to the greater tuberosity, respectively. Large tears of the supraspinatus tendon may extend posteriorly to involve the infraspinatus tendon or anteriorly to involve the biceps tendon and the subscapularis tendon. Smaller fullthickness tears (Fig. 6–8) appear as a localized absence of the cuff with the subdeltoid bursa touching the humeral surface. The most common location of such smaller tears is the anterolateral portion of the supraspinatus tendon in the "critical zone." Even smaller tears appear as a discontinuity of the cuff filled with hypoechoic joint fluid or hyperechoic reactive tissue highlighting the defect (Fig. 6–9).

Abnormalities of cuff echogenicity may be diffuse or focal. Diffuse abnormality of cuff echogenicity is an unreliable sonographic sign for cuff tear but may indicate diffuse cuff degeneration or fibrosis. Although diffuse abnormality of cuff echogenicity is unreliable in the detection of full-thickness tears, significant disparity of cuff thickness suggests cuff attrition. Significant degrees of cuff attrition are associated with partial-thickness tears and also suggest that progressive cuff changes are present. In addition to the major criteria just described, several minor sonographic findings may prove helpful; subdeltoid bursal effusion, concavity of the subdeltoid bursal contour, elevation of the humeral head relative to the acromion, and obliteration of the space normally occupied by the supraspinatus tendon are all associated with defects in the cuff.

Sonography also plays an important role in the evaluation of patients who have had acromioplasty, and especially those who have had surgical repair of a full-thickness

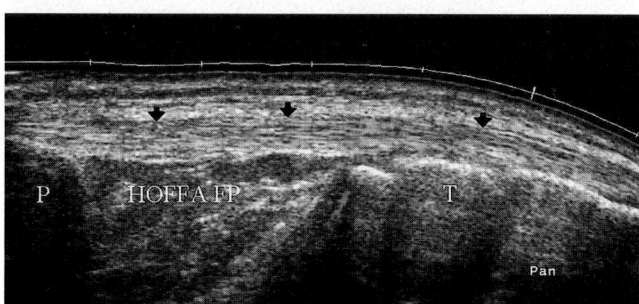

**Figure 6–7.** Patellar tendon. A longitudinal extended field of view of a normal patellar tendon shows a well-defined hyperechoic tendon with a fine intrasubstance fibrillar pattern *(arrows)*. Note the infrapatellar fat pad (Hoffa's FP), the inferior pole of the patella (P), and the tibial tubercle (T).

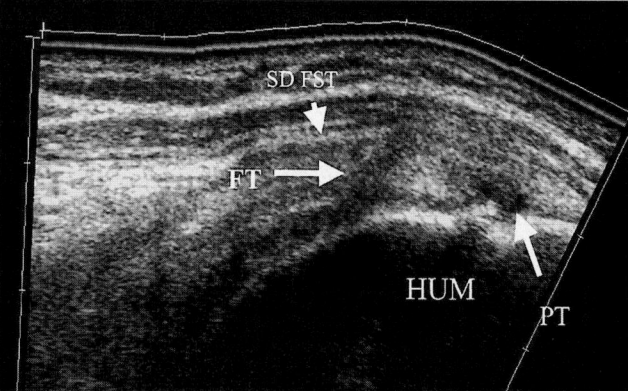

**Figure 6–8.** Rotator cuff tear. A longitudinal view of the supraspinatus tendon demonstrates a focal full-thickness tear (FT) with tendon discontinuity, as well as a partial articular surface tear (PT) near the site of the tendon attachment. Note the mild inferior migration of the subdeltoid fat strip (SD FST) into the defect. HUM, humerus.

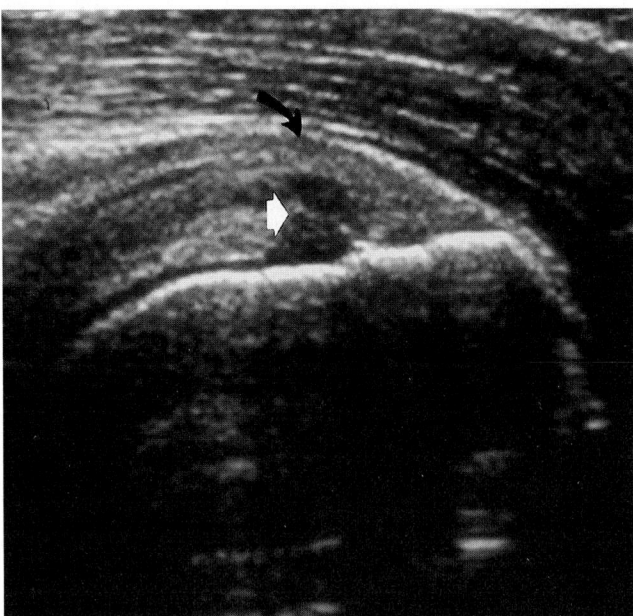

**Figure 6–9.** Rotator cuff tear. A longitudinal view of the infraspinatus tendon shows a discrete irregular hypoechoic focus at the articular margin *(white arrow)*, consistent with a partial articular surface tear. Note the intact superficial fibers *(curved arrow)*.

tear (Fig. 6–10). Postoperatively, the tendons of the cuff, especially the supraspinatus, are often echogenic and thinned when compared with those in the contralateral normal shoulder.

## Ankle and Foot

Because of its superficial location, clinical examination of the Achilles tendon is often sufficient to diagnose acute disruption. The Achilles tendon is best examined with the patient prone and the feet extending beyond the

table. Use of an acoustic standoff helps compensate for the geometry of the region. The normal tendon appears in longitudinal section as a superficial, hyperechoic structure surrounded by the echogenic paratenon. In transverse section, the tendon is elliptic in shape, with broadening in its more caudal aspects. Deep to the tendon, the pre-Achilles fat pad is visualized as an area of low heterogeneous echogenicity. Superficial to the tendon at its insertion in the calcaneus, the superficial bursa may be observed when distended by fluid but not when normal.

Complete rupture of the Achilles tendon appears as discontinuity with retraction of the upper fragment, small amounts of adjacent fluid, and an echogenic clot in the tear. Partial tears have been described as hypoechoic areas within the tendon or as heterogeneous tendon echogenicity (Fig. 6–11). The sonographic appearance of tendinosis is more controversial; however, the thicker the Achilles tendon appears, the more likely is the diagnosis of tendinosis.

In patients with heterozygous familial hypercholesterolemia, the Achilles tendon is the most common location for xanthomas. These lesions appear as thickening of the tendon, with a decrease in overall echogenicity. Focal areas of heterogeneous echogenicity may also be seen. The Achilles tendon is but one of the many tendons about the ankle and foot that can be evaluated with ultrasonography. Ganglion cysts, plantar fasciitis, and Morton's neuromas can also be investigated with sonography.

## Hand, Wrist, and Elbow

The sonographic features of masses of the hand and fingers, including ganglion cysts, angiomas, and glomus tumors, have been described. Ganglion cysts are anechoic or hypoechoic; angiomas are minimally hyperechoic; and the remainder of focal masses are often hypoechoic. Inflammatory abnormalities, including foreign bodies and tenosynovitis, can be visualized with ultrasonography. Sonography has also been used in the evaluation of carpal tunnel syndrome and ganglia.

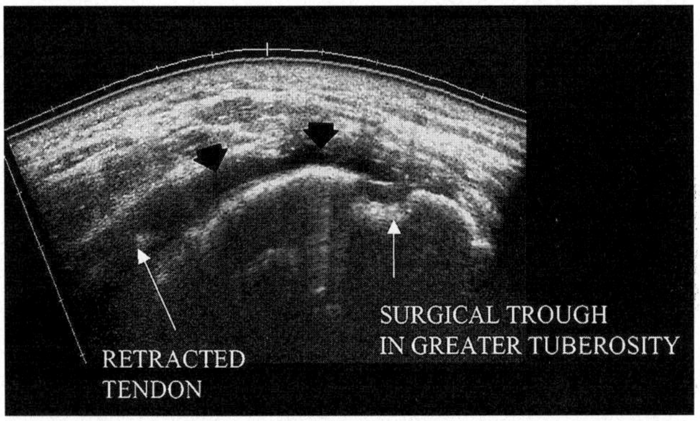

**Figure 6–10.** Rotator cuff retear following surgery. Ultrasonography can be used to evaluate a possible retear after rotator cuff repair. This long axis view of the supraspinatus tendon in a patient who had a rotator cuff repair clearly demonstrates the surgical trough in the greater tuberosity, as well as the retracted tendon edge. Note the large region of tendon discontinuity at the site of repair *(black arrows)*.

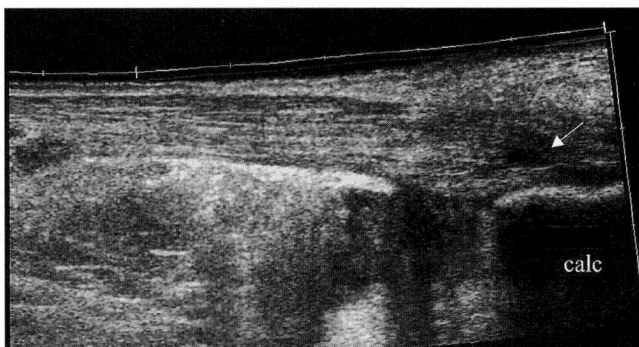

**Figure 6–11.** Achilles tendinosis and tendon tear. A longitudinal extended field of view demonstrates an enlarged, ill-defined Achilles tendon with decreased echogenicity, consistent with underlying tendinosis, as well as a superimposed deep-surface partial tear *(arrow)* near its attachment to the calcaneus (calc).

Ganglia, which are the most common soft tissue masses in this region, are seen as well-marginated, multiloculated, hypoechoic lesions that are easily differentiated from other abnormalities such as lipomas or aneurysms.

Newer applications in infants and children, including delineation of transphyseal fractures and other occult fractures, joint effusions, and cellulitis, have been described (Fig. 6–12). Characteristic findings in lateral epicondylitis ("tennis elbow") include hypoechoic extratendinous collections in muscle tears, fluid collections adjacent to the extensor carpi radialis brevis, bursitis, alterations of tendon echogenicity and size, enthesopathy, and tendinosis.

Neurovascular structures, especially the ulnar nerve, can also be assessed with ultrasonography. Normally, the ulnar nerve is located in the cubital tunnel and, in the longitudinal plane, contains linear hyperechoic strands. Focal enlargement of the nerve and decreased echogenicity are typical of neuritis, and subluxation of the ulnar nerve can be promoted when provocative positions of the elbow are used.

## Tumors of Bone and Soft Tissue

Although sonography easily catalogs mass lesions into cystic or solid groupings, little histologic specificity is obtained from the sonographic appearance alone. In fact, strict adherence to usually reliable sonographic criteria can result in interpretive errors. Soft tissue tumors of neural or nerve sheath origin can mimic the findings classically associated with cystic lesions, even though these are solid neoplasms. Fatty tissue is often, although not invariably, extremely echogenic, and lipomatous

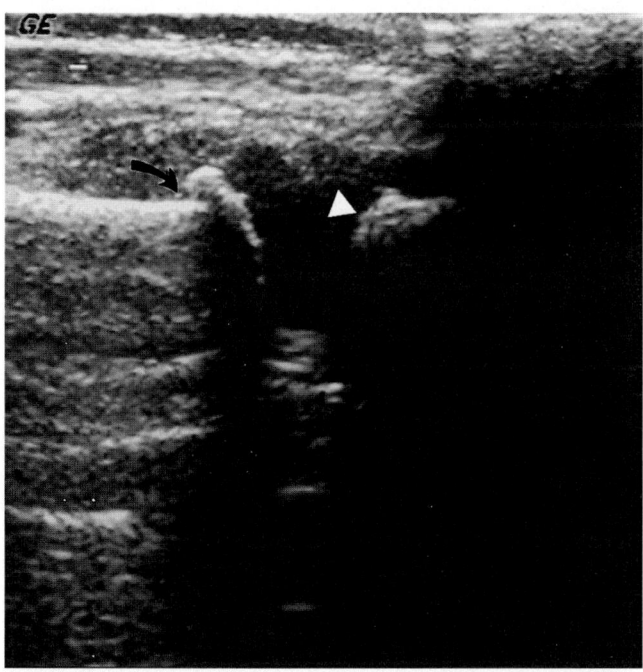

**Figure 6–12.** Fracture of the radial head. A lateral image of the radiocapitellar joint in a child reveals focal cortical irregularity and impaction of the radial head with overriding fragments, consistent with a fracture *(curved arrow)*. Note that the radial head articulates normally with the capitulum *(arrowhead)*.

tumors can appear quite hyperechoic. Neoplasms of lymphatic origin typically contain extensive cystic areas. Highly vascular tumors (e.g., hemangiomas) can also have numerous fluid regions. Color Doppler imaging may be helpful in defining vascular anatomy as well as in confirming the solid nature of such lesions.

Ultrasonography has negligible success in visualizing intraosseous structures, and its role in this setting is limited. However, this technique may be helpful in the evaluation of cartilage-bone relationships in cases of osteochondroma (see Chapter 70).

## Infections of Bone and Soft Tissue

Sonographic features of soft tissue abscesses vary considerably. A typical abscess contains predominantly fluid but frequently has debris that is manifested as fine, low-level echoes within the cystic mass. This material sometimes accumulates in the dependent portion of the abscess, a phenomenon that can be documented by changing the patient's position. The margins of an abscess are usually indistinct, in contrast to those of a simple cyst. The anechoic or hypoechoic regions are often surrounded by regions of increased echogenicity, representing adjacent soft tissue edema. Many abscesses, notably chronic or partially treated lesions, are complex in appearance and can be difficult to distinguish from surrounding soft tissue. Gas-containing abscesses can be quite echogenic on sonograms, an appearance thought to result from the numerous highly reflective interfaces engendered by "microbubbles."

Characteristic sonographic findings have been described in osteomyelitis. Although such infections typically begin in the medullary region of bone, they rapidly progress to involve adjacent soft tissues. Visualization of anechoic fluid collections adjacent to bone is considered highly suggestive of osteomyelitis. Elevation of the periosteum may also be observed, and periosteal elevation of greater than 2 mm is typically associated with subperiosteal pus.

## Foreign Bodies

Sonographic detection of foreign bodies depends on differences in acoustic impedance between adjacent tissues and the foreign body (Fig. 6–13). Because all reported foreign bodies are hyperechoic, they are best visualized in slightly hypoechoic tissues such as subcutaneous fat, muscle, or inflammatory tissue. The foreign body itself is usually echogenic and, if embedded in a tendon, can be difficult to visualize. The foreign body, however, often incites an adjacent inflammatory reaction with vascular granulation tissue, which forms a hypoechoic rim about the hyperechoic foreign body, increasing its conspicuity. Some degradable foreign bodies (e.g., wood) may decrease in echogenicity over time and may disappear within an inflammatory collection.

## Spine

Occult spinal dysraphism in infants can be evaluated with sonography. In about half of the children affected, the spinal defect is signaled by a cutaneous marker, such as

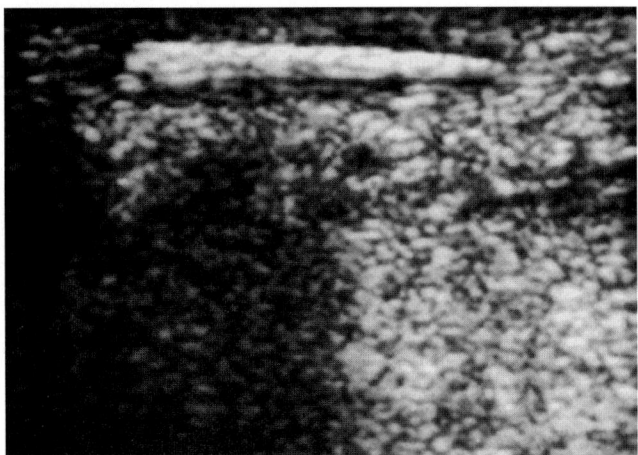

**Figure 6–13.** Foreign body. Scan of the foot demonstrates a foreign body as hyperechoic compared with adjacent soft tissue. The plain film results were negative. A splinter was removed with sonographic localization.

hairy nevi, hemangiomas, or sinus tracts. Children at risk can be screened with sonography for cord tethering, because in the first year of life, ossification of the posterior elements of the spine is incomplete. This provides a window for scanning from a posterior approach. The spinal cord and abnormalities affecting it can be imaged with striking clarity.

### Intraoperative Spinal Sonography

With appropriate care to maintain sterile conditions, many real-time sonographic systems can be adapted for use in the operating room, and instruments now exist that are designed specifically for this purpose. One of the major advantages of sonography is delineation of the extent of a particular problem before opening the dura, which reduces the time and risk of a surgical procedure. Also, processes anterior to the spinal cord—an area that normally cannot be seen without manipulation of the cord—can be identified easily. Localization and drainage of an intramedullary cyst or syrinx, whether idiopathic or related to trauma or an adjacent neoplasm, are relatively straightforward with ultrasonic guidance. The effectiveness of decompression can be assessed before the operation is terminated. Additional applications of intraoperative spinal sonography include the evaluation of patients with trauma; for the identification of bone fragments, foreign bodies, and cord compression; as well as determination of spinal alignment.

### Metabolic Disease

The parathyroid glands are intimately involved in calcium homeostasis and therefore exert considerable influence on bone metabolism. It is the parathyroid glands themselves, however, rather than the osseous changes, that are of interest to sonographers. Normal parathyroid glands measure approximately 3 by 4 by 5 mm, and until the advent of high-resolution, real-time sonography, they could not be imaged. Parathyroid gland enlargement is

important for diagnosis and management, and ultrasonography is now accepted as the procedure of choice. Accuracy rates of approximately 90% have been reported from several centers. Should sonography fail to confirm parathyroid gland enlargement in the neck, CT scanning, MR imaging, or thallium-technetium scans may be useful. Approximately 5% of the population harbors ectopic parathyroid tissue, which is usually situated in the superior mediastinum along the embryologic pathway of thymic descent.

### Hemophilia and Altered Coagulability States

The relative ease with which ultrasonography detects fluid collections such as hematomas makes it an attractive method for evaluating patients with hemophilia and altered coagulability states. Sonography has proved efficacious in this clinical setting, both in diagnosing areas of hemorrhage and in monitoring the natural history of the bleeding. Rectus sheath hematoma is a specific clinical entity that is misdiagnosed in as many as 60% of cases. Signs and symptoms often mimic those of acute abdominal or pelvic conditions, such as intestinal obstruction or hernia, twisted ovarian cyst, or perivesicular inflammatory disease. The sonographic appearance of a rectus sheath hematoma is characteristic and consists of an ellipsoid or spindle-shaped fluid collection in the superficial anterior abdominal wall. The tight boundaries of the rectus sheath confine the bleeding, and the process does not cross the midline unless it occurs low, where the posterior portion of the sheath is deficient.

Iliopsoas hematoma is a common complication of hemophilia. A somewhat typical syndrome of pain and nerve deficit occurs, with bleeding isolated to the closed iliacus compartment that contains the femoral nerve. The psoas fascia is looser and allows more extensive hemorrhage to take place. When this occurs on the right side, differentiation from acute appendicitis may be difficult clinically. Sonography is capable of detecting hemorrhage in both of these muscle compartments.

Depending on the age and chronicity of the hemorrhage, hematomas display a spectrum of appearances on gray-scale sonograms. When fresh and composed of liquid blood, a hematoma is homogeneous and appears virtually echo free. Internal echoes appear when a clot begins to organize and then fragment, resulting in a more complex sonographic appearance. Liquefaction of a clot may then lead once again to a variable fluid pattern on sonography. Considerable overlap exists, with similar features demonstrated, for example, by abscesses or tumors.

### Interventional Ultrasonography

As noted earlier, ultrasonography can be used as a supplementary method in the treatment of a variety of disorders that affect the musculoskeletal system. Therapeutic injections of tendon sheaths, bursae, ganglion cysts, and joints can be performed under sonographic guidance. Similar injections in cases of plantar fasciitis, calcific tendinitis, and interdigital neuromas can also be monitored with ultrasonography, and synovial biopsies and abscess aspirations may require such monitoring.

# FURTHER READING

Craig J: Infection: Ultrasound-guided procedures. Radiol Clin North Am 37:669, 1999.

Harcke HT, Grisson LE, Finkelstein MS: Evaluation of the musculoskeletal system with sonography. AJR 150:1253, 1988.

Kaftori JK, Rosenberger A, Pollack S, et al: Rectus sheath hematoma: Ultrasonographic diagnosis. AJR 128:283, 1977.

Kottle SP, Gonzalez AC, Macon EJ, et al: Ultrasonographic evaluation of vascular access complications. Radiology 129:751, 1978.

Little CM, Parker MG, Callowich MC, et al: The ultrasonic detection of soft tissue foreign bodies. Invest Radiol 21:275, 1986.

Loyer EM, DuBrow RA, David CL, et al: Imaging of soft-tissue infections: Sonographic findings in cases of cellulitis and abscess. AJR Am J Roentgenol 166:149, 1996.

Mack LA, Matsen FA, Kilcoyne RF, et al: US evaluation of the rotator cuff. Radiology 157:205, 1985.

McDonald DG, Leopold GR: Ultrasound B-scanning in the differentiation of Baker's cyst and thrombophlebitis. BR J Radiol 45:729, 1972.

Novick G, Ghelman B, Schneider M: Sonography of the neonatal and infant hip. AJR 141:639, 1983.

Scheible W, James HE, Leopold GR, et al: Occult spinal dysraphism in infants: Screening with high-resolution real-time ultrasound. Radiology 146:743: 1983.

Shiels WE II, Babcock DS, Wilson JL, et al: Localization and gided removal of soft-tissue foreign bodies with sonography. AJR 155:1277, 1990.

Shirkhoda A, Mauro MA, Staab EV, et al: Soft tissue hemorrhage in hemorrhage in hemophiliac patients: Computed tomography and ultrasound study. Radiology 147:811, 1983.

Silver TM, Washburn RL, Stanley JC, et al: Gray scale ultrasound evaluation of popliteal artery aneurysms. AJR 129:1003, 1977.

Sofka CM, Collins AJ, Adler RS: Utilization of ultrasound guidance in interventional musculoskeletal procedures. J Ultrasound Med 19:62, 2000.

Teefey SA, Hasan SA, Middleton WD, et al: Ultrasonography of the rotator cuff: A comparison of ultrasonographic and arthroscopic findings in one hundred consecutive cases. J Bone Joint Surg Am 82:498, 2000.

Weiner SN, Seitz WH: Sonography of the shoulder in patients with tears of the rotator cuff: Accuracy and value for selecting surgical options. AJR 160:103, 1993.

# CHAPTER 7

## Radionuclide Techniques

### Robert Schneider

## SUMMARY OF KEY FEATURES

This chapter contains a survey of the imaging and therapeutic aspects of various radionuclide methods. Despite the availability of many other imaging techniques, the importance of radionuclide examinations remains unchallenged.

## INTRODUCTION

Radioactive materials are used for diagnosis, therapy, and research in musculoskeletal disease. Initially, after the discovery of radioactivity, radioactive materials were used in musculoskeletal disease mainly for treatment. Later, radioactive materials were used for research in bone metabolism and various bony abnormalities, which eventually led to widespread clinical use in diagnosis.

## RADIOPHARMACEUTICALS

In nuclear medicine, the terms *radionuclide, radioisotope, radiopharmaceutical,* and *radiotracer* are often used synonymously for the radioactive materials used. Isotopes are atoms with the same atomic number, but different atomic weights. A nuclide is the nucleus of a particular isotope, characterized by its atomic number and atomic weight. Nuclides or isotopes with significant differences in the number of protons and neutrons tend to be unstable and give off particles (alpha or beta) or electromagnetic radiation (gamma rays) in a transition toward stability (radioactive decay). Those nuclides and isotopes that undergo radioactive decay are called radionuclides and radioisotopes. Radiopharmaceuticals and radiotracers are radionuclides or radioisotopes that are used alone or combined with other materials for diagnosis, therapy, or research.

Diagnostic imaging in nuclear medicine depends on gamma radiation. Beta radiation is used in therapy and in autoradiography for research. The intensity of the radioactivity is determined by the number of nuclear transitions per unit time. Historically, radioactive intensity was expressed in curies (Ci). One curie equals $3.7 \times 10^{10}$ transitions per second. A newer terminology for radioactive intensity, the becquerel (Bq), is now used. One becquerel is equal to one transition per second. The intensity of the radiopharmaceuticals used in nuclear medicine is usually stated as millicuries (mCi). One millicurie equals 37 megabecquerels (MBq). Radiation dose is measured in rads per millicurie or milligrays per megabecquerel. Radiation dose has to be considered in terms of the whole body dose and the dose to specific organs. The whole body dose for a bone scan with technetium-99m methylene diphosphonate ($^{99m}$Tc MDP) is 0.0065 rad/mCi, or about 0.13 to 0.19 rad for a scan. The greatest dose is to the bladder: 0.13 rad/mCi, or about 2.62 to 3.90 rads. The accumulation of radioactivity in the urine in the bladder is one of the reasons why the bladder should be emptied frequently during and after a scan.

## Use in Bone Scanning

Various isotopes of many different elements localize in bone. Fluorine-18 ($^{18}$F) has many excellent properties as a bone scanning agent. It has a high bone uptake at 50% to 60% of the dose—the highest among any of the bone scanning agents. It has a rapid soft tissue clearance through the kidneys. It decays by positron emission, producing gamma energy of 511 keV. It has a short half-life of 1.85 hours. It is relatively expensive due to its cyclotron production and short half-life. The energy of 511 keV is not ideal for a gamma camera, but relatively good counting efficiency can be obtained with rectilinear scanners. $^{18}$F has become an important radioisotope in nuclear medicine; it is used to tag fluorodeoxyglucose (FDG), a glucose analogue that measures metabolic activity, and is used in positron emission tomography (PET) scanning. $^{18}$F can be used alone for bone scanning by coincidence imaging with PET, producing high-quality tomographic images.

$^{99m}$Tc phosphonates are routinely used for bone scanning. $^{99m}$Tc is an ideal scanning agent because of its short physical half-life of 6 hours and gamma energy of 141 keV, which is ideal for a gamma camera. It decays by isomeric transition. It is readily available at low cost. The phosphonate scanning agent routinely used is MDP.

## Mechanism of Uptake

Blood flow to the bone is a necessary requirement for uptake of radiopharmaceuticals on a bone scan. If there is no blood flow to the bone, there will be no uptake, and a cold, or photopenic, area will be present. After injection, the radionuclide flows through the arteries and into the capillaries, with leakage into the extracapillary or extravascular space. In normal bone, the uptake is roughly proportional to the blood flow to the bone. However, in abnormal conditions, such as bony lesions or conditions accompanied by high bone vascularity, this is not the case, and uptake is not directly proportional to blood flow. Studies indicate that blood flow has an influence on bone uptake in bone scanning agents, but this influence is limited. Other factors intrinsic to the bone play a larger role in radionuclide uptake in areas of bony abnormalities.

The exact location in bone of $^{99m}$Tc phosphonates is controversial. For the interpretation of bone scans, it does not matter whether the uptake is in the bone mineral, bone matrix, or both. The most important factor in the uptake of bone-seeking radiopharmaceuticals is new bone formation. Bone destruction without new bone formation does not lead to increased uptake. Increased vascularity also plays a role. Increased blood pool in the extravascular space can be caused by increased capillary permeability. Increased capillary permeability may be due to infection, trauma, or neovascularity found in tumors. In the early phases of the bone scan, the blood flow and blood pool studies measure vascularity and capillary permeability, whereas the uptake on delayed static images obtained 2 or more hours after injection is determined by a combination of new bone formation and vascularity.

## Other Radiopharmaceuticals Used in Musculoskeletal Disease

Gallium-67 ($^{67}$Ga) is used for imaging infection and neoplasms. $^{67}$Ga has a physical half-life of 3.26 days. It binds to some of the iron-binding molecules, including transferrin, lactoferrin, ferritin, and siderophores, which may be important in its uptake in tumors and inflammatory lesions. In infection, increased vascular permeability allows leakage of gallium into the soft tissues, where it is bound to acid mucopolysaccharide. Accumulation in neutrophils may not play a major role. Shortly after injection, gallium is bound to serum proteins, mainly transferrin. About two-thirds remains in the body, and the rest is excreted by the kidney and bowel in about equal amounts. There is prominent uptake in the liver. Gallium in the bowel may interfere with interpretation of the scan. Gallium uptake varies with tumor type and has been used mostly in cases of lymphoma.

Indium-111 ($^{111}$In) is used to label white blood cells for imaging inflammation. It can also be used to label colloid for bone marrow imaging. It has a physical half-life of 2.83 days.

Fluorine-18 2-deoxy-2-fluoro-D-glucose is a scanning agent used with PET. The mechanism of uptake is that it acts like glucose and is transported into cells, where it is converted into FDG-6-phosphate and trapped. In tissues with low rates of dephosphorylation, such as tumors, the amount of uptake of FDG is proportional to the rate of glycolysis. Malignant tumors and other conditions such as inflammation with high metabolic activity have increased glycolysis and increased uptake of FDG. The more malignant the tumor and the more rapid its growth, the higher the rate of glycolysis.

Thallium-201 ($^{201}$Tl) is used in tumor imaging to help differentiate benign from malignant abnormalities and assess the results of therapy. It has a half-life of 3.05 days. It has biologic properties similar to those of potassium. Its uptake in tumors is related to perfusion and cellular metabolic activity. There is uptake in viable tumor and little uptake in necrotic tissue. $^{99m}$Tc methoxyisobutyl isonitrile (sestamibi, or MIBI) is used in a manner similar to that of thallium. It is taken up in the mitochondria of tumors, owing to differences in cell membrane gradient. Both radionuclides have been used in myocardial perfusion imaging, and they have been used in musculoskeletal scintigraphy to help differentiate benign from malignant

lesions and necrotic from viable malignant tumor tissue after therapy. High-grade malignant tumors have higher uptake than do low-grade malignant tumors or benign tumors.

## TECHNIQUES

Several guidelines or reviews of techniques for optimal bone scanning are available. Techniques may vary based on the available equipment or on the clinical situation.

Early-phase imaging (flow and blood pool) was originally emphasized for the diagnosis of infection; however, it also provides information about other abnormalities, including stress and traumatic fractures, tumors, reflex sympathetic dystrophy, synovitis, and arthritis. It helps in determining the chronicity of abnormalities, because increased vascularity returns to normal sooner than increased uptake evident on the delayed images. When pain is localized to a specific area, early-phase scanning should be done, especially for the appendicular skeleton, pelvis, and hips. Early-phase imaging is less useful in the spine, thorax, and skull. Another choice is between a whole body scan and a limited scan of one or more parts of the musculoskeletal system. A limited scan is less expensive and takes less time but may not show widespread abnormalities that are unsuspected. A whole body sweep, done with a moving table or moving camera, does not provide as good resolution as do individual spot scans (Fig. 7–1). In evaluating localized pain, spot scans are preferred. Another decision is whether a single photon emission computed tomography (SPECT) scan should be done. SPECT is most useful in the spine to detect stress fractures of the pars interarticularis (Fig. 7–2) and in a variety of other spinal abnormalities, as well as to detect avascular necrosis about the hips and knees.

There are few contraindications to bone scanning. Allergic reactions are extremely rare. Although bone scanning is not definitely contraindicated in pregnancy, the procedure should be deferred if not absolutely necessary. Breastfeeding should be discontinued for 24 hours after radionuclide injection. For adults, the injected dose of $^{99m}$Tc phosphonates is 20 to 30 mCi (740 to 1110 MBq). For children, the dose is 250 to 500 µCi/kg (9.25 to 18.5 MBq/kg). The patient should drink at least 16 ounces of fluid, preferably more, after the injection.

## NORMAL BONE SCAN

The appearance of a radionuclide bone scan depends on a variety of factors, including the size and age of the patient, degree of hydration, renal status, vascular sufficiency, medications used by the patient, equipment, and technique. Blood flow studies are intravenous radionuclide angiograms that show radionuclide in the arterial, capillary, and venous phases. Variations may occur in blood flow to the extremities, depending on the vascular status and activity. The blood pool scans show radionuclide in the extravascular space. Vascular structures such as kidneys, liver, spleen, and uterus are seen and should not be mistaken for sites of abnormality.

The delayed images obtained 2 to 4 hours after injection show radionuclide in the skeleton and soft tissue.

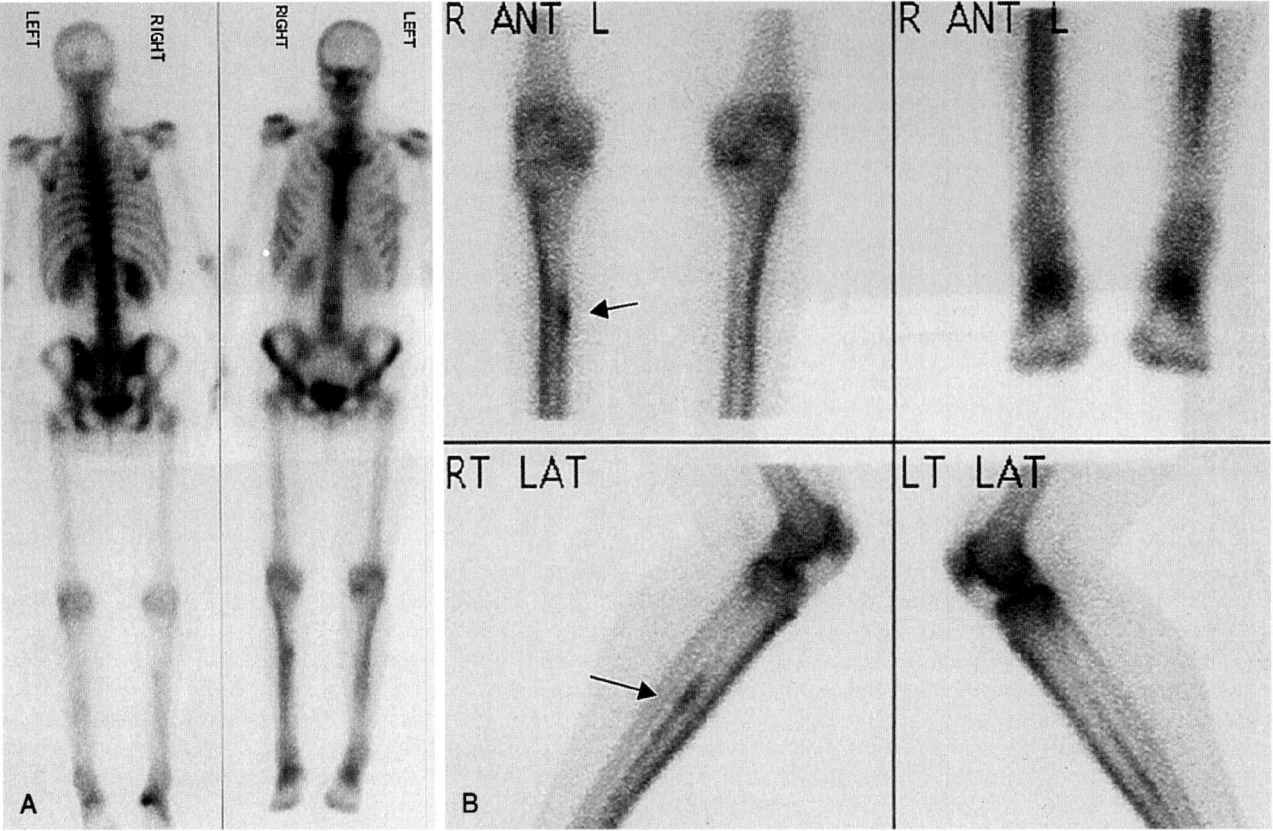

**Figure 7–1.** Comparison of resolution. Whole body sweep *(A)* does not show the increased uptake in the right tibia *(B, arrow)*, due to a stress reaction, as well as the spot scans of the lower legs do.

The metaphyseal regions of long bones show higher uptake than do the diaphyses, where only mild uptake is present. This is due to the higher bone turnover rate in the metaphyses. The areas of highest uptake in the normal bone scan are the sternum and the sacroiliac joints. The anterior wings of the iliac bones and the coracoid processes normally show considerable uptake of the radionuclide. The patellae may show higher uptake than the remainder of the bones about the knees, which may be due to their greater vascularity.

Uptake in calcification of the costal cartilage may be seen as areas of radionuclide accumulation on the anterior scan of the chest. Uptake may normally be present in the soft tissues of the breast. Hyperostosis frontalis interna causes increased uptake in both frontal bones and can be recognized by its characteristic pattern on anterior and lateral views. With scoliosis, the concave side of the spine appears hotter than the convex side does. Thoracic kyphosis and lumbar lordosis may cause some areas of the spine to be farther from the camera, and they will not appear as hot as areas that are closer to the spine.

The radionuclide is excreted through the kidneys, which normally should be visible. If no uptake is seen in the kidneys, either there is renal failure or absent kidneys or a superscan is present, characterized by such high uptake in bone that little radioactivity is excreted by the kidneys. Hydronephrosis may be detected by the appearance of a dilated ureter and renal collecting system. An accessory renal pelvis can accumulate considerable radionuclide and give a false appearance of hydronephrosis. Bladder diverticula or the lateral aspects of a normal bladder may overlie the pubic bones, giving a false appearance of lesions. Urine leakage may occur, producing hot spots that overlie the skeleton and simulate lesions. Unbound $^{99m}$Tc is taken up in the salivary glands, thyroid, and stomach. Thyroid and laryngeal cartilage uptake can be differentiated from abnormalities in the cervical spine, because they will be hotter on the anterior scan than on the posterior scan, whereas the reverse is true for cervical spine lesions. The tips of the scapulae may appear hot and overlie the ribs, simulating rib lesions. Views done with the scapulae raised and the arms brought across the chest may displace the scapulae from the ribs, eliminating this potential diagnostic problem.

The age of the patient may affect the appearance of the bone scan. Children have high, diffuse bone uptake and prominent uptake around the growth plates, owing to new bone formation in the growing skeleton. Elderly patients tend to have poor-quality bone scans. Heavy patients have poor-quality bone scans owing to the greater amount of soft tissue, which causes more scatter and higher attenuation of the photons in the soft tissues because of the greater distance of the detectors from the skeleton. Poor hydration prevents optimal clearance of the radionuclide from the soft tissues. Renal failure also prevents good soft tissue clearance.

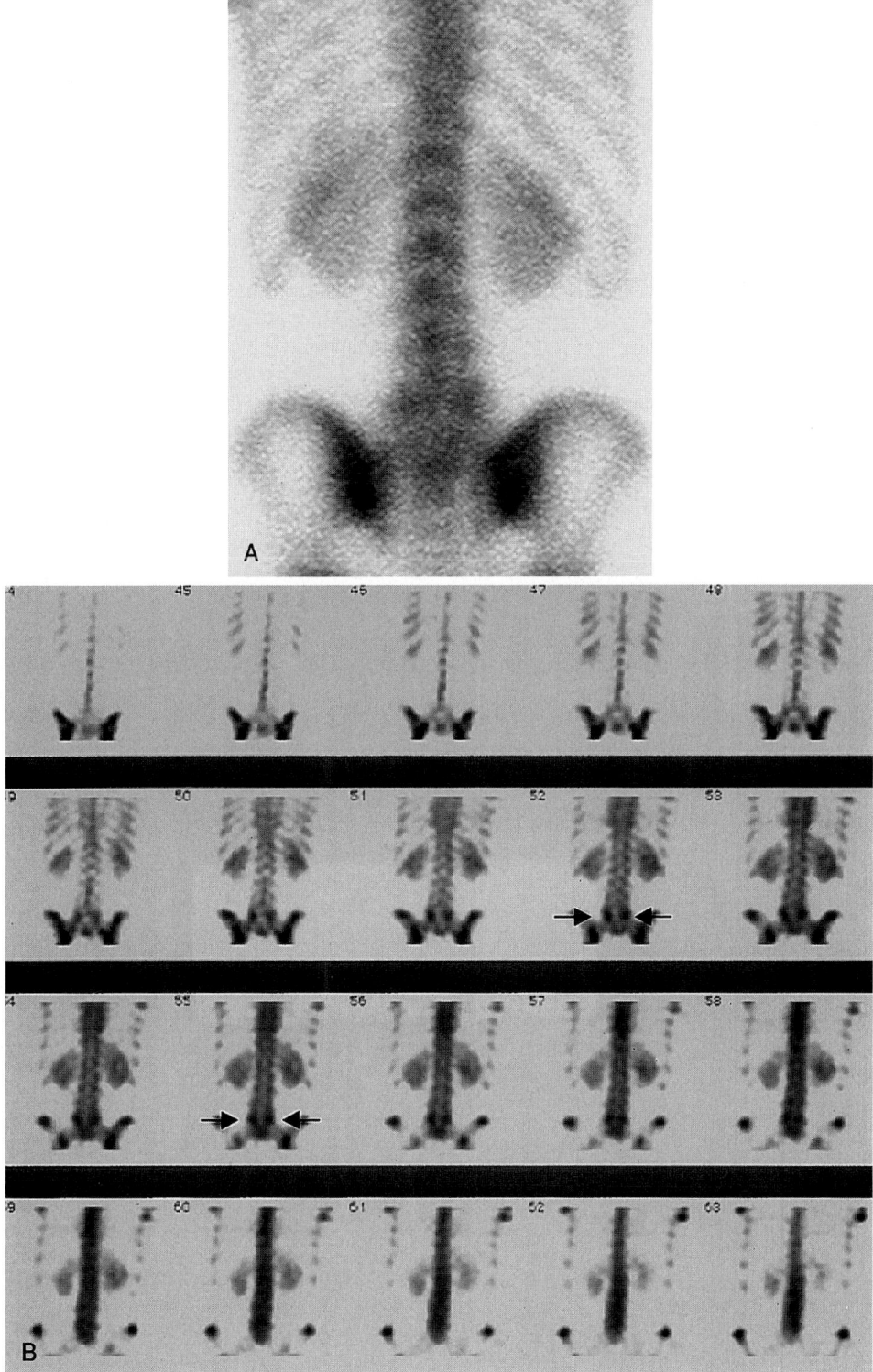

**Figure 7–2.** Stress fractures of the right and left pars of L5. On a posterior planar scan *(A)*, there is a suggestion of faint increased uptake in the posterior elements of L5, but the scan is not diagnostic. On a SPECT scan with coronal reconstructions *(B)*, hot spots are seen in the right and left pars of L5 *(arrows)*.

## METABOLIC BONE DISEASE

### High Bone Turnover Conditions

A number of conditions, including osteomalacia, hyperparathyroidism, and renal osteodystrophy, are frequently associated with increased bone turnover. Increased bone resorption by itself does not cause increased uptake on a radionuclide bone scan; however, such increased resorption is often accompanied by increased formation of bone, which does cause increased uptake. Multiple hot spots in adjacent ribs on both sides of the body in a patient with no history of trauma are suggestive of osteomalacia, as are hot spots in the inferior tips of the scapulae (Fig. 7–3). Insufficiency fractures in metabolic bone disease may also be seen in the pubic rami, femoral necks, femoral condyles, metaphyses of the proximal and distal portions of the tibia, sacrum, and calcaneus.

Bone scanning for detection of osteomalacia, renal osteodystrophy, and, to a lesser degree, primary hyperparathyroidism has been shown to be more sensitive than radiography. Bone scans in patients with osteoporosis do not show these metabolic features, except when accompanied by fractures. A flare response on the bone scan has been reported after treatment for osteomalacia. This response is most likely caused by increased osteoblastic activity due to bone healing and should not be mistaken for progressive disease. In patients with osteomalacia whose symptoms are not improved after 6 months or more of therapy, the possibility of oncogenic osteomalacia should be considered. The cause of this condition is thought to be production of a substance by an osseous

or soft tissue tumor that initiates biochemical change, causing osteomalacia. Most of these tumors are benign, fibrous, and highly vascular and include giant cell granulomas, cavernous hemangiomas, fibroangiomas, nonossifying fibromas, and, rarely, malignant tumors.

Secondary amyloidosis occurs in chronic renal failure, particularly when treated with hemodialysis. There is deposition of $\beta_2$-microglobulin amyloid in and around bones and joints, as well as in other locations. Increased uptake of $^{99m}$Tc phosphonates may occur in the articular and periarticular regions in some (but not all) cases of amyloid deposition, and this uptake may precede radiographic changes. Uptake of $^{67}$Ga and $^{201}$Tl may also be seen in the articular regions of patients with such amyloid deposition. Increased uptake of Tc phosphonates is present in the brown tumors of hyperparathyroidism and may mimic metastatic disease. $^{99m}$Tc sestamibi is often used to localize parathyroid adenomas and also shows increased uptake in brown tumors.

### Generalized Osteoporosis

If all other conditions are equal, a greater quantity of bone in any region shows proportionately more uptake of Tc phosphonates than does a smaller quantity. However, the uptake in a volume of bone is determined not only by the quantity of bone but also by the rate of bone turnover and bone vascularity. Thus, a bone scan cannot be used to measure bone density. Bone scanning in patients with osteoporosis is useful for the evaluation of compression fractures of the spine, insufficiency fractures at any site, and other causes of bone and joint pain. The typical appearance of a compression fracture is a bandlike area of increased uptake in the vertebral body (Fig. 7–4). The bone scan may be positive before vertebral collapse is seen radiographically. If the bone scan is normal in the presence of a compression fracture that is visible on conventional radiographs, the fracture is not new. Bone scans following fracture return to normal in 59% of patients by 1 year, 90% by 2 years, and 97% by 3 years.

Insufficiency fractures associated with osteoporosis may occur in the sacrum, pubis, femoral neck, metaphyses of the proximal and distal portions of the tibia, calcaneus, and ribs, especially the anterior aspect of the ribs. In osteoporosis, there is not the same tendency toward bilateral and symmetrical fractures that is seen in osteomalacia.

### Disuse Osteoporosis

Disuse can cause increased bone turnover and increased uptake on a bone scan. In patients with fractures of the shafts of long bones, diffuse increased uptake is often seen about the joint distal to the fracture. In patients who have bone scans for suspicion of fracture and who are using crutches, the bone scan sometimes shows decreased vascularity and uptake in the limb because of decreased blood flow due to immobilization. In a study of patients with hemiplegia from cerebrovascular accidents, it was found that 65% showed decreased uptake of the radionuclide in the blood flow and blood pool images and normal uptake on delayed images in the affected hand as a result

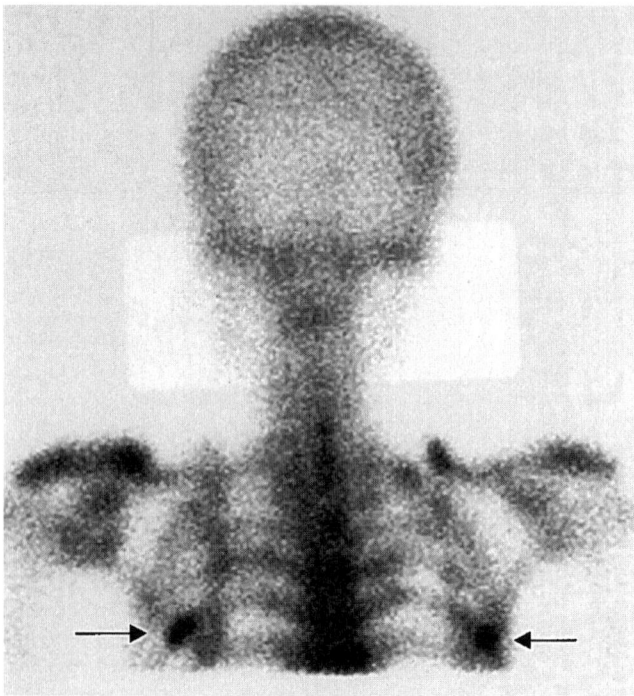

**Figure 7–3.** Osteomalacia. Hot spots in the inferior scapulae bilaterally (*arrows*), in a patient who presented with a clavicle fracture, suggested the diagnosis of osteomalacia, which was confirmed by biochemical tests and bone biopsy.

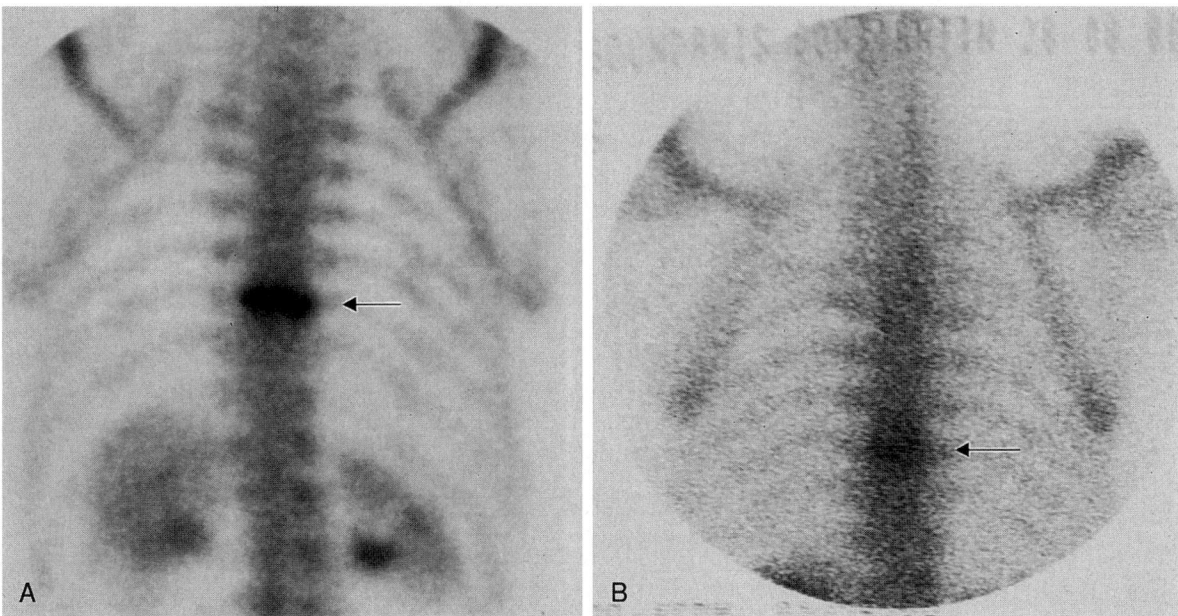

**Figure 7–4.** Vertebral compression fracture. Bandlike high uptake in the T9 vertebral body *(arrow)* on the posterior scan *(A)* was caused by a compression fracture that was also seen on a radiograph. Twelve months later *(B)*, there is only minimal increased uptake in T9 *(arrow)*.

of paralysis or disuse; 25% had diffuse increased uptake on delayed images, which was thought to represent reflex sympathetic dystrophy.

## Reflex Sympathetic Dystrophy

Reflex sympathetic dystrophy (RSD) has also been designated complex regional pain syndrome, sympathetically mediated pain syndrome, algodystrophy, Sudeck's atrophy, and causalgia. Diagnostic criteria for RSD include pain and tenderness in an extremity, soft tissue swelling, dystrophic skin changes, vasomotor instability, functional impairment, and patchy osteoporosis. RSD may demonstrate three scintigraphic patterns, which roughly correlate with three clinical stages.

**Stage I (Inflammatory).** Pain, swelling, and erythema are present. Increased vascularity is seen on the blood flow and blood pool images, and there is increased uptake on the delayed static scans.

**Stage II (Dystrophic).** This stage is characterized by burning and throbbing pain, a reduced range of joint motion, and skin thickening. The blood flow and blood pool images are normal, and there is increased uptake in the delayed images.

**Stage III (Atrophic).** The skin temperature is decreased, joint function is decreased, and contractures are present. Severe osteoporosis may be evident on radiographs. Bone scanning shows decreased uptake on blood flow and blood pool images and normal or decreased uptake on delayed static images.

In RSD, the scintigraphic abnormalities are diffuse, not focal, with widespread increased uptake on delayed images and prominent periarticular uptake (Fig. 7–5). In some cases, other joints of the ipsilateral extremity may also show diffuse increased uptake. Abnormalities other than RSD, however, can cause similar scintigraphic findings. These include synovitis and arthritis, cellulitis, soft tissue trauma, and disuse osteoporosis. The bone scan may also be helpful in patients with suspected RSD by showing a focal abnormality that may be due to trauma or neoplasm. The scintigraphic diagnosis of RSD is most accurate in the early stages of the disorder, with a duration of less than 6 months.

## Transient Osteoporosis

Transient osteoporosis of the hip, also called transient bone marrow edema syndrome, is characterized by markedly increased uptake in the entire femoral head and increased uptake extending down the femoral neck to the intertrochanteric region or proximal shaft of the femur (Fig. 7–6). Increased activity on blood flow and blood pool scans is characteristic. The hypothesis for the cause of transient osteoporosis is an episode of ischemia of the femoral head that does not lead to osteonecrosis. Reactive hyperemia and repair of the ischemic bone occur, accounting for the scintigraphic findings. In transient osteoporosis, intense and homogeneous uptake of the radionuclide agent with femoral head and femoral neck involvement is typical. Insufficiency fractures involving the femoral neck, subchondral portion of the femoral head, or both, may have a scintigraphic appearance similar to that of transient osteoporosis.

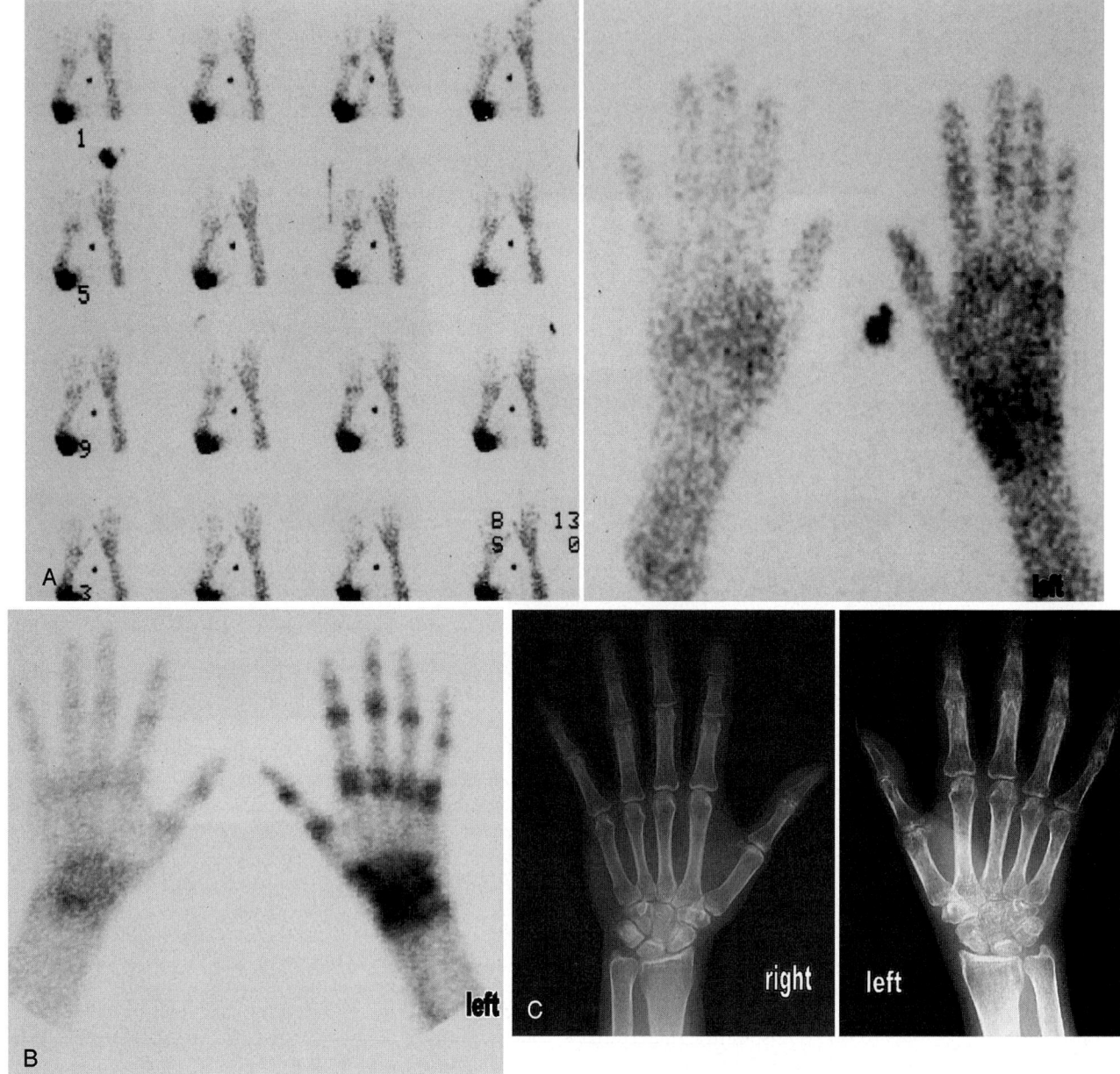

**Figure 7–5.** Reflex sympathetic dystrophy of the left hand. *A,* Mildly increased activity in the blood flow (left) and blood pool (right) phases are noted in the left hand. *B,* Diffuse increased uptake is seen in the left hand and wrist, with prominent periarticular uptake. *C,* Radiograph shows osteoporosis in the left hand and wrist.

## Paget's Disease

Paget's disease results in high bone turnover with intense osteoclastic and osteoblastic activity and increased vascularity. Although in the early stages it may be osteolytic, the osteoblastic activity eventually produces osteosclerosis. Both osteolytic and osteoblastic lesions of Paget's disease produce high uptake on a bone scan. Late in the course, the disease may become quiescent, and relatively little or no increased uptake may be present on the bone scan. Bone scanning is more sensitive than radiography in the detection of lesions of Paget's disease. Symptomatic lesions in Paget's disease are almost always characterized by increased uptake. Pagetic lesions that are positive on radiographs and negative on bone scans are usually asymp-

tomatic and sclerotic. In osteolytic Paget's disease of the skull (osteoporosis circumscripta), high uptake of the radionuclide may be noted only at the edge or margin of the lesion.

Pagetic lesions are most common in the pelvis, spine, femur, skull, and tibia, but can be present anywhere in the skeleton (Fig. 7–7). The characteristic scintigraphic appearance is high uptake involving a large area of bone. In the long bones, the end of the bone is involved, although an exception is sometimes seen in the tibia. In the spine, there is involvement in the vertebral body and, sometimes, in the posterior elements, including the spinous process. This may give a characteristic appearance described as the "Mickey Mouse sign" (see Fig. 7–7).

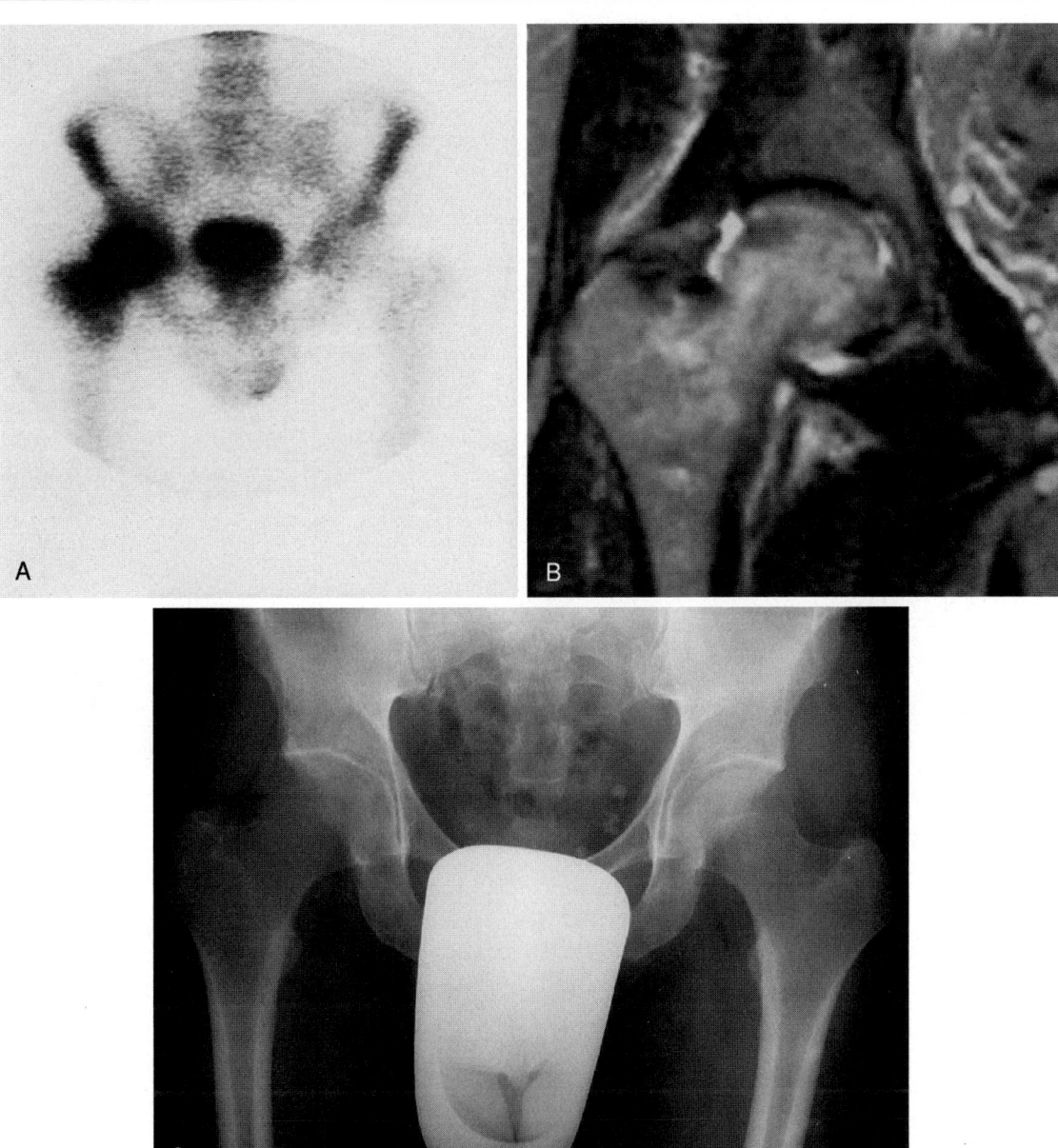

**Figure 7–6.** Transient osteoporosis of the hip. *A,* Increased radionuclide uptake in the right femoral head, extending into the femoral neck, is seen. *B,* Coronal T2-weighted MR image shows diffuse increased signal in the right femoral head. *C,* Radiograph of the pelvis shows osteoporosis in the right femoral head.

Malignant transformation is a complication of Paget's disease. In such transformation, the most common scintigraphic finding is a cold area within the region of high uptake. In some cases, there may be no cold area, and the presence of bone destruction related to the sarcoma may be obscured by the high uptake of the adjacent pagetic bone. Uptake in the soft tissues adjacent to a pagetic lesion is another sign that is suspicious for malignant transformation.

## NEOPLASTIC DISEASE

### Metastatic Disease

Radionuclide bone scanning is the procedure of choice for the evaluation of metastatic disease to the skeleton,

except for the assessment of multiple myeloma. The bone scan provides information about the presence, location, extent, and response to therapy of bony metastases; allows the evaluation of equivocal radiographic findings; and provides guidance regarding the site of biopsy. Abnormalities on bone scans alone, however, should not alter therapy unless metastatic disease is confirmed by other methods.

Bone scintigraphy or another imaging method is indicated in patients with cancer who have musculoskeletal pain. Although metastatic disease should be the first consideration, in the majority of cancer patients without known metastatic disease, the cause of musculoskeletal pain is not malignancy. Bone scans detect metastatic disease that is not seen radiographically. Another issue is the use of serial bone scans to follow patients with malig-

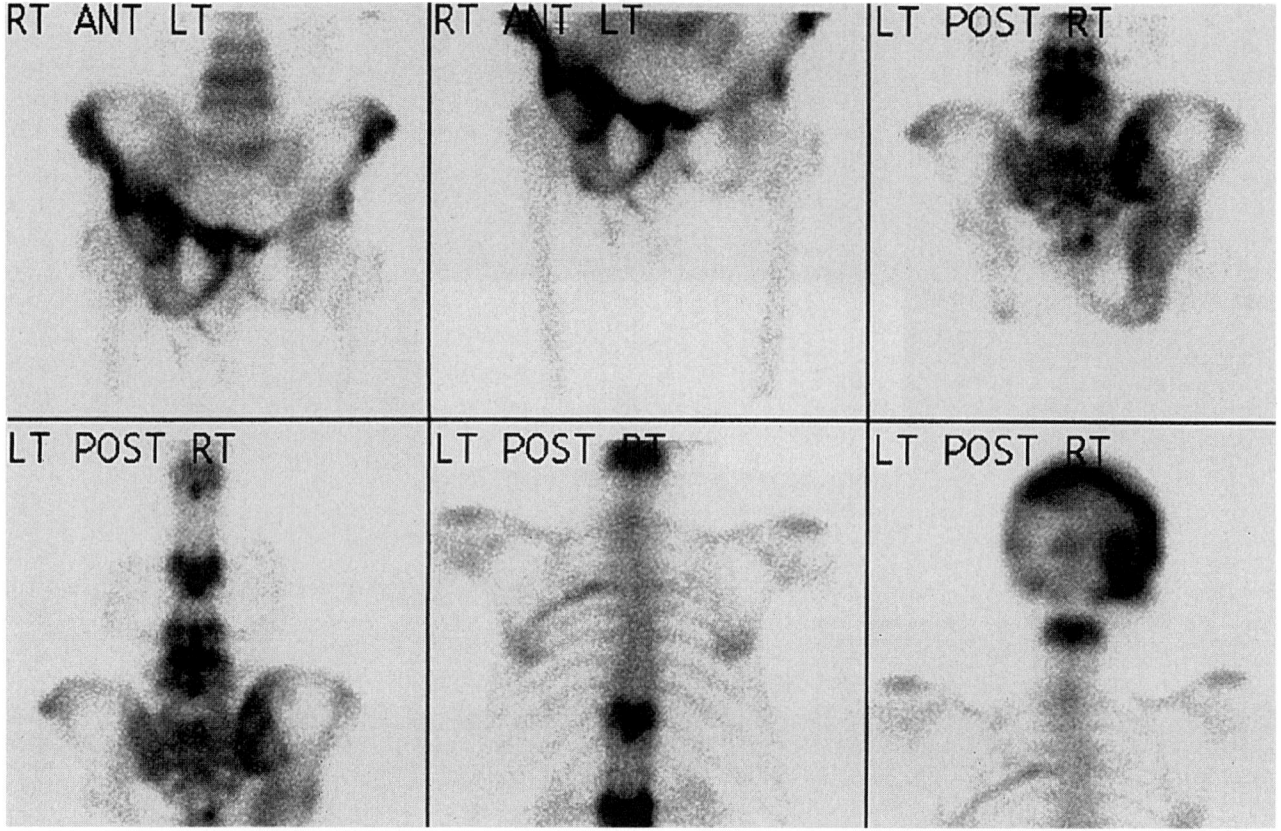

**Figure 7–7.** Paget's disease. High uptake is seen in the cervical, thoracic, and lumbar vertebrae; sacrum; pelvic bones; skull; and a left rib.

nant tumors. Early diagnosis of asymptomatic skeletal metastases does not necessarily lead to increased survival or benefit to the patient.

Metastatic lesions to the skeleton occur through the venous, arterial, or, less commonly, lymphatic circulation. The vertebral venous plexus of Batson has an important role in the spread of metastases to areas in the axial skeleton. In patients with osseous metastases, the vertebrae and thorax are involved in up to 50% of cases, the pelvis in 38%, the extremities in 34%, and the skull in 22%.

Blastic, mixed, and lytic lesions usually show increased uptake on a bone scan. In blastic lesions, this is related to the tumor stimulating the osteoblasts. With lytic lesions, there is usually an osteoblastic repair response to the osteoclastic resorption caused by the tumor. If there is no repair response, a cold, or photopenic, lesion will occur (Fig. 7–8). Although the exact incidence of cold metastatic lesions is not certain, because they may be difficult to detect, they are relatively uncommon. Most multifocal or metastatic tumors, except for multiple myeloma and some highly aggressive anaplastic tumors, are associated with a repair response. Cold lesions are sometimes seen in metastatic lesions arising from bronchogenic carcinoma.

Multiple areas of increased uptake in a random pattern, predominantly in the axial and the proximal appendicular skeleton, are typical of metastatic disease. Increased vascularity is often present on early-phase images, owing to tumor-induced neovascularity with increased capillary

permeability. Scintigraphic abnormalities that are usually related to benign causes include a pattern of focal round areas of increased uptake in adjacent ribs at the same location, which is typical of fracture; hot spots in the anterior ribs near the costochondral junctions and at the posterior costovertebral margins, which are often asso-

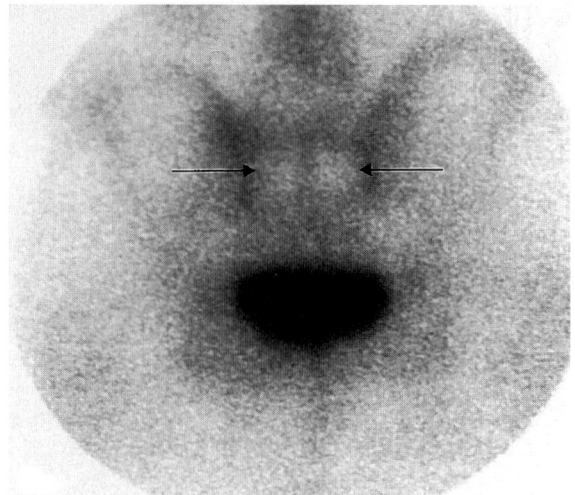

**Figure 7–8.** Metastatic lesions. A large lytic lesion in the sacrum from metastatic melanoma shows decreased uptake, or photopenia *(arrows)*, on a posterior image of the pelvis.

ciated with osteoporosis; and uptake in the periarticular regions, especially involving both sides of the joint, usually due to arthritic disease. Isolated uptake in the peripheral appendicular skeleton is rarely caused by metastases. Occasionally, lung cancer metastasizes to the hands or feet.

Metastatic disease in the spine typically involves the vertebral body or the vertebral body and the pedicle. The pedicle is rarely involved alone. SPECT scanning is more sensitive than planar imaging in detecting vertebral metastases and helps in differentiating benign from malignant disease. Using SPECT, focal uptake confined to the vertebral body is typically benign, as is diffuse uptake confined to the vertebral body. In contradistinction, when there is uptake in both the vertebral body and the pedicle, the responsible tumor is typically malignant.

In lymphoma, bone scans show abnormal uptake, but the pattern may differ from that of metastatic disease. There may be multiple subtle and often asymptomatic lesions, with frequent involvement of the bones of the extremity (Fig. 7–9). Diffuse, patchy uptake may reflect marrow involvement. Some lesions involving the bone marrow, without cortical extent, may not be positive on a bone scan. In leukemia, bone scans are usually normal. In multiple myeloma, bone scanning shows only about 50% of the lesions that are evident on radiography and underestimates the extent of the disease, compared with a radiographic skeletal survey. Radiographic skeletal surveys rather than bone scans are used to follow the course of multiple myeloma.

In following the course of treatment of metastatic disease with serial bone scans, the flare response may be seen. This is characterized by an increase in the intensity and number of focal areas of increased uptake on bone scans performed within the first 3 months after treatment, followed by decreased uptake on later scans. This finding is believed to predict successful therapy and is thought to be due to an osteoblastic response. Radiographs may show osteosclerosis developing in the bony lesions.

Magnetic resonance (MR) imaging has higher sensitivity and specificity than does planar bone scanning for the evaluation of metastatic lesions. Whole body MR imaging with fast spin echo and fast short tau inversion recovery (STIR) sequences, covering the whole skeleton or only the axial skeleton, takes less than 1 hour and has been shown to be an effective method that demonstrates

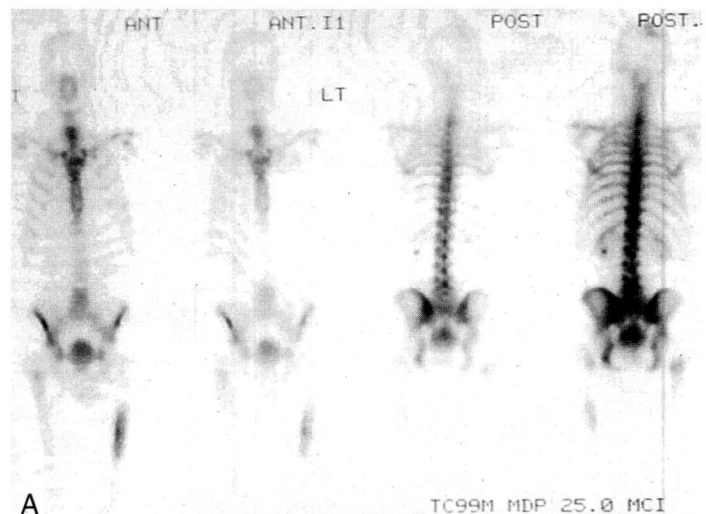

**Figure 7–9.** Non-Hodgkin's lymphoma. The patient presented with a long lesion in the shaft of the left femur. *A*, Bone scan shows abnormalities in the shaft of the left femur, left and right iliac bones, and L4. *B*, T2-weighted MR image with fat suppression reveals the lesion in the left femur but also shows multiple areas of increased signal in the marrow in other locations, including the right femur, both iliac bones, and L3, L4, and L5. Many of the large and small marrow lesions are not visible on the bone scan.

more metastatic lesions than does bone scanning. At this time, however, bone scintigraphy remains the initial procedure used most frequently to screen for skeletal metastases. MR imaging is usually used as a complementary technique when the scintigraphic findings are not diagnostic.

PET scanning with [18]F has been used to evaluate skeletal metastases and other benign and malignant osseous lesions. In comparison to radionuclide bone scanning, PET has been found to be more sensitive. The sensitivity of [18]F PET is similar to that of MR imaging. PET scanning with FDG has been used for the detection of skeletal as well as soft tissue metastases (Fig. 7–10). With FDG, uptake occurs in the metabolically active zones of the tumor because of increased glucose metabolism, whereas with scanning using bone-seeking radionuclides, uptake is due to new bone formation. A recent study found that FDG-PET was superior to Tc MDP bone scanning in the detection of osteolytic metastases but was inferior in the detection of osteoblastic metastases. The osteoblastic lesions apparently had lower metabolic activity and so were less detectable with FDG. FDG-PET, when compared with bone scanning, had a lower sensitivity for the detection of osseous metastases in prostate cancer. FDG-PET was found to be superior to bone scanning in the detection of skeletal lesions in lymphoma.

Iodine-131 ([131]I) is used to detect metastases, including those to bone, from differentiated thyroid carcinoma. The image quality and ability to localize abnormalities are not as good as with bone scanning. Metastases from more aggressive thyroid cancers that do not accumulate radioactive iodine cannot be detected with [131]I scanning but usually can be detected with bone scans.

[99m]Tc sestamibi (MIBI) localizes in bone marrow that is involved with malignancy. This method has been used to detect lesions in multiple myeloma, leukemia, lymphoma, and skeletal metastases. It may be most useful in detecting and showing the extent of conditions with diffuse marrow involvement that may not be seen with bone scanning. [201]Tl acts in a manner similar to MIBI. Malignant bone marrow lesions reveal increased uptake.

[67]Ga scanning is similar to bone scanning with regard to sensitivity in detecting bony lesions in lymphoma, and it allows the detection of extraosseous involvement. For bone lesions related to lymphoma, [67]Ga scanning can be used to monitor the response to therapeutic intervention.

## Primary Malignant Bone and Soft Tissue Tumors

Almost all primary malignant bone tumors reveal increased uptake on a bone scan, owing to tumor neovascularity, increased capillary permeability, and increased bone turnover from bone destruction and repair. This finding cannot be used to differentiate between benign and malignant lesions with certainty. However, primary malignant bone tumors tend to be associated with characteristic scintigraphic patterns, although overlap occurs and there is no unique pattern of features (Fig. 7–11). Soft tissue sarcomas have increased blood flow, as seen on early-phase images of a bone scan (Fig. 7–12). Delayed images often show mild increased uptake in soft tissue lesions. Higher uptake of the radionuclide on delayed images

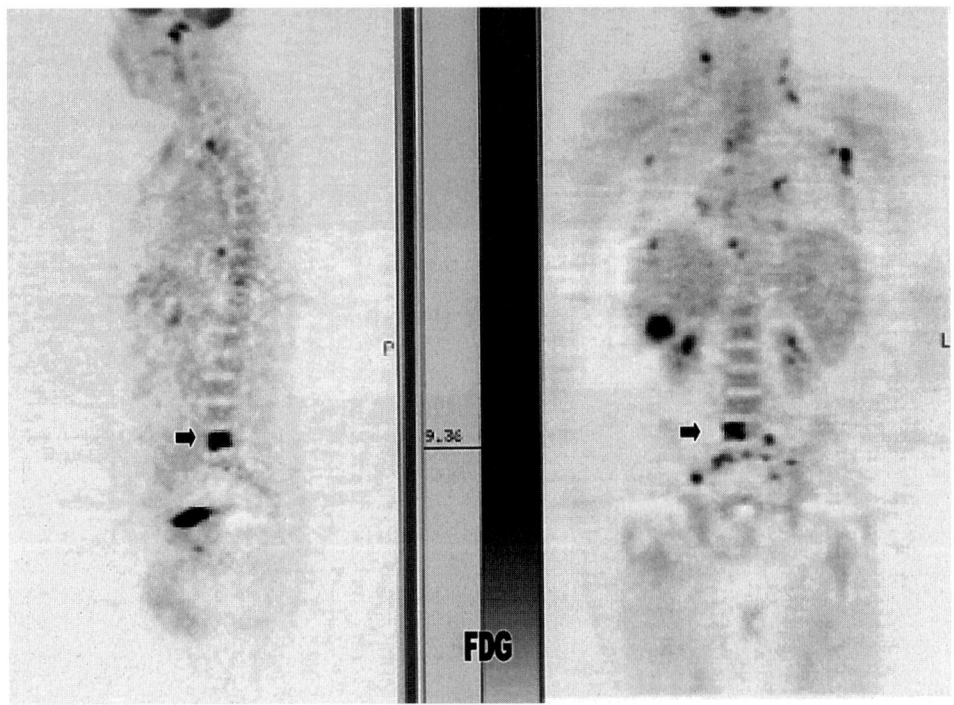

**Figure 7–10.** An FDG-PET scan, with sagittal and coronal tomographic images, shows increased uptake (*arrows*) in a bony metastasis in L5 from colon cancer, as well as multiple soft tissue metastases in lymph nodes. (Courtesy of R. Katz, MD, New York, NY.)

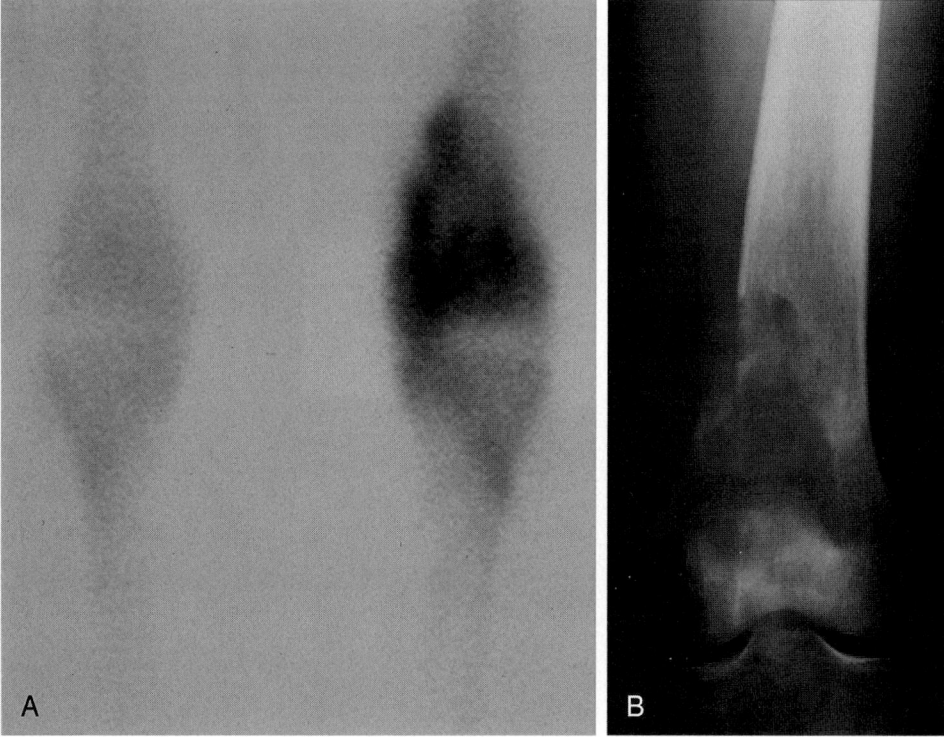

**Figure 7–11.** Osteosarcoma of the left femur. *A*, Bone scan of an osteosarcoma of the left distal femur shows patchy, inhomogeneous high uptake and lower uptake in the center. *B*, On the radiograph, a lytic lesion is present, with cortical destruction and extension into the soft tissues.

may be present if calcification or ossification is present within the tumor.

High-grade malignant lesions tend to have high uptake of radionuclides, and benign tumors tend to have lower uptake. Low-grade malignant tumors cannot always be differentiated from benign tumors, however.

### Benign Bone Tumors and Tumor-Like Conditions

In benign bone tumors, the uptake of $^{99m}$Tc phosphate bone scanning agents varies with the type of tumor; normal, mildly increased, markedly increased, and even decreased uptake may be present. The vascularity on

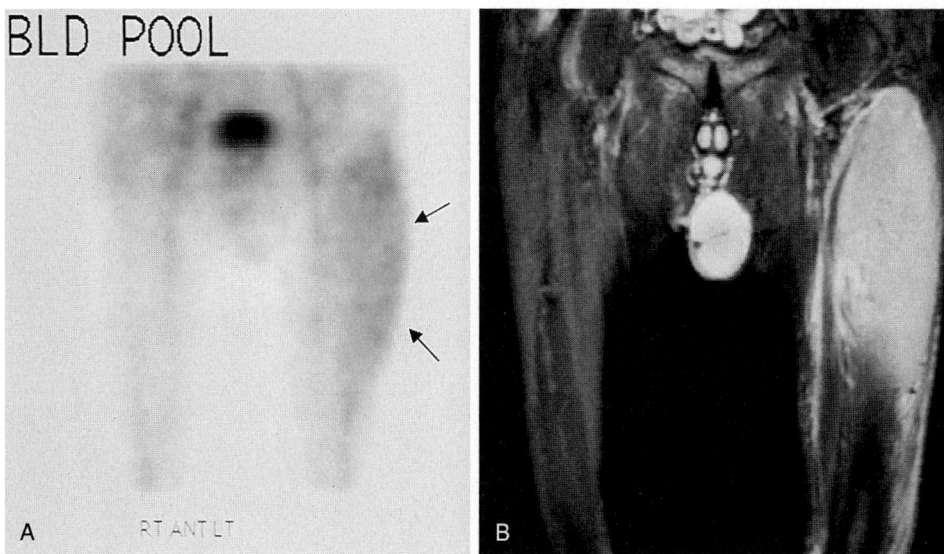

**Figure 7–12.** Soft tissue sarcoma. *A*, Increased activity *(arrows)* is noted in the left thigh on the blood pool scan. *B*, STIR MR image shows high signal in the soft tissues of the thigh.

early-phase imaging may also vary. Bone scanning is very helpful in the diagnosis of osteoid osteomas, especially when radiographs are normal or nondiagnostic. This often occurs when the lesion is in the spine, pelvis, or hip (Fig. 7–13). The characteristic scintigraphic appearance is a small, round, focal area of high uptake. There may be increased vascularity on early-phase scans, but this is often not present. A computed tomography (CT) scan is necessary to confirm the diagnosis of osteoid osteoma and to localize it for removal, either by open surgery or percutaneously under CT guidance.

Most cases of enchondroma are "warm" or "hot" on bone scans; however, bone scanning cannot differentiate enchondroma from chondrosarcoma. In Ollier's disease (enchondromatosis), the sites of multiple enchondromas can be detected. In giant cell tumors, bone scanning shows high uptake on both the early and delayed images, most intensely in the periphery of the lesion. A "donut" appearance is frequent, with a rim of high uptake surrounding a central area of lower uptake (Fig. 7–14). A similar appearance can be seen in other tumors, however.

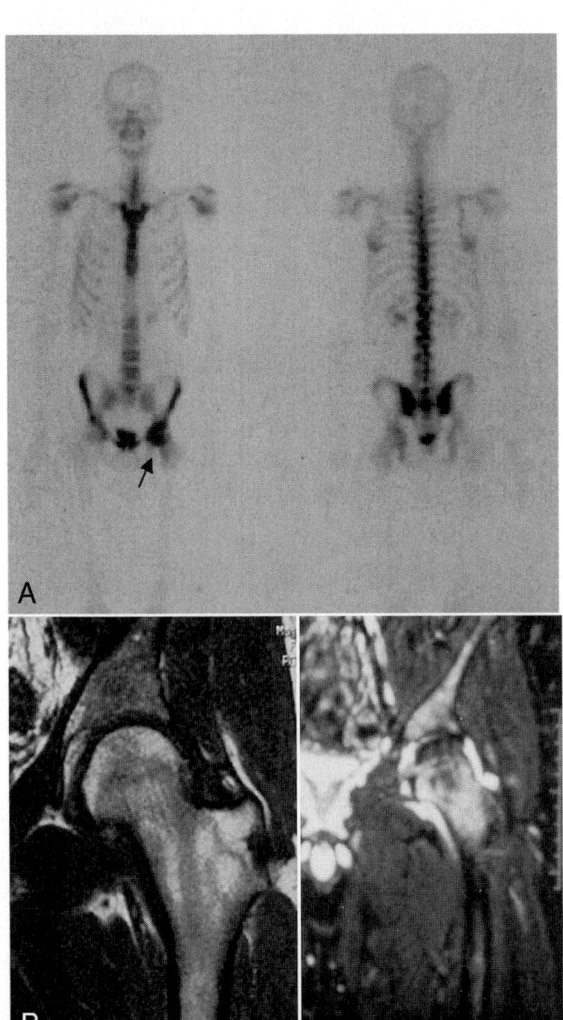

**Figure 7–13.** Osteoid osteoma. *A,* Bone scan shows a focal area of increased uptake in the left femoral neck *(arrow).* *B,* T1-weighted spin echo (left) and STIR (right) MR images show bone marrow edema in the left femoral neck and acetabulum and a synovial effusion. The nidus of an osteoid osteoma is not seen. *C,* Radiograph taken at the time of the bone scan shows mild cortical thickening of the medial femoral neck. *D,* CT scan shows an osteoid osteoma with a calcified nidus in the anterior aspect of the femoral neck.

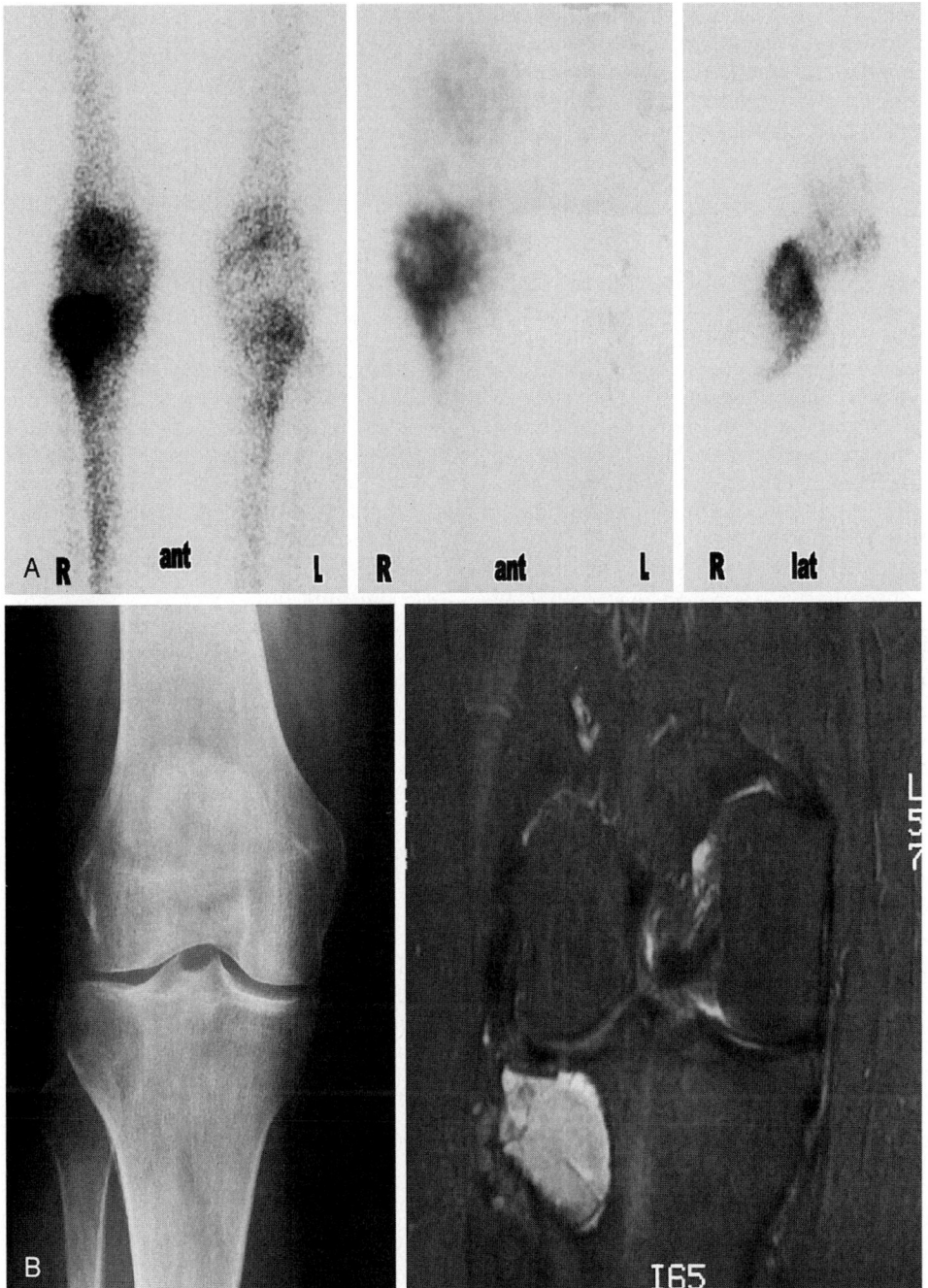

**Figure 7–14.** Giant cell tumor. *A,* High uptake is seen in the right lateral tibial plateau. Lighter anterior and right lateral images show a rim of high uptake surrounding an area of lower uptake. *B,* A lytic lesion is present in the lateral tibial plateau on the radiograph. The fat-suppressed intermediate-weighted spin echo MR image shows mixed high signal in the lesion.

Increased uptake on bone scanning is present in aneurysmal bone cysts, with most revealing a rim of increased uptake around the periphery of the cyst and lower uptake in its center. The intensity of the uptake may vary; however, some aneurysmal bone cysts may show only mild or, rarely, normal uptake. Early-phase scans may show increased radionuclide uptake, reflecting marked hyperemia in the center of the lesion. Unicameral bone cysts have normal or sometimes decreased uptake, except when they are fractured, in which case high uptake is present. The scintigraphic appearance of hemangiomas of bone varies, depending on the biologic activity of the tumor, its site, and the resolution of the equipment.

Fibrous dysplasia is a condition in which there is replacement of normal bone by abnormal fibro-osseous tissue with rapid bone turnover. The bone scan in fibrous dysplasia shows areas of high uptake. The role of bone scanning in patients with Langerhans' cell histiocytosis is controversial, with variable sensitivity. Most bone islands have normal uptake on a bone scan. Growing bone islands may also have normal uptake. However, increased uptake has been reported in large bone islands. Bone scans show normal findings in osteopoikilosis and osteopathia striata but show increased uptake in melorheostosis.

## TRAUMA

### Traumatic Fractures

Bone scanning may be used to detect fractures when radiographs are normal or nondiagnostic, especially in areas that are difficult to evaluate radiographically. Fractures can be detected by bone scan within 24 hours in 95% of patients younger than 65 years. By 72 hours, 95% of fractures in all patients are abnormal on bone scan. Increased blood flow, growth of new blood vessels, and callus formation by osteoblasts occur within hours after the fracture. There are differences in the magnitude of uptake in fractures at different sites. Fractures in periarticular locations reveal high uptake within the first day after trauma. Fractures in the axial skeleton and shafts of the long bones reveal a slower increase in the intensity of uptake, with some requiring 12 days to appear positive on a bone scan. Skull fractures are usually not detected on a bone scan. After the traumatic episode, all fractures have increasing uptake of the radionuclide bone scanning agent, with peak accumulation at 2 to 5 weeks. By 1 year following trauma, the bone scans in 79% of rib fractures, 64% of long bone fractures, and 59% of vertebral fractures return to normal. By 2 years, bone scans in 90% of all fractures are normal.

The diagnosis of a fracture of the femoral neck in patients with normal or nondiagnostic radiographs can be made by radionuclide bone scanning or by MR imaging. Recent evidence suggests that MR imaging has greater sensitivity and specificity for the diagnosis of hip fractures. Bone scanning is often used in the diagnosis of occult scaphoid fractures (Fig. 7–15).

### Stress Fractures

Stress fractures are caused by focal areas of bone resorption occurring as a response to stress, with ultimate weakening of the bone that may lead to fracture. Bone scans are almost always abnormal in stress fractures at the time of onset of pain, whereas radiographs are often normal at this time. The scintigraphic appearance of stress fractures depends on the location, type of bone, and chronicity. Stress fractures can be divided into three types: (1) fatigue fractures due to excessive stress on normal bone, usually found in athletes; (2) insufficiency fractures, due to stress on weakened bone, found in metabolic bone disease; and (3) pathologic fractures caused by neoplasms.

In the early stages of a stress fracture, radiographs may be normal; subsequently, periostitis is observed, and eventually a fracture line is evident. With scintigraphy, the blood flow and blood pool scans are abnormal in recent stress fractures, with first the blood flow and then the blood pool scans returning to normal by about 2 months. The delayed images return to normal more slowly and may still show mild increased uptake 8 to 10 months after the time of clinical presentation. Focal areas of increased uptake are often found in the feet in symptomatic or asymptomatic athletes and should be regarded as stress changes. A focal area of markedly increased uptake in vascular and delayed phases of the bone scan should be considered a stress fracture in a patient with the sudden onset of foot pain.

Femoral neck stress fractures are seen as focal increased uptake in the medial or lateral aspects of the femoral neck or as a bandlike area through the entire femoral neck (Fig. 7–16). Recent articles have also described insufficiency fractures of the subchondral portion of the femoral head. These may simulate osteonecrosis or transient osteoporosis on clinical assessment and imaging studies. Sacral fractures are a frequent cause of low back pain in osteoporotic patients. Such fractures may involve both sacral alae and the body of the sacrum, giving a characteristic

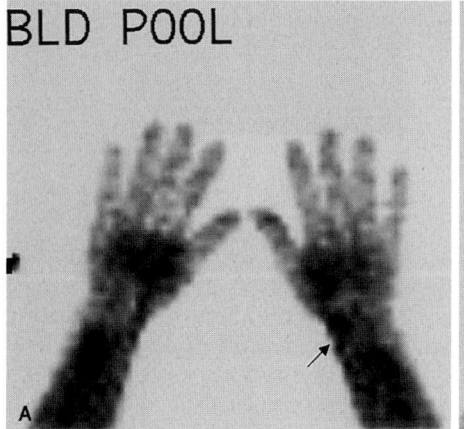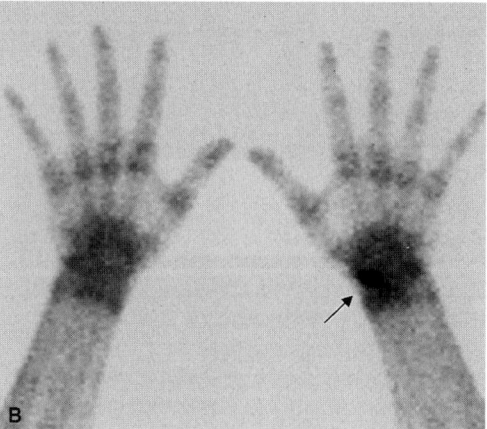

**Figure 7–15.** Scaphoid fracture. The blood pool *(A)* and delayed 3-hour bone scan *(B)* images show increased activity in the scaphoid *(arrows)*, consistent with a fracture, in a patient who had wrist trauma and normal radiographs.

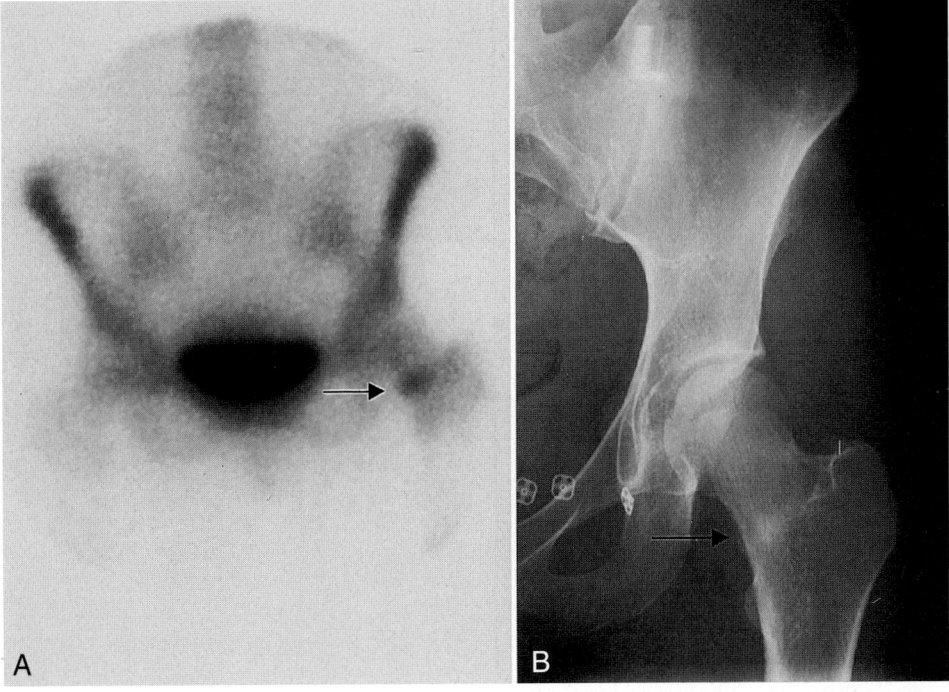

**Figure 7–16.** Stress fracture of the femoral neck. *A,* Focal area of increased uptake is present in the medial aspect of the left femoral neck on the bone scan *(arrow). B,* Radiograph taken 2 weeks after the bone scan shows an area of sclerosis in the medial aspect of the femoral neck *(arrow),* confirming the presence of a stress fracture.

H appearance on the bone scan, which is diagnostic (Fig. 7–17). They may also involve only one sacral ala, giving the appearance of high uptake in the region of the sacroiliac joint, which must be differentiated from sacroiliitis. High-dose radiation therapy that includes the bones of the pelvis may cause sacral and pubic bone insufficiency fractures.

Stress fractures of the pars interarticularis (i.e., spondylolysis) may be a cause of back pain in athletes. SPECT scanning is more sensitive than planar imaging for the detection of spondylolysis and also provides better localization of the defect. Radiographs are often normal. CT scanning may help visualize the fracture, which may be unilateral or bilateral. Increased uptake at the site of spondylolysis suggests that it is the cause of the patient's symptoms of back pain.

The location of the stress fracture depends on the sport or activity and the type of stress that is present. The most frequent site of a stress fracture in runners is the tibial shaft, followed by the metatarsal shaft. Other sites include the calcaneus, femoral shaft, femoral neck, pubic bone, fibula, tarsal navicular bone, posterior elements of the spine, and sacrum. Gymnasts, weight lifters, and tennis players tend to get stress fractures in the posterior elements of the spine because of the hyperextension of the vertebral column that accompanies participation in these activities.

*Shin splints* is a term that has been used to describe chronic exertional shin pain in athletes, which can be caused by a variety of abnormalities. The medial tibial stress syndrome is the most frequent type of exertional shin pain in athletes. Pain in the posteromedial aspect of the tibia may be caused by tibial periostitis, tibial stress fracture or stress reaction, or distal deep chronic posterior compartment syndrome. Blood flow and blood pool scans are normal in cases of shin splints. The location of the uptake suggests that it is related to the attachment site of the soleus muscle. The posterior and anterior tibialis muscles may also be involved in shin splints (Fig. 7–18). The cause of the pain is thought to be periostitis occurring along the tibia caused by muscular and tendinous strain associated with inflammation.

## Soft Tissue Injuries

The scintigraphic appearance of exertional compartment syndrome is an area of decreased uptake in the tibial shaft with increased uptake superiorly and inferiorly. The decreased uptake is most likely due to decreased blood flow from increased pressure in the compartment. $^{201}$Tl chloride is reported to be effective for the diagnosis of exertional compartment syndrome in the lower legs. Bone scans may show evidence of muscle injury. Long-distance runners show increased uptake in the muscles on bone scans obtained within 48 hours of a race, with return to normal by 1 week. The muscles that show increased uptake are the ones used most during the exercise, due to exercise-induced rhabdomyolysis.

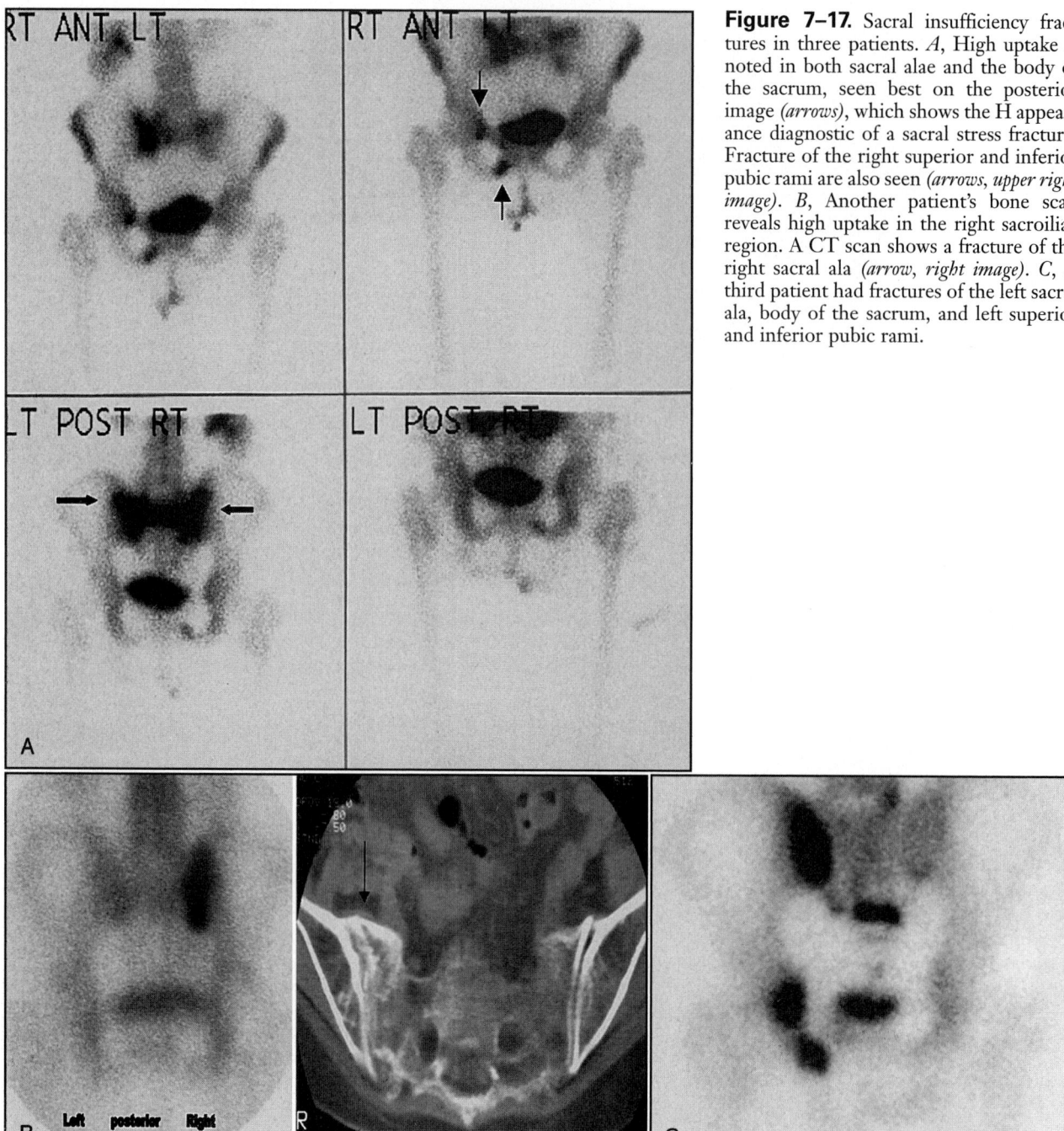

**Figure 7–17.** Sacral insufficiency fractures in three patients. *A,* High uptake is noted in both sacral alae and the body of the sacrum, seen best on the posterior image *(arrows),* which shows the H appearance diagnostic of a sacral stress fracture. Fracture of the right superior and inferior pubic rami are also seen *(arrows, upper right image). B,* Another patient's bone scan reveals high uptake in the right sacroiliac region. A CT scan shows a fracture of the right sacral ala *(arrow, right image). C,* A third patient had fractures of the left sacral ala, body of the sacrum, and left superior and inferior pubic rami.

## INFECTION

Three-phase bone scanning with $^{99m}$Tc phosphonates is an important imaging method in the diagnosis of musculoskeletal infection. The use of early-phase imaging allows cellulitis to be diagnosed and differentiated from osteomyelitis and septic arthritis in cases of suspected infection. Increased activity in blood flow and blood pool phases of the examination, without increased uptake or only mild, diffuse increased uptake in the delayed phases is consistent with cellulitis (Fig. 7–19). A fourth phase, a 24-hour scan, may be helpful when the diagnosis is uncertain. Increased uptake within the bone on all three

or four phases of the bone scan is consistent with the diagnosis of osteomyelitis; however, this pattern is not specific, as fractures, tumors, and other abnormalities may have a similar or identical scintigraphic appearance (Fig. 7–20).

Septic arthritis is characterized by hyperemia on early-phase images and diffuse increased uptake around the joint on delayed images. This is not specific for infection, as noninfectious inflammatory arthritis has similar findings. Osteomyelitis may coexist with septic arthritis. In osteomyelitis, there may also be decreased uptake, or even cold areas, within the bone, most likely due to ischemia

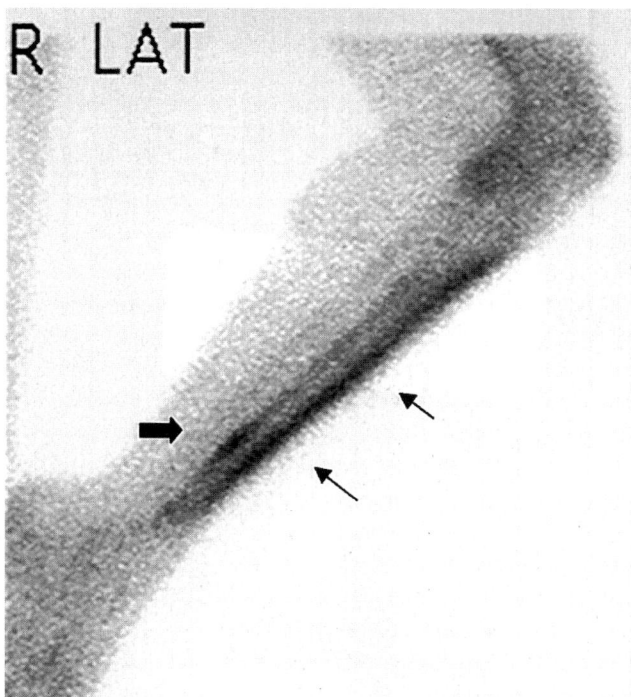

R LAT

**Figure 7–18.** Stress fracture of the tibia and anterior shin splint. A short fusiform area of increased uptake in the posterior aspect of the distal shaft of the tibia represents a stress fracture *(large arrow)*. A long longitudinal area of increased uptake in the anterior aspect of the tibial shaft is consistent with a shin splint *(small arrows)*.

caused by increased pressure in the medullary cavity, beneath the periosteum, or in the soft tissue from the infection. Newer imaging methods, however, including inflammatory scanning agents and FDG-PET, have been shown to be more accurate for the evaluation of musculoskeletal sepsis complicating orthopedic implants, owing to the low specificity of standard bone scanning in this clinical setting. MR imaging has been shown to be more accurate than bone scanning in cases of chronic osteomyelitis, but metal artifact makes it less useful in the presence of many orthopedic implants.

Although gallium scanning is moderately accurate for diagnosing low-grade musculoskeletal infection, including infection of joint prostheses, $^{111}$In-labeled white blood cell (leukocyte) scanning has had superior results and has replaced gallium scanning in most cases. Gallium scanning may be preferred in children, however, in whom the higher radiation dose of $^{111}$In-labeled leukocyte scans has to be considered.

Radiolabeled leukocyte scanning is the predominant inflammatory scanning method for musculoskeletal infection at this time. The labeling process is time consuming and is relatively expensive if done by a commercial laboratory. A lower radiation dose, higher photon flux, and earlier imaging at 2 and 4 hours after preparation, are advantages of $^{99m}$Tc HMPAO–labeled leukocytes. With $^{111}$In-labeled leukocytes, there is a higher radiation dose, imaging is accomplished at 3 and 24 hours, and a smaller dose is injected, resulting in images of poorer quality. Because musculoskeletal infection, especially

with orthopedic implants, is often low grade and chronic in nature, $^{111}$In labeling is usually preferred to $^{99m}$Tc HMPAO labeling, as it allows more time for the leukocytes to migrate to the site of infection.

The FDG-PET method has a high sensitivity for the diagnosis of musculoskeletal infection (Fig. 7–21). It is useful in the assessment of the axial as well as the peripheral skeleton. FDG-PET is not specific, however, because inflammation, tumors, and other causes of increased glucose metabolism may cause greater uptake of this agent. In the early postoperative period, it is difficult to distinguish between postoperative reactive changes and infection.

Identifying osteomyelitis in joints with neuropathic arthropathy may be difficult. Bone scans show increased vascularity and radionuclide uptake in both conditions. Radiolabeled leukocyte scans may show increased uptake in noninfected neuropathic arthropathy. Combined leukocyte and bone scans may produce false-positive scans for infection with spatial or intensity mismatching. Combined leukocyte and bone marrow scans improve the specificity for infection (Fig. 7–22). With infection, increased uptake may be seen on the 24-hour leukocyte scan as compared with the 4-hour scan, which is not true in noninfected neuropathic arthropathy. Neuropathy demonstrates mild, diffuse increased uptake in noninfected cases, compared with focal intense uptake with osteomyelitis. It may also be difficult to distinguish osteomyelitis from soft tissue infection. Soft tissue infection adjacent to bone may cause increased uptake on delayed images of a bone scan. Increased activity in the arterial phase of the blood pool scan occurs in osteomyelitis, whereas only venous hyperemia is present in soft tissue infection.

## PAINFUL JOINT PROSTHESES

Radionuclide scanning may help detect the cause of pain in patients with joint prostheses, including infection, mechanical loosening, and fracture. In asymptomatic patients with cemented hip prostheses, increased uptake may be seen following surgery. Six months after surgery, activity around the lesser trochanter and femoral shaft becomes insignificant. By 2 years, activity around the acetabulum, greater trochanter, and tip of the femoral stem has stabilized; however, 10% of prostheses are characterized by continued uptake at these sites. With total knee prostheses, persistent increased uptake of the radionuclide may be present in asymptomatic patients, especially around the tibial component. Early studies of bone scanning in painful hip prostheses suggested that focal increased uptake at the tip of the femoral stem and greater and lesser trochanters indicates mechanical loosening (Fig. 7–23), whereas diffuse increased uptake indicates that the prosthesis is infected (Fig. 7–24). These patterns were not found to be specific for differentiating infection from mechanical loosening, however.

Joint aspiration has been shown to be a cost-effective and accurate method of detecting infected prostheses. Wide variations in sensitivity and specificity have been reported in different centers; however, these findings are most likely due to differences in technique and interpretation.

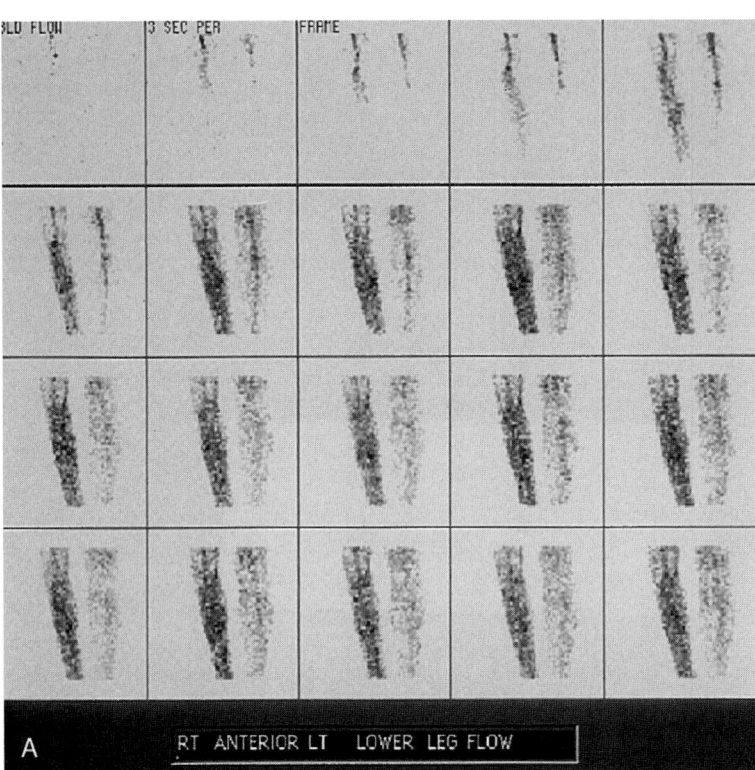

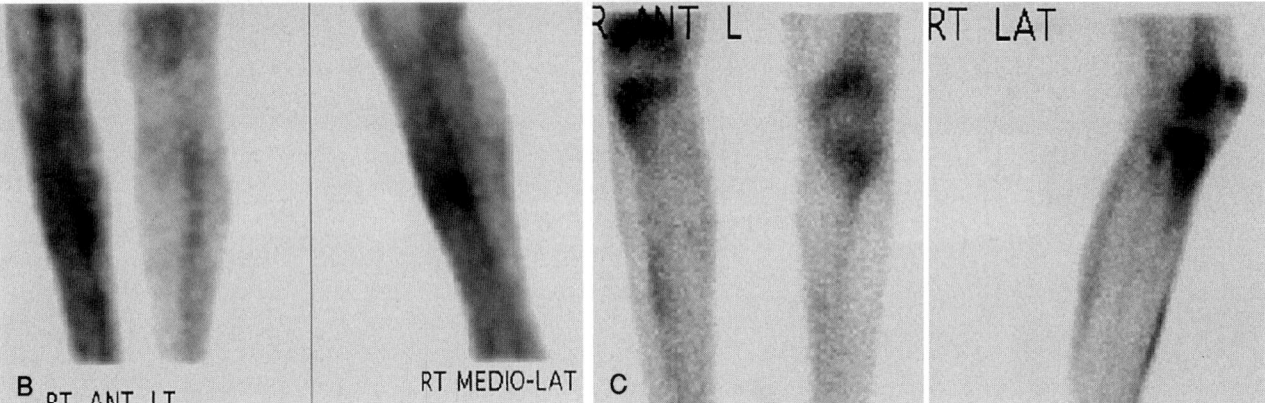

**Figure 7–19.** Cellulitis. Blood flow *(A)* and blood pool *(B)* scans show increased activity in the right lower leg. The delayed 3-hour images *(C)* show mild increased activity in the soft tissues of the anterior aspect of the right lower leg, but the activity is less intense than that in the blood flow and blood pool scans.

Combined $^{99m}$Tc phosphate bone scanning and $^{67}$Ga citrate scanning has been used for diagnosing prosthetic infection. Normal scans are accurate in ruling out infection. The patterns of spatial mismatch of bone and gallium scans and the higher uptake of gallium compared with that of bone scan are specific for infection but are not sensitive. Radiolabeled leukocyte scans have a high sensitivity for the diagnosis of infected prostheses. Specificity is increased by comparison with bone scans, to determine mismatch, or with bone marrow scans, which increases the specificity even more.

Radionuclide arthrography (i.e., arthroscintigraphy) has been used to determine loosening of hip and knee prostheses. Radionuclide arthrography is done by injecting radiolabeled colloid into the joint at the time of a joint aspiration and radiographic contrast arthrogram. A scan is obtained about 2 hours later to determine leakage of the radionuclide into the prosthetic interface, which would indicate loosening. Radionuclide arthrography performs better than radiographic contrast arthrography for the detection of femoral component loosening in patients with hip prostheses, but it does not adequately evaluate the acetabular component.

## ARTHRITIS AND PAIN AROUND JOINTS

### Arthritis

Synovitis is demonstrated by abnormalities in the early phases of a $^{99m}$Tc MDP bone scan that indicate diffuse increased blood flow around a joint. In cases of arthritis, uptake on the delayed (3-hour) scans is related to increased blood flow to the juxta-articular bone that results from synovitis. Uptake is also related to bony changes associated with arthritis, including erosions, sclerosis, osteophytes, and subchondral cysts. A number of new scanning agents that target inflammation are being used for the evaluation of arthritis. One approach is the use of radiolabeled monoclonal antibodies to antigens within the arthritic joint.

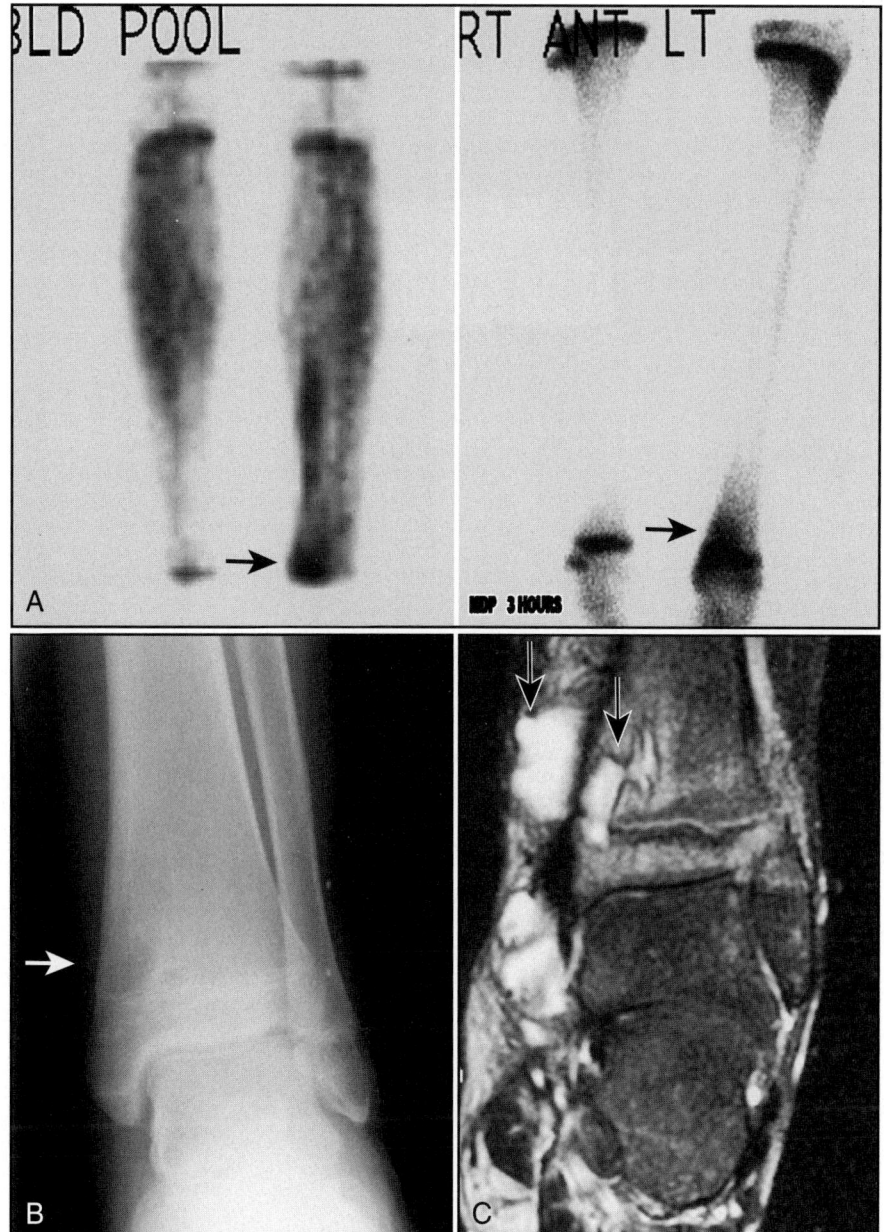

**Figure 7–20.** Osteomyelitis. *A*, Blood pool and delayed 3-hour images of a bone scan show increased activity in the metaphyseal region of the medial aspect of the left distal tibia *(arrows)*. *B*, Radiograph shows a lytic lesion in the medial metaphyseal region of the distal tibia *(white arrow)*. *C*, STIR MR image demonstrates high signal in the lesion in the medial aspect of the distal tibia and shows that the lesion crosses the growth plate from the metaphysis into the epiphysis and extends into the soft tissues *(arrows)*.

In patients with polyarthralgia, a normal bone scan excludes inflammatory joint disease, whereas an abnormal bone scan suggests that inflammatory disease is present, which may affect treatment. The appearance of inflammatory arthritis on a bone scan includes abnormal early and late phases of the examination (Fig. 7–25). Any monarticular process must be considered septic arthritis until proved otherwise. Polyarthritis with involvement of the hands and feet is consistent with rheumatoid arthritis (Fig. 7–26). Uptake at sites of tendon insertion in the feet suggests psoriatic arthritis or Reiter's syndrome.

Osteoarthritis tends to have focal uptake in a joint rather than diffuse uptake. These patterns on the bone scan underscore the well-known morphologic findings of various articular disorders, but differences in severity of involvement may be shown on bone scans versus radiographs.

## Other Causes of Pain around Joints

Occult malignancy, even in patients with no history of cancer, may be a cause of pain around joints. The yield for identification of occult malignancy on bone scans in

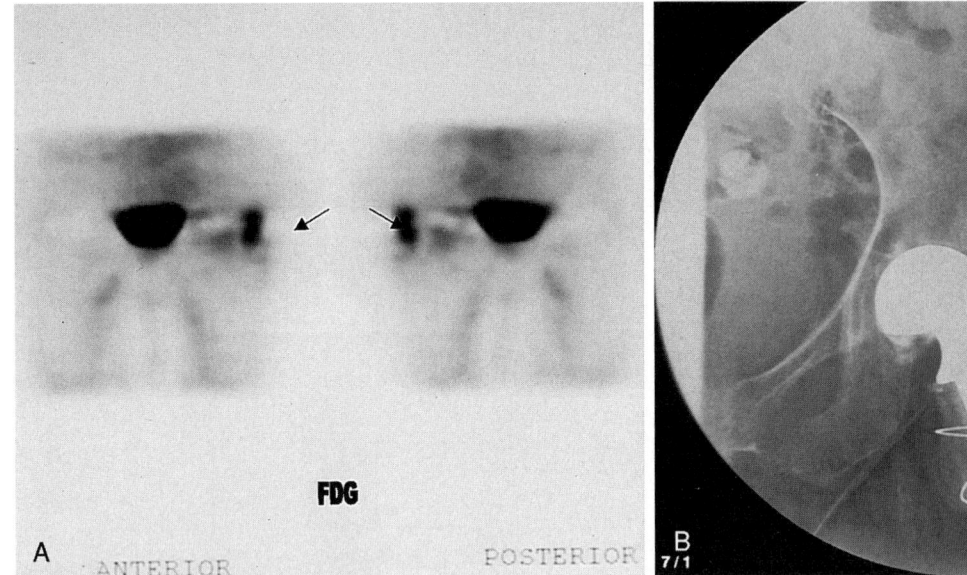

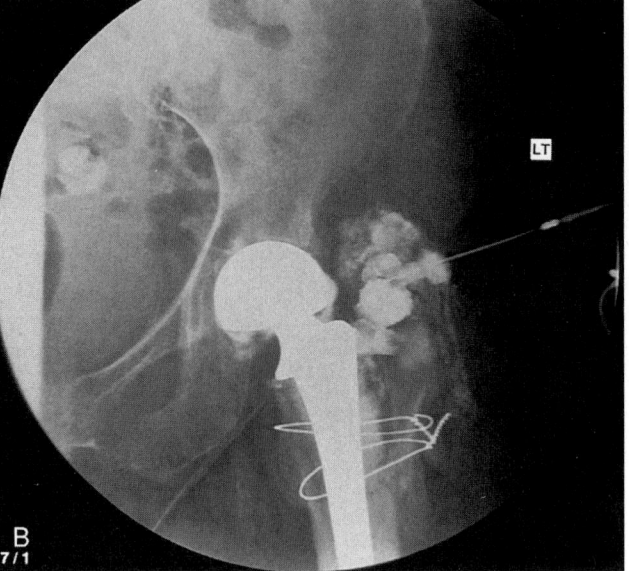

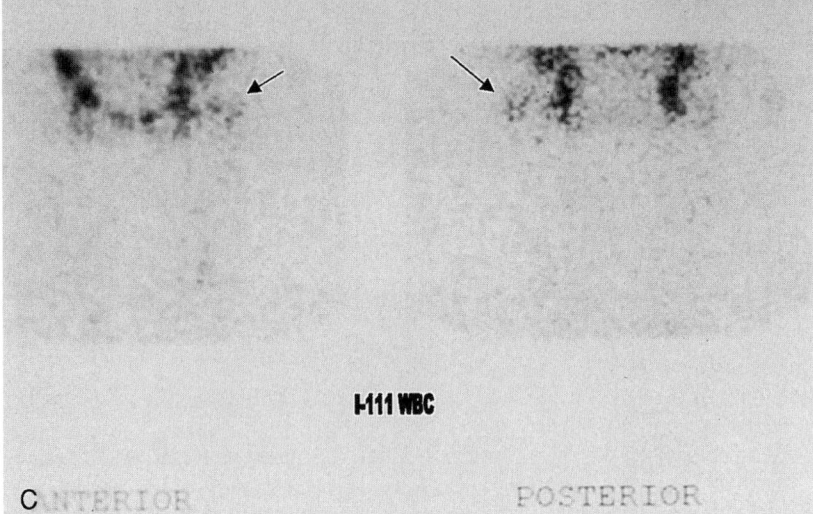

**Figure 7–21.** FDG-PET scan and [111]In-labeled leukocyte scan in a patient with an infected hip prosthesis. *A*, FDG-PET scan shows high uptake *(arrows)* lateral to the left hip. *B*, This area corresponds to the site of an abscess cavity that communicated with the left femoral hemiarthroplasty. *C*, The 24-hour [111]In-labeled leukocyte scan shows mildly increased uptake at this site *(arrows).*

patients aged 50 years or older is 9%. In patients with a history of cancer, metastatic disease should be ruled out as a cause of periarticular pain through the use of a bone scan, before the patient undergoes an extensive workup.

Bone scans are often ordered to evaluate foot pain, because the cause of pain may not be clear clinically or on radiographic examination. Common abnormalities that cause foot pain include plantar fasciitis, stress fractures, degenerative and inflammatory arthritis, sesamoid abnormalities, osteoid osteoma, and tendinosis and tenosynovitis. Coregistration of the abnormalities delineated on the bone scan with those found on radiographs has been suggested when it is difficult to localize the site of radionuclide uptake anatomically, as may occur in the tarsal bones. Plantar fasciitis may cause a focal area of increased uptake on the plantar aspect of the calcaneus at the medial calcaneal tubercle, due to periostitis at the site of insertion of the plantar fascia (Fig. 7–27). Heel "spurs" due to enthesopathic changes at the insertion of the short flexor tendons may also cause increased uptake in the

plantar aspect of the calcaneus and are not necessarily symptomatic.

Focal increased uptake in the patella on a bone scan may be present in some cases of chondromalacia patellae (Fig. 7–28). Focal uptake in the patella is not specific for chondromalacia and could be due to arthritis or osteochondral injury.

Bone scans show abnormalities in both secondary and primary hypertrophic osteoarthropathy. The typical scintigraphic pattern is circumferential uptake around the bones of the wrists, knees, and ankles (Fig. 7–29). After treatment, improvement can be seen in the scan's appearance. Clinical improvement precedes improvement seen scintigraphically, which precedes radiographic signs of improvement.

## OSTEONECROSIS

The scintigraphic appearance of osteonecrosis depends on the cause and stage of the disease, as well as on the scintigraphic equipment and technique used. Osteonecrosis

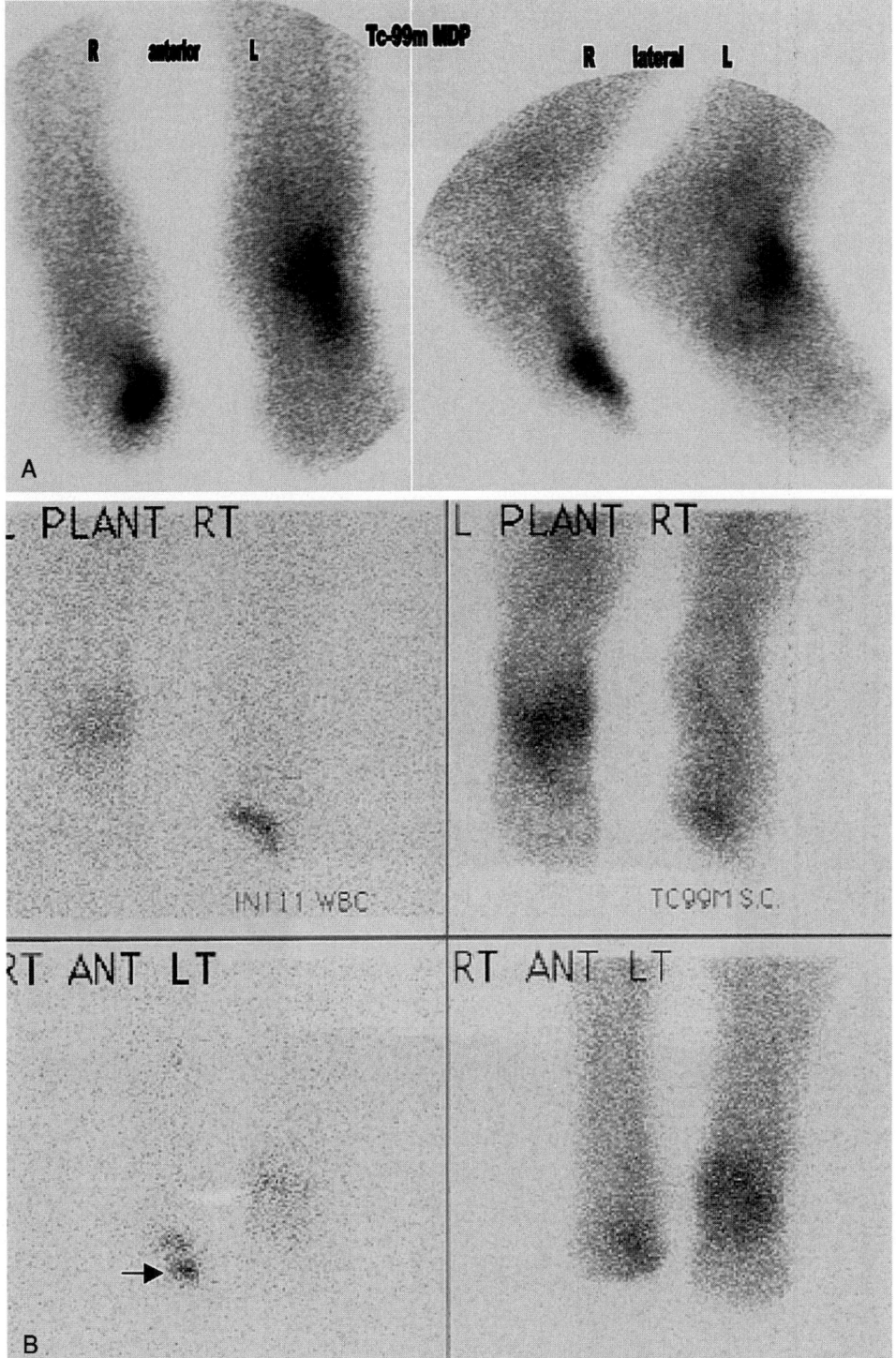

**Figure 7–22.** Infection and neuropathic osteoarthropathy in a diabetic patient. *A,* Bone scan shows increased uptake in the right first toe and in the left midfoot. *B,* Simultaneous 24-hour [111]In-labeled leukocyte scan (left) and 1-hour [99m]Tc sulfur colloid bone marrow scan (right) show increased leukocyte uptake in the right first toe *(arrow)* that is not matched by bone marrow uptake, indicating infection. There was matched leukocyte and bone marrow uptake in the left midfoot, consistent with neuropathic osteoarthropathy.

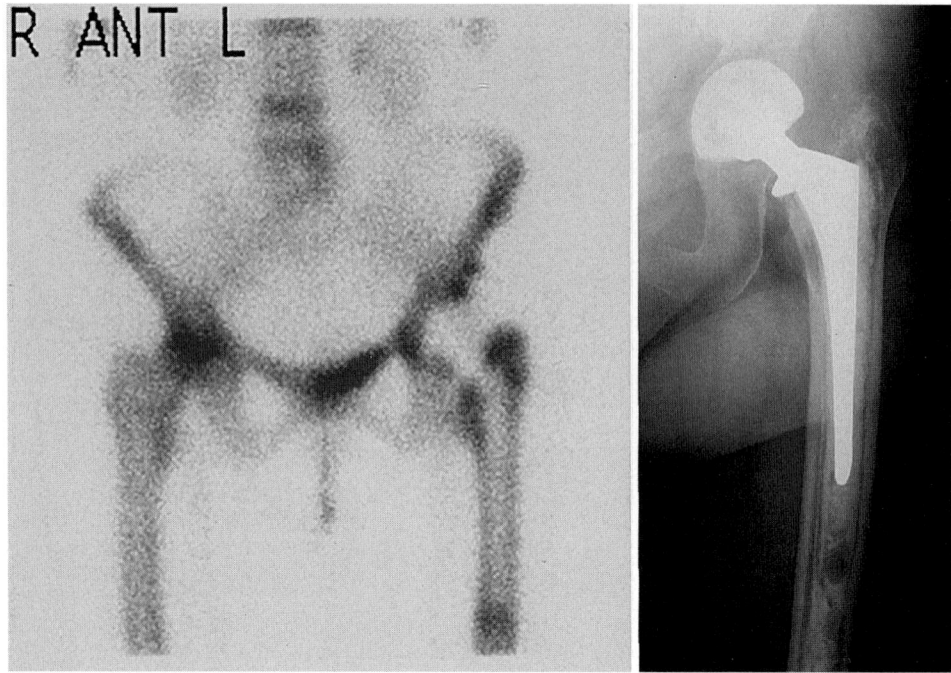

**Figure 7–23.** Bone scan in a case of mechanical loosening of the femoral component of a total hip prosthesis. The 3-hour image shows increased uptake around the tip of the femoral stem and around the greater and lesser trochanters, consistent with mechanical loosening. Increased uptake in the right femoral head was due to osteonecrosis. The radiograph shows a prominent lucency at the cement-bone interface around the entire femoral component, consistent with loosening.

can be divided into septic and aseptic and traumatic and nontraumatic types.

Nontraumatic osteonecrosis is usually associated with one or more risk factors. The most frequent risk factors are use of corticosteroids and increased alcohol intake. Others include sickle cell anemia and dysbarism. Bone scanning has been shown to be more sensitive than radio-

graphy for the detection of osteonecrosis. The characteristic scintigraphic appearance of nontraumatic osteonecrosis in the femoral head is the cold-in-hot lesion (Fig. 7–30). This is a photopenic area caused by the necrotic bone, surrounded by a rim of increased uptake caused by the apposition of viable bone on the periphery of the dead bone, which occurs during the revasculariza-

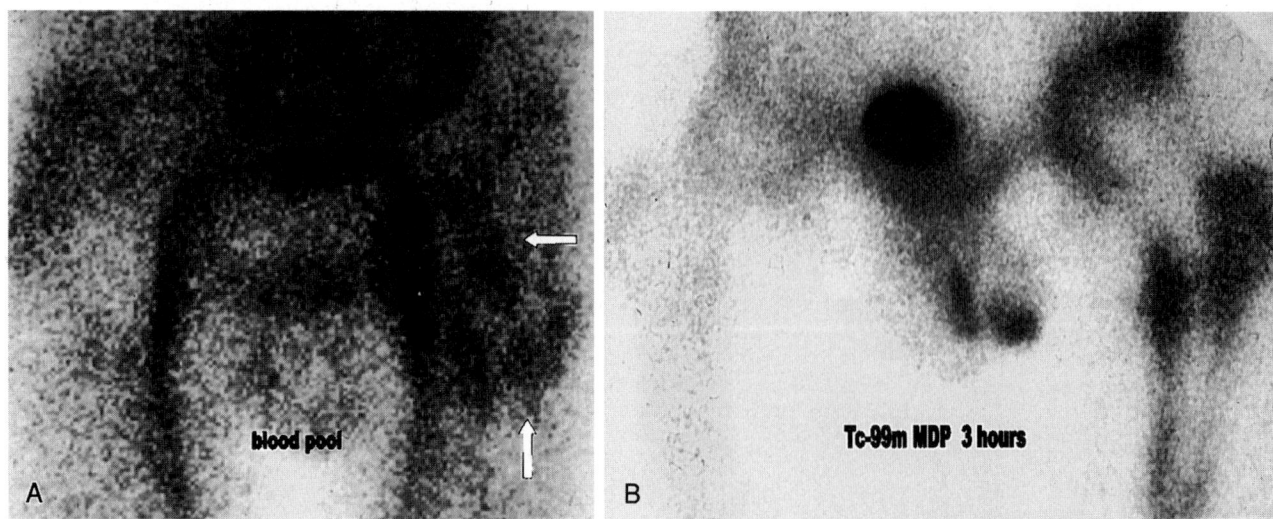

**Figure 7–24.** Bone scan in a patient with an infected total hip prosthesis. *A,* Blood pool scan shows increased activity around the left total hip prosthesis *(arrows). B,* The 3-hour image shows diffuse increased uptake around the femoral and acetabular components, consistent with infection.

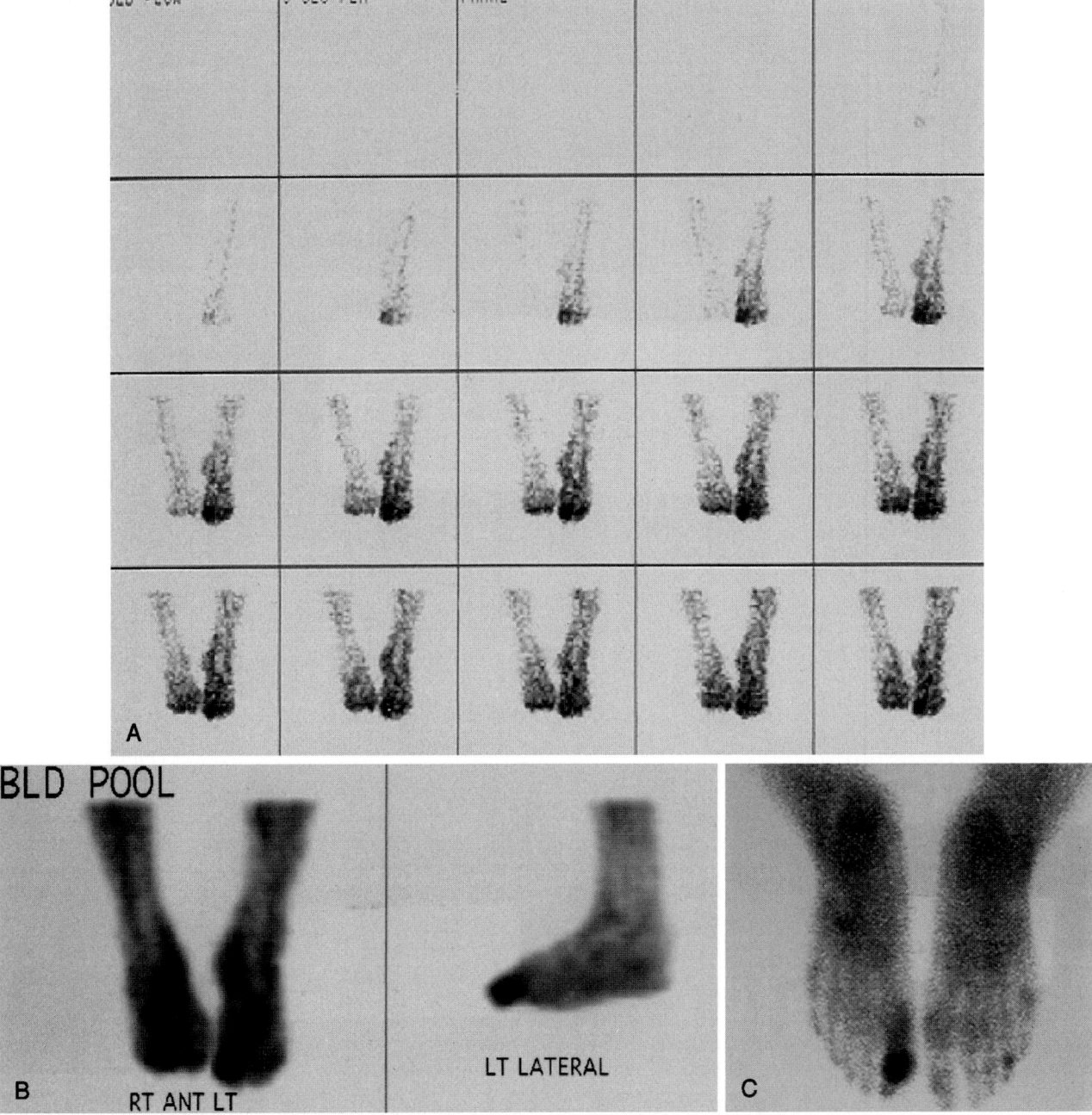

**Figure 7–25.** Gouty arthritis of the first toe. The patient presented with pain and swelling of the first toe but had normal radiographs. The scan was ordered to rule out infection. Blood flow *(A)* and blood pool *(B)* scans show increased activity in the left first toe. A 3-hour plantar bone scan *(C)* shows increased uptake around the left first interphalangeal joint. The scintigraphic findings are consistent with inflammation and arthritis of the joint, which could be infectious or noninfectious. On aspiration of the interphalangeal joint, urate crystals were obtained, indicating gout.

tion and healing phases of the process. The scintigraphic appearance may change as the stages of osteonecrosis progress to bone collapse and secondary osteoarthritis. New areas of increased uptake result from femoral head fragmentation and collapse. With secondary osteoarthritis, increased uptake is present on both sides of the joint. If bone collapse and secondary osteoarthritis do not occur,

the bone scan may become normal; however, this is not commonly seen. Small areas of osteonecrosis may not be detected on scintigraphy. MR imaging is more sensitive than scintigraphy in detecting osteonecrosis.

In traumatic osteonecrosis, which may result from femoral neck fracture, hip dislocation, or scaphoid or talar fracture, there is disruption of the blood supply at

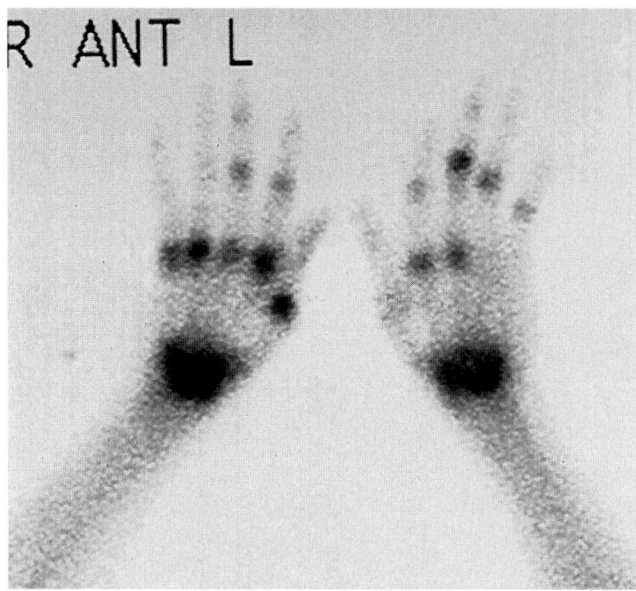

**Figure 7–26.** Rheumatoid arthritis of the hands and wrists. Increased uptake is noted in the radiocarpal, metacarpophalangeal, and proximal interphalangeal joints in a pattern consistent with rheumatoid arthritis.

the time of injury. This can often be identified on three-phase bone scanning as absent uptake during the vascular and delayed phases of the examination. With regard to traumatic osteonecrosis of the femoral head, bone scans can show avascularity at the time of presentation (Fig. 7–31). Evidence of post-traumatic avascular necrosis of the femoral head has been detected by MR imaging 1 month after femoral neck fracture, but not at the time of the fracture. Dynamic MR imaging with a gadolinium-based contrast material may show evidence of avascularity shortly after fracture.

Spontaneous (idiopathic) osteonecrosis about the knee usually involves the weight-bearing aspect of the medial femoral condyle. The scintigraphic findings reflect increased vascularity on the early-phase images and a focal area of markedly increased uptake in the femoral condyle on delayed images. Photopenic areas are not seen in spontaneous osteonecrosis, unlike in other causes of osteonecrosis. Radiographs may be normal initially and show the characteristic focal bony lesion later, or they may never become abnormal. There is evidence that spontaneous osteonecrosis about the knee may be the result of an initial subchondral insufficiency or impaction fracture.

A bone infarct is an area of osteonecrosis in the metaphysis or diaphysis, as opposed to the epiphysis, of a long bone. Bone scans may show decreased uptake; mild, diffuse increased uptake; or normal findings. The pattern may change over the course of the process, with initially decreased uptake, followed by increased uptake, and then normal uptake.

## PEDIATRIC CONDITIONS

The region of the normal growth plate shows high uptake on bone scans in children. The uptake actually corre-

sponds to the zone of provisional calcification in the metaphyseal region of the bone rather than to the cartilage of the growth plate. In infants, this area of high uptake may appear globular, but with increasing age it becomes more linear. Blurring of this region of radionuclide uptake may signify an abnormality adjacent to the growth plate. With maturity of the skeleton and closure of the growth plate, the activity on the bone scan gradually diminishes; however, increased uptake may remain for some time after the growth plate has closed.

Legg-Calvé-Perthes disease (LCP) represents idiopathic avascular necrosis of the femoral head in a child. Bone scanning is highly sensitive for the diagnosis of early LCP. The characteristic scintigraphic appearance of early LCP is absent uptake in the entire femoral head. This can best be seen on pinhole views. Revascularization of the femoral head can also be evaluated on bone scan. Uptake in the ossification center correlates with more rapid healing than does uptake in the region of the growth plate or metaphysis (Fig. 7–32). Meyer's dysplasia is characterized by normal uptake in the femoral heads on bone scans, which differentiates this disorder from LCP.

Transient synovitis of the hip, also called toxic synovitis or irritable hip syndrome, has a variable scintigraphic appearance. Bone scans may be normal in hips of patients with synovitis, or they may show diffuse increased uptake. Diffuse increased uptake and hyperemia may also be present in septic arthritis of the hip, and joint aspiration may be needed to rule out infection. Septic arthritis may also cause absent or decreased uptake in the femoral head because of high pressure from the fluid in the joint.

Concomitant osteomyelitis of the femoral neck carries a worse prognosis for hip involvement than does infection confined to the hip joint alone. Metaphyseal osteomyelitis without joint infection may cause avascularity of the femoral head, as shown by bone scanning (Fig. 7–33). Bone scanning is usually not necessary for the diagnosis of slipped femoral capital epiphysis; however, scintigraphic findings may include increased uptake in the region of the physis and metaphysis. Less commonly, decreased uptake may be seen in the femoral head at the time of presentation.

Bone scanning is especially helpful in a young child with a limp or vague pain, in whom the site of abnormality cannot easily be determined. Occult fractures may be present in the tibia (toddler's fracture), calcaneus, or cuboid. Bone scanning is more sensitive than radiography in detecting fractures in cases of child abuse. Rib fractures in an infant, which may be detected in this fashion, should be an alert for possible child abuse. Bone scanning and radiography are complementary studies for detecting findings of child abuse.

## SOFT TISSUE UPTAKE

There are numerous conditions in which soft tissue or visceral uptake is found on bone scans. In some cases, these findings have no clinical significance; in others, they may indicate a significant pathologic condition. Calcific tendinitis may show focal increased uptake, suggesting the source of pain around a joint (Fig. 7–34). This should be confirmed with radiographs, CT scans, or ultrasono-

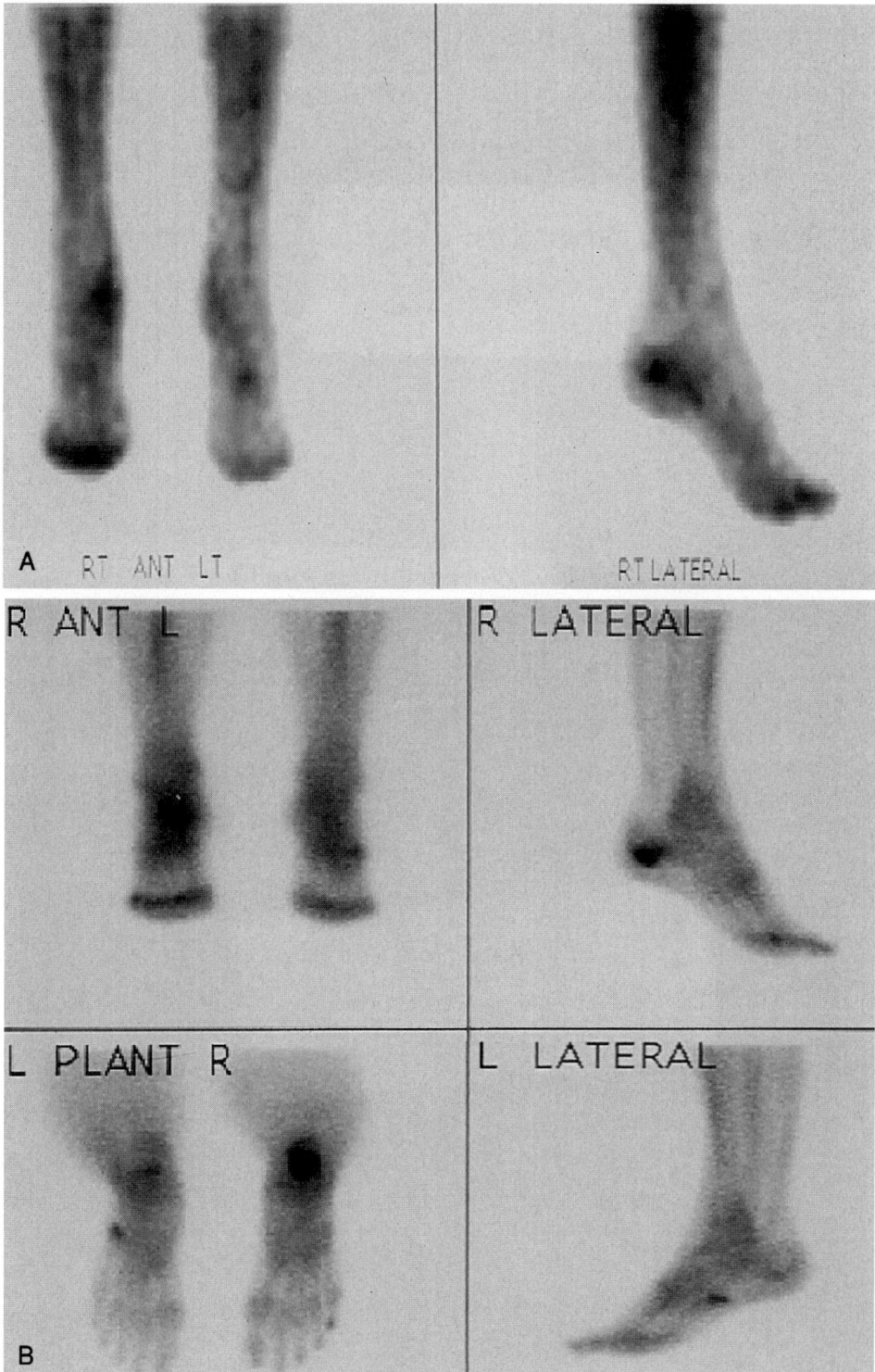

**Figure 7–27.** Plantar fasciitis. The blood pool *(A)* and delayed *(B)* images of a bone scan show focally increased activity in the plantar aspect of the right calcaneus.

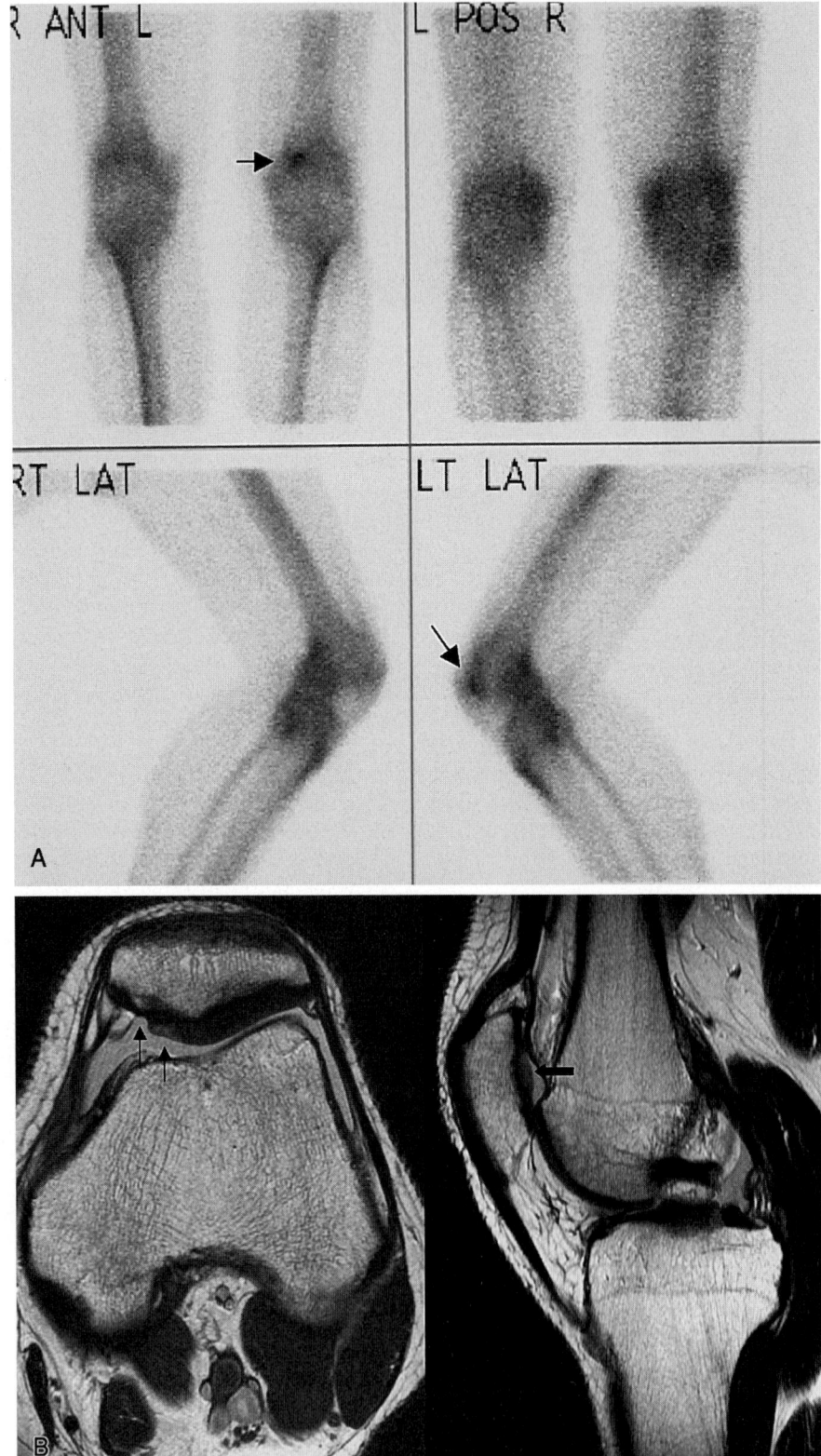

**Figure 7–28.** Chondromalacia patellae. *A,* Bone scan shows a focal area of increased uptake in the medial aspect of the left patellofemoral joint *(arrows).* *B,* Intermediate-weighted spin echo MR image shows abnormal signal and erosion in the medial aspect of the patellar cartilage *(arrows).*

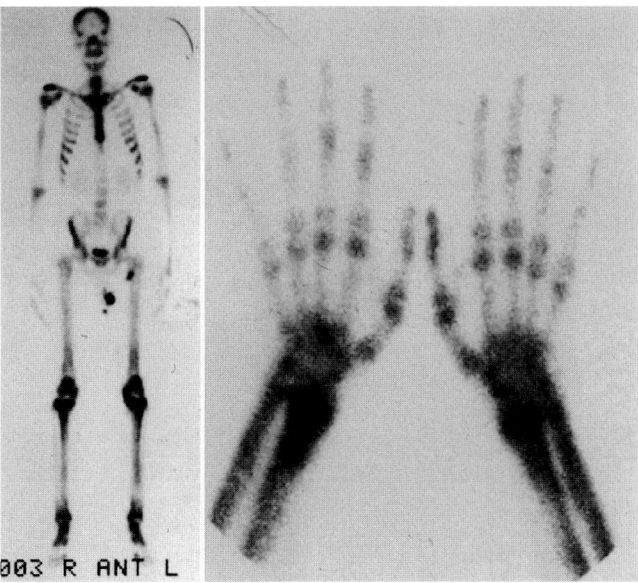

**Figure 7–29.** Secondary hypertrophic osteoarthropathy. The patient had a bone scan because of joint pain. There is increased uptake along the borders of the bones near the knee, ankle, and wrist joints. The diagnosis of hypertrophic osteoarthropathy was made based on the appearance of the bone scan. A chest radiograph showed a mass that was a bronchogenic carcinoma.

grams. This has been seen in the thigh at tendon insertions on the linea aspera in cases of calcific tendinitis of the gluteus maximus or vastus lateralis muscles, and in the proximal portion of the humerus from calcification in the pectoralis major muscle.

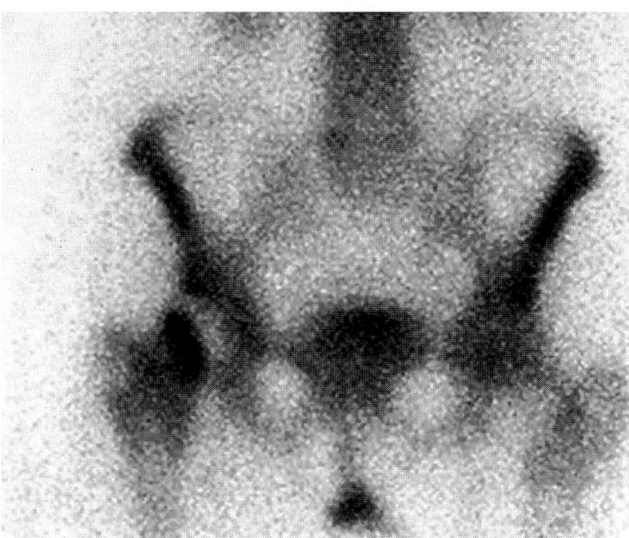

**Figure 7–31.** Post-traumatic osteonecrosis of the femoral head. Bone scan shows a band of increased uptake in the right femoral neck due to a recent subcapital fracture. Decreased uptake in the entire right femoral head indicates avascularity.

Bone scanning has been used for the early diagnosis of heterotopic ossification and for help in determining when surgical resection should be done. The earliest scintigraphic finding is increased activity in the blood flow and blood pool phases, which antedates radiographic changes. This pattern is followed in 2 to 4 weeks by increased uptake on delayed static images and radiographic findings of soft tissue ossification. Sites of heterotopic ossification are considered to be quiescent and amenable to resection

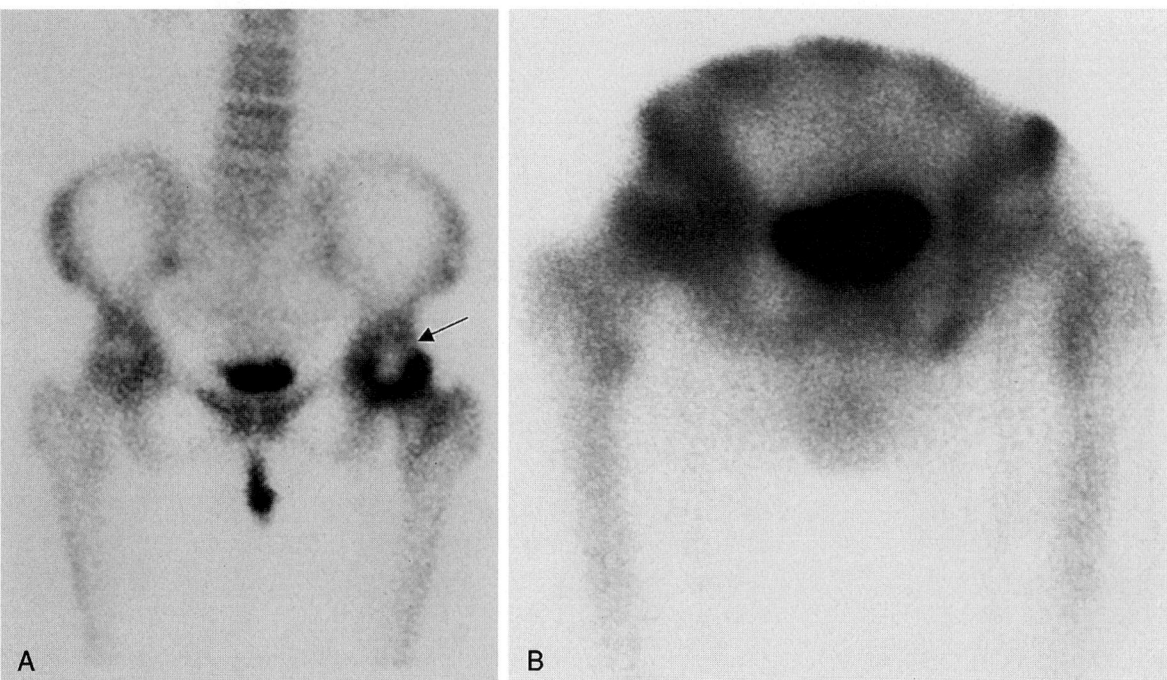

**Figure 7–30.** Osteonecrosis of the femoral head. *A,* A rim of high uptake surrounding an area of lower uptake in the left femoral head *(arrow)* demonstrates the typical "donut" pattern of osteonecrosis. *B,* Scan from a different patient shows increased uptake in the right femoral head with only a small area of decreased uptake.

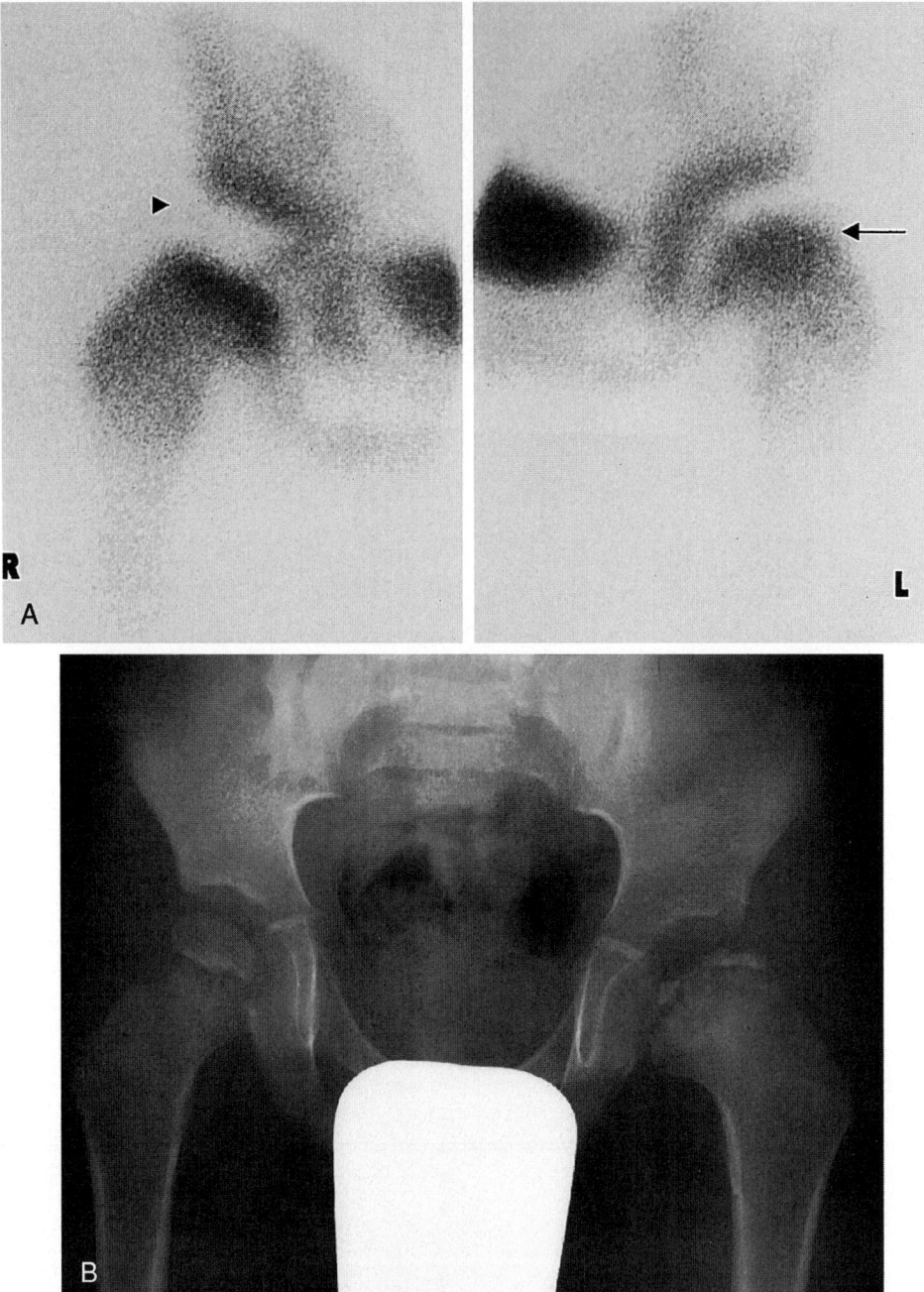

**Figure 7–32.** Legg-Calvé-Perthes disease. *A*, Bone scan shows decreased uptake in virtually the entire right femoral head. There is slight uptake in the lateral column *(arrowhead)*. On the left, there is increased uptake in the metaphysis of the proximal femur *(arrow)* and decreased uptake in the femoral head, with no lateral column uptake. *B*, Radiograph of the pelvis shows a normal contour of the right femoral head. There is collapse of the left femoral head.

without high risk of recurrence when there is normal uptake on a bone scan. However, increased uptake may be present for years. Serial bone scans are needed to determine the maturity of heterotopic ossification.

## RADIONUCLIDES FOR THERAPY

### Radiation Synovectomy

Radiation synovectomy is a nonsurgical method of treating chronic synovitis whose results are comparable to

those of open and arthroscopic synovectomy. It is used in the treatment of hemophilia, rheumatoid arthritis and other inflammatory arthritides, and pigmented villonodular synovitis. Beta radiation–producing radionuclides are injected into a joint to destroy the synovial lining, which causes the inflammation to decrease, or, in hemophilia, to decrease the bleeding into the joint. The radionuclides used for synovectomy are listed in Table 7–1.

These radionuclides have a soft tissue penetrance of less than 1 cm, which leads to effective radiation of the

| TABLE 7–1 | | |
|---|---|---|
| **Radionuclides Used for Synovectomy** | | |
| **Radionuclide** | **Half-life (days)** | **Range (mm)** |
| $^{32}$P | 14.0 | 7.9 |
| $^{165}$Dy | 0.1 | 5.7 |
| $^{90}$Y | 2.7 | 11.1 |
| $^{198}$Au | 2.7 | 3.8 |
| $^{186}$Re | 3.7 | 4.5 |
| $^{153}$Sm | 1.9 | 0.8 |

synovium but not of the rest of the body. Harm to the articular cartilage or an increased frequency of malignancy has not been shown. In hemophilia, fibrosis of the synovium by radiation synovectomy decreases the likelihood of hemarthrosis and the destruction of articular cartilage caused by the chronic synovitis induced by blood in the joint. Radiation synovectomy is much less expensive than open surgical or arthroscopic synovectomy. Radiation synovectomy works best in large joints without marked radiographic changes of cartilage destruction.

## Treatment of Pain from Bone Metastases

Intravenous injection of bone-seeking radionuclides that produce beta radiation has been used for palliation of metastatic disease to bone. This treatment can be used only for lesions that show increased uptake on bone scan. The exact mechanism by which such treatment reduces pain is uncertain. The treatment is palliative and is not

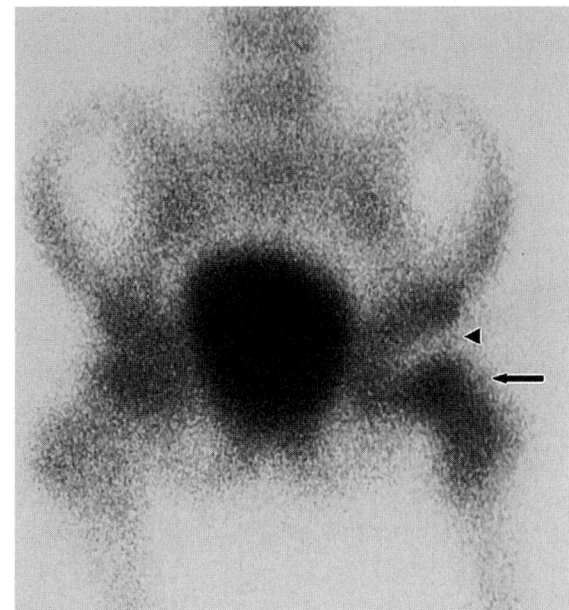

**Figure 7–33.** Osteomyelitis of the proximal femur and septic necrosis of the femoral head. Bone scan shows increased uptake in the femoral neck *(arrow)* and decreased uptake in the femoral head *(arrowhead)*, indicating avascularity.

curative, and it is used in conjunction with other therapies in patients with metastatic disease. Pain reduction occurs within several days to weeks and may last for as long as 6 months; however, such pain relief is often short term, and a flare response, with increased pain, may occur

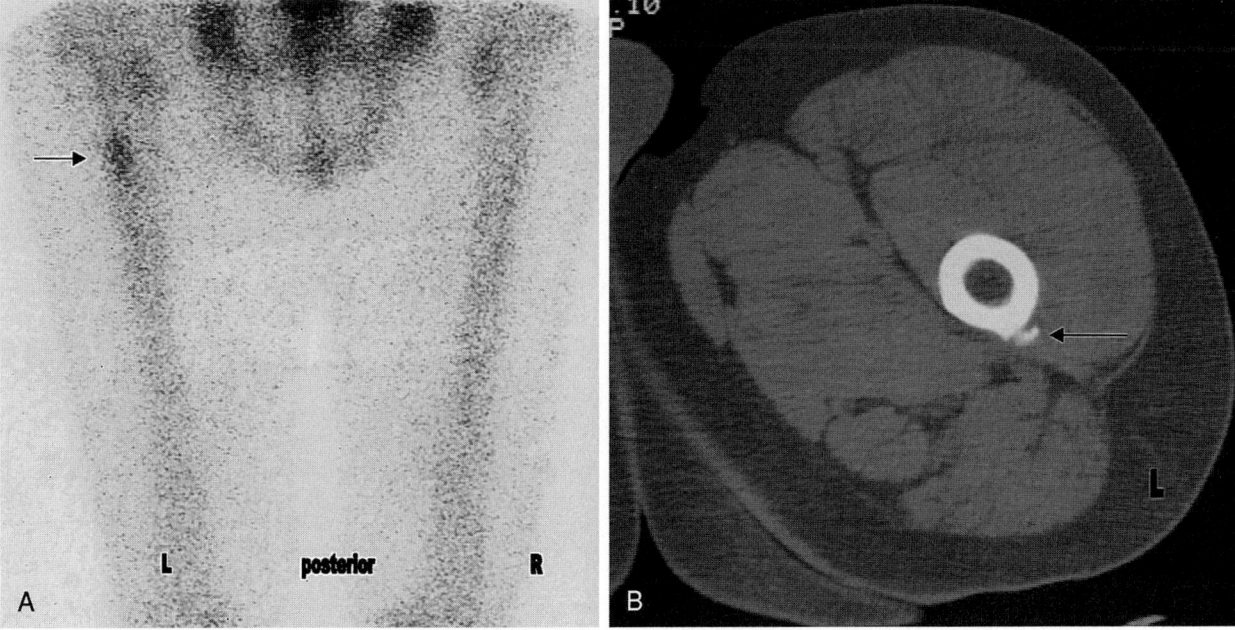

**Figure 7–34.** Calcific tendinitis of the thigh. A bone scan was done because of pain in the left proximal thigh. The posterior bone scan *(A)* shows a focal area of increased uptake overlying the proximal femur *(arrow)*. A CT scan *(B)* shows calcification in the soft tissues of the thigh in the vastus lateralis or gluteus maximus tendon *(arrow)*.

shortly after treatment. The treatment is not useful for relieving pain from pathologic fracture or nerve or spinal cord involvement. The radioisotopes that have been approved for this purpose by the U.S. Food and Drug Administration are phosphorus-32, strontium-89, and samarium-153.

## FURTHER READING

Abe H, Nakamura M, Takahashi S, et al: Radiation-induced insufficiency fractures of the pelvis: Evaluation with 99mTc-methylene diphosphonate scintigraphy. AJR Am J Roentgenol 158:599, 1992.

Alazraki NP: Radionuclide imaging in the evaluation of infections and inflammatory disease. Radiol Clin North Am 31:783, 1993.

Algra PR, Bloem JL, Tissing H, et al: Detection of vertebral metastases: Comparison between MR imaging and bone scintigraphy. Radiographics 11:219, 1991.

Aliabadi P, Tumeh SS, Weissman BN, et al: Cemented total hip prosthesis: Radiographic and scintigraphic evaluation. Radiology 173:203, 1989.

Bahk YW, Park YH, Chung SK, et al: Bone pathologic correlation of multimodality imaging in Paget's disease. J Nucl Med 36:1421, 1995.

Bauer GH: The use of radionuclides in orthopaedics. Part IV. Radionuclide scintimetry of the skeleton. J Bone Joint Surg Am 50:168, 1968.

Brown ML: Bone scintigraphy in benign and malignant tumors. Radiol Clin North Am 31:731, 1993.

Caner B, Kitapcl M, Unlu M, et al: Technetium-99m-MIBI uptake in benign and malignant bone lesions: A comparative study with technetium-99m-MDP. J Nucl Med 33:319, 1992.

Collier BD, Carrera GF, Johnson RP, et al: Detection of femoral head avascular necrosis in adults by SPECT. J Nucl Med 26:979, 1985.

Collier BD, Carrera GF, Messer EJ, et al: Internal derangement of the temporomandibular joint: Detection by single-photon emission computed tomography. Work in progress. Radiology 149:557, 1983.

Collier BD, Johnson RP, Carrera GF, et al: Painful spondylolysis or spondylolisthesis studied by radiography and single-photon emission computed tomography. Radiology 154:207, 1985.

Conway JJ, Collins M, Tanz RR, et al: The role of bone scintigraphy in detecting child abuse. Semin Nucl Med 23:321, 1993.

Cuartero-Plaza A, Martinez-Miralles E, Benito-Ruiz P, et al: Abnormal bone scintigraphy and silent radiography in localized reflex sympathetic dystrophy syndrome. Eur J Nucl Med 19:330, 1992.

Delbeke D: Oncological applications of FDG PET imaging. J Nucl Med 40:1706, 1999.

Demangeat JL, Constantinesco A, Brunot B, et al: Three-phase bone scanning in reflex sympathetic dystrophy of the hand. J Nucl Med 29:26, 1988.

Eggli DF, Tulchinsky M: Normal Planar Bone Scan. St Louis, Mosby, 1996, p 23.

Elgazzar AH, Abdel-Dayem HM, Clark JD, et al: Multimodality imaging of osteomyelitis. Eur J Nucl Med 22:1043, 1995.

Fogelman I, Carr D: A comparison of bone scanning and radiology in the assessment of patients with symptomatic Paget's disease. Eur J Nucl Med 5:417, 1980.

Fogelman I, Carr D: A comparison of bone scanning and radiology in the evaluation of patients with metabolic bone disease. Clin Radiol 31:321, 1980.

Gaucher A, Colomb JN, Naoun A, et al: The diagnostic value of 99m Tc-diphosphonate bone imaging in transient osteoporosis of the hip. J Rheumatol 6:574, 1979.

Glithero PR, Grigoris P, Harding LK, et al: White cell scans and infected joint replacements: Failure to detect chronic infection. J Bone Joint Surg Br 75:371, 1993.

Graham GD, Lundy MM, Frederick RJ, et al: Scintigraphic detection of osteomyelitis with Tc-99m MDP and Ga-67 citrate: Concise communication. J Nucl Med 24:1019, 1983.

Hauzeur JP, Pasteels JL, Schoutens A, et al: The diagnostic value of magnetic resonance imaging in non-traumatic osteonecrosis of the femoral head. J Bone Joint Surg Am 71:641, 1989.

Hawkins RA, Choi Y, Huang SC, et al: Quantitating tumor glucose metabolism with FDG and PET [editorial; comment]. J Nucl Med 33:339, 1992.

Holder LE, Schwarz C, Wernicke PG, Michael RH: Radionuclide bone imaging in the early detection of fractures of the proximal femur (hip): Multifactorial analysis. Radiology 174:509, 1990.

Jacobson AF: Bone scanning in metastatic disease. In Collier BD, Fogelman I, Rosenthall L (eds): Skeletal Nuclear Medicine. St Louis, Mosby, 1996, p 87.

Kashyap R, Bhatnagar A, Mondal A, et al: 24 Hour/3 hour radio-uptake technique for differentiating degenerative and malignant bony lesions in bone scanning. Australas Radiol 37:198, 1993.

Matin P: The appearance of bone scans following fractures, including immediate and long-term studies. J Nucl Med 20:1227, 1979.

Murray IP: The evaluation of malignancy: Primary bone tumors. In Murray IP, Ell PJ (eds): Nuclear Medicine in Clinical Diagnosis and Treatment, vol 2. New York, Churchill Livingstone, 1994, p 935.

Palestro CJ, Kim CK, Swyer AJ, et al: Radionuclide diagnosis of vertebral osteomyelitis: Indium-111-leukocyte and technetium-99m-methylene diphosphonate bone scintigraphy. J Nucl Med 32:1861, 1991.

Palestro CJ, Swyer AJ, Kim CK, et al: Infected knee prosthesis: Diagnosis with In-111 leukocyte, Tc-99m sulfur colloid, and Tc-99m MDP imaging. Radiology 179:645, 1991.

Palestro CJ, Torres MA: Radionuclide imaging in orthopedic infections. Semin Nucl Med 27:334, 1997.

Rizzo PF, Gould ES, Lyden JP, et al: Diagnosis of occult fractures about the hip: Magnetic resonance imaging compared with bone-scanning. J Bone Joint Surg Am 75:395, 1993.

Rupani HD, Holder LE, Espinola DA, et al: Three-phase radionuclide bone imaging in sports medicine. Radiology 156:187, 1985.

Ryan PJ, Fogelman I: Bone scintigraphy in metabolic bone disease. Semin Nucl Med 27:291, 1997.

Ryan PJ, Fogelman I: Osteoporotic vertebral fractures: Diagnosis with radiography and bone scintigraphy. Radiology 190:669, 1994.

Schauwecker DS: Osteomyelitis: Diagnosis with In-111-labeled leukocytes. Radiology 171:141, 1989.

Subramanian G: Radiopharmaceuticals for bone scanning. In Collier BD, Fogelman I, Rosenthall L (eds): Skeletal Nuclear Medicine. St Louis, Mosby, 1996, p 9.

Sy WM, Westring DW, Weinberger G: "Cold" lesions on bone imaging. J Nucl Med 16:1013, 1975.

Tigges S, Stiles RG, Meli RJ, et al: Hip aspiration: A cost-effective and accurate method of evaluating the potentially infected hip prosthesis. Radiology 189:485, 1993.

Utz JA, Lull RJ, Galvin EG: Asymptomatic total hip prosthesis: Natural history determined using Tc-99m MDP bone scans. Radiology 161:509, 1986.

Van Nostrand D, Abreu SH, Callaghan JJ, et al: In-111-labeled white blood cell uptake in noninfected closed fracture in humans: Prospective study. Radiology 167:495, 1988.

Weber DA: Radiotracers used in skeletal procedures: Physical and biologic properties. In Galasko C, Weber DA: Radionuclide Scintigraphy in Orthopaedics. New York, Churchill Livingstone, 1984, p 1.

# CHAPTER 8

## Magnetic Resonance Imaging: Practical Considerations

### David A. Rubin

## SUMMARY OF KEY FEATURES

In its relatively short existence, magnetic resonance (MR) imaging has emerged as the most powerful imaging technique for the noninvasive diagnosis of a host of traumatic, degenerative, rheumatologic, infectious, and neoplastic conditions in the musculoskeletal system. The gross and histologic anatomy of different tissues predicts their MR imaging appearances in both healthy and diseased states. An understanding of the available pulse sequences and imaging options enhances a radiologist's ability to distinguish normal from abnormal tissues. The true utility of MR imaging, however, stems from its depiction of fine anatomic detail. An appreciation of these findings, in turn, helps guide the clinical management of musculoskeletal conditions.

## INTRODUCTION

In the past decade, MR imaging has been widely applied clinically and has become the study of choice for the diagnosis of many bone, joint, and soft tissue disorders. The modality provides the radiologist with an unparalleled, noninvasive look at the detailed anatomy and subtle pathology in the living body, without the use of ionizing radiation. MR imaging can also be cost-effective for applications ranging from diagnosing radiographically occult hip fractures to reducing the number of unnecessary diagnostic knee arthroscopies, staging musculoskeletal infections, and guiding biopsies in patients with inflammatory myopathies. Its superior accuracy in comparison to clinical evaluation has also made MR imaging the optimal technique for the diagnosis of conditions as diverse as meniscal tears in the knee and disc disease in the spine.

## TECHNICAL CONSIDERATIONS

The use of MR imaging for the pathologic diagnosis of musculoskeletal conditions relies on signal intensity and morphologic changes in the tissues being studied. Detecting subtle alterations in these features requires both high contrast resolution (different signal intensities in normal and abnormal structures) and high spatial resolution. To meet these goals, the signal-to-noise ratio (SNR) of the images must be as high as possible. The best way to increase the SNR in musculoskeletal MR imaging is by using local coils. Ideally, the coil surrounds the entire limb, which is possible for the knee, ankle, wrist, and elbow, but not for the hip or shoulder.

Imaging artifacts arise from many sources, including imperfections in the instrumentation and magnetic fields, inherent properties of the mathematics used to reconstruct the images, and tissue interfaces and foreign bodies. The most readily preventable source of artifacts, however, is involuntary patient motion. Carefully positioning the patient to ensure comfort prevents motion artifacts better than forcibly restraining the examined body part.

## BONE MARROW

MR imaging is the most sensitive, noninvasive test for identifying pathologic states within marrow, whether they be infectious, ischemic, traumatic, or neoplastic.

### Normal Appearance and Technique

Hematopoietic or red marrow consists of approximately 40% fat, 40% water, and 20% protein, whereas fatty or yellow marrow is composed of approximately 80% fat, 15% water, and 5% protein. MR pulse sequences can exploit these differences. Because yellow marrow contains a higher percentage of fat than red marrow does, yellow marrow has a shorter T1 and appears brighter on T1-weighted images. Normally, yellow marrow is isointense with subcutaneous fat on T1-weighted images, whereas the signal intensity of normal red marrow falls between that of subcutaneous fat and skeletal muscle (Fig. 8–1A). On T2-weighted images, both yellow marrow and red marrow have similar signal intensities and appear hyperintense in comparison to muscle, but less intense than water. Yellow and red marrow (of which fat is still a major constituent) both appear darker when fat suppression is applied (see Fig. 8–1B). T2-weighted sequences performed with spectral fat suppression are sensitive to small increases in water content and thus easily detect processes that replace normal marrow. Short tau inversion recovery (STIR) sequences, which null the signal from fat based on its T1 value, are even more sensitive to subtle changes in marrow composition. Gradient recalled sequences are less useful for examining marrow.

In the neonate, most of the body's marrow is hematopoietic (Fig. 8–2). As the child grows and develops, red marrow in the appendicular skeleton is converted to fatty marrow in an orderly progression, from distal to proximal. The conversion begins relatively early in infancy. In children, marrow contains a mixture of fat cells and hematopoietic cells and thus exhibits heterogeneous, patchy signal intensity on T1-weighted images. Beyond adolescence, only portions of the axial skeleton and the proximal ends of the femora and humeri contain significant amounts of red marrow. Even in these regions, though, steady replacement of the hematopoietic elements by fat occurs throughout adulthood.

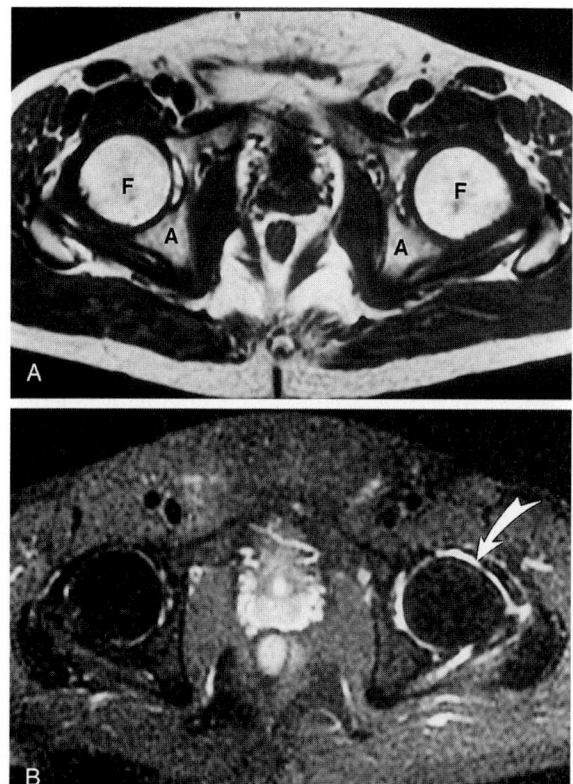

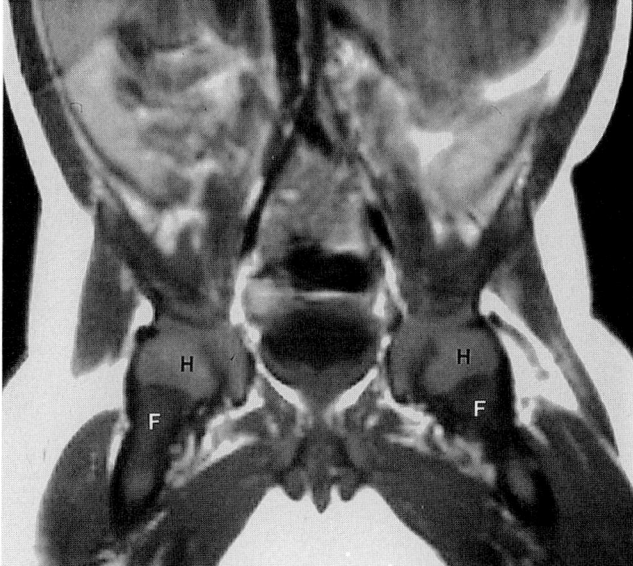

**Figure 8–2.** Normal neonatal bone marrow in an 8-week-old boy. Coronal T1-weighted (TR/TE, 400/12) spin echo MR image. No fatty marrow is present in the proximal metaphysis of the femora (F). The femoral heads (H) are entirely cartilaginous. (Courtesy of W. Totty, MD, St. Louis, Mo.)

**Figure 8–1.** Normal adult bone marrow. *A*, Transaxial T1-weighted (TR/TE, 600/8) spin echo MR image of the pelvis. Yellow marrow within the femoral heads (F) is isointense to subcutaneous fat. Red marrow within the acetabula (A) has signal intensity between that of muscle and fat. *B*, Transaxial fat-suppressed T2-weighted (TR/TEeff, 4000/60) fast spin echo MR image. The signal intensity of both yellow and red marrow decreases. A small effusion is seen in the left hip *(arrow)*.

## Changes in Marrow Composition

The amount of adipose tissue in marrow has an inverse relationship to the degree of ongoing red blood cell production. In times of stress, fatty marrow may be reconverted into hematopoietic marrow. This reconversion follows a progression opposite that of the normal yellow-to-red marrow conversion, in that it occurs in a proximal-to-distal direction. Physiologic reconversion may occur in patients who are heavy cigarette smokers, obese, or chronically anemic or in those who live at high altitudes.

Differentiating physiologic red marrow expansion from pathologic marrow replacement is important. Expanded red marrow should have higher signal intensity than muscle on T1-weighted images and should never be as bright as fluid on fat-suppressed T2-weighted images (Fig. 8–3). Islands of red marrow have a lobulated contour. Under physiologic conditions, red marrow expansion should not extend distal to the wrists or ankles and should not cross the physes into the epiphyses or apophyses of the long bones. (One exception is the subchondral region of the humeral head, which may be a site of physiologic red marrow expansion, especially in young and middle-aged women.)

In patients with severe, chronic anemia such as that associated with sickle cell disease, marrow hyperplasia can be extensive. On MR images, the expanded red marrow still has the signal characteristics of normal hematopoietic marrow. Just as expansion of red marrow reflects an increase in hematopoiesis, disorders that deplete the marrow myeloid elements result in an increase in fatty marrow content. Conversion of red marrow to yellow marrow is seen in patients with untreated aplastic anemia and in patients undergoing some chemotherapy regimens. The edge of radiation ports produces a characteristic, sharply defined margin between normal and treated marrow (Fig. 8–4). Fibrotic marrow (occurring in idiopathic myelofibrosis or in the late, burned-out stage of myeloproliferative disorders such as polycythemia vera) demonstrates low signal intensity on all pulse sequences.

## Hyperemia, Ischemia, and Infarction

Marrow hypervascularity is thought to cause an increase in water content. A pattern of marrow "edema" emerges, with decreased signal intensity seen on T1-weighted images and increased signal intensity noted on fat-suppressed T2-weighted or STIR images. It is likely that the self-limited, painful conditions of reflex sympathetic dystrophy, transient osteoporosis of the hip, regional migratory osteoporosis, and painful tibial edema syndrome are due to changes in intramedullary pressure, blood flow, or both.

Marrow ischemia may also cause signal intensity changes. If the damage is irreversible, infarction ensues. However, transient ischemia can also occur, with the marrow returning to normal after a period of weeks or months. Marrow infarction in subchondral bone is called avascular necrosis (see Chapter 67).

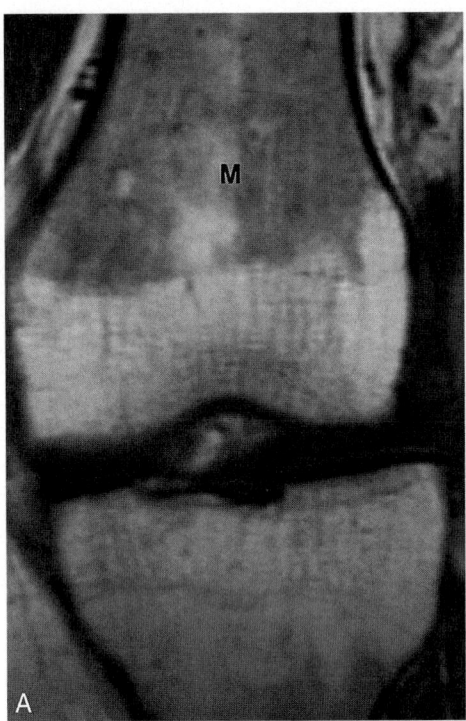
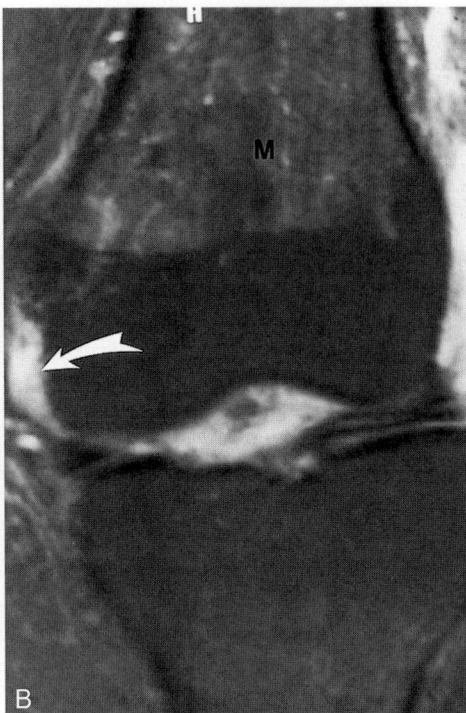

**Figure 8–3.** Physiologic red marrow hyperplasia in a healthy 47-year-old woman. *A*, Coronal T1-weighted (TR/TE, 450/12) spin echo MR image. Hematopoietic marrow (M) in the distal part of the femur is hyperintense in comparison to muscle. Note that the red marrow occurs in confluent islands interspersed with yellow marrow and does not cross into the epiphysis. *B*, Coronal fat-suppressed T2-weighted (TR/TEeff, 3200/54) fast spin echo MR image. The red marrow (M) is hypointense in comparison to joint fluid *(arrow)*.

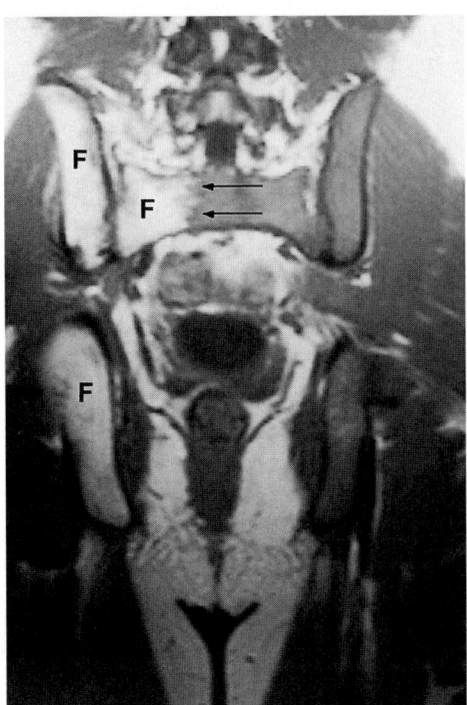

**Figure 8–4.** Effect of radiation therapy. Coronal T1-weighted (TR/TE, 572/12) spin echo MR image. After treatment for Ewing's sarcoma, fatty replacement of the marrow (F) has developed in the right side of the sacrum and pelvis. Observe the characteristic sharp demarcation *(arrows)* between normal and fatty marrow, which corresponds to the boundary of the radiation port.

## Trauma

Bone marrow can be injured either by a single blunt force or by repetitive, cumulative insults. A direct blow to a bone may produce a marrow contusion, or bone "bruise." These radiographically occult injuries probably reflect microfractures of the trabeculae, with resultant marrow edema and hemorrhage. Common examples include bruises in the lateral knee compartment experienced after a tear of the anterior cruciate ligament (ACL) and bruises in the anterolateral femoral condyle and medial patella suffered after a patellar dislocation-relocation injury (Fig. 8–5).

On MR images, bone contusions appear as geographic or reticulated areas of low signal intensity within the fatty marrow on T1-weighted images. The lesions have high signal intensity on fat-suppressed, T2-weighted or STIR images. These findings typically resolve over a period of 6 weeks to 4 months. In addition to bone bruises (which are essentially microfractures), nondisplaced macroscopic fractures can be radiographically occult. MR imaging is exquisitely sensitive to these injuries—more so than bone scintigraphy—and it has the added benefit of directly demonstrating the number, completeness, and position of the fracture plane or planes. Fracture lines appear as linear areas of very low signal intensity in the marrow (Fig. 8–6), typically within an area of more generalized edema. Both T1-weighted images and STIR or fat-suppressed T2-weighted images can demonstrate fractures.

Marrow changes also occur in patients with chronic repetitive trauma. Stress fractures, both the fatigue type and the insufficiency type, demonstrate a pattern of marrow edema surrounding a fracture line. Stress fracture lines are usually linear and have low signal intensity on all

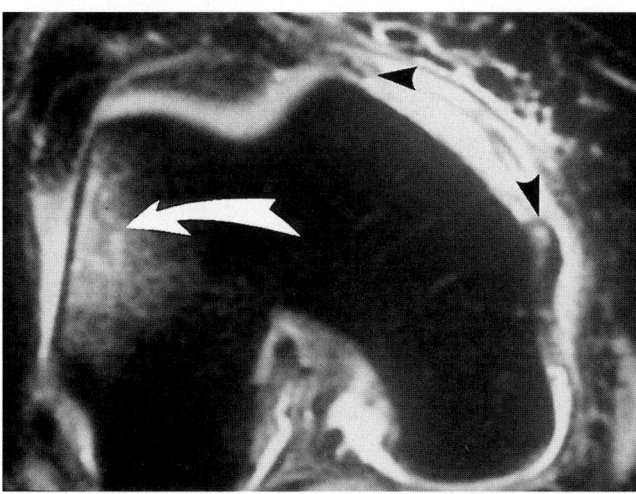

**Figure 8–5.** Bone bruise from patellar dislocation-relocation injury. Transverse fat-suppressed intermediate-weighted (TR/TEeff, 3500/12) fast spin echo MR image. A high-signal-intensity contusion *(arrow)* is apparent in the lateral femoral condyle. Also note the torn medial patellofemoral ligament *(arrowheads)*.

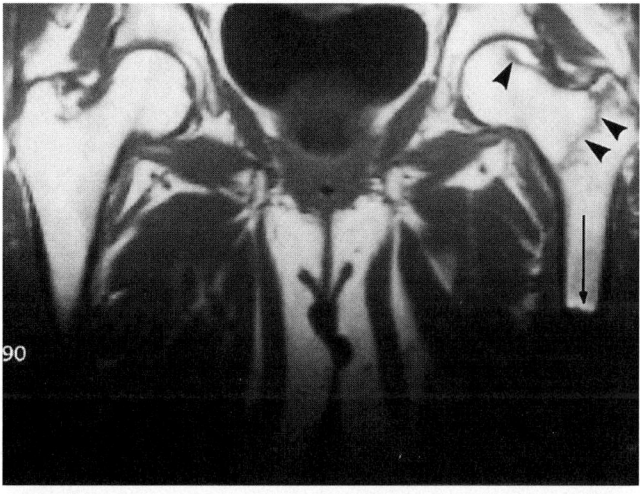

**Figure 8–6.** Occult proximal femoral fracture. Coronal T1-weighted (TR/TE, 500/12) spin echo MR image. Nondisplaced, low-signal-intensity fracture lines *(arrowheads)* are visible in the left intertrochanteric region of the femur and greater trochanter. The fractures were not visible radiographically. An intramedullary rod, placed retrograde to treat a previous distal femoral fracture, produces signal loss in the midfemoral shaft *(arrow)*.

pulse sequences. A spectrum of stress injuries exists. One extreme is a stress fracture that has become a complete, displaced fracture. At the other extreme are ill-defined regions of marrow edema without visible fracture lines, which represent radiographically occult "stress responses" or "stress reactions."

## Marrow Replacement

Alterations in marrow MR signal intensity are sensitive indicators of osteomyelitis, but they are not specific.

Active osteomyelitis produces decreased signal intensity on T1-weighted images and increased signal intensity on T2-weighted or STIR images. However, these signal characteristics also occur in traumatic, ischemic, and neoplastic conditions. In some cases, the signal intensity changes may simply represent marrow hyperemia and edema in response to an adjacent soft tissue infection or septic arthritis. Conversely, the lack of marrow signal changes has a very high negative predictive value. Cortical destruction, a sinus tract, or an adjacent abscess or ulcer increases the likelihood that signal changes within the bone marrow represent active infection. The use of intravenous contrast in cases of bone and soft tissue infection can help stage the process and direct treatment. Within the infected bone, identifying a nonenhancing, nonviable region (whether an intraosseous abscess in an acute case or a sequestrum in a chronic one) may direct treatment toward early surgical débridement in addition to antibiotic administration. Similarly, mapping out deep soft tissue abscesses for drainage results in faster and more cost-effective treatment of the infection.

For primary bone tumors, radiographs are more useful than MR images for lesion characterization. Frequently, MR imaging cannot distinguish benign from malignant causes of marrow replacement. Complex, dynamic gadolinium-enhanced MR techniques have been described to assess very early enhancement (which favors malignant over benign lesions), but overlap between the enhancement features of various processes means that the pattern of enhancement cannot obviate biopsy.

Two other uses of MR imaging for primary bone tumors are local staging and assessing response to chemotherapy. For staging, MR imaging accurately demonstrates intraosseous tumor extent, soft tissue involvement, and proximity to neurovascular bundles, all of which affect surgical management. Early investigators suggested that MR imaging could stage primary tumors more accurately than was possible with computed tomography (CT), but a recent multi-institutional study found that the two modalities are comparable for local staging. For gauging response to neoadjuvant chemotherapy in osteosarcoma and Ewing's tumor, standard MR examination is not useful. However, assessment of dynamic enhancement patterns may accurately predict tumor response to neoadjuvant chemotherapy.

MR imaging is more sensitive than radiography and more specific than bone scintigraphy for the detection of osseous metastatic disease (Fig. 8–7). Additionally, MR imaging may be more sensitive than bone scintigraphy in a defined anatomic location or in cases of diffuse metastatic marrow replacement in children. Scintigraphy is a better screening test for metastases. MR imaging has also been used to evaluate the bone marrow of patients with multiple myeloma, lymphoma, and leukemia (see Chapters 49 and 51).

## CORTICAL BONE, PERIOSTEUM, AND ARTICULAR CARTILAGE

Modalities such as radiography and CT, which differentiate tissues on the basis of attenuation differences, are ideal for the imaging of cortical bone. Although periosteal new bone formation is also visible radiographically, earlier

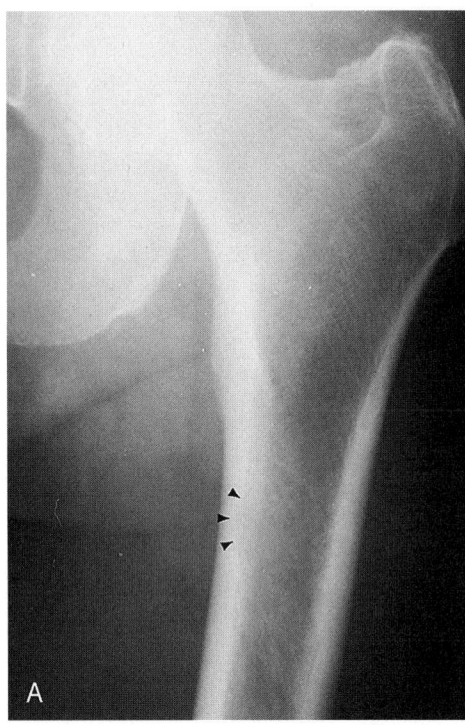 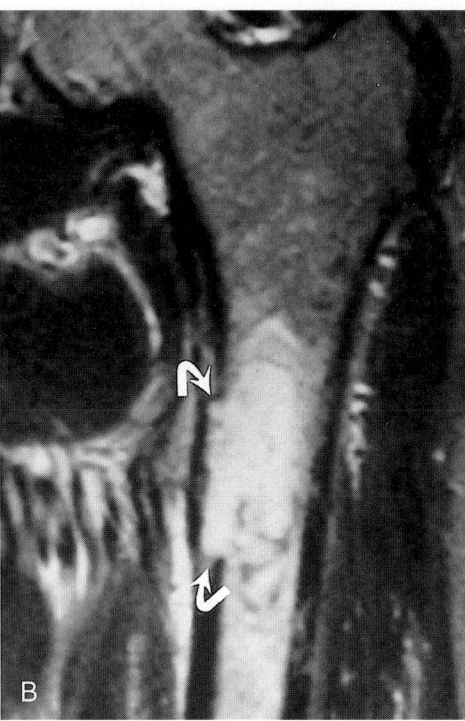

**Figure 8–7.** Metastatic lesion from renal cell carcinoma. *A*, Anteroposterior femur radiograph. Slight endosteal scalloping *(arrowheads)* is the only clue to an underlying lytic lesion. *B*, Coronal fat-suppressed T2-weighted (TR/TEeff, 5000/90) fast spin echo MR image. The high-signal-intensity metastasis is easily seen. The size of the lesion and involvement of the medial femoral cortex *(arrows)* place the bone at risk for pathologic fracture.

stages of periosteal reaction (before mineralization is apparent) may be seen with MR imaging. MR imaging is emerging as the dominant noninvasive modality to assess articular cartilage disorders, whether they result from traumatic, inflammatory, or degenerative causes.

### Normal Appearance and Technique

Cortical (compact) bone has few mobile protons, which results in low signal intensity on all pulse sequences. At bone–soft tissue interfaces, cortical bone appears artifactually thicker when using techniques such as gradient recalled sequences. In the cervical spine, "blooming" of bone size can cause overestimation of the amount of foraminal stenosis. Using the shortest possible TE and higher matrix sizes minimizes the effect. Chemical shift misregistration affects the apparent cortical thickness in the frequency-encoding direction, and the cortex appears artifactually thickened on one side and thinner on the opposite side. This artifact can be reduced by swapping the phase and frequency encoding, decreasing the field of view, or increasing the sampling bandwidth. The use of fat suppression eliminates chemical shift artifacts without necessitating an increase in bandwidth (which decreases the SNR). The periosteum is a thin, fibrous membrane closely apposed to the nonarticular surfaces of bones. Normally, it is not visible on MR images.

The imaging characteristics of normal cartilage reflect its chemical composition and three-dimensional histologic organization. Currently, there is no consensus on the single best articular cartilage sequence. In high-resolution clinical images, a trilaminar appearance may be seen, with the central layer being darker than the superficial and deep ones. However, in these cases, the layering is mostly due to truncation, magic angle, and chemical shift arti-

facts and not to the underlying ultrastructural composition of the cartilage. On T1- and proton density-weighted spin echo images, articular cartilage has intermediate signal intensity, between that of muscle and fat. On T2-weighted images, cartilage has low signal intensity, which contrasts with the high signal intensity of joint fluid. Within cartilage, the T2 progressively increases when moving from the deep to the superficial layers. T2 changes reflect variations in water concentration, under the influence of the surrounding collagen fiber matrix, and, to a lesser extent, variations in proteoglycan concentration. On gradient recalled MR images, articular cartilage has intermediate signal intensity, which becomes progressively darker close to the subchondral plate. When fat suppression is added to a T1-weighted sequence, the cartilage appears bright when compared with the intermediate signal intensity of joint fluid, the dark subchondral plate, and the suppressed marrow fat.

### Traumatic Disorders

MR imaging can also play a role in fractures that are visible radiographically. For example, in tibial plateau fractures, the treating physician often needs to visualize the number and orientation of fracture lines, the size and position of articular fragments, and the status of the articular surface in multiple planes. Although this task can be accomplished equally well with reformatted CT examination, MR imaging has the advantage of also showing associated soft tissue injuries such as meniscal tears and ligament injuries (Fig. 8–8), which have a direct impact on patient management.

A visible fracture line, periosteal new bone formation, or both, distinguish a stress fracture from other stress injuries. The fracture line may be seen in the cancellous

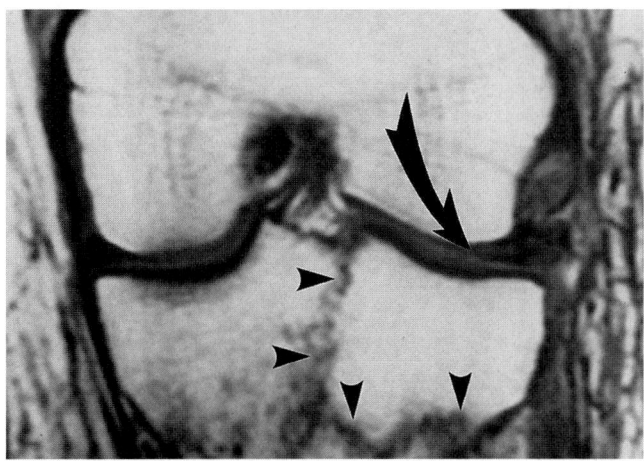

**Figure 8–8.** Tibial plateau fracture. Coronal T1-weighted (TR/TE, 500/17) spin echo MR image. In addition to showing the number and orientation of the fracture lines *(arrowheads)* and the position of the fragments, the image reveals a horizontal tear of the lateral meniscus *(arrow)*.

bone or in the cortex on MR images. Within the cortex, fracture lines are hyperintense on T2-weighted images when compared with the low signal intensity of compact bone. Periosteal reaction can be visualized earlier with MR imaging than with radiography. With stress fractures, a focus of subperiosteal hemorrhage or ill-defined high signal intensity may surround the bone and represents the elevated periosteum, before any mineralization is visible radiographically. Lesser degrees of stress injury, such as shin splints in the tibia, can also demonstrate periosteal high signal intensity on T2-weighted images. MR imaging is also ideal for the evaluation of osteochondral fractures, osteochondritis dissecans, and cartilage defects.

## Degenerative Lesions

Idiopathic chondromalacia begins with softening in the deepest layers of cartilage; eventually, fissuring develops and extends upward to the articular surface. Superficial degeneration starts as fibrillation and fragmentation of the superficial cartilage and extends progressively deeper. Although chondromalacia and superficial degeneration differ in their initial stages, once the articular surface is involved, they appear similar both grossly and on MR images.

MR imaging reliably shows degenerative chondrosis only when macroscopic fissuring, fibrillation, and ulceration reach the articular surface. Focal defects appear in the usually smooth articular surface (Fig. 8–9). Unlike traumatic lesions, degenerative defects do not have a sharp demarcation from the adjacent unaffected cartilage. As long as adequate contrast is present between the joint fluid (or injected contrast) and the cartilage surface, the ability to detect degenerative lesions depends on the spatial resolution of the study. In clinical studies, the sensitivity for showing chondral degeneration is best for lesions that involve at least half the depth of the cartilage. Preliminary data suggest that MR arthrography using a dilute gadolinium solution may perform better than conventional MR imaging for some stages of cartilage degeneration.

## Inflammatory Lesions

In inflammatory arthritides such as rheumatoid arthritis, MR imaging is able to show more erosions than can be seen on standard radiographs. Erosions appear as defects in the subchondral plate and overlying articular cartilage and contain high-signal-intensity pannus or joint fluid on T2-weighted images. Because it can also quantify synovial inflammation, MR imaging with intravenous contrast (Fig. 8–10) is an evolving tool for the early diagnosis and long-term prognostication of patients with inflammatory arthritis.

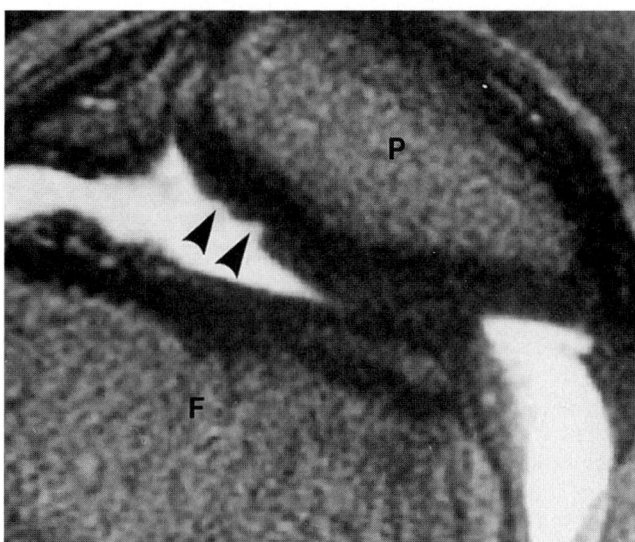

**Figure 8–9.** Degenerative chondrosis. Transaxial T2-weighted (TR/TEeff, 4066/138) fast spin echo MR image. Two shallow, superficial ulcers *(arrowheads)* are evident along the medial patellar articular surface. This high-resolution MR image was obtained with a 10-cm field of view and 256 × 256 imaging matrix. F, femur; P, patella.

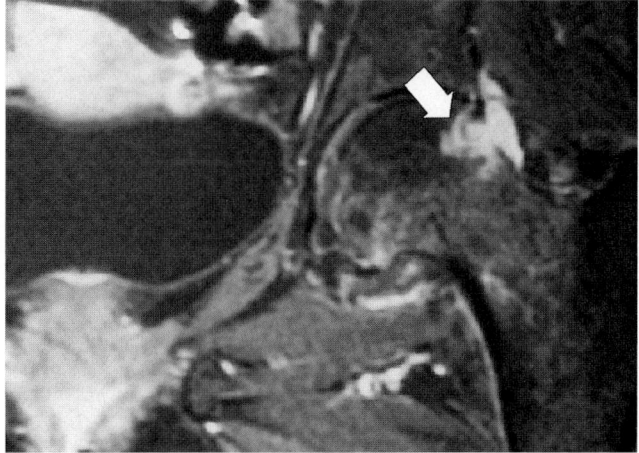

**Figure 8–10.** Rheumatoid arthritis. Coronal fat-suppressed T1-weighted (TR/TE, 800/14) spin echo MR image of the pelvis after the intravenous administration of contrast. Enhancing pannus is eroding the lateral aspect of the femoral head *(arrow)*.

## Neoplasms

MR imaging can show tumors that involve the surface of bone, whether they arise from the cortex, periosteum, or articular cartilage. MR imaging is invaluable for determining the presence and amount of intramedullary extension of surface tumors, as well as the presence and size of associated soft tissue masses. Both of these characteristics affect prognosis and treatment. MR imaging is probably the best study to evaluate symptomatic osteochondromas. MR images can directly demonstrate complications such as stalk fractures and the development of overlying bursae and can show the thickness of the cartilaginous cap.

## SYNOVIAL-LINED STRUCTURES

A synovial membrane lines the diarthrodial (movable) joints in the body, as well as bursae and tendon sheaths. This specialized vascular tissue produces synovial fluid, which has lubricating, nourishing, and shock-absorbing properties.

### Normal Appearance and Technique

The inner lining of the joint capsule is a thin, smooth, delicate synovial membrane. Joints may also have normal extensions (recesses) that are similarly lined. A typical example is a popliteal cyst in the knee, which represents a distended semimembranosus-gastrocnemius recess (Fig. 8–11). A bursa is a synovial-lined space that arises embryologically separate from a joint, typically to provide cushioning between a bony protuberance and the overlying soft tissues. Tendons whose courses change direction around an osseous structure (such as the malleoli in the ankles) or under a retinaculum or pulley (such as the finger flexor tendons) are surrounded by a synovial sheath to ensure low-friction gliding. For tendons that run from the inside of a joint outward (such as the long head of the biceps brachii in the shoulder), the tendon sheath is actually an outpouching of the joint.

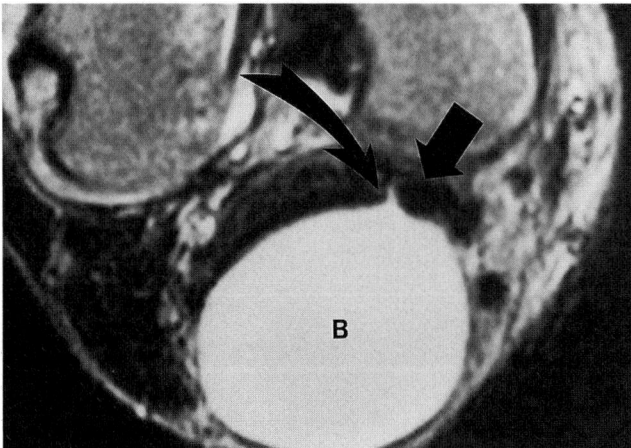

**Figure 8–11.** Baker's cyst. Transverse T2-weighted (TR/TE, 2500/80) spin echo MR image of the knee. Fluid distends the semimembranosus-gastrocnemius recess (B). The neck of the popliteal cyst is located between the tendons of the medial gastrocnemius *(curved arrow)* and semimembranosus *(straight arrow)* tendons.

The normal synovial membrane is usually too thin to visualize on routine MR images. However, together with the more robust fibrous joint capsule, the synovial membrane may occasionally be seen as a thin, low-signal-intensity structure. A nondiseased synovial membrane either does not enhance after the administration of intravenous contrast or enhances only faintly. Normal joints, recesses, bursae, and tendon sheaths also typically contain a small amount of synovial fluid.

### Joint Effusions

An effusion exists when a synovial-lined structure contains more than a physiologic amount of fluid. Nevertheless, the question "how much fluid is normal?" is a difficult one to answer. Although quantitative guidelines for some joints have been published, few radiologists use measurements to determine the presence of an effusion. Most effusions are the result of traumatic, degenerative, or inflammatory conditions. Tendon sheaths normally contain only a trace amount of fluid; however, tendon sheaths that communicate with a joint will be distended passively if an effusion is present in the joint. Bursae, too, normally contain only a trace amount of fluid and thus may not be visible.

When an effusion represents simply increased production of synovial fluid, its signal characteristics will be those of normal joint fluid. However, if synovial fluid contains proteinaceous debris or blood products, its signal intensity will differ. Recent hemorrhage may result in a layering effect, with supernatant fluid floating on top of cellular debris. If a hemarthrosis is due to an intra-articular fracture, a third layer representing fat (lipohemarthrosis) may be seen, with the signal characteristics of adipose tissue. Effusions that represent the subacute phase of a hemarthrosis after cell lysis or exudates from infection or inflammation typically have higher signal intensity than water on T1-weighted images, but they usually remain isointense to fluid on T2-weighted images. Repetitive bleeding into a joint, as might occur with hemophilia or juvenile arthritis, can result in intra-articular hemosiderin deposition. Hemosiderin-laden tissues appear low in signal intensity on all pulse sequences and may demonstrate "blooming"—an apparent increase in size because of the local susceptibility effects of paramagnetic substances—on gradient recalled images.

### Synovial Inflammation

Synovitis is caused by infection, trauma, seropositive or seronegative arthritis, or miscellaneous conditions such as hemophilia. The inflamed synovial membrane (called pannus in inflammatory arthritides) is thicker than normal. It may be nodular or masslike and, especially in chronic cases, may shed hypertrophied particles and form rice bodies (Fig. 8–12). Pannus has variable signal characteristics, depending on the stage of the disease. In chronic or burned-out cases, the synovium demonstrates low signal intensity on both T1- and T2-weighted images. With active inflammation, the MR signal of synovium approximates that of joint fluid on all pulse sequences. Most important, however, is that unlike simple joint fluid,

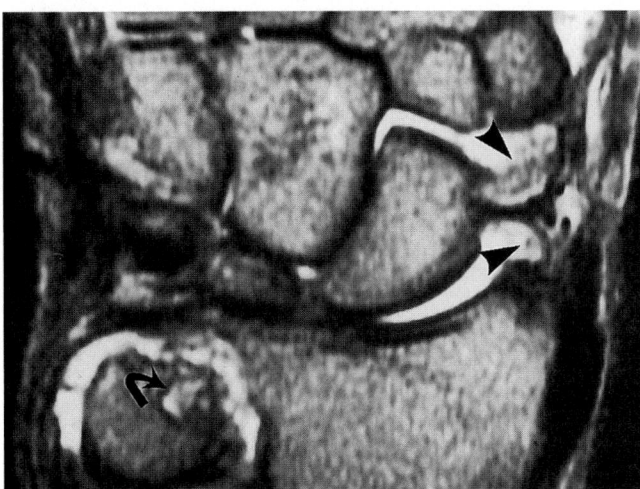

**Figure 8–12.** Erosive rheumatoid arthritis. Coronal T2-weighted (TR/TE, 2500/80) spin echo MR image of the wrist. Pannus with heterogeneous signal intensity is present within an erosion of the ulnar head *(arrow)*. Also note the synovitis with rice bodies *(arrowheads)* in the midcarpal and radiocarpal compartments.

synovitis enhances rapidly after intravenous contrast administration. MR imaging can also be used to evaluate tenosynovitis in inflammatory arthritides or infections. In wrists affected by rheumatoid arthritis, MR imaging demonstrates more tendon sheath involvement than physical examination does and can be used to establish or confirm a diagnosis of extensor tendon rupture.

### Synovial Neoplasm

Proliferative, noninflammatory disorders of the synovium can also occur. These include primary synovial (osteo)-chondromatosis, pigmented villonodular synovitis, and diffuse synovial lipoma (lipoma arborescens). These lesions can have a characteristic appearance on MR imaging (see Chapter 71).

### FIBROCARTILAGE

Several specialized supporting structures within joints are composed of fibrocartilage. Between two articulating bones, they are called discs if they completely separate two joint compartments, and they are called menisci if they partly separate compartments. Examples of discs include the triangular fibrocartilage in the wrists and the articular discs in the temporomandibular, acromioclavicular, and sternoclavicular joints. Menisci occur in the knees and elbows.

### Normal Appearance and Technique

Fibrocartilage is composed of mostly type I collagen interspersed with small amounts of elastin, proteoglycans, and vascular tissue. The articulating surfaces of the knee meniscus, for example, are covered by a thin layer of parallel fibers that permit smooth gliding. Conversely, the bulk of the meniscus is composed of circumferential

strands, joined by a few perpendicular radial tie fibers, to provide the hoop stress necessary to withstand the force of the femoral condyle on the tibial plateau. Vessels are located only in the outer 10% to 30% of the meniscal periphery.

Normal fibrocartilage has low signal intensity on most MR imaging pulse sequences. Some important exceptions exist, however. First, in regions where large numbers of nearly parallel fibers are oriented obliquely to the main magnetic field, the magic angle phenomenon may artifactually increase the internal signal intensity. Second, vascularized regions of fibrocartilage may be relatively hyperintense on MR images. Such regions include the periphery of the knee menisci and the ulnar attachments of the triangular fibrocartilage in the wrist.

Several MR pulse sequences can be used for examining fibrocartilage, and each has unique advantages and disadvantages. For the knee menisci, proton density-weighted images are the most useful. Spin echo technique is preferred to fast spin echo because of the inherent blurring that occurs when fast spin echo images are acquired with a short effective TE. Reducing the interecho spacing, increasing the matrix size, and decreasing the echo train length (turbo factor) can make fast spin echo imaging nearly as sensitive as spin echo imaging for meniscal abnormalities while still maintaining a slight advantage in acquisition time. Regardless of the sequence chosen, sagittal and coronal images should be obtained with slices 3 to 4 mm thick and a field of view of no more than 16 cm.

T1-weighted MR imaging after arthrography with a gadolinium-based contrast agent is most often used in knees that have undergone meniscal surgery. MR arthrography is the most sensitive study for examining the labra in the shoulders and hips and probably for the wrist triangular fibrocartilage as well.

### Traumatic Disorders

In the knee, two MR imaging criteria are used for diagnosing meniscal tears. The first is the presence of intra-meniscal signal on a short TE image that unequivocally extends to one or both articular surfaces of the meniscus (Fig. 8–13). Hyperintense signal that is contained entirely within the meniscus or possibly extends to the surface should not be interpreted as a tear. Hyperintense signal on T2-weighted images peripheral to the meniscal outer margin was once thought to represent meniscocapsular separation, but this finding correlates poorly with true pathology seen at arthroscopy. The second criterion is abnormal meniscal shape: a tear is present if any alteration of the usual cross-sectional triangular or bow-tie shapes is noted. These rules do not apply after meniscal surgery.

In a postoperative knee, a recurrent meniscal tear can be diagnosed confidently only if an abnormality occurs in a region separate from the initial meniscal tear, if fragmentation or displaced fragments are seen, or if a fluid-containing cleft is present within the substance of the meniscus. Intra-articular contrast seen tracking into the substance of the postoperative meniscus on an MR arthrogram is the most specific finding indicating a new meniscal tear or a repaired tear that has not healed (Fig. 8–14).

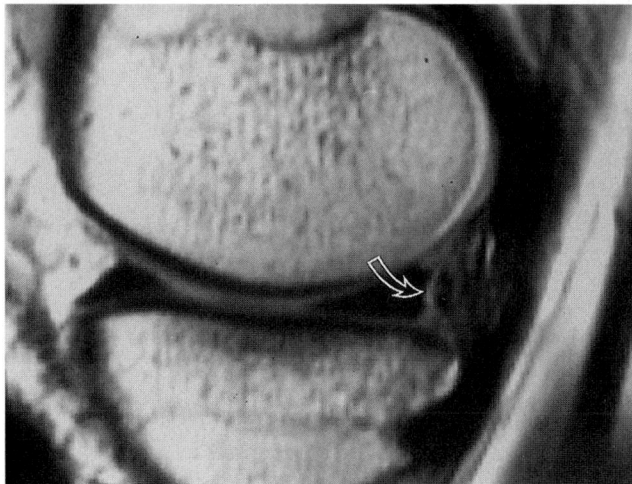

**Figure 8–13.** Full-thickness longitudinal tear of the medial meniscus. Sagittal intermediate-weighted (TR/TE, 2300/20) spin echo MR image. Vertically oriented intrameniscal signal *(arrow)* unequivocally contacts the superior and inferior meniscal surfaces.

An acetabular or glenoid labrum that is absent, detached from the underlying bone (except in the anterosuperior quadrant of the shoulder joint), or fragmented represents a torn structure. Tears of the acetab-

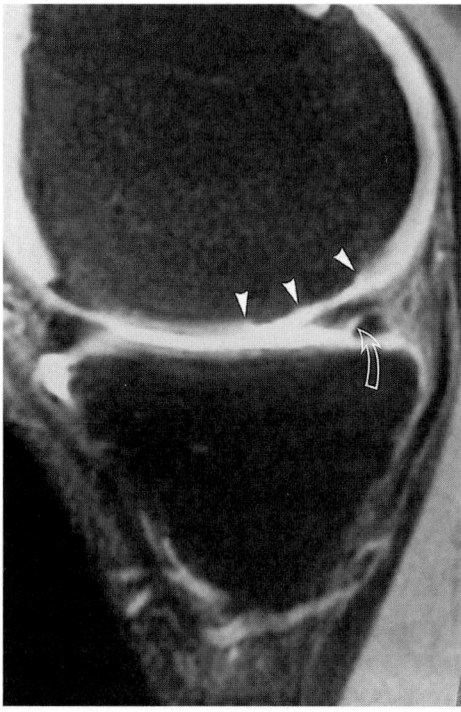

**Figure 8–14.** Recurrent meniscal tear after partial medial meniscectomy. Sagittal fat-suppressed T1-weighted (TR/TE, 800/15) spin echo MR image after a knee arthrogram performed with a dilute gadolinium mixture. Injected contrast enters the substance of a new meniscal tear *(arrow)* in the remnant of the posterior horn. Also note the degenerative cartilage loss along the medial femoral surface *(arrowheads)*.

ular or glenoid labrum can also be diagnosed when the labrum is misshapen or when the internal signal intensity seen on a T2-weighted image extends to the articular surface. Imbibition of injected contrast material into the substance of the labrum also indicates a tear, and the sensitivity of MR arthrography exceeds that of standard MR imaging.

## Nontraumatic Disorders

A discoid meniscus is a meniscus that is larger than normal. A complete discoid meniscus separates a joint into two compartments (like a joint disc); in the case of a partial discoid meniscus, there is still a central opening. Discoid menisci in the knee are more common laterally than medially. When compared with normal menisci, they have an increased propensity to tear. In the elbow, a discoid meniscus can impinge between the posterior of the capitellum and the radial head, blocking extension. On MR imaging examinations, discoid menisci appear larger than normal and often lack the usual triangular cross-sectional shape.

With aging, the fibrocartilage in the body can degenerate. On MR images, degenerated menisci, labra, and discs often contain increased internal signal intensity that may be globular or linear. Degenerative signal extending to the surface of the structure represents a degenerative tear that can be visualized arthroscopically. Chondrocalcinosis can also occur within fibrocartilage with aging, and occasionally, the calcification may be high in signal intensity on short TE images. In cases in which the calcification extends to the articular surface of a meniscus (and presumably in a labrum or disc), the MR appearance may mimic that of a tear.

A para-articular cyst forms when a fibrocartilage tear (either traumatic or degenerative) creates a channel through which fluid can travel to the joint periphery. A one-way valve mechanism allows the cyst to grow. In the knee, meniscal cysts become symptomatic because of their size or from entrapment or compression of surrounding structures. In the shoulder, labral cysts tend to extend into the spinoglenoid or suprascapular notches, where they can compress the suprascapular nerve. On MR imaging studies, cysts may be unilocular or multilocular and should have high signal intensity on T2-weighted images. Because the cysts often contain gelatinous or fibrous material, the contents may be hyperintense in relation to fluid on T1-weighted images. The diagnosis of meniscal cyst should be made only if the cyst abuts a meniscal tear or the site of a healed tear (Fig. 8–15).

## TENDONS

Tendons are highly specialized tissues that provide the mechanical linkage between muscle and bone. As such, they are subject to large stresses when a muscle contracts violently. More important, repetitive, submaximal muscle contractions produce cumulative microscopic tendon damage that results in a spectrum of tendon abnormalities ranging from chronic degeneration (tendonopathy) to complete tendon rupture.

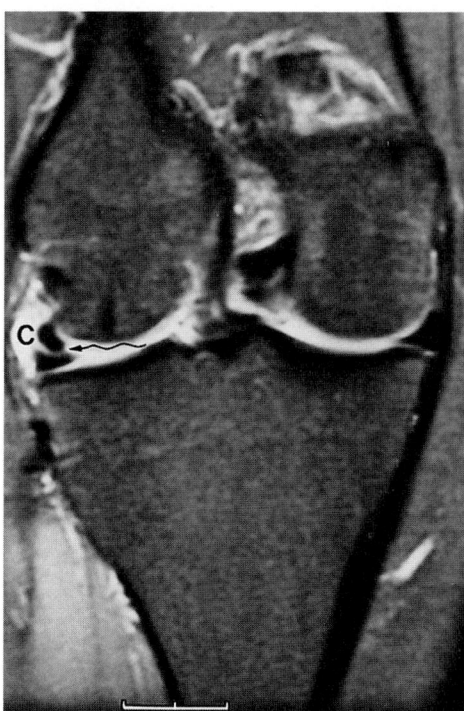

**Figure 8–15.** Lateral meniscal cyst and recurrent meniscal tear after partial meniscectomy. Coronal fat-suppressed intermediate-weighted (TR/TEeff, 3500/16) fast spin echo MR image after the intra-articular injection of a dilute gadolinium mixture. A meniscal cyst (C) communicates with a recurrent horizontal tear of the meniscus, through which gadolinium tracks *(arrow)*. The inner tip of the meniscus is absent because of a partial meniscectomy.

## Normal Appearance and Technique

Type I collagen forms the bulk of a tendon and is arranged in tightly wound parallel fibers to provide tensile strength. Normal tendon is relatively avascular, and vessels do not penetrate the individual tendon fascicles. Tendons that change course by turning around a bony prominence or under a retinaculum or pulley are surrounded by a synovial sheath. Tendons without a sheath are surrounded by a thin, vascular membrane—the paratenon—that provides nutrients and allows the tendon to glide.

Normal tendons have a very short T2 and thus appear uniformly dark on all clinical imaging sequences. There is one exception: the magic angle phenomenon can artifactually increase the internal signal intensity of normal tendons. When a tendon is oriented at approximately 55 degrees with respect to the static magnetic field, T2 decay is greatly retarded, so the intratendinous signal dramatically increases on short TE (T1-weighted, proton density-weighted, and gradient recalled) images. The critical TE above which there is no contribution from the magic angle phenomenon is 37 msec on both 1.0- and 1.5-T scanners. For practical purposes, however, the effect is so slight with TEs of greater than 20 msec that it is not noticeable. Tendons that travel a curved course in the body are the ones most likely to pass through the magic

angle. Common examples include the supraspinatus tendon in the shoulder, the flexor and extensor tendons of the hand, the patellar tendon in the knee, and the medial, lateral, and anterior tendons of the ankle. The peroneus brevis tendon in the ankle seems to be the most frequently affected. To avoid mistaking the increased signal intensity for pathology, abnormal signal intensity should be confirmed on T2-weighted images, which are not affected by the artifact. If the tendon in question is dark on T2-weighted images, a tendon disorder should be diagnosed only when morphologic changes in tendon size or contour accompany increased signal intensity on the short TE images.

Short-axis cross sections (typically in the transverse plane) are used to evaluate tendon size, contour, and internal signal, as well as the surrounding sheath or paratenon. Longitudinal images provide an overview of the tendon from the myotendinous junction to the osseous insertion. These long-axis projections show focal changes in tendon size, and any retraction of the myotendinous origin is due to stretching of the tendon. In cases of complete tendon rupture, longitudinal images demonstrate the size of the tendon gap, the position of the separated fragments, and the quality of the torn tendon ends. Gradient echo images obtained as a three-dimensional acquisition are occasionally useful for evaluating tendons that follow an oblique or curved course, such as the finger flexors.

On MR images, normal tendons are sharply marginated and are typically round, oval, or flat in cross section. The radiologist should be familiar with the normal size range of each tendon, which is often determined by comparing tendons in the same part of the body. For example, the tendon of the normal posterior tibialis is roughly twice as large as the flexor digitorum longus tendon, whose size approximately equals that of the flexor hallucis longus tendon. Throughout its course, a normal tendon should not change in caliber, except at its insertion, where it may widen into a broad osseous attachment. At the insertion, the signal intensity may become heterogeneous as well, representing an admixture of tendon, fibrocartilage, and ossification.

## Tendon Degeneration

Tendon degeneration is the main risk factor for tendon rupture. At least one third of asymptomatic subjects older than 35 years show some histologic evidence of degeneration. Probably more important than the changes of normal aging, however, are the cumulative effects of chronic repetitive injury and inefficient repair. Although the term *tendinitis* may be applied clinically, the condition is not inflammatory, so the terms *tendinopathy* or *tendinosis* are preferred. In clinical practice, the tendons that degenerate most frequently are the rotator cuff, long head of the biceps, extensor carpi radialis brevis, gluteus medius, patellar, posterior tibialis, and Achilles tendons.

On MR images, tendon degeneration is recognized by changes in tendon size, contour, internal signal intensity, or any combination of these factors. The most common finding is focal or diffuse tendon hypertrophy, which probably reflects the disordered collagen fiber arrangement. Tendinopathy of the Achilles and patellar tendons is typically hypertrophic (Fig. 8–16). Less commonly, as degeneration progresses, the tendon loses its viscoelasticity and elongates under the influence of its contracting muscle. The result is an atrophic tendon that has been stretched like taffy. This form of degeneration may be seen in the posterior tibial tendon (Fig. 8–17). Indistinctness of the tendon contour is a second finding in tendinopathy. For example, loss of the usual sharp contour between the posterior fibers of the patellar tendon and the infrapatellar fat in Hoffa's pad signals early degeneration (see Fig. 8–16).

In tendinopathy, the increased signal on T2-weighted images should be less intense than that of fluid. Signal that is isointense to fluid or signal that is less intense but reaches the outer tendon surface probably represents macroscopic tearing. Remember, however, that a degenerated tendon that is not visibly torn still contains microscopic fiber separation and may be just as dysfunctional as a ruptured tendon, especially if it has lost its springiness. Further, a degenerated but intact tendon can still produce pain. To emphasize this, the phrase "tendinopathy without a macroscopic tear" is used by some authors.

## Tendon Tears

Tendon tears occur after penetrating injury, from stretching insults, or spontaneously. Penetrating wounds, typically from glass or knives, produce tendon lacerations that are usually clinically apparent. The wrists, hands, and fingers are most vulnerable. When complete transection has

occurred, MR imaging can be used to identify the location of the retracted proximal and distal tendon ends for surgical planning. After repair, MR imaging may be needed to evaluate complications, including tendon rerupture, and peritendinous scar formation. A normally healed tendon should have a uniform caliber throughout. Nodules at the repair site appear as focal bulbous swellings. Recurrent tears are recognized by a gap between the tendon fibers. Once it has matured, peritendinous scar has low signal intensity on all sequences and typically obliterates the normal surrounding fat planes.

MR imaging is commonly used to diagnose tendon ruptures not caused by penetrating trauma. In the lower extremities, these injuries most frequently involve the distal quadriceps, proximal hamstring, patellar, and Achilles tendons; in the upper limb, the rotator cuff and biceps long head are most commonly affected. Whether these tears are preceded by a recognized acute injury or occur spontaneously, one fact is clear: normal tendons do not tear. Analysis of nearly 900 "spontaneous" tendon ruptures showed that all occurred in histologically diseased tendons, even though two thirds of the patients never had previous symptoms. Because tears occur in diseased tendons, on MR imaging, the signs of a tendon tear are typically superimposed on those of hypertrophic or atrophic tendinopathy (Fig. 8–18). The signal intensity and morphologic changes that distinguish a low-grade, partial-thickness tear from severe tendinopathy may be subtle, because the two conditions are points on a spectrum. Microscopic splitting of collagen strands coalesces into macroscopically recognizable fiber disruption. At this point, the MR signal within the tendon approaches that

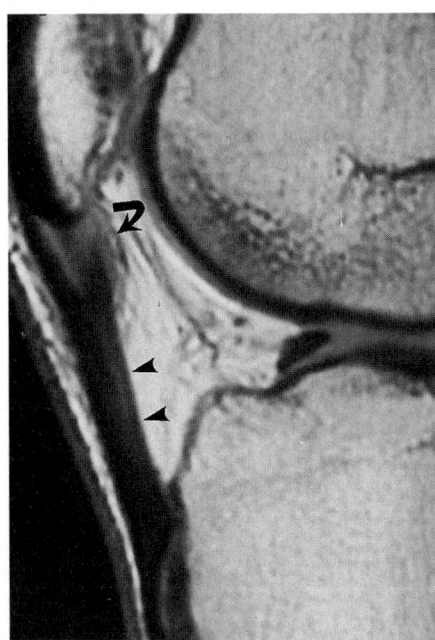

**Figure 8–16.** Proximal patellar tendinopathy in a professional baseball player. Sagittal intermediate-weighted (TR/TE, 2300/14) spin echo MR image of the knee. The proximal patellar tendon is thickened, with increased internal signal intensity. Note the indistinctness of the posterior margin (*arrow*) when compared with the normally sharp interface seen in the lower tendon (*arrowheads*).

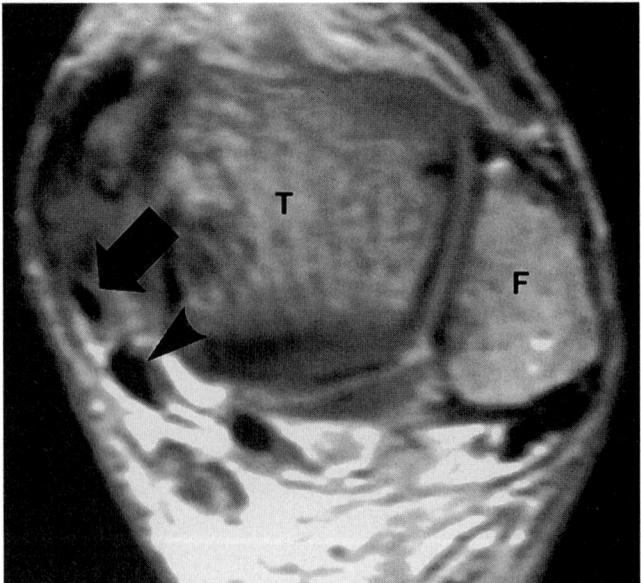

**Figure 8–17.** Atrophic posterior tibial tendinopathy. Transaxial intermediate-weighted (TR/TE, 2500/20) spin echo MR image through the ankle. The posterior tibial tendon (*arrow*) has a smaller diameter than the flexor digitorum longus tendon (*arrowhead*). Normally, the posterior tibial tendon is approximately twice as large as the other tendon. F, fibula; T, talus.

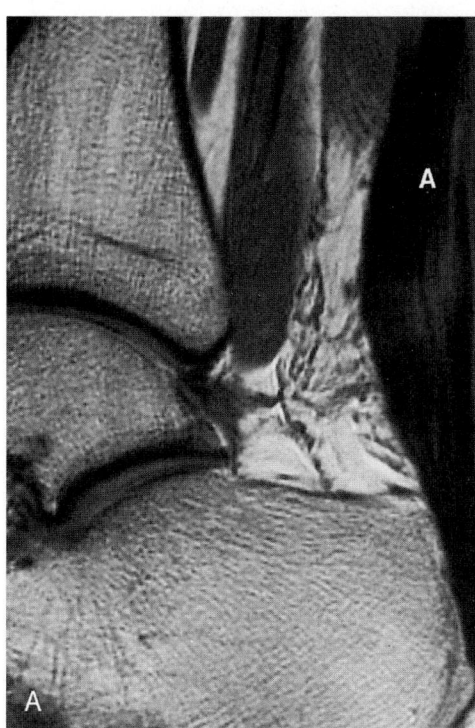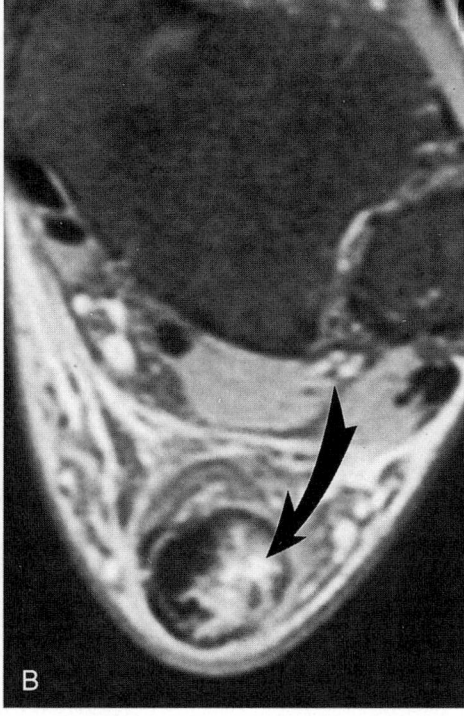

**Figure 8–18.** Partial Achilles tendon tear superimposed on severe tendinopathy. *A,* Sagittal intermediate-weighted (TR/TE, 1000/23) spin echo MR image of the ankle. The Achilles tendon (A) is markedly thickened. *B,* Transverse fat-suppressed T2-weighted (TR/TEeff, 3000/63) fast spin echo MR image. Signal intensity that is nearly isointense with fluid *(arrow)* is seen within the hypertrophied tendon.

of fluid on a T2-weighted image (see Fig. 8–18). A tendon that has split along its long axis appears fragmented in cross section (Fig. 8–19). An abrupt decrease in tendon diameter is another finding indicating a partial tendon tear.

In complete or full-thickness tears, MR images demonstrate a total loss in continuity of the tendon fibers. T2-weighted images show a high-signal-intensity defect if the resultant gap is fluid-filled. However, if scar or granulation tissue fills the gap (which is especially common after tendon repair), the defect will not necessarily contain high-signal-intensity material. This appearance is common in long-standing, massive rotator cuff tears, in which complete absence of any visible tendon is the predominant MR imaging finding. MR images also provide important ancillary information that affects treatment decisions. Assessment of the quality of the torn tendon ends is important, because if they are severely degenerated, they will probably not hold sutures (Fig. 8–20). Severe fatty atrophy of muscle associated with a complete tendon tear indicates chronicity and suggests that although repair or reconstruction of the tendon may improve pain or function, it will probably not improve strength.

MR arthrography has a role in the diagnosis of tears in tendons that form part of the joint capsule, such as the rotator cuff. Performing MR arthrography increases sensitivity for the diagnosis of partial-thickness tears of the tendon surface facing the injected joint. Specificity is also increased for the diagnosis of full-thickness tears, which allow injected contrast to extravasate through the tendon defect. For repaired tendons, MR arthrography differentiates healing or healed repairs from recurrent partial- or full-thickness tears.

In addition to rupture, tendons that course around a bony protuberance or run within a fibro-osseous groove

are at risk for dislocation and subluxation. These injuries commonly involve the long head of the biceps brachii, although dislocation of the peroneal tendons, posterior tibial tendon, and extensor carpi ulnaris tendon can occur

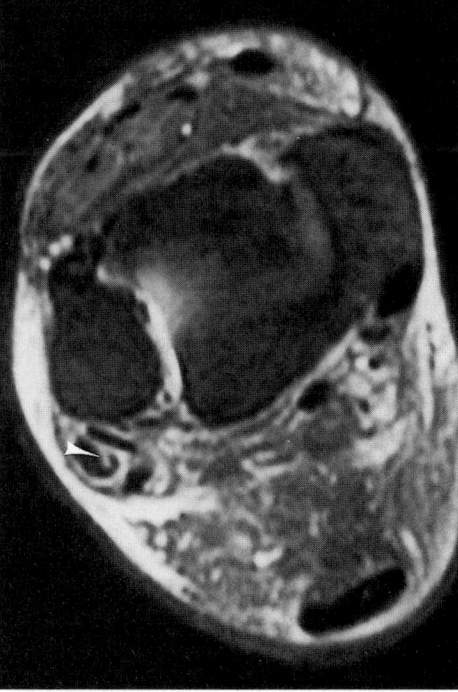

**Figure 8–19.** Sagittal split of the peroneus longus tendon. Transverse fat-suppressed T2-weighted (TR/TEeff, 3000/42) fast spin echo MR image. The normally oval tendon has lost its usual smooth contour because of a high-signal-intensity longitudinal tear *(arrowhead).*

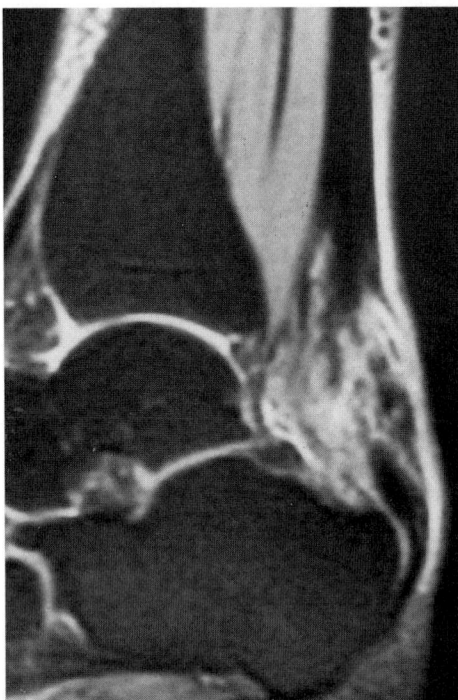

**Figure 8–20.** Complete Achilles tendon tear with degenerated tendon ends. Sagittal fat-suppressed intermediate-weighted (TR/TEeff, 3000/14) fast spin echo MR image. Note the "mop end" configuration of the tendon stumps. Primary repair of a degenerated tendon may be difficult, and a tendon graft is commonly used for reinforcement.

as well. Tendon dislocation or subluxation often indicates an injury to a supporting structure, such as the peroneal retinaculum for the peroneal tendons or the subscapularis muscle for the biceps (Fig. 8–21).

## Inflammatory and Infiltrative Conditions

Inflammatory peritendinitis is less common than degenerative tendinopathy. Insertional enthesitis, which weakens the tendon enthesis and predisposes it to spontaneous rupture, can be seen with rheumatic and collagen vascular diseases. Inflammation can also occur at tendon insertions in athletes without underlying disease and is often associated with an adjacent bursitis. Calcific tendinitis from calcium hydroxyapatite deposition is readily diagnosed with a combination of clinical findings and radiographs showing characteristic fluffy calcifications within a painful tendon. On MR images, the calcium deposits have very low signal intensity on all pulse sequences and may demonstrate "blooming" on gradient recalled images, with high signal intensity in the adjacent tissues on T2-weighted images.

## LIGAMENTS

Ligaments and capsules connect bones together. Retinacula are attached on one or both ends of bone and act as slings for passing tendons. Fasciae typically anchor other soft tissues such as skin, tendon sheaths, or ligaments.

## Normal Appearance and Technique

Ligaments, capsules, retinacula, and fasciae are similar in composition to tendons. Ligaments are hypovascular but not avascular structures. They have more ground substance and less collagen than tendons do. Superficial ligament fibers insert onto the periosteum, which is tightly attached to the underlying osseous cortex via Sharpey's fibers. The deep fibers insert directly into bone, with an orderly histologic transition from ligament tissue to fibrocartilage, to mineralized fibrocartilage, and then to cortical bone.

Ligaments confer low signal intensity on all pulse sequences, except on short TE images in ligaments oriented close to the magic angle. For ligaments composed of distinct bundles, such as the ACL in the knee or the deep deltoid in the ankle, separate fascicles may be visualized with fat or synovium between the bundles. With fibrocartilaginous insertion into bone or insertion into a developing enthesis, the dark ligament fibers blend gradually into the intermediate signal intensity of the underlying tissues. Ligament evaluation should include T2-weighted images; the addition of fat suppression may make subtle abnormalities in signal intensity more conspicuous for ligaments that are surrounded by fat or ligaments that contain fat between their fascicles.

A normal ligament should be visualized in continuity from one osseous attachment to the other; however, depending on the orientation of the structure, the imaging plane, and section thickness, such visualization may not be possible on a single image. Most ligaments appear taut because they are stretched to their full length when the extremity is positioned for MR imaging. Common

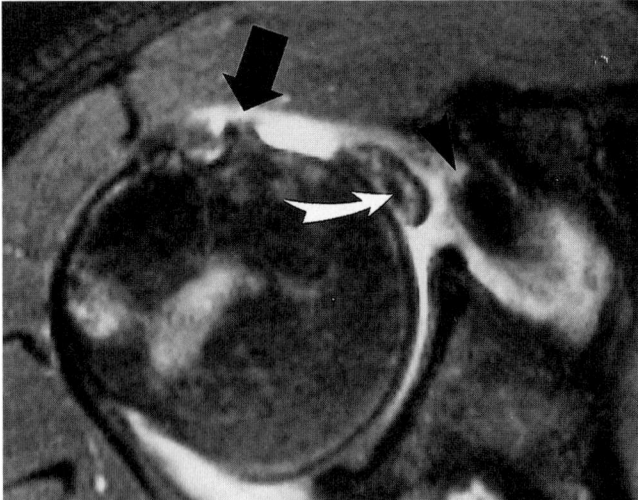

**Figure 8–21.** Tear and dislocation of the long head of the biceps associated with a subscapularis tendon tear. Transaxial fat-suppressed T2-weighted (TR/TEeff, 3120/54) fast spin echo MR image. The enlarged, high-signal-intensity biceps tendon *(curved arrow)* is dislocated medially into the glenohumeral joint. The torn subscapularis tendon end *(arrowhead)* has retracted from its lesser tuberosity insertion *(straight arrow)*. Evidence of subscapularis tendon rupture should be carefully sought whenever intra-articular dislocation of the biceps is found.

examples include the collateral ligaments of the knee, elbow, and digits. For these structures, any waviness or laxity indicates pathology. Others, such as the posterior cruciate ligament in the extended knee, are normally imaged in a lax position, but they should still be visualized in continuity from one bone to the next. For each commonly injured ligament, the radiologist should be familiar with its normal orientation and thickness, because changes in position or size may be the only clues to a chronic tear or previously injured structure.

### Acute Injuries

Acute ligament injuries are called sprains, and they cause joint pain and instability. Sprains occur in the substance of the ligament or at its bony attachments. Grade I sprains represent overstretched fibers that contain microscopic hemorrhage and tearing, without macroscopic disruption of fibers. In grade II injuries, the ligament is partly torn, whereas in grade III sprains, complete ligament disruption is observed. Clinically, higher-grade injuries are associated with increasing laxity of the joint under stress testing.

MR imaging plays a role in confirming the injury, estimating its severity, and identifying associated pathology (Fig. 8–22). Complete tears are characterized by total discontinuity of the ligament fibers, with high-signal-intensity material in the resultant gap on T2-weighted images. Acutely, the torn ligament ends may have a "mop end" appearance, representing unraveled individual fibers that are separated by hemorrhage and edema. Within weeks, the fibers coalesce, and the torn ends can be better defined. Grade II partial tears (or partly healed complete tears) show some intact fibers and some disrupted ones. Ligaments with grade I injuries (interligamentous sprains) appear thickened and contain high signal intensity on T2-weighted images.

In several special circumstances, MR imaging has a direct impact on the clinical management of ligament injuries. For example, whereas physical examination can indicate that the ulnar collateral ligament in the thumb is torn, MR images can demonstrate whether a Stener lesion is present and surgery is necessary (Fig. 8–23). The accuracy of MR imaging is lower in knees with several torn ligaments than in knees with a single torn ligament. Similarly, in severe ankle sprains, MR imaging can demonstrate injuries that involve the tibiofibular (syndesmotic) ligaments, in addition to the anterior talofibular and calcaneofibular ligaments. In cases in which a ligament is shown to be intact, MR imaging often suggests an alternative diagnosis that accounts for the patient's symptoms.

### Chronic and Treated Injuries

As a torn ligament attempts to heal, fibrotic scar tissue forms and has low signal intensity on MR images. A ligament that has successfully healed, after either conservative treatment or repair, is thickened but low in signal intensity on T2-weighted images. Any areas of ossification within the ligament have the signal characteristics of marrow on all pulse sequences. When normal healing

does not occur, the tear is said to be chronic, and patients may have continued instability or nonspecific pain.

The MR imaging appearance of a chronic ligament tear is more variable than that of an acute tear. Occasionally, complete absence of visible ligament tissue is noted. At other times, low-signal-intensity scar is present but does not have the morphology of the normal ligament. This occurrence is common for chronic ACL tears, which may become scarred to the posterior cruciate ligament. The scarred ligament may appear focally angulated or buckled, or it may lie relatively horizontally in the intercondylar notch. Despite scarring between the cruciate ligaments, the scar does not confer stability to the knee. In the lateral ligaments of the ankle, torn ligaments typically scar in their usual locations. It may be difficult to distinguish a healed ligament from a scarred, incompetent one without MR arthrography.

The role of MR imaging in chronic ligament tears is severalfold. In addition to identifying the abnormal ligament itself, MR imaging is used to identify other pathology that may coexist with or mimic a chronically torn ligament. This situation is particularly common in the ankle, where peroneal tendon tears, retinacular injuries, talar dome osteochondral lesions, stress fractures, sinus tarsi syndrome, and soft tissue impingement can all mimic the symptoms of chronic lateral instability.

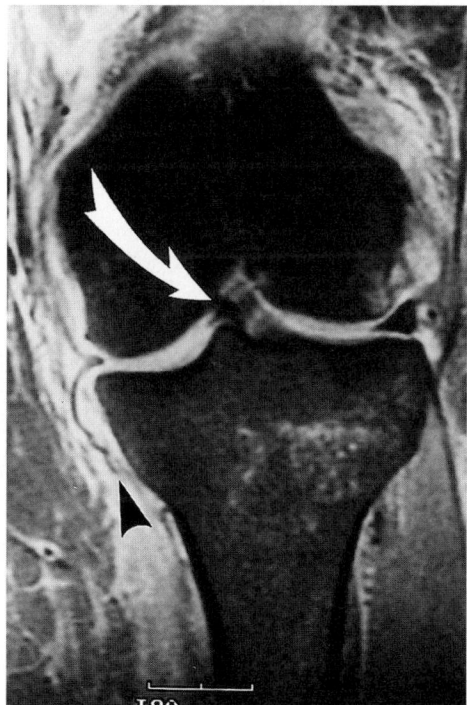

**Figure 8–22.** Complete, acute medial collateral ligament tear. Coronal fat-suppressed intermediate-weighted (TR/TEeff, 3500/20) fast spin echo MR image of the knee. The fibers of the medial collateral ligament are completely disrupted (*arrowhead*). Also note the displacement of an avulsed medial meniscus into the intercondylar notch (*arrow*). Tears that involve the deep medial collateral ligament can also separate the meniscus from its peripheral attachments.

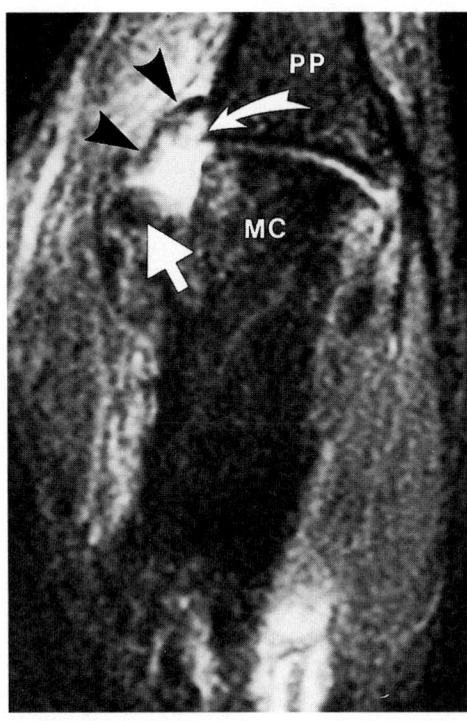

**Figure 8–23.** Thumb ulnar collateral ligament tear and a Stener lesion. Coronal fat-suppressed T2-weighted (TR/TEeff, 3000/44) fast spin echo MR image. The avulsed ulnar collateral ligament is balled up proximally *(straight arrow)* and separated from its distal attachment site *(curved arrow)* by the interposed adductor aponeurosis *(arrowheads)*. MC, metacarpal; PP, proximal phalanx.

## FURTHER READING

Anderson MW, Greenspan A: Stress fractures. Radiology 199: 1, 1996.

Anzel SH, Convey KW, Weiner AD, et al: Disruption of muscles and tendons: An analysis of 1014 cases. Surgery 45:406, 1959.

Cohen MD, Klatte EC, Baehner R, et al: Magnetic resonance imaging of bone marrow disease in children. Radiology 151:715, 1984.

Crues JV 3d, Mink J, Levy TL, et al: Meniscal tears of the knee: Accuracy of MR imaging. Radiology 164:445, 1987.

De Smet AA, Norris MA, Yandow DR, et al: MR diagnosis of meniscal tears of the knee: Importance of high signal in the meniscus that extends to the surface. AJR Am J Roentgenol 161:101, 1993.

Deutsch AL, Mink JH, Waxman AD: Occult fractures of the proximal femur: MR imaging. Radiology 170:113, 1989.

Dooms GC, Fisher MR, Hricak H, et al: Bone marrow imaging: Magnetic resonance studies related to age and sex. Radiology 155:429, 1985.

Ehman RL: MR imaging of medullary bone. Radiology 167:867, 1988.

el-Khoury GY, Wira RL, Berbaum KS, et al: MR imaging of patellar tendinitis. Radiology 184:849, 1992.

Gagliardi JA, Chung EM, Chandnani VP, et al: Detection and staging of chondromalacia patellae: Relative efficacies of conventional MR imaging, MR arthrography, and CT arthrography. AJR Am J Roentgenol 163:629, 1994.

Jones RJ: The role of bone marrow imaging. Radiology 183:321, 1992.

Lecouvet FE, Malghem J, Michaux L, et al: Vertebral compression fractures in multiple myeloma. Part II. Assessment of fracture risk with MR imaging of spinal bone marrow. Radiology 204:201, 1997.

Lecouvet FE, Vande Berg BC, Michaux L, et al: Stage III multiple myeloma: Clinical and prognostic value of spinal bone marrow MR imaging. Radiology 209:653, 1998.

Lynch TC, Crues JV 3d, Morgan FW, et al: Bone abnormalities of the knee: Prevalence and significance at MR imaging. Radiology 171:761, 1989.

Mink JH, Deutsch AL: Occult cartilage and bone injuries of the knee: Detection, classification, and assessment with MR imaging. Radiology 170:823, 1989.

Moore SG, Dawson KL: Red and yellow marrow in the femur: Age-related changes in appearance at MR imaging. Radiology 175:219, 1990.

Morrison WB, Schweitzer ME, Batte WG, et al: Osteomyelitis of the foot: Relative importance of primary and secondary MR imaging signs. Radiology 207:625, 1998.

Noonan TJ, Garrett WE: Injuries at the myotendinous junction. Clin Sports Med 11:783, 1992.

Olson DO, Shields AF, Scheurich CJ, et al: Magnetic resonance imaging of the bone marrow in patients with leukemia, aplastic anemia, and lymphoma. Invest Radiol 21:540, 1986.

Palmer WE, Kuong SJ, Elmadbouh HM: MR imaging of myotendinous strain. AJR Am J Roentgenol 173:703, 1999.

Panicek DM, Gatsonis C, Rosenthal DI, et al: CT and MR imaging in the local staging of primary malignant musculoskeletal neoplasms: Report of the Radiology Diagnostic Oncology Group. Radiology 202:237, 1997.

Peterfy CG, Janzen DL, Tirman PF, et al: "Magic-angle" phenomenon: A cause of increased signal in the normal lateral meniscus on short-TE MR images of the knee. AJR Am J Roentgenol 163:149, 1994.

Resnick D: Common disorders of synovium-lined joints: Pathogenesis, imaging abnormalities, and complications. AJR Am J Roentgenol 151:1079, 1988.

Rosen MA, Jackson DW, Berger PE: Occult osseous lesions documented by magnetic resonance imaging associated with anterior cruciate ligament ruptures. Arthroscopy 7:45, 1991.

Rubin DA: Magnetic resonance imaging of chondral and osteochondral injuries. Top Magn Reson Imaging 9:348.

Rubin DA: MR imaging of the knee menisci. Radiol Clin North Am 35:21, 1997.

Rubin DA, Kettering JM, Towers JD, et al: MR imaging of knees having isolated and combined ligament injuries. AJR Am J Roentgenol 170:1207, 1998.

Schweitzer ME, van Leersum M, Ehrlich SS, et al: Fluid in normal and abnormal ankle joints: Amount and distribution as seen on MR images. AJR Am J Roentgenol 162:111, 1994.

Stafford SA, Rosenthal DI, Gebhardt MC, et al: MRI in stress fracture. AJR Am J Roentgenol 147:553, 1986.

Vahey TN, Broome DR, Kayes KJ, et al: Acute and chronic tears of the anterior cruciate ligament: Differential features at MR imaging. Radiology 181:251, 1991.

Volger JB III, Murphy WA: Bone marrow imaging. Radiology 168:679, 1988.

# CHAPTER 9

## Needle Biopsy of Bone and Soft Tissue

### SUMMARY OF KEY FEATURES

Advances in radiology, including image intensification, biplane videofluoroscopy, computed tomography (CT), ultrasonography, magnetic resonance (MR) imaging, and high-resolution radionuclide bone scanning, have emphasized that radiologists are in a unique position to perform such image-guided needle biopsies. In many cases, such procedures are a cost-effective alternative to open biopsy, and they have become the accepted surgical procedure for the diagnosis of a variety of skeletal disorders, including neoplastic, inflammatory, and metabolic conditions.

### INTRODUCTION

Biopsy specimens can be obtained in one of two ways: aspiration by needle, or removal of a core of tissue by trephine. Tissue obtained by needle aspiration is small in quantity and distorted, with loss of cellular configuration; tissue obtained by trephine biopsy is greater in quantity and intact, although this technique requires a larger needle. Needle aspiration is most useful for tissue culture to exclude infection, although some investigators report the value of needle aspiration in establishing a wide variety of clinical diagnoses; trephine biopsy is a better technique for histologic diagnosis. Use of both methods together, however, has been emphasized in some reports. This combined approach requires little extra time and has been found to minimize false-negative results and increase specificity.

### GENERAL CONSIDERATIONS

Although the treatment of tumors of bone and soft tissue has changed dramatically in recent years because of the increasing use of limb salvage procedures as an option for malignant neoplasms, establishing an accurate diagnosis before instituting therapy remains an important consideration. Whether the procedure is performed directly as an open biopsy by an experienced orthopedic surgeon or indirectly as a percutaneous procedure by a qualified radiologist, it must be done correctly. A biopsy needle or a scalpel creates a pathway through which tumor cells can disseminate. Tissues exposed at the time of an incisional biopsy or during a percutaneous procedure must be removed later during definitive operative excision of a malignant tumor. Clearly, the shortest route to a lesion may not be the best one, and care must be exercised in choosing an appropriate entrance point for either needle aspiration or trephine biopsy. As a general rule for image-guided pro-

cedures, all biopsies must be coordinated with the surgeon who will perform the definitive surgery (Fig. 9–1).

### CLOSED VERSUS OPEN BIOPSY: ADVANTAGES AND DISADVANTAGES

Some of the advantages of closed needle biopsy of bone or soft tissue over open biopsy are obvious and include the following: (1) procedures can be accomplished quickly, usually within 45 minutes; (2) general anesthesia is not required, and the technique can be done as an outpatient procedure; (3) the procedure is safe, and local complications are infrequent; and (4) the use of modern image guidance facilitates accurate needle placement.

The major disadvantages of closed needle biopsy are the following: (1) a relatively small amount of material is obtained, which may not be representative; (2) the success of the procedure requires an experienced pathologist in close cooperation with a radiologist; (3) closed biopsy of a tumor could lead to tumor dissemination in neighboring and distant tissue; and (4) needle biopsy often cannot provide sufficient tissue for cytogenetic analysis, required by certain treatment protocols.

### INDICATIONS AND CONTRAINDICATIONS

Indications for needle biopsy of bone and soft tissue vary from one institution to another; however, certain general guidelines do exist.

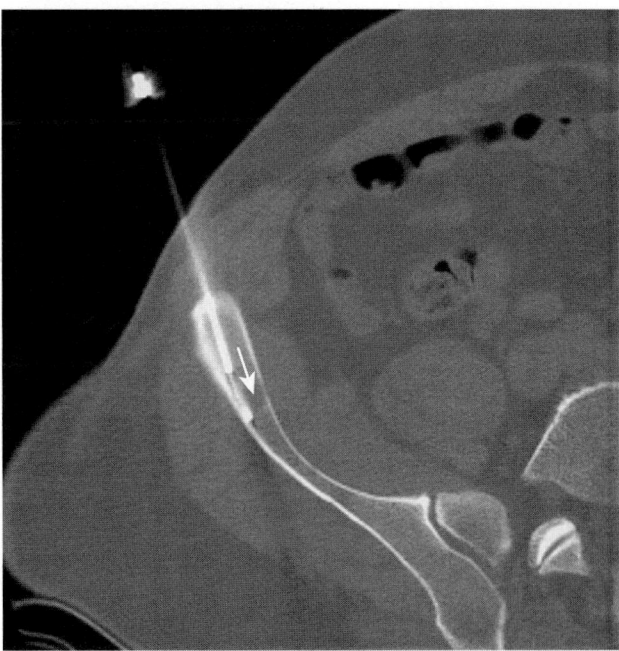

**Figure 9–1.** Biopsy with CT guidance in a patient with a small lytic lesion in the ilium *(arrow)*. Although a path through the gluteal muscles would be more direct, such an approach would violate the tissue planes required for definitive surgery for a primary lesion.

## Neoplastic Disease

With regard to patients with suspected or proven skeletal metastasis, potential indications for closed bone biopsy include the following:

1. Patients with a known primary tumor who have a solitary bone lesion detected by conventional radiography, CT, MR imaging, scintigraphy, or any combination of these, in whom verification of the nature of the lesion will influence treatment.

2. Patients without a known primary tumor who have solitary or multiple osteolytic or osteoblastic lesions and in whom the most probable diagnosis is metastatic disease. In such persons, bone biopsy represents a direct method of quickly establishing the cellular characteristics of the metastatic focus.

3. Patients with known multiple primary tumors who have one or more bone lesions.

4. Patients with a known primary tumor in whom it must be determined whether viable tumor cells are present in a radiographically stable metastatic bone lesion.

5. Patients with a known primary tumor that is in clinical remission and in whom a new bone lesion has developed.

6. Patients who have received radiation therapy for a primary tumor, metastatic bone lesion, or both and in whom osseous abnormalities of an unclear nature have developed in the irradiated skeleton.

7. Patients with a non-neoplastic skeletal problem (e.g., Paget's disease, osteomyelitis) that may predispose to metastatic seeding and in whom a new aggressive lesion of an unclear nature has developed at the site of bone involvement.

## Metabolic Disease

To accurately establish the presence and type of metabolic disease, open wedge resection or percutaneous biopsy of the iliac crest should be accomplished. Large-core biopsy needles are used for this procedure and provide adequate material for qualitative and quantitative histologic evaluation.

## Infectious Disease

Closed needle biopsy or aspiration can be useful in establishing a diagnosis of osteomyelitis or septic arthritis. Material should be obtained for both histologic diagnosis and appropriate tissue culture. The influence of iodinated contrast material and pain medications (e.g., lidocaine) on the successful identification of causative organisms obtained from cultures of removed tissue is controversial, although concentrated mixtures of these agents should probably be avoided.

## Articular Disease

Although closed bone biopsy is usually not necessary in the diagnosis of articular disorders, it may be used to evaluate patients with subchondral cystic lesions in whom the exact diagnosis is in doubt.

## Miscellaneous Diseases

Closed bone biopsies can provide information in numerous other diseases, including Paget's disease, fibrous dysplasia, eosinophilic granuloma, and sarcoidosis.

## BIOPSY SITES

Use of imaging studies in the localization of appropriate biopsy sites is important. Scintigraphy may identify additional lesions that are more accessible to closed needle biopsy than the initially detected abnormality. Closed needle biopsy of radiographically and scintigraphically positive lesions is more successful than biopsy of lesions that are apparent only on radionuclide scans, although definite diagnoses may be established in the latter situation as well. Abnormalities evident with CT scanning and not by routine radiography are best sampled when the former method is used to ensure accurate needle placement. MR imaging can also be used for the detection of lesions that are not apparent on routine radiographs, and with attention to the choice of a specific needle, its orientation, and specific pulse sequences, this method can be used to monitor the biopsy procedure. The preferred biopsy site is a prominent area of a non–weight-bearing bone. Additional accessible areas for biopsy are the pelvis and extremities. Biopsy of the lumbar spine is performed more easily than biopsy of the thoracic spine.

## NEEDLES: TYPES AND TECHNIQUES

A variety of needles is available for both trephine and aspiration biopsy. Trephine needles are of two basic types: (1) needles with narrow, paired cutting blades that engage the tissue, and (2) round tubes with serrated edges that cut the tissue. With a to-and-fro twisting motion and a variable amount of pressure, the cutting needle is driven into the bone, and its position is verified. The needle is moved back and forth to dislodge the specimen from surrounding osseous tissue. The cutting needle is then removed, and the cannula is left in place. The cannula can subsequently be moved to a different location if a second biopsy specimen is required. The tissue is removed from the cutting needle with a long, thin probe and placed in an appropriate specimen container.

Aspiration needles are available in different sizes. For many lesions, an 18- or 20-gauge needle may be sufficient. The needle with stylet is guided into the lesion with gentle pressure under imaging control. The stylet is removed, and a syringe is used for tissue aspiration. It has been suggested that rotation of the syringe allows more adequate biopsy samples. The material is placed on appropriate slides for cytologic examination and, if required, placed in laboratory containers for culture and bacteriologic identification.

## ADDITIONAL TECHNIQUES OF NEEDLE BIOPSY

Although CT, with its cross-sectional display and excellent density resolution, has been used successfully to monitor closed biopsy procedures of the musculoskeletal system, it is not needed in many cases. Ultrasonographically guided biopsy procedures are best reserved for superficial lesions and aspiration of lesions suspected of containing fluid. Biopsies of solid soft tissue masses can likewise be accomplished with ultrasonographic guidance, and this imaging method has been used to guide bone biopsies as well. Localization of subperiosteal abscesses and investigation of diffuse or focal muscle abnormalities can be accomplished with ultrasonic guidance, and this method allows the localization and removal of some foreign bodies. The role of MR imaging–guided biopsy techniques is not yet established, although open-configuration magnets and specially designed needles are important advances.

## BIOPSY OF VERTEBRAE

The techniques for obtaining biopsies of vertebral bodies under fluoroscopic or CT guidance have been well outlined, and the choice of technique depends on the level of the lesion as well as its position within the vertebra. With regard to the thoracic and lumbar vertebrae, two basic methods exist: the transpedicular approach and the posterolateral approach.

### Transpedicular Biopsy

This approach is safe and accurate and well suited for the thoracolumbar spine. C-arm fluoroscopy or CT scanning can be used to guide needle placement. The patient is typically placed prone. Then, using a posterior approach, the needle is advanced into the pedicle and subsequently into the vertebral body (Fig. 9–2).

### Posterolateral Biopsy

The patient is placed in the prone position on the table. The point of needle entrance is lateral to the spinous process of the vertebra to be sampled. A more lateral approach is used in the lower thoracic and lumbar spine (Fig. 9–3). The patient can be left prone or turned to a prone oblique or lateral position during the biopsy procedure. Whereas fluoroscopic guidance may be used with a transpedicular approach, the posterolateral approach is best accomplished with CT guidance.

### Biopsy of the Cervical Vertebrae

The patient is placed supine, and an anterolateral approach is used to avoid the larynx and large vessels. Under fluoroscopic or CT guidance, the needle is advanced at an angle of approximately 20 degrees to the patient's sagittal plane. Because of the complex regional anatomy, however, the use of large trephines is difficult, and aspiration is more easily accomplished with a percutaneous approach to the cervical spine.

### PROCESSING OF THE BIOPSY SPECIMEN

It is always advisable to contact the pathology department before performing the biopsy to ensure correct handling of the specimen. Fluid aspirates should be transferred immediately to culture tubes or rapidly delivered to the laboratory for plating. In cases of suspected articular infection in which no fluid is recovered spontaneously,

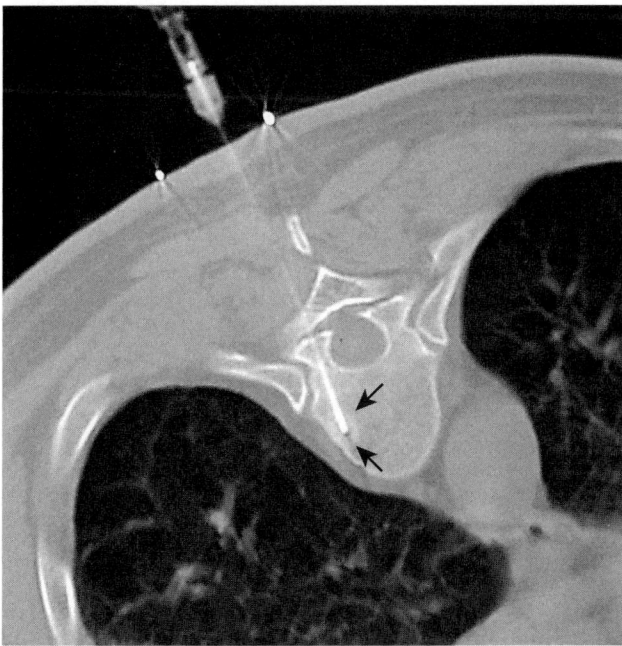

**Figure 9–2.** Transpedicular biopsy of the T7 vertebral body. In this 62-year-old man with newly diagnosed prostate carcinoma, scintigraphy showed a single focus of increased tracer accumulation in the spine. CT demonstrates the tip of the biopsy needle within a small sclerotic lesion *(arrows)*, which documented the presence of metastasis.

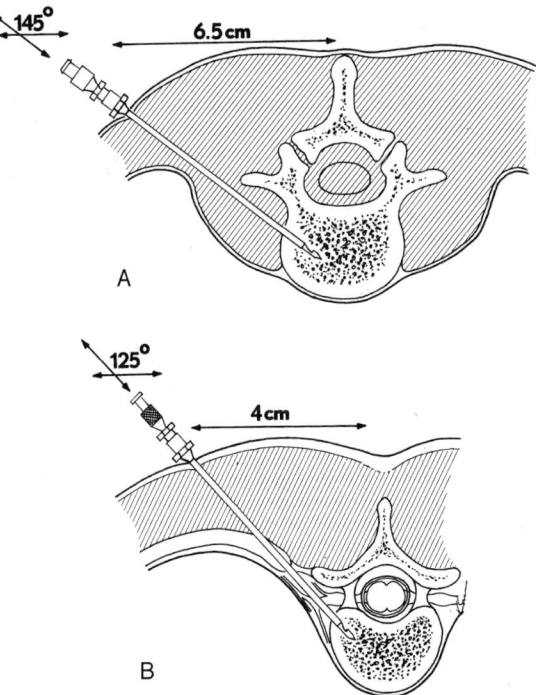

**Figure 9–3.** Technique of spinal biopsy. *A,* Lower thoracic and lumbar vertebrae. The needle is inserted 6.5 cm from the spinous process at a 145-degree angle from the horizontal. *B,* Upper thoracic vertebrae. The needle is inserted approximately 4 cm from the midline, over the rib, at a 125-degree angle from the horizontal.

the instillation of nonbacteriostatic, sterile saline solution should be followed by reaspiration of the joint contents.

Blood that is aspirated from an osseous lesion should not be discarded, because it frequently provides an accurate diagnosis. The blood is allowed to clot in a syringe or plastic cap and then sent to the laboratory as a tissue specimen in formalin and processed separately from the removed tissue. Smears can also be made from small drops of blood. If electron microscopy is being considered as an adjunct to routine histologic analysis, a portion of the tissue should be placed in glutaraldehyde, not formaldehyde. Less commonly used tissue examinations include cytologic studies, tissue imprints, and immunofluorescence.

## COMPLICATIONS

Image-guided percutaneous biopsy is usually performed without significant complications. Mild pain and discomfort are common. Hemorrhage can result when biopsy specimens are obtained from patients with vascular tumors or when a venous or arterial structure is injured, particularly in biopsies of the spine (Fig. 9–4). Other reported

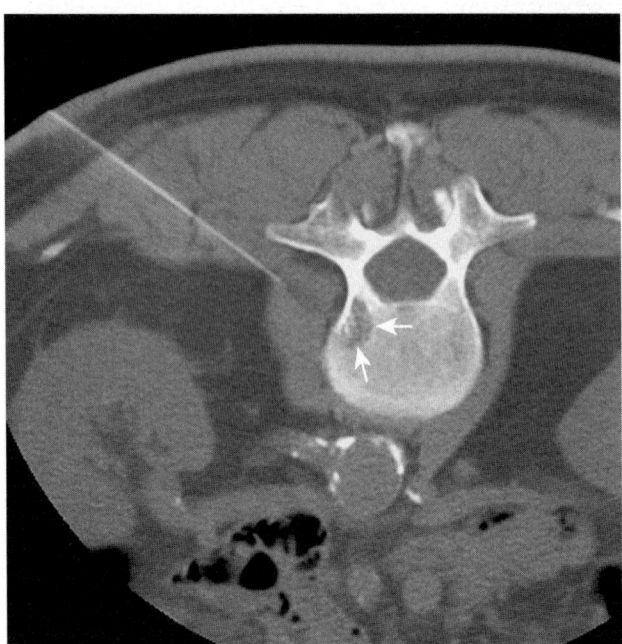

**Figure 9–4.** Biopsy complication—hematoma. In this 73-year-old man with a history of lung carcinoma, spinal MR images obtained for back pain revealed a focal lesion in the L2 vertebral body. A subsequent CT-guided biopsy was done using a posterolateral approach. The image obtained during placement of the needle shows a hematoma forming in the right psoas muscle. Although the hematoma had markedly enlarged on a subsequent scan, conservative treatment was successful.

complications include paresis, pneumothorax, sinus tract, footdrop, pneumonia, pneumoretroperitoneum, meningitis, and even death, but these complications are extremely rare. Because of the potential for local or systemic spread of tumor during or after the biopsy, the procedure should be accomplished in such a way that the needle tract can be resected along with the specimen.

## FURTHER READING

Carces J, Hidalgo G: Lateral access for CT-guided percutaneous biopsy of the lumbar spine. AJR Am J Roentgenol 174:425, 2000.

Craig FS: Vertebral body biopsy. J Bone Joint Surg [Am] 38:93, 1956.

Debnam JW, Staple TW: Needle biopsy of bone. Radiol Clin North Am 13:157, 1975.

Debnam JW, Staple TW: Trephine bone biopsy by radiologists. Results of 73 procedures. Radiology 116:607, 1975.

Kattapuram SV, Rosenthal DI: Percutaneous biopsy of the cervical spine using CT guidance. AJR 149:539, 1987.

Murphy WA, Destouet JM, Gilula LA: Percutaneous skeletal biopsy 1981: A procedure for radiologists—results, review, and recommendations. Radiology 139:545, 1981.

Ottolenghi CE: Aspiration biopsy of the spine. J Bone Joint Surg [Am] 51:1531, 1969.

Pierot L, Boulin A: Percutaneous biopsy of the thoracic and lumbar spine: Transpedicular approach under fluoroscopic guidance. AJNR 20:23, 1999.

Robertson WW Jr, Janssen HF, Pugh JL: The spread of tumor-cell-sized particles after bone biopsy. J Bone Joint Surg [Am] 66:1243, 1984.

Simon MA, Biermann JS: Biopsy of bone and soft-tissue lesions. J Bone Joint Surg [Am] 75:616, 1993.

Stoker DJ, Cobb JP, Pringle JAS: Needle biopsy of musculoskeletal lesions. A review of 208 procedures. J Bone Joint Surg [Br] 73:498, 1991.

Stoker DJ, Kissin CM: Percutaneous vertebral biopsy: A review of 135 cases. Clin Radiol 36:569, 1985.

Tehranzadeh J, Freiberger RH, Ghelman B: Closed skeletal needle biopsy: Review of 120 cases. AJR 140:113, 1983.

# Imaging and Interventional Procedures of the Spine

# CHAPTER 10

## Spinal Imaging

### Jeffrey S. Ross

## SUMMARY OF KEY FEATURES

A variety of diseases affects the osseous and soft tissue structures of the spine. Accurate diagnosis is often challenging, although a number of imaging methods are available for this purpose. Of these, magnetic resonance (MR) imaging is currently receiving the greatest attention.

## INTRODUCTION

A revolution in the diagnosis and management of spinal disorders has occurred in the past 10 to 15 years. Powerful imaging methods can be applied to delineate the complexities of pathologic conditions in the spine. MR imaging has quickly emerged as the method of choice for the assessment of virtually all disorders of the spine, with computed tomography (CT) scanning continuing to play a key ancillary role. This chapter reviews the basic imaging approaches to the spine and their usefulness in specific disease entities.

## IMAGING TECHNIQUES

### Routine Radiography

Routine films are universally available and relatively inexpensive, but they are limited by an inability to allow direct visualization of neural structures and neural compression. The presence of degenerative changes within the cervical and lumbar spine has been shown to be related to age, and such changes can be found in both asymptomatic and symptomatic persons. Twenty-five percent of asymptomatic patients have degenerative changes in the intervertebral disc spaces by the fifth decade of life. By the seventh decade of life, 75% have such degenerative changes.

The goal of spinal fusion is to produce a solid arthrodesis to correct or prevent spinal instability. Bone grafts can be placed posterior to, posterolateral to, or within the disc space for anterior interbody fusion or can be used to fill cages to promote such anterior fusion. Instrumentation is used to increase the success rate of bone fusion by providing purchase to an individual level and rigid linkage to other levels. It usually takes 6 to 9 months for routine radiographs to document solid spinal fusion and 3 years to confirm complete remodeling at the fusion site. Pseudarthrosis or fibrous union is a common complication of spinal fusion. Reabsorption of bone can occur around screws and under implants where there is direct contact with bone, and this is usually associated with vertebral motion.

### Myelography

The diagnosis of extradural neural compression by myelography is inferred by changes in the contour of the normal contrast-filled thecal sac and root sleeves rather than by direct visualization of the lesion (Figs. 10–1 to 10–3). The current nonionic water-soluble agents used in myelography are associated with only mild side effects; significant adverse reactions, such as hallucinations, confusion, or seizures, occur rarely. The major disadvantages of myelography are its invasive nature and lack of diagnostic specificity. The technique of myelography involves instillation of a contrast agent through either lumbar puncture or lateral C1–C2 puncture. Adequate visualization of spinal structures depends on pooling of a sufficient amount of contrast agent in the region of interest.

Accuracy rates for water-soluble nonionic cervical myelography in the diagnosis of nerve root compression range between 67% and 92%. Because the diagnosis of extradural neural compression is indirectly inferred by changes in the contour of the contrast-filled subarachnoid space, the exact nature of the compressing lesion may be uncertain. Central indentation of the contrast agent column at the level of the disc space may be due to compression either by the disc itself or by marginal osteophytes. Similarly, incomplete filling of a nerve root sleeve may be due to either lateral disc herniation or bony foraminal narrowing; the distinction is sometimes difficult to make without the use of ancillary diagnostic methods such as postmyelographic CT.

### Computed Tomography

CT scanning permits direct visualization of potential neural-compressing structures and provides better visualization of lateral pathologic entities, such as foraminal stenosis. CT can also distinguish neural compression by soft tissue from compression by bone. CT scanning is still relatively limited, compared with MR imaging, for visualizing the neural structures below a complete myelographic block. Disadvantages of CT scanning include the effects of partial volume averaging, streak artifacts caused by the dense bone of the shoulder girdle, and changes in

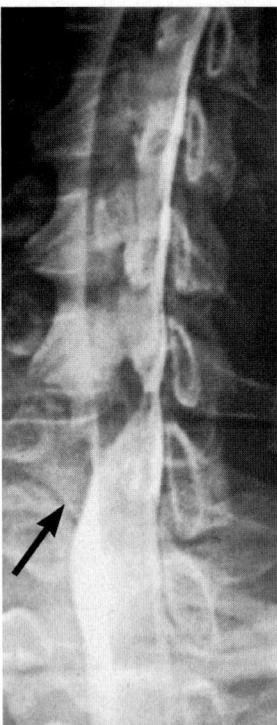

**Figure 10–1.** Extradural disease on myelography. Oblique view of a cervical myelogram via C1–C2 puncture shows marked cutoff of the exiting C6–C7 roots and effacement of the thecal sac by an extradural defect *(arrow)*. Although the root deformity is well defined, the underlying disc herniation is not.

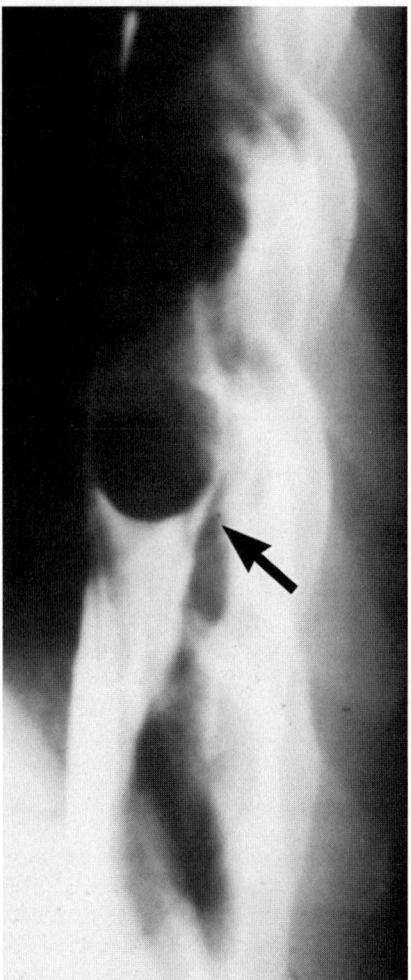

**Figure 10–2.** Intradural extramedullary disease on myelography. Lateral view of the thoracolumbar junction after instillation of intrathecal contrast material shows displacement of the cord by an intradural extramedullary lesion, which is capped by contrast material inferiorly *(arrow)*, with expansion of the cerebrospinal fluid space.

the configuration of the spine between successive motion segments. Many of the limitations can be obviated by obtaining multiple thin sections (1.5 to 3 mm) with the gantry tilted to permit imaging parallel to the plane of the disc. Greater accuracy is obtained by routinely imaging the spine with CT after the introduction of water-soluble contrast agents (intrathecal contrast-enhanced CT) (Figs. 10–4 and 10–5).

## Magnetic Resonance Imaging

**Protocols.** Designing specific imaging protocols for evaluation of the spine involves the consideration of many variables. A careful balance must be reached between disease sensitivity or image quality and patient throughput, because optimization of one of these factors often adversely affects attainment of the other. For the great majority of patients who undergo evaluation for suspected degenerative disease, sagittal spin echo T1-weighted and fast spin echo (FSE) T2-weighted images and transverse T1-weighted images will suffice. If contrast between the disc and cerebrospinal fluid is inadequate on the transverse images, an FSE T2-weighted transverse study may be useful. If the

patient has a history of previous low back surgery, a gadolinium-based contrast agent such as diethylenetriamine pentaacetic acid (Gd-DTPA) is administered intravenously, and T1-weighted sagittal and transverse images are included, the latter of which may be obtained with fat suppression. Patients with possible vertebral osteomyelitis can undergo the routine study noted earlier. If the study shows an area that suggests disc space infection, T1-weighted sagittal and transverse images obtained after intravenous gadolinium administration are often helpful in defining the extent of disease and characterizing epidural inflammatory involvement.

**Gradient Echo.** For images with a transverse orientation, low flip angle two- or three-dimensional gradient echo (GE) sequences producing "myelographic" contrast are a

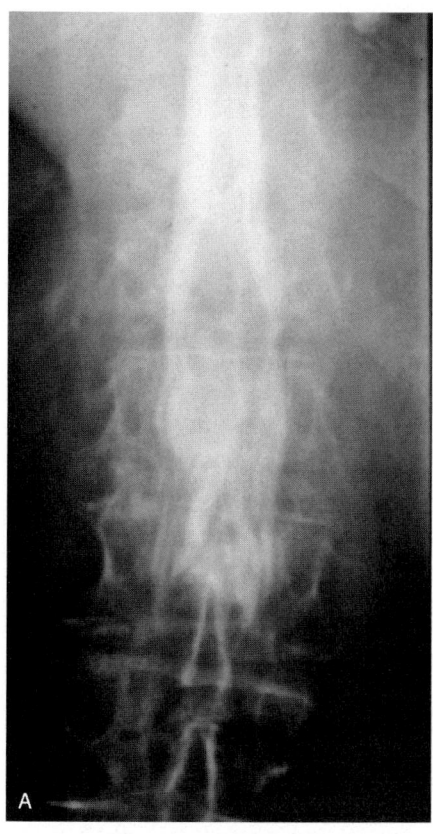

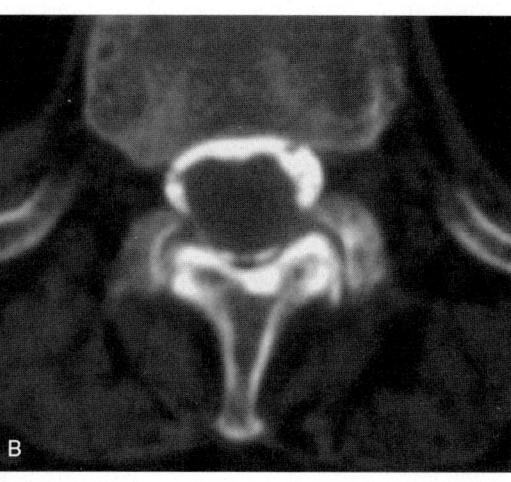

**Figure 10–3.** Intramedullary disease on myelography. *A,* Anteroposterior view of the thoracolumbar junction after instillation of an intrathecal contrast agent via C1–C2 puncture shows marked expansion of the conus medullaris and proximal cauda equina by an intramedullary mass. *B,* Transverse CT scan after myelography better demonstrates the degree of expansion of the conus. At surgery, an ependymoma was found.

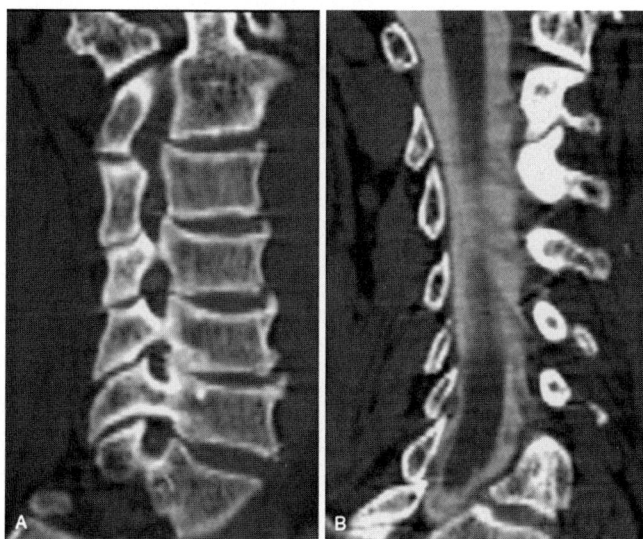

**Figure 10–4.** High-resolution CT myelogram reformations. *A,* Oblique reformatted image perpendicular to the exiting nerve rootlets demonstrates the bony neural foramina well with the use of 1-mm sections and a multirow detector CT. *B,* Reformatted image parallel to the exiting rootlets shows individual rootlets at multiple levels outlined by the intrathecal contrast agent.

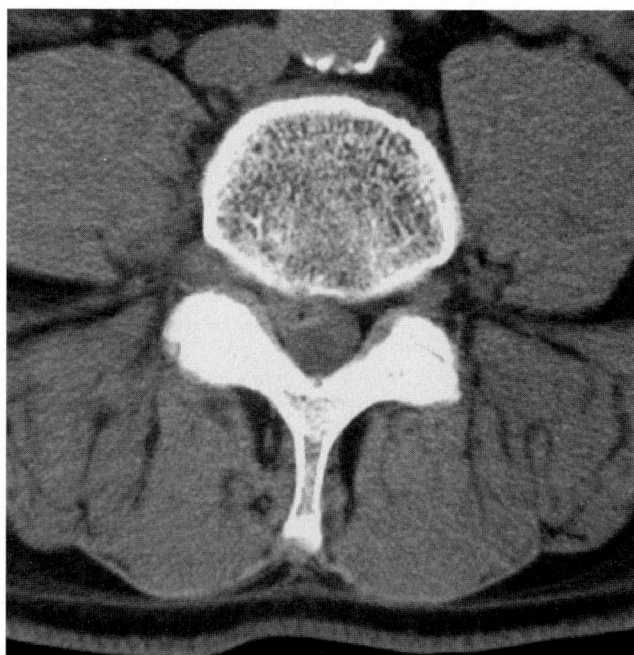

**Figure 10–5.** Lumbar disc herniation. Transverse CT section at the L4–L5 level shows a well-defined soft tissue structure within the anterior and right lateral epidural space that is effacing the thecal sac, a finding indicative of disc herniation.

reasonable baseline standard of comparison, as long as it is acknowledged that these sequences were developed to detect disc herniations and generally perform relatively poorly in detecting intramedullary cord lesions. The advantages of these sequences over T2-weighted spin echo scans when used for transverse imaging are speed, resolution, slice coverage, and suppression of cerebrospinal fluid flow and other motion artifacts. Three-dimensional versions of GE scans are available that have both "myelographic" and T1-weighted image contrast; they produce favorable image quality, sampling speed, resolution, and multiplanar reconstruction.

**Fast Spin Echo.** In routine spin echo imaging, image contrast is controlled by adjustments in TR and TE. New parameters were added with FSE, such as echo train length and echo spacing, which can be manipulated to alter image contrast. New artifacts and appearances are also created by these techniques, such as T2 filtering (imaging blurring), bright (i.e., high-signal-intensity) fat, and diminished sensitivity to susceptibility effects. Because multiple echoes are obtained at different TEs in the FSE sequence, the overall image has not one true TE but an effective TE.

**Fluid-Attenuated Inversion Recovery.** FSE is the gold standard for sagittal T2-weighted and spin density-weighted spinal imaging, driven primarily by the overall image quality and time savings associated with the technique. Other sequences are available, however, with unique image contrast that can be useful for intramedullary (cord) disease. For cord disease, the primary sequence goal is contrast, with resolution assuming much less importance. Fluid-attenuated inversion recovery (FLAIR) is a spin echo sequence that uses a long inversion time to suppress the signal from cerebrospinal fluid. This pulse, when coupled with a long TR/TE, gives the benefits of a T2-weighted image without the interference of high signal from cerebrospinal fluid. FLAIR has been used with considerable success for the evaluation of a wide variety of intracranial disorders. The application of FLAIR in the assessment of the spinal cord has not been as straightforward as its application in the assessment of the brain, and a conservative interpretation of relevant reports suggests that FLAIR should not be used to evaluate spinal cord disease.

**Short Tau Inversion Recovery.** Short tau inversion recovery (STIR) methods have shown high sensitivity for musculoskeletal disease as a result of the synergistic effects of prolonged T1 and T2 times in abnormal tissue, coupled with the improved contrast-to-noise ratio with fat suppression. STIR (especially fast STIR) images may also be used for the diagnosis of intramedullary disease. Fast STIR sequences may be best for detecting multiple sclerosis lesions and may demonstrate lesions missed with other more routine techniques, such as FSE. Overall image quality tends to be rather noisy, but an advantage is its high contrast-to-noise ratio. This technique appears to be very useful for cervical cord disease, but it is prone to motion artifact and has shortcomings in the evaluation of thoracic cord disease.

**Cerebrospinal Fluid Myelogram Effect.** Evaluation of the neural foramina for osteophytes or lateral disc herniation by two-dimensional imaging is best accomplished in the transverse plane. Sequences that lead to high signal intensity of cerebrospinal fluid are generally preferred, because visualizing low-signal-intensity ligaments or osteophytes on T1-weighted imaging in which such fluid is of low signal intensity creates a diagnostic problem. The partial flip angle GE technique for the detection of cervical disc disease uses a small flip angle (3 to 8 degrees) and provides the best contrast among disc, cord, and cerebrospinal fluid.

**Artifacts.** Stainless steel implants are known to generate substantial metal artifact with MR and CT techniques. On CT, metal causes severe x-ray attenuation (missing data) in selected planes. These missing data, or hollow projections, cause classic "starburst" or streak artifacts during image reconstruction (Fig. 10–6). Materials with lower x-ray attenuation coefficients (plastic < titanium < tantalum < stainless steel < cobalt chrome) produce fewer artifactual distortions. Software strategies for artifact reduction exist, and thin-section spiral imaging has shown improvement over conventional discrete slices.

MR imaging in the presence of stainless steel, though safe, leads to severe artifacts, especially if the steel has a low nickel content. When metal is placed in an imaging field, artifacts are produced by differences in the magnetic susceptibility of the metal and adjacent tissue. Magnetic susceptibility is the phenomenon by which material becomes partially magnetized in the presence of an applied external magnetic field, and nonferromagnetic metals may produce local electrical currents induced by the changing magnetic field of the scanner. When tissues with greatly different magnetic susceptibility are placed within a uniform mag-

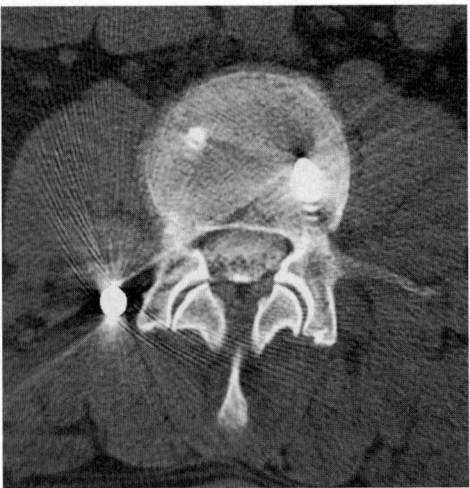

**Figure 10–6.** Metal artifact with CT scanning. Transverse scan at the L3 level shows a mild amount of streak artifact from the right-sided posterior rod, as well as from the tips of the pedicle screws within the vertebral bodies. Nevertheless, the thecal sac is well defined, as are the roots of the cauda equina after intrathecal contrast administration.

netic field, the difference in susceptibility causes distortion in the magnetic field, which results in distortion on the MR image. A number of strategies can be used to reduce susceptibility artifacts on MR imaging, including the use of spin echo techniques, especially FSE and its variants, over GE; larger fields of view; higher readout bandwidths; smaller voxel sizes; and appropriate geometric orientation of the frequency-encoded direction in relation to metallic objects. Imaging at lower field strength also reduces susceptibility artifact but is not an operator-selectable parameter in routine practice. Geometric orientation of the metallic object with respect to the magnetic field is especially important in the case of pedicle screws (Fig. 10–7). Less apparent widening of the short axis of screws is seen when the direction of the frequency-encoded gradient is parallel as opposed to perpendicular to the long axis of the screw.

## Spinal Angiography

Spinal angiography is no longer used for the initial assessment of spinal column disease, given the power of MR imaging and CT. Spinal angiography is extremely useful in evaluating spinal vascular malformations, both for delineation of vascular supply and for therapeutic treatment (Fig. 10–8). Spinal angiography is also used in the pretherapeutic workup of suspected vascular neoplasms involving the vertebral bodies, posterior elements, and spinal canal and is coupled with preoperative or palliative embolization.

## Discography

Discography was originally conceived as a technique for the study of disc herniation. Today, it is considered a useful but limited test that relies on pain provocation to determine the anatomic source of a patient's symptoms. By one definition, discography is a physiologic evaluation of the disc that consists of volumetric, manometric, and radiographic studies plus a pain provocation challenge. This procedure remains quite controversial and has generated voluminous literature. Discography is an invasive procedure and is not performed as a screening technique. The main complication associated with this technique is disc space infection. The risk of discitis is on the order of 0.1% to 0.2%; therefore, a prophylactic broad-spectrum antibiotic is often administered.

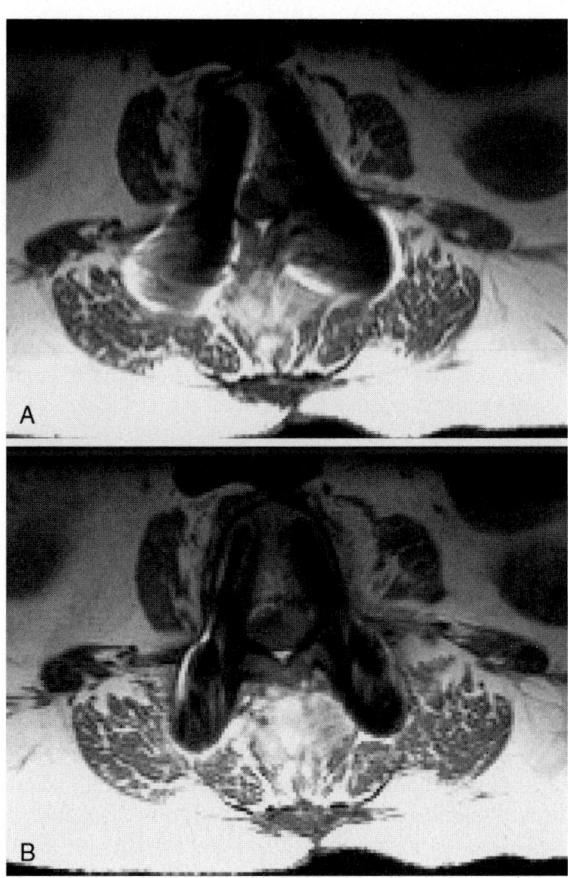

**Figure 10–7.** Metal artifact with MR imaging. *A,* Transverse T1-weighted spin echo MR image with the frequency-encoded direction extending from right to left shows the greatest amount of distortion in that direction; the distortion is obscuring the boundary of the thecal sac. *B,* Transverse T1-weighted spin echo MR image, now with the frequency-encoded direction extending in an anteroposterior direction, shows minimal artifact.

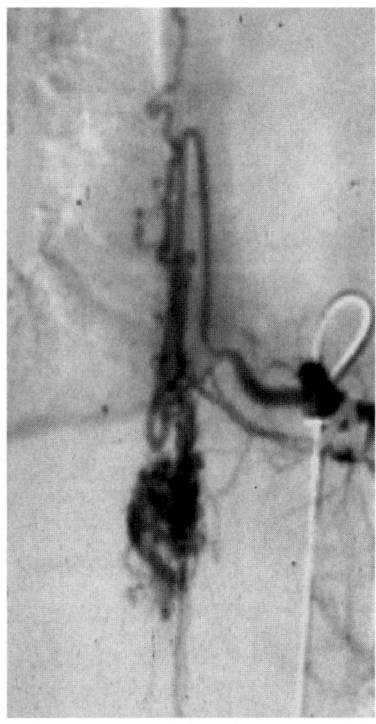

**Figure 10–8.** Spinal arteriovenous malformation. Anteroposterior view of the thoracic spine after injection of the left intercostal artery at the T7 level shows a markedly enlarged anterior spinal artery with a typical "hairpin" turn (artery of Adamkiewicz). The artery is supplying an intramedullary arteriovenous malformation that was of the glomus type histologically.

# ANATOMY

## Vertebrae

As a person ages, red (hematopoietic) marrow is gradually replaced by yellow (fatty) marrow, so that the signal intensity of the vertebral bodies gradually increases from low-intermediate to high on conventional T1-weighted spin echo images. The posterior elements generally contain sufficient marrow to approximate the signal intensity of the vertebral bodies. Often, focal fatty deposits are seen in the vertebral body marrow as rounded regions of high signal intensity on T1-weighted spin echo images. These deposits are of no clinical significance. The basivertebral veins are well seen on midsagittal images. Their signal intensity depends on the pulse sequence, rate of venous flow, amount of perivenous fat, and presence of flow displacement or chemical shift artifact.

## Intervertebral Discs

The intervertebral disc is composed of three parts: cartilaginous endplate, anulus fibrosus, and nucleus pulposus. The height of the lumbar disc space generally increases as one progresses caudally. The anulus fibrosus consists of concentrically oriented collagenous fibers that serve to contain the central nucleus pulposus. These fibers insert into the vertebral cortex via Sharpey's fibers and also attach to the anterior and posterior longitudinal ligaments. The normal contour of the posterior aspect of the anulus fibrosus is dependent on the contour of its adjacent endplate. Typically, the contour is slightly concave on MR images in the transverse plane, although at L4–L5 and L5–S1, these posterior margins are commonly flat or even convex. A convex shape on transverse MR images alone should not be interpreted as degenerative bulging. Within the nucleus pulposus, T2-weighted sagittal images often reveal a linear hypointense region coursing in an antero-posterior direction—the intranuclear cleft. This region of more prominent fibrous tissue should not be interpreted as intradiscal gas or calcification.

## Spinal Canal

The spinal canal surrounds the epidural space and the thecal sac and its contents. The epidural space contains epidural veins, fat, and the proximal spinal nerve root sleeves. The thickness of the epidural fat gradually increases at more caudal levels. The thecal sac contains the cord, nerve roots, and cerebrospinal fluid. Each spinal nerve consists of a dorsal and ventral root. In the lumbar spine, the rootlets are typically loosely clustered posteriorly on transverse MR images and gradually course anterolaterally to enter their respective root sleeves as one progresses caudally. On sagittal images, the roots of the cauda equina occasionally appear clumped, which may falsely suggest the presence of arachnoiditis or a tethered cord. Evaluation of the transverse MR images can prevent this misinterpretation.

## Intervertebral Foramina

The lumbar intervertebral foramen is shaped like an upside-down pear that is bordered anteriorly by the posterior aspect of the vertebral body and intervertebral disc, posteriorly by the superior and inferior articular processes, and cranio-caudally by the pedicles. The nerve roots and dorsal root ganglia, along with small arteries and veins, exit through the foramen in the wider upper portion. The lumbar spinal nerves are numbered in a fashion corresponding to the pedicle above. A 5-mm segment of the spinal nerve immediately distal to the large, solid-appearing dorsal root ganglia normally appears as numerous small fascicles interspersed with fat. Distal to these fascicles, the ventral roots appear as two small ovoid structures.

# DEGENERATIVE DISEASES

## Natural History and Usefulness of Imaging

Back pain is not indicative of a single disorder, and the prognosis of such pain is variable even within clinically homogeneous subgroups (e.g., those with positive straight leg-raising tests). With conservative care, 67% of patients report good outcomes after 7 weeks, and 71% are satisfied with their condition 1 year later. Total remission of back pain is achieved in substantially less than 50% of patients within 1 month, and by 3 months, 40% of patients are still experiencing some discomfort. In general, the course of back pain seems to be characterized by variability and change rather than predictability and stability.

Low back pain with radiculopathy is characteristic of a group of patients with disorders that are less diverse, because the symptoms suggest nerve root compression, often sciatica. Although most patients improve with conservative management, many—up to 20%—experience poor outcomes at 1 year. Fifty percent to 70% of patients recover within 6 weeks, and at 1 year, 60% to 90% have achieved good recovery with conservative treatment. Numerous authors suggest that an imaging study is indicated in the evaluation of a patient with sciatica when (1) true radicular symptoms are present, (2) evidence of nerve root irritation is noted on physical examination (i.e., positive straight leg raising test), and (3) "conservative management" of 4 to 6 weeks' duration has failed.

Any study investigating the prognostic value of morphologic changes in the intervertebral disc will be confounded by the high prevalence of similar changes in the asymptomatic population. In general, studies have demonstrated that many morphologic or pathologic findings have enhanced signal intensity after intravenous gadolinium administration, including peridiscal scar tissue, annular tears, the intervertebral disc itself, and nerve roots. However, most of these reports have not correlated such enhancement with signs and symptoms or outcome. For instance, nerve root enhancement has been described in association with nerve root compression, but it has been difficult to correlate these changes with clinical symptoms. The significance of the findings is further complicated by the observation that normal nerve roots can be enhanced with high doses of contrast medium.

Studies of the usefulness of qualitative assessment of the morphologic features of herniated discs in the spinal canal have had mixed results. In some cases, they have not proved helpful in predicting outcomes in patients with low back pain and sciatica and have not correlated well with clinical signs and severity of symptoms. All these studies leave unanswered the question of the significance of the observed morphologic abnormalities and fail to adequately explain the role that disc herniation plays in the symptomatic population. In fact, the commonly held belief that nerve root compression on imaging studies is a criterion for surgery has not been borne out.

## Disc Degeneration

Irrespective of the various theories proposed to explain its cause, degeneration of the intervertebral disc initiates a complex cascade of morphologic and biochemical changes. These changes may ultimately lead to one or a combination of four morphologic abnormalities: disc degeneration and its sequelae, spinal stenosis, facet arthrosis, and malalignment and instability.

With aging and degeneration come gradual narrowing of the disc space and loss of the normal high intradiscal signal intensity on T2-weighted MR images. As degeneration progresses, small fluid-filled fissures, or cracks, may develop and appear as intradiscal areas of linear high signal intensity on T2-weighted images. Gas and calcification can also develop within a degenerating disc. In addition to these changes, vertebral marrow signal abnormalities adjacent to the degenerating disc are commonly seen. These changes are divided into three types. Type I endplate change is manifested as decreased marrow signal paralleling the endplate or endplates on T1-weighted images and increased signal intensity on T2-weighted images (Fig. 10–9). These changes reflect replacement of normal fatty marrow with

fibrovascular marrow, which has greater water content. Type II endplate changes are slightly more common than type I changes and demonstrate increased signal on T1-weighted images and isointense to slightly increased signal on T2-weighted images (Fig. 10–10). Histologically, this finding correlates with fatty marrow replacement. These changes may be preceded by type I changes, and the changes often exist in combination at the same level or different levels. Type III endplate changes demonstrate decreased marrow signal on both T1- and T2-weighted images, a finding that correlates with endplate sclerosis seen radiographically (see Chapter 30).

No classification system for describing degenerative disc disease is universally accepted. A widely accepted method classifies discs as either normal, bulging, or herniated (Fig. 10–11). A bulging disc is one that extends in a diffuse fashion beyond the margin of the vertebral endplates. Annular bulges are extremely common, and most bulging discs show signal changes indicating underlying degeneration. Herniation is defined as localized displacement of disc material beyond the limits of the intervertebral disc space. Herniations are subclassified into disc protrusions, extrusions, and free (sequestered) fragments. A disc protrusion is a type of herniation in which nuclear material extends focally through a defect in the anulus fibrosus. The outer annular fibers remain intact. The ability of CT and MR imaging to define an intact or partially disrupted anulus is limited. A reasonable imaging definition of protrusion is a herniation that maintains contact with the disc of origin by a bridge as wide as or wider than any diameter of the displaced material. An extruded disc is a larger pattern of disc herniation that extends through the entire

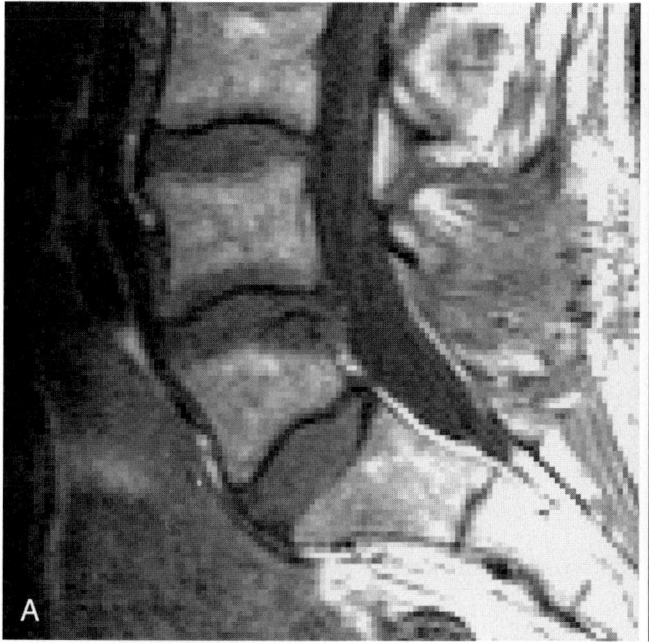 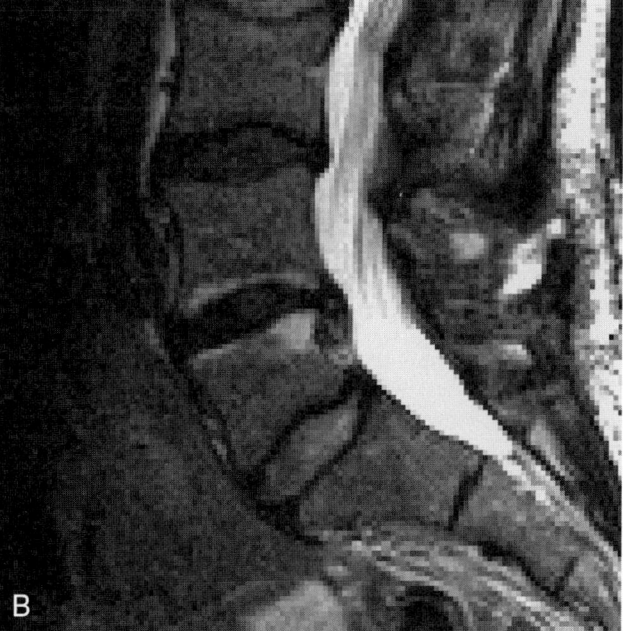

**Figure 10–9.** Type I vertebral endplates. Sagittal T1-weighted spin echo MR image *(A)* of the lumbar spine shows regions of low signal within the adjacent endplates at the L4–L5 level. These regions have increased signal intensity on a sagittal T2-weighted image *(B)*. The L4–L5 intervertebral disc is degenerated, with a decrease in disc space height and loss of disc signal in *(B)*. Note the recurrent disc herniation at this level.

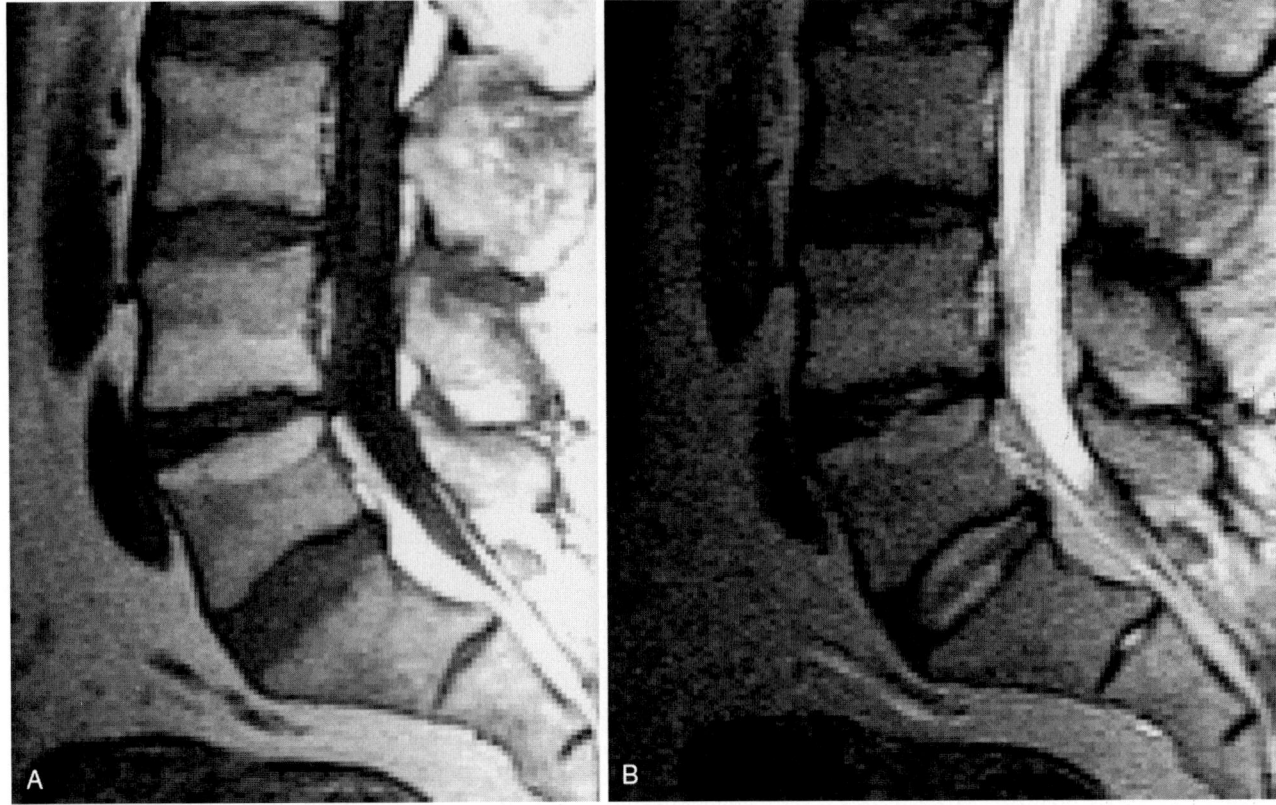

**Figure 10–10.** Type II vertebral endplates. Sagittal T1-weighted *(A)* and T2-weighted *(B)* spin echo MR images of the lumbar spine show signal intensity changes at the L4–L5 level that are typical of a type II endplate. The signal intensity of subchondral bone at this level is identical to that of fat. There is also evidence of degeneration of the intervertebral disc at this level, with a decrease in disc space height and loss of disc signal on the T2-weighted image.

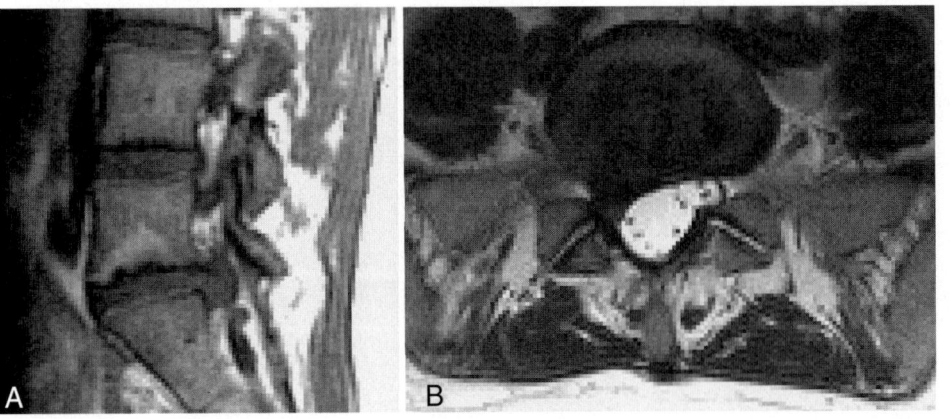

**Figure 10–11.** Disc herniation. Sagittal T1-weighted *(A)* and transaxial T2-weighted *(B)* spin echo MR images show a large extrusion at the L5–S1 level that is extending into the anterior epidural space. Also note the type II degenerative changes of the endplate. The transverse image confirms the right-sided disc herniation, which is affecting the exiting right S1 root as well as the right lateral margin of the thecal sac.

anulus. The extrusion remains attached to the parent nuclear material. A reasonable imaging definition of extrusion is a situation in which the diameter of the disc material beyond the interspace is wider than the bridge, if any, that connects it to the disc of origin. A free (sequestered) disc fragment is an extrusion that is no longer contiguous with the parent disc. A free fragment may be located at the disc level or may migrate superiorly or inferiorly.

## Spinal Stenosis

Spinal stenosis refers to narrowing of the central spinal canal, neural foramina, or lateral recesses. Most commonly it is acquired secondary to degenerative disease of the intervertebral disc, articular facets, or both structures, although developmentally shortened pedicles are an important component of symptomatic spinal stenosis in patients with otherwise mild degenerative changes (Figs. 10–12 and 10–13). MR imaging accurately depicts the degree and cause of thecal sac narrowing in patients with central canal stenosis. Such narrowing is most commonly related to bony and ligamentous hypertrophy.

In addition to central canal stenosis, stenosis of the lateral recess is an important cause of lower extremity pain and paresthesias. The lateral recess is bordered anteriorly by the posterior aspect of the vertebral body and disc, laterally by the pedicle, and posteriorly by the superior articular facet. The root sleeve within the lateral recess is often compressed by bony hypertrophy of the superior facet, frequently in combination with disc bulging and osteophytes along the anterior border of the lateral recess.

## Facet Disease

Degenerative disease of the facet joints typically occurs in combination with degenerative disc disease, although facet disease alone may be responsible for symptoms of pain and radiculopathy. Because of the richly innervated synovium and joint capsule, these changes alone can be a source of pain; alternatively, they can contribute to nerve root impingement by causing spinal stenosis or foraminal compromise. On MR images, degenerated facets appear hypertrophied, sclerotic, and irregular. Enlarged ligamenta flava are commonly present. Facet degeneration can lead to the formation of synovial cysts, which can compress the thecal sac and roots from a posterior direction. Synovial cysts are best depicted on transverse MR images and appear as posterolateral epidural masses adjacent to a

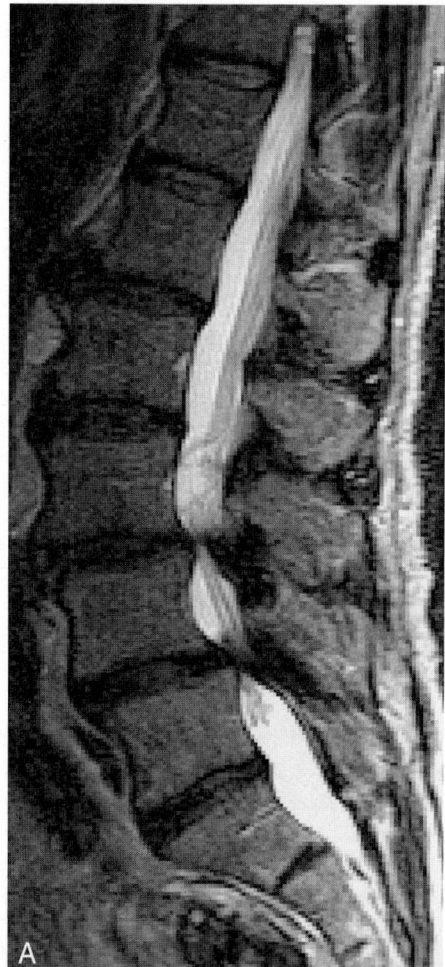

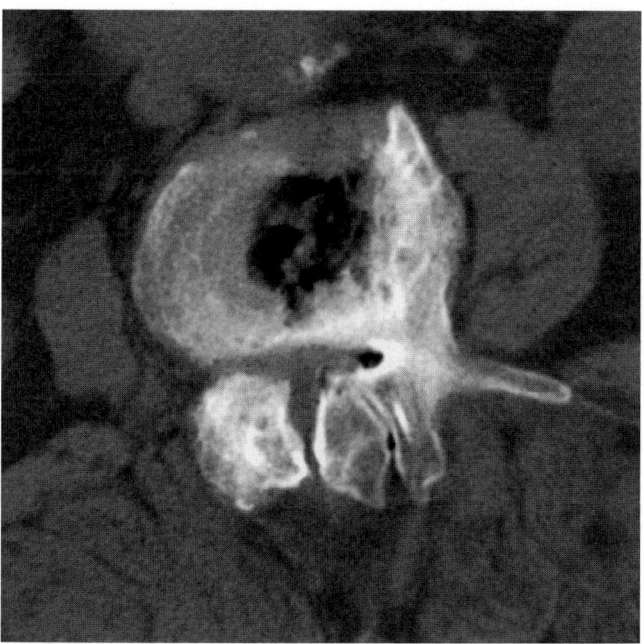

**Figure 10–12.** Severe bony central canal stenosis. Transverse CT image at the L3–L4 level demonstrates marked central canal stenosis related primarily to hypertrophic degenerative changes of the facet joints and their mass effect on the posterior margin of the thecal sac. Severe degeneration of the disc is manifested as a vacuum phenomenon.

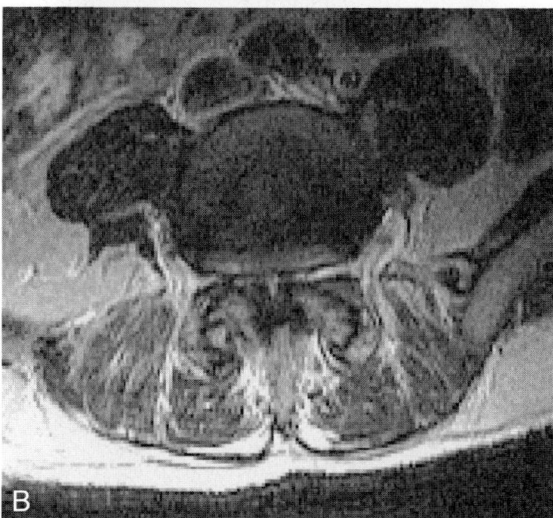

**Figure 10–13.** Lumbar canal stenosis. *A,* Sagittal T2-weighted fast spin echo MR image of the lumbar spine shows severe central canal stenosis at the L3–L4 and L4–L5 levels. This stenosis is related to a combination of bulging of the anulus fibrosus anteriorly and degenerative facet and ligamentous changes posteriorly. Note the tortuous nerve roots and intradural vessels superior to the site of canal stenosis. *B,* Transverse T2-weighted spin echo MR image confirms the severe nature of the canal stenosis, with nearly no recognizable thecal sac.

degenerated facet, most commonly at the L4–L5 level (Fig. 10–14). Synovial cysts have somewhat variable signal characteristics secondary to modifications in the composition of the cystic fluid and to associated hemorrhage, calcification, or gas within the cyst.

## Malalignment and Instability

The most frequently seen alignment abnormality is spondylolisthesis, which is defined as ventral slippage of a vertebra relative to the vertebra below. A commonly used classification system defines four grades of spondylolisthesis, with more than 90% of all cases being classified as grade I. The two most common causes of spondylolisthesis relate to bilateral defects in the pars interarticularis (isthmic or spondylolytic spondylolisthesis) and facet disease (degenerative spondylolisthesis) (Fig. 10–15).

MR imaging is believed to be the most accurate method of diagnosing spondylolisthesis. However, detection of spondylolysis with MR imaging is more problematic, and it is generally agreed that routine radiography and CT are more reliable in this regard.

## Cervical Radiculopathy and Myelopathy

The pathogenesis of cervical radiculopathy and myelopathy is cord impression from multiple morphologic changes related to degenerative disease. These causes include abnormalities of the osseous and soft tissue structures surrounding the cord; disc degeneration with bulging, herniation, or both; and hyperostosis with spondylotic bars (Fig. 10–16). As degenerative disc disease progresses and disc space height is lost, overriding of the

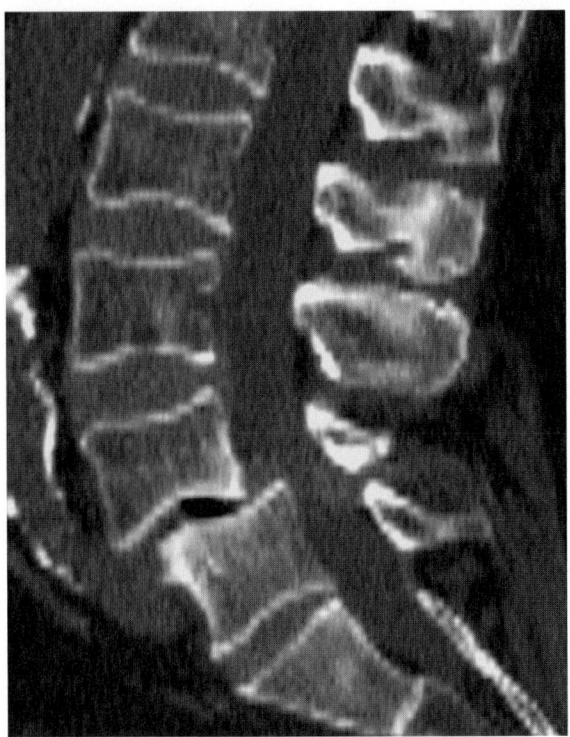

**Figure 10–15.** Degenerative spondylolisthesis. Sagittal reformatted image derived from transverse CT scans of the lumbar spine shows degeneration at the L4–L5 level with a vacuum phenomenon. A grade II spondylolisthesis at the L4–L5 level is due to osteoarthritis of the facet joints.

structures about the uncovertebral joints may occur. Osteoarthritis of the facet joints produces osteophytes, which can contribute to canal and foraminal narrowing. Finally, the ligamentum flavum can hypertrophy and invaginate, contributing to canal narrowing in the cervical spine.

Areas of increased signal intensity on T2-weighted images within the cervical cord secondary to extradural compression reflect myelomalacia, gliosis, or demyelination and edema. Patients who have areas of abnormal signal within the cord tend to have worse clinical manifestations than do those with normal cord signal intensity.

## Ossification of the Posterior Longitudinal Ligament

Ossification of the posterior longitudinal ligament (OPLL) is usually first noted in the upper regions of the cervical spine (C3–C4 or C4–C5) and then progresses inferiorly to involve the lower cervical levels and the upper portion of the thoracic spine. OPLL that is evident on plain films of the cervical spine is rare in asymptomatic North Americans and is seen in approximately 2% of the Japanese population. With clinical myelopathy, the frequency of OPLL increases to 20% to 23% in the United States and 27% in Japan. OPLL is discussed in detail in Chapter 32.

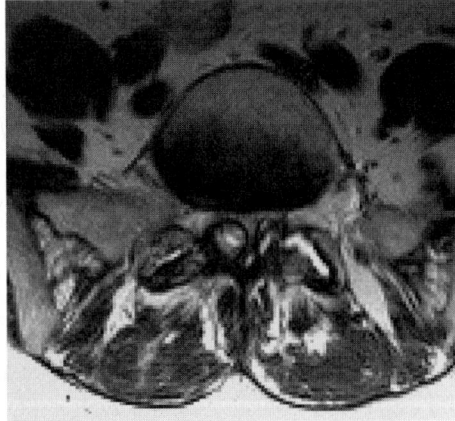

**Figure 10–14.** Lumbar synovial cyst. Transverse T2-weighted fast spin echo MR image shows evidence of bilateral facet effusions at L5–S1, which appear as linear areas of high signal intensity within the apophyseal joints. More heterogeneous areas of high signal intensity are also seen about the ligamentum flavum bilaterally. The area on the right side is larger than that on the left. These regions represent synovial cysts, which have led to severe central canal stenosis.

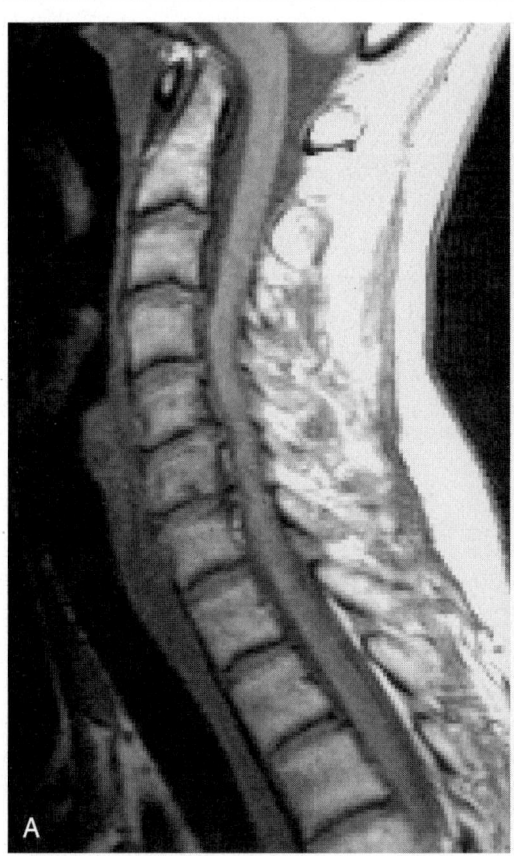 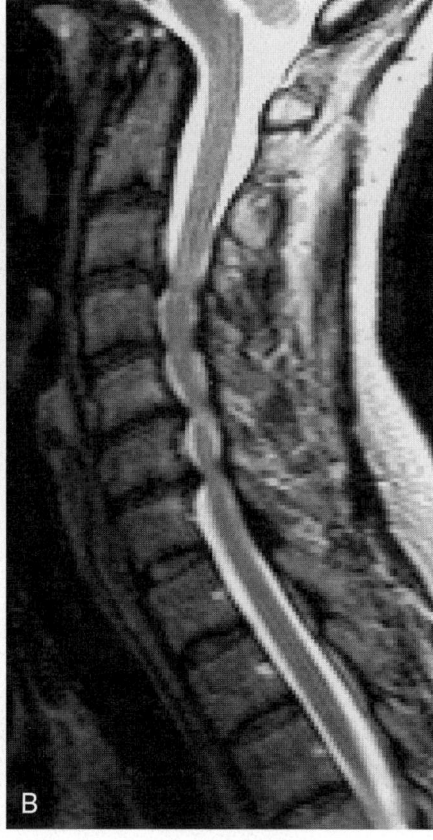

**Figure 10–16.** Cervical spondylosis. Sagittal T1-weighted spin echo *(A)* and sagittal T2-weighted fast spin echo *(B)* MR images of the cervical spine demonstrate disc degeneration at essentially every cervical level, in addition to loss of disc space height and, in *(B)*, diminished signal intensity. Severe central canal stenosis is related to both anterior disc herniation with osteophytes and posterior ligamentous hypertrophy at most of the cervical levels. A focal area of high signal intensity within the cord at the C5–C6 level reflects posttraumatic myelomalacia.

## POSTOPERATIVE COMPLICATIONS

Causes of early and delayed failure of surgical procedures of the lumbar spine are listed in Tables 10–1 and 10–2.

Caution must be used in the interpretation of MR images acquired within the first 6 weeks after surgery. A large amount of tissue disruption with resultant edema may occur following surgery, and these morphologic changes may produce a mass effect on the anterior aspect of the thecal sac. MR imaging can be used in the immediate postoperative period for analysis of the thecal sac and epidural space to exclude significant postoperative hemorrhage, pseudomeningocele, or disc space infection at the laminectomy site. Small fluid collections are not uncommon in the posterior tissues after laminectomy. The distinction between small sterile postoperative fluid collections and infected collections cannot be made on the basis of MR imaging findings related to tissue morphology or signal intensity. Acute hemorrhage is typically characterized by isointensity to increased signal in the epidural space on T1-weighted images and diminished signal on GE or T2-weighted images. Very acute blood collections, however, may have different signal intensity characteristics.

### Epidural Scar and Disc Herniation

The use of Gd-DTPA–enhanced MR imaging for the differentiation of scar tissue and disc material in the postoperative spine is well established. Epidural fibrosis consistently enhances immediately after the intravenous injection of contrast material (Fig. 10–17). In some cases, epidural scars have enhanced in patients more than 20

**TABLE 10–1**

**Causes of Early Failure of Spine Surgery**

Hematoma
Infection
Insufficient decompression of bony foraminal or central
  stenosis
Insufficient removal of disc herniation
Nerve root trauma
Unrecognized free disc fragment (sequestered)
Surgery at the wrong level

**TABLE 10–2**

**Causes of Delayed Recurrence of Low Back Pain, Sciatic Pain, or Both**

Arachnoiditis
Epidural fibrosis (scar)
Facet degenerative disease
Instability (failed fusion or spondylolisthesis)
New disc herniation (different level from the one surgically
  treated)
Recurrent disc herniation (same level as the one surgically
  treated)
Pseudomeningocele
Spinal stenosis (lateral or central stenosis from postoperative
  bony overgrowth)
Vertebral osteomyelitis (disc space infection)

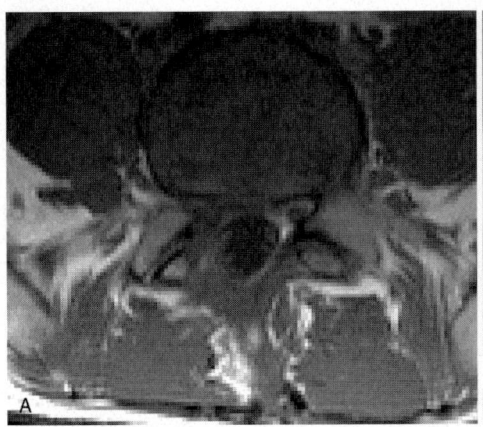 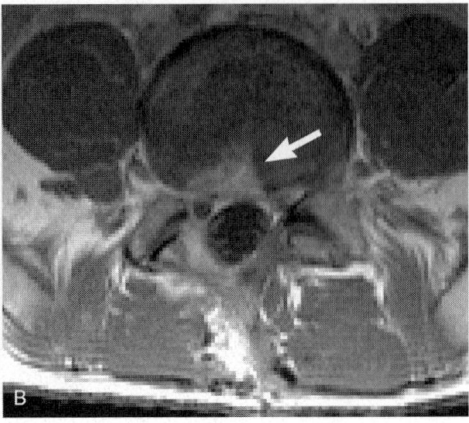

**Figure 10–17.** Epidural scar. Transverse T1-weighted spin echo MR images obtained before (*A*) and after (*B*) intravenous injection of a gadolinium-containing contrast agent show homogeneously enhancing soft tissue (representing epidural fibrosis) along the right lateral and dorsal aspects of the thecal sac and surrounding the exiting right-sided L5 root. Evidence of enhancement can also be seen within the posterior aspect of the anulus fibrosus and is related to scarring at the site of surgical curettage (*arrow*).

years after surgery, so the amount of time that has elapsed since surgery should not dissuade one from using intravenous contrast material in the postoperative state. Disc material does not enhance on early postinjection images because such material is avascular (Fig. 10–18). The addition of fat suppression to gadolinium-enhanced T1-weighted images improves the visualization of enhancing scar; this method aids in differentiating scar from recurrent herniated disc material and more clearly shows the relationship of scar to the nerve roots and thecal sac.

## Spinal Stenosis

Spinal stenosis related to osseous abnormalities has been implicated as a cause of failed back surgery in up to 60% of cases. Various mechanisms can lead to stenotic changes in the canal or foramina (Table 10–3). Many of these stenoses are not symptomatic.

## Arachnoiditis

Arachnoiditis can be classified into three categories, or patterns, and this method of classification can be applied to MR imaging, CT, and myelography. The first pattern is one of central adhesion of the nerve roots within the thecal sac, leading to a central "clump" of soft tissue signal. This pattern is most easily identified on transverse images. The second pattern is adhesion of the nerve roots to the meninges, which gives rise to an "empty" thecal sac. In the third pattern, which can be considered the end stage of the inflammatory response, arachnoiditis appears as an inflammatory mass that fills the thecal sac. On myelography, this type of arachnoiditis gives rise to a spinal block with an irregular "candle-dripping" appearance. MR imaging shows a nonspecific-appearing soft tissue mass, as does CT-myelography (Figs. 10–19 and 10–20).

## INFECTION

### Epidemiology

Sources of the bacterial seeding that causes vertebral osteomyelitis include genitourinary, dermal, and respiratory infections. In children, the bacteria (or other microorganisms) find their way to the vascularized disc, and

subsequent disc destruction causes a loss of disc space height. As the infection spreads to the adjacent vertebral endplates, routine radiographs show characteristic irregularity of bone. Hematogenous spread also occurs in adults, even though the disc has lost a great deal of its vascularity. The seeding of microorganisms occurs in the vascularized endplate, with the disc and opposite endplate becoming infected secondarily.

Because radiographic abnormalities are usually delayed for days to weeks, radionuclide studies have been the traditional imaging method for the early diagnosis of vertebral osteomyelitis. The radionuclides most commonly used to detect inflammatory changes of the spine are technetium-99m–labeled phosphonates, gallium citrate, and indium-111–labeled white blood cells. Indium-111 has several advantages over the other radionuclides, including higher target-to-background ratios, better image quality (compared with gallium), and more intense uptake by abscesses. Its main disadvantage is its accumulation within any inflammatory lesion, whether infectious or not. MR imaging appears to have a sensitivity that exceeds that of radiographs and CT and approaches or equals that of radionuclide studies. T1-weighted spin echo images can detect the increased water content or marrow fluid seen with inflammatory exudates or edema. Like most pathologic processes, disc space infection or vertebral osteomyelitis results in increased signal intensity on T2-weighted images. The diagnostic specificity of MR imaging is provided by the signal intensity changes on T1- and T2-weighted images, as well as by the anatomic pattern of disease involvement and the appropriate clinical data.

### Pyogenic Disc Space Infection

On T2-weighted images, the normal intervertebral disc usually shows increased signal intensity within its central portion, that is bisected by a thin horizontal line of decreased signal, termed the intranuclear cleft. After age 30 years, the cleft of normal intervertebral discs is seen almost universally. On T1-weighted MR images, disc space infections typically produce decreased signal intensity of the adjacent vertebral bodies and the involved intervertebral disc space. A well-defined vertebral endplate cannot be defined. T2-weighted images show increased signal intensity in the

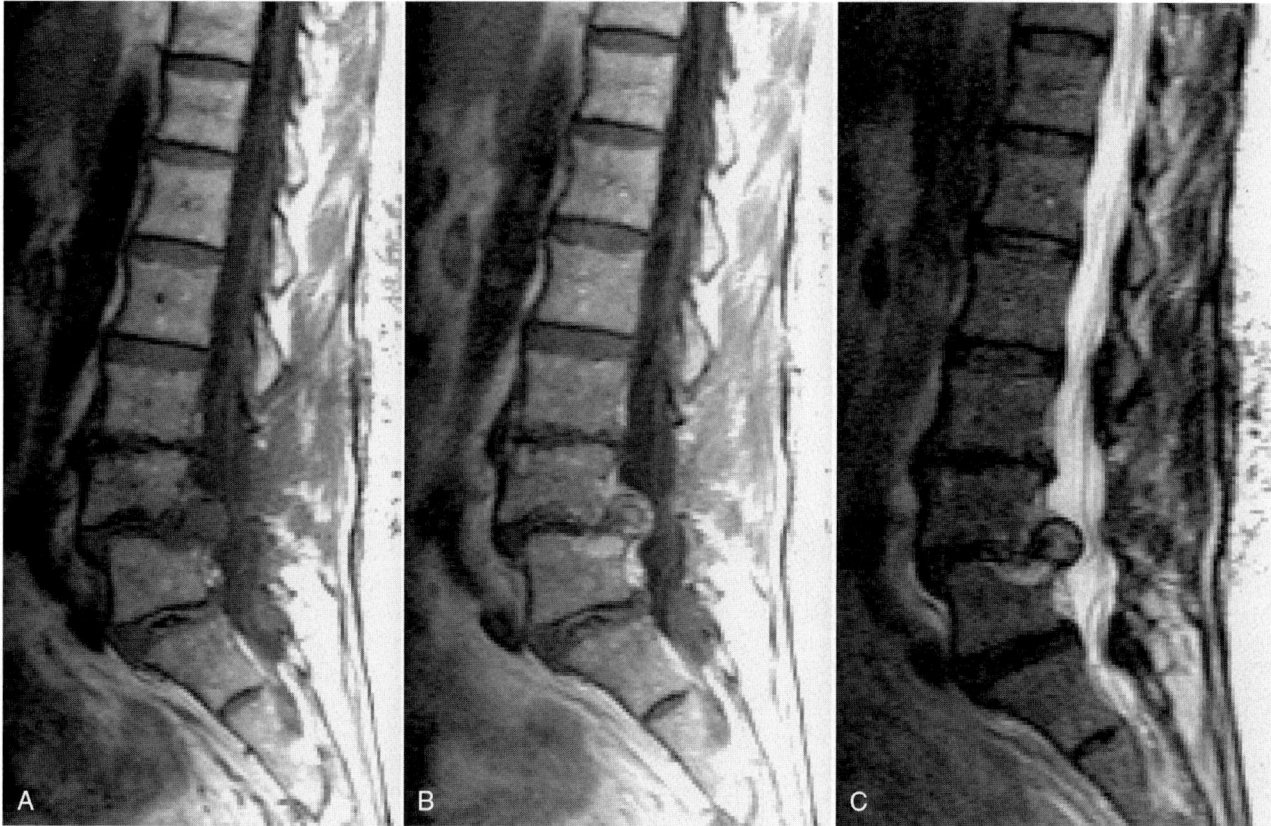

**Figure 10–18.** Recurrent lumbar disc herniation. This patient had undergone laminectomy at the L3–L4 and L4–L5 levels. Sagittal T1-weighted spin echo MR images obtained before *(A)* and after *(B)* intravenous gadolinium administration and a sagittal T2-weighted fast spin echo MR image *(C)* all demonstrate a large soft tissue mass within the anterior epidural space at the L4–L5 level contiguous with the disc space. This mass shows peripheral low signal intensity in *(C)* and patchy enhancement in *(B)*. These findings indicate the presence of a recurrent disc herniation associated with a large amount of granulation tissue.

**TABLE 10–3**

**Mechanisms of Postoperative Spinal Stenosis**

After facetectomy, bony overgrowth may compromise a lateral recess

After posterior fusion, late overgrowth of bone may extend into the posterior or lateral canals

After anterior fusion, a piece of bone may extend into the canal or foramen

After discectomy, narrowing of the space between two contiguous vertebral bodies may allow sufficient overriding of the articular facets to decrease the size of the recesses or foramina

Postoperative spondylolisthesis may produce focal stenosis

vertebral bodies adjacent to the involved disc and an abnormal morphology and increased signal intensity in the disc itself, with absence of the normal intranuclear cleft.

Approximately 95% of infected disc spaces are associated with typical vertebral body changes on T1-weighted images, and 90% have increased "nonanatomic" signal of the disc on T2-weighted images. However, only slightly more than half demonstrate increased signal of the vertebral bodies on T2-weighted images. When faced with the typical T1-weighted changes in the vertebral body and disc and T2-weighted changes in the signal intensity of the intervertebral disc, the absence of increased vertebral body signal on T2-weighted images should not dissuade one from considering the diagnosis of discitis with associated vertebral osteomyelitis (Fig. 10–21). The typical disc space infection presents no problem in diagnosis, provided that both T1- and T2-weighted images are obtained. However, atypical disc space infections do exist.

On routine radiographs and radionuclide studies, severe degenerative changes of the intervertebral disc can produce alterations similar to those seen in vertebral osteomyelitis. The disc space itself, however, is always distinct from the adjacent vertebral body endplate on T1-weighted images. Also, the degenerative disc almost always shows decreased signal on T2-weighted images, whereas inflammation shows high signal intensity in the involved intervertebral disc. In a postoperative spine, the triad of intervertebral disc space enhancement, annular enhancement, and vertebral body enhancement after intravenous gadolinium administration suggests the diagnosis of disc space infection when correlated with appropriate laboratory findings, such as an elevated erythrocyte sedimentation rate.

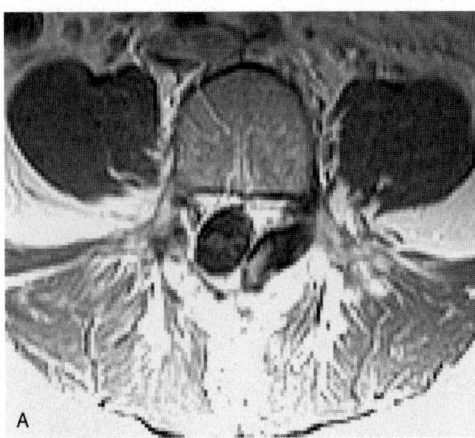
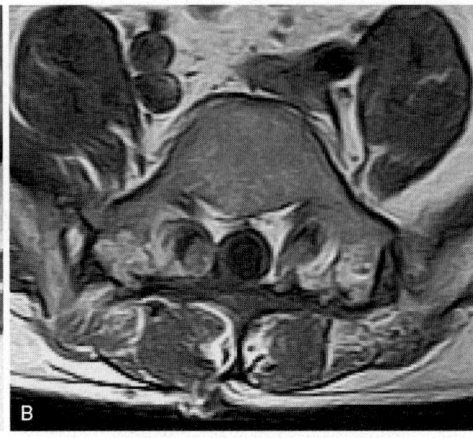

**Figure 10–19.** Arachnoiditis. Transverse T1-weighted spin echo MR images show findings of type I arachnoiditis *(A)*, including central clumping of the nerve roots within the thecal sac, and type II arachnoiditis *(B)*, with peripheral clumping of the nerve roots along the margins of the thecal sac.

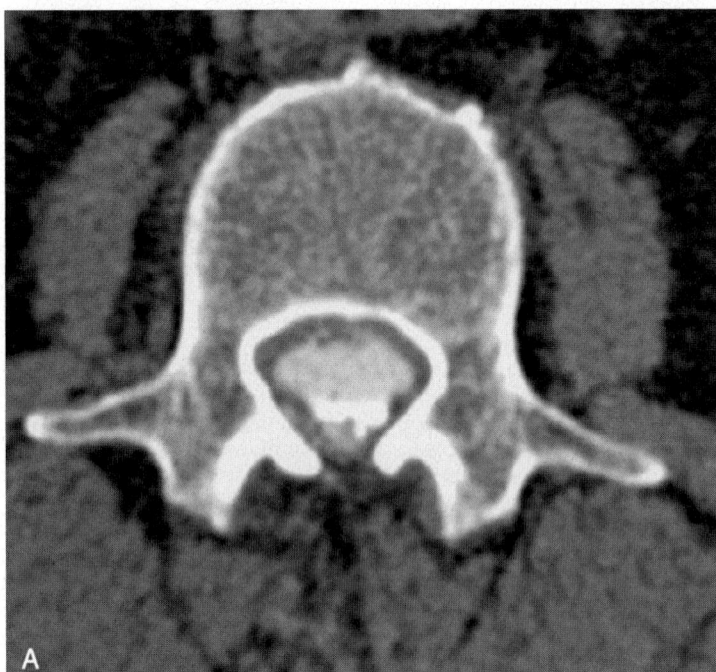
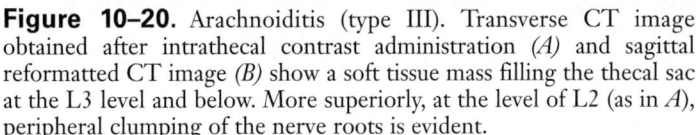
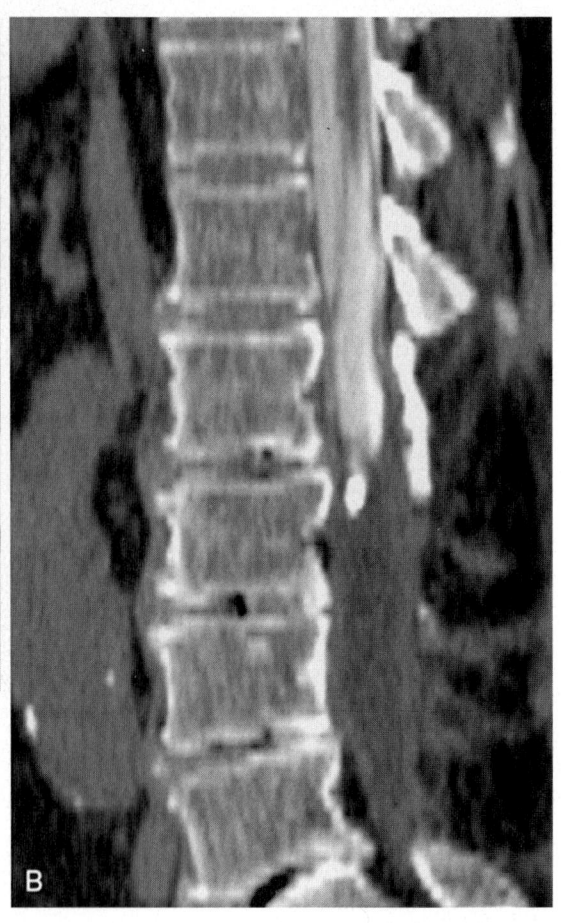

**Figure 10–20.** Arachnoiditis (type III). Transverse CT image obtained after intrathecal contrast administration *(A)* and sagittal reformatted CT image *(B)* show a soft tissue mass filling the thecal sac at the L3 level and below. More superiorly, at the level of L2 (as in *A*), peripheral clumping of the nerve roots is evident.

## Abscess

Risk factors for the development of epidural abscess include altered immune status (e.g., diabetes mellitus), renal failure requiring dialysis, alcoholism, and malignancy. Although intravenous drug abuse is a risk factor for epidural abscess, human immunodeficiency virus infection does not appear to play a role in the overall increasing incidence of the disease. *Staphylococcus aureus*, the organism most commonly associated with epidural abscess, is responsible for approximately 60% of cases. Clinical symptoms classically include back pain, fever, obtundation, and neurologic deficits. Chronic cases are associated with less pain and no elevated temperature.

The primary diagnostic method in the evaluation of epidural abscess is MR imaging. MR imaging of an epidural abscess demonstrates a soft tissue mass in the epidural space with tapered edges and an associated mass effect on the thecal sac and cord (Fig. 10–22). Epidural masses are usually isointense to the cord on T1-weighted images and have increased signal intensity on T2-weighted images.

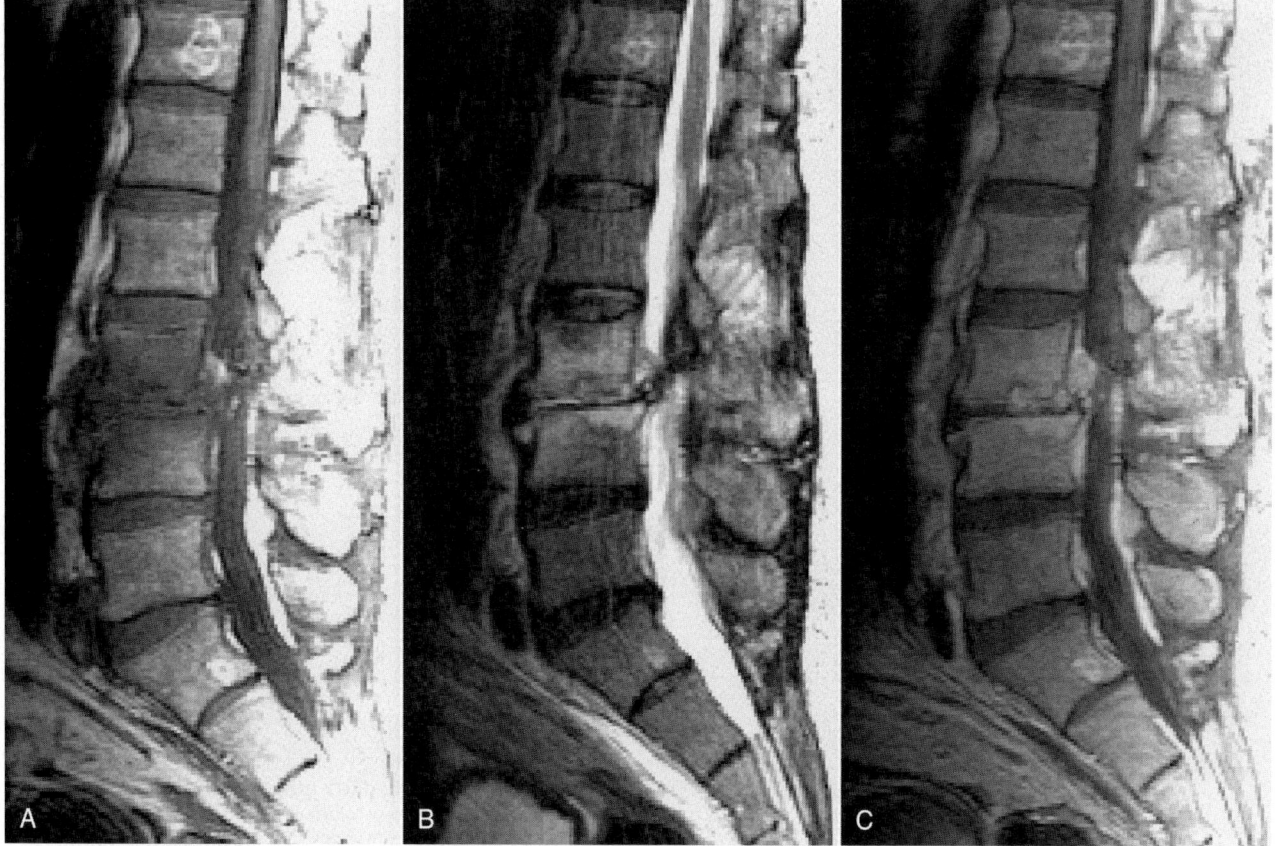

**Figure 10–21.** Disc space infection. Sagittal T1-weighted spin echo MR image *(A)*, sagittal T2-weighted fast spin echo MR image *(B)*, and sagittal T1-weighted spin echo MR image obtained after intravenous gadolinium administration *(C)* demonstrate loss of the endplate margins at the L3–L4 level, associated with high signal within the adjacent vertebral bodies in *(B)* and enhancement of signal intensity within the disc space itself in *(C)*. These findings are consistent with a pyogenic disc space infection. An epidural phlegmon is seen as a mass of homogeneously enhancing tissue posterior to the L3 vertebral body that is effacing the thecal sac.

The patterns of Gd-DTPA enhancement of an epidural abscess include (1) diffuse and homogeneous enhancement, (2) heterogeneous enhancement, and (3) thin peripheral enhancement. Gd-DTPA–enhanced imaging is a useful adjunct for identifying the extent of a lesion when the noncontrast MR images provide equivocal results regarding the activity of an infection. Leptomeningeal infections in the lumbar spine are often secondary to spread from an intracranial source. Intravenous gadolinium administration is essential in suspected cases and shows irregular or linear intradural enhancement.

## NEOPLASMS

Neoplasms involving the lumbar spine are classified by the precise site of involvement into one of three categories: intramedullary, intradural extramedullary, or extradural compartment.

### Intramedullary Lesions

**Tumors.** The most common intramedullary neoplasms are the gliomas, principally astrocytomas and ependymomas. Ependymomas are cited as the most frequent intramedullary tumor in adults. Astrocytomas produce a focal enlargement and, occasionally, an exophytic growth involving the cord. Imaging demonstrates fusiform enlargement of the cord that extends over several segments, and T2-weighted MR images show increased signal intensity, reflecting both tumor and edematous cord.

Although ependymomas may involve any portion of the cord, they most frequently involve the conus medullaris and filum terminale. A typical appearance is that of an intradural extramedullary mass involving the filum terminale and cauda equina, although the tumor can appear as fusiform enlargement of the cord itself. Cervical intramedullary tumors may be seen in patients with neurofibromatosis type 2. These tumors typically enhance following intravenous gadolinium administration and may have intratumoral cysts.

**Inflammatory Myelopathy.** The various causes of inflammatory myelopathies are legion and include multiple sclerosis, postviral demyelination, viral infection, pyogenic infection, and granulomatous disease. The archetypal inflammatory lesion is multiple sclerosis. In this disease, abnormalities in the spinal cord lead to severe motor disability, yet imaging of the spinal cord has always been

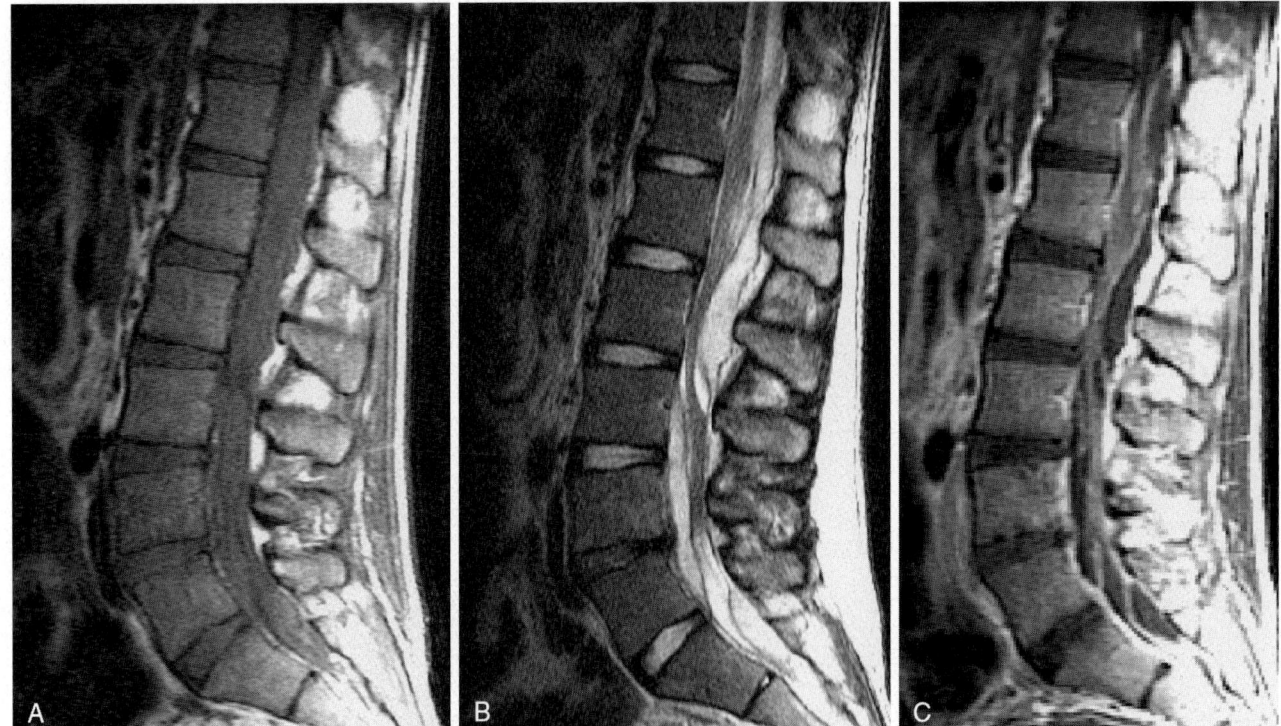

**Figure 10–22.** Epidural abscess. *A*, Sagittal T1-weighted spin echo MR image is remarkable for subtle but abnormal signal located diffusely within the thecal sac. *B*, Sagittal T2-weighted fast spin echo MR image shows a lobulated mass of high signal intensity along the posterior epidural space and extending from the S1 to the T12 levels. *C*, These findings are confirmed on a sagittal T1-weighted spin echo MR image obtained after intravenous gadolinium administration by the demonstration of patchy and irregular enhancement within the extensive posterior epidural abscess.

subordinate to imaging of the brain in clinical investigations of multiple sclerosis. Most focal plaques are less than two vertebral body lengths in size, occupy less than half the cross-sectional diameter of the cord, and are characteristically peripherally located. Approximately 60% to 75% of spinal cord lesions in multiple sclerosis are present in the cervical region, and more than half of patients with multiple sclerosis and cord plaques have multiple plaques. Of patients with cord plaques, 90% have intracranial plaques as well.

**Vascular Abnormalities.** The main arteries that supply the spinal cord include the single anterior spinal artery and the paired posterior spinal arteries. These arteries are contiguous along the longitudinal length of the cord. Contributions from radiculomedullary arteries occur at multiple levels, with the best known and largest being the artery of Adamkiewicz. Cord infarction can be caused by a variety of abnormalities, but it often relates to embolic disease such as that occurring after aortic aneurysm repair. MR findings are nonspecific in many of these vascular abnormalities but include high signal intensity on T2-weighted images. Cord enlargement can sometimes be seen on T1-weighted images. Focal atrophy of the cord is a late finding.

## Intradural Extramedullary Lesions

Intradural extramedullary neoplasms are the largest single group of primary spinal neoplasms and account for approxi-

mately 55% of all primary spinal tumors. The great majority of these tumors are benign, with nerve sheath tumors and meningiomas being the most common lesions. Nerve sheath tumors are the most frequent intraspinal tumors and are histologically divided into two types: schwannomas (also known as neuromas, neurinomas, and neurilemomas) and neurofibromas. Most intraspinal nerve sheath tumors are solitary schwannomas, whereas neurofibromas are almost always associated with neurofibromatosis type 1. Patients with neurofibromatosis type 2, however, more commonly have multiple schwannomas rather than neurofibromas. Nerve sheath tumors are easily recognized on MR imaging as typically isolated, well-circumscribed, solid masses of intermediate signal intensity on T1-weighted images, surrounded by low-signal cerebrospinal fluid. On T2-weighted images, they have variable signal intensity. Schwannomas are more vascular and undergo cystic degeneration, necrosis, and hemorrhage more commonly than do neurofibromas. A variety of local osseous changes, consisting mainly of smooth bony remodeling or foraminal enlargement, is common. Enhancement following intravenous gadolinium administration is almost always present, but the pattern is variable.

Meningiomas most commonly occur in the thoracic spine. As is the case intracranially, these tumors have a female sex predilection, and the lesions occur in a slightly older age group compared with nerve sheath tumors. The great majority are entirely intradural and are typically isointense to the neural elements on T1- and T2-weighted images. Meningiomas enhance intensely after Gd-DTPA administration, which may allow demonstration of the typical broad dural base.

The last category of intradural extramedullary lesions is the so-called leptomeningeal pattern, which includes leptomeningeal metastatic disease and benign granulomatous processes such as sarcoid and tuberculosis. The litany of tumors that may seed cerebrospinal fluid is long, but the main offenders are cranial ependymomas, glioblastomas, and medulloblastomas (especially in the pediatric population). It must be remembered that the overall sensitivity of MR examination is low in patients with proven histologic evidence of neoplastic seeding, so aspiration and study of the cerebrospinal fluid remain the gold standard.

## Extradural Lesions

Primary and secondary tumors in the extradural space are well evaluated by both MR imaging and CT. Metastatic disease to the spine is by far the most common type of extradural tumor. Because of its high contrast sensitivity and spatial resolution, MR imaging is the examination of choice for the detection of osseous metastases. Tumor replacement of fatty marrow is depicted on T1-weighted images as focal or diffuse areas of low signal intensity, and such depiction occurs much earlier than can be achieved with plain radiography or bone scintigraphy. Because many metastatic tumors enhance, the routine use of contrast-enhanced studies alone (i.e., without fat suppression) is not recommended; the resulting signal intensities of metastases and normal marrow fat are similar, occasionally to the point of masking even large metastatic lesions.

## TRAUMA

### Cervical Spine

Radiographs remain the initial study for screening or "clearing" the cervical spine in cases of trauma. The number of views considered adequate for a trauma series varies between three and five (anteroposterior, lateral, and open-mouth odontoid views, with or without supine right and left oblique views). A single lateral view is inadequate, and all seven cervical vertebrae must be visualized. Radiographs are also of primary importance in defining spinal instability in patients with persistent pain or soft tissue swelling but without a definite fracture on the initial plain film evaluation.

CT is indicated in the evaluation of the traumatized cervical spine to further assess definite or possible fractures revealed on plain films and to evaluate areas inadequately seen on plain films. Some studies recommend CT as the primary screening method in patients with multiple areas of spinal trauma. MR imaging allows direct visualization of post-traumatic cord abnormalities that cannot be defined by any other imaging method, and it can define intramedullary hematoma, intramedullary edema and contusion, disc herniation, ligamentous injury, and epidural hemorrhage. Traumatic injuries are discussed in detail in Chapter 58.

## Thoracolumbar Spine

The main area of involvement in the injured lumbar spine is the thoracolumbar junction, which acts as a fulcrum for spine motion and is susceptible to unstable traumatic injuries. The thick, sagittally oriented facets minimize rotational injury, but injuries related to flexion and transverse loading often occur. The forces may combine to produce flexion-compression injuries or the so-called burst fracture. CT remains the method of choice for detecting retropulsed bony fragments and for demonstrating fractures of the posterior elements. A hyperflexion injury occurring in the lumbar spine—the seat-belt or Chance fracture—is associated with motor vehicle accidents involving rapid deceleration. This type of injury is characterized by a horizontal fracture through both the anterior and posterior elements.

Although CT is more sensitive than MR imaging in detecting post-traumatic bony abnormalities, the latter is often superior for evaluating injured soft tissue structures. In particular, the disrupted spinal ligaments show focal discontinuity on T1-weighted images and areas of increased signal intensity on T2-weighted images. The anterior and posterior longitudinal, flaval, interspinous, and supraspinous ligaments can all be evaluated, often most favorably in the sagittal plane. Sagittal and transverse images allow the detection of retropulsed bony fragments and narrowing of the spinal canal. MR imaging excels in the detection of cord compression resulting from bony fragments (see Chapter 58).

## Epidural and Subdural Hemorrhage

Epidural spinal hematomas occur most frequently in the elderly, but they can occur at any age. Clinically, sudden back or neck pain develops that may be radicular in nature. Signs of cord compression can develop immediately or within days. Epidural spinal hematomas are broadly classified into two groups: nonspontaneous and spontaneous. Nonspontaneous epidural spinal hematomas may result from spinal taps, spinal anesthesia, trauma, pregnancy, bleeding diathesis, anticoagulant therapy, spinal hemangioma, vascular malformation, hypertension, and neoplasm. The history is often revealing, but it may consist of merely an episode of sneezing, bending, voiding, turning in bed, or mild trauma. Epidural spinal hematomas can be localized or can spread anywhere along the spinal column (Fig. 10–23).

Subdural hemorrhage is capable of producing severe and irreversible neurologic deficits, and acute surgical intervention may be needed. Subdural spinal hematomas often have a typical configuration. As opposed to epidural hematomas, which tend to be capped by fat, subdural hematomas are located within the thecal sac and are separate from the adjacent extradural fat and the posterior elements of the vertebral bodies (Fig. 10–24). Transverse images are useful in defining the epidural fat surrounding the thecal sac and in delineating the blood in the interior of the sac in subdural hematomas. Subdural hematomas should not extend into the neural foramina; such extension is more typical of an epidural hematoma. Acute hemorrhage can be fairly isointense on T1-weighted images but, over a few days, shows high signal on T1-weighted images. T2-weighted spin echo or GE images are important in

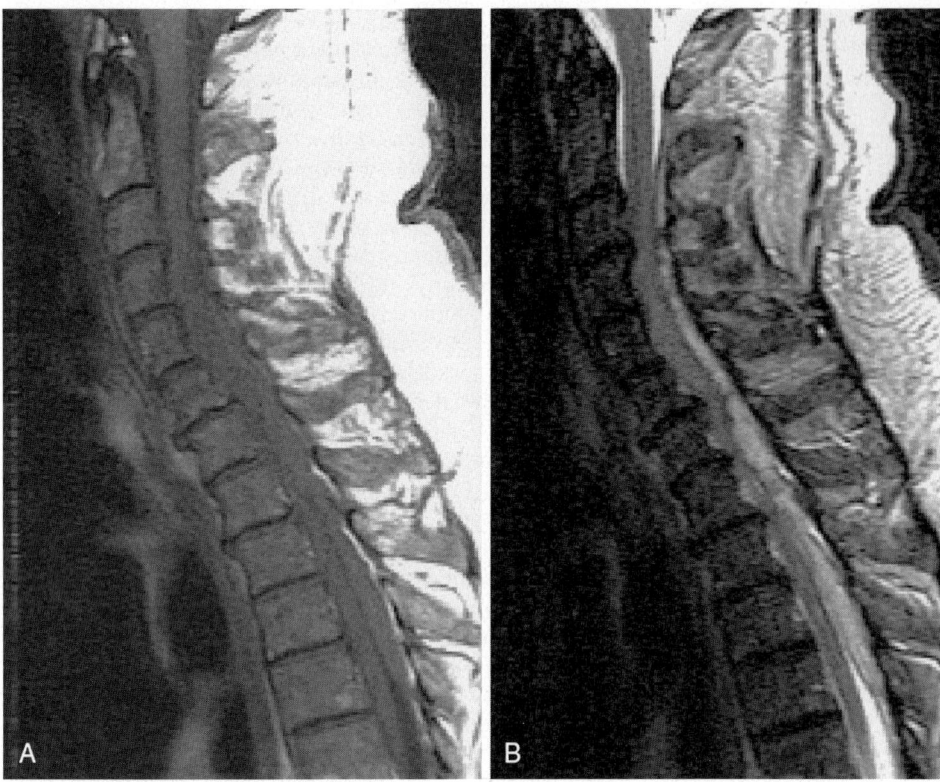

**Figure 10–23.** Epidural hematoma. Sagittal T1-weighted spin echo MR image *(A)* shows an indistinct margin between the spinal cord and cerebrospinal fluid from the C3 level to the upper thoracic spine. A suggestion of a posterior epidural lesion can be seen on this image, but the lesion is better appreciated on a sagittal T2-weighted fast spin echo MR image *(B)*. The signal intensity of the acute hematoma is nearly isointense to the cord in *(A)* and high in *(B)*.

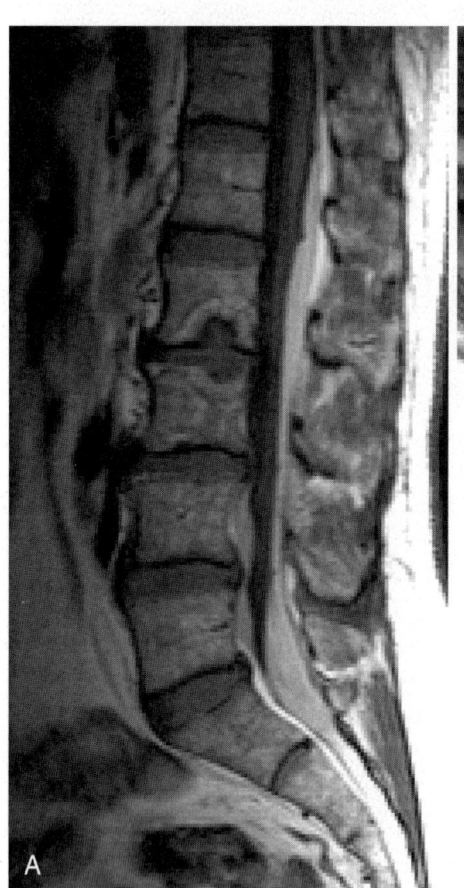

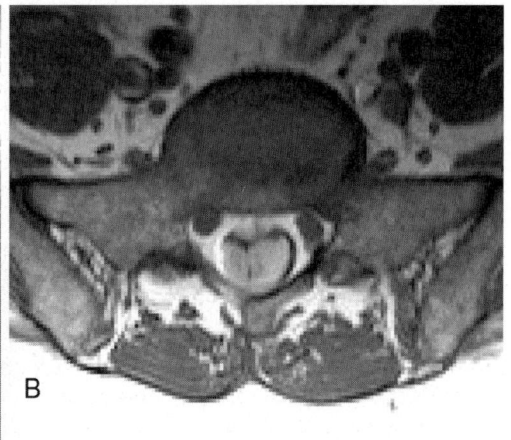

**Figure 10–24.** Subdural hemorrhage. Sagittal *(A)* and transverse *(B)* T1-weighted spin echo MR images show the typical appearance of a subdural hemorrhage. High signal intensity reflects the presence of methemoglobin within the area of hemorrhage. The transverse image shows the "Mercedes Benz" sign, representing the three areas of subdural hemorrhage.

the clinical setting of hemorrhage and show heterogeneous low signal intensity because of the presence of deoxyhemoglobin.

## CONGENITAL ABNORMALITIES

The most common minor congenital variation in the spine relates to the orientation of the facet joints, which may vary from one spinal level to the next or, at the same level, from one side of the body to the other. This arrangement is called facet tropism. The next most common minor congenital variation is an altered number of mobile lumbar segments, the so-called transitional lumbosacral junction. This variant may be characterized by lumbarization of S1, which results in six lumbar-type vertebrae, or sacralization of L5, which produces four lumbar-type vertebrae. Partial sacralization (or lumbarization) of one side of the body may also occur. Partial sacralization (or hemisacralization) has been implicated as a cause of back pain, and this pain is thought to be secondary to increased stress at the L4–L5 spinal level. Congenital hypoplasia of the articular facets or other portions of the vertebra is also encountered (Fig. 10–25).

### Chiari Malformation

The Chiari type I lesion consists of caudal descent of the cerebellar tonsils. The Chiari type II malformation consists of caudal descent of the cerebellar vermis, fourth ventricle, and lower part of the brain stem and is almost always associated with a myelomeningocele. Type III Chiari malformation is an occipital encephalocele of the cerebellum, whereas a type IV lesion is cerebellar hypoplasia (and not herniation). Clinical symptoms in the type II lesion are varied, but brain stem symptoms develop in one third of patients with a myelomeningocele by 5 years of age.

### Syrinx

Hydrosyringomyelia is a term used to describe cavitation of the spinal cord. Syringes are seen in approximately 50% to 75% of Chiari I malformations and 50% to 90%

of Chiari II malformations. The terms *syringomyelia* and *hydromyelia* represent different entities, in that syringomyelia is a cystic lesion lined by glial cells, whereas in hydromyelia, the lining consists of ependymal cells that are in continuity with the central canal. Despite the lack of a comprehensive theory on the pathogenesis of spinal cord cystic cavities, a unifying theme among all the hypotheses put forth to date is the presence of dissecting and moving cerebrospinal fluid shifts.

### Myelomeningocele

Myelomeningocele, the most common form of spinal dysraphism, is characterized by overexpansion of the subarachnoid space, with herniation of neural tissue through a large bony defect dorsally. The cord is tethered at the defect or site of other structural anomalies. Clinically, patients have weakness and paralysis of the lower extremities and a neurogenic bladder. Myelomeningocele is associated with a Chiari II malformation in 99% of cases and can result in hydrocephalus that requires shunting. Other associated anomalies include syringohydromyelia and duplication of the central canal (Fig. 10–26).

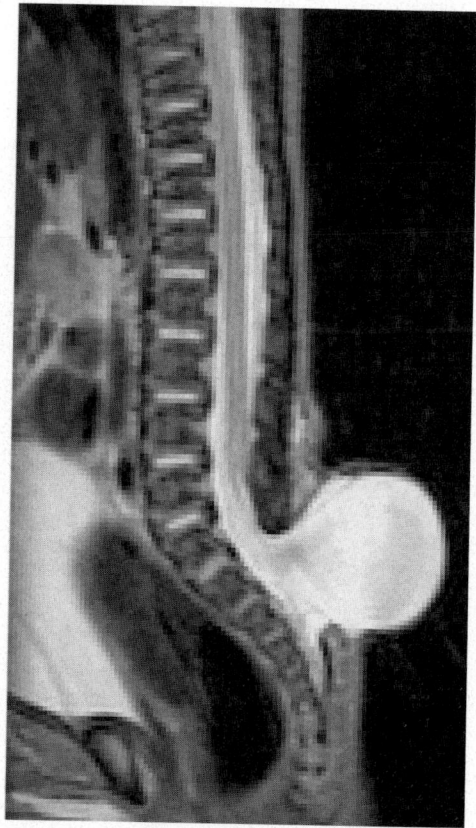

**Figure 10–26.** Myelomeningocele. Sagittal T2-weighted fast spin echo MR images show a myelomeningocele at the lumbosacral junction. The course of the distal end of the cord, the position of the neural placode, and the location of the exiting dorsal and ventral roots that extend from the involved segment are all well demonstrated.

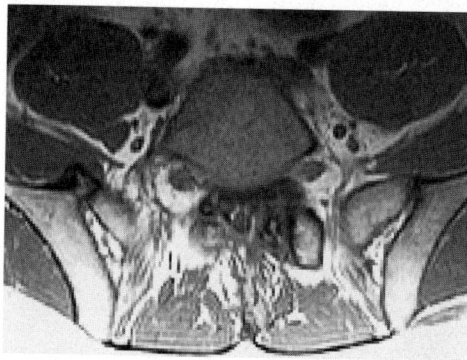

**Figure 10–25.** Hypoplastic facet. Transverse T1-weighted spin echo MR image at the L5–S1 level shows a very small right facet. This hypoplastic facet has led to compensatory hypertrophy of the left facet.

## Diastematomyelia

Diastematomyelia is a form of spinal dysraphism characterized by a partial or complete sagittal cleft of one or more segments of the spinal cord, conus medullaris, or filum terminale. Two hemicords are produced, with one central canal, one dorsal horn, and one ventral horn, each supplying the ipsilateral nerve roots. The term *diastematomyelia* refers to clefting of the cord, not necessarily the fibrous or bony spur. There is a female preponderance (80% to 94% of cases). The bone spur has an inconsistent appearance because it is formed in cartilage and ossifies variably throughout life. Most spurs form in the lower thoracic and lumbar spine. Ninety-one percent of hemicords reunite. Coronal imaging often best demonstrates the cleft, which may be missed on sagittal imaging. The pathognomonic bone finding in diastematomyelia is intersegmental laminar fusion (see Chapter 76).

## Dorsal Dermal Sinus

A dorsal dermal sinus is a midline sinus tract lined by epithelium that extends inward from the skin surface for a variable distance. It may terminate in the subcutaneous tissues or extend deeper and communicate with the conus and cord. The epithelium lining the tract may also produce a dermoid or epidermoid in 30% to 50% of cases. Dorsal dermal sinus occurs most frequently in the sacrococcygeal region. Above this level, it extends into the spinal canal or cord. The sinus is seen with equal frequency in boys and girls. A hypopigmented patch or capillary angioma is usually associated with a skin dimple. Patients can present with signs of infection or of cord or nerve recompression from the intradural dermoid or epidermoid. The intraspinal portion of the tract may be very difficult to visualize with MR imaging.

## Tumor

Intradural extramedullary congenital tumors in children include lipomas, dermoids, epidermoids, and teratomas. Epidermoid tumors should be considered in all cases of a dermal sinus. Acquired epidermoid tumors can result from implantation of epidermoid tissue iatrogenically by spinal needles. It has been estimated that 40% of intraspinal epidermoid tumors are iatrogenic in origin. Clinical features are variable and include back pain, radiculopathy, alteration in gait, and difficulty walking.

# MISCELLANEOUS DISORDERS

## Meningeal Cyst

A confusing array of terms has been used for spinal meningeal cysts. Spinal meningeal cysts are congenital diverticula of the dural sac, root sheaths, or arachnoid and can be classified into three major types. Type I includes extradural cysts without spinal nerve roots, type II includes extradural cysts with spinal nerve roots, and type III consists of intradural cysts. Type I extradural meningeal cysts without roots are diverticula that maintain contact with the thecal sac by a narrow ostium (Fig. 10–27). This

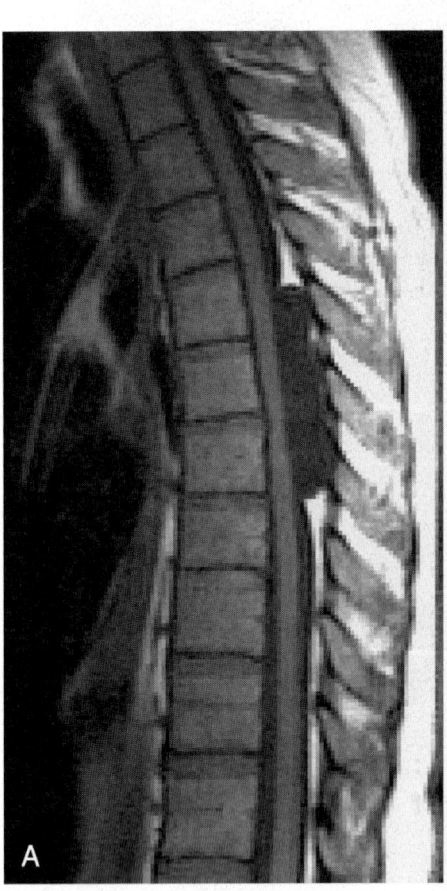
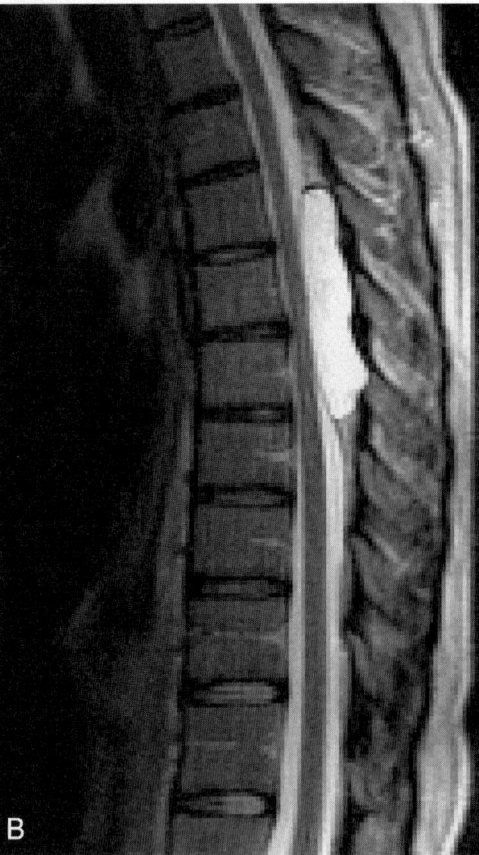

**Figure 10–27.** Type I (extradural) meningeal cyst. Sagittal T1-weighted spin echo *(A)* and T2-weighted fast spin echo *(B)* MR images show a well-defined mass with the signal intensity of cerebrospinal fluid. The mass is extradural in location in the midthoracic spine and is capped by epidural fat both superiorly and inferiorly. Flattening of the posterior margin of the thoracic cord is evident.

type includes extradural cysts, pouches, and diverticula, as well as the so-called occult intrasacral meningoceles. Type I sacral cysts are found in adults and are connected to the tip of the caudal thecal sac by a pedicle. Type II meningeal cysts with nerve roots are extradural lesions previously called Tarlov's cysts, perineural cysts, or nerve root diverticula. These cysts are generally seen incidentally as multiple lesions but are occasionally associated with radiculopathy or incontinence. Type III meningeal cysts are intradural lesions most commonly found in the posterior subarachnoid space; they have been called arachnoid diverticula or arachnoid cysts. These cysts are lined by a single layer of normal arachnoid cells and are filled with cerebrospinal fluid.

## FURTHER READING

Aguila LA, Piraino DW, Modic MT, et al: The intranuclear cleft of the intervertebral disc: Magnetic resonance imaging. Radiology 155:155, 1985.

Amunosen T, Weber H, Lilleas F, et al: Lumbar spinal stenosis: Clinical and radiologic features. Spine 20:1178, 1995.

Bell GR, Modic MT: Radiology of the lumbar spine. In Rothman RH, Simeone FA (eds): The Spine, 3rd ed. Philadelphia, WB Saunders, 1992, p 125.

Byrd SE, Darling CF, McLone DG: Developmental disorders of the pediatric spine. Radiol Clin North Am 29:711, 1991.

Carragee EJ, Kim DH: A prospective analysis of magnetic resonance imaging findings in patients with sciatica and lumbar disc herniation. Spine 22:1650, 1997.

Dwyer AJ, Frank JA, Sank VJ, et al: Short-TI inversion-recovery pulse sequence: Analysis and initial experience in cancer imaging. Radiology 168:827, 1988.

Enzmann DR, Rubin JB: Cervical spine: MR imaging with a partial flip angle, gradient-refocused pulse sequence. Part I. General considerations and disc disease. Radiology 166:467, 1988.

Enzmann DR, Rubin JB: Cervical spine: MR imaging with a partial flip angle, gradient-refocused pulse sequence. Part II. Spinal cord disease. Radiology 166:473, 1988.

Filippi M, Yousry T, Baratti C, et al: Quantitative assessment of MRI lesion load in multiple sclerosis: A comparison of conventional spin echo with fast fluid-attenuated inversion recovery. Brain 119:1349, 1996.

Goldman P, Kulkarni M, MacDugall DJ, et al: Traumatic epidural hematoma of the cervical spine: Diagnosis with magnetic resonance imaging. Radiology 170:589, 1989.

Goske MJ, Modic MT, Yu S: Pediatric spine: Normal anatomy and spinal dysraphism. In Modic MT, Masaryk TJ, Ross JS (eds): Magnetic Resonance Imaging of the Spine. Chicago, Mosby–Year Book, 1994.

Hedberg MC, Drayer BP, Flom RA, et al: Gradient echo (GRASS) MR imaging in cervical radiculopathy. AJR Am J Roentgenol 150:683, 1988.

Hitselberger WE, Witten RM: Abnormal myelograms in asymptomatic patients. J Neurosurg 28:204, 1968.

Holdsworth F: Fractures, dislocations, and fracture-dislocations of the spine. J Bone Joint Surg Am 52:1534, 1970.

Kirshenbaum K, Nadimpalli S, Fantus R, et al: Unsuspected upper cervical spine fractures associated with significant head trauma: Role of CT. J Emerg Med 8:183, 1990.

Lindsey R, Diliberti T, Doherty B, et al: Efficacy of radiographic evaluation of the cervical spine in emergency situations. South Med J 86:1253, 1993.

McCormick PC, Post KD, Stein BM: Intradural extramedullary tumors in adults. Neurosurg Clin N Am 1:591, 1990.

Modic MT: Discography: Science and the ad hoc hypothesis. AJNR Am J Neuroradiol 21:241, 2000.

Modic MT, Masaryk TJ, Ross JS, Carter JR: Imaging of degenerative disc disease. Radiology 168:177, 1988.

Modic MT, Ross JS, Masaryk TJ: Imaging of degenerative disease of the cervical spine. Clin Orthop 239:109, 1989.

Modic MT, Steinberg PM, Ross JS, et al: Degenerative disc disease: Assessment of changes in vertebral body marrow with MRI. Radiology 166:193, 1988.

Post MJD, Quencer RM, Montalvo BM, et al: Spinal infection: Evaluation with MR imaging and intraoperative US. Radiology 169:765, 1988.

Post MJD, Sze G, Quencer RM, et al: Gadolinium-enhanced MR in spinal infection. J Comput Assist Tomogr 14:721, 1990.

Ross JS, Masaryk TJ, Modic MT, et al: MR imaging of lumbar arachnoiditis. AJNR Am J Neuroradiol 8:885, 1987.

Sevick RJ: Cervical spine tumors. Neuroimaging Clin N Am 5:385, 1995.

Sobel DF, Barkovich AJ, Munderloh SH: Metrizamide myelography and postmyelographic computed tomography: Comparative adequacy in the cervical spine. AJNR Am J Neuroradiol 45:385, 1984.

Sze G, Merriam M, Oshio K, Jolesz F: Fast spin echo imaging in the evaluation of intradural disease of the spine. AJNR Am J Neuroradiol 13:1383, 1992.

Takahashi M, Yamashita Y, Sakamoto Y, Kojima R: Chronic cervical cord compression: Clinical significance of increased signal intensity on MR images. Radiology 173:219, 1989.

Tartaglino LM, Friedman DP, Flanders AE, et al: Multiple sclerosis in the spinal cord: MR appearance and correlation with clinical parameters. Radiology 195:725, 1995.

Weinberger E, Shaw DW, White KS, et al: Nontraumatic pediatric musculoskeletal MR imaging: Comparison of conventional and fast-spin-echo short inversion time inversion-recovery technique. Radiology 194:721, 1995.

# CHAPTER 11

## Interventional Spinal Procedures

Brian A. Howard, W. Bonner Guilford,
and James M. Coumas

### SUMMARY OF KEY FEATURES

A number of spinal procedures are increasingly being used in patients with pain, deformity, or both. Radiologists, because of their familiarity with imaging techniques, are in a unique position to perform these procedures. Knowledge of regional anatomy and pathophysiology is fundamental to a successful outcome.

### INTRODUCTION

The cause and natural history of atraumatic mechanical spinal disease are perplexing. The anatomic sites most often responsible for spinal pain are the discs and the zygapophyseal joints (facet joints). Collectively, lumbar zygapophyseal joint pain, internal disc disruption, and sacroiliac joint pain account for nearly 70% of cases of chronic low back pain. Spinal muscles do not appear to be a source of persistent pain.

In symptomatic patients, the incidental age-related, reparative pathoanatomic tissue changes displayed by imaging need to be differentiated from surgically important neurocompressive or neuroirritative lesions. Screening of asymptomatic individuals with magnetic resonance (MR) imaging has shown the presence of disc abnormalities. These structural changes are found in almost 25% of patients younger than 60 years and in more than half of patients older than 60 years. The older group also demonstrates an increased frequency of multilevel disease. In asymptomatic persons, large compressive disc lesions are unusual. Nevertheless, clinical experience shows a high rate of spontaneous resolution of large disc lesions. When monitored by serial MR imaging, one third of disc extrusions disappear by 6 weeks, and two thirds by 6 months.

In adolescents, low back pain is common and episodic in nature, and pain and disability are transient. Persons with disc degeneration occurring soon after the phase of rapid physical growth have an increased risk of recurrent low back pain and also have a long-term risk of recurrent back pain in early adulthood. Imaging confirms that disc disease accompanying low back pain is a key prognostic factor in this age group. Increasing evidence suggests that vascular tissue plays a fundamental role in the pathogenesis of mechanical back pain. Mechanical injury induces an inflammatory response: local tissue reaction with induced endothelial proliferation, vascular dilatation and activation, and collagen proliferation. Pain fibers seem to occur within this proliferating vascular tissue.

### ANALYSIS OF PAIN

Pain perception is a complex sensory response influenced by genetic differences, past experience, and the individual's affect. Perception of pain (nociception) can occur without tissue damage in the presence of nerve injury. In the absence of far lateral or intraforaminal disc extrusion, for example, the sudden onset of severe unilateral radicular pain affecting the buttock and thigh and not associated with a change in position often occurs in diabetic patients and is attributed to small vessel disease.

Neurocompressive conditions, such as disc extrusion, facet cyst, hematoma, and lateral or central canal stenosis, may produce objective neurologic findings. Noncompressive irritative agents or events such as interstitial epidural hemorrhage, ischemia, and local tissue edema may produce severe symptoms with minimal objective neurologic findings.

Acute mechanical pain resulting from tissue injury is transient. Transient pain resolves before and with healing and is associated with a return to normal function. Chronic mechanical pain is triggered and perpetuated by different factors. Chronic pain can be unrelenting and is associated with an inability to restore normal function. In the diagnostic management of spinal pain, a common assumption is that there is always a visible underlying pathoanatomic lesion or lesions acting as a pain generator.

### RATIONALE

Diagnostic assessment of low back pain is based on history and clinical examination rather than imaging studies. The use of laboratory tests and neuromuscular conduction studies may be supportive. The problem with diagnostic imaging in cases of low back pain is related to the high rate of asymptomatic morphologic alterations associated with increasing age. Standard imaging studies (radiography, computed tomography [CT] scanning, and MR imaging) should verify the clinically suspected diagnosis, and the results of these studies may lead to image-guided injection studies (e.g., nerve root block, facet joint block, sacroiliac joint block, provocative discography) to differentiate between symptomatic and asymptomatic morphologic alterations. Both diagnostic and therapeutic effects are possible with the use of long-lasting local anesthetics and steroids.

### Diagnostic Accuracy of Spinal Injections

Although debate continues about the cause of localized spinal pain, the finding of a sensory deficit, loss of reflex, or demonstrable weakness on physical examination is used to identify the level of spinal nerve root compression. Characteristic areas of numbness have also been documented on the medial side of the lower part of the leg in 88% of L4 nerve root blocks, the dorsum of the first digit in 82% of L5 nerve root blocks, and the lateral aspect of the fifth digit in 83% of S1 nerve root blocks. Dermatomal patterns may vary in a substantial minority of patients, however. Transitional segments in the spine can result in inaccurate identification of neural anatomy unless the vertebrae are counted completely from the cervical through the lumbar spine. Various congenital anomalies of the lumbosacral nerve roots have been documented, including a more cranial or caudal origin of a nerve root, a conjoined structure of two roots, and anastomoses between two or more roots, all with restricted mobility. The anomalies are usually unilateral, and the fifth lumbar and first sacral nerve roots are involved most frequently.

Because patient response is dependent on accurate needle placement, fluoroscopic or CT guidance, or both, has been advocated. Visual guidance allows accurate placement of the needle at the correct spinal level and location in the epidural space, as well as confirmation of spread of the anesthetic to the level of the pathologic lesion.

### Therapeutic Efficacy of Spinal Injections

Most patients with back pain and radiculopathy respond to conservative management consisting of education, exercise, medication, physiotherapy, and, increasingly, some form of local injection therapy. Large doses of medication and prolonged bed rest are associated with less patient satisfaction. Underlying disc derangement, neurocompressive stenotic features, and posterior interfacet arthrosis appear to act in concert. Comparative clinical outcome data are insufficient to validate any specific therapeutic approach. Epidural injection or periradicular infiltration of steroids and local anesthetic is commonly used for the management of lumbosacral radicular syndromes. The available well-designed clinical studies show a significantly positive pain-reducing benefit from lumbar epidural steroid injections.

Local anesthetic injections can readily identify sources of pain in soft tissue, scar tissue, nerves, and ligaments. They have particular application in this regard in cases of postsurgical or postinjury back pain in which the normal anatomy or function may be distorted. Local anesthetic blocks can also corroborate or define sites of pain in the posterior facet joints and in torsional annular tears.

### CONTRAINDICATIONS AND COMPLICATIONS

Contraindications to routine elective interventional procedures include active systemic or local infection, pregnancy, documented allergy to corticosteroid medications or contrast agents, and a bleeding diathesis. Preprocedural testing in asymptomatic persons with no bleeding history is not warranted. Informed consent should be obtained after a discussion of the potential benefits and risks associated with needle placement and the injection of contrast agents, corticosteroids, anesthetic agents, and methylmethacrylate cement.

With regard to local tissues, potential complications include neural injury and focal hemorrhage or ischemia. Systemic complications include vasovagal episodes, contrast agent- or drug-induced allergic reactions, and possible cardiorespiratory sequelae. Subacute complications may be associated with a systemic response to injected corticosteroid preparations. Intrathecal injection of corticosteroid may lead to chemical arachnoiditis, development of epidural hematoma, and deep infection. Chronic untoward effects include residual nerve injury and epidural lipomatosis associated with repeated steroid injections.

## GENERAL TECHNIQUE

Accurate selective interventional procedures require image guidance and film confirmation. Overhead or C-arm fluoroscopy with film capture or CT scanning may be used. In general, fluoroscopy results in much higher radiation exposure to patients than do most types of radiographic procedures. A nonionic, iodine-based contrast medium that is regarded as safe for intrathecal use should be chosen. General sedation of the patient may be required. Conventional local anesthetic agents such as 1% to 2% lidocaine and 0.2% to 0.5% bupivacaine in small volumes are used routinely. Systemic effects of steroid preparations that are injected in the epidural space, including dyspepsia and hyperglycemia, are possible because these preparations may interact synergistically with preprocedural oral nonsteroidal anti-inflammatory drugs or recent oral or intramuscular steroid treatments.

## SPECIFIC PROCEDURES

### Apophyseal Joint Injection

Symptoms may originate from multiple elements in the vertebral motion segment, or three-joint, complex. Disorders of the apophyseal joints may give rise to back pain or nerve root irritation and compression. Intra-articular injection of local anesthetic agents with corticosteroids is a common interventional procedure used primarily to identify and treat patients whose back pain arises predominantly from these joints (Fig. 11–1). Facet joint capsular distention has been shown to cause pain and discomfort that can be relieved by selective nerve root blocks or the intra-articular injection of local anesthetic agents. Joint effusions may lead to the formation of synovial cysts, which may produce intermittent or continuous compression of adjacent neurovascular tissue (Fig. 11–2). Multiple facet joints may need to be evaluated with provocative and therapeutic steroid and anesthetic injections. The volume of injected anesthetic varies in reported studies, but the normal capacity of the joint is about 2 mL. Injections of large volumes of solution (3 to 6 mL) may cause capsular rupture posteroinferiorly, periarticularly, or ventrosuperomedially within the epidural space. Early studies of facet joint injection suggested that short-term relief could be obtained in 59% to 94% of patients and long-term relief in 20% to 54% of patients. Long-term studies, however, show that injecting methylprednisolone acetate into the facet joints is of little value in the treatment of patients with chronic low back pain.

### Sacroiliac Joint Injection

The sacroiliac joint is an uncommon but real source of low back pain. The diagnosis of a painful articulation

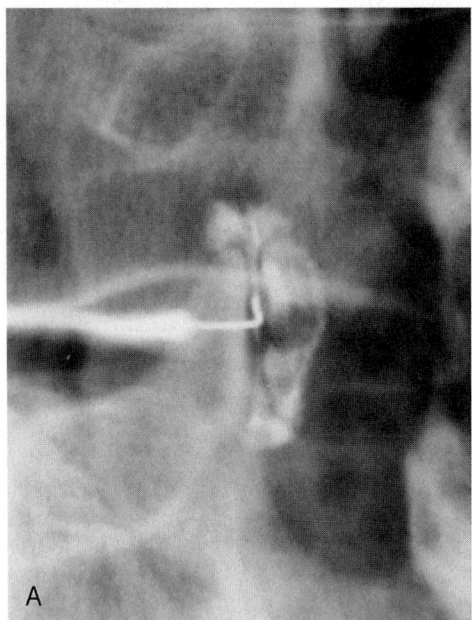
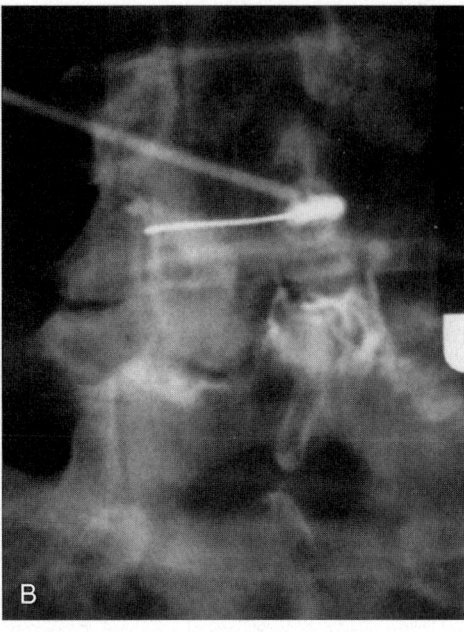

**Figure 11–1.** Apophyseal joint injection. *A,* Postero-oblique view of the lumbar apophyseal joint shows intra-articular placement of a curved needle. The contrast material outlines the superior and inferior recesses, which are alternative puncture sites. *B,* Frontal projection shows that the needle has been placed superiorly, with contrast material extending across the midline to fill the opposite facet joint. Note the posterior interspinous impingement and loss of interlaminar distance, leading to soft tissue impingement and formation of an adventitious interspinous bursa with fistulous communication between the facet joint recesses.

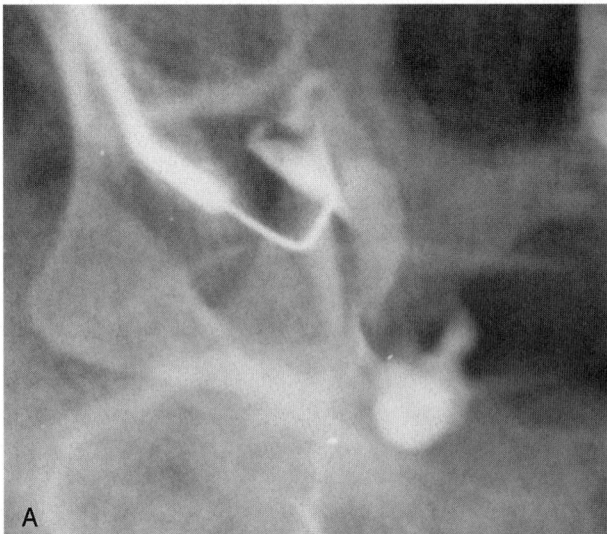
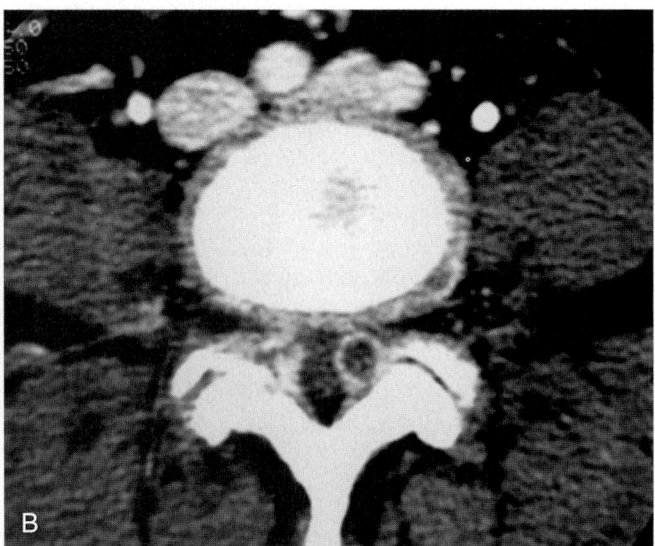

**Figure 11–2.** Synovial cyst. *A,* Postero-oblique view of an opacified facet joint demonstrates a posteroinferior recess of moderate size and a diverticular extension posteromedially. *B,* In a transverse CT image obtained after the intravenous injection of a contrast agent, note the peridiscal enhancement and peripheral enhancement of bilateral synovial cysts about the facet joints that have caused central spinal stenosis. Osteoarthrosis is present in both facet joints.

between a transitional lumbar vertebra and the sacrum can also be confirmed with anesthetic injections.

## Piriformis Muscle Injection

The sciatic nerve may be compressed as it leaves the pelvis through the greater sciatic foramen by the piriformis muscle, and the resultant pain may be increased by muscular contraction, palpation, or prolonged sitting. Diagnostic testing can be used to differentiate piriformis syndrome from other causes of sciatica, lower extremity weakness, and pain. Piriformis muscle injections are performed under CT guidance. Without such guidance, injection into the

midsubstance of the piriformis muscle, with soft tissue extravasation and perisciatic neural leakage, is nonselective and of limited value. Anecdotal evidence suggests that selective anesthetic blockade, combined with local steroid injection at the superficial and deep margins of the distal end of the tendon at its trochanteric attachment site, can resolve symptoms associated with overuse.

## Epidural Injection

Epidural injections used to treat back and limb pain are generally accomplished through a posterior interlaminar, caudal, or transforaminal route. All three techniques are capable of delivering steroid preparations to the epidural space. The interlaminar and caudal methods are imprecise, require substantial volumes of injectant with larger doses of steroids, and may necessitate a series of injections that are expensive and more likely to lead to complications. With the caudal injection technique, the injected solution dissipates mainly in a cephalad direction and seldom crosses the L5–S1 disc space (Fig. 11–3A). The transforaminal route provides precise delivery of a smaller dose of corticosteroids under fluoroscopic guidance. The medication is injected predominantly in the anterior epidural space (see Fig. 11–3B).

Epidural injection of corticosteroids can be used to treat patients with certain radicular pain syndromes of the lower extremity of intermediate duration (2 weeks to 3 months). The short- and long-term benefits of repeated epidural or perineural steroid injections have been evaluated in patients with persistent radicular or low back pain for more than 6 weeks, and long-term improvement has been reported in more than half of patients. A highly variable success rate (23% to 84%) has been reported for epidural injection.

**Selective Lumbosacral Nerve Root Block with Focal Transforaminal Injection.** After sterile preparation and anesthesia of the skin, a 22-gauge short bevel spinal needle is inserted at a point just lateral to the pedicle and below the transverse process. With the patient in a prone oblique

position of 30 to 40 degrees, a straight needle can be directed under fluoroscopic control to the base of the pedicle at its junction with the vertebral body beneath the transverse process. With the patient prone, manipulation of the needle tip around the facet and pedicle requires a needle in which the last centimeter is curved away from the bevel (Fig. 11–4). To reduce the chance of inadvertent dural puncture, the needle tip should not extend beyond the midline of the pedicle. In the upper lumbar levels, the perineural arachnoid sleeve or cysts may extend more laterally (Fig. 11–5).

Access to the S1 nerve root can be obtained through the small posterior sacral foramina; alternatively, a straight needle can be passed directly through the thin posterior cortical bone overlying the S1 nerve root canal just below the S1 pedicle. The patient frequently feels some radicular pain when the needle approaches the nerve. When the needle tip is in the proper position, or when the patient indicates that typical symptoms have been reproduced, contrast medium is injected. Antegrade flow of the contrast material outlines the exiting nerve root. Retrograde flow of the contrast agent extends in a subpedicular direction to the ventral epidural space and to the targeted extrathecal disc space. Fluoroscopy with the patient in a lateral or oblique position ensures accurate placement of the needle. Enough contrast agent should be injected for the operator to recognize intravascular and intrathecal flow. When correct needle position is confirmed and the desired flow

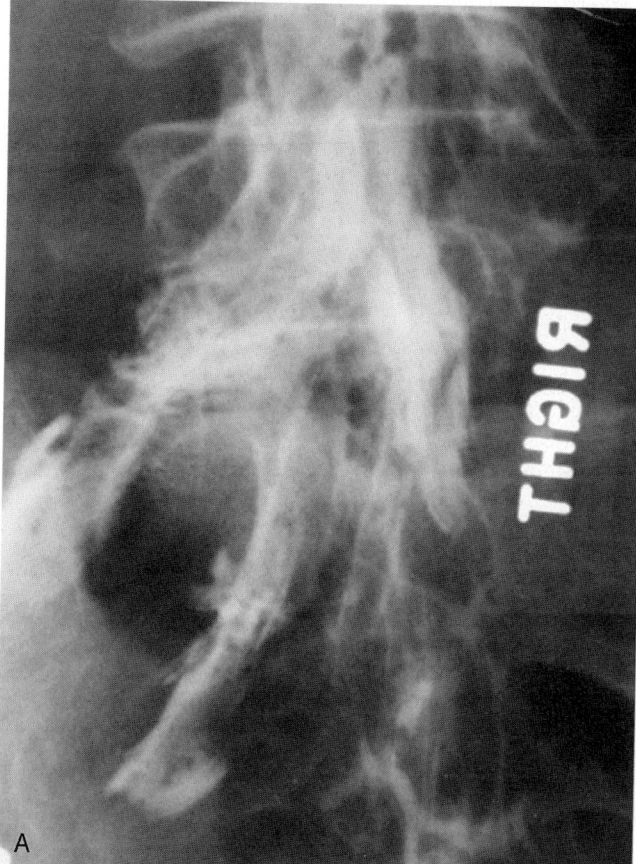

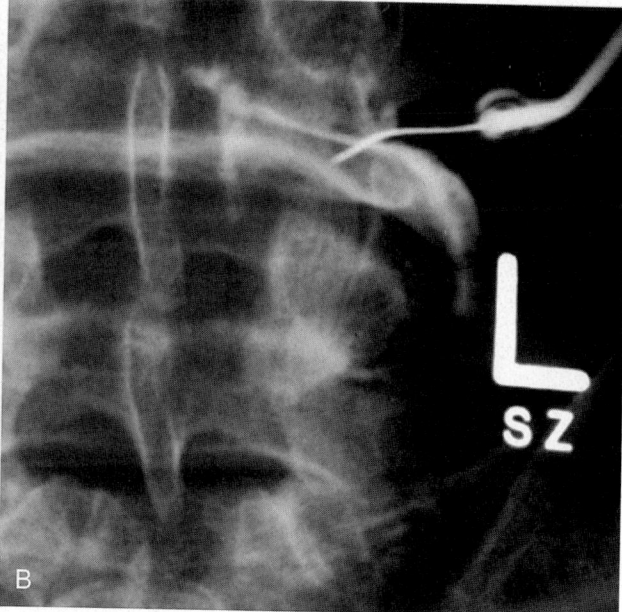

**Figure 11–3.** Epidural injection. *A*, Conventional large-volume epidurogram has been performed via the transsacral hiatus. Contrast opacification of the epidural space and multiple nerve root sleeves on the left is seen. *B*, Selective midtransforaminal needle placement is shown. Note the antegrade and retrograde contrast opacification of the L4 nerve in the lateral nerve root canal. Also note the fusiform swelling of the dorsal nerve root ganglion. The contrast material is perineural and not in the ventral epidural space, as seen in *(A)*.

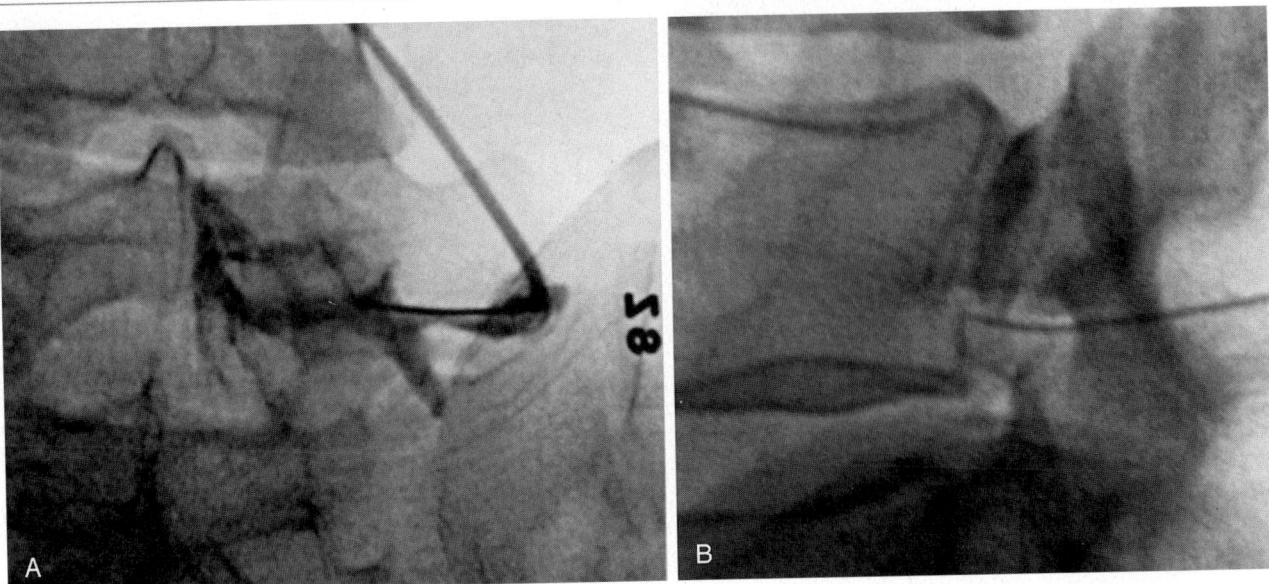

**Figure 11–4.** Epidural injection. *A,* High L5 transforaminal needle placement has resulted in antegrade and retrograde flow of contrast material outlining nerve root divisions and the foraminal floor, with midline flow of contrast agent to the L4–L5 disc margin. *B,* Lateral radiograph confirms the location of the tip of the curved needle, along with retrograde ventral epidural flow of contrast material to the craniad disc space.

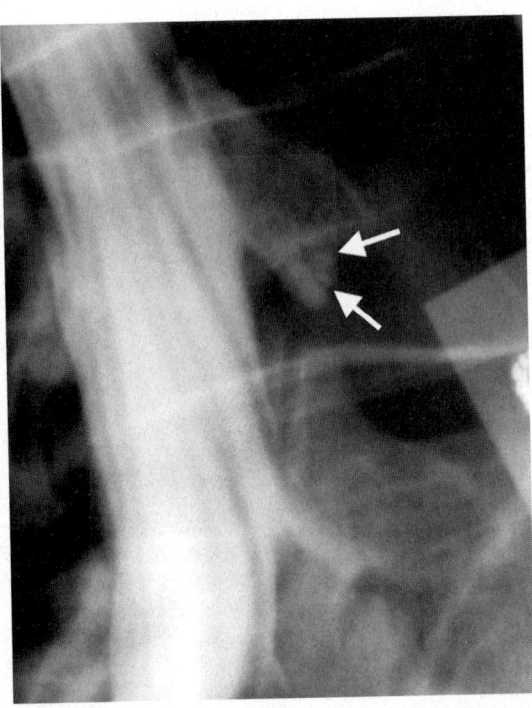

**Figure 11–5.** Tarlov's cysts. Postero-oblique projection during a myelogram outlines the course of an intradural nerve root, elongation of the dural sleeve, and terminal diverticula (Tarlov's cysts) *(arrows).* The presence of long nerve root sleeves and perineural cysts predisposes to inadvertent intrathecal puncture.

pattern is demonstrated, a block is created by injecting 2 to 3 mL of anesthetic and steroid medication. This method delivers about 30 to 40 mg of methylprednisolone or the equivalent dose of betamethasone into the ventral epidural space and achieves a sensory block. The use of bupivacaine with a concentration greater than 0.25% frequently results in loss of motor function for several hours.

**Selective Cervical Nerve Root Block with Focal Transforaminal Injection.** The patient is positioned comfortably in an approximately 45-degree anterior oblique position to enable visualization of the neural foramen fluoroscopically. After sterile preparation and anesthesia of the skin, and with constant fluoroscopic guidance, a 25-gauge spinal needle is directed in an oblique direction from an anterolateral approach until it contacts the anterior aspect of the superior articular process. The needle is "walked off" anteriorly for a distance of 1 to 2 mm into the neural foraminal tissues. Injection of nonionic, low-osmolar myelographic contrast agent is used to confirm opacification of the nerve root and the absence of contrast material in intrathecal or vascular sites (Fig. 11–6). Subsequently, 1 mL of a solution containing 0.25% bupivacaine or 1% lidocaine mixed with 25 mg of methylprednisolone without alcohol or an equivalent dose of betamethasone (Celestone Soluspan) is injected.

**Selective Thoracic Nerve Root Block, Selective Transforaminal Epidural Injection, and Paravertebral Blocks.** Nerve root blocks and transforaminal epidural injections in the thoracic spine are performed under CT guidance (Fig. 11–7). The volume of injected material is 2 mL of 1% lidocaine or 0.25% bupivacaine. Paravertebral sympathetic blocks performed under CT guidance decrease the incidence of pneumothorax and document accurate needle placement. A 20-gauge needle is initially inserted into the paravertebral soft tissues. Subsequent coaxial placement of a 25-gauge needle anterolaterally for induction of an anesthetic block is facilitated by the use of saline infiltration to distend the local tissues between the spine and pleura.

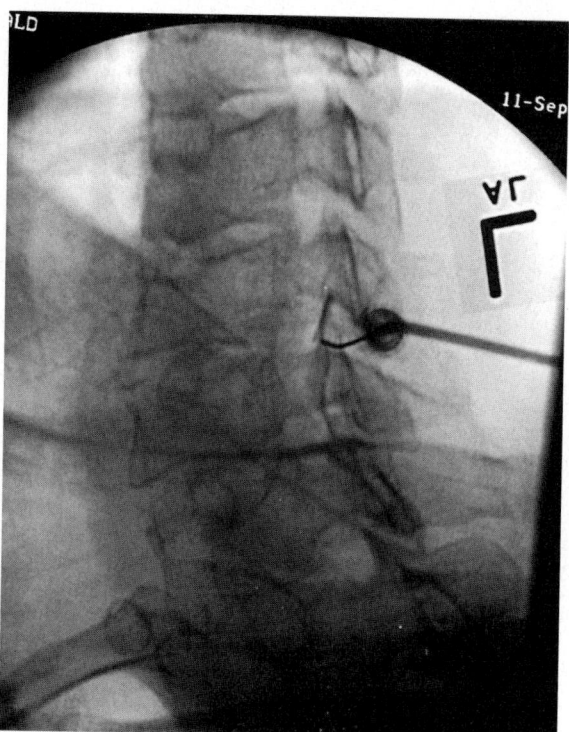

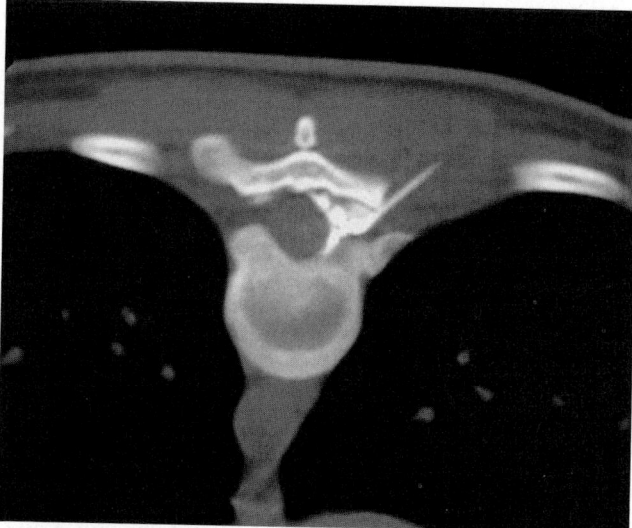

**Figure 11–7.** Thoracic nerve root block. CT image demonstrates the posterolateral transforaminal placement of a 22-gauge spinal needle, with injected contrast material confirming epidural flow in both a ventral and a dorsal direction. Because of the presence of the ribs, CT gantry angulation may aid in proper placement of the needle.

**Figure 11–6.** Selective cervical nerve root block with foraminal injection. Oblique fluoroscopic view confirms placement of a 25-gauge needle in the posterior, lower third of the foramen, with contrast material outlining the C6 nerve.

## Lumbar Discography

Combined with CT, discography has become an established diagnostic procedure that accurately and reliably assesses lumbar disc integrity in patients with persistent low back, buttock, or thigh pain who have failed to respond to conservative therapy or decompressive surgical treatment and for whom spinal fusion is being considered. Discography is usually performed when negative or equivocal results are provided by other diagnostic imaging techniques such as CT scanning, MR imaging, or myelography.

Lumbar discography can be performed via a transdural or posterolateral oblique approach. The transdural approach entails two punctures of the thecal sac for each intervertebral disc that is injected, with a resultant increased propensity for cerebrospinal fluid leakage. The oblique approach can be achieved with a single C-arm fluoroscopic unit or with biplanar imaging. Fluoroscopy allows appropriate needle manipulation and use of the "bevel effect" to ensure optimal penetration of the center of the intervertebral disc. For discography to be performed successfully, the needle tip should be placed in the central third of the disc space (Fig. 11–8). A curved needle can be placed through a larger-bore needle to avoid any osteophytes and to allow access to deeply located L5–S1 discs.

The normal volume that can be injected into a lumbar disc is 1 to 2 mL, and such injection does not produce pain. With injection into an abnormal intervertebral disc,

symptoms may occur when either small (0.5 mL) or large (3.5 mL) volumes of fluid are instilled (Fig. 11–9). Analysis of the location of discomfort, the pattern of pain radiation, the pain severity, and its similarity to the primary pain should be documented carefully. A positive pain response can be terminated by a subsequent controlled intradiscal injection of 1% lidocaine. The patient is observed for 2 hours after the procedure and given medication, if necessary, to resolve any symptoms that were produced or exacerbated during the study.

Contrast opacification of the nuclear space (nucleogram) may reveal a regular or irregular appearance that must be clearly differentiated from contrast material in the anulus fibrosus (annulogram) associated with misplacement of the needle tip. The contrast pattern mirrors the integrity of the nuclear space. Isolated "rim" lesions that do not communicate with the nucleus pulposus represent a small subgroup of lesions leading to discogenic pain that are not well demonstrated by discography. CT scanning after discography allows precise localization and display of the nuclear space, disc extrusions, annular defects, disc fissures, and concomitant nerve root and thecal sac compromise.

External annular disruption results in a bulge in the intervertebral disc that is greater than 2.5 mm beyond the vertebral edge. Discography shows a characteristic "collar stud" extension caused by the rent in the anulus fibrosus, without nuclear extrusion. Such annular disruption results in an inflammatory response consisting of reparative granulation tissue that extends into the cleft. With discography, 65% of patients with severe unresponsive back pain demonstrate a posterolateral annular tear without evidence of an extruded nucleus pulposus.

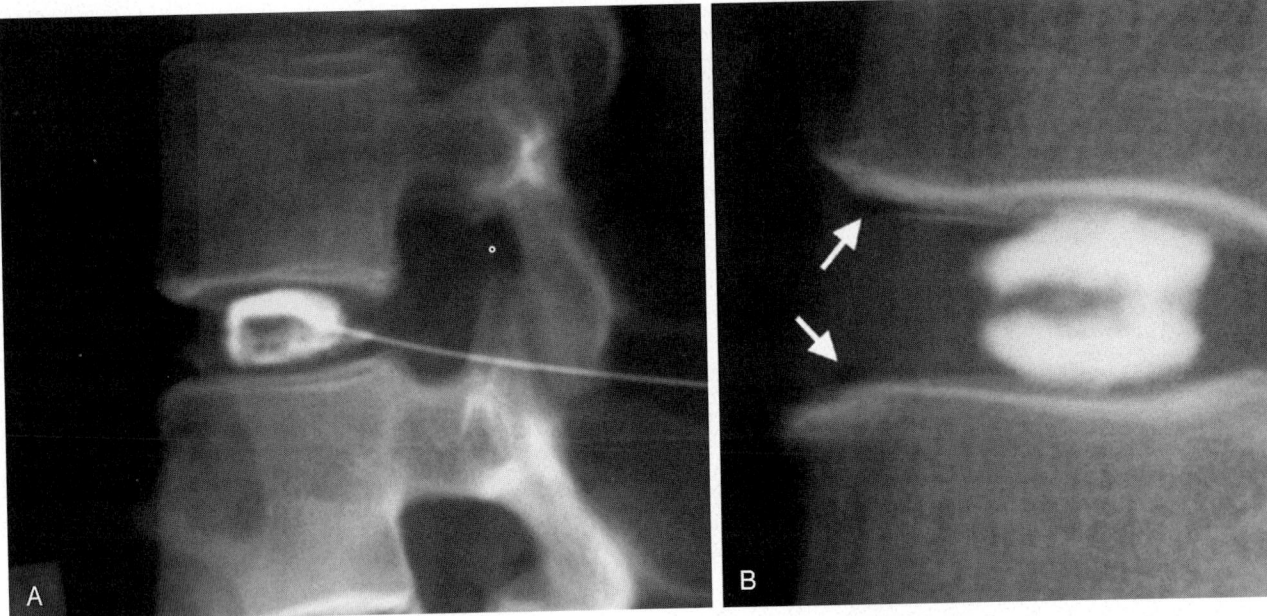

**Figure 11–8.** Lumbar discography. *A,* Lateral lumbar spine with discographic needle entry low in the posterior disc margin. Note the normal unilocular appearance of the nucleogram. *B,* Normal bilocular appearance of the nucleogram. The anterior arrows identify anterior vacuum phenomena in the anulus fibrosus, consistent with peripheral annular tears that were asymptomatic at discography.

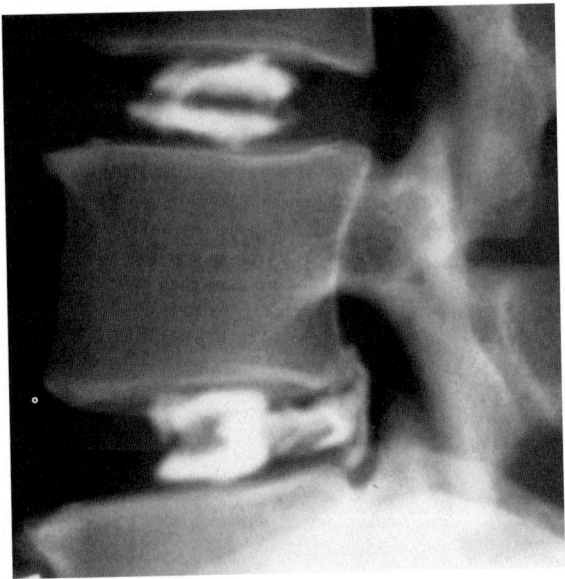

**Figure 11–9.** Lumbar discography. Lateral examination shows a normal L3–L4 bilocular nucleogram. The L4–L5 discogram shows a posterolateral incomplete radial tear with annular enhancement.

## Chemonucleolysis

The role of chemonucleolysis in the management of leg pain related to disc extrusion is controversial. Nucleolysis is produced by the injection of a proteolytic or chondrolytic enzyme, such as chymopapain or collagenase, into the substance of a deranged intervertebral disc. Initial success rates were between 75% and 85%. Although adverse effects of chemonucleolysis are infrequent (<0.1%), they may be more serious (e.g., life-threatening anaphylaxis, infection, bleeding problems, neurologic deficits such as transverse myelitis) than those associated with epidural steroid injection. A mortality rate of 0.02% has been reported.

## Percutaneous Discectomy

Percutaneous discectomy has gained some popularity as a treatment method for an extruded lumbar nucleus pulposus. The reason why percutaneous discectomy is successful is unclear, and no pathophysiologically based explanation is available. There does not appear to be a correlation between the quantity of disc removed and the therapeutic result. Infection is an infrequent complication of percutaneous discectomy, with a prevalence of less than 1%. Morbidity and mortality rates related to this procedure are low. Success rates in carefully chosen patients are between 53% and 87%, compared with 90% in appropriately selected patients undergoing surgical microdiscectomy.

## Laser Disc Therapy

Laser disc therapy entails vaporization of nuclear tissue to relieve or reduce the mechanical deformation effect on the disc contour. The success of this therapy depends on proper patient selection and correct needle placement with appropriate radiologic monitoring. The needle tip must be placed just inside the anulus fibrosus, and the needle itself must be parallel to the axis of the disc and preferably halfway between the superior and inferior endplates.

## Thermocoagulation of the Intervertebral Disc

Intradiscal electrothermal annuloplasty is a relatively new procedure to relieve discogenic pain. It involves heating the intervertebral disc using a specialized flexible catheter with a 6-cm thermoactive tip. Using normal discographic technique, the catheter is inserted via a posterolateral route into the anulus fibrosus or nucleus pulposus with a 17-gauge introducer. The active tip is typically advanced circumferentially around the nuclear tissue and directed circuitously to return posterolaterally, ideally achieving full 360-degree penetration. After appropriate catheter positioning, electrothermal heat is generated at the active tip. Approximately one third of patients feel the same or worse after undergoing electrothermal annuloplasty. Many questions remain regarding the efficacy of this procedure.

## Percutaneous Vertebroplasty

Osteoporosis is a disease of low bone mass that often manifests as a fracture. Hip fractures are the most devastating, but vertebral fractures are the most common and occur in 25% of women older than 50 years and in 40% of those 80 to 85 years of age. Sixty percent of vertebral fractures are clinically silent but are associated with loss in height and spinal deformity. In patients in whom pain management with local and systemic analgesia has failed, vertebroplasty can be effective in controlling pain, obtaining stability of the spine, improving function, and decreasing the likelihood of recurrence, progressive deformity, and disability.

The technique involves percutaneous puncture of the involved vertebrae via a transpedicular approach, followed by injection of polymethylmethacrylate (average injection amount, 7.1 mL) into the vertebral body (Fig. 11–10). Significant pain relief immediately after treatment has been reported in 90% of patients, with a complication rate of about 6%. Careful control of the volume of injected polymethylmethacrylate seems to be the most critical factor for avoiding complications. Injection of opacified polymethylmethacrylate during vertebroplasty may cause compression of adjacent structures and necessitate emergency decompressive surgery; thus, the procedure should be performed only in a surgical center. A multidisciplinary team decision to perform vertebroplasty is based on a number of factors.

## FURTHER READING

Boas RA: Nerve blocks in the diagnosis of low back pain. Neurosurg Clin N Am 2:807, 1991.

Boden P, Davis DO, Dina TS, et al: Abnormal magnetic-resonance scans of the lumbar spine in asymptomatic subjects: A prospective investigation. J Bone Joint Surg Am 72:403, 1990.

Burton AK, Clarke RD, McClune TD, et al: The natural history of low back pain in adolescents. Spine 21:2323, 1996.

Bush K, Cowan N, Katz DE, et al: The natural history of sciatica associated with disc pathology: A prospective study with clinical and independent radiologic follow-up. Spine 17:1205, 1992.

Carette S, Marcoux S, Truchon R, et al: Controlled trial of corticosteroid injections into facet joints for chronic low back pain. N Engl J Med 325:1002, 1991.

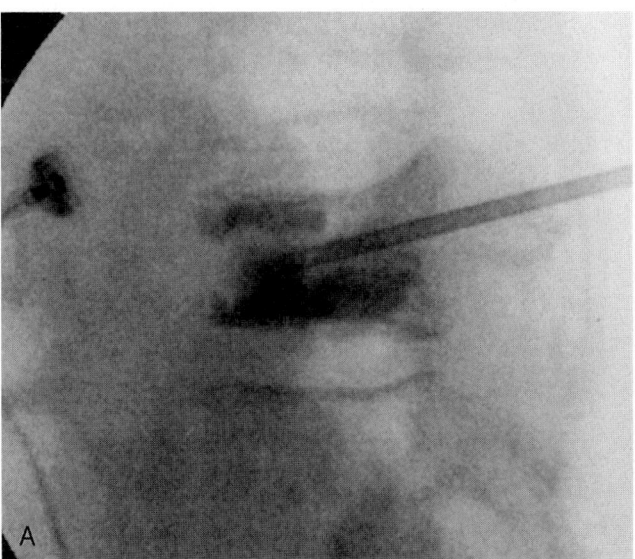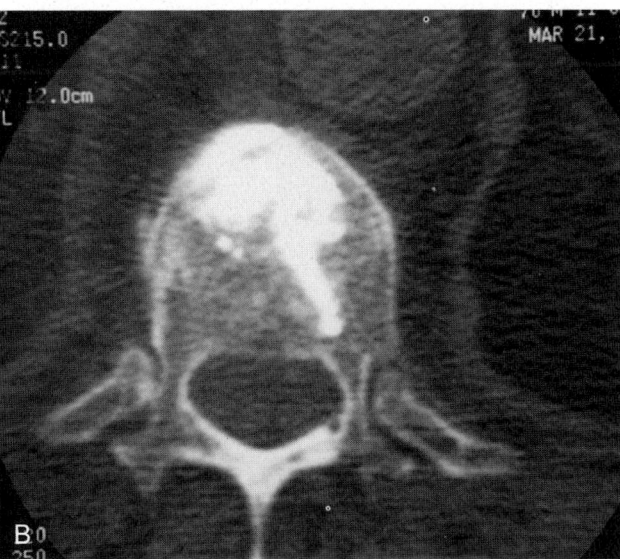

**Figure 11–10.** Percutaneous vertebroplasty. *A,* Lateral fluoroscopic image shows transpedicular placement of a needle into the anterior third of a wedged T12 vertebral body. The opacified cement (methylmethacrylate) is distributed into the lower and upper third of the collapsed vertebral body. No posterior escape of the methylmethacrylate is evident. *B,* CT image demonstrates cement within the anterior third of the vertebral body without extravasation. Minor seepage of the cement is seen along the needle track. (Courtesy of J. B. Vogler, MD, Gainesville, Fla.)

Cotten A, Boutry N, Cortet B, et al: Percutaneous vertebroplasty: State of the art. Radiographics 18:311, 1998.

El-Khoury GY, Renfrew DL: Percutaneous procedures for the diagnosis and treatment of lower back pain: Diskography, facet-joint injection, and epidural injection. AJR Am J Roentgenol 157:685, 1991.

Jensen MC, Brant-Zawadzki MN, Ohuchowski N, et al: Magnetic resonance imaging of the lumbar spine in people without back pain. N Engl J Med 331:69, 1994.

Jensen ME, Evans AJ, Mathis JM, et al: Percutaneous polymethylmethacrylate vertebroplasty in the treatment of osteoporotic vertebral body compression fractures: Technical aspects. AJNR Am J Neuroradiol 18:1897, 1997.

Johansson A, Sjolund B: Nerve blocks with local anesthetics and corticosteroids in chronic pain: A clinical follow-up study. J Pain Symptom Manage 11:181, 1996.

Kaplan PA, Dussault RG: Image guided selective nerve blocks in the spine. Semin Musculoskel Radiol 1:231, 1997.

Kinard RE: Diagnostic spinal injection procedures. Neurosurg Clin N Am 7:151, 1996.

Kirkaldy-Willis WH, Burton CV (eds): Managing Low Back Pain, 3rd ed. New York, Churchill Livingstone, 1992, p 63.

Kraemer J, Ludwig J, Bickert U, et al: Lumbar epidural perineural injection: A new technique. Eur Spine J 6:357, 1997.

Parziale JR, Hudgins TH, Fishman LM: The piriformis syndrome. Am J Orthop 25:819, 1996.

Porzelius J: Memory for pain after nerve-block injections. Clin J Pain 11:112, 1995.

Saifuddin A, Braithwaite I, White J, et al: The value of lumbar spine magnetic resonance imaging in the demonstration of annular tears. Spine 23:453, 1998.

Weinstein JN, Walsh TR, Spratt KF, et al: Lumbar discography: A controlled prospective study of normal volunteers to determine the false positive rate. Proceedings of the International Intradiscal Therapy Society, 1989, Orlando, Fla.

Weinstein SM, Herring SA, Derby R: Contemporary concepts in spine care: Epidural steroid injections. Spine 20:1842, 1995.

# CHAPTER 12

## Imaging after Spinal Surgery

### Mini N. Pathria and Steven R. Garfin

## *SUMMARY OF KEY FEATURES*

Spinal surgery is a rapidly evolving field, with new surgical techniques and hardware being developed continually. Familiarity with the concepts and design principles of surgical instrumentation facilitates interpretation of the placement of and complications associated with spinal hardware. Diagnostic imaging plays an important role in determining the adequacy of surgical intervention and in detecting complications associated with operations on the spine. Advances in computed tomography (CT) scanning and magnetic resonance (MR) imaging have enhanced the ability to monitor both the osseous and soft tissue changes associated with spinal intervention.

## INTRODUCTION

The surgical treatment of low back pain has followed three major trends in the past century. Originally, degenerative or extruded discs were considered the most important cause of low back pain, leading to the development of laminectomy and discectomy. The next major trend was the addition of spinal fusion, because spinal instability was thought to be the cause when a patient continued to have back pain after disc excision. The latest trend is directed toward the treatment of radiculopathy rather than back pain, deformity, or instability alone.

Currently, numerous surgical techniques are used, including percutaneous interventional procedures, osseous resection or decompression, realignment, and fusion. A vast array of spinal hardware systems has been developed to address the full spectrum of spinal disorders.

## DISCECTOMY AND DECOMPRESSION

Resection of bone is performed most commonly for decompression of spinal stenosis, for decompression of traumatic lesions, and to provide access to the disc for discectomy. Only very small amounts of bone need to be removed to perform discectomy in patients without central or foraminal stenosis. Substantial resection, however, may be necessary in patients with severe spinal canal impingement at multiple levels, which typically results from extensive degenerative spinal stenosis.

## Thoracic and Lumbar Spine

Laminotomy and laminectomy are resectional techniques typically used for the removal of an extruded disc in the lumbar spine. Most disc extrusions are posterolateral, and disc material can be easily removed through a unilateral defect known as a laminotomy or hemilaminectomy. In a laminotomy, resection is often limited to the margins of the lamina, whereas the entire lamina is resected during laminectomy. During laminotomy, the spinous process and interspinous ligaments are preserved. A laminotomy defect can usually be recognized on the anteroposterior radiograph by noting unilateral widening of the interlaminar space, but it is often difficult to identify on transaxial CT scans and MR images because of the limited nature of the bone resection. Even if the osseous defect is not apparent with cross-sectional imaging, loss of portions of the ligamentum flavum underlying the resection and distortion of the overlying soft tissues may be recognized. Hemilaminectomy is readily apparent with conventional radiography, CT scanning, and MR imaging because of the presence of a unilateral defect in the laminar bone.

Total laminectomy with foraminotomy or facetectomy is a more extensive resection than that required for simple disc excision. This procedure is commonly used for the treatment of symptomatic lumbar stenosis. It is often bilateral and includes resection of the spinous process, which results in unroofing of the spinal canal and removal of the ligamentum flavum. Foraminotomies typically involve removal of the medial half of the facet, with preservation of the interfacet joint and the pars interarticularis. Foraminotomy results in loss of the normal width and obliquity of the inner margin of the facet. The inferior tip of the facet may be truncated, or the facet may be completely absent (facetectomy) when extensive resection has been performed (Fig. 12–1). The facet joints and posterior intervertebral ligaments are the spine's principal posterior stabilizers; complete resection of the facet leads to an increased likelihood of instability if an arthrodesis is not carried out simultaneously. Patients with underlying degenerative spondylolisthesis or degenerative scoliosis appear to be at highest risk for progressive instability after decompressive surgery.

Thinning of the inferior articular facet at the site of facetectomy predisposes this structure to the development of a postoperative stress fracture. It has been suggested that excessive removal of bone immediately cephalad to the flare of the inferior articular process leads to this type of fracture. The most common locations for postfacetectomy fractures are the pars interarticularis and the inferior tip of the facet. Postoperative fractures are seen in 15% of patients with the postsurgical failed back syndrome. Fractures following facetectomy are difficult to visualize radiographically and may be confused with each other on CT scans unless careful attention is paid to the exact site and orientation of the fracture line. The

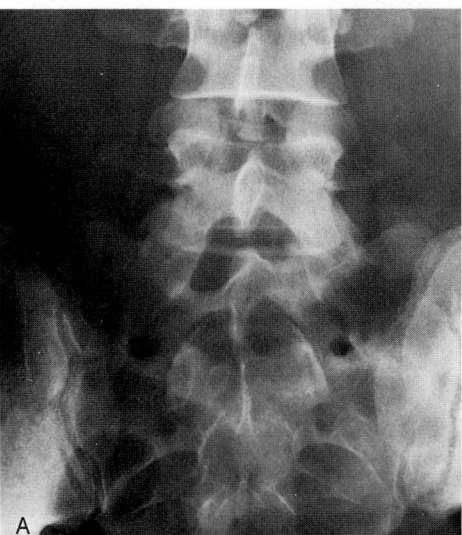

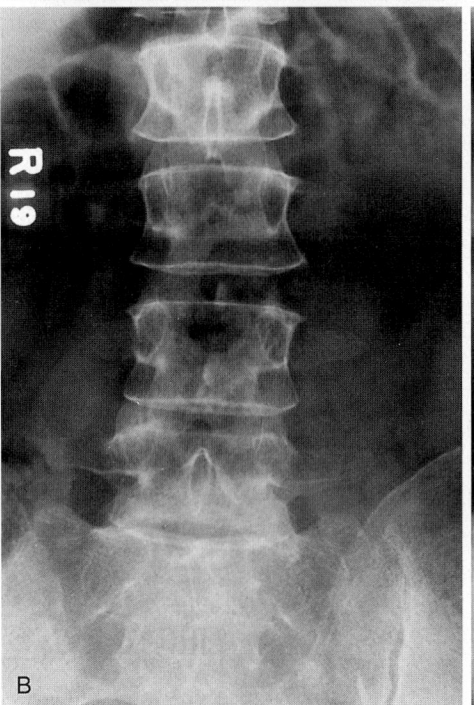

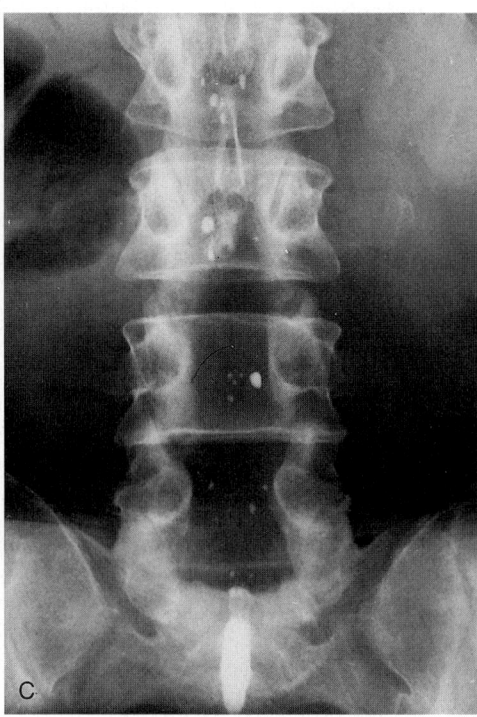

**Figure 12–1.** Resection and decompression procedures. *A*, Hemilaminotomy defect at the cranial aspect of the right lamina of a transitional L5 vertebra. *B*, The inferior facet of L3 has been resected on the left side, and the tip of the superior facet of L4 has become truncated after foraminotomy of the left L3–L4 neural foramen for stenosis. *C*, Extensive resection of the posterior elements, with unroofing of the spinal canal, for spinal stenosis. Note the absence of the spinous processes, laminae (laminectomy), and large portions of the facets in the lower lumbar spine.

CT diagnosis of both pars and facet fractures is facilitated with reformatted images.

In patients with single-level stenosis, adequate surgical treatment includes removal of sufficient portions of the laminae, and often the medial aspects of the facet joints, to cause decompression. Laminotomies of the superior and inferior vertebrae may be adequate; in selected cases, a complete laminectomy can be avoided. Multilevel stenosis necessitates more extensive surgery, with resection of all laminar and facet bone in the areas of stenosis. Most patients with lumbar stenosis severe enough to warrant surgery require multilevel decompression. Postoperative vertebral subluxation is the most common complication encountered in patients after extensive decompressive surgery of the posterior thoracic or lumbar region. In skeletally immature individuals, there is a 50% rate of occurrence of cervicothoracic or thoracic kyphosis after posterior decompressive surgery. In adults, risk factors for postoperative instability include underlying degenerative spondylolisthesis, advanced age, a primary neural disorder, rheumatoid arthritis, or recurrent trauma. Underlying degenerative spondylolisthesis appears to be the most significant risk factor. Patients deemed to be at high risk for instability after decompressive lumbar laminectomy typically undergo fusion with posterolateral or intertransverse bone grafting at the time of surgery. Numerous internal fixation devices have been designed to prevent further subluxation while the bone fusion is consolidating. Despite high rates of pseudarthrosis following fusion, long-term follow-up shows significantly better overall results, with less leg pain and less progression of anterolisthesis, in patients undergoing fusion.

Tears of the dura are not uncommon during resectional surgery and occur more frequently during revision surgery because of the presence of scar adherent to the dura. Dural tears are generally detected and repaired at the time of surgery; small undetected dural leaks typically heal spontaneously, but large leaks may persist and form prominent paraspinal fluid collections (Fig. 12–2). Postoperative pseudomeningocele is an uncommon complication resulting from a chronic unrecognized or incompletely repaired dural tear. With CT, a pseudomeningocele appears as a rounded mass of low attenuation posterior to the thecal sac; the margin typically consists of a well-defined rim of higher attenuation that can be attributed to pseudocapsule formation. With MR imaging, the signal intensity of the collection corresponds to that of cerebrospinal fluid, although increased signal intensity may be seen in cases complicated by hemorrhage.

Decompression is also used occasionally for the management of fractures and dislocations leading to spinal canal compromise. Realignment alone may obviate the need for decompressive surgery in most cases. Considerable controversy exists over the relative merits of anterior versus posterior approaches and over the benefits of concomitant fusion and instrumentation if decompression is necessary. Nowhere is this controversy more evident than in the debate over optimal management of a burst fracture with neurologic deficit caused by retropulsed bone.

## Cervical Spine

Unlike in the lumbar region, access to extruded cervical discs via the posterior approach is significantly limited because of the presence of the spinal cord. The anterior approach is preferred for the management of cervical disc disease when concomitant discectomy and fusion are performed. Laminectomy is typically reserved for patients requiring decompression for cervical spinal stenosis and is usually performed at multiple levels. Cervical spondylitic myelopathy is multifactorial, in that it is due to a combination of progressive degenerative cervical spondylosis, direct spinal cord compression, cord ischemia, and, often, an underlying congenitally narrow spinal canal.

Extensive cervical laminectomy for decompression of myelopathy without adequate fusion can lead to progressive subluxation and kyphosis and produce a "swan-neck" deformity (Fig. 12–3). This deformity is rarely seen after a single-level laminectomy or after multiple unilateral hemilaminectomies. Presumably, it is a result of the loss of posterior ligamentous and osseous stability, aggravated by concomitant muscle weakness. Laminoplasty was developed to prevent this postoperative complication; this technique widens the canal and theoretically maintains stability. Anterior fusion is typically necessary for correction of symptomatic unstable kyphosis. Unlike posterior arthrodesis, anterior fusions are not subject to significant tensile forces during spinal flexion and are therefore more likely to successfully correct the deformity.

Severe cervical spondyloarthropathy can also be treated by anterior decompression and fusion. Anterior decompression allows direct removal of the compressive abnormalities, with stabilization provided by concomitant anterior arthrodesis. Anterior decompression is also used for resection of the ossific masses present in patients with ossification of the posterior longitudinal ligament (OPLL). Surgical resection of the ectopic ossification is frequently complicated by its adherence to the dura, leading to the development of dural tears during decompression. Anterior cervical decompression with fusion is

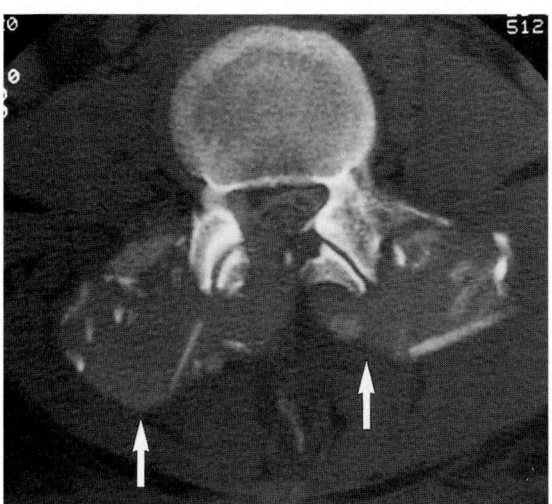

**Figure 12–2.** Dural tear. Transaxial CT scan obtained after the administration of intrathecal contrast agent demonstrates a leak of cerebrospinal fluid into the paraspinal soft tissues (*arrows*). Immature bone graft is present from a recent laminectomy and fusion procedure.

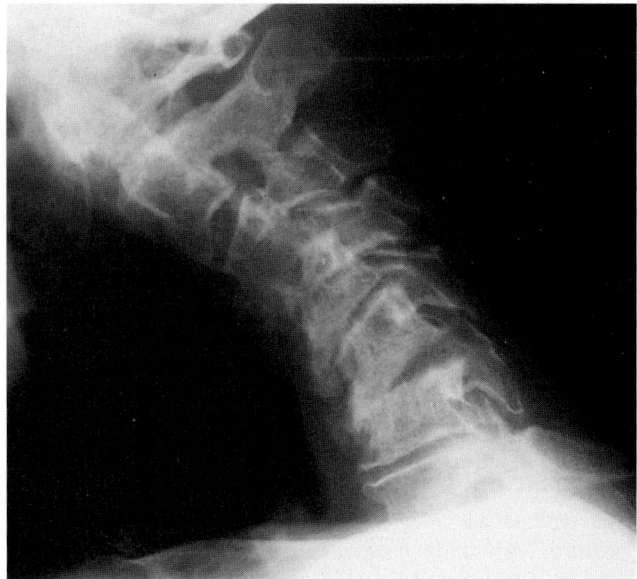

**Figure 12–3.** Postlaminectomy kyphosis. Severe cervical kyphosis has occurred after laminectomies at C5 and C6 for degenerative spondylosis. Disc space loss is seen at multiple cervical levels.

advocated for the management of patients with neurologic deficits after traumatic injury to the cervical region that results in spinal cord compression by anteriorly located bone or disc fragments.

## SPINAL FUSION WITHOUT INSTRUMENTATION

The rationale for spinal arthrodesis is based on the experience with fusion of other articulations of the body, in which arthrodesis has been used to eradicate pain by eliminating motion. Indications for spinal arthrodesis include (1) prevention of progressive spinal deformity, (2) maintenance of corrected deformity, (3) reestablishment of spinal stability, and (4) elimination of pain caused by motion between spinal segments. Spinal fusion may be carried out alone or combined with decompressive surgery, the application of spinal hardware, or both.

### Graft Materials

The graft material used most commonly for achieving spinal fusion is bone, whether it be an autograft or an allograft. An autograft may be obtained from numerous anatomic regions, with the iliac crest being the most common site. The ilium offers a variety of osseous contours and is a source for cortical, corticocancellous, and cancellous graft harvest. The main advantages of an autograft are histocompatibility, availability, and high osteogenic potential because of the presence of viable osteoprogenitor cells. Banked allograft bone is used when the patient's own bone stock is of limited quantity or poor quality, usually as a consequence of metabolic bone disease or previous surgical harvesting. The use of allograft decreases operative time and eliminates the risk of donor site complications. The major disadvantages of allografts are the potential for disease transmission, a slower rate of vascularization, failure of incorporation (nonunion), and higher rates of collapse.

Cortical grafts, though they are stronger mechanically, are revascularized more slowly than cancellous bone. Solid union of cortical grafts may take up to 2 years to develop, and nonunion rates for rib or fibular strut grafts range from 8% to 37%. Major complications related to harvest sites for autologous grafts include fracture of the underlying bone when a large amount of bone has been harvested, infection, and damage to the overlying soft tissue structures. Removal of a large bicortical bone graft, particularly when associated with splitting of the inner and outer tables of the ilium, predisposes the bone to fracture.

Nonosseous sources of graft material include polymethylmethacrylate (PMMA), which is widely used for reconstruction after débridement or resection of spinal neoplasms; bioactive ceramic spacers; and manufactured hydroxyapatite bone graft substitutes. PMMA is a resinous acrylic material formed by mixing its liquid and powder components at the time of surgery. PMMA is used most commonly after corpectomy and débridement of spinal neoplasms, particularly metastatic disease. It is strongest in compression but does not resist tension, so this material is frequently used in the anterior spinal regions. PMMA can be molded to any desired shape, and

its material properties are unaffected by radiation and chemotherapy, both of which are known to inhibit bone healing. The use of PMMA alone or, more typically, in conjunction with metallic internal fixation and bone grafting facilitates early mobilization of patients with malignant lesions.

The major disadvantages of PMMA include increased rates of infection and mechanical loosening. Mechanical loosening is common because the material interdigitates only with native bone and never undergoes incorporation. Gradual resorption at the bone-cement interface, leading to loss of fixation and subsequent extrusion of the construct, is the most frequent complication and accounts for more than 80% of PMMA failures. The substance appears homogeneous and has a density similar to that of soft tissue on conventional radiographs. Radiopaque material, typically barium, is added to the PMMA during manufacture to make it easier to visualize radiographically. PMMA exhibits inhomogeneity on CT scans, and entrapped air bubbles may be apparent in intact noninfected grafts; on MR images, PMMA exhibits signal void with all MR imaging sequences.

Bone graft substitutes consisting of porous hydroxyapatite derived from the calcium carbonate exoskeleton of certain varieties of sea coral are commercially available. Although these implants lack the osteoprogenitor cells and bone-producing factors found in viable autologous bone, they serve as an effective nonantigenic scaffolding for bone ingrowth and incorporation. Some of these constructs have little inherent mechanical stability, which precludes their use in situations in which they must bear large structural loads. On initial radiographs, the implants appear much denser than normal bone and do not exhibit the organized, linear trabecular pattern of bone-based graft materials.

### Thoracic and Lumbar Spine

The posterior approach remains the standard method of obtaining fusion in the thoracic and lumbar regions, but the site of fusion has been modified because of an unacceptably high rate of pseudarthrosis with midline fusion. Currently, most lumbar arthrodeses are performed posterolaterally, adjacent to the posterior elements rather than in the midline. Posterolateral fusions are performed either posterior to the transverse processes (intertransverse fusion) or overlying the posterolateral surfaces of the facet joint and lamina (interlaminar fusion); in some cases, both fusions are done. In a patient with significant spondylolisthesis, fusion is often performed in situ, because reduction of the slippage results in an increased risk of neurologic deficit.

Anterior interbody fusions are performed less frequently than the standard posterolateral arthrodesis. The bone graft is located closer to the center of motion for the vertebral segment, theoretically producing increased stiffness when compared with that derived from posterior fusion alone. Smaller amounts of bone graft are used, and restoration of vertebral body height is achieved with this approach. Interbody grafting of the lumbar spine via a posterior approach, known as a posterior lumbar interbody fusion (PLIF), was developed to provide more stable fixation than could be achieved by a posterior graft alone. The posterior approach to the intervertebral disc avoids complications associated with the anterior transpleural, transperitoneal, and retroperitoneal approaches to the spine.

The most common material used for PLIF is autologous bone in the form of tricortical or cortical cylindrical dowels, usually cut from the ilium. Strut grafts may also be used to obtain more stable immediate fixation. Complications associated with the use of fibular grafts for the fixation of symptomatic high-grade spondylolysis include pseudarthrosis, neurologic deficit, and progression of the grade or angle of the slip. More recently, PLIF using metallic fixation devices placed at the level of the disc space has been described (Fig. 12–4). Anterior interbody fusions via the anterior approach are used when anterior decompression is necessary or when the posterior elements are grossly insufficient.

Single-level intervertebral fusions are typically performed by placement of a cancellous or corticocancellous interbody graft. Anterior interbody grafts tend to show some settling before fusion; this settling may be necessary for successful incorporation. The interbody graft should appear rectangular, because wedge-shaped grafts that are taller anteriorly tend to become extruded upon spinal hyperextension (Fig. 12–5). Minor degrees of graft protrusion anterior to the vertebral margin tend to be resorbed spontaneously. Although immediate postoperative radiographs show restoration of disc height, at long-term follow-up, disc height is typically diminished, along with loss of the initial neuroforaminal distraction. Cortical strut grafts are used when multilevel vertebral body resection is performed. Because of the high mechanical stresses in the anterior aspect of the spinal column in the thoracic and lumbar regions, all types of strut grafts used there have been reported to fracture or collapse.

Metallic and carbon fiber implants filled with nonstructural cancellous bone, referred to as interbody fusion cages, have been found to provide structural support immediately after implantation and to provide a biologic scaffold and substrate that promote fusion. The current generation of metallic cages can be inserted via either an anterior or a posterior approach to the spine with either open or laparoscopic technique. Fusion cages have rapidly gained popularity because of the high fusion rates they afford, without the necessity of performing combined anterior and posterior fusion (circumferential arthrodesis) to achieve spinal stability. Reliable radiographic indicators of fusion include bridging trabecular bone anterior to or surrounding the fusion cage, in conjunction with the absence of motion on flexion-extension radiographs. It is very difficult to identify fusion after interbody cage placement if the bridging trabecular bone is limited to the inside of the cage device.

Anterior thoracic and lumbar approaches are associated with a variety of complications. The rate of major complications associated with such procedures has been reported to range from 1% to 11%. Along with failure of the graft itself, complications related to the adjacent vascular, neural, and visceral structures may be encountered. Vascular complications are rare but are most likely to occur in patients with preexisting vascular abnormalities such as aneurysm, pseudoaneurysm, underlying vascular anomalies, or extensive calcific atherosclerosis.

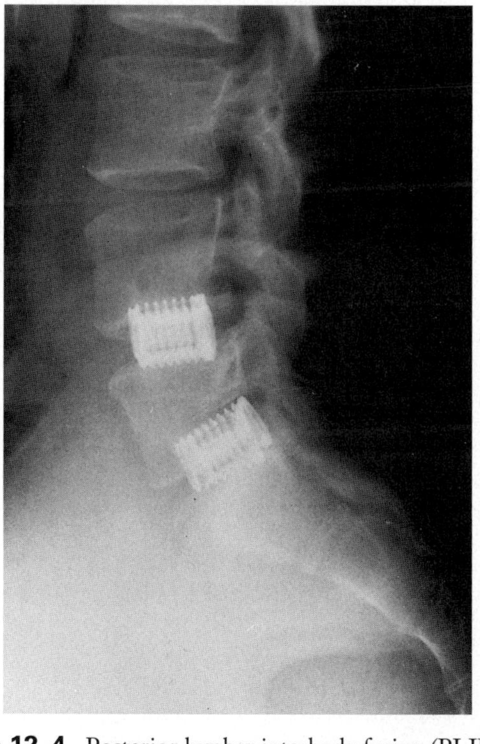

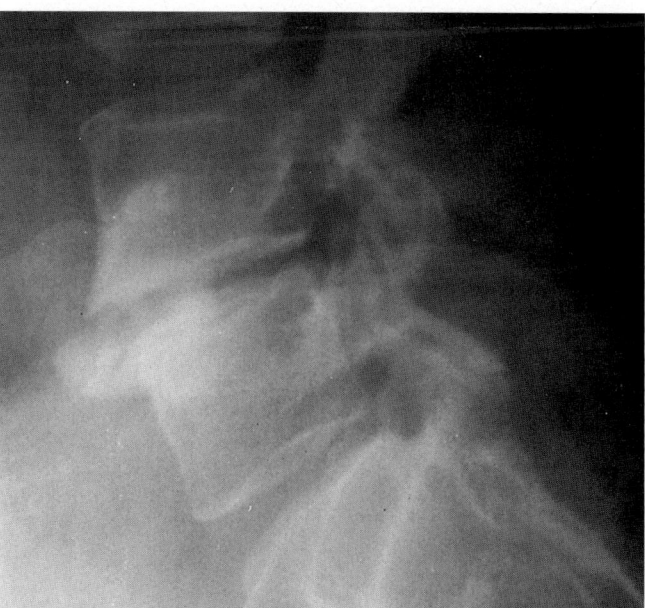

**Figure 12–4.** Posterior lumbar interbody fusion (PLIF). Ray cage PLIFs are seen at L4–L5 and L5–S1. These cylindrical devices are embedded in the vertebral bodies and allow for bone ingrowth.

**Figure 12–5.** Graft extrusion. Anterior extrusion of an L4–L5 interbody graft. This graft was left in situ, with subsequent resorption of the extruded region, followed by fusion.

## Cervical Spine

In contrast to the lumbar region, in the cervical spine, simple bone grafting is used more commonly in an anterior interbody approach rather than a posterior one. Grafting alone is rarely sufficient for posterior stabilization, so posterior grafting is typically combined with the use of some form of metallic hardware to provide stability until the graft is incorporated. The anterior approach is used for removal of degenerated discs and interbody fusion with concomitant removal of symptomatic osteophytes. It can also be used for traumatic lesions, cervical stenosis, inflammatory arthropathies, ligamentous ossification, and many other pathologic cervical conditions requiring anterior decompression.

Some controversy exists over whether single-level discectomy requires interbody fusion, although many surgeons routinely use graft material for such cases. Anterior intervertebral grafting is considered essential to restore spinal stability and function after anterior multilevel decompression. In patients with multiple levels of disc degeneration, interbody grafts can be used at all operated levels, or strut grafting may be performed. Anterior cervical fusion is typically carried out by placing corticocancellous autologous bone grafts in the region of the intervertebral disc after removal of a degenerated disc and any significant osteophytes. The graft functions as a mechanical spacer that maintains or increases disc height; it also distracts the neural foramina and thereby decreases the compressive effect of foraminal osteophytes.

Cervical cortical strut grafts are used after corpectomy and allow for the replacement of one or more vertebral bodies. Anterior strut grafting or augmentation with posterior fusion is often necessary when multilevel decompression is performed in myelopathic patients.

The strut grafts are typically derived from the iliac crest, rib, or fibula. Fibular grafts are stronger but become incorporated slowly; typically, they are reserved for patients undergoing vertebrectomy at more than three levels. Initial incorporation takes place at the ends of the graft, with slowly progressive ingrowth of bone into the medullary portions of the strut graft.

Anterior cervical arthrodesis failure rates of 3% to 20% have been reported. Mechanical causes of failure of anterior cervical grafts include fracture, collapse, resorption, or frank extrusion of the graft (Fig. 12–6). Previous posterior decompression places the anterior graft under increased mechanical stress and significantly increases the failure rate of the anterior fusion. Graft extrusion is a common complication that occurs in 1% to 13% of patients as a result of inadequate compression across the graft, failure of the graft, or failure of its interface with the adjacent vertebrae. Extrusion of the graft typically occurs in an anterior or anterolateral direction, with resultant kyphosis (Fig. 12–7).

It is extremely difficult to determine whether successful interbody fusion for cervical spondylosis accelerates degenerative disease at adjacent disc levels because of diminished motion at the fusion site and increased compensatory motion at adjacent levels. Although many surgeons think that the risk of accelerated spondylosis is increased after spinal fusion, an adequate study that supports this opinion is not available.

## SPINAL INSTRUMENTATION

Hardware was originally developed to allow internal correction of scoliotic deformities and early mobilization of patients. Its applications have since been expanded to

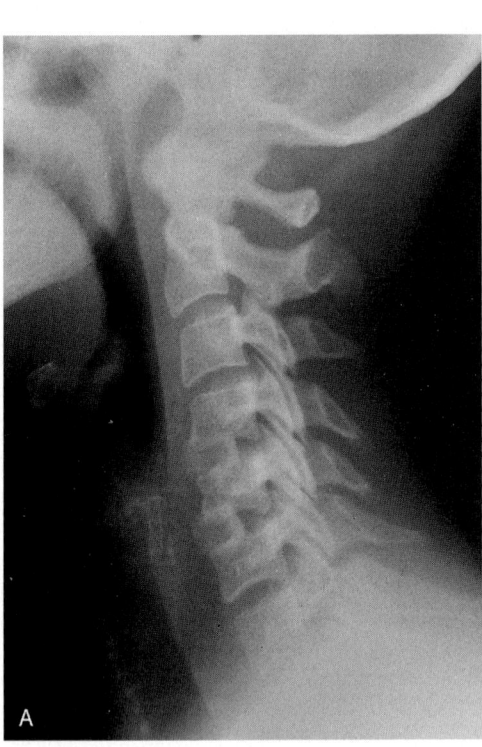
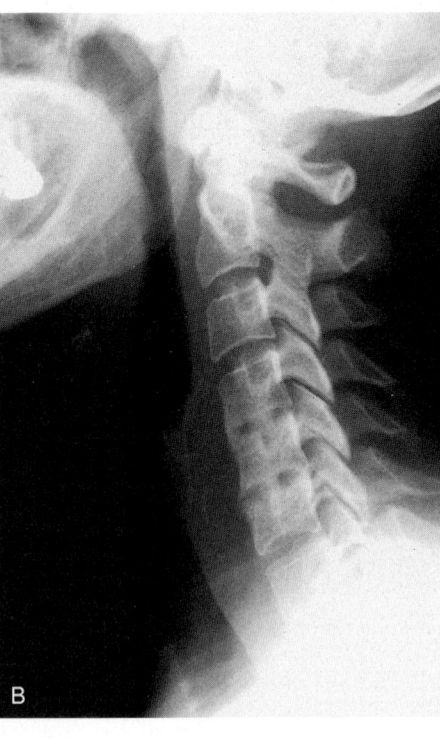

**Figure 12–6.** Graft collapse. *A,* Postoperative radiograph shows grafts at C4–C5 and C5–C6. *B,* Follow-up radiograph demonstrates loss of graft volume as a result of intrabody collapse. Loss of disc space distraction has also occurred.

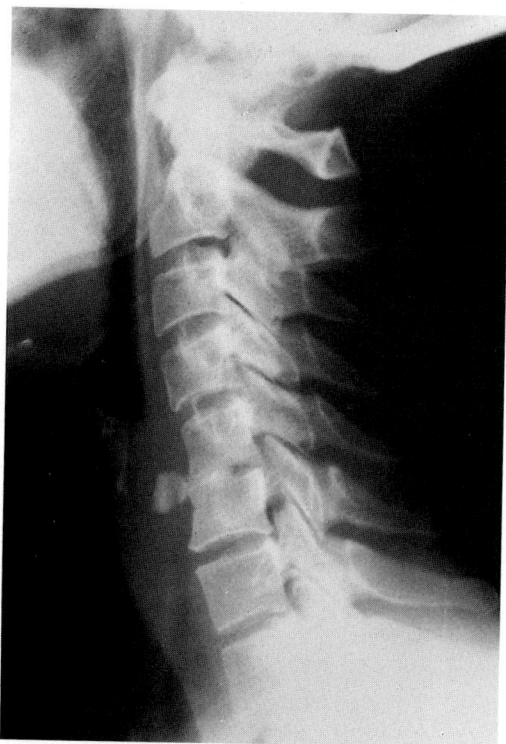

**Figure 12–7.** Graft extrusion. Anterior extrusion of a C5–C6 graft, loss of disc height, and mild focal kyphosis are present at the surgical level.

provide rigid internal fixation for a variety of spinal disorders, such as degenerative spondylosis, spondylolisthesis, fracture, infection, neoplasm, and congenital disorders. Rigid fixation along with bone grafting is used to enhance the likelihood of obtaining bone fusion, prevent pseudarthrosis, correct deformity, provide spinal stabilization, and allow early mobilization. A variety of instruments using combinations of rods, plates, pedicle screws, staples, crosslinks, and hooks and wires is currently available. It must be emphasized that the purpose of instrumentation is to provide temporary, stable fixation and maintain alignment and immobilization until solid bony spinal fusion develops. Metallic devices are unable to bear the long-term repetitive stresses to which the spine is subjected and eventually fail if solid bone fusion is not achieved.

### Thoracic and Lumbar Spine

The first major spinal hardware system was developed by Harrington in the 1950s to treat children with neuromuscular scoliosis induced by poliomyelitis. Although it is rarely used today, it is discussed here because the concepts of its design help in understanding current instrumentation methods. The system is placed posteriorly and involves distraction across the concavity of the deformity and compression along the convexity; the greater the distractive and compressive forces, the more complete the reduction. The major uses for the Harrington system are to effect spinal fusion in the treatment of a single spinal curvature related to idiopathic

thoracic scoliosis and to provide realignment and stabilization of thoracolumbar fractures that have an intact anterior longitudinal ligament. Bone grafting is used at the time of fixation because it is the bone fusion, rather than the hardware system, that is the source of long-term stability.

The stainless steel Harrington distraction rod is 0.625 cm in diameter and is available in a variety of lengths. At the upper end of each distraction rod is a fluted section with a series of circumferential grooves designed so that the upper hook engages on the shoulder of the groove to prevent slippage when axial compression is applied to the hooks. The lower end of the distraction rod has a narrower section (nipple) that fits through a hole in the hub of each hook. Harrington compression rods come in two diameters (3 and 5 mm). The compression rod is fully threaded and can be used with multiple hooks through which it is passed (Fig. 12–8). The use of multiple hooks across the convexity of the curve was probably the earliest form of segmental fixation. A number of different hook designs have been adapted for use with the Harrington rod; these hooks may be placed into the thoracic facet, over the transverse process, or, most commonly, around the edge of the lamina. Dislodgment of the system, which occurs in approximately 2% to 17% of cases, is typically due to hook pullout or hook disengagement from the rod. Fracture of the rods is less common than hook dislodgment.

Use of the Harrington system in the lower lumbar spine is associated with a higher rate of instrument failure and other complications, including hook dislodgment, loss of lumbar lordosis (flat-back deformity), abnormal gait, back pain, disability, and late dural erosion or neurologic complications related to migration of the caudal hook into the spinal canal. The Harrington hardware system has been used extensively for the management of thoracolumbar fractures. Distraction rods are most applicable for injuries related to axial loading of the spine, such as burst fractures whose retropulsed bone fragments cause narrowing of the spinal canal. Use of Harrington hardware is indicated primarily when either the anterior or the posterior longitudinal ligaments are presumed to be intact. The system is difficult to use and potentially dangerous when a grossly unstable translational or rotational injury involving all three vertebral levels is present.

Traditional rod-hook systems apply concentrated vertical stress at the superior and inferior hooks while applying only indirect corrective force to the intervening vertebral bodies. Segmental hardware systems attempt to distribute corrective forces over multiple vertebral segments. Luque hardware uses sublaminar wiring at multiple levels, combined with paired smooth rods, to apply corrective transverse forces over multiple spinal segments (Fig. 12–9). Harrington hardware corrects scoliosis by applying force in a vertical direction, whereas the Luque system corrects scoliosis with multiple horizontal forces. Results from current biomechanical studies suggest that a combination of both distraction and transverse fixation forces is superior to either method alone. Segmental spinal hardware with wiring of the spinous process offers an alternative to the sublaminar wiring technique used by Luque. Fixation of hardware to the

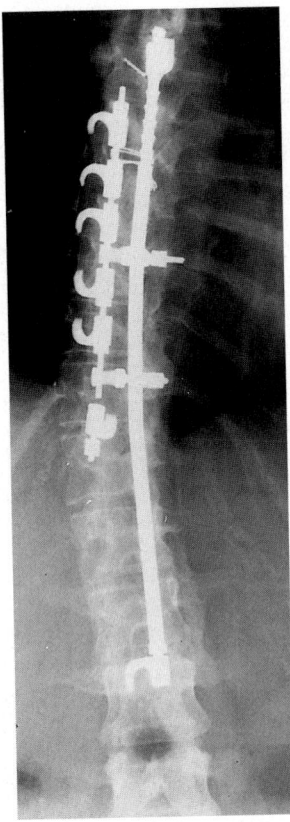

**Figure 12–8.** Harrington hardware system. Anteroposterior view shows a Harrington distraction rod on the left side with single upper and lower hooks. The compression rod on the right has multiple hooks and is fully threaded. Note the fracture of the compression rod above the most caudal hook. Crosslinks have been placed to improve stability.

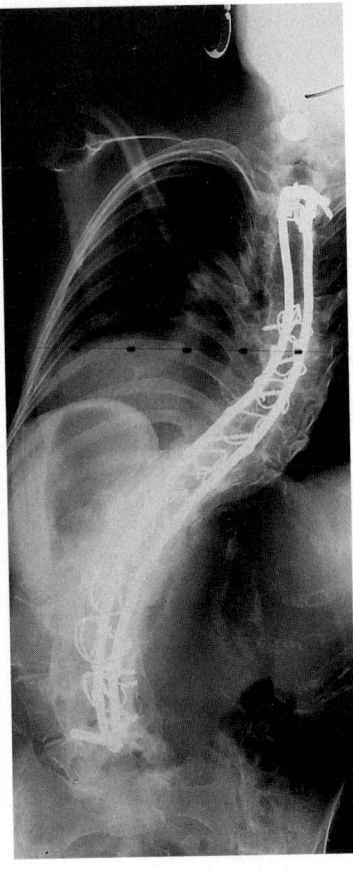

**Figure 12–9.** Luque L-shaped rods. Anteroposterior view shows placement of Luque L-shaped rods for neuromuscular scoliosis. Note the short limb at one end of each rod. Multiple sublaminar wires are present.

spinous process is not as strong as that related to sub-laminar wiring, but it is safer and of adequate strength when multiple fixation points are used.

Attempts to provide segmental hardware for the spine after laminectomy led to the development of transpedicular screw fixation, which is not dependent on an intact posterior arch. Pedicle screw fixation provides stability to all three spinal levels and allows segmental correction of lordosis, kyphosis, scoliosis, and rotation. This type of hardware system is used most frequently for immobilization in patients with painful degenerative arthritis, symptomatic spondy-lolisthesis, post-traumatic deformity, and severe scoliosis and for the prevention or treatment of pseudarthrosis (Fig. 12–10). Pedicle screws are used predominantly in the lumbar region because of the high frequency of degenerative disease in this location, the large size of the lumbar pedicles, and the difficulty of achieving immobilization of the low lumbar region with other systems. Unlike conventional hooks, pedicle screws can be securely fixed to the sacrum, and they can be used after laminectomy. Less commonly, pedicle screw systems are used in the thoracolumbar or upper thoracic region for the management of scoliosis or post-traumatic deformities. Preoperative CT scanning can be used to accurately measure the outer cortical and inner cancellous diameters of the pedicle to select the largest acceptable screw size.

The screws connect to rods or plates either through rigid constrained linkages (as in almost all plate systems, fixators, and most of the rod systems) or through a mobile semiconstrained coupling (usually to a rod) that allows for some motion but offers the capability of reducing spinal malalignment. Most of the newer pedicle screw systems use rods rather than plates to obtain rigid spinal fixation. Rigid connections between the screws and the plate or rod result in a high concentration of stress, which may lead to increased risk of screw loosening, hardware breakage, and stress shielding; fractures of the vertical rods are rare. One of the most important risk factors for loosening is underlying osteoporosis, which makes it difficult to obtain purchase of the screw within the vertebral body. Correct placement is essential to provide adequate purchase and to avoid the neural structures that course alongside the pedicle. Neurologic compromise develops in about 3% of patients after placement of a pedicle screw system. Both rods and plates may be used with pedicular fixation. The use of rods

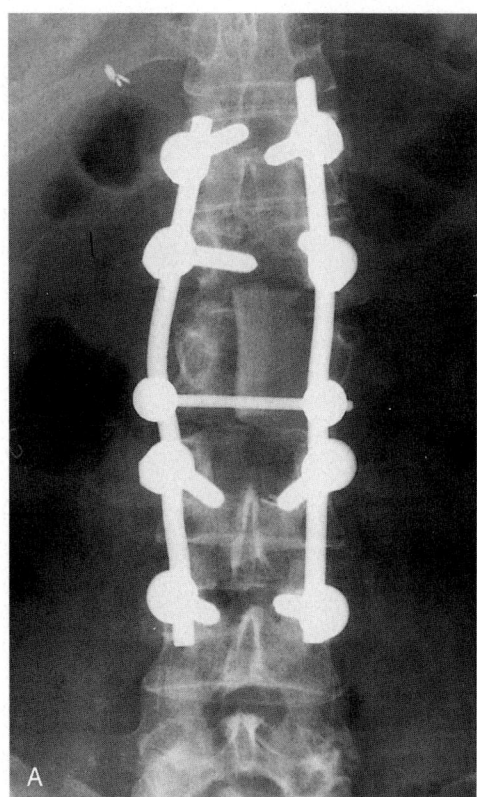
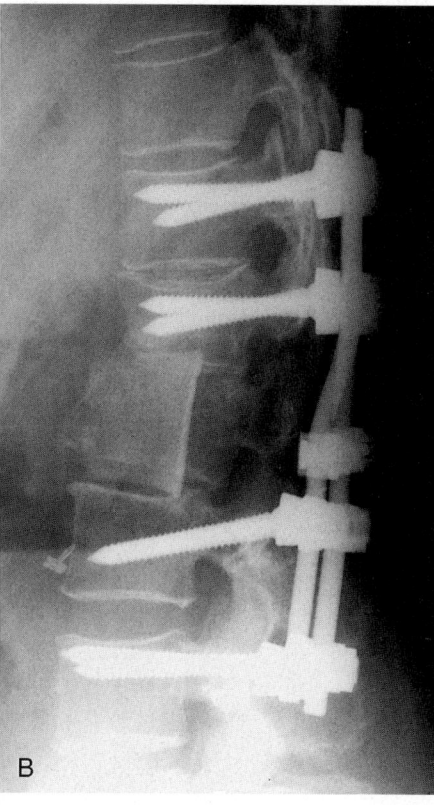

**Figure 12–10.** Pedicle screw fixation system. *A,* Anteroposterior view of pedicle screw fixation of the thoracolumbar spine with universal rods and pedicle screws. *B,* Semiconstrained pedicle connectors seen on the lateral view allow limited motion. An L2 corpectomy with placement of a large corticocancellous graft has been performed.

rather than plates results in more active correction of deformity. Rigid rod-screw systems have also been used successfully to treat defects of the pars interarticularis (i.e., spondylolysis) that produce spondylolisthesis; they result in high fusion rates, even in older patients.

More modular systems of pedicle screw–rod fixation attempt to provide flexibility in the construct to permit some motion, thereby decreasing the degree of stress shielding of the bone graft. The newest development in spinal hardware is the introduction of derotational systems that can be used to apply rigid segmental fixation while also allowing for multidirectional control and correction of deformity in all three planes. These derotational systems, represented by the Cotrel-Dubousset (CD) and Texas Scottish Rite Hospital (TSRH) systems, are adaptable modular systems that can be used for multiple indications. These systems are biomechanically complex, technically demanding to insert, bulky, and expensive, but they are a major advance in spinal hardware.

CD hardware is designed to provide bilateral segmental spinal fixation and selective distraction and compression at different levels, as well as improve alignment in all three planes. The system applies mechanical correction primarily by rotation of the coronal deformity into the sagittal plane, thereby converting scoliotic deformity into a more physiologic kyphosis or lordosis. The introduction of a rotational maneuver to correct spinal deformity was a major evolutionary change in the

management of scoliosis. The correction achieved is not as anatomic as initially believed, but it is still better than that obtained with the previous hardware systems. The CD instrument consists of a pair of 7-mm stainless steel rods that have their entire surface serrated with diamond-shaped irregularities (Fig. 12–11). The rods are connected by slender threaded crosslinks. Hooks, pedicle screws, or both can be applied anywhere along the length of the rods and can face in any direction. Typically, each rod is attached to four or more laminar hooks or pedicle screws. Rotational correction is accomplished by rotating the contoured rod after its insertion into hooks placed at critical points in the spine. Hooks on the same rod can be placed to act in compression or in tension.

The TSRH system has the same fundamental function as CD hardware, but its design modifications allow for easier implantation and, more important, greater ease of removal or revision once the instrument is in place. The system has evolved from the initial develop-ment of a crosslinkage plate to a complete hardware system consisting of rods, hooks, pedicle screws, and crosslinks (Fig. 12–12). TSRH rods are roughened rather than serrated and are available in three levels of stiffness. The TSRH system allows for the placement of both standard pedicle screws (perpendicular to the rod) and pedicle screws at variable angles relative to the rod. The hooks come in a wide array of configurations and sizes. Anterior fixation in the thoracic and lumbar spine is used far less frequently than is posterior fixation hardware.

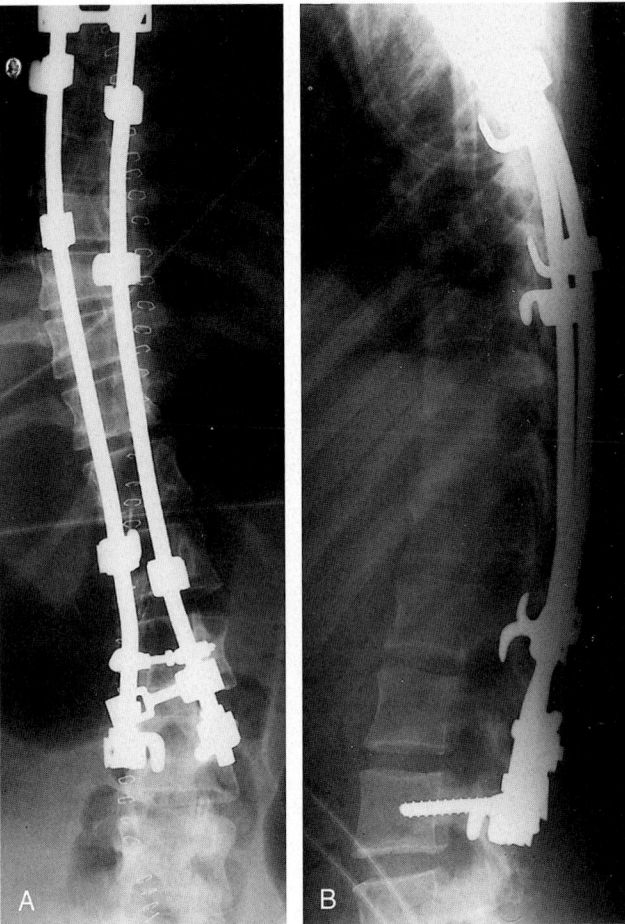

**Figure 12–11.** Cotrel-Dubousset (CD) hardware. *A*, Antero-posterior view shows CD hardware placed for scoliosis correction. The serrated rods are crosslinked with both CD and Texas Scottish Rite Hospital crosslinks. *B*, Lateral view shows the C-shaped hooks and the cut setscrews characteristic of CD hardware.

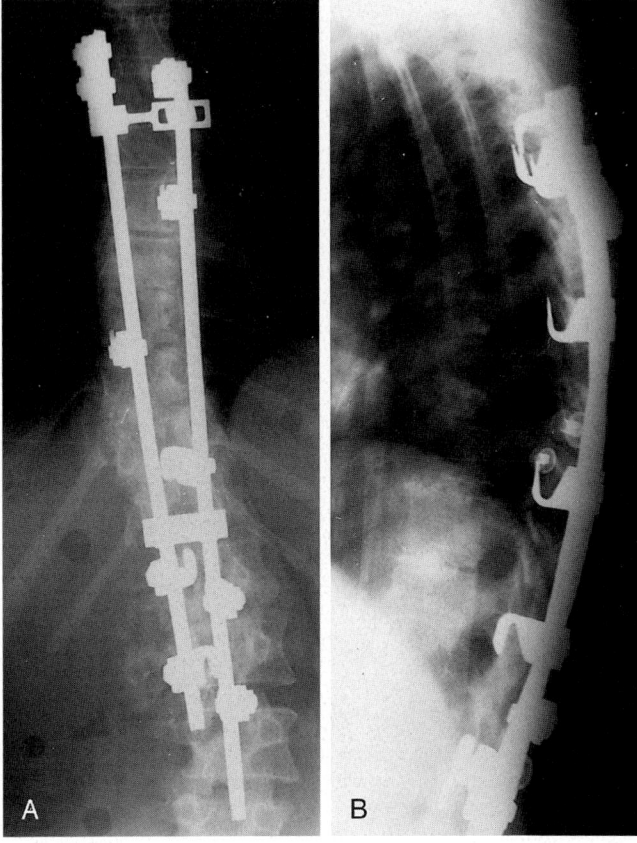

**Figure 12–12.** Texas Scottish Rite Hospital (TSRH) hardware. *A*, Anteroposterior view shows TSRH rods with multiple hooks and crosslinks. *B*, Lateral view shows the anatomic configuration of the thoracic hooks. The uppermost vertebra is engaged by two hooks directed toward each other in a "claw" configuration.

## Cervical Spine

Posterior cervical hardware is used widely, primarily to obtain fusion in patients with spinal deformity and ligamentous insufficiency. Posterior cervical fusions have a relatively low complication rate. The most common complication associated with posterior cervical hardware is loss of fixation and recurrence of deformity. Hardware breakage, loosening, and pulling out of wires from bone are typically due to repetitive stress applied to the fixation.

Almost all fusions at the occipitocervical junction are performed via a posterior approach. In the lower cervical spine, both anterior and posterior hardware systems are used. Anterior approaches to the cervicocranium require temporomandibular joint dislocation, mandibular osteotomy, transoral access (which has a high infection rate), or extensive retropharyngeal dissection.

Occipitocervical fusion is performed primarily for craniocervical or C1–C2 instability produced by acquired abnormalities, such as infection, inflammatory arthritis, and post-traumatic instability, or for the management of unstable congenital anomalies of the occipitoatlantoaxial junction (Fig. 12–13). Like occipitocervical fusion, fixation at C1–C2 typically uses a combination of posterior wiring and bone graft. Recently, fixation screws that pass anterosuperiorly from the lateral mass of C2 into the lateral mass of C1 have been developed.

In the lower cervical spine, both anterior and posterior hardware systems are used to achieve immobilization. Posterior fusion is used most commonly when disruption or instability of the posterior ligamentous structures has occurred after trauma or extensive laminectomy. Both wiring and metal hardware application, combined with bone grafting, are used widely for posterior fusion. Wiring is most effective in limiting flexion, is less effective in limiting extension, and is least effective in controlling rotation. All the posterior elements, including the spinous processes, laminae, facets, and lateral masses, can be used to affix hardware.

Sublaminar or facet fusion must be performed when the spinous processes are absent or insufficient. A variety of sublaminar and facet fusion procedures is used. One technique of sublaminar fusion consists of wiring two

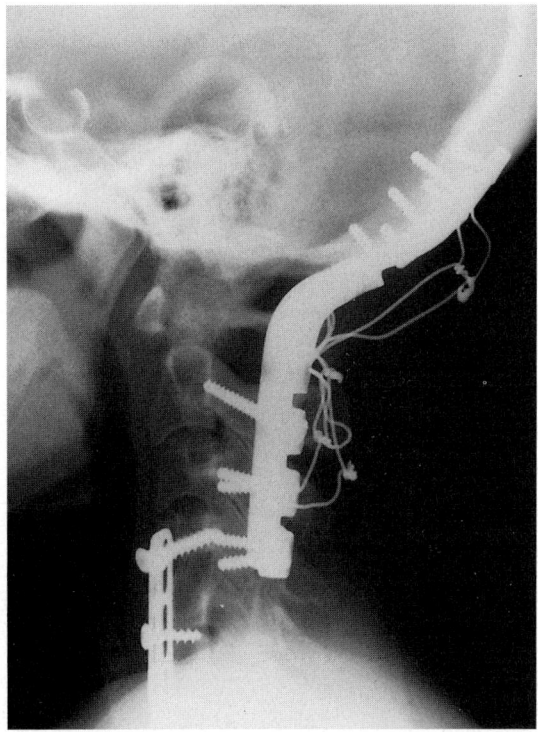

**Figure 12–13.** Occipitocervical fusion. This patient underwent occipitocervical fusion with Roy-Camille plates, bone graft, and wires for occipitocervical dislocation. Note the residual malalignment between the basion and the occiput. Also note the bulky plate reinforcement at each screw hole, characteristic of the Roy-Camille plate. An anterior cervical Caspar plate for another fracture is present at C6.

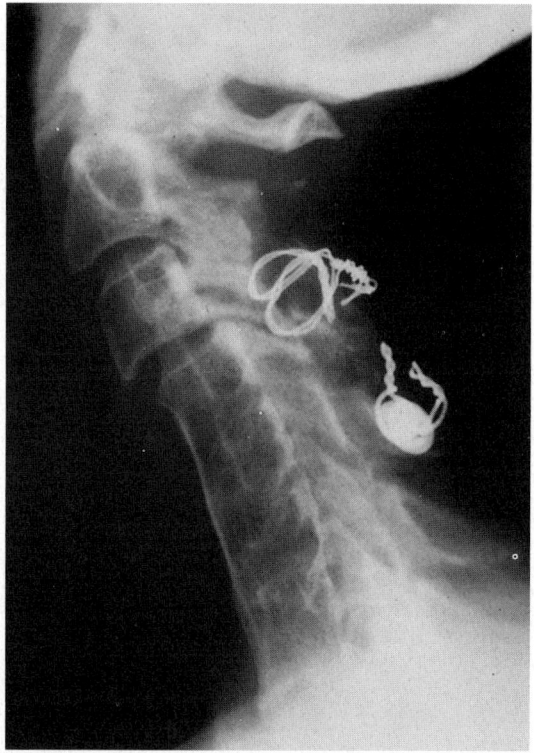

**Figure 12–14.** Posterior cervical fusion. Lateral view shows posterior fusion of C4–C7. A laminectomy was performed at C2–C3. Interfacet wires are present at the C2–C3 level, and there is spinous process wiring at C5 with buttons. The posterior bone graft from C3 to C5 is intact.

adjacent laminae with a stainless steel wire; another incorporates a single wire to connect several consecutive laminae. Because the lower cervical spine allows little room for error, sublaminar wiring is usually reserved for fixation at the C1 and C2 levels. Facet fusions are typically performed when the patient has had multiple laminectomies that preclude spinous process fusion (Fig. 12–14).

Other instruments available for posterior cervical fixation include posterior cervical plates. The use of rigid posterior cervical hardware is technically demanding and is associated with numerous complications, including injury to the vertebral arteries, nerve roots, and spinal cord. Anterior cervical hardware was developed because of the difficulty of achieving cervical fusion with anterior grafting techniques in patients with posterior cervical instability. Indications for the use of anterior hardware remain controversial, and it is generally not used in single-level discectomy; its main utility is in patients undergoing multilevel decompression for spondylotic myelopathy or multilevel fusion. Anterior plates are affixed with screws, which should be placed solidly in the bone. Positioning of the screws within the disc space predisposes to backing out of the pedicle screws, loosening of the hardware, and subsequent breakage of the hardware (Fig. 12–15).

## COMPLICATIONS

The failed back surgery syndrome is produced by a spectrum of disorders characterized by intractable postoperative pain and varying degrees of functional incapacitation. This syndrome develops in approximately 15% of patients after spinal surgery. Although no specific anatomic lesion can be identified in a large number of patients with the failed back surgery syndrome, the most common structural lesions responsible for this syndrome are recurrent or persistent disc extrusion, inadequate decompression of spinal stenosis, arachnoiditis, and epidural fibrosis. Less common causes include facet instability, pseudarthrosis, nerve injury, and surgery at the wrong level.

### Pseudarthrosis

Pseudarthrosis or nonunion of spinal grafts is one of the major causes of failed spinal surgery. Pseudarthrosis is defined broadly as documented failure of solid osseous union 1 year after surgery. The lack of osseous union may result from fibrous tissue bridging the gap (fibrous nonunion) or from abnormal excessive motion caused by the absence of any solid bridging tissue. Fibrous nonunion may be asymptomatic, in which case no intervention is required. Because no uniform method is available to

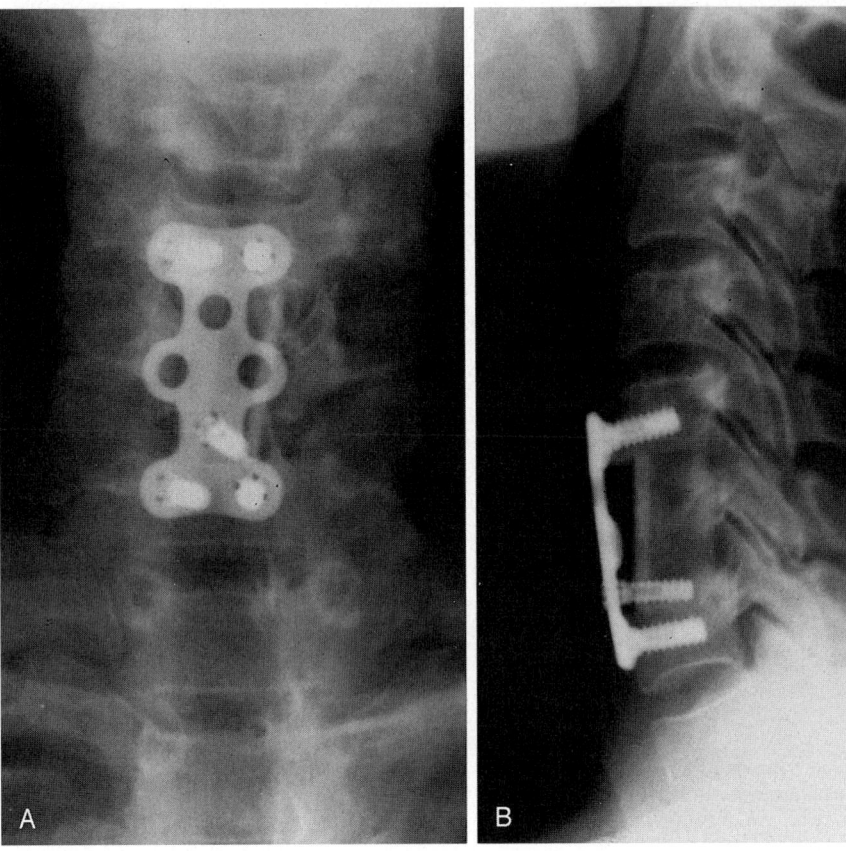

**Figure 12–15.** Morscher AO plate. *A*, Anteroposterior view shows an AO plate with a double-H configuration. *B*, Lateral view shows a corpectomy of C6, with a strut graft extending from C5 to C7. The plate is affixed with Morscher screws, which are cannulated and require purchase only in the anterior cortex.

diagnose nonunion of the fusion mass, there is considerable disparity in the reported rate of pseudarthrosis after bone grafting. The prevalence of pseudarthrosis after attempted fusion ranges from 3% to 30%. Higher rates of pseudarthrosis are encountered in patients undergoing simultaneous multilevel fusion.

The rate of nonunion for anterior cervical fusion ranges from 0% to 26%. Anterior interbody fusions have a higher rate of nonunion than do posterior or posterolateral fusions. Of the various posterolateral fusions used, intertransverse fusion is reportedly less likely to undergo nonunion. In general, the prevalence of pseudarthrosis after posterolateral spinal fusion without instrumentation increases with the number of motion segments included in the arthrodesis. Iliac strut grafts become incorporated more frequently and more rapidly than do fibular struts, which show nonincorporation in as many as 50% of cases. Hardware systems are designed to immobilize the spine to enhance osseous fusion, but they are not always successful.

In some studies, direct current electrical stimulation has been demonstrated to increase the rate of osseous spinal fusion. Implantable direct current stimulators have been shown by some investigators to enhance bone fusion radiographically and histologically in primary lumbar fusions. Externally applied pulsed electromagnetic coils are also available and appear to be as effective at stimulating bone growth as implantable units. The need for routine electrical stimulation has not been established,

and its role remains controversial; at this time, electrical stimulation is considered to be an adjunct to bone grafting in patients with established previous pseudarthrosis or in those patients deemed at high risk for pseudarthrosis.

Numerous imaging methods are used for the detection of pseudarthrosis; these methods can be divided into those that assess the morphologic structure of the grafted material and those that assess the graft functionally. Structural integrity is evaluated by conventional radiography and CT scanning. Functional integrity is assessed with stress views (typically, lateral flexion and extension views).

The initial diagnostic test for the evaluation of spinal fusion consists of conventional radiographs. Solid fusion results in a continuous, organized trabecular pattern across the entire grafted segment (Fig. 12–16). Typically, 6 to 9 months is required for the graft material to appear solid and continuous radiographically. During the early postoperative period, pseudarthrosis is difficult to detect unless gross graft or hardware failure develops. Persistent halos or lucent areas around the graft or hardware suggest failure of incorporation and should be further evaluated with flexion-extension views. The accuracy of radiography for assessing spinal fusion has been questioned in several studies that demonstrate considerable discrepancy between the radiographic appearance of the graft and the surgical findings. The complex anatomy of the bone graft and the overlying osseous structures frequently make it difficult to assess the graft material,

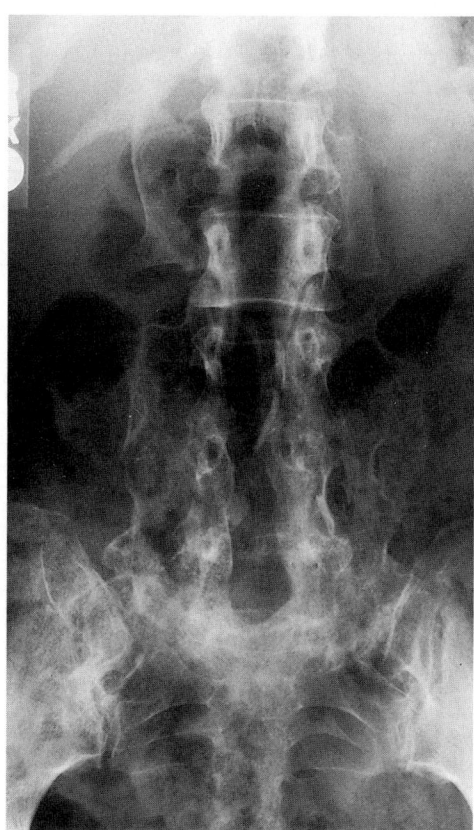

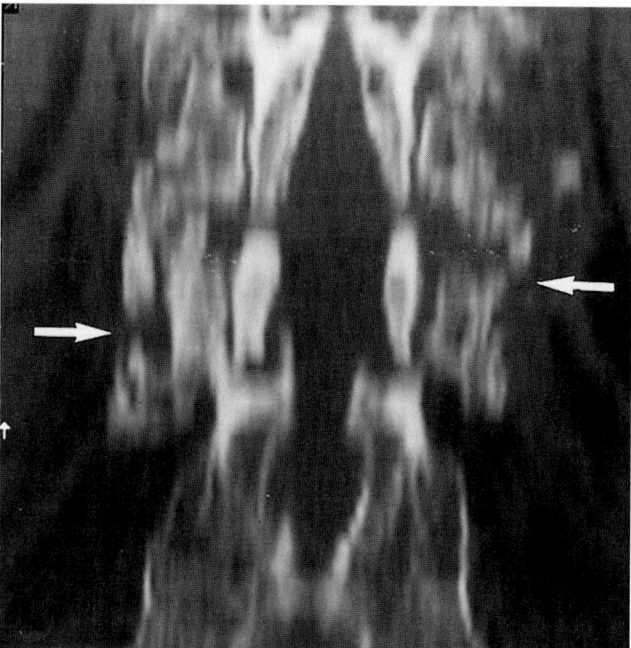

**Figure 12–17.** Pseudarthrosis. Curved coronal reformatted CT scan confirms discontinuity of graft material adjacent to the transverse processes *(arrows)*.

**Figure 12–16.** Intertransverse fusion. Solid osseous fusion with continuous trabeculae and loss of the cortical margins of the transverse processes is present at L1–L2 and at L3 to L5. The L2–L3 level was not fused in this patient. Note the extensive laminectomy and foraminotomy defects. The osteoporosis across the grafted segment is due to stress shielding of the vertebral bodies.

particularly in the presence of hardware. In general, radiographs tend to underestimate the extent of fusion as compared with second-look surgery.

Transaxial CT scans are useful for detecting discontinuity between the bone graft and the underlying vertebrae, but the slices must be thin enough to ensure accurate assessment. CT scans of the graft are generally obtained at 1- or 1.5-mm increments to ensure visualization of thin clefts of nonosseous union. On transaxial images, the bone graft must be identified and followed across sequential slices to ensure that solid graft is present. Reformatted images are especially helpful in this regard (Fig. 12–17). Caution is required, however, in that solid graft is not seen for several months after surgery. Ankylosis of the facet joints is also present as a late finding after successful arthrodesis.

With functional assessment of graft integrity, the absence of significant motion at the fusion site is the criterion for successful fusion. Segmental motion on flexion and extension views is frequently used as the standard diagnostic criterion for pseudarthrosis. Typically, lateral bending views are obtained in full flexion and extension. Despite solid posterior fusion and intact posterior hardware, a considerable amount of movement

at the disc space may still be present. An anterior disc height greater than 2 mm, more than 10 degrees of angular motion, or horizontal vertebral translation greater than 3 mm has been suggested as a reliable criterion for excessive movement across a fused spinal motion segment. Minor degrees of intervertebral movement, the formation of an intradiscal vacuum phenomenon in extension, and the development of osteoporosis are unreliable criteria for pseudarthrosis.

Despite the plethora of imaging methods available, confident diagnosis of pseudarthrosis remains a problem in a large proportion of cases. The five criteria that appear to be most reliable in establishing nonunion are (1) lack of trabecular continuity, (2) collapse of graft height with a gap between the vertebral endplate and graft material, (3) shift in graft position after healing is expected to have occurred, (4) dislodgment or fracture of internal hardware after healing is expected to have occurred, and (5) unexplained pain in the area of the fusion.

## Infection

Postoperative infection is a serious complication of any type of spinal surgery and occurs in approximately 1% to 3% of patients. Risk factors for postoperative spinal infection include advanced age of the patient, prolonged bed rest and hospitalization, obesity, diabetes mellitus, malnutrition, immunosuppression, steroid use, and infection at remote sites. The complexity and duration of the operation are also correlated with the prevalence of infection. Laminotomy and discectomy are rarely associated with infection, spinal fusion without the use of hardware carries a 1% to 5% risk, and fusion with hardware has an average prevalence of infection of 6% or more. The most common organism implicated is *Staphylococcus aureus*, which accounts for approximately 50% of all postoperative spinal infections, although infection with a variety of other organisms (single or multiple) may be encountered.

Early conventional radiographic findings of disc space loss, osteopenia, and vertebral endplate erosion may be difficult to distinguish from some postoperative changes. With progressive infection, vertebral destruction, osseous fragmentation, and reactive sclerosis may occur (Fig. 12–18). Loss of fixation and loosening of spinal hardware are seen if the infection cannot be controlled adequately with débridement, irrigation, and antibiotics. Similarly, in the early stages of infection, CT is not reliable. Scintigraphy is nonspecific, particularly in the early postoperative period. Bone scans using technetium-99m diphosphonate show mild to moderately increased activity within the first 3 weeks after surgery in approximately 50% of patients undergoing laminectomy and discectomy. The gallium scan also becomes abnormal in 89% of patients postoperatively. Increased activity on both bone and gallium scans is related to postoperative alterations in bone and soft tissue and typically persists for several months; the bone scan may remain abnormal up to 1 year after surgery. The normally increased activity seen on scintigraphic studies limits their usefulness in detecting postoperative spinal infection.

The MR imaging findings of postoperative discitis overlap with changes related to uncomplicated surgery. The most reliable finding in postoperative infective discitis on MR images is decreased signal intensity in the vertebral marrow of both adjacent endplates in T1-weighted images, with enhancement of these areas after the intravenous administration of a gadolinium-containing contrast agent.

Postoperative spinal epidural empyema is a rare complication encountered in less than 1% of patients undergoing elective spinal surgery. Patients frequently have a paucity of clinical symptoms or signs to suggest the diagnosis of infection. The frequent presence of an associated laminectomy allows the abscess to dissect posteriorly through the split retrospinal muscles, thereby minimizing compression on adjacent neural structures. The CT appearance of the infected collection is very similar to that of a post-traumatic pseudomeningocele, although the presence of gas bubbles, loss of definition of the fat planes between the collection and the dural sac or the paraspinal muscles, and irregular enhancement of thickened walls are all suggestive of infection.

## FURTHER READING

An HS: Surgical exposure and fusion techniques of the spine. In An HS, Cotler JM (eds): Spinal Instrumentation. Baltimore, Williams & Wilkins, 1992, p 1.

Berchuck M, Garfin SR, Bauman T, Abitbol JJ: Complications of anterior intervertebral grafting. Clin Orthop 284:54, 1992.

Boden SD, Davis DO, Dina TS, et al: Postoperative diskitis: Distinguishing early MR imaging findings from normal postoperative disk space changes. Radiology 184:765, 1992.

Bohlman HH, Emery SE: The pathophysiology of cervical spondylosis and myelopathy. Spine 13:843, 1988.

Brown MD, Malinin TI, Davis PB: A roentgenographic evaluation of frozen allografts versus autografts in anterior cervical spine fusions. Clin Orthop 119:231, 1976.

Cleveland M, Bosworth DM, Thompson FR: Pseudarthrosis in the lumbosacral spine. J Bone Joint Surg Am 30:302, 1948.

Cotler JM, Simpson JM, An HS: Principles, indications, and complications of spinal instrumentation: A summary chapter. In An HS, Cotler JM (eds): Spinal Instrumentation. Baltimore, Williams & Wilkins, 1992, p 435.

Djukic S, Lang P, Morris J, et al: The postoperative spine: Magnetic resonance imaging. Orthop Clin North Am 21:603, 1990.

Edwards CC: Edwards instrumentation: A modular spinal system. In An HS, Cotler JM (eds): Spinal Instrumentation. Baltimore, Williams & Wilkins, 1992, p 303.

Garfin SR, Glover M, Booth RE, et al: Laminectomy: A review of the Pennsylvania Hospital experience. J Spinal Disord 1:116, 1988.

Garfin SR, Herkowitz HN, Mirkovic S: Spinal stenosis. J Bone Joint Surg Am 81:572, 1999.

Grabias S: The treatment of spinal stenosis. J Bone Joint Surg Am 62:308, 1980.

Johnsson K, Willner S, Johnsson K: Postoperative instability after decompression for lumbar spinal stenosis. Spine 11:107, 1986.

Kaneda K: Kaneda anterior spinal instrumentation for the thoracic and lumbar spine. In An HS, Cotler JM (eds): Spinal Instrumentation. Baltimore, Williams & Wilkins, 1992, p 413.

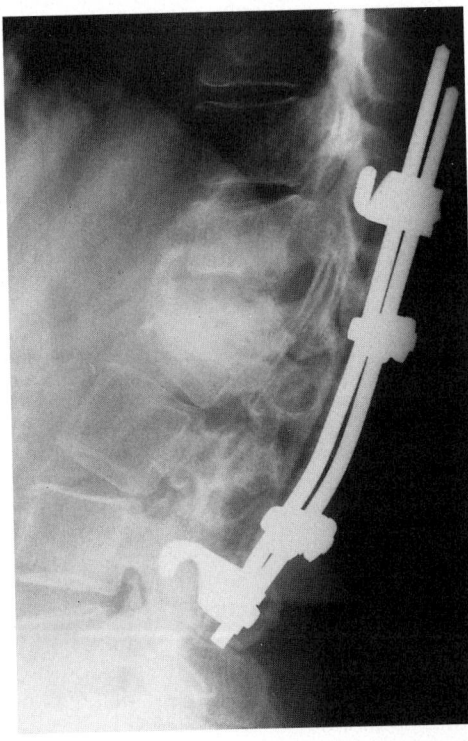

**Figure 12–18.** Postoperative infection. Deep infection of the L1–L2 disc and adjacent vertebrae has occurred after TSRH rodding for a burst fracture of L2. The endplates are eroded, with kyphosis and sclerosis resulting from chronic pyogenic infection.

Lenke LG, Bridwell KH, Blanke K, et al: Radiographic results of arthrodesis with Cotrel-Dubousset instrumentation for the treatment of adolescent idiopathic scoliosis. J Bone Joint Surg Am 80:807, 1998.

Lonstein JE: Post-laminectomy kyphosis. Clin Orthop 128:93, 1977.

Marshall LF: Complications of surgery for degenerative cervical and lumbar disc disease. In Garfin SR (ed): Complications of Spine Surgery. Baltimore, Williams & Wilkins, 1989, p 75.

McAfee PC: Interbody fusion cages in reconstructive operations on the spine. J Bone Joint Surg Am 81:859, 1999.

McAfee PC, Yuan HA, Lasda NA: The unstable burst fracture. Spine 7:365, 1982.

Meyer PR Jr, Rusin JJ, Haak MH: Anterior instrumentation of the cervical spine. In An HS, Cotler JM (eds): Spinal Instrumentation. Baltimore, Williams & Wilkins, 1992, p 49.

Puno RM, Byrd JA III: The Puno-Byrd (PWB) spinal system for transpedicular fixation of the lumbar spine. In An HS, Cotler JM (eds): Spinal Instrumentation. Baltimore, Williams & Wilkins, 1992, p 281.

Rothman SLG, Glenn WV, Kerber CW: Postoperative fractures of lumbar articular facets: Occult cause of radiculopathy. AJR Am J Roentgenol 145:779, 1985.

Sartoris DJ, Gershuni DH, Akeson WH, et al: Coralline hydroxyapatite bone graft substitutes: Preliminary report of radiographic evaluation. Radiology 159:133, 1986.

Slone RM, Heare MM, Griend RAV, et al: Orthopedic fixation devices. Radiographics 11:823, 1991.

Slone RM, MacMillan M, Montgomery WJ: Spinal fixation. Part 1. Principles, basic hardware, and fixation techniques for the cervical spine. Radiographics 13:341, 1993.

Slone RM, MacMillan M, Montgomery WJ, Heare M: Spinal fixation. Part 2. Fixation techniques and hardware for the thoracic and lumbosacral spine. Radiographics 13:521, 1993.

Slone RM, MacMillan M, Montgomery WJ: Spinal fixation. Part 3. Complications of spinal instrumentation. Radiographics 13:797, 1993.

Spivak JM: Degenerative lumbar spinal stenosis. J Bone Joint Surg Am 80:1953, 1998.

Steinmann JC, Herkowitz HN: Pseudarthrosis of the spine. Clin Orthop 284:80, 1992.

Teplick JG, Haskin ME: Computed tomography of the postoperative lumbar spine. AJR Am J Roentgenol 141:865, 1983.

Wang JC, Bohlman HH, Riew KD: Dural tears secondary to operations on the lumbar spine. J Bone Joint Surg Am 80:1728, 1998.

# CHAPTER 13

## Imaging after Surgery in Extraspinal Sites

Barbara N. Weissman

### SUMMARY OF KEY FEATURES

Knowledge of orthopedic devices and techniques is a prerequisite for the accurate interpretation of postoperative radiographs. A number of internal fixation devices, including pins, nails, rods, screws, and plates, in addition to external fixation devices and polymethylmethacrylate (PMMA) cement, are used in fracture fixation. Electrical stimulation may be used to promote fracture healing, and numerous techniques of bone grafting are advocated in the treatment of many skeletal processes. Resection arthroplasty, arthrodesis, and osteotomy represent additional orthopedic methods.

### INTRODUCTION

This chapter describes some of the commonly encountered orthopedic devices and techniques. In each instance, principles that are fundamental to the correct interpretation of pertinent imaging studies are provided, but because of the complexity of the subject, interested readers may wish to consult additional sources.

### FRACTURE FIXATION

Fixation refers to maintenance of the position of fracture fragments during healing. Hardware may be placed directly across the fracture site (internal fixation), or the area may be immobilized by casts or appliances fixed to the adjacent bone (external fixation).

#### Internal Fixation Devices

Internal fixation devices are usually inserted after open reduction of the fracture fragments. In some cases, however, percutaneous placement of internal fixation devices may follow closed fracture reduction.

**Wires and Pins.** Wires, pins, nails, and rods are generally distinguished on the basis of size. Wires are the thinnest. Kirschner wires have spatulate ends and are thin (0.028 to 0.062 inch). The soft tissue end of the wire may be cut off beneath the skin, or its protruding end may be bent or capped to prevent injury. Steinmann pins are thicker than

Kirschner wires; both may be smooth or threaded. Kirschner wires may also serve as guides over which cannulated screws are placed.

**Intramedullary Nails and Rods.** Nails are thicker than pins, and rods are generally thicker than nails. Clinically, however, these terms are often used interchangeably. Intramedullary rods are used primarily for the treatment of closed transverse or short oblique midshaft fractures of the long bones. Compression can occur at the fracture site, with telescoping along the rod, unless proximal and distal interlocking screws are used. Intramedullary rod insertion damages the blood supply to the endosteum; therefore, healing occurs exclusively by periosteal new bone formation and organization of the hematoma formed around the fracture site (Fig. 13–1). Complications of intramedullary pins, rods, and nails include splitting of the shaft of the bone; inability to advance or withdraw the nail; separation of fracture fragments; penetration of the nail into an adjacent joint; pain from a prominent end of the fixation device; inadequate immobilization of the fracture (leading to nonunion); fracture, bending, or loosening of the rod; migration of the rod; fracture at the site of Ender nail insertion; fat embolization; rod corrosion; and spread of infection along the shaft of the bone.

Intramedullary fixation is generally contraindicated in open or compound wounds. Locking intramedullary nails have holes in them that allow screws (transfixation screws) to be inserted to fix the rod within the bone. Interlocking screws placed both proximal and distal to the fracture site inhibit compression and rotation and are used primarily for the treatment of comminuted diaphyseal femoral and tibial fractures. Inserting screws into only one end of the intramedullary nail provides "dynamic" fixation, in which compression at the fracture site may occur, but rotation of the nail in the medullary canal is controlled by the transfixation screw.

**Wires.** Wires may be placed around the fracture fragments (cerclage) for compression. The surgical exposure necessary for the placement of cerclage wires may interfere with periosteal circulation and fracture healing. Tension band wiring eliminates eccentric loading of bone, thereby neutralizing tensile forces on a bone and allowing compression alone at the fracture site. A plate or wire along the convex side is used to absorb the tensile forces and allow compression forces alone to act on the fracture site (Fig. 13–2).

**Screws.** Cortical screws are threaded over their length. They are used primarily to secure plate devices to bone, and they should penetrate both the near and the far cortices. Cancellous lag screws are threaded distally and have smooth proximal shafts (Fig. 13–3). The threads are wider than those of cortical screws, so they hold better in

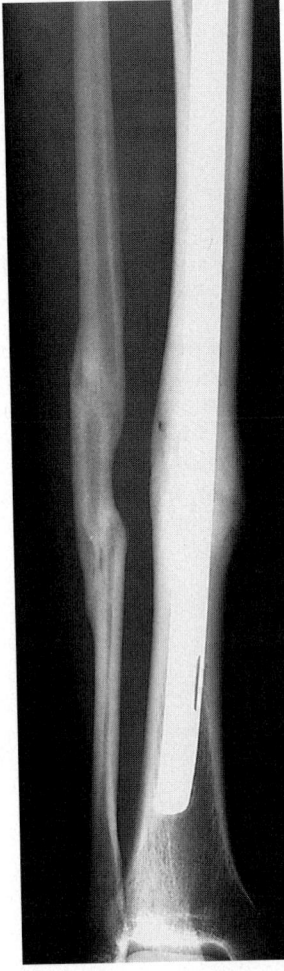

**Figure 13–1.** Healing tibial fracture. An intramedullary rod has maintained essentially anatomic alignment of the tibia during healing. Because the endosteal blood supply is damaged, healing is due largely to periosteal callus formation.

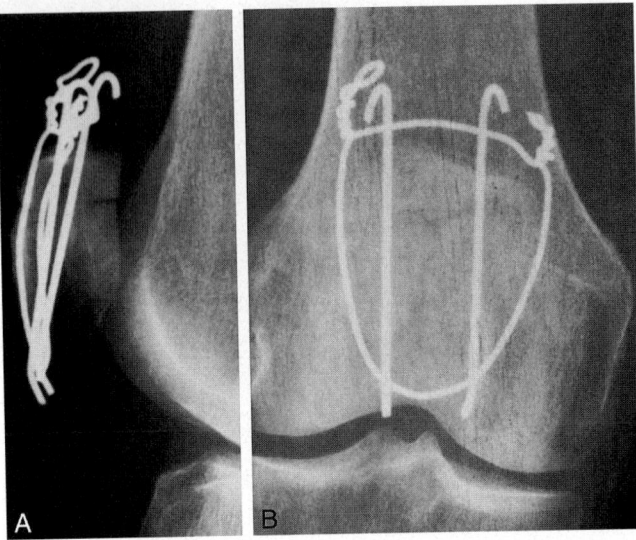

**Figure 13–2.** Tension band wiring for nondisplaced transverse fracture of the superior pole of the patella. Lateral (*A*) and anteroposterior (*B*) views show tension band wiring resulting in a marked improvement in alignment.

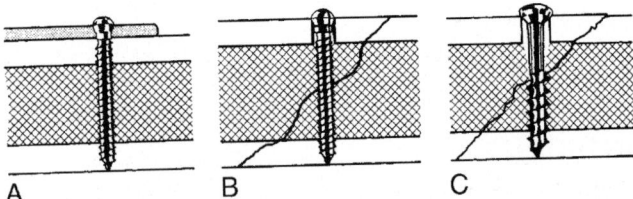

**Figure 13–3.** Cortical and cancellous screws. *A*, A cortical screw is often used to secure plates to bone. *B*, Cortical screws may function as lag screws by overdrilling the proximal cortex so that only the distal threads engage bone. *C*, A cancellous (lag) screw has distal threads and a smooth proximal shaft. The threads are more widely spaced than are those of a cortical screw.

cancellous bone. When cancellous screws are used to produce compression across a fracture, the threaded portion of the screw should be completely within the distal fracture fragment, and the screw threads should not cross the fracture line. Cannulated screws have a central channel so that they can be inserted over a wire or pin for accurate placement. The Herbert screw is a cannulated screw that is threaded proximally and distally but not centrally. The pitch of the threads differs proximally and distally so that as the screw is tightened, the fracture fragments are drawn together. This type of screw is used primarily in the treatment of nonunion of the scaphoid bone and serves to hold the bone graft between the fracture fragments (Fig. 13–4). Interference screws are short, fully threaded screws with a cancellous thread pattern and a recessed head. They are used in cruciate ligament reconstructions, and they wedge the bone of a bone-tendon-bone graft unit against the wall of the tunnel (Fig. 13–5).

The sliding screw plate (dynamic compression screw, dynamic hip screw) is used primarily in the treatment of intertrochanteric fractures, but it is also used in cases of femoral neck and subtrochanteric fractures. This device provides fixation while allowing impaction to occur at the fracture site during healing and weight bearing. The sliding screw plate apparatus consists of a lag screw and a side plate with a barrel. The threaded portion of the screw is placed in the femoral head, and its shaft is inserted into the barrel of the side plate. The tip of the lag screw should be located centrally within the femoral head. The threads of the lag screw should be in subchondral bone, with the screw tip optimally about 0.5 inch from the articular surface. The side plate should lie flush with the femoral shaft, and the screws attaching it to the cortex should just penetrate the far cortex.

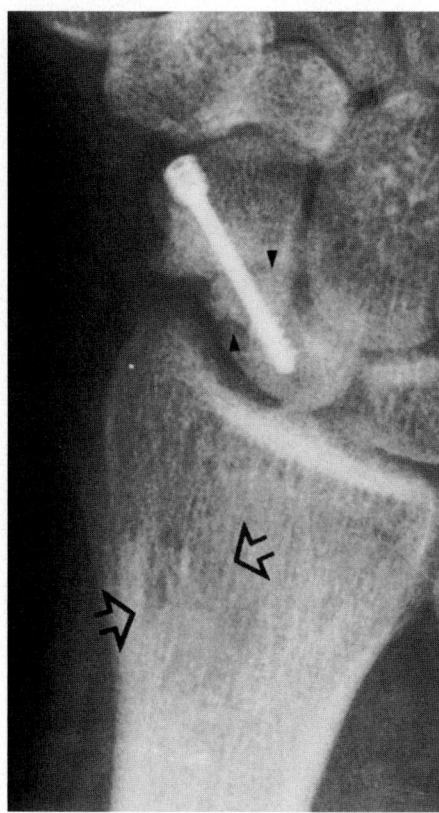

**Figure 13–4.** Bone grafting for nonunion of a scaphoid fracture. A bone graft *(arrowheads)* is held in place by a Herbert screw. The radial donor graft site is faintly visible *(open arrows)*.

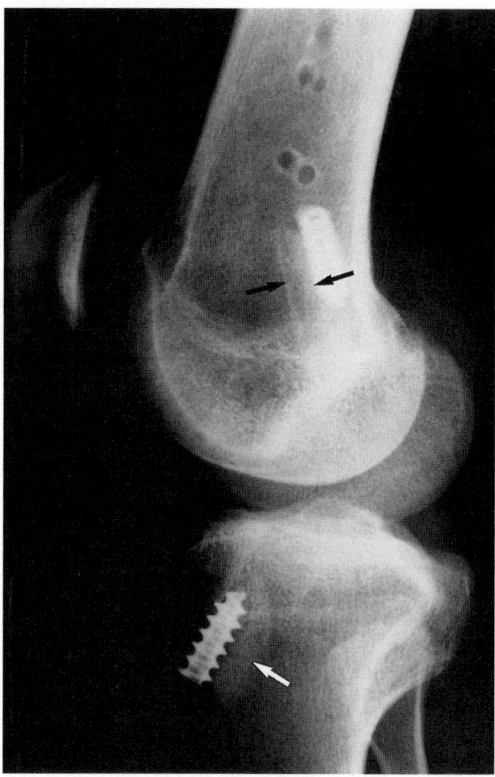

**Figure 13–5.** Interference screw. A lateral view of the knee after anterior cruciate ligament reconstruction shows interference screws holding the bone graft *(arrows)* of a bone-tendon-bone graft preparation in the surgically created tunnels. (Courtesy of A. Newberg, MD, Boston, Mass.)

**Plates.** A plate can be used to provide one or more of the following functions: static or dynamic compression, neutralization, and buttressing (Fig.13–6). Static compression refers to the production of axial compression along fractures. Compression can be achieved either by attaching a tension device to a plate at the time of internal fixation or by using a particular type of plate, the dynamic compression plate. A dynamic compression plate has screw holes with sloped sides that correspond to the slope of the undersurface of the screw. As the screws are tightened, the screw head glides down the incline of the screw hole, toward the center of the plate, thus producing compression at the fracture line. A plate that is used for neutralization bridges a comminuted fracture and transmits bending or torsional forces from the proximal to the distal fragment, thereby protecting the intervening fracture fragments from these forces. When applied to a cortical surface that is concave, the plate is bent slightly so that its central portion is not in contact with the bone. Plates used for buttressing support an area of thin cortex or cancellous bone graft and prevent collapse. These plates are under compression (rather than tension) and are used near joints, such as the tibial metaphysis, to prevent deformity after fracture fixation and grafting.

Plates are categorized into straight plates and plates with special shapes. Straight plates include those with round holes, dynamic compression plates, tubular plates,

and reconstruction plates. Dynamic compression plates are recognizable on radiographs by their oval holes. Tubular plates have a concave inner surface to conform to the curvature of the underlying bone. Reconstruction plates can be bent to conform to the shape of the underlying bone (Fig. 13–7).

## External Fixation Devices

External fixation provides immobilization of fractures while maintaining the potential to adjust the fracture position. In addition, external fixators may be used for compression at sites of attempted fusion (Fig. 13–8) and for distraction during attempted limb lengthening. Several devices are available that consist of one or more frames anchored to the bone with pins. Some indications for external fixation of fractures include open fractures in which comminution is present, especially in cases of segmental bone loss and soft tissue damage; the presence of major vascular damage requiring repair; severe osteoporosis; and extensive epiphyseal and metaphyseal comminution. External fixators are also used in the treatment of infected, nonunited fractures and during healing of free vascularized bone grafts. Complications associated with the use of external fixation include pin tract infections, soft tissue contracture, and delayed union or nonunion.

The Ilizarov frame consists of circular rings that surround the limb and are connected by a series of longitu-

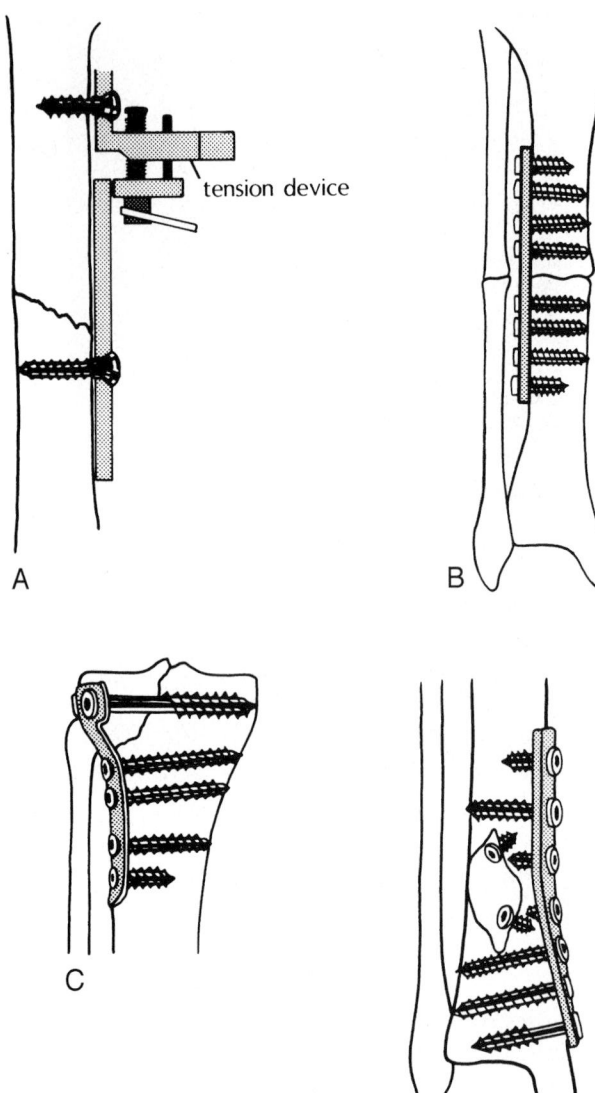

A

B

C

D

**Figure 13–6.** Functions of plates. *A*, Static compression. *B*, Dynamic compression after correction of nonunion with varus deformity. *C*, Buttressing. *D*, Neutralization. (Redrawn from Müller ME, Allgower M, Schneider R, Willenegger H: Manual of Internal Fixation: Technique Recommended by the AO Group. New York, Springer-Verlag, 1979.)

tension device

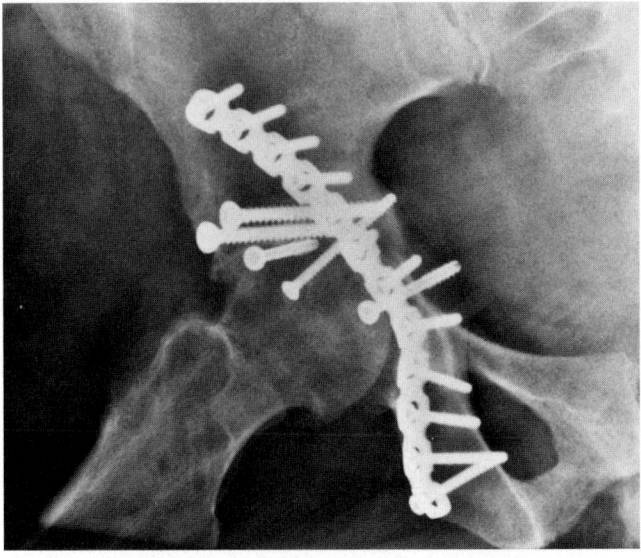

**Figure 13–7.** Reconstruction plate. This patient suffered transverse and posterior acetabular rim fractures. The reconstruction plate has been contoured to fit the posterior column of the acetabulum.

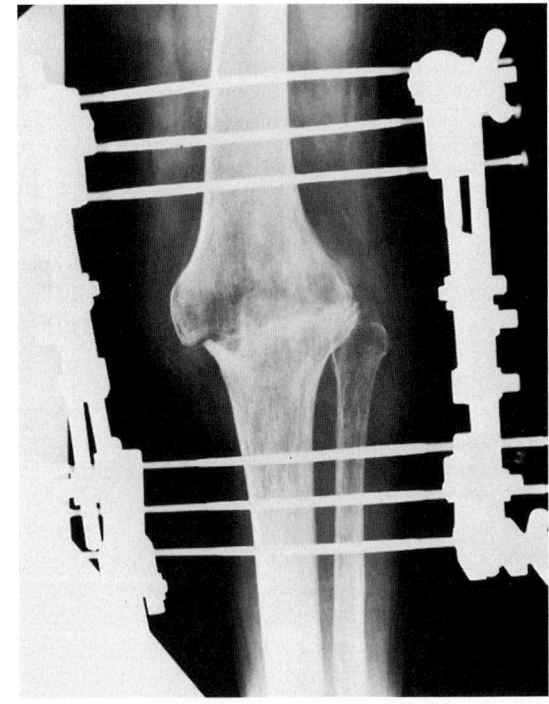

**Figure 13–8.** External fixation apparatus used for compression. An infected prosthesis has been removed. The external fixation (Hoffman) apparatus maintains compression at the site of attempted fusion.

dinal bars with adjustable thread and nut distraction points. Traction wires provide fixation to bone. The system is both strong and adaptable. It is used most often for limb lengthening or for the treatment of limb deformities associated with malunion, nonunion, or congenital disorders. A "corticotomy" procedure in which a metaphyseal osteotomy is performed is used to divide the bone without disturbing the nutrient vessels in the marrow. Bone formation develops at the distraction site within 15 weeks and appears initially as hazy opacity within the gap. Sonography may be useful for detecting bone formation in the gap earlier than on radiographs and for detecting the cystlike collections that occasionally develop.

## Polymethylmethacrylate

In patients with metastatic disease of the long bones or pelvis, PMMA has been used as an adjunct to internal fixation so that prompt weight bearing and pain relief can be achieved (Fig. 13–9). Accepted criteria for the prophylactic fixation of impending pathologic fractures include (1) a well-defined osteolytic lesion greater than 3 cm in diameter, (2) an osteolytic lesion that has destroyed 50% or more of the cortex, and (3) persistent pain in the area of an osteolytic focus. PMMA instilled into an area of cortical destruction increases the strength of that bone.

In addition to using PMMA for the treatment of pathologic fractures, cement has been used to improve fracture fixation in osteoporotic patients. Antibiotics in powder form may be added to the powdered polymer before it is mixed with the liquid monomer at the time of surgery. The cement elutes antibiotics at a greater concentration than can be achieved by systemic administration, and this form of treatment is without hazard when appropriate amounts of antibiotics are administered.

The prosthesis of antibiotic-loaded acrylic cement (PROSTALAC) temporary prosthesis system also uses PMMA. In this system, a one-piece modular femoral stem and polyethylene acetabular component are implanted with antibiotic-impregnated PMMA. The system is designed to serve as a short-term facsimile of a total hip, which allows effective treatment while maintaining patient lifestyle (Fig. 13–10). In recent years, PMMA has been used during vertebroplasties in patients with vertebral body collapse related to osteoporosis and other disorders.

## ELECTRICAL STIMULATION

Application of electrical currents of 5 to 20 μA has been shown to stimulate bone formation at the cathode. In general, two methods of electrical stimulation of bone formation are currently available: direct current stimulation and pulsing electromagnetic fields.

Direct current stimulation requires placement of the cathode in the fracture or nonunion site. The use of pulsing electromagnetic fields to stimulate bone formation involves the application of an external apparatus over the fracture site. The apparatus is connected to household current for 10 to 12 hours per day. Fracture healing after electrical stimulation occurs in about 80% of cases, a rate of healing similar to that of bone graft surgery.

## BONE GRAFTS

### Terminology

Bone grafts are described according to their origins, the type of bone used for grafting, and the method of graft placement (Table 13–1). Types of bone used for grafting include cortical bone, cancellous bone, or both (Table 13–2). Cancellous bone grafts are used primarily to promote osteogenesis, whereas cortical bone grafts are used to pro-

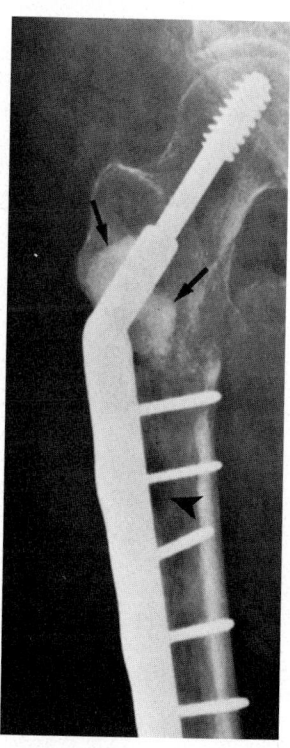

**Figure 13–9.** Polymethylmethacrylate (PMMA) as an adjunct in the treatment of a fracture. This patient suffered a pathologic fracture through a metastatic focus arising from renal carcinoma. A sliding screw plate device was inserted, with PMMA instilled into the medullary canal (*arrows*). Several areas of lytic bone destruction remain (one indicated by an *arrowhead*).

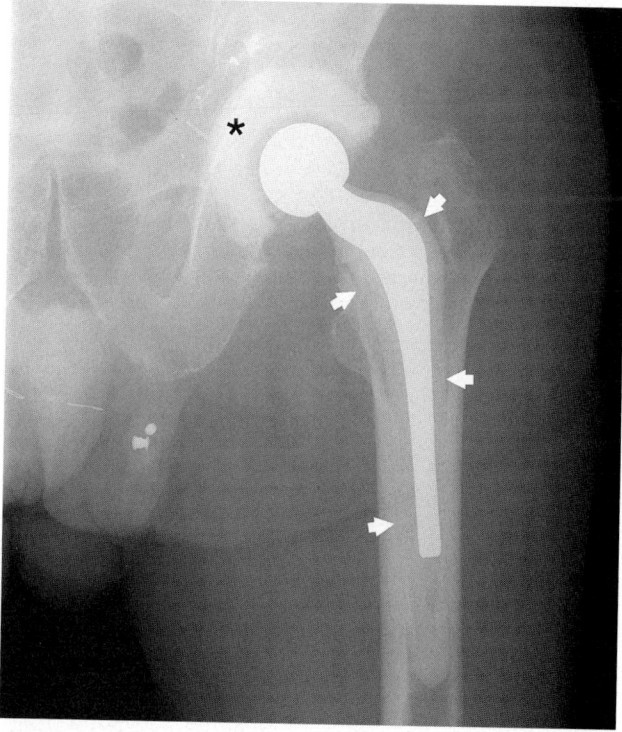

**Figure 13–10.** Prosthesis of antibiotic-loaded acrylic cement (PROSTALAC) temporary hip prosthesis system. Antibiotic-impregnated polymethylmethacrylate (PMMA) marked by *white arrows* and *black asterisk* surround the femoral stem and polyethylene component.

vide structural stability. When corticocancellous bone grafts are used, they are positioned so that the cancellous surface abuts the soft tissues, to facilitate vascular ingrowth.

Grafts may also be described according to their composition, position, and shape. Onlay grafts consist of cortical bone that is placed across a bony defect (such as a nonunion) and held by screws to a surgically denuded or drilled surface of the host bone. A sliding inlay graft consists of bone cut from the proximal fragment and slid distally across the bony defect. A dowel graft consists of a core of cancellous bone that is inserted into a surgically created channel to stimulate osteogenesis. Strut grafts, often composed of a rib or fibula, provide stability and stimulate osteogenesis; these grafts are used most often in the spine (Fig. 13–11).

## Indications

Bone grafts are generally used to promote healing, provide stability, or both. Possible situations in which bone grafting may be used include filling of bony defects or cavities; bridging of joints for arthrodesis; bridging of large defects in a long bone; promoting healing in cases of nonunion; and promoting union or filling defects in cases of delayed union, malunion, fresh fracture, or osteotomy.

## Bone Formation after Grafting

Cancellous bone grafts have a greater capacity to induce new bone formation than cortical grafts do. If the cancellous graft is immobile, a process of "creeping substitution" takes place in which new bone is deposited on the scaffold of dead trabeculae. Allografts are generally less satisfactory than autografts, in that new bone formation is slower, vascular penetration is slower and less dense, and bone replacement tends to be superficial. Rejection of allografts because of sensitization of the host by antigens in the graft is a major reason for their inferiority to autografts.

## Vascularized Bone Grafts

Microsurgical techniques allow bone grafts and their associated vasculature to be transplanted so that the grafts remain viable. Currently, the success rate of this procedure is greater than 90% (Fig. 13–12). This procedure is usually reserved for cases of massive bone loss (>12 cm), patients in whom more conventional techniques have failed, or those in whom an inadequate soft tissue bed is present.

## Massive Cadaver Allografts

Massive cadaver allografts are used for limb salvage in the treatment of primary bone tumors and for reconstruction in patients with severe bone loss after failed joint replacement. In selected cases, such as after resection of aggressive benign bone tumors or bone sarcomas, reconstruction is performed by inserting a massive bone graft consisting of bone, articular cartilage, and accompanying tendons or ligaments. Bone formation (by creeping substitution) occurs at the host-graft junction and is presumed to require many years before remodeling of the entire graft takes place. The graft therefore functions largely as a spacer. Failure of massive allografts is most often due to infection or fracture.

## Donor Sites

The most frequently used donor sites for bone grafting are the iliac crest, tibia, fibula, greater trochanter, distal

---

**TABLE 13–1**

**Bone Graft Types by Origin**

| Type of Graft | Description |
| --- | --- |
| Autograft | Transplanted bone derived from the same person |
| Allograft | Transplanted material derived from another person of the same species |
| Xenograft | Transplanted material derived from a member of a different species |

---

**TABLE 13–2**

**Comparison of Cancellous and Cortical Bone Grafts**

| Cancellous Graft | Cortical Graft |
| --- | --- |
| Better survival of osteogenic cells because the structure allows diffusion and early microvascular anastomoses | Dense bone is a barrier to diffusion |
| Large endosteal surface supplies osteoprogenitor cells | Small endosteal surface |
| Abundant red marrow supplies many osteoprogenitor cells | Fewer osteoprogenitor cells |
| Healing by creeping substitution; new bone is deposited on dead trabeculae, followed by removal of necrotic matrix | Removal of necrotic matrix from around the central canals of osteons occurs first, followed by new bone formation |
| Relatively weak | Relatively strong |

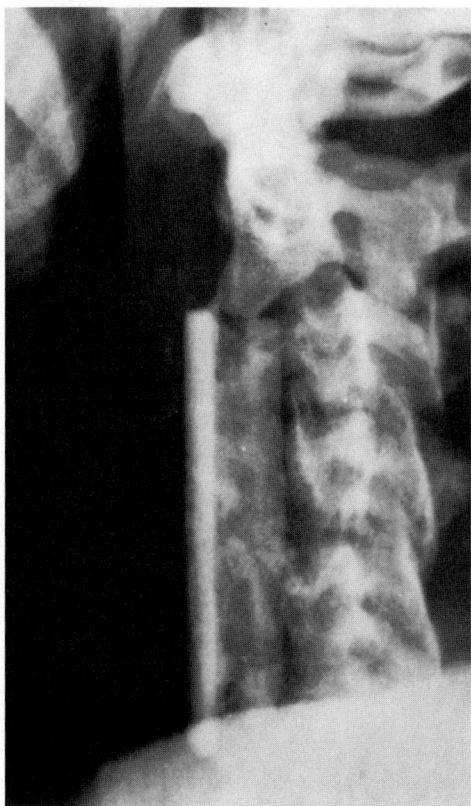

**Figure 13–11.** Strut graft. Anterior fusion was performed, with insertion of a cadaveric fibular allograft. Vertebral alignment is improved. (Courtesy of T. Cochran, MD, West Roxbury, Mass.)

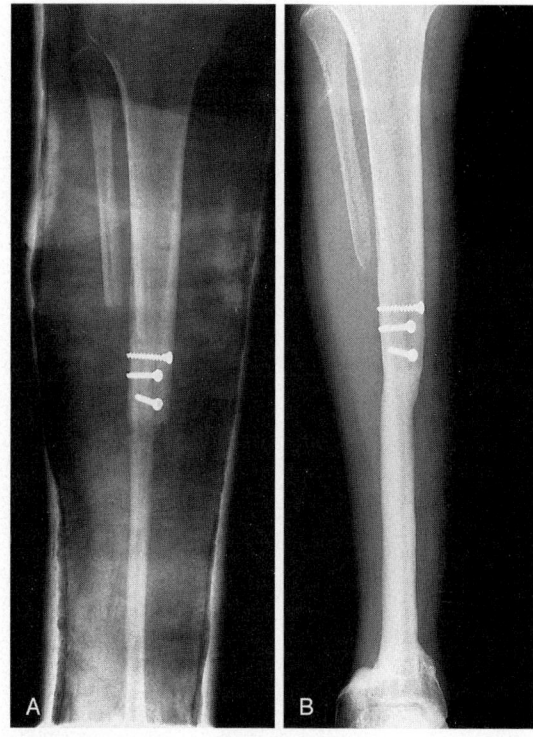

**Figure 13–12.** Vascularized fibular graft. *A*, After removal of a long segment of the distal portion of the tibia owing to tumor, a vascularized segment of fibula was used to bridge the defect. *B*, Bony union occurred proximally and distally between the graft and the tibia; subsequently, hypertrophy of the graft occurred.

portion of the radius, and posterior elements of the spine. The ilium is a good source of cancellous bone grafts. When the patient is supine, cancellous bone is removed from the area below the anterior superior iliac spine. The inner table of bone is left intact to avoid the development of a muscular hernia. If more cancellous bone is needed, the dissection is extended posteriorly. Fibular grafts are obtained from the middle third to half of the bone, because this area can be excised without adverse effects. The distal quarter as well as the proximal segment of the fibula should remain intact to ensure stability at the ankle and knee. Complications at donor graft sites appear to be few. Nonetheless, fracture may occur after cortical graft removal, and intraoperative bleeding and postoperative pain may follow iliac crest biopsy. Stress fractures, hernias through an iliac donor site, and gait problems have also been reported.

### Radiologic Examination

Healing of iliac donor sites is evidenced by sclerosis at the margins of the osseous defects. Bony excrescences from the donor site may appear and be accompanied by pain. Radiographic evaluation of rib and iliac donor sites shows regeneration occurring in children and in adults younger than 30 years, but this is not observed in those older than 30 years. Graft healing is generally documented by the loss of sharp margins between the graft and the host bone, eventually leading to osseous union, with bone continuity across the host-graft junction. Fibrous union is suggested by the persistence of a thin residual radiolucent area between the graft and the host bone. The time required to achieve union depends on the size and type of graft, the local conditions, and the site of surgery.

With regard to vascularized bone grafts, accumulation of the bone scanning agent in the area of the graft within the first week after transplantation indicates both intact vasculature and metabolically viable bone; conversely, the absence of uptake of the bone scanning agent on serial radionuclide examinations suggests segmental nonviability (Fig. 13–13). Accumulation of the bone-seeking radionuclide after this 1-week period, however, may be due to the deposition of new bone on the surface of dead trabeculae and does not indicate either vascular patency or the presence of viable graft. Blood perfusion and blood pool scans are helpful in confirming vascular patency in the first 2 weeks after surgery.

Magnetic resonance (MR) imaging has been used to evaluate arterial anatomy before vascularized fibular grafting, as well as to determine the length of scaphoid bone grafts needed to correct humpback deformity of the scaphoid.

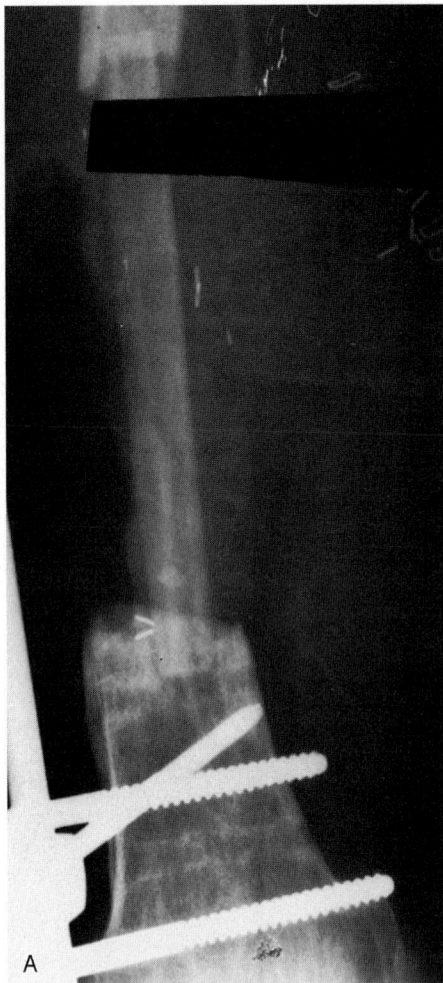

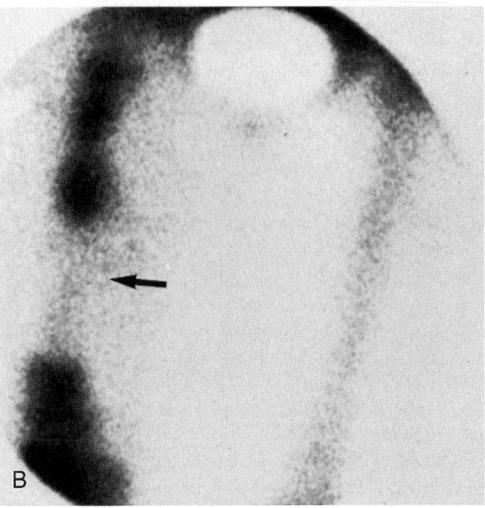

**Figure 13–13.** Absent blood flow to a vascularized graft. *A*, Vascularized bone graft was used to bridge a defect created by the removal of a long segment of bone affected by chronic osteomyelitis. *B*, Bone scan shows absent isotope uptake in the graft *(arrow)*, suggesting nonviability.

At the same time, the vascularity of the scaphoid and the integrity of the adjacent ligaments can be assessed.

### Complications

Delayed union in cortical grafts is defined as the absence of healing 12 months after surgery (Fig. 13–14). Graft failure may be associated with progressive bone resorption, leading to a decrease in the size and density of the graft and ultimately resulting in its disappearance. Similar graft resorption may be due to recurrent tumor or infection.

Stress fractures within cortical grafts are not uncommon. Stress fractures usually occur only after union of the graft and host bone is seen, and they may fail to heal without operative treatment.

### RESECTION ARTHROPLASTY

Resection arthroplasty consists of the removal of one or both articular surfaces of a joint. Currently, this technique is used primarily as a salvage procedure after failed total joint replacement surgery.

### Girdlestone Arthroplasty

The term *Girdlestone arthroplasty* is currently applied in a general sense to any hip joint resection. It is used as a salvage procedure, performed when an infected total hip prosthesis is removed. It is also used in some instances of infectious arthritis in preference to hip fusion. The indications for Girdlestone arthroplasty are listed in Table 13–3. The results of Girdlestone arthroplasty after removal of an infected hip prosthesis have not been as dismal as might be expected, and pain relief and control of infection occur in more than 80% of patients.

Shortening of the affected extremity, a Trendelenburg gait, and joint instability are invariable sequelae that make walking difficult and tiring. Radiographs confirm complete removal of the femoral neck, acetabular rim, and PMMA cement (Fig. 13–15). Optimally, all cement is removed; however, residual cement does not necessarily result in continued infection.

### ARTHRODESIS (JOINT FUSION)

Arthrodesis refers to the surgical stiffening of a joint. Such surgery is usually performed to provide stability or

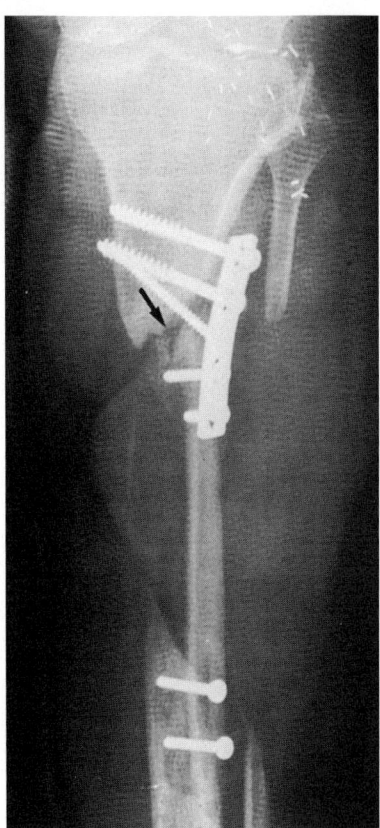

**Figure 13–14.** Failure of bone grafting. A vascularized fibular graft was used to bridge a tibial defect caused by removal of an infected, nonunited fracture. Previous vascular injury and repair had occurred. Despite multiple attempts at supplemental grafting, union never occurred proximally *(arrow)*, and the patient eventually underwent amputation.

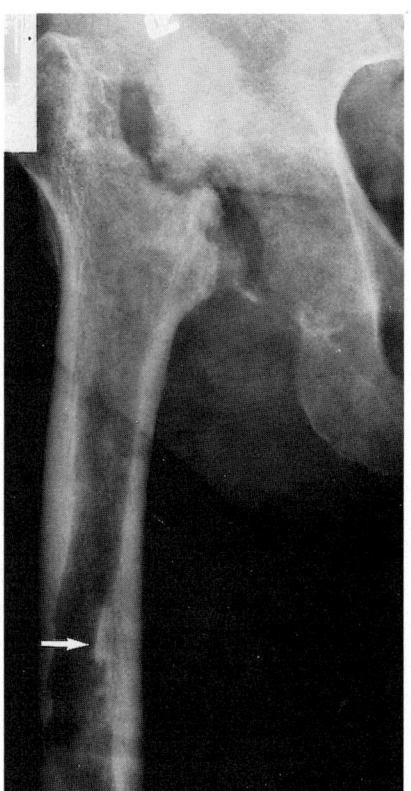

**Figure 13–15.** Girdlestone arthroplasty. This patient had an infected total hip prosthesis that necessitated Girdlestone arthroplasty. Some cement remains in the femoral canal *(arrow)*. Infection recurred at the area of retained cement.

---

**TABLE 13–3**

### Indications for Girdlestone Arthroplasty

Presence of virulent, resistant organisms
Presence of gram-negative organisms
Presence of two or more strains of organisms
Unhealthy and edematous soft tissues
Draining sinus
Radiographic evidence of well-established osteomyelitis with
  bone erosion
Severe loss of bone substance

---

to relieve pain resulting from joint damage caused by previous infection, injury, or failed joint replacement surgery. The bony fusion performed may be intra-articular, extra-articular, or a combination of the two.

### Ankle

Ankle arthrodesis remains a valuable procedure for the alleviation of pain from arthritis, the treatment of paralytic instability, and salvage after a failed total ankle replace-

ment. Results after ankle fusion are surprisingly good. The adequacy of function after ankle fusion is believed to be attributable to compensatory motion of the small joints of the ipsilateral foot; altered motion of the ankle of the contralateral limb, making the gait symmetrical; and the use of footwear with an appropriate heel height (Fig. 13–16). Radiographically identifiable complications of ankle arthrodesis include pseudarthrosis, malunion, infection, hardware impingement of the subtalar joint, and osteoarthritis of the small joints of the foot.

### Hip

Successful hip arthrodesis results in a painless, stable hip and the ability to engage in strenuous activity. It is therefore a procedure that should be considered in young patients with incapacitating pain from unilateral hip damage. The procedure can "buy time" and later be revised to a total hip replacement. Intra-articular arthrodesis includes removing the surface of the femoral head and acetabulum and then maintaining the femoral head in contact with the acetabulum by means of external or internal fixation or both. Graft material may also be used. The results of hip fusion are generally good. The major complications of hip arthrodesis are related to the inability to achieve solid fusion and the long-term effect of such surgery on other joints.

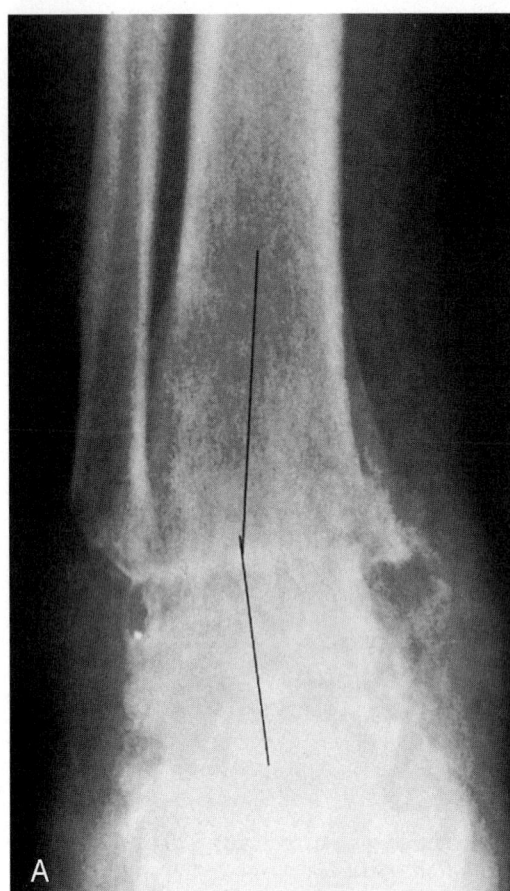 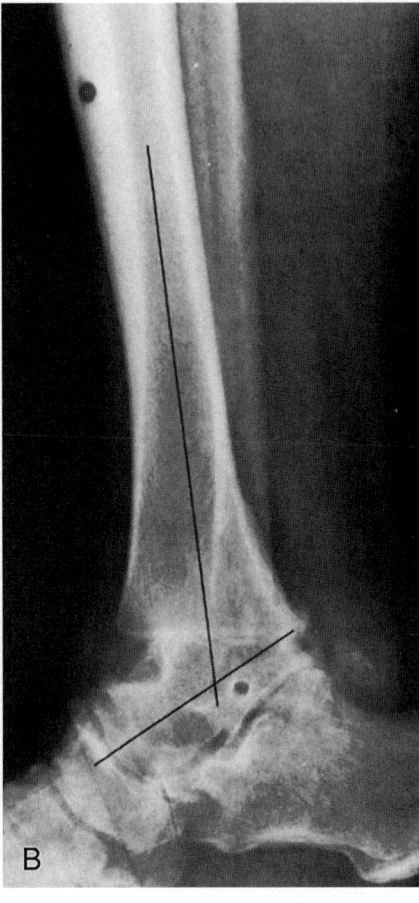

**Figure 13–16.** Ankle fusion. *A*, Anteroposterior view shows no remaining radiolucency along the tibiotalar surface, a sign of healing. Varus alignment is present between the long axis of the tibia and that of the talus. *B*, Lateral view does not include the bottom of the foot. The angle between the long axis of the tibia and the long axis of the talus (through its midportion) has been used to determine the degree of plantar flexion.

## OSTEOTOMY

The term *osteotomy* refers to the surgical cutting of bone. Osteotomies are usually performed to correct or reduce deformity. A closing wedge osteotomy refers to the removal of a triangular bony wedge from one side and approximation of the resection margins; an example is the intertrochanteric varus osteotomy. An opening wedge osteotomy is performed by cutting the bone at an angle to cause one side to open. The defect is then filled with bone graft. A rotational osteotomy consists of rotating the distal fragment on its long axis. A displacement osteotomy involves a shift in position of the distal fragment in relation to the proximal one. "Shish kebab" osteotomies are used to correct severe bowing deformities of the long bones, such as may occur in osteogenesis imperfecta. The shaft is cut in several places, and the fragments are threaded on an intramedullary rod.

### High Tibial Osteotomy

High tibial osteotomy is generally used in active patients younger than 65 years who have knee pain caused by osteoarthritis. Osteotomy allows patients to continue vigorous activities, including sports, and may be used as an interim procedure before total knee replacement is necessary. Surgical correction of the angular deformity by high tibial osteotomy is aimed at restoring the normal mechanical axis with overcorrection of about 3 to 5 degrees (Fig. 13–17).

### Proximal Femoral Osteotomy

High femoral osteotomy has been used effectively in relatively young patients for the treatment of osteoarthritis of the hip.

**Medial Displacement Osteotomy.** An oblique intertrochanteric osteotomy with maximum medial displacement of the distal fragment (Lorenz's osteotomy) transmits body weight directly from the pelvis to the distal femoral fragment. Rotation of the proximal fragment occurs inadvertently in some cases and produces better clinical results than those observed when displacement is unaccompanied by rotation. A displacement osteotomy with inadvertent rotation of the proximal fragment is similar to a varus osteotomy with medial displacement of the distal fragment.

**Adduction (Varus) and Abduction (Valgus) Osteotomy.** A varus osteotomy (Fig. 13–18*A*) is performed when the femoral head is essentially hemispherical, cartilage loss is evident in the superior and lateral portions of the joint, and the articulation is more congruent with the hip in abduction. In this procedure, a carefully measured wedge of bone, wider medially, is removed, and the femoral head is rotated medially (15 to 40 degrees) until the articular surfaces are congruent. The distal femoral fragment is displaced medially so that it is aligned with the mechanical axis of the leg.

A valgus osteotomy (see Fig. 13–18*B*) is considered when the femoral head is not hemispherical and when

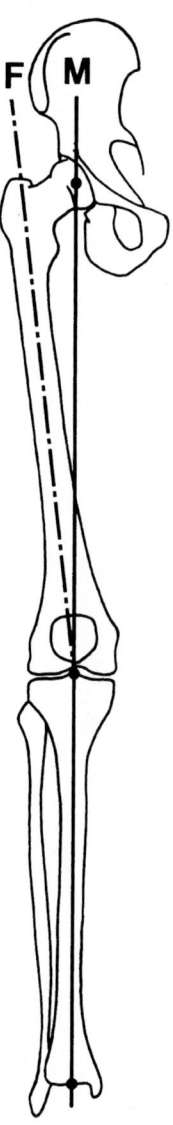

**Figure 13–17.** The mechanical axis. Normally, a straight line can be drawn from the center of the femoral head through the center of the knee to the center of the ankle. This line is the mechanical axis (M). The femoral shaft axis (F) normally deviates from the mechanical axis.

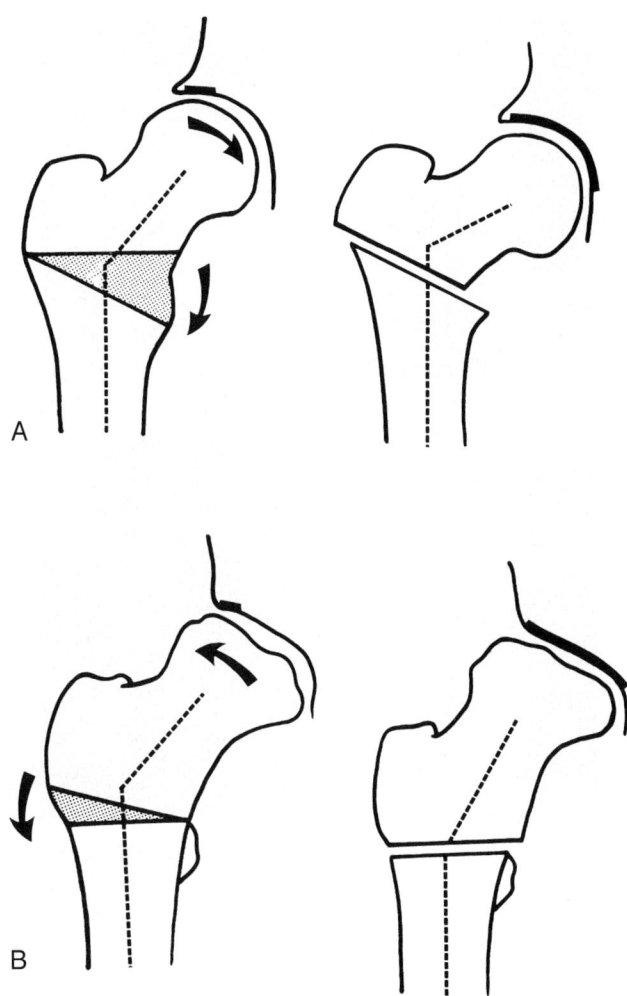

**Figure 13–18.** Femoral osteotomy. *A*, Varus osteotomy. *B*, Valgus osteotomy. (From Weissman BN, Sledge CB: Orthopedic Radiology. Philadelphia, WB Saunders, 1986.)

adduction improves congruency. A wedge of bone is removed that is wider laterally. The lower margin of the removed segment is at the level of the lesser trochanter and perpendicular to the femoral shaft. The femoral head is rotated laterally with some overcorrection so that the cartilage space is about 2 mm wider at the lateral acetabular margin than centrally. The distal fragment is displaced laterally.

### Radiologic Examination

In patients with eccentric loading (such as those with acetabular dysplasia), focal areas of subchondral sclerosis develop (Fig. 13–19). With a marked increase in stress, bone resorption and cyst formation occur. Thus, radiographs document uneven stress distribution, and if loading is improved postoperatively, these abnormal findings should regress. Postoperative radiographs document the degree of correction provided by the osteotomy, healing of the osteotomy site, and any regression of the preoperative osteoarthritic changes. The osteotomy site heals gradually,

with trabecular continuity normally achieved about 4 months after surgery. Evidence of bone resorption adjacent to the orthopedic appliances may be due to abnormal motion or infection (Fig. 13–20). Nonunion is indicated by the development of bone sclerosis and irregular bone resorption along the osteotomy surfaces.

### PROCEDURES FOR ISCHEMIC NECROSIS OF THE FEMORAL HEAD

Treatment strategies for ischemic necrosis of the femoral head are used before osseous collapse and include core decompression, bone grafting, rotational osteotomy, and angular osteotomy. Core decompression is a procedure in which a core of bone is removed, beginning in the lateral cortex of the femur just distal to the greater trochanter and terminating in the anterolateral segment of the femoral head. The rationale for core decompression is the finding of elevated bone marrow pressure in patients suspected of having ischemic necrosis, even when radiographs are normal.

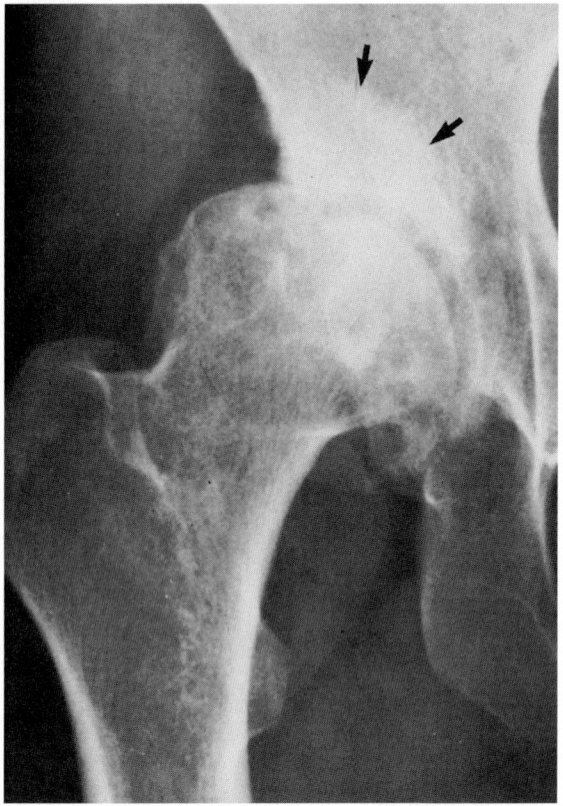

**Figure 13–19.** Acetabular dysplasia with secondary osteo-arthritis. Severe cartilage loss is accompanied by hypertrophic lipping. The abnormal stress on the acetabulum is reflected by the zone of bone sclerosis *(arrows)*.

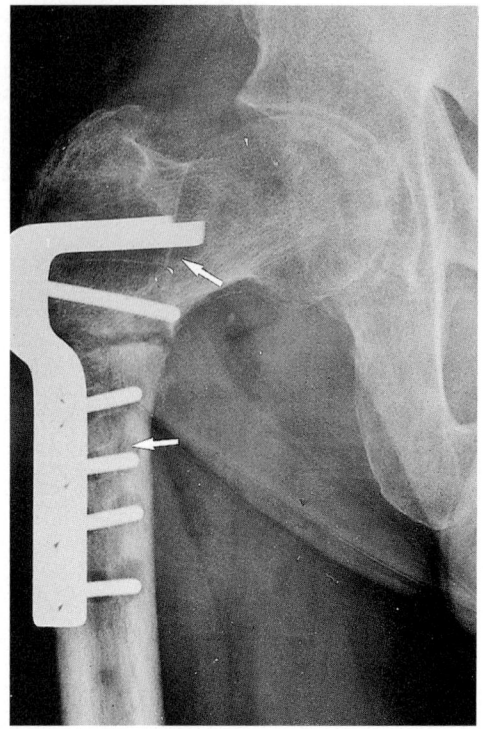

**Figure 13–20.** Delayed union of an intertrochanteric osteotomy. After intertrochanteric osteotomy, loosening of the hardware occurred, with subsequent areas of bone resorption evident *(arrows)*. No infection was found, and healing occurred after reoperation and immobilization.

Bone grafting is a procedure in which a core of bone is removed (as in the core decompression procedure), and the defect is filled with bone graft. Vascularized iliac or fibular grafts may be used in an attempt to revascularize a necrotic femoral head. The femoral head is reamed out and packed with cancellous bone graft. A fibular graft is then placed as far as possible into a tunnel drilled in the femoral head and neck for decompression and curettage. The vascularized fibular graft, its vascular supply, and a surrounding muscle cuff are positioned within the tunnel; thus, the graft alone does not entirely fill the tunnel. Follow-up radiographs should show incorporation of the proximal fibular graft, as evidenced by blurring of its margins, usually an average of 6 months after surgery.

## FURTHER READING

Barr JS, Record EE: Arthrodesis of the ankle joint: Indications, operative technique and clinical experience. N Engl J Med 248:53, 1953.

Bassett CAL: The development and application of pulsed electromagnetic fields (PEMFs) for ununited fractures and arthrodeses. Orthop Clin North Am 15:61, 1984.

Berrey BH, Lord CF, Gebhardt MC, et al: Fractures of allografts: Frequency, treatment and end results. J Bone Joint Surg Am 72:825, 1990.

Bowerman JW, Hughes JL: Radiology of bone grafts. Radiol Clin North Am 13:467, 1975.

Browner BD, Mast J, Mendes M: Principles of internal fixation. In Browner BD, Jupiter JB, Levine AM, et al (eds): Skeletal Trauma. Philadelphia, WB Saunders, 1992, p 243.

Buchholz HW, Elson RA, Heiner K: Antibiotic-loaded acrylic cement: Current concepts. Clin Orthop 190:96, 1984.

Chandler HP, Reineck FT, Wixson RL, et al: Total hip replacement in patients younger than thirty years. J Bone Joint Surg Am 63:1426, 1981.

Edmonson AS: Surgical techniques. In Edmonson AS, Crenshaw AH (eds): Campbell's Operative Orthopedics. St Louis, CV Mosby, 1980, p 19.

Enneking WF, Eady JL, Burchardt H: Autogenous cortical bone grafts in the reconstruction of segmental skeletal defects. J Bone Joint Surg Am 62:1039, 1980.

Girdlestone GR: Acute pyogenic arthritis of the hip: An operation giving free access and effective drainage. Clin Orthop 170:4, 1982.

Harrington KD, Johnston JO, Turner RH, et al: The use of methylmethacrylate as an adjunct in the internal fixation of malignant neoplastic fractures. J Bone Joint Surg Am 54:1665, 1972.

Harrington KD, Sim FH, Enis JE, et al: Methylmethacrylate as an adjunct in internal fixation of pathological fractures. J Bone Joint Surg Am 58:1047, 1976.

Hungerford DS, Zizic TM: Pathogenesis of ischemic necrosis of the femoral head. Hip 249, 1983.

Insall JN, Joseph DM, Msika C: High tibial osteotomy for varus gonarthrosis: A long-term follow-up study. J Bone Joint Surg Am 66:1040, 1984.

Kandel RA, Pritzker KPH, Langer F, et al: The pathologic features of massive osseous grafts. Hum Pathol 15:141, 1984.

Laros GS, Moore JF: Complications of fixation in intertrochanteric fractures. Clin Orthop 101:110, 1974.

Manaster BJ, Coleman DA, Bell DA: Pre- and postoperative imaging of vascularized fibular grafts. Radiology 176:161, 1990.

Mankin HJ, Doppelt S, Tomford W: Clinical experience with allograft implantation: The first ten years. Clin Orthop 174:69, 1983.

Masri BA, Duncan CP, Beauchamp CP: Long-term elution of antibiotics from bone-cement: An in vivo study using the prosthesis of antibiotic-loaded acrylic cement (PROSTALAC) system. J Arthroplasty 13:331, 1998.

Mears DC: External Skeletal Fixation. Baltimore, Williams & Wilkins, 1983.

Müller ME, Allgower M, Schneider R, et al: Manual of Internal Fixation: Technique Recommended by the AO Group. New York, Springer-Verlag, 1991.

Murray WR: Use of antibiotic-containing bone cement. Clin Orthop 190:89, 1984.

Sisk TD: Fractures. In Edmonson AS, Crenshaw AH (eds): Campbell's Operative Orthopedics. St Louis, CV Mosby, 1980, p 509.

Slone RM, Heare MM, Vander Griend RA, et al: Orthopedic fixation devices. Radiographics 11:823, 1991.

Stewart M: Arthrodesis. In Edmonson AS, Crenshaw AH (eds): Campbell's Operative Orthopedics. St Louis, CV Mosby, 1980, p 1113.

Wagner H: Principles of corrective osteotomies in osteoarthrosis of the knee. In Weil UH (ed): Progress in Orthopedic Surgery, vol 4. Joint Preserving Procedures of the Lower Extremities. New York, Springer-Verlag, 1980, p 75.

Weissman BN, Reilly DT: Diagnostic imaging evaluation of the postoperative patient following musculoskeletal trauma. Radiol Clin North Am 27:1035, 1989.

Young JWR, Kovelman H, Resnik CS, et al: Radiologic assessment of bones after Ilizarov procedures. Radiology 177:89, 1990.

# CHAPTER 14

## Imaging of Joint Replacement

### Barbara N. Weissman

## SUMMARY OF KEY FEATURES

As advances and improvements are made in joint replacement technology and surgical technique, imaging remains an important means of monitoring the patient's postoperative progress and identifying complications. Radiographs provide a permanent record of the procedure and can document success or failure of the operation. This chapter presents the information required for accurate interpretation of radiographs after various fixation devices and cement materials have been used. It also reviews the expected findings, both normal and abnormal, of total hip replacement, as well as replacement of the knee and shoulder. Complications of each operation are discussed, as are the uses of various imaging methods.

## INTRODUCTION

The modern era of total joint replacement began in the early 1960s with the introduction of metal-to-plastic hip prostheses embedded in methylmethacrylate cement. Changes over the years have included metal backing of the acetabular component, the development of modular design components and the bipolar prosthesis, the introduction of improved cement fixation, and the development of noncemented fixation.

## TOTAL HIP REPLACEMENT

### Radiographic Technique

Radiographs are critical for monitoring patients with total joint replacements. The standard radiographic series consists of an anteroposterior view of the pelvis centered at the pubis and an anteroposterior and frog-leg lateral view of the affected hip. Enough of the femoral shaft must be included to allow assessment of the size of the medullary canal preoperatively and the entire femoral component and adjacent bone postoperatively.

### Component Position

1. Acetabular inclination indicates the tilt of the acetabular component in relation to a horizontal baseline (Fig. 14–1A). An angle of inclination of 40 to 50 degrees has been classified as neutral, with lower measurements indicating a relatively horizontal orientation and greater measurements indicating a more vertical one.

2. Measurement of the position of the center of the hip is determined as the perpendicular distance from the center of the femoral head to a line connecting the teardrop shadows of both hips (interteardrop line; see Fig. 14–1B).

3. The distance along the interteardrop line from the intersection with a perpendicular line from the center of the femoral head to the teardrop allows comparison of the mediolateral position of the hip over time (see Fig. 14–1B). Changes of more than 2 mm are considered significant with 10% magnification.

4. Anteversion is usually determined from the true lateral view of the hip. A line parallel to the table or film edge provides the baseline in the coronal plane. The angle between a perpendicular to the baseline and the axis of the acetabular marker wire is the angle of anteversion (Fig. 14–2).

5. The tip of the femoral stem should appear on the frontal radiograph to be centered in the medullary canal or to be directed medially (valgus).

6. Leg length is compared on the two sides by noting the distances between the proximal edge of the lesser trochanters and a baseline through the ischial tuberosity on each side.

### Component Fixation

Four major methods of component fixation to bone are currently used: (1) press fitting, (2) fixation with polymethylmethacrylate (PMMA) cement; (3) bone ingrowth into porous surfaces, and (4) hydroxyapatite coating.

### Press Fitting

With press fitting of components, the surgically created bed for the prosthesis is made smaller than the prosthesis itself, which is then forced into the defect.

### Polymethylmethacrylate Cement Fixation

Cement provides immediate stable fixation and functions to distribute load more evenly to the bone. Improvements in cementing techniques have lowered the rates of loosening on the femoral side. On the acetabular side, however, a nearly linear increase in acetabular loosening has been reported, and improvements in cement technique are less applicable to the acetabular component. Currently, porous-coated acetabular implants are often matched with cemented femoral components for older, less active patients.

#### Radiologic Evaluation

Various radiologic methods are used to evaluate PMMA cement fixation.

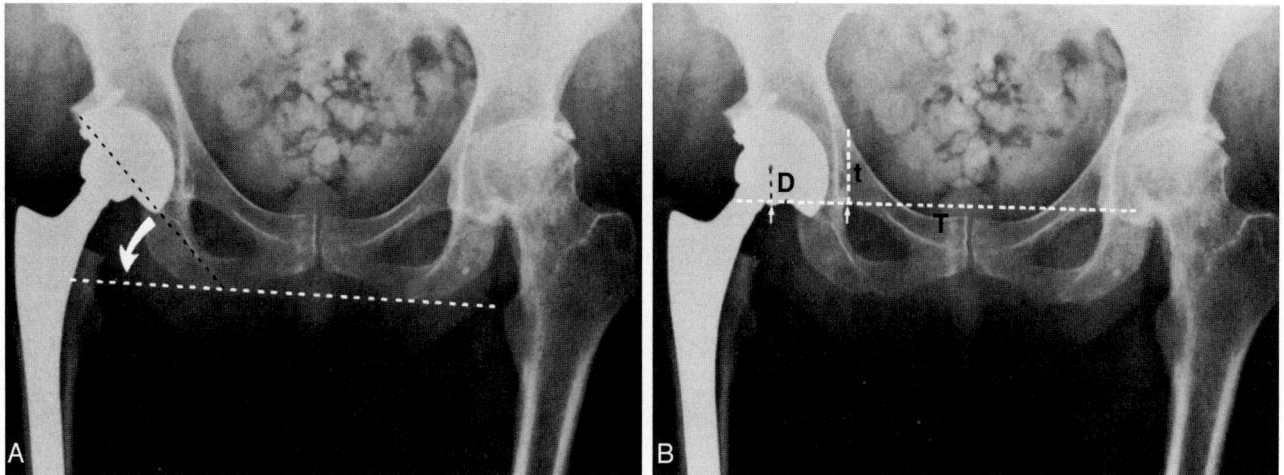

**Figure 14–1.** Component position. *A*, Angle of acetabular inclination. The angle between the baseline and the acetabular orifice *(curved arrow)* describes the tilt of the acetabular component in relation to the horizontal. *B*, Vertical and mediolateral position. The vertical position of the hip is measured as the perpendicular distance (D) from the center of the femoral head to the interteardrop line (T). The mediolateral position of the hip *(between arrows)* is measured as the distance along the interteardrop line from the teardrop (t) to the intersection with a perpendicular from the center of the femoral head.

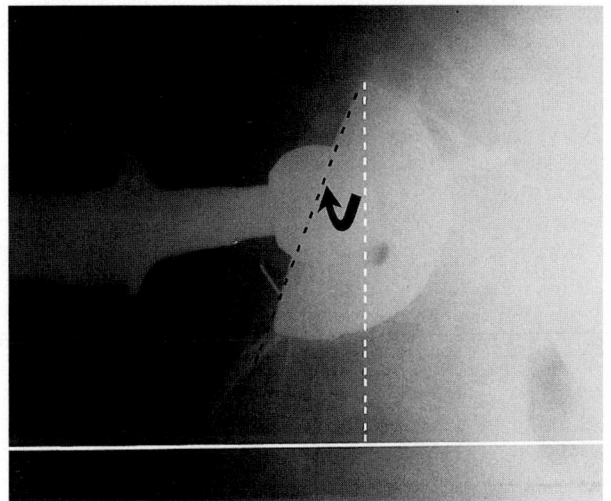

**Figure 14–2.** Acetabular anteversion. The angle *(curved arrow)* between the axis of the acetabular marker wire and a perpendicular to the baseline (parallel to the edge of the film) is the angle of acetabular anteversion.

**Radiography.** Methylmethacrylate transmits stress evenly to the underlying bone via interdigitation of the bone with the cement. On radiographs, thin lucent lines are often seen along the cement-bone interface (Fig. 14–3). These lucent lines generally represent the formation of a fibrous membrane without inflammation. The appearance usually becomes stable by 2 years, with a visible radiolucent zone 0.1 to 1.5 mm wide. Conventional nomenclature has been adapted to describe the regions of the prosthetic components (Fig. 14–4). The interface areas of the acetabulum are described as three zones, and the femoral zones are divided into seven regions.

**Arthrography.** Arthrography is performed most often to confirm intra-articular needle location at the time of attempted aspiration rather than to specifically identify component loosening. When the needle is placed at the medial margin of the head-neck junction, fluid is usually obtained. Instillation of nonbacteriostatic saline solution followed by reaspiration may be done when no fluid is forthcoming. Some authors suggest reaspiration of injected contrast medium, but this practice is controversial. After aspiration of fluid, contrast medium is usually injected until the patient has discomfort, lymphatic filling occurs, or contrast medium is seen along the cement-bone interface.

Theoretically, injected contrast material should remain confined the joint space (Fig. 14–5). Capsular extensions taking the form of bursae and cavities are not uncommon. Bursae are most frequently located adjacent to the greater trochanter and are usually large, smooth-walled extensions of the capsule. Infected cavities are typically irregular and have synovial proliferation and a narrow, irregular line of communication with the joint.

**Bone Scan.** Approximately 10% of asymptomatic patients display increased uptake in the acetabular region for more than 3 years. Uptake of the radiopharmaceutical agent stabilizes at the tip of the femoral stem by 10 to 12 months. Thereafter, an increase in uptake of the radionuclide at the tip of the femoral stem is thought to represent loosening.

### Complications

The major complications of cemented prostheses include loosening, infection, aggressive granulomatous disease, acetabular wear, dislocation, dissociation of components, heterotopic bone formation, and tumor.

**Loosening.** Loosening is the most common cause of failure of cemented prostheses. Improvements in cement technique have reduced loosening rates on the femoral side, but acetabular loosening has been found to increase

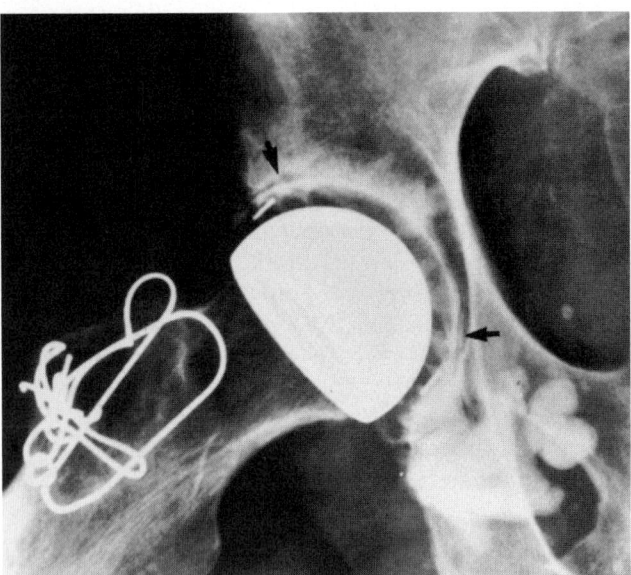

**Figure 14–3.** Lucent lines. A "normal," thin lucent line is present along a portion of the acetabular cement (*arrows*) of this surface replacement.

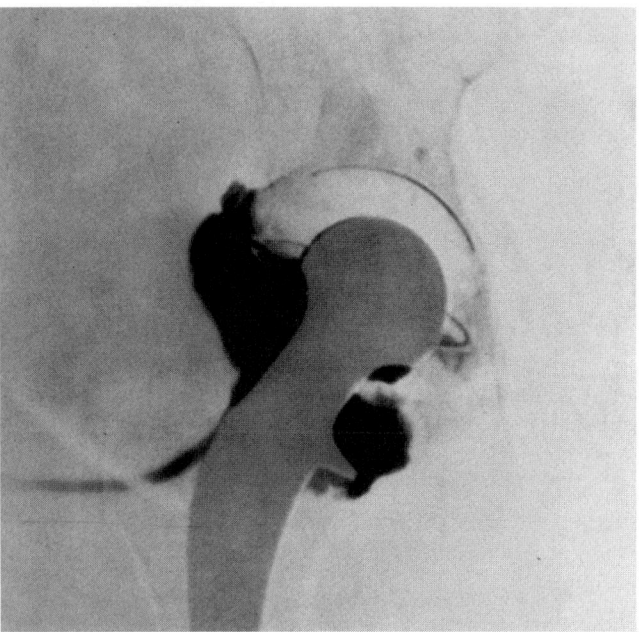

**Figure 14–5.** Subtraction arthrogram. No contrast material is present along the cement-bone interface of either component. The joint capsule is a little larger than usual.

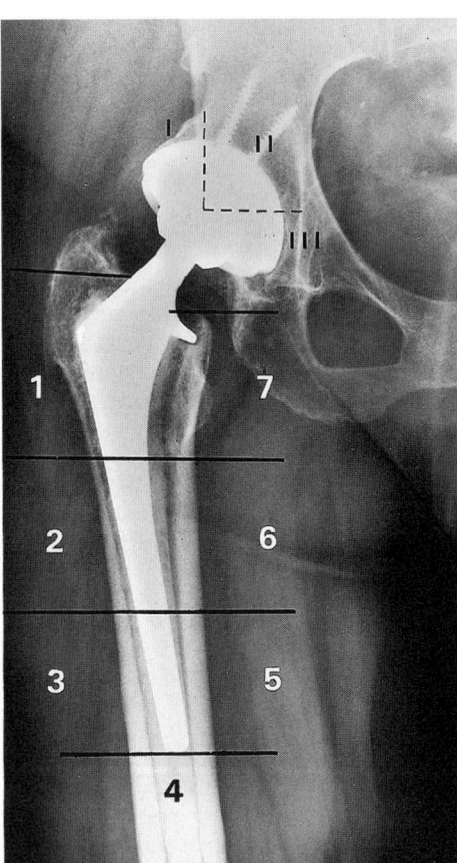

**Figure 14–4.** Reference zones. The zones of the acetabulum are described according to DeLee and Charnley, and those of the femur are described according to Gruen and coworkers. Additional zones are added for evaluation of the lateral radiograph.

with time, and efforts at improving cement fixation there have been less successful. The radiographic findings that suggest loosening of a cemented total hip prosthesis are listed in Table 14–1. Cement-bone lucent zones that are greater than 2 mm thick or zones that are increasing in thickness suggest component loosening. The finding of a wide lucent zone is thought to be more accurate in diagnosing loosening on the femoral side than on the acetabular side. The progressive development of a lucent line, however, indicates component motion. This appearance of loosening is termed subsidence; it represents sinking of the femoral component inferiorly and medially. Cement fracture is also indicative of prosthetic loosening (Fig. 14–6).

Definite loosening of the acetabulum is identified by component migration, and impending loosening is identified when a 2-mm continuous lucent zone is seen. Acetabular loosening that occurs relatively early (within 10 years) is thought to be the result of deficient bone support, whereas late loosening is probably the result of component wear. Femoral component loosening has been described as definite when radiographic evidence of component or cement migration is present, probable when a complete radiolucent zone is noted, and possible when a radiolucent line can be seen at the cement-bone interface and involves 50% to 100% of its interface.

Arthrography can be a useful adjunct in prosthesis evaluation. In general, arthrography is more useful for detecting femoral component loosening than acetabular component loosening. The accuracy of arthrography is decreased when the pseudocapsule is large or bursae are present. Reported arthrographic criteria for loosening of cemented components are widely used (Tables 14–2 and 14–3). Arthrography has a sensitivity and a specificity of more than 90% for the femoral component. On the

**TABLE 14–1**

### Radiographic Findings that Suggest Loosening, Infection, or Both, of Cemented Total Hip Prostheses

Cement–bone lucent zone of 2 mm or more
Widening of the cement–bone lucent zone
Migration of prosthetic components
Development or widening of metal-cement lucent zone
Cement fracture
Periosteal reaction
Motion of components demonstrable on stress views or fluoroscopy

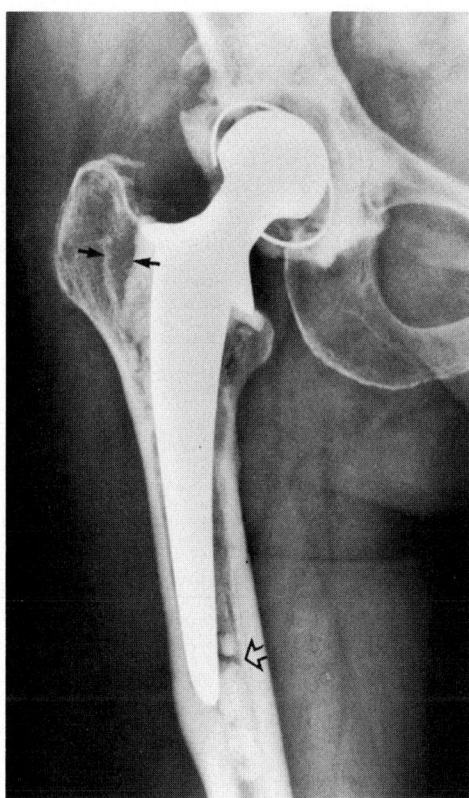

**Figure 14–6.** Loosening of a cemented femoral component with a cement fracture. Subsidence of the femoral stem has occurred, with settling of the stem into a varus position, development of a wide cement-bone interface laterally *(solid arrows)* and a cement fracture distally *(open arrow),* and thickening and remodeling of the femoral cortex near the tip of the prosthesis.

acetabular side, the sensitivity is greater than 90%, but specificity falls to approximately 68% (Fig. 14–7).

Anesthetic injection into a painful postoperative hip may help differentiate pain originating in the hip from that related to extra-articular sources. Lack of pain relief is nonspecific, but significant improvement in pain suggests an intra-articular cause.

**Infection.** Generally, infection or prosthetic loosening should be considered in all cases of painful cemented hip

**TABLE 14–2**

### Arthrographic Criteria for Acetabular Component Loosening

Contrast material in all zones (90%)*
Contrast material in zones I and II or in zones II and III
Contrast material in zones I and III with a medium or large pseudocapsule or bursa (57%)
Contrast material more than 2 mm thick in any zone (95%)
Positive signs on radiographs in a patient with a medium or large pseudocapsule or bursa

*Number in parentheses indicates the percentage of cases with this finding that exhibited prosthetic loosening at surgery.
From Maus TP, Berguist TH, Bender CE, et al: Arthrographic study of painful total hip arthroplasty: Refined criteria. Radiology 162:721, 1987.

**TABLE 14–3**

### Arthrographic Criteria for Femoral Component Loosening

Contrast material in prosthesis–cement interface below the intertrochanteric line (95%)*
Contrast material in the bone-cement interface extending below the intertrochanteric line in regular components or to the midcomponent level in long-stem prostheses (98%)

*Number in parentheses indicates the percentage of components that were loose at the time of surgery.
From Maus TP, Berguist TH, Bender CE, et al: Arthrographic study of painful total hip arthroplasty: Refined criteria. Radiology 162:721, 1987.

replacements in which extra-articular causes of pain have been excluded. Radiographic features of a rapidly developing, wide cement-bone lucent zone within the first postoperative year; endosteal scalloping; and periosteal reaction may indicate infection. The prevalence of infection in revision total hip arthroplasty is about four times as high as in primary hip replacement. In many institutions, therefore, aspiration arthrography is performed in virtually all cases before prosthetic revision. The results of aspiration arthrography vary, and both false-negative and false-positive results may occur.

Despite initial enthusiasm for bone scanning in the evaluation of complications of total hip replacement, recent studies indicate a more limited role for this examination. A normal bone scan does not necessarily exclude complications. The pattern of uptake on bone scanning has also turned out to be of less diagnostic value than originally thought, although a focal pattern of uptake (uptake at the proximal and distal ends of the femoral prosthesis) suggests loosening, whereas diffuse uptake suggests infection (Fig. 14–8). White blood cell scanning with [111]In labeling may improve the ability to diagnose infection, with an accuracy approaching 95%.

**Aggressive Granulomatous Disease (Cement Disease).** Descriptions of extensive localized areas of bone resorption around the femoral stems in patients with cemented total hip replacements led to the concept of "cement

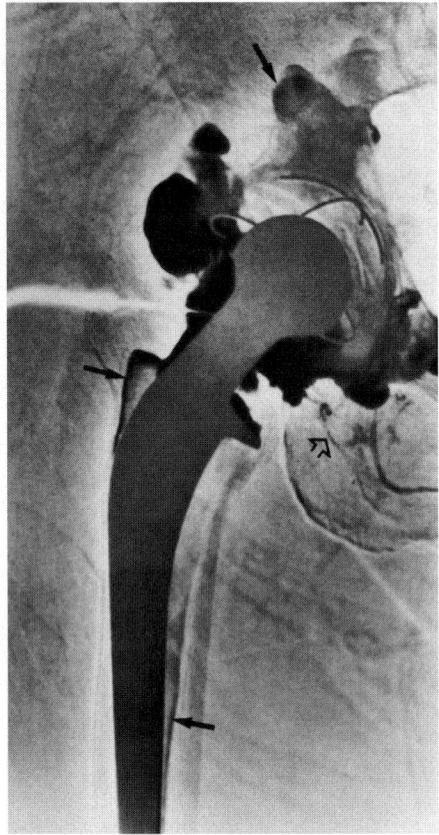

**Figure 14–7.** Loose cemented acetabular and femoral components shown on arthrography. The subtraction arthrogram shows the contrast medium (appearing dark) tracking along the cement around the femoral and acetabular components *(solid arrows)*. Faint lymphatic filling is present *(open arrow)*.

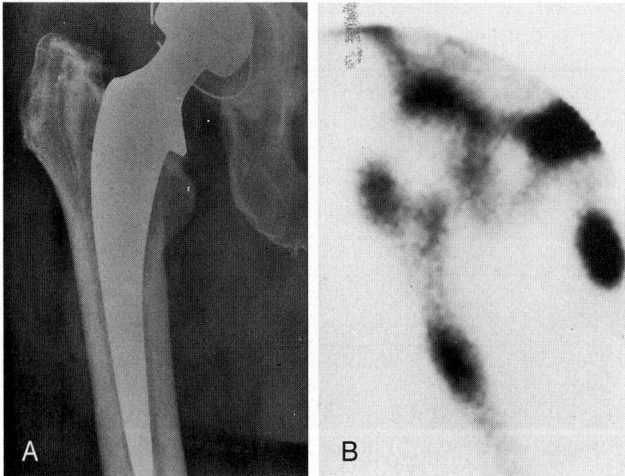

**Figure 14–8.** Focal uptake on bone scan. *A,* Note the radiographic evidence of loosening of the femoral component, with a wide metal-cement lucent zone. *B,* Bone scan demonstrates focal isotope uptake at the proximal and distal ends of the femoral component and along the acetabular component. (From Weissman BN: Current topics in the radiology of joint replacement surgery. Radiol Clin North Am 28:1111, 1990.)

disease," related to hypersensitivity and giant cell reaction to cement particles released during micromotion of the prosthesis. Prosthetic fixation without cement did not alleviate the problem, however. This condition has been reported in association with wear of both the methyl-methacrylate and polyethylene components, with and without prosthetic loosening, with and without cement fixation, with polyethylene particles alone, and without either cement or polyethylene. It appears that either PMMA cement or polyethylene can incite a giant cell response if the size, surface area, and rate of particle production are suitable. Osteolytic lesions appear on radiographs as well-defined focal areas of bone resorption that do not conform to the shape of the prosthesis. They occur most often near the tip of the femoral component or along its medial border but may also be seen adjacent to the acetabular component. Computed tomography may be a useful adjunct in evaluating the extent of aggressive granulomatous disease (Fig. 14–9).

**Acetabular Wear.** Most currently used prostheses consist of a combination of metal and high-density polyethylene. The decreased thickness of the acetabular polyethylene component seen on radiographs is thought to reflect a combination of abrasive wear, creep, and plastic deformation. Usually, however, the change in thickness of the polyethylene is taken as an indicator of wear and, therefore, an indicator of the production of wear debris.

**Prosthetic Dislocation.** Radiographs are essential for confirming prosthetic dislocation, defining any underlying cause, and disclosing any complications or conditions that may interfere with reduction. Generally, the diagnosis of prosthetic dislocation is readily apparent. Such dislocation is reported in as many as 6% of total hip or bipolar prostheses and occurs most often in the immediate postoperative period. When prosthetic dislocation occurs more than 3 months after surgery, malposition of an underlying component should be suspected.

**Dissociation of Prosthetic Components.** The original total hip prosthesis consisted of a high-density polyethylene acetabular component matched with a one-piece femoral head–stem component. Modifications to that design have included metal backing of the acetabular component (introduced in the 1970s to allow replacement of the worn acetabular liner), screws to stabilize the metal-backed components, modular femoral head and neck-stem components, attachable collars, distal and proximal sleeves, and a porous-coated surface. Complications may occur at each of the modular interfaces; they include metal debris from screw fretting, corrosion at the head-neck taper when different metals are used, dissociation of the femoral head from the neck, cracking of polyethylene liners at their superior surface, and separation and inferior rotation of the acetabular liner (Fig. 14–10).

**Heterotopic Bone Formation.** The cause of heterotopic bone formation after total hip replacement is unknown, although it is not uncommon. There is an increased prevalence in men with hypertrophic osteoarthrosis, previous heterotopic ossification or contralateral ossification, ankylosing spondylitis, diffuse idiopathic skeletal hyperostosis, post-

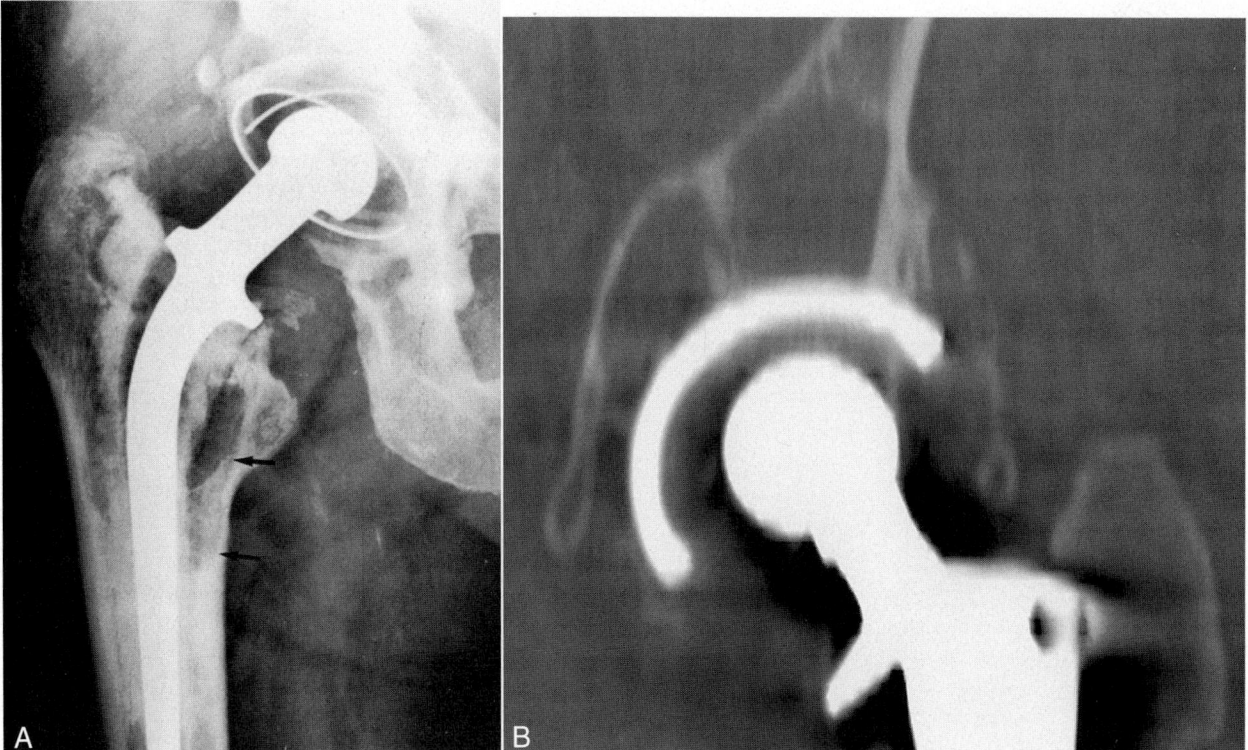

**Figure 14–9.** Aggressive granulomatous disease. *A*, Loosening of the cemented femoral stem is present, as shown by wide metal-cement lucent zones. Well-defined focal areas of bone destruction *(arrows)* indicate aggressive granulomatous disease. *B*, In another patient, a coronal reformatted computed tomography image shows extensive, aggressive granulomatous disease adjacent to the acetabular component. Note thinning of the polyethylene liner in the weight-bearing portion of the joint, indicative of polyethylene wear. (*A*, From Weissman BN: Current topics in the radiology of joint replacement surgery. Radiol Clin North Am 28:1111, 1990.)

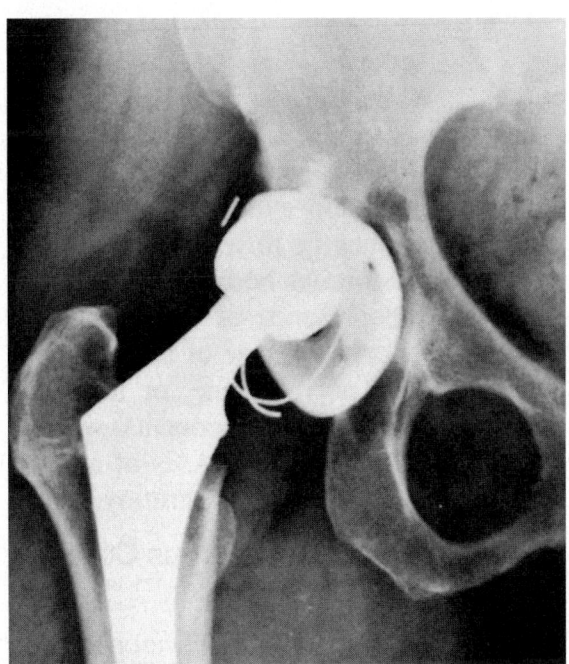

**Figure 14–10.** Acetabular disruption. Radiograph shows displacement of the bone ingrowth acetabular component from the bone and displacement of the acetabular liner (as shown by the marker wire).

traumatic arthritis, previous surgery, or extensive operative trauma. Radiographically, the ossification is usually visible by 2 to 4 weeks after surgery. The classification by Brooker and associates is a convenient method for grading the quantity of bone formed (Table 14–4).

**Tumor.** On rare occasion, malignant tumors have been associated with total hip replacements. Malignant lesions in patients with total joint replacement are of particular concern because of the possible carcinogenic effect of metals, polyethylene, and methylmethacrylate.

### Bone Ingrowth (Porous-Coated, Biologic) Fixation

Cementless fixation was developed with the goal of providing a durable arthroplasty with a lasting, satisfactory clinical result while avoiding cement and maintaining bone stock. The initial porous coatings made of ceramics and polymers have largely been replaced by porous metallic coatings applied to solid metal components (Fig. 14–11). Stabilization of bone ingrowth components may occur as a result of either bone or fibrous tissue ingrowth. Stabilization by bone ingrowth is indicated by the absence of reactive lines around the porous part of the implant and the presence of new bone filling the area between the endosteal surface and the porous portion of the implant (Fig. 14–12). When stabilization by fibrous tissue occurs,

### TABLE 14–4

**Grading of Heterotopic Ossification about the Hip**

| | |
|---|---|
| Class I | Islands of bone within soft tissue |
| Class II | Bone about the pelvis or proximal end of the femur, with at least 1 cm left between apposing bony surfaces |
| Class III | Bone about the pelvis or proximal end of the femur reducing the space between apposing bone surfaces to <1 cm |
| Class IV | Apparent bony ankylosis |

From Brooker AF, Bowerman JW, Robinson RA, Riley LH: Ectopic ossification following total hip replacement. Incidence and a method of classification. J Bone Joint Surg Am 55:1629, 1973

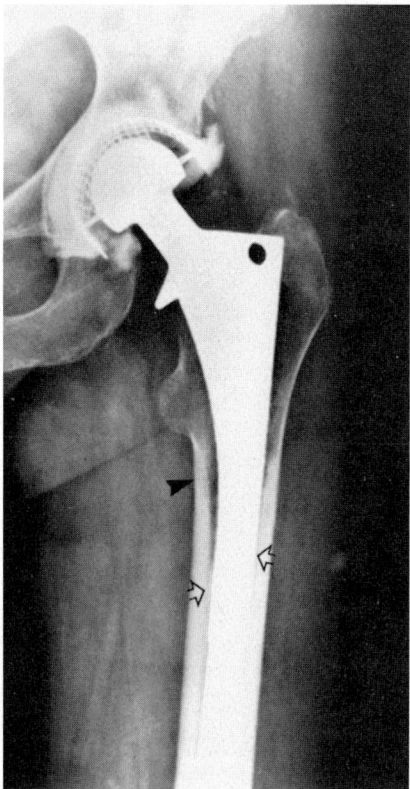

**Figure 14–12.** Stable porous-coated femoral stem with bone ingrowth. At a 4.5-year follow-up radiographic examination, new bone fills the gap from the cortex to the end of the bone ingrowth area *(arrows)*. Loss of bone has occurred proximally, with thinning of the cortices, bone loss from the medial femoral cortex, and loss of density of the cortex medially *(arrowhead)*, a process termed corticocancellization.

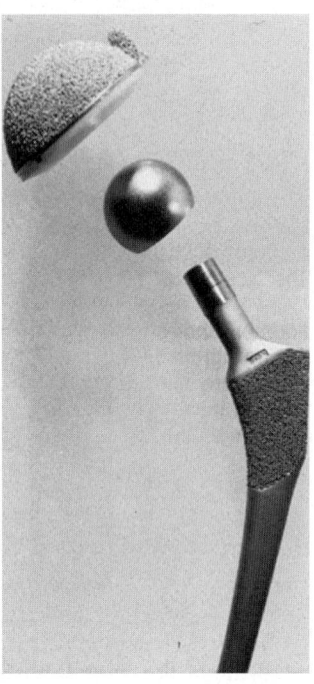

**Figure 14–11.** Bone ingrowth components. A polyethylene acetabular component is covered with a metallic cap. Note the irregularly coated portions of the acetabular and femoral components. The femoral head component is interchangeable, so some adjustment can be made in the length of the neck of the femoral component.

it is evident on radiographs obtained 1 year after surgery by the presence of thin sclerotic lines (demarcation lines) paralleling the porous surface of the implant and separated from it by a thin lucent zone. Stabilization of the prosthesis can be assessed in these cases only by further follow-up. If this interface remains unchanged and no change has occurred in the position of the prosthesis by 2 years after surgery, the component is probably held firm by strong fibrous tissue ingrowth and bone formation beneath the collar and at the stem tip. Conversely, if further migration of the prosthesis occurs, the prosthesis is unstable.

Several radiographic signs should be assessed when evaluating a bone ingrowth component, including (1) signs of bone or fibrous tissue ingrowth (spot welding and demarcation lines), (2) signs of stability or motion, and (3) signs of remodeling occurring as a result of changing stress (rounding, bone resorption or corticocancellization of the medial femoral cortex, hypertrophy of endosteal cancellous bone at the margin of the bone ingrowth surface, and cortical hypertrophy near the distal aspect of the stem). As indicated earlier, thin lucent zones with adjacent thin sclerotic lines (demarcation lines) may appear along the porous-coated portion of the prosthesis. Progression of lucent zones in either width or length has been noted to occur even in asymptomatic persons.

Evidence of bone ingrowth or the absence of signs of loosening indicates stability of the prosthetic components. Even in well-fixed prostheses, however, relative motion may occur between the prosthesis and the bone because of differences in their stiffness. A high frequency of radiolucent lines (bordered by thin sclerotic lines) has been noted along the smooth, uncoated portion of bone ingrowth prostheses and at the proximal portion of the femoral component laterally in the region of the greater trochanter.

Change in femoral component position over time may be more difficult to determine. Subsidence of more than 10 mm or that continuing after the first year are poor prognostic indicators. The significance of displacement of beads into the adjacent soft tissue depends on its chronology. Progressive displacement of beads suggests an unstable component.

Focal thickening of the femoral cortex may be generated by a number of mechanisms. It may reflect poor fixation of the prosthesis proximally and medially, with varus migration of the prosthesis. Loosening with mediolateral toggle produces a windshield wiper effect that results in thickening of the cortex both medially and laterally.

Stress shielding refers to loss of bone adjacent to a prosthesis when stress is diverted from the area. The presence of stress shielding therefore indicates that bone ingrowth has occurred. Bone loss caused by stress shielding is manifested on radiographs as intracortical tunneling (corticocancellization), rounding or bone resorption in the medial aspect of the femoral neck, and "periosteal atrophy," usually most prominent in the medial femoral cortex. Bone resorption as a consequence of wear debris and granuloma formation occurs late and is often progressive, whereas stress shielding occurs within the first year after surgery and stabilizes by the second postoperative year.

A pedestal is a shelf of new bone that develops at the tip of the femoral stem in response to increased load in the area. It may be associated with stable or unstable components. When the components are stable, no new radiolucent zones or reactive lines are present at the tip of the stem.

### Bipolar Prostheses

Bipolar hip prostheses were introduced as alternatives to hemiarthroplasty (e.g., Moore and Thompson prostheses). Theoretically, the increased motion at the articulation between the acetabular component and the femoral head allows less motion at the prosthesis-acetabular articulation and thus decreases acetabular wear. Other theoretical advantages of bipolar prostheses include a lower frequency of prosthetic dislocation and the ability to revise the acetabular component of a total hip replacement if the need arises. Complications of bipolar prostheses include fracture of the ipsilateral femur, component fracture and separation, abnormal wear of the acetabulum, and wear of the acetabular liner (Fig. 14–13).

The unipolar prosthesis has replaced the bipolar prosthesis in some cases. A unipolar prosthesis functions as a hemiarthroplasty but has modular components to allow adjustment of neck length.

### Hydroxyapatite-Coated Prostheses

Hydroxyapatite coating of prostheses allows chemical bonds to form with the adjacent bone and promotes bone apposition. It allows direct bone apposition without interposition of a fibrous membrane; therefore, radiographs can be expected to show bone in direct apposition to the prosthetic surface without an intervening lucent line. Follow-up evaluation 2 years or longer after the insertion of hydroxyapatite-coated prostheses has shown areas of new bone formation adjacent to the junction of the coated and uncoated segments of the prosthesis. Resorption of the calcar, presumably from stress shielding, occurs in almost half the cases. Cortical thickening of the femur occurs most often in zones 3 and 5. Remodeling generally occurs within the first postoperative year.

## TOTAL KNEE REPLACEMENT

Total knee replacement is used to alleviate pain and disability not responsive to medical management, particularly in cases of rheumatoid arthritis and osteoarthritis. Osteotomy is often preferred over total joint replacement in younger patients with osteoarthritis.

The term *total knee replacement* refers to the resurfacing of either the femorotibial compartments or the femorotibial and patellofemoral compartments. Three categories of total knee prostheses are described, according to the degree of stability (or constraint to knee motion) they provide. Nonconstrained components provide no inherent stability and allow considerable motion. Constrained prostheses provide inherent stability, so the cruciate or collateral ligaments of the knee need not be intact. These components limit motion of the joint. Semiconstrained prostheses are the most common. These types of prostheses include a group of cruciate-sparing prostheses, in which a posterior cutout allows the intact posterior cruciate ligament to remain in position, as well as a group of cruciate-sacrificing prostheses.

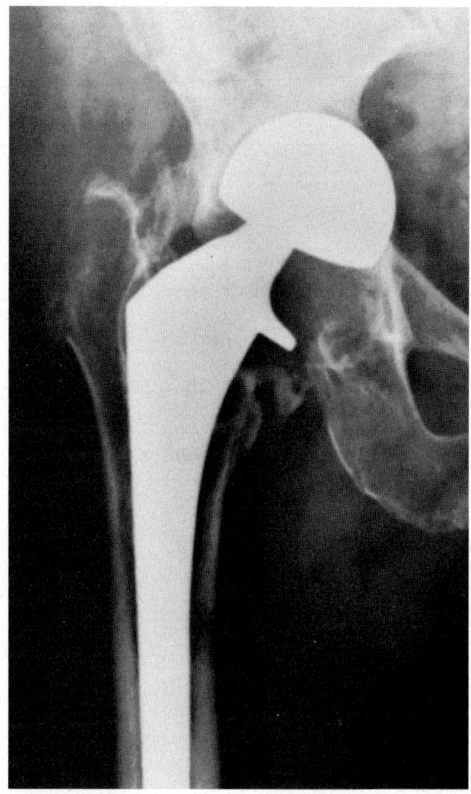

**Figure 14–13.** Bipolar prosthesis with acetabular protrusion. The bipolar prosthesis has migrated superomedially.

Unicompartmental (unicondylar) prostheses resurface both the femoral and the tibial sides of a damaged compartment (Fig. 14–14). They are used only in cases of osteoarthritis in which damage is limited to a single compartment and the ligaments are intact.

Total knee arthroplasty is an exacting operation that requires attention to the details of component positioning and the balance of soft tissue structures. The final tibiofemoral angulation of the knee should be 7 to 9 degrees of valgus, which should re-create the normal mechanical axis of the leg (determined by constructing a line from the center of the femoral head through the center of the knee and the center of the ankle).

## Postoperative Appearance

Anteroposterior views of the knee taken in the supine and standing positions, along with lateral and tangential patellar views, are routinely obtained for the follow-up of patients with total knee replacements. Fluoroscopy may be a useful adjunct for viewing the cement-bone interface in profile. In the normal situation, anteroposterior views show femorotibial alignment of 7 to 9 degrees of valgus. If standing views of the knee are obtained, the center of the knee should lie on the mechanical axis of the leg. The tibial component should be perpendicular in relation to the tibial shaft or in up to 2 degrees of varus alignment. Varus position of the tibial component refers to relative tilting of the component medially. On the lateral view, evaluation often includes assessment of the distance of the tibial component from the anterior and posterior tibial margins, the tilt of the tibial and femoral components in relation to the respective shafts of the tibia and femur, the distance from the center of the tibial component to the center of the tibia, and the height of the joint line. The position of the patellar component is judged on lateral and tangential patellar views.

A normal area of bone rarefaction occurs in the anterior portion of the femur, beneath the femoral component, in about two thirds of cases after total knee arthroplasty. This rarefaction represents bone loss in response to stress shielding and is not evidence of prosthetic loosening (Fig. 14–15).

## Complications

**Patellar Complications.** Revision surgery after total knee arthroplasty is most commonly necessitated by patellar complications. Stress fracture of the patella (Fig. 14–16), loosening of the patellar component, and dislocation or subluxation of the patellar component are the most common problems encountered.

**Prosthetic Loosening.** The incidence of prosthetic loosening seems to be less in the knee than in the hip. The tibial component is involved most often, and loosening develops most frequently at the cement-bone interface. A wide (≥2 mm) or enlarging lucent zone, collapse of subjacent trabecular bone, fragmentation of underlying cement, change in component position, development of a metal-cement lucent region, and change in the angulation of the knee on weight-bearing radiographs are indications of loosening of cemented components (Fig. 14–17). In addition, continued shedding of beads from the surface of bone ingrowth components after the first 3 to 6 months postoperatively suggests prosthetic loosening. Arthrography may confirm loosening of components by showing contrast agent insinuation within the cement-bone interface (Fig. 14–18).

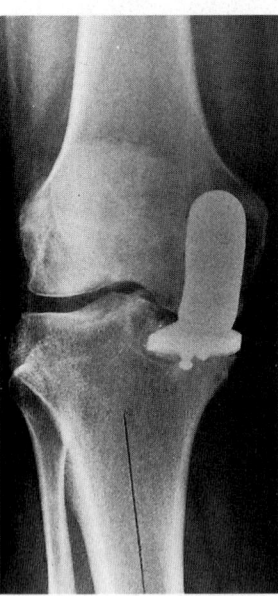

**Figure 14–14.** Loose unicondylar prosthesis. Radiography of the knee (obtained with the patient erect) shows a unicondylar replacement with overall varus alignment of the knee. Settling of the tibial component into the tibia has occurred, and a 1-mm cement-bone lucent zone is visible beneath the tibial component cement. Probable wear of the tibial articular surface is present.

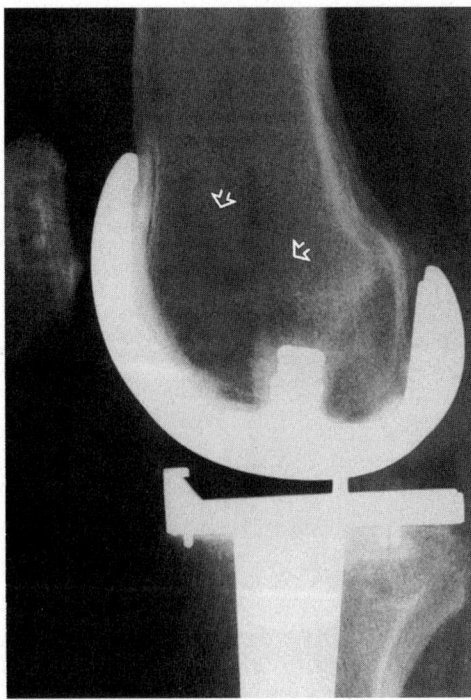

**Figure 14–15.** Stress changes in the femur after total knee replacement. A poorly defined area of osteopenia without a sclerotic margin is noted in the anterior aspect of the femur (*arrows*).

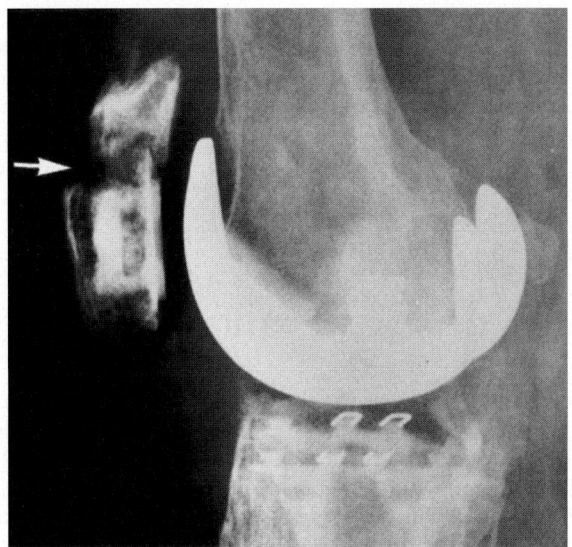

**Figure 14–16.** Patellar fracture. Transverse fracture has occurred at the bone-prosthesis interface. (From Weissman BN, Sledge CB: Orthopaedic Radiology. Philadelphia, WB Saunders, 1986, p. 580.)

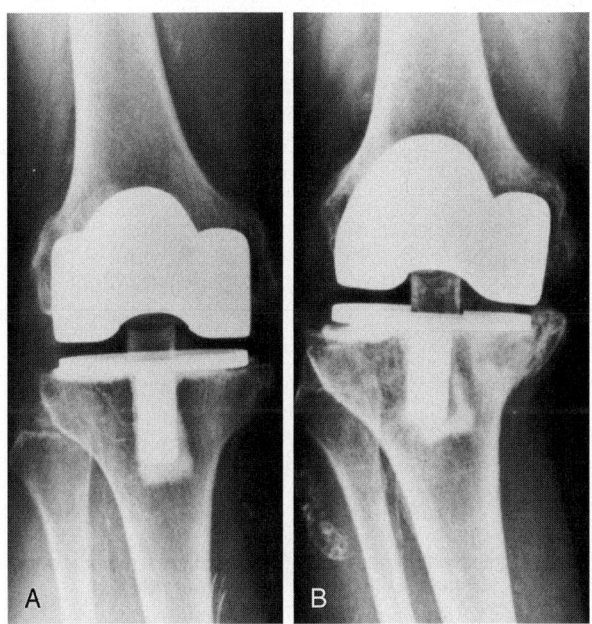

**Figure 14–17.** Tibial component loosening. *A,* The initial standing radiograph shows the knee in slight varus alignment. The tibial component is small in comparison to the width of the tibial plateau. *B,* Standing radiograph 7 years later documents shift of the tibial component position, with sinking of its medial aspect, metal-cement lucent areas laterally and at the tibial stem, increased varus alignment, and thinning of the medial polyethylene liner consistent with wear.

**Prosthetic Wear.** Deposition of metal in the joint after total knee replacement may be caused by wear of a metal-to-metal hinge or wear of polyethylene articular surfaces. The consequent shedding of metal into the joint may be visible as a curvilinear radiodense line outlining the joint capsule ("metal line" sign) or as diffuse opacity of the

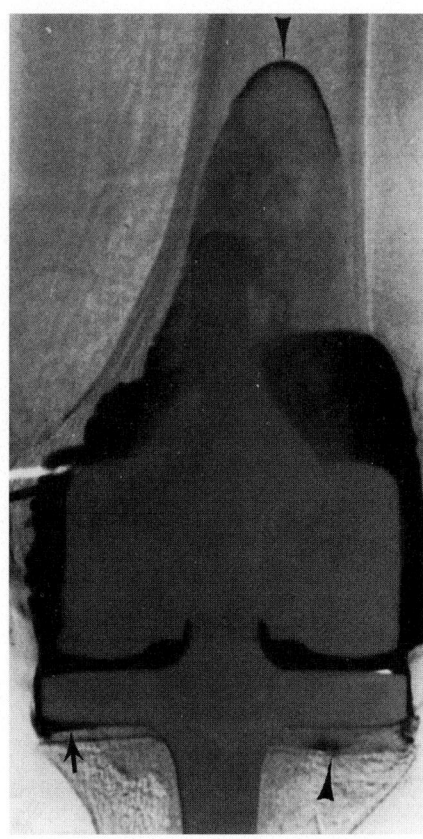

**Figure 14–18.** Prosthetic loosening demonstrated at arthrography. Subtraction arthrogram demonstrates contrast material entering the metal-cement interface of the tibial component *(arrow),* as well as the bone-cement interface of both components *(arrowheads).*

joint fluid (Fig. 14–19). Titanium is particularly prone to such wear. Wear debris consisting of polyethylene, metal, or both may result in the formation of a hypertrophic synovium-like membrane capable of producing substances that induce bone resorption. In the knee, as in the hip, bone cement is not necessary for a foreign body membrane to form or for osteolysis to occur.

**Infection.** Infection is the most frequent reason for failure of a total knee prosthesis. Although infections may occur early in the postoperative course, their appearance may be delayed for several years, particularly in patients with rheumatoid arthritis.

## TOTAL SHOULDER REPLACEMENT

Total shoulder prostheses restore the normal anatomic relationships and provide functional stability. A number of shoulder prostheses have been developed. Loosening of the glenoid component and component instability seem to be the complications that necessitate revision most often. Superior subluxation of the humeral head occurs quite often, particularly in patients with rheumatoid arthritis and nonconstrained components, but it may not result in a poor clinical outcome. The posterior oblique radiograph with the humerus in external rotation is the single most

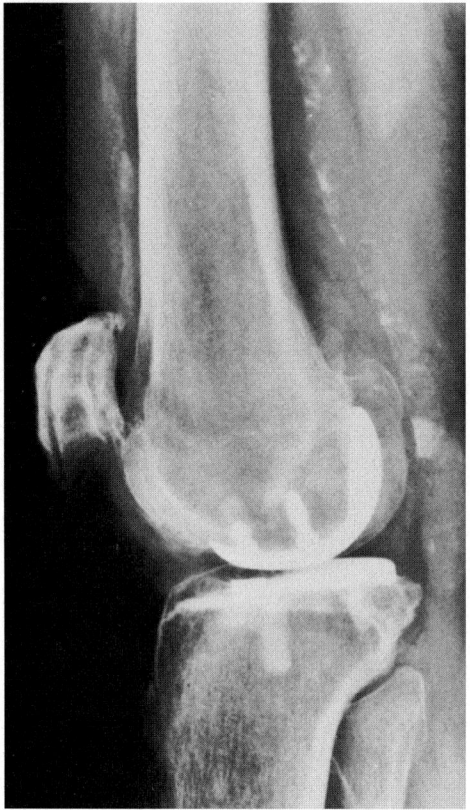

**Figure 14–19.** Metal synovitis. Lateral radiograph of a patient with a medial unicondylar prosthesis shows a dense white line in the suprapatellar pouch, indicative of metal synovitis ("metal line" sign). This finding resulted from wear of the tibial component.

informative postoperative radiograph. An internal rotation view of the shoulder is usually added to complete the routine examination. Lucent zones delineated by thin lines of sclerosis occur more often along the glenoid

components of total shoulder prostheses than along the humeral components. Cement-bone lucent zones wider than 2 mm raise the suspicion of component loosening. The glenoid component may become completely dislodged from the underlying bone and lie free within the joint. Subluxation or dislocation may occur early or late in the postoperative course. Infection is a less common complication than joint instability or prosthetic loosening.

## SILICONE RUBBER PROSTHESES

Silicone rubber elastomer prostheses have been used for replacement of the metacarpophalangeal and interphalangeal joints, radiocarpal articulation, carpal bones (especially the scaphoid), ulnar styloid, radial head, disc of the temporomandibular joint, and first metatarsophalangeal joint. Silicone rubber prostheses are only slightly denser than soft tissue on radiographs, making the components difficult to identify. Complications associated with silicone prostheses include fracture, silicone-induced synovitis, infection, implant dislocation, and recurrent deformity. Fractures of silicone rubber prostheses are quite frequent in some locations.

Silicone synovitis is a response to the shedding of silicone particles from prostheses that are damaged by shear and compressive forces. The radiographic appearance of silicone synovitis is typical. Deformity or fracture of the prosthesis may be visible but is not always apparent. Well-defined subchondral lucent defects and erosions (often with thin sclerotic margins), preservation of cartilage spaces, and soft tissue swelling are typical features. Osteoporosis is not a prominent finding, allowing differentiation of this condition from infection. Magnetic resonance imaging may theoretically play a role in the diagnosis of this condition; these prostheses and their particles are low in signal intensity on T1- and T2-weighted images (Fig. 14–20).

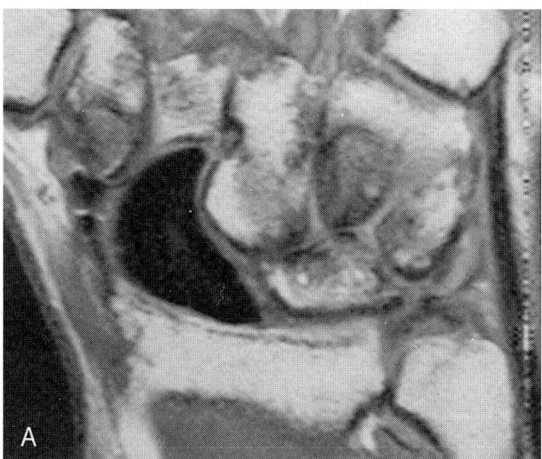
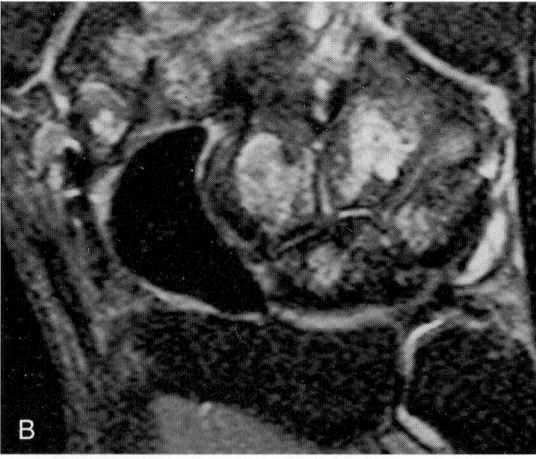

**Figure 14–20.** Silicone synovitis. A Silastic implant was used to replace a fractured scaphoid bone. *A,* Coronal T1-weighted (TR/TE, 733/20) spin echo magnetic resonance (MR) image shows the signal void of the scaphoid implant. Note the regions of intermediate signal intensity in multiple carpal bones, corresponding to fluid within cystic lesions. The lunate-capitate joint space is narrowed. *B,* Coronal short tau inversion recovery (STIR) MR image (TR/TE, 2000/30; inversion time, 140 msec) reveals the implant of low signal intensity and carpal cysts and joint fluid of high signal intensity. Small particles of Silastic are evident in the radial aspect of the wrist. (Courtesy of S. Eilenberg, MD, San Diego, Calif.)

# FURTHER READING

Barrack RL, Harris WH: The value of aspiration of the hip joint before revision total hip arthroplasty. J Bone Joint Surg Am 75:66, 1993.

Barrack RL, Tanzer M, Kattapuram SV, et al: The value of contrast arthrography in assessing loosening of symptomatic uncemented total hip components. Skeletal Radiol 23:37, 1994.

Bergstrom B, Lidgren L, Lindberg L: Radiographic abnormalities caused by postoperative infection following total hip arthroplasty. Clin Orthop 99:95, 1974.

Charnley J: Arthroplasty of the hip: A new operation. Lancet 1:1129, 1961.

Chew FS, Lev MH: Polyethylene osteolysis. AJR Am J Roentgenol 159:1254, 1992.

Dussault RG, Goldman AB, Ghelman B: Radiologic diagnosis of loosening and infection in hip prostheses. J Can Assoc Radiol 28:119, 1977.

Fackler CD, Poss R: Dislocation in total hip arthroplasties. Clin Orthop 151:169, 1980.

Gruen MS, McNeice GM, Amstutz HC: "Modes of failure" of cemented stem-type femoral components. Clin Orthop 141:17, 1979.

Harris WH, Barrack RL: Contemporary algorithms for evaluation of the painful total hip replacement. Orthop Rev 22:531, 1993.

Harris WH, Barrack RL: Developments in diagnosis of the painful total hip replacement. Orthop Rev 22:439, 1993.

Insall JN: Presidential address to the Knee Society: Choices and compromises in total knee arthroplasty. Clin Orthop 226:43, 1988.

Jaffe WL, Scott DF: Total hip arthroplasty with hydroxyapatite-coated prostheses. J Bone Joint Surg Am 78:1918, 1996.

Johnston RC, Fitzgerald RH, Harris WH, et al: Clinical and radiographic evaluation of total hip replacement. J Bone Joint Surg Am 72:161, 1990.

Kattapuram SV, Lodwick GS, Chandler H, et al: Porous-coated anatomic total hip prostheses: Radiographic analysis and clinical correlation. Radiology 174:861, 1990.

Lieberman JR, Huo MH, Schneider R, et al: Evaluation of painful hip arthroplasties. J Bone Joint Surg Br 75:475, 1993.

Lindstrand A, Stenström A: Polyethylene wear of the PCA unicompartmental knee. Acta Orthop Scand 63:260, 1992.

Maus TP, Berquist TH, Bender CE, et al: Arthrographic study of painful total hip arthroplasty: Refined criteria. Radiology 162:721, 1987.

Mian SW, Truchly G, Pflum FA: Computed tomography measurement of acetabular cup anteversion and retroversion in total hip arthroplasty. Clin Orthop 276:206, 1992.

O'Neill DA, Harris WH: Failed total hip replacement: Assessment by plain radiographs, arthrograms, and aspiration of the hip joint. J Bone Joint Surg Am 66:540, 1984.

Oswald SG, Van Nostrand D, Savory CG, et al: Three-phase bone scan and indium white blood cell scintigraphy following porous coated hip arthroplasty: A prospective study of the prosthetic tip. J Nucl Med 30:1321, 1989.

Resnick D, Kerr R, André M, et al: Digital arthrography in the evaluation of painful joint prostheses. Invest Radiol 19:432, 1984.

Thomas BJ: Heterotopic bone formation. In Harlan CA (ed): Hip Arthroplasty. New York, Churchill Livingstone, 1991, p 405.

Tigges S, Stiles RG, Meli RJ, et al: Hip aspiration: A cost-effective and accurate method of evaluating the potentially infected hip prosthesis. Radiology 189:485, 1993.

Weissman BN: Current topics in the radiology of joint replacement surgery. Radiol Clin North Am 28:1111, 1990.

Weissman BN: Radiographic evaluation of total joint replacement. In Kelley WN, Harris ED, Ruddy S, Sledge CB (eds): Textbook of Rheumatology, 4th ed. Philadelphia, WB Saunders, 1993, p 1881.

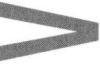
# Rheumatoid Arthritis and Related Diseases

# CHAPTER 15

## Rheumatoid Arthritis and the Seronegative Spondyloarthropathies: Radiographic and Pathologic Concepts

## SUMMARY OF KEY FEATURES

The pathologic and radiographic abnormalities associated with articular involvement in rheumatoid arthritis and the seronegative spondyloarthropathies (ankylosing spondylitis, psoriatic arthritis, Reiter's syndrome) are similar in many respects. Involvement of synovial and cartilaginous joints, bursae, tendon sheaths, entheses, tendons, ligaments, soft tissues, and bones can be encountered in any of these disorders. The distribution and extent of abnormalities differ among these diseases, however. In rheumatoid arthritis, alterations in synovium-lined articulations, bursae, and tendon sheaths frequently overshadow those in cartilaginous joints and sites of tendon and ligament attachment to bone. In ankylosing spondylitis, psoriatic arthritis, and Reiter's syndrome, abnormalities can be severe at cartilaginous articulations, including the discovertebral and manubriosternal joints and symphysis pubis. In addition, in those three conditions, a peculiar enthesopathy produces bone erosion and proliferation at tendo-osseous junctions.

## INTRODUCTION

Rheumatoid arthritis and the seronegative spondyloarthropathies (ankylosing spondylitis, psoriatic arthritis, and Reiter's syndrome) have many radiographic and pathologic characteristics in common. They affect synovium-lined joints, bursae, and tendon sheaths; cartilaginous articulations; entheses, or sites of ligamentous and tendinous attachment to bone; soft tissues; and bones. They lead to inflammation in a variety of tissues, and although the distribution and extent of abnormalities at specific target areas in the body vary among the disorders, the musculoskeletal effects of this inflammation are fundamentally similar.

## RHEUMATOID ARTHRITIS

### Overview

The major abnormalities of rheumatoid arthritis appear in synovial articulations of the appendicular skeleton, particularly the small joints of the hand and foot, the wrist, the knee, the elbow, and the glenohumeral and acromioclavicular joints. The synovial articulations of the axial skeleton may also be affected, especially the apophyseal and atlantoaxial joints of the cervical spine. In most of these synovium-lined cavities, changes are distributed symmetrically on the right and left sides of the body and consist of fusiform soft tissue swelling, regional osteoporosis, diffuse loss of joint space, marginal and central erosions, and fibrous ankylosis. The synovium of bursae and tendon sheaths is also affected. Abnormalities of cartilaginous articulations and entheses are less frequent and extensive, with the exception of the discovertebral joints of the cervical spine.

### Synovial Joints

**General Enzymatic Factors.** The fundamental target area in rheumatoid arthritis is the synovium, which lines the articulation. Rheumatoid synovitis is the result of a cellular immune response to an antigen present in the synovial membrane. The precise identity of this antigen is not clear; however, the response to it includes the production of a number of factors that lead to the formation of an erosive pannus and inflammatory mediators that induce joint destruction (Table 15–1).

**Synovial Membrane.** The earliest recognizable pathologic abnormality in rheumatoid arthritis is acute synovitis, which is associated with congestion and edema of the synovial membrane (Fig. 15–1). Capillary proliferation

---

**TABLE 15–1**

**Abnormalities of Synovial Joints in Rheumatoid Arthritis**

| Pathologic | Radiologic |
|---|---|
| Synovial inflammation and production of fluid | Soft tissue swelling and widening of joint space |
| Hyperemia | Osteoporosis |
| Pannus destruction of cartilage | Narrowing of joint space |
| Pannus destruction of "unprotected" bone at margin of joint | Marginal bony erosions |
| Pannus destruction of subchondral bone | Bony erosions and formation of subchondral cysts |
| Fibrous and bony ankylosis | Bony ankylosis |
| Laxity of capsule and ligaments and muscular contraction and spasm | Deformity, subluxation, dislocation, fracture, fragmentation, and sclerosis |

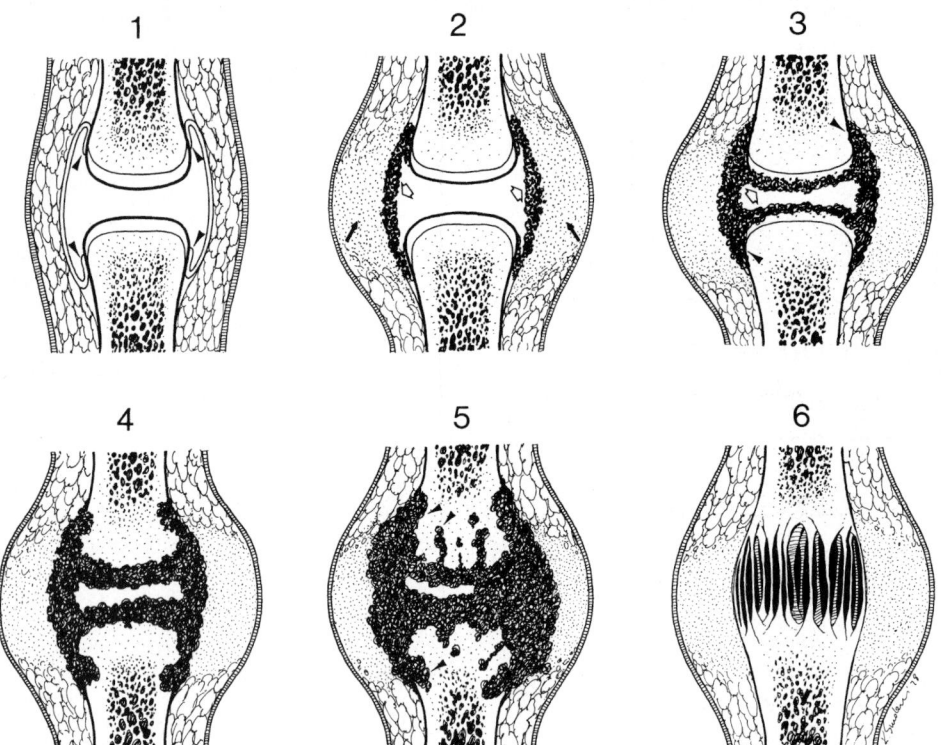

**Figure 15–1.** Synovial joint abnormalities in rheumatoid arthritis: pathologic overview. In a normal joint (1), observe the articular cartilage and synovial membrane. At the edges of the articulation *(arrowheads)*, synovium abuts on bone that does not possess protective cartilage. The very early abnormalities of rheumatoid arthritis (2) consist of synovial proliferation *(open arrows)*, soft tissue edema *(solid arrows)*, and osteoporosis. At a slightly later stage (3), the inflamed synovial tissue or pannus *(open arrow)* has extended across the cartilaginous surface and is leading to chondral erosion. Capsular distention, soft tissue edema, and osteoporosis are seen. Small osseous erosions at the margins of the joint are appearing *(arrowheads)*. In more advanced stages (4, 5), large marginal and central erosions and "cysts" are noted *(arrowheads)*. In advanced rheumatoid arthritis (6), fibrous ankylosis of the joint is typical.

and abnormal permeability are accompanied by exudation of plasma and fibrin precipitation. Accumulation of erythrocytes results from altered capillary permeability, and phagocytosis of these cells leads to hemosiderin deposition. These microscopic abnormalities result in a macroscopically evident thickened and injected synovial membrane. Continued proliferation may produce a bulky, hypervascular synovial tissue that superficially resembles a tumor. This tissue projects into the joint lumen as villous fronds containing many cells that maintain contact with the synovial fluid.

The pathologic findings described occur in the "synovial" stage of rheumatoid arthritis and are accompanied by characteristic radiographic abnormalities (Fig. 15–2). Accumulation of synovial inflammatory tissue within the joint, an increase in intra-articular fluid, capsular distention, and surrounding soft tissue edema lead to one early radiographic finding of the disease—soft tissue swelling. The periarticular soft tissue prominence is generally distributed symmetrically or is fusiform in configuration. In response to the hyperemia provoked by synovial inflammation, regional or periarticular osteoporosis—the second

early radiographic sign of rheumatoid arthritis—can be demonstrated. This finding, which is not invariable, produces thinning and small areas of discontinuity or gaps (dot-dash pattern) in the subchondral bone plate.

**Articular Cartilage.** After an acute inflammatory episode, the inflamed synovium soon spills from the peripheral portion and marginal pockets of the joint and grows toward the cartilaginous tissue. The synovial tissue applied to the articular cartilaginous surface causes morphologic changes. These changes result from enzymatic destruction of cartilage, interference with proper cartilaginous nutrition, or both. Cartilage destruction may ultimately become widespread and severe; when the cartilaginous surface on two apposing bones is significantly compromised, granulation tissue may bridge the articular cavity.

The radiographic counterpart of this "cartilaginous" stage of rheumatoid arthritis is loss of the articular space (see Fig. 15–2). Classically, joint space diminution is a relatively early finding in the disease, and it may appear within a period of weeks or months in some patients. Along with soft tissue swelling and periarticular osteoporosis, joint

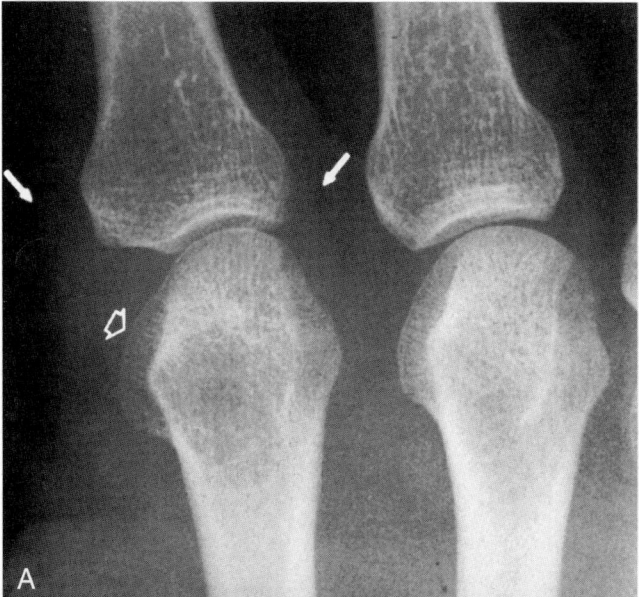

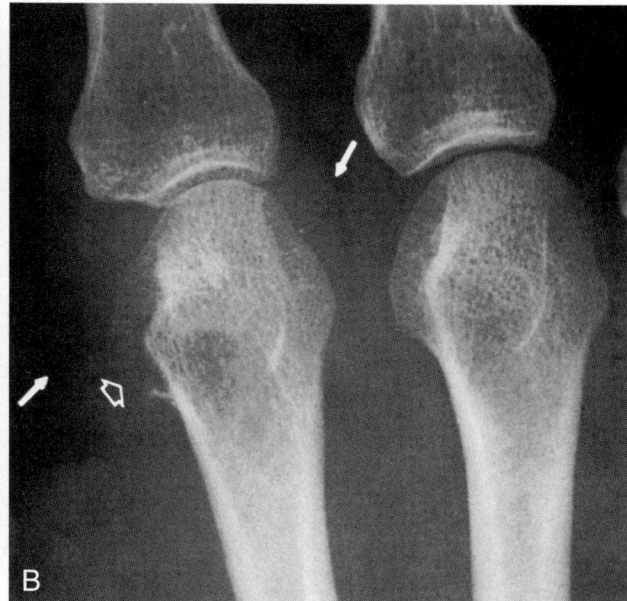

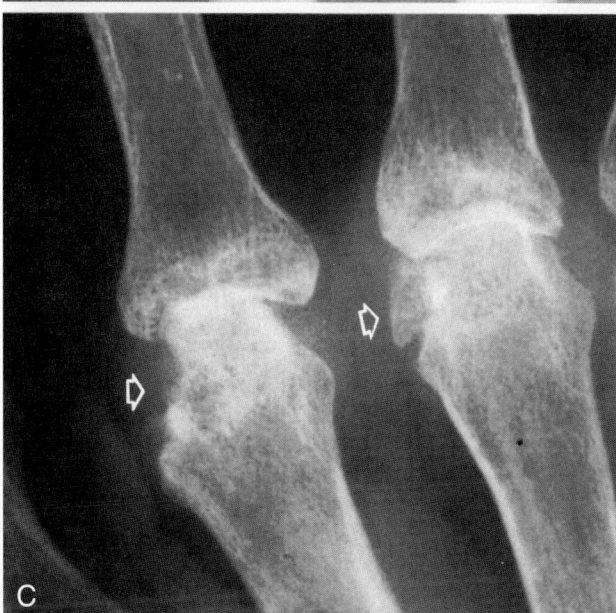

**Figure 15–2.** Synovial joint abnormalities in rheumatoid arthritis: sequential radiographic changes in metacarpophalangeal joints. *A*, The earliest abnormalities consist of soft tissue swelling *(solid arrows)*, periarticular osteoporosis, loss of a portion of the subchondral bone plate on the metacarpal head *(open arrow)*, and minimal joint space narrowing. *B*, With progression, increases in soft tissue swelling *(solid arrows)* and osteoporosis are associated with marginal erosions of the metacarpal heads *(open arrow)*. *C*, The later stages of rheumatoid arthritis are characterized by complete obliteration of the articular space and large central and marginal osseous erosions *(open arrows)*.

space narrowing is one of three early radiographic characteristics of rheumatoid arthritis. Loss of the articular space is usually diffuse or widespread because of the generalized nature of the cartilaginous destruction. This pattern of articular space diminution differs from the focal, segmental, or asymmetrical type of joint space loss that occurs in osteoarthritis.

**Subchondral Bone.** Two alterations in subchondral bone that occur in the early stages of rheumatoid arthritis are osteoporosis and marginal erosion. Osteoporosis, which can progress with time and eventually extend along the adjacent diaphyses, is related to a combination of disuse of the articulation, osteoclastic resorption of the subchondral spongy trabeculae, and steroid-induced bone changes.

The initial erosions in rheumatoid arthritis occur at the margins or unprotected areas of the articulation, where pannus is intimate with osseous tissue that does not possess protective cartilage. Symmetrically distributed defects appear on both the proximal and distal bones that constitute the articulation; they are usually, but not invariably, accompanied by soft tissue swelling, periarticular osteoporosis, and joint space narrowing. Such erosions may be a very early manifestation of the disease and occur within 1 or 2 years of the onset of joint symptoms.

The radiographic appearance of multiple subchondral lucent areas throughout the articulation in patients with early or more advanced rheumatoid arthritis is well recognized. These lesions may develop in several different fashions, including intraosseous extension of pannus, nutritional and metabolic injury of bone, and true intraosseous rheumatoid nodules. Large radiolucent cystic areas have been noted in patients with rheumatoid arthritis who maintain a high level of physical activity. In this peculiar cystic pattern, which has been termed rheumatoid arthritis of the robust reaction type, magnetic resonance (MR) imaging indicates that the subchondral cystlike lesions may contain fluid, inflamed synovium, or both, and they may or may not reveal obvious communications with the joint (Fig. 15–3).

It is interesting to speculate that cyst formation represents one mechanism of joint decompression (Fig. 15–4). Whatever their pathogenesis, subchondral lucent areas are an important radiographic manifestation of rheumatoid arthritis. Pathologically, these cysts do not possess a true epithelial cystic lining, which accounts for the variety of terms applied to these lesions, including cysts, pseudocysts, granulomas, and geodes. They are usually multiple, distributed symmetrically, of small size, and without sclerotic margins. Subchondral cysts are sometimes observed in the absence of classic marginal bone erosions, articular space loss, and osteopenia. In these instances, the radiographic manifestations resemble those of gout.

**Fibrous Capsule.** The fibrous capsule of the synovial joint reveals only minor alterations in patients with rheumatoid arthritis. After prolonged inflammation, capsular contraction can aggravate the malalignment and subluxation provoked by changes in supporting structures.

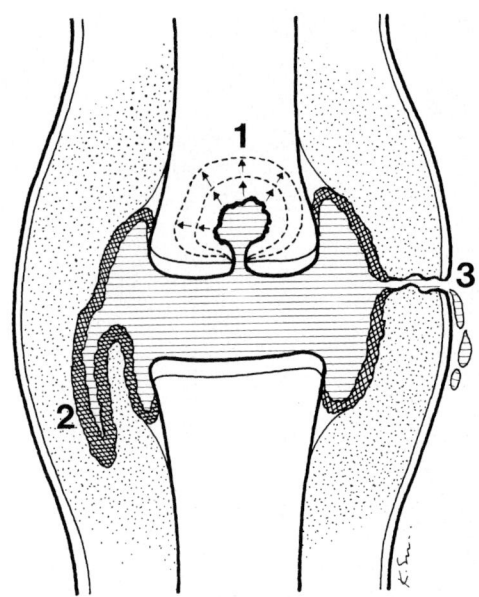

**Figure 15–4.** Mechanism of decompression of joints with raised intra-articular pressure. The three potential pathways are subchondral cystic lesions (1), synovial cysts (2), and fistulas or sinus tracts (3).

**Synovial Membrane, Cartilage, and Bone in Advanced Rheumatoid Arthritis.** The pathologic and radiographic changes in the synovial joints of patients with rheumatoid arthritis do not always progress relentlessly. Even in later phases, after irreversible damage has occurred, the changes may remain static for an indefinite period. In the late stage of rheumatoid arthritis, the total synovial surface area is dramatically increased by the proliferation and hypertrophy of synovial villi during the course of articular inflammation. Once the villi have appeared, they persist even when the synovitis has subsided. As a terminal event, very elongated villi may become detached and appear in the joint cavity as "rice bodies," so called because of their resemblance to grains of polished rice.

Fragments of cartilage and bone are found embedded in the synovial tissue. Although the exact pathogenesis of such fragments is unclear, they probably arise from the erosive process that destroys cartilage and bone. The fate of the detached spicules varies. The radiographic appearance associated with bone fragmentation in rheumatoid arthritis is characterized by well-defined, separated osseous densities resembling those in neuropathic osteoarthropathy, osteoarthritis, gout, osteochondritis dissecans, osteonecrosis, and idiopathic synovial osteochondromatosis, although the number of fragmented bony particles in rheumatoid arthritis is generally limited.

Osteoarthritis can be a prominent secondary phenomenon in the synovial joints of patients with rheumatoid arthritis. When prominent, osteoarthritic abnormalities can obscure the underlying rheumatoid process on both pathologic and radiographic examinations. The possibility of underlying rheumatoid arthritis (or other processes characterized by synovial inflammation) should be considered whenever radiographs reveal osteoarthritis with unusual features or in unusual sites (Fig. 15–5).

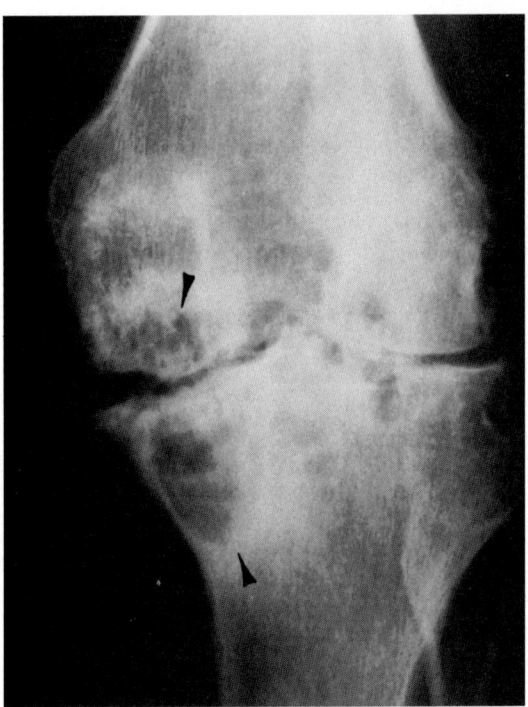

**Figure 15–3.** Pseudocystic rheumatoid arthritis. In some patients with rheumatoid arthritis, particularly men, multiple large radiolucent lesions *(arrowheads)* about involved articulations can simulate the appearance of gout or neoplasm.

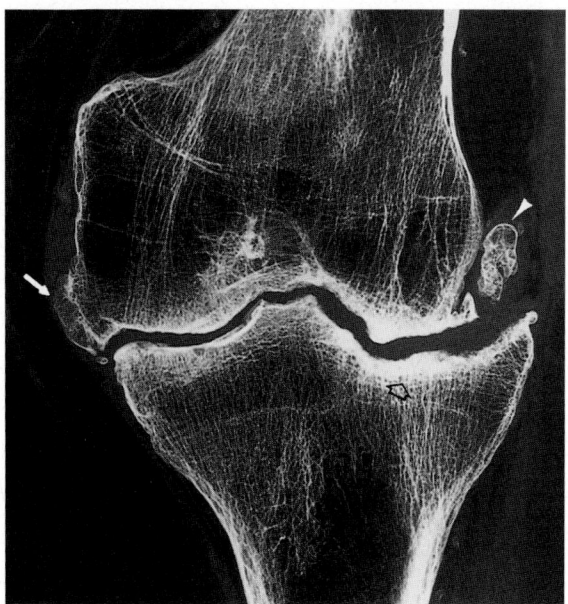

**Figure 15–5.** Synovial joint abnormalities in rheumatoid arthritis: productive changes in bone. On a radiograph of a coronal section of the knee, observe the abnormalities related to bone production in the form of osteophytes *(solid arrow)* and subchondral sclerosis *(open arrow)*. These findings should not be regarded as evidence of a diagnosis other than rheumatoid arthritis. In this case, involvement of both the medial femorotibial space and lateral femorotibial space, with predominant involvement of the latter area, aids in the accurate diagnosis of rheumatoid arthritis. Fragmentation of the articular surface, with the formation of a large intra-articular body *(arrowhead)*, is seen.

## Bursae and Tendon Sheaths

Synovial inflammation in rheumatoid arthritis is not confined to the intra-articular structures; similar inflammation occurs in the synovial lining of tendon sheaths and bursae, but usually to a lesser extent (Table 15–2). Bursal involvement in this disease may occur in more than 5% of patients, particularly in the popliteal region of the knee and in the olecranon, subacromial (subdeltoid) bursa, and retrocalcaneal bursa, but also about the wrist and foot (Fig. 15–6). Tenosynovitis is especially prominent in the dorsum of the hand, the fingers, and the foot (Fig. 15–7). Bursitis and tenosynovitis can be coupled with typical involvement of adjacent articulations, although they can also occur as isolated or predominant manifestations of the disorder. In association with tenosynovitis, the tendon

**TABLE 15–2**

**Abnormalities of Bursae and Tendon Sheaths in Rheumatoid Arthritis**

| Pathologic | Radiologic |
| --- | --- |
| Synovial inflammation and production of fluid | Soft tissue swelling |
| Hyperemia | Osteoporosis |
| Pannus destruction of subjacent bone | Surface resorption of bone |

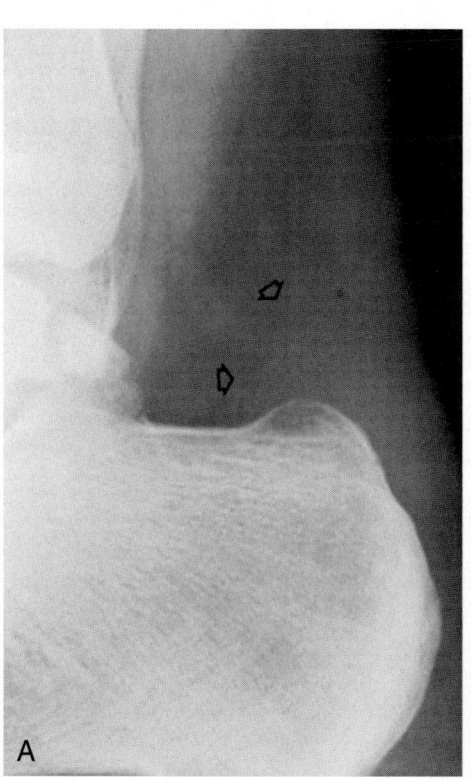
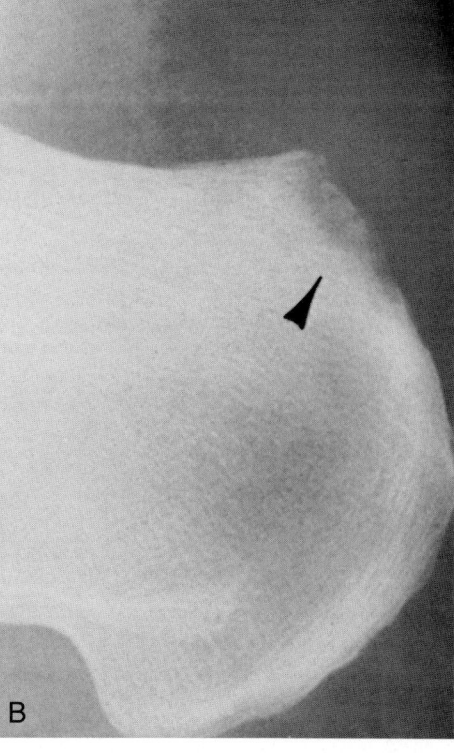

**Figure 15–6.** Abnormalities of bursae in rheumatoid arthritis. *A* and *B*, Retrocalcaneal bursitis. Soft tissue swelling *(open arrows)* represents a fluid-filled, distended retrocalcaneal bursa. Subjacent osseous erosion *(arrowhead, B)* can be seen.

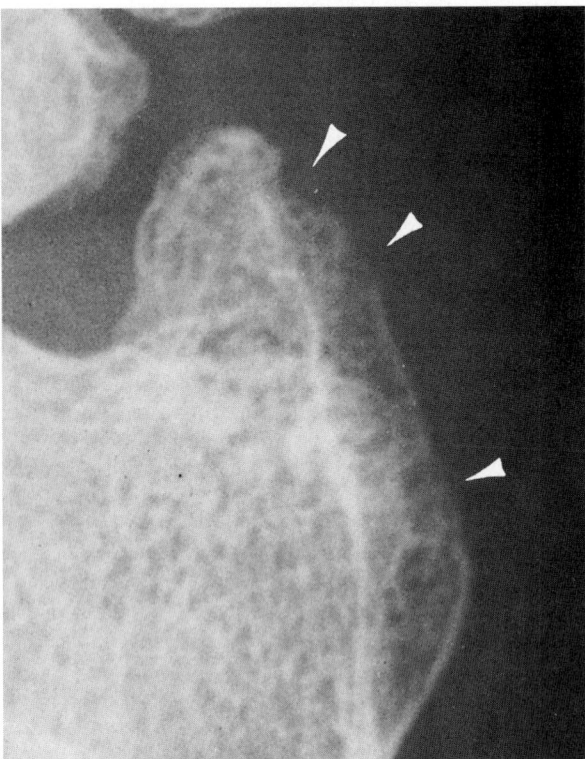

**Figure 15–7.** Abnormalities of tendon sheaths and bursae in rheumatoid arthritis. Surface resorption of bone beneath an inflamed extensor carpi ulnaris tendon sheath produces typical defects along the outer aspect of the ulnar styloid *(arrowheads)*.

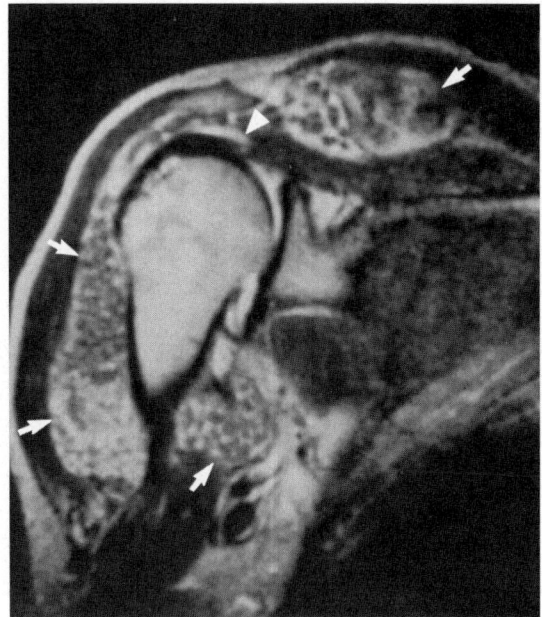

**Figure 15–8.** Abnormalities of bursae in rheumatoid arthritis. Subdeltoid-subacromial bursitis. T2-weighted (TR/TE, 2000/80) coronal oblique spin echo MR images reveal a markedly distended bursa *(arrows)*. Note the increase in signal intensity of fluid in the joint and in the bursa; however, regions of low signal density remain in the bursa. At surgery, these areas were found to represent small fibrous nodules, or rice bodies. Also note the tear of the supraspinatus tendon *(arrowhead)*, which may represent a complication of rheumatoid arthritis. (Courtesy of J. Hodler, MD, Zurich, Switzerland.)

itself may be affected and become disposed to a variety of complications, including weakening, subluxation, entrapment, and rupture.

The most common radiographic finding associated with tenosynovitis and bursitis is soft tissue swelling. Erosion of subjacent bone can be observed, particularly in the posterosuperior aspect of the calcaneus (in relation to retrocalcaneal bursitis), the olecranon process (in relation to olecranon bursitis), and the inferior surface of the acromion and distal end of the clavicle (in relation to subacromial bursitis). In addition, surface resorption of bone beneath inflamed tendon sheaths is characteristic, particularly in the outer aspect of the distal portion of the ulna (extensor carpi ulnaris tenosynovitis) (see Fig. 15–7). Arthrography, bursography, tenography, ultrasonography, and MR imaging (Fig. 15–8) can be used to directly delineate the nature of the soft tissue swelling and the extent of synovial inflammation.

## Cartilaginous Joints and Entheses

Although involvement of cartilaginous joints, such as the symphysis pubis and manubriosternal and discovertebral articulations, and of entheses, such as those related to the spinous processes of the vertebrae, the inferior surface of the calcanei, the iliac wings, the ischial tuberosities, and the femoral trochanters, is observed in rheumatoid arthritis,

the frequency and severity of such involvement are far less striking than in the seronegative spondyloarthropathies. Of the cartilaginous joints, the alterations of the discovertebral junction in rheumatoid arthritis receive the most attention (Table 15–3). Such changes predominate in the cervical region, although the pathogenesis of these alterations is unclear. Various schools of thought have advanced the following suggestions (Fig. 15–9): (1) dis-

**TABLE 15–3**

**Abnormalities of Discovertebral Cartilaginous Joints in Rheumatoid Arthritis**

| Potential Mechanism | Pathogenesis |
| --- | --- |
| Synovial inflammation | "Pannus" is derived from joints of Luschka (cervical region) and costovertebral articulations (thoracic region) |
| Trauma | Apophyseal joint instability leads to traumatic disruption of the discovertebral junction with cartilaginous node formation |
| Enthesopathy | Inflammation at ligamentous and capsular attachments leads to adjacent osseous erosion |

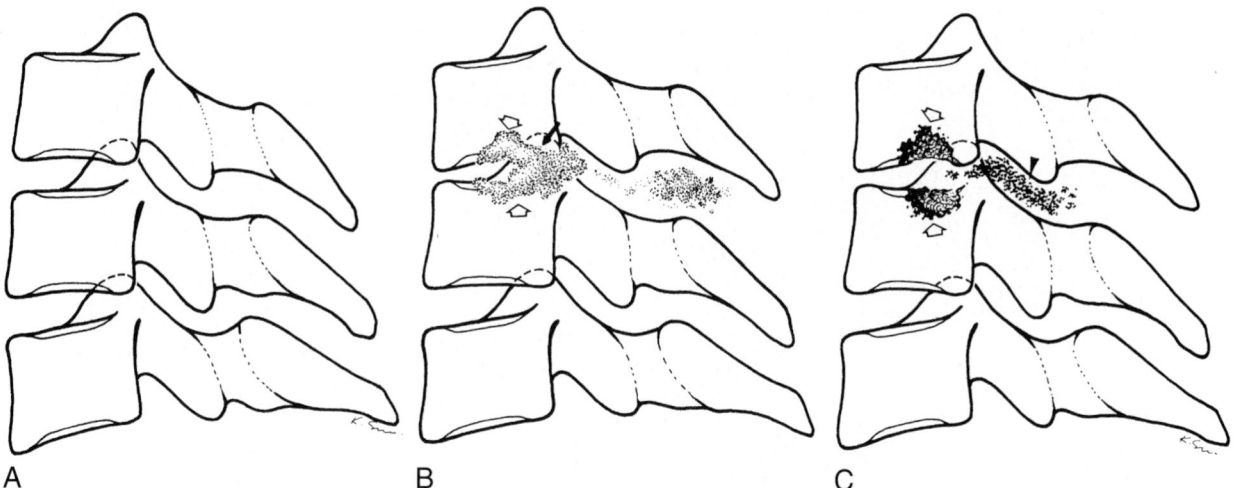

**Figure 15–9.** Abnormalities of the discovertebral junctions of the cervical spine in rheumatoid arthritis. *A,* The normal situation. *B,* Proponents of the synovial school of thought suggest that inflammatory tissue in the neurocentral joints of Luschka *(solid arrow)* spreads across the discovertebral junction, a process leading to osseous erosion *(open arrows).* *C,* Proponents of the traumatic school of thought believe that instability of the apophyseal joints resulting from synovial inflammation *(arrowhead)* produces recurrent discovertebral trauma, which leads to cartilaginous nodes with surrounding sclerosis *(open arrows).*

covertebral abnormalities occur as a secondary manifestation of synovial inflammation in the adjacent neurocentral articulations (joints of Luschka) in the cervical spine and the neighboring costovertebral articulations in the thoracic spine (the synovial school); (2) discovertebral alterations relate to traumatic insults produced by instability of the posterior elements of the spine (the traumatic school); or (3) discovertebral alterations in rheumatoid arthritis, as in ankylosing spondylitis, are produced by a primary enthesopathy (the enthesopathic school). The resulting abnormalities are characteristic (Fig. 15–10). Erosion and reactive sclerosis of the spinous processes of the cervical vertebrae appear to be related to two mechanisms: an inflammatory process at the sites of ligament attachment to bone, consistent with the enthesopathy, and a synovial inflammation in interspinous bursae.

## Tendons and Ligaments

Inflammatory and degenerative changes and laxity resulting from distortion of tendons and ligaments by the intra-articular process contribute to the typical joint deformities that accompany long-standing rheumatoid arthritis. "Spontaneous" tendon ruptures are a known manifestation of rheumatoid arthritis. They are encountered most frequently in the hand and wrist, although ruptures of other tendons can occur, including the Achilles, infra-patellar, tibialis posterior, and rotator cuff tendons. Joint subluxation, malalignment, and deformity in rheumatoid arthritis can be attributed to numerous factors. Inflammatory destruction of intra-articular structures leading to surface incongruity, capsular and ligamentous weakening leading to laxity, tendinosis and tenosynovitis leading to contracture and rupture, and muscular contraction are all influential in this regard. Articular deformity is most characteristic at the wrist; the metacarpophalangeal,

metatarsophalangeal, and interphalangeal articulations of the hand and foot; and the atlantoaxial region. Subluxation is combined almost invariably with typical intra-articular alterations. Infrequently, a deforming, nonerosive joint disease is apparent and must be distinguished from the arthropathy of Jaccoud or from systemic lupus erythematosus (Fig. 15–11).

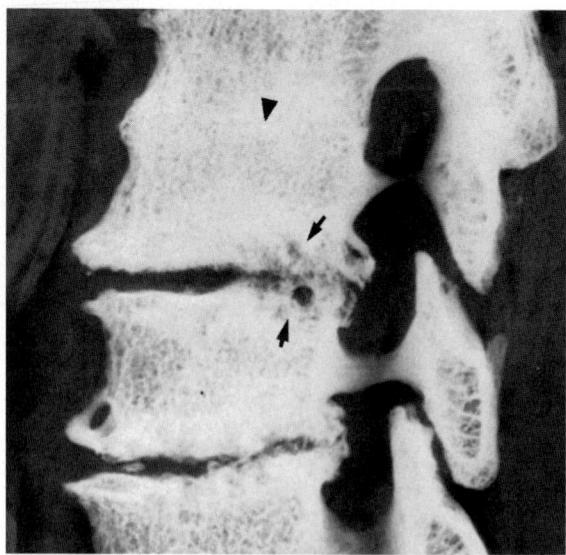

**Figure 15–10.** Discovertebral lesions in the cervical spine in rheumatoid arthritis. Sagittal sectional radiograph reveals, at one discovertebral level, prominent erosions about the neuro-central joints *(arrows).* At a lower level, widespread discovertebral erosions and disc space loss are apparent. Above, bone ankylosis *(arrowhead)* has led to obliteration of an intervertebral disc. The apophyseal joints are not well evaluated in this radiograph.

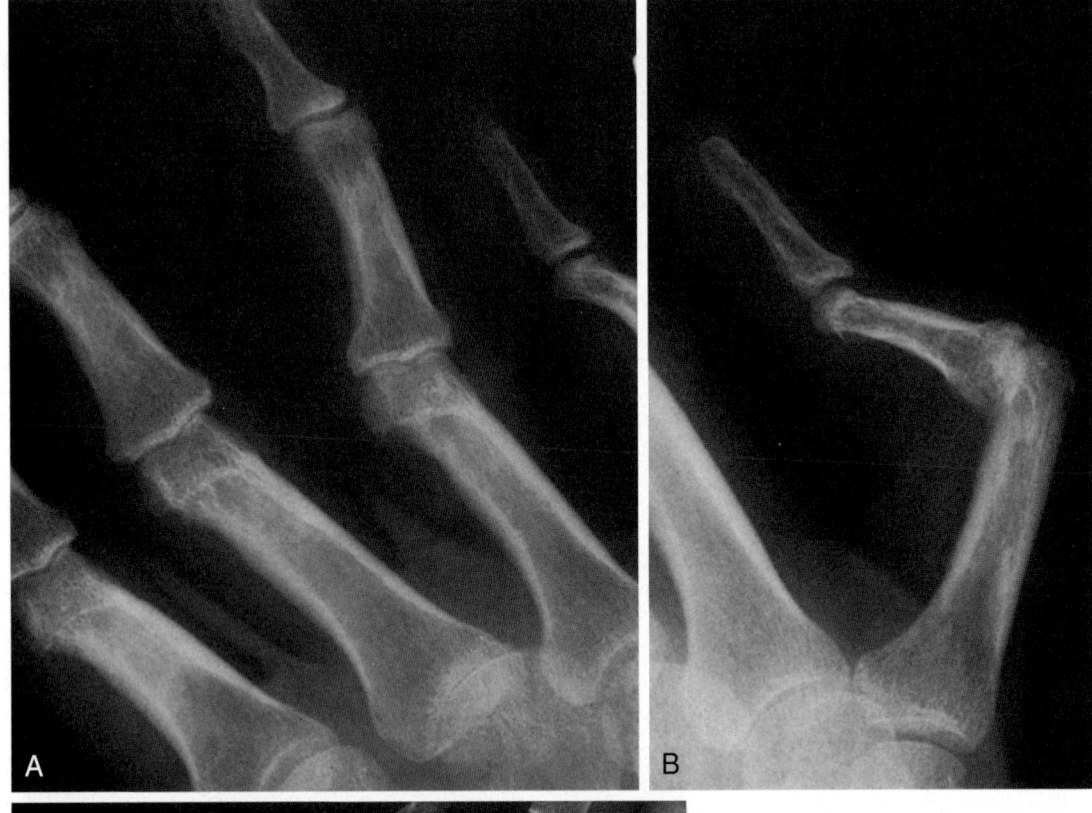

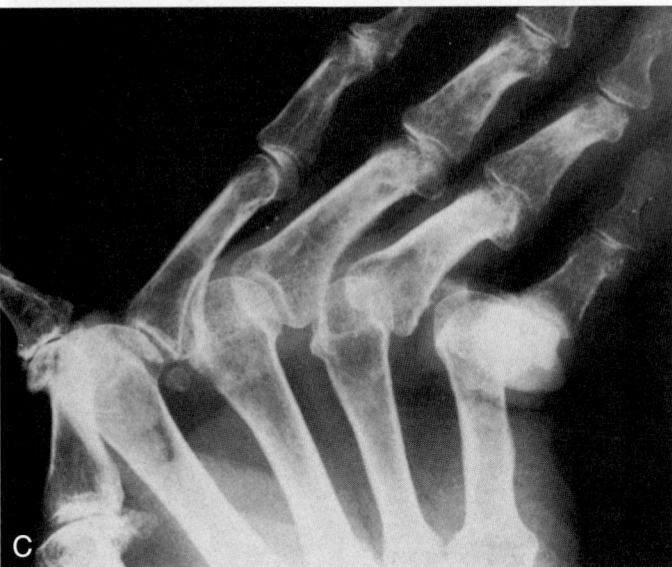

**Figure 15–11.** Joint malalignment in rheumatoid arthritis: typical digital deformities of the hand. *A*, Swan-neck deformity (hyperextension at the proximal interphalangeal joint and flexion at the distal interphalangeal joint). *B*, Boutonnière deformity (flexion at the proximal interphalangeal joint and hyperextension at the distal interphalangeal joint). *C*, Rarely, severe subluxation of the hand in rheumatoid arthritis is associated with only minor intra-articular abnormality. Note the ulnar deviation and flexion at the metacarpophalangeal joints with swan-neck deformities. Minor degrees of joint space narrowing are evident, but erosions are not prominent.

## Soft Tissues

**Edema.** In patients with rheumatoid arthritis, widespread peripheral edema can occur in association with generalized factors such as anemia, fluid retention, and hypoalbuminemia. Localized factors, including obstruction of venous and lymphatic channels, reduced numbers of lymphatic vessels, and increased capillary permeability, have also been implicated. Although the precise cause of the lymphatic involvement in rheumatoid arthritis is not clear, it may relate to extension of inflammation from a joint to the surrounding soft tissue.

Clinically, lymphedema in patients with rheumatoid arthritis affects men and women with equal frequency and usually involves an entire limb, especially an upper extremity. The appearance of lymphedema in rheumatoid arthritis assumes diagnostic significance because of the recent identification of a syndrome in elderly patients consisting of peripheral seronegative inflammatory polyarthritis with pitting edema. This condition, termed remitting seronegative symmetrical synovitis with pitting edema (RS₃PE) syndrome, is discussed in more detail in Chapter 16.

**Rheumatoid Nodules.** The most frequent soft tissue lesion in rheumatoid arthritis is a subcutaneous nodule. Although a subcutaneous nodule was once considered virtually diagnostic of rheumatoid arthritis, it is now recognized that such nodules are associated with a wide variety of disorders, including rheumatic fever, collagen vascular disorders, sarcoidosis, Weber-Christian disease, gout, dermatologic processes, xanthomatosis, and various infections.

One or more subcutaneous nodules are detectable in approximately 20% to 35% of patients with rheumatoid arthritis. The nodules are most commonly located between the skin and an underlying bony prominence. Typical locations include the olecranon, the proximal portion of the ulna (Fig. 15–12), the lateral aspects of the fingers, the gluteal and Achilles tendon regions, and the areas about the femoral trochanters and ischial tuberosities. Almost invariably, rheumatoid nodules are associated with seropositivity for rheumatoid factor. Their presence also suggests a propensity for severe erosive disease and vasculitis. They may be identified before the clinical onset of arthritis.

Subcutaneous nodules vary in size from a few millimeters to greater than 5 cm. Usually, they are firm and nontender. Nodules are frequently attached to the deep fascia or the periosteum, but they can be freely movable. Most commonly, they are asymptomatic.

Radiographically, subcutaneous rheumatoid nodules are associated with lobulated, eccentric soft tissue masses (see Fig. 15–12). These masses infrequently calcify, a diagnostic point that may be helpful in distinguishing them from gouty tophi, which can contain calcification. In unusual instances, rheumatoid nodules can lead to erosion of subjacent bone. In this regard, scalloped defects in the cortex of the proximal portion of the ulna, metacarpals, metatarsals, or other bones in rheumatoid arthritis can simulate the appearance of a variety of benign soft tissue neoplasms, as well as gout, giant cell tumor of a tendon sheath, ganglion cyst, and xanthoma. With MR imaging, rheumatoid nodules typically demonstrate a nonspecific low to intermediate signal intensity on T1-weighted spin echo images and heterogeneous low to high signal intensity on T2-weighted spin echo images, and they show enhancement of signal intensity after the intravenous administration of a gadolinium-containing agent (Fig. 15–13).

An atypical variant of rheumatoid disease, rheumatoid nodulosis, is characterized by the presence of multiple subcutaneous nodules and the absence of significant synovitis or systemic manifestations. Men are usually affected. In addition to nodular soft tissue masses, radiographs may reveal intra-articular cystic osseous defects with or without

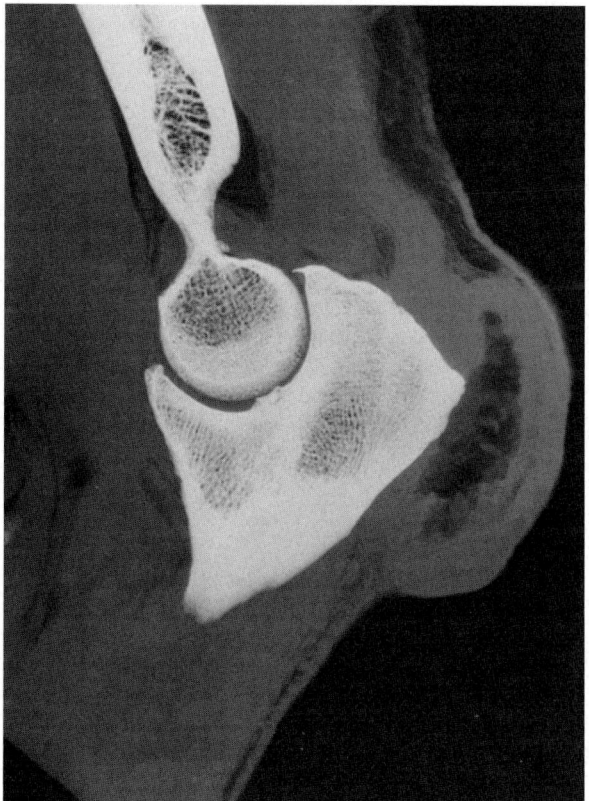

**Figure 15–12.** Soft tissue nodules in rheumatoid arthritis. A typical site of involvement is about the proximal portion of the ulna, as shown in this sagittal section radiograph. The olecranon bursa is also inflamed.

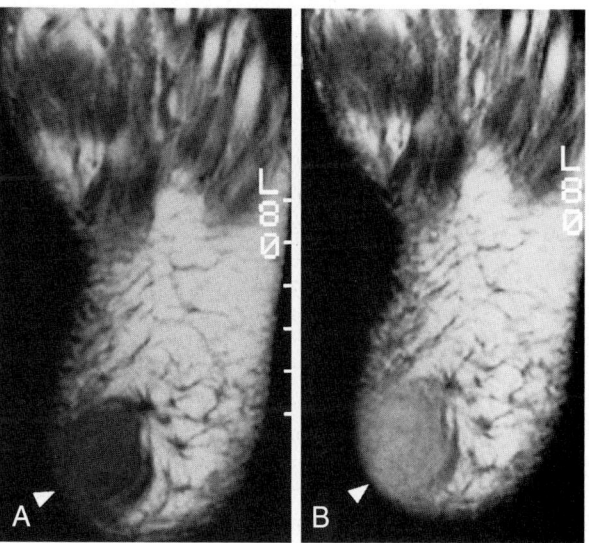

**Figure 15–13.** Soft tissue nodules in rheumatoid arthritis: MR imaging. This 65-year-old woman with rheumatoid arthritis had multiple subcutaneous nodules, including one in the plantar aspect of the left heel. *A,* T1-weighted (TR/TE, 600/20) transverse MR image reveals the soft tissue nodule in the left heel *(arrowhead),* surrounded by fat. *B,* After the intravenous injection of gadolinium-containing contrast agent, an identical T1-weighted MR image shows diffuse enhancement of the nodule *(arrowhead).* (Courtesy of S. Moreland, MD, San Diego, Calif.)

joint space narrowing or osteoporosis. Serologic tests for rheumatoid factor are commonly positive in these persons, and biopsy of the nodules and synovium reveals typical histologic changes of rheumatoid arthritis.

**Calcification.** Soft tissue calcification is rare in rheumatoid arthritis. Calcific deposits within rheumatoid nodules and within periarticular subcutaneous tissue have occasionally been described in persons with this disease. In all such cases, the possibility of mixed connective tissue disease or collagen vascular overlap syndromes must be considered.

**Synovial Cysts.** Synovial cysts are a well-known manifestation of rheumatoid arthritis (Fig. 15–14). Although synovial cysts may arise as a result of rupture of the joint capsule, with extravasation of fluid and secondary encapsulation, or as a result of herniation of the synovial membrane, most authorities now believe that these lesions represent abnormal distention of various bursae that communicate with the adjacent articulation. These communicating channels have been well documented in the knee and frequently possess a valvular mechanism, allowing the flow of synovial fluid to proceed in only one direction (from the articulation to the cyst, not from the cyst to the articulation). Clinically, it may be difficult to differentiate signs and symptoms related to synovial cysts about the knee from those caused by thrombophlebitis. Rupture of a synovial cyst is accompanied by swelling and edema that may lead to stasis, inflammation of the wall of the vein, and thrombophlebitis; alternatively, the soft tissue swelling accompanying thrombophlebitis may produce an increase in pressure within a synovial cyst and predispose it to rupture.

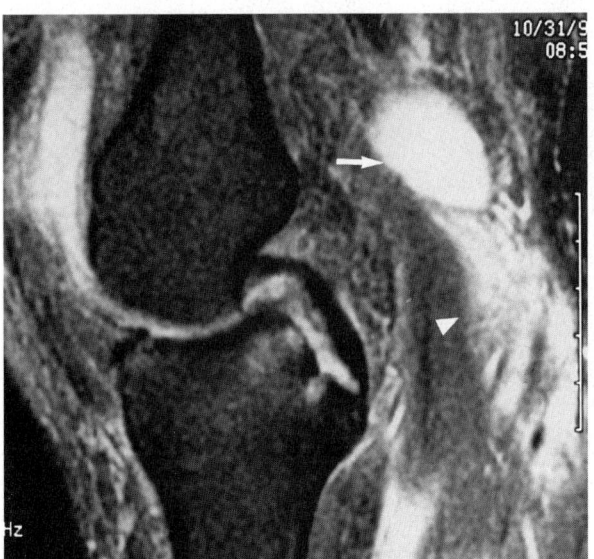

**Figure 15–14.** Synovial cysts in rheumatoid arthritis: MR imaging. This sagittal, fat-suppressed, fast spin echo (TR/TE, 2900/34) MR image reveals a synovial cyst (*arrow*) with extravasation of fluid (*arrowhead*), indicative of rupture.

Although rheumatoid synovial cysts are observed most frequently in the popliteal region, they have been described at other sites, including the calf, knee, ankle, plantar aspect of the foot, hip, hand and wrist, elbow, and shoulder. Presumably, an extra-articular synovial mass can arise around any involved articulation in this disease.

**Sinus Tracts.** Cutaneous-articular sinus tracts are recognized as an occasional feature of rheumatoid arthritis. Classic "fistulous" rheumatism is related to the appearance of chronic skin sinuses near affected joints in patients with rheumatoid arthritis. In these patients, erythematous periarticular nodules erupt and form draining sinuses, often multiple, in the vicinity of the hands and feet. Synovial cyst formation with sinus tract formation is a rare complication of fistulous rheumatism. Although spontaneous cutaneous drainage of popliteal cysts has been reported in patients with rheumatoid arthritis, this complication is more frequent after direct aspiration.

## Muscles

In rheumatoid arthritis, generalized muscle weakness is common, although other symptoms and signs related to muscle involvement are rare. Possible causes of muscle involvement in this disease include muscle atrophy, steroid myopathy, peripheral neuropathy, and acute or chronic myositis. Toxic myopathy precipitated by various therapeutic agents is also well recognized.

## Digital Vessels

Necrotizing arteritis in mesenteric, renal, and cerebral locations; subacute arteritis in skeletal muscles; and fibromuscular hyperplasia in peripheral vessels are all recognized in rheumatoid arthritis. Vasculitis complicated by digital gangrene and acro-osteolysis can be seen in rheumatoid arthritis as well as in other collagen vascular disorders. In patients with rheumatoid arthritis, such acro-osteolysis is almost invariably associated with severe erosive arthritis and is usually associated with peripheral neuropathy. Vasculitis in rheumatoid arthritis has been suggested as a potential cause of ischemic necrosis.

## Bones

Generalized or periarticular osteoporosis is a common manifestation in patients with rheumatoid arthritis. The pathogenesis of periarticular osteoporosis appears to be related to the adjacent synovial inflammation with hyperemia; however, the cause of the generalized osteoporosis in this disease is not entirely clear.

Osteoporosis producing bone weakening contributes to the fractures that are not uncommonly encountered in patients with rheumatoid arthritis (Table 15–4; Fig. 15–15). These fractures may occur after minimal trauma or spontaneously in either spinal sites (compression fractures of vertebral bodies) or extraspinal locations. Typical locations include the femur, tibia, fibula, sacrum, and para-acetabular and symphyseal regions. Accurate diagnosis of

**TABLE 15–4**

**Mechanisms and Sites of Pathologic Fractures in Rheumatoid Arthritis**

| Mechanism | Typical Sites |
| --- | --- |
| Synovial inflammation with erosion of bone | Odontoid process, carpal scaphoid bone, distal portion of ulna |
| Mechanical erosion of bone | Ribs, articular surfaces of small bones in hands and feet, medial aspect of humeral neck |
| Intraosseous cystic lesions | Proximal portion of ulna, femoral neck, femur and tibia about the knee |
| Bone deformation | Acetabulum |
| Generalized osteopenia | Insufficiency fractures of vertebral bodies, pelvis, tubular bones of lower extremity, small bones of foot |
| Ischemic necrosis | Femoral head, vertebral bodies |
| Osteomyelitis | Variable |

insufficiency fractures can be difficult and requires a high index of clinical suspicion, quality radiographs, and even scintigraphy, computed tomography, or MR imaging (Fig. 15–16).

Erosive abnormality of bone related to the rheumatoid process itself can also lead to fracture and deformity. Thus, pathologic fractures through the odontoid process and olecranon process and acetabular weakening and fracture leading to protrusion deformity are observed. Other sites include the scaphoid and humeral neck (Fig. 15–17), as well as the phalanges of the hand.

## SERONEGATIVE SPONDYLOARTHROPATHIES

### Overview

The three major seronegative spondyloarthropathies—ankylosing spondylitis, psoriatic arthritis, and Reiter's syndrome—share many radiologic and pathologic features with rheumatoid arthritis. They, too, involve synovial joints and are associated with considerable inflammation of the synovial membrane. Fundamental differences exist between the spondyloarthropathies and rheumatoid arthritis, however, especially in the distribution and morphology of osteoarticular lesions (Table 15–5).

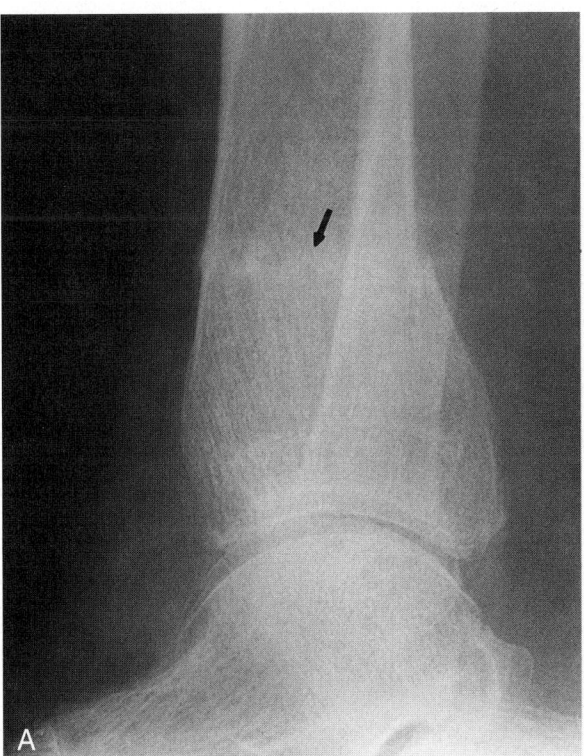
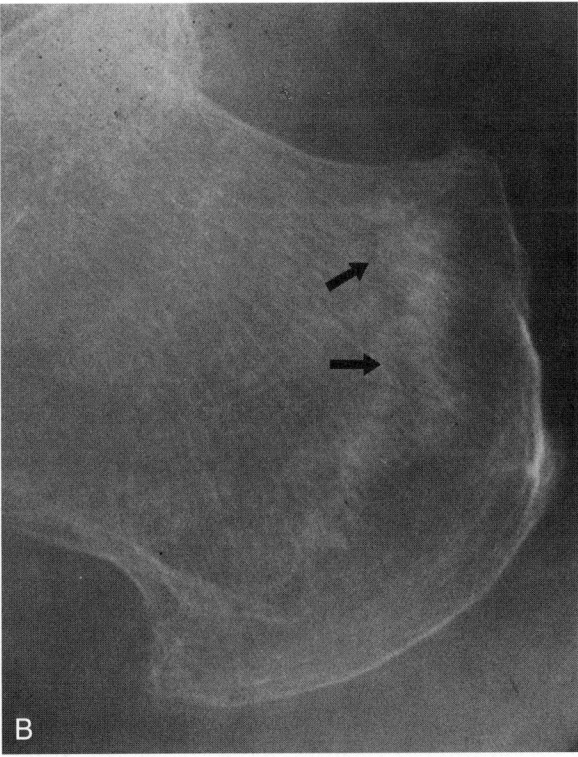

**Figure 15–15.** Insufficiency (stress) fractures in rheumatoid arthritis. *A*, Radiograph demonstrates a pathologic fracture of the distal portion of the tibia *(arrows)* that arose from fatigue of the osteoporotic bone. *B*, In another patient with rheumatoid arthritis, a classic insufficiency fracture of the calcaneus *(arrows)* has produced vertically oriented bony sclerosis.

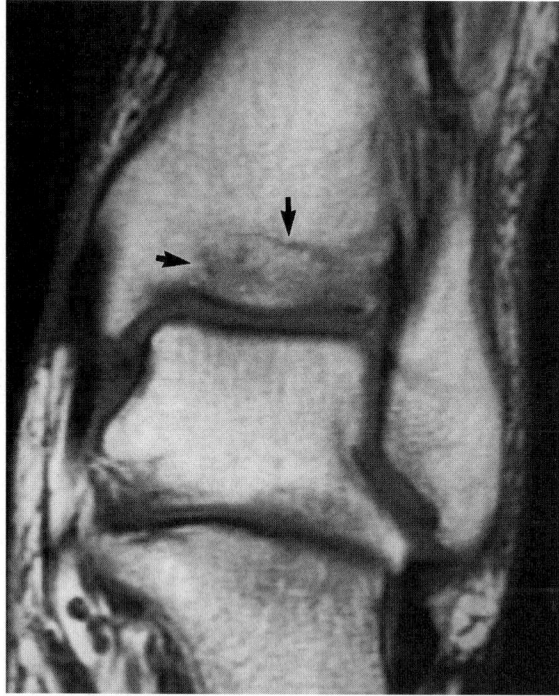

**Figure 15–16.** Insufficiency (stress) fractures in rheumatoid arthritis: MR imaging. This coronal T1-weighted (TR/TE, 500/18) spin echo MR image reveals insufficiency fractures *(arrows)* in the distal portion of the tibia.

**TABLE 15–5**

**Rheumatoid Arthritis versus the Seronegative Spondyloarthropathies**

| Characteristic | Rheumatoid Arthritis | Seronegative Spondylo-arthropathies |
| --- | --- | --- |
| Synovial joint involvement | + | + |
|   Soft tissue swelling | + | + |
|   Osteoporosis | + | ± |
|   Marginal erosions | + | + |
|   Central erosions and cysts | + | + |
|   Bony ankylosis | ± | + |
|   Bony proliferation | – | + |
|   Malalignment and subluxation | + | ± |
| Bursal and tendon sheath involvement | + | + |
|   Soft tissue swelling | + | + |
|   Bony erosions | + | + |
|   Bony proliferation | – | + |
| Cartilaginous joint involvement | ± | + |
|   Bony erosions | ± | + |
|   Bony proliferation | ± | + |
|   Bony ankylosis | ± | + |
| Enthesopathy | ± | + |
|   Bony erosions | ± | + |
|   Bony proliferation | ± | + |

+, common; ±, less common; –, rare or absent.

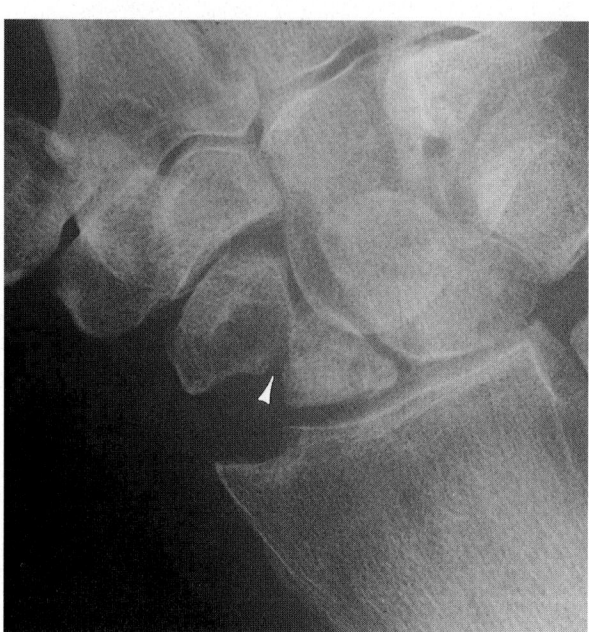

**Figure 15–17.** Fractures through sites of bone erosion in rheumatoid arthritis. This radiograph documents a fracture of the carpal scaphoid bone through a site of erosion *(arrowhead)*. Ischemic necrosis of the proximal pole of the bone is evident.

(From Resnick D, Cone R: Pathological fractures in rheumatoid arthritis: Sites and mechanisms. Radiographics 4:549, 1984.)

All three of these spondyloarthropathic processes produce significant abnormalities in the cartilaginous joints and entheses, as well as in the synovial articulations. The discovertebral junctions throughout the spine, the symphysis pubis, the manubriosternal joint, and the tendinous and ligamentous attachments in the calcaneus, pelvis, trochanters of the femur, tuberosities of the humerus, and patella are altered to a much greater extent in ankylosing spondylitis, psoriatic arthritis, and Reiter's syndrome than in rheumatoid arthritis. Ankylosing spondylitis affects primarily the synovial and cartilaginous joints and entheses of the axial skeleton, with less consistent and severe changes in the appendicular skeleton. The distribution of psoriatic arthritis is somewhat variable, although a polyarticular disorder of the synovial joints of the appendicular skeleton, with prominent involvement of the interphalangeal articulations of the hand and foot, combined with changes at the synovial and cartilaginous joints of the axial skeleton and entheses of the axial and appendicular skeleton, is distinctive. In Reiter's syndrome, asymmetrical and "spotty" abnormalities of the synovial articulations of the lower extremities are frequently coupled with sacroiliitis, spondylitis, and enthesopathy of the inferior surface of the calcaneus.

In addition to these differences in the distribution of articular abnormalities, differences in the morphology of the lesions may be evident. In this regard, the radiographic and pathologic characteristics of joint involvement in ankylosing spondylitis, psoriatic arthritis, and Reiter's syndrome are fundamentally similar and can be distinguished from those in rheumatoid arthritis. In synovial articulations, the absence of osteoporosis and the presence of bony proliferation and intra-articular bony ankylosis in the seronegative spondyloarthropathies are most helpful in differentiating the changes from those of rheumatoid arthritis. In cartilaginous joints, the extent of osseous erosion and bone proliferation in the former disorders is also helpful in the differential diagnosis. At sites of tendon and ligament attachment to bone, an inflammatory enthesopathy leading to osseous destruction and repair is characteristic of the spondyloarthropathies.

## Synovial Joints

The predominant target area in the synovial joints in the seronegative spondyloarthropathies appears to be the synovial membrane (Table 15–6; Fig. 15–18). Compared with the situation in rheumatoid arthritis, however, the inflammatory changes in ankylosing spondylitis, psoriatic arthritis, and Reiter's syndrome are less intense. Fibroplasia, which is followed by cartilaginous metaplasia and chondro-ossification, can lead to intra-articular bony ankylosis, a feature that may be apparent in any of the spondyloarthropathies but is most typical of ankylosing spondylitis and psoriatic arthritis. Detection of osseous fusion at sites other than the carpal and tarsal areas is relatively unusual in rheumatoid arthritis. The propensity of the seronegative spondyloarthropathies (especially ankylosing spondylitis) to lead to intra-articular bony ankylosis is a remarkable characteristic whose cause is not clear, although the tendency to produce new bone in these disorders is associated with the histocompatibility antigen HLA-B27.

The proclivity for osseous fusion of certain synovial joints, such as the apophyseal and sacroiliac articulations, especially in ankylosing spondylitis, can also be related to abnormalities occurring at the capsuloligamentous attachments, perhaps reflecting another manifestation of a generalized enthesopathy. Capsular ossification can apparently lead to interosseous bridging at the periphery of an involved articulation. Subsequent removal of the cartilaginous surface may occur by the process of endochondral ossification.

In the seronegative spondyloarthropathies, subchondral eburnation, irregular excrescences ("whiskers") at the margins of the joint, and periostitis of adjacent diaphyses, particularly in the phalanges and the metacarpal and metatarsal bones, are distinctive (Fig. 15–19). Bone erosion in ankylosing spondylitis, psoriatic arthritis, and Reiter's syndrome may be superficial and quickly obscured by the profound tendency toward bone proliferation. Further, osteoporosis is not commonly a significant finding in the seronegative spondyloarthropathies. Some patients, however, particularly those with psoriatic arthritis, can exhibit striking osteolysis.

## Bursae and Tendon Sheaths

Inflammation in synovium-lined bursae and tendon sheaths occurs less often in the seronegative spondyloarthropathies than in rheumatoid arthritis. Retrocalcaneal bursitis in ankylosing spondylitis, psoriatic arthritis, or Reiter's syndrome produces pre-Achilles soft tissue swelling and indistinctness, as well as osseous erosion of the subjacent

---

**TABLE 15–6**

### Abnormalities of Synovial Joints in the Seronegative Spondyloarthropathies

| Pathologic | Radiologic |
|---|---|
| Synovial inflammation and production of fluid | Soft tissue swelling and widening of the joint space |
| Mild to moderate hyperemia | Variable osteoporosis |
| Pannus destruction of cartilage | Narrowing of the joint space |
| Pannus destruction of "unprotected" bone at the margin of a joint | Marginal bony erosions |
| Pannus destruction of subchondral bone | Bony erosions and formation of subchondral cysts |
| Fibroplasia, cartilaginous metaplasia, chondro-ossification, capsular ossification | Bony ankylosis |
| Bony proliferation in response to damage | Marginal "whiskering," periostitis, subchondral sclerosis |
| Noninflammatory proliferation of the periosteum | Cortical atrophy, osteolysis |

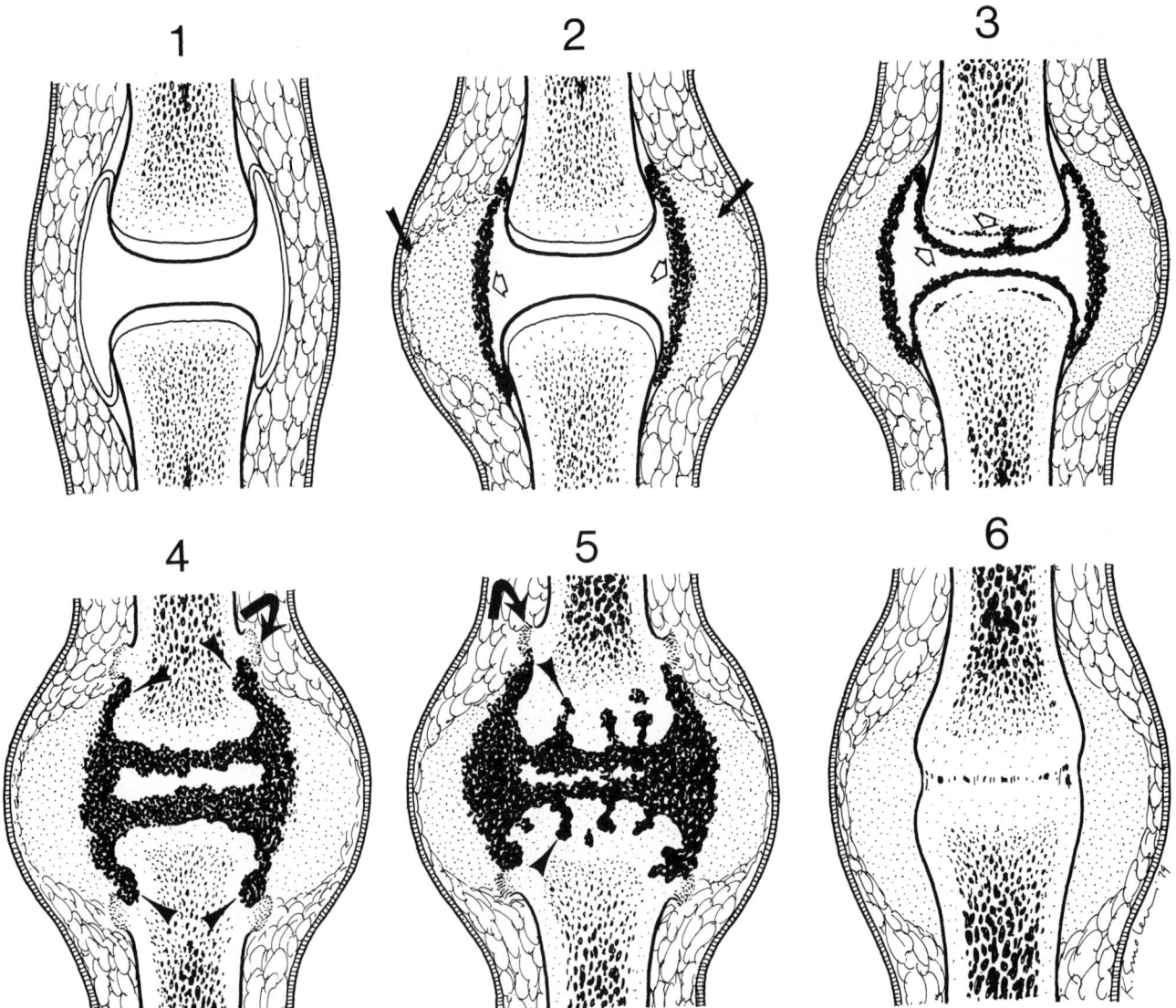

**Figure 15–18.**  Synovial joint abnormalities in seronegative spondyloarthropathies: pathologic overview. Normal synovial joint is depicted at the upper left (1). Early changes (2) consist of synovial inflammation *(open arrows)* and soft tissue edema *(solid arrows)*. Osteoporosis may not be evident. Subsequently (3), synovial inflammatory tissue, or pannus, extends across and beneath the chondral surface *(open arrows)* and leads to cartilaginous erosion or disruption. At later stages (4, 5), marginal and central osseous erosions develop *(arrowheads)*. Associated bony proliferation *(curved arrows)* becomes evident. Finally (6), intra-articular bony ankylosis may develop.

calcaneal surface (Fig. 15–20). In some patients, proliferation about the bony erosions can create poorly defined margins. Tenosynovitis, a frequently encountered manifestation of rheumatoid arthritis, may occasionally be a prominent feature in the seronegative spondyloarthropathies. Considerable soft tissue swelling in this clinical situation can produce a sausage-shaped finger or toe (Fig. 15–21).

## Cartilaginous Joints and Entheses

The tendency for ankylosing spondylitis, psoriatic arthritis, and Reiter's syndrome to affect cartilaginous articulations and the sites of tendon and ligament attachment to bone is well known (Table 15–7). At the manubriosternal joint and symphysis pubis, progressive fibrosis and bone formation lead to bone trabecular thickening and intra-articular ossification. Similar abnor-

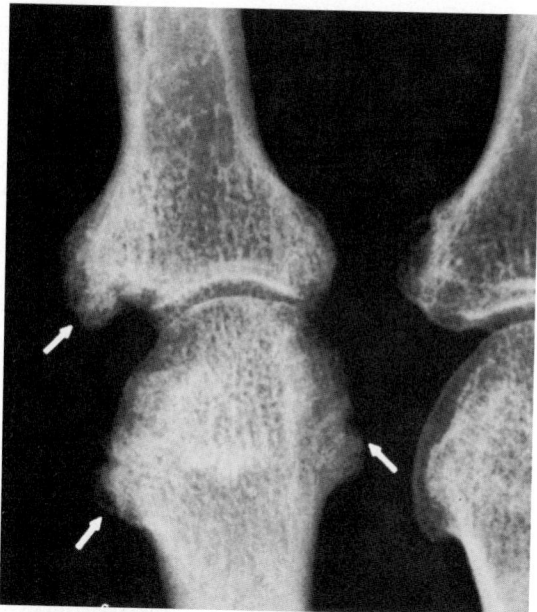

**Figure 15–19.** Synovial joint abnormalities in seronegative spondyloarthropathies: radiographic changes of bony proliferation, or "whiskering." In a cadaver with ankylosing spondylitis, observe the irregular osseous outline caused by superficial osseous erosion with adjacent bony proliferation *(arrows)*. Osteoporosis is not apparent.

malities in the discovertebral joint produce "osteitis" of the anterior vertebral margin, which is accompanied by erosion and sclerosis of bone and the progressive discal ossification associated with syndesmophyte formation (Fig. 15–22). At each of the cartilaginous articulations (manubriosternal joint, symphysis pubis, discovertebral junction), the changes may relate not only to true chondro-osseous inflammation but also to an enthesopathy at the peripheral capsular attachments.

The pathogenesis of destructive lesions at single or multiple discovertebral junctions during the course of ankylosing spondylitis is not clear, and several mechanisms probably contribute to these lesions. These include an increasing enthesopathy, pressure destruction of the intervertebral disc related to kyphosis, cartilage node formation, and pseudarthrosis about a fracture site. The last-mentioned mechanism is expected in long-standing disease in which a rigid vertebral column, caused by widespread bony ankylosis, is predisposed to fracture in a manner similar to that of a long tubular bone. Continued motion at the fracture site leads to improper fracture healing, often designated a pseudarthrosis, in which callus formation, hemorrhage, fibrous proliferation, and mild inflammatory changes are seen.

An enthesopathy occurring at other tendinous and ligamentous connections to bone in patients with seronega-

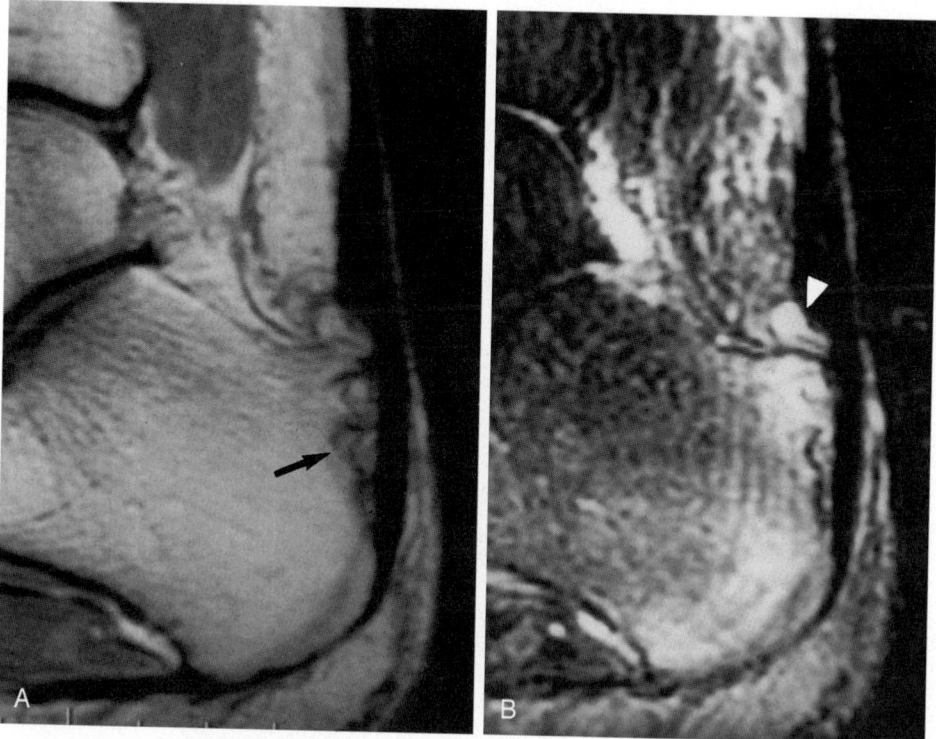

**Figure 15–20.** Abnormalities of bursae in seronegative spondyloarthropathies. In this patient with probable Reiter's syndrome, sagittal intermediate-weighted (TR/TE, 3000/24) *(A)* and fat-suppressed T2-weighted (TR/TE, 3500/114) *(B)* fast spin echo MR images reveal erosion of the posterior surface of the calcaneus *(arrow)* and fluid in the retrocalcaneal bursa *(B, arrowhead)*, with reactive edema in the posterosuperior aspect of the bone. Additional findings include focal thickening of the Achilles tendon, calcaneal edema adjacent to the attachment site of the plantar fascia, and superficial bursitis posterior to the Achilles tendon.

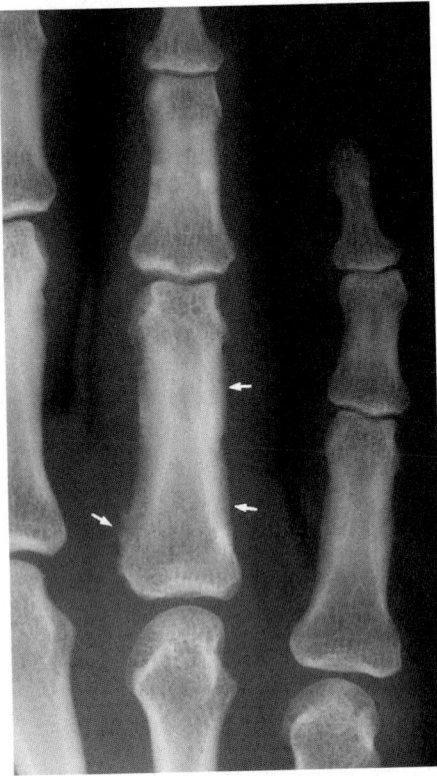

**Figure 15–21.** Abnormalities of tendon sheaths in seronegative spondyloarthropathies. The soft tissue swelling and periostitis *(arrows)* involving the proximal phalanx of the fourth finger are entirely consistent with tenosynovitis, a characteristic finding of the seronegative spondyloarthropathies. (Courtesy of D. Goodwin, MD, Hanover, N.H.)

**TABLE 15–7**

**Abnormalities of Cartilaginous Joints and Entheses in the Seronegative Spondyloarthropathies**

| Pathologic | Radiologic |
|---|---|
| Inflammation of subchondral bone | Bony erosion and sclerosis |
| Bony proliferation | Bony ankylosis |
| Inflammation of capsular, ligamentous, and tendinous attachments | Bony erosion and sclerosis |

tive spondyloarthropathies is responsible for the prominent clinical and radiographic manifestations in the plantar aspect of the calcaneus, pelvis, patella, iliac crest, ischial and humeral tuberosities, and femoral trochanters (Fig. 15–23). At these sites, edema, a decrease in hematopoietic tissue, and cellular deposits in the adjacent bone marrow are associated with osseous erosion and sclerosis. Bony deposition can eventually obscure the eroded surface and produce a poorly defined or "fluffy" osseous contour.

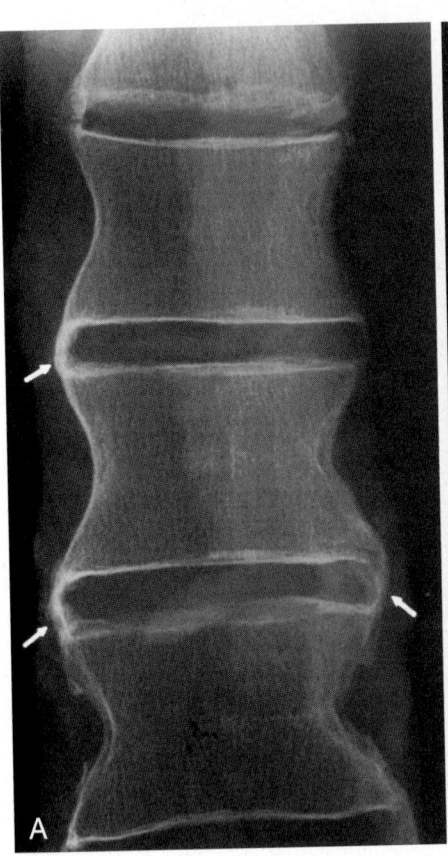

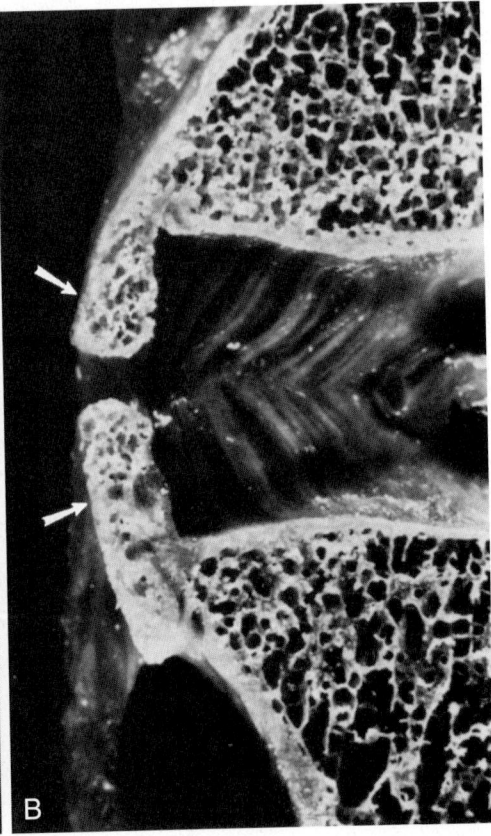

**Figure 15–22.** Cartilaginous joint (discovertebral junction) abnormalities in seronegative spondyloarthropathies. *A,* Radiograph of a coronal section of the spine in a cadaver with ankylosing spondylitis reveals typical syndesmophytes extending as linear osseous bridges from one vertebral body to the next *(arrows). B,* In a photograph of a corresponding section from another cadaver with ankylosing spondylitis, the nature of the syndesmophytes is evident *(arrows)*—they represent chondrification and ossification of the anulus fibrosus.

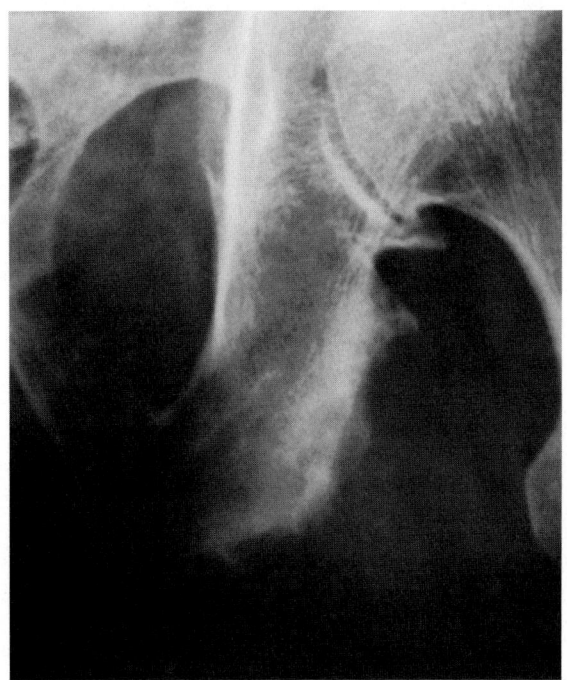

**Figure 15–23.** Abnormalities of entheses in seronegative spondyloarthropathies. Observe the poorly defined erosion and reactive bone formation in the ischial tuberosity in a patient with ankylosing spondylitis. (Courtesy of V. Vint, MD, San Diego, Calif.)

## FURTHER READING

Ball J: Enthesopathy of rheumatoid and ankylosing spondylitis. Ann Rheum Dis 30:213, 1971.

Bywaters EGL: Pathology of the spondyloarthropathies. In Calin A (ed): Spondyloarthropathies. New York, Grune & Stratton, 1984.

Bywaters EGL: Rheumatoid and other diseases of the cervical interspinous bursae and changes in the spinous processes. Ann Rheum Dis 41:360, 1982.

Cruickshank B: Pathology of ankylosing spondylitis. Clin Orthop 74:43, 1971.

Fassbender HG: Pathology of Rheumatic Diseases. New York, Springer-Verlag, 1975, p 79.

Gardner DL: Pathology of rheumatoid arthritis. In Copeman's Textbook of the Rheumatic Diseases, 5th ed. Edinburgh, Churchill Livingstone, 1978, p 273.

Ginsberg MH, Genant HK, Yu TF, et al: Rheumatoid nodulosis: An unusual variant of rheumatoid disease. Arthritis Rheum 18:49, 1975.

Goupille P, Roulot B, Akoka S, et al: Magnetic resonance imaging: A valuable method for the detection of synovial inflammation in rheumatoid arthritis. J Rheumatol 28:35, 2001.

Jaffe HL: Metabolic, Degenerative and Inflammatory Diseases of Bones and Joints. Philadelphia, Lea & Febiger, 1972, p 779.

Kaye BR, Kaye RL, Bobrove A: Rheumatoid nodules: Review of the spectrum of associated conditions and proposal of a new classification, with a report of four seronegative cases. Am J Med 76:279, 1984.

Martel W: Pathogenesis of cervical discovertebral destruction in rheumatoid arthritis. Arthritis Rheum 20:1217, 1977.

Martel W, Hayes JT, Duff IF: The pattern of bone erosion in the hand and wrist in rheumatoid arthritis. Radiology 84:204, 1965.

Rapoport AS, Sosman JL, Weissman BN: Lesions resembling gout in patients with rheumatoid arthritis. AJR Am J Roentgenol 126:41, 1976.

Rauschning W: Popliteal cysts and their relation to the gastrocnemiosemimembranosus bursa: Studies on the surgical and functional anatomy. Acta Orthop Scand 179(Suppl):9, 1979.

Resnick D: Inflammatory disorders of the vertebral column: Seronegative spondyloarthropathies, adult-onset rheumatoid arthritis, and juvenile chronic arthritis. Clin Imaging 13:253, 1989.

Resnick D: Radiology of seronegative spondyloarthropathies. Clin Orthop 143:38, 1979.

Resnick D, Cone R: Pathological fractures in rheumatoid arthritis: Sites and mechanisms. Radiographics 4:549, 1984.

Resnick D, Feingold ML, Curd J, et al: Calcaneal abnormalities in articular disorders: Rheumatoid arthritis, ankylosing spondylitis, psoriatic arthritis and Reiter's syndrome. Radiology 125:355, 1977.

Resnick D, Niwayama G: On the nature and significance of bony proliferation in "rheumatoid variant" disorders. AJR Am J Roentgenol 129:275, 1977.

Resnick D, Niwayama G, Coutts R: Subchondral cysts (geodes) in arthritic disorders: Pathologic and radiographic appearance of the hip joint. AJR Am J Roentgenol 128:799, 1977.

Schils JP, Resnick D, Haghighi PN, et al: Pathogenesis of discovertebral and manubriosternal joint abnormalities in rheumatoid arthritis: A cadaveric study. J Rheumatol 16:291, 1989.

Schneider R, Kaye JJ: Insufficiency and stress fractures of the long bones occurring in patients with rheumatoid arthritis. Radiology 116:595, 1975.

Sokoloff L: The pathology of rheumatoid arthritis and allied disorders. In Hollander JL, McCarty DJ Jr (eds): Arthritis and Allied Conditions, 8th ed. Philadelphia, Lea & Febiger, 1972, p 309.

Sugimoto H, Takeda A, Hyodoh K: Early stage rheumatoid arthritis: Prospective study of the effectiveness of MR imaging for diagnosis. Radiology 216:569, 2000.

Wu PC, Fang D, Ho EKW, et al: The pathogenesis of extensive discovertebral destruction in ankylosing spondylitis. Clin Orthop 230:154, 1988.

# CHAPTER 16

## Rheumatoid Arthritis

### SUMMARY OF KEY FEATURES

Rheumatoid arthritis is a common articular disorder with a characteristic radiographic picture. A symmetrical polyarticular disease of the synovial joints of the appendicular skeleton is apparent, with prominent abnormalities of the proximal interphalangeal and metacarpophalangeal joints of the hand, the wrist, the metatarsophalangeal joints of the foot, the posterior and plantar aspects of the calcaneus, the knee, the elbow, the glenohumeral and acromioclavicular joints, the ankle, and the hip; these abnormalities are commonly combined with changes in the cervical spine. This distribution of synovial joint involvement generally allows an accurate diagnosis, especially when the involvement is characterized by fusiform soft tissue swelling, regional or periarticular osteoporosis, marginal and central osseous erosions and cysts, and diffuse loss of interosseous space.

### INTRODUCTION

Rheumatoid arthritis is an "everyday" disease whose general clinical, pathologic, and radiologic features are well known to most physicians. An in-depth inspection of the radiographic and pathologic characteristics of rheumatoid arthritis provides a standard by which the other rheumatologic conditions can be measured. Such an inspection must initially consider the basic pathology and radiology of rheumatoid involvement of musculoskeletal tissue. This essential background information was presented in Chapter 15. This chapter analyzes the changes produced by rheumatoid arthritis in specific locations of the body.

### DIAGNOSTIC CRITERIA

Accurate diagnosis of rheumatoid arthritis is made without difficulty in a patient with a generalized symmetrical, peripherally located polyarthritis associated with (1) clinically detectable severe morning stiffness, synovial inflammation, and subcutaneous nodules; (2) radiologic evidence of an erosive articular process; (3) laboratory parameters of the disease, including a positive serologic test for rheumatoid factor and an elevated erythrocyte sedimentation rate; and (4) pathologic documentation of typical rheumatoid lesions of the synovium and soft tissues. More troublesome, however, is establishing the presence of this disease in a person who has atypical clinical and radiologic features. Because of this difficulty, diagnostic criteria have been proposed:

1. Morning stiffness in and around joints lasting at least 1 hour before maximal improvement

2. Soft tissue swelling (arthritis) of three or more joint areas observed by a physician

3. Swelling (arthritis) of the proximal interphalangeal, metacarpophalangeal, or wrist joints

4. Symmetrical swelling (arthritis)

5. Rheumatoid nodules

6. Presence of rheumatoid factor

7. Radiographic erosions, periarticular osteopenia, or both, in the hand, wrist, or both joints

Criteria 1 through 4 must have been present for at least 6 weeks. Rheumatoid arthritis is defined by the presence of four or more criteria, and no further qualification (e.g., classic, definite, probable) or list of exclusions is required.

### CLINICAL ABNORMALITIES

#### General Features

Although rheumatoid arthritis can occur in persons of all ages, it predominates in those between the ages of 25 and 55 years. Women are affected more commonly than men, with the female-to-male ratio being approximately 2:1 to 3:1. Various prodromal symptoms have been noted in rheumatoid arthritis, including fatigue, anorexia, weight loss, malaise, and muscular pain and stiffness. These findings can be obscured by prominent articular complaints, which are frequently an early manifestation of the disease. Joint pain and stiffness may initially involve a single joint for a period of weeks or months before more generalized articular findings become evident. In these instances of monoarthritis, clinical diagnosis can be extremely difficult. With the appearance of polyarticular disease, the correct diagnosis becomes more apparent. The eventual outcome of the joint disease is variable. Some patients demonstrate mild clinical manifestations for a long time, whereas others rapidly develop severe, disabling arthritis.

#### Articular Involvement

Articular involvement manifests as pain that is aggravated by motion, swelling, stiffness, and limitation of movement. Periarticular soft tissue swelling is fusiform or spindle shaped, as a result of increased intra-articular fluid, synovial hypertrophy, and thickening of adjacent soft tissues.

The most typically affected joints are the proximal interphalangeal and metacarpophalangeal joints of the hand, the wrist, the metatarsophalangeal joints of the foot, the knee, the joints of the shoulder, the ankle, and, to a lesser extent, the hip; any joint can be involved, however. Although symmetry is the hallmark of joint involvement, some exceptions exist:

1. Symmetrical abnormalities of groups of joints (e.g., metacarpophalangeal and metatarsophalangeal articulations) may be seen, but the same digits may not be affected on both sides of the body.

2. Initially, monoarticular or pauciarticular abnormalities may be noted that do not obey the rule of symmetry.

3. A markedly asymmetrical or unilateral distribution may be seen in patients with neurologic deficits. Unilateral muscle weakening or paralysis protects the ipsilateral side from the effects of the articular disease.

4. Differences in the distribution of rheumatoid arthritis are occasionally related to the sex of the patient. A symmetrical distribution in the small peripheral joints of the extremities is more typical in women than in men.

5. Atypical cases of "rheumatoid arthritis" (those that do not meet all the necessary criteria for the disease) are often characterized by asymmetrical joint alterations.

## Soft Tissue, Muscular, and Vascular Involvement

Subcutaneous nodules are evident in approximately one fourth of patients with rheumatoid arthritis. They appear at pressure points, especially the juxta-articular regions of the elbow, although they may appear in distant body sites, including the lungs, pleurae, and abdominal wall. Subcutaneous nodules usually have an insidious onset and persist unchanged for months or years. Ulceration, drainage, and sepsis can occur in association with these lesions.

Muscular weakness and atrophy may be prominent in patients with rheumatoid arthritis. These muscular abnormalities may be related to disuse or inflammatory changes. Inflammatory and noninflammatory vascular lesions also occur and can lead to complications, including peripheral neuropathy, bowel perforation, myocardial infarction, Raynaud's phenomenon, gangrene, and pulmonary hypertension.

## Systemic Involvement

**Neuropathies.** Several types of peripheral neuropathies occur in this disease. A mild or severe sensory and motor neuropathy has been noted. Its manifestations include a symmetrical distribution, involvement of the upper or lower extremities, a "stocking" distribution of sensory impairment, and wristdrop and footdrop. Entrapment or compressive neuropathies are also observed. These neuropathies, which relate to mechanical irritation of a specific peripheral nerve at a vulnerable anatomic site (within fibrous or osseofibrous canals), can affect the median nerve (carpal tunnel syndrome, "double crush" syndrome, anterior interosseous syndrome), ulnar nerve (cubital canal syndrome, canal of Guyon syndrome, double crush syndrome), and radial nerve (posterior interosseous syndrome) in the upper extremity and the sciatic nerve (tibial or common peroneal entrapment by a Baker's cyst), common peroneal nerve (pressure palsy), and tibial nerve (tarsal tunnel syndrome, medial plantar syndrome, lateral plantar syndrome) in the lower extremity.

**Felty's Syndrome.** This syndrome consists of rheumatoid arthritis, splenomegaly, and leukopenia. Additional clinical manifestations include a typical onset in the fifth, sixth, or seventh decade of life, weight loss, anemia, lymphadenopathy, chronic leg ulceration, and abnormal skin pigmentation. Women are affected more frequently than men, and the disease is rare in black persons. The articular manifestations of Felty's syndrome are similar to those of severe rheumatoid arthritis.

**Metabolic Bone Disorders.** Osteopenia is a well-recognized manifestation of rheumatoid arthritis. In almost all patients, such osteopenia relates to osteoporosis. In addition, osteomalacia may contribute to osteopenia in some patients.

**Sjögren's Syndrome.** Sjögren's syndrome is a triad consisting of keratoconjunctivitis sicca, xerostomia, and connective tissue disease. The last feature is evident in 50% to 70% of patients with Sjögren's syndrome and may be identical to rheumatoid arthritis.

## LABORATORY ABNORMALITIES

A moderate normochromic or hypochromic normocytic anemia is common in this disease. The leukocyte count can be normal, elevated, or, infrequently, decreased. The erythrocyte sedimentation rate is commonly markedly elevated and tends to parallel the activity of the disease. C-reactive protein is evident in almost all patients with clinical evidence of disease activity, and the presence of this protein parallels the elevation in the erythrocyte sedimentation rate. Rheumatoid factors are generally present in high titer in the serum of patients with this disease. They are also evident in a variety of chronic inflammatory conditions but are not detected in great concentration in most other articular disorders. Seropositivity is generally associated with a poorer prognosis in rheumatoid arthritis.

## ABNORMALITIES AT SPECIFIC LOCATIONS
### General Distribution

A symmetrical arthritis showing a predilection for the hands, wrists, feet, knees, shoulders, elbows, ankles, and hips is typical (Fig. 16–1). In the axial skeleton, the articulations of the cervical spine are the only sites that are consistently affected, although changes in the thoracolumbar spine and sacroiliac joints are occasionally encountered.

## Hand

### Clinical Abnormalities

The joints of the hand are affected in almost all persons with rheumatoid arthritis. Metacarpophalangeal and proximal interphalangeal joint alterations predominate. Clinical (as well as radiologic) evidence of distal interphalangeal joint disease is less common and is infrequently severe. In long-standing disease, swan-neck deformities (hyperextension at the proximal interphalangeal joints and flexion at the distal interphalangeal joints), boutonnière deformities (flexion at the proximal interphalangeal joints and hyperextension at the distal interphalangeal joints), and hitchhiker's, or Z-shaped, deformity of the thumb (flexion at the metacarpophalangeal joint and hyperextension at the interphalangeal joint) can be observed.

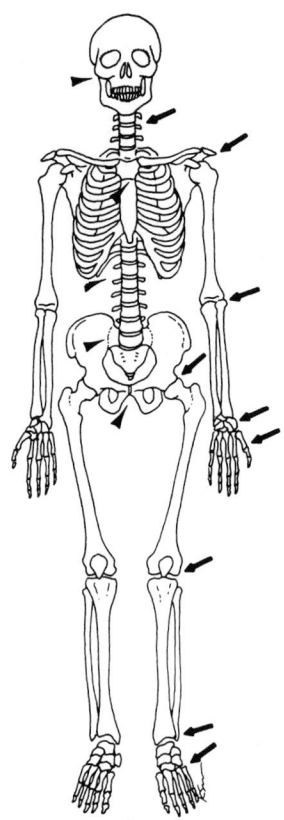

**Figure 16–1.** General distribution of disease in rheumatoid arthritis. Rheumatoid arthritis is characteristically a symmetrical arthritis of the small joints of the hands (proximal interphalangeal and metacarpophalangeal joints), feet (metatarsophalangeal joints and interphalangeal joint of the great toe), wrists (all compartments), knees, ankles, elbows, glenohumeral and acromioclavicular joints, and hips *(arrows)*. In the axial skeleton, the articulations of the cervical spine are typically affected *(arrow)*. Less consistent involvement occurs in the thoracolumbar spine, sacroiliac and temporomandibular joints, symphysis pubis, and manubriosternal joint *(arrowheads)*.

Spontaneous rupture of the extensor tendons of the digits is a well-recognized complication of this disease.

## Radiographic-Pathologic Correlation

### Early Abnormalities

Radiographic abnormalities of the interphalangeal and metacarpophalangeal joints in rheumatoid arthritis are well described. The second and third metacarpophalangeal joints and the third proximal interphalangeal joint may reveal the earliest abnormalities (Figs. 16–2 to 16–4). Fusiform soft tissue swelling, periarticular osteoporosis, concentric loss of articular space, and marginal erosions become evident at many or all of the proximal interphalangeal and metacarpophalangeal joints.

Marginal erosions about the distal interphalangeal joints are generally small in comparison to those at the more proximal digital joints. In addition to marginal erosions, two other types of bone erosion have been noted in the hands of patients with rheumatoid arthritis: compressive (pressure) erosions and superficial surface resorption (Table 16–1).

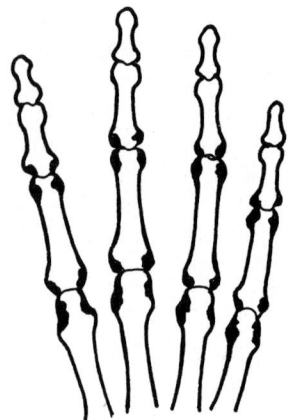

**Figure 16–2.** Metacarpophalangeal and proximal interphalangeal joints: target areas. In the four ulnar digits, early osseous erosions may appear at the radial and ulnar aspects of the metacarpophalangeal and proximal interphalangeal joints. The initial changes occur on the radial aspect of the phalanges and metacarpal bones at the second and third metacarpophalangeal joints and on the radial and ulnar aspects of the phalanges at the third proximal interphalangeal articulation. Distal interphalangeal joint changes are less common and less severe.

### Continued Abnormalities

With further destruction of cartilage and bone, the articular space may be obliterated completely. Erosion of central portions of the joint can lead to apparently enclosed radiolucent defects. In some patients, particularly those with rheumatoid nodulosis, prominent cystic lesions of the phalanges may be unaccompanied by joint space narrowing or significant synovitis.

Although fibrous ankylosis is characteristically the ultimate fate of severe arthritis of the metacarpophalangeal and proximal interphalangeal joints, occasional examples of intra-articular osseous fusion can be seen in these locations. In almost all such instances, the proximal interphalangeal joint is ankylosed; bony ankylosis of the metacarpophalangeal articulation is exceedingly unusual, with the exception of that in the thumb.

### Finger Deviations and Deformities

Deviation and deformity of the fingers are common complications of rheumatoid arthritis.

**Mallet Finger.** Loosening or disruption of the distal attachment of the extensor tendon to the terminal phalanx may result in the development of a typical mallet or drop finger. With progressive loosening of the collateral ligaments, combined with the detrimental effect of the intra-articular inflamed synovial tissue on cartilage and bone, instability of the distal interphalangeal joint can appear. This is relatively uncommon.

**Boutonnière Deformity.** In normal situations, the balanced tendon mechanism and ligamentous restriction prevent collapse deformity of the digits, but in rheumatoid arthritis, this vulnerable balance is compromised by the direct

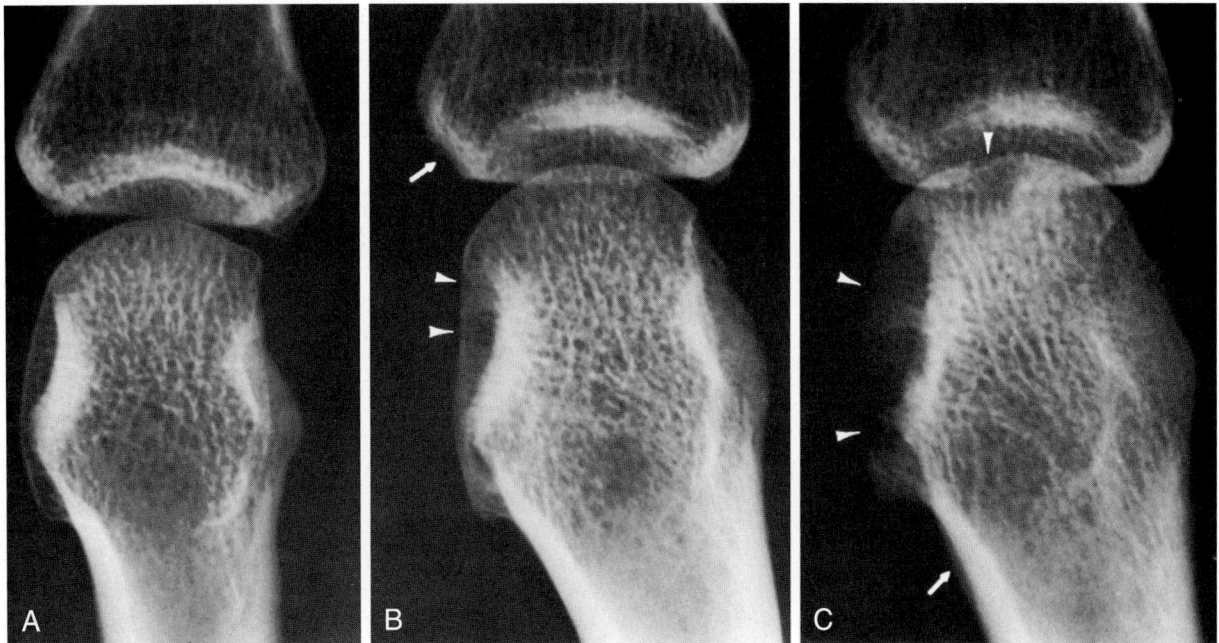

**Figure 16–3.** Metacarpophalangeal joint abnormalities: early changes. *A,* Initially, the bones appear normal, with preservation of the subchondral bone plate on the radial aspect of the metacarpal head. *B,* Subsequently, small radiolucent areas appear beneath the metacarpal head and are related to thinning of the bone plate with focal discontinuity or gaps *(arrowheads).* Tiny erosions and surface irregularity of the proximal phalanx are also evident *(arrow).* *C,* At a later stage, obvious osseous defects are seen *(arrowheads).* Note the mild periosteal proliferation *(arrow).*

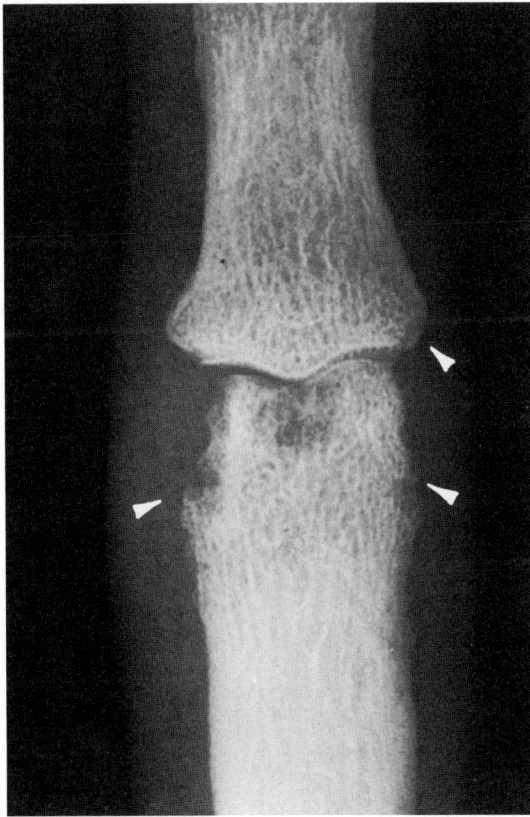

**Figure 16–4.** Proximal interphalangeal joint abnormalities: early changes. Initial radiographic changes include soft tissue swelling, joint space narrowing, and marginal erosions *(arrowheads).* Note that the erosive changes are more extensive on the proximal phalanx than on the middle phalanx.

effect of the disease on articulations, tendons, and ligaments. Flexion of the proximal interphalangeal joint combined with hyperextension at the distal interphalangeal joint produces a boutonnière deformity of the digit (Fig. 16–5).

**Swan-Neck Deformity.** Swan-neck deformity (see Fig. 16–5) consists of hyperextension of the proximal interphalangeal joint and flexion of the distal interphalangeal joint. Although synovitis of the proximal interphalangeal joint, hyperextension of the long extensor tendons, deformity of the metacarpophalangeal articulation, and carpal collapse may be contributory factors, the primary cause of the deformity is synovitis of the flexor tendon sheath, which restricts interphalangeal joint flexion.

**Deformities of the Metacarpophalangeal Joint.** A variety of metacarpophalangeal articular deformities and deviations (Fig. 16–6) may appear in rheumatoid hands, including ulnar drift, extensor tendon subluxation, and palmar subluxation and flexion of the joint. Ulnar deviation has been recorded in 25% to 65% of hands in patients with rheumatoid arthritis, and palmar subluxation has been noted in 20% to 68%. A relationship between radial deviation of the wrist and ulnar deviation at the metacarpophalangeal joints has been noted to produce the zigzag deformity of the hand in rheumatoid arthritis.

**Thumb Deformities.** The thumb malalignments encountered most frequently in rheumatoid arthritis are collapse deformities (boutonnière deformity) related to disturbance of function at the first metacarpophalangeal joint; swan-neck deformity, related to disturbance of function at the first carpometacarpal joint; and instability, stiffness,

TABLE 16-1

### Types of Bony Erosion in the Hand and Wrist in Rheumatoid Arthritis

| Type | Mechanism | Common Sites |
|------|-----------|--------------|
| Marginal erosion | Pannus destruction of bare areas (without protective cartilage) of bone | Metacarpophalangeal and proximal interphalangeal joints, radial styloid, midportion of scaphoid, triquetrum, capitate, trapezium |
| Compressive erosion | Collapse of osteoporotic bone by muscular forces | Metacarpophalangeal joints |
| Surface resorption | Erosion of bone beneath inflamed tendons | Outer aspect of distal end of ulna, dorsal aspect of first metacarpal bone, proximal phalanx of first digit |

or pain of the interphalangeal, metacarpophalangeal, and carpometacarpal joints. Boutonnière deformity (Z-shaped deformity, or hitchhiker's thumb) is the most common collapse deformity of the thumb in patients with rheumatoid arthritis.

## Wrist

### Clinical Abnormalities

Although generally accompanied by abnormalities in the fingers, clinical (and radiologic) involvement of the wrist may initially appear in the absence of significant digital alterations. Clinical findings may be related to synovitis in any of the compartments of the wrist, adjacent tenosynovitis, and attenuation or injury of several soft tissue, tendinous, and ligamentous structures. Extensor carpi ulnaris tenosynovitis creates a painless swelling on the ulnar aspect of the wrist. Subsequent clinical features in rheumatoid arthritis relate to dorsal subluxation of the distal portion of the ulna; carpal tunnel syndrome, attributable to synovitis in the carpal tunnel, with dysesthesias along the course of the median nerve; and rupture of one or more extensor tendons. Further, synovial cysts arising during the disease can create local soft tissue masses.

### Radiographic-Pathologic Correlation

#### Early Abnormalities

The early radiographic and pathologic findings of rheumatoid wrist disease have been well delineated.

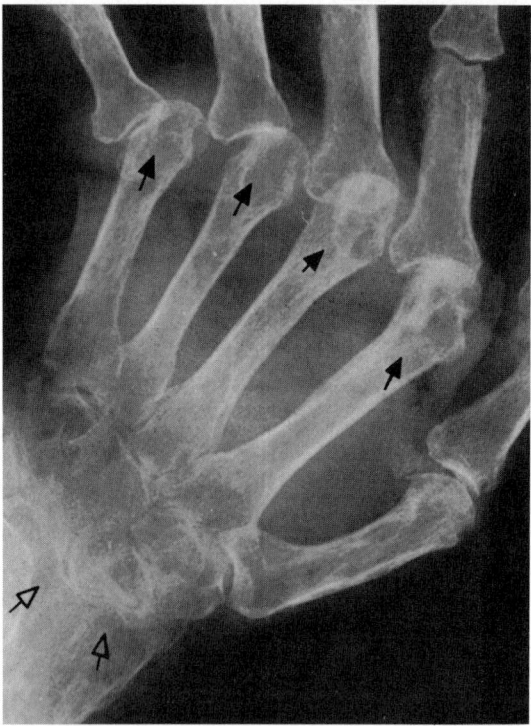

**Figure 16–6.** Metacarpophalangeal joint deformities: ulnar deviation. The simultaneous occurrence of ulnar deviation at the metacarpophalangeal joints (*solid arrows*) and radial deviation at the radiocarpal joint of the wrist (*open arrows*) is obvious in this patient. The resulting appearance is termed the zigzag deformity.

**Figure 16–5.** Boutonnière and swan-neck deformities of the digits. A typical swan-neck deformity of the third and fourth digits (*open arrows*) and boutonnière deformity of the second digit (*closed arrow*) are evident in this patient with rheumatoid arthritis.

**Distal End and Styloid Process of the Ulna.** Erosion and swelling around the distal end of the ulna and the ulnar styloid process are early manifestations of rheumatoid arthritis and are related to abnormalities of the prestyloid recess of the radiocarpal compartment, the inferior radioulnar compartment, and the extensor carpi ulnaris tendon and sheath (Figs. 16–7 and 16–8). The prestyloid recess of the radiocarpal compartment is intimate with the ulnar styloid process. The inflamed synovial tissue within the prestyloid recess is in contact with and may produce erosions of the tip of the ulnar styloid process. As erosion progresses, the ulnar styloid tip becomes increasingly irregular. Proliferative synovitis within the inferior radioulnar compartment is frequently coincident with rheumatoid arthritis and results in localized prominence of the soft tissues. Tendinosis and tenosynovitis of the extensor carpi ulnaris tendon and its sheath also contribute to the abnormality of the distal end of the ulna and the ulnar styloid process.

**Radial Styloid Process and Scaphoid.** Synovial inflammation within the radiocarpal compartment leads to rheumatoid erosion of the distal end of the radius (i.e., radial styloid process) and the adjacent scaphoid bone (Fig. 16–9). Alterations in the lateral midportion of the scaphoid bone are characteristic, although surface irregularity at this site must be distinguished from a normal degree of notching of the scaphoid.

**Palmar Aspect of the Distal End of the Radius.** Radiographs of rheumatoid wrists frequently reveal erosions that appear as irregular radiolucent shadows overlying the midportion of the distal end of the radius in posteroanterior views.

**Triquetrum and Pisiform Bones.** Erosion of the triquetrum and pisiform bones is common in early rheumatoid arthritis and occurs at three sites: the proximal medial portion of

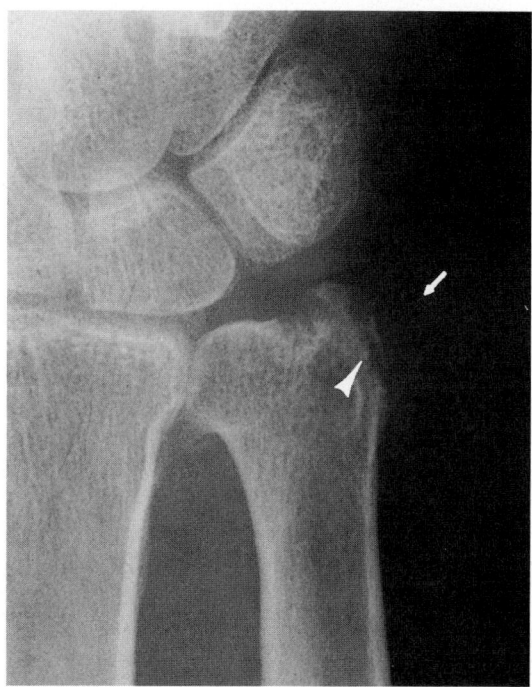

**Figure 16–8.** Abnormalities of the distal end and styloid process of the ulna: extensor carpi ulnaris tendon and tendon sheath. The wrist of a rheumatoid patient shows soft tissue swelling *(arrow)* and subjacent resorption of bone with periosteal proliferation *(arrowhead)*. Additional alterations include changes on apposing surfaces of the distal ends of the radius and ulna.

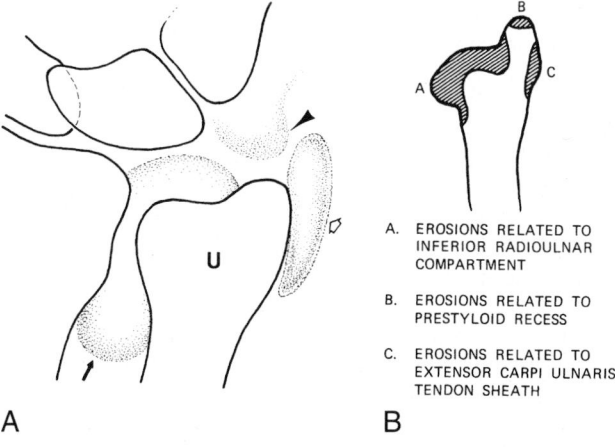

**Figure 16–7.** Abnormalities of the distal end and styloid process of the ulna: sites of early soft tissue swelling and osseous erosion. *A,* Soft tissue swelling about the distal end of the ulna (U) may appear as distention of the prestyloid recess of the radiocarpal compartment *(arrowhead)*, the inferior radioulnar compartment *(solid arrow)*, or the extensor carpi ulnaris tendon sheath *(open arrow)*. *B,* Early osseous erosions appear at three distinct areas in the distal portion of the ulna.

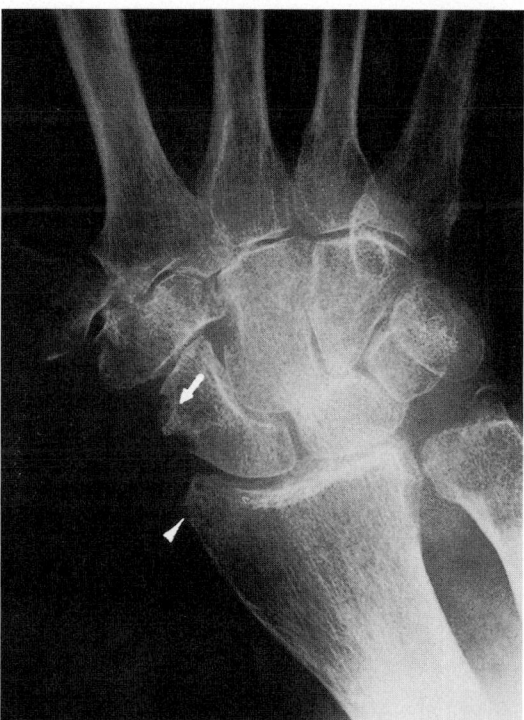

**Figure 16–9.** Abnormalities of the radial styloid process and scaphoid. Radiograph of a rheumatoid wrist shows erosion of the radial styloid process *(arrowhead)* and lateral midportion of the scaphoid bone *(arrow)*, characteristic of rheumatoid arthritis. Widespread abnormalities are present throughout the wrist.

the triquetrum, the distal medial portion of the triquetrum, and the adjacent surfaces of the triquetrum and the pisiform (Fig. 16–10). The pisiform-triquetral compartment is seen tangentially in "reverse" oblique radiographs made with the wrist in a semisupinated position. Because these abnormalities may occur early and are not visible on posteroanterior radiographs, radiography in the reverse oblique projection is suggested for evaluation of the wrist in rheumatoid arthritis.

**Midcarpal, Carpometacarpal, and Intermetacarpal Compartments.** Marginal erosion of the trapezium adjacent to the attachment of the radial collateral ligament and on the radial aspect of the capitate bone has been noted. Marginal erosion of the radial aspect of the base of the first metacarpal bone indicates rheumatoid involvement of the first carpometacarpal compartment.

### Continued Abnormalities

Continued synovial inflammation within the wrist soon results in significant alteration in all the compartments, characterized by progressive loss and obliteration of the articular space, further osseous erosion, and bony ankylosis (Fig. 16–11). This pancompartmental distribution is characteristic of rheumatoid arthritis and allows differentiation from the selective compartmental changes encountered in a variety of other disease processes affecting the wrist. Intra-articular osseous fusion can lead to carpal masses of variable size.

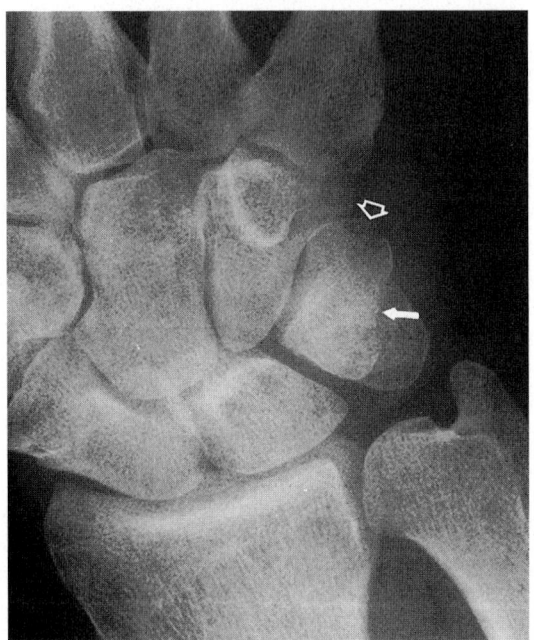

**Figure 16–10.** Abnormalities of the triquetrum and pisiform: radiocarpal and midcarpal compartments. Radiograph of the wrist in a patient with rheumatoid arthritis shows marginal erosions *(open and solid arrows)* of the triquetrum. The erosions are related to abnormality at the ulnar, or medial, limit of the midcarpal compartment and, to a lesser extent, the ulnar limit of the radiocarpal compartment.

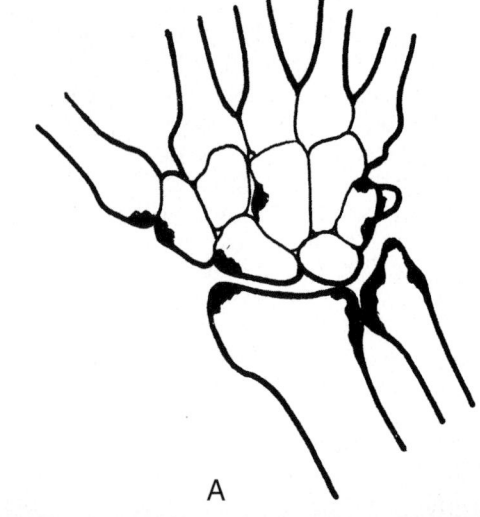

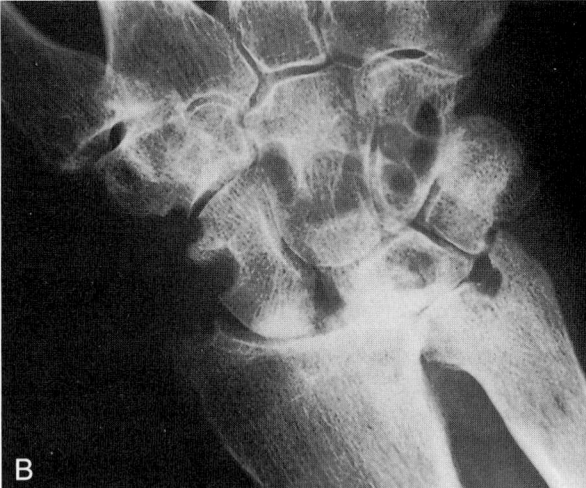

**Figure 16–11.** Pancompartmental abnormalities of a rheumatoid wrist. *A*, Some of the typical sites of osseous erosion in rheumatoid arthritis are indicated. Note that all the compartments in the wrist are soon involved. *B*, Radiograph demonstrates typical pancompartmental osseous erosions in rheumatoid arthritis.

### Wrist Malalignment and Deformity

Incongruity in cartilaginous and osseous surfaces, laxity of the articular capsule and ligaments, and muscular and tendinous imbalance can cause malalignment of the wrist in rheumatoid arthritis.

**Radiocarpal Malalignment.** Destruction of the triangular fibrocartilage and dorsal subluxation of the distal end of the ulna disrupt the normal concavity of the radiocarpal compartment (Fig. 16–12). The proximal row of carpal bones migrates in a medial (ulnar) and palmar direction along the inclined articular surface of the distal end of the radius. The radial deviation at the radiocarpal compartment that results from medial migration of the scaphoid and lunate may be apparent in as many as 70% of wrists of patients with rheumatoid arthritis. Imbalance of the muscles and tendons contributes to radial deviation at the wrist, and imbalance of the tendons may also be asso-

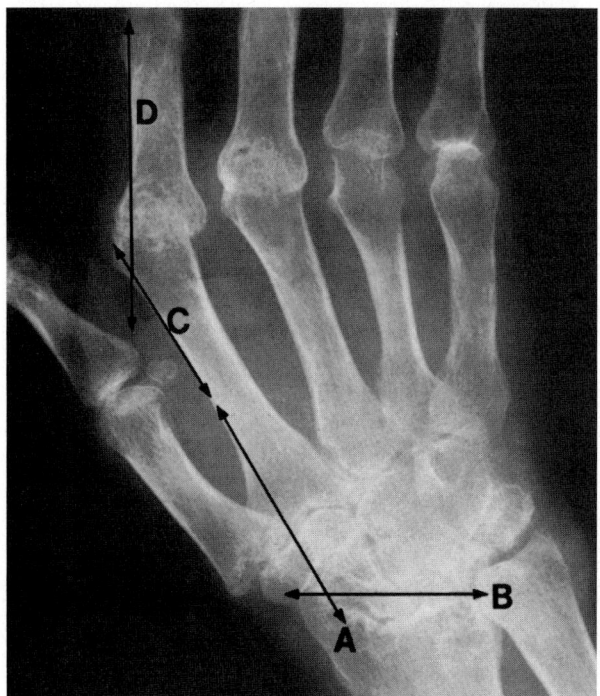

**Figure 16–12.** Wrist malalignment and deformity: radiocarpal malalignment. Radiograph shows a typical zigzag deformity caused by radial deviation at the wrist (angle created by the intersection of lines A and B) and ulnar deviation at the metacarpophalangeal joints (angle created by the intersection of lines C and D).

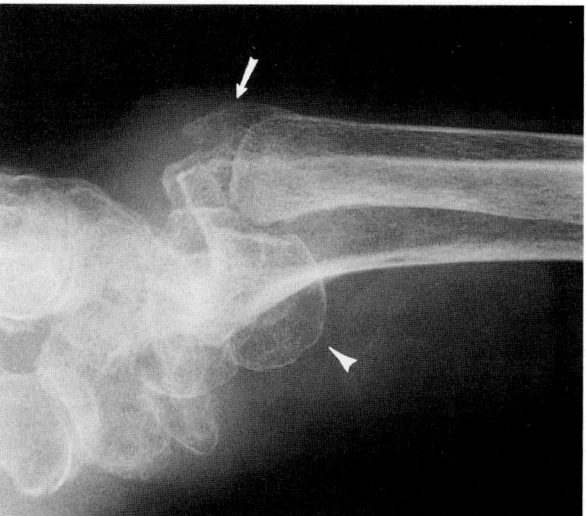

**Figure 16–13.** Wrist malalignment and deformity: inferior radioulnar and distal ulnar malalignment. Lateral radiograph reveals severe dorsal subluxation of the distal part of the ulna (*arrow*), in addition to significant and widespread osseous and articular changes. Note the abnormal position of the lunate (*arrowhead*) overlying the distal end of the radius.

ciated with ulnar deviation at the metacarpophalangeal joints, producing a zigzag deformity of the hand.

**Intercarpal Malalignment.** Both palmar flexion instability (palmar, or volar, intercalated segment instability) and dorsiflexion instability (dorsal intercalated segment instability) occur in the wrist in rheumatoid arthritis, although the latter is more frequent. Palmar flexion instability is manifested by medial migration of the proximal row of carpal bones, with resulting palmar flexion of the lunate and scaphoid bones. Dorsiflexion instability is sometimes related to abnormality of the distal attachment of the palmar radiocarpal ligaments and disruption of the scapholunate ligament.

**Inferior Radioulnar and Distal Ulnar Malalignment.** Rheumatoid arthritis deformities on the ulnar aspect of the wrist include distal and dorsal subluxation of the ulna and diastasis of the inferior radioulnar compartment (Fig. 16–13). The caput ulnae syndrome consists of pain, limited motion, and dorsal prominence of the distal end of the ulna. The abnormally located, eroded head of the ulna projects into the compartments of the extensor tendons on the dorsum of the wrist and produces fraying of the tendon surfaces. Mechanical attrition in association with tenosynovitis may lead to weakening of these tendons and rupture.

## Elbow

### Clinical Abnormalities

The elbow is frequently involved in rheumatoid arthritis. Involvement is commonly bilateral but may be more marked in the dominant extremity, and it is usually associated with polyarthritis. Clinical symptoms and signs are variable but can lead to considerable disability as a result of limitation of both flexion and extension of the joint. Additional clinical manifestations include mild to moderate pain and tenderness, swelling over the lateral aspect of the joint between the radial head and the olecranon, antecubital soft tissue masses related to synovial cysts with compression of adjacent nerves, and paraolecranon nodules, synovial cysts, or bursitis. Olecranon bursitis is seen not only in rheumatoid arthritis but also in gout and in association with trauma or infection.

### Radiographic-Pathologic Correlation

Synovial inflammation in the elbow with progressive destruction of cartilage and bone produces soft tissue swelling with a positive "fat pad" sign, periarticular osteoporosis, joint space narrowing, and bone erosions. Erosion and deformity of the radial head, the coronoid process of the ulna, and the distal portion of the humerus are most typical. More severe changes are characterized by extensive osteolysis of large portions of the humerus, radius, and ulna. Prominent cystic lesions of the olecranon process can fracture spontaneously or after minor trauma (Fig. 16–14).

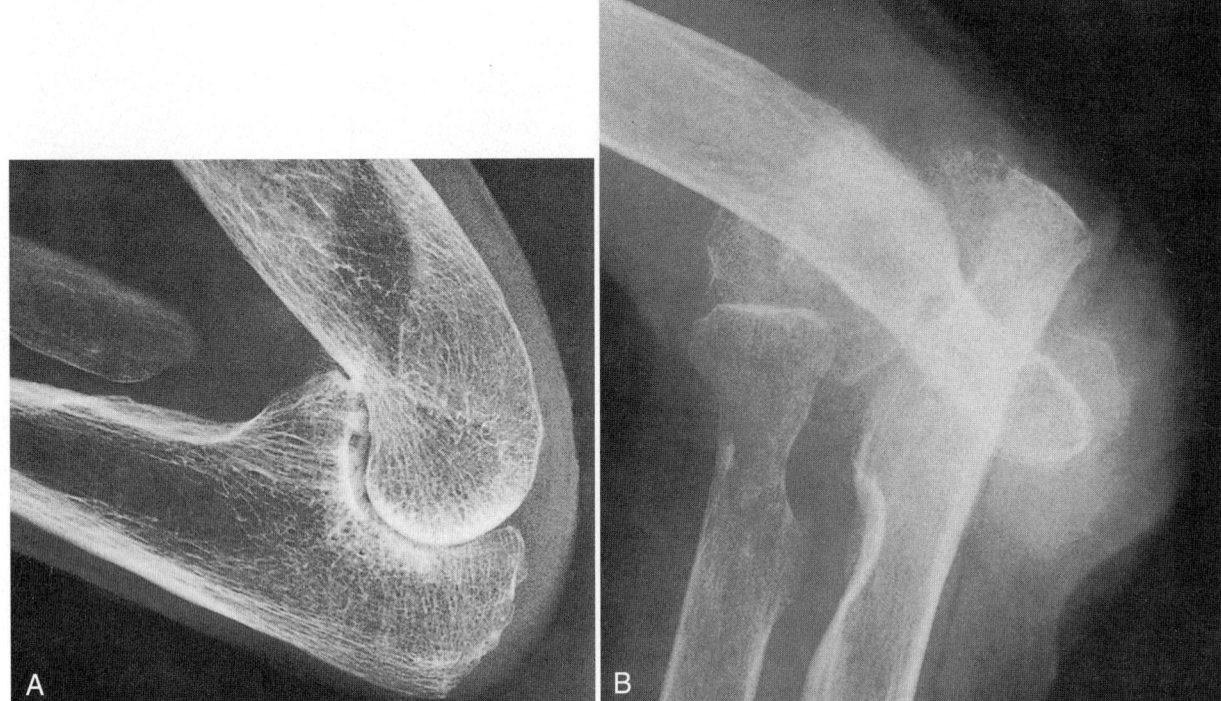

**Figure 16–14.** Abnormalities of the elbow: articular destruction. *A*, Radiograph of a sagittal section of a rheumatoid elbow joint indicates considerable narrowing and bony eburnation of the humeroulnar space. *B*, Lateral radiographs of the elbow in a different patient with rheumatoid arthritis demonstrate a fracture of the distal portion of the humerus that occurred after minor trauma. The fragment and the radius and ulna are displaced, predominantly in a proximal, radial, and posterior direction.

## Glenohumeral Joint

### Clinical Abnormalities

Clinical symptoms of disability related to glenohumeral joint involvement in rheumatoid arthritis are not infrequent. Pain, tenderness, and restricted motion may be evident. Associated subacromial bursitis may result in prominent soft tissue swelling. Acute tearing of the rotator cuff in rheumatoid arthritis may produce clinical findings simulating infection.

### Radiographic-Pathologic Correlation

Progressive destruction of the chondral surface of the glenoid cavity and humeral head leads to diffuse loss of joint space, which may be accompanied by marginal erosions and by subchondral cystic lesions and sclerosis of apposing surfaces of the glenoid and humerus. In this joint, osteophytes are a prominent radiographic finding. Particularly characteristic are superficial irregularities, deep erosive changes, and cystic changes on the superolateral aspect of the humeral head adjacent to the greater tuberosity. These osseous abnormalities resemble a Hill-Sachs compression fracture occurring after anterior glenohumeral joint dislocation (although the Hill-Sachs lesion is localized in the posterolateral aspect of the humeral head) and the marginal erosions of other synovial processes, such as ankylosing spondylitis. A deep bone erosion may develop on the medial aspect of the surgical

neck of the humerus as a result of the abnormal pressure exerted by the adjacent glenoid margin. It is usually accompanied by elevation of the humerus with respect to the glenoid cavity secondary to rotator cuff atrophy and may eventually lead to a pathologic fracture of the humeral neck.

Rotator cuff atrophy or tear is common in long-standing rheumatoid arthritis and is caused by the damaging effect of the inflamed synovial tissue on the undersurface of the tendons adjacent to the greater tuberosity (Fig. 16–15). This complication can be visualized radiographically as progressive elevation of the humeral head with respect to the glenoid cavity, narrowing of the space between the top of the humerus and the inferior surface of the acromion, sclerosis and cyst formation on adjacent portions of the humeral head and acromion, reversal (or concavity) of the normal convex shape of the inferior acromion, and accentuation of cystic and sclerotic changes on the superolateral aspect of the head of the humerus as a result of abutment of this surface against the acromion on abduction of the shoulder.

## Acromioclavicular Joint

Pain, tenderness to direct palpation, and local soft tissue swelling can indicate rheumatoid involvement of the acromioclavicular joint (Fig. 16–16). Soft tissue swelling superior to the joint and subchondral osteoporosis and erosions predominating on the clavicle, especially its

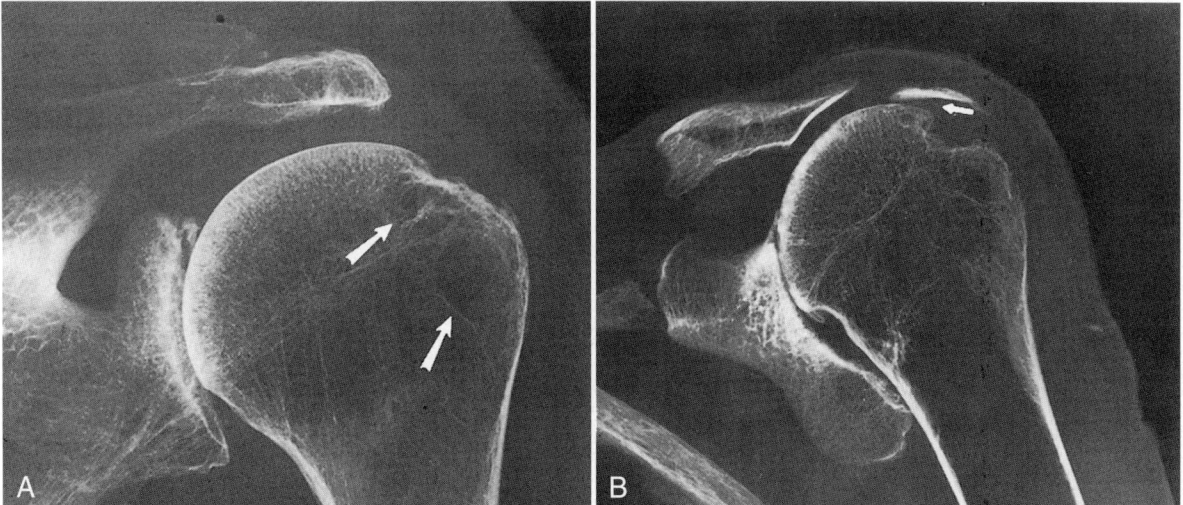

**Figure 16–15.** Abnormalities of the glenohumeral joint: articular destruction and rotator cuff tear and atrophy. *A,* Radiograph of a coronal section of the articulation illustrates joint space narrowing, bony eburnation, and erosive and cystic changes, predominantly on the lateral aspect of the humeral head *(arrows).* *B,* Radiograph of a coronal section of a rheumatoid glenohumeral joint indicates the presence of severe articular changes and rotator cuff atrophy. Note the joint space narrowing and sclerosis, erosion of the superolateral aspect of the humeral head, elevation of the humeral head with respect to the glenoid, and narrowing of the acromiohumeral head distance *(arrow).* The rotator cuff is atrophic.

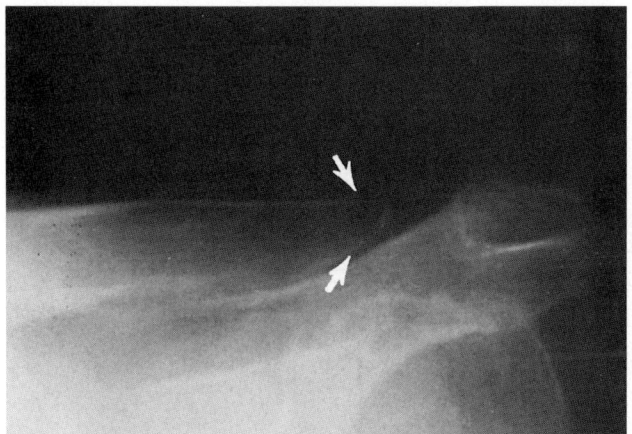

**Figure 16–16.** Abnormalities of the acromioclavicular joint. Radiograph shows tapering of the distal end of the clavicle *(arrows)* with widening of the acromioclavicular joint.

inferior margin, are early findings. Subsequently, larger erosive changes are detected and may progress to extensive osteolysis of the outer third of the clavicle, disruption of adjacent ligamentous and capsular structures, and subluxation.

## Coracoclavicular Joint

An elongated, shallow erosion can be seen along the undersurface of the distal end of the clavicle in rheumatoid arthritis (Fig. 16–17). The pathogenesis of this erosive change is not clear.

## Sternoclavicular and Manubriosternal Joints

Although clinical evidence of abnormalities in one or both sternoclavicular joints may be elicited by a careful history and physical examination, particularly in long-standing disease, radiologic evidence of sternoclavicular changes is more difficult to detect because of the inadequacies of routine sternoclavicular joint radiography. Infrequently, extensive osteolysis of the medial end of the clavicle, with or without associated osteolysis of the distal end of the clavicle, can be seen. Radiographic features include osteo-

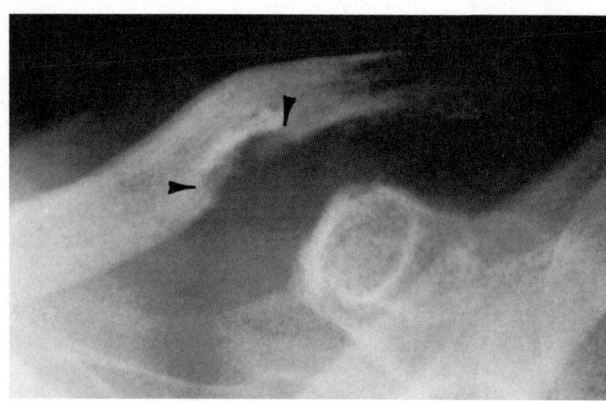

**Figure 16–17.** Abnormalities of the coracoclavicular joint. Scalloped erosions *(arrowheads)* on the undersurface of the distal end of the clavicle may be seen in rheumatoid arthritis. A similar finding may occur in ankylosing spondylitis and hyperparathyroidism.

(From Resnick D, Niwayama G: Resorption of the undersurface of the distal clavicle in rheumatoid arthritis. Radiology 120:75, 1976.)

porosis, slight irregularity of the osseous surfaces, eburnation, decreased height of the intervening fibrocartilage, and bony ankylosis, but these changes are less frequent and less severe than in ankylosing spondylitis.

## Forefoot

### Clinical Abnormalities

Clinical abnormalities of the forefoot are especially common in rheumatoid arthritis (80% to 90% of patients) and may be the initial manifestation of the disease (10% to 20% of patients). The metatarsophalangeal joints of the lateral digits are affected most frequently. Intermittent or constant pain, tenderness, and soft tissue swelling can be prominent findings. Characteristic deformities include spreading of the metatarsal bones, hallux valgus, lateral deviation of the toes at the metatarsophalangeal joints, hammer toe, and "cock-up" toe. Additional findings in rheumatoid arthritis include insufficiency (stress) fractures, peripheral neuropathy, tendon injury and rupture, widespread edema, rheumatoid nodules, and hallux rigidus.

### Radiographic-Pathologic Correlation

Radiologic abnormalities of the forefoot are also frequent and are commonly the initial manifestation of the disease.

The earliest alterations appear at the metatarsophalangeal joints, particularly the fifth. Changes predominate on the medial aspect of the metatarsal head, with the exception of the fifth digit, where soft tissue swelling and subjacent osseous erosion on the lateral aspect of the bone can be very early and important findings (Fig. 16–18).

Early radiographic alterations at the metatarsophalangeal joints consist of soft tissue swelling, periarticular osteoporosis, concentric joint space narrowing, and marginal and central osseous defects. In the great toe, changes in the metatarsal head and the proximal phalanx about the metatarsophalangeal joint are accompanied by osteoporosis, joint space loss, and erosion of the adjacent sesamoids. The frequency of hallux valgus deformity rises with increasing duration of the disease. Especially characteristic is an elongated surface irregularity that appears on the medial margin of the proximal phalanx adjacent to the interphalangeal joint; this irregularity may be associated with smaller erosions on the medial aspect of the adjacent distal phalanx. The radiographic characteristics of a deformed forefoot in rheumatoid arthritis include fibular deviation of the toes (with the exception of the fifth digit) and dorsiflexion and lateral subluxation or dislocation of the proximal phalanges at the metatarsophalangeal articulations (Fig. 16–19).

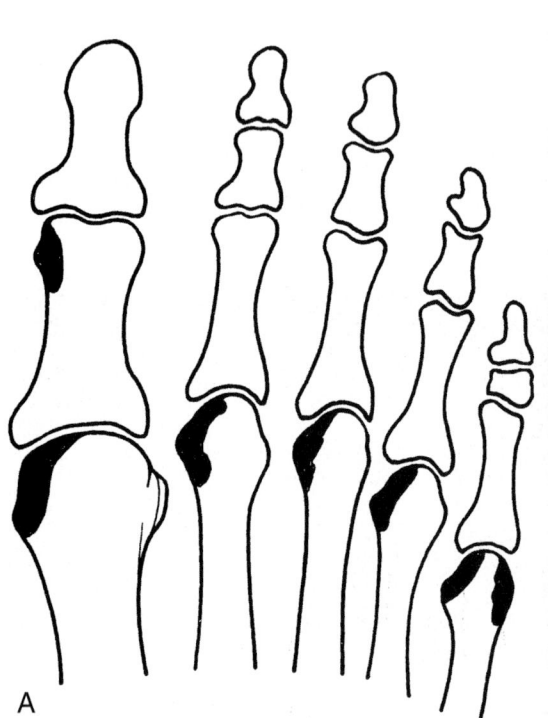
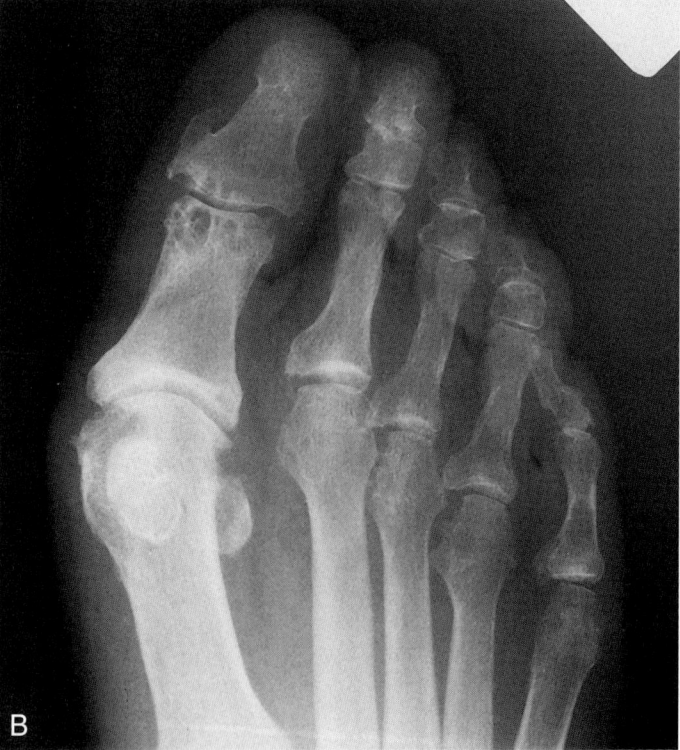

**Figure 16–18.** Abnormalities of the forefoot: target areas. *A*, Early osseous erosions of rheumatoid arthritis appear on the medial aspect of the first to fourth metatarsal bones, the medial and lateral aspects of the fifth metatarsal bone, and the medial aspect of the distal portion of the proximal phalanx of the great toe. *B*, Radiograph reveals early erosions. All the metatarsal heads are involved, particularly the medial aspects. Note the prominent changes at the interphalangeal joint of the great toe and the relative absence of findings in other interphalangeal articulations.

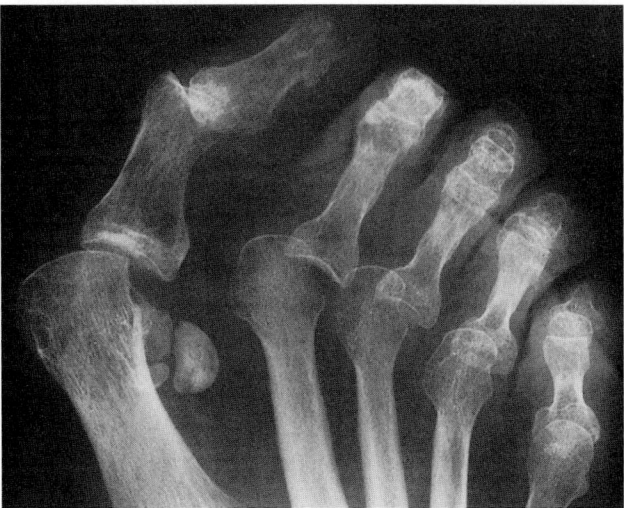

**Figure 16–19.** Forefoot deformities. Fibular deviation and subluxation of the phalanges typically occur at the first to fourth digits. The relatively mild nature of the osseous erosions in comparison to the degree of deformity evident in this patient is somewhat unusual.

## Midfoot

### Clinical Abnormalities

The most frequent midtarsal deformity in rheumatoid arthritis is pes planovalgus. This deformity may be related to rupture of an inflamed tibialis posterior tendon.

### Radiographic-Pathologic Correlation

Radiographic changes in the midfoot in rheumatoid arthritis are common, with a predilection for the talocalcaneonavicular joint. Radiographs may reveal diffuse joint space loss, focal sclerosis, and osteophytosis. Erosions are infrequent and small, and osseous fusion is occasionally seen. Adjacent sesamoid bones can be affected. The cuneonavicular, intercuneiform, cuneocuboid, and cuboideonavicular joints are often altered concurrently (Fig. 16–20).

## Heel

### Clinical Abnormalities

Clinical lesions of the heel encountered in rheumatoid arthritis and the seronegative spondyloarthropathies are retrocalcaneal bursitis, Achilles tendinosis, peritendinitis and paratendinitis, and plantar fasciitis. Retrocalcaneal bursitis is characterized by a fluctuating mass that falls to the sides of the Achilles tendon. Achilles tendinosis is associated with pain, local tenderness to palpation, and a thickened or swollen tendinous structure. Plantar fasciitis can lead to redness, swelling, and tenderness of the plantar surface of the calcaneus.

### Radiographic-Pathologic Correlation

Retrocalcaneal bursitis can produce a soft tissue mass on the posterosuperior aspect of the calcaneus that obliterates the normal radiolucent region extending between

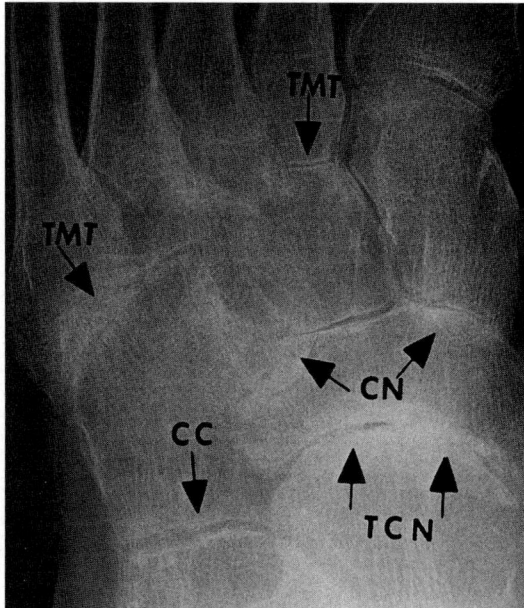

**Figure 16–20.** Abnormalities of the tarsometatarsal joints. Joint space loss in the lateral and intermediate tarsometatarsal (TMT) cavities is associated with diffuse alterations of the talonavicular portion of the talocalcaneonavicular (TCN) joint and cuneonavicular (CN) and calcaneocuboid (CC) joints.
(From Resnick D: Roentgen features of the rheumatoid mid- and hindfoot. J Can Assoc Radiol 27:99, 1976.)

the top of the bone and the Achilles tendon and projecting into the inferior portion of the pre-Achilles fat pad (Fig. 16–21). Subjacent well or poorly defined erosion of the calcaneus on both its posterior and superior aspects is characteristic. Achilles tendinosis leads to enlargement and blurring of the tendon.

Well-defined calcaneal excrescences are also observed on the plantar aspect of the bone in patients with rheumatoid arthritis. Poorly marginated plantar outgrowths with adjacent sclerosis, as seen in the seronegative spondyloarthropathies, are rare in rheumatoid arthritis. Spontaneous Achilles tendon rupture has been described in patients with rheumatoid arthritis.

## Ankle

Clinical and radiologic abnormalities are less frequent in the ankle than in the knee and the articulations of the hand, wrist, and foot. In the presence of synovitis of the ankle, soft tissue swelling, limitation of motion, and pain may be evident. Diffuse loss of joint space is typical. With continued disease activity, extensive erosions and subchondral cysts become apparent.

## Knee

### Clinical Abnormalities

The knee is frequently affected in rheumatoid arthritis, often at an early stage of the disease. Pain and swelling appear. The presence of a joint effusion can be substantiated by radiography (Fig. 16–22). Increased fluid accu-

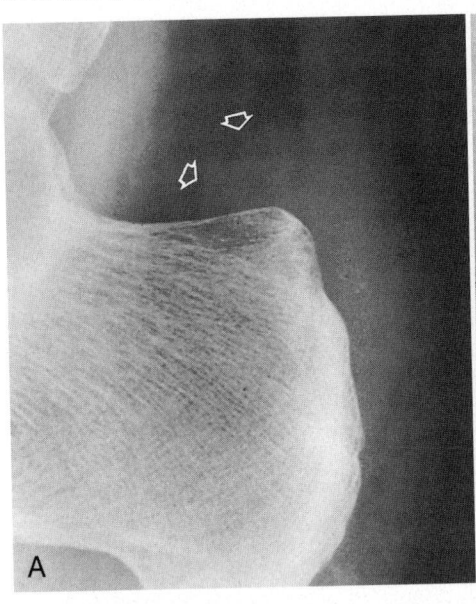

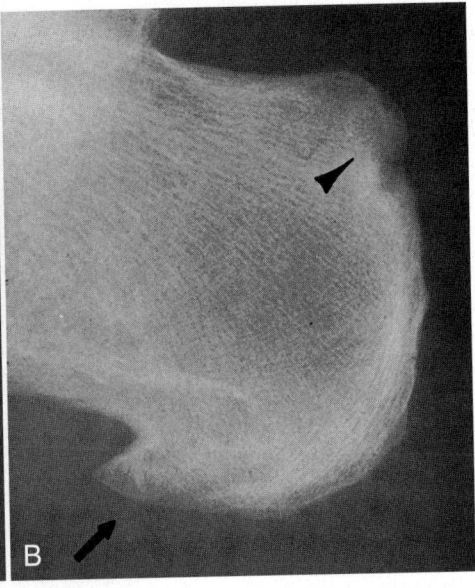

**Figure 16–21.** Abnormalities of the calcaneus: posterosuperior and inferior aspects. *A,* Low-kV soft tissue radiograph defines a thickened Achilles tendon and a fluid-filled retrocalcaneal bursa *(open arrows)* that projects into the pre-Achilles fat pad. Focal osteoporosis of the neighboring calcaneus is evident. *B,* Observe the erosion of the posterosuperior aspect of the calcaneus *(arrowhead)* and a well-defined plantar calcaneal enthesophyte *(arrow).* (*A,* Courtesy of J. Weston, MD, Lower Hutt, New Zealand.)

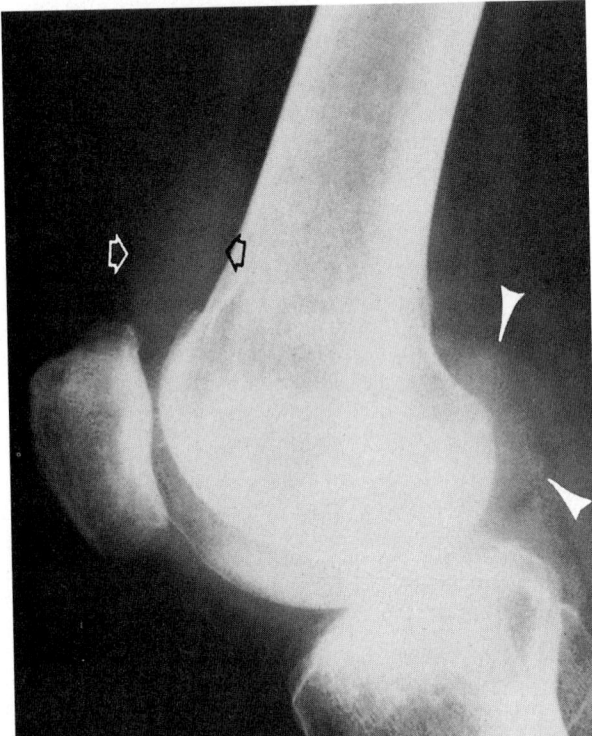

**Figure 16–22.** Abnormalities of the knee: synovial effusion. On a lateral radiograph, an effusion is indicated by an enlarged (>10 mm thick) suprapatellar pouch *(arrows)* between two radiolucent fat collections—one above the patella and one anterior to the distal end of the femur—and by increased radiodensity in the posterior recesses *(arrowheads).*

mulation in the joint may be accompanied by small or large synovial cysts, especially on the posterior aspect of the knee.

### Radiographic-Pathologic Correlation

Characteristically, symmetrical abnormalities occur in both the medial and the lateral femorotibial compart-

ments (Fig. 16–23) and may be combined with similar changes in the patellofemoral compartment. This bicompartmental or tricompartmental distribution, which can be depicted on radiography, is an important clue to the correct diagnosis. Occasionally, the lateral femorotibial compartment is involved more severely than the medial one and may lead to a valgus deformity of the knee. Small erosions on the medial and lateral margins of the tibia and femur may be the first radiographic findings. These lesions are occasionally preceded or soon accompanied by diffuse loss of the interosseous distance between the femur and tibia in both the medial and lateral compartments and by the development of subchondral erosions and cysts.

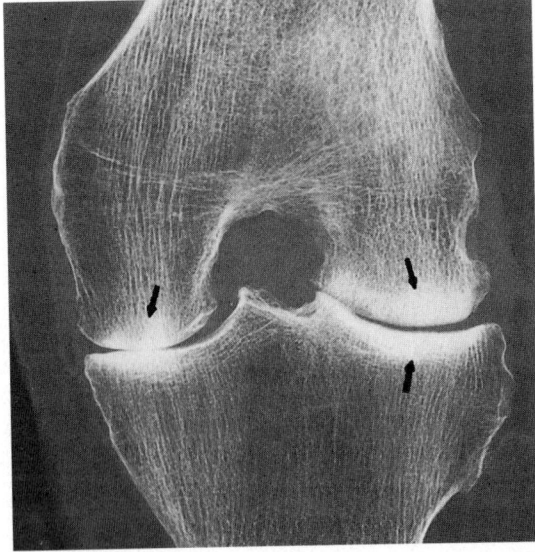

**Figure 16–23.** Abnormalities of the knee: femorotibial compartments. Radiograph of a macerated coronal section of the knee demonstrates diffuse loss of articular space in both the medial and lateral femorotibial compartments, associated with subchondral sclerosis *(arrows).*

## Proximal Tibiofibular Joint

Approximately one third of rheumatoid arthritis patients with knee joint involvement have additional changes in the proximal tibiofibular articulation consisting of joint space loss and osseous erosion.

## Hip

### Clinical Abnormalities

Abnormalities of the hip are far less frequent than those of the knee and increase with the duration and severity of rheumatoid arthritis. Pain, tenderness, shortening of the limb, gait abnormalities, and decreased range of motion, particularly internal rotation, extension, and abduction, are observed. Soft tissue swelling on the anterior aspect of the joint and over the greater trochanter (secondary to bursitis) may be evident.

### Radiographic-Pathologic Correlation

Radiographic abnormalities of the hip are generally bilateral and symmetrical. The most typical early abnormality is loss of joint space (Fig. 16–24). In almost all patients, diminution of articular space is concentric and reflects thinning and loss of the cartilaginous coat over much of the femoral and acetabular surfaces. The femoral head moves centrally along the axis of the femoral neck (axial migration). Much less frequently, greater loss of joint space appears on the superior aspect of the joint and produces upward or superior migration of the femoral head with respect to the acetabulum, similar to that accompanying osteoarthritis. Eventually, this space may be completely obliterated, and the femoral head and acetabulum protrude into the pelvis (Fig. 16–25). Acetabular protrusion—defined as inward movement of the acetabular

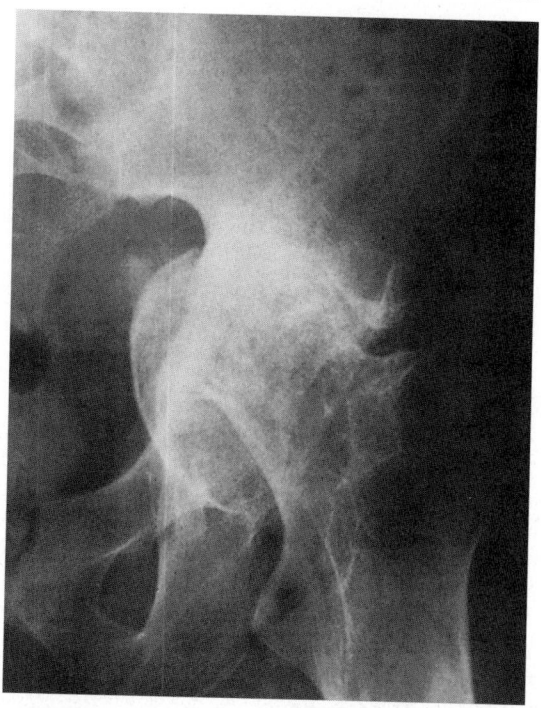

**Figure 16–25.** Abnormalities of the hip: late changes with acetabular protrusion. Protrusion deformity with acetabular fragmentation is shown. Observe the small size of the femoral head.

line so that the distance between this line and the laterally located ilioischial line is 3 mm or more in men and 6 mm or more in women—is particularly characteristic of rheumatoid arthritis. The deformity is commonly bilateral and is associated with subchondral cystic lesions, osseous collapse of the acetabular roof and femoral head, and osteoporosis.

Radiographically, the earliest lucent zones appear at the chondro-osseous margin of the femoral head near the femoral neck. Additional lesions are observed as surface irregularities throughout the femoral head and, to a lesser degree, the acetabulum. Some degree of sclerosis may appear about the hip after a considerable length of time. The eventual outcome of rheumatoid hip disease is often complete obliteration of the articular space and fibrous ankylosis. Bony ankylosis is exceedingly rare.

Osteonecrosis of the femoral head is not uncommon and generally occurs in patients with rheumatoid arthritis who are being treated with corticosteroids. The radiographic appearance of osteonecrosis of the femoral head in a relatively normal joint with osseous collapse, cyst formation, and sclerosis without joint space loss is identical to that of osteonecrosis occurring in patients without rheumatoid disease.

## Sacroiliac Joint

As opposed to the frequent and severe clinical and radiologic abnormalities that characterize sacroiliac joint disease in ankylosing spondylitis, changes in this location are relatively infrequent and mild in rheumatoid arthritis.

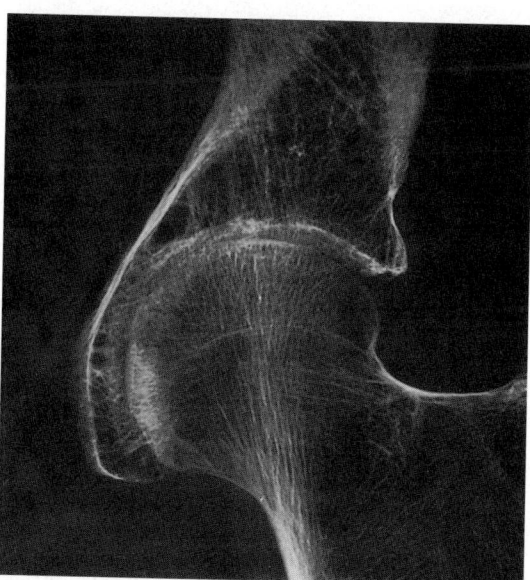

**Figure 16–24.** Abnormalities of the hip: early changes. Radiograph of a coronal section of a rheumatoid cadaveric hip indicates diffuse loss of articular space, with migration of the femoral head axially along the axis of the femoral neck.

Asymptomatic radiographic abnormalities of the sacroiliac joint may be present in as many as 25% to 35% of patients with severe, long-standing disease. Abnormalities, which may be more frequent in women than in men, can be bilateral or unilateral in distribution, but symmetrical alterations, which are the rule in ankylosing spondylitis, are not frequent in rheumatoid arthritis. Joint space narrowing is often mild. Osseous erosions have a predilection for the iliac aspect of the joint; they are superficial and well marginated and are associated with absent or only mild sclerosis.

## Symphysis Pubis

The symphysis pubis, which is frequently affected in the seronegative spondyloarthropathies, is not commonly altered in rheumatoid arthritis. Occasionally, radiographic abnormalities are detected in patients with chronic disease, but they are generally clinically silent. These abnormalities include subchondral erosion, mild eburnation, and narrowing of the interosseous space. Parasymphyseal insufficiency fractures of the os pubis have been described in patients with rheumatoid arthritis, as well as in those with postmenopausal osteoporosis.

## Ribs

Abnormalities of the thoracic cage in patients with rheumatoid arthritis can include erosions on the superior margin of the posterior aspect of the upper ribs. They are identical to those encountered in other collagen vascular disorders, neurologic processes, and chronic obstructive lung disease. Rib erosions in rheumatoid arthritis, as well as in some other processes, are probably due to a pressure effect from the scapula.

## Thoracic and Lumbar Spine

When compared with the distinctive alterations of the cervical spine, which represent a common and well-known manifestation of rheumatoid arthritis, abnormalities of the thoracic and lumbar spine are relatively uncommon. Rheumatoid arthritic changes in the apophyseal joints of the thoracic and lumbar spine are reported only infrequently. Alterations at the discovertebral junction of the thoracic and lumbar spine are also infrequent. Intervertebral disc space narrowing, irregularity of the subchondral margins of the vertebral bodies, "erosion," and sclerosis may be evident on radiography of these sites (Fig. 16–26).

Patients with rheumatoid arthritis who are receiving corticosteroid medication are predisposed to ischemic necrosis of bone. Although the femoral head is the typical site of this complication, vertebral bodies in the thoracic and lumbar segments of the spine can be affected. Radiographic abnormalities include vertebral collapse and fragmentation. Radiolucent fracture lines, which may accumulate gas from surrounding tissues (vacuum vertebral body), are an important clue that allows a correct diagnosis.

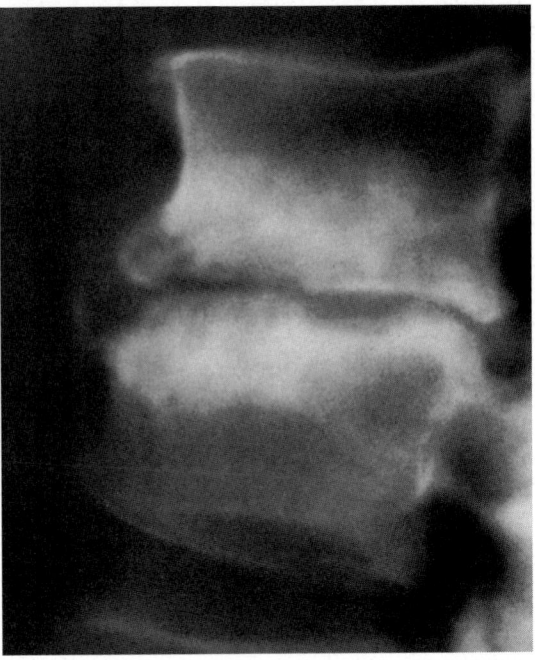

**Figure 16–26.** Abnormalities of the thoracolumbar spine: discovertebral lesions. Lateral conventional tomogram of the lumbar spine in a rheumatoid arthritis patient shows disc space narrowing, poorly defined osseous erosion, and sclerosis, which resemble the findings in infection and intervertebral osteochondrosis.

## Cervical Spine

### Clinical Abnormalities

Cervical spine involvement is common in rheumatoid arthritis and can lead to severe pain and disability, as well as a variety of neurologic manifestations, although some patients with significant radiographic evidence of disease may be entirely asymptomatic. Initial or predominant involvement of the cervical spine can occur without obvious clinical (or radiographic) abnormalities at other locations.

Symptoms and signs related to cervical spine abnormalities develop in approximately 60% to 80% of rheumatoid arthritis patients at some time during their illness. Pain is the most common clinical manifestation. Weakness and abnormal mobility may also be evident. Neurologic manifestations include paresthesias, paresis, and muscle wasting; in some instances, quadriplegia and death can occur.

### Radiographic-Pathologic Correlation

**General Features.** The entire cervical spine is affected by the rheumatoid process; changes may be evident as far cephalad as the base of the occiput and as far caudad as the C7–T1 junction (Table 16–2). Further, synovial and cartilaginous articulations, the joints of Luschka, tendinous and ligamentous attachments, and soft tissues of the cervical region can exhibit significant abnormalities in this disease. In patients who can undergo complete radiographic evaluation, the frequency of radiographic

| **TABLE 16-2** |
| :--- |

**Cervical Spine Abnormalities in Rheumatoid Arthritis**

**Occipitoatlantoaxial Articulations**
   Atlantoaxial subluxation
   Odontoid erosion and fracture
   Apophyseal joint erosion, sclerosis, and fusion

**Subaxial Articulations**
   Subaxial subluxation
   Apophyseal joint erosion, sclerosis, and fusion
   Intervertebral disc space narrowing
   Erosion and sclerosis of vertebral body margins
   Spinous process erosion
   Osteoporosis

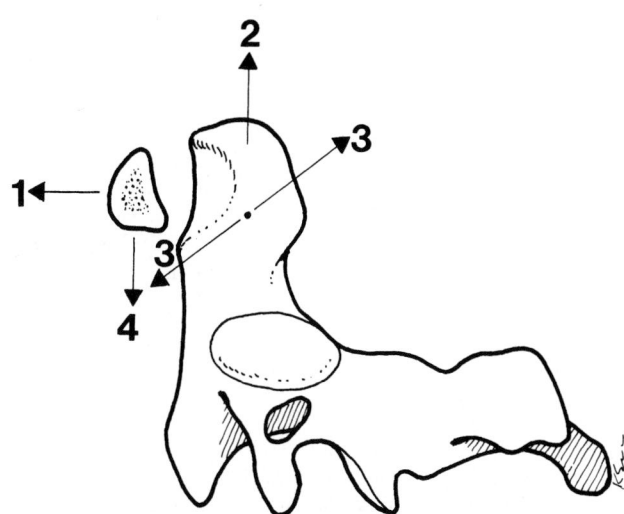

**Figure 16–27.** Abnormalities of the cervical spine: directions of atlantoaxial subluxation. Varying types of subluxation may occur at the atlantoaxial articulations in patients with rheumatoid arthritis. Most typically, anterior movement of the atlas with respect to the axis (1) is seen. Vertical translocation of the odontoid process, or cranial settling (2), can also occur. Lateral subluxation (3) can be recorded on frontal radiographs as asymmetry becomes apparent between the odontoid process and the lateral masses of the atlas. In addition, the anterior arch of the atlas can move inferiorly (4) with respect to the odontoid process, a finding associated with cranial settling. Finally, in the presence of severe erosion of the odontoid process, the anterior arch can move posteriorly against the eroded bone or, rarely, behind the eroded odontoid process.

changes of the cervical spine is consistently high and may reach 85%. Radiographic abnormalities in the cervical spine have been reported to correlate with those in the peripheral joints and with the presence of serum rheumatoid factor and subcutaneous nodules. Careful radiographic technique is important; in an apparently normal cervical spine, considerable subluxation at the C1–C2 junction can be revealed with the addition of a lateral view of the flexed neck. When all radiographic parameters are used, demonstration of abnormalities throughout the cervical spine is frequent, although they usually predominate in the upper cervical region.

**Occipitoatlantoaxial Articulations.** Various types of malalignment in the atlantoaxial region have been described in rheumatoid arthritis (Fig. 16–27). The major types include anterior atlantoaxial subluxation, vertical subluxation (also known as cranial settling and atlantoaxial impaction), lateral subluxation, and posterior subluxation. Subluxations of all types have been noted in 40% to 85% of patients with rheumatoid arthritis.

Abnormal separation between the anterior arch of the atlas and the odontoid process (dens) of the axis, designated anterior atlantoaxial subluxation, is a characteristic finding in rheumatoid arthritis that may be evident at an early stage of the disease, when other cervical spine abnormalities, including odontoid erosion, are not apparent. Generally, the interosseous distance between the posterior aspect of the anterior arch of the atlas and the anterior aspect of the odontoid process does not exceed 2.5 mm in adults. Measurement of the inferior aspect of this articulation is used most often. Anterior atlantoaxial subluxation occurs in 20% to 25% of patients with rheumatoid arthritis (Fig. 16–28). The pathogenesis of anterior atlantoaxial subluxation relates to the presence of transverse ligament laxity caused by synovial inflammation and hyperemia of the adjacent articulations.

Vertical subluxation at C1–C2 can also be observed in patients with rheumatoid arthritis and, when extensive, can be fatal (see Fig. 16–28). This complication has been associated with neurologic symptoms and signs related to entrapment of the first and second cervical nerve roots, impairment of cranial nerves, bulbomedullary compression, occlusion of the branches of the spinal and vertebral

arteries, and hydrocephalus. Atlantoaxial impaction is diagnosed by applying one or more radiographic measurements that assess the relationship of the tip of the odontoid process to landmarks at the base of the skull. When severe, such settling is easily diagnosed on radiographs obtained in a lateral projection or on conventional tomograms or computed tomography (CT) scans. Cranial settling has been observed in 5% to 22% of patients with rheumatoid arthritis. In general, vertical translocation of the dens results from disruption and collapse of the osseous and articular structures that exist between the occiput and the atlas and between the atlas and the axis. Magnetic resonance (MR) imaging (Fig. 16–29) is an effective method for the further evaluation of such subluxation, as well as its effects on the spinal cord.

Lateral subluxation of the atlantoaxial joints has also been observed in patients with rheumatoid arthritis. In these patients, asymmetry is recorded between the odontoid process (and body of the axis) and the atlas. This complication is diagnosed when the lateral masses of the atlas are displaced more than 2 mm with respect to those of the axis, and it is observed in 10% to 20% of patients with rheumatoid arthritis (Fig. 16–30). The sequence of events that leads to lateral subluxation of the atlantoaxial joints includes articular space narrowing, bone erosion, disruption of the articular capsules, and, in severe cases, collapse of the lateral masses of the axis. Bone erosion may be the most important factor in the development of this deformity.

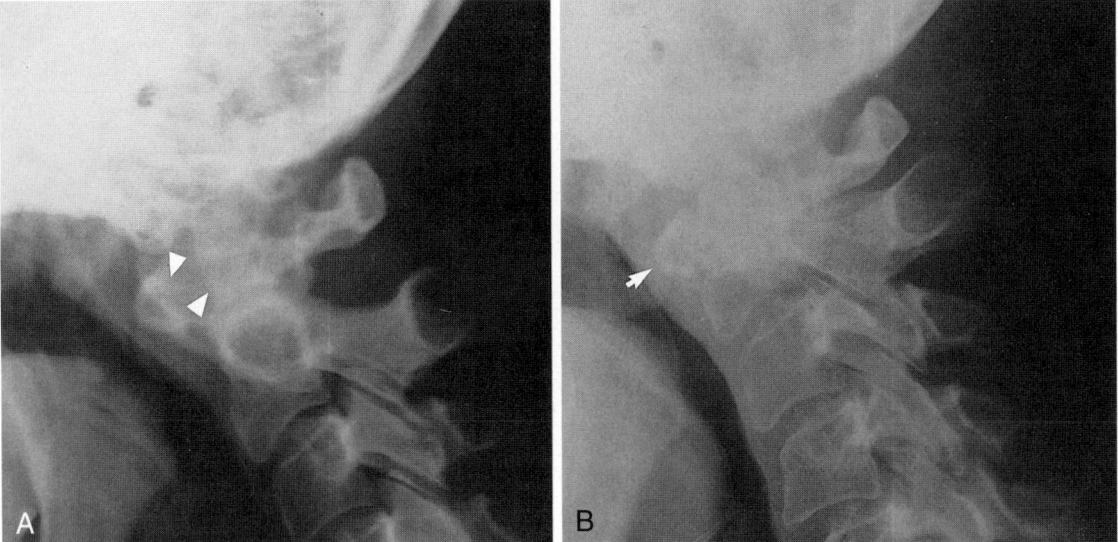

**Figure 16–28.** Abnormalities of the cervical spine: anterior atlantoaxial subluxation and vertical translocation of the odontoid process (cranial settling). *A* and *B*, Lateral radiographs of the cervical spine in a patient with rheumatoid arthritis obtained 9 years apart. In the earlier study *(A)*, anterior atlantoaxial subluxation *(arrowheads)* is evident. In the later study *(B)*, cranial settling has occurred, with the anterior arch of the atlas *(arrow)* having moved inferiorly with respect to the axis. Note that the apparent absence of anterior atlantoaxial subluxation in *(B)* suggests improvement in the radiographic findings, but this is definitely not the case.

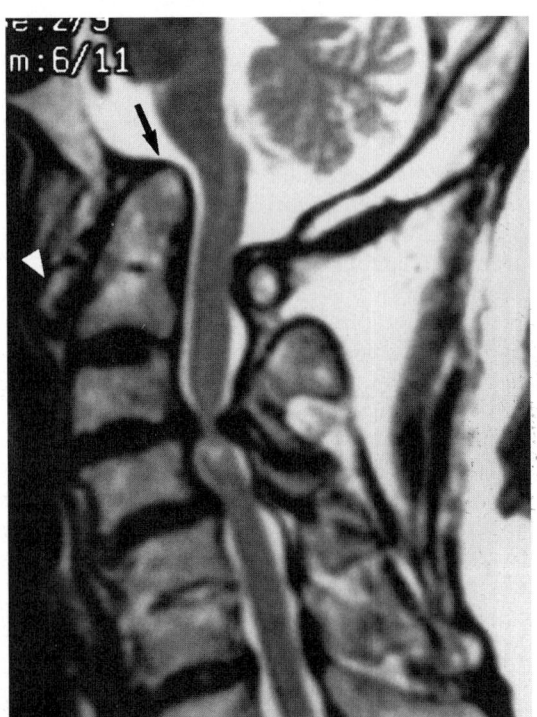

**Figure 16–29.** Abnormalities of the cervical spine: vertical translocation of the odontoid process (cranial settling). This sagittal T2-weighted (TR/TE, 3500/91) spin echo MR image shows that the odontoid process *(arrow)* extends through the foramen magnum, and the anterior arch of the atlas *(arrowhead)* articulates too low on the odontoid process. Also note the multiple subaxial cervical subluxations, posterior disc displacements, impingement on the spinal cord with spinal stenosis, and abnormal signal intensity in the cord. (Courtesy of C. Chen, MD, Kaohsiung, Taiwan.)

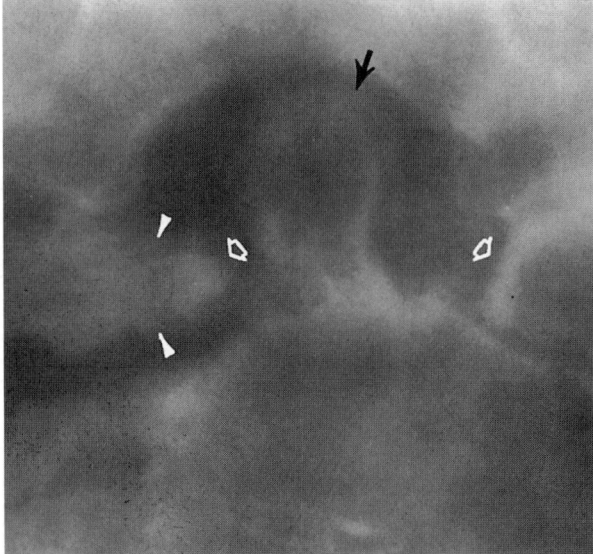

**Figure 16–30.** Abnormalities of the cervical spine: lateral atlantoaxial subluxation. Frontal conventional tomogram of the upper portion of the cervical spine demonstrates lateral subluxation of the odontoid process *(solid arrow)* with respect to the lateral masses of the atlas *(open arrows)*. Note the erosion of the base of the odontoid process and severe abnormalities in the occipitoatlantal and lateral atlantoaxial joints. The right lateral mass of the atlas *(arrowheads)*, as well as the axis, is collapsed, and the head is tilted to the right.

The clinical course of patients with atlantoaxial subluxation is variable. In some persons, only mild symptoms and signs appear, and they do not progress. In others, clinical and radiographic deterioration becomes evident, and disabling neurologic abnormalities may develop that require operative intervention to ensure stability.

In general, vertical subluxation (cranial settling) is a later manifestation than anterior atlantoaxial subluxation. With descent of the anterior process of the atlas with respect to the odontoid process during cranial settling, the degree of anterior atlantoaxial subluxation diminishes, and even the pannus of the area may decrease. This situation is sometimes referred to as stable atlantoaxial subluxation and may be accompanied by spontaneous atlantoaxial fusion.

Odontoid process erosions have been detected in 14% to 35% of patients with rheumatoid arthritis. Erosions occur as a natural consequence of synovial inflammation in adjacent articulations (Fig. 16–31). Thus, they predominate in the osseous portions that are intimate with the synovium-lined spaces between the anterior arch of C1 and the anterior aspect of the odontoid process and between the posterior surface of the odontoid process and the transverse ligament. Defects of the odontoid tip at sites of ligamentous attachment and defects of the base of the odontoid process related to the nearby lateral atlantoaxial joints can also be seen. Further erosion of the odontoid process, which is usually associated with atlantoaxial subluxation, can lead to considerable osteolysis. The dens may be reduced to a small osseous spicule (Fig. 16–32).

**Subaxial Articulations.** Subluxation and dislocation are observed at one or more subaxial levels in patients with rheumatoid arthritis. These abnormalities have been noted in 9% of patients with chronic and severe articular disorders. Associated myelopathy occurs but is uncommon; it may be related in some cases to cervical cord compression. When localized to one area, changes are particularly characteristic at the C3–C4 and C4–C5 levels;

however, multilevel subluxations are more typical and produce a "doorstep" or "stepladder" appearance on lateral radiographs (Fig. 16–33). Anterior subluxation is far more frequent than posterior subluxation.

Apophyseal joint abnormalities in the subaxial region, including joint space narrowing and superficial erosions, are common (see Fig. 16–33). During flexion of the neck, instability produces tilting of the lateral masses of one vertebra on the next, with abnormal widening of the articular spaces. Generally, fibrous ankylosis is the terminal event; however, bony ankylosis of one or more articulations may be seen.

Discovertebral joint abnormalities observed in the cervical spine in rheumatoid arthritis include intervertebral disc space narrowing, subchondral osseous irregularity, and adjacent eburnation (Fig. 16–34). Erosions can be confined to one aspect of the junction, usually the posterior, or involve the entire joint. Surrounding eburnation can also be localized or generalized in distribution. Multiple levels of the cervical spine are typically affected. A characteristic manifestation of rheumatoid discitis is the absence of osteophytosis, which distinguishes the cervical spinal abnormalities of rheumatoid arthritis from those of degenerative disc disease.

Spinous process erosions and destruction of one or more spinous processes may be detected, particularly in the lower cervical (and upper thoracic) region. Tapered and sharpened spinous elements may be related to inflammation of the adjacent supraspinous ligaments or neighboring bursae.

**Diffuse Locations.** Diffuse involvement of the entire cervical spine is common, particularly in long-standing rheumatoid arthritis (see Table 16–2). The resulting radiographic picture, which consists of atlantoaxial subluxation, odontoid and apophyseal joint erosions, subaxial

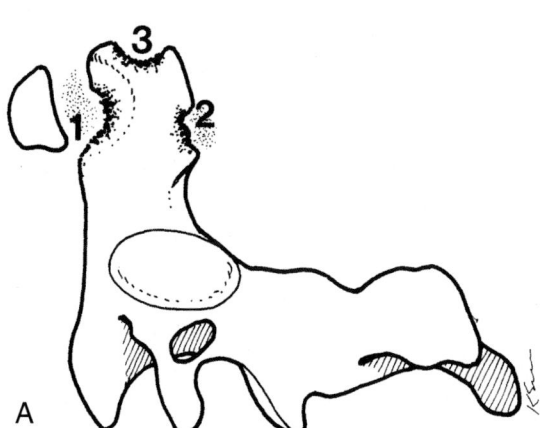
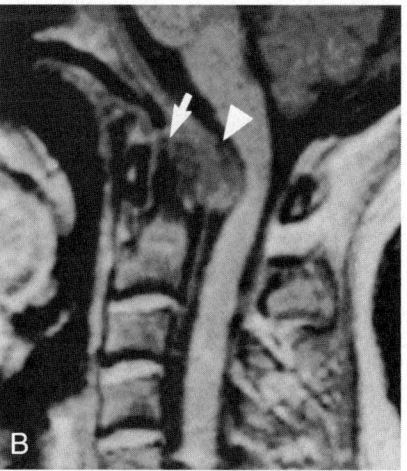

**Figure 16–31.** Abnormalities of the cervical spine: odontoid process erosions. *A,* Odontoid process erosions occur in areas that are intimate with the synovial articulations between the anterior arch of the atlas and the dens (1) and between the dens and the transverse ligament of the atlas (2), and in areas that are intimate with the ligamentous attachments (3) at the tip of the odontoid process. *B,* Sagittal MPGR (TR/TE, 300/9; flip angle, 15 degrees) MR image reveals prominent synovial inflammation in the posterior median atlantoaxial joint *(arrowhead),* along with erosion of the odontoid process *(arrow)* and compression of the spinal cord. (Courtesy of S. Moreland, MD, San Diego, Calif.)

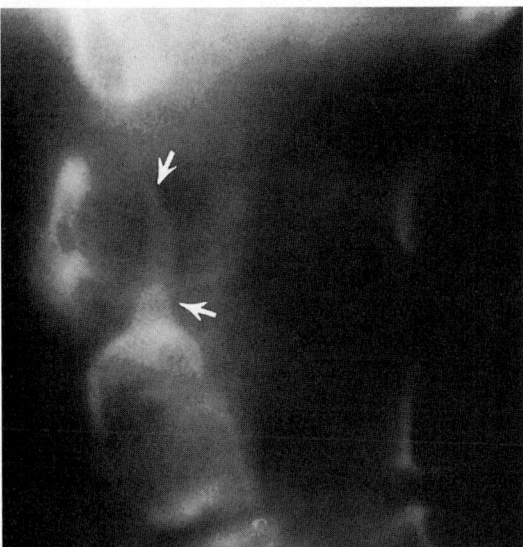

**Figure 16–32.** Abnormalities of the cervical spine: odontoid process erosions. Lateral conventional tomogram reveals severe destruction of the odontoid process *(arrows)*, which has been reduced to an irregular, pointed protuberance.

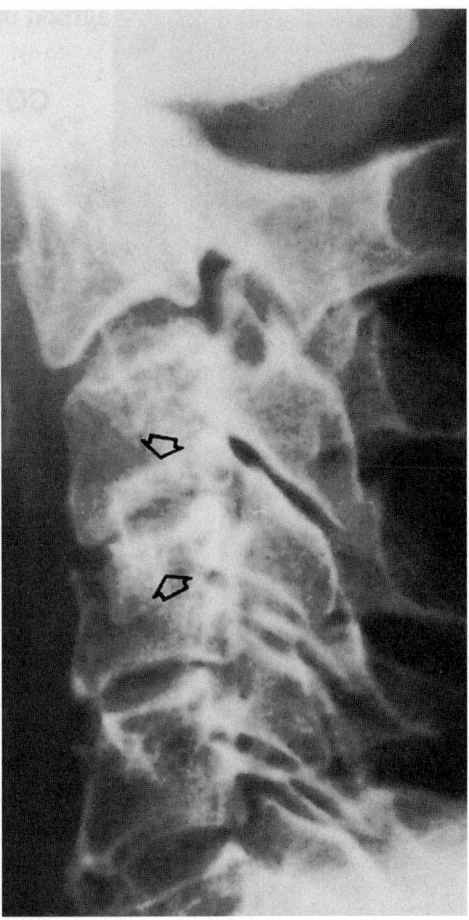

**Figure 16–34.** Abnormalities of the cervical spine: discovertebral joint changes. On this lateral radiograph, observe the narrowing of multiple intervertebral discs and irregularity and sclerosis of adjacent vertebral surfaces *(arrows)*. These findings, in the absence of osteophytes, strongly suggest the diagnosis of rheumatoid arthritis.

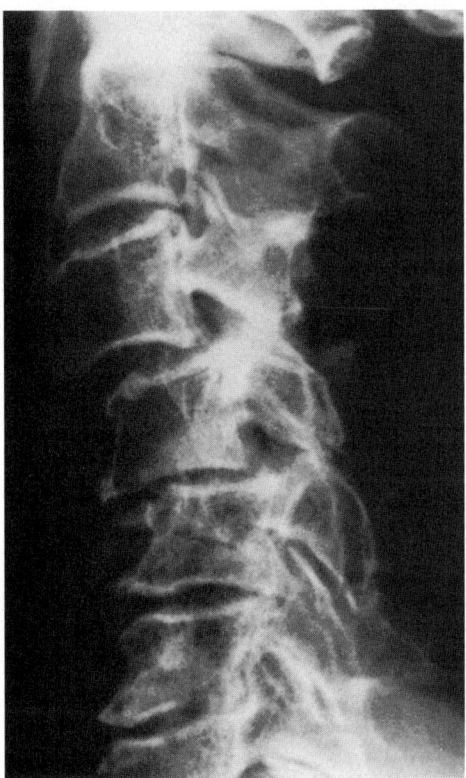

**Figure 16–33.** Abnormalities of the cervical spine: subaxial subluxation and apophyseal joint changes. Note the "step-ladder" appearance caused by subluxation at multiple cervical levels in association with narrowing of the intervertebral disc spaces and narrowing, sclerosis, and subluxation of the apophyseal joints.

subluxation, intervertebral disc space narrowing, marginal sclerosis of vertebrae, and spinous process destruction, is virtually pathognomonic of this disease.

## COEXISTENT OSSEOUS AND ARTICULAR DISEASE

### Septic Arthritis

Infections are frequent in patients with rheumatoid arthritis, especially after the introduction of steroids and immunosuppressive agents. Pulmonary infections, skin infections, osteomyelitis, and septic arthritis have all been noted. The cause of the increased susceptibility to infection in patients with rheumatoid arthritis is not known. The reported frequency of suppurative arthritis in patients with rheumatoid disease varies from less than 1% to 12% or higher. Indeed, rheumatoid arthritis appears to be the most common predisposing factor to septic arthritis. Pyarthrosis is more frequent in elderly rheumatoid arthritis patients with severe disability. The most frequently reported infecting organism is *Staphylococcus aureus*.

Septic arthritis complicating rheumatoid disease often affects multiple joints; it is more unusual to find polyarticular involvement in uncomplicated septic arthritis in adult patients. The onset of pyarthrosis in a person with rheumatoid arthritis may produce only subtle clinical changes; a source of infection, onset of chills, or any deterioration in the clinical state should arouse suspicion of a superimposed articular infection. Joint aspiration to demonstrate a specific organism and to determine its response to antibiotics is essential for correct diagnosis and treatment. The importance of early diagnosis is underscored by the fact that infection is the most common cause of death in patients with rheumatoid arthritis. Certain radiographic observations are diagnostic aids (Table 16–3). Radiographic evidence of any rapid deterioration of a joint should be suspect. Asymmetrical joint disease and poorly defined and rapid destruction of bone are other useful signs of infection in a patient with rheumatoid arthritis.

## Amyloidosis

Disorders characterized by paraproteinemia, such as multiple myeloma, macroglobulinemia, and amyloidosis, may develop in patients with rheumatoid arthritis. Amyloid deposits are commonly noted within joints in rheumatoid arthritis. Alternatively, articular manifestations of amyloid disease with or without multiple myeloma can simulate rheumatoid arthritis.

## Gout

The coexistence of rheumatoid arthritis and gout is not common, although it is being reported with increasing frequency. Typically, men are affected. Gout is the initial disease, and rheumatoid arthritis develops years later.

## Calcium Pyrophosphate Dihydrate Crystal Deposition Disease

The coexistence of rheumatoid arthritis and calcium pyrophosphate dihydrate (CPPD) crystal deposition disease is encountered occasionally. It appears likely that the coexistence of true rheumatoid arthritis and CPPD crystal deposition disease is merely a chance occurrence. Radiographic examination outlines changes compatible with crystal deposition disease and other changes indicative of an erosive articular process. Accurate interpretation of the radiograph is not difficult. Bone erosion is not

---

**TABLE 16-3**

**Radiographic Features of Septic Arthritis Complicating Rheumatoid Arthritis**

Monoarticular or polyarticular distribution
Predilection for knee involvement
Asymmetrical changes
Progressive soft tissue swelling and joint effusion
Rapid and poorly defined bony erosion

---

a manifestation of CPPD crystal deposition disease and, when present, should arouse suspicion of a superimposed articular process. Similarly, calcification and an arthropathy resembling degenerative disease are not features of rheumatoid arthritis.

## Ankylosing Spondylitis

Rheumatoid arthritis and ankylosing spondylitis may coexist in the same patient. In these persons, clinical and radiologic manifestations of rheumatoid arthritis are combined with those of ankylosing spondylitis and presence of the HLA-B27 antigen.

## Diffuse Idiopathic Skeletal Hyperostosis

Not surprisingly, rheumatoid arthritis and diffuse idiopathic skeletal hyperostosis—both common disorders in middle-aged and elderly patients—may occur together. In patients with both disorders, atypical clinical features include a high frequency of flexion contractures of the elbows, ankles, wrists, or knees; atypical radiologic features include the absence of osteoporosis and the presence of bony sclerosis and proliferation about erosions, osteophytes, and intra-articular bony ankylosis.

## Psoriasis and Pemphigoid

True rheumatoid arthritis, with all its clinical and radiologic manifestations, can develop in persons with psoriatic skin disease. These patients must be distinguished from those with psoriatic arthritis, who have a symmetrical rheumatoid arthritis–like distribution of articular disease and negative serologic test results for rheumatoid factor.

Another skin disease, pemphigoid, has been noted in association with rheumatoid arthritis. In pemphigoid, which is a bullous cutaneous disorder occurring mainly in older persons, immunoglobulins and complement are bound in the dermoepidermal junction. In this regard, coexistence of pemphigoid with rheumatoid arthritis and other collagen vascular disorders may be more than a chance occurrence.

## Collagen Vascular Disorders

Rheumatoid arthritis can be combined with other collagen vascular disorders in various overlap syndromes and in mixed connective tissue disease. In some of these disorders, specific laboratory parameters allow an accurate diagnosis. In others, the exact nature of the disease is more perplexing, and diagnosis is complicated by the occurrence of rheumatoid arthritis–like clinical and radiographic features in patients with "pure" collagen vascular disorders.

## RADIOLOGIC ASSESSMENT OF DISEASE EXTENT AND PROGRESSION

Despite the sensitivity of newer techniques, particularly MR imaging, in detecting the very early structural abnormalities of rheumatoid arthritis, conventional radiography remains the dominant imaging method for evaluating the disease. The presence or absence of bone erosions appears to have profound implications for treatment and prognosis. Many patients have such erosions when first examined, and in most patients who eventually develop bone erosions, they occur during the first 2 years of clinically evident disease. As many as 25% of patients with rheumatoid arthritis, however, have no bone erosions even when closely monitored for 5 years or more. Whether these latter patients would have had bone erosions without early and aggressive therapy is not clear. Because of the clinical importance of the early detection of bone erosions, most experts recommend that serial radiographs of classic target sites in patients with early polyarthritis be an integral part of their treatment. Accurate radiographic diagnosis of rheumatoid arthritis lies in analysis of the hands, wrists, and feet.

Because osteoporosis, joint space narrowing, and bone erosion are considered characteristic radiographic features of rheumatoid arthritis, most attempts at grading the severity of articular involvement emphasize one or more of these features. In some cases, problems arise as a result of the independence of one radiographic feature with respect to another (e.g., progression of bone erosion with lack of progression of joint space loss) or the independence of one joint with respect to another (e.g., progression of disease in the second metacarpophalangeal joint and absence of progression in the third metacarpophalangeal joint), and as a result of the difficulty in defining the changing size of an osseous erosion or the extent of joint space loss, especially in the presence of effusion, subluxation, or deformity.

In general, radiographically evident bone erosions show little change in patients with significant clinical improvement; in these persons, the lack of progression of such erosions on radiographs may be a more reliable indicator of therapeutic success. Although radiographic evidence of healing of bone erosions, characterized by decreased size and a sclerotic margin, has been recorded, it is infrequent and requires a long period of observation—usually years. Therefore, when planning a radiologic protocol that is appropriate in patients receiving treatment for rheumatoid arthritis, physicians should use longer intervals between examinations and standardize the radiographic technique. Further investigation is required to delineate the ideal use of conventional radiographs as well as other diagnostic methods, particularly scintigraphy and MR imaging.

## OTHER DIAGNOSTIC TECHNIQUES

### Fine-Detail Radiography with Magnification

Fine-detail radiography with magnification allows the identification of subtle abnormalities, especially about the small joints of the hand and foot and about the calcaneus, at a time when conventional radiographs are negative or equivocal.

### Arthrography

Arthrography has a limited role in the routine evaluation of rheumatoid arthritis patients and has generally been replaced by MR imaging. Arthrography can delineate the presence and extent of synovial hypertrophy and inflammation, showing an irregular or corrugated appearance of the contrast material and lymphatic filling. Rotator cuff disruption, synovial cysts (Fig. 16–35), and sinus tracts are also definitively delineated during arthrographic examination.

### Scintigraphy

As in other articular disorders, radionuclide examination using bone- or joint-seeking pharmaceutical agents is a sensitive method for evaluating disease activity in rheumatoid arthritis. Technetium pertechnetate and technetium phosphate scans outline joint inflammation that may antedate clinical activity, and these studies can be used to monitor response to therapy. A typical abnormal radionuclide pattern in rheumatoid arthritis consists of a symmetrically distributed peripheral joint process most prominent in the wrist, the metacarpophalangeal and proximal interphalangeal (and occasionally distal interphalangeal) joints of the hand, the metatarsophalangeal and interphalangeal joints of the foot, the knee, and the elbow (Fig. 16–36). Enhanced uptake has been observed in the cervical spine, atlantoaxial region, and temporomandibular joint.

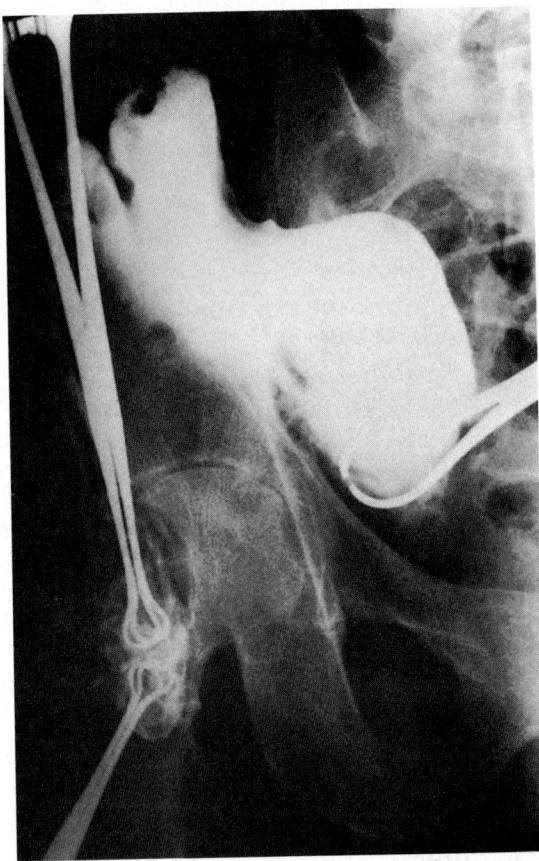

**Figure 16–35.** Arthrography in rheumatoid arthritis. Intraoperative arthrogram in a 50-year-old man with rheumatoid arthritis and a mass in the groin confirms the existence of a large synovial cyst arising from an abnormal hip and extending into the pelvis. (Courtesy of J. Scavulli, MD, San Diego, Calif.)

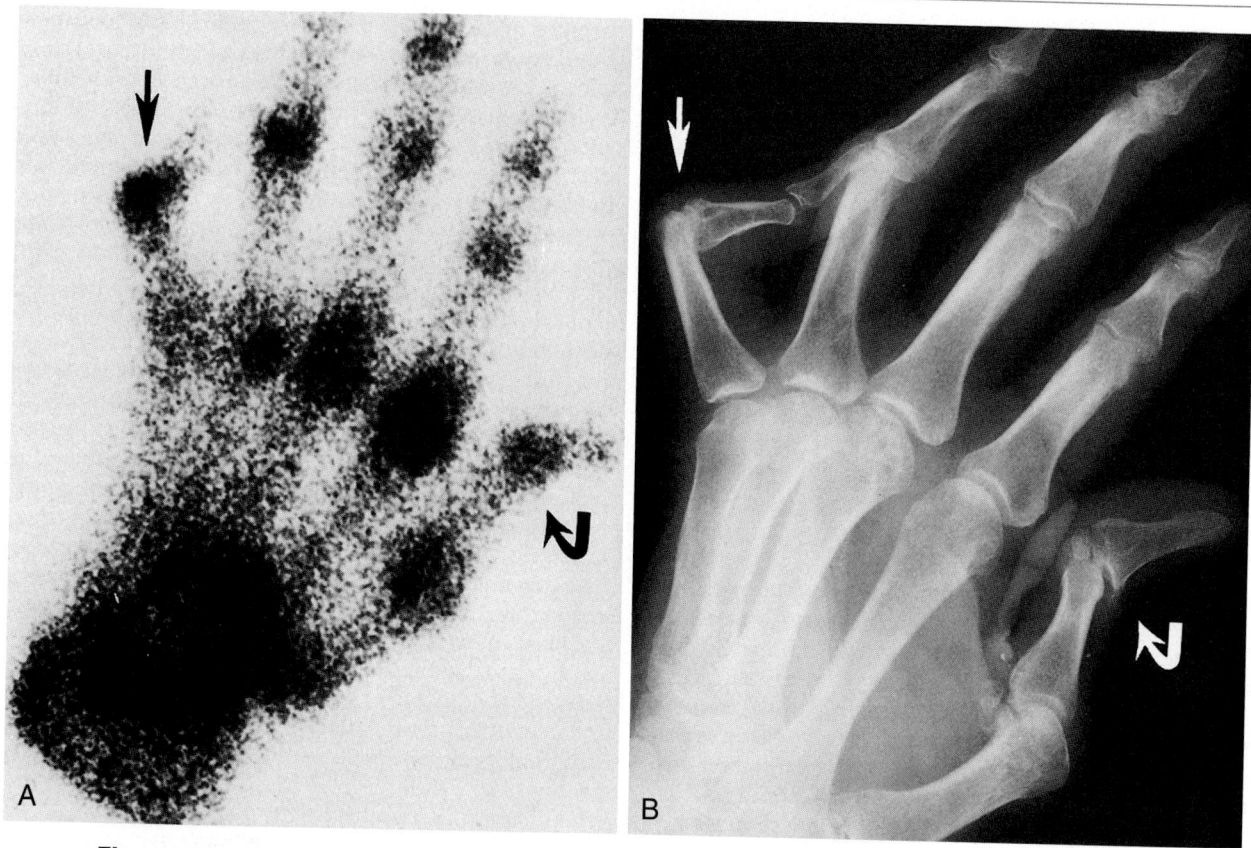

**Figure 16–36.** Scintigraphy in rheumatoid arthritis. *A*, Radionuclide scan of the right hand demonstrates uniform wrist activity and greater proximal than distal joint involvement. Note the deformities of the first *(curved arrow)* and fifth *(arrow)* digits. *B*, Radiograph of same hand shows typical deformities. Areas of greatest radionuclide activity correlate well with radiographic changes.
(From Weissberg D, Resnick D, Taylor A, et al: Rheumatoid arthritis and its variants: Analysis of scintiphotographic, radiographic, and clinical examinations. AJR Am J Roentgenol 131:665, 1978.)

## Computed Tomography

CT is generally not required when assessing the distribution and extent of joint involvement in this disease. Acetabular protrusion and ischemic necrosis of the femoral head are two examples of problems seen in patients with rheumatoid arthritis that can be evaluated with CT. It is clear, however, that ischemic necrosis of the femoral head cannot be diagnosed at an earlier stage with CT than with MR imaging. CT is well suited to the evaluation of para-articular masses, which in rheumatoid arthritis are commonly related to synovial cyst formation.

CT has been advocated as a useful noninvasive method in the diagnosis and management of cervical spine abnormalities in rheumatoid arthritis patients. The craniocervical junction and atlantoaxial region are well displayed in the transaxial and reformatted images obtainable with CT.

## Ultrasonography

With regard to rheumatoid arthritis, ultrasonography has proved capable in the analysis of para-articular masses such as synovial cysts and tendon sheath and joint involvement (especially in the hands and wrists). Abnormalities of the flexor tendons of the hand detectable with ultrasonography include loss of normal texture, tenosynovial cysts, tenosynovitis, and tendon (i.e., rheumatoid) nodules.

## Magnetic Resonance Imaging

General applications of MR imaging in the evaluation of rheumatoid arthritis include detection of articular disease, assessment of such disease activity, determination of the nature of some complications, and analysis of the extent of articular and para-articular changes in specific locations.

MR imaging is a very sensitive imaging method for the detection of articular diseases and has been used to assess the activity of rheumatoid arthritis, as well as its response to a variety of therapeutic regimens. It should be noted, however, that differentiating synovial fluid and inflammatory synovial tissue, or pannus, in a rheumatoid joint on standard spin echo and gradient echo sequences may be difficult (but possible) and that modification of the MR imaging technique may be required. Imaging following intravenous administration of gadolinium-containing contrast agents is useful in differentiating synovial inflammatory tissue and fluid.

On routine spin echo studies without such injection, low-intensity signal is derived from both fluid and pannus on T1-weighted images, whereas high-intensity signal characterizes both fluid and pannus on T2-weighted images. Immediately after the intravenous injection of a gadolinium-containing agent, the effusion remains of low signal intensity on T1-weighted spin echo images, and the synovium demonstrates enhancement with increased signal intensity on these images (Fig. 16–37). Synovial enhancement is greater in regions of hypervascular proliferative pannus and less in areas of fibrotic synovial tissue. Delayed imaging after intravenous injection of the contrast medium is characterized by seepage of contrast agent across the inflammatory pannus, with an increase in the signal intensity of joint fluid on T1-weighted spin echo images. The enhancement of joint fluid occurs within minutes, reaches a plateau in about 30 minutes, and persists for at least 60 minutes.

A variety of musculoskeletal complications of rheumatoid arthritis can be well evaluated with MR imaging. These include ischemic necrosis of bone, bursitis, synovial cyst formation, rheumatoid nodules, carpal tunnel syndrome and other entrapment neuropathies, tendon injury and disruption, and insufficiency fractures. Fluid collections and abnormal synovium within the iliopsoas, subdeltoid-subacromial, retrocalcaneal, olecranon, and prepatellar bursae are easily demonstrated with this technique (Fig. 16–38). Similarly, synovial cysts around any involved joint can be delineated with MR imaging. In superficial articulations such as the knee, ultrasonography is equally effective in the assessment of synovial cysts, although in deeper locations, including the hip and spine, MR imaging has distinct advantages. Tendon injury and

rupture, which may affect the hand, foot, knee, and shoulder in patients with rheumatoid arthritis, are best assessed with MR imaging.

Insufficiency fractures, an important complication of rheumatoid arthritis that occurs in the sacrum, femoral neck, parasymphyseal bone, tubular bones of the lower extremity, and elsewhere, reveal characteristic signal intensity abnormalities with MR imaging. With standard spin echo techniques, such fractures demonstrate serpentine linear shadows of low signal intensity surrounded by larger regions of intermediate signal intensity on T1-weighted images. The areas of intermediate signal, presumably representing surrounding edematous foci, become brighter on T2-weighted images (Fig. 16–39).

Evaluation of rheumatoid spines with MR imaging deserves special emphasis (Fig. 16–40). Although this technique can be used to assess any spinal segment, most reports have emphasized changes in the cervical region, especially the craniocervical junction. MR imaging allows assessment of the relationship of the occiput, atlas, and axis and is therefore useful in delineating the extent of subluxation in this spinal segment. MR imaging allows direct visualization of the spinal cord so that sites of physical distortion of the cord by displaced vertebrae, inflammatory masses, or both can be detected. The severity of myelopathy correlates better with MR imaging findings than with findings on conventional radiography. Medullary compression by the tip of the odontoid process in instances of cranial settling is far better appreciated on MR images than on standard radiographs. In instances of cord compression, areas of abnormal signal intensity within the spinal cord itself, perhaps reflecting edema, have been detected in rheumatoid arthritis patients by MR imaging.

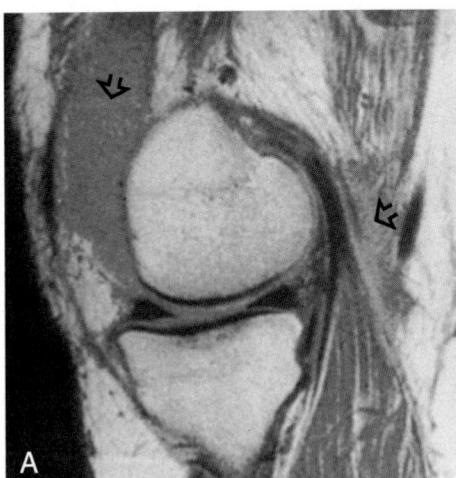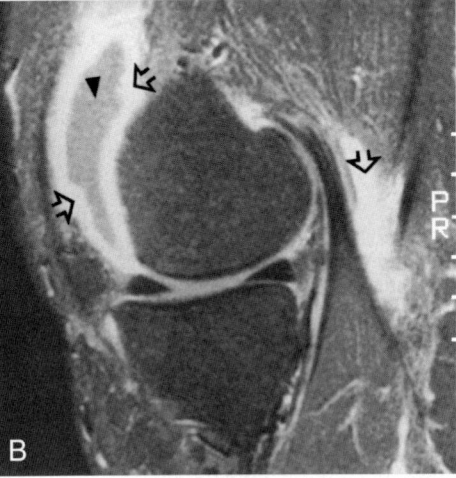

**Figure 16–37.** MR imaging in rheumatoid arthritis: differentiation of effusion and pannus with an intravenous gadolinium contrast agent. *A,* Initial intermediate-weighted (TR/TE, 1200/30) parasagittal spin echo MR image before the intravenous injection of a gadolinium compound reveals relatively low signal intensity of fluid, pannus, or both in the knee joint and within a synovial cyst *(open arrows). B,* Immediately after intravenous injection of the gadolinium agent, an intermediate-weighted (TR/TE, 1600/30) parasagittal spin echo MR image obtained with fat suppression reveals enhancement of the inflamed synovial membrane in the joint and bursa *(open arrows).* The fluid *(arrowhead)* remains of low signal intensity.

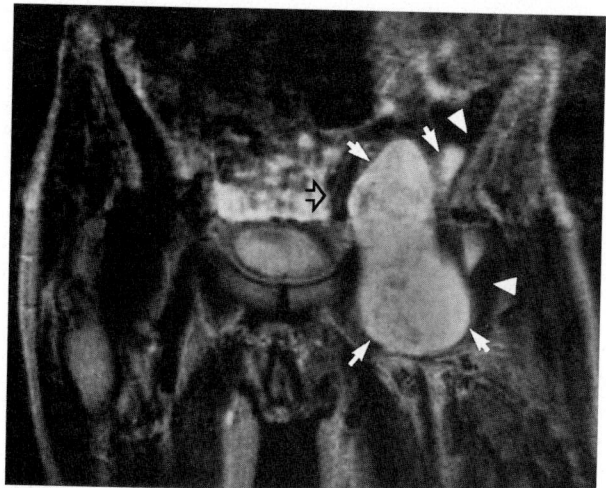

**Figure 16–38.** MR imaging in rheumatoid arthritis: iliopsoas bursitis. A progressively enlarging, painful mass developed in the left inguinal region in a 64-year-old man with long-standing rheumatoid arthritis. Coronal T2-weighted (TR/TE, 2000/90) spin echo MR image shows the cyst *(solid arrows)* medial to the psoas muscle *(arrowheads)* and lateral to the external iliac vessels *(open arrow)*. At surgery, a grossly dilated, fluid-filled iliopsoas bursa with chronically inflamed synovium was identified.

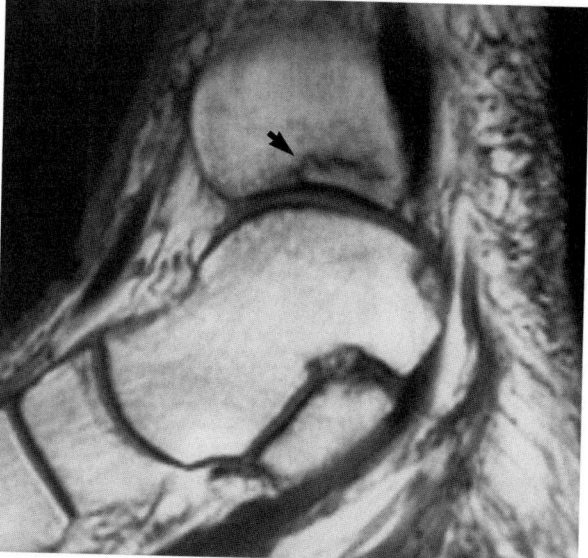

**Figure 16–39.** MR imaging in rheumatoid arthritis: insufficiency fractures. In this elderly man with both rheumatoid arthritis and diabetes mellitus, sagittal T1-weighted (TR/TE, 500/16) spin echo MR images show an insufficiency fracture of the distal portion of the tibia *(arrow)* as a serpentine region of low signal intensity.

## DIFFERENTIAL DIAGNOSIS

### General Abnormalities

The diagnosis of rheumatoid arthritis is obvious when radiographic examination reveals a symmetrically distributed articular disorder characterized by osteoporosis, fusiform soft tissue swelling, concentric joint space loss, and marginal and central erosions affecting the proximal interphalangeal and metacarpophalangeal joints of the hands, the wrists, the metatarsophalangeal joints of the feet, the knees, and the elbows. When radiographs disclose some degree of asymmetry, mild or absent osteoporosis, or preservation of joint space, an accurate appraisal is much more difficult.

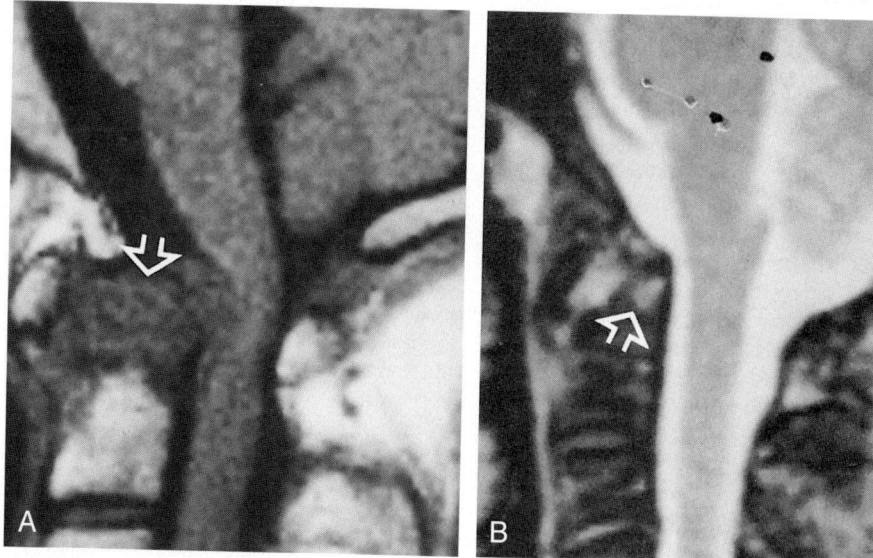

**Figure 16–40.** MR imaging in rheumatoid arthritis: evaluation of spinal involvement—periodontoid disease. *A,* Sagittal T1-weighted (TR/TE, 450/30) spin echo MR image of the upper cervical spine reveals a mass of intermediate signal intensity *(arrow)* that is eroding the odontoid process and causing cord compression. *B,* Periodontoid disease in a different patient with rheumatoid arthritis. Erosion is seen to better advantage *(arrow)* on a sagittal MPGR image (TR/TE, 450/15; flip angle, 15 degrees). Note the bright signal between the anterior arch of the atlas and the eroded dens, a sign of abnormality in the median anterior atlantoaxial joint. (*A,* From Neuhold A, Seidl G, Wicke L, et al: Medicamundi 32:38, 1987.)

**Seronegative "Rheumatoid" Arthritis.** Many patients with polyarticular inflammatory disease are serologically negative (seronegative) for rheumatoid factor, and the precise nature of their joint abnormality is variable and often unclear. Patients who have seronegative "rheumatoid" arthritis can generally be divided into two major groups: those with otherwise typical rheumatoid arthritis who are serologically negative for rheumatoid factor, and those with some other form of arthritis. In the former group, some patients will become seropositive, and some have become seronegative as a result of therapy. In the latter group, certain patients share clinical and radiologic features that will eventually allow their placement into a more homogeneous disease category. With respect to radiologic abnormalities, many persons with seronegative "rheumatoid" arthritis have atypical features, and in fact, an observer can often predict such seronegativity when reviewing the radiographs. One such feature is the asymmetry of articular involvement.

The presence of one or more radiographic features that are otherwise atypical for rheumatoid arthritis should alert the observer that the patient is probably seronegative for rheumatoid factor. The greater the number of such features, the greater the likelihood of seronegativity. The disease in such patients is best regarded as "rheumatoid-like" arthritis, an indication that the radiographic abnormalities are explained by a pathologic process resembling that of true rheumatoid arthritis.

**Remitting Seronegative Symmetrical Synovitis with Pitting Edema (RS₃PE Syndrome).** Patients with RS₃PE syndrome are generally elderly with an acute onset of bilateral and symmetrical synovitis involving predominantly the hands and wrists, along with evidence of tenosynovitis and pitting edema of the dorsum of the hands. Patients are typically seronegative for rheumatoid factor, and most possess the HLA-B27 antigen. Other clinical features include the involvement of large joints and flexion contractures of the wrists, fingers, and elbows. Although the remitting course and absence of joint destruction are clearly different from the characteristics of rheumatoid arthritis, many similarities exist between RS₃PE syndrome and polymyalgia rheumatica. Clearly, the final word regarding RS₃PE syndrome has yet to be written.

**Spondyloarthropathies.** Rheumatoid arthritis characteristically has articular lesions that differ in distribution and morphology from those of the seronegative spondyloarthropathies. Ankylosing spondylitis (which shows a predilection for the axial skeleton, although it may also produce appendicular articular disease), psoriatic arthritis (which may affect the axial and appendicular skeleton as well as the distal interphalangeal articulations), and Reiter's syndrome (which leads to asymmetrical arthritis of the lower extremity, with or without sacroiliac and spinal alterations) may each be associated with prominent findings in synovial and cartilaginous joints and entheses. In the synovial joints, the absence of osteoporosis and the presence of bony proliferation and intra-articular osseous fusion are commonly encountered in the seronegative spondyloarthropathies, findings that differ from the features of rheumatoid arthritis. Similarly, ankylosing spondylitis, psoriatic arthritis, and Reiter's syndrome can produce significant and extensive abnormalities of the cartilaginous joints and entheses; these sites are much less frequently and severely affected in rheumatoid arthritis. Widespread spondylitis and sacroiliitis are also characteristic of the seronegative spondyloarthropathies.

**Gout.** Gouty arthritis is associated with a form of asymmetrical articular disease of the appendicular skeleton that is characterized by soft tissue masses, asymmetric osseous erosions, bony proliferation, preservation of joint space, and absence of osteoporosis. Generally, the features are easily differentiated from those of rheumatoid arthritis.

**Collagen Vascular Disorders.** The arthropathy of systemic lupus erythematosus is a deforming, nonerosive process that is initially reversible. Cartilaginous destruction caused by pressure erosion at areas of contact between malpositioned osseous structures, as well as periarticular bony "hook" erosions caused by capsular and ligamentous changes, can be observed in systemic lupus erythematosus, but marginal and central osseous defects and diffuse joint space narrowing are unusual in this disease unless coexistent rheumatoid arthritis is present. In contrast, the deformities in rheumatoid arthritis are almost universally associated with joint space narrowing and bone erosion.

In scleroderma, articular changes may be especially prominent in the distal interphalangeal joints of the fingers and the first carpometacarpal and inferior radioulnar compartments of the wrist. They are generally associated with tuft resorption and soft tissue and capsular calcification. Mixed connective tissue disease and overlap syndromes can lead to radiographic abnormalities common to more than one collagen vascular disorder. Thus, detection of rheumatoid arthritis–like alterations as well as those of scleroderma or systemic lupus erythematosus can provide a clue to the mixed nature of the collagen disease.

**Calcium Pyrophosphate Dihydrate Crystal Deposition Disease.** This articular disorder is radiographically manifested as articular and periarticular calcification and pyrophosphate arthropathy. The calcification involves various structures, including cartilage (chondrocalcinosis), and is most prominent in the knees, wrists, metacarpophalangeal joints, and symphysis pubis. Pyrophosphate arthropathy leads to joint space narrowing, eburnation, cyst formation, collapse, and fragmentation. The resulting radiographic picture does not resemble that of rheumatoid arthritis. The arthropathy of hemochromatosis is very similar to that of idiopathic CPPD crystal deposition disease.

## Abnormalities at Specific Sites

**Hand and Wrist.** Symmetrical changes at the metacarpophalangeal and proximal interphalangeal joints are common in rheumatoid arthritis (Table 16–4). Psoriatic arthritis leads to significant abnormalities of the distal interphalangeal joints, as well as the more proximal articulations. Osteoarthritis (inflammatory or noninflammatory) most typically affects the distal interphalangeal, proximal interphalangeal, and metacarpophalangeal joints. Gouty arthritis

**TABLE 16-4**

## Compartmental Analysis of Hand and Wrist Disease*

| | DIP Joints | PIP Joints | MCP Joints | Radiocarpal Joint | Inferior Radioulnar Joint | Midcarpal Joint | Pisiform-Triquetral Joint | Common Carpometacarpal Joint | First Carpometacarpal Joint |
|---|---|---|---|---|---|---|---|---|---|
| Rheumatoid arthritis | | + | + | + | + | + | + | + | + |
| Osteoarthritis | + | + | + | | | +† | | | + |
| Inflammatory osteoarthritis | + | + | ± | | | +† | | | + |
| Calcium pyrophosphate dihydrate crystal deposition disease | | + | | + | | +† | | | + |
| Gouty arthritis | + | + | + | + | + | + | | +‡ | + |
| Scleroderma§ | + | + | | | + | | | | + |
| | | | | | + | | | | + |

*Only the typical locations for each disease are indicated.

†Has a predilection for trapezioscaphoid area of the midcarpal joint.

‡Very severe abnormalities may be present in this compartment.

§Some patients have coexistent rheumatoid arthritis.

DIP, distal interphalangeal; MCP, metacarpophalangeal; PIP, proximal interphalangeal.

can involve any joint of the hand, including the distal interphalangeal joints. CPPD crystal deposition disease has a predilection for the metacarpophalangeal articulations.

Rheumatoid arthritis can manifest initially as soft tissue swelling, joint space narrowing, and osseous erosions in one or two locations of the wrist. Soon, however, pancompartmental alterations become evident. In patients without a significant history of accidental or occupational trauma, osteoarthritis leads to articular abnormalities that are invariably confined to the first carpometacarpal compartment, the trapezioscaphoid space of the midcarpal compartment, or both. CPPD crystal deposition disease favors the radiocarpal compartment; scleroderma may selectively involve the first carpometacarpal and inferior radioulnar compartments; and gout produces pancompartmental disease, with predominant involvement of the common carpometacarpal compartment.

**Elbow.** Radiographic abnormalities of the elbow in rheumatoid arthritis are sufficiently characteristic in most instances to allow an accurate diagnosis. Joint space narrowing, osseous erosions, and cysts are frequently accompanied by soft tissue prominence related to rheumatoid nodules and olecranon bursitis. The elbow is involved in other polyarticular disorders, but differences in radiographic findings between these diseases and rheumatoid arthritis are usually obvious.

**Glenohumeral Joint.** Marginal erosions of the humeral head are seen in rheumatoid arthritis, ankylosing spondylitis, and infection, as well as in other disorders. In ankylosing spondylitis, the size of the defect may be considerably larger than that in rheumatoid arthritis. Septic arthritis of the glenohumeral joint is usually monoarticular.

**Acromioclavicular Joint.** Resorption of the distal end of the clavicle and widening of the acromioclavicular joint are observed in rheumatoid arthritis, ankylosing spondylitis, infection, other collagen vascular disorders, and hyperparathyroidism, as well as after trauma. When the changes are secondary to an articular process, prominent acromial abnormalities may accompany the clavicular alterations. In hyperparathyroidism, subchondral resorption of bone is evident on both the acromial and the clavicular aspects of the articulation, but the acromial alterations are relatively mild. Post-traumatic osteolysis of the distal end of the clavicle is accompanied by a pertinent clinical history of acute or chronic injury.

**Coracoclavicular Joint.** Resorption of the undersurface of the distal portion of the clavicle is seen in rheumatoid arthritis, hyperparathyroidism, and ankylosing spondylitis. In ankylosing spondylitis, bone proliferation is an associated radiographic manifestation.

**Sternoclavicular and Manubriosternal Joints.** Changes in the sternoclavicular and manubriosternal joints are not specific for rheumatoid arthritis. Similar abnormalities accompany the seronegative spondyloarthropathies.

**Forefoot.** The most common sites of articular disease of the forefoot in rheumatoid arthritis are the metatarsophalangeal joints and the interphalangeal joint of the great toe. Although these same articulations are involved in psoriatic arthritis, Reiter's syndrome, and gout, extensive abnormalities of other interphalangeal joints in one or more digits should be evident in these disorders (Table 16–5). Further, forefoot abnormalities are usually symmetrical in distribution in rheumatoid arthritis and asymmetrical in psoriatic arthritis, Reiter's syndrome, and gouty arthritis.

**Midfoot**. Diffuse changes with a predilection for the talonavicular portion of the talocalcaneonavicular joint characterize midfoot involvement in rheumatoid arthritis. The talonavicular space is also affected in CPPD crystal deposition disease and neuropathic osteoarthropathy, but both of these disorders are associated with bony sclerosis and fragmentation. In gout, abnormalities often predominate at the tarsometatarsal joints.

**Heel**. Retrocalcaneal bursitis producing soft tissue swelling and subjacent osseous erosion occurs not only in rheumatoid arthritis but also in ankylosing spondylitis, psoriatic arthritis, and Reiter's syndrome (Table 16–6). The changes are virtually indistinguishable in these four disorders, and tendon thickening can be seen in any one of them. Nodular prominence of the Achilles tendon can also be encountered in gout (as a result of tophi) and hyperlipoproteinemia (secondary to xanthoma).

**Knee**. In rheumatoid arthritis, symmetrical involvement of the medial and lateral femorotibial compartments is seen, with or without patellofemoral compartment changes. In osteoarthritis, asymmetrical alterations of the medial and lateral femorotibial compartments (the medial side is usually the dominant side of involvement, especially in men) can be combined with patellofemoral compartment disease. In CPPD crystal deposition disease, patellofemoral abnormalities, occurring alone or in combination with asymmetrical medial and lateral femorotibial alterations, are typical. A varus deformity is especially characteristic of osteoarthritis, whereas valgus deformity is not uncommon in rheumatoid arthritis and CPPD crystal deposition disease. Marginal erosions of the femur and tibia are evident in rheumatoid arthritis, the seronegative spondyloarthropathies, gout, and infection, especially tuberculosis. In gout and tuberculosis, such erosions may be unaccompanied by joint space narrowing.

**Hip**. Concentric loss of the articular space and axial migration of the femoral head with respect to the acetabulum are typical of rheumatoid involvement of the hip. In osteoarthritis, superior or medial migration is more frequent than axial migration, a finding reflecting the asymmetrical nature of the cartilaginous destruction. Axial migration of the femoral head can accompany the hip alterations of CPPD crystal deposition disease and ankylosing spondylitis, although both of these disorders are associated with osteophytes and sclerosis. In long-standing rheumatoid arthritis, however, osteophytes may appear as a manifestation of secondary degenerative joint disease.

Acetabular protrusion is a common manifestation of severe rheumatoid hip disease. It is associated with diffuse loss of the interosseous space and an eroded and often diminutive femoral head. Protrusio acetabuli can also be encountered in patients with osteoarthritis, familial or idiopathic protrusion deformities (Otto pelvis), ankylosing spondylitis, infection, osteomalacia, and Paget's disease (Table 16–7).

**Sacroiliac Joint**. Sacroiliac joint abnormalities are not common or prominent in rheumatoid arthritis. When evident, they are generally asymmetrical in distribution

---

**TABLE 16-5**

**Compartmental Analysis of Forefoot Disease***

|  | Metatarsophalangeal Joints | Interphalangeal Joint of Great Toe | Other Interphalangeal Joints |
|---|---|---|---|
| Rheumatoid arthritis | + | + |  |
| Gouty arthritis | + | + | + |
| Psoriatic arthritis | + | +[†] | + |
| Reiter's syndrome | + | +[†] | + |
| Osteoarthritis | +[‡] |  |  |

*Only the typical locations of each disease are indicated.

[†]Severe destructive changes may be observed.

[‡]Has a predilection for the metatarsophalangeal joint of the first digit.

---

**TABLE 16-6**

**Abnormalities of the Heel**

|  | Retrocalcaneal Bursitis with Posterosuperior Calcaneal Erosion | Achilles Tendinosis | Enthesophyte at Posterior Attachment of Achilles Tendon | Well-Defined Plantar Calcaneal Enthesophyte | Poorly Defined Plantar Calcaneal Enthesophyte |
|---|---|---|---|---|---|
| Rheumatoid arthritis | + | + | + | + |  |
| Ankylosing spondylitis | + | + | + |  | +* |
| Psoriatic arthritis | + | + | + |  | +* |
| Reiter's syndrome | + | + |  |  | +* |
| Gouty arthritis | +[†] | +[‡] |  |  |  |
| Xanthoma | +[†] | +[‡] |  |  |  |

*Poorly defined enthesophytes may become better defined with healing.

[†]Erosion of the calcaneus can occur beneath a tophus or xanthoma.

[‡]Nodular thickening of the tendon may be seen.

and consist of minor subchondral erosions, minimal eburnation, and absent or focal intra-articular bony ankylosis (Table 16–8). These characteristics differ from those of ankylosing spondylitis (bilateral symmetrical disease with extensive erosions, sclerosis, and bony fusion), psoriatic arthritis and Reiter's syndrome (bilateral symmetrical or asymmetrical disease or unilateral disease with changes identical to those of ankylosing spondylitis), gout (bilateral or unilateral abnormalities with large erosions), degenerative joint disease (bilateral or unilateral disease with prominent subchondral sclerosis), osteitis condensans ilii (bilateral symmetrical alterations of the lower part of the ilium with significant bony eburnation), hyperparathyroidism (bilateral symmetrical abnormalities with widening of the interosseous space, erosions, and sclerosis), and infection (unilateral disease with poorly defined osseous defects and reactive sclerosis).

**Spine.** Rheumatoid arthritis produces infrequent abnormalities of the thoracic and lumbar spine. Rheumatoid changes in the cervical spine consisting of apophyseal joint erosion and malalignment, intervertebral disc space narrowing with adjacent eburnation and without osteophytes, and multiple subluxations (including at the atlantoaxial junction) are virtually diagnostic when they occur as a group. They differ from the cervical alterations of ankylosing spondylitis (widespread apophyseal joint ankylosis and syndesmophytes), psoriatic arthritis (apophyseal joint narrowing, eburnation, and prominent anterior vertebral bone formation), diffuse idiopathic skeletal hyperostosis (flowing ossification and excrescences along the anterior aspect of the spine, with preservation of intervertebral disc height), and juvenile chronic arthritis (apophyseal joint ankylosis with hypoplasia of the vertebral bodies and intervertebral discs). Atlantoaxial subluxation alone is not a pathognomonic sign of rheumatoid arthritis, however. It is also observed in ankylosing spondylitis, psoriatic arthritis, Reiter's syndrome, and juvenile chronic arthritis, as well as after trauma or local infection (Grisel's syndrome).

## FURTHER READING

Adams ME, Li DKB: Magnetic resonance imaging in rheumatology. J Rheumatol 12:1038, 1985.

Berens DL, Lin RK: Roentgen Diagnosis of Rheumatoid Arthritis. Springfield, Ill, Charles C Thomas, 1969.

Braunstein EM, Weissman BN, Seltzer SE, et al: Computed tomography and conventional radiographs of the craniocervical region in rheumatoid arthritis: A comparison. Arthritis Rheum 27:26, 1984.

Castillo BA, El Sallab RA, Scott JT: Physical activity, cystic erosions, and osteoporosis in rheumatoid arthritis. Ann Rheum Dis 24:522, 1965.

Currey HLF: Aetiology and pathogenesis of rheumatoid arthritis. In Scott JT (ed): Copeman's Textbook of the Rheumatic Diseases, 5th ed. Edinburgh, Churchill Livingstone, 1978, p 261.

El-Khoury GY, Larson RK, Kathol MH, et al: Seronegative and seropositive rheumatoid arthritis: Radiographic differences. Radiology 168:517, 1988.

El-Khoury GY, Wener MH, Menezes AH, et al: Cranial settling in rheumatoid arthritis. Radiology 137:637, 1980.

Felty AR: Chronic arthritis in the adult associated with splenomegaly and leukopenia: A report of 5 cases of an unusual clinical syndrome. Johns Hopkins Hosp Bull 35:16, 1924.

Fries JF, Bloch DA, Sharp JT, et al: Assessment of radiologic progression in rheumatoid arthritis: A randomized controlled trial. Arthritis Rheum 29:1, 1986.

Gasson J, Gandy SJ, Hutton CW, et al: Magnetic resonance imaging of rheumatoid arthritis in metacarpophalangeal joints. Skeletal Radiol 29:324, 2000.

Gelman MI, Ward JR: Septic arthritis: A complication of rheumatoid arthritis. Radiology 122:17, 1977.

Heywood AWB, Meyers OL: Rheumatoid arthritis of the thoracic and lumbar spine. J Bone Joint Surg Br 68:362, 1986.

Kaye JJ, Callahan LF, Nance EP Jr, et al: Rheumatoid arthritis: Explanatory power of specific radiographic findings for patient clinical status. Radiology 165:753, 1987.

Kelley WN, Harris ED Jr, Ruddy S, et al (eds): Textbook of Rheumatology, 5th ed. Philadelphia, WB Saunders, 1997.

Kursunoglu-Brahme S, Riccio T, Weisman MH, et al: Rheumatoid knee: Role of gadopentetate-enhanced MR imaging. Radiology 176:831, 1990.

Martel W: Pathogenesis of cervical discovertebral destruction in rheumatoid arthritis. Arthritis Rheum 20:1217, 1977.

Martel W: The pattern of rheumatoid arthritis in the hand and wrist. Radiol Clin North Am 2:221, 1964.

McAfee PC, Bohlman HH, Han JS, et al: Comparison of nuclear magnetic resonance imaging and computed tomography in the diagnosis of upper cervical spinal cord compression. Spine 11:295, 1986.

Monsees B, Destouet JM, Murphy WA, et al: Pressure erosions of bone in rheumatoid arthritis: A subject review. Radiology 155:53, 1985.

---

**TABLE 16-7**

### Causes of Protrusio Acetabuli

Rheumatoid arthritis
Ankylosing spondylitis
Osteoarthritis (medial migration pattern)
Infection
Paget's disease
Osteomalacia
Irradiation
Acetabular trauma

---

**TABLE 16-8**

### Comparison of Sacroiliac Joint Abnormalities in Rheumatoid Arthritis and Ankylosing Spondylitis

|  | Rheumatoid Arthritis | Ankylosing Spondylitis |
|---|---|---|
| Distribution | Asymmetrical or unilateral | Bilateral and symmetrical |
| Erosions | Superficial | Deep |
| Sclerosis | Mild or absent | Moderate or severe* |
| Bony ankylosis | Rare, segmental | Common, diffuse |

*Sclerosis may disappear in long-standing disease.

Park WM, O'Neill M, McCall IW: The radiology of rheumatoid involvement of the cervical spine. Skeletal Radiol 4:1, 1979.

Resnick D: Patterns of migration of the femoral head in osteoarthritis of the hip: Roentgenographic-pathologic correlation and comparison with rheumatoid arthritis. AJR Am J Roentgenol 124:62, 1975.

Resnick D: Rheumatoid arthritis of the wrist: The compartmental approach. Med Radiogr Photogr 52:50, 1976.

Resnick D, Feingold ML, Curd J, et al: Calcaneal abnormalities in articular disorders: Rheumatoid arthritis, ankylosing spondylitis, psoriatic arthritis and Reiter's syndrome. Radiology 125:355, 1977.

Ropes MW, Bennett GA, Cobb S, et al: Diagnostic criteria for rheumatoid arthritis, 1958 revision. Ann Rheum Dis 18:49, 1959.

Schils JP, Resnick D, Haghighi PN, et al: Pathogenesis of discovertebral and manubriosternal joint abnormalities in rheumatoid arthritis: A cadaveric study. J Rheumatol 16:291, 1989.

Scott JT (ed): Copeman's Textbook of the Rheumatic Diseases, 5th ed. Edinburgh, Churchill Livingstone, 1978.

Sharp JT: An overview of radiographic analysis of joint damage in rheumatoid arthritis and its use in metaanalysis. J Rheumatol 27:254, 2000.

Sharp JT, Young DY, Bluhm GR, et al: How many joints in the hands and wrists should be included in a score of radiologic abnormalities used to assess rheumatoid arthritis? Arthritis Rheum 28:1326, 1985.

Stiskal MA, Neuhold A, Szolar DH, et al: Rheumatoid arthritis of the craniocervical region by MR imaging: Detection and characterization. AJR Am J Roentgenol 165:585, 1995.

Sugimoto H, Takeda A, Hyodoh K: Early-stage rheumatoid arthritis: Prospective study of the effectiveness of MR imaging for diagnosis. Radiology 216:569, 2000.

Swanson AB, Swanson GG: Pathogenesis and pathomechanics of rheumatoid deformities in the hand and wrist. Orthop Clin North Am 4:1039, 1973.

Weissberg D, Resnick D, Taylor A, et al: Rheumatoid arthritis and its variants: Analysis of scintiphotographic, radiographic, and clinical examinations. AJR Am J Roentgenol 131:665, 1978.

Weissman BNW, Alibadi P, Weinfeld MS, et al: Prognostic features of atlanto-axial subluxation in rheumatoid arthritis. Radiology 144:745, 1982.

Wolfe BK, O'Keeffe D, Mitchell DM, et al: Rheumatoid arthritis of the cervical spine: Early and progressive radiographic features. Radiology 165:145, 1987.

# CHAPTER 17

## Juvenile Chronic Arthritis

## SUMMARY OF KEY FEATURES

Juvenile chronic arthritis is a disorder encompassing a variety of conditions that affect articular structures in children. Although the specific radiographic features of juvenile chronic arthritis depend on the subgroup of patients being evaluated, certain characteristics are sufficiently common in most patients to allow differentiation of juvenile chronic arthritis from various adult diseases. Loss of articular space and osseous erosions are relatively late manifestations of juvenile disease. Metaphyseal radiolucency, periostitis, intra-articular bony ankylosis, epiphyseal compression fractures, subluxation or dislocation, and growth disturbances are common. Although changes may be observed in many different skeletal sites, abnormalities of the hand, wrist, foot, knee, hip, cervical spine, mandible, and temporomandibular joint are especially characteristic.

The differential diagnosis of juvenile chronic arthritis includes hemophilia, idiopathic multicentric osteolysis, mucopolysaccharidoses, epiphyseal dysplasias, multicentric reticulohistiocytosis, and infection.

## INTRODUCTION

In 1897, Still, an English pediatrician, described in detail an articular condition in 22 children that appeared to be distinct from the adult type of rheumatoid arthritis because of its predilection for large joints rather than small ones, its propensity for producing joint contractures and muscle wasting, and its association with significant extra-articular manifestations such as splenomegaly, lymphadenopathy, anemia, fever, pleuritis, and pericarditis. Since that report, the term *Still's disease* has frequently been used to describe rheumatoid arthritis in children. It is now recognized that a number of separate disorders can lead to chronic arthritis in children and that in many patients, scrutiny of the clinical and radiographic features allows a more precise diagnosis.

## CLASSIFICATION

In the classification of articular disease in children, certain groups of disorders with characteristic features must be excluded. Infectious diseases; bleeding diatheses; neoplasms such as leukemia and neuroblastoma; collagen vascular disorders, including scleroderma, systemic lupus erythematosus, and dermatomyositis; Sjögren's syndrome; rheumatic fever; postdysenteric arthritis; and some rarer conditions are all eliminated in this fashion. The remaining group of diseases is designated juvenile chronic arthritis (or polyarthritis) or, more recently, juvenile idiopathic arthritides (Tables 17–1 and 17–2). At the time of the initial examination, however, it is often impossible to classify childhood arthritis into one specific subgroup of juvenile chronic arthritis.

### Juvenile-Onset Adult-Type (Seropositive) Rheumatoid Arthritis

An articular disease that resembles and behaves like its adult counterpart has been noted in 10% of children with juvenile chronic arthritis (Fig. 17–1*A*). This subtype is more common in girls than in boys and is more common after the age of 10 years. The clinical onset is usually polyarticular (involvement of five or more joints), with early involvement of the interphalangeal and metacarpophalangeal joints of the hand, the wrist, the knee, and the metatarsophalangeal and interphalangeal joints of the foot. Subcutaneous nodules, particularly about the elbow, can be detected in approximately 10% to 20% of children. Iridocyclitis is not present.

Radiologic changes in juvenile-onset adult-type rheumatoid arthritis include soft tissue swelling, periarticular osteoporosis, and periostitis in the hands and feet. Periosteal bone formation can involve large segments of the metaphyses of the phalanges, metacarpals, and metatarsals. The frequency and severity of periostitis account for the fundamental difference between juvenile-onset and adult-onset disease. Significant osseous erosions are also encountered in children with this subtype of disease, unaccompanied by loss of the interosseous space. The appearance of significant erosive abnormality in the absence of joint space loss is an important diagnostic sign of juvenile-onset rheumatoid arthritis. The prognosis of polyarthritis in children who become seropositive for rheumatoid factor is generally poor.

### Seronegative Chronic Arthritis (Still's Disease)

In this most common (approximately 70%) subtype of juvenile chronic arthritis, systemic or articular (or both)

### TABLE 17–1

**Juvenile Chronic Arthritis: Classification**

Juvenile-onset adult-type (seropositive) rheumatoid arthritis
Seronegative chronic arthritis (Still's disease)
Classic systemic disease
Polyarticular disease
Pauciarticular or monoarticular disease
Juvenile-onset ankylosing spondylitis
Psoriatic arthritis
Arthritis of inflammatory bowel disease
Other seronegative spondyloarthropathies
Miscellaneous arthritis

**TABLE 17–2**

## Juvenile Chronic Arthritis: Clinical and Radiographic Features

| Disorder | Clinical Features | Sites of Articular Involvement | Radiographic Features |
|---|---|---|---|
| Juvenile-onset adult-type (seropositive) rheumatoid arthritis | Female predominance<br>>10 yr old<br>Polyarticular involvement<br>± Subcutaneous nodules<br>± Vasculitis<br>Seropositive for rheumatoid factor | MCP and IP joints of the hand<br>Wrist<br>Knee<br>MTP and IP joints of the foot<br>Cervical spine | Soft tissue swelling<br>Osteoporosis<br>Periostitis<br>Erosions<br>± Joint space loss<br>Atlantoaxial subluxation |
| Still's disease<br>  Systemic disease | Affects males and females equally <5 yr old<br>Systemic manifestations<br>Mild articular manifestations | Unusual and mild joint involvement* | |
| Polyarticular disease | Affects males and females equally<br>Variable age<br>Polyarticular involvement<br>Symmetrical | MCP and IP joints of the hand<br>Wrist<br>Knee<br>Ankle<br>Intertarsal, MTP, and IP joints of the foot<br>Cervical spine | Soft tissue swelling<br>Osteoporosis<br>Periostitis<br>Growth disturbances<br>± Erosions<br>± Joint space loss<br>Intra-articular bony ankylosis<br>Apophyseal joint ankylosis with hypoplasia of the cervical vertebrae and discs<br>Scoliosis |
| Pauciarticular or monoarticular disease | Female predominance<br>Young age<br>Iridocyclitis<br>± Systemic manifestations<br>Asymmetrical | Knee<br>Ankle<br>Elbow<br>Wrist | Soft tissue swelling<br>Osteoporosis<br>Growth disturbances<br>± Joint space loss<br>± Erosions |
| Juvenile-onset ankylosing spondylitis | Male predominance<br>10–12 yr old<br>Polyarticular or pauciarticular involvement<br>Predilection for the lower extremity<br>Asymmetrical<br>± Back pain<br>± Iridocyclitis<br>± Family history<br>HLA-B27 positive | Ankle<br>Knee<br>Intertarsal joints<br>Calcaneus<br>Hip<br>± Sacroiliac joint<br>± Spine | ± Sacroiliitis<br>± Spondylitis<br>Joint space loss<br>Intra-articular bony ankylosis<br>Erosions<br>Bony proliferation |

*When present, findings are similar to those of polyarticular or pauciarticular disease.
IP, interphalangeal; MCP, metacarpophalangeal; MTP, metatarsophalangeal.

symptoms and signs develop in the absence of positive serologic test results for rheumatoid factor. Within this subgroup are certain clinical varieties, such as classic systemic disease, polyarticular disease, and pauciarticular or monoarticular disease.

**Classic Systemic Disease.** This pattern, which is usually seen in boys and girls younger than 5 years and represents approximately 20% of cases of juvenile chronic arthritis, is associated with severe extra-articular clinical manifestations. An acute febrile onset may or may not be accompanied by arthritis. Affected children have toxic symptoms along with irritability, listlessness, anorexia, and weight loss. A rash accompanies the fever in approximately 80% to 90% of children. Generalized lymphadenopathy and hepatosplenomegaly can simulate findings in leukemia or lymphoma. Pericarditis and myocarditis represent serious manifestations of Still's disease. Although joint manifestations are common, they are generally mild. Myalgia and arthralgia may precede actual arthritis. Radiologic findings are unusual, although chronic and disabling articular changes occasionally become evident.

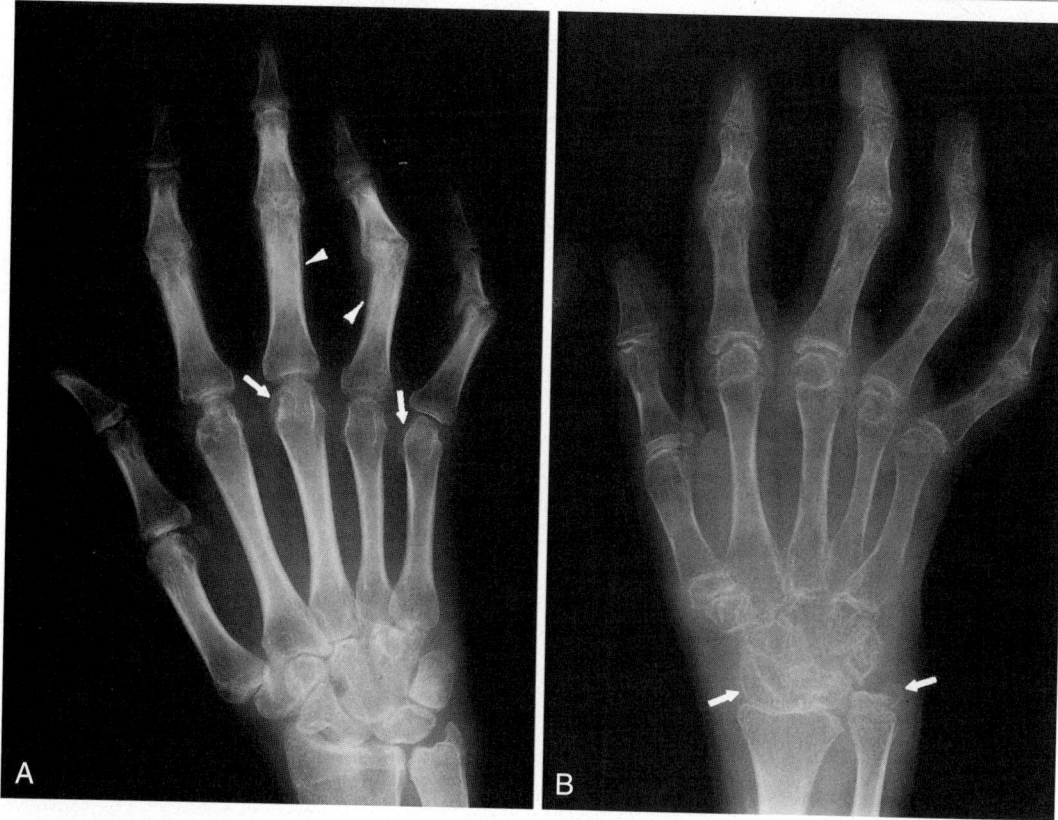

**Figure 17–1.** Juvenile chronic arthritis: subtypes of disease. *A,* Juvenile-onset adult-type (seropositive) rheumatoid arthritis in an 18-year-old girl with seropositive rheumatoid arthritis for approximately 6 years. Observe that the radiographic abnormalities are similar to those seen in adult-onset disease. Involvement occurs in all the compartments of the wrist and in the metacarpophalangeal and proximal interphalangeal joints, with less striking changes in the distal interphalangeal joints. Radiographic changes include soft tissue swelling, periarticular osteoporosis, joint space narrowing, and marginal erosions. At some metacarpophalangeal joints, considerable erosive alterations are not accompanied by severe loss of joint space *(arrows).* Also note the intra-articular osseous fusion at several proximal interphalangeal joints and periostitis of the phalangeal shafts *(arrowheads). B,* Seronegative chronic arthritis (Still's disease): polyarticular disease. An 11-year-old girl, seronegative for rheumatoid factor, had symmetrical articular disease of the hands, wrists, knees, feet, and cervical spine. The radiograph outlines considerable generalized osteoporosis, periarticular soft tissue swelling, superficial erosions of carpal bones and metacarpal heads with shape irregularities, joint space narrowing, epiphyseal collapse, and enlargement of the epiphyses, particularly those of the distal end of the radius and distal portion of the ulna *(arrows).* The crenated or "crinkled" appearance of the carpus and metacarpal heads is distinctive. Flexion contractures of several digits are evident.

**Polyarticular Disease.** Polyarticular arthritis (see Fig. 17–1*B*) may occur at the onset of Still's disease or as a later complication in a child with systemic manifestations. This pattern is evident in approximately 20% of patients with juvenile chronic arthritis. Boys and girls are affected in equal numbers. Symmetrical or asymmetrical involvement of the metacarpophalangeal and proximal interphalangeal joints of the hands, the wrists, the knees, the ankles, and the intertarsal, metatarsophalangeal, and interphalangeal joints of the feet is typical. The cervical spine is frequently a site of early abnormality and is characteristically the only region of the vertebral column affected.

In the initial stages of polyarthritis, radiographic findings are soft tissue swelling, osteoporosis, and advanced skeletal maturation. In the hands and feet, abnormalities in the shape (squaring) of the carpal and tarsal bones are frequently combined with initial loss of joint space and sub-sequent intra-articular bony ankylosis. Synovitis of the flexor tendon sheaths may produce periostitis of the diaphyses and metaphyses of the phalanges, metacarpals, and metatarsals. Premature fusion of the epiphyses of the bones is not uncommon and accounts for the characteristic growth defects. The epiphyses may appear enlarged or ballooned in relation to the diaphyses, and a decrease in bone length is characteristic. Osseous erosion is unusual.

In larger articulations such as the knee, osteoporosis and epiphyseal overgrowth are more typical. In the hip, enlargement and osteoporosis of the femoral capital epiphysis, failure of growth and premature fusion of the femoral neck, coxa valga deformity, hypoplasia of the iliac bones, and protrusio acetabuli are seen. Apophyseal joint erosions, narrowing, and bony ankylosis predominate in the upper cervical region. Associated hypoplasia of the vertebral bodies and intervertebral discs is characteristic.

**Pauciarticular or Monoarticular Disease.** This pattern, which is observed in young children and may represent 30% to 70% of all cases of juvenile chronic arthritis, is generally confined to the large joints, most frequently the knees, ankles, elbows, and wrists. This clinical pattern of arthritis carries with it a serious threat of blindness from iridocyclitis. Additional systemic manifestations are infrequent, although lymphadenopathy, splenomegaly, fever, and rash are occasionally observed. In recent years, two distinct subtypes of this disease pattern have been identified on the basis of clinical and immunogenetic evidence. Pauciarticular disease type I affects children 5 years or younger, predominantly girls. Chronic iridocyclitis is frequent, as are positive tests for antinuclear antibodies. Sacroiliitis and spondylitis are absent, and the prognosis for ultimate joint function is good. Pauciarticular disease type II affects children who are older at the time of disease onset, and principally boys are affected. The peripheral joints in the lower extremities are characteristically involved. Iridocyclitis may be observed, and sacroiliitis may become apparent at follow-up evaluation.

A monoarticular type of juvenile chronic arthritis has been reported in 5% to 35% of patients. In children who initially exhibit monoarticular disease, pauciarticular disease or, infrequently, polyarthritis may develop. In general, it cannot be predicted whether more widespread articular abnormality will develop in children with monoarthritis.

In monoarticular or pauciarticular Still's disease, radiographically demonstrable abnormalities of bone growth may appear at an early stage. Increased size and accelerated maturation of epiphyseal ossification centers, longitudinal overgrowth of bones adjacent to an affected articulation, and regional atrophy and remodeling of bone are observed. Soft tissue swelling and osteoporosis are seen, but bone erosion is a late manifestation.

### Juvenile-Onset Ankylosing Spondylitis

In children with ankylosing spondylitis, particularly boys, sacroiliitis and spondylitis develop in the presence of the histocompatibility antigen HLA-B27. The mean age at disease onset is 10 to 12 years. An asymmetrical arthritis is generally observed, and the articulations of the lower limbs are affected. Clinical manifestations may be encountered in the sacroiliac joints, but radiographic changes in these articulations and those of the spine are difficult to interpret in young children and are frequently delayed until the latter part of the second decade of life. Acute iridocyclitis is not a common initial feature of the disease but subsequently becomes apparent in as many as 25% of patients.

Radiographic abnormalities in juvenile-onset ankylosing spondylitis are virtually indistinguishable from those of adult-onset disease. Sacroiliac joint alterations appear as the disease progresses. Articular space widening, indistinct joint margins, erosions, and sclerosis may be noted. Eventually, joint space diminution and osseous ankylosis become evident. Osteitis or sclerosis of vertebral corners, squaring of the anterior vertebral surface, syndesmophytosis, and apophyseal joint bony ankylosis may be seen.

### Psoriatic Arthritis

In a small subgroup of children with juvenile chronic arthritis, articular involvement antedates psoriatic skin disease and can be characterized by severe and progressive joint destruction. Radiographic abnormalities can simulate those in adults with psoriatic arthritis, including distal interphalangeal joint destruction, phalangeal tuft resorption, and sacroiliitis. Juvenile-onset psoriatic arthritis usually has an oligoarticular onset.

### Arthritis of Inflammatory Bowel Disease

In this type, spinal, sacroiliac, and peripheral articular findings accompany enteritis and colitis, although such findings may also develop in a child before the recognition of inflammatory bowel disease.

### Other Seronegative Spondyloarthropathies

Other seronegative spondyloarthropathies, including Reiter's syndrome and reactive arthritis, can affect children.

## RADIOGRAPHIC ABNORMALITIES

The radiographic abnormalities associated with juvenile chronic arthritis depend on the specific subgroup being investigated. In the following discussion, emphasis is placed on features that can be encountered in juvenile-onset adult-type (seropositive) rheumatoid arthritis and the polyarticular and pauciarticular types of seronegative chronic arthritis (Still's disease). The many similarities among these forms of arthritis facilitate their discussion as a group in the following analysis.

### General Features

The general radiographic characteristics of juvenile chronic arthritis in comparison to adult-onset disease are shown in Table 17–3 (Fig. 17–2).

**Soft Tissue Swelling.** Periarticular fusiform soft tissue swelling is a common early manifestation of arthritis. Large joint effusions are sometimes apparent. Eccentric soft tissue prominence can relate to tenosynovitis.

**Osteopenia.** Juxta-articular or diffuse osteoporosis may be encountered. In addition, bandlike metaphyseal lucent zones may be seen, particularly in the distal end of the femur, proximal portion of the tibia, and distal ends of the radius, tibia, and fibula. They are identical to those seen in childhood leukemia. Subsequent development of transverse radiodense "growth recovery" lines has been noted.

Osteoporosis in children with juvenile chronic arthritis may lead to fractures, including compression fractures of the epiphyses, diaphyseal and metaphyseal fractures of tubular bones, and compression fractures of vertebral bodies.

**Joint Space Abnormalities.** Diminution of the interosseous space in juvenile chronic arthritis is less frequent than in adult-onset rheumatoid arthritis. The combination of osteo-

**TABLE 17–3**

**Juvenile Chronic Arthritis versus Adult-Onset Rheumatoid Arthritis: General Radiographic Characteristics***

| Finding | Juvenile Chronic Arthritis | Adult-Onset Rheumatoid Arthritis |
|---|---|---|
| Soft tissue swelling | Common | Common |
| Osteoporosis | Common | Common |
| Joint space loss | Late manifestation | Early manifestation |
| Bony erosions | Late manifestation | Early manifestation |
| Intra-articular bony ankylosis | Common | Rare |
| Periostitis | Common | Rare |
| Growth disturbances | Common | Absent |
| Epiphyseal compression fractures | Common | Less common |
| Joint subluxation | Common | Common |
| Synovial cysts | Uncommon | Common |

*Characteristics depend on the specific subgroups of juvenile chronic arthritis.

porosis and soft tissue swelling without cartilaginous (or osseous) destruction is an important radiographic characteristic of this disease. Preservation of the joint space is especially characteristic of monoarticular disease. In later stages of juvenile chronic arthritis, intra-articular bony ankylosis is frequent, especially in the small joints of the hands and wrists.

**Bone Erosion.** Destruction of bone is also a relatively late manifestation of juvenile chronic arthritis. Osseous erosions may occur at the margins of the articulation (as in adult-onset rheumatoid arthritis) or along the entire articular surface of the bone.

**Periostitis.** Periosteal bone formation is a frequent and prominent manifestation of juvenile chronic arthritis. It is most common in the periarticular regions of the phalanges, metacarpals, and metatarsals. Periostitis can appear early in the course of the disease in combination with osteoporosis and soft tissue swelling, much like the appearance of osteomyelitis.

**Growth Disturbances.** Growth disturbances are a remarkable feature of juvenile chronic arthritis. Epiphyseal enlargement from accelerated growth stimulated by hyperemia is frequent about the small and large articulations. This overgrowth is accentuated by the adjacent constricted appearance of the metaphysis and diaphysis. Accelerated osseous growth and maturation lead to an increase in the number and size of the carpal and tarsal bones.

Disturbance of the normal growth of the diaphysis leads to a variety of bone abnormalities in juvenile chronic arthritis. Bone atrophy with osteoporosis and a reduction in diameter, overgrowth, or undergrowth may be seen. In the hands and feet, short, broad phalanges, metacarpals, and metatarsals simulate the changes in various bone dysplasias. In the lower extremities, leg length discrepancies are seen.

**Epiphyseal Compression Fractures.** Epiphyseal compression fractures are evident in the weight-bearing epiphyses of the lower extremities, as well as the epiphyses of the hands and feet. They are produced by abnormal stress

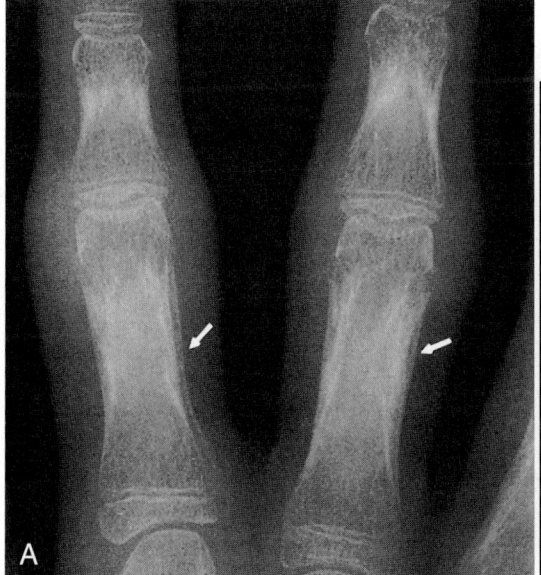
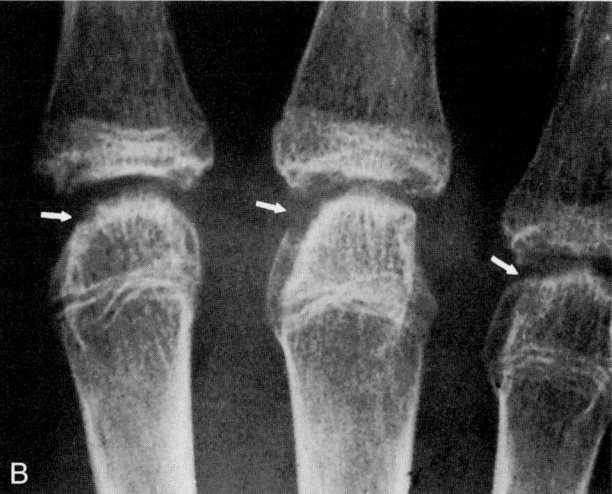

**Figure 17–2.** Juvenile chronic arthritis: general radiographic abnormalities. *A,* Periostitis. Prominent periosteal proliferation of numerous phalanges *(arrows)* is associated with osteoporosis and periarticular soft tissue swelling. Joint space diminution and erosions are not significant features in this child. *B,* Epiphyseal compression fractures. The irregular outline of the metacarpal heads *(arrows)* is produced by compression of weakened osteoporotic bones.

(resulting from muscle spasm and joint subluxation) acting on weakened osteoporotic bone. Flattening and deformity of the epiphyseal ossification centers and formation of dense intraosseous foci as a result of trabecular compression are evident.

**Joint Subluxation.** Subluxation and dislocation can be observed in any articulation but are most common in the hip. These complications result from large intra-articular effusions or, more importantly, from ligamentous destruction and muscle foreshortening secondary to fibrosis.

**Soft Tissue Calcification.** Periarticular soft tissue calcific deposits may be recorded in this disease. They appear to be located in the joint capsule, ligament, or muscle. The exact cause of periarticular calcification in juvenile chronic arthritis is not known, although an association with intra-articular corticosteroid therapy or other forms of intra-articular treatment has been reported.

## Abnormalities in Specific Locations

A comparison of the radiographic abnormalities of chronic juvenile arthritis and those of similar diseases is presented in Table 17–4.

**Hand.** Any articulation of the hand may be affected (Fig. 17–3). Asymmetrical abnormalities of both hands are most typical. Swelling and regional osteoporosis can develop about the distal interphalangeal, proximal interphalangeal, and metacarpophalangeal joints. Periostitis of the metacarpal and phalangeal shafts, preservation of the joint space, and absence of significant erosions are most common. Epiphyseal collapse and deformity are also characteristic. A variety of finger deformities may eventually appear, including boutonnière deformity (characterized by flexion at the proximal interphalangeal joint and hyperextension at the distal interphalangeal joint), flexion deformity (characterized by flexion at both the proximal interphalangeal and distal interphalangeal joints), and, less frequently, swan-neck deformity (characterized by hyperextension at the proximal interphalangeal joint and flexion at the distal interphalangeal joint).

**Wrist.** Abnormalities of the wrist are extremely common (Fig. 17–4). Soft tissue prominence, osteoporosis, and irregular carpal ossification centers are seen. Intra-articular osseous ankylosis of the compartments of the wrist may be prominent. Growth disturbances and articular destruction can lead to significant wrist deformities. The ulna may be relatively short in comparison to the radius and produce ulnar deviation at the wrist.

**Knee.** Radiographic abnormalities of the knee in juvenile chronic arthritis include osteoporosis, soft tissue swelling, enlargement with ballooning of the distal femoral and proximal tibial epiphyses, flattening of the femoral condyles, widening of the intercondylar notch, joint space narrowing, and marginal or central osseous erosions (Fig. 17–5). These findings are virtually identical to those in hemophilia. Alterations in patellar shape consist of flattening of the inferior pole of the patella, which results in squaring of the bone.

**Hip.** Involvement of the hip is common and is radiographically evident in approximately 35% to 45% of patients (Fig. 17–6). In younger patients, impairment of iliac bone development and coxa valga deformity are not uncommon. The femoral capital epiphysis may be enlarged and irregular in outline, and premature fusion of the growth plate may

---

**TABLE 17–4**

**Comparison of Radiographic Abnormalities**

| Finding | Juvenile Chronic Arthritis* | Adult-Onset Rheumatoid Arthritis | Juvenile-Onset Ankylosing Spondylitis | Adult-Onset Ankylosing Spondylitis |
|---|---|---|---|---|
| Cervical spine | | | | |
|   C1–C2 subluxation | + | ++ | + | + |
|   Apophyseal joint ankylosis | ++ | ± | ++ | ++ |
|   Hypoplasia of the vertebral bodies and intervertebral discs | ++ | – | ± | – |
| Thoracolumbar spine | | | | |
|   Apophyseal joint ankylosis | ± | – | ++ | ++ |
|   Syndesmophytes | – | – | ++ | ++ |
| Sacroiliac joints | | | | |
|   Erosions | + | + | ++ | ++ |
|   Ankylosis | ± | ± | ++ | ++ |
| Peripheral joints | | | | |
|   Early involvement | ++ | ++ | ++ | ± |
|   Erosions | ± | ++ | + | + |
|   Joint space narrowing | ± | ++ | + | + |
|   Bony proliferation and periostitis | ++ | ± | ++ | ++ |

*Characteristics of juvenile-onset adult-type rheumatoid arthritis and Still's disease.
++, very common; +, common; ±, uncommon; –, rare or absent.

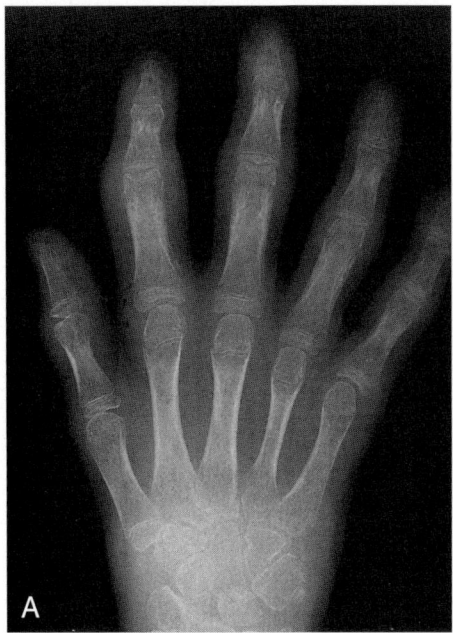 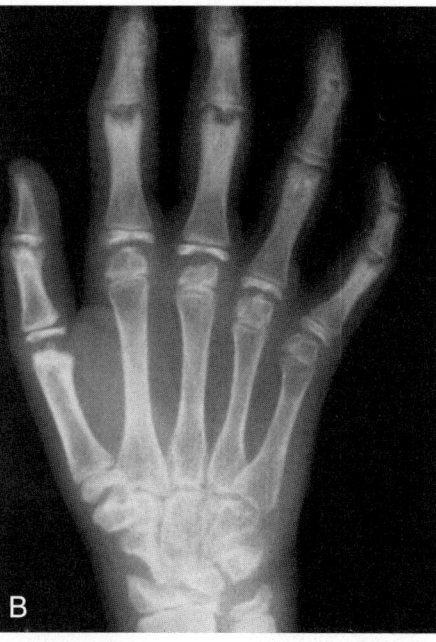

**Figure 17–3.** Abnormalities of the hand. *A*, Typical changes in this child with polyarticular Still's disease include periarticular soft tissue swelling and osteoporosis about the metacarpophalangeal and proximal interphalangeal joints and the wrist, mild joint space narrowing and erosive abnormalities, and periosteal bone formation in the phalanges. *B*, Note the extent of epiphyseal compression about the metacarpophalangeal and proximal interphalangeal joints, combined with osteoporosis, soft tissue swelling, and carpal involvement.

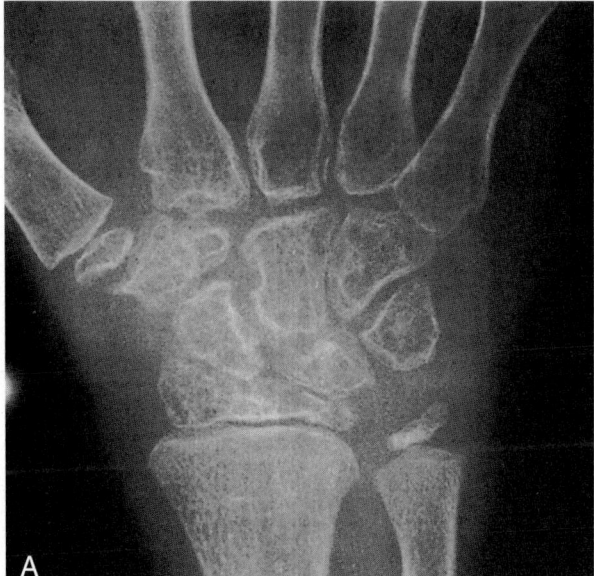 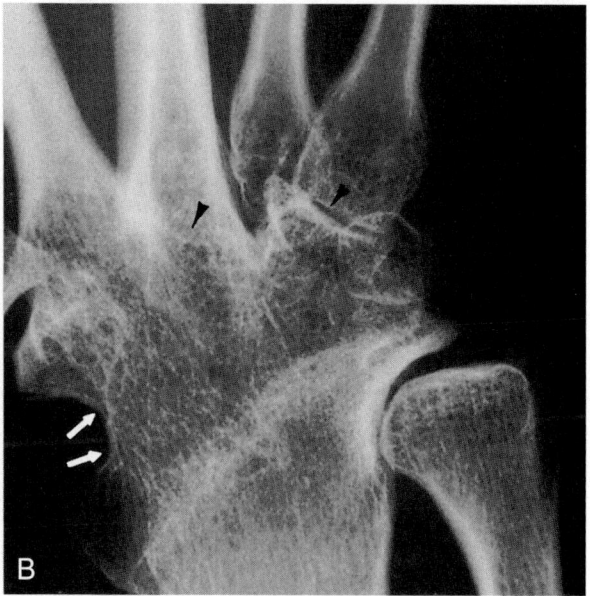

**Figure 17–4.** Abnormalities of the wrist. *A*, In this young child, erosions of multiple carpal bones have led to crenated osseous contours. Joint space narrowing and acceleration of bone maturation are seen. *B*, In this patient, bony ankylosis of the radiocarpal and midcarpal compartments is prominent *(arrows)*. Joint space narrowing and partial ankylosis at the common carpometacarpal joint are also apparent *(arrowheads)*.

be evident. Articular space narrowing and osseous erosion may also develop as a joint deteriorates, and osteophytosis may appear. Protrusio acetabuli is more frequent in older children.

**Foot and Ankle.** The radiographic abnormalities of the tarsus are similar to those in the carpus. Enlargement and irregularity of the tarsal bones, joint space narrowing, and intra-articular bony ankylosis can be seen. Metatar-

sophalangeal and interphalangeal joint alterations consist of osteoporosis, epiphyseal enlargement, brachydactyly, and periostitis (Fig. 17–7). Late deformities include clawing of the toes, hammer toes, hindfoot varus or valgus, pes cavus, and hallux valgus.

**Other Articulations of the Appendicular Skeleton.** Alterations of the humeral head parallel those of the femoral head, including osteoporosis, bone enlargement, joint

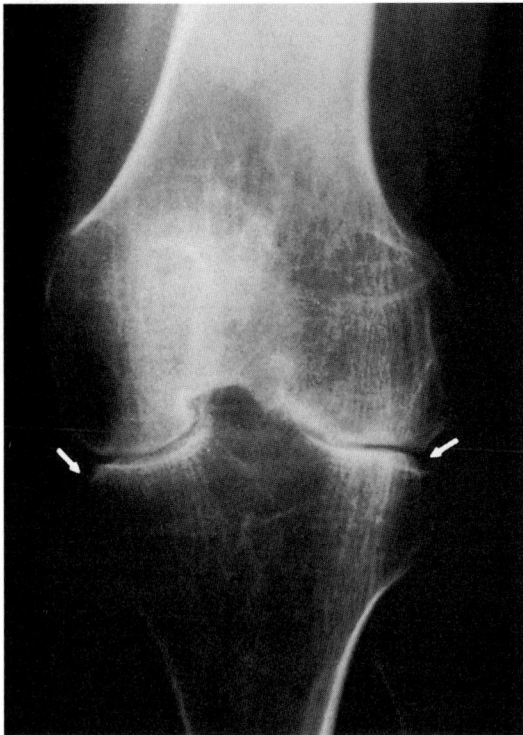

**Figure 17–5.** Abnormalities of the knee. The major radiographic abnormalities in this 23-year-old woman who has had arthritis for approximately 10 years consist of diffuse joint space narrowing and marginal erosions *(arrows)*. These simulate the findings in adult-onset rheumatoid arthritis, but slight overgrowth of the femoral epiphysis indicates that the disease began at a relatively young age.

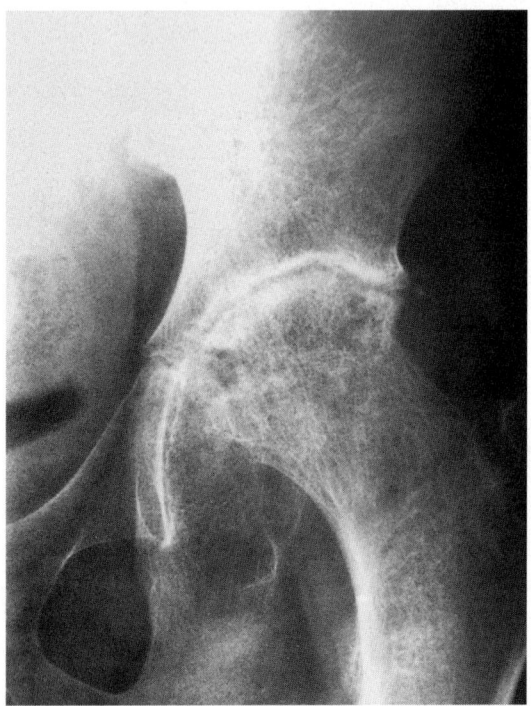

**Figure 17–6.** Abnormalities of the hip. In a child with juvenile-onset adult-type (seropositive) rheumatoid arthritis, note diffuse joint space narrowing, significant erosions of the femoral head and acetabulum, and osteoporosis.

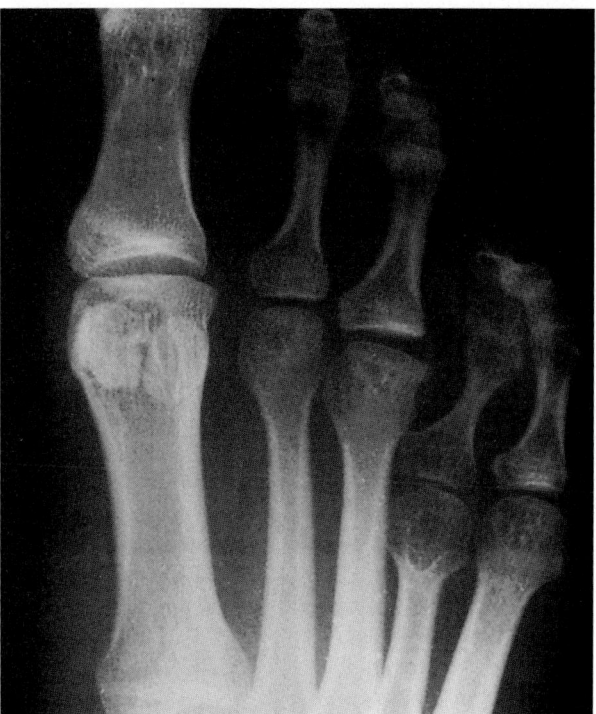

**Figure 17–7.** Abnormalities of the foot. Prominent growth disturbances such as these may accompany Still's disease. Shortening of the metatarsal bones and deformity of some of the metatarsophalangeal joints are the most prominent findings.

space narrowing, erosions, and subluxation. In the elbow, the radial head may become significantly enlarged, a finding that is also seen in hemophilia.

**Sacroiliac Joint.** Although children with juvenile-onset ankylosing spondylitis, psoriatic arthritis, and inflammatory bowel disease can have significant sacroiliac joint abnormalities (see Table 17–4), changes in this articulation in other varieties of juvenile chronic arthritis are relatively infrequent. Further, documenting the presence of an abnormal sacroiliac joint can be difficult because of the widened articular space and indistinct subchondral bone that characterize the normal sacroiliac joint in the pediatric age group.

**Cervical Spine.** Radiographic abnormalities of the cervical spine are a significant feature of juvenile chronic arthritis (see Table 17–4; Fig. 17–8). Subluxation may develop in any vertebral segment but is most characteristic at the atlantoaxial level. Atlantoaxial instability in a child is not diagnostic of juvenile chronic arthritis; it is also observed in trauma and in a variety of other conditions, including those causing hypoplasia of the odontoid process and congenital weakening of the surrounding ligaments, such as Down's syndrome, and those associated with inflammation in the neck.

Erosions of the anterior, posterior, and superior surfaces of the odontoid process may also be seen. Apophyseal joint space narrowing and bony ankylosis in association with subchondral erosions predominate in the upper cervical

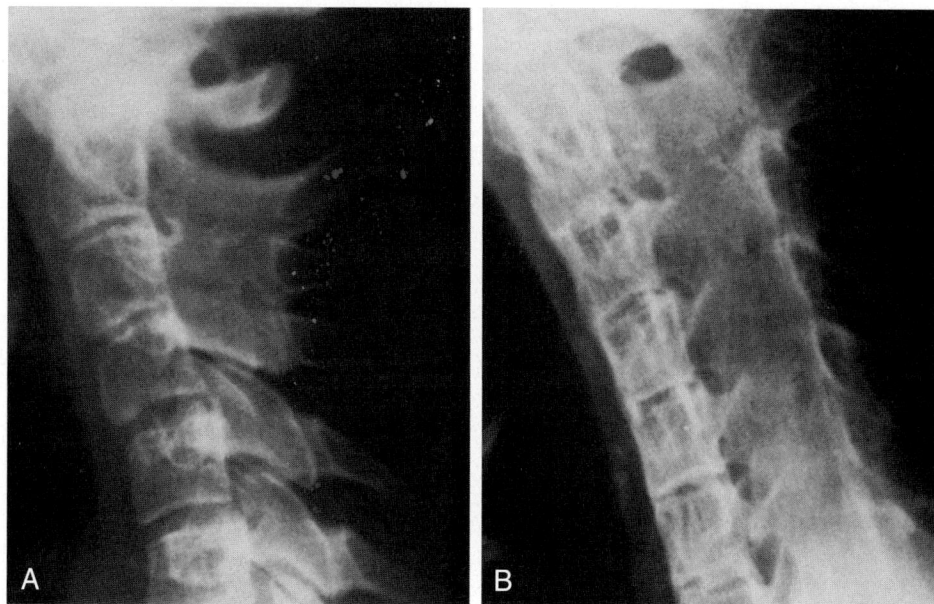

**Figure 17–8.** Abnormalities of the cervical spine: apophyseal joint bony ankylosis. *A* and *B*, In two children with Still's disease, apophyseal joint ankylosis is evident. The process is usually first apparent in the upper cervical region and progresses to the lower vertebrae. Hypoplasia of the vertebral bodies and intervertebral discs is prominent in both cases. Atlantoaxial subluxation is also evident in *(A)*.

spine. Growth disturbances consist of decreased vertical and anteroposterior diameters of the vertebral bodies at the levels of apophyseal joint ankylosis. The adjacent intervertebral discs are also diminished in height (or completely obliterated) and may contain calcification.

The resulting radiographic appearance in juvenile chronic arthritis is distinctive, with dwarflike alterations of both the vertebral bodies and the intervertebral discs and apophyseal joint ankylosis. Although apophyseal joint ankylosis can be seen in ankylosing spondylitis, the vertebral bodies are not significantly diminished in size in that disease, nor are the intervertebral discs diminutive, because disease onset generally occurs at a more advanced age. Further, in ankylosing spondylitis, syndesmophytes are characteristic. Congenital fusion of vertebral bodies (Klippel-Feil deformity) may simulate the changes in juvenile chronic arthritis, although in the former disorder, the spinous processes of several vertebrae may also be incorporated into a single ossific mass. Fibrodysplasia ossificans progressiva can be accompanied by vertebral alterations, but additional abnormalities, such as soft tissue ossification, ensure an accurate diagnosis of that condition.

**Thoracic and Lumbar Spine.** The thoracolumbar spine is not commonly affected (see Table 17–4). Compression fractures of vertebral bodies may be observed, particularly in patients who have received steroid medication. Scoliosis, which may appear rapidly, has also been noted.

**Mandible, Temporomandibular Joint, and Other Facial Structures.** Underdevelopment of the jaw (micrognathia) is not uncommon, occurring in approximately 10% to 20% of patients, and frequently occurs in association with temporomandibular joint abnormalities. Radiographic abnormalities include shortening of the body and vertical rami of the mandible, with widening of the mandibular notches. Both mandibular condyles are frequently flattened and poorly differentiated, although the temporomandibular joints themselves may appear normal. Articular space narrowing, bone erosion, and abnormal joint motion may be encountered in some persons.

Antegonial notching of the mandible has been emphasized as an additional radiographic manifestation of juvenile chronic arthritis. This notching represents a concavity on the undersurface of the mandibular body just anterior to the angular process (gonion) (Fig. 17–9).

## OTHER DIAGNOSTIC TECHNIQUES

### Scintigraphy

The major application of bone scintigraphy in persons with juvenile chronic arthritis relates to the determination of disease distribution. This method allows simultaneous assessment of all major articulations of the body, and monoarticular, oligoarticular, or polyarticular patterns of disease can be identified.

### Computed Tomography

Computed tomography scanning is best applied in regions with complex anatomy, such as the hip, shoulder, spine, and temporomandibular joint. The value of computed tomography in the evaluation of children with juvenile chronic arthritis is limited.

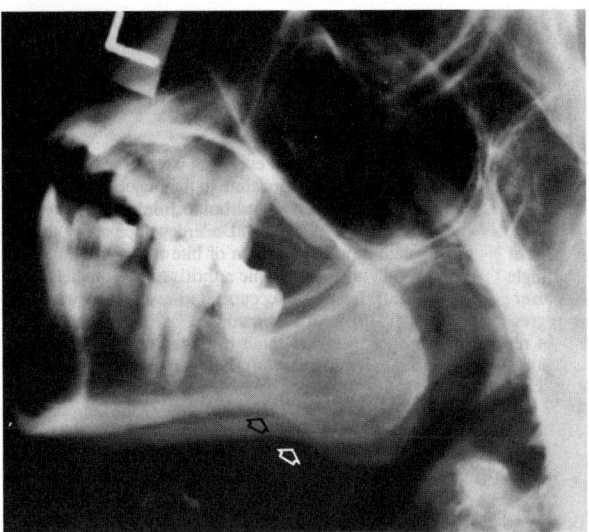

**Figure 17–9.** Abnormalities of the mandible. In this child with juvenile chronic arthritis, note the short antegonial notches *(arrows)*. Additional findings are articular changes in the temporomandibular joints (not well shown here).

## Ultrasonography

Ultrasonography has been used to detect joint effusions in children with juvenile chronic arthritis. This modality is particularly helpful in the assessment of periarticular swelling in this disease, which may relate to bursitis, tenosynovitis, or synovial cysts.

## Magnetic Resonance Imaging

Magnetic resonance (MR) imaging is an effective method for evaluating pediatric joint disease, primarily because of its ability to allow direct visualization of nonossified portions of epiphyseal cartilage. In children with juvenile chronic arthritis, it can detect alterations in the articular cartilage, although many of the standard imaging sequences used in the analysis of chondral defects may be deficient in this regard (Fig. 17–10). Differentiation of joint fluid and synovial inflammatory tissue in juvenile chronic arthritis remains a difficult task when standard spin echo imaging sequences are used, although the addition of intravenously administered gadolinium compounds improves such differentiation.

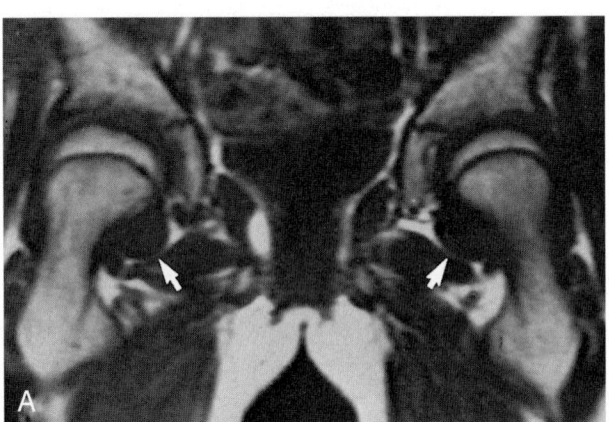

**Figure 17–10.** Juvenile chronic arthritis: MR imaging. *A*, Hip involvement in a 10-year-old girl. Coronal T1-weighted (TR/TE, 400/20) spin echo MR image reveals mild flattening of both femoral heads and acetabula and bilateral joint effusions *(arrows)*. *B* and *C*, Knee involvement in a 12-year-old girl. T1-weighted (TR/TE, 920/17) spin echo MR image *(B)* shows a large joint effusion and marrow edema in the femoral and tibial epiphyses. The articular cartilage is not well seen because its signal intensity is only slightly higher than that of the fluid. A posterior lymph node is observed, but it is more evident in *(C)*, a sagittal fat-suppressed fast spin echo (TR/TE, 4226/99) MR image in which both the fluid and the edema are of high signal intensity. The lateral meniscus appears slightly hypoplastic. (*B* and *C*, Courtesy of J. Kramer, MD, Vienna, Austria.)

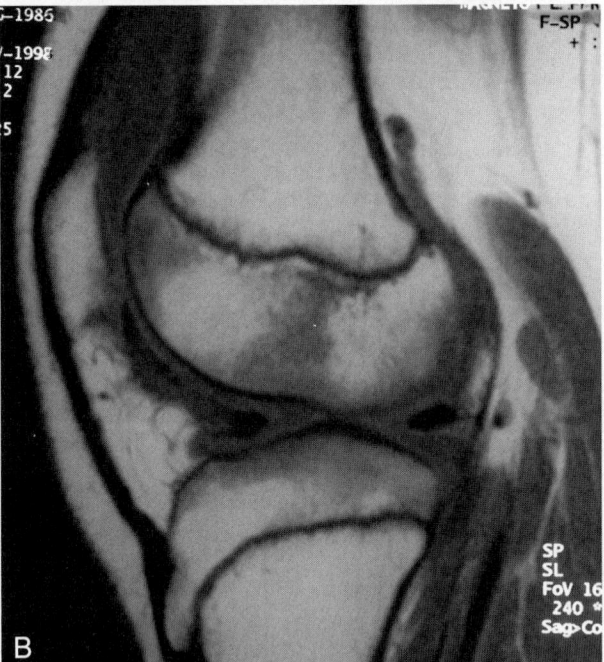

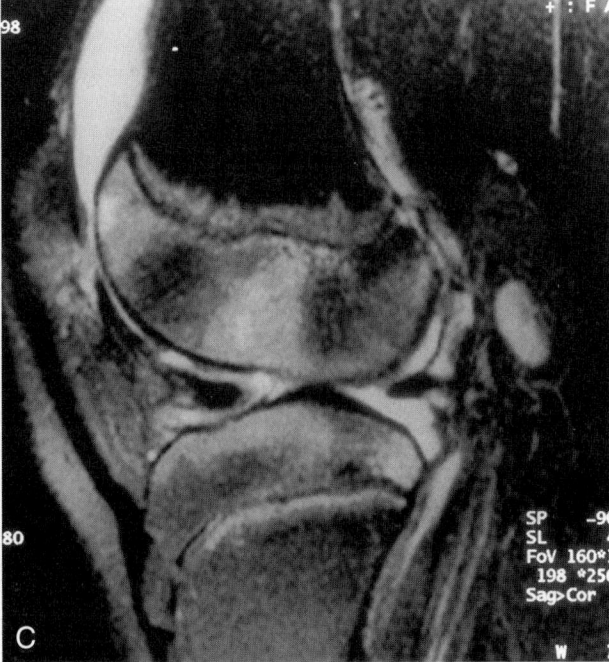

Additional applications of MR imaging in children with juvenile chronic arthritis include analysis of the temporomandibular and sacroiliac joints and assessment of such complications as ischemic necrosis of bone and growth disturbances. The technique is also useful in the evaluation of the spine.

## PATHOLOGIC ABNORMALITIES

Synovial inflammation in juvenile chronic arthritis resembles that in adult-onset rheumatoid arthritis. Macroscopically evident villous hypertrophy of the synovial membrane may be associated with varying degrees of fibrin accumulation in the lining and subintimal layers, cellular hyperplasia, and an inflammatory cellular response. Subcutaneous nodules are identified in 10% to 20% of patients with juvenile chronic arthritis.

## SPECIAL TYPE OF JUVENILE CHRONIC ARTHRITIS: ADULT-ONSET STILL'S DISEASE

Some adults may develop a disorder that is indistinguishable from Still's disease, designated adult-onset Still's disease. Pauciarticular abnormalities predominate, with a predilection for the knees, fingers, and wrists. Radiographic alterations develop in only a few patients. A distinctive radiographic pattern of articular disease of the wrist has been noted: narrowing of portions of the common carpometacarpal and midcarpal compartments without osseous erosions, which may culminate in bony ankylosis (Fig. 17–11). Similar patterns of ankylosis of the carpal (and tarsal) bones can be observed in children with juvenile chronic arthritis.

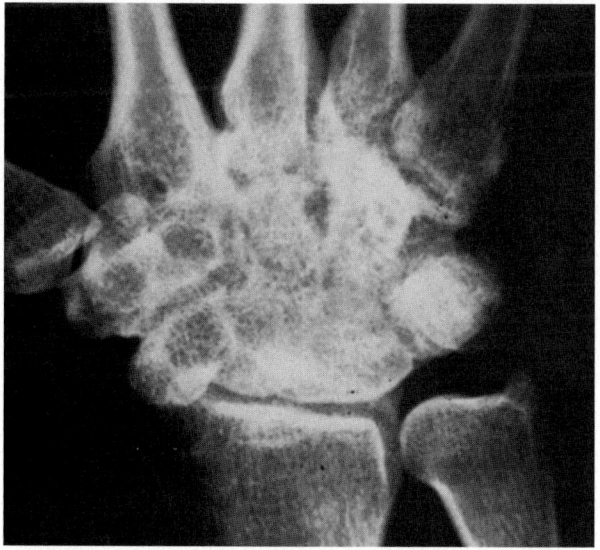

**Figure 17–11.** Adult-onset Still's disease: wrist involvement. This 44-year-old woman has had Still's disease since age 25 years. A frontal radiograph shows bony ankylosis of the midcarpal, common carpometacarpal, and intermetacarpal compartments of the wrist. The radiocarpal compartment is moderately narrowed. (Courtesy of J. Esdaile, MD, Montreal, Quebec, Canada.)

## DIFFERENTIAL DIAGNOSIS

### Hemophilia

Differentiating juvenile chronic arthritis and hemophilia can be difficult. Soft tissue swelling, osteoporosis, subchondral osseous irregularity, interosseous space diminution, and growth disturbances may be evident in both disorders. In the knee, ankle, and elbow, the resulting radiographic picture may be identical in the two conditions. Polyarticular disease and significant involvement of the small joints of the hand and wrist are less frequent in hemophilia than in juvenile chronic arthritis, whereas radiodense joint effusions and multiple subchondral cystic lesions are somewhat more common in hemophilic arthropathy. Squaring or flattening of the inferior pole of the patella may be more characteristic of juvenile chronic arthritis.

### Idiopathic Multicentric Osteolysis

Idiopathic multicentric osteolysis is a disorder characterized by multifocal articular destruction beginning in infancy or childhood (see Chapter 83). Although the clinical and radiographic features of idiopathic multicentric osteolysis are somewhat variable, pain and swelling of the hands, wrists, feet, ankles, and elbows are typical. Because of a remarkable predilection for the carpal and tarsal bones, the disorder is also referred to as carpal and tarsal osteolysis or disappearing carpal bones. Radiographic characteristics include osteoporosis, progressive osteolysis, and deformity, findings that may simulate the changes in juvenile chronic arthritis.

### Mucopolysaccharidoses and Related Disorders

Articular abnormalities accompanying mucopolysaccharidoses may simulate those in juvenile chronic arthritis, although characteristic findings are noted on skeletal surveys in patients with mucopolysaccharidoses (see Chapter 75). In many of these syndromes, periarticular involvement is apparent and leads to alterations in ligamentous and tendinous structures.

### Familial Arthropathy and Congenital Camptodactyly

Several inherited disorders can lead to flexion deformities of the fingers and arthropathy, but the patterns of inheritance are not uniform or clear. The radiographic abnormalities, consisting mainly of osteoporosis and deformity (flattening of the metacarpal and metatarsal heads, coxa vara, and contractures of the fingers, wrists, and elbows), are easily distinguishable from those of juvenile chronic arthritis.

### Other Disorders

Multiple epiphyseal dysplasia (and spondyloepiphyseal dysplasia) can lead to irregularity of many epiphyses and secondary degenerative joint abnormalities that could be confused with the changes of juvenile chronic arthritis (see Chapter 74). Progressive pseudorheumatoid arthritis of childhood (i.e., progressive pseudorheumatoid chondrodysplasia) is a term applied to a hereditary arthropathy affecting the major and minor joints; findings include restricted articular motion, swelling about the interphalangeal articulations, platyspondyly, and irregularities of vertebral bodies. Infection or synovial hemangiomas can produce abnormalities of single articulations, which also simulate the findings of juvenile chronic arthritis. Similarly, neuromuscular disorders may lead to skeletal abnormalities of certain articulations that are indistinguishable from those of juvenile chronic arthritis. Other entities to be considered in the differential diagnosis of juvenile chronic arthritis include multicentric reticulohistiocytosis (see Chapter 50).

## FURTHER READING

Ansell BM: Chronic arthritis in childhood. Ann Rheum Dis 37:107, 1978.

Ansell BM, Kent PA: Radiological changes in juvenile chronic polyarthritis. Skeletal Radiol 1:129, 1977.

Brill PW, Kim HJ, Beratis NG, et al: Skeletal abnormalities in the Kniest syndrome with mucopolysacchariduria. AJR Am J Roentgenol 125:731, 1975.

Bywaters EGL: Still's disease in the adult. Ann Rheum Dis 30:121, 1971.

Cassidy JT, Levinson JE, Bass JC, et al: A study of classification criteria for a diagnosis of juvenile rheumatoid arthritis. Arthritis Rheum 29:274, 1986.

Chlosta EM, Kuhns LR, Holt JF: The "patellar ratio" in hemophilia and juvenile rheumatoid arthritis. Radiology 116: 137, 1975.

Cohen PA, Job-Deslandre CH, Lalande G, et al: Overview of the radiology of juvenile idiopathic arthritis (JIA). Eur J Radiol 33:94, 2000.

Hervé-Somma CMP, Sebag GH, Prieur A-M, et al: Juvenile rheumatoid arthritis of the knee: MR evaluation with Gd-DOTA. Radiology 182:93, 1992.

Martel W, Holt JF, Cassidy JT: Roentgenologic manifestations of juvenile rheumatoid arthritis. AJR Am J Roentgenol 88:400, 1962.

Martinez-Lavin M, Buendia A, Delgado E, et al: A familial syndrome of pericarditis, arthritis, and camptodactyly. N Engl J Med 309:224, 1983.

Medsger TA Jr, Christy WC: Carpal arthritis with ankylosis in late onset Still's disease. Arthritis Rheum 19:232, 1976.

Parke WW, Rothman RH, Brown MD: The pharyngovertebral veins: An anatomical rationale for Grisel's syndrome. J Bone Joint Surg Am 66:568, 1984.

Poznanski AK, Hernandez RJ, Guire KE, et al: Carpal length in children—a useful measurement in the diagnosis of rheumatoid arthritis and some congenital malformation syndromes. Radiology 129:661, 1978.

Richardson ML, Helms CA, Vogler JB III, et al: Skeletal changes in neuromuscular disorders mimicking juvenile rheumatoid arthritis and hemophilia. AJR Am J Roentgenol 143:893, 1984.

Schaller J, Wedgwood RJ: Juvenile rheumatoid arthritis: A review. Pediatrics 50:940, 1972.

Schnedl WJ, Lipp RW, Trinker M, et al: Bone scintigraphy and magnetic resonance imaging in adult-onset Still's disease. Scand J Rheumatol 28:257, 1999.

Senac MO Jr, Deutsch D, Bernstein BH, et al: MR imaging in juvenile rheumatoid arthritis. AJR Am J Roentgenol 150:873, 1988.

Spranger J, Albert C, Schilling F, et al: Progressive pseudorheumatoid arthropathy of childhood (PPAC): A hereditary disorder simulating juvenile rheumatoid arthritis. Am J Med Genet 14:399, 1983.

Stabrun AE, Larheim TA, Höyeraal HM, et al: Reduced mandibular dimensions and asymmetry in juvenile rheumatoid arthritis: Pathogenetic factors. Arthritis Rheum 31:602, 1988.

Still GF: On a form of chronic joint disease in children. Med Chir Trans 80:47, 1897.

Tyler T, Rosenbaum HD: Idiopathic multicentric osteolysis. AJR Am J Roentgenol 126:23, 1976.

Winchester P, Grossman H, Lim WN, et al: A new acid mucopolysaccharidosis with skeletal deformities simulating rheumatoid arthritis. AJR Am J Roentgenol 106:121, 1969.

# CHAPTER 18

## Ankylosing Spondylitis

### SUMMARY OF KEY FEATURES

Ankylosing spondylitis is a disease with widespread musculoskeletal manifestations. Abnormalities are detected at the synovial and cartilaginous joints and at sites of tendinous and ligamentous attachment to bone in spinal and extraspinal locations. The hallmark of the disorder is sacroiliitis, which is typically bilateral and symmetrical in distribution. Spondylitis leads to significant abnormalities at the discovertebral junction, apophyseal and costovertebral joints, and posterior ligamentous attachments. Accurate differentiation of ankylosing spondylitis from rheumatoid arthritis is not difficult, but distinguishing the articular abnormalities of ankylosing spondylitis from those of psoriatic arthritis and Reiter's syndrome is more troublesome.

### INTRODUCTION

Ankylosing spondylitis is a chronic inflammatory disorder of unknown cause that principally affects the axial skeleton, although the appendicular skeleton may also be significantly involved. Alterations occur in synovial and cartilaginous joints and in sites of tendon and ligament attachment to bone. Although ankylosing spondylitis is now the accepted name for this disease, many synonyms and eponyms have been used in the past, including Marie-Strümpell disease, von Bechterew's syndrome, and rheumatoid spondylitis.

It is difficult to determine the true prevalence; however, ankylosing spondylitis is a common cause of back pain and disability, especially in young men. The prevalence of this disease in the general population is more difficult to determine, although a figure of approximately 0.1% is commonly quoted. The precise ratio of the disease in men versus women is not known, with reports varying from 4:1 to 10:1. The true prevalence of ankylosing spondylitis in women may be much higher than these reports indicate, as the disease may be more subtle and difficult to diagnose in female patients.

### CLINICAL ABNORMALITIES
#### General Features

The onset of ankylosing spondylitis generally occurs between the ages of 15 and 35 years (average age of onset, 26 to 27 years) in both men and women, although an earlier onset has been noted in some female patients. An insidious onset of disease, which occurs in 75% to 80% of patients, can lead to considerable delay in accurate diagnosis. Early clinical manifestations are generally noted in the back (70% to 80% of patients), although they may appear in the peripheral joints (10% to 20% of patients) or in the chest. Sciatic pain may be the initial symptom in 5% to 10% of patients. Constitutional findings include anorexia, weight loss, and low-grade fever. The consensus is that in less than 20% of patients with adult-onset ankylosing spondylitis does the disease progress to a condition of significant disability.

### Axial Skeletal Symptoms and Signs

Clinical manifestations related to the spine and sacroiliac joints are characteristic of ankylosing spondylitis. Initially, transient aching pain and stiffness of variable intensity are observed in the low back region, but these symptoms may subsequently become persistent. With evolution of the disease, spread to higher levels of the vertebral column is frequent.

Local pain and tenderness over the sacroiliac joints can be prominent in the early phases of the disease. With ankylosis of these joints, the clinical manifestations may become milder or disappear completely. Pain radiating into the lower extremities, not unlike sciatica, can be observed in approximately 50% of patients at some stage of the disorder. In the lumbar spine, paravertebral muscle spasm, straightening of the vertebral column, tenderness to percussion, and muscle atrophy are observed; in the thoracic spine, similar abnormalities may be accompanied by diminished chest expansion and exaggeration of the normal kyphotic curvature. Slight, moderate, or marked limitation of movement may be evident in the cervical spine. The head and neck protrude forward, and the patient may eventually be forced to constantly gaze at the floor.

The cauda equina syndrome can be observed in patients with ankylosing spondylitis. Although its pathogenesis in this disease is not clear, the occurrence of loss of cutaneous sensation in the sacral and lower lumbar dermatomes, muscle weakness, and disturbed sphincter function may be related to arachnoiditis with subsequent loss of meningeal elasticity.

### Peripheral Skeletal Symptoms and Signs

Peripheral articular manifestations are initially apparent in approximately 10% to 20% of patients and eventually occur in as many as 50%. In most persons, the manifestations are mild and transient, and asymmetrical involvement of a few joints is typical. Asymmetry is more frequent, and residual destruction and deformity are less frequent, in ankylosing spondylitis than in rheumatoid arthritis. Involvement of the proximal or "root" joints (hips and shoulders) is particularly characteristic and may lead to severe clinical disability. Typical findings include regional pain, limitation of motion, muscle atrophy, and flexion contractures.

### Extraskeletal Symptoms and Signs

Iritis occurs in 20% of patients with ankylosing spondylitis and may be the initial feature of the disease. Spondylitic heart disease can lead to cardiac enlargement, conduction defects, and pericarditis, particularly in patients with chronic disease. Typically, aortic insufficiency caused by inflammation of the aortic valve and aorta resembles the finding in syphilitic aortitis. Pulmonary involvement in ankylosing spondylitis can manifest as a peculiar fibrosis and cavitation in the upper lobes that simulate the findings in tuberculosis. Additional systemic manifestations of ankylosing spondylitis include associations with inflammatory bowel disease (see Chapter 21) and amyloidosis.

## Laboratory Findings

Many patients with ankylosing spondylitis possess the histocompatibility antigen HLA-B27. The erythrocyte sedimentation rate is frequently elevated during the active phase and may become normal in later phases.

## RADIOGRAPHIC-PATHOLOGIC CORRELATION

### General Distribution

Ankylosing spondylitis affects synovial and cartilaginous joints, as well as sites of tendon and ligament attachment to bone (entheses). An overwhelming predilection exists for involvement of the axial skeleton, especially the sacroiliac, apophyseal, discovertebral, and costovertebral articulations (Fig. 18–1).

Classically, changes are noted initially in the sacroiliac joints and next appear at the thoracolumbar and lumbosacral junctions; with disease chronicity, the midlumbar, upper thoracic, and cervical vertebrae may become involved. Radiographic abnormalities of the sacroiliac joint without vertebral changes are unusual. The combination of sacroiliac joint and cervical spine abnormalities without significant thoracic or lumbar spine changes appears to be more common in female patients than in male patients. Spinal alterations without sacroiliac joint changes are unusual in classic ankylosing spondylitis in either men or women.

The frequency of radiographically evident abnormalities in peripheral locations in cases of long-standing ankylosing spondylitis is greater than 50% if all articulations are included. Radiographic changes predominate in the hips and glenohumeral joints, followed in descending order of frequency by the knees, hands, wrists, and feet, including the calcaneus. Bilateral abnormalities are common, although the degree of symmetry is less striking than in cases of rheumatoid arthritis.

Radiographic abnormalities can be encountered in the symphysis pubis and in the manubriosternal, acromioclavicular, sternoclavicular and temporomandibular joints. Changes are also evident at tendinous and ligamentous attachments to bone.

### General Radiographic and Pathologic Abnormalities

**Synovial Articulations.** In general, the inflammatory process in ankylosing spondylitis is similar to that in rheumatoid arthritis; however, it is more discrete and of lower intensity. Marked fibroplasia may be followed by cartilaginous

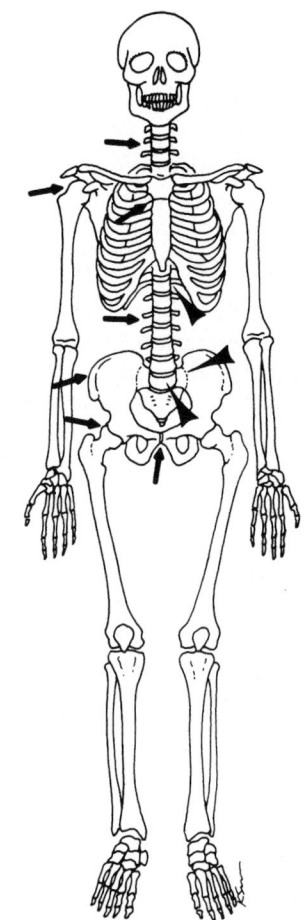

**Figure 18–1.** Ankylosing spondylitis: distribution of articular disease. Initial abnormalities are most frequent in the sacroiliac joint and the thoracolumbar and lumbosacral junctions (*arrowheads*). Subsequent abnormalities are common in the entire vertebral column, tendinous insertions in the pelvis and proximal end of the femur, sternal joints, symphysis pubis, hips, and glenohumeral joints (*arrows*).

metaplasia with chondral ossification. Intra-articular bony ankylosis may be evident. This ankylotic process in the small articulations of the axial skeleton can also result from ossification of the joint capsule.

The basic similarity of the pathologic alterations in synovial joints in ankylosing spondylitis and rheumatoid arthritis accounts for the overlap in their radiographic features. Both cause some degree of osteoporosis, joint space narrowing, and osseous erosion. Certain findings are more characteristic of ankylosing spondylitis than of rheumatoid arthritis, however. Prominent periarticular osteoporosis is not common in ankylosing spondylitis. In fact, subchondral eburnation is typical. Periostitis is also observed and results in irregular or shaggy periarticular osseous surfaces. Extensive and diffuse joint space diminution is more frequent in rheumatoid arthritis than in ankylosing spondylitis. In ankylosing spondylitis, intra-articular bony ankylosis is common in the synovial joints of both the axial skeleton (sacroiliac, costovertebral, and apophyseal joints) and the extra-axial skeleton (hip, wrist, and articulations of the midfoot). In adult-onset rheumatoid arthritis, fibrous ankylosis is more characteristic, except in the carpal and tarsal areas.

**Cartilaginous Articulations.** In the cartilaginous joints of the axial skeleton (discovertebral junction, symphysis pubis, and manubriosternal articulation), the fundamental process appears to be inflammatory in nature. At the junction of the intervertebral disc and the vertebral edge, chondrocytes undergo calcification and become vascularized and subsequently ossified, with production of syndesmophytes that extend from one vertebral body to another (Fig. 18–2). Eventually, extensive bony ankylosis of the entire articulation may be evident. These alterations in cartilaginous joints are typical of the seronegative spondyloarthropathies and are not characteristic of the skeletal involvement in rheumatoid arthritis.

**Entheses.** Abnormalities in ligamentous attachments (enthesopathy) are a prominent feature of ankylosing spondylitis and the other seronegative spondyloarthropathies. Inflammation with cellular infiltration is associated with erosion and eburnation of the subligamentous bone. On radiographs, poorly defined erosive abnormalities with surrounding sclerosis are observed. As the lesions heal, the sclerosis decreases, the osseous surface becomes less irregular, and well-defined bony excrescences appear (Fig. 18–3).

## Radiographic and Pathologic Abnormalities at Specific Sites

### Sacroiliac Joint

Sacroiliitis is the hallmark of ankylosing spondylitis. It occurs early in the course of the disease. Although an asymmetrical or unilateral distribution may be evident on the initial radiographic examination, radiographic changes at later stages of the disease are almost invariably bilateral and symmetrical (Fig. 18–4).

Changes in the sacroiliac joint occur in both the synovial and ligamentous (superior and posterior) portions. They predominate in the ilium. Preferential involvement of the ilium likely results from mechanical or anatomic features. These include thinner iliac cartilage (compared with the sacrum) and the presence of degenerative clefts through which inflammatory synovial tissue may gain access to the subchondral bone of the ilium. Initial changes consist of patchy periarticular osteoporosis, loss of definition, superficial erosion, and focal sclerosis of subchondral bone. A poorly defined subchondral bone plate is an important radiographic sign of sacroiliitis that is not observed in degenerative sacroiliac joint disease. Further erosive changes lead to considerable fraying of the osseous surface and widening of the interosseous space. As proliferative bony changes in the sacroiliac joint become more prominent, irregular bony bridges traverse the articular cavity. This process of osseous fusion is initially incomplete.

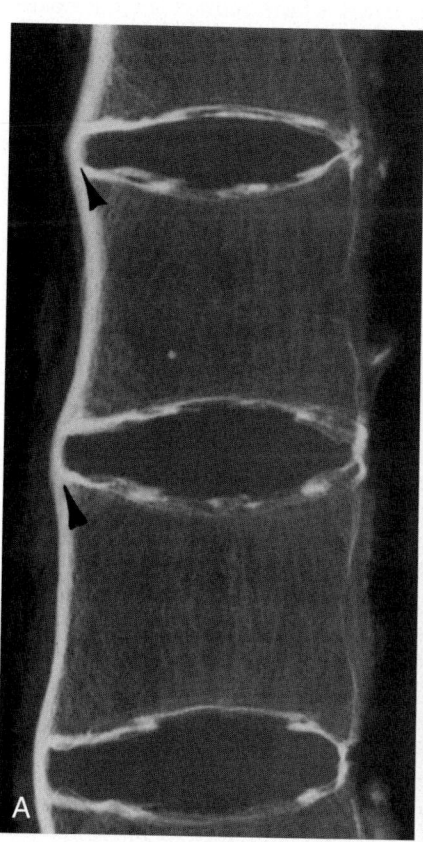
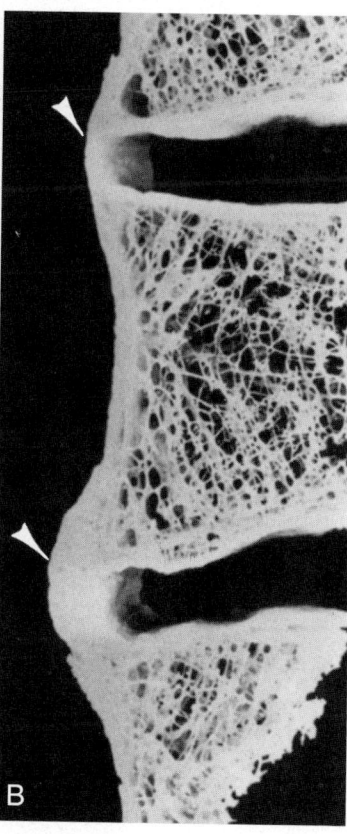

**Figure 18–2.** Cartilaginous articulations: general radiographic and pathologic abnormalities of the discovertebral junction. Radiograph *(A)* and photograph *(B)* of a sagittal section of the spine (the left side of each picture is anterior) reveal typical syndesmophytes *(arrowheads)* extending from one vertebral body to another. Note their vertical direction and slender configuration.

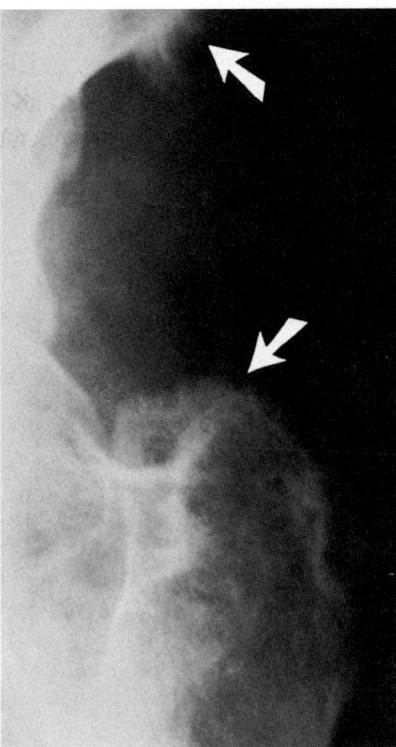

**Figure 18–3.** Entheses: general radiographic abnormalities of the femoral trochanter. Radiographic findings include irregular hyperostosis of the trochanter and iliac crest *(arrows)*.

Later, complete ankylosis can be observed, and the entire joint cavity is obliterated. Periarticular eburnation can subsequently become diminished, and the radiodensity of the bone may return to normal.

## Spine

Abnormalities of the spine (Table 18–1) can be seen in the discovertebral junction, apophyseal joint, costovertebral joints, posterior ligamentous attachments, and atlantoaxial joints. Although initially apparent at the thoracolumbar and lumbosacral junctions, changes can eventually be noted throughout the vertebral column.

### Discovertebral Junction

Lesions affecting the discovertebral junction include osteitis, syndesmophytosis, erosions, discal calcification, and osteoporosis and discal ballooning.

**Osteitis.** Focal destructive areas along the anterior margin of the discovertebral junction at the superior and inferior portions of the vertebral body are an early and significant feature of ankylosing spondylitis and have been termed Romanus lesions. Osseous erosion (osteitis) of the corners of the vertebral body (Fig. 18–5), when combined with bone formation, results in loss of the normal concavity of the anterior vertebral surface and thus creation of a squared

contour. This change in vertebral configuration is much easier to assess in the lumbar spine. As the erosions heal, reactive sclerosis produces "whitening" or a "shiny corner" configuration.

**Syndesmophytosis.** Erosive vertebral abnormalities are associated with bone formation that extends across the margin of the intervertebral disc (Fig. 18–6). Thin vertical outgrowths are termed syndesmophytes and represent ossification of the anulus fibrosus itself. As the syndesmophytes enlarge, ossification can involve the adjacent anterior longitudinal ligament and paravertebral connective tissue. Syndesmophytes predominate on the anterior and lateral aspects of the spine. The vertical nature of the outgrowths and their connection to the vertebral edges allow their differentiation from spinal osteophytes (which are triangular in shape and arise several millimeters from the discovertebral junction) and from the paravertebral ossification of psoriatic arthritis and Reiter's syndrome (which begins at a distance from the vertebral body and intervertebral disc). In the later phases of ankylosing spondylitis, extensive syndesmophytes produce the undulating vertebral contour that is called bamboo spine.

**Discovertebral Erosions and Destruction.** Destructive foci that appear throughout the discovertebral junction in ankylosing spondylitis can be localized to one or two areas or can involve the entire junction (Fig. 18–7). Lesions localized to the central subchondral portions of the discovertebral junction can be observed in ankylosed and nonankylosed spines. Histologic evaluation confirms the presence of intraosseous discal displacement (Schmorl's or cartilaginous nodes) in many cases. Radiographic examination outlines irregularity of the central portion of the superior and inferior vertebral margins, and radiolucent areas with surrounding sclerosis are present in the vertebral bodies. The appearance is similar or identical to that associated with cartilaginous nodes from any cause. Localized peripheral discovertebral lesions can also be caused by discal displacement, although other mechanisms may be important in the production of these peripheral discovertebral lesions in ankylosing spondylitis. Inflammation in the outer fibers of the anulus fibrosus related to the spondylitic process may play a role in the development of these lesions (Fig. 18–8).

Destruction of the entire discovertebral junction of two neighboring vertebral bodies occurs almost exclusively in patients with advanced ankylosis (Fig. 18–9). Many patients relate a history of significant trauma, and radiographs obtained at the time of injury may reveal an associated fracture through the ankylosed apophyseal articulations, the neighboring articular processes, or, infrequently, the laminae or spinous process. Serial radiographs indicate an initial fracture of the spine and the subsequent development of bone destruction and sclerosis.

An ankylosed spine in the later stages of this disease is prone to fracture, a vulnerability that is accentuated by adjacent vertebral osteoporosis (Fig. 18–10). The cervical spine is especially susceptible to fracture (60% to 75% of fractures), and neurologic complications or death may result. Conversely, fractures in the thoracic and lumbar spine in ankylosing spondylitis are often unrecognized

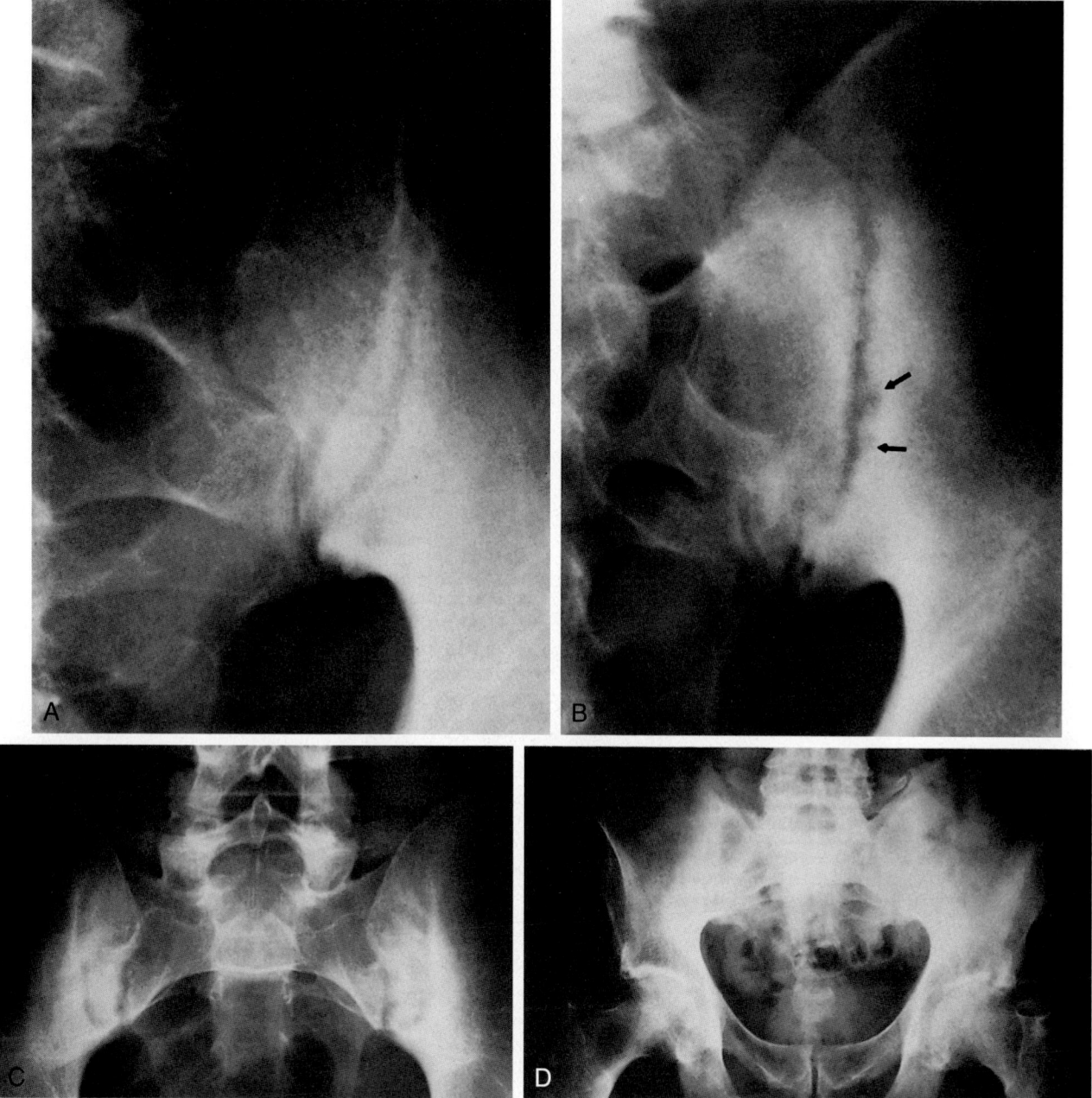

**Figure 18–4.** Abnormalities of the sacroiliac joint: radiographic stages (four different patients). *A,* Initial abnormalities consist of superficial bony erosion and eburnation, predominantly in the ilium. *B,* At a slightly later stage, note the larger erosions *(arrows),* progressive sclerosis, and focal narrowing of the articular space. *C,* At a more advanced stage, bilateral symmetrical changes consist of extensive sclerosis and focal ankylosis. *D,* Eventually, complete ankylosis of the synovial and ligamentous portions of the sacroiliac space on both sides is evident. The sclerosis has diminished.

clinically. Hyperextension injuries lead to spinal fractures that begin anteriorly in the vertebral body or, more commonly, the intervertebral disc; hyperflexion injuries produce spinal fractures that commence in the posterior osseous elements of the vertebra. Many of the resulting fractures become displaced. With continued movement at the fracture site, however, fibrous union can occur and result in what has been labeled a pseudarthrosis.

**Discal Calcification.** Central or eccentric circular or linear calcific collections may appear within the intervertebral disc at single or multiple sites (Fig. 18–11). Calcifications are accentuated by osteoporosis of the surrounding vertebral bodies. Similar deposits accompany other conditions of the vertebral column that are characterized by ankylosis, such as diffuse idiopathic skeletal hyperostosis (DISH) and juvenile chronic arthritis.

**TABLE 18–1**

**Terminology Commonly Applied to Spinal Abnormalities in Ankylosing Spondylitis**

| Term | Definition |
|---|---|
| Osteitis | Enthesopathy occurring at the discovertebral junction associated with erosion, sclerosis, and syndesmophytosis |
| "Shiny corner" sign | Increased radiodensity of the corners of the vertebral body related to "osteitis" |
| Squaring | Straightened or convex anterior margin of the vertebral body related to erosion |
| Syndesmophyte | Ossification within the anulus fibrosus leading to thin, vertical, radiodense areas |
| Bamboo spine | Undulating vertebral contour caused by extensive syndesmophytosis |
| Discitis | "Erosive" abnormalities of the discovertebral junction related to several mechanisms |
| Discal ballooning | Biconvex shape of the intervertebral disc related to osteoporotic deformity of the vertebral body |
| Trolley-track sign | Three vertical radiodense lines on frontal radiographs related to ossification of the supraspinous and interspinous ligaments and apophyseal joint capsules |
| Dagger sign | Single central radiodense line on frontal radiographs related to ossification of the supraspinous and interspinous ligaments |

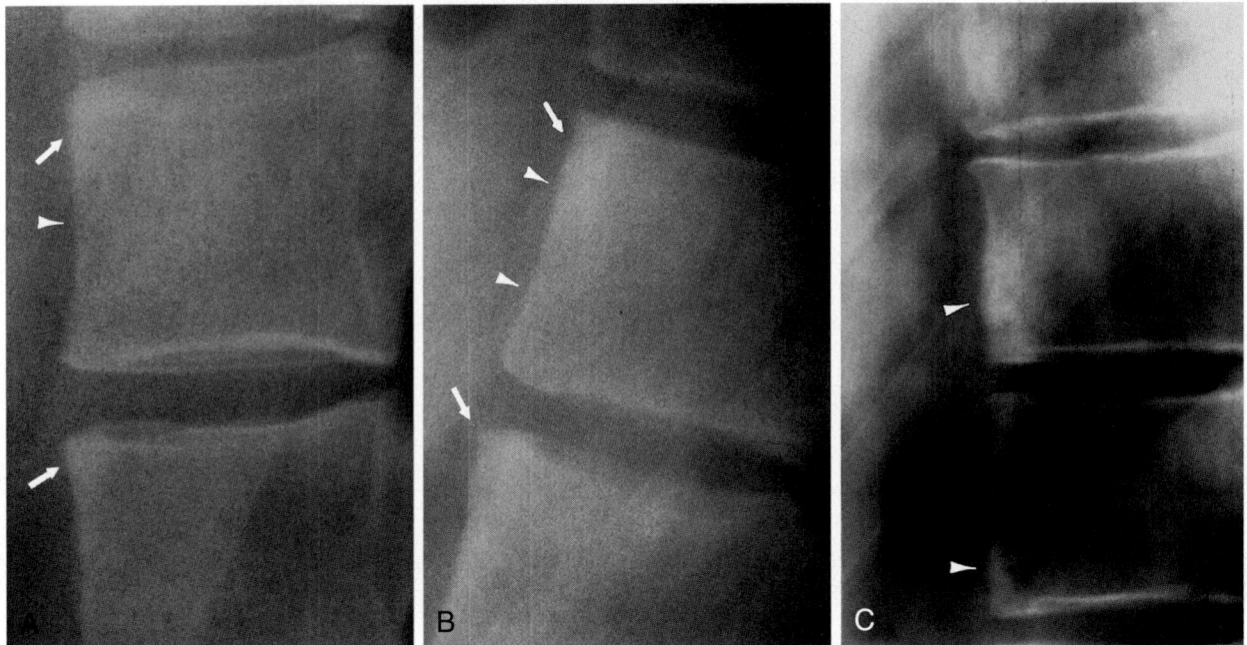

**Figure 18–5.** Osteitis: radiographic abnormalities (three different patients). *A,* Osseous erosion and sclerosis have produced whitening of the corners and margins along the anterior surfaces of the vertebrae *(arrows).* Note the straightening of the vertebral surface *(arrowhead). B,* Considerable straightening *(arrowheads)* and bone formation *(arrows)* along the anterior vertebral surface are observed. *C,* Convex anterior margin *(arrowheads)* of the vertebral bodies is associated with eburnation.

**Osteoporosis and Discal Ballooning.** In many patients with ankylosing spondylitis of long duration, osteoporosis of the vertebral bodies becomes apparent and may reach severe proportions. In some persons, typical biconcave deformities of the vertebral bodies ("fish vertebrae") lead to biconvex or ballooned intervertebral discs (see Fig. 18–11).

### Apophyseal Joint

Apophyseal joint inflammation is an essential abnormality in ankylosing spondylitis, and some investigators believe that apophyseal joint disease, including ankylosis, occurs before syndesmophyte formation. Further, an inverse relationship may exist between the extent of apophyseal

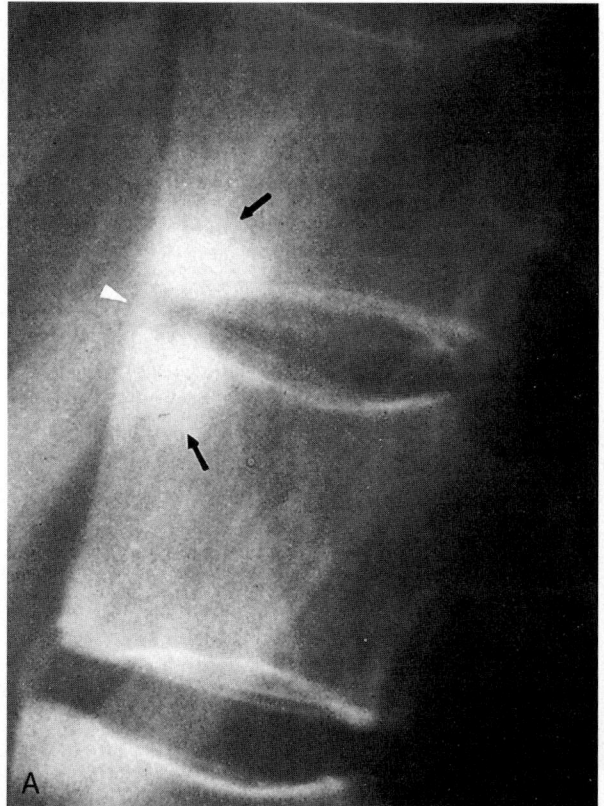

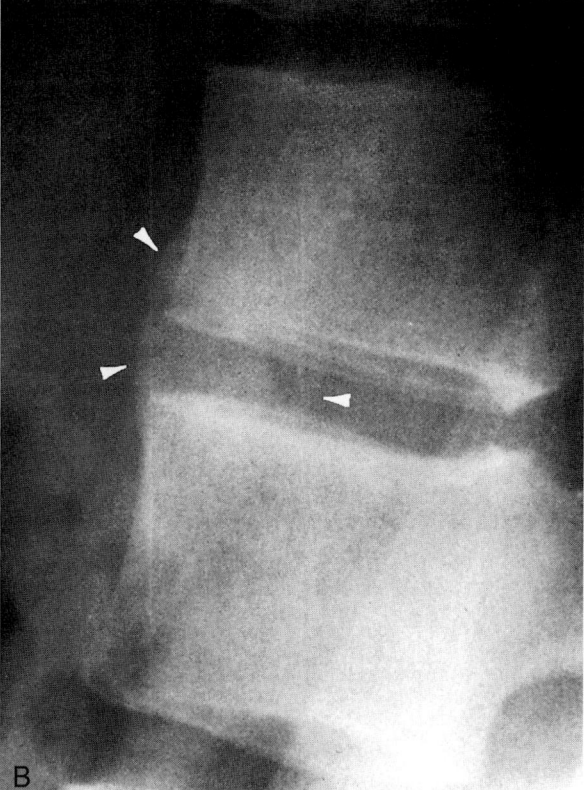

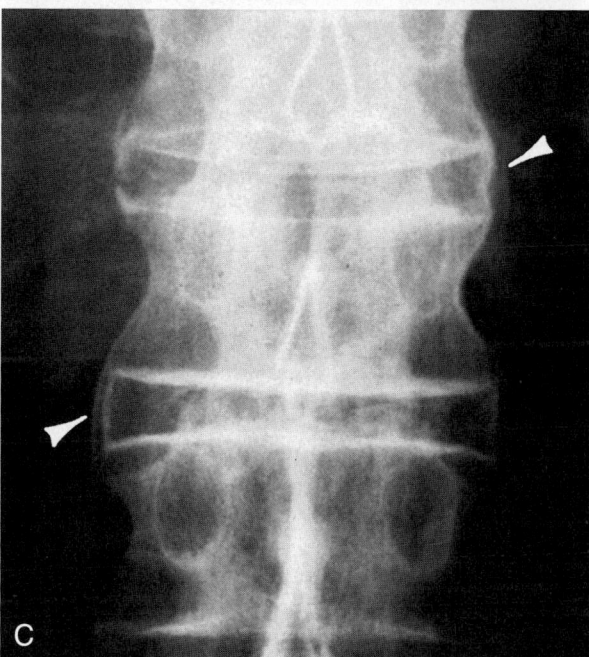

**Figure 18–6.** Syndesmophytosis: radiographic abnormalities. *A*, In association with osteitis of the corners of the vertebral bodies *(arrows)*, early syndesmophyte formation has produced blurring of the margin of the intervertebral disc *(arrowhead)*. *B*, In a different patient, more extensive syndesmophyte formation *(arrowheads)* is apparent. *C*, Frontal radiograph reveals typical syndesmophytes *(arrowheads)*. They extend in a vertical fashion from one vertebral body to the next.

joint involvement and the size of the syndesmophytes at the corresponding spinal level.

**Erosion and Sclerosis.** Poorly defined erosions of apophyseal joints in the lumbar, thoracic, and cervical segments of the spine are accompanied by reactive subchondral bone formation. In the cervical spine, such abnormalities are readily apparent on lateral radiographs. In any segment of the spine, apophyseal joint space narrowing is common as the disease process continues.

**Bony Ankylosis.** Apophyseal joint osseous fusion and capsular ossification are frequent in the lumbar, thoracic, and cervical spine in this disease (Fig. 18–12). These findings

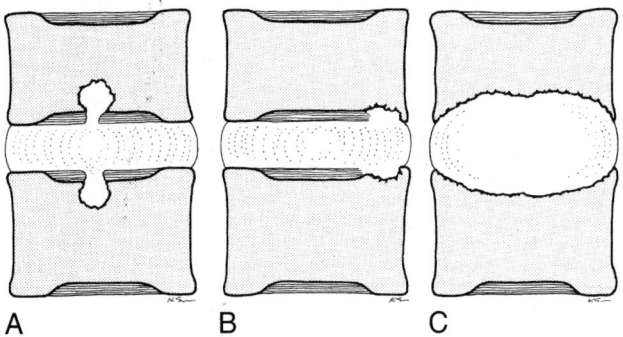

**Figure 18–7.** Discovertebral erosion and destruction: types of lesions. *A,* Localized central discovertebral lesions. Defects with surrounding eburnation in the central portion of the discovertebral junction may reflect intraosseous displacement of disc material (cartilaginous nodes). *B,* Localized peripheral discovertebral lesions. Defects may occur on the anterior or posterior aspect of the discovertebral junction. Their cause is obscure; they may be related to kyphosis with discal injury, cartilaginous node formation, or enthesopathy. *C,* Extensive central and peripheral discovertebral lesions. Destruction of the entire discovertebral junction is frequently the result of improper fracture healing.

are less common in psoriatic spondylitis and Reiter's syndrome. Apophyseal joint ankylosis can be very striking in the cervical spine (Fig. 18–13). Complete obliteration of the articular spaces between the posterior elements of the second through seventh vertebrae results in a true column, or pillar, of bone. The appearance is reminiscent of that

in juvenile chronic arthritis, although hypoplasia of the vertebral bodies and intervertebral disc spaces, a prominent finding in juvenile chronic arthritis, is not observed in ankylosing spondylitis.

### Costovertebral Joints

The costovertebral joints may demonstrate erosion, sclerosis, and ankylosis (Fig. 18–14). Indistinctness and erosion of subchondral bone, sclerosis, and partial or complete osseous fusion are more easily defined with computed tomography (CT) scanning.

### Posterior Ligamentous Attachments

Lesions affecting the posterior ligamentous attachments include calcification, ossification, and subligamentous erosion (Fig. 18–15).

### Atlantoaxial Articulations

Inflammatory changes of the synovial and adjacent ligamentous structures can lead to erosion of the dens. Similar abnormalities may be evident in rheumatoid arthritis. Although atlantoaxial subluxation can be observed in patients with ankylosing spondylitis, the frequency of this complication appears to be less than that in rheumatoid arthritis. When present, atlantoaxial subluxation is generally observed in the later stages of the disease.

### Complications of Spinal Involvement

Neurospinal complications, including spinal cord compression and even death, are a recognized though infrequent manifestation of ankylosing spondylitis. Vertebral fractures, especially in the cervical region, are associated with significant morbidity and mortality related to deformity of the cord produced by osseous surfaces, as well as hematomas. Atlantoaxial instability, in either a horizontal or a vertical direction, can produce neurologic deficit and may be fatal. Spondylodiscitis has been associated with compression of the cord or nerve roots, especially in the lumbar segment.

Although the mechanism is not clear, spinal stenosis is being recognized with increasing frequency in patients with ankylosing spondylitis. The cauda equina syndrome is also observed in some patients with ankylosing spondylitis. This syndrome occurs late in the course of the disease. Typical clinical findings include cutaneous sensory impairment of the lower limbs and perineum with sphincter disturbances. Widening of the neural canal in the lumbar segment, dilatation of the dural sac, and thecal diverticula may also be seen (Fig. 18–16).

### Symphysis Pubis

Alterations of the symphysis pubis (Fig. 18–17) have been described in 16% to 23% of patients with ankylosing spondylitis. Erosion and blurring of the subchondral bone on both sides of the joint are combined with adjacent eburnation. Articular space narrowing and bony ankylosis may be noted.

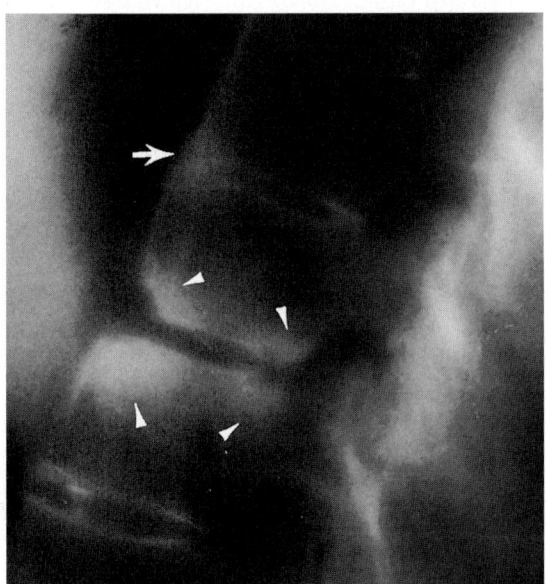

**Figure 18–8.** Discovertebral erosion and destruction. Localized central and peripheral defects with bony sclerosis *(arrowheads)* are observed on a lateral conventional tomogram of the thoracolumbar junction. Syndesmophytosis *(arrow)* is also seen. The apophyseal joint at this level is only partially ossified. (Courtesy of V. Vint, MD, San Diego, Calif.)

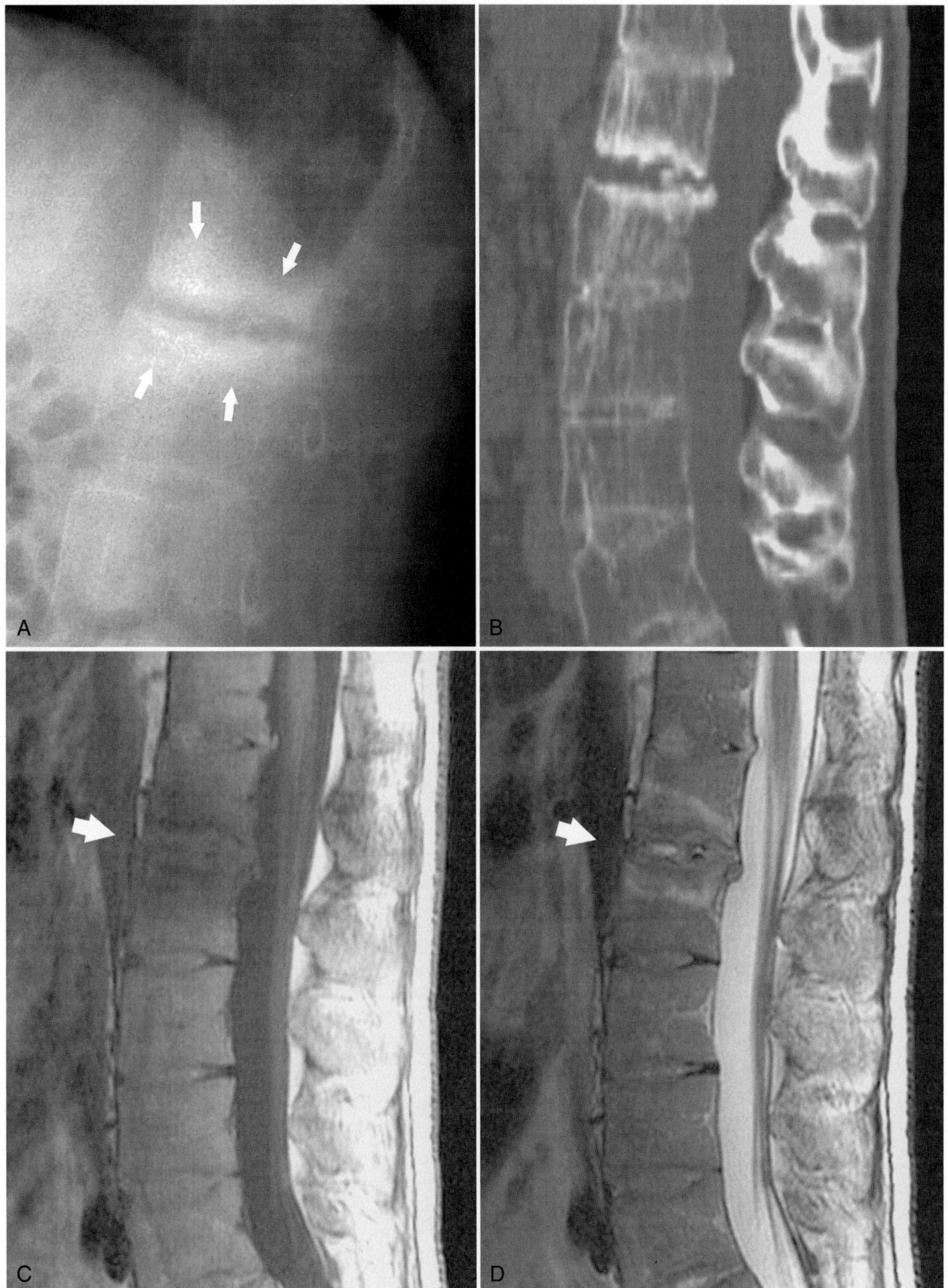

**Figure 18–9.** Discovertebral erosion and destruction: central and peripheral lesions—improper fracture healing or pseudarthrosis. *A,* Lateral radiographs reveal a typical pseudarthrosis of the lower thoracic spine characterized by extensive osseous resorption and sclerosis *(arrows).* The appearance simulates that of an infection. *B,* Sagittal reformatted CT scan shows the fracture to better advantage. *C* and *D,* Corresponding sagittal T1-weighted (TR/TE, 500/14) spin echo MR image *(C)* and fast T2-weighted (TR/TE, 4000/108) MR image *(D)* show nonspecific abnormal signal intensity adjacent to the pseudarthrosis *(arrow).*

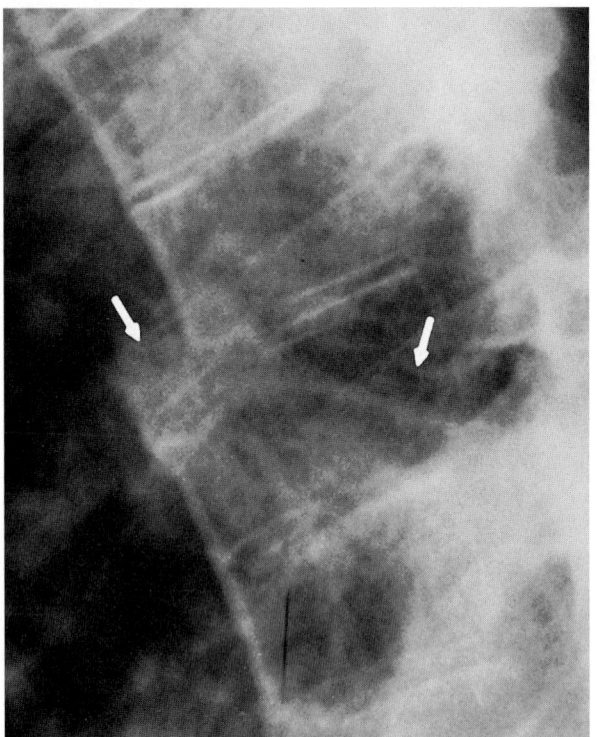

**Figure 18–10.** Spinal fractures. Acute midthoracic spinal fracture *(arrows)* is associated with subluxation. Conventional tomography revealed that the laminae were also disrupted.

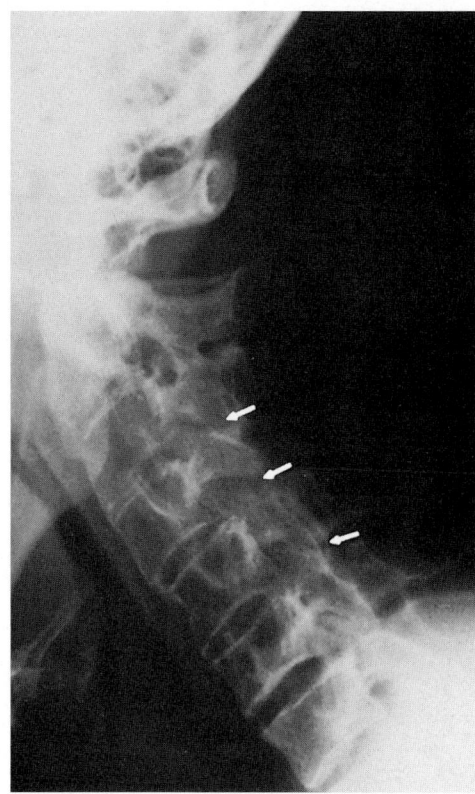

**Figure 18–12.** Apophyseal joint ankylosis. In the cervical spine, note the apophyseal joint narrowing and fusion *(arrows)* extending from C2 to C7. Syndesmophytes, osteoporosis, and mild subluxation at C4–C5 are seen.

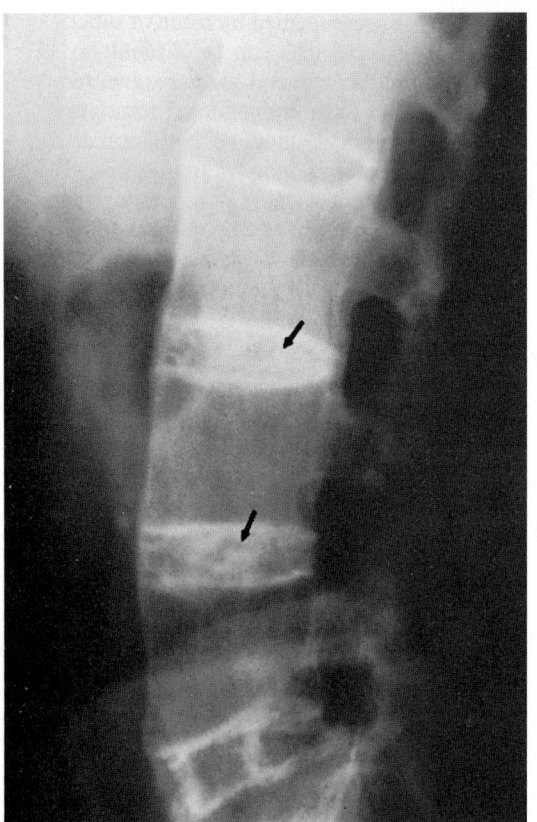

**Figure 18–11.** Discal calcification and ballooning. Long-standing ankylosing spondylitis is characterized by syndesmophytosis, apophyseal joint ankylosis, discal calcification *(arrows)*, osteoporosis, and ballooning, or biconvexity, of the intervertebral disc.

## Additional Pelvic Sites

Enthesopathy is especially prominent in certain pelvic sites, such as the ischial tuberosities, iliac crests, and sacroiliac spaces above the true synovial joints; similar abnormalities occur at extrapelvic sites, such as the femoral trochanters, humeral tuberosities, inferior clavicular margin at the site of attachment of the coracoclavicular ligament, anterior surface of the patella, and plantar aspect of the calcaneus. Osteoporosis, osseous erosion with poorly defined subchondral bony margins, and reactive sclerosis are the observed radiographic alterations; they are similar to those occurring in psoriatic arthritis, Reiter's syndrome, and inflammatory bowel disease.

## Manubriosternal Joint

Involvement of the manubriosternal joint generally occurs in patients with long-standing disease and severe sacroiliitis. Bony proliferation leads to sclerosis and intra-articular ankylosis, and soft tissue masses about the affected joint have been described.

## Hip

A bilateral (93%) and symmetrical (73%) distribution, with concentric joint space narrowing (50%) and osteophy-

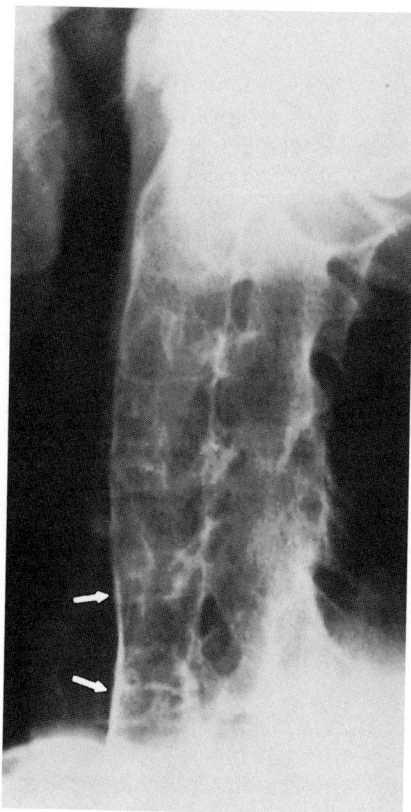

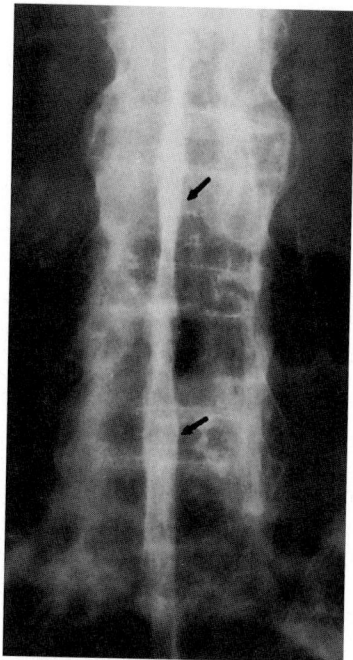

**Figure 18–15.** Posterior spinal ligamentous ossification. Frontal radiograph of the lumbar spine reveals ossification of the interspinous and supraspinous ligaments, which is producing a vertical central radiodense shadow *(arrows)*, the dagger sign.

**Figure 18–13.** Cervical apophyseal joint ankylosis and vertebral body resorption. Severe abnormalities of ankylosing spondylitis (apophyseal joint ankylosis, syndesmophytosis) include osseous resorption along the anterior aspect of the lower cervical vertebral bodies *(arrows)*.

tosis (58%), is characteristic (Table 18–2). An early and distinctive abnormality is an osteophyte, or "bump," on the lateral aspect of the femoral head. Osteophytes subsequently progress and create a collar around the femoral neck at the margin of the articular surface. Subsequent diffuse or concentric joint space narrowing produces axial migration of the femoral head with respect to the acetabulum. Protrusio acetabuli can eventually occur (Fig. 18–18). The combination of concentric diminution of the articular space and osteophytosis is characteristic of hip disease in ankylosing spondylitis, although it may also be observed in calcium pyrophosphate dihydrate crystal deposition disease, Paget's disease, and, infrequently, uncomplicated osteoarthritis. Concentric joint space narrowing is also seen in rheumatoid arthritis, but osteophytosis is not generally a prominent feature of this disease.

Intra-articular bony ankylosis has been emphasized as a complication of spondylitic hip disease. Subchondral cysts can also be observed. These cysts are generally multiple and of variable size and predominate in the acetabulum.

The radiographic course of spondylitic hip disease is variable, and some patients may require arthroplasty. Restricted motion and periarticular bone formation develop in the postoperative period in some patients with ankylosing spondylitis who require arthroplasty for hip disease.

### Shoulder

With the exception of the hip, the glenohumeral joint is the peripheral articular site most frequently affected in patients with long-standing ankylosing spondylitis (32%

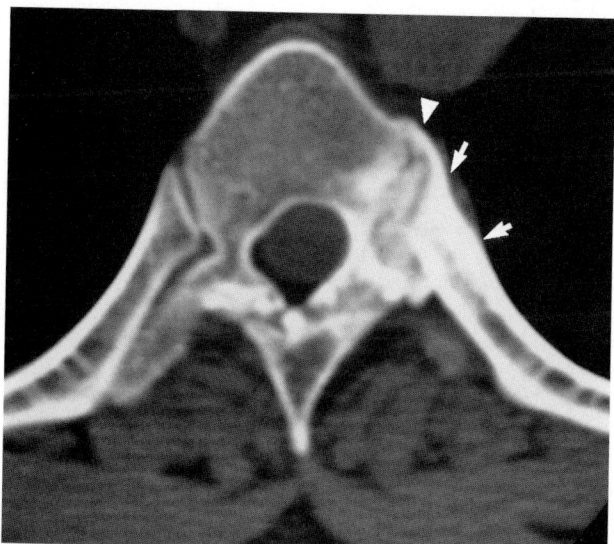

**Figure 18–14.** Costovertebral joint ankylosis. Transaxial CT scan of a thoracic vertebra in a patient with ankylosing spondylitis reveals bone erosions and partial ankylosis *(arrowhead)* of the costovertebral joints on one side. Note the involvement of the ipsilateral rib with cortical thickening *(arrows)*.

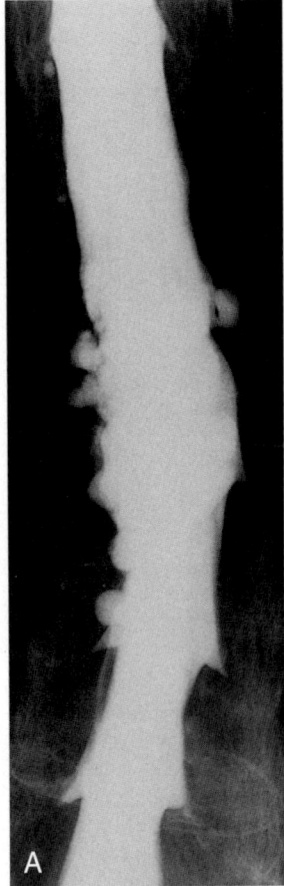

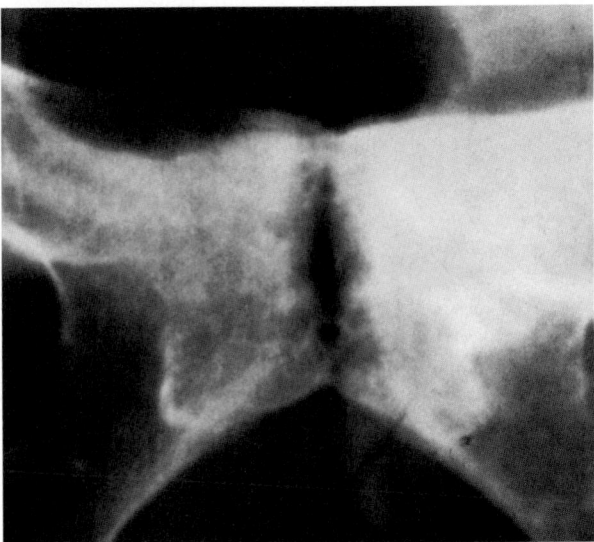

**Figure 18–17.** Abnormalities of the symphysis pubis. Note the narrowing, osseous fusion, and sclerosis of the symphysis pubis.

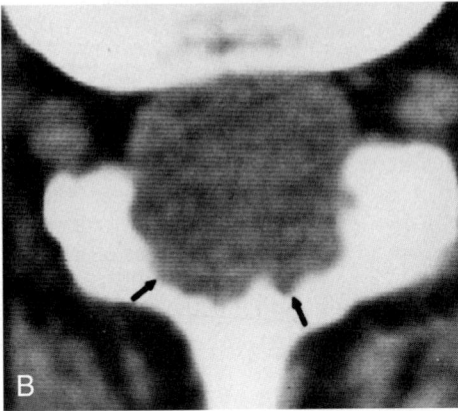

**Figure 18–16.** Thecal diverticula. *A*, Frontal radiographs during myelography in an elderly man with ankylosing spondylitis and cauda equina syndrome outline multiple arachnoid diverticula. *B*, Transaxial CT scan at the level of the third lumbar vertebra in a different patient demonstrates asymmetrical erosion of the lamina and spinous process *(arrows)*. (*A*, Courtesy of D. Moody, MD, Winston-Salem, N.C.; *B*, from Mitchell MJ, Sartoris DJ, Moody D, et al: Cauda equina syndrome complicating ankylosing spondylitis. Radiology 175:521, 1990.)

of patients). The abnormalities are more commonly bilateral than unilateral and may appear without changes in any other appendicular skeletal site. Osteoporosis, diffuse joint space narrowing, and erosive changes predominantly in the superolateral aspect of the humeral head simulate the changes seen in rheumatoid arthritis. In some spondylitic

patients, the entire outer aspect of the humerus is destroyed—the "hatchet" sign (Fig. 18–19). Destructive acromioclavicular joint abnormalities and articular changes in this location, which are commonly bilateral in distribution, are identical to those in rheumatoid arthritis.

### Sternoclavicular Joint

Bilateral or, less commonly, unilateral abnormalities of the sternoclavicular joint in ankylosing spondylitis consist of erosion and sclerosis of the sternum and the medial aspect of the clavicle, findings mimicking those in rheumatoid arthritis or infection. Osseous fusion may eventually occur.

### Hand and Wrist

Asymmetrically distributed abnormalities of the small joints of the hands and wrists (Fig. 18–20) are not infrequent (approximately 30% of patients with severe disease). Periarticular swelling, juxta-articular osteoporosis, joint space narrowing, and osseous erosions are observed. The metacarpophalangeal, proximal interphalangeal, and distal interphalangeal joints; all the compartments of the wrist; and the ulnar styloid can be affected. In general, erosive abnormalities are less prominent than in rheumatoid arthritis and are associated with adjacent periarticular bone proliferation, which produces a poorly defined and fuzzy osseous contour.

### Knee

In approximately 30% of patients with ankylosing spondylitis of long duration, radiographic abnormalities appear in the knees. Typically, bilateral and symmetrical changes in the three compartments of the knee include

**TABLE 18–2**

## Differential Diagnosis of Hip Involvement

| Disease | Typical Distribution | Femoral Head Migration | Osteophytosis | Miscellaneous Findings |
|---|---|---|---|---|
| Ankylosing spondylitis | Bilateral, symmetrical | Axial | Lateral aspect of femur, collar at femoral head-femoral neck junction | Cysts, bony ankylosis, protrusion deformity, postoperative heterotopic ossification |
| Rheumatoid arthritis | Bilateral, symmetrical | Axial | Rare | Osteoporosis, erosions, protrusion deformity |
| Osteoarthritis | Unilateral or bilateral | Superior or medial | Lateral and medial Femoral and acetabular | Sclerosis, cysts, buttressing |
| Calcium pyrophosphate dihydrate crystal deposition disease | Bilateral, symmetrical or asymmetrical | Axial | Lateral and medial Femoral and acetabular | Sclerosis, cysts, collapse, fragmentation, calcification |

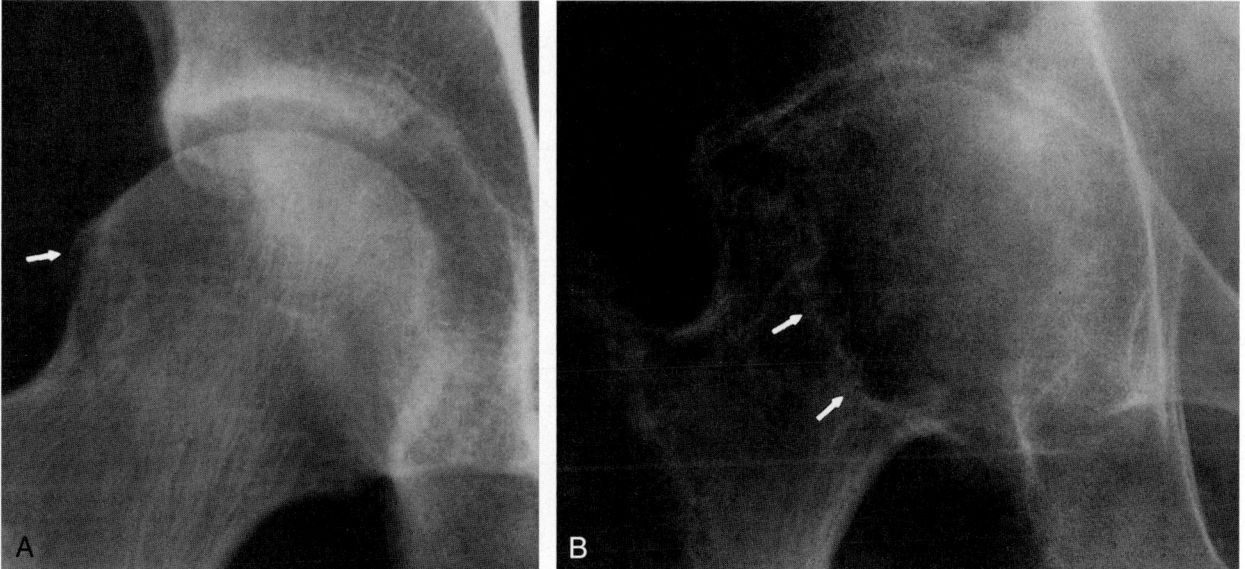

**Figure 18–18.** Abnormalities of the hip: osteophytosis. *A,* Observe the bone formation on the lateral margin of the femoral head *(arrow),* which has resulted in a bumpy contour. *B,* The osteophytes have formed a collar about the femoral neck *(arrows).* Extensive concentric joint space narrowing has occurred.
(From Dwosh IL, Resnick D, Becker MA: Hip involvement in ankylosing spondylitis. Arthritis Rheum 19:683, 1976.)

effusions, osteoporosis, and joint space narrowing. Additional manifestations are marginal erosions, subchondral cysts, and juxta-articular periostitis.

### Forefoot and Midfoot

Bilateral symmetrical or asymmetrical abnormalities of the feet, which may be evident in approximately 15% of patients with long-standing ankylosing spondylitis, show a predilection for the metatarsophalangeal and first tarsometatarsal joints and for the interphalangeal joint of the great toe. Soft tissue swelling, diffuse joint space narrowing, erosions with adjacent bony proliferation predominantly on the medial aspect of the metatarsal heads, periostitis of the phalangeal and metatarsal shafts, and intra-articular bony ankylosis can be detected. Subluxation at the metatarsophalangeal joints consisting of fibular deviation of the toes is less frequent and severe than in rheumatoid arthritis.

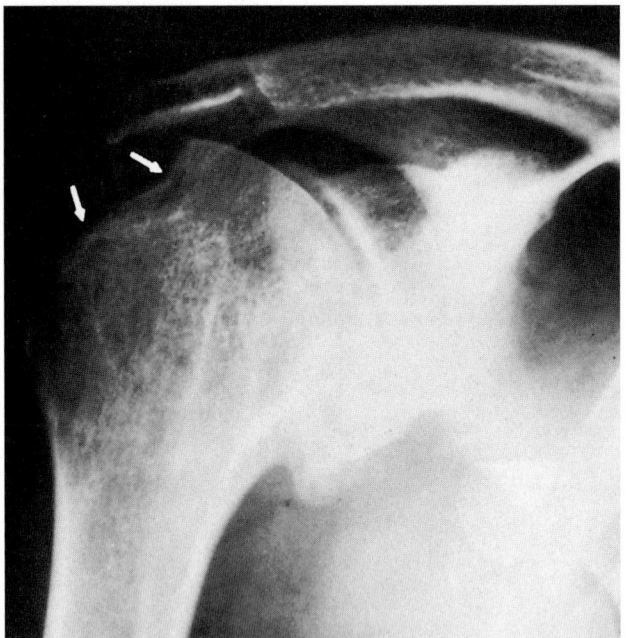

**Figure 18–19.** Abnormalities of the shoulder: glenohumeral joint. Observe the joint space narrowing, mild osteoporosis, and large erosive abnormality along the lateral aspect of the humeral head *(arrows)*.

## Calcaneus

Although clinically manifested heel abnormalities are infrequent in ankylosing spondylitis, radiographic changes of the calcaneus are common (Fig. 18–21). Bilateral abnormalities predominate. Well-defined plantar or posterior calcaneal enthesophytes are a common manifestation but are similar in appearance to those in a "normal" population. Retrocalcaneal swelling (related to bursitis), posterior calcaneal erosion, and Achilles tendon thickening are also frequent findings. Bony erosion and proliferation resulting in poorly defined enthesophytes at the site of ligamentous attachment to bone on the inferior surface of the calcaneus are identical to the findings of psoriatic arthritis and Reiter's syndrome.

## Temporomandibular Joint

Clinical and radiographic manifestations result from temporomandibular joint arthritis in patients with ankylosing spondylitis. Asymmetrical or unilateral involvement is frequent. Erosions predominate on the mandibular condyle.

## COEXISTENCE WITH OTHER DISORDERS
### Rheumatoid Arthritis

The concept that ankylosing spondylitis and rheumatoid arthritis are separate and distinct diseases is seldom challenged today. Uncommonly, both ankylosing spondylitis and rheumatoid arthritis appear to develop in the same person. Typically, ankylosing spondylitis develops in a male patient at a young age; subsequently, when his spondylitic process is largely inactive, rheumatoid arthritis develops.

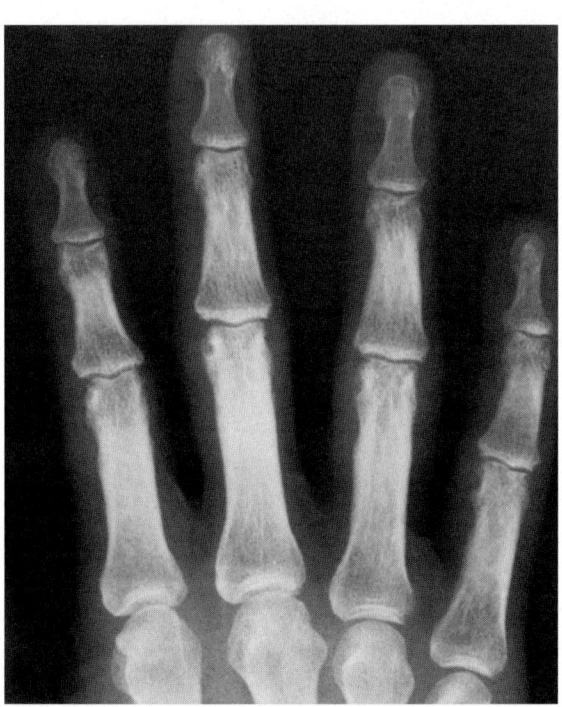

**Figure 18–20.** Abnormalities of the hand. Abnormalities consist of fusiform periarticular soft tissue swelling, mild joint space diminution, and marginal erosion of the proximal interphalangeal and distal interphalangeal joints.

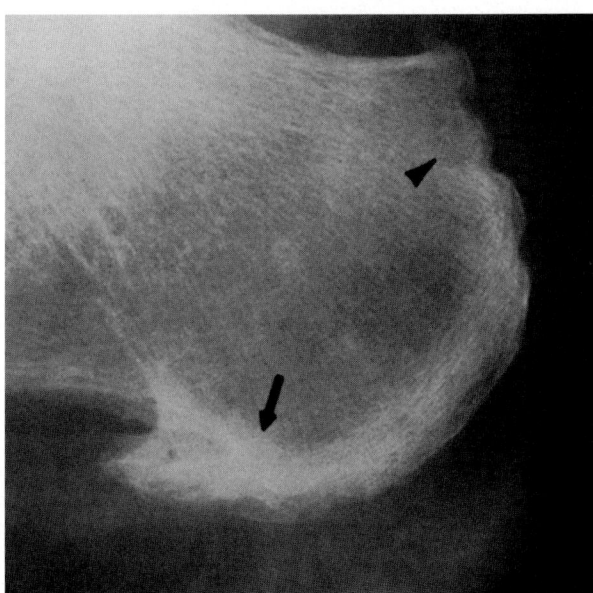

**Figure 18–21.** Abnormalities of the calcaneus. Findings include erosion of the posterosuperior aspect of the bone *(arrowhead)* related to retrocalcaneal bursitis, as well as erosive and proliferative changes of the plantar aspect of the bone *(arrow)* related to an enthesopathy at the ligamentous attachments.

## Diffuse Idiopathic Skeletal Hyperostosis

During the radiographic examination of older persons with long-standing ankylosing spondylitis, it is not unusual to document the presence of DISH as well. In this situation, widespread intra-articular bony ankylosis of both sacroiliac joints, syndesmophytosis, and apophyseal joint space narrowing or osseous fusion are combined with "flowing" ossification along the anterior aspect of a portion of the spine, particularly in the thoracic segment. Although it is a natural tendency to attribute all the radiographic findings to one disease, careful analysis ensures an accurate diagnosis of both disorders. The anteriorly distributed, broad osseous excrescences of DISH differ considerably from the thin vertical syndesmophytes of ankylosing spondylitis, which hug the outer portion of the intervertebral disc. The intra-articular bony ankylosis of the sacroiliac and apophyseal joints, which is typical of ankylosing spondylitis, is easily differentiated from the para-articular osteophytic changes of DISH.

## Inflammatory Bowel Disorders

The well-documented association of ankylosing spondylitis and certain inflammatory bowel disorders, such as ulcerative colitis and Crohn's disease, is discussed in Chapter 21.

## OTHER DIAGNOSTIC TECHNIQUES

### Scintigraphy

Sacroiliac and spinal abnormalities in ankylosing spondylitis can be evaluated with radionuclide scintigraphy. Qualitative analysis of the accumulation of bone-seeking radiopharmaceutical preparations in the sacroiliac region is often difficult, however, because of the normal radionuclide activity in this location. In addition, uptake of the radionuclide in the sacrum and the joint is influenced by the age and sex of the patient, and ratios are not always uniform for the two sides of the body in normal persons. In patients with advanced disease, radionuclide uptake in the sacroiliac joints (as well as the spine) may not be abnormal. Single photon emission computed tomography (SPECT) can also be used for the detection of sacroiliitis. Increased accumulation of radionuclide in spinal and peripheral articulations and at entheses may be observed. Focal areas of augmented radionuclide accumulation in the spine may indicate the site of an acute fracture or chronic pseudarthrosis (Fig. 18–22).

### Computed Tomography

Because of the difficulty in detecting sacroiliitis by conventional radiography and the controversy regarding the

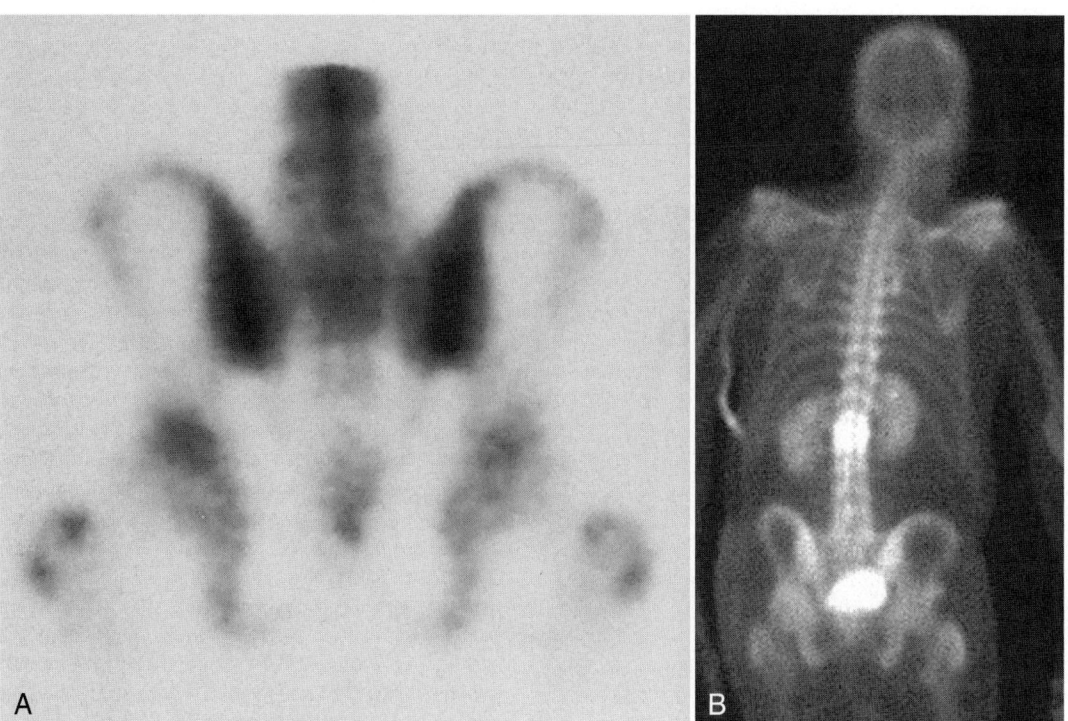

**Figure 18–22.** Scintigraphic abnormalities in ankylosing spondylitis. *A*, In this patient with typical spondylitic changes in the sacroliac joints, $^{99m}$Tc pyrophosphate radionuclide scintigraphy shows marked increased focal uptake. Uptake in the hip corresponds to entheses. *B*, In another patient with long-standing ankylosing spondylitis who had been injured in a fall, a focal area of markedly increased activity on bone scan corresponds to the site of a fracture and pseudarthrosis. The sacroiliac joints are ankylosed and are normal on scintigraphy.

role of scintigraphy, CT scanning has been used by some investigators in an effort to delineate early abnormalities of the sacroiliac joint in ankylosing spondylitis. CT scans must be accomplished using meticulous technique and should be interpreted by those who are knowledgeable about the normal variations of the sacroiliac joint that can simulate the findings of inflammation. In this regard, severe joint space loss, subchondral bone sclerosis in subjects younger than 40 years, osseous erosions, and intra-articular bone ankylosis are more valuable CT indicators of sacroiliitis than are nonuniform iliac sclerosis and focal joint space narrowing in patients older than 30 years. In addition to standard axial images, reformatted or directly acquired oblique coronal and transaxial images may be useful imaging planes (Fig. 18–23).

CT scanning can also be used to accurately guide an intra-articular injection of corticosteroid medication into the sacroiliac joint. Additional indications for CT scanning in patients with ankylosing spondylitis include detection of spinal fractures, spinal stenosis, thecal diverticula, atlantoaxial instability, and manubriosternal and costovertebral disease.

## Magnetic Resonance Imaging

Magnetic resonance (MR) imaging may prove useful in certain manifestations and complications of ankylosing spondylitis. Although the technique has been applied to the assessment of discovertebral disease activity in a relatively early stage of ankylosing spondylitis, at present, this use appears to be a minor indication for MR imaging. In T2-weighted spin echo sequences, increased signal intensity within the vertebral body marrow, adjacent to abnormal intervertebral discs, is consistent with the presence of edema (Fig. 18–24); a similar observation occurs when contrast-

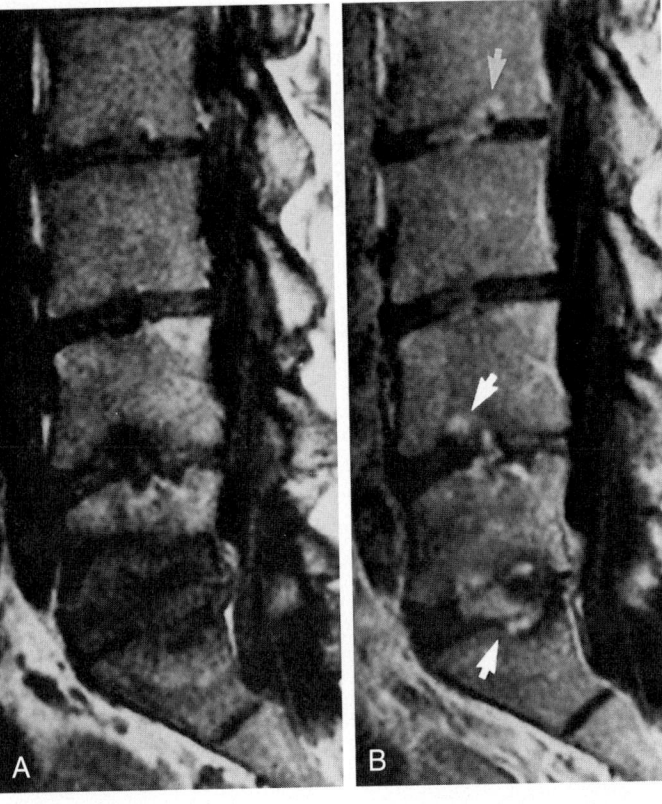

**Figure 18–24.** MR imaging in ankylosing spondylitis: spondylodiscitis. Sagittal T1-weighted (TR/TE, 650/20) spin echo MR images obtained before *(A)* and after *(B)* the intravenous injection of a gadolinium contrast agent reveal irregular discovertebral junctions with enhancement of signal intensity *(B, arrows)*. (Courtesy of J. Hodler, MD, Zurich, Switzerland.)

enhanced MR imaging is used. This finding is not unexpected with active spondylodiscitis. Complicating the assessment of discovertebral changes in ankylosing spondylitis is the variable signal intensity typical of discal calcification, a common finding in the disease. Increased signal intensity at the site of calcification may occur on T1-weighted spin echo MR images.

MR imaging has been applied successfully to the evaluation of spondylitic patients with the cauda equina syndrome. Dorsally situated arachnoid diverticula are directly visualized with this method. The fluid contents of the diverticula are well demonstrated, as are the accompanying osseous erosions of the posterior elements and bodies of affected vertebrae.

In the analysis of sacroiliac joint inflammation, MR imaging reveals variable patterns of altered signal intensity. Most frequently, low signal intensity is evident in all sequences. Less often, there is low signal intensity in the subchondral bone marrow on T1-weighted spin echo images and high signal intensity on T2-weighted spin echo images (Fig. 18–25). Recent studies of the role of MR imaging in the assessment of sacroiliitis have confirmed the sensitivity of the technique, particularly with regard to changes in subchondral bone (Fig. 18–26), as well as the benefits of using intravenous gadolinium-containing contrast agents combined with fat-suppressed imaging.

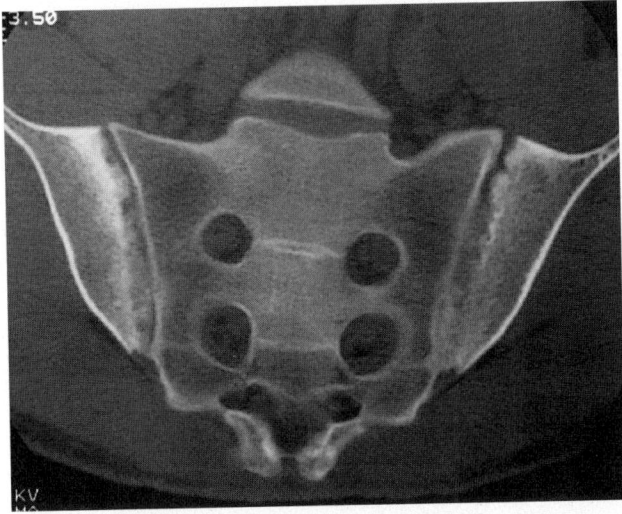

**Figure 18–23.** CT scanning in ankylosing spondylitis: sacroiliitis. An oblique transaxial image through the lower portion of the sacroiliac joint shows bilateral articular abnormalities, greater on the right side. These abnormalities consist of joint surface irregularity and erosion in the ilium, along with associated new bone formation. (Courtesy of T. Learch, MD, Los Angeles, Calif.)

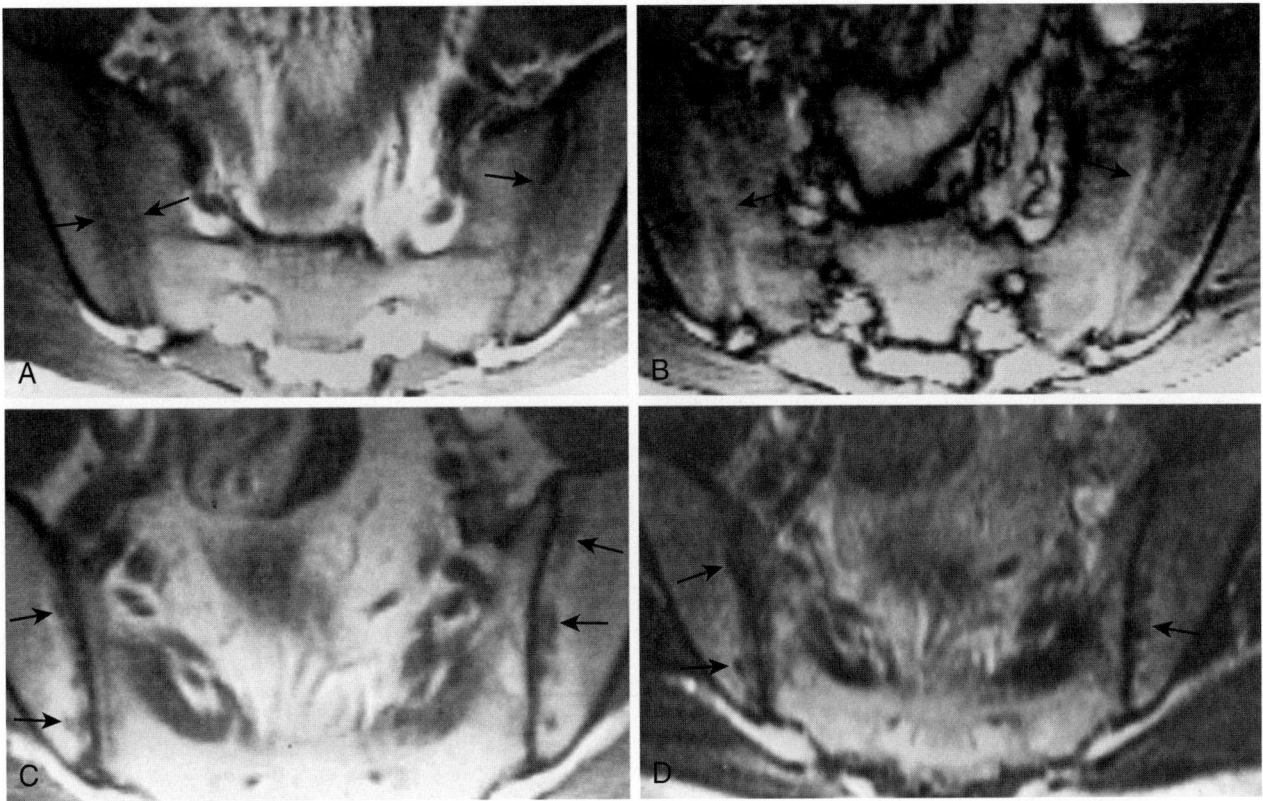

**Figure 18–25.** MR imaging in ankylosing spondylitis: sacroiliitis. *A* and *B*, In this 17-year-old patient with suspected sacroiliitis, conventional radiography and CT failed to reveal any abnormalities. Transaxial T1-weighted (TR/TE, 500/22) spin echo MR image *(A)* shows regions of low signal intensity about both sacroiliac joints *(arrows)*. In a transaxial intermediate-weighted (TR/TE, 1500/37) spin echo MR image *(B)*, the signal intensity in the periarticular bone marrow is increased *(arrows)*. *C* and *D*, In a different patient with confirmed ankylosing spondylitis, a transaxial T1-weighted (TR/TE, 500/22) spin echo MR image *(C)* reveals low signal intensity within periarticular bone marrow *(arrows)*. A similar T2-weighted (TR/TE, 2000/90) MR image *(D)* shows persistent low signal intensity in these regions *(arrows)*.

(From Ahlström H, Feltelius N, Nyman R, Hallgren R: Magnetic resonance imaging of sacroiliac joint inflammation. Arthritis Rheum 33:1763, 1990.)

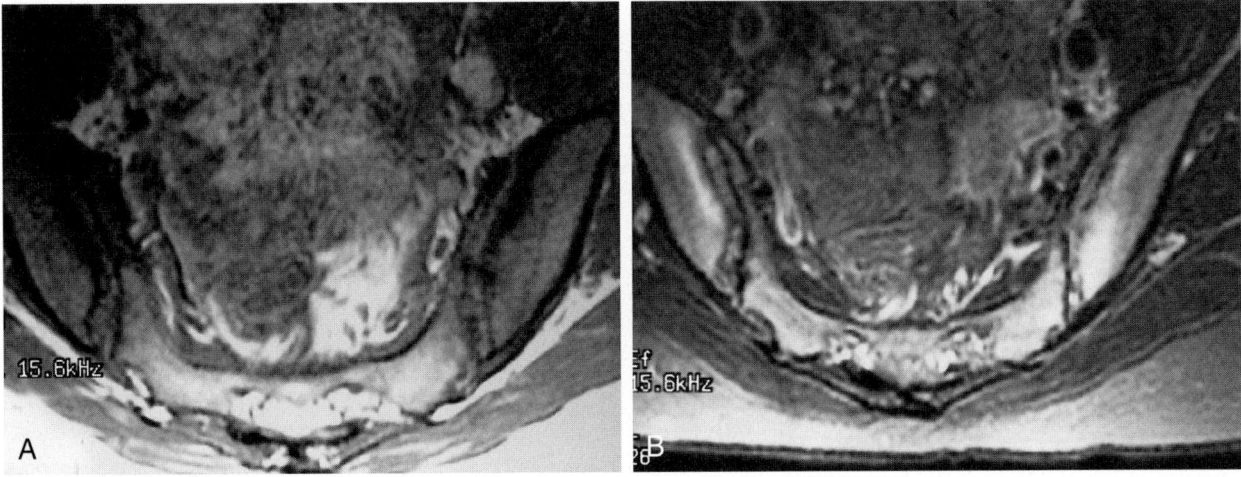

**Figure 18–26.** MR imaging in ankylosing spondylitis: sacroiliitis. As shown in these transaxial T1-weighted (TR/TE, 600/20) spin echo *(A)* and fat-suppressed T2-weighted (TR/TE, 4000/104) fast spin echo *(B)* MR images, abnormalities of subchondral bone may be the most prominent finding of active sacroiliitis. The subchondral bone in the sacrum and ilium is of low signal intensity in *(A)* and high signal intensity in *(B)*. (Courtesy of S. Lee, MD, Orange, Calif.)

Patterns of enhancement of signal intensity after contrast agent administration may provide information with regard to disease activity. The specificity of MR imaging in the differentiation of inflammatory and degenerative conditions of the sacroiliac joint is not yet clear, however.

## CAUSE AND PATHOGENESIS

A strikingly high frequency of the HLA-B27 antigen has been documented in patients with ankylosing spondylitis. In most reports, more than 90% of white spondylitic patients possess the B27 gene; the frequency of this gene in whites who do not have ankylosing spondylitis is approximately 6% to 8%. To date, this finding is the most significant association between a readily detectable HLA antigen and a well-defined disease, and it underscores the importance of genetics in the causation of ankylosing spondylitis.

## DIFFERENTIAL DIAGNOSIS

### Sacroiliitis

The sacroiliac joint abnormalities in ankylosing spondylitis must be differentiated from those accompanying other disorders (Table 18–3). This can be accomplished by analyzing both the distribution and the morphology of the articular changes. Classically, a bilateral and symmetrical distribution is observed in ankylosing spondylitis. Although a similar pattern may be evident in other seronegative spondyloarthropathies, such as psoriatic arthritis and Reiter's syndrome, asymmetrical or, infrequently, unilateral alterations may accompany these latter disorders. A bilateral and symmetrical distribution, identical in every regard to that of classic ankylosing spondylitis, is also associated with the sacroiliitis of inflammatory bowel disease (ulcerative colitis, Crohn's disease, Whipple's disease). In rheumatoid arthritis, minor sacroiliac articular abnormalities are commonly bilateral but may be asymmetrical in appearance. Bilateral and symmetrical alterations are also noted in hyperparathyroidism (and renal osteodystrophy), osteitis condensans ilii, gouty arthritis, and degenerative joint disease, although in the last two conditions, an asymmetrical or unilateral distribution is not uncommon. Unilateral abnormalities are most typical in infection.

Poorly defined erosive abnormality with adjacent sclerosis (particularly in the ilium), associated joint space narrowing, intra-articular osseous fusion, and ligamentous ossification is the characteristic appearance of sacroiliac joint disease in classic ankylosing spondylitis and in the sacroiliitis of inflammatory bowel disease. In psoriatic arthritis and Reiter's syndrome, extensive bony eburnation may be unaccompanied by intra-articular osseous fusion. Sacroiliac joint involvement in rheumatoid arthritis is usually manifested as superficial erosions, minimal sclerosis, and absence of significant bony ankylosis. Subchondral resorption of bone, predominantly in the ilium, in conjunction with primary or secondary hyperparathyroidisms leads to irregularity of the osseous surface, adjacent sclerosis, and widening of the interosseous joint space. In osteitis condensans ilii, a triangular segment of bony sclerosis is evident in the inferior aspect of the ilium. The joint surface is well defined, and the articular space is not diminished. In chronic tophaceous gouty arthritis, large, gouged-out defects with surrounding sclerosis are observed, whereas in degenerative arthritis, joint space narrowing, bony sclerosis, and anterior osteophytes are associated with a noneroded, smooth subchondral bony margin. Calcification and ossification of the interosseous ligament above the synovial sacroiliac joint can be encountered in degenerative joint disease and DISH. Cartilage atrophy accompanying paralysis or disuse produces diffuse loss of articular space with surrounding osteoporosis.

### Spondylitis

Spinal abnormalities in classic ankylosing spondylitis initially appear in the thoracolumbar and lumbosacral junctions and may subsequently extend throughout the thoracic and lumbar spine and into the cervical region. An identical distribution is encountered in the spondylitis of inflammatory bowel disease. Although the entire vertebral column

---

**TABLE 18–3**

**Distribution of Sacroiliac Joint Abnormalities in Various Disorders***

| Disorder | Bilateral, Symmetrical Distribution | Bilateral, Asymmetrical Distribution | Unilateral Distribution |
|---|---|---|---|
| Ankylosing spondylitis | + | − | − |
| Psoriatic spondylitis | + | + | + |
| Reiter's syndrome | + | + | + |
| Inflammatory bowel disease | + | − | − |
| Rheumatoid arthritis | − | + | + |
| Osteitis condensans ilii | + | − | − |
| Hyperparathyroidism | + | − | − |
| Gouty arthritis | + | + | + |
| Osteoarthritis | + | + | + |
| Infection | − | − | + |

*Only the most typical patterns of distribution are indicated.

may be altered in psoriatic arthritis and Reiter's syndrome, spotty involvement and absence of severe cervical spinal changes are typical of the latter disorder. This same distribution can be encountered in patients with psoriatic arthritis. Spondylitis without sacroiliitis is relatively rare in classic ankylosing spondylitis, although it may be observed in both psoriatic arthritis and Reiter's syndrome.

The thin, vertically oriented syndesmophytes that are evident in most patients with classic ankylosing spondylitis and the spondylitis of inflammatory bowel disease differ considerably in appearance from the broad, asymmetrical bony outgrowths seen in most patients with the spondylitis of psoriatic arthritis and Reiter's syndrome, the triangular outgrowths of spondylosis deformans, and the flowing anterolateral ossification of DISH (Table 18–4). The bony excrescences accompanying neuropathic osteoarthropathy, acromegaly, and fluorosis cannot be confused with the syndesmophytes of ankylosing spondylitis. Vertebral (and sacroiliac joint) abnormalities in X-linked hypophosphatemic vitamin D–resistant osteomalacia may simulate those in ankylosing spondylitis (see Chapter 42).

Osteitis with sclerosis and erosion of the anterior corners of the vertebral bodies and squaring are encountered much more commonly in classic ankylosing spondylitis and the spondylitis of inflammatory bowel disease than in psoriatic arthritis and Reiter's syndrome. Discovertebral erosions and sclerosis, which are seen in ankylosing spondylitis, are also observed in psoriatic arthritis. Similar lesions are evident in the cervical spine in patients with rheumatoid arthritis and throughout the spine in many disorders that are associated with cartilaginous (Schmorl's) nodes. When severe, spondylitic erosions can simulate the findings in infection, although more widespread osseous destruction and rapid disc space loss are more characteristic of infectious lesions of the spine.

Odontoid erosion and atlantoaxial subluxation are encountered in ankylosing spondylitis, usually in patients with long-standing disease. Similar findings are observed in psoriatic arthritis and, less commonly, in Reiter's syndrome. In rheumatoid arthritis, these findings are combined with other diagnostic features in the cervical spine.

In the cervical spine, the widespread apophyseal joint ankylosis accompanying ankylosing spondylitis resembles the findings in juvenile chronic arthritis. In the latter disorder, associated hypoplasia of the vertebral bodies and intervertebral discs is distinctive. Abnormalities of the cervical spine in other diseases can generally be differentiated from those in ankylosing spondylitis (Fig. 18–27).

## Abnormalities of Extraspinal Synovial Articulations

The absence of symmetrical changes and osteoporosis and the presence of bony proliferation and intra-articular osseous fusion are features that are common to all three seronegative spondyloarthropathies (ankylosing spondylitis, psoriatic arthritis, and Reiter's syndrome) and differ from the characteristics of rheumatoid arthritis (symmetry, osteoporosis, fibrous ankylosis, and absence of bony proliferation). Differentiating among the seronegative spondyloarthropathies on the basis of abnormalities in the synovial joints in the appendicular skeleton can be difficult (Table 18–5).

## Abnormalities of Extraspinal Cartilaginous Articulations

The seronegative spondyloarthropathies are frequently associated with significant abnormalities of the symphysis pubis and the manubriosternal joint. Although similar changes appear in rheumatoid arthritis, their frequency and severity are less striking.

---

**TABLE 18–4**

**Bony Outgrowths of the Spine**

| Outgrowth | Definition | Representative Disorders | Appearance |
|---|---|---|---|
| Syndesmophyte | Ossification of the anulus fibrosus | Ankylosing spondylitis Alkaptonuria | Vertical outgrowth extending from the edge of one vertebral body to the next |
| Osteophyte | Hyperostosis at the attachment of annular fibers | Spondylosis deformans | Triangular outgrowth located several millimeters from the edge of the vertebral body |
| Flowing anterior ossification | Ossification of the intervertebral disc, anterior longitudinal ligament, and paravertebral connective tissue | Diffuse idiopathic skeletal hyperostosis | Undulating outgrowth along the anterior aspect of the spine |
| Paravertebral ossification | Ossification of paravertebral connective tissue | Psoriatic spondylitis Reiter's syndrome | Poorly defined or well-defined outgrowth separated from the edge of the vertebral body and the intervertebral disc |

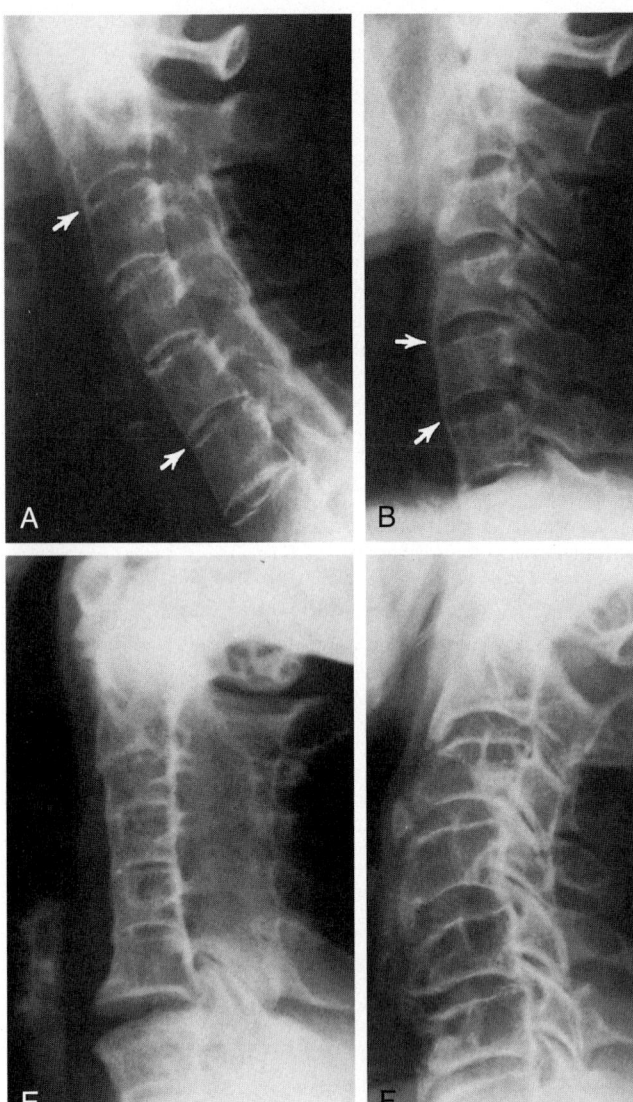

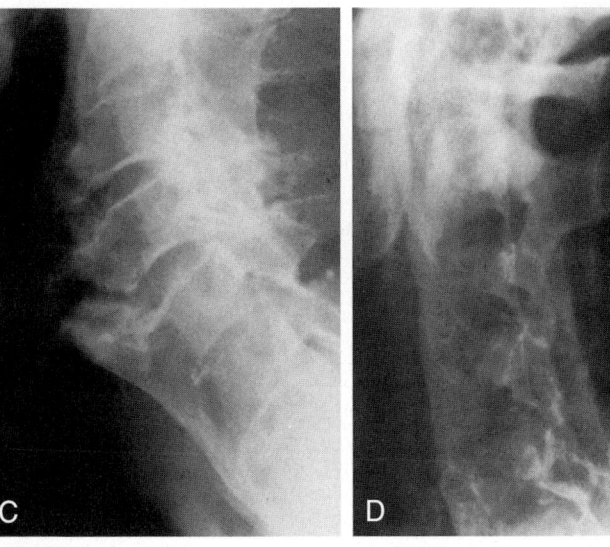

**Figure 18–27.** Differential diagnosis of cervical spine abnormalities. *A*, Ankylosing spondylitis is characterized by syndesmophytes *(arrows)* and apophyseal joint ankylosis. *B*, Psoriatic spondylitis leads to bony outgrowths *(arrows)* that predominate in the lower cervical spine. The apophyseal joints appear normal. *C*, Diffuse idiopathic skeletal hyperostosis is accompanied by extensive bone deposition on the anterior portion of the vertebral column. *D*, Sternocostoclavicular hyperostosis is characterized by exuberant bone formation anteriorly and centrally, which obliterates the interface between vertebral bodies and intervertebral discs, and by apophyseal joint ankylosis. *E*, Juvenile chronic arthritis is associated with hypoplasia of the vertebral bodies and intervertebral discs, apophyseal joint ankylosis, and a predilection for the upper cervical region. *F*, Acromegaly leads to bone deposition that resembles that of spondylosis deformans and an increase in the anteroposterior dimension of the vertebral bodies.

---

**TABLE 18–5**

### Abnormalities of Synovial Articulations

| Disease | Symmetrical Involvement | Soft Tissue Swelling | Osteoporosis | Joint Space Narrowing | Bony Ankylosis | Erosions, Cysts | Bony Proliferation or "Whiskering" |
|---|---|---|---|---|---|---|---|
| Ankylosing spondylitis | ± | + | ± | + | + | + | + |
| Rheumatoid arthritis | + | + | + | + | ± | + | − |
| Psoriatic arthritis | ± | + | − | + | + | + | + |
| Reiter's syndrome | − | + | ± | + | + | + | + |
| Gouty arthritis | ± | + | − | ± | − | + | +* |
| Septic arthritis | − | + | + | + | + | + | +† |

*Irregular lips of bone are apparent.
†Poorly defined "fraying" of bone is seen.

---

## Enthesopathy

Bony erosion with proliferation at the site of the osseous attachment of ligaments and tendons is a typical lesion of ankylosing spondylitis, psoriatic arthritis, and Reiter's syndrome. In all locations, an irregular frayed surface may be created that is virtually diagnostic of one of these three conditions. Enthesopathic alterations are less prominent in rheumatoid arthritis, but when present, they are usually not associated with severe bony proliferation.

# FURTHER READING

Berens DL: Roentgen features of ankylosing spondylitis. Clin Orthop 74:20, 1971.

Cawley MID, Chalmers TM, Kellgren JH, et al: Destructive lesions of vertebral bodies in ankylosing spondylitis. Ann Rheum Dis 31:345, 1972.

Cruickshank B: Pathology of ankylosing spondylitis. Bull Rheum Dis 10:211, 1960.

Dwosh IL, Resnick D, Becker MA: Hip involvement in ankylosing spondylitis. Arthritis Rheum 19:683, 1976.

Forestier J, Jacqueline F, Rotes-Querol J: Ankylosing Spondylitis. Springfield, Ill, Charles C Thomas, 1956.

Gelman MI, Umber JS: Fractures of the thoracolumbar spine in ankylosing spondylitis. AJR Am J Roentgenol 130:485, 1978.

Ginsburg WN, Cohen MD, Miller GM, et al: Posterior vertebral body erosion by cauda equina syndrome: An unusual manifestation of ankylosing spondylitis. J Rheumatol 24:1417, 1997.

Goldberg RP, Genant HK, Shimshak R, et al: Applications and limitations of quantitative sacroiliac joint scintigraphy. Radiology 128:683, 1978.

Jevtic V, Kos-Golja M, Rozman B, et al: Marginal erosive discovertebral "Romanus" lesions in ankylosing spondylitis demonstrated by contrast enhanced Gd-DTPA magnetic resonance imaging. Skeletal Radiol 29:27, 2000.

Kozin F, Carrera GF, Ryan LM, et al: Computed tomography in the diagnosis of sacroiliitis. Arthritis Rheum 24:1479, 1981.

McEwen C, DiTata D, Lingg C, et al: Ankylosing spondylitis and the spondylitis accompanying ulcerative colitis, regional enteritis, psoriasis, and Reiter's disease: A comparative study. Arthritis Rheum 14:291, 1971.

Mitchell MJ, Sartoris DJ, Moody D, et al: Cauda equina syndrome complicating ankylosing spondylitis. Radiology 175:521, 1990.

Murphey MD, Wetzel LH, Bramble JM, et al: Sacroiliitis: MR imaging findings. Radiology 180:239, 1991.

Olivieri I, Ciancio G, Scarano E, et al: The extension of the ankylosing spondylitis "dagger sign" into the sacrum. J Rheumatol 27:2944, 2000.

Oostveen J, Prevo R, den Boer J, et al: Early detection of sacroiliitis on magnetic resonance imaging and subsequent development of sacroiliitis on plain radiography: A prospective, longitudinal study. J Rheumatol 26:1953, 1999.

Resnick D: Inflammatory disorders of the vertebral column: Seronegative spondyloarthropathies, adult-onset rheumatoid arthritis, and juvenile chronic arthritis. Clin Imaging 13:253, 1989.

Resnick D, Dwosh IL, Goergen TG, et al: Clinical and radiographic "reankylosis" following hip surgery in ankylosing spondylitis. AJR Am J Roentgenol 126:1181, 1976.

Trent G, Armstrong GWD, O'Neil J: Thoracolumbar fractures in ankylosing spondylitis: High-risk injuries. Clin Orthop 227:61, 1988.

Volger JB III, Brown WH, Helms CA, et al: The normal sacroiliac joint: A CT study of asymptomatic patients. Radiology 151:433, 1984.

Vyas K, Eklem M, Seto H, et al: Quantitative scintigraphy of sacroiliac joints: Effect of age, gender, and laterality. AJR Am J Roentgenol 136:589, 1981.

Wilkinson M, Bywaters EGL: Clinical features and course of ankylosing spondylitis as seen in a follow up of 222 hospital referred cases. Ann Rheum Dis 17:209, 1958.

# CHAPTER 19

## Psoriatic Arthritis

### SUMMARY OF KEY FEATURES

Psoriatic arthritis produces distinctive abnormalities of synovial and cartilaginous joints, as well as abnormalities of the tendon and ligament attachments to bone. Although the classic manifestation is that of a polyarticular disorder with a predilection for the distal interphalangeal joints of the fingers, a variety of other clinical patterns may be observed, including a symmetrical seronegative polyarthritis identical in distribution to rheumatoid arthritis, arthritis mutilans, oligoarthritis or monoarthritis, and sacroiliitis and spondylitis. In most instances, the diagnosis is not difficult and is based on the characteristic radiographic features, which include some degree of asymmetry, progressive intra-articular erosive changes with separation of the subchondral margins of adjacent bones, periosteal proliferation, intra-articular osseous fusion, and absence of osteoporosis in synovial articulations; also included are bilateral symmetrical or asymmetrical sacroiliac joint abnormalities and paravertebral ossification, erosion and sclerosis in cartilaginous articulations, erosion and bone proliferation at sites of tendon and ligament attachment to bone, and osteolysis of the terminal phalanges.

### INTRODUCTION

For many years after the original descriptions of psoriatic arthritis in the late 19th century, the joint abnormalities associated with psoriasis were considered to be part of the spectrum of rheumatoid arthritis. The distinctive alterations of psoriatic arthritis were gradually recognized, however, and today the concept of a specific type of arthritis in patients with psoriasis is seldom challenged. Psoriatic arthritis has a wide clinical and radiographic spectrum, which is emphasized here.

### PREVALENCE AND SPECTRUM

The most accurate estimates of the frequency of arthritis in patients with psoriasis range from 2% to 6%. Conversely, the reported prevalence of psoriasis among patients with polyarticular arthritis ranges from 3% to 5%. Five broad clinical varieties of psoriatic arthritis have been recognized: (1) polyarthritis characterized by distal interphalangeal joint involvement; (2) a deforming type of arthritis characterized by widespread ankylosis and, occasionally, arthritis mutilans; (3) a symmetrical seronegative polyarthritis simulating rheumatoid arthritis but without its laboratory parameters; (4) monoarthritis or asymmetrical oligoarthritis; and (5) sacroiliitis and spondylitis resembling ankylosing spondylitis (Table 19–1).

---

**TABLE 19-1**

**Varied Patterns of Psoriatic Arthritis***

Polyarthritis with distal interphalangeal joint involvement
Symmetrical seronegative polyarthritis simulating rheumatoid arthritis
Monoarthritis or asymmetrical oligoarthritis
Sacroiliitis and spondylitis
Arthritis mutilans

---

*In addition, patients with psoriatic arthritis may have coincidental rheumatoid arthritis.

---

Although radiographic abnormalities accompany these five types of disease, features in certain groups are much more specific than those in other groups, and in some patients, a diagnosis of psoriatic arthritis cannot be made on the basis of radiographic changes.

### CLINICAL ABNORMALITIES

The age of onset of psoriatic arthritis does not differ significantly from that of rheumatoid arthritis, although children with psoriatic arthritis are increasingly being recognized. In most adult patients, a long history of psoriatic skin disease is evident, although in a few persons, the articular abnormalities coincide with or even antedate the appearance of skin lesions. Articular disease is much more prevalent in patients with moderate or severe skin abnormalities. Nail abnormalities appear to correlate most closely with articular disease. These nail changes are generally apparent in the same digit that has a significant distal interphalangeal articular abnormality.

The clinical nature of the articular disease is variable. A monoarticular, pauciarticular, or polyarticular distribution may be encountered, and virtually any joint can be affected, although the small joints of the hands and feet are reportedly involved in 25% to 75% of patients with arthritis. In some patients, low back complaints predominate as a result of involvement of the spine and the sacroiliac joints. Soft tissue swelling can be prominent, and in some patients an entire digit is enlarged (sausage digit) because of abnormalities of the distal interphalangeal and proximal interphalangeal joints and tendon sheath. Subcutaneous nodules are characteristically not evident.

Laboratory analysis confirms the absence of serologically detectable rheumatoid factor in most patients. Additional laboratory parameters may include mild anemia, an elevated erythrocyte sedimentation rate, and, occasionally, elevated serum uric acid levels (related to cellular turnover in psoriatic cutaneous lesions). The histocompatibility antigen HLA-B27 is often present in patients with psoriatic arthritis and sacroiliitis.

# RADIOGRAPHIC ABNORMALITIES

The characteristic radiographic features of psoriatic arthritis are well described (Table 19–2).

## Initial Radiographic Abnormalities

In the initial phase of psoriatic arthritis, radiographs may be entirely normal. Early radiographic abnormalities, which include soft tissue swelling and some degree of osteoporosis, may resolve without any permanent sequelae. With clinical progression of articular problems, more extensive radiographic abnormalities appear and may worsen at a variable rate. Significant joint destruction and deformity are more characteristic of psoriatic arthritis than of Reiter's syndrome.

## Distribution of Radiographic Abnormalities

Psoriatic arthritis can affect synovial and cartilaginous joints and sites of tendon and ligament attachment to bone in both the appendicular and the axial skeleton (Fig. 19–1). Although the articular distribution of psoriatic arthritis is somewhat variable, an asymmetrical or even unilateral appearance is much more common in psoriatic arthritis than in rheumatoid arthritis, although widespread involvement of one side of the body is almost invariably associated with changes on the other side. Both upper extremity and lower extremity joints are affected in psoriatic arthritis; in contrast, Reiter's syndrome involves predominantly the joints of the lower extremity. The distal interphalangeal and proximal interphalangeal joints (as well as the metacarpophalangeal and metatarsophalangeal joints) of the hand and foot are commonly affected. Abnormalities of the phalangeal tufts and calcaneus are also characteristic. Significant abnormalities of the hip and shoulder are relatively uncommon. In the axial skeleton, sacroiliac joint and spinal abnormalities predominate.

## General Radiographic Abnormalities
(Fig. 19–2)

**Soft Tissue Swelling.** Fusiform soft tissue swelling is frequently evident about involved joints and reflects the presence of synovial effusions of variable size and soft tissue edema. Sausage-like swelling of entire digits or

diffuse swelling of all or part of an extremity may also be encountered.

**Osteoporosis.** Osteoporosis is not a prominent feature of psoriatic arthritis, although it may be demonstrated in early phases of the disease.

**Joint Space Narrowing or Widening.** The articular space may be narrowed or widened. In large joints, such as the knee, ankle, elbow, and hip, diffuse loss of joint space is identical to that observed in rheumatoid arthritis. In the small joints of the fingers and toes, severe destruction of marginal and subchondral bone can lead to considerable widening of the articular space. This finding is uncommon in rheumatoid arthritis but may be seen in gout and multicentric reticulohistiocytosis.

**Bone Erosion.** Erosive abnormalities are prominent in psoriatic arthritis. Initially, erosions predominate in the marginal areas of the articulation, but as they progress, central areas are also affected. In the small joints of the hands and feet, destruction or whittling of the head of

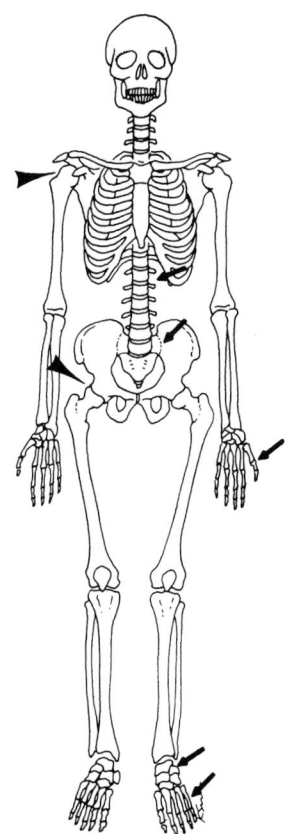

**Figure 19–1.** Psoriatic arthritis: distribution of radiographic abnormalities. The most typical sites of abnormality are the interphalangeal joints of the hand and foot, metacarpophalangeal and metatarsophalangeal joints, calcaneus, sacroiliac joint, and spine (*arrows*). Not uncommon are changes in the knee; ankle; manubriosternal, sternoclavicular, acromioclavicular, and costovertebral joints; symphysis pubis; and tendinous connections of the pelvis, elbow, and wrist. Significant alterations of the hip and glenohumeral joint are relatively unusual (*arrowheads*).

---

**TABLE 19-2**

### Characteristics of Psoriatic Arthritis

Involvement of synovial and cartilaginous joints and entheses
Asymmetrical distribution more common than symmetrical distribution
Involvement of interphalangeal joints of the hands and feet
Sacroiliitis and spondylitis with paravertebral ossification
Bony erosion with adjacent proliferation
Intra-articular bony ankylosis
Destruction of phalangeal tufts
Enthesitis

one phalanx may produce a small, blunt osseous surface that projects into the expanded base of a neighboring phalanx, reminiscent of a pencil-and-cup or cup-and-saucer arrangement. Similar changes are encountered at metacarpophalangeal and metatarsophalangeal locations. In some patients with psoriatic arthritis, complete dissolution of large segments of apposing bones, fragmentation with osseous debris, and disorganization of the joint resemble the changes of neuropathic osteoarthropathy.

**Bone Proliferation.** As in the other seronegative spondyloarthropathies, proliferation of bone is a striking feature of psoriatic arthritis. Irregular excrescences create a spiculated, frayed, or "paintbrush" appearance. Bone proliferation probably relates to an exaggerated healing response of the injured bone. The osseous erosion in rheumatoid arthritis is generally not associated with adjacent bony deposition. Although bone proliferation may accompany erosions in gouty arthritis, the resulting excrescences are generally well defined.

Periostitis in the metaphyses and diaphyses of bones is not uncommon in psoriatic arthritis, particularly in the hands and feet. In these locations, periosteal bone formation, probably related to tenosynovitis, may lead to significant "cloaking" of an entire phalanx or a portion of a metacarpal or metatarsal bone. This change may appear early in the disease course, in association with soft tissue swelling, before significant abnormalities occur in the adjacent articulations. Condensation of bone on the periosteal and endosteal surfaces of the cortex and trabecular thickening in the spongiosa can cause an entire phalanx to appear radiodense. This latter appearance is termed the ivory phalanx and is most common in the terminal phalanges of the toes.

Intra-articular osseous fusion is another manifestation of bone proliferation in psoriatic arthritis, and it is particularly prominent in the hands and feet. Although intra-articular osseous fusion is also observed in inflammatory (erosive) osteoarthritis, septic arthritis, and even rheumatoid arthritis (carpal and tarsal areas), it is an important radiographic sign of the seronegative spondyloarthropathies.

Bone proliferation occurs at sites where tendons and ligaments insert on bones. These locations include the posterior and inferior surfaces of the calcaneus, femoral trochanters, ischial tuberosities, medial and lateral malleoli, ulnar olecranon, and anterior surface of the patella.

**Tuft Resorption.** Resorption of the tufts of the distal phalanges of the hands and feet is characteristic of psoriatic arthritis. Soft tissue swelling and adjacent interphalangeal joint abnormalities are frequent. The nail of the involved digit is almost always affected.

**Malalignment and Subluxation.** Deformities of the hands and feet can be encountered in some patients with psoriatic arthritis. Telescoping of one bone on its neighbor may lead to the "opera-glass hand." In this situation, excess skin may be folded over the involved joints and produce a concertina-like appearance. Ulnar deviation at the metacarpophalangeal joints, fibular deviation at the metatarsophalangeal joints, and boutonnière and swan-neck deformities are not as common in psoriatic arthritis as in rheumatoid arthritis.

## Radiographic Abnormalities at Specific Sites

**Hand.** The destructive arthritis of the distal interphalangeal joints of the hand (Figs. 19–2 and 19–3) is the best-known manifestation of psoriatic arthritis. At these sites, bilateral symmetrical or asymmetrical changes or unilateral changes are observed. Initial erosions occur at the margins of the articulation and proceed centrally. The resulting irregular osseous surfaces may become separated from each other as a consequence of the extensive nature of the erosive process. This lack of apposition of adjacent bony margins distinguishes the radiographic picture of psoriatic arthritis from that of osteoarthritis, in which closely applied undulating osseous surfaces are the rule. The adjacent proximal interphalangeal joints are frequently affected. The metacarpophalangeal joints may be relatively spared.

At any altered interphalangeal site, radiographic findings may include separated, eroded, well-demarcated bone margins; protrusion of a blunted and distorted osseous surface into an adjacent expanded one (pencil-and-cup appearance); irregular periosteal bone proliferation (whiskering); and intra-articular osseous fusion. Tuft resorption may be evident in one or more terminal phalanges. Both phalangeal resorption and destructive arthritis of the distal interphalangeal joints are generally associated with significant nail changes in the same digit.

**Wrist.** Abnormalities in the wrist in psoriatic arthritis (Fig. 19–4) are not as frequent as those in the fingers and are rarely encountered without more typical distal changes.

**Other Upper Extremity Sites.** Psoriatic arthritis can lead to changes in the elbow and glenohumeral, acromioclavicular, and sternoclavicular joints.

**Forefoot.** The forefoot is commonly affected in psoriatic arthritis (Fig. 19–5). Bilateral asymmetrical changes predominate in the interphalangeal and metatarsophalangeal joints and are characterized by marginal erosions, bony proliferation, alterations in joint space (narrow or wide), and lack of osteoporosis. Extensive destruction of the interphalangeal joint of the great toe is more characteristic of this articular disorder than of any other disease. Osteolysis of tufts and the phalangeal and metatarsal shafts may be encountered. In the terminal phalanges, extensive new bone formation may lead to increased osseous density of the entire bone (ivory phalanx).

**Calcaneus.** As in the other seronegative spondyloarthropathies, erosion and proliferation of the posterior or inferior surface of the calcaneus, or both, may be prominent in psoriatic arthritis (Fig. 19–6). Retrocalcaneal bursitis creates a radiodense area adjacent to the posterosuperior aspect of the bone that may extend into the pre-Achilles fat pad. Subjacent erosion of the calcaneus is associated with surrounding bony proliferation.

**Other Lower Extremity Sites.** Articular involvement in psoriatic arthritis may be apparent in the midfoot or

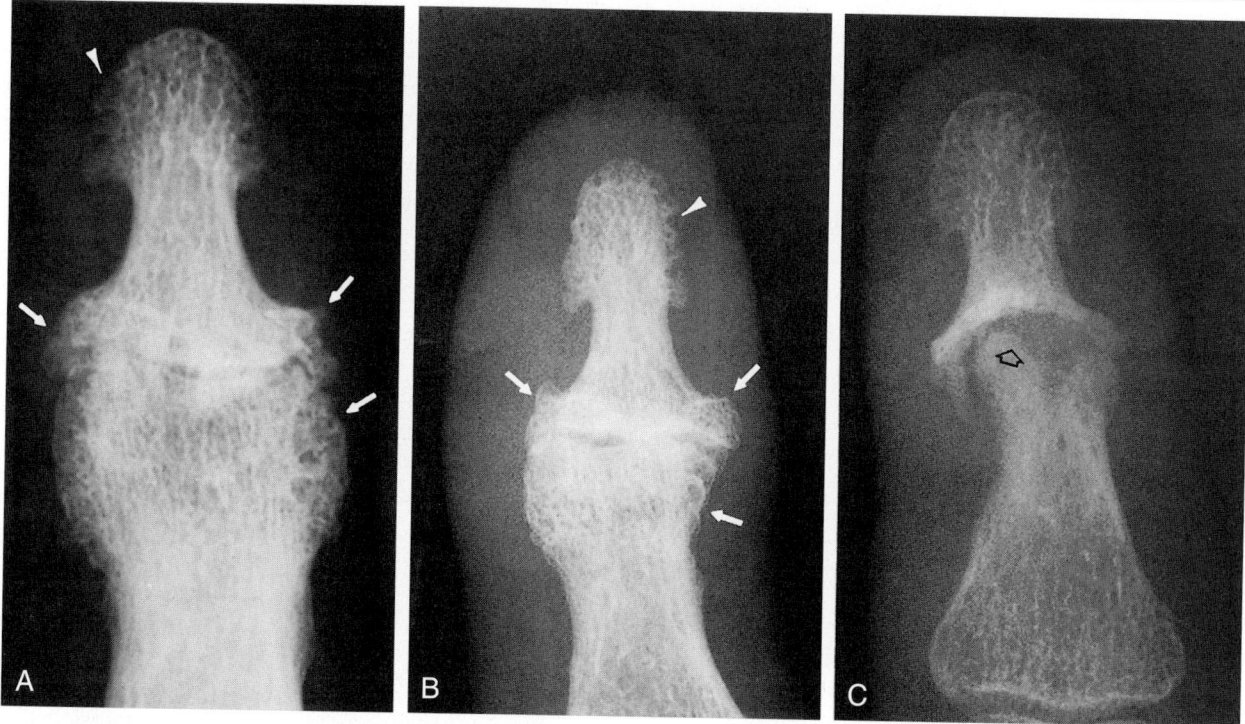

**Figure 19–2.** General radiographic abnormalities. *A to C*, Classic radiographic changes are depicted about the distal interphalangeal joints in three patients with psoriatic arthritis. These changes include soft tissue swelling, lack of osteoporosis, joint space narrowing, osseous erosions with accompanying proliferation *(solid arrows)*, osteolysis with a pencil-and-cup appearance *(open arrow)*, and tuft resorption *(arrowheads)*.

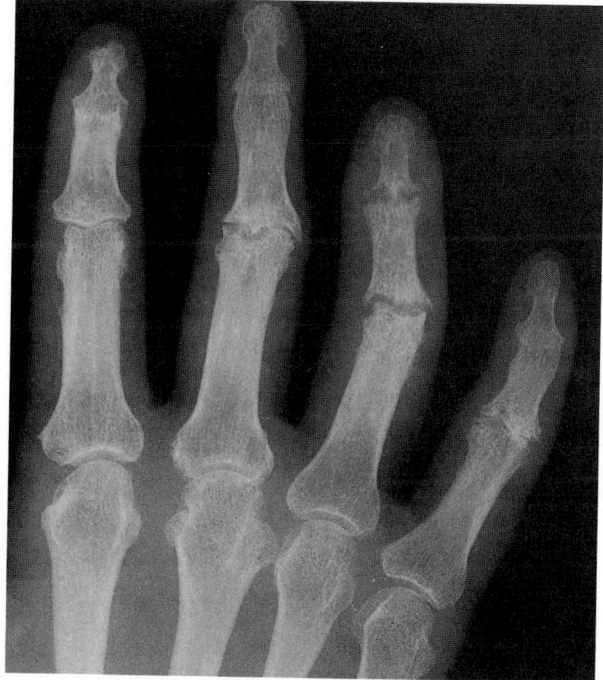

**Figure 19–3.** Radiographic abnormalities of the hand. Interphalangeal joint changes consist of articular space narrowing, intra-articular bony ankylosis, marginal and central erosions, flexion contractures, and osteolysis of the phalangeal tufts. Metacarpophalangeal joint abnormalities, although less marked, include joint space narrowing, marginal erosions, and bony proliferation.

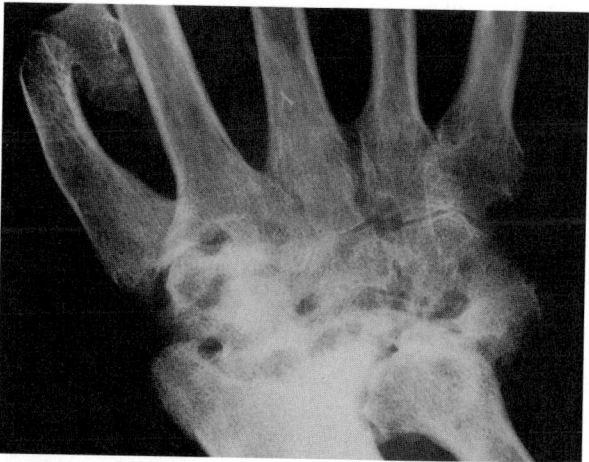

**Figure 19–4.** Radiographic abnormalities of the wrist. Severe pancompartmental involvement of the wrist is characterized by joint space narrowing, intra-articular osseous fusion, erosions, bony proliferation, and the absence of osteoporosis. Considerable destruction about the first metacarpophalangeal joint is also seen.

hindfoot, ankle, or knee. Abnormality of the hip is relatively unusual.

**Sacroiliac Joint.** Approximately 10% to 25% of patients with moderate or severe psoriatic skin disease have sacroiliac joint changes on radiographic examination. It also appears that such changes develop in approximately

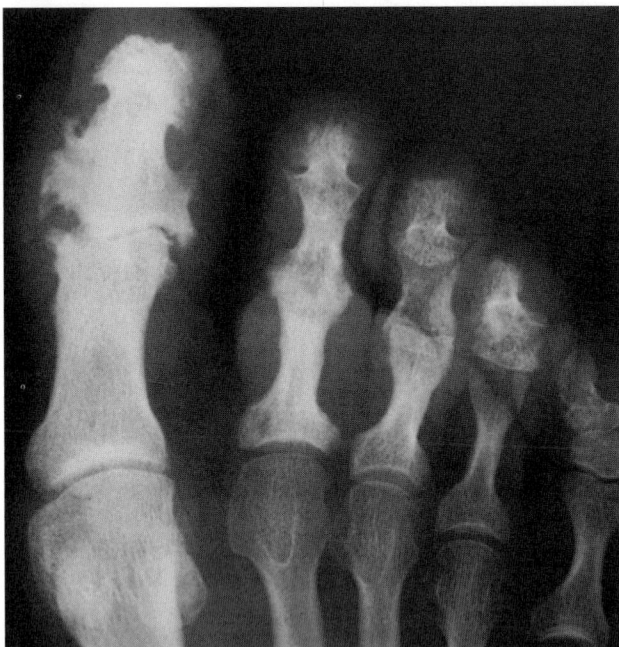

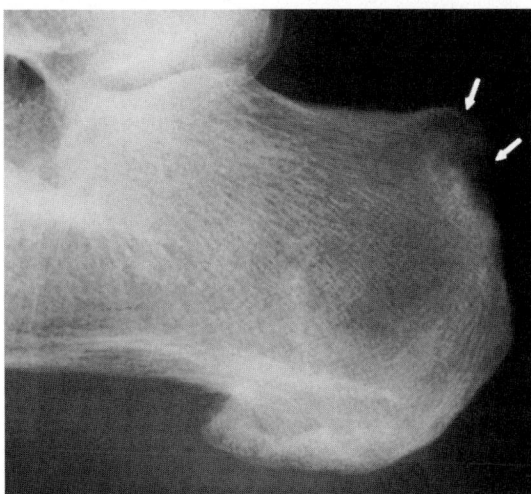

**Figure 19–6.** Abnormalities of the calcaneus. Retrocalcaneal bursitis is manifested as erosion of the posterosuperior aspect of the calcaneus (*arrows*). A large plantar calcaneal enthesophyte is identified.

**Figure 19–5.** Radiographic abnormalities of the forefoot. Findings include joint space narrowing and bony ankylosis of multiple interphalangeal joints and osseous erosion and proliferation, particularly about the interphalangeal joint of the great toe. Note the tuftal osteolysis and sclerosis of bone in multiple digits.

30% to 50% of patients with psoriatic arthritis. Bilateral abnormalities of the sacroiliac joint are much more frequent than unilateral changes in psoriatic arthritis. Although asymmetrical findings may be apparent, symmetrical abnormalities predominate. Sacroiliitis can appear without spondylitis. Radiographic sacroiliac joint changes include erosions and sclerosis, predominantly in the ilium, and widening of the articular space (Fig. 19–7). Although significant joint space diminution and bony ankylosis can occur, these findings (particularly ankylosis) are less prevalent than in classic ankylosing spondylitis or the spondylitis associated with inflammatory bowel disease.

**Spine.** As in Reiter's syndrome, paravertebral ossification about the lower thoracic and upper lumbar segments can occur in psoriatic arthritis (Fig. 19–8). Initially, ossification appears as a thick and fluffy, or thin and curvilinear, radiodense region on one side of the spine that parallels the lateral surface of the vertebral bodies and the intervertebral discs. It extends progressively at a variable rate and eventually may produce a large and bulky outgrowth that merges with the underlying osseous and discal tissue. Its greater size, its unilateral or asymmetrical distribution, and its location farther away from the vertebral column distinguish paravertebral ossification from the typical syndesmophytosis of ankylosing spondylitis and the spondylitis in inflammatory bowel disease.

In addition to the pattern and distribution of bony outgrowths, other features of psoriatic spondylitis differ from those of classic ankylosing spondylitis. Osteitis and squaring of the anterior surfaces of the vertebral bodies

are relatively infrequent in psoriatic arthritis. Although apophyseal joint space narrowing, sclerosis, and bony ankylosis may be seen, the frequency of these findings is much less than that in ankylosing spondylitis.

Cervical spine abnormalities (Fig. 19–9) may become striking in patients with psoriatic arthritis. These abnormalities include apophyseal joint space narrowing and sclerosis, osseous irregularity at the discovertebral joint, and extensive proliferation along the anterior surface of the spine. Atlantoaxial subluxation may also be evident.

**Other Sites.** The manubriosternal joint can reveal severe alterations, almost invariably in association with changes in other skeletal sites. Osteoporosis, subchondral erosion, eburnation, and synostosis are seen. Adjacent soft tissue swelling may be prominent. The temporomandibular joint can also be significantly affected in psoriatic arthritis.

## OTHER DIAGNOSTIC TECHNIQUES

Scintigraphy with bone-seeking radiopharmaceutical agents can delineate an articular abnormality of psoriatic arthritis before its appearance on radiographic examination. Increased radionuclide accumulation predominates at the interphalangeal, metacarpophalangeal, and metatarsophalangeal joints of the hands and feet; however, calcaneal, sacroiliac joint, and spinal uptake can be considerable (Fig. 19–10). The asymmetrical nature of the scintigraphic alterations in psoriatic arthritis frequently permits its differentiation from rheumatoid arthritis.

The role of ultrasonography in the assessment of psoriatic arthritis is limited to superficial structures. Tenosynovitis, tendon disruption, dactylitis, soft tissue edema, and bursitis are processes that can be evaluated with this method.

The application of magnetic resonance (MR) imaging to the analysis of psoriatic arthritis has received little

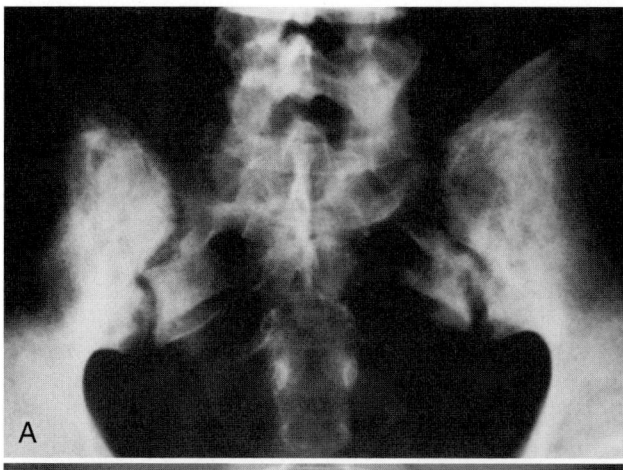

A

**Figure 19–7.** Abnormalities of the sacroiliac joint. *A,* Bilateral and symmetrical changes consist of erosions and sclerosis, predominantly in the ilium. Intra-articular bony ankylosis is not seen. *B,* In this patient, asymmetrical abnormalities are present. The left sacroiliac joint reveals sclerosis with extensive erosive change, giving the joint space a widened appearance. Minimal changes are present on the right side. *C,* Axial noncontrast computed tomographic scan shows extensive sclerosis and erosion of the left sacroiliac joint. Milder changes are seen on the right.

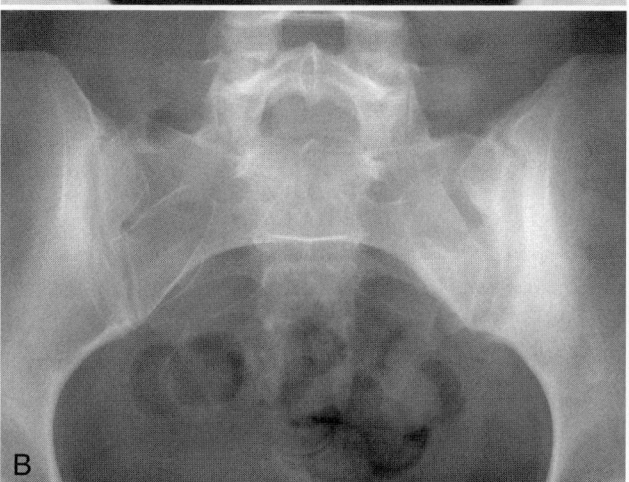

B

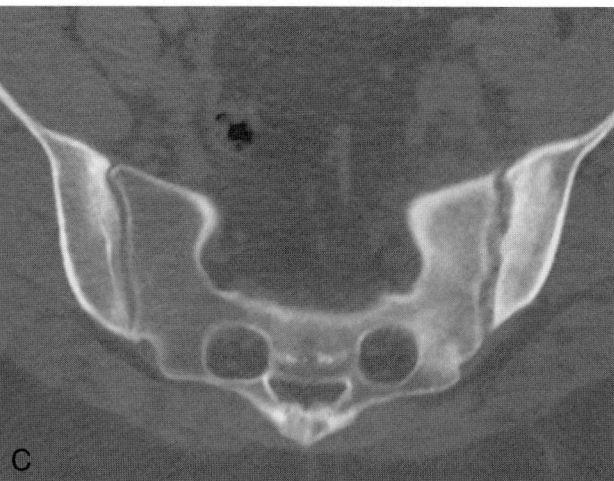

C

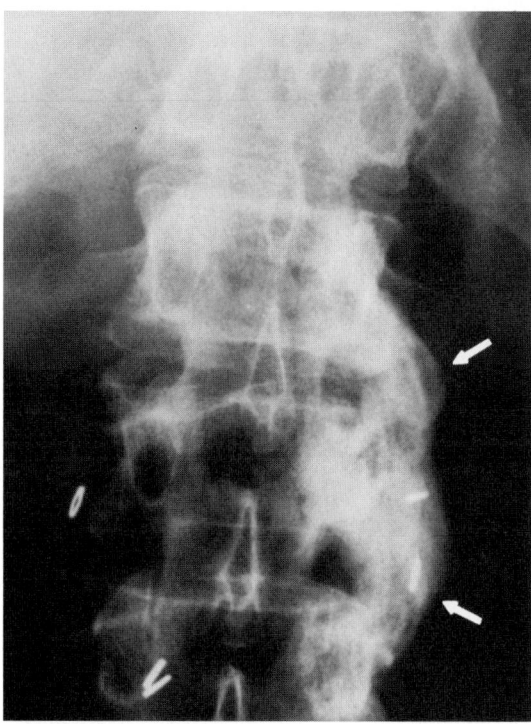

**Figure 19–8.** Radiographic abnormalities of the thoracic and lumbar spine. Bulky outgrowths appear *(arrows)* and merge with the underlying vertebral bodies and intervertebral discs. Note the asymmetrical distribution and absence of significant sacroiliac joint disease. Surgical clips are evident.

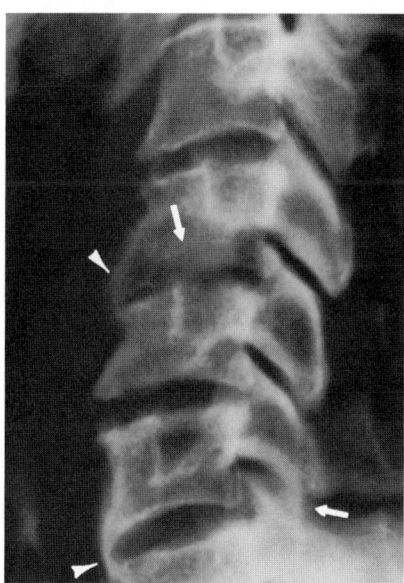

**Figure 19–9.** Radiographic abnormalities of the cervical spine. Note the erosions at the discovertebral junction and apophyseal joints *(arrows)* and syndesmophytes *(arrowheads).*

emphasis. The degree of marrow edema in psoriatic arthritis can be profound, perhaps related to inflammation; this may account for the tendency toward bone formation that is seen in this disease (Fig. 19–11). Similar

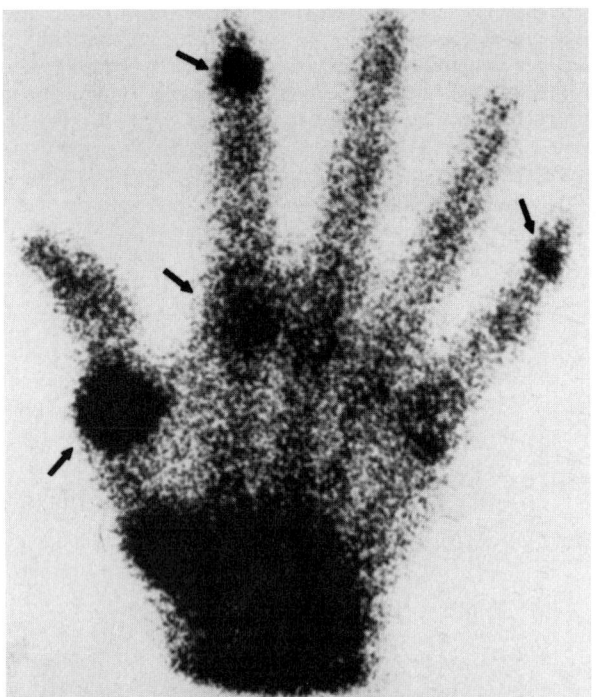

**Figure 19–10.** Scintigraphic abnormalities. Radionuclide imaging using a bone-seeking pharmaceutical preparation in a patient with psoriatic arthritis outlines uptake in the metacarpophalangeal and interphalangeal joints of the hand (*arrows*). Although the other side was involved, the distribution of abnormalities was asymmetrical.

(From Weissberg D, Resnick D, Taylor A, et al: Rheumatoid arthritis and its variants: Analysis of scintiphotographic, radiographic, and clinical examinations. AJR Am J Roentgenol 131:665, 1978.)

edema at entheses, such as the joint capsule, may also be evident; therefore, MR imaging may allow the differentiation of psoriatic arthritis and rheumatoid arthritis. When dactylitis is present, MR imaging reveals distention of the flexor tendon sheaths as a consequence of the tenosynovitis.

## PATHOLOGIC ABNORMALITIES

### Synovial Articulations

Although the pathologic changes of psoriatic arthritis are basically similar to those of rheumatoid arthritis, some pathologic characteristics of psoriatic arthritis are distinctive: (1) synovial inflammation is encountered, but the degree of cellular infiltration with lymphocytes and plasma cells is much less marked than in rheumatoid arthritis; (2) inflammatory synovial tissue, or pannus, is prominent only on the surface of the cartilage, whereas in rheumatoid arthritis, hyperplastic synovium is seen in both the superficial and the deep layers of cartilage; (3) bone proliferation is evident in the periarticular regions; (4) fibrous ankylosis of the articulation may be noted, as in rheumatoid arthritis, but in psoriatic arthritis, bony ankylosis is also prominent.

### Discovertebral Junction

Details of the histologic findings related to paravertebral ossification in psoriatic arthritis (and Reiter's syndrome) are lacking. An inflammatory process in the paravertebral connective tissue or a periosteal reaction at the site of osseous attachment of the ligaments and tendons may be significant in this regard.

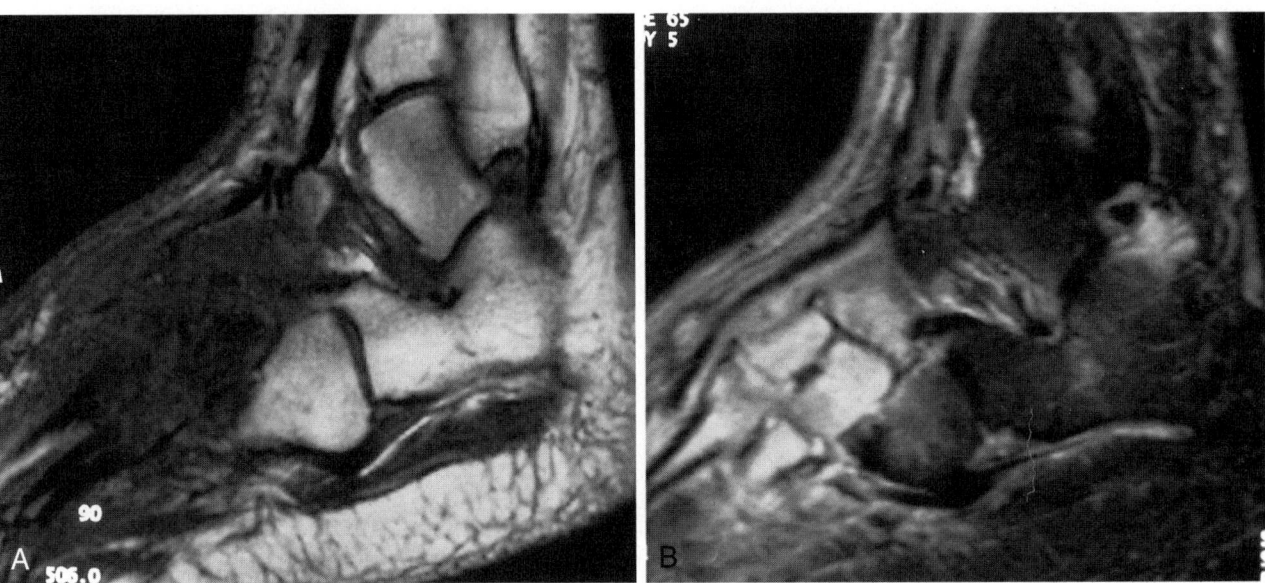

**Figure 19–11.** MR imaging abnormalities. Marrow and soft tissue edema are seen in this patient with psoriatic arthritis and a swollen, hot foot. *A,* Sagittal T1-weighted (TR/TE, 506/12) spin echo MR image shows marrow edema of low signal intensity principally involving the navicular, cuneiform, and metatarsal bones. Dorsal soft tissue edema is also seen. B, Sagittal short tau inversion recovery (STIR) MR image (TR/TE, 7268/60; inversion time, 150 msec) reveals high signal intensity at these same sites, as well as an ankle effusion, increased signal intensity in the sinus tarsi, and subtle calcaneal edema. Biopsy of the bone excluded the presence of infection. (Courtesy of T. Learch, MD, Los Angeles, Calif.)

## Osteolysis

Tapering and dissolution of the terminal phalanges are characteristic alterations in psoriatic arthritis. Initially, thinning or loss of the cortex is related to irregular rapid removal and synthesis of bone. The surrounding periosteal membrane demonstrates noninflammatory cellular proliferation, although the periosteal process ceases with time.

## CAUSE AND PATHOGENESIS

Hereditary factors appear to be important in the pathogenesis of uncomplicated psoriatic arthritis, but the exact mode of inheritance is not known. The role of heredity in the articular manifestations of this disease has also been emphasized. Histocompatibility typing in patients with psoriatic arthritis has revealed a high frequency (approximately 25% to 60%) of HLA-B27 antigen, particularly in patients with sacroiliitis or spondylitis.

## ADDITIONAL DISEASES OF SKIN AND JOINTS

Certain cutaneous disorders are associated with clinical and radiographic findings of arthritis, which in some cases simulate those of psoriatic arthritis. In acne fulminans, arthritis typically occurs in male adolescents. Musculoskeletal symptoms typically begin at the same time as skin abnormalities. Findings may include sacroiliitis and synovitis in the peripheral joints, associated with osteopenia and periostitis. Osteolytic lesions of the cervical vertebral bodies and intervertebral discs may be multiple in about 50% of patients and are commonly accompanied by periosteal reaction. The clavicle, sternum, and tubular bones are frequent sites of involvement.

In acne conglobata and hidradenitis suppurativa, articular disease is seen in adults. Bone erosion about the small joints of the hand, wrist, and foot; periostitis; soft tissue swelling; and osteoporosis are noted. In the axial skeleton, unilateral or, less commonly, bilateral sacroiliitis and syndesmophytosis, particularly in an asymmetrical distribution in the lumbar and thoracic segments, are the reported manifestations.

Pyoderma gangrenosum is characterized by painful skin ulcers and occurs as an isolated event or in combination with ulcerative colitis, Crohn's disease, myeloproliferative disorders, and paraproteinemias. Articular manifestations develop in approximately 30% of patients with this skin disease. Although the joint alterations are variable, pyoderma gangrenosum may be accompanied by a seronegative polyarthritis that is similar or identical to rheumatoid arthritis.

Pustular lesions of the skin in the hand and foot (pustulosis palmaris et plantaris) are observed in some persons with hyperostosis of the clavicles, upper ribs, and sternum. This syndrome, which is termed sternocostoclavicular hyperostosis, and related syndromes, including chronic recurrent multifocal osteomyelitis (CRMO) and synovitis, acne, pustulosis, hyperostosis, and osteitis (SAPHO) syndrome, are discussed in Chapter 82.

Acro-osteolysis may accompany a variety of dermatologic conditions in addition to psoriatic arthritis; they include mycosis fungoides, pityriasis rubra pilaris, epidermolysis bullosa, erythema elevatum diutinum, and ichthyosiform erythroderma.

## DIFFERENTIAL DIAGNOSIS

### Other Seronegative Spondyloarthropathies (Ankylosing Spondylitis, Reiter's Syndrome)

The radiographic findings in psoriatic arthritis are fundamentally similar to those in the other two seronegative spondyloarthropathies, ankylosing spondylitis and Reiter's syndrome (Table 19–3). In all three disorders, synovial joint involvement is characterized by the absence of osteoporosis and the presence of soft tissue swelling, joint space abnormality, osseous erosion, and bony proliferation. In psoriatic arthritis and ankylosing spondylitis, intra-articular bony ankylosis is not uncommon; in Reiter's syndrome, such ankylosis is less frequent. In psoriatic arthritis, the extent of osteolysis of juxta-articular bone is greater than in Reiter's syndrome and ankylosing spondylitis.

In each of these seronegative spondyloarthropathies, abnormalities of the cartilaginous joints, consisting of erosion and bony proliferation, may be observed. Similarly, each of these diseases may be associated with abnormalities at tendon and ligament attachments to bone. In psoriatic arthritis, osteolysis of the terminal phalanges is characteristic.

The distribution of articular abnormalities differs among psoriatic arthritis, Reiter's syndrome, and ankylosing spondylitis. In psoriatic arthritis, an asymmetrical polyarticular disorder involving the upper and lower extremities, with a predilection for the interphalangeal joints of the hands and the metatarsophalangeal and interphalangeal joints of the feet, is observed. In Reiter's syndrome, asymmetrical disease of the articulations of the lower extremity is most characteristic, whereas in ankylosing spondylitis, appendicular skeletal involvement is less prominent than axial skeletal involvement.

Spinal and sacroiliac joint alterations occur in psoriatic arthritis, Reiter's syndrome, and ankylosing spondylitis. In the first two disorders, symmetrical or asymmetrical abnormalities of the sacroiliac joints and large, broad excrescences of the spine may be seen; however, the prevalence and severity of spinal changes, particularly in the cervical spine, are less in Reiter's syndrome than in psoriatic arthritis. In ankylosing spondylitis (as well as in the sacroiliitis and spondylitis of inflammatory bowel disease), bilateral symmetrical sacroiliac joint abnormalities are almost universal, and spinal changes typically consist of thin, linear, and symmetrically distributed outgrowths.

### Rheumatoid Arthritis

In some patients with psoriatic arthritis, the distribution of articular abnormalities in the appendicular skeleton is similar to that in rheumatoid arthritis, whereas in others, asymmetry and extensive distal interphalangeal articular alterations facilitate differentiation from rheumatoid arthritis. In the latter disease, osteoporosis, diffuse joint space narrowing, marginal erosions, and fibrous anky-

**TABLE 19-3**

**Differential Diagnosis of Psoriatic Arthritis**

| | Psoriatic Arthritis | Reiter's Syndrome | Rheumatoid Arthritis |
|---|---|---|---|
| Types of involved articulations | Synovial joints<br>Symphyses<br>Entheses | Synovial joints<br>Symphyses<br>Entheses | Synovial joints* |
| Distribution of arthritis | Appendicular and axial<br>  skeleton<br>Polyarticular or pauciarticular<br>Symmetrical, asymmetrical,<br>  or unilateral<br>Upper and lower extremities<br>Sacroiliac joints and entire<br>  spine | Appendicular and axial<br>  skeleton<br>Polyarticular or pauciarticular<br>Assymmetrical<br><br>Lower extremities<br>Sacroiliac joints and, less<br>  commonly, spine | Appendicular and axial<br>  skeleton<br>Polyarticular<br>Symmetrical<br><br>Upper and lower extremities<br>Cervical spine |
| Nature of lesions[†] | | | |
| Osteoporosis | + | + | ++ |
| Soft tissue swelling | ++ | ++ | ++ |
| Joint space narrowing | + | + | ++ |
| Severe periarticular osteolysis | ++ | + | + |
| Intra-articular bony ankylosis | ++ | ++[‡] | + |
| Bone proliferation and<br>  periostitis | ++ | ++ | –[§] |
| Tuft resorption | ++ | – | – |

*Symphyses and entheses are less commonly and less extensively involved in rheumatoid arthritis than in psoriatic arthritis or Reiter's syndrome.

[†]–, absent; +, occasionally present; ++, commonly present.

[‡]Less frequent than in psoriatic arthritis.

[§]Occassionally seen in male patients with rheumatoid arthritis and in those with both rheumatoid arthritis and diffuse idiopathic skeletal hyperostosis.

**TABLE 19-4**

**Causes of Erosive Arthritis of Distal Interphalangeal Joints**

Psoriatic arthritis
Inflammatory (erosive) osteoarthritis
Gout
Hyperparathyroidism
Multicentric reticulohistiocytosis
Scleroderma
Thermal injuries

losis are most characteristic. In psoriatic arthritis, severe marginal and central erosions, bony ankylosis, and absence of osteoporosis are typical. Further, in psoriatic arthritis, bony proliferation leads to fraying or irregularity of the periarticular bony surfaces, a finding not evident in rheumatoid arthritis.

## Other Disorders

Erosive arthritis of the distal interphalangeal joints can be observed in many disease processes (Table 19–4). Several features of hand and wrist involvement in psoriatic arthritis allow its differentiation from other disorders, especially inflammatory (erosive) osteoarthritis. These features include a tendency to involve articulations of a single ray (ray pattern) or to affect many joints of one hand with sparing of the other (polyarticular unilateral pattern), marginal osseous erosions resembling mouse ears, and the presence or absence of soft tissue swelling.

## FURTHER READING

Avila R, Pugh D, Slocumb CH, et al: Psoriatic arthritis: A roentgenologic study. Radiology 75:691, 1960.

Battistone MJ, Manaster BJ, Reda DJ, et al: The prevalence of sacroiliitis in psoriatic arthritis: New perspectives from a large, multicenter cohort. Skeletal Radiol 28:196, 1999.

Forrester DM: The "cocktail sausage" digit. Arthritis Rheum 26:664, 1983.

Gladman DD: Psoriatic arthritis. In Kelley WW, Harris ED Jr, Ruddy S, et al (eds): Textbook of Rheumatology, 5th ed. Philadelphia, WB Saunders, 1997, p 999.

Hanly JG, Russell ML, Gladman DD: Psoriatic spondyloarthropathy: A long term prospective study. Ann Rheum Dis 47:386, 1988.

Helliwell PS, Hickling P, Wright V: Do the radiological changes of classic ankylosing spondylitis differ from the changes found in the spondylitis associated with inflammatory bowel disease, psoriasis, and reactive arthritis? Ann Rheum Dis 57:135, 1998.

Houben HHML, Lemmens JAM, Boerbooms AMT: Sacroiliitis and acne conglobata. Clin Rheumatol 4:86, 1985.

Knitzer RH, Needleman BW: Musculoskeletal syndromes associated with acne. Semin Arthritis Rheum 20:247, 1991.

Martel W, Stuck KJ, Dworin AM, et al: Erosive osteoarthritis and psoriatic arthritis: A radiologic comparison in the hand, wrist, and foot. AJR Am J Roentgenol 134:125, 1980.

McEwen C, Ditata D, Lingg C, et al: Ankylosing spondylitis and spondylitis accompanying ulcerative colitis, regional enteritis, psoriasis, and Reiter's disease. Arthritis Rheum 14:291, 1971.

McGonagle D, Gibbon W, O'Connor P, et al: Characteristic magnetic resonance imaging entheseal changes of knee synovitis in spondyloarthropathy. Arthritis Rheum 41:694, 1998.

Meaney TF, Hays RA: Roentgen manifestations of psoriatic arthritis. Radiology 68:403, 1957.

Moll JMH, Wright V: Psoriatic arthritis. Semin Arthritis Rheum 3:55, 1973.

Resnick D, Niwayama G: On the nature and significance of bony proliferation in "rheumatoid variant" disorders. AJR Am J Roentgenol 129:275, 1977.

Sundaram M, Patton JT: Paravertebral ossification in psoriasis and Reiter's disease. Br J Radiol 48:628, 1975.

# CHAPTER 20

## Reiter's Syndrome

## SUMMARY OF KEY FEATURES

Reiter's syndrome has a distinctive radiographic appearance. Involvement of the synovial and cartilaginous joints, as well as the sites of tendon and ligament attachment to bone, is observed. In the appendicular skeleton, an asymmetrical arthritis of the articulations of the lower extremity distal to the hip is most typical. Extensive changes may be observed in the foot and the posterior and plantar aspects of the calcaneus. Widespread and severe changes in the upper extremity are unusual. In the axial skeleton, bilateral symmetrical or asymmetrical (or even unilateral) sacroiliac joint abnormalities are seen. Paravertebral ossification may produce bulky outgrowths, particularly in the thoracolumbar region. The symphysis pubis and manubriosternal joint can reveal significant erosion and sclerosis. The findings of Reiter's syndrome are similar to those of the other two seronegative spondyloarthropathies—ankylosing spondylitis and psoriatic arthritis—although their distribution usually allows an accurate diagnosis.

## INTRODUCTION

The classic triad of Reiter's syndrome consists of urethritis, arthritis, and conjunctivitis. Currently, it is recognized that many patients who apparently have Reiter's syndrome do not demonstrate all three elements. Until the cause of Reiter's syndrome is firmly established, however, it cannot be said with certainty that patients with an incomplete syndrome suffer from the same disorder as patients with the triad of urethritis, arthritis, and conjunctivitis. Although radiographic findings may not be an essential part of these criteria, few investigators would dispute that radiographs are important in the evaluation of patients with this syndrome.

Reiter's syndrome is accompanied by typical radiographic features, which it shares with the other seronegative spondyloarthropathies—psoriatic arthritis and ankylosing spondylitis. It is the distribution of articular abnormalities that allows a firm radiographic diagnosis in many patients with Reiter's syndrome. This chapter delineates the radiographic characteristics and distribution of the syndrome.

## CLINICAL ABNORMALITIES

### Age and Sex

Reiter's syndrome is a relatively uncommon articular disorder. It appears likely that the disease can be transmitted in association with either epidemic dysentery or sexual intercourse. Most patients with Reiter's syndrome are between 15 and 35 years of age. At any age, the disease is much more common in men than in women, with the cited male-female ratio ranging from 5:1 to 50:1. Reiter's syndrome in female patients is especially common after dysentery and may consist of arthritis, conjunctivitis, and cystitis. The intestinal variety of the disease usually follows bacillary dysentery, although the syndrome may occur after amebic dysentery, shigellosis, and other gastrointestinal disorders.

### General Symptoms and Signs

Urethritis is frequently the initial manifestation of the disease. Circinate balanitis has been noted in 20% to 80% of patients with the dysenteric and venereal forms of Reiter's syndrome. Early and transient conjunctivitis frequently accompanies acute attacks. Mild bilateral involvement is characteristic, with burning and itching of the eyes. Later and more severe ocular involvement may include episcleritis, keratitis, uveitis, iritis, retrobulbar neuritis, corneal ulceration, and intraocular hemorrhage.

The characteristic skin lesion, which occurs in 5% to 30% of patients, is termed keratoderma blennorrhagicum. It is most commonly noted on the soles of the feet and the palms of the hands. The skin lesions pass through various stages: macular, papular, vesicular, and pustular. Keratosis of the nails may also be observed and simulate the findings of psoriasis.

On the buccal mucosa and the tongue, superficial erythematous ulcerations may be evident in 5% to 10% of patients. Reiter's syndrome may involve other organ systems, including the gastrointestinal tract (diarrhea, dysentery) and the cardiovascular (palpitations, valvular damage), neurologic (encephalitis, peripheral neuropathy), and pulmonary (pneumonia, fibrosis, pleurisy) systems. Additional clinical findings in Reiter's syndrome include fever, weight loss, thrombophlebitis, amyloidosis, and rheumatoid arthritis. The serum histocompatibility antigen HLA-B27 may be present in as many as 75% of patients.

### Articular Symptoms and Signs

Characteristically, an asymmetrical arthritis of the lower extremity becomes evident in Reiter's syndrome, often within 1 to 3 weeks of the inciting episode of urethritis or diarrhea. Initially, the most commonly affected joints are the knee and the ankle, followed in descending order of frequency by the metatarsophalangeal joints, heel, shoulder, wrist, hip, and lumbar spine. The occurrence of heel pain and tenderness should be stressed as a common manifestation of Reiter's syndrome. The pain, which may be located posteriorly (in the region of the retrocalcaneal bursa or Achilles tendon) or inferiorly (at the site of attachment of the aponeurosis on the plantar surface of the calcaneus), can be the initial symptom of the disease, even preceding the ocular and urethral findings. The arthritic attacks of Reiter's syndrome are usually self-limited and of short duration, although recurrences are frequent. Residual disability and deformity occur in approximately 5% of patients.

## RADIOGRAPHIC ABNORMALITIES

The radiographic features of Reiter's syndrome have received considerable emphasis in the literature (Table 20–1).

### Frequency and Distribution of Radiographic Abnormalities

Sixty percent to 80% of patients with Reiter's syndrome will develop radiographic alterations. In the early phases of the disease, radiographs may be entirely normal. Acute attacks of arthritis may be accompanied by soft tissue swelling and osteoporosis, but these findings may disappear completely, without residual abnormalities. With repeated episodes of arthritis, however, permanent radiographic abnormalities are common.

The synovial joints, symphyses, and entheses are affected. Typically, an asymmetrical distribution, with a predilection for articulations of the lower extremity, is seen (Fig. 20–1). The most characteristic sites of abnormality are the small articulations of the foot, the calcaneus, the ankle, and the knee. Joint alterations in the upper extremity are less frequent, and abnormalities of the hip are uncommon. In the axial skeleton, the sacroiliac joints, spine, symphysis pubis, and manubriosternal articulation are frequent targets.

### General Radiographic Abnormalities

The general radiographic characteristics of articular involvement in Reiter's syndrome are similar to those in the other seronegative spondyloarthropathies (ankylosing spondylitis and psoriatic arthritis) and differ from those of rheumatoid arthritis (Fig. 20–2).

**Soft Tissue Swelling.** Soft tissue prominence is related to intra-articular effusion, periarticular edema, and inflammation of bursal and tendinous structures. This finding, which is not specific, is frequent in the interphalangeal joints of the toes and the fingers and may result in sausage-like swelling of an entire digit.

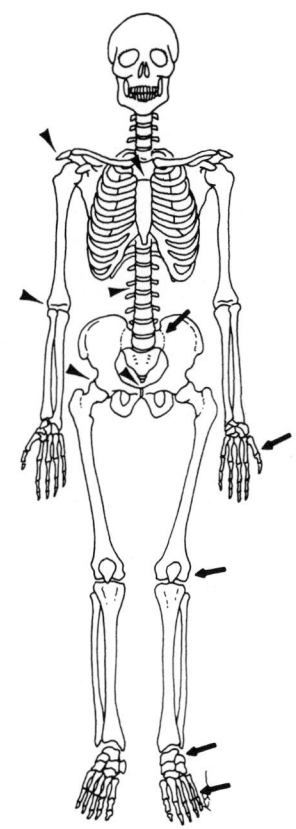

**Figure 20–1.** Reiter's syndrome: distribution of articular abnormalities. The most characteristic sites of involvement are the small articulations of the foot, calcaneus, ankle, knee, hand, and sacroiliac joint (*arrows*). Less commonly, the shoulder, elbow, hip, spine, symphysis pubis, and manubriosternal joint are affected (*arrowheads*).

**Osteoporosis.** Regional or periarticular osteoporosis accompanies acute episodes of arthritis. With recurrent or prolonged bouts of articular disease, osteoporosis may decrease in extent and severity, and it is not uncommon to detect severe cartilaginous and osseous lesions without adjacent osteoporosis.

**Joint Space Narrowing.** Loss of the interosseous space is more frequent in the small articulations of the foot, hand, and wrist than in the knee and ankle. This finding may be observed in, the acute or chronic phases of the disease. Diffuse loss of articular space is more characteristic than focal joint space diminution.

**Bone Erosion.** Erosion of articular surfaces may be noted in both the appendicular and the axial skeleton. The most frequent sites of osseous erosion are the small joints of the foot, hand, and wrist; the knee; and the sacroiliac joint. Erosions initially appear at the joint margins and may later progress to involve the subchondral bone in the central portion of the articulation. Superficial resorption of the osseous surface may also occur beneath inflamed bursae and tendon sheaths.

**Bony Proliferation.** Bony proliferation is particularly characteristic of all three seronegative spondyloarthro-

---

**TABLE 20-1**

**Characteristics of Arthritis in Reiter's Syndrome**

Involvement of synovial joints, symphyses, and entheses
Asymmetrical arthritis of the lower extremities
Predilection for the small articulations of the foot, calcaneus, ankle, knee, and sacroiliac joint
Bone erosion with adjacent proliferation
Paravertebral ossification

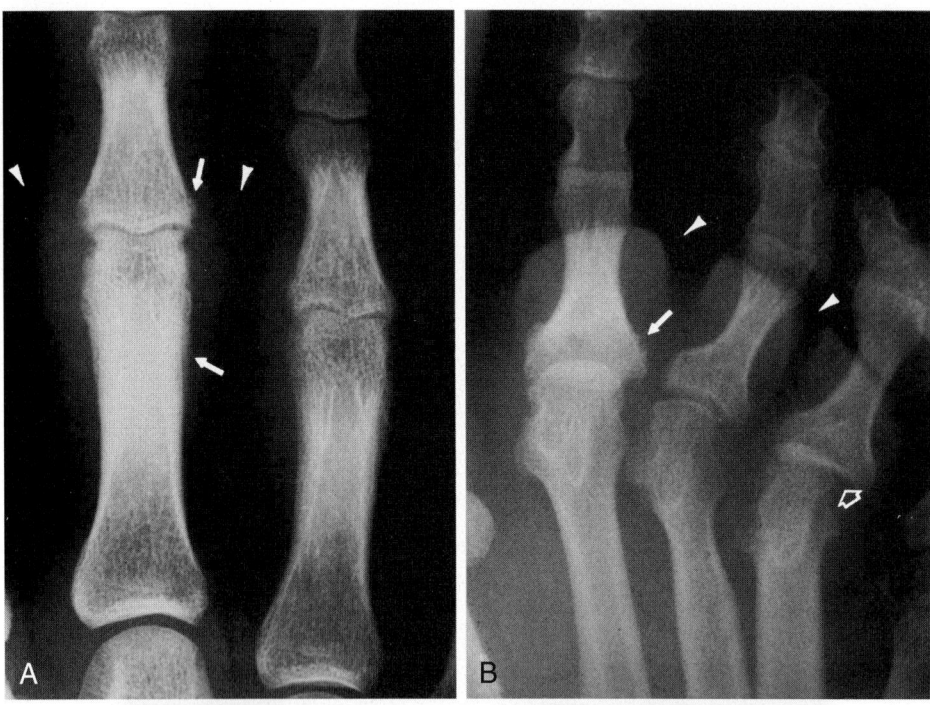

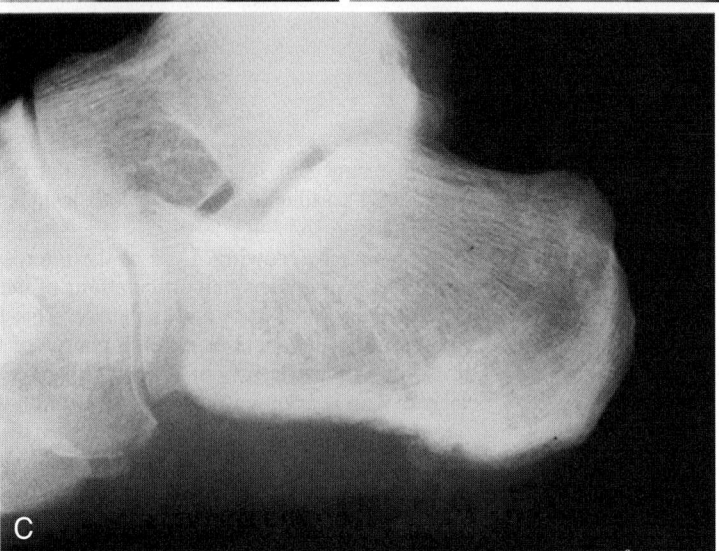

**Figure 20–2.** General radiographic abnormalities of Reiter's syndrome in three different patients. Note the absence of osteoporosis and the presence of soft tissue swelling *(arrowheads)*, periostitis and "whiskering" *(A and B, solid arrows)*, osseous erosions, subluxation *(B, open arrow)*, and bone production along the plantar aspect of the calcaneus *(C)*.

pathies and is the most helpful radiographic feature in distinguishing these conditions from rheumatoid arthritis. Linear or fluffy periosteal bony proliferation is not uncommon in Reiter's syndrome, especially in the metacarpal, metatarsal, and phalangeal shafts; the malleolar region; and the knee. At sites of tendon and ligament attachment to bone (e.g., plantar aspect of calcaneus, ischial tuberosity), osseous surfaces frequently appear poorly defined or frayed. The eroded bony surfaces appear irregular, fuzzy, or blurred in outline, and the articular bone may be enlarged. Subchondral sclerosis and eburnation and adjacent periostitis are associated radiographic findings. Intra-articular bony ankylosis has been recorded in the small joints of the hands and feet, but this complication is far less frequent.

**Tendinous Calcification and Ossification.** Tendinous calcification and ossification are frequent about the knee, where the findings can resemble Pellegrini-Stieda syndrome (posttraumatic calcification of the medial collateral ligament).

## Specific Sites of Abnormality

**Forefoot.** Radiographs of the feet frequently reveal asymmetrical involvement of the metatarsophalangeal and interphalangeal joints (Fig. 20–3); the reported prevalence of these findings varies from 40% to 55%. At any location in the foot, osteoporosis, joint space loss, and marginal erosions with adjacent proliferation can be observed. The sesamoid bones can undergo significant erosion and proliferation. Subluxation and deformity of

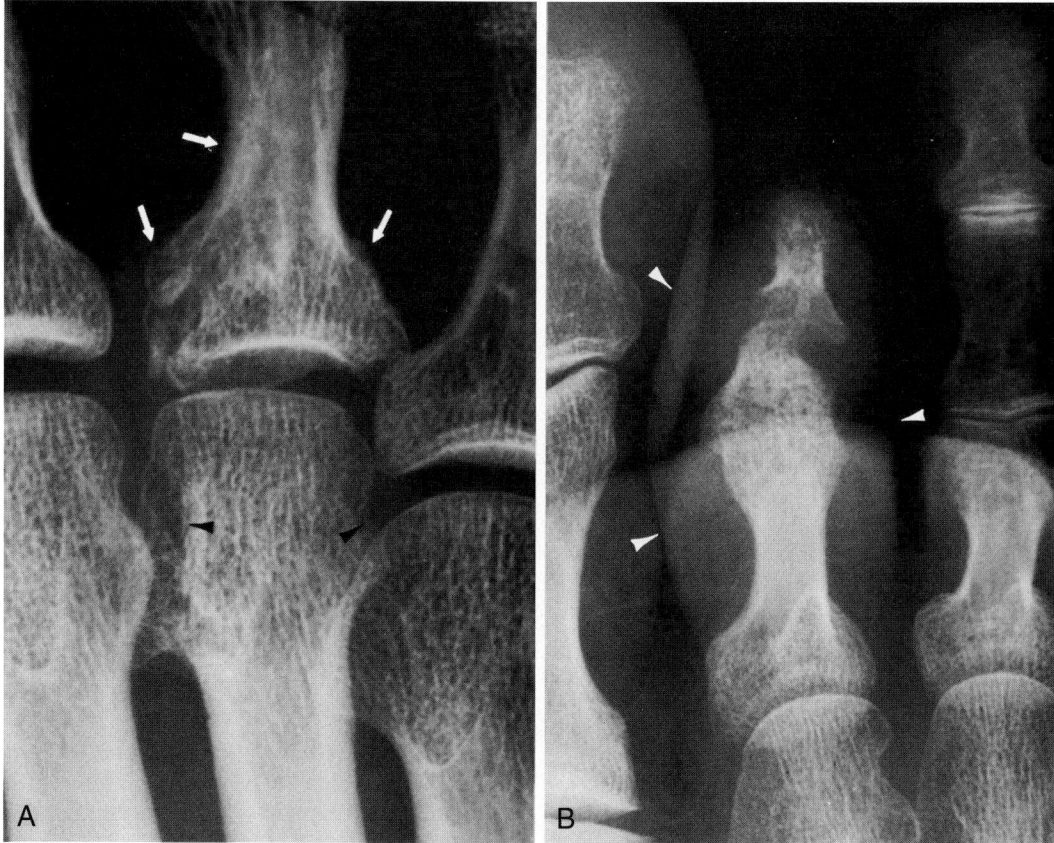

**Figure 20–3.** Abnormalities of the forefoot. *A*, Magnification radiograph of the third metatarsophalangeal joint outlines erosions of the metatarsal head *(arrowheads)* and adjacent bony proliferation *(arrows)*. The joint space is not narrowed. *B*, Radiograph of the forefoot reveals soft tissue swelling of the second digit *(arrowheads)*, destruction of the distal interphalangeal joint, and intra-articular bony ankylosis of the proximal interphalangeal joint. Note the absence of osteoporosis.

the metatarsophalangeal articulations may be evident, an appearance that has been termed Launois' deformity.

**Calcaneus.** Calcaneal alterations are characteristic of Reiter's syndrome (25% to 50% of patients). Both the posterior (Fig. 20–4) and the plantar (see Fig. 20–2C) aspects of the bone are affected. Bilateral changes are frequent. Retrocalcaneal bursitis with fluid accumulation creates a radiodense shadow that, on lateral radiographs, obliterates the normal lucent area between the top of the calcaneus and the adjacent Achilles tendon and projects into the pre-Achilles fat pad. Subsequently, poorly defined calcaneal erosions appear on the posterior and postero-superior aspects of the bone. The Achilles tendon is frequently thickened. Posterior calcaneal enthesophytes at the site of attachment of the Achilles tendon to the calcaneus are rare in Reiter's syndrome.

**Ankle and Tarsal Areas.** In approximately 25% of patients, erosive and proliferative changes are evident, with irregular or fluffy exuberant new bone formation in response to erosion. Radiographic abnormalities about one or both ankles can be recognized in 30% to 50% of patients, including soft tissue swelling, linear or fluffy periostitis, articular space loss, and, less frequently, marginal erosions.

**Hand and Wrist.** Severe and widespread radiographic abnormalities of the upper extremity are distinctly unusual in Reiter's syndrome. In 10% to 30% of patients, however, one or more fingers of one or both hands reveal significant radiographic changes (Fig. 20–5). Proximal interphalangeal joint abnormalities are more frequent than metacarpophalangeal or distal interphalangeal joint alterations. Fusiform or sausage-like soft tissue swelling, regional or periarticular osteoporosis, and joint space narrowing may be evident. The erosive changes are accompanied by fluffy new bone formation. Wrist involvement is usually asymmetrical (Fig. 20–6).

**Manubriosternal Joint and Symphysis Pubis.** Osseous erosion and adjacent bony proliferation at the manubriosternal articulation are not rare in Reiter's disease. Similar abnormalities occur at the symphysis pubis, and at this location, apposing margins of the pubic bones may appear eroded and sclerotic.

**Sacroiliac Joint.** Sacroiliitis is common in Reiter's syndrome (Fig. 20–7). Initially, abnormalities may be detected in only 5% to 10% of patients, but after several years, sacroiliac joint alterations may affect 40% to 60%. Bilateral symmetrical or asymmetrical changes are typical;

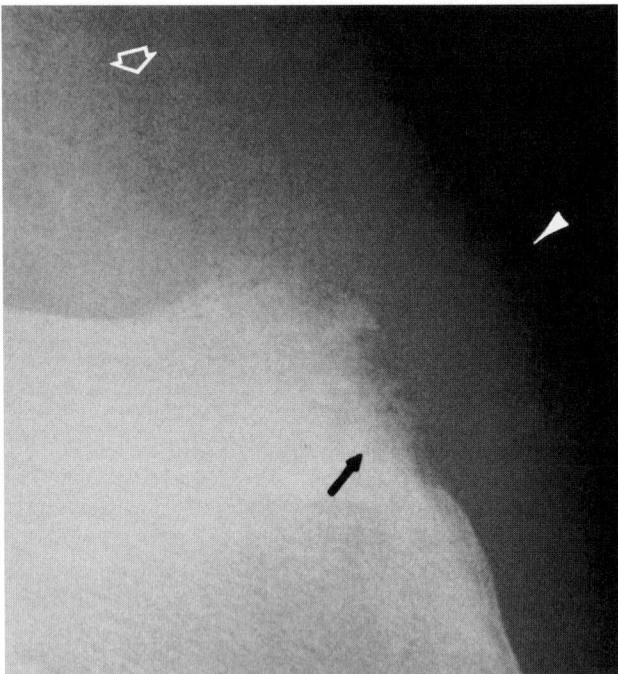

**Figure 20–4.** Abnormalities of the calcaneus: posterior aspect. Soft tissue swelling *(arrowhead)*, retrocalcaneal bursitis *(open arrow)*, and irregular osseous erosion and proliferation *(solid arrow)* are apparent.

however, asymmetrical and, less commonly, unilateral sacroiliac joint abnormalities do occur, particularly early in the disease process.

Osseous erosion on the iliac surface predominates over that on the sacral surface. Adjacent sclerosis varies from mild to severe. Early joint space widening may later be replaced by narrowing of the space between the sacrum and ilium. Although intra-articular osseous fusion may eventually appear, this finding is less frequent in Reiter's syndrome (and psoriatic arthritis) than in classic ankylosing spondylitis and the sacroiliitis of inflammatory bowel disease.

**Spine.** Although abnormalities of the spine occur in Reiter's syndrome, their frequency and extent are less than in classic ankylosing spondylitis and psoriatic arthritis. When present, these changes may resemble those of ankylosing spondylitis, although specific radiographic features allow accurate differentiation of the two conditions in some cases.

An early finding in Reiter's syndrome (and psoriatic arthritis) is the appearance of paravertebral ossification about the lower three thoracic and upper three lumbar vertebrae (Fig. 20–8). On frontal radiographs, elongated vertical osseous bridges extend across the intervertebral disc but are separated by a clear space from the lateral margins of both the disc and the vertebral body. The outgrowths may be either well defined and linear or thick and fluffy. Their course is also variable, although many of the ossifications eventually fuse with the underlying intervertebral disc and vertebral body, simulating the appearance of bulky osteophytes (spondylosis deformans). Involvement of large segments of the thoracic and lumbar spine, as well as the cervical spine, may eventually be noted.

The importance of recognizing paravertebral ossification is twofold: the finding may be an initial manifestation of the disease, and the abnormality is more diagnostic of Reiter's syndrome or psoriatic arthritis than of

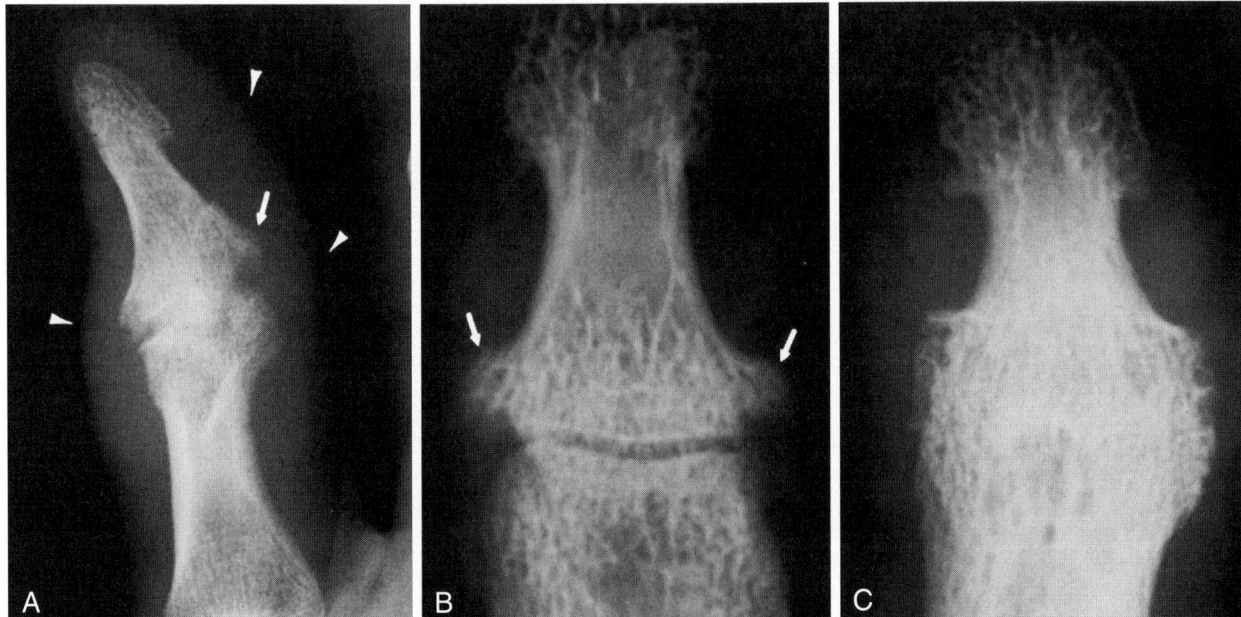

**Figure 20–5.** Abnormalities of the hand. *A,* Soft tissue swelling *(arrowheads)*, erosion, and bony proliferation *(arrow)* are the radiographic findings. *B,* Note joint space narrowing and irregular excrescences, or "whiskers" *(arrows)*, at the margins of the distal interphalangeal joint. *C,* In another patient, intra-articular bony ankylosis is evident.

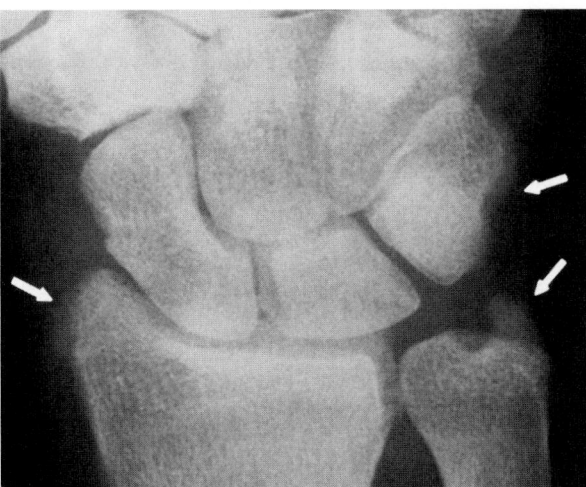

**Figure 20–6.** Abnormalities of the wrist. The major radiographic abnormality is bony proliferation *(arrows)* about several compartments of the wrist. Soft tissue swelling is also evident.

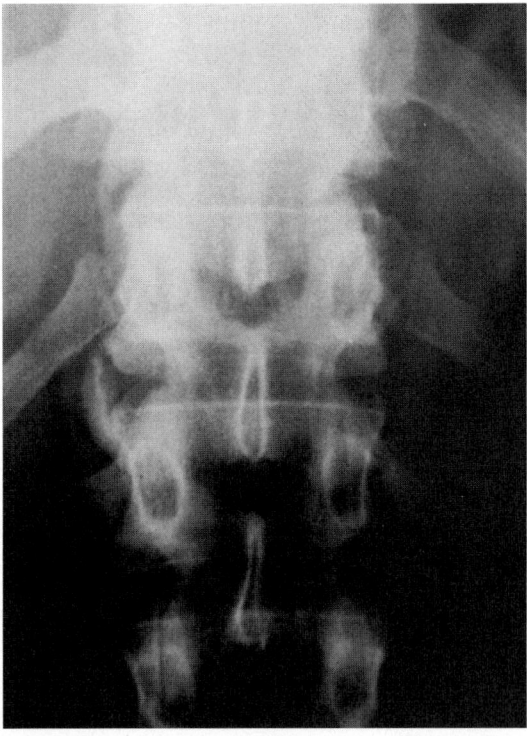

**Figure 20–8.** Abnormalities of the spine. Radiograph of the thoracolumbar spine shows paravertebral ossification. Note the asymmetrical nature and lateral location of the outgrowths.

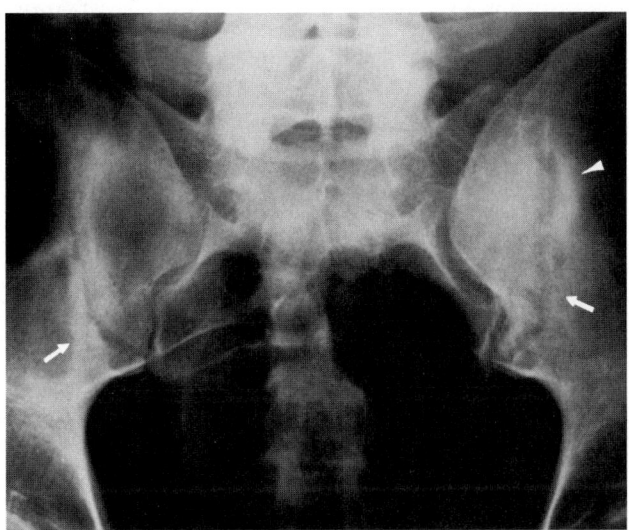

**Figure 20–7.** Abnormalities of the sacroiliac joint. Bilateral and asymmetrical alterations are observed in Reiter's syndrome. Erosions and reactive eburnation predominate in the ilium *(arrows)*. Also, hyperostosis can be seen at the superior aspect of the joint *(arrowhead)*.

classic ankylosing spondylitis or the spondylitis associated with inflammatory bowel disease. In the latter regard, the asymmetrical distribution (right and left sides), the broader or bulkier nature of the radiodense areas, and their relatively distant position from the spine are characteristic of paravertebral ossification. Some patients with Reiter's syndrome and psoriatic arthritis develop typical syndesmophytes of the spine. Further, apophyseal joint erosion, sclerosis, and osseous fusion may be apparent in Reiter's syndrome, although the frequency of these findings is less than in classic ankylosing spondylitis.

Cervical spine abnormalities are not frequent in Reiter's syndrome. Atlantoaxial subluxation and odontoid erosion, although rare, have been observed in patients with Reiter's syndrome.

## OTHER DIAGNOSTIC TECHNIQUES

Scintigraphy with bone-seeking radiopharmaceutical agents may allow the early diagnosis of Reiter's syndrome. Asymmetrical involvement of the articulations of the lower extremity is typically seen. Increasing radioactivity related to the plantar and posterior aspects of the calcaneus may be striking. Asymmetrical accumulation about the sacroiliac joints also facilitates the diagnosis of sacroiliitis (Fig. 20–9).

As in rheumatoid arthritis and other synovial inflammatory diseases, magnetic resonance imaging in Reiter's disease can reveal information about the extent of the process; the presence of bursitis, tenosynovitis, and sacroiliitis; and the occurrence of such complications as synovial cysts (Fig. 20–10).

## CAUSE AND PATHOGENESIS

Of all the rheumatic diseases, Reiter's syndrome is most likely to have an infectious cause. The syndrome frequently follows an infection of the bowel or lower genitourinary tract, and it seems likely that these sites are the portals of entry for the causative agent. Considerable

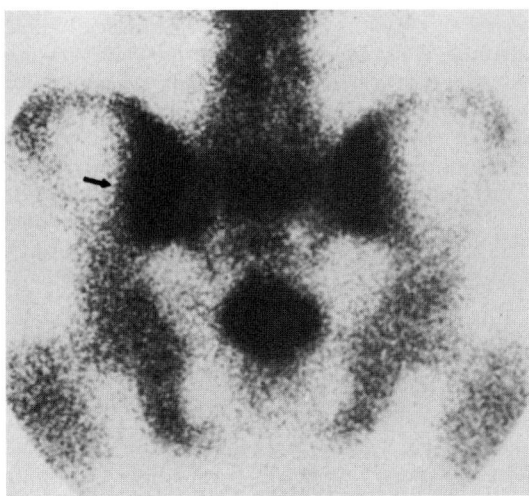

**Figure 20–9.** Radionuclide abnormalities. Asymmetrical sacroiliitis, greater on the right side, is evident with scintigraphy (*arrow*).

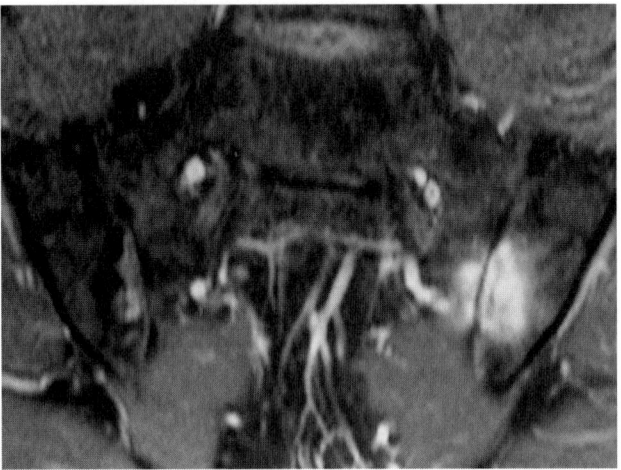

**Figure 20–10.** Magnetic resonance (MR) imaging abnormalities: sacroiliitis. Oblique, transverse, fat-suppressed T1-weighted spin echo MR image obtained after intravenous gadolinium administration reveals high signal intensity in the left sacrum and ilium, indicating sacroiliitis. (Courtesy of G. Sandrini De Toni, MD, São Paulo, Brazil.)

difficulty has been encountered in attempting to isolate a specific infective agent in Reiter's syndrome.

An alternative explanation for the association of Reiter's syndrome and bowel or genitourinary infection is that Reiter's syndrome is related not to purulent arthritis but to the reaction of a joint (or other target site) to infection elsewhere in the body. The concept of reactive arthritis is discussed in Chapters 21 and 53, with rheumatic fever, initiated by a beta-hemolytic streptococcal infection in the throat, being a classic example.

The increased frequency (up to 96%) of the histocompatibility antigen HLA-B27 in this disorder is well recognized. Possession of this antigen may predispose patients to Reiter's syndrome after exposure to an infectious agent.

## DIFFERENTIAL DIAGNOSIS

### Other Seronegative Spondyloarthropathies

Although its general features resemble those of the other two seronegative spondyloarthropathies (ankylosing spondylitis and psoriatic arthritis), Reiter's syndrome has a sufficiently characteristic articular distribution to allow accurate diagnosis. This syndrome is associated with an asymmetrical arthritis of the lower extremity, sacroiliitis, and, less commonly, spondylitis. Ankylosing spondylitis has a similar axial skeletal appearance, but significant peripheral articular changes are less frequent. Psoriatic arthritis may lead to considerable alterations in the articulations of both the appendicular and the axial skeleton. In psoriatic arthritis, however, widespread involvement of the upper extremity may be apparent. In all three spondyloarthropathies, the presence of soft tissue swelling, joint space narrowing, erosions, and bony proliferation in synovial articulations is typical. In Reiter's syndrome, the frequency of osteoporosis in the acute phase of the disease appears to be greater than in psoriatic arthritis and ankylosing spondylitis, and the frequency of intra-articular bony ankylosis is less than in the other two diseases.

The sacroiliac and spinal changes of Reiter's syndrome are virtually identical to those of psoriatic arthritis, although the prevalence and severity of these abnormalities and the tendency to involve the cervical spine are greater in psoriatic arthritis. Symmetrical, asymmetrical, or unilateral sacroiliac articular changes and broad asymmetrical spinal outgrowths occur in both Reiter's syndrome and psoriatic arthritis. In classic ankylosing spondylitis, symmetrical sacroiliac joint changes and symmetrical slender bony outgrowths of the spine are typical. Further, in ankylosing spondylitis, vertebral body osteitis, apophyseal joint ankylosis, and intra-articular osseous fusion of the sacroiliac joint are more frequent than in Reiter's syndrome or psoriatic arthritis. The spondylitis and sacroiliitis of inflammatory bowel disease are identical to those of classic ankylosing spondylitis.

### Rheumatoid Arthritis

The radiographic features of rheumatoid arthritis differ considerably from those of Reiter's syndrome. Rheumatoid arthritis is associated with bilateral and symmetrical alterations. Osteoporosis, early joint space narrowing, and marginal erosions are observed. Bony proliferation is unusual, and the irregular, proliferative, erosive changes of the spondyloarthropathies are not seen in rheumatoid arthritis. Widespread and severe sacroiliac and thoracolumbar spinal changes are very uncommon in rheumatoid arthritis.

### Septic Arthritis and Osteomyelitis

The early localized abnormalities of Reiter's syndrome may resemble the findings of osseous and articular infection. Soft tissue swelling, osteoporosis, bony and cartilaginous destruction, and periostitis are evident in both Reiter's syndrome and infectious disease. Eventually, the polyarticular nature of Reiter's syndrome allows its accurate differentiation from infectious disease.

## FURTHER READING

El-Khoury GY, Kathol MH, Brandser EA: Seronegative spondyloarthropathies. Radiol Clin North Am 34:343, 1996.

Fan PT, Yu DTY: Reiter's syndrome. In Kelley WN, Harris ED Jr, Ruddy S, et al (eds): Textbook of Rheumatology, 5th ed. Philadelphia, WB Saunders, 1997, p 983.

Helliwell PS, Hickling P, Wright V: Do the radiological changes of classic ankylosing spondylitis differ from the changes found in the spondylitis associated with inflammatory bowel disease, psoriasis, and reactive arthritis? Ann Rheum Dis 57:135, 1998.

Keat A: Reiter's syndrome and reactive arthritis in perspective. N Engl J Med 309:1606, 1983.

Kransdorf MJ, Wehrle PA, Moser RP Jr: Atlantoaxial subluxation in Reiter's syndrome: A report of three cases and review of the literature. Spine 13:12, 1988.

Martel W, Braunstein EM, Borlaza G, et al: Radiologic features of Reiter's disease. Radiology 132:1, 1979.

McEwen C, Di Tata D, Lingg C, et al: Ankylosing spondylitis and spondylitis accompanying ulcerative colitis, regional enteritis, psoriasis and Reiter's disease. Arthritis Rheum 14:291, 1971.

Peterson CC Jr, Silbiger ML: Reiter's syndrome and psoriatic arthritis: Their roentgen spectra and some interesting similarities. AJR Am J Roentgenol 101:860, 1967.

Resnick D, Feingold ML, Curd J, et al: Calcaneal abnormalities in articular disorders: Rheumatoid arthritis, ankylosing spondylitis, psoriatic arthritis and Reiter's syndrome. Radiology 125:355, 1977.

Sholkoff SD, Glickman MG, Steinback HL: Roentgenology of Reiter's syndrome. Radiology 97:497, 1970.

Sundaram M, Patton JT: Paravertebral ossification in psoriasis and Reiter's disease. Br J Radiol 48:628, 1975.

Weinberger HW, Ropes MW, Kulka JP, et al: Reiter's syndrome: Clinical and pathological observations—a long term study of 16 cases. Medicine 41:35, 1962.

Weldon WV, Scalettar R: Roentgen changes in Reiter's syndrome. AJR Am J Roentgenol 86:344, 1961.

# CHAPTER 21

## Enteropathic Arthropathies

## SUMMARY OF KEY FEATURES

Musculoskeletal manifestations are frequently associated with disorders of the gastrointestinal system. Peripheral joint arthralgias and arthritis accompany ulcerative colitis, Crohn's disease, and Whipple's disease, although radiographic findings are generally minimal and nonspecific. In addition, these three disorders may be associated with sacroiliac and spinal abnormalities that are identical to those of classic ankylosing spondylitis. Intestinal infections related to *Salmonella*, *Shigella*, and *Yersinia* organisms can lead to polyarthritis and, in rare circumstances, sacroiliitis and spondylitis. Intestinal bypass surgery may provoke a similar response in joints of the appendicular and axial skeletons. Joint manifestations also accompany Laënnec's cirrhosis, viral hepatitis, chronic active hepatitis, and biliary cirrhosis. In biliary cirrhosis, xanthomas and a peculiar type of erosive arthritis may be evident. Pancreatic disorders can manifest as subcutaneous nodules, skin lesions, and polyarthritis, probably related to fat necrosis; epiphyseal and diametaphyseal infarction; and skeletal metastasis. Bone resorption in association with carcinoid tumors simulates the findings of hyperparathyroidism.

## INTRODUCTION

The appearance of musculoskeletal abnormalities in patients with gastrointestinal disorders has been recognized with increasing frequency in recent years. These abnormalities have been designated enteropathic arthropathies because of the close association of articular and intestinal findings (Table 21–1). Ulcerative colitis, Crohn's disease (regional enteritis), and Whipple's disease are three intestinal diseases whose rheumatologic manifestations are now well known. In addition, musculoskeletal abnormalities can occur after certain intestinal infections, specifically, those associated with *Salmonella*, *Shigella*, or *Yersinia* organisms; after intestinal bypass surgery; and as a complication of extraintestinal disorders, including Laënnec's and biliary cirrhosis, hepatitis, and pancreatic disease.

The relationship between inflammatory intestinal diseases and arthritis is not fully understood. Several theoretical possibilities could explain this relationship. An infectious cause has been postulated, as has an immune mechanism. Evidence also indicates that genetic factors play an important role in the development of enteropathic arthropathies. Approximately 90% of patients with ulcerative colitis and Crohn's disease in whom spondylitis or sacroiliitis develops demonstrate the genetically determined histocompatibility antigen HLA-B27 on their cells.

## ULCERATIVE COLITIS

### General Abnormalities

Ulcerative colitis is a chronic inflammatory disease of unknown cause that has a predilection for the young. Clinical findings associated with colon involvement include malaise, anorexia, weight loss, and a change in stool consistency. The severity of the disorder differs from one person to another, but significant complications may be encountered, including intestinal obstruction, perforation, fistulas, and perianal abnormalities. Musculoskeletal abnormalities are the most common extraintestinal manifestation of the disease. The type of articular disease can be categorized as peripheral joint arthralgia and arthritis (50% to 60%), sacroiliitis and spondylitis (20% to 30%), and miscellaneous abnormalities (10% to 20%).

### Peripheral Joint Arthralgia and Arthritis

The reported frequency of peripheral joint abnormalities in ulcerative colitis varies from 0 to 25%, although a frequency of 10% to 12% seems most typical. Adults are usually affected. Although bowel disease is usually clinically evident before the onset of arthritis, articular abnormalities may appear before intestinal abnormalities in 10% to 15% of patients. A close temporal association exists between exacerbations of intestinal disease and joint inflammation.

The articular findings can be categorized as an acute synovitis that is predominantly monoarticular or pauciarticular in distribution, although it can be polyarticular. The knees are involved most commonly, followed by the ankles, elbows, wrists, shoulders, and small joints of the hands and feet. Asymmetrical inflammation of the proximal interphalangeal joints of the toes is suggestive of "colitic arthritis." Joints in the lower extremity are affected more frequently than those in the upper extremity. The attacks are usually self-limited, frequently resolving within 1 to 3 months. Permanent joint abnormalities are infrequent, even in the setting of recurrent clinical attacks of arthritis. Although cartilaginous and osseous changes can develop, joint deformities are exceedingly rare.

The radiographic analysis is nonspecific. Soft tissue swelling and periarticular osteoporosis are the two most common radiographic characteristics (Fig. 21–1). Radiographic evidence of osseous and cartilaginous destruction is unusual, but when present, the findings can simulate those of rheumatoid arthritis. The cause and pathogenesis of peripheral joint disease in ulcerative colitis are not known.

### Sacroiliitis and Spondylitis

The reported frequency of ankylosing spondylitis in patients with ulcerative colitis varies from 1% to about 30%. Conversely, estimates of the frequency of chronic inflammatory bowel disease in ankylosing spondylitis

**TABLE 21–1**

### Radiographic Manifestations of Enteropathic Arthropathies

| Disorder | Sacroiliitis | Spondylitis | Peripheral Joints | Other Manifestations |
|---|---|---|---|---|
| Ulcerative colitis | + | + | Soft tissue swelling<br>Osteoporosis<br>Joint space narrowing (r)<br>Erosions, cysts (r) | Periostitis (r) |
| Crohn's disease | + | + | Soft tissue swelling<br>Osteoporosis<br>Joint space narrowing (r)<br>Erosions, cysts (r)<br>Septic arthritis (r) | Periostitis (r)<br>Osseous granulomas (r)<br>Osteomyelitis (r) |
| Whipple's disease | + | + | Soft tissue swelling<br>Osteoporosis<br>Joint space narrowing (r)<br>Erosions, cysts (r) | Subcutaneous nodules (r) |
| *Salmonella, Shigella,* and *Yersinia* infections | + | + | Soft tissue swelling<br>Osteoporosis<br>Septic arthritis | |
| Intestinal bypass surgery | + | + | Soft tissue swelling<br>Osteoporosis<br>Gout (r) | Osteomalacia (r) |
| Laënnec's cirrhosis | | | Soft tissue swelling<br>Osteoporosis | Soft tissue calcification (r) |
| Biliary cirrhosis | | | Soft tissue swelling<br>Joint space narrowing<br>Erosions<br>Destruction<br>Chondrocalcinosis (r) | Osteomalacia<br>Xanthoma<br>Periostitis (r) |
| Viral hepatitis | | | Soft tissue swelling (r) | Subcutaneous nodules |
| Pancreatic disease | | | Soft tissue swelling (r)<br>Osteoporosis<br>Erosions, cysts (r)<br>Osteonecrosis | Subcutaneous nodules<br>Osteolysis<br>Periostitis<br>Metastasis |

+, present; r, rare.

range from 2% to 18%. Spondylitis in ulcerative colitis is poorly correlated with activity of the bowel disease. Further, spinal abnormalities may manifest before, at the same time as, or after the onset of intestinal changes. The clinical features of ankylosing spondylitis in patients with ulcerative colitis are identical to those of classic ankylosing spondylitis, although the male predilection may be less striking. Laboratory evaluation reveals an increased frequency of the histocompatibility antigen HLA-B27, although not as great as in classic ankylosing spondylitis. This antigen is not commonly detected in patients with inflammatory bowel disease.

On radiographic examination, the spinal and sacroiliac joint abnormalities in ulcerative colitis are virtually indistinguishable from those in classic ankylosing spondylitis. Sacroiliac joint involvement is usually bilateral and symmetrical in distribution (Fig. 21–2). Osseous erosion and sclerosis are evident, as well as joint space alterations. Initially, the articular space may appear widened, although joint space narrowing and bony ankylosis are common in later stages of the disease. Additional pelvic abnormalities include bone erosion and sclerosis about the symphysis pubis and bone erosion and proliferation at the ischial tuberosities and iliac crests. In the spine, vertebral body erosions with alterations in vertebral shape (squaring) are seen. Eventually, a bamboo spine may be evident. In the apophyseal joints, articular space narrowing, erosion, sclerosis, and bony ankylosis are identical to changes in classic ankylosing spondylitis.

The sacroiliitis and spondylitis of classic ankylosing spondylitis and ulcerative colitis (as well as Crohn's disease) are readily differentiated from the sacroiliitis and spondylitis of psoriatic arthritis and Reiter's syndrome. Bilateral, symmetrical sacroiliac joint changes with eventual intra-articular bony ankylosis are more common in classic ankylosing spondylitis and colitic disease than in psoriatic arthritis and Reiter's syndrome. In the spine, vertical syndesmophytes, significant apophyseal joint abnormalities, and vertebral squaring are also more typical of classic ankylosing spondylitis and colitic disorders.

### Miscellaneous Abnormalities

Clubbing of the fingers is a recognized complication of ulcerative colitis. On rare occasion, hypertrophic osteoarthropathy leading to periosteal bone formation in

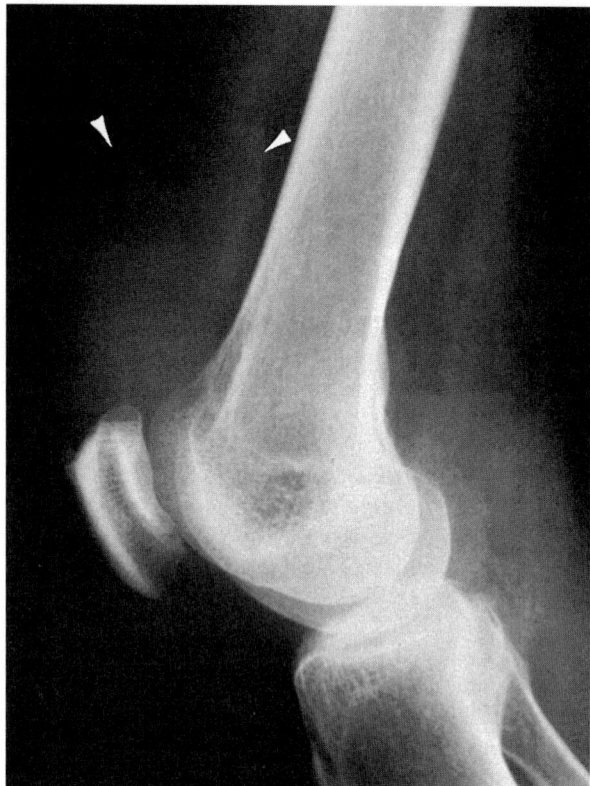

**Figure 21–1.** Ulcerative colitis: peripheral joint abnormalities. Observe a large joint effusion of the knee with displacement of the fat pads and prominence of the suprapatellar pouch *(arrowheads)*.

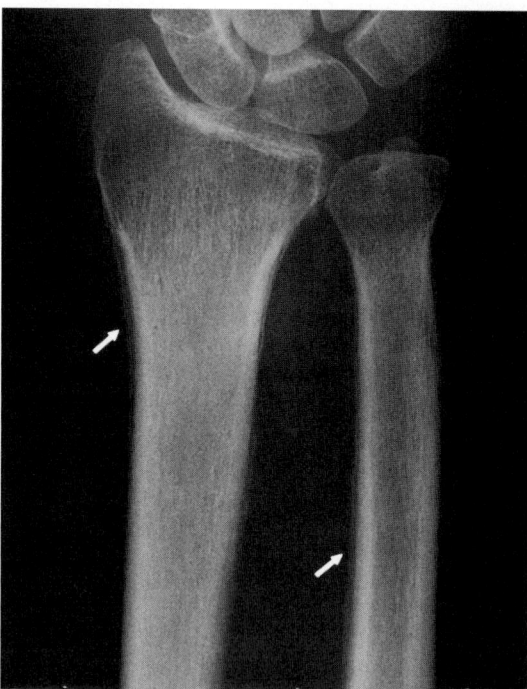

**Figure 21–3.** Ulcerative colitis: hypertrophic osteoarthropathy: Note the periostitis *(arrows)* of the diaphyses and metaphyses of the radius and ulna.

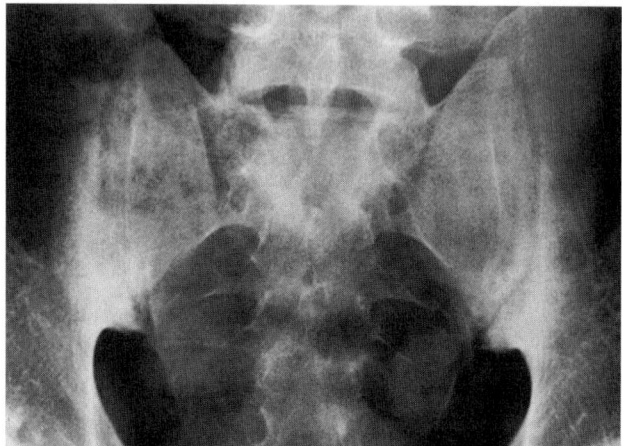

**Figure 21–2.** Ulcerative colitis and ankylosing spondylitis: sacroiliac joint abnormalities. Bilateral, symmetrical sacroiliac articular abnormalities are characterized by erosion and sclerosis, predominantly in the ilium.

the tibia, fibula, radius, and ulna may also be apparent (Fig. 21–3).

## Differential Diagnosis

Radiographic features of peripheral joint arthritis in patients with ulcerative colitis are not specific. Although the appearance of joint space narrowing, erosions, and cysts can simulate the changes in rheumatoid arthritis, these abnormalities are not frequent in the arthritis of ulcerative colitis. The spondylitis and sacroiliitis in ulcerative colitis are identical to the changes in classic ankylosing spondylitis. Bilateral, symmetrical sacroiliac joint involvement and syndesmophytosis are seen in both disorders. In psoriatic arthritis and Reiter's syndrome, sacroiliac joint abnormalities may be asymmetrical or even unilateral in distribution, whereas spinal alterations include broad, asymmetrical bony excrescences that differ in appearance from typical syndesmophytes.

## CROHN'S DISEASE

### General Abnormalities

Crohn's disease is a chronic and recurrent granulomatous process of unknown cause that involves principally the terminal ileum and proximal portion of the colon. Crohn's disease is associated with a variety of clinical findings, including abdominal pain, tenderness, diarrhea, weight loss, and fever. Complications include intestinal hemorrhage, obstruction, draining sinuses, and fistulas. Crohn's disease is most frequent in young adults, although patients of all ages can be affected. Musculoskeletal manifestations in Crohn's disease can take several forms: peripheral joint arthralgia and arthritis, sacroiliitis and spondylitis, and miscellaneous abnormalities.

## Peripheral Joint Arthralgia and Arthritis

The reported frequency of enteropathic arthritis in patients with Crohn's disease varies from less than 1% to 22%. Peripheral joint abnormalities in Crohn's disease are equally frequent in men and women. The pattern of articular involvement is typically a mild, migratory synovitis of one or, less commonly, several joints that involves the lower extremity more frequently than the upper extremity. The knee is the most common site of abnormality, followed by the ankle, shoulder, wrist, elbow, and small joints of the hands and feet. Arthritis, which may be associated with erythema nodosum, can occur simultaneously with the onset of bowel disease or at any time during its course. Infrequently, it may precede intestinal alterations. The recrudescence of arthritis is commonly associated with an exacerbation of intestinal disease.

Radiographic abnormalities are nondistinctive. Soft tissue swelling and regional osteoporosis may be observed. Permanent cartilaginous and osseous changes are present infrequently. The cause of the enteropathic arthritis accompanying Crohn's disease is not known.

## Sacroiliitis and Spondylitis

Sacroiliac joint and spinal changes develop in a significant number of patients with Crohn's disease (3% to 16%);

conversely, a high frequency of Crohn's disease occurs in patients with ankylosing spondylitis. Men and women are affected with equal frequency. Symptoms and signs may antedate or follow the onset of bowel disease. Exacerbation of these findings does not appear to be related to activity of the bowel disease, nor does treatment of the intestinal disorder influence the progress of the arthritis. Serologic testing for the presence of HLA-B27 antigen is positive in approximately 50% of patients with Crohn's disease and sacroiliitis or spondylitis.

The radiographic features of the spinal and sacroiliac articular abnormalities in Crohn's disease are identical to those of classic ankylosing spondylitis. Bilateral sacroiliac joint narrowing and erosion and sclerosis of the ilium and sacrum are evident (Figs. 21–4 and 21–5). Spinal involvement can include syndesmophytosis; vertebral erosion, sclerosis, and squaring; and apophyseal joint erosion, sclerosis, and narrowing. Progressive alterations can lead to a bamboo spine.

## Miscellaneous Abnormalities

Digital clubbing has been detected in as many as 40% of patients with Crohn's disease. Bilateral, symmetrical periostitis, which is a manifestation of hypertrophic osteoarthropathy, is an extremely rare complication of Crohn's disease.

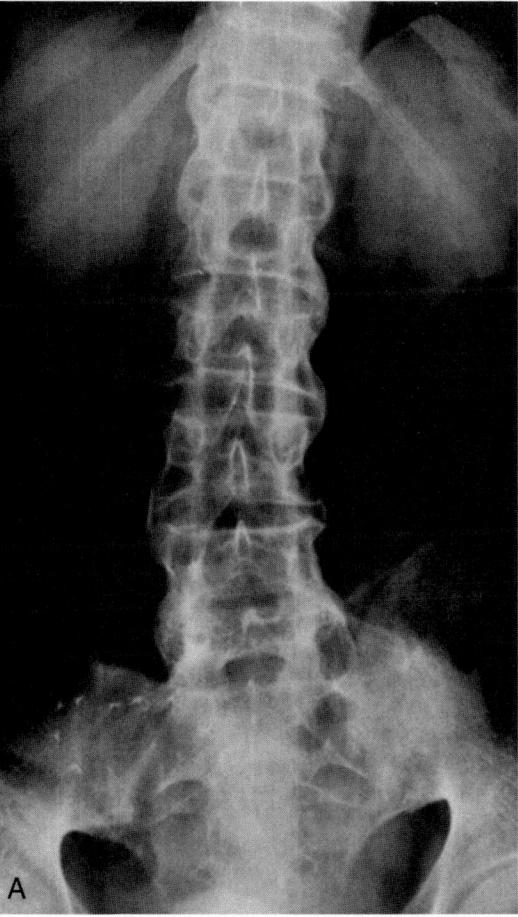

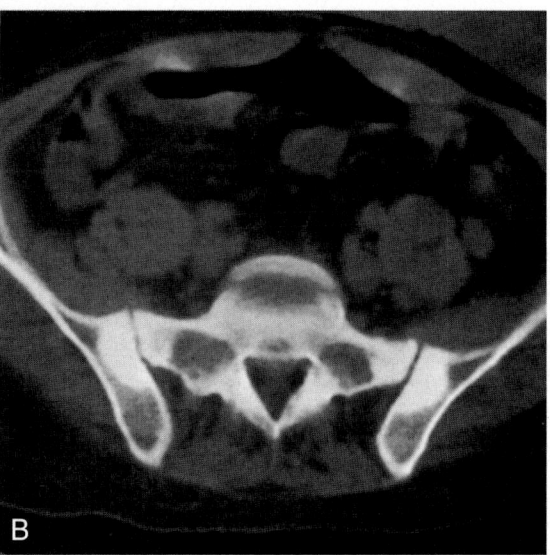

**Figure 21–4.** Crohn's disease and ankylosing spondylitis: sacroiliac joint and spinal abnormalities. *A,* Frontal radiograph reveals bilateral, symmetrical sacroiliac joint changes with intra-articular bone fusion. Syndesmophytes are seen in the spine. *B,* In a different patient, transaxial computed tomography scanning demonstrates bilateral, symmetrical sacroiliitis characterized by an extreme degree of bone sclerosis in both the ilium and the sacrum. (Courtesy of P. Ellenbogen, MD, Dallas, Tex.)

A

B

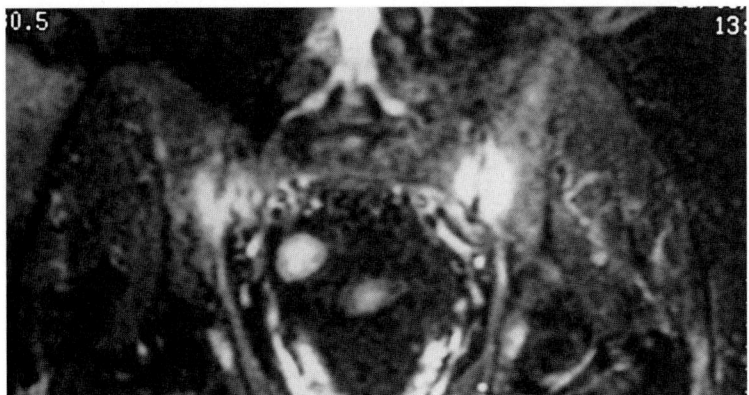

**Figure 21–5.** Crohn's disease and ankylosing spondylitis. Coronal short tau inversion recovery (STIR) (TR/TE, 4300/52; inversion time, 150 msec) MR image shows regions of high signal intensity in the subchondral bone of the ilium and sacrum about both sacroiliac joints, consistent with sacroiliitis. Bilateral small hip effusions and abnormal high signal intensity about both greater trochanters are also evident.

Granulomatous and infectious processes of bone have been reported in association with Crohn's disease. Although an abscess of the psoas muscle is an infrequent complication of Crohn's disease, with a prevalence of approximately 3% to 5%, some investigators regard Crohn's disease as the leading cause of psoas abscesses.

## Differential Diagnosis

The radiographic abnormalities in the peripheral joints of patients with Crohn's disease lack specificity. Soft tissue swelling and osteoporosis are observed, but permanent cartilaginous and osseous changes are unusual. Thus, the presence of joint space narrowing and erosions virtually eliminates the diagnosis of enteropathic arthritis.

The axial skeletal abnormalities in this disease cannot be differentiated from those of classic ankylosing spondylitis or the spondylitis of ulcerative colitis. The presence of bilateral and symmetrical sacroiliac joint changes and syndesmophytosis of the spine is typical of these disorders.

## WHIPPLE'S DISEASE

### General Abnormalities

Whipple's disease (intestinal lipodystrophy) is a rare progressive disorder that affects predominantly men in the fourth and fifth decades of life and leads to fever, weight loss, lymphadenopathy, peripheral edema, hypotension, brown pigmentation of the skin, polyserositis, and polyarthritis. Pathologically, the major feature is the accumulation of periodic acid-Schiff–positive inclusions in macrophages of the lamina propria of the small intestine, lymph nodes, and other tissues. The cause of the disease appears to be related to a bacterial organism, inasmuch as antibiotic therapy can effect a cure.

Musculoskeletal manifestations are an important feature of the disease. These manifestations can be divided into peripheral joint arthralgia and arthritis, sacroiliitis and spondylitis, and miscellaneous abnormalities.

### Peripheral Joint Arthralgia and Arthritis

Acute migratory episodic arthralgia and arthritis are apparent in 60% to 90% of patients with Whipple's disease. These findings may antedate other changes of the disease. With the onset of gastrointestinal findings, the pattern of arthritis generally remains unaltered, although occasionally, joint symptoms and signs may decrease in intensity. Articular abnormalities are usually transient and last hours to days. The findings generally subside and subsequently recur after periods of remission of variable length. Residual joint deformities are rare. Characteristically, the ankles, knees, shoulders, and wrists are affected. Polyarthritis is more frequent than monoarthritis. Clinical findings include mild to severe joint pain, swelling, warmth, and restrictive motion. Stiffness is usually not a prominent manifestation of the disease.

Radiographic examination of involved peripheral joints may yield entirely normal results. Soft tissue swelling, osteoporosis, and joint space narrowing are occasionally evident (Fig. 21–6). These findings are most common in the metacarpophalangeal and metatarsophalangeal joints, wrist, ankle, hip, and knee.

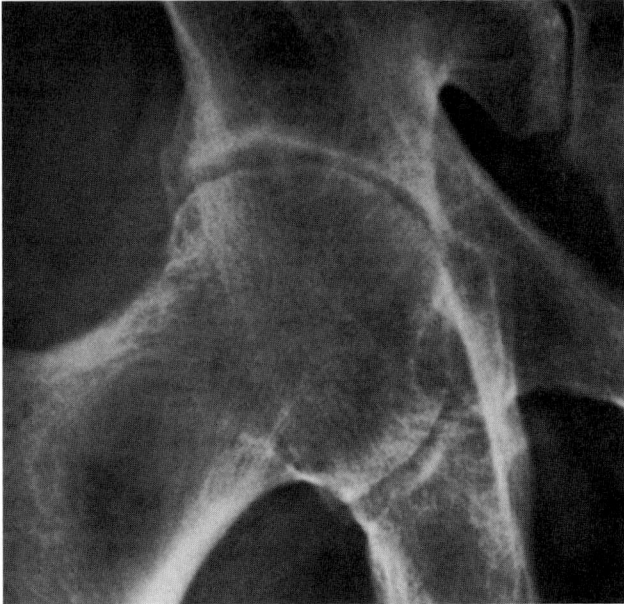

**Figure 21–6.** Whipple's disease: peripheral joint abnormalities. Observe the hip joint space narrowing and osseous cysts. Similar changes were seen in the contralateral hip.

(From Chevallier PL, Vallat JP, Luthier F, et al: Bilateral coxopathy revealing Whipple disease. Apropos of a case. Article in French.) Rev Rhum Mal Osteoartic 43:663, 1976.)

## Sacroiliitis and Spondylitis

Sacroiliitis and spondylitis have been described in patients with Whipple's disease. The exact frequency of these abnormalities is not known. In most cases, the spinal and sacroiliac joint alterations resemble those of classic ankylosing spondylitis. Approximately one quarter to one third of patients with Whipple's disease have been reported to possess the HLA-B27 antigen.

## Miscellaneous Abnormalities

Subcutaneous nodules, particularly on extensor surfaces of the extremities, are evident in some patients with joint symptoms. Additional manifestations include clubbing of the fingers, hypertrophic osteoarthropathy, reflex sympathetic dystrophy, and myalgias.

## Differential Diagnosis

The peripheral joint abnormalities in Whipple's disease are entirely nonspecific on radiographic evaluation. In the axial skeleton, sacroiliac joint and spinal changes, when present, are identical to those found in classic ankylosing spondylitis and the spondylitis of ulcerative colitis and Crohn's disease. Although clinical features permit the separation of these disorders, the radiographic changes do not allow an accurate differential diagnosis.

## INTESTINAL INFECTIONS AND REACTIVE ARTHRITIS

A variety of infectious agents can initiate or trigger a synovial reaction at one or more sites distant to the area of infection. The phenomenon, which is unrelated to direct contamination of the joint, is referred to as reactive arthritis (Table 21–2). The diagnostic criteria for reactive arthritis are not agreed on, although emphasis has been placed on evidence of a preceding infection and asymmetrical articular disease of the lower limbs. Certain genetic factors, such as presence of the HLA-B27 antigen, appear to impart susceptibility to reactive arthritis in some persons.

Four possible mechanisms are postulated by which an enteric infectious agent may initiate or perpetuate articular inflammation: (1) altered bowel anatomy (e.g., the intestinal bypass syndrome), (2) autoimmunity as a result of molecular mimicry (e.g., postdysenteric reactive arthritis and ankylosing spondylitis), (3) altered bowel permeability (e.g., inflammatory bowel disorders, milk allergy, and celiac disease), and (4) toxin-mediated synovitis (e.g., pseudomembranous enterocolitis). Recent investigations support the third of these possible mechanisms: altered bowel permeability.

General clinical characteristics of reactive arthritis include a symptom-free interval between the initiation of infection and the rheumatic reaction; a self-limited clinical course, usually associated with the acute onset of a migratory polyarthritis and fever; a tendency in some patients toward involvement of the heart; and a negative serologic test for rheumatoid factor. Although the location of the inciting infection varies, three portals of entry are most common: the oronasopharynx (e.g., tonsillitis, dental infection), the urogenital tract (e.g., urethritis), and the intestinal tract.

Seronegative sterile arthritis may follow intestinal infections related to *Salmonella*, *Shigella*, *Yersinia*, or *Campylobacter* organisms. The frequency of arthritis in patients after *Salmonella* or *Shigella* infection is 1% to 2%; that occurring after *Yersinia* infection may be as high as 30%.

The various forms of sterile arthritis can be associated with soft tissue swelling and joint effusions, but other radiographic features are generally lacking. Infrequently, erosive bone changes are seen. After bowel disease caused by *Yersinia*, sacroiliitis and spondylitis have been noted. In this regard, it is significant that HLA-B27 antigen has been detected in approximately 90% of patients in whom sterile arthritis develops after bowel infection with *Salmonella*, *Shigella*, or *Yersinia* organisms. A true septic arthritis is a definite and serious complication of *Salmonella* infection, particularly in children. *Yersinia enterocolitica* infection has also been associated with septic arthritis, as well as osteomyelitis and psoas muscle abscess.

## ARTHROPATHY AFTER INTESTINAL BYPASS SURGERY

Intestinal bypass surgery has been performed for many years for the treatment of intractable obesity. Rheumatologic manifestations in the postoperative period predominate in women and include polymyalgia, polyarthralgia, acute or subacute arthritis, and tenosynovitis. The prevalence of these manifestations in patients undergoing such surgery has decreased in recent years as a result of improved technology and professional awareness. The symptoms and signs are usually transient, although they occasionally persist. They generally develop within 2 years after surgical intervention and resolve within 1 to 2 years. Symmetrical polyarthritis is the rule. Articular involvement is most frequent in the knees, ankles, fingers, and wrists.

Radiographic evaluation demonstrates soft tissue swelling and osteoporosis. On rare occasion, osseous erosions are evident. Sacroiliitis and spondylitis have also been observed in patients undergoing jejunocolic-type bypass procedures (Fig. 21–7). The cause and pathogenesis of the

---

**TABLE 21–2**

**Mechanisms of Infection-Induced arthritis**

| Mechanism | Example |
|---|---|
| Direct penetration and subsequent multiplication of viable organisms | Bacterial arthritis |
| "Reactive" arthritis as a response to a distant infection | Rheumatic fever |
| Immune-mediated response to an antigen in the joint or blood | Hepatitis |
| Direct toxin released by the infectious agent | None known |

Modified from Goldenberg DL: "Postinfectious" arthritis: New look at an old concept with particular attention to disseminated gonococcal infection. Am J Med 74:625, 1983.

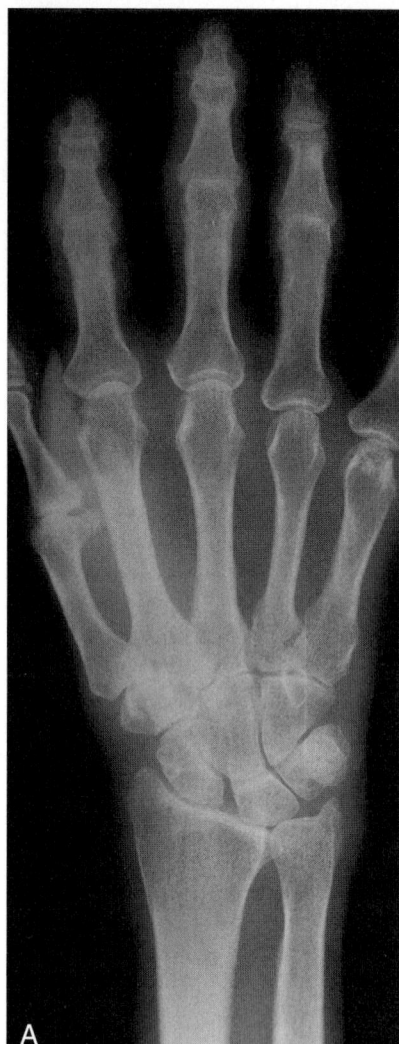

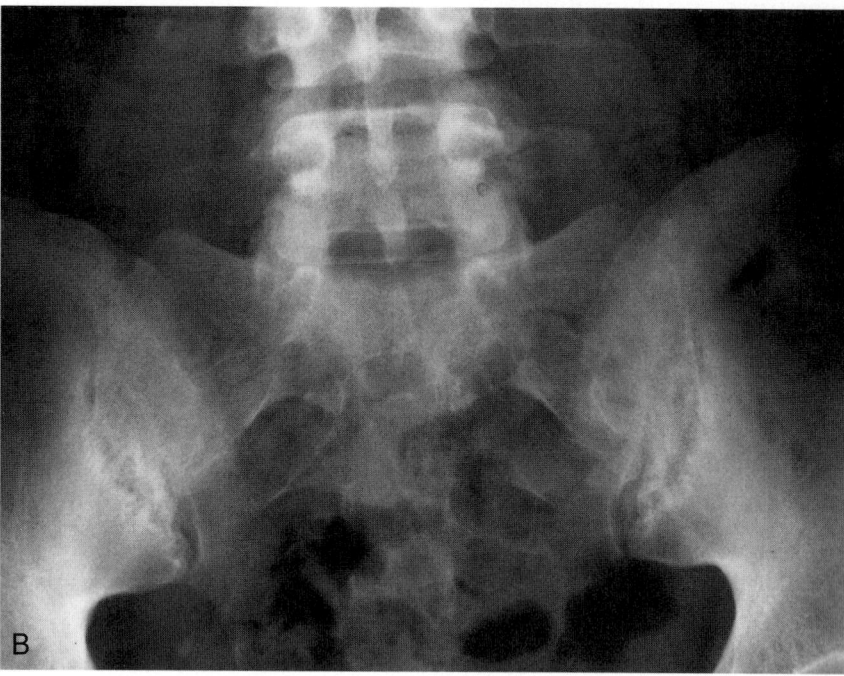

**Figure 21–7.** Intestinal bypass surgery: peripheral joint disease and sacroiliitis. Fourteen years after a jejunocolic bypass, peripheral joint disease is noted. It is characterized by osteopenia; soft tissue swelling, especially about the proximal interphalangeal and metacarpophalangeal joints; and joint space narrowing in the wrist, particularly the radiocarpal and ulnocarpal regions (*A*). Bilateral sacroiliitis is also evident (*B*).

arthropathy after intestinal bypass procedures have not been clearly delineated. Apparently, the type of bowel surgery influences the pattern and distribution of arthritis. Additional radiographic findings seen after intestinal bypass surgery include gout, osteomalacia, and osteoporosis.

## LAËNNEC'S CIRRHOSIS

Inflammatory polyarthritis can occur in patients with Laënnec's cirrhosis during the recovery period, when liver function tests are showing improvement. Most commonly the shoulders, elbows, and knees are affected. Clinical findings include pain, swelling, tenderness, and limitation of motion. Radiographs reveal osteoporosis and a possible proclivity toward the development of calcific periarthritis. The condition appears to be self-limited, with improvement usually occurring within 1 year. The pathogenesis of these arthritic alterations is unknown.

## PRIMARY BILIARY CIRRHOSIS

Primary biliary cirrhosis is a rare disorder that affects women almost exclusively. Immune mechanisms appear

to be fundamental to its pathogenesis. Clinical findings include the insidious onset of jaundice, pruritus, hepatomegaly, and abnormal liver function. The diagnosis is confirmed by the presence of antimitochondrial antibodies and characteristic findings on liver biopsy.

Musculoskeletal complaints can relate to osteomalacia and osteoporosis, arthralgia or arthritis, hypertrophic osteoarthropathy, or the coexistence of a connective tissue disease such as scleroderma or Sjögren's syndrome. The osteomalacia and osteoporosis in this disorder are probably due to a combination of steatorrhea, cholestasis, and hepatic dysfunction. Hypercholesterolemia can lead to xanthoma formation in soft tissues and in subperiosteal and intramedullary sites. Associated radiographic findings include nodular soft tissue masses, subperiosteal erosion of bone, and cystic lesions. Of particular interest is the appearance of erosive arthritis of the hands and wrists in patients with primary biliary cirrhosis Erosions are well defined, of varying size, and marginal in location, and they are distributed predominantly in an asymmetrical fashion in the distal interphalangeal and proximal interphalangeal joints (Fig. 21–8).

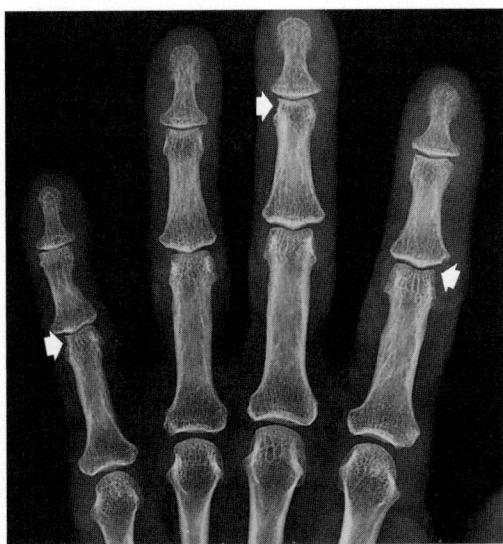

**Figure 21–8.** Primary biliary cirrhosis: peripheral joint abnormalities. Note the small marginal erosions in the proximal interphalangeal and distal interphalangeal joints *(arrows)*.

(From O'Connell DJ, Marx WJ: Hand changes in primary biliary cirrhosis. Radiology 129:31, 1978.)

## VIRAL HEPATITIS

Articular manifestations can occur during the course of hepatitis B (serum hepatitis) and, less commonly, hepatitis A (infectious hepatitis) and hepatitis C. A symmetrical, polyarticular pattern of joint disease is observed and most commonly involves the hands, wrists, elbows, knees, and ankles. Clinical findings include pain and stiffness, which may persist for a few days to more than 1 month and may decrease as jaundice develops. Joint destruction and deformity are not seen.

## PANCREATIC DISEASE

### Fat Necrosis

Pancreatic disorders can be complicated by fat necrosis at multiple distant sites, with subsequent subcutaneous nodular skin lesions, polyarthritis, and medullary fat necrosis. These manifestations appear most frequently in older men in association with carcinoma of the pancreas, although they can also occur with acute pancreatitis caused by either abdominal trauma or alcohol abuse, pancreatic pseudocysts, and pancreatic duct calculi. In many patients, joint pain and nodules precede abdominal pain. Articular abnormalities are characterized by a symmetrical or asymmetrical polyarthritis, which can be associated with pain, swelling, tenderness, warmth, and effusion. A predilection for the ankles, elbows, knees, wrists, and small joints of the hands and feet is seen.

Radiographic findings related to joint disease are absent or minimal; osteoporosis and soft tissue swelling may be seen, but joint space narrowing and osseous erosion are reported infrequently. Bone involvement can occur simultaneously with subcutaneous nodules and polyarthritis,

or it can represent an isolated phenomenon. Osteolytic lesions with moth-eaten bone destruction and periostitis of the tubular bones of the extremities resemble the findings in osteomyelitis or osteonecrosis (Fig. 21–9). These changes occur in the long bones of the extremities, in the small bones of the hands and feet, or in both locations. In the bones of the hands and feet, cystic defects and a coarsened trabecular pattern may be apparent, and the epiphyses may be unaffected. Magnetic resonance (MR) imaging is sensitive to the early changes of intraosseous fat necrosis and shows multiple foci of abnormal signal (Fig. 21–10).

Although the exact pathogenesis of the articular and osseous findings associated with pancreatic disorders has not been delineated accurately, it appears probable that widespread fat necrosis is responsible for these abnormalities. Obstruction of pancreatic ducts by edema, calculi, or tumor or hormonal hypersecretion by acinar cell carcinomas and functioning metastases can lead to the release of excess circulating lipase into the bloodstream, which results in autodigestion of fat deposits at distant sites.

### Osteonecrosis

Osteonecrosis is a recognized manifestation of pancreatic disease. This complication is most frequently associated with chronic or inactive pancreatitis. Abnormalities of the

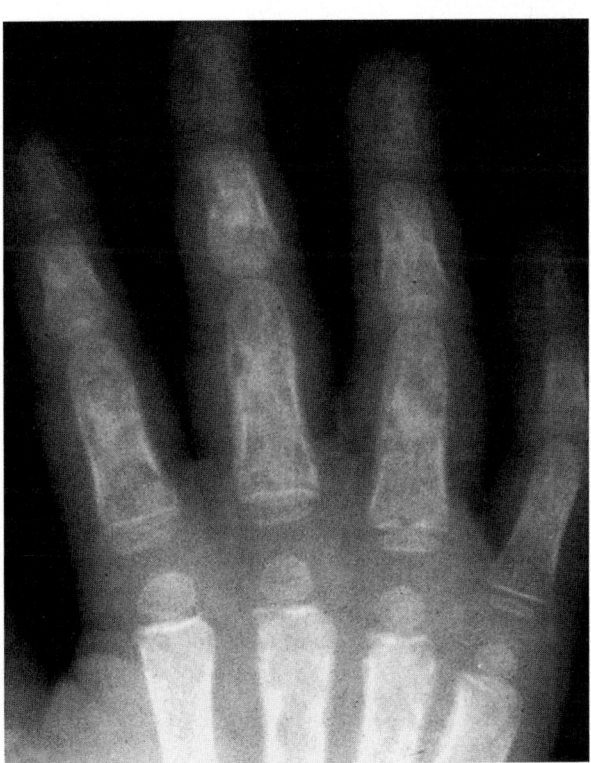

**Figure 21–9.** Pancreatic disease: fat necrosis. Radiographic abnormalities include lytic defects of the metacarpals, phalanges, and metatarsals, with associated periostitis. Soft tissue swelling is also evident. (Courtesy of A. Brower, MD, Norfolk, Va.)

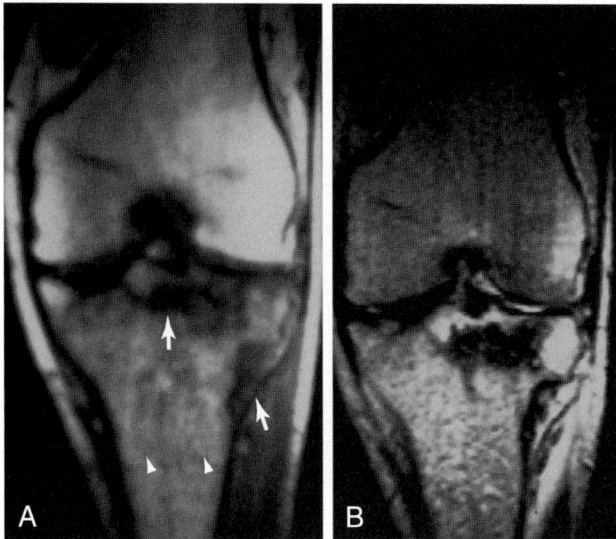

**Figure 21–10.** Pancreatic disease: fat necrosis. MR imaging abnormalities include joint swelling and subcutaneous nodules in the upper and lower extremities in this 44-year-old man with alcoholic pancreatitis. Osteolysis is apparent at multiple sites, including the left tibia. Biopsy of a skin nodule confirmed the presence of fat necrosis. *A,* Coronal T1-weighted (TR/TE, 600/28) spin echo MR image shows inhomogeneous signal intensity in the metaphysis of the tibia *(arrowheads).* The adjacent epiphysis and a small portion of the metaphysis are characterized by decreased signal intensity *(arrows). B,* Coronal T2-weighted (TR/TE, 2025/120) spin echo MR image reveals a considerable increase in signal intensity in the metaphysis and the epiphysis of the tibia, compatible with the presence of bone marrow edema and necrosis. (Courtesy of G. Greenway, MD, Dallas, Tex.)

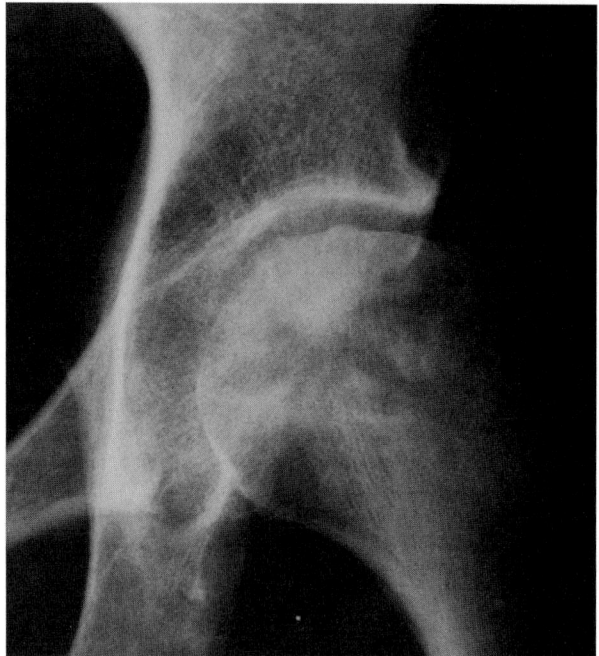

**Figure 21–11.** Pancreatic disease: osteonecrosis. In this alcoholic patient with a history of acute and chronic pancreatitis, observe osteonecrosis of the femoral head, along with cystic lesions and articular collapse.

femoral and humeral heads are typical, although diaphyseal and metaphyseal infarction in long tubular bones may be seen. Radiographically, epiphyseal involvement is characterized by mottled lysis and sclerosis, subchondral radiolucent areas, and partial or complete collapse of bone (Fig. 21–11); diaphyseal and metaphyseal involvement, which is most frequent in the distal end of the femur and proximal portion of the tibia, is associated with radiolucency, calcification, and periosteal bone formation.

### Skeletal Metastasis

Osteolytic or osteoblastic lesions can occur in patients with skeletal metastasis from adenocarcinoma of the pancreas. Changes, particularly those that are osteoblastic in nature, are most common in the vertebral column. Frequent involvement of the upper lumbar spine could conceivably indicate direct invasion by neoplasm rather than hematogenous spread in some patients with pancreatic carcinoma.

### Differential Diagnosis

The osseous changes of fat necrosis in patients with pancreatic disease simulate those of osteomyelitis and osteonecrosis. Lytic lesions and periostitis on radiographic examination and areas of increased radionuclide uptake

on scintigraphic examination are common manifestations of these disorders. In fact, fat necrosis, osteonecrosis, and osteomyelitis can occur together in these patients. Although some reports indicate an absence of periostitis in cases of intraosseous fat necrosis, the diagnostic value of this sign is questionable. The combination of osteolysis, periosteal bone formation, calcification of medullary bone, and epiphyseal osteonecrosis should stimulate a clinical investigation to exclude a pancreatic origin of these findings.

### FURTHER READING

Arlart IP, Maier W, Leupold D, et al: Massive periosteal new bone formation in ulcerative colitis. Radiology 144:507, 1982.

Baron M, Paltiel H, Lander P: Aseptic necrosis of the talus and calcaneal insufficiency fractures in a patient with pancreatitis, subcutaneous fat necrosis, and arthritis. Arthritis Rheum 27:1309, 1984.

Bjorkengren AG, Resnick D, Sartoris DJ: Enteropathic arthropathies. Radiol Clin North Am 25:189, 1987.

Clark RL, Muhletaler CA, Margulies SI: Colitic arthritis: Clinical and radiographic manifestations. Radiology 101:585, 1971.

Genant HK, Mall JC, Wagonfeld JB, et al: Skeletal demineralization and growth retardation in inflammatory bowel disease. Invest Radiol 11:541, 1976.

Goldenberg DL: "Postinfectious" arthritis: New look at an old concept with particular attention to disseminated gonococcal infection. Am J Med 74:925, 1983.

Haller J, Greenway G, Resnick D, et al: Intraosseous fat necrosis associated with acute pancreatitis: MR imaging. Radiology 173:193, 1989.

Hirondel JL, Fournier L, Fretille A, et al: Intraosseous fat necrosis and metaphyseal osteonecrosis in a patient with chronic pancreatitis: MR imaging and CT scanning. Clin Exp Rheumatol 12:191, 1994.

Joffe N, Antonioli DA: Osteoblastic bone metastases secondary to adenocarcinoma of the pancreas. Clin Radiol 29:41, 1978.

Karasick D, Schweitzer ME: Case 4: Intraosseous fat necrosis associated with pancreatitis. Radiology 209:521, 1998.

Khan MA: Axial arthropathy in Whipple's disease. J Rheumatol 9:928, 1982.

McEwen C, DiTata D, Lingg C, et al: Ankylosing spondylitis and spondylitis accompanying ulcerative colitis, regional enteritis, psoriasis and Reiter's disease. Arthritis Rheum 14:291, 1971.

Mueller CE, Seeger JF, Martel W: Ankylosing spondylitis and regional enteritis. Radiology 112:579, 1974.

O'Connell DJ, Marx WJ: Hand changes in primary biliary cirrhosis. Radiology 129:31, 1978.

Orchard TR, Jewell DP: The importance of ileocaecal integrity in the arthritic complications of Crohn's disease. Inflamm Bowel Dis 5:92, 1999.

Radin DR, Colletti PM, Forrester DM, et al: Pancreatic acinar carcinoma with subcutaneous and intraosseous fat necrosis. Radiology 158:67, 1986.

Slovis TL, Berdon WE, Haller JO, et al: Pancreatitis and the battered child syndrome: Report of 2 cases with skeletal involvement. AJR Am J Roentgenol 125:456, 1975.

Stein HB, Schlappner OLA, Boyko W, et al: The intestinal bypass arthritis-dermatitis syndrome. Arthritis Rheum 24:684, 1981.

# CHAPTER 22

## Periodic, Relapsing, and Recurrent Disorders

## SUMMARY OF KEY FEATURES

Familial Mediterranean fever, relapsing polychondritis, and Behçet's syndrome are three uncommon disorders that may be associated with periodic, relapsing, or recurrent clinical manifestations. In each disease, synovitis occasionally leads to soft tissue swelling and periarticular osteoporosis, and in rare instances, cartilaginous and osseous destruction can become evident. Each of these three disorders has also been associated with sacroiliitis, although this association is not frequent, nor is it without controversy in some cases.

## INTRODUCTION

Discussed in this chapter are three diseases that are characterized clinically by intermittent periods of activity separated by disease-free intercritical periods. Their causes are generally unclear or unknown. These three diseases are relatively uncommon and are associated with a nonspecific or unremarkable radiographic appearance.

## FAMILIAL MEDITERRANEAN FEVER
### Clinical Abnormalities

Familial Mediterranean fever (familial recurrent poly-serositis) is an uncommon disease that affects predominantly Sephardic (non-Ashkenazic) Jews, Armenians, and Arabs. It is inherited as an autosomal recessive trait with complete penetrance. Men are affected more commonly than women. Symptoms and signs of the disorder usually appear in childhood or adolescence and subsequently recur throughout the remainder of life. Typical manifestations include episodes of fever with abdominal, thoracic, or joint pain caused by inflammation of the peritoneum, pleura, and synovial membrane. Amyloidosis, a recognized complication of the disease, can produce the nephrotic syndrome and renal failure and can result in early death.

Attacks of familial Mediterranean fever are usually brief in duration and occur at irregular intervals without periodicity, with widely varying breaks between episodes that may last for years. Musculoskeletal manifestations occur in 30% to 70% of patients. Arthritis may be the initial or sole feature of the disease in 25% of patients. Asymmetrical arthritis in the larger joints of the lower extremity is most typical; the affected sites, in order of decreasing frequency, are the knees, ankles, hips, shoulders, feet, elbows, and hands and wrists. Monoarticular arthritis is more common than polyarticular arthritis.

### Radiographic Abnormalities

Osteoporosis can develop rapidly and become profound. In children, hyperemia can lead to epiphyseal overgrowth, which, when combined with soft tissue swelling and effusion, can simulate the findings of juvenile chronic arthritis or hemophilia. Chronicity leads to joint space narrowing and juxta-articular erosions (Fig. 22–1), changes that are most evident in the hip and the knee.

Sacroiliac joint abnormalities have also been described in familial Mediterranean fever (Table 22–1). The reported frequency of these abnormalities varies from about 2% to 15%. Widening of the articular space, loss of normal subchondral bone definition, sclerosis with or without erosions, and bony ankylosis can appear in one or both sacroiliac joints; asymmetrical abnormalities predominate (Fig. 22–2). Unilateral sacroiliac joint changes are also encountered. HLA-B27 antigen is absent in patients with familial Mediterranean fever and sacroiliitis.

### Differential Diagnosis

The radiographic findings in familial Mediterranean fever are not diagnostic. In children, soft tissue swelling, osteoporosis, and epiphyseal overgrowth are evident in other articular disorders as well, such as juvenile chronic arthritis and hemophilia. In children and adults, joint space narrow-

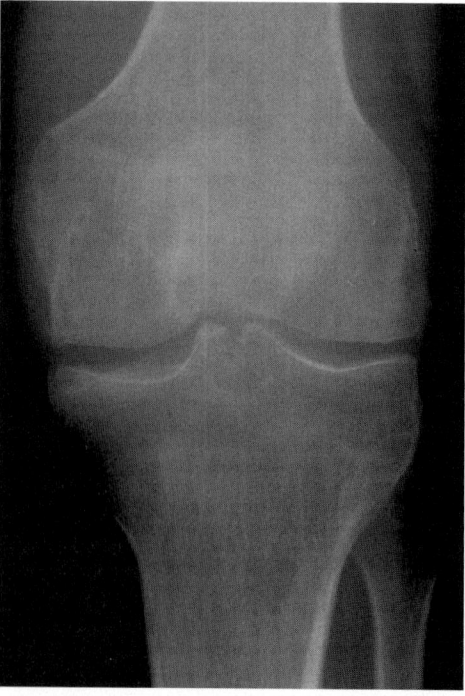

**Figure 22–1.** Familial Mediterranean fever: peripheral joint abnormalities. Note the mild joint space loss in the knee, plus marginal erosions of the femur and tibia. (Courtesy of J. Hodler, MD, Zurich, Switzerland.)

**TABLE 22-1**

**Sacroiliac Joint Abnormalities**

| | Distribution | | |
| --- | --- | --- | --- |
| *Disorder* | *Bilateral Symmetrical* | *Bilateral Asymmetrical* | *Unilateral* |
| Familial Mediterranean fever | x | x* | x |
| Relapsing polychondritis | x | x* | x |
| Behçet's syndrome† | x | x | x |

*Probably the predominant pattern of involvement.

†Questionable association with sacroiliitis.

ing and osseous erosion can simulate the findings of arthritides associated with synovial inflammation, such as rheumatoid arthritis and septic arthritis. The sacroiliitis in familial Mediterranean fever simulates that of ankylosing spondylitis and the other seronegative spondyloarthropathies.

## RELAPSING POLYCHONDRITIS

### Clinical Abnormalities

Relapsing polychondritis is an uncommon disorder characterized by episodic inflammation of cartilaginous tissue and special sense organs; abnormalities are especially prominent in the external ear, nose, trachea, larynx, sclera, ribs, and articular cartilage. Relapsing polychondritis appears in all age groups, with a maximal frequency in the fourth decade of life. Men and women are affected in equal numbers. The initial clinical findings are usually auricular chondritis and arthritis; less typically, respiratory

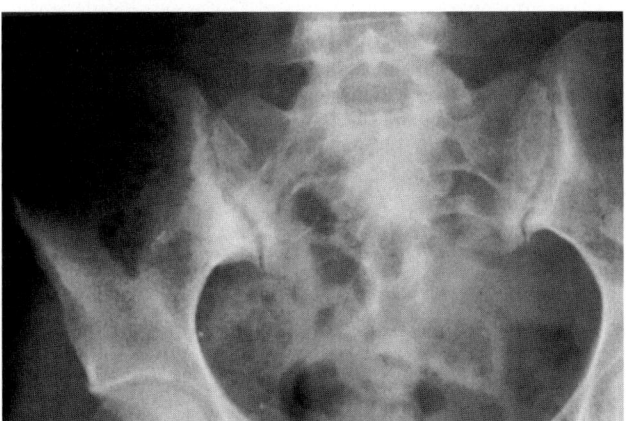

**Figure 22–2.** Familial Mediterranean fever: sacroiliitis. Bilateral, asymmetrical sacroiliac joint disease is characterized by osseous erosions and reactive sclerosis, predominantly in the ilium.

(From Brodey PA, Wolff SM: Radiographic changes in the sacroiliac joints in familial Mediterranean fever. Radiology 114:331, 1975.)

tract involvement, nasal chondritis, and ocular involvement are evident at the outset of the disease. Auricular chondritis leads to painful erythematous swelling of the cartilaginous portion of one or both external ears, lasting from 5 to 10 days. Arthralgia and arthritis occur in as many as 80% of patients and generally affect more than one joint, including the hips, knees, manubriosternal and sternoclavicular articulations, costochondral junctions, and small and large joints of the upper extremity.

Respiratory tract involvement is a potentially serious manifestation of the disease that may require a tracheostomy. Nasal chondritis may be sudden in onset and painful, and chronic involvement can lead to a characteristic saddle nose deformity. Additional manifestations include back pain as a result of spinal alterations, chest pain related to costochondritis, hearing loss attributable to obstruction of the external auditory meatus, fever, anorexia and weight loss, and cardiovascular abnormalities. Clinical manifestations, in their order of frequency, include auricular chondritis (89%), polyarthritis (81%), nasal chondritis (72%), ocular inflammation (65%), respiratory tract chondritis (56%), audiovestibular damage (46%), cardiovascular involvement (24%), and cutaneous lesions (17%).

### Radiographic Abnormalities

In most cases, the radiographic features of joint involvement in relapsing polychondritis are not striking, although extra-articular findings may be present, such as tracheal narrowing or stenosis, calcification of the auricular cartilage, and aortic alterations after repeated attacks. Periarticular osteoporosis may or may not be evident. Typically, a nonerosive, nondeforming arthropathy appears. The presence of joint space narrowing in the absence of bone erosions is reported to be characteristic of relapsing polychondritis (Fig. 22–3).

Sacroiliitis may be evident in some patients with relapsing polychondritis, although the prevalence is probably not high (see Table 22–1). Unilateral or bilateral abnormalities characterized by the presence of joint space loss, erosion, and eburnation and by the absence of spinal alterations predominate (Fig. 22–4). HLA-B27 antigen does not appear to be associated with the arthropathy of relapsing polychondritis.

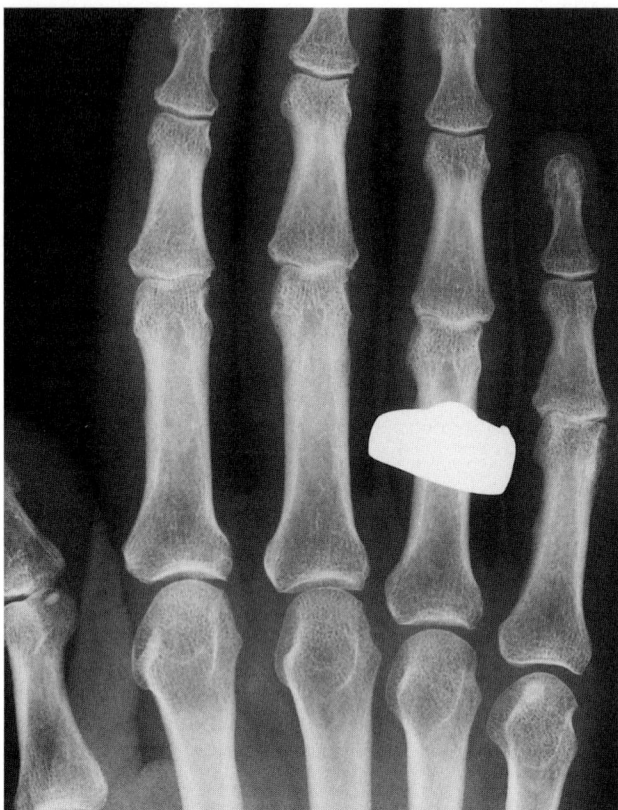

**Figure 22–3.** Relapsing polychondritis: peripheral joint abnormalities. Note the marked reduction in the joint spaces of the proximal interphalangeal joints and, to a lesser extent, the metacarpophalangeal joints.

(From Booth A, Dieppe PA, Goddard PL, et al: The radiological manifestations of relapsing polychondritis. Clin Radiol 40:147, 1989.)

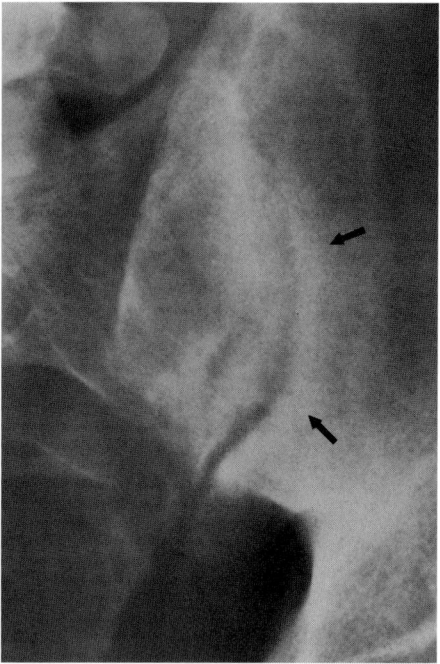

**Figure 22–4.** Relapsing polychondritis: sacroiliac joint abnormalities. Moderate osseous erosions and reactive sclerosis are seen *(arrows)*. (From Braunstein EM, Martel W, Stillwell E, et al: Radiological aspects of the arthropathy in relapsing polychondritis. Clin Radiol 30:444, 1979.)

## Differential Diagnosis

The radiographic features of articular involvement in this disease lack specificity. Periarticular osteoporosis and soft tissue swelling about synovial articulations simulate changes in a variety of disorders. With the occurrence of diffuse joint space narrowing and osseous erosions in these sites, the radiographic picture is almost identical to that of rheumatoid arthritis, although symmetry and more extensive cartilaginous and osseous destruction with deformities are more characteristic of the latter disease. Sacroiliitis in relapsing polychondritis is similar to that in ankylosing spondylitis or the other seronegative spondyloarthropathies. Calcification of ear cartilage is seen not only in relapsing polychondritis but also in adrenal insufficiency, acromegaly, alkaptonuria, hyperparathyroidism, and diabetes mellitus and after injury.

## BEHÇET'S SYNDROME

### Clinical Abnormalities

Behçet's syndrome is a multisystem vasculitis that was initially described as a triad of painful, recurrent oral and genital ulcerations and ocular inflammation. It is now recognized that many additional systems can be affected, including the skin, joints, and cardiovascular, neurologic, and gastrointestinal organs. The age of onset of Behçet's syndrome varies from 5 to 70 years, with a mean age of approximately 25 to 30 years; men are affected more commonly than women.

More than 90% of patients have ulcerations in portions of the mouth or pharynx. Ophthalmic lesions are evident in approximately 80% of patients, and genital lesions appear in approximately 60% of cases. Skin lesions are observed in approximately 75% of cases and consist of pyoderma with pustules of varying size and erythema nodosum–like abnormalities of the lower extremity.

Articular alterations appear in more than 50% of patients and are very common in children with the disease. Monoarticular or oligoarticular involvement predominates, with the knees principally affected; the ankles, wrists, elbows, and sacroiliac and manubriosternal articulations may also be involved. An insidious onset, variable duration, and recurrence after the disappearance of findings typify the bouts of arthralgia or arthritis. Joint effusion, stiffness, warmth, and tenderness are observed, but permanent changes are rare. An increased frequency of the tissue-typing antigen HLA-B5 has been found in some series.

### Radiographic Abnormalities

Radiographic findings in the skeleton are usually mild. Osteoporosis and soft tissue swelling can be seen, but joint space narrowing and osseous erosions are encountered only infrequently (Fig. 22–5). When present,

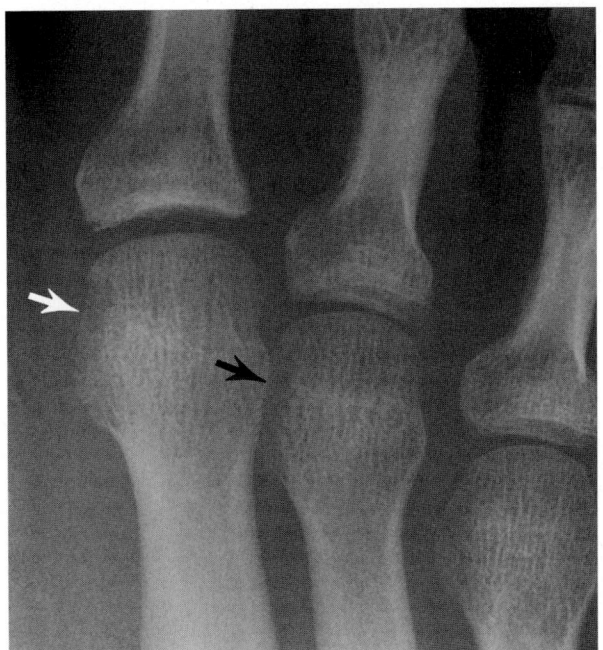

**Figure 22–5.** Behçet's syndrome: peripheral joint abnormalities. Observe the small osseous erosions of the metatarsal heads *(arrows)* and osteoporosis. (Courtesy of A. Brower, MD, Norfolk, Va.)

sacroiliac joint changes can include bone erosion, sclerosis, and joint space narrowing in a patchy or asymmetrical distribution. Bony ankylosis is unusual (see Table 22–1).

## Differential Diagnosis

When they are radiographically evident, the joint alterations in Behçet's syndrome may resemble those of rheumatoid arthritis or related disorders. Sacroiliitis can simulate the changes in ankylosing spondylitis or the other seronegative spondyloarthropathies.

## FURTHER READING

Barnes CG, Yazici H: Behçet's syndrome. Rheumatology 38: 1171, 1999.

Ben-Dov I, Zimmerman J: Deforming arthritis of the hands in Behçet's disease. J Rheumatol 9:617, 1982.

Booth A, Dieppe PA, Goddard PL, et al: The radiological manifestations of relapsing polychondritis. Clin Radiol 40:147, 1989.

Braunstein EM, Martel W, Stillwell E, et al: Radiological aspects of the arthropathy in relapsing polychondritis. Clin Radiol 30:441, 1979.

Brodey PA, Wolff SM: Radiographic changes in the sacroiliac joints in familial Mediterranean fever. Radiology 114:331, 1975.

Chajek T, Fairnaru M: Behçet's disease: Report of 41 cases and review of the literature. Medicine 54:179, 1975.

Johnson TH, Mital N, Rodnan GP, et al: Relapsing polychondritis. Radiology 106:313, 1973.

Koss JC, Dalinka MK: Atlantoaxial subluxation in Behçet's syndrome. AJR Am J Roentgenol 134:392, 1980.

McAdam LP, O'Hanlan MA, Bluestone R, et al: Relapsing polychondritis: Prospective study of 23 patients and a review of the literature. Medicine 55:193, 1976.

O'Hanlan M, McAdam LP, Bluestone R, et al: The arthropathy of relapsing polychondritis. Arthritis Rheum 19:191, 1976.

Schirmer M, Calamia KT, Direskeneli H: Ninth International Conference on Behçet's disease. Seoul, Korea, May 27-29, 2000. J Rheumatol 28:636, 2001.

Schwabe AD, Peters RS: Familial Mediterranean fever in Armenians: Analysis of 100 cases. Medicine 53:453, 1974.

Shahin N, Sohar E, Dalith F: Roentgenologic findings in familial Mediterranean fever. AJR Am J Roentgenol 84:269, 1960.

Sohar E, Gafni J, Pras M, et al: Familial Mediterranean fever: A survey of 470 cases and review of the literature. Am J Med 43:227, 1967.

Yazici H, Tuzlaci M, Yurdakul S: A controlled survey of sacroiliitis in Behçet's disease. Ann Rheum Dis 40:558, 1981.

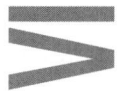
# Connective Tissue Disease

# CHAPTER 23

## Systemic Lupus Erythematosus

## SUMMARY OF KEY FEATURES

Musculoskeletal abnormalities represent a significant part of the clinical and radiographic picture of systemic lupus erythematosus. These abnormalities include myositis, symmetrical polyarthritis, deforming nonerosive arthropathy, spontaneous rupture of tendons, osteonecrosis, soft tissue calcification, osteomyelitis and septic arthritis, and terminal phalangeal sclerosis and erosion. Many of these abnormalities resemble the changes that occur in other collagen vascular disorders and rheumatoid arthritis. In addition, findings of systemic lupus erythematosus may be combined with those of other collagen vascular diseases in various overlap syndromes and in mixed connective tissue disease, and they may also be evident in the antiphospholipid syndrome.

## INTRODUCTION

Systemic lupus erythematosus is a relatively common connective tissue disorder characterized by significant immunologic abnormalities and involvement of multiple organ systems. The musculoskeletal system is frequently affected, and a number of clinical, pathologic, and radiographic findings have been noted.

## GENERAL CLINICAL ABNORMALITIES

Systemic lupus erythematosus is much more common in women than in men and is more common in blacks than in whites. Its familial nature is also well recognized. Although disease onset can occur at any age, it is most frequent in women during the childbearing years. The disease is rare in persons older than 45 years. Symptoms and signs are variable and depend on the distribution and extent of systemic alterations. Initial clinical manifestations most frequently include constitutional symptoms and signs (malaise, weakness, fever, anorexia, and weight loss) and articular (polyarthritis) and cutaneous (skin rash) findings. Subsequently, major clinical abnormalities may involve the musculoskeletal, cutaneous, neurologic, renal, pulmonary, and cardiac systems.

Skin manifestations are variable and include a typical butterfly eruption on the face; erythematous rashes on the eyelids, forehead, and neck; subungual erythema; urticaria; vasculitis with livedo reticularis; and alopecia. Skin nodules resembling those of rheumatoid arthritis may be observed in 5% to 10% of patients with systemic lupus erythematosus. Additional clinical abnormalities may involve the gastrointestinal system (peritonitis, pancreatitis, perihepatitis, intestinal arteritis), the reticulo-endothelial system (splenomegaly, lymphadenopathy), and the peripheral vasculature (gangrene, thrombophlebitis). Infections may develop in patients with systemic lupus erythematosus, perhaps related to decreased complement levels, impairment of delayed hypersensitivity, and defective phagocytosis.

## MUSCULOSKELETAL ABNORMALITIES

Characteristic and significant musculoskeletal abnormalities are encountered in patients with systemic lupus erythematosus (Table 23–1). These abnormalities may include myositis, symmetrical polyarthritis, deforming nonerosive arthropathy, subchondral cysts, spontaneous tendon weakening and rupture, osteonecrosis, soft tissue calcification, osteomyelitis and septic arthritis, and other abnormalities.

### Myositis

Muscle involvement has been observed in 30% to 50% of persons with systemic lupus erythematosus. Possible causes include pain referred to muscles from adjacent involved joints, corticosteroid-induced myopathy, and myositis. Myositis, which has been reported in 4% of patients with systemic lupus erythematosus, may be associated with diffuse muscular tenderness and weakness, with or without elevated serum levels of muscle enzymes.

---

**TABLE 23–1**

**Musculoskeletal Manifestations of Systemic Lupus Erythematosus**

Myositis
Polyarthritis
Deforming nonerosive arthropathy
Subchondral cysts
Tendon weakening and rupture
Osteonecrosis
Soft tissue calcification
Osteomyelitis and septic arthritis
Acrosclerosis
Tuft resorption
Insufficiency fracture

## Symmetrical Polyarthritis

Articular symptoms and signs are among the most common clinical manifestations of the disease and are present in 75% to 90% of patients. Articular involvement is most frequently bilateral and symmetrical, affecting predominantly the small joints of the hand as well as the knee, wrist, and shoulder; the findings include morning stiffness, pain, tenderness, and soft tissue swelling. Joint effusions are detected but are not large. Synovial membrane biopsy may reveal a thick layer of superficial fibrin-like material and signs of synovial inflammation.

Radiographic abnormalities accompanying uncomplicated synovitis in systemic lupus erythematosus consist of soft tissue swelling and periarticular osteoporosis; cartilaginous and osseous destruction is rare in the absence of coexistent osteonecrosis. In the hand, the findings of fusiform soft tissue prominence and regional osteoporosis about the proximal interphalangeal and metacarpophalangeal joints simulate the abnormalities of rheumatoid arthritis. Well-defined lytic lesions or cysts in periarticular bone have occasionally been recorded. The joint space is generally not narrowed (Fig. 23–1).

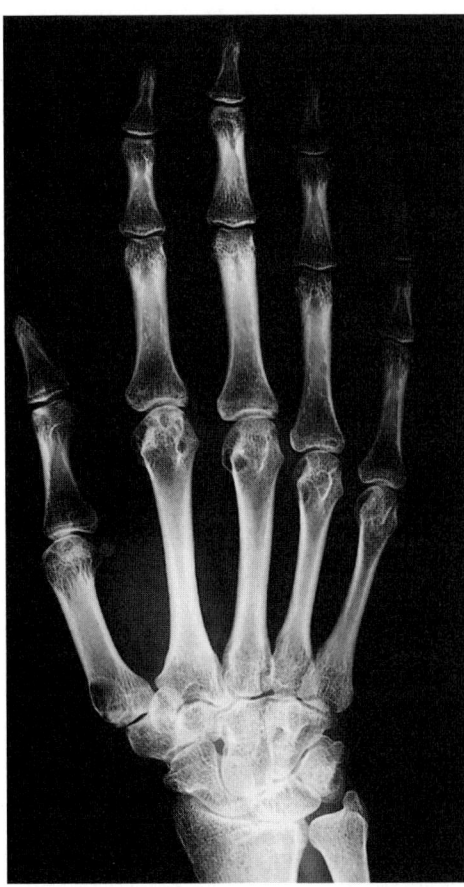

**Figure 23–1.** Polyarthritis: radiographic abnormalities. Although soft tissue swelling and osteoporosis are usually the only radiographic manifestations of acute polyarthritis in systemic lupus erythematosus, multiple well-defined subchondral cysts may be seen. Note that the joint spaces are preserved.

(From Leskinen RH, Skrifvars BV, Laasonen LS, et al: Bone lesions in systemic lupus erythematosus. Radiology 153:349, 1984.)

## Deforming Nonerosive Arthropathy

A deforming nonerosive arthropathy may be evident in as many as 5% to 40% of patients with articular abnormalities. Characteristically, the deformities cause little functional disability and are completely reducible; in fact, they may disappear when the hand is placed firmly on the cassette during radiography. In some instances, chronic fixed deformities can appear. Symmetrical involvement of the interphalangeal joints of multiple digits of the hand is most typical. Hyperextension at the proximal interphalangeal joints and flexion at the distal interphalangeal joints create swan-neck deformities (Fig. 23–2). Boutonnière deformities, with flexion at the proximal interphalangeal joints and hyperextension at the distal interphalangeal joints, can also be seen. Hyperextension at the interphalangeal joint of the thumb is characteristic. Additional deformities include subluxation with ulnar drift at the metacarpophalangeal joints and subluxation at the first carpometacarpal joint (Fig. 23–3). Associated abnormalities in the foot include hallux valgus, subluxation at the metatarsophalangeal joints, and widening of the forefoot. Instability in the knee or shoulder has also been encountered. Of further interest, atlantoaxial subluxation has been reported in approximately 10% of patients with systemic lupus erythematosus.

It is important to stress that joint space narrowing and osseous erosion are not prominent in this deforming arthropathy, a characteristic that distinguishes it from the articular abnormalities of rheumatoid arthritis. Infrequently, cartilaginous and osseous alterations do become evident in lupus arthropathy. Diminution of cartilage may

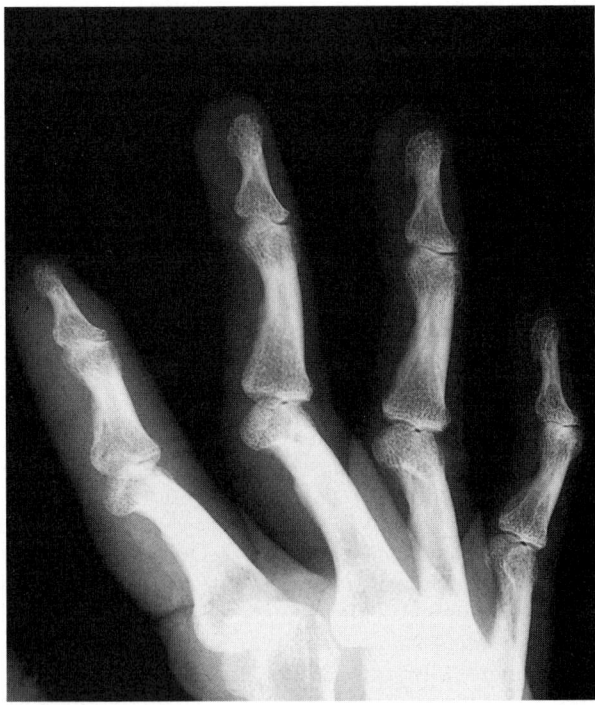

**Figure 23–2.** Lupus arthropathy. Severe (and reversible) swan-neck deformities of all the digits are characterized by hyperextension at the proximal interphalangeal joints and flexion at the distal interphalangeal joints.

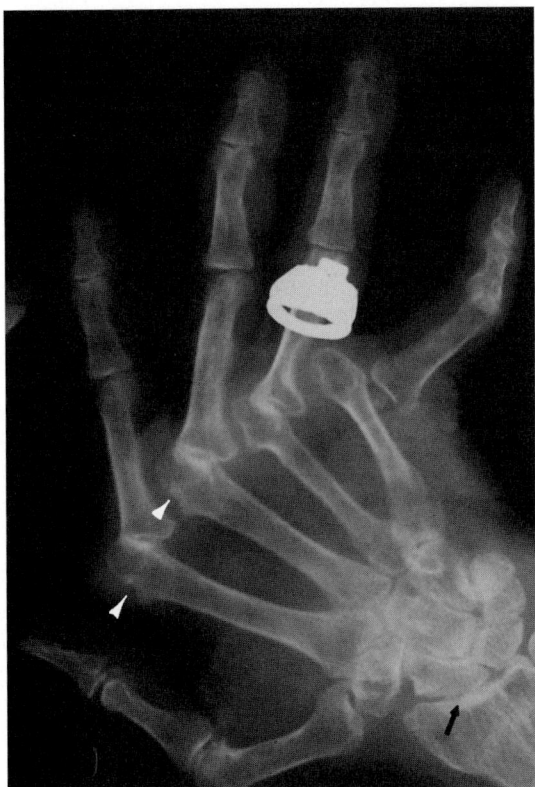

**Figure 23–3.** Lupus arthropathy: severe manifestations. Findings include radial deviation at the radiocarpal joint, ulnar deviation and subluxation at multiple metacarpophalangeal joints, and boutonnière and swan-neck deformities. Observe the joint space narrowing in the radiocarpal compartment *(arrow)* and hook erosions of the metacarpal heads *(arrowheads)*.

metacarpal and metatarsal heads (see Fig. 23–1). The cystic lesions occur beneath cartilage that is relatively normal, and they appear to represent a remodeling phenomenon.

## Spontaneous Tendon Weakening and Rupture

Spontaneous rupture of tendons is observed in patients with systemic lupus erythematosus, almost invariably in association with systemically or locally administered steroids (Fig. 23–4). In general, tendons in weight-bearing locations are affected. A tendency for the development of this complication in older patients and in men has been suggested. Weakening or rupture of the Achilles, quadriceps, and patellar tendons, as well as the extensor tendons of the hand, is encountered. Infrequently, the triceps or biceps tendon is involved.

## Osteonecrosis

Osteonecrosis is observed in approximately 5% of patients with systemic lupus erythematosus, with some estimates as high as 40%. Although the femoral head is the most common site of abnormality, involvement of other and multiple sites has been confirmed; osteonecrosis is not uncommon in the humeral head, femoral condyle, tibial plateau, and talus. The pathogenesis of osteonecrosis in this disease has not been fully delineated. Although it is

be related to either atrophy of disuse or pressure erosion from apposing bone in subluxed articulations. Bilateral or unilateral defects on the metacarpal (and infrequently the metatarsal) heads are occasionally evident. The erosions, which are designated hook erosions and predominate on the radial aspect of the bone, are probably produced by capsular pressure and deformity and may represent an adaptive change related to altered stress across the involved articulation (see Fig. 23–3). They are not associated with pannus erosion of bone.

The articular deformities of lupus arthropathy are related to capsular and ligamentous laxity and contracture and to muscular imbalance. Similar abnormalities occur in other deforming nonerosive arthropathies but are particularly apparent in patients with rheumatic fever. The alterations are distinct from those of rheumatoid arthritis, in which severe intra-articular inflammatory changes produce permanent cartilaginous and osseous destruction, leading to instability and subluxation.

## Subchondral Cysts

Osteoporosis and cyst formation within subchondral bone can occur in systemic lupus erythematosus. The most common sites of involvement are the bones in the hand, wrist, and foot, particularly the carpus and

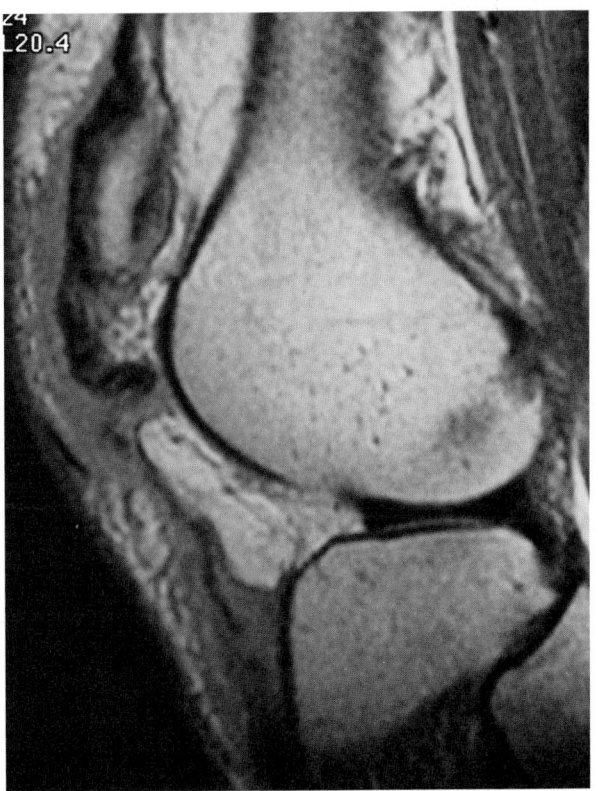

**Figure 23–4.** Tendon weakening and rupture. Sagittal intermediate-weighted (TR/TE, 1600/30) spin echo MR images show complete rupture of the patellar tendon, surrounding edema, and an elevated patella.

usually attributable to steroid administration, the development of osteonecrosis may be multifactorial, related to both the basic disease process and the previous administration of steroids.

The radiographic and pathologic features of osteonecrosis in patients with systemic lupus erythematosus are identical to those in patients who do not have this disease (see Chapter 67). The occurrence of bone necrosis in unusual sites, such as the metacarpal heads, carpal bones, tarsus, and metatarsal heads, however, should suggest systemic lupus erythematosus as a potential diagnosis (Figs. 23–5 and 23–6). Detection of osteonecrosis at any site is accomplished with more sensitivity and specificity with magnetic resonance (MR) imaging than with routine radiography.

## Soft Tissue Calcification

Soft tissue calcification is occasionally observed in systemic lupus erythematosus. Several patterns of calcification are reported: diffuse linear, streaky, or nodular calcification in the subcutaneous and deeper tissues, particularly in the lower extremities; focal or localized plaquelike calcification; periarticular calcification; and arterial calcification. Diffuse or focal calcific deposits may be associated with adjacent skin ulceration, inflammation, and necrosis. Juxta-articular calcifications appear as single or multiple deposits of varying size, with or without adjacent joint disease (Fig. 23–7).

## Osteomyelitis and Septic Arthritis

An unusually high frequency of bacterial and mycotic infections is found in patients with systemic lupus erythematosus. Two major factors contribute to this susceptibility to infection: steroid administration and renal disease. The respiratory tract, urinary tract, skin, and soft tissues are the sites commonly infected. The occurrence of bone and joint infection in systemic lupus erythematosus is less frequent. Monoarticular infection of the knee, hip, and ankle appears to be most typical. Implicated organisms include *Neisseria gonorrhoeae*, *Neisseria meningitidis*, *Staphylococcus aureus*, gram-negative bacilli, atypical mycobacteria, *Mycobacterium tuberculosis*, and *Salmonella* species. Radiographic findings of a large or increasing joint effusion and progressive cartilaginous and osseous destruction should raise the possibility of articular infection.

## Sacroiliitis

Rarely in patients with systemic lupus erythematosus, imaging studies reveal alterations about the sacroiliac joints. Radiographic changes include joint space narrowing, bone erosion, and reactive sclerosis in a unilateral or bilateral distribution. These changes are similar to those seen in osteoarthritis, so caution is required in assuming that they are signs of sacroiliitis.

## Miscellaneous Abnormalities

Osteopenia, presumably representing osteoporosis, is observed in some patients with systemic lupus erythematosus. Potential causes include debilitation and corti-

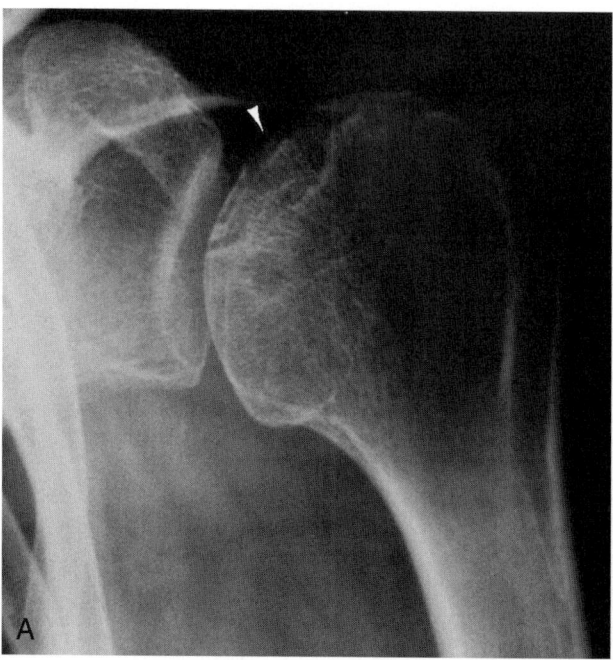
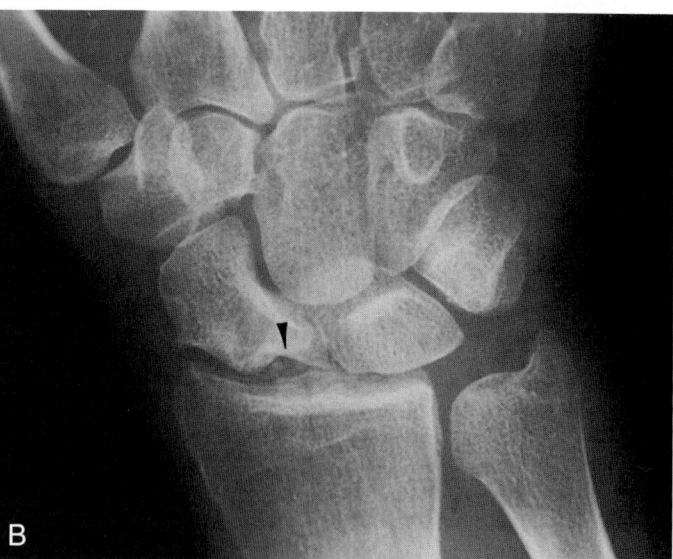

**Figure 23–5.** Osteonecrosis: multiple sites. In a young female patient with systemic lupus erythematosus, osteonecrosis developed at multiple sites after corticosteroid therapy. *A*, In the shoulder, typical changes are seen, including fragmentation of the humeral head with depression of the subchondral bone *(arrowhead)*. *B*, Changes in this wrist related to osteonecrosis include fragmentation and collapse of the proximal portion of the scaphoid *(arrowhead)* and intra-articular debris. (*B*, Courtesy of I. Dwosh, MD, Toronto, Ontario, Canada.)

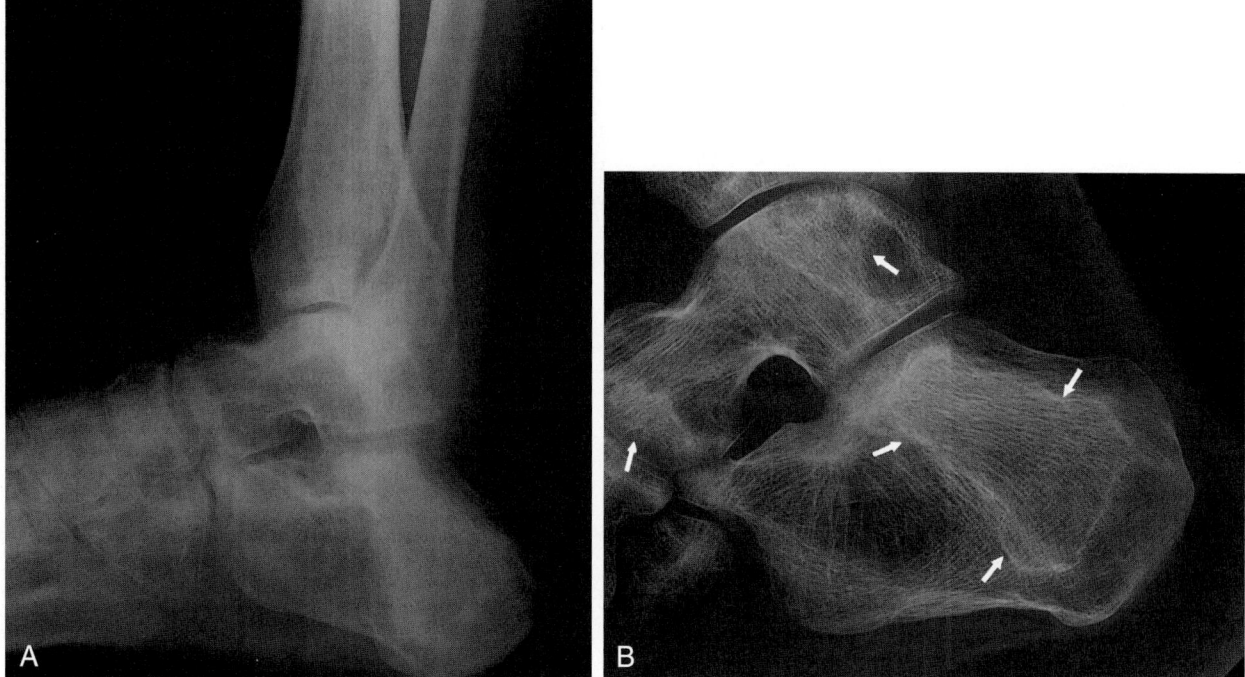

**Figure 23–6.** Osteonecrosis: ankle and foot. This young man with systemic lupus erythematosus developed vasculitis, which necessitated amputation of the leg. He had been treated with corticosteroids. *A,* Lateral radiograph reveals evidence of ischemic necrosis of bone, manifested as serpentine calcification in the tibia and calcaneus. Increased radiodensity of the proximal and distal articular surfaces of the talus, navicular, and cuboid is evident. *B,* Radiograph of a sagittal section of the hindfoot documents regions of bone infarction in the talus, calcaneus, and cuboid *(arrows)* that are associated with peripheral calcification.

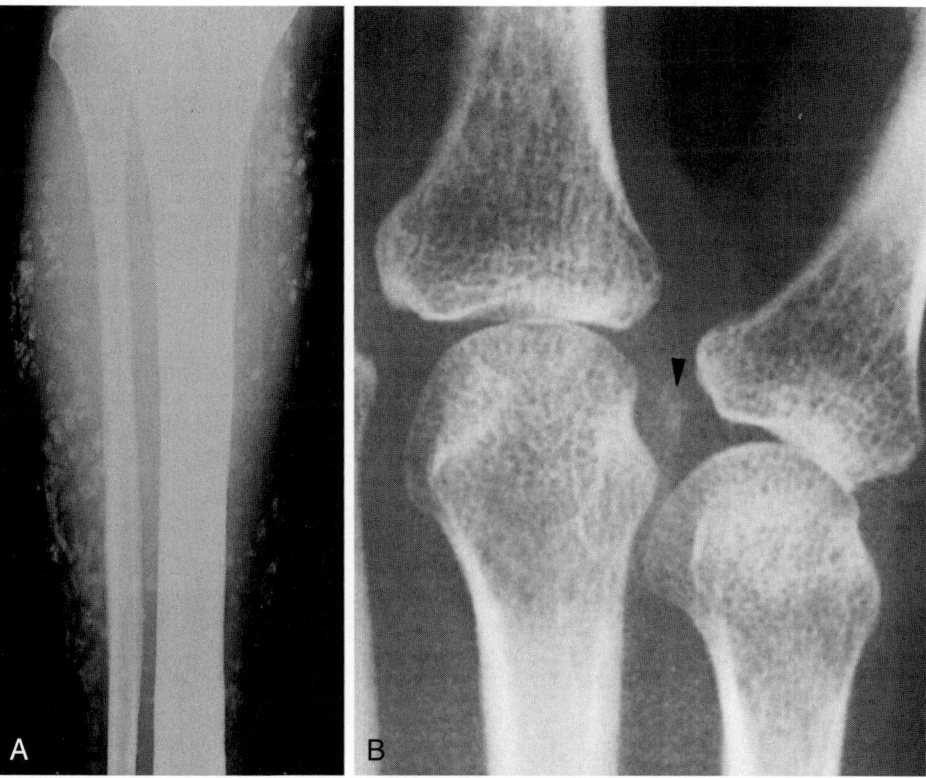

**Figure 23–7.** Patterns of soft tissue calcification in systemic lupus erythematosus. *A,* Widespread soft tissue calcification is evident in the lower part of the leg. *B,* Periarticular calcific (or ossific) dense shadow is seen about the metacarpophalangeal joint *(arrowhead).*

costeroid therapy. Insufficiency fractures are caused by normal or abnormal forces on weakened bone, and their distribution in systemic lupus erythematosus is similar to that in rheumatoid arthritis (Fig. 23–8).

Reported alterations of the terminal tufts of the phalanges in systemic lupus erythematosus include osteosclerosis and resorption (Fig. 23–9). The appearance of sclerosis at this site (acral sclerosis) must be evaluated with caution, because focal sclerotic lesions of one or several phalanges may be an incidental finding, especially in women. The detection of diffuse sclerosis of multiple digits may be more significant; this abnormality has been seen in a variety of collagen vascular disorders, including rheumatoid arthritis, and in sarcoidosis. The pattern of resorption of the phalangeal tufts in this disease is identical to that in scleroderma.

The occurrence of clinical and radiographic features of systemic lupus erythematosus in patients with other collagen vascular diseases has been documented in various overlap syndromes, as well as in mixed connective tissue disease. In patients with mixed connective tissue disease, high titers of antibodies to extractable nuclear antigen are present in the serum. In both mixed connective tissue disease and overlap syndromes, musculoskeletal manifestations of systemic lupus erythematosus may be combined with those of scleroderma, dermatomyositis, or rheumatoid arthritis.

## ANTIPHOSPHOLIPID SYNDROME

The antiphospholipid syndrome is characterized by venous and arterial thrombosis (often multiple) and recurrent fetal loss, frequently accompanied by thrombocytopenia and antiphospholipid antibodies. This syndrome may

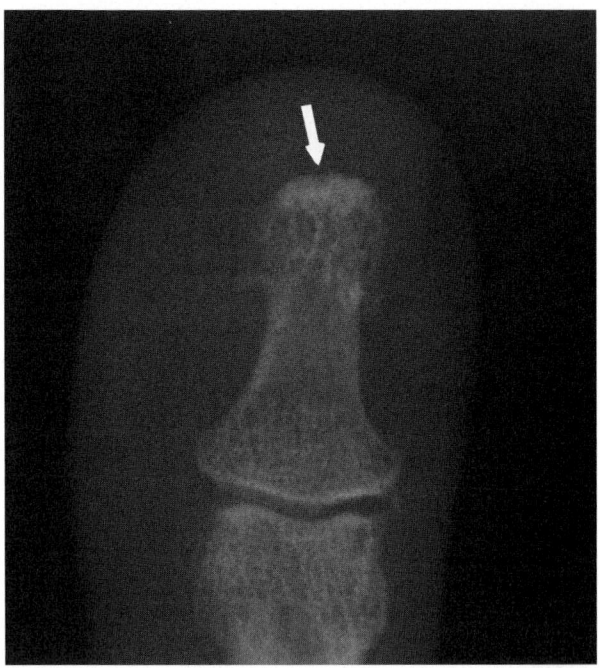

**Figure 23–9.** Tuft sclerosis. Focal bone sclerosis is evident in the tuft *(arrow)*. (Courtesy of A. Brower, MD, Norfolk, Va.)

occur without evidence of any other condition (primary antiphospholipid syndrome) or with findings of another disease (secondary antiphospholipid syndrome) such as systemic lupus erythematosus, other autoimmune disorders (e.g., vasculitides, idiopathic thrombocytopenic purpura, Crohn's disease), malignant tumors, and infections (e.g., human immunodeficiency virus), as well as after exposure to certain drugs. Clinical manifestations of the antiphospholipid syndrome are dependent on the site and extent of thrombosis.

Osteonecrosis is a well-recognized manifestation of the antiphospholipid syndrome. Involved sites include the femoral head and, less commonly, the humeral head, femoral condyles, bones about the ankle, and small bones of the wrist, hand, and foot. Extensive osteonecrosis is described more often in cases of secondary antiphospholipid syndrome when it is associated with systemic lupus erythematosus.

## DIFFERENTIAL DIAGNOSIS

The symmetrical polyarthritis associated with systemic lupus erythematosus produces nonspecific radiographic findings, including soft tissue swelling and osteoporosis. The deforming nonerosive arthropathy of the hands and wrists (and, less commonly, the feet) in systemic lupus erythematosus is similar to Jaccoud's arthropathy, which usually follows rheumatic fever (Table 23–2). In the classic descriptions of Jaccoud's arthropathy, involvement of the ulnar digits (fourth and fifth fingers) is stressed, although a more extensive distribution may be encountered; in the arthropathy of systemic lupus erythematosus, often all the digits, including the thumb, are affected. A deforming arthropathy without significant erosive abnormality may also be seen in such rare disorders as Ehlers-Danlos

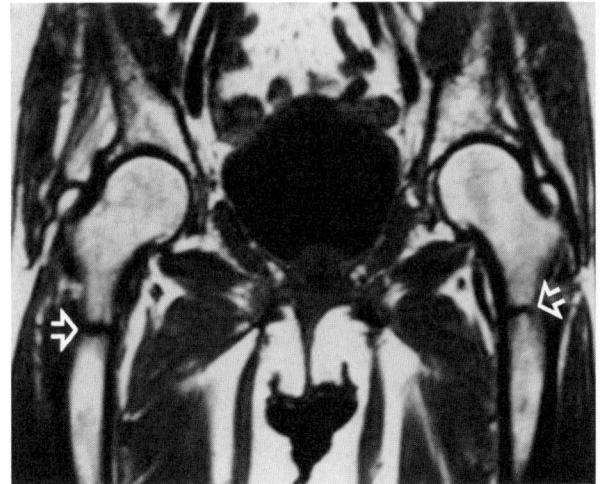

**Figure 23–8.** Insufficiency fractures. In this 48-year-old woman with systemic lupus erythematosus, insufficiency fractures occurred in both femora. A coronal T1-weighted (TR/TE, 500/20) spin echo MR image reveals these fractures as linear areas of low signal intensity *(arrows)*. More diffuse regions of decreased signal intensity about the fractures represent foci of bone marrow edema. (Courtesy of A. Motta, MD, Cleveland, Ohio.)

**TABLE 23–2**

**Differential Diagnosis of Radiographic Abnormalities in the Hand**

| Diagnosis | Distribution | Deformities | Erosions | Joint Space Narrowing |
|---|---|---|---|---|
| Lupus arthropathy | MCP and IP joints of all the digits; prominent abnormalities of the thumb | Initially reversible; may subsequently become fixed | Hook erosions on the radial and volar aspects of the metacarpal heads (uncommon) | Cartilage atrophy and pressure erosion in subluxed articulations (uncommon) |
| Classic Jaccoud's arthropathy | MCP and IP joints of the ulnar digits, particularly the fourth and fifth fingers | Initially reversible; may subsequently become fixed | Hook erosions on the radial and volar aspects of the metacarpal heads (uncommon) | Cartilage atrophy and pressure erosion in subluxed articulations (uncommon) |
| Rheumatoid arthritis | MCP and PIP joints of all the digits; prominent abnormalities | Progressive | Widespread marginal and central erosions at involved sites (common) | "Pannus" destruction of cartilage in subluxed and nonsubluxed articulations (common) |

IP, interphalangeal; MCP, metacarpophalangeal; PIP, proximal interphalangeal.

syndrome and hypogammaglobulinemia. In rheumatoid arthritis, joint space narrowing and bone erosion are characteristic, although occasionally, digital deformity may occur in the absence of cartilaginous and osseous abnormalities. In these instances, accurately distinguishing the joint disease of systemic lupus erythematosus from that of rheumatoid arthritis is difficult. Further, the appearance of joint space narrowing, hook erosions, and cyst formation in some patients with lupus arthropathy complicates this differentiation. The thumb deformities in systemic lupus erythematosus can be extensive; hyperextension of the interphalangeal joint and subluxation at the first carpometacarpal joint are particularly characteristic. Significant thumb deformity (as well as changes at the first carpometacarpal joint) is also evident, however, in other collagen vascular disorders such as scleroderma.

Spontaneous tendon rupture, which has been noted in patients with systemic lupus erythematosus, also occurs without an obvious precipitating event in hyperparathyroidism and in patients who have received steroid medication.

Osteonecrosis complicating systemic lupus erythematosus generally cannot be differentiated from that accompanying a variety of disease processes. Involvement of the metacarpal and metatarsal heads and the tarsal and carpal bones, however, appears to be especially characteristic of systemic lupus erythematosus. Soft tissue calcification is observed in systemic lupus erythematosus, but it also accompanies other collagen vascular disorders, particularly scleroderma and dermatomyositis. Differentiation among these disorders on the basis of the appearance of soft tissue calcific deposits is extremely difficult. Further, phalangeal tuft resorption or sclerosis has been identified in many collagen vascular diseases, as well as in sarcoidosis.

**FURTHER READING**

Babini SM, Cocco JAM, Babini JC, et al: Atlantoaxial subluxation in systemic lupus erythematosus: Further evidence of tendinous alterations. J Rheumatol 17:173, 1990.
Budin JA, Feldman F: Soft tissue calcifications in systemic lupus erythematosus. AJR Am J Roentgenol 124:358, 1975.
Bywaters EGL: Jaccoud's syndrome: A sequel to the joint involvement in systemic lupus erythematosus. Clin Rheum Dis 1:125, 1975.
Fishel B, Caspi D, Eventov I, et al: Multiple osteonecrotic lesions in systemic lupus erythematosus. J Rheumatol 14:601, 1987.
Houssiau FA, Toukap AN, Depresseux G, et al: Magnetic resonance imaging–detected avascular osteonecrosis in systemic lupus erythematosus: Lack of correlation with antiphospholipid antibodies. Br J Rheumatol 37:448, 1998.
Khan MA, Ballou SP: Tendon rupture in systemic lupus erythematosus. J Rheumatol 8:308, 1981.
Klipper AR, Stevens MB, Zizic TM, et al: Ischemic necrosis of bone in systemic lupus erythematosus. Medicine 55:251, 1976.
Leskinen RH, Skrifvars BV, Laasonen LS, et al: Bone lesions in systemic lupus erythematosus. Radiology 153:349, 1984.
Leventhal GH, Dorfman HD: Aseptic necrosis of bone in systemic lupus erythematosus. Semin Arthritis Rheum 4:73, 1974.
Myones BL, McCurdy D: The antiphospholipid syndrome: Immunologic and clinical aspects. Clinical spectrum and treatment. J Rheumatol 27:20, 2000.
Okada J, Nomura M, Shirataka M, et al: Prevalence of soft tissue calcifications in patients with SLE and effects of alfacarcidol. Lupus 8:456, 1999.
Sugimoto H, Hyodoh K, Kikuno M, et al: Periarticular calcification in systemic lupus erythematosus. J Rheumatol 26:574, 1999.
Weissman BN, Rappoport AS, Sosman JL, et al: Radiographic findings in the hands in patients with systemic lupus erythematosus. Radiology 126:313, 1978.

# CHAPTER 24

## Scleroderma (Progressive Systemic Sclerosis)

## SUMMARY OF KEY FEATURES

Scleroderma (progressive systemic sclerosis) leads to characteristic musculoskeletal abnormalities caused by the involvement of skin, subcutaneous tissues, muscles, bones, and joints. Many of the diverse clinical manifestations of this disease are represented on radiographs as soft tissue atrophy and calcification and bone resorption. Changes frequently predominate in the phalanges of the hand, although diffuse subcutaneous calcification, widespread periarticular calcification, and bone resorption are encountered at other sites such as the mandible, ribs, and clavicles. Major articular alterations consist of an erosive arthritis, particularly in the distal interphalangeal, proximal interphalangeal, metacarpophalangeal, first carpometacarpal, and inferior radioulnar joints, which may terminate as bony ankylosis and intra-articular calcific collections.

## INTRODUCTION

Scleroderma is an uncommon generalized disorder of connective tissue that affects various organ systems, principally the skin, lungs, gastrointestinal tract, heart, kidneys, and musculoskeletal system. Its pathologic characteristics include severe fibrosis and alterations of small blood vessels. The cause and pathogenesis of scleroderma are not known.

## NOMENCLATURE

The many reports of scleroderma and the difficulty in distinguishing it from other disorders associated with induration of the skin have led to a variety of descriptive terms and classification systems for the disease. Additional nomenclature that is commonly encountered includes the following:

**Raynaud's Phenomenon or Syndrome.** Paroxysmal occlusion of the digital arteries that is precipitated by cold or emotional stress and relieved by heat. This syndrome, which is associated with local pallor, cyanosis, pain, burning, numbness, swelling, and hyperhidrosis, is caused by a change in the diameter of the digital, palmar, and plantar arteries. It can be further classified as primary (or idiopathic) or secondary. Diseases leading to secondary Raynaud's syndrome include collagen vascular disorders, other vasculitides, obstructive arterial disorders, drug intoxication, neurologic and neoplastic processes, and thermal or occupational trauma.

**Acrosclerosis.** Sclerosis of facial structures and fingers that is associated with Raynaud's phenomenon.

**Diffuse Systemic Sclerosis.** Involvement of the skin of the trunk that is commonly associated with systemic abnormalities and may be associated with peripheral skin involvement.

**CRST Syndrome.** The association of subcutaneous calcinosis, Raynaud's phenomenon, sclerodactyly, and telangiectasia.

**CREST Syndrome.** The association of CRST syndrome with esophageal abnormalities.

**Thibierge-Weissenbach Syndrome.** The combination of calcinosis and digital ischemia.

**Scleroderma Circumscriptum, Scleroderma Diffusum, Scleroderma Morphea, Scleroderma en Bande.** Dermatologic variants of the disease.

**Shulman's Syndrome.** Scleroderma-like syndrome with eosinophilia and hypergammaglobulinemia, but without systemic or vascular involvement. This syndrome is also called eosinophilic fasciitis.

**Scleroderma Adultorum.** A benign, self-limited condition unrelated to true scleroderma that occurs after acute infections and is characterized by nonpitting edema of the skin and spontaneous resolution within a few months.

## CLINICAL ABNORMALITIES

### General Features

Scleroderma affects women more frequently than men and usually becomes apparent in the third to fifth decades of life. The onset of the disease is usually insidious. A common initial manifestation is intermittent pallor of the digits (fingers or toes) on exposure to cold (Raynaud's phenomenon). Other initial symptoms may include gradual thickening of the skin and edema in the distal portion of the extremities and pain and stiffness in the small joints of the hands and knees. The natural history of systemic sclerosis is variable. Although a fulminant, rapidly progressive disorder is occasionally evident, a protracted disease course with survival for 20 years or more is typical. As the disease advances, skin changes frequently represent the most characteristic clinical feature. Melanotic hyperpigmentation, vitiligo, and telangiectasis may be observed. Small or large calcific collections develop in subcutaneous tissue, predominantly in women. Systemic involvement in scleroderma can lead to a variety of symptoms and signs, depending on the site of abnormality, and include gastrointestinal, pulmonary, renal and cardiac alterations.

## Rheumatologic Features

Articular involvement has been described as an initial manifestation in 12% to 65% of patients with scleroderma and as an eventual manifestation in 46% to 97% of patients. The fingers, wrists, and ankles are commonly affected. The mode of onset can be acute or insidious, and the course is generally intermittent. Oligoarticular and polyarticular patterns predominate. Tendon and tendon sheath involvement is also common, especially in the knees, fingers, wrists, ankles, and feet.

Laboratory analysis indicates elevation of the erythrocyte sedimentation rate in approximately 60% to 70% of patients, positive serologic test results for rheumatoid factor in approximately 30% to 40% of patients, and the presence of antinuclear antibodies in 35% to 96% of patients.

## Overlap Syndromes

Some patients with scleroderma have clinical patterns that suggest the presence of more than one collagen vascular disease; findings may indicate an overlap condition consisting of scleroderma and dermatomyositis or scleroderma and systemic lupus erythematosus.

## RADIOGRAPHIC ABNORMALITIES

### Bone and Soft Tissue Involvement

**Hand.** Abnormalities of the hand (Fig. 24–1) are characterized by resorption of soft tissue, subcutaneous calcification, and osseous destruction. One or more of these changes were evident in 63% of patients in a large series of persons with scleroderma. Soft tissue resorption of the fingertips is a common finding in scleroderma. Its frequency varies from 15% to 80%, according to previous reports, and increases dramatically in patients with accompanying Raynaud's phenomenon. Resorption of soft tissue produces a conical shape of the fingertips. Its presence can be verified by measuring the vertical distance between the phalangeal tip and the skin surface on a frontal radiograph of the digit. If this distance is less than 20% of the transverse diameter of the base of the same distal phalanx, soft tissue resorption is present.

Amorphous calcification is common in patients with scleroderma, especially in the hand. The reported frequency of digital calcification in patients with scleroderma is approximately 10% to 30%. Digital calcification can involve either subcutaneous or capsular tissue. The appearance includes small punctate deposits at the phalangeal tip, focal conglomerate deposits with a wider distribution, sheetlike or tumoral collections, and curvilinear deposits within the joint capsule.

Bony erosion of the phalanges in the hand occurs in 40% to 80% of patients with scleroderma. It commences on the tuft, particularly on the palmar aspect of the bone. Continued resorption leads to "penciling" or sharpening of the phalanx, and in severe cases, much or all of the distal phalanx can be destroyed, with subsequent tapering of the entire digit.

**Foot.** Abnormalities of the bones and soft tissues of the foot are less frequent and less pronounced than those in the hand.

**Mandible.** A relatively specific dental sign of scleroderma is thickening of the periodontal membrane (Fig. 24–2); the frequency of this radiographic finding is reportedly

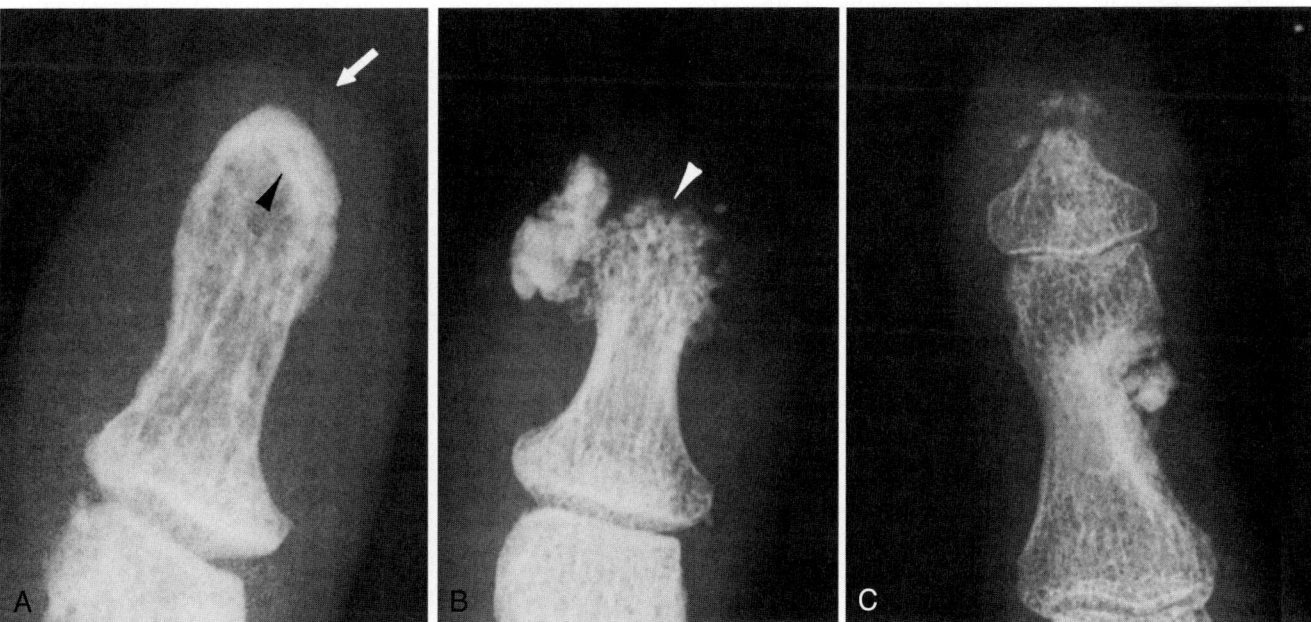

**Figure 24–1.** Bone and soft tissue abnormalities: digits of the hand. *A*, Observe the atrophy of the soft tissue *(arrow)* and hyperostosis of the phalangeal tuft *(arrowhead)*. *B*, In this digit, findings include resorption of the tuft *(arrowhead)* and adjacent calcification. *C*, Soft tissue swelling, tuft resorption, and calcification are seen. Note the deformity of the nail.

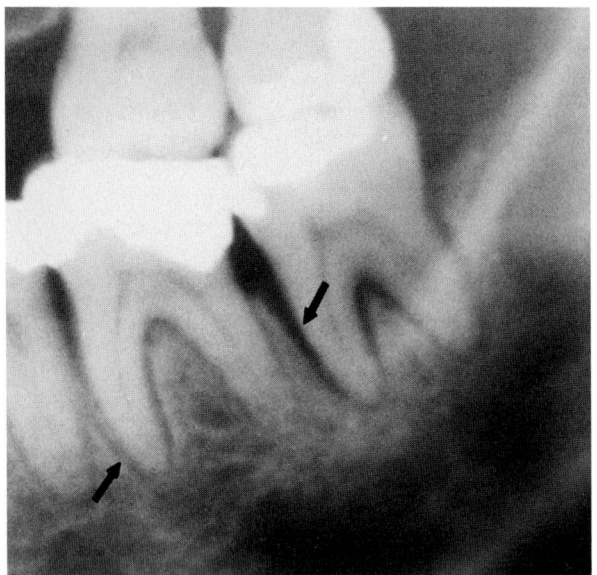

**Figure 24–2.** Bone and soft tissue abnormalities: mandible. Observe the exaggerated radiolucent area between the teeth and the mandible *(arrows)*, corresponding to the location of a thickened periodontal membrane.

20% to 33%. The enlarged membrane creates an exaggerated radiolucent area between the tooth and the mandibular bone that is best detected on dental films.

**Ribs.** Symmetrically distributed erosions of the superior aspect of multiple ribs are seen (Fig. 24–3). The changes predominate along the posterior aspects of the third to sixth ribs and may occur in the absence of bone resorption at other sites. Evidence suggests that the rib resorption in scleroderma is related to intercostal muscle atrophy, with resultant loss of mechanical stress on the cortical bone at the muscle insertions, leading to osseous resorption.

**Spine.** Paraspinal calcification has been emphasized as an additional manifestation of scleroderma (Fig. 24–4). Such calcification, which may become massive, has been observed in all spinal segments and may lead to local pain, discomfort, stiffness, dysphagia, and spinal cord or nerve root compression.

**Other Sites and Manifestations.** Soft tissue calcification in scleroderma occurs not only in the digits but also in the face, axilla, forearms, lower legs, and pressure areas such as the ischial tuberosities. In addition, periarticular "tumoral" collections can appear at single or multiple sites and simulate the findings in milk-alkali syndrome, hypervitaminosis D, and renal osteodystrophy (Fig. 24–5). Bone resorption in scleroderma may also be apparent at other sites (Table 24–1).

## Articular Involvement

In addition to the "articular" abnormalities that result from primary osseous resorption in scleroderma, several other articular manifestations occur (Table 24–2):

**Interphalangeal Joints.** Alterations at the distal interphalangeal joints are usually confined to regional or periarticular osteoporosis and swelling and thickening of adjacent soft tissue, without evidence of joint space narrowing or osseous erosion. Occasionally, however, joint manifestations in scleroderma closely resemble those of rheumatoid arthritis, with osteoporosis, joint space narrowing, and osseous erosion in typical "target" areas. In some patients with scleroderma, alterations occur at the distal interphalangeal joints, articulations that are not commonly involved in rheumatoid arthritis (Fig. 24–6).

**First Carpometacarpal Joints.** Selective involvement of the first carpometacarpal joint of the wrist may be apparent in scleroderma. Distinctive bilateral resorption of the trapezium and adjacent metacarpal bone is observed, with varying degrees of radial subluxation of the metacarpal base. Intra-articular calcification may be seen (Fig. 24–7). Preferential involvement of the first carpometacarpal joint is the distinctive feature of this arthropathy. Its pathogenesis is unknown, but a similar arthropathy may be

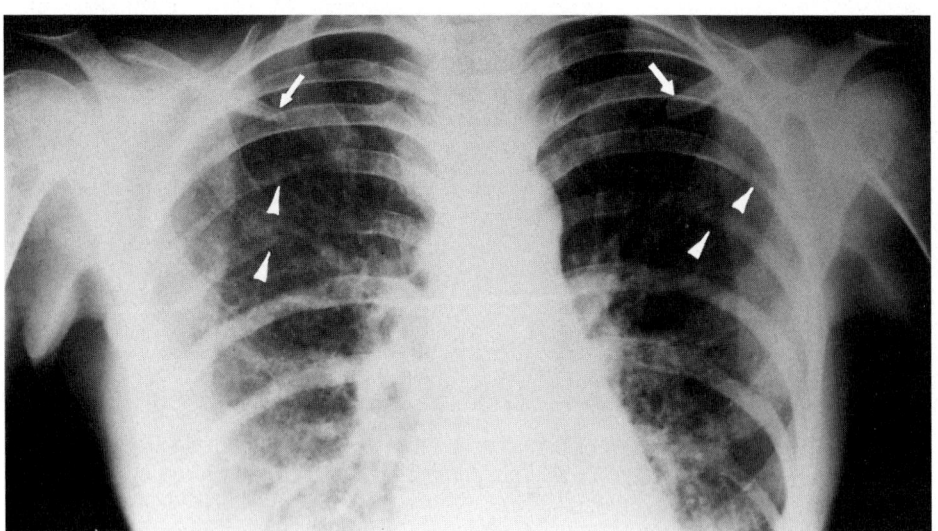

**Figure 24–3.** Bone and soft tissue abnormalities: ribs and clavicle. Note resorption of the clavicles *(arrows)* and ribs *(arrowheads)*. Observe the peripheral abnormalities in the lower lobes of the lungs. (Courtesy of P. Kline, MD, San Antonio, Tex.)

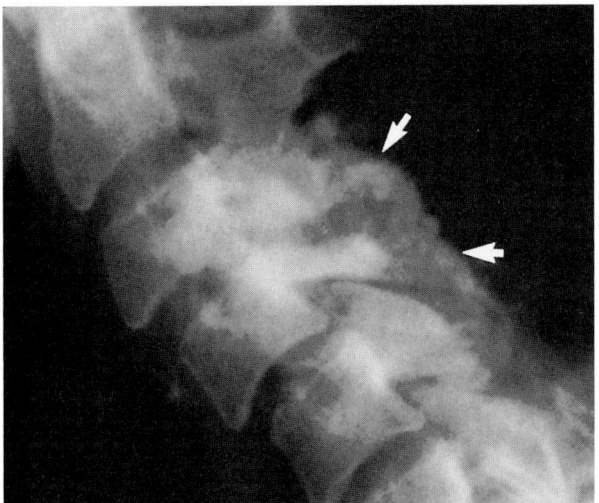

**Figure 24–4.** Bone and soft tissue abnormalities: cervical spine. Lateral radiograph shows calcific masses about the apophyseal joints *(arrows)* between the third and sixth cervical levels. (Courtesy of W. Peck, MD, Orange, Calif.)

apparent in other disorders that alter muscle and tendon balance, such as systemic lupus erythematosus, Jaccoud's arthropathy, dermatomyositis, and Ehlers-Danlos syndrome.

**Other Sites and Manifestations.** In addition to soft tissue and periarticular calcific deposition, intra-articular (free or intrasynovial) calcification may become evident in

---

### TABLE 24-1

**Sites of Osteolysis in Scleroderma**

Phalanges of the hand and foot
Carpal bones
Distal portions of the radius and ulna
Mandible
Ribs
Clavicle
Humerus
Acromion
Cervical spine

---

### TABLE 24-2

**Sites of Erosive Articular Disease in Scleroderma**

Metacarpophalangeal joints
Proximal and distal interphalangeal joints
First carpometacarpal joint
Inferior radioulnar joint
Metatarsophalangeal joints

---

scleroderma (Fig. 24–8). Radiographs reveal cloudlike radiodense regions conforming to a portion of the joint or the entire articulation (see Fig. 24–7). Intra-articular calcification is most frequent in the elbow, the inferior radioulnar and first carpometacarpal joints of the wrist,

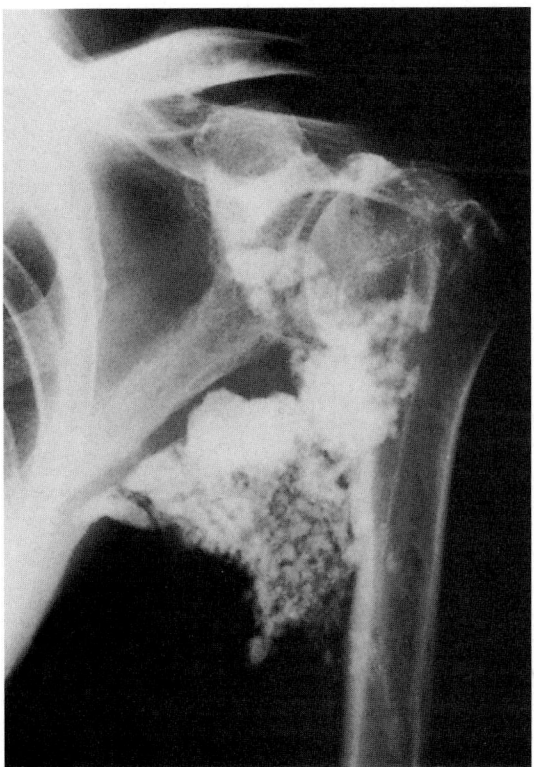

**Figure 24–5.** Bone and soft tissue abnormalities: periarticular calcification. Periarticular deposits are evident about the shoulder.

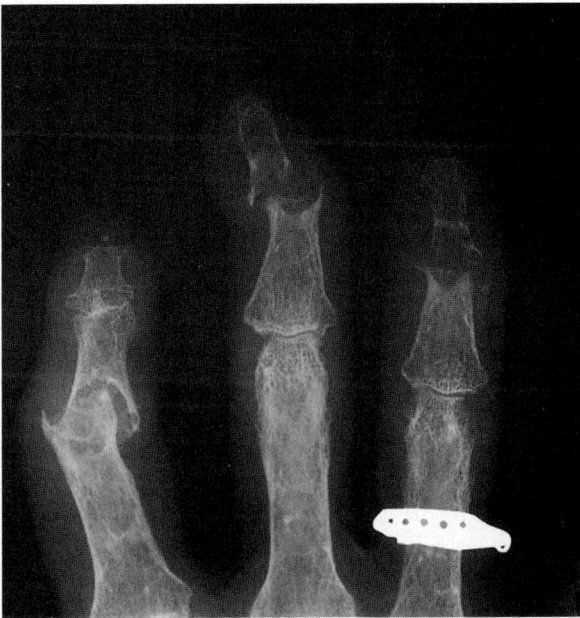

**Figure 24–6.** Articular involvement: interphalangeal joints. Extensive bone erosion about the distal interphalangeal and proximal interphalangeal joints can be observed. Note the separation of the osseous margins and the sharply demarcated irregular surfaces. Subluxation is also apparent. The findings are reminiscent of psoriatic arthritis.

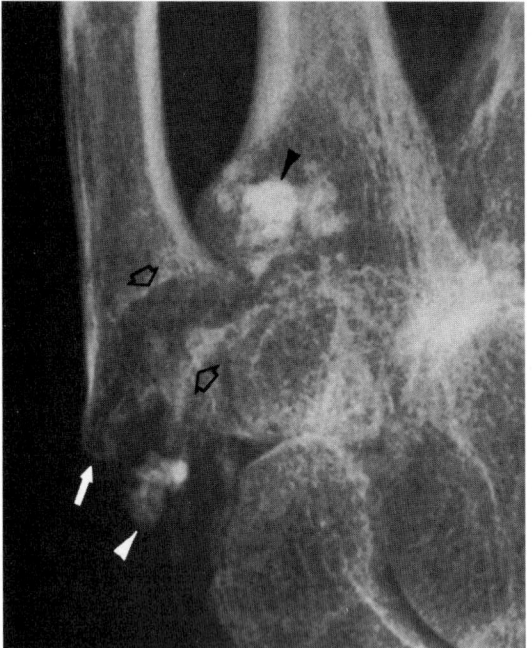

**Figure 24–7.** Articular involvement: wrist. Selective involvement of the first carpometacarpal joint in scleroderma. Observe the scalloped erosions of the trapezium and base of the metacarpal *(open arrows)*, radial and proximal subluxation of the metacarpal base *(solid arrow)*, and intra-articular calcification *(arrowhead)*.

(From Resnick D, Greenway G, Vint VC, et al: Selective involvement of the first carpometacarpal joint in scleroderma. AJR Am J Roentgenol 131:283, 1978.)

the metacarpophalangeal and metatarsophalangeal joints, the knee, and the hip (Fig. 24–9). Synovial calcification may be apparent within tendon sheaths or bursae in scleroderma. Such calcification is seen most frequently about the heel, elbow, knee, hip, and shoulder. Extensive linear radiodense regions conforming to the location of the tendon sheath and cloudlike calcification conforming to the location of the bursa are seen (Fig. 24–10).

## Vascular Involvement

Arteriography confirms the presence of vascular abnormalities in patients with Raynaud's phenomenon. Vasospasm, narrowing, and obstructive lesions of the digital arteries are observed, although the extent and severity of the occlusive lesions do not always correlate with the clinical severity of digital ischemia, the duration of the disease, or the presence of Raynaud's phenomenon. Additional arteriographic findings include incomplete, poorly formed, or absent palmar arterial arches and ulnar artery.

## PATHOLOGIC ABNORMALITIES

The pathologic changes in the skin of patients with scleroderma consist of a low-grade inflammatory reaction characterized by perivascular cellular infiltration. Subsequently, a progressive increase in compact collagen fibers in the dermis, thinning of the overlying epidermis, and atrophy of dermal appendages are evident, as well as thickening of the intima, medial fibrosis, and thrombotic occlusion of arterioles. Abnormalities of the synovial membrane consist of inflammatory changes characterized by hyperemia, cellular infiltration, vascular sclerosis, and

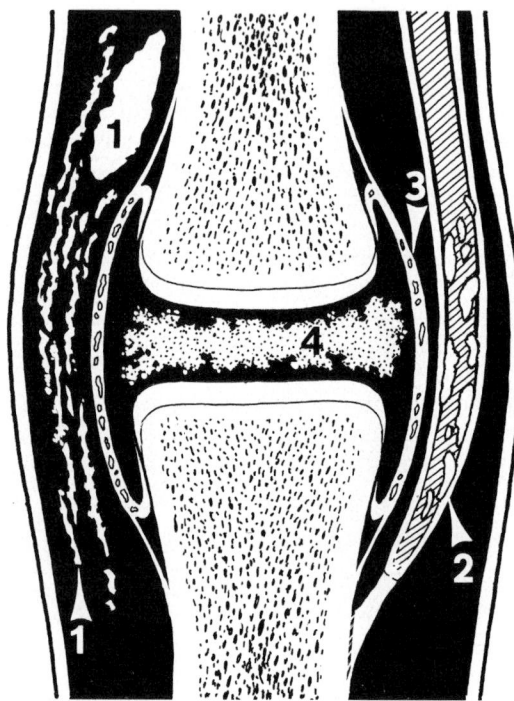

**Figure 24–8.** Sites of calcification in scleroderma. Deposits may occur in the soft tissues (1), tendons and tendon sheaths (2), and capsule (3), as well as within the joint (4).

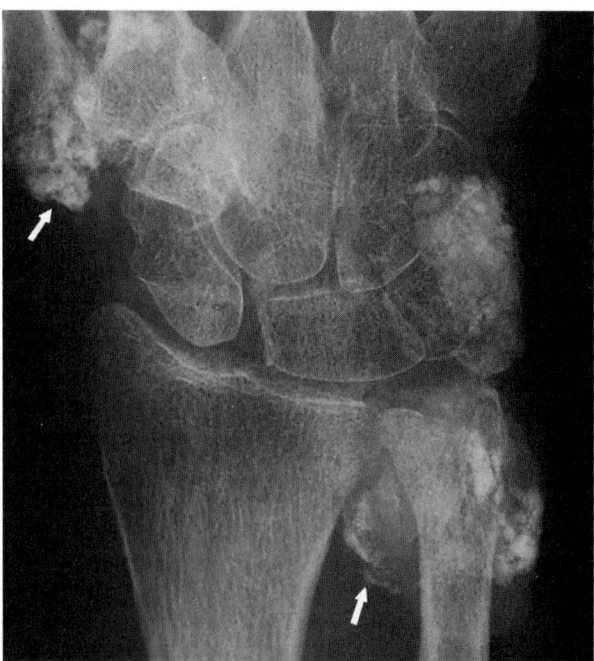

**Figure 24–9.** Articular involvement: juxta-articular calcification. Intra-articular calcification is particularly evident at the first carpometacarpal and inferior radioulnar joints *(arrows)*.

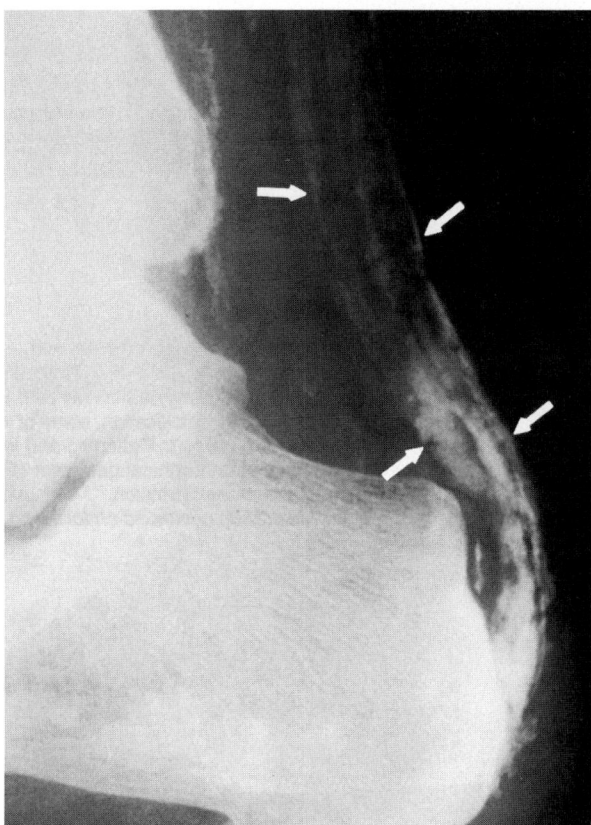

**Figure 24–10.** Articular involvement: tendon and bursal calcification. Striking example of diffuse calcification about the Achilles tendon *(arrows)*.

surface fibrin deposition. Subsequently, intense fibrosis of the superficial or all layers of the synovium becomes evident.

## OTHER SYNDROMES AND CONDITIONS ASSOCIATED WITH SCLERODERMA

### Chemically Induced Scleroderma-Like Conditions

Certain chemicals, including vinyl chloride, pentazocine, and bleomycin, can induce cutaneous abnormalities simulating those of scleroderma. Raynaud's phenomenon and pulmonary fibrosis, along with a distinctive pattern of acro-osteolysis, are evident in workers who clean reactor vessels and are exposed to the polymerizing agent vinyl chloride (see Chapter 83). Scleroderma-like changes are also observed with other chemical agents, including solvents, paraffin and silicone implants, and cocaine. A toxic epidemic syndrome (toxic oil syndrome) has been associated with the consumption of adulterated rapeseed oil, marketed illegally and sold as a cheap cooking oil.

### Rheumatic Diseases Associated with Silicone Breast Implants

The precise relationship between silicone breast implants and rheumatic disease is controversial. Despite numerous reports (some better documented than others) of rheu-matic disorders occurring after breast augmentation with silicone, a true association has not been firmly established. The observed disorders often lack specificity, although scleroderma-like clinical manifestations have been noted in 10% to 25% of cases. At this time, a proven relationship between silicone implants and rheumatic disease does not exist.

### Eosinophilic Fasciitis

Eosinophilic fasciitis, also known as Shulman's syndrome, is seen predominantly in adults. It is associated with inflammation and induration of the skin and subcutaneous tissues of the hands, forearms, feet, and legs, usually after an episode of physical exertion. Polyarthralgia, polyarthritis, muscle atrophy, and carpal tunnel syndrome have been observed. Arthritis is common in the joints of the hands and wrists and in the knees, and clinical findings resemble those of rheumatoid arthritis. Joint contractures, related to induration and sclerosis of subcutaneous tissue, are seen especially in the elbows, wrists, ankles, knees, and hands. The disorder is associated with peripheral blood eosinophilia, especially during the early stages; hypergammaglobulinemia (IgG); and an elevated erythrocyte sedimentation rate. Raynaud's phenomenon and visceral manifestations of progressive systemic sclerosis are conspicuously absent. Improvement in clinical and laboratory parameters follows the systemic administration of corticosteroids.

Because the pathologic alterations involve the lower subcutaneous tissues and the fascia, a deep wedge biopsy that extends through these tissues, as well as through muscle, is required for diagnosis. Radiographic abnormalities are generally confined to osteopenia, although additional findings may include bone erosions and periostitis. Magnetic resonance (MR) imaging has been used to study the soft tissue abnormalities of eosinophilic fasciitis. Findings include thickening of the fascia and increased signal intensity in the fascia, subcutaneous tissue, and superficial muscle fibers on fluid-sensitive sequences, as well as contrast enhancement (Fig. 24–11). Increased attenuation values of the superficial and deep fasciae have been evident with computed tomography.

The cause of eosinophilic fasciitis is unknown. It most resembles scleroderma, and some investigators believe that it may not be a separate disorder at all; however, it is generally self-limited and without systemic manifestations. Eosinophilia, raised serum IgG levels, and the identification of immunoglobulin in the inflamed fascia suggest that a humoral or cellular immune mechanism is involved in eosinophilic fasciitis.

### Eosinophilia-Myalgia Syndrome

The eosinophilia-myalgia syndrome has been related to ingestion of the amino acid L-tryptophan and bears a close resemblance to eosinophilic fasciitis. Initial clinical abnormalities include fatigue, fever, and diffuse myalgia of the proximal muscles. The disease continues to unfold over a period of several weeks or months, and eventually, an impressive list of organs may be involved. Arthralgia (10% to 50% of cases) or, less commonly, arthritis (10%

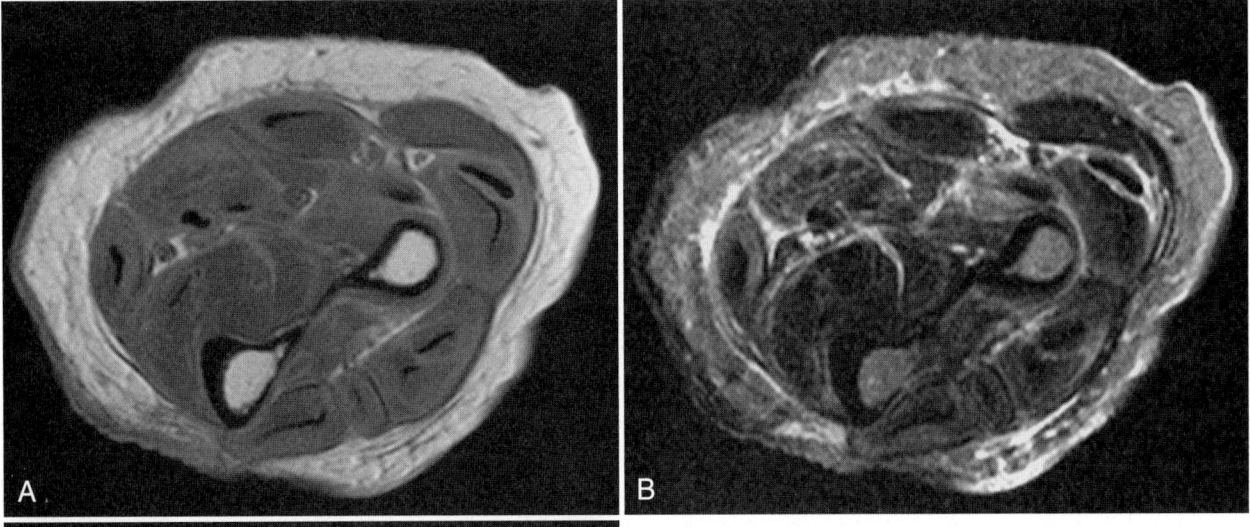

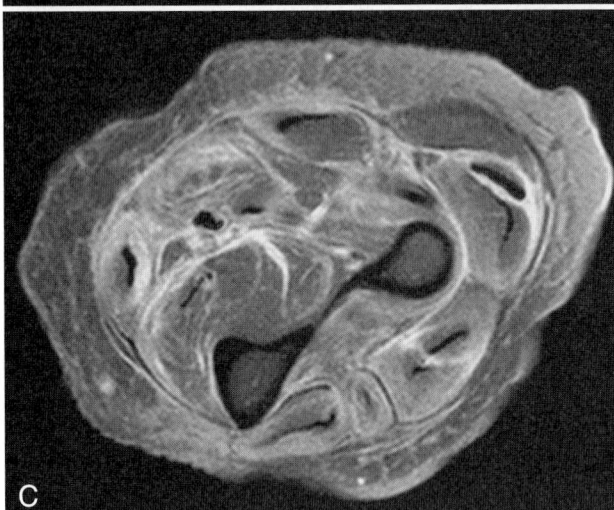

**Figure 24–11.** Eosinophilic fasciitis: MR imaging features. *A* and *B*, Axial T1-weighted (TR/TE, 622/17) *(A)* and T2-weighted (TR/TE, 2250/80) *(B)* spin echo MR images of the forearm show thickening of the fascia and increased signal intensity in the fascia and adjacent muscle on fluid-sensitive sequences. *C*, Corresponding axial fat-suppressed T1-weighted (TR/TE, 665/17) spin echo MR image following intravenous contrast shows enhancement of the thickened fascia and adjacent muscle.

to 20% of cases) is seen, usually involving the large joints. Progressive contracture of the knees and elbows may develop, and limited mobility of the ankles and wrists has been evident in some cases.

The natural history of this syndrome is variable. Corticosteroid therapy is not effective in most patients, and the mortality rate varies from 2% to 6%. The relationship of the eosinophilia-myalgia syndrome to eosinophilic fasciitis has been the subject of speculation; evidence suggests that the two diseases are not identical and that the eosinophilia-myalgia syndrome is a more severe disorder.

### Graft-versus-Host Disease

Graft-versus-host disease occurs when immunologically competent cells engrafted onto a foreign host attack the tissues of that host. In current practice, this disease usually appears after allogeneic bone marrow transplantation. The specific prerequisites for identifying graft-versus-host disease are the following: the graft must contain immunocompetent cells, the host must be sufficiently genetically different from the graft for it to be perceived

as antigenically foreign, and the host must be unable to reject the graft effectively.

Graft-versus-host disease occurs in either an acute or a chronic form, the former appearing before 100 days after the transplant and the latter generally after 100 days. It is the chronic form of graft-versus-host disease that resembles a collagen vascular disease, specifically, scleroderma. Chronic graft-versus-host disease develops in 10% to 30% of patients undergoing bone marrow transplantation. In untreated cases, tightly bound skin, contractures, and tissue wasting are observed. Laboratory aberrations include anemia, leukopenia, thrombocytopenia, eosinophilia, elevated serum levels of immunoglobulins, and the presence of circulating autoantibodies.

## DIFFERENTIAL DIAGNOSIS
### Bony Abnormalities

Generalized resorption of the terminal phalanges of the hand, foot, or both in scleroderma is characterized by "penciling" of the tuft (Fig. 24–12). A similar finding can be seen in other disorders, such as Raynaud's disease

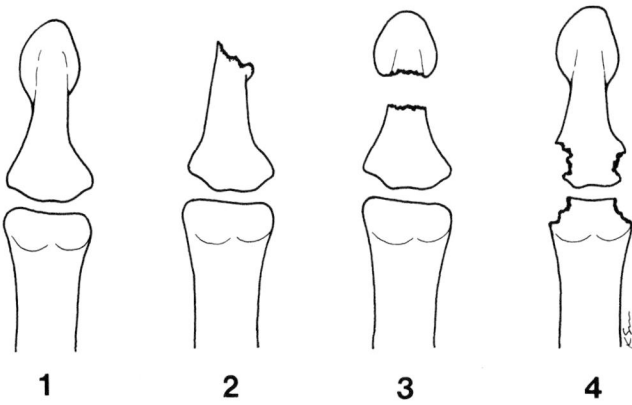

**1        2        3        4**

**Figure 24–12.** Phalangeal resorption: differential diagnosis. The normal situation is depicted in diagram 1. Resorption of the tuft (2) can be seen in scleroderma, other collagen vascular disorders, thermal injuries, hyperparathyroidism, psoriatic arthritis, and epidermolysis bullosa. Bandlike resorption of the terminal phalanx (3) is seen in familial and occupational acro-osteolysis, collagen vascular disorders, and hyperparathyroidism. Erosions about the distal interphalangeal joint (4) can be noted in psoriatic arthritis, multicentric reticulohistiocytosis, gout, thermal injuries, scleroderma, and hyperparathyroidism.

without scleroderma, thermal injuries (burn, frostbite, electrical), trauma, other collagen vascular diseases (dermatomyositis), neuropathic diseases (congenital indifference to pain, leprosy, diabetes mellitus, meningomyelocele), articular disorders (psoriatic arthritis, Lesch-Nyhan syndrome), hyperparathyroidism, progeria, and epidermolysis bullosa. In most of these diseases, the distribution of changes and the presence of additional abnormalities usually allow an accurate diagnosis (Table 24–3). Further, the association of tuft resorption, skin atrophy, and soft tissue calcification in scleroderma is of great diagnostic significance.

Tuft resorption in scleroderma should not be confused with congenital disorders associated with hypoplasia of the terminal phalanges. In addition, the type of bone resorption in scleroderma is usually easily differentiated from disorders characterized by bandlike resorption of the distal phalangeal shafts (polyvinyl chloride–associated acro-osteolysis, familial acro-osteolysis, and hyperparathyroidism) and from those characterized by intraosseous or eccentric destruction of the terminal phalanx (inclusion cyst, glomus tumor, enchondroma, osteomyelitis, and skeletal metastasis). The combination of tuft resorption and erosive arthritis of the distal interphalangeal joints may be apparent in scleroderma as well as in hyperparathyroidism, psoriatic arthritis, thermal injuries, and multicentric reticulohistiocytosis.

## Soft Tissue Abnormalities

Atrophy of the distal phalangeal soft tissue is a finding in scleroderma that can be observed in other collagen vascular diseases, thermal injuries, vascular disorders, Raynaud's disease, and epidermolysis bullosa, as well as other conditions. Scleroderma-like skin changes can also be evident in graft-versus-host disease after allogeneic bone marrow transplantation, in eosinophilic fasciitis, and after exposure to certain chemicals.

Calcification of the phalangeal soft tissues may be apparent in other collagen vascular diseases. More diffuse calcification in muscles and subcutaneous tissue is observed in many collagen vascular disorders, renal osteodystrophy, hypoparathyroidism, pseudohypoparathyroidism, fat necrosis, hypervitaminosis D, idiopathic hypercalcemia, milk-alkali syndrome, parasitic infections, Ehlers-Danlos syndrome, and idiopathic tumoral calcinosis. In many of these disorders, the pattern of calcification is distinctive and differs from the punctate or linear deposits observed in scleroderma. Scleroderma may be associated with "tumoral" periarticular calcifications, an appearance that

---

**TABLE 24-3**

**Characteristic Sites of Distal Phalangeal Resorption in Various Disorders***

| | Site | | |
| --- | --- | --- | --- |
| **Disorder** | **Tuft** | **Midportion or Waist** | **Periarticular** |
| Scleroderma | + | | + |
| Hyperparathyroidism | + | + | + |
| Thermal injury | + | | + |
| Psoriatic arthritis | + | | + |
| Epidermolysis bullosa | + | | |
| Polyvinyl chloride acro-osteolysis | | + | |
| Multicentric reticulohistiocytosis | + | | + |
| Inflammatory (erosive) osteoarthritis | | | + |
| Lesch-Nyhan syndrome | + | | |
| Progeria | + | | |

*Only the characteristic sites of bone resorption are indicated, although in any single disease, considerable variability in these sites may exist.

may also be apparent in other collagen vascular diseases, renal osteodystrophy, milk-alkali syndrome, hypervitaminosis D, calcium hydroxyapatite crystal deposition disease, and sarcoidosis.

## Articular Abnormalities

An erosive arthritis of the distal interphalangeal joints accompanies scleroderma, inflammatory (erosive) osteoarthritis, psoriatic arthritis, multicentric reticulohistiocytosis, gout, and thermal injuries. In most patients with scleroderma, erosions of these joints are mild, although uncommonly, larger erosions with extensive phalangeal destruction and intra-articular bony ankylosis may be indistinguishable from psoriasis or inflammatory (erosive) osteoarthritis. Associated radiographic findings, including intra-articular calcification, allow an accurate diagnosis of scleroderma in some cases.

The intra-articular cloudlike calcification in scleroderma differs in radiographic appearance from that of calcium pyrophosphate dihydrate crystal deposition disease, calcium hydroxyapatite crystal deposition disease, idiopathic synovial osteochondromatosis, intra-articular osseous bodies, gout, and synovioma or hemangioma.

## FURTHER READING

Barnett AJ: Scleroderma (Progressive Systemic Sclerosis). Springfield, Ill, Charles C Thomas, 1974.

Bassett LW, Blocka KLN, Furst DE, et al: Skeletal findings in progressive systemic sclerosis (scleroderma). AJR Am J Roentgenol 136:1121, 1981.

Edworthy SM, Martin L, Barr S, et al: A clinical study of the relationship between silicone breast implants and connective tissue disease. J Rheumatol 25:254, 1998.

Ishakawa O, Akimoto S, Sato M, et al: Multiple bursitis in systemic sclerosis. J Rheumatol 24:1189, 1997.

Keats TE: Rib erosions in scleroderma. AJR Am J Roentgenol 100:530, 1967.

Lakhanpal S, Ginsburg WW, Michet CJ, et al: Eosinophilic fasciitis: Clinical spectrum and therapeutic response in 52 cases. Semin Arthritis Rheum 17:221, 1988.

Martin L: Silicone breast implants: The saga continues. J Rheumatol 26:1020, 1999.

Monsees B, Murphy WA: Distal phalangeal erosive lesions. Arthritis Rheum 27:449, 1984.

Moore TL, Zuckner J: Eosinophilic fasciitis. Semin Arthritis Rheum 9:228, 1980.

Rabinowitz JG, Twersky J, Guttadauria M: Similar bone manifestations of scleroderma and rheumatoid arthritis. AJR Am J Roentgenol 121:35, 1974.

Resnick D, Greenway G, Vint VC, et al: Selective involvement of the first carpometacarpal joint in scleroderma. AJR Am J Roentgenol 131:283, 1978.

Resnick D, Scavulli JF, Goergen TG, et al: Intra-articular calcification in scleroderma. Radiology 124:685, 1977.

Rocco VK, Hurd ER: Scleroderma and scleroderma-like disorders. Semin Arthritis Rheum 16:22, 1986.

Roubenoff R, Coté T, Watson R, et al: Eosinophilia-myalgia syndrome due to L-tryptophan ingestion. Arthritis Rheum 33:930, 1990.

Rush PJ, Bell MJ, Fam AG: Toxic oil syndrome (Spanish oil disease) and chemically induced scleroderma-like conditions. J Rheumatol 11:262, 1984.

Schweitzer ME, Cervilla V, Manaster BJ, et al: Cervical paraspinal calcification in collagen vascular diseases. AJR Am J Roentgenol 157:523, 1991.

Spielvogel RL, Goltz RW, Kersey JH: Scleroderma-like changes in chronic graft vs host disease. Arch Dermatol 113:1424, 1977.

Vasey FB, Seleznick MJ: Epidemiology versus outcome: The silicone breast implant controversy. J Rheumatol 26:1018, 1999.

Ward M, Curé J, Schabel S, et al: Symptomatic spinal calcinosis in systemic sclerosis (scleroderma). Arthritis Rheum 40:1892, 1997.

# CHAPTER 25

## Dermatomyositis, Polymyositis, and Other Inflammatory Myopathies

## *SUMMARY OF KEY FEATURES*

Dermatomyositis and polymyositis are disorders of unknown cause characterized by inflammation and degeneration of muscle. A variety of clinical patterns may be observed in both children and adults affected by these disorders. The radiographic features of musculoskeletal involvement consist of soft tissue edema, atrophy, contracture, and calcification; bone resorption (phalangeal tufts); and, possibly, articular erosion and subluxation. These features most resemble the abnormalities accompanying other collagen vascular diseases, including scleroderma and systemic lupus erythematosus. Magnetic resonance (MR) imaging is an effective method of studying the muscular abnormalities that characterize these diseases.

## INTRODUCTION

Dermatomyositis and polymyositis are disorders of striated muscle characterized by diffuse, nonsuppurative inflammation and degeneration. In dermatomyositis, both skeletal muscle and the skin are involved, whereas in polymyositis, skeletal muscle alone is affected. The cause of these disorders is unknown, and they affect patients of all ages, although they are most frequent in middle-aged women. They are but two of a number of inflammatory diseases of muscle—the inflammatory myopathies—characterized by proximal muscle weakness and muscle inflammation without suppuration. Such myositis can accompany other collagen vascular diseases and may occur in a variety of viral and bacterial infections. Although dermatomyositis and polymyositis are well recognized, the recent development of more sophisticated histologic and immunologic tests has allowed the identification of other types of inflammatory myopathies (Table 25–1).

## NOMENCLATURE AND CLASSIFICATION

The variability in the clinical and laboratory features of dermatomyositis and polymyositis has made it difficult to classify these diseases. To better define these disorders, five diagnostic criteria have been proposed: (1) proximal symmetrical muscle weakness that progresses over a period of weeks to months, (2) elevated serum levels of muscle enzymes or elevated urinary creatinine excretion, (3) an abnormal electromyogram, (4) abnormal muscle biopsy findings that are consistent with myositis, and (5) the presence of cutaneous disease typical of dermatomyositis.

### TABLE 25-1

**Inflammatory Diseases of Muscle**

Idiopathic inflammatory myopathies
  Polymyositis
  Dermatomyositis
  Juvenile (childhood) dermatomyositis
  Myositis associated with malignancy
  Inclusion body myositis
Other inflammatory myopathies
  Myositis associated with eosinophilia
  Myositis ossificans
  Localized (focal) myositis
Myopathies caused by infection
Myopathies caused by drugs and toxins

From Wortmann RL: Inflammatory diseases of muscle and other myopathies. In Kelley WN, Harris ED Jr, Ruddy S, Sledge CB (eds): Textbook of Rheumatology, 5th ed. Philadelphia, WB Saunders, 1997, p 1177.

### Type I: Typical Polymyositis

Type I is the most common type and represents approximately 35% of cases. It is most frequent in the third, fourth, and fifth decades of life and affects women more commonly than men (2:1). Cases are generally sporadic. Polymyositis is characterized by gradually increasing muscle weakness, first appearing in the musculature of the thighs and pelvic girdle and later affecting the upper extremity. Dermal manifestations are inconstant. Joint manifestations include arthralgias and arthritis, which may be accompanied by joint effusion and positive serologic tests for rheumatoid factor.

### Type II: Typical Dermatomyositis

Type II is present in approximately 25% of patients, more frequently women, and is characterized by muscle weakness and a diffuse erythematous skin rash on the face, neck, chest, shoulders, and arms. Adults in the fifth or sixth decade are typically affected. Dermal and muscular abnormalities may occur simultaneously. Additional clinical features include malaise and joint pain.

### Type III: Typical Dermatomyositis with Malignancy

In patients older than 40 years, particularly men, type III dermatomyositis is characterized by the presence of skin rash, muscle weakness, and malignancy. Reports suggest that malignancy becomes evident in approximately 15% to 25% of patients with dermatomyositis and that this prevalence increases with the age of the patient. Polymyositis without dermatologic abnormalities is associated less frequently with malignancy. Muscular and dermal manifestations usually antedate the appearance of malignancy by months to years. The most commonly associated tumors arise from the lungs, prostate, female pelvic organs, breast, and gastrointestinal tract. The prognosis in patients with type III dermatomyositis is guarded.

## Type IV: Childhood Dermatomyositis

Dermatomyositis or, less commonly, polymyositis affects children or adolescents in approximately 20% of cases. Girls are affected more commonly than boys, most often between the ages of 5 and 10 years. Clinical findings include proximal muscle weakness, extensive edema and calcification of the skin and subcutaneous tissue, vasculitis, lipodystrophy, and joint contractures. Although the mortality in this disease is approximately the same in children and adults, the interval between the onset of myositis and death is shorter and the degree of soft tissue calcification is more extensive in childhood dermatomyositis. With regard to prognosis, two types of dermatomyositis occurring in children have been identified: an acute fulminant pattern (Banker type) associated with vasculitis, little calcinosis, and a poor prognosis, and a slowly progressive pattern (Brunsting type) associated with calcinosis without vasculitis and a good prognosis.

## Type V: Acute Myolysis

Type V disease, which is present in approximately 3% of patients, is characterized by the sudden onset of myolysis, particularly in patients in the first or second decade of life. Clinical manifestations include diffuse muscle weakness involving the facial, proximal, and distal musculature. A fatal outcome is not infrequent.

## Type VI: Polymyositis in Sjögren's Syndrome and Other Connective Tissue Diseases

In some patients with Sjögren's syndrome, slowly progressive weakness of the proximal musculature is evident. This type of polymyositis, which represents approximately 5% of all cases, is not generally accompanied by skin abnormalities. Myositis accompanies other connective tissue diseases as well, including scleroderma, systemic lupus erythematosus, rheumatoid arthritis, and overlap syndromes.

## CLINICAL ABNORMALITIES

The most constant clinical finding is muscle weakness, which eventually appears in virtually all persons with the disease; this manifestation is the initial symptom in approximately 50% of patients. Symmetrical involvement of proximal muscles is most characteristic. Fatigue, inability to walk or climb stairs, and aching are frequent. Typical or atypical skin rashes eventually occur in 40% to 60% of patients and are an initial manifestation of the disease in 20% to 25%. Raynaud's phenomenon occurs in about one third of patients with polymyositis. It appears more commonly in persons who exhibit clinical features of scleroderma or acrosclerosis, and it is generally mild in nature.

Arthralgias and arthritis are present in 20% to 50% of patients. Typically, the wrists, knees, and small joints of the fingers are affected symmetrically. Permanent joint damage is unusual (see discussion later in this chapter). Clinical manifestations of visceral involvement in dermatomyositis and polymyositis include cardiac (arrhythmia, pericarditis), pulmonary (pneumonitis, fibrosis), gastrointestinal (dysphagia, abdominal pain, constipation), renal, neurologic, and ocular abnormalities.

## RADIOGRAPHIC ABNORMALITIES

Radiographic abnormalities of the musculoskeletal system in dermatomyositis and polymyositis can be divided into soft tissue and articular abnormalities.

### Soft Tissue Abnormalities

Although soft tissue abnormalities occur in both children and adults, findings in children occur with greater frequency and severity. The initial soft tissue manifestation is edema of the subcutaneous tissue and muscle, which produces increased muscular bulk and radiodensity, thickening of subcutaneous septa, and poor delineation of the subcutaneous tissue–muscle interface (Fig. 25–1). The changes are more prominent in the proximal musculature, axilla, chest wall, forearms, thighs, and calves. After effective treatment, tissue edema may decrease or disappear entirely, although in many patients, fibrosis and muscle atrophy and contracture become apparent in the later stages of the disease. In these stages, decreased soft tissue and muscular bulk, increased soft tissue lucency, contractures, and associated osteoporosis are evident.

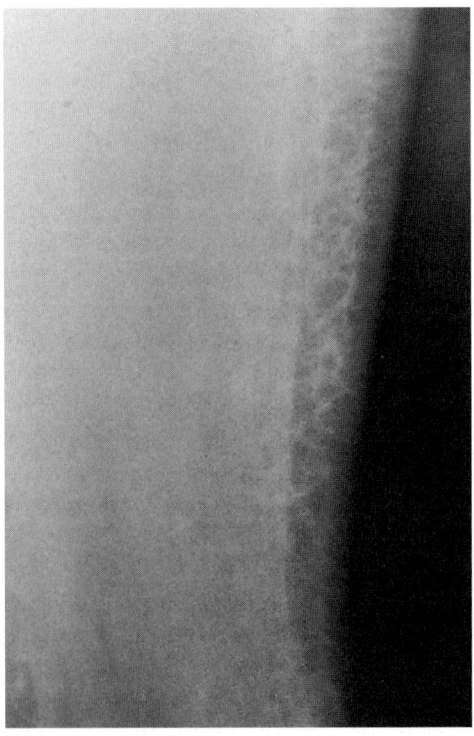

**Figure 25–1.** Dermatomyositis and polymyositis: early soft tissue edema. Observe the extensive edema of the subcutaneous tissue septa. (From Ozonoff MB, Flynn FJ Jr: Roentgenologic features of dermatomyositis of childhood. AJR Am J Roentgenol 118:206, 1973.)

The most characteristic soft tissue abnormality in dermatomyositis and polymyositis is calcification. The frequency of this finding in children is high. Calcification may occur within the first year of illness. The extent of calcification, particularly within musculature, appears to increase with the severity of the disease. Small or large calcareous intermuscular fascial plane calcification is distinctive (Fig. 25–2), although it may not be as common as subcutaneous calcification (Fig. 25–3). The favorite sites of intermuscular calcification are the large muscles in the proximal portion of the limbs. The appearance and distribution of subcutaneous calcification in dermatomyositis and polymyositis simulate those in scleroderma. Fingertip calcification can be associated with terminal phalangeal erosion, which further complicates the radiographic differentiation of these two disorders.

Four distinct patterns of soft tissue calcification are described in childhood dermatomyositis: deep calcareous masses; superficial calcareous masses; deep linear deposits; and lacy, reticular, subcutaneous collections encasing the torso. Of these, the first and third patterns, evident in deeper tissues, are more common; the fourth, though infrequent, appears to identify a subgroup of children in whom the disorder has a severe clinical course.

### Articular Abnormalities

The arthralgia and arthritis of dermatomyositis and polymyositis are usually unaccompanied by radiographic

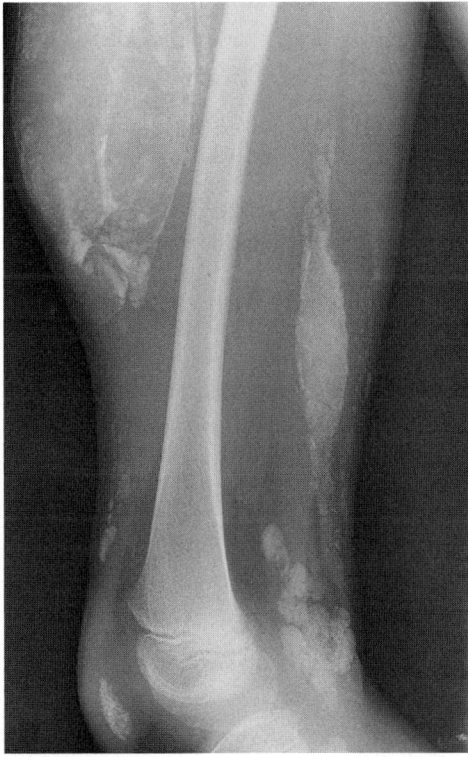

**Figure 25–2.** Dermatomyositis and polymyositis: intermuscular fascial plane calcification. Large calcareous muscular masses have produced nodular deformity of the overlying skin. Note the "tumoral" nature of the calcifications. (From Ozonoff MB, Flynn FJ Jr: Roentgenologic features of dermatomyositis of childhood. AJR Am J Roentgenol 118:206, 1973.)

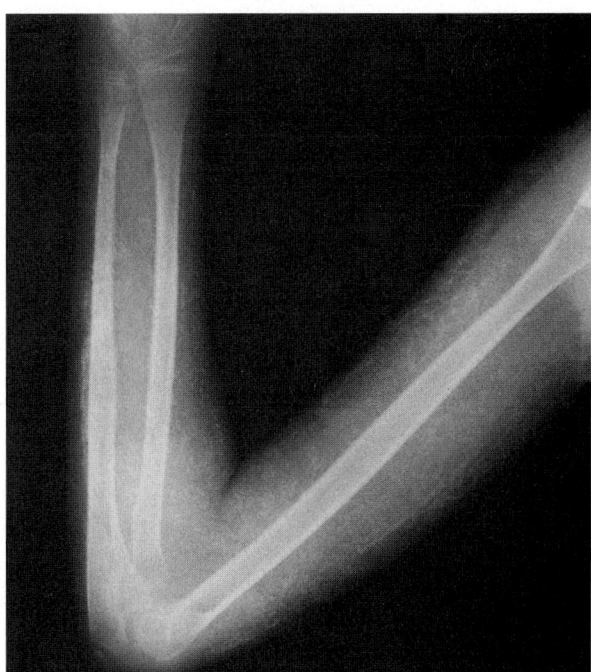

**Figure 25–3.** Dermatomyositis and polymyositis: subcutaneous calcification. In this child, diffuse linear subcutaneous calcinosis is evident.

abnormalities or are associated with transient radiographic features, including soft tissue swelling and periarticular osteoporosis. Destructive joint changes have occasionally been noted. Reported radiographic changes include soft tissue swelling (particularly in the metacarpophalangeal and interphalangeal joints), periosteal and soft tissue calcification in the form of flecks or small clumps in these same joints, bone erosion (inferior radioulnar, metacarpophalangeal, proximal interphalangeal, and distal interphalangeal joints, as well as the ulnar styloid), and alignment abnormalities (flexion deformities of the metacarpophalangeal joints, swan-neck deformities) (Fig. 25–4). Particularly characteristic is radial subluxation or dislocation at the interphalangeal joint of the thumb ("floppy thumb" sign).

### SCINTIGRAPHIC ABNORMALITIES

Technetium polyphosphate and similar agents may accumulate in abnormal muscle in patients with dermatomyositis and polymyositis. This abnormal accumulation demonstrates some correlation with the severity of muscle weakness and may improve after corticosteroid therapy. Gallium may also be used in this clinical situation.

### MAGNETIC RESONANCE IMAGING ABNORMALITIES

MR imaging is well suited to the analysis of a variety of muscle disorders, including dermatomyositis and polymyositis. Muscle atrophy, fatty replacement of muscle, and intramuscular regions of abnormal signal intensity that correlate with fibrosis and inflammation are noted. At the outset of the disease, a significant increase in

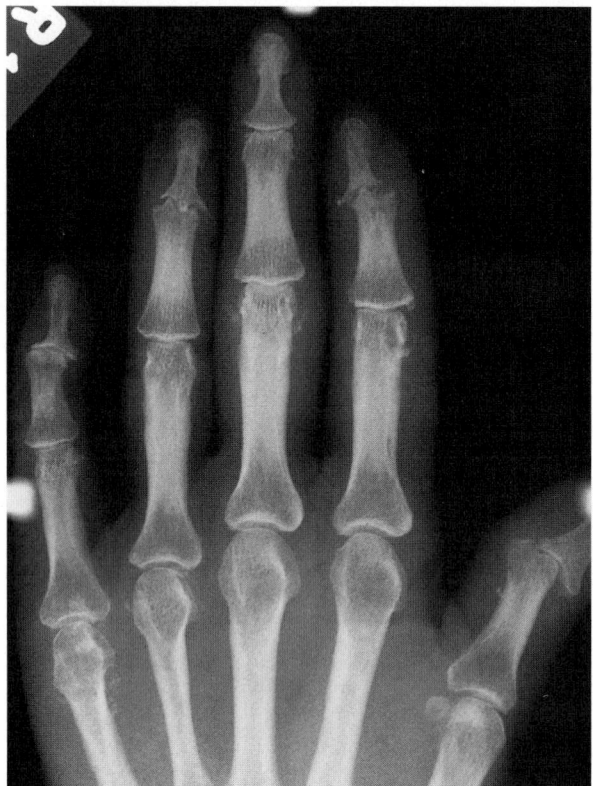

**Figure 25–4.** Dermatomyositis and polymyositis: destructive articular abnormalities. In this 50-year-old woman with well-documented polymyositis, note the bilateral articular abnormalities consisting of erosions of multiple distal interphalangeal joints, periarticular calcifications, and subluxation of the interphalangeal joint of the right thumb.

signal intensity in T2-weighted MR images occurs in the involved muscle groups. With clinical improvement, this signal intensity returns to normal, and with the recurrence of clinically evident disease activity, increased signal intensity at sites of muscle involvement is again noted on T2-weighted images. Predominant involvement of the vastus lateralis muscle is seen, with lesser involvement of the vastus intermedius and vastus medialis muscles. The rectus femoris and biceps femoris muscles are relatively spared (Figs. 25–5 and 25–6).

The value of MR imaging in the assessment of inflammatory muscle disease is now well established. Reported experience with MR imaging in the assessment of inflammatory myopathies has shown that signal intensity alterations in muscle correlate with disease activity. Accordingly, changes in signal patterns can be used to monitor response to therapy and identify muscle sites suitable for biopsy. MR imaging may allow the correct diagnosis of dermatomyositis or polymyositis in cases in which muscle involvement is not evident clinically. It may also allow the differentiation of either of these two diseases from noninflammatory myopathies, such as fibromyalgia.

## PATHOLOGIC ABNORMALITIES

The microscopic aberrations in involved musculature include focal or extensive degeneration of muscle fibers, regenerative activity, infiltration with chronic inflammatory cells, interstitial fibrosis, phagocytosis of necrotic fibers, and variation in the cross-sectional diameter of adjacent muscle fibers. These histologic aberrations vary little among the various subgroups of the disease.

## CAUSE AND PATHOGENESIS

Although the cause of dermatomyositis and polymyositis is unknown, evidence indicates that a cell-mediated immune mechanism is responsible for this damage by affecting either the muscle or the adjacent blood vessels. A genetic predisposition to such immunologic mechanisms has been suggested, as has an infectious cause. The association of dermatomyositis and neoplasm has raised the additional possibility that tumor may precipitate inflammatory muscle disease.

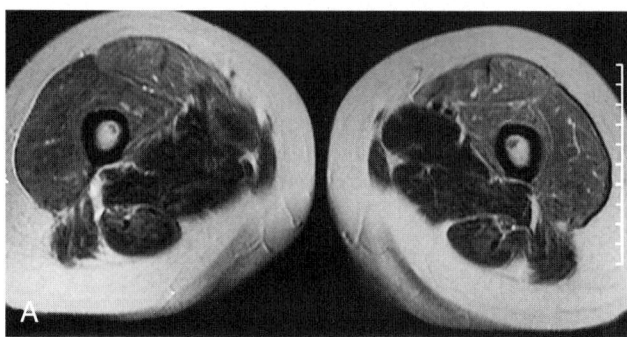
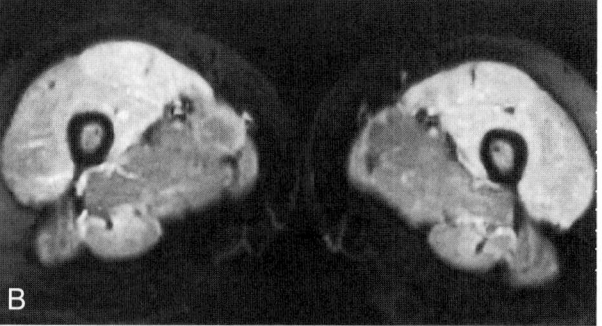

**Figure 25–5.** Dermatomyositis and polymyositis: MR imaging abnormalities. This 36-year-old woman with dermatomyositis had been symptomatic for 2 years with anterior thigh pain. Transaxial T2-weighted (TR/TE, 3700/96) spin echo *(A)* and short tau inversion recovery (STIR) (TR/TE, 5320/30; inversion time, 150 msec) *(B)* MR images reveal signal intensity alterations in the anterior musculature of both thighs. The changes, characterized by increased signal intensity, are more prominent in *(B)*. (Courtesy of J. Hodler, MD, Zurich, Switzerland.)

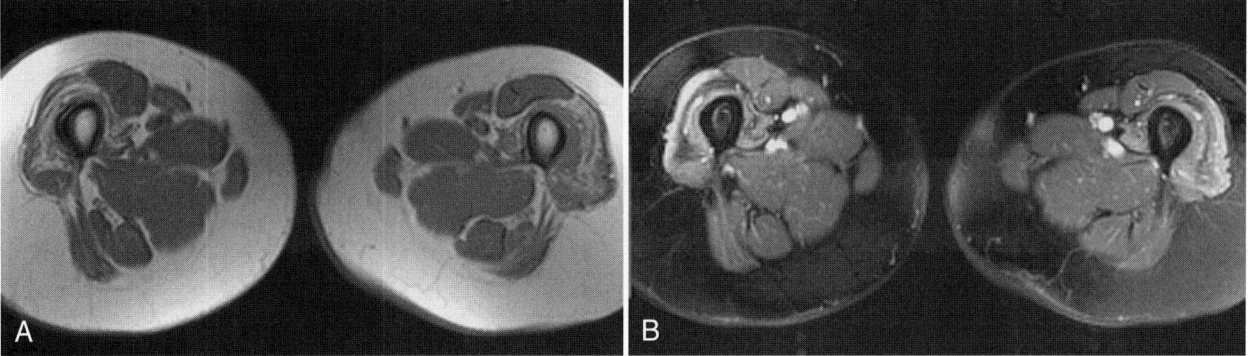

**Figure 25–6.** Dermatomyositis and polymyositis: MR imaging abnormalities. Long-standing disease in a 67-year-old woman. Transaxial T1-weighted (TR/TE, 616/17) spin echo *(A)* and STIR (TR/TE, 4000/55; inversion time, 150 msec) *(B)* MR images reveal signal intensity alterations in the anterior musculature of both thighs compatible with atrophy, fatty infiltration, fibrosis, and inflammation. Based on imaging, a biopsy specimen was taken from the area of high signal in the vastus lateralis. Note marked involvement of the vastus lateralis, vastus intermedius, and vastus medialis muscles, with relative sparing of the rectus femoris.

## OTHER INFLAMMATORY DISEASES OF MUSCLE

### Inclusion Body Myositis

Inclusion body myositis is a rare disease occurring predominantly in men. The age of onset is variable; however, the disease typically affects older patients and is the most frequently occurring progressive myopathy in adults older than 55 years. Clinical findings resemble those of polymyositis. The course of the disease is variable; muscle weakness may progress slowly or reach a plateau. In contrast to polymyositis, there is little or no association with malignancy or connective tissue disease, and patients with inclusion body myositis show resistance to high-dose corticosteroid therapy. Most important, however, in the differentiation of inclusion body myositis and polymyositis are the distinctive pathologic features of the former disease, including the identification of large intranuclear and intracytoplasmic inclusions by light microscopy and characteristic microtubular elements by electron microscopy.

### Focal Myositis

Focal (or localized) myositis is a benign inflammatory disorder of muscle leading to one or more nodules or pseudotumors with histologic features similar or identical to those of polymyositis. Other names for this disorder include localized nodular myositis, focalized interstitial polymyositis, interstitial nodular myositis, and focal nodular myositis. The typical site of involvement is the musculature of the thigh or lower extremity (75% of cases). Focal myositis can occur in children or adults, with equal frequency in male and female subjects. Patients present with a painful localized intramuscular soft tissue mass (Fig. 25–7) that may enlarge rapidly over a period of weeks. The lesion may progress over days or weeks

to a more generalized distribution that is typical of polymyositis.

MR imaging confirms the intramuscular location of the mass, which has a signal intensity similar to that of muscle on T1-weighted spin echo images and poorly defined increased signal intensity on T2-weighted spin echo images; it is confined to a single muscle or muscle group. MR imaging findings have been reported to correlate with the severity of clinical and histologic abnormalities, suggesting that this imaging method may provide prognostic criteria in cases of focal myositis.

### Eosinophilic Myositis

Eosinophilic myositis is a rare disorder characterized by the subacute onset of weakness of proximal muscles, elevated serum levels of muscle enzymes, abnormal electromyographic findings, and, on histologic analysis, an eosinophilic inflammatory infiltrate in skeletal muscle. It may occur as a localized disorder or be evident in eosinophilic fasciitis and in the eosinophilia-myalgia syndrome.

### Drug-Related Myositis

A large number of drugs have been reported to lead to myopathic changes, including alcohol, aspirin, penicillin, and sulfonamides. No single mechanism explains the association of drug use and myopathies. Immune-mediated responses, toxic effects, and metabolic or electrolyte imbalances are potentially important factors. Further, the types of myopathy caused by these drugs vary and include both acute inflammatory changes and chronic fibrosis. Fibrotic myopathy is a well-recognized complication of direct intramuscular injection of drugs and affects principally the deltoid and quadriceps muscles. MR imaging findings are variable and include intramuscular regions with abnormally low or high signal intensity.

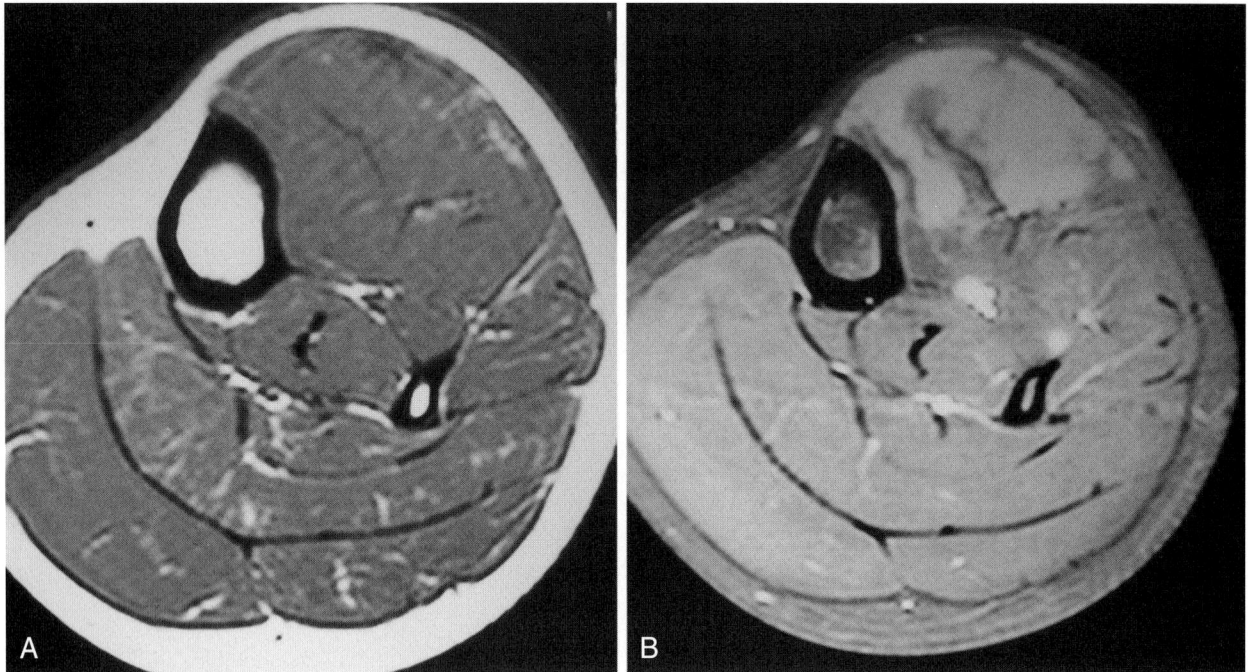

**Figure 25–7.** Focal myositis. In a 13-year-old girl, a transaxial T1-weighted (TR/TE, 577/11) spin echo MR image *(A)* shows enlargement of the anterior tibialis muscle. After the intravenous administration of a gadolinium-containing agent, a transaxial fat-suppressed T1-weighted (TR/TE, 500/8) spin echo MR image *(B)* shows enhancement of signal intensity in the intramuscular mass. (Courtesy of J. Jacobson, MD, Ann Arbor, Mich.)

## DIFFERENTIAL DIAGNOSIS

### Soft Tissue Abnormalities

Soft tissue calcification is a common feature of various collagen vascular diseases, particularly dermatomyositis (polymyositis) and scleroderma. Calcific deposits may appear in the intermuscular fascial planes and exhibit distinctive radiographic features that are seen more frequently in dermatomyositis and polymyositis than in other collagen vascular diseases. A second pattern of calcification in dermatomyositis and polymyositis relates to deposition in subcutaneous tissue. This appearance has not been emphasized in these disorders, although it is well recognized in scleroderma. Subcutaneous calcification may also be evident in systemic lupus erythematosus, mixed collagen vascular disease, and overlap syndromes. Periarticular calcific deposits in dermatomyositis and polymyositis are generally linear or punctate, a characteristic that usually allows differentiation from the "tumoral" deposits associated with hyperparathyroidism, hypervitaminosis D, and the milk-alkali syndrome.

### Articular Abnormalities

Severe deformity of the interphalangeal joint of the thumb may be apparent in other collagen vascular disorders, especially systemic lupus erythematosus. The interphalangeal joint erosions (with or without metacarpophalangeal joint and wrist abnormalities) in polymyositis may also occur in scleroderma, rheumatoid arthritis, psoriatic arthritis, multicentric reticulohistiocytosis, and gout, as well as after thermal injuries.

### Muscle Abnormalities

MR imaging is very sensitive for the detection of myositis. The absence of a focal mass on MR imaging in most cases of polymyositis generally allows differentiation from pyomyositis and tumors, although certain tumors and tumor-like lesions, such as lymphoma and sarcoidosis, may be associated with MR imaging findings simulating those of polymyositis. Other diagnostic considerations include denervation, physical injury, rhabdomyolysis, and muscle infarction (especially in diabetic patients).

## FURTHER READING

Adams EM, Chow CK, Premkumar A, et al: The idiopathic inflammatory myopathies: Spectrum of MR imaging findings. Radiographics 15:563, 1995.

Banker BQ, Victor M: Dermatomyositis (systemic angiopathy) of childhood. Medicine 45:261, 1966.

Black KA, Zilko PJ, Dawkins RL, et al: Cancer in connective tissue disease. Arthritis Rheum 25:1130, 1982.

Blane CE, White SJ, Braunstein EM, et al: Patterns of calcification in childhood dermatomyositis. AJR Am J Roentgenol 142:397, 1984.

Bunch TW, O'Duffy JD, McLeod RA: Deforming arthritis of the hands in polymyositis. Arthritis Rheum 19:243, 1976.

Fleckenstein JL, Reimers CD: Inflammatory myopathies: Radiologic evaluation. Radiol Clin North Am 34:427, 1996.

Greenway G, Weisman MH, Resnick D, et al: Deforming arthritis of the hands: An unusual manifestation of polymyositis. AJR Am J Roentgenol 136:611, 1981.

Ozonoff MB, Flynn FJ Jr: Roentgenologic features of dermatomyositis of childhood. AJR Am J Roentgenol 118:206, 1973.

Park JH, Vansant JP, Kumar NG, et al: Dermatomyositis: Correlative MR imaging and P-31 MR spectroscopy for quantitative characterization of inflammatory disease. Radiology 177:473, 1990.

Rider LG, Miller FW: Classification and treatment of the juvenile idiopathic inflammatory myopathies. Rheum Dis Clin North Am 23:619, 1997.

Sayers ME, Chou SM, Calabrese LH: Inclusion body myositis: Analysis of 32 cases. J Rheumatol 19:1385, 1992.

Schumacher HR, Schimmer B, Gordon GV, et al: Articular manifestations of polymyositis and dermatomyositis. Am J Med 67:287, 1979.

Steiner RM, Glassman L, Schwartz MW, et al: The radiological findings in dermatomyositis of childhood. Radiology 111: 385, 1974.

Steinfeld JR, Thorne NA, Kennedy TF: Positive [99mTc] pyrophosphate bone scan in polymyositis. Radiology 122:168, 1977.

Wortmann RL: Inflammatory disease of muscle and other myopathies. In Kelley WN, Harris ED Jr, Ruddy S, Sledge CB (eds): Textbook of Rheumatology, 5th ed. Philadelphia, WB Saunders, 1997, p 1177.

# CHAPTER 26

## Polyarteritis Nodosa and Other Vasculitides

## SUMMARY OF KEY FEATURES

Vasculitis occurs in a number of disorders and may be associated with musculoskeletal manifestations. Although arteriography can reveal characteristic alterations in these disorders, radiographic abnormalities are unimpressive. In polyarteritis nodosa, periosteal bone formation may be seen, particularly in the lower extremity. Articular abnormalities in giant cell (temporal) arteritis relate to its association with polymyalgia rheumatica and include soft tissue swelling and osteoporosis. In Henoch-Schönlein purpura and erythema nodosum, joint effusions are the only characteristic radiographic abnormality. Cryoglobulinemia is occasionally accompanied by cystic and erosive lesions of bone in both the axial and the appendicular skeletons.

## INTRODUCTION

A number of disorders are characterized by inflammation of blood vessels. Clinical symptoms and signs in these disorders are protean and depend on the distribution, extent, and severity of the vascular lesions; although musculoskeletal abnormalities may be encountered, they are usually overshadowed by findings related to the involvement of other organ systems. Characteristic radiographic findings are detected most reliably by arteriography. Abnormalities on radiographs related to articular and osseous involvement are generally infrequent and nonspecific.

## CLASSIFICATION OF VASCULITIDES

The limitations of classification systems for the vasculitides have become increasingly obvious in the last 40 years because of the growing spectrum of disorders. Histologic characteristics of the vascular lesions have been used as guidelines for classification of the various systemic vascular disorders, despite the overlap of certain clinical and pathologic features. Three major groups of vasculitides are recognized: (1) inflammatory vascular lesions (necrotizing angiitis), including polyarteritis nodosa, hypersensitivity angiitis, granulomatous angiitis, and Wegener's granulomatosis; (2) vasculitides accompanied by granuloma formation, including granulomatous angiitis, Wegener's granulomatosis, temporal arteritis, and Takayasu's arteritis; and (3) vasculitides associated with intimal hyperplasia, necrosis of the media and elastic lamina, and varying degrees of inflammation in the adventitia and vasa vasorum, including temporal arteritis, Takayasu's arteritis, and scleroderma.

The vasculitides can also be divided into three groups on the basis of both pathologic characteristics and the size of affected vessels: (1) polyarteritis nodosa group, (2) small vessel vasculitides, and (3) giant cell arteritides. Characteristics of the first group are involvement of medium-sized (and, to a lesser extent, small-sized) arteries, the presence of microaneurysms, the sequential initiation of arterial damage, and histologic findings varying from acute inflammation to scarring. Included in the polyarteritis nodosa group are generalized or classic disease, localized disease (to pulmonary, mesenteric or other vessels), and Kawasaki's disease (with prominent coronary involvement). Small vessel vasculitides are characterized by involvement of arterioles and venules and, commonly, by prominent skin involvement. Disorders in this group may produce a granulomatous reaction (Churg-Strauss syndrome, Wegener's granulomatosis). Giant cell arteritides affect large arteries and consist principally of two diseases: cranial (temporal) arteritis and Takayasu's arteritis.

## POLYARTERITIS NODOSA

### General Features

Polyarteritis nodosa is an uncommon disorder of unknown cause characterized by inflammation and necrosis in the walls of medium-sized and small arteries. It affects men more frequently than women and occurs predominantly in young and middle-aged adults. Ten diagnostic criteria for polyarteritis nodosa have been identified by the subcommittee of the American College of Rheumatology: weight loss of 4 kg or more; livedo reticularis (mottled reticular pattern in the skin of portions of the extremities or torso); testicular pain or tenderness (not resulting from infection, trauma, or other causes); myalgias, weakness, or leg tenderness; mononeuropathy or polyneuropathy; diastolic blood pressure greater than 90 mm Hg; elevated levels of blood urea nitrogen or creatinine; presence of hepatitis B surface antigen or antibody in serum; arteriographic abnormality (characterized by aneurysms or occlusion of visceral arteries not caused by arteriosclerosis, fibromuscular dysplasia, or other noninflammatory conditions); and histologic changes (obtained from a biopsy of a small or medium-sized artery) showing the presence of granulocytes or granulocytes and mononuclear leukocytes in the arterial wall. A patient is considered likely to have polyarteritis nodosa if at least 3 of these 10 criteria are met.

### Clinical Abnormalities

The clinical manifestations of polyarteritis nodosa relate to the distribution and extent of the vascular lesions. The spectrum of disease varies from a mild and limited form to a fulminating and rapidly fatal process. Fever, weight loss, tachycardia, anemia, and leukocytosis are frequent. Renal involvement, which occurs in approximately 75% to 80% of patients, can lead to blood and protein in the urine, hypertension, and renal failure with uremia. Acute vascular episodes involving other abdominal viscera can produce severe abdominal pain and gastrointestinal hemorrhage or perforation. Cardiac manifestations, peripheral vascular involvement, and pulmonary arteritis may be seen. Cutaneous manifestations are common and include ulceration, subcutaneous nodules, maculopapules, purpura, and necrotic lesions.

The most prominent articular manifestation in polyarteritis nodosa is pain, which frequently occurs simultaneously with muscle tenderness. Migratory polyarthralgia is characteristic. Larger joints in the lower extremity are typically affected. Actual synovitis with joint effusion is rare and appears in 10% to 15% of patients who have articular symptoms. An association between polyarteritis and rheumatoid arthritis has been emphasized.

### Radiographic Abnormalities

Radiographic manifestations of polyarteritis nodosa are unusual. Soft tissue swelling may accompany arthritis, but cartilaginous and osseous destruction is not apparent. Periosteal bone formation has been observed in some patients with this disease. Such periosteal bone formation, similar to that seen in other types of arteritis, is more common in men and has a predilection for the lower extremities (Fig. 26–1). It may be bilateral or unilateral and is associated with pain and swelling. Digital clubbing is uncommon, and symptoms and signs may improve dramatically with corticosteroid therapy. Periostitis in this disease is generally identical to that in hypertrophic osteoarthropathy, although more extensive undulating new bone formation has been observed in a few instances. Arteriography of involved areas may demonstrate small aneurysms, an important diagnostic feature (Fig. 26–2). Such aneurysms may later disappear, apparently as a result of healing.

### Pathologic Abnormalities

Medium- and small-caliber arteries from involved tissues reveal characteristic abnormalities. Initial changes are most common in the tunica media, with subsequent extension into the intima and adventitia and disruption of the internal elastic lamina. Necrosis, fibrinoid change, and cellular infiltration are observed. Weakening of the vessel wall can lead to aneurysm formation, rupture, and hemorrhage. In later stages of the disease, thrombosis and infarction may be observed. Arterial involvement is segmental, affecting only a portion of an artery along its length, and a normal artery may be found adjacent to one that is severely affected.

## MICROSCOPIC POLYANGIITIS

Although it is clear that cases of microscopic polyangiitis were included in previous reports of polyarteritis nodosa, microscopic polyangiitis is now considered a distinct syndrome characterized by necrotizing vasculitis affecting predominantly the small vessels, especially in the kidney

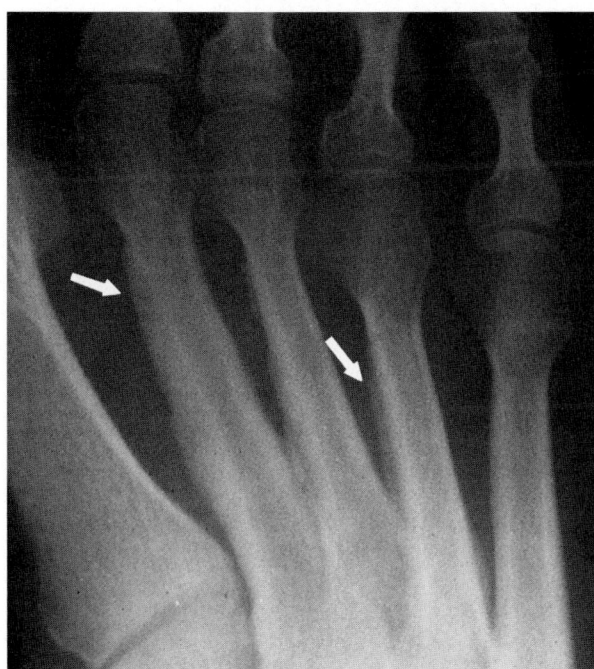

**Figure 26–1.** Polyarteritis nodosa: periostitis in the lower extremity. Observe the periosteal new bone formation predominating on the medial aspect of multiple metatarsal bones *(arrows)*. (Courtesy of M. Dalinka, MD, Philadelphia, Pa.)

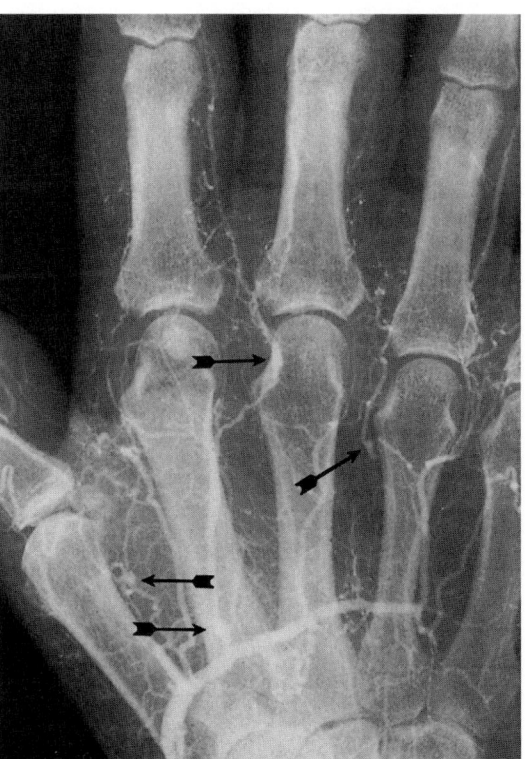

**Figure 26–2.** Polyarteritis nodosa: arteriography. Multiple proper digital arteries and the ulnar artery are occluded. The presence of a number of small aneurysms *(arrows)* suggests the possibility of a necrotizing arteritis. (Courtesy of J. J. Bookstein, MD, San Diego, Calif.)

but also in the skin and lung. This syndrome is characterized by the presence of autoantibodies to neutrophil cytoplasm antigens and the absence of immune deposits in involved vessels. Men are affected more often than women. Patients are typically between 40 and 60 years and usually have renal disease. Angiography generally fails to reveal evidence of aneurysms.

## CHURG-STRAUSS SYNDROME

Churg-Strauss syndrome, also called allergic granulomatosis and angiitis, is characterized by the combination of asthma, eosinophilia, vasculitis, and extravascular granulomas. It is a rare disease that is more frequent in men than in women and affects patients of different ages. The cause of the syndrome is not clear, although immunoglobulins and complement have been found in the walls of vessels. The basic pathologic lesion is a necrotizing vasculitis involving the small arteries and veins that results in granulomas. Regardless of which organs are involved, the two essential findings in this syndrome are angiitis and extravascular necrotizing granulomas, usually with eosinophilic infiltrates. Subcutaneous nodules may be observed. Polyarthralgias are uncommon, and arthritis is rare. Diagnostic criteria emphasize six findings: asthma, eosinophilia, mononeuropathy or polyneuropathy, pulmonary infiltrates, abnormalities of the paranasal sinuses, and a biopsy specimen containing a blood vessel with extravascular eosinophils.

## WEGENER'S GRANULOMATOSIS

Wegener's granulomatosis is associated with necrotizing granulomatous lesions of the respiratory tract, vasculitis, and glomerulonephritis. Patient age at disease onset ranges from very young to aged; the disease is slightly more common in men than in women. Clinical features include acute or chronic sinusitis, chronic rhinitis, nasal ulceration, anorexia, weight loss, and fever. Arthralgias and arthritis are evident in approximately half the cases; they are generally not associated with significant radiographic changes. Infrequently, bone erosions are seen, although they may be related to chronic renal disease (Fig. 26–3). The precise cause of Wegener's granulomatosis is unknown, but hypersensitivity is a leading candidate. Diagnostic criteria, as proposed by the American College of Rheumatology, include abnormal urinary sediment, abnormal findings on chest radiography (nodules, cavities, or fixed infiltrates), oral ulcers or nasal discharge, and granulomatous inflammation on biopsy.

## MIDLINE GRANULOMA

Midline granuloma is a disease associated with destructive lesions of the nose, midface, and upper airway. Pulmonary and renal involvement is typically lacking. Soft tissues and adjacent bones are affected by a pathologic process that is associated with dense cellular infiltrates consisting of lymphocytes, plasma cells, histiocytes, and immunoblasts in an angiocentric distribution. Symptoms and signs are related to abnormalities in the mouth, nose, and upper airway.

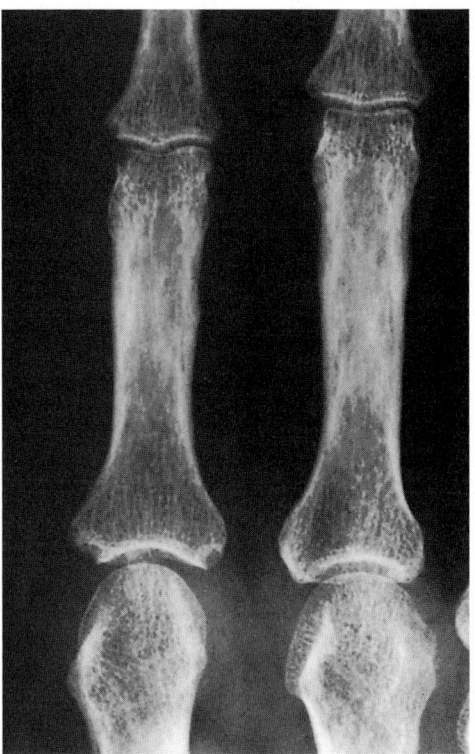

**Figure 26–3.** Wegener's granulomatosis: articular abnormalities. In this patient with well-established disease, osteoporosis and subtle periarticular bone erosions are present about the interphalangeal and metacarpophalangeal joints. The nature and significance of these findings are unknown. (Courtesy of A. Brower, MD, Norfolk, Va.)

## GIANT CELL (TEMPORAL) ARTERITIS AND POLYMYALGIA RHEUMATICA

Giant cell (temporal) arteritis is characterized by granulomatous inflammation of large arteries, particularly the internal and external carotid, occipital, temporal, and ophthalmic arteries. Typically, patients older than 50 years are affected. The arteritis is more frequent in women than in men, with a ratio of approximately 2:1. Clinical findings include painful swelling of the temporal arteries, headaches, visual disturbances, and peripheral neuropathy. The diagnosis is supported by characteristic findings on temporal artery biopsy or angiography. Diagnostic criteria recommended by the American College of Rheumatology include disease onset at age 50 years or older, new onset of localized headache, tenderness of the temporal artery or decreased temporal artery pulse, elevation of the erythrocyte sedimentation rate, and a biopsy sample of an artery showing necrotizing arteritis.

Synovitis is detected in approximately 15% of biopsy-proven cases of giant cell arteritis. Clinical findings related to articular involvement are usually confined to soft tissue swelling, although an erosive, seronegative polyarthritis may appear before or after the onset of arteritis. Coexistent rheumatoid arthritis has also been documented.

An association has been suggested between giant cell arteritis and polymyalgia rheumatica. The latter condition is encountered most frequently in elderly patients, particularly women, and is associated with progressive pain in the back, thighs, neck, and shoulders. Transient inflammatory synovitis may develop in the knee, shoulder, hip, wrist, and, infrequently, small joints of the fingers. Chronic inflammatory changes are evident when the synovial membrane is examined. Significant cartilaginous and bony abnormalities are generally not encountered. In some cases, involvement of the axial skeleton, the sterno-clavicular and sternomanubrial joints, and the shoulder region is consistent with a "central" synovitis in this disease. Approximately 50% of patients with giant cell arteritis experience a prodromal phase with features of polymyalgia rheumatica, and approximately 30% of patients with polymyalgia rheumatica have symptoms and signs of giant cell arteritis.

## HENOCH-SCHÖNLEIN (ANAPHYLACTOID) PURPURA

This syndrome, which consists of nonthrombocytopenic purpura, arthralgia or arthritis, abdominal pain, and renal disease, is related to a generalized leukocytoclastic or necrotizing angiitis involving the arterioles and capillaries. Increased vascular permeability is associated with edema and hemorrhage. The cause of this condition is unknown, although an allergic phenomenon has been suggested. The disease is more frequent in children than in adults, with a peak incidence at age 3 to 10 years. Diagnostic criteria proposed by the American College of Rheumatology are disease onset at age 20 years or younger, palpable purpura, acute abdominal pain, and a biopsy specimen showing granulocytes in the walls of small arterioles or venules.

The classic triad of findings, observed in 70% to 80% of cases, consists of purpura, abdominal pain, and arthritis. Articular manifestations consisting of pain, tenderness, and swelling develop in approximately 60% to 70% of patients with Henoch-Schönlein purpura. The joints involved most commonly are the knees, ankles, hips, wrists, and small joints of the hand. Periarticular soft tissue swelling, the only radiographic abnormality, is related to synovial effusion. Complete resolution of clinical and radiographic joint abnormalities is characteristic.

## CRYOGLOBULINEMIA

Essential cryoglobulinemia is a distinct type of disease that manifests as arthralgia or arthritis; the skin, lungs, kidneys, nervous system, and gastrointestinal tract are involved. The disorder may follow a chronic course, with minimal symptoms, or death may result from renal abnormalities. Intermittent arthralgia is observed in 20% to 75% of patients, whereas arthritis is evident in only 5% to 25% of cases. Most commonly, joints in the hands, knees, ankles, and elbows are involved. Although the radiographic features in these locations are not dramatic (Fig. 26–4), well-defined subchondral cystic lesions have been identified.

## TAKAYASU'S ARTERITIS

Takayasu's arteritis is a chronic, nonarteriosclerotic inflammatory disease of the aorta and its main branches

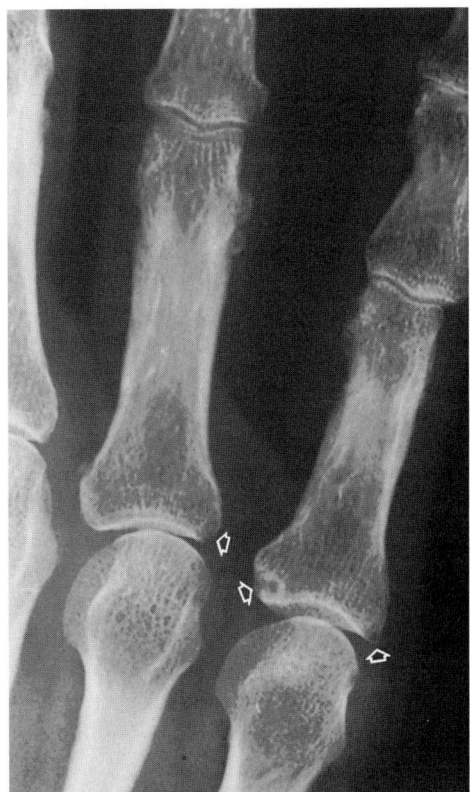

**Figure 26–4.** Cryoglobulinemia: articular abnormalities. In this 55-year-old man, small discrete osteolytic foci (*arrows*) are seen in the phalanges. Bone proliferation involves the proximal phalanx of the fourth finger. (Courtesy of V. Vint, MD, San Diego, Calif.)

and the elastic pulmonary arteries. It is observed most commonly in young women between the ages of 15 and 45 years and is most prevalent in Asia. Initial symptoms are not specific and include weight loss, fever, arthralgia, myalgia, and anemia. The disorder progresses at a variable rate, with gradual obliteration of the involved vessels. Aortic arch syndrome, pulseless disease, renovascular hypertension, and claudication are among the later manifestations. Diagnostic criteria include disease onset at age 40 years or younger, claudication of an extremity, decreased pulse in the brachial artery, a greater than 10 mm Hg difference in systolic pressure between arms, a bruit over the subclavian arteries or the aorta, and arteriographic evidence of narrowing or occlusion of the entire aorta, its primary branches, or large arteries in the proximal portion of the upper or lower extremities. Although arthralgias may be observed in more than 50% of patients, radiographic findings of joint disease are lacking.

## BUERGER'S DISEASE

Buerger's disease, or thromboangiitis obliterans, is a segmental, inflammatory, occlusive, nonatherosclerotic vascular disease. It is more common in men than in women and typically occurs in adult smokers. Buerger's disease always affects two or more limbs, beginning distally with proximal progression. The lower extremities are involved more frequently than the upper extremities, but both the lower and upper extremities may be affected together. Claudication of the calf or ankle is a common initial feature. Small and medium-sized arteries and veins are affected more often than large vessels. Buerger's disease may progress rapidly unless the use of tobacco (smoking or chewing) is eliminated. Angiography reveals multiple, bilateral focal segments of arterial stenosis or occlusion, particularly in the digital, palmar, plantar, ulnar, radial, tibial, and peroneal vessels, without evidence of atherosclerosis. Intermittent arthralgias, especially in the large joints, have been reported.

## ERYTHEMA NODOSUM

Erythema nodosum is a disorder characterized by red, tender, warm nodular cutaneous lesions (particularly in the lower legs) that on biopsy demonstrate vasculitis and cellular infiltration. The disorder may be an allergic or hypersensitivity response to a number of precipitating factors, such as infection or drugs. Erythema nodosum occurs in some patients with ulcerative colitis, Crohn's disease, sarcoidosis, and Behçet's syndrome.

Approximately three fourths of patients with erythema nodosum experience recurrent episodes of arthralgia and arthritis. Joint findings are usually symmetrical in distribution, with a predilection for the knees, ankles, elbows, wrists, and small joints of the hands. Soft tissue swelling related to joint effusion is the only prominent radiographic abnormality.

## FURTHER READING

Alarcón-Segovia D: Classification of the necrotizing vasculitides in man. Clin Rheum Dis 6:223, 1980.

Albert DA, Rimon D, Silverstein MD: The diagnosis of polyarteritis nodosa. Arthritis Rheum 31:1117, 1988.

Fauchald P, Rygvold O, Oystese B: Temporal arteritis and polymyalgia rheumatica—clinical and biopsy findings. Ann Intern Med 77:845, 1972.

Gonzalez-GA Ma, Garcia-Porrura C, Vazquez-Caruncho M: Polymyalgia rheumatica in biopsy proven giant cell arteritis does not constitute a different subset but differs from isolated olymyalgia rheumatica. J Rheumatol 25:1750, 1998.

Guillevin L, Cohen P, Gayraud M, et al: Churg-Strauss syndrome: Clinical study and long-term follow-up of 96 patients. Medicine (Baltimore) 78:26, 1999.

Hamidou MA: Periosteal new bone formation in Wegener's granulomatosis. J Rheumatol 24:814, 1977.

Lightfoot RW Jr, Michel BA, Bloch DA, et al: The American College of Rheumatology 1990 criteria for the classification of polyarteritis nodosa. Arthritis Rheum 33:1088, 1990.

Moncada R, Baker D, Rubinstein H, et al: Selective temporal arteriography and biopsy in giant cell arteritis: Polymyalgia rheumatica. AJR 122:580, 1974.

Salvarani C, Hunder GG: Musculoskeletal manifestations in a population-based cohort of patients with giant cell arteritis. Arthritis Rheum 42:1259, 1999.

Truelove LH: Articular manifestations of erythema nodosum. Ann Rheum Dis 19:174, 1960.

Valente RM, Hall S, O'Duffy JD, et al: Vasculitis and related disorders. In Kelley WN, Harris Jr, ED, Ruddy S, Sledge CB (eds): Textbook of Rheumatology, 5th ed. Philadelphia, WB Saunders, 1997, p 1079.

Weinberger A, Berliner S, Pinkhas J: Articular manifestations of essential cryoglobulinemia. Semin Arthritis Rheum 10:224, 1981.

Woodward AH, Andreini PH: Periosteal new bone formation in polyarteritis nodosa. A syndrome involving the lower extremities. Arthritis Rheum 17:1017, 1974.

Zvaifler NJ: Vasculitides: Classification and pathogenesis. Aust N Z J Med 8(Suppl 1):134, 1978.

# CHAPTER 27

## Mixed Connective Tissue Disease and Collagen Vascular Overlap Syndromes

## *SUMMARY OF KEY FEATURES*

Mixed connective tissue disease (MCTD) is an overlap syndrome defined serologically by the presence of a ribonuclease-sensitive extractable nuclear antigen. It demonstrates clinical features of several collagen vascular diseases. The radiographic characteristics of MCTD also underscore the mixed character of the disease. Changes compatible with rheumatoid arthritis (articular erosion, joint space narrowing, periarticular osteoporosis), scleroderma (tuft resorption, soft tissue calcification), and systemic lupus erythematosus (deforming nonerosive arthropathy) may be observed. Radiographic detection of skeletal abnormalities characteristic of more than one collagen vascular disease should raise the possibility of MCTD, although other overlap syndromes may result in similar findings.

## INTRODUCTION

Diagnosis of the collagen vascular disorders described in Chapters 23 to 26 is based on a composite evaluation of clinical, laboratory, radiographic, and pathologic data and the application of a variety of selective and non-selective disease criteria. In many patients, this diagnostic exercise provides a single answer—that is, the constellation of findings fits one of the five diffuse connective tissue diseases (systemic lupus erythematosus, scleroderma, dermatomyositis, polymyositis, and rheumatoid arthritis). In other patients, however, the manifestations of the disease process are incompatible with a single diagnosis. These patients, as well as many others, appear to have more than one collagen vascular disease, and the diagnosis of an overlap syndrome or MCTD is offered as an explanation for the diverse clinical, radiographic, and laboratory aberrations. It has been suggested that as many as 25% of cases of connective tissue disease fall into the category of an overlap syndrome.

## MIXED CONNECTIVE TISSUE DISEASE

MCTD is characterized by clinical features that suggest an overlap of systemic lupus erythematosus, scleroderma, dermatomyositis, and rheumatoid arthritis. The presence of antibodies to a saline-soluble extractable nuclear antigen is fundamental to the diagnosis of MCTD. The existence of MCTD as a definite entity is not universally accepted, despite the recent emphasis placed on its clinical and radiographic features. It has been suggested MCTD represents systemic lupus erythematosus that has been altered or modified by the presence of ribonucleoprotein antibodies. Other authorities believe that MCTD is a specific disease because of its distinctive genetic, serologic, and clinical characteristics and that it should not be considered an undifferentiated connective tissue disease. Some reports indicate that MCTD infrequently evolves into systemic lupus erythematosus or progressive systemic sclerosis.

### Clinical Abnormalities

MCTD is characterized by overlapping clinical features of scleroderma, systemic lupus erythematosus, dermatomyositis, and rheumatoid arthritis and by the presence in the serum of high titers of antibodies to ribonucleoprotein. Both adults and children can be affected. The variable clinical features of MCTD include fatigue, weight loss, fever, myalgia and myositis, lymphadenopathy, sclerodactyly, digital swelling, Raynaud's phenomenon, dyspnea, dysphagia, diarrhea, skin rash, and neuralgia. In general, the prognosis of the disease is good, although serious gastrointestinal, neurologic, or renal manifestations may occur.

Clinically detectable joint abnormalities in MCTD are common. Any joint can be affected, but involvement of the small joints of the hand and foot, as well as the wrist, is typical. Intermittent arthralgia may progress to arthritis, with considerable pain, stiffness, and swelling. Subcutaneous and peritendinous nodules may also be evident, particularly in the forearms and on the dorsum of the hands; on biopsy, these may demonstrate the characteristic features of a rheumatoid nodule. Joint deformities simulating those of rheumatoid arthritis can appear in MCTD. The most important laboratory finding is the presence of ribonucleoprotein antibodies in serum. In addition, patients may have positive serologic test results for rheumatoid factor, elevation of the erythrocyte sedimentation rate, and anemia.

### Radiographic Abnormalities

On radiographs, osseous, articular, and soft tissue abnormalities confirm the overlapping nature of MCTD; bone and soft tissue findings may be identical to those in scleroderma, whereas the articular abnormalities are more variable. Radiographic alterations in the hands, wrists, and feet can include the following characteristics (Figs. 27–1 to 27–3).

**Joint Distribution.** Radiographic abnormalities are most frequent in the proximal interphalangeal and metacarpophalangeal joints of the hands, midcarpal and radiocarpal compartments of the wrist, and metatarsophalangeal and interphalangeal joints of the feet. Distal interphalangeal joint changes are also encountered. The distribution of abnormalities may be either symmetrical or asymmetrical.

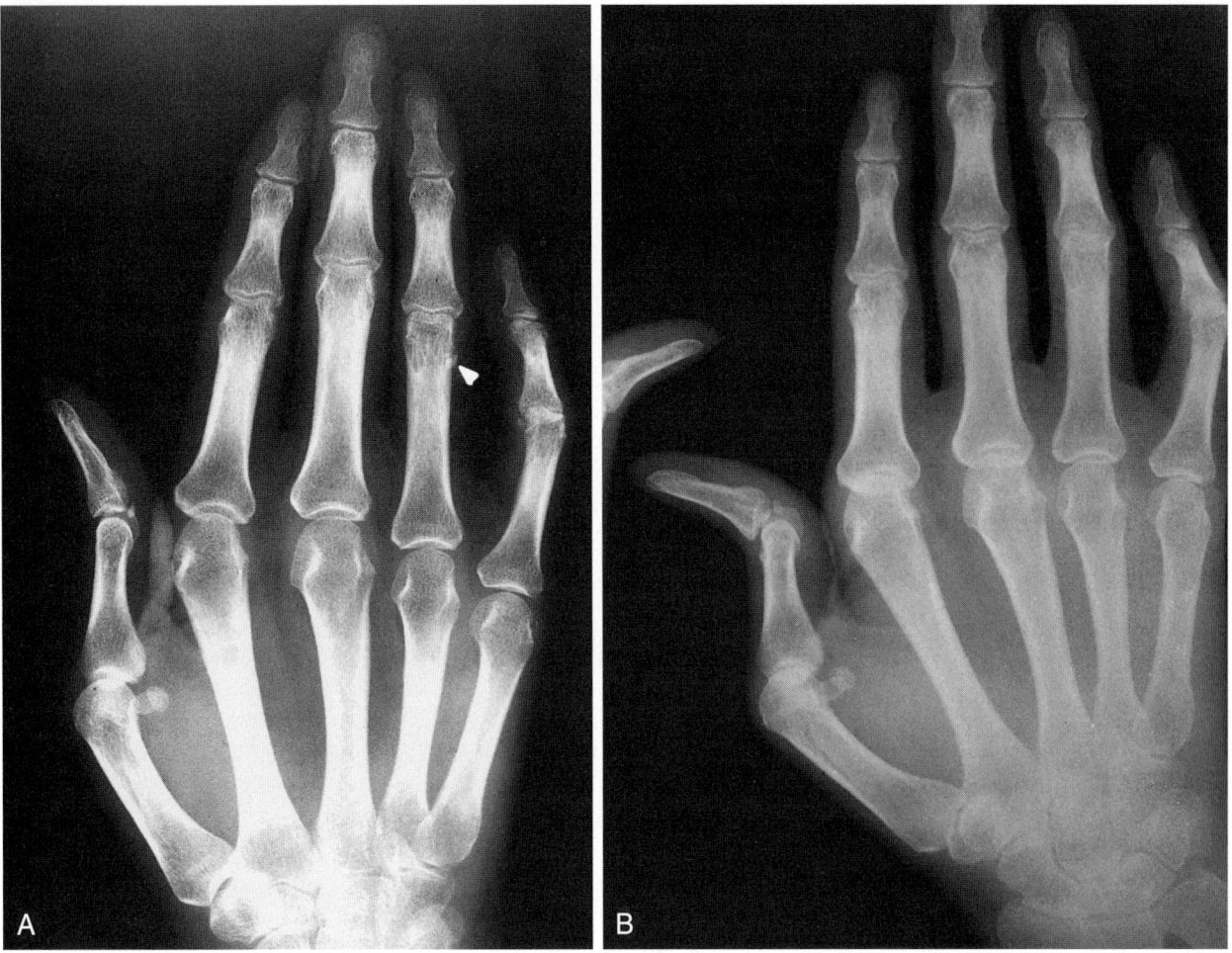

**Figure 27–1.**   Mixed connective tissue disease: deforming nonerosive arthropathy. A 32-year-old woman had progressive deformities of the hand. *A,* The initial radiograph outlines periarticular osteoporosis, capsular calcification *(arrowhead),* and a minor degree of ulnar deviation at the metacarpophalangeal joints. *B,* Nine years later, the joint deformities have progressed. Observe the flexion at the first metacarpophalangeal joint and hyperextension of the interphalangeal joint of the same digit. Also note the radial deviation at the wrist, ulnar deviation and flexion at the metacarpophalangeal joints, and flexion at the proximal interphalangeal joints. The width of the joint spaces is difficult to evaluate because of the associated deformities. (Courtesy of M. Dalinka, MD, Philadelphia, Pa.)

**Osteoporosis.** Diffuse or periarticular osteoporosis is common (10% to 100% of patients). In this regard, the findings simulate those of rheumatoid arthritis.

**Soft Tissue Swelling.** Symmetrical soft tissue swelling is common about the involved articulations (65% to 75% of patients). Diffuse swelling of the hand related to widespread edema is also apparent.

**Joint Space Narrowing.** Diffuse narrowing of the articular space is also common (10% to 100% of patients). Intra-articular bony ankylosis has also been noted.

**Bone Erosions.** The osseous erosions in MCTD (found in 25% to 75% of patients) are similar to those in rheumatoid arthritis. Erosions of the distal interphalangeal joints of the fingers may be observed in MCTD. In addition, in an occasional patient with MCTD, severe destructive arthritis can simulate the appearance of psoriatic arthritis.

**Changes in Phalangeal Tips.** Soft tissue atrophy, soft tissue calcification, and resorption of the terminal tufts of the phalanges (detected in 25% to 70% of patients) simulate the findings of scleroderma. Osseous resorption leads to typical "penciling" of the phalanges.

**Joint Subluxation.** Joint subluxation (present in 12% to 100% of patients) is identical to that in rheumatoid arthritis or systemic lupus erythematosus.

Although clinical involvement of other joints is not uncommon, radiographic changes in these locations are recorded infrequently. Periarticular osteoporosis and, uncommonly, calcification may be seen about the knee, elbow, or hip (Fig. 27–4). The erosive arthritis of MCTD is generally indistinguishable from rheumatoid arthritis. In patients with MCTD who demonstrate erosive arthritis, serologic testing for rheumatoid factor may yield positive or negative results. The soft tissue calcifications detected in patients with MCTD are generally indistin-

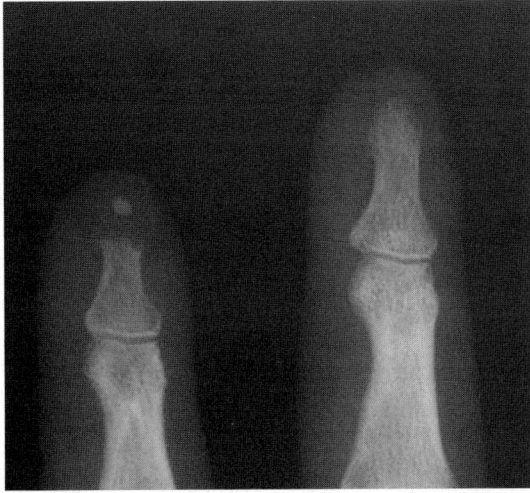

**Figure 27–2.** Mixed connective tissue disease: bone erosions and phalangeal tuft resorption. Observe the osteolysis of the terminal phalangeal tuft of the second finger and, to a lesser extent, the third finger. Punctate calcification is evident in the second digit. (Courtesy of D. Alarcón-Segovia, MD, Mexico City, Mexico.)

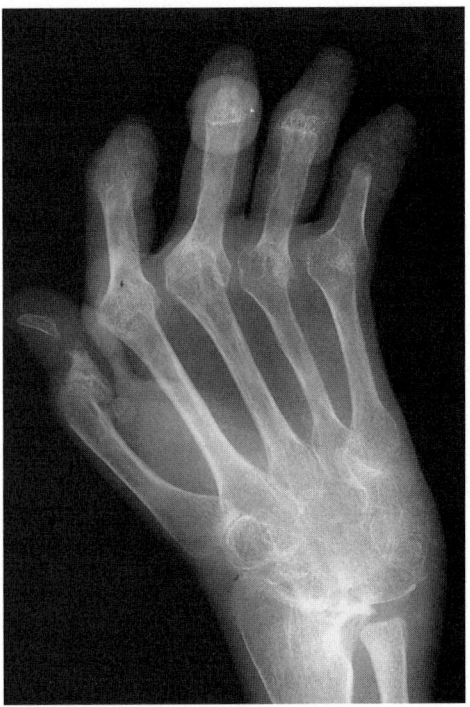

**Figure 27–3.** Mixed connective tissue disease: arthritis mutilans. The severe destructive arthropathy involving multiple locations in the hand and wrist resembles psoriatic arthritis. The opposite side (not shown) was similarly involved. (Courtesy of D. Alarcón-Segovia, MD, Mexico City, Mexico.)

guishable from those in scleroderma. Intra-articular calcifications, related to calcium hydroxyapatite crystal deposition, have also been observed in the hands and wrists of patients with MCTD. Soft tissue swelling in periarticular locations in MCTD is also nonspecific. Diffuse swelling in the hands corresponding to edema is suggestive of MCTD.

The diagnosis of MCTD is suggested when radiographic examination of the skeleton reveals features typical of more than one collagen vascular disease (Table 27–1). A variety of overlap syndromes can have a similar radiographic appearance.

## COLLAGEN VASCULAR OVERLAP SYNDROMES

As indicated previously, in many patients with collagen vascular disorders, the clinical features cannot be pre-cisely classified as those of a specific disease; instead, they are consistent with more than one disease. Such overlap syndromes include dermatomyositis and scleroderma, rheumatoid arthritis and scleroderma, systemic lupus erythematosus and dermatomyositis, rheumatoid arthritis and systemic lupus erythematosus, and scleroderma and systemic lupus erythematosus. This overlap of clinical manifestations does not clarify whether a single rheumatic disease syndrome with wide clinical expression is present or whether there are two coexistent disorders. The clinical and radiographic features of other overlap syndromes simulate the findings of MCTD.

**TABLE 27-1**

**Radiographic Features of Mixed Connective Tissue Disease**

| Scleroderma-Like Features | Lupus Erythematosus–Like Features | Rheumatoid Arthritis–Like Features | Dermatomyositis-Like Features |
|---|---|---|---|
| Soft tissue atrophy | Deforming nonerosive arthropathy | Symmetrical soft tissue swelling | Soft tissue calcification |
| Soft tissue or capsular calcification | Osteonecrosis | Periarticular osteoporosis | |
| Phalangeal tuft erosion | | Diffuse joint space narrowing | |
| Distal interphalangeal joint erosion | | Marginal bone erosion | |
| | | Soft tissue nodule | |

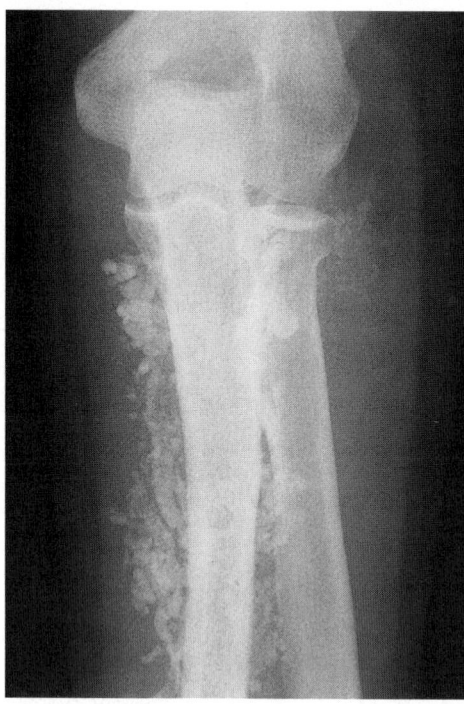

**Figure 27–4.** Mixed connective tissue disease: periarticular calcification. A 38-year-old woman complained of elbow pain. A frontal radiograph delineates extensive circular and linear collections of calcification about the elbow. (Courtesy of M. Dalinka, MD, Philadelphia, Pa.)

## FURTHER READING

Alarcón-Segovia D, Uribe-Uribe O: Mutilans-like arthropathy in mixed connective tissue disease. Arthritis Rheum 22:1013, 1979.

Baron M, Srolovitz H, Lander P, et al: The coexistence of rheumatoid arthritis and scleroderma: A case report and review of the literature. J Rheumatol 9:947, 1982.

Bennett RM: Mixed connective tissue disease and other overlap syndromes. In Kelley WN, Harris ED Jr, Ruddy S, Sledge CB (eds): Textbook of Rheumatology, 5th ed. Philadelphia, WB Saunders, 1997, p 1065.

Cervera R, Khamashta MA, Hughes GRV: "Overlap" syndromes. Ann Rheum Dis 49:947, 1990.

Cohen MG, Webb J: Concurrence of rheumatoid arthritis and systemic lupus erythematosus: Report of 11 cases. Ann Rheum Dis 46:853, 1987.

Fischman AS, Abeles M, Zanetti M, et al: The coexistence of rheumatoid arthritis and systemic lupus erythematosus: A case report and review of the literature. J Rheumatol 8:405, 1981.

Hoffman RW, Greidinger EL: Mixed connective tissue disease. Curr Opin Rheumatol 12:386, 2000.

LeRoy EC: Overlap features of connective tissue disease. Arthritis Rheum 25:889, 1982.

Ramos-Niembro F, Alarcón-Segovia D, Hernandez-Ortiz J: Articular manifestations of mixed connective tissue disease. Arthritis Rheum 22:43, 1979.

Sharp GC, Irvin WS, Tan EM, et al: Mixed connective tissue disease—an apparently distinct rheumatic disease syndrome associated with a specific antibody to an extractable nuclear antigen (ENA). Am J Med 52:148, 1972.

Silver TM, Farber SJ, Bole GG, et al: Radiological features of mixed connective tissue disease and scleroderma–systemic lupus erythematosus overlap. Radiology 120:269, 1976.

Smolen JS, Steiner G: Mixed connective tissue disease: To be or not to be? Arthritis Rheum 41:768, 1998.

Udoff EJ, Genant HK, Kozin F, et al: Mixed connective tissue disease: The spectrum of radiographic manifestations. Radiology 124:613, 1977.

# CHAPTER 28

## Rheumatic Fever

## SUMMARY OF KEY FEATURES

Articular involvement in rheumatic fever typically appears as polyarthritis, particularly in large joints, and as Jaccoud's arthropathy. Jaccoud's arthropathy is associated with deforming nonerosive articular changes. It shows a predilection for the ulnar digits of the hand and leads to deviation and subluxation at the metacarpophalangeal joints, which may be accompanied by deformities of the interphalangeal joints of the fingers and the metatarsophalangeal joints of the feet. The hand abnormalities, which resemble the changes in systemic lupus erythematosus and other collagen vascular diseases, can usually be differentiated from rheumatoid arthritis, in which early and significant cartilaginous and osseous destruction is apparent.

## INTRODUCTION

Rheumatic fever is clinically characterized by fever, carditis, and polyarthritis; the patient history typically includes a previous episode of group A beta-hemolytic streptococcal infection. Although rheumatic fever affects many tissues of the body, cardiac involvement is most significant to the patient and has received considerable attention over the years. Rheumatic fever, however, can also cause articular abnormalities.

A report of post–rheumatic fever arthropathy first appeared in 1867 when Jaccoud described a young man with rheumatic fever and recurrent bouts of polyarthritis in whom a chronic deforming arthropathy developed. The arthropathy was characterized by muscle atrophy, ulnar deviation with flexion and subluxation at multiple metacarpophalangeal joints, and hyperextension of the distal interphalangeal joints. Subsequent reports of Jaccoud's arthropathy indicated that it can also involve the feet, that it is correctable initially but may later become fixed, and that it is not confined to patients with rheumatic fever but may also appear in those with collagen vascular disorders such as systemic lupus erythematosus.

## ARTICULAR ABNORMALITIES

Classically, an attack of rheumatic fever occurs several days to several weeks after a streptococcal throat infection. Symptoms and signs of the clinical attack are variable. An acute onset may be characterized by fever, night sweats, headaches, and joint pain, whereas an insidious onset may be accompanied by pallor, fatigue, anorexia, weight loss, and muscular pain.

## Polyarthritis

Joint involvement is the most common clinical manifestation of rheumatic fever and frequently appears early during the course of a rheumatic attack. It occurs in approximately 75% of patients and is more frequent with increasing patient age. The involvement varies in severity from arthralgia to arthritis. Multiple joints are usually affected, particularly large joints such as the knees and ankles. Many joints may be affected simultaneously or in quick succession. Without treatment, joint inflammation may persist for several days to a week. Radiographs reveal soft tissue swelling without evidence of cartilaginous or osseous destruction. Mild osteoporosis may be apparent.

## Deforming Nonerosive (Jaccoud's) Arthropathy

Jaccoud's arthropathy appears to result from capsular inflammation and fibrosis. As already mentioned, it may occur in association with systemic lupus erythematosus and scleroderma, as well as with rheumatic fever. The clinical findings are characteristic, with a history of previous attacks of rheumatic fever, combined with symptoms and signs of residual heart lesions. Symptomless and reversible joint deformities become evident, particularly in the hands but also in the feet. Typically, ulnar deviation and flexion deformities are apparent at the metacarpophalangeal joints, predominantly in the fourth and fifth digits, and may be combined with hyperextension at the interphalangeal joints. In the foot, fibular deviation and subluxation at the metatarsophalangeal joints may be observed. In the hands and feet, the reversible nature of the articular deformity is striking. During radiography, pressing the hand against the cassette may result in an entirely normal posteroanterior radiograph (Fig. 28–1).

The clinical manifestations necessary for a diagnosis of Jaccoud's arthropathy are listed in Table 28–1. On radiographic evaluation, joint deformities may be apparent (Table 28–2). In most patients, articular space narrowing and osseous erosions are not evident, thereby allowing the differentiation of Jaccoud's arthropathy from rheumatoid arthritis and other inflammatory synovial processes. Occasionally, however, articular space diminution is encountered; this probably represents cartilaginous atrophy caused by disuse and cartilaginous erosion secondary to closely applied subluxed osseous surfaces. Hook erosions on the radial and palmar aspects of the metacarpal heads, which can appear in Jaccoud's arthropathy, superficially resemble the marginal erosions of rheumatoid arthritis (Fig. 28–2).

## DIFFERENTIAL DIAGNOSIS

Jaccoud's deforming arthropathy is a descriptive term for characteristic joint subluxation and malalignment in the hands (and feet); it frequently occurs without clinical findings of synovial disease and without radiographic find-

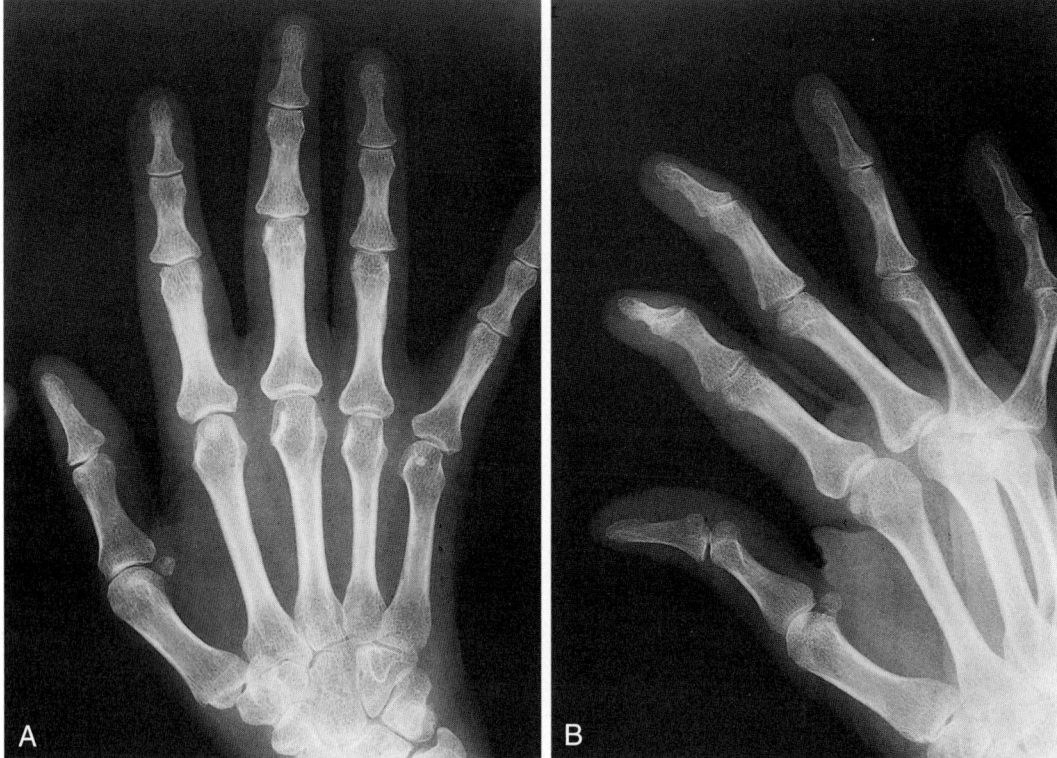

**Figure 28–1.**  Rheumatic fever: Jaccoud's arthropathy.  *A,* On a posteroanterior radiograph with the hand pressed firmly against the cassette, the only striking deformity is ulnar deviation of the fifth finger at the metacarpophalangeal joint. Mild periarticular osteoporosis is seen. No evidence of osseous erosion is apparent. *B,* On the oblique radiograph, the hand has been lifted from the cassette. Boutonnière and swan-neck deformities of all the digits can be seen.

ings of joint space narrowing and osseous erosion. The deforming nonerosive arthropathy of rheumatic fever is similar to that of systemic lupus erythematosus and, more infrequently, other collagen vascular diseases and vasculitides (Table 28–3). Although classically the ulnar digits are more commonly affected in rheumatic fever, and all the digits (including the thumb) are affected in systemic

**TABLE 28-1**

**Clinical Manifestations Necessary for a Diagnosis of Jaccoud's Arthropathy**

History of recurrent attacks of acute rheumatic fever

Delayed recovery after joint inflammation with subsequent deformity, particularly the MCP joints

Characteristic articular deformity consisting of flexion and ulnar deviation at the MCP, particularly in the fourth and fifth digits

Elicitation of tendon crepitus

Joint disease that is generally asymptomatic

MCP, metacarpophalangel.

**TABLE 28-2**

**Radiographic Characteristics of Jaccoud's Arthropathy**

Flexion and ulnar deviation of the metacarpophalangeal joints, particularly in the fourth and fifth digits

Flexion and fibular deviation of the metatarsophalangeal joints

Periarticular osteoporosis

Joint space narrowing (rare)

Hook erosions on the radial and palmar aspects of the metacarpal heads (rare)

**TABLE 28-3**

**Diseases That May Lead to Deforming Nonerosive Arthropathy**

Rheumatic fever

Collagen vascular disorders, particularly systemic lupus erythematosus

Rheumatoid arthritis (rare)

Agammaglobulinemia (rare)

Ehlers-Danlos syndrome (rare)

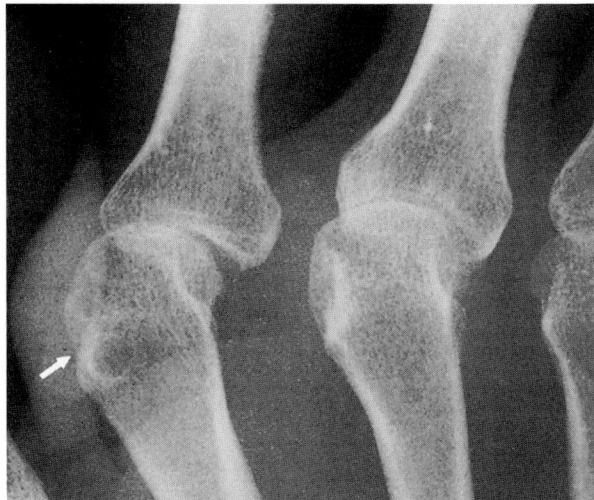

**Figure 28–2.** Jaccoud's arthropathy of unknown cause, with joint space narrowing and osseous erosion. A 45-year-old man had long-standing articular deformities of the hands without significant symptoms. An extensive workup failed to document the cause of the abnormalities. Rheumatoid factor was not present in the serum. A frontal radiograph reveals ulnar deviation of the second to fourth metacarpophalangeal joints, with articular space narrowing. A cystic lesion *(arrow)* can be seen on the radial aspect of the second metacarpal head. Associated soft tissue swelling and osteoporosis are evident.

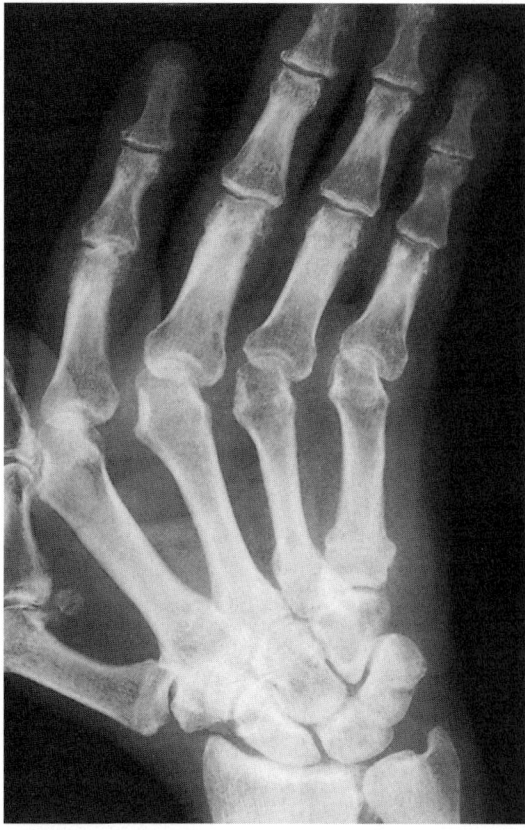

**Figure 28–3.** Rheumatoid arthritis. In this patient with classic seropositive rheumatoid arthritis, radial deviation at the radiocarpal joint and ulnar deviation at the metacarpophalangeal joints have occurred without significant osseous erosion. Periarticular osteoporosis can be noted.

lupus erythematosus, the patterns of distribution are variable and may be identical in both disorders. Deforming nonerosive arthropathies may also be encountered in agammaglobulinemia (hypogammaglobulinemia), Ehlers-Danlos syndrome, sarcoidosis, and, infrequently, rheumatoid arthritis (Fig. 28–3).

## FURTHER READING

Bisno AL: Rheumatic fever. In Kelley WN, Harris ED Jr, Ruddy S, Sledge CB (eds): Textbook of Rheumatology, 5th ed. Philadelphia, WB Saunders, 1997, p 1225.

Bywaters EGL: The relation between heart and joint disease including "rheumatoid heart disease" and chronic postrheumatic arthritis (type Jaccoud). Br Heart J 12:101, 1950.

Jaccoud S: Leçons de Clinique Médicale faites à l'Hôpital de la Charité. Vingt-troisième leçon, sur une forme de rhumatisme chronique. Paris, Adrien Delahaye, 1867, p 598.

Murphy WA, Staple TW: Jaccoud's arthropathy reviewed. AJR Am J Roentgenol 118:300, 1973.

Pastershank SP, Resnick D: "Hook" erosions in Jaccoud's arthropathy. J Can Assoc Radiol 31:174, 1980.

Zvaifler NJ: Chronic postrheumatic-fever (Jaccoud's) arthritis. N Engl J Med 267:10, 1962.

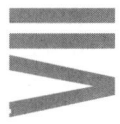
# Degenerative Diseases

# C H A P T E R  2 9

## Degenerative Diseases of Extraspinal Locations

### *SUMMARY OF KEY FEATURES*

Degenerative joint disease is widespread and common. In synovial joints, the process is termed osteoarthritis. At these sites, abnormalities predominate in the cartilaginous and osseous tissues, whereas alterations in the synovial membrane generally are mild. Typical findings include joint space loss, eburnation, cyst formation, and osteophytosis. Subluxation, malalignment, fibrous ankylosis, and intra-articular osseous and cartilaginous bodies may complicate osteoarthritis.

The most common sites of extraspinal osteoarthritis are the interphalangeal and metacarpophalangeal joints of the hand, first carpometacarpal and trapezioscaphoid areas of the wrist, acromioclavicular and sternoclavicular articulations, hip, knee, and tarsometatarsal and metatarsophalangeal joints of the great toe. At each of these sites, radiographic features of the disease are sufficiently characteristic to allow their differentiation from the features of other articular disorders.

Two special varieties of osteoarthritis have been described, although their existence as discrete entities is not universally accepted. Generalized osteoarthritis may be a particular form of degenerative joint disease in which multiple articulations are affected. Inflammatory (erosive) osteoarthritis is associated with clinical and pathologic features of joint inflammation. Although its distribution is virtually identical to that of noninflammatory digital osteoarthritis, certain radiographic features, such as erosions and intra-articular bony ankylosis, appear to be more typical of inflammatory osteoarthritis.

### INTRODUCTION

Degenerative joint disease is the most frequent articular affliction. Despite its common occurrence, degenerative arthritis did not receive a great deal of attention in the past, because many considered the disorder to be the dull and inevitable accompaniment of advancing age. More recently, a new curiosity and an enthusiasm to learn about degenerative arthritis have stimulated the considerable investigation that this common and significant condition deserves.

### TERMINOLOGY AND CLASSIFICATION

Degenerative joint disease is the best general phrase to describe degenerative alterations in any type of articulation. These alterations may appear in fibrous, cartilaginous, or synovial articulations. Their pathologic and radiographic appearances vary from one location to another, but at any site, the abnormalities appear to be related to degeneration of some articular structure. The terms *osteoarthrosis* and *osteoarthritis* are reserved for degenerative disease of synovial joints. Although inflammatory changes are not pronounced in most of these joints (making the suffix "-osis" more appropriate than "-itis"), the term *osteoarthritis* is used throughout this chapter, as this designation is widely accepted in the United States. Furthermore, when significant synovial inflammatory abnormalities do accompany degenerative joint disease, osteoarthritis is the more accurate description of the disorder.

Degeneration may also affect fibrous joints or entheses. An enthesis is a site of attachment of a tendon, ligament, or joint capsule to bone. An enthesopathy is an abnormality at this site, and a degenerative enthesopathy is the proper term for degeneration at this site. Degeneration of a cartilaginous joint is also recognized, especially at the discovertebral junction, where it is termed intervertebral osteochondrosis and spondylosis deformans (see Chapter 30).

Traditionally, degenerative joint disease was classified into primary (idiopathic) and secondary types. Primary degenerative joint disease was regarded as a process in which articular degeneration occurs in the absence of any obvious underlying abnormality, whereas secondary degenerative joint disease was regarded as articular degeneration produced by alterations from a preexisting affliction. This classification into primary and secondary degenerative joint disease is misleading. Careful evaluation of many examples of so-called primary degenerative joint disease discloses some mechanical deviation in the involved articulation that has led to secondary degeneration of the joint. It appears likely, therefore, that primary degenerative joint disease does not exist, and use of such a designation only underscores our limited diagnostic capabilities.

Articular degeneration may result from either an abnormal concentration of force across a joint with a normal articular cartilage matrix or a normal concentration of force across an abnormal joint (one with cartilaginous or subchondral osseous alterations) (Table 29–1). Eventually, abnormalities of force and articular structure appear together.

## TABLE 29–1

### Classification of Degenerative Joint Disease

A. Abnormal concentration of force on normal joint
  1. Intra-articular malalignment
    a. Epiphyseal injuries
    b. Epiphyseal dysplasia
    c. Neuromuscular imbalance
  2. Extra-articular malalignment
    a. Inequality of leg length
    b. Congenital and acquired varus or valgus deformities
    c. Malunited fractures
    d. Ligamentous abnormalities
  3. Loss of protective sensory feedback
    a. Neuropathic osteoarthropathy
    b. Intra-articular injection of steroids
  4. Miscellaneous
    a. Obesity
    b. Occupational
B. Normal concentration of force on abnormal joint
  1. Normal concentration of force on abnormal cartilage
    a. Transchondral fractures
    b. Meniscal tears and discoid menisci
    c. Loose bodies
    d. Preexisting arthritis
    e. Metabolic abnormalities (gout, calcium pyrophosphate dihydrate crystal deposition disease, acromegaly, alkaptonuria, mucopolysaccharidoses)
  2. Normal concentration of force on normal cartilage supported by weakened subchondral bone
    a. Osteonecrosis
    b. Osteoporosis
    c. Osteomalacia
    d. Osteitis fibrosa cystica (hyperparathyroidism)
    e. Neoplasm
  3. Normal concentration of force on normal cartilage supported by stiffened subchondral bone
    a. Osteopetrosis
    b. Paget's disease

## CAUSE

Many diverse factors appear to be important in the causation of degenerative joint disease (Table 29–2).

### Systemic Factors

**Genetics.** Although genetic patterns have been recognized in some forms of degenerative joint disease (e.g., generalized osteoarthritis with Heberden's nodes), they are not identifiable in most varieties of the disease.

**Obesity.** The role of obesity in the development of articular degeneration remains controversial. Studies of large populations of patients with degenerative joint disease reveal a great number of obese patients. Accumulating data strongly support an association between obesity and osteoarthritis of the knee; such an association for osteoarthritis of the great toe and hand appears likely, but despite evidence to the contrary, an association between obesity and osteoarthritis of the hip has not been established. Although it appears logical that excessive body weight should accentuate stresses across weight-bearing articulations, extreme obesity may lead to patient immobility and decreased active joint motion, thereby diminishing any predisposition to develop degenerative articular alterations.

**Age.** Strong evidence exists that degenerative joint disease occurs with increasing frequency in older persons, perhaps related to aging cartilage's diminished capacity to resist mechanical stress due to changing physical and biochemical properties. The correlation of joint degeneration and advancing age is not linear. Rather, an age-related predisposition to degenerative joint disease appears to increase exponentially after the age of 50 or 60 years.

**Sex.** The pattern of degenerative joint disease is also influenced by the sex of the patient. Although the fre-

## TABLE 29–2

### Main Causative Factors According to Location of Osteoarthritis

| Affected Joint(s) | Intrinsic Factors | | | | | Extrinsic Factors | | |
| --- | --- | --- | --- | --- | --- | --- | --- | --- |
| | Age | Female Sex | Heredity | Obesity | Inflammation | Trauma | Minor Mechanical Disturbance | Dysplasia or Angulation |
| Fingers: DIP and nodal generalized osteoarthritis | + | ++ | ++ | | | | | |
| Fingers: PIP and non-nodal generalized osteoarthritis | + | | | + | ++ | | | |
| First carpometacarpal | + | + | | | | | | |
| First metatarsophalangeal | (+) | | | | | | + | |
| Hip | (+) | | | | | | | ++ |
| Knee | (+) | + | | + | | | + | ++ |
| Shoulder | (+) | | | | | + | + | |
| Ankle | | | | | | + | | |
| Wrist | | | | | | + | | |

DIP, distal interphalangeal; PIP, proximal interphalangeal.
From Peyron JG: Semin Arthritis Rheum 8:288, 1979.

quency of the disease is approximately equal in both sexes, men younger than 45 years are affected more commonly than are women of this age. In addition, women demonstrate severe disease more frequently than men and are more commonly afflicted with primary generalized osteoarthritis, Heberden's nodes, and inflammatory osteoarthritis.

**Activity and Occupation.** Although normal use of a joint is believed to be beneficial to its integrity, it is generally assumed that either inactivity or excessive activity leads to articular degeneration. Certain occupations that are associated with chronic and repetitive articular abuse are reportedly associated with degenerative joint disease at specific locations. Ballet dancers may develop degenerative alterations in the ankles and joints of the feet. Degenerative disease has also been reported in the knees of football players, the patellofemoral joints of cyclists, and the hips of farmers. The deleterious effects of excessive repetitive impulse loading on joints (and bones) are perhaps best exemplified by the articular abnormalities in workers using vibrating tools (Fig. 29–1).

**Nutritional and Metabolic Status.** The recognition of degenerative joint abnormalities in Kashin-Beck disease has stimulated interest in the role of nutritional factors in the development of articular degeneration. In this disease, which is endemic in Siberia and other parts of the Far East, defective growth and maturation of epiphyses are associated with osteonecrosis and the appearance of osteoarthritis-like aberrations. Although the exact cause of Kashin-Beck disease is not known, it has been attributed to the toxic effects of fungus-contaminated grain, to sele-

nium deficiency, to chronic ingestion of excessive quantities of iron, and to defective mineral content of grain.

An increased frequency of degenerative joint disease has been described in patients with a variety of endocrine disorders, such as diabetes mellitus and acromegaly. Degenerative joint disease can also complicate various metabolic disorders, including Paget's disease, alkaptonuria, hemochromatosis, Wilson's disease, gout, idiopathic calcium pyrophosphate dihydrate crystal deposition disease, mucopolysaccharidoses, and osteopetrosis.

**Osteoporosis.** Although osteoporosis and degenerative joint disease are both common in older persons, increasing evidence supports an inverse correlation between the two processes. Secondary evidence of this dissociation is provided by reports that indicate differences in the patient populations affected by osteoporosis and osteoarthritis; the former condition is evident in short and slender women, the latter in obese women. A reduction in bone mass in subchondral locations may lead to an increase in the tissue's ability to absorb stress and a decrease in degenerative abnormalities.

## Local Factors

**Trauma.** Major or minor traumatic episodes appear to be important in producing abnormal stress across a joint, leading to its degeneration. Repetitive trauma is significant in athletic and occupation-induced degenerative joint disease. It is also implicated in the appearance of joint degeneration in association with ligament laxity (Ehlers-Danlos syndrome), loss of protective sensory feedback (neuropathic osteoarthropathy), extra-articular malalignment, and intra-articular malalignment (epiphyseal injury or slipping). Single episodes of trauma can also lead to incongruity of apposing articular surfaces, with resultant degenerative joint disease. Traumatic factors may explain the presence of more severe articular degeneration in the upper extremity on the dominant side than on the nondominant side, the lesser frequency of osteoarthritis in joints that are located ipsilateral to and immediately above the site of amputation of a portion of the leg, and the absence of significant joint degeneration in an immobilized or paralyzed limb.

**Preexisting Articular Disease or Deformity.** Degenerative changes in cartilage and bone may be superimposed on any primary articular process that has led to incongruity of and abnormal stress on the joint surfaces. Thus, degenerative arthritis may follow inflammatory joint disease (such as rheumatoid arthritis and septic arthritis). Similarly, degenerative joint abnormalities may accompany hemophilia and other bleeding disorders, crystal-induced arthropathy, osteonecrosis, and congenital disorders (such as acetabular dysplasia or spondyloepiphyseal dysplasia).

## PATHOGENESIS

The previous discussion makes it clear that numerous factors can initiate the pathologic and radiologic features of degenerative joint disease. One way or another, these

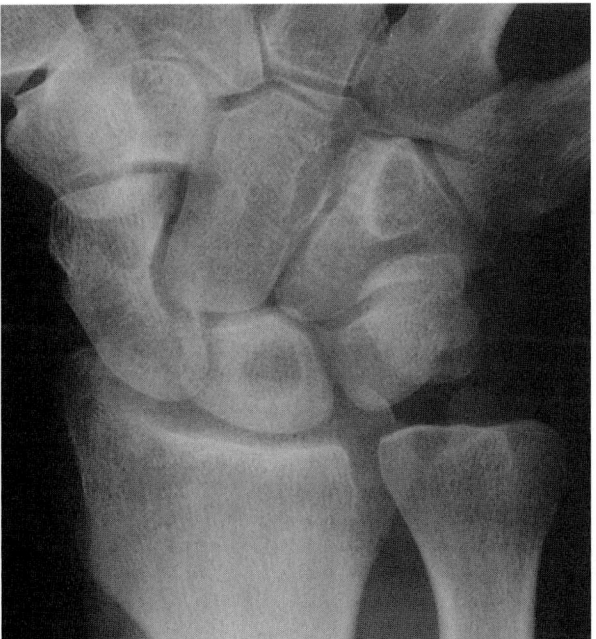

**Figure 29–1.** Occupation-induced degenerative joint disease. In this pneumatic driller with 10 years of professional experience, cystic lesions are seen in the lunate and scaphoid. (Courtesy of S. Sintzoff, MD, Brussels, Belgium.)

factors create a situation in which the intra-articular structures can no longer resist the physical forces being applied to the joint. In some instances, it is the force itself that is abnormal, whereas in other instances, weakened cartilage or subchondral bone is unable to combat the normal forces acting across the articulation.

Traditionally, degenerative alterations are thought to begin in the articular cartilage. Physical forces apparently disrupt the cartilage matrix and adversely affect the chondrocytes. The alterations in the matrix are almost certainly related to enzymatic destruction. An alternative theory emphasizes the initial role of subchondral bony abnormalities in the pathogenesis of degenerative joint disease. According to this theory, overload produces microfractures in the subchondral bony trabeculae. Repair of these fractures leads to increased stiffness of the bone, a reduction in its shock-absorbing efficiency, and exposure of overlying cartilage to increased force. This theory gains support from the clinical observations that some patients with osteoarthritis demonstrate increased bone density when radiography, computed tomography (CT), or photon absorption techniques are used; that persons with disorders characterized by increased bone density (Paget's disease, osteopetrosis) may have degeneration of neighboring articulations; and that patients with osteoporosis of the femoral head may have a lower rate of occurrence of osteoarthritis of the hip.

There is no convincing evidence that alterations in the synovial membrane and joint lubrication play important roles in the initiation of degenerative joint disease. After the appearance of degeneration in the cartilage or subchondral bone, a vicious circle of events occurs that aggravates the articular insult, resulting in progression of disease. Cartilaginous destruction increases joint instability, provoking further stress on cartilage and bone. In synovium-lined joints, damage confined to cartilage generally shows a poor reparative response, whereas that extending to subchondral bone is accompanied by the appearance of cartilaginous tissue formed by vascular invasion. This tissue is not as sound mechanically as the original hyaline surface; it resembles fibrocartilage and accounts for such events as restoration of joint space, disappearance of bone eburnation and cysts, and improved joint congruity.

## RADIOGRAPHIC-PATHOLOGIC CORRELATION
### Synovial Joints

The concept that excessive wear and tear initiates articular degeneration in the stressed (pressure) areas of a joint is a valuable one that has been emphasized repeatedly in the literature. It is also important to recognize that changes are common in the nonstressed (nonpressure) segments of the joint. In general, the type and severity of cartilaginous and osseous abnormalities are different in the pressure and nonpressure segments of the articulation. In fact, the segmental nature of the alterations is an important characteristic of degenerative joint disease, allowing its pathologic and radiographic differentiation from other disorders. In the pressure segment, progressive thinning and denudation of the cartilaginous

surface are pathologically evident, and vascular invasion, infarction, and necrosis of the subchondral trabeculae account for joint space loss, bony sclerosis, and cyst formation, which are apparent on radiographs; in the nonpressure segment, pathologically evident hypervascularity of marrow and cartilage leads to radiographically detectable osteophytosis. These findings emphasize the simultaneous occurrence of both destructive and reparative processes in this disease (Table 29–3).

## Cartilaginous Abnormalities

Characteristic changes in articular cartilage accompany degenerative joint disease (Fig. 29–2). Involved cartilage appears discolored (brown-gray or yellow-gray) and thinned. Irregular crevices or cracks and larger areas of

---

### TABLE 29–3

**Degenerative Joint Disease of Synovial Articulations (Osteoarthritis): Radiographic-Pathologic Correlation**

| Pathologic Abnormality | Radiographic Abnormality |
| --- | --- |
| Cartilaginous fibrillation and erosion | Localized loss of joint space |
| Increased cellularity and hypervascularity of subchondral bone | Bony eburnation |
| Synovial fluid intrusion or bony contusion | Subchondral cysts |
| Revascularization of remaining cartilage and capsular traction | Osteophytes |
| Periosteal and synovial membrane stimulation | Osteophytes and buttressing |
| Compression of weakened and deformed trabeculae | Bony collapse |
| Fragmentation of osteochondral surface | Intra-articular osseous bodies |
| Disruption and distortion of capsular and ligamentous structures | Deformity and malalignment |

---

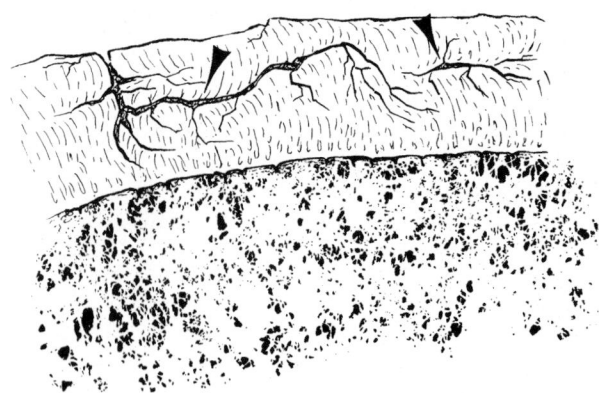

**Figure 29–2.** Cartilaginous abnormalities: pathologic findings. Drawing depicts the irregular cracks or crevices (*arrowheads*) that may appear in the chondral surface.

erosion develop, and ulcers of variable depth are seen, some of which are deep enough to expose the subchondral bone. Denuded areas appear, uncovering the subchondral bone. Eventually, loss of entire segments of the cartilaginous coat may be evident.

It is this progressive loss of cartilage, evident on pathologic examination, that accounts for one fundamental radiographic sign of degenerative joint disease: diminution of the articular space. Characteristically, the loss of joint space is localized predominantly in the area of the joint that has been subject to excessive pressure. Thus, joint space narrowing is apparent in the superolateral aspect of an osteoarthritic hip and in the medial femorotibial space of an osteoarthritic knee. In certain sites, articular space diminution may be more diffuse (osteoarthritis of the interphalangeal or metacarpophalangeal joints), and joint space loss may involve the entire articulation. With these few exceptions, however, it is the focal nature of the cartilaginous destruction and resulting loss of the interosseous space that allow the differentiation of osteoarthritis from processes, such as rheumatoid arthritis, that lead to diffuse chondral alterations.

## Subchondral Bony Abnormalities

Subchondral bony abnormalities accompany degenerative joint disease and can be divided into a destructive phase (regressive remodeling) and a productive phase (progressive remodeling). Characteristics of the destructive phase are bony eburnation, cyst formation, flattening, and deformity, which predominate in the pressure segment of the joint; characteristics of the productive phase are osteophytes, which predominate in the nonpressure segment of the joint.

### Eburnation

After cartilage loss, bony eburnation becomes evident in the closely applied osseous surfaces, apparently related to deposition of new bone on preexisting trabeculae and to trabecular compression and fracture with callus formation. The weakened hyperemic subchondral bone in the pressure segment of the joint is vulnerable to further deformity. The loss of resilient cartilage and the restriction of joint motion heighten and localize the abnormal stress on the bone, leading to trabecular fracture, flattening, and collapse.

On radiographic examination, sclerosis and joint space diminution are closely related. Generally, radiographic evidence of loss of articular space is present before significant eburnation becomes apparent. With progressive obliteration of this space, sclerosis becomes more prominent, extending vertically into deeper regions of the subchondral bone and horizontally into adjacent osseous segments.

### Cyst Formation

Cysts are an important and prominent finding in osteoarthritis (as well as in other articular disorders) (Fig. 29–3). These lesions have been termed subchondral cysts, subarticular pseudocysts, and geodes. Any desig-

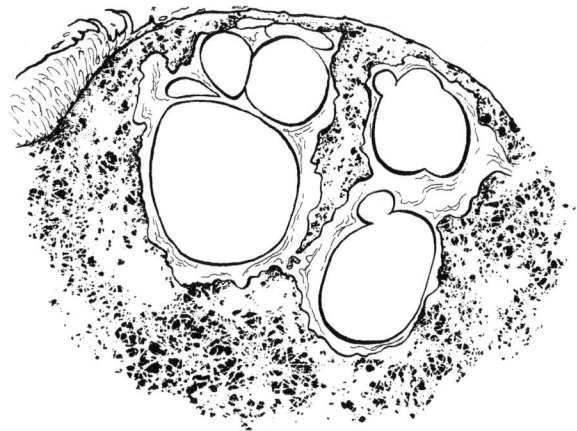

**Figure 29–3.** Subchondral bone cysts: pathologic findings. Drawing reveals the typical appearance of multiple subchondral cysts of varying size in areas of cartilaginous degeneration or disappearance. They are surrounded by sclerotic bone.

nation using the term *cyst* is not entirely accurate, in that a cyst implies a cavitary lesion with an epithelial lining. Subchondral cysts are not surrounded by such a lining, nor are they uniformly cavitary. The term *geode*, which is popular in Europe, is a geologic term and is likewise not very appropriate; geodes are small, hollow rocks lined with crystals. Here, the designation subchondral cyst is used despite its obvious inadequacies.

Within the pressure segment of the subchondral bone in osteoarthritis, cystic spaces appear between thickened trabeculae. These cysts commonly are multiple, of variable size, and piriform in shape. On pathologic examination, some cysts are noncavitary, containing myxoid and adipose tissue mixed with loose fibrous elements; others possess central cavitation containing proteinaceous material, are surrounded by fibrous tissue, and are well demarcated by adjacent eburnated bone. On radiographic examination, cysts appear in association with joint space loss and bony eburnation. Communication with the articular space may or may not be identifiable; when present, such communication may allow gas to pass from the joint into the cyst, creating a pneumatocyst.

The pathogenesis of cystic lesions in degenerative joint disease has received a great deal of attention. Although all reports emphasize the importance of concentrated pressure or stress on the articular cartilage and subchondral bone in the development of these lesions, two fundamental theories of pathogenesis have been proposed: synovial fluid intrusion and bony contusion (Fig. 29–4). Recent evidence indicates that both elements are operating together in the pathogenesis of cystic lesions. Although the pathogenesis of subchondral cysts is contested, their occurrence in degenerative joint disease is not. In this disease, the cystic lesions create multiple radiolucent areas of varying size on apposing surfaces of bone in the pressure segment of the joint, which must be differentiated from the subchondral lucent lesions that may accompany other disorders (Table 29–4).

In rheumatoid arthritis, cysts occur initially at chondro-osseous junctions as a result of erosion of cartilage-free bone by inflammatory synovial tissue or

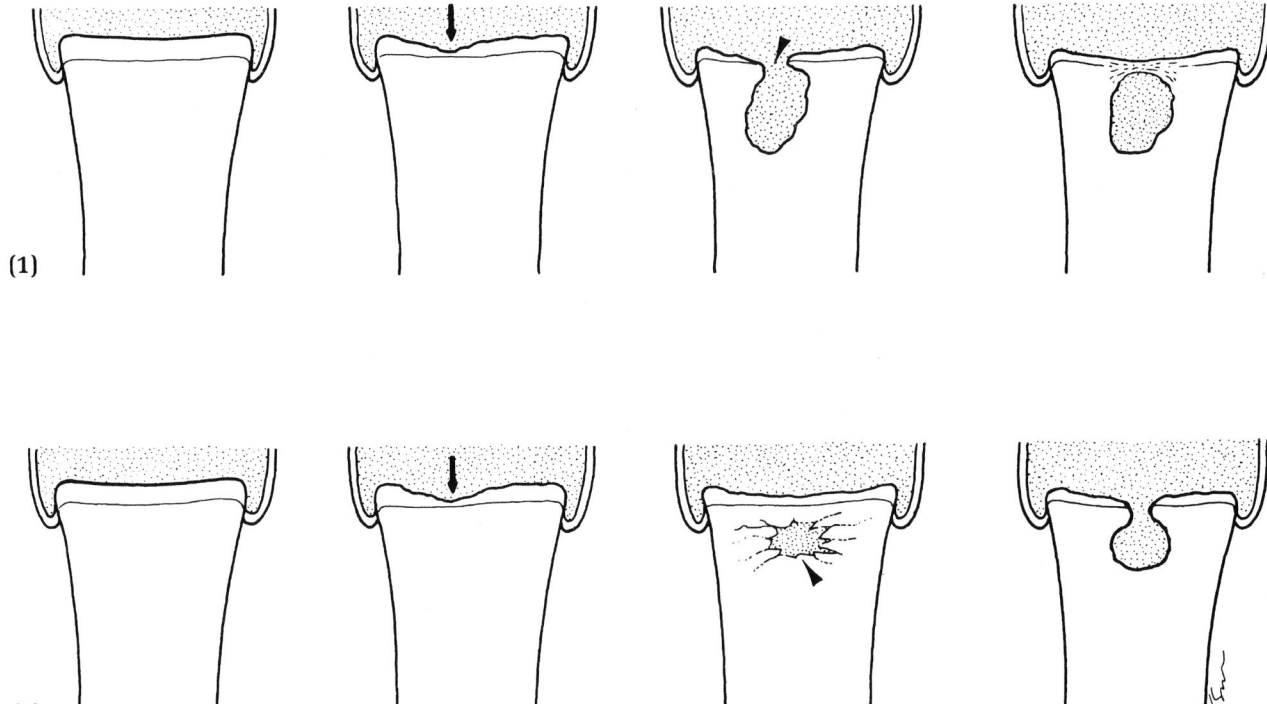

**Figure 29–4.** Pathogenesis of subchondral cysts. Two fundamental theories are illustrated. The theory of synovial intrusion (1) states that abnormal stress on cartilage *(arrow)* leads to cartilaginous degeneration. Synovial fluid is driven into the subchondral bone through gaps in the chondral surface and bone plate *(arrowhead)*, producing cysts that initially communicate with the joint and subsequently may become occluded with fibrous tissue. The theory of bony contusion (2) also holds that cartilage loss occurs due to abnormal stress *(arrow)*. Subsequently, fracture and vascular insufficiency of the bone itself *(arrowhead)* produce cysts, which may communicate with the joint secondarily.

pannus and are accompanied by early loss of articular space. They frequently are multiple, lack sclerotic margins, and subsequently extend over large segments of the joint surface. In calcium pyrophosphate dihydrate crystal deposition disease, multiple, large, and widespread cystic lesions are characteristic. They resemble the cysts in degenerative joint disease, except that they are larger, more numerous, and more frequently associated with disruption, collapse, and fragmentation of the subchondral bone plate. In osteonecrosis, cysts appear within the pressure segment of the articulation, related to osteoclastic resorption of necrotic trabeculae, with fibrous replacement of bone. Collapse of the subchondral bone plate and preservation of the joint space are additional characteristic features of osteonecrosis.

Subchondral cyst formation is occasionally a sequela of bone injury, although its precise mechanism is not known. A radiolucent lesion of variable size becomes evident over a period of months after the traumatic episode. The lesion, which is observed most commonly about the ankle, knee, or hip, is well marginated by a rim of bony sclerosis and may communicate with the articular cavity (Fig. 29–5). It resembles a degenerative cyst, although its larger size and the relatively normal appearance of the joint itself are useful diagnostic features.

An intraosseous ganglion is another subchondral radiolucent lesion that may simulate a degenerative cyst (Fig. 29–6), although there is debate regarding the existence of this lesion as an entity that can be separated from post-traumatic and degenerative cysts of bone. This lesion, which is commonly encountered in middle-aged adults, is characterized by mild, localized pain and the absence of a significant history of trauma. The ganglion is generally solitary and is located in the epiphysis of a long bone (particularly the medial malleolus and femoral head), a carpal bone, or a subarticular region of a flat bone (particularly the acetabulum). It is apparent that the radiographic and pathologic characteristics of intraosseous ganglia and degenerative cysts are similar, although some differences may be encountered. Characteristics of an intraosseous ganglion that may be distinctive include its occurrence in nonpressure areas of a joint, its association with a relatively normal adjacent articulation, its lack of communication with the nearby joint, and its relatively large size. In fact, some investigators emphasize that these ganglionic cysts do not originate from an articular disorder; degenerative or inflammatory changes are usually absent in the adjacent articulation.

Subchondral cysts in degenerative joint disease must also be distinguished from a variety of primary and secondary neoplasms of bone. These include chondroblastoma (10- to 30-year-old age group, solitary lesion), giant cell tumor (20- to 40-year-old age group, solitary eccentric trabeculated lesion), and skeletal metastasis (older patients, single or multiple lesions of variable appearance). In general, this differentiation is not difficult.

**TABLE 29–4**

**Differential Diagnosis of Subchondral Cystic Lesions**

| Disorder | Probable Mechanism of Cyst Formation | Radiographic Appearance |
|---|---|---|
| Osteoarthritis | Synovial fluid intrusion<br>Bony contusion | Multiple radiolucent lesions within pressure segment of joint<br>Surrounding sclerotic margin<br>Accompanying joint space narrowing and bony sclerosis |
| Rheumatoid arthritis | Pannus invasion of bone | Multiple radiolucent lesions begin at chondro-osseous junction and become widespread<br>No surrounding sclerotic margin<br>Accompanying joint space narrowing and osteoporosis |
| Calcium pyrophosphate dihydrate crystal deposition disease | Synovial intrusion<br>Bone contusion | Widespread radiolucent lesions, frequently large<br>Surrounding sclerotic margin<br>Accompanying joint space narrowing, bony sclerosis, collapse, and fragmentation |
| Osteonecrosis | Osteoclastic resorption of necrotic trabeculae | Single or multiple radiolucent lesions within pressure segment of joint<br>Accompanying bony sclerosis, collapse, and fragmentation |
| Intraosseous ganglion | Intraosseous penetration of a soft tissue ganglion<br>Primary intraosseous process, perhaps related to synovial intrusion, synovial rests, or intramedullary mucoid degeneration due to vascular insufficiency resulting from trauma | Single or loculated radiolucent lesion in pressure or nonpressure segment of joint<br>Surrounding sclerotic margin<br>Accompanying soft tissue mass |
| Neoplastic disorders<br>Chondroblastoma<br>Giant cell tumor<br>Clear cell chondrosarcoma<br>Skeletal metastasis | Neoplastic proliferation with destruction and displacement of trabeculae | Variable, depending on the nature of the neoplasm |

Features of degenerative cysts such as multiplicity, segmental distribution, surrounding sclerosis, and adjacent abnormal joint are of great diagnostic aid.

*Osteophytosis*

Osteophytes are considered by many physicians to be the most characteristic abnormality of degenerative joint disease. Osteophytes develop in areas of a joint that are subjected to low stress; they may be marginal (peripheral), although they may become apparent at additional locations (Table 29–5).

**Marginal Osteophytes.** At the peripheral portions of involved joints, characteristic outgrowths develop in degenerative joint disease (Fig. 29–7). Vascularization of the subchondral bone marrow in this region produces calcification of the adjacent cartilage and stimulates endochondral ossification. As it grows, it leaves behind remnants of the original calcified cartilage (and subchondral bone plate) as a telltale indicator of the location of the original joint surface, which can be identified histologically and radiographically.

Radiographically, marginal osteophytes appear as lips of new bone around the edges of the joint. They may be smooth, pitted, or undulating and are of variable size.

The excrescences frequently predominate on one side of the joint. Marginal osteophytes develop initially in areas of relatively normal joint space and usually are unassociated with significant adjacent sclerosis or cyst formation; articular space loss, eburnation, and subchondral cysts are findings that are characteristic of pressure segments of the joint.

**Central (Interior) Osteophytes.** The presence of osteophytic outgrowths in the central or interior portions of the articular space is a less well recognized manifestation of osteoarthritis (Fig. 29–8). In central areas where remnants of articular cartilage still exist, hypervascularity of subchondral bone stimulates endochondral ossification. The resulting excrescences (which are most prominent in the hip and knee) are button-like or flat and are often demarcated at their bases by remnants of the original calcified cartilage.

Central osteophytes frequently lead to a bumpy articular contour on radiographic examination. The small excrescences can be misinterpreted as evidence of intra-articular osseous (loose) bodies (Fig. 29–9) or cartilage calcification (chondrocalcinosis). The presence of continuity between the osteophyte and the underlying bone and of ossification rather than calcification should lead to the correct analysis of the radiographs.

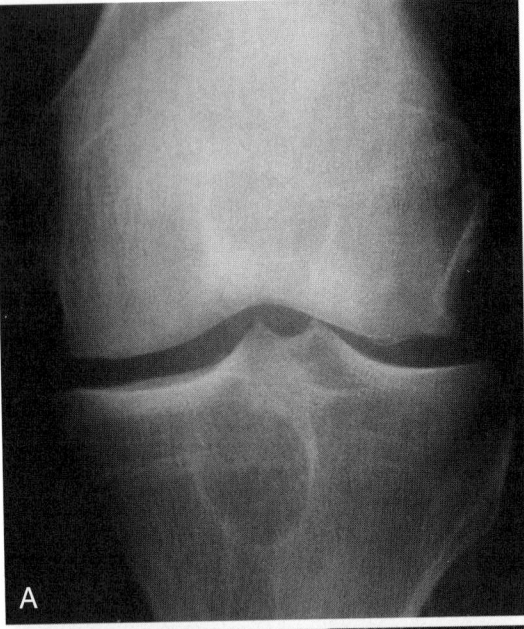

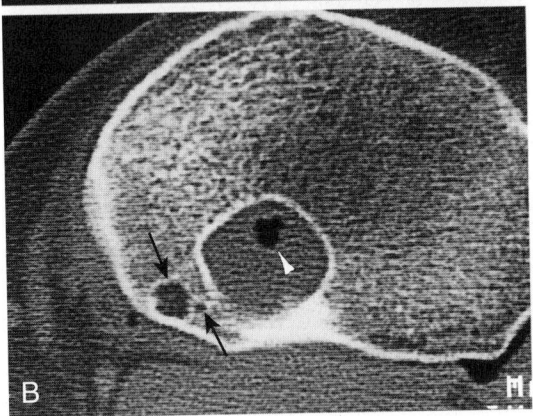

**Figure 29–5.** Post-traumatic subchondral cyst. This 38-year-old man developed knee pain and swelling after a fall. An enlarging lesion in the proximal end of the tibia was evident over a 2-year period. Subsequently, the lesion stabilized and the symptoms disappeared. *A*, Anteroposterior radiograph reveals a well-circumscribed radiolucent area in the proximal portion of the tibia. *B*, CT was accomplished after the introduction of air into the articular cavity. This transaxial section at the level of the proximal end of the tibia demonstrates a large cyst containing air *(arrowhead)* and one or two smaller lesions *(arrows)*. The air within the cyst documents that it communicated with the joint cavity.

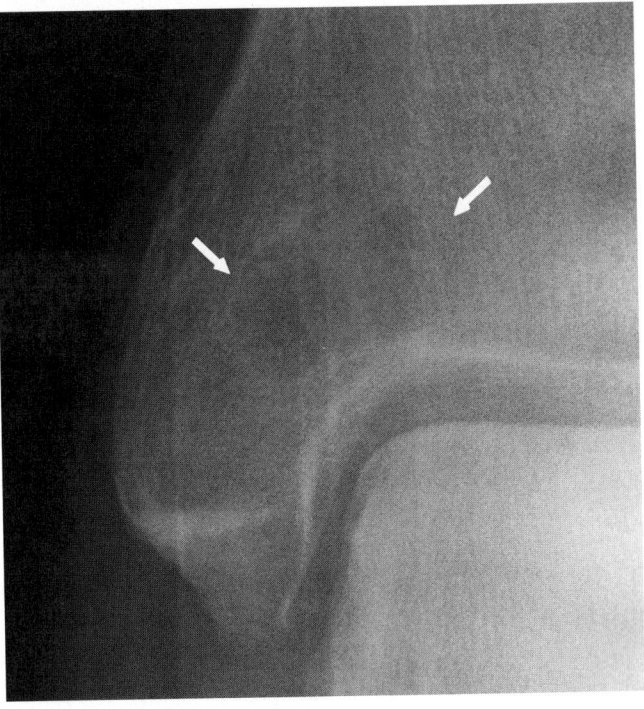

**Figure 29–6.** Intraosseous ganglion. An intraosseous ganglion, confirmed at surgery, is located adjacent to the ankle near the medial malleolus *(arrows)*. It is lucent and surrounded by a thin rim of sclerosis and apparently does not communicate with the articular cavity.

**Periosteal and Synovial Osteophytes.** In certain articulations, bone may develop from the periosteum or synovial membrane (Fig. 29–10). This phenomenon is most characteristic in the femoral neck, where it is termed buttressing. In the degenerative hip joint, buttressing predominates on the medial aspect of the femoral neck. On radiographs, a radiodense line of variable thickness extends along a part or all of the femoral neck. Associated excrescences may project circumferentially, producing a radiodense line across the neck that simulates a fracture.

**Capsular Osteophytes.** Osteophytes accompanying degenerative joint disease may develop at the site of bony attachment of the joint capsule (and articular ligaments) (Fig. 29–11). This phenomenon is particularly charac-

**TABLE 29–5**

### Types of Osteophytes

| Type | Mechanism | Radiographic Appearance |
|---|---|---|
| Marginal osteophyte | Endochondral ossification due to vascularization of subchondral bone marrow | Outgrowth at margins (nonpressure segments) of joint, producing lips of bone |
| Central osteophyte | Endochondral ossification due to vascularization of subchondral bone marrow | Outgrowth at central areas of joint, producing bumpy contour |
| Periosteal (synovial) osteophyte | Intramembranous type of ossification due to stimulation of periosteal (synovial) membrane with appositional bone formation | Thickening of intra-articular "cortices," producing buttressing |
| Capsular osteophyte | Capsular traction | Lips of bone extending along the direction of capsular pull |

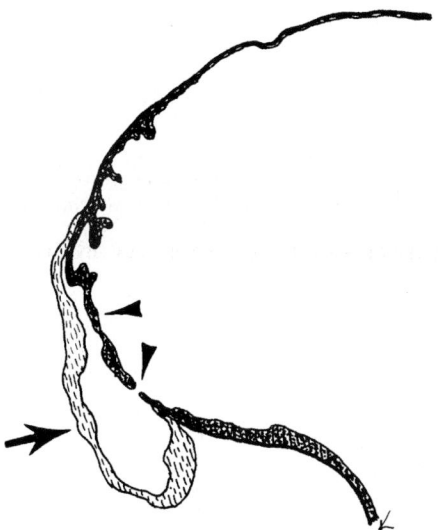

**Figure 29–7.** Marginal osteophytes: pathologic findings. The marginal osteophyte develops as a lip of bone *(arrow)* as a result of vascularization of the subchondral marrow with the inception of endochondral ossification. As it grows, it leaves behind a remnant of the original calcified cartilage *(arrowheads)*.

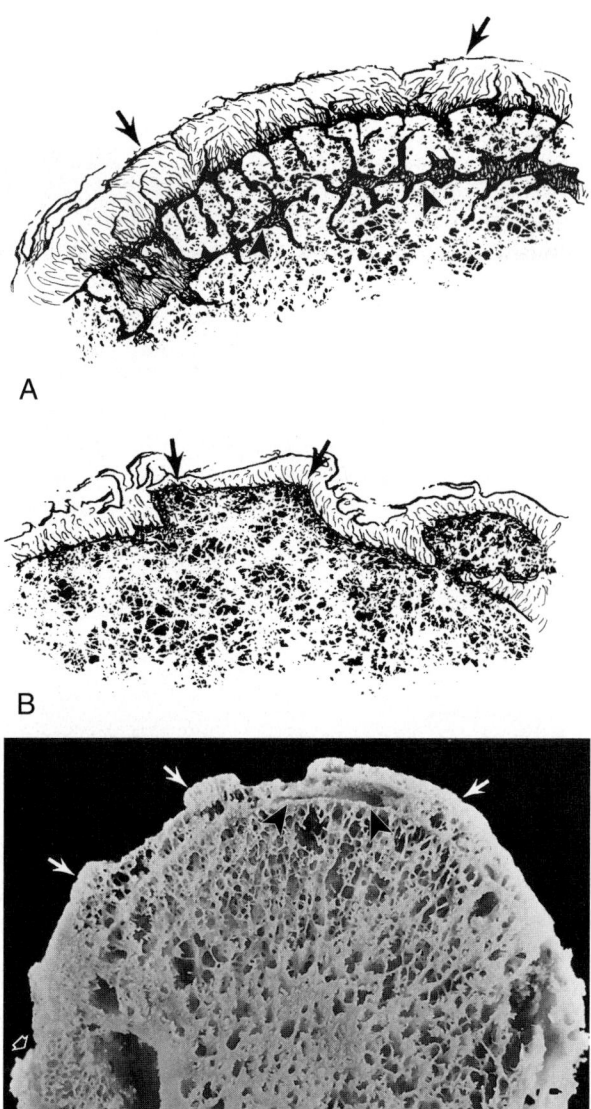

**Figure 29–8.** Central osteophytes: pathologic findings. *A,* Reduplication of cartilage and bone. In the central portions of the articulation, hypervascularity of subchondral bone can lead to stimulation of remnants of cartilage, producing endochondral ossification. The flat outgrowths that develop *(arrows)* are often demarcated by the original zone of calcified cartilage *(arrowheads)*. *B,* Shifting of cartilage and bone border. In this situation, the osteophyte develops *(arrows)* without leaving behind a zone of calcified cartilage. *C,* On a photograph of a macerated coronal section of the femoral head in a patient with osteoarthritis, the osteophytes *(solid arrows)* are developing by reduplication and shifting of the cartilage-bone junction. In places, a calcified zone of cartilage is identified *(arrowheads)*. A marginal osteophyte is also apparent *(open arrow)*.

teristic in the interphalangeal joints. At these sites, the resulting excrescences extend proximally, resembling the wings of a seagull (seagull sign).

### *Osteonecrosis*

The frequency and significance of osteonecrosis (Fig. 29–12) in osteoarthritis have not been fully delineated. Bone necrosis may be apparent on histologic examination of the eburnated surface in the pressure segment of the joint. The changes of necrosis become more exaggerated as the disease process becomes more advanced; however, bone necrosis is generally a localized microscopic process in osteoarthritis and usually cannot be detected on radiographic examination. Further, flattening and collapse may be apparent in osteoarthritis without indicating the presence of significant osteonecrosis. The radiographic differentiation of osteoarthritis (with or without osteonecrosis) from osteonecrosis with secondary joint degeneration can be extremely difficult, however.

### Synovial Membrane Abnormalities

Synovial membrane alterations are not prominent in most cases of osteoarthritis. With increasing severity of cartilaginous and osseous alterations, the changes in the synovial membrane may become more prominent. Cartilaginous and osseous debris that originated from the articular surfaces may become embedded in the synovial membrane, acting as a local irritant and producing proliferative changes.

Infrequently, synovial abnormalities in osteoarthritis may become so severe that they resemble the changes of rheumatoid arthritis. In the interphalangeal joints of the fingers, such synovial inflammation is present in inflam-

matory (erosive) osteoarthritis (see the later discussion in this chapter). Small synovial effusions may be encountered in osteoarthritis. Sizable joint effusions that occur in the absence of trauma or osseous collapse should stimulate an investigation to exclude a superimposed articular process, such as infection or crystal deposition disease.

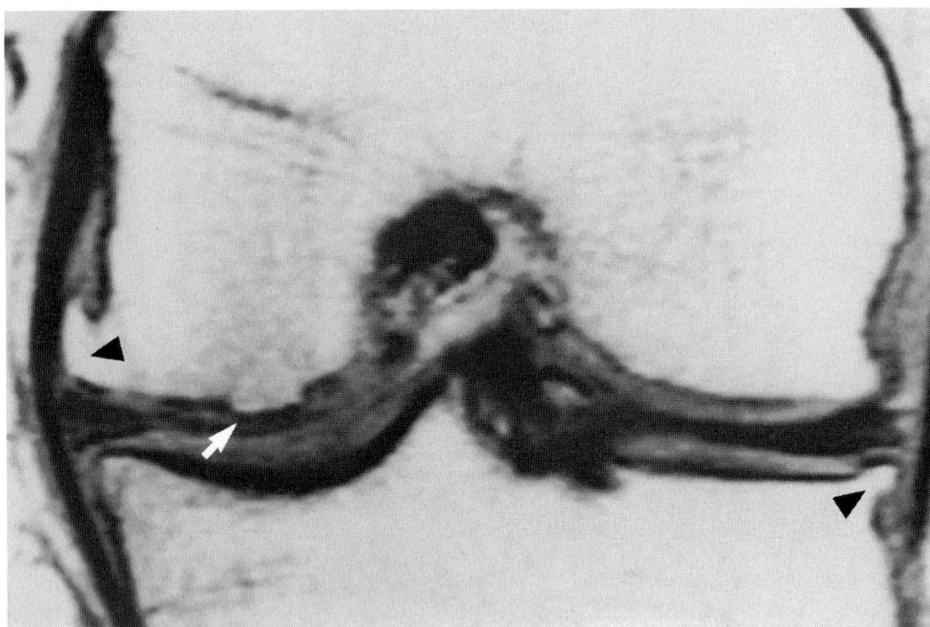

**Figure 29–9.** Central osteophytes: resemblance to intra-articular osseous bodies. Coronal T1-weighted (TR/TE, 800/20) spin echo MR image reveals a central osteophyte *(arrow)* in the medial femoral condyle and marginal osteophytes *(arrowheads)*. (Courtesy of A. Motta, MD, Cleveland, Ohio.)

## Abnormalities of Other Articular Structures

In certain joints (knee, wrist, and sternoclavicular, acromioclavicular, and temporomandibular joints), fibrocartilaginous discs or menisci are present that may show considerable degeneration, particularly in older persons or after significant trauma (see Chapter 59). Degeneration and calcification may also appear in the fibrocartilaginous labrum of the hip and glenohumeral joint. In some instances, these changes occur in the absence of any other articular abnormalities, whereas in other instances, findings of osteoarthritis are evident.

## Differential Diagnosis

Osteoarthritis is associated with joint space loss, bony sclerosis, and cyst formation in the pressure (or stressed) segment of the joint and with osteophytes in the non-pressure segment (Table 29–6). Osteoporosis, osseous erosion, and sizable joint effusions are not typical of this disease.

In rheumatoid arthritis, joint effusion, osteoporosis, and uniform joint space loss are characteristic. In the seronegative spondyloarthropathies (ankylosing spondylitis, psoriatic arthritis, and Reiter's syndrome), bone formation may be seen, but it does not resemble the well-defined subchondral sclerosis or osteophytosis of osteoarthritis. Rather, in the seronegative spondyloarthropathies, irregular, poorly defined proliferation and intra-articular bony ankylosis may be noted.

In gouty arthritis, bulky asymmetrical masses, eccentric well-circumscribed osseous erosions, and preservation of the articular space are common. In calcium pyrophosphate dihydrate crystal deposition disease (idiopathic or that associated with hemochromatosis), findings are very similar to those of osteoarthritis. Diagnostic aids in the

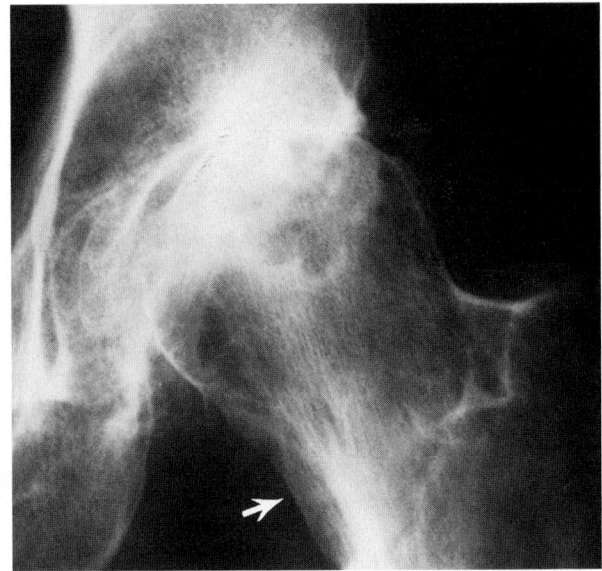

**Figure 29–10.** Periosteal and synovial osteophytes: buttressing. Note the bone formation along the medial aspect of the femoral neck *(arrow)* in addition to other changes of osteoarthritis, including joint space narrowing, sclerosis, and cyst formation.

former disorder are intra-articular and extra-articular calcification, involvement of unusual joints, large tumor-like cystic lesions, progressive abnormalities with fragmentation and collapse of bone, and absence of osteophytosis.

Osteonecrosis may produce considerable collapse of subchondral bone while the joint space is maintained. This combination is not evident in osteoarthritis. The subsequent appearance of secondary degenerative joint

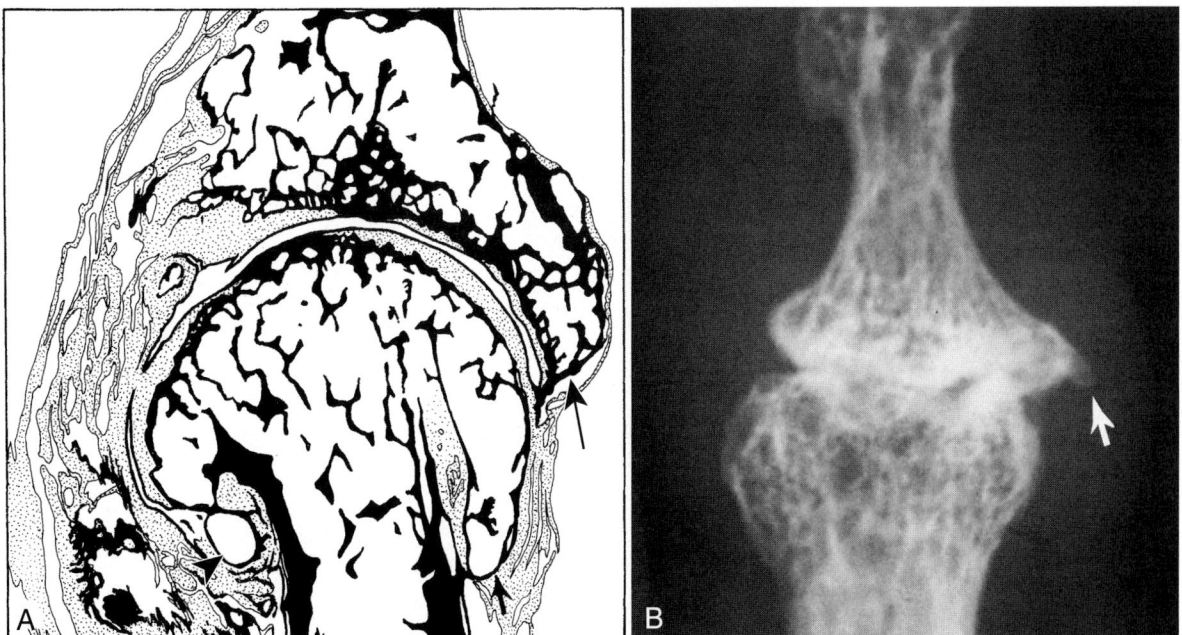

**Figure 29–11.** Capsular osteophytes: pathologic and radiographic findings. *A,* Drawing of a section through an osteoarthritic distal interphalangeal joint reveals capsular osteophytes *(arrows)* arising from the distal and middle phalanges. Note that the outgrowths extend proximally and are associated with small ossicles *(arrowhead).* Additional findings include cartilaginous destruction and subchondral sclerosis. *B,* Radiograph shows the capsular osteophyte *(arrow)* arising from the distal phalanx. Joint space narrowing and sclerosis are also seen.

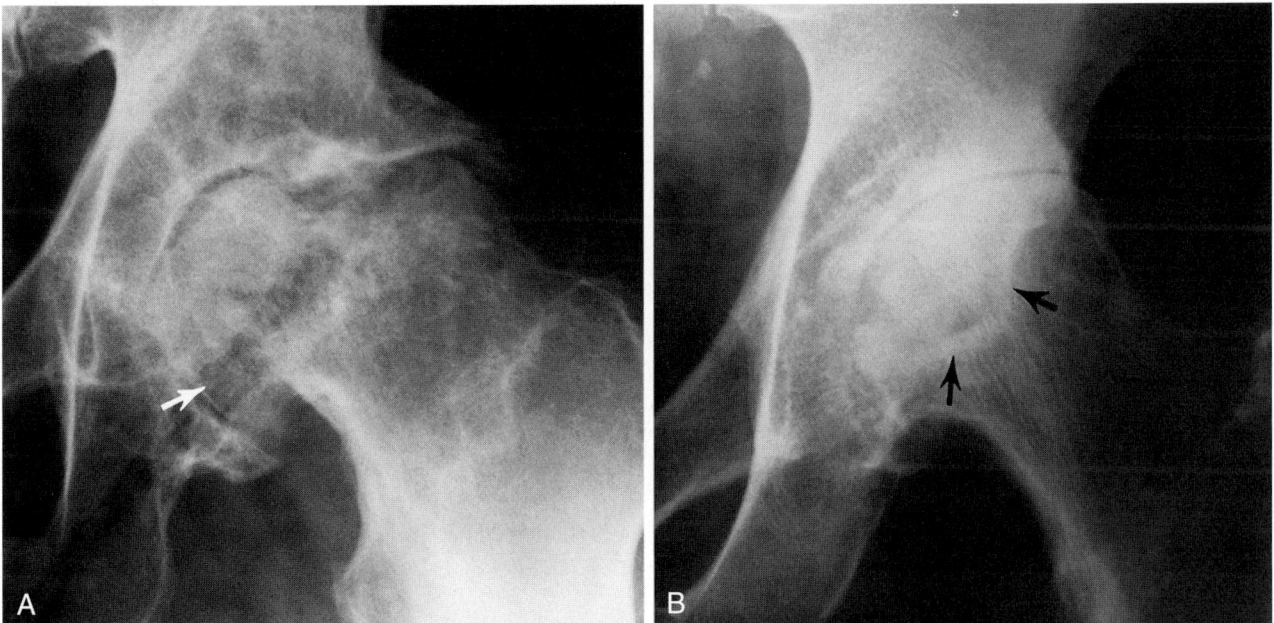

**Figure 29–12.** Osteoarthritis versus osteonecrosis. *A,* Osteoarthritis with collapse and fragmentation. In this patient with long-standing disease, considerable collapse of the weight-bearing surface of the femoral head is evident. Note superior or upward migration of the femoral head with respect to the acetabulum, a large medial osteophyte *(arrow),* acetabular osteophytes, and buttressing. The changes are those of osteoarthritis; the extent of bony collapse, though perhaps indicating secondary osteonecrosis, should not lead to an erroneous diagnosis of primary osteonecrosis. *B,* Osteonecrosis with secondary cartilaginous destruction. In this patient, segmental collapse of the femoral head *(arrows)* is evident. Note diffuse loss of joint space, related either to secondary osteoarthritis or to chondrolysis. Although sclerosis and buttressing are evident, the findings do not resemble those of primary osteoarthritis.

**TABLE 29-6**

## Differential Diagnosis of Osteoarthritic Changes

| | Osteoporosis | Joint Space Narrowing | Osseous Erosions | Osseous Cysts | Sclerosis | Osteophytosis | Bone "Whiskering" | Intra-articular Osseous Fusion | Osseous Fragmentation, Collapse | Typical Location |
|---|---|---|---|---|---|---|---|---|---|---|
| Osteoarthritis | – | Focal | – | + | + | + | – | – | In large joints | DIP, PIP, MCP joints of hand; first CMC and trapezioscaphoid joints of wrist; first MTP, TMT joints of foot; knee; hip; apophyseal joints of spine |
| Inflammatory osteoarthritis | – | Focal | + | + | + | + | – | DIP, PIP joints | – | DIP, PIP, MCP joints of hand; first CMC and trapezioscaphoid joints of wrist |
| Rheumatoid arthritis | + | Diffuse | + | + | – | – | – | Carpal, tarsal areas | Rare | PIP, MCP joints of hand; wrist; MTP joints of foot; knee; elbow; glenohumeral joint; cervical spine |
| Gouty arthritis | – | May be absent | + | + | + | + | – | Rare | ± | MTP, IP joints of foot; DIP, PIP, MCP joints of hand; wrist; elbow; knee |
| Pyrophosphate arthropathy | – | Diffuse | – | + | + | ± | – | – | + | MCP joints of hand; radiocarpal joint of wrist; knee |
| Seronegative spondyloarthropathies | ± | Diffuse | + | + | + | – | + | + | – | Spine; sacroiliac joint; various articulations of the appendicular skeleton |
| Osteonecrosis | – | Absent until late | – | + | + | – | – | – | + | Hip; glenohumeral joint; knee; sites of trauma |
| Neuropathic osteoarthropathy | – | Variable | – | ± | + | ± | – | – | + | Sites depend on underlying disorder |

CMC, carpometacarpal; DIP, distal interphalangeal; IP, interphalangeal; MCP, metacarpophalangeal; MTP, metatarsophalangeal; PIP, proximal interphalangeal; TMT, tarsometatarsal.

disease in osteonecrosis can lead to difficulty in making a diagnosis. Neuropathic osteoarthropathy is characterized by severe fragmentation and collapse of the articular surfaces, extensive bony sclerosis, multiple cartilaginous and osseous intra-articular bodies, large joint effusions, subluxation, and malalignment.

## Cartilaginous Joints

Two major extraspinal symphyses are the symphysis pubis and the manubriosternal joint. In the symphysis pubis, cleftlike cavities appear in the central portion of the joint, usually after the age of 10 to 20 years (Fig. 29–13). They subsequently widen and become more irregular and may contain gas, leading to a vacuum phenomenon. Age-related degenerative changes in the manubriosternal joint are similar.

## Syndesmoses and Entheses

At syndesmoses (e.g., tibiofibular and radioulnar interosseous membranes and ligaments), fibrous degeneration and bone proliferation may become apparent. At osseous sites of tendon attachment, a degenerative enthesopathy becomes apparent (Fig. 29–14). The degree of bone proliferation may be considerable, resulting in radiographically detectable excrescences (e.g., ischial tuberosity, trochanters) and enthesophytes (e.g., calcaneus, ulnar olecranon, patella). Tendon and ligament calcification may also be noted (e.g., sacrospinous and sacrotuberous ligaments). These changes are accelerated in the presence of trauma or chronic stress and may be generalized in diffuse idiopathic skeletal hyperostosis. Inflammatory enthesopathies are common in ankylosing spondylitis and other spondyloarthropathies.

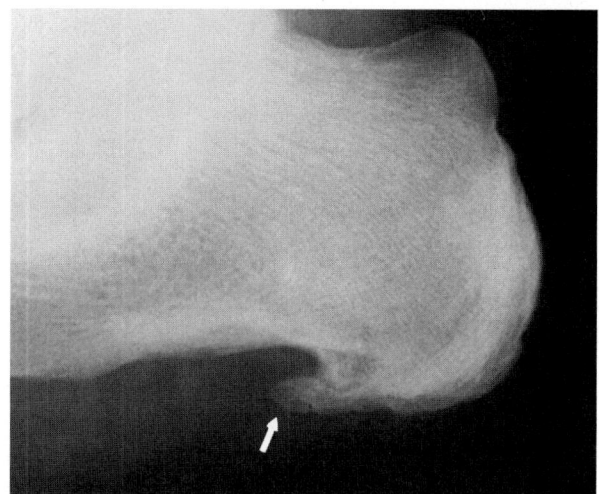

**Figure 29–14.** Degenerative enthesopathy: calcaneus. Radiograph depicts the irregular osseous proliferation that can occur at sites of tendon and ligament attachment to bone. One such site is the plantar aspect of the calcaneus *(arrow)*.

## COMPLICATIONS OF DEGENERATIVE JOINT DISEASE

Although there are numerous local complications of degenerative joint disease, several complications are particularly well known and deserve special emphasis.

## Malalignment and Subluxation

Angular deformity in osteoarthritis is not unexpected in view of the nonuniform nature of the joint involvement. Focal loss of articular space is characteristic and may produce, for example, varus (and, less commonly, valgus) deformity of the knee (Fig. 29–15). Changes in bone, capsule, and supporting tissue allow progressive subluxation, examples of which are lateral displacement of the tibia on the femur, lateral displacement of the femoral head in the acetabulum, and radial and proximal displacement of the first metacarpal base on the trapezium.

## Fibrous and Bony Ankylosis

Although fibrous ankylosis may be prominent at some sites of osteoarthritis (sacroiliac joint), bony ankylosis is unusual. An exception to this is the occasional appearance of intra-articular bony ankylosis in association with inflammatory (erosive) osteoarthritis of the interphalangeal joints of the hand. Para-articular bony ankylosis related to prominent osteophytes or overriding osseous surfaces related to malalignment may simulate intra-articular osseous fusion.

## Intra-articular Cartilaginous and Osseous Bodies ("Joint Mice")

Osteocartilaginous bodies within a joint can arise from several sources: transchondral fractures, disintegration of the articular surface, and synovial metaplasia (Fig. 29–16). Fragmentation of the joint surface can accompany a

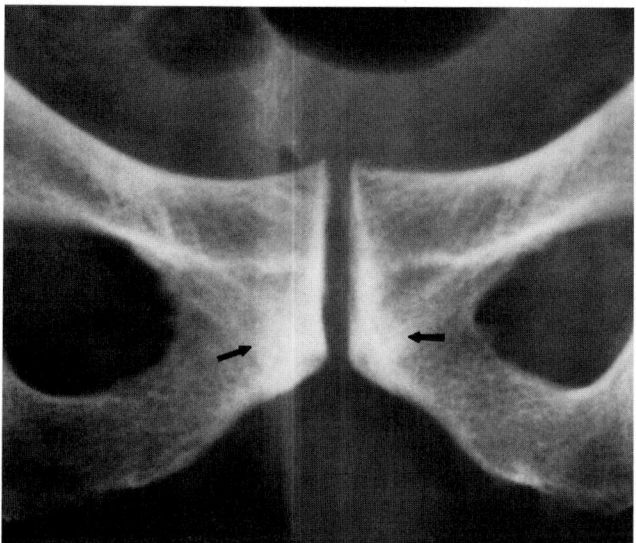

**Figure 29–13.** Symphyseal degeneration. Radiograph of a symphysis pubis reveals subchondral sclerosis *(arrows)* and superior beaking, consistent with mild degenerative arthritis.

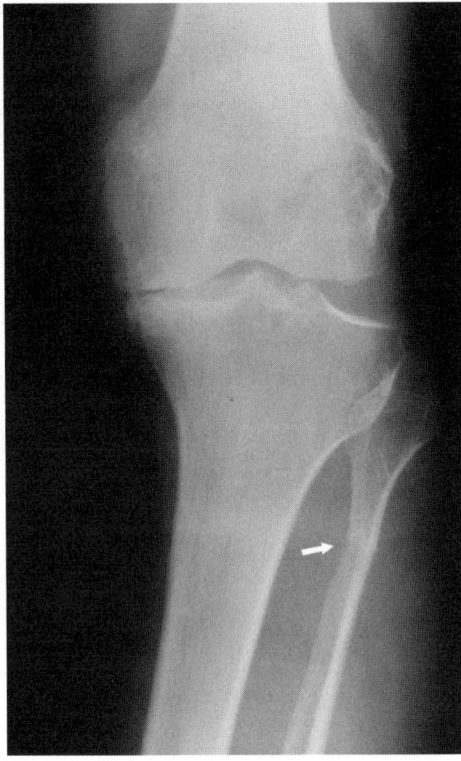

**Figure 29–15.** Complications of degenerative joint disease: malalignment with stress fracture. Severe varus deformity of an osteoarthritic knee is associated with a subtle stress fracture of the proximal end of the fibula *(arrow).*

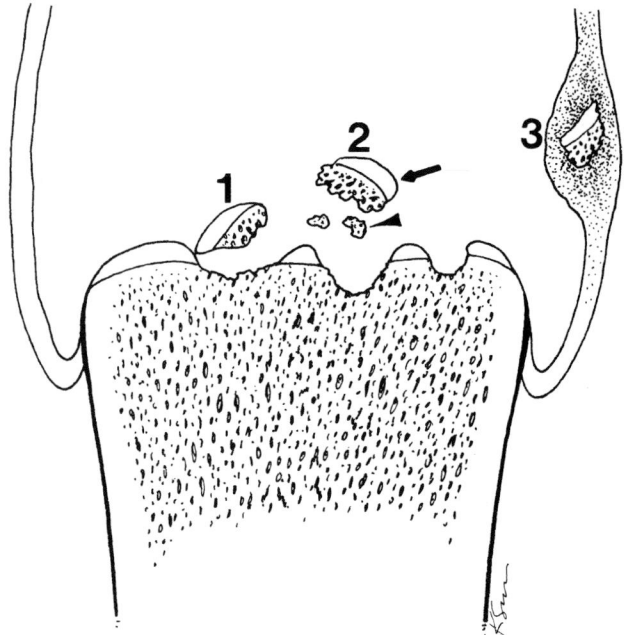

**Figure 29–16.** Complications of degenerative joint disease: intra-articular osteocartilaginous bodies. In osteoarthritis, fragmentation of the cartilaginous or osseous surface, or both, can produce intra-articular bodies that remain on the joint surface (1), become dislodged or loose in the joint cavity (2), or become embedded in the synovial membrane at a distant site, evoking a local inflammatory response (3). Fragments can consist of degenerative cartilage and subchondral bone *(arrow)* or subchondral bone alone *(arrowhead).*

variety of disease processes, including osteoarthritis. Cartilaginous and osseous debris may remain on the joint surface or become dislodged or loose in the joint cavity. Debris subsequently may become embedded at a distant synovial site, eliciting a local inflammatory response.

On radiographs, the osteocartilaginous bodies can increase or decrease in size, disappear, or remain unchanged. Osteochondral bodies commonly migrate to and become lodged in saclike articular regions, such as the acetabular fossa of the hip, olecranon fossa of the elbow, or subscapular recess and axillary pouch of the glenohumeral joint (Fig. 29–17). They must be differentiated from the osteophytes and fibrocartilaginous (meniscal) calcification and ossification that may accom-

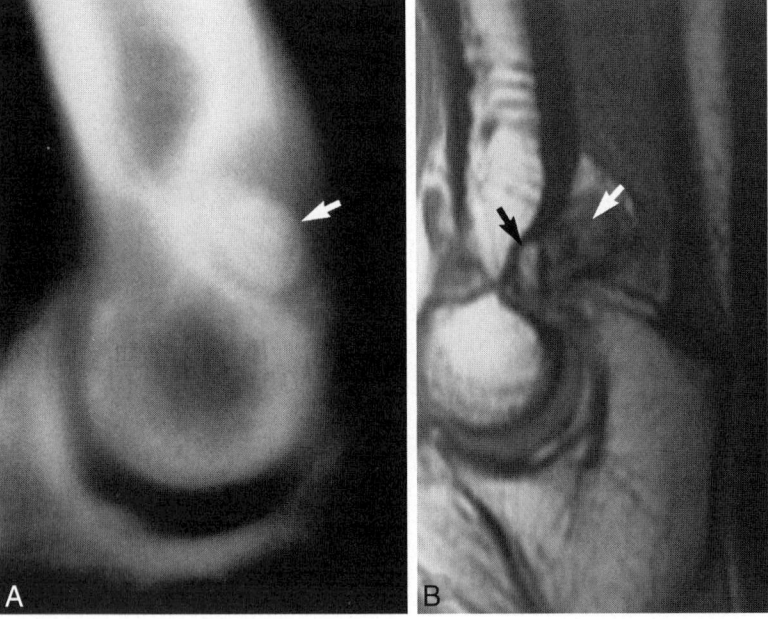

**Figure 29–17.** Intra-articular osteocartilaginous bodies: olecranon fossa of elbow. *A,* Conventional tomography in a 20-year-old man with limited elbow extension shows an ossified body *(arrow)* in the olecranon fossa. It was removed surgically. *B,* Sagittal T1-weighted (TR/TE, 800/20) spin echo MR image in a 36-year-old man with a similar history reveals smaller bone fragments *(arrows)* in the olecranon fossa. Abnormal signal intensity in the brachialis muscle and tendon is also present. (*A,* Courtesy of G. Greenway, MD, Dallas, Tex.)

pany other disease processes, such as idiopathic synovial osteochondromatosis, transchondral fractures, or osteochondritis dissecans. Differentiation is usually not difficult when osseous or cartilaginous dense lesions are seen in joints that do not reveal any manifestations of osteoarthritis (as in idiopathic synovial osteochondromatosis or osteochondritis dissecans). Furthermore, idiopathic synovial osteochondromatosis is commonly associated with a large number of osteocartilaginous bodies of approximately equal size, whereas secondary synovial osteochondromatosis (as is evident in osteoarthritis) leads to fewer bodies (generally <10) of varying size. Distinguishing intra-articular osseous and cartilaginous bodies from osteophytes or meniscal calcification (or ossification) can be difficult, however.

## DEGENERATIVE JOINT DISEASE IN SPECIFIC LOCATIONS

### Interphalangeal Joints of the Hand

#### Clinical Abnormalities

Osteoarthritis of the distal and proximal interphalangeal joints of the hand (including the interphalangeal joint of the thumb) is extremely common, particularly in middle-aged, postmenopausal women (Fig. 29–18). Clinically detectable bony enlargements about the distal interphalangeal joints are designated Heberden's nodes; similar alterations at the proximal interphalangeal joints are termed Bouchard's nodes. Involvement of multiple digits of both hands is characteristic. Occasionally, small gelatinous cysts of the soft tissues appear on the dorsal aspects of involved distal interphalangeal joints or, more uncommonly, proximal interphalangeal joints.

The clinical differentiation of osteoarthritis and rheumatoid arthritis in the hand usually is not difficult. The finger deformities in the former disease are characterized by horizontal instability (medial-lateral), whereas in rheumatoid arthritis, vertical subluxations (swan-neck and boutonnière deformities) are apparent.

#### Radiographic-Pathologic Correlation

Distal and proximal interphalangeal joints are frequently affected simultaneously; however, extensive alterations at distal interphalangeal joints may occur in the absence of proximal interphalangeal joint abnormalities (Fig. 29–19). Some degree of symmetry in the location of alterations in the two hands is the rule.

Radiographs reveal prominent osteophytes and joint space narrowing, providing close apposition of adjacent enlarged osseous surfaces. It is the closely applied, undulating articular surfaces that produce the diagnostic radiographic appearance of the disease, allowing its differentiation from erosive disorders, which cause separation of the involved bones. In osteoarthritis, the wavy contour of the base of the distal phalanx resembles the wings of a bird, the seagull sign. On frontal radiographs, the involved digits frequently reveal mild to moderate radial and ulnar subluxation at distal or proximal interphalangeal joints, producing a zigzag contour. At the margins of the affected joint, focal radiodense

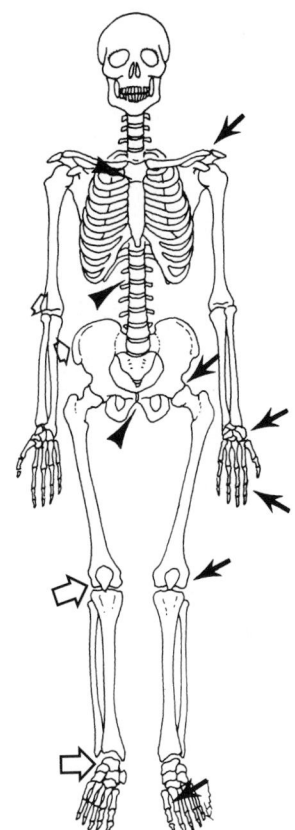

**Figure 29–18.** Distribution of degenerative joint disease. The most characteristic sites of synovial joint degeneration (osteoarthritis) are the distal and proximal interphalangeal joints of the hand, the first carpometacarpal (trapeziometacarpal) and trapezioscaphoid areas of the wrist, the acromioclavicular joint, the hip, the knee, and the articulations of the first ray of the foot *(solid arrows)*. The most typical sites of degeneration of cartilaginous joints are the intervertebral disc, symphysis pubis, and manubriosternal joint *(arrowheads)*. Degenerative enthesopathy is most common on the plantar aspect of the calcaneus, the pelvis, the ulnar olecranon, and the anterior surface of the patella *(open arrows)*.

lesions, or ossicles, are apparent overlying the joint capsule; they resemble intra-articular osseous bodies.

#### Differential Diagnosis

Occasionally, the undulating, irregularly enlarged subchondral or marginal bone may contain small pockets that can be misinterpreted as osseous erosion (Fig. 29–20), leading to an erroneous diagnosis of inflammatory (erosive) osteoarthritis. Erosive abnormalities of distal (and proximal) interphalangeal joints accompany various other disorders, including psoriatic arthritis, gout, multicentric reticulohistiocytosis, thermal injuries, hyperparathyroidism, and rheumatoid arthritis.

### Metacarpophalangeal Joints

Metacarpophalangeal joint involvement in osteoarthritis is almost invariably associated with more prominent abnormalities at distal and proximal interphalangeal joints.

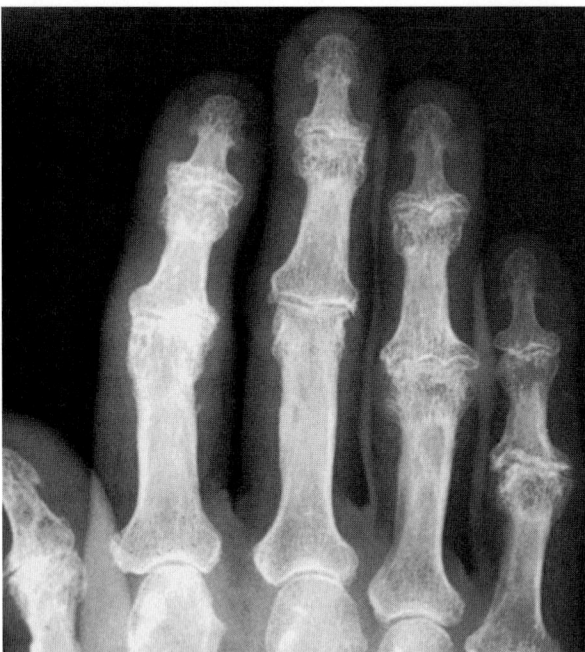

**Figure 29–19.** Osteoarthritis of the interphalangeal joints of the hand: typical distribution. Findings are apparent in distal interphalangeal, proximal interphalangeal, and, to a lesser extent, metacarpophalangeal joints. The interphalangeal joint of the thumb is also affected.

Uniform narrowing of one or more metacarpophalangeal interosseous spaces is evident in 90% to 95% of patients with interphalangeal joint osteoarthritis (see Fig. 29–19). Cystic lesions and osteophytes may also be apparent. Nonuniform loss of interosseous space is unusual, and erosions are absent. It is the combination of uniform loss of joint space and absence of marginal erosions that allows differentiation of osteoarthritis from rheumatoid arthritis at these articulations. Osteophytosis is an additional manifestation of metacarpophalangeal joint degeneration. The outgrowths generally are small and may be distributed on either the metacarpal head or the phalanx.

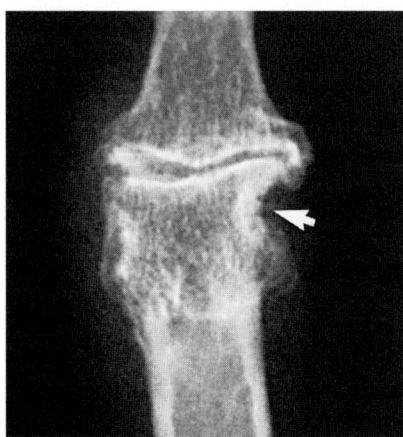

**Figure 29–20.** Osteoarthritis of the interphalangeal joints of the hand: pseudoerosions. Irregularity of marginal bone (*arrow*) related to osteophytes may simulate the appearance of a true erosion.

They occur on the margins of the articular surface, particularly the radial aspect of the head of the metacarpal.

The metacarpophalangeal joint abnormalities in osteoarthritis usually can be differentiated from those accompanying other articular disorders such as rheumatoid arthritis (periarticular osteoporosis, marginal erosions, subluxations, lack of osteophytosis); idiopathic calcium pyrophosphate dihydrate crystal deposition disease or hemochromatosis (large cystic lesions, collapse and fragmentation of the metacarpal heads, prominent hook-like osteophytes, intra-articular and periarticular calcification and debris); gouty arthritis (asymmetrical masses, eccentric erosions, preservation of interosseous space); and Wilson's disease (peculiar brushlike spiculation). The metacarpophalangeal joint changes in osteoarthritis are identical to those accompanying inflammatory osteoarthritis.

## Wrist

The radial distribution of osteoarthritis of the wrist is well known. In the absence of significant accidental or occupational trauma, changes are usually confined to the trapeziometacarpal (first carpometacarpal) joint and trapezioscaphoid space of the midcarpal joint.

**Trapeziometacarpal (First Carpometacarpal) Joint.** Involvement of the trapeziometacarpal joint can lead to prominent clinical abnormalities. These include pain that is aggravated by twisting and gripping motions, restricted movement, crepitus, and instability. The radiographic features of degenerative trapeziometacarpal joint disease include increasing radial subluxation of the metacarpal base, narrowing of the interosseous space, sclerosis and cystic changes in the subchondral bone, osteophytosis, and bony fragmentation. Bony excrescences extend from the trapezium in a distal direction between the first and second metacarpal bones (Fig. 29–21).

**Trapezioscaphoid Space.** Osteoarthritis in the trapezioscaphoid space of the midcarpal compartment of the wrist is frequently combined with degenerative changes at the trapeziometacarpal joint (see Fig. 29–21). Isolated abnormalities at this space are also reported, but predominant and severe changes resembling those of degenerative joint disease at this articulation can indicate the presence of calcium pyrophosphate dihydrate crystal deposition disease. Typical radiographic features of osteoarthritis are apparent in a unilateral or bilateral distribution, including joint space narrowing and sclerosis of apposing surfaces of the trapezium, trapezoid, and scaphoid.

**Other Joints.** Osteoarthritis localized to other compartments of the wrist is distinctly unusual in the absence of a history of trauma. Fracture, subluxation, dislocation, or osteonecrosis about the wrist can lead to altered joint motion, however, resulting in secondary osteoarthritis. Typical examples include degenerative disease of the radiocarpal and midcarpal compartments after scaphoid injuries, degenerative joint disease of the radiocarpal and inferior radioulnar compartments after osteonecrosis

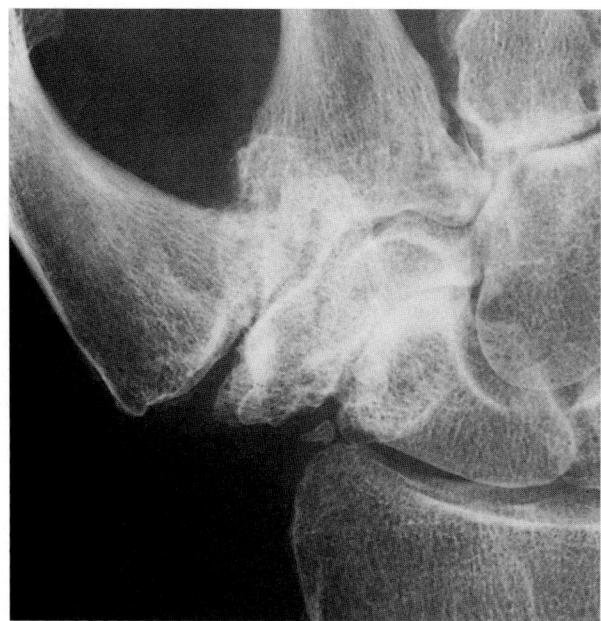

**Figure 29–21.** Osteoarthritis of the trapeziometacarpal (first carpometacarpal) joint. Radiograph illustrates pantrapezial osteoarthritis with degenerative changes in the trapezium–first metacarpal, trapezioscaphoid, trapeziotrapezoid, and trapezium–second metacarpal spaces. Observe joint space narrowing, eburnation, osteophytes, and radial subluxation of the base of the metacarpal. The additional alterations of the common carpometacarpal compartment at the bases of the second and third metacarpals can be accepted as evidence of osteoarthritis in the presence of extensive disease along the radial aspect of the wrist.

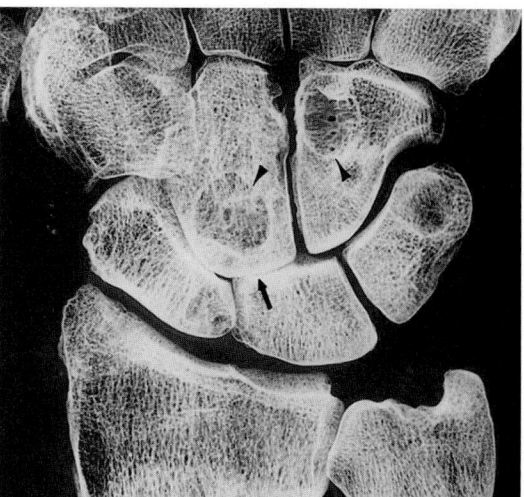

**Figure 29–22.** Lunate-capitate arthrosis: scapholunate advanced collapse (SLAC). Post-traumatic abnormalities include prominent narrowing of the lunate-capitate portion of the midcarpal compartment and, to a lesser extent, the scapho-capitate space, with cartilage loss (*arrow*) and cyst formation (*arrowheads*). This is an infrequent pattern of osteoarthritis in the wrist and is also observed in other articular disorders.

of the lunate (Kienböck's disease), and degenerative joint disease of the inferior radioulnar compartment after subluxation of the distal portion of the ulna. After scaphoid fractures complicated by nonunion at the fracture site, a degenerative-like arthropathy affecting the space between the distal pole of the scaphoid and radius may be seen.

Arthrosis of the lunate-capitate space, leading to interosseous narrowing, sclerosis, and cyst formation, has been emphasized as a post-traumatic degenerative condition (Fig. 29–22). Seen infrequently in isolation, this abnormality is usually combined with scapholunate separation or dissociation and narrowing of the radioscaphoid space. The resulting radiographic changes are termed the scapholunate advanced collapse pattern, or SLAC wrist.

## Elbow

Osteoarthritis of the elbow is not common. When present, it usually follows accidental or occupational trauma. Radiographic findings include joint space narrowing, sclerosis, cysts, and osteophytes. These predominate in the radiohumeral space. Olecranon enthesophytes at the attachment of the triceps tendon may accompany these alterations.

## Shoulder

**Glenohumeral Joint Osteoarthritis.** Significant osteoarthritis of the glenohumeral joint is unusual in the absence of

local trauma, and the detection of considerable degenerative changes in patients without known accidental or occupational trauma requires a search for other disorders, such as alkaptonuria, acromegaly, epiphyseal dysplasia, calcium pyrophosphate dihydrate or hydroxyapatite crystal deposition disease, or hemophilia. The most frequent abnormality accompanying osteoarthritis in this site is the formation of osteophytes along the articular margin of the humeral head and the line of attachment of the labrum to the glenoid fossa. These osteophytes predominate in the anterior and inferior aspects of the joint margin and commonly are most evident in the inferomedial aspect of the humeral head (Fig. 29–23). Focal or global eburnation of the articular surface of the humeral head may also be seen, manifested radiographically as subchondral sclerosis (Fig. 29–24).

**Deterioration and Disruption of the Rotator Cuff.** Rotator cuff abnormalities are common, especially in elderly persons. They result in characteristic radiographic findings, including elevation of the humeral head with respect to the glenoid cavity, narrowing of the acromiohumeral space, eburnation and cysts of apposing bony surfaces of the humeral head and acromion, cystic and notchlike defects in the humeral surface near the bicipital groove, and reversal of the normal inferior convexity of the acromion. Glenohumeral joint arthrography demonstrates communication between the articular cavity and the subacromial bursa. Magnetic resonance (MR) imaging and ultrasonography may also be used to evaluate the rotator cuff (see Chapters 6 and 59).

Pitfalls exist in the accurate diagnosis of rotator cuff disruption. Narrowing of the acromiohumeral space, a characteristic alteration of cuff disruption, can be simulated by faulty patient positioning during radiography and can accompany atrophy of the cuff in the absence of

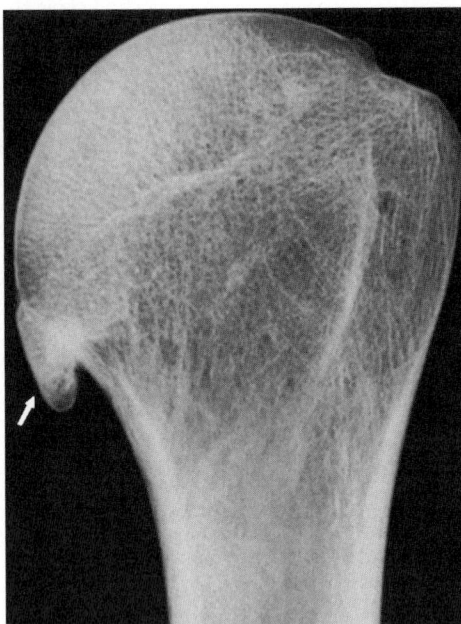

**Figure 29–23.** Osteoarthritis of the glenohumeral joint: osteophytosis of the humeral head. Radiograph of a humeral specimen in external rotation documents an osteophyte *(arrow)* arising at the articular margin.

a full-thickness tear. Even with ideal radiographic technique, the acromiohumeral space varies according to the patient's sex and age; it typically measures between 9 and 10 mm, is larger in men than in women, and decreases slightly with advancing age. A measurement of less than 6 mm in middle-aged patients should be regarded as pathologic, generally indicating disruption of the supraspinatus tendon. A significant association appears to exist between osteoarthritis of the glenohumeral joint and rotator cuff degeneration; however, it is not clear whether these two entities represent independent and somewhat frequent phenomena of aging or a common pathogenetic mechanism connects them (Fig. 29–25).

**Shoulder Impingement Syndrome.** The most common type of shoulder impingement exists when there is encroachment on the subacromial space, with loss of the normal gliding mechanism between the superior periarticular soft tissues about the glenohumeral joint and the coracoacromial arch. Entrapment of the soft tissue structures between this arch and the greater tuberosity of the proximal end of the humerus during abduction and elevation or forward flexion and internal rotation of the arm results in subacromial bursitis and tendinosis of the rotator cuff, with eventual progression to cuff fibrosis and rupture. Although the diagnosis of impingement syndrome can generally be made by careful physical examination, various imaging studies are occasionally required. Radiographic alterations include bony proliferation, eburnation, and cystic change in the greater tuberosity. A well-defined osseous excrescence, termed a subacromial enthesophyte, is evident in some patients with this syndrome (Fig. 29–26). The excrescence arises at the site of osseous attachment of the coracoacromial ligament and is of variable size (Fig. 29–27).

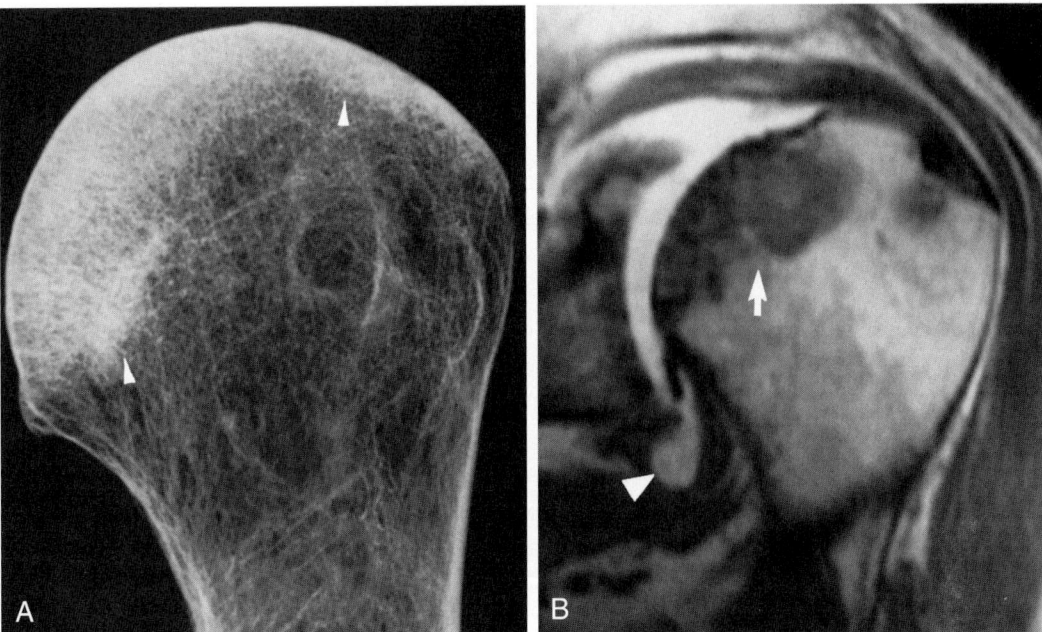

**Figure 29–24.** Osteoarthritis of the glenohumeral joint: subchondral sclerosis in the humeral head. *A,* Radiograph demonstrates focal eburnation involving the mid-superior portion of the humeral head, with radiographic evidence of bony sclerosis *(arrowheads)*. *B,* Coronal oblique T1-weighted (TR/TE, 650/20) spin echo MR image after the intra-articular injection of gadolinium compound reveals sclerosis, with low signal intensity, in the humeral head *(arrow)*. The rotator cuff is intact, there is sclerosis in the glenoid, and debris *(arrowhead)* is present in the axillary pouch.

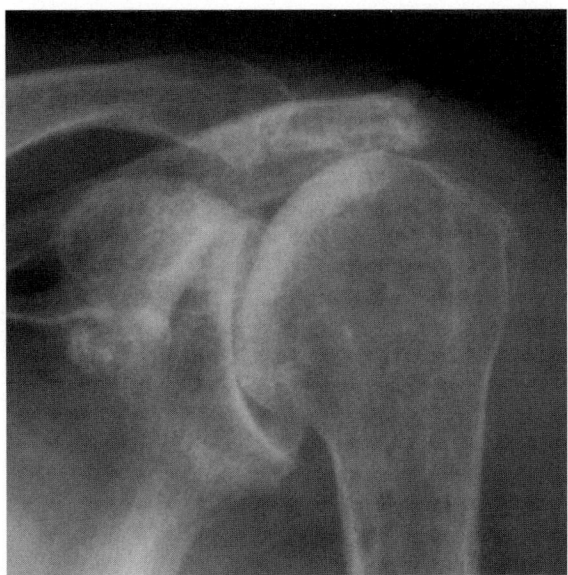

**Figure 29–25.** Cuff tear arthropathy. This radiograph of the shoulder in a man with an arthrographically proven full-thickness tear of the rotator cuff reveals focal subchondral eburnation and elevation of the humeral head with respect to the glenoid cavity. An intra-articular body is present in the subscapular recess.

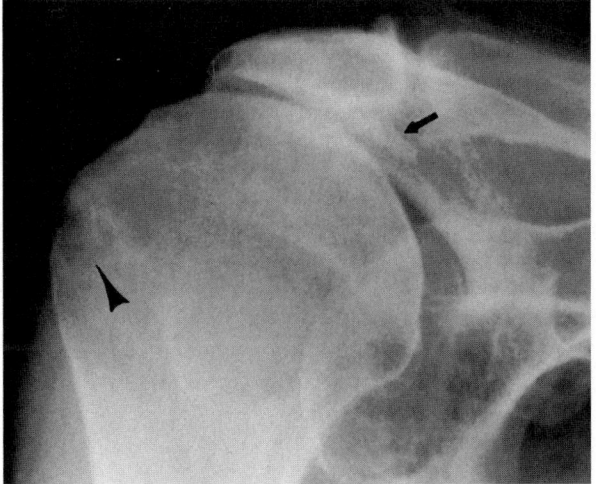

**Figure 29–26.** Shoulder impingement syndrome: subacromial enthesophyte. Radiograph reveals a prominent subacromial enthesophyte *(arrow)*, sclerosis, and cyst formation *(arrowhead)* in the greater tuberosity, with progressive elevation of the humeral head, indicative of disruption of the rotator cuff.

## Acromioclavicular Joint

Degenerative changes in this synovial articulation are almost universal in elderly persons. Diffuse discomfort in the shoulder region, radiating to the upper arm and aggravated by motion, is suggestive of osteoarthritis in the acromioclavicular joint. Radiographic examination of the degenerating acromioclavicular joint reveals joint space diminution, sclerosis of apposing osseous surfaces, marginal osteophytes, hypertrophy and inferior subluxation of the acromial end of the clavicle, and osseous proliferation on the superior surface of the acromion. It

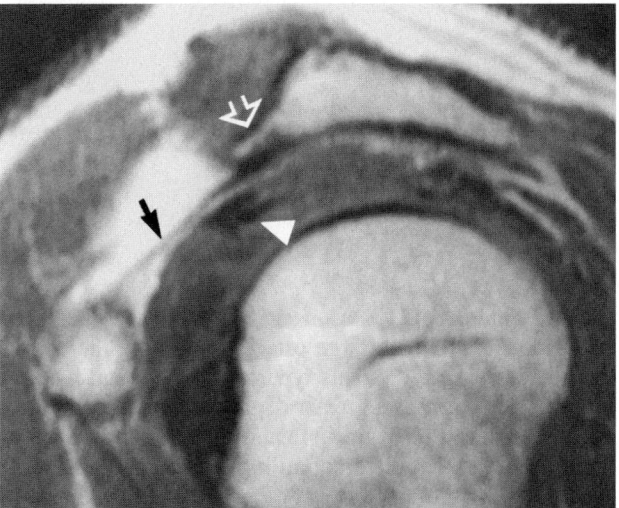

**Figure 29–27.** Shoulder impingement syndrome: subacromial enthesophyte. Sagittal oblique T1-weighted (TR/TE, 800/20) spin echo MR image shows the enthesophyte *(open arrow)*, which is intimate with the coracoacromial ligament *(solid arrow)* and supraspinatus tendon *(arrowhead)*.

has been suggested that distally pointed osteophytes about this joint are important in the pathogenesis of ruptures of the supraspinatus tendon. An os acromiale, representing a separate fragment of the acromion, may have a similar deleterious effect on the rotator cuff.

## Sternoclavicular Joint

Osteoarthritis of the sternoclavicular joint is not uncommon. Its clinical manifestations include pain, tenderness, and palpable enlargement of the articulating bone. Radiographic findings include unilateral or bilateral joint space narrowing, sclerosis, and osteophytosis.

## Sacroiliac Joint

Degenerative changes in the sacroiliac joint can be demonstrated pathologically in middle-aged and elderly persons. The pathologic abnormalities become prominent, particularly in the ilium, and include cartilage fibrillation and erosion, denudation of cartilaginous surfaces, and partial or complete fibrous ankylosis of the joint. Subchondral eburnation and osteophytes become apparent. Changes may be unilateral or bilateral in distribution and may be associated with significant clinical findings, including pain and tenderness.

Radiographic manifestations include loss of articular space and well-defined subchondral bony sclerosis (Fig. 29–28). Although erosion of subchondral bone is infrequent in degenerative disease of the sacroiliac joint, osteophytes are common. Osteophytes can occur at any level in the joint but are most characteristic at the anterosuperior and anteroinferior limits of the articular cavity. They may produce prominent focal radiopaque lesions, which can simulate the appearance of osteoblastic skeletal metastasis (Fig. 29–29). On frontal radiographs, these anterior osteophytes are superimposed on the interosseous space, simulating intra-articular bony ankylosis.

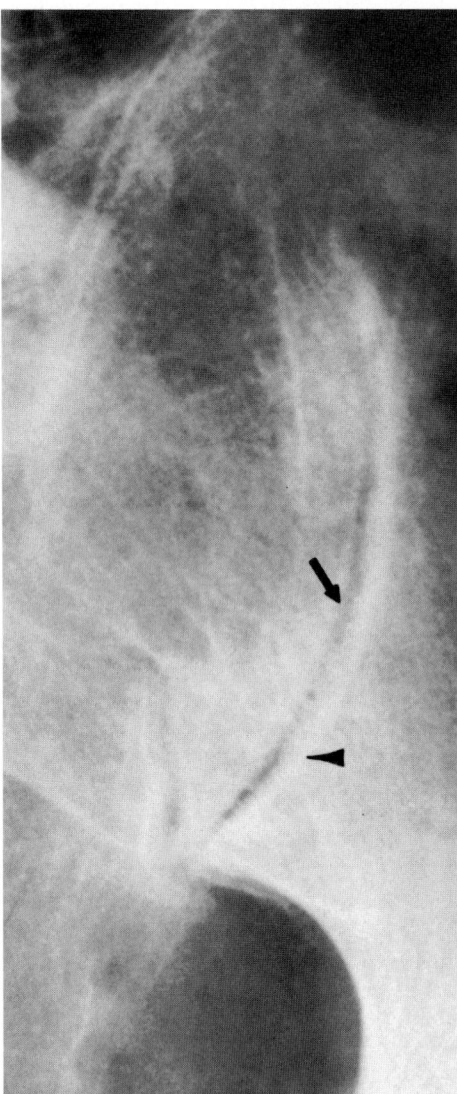

CT or MR imaging can exquisitely demonstrate the bony excrescences that bridge the articular cavity (Fig. 29–30). Although fibrous ankylosis within the joint is typical of advanced osteoarthritis of the sacroiliac joint, intra-articular bony ankylosis is unusual.

One additional radiographic manifestation of degenerative sacroiliac joint disease is a vertical radiolucent line overlying the articulation. This finding apparently represents a vacuum phenomenon analogous to that which occurs in other joints. It is not a specific sign of osteoarthritis, as it is also observed in other disorders. Gas may extend from the joint into subchondral cysts (pneumatocysts) (Fig. 29–31).

The radiographic characteristics of degenerative disease of the sacroiliac joint may be confused with those of ankylosing spondylitis (Table 29–7). Joint space narrowing occurs in both diseases. When it accompanies degenerative disease, it may be focal and either asymmetrical or symmetrical. The adjacent subchondral bone is usually well defined. Joint space diminution in ankylosing spondylitis is commonly widespread and symmetrical. The surrounding bone is frayed or irregular in outline. In degenerative disease, such ankylosis results from periarticular bridging osteophytes, whereas in ankylosing spondylitis, true intra-articular ankylosis is characteristic. Subchondral erosions, a prominent feature of ankylosing spondylitis, are infrequent and superficial in osteoarthritis.

## Hip

### Clinical Abnormalities

Osteoarthritis of the hip may produce significant clinical symptoms confined to the hip region or referred to other sites, such as the knee, buttock, thigh, groin, or greater trochanter. Restriction of motion, particularly rotation and extension, is also common. Flexion deformities are frequent in many patients with long-standing osteoarthritis of the hip.

### Radiographic-Pathologic Correlation

Degenerative hip disease may demonstrate several distinct patterns on frontal radiographs, based on the relative

**Figure 29–28.** Degenerative disease of the sacroiliac joint: joint space narrowing and bony sclerosis. The joint space is uniformly narrowed *(arrow)*, with linear condensation of bone in the ilium *(arrowhead)*. Note the sharp definition of the subchondral bone. A vacuum phenomenon is apparent within the inferior aspect of the joint.

---

**TABLE 29–7**

**Differential Diagnosis of Degenerative Disease of the Sacroiliac Joint**

|  | Osteoarthritis | Ankylosing Spondylitis | Osteitis Condensans Ilii |
|---|---|---|---|
| Age | Older patients | Younger patients | Younger patients |
| Sex | Men and women | Men > women | Women > men |
| Distribution | Bilateral or unilateral | Bilateral, symmetrical | Bilateral, symmetrical |
| Sclerosis | Iliac | Iliac | Iliac |
|  | Mild, focal | May be extensive | Triangular in shape |
| Erosions | Absent | Common | Absent |
| Intra-articular bony ankylosis | Rare | Common | Absent |
| Para-articular osteophytosis | Common | Rare | Rare |
| Ligamentous ossification | Less common | Common | Absent |

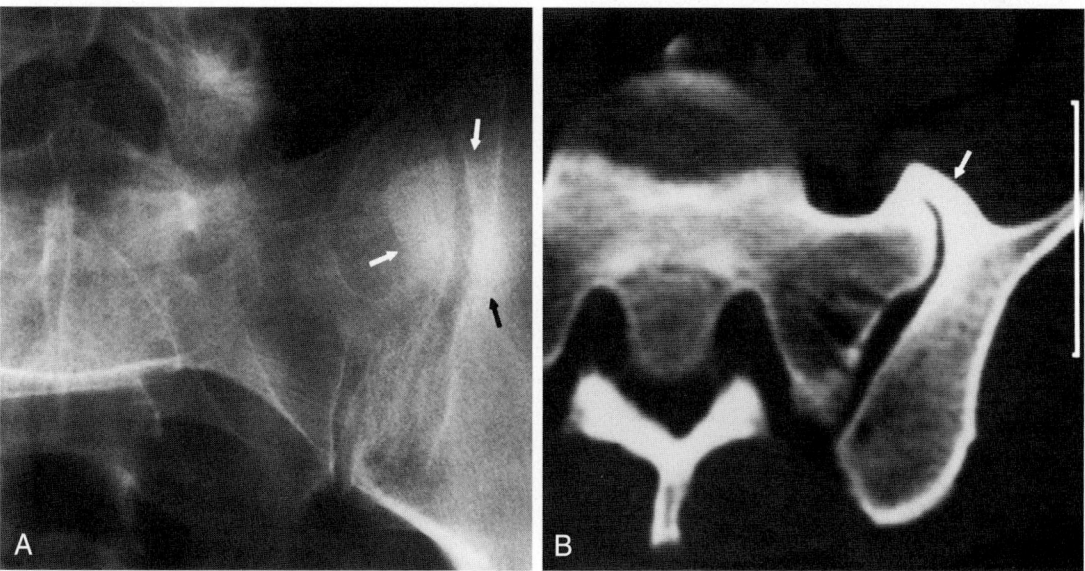

**Figure 29–29.** Degenerative disease of the sacroiliac joint: osteophytosis. *A*, Frontal radiograph demonstrates a radiodense lesion *(arrows)* overlying the superior aspect of the synovium-lined portion of the sacroiliac joint. *B*, With CT, which provided a transaxial section through this lesion, it is apparent that bony sclerosis and a bridging osteophyte *(arrow)* are the cause of the abnormal density seen in the plain film. *(B*, Courtesy of J. Scavulli, MD, San Diego, Calif.)

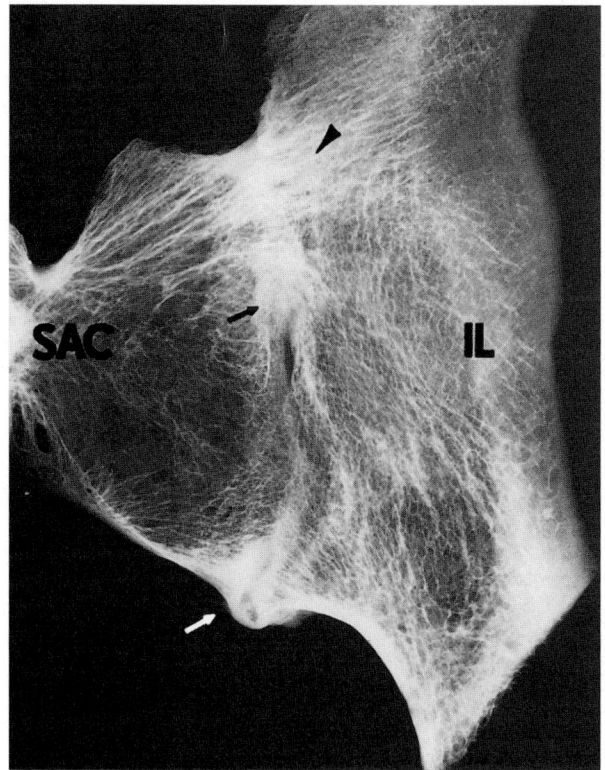

**Figure 29–30.** Degenerative disease of the sacroiliac joint: ligamentous calcification and ossification. Radiograph of a macerated sacroiliac joint (SAC) reveals prominent calcification and ossification *(arrowhead)* of the interosseous ligament (IL) above the synovial joint. Bridging osteophytes *(arrows)* are also evident.

positions of the femoral head and the acetabulum (Fig. 29–32). With the onset of joint space narrowing, the femoral head moves, or migrates, toward the acetabulum in one of three basic patterns: superior migration, in which articular space loss is most prominent on the upper aspect of the joint, and the femoral head moves in a vertical or upward direction; medial migration, in which joint space loss is most marked on the inner aspect of the joint, and the femoral head moves in a medial direction; and axial migration, in which diffuse joint space loss occurs throughout the articular cavity, and the femoral head moves inward and centrally along the axis of the femoral neck. It should be emphasized that this classification system relies on changes on the frontal radiograph; anterior and posterior patterns of migration, as evident on lateral radiographs and axial imaging, have not been used routinely to classify osteoarthritis of the hip.

**Superior Migration Pattern.** The most common location of joint space loss in osteoarthritis is the superior aspect of the joint, resulting in superior migration of the femoral head with respect to the acetabulum. This pattern can be further classified into a superolateral pattern and a superomedial pattern.

Superolateral migration of the femoral head is more frequent in women and is usually unilateral or asymmetrical (Fig. 29–33). This pattern may be identified in 15% to 50% of patients with osteoarthritis of the hip. Superolateral migration has been attributed to acetabular dysplasia. On radiography, the femoral head moves superiorly in conjunction with diminution of the interosseous space. Sclerosis and subchondral cystic lesions predomi-

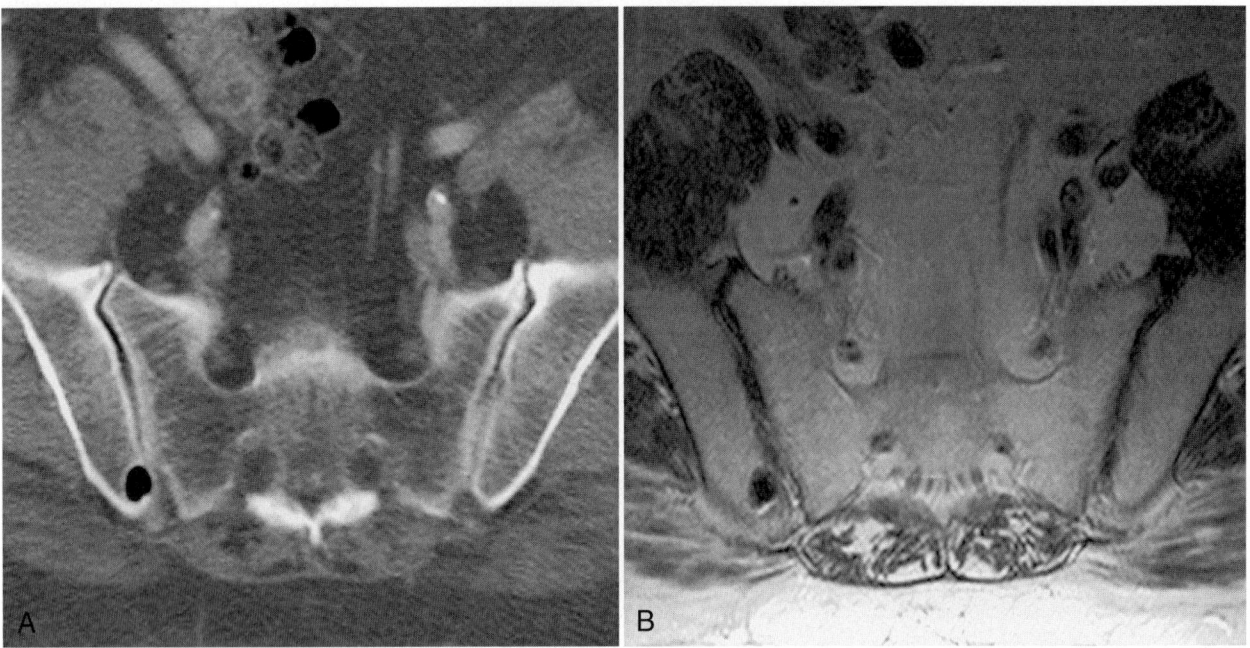

**Figure 29–31.** Degenerative disease of the sacroiliac joint: pneumatocyst. *A*, Transaxial CT scan shows the well-defined gas-filled iliac cyst. *B*, Corresponding axial T2-weighted (TR/TE, 5710/120) fast spin echo MR image shows a prominent signal void. Although the location is atypical, a bone island could exhibit a similar signal void.

nate on the outer aspect of the femoral head and the acetabulum. In some instances, the acetabular cysts become large, contain gas, and are associated with tears and mucinous degeneration of the labrum (Fig. 29–34).

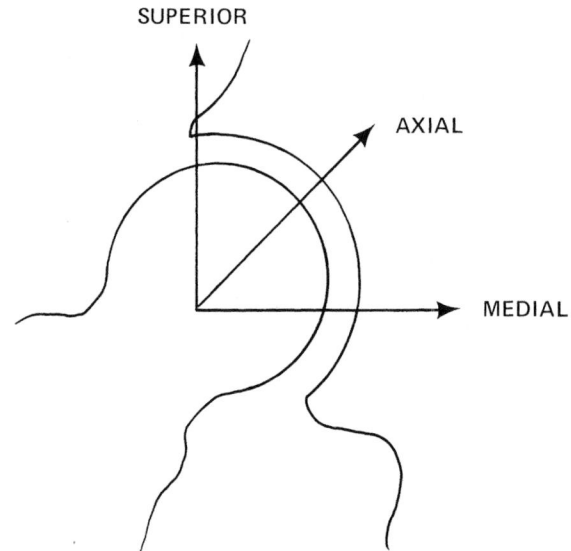

**Figure 29–32.** Patterns of migration of the femoral head with respect to the acetabulum for the right hip. Three directions can be identified. When superior joint space loss predominates, the femoral head moves in an upward, or superior, direction with respect to the acetabulum. When joint space loss is confined to the inner one third of the joint, a medial migration pattern is evident. With diffuse loss of articular space, the femoral head migrates axially along the axis of the femoral neck. (Redrawn from Graham J, Harris WH: Paget's disease involving the hip joint. J Bone Joint Surg Br 53:651, 1971.)

Superomedial migration (tilt deformity) of the femoral head, which may be detected in 35% to 50% of patients with osteoarthritis, is more frequent in men than in women and is commonly bilateral (Fig. 29–35). Patients with this pattern of disease may become symptomatic at a relatively young age. Its cause is unknown; however, in most patients, it is unrelated to previous epiphysiolysis. Early radiographic abnormalities consist of superior displacement of the femoral head, associated with joint space narrowing in the outer one third of the articular cavity. Progressive joint space loss results in close apposition of the superior and middle surfaces of the femoral head and acetabulum. With continued deformity along the outer one third of the femoral head, osteophytosis on its medial and inferior surface is seen. These osteophytes begin as broad-based shallow outgrowths that fill in the free space on the medial aspect of the joint cavity. With further growth along its inferomedial aspect and resorption along its superolateral aspect, the femoral head assumes an altered relationship with the femoral neck. Careful examination of radiographs often reveals the presence of a curvilinear radiodense area on the inner aspect of the femoral head. This represents the original calcified zone of articular cartilage, allowing accurate appraisal of the position of the femoral head before its remodeling.

This description of the tilt deformity (superomedial pattern of migration) emphasizes its similarity to the superolateral pattern of femoral head migration. In both situations, the femoral head is displaced laterally until restraining osteophytes are formed on the lateral aspect of the acetabulum, at which time subluxation ceases. Osteophyte formation is then noted on the inferomedial aspect of the femoral head. With the tilt deformity, the

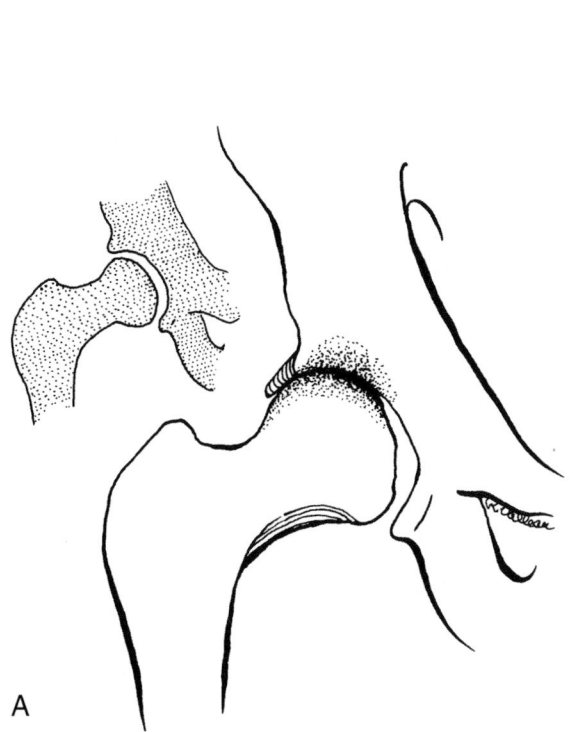
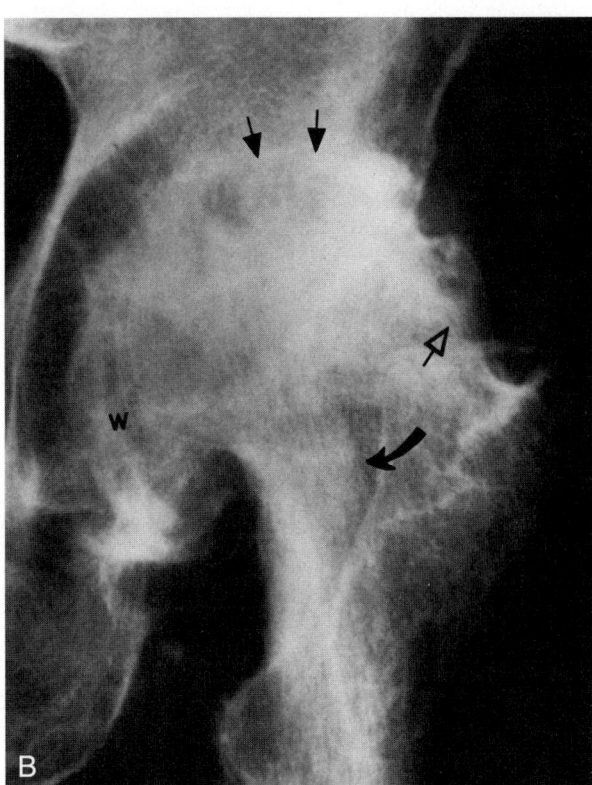

**Figure 29–33.** Osteoarthritis of the hip: superolateral migration pattern. *A,* Progressive narrowing of the outer one third of the joint space results in upward migration of the femoral head with respect to the acetabulum. Associated findings include eburnation, lateral acetabular osteophytes, and medial femoral buttressing. *B,* In this patient, joint space narrowing and sclerosis *(solid straight arrows)* along the superior articulating surface are associated with subchondral collapse of the adjacent femoral head. A lateral osteophyte *(open arrow)*, widened inferomedial joint space (W), and medial femoral neck buttressing *(curved arrow)* are noted.

acetabular depth is normal grossly, and although minor degrees of lateral movement occur, acetabular outgrowths develop, which resist considerable lateral subluxation of the head. Intermediate varieties of superior migration exist (10% to 15% of patients) in which the degree of lateral subluxation is less than that associated with superolateral migration but greater than that associated with superomedial migration.

The tilt deformity resulting from remodeling in the osteoarthritic hip can be differentiated from a similar deformity accompanying epiphysiolysis with secondary degeneration. In the latter case, because of true slipping of the femoral head in relation to the femoral neck, the original zone of calcified cartilage, along with the remainder of the head, becomes displaced posteromedially.

**Medial Migration Pattern.** In 10% to 35% of patients with osteoarthritis of the hip, a pattern of medial migration of the femoral head is evident (Fig. 29–36). This pattern is commonly bilateral and symmetrical and is more frequent in women. It is interesting to speculate that specific idiosyncrasies in the acetabular structure produce stress in what would otherwise be a medial nonpressure area, leading to degenerative alterations.

Radiographic analysis indicates medial displacement of the femoral head, with narrowing of the medial joint space and associated widening of the lateral joint space. Mild to moderate protrusio acetabuli deformities may become evident with increased bone density of the central and inferior aspects of the acetabulum. Osteophyte formation occurs on both the acetabulum and the femur.

**Axial Migration Pattern.** Axial migration of the femoral head due to diffuse or concentric loss of articular space is infrequent. When radiographs reveal a degenerative-type articular disease associated with diffuse loss of joint space, other primary diagnoses must be considered before attributing the abnormalities to osteoarthritis. When axial migration is present in degenerative joint disease, the pattern of joint space loss is similar to that in rheumatoid arthritis. The presence of osteophytes and sclerosis and the absence of erosions, osteoporosis, and severe acetabular protrusion, however, allow the differentiation of osteoarthritis and rheumatoid arthritis.

**Miscellaneous Migration Patterns.** The previously described patterns of migration are based on data derived from frontal radiographs. CT images used to study osteo-

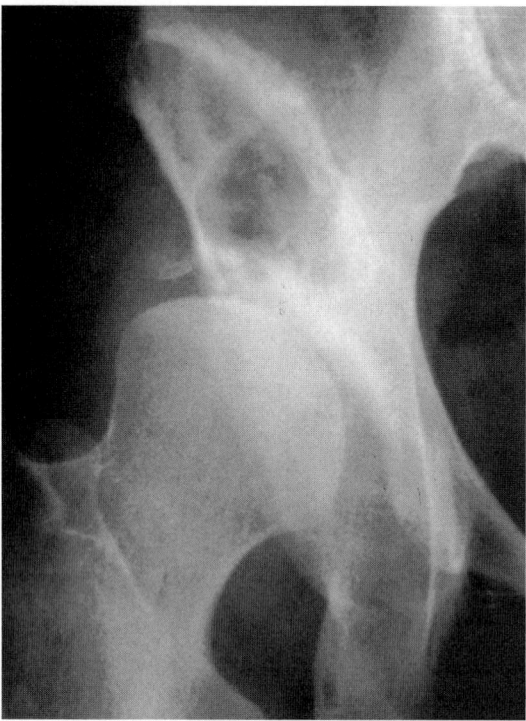

**Figure 29–34.** Osteoarthritis of the hip: superolateral migration pattern. Developmental dysplasia of the hip with cyst (or ganglion) formation. In this 40-year-old woman, a frontal radiograph shows a dysplastic hip, flattening and vertical inclination of the acetabulum, lateral displacement with uncovering of the femoral head, bone fragmentation, joint space loss, and a septated acetabular cyst (or ganglion).

arthritis of the hip show superior migration patterns that are accompanied by anterior migration of the femoral head; these can be considered to represent anterosuperior migration patterns (Fig. 29–37). The medial migration pattern is accompanied by posterior migration of the femoral head and can be considered to represent a posteromedial migration pattern (Fig. 29–38).

Other patterns of femoral head migration in osteoarthritis are exceedingly rare. In addition, in some instances, a similar pattern may appear when degenerative joint disease is superimposed on primary osteonecrosis of the femoral head. Descriptions also exist of a rapidly progressive variety of osteoarthritis, affecting older persons, in which atrophic changes occur on both the femoral and acetabular sides of the joint (Fig. 29–39). Acetabular protrusion deformity is an associated feature, and disintegration of the involved joint usually occurs in less than a year. Because other articulations, such as the glenohumeral joint, wrist, and knee, may be affected simultaneously, this rapidly progressive disease may not represent osteoarthritis at all. Indeed, it resembles calcium hydroxyapatite crystal deposition disease (see Chapter 35) and may be the hip equivalent of the Milwaukee shoulder syndrome.

## Differential Diagnosis

**Patterns of Migration.** Osteoarthritis is associated with superior or, less commonly, medial migration of the femoral head with respect to the acetabulum (Table 29–8). Axial migration is unusual. Thus, the appearance of diffuse

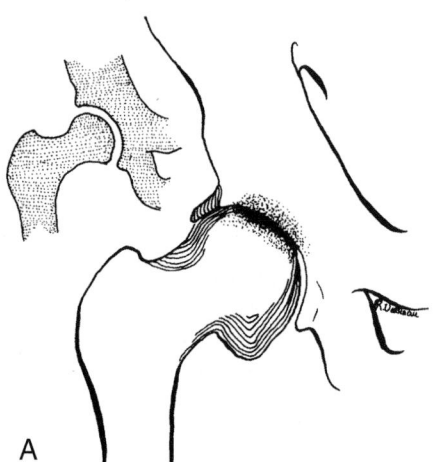
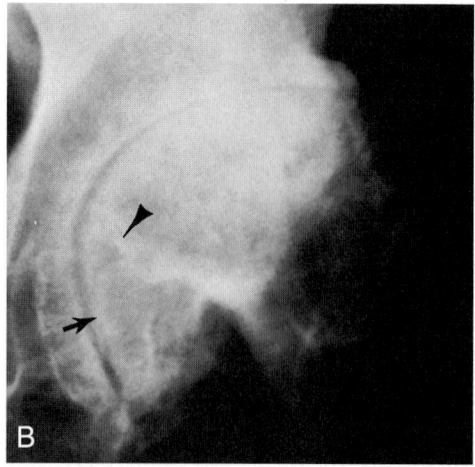

**Figure 29–35.** Osteoarthritis of the hip: superomedial migration pattern (tilt deformity). *A,* Progressive resorption of bone along the lateral femoral head and deposition along its medial aspect result in a tilt deformity. *B,* Hip radiograph demonstrates superior and middle joint space loss and subchondral sclerosis, medial femoral neck buttressing, and small lateral acetabular and massive medial femoral osteophytes *(arrow).* The original calcified cartilaginous zone *(arrowhead)* is faintly visible.

(From Resnick D: Patterns of migration of the femoral head in osteoarthritis of the hip: Roentgenographic-pathologic correlation and comparison with rheumatoid arthritis. AJR Am J Roentgenol 124:62, 1975.)

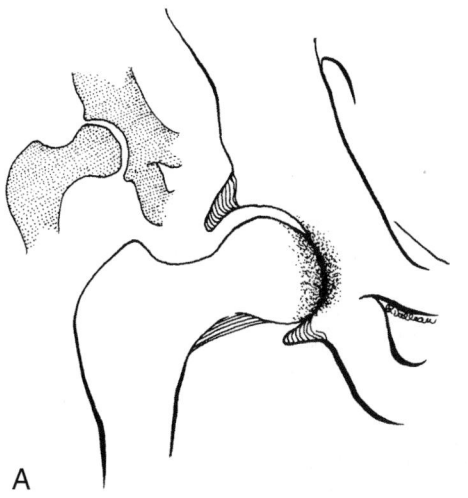

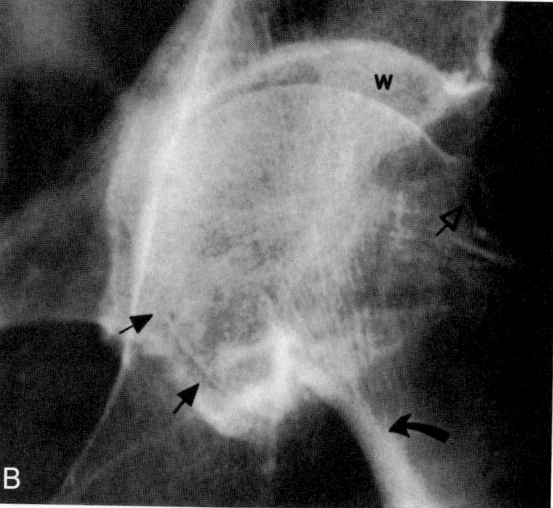

**Figure 29–36.** Osteoarthritis of the hip: medial migration pattern. *A,* As the femoral head migrates medially, joint space narrowing and sclerosis of the inferomedial aspect of the articular surface result, and the superior joint space widens. *B,* Medial joint space loss *(solid arrows)* and a widened lateral joint space (W) have resulted from this pattern of migration. A lateral femoral osteophyte *(open arrow)* and medial femoral neck buttressing *(curved arrow)* are evident. Mild protrusion deformity is seen.

joint space loss with axial migration often indicates another disease process, such as rheumatoid arthritis, infection, or cartilage atrophy due to disuse or immobilization. If axial migration of the femoral head is accompanied by sclerosis and osteophyte formation, additional diseases should be considered, including ankylosing spondylitis, calcium pyrophosphate dihydrate crystal deposition

disease, and alkaptonuria. Further, secondary degenerative joint disease superimposed on another primary process can lead to symmetrical loss of joint space, osteophytosis, and eburnation; these processes include trauma with acetabular fracture, synovial disorders such as rheumatoid arthritis, Paget's disease, chondrolysis, epiphyseal dysplasia, and osteonecrosis.

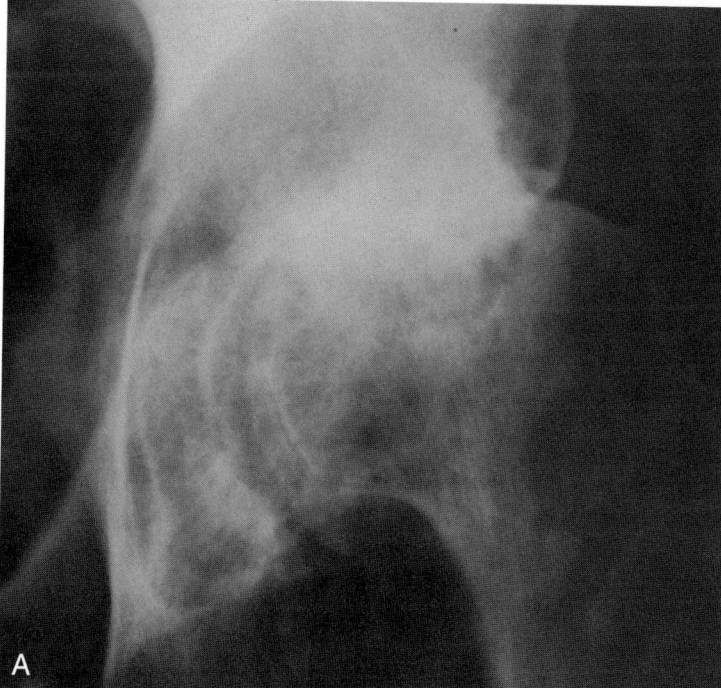

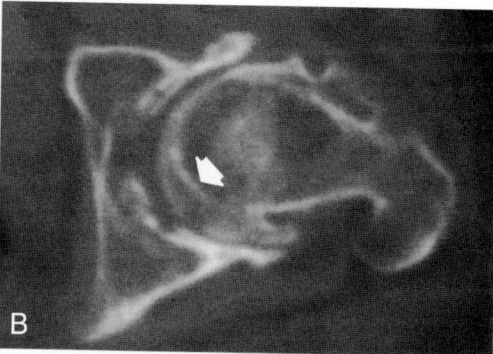

**Figure 29–37.** Osteoarthritis of the hip: anterosuperior migration pattern. *A,* Radiograph shows classic features of osteoarthritis, with superior migration of the femoral head and a medial femoral osteophyte. *B,* Transaxial CT scan shows anterior migration of the femoral head with a large osteophyte posterior to the original cortex *(arrow),* filling in the posterior portion of the articular space.
(*B,* From Hayward I, Bjorkengren AG, Pathria MN, et al: Patterns of femoral head migration in osteoarthritis of the hip: A reappraisal with CT and pathologic correlation. Radiology 166:857, 1988.)

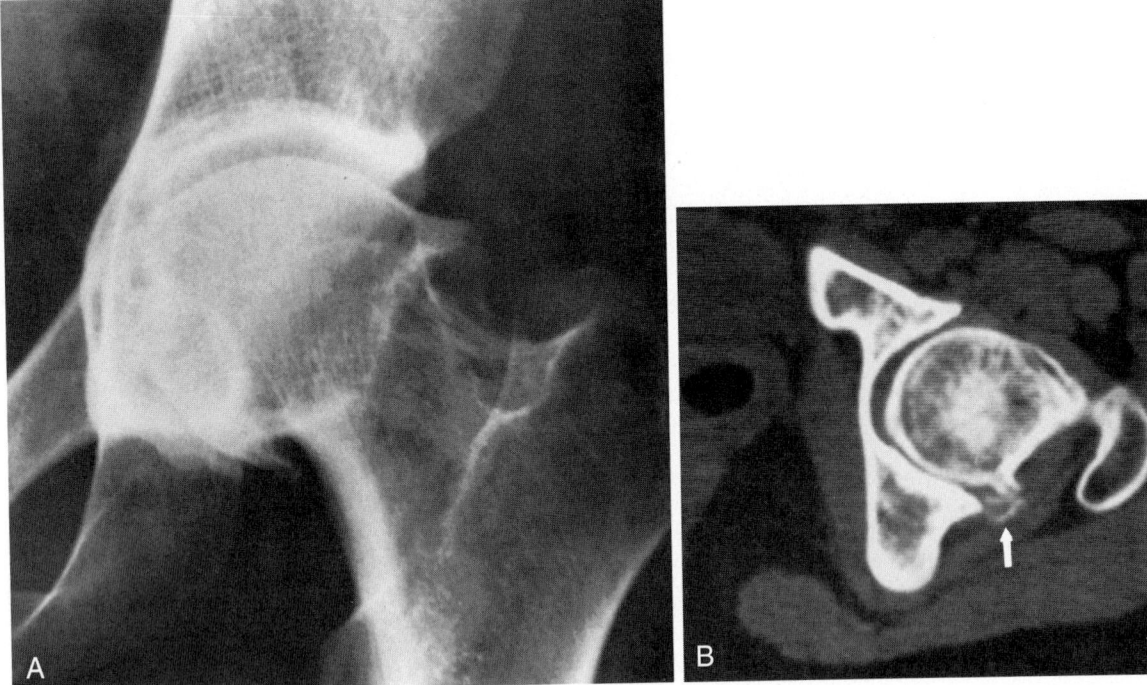

**Figure 29–38.** Osteoarthritis of the hip: posteromedial migration pattern. *A,* Frontal radiograph reveals mild medial migration of the femoral head and slight acetabular protrusion. Osteophytes are seen. *B,* Transaxial CT scan shows that the femoral head is closely applied to the posterior surface of the acetabulum and possesses a prominent posterior osteophyte *(arrow).* (*B,* Courtesy of D. Haselwood, MD, Sacramento, Calif.)

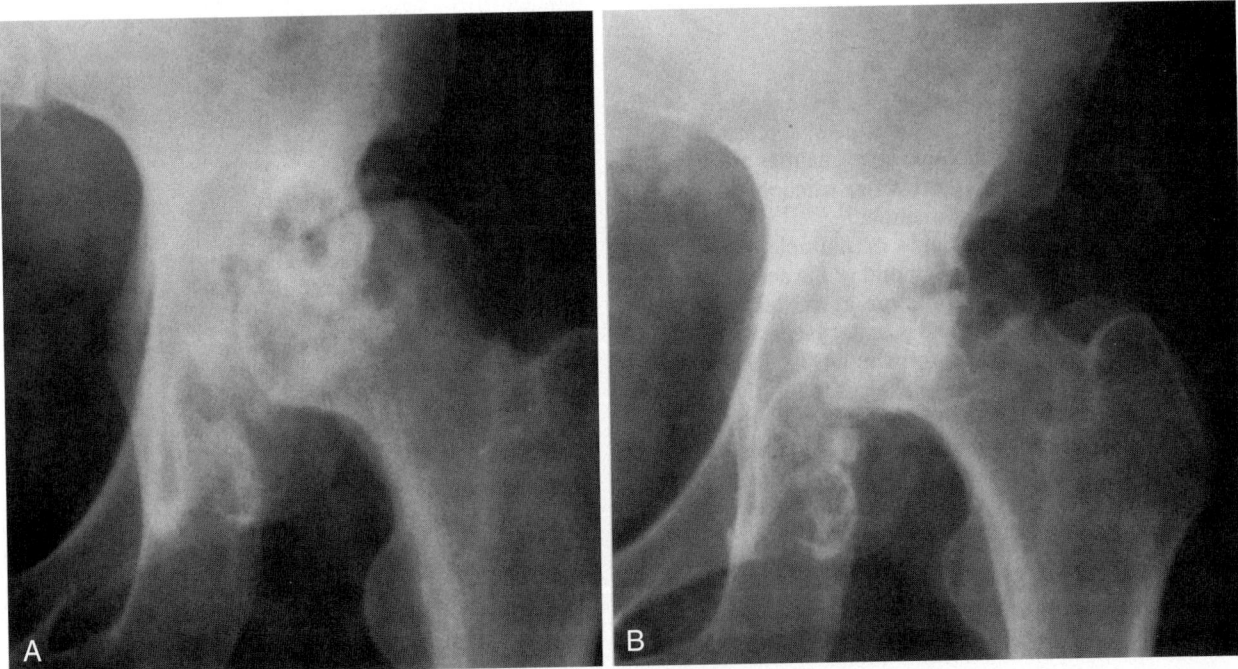

**Figure 29–39.** Osteoarthritis of the hip: rapidly progressive disease. *A* and *B,* Radiographs obtained several months apart indicate progressive compression and deformity of the femoral head, presumably related to the collapse of subchondral cysts. The severity, rapidity, and morphology of the changes are distinctly unusual for uncomplicated osteoarthritis. A thorough investigation for other causes of the articular disease, such as crystal- or steroid-induced arthropathy and infection, was unrewarding in this patient.

**TABLE 29–8**

**Differential Diagnosis of Patterns of Femoral Head Migration**

|  | Superior | Axial | Medial |
|---|---|---|---|
| Osteoarthritis | + | Rare | + |
| Rheumatoid arthritis | Rare | + | |
| Ankylosing spondylitis | Rare | + | |
| Calcium pyrophosphate dihydrate crystal deposition disease | Rare | + | |
| Chondrolysis | | + | |
| Paget's disease with secondary joint degeneration | + | + | + |
| Osteonecrosis with secondary cartilage loss | + | + | |

+, common.

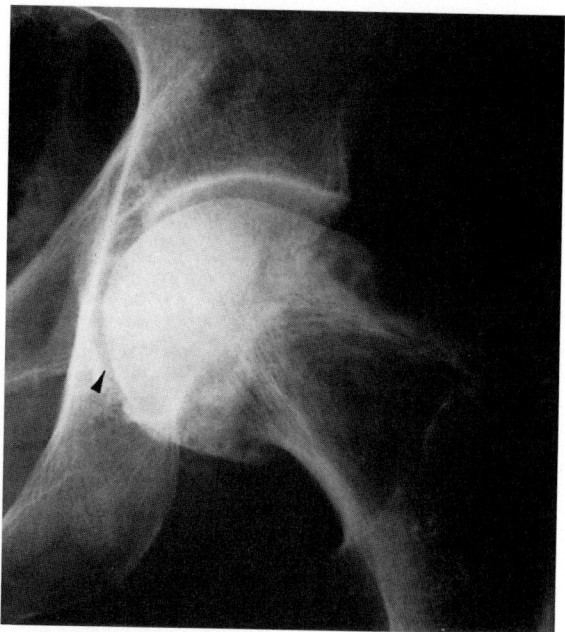

**Figure 29–40.** Paget's disease with medial migration of the femoral head. Observe the coarse trabecular pattern within the femoral head and femoral neck and narrowing of the medial joint space *(arrowhead)*. The axial and lateral spaces appear relatively normal.

Superior migration of the femoral head associated with sclerosis, cysts, and osteophytes usually ensures the diagnosis of osteoarthritis. Medial migration of the femoral head is observed in "primary" osteoarthritis but also in degenerative joint disease superimposed on other disorders, such as Paget's disease and osteomalacia (Fig. 29–40).

**Sclerosis, Cyst Formation, and Osteophytosis.** Calcium pyrophosphate dihydrate crystal deposition disease can be accompanied by significant sclerosis and prominent cyst formation. Osteophytes may or may not be evident. In this disease, fragmentation and collapse of the femoral head are more prominent than in osteoarthritis. Neuropathic osteoarthropathy leads to severe bony eburnation; however, the findings of considerable collapse and fragmentation with or without exuberant osteophytes are helpful clues to its proper diagnosis. The hip disease of ankylosing spondylitis is associated with the presence of a characteristic lateral femoral osteophyte, which subsequently extends across the femoral head–femoral neck junction; diffuse loss of articular space is typical of this disease. Osteonecrosis is accompanied by prominent cysts and sclerosis of the femoral head, but is usually associated with maintenance of the articular space until late in the disease. Acromegaly leads to large osteophytes, but the interosseous space is usually preserved or even widened until secondary cartilage degeneration supervenes.

**Buttressing.** Thickening of bone along the femoral neck, particularly medially, is characteristic of osteoarthritis, but can also be seen in osteonecrosis.

**Acetabular Protrusion.** Acetabular protrusion in osteoarthritis is associated most typically with medial migration of the femoral head. The degree of protrusion is usually mild. Moderate to severe acetabular protrusion, which is accompanied by diffuse loss of articular space (axial migration), can be observed in a variety of disorders, including rheumatoid arthritis, ankylosing spondylitis, other processes such as Paget's disease, and infection.

## Knee

### Cause

The knee joint is the most common site of degenerative changes. Many factors appear to contribute to osteoarthritis in this articulation, including previous surgery or trauma, angular deformity, osteonecrosis, osteochondritis dissecans, and obesity. Under normal circumstances, with the patient standing, the line of weight bearing passes from the center of the femoral head through the centers of both the knee and the ankle. In the presence of genu varum, the weight-bearing forces pass through the medial side of the joint, and with genu valgum, these forces pass through the lateral side of the knee. Therefore, any condition leading to angular deformity will result in a shift of stress to one compartment of the joint and can predispose to the development of osteoarthritis.

The role of meniscal abnormality or removal in the appearance and progression of osteoarthritis of the knee has received a great deal of emphasis. In view of the importance of the menisci in cushioning forces at the knee joint, it appears that meniscal changes might lead to degeneration of articular cartilage. Owing to the accumulation of increasing data that support the occurrence of articular cartilage degeneration after complete or partial meniscectomy, the general trend in arthroscopic surgery is to preserve as much of the meniscal tissue as possible.

### Clinical Abnormalities

Pain is usually the presenting symptom, and it is typically aggravated by walking or exercise and persists even while resting. Stiffness, tenderness, swelling, and warmth may also be recorded. Symptoms and signs of synovitis are generally less striking in osteoarthritis than in rheumatoid arthritis, although patients occasionally have large joint effusions and masses related to synovial rupture and popliteal cysts. Angular deformity (usually varus), instability, and soft tissue atrophy are late manifestations of the disease.

## Radiographic-Pathologic Correlation

**Compartmental Distribution.** When interpreting the radiographic and pathologic changes in an osteoarthritic knee, it is useful to regard the joint as consisting of three compartments or spaces: medial femorotibial, lateral femorotibial, and patellofemoral (Fig. 29–41). Radiographic abnormalities usually predominate in one or two of the three compartments, although pathologic aberrations are evident in all three areas. Typical pathologic changes include cartilage fibrillation and denudation of the osseous surfaces, eburnation, subchondral cystic lesions, and osteophytosis.

The ability of radiographs to detect pathologic abnormalities depends on the method of examination. Routine techniques are limited in their sensitivity to delineate early alterations, although some degree of joint space narrowing, sclerosis, cysts, and osteophytes are usually detected in the more involved weight-bearing compartment (medial or lateral femorotibial compartment). "Tunnel" projections obtained during knee flexion may reveal cartilaginous and osseous lesions that are not evident on routine radiographs. Radiographs obtained during stress or weight bearing provide a better assessment of cartilage loss as the joint space collapses under the body weight (Fig. 29–42). They also allow more accurate delineation of subluxation of the femur and tibia and of varus or valgus angulation. Patellofemoral compartment analysis requires special radiographic projections, including tangential and oblique views.

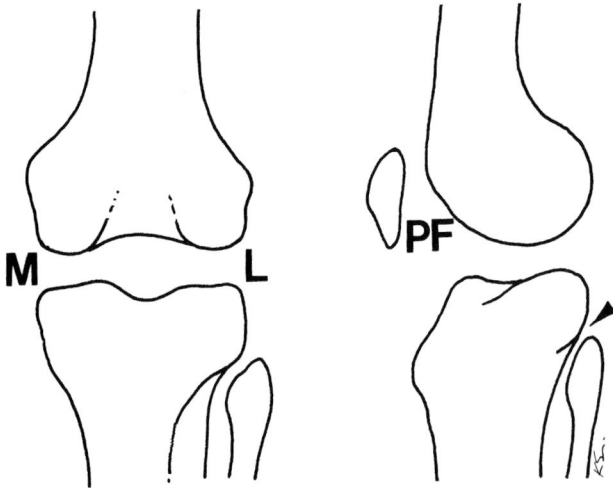

**Figure 29–41.** Compartmental analysis of knee disease. Evaluation of the medial femorotibial (M), lateral femorotibial (L), and patellofemoral (PF) compartments should be accomplished on all knee radiographs. A fourth area, the proximal tibiofibular joint (*arrowhead*), may also be affected.

**Femorotibial Compartments.** Bilateral or unilateral alterations may be evident. Radiographic findings are usually more prominent on the medial aspect of the joint (see Fig. 29–42). Unicompartmental (medial or, less frequently, lateral femorotibial compartment) or bicompartmental (medial femorotibial and patellofemoral compartments or, less often, lateral femorotibial and patellofemoral compartments) involvement is more typical than tricompartmental involvement in patients with osteoarthritis. The discovery of alterations confined to or predominantly in the medial femorotibial compartment is most consistent with osteoarthritis. Similar abnormalities in the lateral femorotibial compartment are compatible with this disease, especially in women, and may even be characteristic after certain injuries, such as those resulting in laxity of the anterior cruciate ligament; however, this pattern requires that rheumatoid arthritis and calcium pyrophosphate dihydrate crystal deposition disease be given careful consideration as alternative diagnoses. Symmetrical changes in both the medial and lateral femorotibial compartments generally indicate a disorder other than osteoarthritis.

Joint space narrowing, which corresponds to cartilaginous erosion, varies from mild to severe, with complete obliteration of the articular space (Fig. 29–43). Sclerosis of subchondral bone is more frequent in the tibia; isolated sclerosis of the femur is unusual. Sclerotic bone is found consistently in compartments with articular space narrowing. Most commonly it is localized to the immediate subchondral regions. Subchondral cysts are less frequent in the knee than in the hip. Osteophytes are frequent and predominate at the margins of the articulation in both the femur and the tibia. Central, or interior, osteophytes simulating intra-articular bodies may also be observed, especially on the femoral condyles. Marginal or central osteophytes contribute to intra-articular surface irregularity, as well as to sharpening of the tibial spines.

**Patellofemoral Compartment.** The patellofemoral compartment is frequently affected in osteoarthritis. Abnormalities in this area are best detected on axial projections. The ideal projection, particularly for the evaluation of possible patellar subluxation, is obtained with only a moderate amount of knee flexion. In osteoarthritis, cartilaginous fibrillation and erosion and subchondral bony eburnation are detected. In the patella, these changes predominate in the lateral facet, probably related to the large articular surface and the lateral vector of forces resulting from physiologic valgus.

On radiographs, patellofemoral compartment alterations are usually combined with abnormalities of the femorotibial compartments. Most typically, the medial femorotibial compartment is altered, although occasionally, lateral femorotibial and patellofemoral compartment changes occur together. It is unusual to see extensive changes in the patellofemoral compartment without significant abnormality of one of the femorotibial compartments. Thus, the finding of abnormalities resembling degenerative joint disease isolated to the patellofemoral area should lead to a search for another disease process, such as calcium pyrophosphate dihydrate crystal deposition disease, Wilson's disease, or hyperparathyroidism.

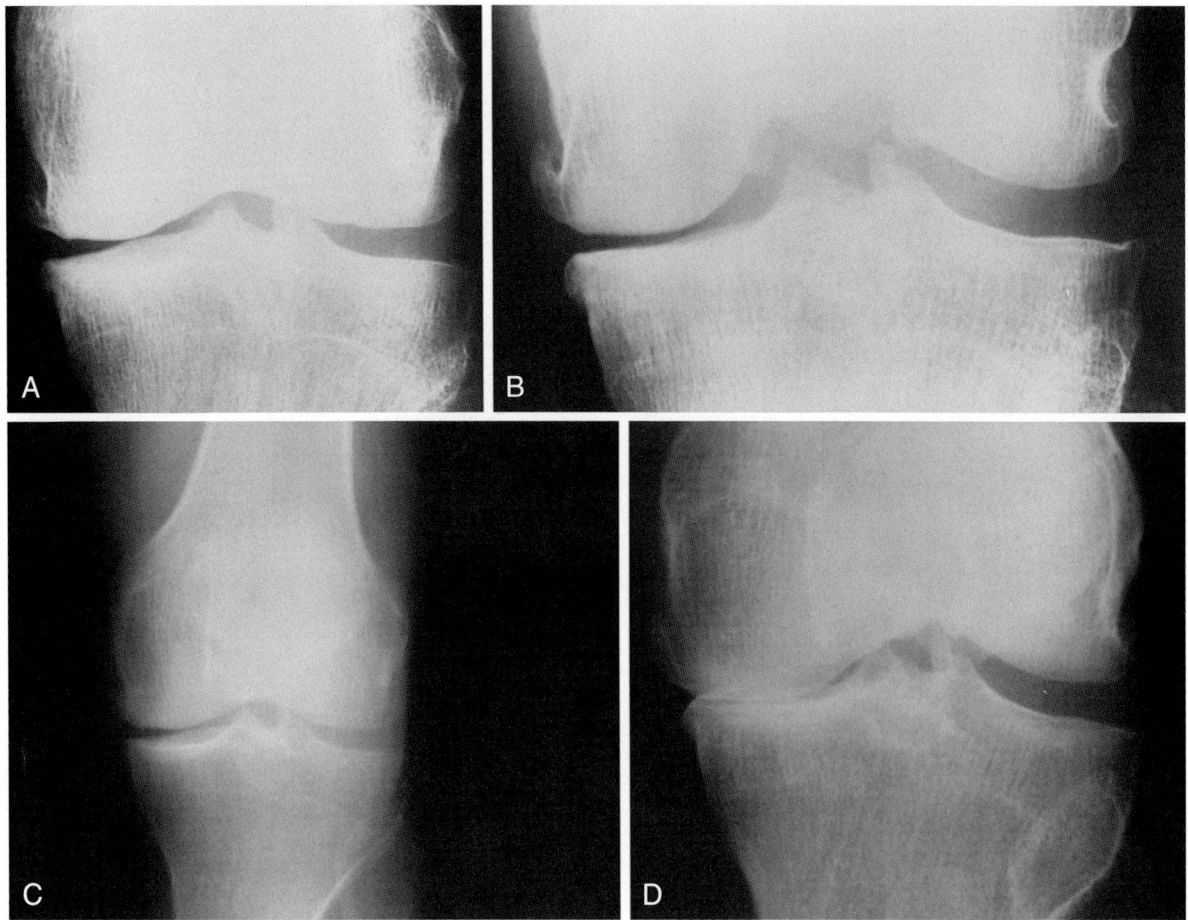

**Figure 29–42.** Osteoarthritis of the knee: supplementary views. *A*, Standard non–weight-bearing antero-posterior radiograph shows mild medial femorotibial compartment narrowing. *B*, Standard non–weight-bearing "tunnel" radiograph shows moderate joint space loss in the medial femorotibial compartment. *C*, Standard weight-bearing radiograph of the fully extended knee reveals moderate to severe joint space loss in the medial femorotibial compartment. *D*, Weight-bearing radiograph of the slightly flexed knee ("standing tunnel projection") shows severe joint space loss in the medial femorotibial compartment.

Radiographic features of patellofemoral osteoarthritis include joint space narrowing, sclerosis, and osteophytes, particularly on the patellar side of the space. Associated scalloped defects of the anterior cortex of the femur may become prominent in osteoarthritis (Fig. 29–44). This finding appears to arise from pressure erosion of the femoral cortex, generally by the adjacent patella; the femoral defect is located at the level that the patella assumes in full extension of the knee. Abnormal tilting and posterior angulation of the superior pole of the patella due to quadriceps dysfunction probably contribute to the lesion.

An additional degenerative phenomenon that occurs on the anterior surface of the patella consists of bony proliferation at the site of osseous attachment of the quadriceps apparatus. This is not a manifestation of osteoarthritis but rather is an enthesopathic alteration probably related to abnormal stress on the ligamentous connection to the bone (Fig. 29–45). It produces irregular excrescences that are detected radiographically as hyperostosis or "whitening" of the anterior patellar surface, termed the "tooth" sign or patellar "whiskering."

**Angulation and Subluxation.** Angulation and subluxation at the knee joint may accompany the ligamentous changes evident in severe osteoarthritis. Varus angulation is more frequent than valgus angulation. Translation or subluxation of the tibia on the femur laterally with varus angulation and medially with valgus angulation is typical, although the magnitude of displacement is generally less than 10 mm.

**Synovitis, Synovial Cyst Formation, and Intra-articular Osteocartilaginous Bodies.** Joint effusions are generally small in osteoarthritis of the knee. Localized cartilaginous and osseous debris arises from the disintegrating articular surfaces of the femur, tibia, and patella. Such debris may exist as loose bodies, or "joint mice," before its incorporation into the synovial membrane (Fig. 29–46). Arthrography, CT scanning, MR imaging or CT or MR arthrography can also be used in the assessment of intra-articular bodies in the knee (Fig. 29–47).

**Sesamoid Involvement.** In osteoarthritis of the knee, cartilaginous fibrillation and erosion and osseous prolifera-

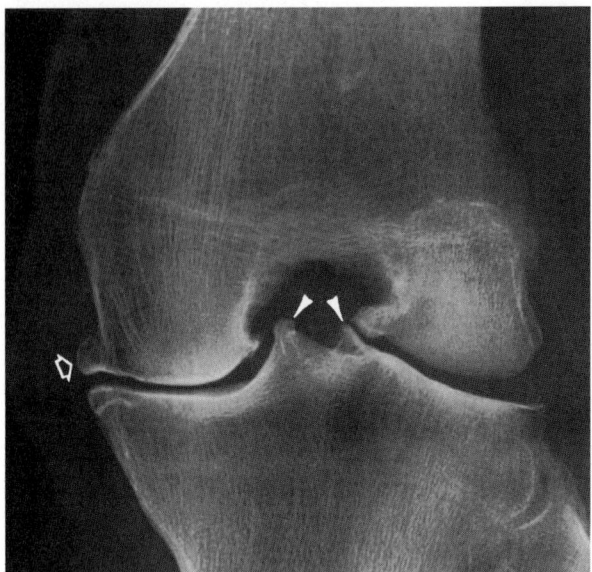

**Figure 29–43.** Osteoarthritis of the knee: femorotibial compartment abnormalities. Radiograph of a coronal section of a cadaveric knee indicates osteoarthritic changes that are more prominent in the medial femorotibial compartment. Findings include joint space narrowing related to cartilage erosion, subchondral bony sclerosis, osteophytosis *(open arrow)*, and sharpening of the tibial spines *(arrowheads)*. Degeneration of both the medial meniscus and the lateral meniscus is evident.

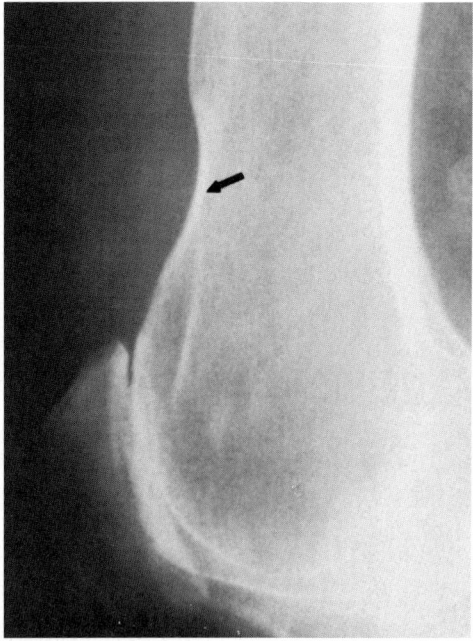

**Figure 29–44.** Osteoarthritis of the knee: patellofemoral compartment abnormalities. Lateral radiograph of the knee indicates extensive narrowing of the patellofemoral space, with eburnation of both the patella and the femur. Note the scalloped defect on the anterior aspect of the distal end of the femur *(arrow)* due to mechanical attrition from contact with the diseased patella.

tion can be observed in the fabella. On radiographs, the anterior surface of the fabella may reveal flattening and sclerosis.

## Other Diagnostic Methods

Contrast opacification of the knee joint provides a more direct method of evaluating the cartilaginous surfaces. This technique is difficult to perform in elderly osteoarthritic patients, however, and allows visualization of only those portions of the articular surface that are tangential to the x-ray beam. Radionuclide examination with bone-seeking pharmaceutical agents is a more sensitive but less specific technique than radiography. Both CT and MR imaging have proved effective in accurately assessing the state of articular cartilage (see Chapter 59).

## Chondromalacia Patellae and Other Patellar Syndromes

Chondromalacia patellae is a term applied to a syndrome of pain and crepitus over the anterior aspect of the knee, especially in flexion, which occurs in adolescents and young adults. The patella consists of three facets: the lateral facet, the medial facet, and a more medially located odd facet (Fig. 29–48). Classically, it is stated that the medial facet of the patella is the typical site of chondromalacia, particularly about the ridge that separates the medial and odd facets of the bone. The pathologic findings accompanying chondromalacia of the medial facet of the patella consist of swelling and edema of the cartilaginous surface.

Radiographs play a small role in accurately diagnosing the classic varieties of chondromalacia, with pathologic aberrations confined to cartilage. Although osteopenia is evident occasionally, other radiographic changes are lacking. A more direct assessment of cartilage integrity is provided by arthrography, especially when combined with CT scanning. CT can also be effective in assessing the relationship of the patella and femur and subluxation of the patella. MR imaging may also be used in the evaluation of chondromalacia and patellar subluxation (see Chapters 57 and 59). The possible relationship of chondromalacia patellae and osteoarthritis of the patellofemoral compartment has not been defined.

## Differential Diagnosis

**Compartmental Analysis.** Osteoarthritis does not involve the three compartments of the knee to an equal extent (Table 29–9). Most typically, radiographic changes are predominantly in one of the two femorotibial compartments, usually the medial one in men and either the medial or the lateral compartment in women. These changes may be combined with significant abnormalities of the patellofemoral compartment. Symmetrical medial and lateral femorotibial compartment disease and isolated patellofemoral compartment disease are unusual manifestations of osteoarthritis.

The medial and lateral femorotibial compartments are commonly affected to the same degree in rheumatoid arthritis, the seronegative spondyloarthropathies, septic arthritis, and cartilage atrophy (as in paralysis or disuse).

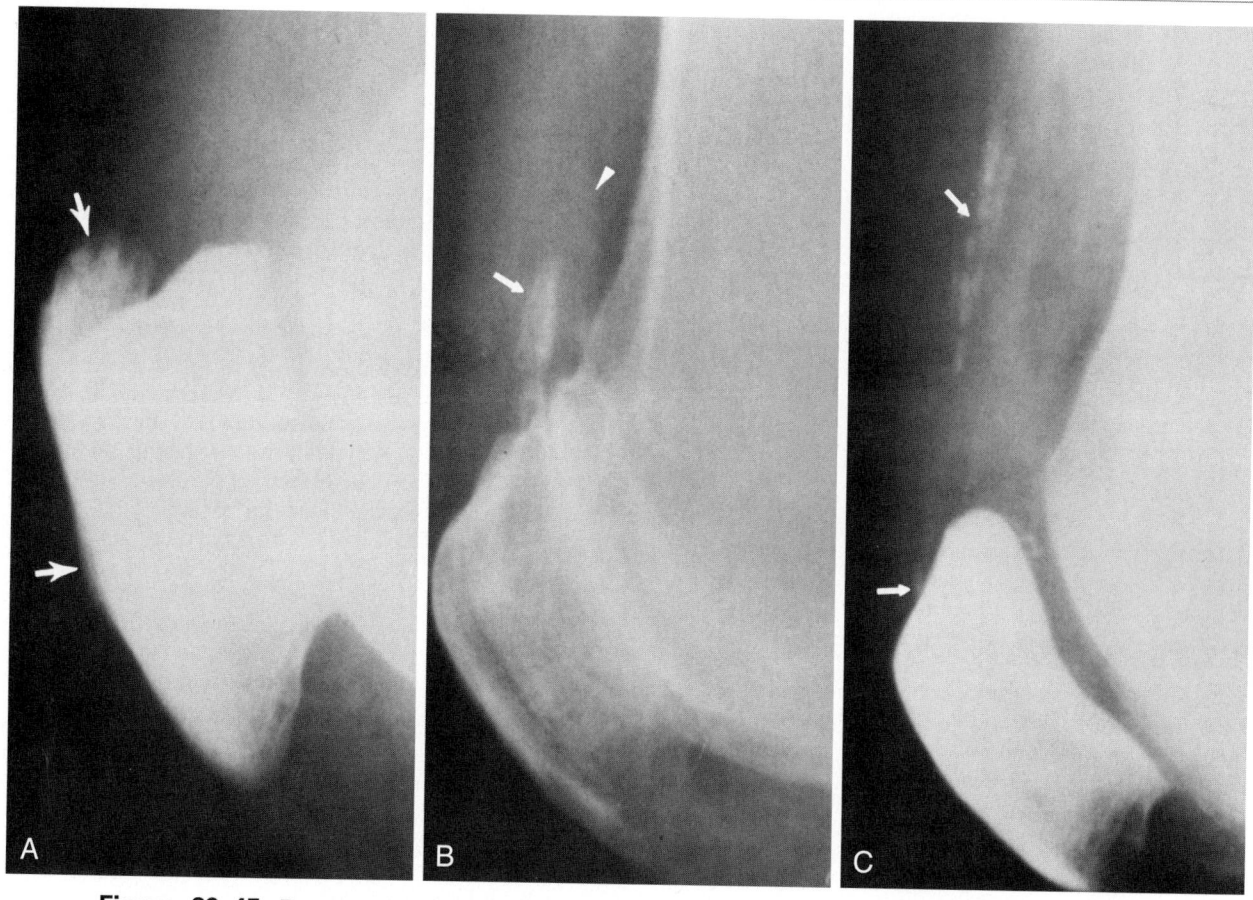

**Figure 29–45.** Degenerative disease of the knee: enthesopathy and differential diagnosis. Patellar excrescences and radiodense lesions may have several causes. *A*, Enthesopathy. Typical osseous excrescences are developing at the quadriceps attachment to the anterior surface of the patella *(arrows)*. This is not a manifestation of osteoarthritis. *B*, Osteoarthritis. Osteophytes are evident *(arrow)* at the superior articular surface of the patella. Note patellofemoral compartment narrowing and an effusion *(arrowhead)*. *C*, Calcific tendinitis. Linear radiodense areas *(arrows)* in the tendon are related to calcific tendinitis. Calcium hydroxyapatite or calcium pyrophosphate dihydrate crystal deposition can create this appearance.

Isolated patellofemoral compartment abnormalities are encountered in calcium pyrophosphate dihydrate crystal deposition disease, Wilson's disease, and hyperparathyroidism. Uncommonly, such changes are noted in osteoarthritis.

**Sclerosis, Cyst Formation, and Osteophytosis.** Crystal-induced arthropathies (gout or calcium pyrophosphate dihydrate crystal deposition disease) can also be associated with sclerosis, cysts, and osteophytes; however, the presence of osseous erosions and the absence of articular

## TABLE 29-9

**Compartmental Analysis of Knee Disease**

| | Femorotibial Compartments | Patellofemoral Compartment |
|---|---|---|
| Osteoarthritis | Medial > lateral | Commonly involved in conjunction with medial or lateral femorotibial disease |
| Rheumatoid arthritis | Medial = lateral | Commonly involved in conjunction with medial and lateral femorotibial disease |
| Calcium pyrophosphate dihydrate crystal deposition disease | Medial > lateral | Commonly involved alone or in conjunction with medial or lateral femorotibial disease |
| Hyperparathyroidism | Medial = lateral* | Involved owing to subchondral resorption, crystal-induced arthropathies, or unknown mechanism |

*Subchondral resorption can produce collapse of bone in the medial or lateral femorotibial compartment, or both.

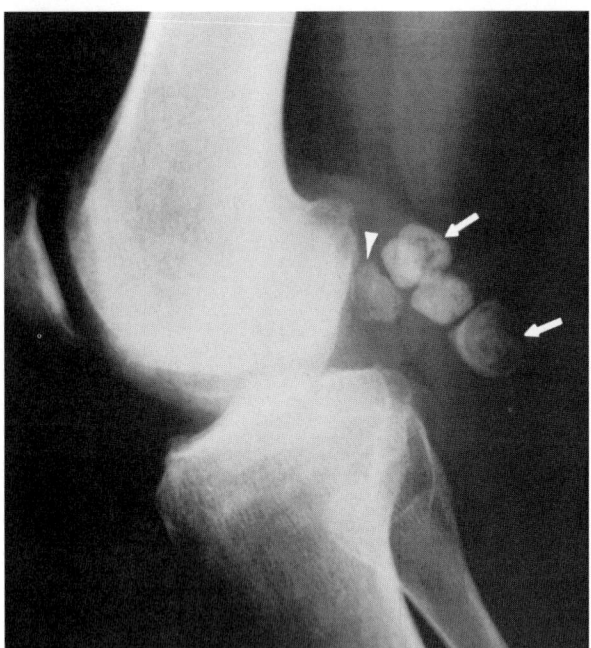

**Figure 29–46.** Osteoarthritis of the knee: intra-articular osseous bodies. Numerous radiodense lesions are grouped together *(arrows)* posterior to the knee joint. This is the typical appearance of osteocartilaginous bodies within a synovial (popliteal) cyst. One of the radiodense lesions *(arrowhead)* represents the fabella, with its typical flattened anterior surface. Osteoarthritis of the patellofemoral joint probably indicates that the bodies arose from a degenerative knee joint and passed into the synovial cyst.

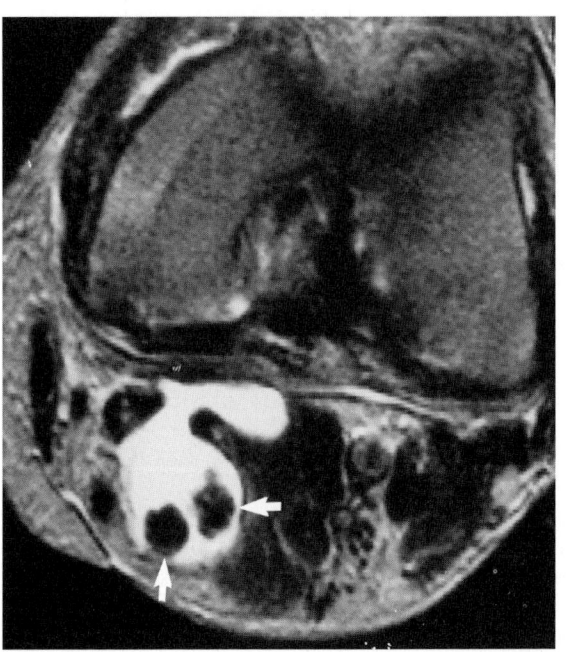

**Figure 29–47.** Osteoarthritis of the knee: intra-articular osteocartilaginous bodies. Transaxial T2-weighted (TR/TE, 1800/90) spin echo MR image reveals a joint effusion, medial meniscal degeneration, cartilage loss, and a large synovial cyst containing ossified bodies *(arrows)*.

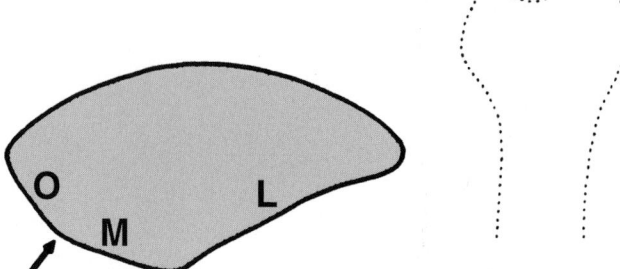

**Figure 29–48.** Chondromalacia patellae: distribution of abnormalities. The lateral facet (L), medial facet (M), and odd facet (O) of the patella are indicated on this illustration of the tangential appearance of the bone. Classically, chondromalacia is located on the osseous ridge *(arrow)* that separates the medial and odd facets. In the global pattern of chondromalacia, cartilaginous changes are apparent on the medial and lateral facets. A similar distribution is seen in osteoarthritis. Surface degeneration of cartilage on the odd facet has also been observed.

space loss are typical of gout, whereas extreme sclerosis, large cystic lesions, and considerable fragmentation and deformity are observed in calcium pyrophosphate dihydrate crystal deposition disease. In osteonecrosis, the joint space is maintained, and depression and fragmentation of the osseous surface are recognized in association with sclerosis and cyst formation.

**Other Findings.** Varus deformity is more frequent than valgus deformity in osteoarthritis of the knee, especially in men. Severe valgus angulation is not uncommon in calcium pyrophosphate dihydrate crystal deposition disease and in rheumatoid arthritis, and it may also be observed in women with osteoarthritis.

## Ankle

In the absence of significant trauma, osteoarthritis of the ankle is infrequent. It may occur after fracture of the neighboring bones or ligamentous injury, particularly when the ankle mortise is disrupted (Fig. 29–49). Capsular traction can produce a talar beak on the dorsal aspect of the bone, which, although reminiscent of the beak that accompanies tarsal coalition, is distinctive in appearance.

## Tarsal Articulations

Significant degenerative changes may develop at the first tarsometatarsal joint (Fig. 29–50). In this location, joint space narrowing and sclerosis related to osteoarthritis simulate the findings of gouty arthritis. Alterations at additional tarsal locations may develop after trauma. Persistent hindfoot pain occurring after a calcaneal fracture is a potential complication of osteoarthritis in one or both subtalar joints. Radiographs are generally inadequate for delineating the degenerative abnormalities; these are seen to better advantage on CT scans (Fig. 29–51).

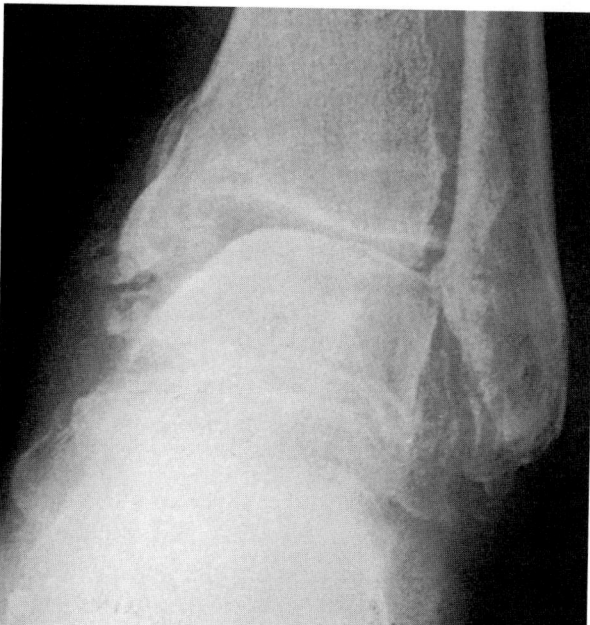

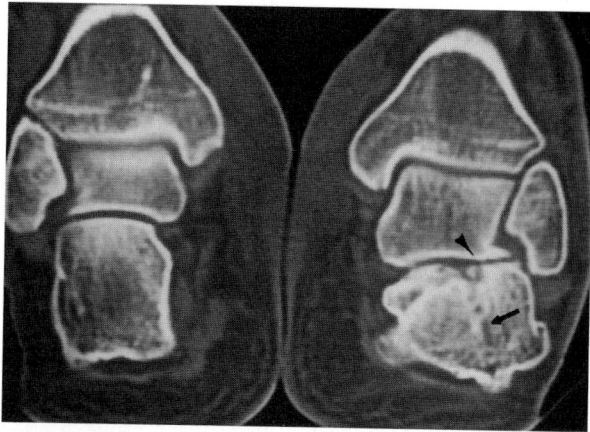

**Figure 29–51.** Osteoarthritis of the posterior subtalar joint after calcaneal fracture. In this 58-year-old man, hindfoot pain began approximately 4 years after a fracture of the calcaneus. A coronal CT scan reveals depression of the posterosuperior surface of the calcaneus and the site of previous fracture *(arrow)*. Note the narrow posterior subtalar joint *(arrowhead)*, with osteophytes and bone fragmentation, and the close relationship of the fibula and the calcaneus. Compare the opposite normal side.

**Figure 29–49.** Osteoarthritis of the ankle. This middle-aged man developed progressive pain and swelling of the ankle after an injury many years ago. Neurologic examination was normal. Anteroposterior radiograph of the ankle delineates joint space narrowing, sclerosis, fragmentation, and osteophytosis. Note the tilting of the talus with respect to the tibia.

Plantar and posterior calcaneal enthesophytes are frequent radiographic findings that may be unassociated with clinical abnormalities. These excrescences develop at or close to the osseous sites of attachment of the Achilles tendon, plantar aponeurosis, and long plantar ligament. A poorly defined or fluffy plantar calcaneal bony outgrowth can be an important radiographic finding of ankylosing spondylitis, psoriatic arthritis, and Reiter's syndrome.

### Metatarsophalangeal and Interphalangeal Joints

Osteoarthritis of the first metatarsophalangeal joint (hallux rigidus) is very common (Fig. 29–52). This condition may lead to painful restriction of dorsiflexion of the great toe. Radiographic evaluation reveals joint space loss, bony sclerosis, and osteophytes, particularly on the dorsal aspect of the metatarsal head.

Another common lesion of the first metatarsophalangeal joint is hallux valgus. The essential intrinsic lesion of this condition may be stretching of the ligaments about the metatarsophalangeal joint that attach the medial sesamoid and basal phalanx to the metatarsal bone, with erosion of the ridge that separates the grooves for the sesamoids on the metatarsal head. On radiographs, valgus angulation is frequently associated with pronation of the great toe and bony hypertrophy or osteophytosis, particularly on the medial aspect of the metatarsal head. The enlarged and irregular medial portion of the metatarsal bone may contain cystic lesions and thickened trabeculae, findings that can simulate those of gout. An angular deformity of the fifth metatarsophalangeal joint with medial deviation of the fifth toe is designated a tailor's bunion, or bunionette. This condition is accompanied by an inflamed and thickened adventitious bursa and hypertrophic keratoses or calluses.

Osteoarthritis of the interphalangeal joints of the toes may be an incidental finding on radiographs. These changes are frequently obscured by curling or deformity

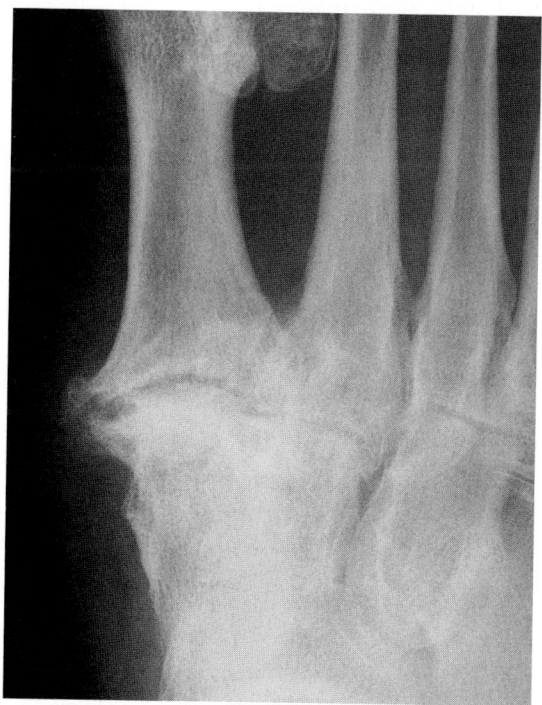

**Figure 29–50.** Osteoarthritis of the first tarsometatarsal joint. Findings include joint space narrowing, sclerosis, and osteophytes at the first (medial) tarsometatarsal joint and, to a lesser extent, the second tarsometatarsal space.

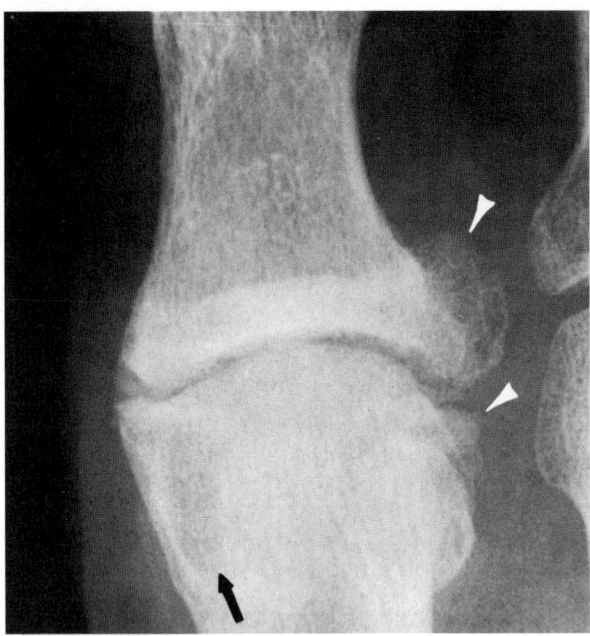

**Figure 29–52.** Osteoarthritis of the first metatarsophalangeal joint: hallux rigidus. Frontal radiograph reveals considerable joint space narrowing, sclerosis, and osteophytosis *(arrowheads)* about the first metatarsophalangeal joint. Observe the flattening of the metatarsal head and a large metatarsal cyst *(arrow)*.

of the digits. Four types of deformity of the toes have been defined: claw toe, characterized by hyperextension of the metatarsophalangeal joint and flexion of the proximal and distal interphalangeal joints; hammer toe, in which there is hyperextension of the metatarsophalangeal joint, flexion of the proximal interphalangeal joint, and hyperextension of the distal interphalangeal joint; mallet toe, with flexion of the distal interphalangeal joint; and curly toe, in which the metatarsophalangeal joint is in a neutral position and there is flexion of the proximal and distal interphalangeal joints.

## SPECIAL TYPES OF DEGENERATIVE JOINT DISEASE

### Generalized Osteoarthritis

The concept of generalized or polyarticular osteoarthritis is not universally accepted. When radiographs reveal evidence of degenerative changes in multiple sites, diagnoses other than generalized osteoarthritis must be considered. Multiple epiphyseal dysplasia, spondyloepiphyseal dysplasia, osteonecrosis, alkaptonuria, Paget's disease, acromegaly, occupation-induced articular disorders, calcium pyrophosphate dihydrate or calcium hydroxyapatite crystal deposition disease, gout, hemophilia, and inflammatory arthritides all may lead to similar changes at multiple articular locations. In some of these disorders (osteonecrosis, gout, hemophilia, inflammatory arthritides), secondary degenerative abnormalities related to altered joint mechanics can obscure the more diagnostic radiographic features; in others (calcium pyrophosphate dihydrate crystal deposition disease, alkaptonuria), abnormalities resembling those of degenerative joint disease are part of the basic disease process.

## Inflammatory (Erosive) Osteoarthritis

### Historical Aspects

Inflammatory (erosive) osteoarthritis is a peculiar form of osteoarthritis occurring predominantly in middle-aged women and characterized by interphalangeal joint involvement and acute inflammatory episodes. The term *erosive osteoarthritis* has been used to emphasize the juxta-articular and intra-articular erosions that are evident on radiographic examination of these patients; the term *inflammatory osteoarthritis* has been used to emphasize the clinical and pathologic characteristics of the joint disease. The latter term may be preferable, because patients with typical clinical findings of inflammatory osteoarthritis may not reveal erosive alterations on radiographs of the digits.

### Clinical Abnormalities

The onset of the disease may be abrupt. Painful nodules of the distal and proximal interphalangeal joints of the fingers are associated with edema and redness of the overlying skin, as well as tenderness and restricted motion. Interphalangeal joints are affected most commonly, although abnormalities of the metacarpophalangeal and carpometacarpal joints, trapezioscaphoid area of the midcarpal joints, knees, and hips may become apparent. The course of the disease is variable. In some patients, the inflammatory signs subside with conservative therapeutic measures after a period of months to years. In others, the inflammatory signs progress and the clinical manifestations resemble or become identical to those of rheumatoid arthritis (see the later discussion in this chapter).

### Radiographic Abnormalities

The radiographic changes are often characterized by a combination of bone proliferation and erosion. Typically, osteophytosis resembles that in noninflammatory osteoarthritis, predominating at the articular margins of the distal and proximal interphalangeal joints. At these sites, joint space narrowing is common, with associated subchondral sclerosis. Interosseous space diminution also becomes evident at the interphalangeal joint of the thumb, the metacarpophalangeal and first carpometacarpal joints, and the trapezioscaphoid space of the midcarpal articulation.

In some involved joints, erosions may become prominent. They are particularly frequent in interphalangeal articulations (Fig. 29–53). The erosions commonly begin at the central portion of the joint in the form of sharply marginated, etched defects. This central location is characteristic, differing from the marginal location of erosions in rheumatoid arthritis, psoriatic arthritis, and related disorders. Although the exact pathogenesis of erosions in inflammatory osteoarthritis is not clear, they may be related to collapse or pressure atrophy of subchondral bone rather than to synovial inflammation. Intra-articular bony ankylosis is also evident in many patients with inflammatory osteoarthritis. This finding is virtually confined to one or several interphalangeal joints; after ankylosis, osteophytosis and sclerosis about the involved joint may disappear. Radiographic abnormalities in ar-

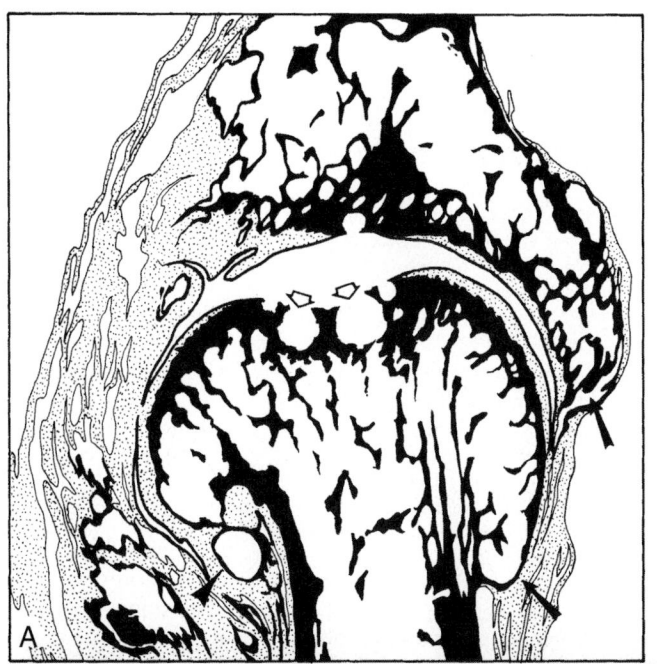

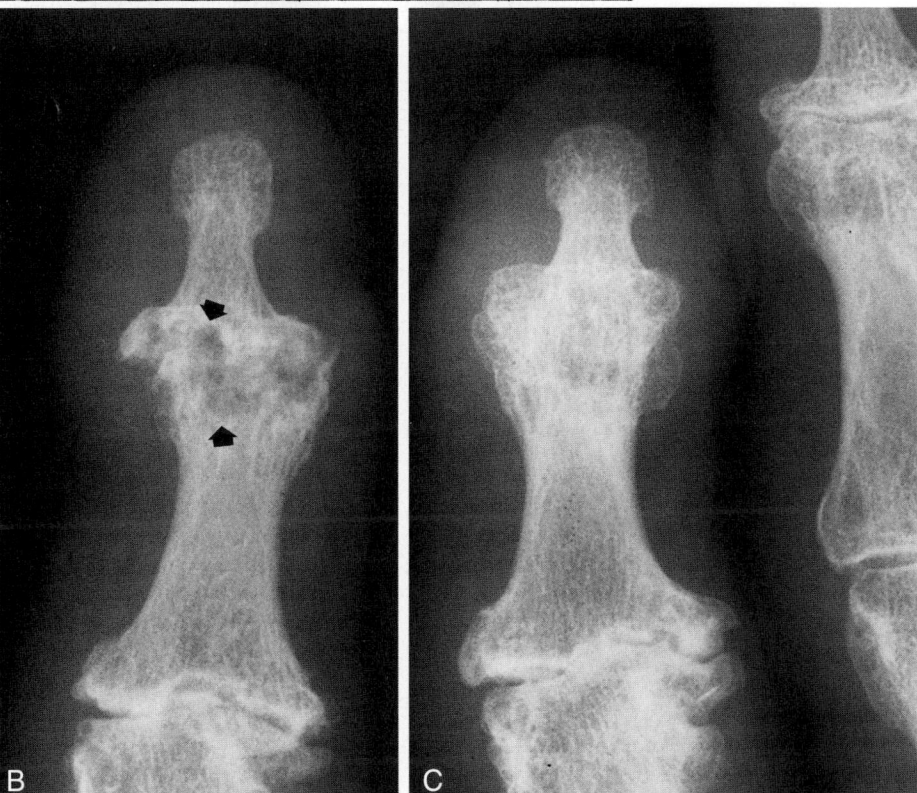

**Figure 29–53.** Inflammatory (erosive) osteoarthritis: interphalangeal joint abnormalities. *A,* Drawing depicts the usual appearance of inflammatory osteoarthritis of the interphalangeal joints. Findings resemble those of noninflammatory osteoarthritis, including traction osteophytes *(solid arrows),* ossicles *(arrowhead),* and eburnation. Erosive changes are also apparent, particularly in the central aspect of the joint *(open arrows)* (compare with Fig. 29–11). *B,* In a more advanced case, disruption of the entire central aspect of the joint *(arrows)* is typical. Note the changes in the proximal interphalangeal joint, which are identical to those of noninflammatory osteoarthritis. *C,* The eventual result may be intra-articular osseous fusion, as seen in the distal interphalangeal joint.

ticular sites other than those in the hands are recorded infrequently. The findings are identical to those in noninflammatory osteoarthritis.

## Pathologic Abnormalities

Synovial biopsies have revealed tissue that is mildly to severely inflamed, although in some cases, synovial, cartilaginous, and osseous changes are identical to those of noninflammatory osteoarthritis. Degeneration of cartilage and bony proliferation are evident.

## Relationship to Other Articular Disorders

**Rheumatoid Arthritis.** In approximately 15% of patients with inflammatory osteoarthritis, clinical, laboratory, and radiographic findings of rheumatoid arthritis may be seen. In all reported patients with both rheumatoid arthritis and inflammatory osteoarthritis, the osteoarthritic alterations preceded those of rheumatoid arthritis.

**Osteoarthritis.** The relationship of inflammatory and noninflammatory osteoarthritis is not clear. The distribution of affected joints is almost identical in both diseases. The major differences between inflammatory and noninflammatory osteoarthritis are the clinical signs of joint inflammation and the radiographic findings of bone erosion and ankylosis in the former disorder. Inflammatory osteoarthritis may represent one extreme in the spectrum of degenerative joint disease, however, rather than being a separate entity.

**Calcium Hydroxyapatite Crystal Deposition Disease.** Abnormal accumulation of calcium hydroxyapatite crystals in the interphalangeal joints of the hand, manifested as cloudlike radiodense lesions, may be seen. This pattern of calcification can occur in the absence of additional radiographic alterations, although in some cases, it arises in a joint that is already affected by osteoarthritis.

**Gout.** The deposition of monosodium urate crystals in osteoarthritic joints of the fingers, leading to articular inflammation, may also be seen. Patients are generally elderly; indeed, they are older than the typical population with gout. Many of them are receiving diuretic therapy. The radiographic diagnosis of secondary gout in patients with osteoarthritis of the interphalangeal joints of the fingers may be difficult.

## Differential Diagnosis

Inflammatory osteoarthritis is associated with proliferative and erosive abnormalities of interphalangeal joints. If proliferative changes predominate, the resulting radiographic appearance is identical to that of noninflammatory osteoarthritis. In the presence of erosions or bony ankylosis, the differentiation of inflammatory from noninflammatory osteoarthritis is facilitated. The erosions of inflammatory osteoarthritis are unusual in their distribution within an involved joint; they frequently predominate in the central portion. This central localization differs from the marginal localization associated with other erosive arthritides of the interphalangeal joints, such as rheumatoid arthritis, psoriatic arthritis, multicentric reticulohistiocytosis, and gout.

The most difficult aspect of the differential diagnosis is distinguishing inflammatory osteoarthritis and psoriatic arthritis. In addition to the central location of erosions, a widespread and symmetrical distribution characterizes inflammatory osteoarthritis. This differs from psoriatic arthritis, in which marginal erosions and poorly defined bony proliferation may be distributed in an asymmetrical, unilateral, or even raylike pattern. Intra-articular bony ankylosis, which accompanies inflammatory osteoarthritis, may also be evident in psoriatic arthritis and, less commonly, in rheumatoid arthritis. In the latter disease, intra-articular ankylosis may be encountered at proximal interphalangeal joints, whereas in psoriatic arthritis, either distal or proximal interphalangeal joints may become ankylosed. Intra-articular osseous fusion is not regarded as a characteristic manifestation of noninflammatory osteoarthritis, gout, or multicentric reticulohistiocytosis. Finally, in patients with nodal osteoarthritis who develop inflammatory clinical manifestations, the possibility of secondary crystal deposition, including calcium

hydroxyapatite, monosodium urate, and even calcium pyrophosphate dihydrate crystals, should be considered.

## FURTHER READING

Arnoldi CC, Linderholm H, Mussbichler H: Venous engorgement and intra-osseous hypertension in osteoarthritis of the hip. J Bone Joint Surg Br 54:409, 1972.

Bock GW, Garcia A, Weisman MH, et al: Rapidly destructive hip disease: Clinical and imaging abnormalities. Radiology 186:461, 1993.

Boegård T, Jonsson K: Radiography in osteoarthritis of the knee. Skeletal Radiol 28:605, 1999.

Boegård T, Rudling O, Dahlstrom J, et al: Bone scintigraphy in chronic knee pain: Comparison with magnetic resonance imaging. Ann Rheum Dis 58:20, 1999.

Boegård T, Rudling O, Petersson IF, et al: Correlation between radiographically diagnosed osteophytes and magnetic resonance detected cartilage defects in the tibiofemoral joint. Ann Rheum Dis 57:401, 1998.

Burke MJ, Fear EC, Wright V: Bone and joint changes in pneumatic drillers. Ann Rheum Dis 36:276, 1977.

Conway WF, Destouet JM, Gilula LA, et al: The carpal boss: An overview of radiographic evaluation. Radiology 156:29, 1985.

Crain DC: Interphalangeal osteoarthritis characterized by painful inflammatory episodes resulting in deformity of the proximal and distal articulations. JAMA 175:1049, 1961.

Dalinka MK, Kricun ME, Zlatkin MB, et al: Modern diagnostic imaging in joint disease. AJR Am J Roentgenol 152:229, 1989.

DePalma AF: Degenerative Changes in Sternoclavicular and Acromioclavicular Joints in Various Decades. Springfield, Ill, Charles C Thomas, 1957.

Dihlmann W, Hering L: Dense bone about the sacroiliac joint: A radiological review of the differential diagnosis. Eur J Radiol 27:241, 1998.

Dixon T, Benjamin J, Lund P, et al: Femoral neck buttressing: A radiographic and histologic analysis. Skeletal Radiol 29:587, 2000.

Ehrlich GE: Inflammatory osteoarthritis. II. The superimposition of rheumatoid arthritis. J Chronic Dis 25:635, 1972.

Feldman F, Johnston A: Intra-osseous ganglion. AJR Am J Roentgenol 118:328, 1973.

Ficat RP, Hungerford DS: Disorders of the Patello-Femoral Joint. Baltimore, Williams & Wilkins, 1977.

Hayes CW, Conway WF: Evaluation of articular cartilage: Radiographic and cross-sectional imaging techniques. Radiographics 12:409, 1992.

Jaffe HL: Metabolic, Degenerative and Inflammatory Diseases of Bones and Joints. Philadelphia, Lea & Febiger, 1972.

Karasick D, Wapner KL: Hallux rigidus deformity: Radiologic assessment. AJR Am J Roentgenol 157:1029, 1991.

Kellgren JH, Moore R: Generalized osteoarthritis and Heberden's nodes. BMJ 1:181, 1952.

Kindynis P, Haller J, Kang HS, et al: Osteophytes of the knee: Anatomic, radiologic, and pathologic investigation. Radiology 174:841, 1990.

Mankin HJ: The reaction of articular cartilage to injury and osteoarthritis. Part 1. N Engl J Med 291:1285, 1974.

Mankin HJ: The reaction of articular cartilage to injury and osteoarthritis. Part 2. N Engl J Med 291:1335, 1974.

Martel W, Braunstein EM: The diagnostic value of buttressing of the femoral neck. Arthritis Rheum 21:161, 1978.

Martel W, Snarr JW, Horn JR: The metacarpophalangeal joints in interphalangeal osteoarthritis. Radiology 108:1, 1973.

Martel W, Stuck KJ, Dworin AM, et al: Erosive osteoarthritis and psoriatic arthritis: A radiologic comparison in the hand, wrist, and foot. AJR Am J Roentgenol 134:125, 1980.

McCarty DJ, Halverson PB, Carrera GF, et al: "Milwaukee shoulder"—association of microspheroids containing hydroxyapatite crystals, active collagenase, and neutral protease with rotator cuff defects. I. Clinical aspects. Arthritis Rheum 24:464, 1983.

Milgram JW: The development of loose bodies in human joints. Clin Orthop 124:292, 1977.

Neer CS: Anterior acromioplasty for the chronic impingement syndrome in the shoulder. J Bone Joint Surg Am 54:41, 1972.

Prassopoulos PK, Faflia CP, Voloudaki AE, et al: Sacroiliac joints: Anatomical variants on CT. J Comput Assist Tomogr 23:323, 1999.

Radin E: Chondromalacia of the patella. Bull Rheum Dis 34:1, 1984.

Resnick D: Patterns of migration of the femoral head in osteoarthritis of the hip: Roentgenographic-pathologic correlation and comparison with rheumatoid arthritis. AJR Am J Roentgenol 124:62, 1975.

Resnick D, Niwayama G: Entheses and enthesopathy: Anatomical, pathological, and radiological correlation. Radiology 146:1, 1983.

Resnick D, Niwayama G, Coutts RD: Subchondral cysts (geodes) in arthritic disorders: Pathologic and radiographic appearance of the hip joint. AJR Am J Roentgenol 128:799, 1977.

Resnick D, Niwayama G, Goergen TG: Comparison of radiographic abnormalities of the sacroiliac joint in degenerative disease and ankylosing spondylitis. AJR Am J Roentgenol 128:189, 1977.

Rose CP, Cockshott WP: Anterior femoral erosion and patellofemoral osteoarthritis. J Can Assoc Radiol 33:32, 1982.

Sokoloff L: Kashin-Beck disease. Rheum Clin North Am 13:101, 1987.

Thomas RH, Resnick D, Alazraki NP, et al: Compartmental evaluation of osteoarthritis of the knee: A comparative study of available diagnostic modalities. Radiology 116:585, 1975.

Trueta J: Studies of the Development and Decay of the Human Frame. Philadelphia, WB Saunders, 1968.

Watson HK, Ballet FL: The SLAC wrist: Scapholunate advanced collapse pattern of degenerative arthritis. J Hand Surg [Am] 9:358, 1984.

Yoshimura N, Sasaki S, Iwasaki K, et al: Occupational lifting is associated with hip osteoarthritis: A Japanese case-control study. J Rheumatol 27:434, 2000.

Zhang Y, Hannan MT, Chaisson CE, et al: Bone mineral density and risk of incident and progressive radiographic knee osteoarthritis in women: The Framingham study. J Rheumatol 27:1032, 2000.

# CHAPTER 30

## Degenerative Disease of the Spine

### *SUMMARY OF KEY FEATURES*

A variety of degenerative processes involve the spine, each of which is characterized by distinctive radiographic manifestations. Intervertebral (osteo)chondrosis is associated with vacuum phenomena, disc space narrowing, and reactive sclerosis of the vertebral body; spondylosis deformans is associated with osteophytosis; osteoarthritis leads to joint space narrowing, bone sclerosis and hypertrophy, and, infrequently, osseous fusion; and ligamentous degeneration can be associated with calcification and ossification. Although any one degenerative process may predominate in a patient, frequently, all occur together.

Several complications may appear during the course of degenerative disorders of the spine, including abnormalities of vertebral alignment (segmental instability, degenerative anterior spondylolisthesis, degenerative retrolisthesis, senile thoracic kyphosis, and degenerative lumbar scoliosis and kyphosis), intervertebral disc displacement (cartilaginous nodes, intraspinal displacement), disc calcification and ossification, and spinal stenosis. Plain-film radiographic examination in patients with such complications may be supplemented with conventional tomography, myelography, discography, computed tomography, and magnetic resonance imaging.

### INTRODUCTION

The convenient label "degenerative disease" is carelessly applied to a variety of distinct processes of the spinal joints. Because the joints of the spine have fundamental anatomic differences, it is incorrect to assume that they deteriorate in an identical fashion. Rather, the synovial joints, the symphyses, the syndesmoses, and the entheses (sites of ligamentous attachment to bone) each degenerate in a specific fashion that is associated with characteristic clinical, pathologic, and imaging aberrations.

### MAJOR TYPES OF SPINAL ARTICULATIONS

Below the level of the second cervical vertebra, the vertebrae are united principally by a series of cartilaginous joints (intervertebral discs) between the vertebral bodies and a series of synovial joints (apophyseal joints) between the vertebral arches. In addition, ligamentous connections exist both anteriorly (anterior longitudinal ligament, posterior longitudinal ligament) and posteriorly (ligamenta flava and interspinous, supraspinous, and intertransverse ligaments).

The central portion of the intervertebral disc, the nucleus pulposus, is soft and gelatinous at birth and consists mainly of mucoid material. Gradually, the mucoid substance is replaced by fibrocartilage. The anulus fibrosus surrounds the nucleus pulposus and contains an outer zone of collagenous fibers and an inner zone of fibrocartilage. Anteriorly, the anulus fibrosus is anchored to the cartilaginous endplate, vertebral rim, and periosteum of the vertebral body; the last site of attachment consists of strong fibers termed Sharpey's fibers (Fig. 30–1). Cartilaginous endplates are closely applied to the central depressions present on the superior and inferior surfaces of the vertebral body.

Apophyseal articulations are situated between the articular facets of adjacent vertebrae. They possess a synovial membrane, meniscus-like structures, and thin and loose articular capsules.

The anterior longitudinal ligament, which extends along the anterior surface of the vertebral column, is particularly adherent to the edge of the vertebral body adjacent to the discovertebral junction. The posterior longitudinal ligament extends along the inside of the vertebral column and is intimate with the posterior surfaces of the vertebral bodies and intervertebral discs.

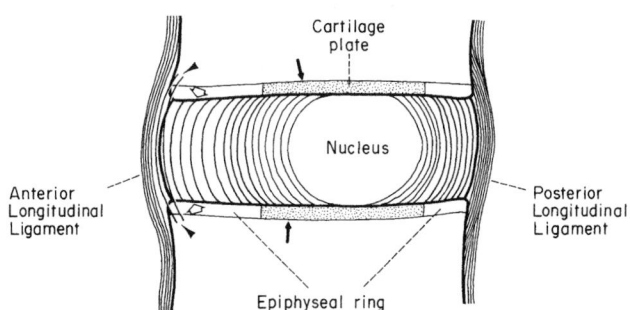

**Figure 30–1.** Anatomy of the discovertebral junction. Drawing of a sagittal section of a normal discovertebral joint indicates its major constituents. Observe the nucleus pulposus, located slightly posterior to the midportion of the intervertebral disc. It is surrounded by the concentric fibers of the anulus fibrosus. Each vertebral body possesses elevated cortical rims, related to fusion of the marginal apophyseal (epiphyseal) rings, and a central depression that is covered by a cartilaginous endplate. Beneath the endplate is a subchondral bone plate (*solid arrows*). The anulus fibrosus is attached to the bony rims through calcified cartilage connected to osseous tissue (*open arrows*). The outer fibers of the anulus fibrosus, occasionally termed perivertebral ligaments, anchor to the cortex of the vertebral body by strong Sharpey's fibers (*arrowheads*). The anterior longitudinal ligament attaches to the anterior surface of the vertebral body and is less adherent to the intervertebral disc. The posterior longitudinal ligament is applied to the back of the intervertebral discs and vertebral bodies.

(From Resnick D: Degenerative diseases of the vertebral column. Radiology 156:3, 1985.)

Additional ligaments are the ligamenta flava (connecting the laminae of adjacent vertebrae), supraspinous ligaments (connecting the apices of the spinous processes), interspinous ligaments (connecting adjoining spinous processes), intertransverse ligaments (connecting transverse processes), and ligamentum nuchae (connecting the occipital protuberance and external occipital crest to the spine of the seventh cervical vertebra).

## MAJOR TYPES OF DEGENERATIVE DISEASES OF THE SPINE

Tables 30–1 and 30–2 list degenerative diseases of the spine.

### Cartilaginous Joints

The major components of the cartilaginous joints, the nucleus pulposus, anulus fibrosus, and cartilaginous endplates (see Fig. 30–1), are intimately related both anatomically and physiologically. A vascular network that supplies blood to the cartilaginous endplate and intervertebral disc in infants and young children soon atrophies and may disappear by the age of 8 to 12 years. The metabolism of the intervertebral disc becomes primarily anaerobic and is dependent on diffusion of fluid either from the marrow of the vertebral bodies across the subchondral bone and cartilaginous endplate or through the anulus fibrosus from the surrounding blood vessels.

Magnetic resonance (MR) imaging is a noninvasive means of determining the integrity of the intervertebral disc. Although considerable data indicate that the signal characteristics of a healthy disc differ from those of a diseased one, it is not entirely clear which components of the intervertebral disc contribute most significantly to these signal characteristics. Because degenerative changes of the disc are accompanied by alterations in both the water and proteoglycan content of the tissue, either or both could be responsible for alterations in signal intensity. MR imaging can be used to provide qualitative and quantitative data that depend primarily on the water content of the intervertebral disc; therefore, it can monitor the biochemical aberrations that accompany the major degenerative diseases of the intervertebral disc.

**Intervertebral (Osteo)Chondrosis.** Aging results in dehydration and loss of tissue resiliency in the intervertebral disc, particularly in the nucleus pulposus. This process has been termed intervertebral chondrosis or intervertebral (osteo)chondrosis (Fig. 30–2). The cause of intervertebral (osteo)chondrosis is not known. Changes are observed in the nucleus pulposus, anulus fibrosus, and hyaline cartilage endplate, although the findings in the nucleus pulposus are most striking. The nucleus pulposus appears desiccated and friable, related to loss of water and proteoglycans. Clefts or crevices appear and extend in an oblique or transverse fashion from the nucleus into the anulus fibrosus.

Even in the early stages of intervertebral (osteo)chondrosis, radiographic findings of linear or circular radiolucent collections—vacuum phenomena—appear within the intervertebral discs. This finding is accentuated in extension and may disappear in flexion. Distraction of the intervertebral disc (which occurs in extension) increases the disc space and attracts gas from the surrounding extracellular fluid. In flexion, the space is obliterated and the gas is resorbed. Vacuum phenomena are a reliable indicator of disc degeneration; they are very rare in the presence of disc infection.

As the process of intervertebral (osteo)chondrosis progresses, the clefts or cavities enlarge and involve both the

---

**TABLE 30–1**

**Major Types of Degenerative Diseases of the Spine**

Cartilaginous joints (discovertebral junction)
  Intervertebral (osteo)chondrosis
  Spondylosis deformans
Uncovertebral (neurocentral) joints
  Arthrosis
Synovial joints
  Apophyseal joint osteoarthritis
  Costovertebral joint osteoarthritis
Fibrous joints and entheses
  Diffuse idiopathic skeletal hyperostosis
  Ossification of the posterior longitudinal ligament
  Degeneration of the ligamenta flava and the supraspinous, interspinous, and iliolumbar ligaments

---

**TABLE 30–2**

**Degenerative Disorders of the Spine**

| | Intervertebral (Osteo)Chondrosis | Spondylosis Deformans | Osteoarthritis |
|---|---|---|---|
| Major site of abnormality | Nucleus pulposus | Anulus fibrosus | Apophyseal and costovertebral joints |
| Intervertebral disc | Moderate to severe decrease in height, vacuum phenomena | Normal or slight decrease in height | Normal |
| Vertebral body | Sclerosis of superior and inferior surfaces; cartilaginous nodes | Osteophytosis | Normal |
| Apophyseal and costovertebral joints | Normal | Normal | Joint space narrowing, sclerosis |

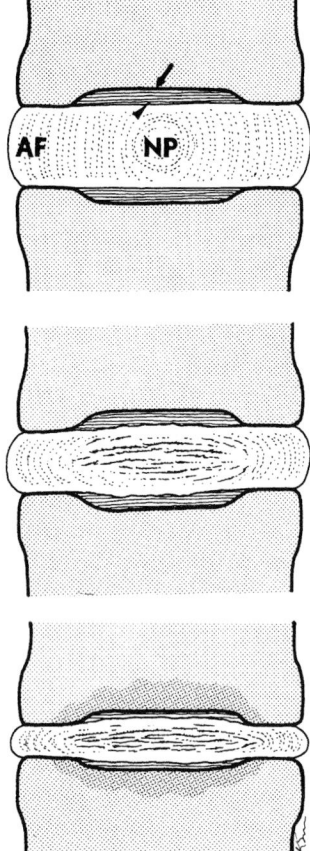

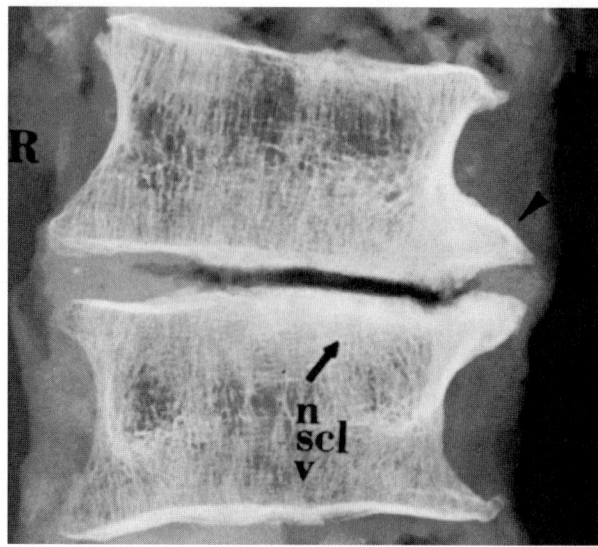

**Figure 30–3.** Intervertebral (osteo)chondrosis: later radiographic abnormalities. On a radiograph of a coronal section of the spine, observe the vacuum phenomena, disc space narrowing, sclerosis *(arrow)*, and osteophytosis *(arrowhead)*.

**Figure 30–2.** Intervertebral (osteo)chondrosis: progressive stages of the disease. *Top*, Normal situation. The cartilaginous endplate *(arrowhead)* and subchondral bone plate *(arrow)* are shown. *Middle*, Early abnormalities of intervertebral (osteo)chondrosis consist of enlarging clefts within the nucleus pulposus (NP), degeneration of the cartilaginous endplate, and loss of intervertebral disc height. *Bottom*, Clefts appear in both the nucleus pulposus and anulus fibrosus (AF). The degenerative changes of the cartilaginous endplate have progressed, and further disc space loss is apparent. Reactive sclerosis of adjacent vertebral bodies can be seen.

nucleus pulposus and anulus fibrosus, and the intervertebral disc diminishes in height. The cartilaginous endplates reveal concomitant degeneration. Radiographically, at this stage, disc space loss and bony eburnation are characteristic (Fig. 30–3). Sclerosis is generally well defined, linear, or triangular and extends to the intervertebral disc. Subchondral condensation of bone in both vertebral bodies bordering the intervertebral disc is typical. Although they may be homogeneous, the sclerotic areas can contain radiolucent lesions of variable size that reflect intraosseous disc displacement; these lesions are termed cartilaginous (Schmorl's) nodes.

The radiographic characteristics of disc space loss and reactive sclerosis in this condition are similar to changes accompanying other spinal disorders (Table 30–3). Infection also produces this combination of findings; however, clinical signs of sepsis, fraying or a poorly defined vertebral outline, and a soft tissue mass may be apparent.

In general, neoplasms do not produce significant alterations in the intervertebral disc, although osseous lesions with disruption of the cartilaginous endplate and subchondral bone plate may lead to cartilaginous node formation with disc space loss, thereby simulating intervertebral (osteo)chondrosis or infection. Intervertebral disc space loss and bony eburnation are also seen in association with trauma, rheumatoid arthritis, neuropathic osteoarthropathy, sarcoidosis, and renal osteodystrophy. In ankylosing spondylitis and, less commonly, the other seronegative spondyloarthropathies, inflammatory changes at the discovertebral junction are associated with loss of disc height and erosions and eburnation of adjacent vertebral bodies. The presence of additional clinical and radiographic findings in ankylosing spondylitis and related disorders provides diagnostic accuracy.

Vacuum phenomena are characteristic but are not a pathognomonic radiographic sign of intervertebral (osteo)chondrosis. Vacuum phenomena represent radiolucent collections of gas, principally nitrogen, that appear at sites of negative pressure produced by abnormal spaces or clefts. In the case of intervertebral (osteo)chondrosis, these sites predominate in the nucleus pulposus of the disc, although vacuum phenomena are well recognized in synovial joints, where stress distracts the apposing articular surfaces. If no fluid is present within the articular cavity, the increasing joint space that results creates a negative pressure that causes gas to collect from surrounding extracellular spaces. Vacuum phenomena isolated in the outer portions of the anulus fibrosus have a different significance. In some instances, they correspond in position to the annular defects seen in spondylosis deformans. Similar gaseous collections have been noted in the discs of the cervical spine after trauma, presumably related to the defect created by avulsion of peripheral disc fibers from the vertebral rim.

**TABLE 30-3**

**Intervertebral Disc Space Loss and Adjacent Sclerosis**

| Disease | Mechanism | Radiographic Appearance |
|---|---|---|
| Intervertebral (osteo)chondrosis | Degeneration of the nucleus pulposus and cartilaginous endplate<br>Cartilaginous nodes | Disc space narrowing<br>Vacuum phenomena<br>Well-defined sclerotic vertebral margins |
| Infection | Osteomyelitis and "discitis" | Disc space narrowing<br>Poorly defined sclerotic vertebral margins<br>Soft tissue mass |
| Trauma | Disc injury and degeneration<br>Cartilaginous nodes | Disc space narrowing<br>Well-defined sclerotic vertebral margins<br>Fracture<br>Soft tissue mass |
| Neuropathic osteoarthropathy | Loss of sensation and proprioception with repetitive trauma | Disc space narrowing<br>Extensive sclerosis of vertebrae<br>Osteophytosis<br>Fragmentation<br>Malalignment |
| Rheumatoid arthritis* | Apophyseal joint instability with recurrent discovertebral trauma<br>or<br>Inflammatory tissue extending from neighboring articulations | Disc space narrowing<br>Poorly or well-defined sclerotic vertebral margins<br>Subluxation<br>Apophyseal joint abnormalities |
| Calcium pyrophosphate dihydrate crystal deposition disease | Crystal deposition in cartilaginous endplate and intervertebral disc with degeneration | Disc space narrowing<br>Calcification<br>Poorly or well-defined sclerotic vertebral margins<br>Fragmentation<br>Subluxation |
| Alkaptonuria | Crystal deposition in cartilaginous endplate and intervertebral disc with degeneration | Disc space narrowing<br>Vacuum phenomena<br>Well-defined sclerotic vertebral margins<br>Calcification |

*Usually involves the cervical spine.

With disc displacement through the endplate, fissures may appear within the affected disc. These fissures course horizontally through the disc and extend vertically into the osseous defect. Gas collections within these clefts demonstrate a branching pattern, with both horizontal and vertical components, and gas may extend into the vertebral body at the site of displacement in a linear or arclike form. Detection of the branching nature of the vacuum phenomenon and its vertical component suggests the presence of intervertebral disc displacement even when the osseous defect itself is not apparent. Displacement of portions of a degenerating intervertebral disc into the spinal canal can be associated with gas formation in both the disc and the canal, a finding that is readily apparent with the use of computed tomography (CT) or MR imaging. The observation of gas overlying the spinal canal adjacent to a degenerative intervertebral disc strongly supports the diagnosis of intraspinal disc displacement.

Fracture and fragmentation of vertebrae with intraosseous vacuum phenomena have been described in cases of ischemic necrosis, particularly in patients taking steroid medications. Visualization of the crescent sign, a radiolucent region at the site of a linear or semicircular fracture through the subchondral bone, is suggestive of bone necrosis (Fig. 30–4) and is reminiscent of that accompanying ischemic necrosis of the femoral or humeral head. Intraosseous gas collections in collapsed vertebral bodies, however, may occur in the absence of bone necrosis. Radiolucent areas representing gas in the apophyseal joints of the spine, especially in the lumbar region, are occasionally present in patients with osteoarthritis in this location (Fig. 30–5). Similar areas have been noted in other degenerative joints, such as the sacroiliac articulations.

Vacuum phenomena are a frequent finding in the vertebral column and can be localized to the intervertebral disc or, less commonly, the spinal canal, apophyseal joints,

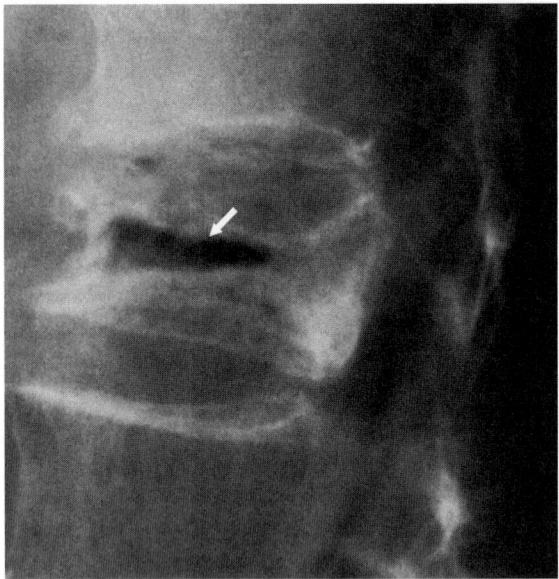

**Figure 30–4.** Types of vacuum phenomena: vacuum vertebral body. Note the intraosseous gas collection *(arrow)*. This finding is virtually diagnostic for non-neoplastic, noninfectious vertebral collapse, presumably related to ischemic necrosis.

(From Resnick D: Degenerative diseases of the vertebral column. Radiology 156:3, 1985.)

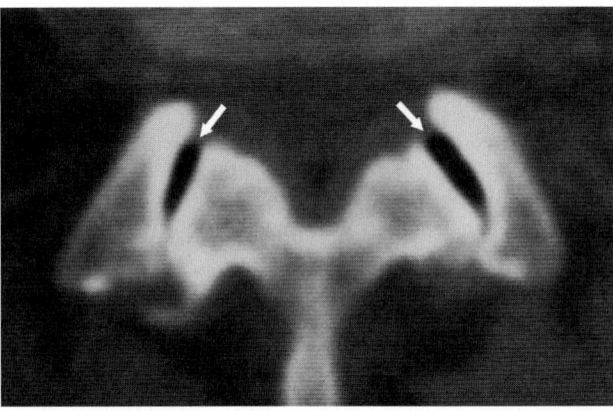

**Figure 30–5.** Types of vacuum phenomena: osteoarthritis of the apophyseal joints. Transaxial CT scan of the apophyseal joints of a lumbar vertebra shows bilateral vacuum phenomena *(arrows)* and minor changes of osteoarthritis.

soft tissues, and vertebral bodies (Table 30–4). The presence of radiolucent collections within an intervertebral disc or vertebra militates against the diagnosis of infection. In cases in which the cause of destruction in two adjacent vertebral bodies with narrowing of the intervertebral disc or vertebral collapse is unknown, radiographic elicitation of a vacuum phenomenon in the disc or bone obtained during trunk extension (Fig. 30–6) virtually excludes the possibility of infection and makes the presence of tumor highly unlikely.

### TABLE 30–4

**Types of Spinal Vacuum Phenomena**

| Disease or Condition | Location of Vacuum Phenomenon |
| --- | --- |
| Intervertebral (osteo)chondrosis | Nucleus pulposus, anulus fibrosus |
| Spondylosis deformans | Anulus fibrosus |
| Cartilaginous node | Intervertebral disc within vertebral body |
| Intraspinal disc displacement | Intervertebral disc within spinal canal or epidural space |
| Osteoarthritis | Apophyseal joint |
| Ischemic necrosis | Vertebral body |

Routine radiographs are relatively insensitive in detecting the early stages of intervertebral (osteo)chondrosis, and MR imaging has been shown to be useful in this regard. The MR imaging signal characteristics of a normal intervertebral disc and those accompanying intervertebral (osteo)chondrosis are well summarized by Modic and coworkers. In the normal situation, the region of the vertebral endplate has decreased signal intensity on both T1- and T2-weighted images. On T1-weighted images, the central portion of the intervertebral disc has slightly decreased signal intensity in comparison to the peripheral portion, which blends with an area of even further decreased signal intensity in the region of the outer fibers of the anulus fibrosus. On T2-weighted spin echo sequences, the normal intervertebral disc consists of a central region of high signal intensity and a peripheral region of decreased signal intensity. As a general rule, the signal intensity of a normal intervertebral disc is lower than that of the vertebral body on T1-weighted spin echo images and is higher than that of the vertebral body on T2-weighted spin echo or gradient echo images and other fluid-sensitive sequences (Fig. 30–7).

Intervertebral (osteo)chondrosis is associated with modifications of the normal signal patterns. In the intervertebral disc, loss of signal intensity is evident on T2-weighted spin echo sequences; this is believed to be secondary to changes in hydration. Loss of disc height accompanies these changes in signal intensity. Vacuum phenomena, as well as calcification, in such discs typically (but not invariably) appear as areas of signal void. Fluid collecting within clefts at the site of a vacuum phenomenon causes these regions to appear as sites of high signal intensity on T2-weighted spin echo MR images. Disc calcification occasionally reveals high signal intensity on T1-weighted spin echo MR images.

Alterations in signal intensity of the vertebral body marrow in patients with disc degeneration were first emphasized by Modic and Ross and their coworkers. Three types of changes commonly accompany intervertebral (osteo)chondrosis:

*Type I.* These changes, which consist of decreased signal intensity on T1-weighted images and increased signal intensity on T2-weighted images, occur in approxi-

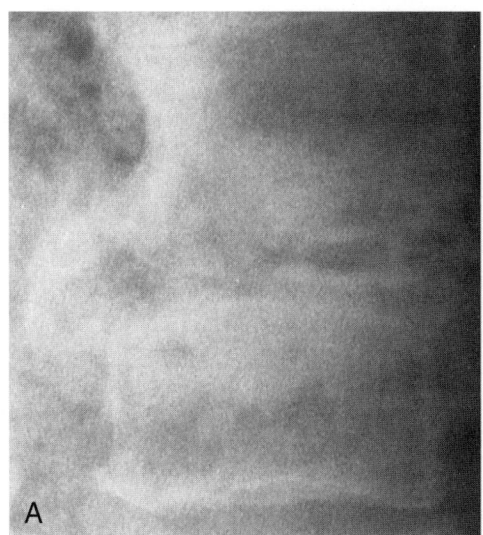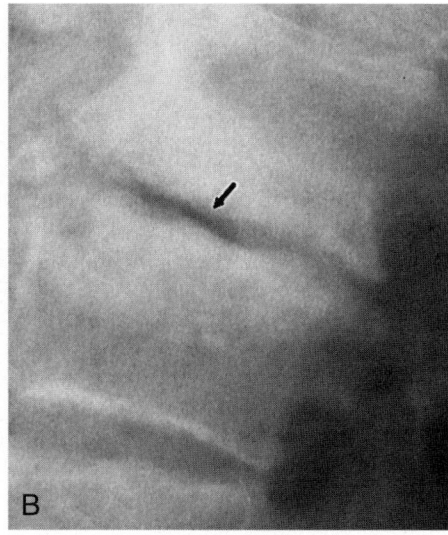

**Figure 30–6.** Disc vacuum phenomenon produced by trunk extension. Lateral radiographs of the lumbar spine obtained with the patient in the neutral position *(A)* and with the trunk hyperextended *(B)* reveal an intradiscal gas collection *(arrow* in *B)*, which virtually eliminates the diagnosis of spinal infection.

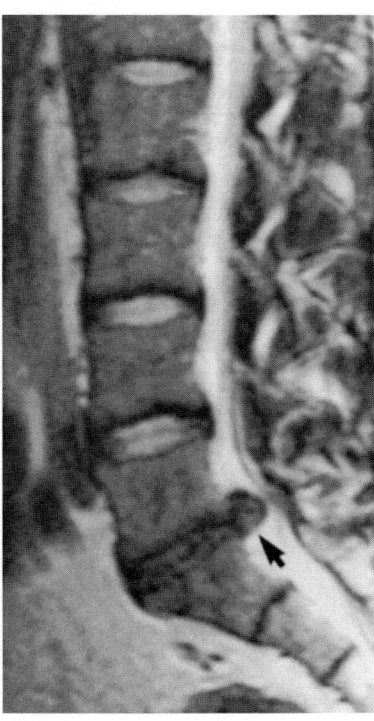

**Figure 30–7.** Normal and abnormal intervertebral disc: sagittal T2-weighted (TR/TE, 3400/96) spin echo MR imaging technique. In discs that are relatively normal (L1–L2, L3–L4, and L4–L5), a central portion of high signal intensity containing a horizontal line of low signal intensity is evident. In the disc (L2–L3) with mild intervertebral (osteo)chondrosis, minimal loss of signal intensity is seen, particularly in its anterior third. With severe intervertebral (osteo)chondrosis (L5–S1), the disc is of low signal intensity and diminished in height. A large posterior extruded disc *(arrow)* with low signal intensity is also evident.

mately 4% of patients undergoing MR imaging for lumbar disc disease. Type I abnormalities are histologically characterized by replacement of normal cellular vertebral body marrow with fibrovascular marrow (Fig. 30–8).

*Type II.* These changes are manifested as increased signal intensity on T1-weighted images and as isointensity or slightly increased signal intensity on T2-weighted images. They occur in approximately 16% of patients undergoing MR imaging examination for lumbar disc disease. Histologically, these changes correspond to conversion sites of hematopoietic marrow to fatty marrow (Fig. 30–9).

*Type III.* These changes are represented by decreased signal intensity on both T1- and T2-weighted images and, unlike type I and II changes, are associated with sclerosis in the vertebral bodies. Type III changes reflect the absence of marrow in regions of considerable bone sclerosis (Fig. 30–10).

## Spondylosis Deformans

The most obvious pathologic and radiographic degenerative disease of the spine is associated with bone production, particularly along the anterior and lateral aspects of the vertebral column. The outgrowths are termed osteophytes, although spondylosis deformans is currently the most popular and accurate designation. Spinal osteophytosis is extremely common. By the age of 50 years, approximately 60% of women and 80% of men have such excrescences. These bony outgrowths are more frequent in men than in women and are more common in the older population. Any segment of the vertebral column can be affected; in the thoracic spine, right-sided out-

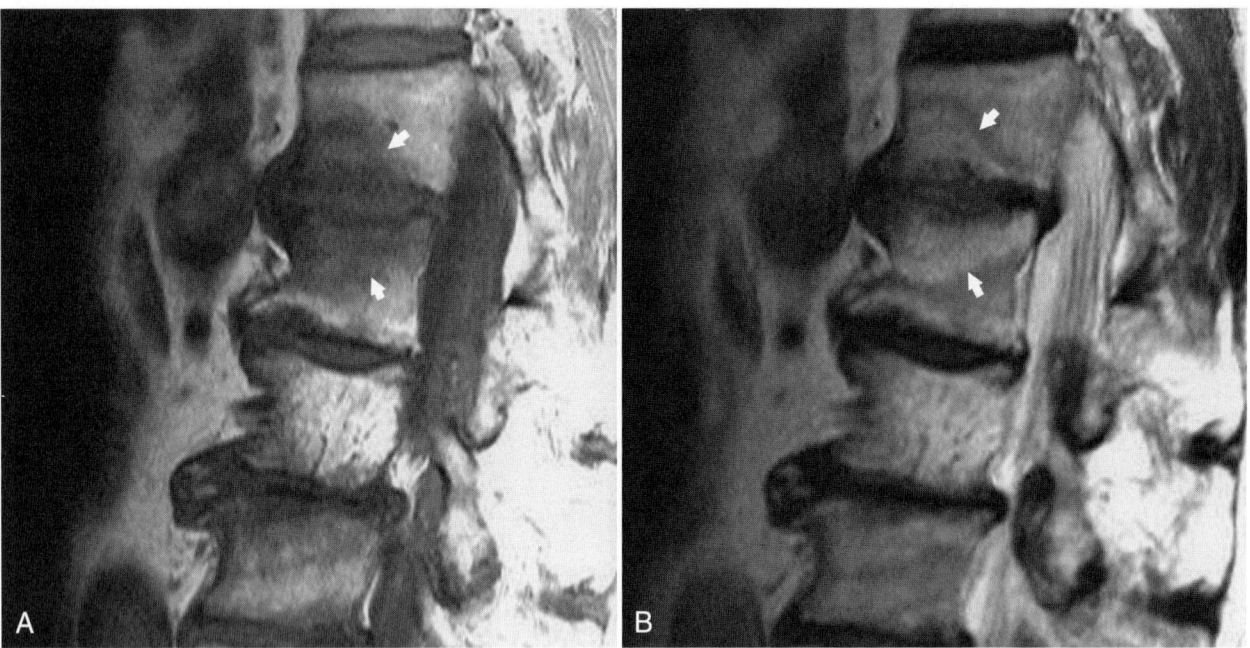

**Figure 30–8.** Abnormal intervertebral disc: Modic type I change. *A*, Sagittal T1-weighted (TR/TE, 650/15) spin echo MR image shows decreased signal intensity *(arrows)*. B, Sagittal T2-weighted (TR/TE, 4400/108) spin echo MR image shows increased signal intensity *(arrows)*.

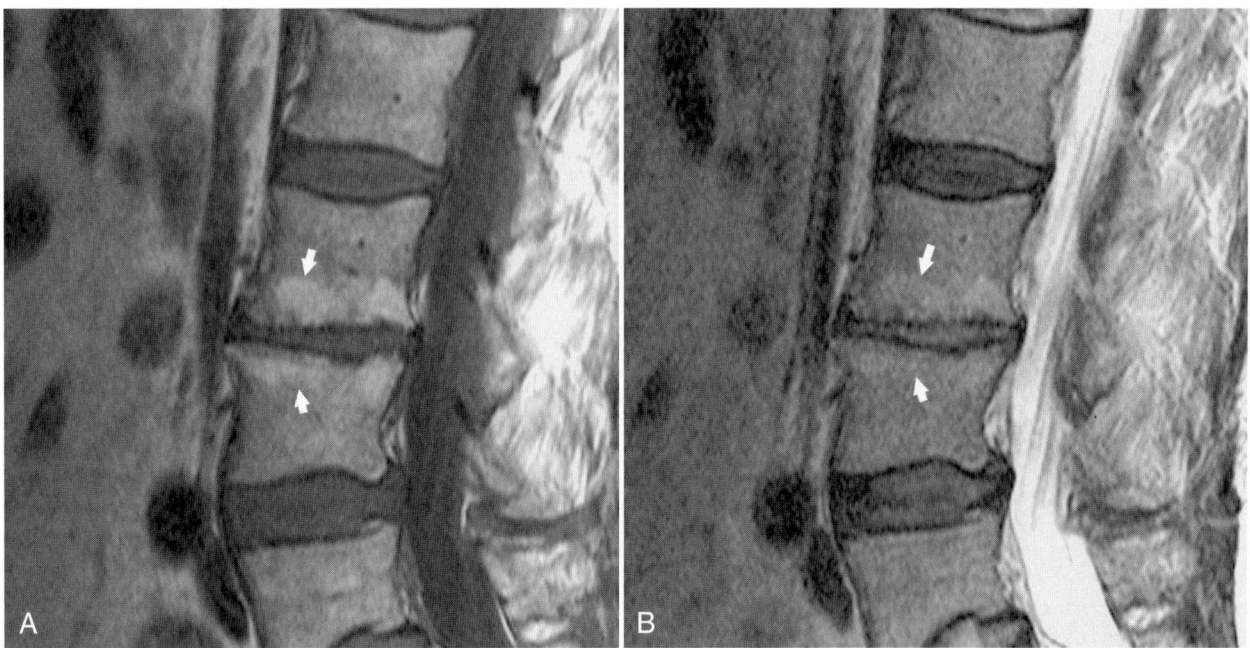

**Figure 30–9.** Abnormal intervertebral disc: Modic type II change. *A*, Sagittal T1-weighted (TR/TE, 663/12) spin echo MR image shows increased signal intensity *(arrows)*. B, Sagittal T2-weighted (TR/TE, 4630/138) spin echo MR image shows isointense or slightly increased signal intensity *(arrows)*.

growths predominate, presumably related to pulsations of the descending aorta on the left side.

Schmorl's concept of the pathogenesis of spondylosis deformans, with some modification, is generally accepted today (Fig. 30–11). This concept emphasizes abnormalities in the peripheral fibers of the anulus fibrosus as the initiating factor in this disorder. Once the attachment between the anulus fibrosus and the vertebral rim is disrupted, even though this attachment is related to the presence of calcified cartilage, minor degrees of anterior and anterolateral disc displacement are possible and may lead to traction at the site of osseous attachment of the

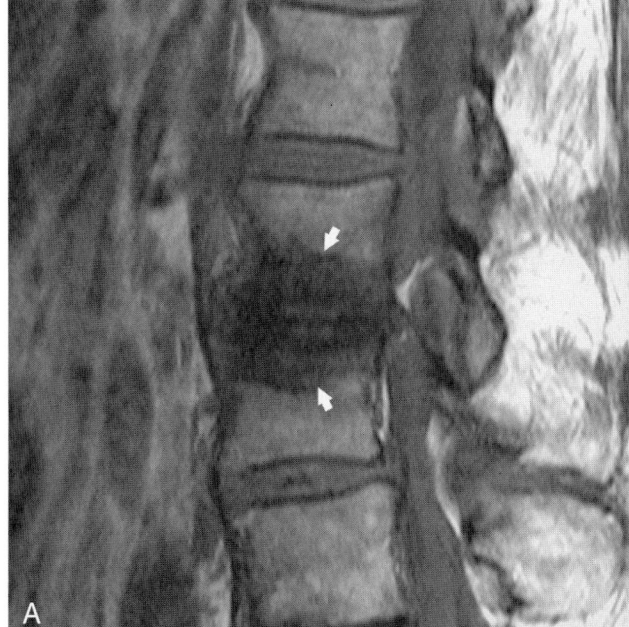
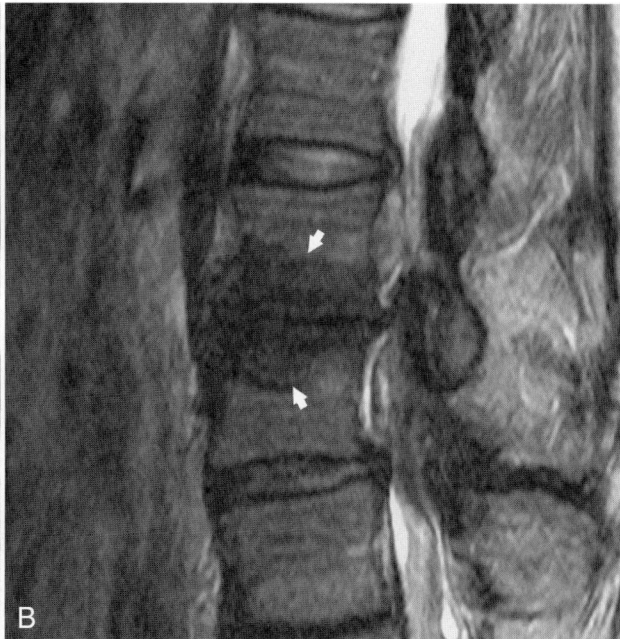
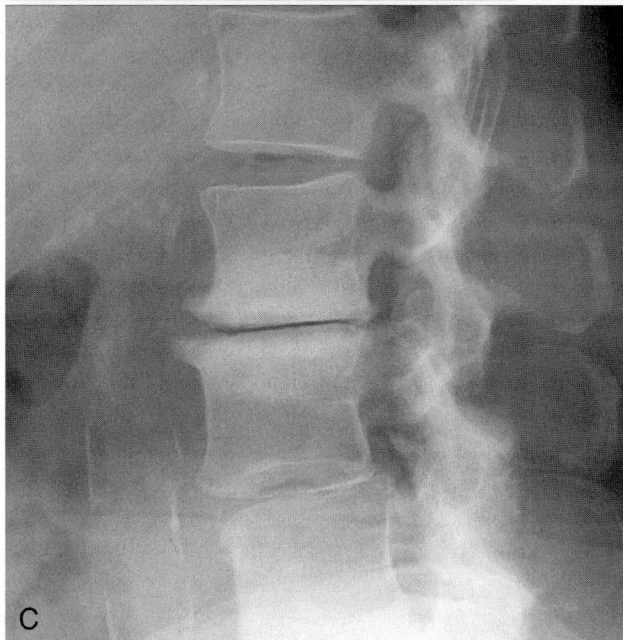

**Figure 30–10.** Abnormal intervertebral disc: Modic type III change. *A* and *B*, Sagittal T1-weighted (TR/TE, 533/20) *(A)* and T2-weighted (TR/TE, 4000/102) *(B)* spin echo MR images both show decreased signal intensity *(arrows)*. *C*, Lateral radiograph shows considerable bone sclerosis in areas of decreased signal intensity. Note the vacuum disc.

outermost fibers of the anulus fibrosus or short perivertebral ligaments to the vertebral surfaces. Osteophytes develop at this location, several millimeters from the discovertebral junction (Fig. 30–12). The type and severity of clinical manifestations related to spinal osteophytes depend on the size and location of the outgrowths and their relationship to adjacent soft tissue and neurologic structures. Dysphagia, stiffness, restricted motion, and even pain can probably be attributed to spinal osteophytes in some patients. Neurologic deficits produced by bony impingement on the spinal cord are unusual.

Spinal osteophytes accompanying spondylosis deformans must be differentiated from other bony outgrowths of the vertebral column (Fig. 30–13). Small triangular osteophytes are encountered in intervertebral (osteo)-

chondrosis. In this condition, enlarging tears of the nucleus pulposus may extend into the anulus fibrosus and eventually lead to the disruption of annular attachments to bone. The changes of spondylosis deformans are then superimposed on those of intervertebral (osteo)chondrosis. Additional findings of intervertebral (osteo)chondrosis are seen, including loss of disc integrity with diminution of intervertebral disc height, approximation of adjacent osseous surfaces, and reactive sclerosis and bone formation. Diffuse idiopathic skeletal hyperostosis is associated with extensive ossification along the anterior and lateral aspects of the vertebral column, resembling the features of severe spondylosis deformans. Ankylosing spondylitis is characterized by ossification within the outer portion of the anulus fibrosus, resulting in outgrowths (syndesmo-

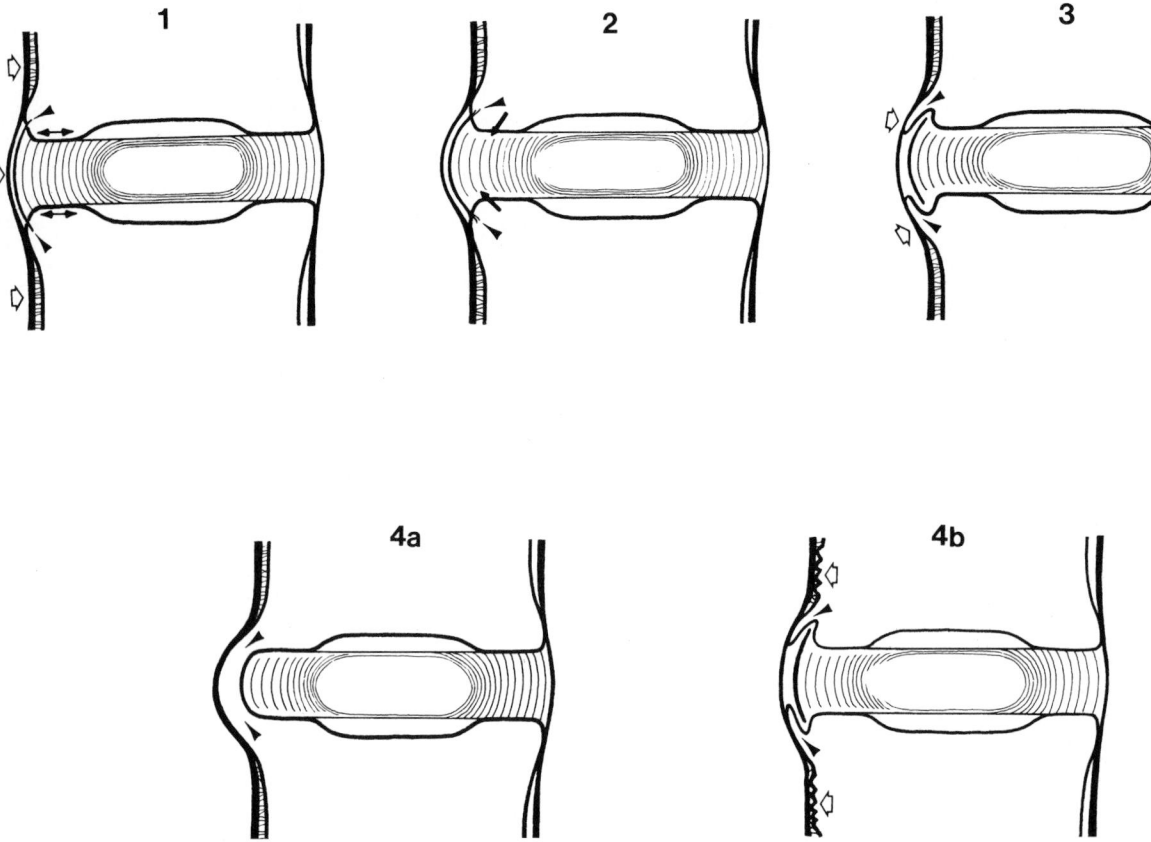

**Figure 30–11.** Spondylosis deformans: progressive stages. The normal situation is depicted in (1). The anulus fibrosus is attached to the vertebral rim by calcified cartilage *(double-headed arrows)* and to the anterior vertebral surface by Sharpey's fibers *(arrowheads)*. The anterior longitudinal ligament *(open arrows)* is connected to the anterior vertebral surface. In (2), breakdown in sites of attachment of the anulus fibrosus to the vertebral rim is evident *(arrows)*, although Sharpey's fibers *(arrowheads)* are intact. Mild anterior disc displacement is seen. With progression of disease, as shown in (3), osteophytes *(arrowheads)* develop at the site of attachment of Sharpey's fibers to the anterior vertebral surface. The anterior longitudinal ligament *(open arrows)* is stretched by the displaced intervertebral disc. With still further progression, as in (4a), an osteophyte may bridge the intervertebral disc *(arrowheads)*. Alternatively, as in (4b), continued traction on the anterior longitudinal ligament may lead to proliferative enthesopathy, with the production of new bone *(open arrows)* at its site of attachment to the anterior vertebral surface, combined with more typical osteophytes *(arrowheads)*.

(3, From Resnick D: Degenerative diseases of the vertebral column. Radiology 156:3, 1985.)

phytes) that are typically thin and vertically oriented as they extend from one vertebral body to the next. Bony outgrowths in psoriasis and Reiter's syndrome may resemble the typical syndesmophytes of ankylosing spondylitis or appear as distinct paravertebral ossifications. In the latter circumstance, they are separated from the vertebral surface and, initially, possess a poorly defined or irregular contour.

Osseous excrescences of the spine accompanying neuropathic osteoarthropathy and ochronosis do not resemble the outgrowths of spondylosis deformans. Spinal infection or trauma can produce outgrowths that are identical to those of spondylosis deformans; however, they are usually localized to one (or two) sites. Fluorosis leads to osteophytosis identical to that in spondylosis deformans, but additional radiographic findings (e.g., increased osseous density and ligamentous ossification) allow an accurate diagnosis. Additional causes of bony excrescences of the spine that may resemble or are identical to the osteophytes of spondylosis deformans are hypoparathyroidism, sternocostoclavicular hyperostosis, acne conglobata, paralysis, and certain medications such as vitamin A derivatives.

## Uncovertebral (Neurocentral) Joint Arthrosis

The five lowest cervical vertebral bodies (C3 to C7) contain bony ridges extending from each side—the uncinate, or lunate, processes. Between the superior process of the lower vertebral body and the inferior process of the upper vertebral body is a joint termed the uncovertebral or neurocentral joint, or joint of Luschka.

With increasing intervertebral disc degeneration, progressive loss of disc space height occurs, and the bony

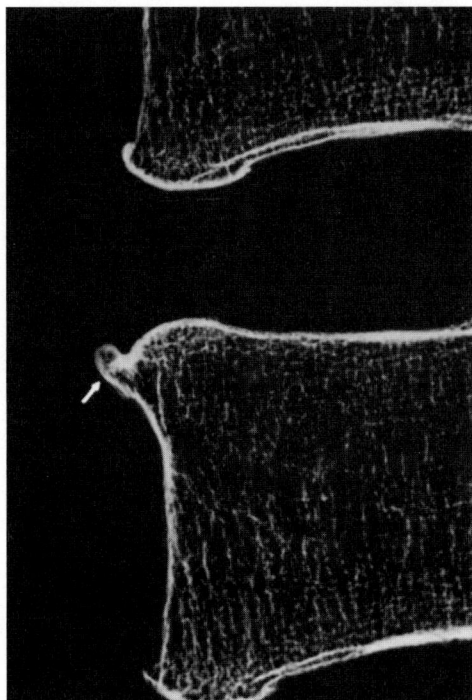

**Figure 30–12.** Spondylosis deformans: radiographic-pathologic correlation. Radiograph of a macerated sagittal section of a lumbar spine reveals the characteristics of an osteophyte *(arrow)*. Note that it develops several millimeters from the vertebral rim and extends first in a horizontal direction and then in a vertical one.

(From Resnick D: Degenerative diseases of the vertebral column. Radiology 156:3, 1985.)

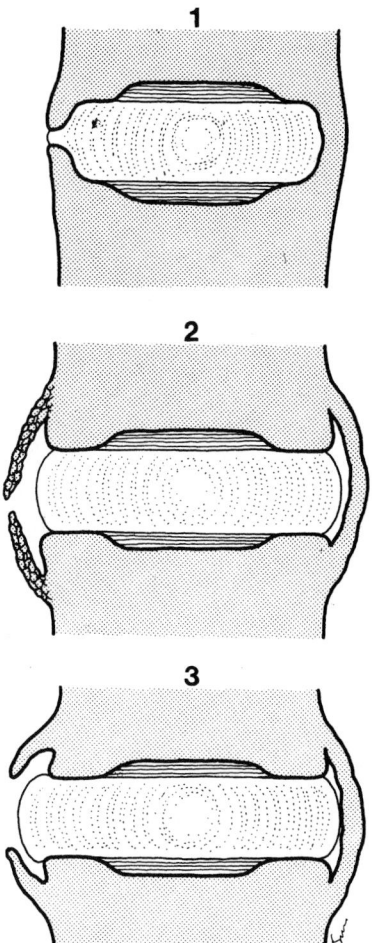

**Figure 30–13.** Bony outgrowths of the spine: differential diagnosis. A variety of conditions can lead to bony outgrowths of the vertebral column. Illustrated here are ankylosing spondylitis (1), psoriatic arthritis and Reiter's syndrome (2), and spondylosis deformans (3). In each drawing, the early appearance of the outgrowth is depicted on the left and the later appearance on the right. In ankylosing spondylitis, ossification occurs within the anulus fibrosus in the form of a syndesmophyte, which may eventually bridge the intervertebral disc space; observe the vertical configuration of the syndesmophyte. In psoriatic arthritis and Reiter's syndrome, paravertebral ossification forms in the connective tissue at some distance from the spine. Initial irregular or poorly defined outgrowths may subsequently become better defined and merge with the vertebral bodies. In spondylosis deformans, the osteophytes begin as triangular outgrowths located several millimeters from the edge of the vertebral body. These, too, may eventually bridge the intervertebral disc space.

protuberances about the uncovertebral joints approach each other. With further disc deterioration, the articular processes are pressed firmly together, and the intervening joint degenerates. Osteophytes produce humplike or pointed outgrowths that enlarge the articular surface. They project from the posterior edge of the vertebral body into the disc space and into the intervertebral foramina (Fig. 30–14). At the latter site, they compromise the adjacent nerve roots. On frontal projections, the rounded uncinate processes and the narrowed joint space are readily apparent. On the lateral projection, a radiolucent line extending in an anteroposterior direction, overlying the vertebral body, is easily misinterpreted as a fracture.

## Synovial Joints

**Apophyseal Joint Osteoarthritis (Osteoarthrosis).** The apophyseal joints of the vertebral column are a frequent site of degenerative joint disease. Changes commonly predominate in the middle and lower cervical spine, mid and upper thoracic spine, and the lower lumbar spine. Fibrillation and erosion of articular cartilage, progressing to irregularity, and partial or complete denudation of the cartilaginous surface are accompanied by radiographically detectable joint space narrowing. Bony eburnation and osteophytes are frequent and may be associated with intra-articular osseous and cartilaginous bodies (Fig. 30–15). Capsular laxity allows malalignment and subluxation of one vertebra on another, a process that has been termed degenerative spondylolisthesis or pseudospondylolisthesis. Occasionally, especially in the cervical spine, intra-articular bony ankylosis can result, simulating the appearance of ankylosing spondylitis or juvenile chronic arthritis.

CT or MR imaging, with its cross-sectional display, is ideal for delineating osseous and soft tissue alterations of degenerative disease of the apophyseal joints; in addition,

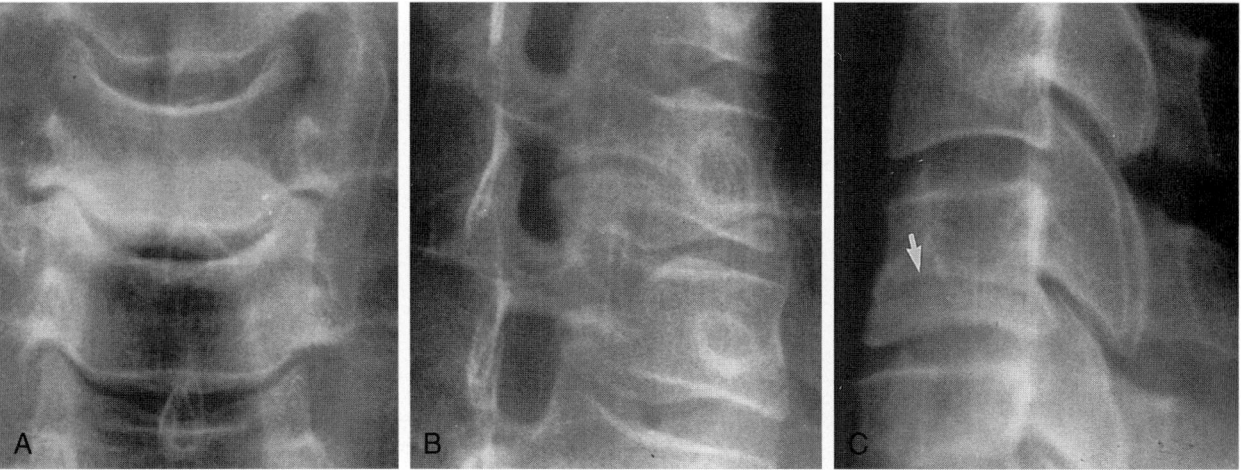

**Figure 30–14.** Uncovertebral (neurocentral) joint arthrosis: radiographic abnormalities. Frontal *(A)*, oblique *(B)*, and lateral *(C)* radiographs show arthrosis of the uncovertebral joints, particularly at the C5–C6 level, that has led to narrowing of the corresponding intervertebral foramen *(B)* and a radiolucent line *(arrow in C)* simulating a fracture.

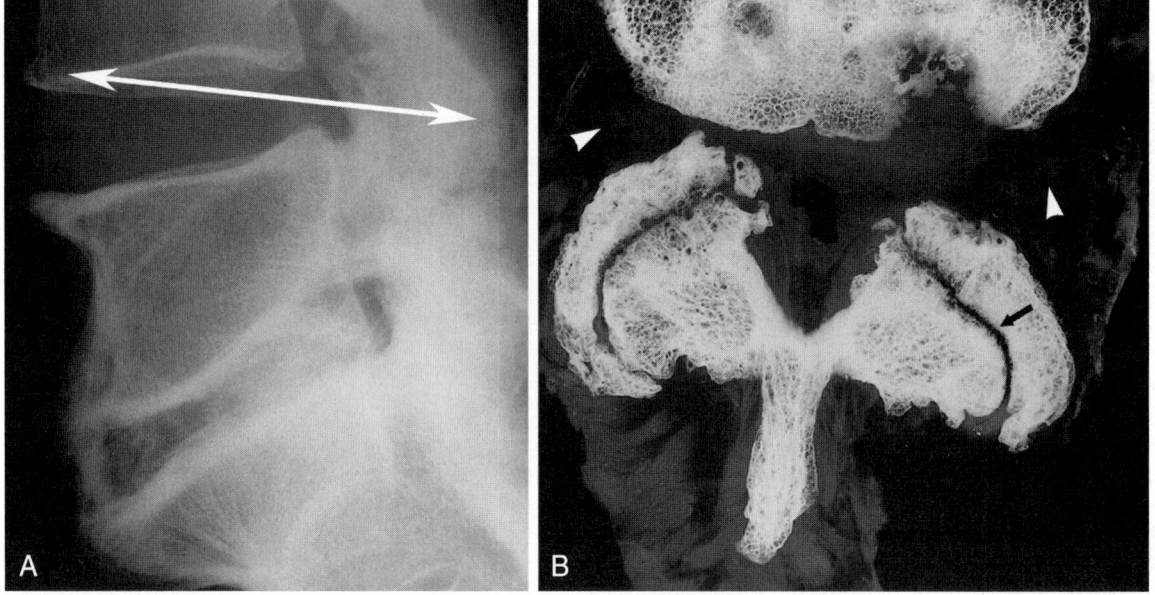

**Figure 30–15.** Apophyseal joint osteoarthritis: lumbar spine. *A*, Lateral radiograph of a cadaveric spine shows considerable alterations of osteoarthritis involving the apophyseal joints between the fourth and fifth lumbar vertebrae and between the fifth lumbar vertebra and the sacrum. Joint space narrowing, bone sclerosis, and osteophytes are apparent. *B*, Radiograph of a transverse section at the approximate level indicated by the double-headed arrow in *(A)* reveals the osteoarthritic changes to better advantage. Findings include joint space narrowing, vacuum phenomenon *(arrow)*, and bone fragmentation in the articular processes. Although the neural foramina are narrowed, there is no impingement on the nerve roots *(arrowheads)*, which have passed through the foramina at a higher level.

(B, From Resnick D: Degenerative diseases of the vertebral column. Radiology 156:3, 1985.)

the relationship of bone proliferation to the central spinal canal, lateral recesses, and neural foramina can be defined. The presence of a vacuum phenomenon in the osteoarthritic apophyseal joint leads to an arclike radiolucent collection between the articular processes. In some patients with osteoarthritis of the apophyseal joints, MR imaging reveals altered signal intensity in the adjacent pedicle,

presumably related to stress-induced marrow edema. Prominent clinical symptoms and signs may accompany osteoarthritis of the apophyseal joints. The synovial membrane, capsules, and ligaments of these articulations are richly supplied with nerves, which may explain the common but controversial occurrence of pain in patients with degenerative joint disease at these sites.

**Costovertebral Joint Osteoarthritis (Osteoarthrosis).** The costovertebral joints are located between the heads of the ribs and the vertebral bodies and between the necks and tubercles of the ribs and the transverse processes of the vertebrae (costotransverse joints). Degenerative changes predominate in the articulations of the 11th and 12th ribs. Joint space narrowing, bony eburnation, and osteophytosis are the expected alterations (Fig. 30–16), although radiographic demonstration of these changes is difficult because of the adjacent osseous shadows of the vertebral bodies and ribs. Osteoarthritis of the costovertebral joints may lead to partial or complete bone bridging between the vertebrae and ribs This finding is associated with pagetoid, or Paget's disease–like, cortical thickening and hyperostosis of the posterior portion of the affected ribs. The pathogenesis of these bone changes appears to be stress exerted by muscles affixed to ribs made hypomobile or immobile by the exuberant osteophytosis.

**Osteoarthritis (Osteoarthrosis) of Transitional Lumbosacral Joints.** Congenital variations at the lumbosacral junction are frequent, and many transitional patterns are encoun-tered. Newly formed articulations may exist between the enlarged transverse process of the involved vertebra and the wings of the sacrum (or, infrequently, the ilium). These articulations have a bilateral or unilateral distribution. Osteoarthritis can result from abnormal stress and move-ment at the various joints. Articular space narrowing, scle-rosis, and osteophytosis are evident. Bony ankylosis may eventually occur. The relationship of back pain to congenital transitional vertebrae at the lumbosacral junc-tion is not clear. The relationship between transitional lumbosacral joints and posteriorly extruded discs is also debated.

**Osteoarthritis (Osteoarthrosis) of Median and Lateral Atlantoaxial Joints.** Degenerative abnormalities in the anterior median atlantoaxial joint (Fig. 30–17) are reported infrequently. They are generally regarded as incidental findings. On radiographs and conventional tomograms in the lateral projection, narrowing of the interosseous space is observed between the anterior arch of the atlas and the odontoid process, frequently combined with cortical thickening and osteophytosis. CT findings of osteoarthritis of the anterior median atlantoaxial joint include osteo-phytes of the median facet of the atlas, small ossicles, and calcification of the transverse ligament. Such ligament calci-fication may also be a manifestation of calcium pyrophos-phate dihydrate crystal deposition disease.

## Fibrous Joints and Entheses

**Ligamentous Degeneration.** Degenerative abnormalities may become evident in various spinal ligaments, including the anterior longitudinal ligament; posterior longitudinal ligament; ligamenta flava; interspinous, supraspinous, and intertransverse ligaments; ligamentum nuchae; and iliolumbar ligaments. Because ligaments con-tain a rich supply of nerves, these processes are associated with pain and tenderness. Calcification and ossification within the anterior longitudinal ligament are characteristic of the ossifying diathesis that is present in diffuse idio-pathic skeletal hyperostosis; ossification of the posterior longitudinal ligament is also well recognized.

Supraspinous and interspinous ligament abnormalities frequently coexist. Excessive lordosis or extensive disc space loss leads to close approximation and contact of the

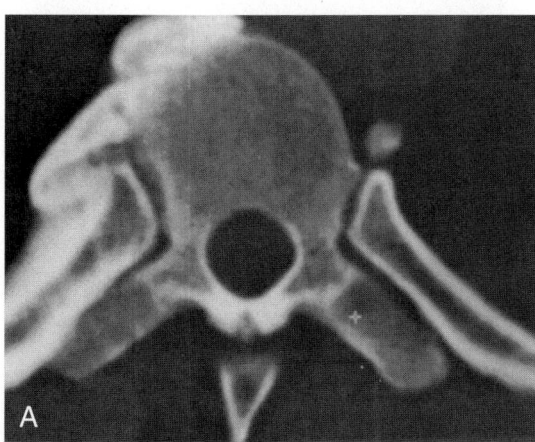

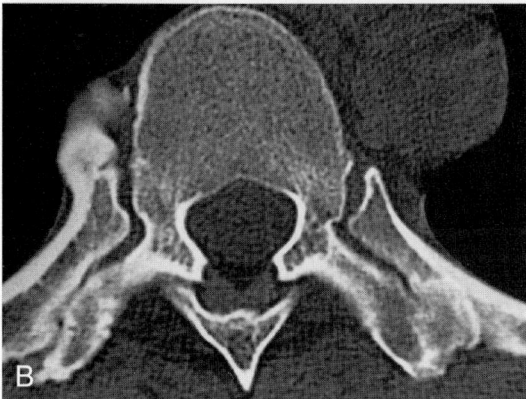

**Figure 30–16.** Costovertebral joint osteoarthritis: hyperos-tosis of adjacent ribs. *A,* Transaxial CT scan reveals a bridge of bone extending from the rib to the anterior surface of the ver-tebral body. Note the cortical thickening of the right rib. *B,* In a different patient, transaxial CT scan shows severe disease of both costotransverse joints, with bone ankylosis on the left and costovertebral bone proliferation on the right. (*A,* Courtesy of J. Haller, MD, Vienna, Austria.)

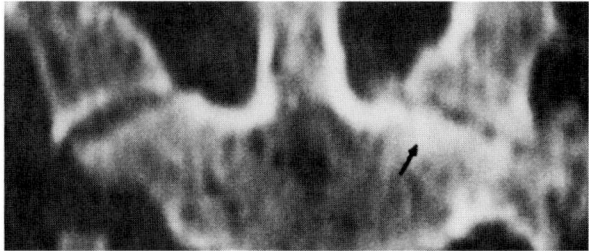

**Figure 30–17.** Osteoarthritis of the atlantoaxial joints. Reformatted coronal CT image reveals a minor offset between the atlas and the axis and considerable joint space narrowing and bone sclerosis in the left lateral atlantoaxial joint (*arrow*). (Courtesy of L. Kaseff, MD, Burlingame, Calif.)

spinous processes and to degeneration of the intervening ligaments, changes that can be evaluated with contrast examination. The "kissing spines" are subject to reactive eburnation (Baastrup's disease) and may be associated with considerable pain. Abnormal contact of apposing spinous processes, when combined with sclerosis in the superior and inferior portions of adjacent processes, is the characteristic radiographic abnormality. The spinous processes may appear enlarged (Fig. 30–18).

Ossification of varying degrees (or the presence of sesamoid bones) within the ligamentum nuchae is common and has no clinical significance. The iliolumbar ligament, which extends from the tip of the transverse process of the lowest lumbar vertebra to the iliac crest, sometimes calcifies, producing a horizontal radiodense band on radiographic examination. The pathogenesis of such ossification is unknown; however, it may be related to traumatic or congenital factors, and it is particularly common in patients with diffuse idiopathic skeletal hyperostosis. It may be associated with calcification in the sacrotuberous and interosseous sacroiliac ligaments.

## DEGENERATIVE DISEASES OF THE SPINE BY SEGMENT

### Cervical Spine

Degenerative changes of the intervertebral discs of the cervical spine (Fig. 30–19) are common after the age of 40 years and affect more than 70% of patients older than 70 years. Usually, multiple levels are altered, and changes

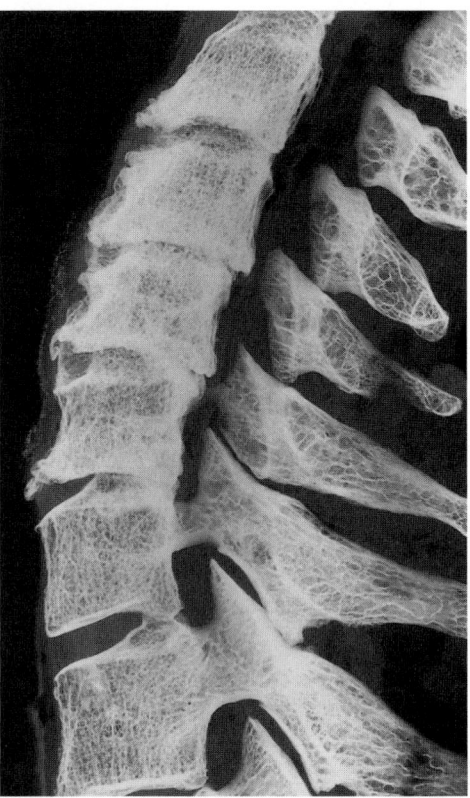

**Figure 30–19.** Degenerative disease of the cervical spine: intervertebral (osteo)chondrosis and ligamentous hypertrophy. In this radiograph of a sagittal section of the cervical spine, findings include widespread intervertebral (osteo)chondrosis, characterized by significant narrowing of multiple intervertebral discs, and ligamentous hypertrophy, leading to impingement on the spinal cord.

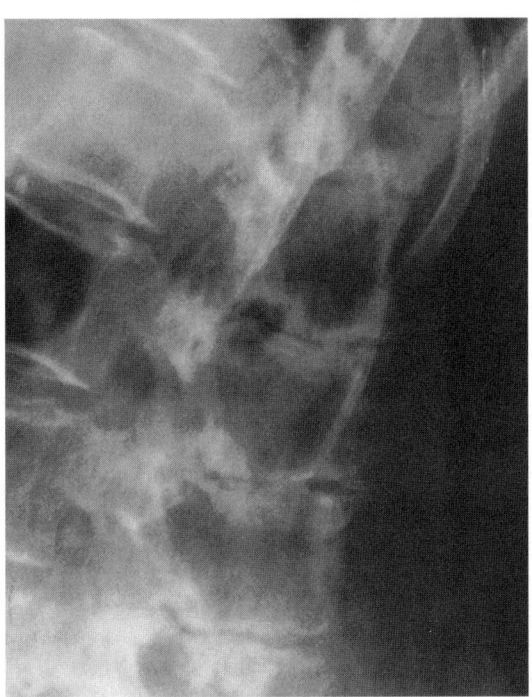

**Figure 30–18.** Baastrup's disease. Massive enlargement and prominent sclerosis of the spinous processes are evident. (Courtesy of C. Boles, MD, Hillside, Ill.)

predominate in the lower cervical spine. The most commonly involved site is the intervertebral disc at the C5–C6 level, followed by the C6–C7 level. Associated changes in the joints of Luschka show a predilection for these same levels. Osteoarthritis of the apophyseal joints is also most common in the middle and lower cervical spine.

### Thoracic Spine

Degenerative diseases of the lumbar and cervical spine have received more attention than those of the thoracic spine. Spondylosis deformans predominates in the middle and lower thoracic region, whereas intervertebral (osteo)chondrosis has a predilection for the midthoracic area. Obviously, costovertebral osteoarthritis is confined to the thoracic region.

### Lumbar Spine

Degenerative changes in the lumbar spine are frequent. Intervertebral (osteo)chondrosis, spondylosis deformans, or osteoarthritis of the apophyseal joints is detected on pathologic examination in 60% to 80% of men and women by the sixth decade of life and in about 100% of subjects by age 70 years. These changes predominate in the lower lumbar region, particularly between the fourth lumbar and first sacral segments. Disc space narrowing is very common in these areas, although assessment of disc space loss at the L5–S1 level is difficult because of the common occurrence of anatomic variations at this segment and discrepancies in the height of the anterior and posterior portions of the L5–S1 disc (posterior disc height is a more reliable indicator of the status of the disc). The clinical significance of radiographic evidence of degenerative disease in the lumbar spine is debated.

## COMPLICATIONS OF DEGENERATIVE DISEASES OF THE SPINE

### Alignment Abnormalities

**Segmental Instability.** Assessment of the degree and pattern of motion in the lumbar spine is possible with appropriate radiographs. In general, lateral radiographs with the patient in the neutral position and during spinal flexion and extension are obtained. Some investigators suggest the addition of frontal radiographs in the neutral attitude and with the patient bent to either side. General radiographic findings suggestive of instability include the presence of gas within the intervertebral disc, osteophytes on adjacent vertebral bodies below the rims of the end-plate (traction osteophytes), and evidence of a radial fissure in the intervertebral disc during discography. Lateral radiographs obtained in flexion and extension should be regarded as positive when they reveal forward or backward displacement of one vertebra with respect to another (Fig. 30–20), an abrupt change in the length of the pedicles, narrowing of the intervertebral foramina, and loss of height of an intervertebral disc. On frontal radiographs obtained with the patient bending first in one direction and then in the other, additional abnormalities include

asymmetry in the ability to bend in both directions, loss of normal vertebral rotation and tilt, abnormal degree of disc closure or opening, malalignment of spinous processes and pedicles, and lateral translation of one vertebra on another because of an abnormal degree of rotation. The traction osteophyte is an important sign of spinal instability (Fig. 30–21). This osseous excrescence arises on the anterior surface of the vertebral body, several millimeters from the discovertebral junction, and extends in a horizontal direction, developing at the site of attachment of the strong outermost fibers of the anulus fibrosus to the vertebral surface.

**Degenerative Anterior Spondylolisthesis.** The term *spondylolysis* refers to an interruption of the pars interarticularis of the vertebra. Although the cause of spondylolysis (Table 30–5) has been debated, most investigators now believe that it is an acquired abnormality characterized by a mechanical failure of bone related to abnormal vertebral stress. The term *spondylolisthesis* refers to displacement of one vertebra on another. Although spondylolisthesis often occurs with spondylolysis (Fig. 30–22), it may occur without it, often in association with degenerative disease.

Degenerative anterior spondylolisthesis occurs in approximately 4% of elderly patients and predominates at the interspace between the fourth and fifth lumbar vertebrae in older women. The facets at the L4–L5 level are oriented more sagittally than those at the L5–S1 level and are therefore more capable of allowing anterior movement. In the presence of degenerative joint changes, this sagittal orientation may become even more striking because of bone remodeling about the degenerative apophyseal joint. The check of one facet lying behind the other becomes deficient, and the inferior facets of the fourth lumbar vertebra gradually erode between the superior facets of the fifth lumbar vertebra and produce forward

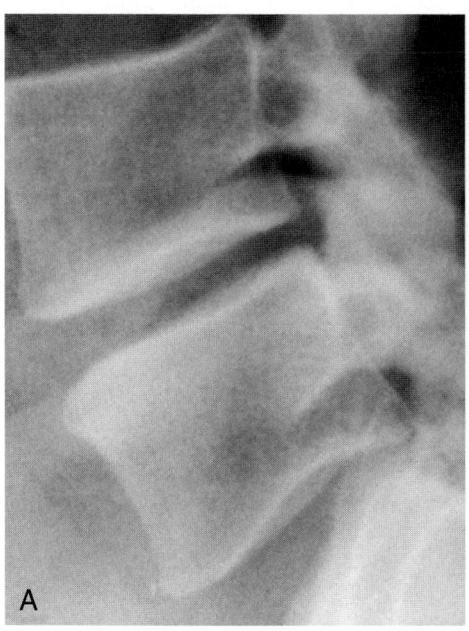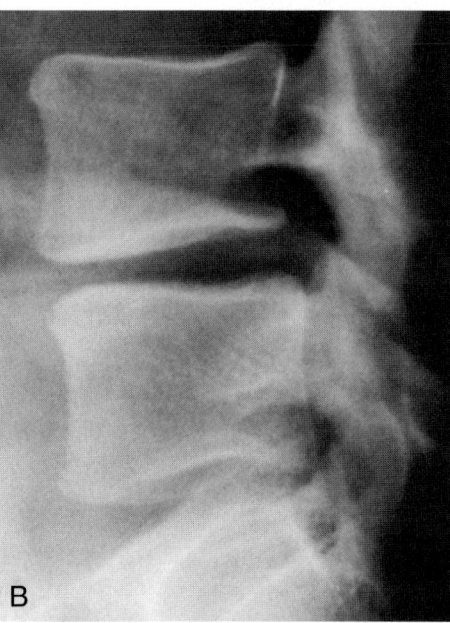

**Figure 30–20.** Segmental instability: abnormal vertebral movement. In these lateral radiographs obtained in extension *(A)* and flexion *(B)* of the lower part of the back, observe the narrowing of the intervertebral disc at the L4–L5 level. In *(B)*, note the abrupt change in the configuration of this disc and the anterior displacement of L4 with respect to L5. Bone sclerosis and early osteophytosis of the anterosuperior portion of L5 are also seen.

A    B

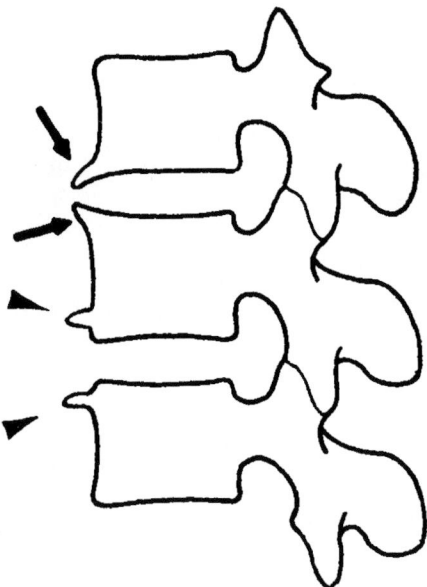

**Figure 30–21.** Segmental instability: traction versus claw osteophyte. A traction osteophyte *(arrowheads)* develops 2 to 3 mm from the edge of the intervertebral disc and projects in a horizontal direction. A claw osteophyte *(arrows)* develops closer to the disc margin and has a sweeping configuration. (Modified from Macnab I: The traction spur: An indicator of segmental instability. J Bone Joint Surg Am 53:663, 1971.)

displacement of L4 (Fig. 30–23). Clinical patterns associated with degenerative anterior spondylolisthesis include backache with or without leg pain, sciatica with or without backache but with signs of nerve root compression, and intermittent claudication of the cauda equina. Symptoms and signs related to bulged or extruded intervertebral discs are not uncommon. Radiographic findings of degenerative anterior spondylolisthesis include osteoarthritis of the apophyseal joints (articular space narrowing, sclerosis, and osteophytes), forward slipping of the superior vertebra on the inferior one, and, in some instances, intervertebral (osteo)chondrosis (vacuum phenomena, disc space narrowing, and vertebral body sclerosis).

**Degenerative Retrolisthesis.** Another pattern of spondylolisthesis without spondylolysis is a degenerative type associated with intervertebral (osteo)chondrosis. In this pattern, the characteristic posterior displacement of the superior vertebra led to the designation retrolisthesis (Fig. 30–24). The cause of degenerative retrolisthesis appears to be degeneration of the intervertebral disc (intervertebral [osteo]chondrosis), which results in decreased height of the involved disc space, closer approximation of adjacent vertebral bodies, and gliding or telescoping of the corresponding articular processes. Degenerative retrolisthesis is most frequent in mobile portions of the spine, particularly the cervical and lumbar spine. Radiographic findings include the typical changes of intervertebral (osteo)chondrosis (vacuum phenomena, disc space loss, vertebral body marginal sclerosis, and small osteophytes) and apophyseal joint instability and subluxation. Clinical findings include pain, an inability or unwillingness to bend forward or backward, rigidity, and neurologic abnormalities related to spinal cord compression.

**Senile Thoracic Kyphosis.** Exaggerated thoracic kyphosis is a common finding in older persons. This deformity may be related to one of two processes: kyphosis secondary to vertebral osteoporosis (osteoporotic kyphosis) or kyphosis secondary to degeneration of the anulus fibrosus (senile kyphosis). Kyphosis accompanying osteoporosis is noted in the middle and upper thoracic spine. Because of the normal dorsal kyphosis in this area, the anterior aspect of the vertebral bodies bears the greatest stress. In an osteoporotic spine, wedging or collapse of the weakened anterior vertebral surface is encountered. Senile thoracic kyphosis appears in older persons, particularly men, who do not have significant vertebral osteoporosis. The radiographic features of senile thoracic kyphosis resemble those of intervertebral (osteo)chondrosis, although the disc space narrowing and reactive sclerosis are located in a more anterior position in senile kyphosis. Senile thoracic kyphosis and osteoporotic (thoracic) kyphosis are similar in many ways: both occur in older patients, both involve the anterior aspect of the thoracic spine, and both produce progressive kyphosis (Table 30–6). The two processes are related to mechanical failure of vertebral structures: in senile thoracic kyphosis, the failure occurs in the anterior aspect of the intervertebral disc, and in osteoporotic

**TABLE 30–5**

**Spondylolisthesis**

| Type | Initial Cause of Abnormality | Initial Site of Abnormality | Direction of Slippage |
|---|---|---|---|
| Spondylolisthesis with spondylolysis | Trauma (? congenital predisposition) | Pars interarticularis | Anterior slippage of involved vertebra |
| Spondylolisthesis without spondylolysis | | | |
| Degenerative anterior spondylolisthesis | Osteoarthritis | Apophyseal joints | Anterior slippage of upper vertebra |
| Degenerative retrolisthesis | Intervertebral (osteo)chondrosis | Intervertebral disc | Posterior slippage of upper vertebra |

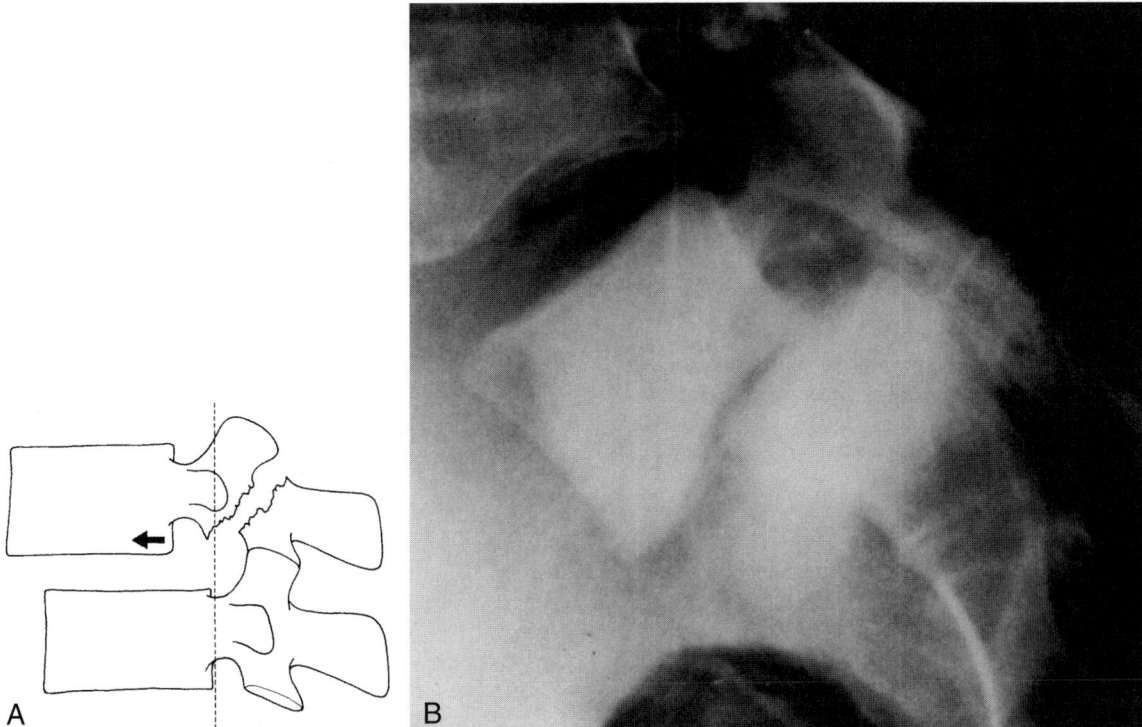

**Figure 30–22.** Spondylolisthesis with spondylolysis. *A*, Bilateral defects through the pars interarticularis allow anterior displacement of the vertebral body with respect to its neighbor. The alignment of the apophyseal joints is normal. *B*, Observe the anterior spondylolisthesis of the fifth lumbar vertebral body on the sacrum. The pars defects are not well delineated. Note the considerable intervertebral disc space narrowing, sclerosis, and fragmentation of the osseous surfaces.

kyphosis, the failure occurs in the weakened vertebral bodies. It is the wedgelike vertebral deformities of osteoporotic kyphosis that prevent the development of disc deterioration. Both senile and osteoporotic thoracic kyphosis can occur in the same patient.

**Degenerative Lumbar Scoliosis.** Scoliosis may occur in the lumbar spine of elderly persons. Degenerative lumbar scoliosis (Fig. 30–25) in elderly patients may progress, generally at a slow rate, although it occasionally develops in a rapid fashion. Its relationship to significant symptoms and signs, as well as to idiopathic scoliosis of adolescence, is debated. Typically, degenerative diseases of the spine do not lead to the development of scoliosis, although they may appear during the course of scoliosis.

**Degenerative Lumbar Kyphosis.** Although the occurrence of increased thoracic kyphosis and decreased lumbar lordosis in older persons is well recognized, marked loss of lordosis or even reversal of lordosis (i.e., kyphosis) in the lumbar spine as a degenerative phenomenon has been emphasized only recently. Affected persons walk in a forward-bending posture and complain of low back pain. Radiographs reveal a marked loss of sacral inclination, marked narrowing of the lumbar intervertebral discs, and

loss of height of the anterior portion of the lumbar vertebral bodies. The initiating event in this condition is not clear.

## Intervertebral Disc Displacement

Normally, the intervertebral disc is a load-bearing structure with hydrostatic properties related to its high water content. The nucleus pulposus consists of about 85% water, and the anulus fibrosus consists of 78% water; these percentages decrease to approximately 70% with degeneration. The anatomic arrangement of a centrally located nucleus pulposus surrounded by concentric lamellae of the anulus fibrosus allows the conversion of axial loading forces to tensile strain on the annular fibers and cartilaginous endplates. Disc pressure becomes elevated in the presence of abnormal externally applied loads. As the nucleus is subjected to elevated pressure, it attempts to prolapse from its confined space. The direction of this prolapse is variable; the intervertebral disc may be displaced anteriorly and laterally (spondylosis deformans), posteriorly or posterolaterally (intraspinal or intraforaminal displacement), or superiorly and inferiorly (cartilaginous nodes) (Table 30–7; Fig. 30–26).

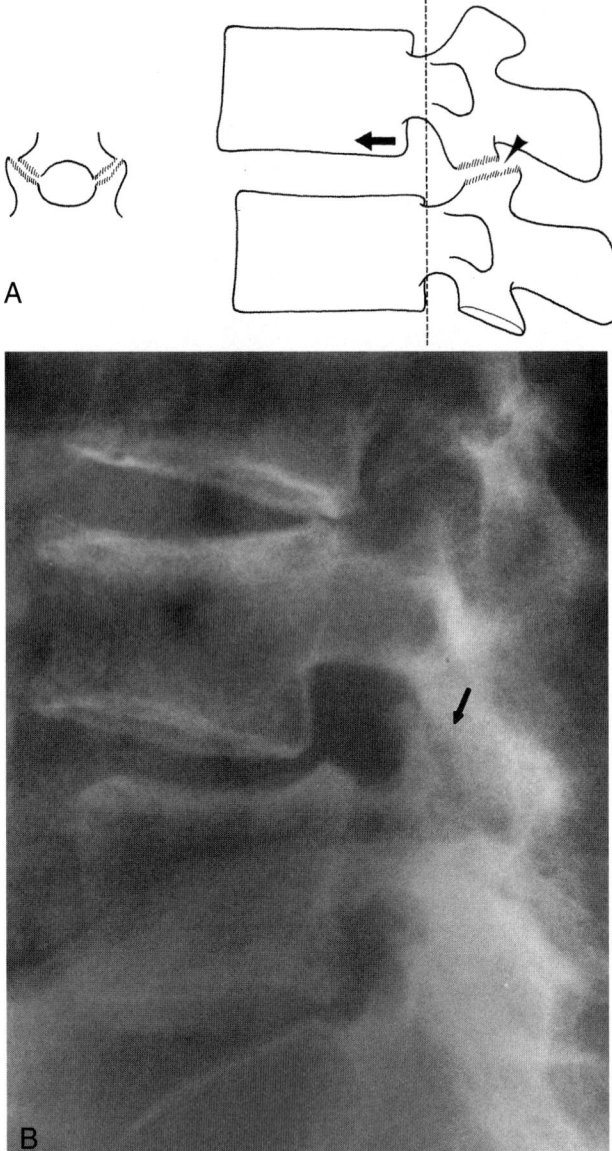

A

B

weaken or disrupt the endplate or subchondral bone (Table 30–8). These processes include Scheuermann's disease (juvenile kyphosis), trauma, infection, metabolic and endocrine disorders, and neoplasm.

The frequency of Schmorl's nodes varies according to the method used to detect them; it is highest (35% to 75% of cases) when careful pathologic inspection of the spine is accomplished and is quite low (approximately 10% of cases) when routine radiography is used. Cartilaginous nodes usually involve the lower cartilaginous plate and are more common in men than in women, especially in younger age groups. The radiographic and pathologic appearance of cartilaginous nodes is fundamentally similar, no matter what the specific cause (Fig. 30–27). A radiolucent lesion within the vertebral body, surrounded by helmet-shaped sclerosis that borders on the intervertebral disc, corresponds to a site of disc displacement contained within eburnated or thickened bony trabeculae. CT and MR imaging are diagnostic tools that can show characteristic features (Fig. 30–28). Cartilaginous nodes associated with enhancement of signal intensity in the adjacent vertebral body after intravenous injection of a gadolinium-containing contrast agent are believed by some authorities to be a cause of back pain.

A distinct type of cartilaginous node formation that may occur in association with intervertebral (osteo)chondrosis is characterized by intraosseous penetration of disc material at the junction of the cartilaginous endplate and the bony rim. This abnormality is observed in children in whom the developing apophyses have not yet fused with the remaining portion of the vertebral body. In these situations, displaced pieces of the intervertebral disc extend along an oblique course toward the outer surface of the vertebral body, with a small segment of bone subsequently isolated (Fig. 30–29). The resulting abnormality, which has been termed a limbus vertebra, is most common at the anterosuperior corner of a single lumbar vertebral body. Traumatically induced posterior limbus vertebrae (Fig. 30–30), especially in the lumbar spine, are associated with disc herniation.

**Posterior Disc Displacement.** Displacement of disc material in a posterior or posterolateral direction may occur suddenly or gradually and is of great clinical significance because of the intimate relationship between the intervertebral disc and important neurologic structures. Anatomic features predisposing to such disc displacement include the somewhat posterior position of the normal nucleus pulposus, the existence of fewer and weaker annular fibers in this region, and a posterior longitudinal ligament that is not as strong as the anterior longitudinal ligament. The extruded disc material may contain not only a portion of the nucleus pulposus but also pieces of the anulus fibrosus and the cartilaginous endplate.

Although the terminology used to indicate the extent of intervertebral disc displacement is not uniform, the following terms are generally accepted and indicate increasing stages of disc displacement (Fig. 30–31):

*Annular bulge:* In this situation, the annular fibers remain intact but protrude in a localized or diffuse fashion into the spinal canal.

**Figure 30–23.** Spondylolisthesis without spondylolysis: degenerative anterior spondylolisthesis. *A,* Apophyseal joint osteoarthritis *(arrowhead)* allows the inferior articular processes to move anteriorly and produce forward subluxation of the superior vertebra on the inferior vertebra. The inset demonstrates the manner in which the abnormal apophyseal joints may allow anterior subluxation. *B,* Osteoarthritis of the apophyseal joints between the fourth and fifth lumbar vertebrae *(arrow)* has led to anterior displacement of the upper vertebra with respect to the lower.

(*B,* From Resnick D: Degenerative diseases of the vertebral column. Radiology 156:3, 1985.)

**Anterolateral Disc Displacement.** Displacement of intervertebral disc material after degeneration of the fibers of the anulus fibrosus produces the pathologic and radiographic features of spondylosis deformans. Usually, the stretched anterior longitudinal ligament prevents complete displacement of disc contents.

**Superior and Inferior Disc Displacement.** Cartilaginous nodes are also apparent in other disease processes that

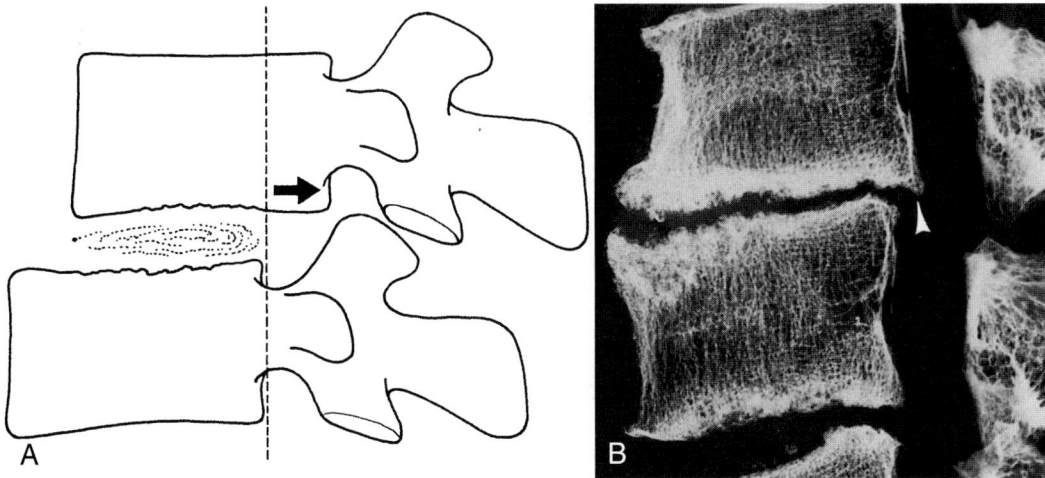

**Figure 30–24.** Spondylolisthesis without spondylolysis: degenerative retrolisthesis. *A,* As the intervertebral disc space narrows because of intervertebral (osteo)chondrosis, telescoping of the apophyseal joints allows backward displacement of the upper lumbar vertebra with respect to the lower one. *B,* Retrolisthesis of L2 in relation to L3 *(arrowhead)* is related to severe intervertebral (osteo)chondrosis in the intervening intervertebral disc.

(*B,* From Resnick D: Degenerative diseases of the vertebral column. Radiology 156:3, 1985.)

**TABLE 30–6**

**Senile versus Osteoporotic Kyphosis**

|  | Age Group | Initial Site of Abnormality | Radiographic Abnormalities |
|---|---|---|---|
| Senile kyphosis | Elderly | Anterior aspect of intervertebral disc | Disc space loss<br>Vertebral body sclerosis<br>Ankylosis of intervertebral disc |
| Osteoporotic kyphosis | Elderly | Anterior aspect of vertebral body | Osteoporosis<br>Wedge-shaped vertebrae |

*Disc protrusion:* The displaced nucleus pulposus extends through some of the fibers of the anulus fibrosus but is still confined by the intact outermost fibers.

*Disc extrusion:* The displaced nucleus pulposus penetrates all the fibers of the anulus fibrosus and lies under the posterior longitudinal ligament.

*Disc sequestration:* The displaced nucleus pulposus penetrates or extends around the posterior longitudinal ligament and lies within the epidural space, or the displaced nucleus pulposus, although not extending through this ligament, migrates for a considerable distance in a cephalad or caudad direction as a fragment that is separate from the remaining portion of the intervertebral disc.

If disc herniation is defined as a situation in which the nucleus pulposus extends through some or all of the fibers of the anulus fibrosus, disc prolapse, extrusion, and sequestration would all be forms of herniation (Fig. 30–32).

The features of disc herniation have been well described. Detection of abnormalities depends on central or lateral localization, as well as the extent of posterior displacement. Centrally located herniated discs that lie beneath the posterior longitudinal ligament (i.e., disc extrusion) produce a smooth, focal, radiodense area that deforms or displaces the dural sac. When nuclear material penetrates this ligament or extends around it (i.e., disc sequestration), a soft tissue mass is evident within the epidural fat. Inferior migration of the sequestered fragment is slightly more common than superior migration is.

Although extension of central disc displacement into a neural foramen is unusual, extreme lateral displacement, which represents approximately 12% of all protrusions and extrusions and is most frequent at the L4–L5 spinal level, presents a diagnostic challenge. MR imaging is ideal to define the type or extent of disc displacement (prolapse, extrusion, or sequestration). Disc protrusions

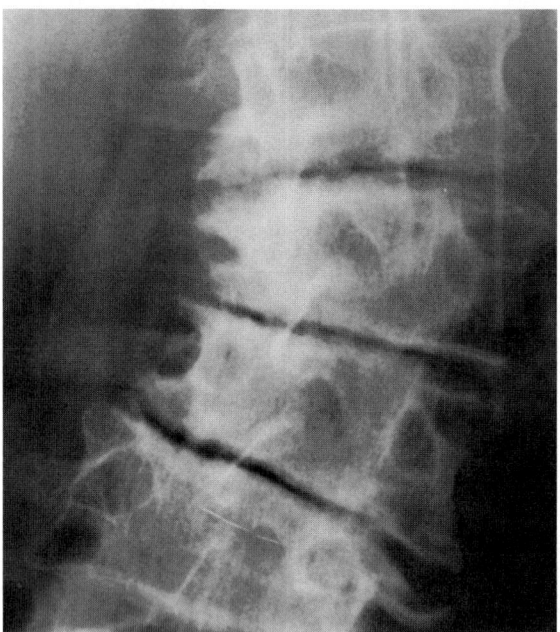

**Figure 30–25.** Degenerative lumbar scoliosis. A scoliotic curve in the lumbar region is associated with intervertebral (osteo)chondrosis (vacuum phenomena, disc space narrowing, sclerosis) and spondylosis deformans (osteophytes). Both processes are more exaggerated on the concave aspect of the curve.

---

**TABLE 30–7**

**Disc Displacement**

| Direction | Resulting Abnormality |
| --- | --- |
| Anterior displacement | Spondylosis deformans |
| Posterior displacement | Intraspinal displacement |
| Superior displacement | Cartilaginous (Schmorl's) node |
| Inferior displacement | Cartilaginous (Schmorl's) node |

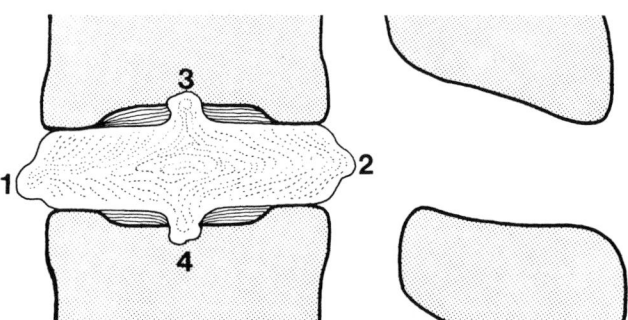

**Figure 30–26.** Intervertebral disc displacement: directions of prolapse. Drawing of a sagittal section of the spine indicates the possible directions of disc displacement. Anterior displacement (1) leads to spondylosis deformans, posterior displacement (2) may produce spinal cord compression, and superior (3) or inferior (4) displacement is associated with cartilaginous node formation.

---

**TABLE 30–8**

**Conditions Associated with Cartilaginous (Schmorl's) Nodes**

Intervertebral (osteo)chondrosis
Scheuermann's disease (juvenile kyphosis)
Trauma
Hyperparathyroidism
Osteoporosis
Infection
Neoplasm

---

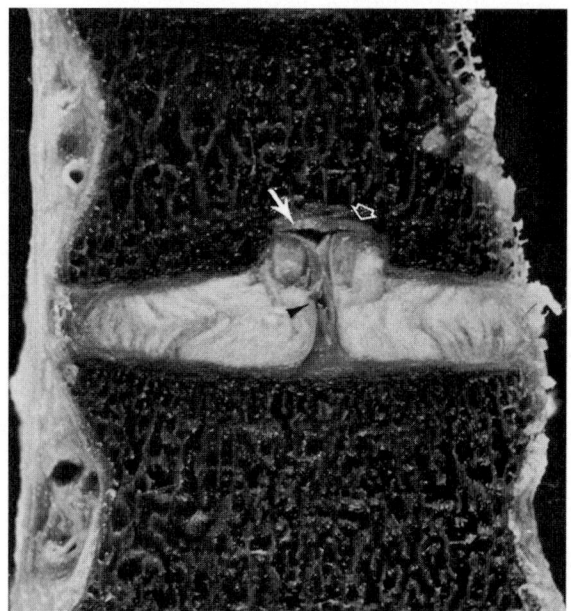

**Figure 30–27.** Intervertebral disc displacement: cartilaginous nodes. In this photograph of a sagittal section of the spine, a cartilaginous node *(open arrow)* is evident. The displaced nucleus pulposus contains vertical *(arrowhead)* and horizontal *(solid arrow)* fissures.

(From Resnick D, Niwayama G, Guerra J Jr, et al: Spinal vacuum phenomena: Anatomical study and review. Radiology 139:341, 1981.)

or extrusions are characterized by focal extension of the disc beyond the margins of the adjacent vertebral endplates in a central or lateral direction, or in both directions (Figs. 30–33 to 30–36). The signal intensity of the displaced disc is similar to that of the parent disc on T1-weighted spin echo MR sequences. On T2-weighted sequences, the signal intensity is decreased relative to that of cerebrospinal fluid in the case of small displacements, and it is increased relative to that of the parent disc in the case of large extrusions or free fragments. MR imaging is also useful in the delineation of foraminal and

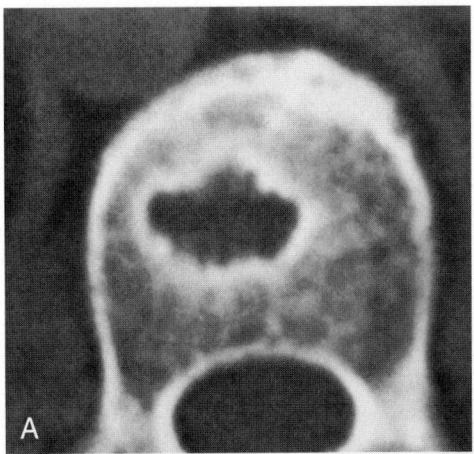

**Figure 30–28.** Intervertebral disc displacement: cartilaginous nodes. *A*, Transaxial CT scan shows a typical lesion—radiolucent with a rim of bone sclerosis. *B* and *C*, In a different patient, sagittal T1-weighted (TR/TE, 682/16) *(B)* and T2-weighted (TR/TE, 400/108) fat-suppressed *(C)* fast spin echo MR images show multiple degenerative discs, along with Schmorl's nodes. Note the Modic type II changes in the vertebral body adjacent to the node at L2. *D*, Corresponding radiograph shows multiple Schmorl's nodes.

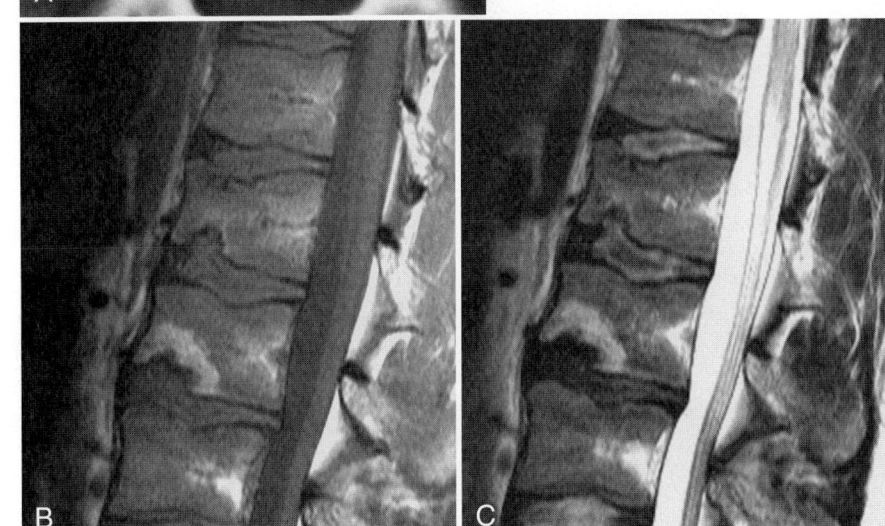

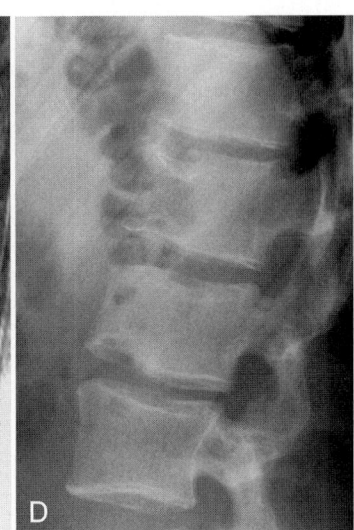

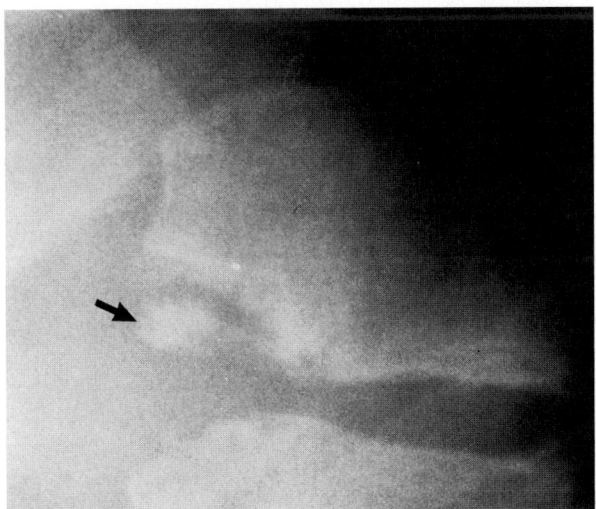

**Figure 30–29.** Intervertebral disc displacement: cartilaginous nodes and anterior limbus vertebra. In this young patient, the disc displacement has isolated a segment of the vertebral rim *(arrow)*. Irregularity of the anterior surfaces of the vertebral bodies is a common associated finding.

extraforaminal (lateral) disc displacements and migrated disc fragments. MR imaging analysis of free disc fragments indicates that fragment migration occurs with equal frequency in superior and inferior directions and that, in more than 90% of cases, migrated fragments are located either to the right or to the left of midline, a localization apparently related to the presence of a sagittally oriented midline septum in the anterior epidural space.

MR imaging's sensitivity for the detection of posterior disc displacement and associated annular tears has been documented by the results of countless investigations; however, such findings have also been documented in asymptomatic persons. Although some reports emphasize that disc extrusion and sequestration, nerve root compression, endplate abnormalities, and osteoarthritis of the apophyseal joints may be predictive of low back pain in symptomatic patients younger than 50 years, this association has not been proved. Intuitively, the more profound the abnormalities displayed by MR imaging (e.g., a large extruded disc with compression of the adjacent thecal sac), the more likely they are to be clinically significant, although the correlation among imaging, surgical, and

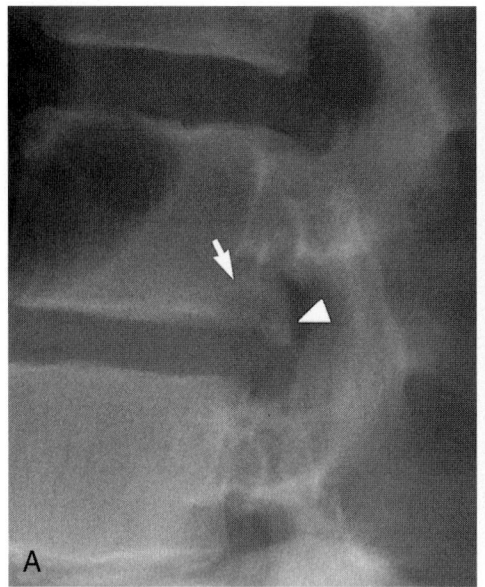

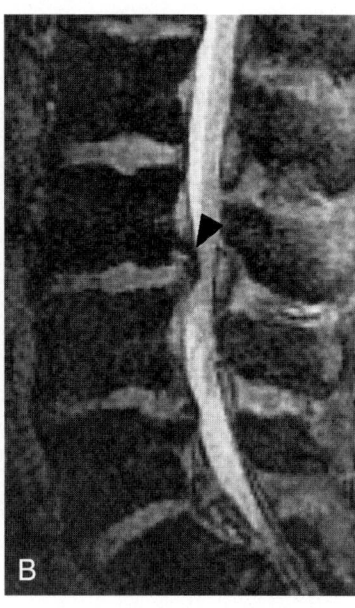

**Figure 30–30.** Intervertebral disc displacement: cartilaginous nodes and posterior limbus vertebra. This 21-year-old man had acute-onset low back and leg pain after heavy lifting. *A*, Lateral radiograph shows narrowing of the L3–L4 intervertebral disc, irregularity of the posteroinferior surface *(arrow)* of the third lumbar vertebral body, and a bone fragment *(arrowhead)* in the spinal canal. *B*, Sagittal gradient echo MR image (TR/TE, 450/17; flip angle, 17 degrees) reveals findings of lumbar disc degeneration at multiple levels. Note the posterior displacement of the discs at the L3–L4 and L4–L5 levels and, at the former site, a posterior ridge of bone *(arrowhead)*.

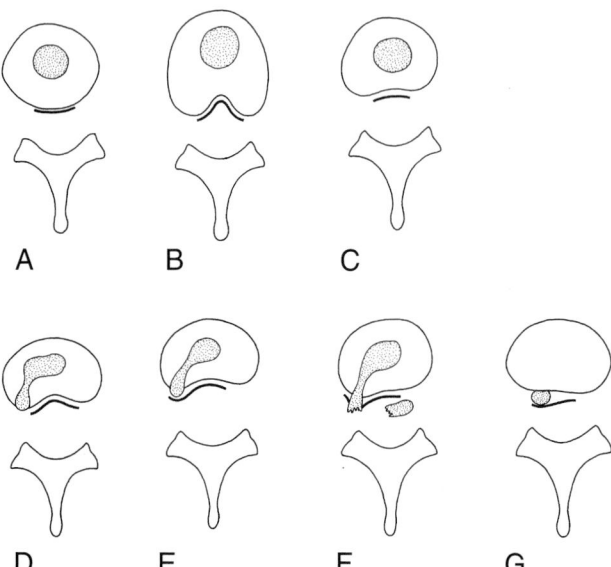

**Figure 30–31.** Posterior disc displacement. *A* to *C*, Annular bulge in three different patterns. *D*, Disc protrusion. The displaced nucleus pulposus is still confined by the outermost annular fibers. *E*, Disc extrusion. The displaced nucleus pulposus has violated the outer fibers of the anulus fibrosus but is still confined by the posterior longitudinal ligament. *F*, Disc sequestration. The displaced nucleus pulposus has penetrated the posterior longitudinal ligament and lies within the epidural space. A nearby disc fragment is seen. *G*, Disc sequestration. A fragment of the displaced disc has migrated beneath the posterior longitudinal ligament in a cephalad or caudad direction and is separated from the remaining portion of the intervertebral disc.

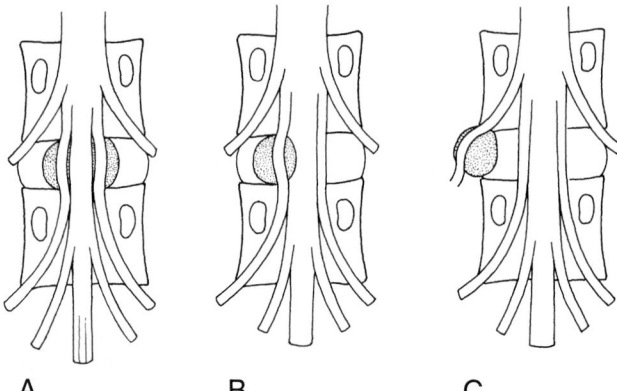

**Figure 30–32.** Posterior disc extrusion. Extrusion of disc material can occur centrally *(A)*, eccentrically *(B)*, or laterally *(C)*. The precise direction of displacement influences the clinical manifestations by affecting different portions of the spinal cord and nerve roots. With lateral extrusions, CT or MR imaging is diagnostically superior to myelography.

pathologic findings is far from perfect. Currently, the consensus is that imaging examinations are most useful in patients who are completely disabled from pain, have objective neurologic findings, or have symptoms that merit consideration of surgery or hospital admission. They are less useful in patients with stable back pain only.

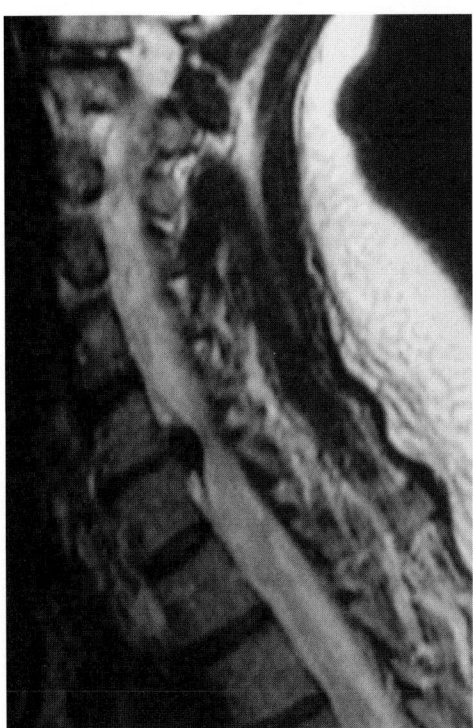

**Figure 30–33.** Posterior disc displacement: MR imaging findings. Sagittal T2-weighted (TR/TE, 2608/96) fast spin echo MR image reveals an extruded paracentral disc of low signal intensity at the C6–C7 spinal level. (Courtesy of D. Goodwin, MD, Hanover, N.H.)

Determining the need for and usefulness of imaging methods in the assessment of posterior disc displacement is also made difficult by the natural history of the condition. Many studies have documented that posterior disc displacements may decrease in size or even disappear, whether they are large or small or contained, extruded, or migrated. This decrease in size is greater with larger disc displacements.

## Synovial Cyst

Intraspinal synovial cysts are more common in women than in men and are rare before age 30 years. Although patients may be asymptomatic, most have clinical manifestations that include motor and sensory deficits and reflex changes. Approximately 90% of reported intraspinal synovial cysts occurred in the lumbar region. Lumbar synovial cysts predominate at the L4–L5 level (about 60%), followed in frequency by the L3–L4 level (about 20%) and the L5–S1 level (about 15%). The vast majority of such cysts arise adjacent to the apophyseal joints with which they commonly communicate, and these joints are frequently involved with osteoarthritis.

Routine radiography findings are nonspecific in cases of intraspinal synovial cysts. Myelography may show a rounded, extradural filling defect that has a posterolateral location and extends cephalad to the intervertebral disc space.

CT provides far more diagnostic information and typically shows a soft tissue mass adjacent to a degenerative apophyseal joint; the mass may contain gas or may have a partially or completely calcified rim (Fig. 30–37). CT scans obtained after the injection of contrast material into the adjacent apophyseal joint may show opacification of the cystic lesion. Indeed, in cases in which the apophyseal joint and synovial cyst communicate freely, injection of corticosteroid medication into the joint may provide effective therapy by passing into the cyst itself. The MR imaging findings of intraspinal synovial cysts include a mass lesion with variable signal intensity, signal void related to the presence of gas, and degenerative changes with fluid or gas collections in the apophyseal joints. Enhancement of signal intensity in the rim of the cyst may be seen after the intravenous injection of a gadolinium-based contrast agent.

## Segmental Sclerosis of Vertebral Bodies

Idiopathic segmental sclerosis of the vertebral body predominates in the lumbar spine in young and middle-aged women. Clinical manifestations indicating infection or tumor and paraspinal abnormalities are lacking. One, two, or, less commonly, several vertebral bodies are affected. The sclerosis involves the portion of the vertebral body that is adjacent to the intervertebral disc (Fig. 30–38); it is a recognized manifestation of intervertebral (osteo)-chondrosis and cartilaginous node formation. In the former situation, additional radiographic manifestations include loss of disc height and vacuum phenomena; in the latter situation, radiolucent foci within the area of vertebral sclerosis are usually evident and reflect sites of displaced disc material.

Radiographic features include bone lysis, bone sclerosis, or both. Lysis has a predilection for the upper portion of the vertebral body, with sparing of the endplate of the adjacent vertebral body. Sclerosis shows selective involvement of the anteroinferior portion of the vertebral body, especially L4 and, less frequently, L3. A hemispheric band of sclerosis extends for a variable distance from the anterior and inferior margins of the vertebral body to its central portion. The increased bone density is commonly well defined, and the bone may be uniformly dense or possess small osteolytic foci. Narrowing of the intervertebral disc space and involvement of the adjacent vertebral body are evident in some instances. MR imaging findings of idiopathic segmental sclerosis include decreased signal intensity in the affected vertebral body on T1-weighted spin echo images in an area that may be slightly larger than the region of bone sclerosis, as well as increased signal intensity in this area on T2-weighted images. The increased signal intensity predominates at the periphery of the lesion. MR imaging findings may include degeneration of the adjacent intervertebral disc, with loss of signal intensity on T2-weighted images. The importance of idiopathic segmental sclerosis of the vertebral body lies in its differentiation from other patterns of vertebral sclerosis (Fig. 30–39).

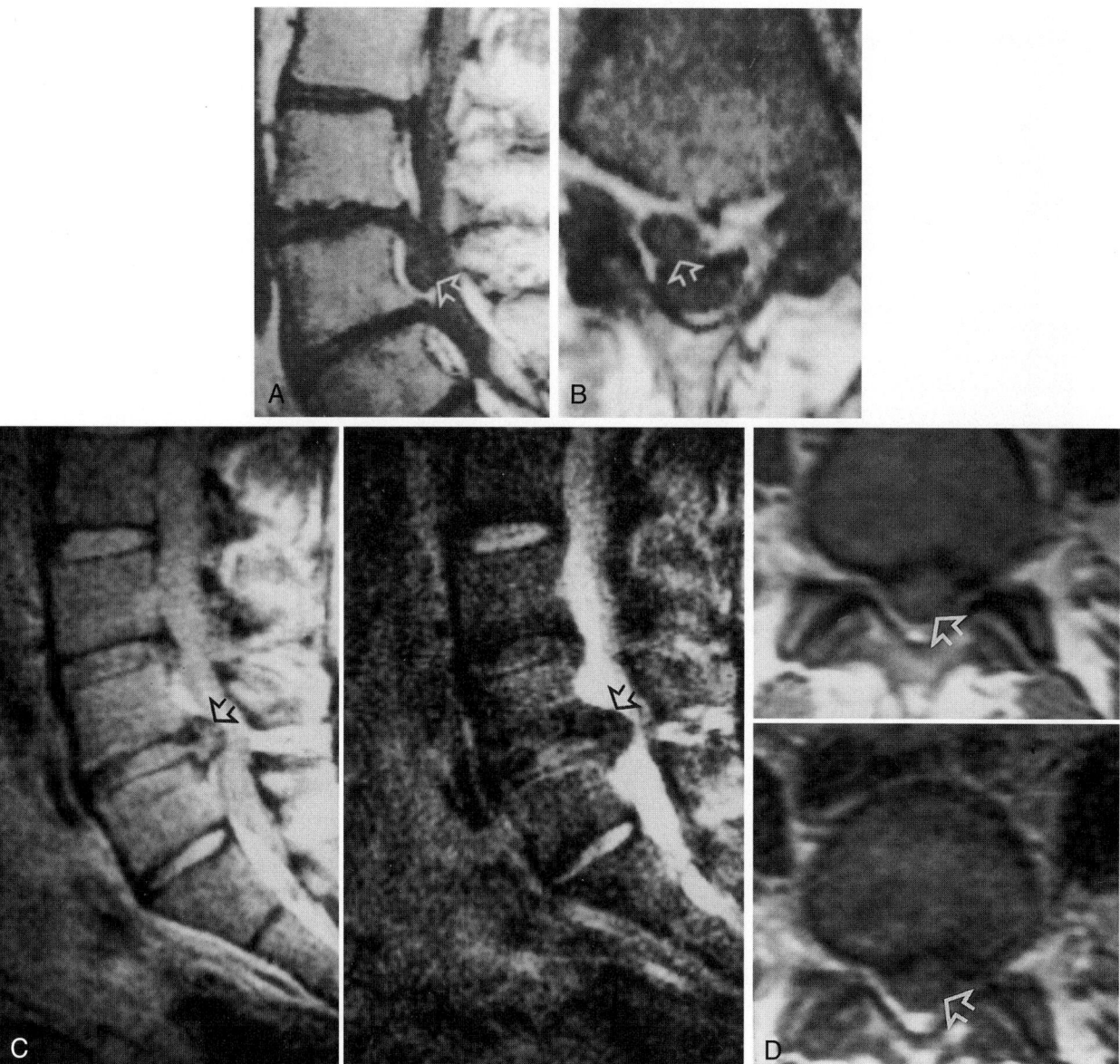

**Figure 30–34.** Posterior disc displacement: MR imaging findings. *A* and *B*, Sagittal *(A)* and transaxial *(B)* T1-weighted (TR/TE, 517/20 and 650/20, respectively) spin echo MR images reveal a large sequestered disc at the L3–L4 spinal level. The displaced disc *(arrows)*, still continuous with the parent disc, has migrated inferiorly and is located behind the fourth lumbar vertebral body. Its signal intensity is similar to that of the parent disc in these images. Degeneration of multiple lumbar intervertebral discs is seen. *C* and *D*, Sagittal intermediate-weighted (TR/TE, 2000/20) (left image in *C*) and T2-weighted (TR/TE, 2000/80) (right image in *C*) spin echo MR images and transaxial intermediate-weighted (TR/TE, 2000/20) (top image in *D*) and T2-weighted (TR/TE, 2000/80) (bottom image in *D*) spin echo MR images reveal massive disc displacement *(arrows)* at the L4–L5 spinal level. Note that the signal intensity of the displaced disc is similar to that of the parent disc on the intermediate-weighted images and is lower than that of cerebrospinal fluid on the T2-weighted images. (*C* and *D*, Courtesy of J. Kirkham, MD, Minneapolis, Minn.)

## Intervertebral Disc Calcification and Ossification

**Calcification.** Disc calcification is common and has been described in approximately 5% of chest radiographs. Many systemic disorders are associated with such deposits, including alkaptonuria, hemochromatosis, idiopathic calcium pyrophosphate dihydrate crystal deposition disease, hyperparathyroidism, poliomyelitis, acromegaly, and amyloidosis. The location, appearance, and chemical nature of the calcific deposits vary from one disorder to the next, although in most of these conditions, multiple intervertebral discs are involved. Calcification of discs

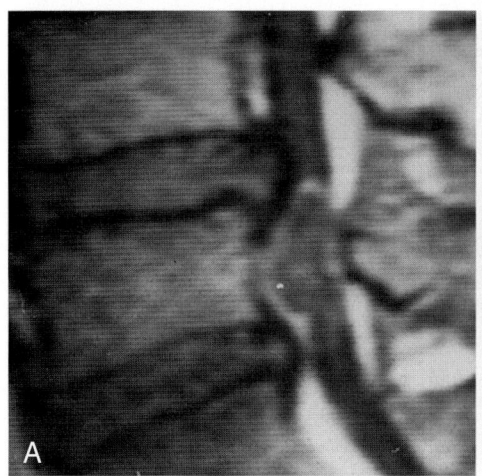 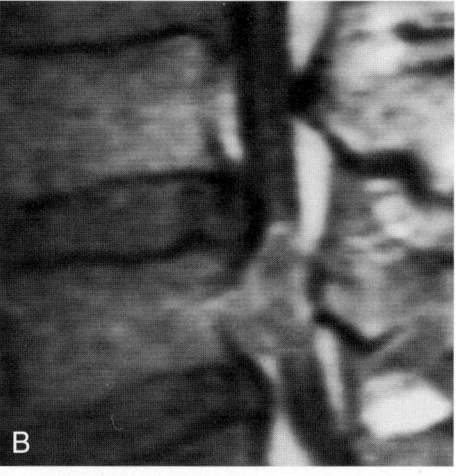

**Figure 30–35.** Posterior disc displacement: MR imaging findings. Sagittal T1-weighted (TR/TE, 600/20) spin echo images obtained before *(A)* and after *(B)* the intravenous administration of gadolinium contrast agent reveal a large sequestered disc at the L4–L5 spinal level, with the disc fragment located behind the fifth lumbar vertebral body. Some peripheral enhancement of the disc fragment is evident in *(B)*. (Courtesy of H.S. Kang, MD, Seoul, Korea.)

may also appear after surgical fusion or spontaneous ankylosis.

Calcification localized to one or two disc levels is encountered in two broad clinical situations. In adults, chronic degenerative calcific deposits may occur in the anulus fibrosus, nucleus pulposus, or cartilaginous endplates, particularly in older men and in the midthoracic and upper lumbar regions of the spine. In an autopsy study, the reported frequency of such calcification in the anulus fibrosus was 71%; in the nucleus pulposus, it was 6.5%.

The second situation associated with disc calcification is observed in children (Fig. 30–40). Such calcification is most common between 6 and 10 years of age, although it may occur at any age from birth to early adulthood. It affects boys and girls with equal frequency. The cervical spine is affected most commonly. Symptoms, which may be evident in as many as 75% of children with disc calcification, include pain, stiffness, limitation of motion, and torticollis. Fever, leukocytosis, and elevation of the erythrocyte sedimentation rate may be apparent. On radiographs, the calcification involves predominantly the nucleus pulposus and produces single or multiple, oval or flat, dense areas. Rupture of these calcific collections into the vertebral bodies (cartilaginous nodes), intervertebral foramina, spinal canal, or adjacent soft tissues may be evident. Anterior displacement of the calcified disc may lead to dysphagia, and posterior and posterolateral displacement may lead to neurologic findings. The displaced and calcified discs may diminish in size with time.

MR imaging reveals expansion of affected discs and inhomogeneity of disc signal intensity, with areas of signal void in regions of calcification. Of interest, disc expansion may also be evident at other spinal levels that do not show radiographically evident calcification (Fig. 30–41). The prognosis of disc calcification in children is excellent. In most cases, pain resolves within a few days to

weeks after only symptomatic treatment. Further, the calcification usually disappears within a few weeks to months.

It is evident that the clinical and radiographic characteristics of localized disc calcification depend on the age of the patient. In adults, calcification predominates in the anulus fibrosus of the thoracic and lumbar intervertebral discs and is usually asymptomatic and permanent; in children, calcification predominates in the nucleus pulposus of the cervical spine and is usually symptomatic and transient. The temporary nature of this phenomenon in children may relate to calcific resorption through vascular channels, which are normally present in the cartilaginous plates in children.

**Fibrosis, Vascularization, and Ossification.** Disc degeneration or trauma may be followed by proliferation of fibrous tissue and blood. Hypervascularity may stimulate ossification (Fig. 30–42) and produce radiodense lesions possessing trabeculae that overlie the intervertebral disc. These ossifications, which appear within the nucleus pulposus or the anulus fibrosus, may be displaced posteriorly into the spinal canal or extend from the adjacent vertebral body, similar to osteophytes (spondylosis deformans).

## Spinal Stenosis

A narrow spinal canal may be present at birth. This stenosis can later be accentuated by developmental narrowing produced by postnatal growth abnormalities and by acquired narrowing associated with various disease processes. Degenerative disorders of the vertebral column (osteoarthritis) lead to hypertrophic alterations about involved joints that may compromise the spinal contents.

Narrowing of the spinal canal may occur in the absence of significant extraspinal alterations in the lumbar, tho-

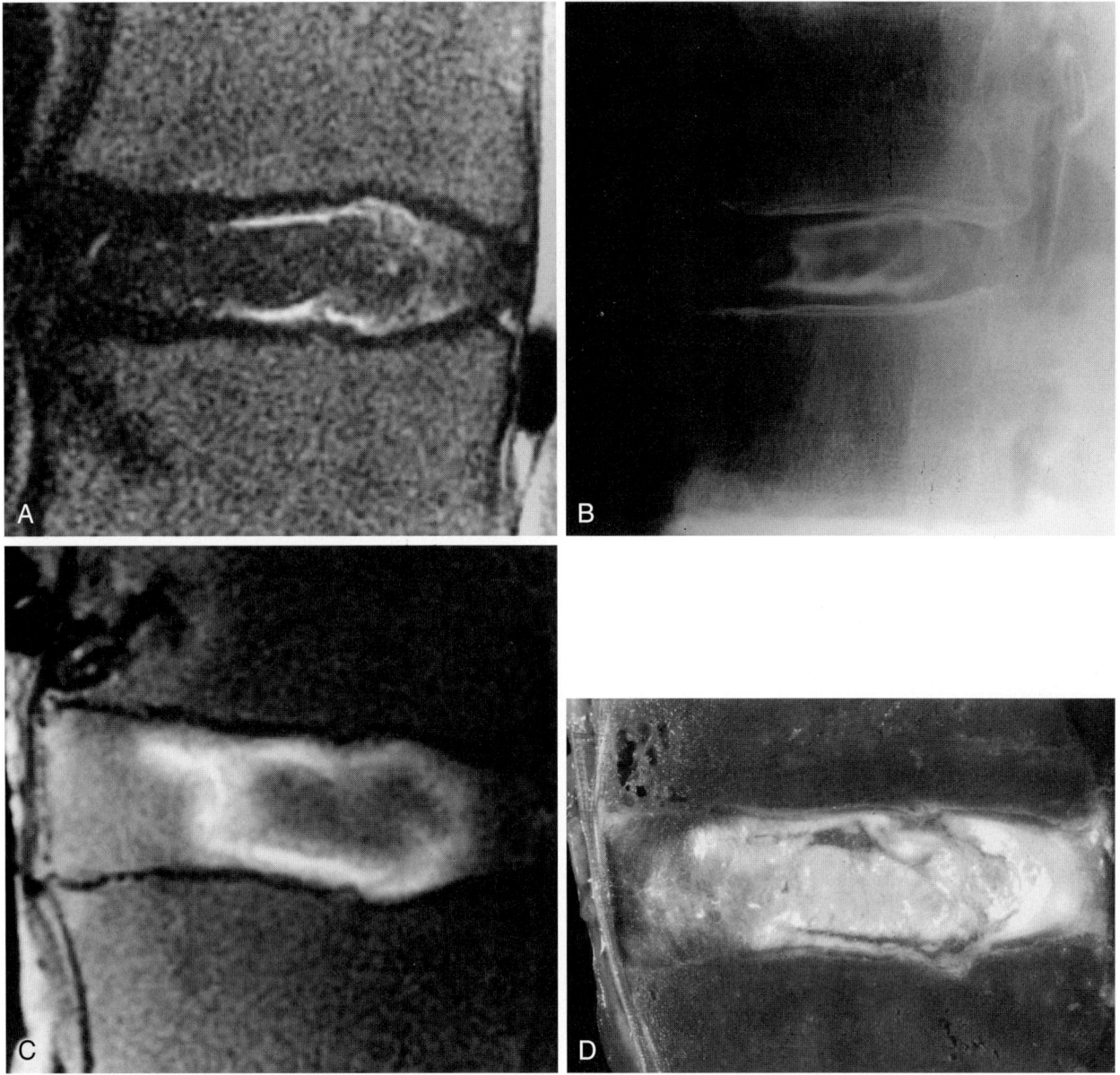

**Figure 30–36.** Annular tears: discographic, MR imaging, and MR discographic findings. *A,* In a cadaveric spine, a sagittal fat-suppressed T2-weighted (TR/TE, 3000/108) fast spin echo MR image of the L1–L2 level reveals linear regions of high signal intensity in the nucleus pulposus near each vertebral endplate. *B,* Conventional discography reveals contrast material collecting in these annular tears. *C,* MR discography using a sagittal fat-suppressed T1-weighted (TR/TE, 500/8) spin echo MR image obtained after the intradiscal injection of a gadolinium-containing contrast agent reveals the full extent of the annular tears. *D,* Photograph of a sagittal section of the spine confirms the presence of these annular tears. (Courtesy of Y. Kakitsubata, MD, Miyazaki, Japan, and D. Theodorou, MD, Ioannina, Greece.)

racic, or cervical segments of the vertebral column in both adults and children. The classification of spinal stenosis takes into account its various causes and includes categories of congenital or developmental stenosis (e.g., idiopathic, achondroplasia, osteopetrosis) and acquired stenosis. The latter is further divided into degenerative stenosis

(e.g., central, lateral recess, or foraminal degenerative spondylolisthesis), iatrogenic stenosis (e.g., following laminectomy, discectomy, or arthrodesis), traumatic stenosis, and miscellaneous causes of stenosis (e.g., acromegaly, Paget's disease, fluorosis, or ankylosing spondylitis) (Fig. 30–43).

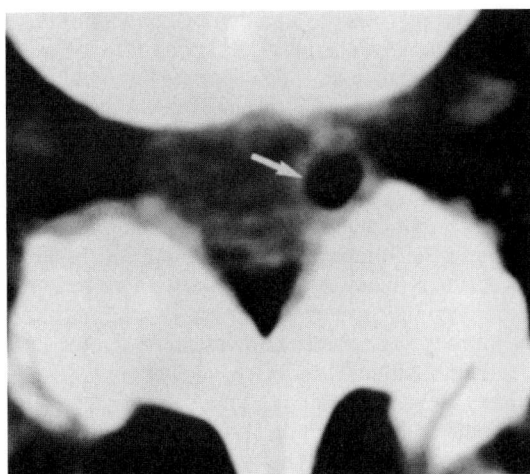

**Figure 30–37.** Intraspinal synovial cyst: lumbar spine. On a CT scan, observe a mass adjacent to the apophyseal joint. It contains gas (*arrow*).

Although symptoms and signs are occasionally encountered in the young, they are far more frequent in middle-aged and elderly persons, in whom degenerative abnormalities may further compromise a congenitally narrowed spinal canal. Clinical manifestations of spinal stenosis likewise vary according to the vertebral segment affected.

**Cervical Spinal Stenosis.** Radiographic measurement of the sagittal diameters of the spine (measured from the posterior surface of the vertebral body to the spinolaminar line) may be used to detect stenosis of the cervical canal; cord compression may occur in adults if this diameter is 10 mm or less and is unlikely to occur if this diameter

is 13 mm or more. Measurement between these osseous landmarks on radiographs does not always provide an accurate appraisal of the width of the spinal cord, however. Further, magnification errors may be introduced during routine radiography. These errors can be eliminated by using a ratio calculated by dividing the anteroposterior diameter of the spinal canal by the anteroposterior diameter of the vertebral body; normally, this ratio is about 1, with a value of 0.8 or less being indicative of developmental canal stenosis. Cervical spinal stenosis can be related to many congenital factors (anomalies, dysplasias, malformations, subluxations) and can be acquired in traumatic, infectious, neoplastic, and metabolic disorders. Cervical spinal stenosis also develops in degenerative articular diseases, such as spondylosis deformans and osteoarthritis, as well as in additional degenerative processes, such as ossification of the posterior longitudinal ligament (see Chapter 32).

**Thoracic Spinal Stenosis.** Significant spinal stenosis in the thoracic segment related to degenerative articular processes is much less frequent than is stenosis in the cervical or lumbar segments. Occasionally, osteophytes developing at the apophyseal joint or discovertebral junction and thickening of the laminae may lead to narrowing of the thoracic spinal canal and encroachment of neural tissue.

**Lumbar Spinal Stenosis.** As in the cervical spine, congenital and developmental factors may lead to a narrowed lumbar spinal canal (see Fig. 30–43), which can be compromised further by acquired alterations related to many disease processes. With developmental stenosis, characteristic alterations include narrowing of the anteroposterior and interpediculate diameters of the lower two or three lumbar vertebrae, vertical orientation of the laminae, and extreme diminution of the interlaminar space. These osseous abnormalities can be detected radiographically by measuring the anteroposterior (midsagittal) diameter

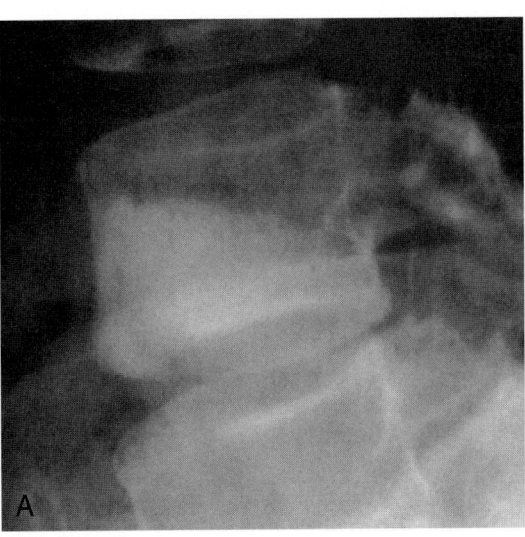
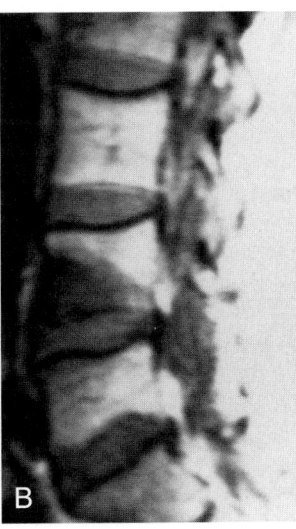

**Figure 30–38.** Segmental sclerosis of the vertebral body. This 46-year-old woman had mild back pain. *A,* Routine radiograph shows well-defined sclerosis involving the anteroinferior portion of the fourth lumbar vertebral body. Focal radiolucent areas are seen in the region of bone sclerosis. The L4–L5 intervertebral disc space is slightly narrowed, and the fifth lumbar vertebral body appears normal. *B,* Sagittal T1-weighted (TR/TE, 600/20) spin echo MR image shows low signal intensity in the region of bone sclerosis. On T2-weighted images (not shown), a slight increase in signal intensity was apparent in this region.

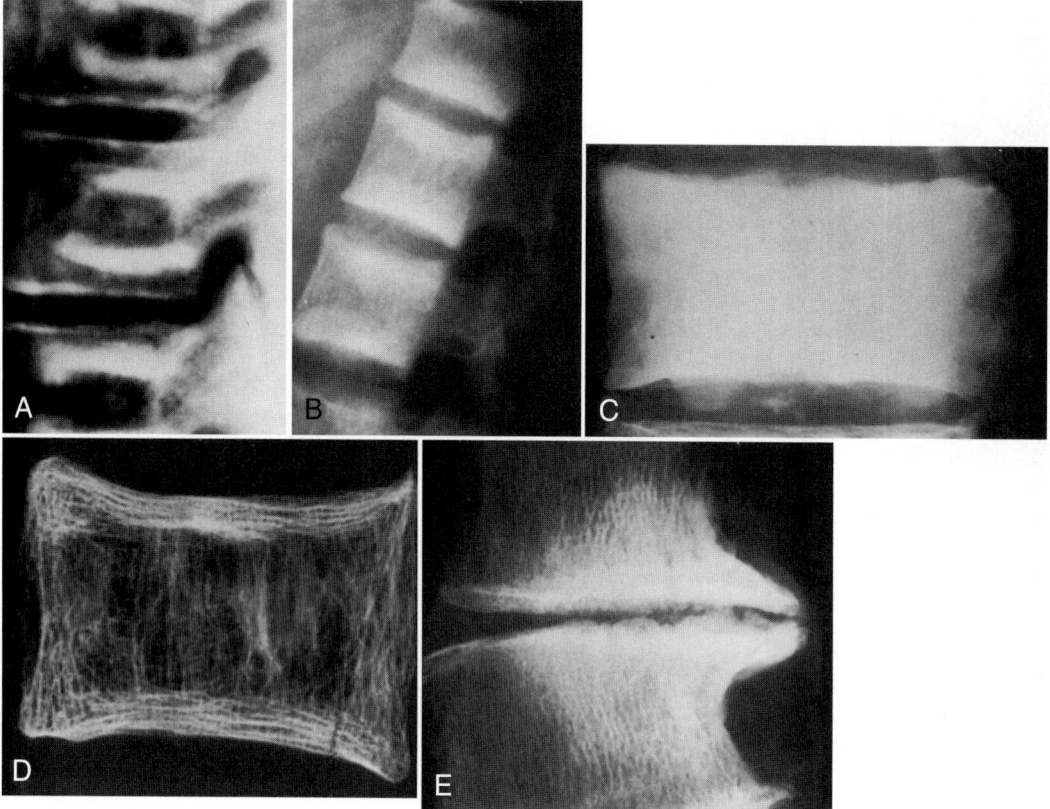

**Figure 30–39.** Patterns of sclerosis of the vertebral body. *A*, Sandwich vertebral body: osteopetrosis tarda. A bone-within-bone appearance is created by well-defined radiodense bands. *B*, Rugger-jersey vertebral body: renal osteodystrophy. Bands of increased radiodensity are evident at the top and bottom of each vertebral body. *C*, Ivory vertebral body: skeletal metastasis (carcinoma of the prostate). The entire vertebral body is radiodense and, on pathologic inspection, contains cartilaginous nodes. *D*, Picture-frame vertebral body: Paget's disease. The peripheral portions of the vertebral body are radiodense in comparison with the central portion. *E*, Marginal condensation: intervertebral (osteo)chondrosis. Triangular region of sclerosis borders on a narrowed intervertebral disc. (*A*, Courtesy of P. Kaplan, MD, Boston, Mass.)

(the distance from the posterior surface of the vertebral body to the base of the superior portion of the spinous process) and the transverse diameter (the distance between the inner aspect of the pedicles) of the spinal canal. The lower limit of normal for the midsagittal diameter of the five lumbar vertebrae in men and women is 15 mm; for the transverse diameter, it is 20 mm. Measurements less than these values indicate the presence of lumbar spinal canal stenosis. Most investigators regard an anteroposterior spinal diameter less than 12 mm as unequivocally pathologic. On CT scans, anteroposterior diameters less than 11.5 mm, interpediculate distances less than 16 mm, and canal cross-sectional areas less than 1.45 cm$^2$ are considered small. Although these CT measurements of the central canal are useful as guidelines, they should not be applied too rigorously.

Degenerative processes contribute to stenosis of the lumbar spinal canal. Ventral osteophytes, prolapse of intervertebral disc material, hypertrophy and subluxation of the articular facets, enlarged laminae, and hyperplasia or ossification of the ligamenta flava lead to further encroachment on the canal and may produce clinical symptoms and signs in a patient whose spine has already been compromised by developmental stenosis. Although these alterations are usually apparent on radiographs, their exact location and extent can be delineated more fully by CT or MR imaging. Using these techniques, spinal stenosis in the lumbar segment can be further divided into three groups on the basis of its anatomic location: stenosis of the central canal; stenosis of the subarticular, or lateral, recesses; and stenosis of the neural foramina.

The central canal is normally round or slightly oval in cross section. CT findings of central canal stenosis include distortion of its normal configuration, compression of the thecal sac in an anteroposterior direction,

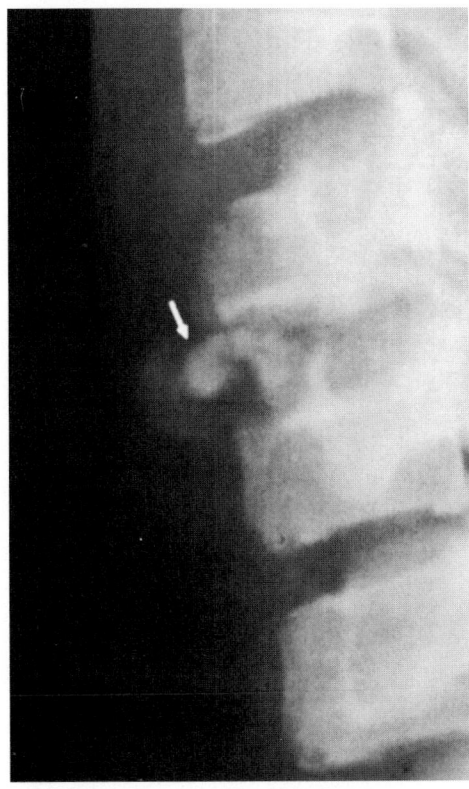

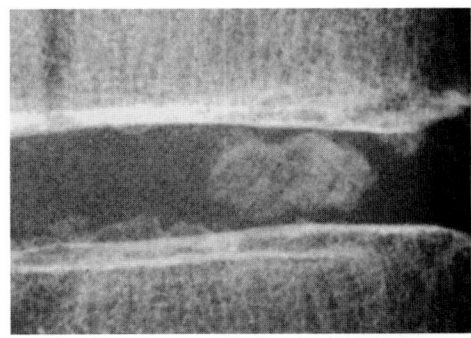

**Figure 30–42.** Intervertebral disc ossification. Magnified sectional radiograph of the spine demonstrates ossific collections in the intervertebral disc.

and obliteration of the adjacent epidural fat. Similar abnormalities are delineated with MR imaging on both sagittal and transaxial images. MR imaging appears to be superior to CT in the demonstration of narrowing of the thecal sac, whereas osseous abnormalities are visualized more easily with CT. Causes of central lumbar spinal stenosis are developmental narrowing of the interpediculate distance (as in achondroplasia), hypertrophic changes related to osteoarthritis in the apophyseal articulations, thickening of the ligamentum flavum, ligamentous calcification or ossification, diffuse bone overgrowth (as in

**Figure 30–40.** Intervertebral disc calcification in a child. Observe the calcified and extruded intervertebral disc *(arrow)*, with adjacent soft tissue swelling. (Courtesy of M. Dalinka, MD, Philadelphia, Pa.)

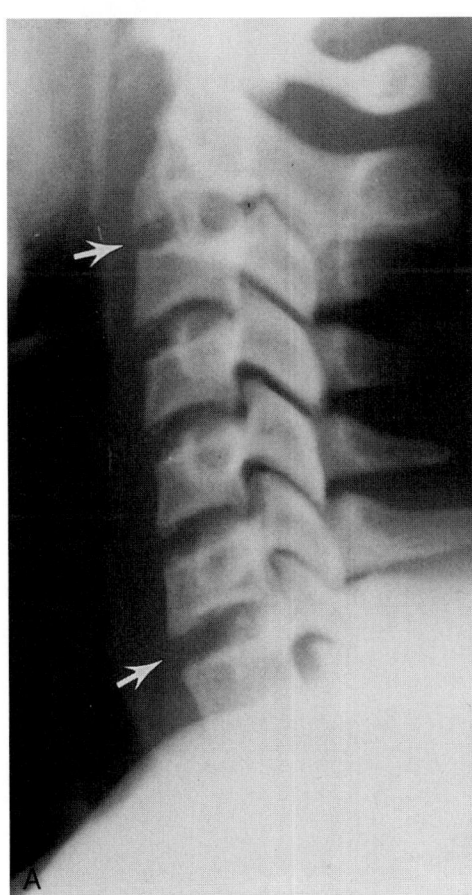

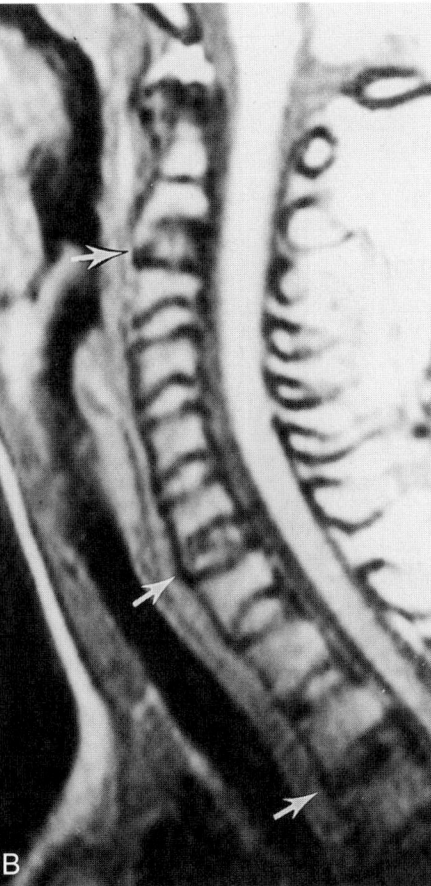

**Figure 30–41.** Intervertebral disc calcification in a 13-year-old girl with back pain. A radiograph of the thoracic spine (not shown) revealed calcification of the intervertebral disc at the T2–T3 level. *A,* Radiograph of the cervical spine shows slightly expanded intervertebral disc spaces at the C2–C3 and C6–C7 levels *(arrows)*. *B,* Sagittal T1-weighted (TR/TE, 500/24) spin echo MR image demonstrates expanded discs at the C2–C3 and C6–C7 levels *(upper two arrows)*; the signal intensity of both discs is inhomogeneous. Additional findings are loss of signal intensity in the anterior portion of the T1–T2 intervertebral disc and signal void in the calcified T2–T3 disc *(lower arrow)*.

(From Swischuk LE, Stansberry SD: Calcific discitis: MRI changes in discs without visible calcification. Pediatr Radiol 21:365, 1991.)

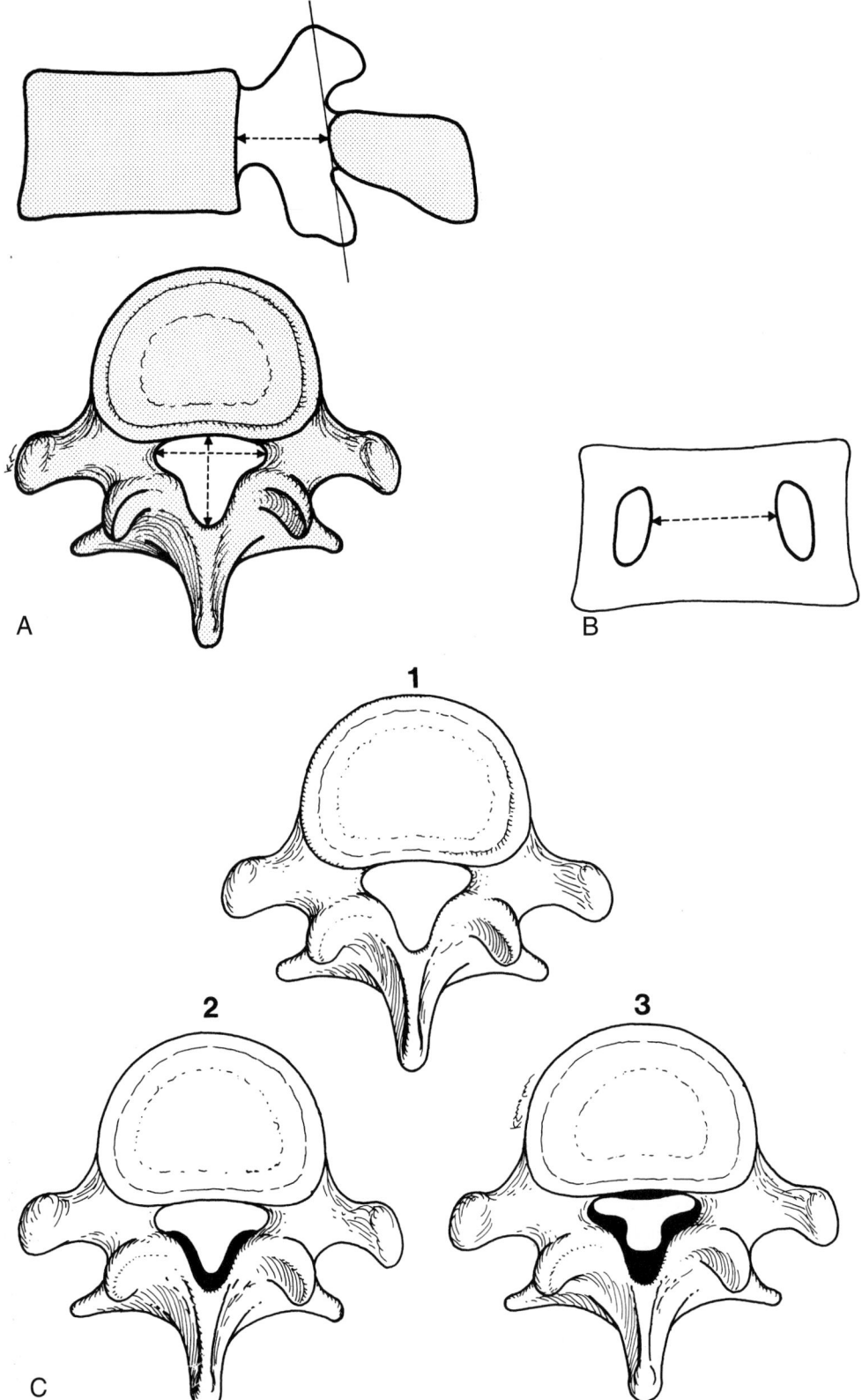

**Figure 30–43.** Patterns of lumbar spinal stenosis. The normal situation is indicated in (1). Observe the stenosis caused by laminar thickening (2) and by both anterior and posterior bony overgrowth (3), a situation resulting in the trefoil, or fleur-de-lis, appearance.

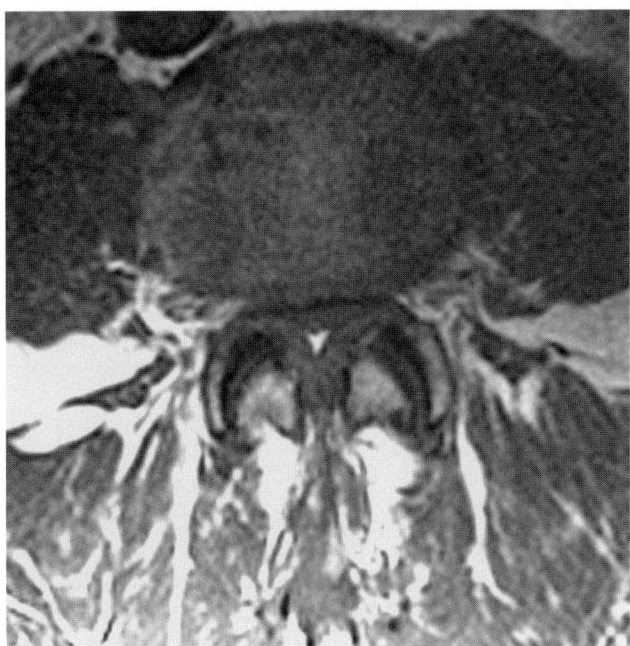

**Figure 30–44.** Central spinal stenosis. Axial T1-weighted (TR/TE, 520/20) spin echo MR image demonstrates narrowing of the anteroposterior and interpediculate diameters, with hypertrophy of the ligamentum flavum, facet hypertrophy, and disc bulging.

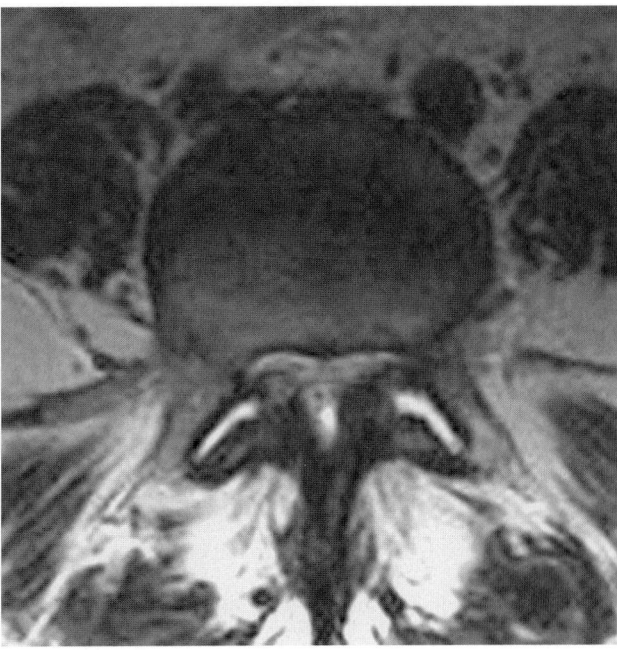

**Figure 30–45.** Lateral recess stenosis. Axial TSE T2-weighted (TR/TE, 4200/110) spin echo MR image shows marked lateral recess stenosis.

Paget's disease), osteophytes in the vertebral body, and, in the postoperative period, hypertrophy of bone grafts and fibrosis (Fig. 30–44).

The subarticular, or lateral, recess lies immediately ventral to the superior articular process and pars interarticularis and is bordered laterally by the medial margin of the pedicle and anteriorly by the posterior surface of the vertebral body. Its anteroposterior dimension, or depth, varies from one spinal level to another, although a measurement of 3 mm or less is definitely abnormal, and one between 3 and 5 mm is highly suggestive of lateral recess stenosis (Fig. 30–45).

The intervertebral foramen is bordered above and below by ipsilateral pedicles at adjacent vertebral levels, anteriorly by the posterior portion of the vertebral body and intervertebral disc, and posteriorly by the pars interarticularis and the superior articular process. Because the lumbar nerve passes laterally just below the pedicle of the upper vertebra, narrowing in this portion of the neural foramen has more significance; diminution of the lower part of the foramen is not as important, because no nerve traverses this region. Causes of foraminal narrowing include disc displacement, osteophytosis involving the vertebral body or articular processes (Fig. 30–46), focal inflammatory disease, tumor, synovial cyst, proximal placement of the dorsal root ganglia, and postoperative fibrosis. Further, spondylolisthesis is commonly associated with distortion of the foramen and may lead to compromise of the exiting nerve.

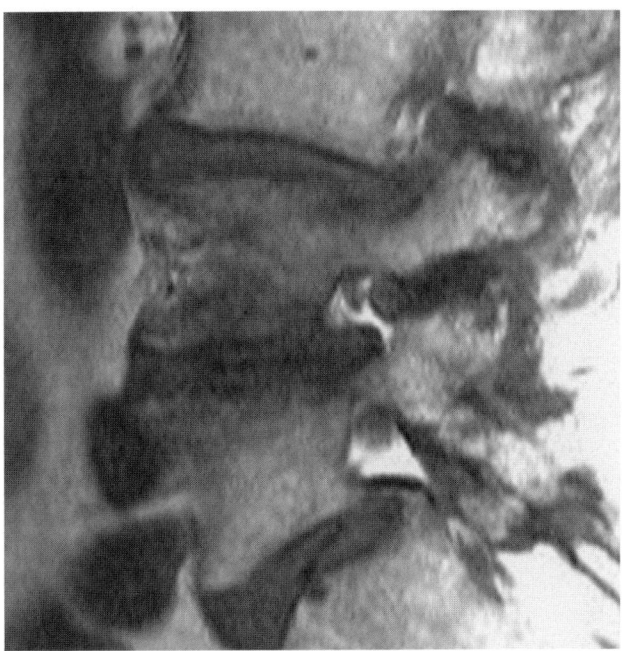

**Figure 30–46.** Foraminal stenosis. Sagittal T1-weighted (TR/TE, 650/15) spin echo MR image shows osteophytosis involving the vertebral body and articular processes.

## FURTHER READING

Adams MS, McNally DS, Dolan P: "Stress" distributions inside intervertebral discs: The effects of age and degeneration. J Bone Joint Surg Br 78:965, 1996.

Bick EM: Vertebral osteophytosis: Pathologic basis of its roentgenology. AJR Am J Roentgenol 73:979, 1955.

De Maeseneer M, Lenchik L, Everaert H, et al: Evaluation of lower back pain with bone scintigraphy and SPECT. Radiographics 19:901, 1999.

DePalma A, Rothman R: The Intervertebral Disc. Philadelphia, WB Saunders, 1970.

Dorwart RH, Vogler JB, Helms CA: Computed tomography of spinal stenosis. Radiol Clin North Am 21:301, 1983.

Edelman RR, Shoukimas GM, Stark DD, et al: High-resolution surface-coil imaging of lumbar disk disease. AJR Am J Roentgenol 144:1123, 1985.

Epstein JA, Epstein BS, Jones MD: Symptomatic lumbar scoliosis with degenerative changes in the elderly. Spine 4:542, 1979.

Francois RJ: Ligament insertions into the human lumbar vertebral body. Acta Anat 91:467, 1975.

Hadley LA: Anatomico-Roentgenographic Studies of the Spine, 2nd ed. Springfield, Ill, Charles C Thomas, 1973, p 447.

Hemminghytt S, Daniels DL, Williams AL, et al: Intraspinal synovial cysts: Natural history and diagnosis by CT. Radiology 145:375, 1982.

Inoue H, Ohmori K, Miyasaka K, et al: Radiographic evaluation of the lumbosacral disc height. Skeletal Radiol 28:638, 1999.

Jacobson HG, Tausend ME, Shapiro JH, et al: The "swayback" syndrome. AJR Am J Roentgenol 79:677, 1958.

Jones RAC, Thomson JLG: The narrow lumbar canal: A clinical and radiological review. J Bone Joint Surg Br 50:595, 1968.

Kirkaldy-Willis WH, Wedge JH, Yong-Hing K, et al: Pathology and pathogenesis of lumbar spondylosis and stenosis. Spine 3:319, 1978.

Knutsson F: The vacuum phenomenon in the intervertebral discs. Acta Radiol 23:173, 1942.

Love TW, Fagan AB, Fraser RD: Degenerative spondylolisthesis: Developmental or acquired? J Bone Joint Surg Br 81:670, 1999.

Macnab I: Spondylolisthesis with an intact neural arch—the so-called pseudospondylolisthesis. J Bone Joint Surg Br 32:325, 1950.

Macnab I: The traction spur: An indicator of segmental instability. J Bone Joint Surg Am 53:663, 1971.

Maldague BE, Noel HM, Malghem JJ: The intravertebral vacuum cleft: A sign of ischemic vertebral collapse. Radiology 129:23, 1978.

Marcelis S, Seragini FC, Taylor JAM, et al: Cervical spine: Comparison of 45 and 55 anteroposterior oblique radiographic projections. Radiology 188:253, 1993.

Martel W, Seeger JF, Wicks JD, et al: Traumatic lesions of the discovertebral junction in the lumbar spine. AJR Am J Roentgenol 127:457, 1976.

McCullough JA: Chemonucleolysis: Experience with 2000 cases. Clin Orthop 145:138, 1980.

Modic MT, Masaryk T, Boumphrey F, et al: Lumbar herniated disk disease and canal stenosis: Prospective evaluation by surface coil MR, CT, and myelography. AJR Am J Roentgenol 147:757, 1986.

Modic MT, Masaryk TJ, Ross JS, et al: Imaging of degenerative disc disease. Radiology 168:177, 1988.

Modic MT, Steinberg PM, Ross JS, et al: Degenerative disk disease: Assessment of changes in vertebral body marrow with MR imaging. Radiology 166:193, 1988.

Morrison JL, Kaplan PA, Dussault RG, et al: Pedicle marrow signal intensity changes in the lumbar spine: A manifestation of facet degenerative joint disease. Skeletal Radiol 29:703, 2000.

Muhle C, Metzner J, Weinert D, et al: Classification system based on kinematic MR imaging in cervical spondylitic myelopathy. AJNR Am J Neuroradiol 19:1763, 1998.

Pech P, Haughton VM: Lumbar intervertebral disk: Correlative MR and anatomic study. Radiology 156:699, 1985.

Resnick D, Niwayama G: Intervertebral disc herniations: Cartilaginous (Schmorl's) nodes. Radiology 126:57, 1978.

Resnick D, Niwayama G, Guerra Jr, et al: Spinal vacuum phenomena: Anatomical study and review. Radiology 139:341, 1981.

Schmorl G, Junghanns H: The Human Spine in Health and Disease, 2nd ed. Trans EF Besemann. New York, Grune & Stratton, 1971, p 138.

Schweitzer ME, El-Noueam KI: Vacuum disc: Frequency of high signal intensity on T2-weighted MR images. Skeletal Radiol 27:83, 1998.

Seidenwurm D, Litt AW: The natural history of lumbar spine disease. Radiology 195:323, 1995.

Silverman FN: Calcification of intervertebral disks in childhood. Radiology 62:801, 1954.

Williams AL, Haughton VM, Daniels DL, et al: Differential CT diagnosis of extruded nucleus pulposus. Radiology 148:141, 1983.

# CHAPTER 31

## Diffuse Idiopathic Skeletal Hyperostosis

### SUMMARY OF KEY FEATURES

The clinical, radiographic, and pathologic features of diffuse idiopathic skeletal hyperostosis (DISH) distinguish it from ankylosing spondylitis, spondylitic variants, acromegaly, hypoparathyroidism, hypervitaminosis A, ochronosis, and fluorosis. Although there is a general tendency to attribute the peculiar pattern of spinal abnormality in DISH to "degenerative" or "discogenic" alterations, this is misleading. DISH differs considerably from intervertebral (osteo)chondrosis, which is the typical degenerative disease of the nucleus pulposus. DISH most resembles spondylosis deformans, although both qualitative and quantitative differences exist between the two entities.

Spondylosis deformans is associated with spinal osteophytosis, and the pathogenesis of these outgrowths probably relates to changes in the anulus fibrosus. Disc protrusion followed by traction osteophytes appears to be the sequence of events in spondylosis deformans. These findings are identical to those occurring as part of the spinal abnormalities of DISH (type II). Spinal ligament calcification and ossification occur in DISH but are not a prominent feature of spondylosis deformans, and an enthesopathy is observed where the anterior longitudinal ligament attaches to the periosteal surface of the vertebral body. These findings could represent true qualitative differences between the two disorders. DISH may represent an ossifying diathesis that causes excessive bone formation at skeletal sites subject to normal or abnormal stress. These sites are generally found at points of tendon and ligament attachment to bone, in both the axial and extra-axial skeletons.

### INTRODUCTION

DISH is a skeletal disorder that produces characteristic alterations in both spinal and extraspinal structures. Although the name is relatively new, the disorder is not; it has been described by many names (Table 31–1). This chapter defines the major clinical, radiographic, and pathologic findings in DISH.

### DIAGNOSTIC CRITERIA

Three strict radiographic features of the spine should serve as a prerequisite for the diagnosis of DISH:

1. The presence of flowing calcification and ossification along the anterolateral aspect of at least four contiguous vertebral bodies, with or without associated localized,

---

**TABLE 31–1**

**Synonyms for Diffuse Idiopathic Skeletal Hyperostosis**

Spondylitis ossificans ligamentosa
Spondylosis hyperostotica
Physiologic vertebral ligamentous calcification
Generalized juxta-articular ossification of vertebral ligaments
(Senile) Ankylosing hyperostosis of the spine
Forestier's disease
Spondylosis deformans
Vertebral osteophytosis

---

pointed excrescences at the intervening vertebral body–intervertebral disc junctions.

2. Relative preservation of intervertebral disc height in the involved vertebral segment and the absence of extensive radiographic changes of "degenerative" disc disease, including vacuum phenomenon and vertebral body marginal sclerosis.

3. The absence of apophyseal joint bony ankylosis and sacroiliac joint erosion, sclerosis, or intra-articular osseous fusion.

All three radiographic criteria must be fulfilled to establish a definitive diagnosis of DISH. Each has been chosen to eliminate other spinal disorders that might be confused with DISH: the first criterion is helpful in separating this condition from typical spondylosis deformans, the second criterion distinguishes DISH from intervertebral (osteo)chondrosis, and the third criterion eliminates patients with ankylosing spondylitis. The choice of four contiguous vertebral bodies as the least extensive ossification that is compatible with the diagnosis of DISH is arbitrary, but it is based on a desire to separate this entity from typical spondylosis deformans. The second criterion insists on relative preservation of disc height and absence of extensive radiographic changes of intervertebral (osteo)chondrosis, which results in some patients who have both DISH and "degenerative" disc disease being eliminated. Finally, sacroiliac joint abnormalities do occur in DISH; however, these abnormalities, which consist of osteophytosis and coexistent osteoarthritis, are usually associated with sacroiliac joint space narrowing and para-articular bony bridging and should not be confused with those in ankylosing spondylitis.

### CLINICAL ABNORMALITIES

DISH has long been regarded as a radiographic entity whose clinical manifestations are minor and of little significance. DISH is a common disease of older persons. The mean age in most study populations is in the seventh decade. In reality, the advanced age of patients with DISH reflects not that the disorder begins in elderly patients but rather that a lengthy period is necessary before the spinal abnormalities progress to such a degree that they fulfill specific radiographic criteria. DISH predominates in men, who represent about two thirds of reported patients.

A variety of symptoms and signs appear in patients with DISH (Table 31–2). Stiffness, restricted motion, and tendinosis in these patients are consistent with the underlying radiographic alterations. In general, the clinical findings are mild in comparison to the spectacular radiographic evidence of the disease. Spinal stiffness and pain usually become evident in middle age and may persist for many years. Cervical dysphagia may be an additional prominent symptom in patients with DISH and is directly related to the presence of prominent cervical osteophytes.

## RADIOGRAPHIC ABNORMALITIES

Distinctive radiographic abnormalities in spinal and extraspinal sites occur in DISH (Table 31–3).

### Spinal Abnormalities

**Thoracic Spine.** The radiographic abnormalities of DISH are encountered most commonly in the thoracic spine (Fig. 31–1). Such abnormalities are most frequently apparent between the 7th and 11th thoracic vertebrae. Laminated calcification and ossification appear along the anterolateral aspect of the vertebral bodies and continue across the intervertebral disc spaces. Such calcification and ossification are most apparent on lateral radiographs of the thoracic spine. The deposited bone varies considerably in thickness; when broad, the deposited bone appears as a radiodense shield in front of the vertebral column. Although ossification may extend to involve both the right and the left lateral aspects of the vertebral column, it is more common and exuberant on the right side of the thoracic spine, presumably related to an inhibiting effect by a left-sided pulsating, descending thoracic aorta. The contour of the involved thoracic spine is generally irregular and bumpy; occasionally, examples of a smooth "pseudospondylitic" pattern of ossification may be seen. The bumpy spinal contour is particularly prominent at the level of the intervertebral discs as a result of two processes: (1) increased deposition of bone at the disc space, frequently merging with bony excres-

---

**TABLE 31–2**

### Clinical Features of Diffuse Idiopathic Skeletal Hyperostosis

Recurrent Achilles tendinosis
Recurrent "tennis elbow"
Progressive restriction of range of motion
Palpable calcaneal enthesophytes
Palpable olecranon enthesophytes
Dysphagia
Restricted motion after total joint replacement

---

**TABLE 31–3**

### Radiographic Abnormalities in Diffuse Idiopathic Skeletal Hyperostosis

**Spinal**
Anterolateral flowing ossification
Bumpy spinal contour
Radiolucent disc extension
Radiolucent area beneath deposited bone

**Extraspinal**
Bony proliferation
Ligament calcification, ossification
Para-articular osteophytes

---

cences on the superior and inferior margins of the vertebra, and (2) a more anterior position of the deposited bone at the level of the intervertebral disc. Radiolucent areas within the ossified mass at the level of the intervertebral discs correspond to anterolateral extension of disc material. An additional radiolucent lesion in the form of a linear defect is present between the newly deposited bone and the subjacent vertebral body. This radiolucent area may not be apparent at each thoracic level but is usually observed at some level. This linear defect ends abruptly at the superior and inferior margins of the vertebral body, where horizontal struts of new bone are deposited. In some persons, an exaggerated concavity along the anterior aspect of the vertebral body produces a semicircular, rather than a linear, radiolucent lesion. Thoracic disc space narrowing is generally mild or absent.

**Cervical Spine.** Cervical spine alterations (Fig. 31–2) are also frequent in DISH. Abnormalities are more common in the lower cervical region (between the fourth and seventh cervical vertebral bodies). The initial finding is hyperostosis of the cortex along the anterior surface of the vertebral body. Gradually, elongated bony outgrowths appear at the anterior margin of the vertebra and extend across the intervertebral disc space. These outgrowths are observed most commonly at the inferior lip of the vertebral body and extend downward. Progressive bony deposition can be either smooth and homogeneous or bumpy and irregular. A flowing pattern of ossification may result, but this ossification is frequently interrupted by radiolucent disc extensions at the level of the intervertebral disc.

The predilection for anterior deposition of bone in the cervical spine follows the general distribution of ossification throughout the vertebral column. In the cervical region, however, posterior vertebral abnormalities are not infrequent and include hyperostosis of the posterior aspect of the vertebra, posterior spinal osteophytosis, and posterior longitudinal ligament calcification and ossification. Elongation of the styloid process at the base of the skull or calcification or ossification of the stylohyoid ligament, or both, may be evident in patients with DISH (Fig. 31–3).

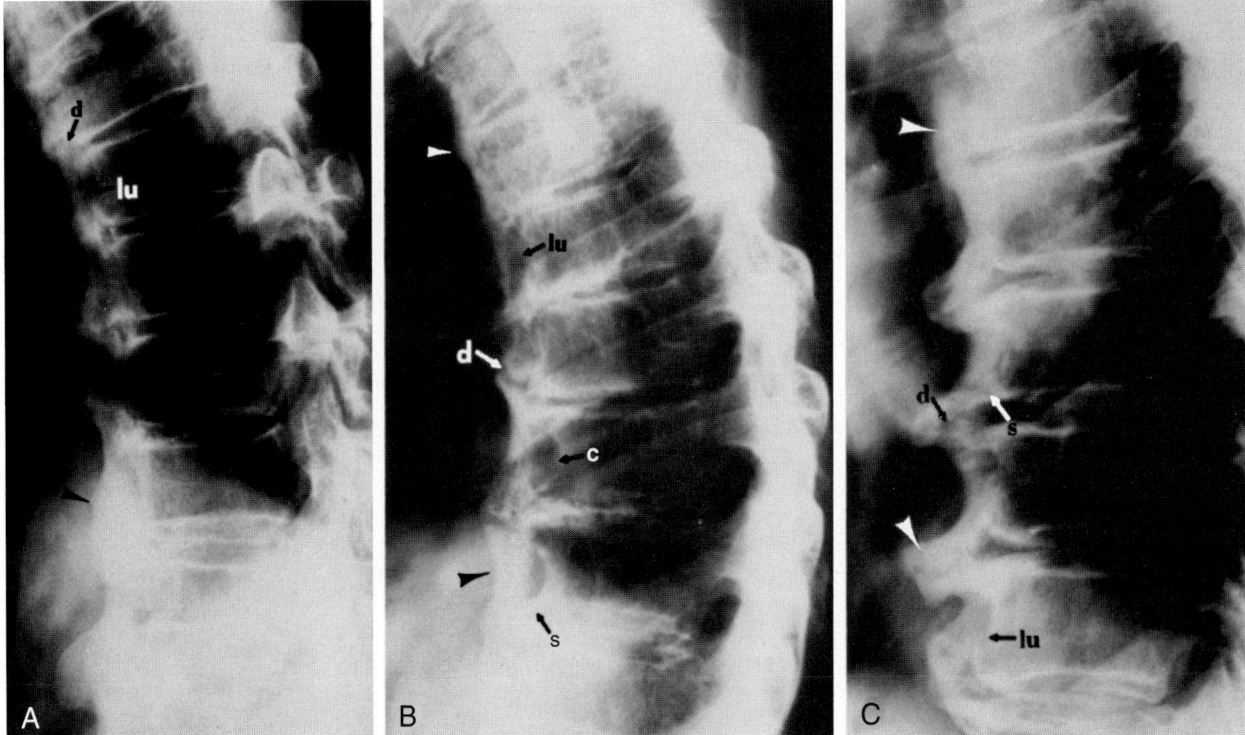

**Figure 31–1.** Thoracic spine abnormalities in DISH. *A,* Findings include flowing anterior ossification *(arrowhead)* with a bumpy spinal contour, radiolucent disc extensions (d), and a radiolucent area between the deposited bone and underlying vertebral bodes (lu). *B,* Note the anterior spinal ossification *(arrowheads),* radiolucent disc extensions (d), radiolucent areas between deposited bone and subjacent vertebrae (lu), exaggerated anterior vertebral concavity (c), and horizontal bony struts (s). *C,* The bumpy spinal contour *(arrowheads)* reflects anterior hyperostosis with radiolucent disc extensions (d), linear radiolucent areas (lu), and horizontal struts of bone (s).

(*A* and *B,* From Resnick D, Shapiro RF, Wiesner KB, et al: Diffuse idiopathic skeletal hyperostosis (DISH) [ankylosing hyperostosis of Forestier and Rotes-Querol]. Semin Arthritis Rheum 7:153, 1978. *C,* From Resnick D, Niwayama G: Radiographic and pathologic features of spinal involvement in diffuse idiopathic skeletal hyperostosis (DISH). Radiology 119:559, 1976.)

**Lumbar Spine.** Lumbar spine abnormalities in DISH are almost as frequent as thoracic spine abnormalities (Fig. 31–4). These findings are usually observed in the upper lumbar region. The lumbar changes resemble alterations in the cervical spine. Initially, hyperostosis is observed along the anterior aspect of the vertebral body. With progression, cloudlike increased bone density and pointed bony excrescences develop. Additional findings include radiolucent anterior disc extension, occasional radiolucent areas between the deposited bone and the subjacent vertebral body, and the rare occurrence of posterior outgrowths. The predilection for right-sided involvement in the thoracic spine is not apparent in the lumbar region.

**Miscellaneous Spinal Abnormalities.** Osteoporosis is not a feature of this disorder, and skeletal radiodensity may appear excessive in view of the patient's advanced age. Additionally, osseous ankylosis is commonly observed in the thoracic spine and less frequently in the cervical and lumbar spine.

**Magnetic Resonance Imaging.** DISH is a frequent incidental finding on spinal magnetic resonance (MR) imaging. The signal intensity of the involved region reflects the nature of the hyperostosis and associated calcification and ossification, ranging from low to an intensity similar to that of marrow fat (Fig. 31–5).

### Extraspinal Abnormalities

The extraspinal radiographic manifestations of DISH are not only frequent but also distinctive (Table 31–4). Although extraspinal radiographic features of DISH can occur at virtually any skeletal site, they are most characteristic in certain locations. Typically, they have a bilateral and symmetrical distribution.

**Pelvis.** Abnormalities of the pelvic bones are common in DISH and consist of bony proliferation or "whiskering," ligament calcification and ossification, and para-articular osteophytes (Fig. 31–6). Proliferation (whiskering) is seen at sites of ligament and tendon attachment to bone, particularly on the iliac crest, ischial tuberosity, and trochanters. Ligament calcification and ossification occur in the iliolumbar and sacrotuberous ligaments. Para-articular osteophytes are noted along the inferior aspect of the sacroiliac joint, lateral aspect of the acetabulum, and superior pubic margins, where they produce para-

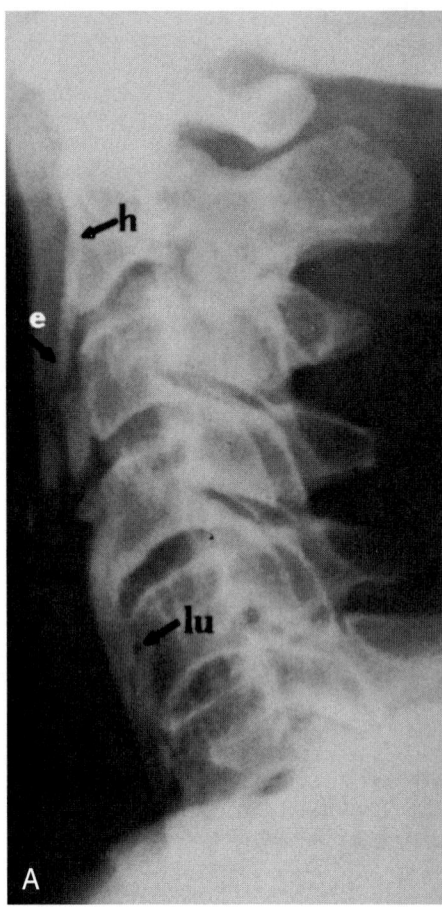
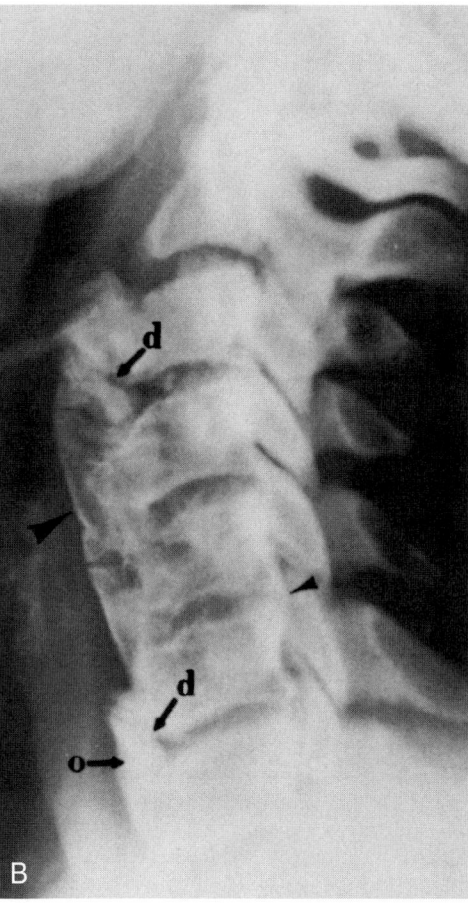

**Figure 31–2.** Cervical spine abnormalities in DISH. *A,* Observe the cortical hyperostosis (h), pointed excrescences (e), and linear ossification with a circular radiolucent area (lu). *B,* A bony shield *(large arrowhead)* is evident along the cervical spine. Also note the radiolucent disc extensions (d), bony ossicle (o) in front of the intervertebral disc, small posterior osteophytes *(small arrowhead),* and relatively intact apophyseal joints.

(*A,* From Resnick D, Shapiro RF, Wiesner KB, et al: Diffuse idiopathic skeletal hyperostosis (DISH) [ankylosing hyperostosis of Forestier and Rotes-Querol]. Semin Arthritis Rheum 7:153, 1978. *B,* From Resnick D, Niwayama G: Radiographic and pathologic features of spinal involvement in diffuse idiopathic skeletal hyperostosis (DISH). Radiology 119:559, 1976.)

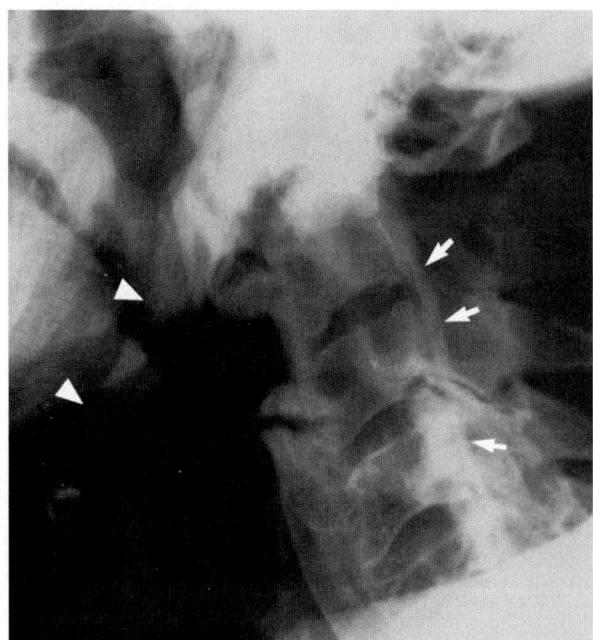

**Figure 31–3.** Cervical spine abnormalities in DISH. Radiographic abnormalities in this patient with DISH include extensive anterior bone formation, ossification of the posterior longitudinal ligament *(arrows),* and ossification of both stylohyoid ligaments *(arrowheads).*

articular osseous bridging. Para-articular fusion is far more common than true intra-articular ankylosis. The most specific abnormalities in DISH are calcification or ossification of ligaments and enthesophyte formation at insertion sites.

**Heel.** Enthesophytes on the posterior and inferior surfaces of the calcaneus are common in patients with DISH (Fig. 31–7). These enthesophytes are well demarcated and irregular in outline, without adjacent reactive bone sclerosis or erosions.

**Foot.** Bony excrescences of the foot in patients with DISH show a predilection for the dorsal surface of the talus, dorsal and medial regions of the tarsal navicular, lateral and plantar aspects of the cuboid, and base of the fifth metatarsal bone. Hyperostosis of the talus may result in a talar beak.

**Patella and Knee.** Patellar and peripatellar alterations occur in DISH (Fig. 31–8), including ligamentous ossification within the quadriceps mechanism with anterior patellar hyperostosis (best evaluated on tangential radiographs) and irregularities of the tibial tuberosity.

**Elbow.** Olecranon enthesophytes are frequent, well defined, and occasionally of considerable size (Fig. 31–9).

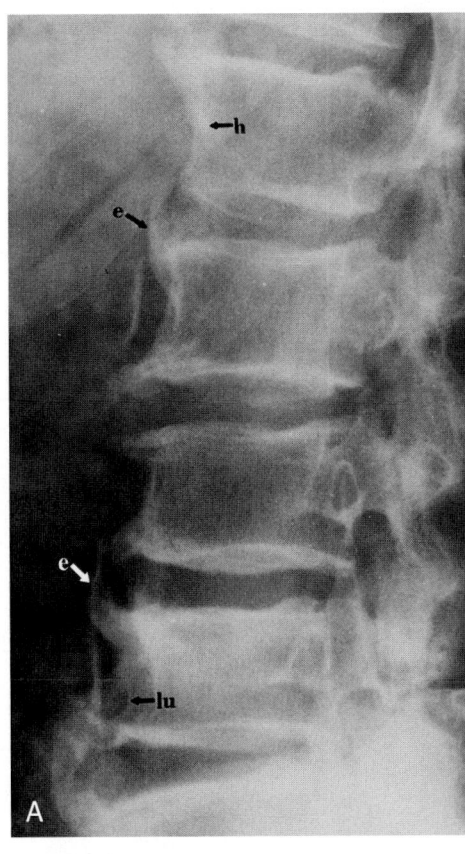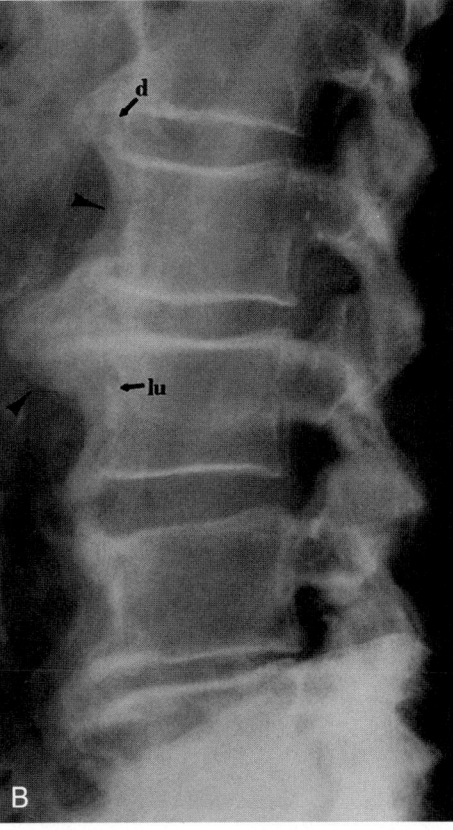

**Figure 31–4.** Lumbar spine abnormalities in DISH. *A,* Radiographic findings include bony excrescences (e), cortical hyperostosis (h), and small radiolucent areas (lu). Note the preservation of the height of the intervertebral discs. *B,* More severe abnormalities in another patient include anterior linear ossification *(arrowheads)* and radiolucent areas, both beneath the deposited bone (lu) and at the level of the intervertebral disc (d).

(*A,* From Resnick D, Niwayama G: Radiographic and pathologic features of spinal involvement in diffuse idiopathic skeletal hyperostosis (DISH). Radiology 19:559, 1976. *B,* From Resnick D, Shapiro RF, Wiesner KB, et al: Diffuse idiopathic skeletal hyperostosis (DISH) [ankylosing hyperostosis of Forestier and Rotes-Querol]. Semin Arthritis Rheum 7:153, 1978.)

**Shoulder and Humerus.** Findings in this location may include prominence and exaggerated bony irregularity along the deltoid tuberosity and greater tuberosity, medial aspect of the humeral shaft, inferior glenoid, inferior distal end of the clavicle, and osseous attachments of the coracoclavicular ligament.

## PATHOLOGIC ABNORMALITIES

**Thoracic Spine.** The pathologic and radiologic aberrations of thoracic spine involvement in DISH are characterized by several distinct types of bone formation, ligamentous ossification, proliferative enthesopathy, and periosteal proliferation (Figs. 31–10 and 31–11). Linear paravertebral and paradiscal bone and osteophytes are evident.

---

**TABLE 31–4**

**Common Sites\* of Extraspinal Abnormality in Diffuse Idiopathic Skeletal Hyperostosis**

---

Pelvis
Heel
Foot
Elbow
Hand, wrist
Knee

---

*\*In order of decreasing frequency.*

The osteophytes develop close to the discovertebral junction and appear identical to those of spondylosis deformans; however, the other abnormalities are not prominent in typical spondylosis deformans, although this difference does not indicate with certainty that DISH and spondylosis deformans are separate entities.

**Lumbar Spine.** In the lumbar spine (and presumably in the cervical spine), the pathologic changes most resemble those of spondylosis deformans. Anulus defects, protrusion of disc material, elevation of the outer annular fibers, and traction osteophytes are sequential abnormalities. Pointed excrescences of variable size develop at the superior and inferior margins of the vertebra adjacent to the intervertebral disc.

**Late Thoracolumbar Abnormalities.** The appearance of a spine that is severely involved is striking. A shell of bone extends across the anterior surface of the vertebral column. In the thoracic spine, it predominates on the right side. In the lumbar spine, both the right and left sides of the vertebral body may be involved equally. Although bony ankylosis is frequent in the thoracic spine, close inspection commonly reveals areas in which true ankylosis is not present; rather, the irregular osseous outgrowths interdigitate, their undulating surfaces separated by thin layers of fibrous tissue representing extension of intervertebral disc material. A bumpy spinal contour reflects the increased thickness of deposited bone at the level of the intervertebral disc. Lucent areas at the level of the intervertebral disc reflect unossified protruded portions

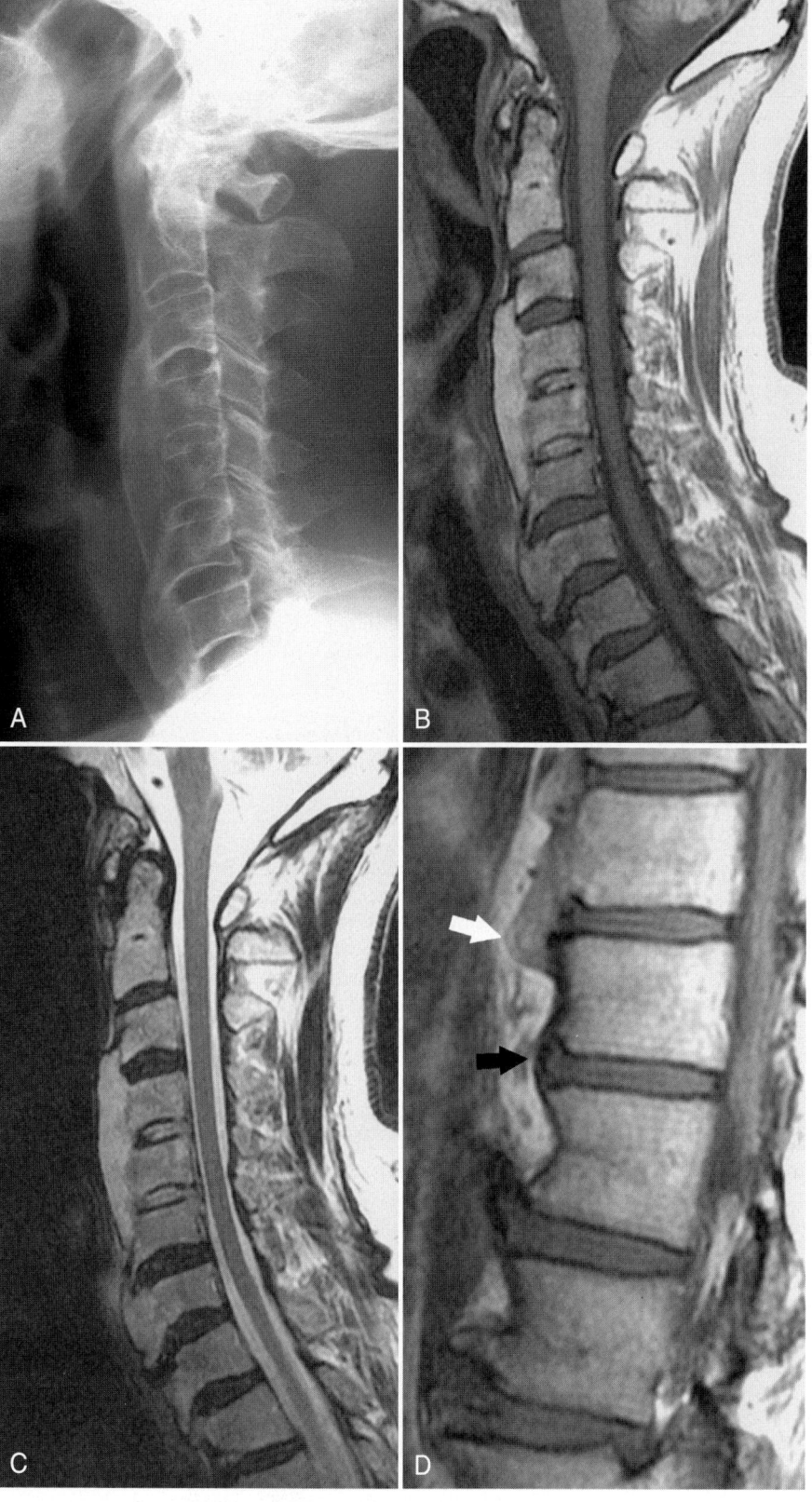

**Figure 31–5.** MR imaging of spinal abnormalities in DISH. *A,* Radiographic abnormalities in this patient with DISH include extensive anterior bone formation. *B* and *C,* Corresponding T1-weighted (TR/TE, 700/15) *(B)* and turbo T2-weighted (TR/TE, 4000/100) *(C)* spin echo MR images show that the anterior ossification has a signal intensity similar to that of the adjacent marrow. *D,* T1-weighted (TR/TE, 600/10) spin echo MR image of the lumbar spine in a different patient shows flowing anterior ossification in the lower thoracic spine with a signal intensity similar to that of marrow fat *(white arrow).* More inferiorly, it shows a markedly decreased signal intensity *(black arrow).*

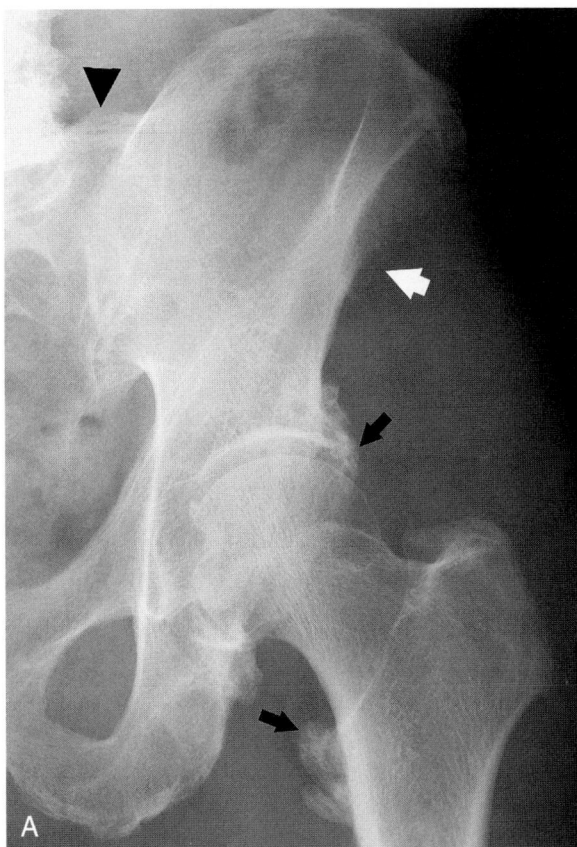

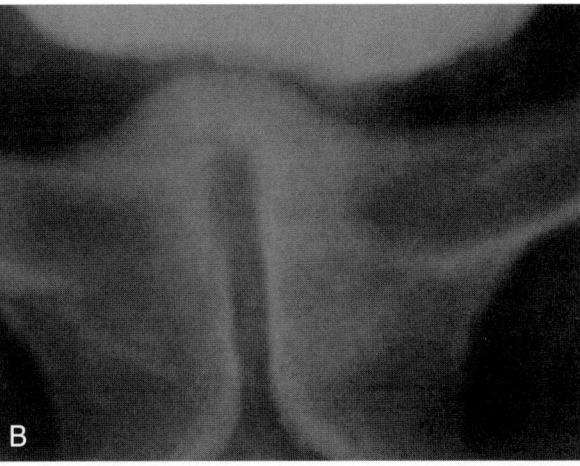

**Figure 31–6.** Pelvic abnormalities in DISH. *A,* Note the iliolumbar ligament mineralization *(arrowhead)*, osseous proliferation or "whiskering" *(white arrow)*, and irregular bony excrescences above the acetabulum and from lesser trochanter *(black arrows).* *B,* In a different patient, an osseous bridge extends across the symphysis pubis.

(*B,* From Resnick D, Shaul S, Robins JM: Diffuse idiopathic skeletal hyperostosis (DISH): Forestier's disease with extraspinal manifestations. Radiology 115:513, 1975.)

of disc material, primarily anulus fibrosus. Characteristic linear lucencies occur when the deeper portion of the anterior longitudinal ligament is not completely ossified or, to a lesser extent, when fibrous material from the disc extends between the anterior longitudinal ligament and vertebral body.

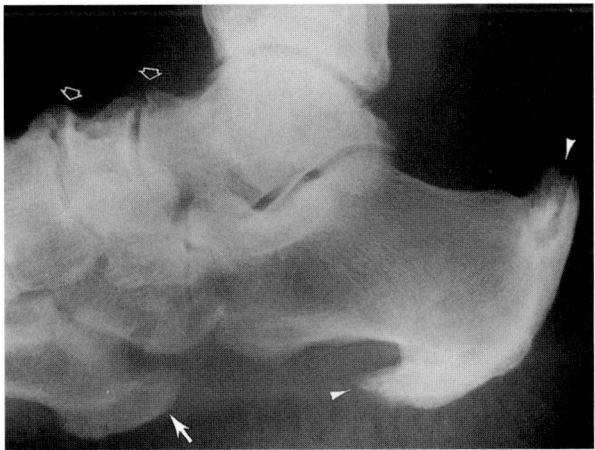

**Figure 31–7.** Heel abnormalities in DISH. Peculiar osseous excrescences *(arrowheads)* project from the plantar and posterior aspects of the calcaneus and are associated with dorsal bone outgrowths *(open arrows)* and irregularity and enlargement of the base of the fifth metatarsal bone *(solid arrow).* (Courtesy of G. Greenway, MD, Dallas, Tex.)

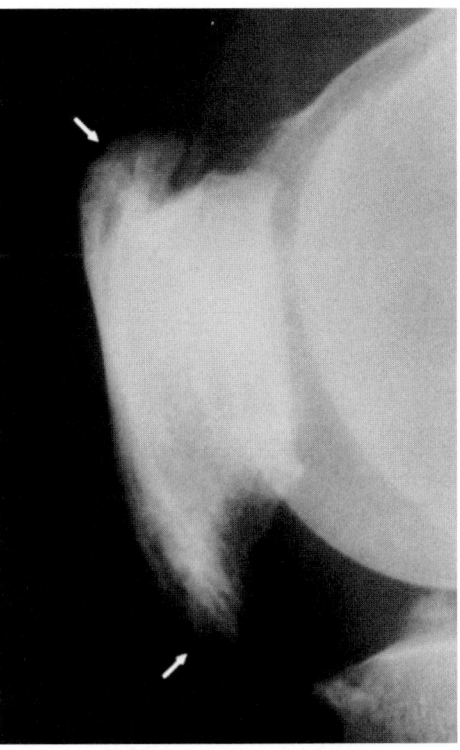

**Figure 31–8.** Patellar abnormalities in DISH. Osseous proliferation has resulted in thickening of the anterior patellar surface, with excrescences extending from its superior and inferior margins into the adjacent tendons *(arrows).*

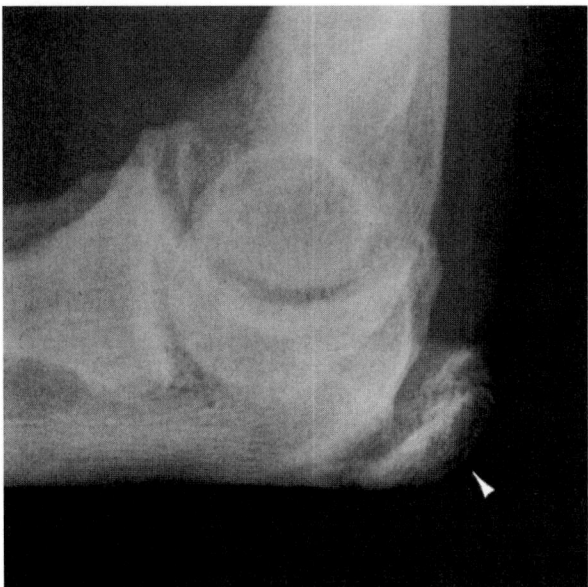

**Figure 31–9.** Elbow abnormalities in DISH. A large olecranon enthesophyte is evident *(arrowhead)*.

(From Resnick D, Shapiro RF, Wiesner KB, et al: Diffuse idiopathic skeletal hyperostosis (DISH) [ankylosing hyperostosis of Forestier and Rotes-Querol]. Semin Arthritis Rheum 7:153, 1978.)

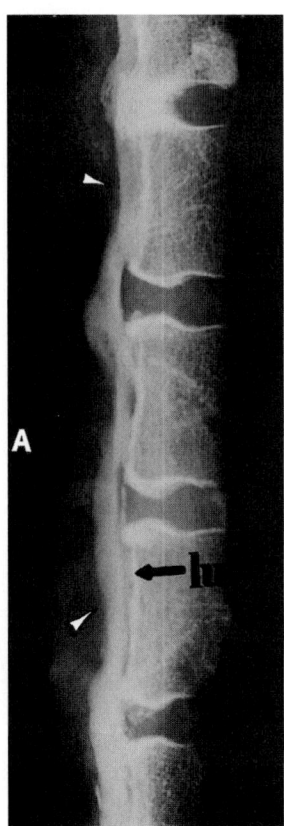

**Figure 31–10.** Pathologic abnormalities of the thoracic spine in DISH. Anterior longitudinal ligament calcification and ossification *(arrowheads)* are observed on the anterior (A) surface of the vertebrae, with subjacent radiolucent areas (lu).

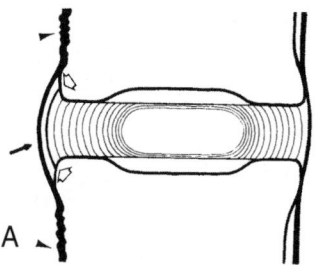

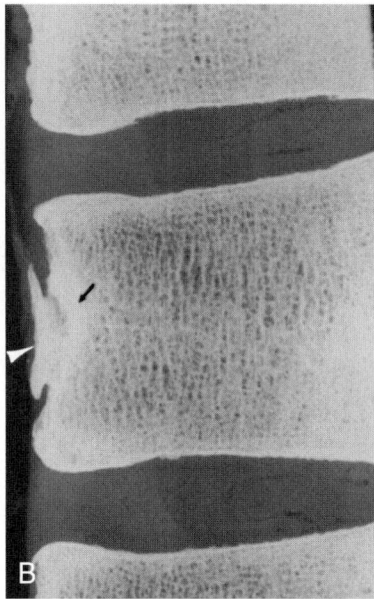

**Figure 31–11.** Pathologic abnormalities of the thoracic spine in DISH. *A,* Bone formation occurs in the middle of the anterior surface of the vertebral body *(arrowheads)*, where the anterior longitudinal ligament *(solid arrow)* is attached to the vertebral surface. *Open arrows* indicate Sharpey's fibers. *B,* Osseous proliferation *(arrowhead)* is seen on the anterior surface of the vertebral body. Mild sclerosis *(arrow)* in the vertebral body is also apparent.

## CLINICAL AND RADIOGRAPHIC COMPLICATIONS

### Postoperative Heterotopic Ossification

The occurrence of excessive heterotopic ossification after hip surgery is seen in some patients with DISH (Fig. 31–12) and may indicate a bone-forming tendency in such patients. A similar tendency for heterotopic bone formation in the postoperative period has been noted in patients with ankylosing spondylitis.

### Rheumatoid Arthritis

Although rheumatoid arthritis and DISH do not appear to be causally related, they are both common disorders and can coexist in the same patient. The radiographic abnormalities of rheumatoid arthritis may be modified in the presence of DISH. Atypical radiographic features of rheumatoid arthritis include the absence of osteoporosis and the presence of bony sclerosis and proliferation about erosions, osteophytes, and intra-articular bony ankylosis.

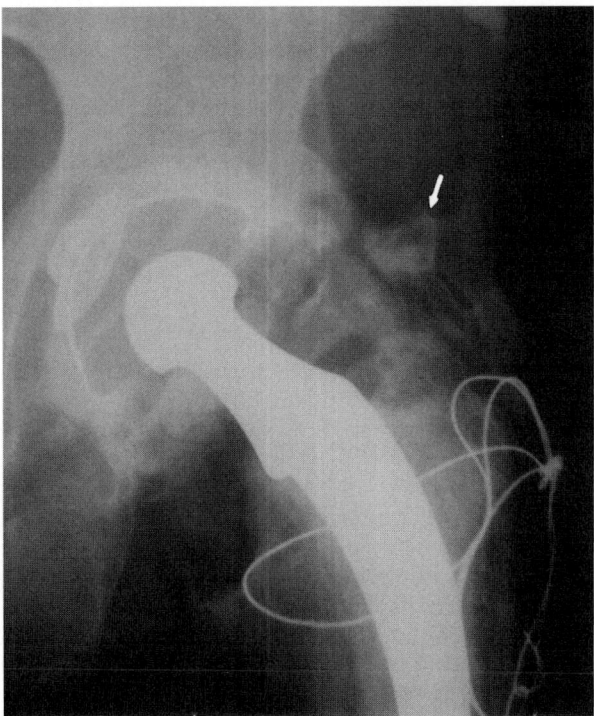

**Figure 31–12.** Heterotopic ossification in DISH. After total hip arthroplasty, extensive ossification is seen lateral to the femoral prosthesis *(arrow)*.

(From Resnick D, Shapiro RF, Wiesner KB, et al: Diffuse idiopathic skeletal hyperostosis (DISH) [ankylosing hyperostosis of Forestier and Rotes-Querol]. Semin Arthritis Rheum 7:153, 1978.)

## Ankylosing Spondylitis

A meaningful association between ankylosing spondylitis and DISH has not been established. In some patients, spinal abnormalities of both disorders are observed; in others, the spinal abnormalities of DISH are combined with the sacroiliac alterations of ankylosing spondylitis. It should be recognized, however, that diagnostic difficulties arise because of the spondylitis-type changes that may occur in some persons with DISH.

## Ossification of the Posterior Longitudinal Ligament

Ossification of the posterior longitudinal ligament, which is discussed in detail in Chapter 32, occurs with increased frequency in patients with DISH (see Fig. 31–3). In almost all instances, the cervical spine is affected. Approximately 50% of patients with DISH have radiographic evidence of calcification or ossification of the posterior longitudinal ligament.

## Spinal Stenosis

Compromise of the cord in the cervical region can relate to hyperostosis or ossification of the spinal ligaments, whereas such compromise in the thoracic and lumbar regions may be secondary to hypertrophy of the ligamen-

tum flavum or bony proliferation about the apophyseal joints.

## Fracture

Ankylosing diseases of the spine theoretically predispose the vertebral column to acute fracture and possible pseudarthrosis. These complications are well recognized in ankylosing spondylitis and, increasingly, in DISH (Fig. 31–13). Fractures occur in moderate to severe cases of DISH in which osseous fusion of long segments of the spine is present. The ankylosed region is vulnerable to fracture, even with relatively minor trauma; transverse fractures are typical. The cervical and thoracic segments appear to be more susceptible than the lumbar segment. Significant neurologic complications, including quadriplegia, are related in part to spinal instability and to delay in both diagnosis and treatment.

## Infective Spondylitis

Although the hyperostotic spine in DISH is apparently not associated with a predisposition to infective spondylitis, the two conditions may occasionally coexist. In such cases, accurate diagnosis of spinal infection may be difficult because of the possibility that the bridging vertebral outgrowths prevent disc space collapse, which is a fundamental radiographic sign of pyogenic spondylitis.

## CAUSE

The cause of DISH is unknown. One common factor in patients with DISH is advanced age. Some patients relate a history of spinal trauma or occupational stress; others have no history of significant accidental or occupational trauma.

Although the occurrence of spinal and extraspinal hyperostosis resembling that of DISH has been reported in various diseases, as well as with the administration of vitamin A derivatives (e.g., 13-*cis*-retinoic acid) to patients with cutaneous disorders, there is no definite evidence connecting the hyperostosis in DISH with any of these other disorders. Because of the apparent similarity between DISH and ankylosing spondylitis, the prevalence of the HLA-B27 antigen has been studied in patients with DISH, but published studies have failed to confirm an increased prevalence of HLA-B27 in patients with DISH.

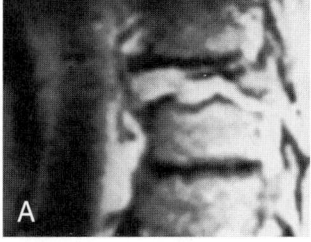
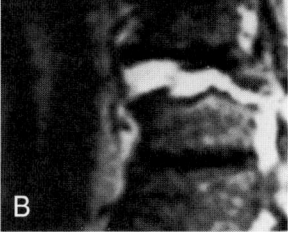

**Figure 31–13.** Spinal fractures and DISH. In this 56-year-old man with DISH, note a transverse fracture of high signal intensity on sagittal intermediate-weighted (TR/TE, 2200/30) *(A)* and T2-weighted (TR/TE, 2200/70) *(B)* spin echo MR images. (Courtesy of C. Gundry, MD, Minneapolis, Minn.)

# DIFFERENTIAL DIAGNOSIS

## Spinal Abnormalities

Although the clinical and radiographic features of DISH are characteristic, DISH must be distinguished from other disorders of the vertebral column associated with hyperostosis (Tables 31–5 and 31–6).

**Intervertebral (Osteo)Chondrosis.** Intervertebral (osteo)chondrosis is a term applied to alterations of the intervertebral disc related to physiologic and pathologic dehydration occurring with advancing age. Cleft formation in the nucleus may extend into the anulus fibrosus and is associated with the so-called vacuum phenomenon on radiographs. Continued destruction of the nucleus pulposus results in flattening of the intervertebral disc and disc space narrowing. With further progression of disease, sclerosis and intravertebral disc displacement (cartilaginous, or Schmorl's, nodes) are observed. These changes differ considerably from those of DISH.

---

**TABLE 31–5**

### Conditions Associated with or Causing Bony Outgrowths of the Spine

DISH
Spondylosis deformans
Ankylosing spondylitis
Spondylitic variant disorders
Acromegaly
Hypoparathyroidism
Fluorosis
Ochronosis
Neuropathic osteoarthropathy
Trauma
Sternocostoclavicular hyperostosis

---

**Spondylosis Deformans.** Spondylosis deformans, a common condition, results in spinal osteophytosis. Some of the spinal findings in DISH resemble those of spondylosis deformans. The degree of disc prolapse, the size and number of osteophytes, the presence of ligamentous calcification or ossification, and the existence of a proliferative enthesopathy generally distinguish DISH from typical spondylosis deformans.

**Ankylosing Spondylitis.** The clinical, radiographic, and pathologic features of ankylosing spondylitis differ from those of DISH. Ankylosing spondylitis affects predominantly young adults and produces considerable signs and symptoms; DISH affects middle-aged and elderly patients and may be asymptomatic or associated with mild to moderate restriction of motion. In ankylosing spondylitis, syndesmophytes are thin, vertical osseous bridges that extend from one vertebral body to the next (Fig. 31–14). DISH is associated with exuberant bone formation encompassing the anulus, anterior longitudinal ligament, and connective tissue. Outgrowths are broad and irregular and have an anterior distribution. Further, ankylosing spondylitis is characterized by vertebral body osteitis and subsequent erosion and reactive sclerosis along the anterior corners of the vertebra; sacroiliac joint erosion, sclerosis, and intra-articular bony ankylosis; and apophyseal joint ankylosis. These manifestations are absent in DISH.

**Spondylitic Variants.** Psoriatic arthritis (Fig. 31–15), Reiter's syndrome, and bowel disorders such as ulcerative colitis, regional enteritis, and Whipple's disease are associated with bony abnormalities of the vertebral column. In psoriatic arthritis and, to a lesser extent, in Reiter's syndrome, such abnormalities consist of (1) outgrowths that may resemble the typical syndesmophytes of ankylosing spondylitis, (2) asymmetrical osteophytes, or (3) paravertebral ossification. In some instances, the bone formation in these two disorders may resemble DISH, although an anterior linear pattern of ossification is not

---

**TABLE 31–6**

### Differential Diagnosis of Radiographic Findings in Diffuse Idiopathic Skeletal Hyperostosis (DISH), Ankylosing Spondylitis, and Intervertebral (Osteo)Chondrosis

| Site | DISH | Ankylosing Spondylitis | Intervertebral (Osteo)Chondrosis |
|---|---|---|---|
| Vertebral bodies | Flowing ossification and hyperostosis; large osteophytes; bony ankylosis frequent radiographically, less frequent pathologically | Thin syndesmophytes, osteitis with "squaring," extensive bony ankylosis radiographically and pathologically | Sclerosis of superior and inferior surfaces |
| Intervertebral discs | Normal or mild decrease in height | Normal or convex in shape | Moderate to severe decrease in height; vacuum phenomena |
| Apophyseal joints | Normal or mild sclerosis, occasional osteophytes | Erosions, sclerosis, bony ankylosis | Normal |
| Sacroiliac joints | Para-articular osteophytes | Erosions, sclerosis, bony ankylosis | Normal |
| Peripheral skeleton | "Whiskering," para-articular osteophytes, ligament calcification and ossification, hyperostosis | "Whiskering," arthritis | Normal |

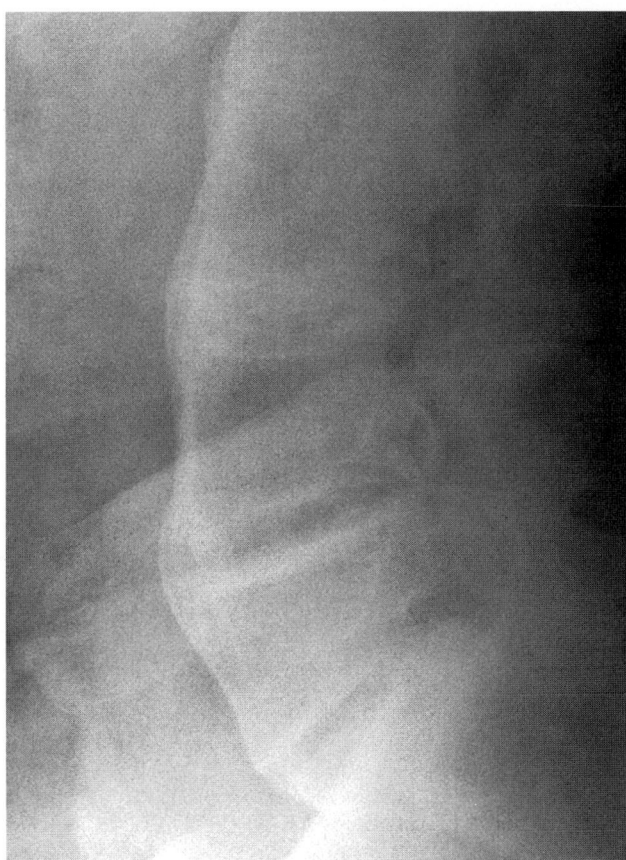

**Figure 31–14.** Ankylosing spondylitis. Classic radiographic features include squaring of the vertebral bodies, osteitis or "whitening" of the vertebral corners, and syndesmophytes.

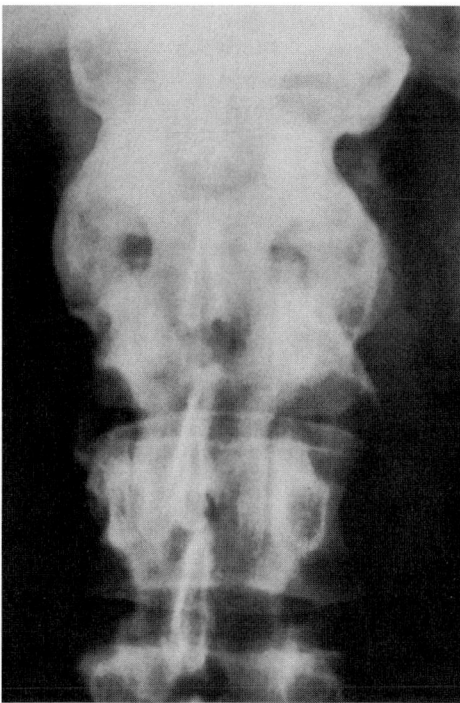

**Figure 31–15.** Psoriatic arthritis. Spinal involvement is characterized by bulky ossification about multiple lumbar intervertebral discs.

(From Resnick D, Shapiro RF, Wiesner KB, et al: Diffuse idiopathic skeletal hyperostosis (DISH) [ankylosing hyperostosis of Forestier and Rotes-Querol]. Semin Arthritis Rheum 7:153, 1978.)

usually apparent. In general, outgrowths in psoriatic arthritis and Reiter's syndrome are better demonstrated on frontal radiographs than on lateral radiographs. In bowel disorders, the spinal alterations resemble typical syndesmophytes. In psoriatic arthritis, Reiter's syndrome, and bowel disorders, sacroiliitis and apophyseal joint alterations allow proper distinction from DISH.

**Acromegaly.** Acromegaly may be associated with osseous outgrowths of the spine. Periosteal new bone formation occurs on the anterior and lateral aspects of the vertebral body and produces apparent flattening of the vertebra related to an increased anteroposterior diameter. Osteophytes may bridge the intervertebral disc space. Additional spinal findings in acromegaly are posterior concavity or scalloping of the vertebral body and increased intervertebral disc space height.

**Hypoparathyroidism.** Hypoparathyroidism may be associated with osteophytes and enthesophytes in the presence of a normal intervertebral disc space, as well as with ossification of muscle and ligamentous insertions. Patients with DISH have no history of tetany or convulsions, and serum levels of calcium, phosphorus, alkaline phosphatase, magnesium, and parathyroid hormone are normal.

**Fluorosis.** Fluorosis is associated with severe osteophytosis of the spine and ligament ossification, particularly ossification of the sacrotuberous ligament. These findings may resemble those of DISH, a similarity that is further accentuated by the appearance of calcification in the para-articular ligaments, musculotendinous attachments, and interosseous membranes in fluorosis. The presence of bone sclerosis in fluorosis is distinctive.

**Ochronosis.** This rare disorder is associated with characteristic spinal changes, including osteophytosis and anterior disc ossification. The presence of extensive disc calcification and vertebral body osteoporosis allows an accurate diagnosis.

**Axial Neuropathic Osteoarthropathy.** Axial neuropathic osteoarthropathy can be noted in syphilis, diabetes mellitus, and syringomyelia. The initial radiographic findings may simulate those of intervertebral (osteo)chondrosis, with loss of intervertebral disc space and vertebral body marginal sclerosis. Progressive alterations are increasing sclerosis, subluxation, fragmentation, and bizarre osteophytosis. The presence of disc space loss, extreme sclerosis, and subluxation creates a disorganized look that differs considerably from the findings of DISH.

**Sternocostoclavicular Hyperostosis.** As described in Chapter 82, this rare syndrome can lead to spinal alterations very similar to those of DISH. In the cervical spine, unique abnormalities consisting of massive new bone formation are occasionally identified. In sternocostoclavicular hyperostosis, ossification also affects the medial aspect of the clavicles, the upper ribs, and the sternum, and pustular skin lesions are common on the palms and soles.

## Extraspinal Abnormalities

The extraspinal manifestations of DISH may be confused with certain disorders that involve both spinal and extraspinal sites. The peripheral skeletal changes in fluorosis and hypoparathyroidism have already been noted. Other disorders must also be considered.

**Ankylosing Spondylitis and Spondylitic Variant Disorders.** These diseases produce abnormalities at sites of tendon and ligament attachment to bone, particularly about the pelvis and proximal ends of the femora. The changes superficially resemble the hyperostosis observed in DISH. In ankylosing spondylitis and spondylitic variant disorders, osseous erosion and sclerosis are more prominent, and the newly formed bone is poorly defined and irregular. In DISH, proliferative changes are frequently sharply demarcated, without signs of erosion or underlying bone sclerosis.

**Hypertrophic Osteoarthropathy.** Hypertrophic osteoarthropathy is characterized by symmetrical periostitis, particularly of the radius, ulna, tibia, and fibula, with lesser involvement of the femur, humerus, metacarpals, metatarsals, and phalanges. Although patients with DISH occasionally demonstrate diaphyseal periostitis, particularly in the femur, humerus, and metacarpals—a finding simulating hypertrophic osteoarthropathy—diaphyseal periostitis is not usually prominent in DISH.

**Pachydermoperiostosis.** Pachydermoperiostosis, a familial disorder, is characterized by the insidious development of digital clubbing; soft tissue thickening of the legs and forearms; thickening and greasiness of the skin, particularly the skin of the face; excessive sweating; and radiographic evidence of symmetrical, irregular, periosteal new bone formation showing a predilection for the radius, ulna, tibia, and fibula. These clinical features are not noted in DISH, nor are the radiographic abnormalities of pachydermoperiostosis strikingly similar to those observed in DISH.

**Hypervitaminosis A.** Although vitamin A intoxication may be associated with extensive bone formation in cats, it does not generally produce changes in humans that resemble DISH. Chronic poisoning may lead to periosteal reaction and no other bone abnormality. Of interest, prolonged therapy with retinoid drugs (which are chemically similar to vitamin A) in patients with dermatologic disorders has been associated with skeletal hyperostosis in both the axial skeleton (especially the cervical spine) and the appendicular skeleton (see Chapter 63).

**Calcium Pyrophosphate Dihydrate Crystal Deposition Disease.** Calcium pyrophosphate dihydrate crystal deposition disease is a common disorder and may coexist with DISH. One of its radiographic features, tendon calcification, superficially resembles the findings of DISH. Other findings of this crystal deposition disease, including chondrocalcinosis and pyrophosphate arthropathy, are characteristic and allow an accurate diagnosis.

**X-Linked Hypophosphatemic Osteomalacia.** This disorder, which is characterized by hypophosphatemia, impaired renal tubular reabsorption of phosphate, and defective calcification of cartilage and bone (see Chapter 42), is associated with an enthesopathy in which exuberant calcification of the joint capsules and tendinous and ligamentous insertions becomes evident. Changes in the spine are infrequent and mild.

## FURTHER READING

Abiteboul M, Arlet J: Retinol-related hyperostosis. AJR Am J Roentgenol 144:435, 1985.

Blasinghame JP, Resnick D, Coutts RD, et al: Extensive spinal osteophytosis as a risk factor for heterotopic bone formation after total hip replacement. Clin Orthop 161:191, 1981.

Bundrick TJ, Cook DE, Resnik CS: Heterotopic bone formation in patients with DISH following total hip replacement. Radiology 155:595, 1985.

DiGiovanna JJ, Helfgott RK, Gerber LH, et al: Extraspinal tendon and ligament calcification associated with long-term therapy with etretinate. N Engl J Med 315:1177, 1986.

Forestier J, Rotes-Querol J: Senile ankylosing hyperostosis of the spine. Ann Rheum Dis 9:321, 1950.

Francois RJ: Vertebral ankylosing hyperostosis: What new bone, where and why? J Rheumatol 10:837, 1983.

Haller J, Resnick D, Miller CW, et al: Diffuse idiopathic skeletal hyperostosis: Diagnostic significance of radiographic abnormalities of the pelvis. Radiology 172:835, 1989.

Hendrix RW, Melany M, Miller F, et al: Fracture of the spine in patients with ankylosis due to diffuse skeletal hyperostosis: Clinical and imaging findings. AJR Am J Roentgenol 162:899, 1994.

Le Hir PX, Sautet A, Le Gars L, et al: Hyperextension vertebral body fractures in diffuse idiopathic skeletal hyperostosis: A cause of intravertebral fluid-like collections on MR imaging. AJR Am J Roentgenol 173:1679, 1999.

Lee SH, Coleman PE, Hahn FJ: Magnetic resonance imaging of degenerative disk disease of the spine. Radiol Clin North Am 26:949, 1988.

Littlejohn GO, Urowitz MB, Smythe HA, et al: Radiographic features of the hand in diffuse idiopathic skeletal hyperostosis (DISH): Comparison with normal subjects and acromegalic patients. Radiology 140:623, 1981.

Mata S, Chhem RK, Fortin PR, et al: Comprehensive radiographic evaluation of diffuse idiopathic skeletal hyperostosis: Development and interrater reliability of scoring system. Semin Arthritis Rheum 28:88, 1998.

Mata S, Wolfe F, Joseph L, et al: Absence of an association of rheumatoid arthritis and diffuse idiopathic skeletal hyperostosis: A case-control study. J Rheumatol 22:2062, 1995.

Meyer PR Jr: Diffuse idiopathic skeletal hyperostosis in the cervical spine. Clin Orthop 359:49, 1999.

Polisson RP, Martinez S, Khoury M, et al: Calcification of entheses associated with X-linked hypophosphatemic osteomalacia. N Engl J Med 313:1, 1985.

Resnick D, Curd J, Shapiro RF, et al: Radiographic abnormalities of rheumatoid arthritis in patients with diffuse idiopathic skeletal hyperostosis. Arthritis Rheum 21:1, 1978.

Resnick D, Guerra J Jr, Robinson CA, et al: Association of diffuse idiopathic skeletal hyperostosis (DISH) and calcification and ossification of the posterior longitudinal ligament. AJR Am J Roentgenol 131:1049, 1978.

Resnick D, Linovitz RJ, Feingold ML: Postoperative heterotopic ossification in patients with ankylosing hyperostosis of the spine (Forestier's disease). J Rheumatol 3:313, 1976.

Resnick D, Niwayama G: Radiographic and pathologic features of spinal involvement in diffuse idiopathic skeletal hyperostosis (DISH). Radiology 119:559, 1976.

Resnick D, Shaul S, Robins JM: Diffuse idiopathic skeletal hyperostosis (DISH): Forestier's disease with extraspinal manifestations. Radiology 115:513, 1975.

Weinfeld RM, Olson PN, Maki DD, et al: The prevalence of diffuse idiopathic skeletal hyperostosis (DISH) in two large American Midwest metropolitan hospital populations. Skeletal Radiol 26:222, 1997.

# CHAPTER 32

## Calcification and Ossification of the Posterior Spinal Ligaments and Tissues

ligament, and ossification of the ligamentum nuchae are additional abnormalities of the posterior spinal tissues.

## SUMMARY OF KEY FEATURES

Calcification and ossification affect a variety of posterior spinal ligaments and tissues. Ossification of the posterior longitudinal ligament is a characteristic disorder of the spine that may be associated with significant neurologic findings. Its radiographic appearance is diagnostic and consists of a linear band of ossification along the posterior margin of the vertebral bodies and intervertebral discs, particularly in the cervical spine. Arachnoiditis ossificans is a rare condition that leads to extensive ossification in the arachnoid membrane, especially in the thoracic spine, and it produces significant symptoms and signs.

Osseous proliferation at the cephalad and caudad attachments of the ligamentum flavum is a frequent finding that is generally of no significance. When extensive, however, such ossification in the thoracic spine leads to neurologic manifestations and is accompanied by involvement of nearby tissues and ligaments and, in some cases, diffuse idiopathic skeletal hyperostosis. Calcification in the ligamentum flavum is usually observed in the cervical spine and is associated with calcium hydroxyapatite crystal deposition or, more infrequently, calcium pyrophosphate dihydrate crystal accumulation. A nodular radiodense collection is the typical radiographic abnormality.

Hyperostosis at the osseous sites of attachment of the supraspinous ligament, calcification in the interspinous

## INTRODUCTION

Chapter 31 discusses diffuse idiopathic skeletal hyperostosis (DISH), a disease is characterized in part by calcification and ossification in the anterior longitudinal ligament of the spine. Although such changes are most frequent in this ligament, other spinal ligaments may calcify or ossify (Table 32–1). A review of these less common processes is provided in this chapter.

## ANATOMIC CONSIDERATIONS

The posterior longitudinal ligament extends from the axis and tectorial membrane above to the sacrum below, within the vertebral canal (Fig. 32–1). It is attached to the intervertebral discs and the margins of the vertebral bodies; it is strung like a bow over the central, concave portion of the vertebral body.

The ligamenta flava are attached to the articular capsule of the apophyseal joints and the laminae. The ligaments from each side approximate each other at the base of the spinous process. The ligamenta flava are thickest in the lumbar segment, somewhat thinner in the thoracic spine, and thinnest in the cervical region.

The interspinous ligaments extend from the root to the apex of each spinous process and connect adjoining processes. They meet the ligamenta flava anteriorly and the supraspinous ligament posteriorly. The latter is a strong fibrous structure connecting the apices of the spinous processes from the level of the seventh cervical vertebra to the sacrum. Above this cervical attachment,

### TABLE 32–1

**Calcification and Ossification of Posterior Spinal Ligaments and Tissues**

| Condition | Most Common Spinal Location | Clinical Manifestations | Associated Conditions |
|---|---|---|---|
| Ossification of posterior longitudinal ligament (OPLL) | Cervical | May be present | DISH, OLF |
| Arachnoiditis ossificans | Thoracic | May be present | |
| Enthesopathy of ligamenta flava | Thoracic | Absent | |
| Calcification of ligamenta flava | Cervical | May be present | CPPD crystal deposition disease |
| Ossification of ligamenta flava (OLF) | Thoracic | May be present | OPLL, DISH |
| Ossification of ligamentum nuchae | Cervical | Absent | DISH |
| Enthesopathy of supraspinous ligament | Lumbar | May be present | Baastrup's disease, DISH |

CPPD, calcium pyrophosphate dihydrate; DISH, diffuse idiopathic skeletal hyperostosis.

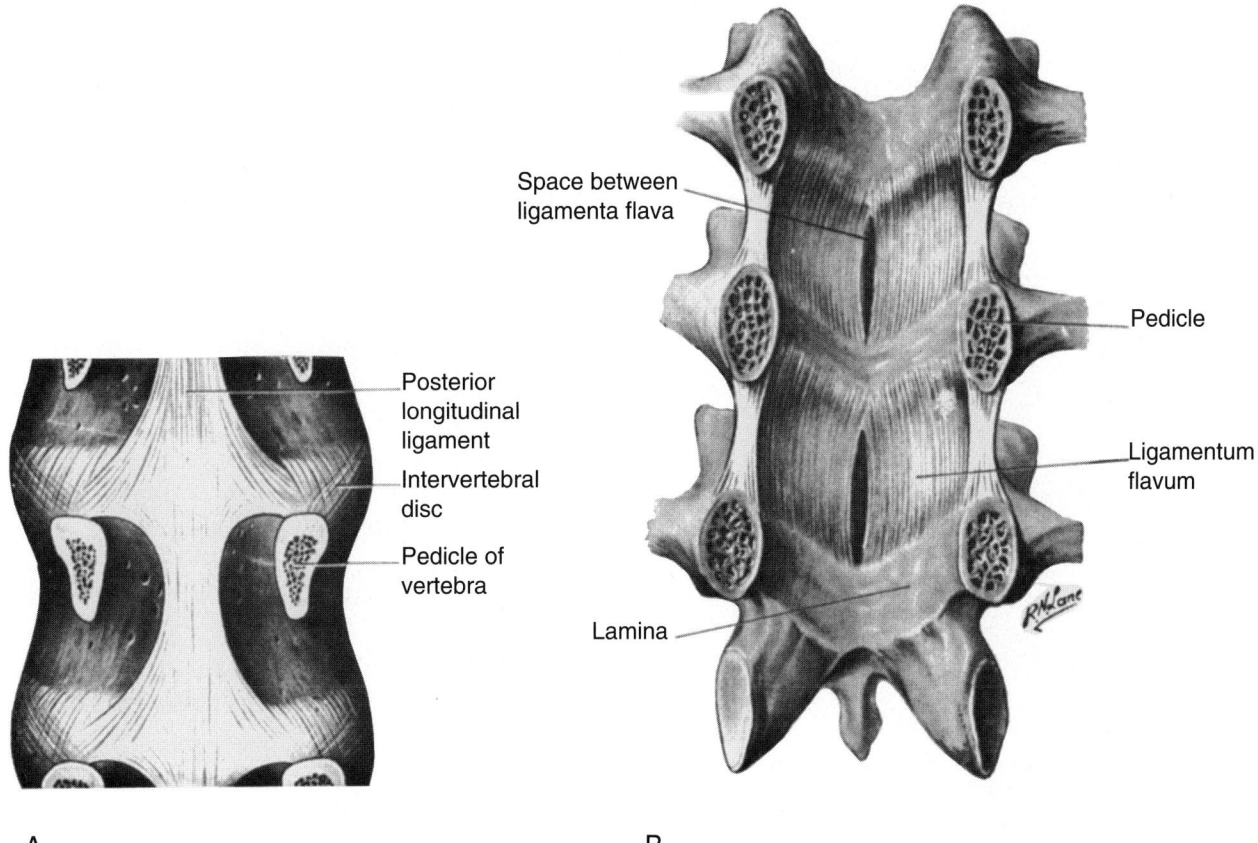

**Figure 32–1.** Posterior spinal ligaments: anatomic considerations. *A*, Posterior longitudinal ligament: lumbar spine. Drawing of the posterior aspect of the vertebral bodies and intervertebral discs shows the position and appearance of the posterior longitudinal ligament. Note that it is narrow at the level of the vertebral bodies and broad at the level of the intervertebral discs. *B*, Ligamenta flava: lumbar spine. Drawing of the anterior aspect of the vertebral arches reveals the position of the paired ligamenta flava. At the bases of the spinous processes, spaces between the ligaments allow passage of veins.
(From Williams PL, Warwick R: Gray's Anatomy, 36th Br ed. Philadelphia, WB Saunders, 1980, p 44.)

the ligament expands to form the ligamentum nuchae, which extends cephalad to the external occipital protuberance. The intertransverse ligaments are located between the transverse processes of the vertebrae.

## OSSIFICATION OF THE POSTERIOR LONGITUDINAL LIGAMENT

### Clinical Abnormalities

Ossification of the posterior longitudinal ligament (OPLL) is more frequent in men than women, with a ratio of approximately 2:1. Diagnosis of the disorder is usually established in the fifth to seventh decades of life. Although persons with OPLL may be entirely asymptomatic, a variety of symptoms and signs have been associated with this disorder. Neurologic symptoms may be divided into three groups: cord signs, which are most common, manifested by dominant motor and sensory disturbances in the lower extremity; segmental signs, manifested by dominant motor and sensory disturbances in the upper extremity; and cervicobrachialgia, which

causes no obvious neurologic deficits and is associated with pain in the neck, shoulder, and arm. Neurologic manifestations are more frequent in patients in whom the thickness of the ligament is greater than 30% to 60% of the sagittal diameter of the cervical spinal canal as measured by radiographs.

The choice of therapy is made difficult by some inconsistency in the relationship between the neurologic manifestations and the degree of ligamentous ossification and by reports of postoperative progression of such ossification.

### Radiographic Abnormalities

The diagnosis of OPLL is established by its characteristic radiographic appearance (Fig. 32–2). In the cervical spine (and, infrequently, in the thoracic and lumbar spine), a dense, ossified strip or plaque of variable thickness (1 to 5 mm) is evident along the posterior margins of the vertebral bodies and the intervertebral discs. It is most common in the midcervical region (C3 to C5), although any cervical level may be affected. The ossified ligament may be confined to one or several vertebral bodies, without

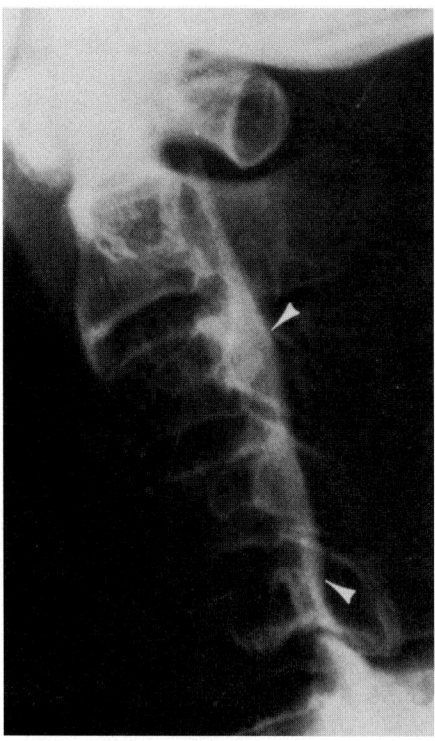

**Figure 32–2.** Ossification of the posterior longitudinal ligament: radiographic abnormalities of the cervical spine. This 53-year-old man complained of clumsiness and numbness in the hands and difficulty walking. OPLL extends from the first through sixth cervical vertebrae *(arrowheads)*.

(From Ono K, Ota H, Tada K, et al: Ossified posterior longitudinal ligament. Spine 2:126, 1977.)

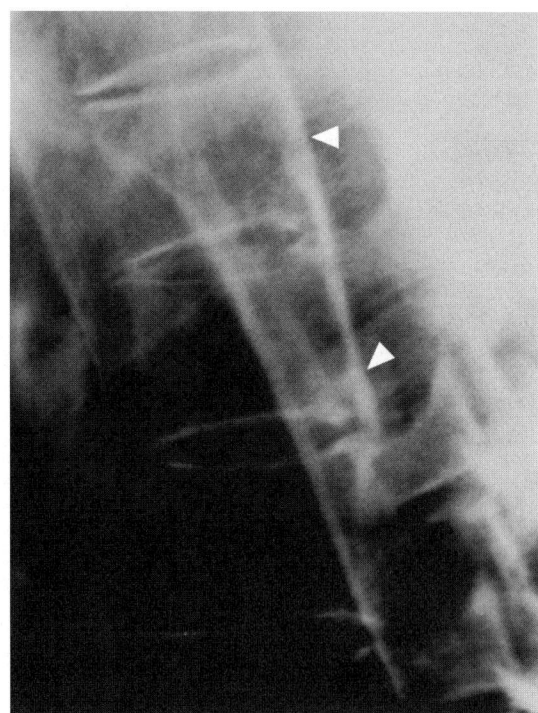

**Figure 32–3.** Ossification of the posterior longitudinal ligament: radiographic abnormalities of the thoracic spine. Note the radiodense stripe *(arrowheads)* applied to the backs of several upper thoracic vertebral bodies. (Courtesy of M. Mitchell, MD, Halifax, Nova Scotia, Canada.)

involvement of the intervening intervertebral discs (segmental distribution), or it may extend in an uninterrupted fashion for several vertebrae (continuous distribution). Often, OPLL is separated from the vertebral body by a thin radiolucent zone. The intervertebral discs in the involved area are generally well preserved, without evidence of disc space narrowing; however, anterior vertebral osteophytes are frequently identifiable (30% to 50% of patients).

OPLL is not confined to the cervical region and may involve the thoracic and lumbar segments as well. In the thoracic spine, OPLL is most common at the fourth to seventh thoracic vertebral levels (Fig. 32–3). Involvement in the lumbar spine can be apparent at any level, although changes predominate in the L1 to L2 region. The extent of OPLL and the degree of spinal encroachment have been further delineated by means of conventional tomography, axial transverse tomography, computed tomography (CT), myelography, and magnetic resonance (MR) imaging (Fig. 32–4).

### Magnetic Resonance Imaging Abnormalities

MR imaging is well suited to the evaluation of patients with OPLL. OPLL is generally seen as a band of low signal intensity between the bone marrow of the vertebral body and the dural sac on T1- and T2-weighted spin echo MR images. Within the area of ossification, an area of increased or intermediate signal intensity, correspond-

ing to that of fat, can be observed in more than half of patients with the continuous type of OPLL and occasionally with segmental OPLL. The degree of spinal cord compression is generally more severe in cases of continuous OPLL, and disc degeneration is a frequently associated feature (see Fig. 32–4).

The differential diagnosis of a lesion around the spinal cord, when characterized by low signal intensity on both T1- and T2-weighted images, includes OPLL, a hypertrophied ligament, hemosiderin deposition, flowing blood or cerebrospinal fluid, and calcified meningioma. When high signal intensity is evident as well, OPLL, osteophyte formation, and disc displacement are diagnostic considerations.

### Pathologic Abnormalities

The bony overgrowth appears as cortical bone composed of lamellar bone with well-developed haversian canals and poorly developed marrow cavities. In places, the ossified mass is firmly attached to the posterior aspect of the vertebral body and intervertebral disc; elsewhere, it is separated from these structures by intervening connective tissue. Closer inspection of the ossification allows the identification of calcific areas within the posterior longitudinal ligament, which suggests that the ossification involves the ligament itself but need not be complete. The exact mechanism leading to mineral deposition in the posterior longitudinal ligament is not clear.

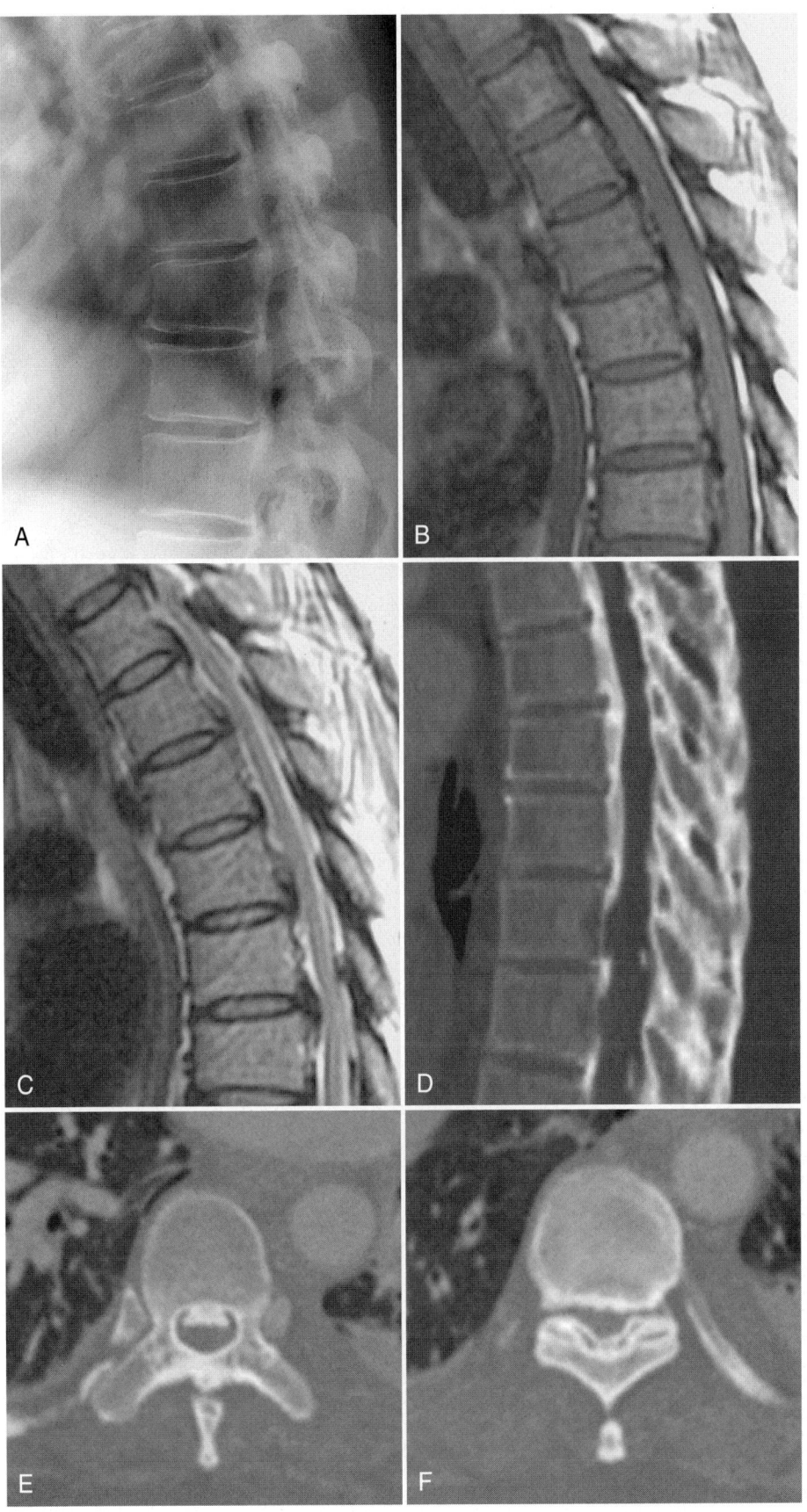

**Figure 32–4.** Ossification of the posterior longitudinal ligament: MR imaging and CT abnormalities of the thoracic spine. The patient is a 47-year-old woman with back pain and leg weakness. *A*, Radiograph shows a dense ossified strip along the posterior margin of the vertebral bodies. Note continuous involvement superiorly and relative preservation of intervertebral disc spaces. *B* and *C*, Corresponding sagittal T1-weighted (TR/TE, 500/9) *(B)* and turbo T2-weighted (TR/TE, 4000/100) *(C)* MR images show that the signal intensity within the posterior longitudinal ligament is equal to or less than that of the adjacent fatty marrow, with the more densely ossified areas showing decreased signal. *D*, Sagittal reformatted noncontrast CT scan shows the ossification to better advantage. Note mineralization of the ligamentum flavum and interspinous and supraspinous ligaments. *E*, Midthoracic axial CT scan at the pedicular level shows extensive ossification of the posterior longitudinal ligament, with significant compromise of the spinal canal. *F*, Axial CT scan at the level of the facet joints shows ligamentum flavum and apophyseal joint capsule mineralization.

## Cause and Pathogenesis

The cause of OPLL is not precisely known. The observation that OPLL is frequent in patients with DISH suggests a common cause and pathogenesis for these conditions. OPLL may be apparent in as many as 50% of patients with DISH; conversely, DISH has been observed in more than 20% of patients with OPLL. The association of OPLL with other forms of spinal hyperostosis has also been recorded. Ossification of the ligamenta flava can accompany OPLL and has been reported in 7% of cases of OPLL, and the coexistence of OPLL, DISH (with both spinal and extraspinal manifestations), and ossification of the ligamenta flava is not rare.

## Differential Diagnosis

When extensive, OPLL creates a radiodense band posterior to the vertebral body and intervertebral disc that bears little resemblance to the bony outgrowths associated with spondylosis deformans or articular disorders such as ankylosing spondylitis. In spondylosis deformans, osteophytes are most common along the anterolateral aspect of the vertebral column; posterior excrescences are absent or small. In addition, osteophytes are usually triangular in shape, arising adjacent to the vertebral edge and extending in a horizontal direction. Their appearance therefore differs from the linear vertical ossification in OPLL. In ankylosing spondylitis, syndesmophytes initially form in the outer fibers of the anulus fibrosus. They are vertical in orientation and extend from one vertebral body to the next. In psoriatic (and Reiter's) spondylitis, larger areas of ossification are apparent about the vertebral column, but, unlike in OPLL, these regions are most readily apparent on frontal radiographs as asymmetrical radiodense areas adjacent to the lateral margins of the vertebrae and intervertebral discs. Similarly, the ossification in DISH bears no resemblance to that of OPLL, although both conditions can occur simultaneously.

## ARACHNOIDITIS OSSIFICANS

Arachnoiditis is an inflammatory process affecting the pia-arachnoid membrane. It is usually observed after spinal surgery or injection of contrast material. Three stages of the disease have been identified: radiculitis, arachnoiditis, and adhesive arachnoiditis. In the adhesive stage, osseous metaplasia may be evident in the dense proliferative collagenous layer, a process called arachnoiditis ossificans. Arachnoiditis ossificans is seen most commonly in one or more regions of the thoracic spine. Symptoms and signs are variable, but back pain and tenderness and paresis may be noted. Radiographs may demonstrate linear calcifications and ossifications within the spinal canal. CT scanning or MR imaging demonstrates the plaquelike ossification in the arachnoid membrane (Fig. 32–5).

## CALCIFICATION OR OSSIFICATION OF THE LIGAMENTUM FLAVUM

Anatomic studies have verified that osseous proliferation (enthesopathy) in both the cephalad and caudad attachments of the ligamentum flavum is frequent and generally of no clinical significance (see Fig. 32–4F). Extensive calcification or ossification (or both) in hypertrophied ligamenta flava is more clinically significant, inasmuch as these alterations have been reported in association with myelopathy or radiculopathy. In the cervical spine, calcification typically occurs in elderly patients, particularly women. The calcific collections consist of calcium hydroxyapatite in most cases; calcium pyrophosphate dihydrate (CPPD) crystals are occasionally encountered. The middle cervical region is the most common site of involvement. A nodular radiodense collection is the characteristic radiographic abnormality. Myelography may reveal generalized hypertrophy of the ligamentum flavum. CT scanning or MR imaging is an excellent means to document and localize the abnormality.

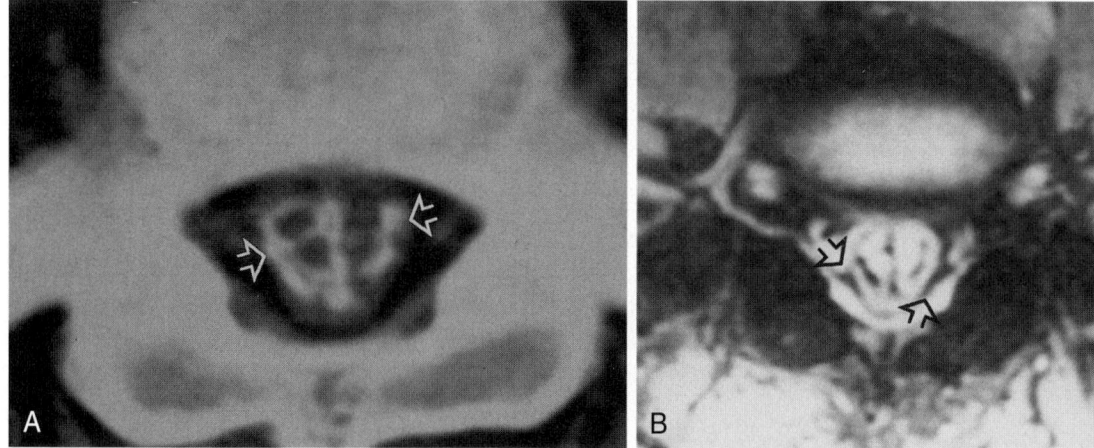

**Figure 32–5.** Arachnoiditis ossificans. *A*, In this transaxial CT scan, observe the extensive ossification *(open arrows)* in the lumbosacral region of the spinal canal. The unossified nerve roots are identifiable. *B*, On a transaxial gradient echo (MPGR) MR image (TR/TE, 1000/15; flip angle, 50 degrees), the calcified areas are of low signal intensity *(open arrows)*. (Courtesy of S. Eilenberg, MD, San Diego, Calif.)

In the thoracic and upper lumbar spine, ossification (rather than calcification) of the ligamentum flavum predominates. Both men and women are affected, typically in the fifth and sixth decades of life. Neurologic manifestations include decreased sensation, paresis, and even neurogenic bladder. Ossification of the ligamentum flavum appears to be an accentuation of the bone spiculation that is observed anatomically at the sites of osseous attachment of the ligamenta flava.

CPPD crystal deposition disease is a recognized cause of calcification in the ligamentum flavum, as well as in other posterior spinal structures such as the posterior longitudinal ligament, interspinous and supraspinous ligaments, and apophyseal joints. Linear or nodular deposits related to CPPD crystal accumulation in the thoracic spine are typical.

## CALCIFICATION OR OSSIFICATION OF OTHER POSTERIOR SPINAL LIGAMENTS

Hyperostosis at the sites of attachment of the supraspinous ligament and calcification and ossification within this ligament occur as isolated abnormalities or in association with DISH. Calcification within the interspinous ligament occurs in CPPD crystal deposition disease. Ossification in the ligamentum nuchae is an incidental and frequent radiographic finding that is also seen in DISH.

## FURTHER READING

Barthelemy CR: Arachnoiditis ossificans. J. Comput Assist Tomogr 6:809, 1982.

Ehara S, Shimamura T, Nakamura R, et al: Paravertebral ligamentous ossification: DISH, OPLL and OLF. Eur J Radiol 27:96, 1998.

Griffiths ID, Fitzjohn TP: Cervical myelopathy, ossification of the posterior longitudinal ligament, and diffuse idiopathic skeletal hyperostosis: Problems in investigation. Ann Rheum Dis 46:166, 1987.

Kudo S, Ono M, Russell WJ: Ossification of thoracic ligamenta flava. AJR 141:117, 1983.

Minagi H, Gronner AT: Calcification of the posterior longitudinal ligament: A cause of cervical myelopathy. AJR 105:365, 1969.

Ono K, Ota H, Tada K, et al: Ossified posterior longitudinal ligament. Spine 2:126, 1977.

Ono K, Yonenobu K, Miyamoto S, et al: Pathology of ossification of the posterior longitudinal ligament and ligamentum flavum. Clin Orthop 359: 18, 1999.

Ono M, Russell WJ, Kudo S, et al: Ossification of the thoracic posterior longitudinal ligament in a fixed population. Radiological and neurological manifestations. Radiology 143:469, 1982.

Resnick D, Pineda C: Vertebral involvement in calcium pyrophosphate dihydrate crystal deposition disease. Radiographic-pathologic correlation. Radiology 153:55, 1984.

Resnick D, Guerra J Jr, Robinson CA, et al: Association of diffuse idiopathic skeletal hyperostosis (DISH) and calcification and ossification of the posterior longitudinal ligament. AJR 131:1049, 1987.

Revilla TY, Ramos A, Gonzalez P, et al: Arachnoiditis ossificans: Diagnosis with helical computed tomography. Clin Imaging 23:1, 1999.

Williams DM, Gabrielsen TO, Latack JT, et al: Ossification in the cephalic attachment of the ligamentum flavum. An anatomical and CT study. Radiology 150:423, 1984.

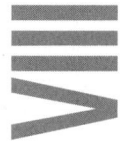
# Crystal-Induced and Related Diseases

# CHAPTER 33

## Gouty Arthritis

## SUMMARY OF KEY FEATURES

Gouty arthritis is characterized by asymmetrical polyarticular involvement, predominantly affecting the feet, hands, wrists, elbows, and knees. Radiographic manifestations occur late in the course of the disease and include lobulated eccentric soft tissue masses, intra-articular and juxta-articular bone erosions, relative preservation of the joint space, subperiosteal apposition of bone, intraosseous calcification, and secondary degenerative alterations. Osteoporosis is generally lacking. In most cases, these radiographic features readily differentiate gouty arthritis from other articular disorders.

## INTRODUCTION

Famous and influential people have suffered from the ravages of gout throughout history. Apparent descriptions of the disorder can be found in the Babylonian Talmud from more than 2000 years ago, as well as in the Bible. The disease was originally called podagra, a Greek derivative from *pous* (foot) and *agra* (attack). The current term gout is derived from the Latin word *gutta* (drop), a reflection of the early belief that an acute attack of the disease was the result of poison (malevolent humor) dropping into the joint.

## CLINICAL FEATURES

The biochemical hallmark of the disease is hyperuricemia, which may develop from excessive production of uric acid, a decrease in renal excretion of uric acid, or a combination of the two. Traditionally, gout has been classified into two types: (1) primary gout, in which the underlying hyperuricemia is the result of an inborn error of metabolism, and (2) secondary gout, in which the hyperuricemia is a consequence of any number of other disorders. More recently, it has been observed that a variety of metabolic defects account for the hyperuricemia and clinical disease in patients with so-called primary gout. These discoveries have caused a reclassification of hyperuricemia and gout. One such classification system is presented in Table 33–1.

Idiopathic gout occurs far more commonly in men than in women (≈20:1). The first attack of arthritis most frequently occurs during the fifth decade of life in men and in the postmenopausal period in women. Premenopausal women with gout usually have a family history of

### TABLE 33–1

**Classification of Hyperuricemia and Gout**

Idiopathic gout
Gout associated with other clinical disorders
  A. Hereditary diseases
    1. With excess purine synthesis
      a. Glycogen storage disease, type I (glucose-6-phosphate deficiency)
      b. X-linked uric aciduria (hypoxanthine-guanine phosphoribosyltransferase [PRT] deficiency)
        i. Lesch-Nyhan syndrome with virtually complete PRT deficiency
        ii. Gout with incomplete PRT deficiency
      c. Possible amidophosphoribosylpyrophosphatetransferase deficiency
      d. Mental retardation with autistic behavior
      e. Encephalopathy
    2. With diminished renal clearance of uric acid
      a. Hereditary nephropathy
      b. Glycogen storage disease, type I
    3. Undetermined
      a. Down's syndrome
      b. Vasopressin-resistant nephrogenic diabetes insipidus
  B. Hematologic disorders
    1. Hemolytic disease
    2. Myeloproliferative disease
  C. Endocrine abnormalities
    1. Hypothyroidism
    2. Hypoparathyroidism
    3. Hyperparathyroidism
  D. Vascular disease
    1. Hypertension
    2. Myocardial infarction
  E. Renal disease
    1. Glomerulonephritis and pyelonephritis
    2. Lead poisoning as a late effect
  F. Miscellaneous disorders—obesity, starvation, psoriasis, idiopathic hypercalciuria
Drug-induced gout

From Seegmiller JE: Diseases of purine and pyrimidine metabolism. In Bondy PK, Rosenberg LE (eds): Metabolic Control and Disease, 8th ed. Philadelphia, WB Saunders, 1979, p 780.

the disease or, infrequently, long-term diuretic use. The hereditary nature of hyperuricemia and gout is well known, with the reported familial prevalence varying from 6% to 80%.

Idiopathic gout can be divided into several stages, distinguishable by the amount and sites of crystal deposition and by the state of the inflammatory response.

## Asymptomatic Hyperuricemia

Many persons have hyperuricemia for prolonged periods, even a lifetime, without any symptoms or signs. Indeed, hyperuricemia has been described in 2.3% to 17.6% of persons, 20% of whom will develop renal calculi or acute gout. The prevalence of gout increases substantially with advancing age and increasing serum urate concentration. Urolithiasis, articular attacks of gout, or both, mark the end of this phase.

## Acute Gouty Arthritis

Early in the course of gouty arthritis, the disorder is usually monoarticular or oligoarticular. Gout has a predilection for the joints of the lower extremity, particularly the first metatarsophalangeal and intertarsal joints, the ankles, and the knees. The first metatarsophalangeal joint is the most common site of initial involvement and may eventually be altered in 75% to 90% of patients with gout. Inflammatory changes in the spine, hip, shoulder, or sacroiliac joint are unusual and generally occur only in long-standing articular disease. The onset and severity of arthritis in acute gout are often dramatic, and the clinical findings of acute gout may simulate those of septic arthritis. Pain, tenderness, and swelling occur within several hours and may persist for days to weeks.

## Interval Phase of Gout (Intercritical Gout)

The asymptomatic period between gouty attacks may last from months to years. With recurring attacks, the arthritis commonly becomes longer in duration, more frequent in occurrence, and polyarticular in distribution. Eventually, recovery between acute attacks becomes incomplete.

## Chronic Tophaceous Gout

Before the advent of effective therapy for hyperuricemia, clinical or radiographic evidence of gout (called tophi) developed in 50% to 60% of patients, but this frequency has now decreased sharply. Tophi (deposits of monosodium urate) commonly occur in the synovium and subchondral bone and are frequently noted on the helix of the ear and in the subcutaneous and tendinous tissues of the elbow, hand, foot, knee, and forearm. These deposits may appear as irregular, hard masses and produce ulceration of the overlying skin, with extrusion of chalky masses or urate crystals.

## GENERAL PATHOLOGIC FEATURES

### Acute Gouty Arthritis

Urate crystals are needle shaped, with strong negative birefringence when examined under polarized light. Their identification is regarded as the major criterion for the diagnosis of gouty arthritis. Modifications may occur in the shape of the urate crystals, with a rodlike appearance being more common than the classic needle-like configuration in subacute and chronic gout. The appearance of urate crystals differs considerably from that of calcium pyrophosphate dihydrate (CPPD) crystals, which are present in the joints of patients with pseudogout; CPPD crystals are more rhomboid and variable in shape and demonstrate weak positive birefringence when examined under polarized light. Microcrystals of sodium urate are capable of evoking an acute inflammatory response in the skin, subcutaneous tissues, and joints.

## Interval Phase of Gout

The morphologic alterations within the joint in the interval phase of gout have not been well documented. Whether the urates that were deposited during acute attacks persist or undergo resorption is not known. Urate crystals may be identified in the synovial fluid between attacks of gout; usually, however, these crystals are extracellular. Similarly, urate crystals can occasionally be recovered from a noninvolved joint in patients with gouty arthritis at other locations and in those with little history of gouty arthritis. It appears that crystalline deposits are often inert, but if disrupted by mechanical factors or altered solubility, the crystals are capable of being released into the joint space and initiating an acute inflammatory response.

## Chronic Tophaceous Gout

In chronic tophaceous gout, urate deposition occurs in the articular cartilage, subchondral bone, synovial membrane, and capsular and periarticular tissues. In cartilage, the initial deposits are located within the superficial layers. These collections may originate from the adjacent synovial fluid. With time, nonspecific cartilaginous degenerative changes occur, with cartilage fibrillation, fragmentation, and erosion. Portions of the cartilage are sloughed into the articular cavity. Urates penetrate the entire thickness of cartilage and collect in subchondral and deeper osseous areas. Additional foci in bone result from direct deposition of urates in bone marrow or from extension of adjacent urate collections within the periosteum, ligaments, tendons, bursae, and soft tissues. These deposits produce focal defects within the bone or erosive changes along the osseous contour.

Urate deposits within the thickened villi are surrounded by connective tissue containing giant cells, macrophages, and other inflammatory cells. Sequestered fragments of cartilage and bone may be embedded within or on the surface of the synovium and produce local irritation. Inflammatory synovial tissue, or pannus, grows from the edges of the joint across the irregular cartilaginous surface. Fibrous ankylosis of the joint has been described, and secondary osteoarthritic alterations are frequent.

Tophaceous deposits also occur in periarticular tissues, such as the joint capsules, tendons, ligaments, and bursae, particularly in the olecranon and prepatellar regions. Extra-articular collections may be noted in the helix or antihelix of the ear, skin of the fingertips, palms, soles, and other regions, including the tarsal plates of the eyelids, nasal cartilage, and cornea or sclerotic coats of the eye. These tophaceous nodules consist of multicentric deposition of urate crystals and intercrystalline matrix, as well as foreign body granulomatous reaction. As they become larger, tophi may calcify or ossify and produce tendon rupture and nerve compression with paralysis.

# GENERAL RADIOGRAPHIC FEATURES

Although radiographic alterations may accompany the initial bouts of acute gouty arthritis, routine radiographic evaluation reveals no abnormalities of the articular structures in a large percentage of patients with clinical evidence of gout and symptoms spanning many years. During the acute attack of arthritis, soft tissue prominence or swelling about the involved joint or joints coincides with the presence of synovial inflammation, capsular distention, and surrounding soft tissue edema. As the attack subsides, these radiographic abnormalities usually disappear. After years of intermittent episodic arthritis, chronic tophaceous gout may lead to permanent radiographic abnormalities. Conversely, radiographic changes of gout may be identified in patients who deny articular symptoms and in those without tophi.

## Soft Tissue Abnormalities

Eccentric nodular soft tissue prominence accompanies soft tissue deposition of urates (Fig. 33–1). This is most frequent in the feet, hands, ankles, elbows, and knees. Calcification of a tophus is unusual but, when present, is preferentially peripheral and may appear irregular or cloudlike and may reflect a coexisting abnormality of calcium metabolism.

## Articular Space Abnormalities

In gout, the joint space is remarkably well preserved in width until late in the course of articular disease (Fig. 33–2); this is an important radiographic characteristic. This distinctive feature relates to the relative integrity of cartilage adjacent to areas of extensive cartilaginous and osseous destruction. In advanced disease, joint space narrowing is frequent and may be uniform, similar to the appearance in rheumatoid arthritis. Bony ankylosis has been observed but is extremely rare, except in the

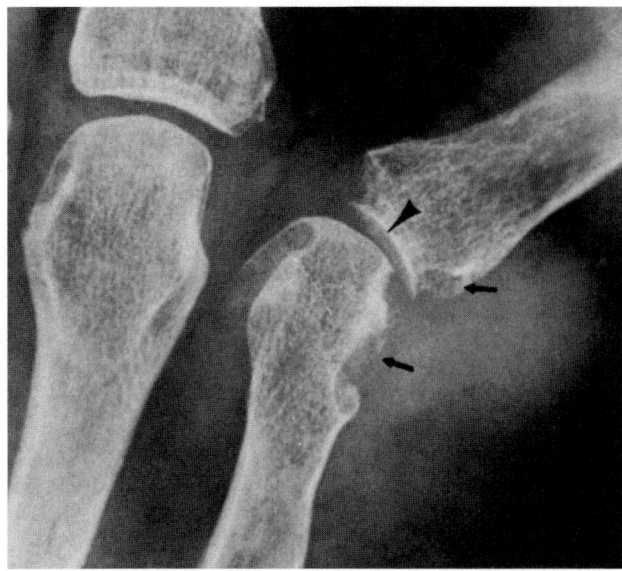

**Figure 33–2.** Radiographic features of gout: articular space abnormalities. Observe that the articular space is only minimally narrowed (*arrowhead*), despite the presence of nodular soft tissue masses and eccentric osseous erosions (*arrows*).

(From Resnick D: The radiographic manifestations of gouty arthritis. CRC Crit Rev Diagn Imaging 9:265, 1977.)

interphalangeal joints of the hands and feet and the intercarpal region.

## Bone Mineralization Abnormalities

Although osteoporosis of subchondral bone can be observed during an acute gouty attack, extensive loss of bone density is not characteristic. Osteoporosis may be mild, even in the presence of widespread articular destruction.

## Bone Erosions

Bone erosions in gout are produced by tophaceous deposits and may be intra-articular, para-articular, or located a considerable distance from the joint (Fig. 33–3). Intra-articular erosions usually commence in the marginal areas of the joint and proceed centrally; para-articular erosions are eccentric in location, frequently beneath soft tissue nodules. Gouty erosions may be surrounded by a sclerotic border and produce a "punched out" appearance.

In about 40% of patients with gouty erosions of bone, an elevated bony margin, or lip, extends outward in the soft tissues, apparently covering the tophaceous nodule (see Fig. 33–3). The overhanging edge may relate to bone resorption beneath the gradually enlarging tophus, with periosteal bony apposition at the outer aspect of the involved cortex. Although the appearance is not pathognomonic, it is strongly suggestive of gouty arthritis.

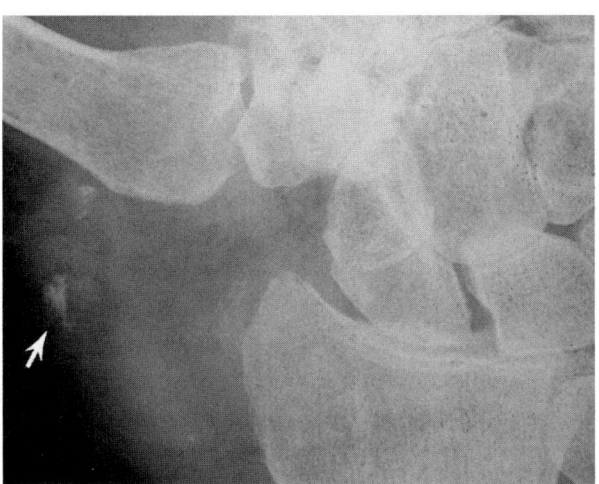

**Figure 33–1.** Radiographic features of gout: soft tissue abnormalities. Partial peripheral calcification (*arrow*) of an eccentric mass (representing a tophus) is evident on the radial aspect of the wrist.

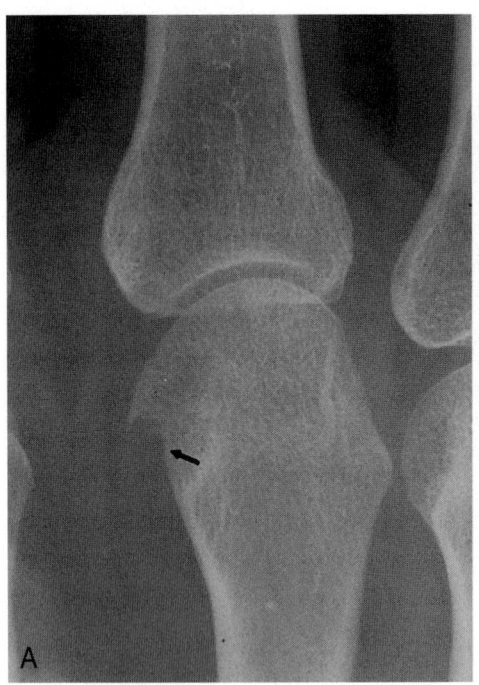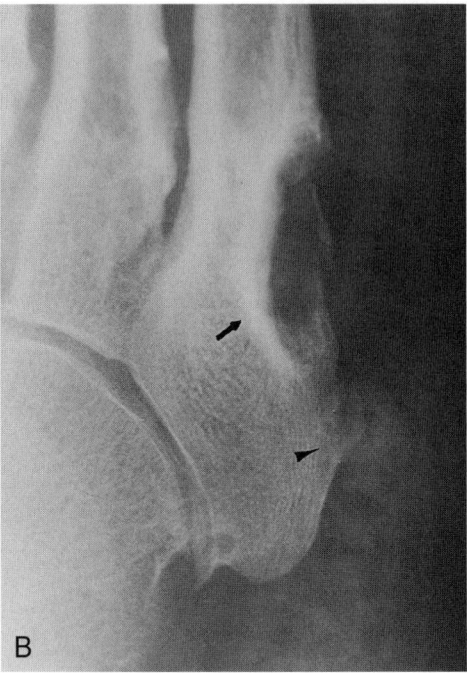

**Figure 33–3.** Radiographic features of gout: erosive bony abnormalities. *A*, Well-defined marginal erosion is evident *(arrow)*, without reactive sclerosis. The articular space is narrowed only minimally. *B*, Well-defined extra-articular erosion *(arrow)* demonstrates surrounding bony eburnation. Additionally, soft tissue calcification and bone proliferation *(arrowhead)* are evident. *C*, Overhanging margin. This lip of bone *(arrowheads)* may be evident in intra- or extra-articular locations.

(From Resnick D: The radiographic manifestations of gouty arthritis. CRC Crit Rev Diagn Imaging 9:265, 1977.)

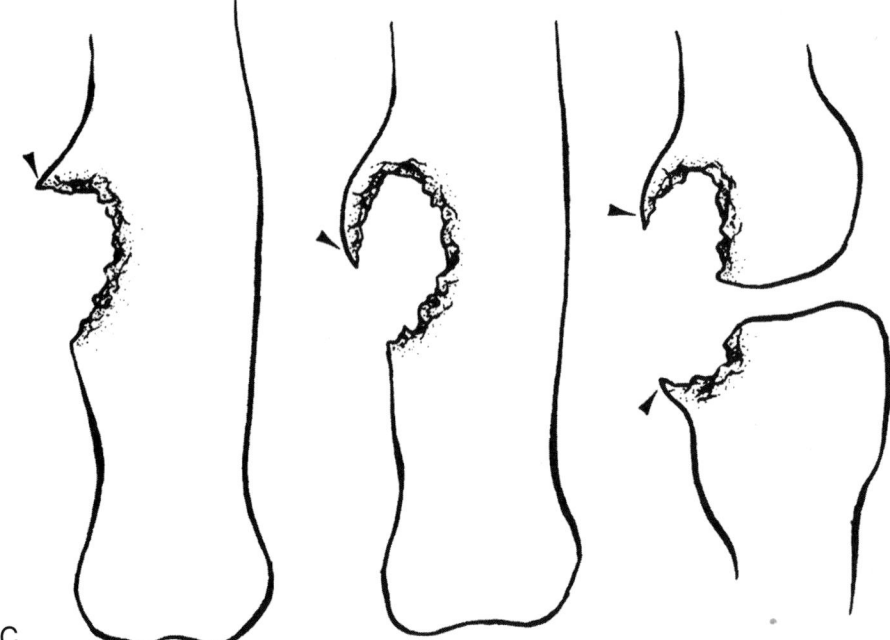

## Subperiosteal Apposition of Bone and Proliferative Changes

Bone proliferation is occasionally observed in gout (Fig. 33–4). Enlargement of the ends and shafts of involved bones can produce club-shaped metacarpal, metatarsal, and phalangeal heads (termed mushrooming), an enlarged ulnar styloid, and thickened diaphyses. Secondary osteoarthritic alterations in gouty joints are common and include subchondral sclerosis and osteophytosis. These findings, which are particularly frequent in the first metatarsophalangeal joint, intertarsal areas, and knees, may obscure other manifestations of the disease.

## Intraosseous Calcification

Intraosseous calcific deposits have been observed in approximately 6% of patients with chronic gouty arthritis. These deposits represent intraosseous urate deposits that, in most cases, arise from the adjacent joint, penetrate the cartilaginous surface, and extend into the adjacent spongiosa. Intraosseous calcification in gout is seen most frequently in the hands and feet. Radiographic findings include focal or diffuse calcific collections, usually involving subchondral or subligamentous bony areas, in association with adjacent joint disease, osseous destruction, and involvement of periarticular tissue (Fig. 33–5).

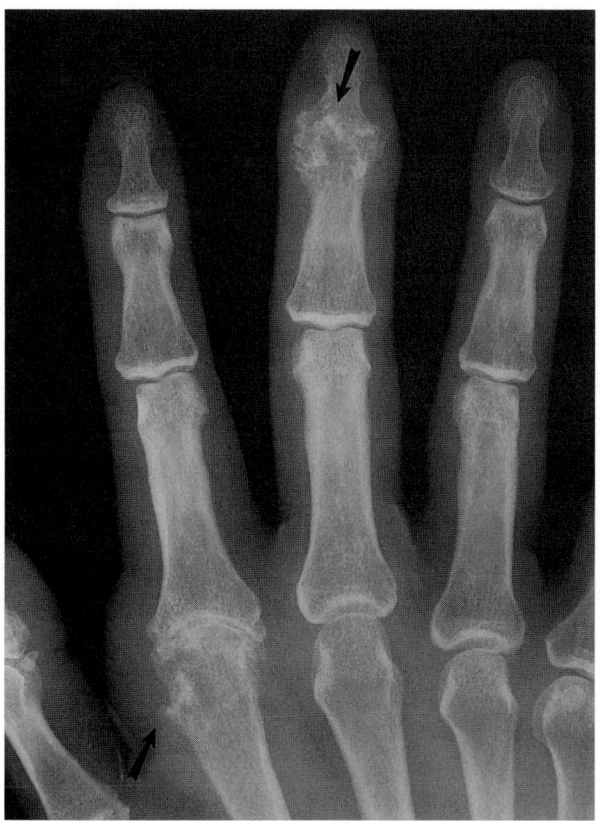

**Figure 33–4.** Radiographic features of gout: proliferative bony abnormalities. Considerable productive changes of bone are apparent at the second metacarpophalangeal and third distal interphalangeal joints *(arrows)*.

The radiographic alterations resemble those of enchondromas or bone infarcts.

## DISTRIBUTION OF ARTICULAR INVOLVEMENT

Although the distribution of radiographic abnormalities in gouty arthritis is somewhat variable, it is generally asymmetrical and polyarticular. There is a predilection for the lower extremity, and involvement is common in the feet, hands, wrists, elbows, and knees.

### Common Sites of Disease

**Foot Abnormalities.** The most characteristic site of abnormality in gout is the first metatarsophalangeal joint (Fig. 33–6). Erosions are particularly frequent on the medial and dorsal aspects of the first metatarsal head. Associated soft tissue swelling and hallux valgus deformity are frequently, but not invariably, present. An enlarged, irregular first metatarsal head is observed. Any of the other metatarsophalangeal joints may be involved, particularly the fifth. The interphalangeal joints may reveal similar abnormalities. Swelling on the dorsum of the foot may be associated with extensive destruction in the tarsometatarsal (Fig. 33–7), intertarsal, and talocalcaneal joints.

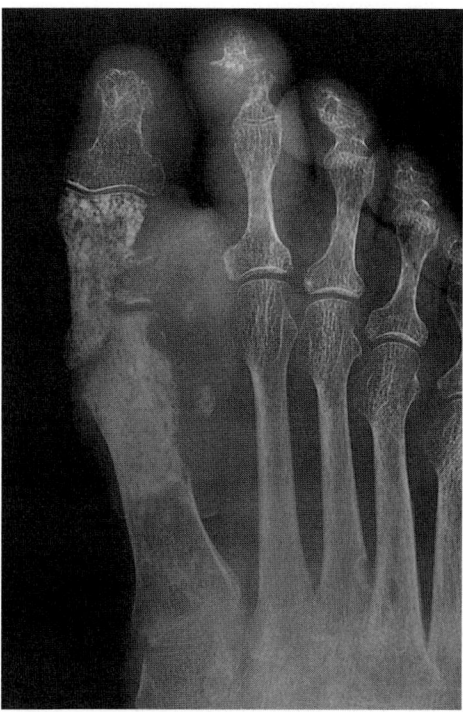

**Figure 33–5.** Radiographic features of gout: intraosseous calcification. Observe the punctate and circular calcifications in the proximal phalanx and metatarsal of the great toe, as well as in the cuneiforms. Extensive soft tissue swelling and calcification about a destroyed first metatarsophalangeal joint are evident.

**Hand and Wrist Abnormalities.** Radiographs of the hands and wrists in patients with gout may reveal widespread articular abnormalities involving the distal interphalangeal, proximal interphalangeal, and, to a lesser extent, metacarpophalangeal joints (Figs. 33–8 and 33–9). These hand and wrist alterations lack the symmetry that is characteristic of rheumatoid arthritis. Large erosions of the intercarpal and carpometacarpal joints occur, and all the compartments in the wrist may eventually be affected.

**Elbow Abnormalities.** Bursal inflammation commonly produces bilateral soft tissue swelling over the extensor surface of the elbow. Erosive and proliferative changes may be seen in the subjacent olecranon process of the ulna (Fig. 33–10).

**Knee Abnormalities.** Marginal erosions in the knee may occur on the medial or lateral aspect of the femur and tibia, or both, in the absence of significant narrowing of the articular space (Fig. 33–11). Focal lesions of the patella or femur caused by intraosseous tophi may simulate neoplasm (Fig. 33–12). Osteolytic lesions of the patella in gout predominate in the superolateral aspect of the bone, may be unilateral or bilateral, and are associated with soft tissue swelling.

### Uncommon Sites of Disease

**Shoulder Abnormalities.** Radiographic changes of the glenohumeral or acromioclavicular joint in gout are not

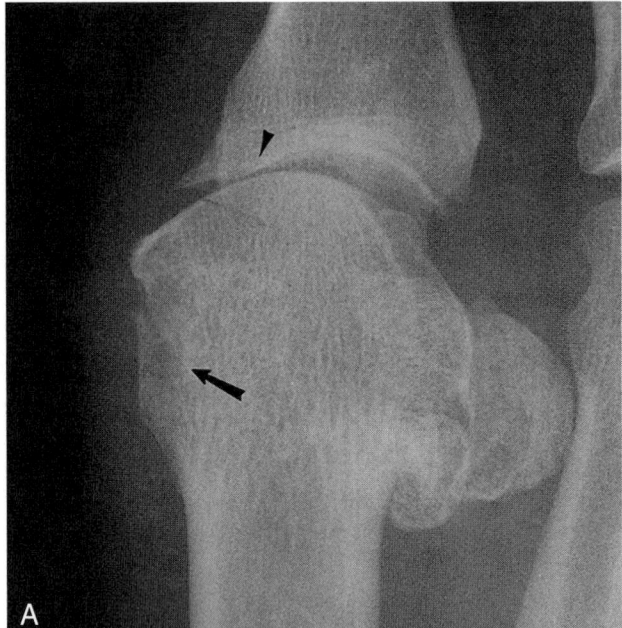

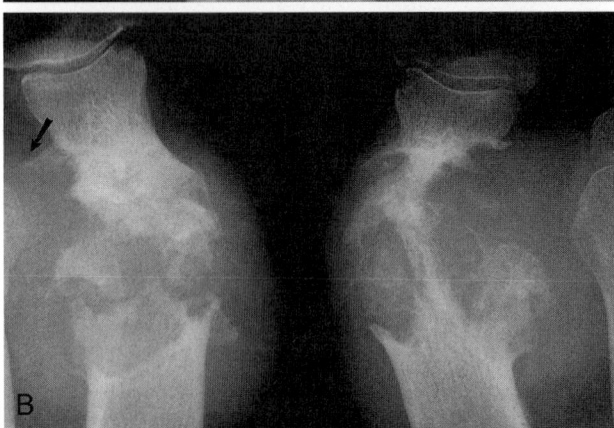

**Figure 33–6.** Forefoot abnormalities in gout. *A*, Early involvement of the first metatarsophalangeal joint. Erosions predominate at the dorsomedial aspect of the metatarsal head *(arrow)* and are associated with soft tissue swelling, articular space narrowing *(arrowhead)*, and osteophyte formation. *B*, Severe forefoot abnormalities. Findings include extensive bony destruction with overhanging margins and pathologic fractures *(arrow)*.

(From Resnick D: The radiographic manifestations of gouty arthritis. CRC Crit Rev Diagn Imaging 9:265, 1977.)

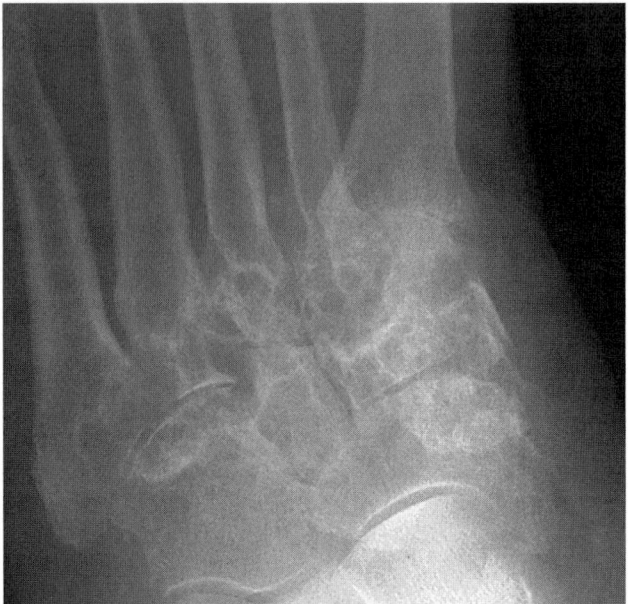

**Figure 33–7.** Midfoot abnormalities in gout. A typical site of alteration is the tarsometatarsal joint, where erosions may be extensive.

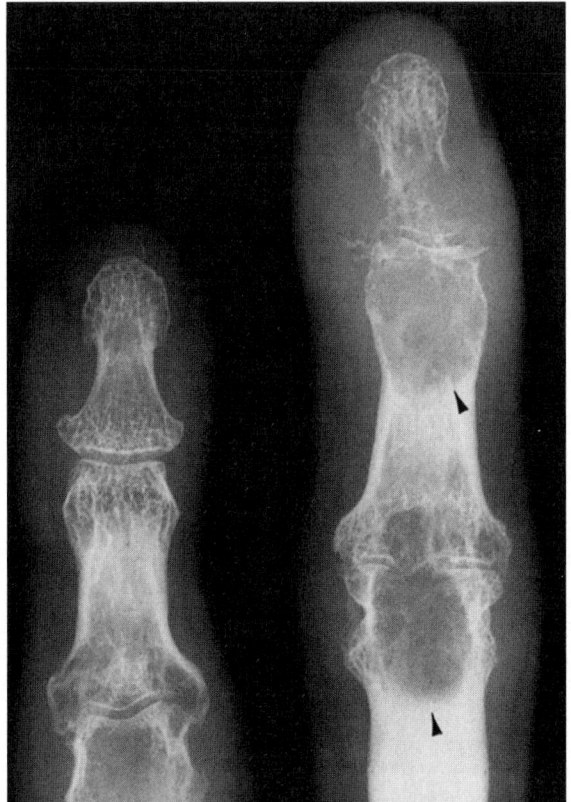

**Figure 33–8.** Hand abnormalities in gout. Interphalangeal joint alterations include bone erosion and intraosseous defects *(arrowheads)*. Soft tissue swelling is seen.

(From Resnick D: The radiographic manifestations of gouty arthritis. CRC Crit Rev Diagn Imaging 9:265, 1977.)

common. Soft tissue swelling, bony erosions, loss of articular space, and secondary proliferative changes are encountered.

**Hip Abnormalities.** Abnormalities of the hip are rare in gout. Some reports have indicated a high frequency of hyperuricemia or gout in patients with osteonecrosis of the femoral head, but in large series of patients with gout, the frequency of osteonecrosis of the femoral head is extremely low, and when present, osteonecrosis is frequently related to concomitant steroid administration.

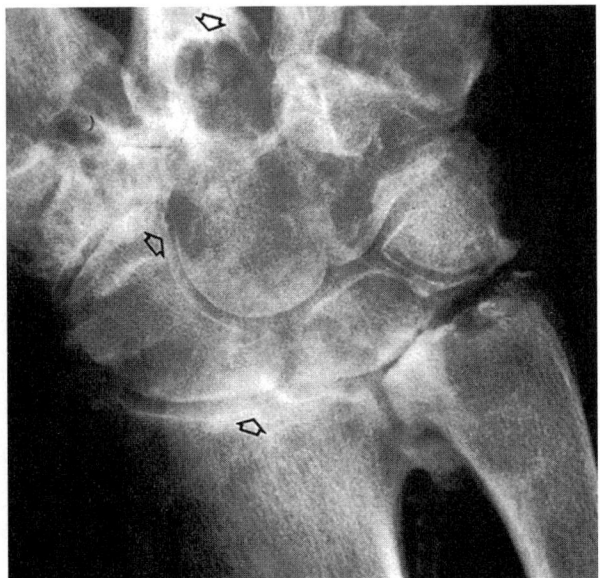

**Figure 33–9.** Wrist abnormalities in gout. Diffuse disease of all compartments of the wrist is evident. Erosions *(arrows)* are most prominent at the common carpometacarpal compartment *(upper arrow)*.
(From Resnick D: The radiographic manifestations of gouty arthritis. CRC Crit Rev Diagn Imaging 9:265, 1977.)

**Sacroiliac Joint Abnormalities.** Sacroiliac joint involvement in gout is infrequent (Fig. 33–13), and many reported cases are not verified histologically. Large areas of erosion in the subchondral bone of the ilium and sacrum are occasionally seen in gout. Sacroiliac joint gout has been noted more frequently in early-onset disease (which may reflect a longer and more severe clinical course).

**Spine Abnormalities.** Spinal manifestations of gout are extremely uncommon. Radiographic abnormalities in the cervical segment include erosions of the odontoid process or endplates of the vertebral bodies, disc space narrowing, and vertebral subluxation. Spinal cord compression at various spinal levels has been reported as a complication of gout.

## COMPUTED TOMOGRAPHY

The role of computed tomography (CT) in gout is limited. Although CT allows determination of the extent of bone and joint involvement, only infrequently is such delineation required. It is especially useful in areas of complex anatomy such as the spine, small bones of the hands and feet, base of the skull, and pelvis. CT scanning has revealed tophaceous deposits with attenuation values similar to those of calcifications, and the differentiation of noncalcified and calcified tophi may be difficult with CT.

## MAGNETIC RESONANCE IMAGING

Magnetic resonance (MR) imaging may be useful in assessing the full extent of the gouty process, especially in anatomically complex regions such as the spine, small

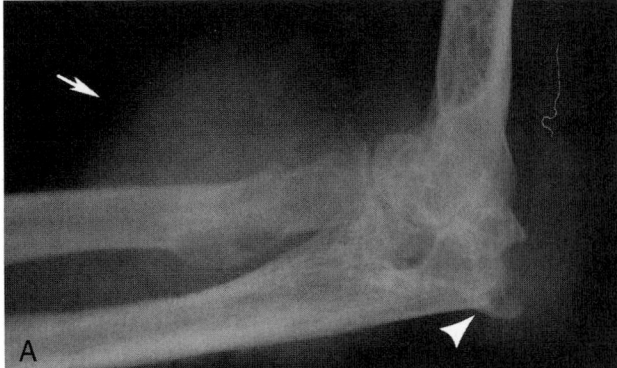

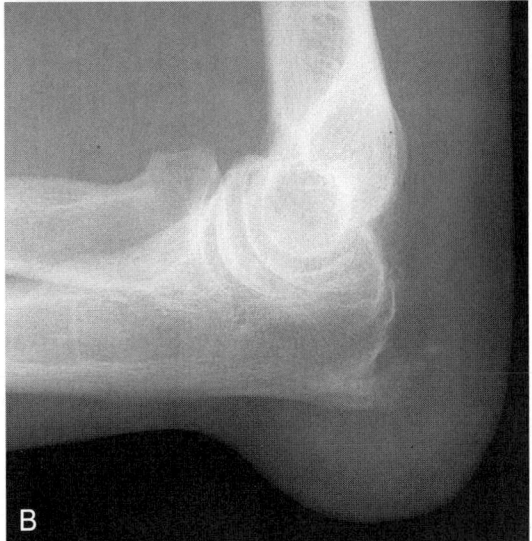

**Figure 33–10.** Elbow abnormalities in gout. *A,* Olecranon changes consisting of soft tissue swelling and subjacent osseous erosion *(arrowhead)* are seen. Additional soft tissue swelling is also evident *(arrow)*. *B,* Similar changes in another patient with a tophus containing calcification.

bones of the hands and feet, and sacroiliac and temporomandibular joints. In the peripheral skeleton, MR imaging allows visualization of the extent of soft tissue, synovial, cartilage, and bone involvement (Fig. 33–14). MR imaging shows intermediate to low signal intensity in noncalcified gouty tophi on both T1-weighted and T2-weighted spin echo images. MR imaging following gadolinium administration shows heterogeneous enhancement, with no enhancement in areas of calcification and amorphous urate deposits and variably intense enhancement in the inflamed synovium (see Fig. 33–14).

## POSITRON EMISSION TOMOGRAPHY

The clinical application of positron emission tomography (PET) is still evolving, and it is currently most valuable in the diagnosis, staging, and restaging of selected malignancies. Although it is unlikely that PET will be used for the evaluation of gout, the disease may be identified as an incidental finding in patients scanned for unrelated

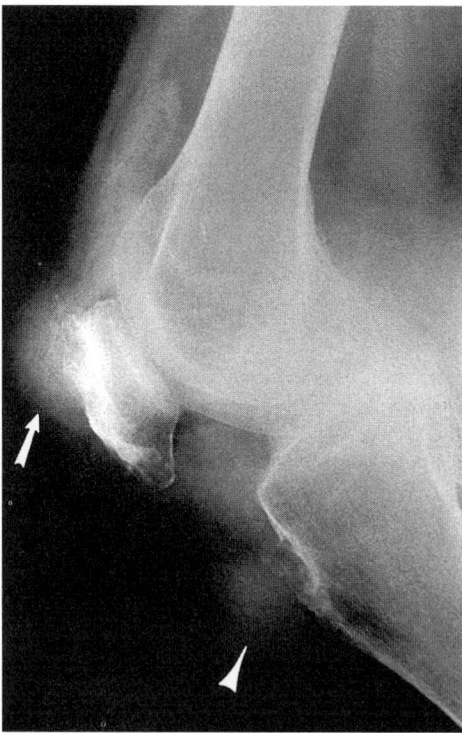

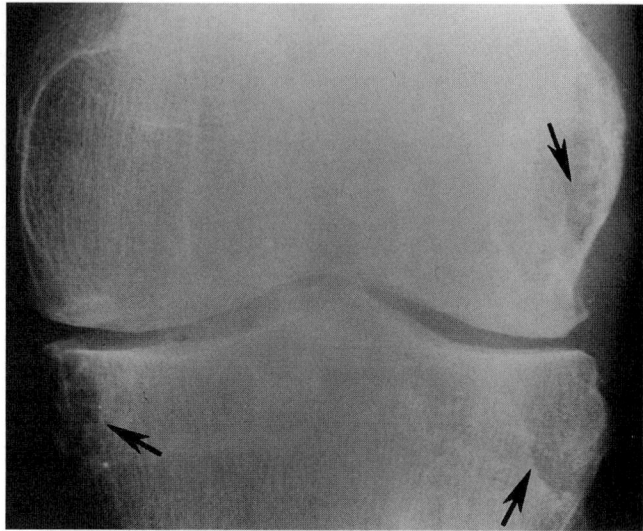

**Figure 33–11.** Knee abnormalities in gout. Large marginal erosions are apparent *(arrows)*. The joint space is narrowed.

(From Resnick D: The radiographic manifestations of gouty arthritis. CRC Crit Rev Diagn Imaging 9:265, 1977.)

**Figure 33–12.** Patellar abnormalities in gout. Observe a prepatellar tophus *(arrow)*, partially calcified, that is producing erosion of the anterior surface of the patella. An additional soft tissue deposit with subjacent bone erosion can be seen *(arrowhead)*.

(From Resnick D: The radiographic manifestations of gouty arthritis. CRC Crit Rev Diagn Imaging 9:265, 1977.)

reasons. Based on anecdotal experience with gout, it demonstrates variable, multiple hypermetabolic foci, reflecting the inflamed synovium associated with tophi (Fig. 33–15).

## COEXISTENT ARTICULAR DISORDERS

### Calcium Pyrophosphate Dihydrate and Hydroxyapatite Crystal Deposition

Chondrocalcinosis can occur in patients with gout. These calcific deposits are usually localized in one or two sets of

joints, particularly within the menisci of the knee, symphysis pubis, and triangular fibrocartilage of the wrist. Hyaline cartilage calcification or widespread chondrocalcinosis is rare in gouty arthritis. Both monosodium urate and CPPD crystals may be obtained from the same joint. Crystals are frequently found in asymptomatic joints. Calcium-containing crystals are found in a large array of clinical situations, and examination of deposits often reveals a mixture of crystalline material.

### Osteoarthritis

In patients with osteoarthritis of the interphalangeal joints of the hand (nodal osteoarthritis) in whom inflammation and radiographically evident erosions develop, diagnostic possibilities include secondary gout, calcium hydroxyapatite crystal deposition, CPPD crystal deposition, and inflammatory (erosive) osteoarthritis.

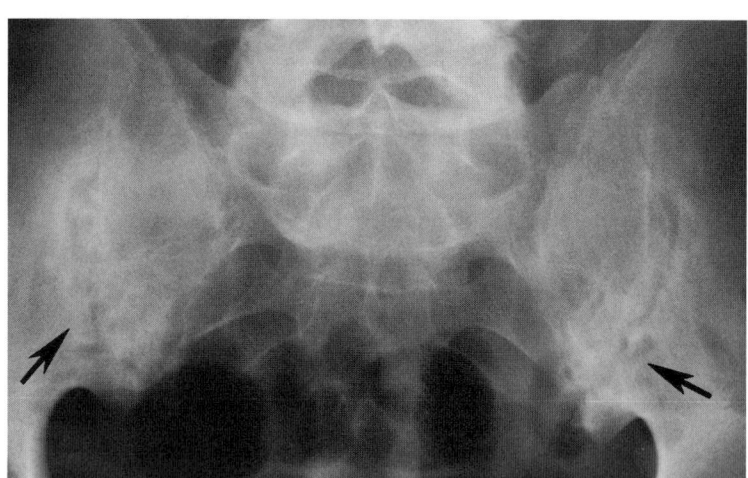

**Figure 33–13.** Sacroiliac joint abnormalities in gout. Bilateral sacroiliac joint alterations *(arrows)* typical of gout include scalloped erosions and adjacent bony sclerosis.

(From Resnick D: The radiographic manifestations of gouty arthritis. CRC Crit Rev Diagn Imaging 9:265, 1977.)

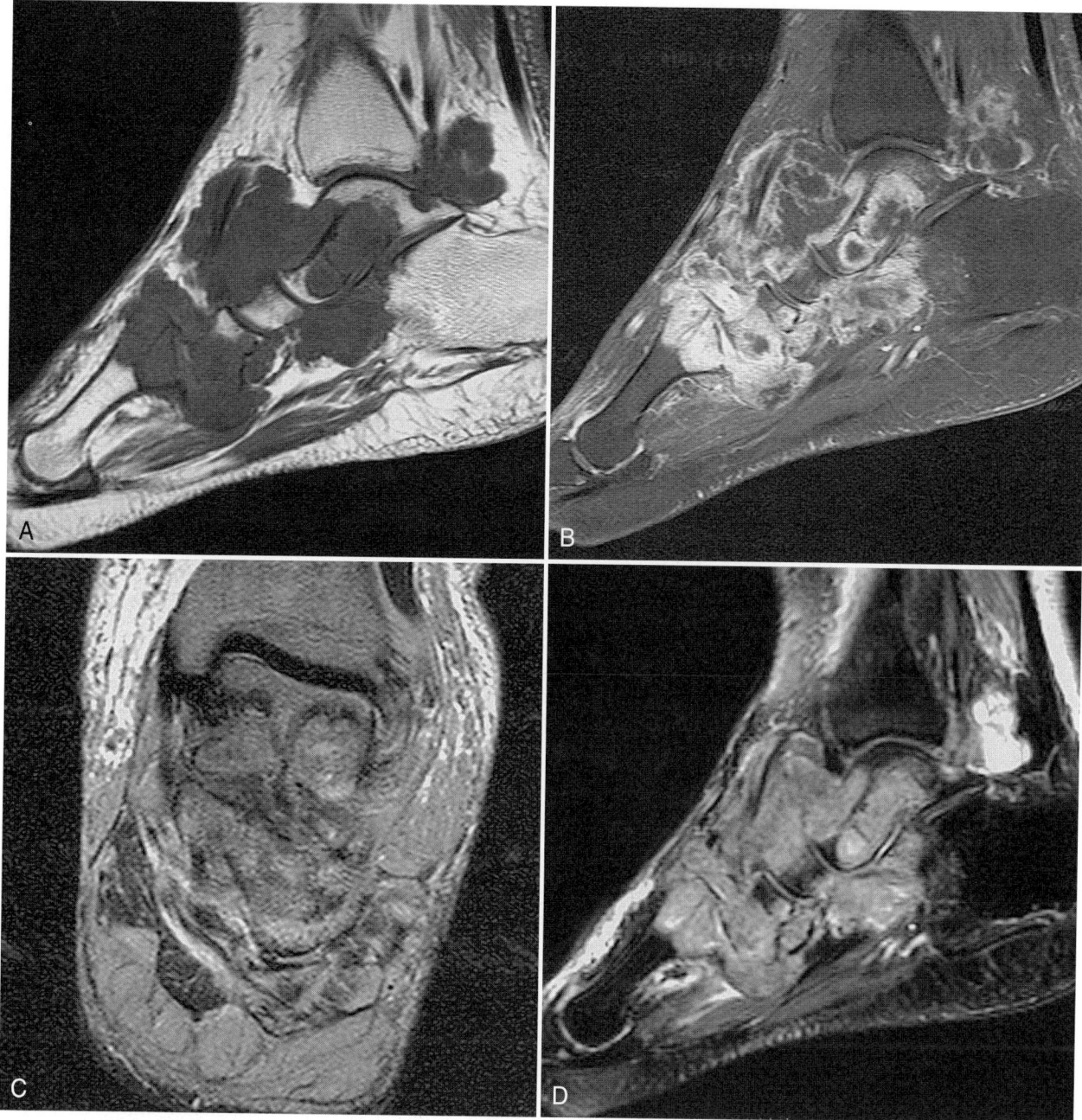

**Figure 33–14.** MR imaging abnormalities in gout. *A,* Sagittal T1-weighted (TR/TE, 537/17) spin echo MR image of the foot shows multiple soft tissue and intra-articular masses of intermediate signal intensity, with extensive osseous involvement. *B,* Corresponding fat-suppressed T1-weighted (TR/TE, 400/17) spin echo MR image following contrast shows intense heterogeneous enhancement, with no enhancement in the areas of calcification and amorphous urate deposits and variably intense enhancement in the inflamed synovium. *C,* Coronal T2-weighted (TR/TE, 2930/80) spin echo MR image shows the tophi to have a heterogeneous intermediate signal intensity. Note subcutaneous edema around the ankle. *D,* Tophi show hyperintense signal on sagittal fat-suppressed T2-weighted (TR/TE, 6000/62) fast spin echo MR image.

## Other Disorders

Although rheumatoid arthritis and gout are not uncommon diseases, their coexistence is extremely rare. With few exceptions, patients are men in whom gout was the initial disease, followed years later by the development of rheumatoid arthritis.

The coexistence of joint infection and gout is also unusual. The association of hyperuricemia and gouty arthritis with other rheumatic disorders, including ankylosing spondylitis and psoriatic arthritis, has been noted, although it is poorly documented in most instances. Further, gout has been encountered in patients with systemic lupus erythematosus and Paget's disease.

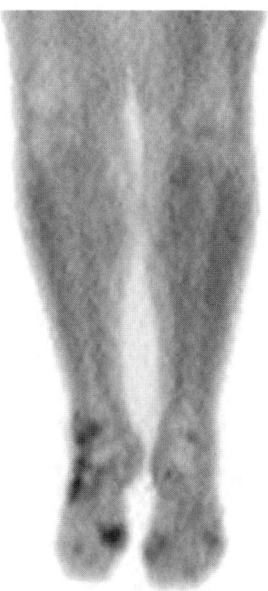

**Figure 33–15.** PET imaging abnormalities in a 52-year-old woman with gout. Anteroposterior image of the lower extremities shows multiple hypermetabolic foci in the feet, corresponding to multiple tophi.

## SPECIAL TYPES OF GOUTY ARTHRITIS

### Early-Onset Idiopathic Gouty Arthritis

The reported peak age of occurrence of idiopathic gout varies from 30 to 50 years. Gout has been reported in early life, but clinical and radiographic abnormalities in idiopathic gout in the first 2 decades of life are uncommon. Radiographic abnormalities in these young patients resemble the changes in adults with gout (Fig. 33–16). The joints involved most frequently are those in the feet and hands.

### Gout Associated with Hereditary Disease

**Type I Glycogen Storage Disease.** Patients with type I glycogen storage disease (glucose-6-phosphatase deficiency), a rare hereditary disorder of childhood, may contract gouty arthritis if they live to adulthood. In some of these patients, arthritis develops in the first decade of life and is extremely disabling.

**Lesch-Nyhan and Kelley-Seegmiller Syndromes.** Lesch-Nyhan syndrome includes spasticity, choreoathetosis, mental retardation, and compulsive self-mutilation manifested as finger and lip biting. Boys are affected, and the

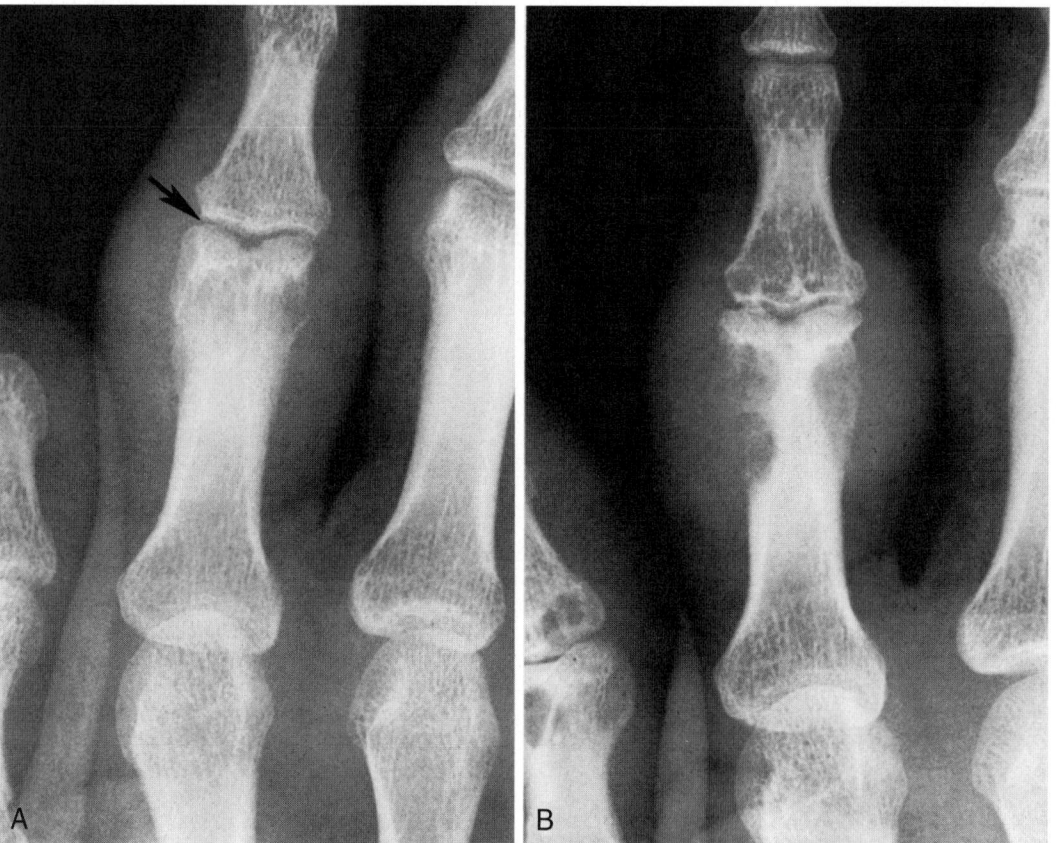

**Figure 33–16.** Early-onset gouty arthritis. Progressive abnormalities occurred over a 2-year period in this 23-year-old man with gout. *A,* Initial film reveals soft tissue swelling and bony destruction of the proximal phalanx *(arrow). B,* Subsequent radiograph demonstrates increased severity of the bony and soft tissue changes.

(From Resnick D: The radiographic manifestations of gouty arthritis. CRC Crit Rev Diagn Imaging 9:265, 1977.)

disorder is X-linked (Fig. 33–17). Complete or virtually complete deficiency of hypoxanthine-guanine phosphoribosyltransferase (HPRT) is associated with Lesch-Nyhan syndrome. Radiographic abnormalities of Lesch-Nyhan syndrome reflect self-mutilation, with amputation of the soft tissues and osseous structures of the hands. Gouty erosions, retarded skeletal maturation, coxa valga deformities with subluxation of the hips, and soft tissue tophi have been described in this disorder. Additional findings include traumatic changes occurring after seizures, cerebral atrophy, and uric acid calculi in the urinary tract.

In Kelley-Seegmiller syndrome, the deficiency of HPRT is incomplete, and patients may have adolescent- or adult-onset gouty arthritis and occasional mild neurologic disease. Radiographic abnormalities are generally limited to gouty arthritis, because most patients are normal neurologically.

## Saturnine Gout

The accidental contamination of alcoholic beverages with lead has been recognized for centuries. In addition, lead was sometimes intentionally added to wine to improve its flavor or prevent spoiling, a practice that was subsequently ruled illegal. Gout occurring as a complication of chronic lead intoxication is called saturnine gout. Currently, this form of gout is principally associated with the ingestion of illegally manufactured alcohol (moonshine). It is caused in large part by decreased urate clearance by the kidneys as a result of lead nephropathy. Saturnine gout accounts for only a small number of cases of gout. Patients are typically male, black, aged 45 to 55 years, often azotemic and anemic, but otherwise asymptomatic except for joint disease. Radiographic findings resemble those of idiopathic gout.

## Gout Associated with Other Clinical Disorders (Secondary Gout)

A number of other disorders may result in hyperuricemia and secondary gout. Myeloproliferative disorders, which are apparent in approximately 5% to 10% of patients with gout, include polycythemia vera, leukemia, lymphoblastoma, myeloid metaplasia, hemolytic anemia, sickle cell anemia, pernicious anemia, thalassemia, multiple myeloma, secondary polycythemia, infectious mononucleosis, and Waldenström's hyperproteinemia, as well as some carcinomas.

Hyperuricemia may be associated with a variety of endocrine disorders, including hyperparathyroidism, hypoparathyroidism, myxedema, and hypoadrenal states. Additional causes of hyperuricemia and gout are obesity, idiopathic hypercalciuria, psoriasis, myocardial infarction and vascular disease, renal disease, and near-starvation states. Drug-induced gout has been noted in association with diuretic, pyrazinamide, and salicylate therapy.

The radiographic manifestations of secondary and idiopathic gout are generally indistinguishable.

## DIFFERENTIAL DIAGNOSIS

Because radiographic abnormalities in gouty joints appear late in the course of the disease, the diagnosis is usually well established clinically, and the radiologist need only document its extent and severity. Occasionally, the disease is not suspected before radiographic examination.

## Rheumatoid Arthritis

Rheumatoid arthritis produces radiographic alterations that differ from those of gout, including symmetrical joint involvement, fusiform soft tissue swelling, and regional osteoporosis (Table 33–2; Fig. 33–18). Early diffuse joint space loss accompanies marginal erosive changes in the bone.

## Psoriatic Arthritis

Psoriatic arthritis may produce radiographic changes that resemble those of gout, and the presence of elevated serum uric acid levels may lead to further diagnostic difficulty. Articular manifestations of psoriatic arthritis include progressive destruction of the peripheral joints of the extremities, periosteal proliferation at the margins of the joint, paravertebral ossification, and sacroiliac disease. Osteoporosis is generally not apparent.

## Calcium Pyrophosphate Dihydrate Crystal Deposition Disease

CPPD crystal deposition disease resulting from the presence of intra-articular crystals can produce an acute arthritis termed the pseudogout syndrome. The clinical symptoms are identical to those of gout, and radiographic abnormalities consist of articular and periarticular calcification and a "degenerative" arthropathy. The cartilage calcification (chondrocalcinosis) accompanying CPPD crystal deposition disease is frequently widespread and involves hyaline cartilage and fibrocartilage; chondro-

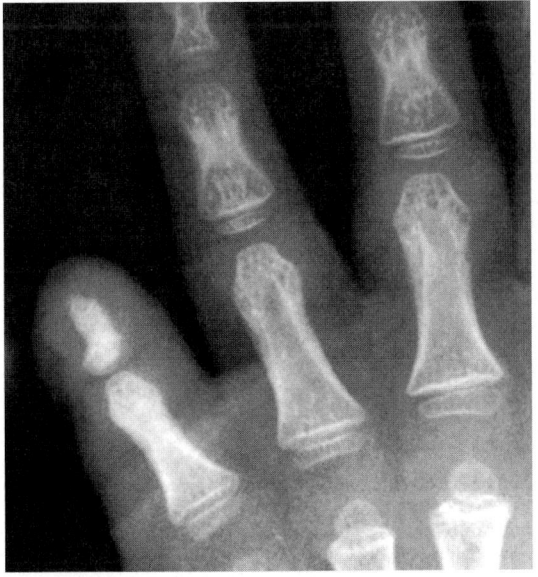

**Figure 33–17.** Lesch-Nyhan syndrome. Destruction and partial amputation of the phalanges in both hands are seen.

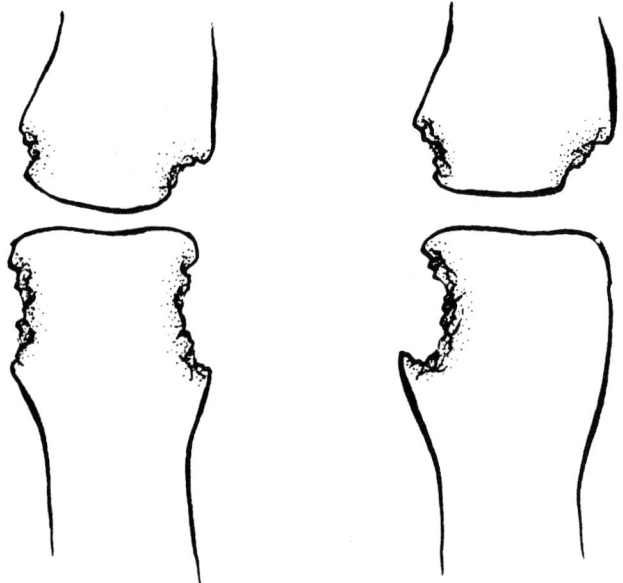

**Figure 33–18.** Rheumatoid arthritis versus gout. In rheumatoid arthritis (left), findings include diffuse loss of articular space and marginal erosions. In gout (right), note the preservation of joint space, eccentric erosions, and an "overhanging edge."

(From Resnick D: The radiographic manifestations of gouty arthritis. CRC Crit Rev Diagn Imaging 9:265, 1977.)

calcinosis in gout is usually localized to one or two joints and involves fibrocartilage alone. The structural joint abnormalities of CPPD crystal deposition disease (termed pyrophosphate arthropathy) demonstrate an unusual predilection for the wrist, metacarpophalangeal joints, and knee; they include joint space narrowing, subchondral sclerosis and cyst formation, bone fragmentation and collapse, and variable osteophyte formation. Although the radiographic manifestations of pyrophosphate arthropathy may resemble those of gout, the presence of lobulated soft tissue masses, intact joint spaces, and osseous erosions in the latter disease usually permits differentiation of the two disorders (Fig. 33–19).

## Sarcoidosis

Sarcoidosis may produce skeletal abnormalities, particularly in the hand. These abnormalities include widening of the medullary portion of the bone, a honeycomb configuration, focal lucent osseous defects, and sclerosis. Although granulomatous involvement of the synovium and juxta-articular bone occurs in the chronic arthritis of sarcoidosis, articular destruction and deformity are unusual.

## Amyloidosis

Amyloidosis, which occurs in a primary form or as a secondary manifestation of another disease, can result in bone or joint lesions. Amyloid infiltration of the articular structures may cause soft tissue masses and focal erosive osseous lesions indistinguishable from those of gout.

## Xanthomatosis

Tendinous xanthomas are particularly frequent on the extensor surface of the hand and foot and in the patellar and Achilles tendon regions. Tuberous xanthomas occur in the subcutaneous tissues of the elbows and knees. Radiographic changes consist of eccentric soft tissue nodular masses with subjacent bone erosion, findings simulating gouty tophi (Fig. 33–20). Hypercholesterolemia in patients with xanthomatosis is an important laboratory abnormality.

## Inflammatory (Erosive) Osteoarthritis and Multicentric Reticulohistiocytosis

Destructive articular abnormalities of the interphalangeal joints, which are noted in both gout and psoriatic arthritis, are also apparent in inflammatory (erosive) osteoarthritis and multicentric reticulohistiocytosis. The former disease affects middle-aged and elderly women and produces symmetrical joint changes, usually confined to the interphalangeal joints of the fingers, the first carpometacarpal joint, and the trapezioscaphoid articulation. The erosions in inflammatory osteoarthritis

---

**TABLE 33–2**

**Radiographic Features of Gouty and Rheumatoid Arthritis**

|  | Gouty Arthritis | Rheumatoid Arthritis |
|---|---|---|
| Distribution | Asymmetrical joint involvement | Symmetrical joint involvement |
| Soft tissue swelling | Eccentric | Fusiform |
| Soft tissue calcification | Occasional | Rare |
| Osteoporosis | Absent or mild | Moderate or severe |
| Joint space loss | Frequently absent | Diffuse; occurs early in disease course |
| Bony erosions | Eccentric | Marginal |
|  | Frequent sclerotic margin | Rare sclerotic margin |
|  | Intra- and extra-articular | Intra-articular |
|  | Overhanging edge | No overhanging edge |
| Malalignment, subluxation | Rare | Common |

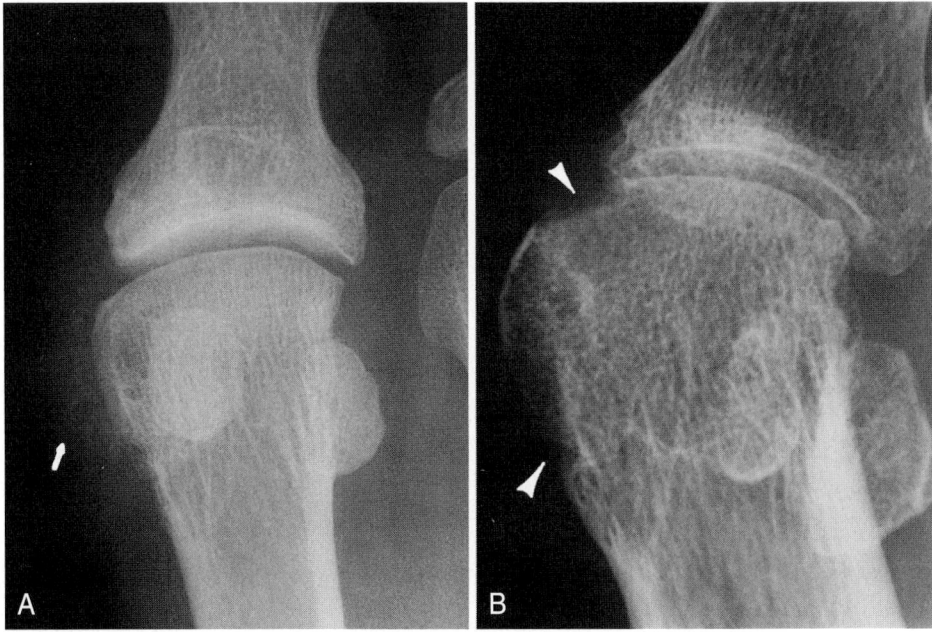

**Figure 33–19.** Calcium pyrophosphate dihydrate (CPPD) crystal deposition disease versus gout. *A*, In CPPD crystal deposition disease, changes at the first metatarsophalangeal joint may consist of soft tissue calcification *(arrow)*. *B*, In gout, typical marginal and central erosions are observed *(arrowheads)*.

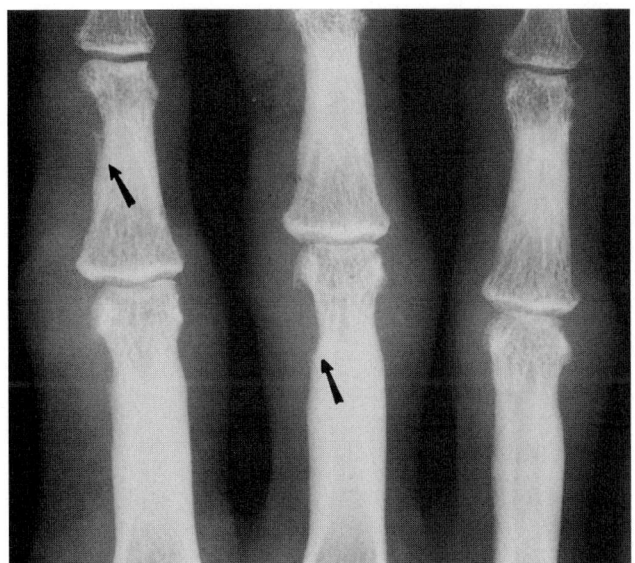

**Figure 33–20.** Xanthomatosis. Note the soft tissue masses with subjacent scalloped erosions of the phalanges *(arrows)*.
(From Resnick D: The radiographic manifestations of gouty arthritis. CRC Crit Rev Diagn Imaging 9:265, 1977.)

frequently commence in the central portion of the joint. The radiographic manifestations in multicentric reticulo-histiocytosis include erosions with sharp margins and lack of osteoporosis. Multicentric reticulohistiocytosis produces symmetrical joint lesions, and the articular space may be narrowed rapidly. These latter features do not commonly occur in gout.

## FURTHER READING

Alarcón-Segovia D, Cetina JA, Diaz-Jouanen E: Sacroiliac joints in primary gout: Clinical and roentgenographic study of 143 patients. AJR Am J Roentgenol 118:438, 1973.

Barthelemy CR, Nakayama DA, Carrera GF, et al: Gouty arthritis: A prospective radiographic evaluation of sixty patients. Skeletal Radiol 11:1, 1984.

Bjelle A: Crystals in joints. Clin Rheumatol 2:103, 1988.

Brailsford JR: The radiology of gout. Br J Radiol 32:472, 1959.

Chen CKH, Chung CB, Yeh L, et al: Carpal tunnel syndrome caused by tophaceous gout: CT and MR imaging features in 20 patients. AJR Am J Roentgenol 175:655, 2000.

Chen CKH, Yeh LR, Pan H-B, et al: Intra-articular gouty tophi of the knee: CT and MR imaging in 12 patients. Skeletal Radiol 28:75, 1999.

Forrester DM, Brown JC, Nesson JW: The Radiology of Joint Disease, 2nd ed. Philadelphia, WB Saunders, 1978.

Good AE, Rapp R: Chondrocalcinosis of the knee with gout and rheumatoid arthritis. N Engl J Med 277:286, 1967.

Halla JT, Ball GV: Saturnine gout: A review of 42 patients. Semin Arthritis Rheum 11:307, 1982.

Jaffe HL: Metabolic, Degenerative and Inflammatory Disease of Bones and Joints. Philadelphia, Lea & Febiger, 1972, p 479.

Kelley WN, Greene ML, Rosenbloom FM, et al: Hypoxanthine-guanine phosphoribosyltransferase deficiency in gout: A review. Ann Intern Med 70:155, 1969.

Kelley WN, Wortmann RL: Gout and hyperuricemia. In Kelley WN, Harris ED Jr, Ruddy S, et al (eds): Textbook of Rheumatology, 5th ed. Philadelphia, WB Saunders, 1997, p 1313.

Lally EV, Zimmermann B, Ho G Jr, et al: Urate-mediated inflammation in nodal osteoarthritis: Clinical and roentgenographic correlations. Arthritis Rheum 32:86, 1989.

Lesch M, Nyhan WL: A familial disorder of uric acid metabolism and central nervous system function. Am J Med 36:561, 1964.

Martel W: The overhanging margin of bone: A roentgenologic manifestation of gout. Radiology 91:755, 1968.

Martin DJ, Merenda G, McDonald DJ, et al: Recurrent hemarthrosis associated with gout. Clin Orthop 277:262, 1992.

Resnick D: The radiographic manifestations of gouty arthritis. CRC Crit Rev Diagn Imaging 9:265, 1977.

Resnick D, Broderick TW: Intraosseous calcifications in tophaceous gout. AJR Am J Roentgenol 137:1157, 1981.

Resnick D, Reinke RT, Taketa RM: Early-onset gouty arthritis. Radiology 114:67, 1975.

Ruiz ME, Erickson SJ, Carrera GF, et al: Monoarticular gout following trauma: MR appearance. J Comput Assist Tomogr 17:151, 1993.

Seegmiller JE: Human aberrations of purine metabolism and their significance for rheumatology. Ann Rheum Dis 39:103, 1980.

Watt I, Middlemiss H: The radiology of gout. Clin Radiol 26:27, 1975.

# CHAPTER 34

## Calcium Pyrophosphate Dihydrate Crystal Deposition Disease

### SUMMARY OF KEY FEATURES

Until recently, calcium pyrophosphate dihydrate (CPPD) crystal deposition disease was a commonly overlooked condition. In the past 3 decades, considerable attention to its various clinical and radiographic manifestations has increased physicians' awareness of this disorder. Chondrocalcinosis can no longer be considered the only significant radiographic feature of CPPD crystal deposition disease. An equally characteristic radiographic finding is the presence of other intra-articular and periarticular calcifications and structural joint damage. The pattern and distribution of structural joint damage (pyrophosphate arthropathy) are especially distinctive and can be differentiated from the features of degenerative joint disease to allow an accurate diagnosis of CPPD crystal deposition disease even in the absence of chondrocalcinosis.

### INTRODUCTION

In 1961 and 1962, McCarty and others discovered nonurate crystals in the joint fluid of patients experiencing goutlike attacks of arthritis. These crystals were subsequently identified as calcium pyrophosphate dihydrate (CPPD) by their x-ray diffraction powder pattern. When clinical and radiographic findings in these patients were analyzed, it was recognized that the same disease had been described as chondrocalcinosis polyarticularis, reflecting the calcific deposits within cartilage. It thus became clear that patients with a distinctive goutlike pattern of arthritis (pseudogout syndrome) had crystal accumulation within joints (CPPD deposition) that could cause cartilage calcification (chondrocalcinosis). Subsequently, other crystals were found to produce calcific collections in the knee (Table 34–1).

### TERMINOLOGY

The variety of names linked to this condition has led to considerable confusion in nomenclature. Articular chondrocalcinosis and pseudogout are but two of these names, and at times they have been used interchangeably. The following related terms are defined in accordance with current usage:

*Calcium pyrophosphate dihydrate (CPPD) crystal deposition disease:* General term for a disorder characterized by the presence of $Ca_2P_2O_7 \bullet 2H_2O$ (CPPD) crystals in or around joints.

*Pseudogout:* Term applied to one of the clinical patterns that may be associated with crystal deposition. This pattern, characterized by intermittent acute attacks of arthritis, simulates that of gout.

### TABLE 34–1

**Reported Prevalence in Early Investigations of Chondrocalcinosis in the Knee**

| Author | Number of Cases | Age of Patients | Selection of Material | Method of Study | Incidence of Chondrocalcinosis |
|---|---|---|---|---|---|
| Tobler (1929) | 1400 | Elderly | Autopsy and surgical specimens | Histologic examination | 30% |
| Wolke (1935) | 12,268 | Wide range | Retrospective | Conventional radiograph | 0.42% |
| Bennett et al (1942) | 63 | Elderly | Cadavers | Histologic study | 4.1% |
| McCarty and Haskin (1963) | 215 | 71 yr (mean) | Cadavers | Specimen radiograph, histologic study, and crystal analysis | 7% total 3.3% CPPD 2.3% DCPD 1.4% HA |
| Bocher et al (1965) | 455 | 80 yr (mean) | Retrospective and prospective surgery | Conventional radiograph | 7% |
| Lagier and Baud (1968) | 320 | Elderly | Cadavers | Histologic study and crystal analysis | 6.8% CPPD |
| Schmied et al (1971) | 97 | 64 yr (mean) | Prospective control and diabetic survey | Conventional radiograph | 4.2% |
| Ellman and Levin (1975) | 58 | 83 yr (mean) | Survey of patients in home for elderly | Industrial film radiograph | 28% |

CPPD, calcium pyrophosphate dihydrate; DCPD, dicalcium phosphate dihydrate; HA, calcium hydroxyapatite.

After Genant HK: Roentgenographic aspects of calcium pyrophosphate dihydrate crystal deposition disease (pseudogout). Arthritis Rheum 19(Suppl)3:307, 1976.

*Chondrocalcinosis:* Term reserved for pathologically or radiographically evident cartilage calcification. In some instances, this calcification may indicate not CPPD crystal deposition but deposits of other crystals.

*Articular and periarticular calcification:* Terms used for pathologically or radiographically evident calcification in and around joints. Chondrocalcinosis is but one of the possible manifestations of such calcification.

*Pyrophosphate arthropathy:* Term used to describe a peculiar pattern of structural joint damage occurring in CPPD crystal deposition disease that simulates, in many ways, degenerative joint disease but is characterized by distinctive features.

## CLINICAL PATTERNS

CPPD crystal deposition disease affects both men and women and is generally observed in middle-aged and elderly patients. Various clinical patterns underscore the ability of this disease to simulate a variety of other conditions, and a patient may demonstrate several different clinical patterns during the course of the disease. Numbers in parentheses below indicate the approximate percentage of symptomatic patients who fall into each category.

### Type A: Pseudogout (10% to 20%)

This pattern of disease is characterized by acute or subacute self-limited attacks of arthritis involving one or several appendicular joints. The attacks, which range in duration from 1 day to several weeks, are generally less painful than attacks of gout and may be provoked by trauma, surgery, intra-articular injection, or medical illness. The knee is the most common site of acute arthritis, but other sites may be involved, such as the hip, shoulder, elbow, wrist, ankle, and acromioclavicular, talocalcaneal, and metatarsophalangeal joints. Occasionally, pain in the heel or spine may be the initial complaint. Inflammation may begin in one joint and spread to another. This pattern of disease may be relieved by colchicine.

### Type B: Pseudo–Rheumatoid Arthritis (2% to 6%)

Characterized by almost continuous acute attacks of arthritis, this pattern is associated with symptoms and signs lasting 4 weeks to several months that consist of morning stiffness, fatigue, synovial thickening, restricted joint motion, and an elevated erythrocyte sedimentation rate.

### Type C: Pseudo-Osteoarthritis (35% to 60%)

In this pattern, chronic progressive arthritis with superimposed acute inflammatory episodes is apparent in large joints such as the knee and hip, as well as in the metacarpophalangeal, elbow, ankle, wrist, and shoulder joints. It is characterized by bilateral symmetrical involvement and flexion contractures, particularly of the knee and elbow.

### Type D: Pseudo-Osteoarthritis (10% to 35%)

This clinical pattern is characterized by chronic progressive arthritis without acute exacerbations. As in type C, the findings resemble those of degenerative joint disease.

### Type E: Asymptomatic Joint Disease

Although reports indicate that symptoms may be absent in 10% to 20% of cases of CPPD crystal deposition disease, the frequency of asymptomatic disease is actually much higher, because many asymptomatic patients are never seen by a physician. Type E is the most common clinical pattern. Cartilage calcification was recently reported in 27.6% of elderly Jewish patients, most of whom were asymptomatic.

### Type F: Pseudo–Neuropathic Osteoarthropathy (0% to 2%)

A less common clinical pattern in CPPD crystal deposition disease simulates neuropathic osteoarthropathy. On radiographic examination, patients with pyrophosphate arthropathy without neurologic deficit may have destructive joint alterations that resemble those of neuropathic osteoarthropathy.

### Type G: Miscellaneous Patterns (0% to 1%)

CPPD crystal deposition disease can produce symptoms that suggest rheumatic fever, psychogenic disease, and trauma. Clinical findings resembling those of ankylosing spondylitis have also been observed.

## CLASSIFICATION

CPPD crystal deposition disease can be conveniently classified into cases that are hereditary, sporadic (idiopathic), or associated with other disorders. Hereditary cases are not associated with other disease processes. Sporadic disease usually occurs in middle-aged and elderly patients, and series with both male and female predominance have been recorded. Other disorders associated with CPPD crystal deposition disease are discussed in the next section.

## ASSOCIATED DISEASES

Many disorders have been reported in association with CPPD crystal deposition (Table 34–2). In most instances, the nature and significance of such associations cannot be assessed, and they may merely represent the chance occurrence of two diseases. The most important disorders associated with CPPD crystal deposition disease are hyperparathyroidism and hemochromatosis.

### Hyperparathyroidism

The reported frequency of hyperparathyroidism in patients with CPPD crystal deposition disease varies from 0% to 15%. The frequency of chondrocalcinosis in patients with hyperparathyroidism is reportedly 18% to 40%. CPPD crystal deposition and pseudogout attacks

**TABLE 34–2**

**Conditions Associated with CPPD Crystal Deposition**

**Group A: True association—high probability**
1. Primary hyperparathyroidism
2. Familial hypocalciuric hypercalcemia
3. Hemochromatosis
4. Hemosiderosis
5. Hypophosphatasia
6. Hypomagnesemia
7. Bartter's and Gitelman's syndromes
8. Hypothyroidism
9. Gout
10. Neuropathic osteoarthropathy
11. Amyloidosis
12. Localized trauma
    a. Surgery for osteochondritis dissecans
    b. Hypermobility syndrome
13. Corticosteroid therapy (long-term)
14. Aging

**Group B: True association—modest probability**
1. Hyperthyroidism
2. Nephrolithiasis
3. Diffuse idiopathic skeletal hyperostosis
4. Ochronosis
5. Wilson's disease
6. Hemophilic arthritis

**Group C: True association unlikely**
1. Diabetes mellitus
2. Hypertension
3. Azotemia
4. Hyperuricemia
5. Gynecomastia
6. Inflammatory bowel disease
7. Rheumatoid arthritis
8. Paget's disease of bone
9. Acromegaly

From McCarty D: Ann Rheum Dis 42:243, 1983.

have also been described in patients with chronic renal failure with or without secondary hyperparathyroidism.

## Hemochromatosis

Chondrocalcinosis has been observed in 41% of patients with hemochromatosis, and structural joint changes simulating pyrophosphate arthropathy are frequently seen in these patients. Chondrocalcinosis may also occur in patients with secondary hemochromatosis related to hereditary spherocytosis.

## PATHOGENESIS OF CRYSTAL DEPOSITION AND SYNOVITIS

CPPD crystal deposition is generally first observed in articular cartilage, although deposits may be recognized in other articular tissues, such as synovium and capsule, as well as periarticular tissues, such as tendons and ligaments. The earliest site of crystal deposition is probably around the chondrocyte lacunae in the midzonal area, although the mechanism by which CPPD crystals are precipitated in cartilage is unknown. In recent years, increasing emphasis has been placed on local tissue damage as a cause of crystal deposition, rather than crystal deposition as a cause of local tissue damage. The initial event leading to crystal deposition may be cartilage damage that is age related, secondary to trauma, or disease induced.

Just as the manner in which CPPD crystals are accumulated in cartilage is not clear, the events leading to joint inflammation after such accumulation are not known precisely. The pathogenesis of the acute synovitis in this disease may be related to a process of crystal shedding in which cartilaginous deposits are cast into the articular cavity. Crystal shedding may also be exaggerated in conditions associated with significant cartilage destruction, such as infection and neuropathic osteoarthropathy.

## GENERAL PATHOLOGIC FEATURES

The pathologic features associated with CPPD crystal deposition disease have not been studied extensively. Observations include crystal deposition in various articular and periarticular tissues and structural joint damage.

### Crystal Deposition

CPPD crystals may be apparent in cartilage, synovium, capsule, tendons, and ligaments.

**Cartilage Abnormalities.** Crystalline deposits can occur in both fibrocartilage and hyaline cartilage (Fig. 34–1). Fibrocartilaginous collections of CPPD crystals are most frequently observed in the menisci of the knee, triangular fibrocartilage of the wrist, acetabular labra, symphysis pubis, and anulus fibrosus of the intervertebral disc. Additional sites of fibrocartilaginous deposition include the articular discs of the acromioclavicular and sternoclavicular joints and the glenoid labra. In the wrist, CPPD crystal deposition in the triangular fibrocartilage has been associated with degenerative tears, as well as with degeneration of articular cartilage in the lunate.

**Synovial Membrane and Synovial Fluid Abnormalities.** Both acute and chronic inflammatory changes may be evident in the synovial membrane. Crystals are generally apparent within the inflamed synovial membrane, but it is not clear whether the crystals are deposited there directly or whether they migrate from the adjacent cartilage. During acute attacks of inflammation, CPPD crystals are observed within leukocytes in the synovial fluid.

**Tendon and Ligament Abnormalities.** In CPPD crystal deposition disease, calcification may occur in tendons and ligaments. These calcifications are most frequently apparent in the Achilles, triceps, quadriceps, gastrocnemius, and supraspinatus tendons but may also be noted in adjacent bursae, such as the subacromial bursa.

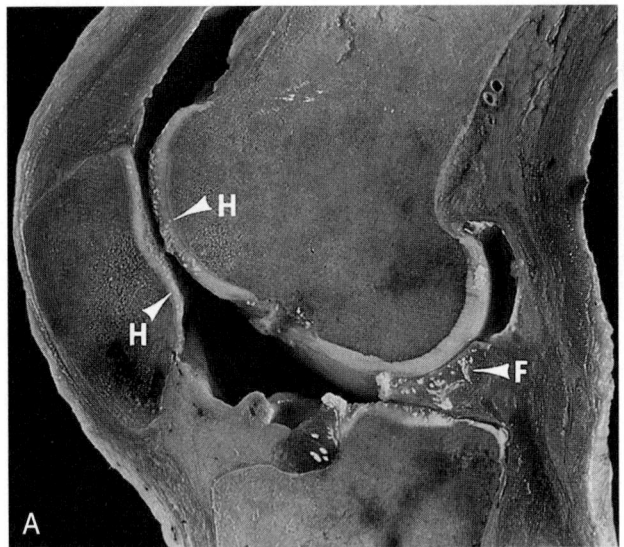

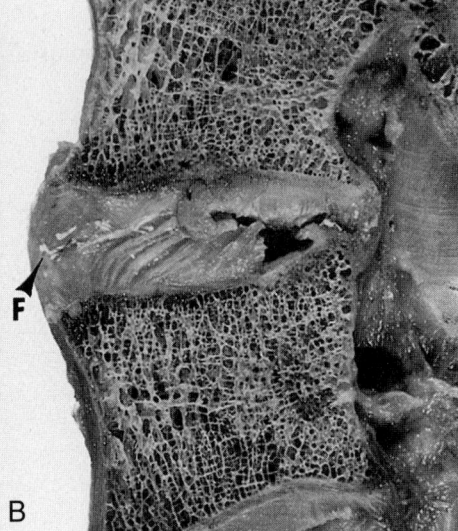

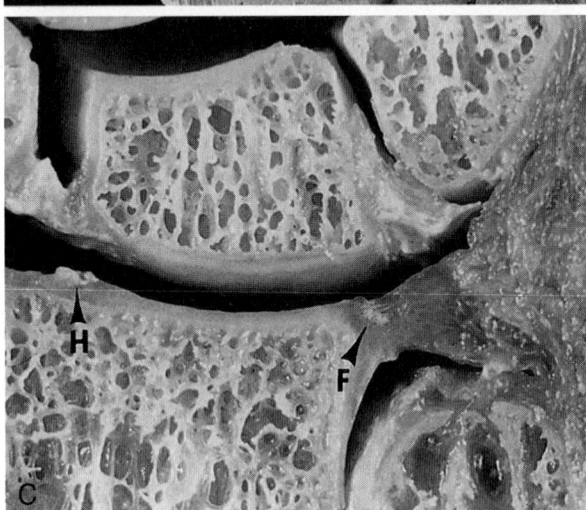

**Figure 34–1.** Pathologic abnormalities: crystal deposition in cartilage. *A*, Fibrocartilage and hyaline cartilage of the knee. Sagittal section reveals CPPD crystal deposition in the fibrocartilage (F) of the menisci and the hyaline cartilage (H) of the patella, femur, tibia, and fibula. *B*, Fibrocartilage of the intervertebral disc. Fibrocartilage (F) calcification is apparent mainly in the anulus fibrosus in this sagittal section of the spine. *C*, Fibrocartilage and hyaline cartilage of the wrist. In a coronal section, both fibrocartilage (F) and hyaline cartilage (H) are calcified.

## Structural Joint Damage

The structural joint damage associated with CPPD crystal deposition disease resembles degenerative joint disease on pathologic as well as radiographic examination (Fig. 34–2). Cartilage fibrillation, erosion, and partial or complete denudation are pathologic findings that correlate with radiographically evident joint space narrowing. Subchondral bone contains thickened trabeculae and multiple cysts. The cysts may or may not communicate with the adjacent articular cavity; in some cases, a narrow neck connects the piriform cystic structure and joint space, whereas in other cases, fibrous tissue or sclerotic bone obliterates this area of communication. When compared with the cystic lesions occurring in degenerative joint disease, the cysts of CPPD crystal deposition disease are larger, more numerous, and more widespread. Bone fragmentation and collapse, which are frequent in this disease, may be related to fracture of these cystic lesions. Intraarticular osseous bodies may be loose within the joint cavity or embedded in the cartilaginous and synovial tissue.

## GENERAL RADIOGRAPHIC FEATURES

The general radiographic features of CPPD crystal deposition disease can be divided into articular and periarticular calcification and pyrophosphate arthropathy.

### Articular and Periarticular Calcification

CPPD crystal deposition disease is associated with calcification of articular and periarticular structures (Fig. 34–3). Articular and periarticular calcific deposits may be located in cartilage, synovium, capsules, tendons, bursae, ligaments, soft tissues, and vessels and may demonstrate some degree of symmetry from one side to the other. The frequency of radiographically demonstrable articular calcification is greatest in the knee, symphysis pubis, wrist, elbow, and hip. In patients who demonstrate calcification of some articulation on complete skeletal surveys, frontal radiographs of the knees alone detect calcification in approximately 90%; frontal radiographs of the knees and symphysis pubis detect calcification in approximately

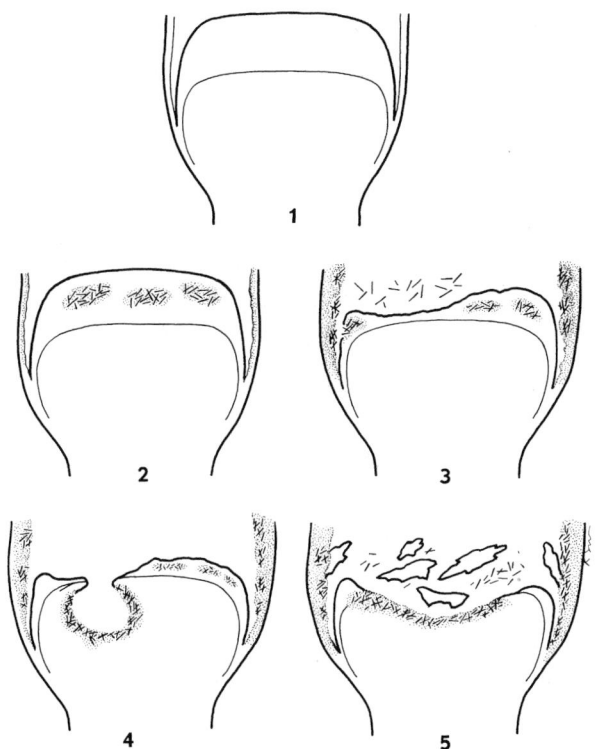

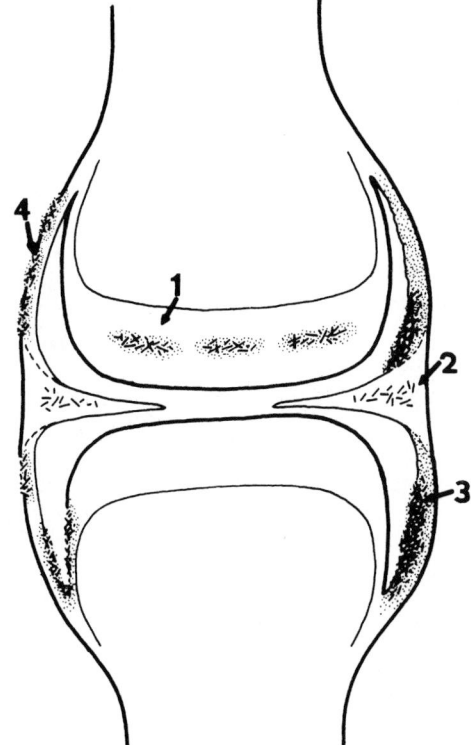

**Figure 34–2.** Pathogenesis of pyrophosphate arthropathy. 1, The normal situation. 2, Crystal deposition in hyaline cartilage is apparent. 3, Cartilage loss, crystal shedding, and synovial deposits are seen, with secondary synovial inflammation. 4, Cystic degeneration and bony sclerosis have occurred. 5, Fragmentation of bone and cartilage may lead to cartilaginous and osseous debris embedded in the synovial membrane.

(Redrawn from McCarty DJ Jr: Calcium pyrophosphate dihydrate crystal deposition disease—1975. Arthritis Rheum 19[Suppl]3:275, 1976.)

98%; and frontal radiographs of the knees, symphysis pubis, and wrists detect calcification in approximately 100%. Thus, an effective screening test for articular calcification consists of a posteroanterior radiograph of each wrist, an anteroposterior radiograph of the pelvis, and an anteroposterior radiograph of each knee.

**Cartilaginous Calcification.** Chondrocalcinosis is most frequent in the knee, wrist, symphysis pubis, elbow, and hip and may involve fibrocartilage or hyaline cartilage (Fig. 34–4). Fibrocartilaginous calcification is most common in the menisci of the knee, triangular cartilage of the wrist, symphysis pubis, anulus fibrosus of the intervertebral disc, and acetabular and glenoid labra. Fibrocartilaginous deposits appear as thick, shaggy, irregular radiodense areas, particularly within the central aspect of the joint cavity.

Hyaline cartilage calcification may occur in many locations but is most common in the wrist, knee, elbow, and hip. These deposits are thin and linear or curvilinear and are parallel to and separated from the subjacent subchondral bone.

**Synovial Calcification.** Calcification within the synovial membrane is a common feature of CPPD crystal deposi-

**Figure 34–3.** Articular and periarticular calcifications. Deposits may be located in the hyaline cartilage (1), fibrocartilage (2), synovial membrane (3), and joint capsule (4).

tion disease (Fig. 34–5). This form of calcification is usually combined with chondrocalcinosis but may sometimes be the dominant radiographic pattern. Synovial deposits are most frequent in the wrist, particularly about the radiocarpal and inferior radioulnar joints; knee; and metacarpophalangeal and metatarsophalangeal joints. These deposits are cloudlike in appearance, particularly at the margins of the joint, and may simulate idiopathic synovial osteochondromatosis.

**Capsular Calcification.** CPPD crystal deposition in joint capsules is most commonly observed in the elbow and metatarsophalangeal joints but is also observed in the metacarpophalangeal and glenohumeral joints (Fig. 34–6). These collections appear as fine or irregular linear calcifications that span the joint. They may be associated with joint contractures, particularly in the elbow.

**Tendinous, Bursal, and Ligamentous Calcification.** Calcification is most often observed in the Achilles, triceps, quadriceps, gastrocnemius, and supraspinatus tendons, as well as in the subacromial bursa (Fig. 34–7). In tendons, calcifications may simulate the findings of idiopathic calcific tendinitis related to calcium hydroxyapatite crystal deposition, except that they may be more extensive. Bursal calcification associated with inflammation is also seen. In shoulders that demonstrate tendinous and bursal calcification, rotator cuff tears are not infrequent.

**Soft Tissue and Vascular Calcification.** In some patients, poorly defined calcific deposits are seen in the soft tissues

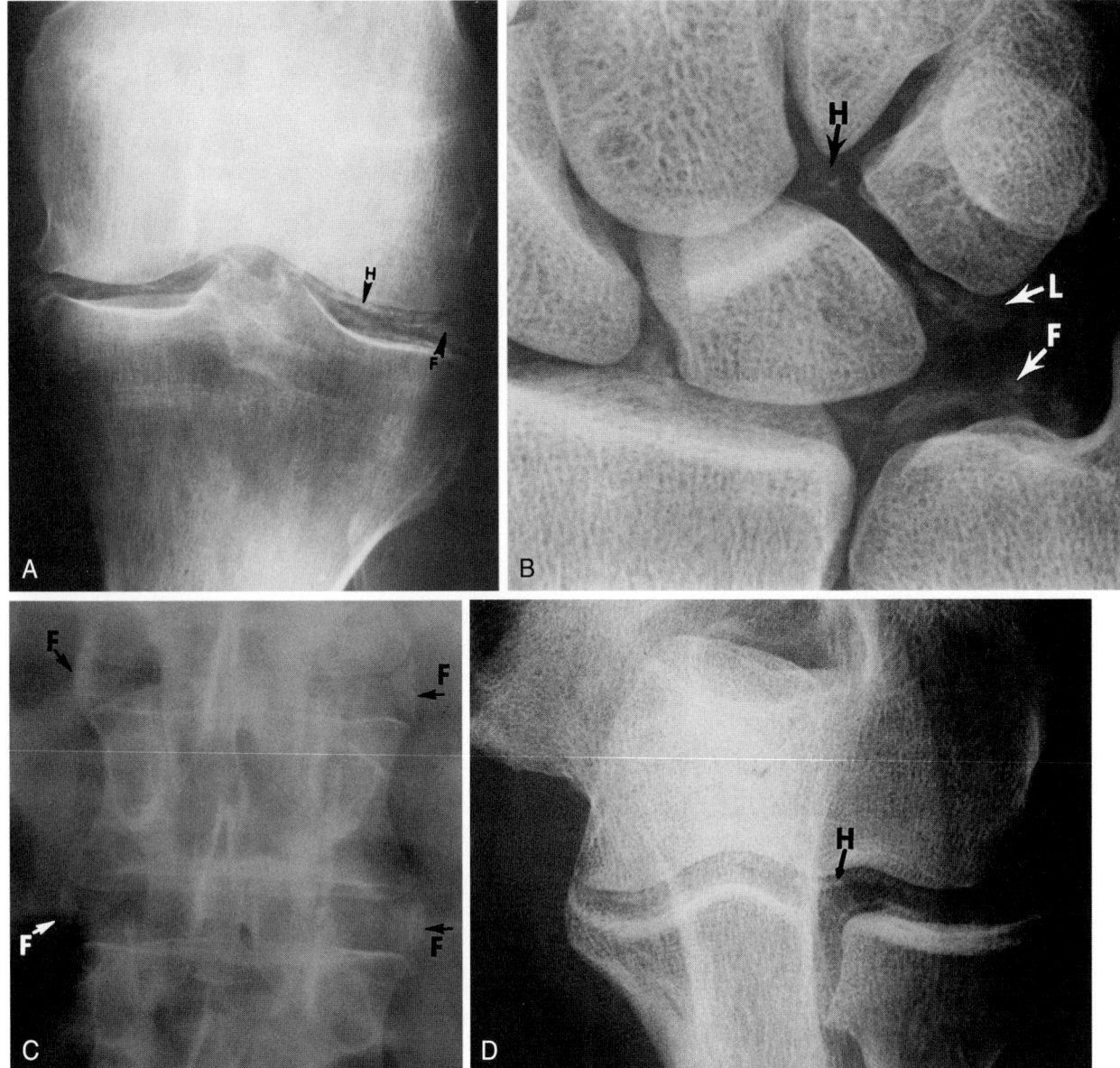

**Figure 34–4.** Radiographic abnormalities: chondrocalcinosis. *A–C*, Chondrocalcinosis of fibrocartilage (F) is apparent in the menisci of the knee, triangular cartilage of the wrist, anulus fibrosus of the intervertebral discs, and meniscus of the acromioclavicular joint. It is thick and shaggy in character. Hyaline cartilage calcification (H), which is seen in the knee and wrist, is thin and parallels the osseous surface. Possible ligamentous calcification (L) is also noted in the wrist. *D*, Hyaline cartilage (H) calcification in the elbow.
    (*A*, From Resnick D, Niwayama G, Goergen TG, et al: Clinical, radiographic and pathologic abnormalities in calcium pyrophosphate dihydrate deposition disease [CPPD]: Pseudogout. Radiology 122:1, 1977.)

and vessels. Soft tissue calcification is most common about the elbow, wrist, and pelvis. Tumorous calcific collections that resemble gouty tophi are occasionally observed (Fig. 34–8). The resulting radiographic findings, which have been designated "tophaceous" pseudogout by some investigators, may resemble the abnormalities of idiopathic synovial (osteo)chondromatosis, soft tissue chondrosarcoma or osteosarcoma, gout, soft tissue chondroma, periosteal or parosteal osteosarcoma, or idiopathic calcium hydroxyapatite crystal deposition.

## Pyrophosphate Arthropathy

The structural joint changes associated with CPPD crystal deposition disease are both common and characteristic. These alterations may appear without adjacent or distant articular calcification. Pyrophosphate arthropathy is most common in the knee, wrist, and metacarpophalangeal joints. The distribution is usually bilateral, although symmetrical changes may not be present. In some ways, pyrophosphate arthropathy is similar to degenerative joint disease with regard to articular space narrowing, bony

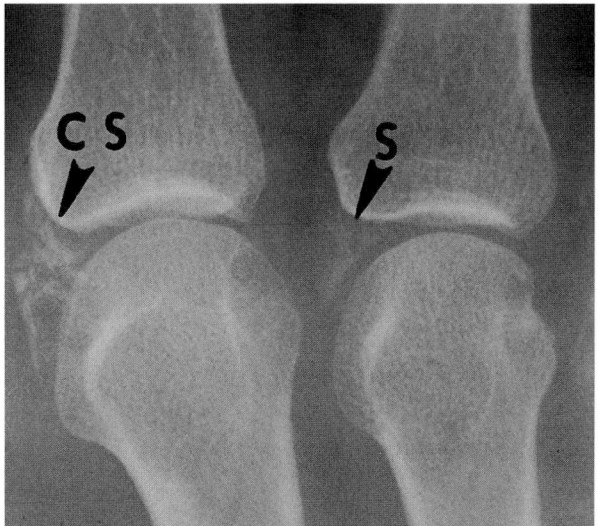

**Figure 34–5.** Radiographic abnormalities: synovial calcification. Observe the synovial (S) and capsular (C) calcification of the metacarpophalangeal joints.

(From Resnick D, Niwayama G, Goergen TG, et al: Clinical, radiographic and pathologic abnormalities in calcium pyrophosphate dihydrate deposition disease [CPPD]: Pseudogout. Radiology 122:1, 1977.)

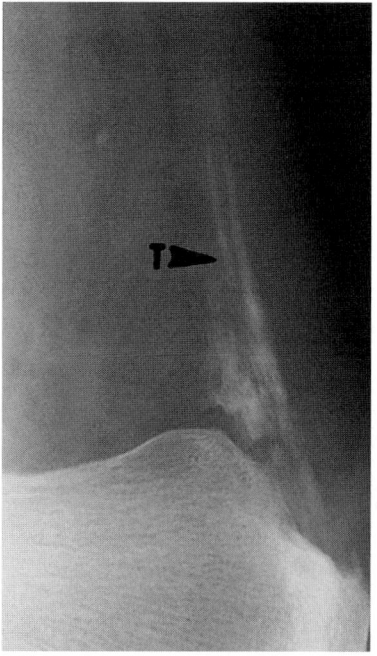

**Figure 34–7.** Radiographic abnormalities: tendinous, ligamentous, and soft tissue calcification. Calcification within the Achilles tendon (T) is apparent.

(From Resnick D, Niwayama G, Goergen TG, et al: Clinical, radiographic and pathologic abnormalities in calcium pyrophosphate dihydrate deposition disease [CPPD]: Pseudogout. Radiology 122:1, 1977.)

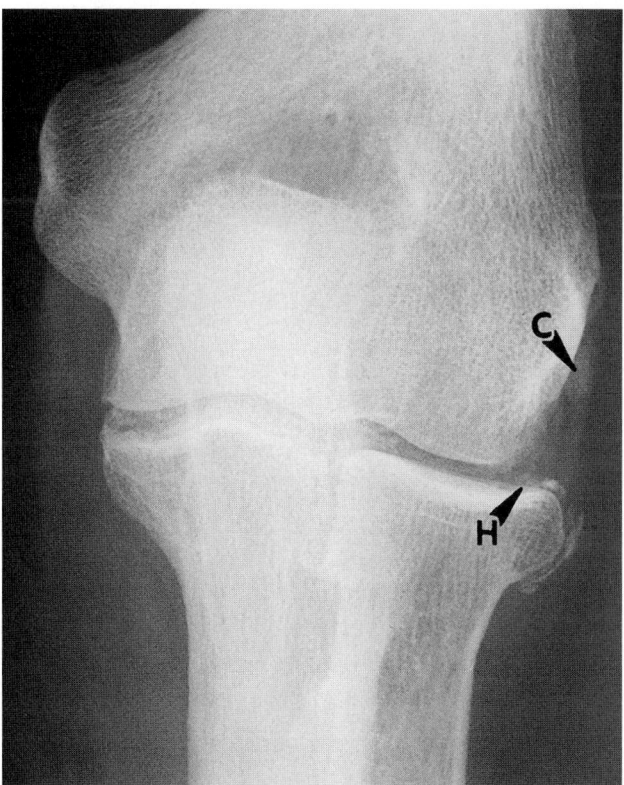

**Figure 34–6.** Radiographic abnormalities: capsular calcification. In the elbow, capsular calcification (C) is associated with hyaline cartilage calcification (H).

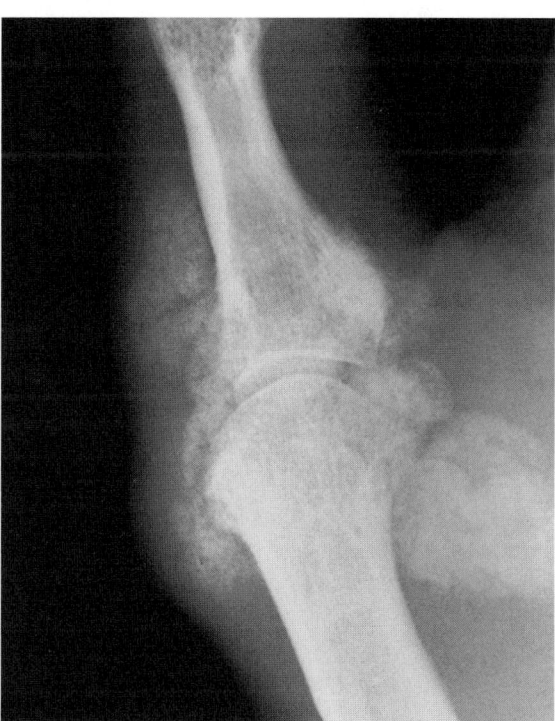

**Figure 34–8.** Radiographic abnormalities: tophaceous pseudogout. Intra-articular and periarticular tumoral deposits are evident at the base of the thumb. (Courtesy of G. El Khoury, MD, Iowa City, Iowa.)

sclerosis, and cyst formation, but it differs from degenerative joint disease in five respects:

1. *Unusual articular distribution.* Although arthropathy is encountered in weight-bearing joints, such as the knee and hip, it is also apparent in sites that are involved less commonly in degenerative joint disease, such as the wrist, elbow, and glenohumeral joint (Fig. 34–9).

2. *Unusual intra-articular distribution.* The distribution of pyrophosphate arthropathy in certain joints is characteristic (Fig. 34–10). Thus, isolated or significant involvement of the radiocarpal or trapezioscaphoid joint of the wrist, patellofemoral compartment of the knee, and talocalcaneonavicular joint of the midfoot may signify CPPD crystal deposition disease.

3. *Prominent subchondral cyst formation.* The cysts associated with pyrophosphate arthropathy are numerous and may reach considerable size. They are typically multiple, subchondral in location, clustered in a group, and surrounded by sclerotic, smudged, and indistinct margins. When large, they may fracture or simulate neoplasm.

4. *Destructive bone changes that are severe and progressive.* Pyrophosphate arthropathy may be associated with extensive and rapid subchondral bone collapse and fragmentation and the appearance of single or multiple intra-articular osseous bodies (Fig. 34–11). These features may resemble those of neuropathic osteoarthropathy.

5. *Variable osteophyte formation.* In some patients, large, irregular bony excrescences are noted about the involved joints; in others, joint space narrowing, sclerosis, and fragmentation may be unaccompanied by osteophyte formation and produce a polished, eburnated bony surface (Fig. 34–12).

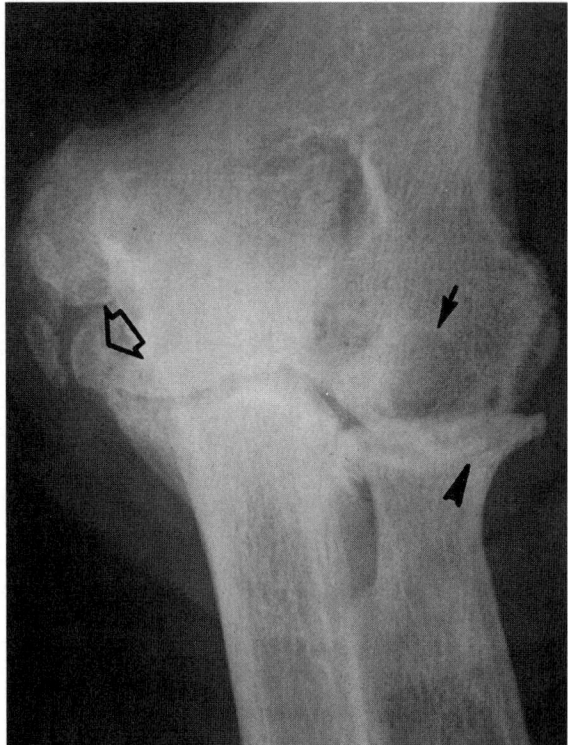

**Figure 34–9.** Characteristics of pyrophosphate arthropathy: unusual articular distribution. Changes in the elbow include joint space narrowing, subchondral cysts *(solid arrow)*, deformity of the radial head *(arrowhead)*, and fragmentation *(open arrow)*.

(From Resnick D, Niwayama G, Goergen TG, et al: Clinical, radiographic and pathologic abnormalities in calcium pyrophosphate dihydrate deposition disease [CPPD]: Pseudogout. Radiology 122:1, 1977.)

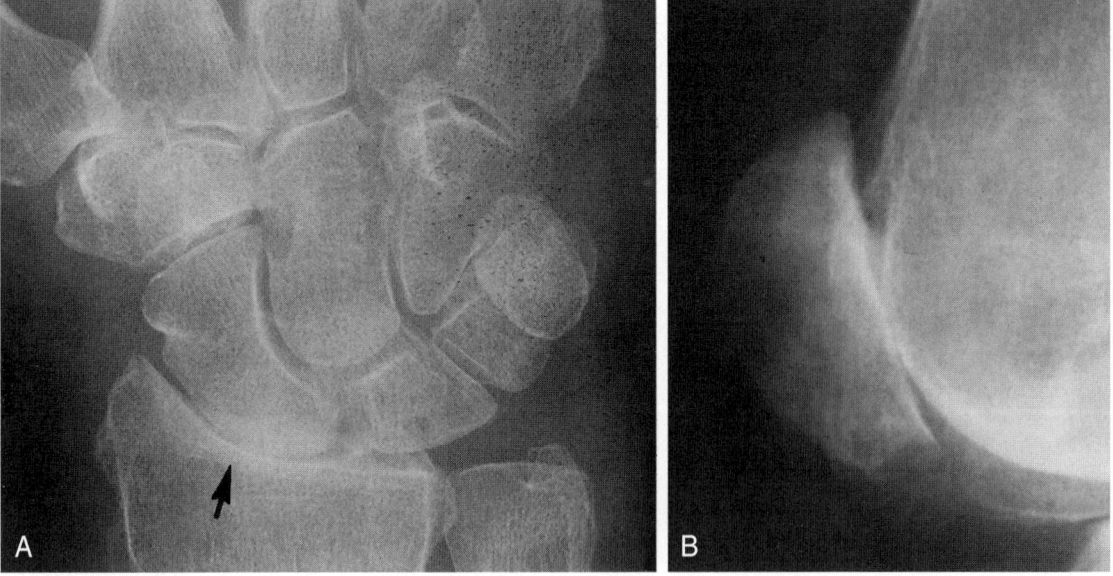

**Figure 34–10.** Characteristics of pyrophosphate arthropathy: unusual intra-articular distribution. *A,* Observe the selective involvement of the radiocarpal compartment of the wrist *(arrow). B,* Predilection for the patellofemoral compartment of the knee is apparent on this lateral radiograph.

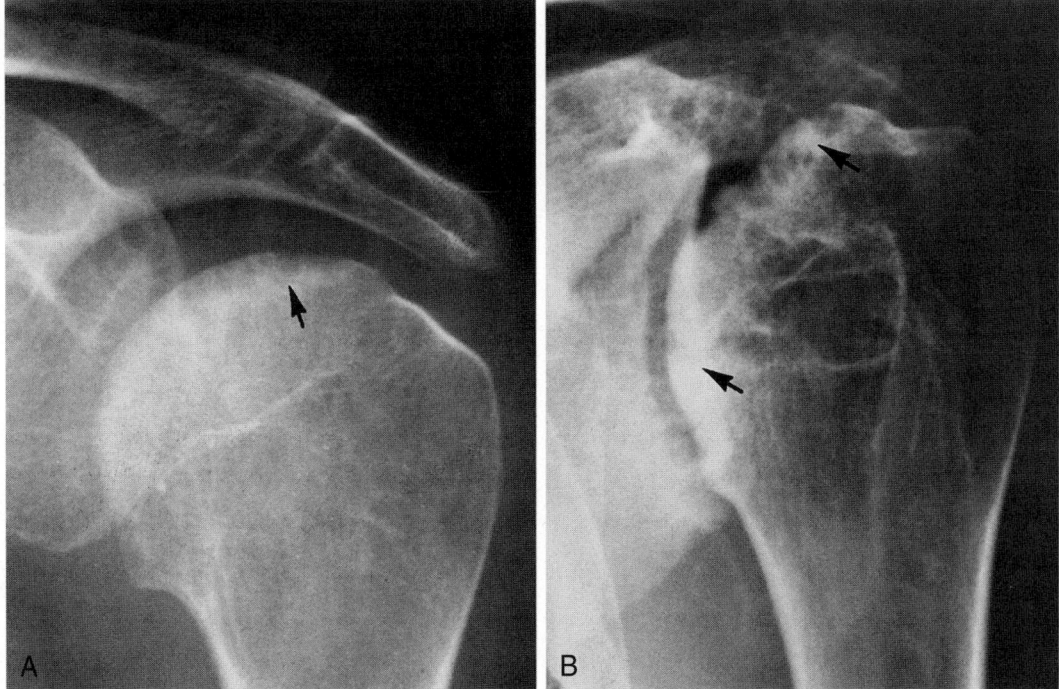

**Figure 34–11.** Characteristics of pyrophosphate arthropathy: destructive bone changes that are severe and progressive. Radiographs of the glenohumeral joint obtained 16 months apart outline the rapidity of joint destruction in this disease *(arrows).*

(From Resnick D, Niwayama G, Goergen TG, et al: Clinical, radiographic and pathologic abnormalities in calcium pyrophosphate dihydrate deposition disease [CPPD]: Pseudogout. Radiology 122:1, 1977.)

## RADIOGRAPHIC FEATURES IN SPECIFIC ARTICULATIONS

### Knee

The knee is the joint involved most commonly (Fig. 34–13; Table 34–3). Chondrocalcinosis and synovial calcification may be combined with tendinous and ligamentous deposits in the quadriceps muscle, gastrocnemius muscle, and collateral and cruciate ligaments. Intra-articular osseous and calcific bodies are frequently observed.

Pyrophosphate arthropathy most commonly involves the medial femorotibial compartment; the patellofemoral compartment is the second most commonly involved area. More important, the distribution of knee compartmental alterations in CPPD crystal deposition disease differs from that of degenerative joint disease. Isolated or severe patellofemoral compartment changes have been stressed as a manifestation of this crystal deposition disease. Isolated lateral compartment alterations (especially in men), severe flattening of either the medial or lateral tibial condyles, and significant varus or valgus angulation are additional characteristics of knee involvement in this disease.

### Wrist

Calcification in the wrist (Fig. 34–14) is observed most commonly in the triangular fibrocartilage; hyaline cartilage of the radiocarpal, midcarpal, and common carpometacarpal joints; synovium; and ligamentous structures, particularly between the scaphoid and lunate and between the lunate and triquetrum. Carpal malalignment with separation of the scaphoid and lunate may be observed, with disruption of the intervening interosseous ligament.

The wrist arthropathy of CPPD crystal deposition disease demonstrates an unusual predilection for the radiocarpal compartment. Joint space narrowing, sclerosis, and discrete subchondral radiolucent lesions are observed between the distal end of the radius and the proximal carpal row. The scaphoid moves proximally, and at the same time, the lunate may move distally and approach

**TABLE 34–3**

**Most Frequent Sites of Clinical and Radiographic Abnormalities in CPPD Crystal Deposition Disease**

|  | Clinical Manifestations | Calcification | Arthropathy |
|---|---|---|---|
| Hand | + |  | + |
| Wrist | + | + | + |
| Elbow |  |  | + |
| Shoulder |  |  | + |
| Hip | + | + |  |
| Knee | + | + | + |
| Ankle | + |  |  |
| Spine |  | + |  |
| Pelvis |  | + |  |

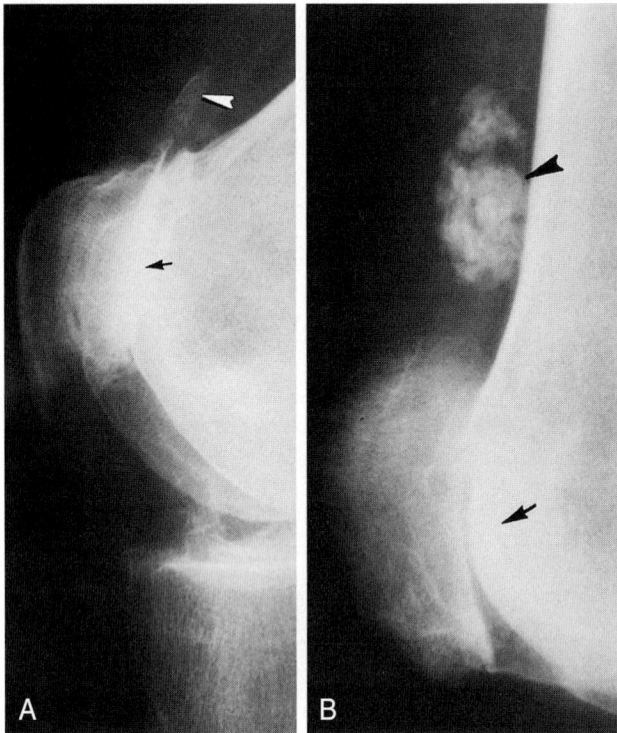

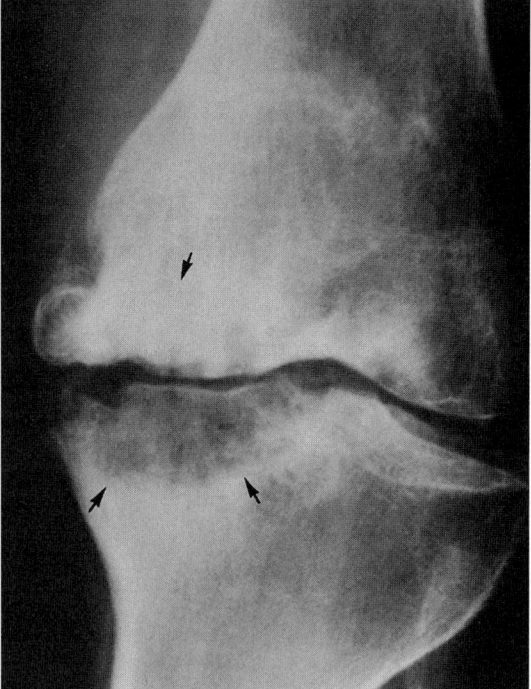

**Figure 34–12.** Characteristics of pyrophosphate arthropathy: variable osteophyte formation. *A*, In some persons, large osteophytes *(arrowhead)* accompany joint space narrowing *(arrow)*. *B*, In other persons, joint space narrowing *(arrow)* occurs without osteophyte formation. Intra-articular bodies are apparent *(arrowhead)*.

(From Resnick D, Niwayama G, Goergen TG, et al: Clinical, radiographic and pathologic abnormalities in calcium pyrophosphate dihydrate deposition disease [CPPD]: Pseudogout. Radiology 122:1, 1977.)

**Figure 34–13.** Knee abnormalities in CPPD crystal deposition disease. Considerable collapse and fragmentation of the medial femorotibial compartment are visualized *(arrows)*.

(From Resnick D, Niwayama G, Goergen TG, et al: Clinical, radiographic and pathologic abnormalities in calcium pyrophosphate dihydrate deposition disease [CPPD]: Pseudogout. Radiology 122:1, 1977.)

the capitate. Such a "stepladder" appearance is very suggestive of this disease. It is similar to what has been termed scapholunate advanced collapse (SLAC) in instances of wrist injury.

The compartmental distribution of CPPD arthropathy differs considerably from that of degenerative joint disease. The latter disorder affects predominantly the first carpometacarpal and trapezioscaphoid areas, with sparing of the radiocarpal compartment. In CPPD crystal deposition disease, the radiocarpal compartment is the most common site of abnormality.

## Metacarpophalangeal Joints

Radiographic abnormalities in this location include cartilaginous, capsular, and synovial calcifications and arthropathy (Fig. 34–15). The structural joint changes show a predilection for the second and third metacarpophalangeal joints and are characterized by joint space narrowing, sclerosis, cyst formation, and bony collapse, particularly of the metacarpal head. Although the second and third metacarpophalangeal joints are also involved in hemochromatosis, changes in the fourth and fifth digits are not infrequent in that disease. Further, the absence of erosions of the metacarpal heads in CPPD crystal deposition disease differs from the findings of rheumatoid arthritis.

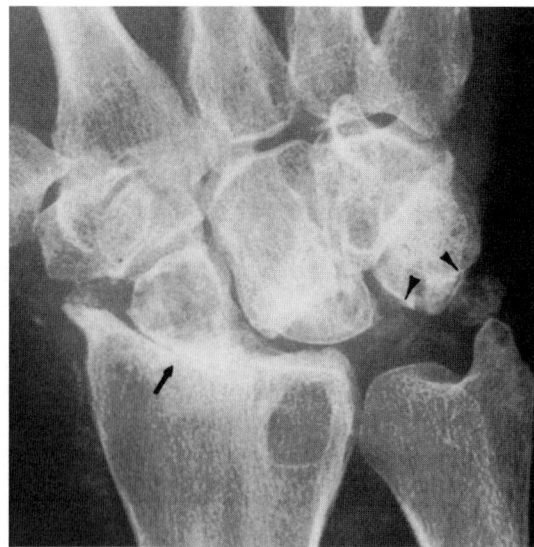

**Figure 34–14.** Wrist abnormalities in CPPD crystal deposition disease. In addition to chondrocalcinosis and synovial and ligamentous calcification *(arrowheads)*, observe the considerable narrowing of the radiocarpal *(arrow)* and midcarpal compartments, with cyst formation and sclerosis. Note the "stepladder" appearance, with proximal migration of the scaphoid and distal migration of the lunate.

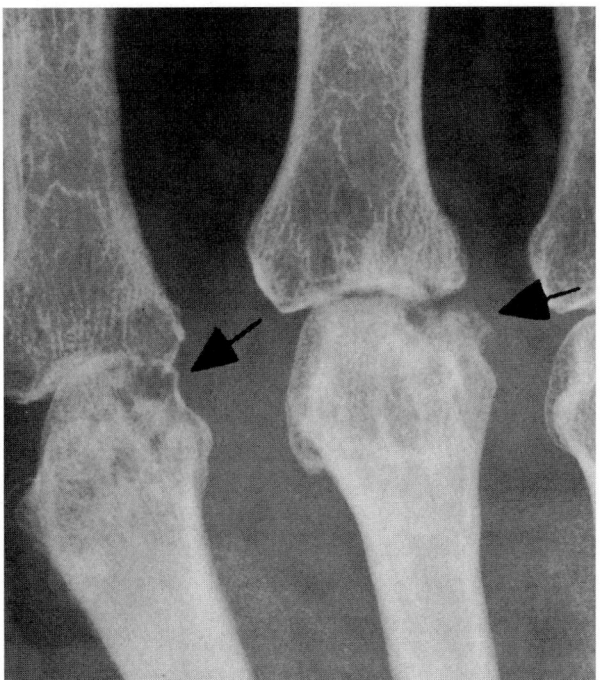

**Figure 34–15.** Metacarpophalangeal joint abnormalities in CPPD crystal deposition disease. Collapse and fragmentation (*arrows*) about the metacarpophalangeal joints are noted.

### Elbow

Radiographic findings in this joint include chondrocalcinosis, capsular and synovial calcification, triceps tendon deposits, and arthropathy. Osseous resorption in the proximal portions of the radius and ulna, joint space narrowing, extensive sclerosis, cyst formation, and bone fragmentation are features of arthropathy of the elbow.

### Hip

Both fibrocartilaginous calcification of the acetabular labra and hyaline cartilage calcification may be seen (Fig. 34–16). Joint space narrowing may involve the entire joint or be confined to its superolateral aspect. In the latter situation, the changes resemble those of osteoarthritis, whereas with diffuse loss of joint space, the findings are similar to those of rheumatoid arthritis. Additional manifestations of hip involvement in CPPD crystal deposition disease are rapid and extensive destruction of the femoral head and acetabulum, fragmentation, protrusio acetabuli deformity, tendon calcification, and large tumor-like lesions (i.e., tophaceous pseudogout).

### Shoulder

Abnormalities in this location include chondrocalcinosis; capsular, tendinous, and bursal deposits; rotator cuff tears; joint space narrowing; bony eburnation; and cysts. Acromioclavicular joint destruction and masses above this joint are also well-known features of CPPD crystal deposition disease.

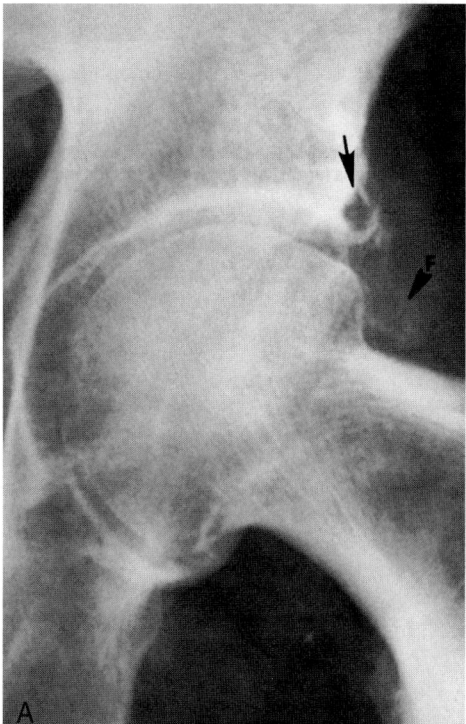

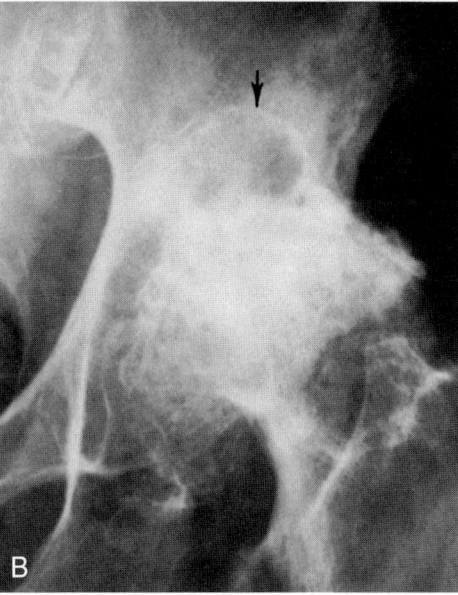

**Figure 34–16.** Hip abnormalities in CPPD crystal deposition disease. *A*, Fibrocartilage (F) calcification of the acetabular limbus is seen adjacent to a small subchondral cystic lesion (*arrow*). *B*, Considerable flattening and deformity of the femoral head are associated with an elongated lateral acetabular osteophyte and new bone formation on the medial aspect of the femoral neck. The articular space is obliterated, and a large subchondral cyst (*arrow*) is evident.

(From Resnick D, Niwayama G, Goergen TG, et al: Clinical, radiographic and pathologic abnormalities in calcium pyrophosphate dihydrate deposition disease [CPPD]: Pseudogout. Radiology 122:1, 1977.)

### Ankle, Hindfoot, and Midfoot

Although articular and periarticular calcification can be seen about the ankle, arthropathy in this site is unusual.

More commonly, the midfoot is altered, particularly the talocalcaneonavicular joint. The findings resemble those of neuropathic osteoarthropathy, particularly that associated with diabetes mellitus.

## Forefoot

Capsular calcification may be apparent about any metatarsophalangeal joint. In unusual circumstances, cartilaginous and synovial calcification and soft tissue swelling at the first metatarsophalangeal joint resemble the changes of gout.

## Spine

In the spine, CPPD crystal deposition disease frequently demonstrates intervertebral disc calcification, with deposits initially appearing in the outer fibers of the anulus fibrosus (Figs. 34–17 and 34–18). The nucleus pulposus is generally not involved. CPPD deposits are detected in other spinal tissues as well, including the ligamentum flavum, posterior longitudinal ligament, interspinous and supraspinous ligaments, and interspinous bursae.

Disc space narrowing is a common finding in CPPD crystal deposition disease. The narrowing may be extensive, widespread, and associated with considerable vertebral sclerosis. In unusual circumstances, severe osseous destruction of the adjacent vertebral bodies is seen. CPPD crystal deposition in the spine is widespread, and destructive abnormalities of the cervical spine are occasionally apparent. In the atlantoaxial joint, tumor-like masses may compress the spinal cord, and the anterior longitudinal ligament may become calcified as well. Complications of involvement include atlantoaxial subluxation and spontaneous fractures of the odontoid process.

## Sacroiliac Joint

Abnormalities in the sacroiliac joint have been observed in 45% to 50% of cases. Calcification of articular cartilage is infrequently identified on radiographic examina-

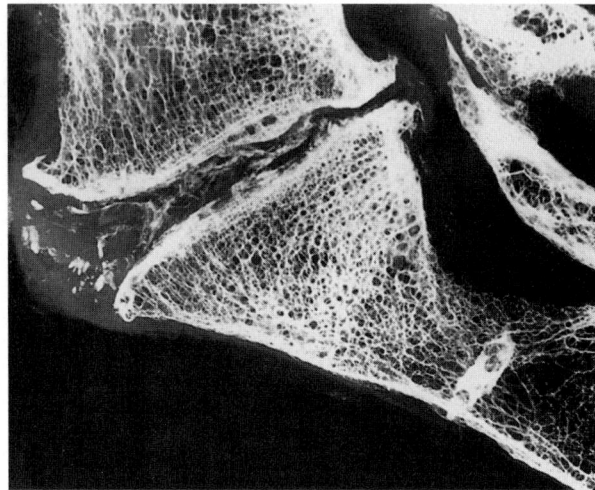

**Figure 34–17.** Spine abnormalities in CPPD crystal deposition disease: alterations of the intervertebral disc. In association with widespread disc calcification, disc space loss and bone eburnation are seen in this sagittal section of the lumbosacral junction.

tion. Unilateral or bilateral subchondral erosions, sclerosis, and cyst formation may be accompanied by joint space narrowing and bridging osteophytosis.

## CLINICAL AND RADIOGRAPHIC CORRELATIONS

Although calcification and arthropathy frequently coexist in the same joint, either radiographic finding can be identified in the absence of the other. More commonly, calcification precedes arthropathy, with calcification beginning in the fibrocartilage and subsequently involving the hyaline cartilage of large joints and eventually the hyaline cartilage of the small joints of the hands and feet. In some instances, however, arthropathy develops in patients who demonstrate neither local (in the same joint) nor distant (in any joint) calcification, and it is unusual to document the initial appearance of calcification after arthropathy.

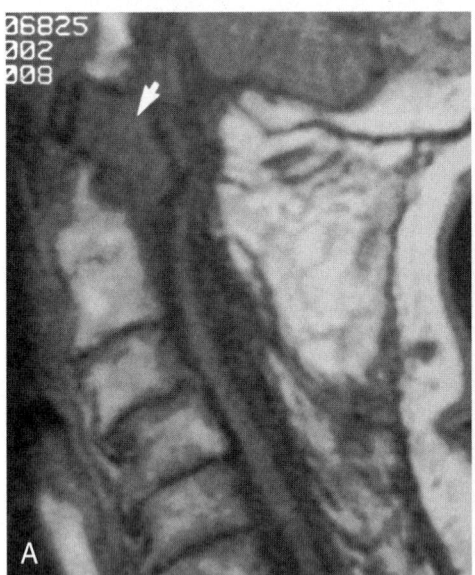
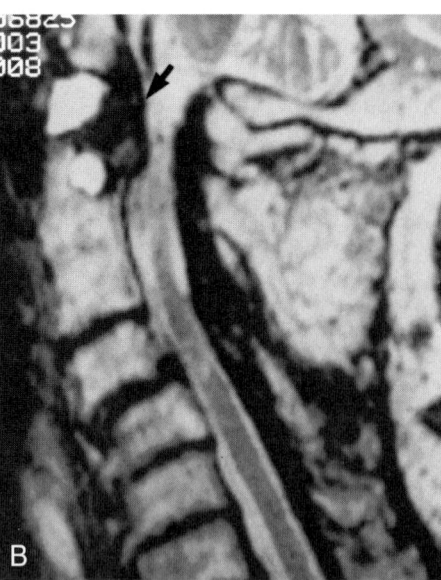

**Figure 34–18.** Spine abnormalities in CPPD crystal deposition disease: alterations about the odontoid process. In this 70-year-old man, sagittal T1-weighted (TR/TE, 500/12) *(A)* and T2-weighted (TR/TE, 3400/96) *(B)* spin echo MR images show a mass *(arrows)* about the eroded odontoid process. Note the adjacent areas of high signal intensity in *(B)*. The spinal cord is displaced. On computed tomography scans (not shown), the mass was found to be calcified. CPPD crystal deposition was documented when the mass was removed surgically.

# MAGNETIC RESONANCE IMAGING ABNORMALITIES

CPPD crystal accumulation typically leads to masses with predominantly low signal intensity, although these masses may show enhancement of signal intensity after the intravenous administration of a gadolinium-containing contrast agent. Small collections of CPPD crystals in the menisci of the knee and the triangular fibrocartilage of the wrist are easily overlooked during magnetic resonance (MR) imaging examinations, as are those within the intervertebral disc. Low signal intensity is characteristic of such calcific collections. In the menisci of the knee, however, regions of intermediate signal intensity may simulate meniscal tears. Similarly, in hyaline cartilage, CPPD crystal deposits appear as hypointense foci. Synovial calcifications and intra-articular debris (often composed of both CPPD and calcium hydroxyapatite crystals) are also apparent on MR imaging.

# DIFFERENTIAL DIAGNOSIS

## Intra-articular Calcification

Chondrocalcinosis, particularly of the menisci of the knee, may relate not only to the presence of CPPD crystals but also to the deposition of other crystalline material, such as dicalcium phosphate dihydrate and calcium hydroxyapatite. Chondrocalcinosis of more than one set of joints usually indicates CPPD crystal deposition.

Additional causes of intra-articular radiodense lesions that may simulate CPPD crystal deposition generally produce abnormalities of a single joint and include meniscal ossicles of the knee; osteochondritis dissecans of the knee, ankle, or elbow; osteonecrosis; and idiopathic synovial osteochondromatosis. Disintegration of articular surfaces with the production of single or multiple calcific and ossific dense areas may be seen in a variety of other articular disorders, including neuropathic osteoarthropathy, steroid-induced arthropathy, infection, gout, and rheumatoid arthritis. In these cases, characteristic signs of the underlying articular disorder are usually apparent. Diagnostic difficulty arises in certain cases of CPPD crystal deposition disease in which homogeneous, tumoral, intra-articular or periarticular calcifications (tophaceous pseudogout), or osteochondral fragments are seen or in cases with both CPPD and calcium hydroxyapatite accumulation (mixed crystal deposition disease).

## Periarticular Calcification

Periarticular radiodense deposits may be associated with metastatic calcification, dystrophic calcification, or calcinosis. Such calcification may be seen in renal osteodystrophy, idiopathic tumoral calcinosis, collagen vascular diseases, milk-alkali syndrome, and hypervitaminosis D.

Calcific periarthritis or peritendinitis may be associated with the deposition of calcium hydroxyapatite crystals in tendons and bursae, particularly about the shoulder. Tendinous calcification in CPPD crystal deposition disease produces similar abnormalities, but the deposits may be more elongated. Differentiation between these two disorders is aided by the absence of chondrocalcinosis in patients with calcific periarthritis.

## Pyrophosphate Arthropathy

The arthropathy of CPPD crystal deposition disease closely resembles degenerative joint disease but, as indicated previously, involves unusual joints and compartments and is associated with extensive sclerosis, multiple cysts, bone fragmentation, osseous debris, and variable osteophyte formation (Table 34–4). The degree of bone fragmentation, sclerosis, and collapse encountered in patients with CPPD crystal deposition disease is reminiscent of the changes accompanying other disorders such as neuropathic osteoarthropathy, steroid-induced arthropathy, osteonecrosis, and infection. The absence of clinical features typical of these other disorders usually ensures an accurate diagnosis of CPPD crystal deposition disease.

**TABLE 34–4**

**Differential Diagnosis of Pyrophosphate Arthropathy**

| | Pyrophosphate Arthropathy | Degenerative Joint Disease | Neuropathic Osteoarthropathy | Rheumatoid Arthritis |
|---|---|---|---|---|
| Common sites | Knee, wrist (radiocarpal), metacarpophalangeal | Hip, knee, interphalangeal of hand, wrist (first carpometacarpal, trapezioscaphoid), first metatarsophalangeal | Tabes: knee, ankle, hip, spine<br>Diabetes: midfoot and forefoot<br>Syringomyelia: upper extremity | Wrist (pancompartmental), metacarpophalangeal, interphalangeal of hand, metatarsophalangeal, knee, shoulder, cervical spine |
| Articular space narrowing | + | + | ± | + |
| Sclerosis | + | + | + | − |
| Osteophytosis | ± | + | ± | − |
| Erosions | − | − | − | + |
| Cysts | + | + | ± | + |
| Fragmentation | + | − | + | − |

Bone erosion is not a feature of CPPD crystal deposition disease. The absence of erosive change usually aids in distinguishing this condition from rheumatoid arthritis and related synovial disorders such as psoriatic arthritis and ankylosing spondylitis. The appearance of joint space narrowing, bony eburnation, osteophytosis, and sclerosis in CPPD crystal deposition disease may resemble the features of gout. Differentiation between gout and CPPD crystal deposition disease is further complicated by the occasional presence of periarticular calcification and chondrocalcinosis in gouty arthritis. In gouty arthritis, however, focal soft tissue swelling and bone erosion—findings not generally seen in CPPD crystal deposition disease—may be noted.

**Knee.** Although the distribution of compartmental abnormalities in the knee in CPPD crystal deposition disease may be identical to that of degenerative joint disease, isolated patellofemoral compartment changes are an important diagnostic clue suggesting the presence of pyrophosphate arthropathy. In degenerative joint disease, patellofemoral changes are frequent, but in most cases they are combined with alterations in the medial femorotibial compartment. Symmetrical loss of joint space in the medial and lateral femorotibial spaces or tricompartmental involvement is common in rheumatoid arthritis and infection. Patellofemoral compartment erosions may be noted in patients with primary hyperparathyroidism or renal osteodystrophy, but additional skeletal findings allow the diagnosis of these conditions.

**Wrist.** Selective involvement of the radiocarpal compartment of the wrist is most characteristic of CPPD crystal deposition disease. Degenerative joint disease in the wrist usually produces changes in the first carpometacarpal and trapezioscaphoid areas rather than in the radiocarpal compartment. After injury, however, osteoarthritis can appear in any region of the wrist, including the radioscaphoid, radiolunate, and lunate-capitate spaces. Radiocarpal compartment changes may occasionally be seen in patients with gout or occupation-related degenerative disease. Rheumatoid arthritis also involves this joint, but additional changes in other compartments of the wrist are generally apparent in this disease. In rheumatoid arthritis, the inferior radioulnar compartment demonstrates extensive abnormalities; this site is not commonly involved in pyrophosphate arthropathy.

The SLAC pattern of osteoarthritis, occurring either spontaneously or after trauma, is characterized by narrowing of both the radioscaphoid and capitolunate spaces. A similar pattern of arthropathy is characteristic of CPPD crystal deposition disease and, in the presence of chondrocalcinosis and the absence of traumatic injury, strongly suggests the diagnosis of CPPD crystal deposition disease.

**Metacarpophalangeal Joints.** The metacarpophalangeal joints are frequently altered in CPPD crystal deposition disease. The changes in this location predominate over changes at the interphalangeal joints, whereas the converse is true in degenerative joint disease. The absence of osseous erosion of the metacarpal heads and proximal phalanges in CPPD crystal deposition disease allows its differentiation from rheumatoid arthritis.

The arthropathies of idiopathic CPPD crystal deposition disease and hemochromatosis are very similar, but subtle differences have been defined. Although both disorders involve the second and third metacarpophalangeal joints, changes in the fourth and fifth digits are more prevalent in hemochromatosis. Peculiar hooklike osteophytes on the radial aspect of the metacarpal heads are also more characteristic of hemochromatosis than idiopathic CPPD crystal deposition disease.

**Hip.** Focal loss of joint space in the superolateral aspect of this joint may occur in patients with CPPD crystal deposition disease and mimic the findings of degenerative joint disease. Diffuse joint space loss may also be seen, simulating the pattern of joint space loss in rheumatoid arthritis and ankylosing spondylitis. The degree of bony sclerosis and osteophytosis in CPPD crystal deposition disease allows its differentiation from rheumatoid arthritis, but the hip involvement of pyrophosphate arthropathy may resemble that of ankylosing spondylitis. The presence of bone fragmentation and collapse and the absence of sacroiliac joint abnormalities in CPPD crystal deposition disease are findings that are not apparent in ankylosing spondylitis.

A rapidly destructive pattern of hip disease has been described, termed *rapidly destructive osteoarthritis*. Rapid progression of hip pain and disability is a consistent clinical feature. Radiographs reveal flattening of the femoral head, joint space loss, subchondral cysts, sclerosis on both sides of the joint, and lateral subluxation of the femoral head. Acetabular protrusion may or may not be present. The resulting imaging features resemble those of neuropathic osteoarthropathy or infection. The features also resemble those of osteonecrosis. A similar pattern of hip destruction may occur in patients with calcium hydroxyapatite or pyrophosphate crystal deposition disease.

**Foot.** Selective involvement of the talonavicular portion of the talocalcaneonavicular joint is observed in some patients with pyrophosphate arthropathy. This distribution of abnormalities is also observed in the neuropathic osteoarthropathy accompanying diabetes mellitus, and differentiation of the midfoot changes in these two disorders may be difficult. The absence of significant erosion of the first metatarsophalangeal joint distinguishes pyrophosphate arthropathy from gouty arthritis.

**Spine.** Disc calcification related to CPPD crystal deposition initially occurs in the outer fibers of the anulus fibrosus. With progressive calcification, widespread disc deposits resemble the changes of alkaptonuria. The resemblance between these two disorders is accentuated by the possible occurrence of both peripheral arthropathy and chondrocalcinosis in patients with alkaptonuria. The disc space narrowing in the thoracic and lumbar spine in CPPD crystal deposition disease is identical to that seen in intervertebral osteochondrosis (degenerative disease of the nucleus pulposus). Vertebral body sclerosis may be observed in both disorders, but the degree of bony eburnation and the possible occurrence of vertebral body destruction in CPPD crystal deposition disease allow an accurate diagnosis.

Cervical spine subluxation, particularly at the atlanto-axial junction, in CPPD crystal deposition disease resembles the findings of rheumatoid arthritis. The absence of discovertebral and apophyseal joint erosions in pyrophosphate arthropathy distinguishes it from rheumatoid arthritis.

## FURTHER READING

Adamson TC III, Resnik CS, Guerra J Jr, et al: Hand and wrist arthropathies of hemochromatosis and calcium pyrophosphate deposition disease: Distinct radiographic features. Radiology 147:377, 1983.

Burke BJ, Escobedo EM, Wilson AJ, et al: Chondrocalcinosis mimicking a meniscal tear on MR imaging. AJR 170:69, 1998.

Chen C, Chandnani VP, Kang HS, et al: Scapholunate advanced collapse: A common wrist abnormality in calcium pyrophosphate dihydrate crystal deposition disease. Radiology 177:459, 1990.

Dieppe PA, Alexander GJM, Jones HE, et al: Pyrophosphate arthropathy: A clinical and radiological study of 105 cases. Ann Rheum Dis 41:371, 1982.

Leisen J: Calcium pyrophosphate dihydrate deposition disease: Tumorous form. AJR 138:962, 1982.

Ling D, Murphy WA, Kyriakos M: Tophaceous pseudogout. AJR 138:162, 1982.

Martel W, Champion CK, Thompson GR, et al: A roentgenologically distinctive arthropathy in some patients with the pseudogout syndrome. AJR 109:587, 1970.

Martel W, McCarter DK, Solsky MA, et al: Further observations on the arthropathy of calcium pyrophosphate crystal deposition disease. Radiology 141:1, 1981.

McCarty DJ, Hollander JL: Identification of urate crystals in gouty synovial fluid. Ann Intern Med 54:452, 1961.

McCarty DJ Jr, Kohn NN, Faires JS: The significance of calcium phosphate crystals in the synovial fluid of arthritis patients: The "pseudogout" syndrome. Ann Intern Med 56:711, 1962.

McCarty DJ, Silcox DC, Coe F, et al: Diseases associated with calcium pyrophosphate dihydrate crystal deposition. Am J Med 56:704, 1974.

Resnick D, Pineda C: Vertebral involvement in calcium pyrophosphate dihydrate crystal deposition disease. Radiographic-pathologic correlation. Radiology 158:55, 1984.

Resnick D, Niwayama G, Goergen TG, et al: Clinical, radiographic and pathologic abnormalities in calcium pyrophosphate dihydrate deposition disease (CPPD): Pseudogout. Radiology 122:1, 1977.

Rosenberg ZS, Shankman S, Steiner GC, et al: Rapid destructive osteoarthritis: Clinical, radiographic, and pathologic features. Radiology 182:213, 1992.

Rynes RI, Merzig EG: Calcium pyrophosphate crystal deposition disease and hyperparathyroidism: A controlled, prospective study. J Rheumatol 5:460, 1978.

Utsinger PD, Zvaifler NJ, Resnick D: Calcium pyrophosphate dihydrate deposition disease without chondrocalcinosis. J Rheumatol 2:258, 1975.

Watt I, Dieppe PA: Medial femoral condyle necrosis and chondrocalcinosis: A causal relationship? Br J Radiol 56:7, 1983.

Zitbrenan D, Sitaj S: Chondrocalcinosis articularis. Section I. Clinical and radiological study. Ann Rheum Dis 22:142, 1963.

# CHAPTER 35

## Calcium Hydroxyapatite Crystal Deposition Disease

## *SUMMARY OF KEY FEATURES*

Calcium hydroxyapatite (HA) crystal deposition can lead to periarticular accumulations that are associated with typical clinical and radiographic findings. The radiographic manifestations are observed most frequently in the shoulder, although similar abnormalities may be apparent at other articular sites. Intra-articular alterations have also been documented as a consequence of calcium HA crystal deposition disease, and the combination of calcium HA and calcium pyrophosphate dihydrate (CPPD) crystal accumulation (mixed calcium phosphate crystal deposition disease) is being identified with greater frequency.

## INTRODUCTION

Over the past 30 years, the development of methods such as polarizing microscopy that can identify crystalline deposits in and around joints has led to the elucidation of several disorders associated with tissue inflammation: needle-shaped crystals of monosodium urate in patients with gout; CPPD crystals in patients who have the pseudogout syndrome; and crystalline depot corticosteroid preparations, which, when injected intra-articularly, can produce acute synovitis. Another group of crystals related to calcium HA or apatite-like crystals has also been identified in periarticular or articular (e.g., synovial fluid, synovial membrane, cartilage) structures or in both. The precise relationship between such crystal deposition and clinical manifestations remains obscure, although evidence is accumulating that both periarticular and articular abnormalities accompany the deposition of these basic calcium phosphate crystals.

Although the presence of calcification in periarticular soft tissues and tendons, particularly about the shoulder, had been observed for many years, it was not until 1966 that calcium HA was implicated as the material deposited in these calcific collections. Calcium HA crystals are currently regarded as a cause of bursitis and other periarticular inflammatory conditions that may be associated with radiographically demonstrable calcification. Some investigators have noted that calcium HA crystals may also be observed in joint fluid and, in this location, can lead to articular manifestations. The identification of individual HA crystals is generally not possible using ordinary polarized light microscopy; this requires electron microscopy, radioisotopic techniques, or x-ray diffusion analysis.

## PERIARTICULAR CRYSTAL DEPOSITION

### Clinical Features

Recurrent painful periarticular calcific deposits in tendons and soft tissues have been described by a variety of names, including calcific tendinitis, peritendinitis and bursitis, and hydroxyapatite rheumatism. Although inflammation about a calcified tendon (peritendinitis) may be noted, degeneration (tendinosis or tendinopathy) rather than inflammation (tendinitis) is evident in the involved tendon. These deposits are usually monoarticular in distribution, although they can be polyarticular. The most frequent site of involvement is the shoulder, although other sites such as the wrist, hand, foot, elbow, hip, neck, and lumbar spine may be involved. The disease affects both men and women and is particularly common between 40 and 70 years of age.

Acute symptoms include pain, tenderness on pressure, local edema or swelling, restricted motion, and mild fever. Chronic symptoms and signs may also be present. In many patients, deposits are detected radiographically in persons who are entirely asymptomatic.

### General Pathologic Features

Granular deposits of calcium material in fibrous connective tissue may be associated with necrosis, loss of fibrous structure, and surrounding inflammatory changes. The deposits appear milky or cheesy in consistency and are inspissated or chalklike in quality.

### General Radiographic Features

The radiographic features of periarticular calcium HA crystal deposition depend on the site of involvement. Initially, the deposits may appear thin, cloudlike, and poorly defined as they blend into the surrounding soft tissues. With time, they may appear denser, homogeneous, and more sharply delineated, with a linear or circular configuration. Adjacent osseous tissues may be entirely normal, although osteoporosis, lytic lesions, reactive sclerosis, and contour irregularities or frank erosions are sometimes apparent.

Sequential radiographic examinations in patients with calcific periarticular deposits reveal varying patterns. In some patients, the deposits remain static for long periods. In other patients, the deposits may enlarge and change shape. Alternatively, the calcification may diminish in size and disappear, in the absence of symptoms. Reappearance of calcification has also been documented. Periarticular amorphous calcific collections in association with some disorders, such as chronic renal disease, may become massive and surround the joint.

### Cause, Pathogenesis, Classification, and Treatment

The cause and pathogenesis of calcium HA crystal deposition in periarticular tissues are unknown. In the past, it was assumed that such collections resulted from the deposition of calcium in degenerated, injured, or necrotic tissue, perhaps related to a change in local pH values as a result of increased alkalinity or decreased carbon dioxide tension. More recently, documentation of familial cases, polyarticular involvement, and an increased frequency of certain histocompatibility antigens in these patients suggest that multiple local, systemic, metabolic, and genetic factors may be involved. Although the precise pathogenesis of calcium HA crystal deposition may vary among these many causes, tissue degeneration is a common theme. Thus, calcium HA crystal deposition occurring in tendons is more accurately termed calcific tendinosis rather than calcific tendinitis, and the former designation is used for the remainder of this chapter.

In the past, many techniques were used to treat calcific tendinosis and bursitis of the shoulder, with varying success. These techniques included heat and cold therapy, ultrasonic and diathermic procedures, needling and aspiration, steroid injections, surgery, and radiotherapy. In certain instances, calcific collections may diminish in size and even disappear; at other times, the calcification may become more extensive or the deposits may remain unchanged in size.

## Calcific Tendinosis and Bursitis at Specific Sites

### Shoulder

The capsular, tendinous, ligamentous, and bursal tissues about the shoulder are the most common sites of calcific deposits. These deposits occur in about 3% of adults, are bilateral in almost 50% of persons, and are most frequently in the supraspinatus tendon. Clinical findings are apparent in about one third of patients.

The radiographic appearance of shoulder calcification depends on the exact location of the abnormal deposits; they are commonly encountered in the tendons of the rotator cuff, adjacent tendons, and bursae. The precise appearance and position of the calcification depend on the disease and the specific tendon in which the deposits are located (Figs. 35–1 and 35–2).

**Supraspinatus Tendon Calcification.** The supraspinatus tendon is the most frequent site of calcification. The deposits are located at the tendinous insertion on the promontory of the greater tuberosity (Fig. 35–3). Radiodense lesions at this site may be seen in profile on external rotation of the shoulder. They may remain in profile on internal rotation, although, as the calcification moves medially in this projection, it may overlie the humeral head.

**Infraspinatus Tendon Calcification.** Calcification within the substance of the infraspinatus tendon may be projected over the lateral aspect of the humeral head in external rotation because of the attachment of this tendon to the posterior aspect of the greater tuberosity. In internal rotation, the calcification moves laterally and may be seen in profile (Fig. 35–4).

**Teres Minor Tendon Calcification.** The teres minor tendon attaches to the posterior aspect of the greater tuberosity below the site of attachment of the infraspinatus tendon. Calcification within this tendon is projected over the humeral head in external rotation and moves laterally in internal rotation, where it may be seen in profile (see Fig. 35–4).

**Subscapularis Tendon Calcification.** The subscapularis tendon attaches mainly to the lesser tuberosity of the humerus. Subscapularis tendon calcification is projected over the humeral head in external rotation because of the anterior position of the lesser tuberosity (see Fig. 35–4). This calcification moves medially on internal rotation and can be seen near the inner surface of the humeral head in this position. Calcification is evident tangentially adjacent to the lesser tuberosity in an axillary projection.

**Bicipital Tendon Calcification.** The long head of the biceps tendon attaches to the superior aspect of the glenoid fossa after passing through the bicipital groove, and calcific tendinosis of this structure appears as a radiodense area that does not move appreciably on external or internal rotation. The short head of the biceps attaches to the coracoid process. Calcification in this tendon is apparent adjacent to the coracoid tip. Calcification in the long head of the biceps is also seen along the shaft of the humerus. In this location, calcification occurs at the junction of the tendon and muscle (Fig. 35–5). Its appearance simulates that of an osseous body trapped in the sheath of the tendon.

**Other Tendon Calcification.** Other sites of tendon calcification about the shoulder are recorded infrequently. These sites include the pectoralis major tendon, the tendon of the long head of the triceps muscle (with calcification adjacent to the inferior margin of the glenoid cavity), the deltoid attachment to the acromion, the trapezius insertion (with calcification adjacent to the acromioclavicular joint), and the subacromial bursa. Subacromial bursa calcification appears as a teardrop-shaped, ulcerated, or "skullcap" radiodense area adjacent to the superolateral aspect of the joint capsule and possibly extending under the greater tuberosity (Fig. 35–6).

### Elbow

Calcification about the elbow may be observed adjacent to the medial and lateral condyles of the humerus, in the area of the collateral ligaments, at the insertion of the triceps tendon to the ulnar olecranon, and within the olecranon bursa.

### Hand and Wrist

Calcification in the wrist is more frequent than in the hand, and deposits may be noted in or near the tendons of the flexor carpi ulnaris (adjacent to the pisiform), flexor carpi radialis (on the volar aspect of the radiocarpal joint), common flexors (near the volar aspect of the wrist), and extensor carpi ulnaris (adjacent to the distal end of the ulna and ulnar styloid). The most common site

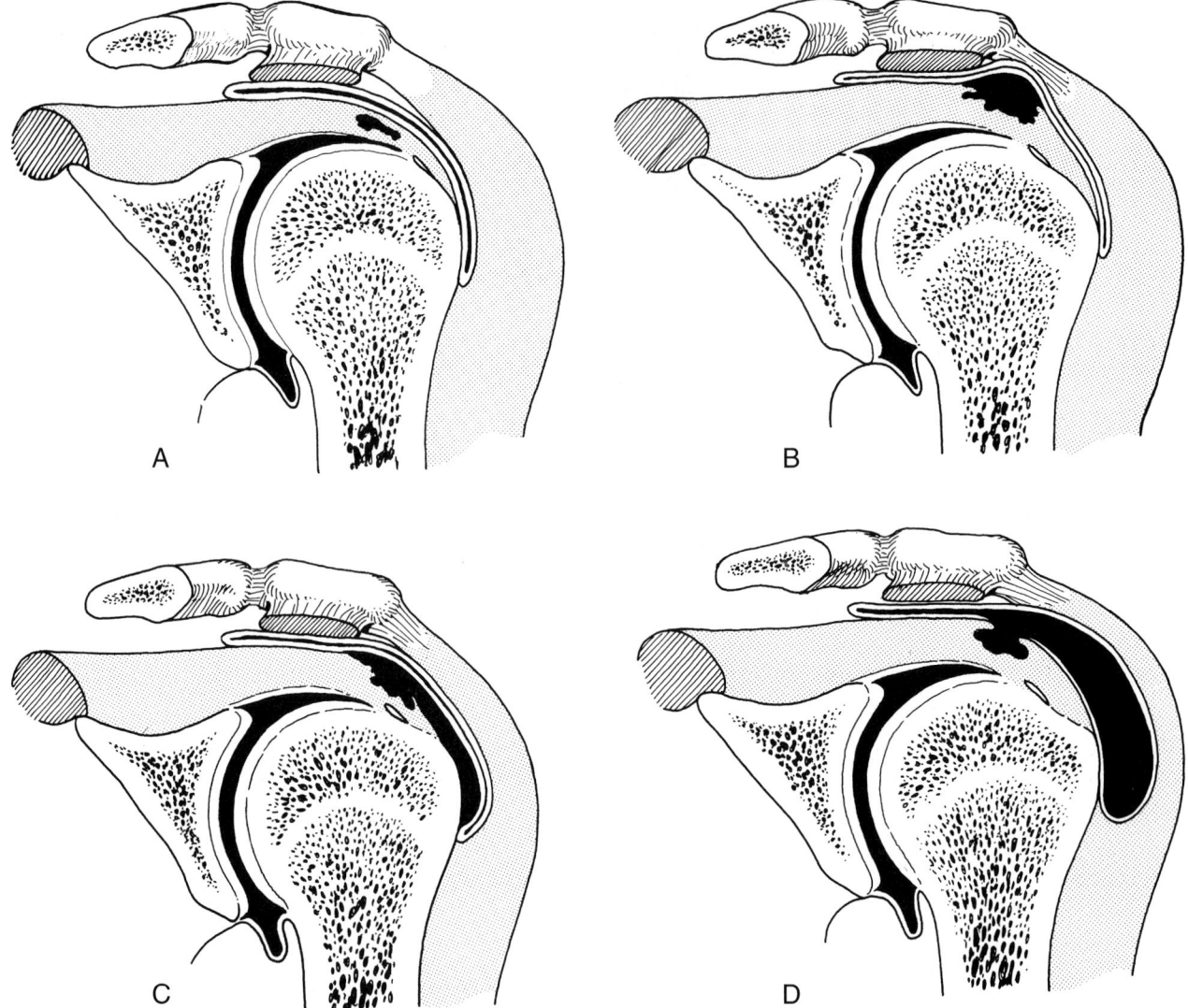

**Figure 35–1.** Periarticular crystal deposition in the shoulder: phases of the disease. *A*, Silent phase. Subclinical deposition of calcium occurs in the substance of the rotator cuff tendons. *B*, Mechanical phase—elevation of bursal floor. As the deposits increase in size, the floor of the subdeltoid (subacromial) bursa is raised. *C*, Mechanical phase–sub-bursal rupture. Observe that rupture of the calcific deposits has occurred beneath the floor of the bursa. *D*, Mechanical phase–intrabursal rupture. The entire deposit is being expelled into the subdeltoid bursa.

of calcification appears to be within the flexor carpi ulnaris tendon (Fig. 35–7). In the hand, deposits show a predilection for the regions of the metacarpophalangeal joints and fingers.

### Hip and Pelvis

Calcific deposits are frequent in the gluteal insertions into the greater trochanter and in the surrounding bursae, where they appear as single or multiple cloudlike linear, triangular, or circular radiodense areas. Calcification in the femoral insertion of the gluteus maximus muscle (Fig. 35–8) is particularly characteristic and leads to a radiodense shadow adjacent to the proximal posterior portion of the femur, best observed in the frog-leg view. Adjacent erosion of the femoral cortex is not unusual at

any location. Calcifications may relate to other tendinous structures, such as the piriformis, rectus femoris, vastus lateralis, adductor magnus, and biceps femoris.

### Knee

Calcific tendinosis and bursitis about the knee have been described, particularly adjacent to the femoral condyles, fibular head, and prepatellar region.

### Ankle, Foot, and Heel

Calcific deposits may occasionally be seen about the ankle, foot, and heel. Involvement may include the tendons of the flexor hallucis brevis, flexor hallucis longus, and peroneus muscles.

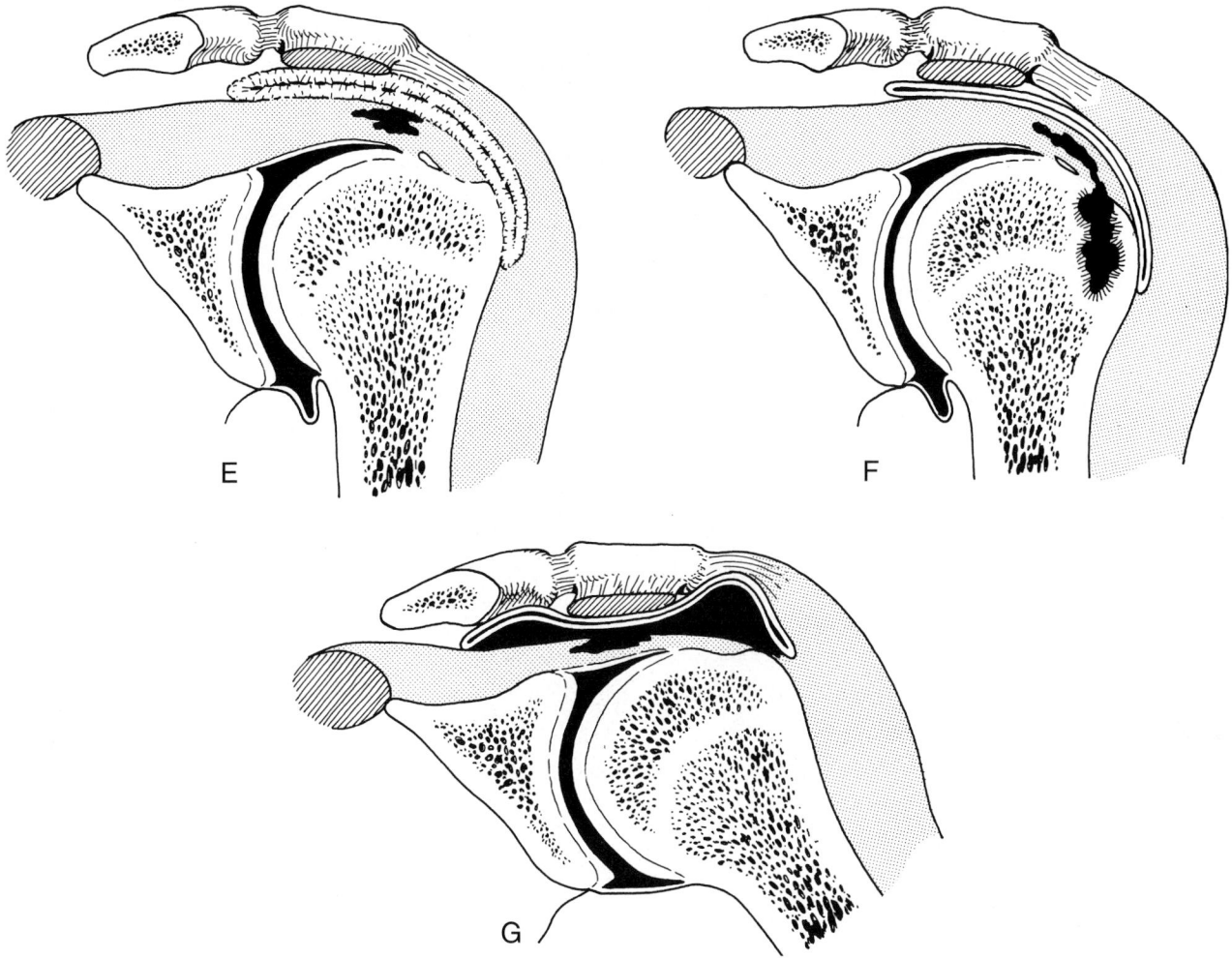

**Figure 35–1.**—Continued *E*, Adhesive periarthritis. Note the adduction of the shoulder with adhesive bursitis. *F*, Intraosseous loculation. The calcific deposit has extended into the bone. *G*, Dumbbell loculation. Rarely, a biloculated deposit may be seen as a result of pressure from the adjacent coracoacromial ligament. (Redrawn from Moseley HF: Shoulder Lesions, 3rd ed. Edinburgh, E&S Livingstone, 1969.)

## Neck

Calcific tendinosis of the neck may appear within the longus colli muscle and tendon, the principal flexor of the cervical spine (Fig. 35–9). Tendinosis and peritendinitis in this region may result in acute neck and occipital pain, rigidity, and dysphagia. Radiographic findings include prevertebral soft tissue swelling, particularly in the upper cervical region, as well as amorphous calcification, which is usually seen anterior to the second cervical vertebra, just inferior to the body of the atlas. Resorption of calcification is common and may be complete in 1 to 2 weeks, with disappearance of the soft tissue swelling.

## Magnetic Resonance Imaging and Computed Tomography Features

The occurrence of pain and swelling at an involved site, indicative of inflammation about calcific tissue, is well documented. This inflammatory response dominates the magnetic resonance (MR) imaging findings of this disorder (Fig. 35–10), and the calcification may be difficult to appreciate on many MR imaging sequences (except for fast spin echo or gradient echo sequences) unless it is large. The calcification is better delineated with routine radiography, although computed tomography (CT) scanning is especially useful in areas where the osseous anatomy is complex. Inflamed and edematous soft tissues and muscles appear as regions of high signal intensity on T2-weighted spin echo and other fluid-sensitive sequences, and signal enhancement after the intravenous administration of gadolinium compounds is to be expected. Bone erosion beneath calcified tendons is well shown by CT and, to a lesser extent, MR imaging, and marrow signal intensity may be altered because of intraosseous edema. The calcified collections are of low signal intensity on all MR imaging sequences, and they may be more apparent as a result of the surrounding inflammatory response.

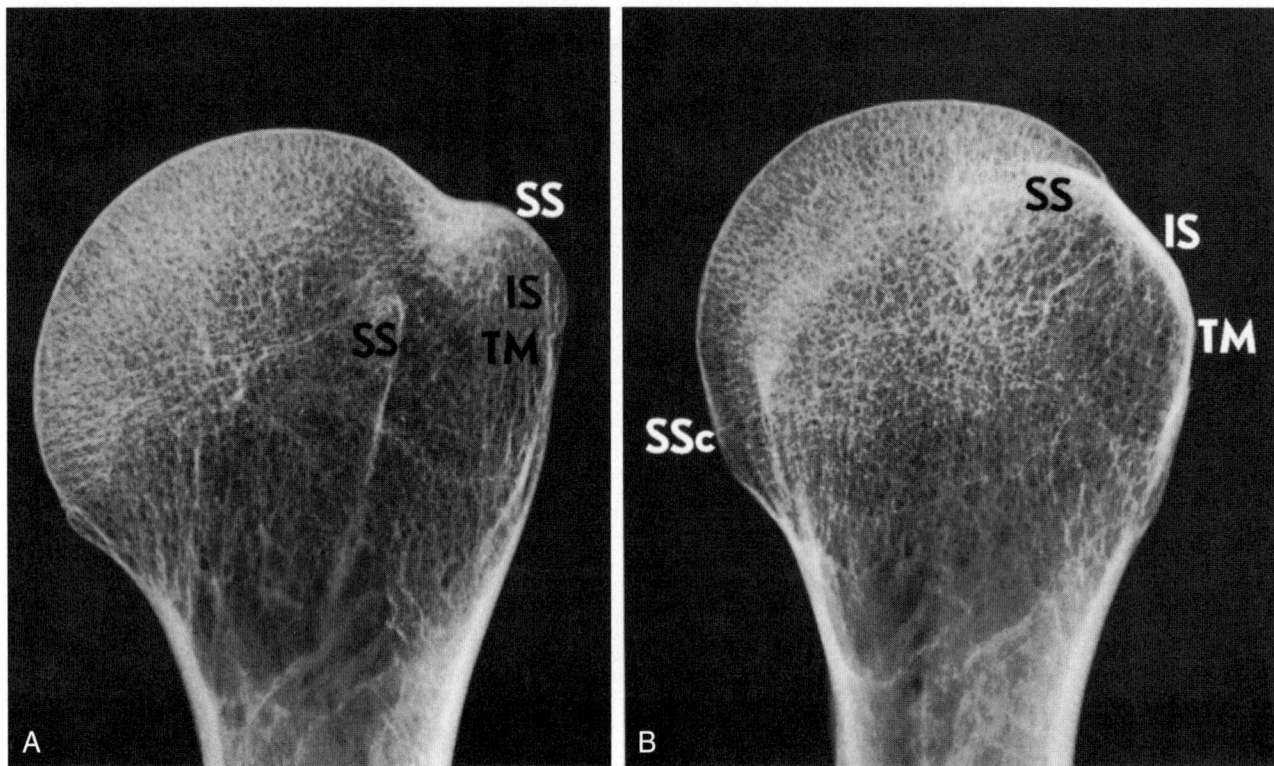

**Figure 35–2.** Periarticular crystal deposition in the shoulder: sites of tendon calcification. *A*, In external rotation, calcification in the supraspinatus (SS) tendon is observed adjacent to the greater tuberosity, whereas that in the infraspinatus (IS) and teres minor (TM) tendons overlies the greater tuberosity. Calcification in the subscapularis (SSc) tendon overlies the lesser tuberosity. *B*, In internal rotation, calcification in the infraspinatus (IS) and teres minor (TM) tendons is seen lateral to the greater tuberosity, calcification in the supraspinatus (SS) tendon is projected over the greater tuberosity, and calcification in the subscapularis (SSc) tendon rotates medially, adjacent to the inner margin of the humeral head.

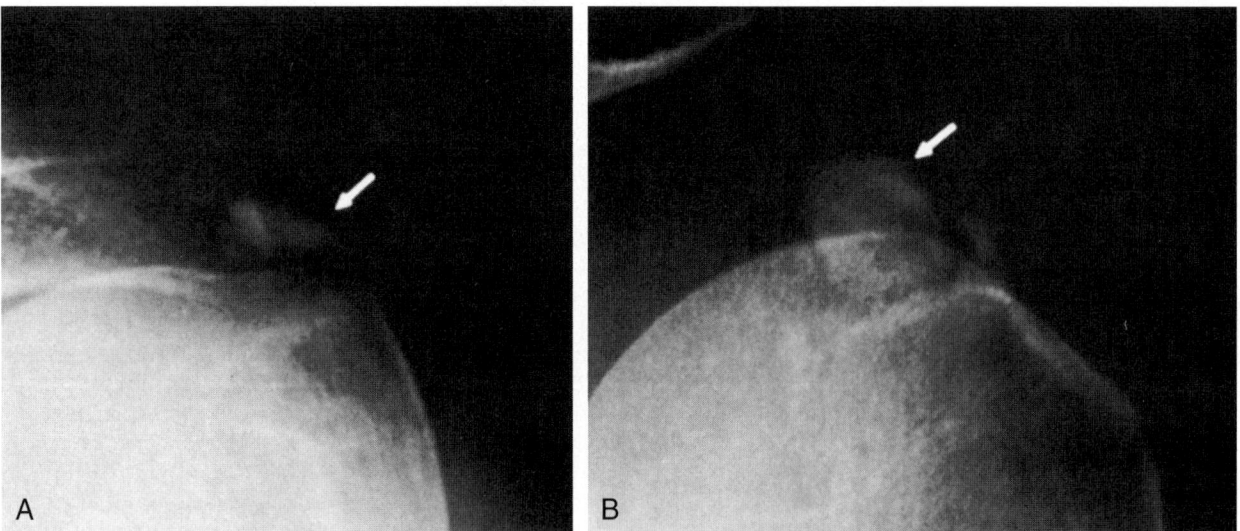

**Figure 35–3.** Periarticular crystal deposition: supraspinatus tendon calcification. *A*, In external rotation, calcification is apparent above the greater tuberosity *(arrow)*. *B*, In internal rotation, the calcification moves medially *(arrow)*.

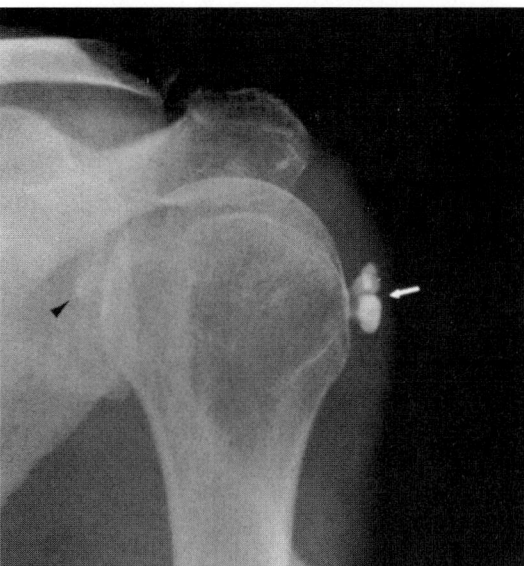

**Figure 35–4.** Periarticular crystal deposition: infraspinatus, teres minor, and subscapularis tendon calcification. In internal rotation, calcific deposits in the infraspinatus and teres minor tendons appear lateral to the humeral head *(arrow)*, and those in the subscapularis tendon are located near the lesser tuberosity, overlying the joint space *(arrowhead)*.

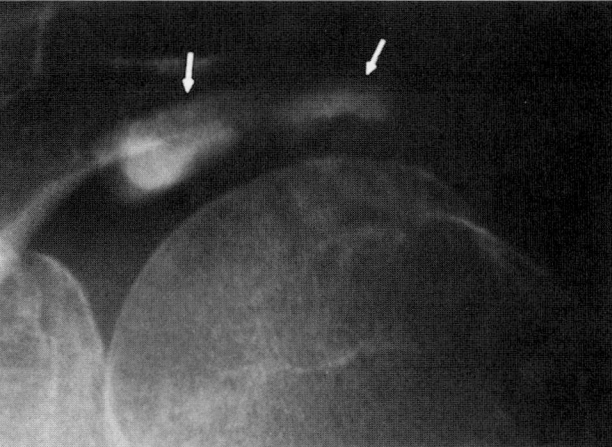

**Figure 35–6.** Periarticular crystal deposition: subdeltoid (subacromial) bursal calcification. Note the extensive calcific deposition *(arrows)* adjacent to the humeral head.

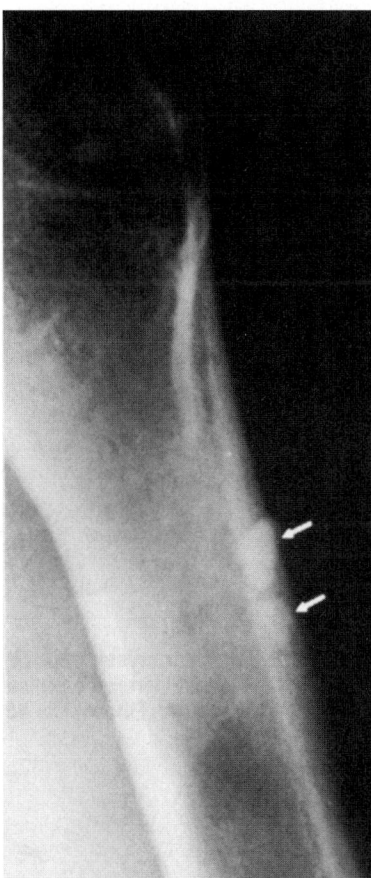

**Figure 35–5.** Periarticular crystal deposition. Calcification in the biceps tendon *(arrows)* is shown in external rotation.

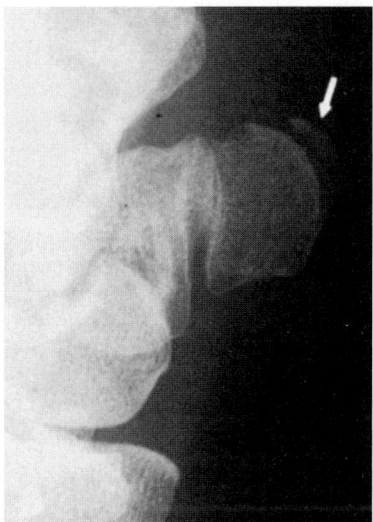

**Figure 35–7.** Periarticular crystal deposition in the wrist. Calcification *(arrow)* is apparent on the undersurface of the pisiform within the tendon of the flexor carpi ulnaris muscle.

## Differential Diagnosis

Tendinosis with peritendinitis and bursitis may produce soft tissue swelling without radiographically recognizable calcification. Stenosing tenosynovitis of the abductor pollicis longus and extensor pollicis brevis muscles (de Quervain's disease) is well known, and similar involvement is recognized at other sites, such as the flexor and extensor digital tendons, flexor carpi radialis tendon, tibialis posterior tendon, common peroneal tendon sheath, and flexor tendons of the wrist within the carpal tunnel. An example of noncalcific bursitis is Haglund's syndrome, characterized by painful soft tissue swelling at the level of the Achilles tendon insertion in the calcaneus. A localized area of soft tissue prominence termed a "pump bump" may be encountered. The condition appears to be

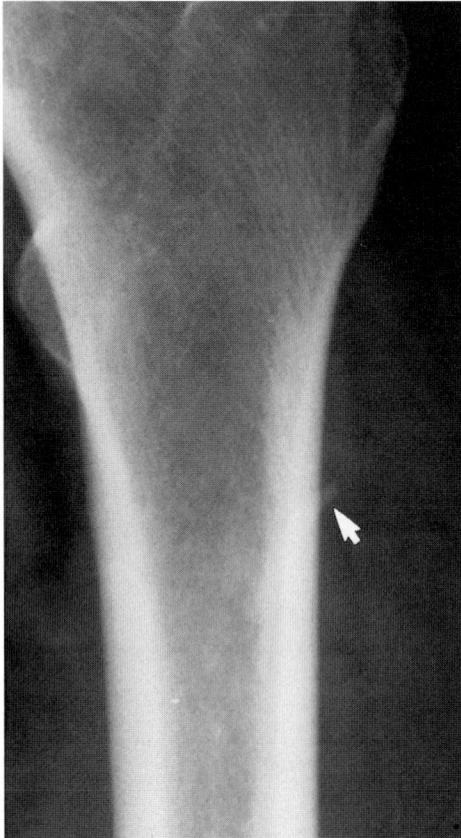

**Figure 35–8.** Periarticular crystal deposition in the hip. Radiograph reveals the typical appearance and location of calcification in the tendon of the gluteus maximus muscle *(arrow)*. Note the elongated shape of the calcified tendon.

produced by compression of the Achilles tendon and adjacent soft tissues between the os calcis and the shoe.

Calcific tendinosis and bursitis must be distinguished from many disorders that produce periarticular calcification (Table 35–1). Such soft tissue deposits may relate to metastatic calcification, in which a disturbance of calcium and phosphorus metabolism is present; calcinosis, in which calcification of the skin and subcutaneous and connective tissues occurs in the presence of normal calcium metabolism (Fig. 35–11); and dystrophic calcification, in which calcium deposition occurs in devitalized tissues. Metastatic calcification is common in renal osteodystrophy (Fig. 35–12) and may also be seen in hypoparathyroidism, sarcoidosis, hypervitaminosis D, milk-alkali syndrome, and numerous other conditions.

Calcific tendinosis and bursitis should be differentiated from causes of soft tissue ossification (Table 35–2). Frequently, such differentiation is possible because ossified masses reveal trabecular patterns. Soft tissue ossification is frequent after trauma (myositis ossificans), neurologic injury (Fig. 35–13), and burns.

## INTRA-ARTICULAR CRYSTAL DEPOSITION

The concept of intra-articular calcium HA crystal deposition has been studied extensively in recent years.

Investigations of elderly women who had painful shoulders with decreased mobility or stability revealed radiographic evidence of disruption of the rotator cuff and demonstration of microspheroids containing calcium HA crystals in synovial fluid. This fluid also revealed activated collagenase and neutral protease activity. These findings led to the concept of Milwaukee shoulder syndrome, in which intra-articular HA crystal deposition is followed by release of enzymes that attack the periarticular tissues, including the rotator cuff, with subsequent cuff disruption.

On the basis of evidence contained in these investigations, as well as others, it can be concluded that calcium HA crystal deposition plays an important role in the degeneration of cartilaginous, osseous, and soft tissue structures in and about joints. Although the initial observations were related to disintegration of the glenohumeral joint, the concept has been applied to other sites, including the knee, elbow, hip, and midtarsal articulations. It must be emphasized, however, that intra-articular accumulation of calcium HA crystals may occur in the absence of joint inflammation, and other factors likely contribute to joint degeneration.

### Radiographic and Pathologic Features

The general radiographic and pathologic abnormalities associated with intra-articular calcium HA crystal deposition disease can be divided into calcification and structural joint damage, or arthropathy.

**Calcification.** Calcium HA crystal accumulation in joints can lead to intra-articular calcification. Although cartilage calcification, or chondrocalcinosis, has been noted occasionally, especially in the knee, other patterns of calcification are more typical. Crystal deposition can involve the synovial membrane, capsule, or both and usually leads to amorphous or cloudlike radiodense areas within the joint (Fig. 35–14).

Calcification related to calcium HA crystal deposition can occur in a joint that is otherwise normal, in which case it may lead to deterioration of the joint, or it can develop in an articulation with preexisting abnormalities. Although usually evident in the small joints of the hand and wrist or foot, calcium HA crystal accumulation can cause calcification in large joints, such as the elbow, hip, knee, and glenohumeral articulation. Women are affected more frequently than men, and adults are affected much more commonly than children.

**Arthropathy.** Structural joint damage is observed in some patients with intra-articular calcium HA crystal accumulation. Such crystal-induced damage has been investigated most extensively in the shoulders of elderly patients, especially women (Milwaukee shoulder syndrome). Radiographic findings in Milwaukee shoulder include loss of joint space, destruction of bone, subchondral sclerosis, intra-articular osseous debris, and joint disorganization (Fig. 35–15). Associated disruption of the rotator cuff allows the humeral head to become displaced in a superior direction. In the presence of a massive tear of the rotator cuff, the displaced humeral head can severely

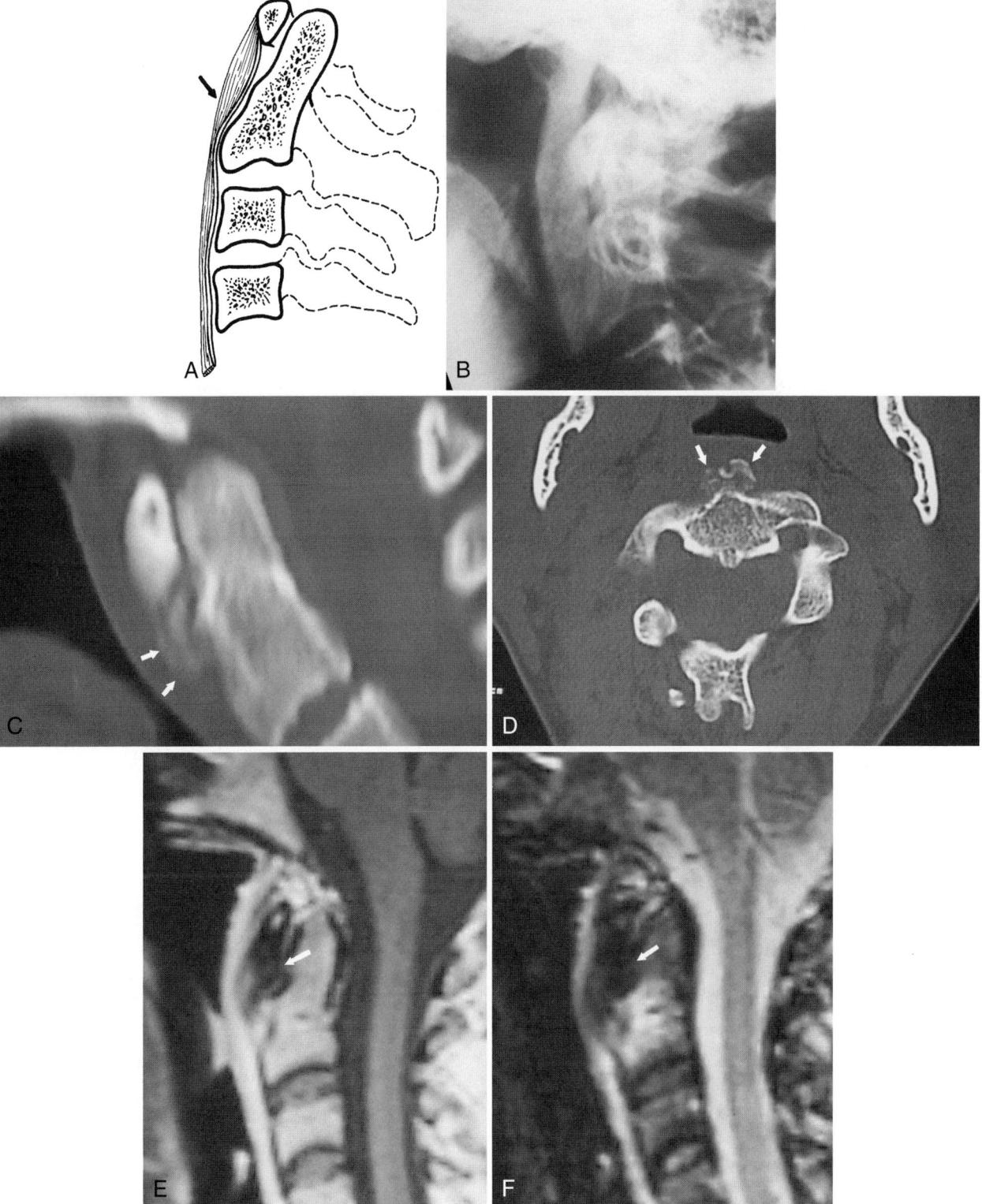

**Figure 35–9.** Periarticular crystal deposition in the longus colli in a 36-year-old woman. *A*, Drawing of a sagittal section of the neck indicates the course of the longus colli muscle *(arrow)*, which attaches to the anterior tubercle of the atlas and the anterior surface of the second through fourth cervical vertebrae. *B*, Lateral radiograph shows soft tissue swelling with calcification immediately below the anterior arch of C1. *C* and *D*, Corresponding reformatted sagittal *(C)* and axial *(D)* CT scans of the spine show the calcification *(arrows)* to better advantage. *E* and *F*, Corresponding sagittal T1-weighted (TR/TE, 500/15) *(E)* and conventional T2-weighted (TR/TE, 2000/90) *(F)* spin echo MR images show the calcification as an area of low signal intensity *(arrow)*. Note the surrounding high signal intensity, on $T_2$-weighted image (F) representing inflammatory changes as well as marrow edema.

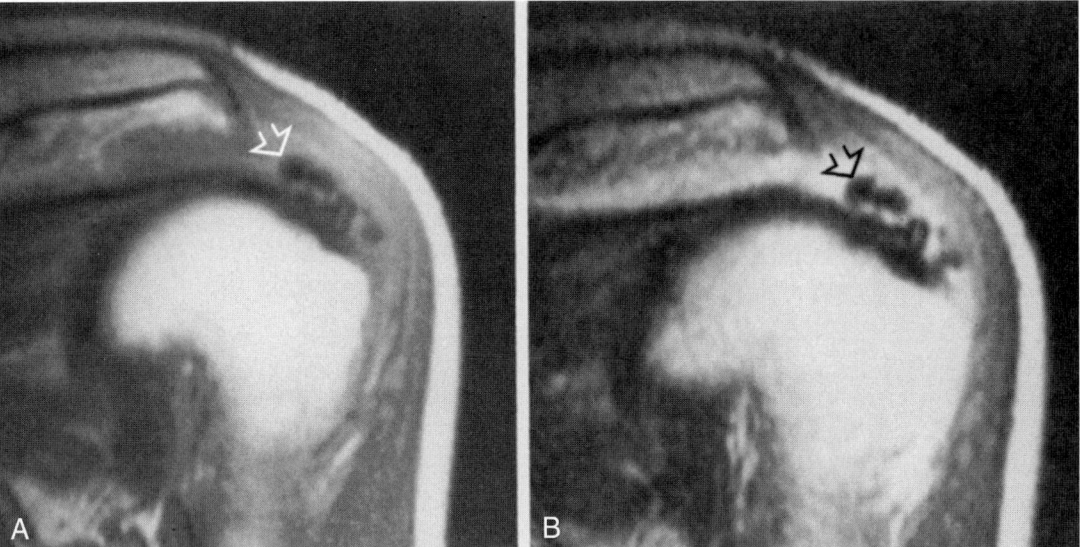

**Figure 35–10.** Periarticular crystal deposition in the subdeltoid bursa: MR imaging abnormalities. Coronal oblique T1-weighted (TR/TE, 700/20) *(A)* and T2-weighted (TR/TE, 1800/80) *(B)* spin echo MR images show areas of low signal intensity, reflecting calcification *(arrows)*, which in *(B)* is associated with surrounding inflammatory tissue and fluid of high signal intensity.

erode the anterior portion of the acromion, distal portion of the clavicle, glenoid cavity, and coracoid process. The resulting articular disease is termed cuff tear arthropathy by some investigators, who believe that the initial alteration is not calcium HA crystal accumulation but rather disruption of the rotator cuff, followed by leakage of synovial fluid, deterioration of cartilage nutrition, and mechanical derangement of the joint.

An association between arthropathy in the shoulder and arthropathy in other joints, especially the knee, has been reported. Typically, unicompartmental alterations are seen in the lateral femorotibial space and lead to joint space narrowing, collapse of the articular surfaces of the tibia and femur, bone sclerosis and fragmentation, and valgus angulation. Additional joints such as the hip and small joints of the hand and feet may be involved (Fig. 35–16).

---

**TABLE 35–1**

**Conditions Associated with Periarticular Calcification**

---

Calcific tendinosis and bursitis
Collagen vascular disease
Hyperparathyroidism and renal osteodystrophy
Hypoparathyroidism
Hypervitaminosis D
Milk-alkali syndrome
Idiopathic tumoral calcinosis
Articular disorders: CPPD crystal deposition disease, gout, infection, synovial chondromatosis
Sarcoidosis
Primary soft tissue tumors (especially synovial sarcoma)

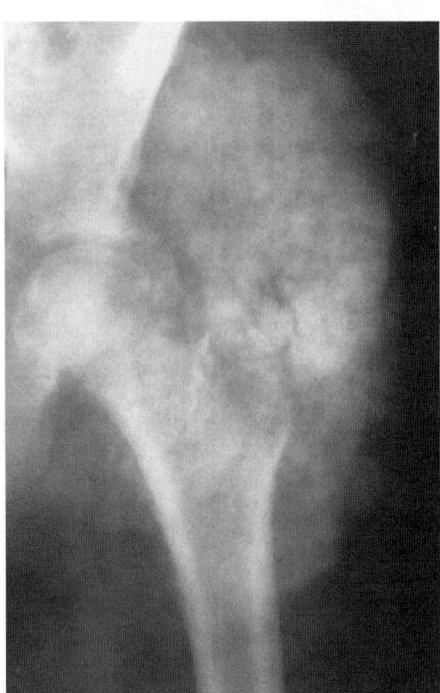

**Figure 35–11.** Idiopathic tumoral calcinosis. Observe the large saclike collection of calcification about the hip.

## Differential Diagnosis

The radiographic manifestations of intra-articular calcium HA crystal deposition disease are similar to those of osteoarthritis and CPPD crystal deposition disease. In the knee, the arthropathy associated with calcium HA crystal accumulation is more aggressive than osteoarthritis. Osteoarthritis of the glenohumeral joint is accompanied

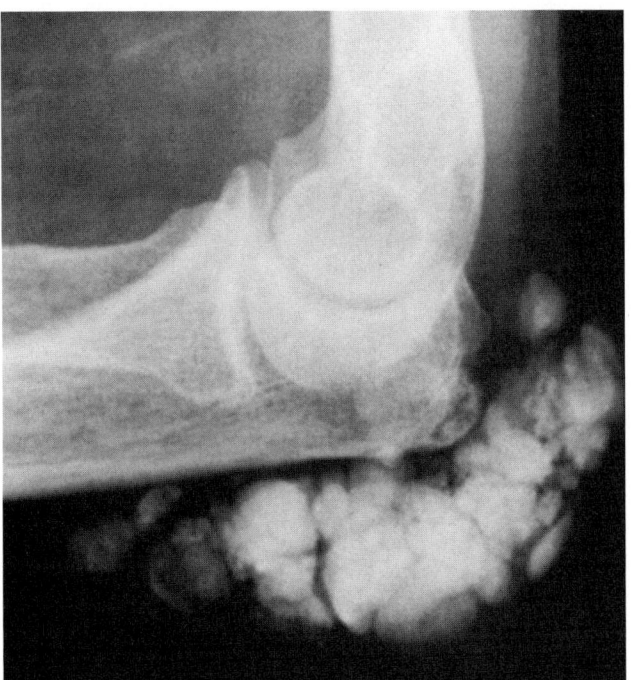

**Figure 35–12.** Renal osteodystrophy. Large radiodense collections about the elbow are typical of calcifications in this disorder.

**TABLE 35–2**

**Conditions Associated with Soft Tissue Ossification**

Myositis ossificans traumatica
Fibrodysplasia (myositis) ossificans progressiva
Neurologic injury
Burn
Pseudomalignant osseous tumor of soft tissue

by minor radiographic alterations, unlike the severe abnormalities of apatite arthropathy. Other disorders of the shoulder, such as alkaptonuria, infection, neuropathic osteoarthropathy, and idiopathic chondrolysis, resemble the arthropathy of calcium HA crystal deposition disease.

Apatite arthropathy most simulates pyrophosphate arthropathy. In general, however, calcium HA crystal accumulation does not produce chondrocalcinosis but leads to homogeneous, cloudlike intra-articular radiodensities.

## MIXED CALCIUM PHOSPHATE CRYSTAL DEPOSITION

Inspection of synovial fluid or cartilage has documented the coexistence of calcium HA and CPPD crystals in

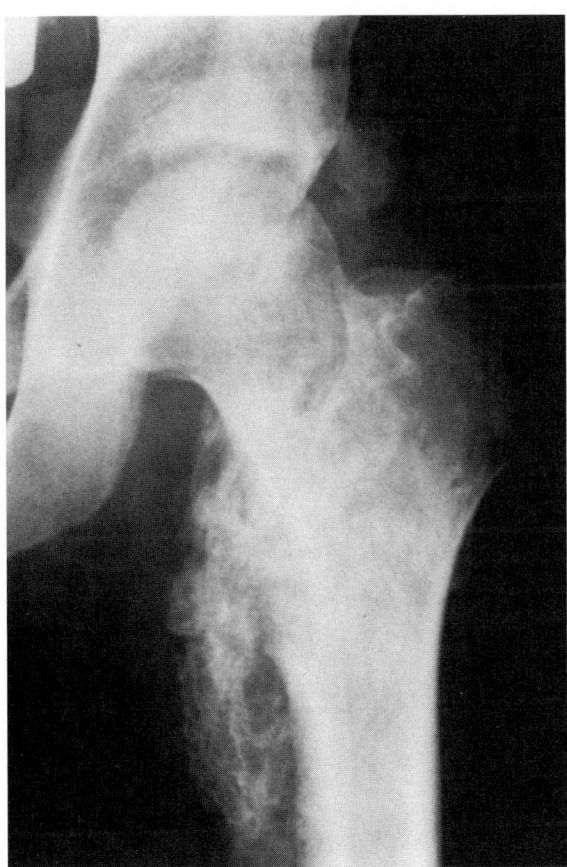

**Figure 35–13.** Heterotopic ossification after neurologic injury. In a paralyzed patient, ossification about the acetabulum and proximal portion of the femur can be seen.

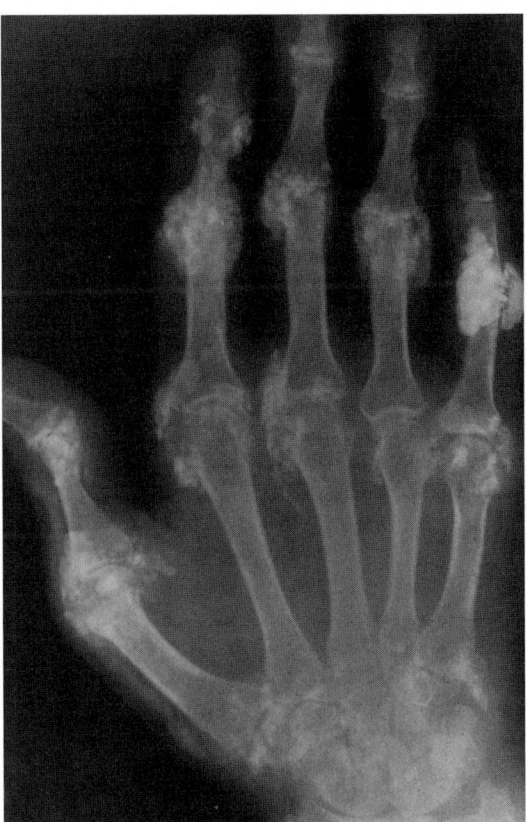

**Figure 35–14.** Intra-articular crystal deposition. Radiograph reveals periarticular and intra-articular calcification involving the hand and wrist. The opposite side was affected similarly. A synovial biopsy of a proximal interphalangeal joint documented the presence of calcium hydroxyapatite crystal deposition.

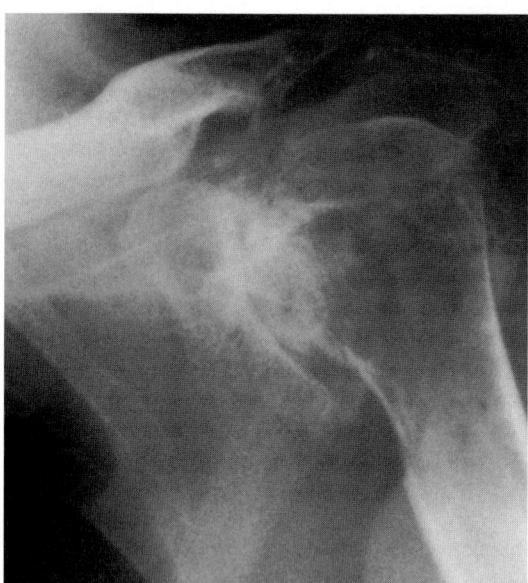

**Figure 35–15.** Intra-articular crystal deposition: Milwaukee shoulder syndrome. Note the joint space narrowing, subchondral sclerosis, and erosion of the undersurface of the clavicle and acromion.

numerous patients. When the crystals occur together, it is difficult to precisely identify their relative roles in the production of joint damage. The radiographic diagnosis of such mixed crystal disease is also difficult. A diagnostic clue is provided by cartilage calcification (chondrocalcinosis), which, when widespread, is much more characteristic of CPPD crystal deposition than calcium HA crystal accumulation. Conversely, in calcium HA crystal deposition, diffuse amorphous calcification within the joint is more typical.

Certain radiographic signs should raise the possibility of mixed calcium phosphate crystal deposition disease. An association appears to exist between intra-articular accumulation of CPPD crystals (in the form of chondrocalcinosis) and periarticular accumulation of calcium HA crystals (in the form of capsular and tendinous calcification). The presence of both disorders should be suspected if radiographs reveal extensive cartilage calcification (indicative of CPPD crystal deposition) and diffuse capsular calcification or dense homogeneous calcific

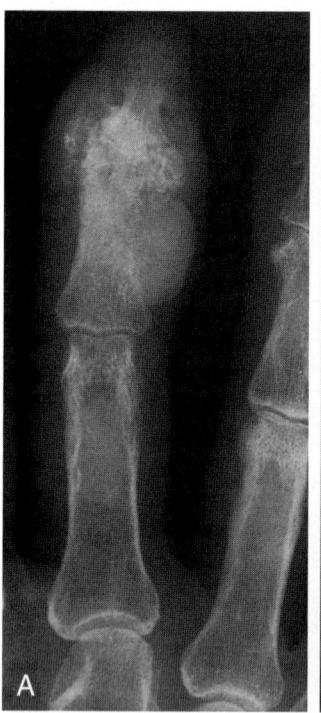
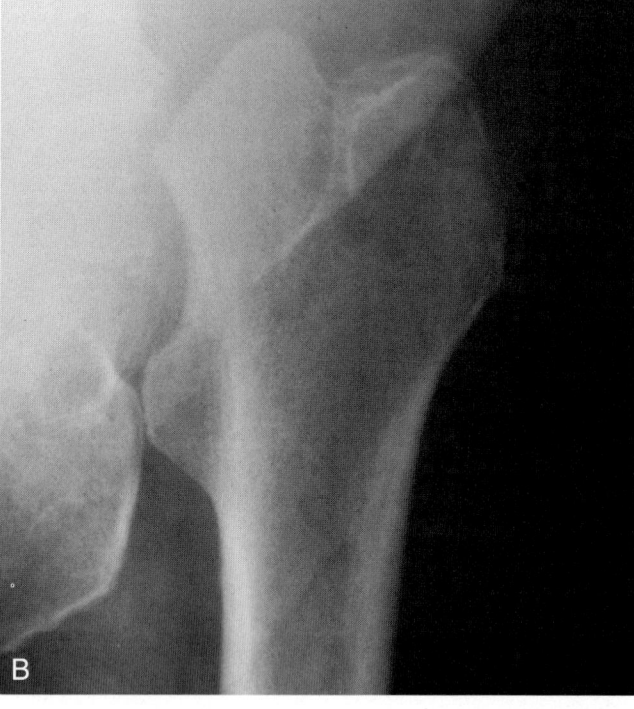

**Figure 35–16.** Intra-articular crystal deposition: arthropathy. *A*, Radiograph of the hand reveals progressive calcification within and around a distal interphalangeal joint associated with joint space narrowing and osteophytosis. *B*, In a different patient, rapidly progressive hip disease resulted in dissolution of a large portion of the femoral head. (*A*, Courtesy of V. Vint, MD, San Diego, Calif.)

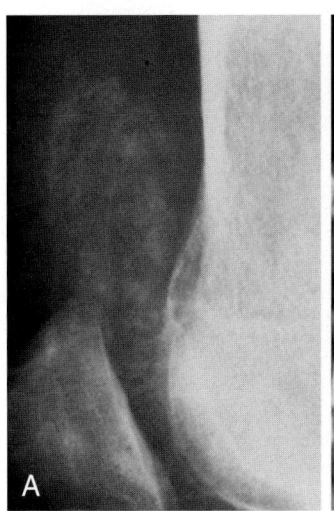 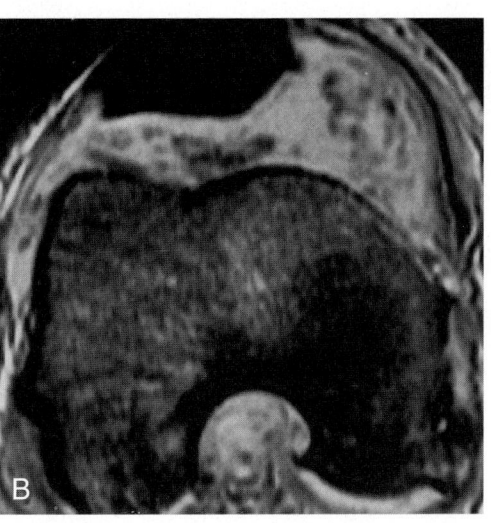

**Figure 35–17.** Mixed calcium phosphate crystal deposition disease. This 83-year-old man had widespread chondrocalcinosis, presumably related to calcium pyrophosphate dihydrate crystal deposition. Intra-articular bodies in the knee were removed and found to be composed of calcium hydroxyapatite crystals. *A*, Routine radiography shows diffuse calcification in the suprapatellar bursa of the knee. *B*, Transaxial gradient echo MR image (TR/TE, 450/15; flip angle, 60 degrees) reveals joint fluid of relatively high signal intensity containing foci of low signal intensity. Calcification within the synovial membrane is also evident.

collections at tendinous insertions (indicative of calcium HA crystal deposition) (Fig. 35–17).

The number of cases of mixed calcium phosphate crystal deposition disease is expected to rise as awareness of the condition increases and diagnostic methods become more readily available. It is evident that the factors necessary for deposition of HA and CPPD crystals are not mutually exclusive. Indeed, it is possible that cases in which both crystals are present are more numerous than those in which one or the other is present alone.

## FURTHER READING

Bonavita JA, Dalinka MK, Schumacher HR Jr: Hydroxyapatite deposition disease. Radiology 134:621, 1980.

Codman EA: The Shoulder. Boston, Thomas-Todd Co, 1934.

Dieppe PA, Doherty M, MacFarlane DG, et al: Apatite associated destructive arthritis. Br J Rheumatol 23:84, 1984.

Fritz P, Bardin T, Laredo J-D, et al: Paradiaphyseal calcific tendinitis with cortical bone erosion. Arthritis Rheum 37:718, 1994.

Goldman AB: Calcific tendinitis of the long head of the biceps brachii distal to the glenohumeral joint: Plain film radiographic findings. AJR 153:1011, 1989.

Halverson PB, McCarty DJ: Clinical aspects of basic calcium phosphate crystal deposition. Rheum Dis Clin North Am 14:427, 1988.

Halverson PB, McCarty DJ: Patterns of radiographic abnormalities associated with basic calcium phosphate and calcium pyrophosphate dihydrate crystal deposition in the knee. Ann Rheum Dis 45:603, 1986.

Halverson PB, McCarty DJ, Cheung HS, et al: Milwaukee shoulder syndrome: Eleven additional cases with involvement of the knee in seven (basic calcium phosphate crystal deposition disease). Semin Arthritis Rheum 14:36, 1984.

Hayes CW, Conway WF: Calcium hydroxyapatite deposition disease. Radiographics 10:1031, 1990.

Hayes CW, Rosenthal DI, Plata MJ, et al: Calcific tendinitis in unusual locations associated with cortical bone erosion. AJR 149:967, 1987.

Kraemer EJ, El-Khoury GY: Atypical calcific tendinitis with cortical erosions. Skeletal Radiol 29:690, 2000.

Martin JF, Brogdon BG: Peritendinitis calcarea of the hand and wrist. AJR 78:74, 1957.

McCarty DJ, Gatter RA: Recurrent acute inflammation associated with focal apatite crystal deposition. Arthritis Rheum 9:804, 1966.

McCarty DJ, Halverson PB, Carrera GF, et al: "Milwaukee shoulder" — association of microspheroids containing hydroxyapatite crystals, active collagenase, and neutral protease with rotator cuff defects. I. Clinical aspects. Arthritis Rheum 24:464, 1981.

Neer CS II, Craig EV, Fukuda H: Cuff-tear arthropathy. J. Bone Joint Surg [Am] 65:1232, 1983.

Newmark H III, Forrester DM, Brown JC, et al: Calcific tendinitis of the neck. Radiology 128:355, 1978.

Pavlov H, Heneghan MA, Hersh A, et al: The Haglund syndrome: Initial and differential diagnosis. Radiology 144:83, 1982.

Rosenberg ZS, Shankman S, Steiner GC, et al: Rapid destructive osteoarthritis: Clinical, radiographic, and pathologic features. Radiology 182:213, 1992.

Schumacher HR, Somlyo AP, Tse RL, et al: Arthritis associated with apatite crystals. Ann Intern Med 87:411, 1977.

Uhthoff HK, Sarkar K, Maynard JA: Calcifying tendinitis. A new concept of its pathogenesis. Clin Orthop 118:164, 1976.

ViGario DG, Keats TE: Localization of calcific deposits in the shoulder. AJR 108:806, 1970.

# CHAPTER 36

## Hemochromatosis and Wilson's Disease

## SUMMARY OF KEY FEATURES

The skeletal manifestations of hemochromatosis include osteoporosis, chondrocalcinosis, and a distinctive arthropathy characterized by joint space narrowing, subchondral cyst formation, and osteophyte formation. These abnormalities resemble the findings of calcium pyrophosphate dihydrate (CPPD) crystal deposition disease but are associated with more uniform loss of joint space and a less progressive course.

Wilson's disease is associated with distinctive skeletal abnormalities, including osteopenia, bone fragmentation and cyst formation, ossicles, poorly defined subchondral bone, and osteochondritis dissecans. These findings superficially resemble the changes in hemochromatosis and idiopathic CPPD crystal deposition disease.

## HEMOCHROMATOSIS

Disorders of iron storage can be conveniently divided into those that are primary or idiopathic, and those that are secondary to iron overload states. Such overload states are associated with an increase in the availability of iron related to parenteral or oral intake, ineffective erythropoiesis, or inherited disease.

Primary hemochromatosis, a rare autosomal recessive disease, is believed to be a consequence of a genetically determined error of metabolism characterized by an unexplained increased absorption of iron from the gastrointestinal tract. The clinical findings include a classic triad of abnormalities: bronze pigmentation of the skin, cirrhosis, and diabetes. Specific clinical manifestations relate to tissue damage at the site of abnormal iron accumulation: iron within the parenchymal cells of the liver is associated with hypertrophy and cirrhosis, iron deposits in the pancreas result in diabetes, iron and melanin accumulations in the skin produce abnormal pigmentation, and cardiac deposition of iron results in heart failure.

Secondary hemochromatosis is associated with an increased intake and accumulation of iron of known cause, such as alcoholic cirrhosis, multiple blood transfusions, refractory anemia, and chronic excess oral iron ingestion. In both primary and secondary hemochromatosis, significant iron overload occurs only after many years, so the onset of disease is generally between 40 and 60 years of age. Hemochromatosis is less frequent in women, presumably because of menstrual blood loss. The disease is diagnosed by detection of an elevated serum iron concentration and increased saturation of the plasma iron-binding protein transferrin, combined with a typical histologic appearance on liver biopsy.

## Clinical Features

Most patients with primary hemochromatosis become symptomatic between the ages of 40 and 60 years. The disorder is 8 to 20 times more frequent in men than in women, and women with this disorder frequently report absent or scanty menses. Initial clinical manifestations relate to the classic triad of the disease: cirrhosis, skin pigmentation, and diabetes. Subsequent complaints relate to ascites and cardiac failure.

The arthropathy associated with hemochromatosis is more frequent in genetic hemochromatosis than in secondary hemochromatosis and is manifested as a noninflammatory condition initially involving the small joints of the hands, particularly the second and third metacarpophalangeal joints, and eventually involving large articulations.

## Pathologic Features

Articular abnormalities consist of two major features: abnormal amounts of hemosiderin granules, and CPPD crystal deposition disease. Both iron and CPPD crystals may accumulate in the same joint.

**Synovial Membrane Abnormalities.** Hemosiderin granules are seen in the synovial membrane. Increased synovial tissue deposition of iron is not limited to hemochromatosis but may be observed in a variety of disorders, including rheumatoid arthritis, degenerative disease, pigmented villonodular synovitis, hemophilia, and hemarthrosis. In these situations, light microscopy has revealed that the iron occurs predominantly in deep macrophages, in contrast to its localization in synovial lining cells in patients with hemochromatosis. CPPD crystals may be seen in the synovium, particularly in the superficial layers of the membrane.

**Cartilage Abnormalities.** Chondrocalcinosis occurs in as many as 30% of patients with hemochromatosis, either as an isolated phenomenon or in association with structural joint damage (Fig. 36–1). Calcification related to CPPD crystal deposition involves predominantly the fibrocartilage and hyaline cartilage of the knee but is also frequent in the symphysis pubis, wrist, and intervertebral disc. Cartilaginous fibrillation and erosion with partial or complete denudation may be observed.

**Bone Abnormalities.** The osseous abnormalities in hemochromatosis are similar to those noted in idiopathic CPPD crystal deposition disease. Specifically, the presence of bony eburnation and cysts and the absence of significant osteophyte formation are findings of pyrophosphate arthropathy. Because CPPD crystal deposition is a documented feature of hemochromatosis, the bone changes in this disease may be related, at least in part, to the presence of these crystals.

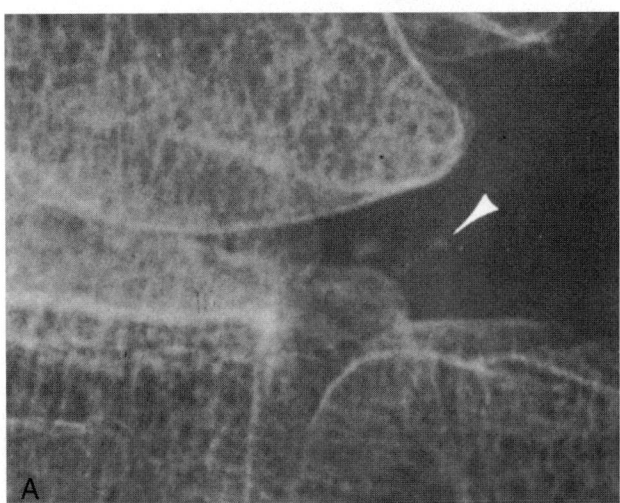

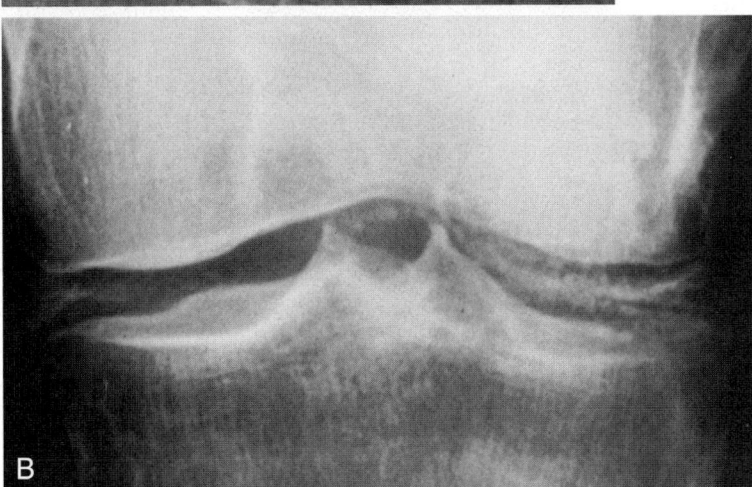

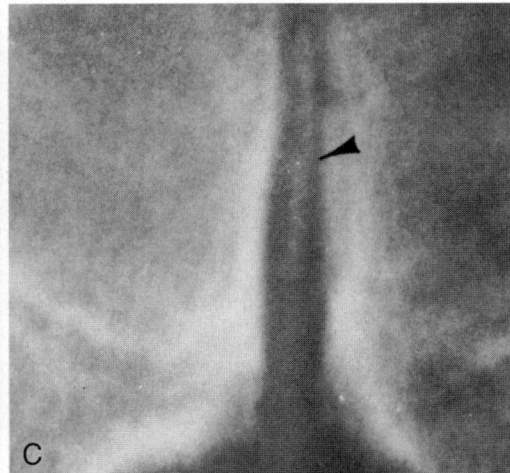

**Figure 36–1.** Radiographic findings in hemochromatosis: chondrocalcinosis. *A*, Magnification radiography outlines calcium deposits *(arrowhead)* in cartilage in the wrist. *B*, Diffuse chondrocalcinosis of both fibrocartilage and hyaline cartilage is present in the knee. *C*, In the symphysis pubis, chondrocalcinosis *(arrowhead)* of fibrocartilage is apparent.

## Radiographic Features

The radiographic features of bone and joint involvement in hemochromatosis can be divided into four categories: osteoporosis; articular calcification; structural joint damage, or arthropathy; and miscellaneous abnormalities.

**Osteoporosis.** The reported frequency of osteoporosis varies from 25% to 58%. It is usually described in primary hemochromatosis, although it has also been observed in secondary hemochromatosis. In the axial skeleton, osteoporosis of the vertebral bodies produces biconcave deformities, or "fish vertebrae," that are identical to those occurring in other forms of osteoporosis. In the appendicular skeleton, diffuse osteoporosis without a predilection for periarticular regions has been seen.

**Articular Calcification.** The reported frequency of chondrocalcinosis related to CPPD crystal deposition in patients with hemochromatosis varies from approximately 20% to 60%. It is most frequently seen in the wrist, knee, symphysis pubis, intervertebral disc, shoulder, and hip, and it may involve fibrocartilage or hyaline cartilage (see Fig. 36–1). The distribution of chondrocalcinosis in hemochromatosis may be identical to that associated with idiopathic CPPD crystal deposition disease, and it has been suggested that there is no difference between the two with regard to the total amount of chondrocalcinosis. However, there is more involvement of the symphysis pubis in hemochromatosis; there is more prominent calcification of the hyaline cartilage in hemochromatosis; and there is good correlation between the severity of arthropathy and the degree of chondrocalcinosis in hemochromatosis, but no such correlation exists in idiopathic CPPD crystal deposition disease.

Fibrocartilage calcification, which is frequent in the triangular fibrocartilage of the wrist, menisci of the knee, symphysis pubis, and intervertebral disc, appears as thick, shaggy, irregular radiodense lesions, commonly within the central portion of the joint. Hyaline cartilage calcification appears as linear or curvilinear radiodense areas paralleling the subchondral osseous surface. In the intervertebral disc, CPPD crystal deposition occurs in the outer fibers of the anulus fibrosus.

**Structural Joint Damage, or Arthropathy.** The reported frequency of arthropathy in hemochromatosis ranges from 24% to 50%. Although the arthropathy superficially resembles degenerative joint disease—with joint space narrowing, sclerosis, and osteophytosis—definite characteristics in its distribution and appearance enable it to be recognized on radiographic examination. The arthropathy in hemochromatosis is almost identical to the arthropathy in idiopathic CPPD crystal deposition disease, and they share the following features:

1. Involvement of unusual articular sites. Arthropathy may produce abnormalities at joints that are not commonly involved in degenerative joint disease, such as the metacarpophalangeal joints, midcarpal and radiocarpal compartments of the wrists, elbows, and glenohumeral articulations.

2. Formation of large subchondral cystic lesions. Arthropathy may be associated with multiple cysts in the subchondral bone, which can occasionally attain a large size.

3. Uniform loss of articular space. Arthropathy may be characterized by diffuse loss of articular space, an unusual finding in degenerative joint disease. The joint space loss is associated with subchondral bony eburnation and cyst formation.

Although it is difficult to differentiate the arthropathy of hemochromatosis and that of idiopathic CPPD crystal deposition disease, several subtle findings appear to be more typical of hemochromatosis:

1. Predilection for the metacarpophalangeal joints. These joints are the most characteristic sites of involvement in hemochromatosis (Fig. 36–2). Abnormalities are particularly frequent in the second and third metacarpophalangeal joints. The first, fourth, and fifth metacarpophalangeal joints and the interphalangeal joints are less commonly abnormal. Involvement of the metacarpophalangeal joints is associated with diffuse or focal loss of articular space, well-defined subchondral bony eburnation, sharply marginated 1- to 3-mm cysts, osteophytes on the medial aspect of the metacarpal head, and flattening or mild collapse of the osseous surface. Although both CPPD crystal deposition disease and hemochromatosis produce structural alterations in the metacarpophalangeal joints, more prevalent narrowing in these articulations (including those in the fourth and fifth digits) and peculiar hook-like osteophytes on the radial aspect of the metacarpal heads are characteristic of hemochromatosis.

2. Widespread abnormalities of the wrist. Involvement of the carpal bones may be noted in 30% to 50% of patients (Fig. 36–3). Findings include joint space narrowing, sclerosis, and cyst formation. Although the radiocarpal compartment may be affected, as in idiopathic CPPD crystal deposition disease, this compartment is occasionally unaffected in the arthropathy of hemochromatosis.

3. Slowly progressive alterations. The arthropathy of hemochromatosis may be slowly progressive. More rapid change, with fragmentation of bone, is more characteristic of idiopathic CPPD crystal deposition disease.

4. Unusual pattern of osteophytosis. Beaklike osteophytes of the metacarpal heads are particularly characteristic (Fig. 36–4). Similarly, osteophytes may be apparent about other involved articulations, such as the hip and glenohumeral joint.

The arthropathy of hemochromatosis may be widespread and occur throughout the skeleton, including involvement of the hand and wrist, elbow, glenohumeral joint, hip, knee, ankle, foot, and spine. Radiographic abnormalities typically include joint space narrowing, bony eburnation, subchondral cyst formation, and osteophytosis. Chondrocalcinosis may or may not be apparent in the involved joint.

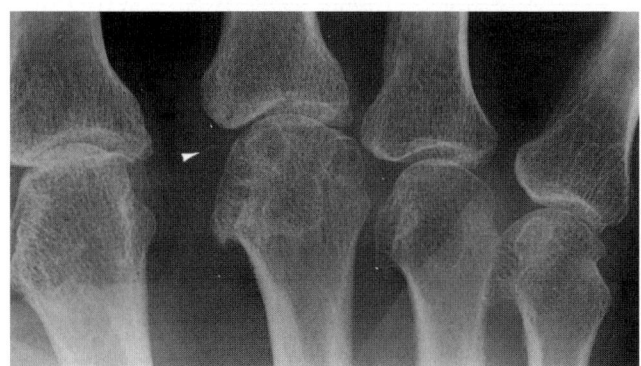

**Figure 36–2.** Radiographic findings in hemochromatosis: metacarpophalangeal joint arthropathy. Involvement of all the metacarpophalangeal joints is characterized by articular space narrowing, surface irregularity, small cystic lesions, beaklike osteophytes, focal calcifications (*arrowhead*), and mild osteoporosis.

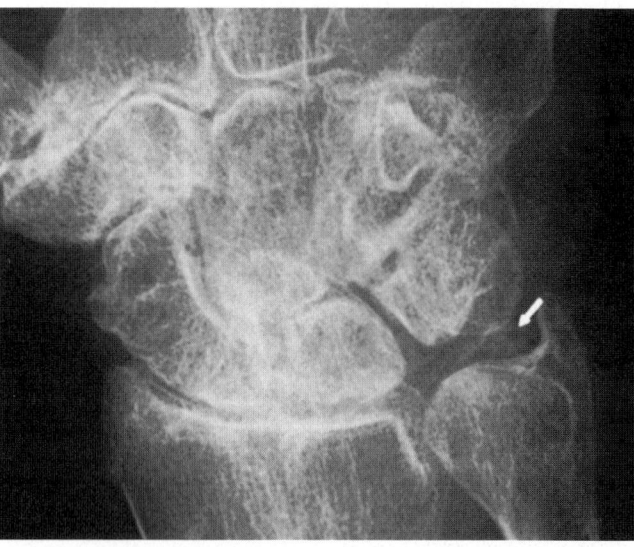

**Figure 36–3.** Radiographic findings in hemochromatosis: wrist arthropathy. Observe the chondrocalcinosis (*arrow*) and diffuse narrowing of the radiocarpal, midcarpal, and first carpometacarpal joints.

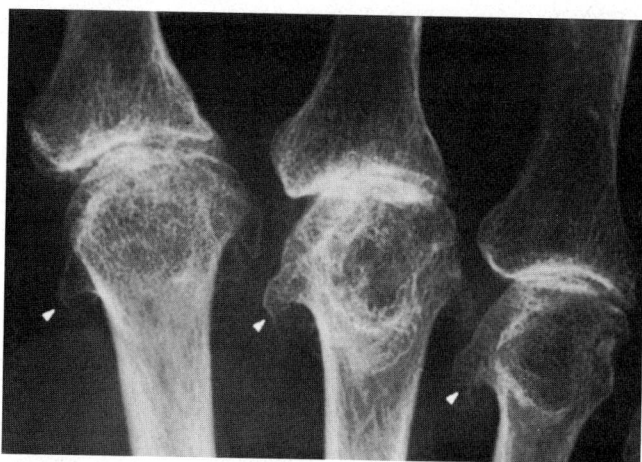

**Figure 36–4.** Radiographic findings in hemochromatosis: unusual pattern of osteophytosis. Note the beaklike excrescences (*arrowheads*), particularly on the radial aspect of the flattened and sclerotic metacarpal heads.

## Magnetic Resonance Imaging

Few data exist with regard to magnetic resonance (MR) imaging in cases of joint involvement in hemochromatosis. Susceptibility artifacts in periarticular locations, perhaps related to ferritin deposits, were noted in one report. To date, however, MR imaging has not proved to be reliable in the detection of intra-articular iron, nor has a correlation been found among serum ferritin levels, severity of the arthropathy, or signal intensity values. MR imaging may reveal meniscal calcification (chondrocalcinosis), with findings simulating those of a meniscal tear.

## Pathogenesis of Chondrocalcinosis and Arthropathy

The mechanism leading to cartilage calcification and arthropathy in hemochromatosis is not known. Some investigators believe that cartilaginous changes are the initial abnormality, followed by calcification. If this is the case, it can be speculated that iron deposition itself may lead to cartilage abnormality. Arthropathy has been described in association with the iron overload of repeated blood transfusions.

For investigators who maintain that CPPD crystal deposition precedes cartilaginous alterations in hemochromatosis, it is attractive to note that iron inhibits pyrophosphatase activity in cartilage in vitro and can thereby lead to the precipitation of CPPD crystals. After such precipitation, sequential abnormalities might lead to the arthropathy of hemochromatosis, much as they might contribute to the arthropathy of idiopathic CPPD crystal deposition disease.

## Differential Diagnosis

In most patients with hemochromatosis, the clinical manifestations of the disease allow an accurate diagnosis. In some patients, articular changes may be the initial or predominant manifestation of the disorder. In these latter patients, it is imperative to differentiate the radiographic manifestations of hemochromatosis from those associated with other disorders so that appropriate therapy can be instituted before the onset of irreversible tissue damage.

**Articular Calcification.** The chondrocalcinosis associated with hemochromatosis is almost identical to that associated with idiopathic CPPD crystal deposition disease and primary hyperparathyroidism. The chondrocalcinosis in hemochromatosis is readily differentiated from the other intra-articular and periarticular calcifications that can be observed in a variety of disorders.

**Arthropathy.** The arthropathy of hemochromatosis is easily differentiated from that of rheumatoid arthritis, the seronegative spondyloarthropathies, and gout. It differs from degenerative joint disease in its distribution and appearance; involvement of unusual joints and the presence of uniform loss of articular space, multiple cystic lesions, distinctive osteophytes, and mild collapse and flattening of bone allow the differentiation of hemochromatosis from degenerative joint disease in most patients. The arthropathy of hemochromatosis is almost identical to that of idiopathic CPPD crystal deposition disease (Table 36–1). Subtle differences in hemochromatosis may include involvement of all the metacarpophalangeal joints, including the fourth and fifth, as well as the midcarpal and common carpometacarpal joints; the presence of osteoporosis and distinctive beaklike osteophytes; and the absence of rapidly progressive neuropathic-like joint damage (Fig. 36–5).

## WILSON'S DISEASE

Wilson's disease (hepatolenticular degeneration) is a rare autosomal recessive disorder characterized by degenerative changes in the brain, particularly the basal ganglia; cirrhosis of the liver; and diagnostic Kayser-Fleischer rings of greenish brown pigment at the limbus of the cornea. The primary abnormality in Wilson's disease is not known. It is certain, however, that the clinical symptoms and signs of Wilson's disease result from the relentless accumulation of copper in the body. The copper concentration is increased in the liver, brain, and other tissues; levels of serum copper and copper-binding protein (ceruloplasmin) are generally decreased.

## Clinical Features

Wilson's disease may be slightly more common in men than in women. Symptoms and signs are usually apparent between the ages of 5 and 40 years, with 50% of patients symptomatic by the age of 15 years. The initial clinical manifestations are hepatic in 42%; neurologic in 34%; psychiatric in 10%; and hematologic, endocrinologic, or renal in less than 10% of patients. Lenticular degeneration leads to neurologic symptoms, which include tremor, rigidity, dysarthria, incoordination, and personality change.

Articular alterations in Wilson's disease are unusual in children but may be observed in as many as 50% of

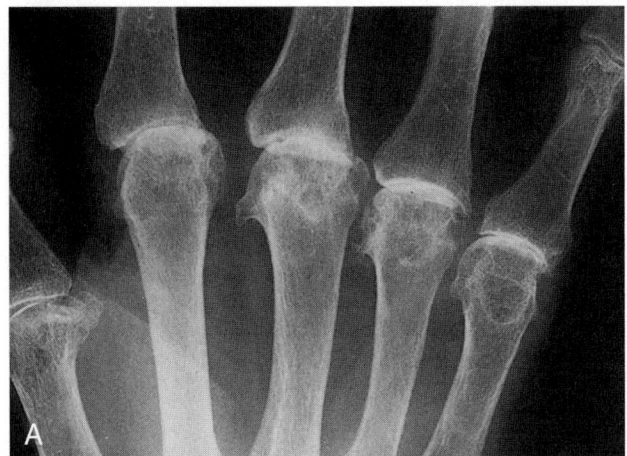

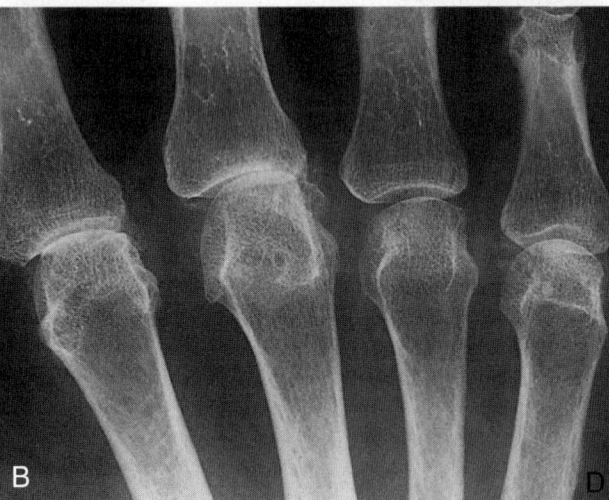

**Figure 36–5.** Hemochromatosis versus idiopathic calcium pyrophosphate dihydrate (CPPD) crystal deposition disease. *A,* Hemochromatosis. Note the uniform loss of joint space at all metacarpophalangeal joints, including the fourth and fifth. Significant "crumbling" of the metacarpal heads is evident, especially in the third digit. Beaklike osseous excrescences are arising from the radial aspect of the metacarpal heads, particularly the third and fourth. Abnormal calcification is not apparent. *B,* Idiopathic CPPD crystal deposition disease. Loss of joint space is evident in the second and third metacarpophalangeal joints, with relative sparing of those in the fourth and fifth digits. Slight flattening of the metacarpal heads and abnormal calcification about the metacarpophalangeal joints are seen. Small osteophytes are arising from the radial aspect of the second and third metacarpal heads, but they are not nearly as apparent as in *(A)*.

adults. Most patients with articular involvement are 20 to 40 years of age. The joint abnormalities are frequently asymptomatic and are detected only by radiographic examination, although pain and swelling may occasionally be observed. Many joints are involved, including those in the hand, wrist, elbow, shoulder, hip, and knee. Osteopenia has also been recognized as a manifestation of Wilson's disease and has been described in 25% to 50% of patients; this may lead to fracture.

## Pathologic Features

The pathologic features of the osseous and articular involvement in Wilson's disease have not been well delineated. Synovial biopsy findings include microvillus formation, with mild lining cell hyperplasia, inflammatory changes, and vasculitis. Copper accumulation is not apparent in these synovial specimens, nor can evidence of CPPD crystal deposition be found. Copper deposition in articular cartilage, however, has been reported.

## Radiographic Features

The radiographic features of the skeleton in Wilson's disease can be divided into osteopenia, chondrocalcinosis, arthropathy, and miscellaneous abnormalities.

**Osteopenia.** Loss of bone density has been described in up to 50% of patients with Wilson's disease. It is most apparent in the hands, feet, and spine and may be associated with a high frequency of fractures. Rickets and osteomalacia, as well as Fanconi's syndrome, have been reported in patients with Wilson's disease.

**Chondrocalcinosis.** Cartilage calcification in Wilson's disease is rare. When present, it is most common in the knee. Although the nature of these calcific deposits has not been studied, some believe that they are related to CPPD crystal accumulation. In view of the frequency of idiopathic CPPD crystal deposition disease and the presence of bone fragmentation in Wilson's disease, which might be confused with chondrocalcinosis, caution must be exercised when reporting a true association between Wilson's disease and CPPD crystal deposition.

**Arthropathy.** Articular manifestations in Wilson's disease reportedly include subchondral bone fragmentation, cyst formation, cortical irregularities, and sclerosis in the wrist, hand, foot, hip, shoulder, elbow, and knee (Fig. 36–6). These abnormalities, which may be apparent in half of persons affected with the disease, are sometimes collectively referred to as osteoarthritis, but they can be readily differentiated from that disorder.

Radiodense lesions occur centrally and at the joint margins and may be associated with articular space narrowing. Distinct ossicles that possess complete cortices may appear (Fig. 36–7). The subchondral bone is irregular and indistinct, and focal areas of fragmentation of the articular surface can be observed in the metacarpophalangeal, interphalangeal, and wrist joints. Larger areas of fragmentation of the osseous surface are also noted, including findings resembling osteochondritis dissecans of the knee and talus (Fig. 36–8).

The cause of the bone fragmentation in Wilson's disease is obscure. Because of their spasticity and tremors, patients with Wilson's disease may be prone to minor injuries producing cartilaginous and osseous damage. Joint hypermobility has also been reported.

Joint space loss confined to the patellofemoral space has been observed in Wilson's disease. This change, which has been compared with chondromalacia patellae, resembles the patellofemoral arthropathy of CPPD crystal deposition disease.

**TABLE 36-1**

**Hemochromatosis, Wilson's Disease, and Idiopathic CPPD Crystal Deposition Disease**

| | Hemochromatosis | Wilson's Disease | Idiopathic CPPD Crystal Deposition Disease |
|---|---|---|---|
| Osteopenia | + | + | − |
| Chondrocalcinosis | +* | ?† | + |
| Additional calcification | ± | ?† | + |
| Joint space narrowing | + | + | + |
| Subchondral cysts | + | + | + |
| Rapid progression | ± | − | + |
| Involvement of unusual articular sites | +‡ | + | + |

*Hemochromatosis may be associated with more prominent hyaline cartilage calcification than noted in idiopathic CPPD crystal deposition disease.

†Bone fragmentation in Wilson's disease may resemble intra-articular and periarticular calcification.

‡Wrist involvement in hemochromatosis may be more diffuse and metacarpophalangeal joint involvement may be more widespread than in idiopathic CPPD crystal deposition disease.

CPPD, calcium pyrophosphate dihydrate.

Additional radiographic characteristics of the arthropathy in Wilson's disease are small joint effusions; peculiar tonguelike osteophytes at bony prominences, such as those about the elbow and ankle; and fluffy periostitis of the trochanters and inferior surface of the calcaneus (Fig. 36–9). These latter changes may reflect periosteal bone formation at osseous sites of tendon and ligament attachment and resemble the alterations apparent in such rheumatoid variant disorders as ankylosing spondylitis, psoriatic arthritis, and Reiter's syndrome.

## Differential Diagnosis

Although reports emphasize that the articular abnormalities in Wilson's disease may be confused with degenerative joint disease, close inspection of the radiographs allows the differentiation of these two disorders. The distribution of articular abnormality in Wilson's disease includes a predilection for the small joints of the hands and wrists, particularly the metacarpophalangeal articulations; this distribution is not observed in osteoarthritis. The bone fragmentation and irregular osseous surfaces in

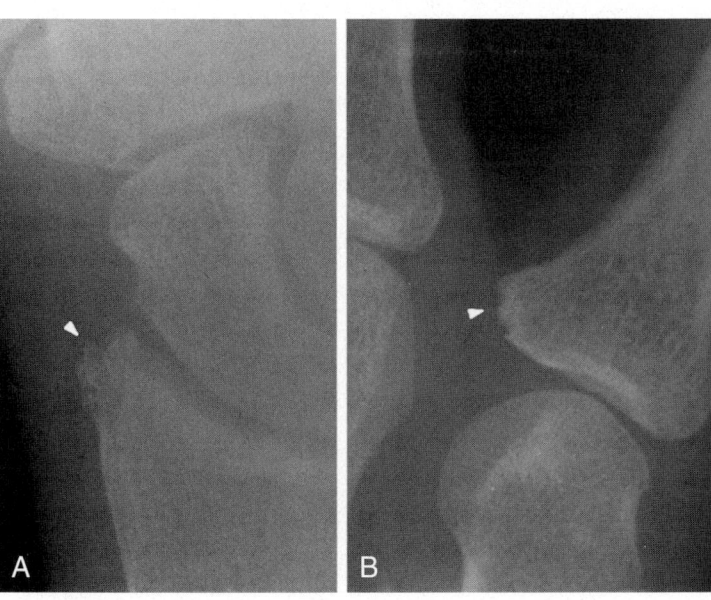

**Figure 36–6.** Radiographic findings in Wilson's disease: bone irregularity and cyst formation. *A* and *B*, Observe the osseous irregularity in the radial styloid process and base of a proximal phalanx *(arrowheads)*. (Courtesy of C. Alexander, MD, Auckland, New Zealand.)

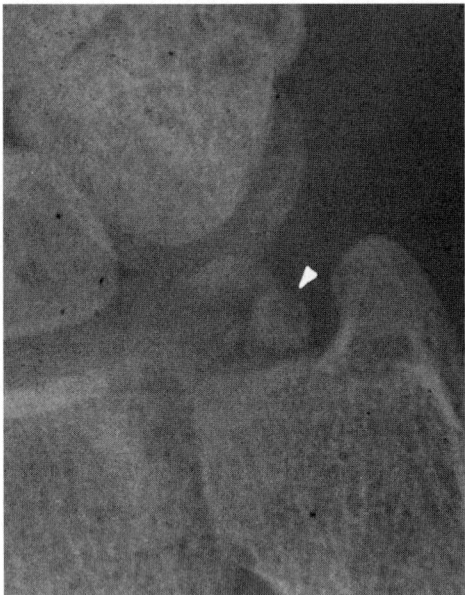

**Figure 36–7.** Radiographic features of Wilson's disease: distinct ossicles. One or more ossicles *(arrowhead)* are present about the distal end of the ulna, a finding resembling chondrocalcinosis. (Courtesy of M. Dalinka, MD, Philadelphia, Pa.)

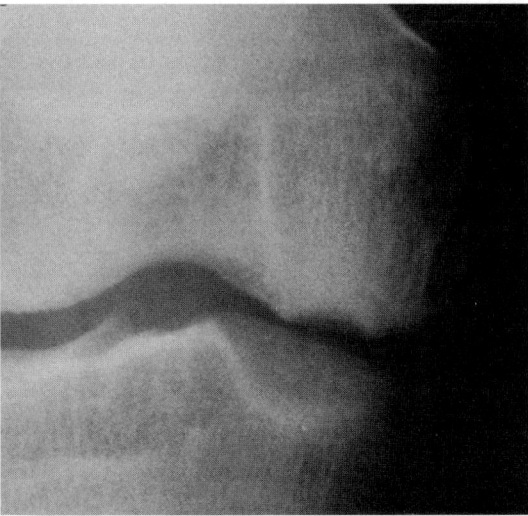

**Figure 36–8.** Radiographic findings in Wilson's disease: osteochondritis dissecans. Flattening of the medial femoral condyle in association with sclerosis can be seen. (From Golding DN, Walshe JM: Arthropathy of Wilson's disease. Study of clinical and radiological features in 32 patients. Ann Rheum Dis 36:99, 1977.)

Wilson's disease differ from the findings in degenerative joint disease, although both disorders are associated with joint space narrowing and subchondral bony eburnation and cyst formation.

The arthropathy of Wilson's disease most resembles that of idiopathic CPPD crystal deposition disease and hemochromatosis. These last two disorders are associated with CPPD crystal deposition manifested as chondrocalcinosis and intra-articular and periarticular calcification; a definite association between Wilson's disease and CPPD crystal deposition has not been proved. In Wilson's disease, distinctive findings are multiple small ossicles and poor definition of the subarticular bone.

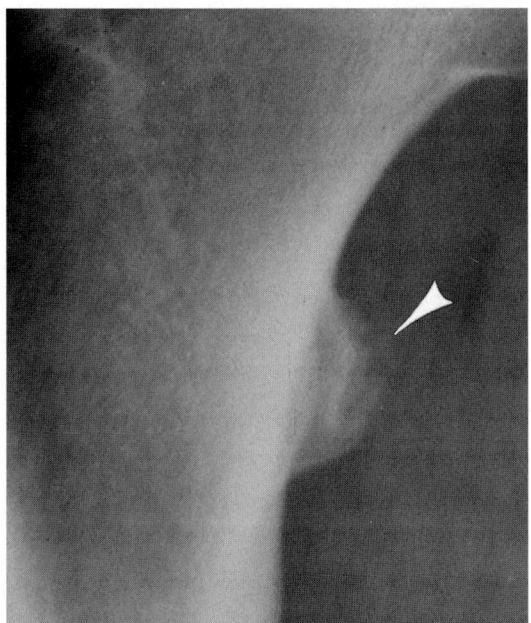

**Figure 36–9.** Radiographic findings in Wilson's disease: bony proliferation. Observe the fluffy bone production on the lesser trochanter *(arrowhead)*. (From Golding DN, Walshe JM: Arthropathy of Wilson's disease. Study of clinical and radiological features in 32 patients. Ann Rheum Dis 36:99, 1977.)

## FURTHER READING

Adamson TC III, Resnik CS, Guerra J Jr, et al: Hand and wrist arthropathies of hemochromatosis and calcium pyrophosphate deposition disease: Distinct radiographic features. Radiology 147:377, 1983.

Atkins CJ, McIvor J, Smith PM, et al: Chondrocalcinosis and arthropathy: Studies in haemochromatosis and in idiopathic chondrocalcinosis. Q J Med 39:71, 1970.

Felitti VJ, Beutler E: New developments in hereditary hemochromatosis. Am J Med Sci 318:257, 1999.

Finby N, Bearn AG: Roentgenographic abnormalities of the skeletal system in Wilson's disease (hepatolenticular degeneration). AJR Am J Roentgenol 79:603, 1958.

Hamilton E, Williams R, Barlow KA, et al: The arthropathy of idiopathic haemochromatosis. Q J Med 37:171, 1968.

Hirsch JH, Killien C, Troupin RH: The arthropathy of hemochromatosis. Radiology 118:591, 1976.

Mindelzun R, Elkin M, Scheinberg IH, et al: Skeletal changes in Wilson's disease: A radiological study. Radiology 94:127, 1970.

Moore EA, Vennart W, Jacoby RK, et al: Magnetic resonance manifestations of idiopathic hemochromatosis in the wrist. Br J Rheumatol 32:917, 1993.

Narvaez J, Alegre-Sancho JJ, Juanola X, et al: Arthropathy of Wilson's disease presenting as noninflammatory polyarthritis. J Rheumatol 24:2494, 1997.

Schumacher HR Jr: Hemochromatosis and arthritis. Arthritis Rheum 7:41, 1964.

Sinigaglia L, Fargion S, Ludovica A, et al: Bone and joint involvement in genetic hemochromatosis: Role of cirrhosis and iron overload. J Rheumatol 24:1809, 1997.

Yarze JC, Martin P, Muoz SJ, et al: Wilson's disease: Current status. Am J Med 92:643, 1992.

Yu-zhang X, Xue-zhe Z, Xian-hao X, et al: Radiologic study of 42 cases of Wilson's disease. Skeletal Radiol 13:114, 1985.

# CHAPTER 37

## Alkaptonuria

### SUMMARY OF KEY FEATURES

Alkaptonuria is a rare hereditary disorder resulting from an inability to metabolize homogentisic acid. Clinical and radiographic findings relate to homogentisic aciduria and ochronosis. The latter feature is accompanied by typical radiographic and pathologic findings in both spinal and extraspinal sites. The most characteristic manifestations of ochronosis are widespread disc calcification, with loss of intervertebral disc height, and a distinctive arthropathy of the axial and extra-axial articulations. Careful evaluation of the radiographs usually allows an accurate diagnosis by differentiating this condition from degenerative joint disease and ankylosing spondylitis, the two disorders with which it is most likely to be confused.

### INTRODUCTION

Alkaptonuria is a rare hereditary metabolic disorder characterized by absence of the enzyme homogentisic acid oxidase. As a result of this defect, homogentisic acid, produced during the metabolism of phenylalanine and tyrosine, accumulates and is excreted in the urine. When the urine of affected persons is allowed to stand, the homogentisic acid is oxidized to a melanin-like product, which causes the urine to gradually turn dark. The term *ochronosis* describes the bluish black pigmentation of connective tissue that may be apparent at such sites as the skin, sclera, and ear in patients with alkaptonuria. Ochronotic arthropathy results from pigment deposition in the joints of the appendicular and axial skeletons of affected individuals.

### PATHOGENESIS

Under normal conditions, the enzyme homogentisate 1,2-dioxygenase metabolizes the homogentisic acid formed from phenylalanine and tyrosine, and the acid is not detectable in either urine or plasma. In alkaptonuria, no enzyme activity is present in either liver or kidney tissue. As a result, homogentisic acid is not metabolized and appears in the urine and plasma. Homogentisic acid can be oxidized when alkali and oxygen are present, such as occurs in the urine. An ochronotic pigment is formed that has a high affinity for cartilage and connective tissue macromolecules.

### TERMINOLOGY

For clarity, it is necessary to define several terms related to this disorder.

*Alkaptonuria:* General name of a disease characterized by the absence of homogentisate 1,2-dioxygenase and the accumulation of homogentisic acid in the urine.

*Ochronosis:* The abnormal pigmentation, brown-black in color, that may be observed in various connective tissues in patients with alkaptonuria.

*Ochronotic arthropathy:* Structural damage that results from the pigmented deposits in the joints of the appendicular and axial skeletons.

### GENERAL CLINICAL FEATURES

Alkaptonuria has a worldwide distribution and affects both men and women. Patterns of inheritance have not been consistent in previous descriptions of the disease. In general, alkaptonuria is asymptomatic until adult life, although in children, discoloration of urine may be detected. Alkaptonuria almost inevitably progresses to ochronosis and arthropathy.

Ochronotic pigmentation is observed infrequently before the age of 20 or 30 years, initially appearing as mild pigmentation of the ears or sclerae, although more widespread ocular abnormality may be apparent. In the ear, cartilage may appear thickened, with slate blue or gray discoloration. Discoloration of skin leading to staining of clothes is caused by perspiration in the axillary and genital areas.

Ochronotic arthropathy is a manifestation of long-standing alkaptonuria. Symptoms and signs usually appear in the fourth decade of life. Initial clinical manifestations such as pain and limitation of motion may be seen in the hip, knee, and shoulder. Acute exacerbations of arthritis may resemble rheumatoid arthritis. Joint effusions result from fragmentation of friable cartilage, with subsequent irritation of the synovial membrane. Stiffness and low back pain, obliteration of the normal lumbar curve, thoracic kyphosis, and restriction of motion are spinal manifestations of the disease, and an elderly person with alkaptonuria may be completely disabled. Symptoms and signs of alkaptonuria may relate to ochronotic deposition in other organs, including the cardiovascular and genitourinary systems and upper respiratory tract.

### GENERAL PATHOLOGIC FEATURES

Abnormal pigmentation of the connective tissue may be observed in the sclera; cornea; laryngeal, tracheal, bronchial, and costal cartilage; tympanic membrane; aortic intima; heart valves; kidney; and prostate. Pigment may also involve articular cartilage, tendons, and ligaments. It appears coal black in some areas, and the chemical characteristics of the pigment resemble those of melanin. In the large diarthrodial joints, the pigment is located in the deeper layers of cartilage. Pigmented necrotic cartilage may become embedded within the marrow, and displaced pieces of cartilage and bone may become lodged in the synovial membrane, where they may stimulate metaplasia of synovial lining cells into chondrocytes. Foreign body reaction, synovial polyp formation, and osteochondral bodies are observed. Inflammatory changes in the synovial membrane are absent or minimal.

In the spine, ochronotic disc deterioration is related to cartilage brittleness, similar to that observed in the cartilage of diseased peripheral joints. Disc fragmentation provokes an adjacent connective tissue reaction that is identical to the reaction noted in the synovial membrane about embedded cartilaginous and osseous debris.

## GENERAL RADIOGRAPHIC FEATURES

The radiographic manifestations of skeletal involvement in alkaptonuria have been well outlined. These findings can be divided into spinal and extraspinal abnormalities (Table 37–1).

### Spinal Abnormalities

Disc calcification is the most characteristic abnormality of the spine (Fig. 37–1). The calcium deposits are found predominantly in the inner fibers of the anulus fibrosus, although they may be distributed diffusely throughout the intervertebral disc in a wafer-like configuration. They consist of apatite crystals and are considered dystrophic in nature. Calcification may appear in any segment of the vertebral column but has a predilection for the intervertebral discs of the lumbar spine; cervical spine alterations are less frequent.

Narrowing of the intervertebral disc space is also a characteristic manifestation of alkaptonuria. The so-called vacuum phenomenon, with linear or circular radiolucent collections of gas overlying the intervertebral disc at mul-

| TABLE 37–1 |
| --- |
| **Diagnostic Features of Ochronotic Arthropathy** |

**Spinal Abnormalities**

  Osteoporosis of vertebral bodies
  Calcification and ossification of intervertebral discs
  Disc space narrowing with vacuum phenomenon
  Small or absent osteophytes
  Loss of lumbar lordosis

**Extraspinal Abnormalities**

  Involvement of sacroiliac joints, symphysis pubis, and large peripheral joints
  Articular space narrowing
  Bony sclerosis
  Collapse and fragmentation with intra-articular osseous bodies
  Small or absent osteophytes
  Tendinous calcification, ossification, and rupture
  Unusual involvement of hand, wrist, foot, elbow, and ankle

tiple levels, is also suggestive of this diagnosis (Fig. 37–2). Progressive ossification of the discs may be seen, with the formation of marginal intervertebral bridges and obliteration of the intervertebral space (Fig. 37–3). These bridges resemble the syndesmophytes of ankylosing spondylitis. Narrowing of the intervertebral disc is associated with bony eburnation of apposing vertebral bodies and small marginal osteophytes.

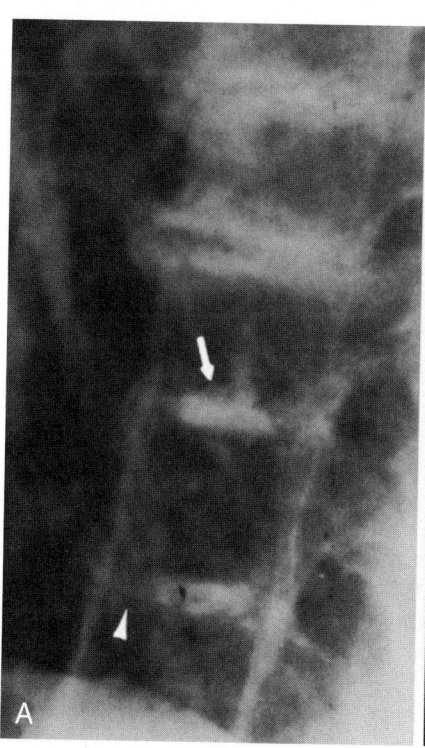
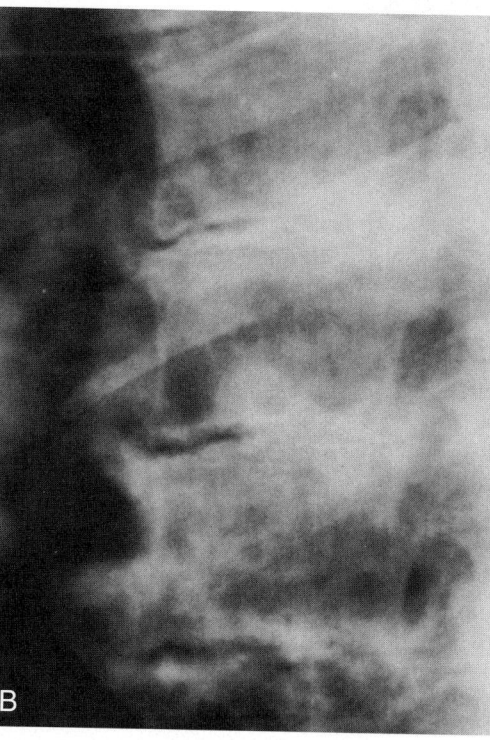

**Figure 37–1.** Radiographic features of alkaptonuria: thoracic spine. *A*, Alterations include disc calcification *(arrow)* and ossification *(arrowhead)*, disc space loss, vertebral body osteoporosis with marginal sclerosis, and mild osteophytosis. *B*, In another patient, the most obvious abnormalities are disc space loss, vertebral body marginal sclerosis, and anterior osteophytes.

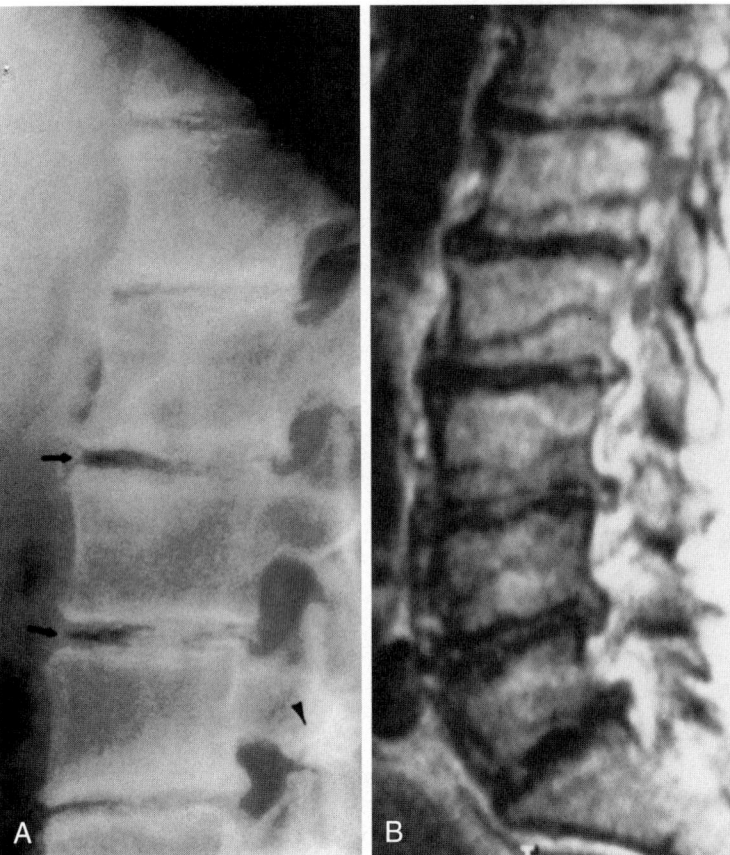

**Figure 37–2.** Radiographic and MR imaging features of alkaptonuria: disc space narrowing and vacuum phenomenon. *A,* Observe the linear radiolucent areas *(arrows)* within multiple narrowed intervertebral discs. Disc calcification is not prominent. Apophyseal joint space narrowing is seen. Note the spondylolysis of a lower lumbar vertebra *(arrowhead). B,* Sagittal intermediate-weighted (TR/TE, 1000/30) spin echo MR image shows diffuse loss of intervertebral disc spaces. Low signal intensity in each of the discs is compatible with the presence of gas, calcification, or both. Posterior disc extensions are also observed. (*B,* Courtesy of P. Katzenstein, MD, Houston, Tex.)

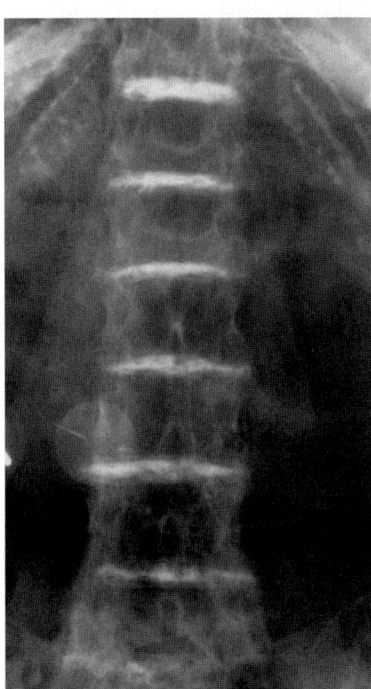

**Figure 37–3.** Radiographic features of alkaptonuria: disc calcification and ossification. Frontal radiograph of the lumbar spine shows osteoporosis, disc calcification, and, at the periphery of the intervertebral disc, ossification simulating the syndesmophytes of ankylosing spondylitis. (Courtesy of J. Loewy, MD, Saskatoon, Saskatchewan, Canada.)

Severe changes may be apparent in long-standing disease and include progressive kyphosis, osteoporosis, obliteration of intervertebral disc spaces, and bony bridging, with a bamboo spine. The appearance of a bamboo spine may lead to an erroneous diagnosis of ankylosing spondylitis. The relationship between alkaptonuria and ankylosing spondylitis is unclear, but it is known that alkaptonuria can lead to spinal alterations whose clinical and radiographic manifestations are virtually indistinguishable from those of ankylosing spondylitis. Further, spondylitis-like changes in the sacroiliac and apophyseal joints, symphysis pubis, and hips have been ascribed to alkaptonuria.

Magnetic resonance (MR) imaging reveals the extent of spinal disease and complications such as disc displacement, but the findings lack specificity, inasmuch as regions of disc calcification may be difficult to identify. Such calcification may appear as foci of either low or high signal intensity.

### Extraspinal Abnormalities

At the symphysis pubis, articular space narrowing, calcification, bony eburnation, and fragmentation may be seen. Similarly, joint space narrowing, sclerosis, and osteophytosis may be apparent at the sacroiliac articulations (Fig. 37–4).

The knee is the most common site of peripheral abnormality (Fig. 37–5). Findings in this location simulate those of uncomplicated degenerative joint disease

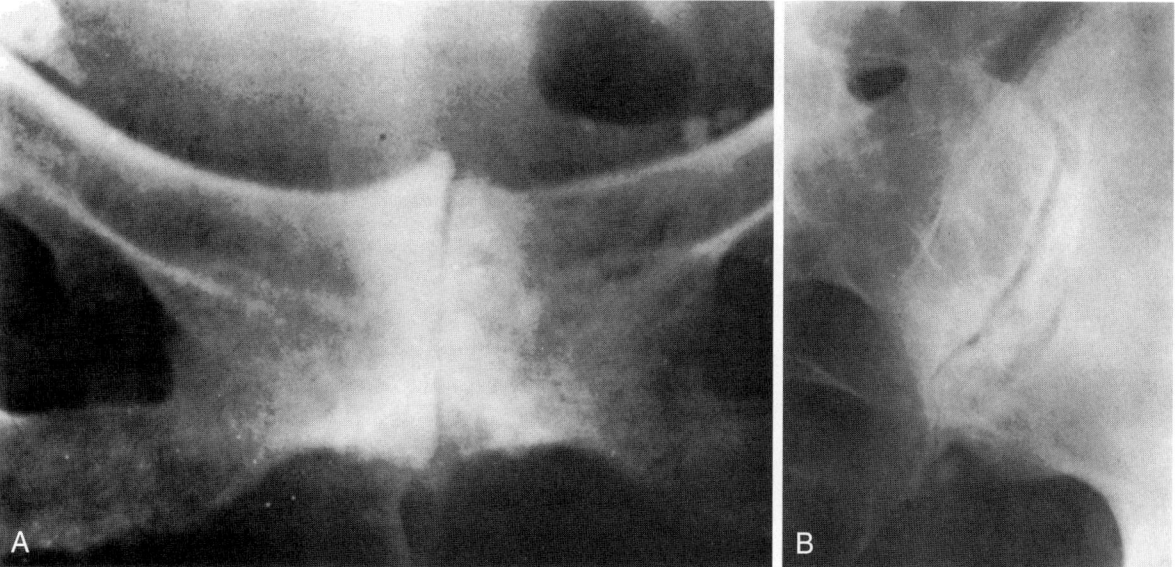

**Figure 37–4.** Radiographic features of alkaptonuria: symphysis pubis and sacroiliac joint. *A,* Symphysis pubis. The findings are extreme narrowing of the joint space and extensive bony sclerosis. Beaklike osteophytes are seen. *B,* Sacroiliac joint. Diffuse narrowing of the articular space is associated with irregularity of subchondral bone and sclerosis. The articular margins are more sharply defined than would be expected in ankylosing spondylitis.

and consist of effusion, articular space narrowing, and bony sclerosis. Differences between these two diseases may include isolated involvement of the lateral femorotibial compartment, relatively symmetrical involvement of both the medial and lateral femorotibial compartments, bony

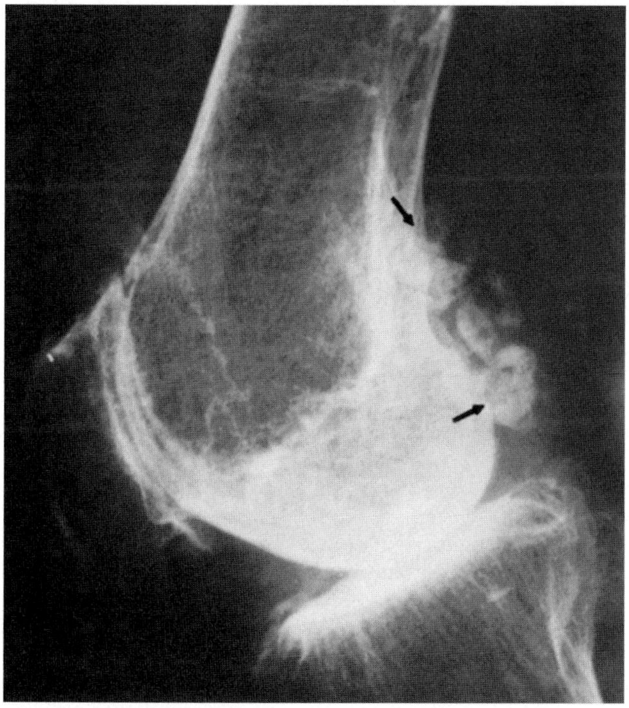

**Figure 37–5.** Radiographic features of alkaptonuria: knee. In this patient, abnormalities include joint space narrowing in the lateral femorotibial and patellofemoral compartments, associated with bony sclerosis, small osteophytes, and multiple intra-articular osseous bodies *(arrows).*

collapse and fragmentation with multiple radiopaque intra-articular bodies, meager osteophytosis, and tendinous calcification in alkaptonuria.

Radiographic findings in the hip may be identical to the changes of degenerative joint disease, with articular space narrowing and sclerosis (Fig. 37–6). In some patients with alkaptonuria, diffuse loss of joint space, severe destruction with fragmentation and formation of intra-articular cartilaginous and osseous bodies, and tendinous calcification and ossification permit differentiation from typical degenerative alterations. Involvement of the glenohumeral joint, small joints of the hands and feet, elbow, and ankle is not common.

## DIFFERENTIAL DIAGNOSIS

### Spinal Manifestations

Disc calcification in alkaptonuria may be confused with that accompanying other disorders (Table 37–2). Dystrophic calcification of the nucleus pulposus is not infrequent. In these instances, the radiodense collections are generally globular and confined to the central portion of the intervertebral disc. This pattern of central disc calcification is generally not widespread and can be readily differentiated from the diffuse disc calcification at multiple levels of the spine in patients with alkaptonuria.

Calcification of the intervertebral disc may be seen as a secondary phenomenon in patients with primary disorders that lead to spinal ankylosis. Thus, disc calcification can be noted in patients with ankylosing spondylitis, diffuse idiopathic skeletal hyperostosis, juvenile-onset rheumatoid arthritis, Klippel-Feil deformities, and surgical fusion of the spine.

Disc calcification is also observed in calcium pyrophosphate dihydrate (CPPD) crystal deposition disease.

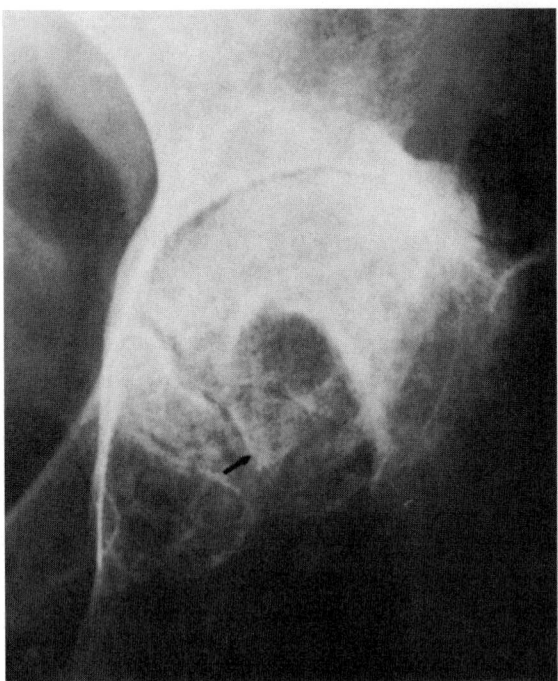

**Figure 37–6.** Radiographic features of alkaptonuria: hip. Extensive resorption and flattening of the femoral head are associated with a bizarre radiographic appearance. Findings include joint space narrowing, mild acetabular protrusion, and bone fragmentation (*arrow*).

In this disorder, the deposits predominate in the outer fibers of the anulus fibrosus, and wafer-like collections are not seen. Disc space loss, vacuum phenomenon, and vertebral body marginal sclerosis accompany intervertebral osteochondrosis. The findings are generally not as pronounced or widespread as in alkaptonuria, and they frequently occur in elderly patients. Nonetheless, the possibility of alkaptonuria must be considered in any patient whose radiographs reveal loss of height of multiple intervertebral discs, particularly if the changes occur in a middle-aged patient and are accompanied by multiple vacuum phenomena, disc calcification, vertebral fusion, and kyphosis.

Disc ossification with fusion of the vertebral bodies, a finding in alkaptonuria, may resemble abnormalities in ankylosing spondylitis. In long-standing alkaptonuria, a bamboo spine may again simulate that in ankylosing spondylitis.

## Extraspinal Manifestations

Involvement of extraspinal sites in patients with alkaptonuria may lead to a radiographic appearance reminiscent of degenerative joint disease. Certain features of ochronotic arthropathy usually permit its identification in these persons (Table 37–3):

1. Involvement of unusual articular sites. Arthropathy of the glenohumeral joint resembling that of severe degenerative articular disease should suggest the diagnosis of alkaptonuria, because considerable findings of degenerative joint disease are unusual in this location without a history of significant trauma. Similarly, severe changes in the sacroiliac or symphyseal joints may be a clue to the presence of ochronotic arthropathy.

2. Unusual patterns of joint space loss. Ochronotic arthropathy of the knee may lead to isolated lateral femorotibial compartment changes or to diffuse loss of articular space in both the medial and lateral femorotibial compartments. These patterns are unusual in degenerative joint disease.

3. Severe abnormalities with extreme sclerosis, fragmentation, and intra-articular cartilaginous and osseous bodies. The severity of the changes accompanying ochronotic arthropathy may be greater than those usually seen in degenerative joint disease. The production of multiple intra-articular bodies is particularly characteristic.

The peculiar pattern of "degenerative" arthropathy that is characteristic of alkaptonuria may be simulated by

### TABLE 37–2

#### Disc Calcification

| Diagnosis | Site of Calcification | Nature of Calcification |
|---|---|---|
| Ochronosis | AF, NP | HA |
| CPPD crystal deposition disease | | |
|   Sporadic | AF | CPPD |
|   Familial | AF, NP | ? |
| Hemochromatosis | AF, NP | CPPD |
| Hyperparathyroidism | AF, NP | CPPD |
| Acromegaly | AF, NP | HA |
| Poliomyelitis | AF, NP | ? |
| Amyloidosis | AF, NP | ? |
| Spinal fusion | NP | ? |

AF, anulus fibrosus; CPPD, calcium pyrophosphate dihydrate; HA, hydroxyapatite; NP, nucleus pulposus.

From Weinberger A, Myers AR: Semin Arthritis Rheum 18:69, 1978.

### TABLE 37–3

#### Ochronotic Arthropathy versus Degenerative Joint Disease

| Ochronotic Arthropathy | Degenerative Joint Disease |
|---|---|
| Involvement of hip, shoulder, knee, sacroiliac joint, and symphysis pubis | Involvement of hip, knee, and hand |
| Focal or diffuse joint space loss | Focal joint space loss |
| Absent or meager osteophytosis | Prominent osteophytosis |
| Small cystic lesions | Small or large cystic lesions |
| Collapse, fragmentation, and intra-articular osseous bodies | No collapse or fragmentation |
| Tendon abnormalities | No tendon abnormalities |

other disorders, such as CPPD crystal deposition disease, calcium hydroxyapatite crystal deposition disease, acromegaly, and epiphyseal and spondyloepiphyseal dysplasias.

## FURTHER READING

Dom K, Pittevils T: Ochronotic arthropathy: The black hip. Case report and review of the literature. Acta Orthop Belg 63:122, 1997.

Hamdi N, Cooke TD, Hassan B: Ochronotic arthropathy: Case report and review of the literature. Int Orthop 23:122, 1999.

Justesen P, Andersen PE Jr: Radiologic manifestations in alcaptonuria. Skeletal Radiol 11:204, 1984.

Lagier R, Sitaj S: Vertebral changes in ochronois: Anatomical and radiological study of one case. Ann Rheum Dis 33:86, 1974.

Lasker RH, Sargison KD: Ochronotic arthropathy: A review with four case reports. J Bone Joint Surg Br 52:653, 1970.

Millea TP, Segal LS, Liss RG, et al: Spine fracture in ochronosis: Report of a case. Clin Orthop 281:208, 1992.

Pomeranx MM, Friedman LJ, Tunick IS: Roentgen findings in alkaptonuric ochronosis. Radiology 37:295, 1941.

Selvi E, Manganelli S, Benucci M, et al: Chronic ochronotic arthritis: Clinical, arthroscopic, and pathologic findings. J Rheumatol 27:2272, 2000.

Thompson MM Jr: Ochronosis. AJR Am J Roentgenol 78:46, 1957.

# CHAPTER 38

## Other Crystal-Induced Diseases

## *SUMMARY OF KEY FEATURES*

Other crystals besides monosodium urate, calcium pyrophosphate dihydrate (CPPD), and calcium hydroxyapatite crystals can lead to soft tissue, articular, and osseous abnormalities. Cholesterol crystals are identified in patients with rheumatoid arthritis, as well as osteoarthritis; they appear to reflect local rather than systemic alterations and may be responsible for low-grade synovial inflammation. When corticosteroid preparations are injected into joints, there is a mild synovial inflammatory response. Accumulation of calcium oxalate crystals is seen in both primary and secondary oxalosis, the latter most typically occurring as a complication of chronic renal disease. Destructive lesions of the metaphyseal regions of tubular bones, discovertebral regions, and sometimes joints become apparent. Cystine, hemoglobin, and Charcot-Leyden crystals can also accumulate in bones or joints, although the precise relationship between such accumulation and structural abnormality is not known. Xanthine and hypoxanthine crystals may be deposited in muscles.

## INTRODUCTION

When synovial fluid is examined with polarizing light microscopy, a variety of crystals can be identified; this may provide an immediate clue to the precise cause of articular symptoms and signs. Previous chapters discussed three basic crystal-induced arthropathies: monosodium urate crystal deposition disease (gout), CPPD crystal deposition disease (pseudogout and other clinical manifestations), and calcium hydroxyapatite crystal deposition disease. This chapter describes several additional crystals, as well as their possible relationship to articular manifestations.

## CHOLESTEROL CRYSTALS

Crystals of cholesterol are frequently identified in the joint effusions of patients with rheumatoid arthritis and, less commonly, in the effusions of those with osteo-arthritis, chronic tophaceous gout, ankylosing spondylitis, and systemic lupus erythematosus. The exact origin of cholesterol crystals within the joint is unknown, although local rather than systemic factors appear to play a more important role in their cause. In certain situations, these crystals may be responsible for low-grade synovial inflammation and the production of articular abnormalities.

## CORTICOSTEROIDS

Corticosteroid preparations for intra-articular injection are suspensions of microcrystals that may persist for some time and be misinterpreted as monosodium urate or CPPD during polarizing microscopy. The use of intra-synovial corticosteroid therapy has been followed inconstantly by local exacerbations of symptoms in the treated joints. This phenomenon, termed a postinjection flare, usually commences within 1 to 3 days after the injection and persists for several days.

## CHARCOT-LEYDEN CRYSTALS

Charcot-Leyden crystals have been identified in a variety of conditions associated with eosinophilia, including allergy, asthma, parasitic disorders, and granulocytic leukemia. They have been noted in synovial fluid, where they demonstrate weakly positive birefringence and are accompanied by turbid joint effusions. It is not certain whether the crystals contribute to acute inflammation.

## CALCIUM OXALATE (OXALOSIS)

Deposition of crystals of calcium oxalate in tissue occurs in two main situations: as a rare primary hereditary process or, more commonly, as a secondary or acquired process, usually in association with chronic renal disease.

### Primary Oxalosis

Inherited as an autosomal recessive trait, primary oxalosis is divided into two types: type 1, glycolic aciduria caused by the absence of $\alpha$-ketoglutarate–glyoxylate carboxylase (or glyoxylate aminotransferase) activity; and type 2, 1-glyceric aciduria caused by a defect in D-glycerate dehydrogenase–glyoxylate reductase. Overproduction of oxalate related to these enzyme defects is accompanied by its accumulation in various tissues. Damage to the kidneys in the form of calcium oxalate nephrolithiasis and nephrocalcinosis produces progressive renal failure and uremia. Extrarenal accumulation of calcium oxalate occurs in the small arteries, eyes, soft tissues, and bones.

Both boys and girls are affected. Clinical manifestations generally become apparent before the age of 5 years and are mainly the result of renal accumulation of calcium oxalate crystals. Calculi and pyelonephritis are observed. Radiographic examination of the genitourinary system may reveal small, contracted kidneys with parenchymal calcification (Fig. 38–1).

The skeletal abnormalities associated with primary oxalosis include irregular transverse sclerotic bands in the metaphyseal segments of tubular bones, including the femur, humerus, tibia, fibula, metacarpals, metatarsals, and phalanges. These bands extend into the epiphyses, and narrow translucent zones, which may replace the radiodense lines, are seen at the level of the physis between the epiphyseal and metaphyseal components (Fig. 38–2A). Similar radiodense regions can appear in subchondral areas in the humeri and femora and resemble the findings of ischemic necrosis. Alternating

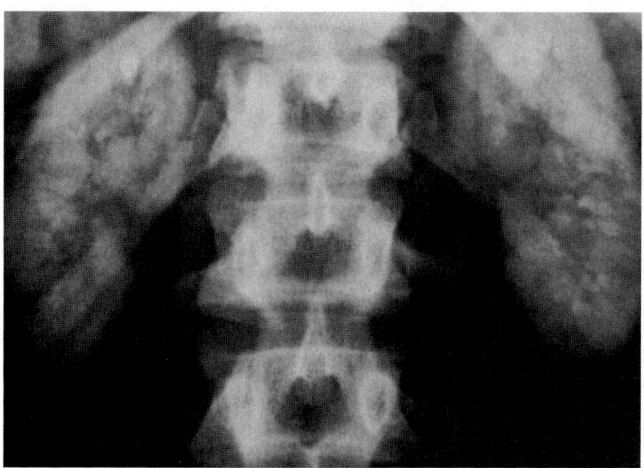

**Figure 38–1.** Primary oxalosis: radiographic abnormalities. In a 27-year-old woman with primary oxalosis, a preliminary film from an intravenous pyelogram, before the injection of contrast material, reveals bilateral diffuse calcification within contracted kidneys. (Courtesy of L. Cooperstein, Pittsburgh, Pa.)

radiolucent and radiodense bands have been identified in the ilium and sternum, whereas in the spine, sclerotic zones at the top and bottom of the vertebral bodies simulate the rugger-jersey appearance of renal osteodystrophy (see Fig. 38–2B). Diffuse osteosclerosis of the vertebrae may also occur, and oxalate crystal deposition in adjacent ligaments and soft tissues may contribute to spinal stenosis. Additional skeletal alterations include a drumstick con-

figuration of the metacarpal bones and patchy sclerosis in the clavicles. Eventually, chronic renal failure can lead to the widespread skeletal abnormalities of renal osteodystrophy.

Histologic investigation of the skeletal abnormalities in both primary and secondary oxalosis indicates that the sclerotic regions in the tubular bones represent, in large part, deposition of calcium oxalate crystals in the marrow. A foreign body giant cell reaction results and stimulates new bone formation. Massive deposits of calcium oxalate are associated with resorption and disappearance of trabeculae, cystic lesions, fracture, and deformities such as acetabular protrusion.

## Secondary Oxalosis

Oxalosis is a recognized complication of other diseases, especially renal disorders; secondary forms of oxalosis are also related to (1) ingestion of substances that either contain the oxalate ion or are metabolized to oxalate (rhubarb, ethylene glycol), (2) thiamine and pyridoxine deficiencies that inhibit glyoxylate metabolism and increase the production of oxalate, (3) formation of oxalate by *Aspergillus niger*, and (4) bowel disorders that cause malabsorption and steatorrhea. Because oxalic acid is excreted by the kidneys, plasma oxalate levels generally rise in proportion to blood urea nitrogen in end-stage renal failure. Deposition of calcium oxalate subsequently occurs in the body's tissues, primarily in the kidney itself; more than 75% of patients with end-stage renal disease of longer than 2 months' duration have significant accumulations of calcium oxalate in the kidney. Other organs that are

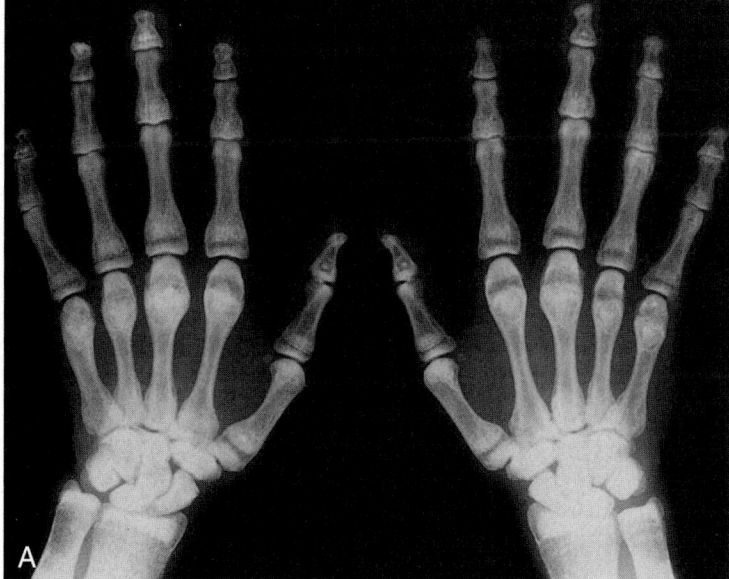

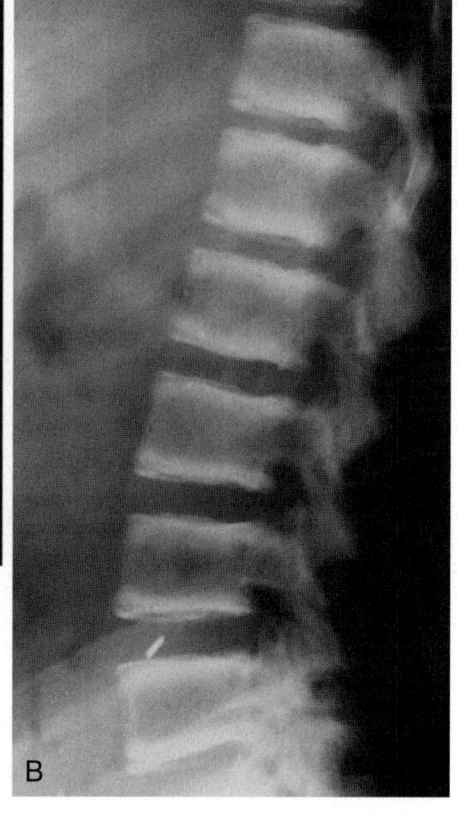

**Figure 38–2.** Primary oxalosis: radiographic abnormalities. In this 32-year-old man, diffuse skeletal abnormalities are present. *A*, Findings include a drumstick configuration of the metacarpal bones, hypoplasia of the terminal phalanges, a coarsened trabecular pattern, and patchy metaphyseal sclerosis. *B*, In the spine, abnormalities include irregularities in vertebral shape and a rugger-jersey appearance in the vertebral bodies. Surgical clips are evidence of previous renal transplantation. (Courtesy of R. Bluestone, MD, Los Angeles, Calif.)

involved include the myocardium, thyroid gland, spleen, liver, lymph nodes, brain, salivary glands, dentin, dental pulp, arteries and veins, and musculoskeletal tissues.

Trabecular condensation or disarray, or both, accounts for the resulting radiodensity and cystic appearance on radiographs. Articular manifestations, which may include effusions, pain, and stiffness, have been reported in multiple locations, including the knee, wrist, and metacarpophalangeal and interphalangeal joints. In addition to juxta-articular osteoporosis, radiographs may reveal capsular and cartilage calcification (chondrocalcinosis), the latter unrelated to CPPD crystal deposition (Fig. 38–3).

The radiographic characteristics of musculoskeletal involvement in secondary oxalosis present diagnostic difficulties. Chondrocalcinosis, as well as calcification in the joint capsule and tendons, may be related to CPPD, calcium hydroxyapatite, or calcium oxalate crystal deposition (or any combination of the three) in patients with chronic renal disease. Bone erosions may be related to any of these crystals or to secondary hyperparathyroidism. Discovertebral destruction, a recognized complication of renal dialysis, may represent an additional manifestation of calcium oxalate crystal accumulation, inasmuch as such crystals have been observed in areas of disc degeneration; however, subchondral resorption resulting from secondary hyperparathyroidism, calcium hydroxyapatite or CPPD crystal deposition, or amyloid deposition can lead to a

similar aberration. Sclerosis in the metaphyseal segments of tubular bones is a finding of secondary (as well as primary) oxalosis, although it can apparently be seen in chronic renal disease without oxalate deposition.

## CYSTINOSIS

Cystinosis is a rare familial disorder characterized by the widespread deposition of cystine crystals in body tissues. Although the cause of this deposition is unknown, cystine accumulates within lysosomes, most prominently in the reticuloendothelial cells of the liver, spleen, lymph nodes, and bone marrow; in peripheral leukocytes; in the medullary, cortical, and glomerular mesangium of the kidney; in the rectal mucosa; and in the uvea and conjunctiva of the eye. The renal deposition is responsible for the secondary tissue damage that results in renal insufficiency and failure in certain forms of the disease.

Three varieties of the disease have been identified: infantile cystinosis, of autosomal recessive inheritance, in which renal insufficiency becomes apparent in the first decade of life and may lead to early death; juvenile or intermediate cystinosis, in which renal disease becomes evident in the second or third decade of life; and adult or benign cystinosis, which is manifested as corneal rather than renal deposition of cystine and is compatible with long survival. In the first two forms of the disease, damage to the tubules and, subsequently, to the glomeruli of the kidneys leads to electrolyte imbalance, anemia, cardiac failure, retinopathy, and rickets. In general, the amount of cystine deposited in the tissues is directly related to the clinical severity of the disorder.

In the infantile variety, polyuria, dehydration, chronic acidosis, vitamin D–resistant rickets, and growth disturbance may antedate progressive uremia and death, all of which may occur before the age of 10 years. In adult cystinosis, ocular manifestations predominate and include burning and itching of the eyes, photophobia, and headache. In the juvenile variety, clinical abnormalities are intermediate between the infantile and adult types and consist of both ocular and renal alterations. Although accumulation of cystine crystals in the bone marrow is a recognized sequela of the disease, osseous and articular manifestations, other than those related to rickets, have not received a great deal of attention. Radiolucent cystic lesions in bone and articular calcification have been reported, but their precise relationship to cystine deposition is not clear.

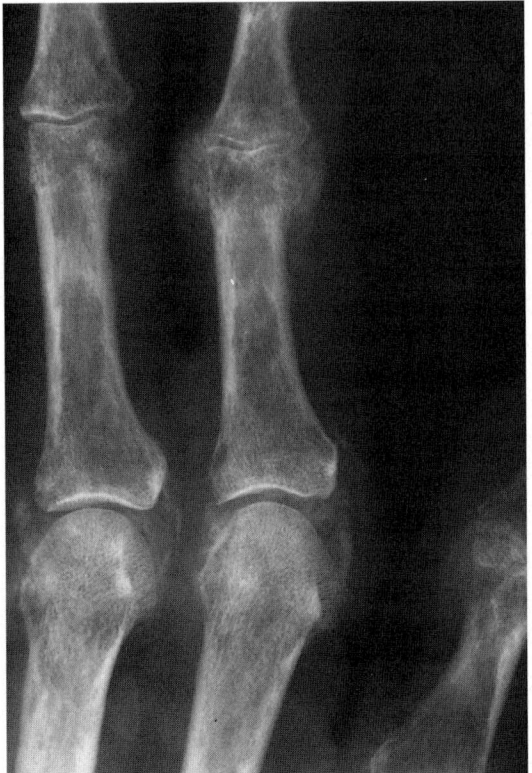

**Figure 38–3.** Secondary oxalosis: radiographic abnormalities. Radiograph reveals periarticular and intra-articular calcification. The latter is within the capsule, the synovium, and, possibly, the cartilage. Minimal subperiosteal bone resorption is suggested.

### FURTHER READING

Brancaccio D, Poggi A, Ciccarelli C, et al: Bone changes in end-stage oxalosis. AJR Am J Roentgenol 136:935, 1981.

Danpure CJ: The molecular basis of alanine glyoxylate aminotransferase mistargeting: The most common single cause of primary hyperoxaluria type 1. J Nephrol 11:8, 1998.

Day DL, Scheinman JI, Mahan J: Radiological aspects of primary hyperoxaluria. AJR Am J Roentgenol 146:395, 1986.

Elmstahl B, Rausing A: A case of hyperoxaluria: Radiological aspects. Acta Radiol 38:1031, 1997.

Fam AG, Sugai M, Gertner E, et al: Cholesterol "tophus." Arthritis Rheum 26:1525, 1983.

Freiberg AA, Fish DN, Louis DS: Hand manifestations of oxalosis. J Hand Surg [Am] 18:140, 1993.

Kemper MJ, Conrad S, Muller-Wiefel DE: Primary hyperoxaluria type 2. Eur J Pediatr 156:509, 1997.

Martijn A, Thijn CJP: Radiologic findings in primary hyperoxaluria. Skeletal Radiol 8:21, 1982.

McCarty DJ Jr, Hogan JM: Inflammatory reaction after intrasynovial injection of microcrystalline adrenocorticosteroid esters. Arthritis Rheum 7:359, 1964.

Milgram JW, Salyer WR: Secondary oxalosis of bone in chronic renal failure: A histopathological study of three cases. J Bone Joint Surg Am 56:387, 1974.

Reginato AF, Falasca GF, Usmani Q: Do we really need to pay attention to the less common crystals? Curr Opin Rheumatol 11:446, 1999.

Zuckner J, Uddin J, Gantner GE Jr, et al: Cholesterol crystals in synovial fluid. Ann Intern Med 60:436, 1964.

# Temporomandibular Manifestations of Articular Disease

# CHAPTER 39

## Temporomandibular Joint

William A. Murphy Jr., Phoebe A. Kaplan,
and Donald Resnick

## SUMMARY OF KEY FEATURES

Temporomandibular joint (TMJ) pain and dysfunction are important clinical problems. Many of these disorders have long been misunderstood or ignored by physicians, who for years had little interest in or opportunity to learn about them. In the past 15 or 20 years, however, radiologists have had a major role in the diagnosis of TMJ disorders because of the explosion of new imaging methods. Foremost among these methods are arthrography, computed tomography (CT), and, more recently, magnetic resonance (MR) imaging. The impact of these imaging techniques on the diagnosis of TMJ disorders is undeniable.

## INTRODUCTION

The TMJ is afflicted by many osseous and soft tissue conditions, as are other joints. Because of its particular anatomy, however, the TMJ is subject to a unique biomechanical environment and set of pathologic conditions.

## ANATOMY

The condylar and temporal bone components of the TMJ are maintained in apposition by muscles, ligaments, and the joint capsule. The capsule attaches about the joint margins and is reinforced laterally by a strong temporomandibular ligament and medially by two weaker ligaments. Branches of the mandibular division of the trigeminal nerve innervate the joint. Similarly, branches of the superficial temporal and maxillary arteries provide the blood supply.

### Osseous Anatomy

Important osseous landmarks in the lateral projection are the cortical and trabecular elements of the condyle, mandibular fossa, temporal eminence, and auditory canal (Fig. 39–1). The long axis of the mandibular condyle is perpendicular to the mandibular ramus. The sagittal surface of the eminence is gently convex, and the combined mandibular fossa and eminence describe a smooth sigmoid curve.

Major osseous landmarks in Towne's projection are portions of the condyle, including its neck and medial and lateral poles (Fig. 39–2). The mandibular fossa is limited by an osseous ridge medially, which is a barrier to medial dislocation of the condyle. In both lateral (sagittal) and frontal (coronal or Towne's) perspectives, the joint surfaces are smooth, and the joint space is of nearly uniform thickness along the articulating surfaces. The condyle rests symmetrically within the fossa. The joint surfaces are covered by fibrocartilage rather than hyaline cartilage, presumably because of the great forces to which they are subjected.

### Soft Tissue Anatomy

The major soft tissue structure of the TMJ is an articular disc (meniscus) that is interposed between the adjacent osseous elements (Fig. 39–3). The disc separates the joint into two synovial articulations—one superior, between the temporal bone and the disc, and the other inferior, between the disc and the condylar head. The disc is thin centrally (the intermediate zone) and ridged or thickened peripherally. It is attached to capsular, ligamentous, and other soft tissue structures about its entire periphery.

The disc is a biconcave fibrocartilage. In the sagittal perspective, the anterior and posterior ridges of the disc are prominent and are termed the anterior and posterior bands; their mediolateral length is much greater than their anteroposterior length. The anterior band of the disc is smaller than the posterior band and attaches to the anterior margin of the articular eminence and to the anteroinferior aspect of the articular margin of the condyle. The posterior band of the disc blends with highly vascular and innervated areolar tissue, termed the bilaminar zone or posterior attachment. These anterior and posterior attachments are continuous medially and laterally and bind the disc to the condyle and the fossa.

With the jaw closed, the disc is positioned between the condyle and the fossa such that the posterior band is located between the apex of the condyle and the depth of the fossa, sometimes termed the 12 o'clock position. As the jaw opens, the disc and condyle move forward in a complex coordinated fashion. The result is that the thin central portion of the disc maintains a position between the juxtaposed articular surfaces of the condyle and eminence.

## IMAGING METHODS
### Radiography

Conventional radiography has long been considered the initial imaging method that is best suited for displaying

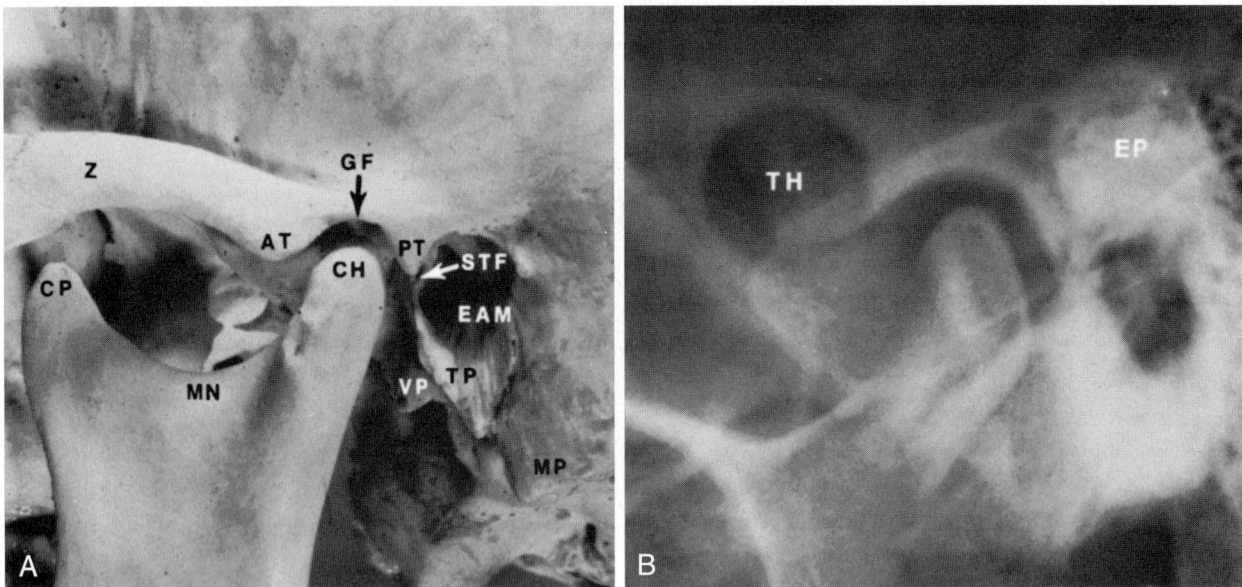

**Figure 39–1.** Lateral perspective of normal adult osseous anatomy. *A*, Surface photograph of the skull. *B*, Magnified lateral projection (closed-mouth position) in a 22-year-old woman. The following anatomic landmarks can be identified: AT, anterior glenoid tubercle (articular eminence); CH, condylar head; CP, coronoid process; EAM, external auditory meatus; EP, ear plug; GF, glenoid (mandibular) fossa; MN, mandibular or sigmoid notch; MP, mastoid process; PT, posterior glenoid tubercle; STF, squamotympanic fissure; TH, threaded hole in the radiographic positioning device; TP, tympanic process; VP, vaginal process; Z, zygoma.

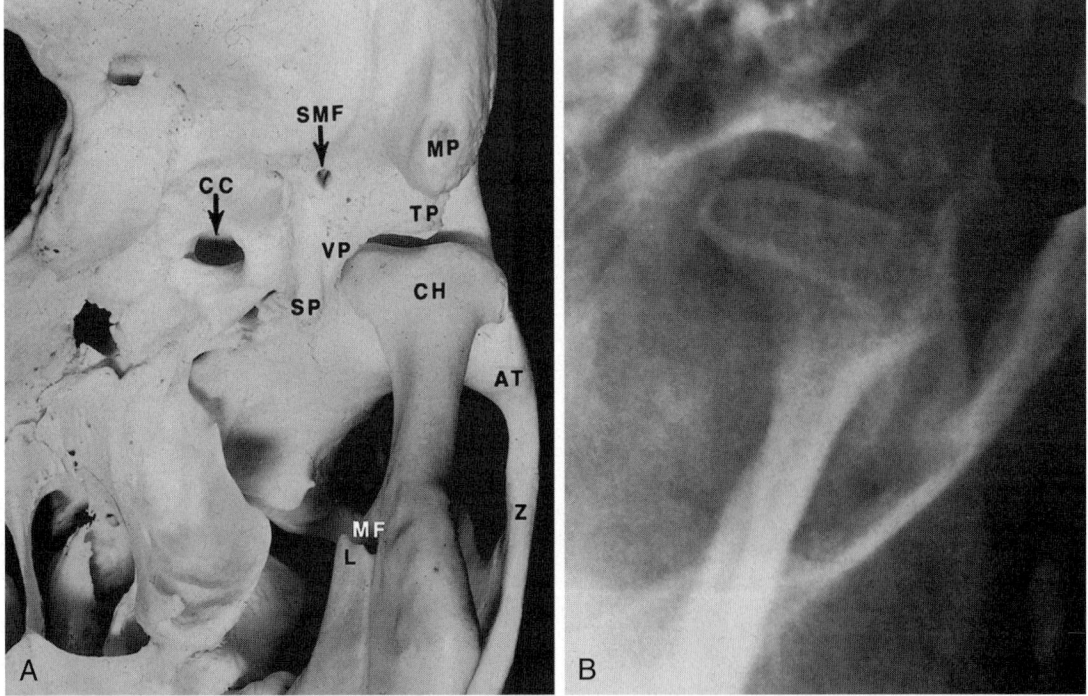

**Figure 39–2.** Frontal (Towne's) perspective of normal adult osseous anatomy. *A*, Surface photograph of the skull. *B*, Magnified Towne's projection (closed-mouth position) in a 23-year-old woman. The following anatomic landmarks can be identified: AT, anterior glenoid tubercle; CC, carotid canal; CH, condylar head; L, lingula; MF, mandibular foramen; MP, mastoid process; SMF, stylomastoid foramen; SP, styloid process; TP, tympanic process; VP, vaginal process; Z, zygoma.

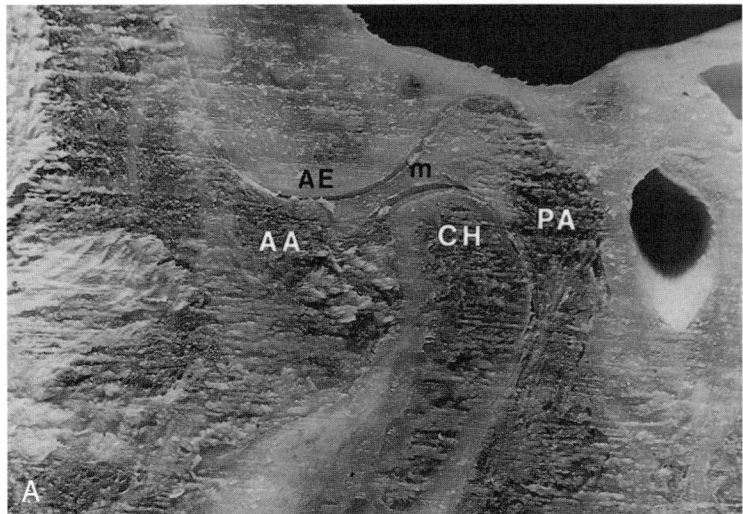
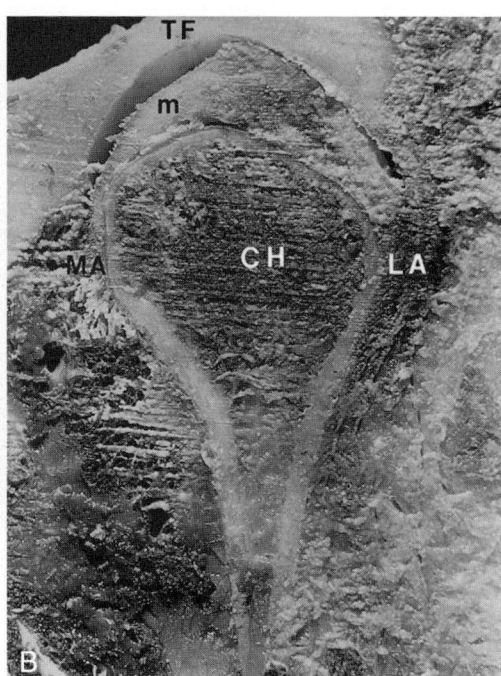

**Figure 39–3.** Normal soft tissue anatomy of the temporomandibular joint. *A*, Sagittal section shows disc or meniscus (m) separating the articular eminence (AE) from the condylar head (CH). Anterior (AA) and posterior (PA) meniscal attachments are broadly based in the adjacent soft tissues. *B*, Coronal section shows the meniscus (m) separating the temporal fossa (TF) from the condylar head (CH). Meniscal attachments to the condylar head are thin medially (MA) and thick laterally (LA).

the osseous anatomy and the general positional relationship of the condyle with respect to the mandibular fossa; however, because of the small size of the joint, its complex anatomic structure, and its location among the other bones of the skull, obtaining optimal images is technically demanding and not always successful.

The panoramic radiographic projection provides an excellent survey of the mandible and dentition. It images both TMJs simultaneously and may reveal disease processes of these joints, the mandible, or the teeth (Fig. 39–4). It provides a relatively lateral projection of both joints and is particularly useful for evaluating symmetry. Panoramic radiography is also an effective method for studying mandibular fractures and tumors.

### Radionuclide Imaging

Two general methods of imaging are used: planar and tomographic. Planar images are generally obtained with a gamma camera having a large field of view and fitted with a high-resolution collimator. Single photon emission computed tomography (SPECT) scans require a special rotating gamma camera device with an appropriate collimator. Planar radionuclide imaging of the TMJ has not had any impact on the detection or management of TMJ disorders. SPECT is more sensitive than the planar method, but it is not more specific.

### Computed Tomography

CT is especially useful for the evaluation of osseous anatomy, including the detection and staging of tumors, arthritic changes, and fractures. Spiral and multidetector scanners have markedly improved the ability to obtain reformatted images (Fig. 39–5). A greater emphasis, however, has been placed on the detection of internal derangement of the disc, and MR imaging has surpassed CT as the noninvasive imaging method used in most institutions.

### Magnetic Resonance Imaging

For TMJ imaging, the sagittal plane has been emphasized. Images obtained in the coronal plane, however, may provide greater accuracy than sagittal MR images alone for diagnosing discs that are displaced mainly medial or lateral to the condyle—an unusual occurrence. Documenting the position of the disc and the status of the osseous structures of the TMJ can be done well with T1-weighted spin echo MR images alone. Identifying fluid or masses within the joint or in the muscles of mastication about the joint requires the use of some type of T2 weighting, especially in the setting of trauma as opposed to routine internal derangements. Fast gradient echo imaging is useful for demonstrating the TMJ in different phases of mouth opening. For the evaluation of routine internal derangements of the TMJ, two sets of sagittal T1-weighted images (one with the mouth closed and the other with the mouth completely open) constitute a standard approach. In the final analysis, however, optimized MR imaging is the leading noninvasive method for determining disc location (Fig. 39–6).

### DISORDERS

Disorders of the TMJ region can be divided into two general categories: extracapsular and intracapsular (Table

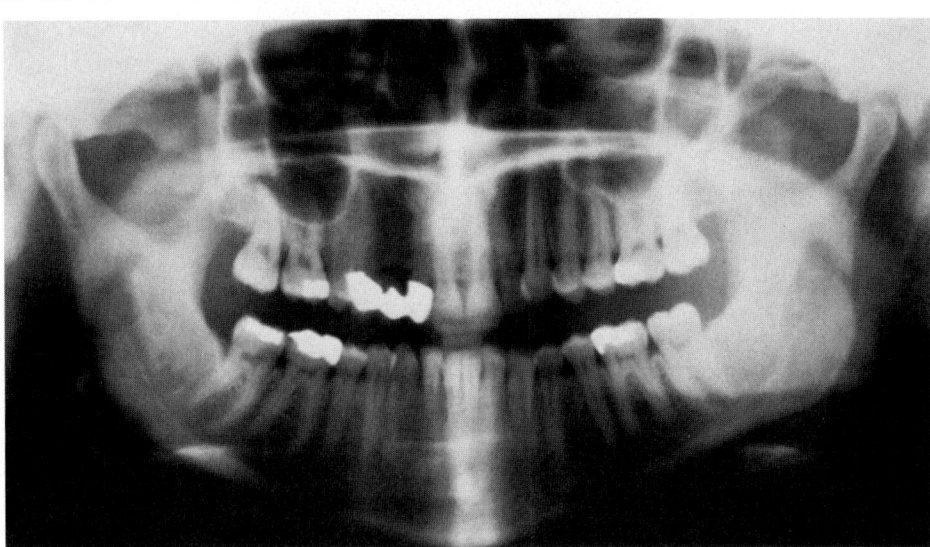

**Figure 39–4.** Panoramic radiograph shows the mandible, dental structures, and temporomandibular joints (TMJs) in a single image—a useful survey for dental or periarticular disease that might manifest as TMJ pain.

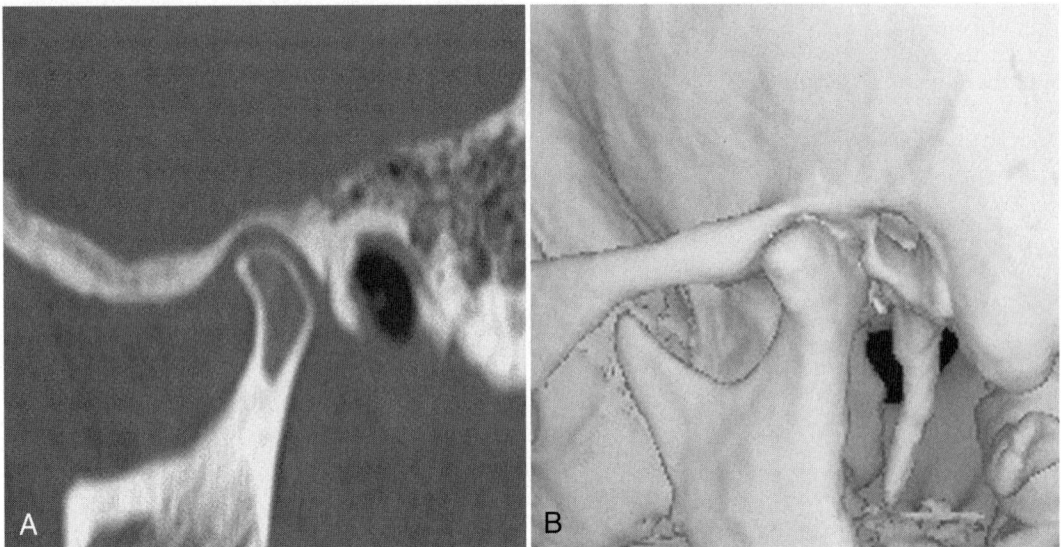

**Figure 39–5.** CT scan of the temporomandibular joint (TMJ). *A*, Reformatted sagittal image of the TMJ displayed at bone window shows the normal anatomy. *B*, Corresponding surface-rendering three-dimensional CT image.

39–1). Both groups of conditions can produce similar symptoms, including pain, the sensation of various noises, and decreased or uncoordinated range of motion.

Extracapsular disorders are seen frequently by clinicians and are often classified as myofascial pain-dysfunction syndrome. Affected patients often complain of some combination of neck and masticatory muscle pain, headache, joint noise, tinnitus, malocclusion, deviation of the mandible, loss of motion, and stress or anxiety. In these extracapsular conditions, the intraoral structures and masticatory muscles may be abnormal on physical examination, but examination of the TMJ is unremarkable. Likewise, the results of radiography, arthrography, and sectional imaging are normal.

Intracapsular disorders may also exhibit similar combinations of symptoms. The physical examination, how-

ever, is more likely to reveal one or more abnormalities, and the imaging workup should disclose a structural or functional abnormality. The combination of symptoms, signs, and imaging findings is usually sufficiently characteristic to allow a specific diagnosis.

## Congenital or Developmental Disorders

Congenital TMJ disturbances generally relate to developmental abnormalities of the first branchial arch and result in agenesis, hypoplasia, or hyperplasia of the mandible. The defects may be focal, diffuse, unilateral, or bilateral. Conventional or panoramic radiographic imaging usually allows the identification of these congenital or developmental conditions and demonstrates features useful for their classification.

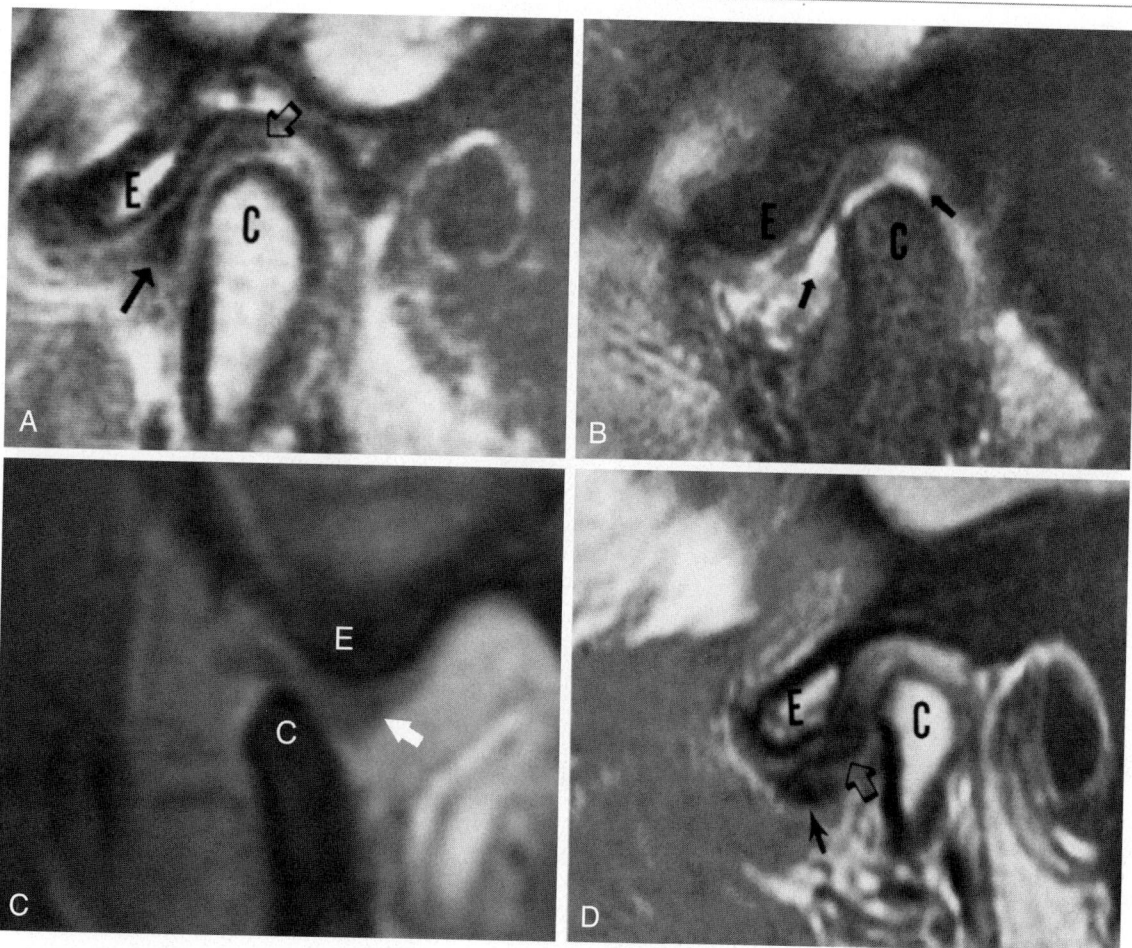

**Figure 39–6.** MR imaging of the temporomandibular joint (TMJ). *A*, T1-weighted sagittal spin echo MR image of a normal TMJ. View with the mouth closed shows high signal intensity from the condylar marrow (C) and articular eminence (E). Surrounding cortical bone is devoid of signal. The disc, of low signal intensity, is interposed between the condyle and the fossa; the intermediate zone articulates with the condyle and eminence where they are most closely apposed. The *solid arrow* points to the anterior band and the *open arrow* to the posterior band of the disc. *B*, Sagittal gradient echo MR image used for fast (pseudodynamic) scanning shows a normal position of the disc with the mouth closed. Marrow becomes low in signal intensity with this sequence, and fluid in the inferior joint space becomes bright *(arrows)*; the disc remains low in signal intensity. C, condyle; E, eminence. *C*, Sagittal gradient image of a normal TMJ with the mouth open. The intermediate zone of the disc maintains its position between the condyle (C) and the eminence (E), whereas the posterior band slides posterior to the condyle *(arrow)*. *D*, T1-weighted sagittal spin echo MR image in a patient with clicking and pain demonstrates internal derangement, with both the anterior *(solid arrow)* and posterior *(open arrow)* bands of the disc displaced anteriorly relative to the condyle (C).

## Tumors and Tumor-Like Disorders

Tumors of the TMJ are rare, although many types of bone or joint neoplasms have been described in this location. Most often, the joint is affected secondarily by extension of a mandibular neoplasm, such as osteosarcoma or metastasis. Intra-articular tumor-like processes include osteocartilaginous bodies, synovial (osteo)chondromatosis (Fig. 39–7), and pigmented villonodular synovitis.

## Traumatic Disorders

Injury to the mandible or a direct blow to the TMJ is a common cause of TMJ pain and dysfunction. The trauma may result in soft tissue injury, fracture, or some combination of soft tissue, bone, and joint injury. Evaluation of the effect of trauma to this region must include an analysis of the mandible, the dental occlusion, and the TMJ. Because of the complex anatomy of the mandible and its articulations, CT scanning is an important diagnostic method for the analysis of mandibular and TMJ trauma. It shows both soft tissue and osseous anatomy and can display complicated fractures and the location of fragments better than other studies can. The mandible is a ringlike structure; therefore, when one fracture is discovered, another mandibular fracture should be sought. A common combination is a condylar fracture associated with a body or ramus fracture. Multiple fractures (more than two) are often associated with facial fractures. When force is applied directly to the chin and the mandible does not fracture, the energy may be dissipated into the TMJ.

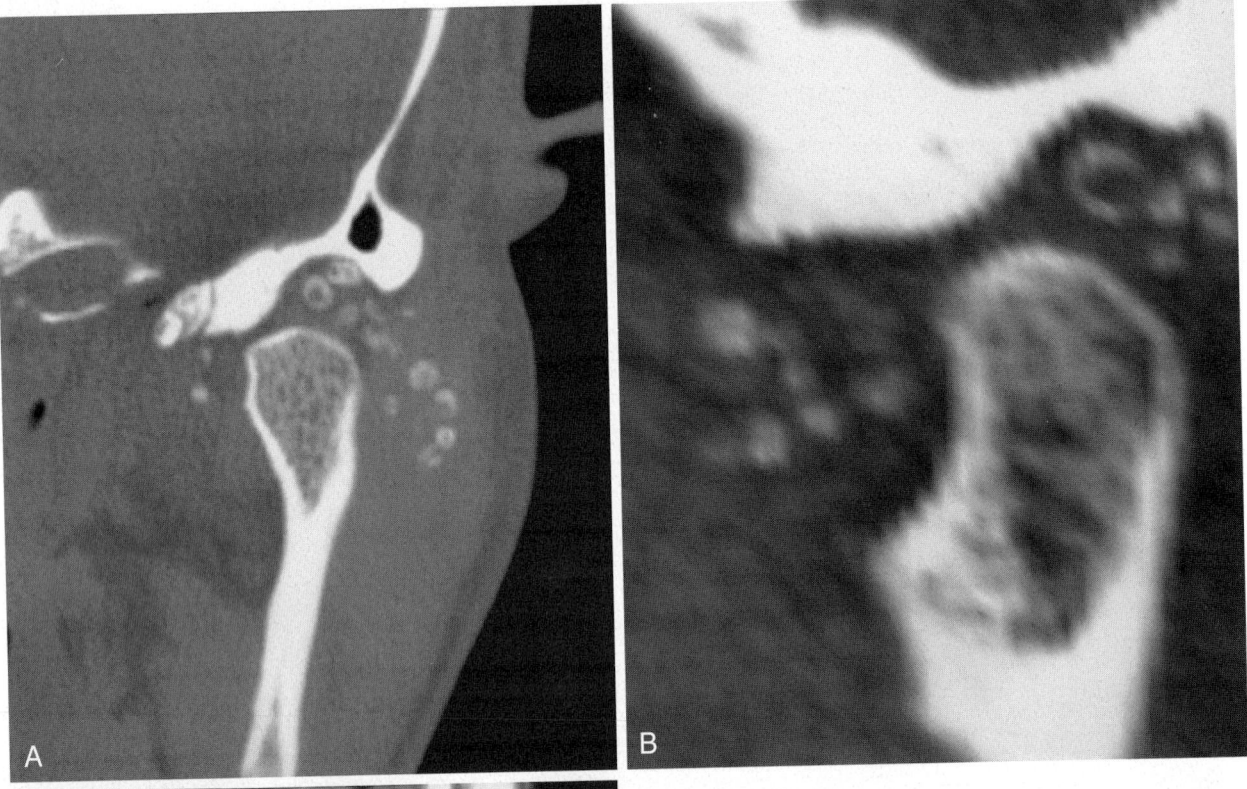

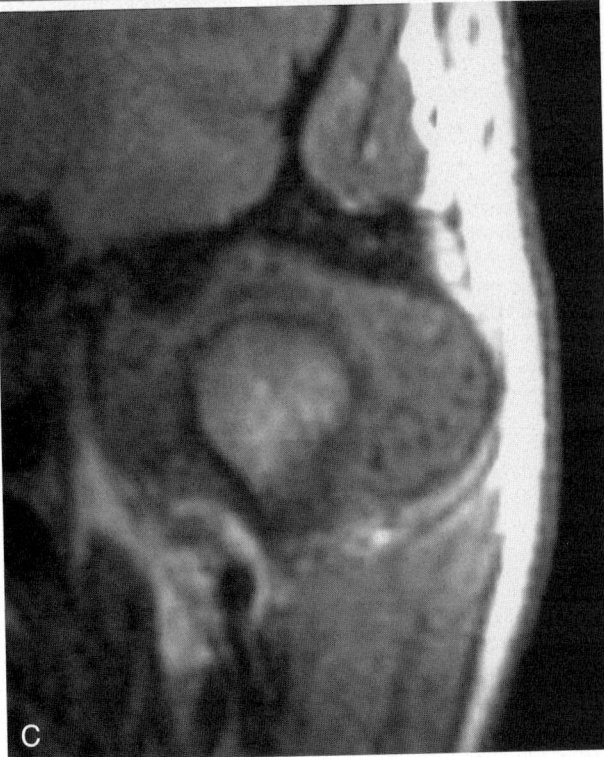

**Figure 39–7.** Idiopathic synovial (osteo)chondromatosis of the temporomandibular joint. Coronal *(A)* and sagittal reformatted *(B)* CT scans show the typical appearance of the lesion, which is characterized by ossified foci of similar size scattered throughout the joint. Coronal T1-weighted (TE/TR, 400/20) spin echo MR image *(C)* shows these foci to be of low signal intensity. (Courtesy of P. Kindynis, MD, Geneva, Switzerland.)

Fractures of the mandible are classified according to their anatomic location, which includes the condylar head, condylar neck, coronoid process, and mandibular ramus, angle, body, and symphysis (Fig. 39–8). Condylar fractures are subdivided according to their intracapsular or extracapsular location, displacement at the fracture site, and position of the condylar head with respect to the mandibular fossa of the temporal bone (Table 39–2). Intracapsular fractures of the condylar head are infrequent. Extracapsular condylar neck fractures may be nondisplaced or displaced, and the condylar head may remain in the mandibular fossa or be dislocated (Fig. 39–9).

| **TABLE 39–1** |
| --- |

**Alderman's Classification of Temporomandibular Joint Disorders**

**Extracapsular Disorders**

*Psychophysiologic:* tension, anxiety, oral habits

*Iatrogenic:* misdirected mandibular nerve block, excessive depression of the mandible during anesthesia or oral procedures

*Traumatic:* blow to face not involving fracture

*Dental:* occlusal abnormalities; periapical or periodontal lesions; mobile, sensitive, or damaged teeth; ulcerations

*Infectious:* secondary, outside the joint

*Otologic:* otitis media or external ear infection

*Neoplastic:* parotid gland, nasopharyngeal tumor

**Intracapsular Disorders**

*Congenital:* agenesis, hyperplastic or hypoplastic condyle

*Infectious:* primary bacterial infection within the joint

*Arthritic:* rheumatoid arthritis, osteoarthritis, psoriatic arthritis, juvenile chronic arthritis

*Traumatic:* fracture, disc tear

*Functional:* subluxation, dislocation, disc derangement, hypermobility, ankylosis

*Neoplastic:* benign or malignant tumor

---

Complications of mandibular fractures include loss of teeth, malunion or nonunion, displacement with deformity, and infection. Secondary complications of trauma are often more severe. The two major secondary complications are malocclusion and TMJ internal derangement, both of which result in pain and malfunction.

## Infectious Disorders

Pyogenic or granulomatous infections of the TMJ are uncommon. They may occur as a result of hematogenous seeding from a distant infection, but more commonly they develop as a direct extension of oral infections or after TMJ surgery. The radiographic findings are similar to those of rheumatoid arthritis, but the clinical course is much more rapid (Fig. 39–10). The history and physical examination should suggest the diagnosis.

## Articular Disorders

TMJ arthritis is a common problem. Many patients have osteoarthritis, usually secondary to internal derangement of the disc. Although it is very rare, calcium pyrophosphate dihydrate crystal deposition or gout may occur in the TMJ.

Rheumatoid arthritis, juvenile chronic arthritis, psoriatic arthritis, ankylosing spondylitis, and systemic lupus erythematosus may all affect the TMJ. All may show a spectrum of radiographic changes, including osteopenia, joint space narrowing, and bone erosion or production (Fig. 39–11).

Osteoarthritis of the TMJ is generally similar in radiographic appearance to osteoarthritis of other joints. Joint space narrowing, bone erosion, osteosclerosis, osteophytosis, and remodeling are seen (Figs. 39–12 and 39–13). Cartilage loss may be the predominant feature. Osteophytes may vary in size from small to large, and they typically develop at the margins of the articular surface. The degree of bone sclerosis and remodeling can be very pronounced. Even with advanced osteoarthritis, a remarkable range of joint mobility may be retained.

It is now well recognized that TMJ osteoarthritis often follows the development of an internal derangement. At least 20% of patients with internal derangement have osteoarthritis at the time of the initial clinical examination. The frequency of osteoarthritis seems to increase with increasing duration of internal derangement. Osteoarthritis is closely associated with disc dislocation, joint locking, disc perforation, and disc fragmentation.

## Internal Derangement

Internal derangement is the most frequent disorder of the TMJ. It is defined as an abnormal relationship of the disc relative to the condyle, fossa, and articular eminence. The disc is usually displaced anteriorly, but infrequently, it may be displaced lateral, medial, or posterior to the

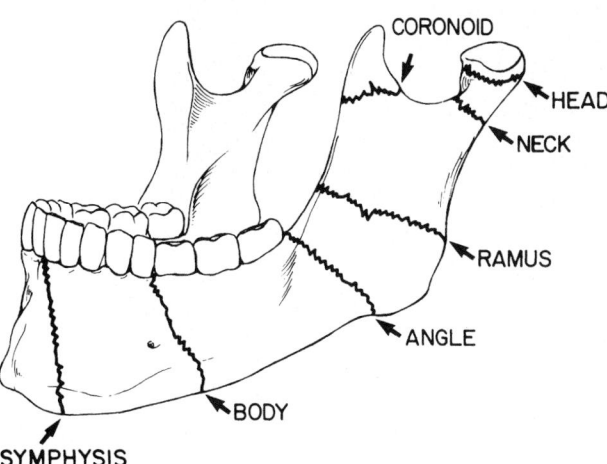

**Figure 39–8.** Diagram shows the location of various mandibular fractures.

| **TABLE 39–2** |
| --- |

**Fractures of the Mandibular Condyle**

I. Intracapsular head fracture
  A. Nondisplaced
  B. Displaced
II. Extracapsular neck fracture
  A. Nondisplaced
  B. Displaced—head not dislocated
  C. Displaced—head dislocated
III. Extracapsular subcondylar fracture
  A. Nondisplaced
  B. Displaced

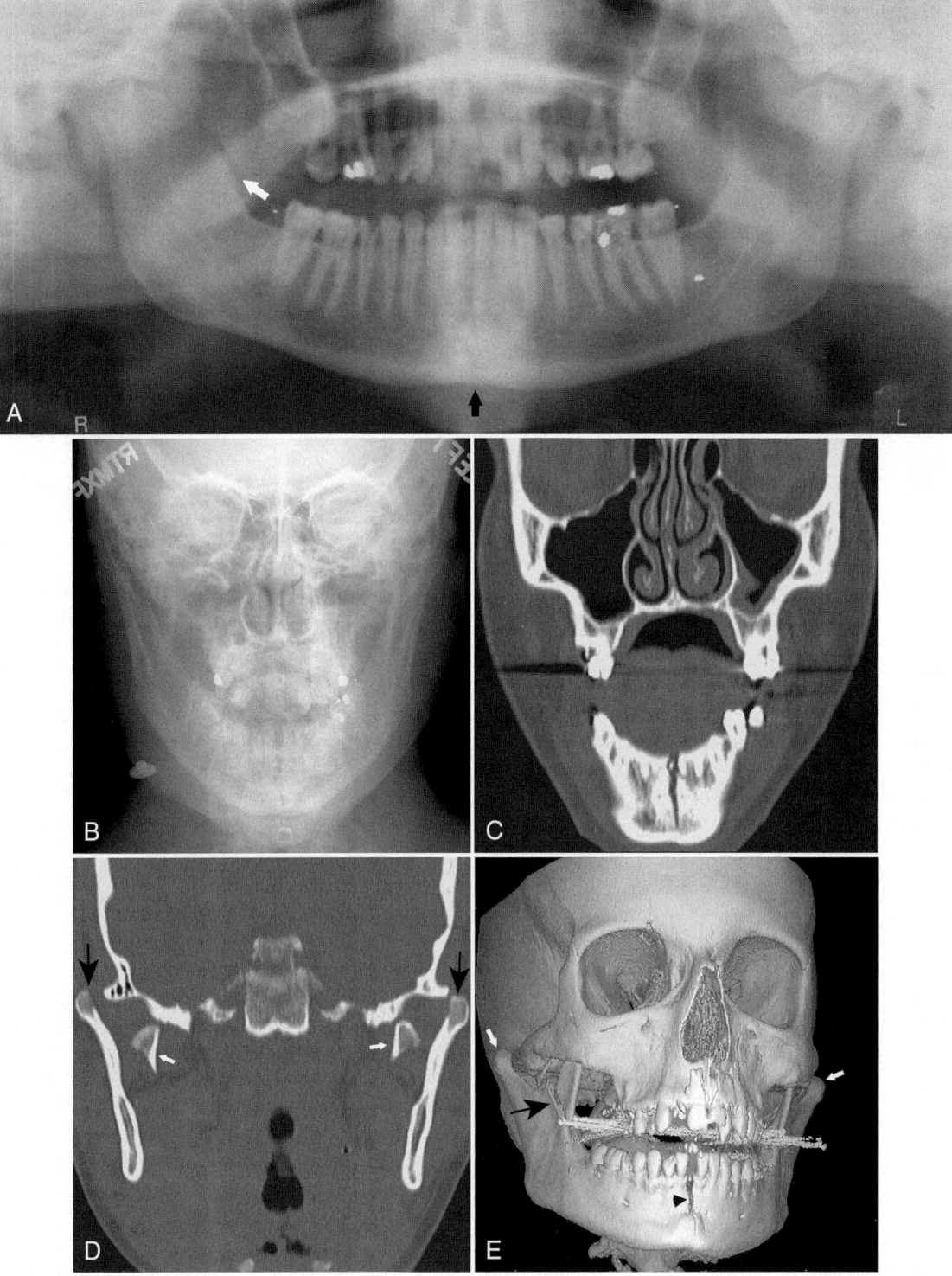

**Figure 39–9.** Multiple mandibular fractures in a 23-year-old woman following a fall. *A,* Panoramic radiograph shows fracture of the symphysis *(black arrow)* and right coronoid process *(white arrow)*. Fractures of both condylar necks with dislocation of both condylar heads are not well seen. *B,* Anteroposterior radiograph shows symphysis and right coronoid fractures. Neck fractures are not as visible, *C,* Reformatted coronal CT scan through the anterior mandible shows the symphysis fracture to better advantage. *D,* Reformatted coronal CT scan through the condyles shows fractures of both condyles, with medial displacement of the displaced fragments *(white arrows)*. Remaining condylar heads are dislocated laterally *(black arrows)*. *E,* Reformatted three-dimensional image shows the fractures of the symphysis *(black arrowhead)* and coronoid *(black arrow)* to better advantage. The lateral displacement of the condylar heads *(white arrows)* is also well seen.

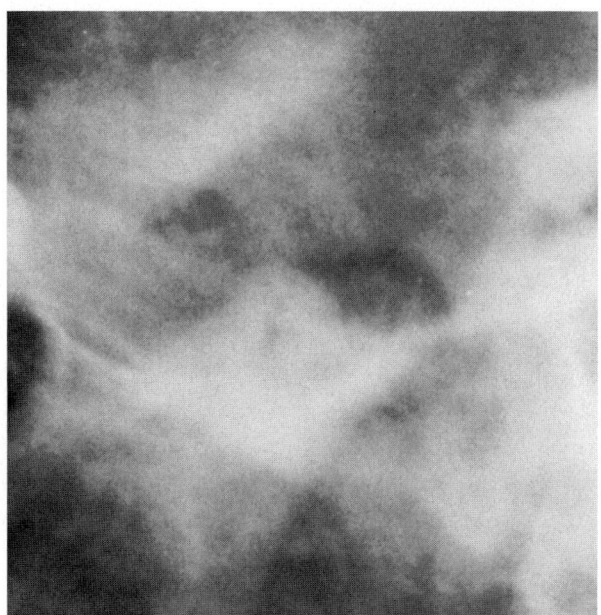

**Figure 39–10.** Pyogenic infection has destroyed the condylar head in this 60-year-old man.

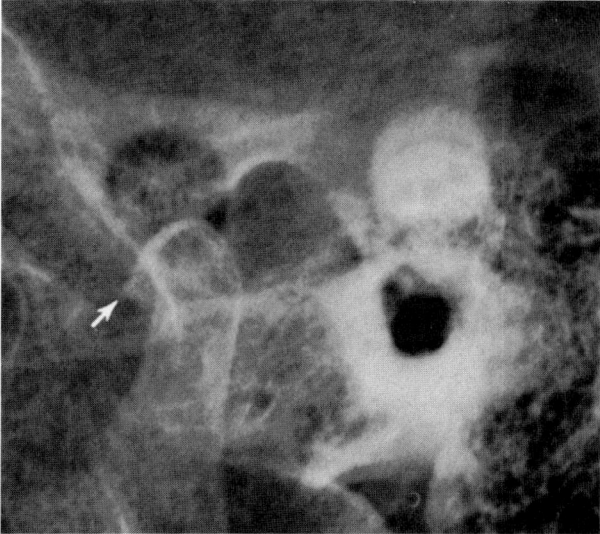

**Figure 39–12.** Osteoarthritis in a 64-year-old woman. With the temporomandibular joint in the open-mouth position, a single small osteophyte *(arrow)* is shown at the anterior margin of the condylar head.

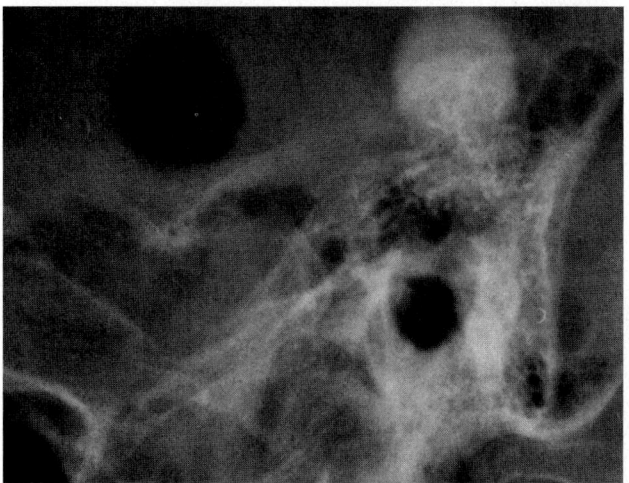

**Figure 39–11.** Seropositive rheumatoid arthritis in a 46-year-old woman. The joint space is very narrow, periarticular osteopenia is advanced, and bone erosions are large and diffuse.

condyle. Although estimates of prevalence vary, most investigators agree that between 20% and 30% of the adult population has signs and symptoms of TMJ internal derangement. Surprisingly, many adolescents have functional disturbances. Women are clinically affected three to five times more frequently than men. The average age at diagnosis in both men and women is in the fourth decade of life.

Knowledge of the dynamic functioning of the TMJ and the position of the disc in different phases of mouth opening is critical for the proper interpretation of imaging studies (Fig. 39–14). Disc position with the mouth closed is classically described as the position of the posterior band with respect to the condyle. The posterior band should lie directly on top of the condyle, or the posterior margin of the band should lie within 10 degrees of the 12 o'clock position on the condyle. Deformation of the inferior joint space during the initial phase of mouth opening allows the condyle to rotate on the disc with a hinge action. Subsequently, the condyle translates anteriorly as a result of deformation of the superior joint space. As the mouth opens and the condyle translates anteriorly under or slightly beyond the eminence, a smooth and coordinated relationship takes place among the disc, condyle, and eminence. The posterior band comes to lie posterior to the condyle with mouth opening (Fig. 39–15). As the mouth closes, the relationships reverse, and the disc is pulled posteriorly by recoil of the elastic posterior attachment.

Internal derangements are attributable primarily to ligamentous laxity (Fig. 39–16). The mildest form of derangement is anterior displacement of the disc and reduction to a normal position with mouth opening. The disc redislocates with mouth closing, and mouth opening is not limited. The second category of derangement occurs when the disc is displaced anteriorly but does not reduce to normal position with mouth opening. The final category is a displaced disc that does not reduce to normal position with mouth opening and in which a perforation occurs, either through the posterior attachment or, less commonly, through the disc itself. The displaced disc is an anatomic impediment to normal function. It results in irregular, hesitant, jerky, deviant, or limited joint movement. Such joint movement is clinically characterized as a click or lock.

A click is a friction event that occurs when the disc and the condyle move in opposite directions momentarily as the disc is pinched between the condyle and the eminence. Clicks are a result of disc malposition that places the thick posterior band anterior to the condyle

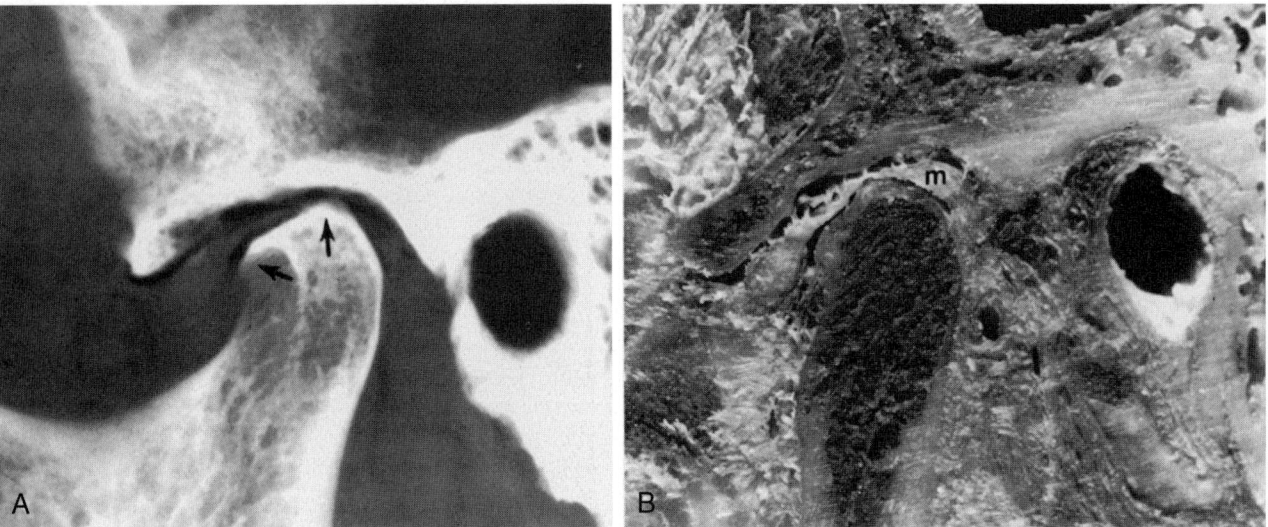

**Figure 39–13.** Osteoarthritis compared in a radiograph *(A)* and photograph *(B)* of a sagittally sectioned specimen. The joint space is narrow, and the disc is dislocated anteriorly, with thinning and fraying of the meniscal (m) posterior attachment or bilaminar zone. The condylar head cortex is thickened, with small osteophytes *(arrows)*. The mandibular fossa is sclerotic and remodeled, and only a shallow concavity is seen where the articular eminence once was.

(Fig. 39–17). During mouth opening, the posterior band moves posteriorly instantaneously, thereby producing an opening click and reducing the dislocation. During closure, the posterior band moves anteriorly, thereby producing a closing click instantaneously and resulting in redislocation of the disc. The phenomenon of combined opening and closing clicks is termed reciprocal clicking.

Locking is the result of a dislocated disc that will not reduce. An acute lock is generally painful and associated with very limited function (Fig. 39–18). With time, the bilaminar zone (retrodiscal tissue) usually stretches, such that pain diminishes and considerable range of motion is regained (Fig. 39–19).

The value of radiographs for diagnosing internal derangement is limited. The abnormalities that may be

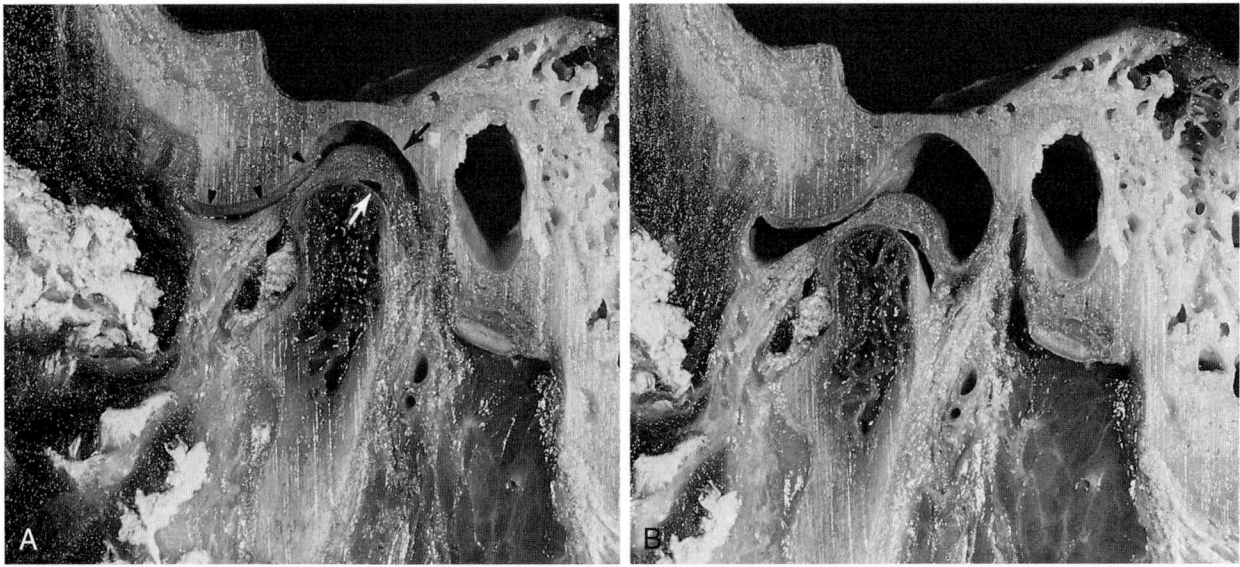

**Figure 39–14.** Functional anatomy of the temporomandibular joint. *A,* Sagittal section of a fresh specimen in a slightly open-mouth position shows posterior sulci *(arrows)* beginning to open. Articular cartilage *(arrowheads)* covers the articular eminence. Note that the posterior band of the disc is at the 12 o'clock position. *B,* In the intermediate open-mouth position, the posterior and anterior superior sulci are open. Note that the thin region of the disc stays between the articular surfaces and that changes in joint shape are primarily a result of changes in the soft tissues about the sulci. Also note that translation is related primarily to motion of the disc and condyle with respect to the eminence.

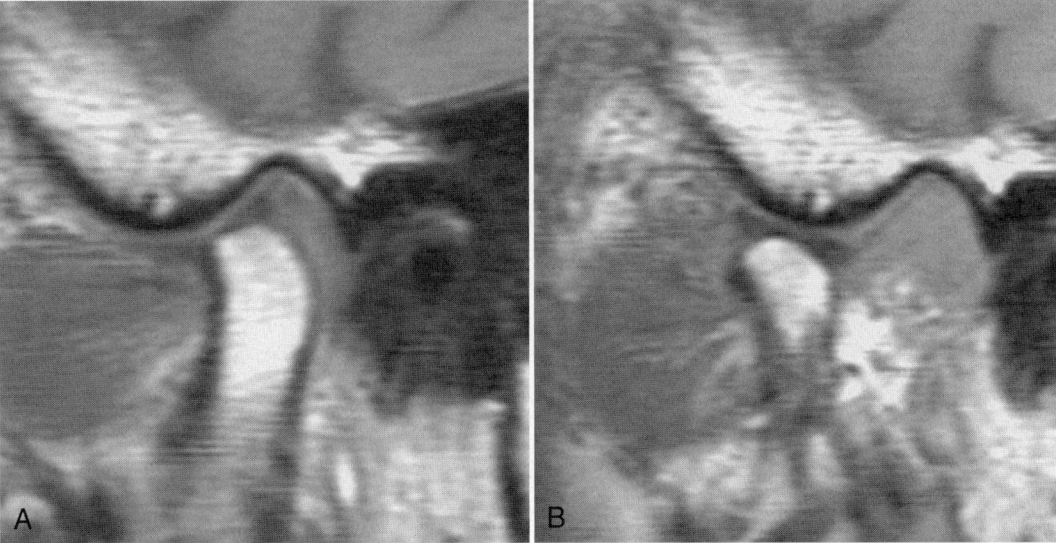

**Figure 39–15.** MR imaging of the normal temporomandibular joint (TMJ). *A,* T1-weighted sagittal spin echo MR image of a normal TMJ. View with the mouth closed shows high signal intensity from the condylar marrow and articular eminence. Surrounding cortical bone is devoid of signal. The disc, of low signal intensity, is interposed between the condyle and the fossa; the intermediate zone articulates with the condyle and eminence where they are most closely apposed. *B,* Sagittal T1-weighted image shows a normal position of the disc with the mouth open. The intermediate zone of the disc maintains its position between the condyle and the eminence, whereas the posterior band slides posterior to the condyle. Note translation of the condyle to the apex of the eminence.

seen are often nonspecific and occur late in the disease process. High-resolution CT with reformatted sagittal and coronal images is the ideal method for evaluating the morphologic osseous abnormalities. Owing to its non-invasive nature, MR imaging is the preferred modality for diagnosing internal derangements, and it is ideal for

demonstrating marrow abnormalities. The sagittal plane is most useful in this assessment, although coronal MR images are often included. Imaging is performed with the mouth both open and closed. Disagreement exists, how-ever, about other specifics of MR imaging methodology, including the choice of spin echo or gradient echo

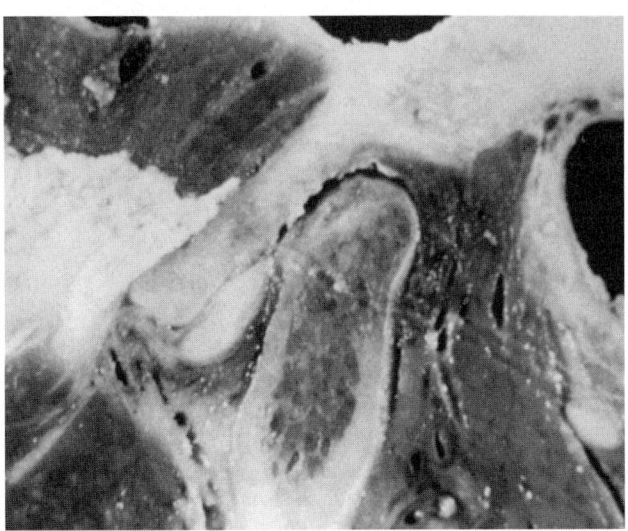

**Figure 39–16.** Sagittal section of a dislocated disc. The deformed disc is located anterior to the condyle. No tissue is interposed between the condyle and the mandibular fossa. Osteoarthritic alterations are present. (Courtesy of J. deGroot, PhD, San Francisco, Calif.)

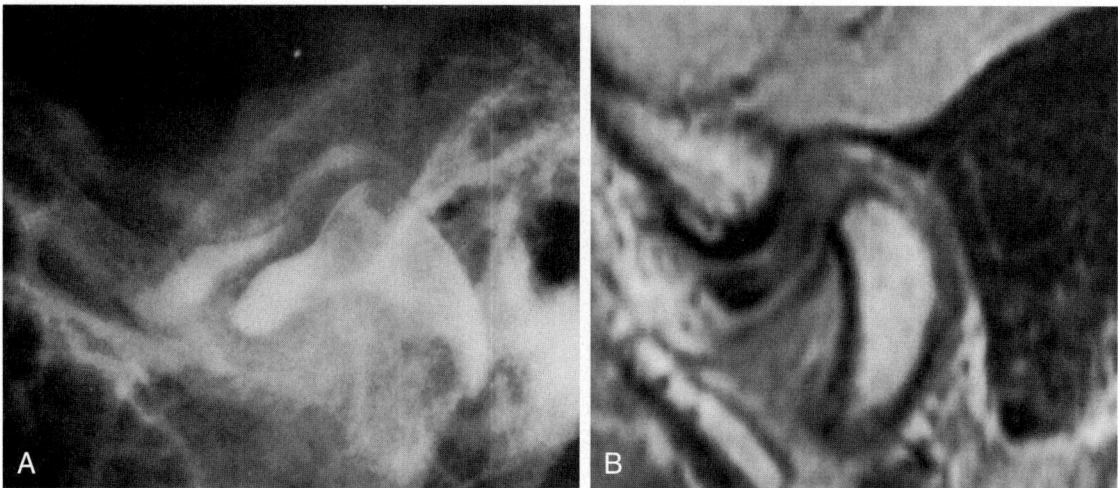

**Figure 39–17.** Anteriorly displaced disc. *A*, Bicompartment arthrogram shows a posterior band anterior to the condyle, which is creating a concave defect in the anterior recess. *B*, Sagittal T1-weighted spin echo MR image in a different patient with a biconcave disc dislocated anterior to the condyle with the mouth closed. Note the normal high signal intensity in the center of the anterior and posterior bands.

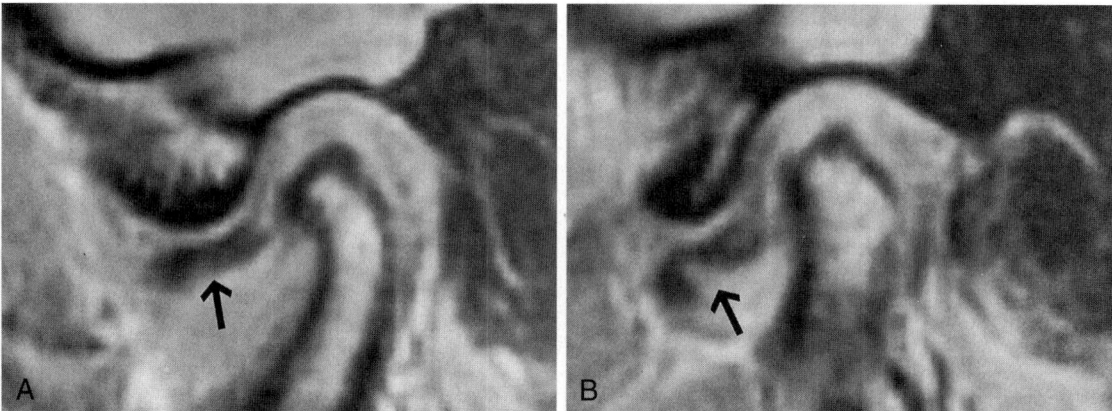

**Figure 39–18.** Acute temporomandibular joint lock from a nonreducing displaced disc. *A*, T1-weighted sagittal spin echo MR image with the mouth closed shows the dislocated disc *(arrow)* anterior to the condyle. *B*, With attempted mouth opening, no appreciable anterior translation of the condyle occurs, but the disc folds on itself in the thin intermediate zone because of increased pressure from the condyle. The normal biconcave configuration of the disc and the normal intradiscal signal intensity are maintained *(arrow)*.

sequences, or both, and whether intravenous contrast agents should be used.

A number of different techniques have been devised for the treatment of internal derangements, including splint therapy, arthroplasty with plication and repositioning of the disc, arthroscopy to distend the joint and break up adhesions, and disc removal with placement of either an alloplastic disc implant or some type of autograft. One complication of such TMJ surgery was a foreign body giant cell reaction to the alloplastic disc implants that were previously in use (Fig. 39–20).

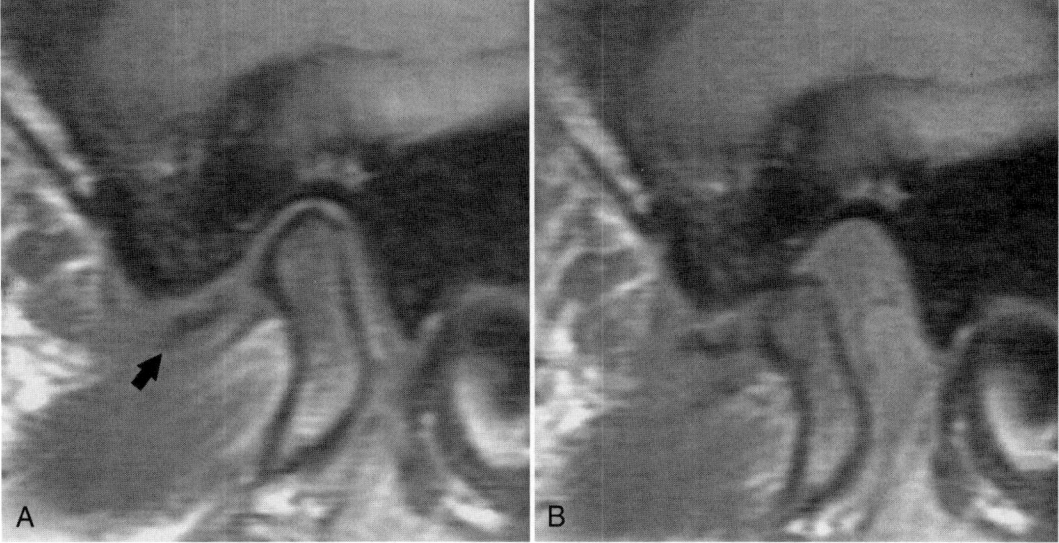

**Figure 39–19.** Nonreducing anteriorly displaced disc. *A*, T1-weighted sagittal spin echo MR image with the mouth closed shows a dislocated disc *(arrow)* anterior to the condyle. *B*, With mouth opening, the disc folds on itself and becomes crumbled. Anterior translation is somewhat reduced. Mild degenerative changes are noted with osteoarthritis.

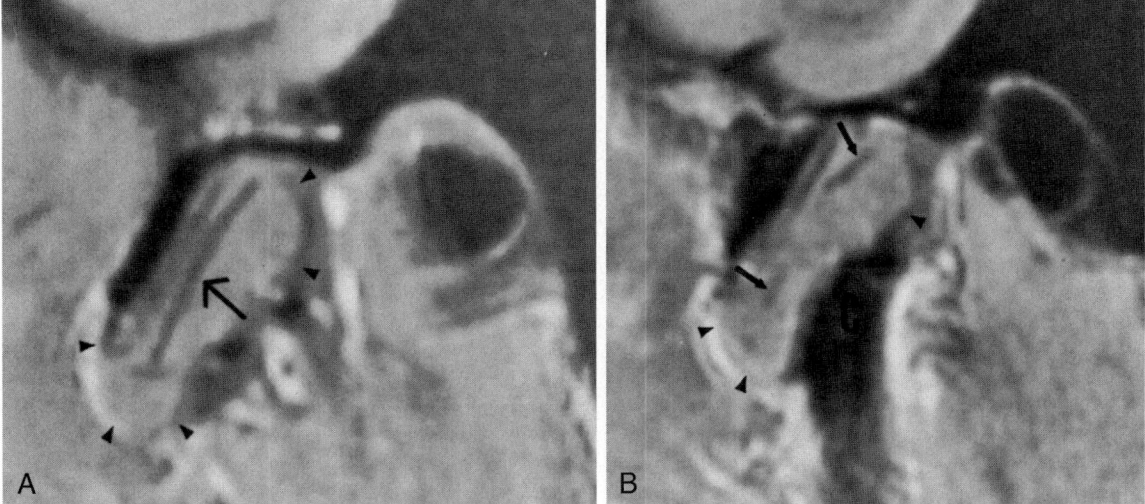

**Figure 39–20.** Foreign body reaction to an allograft disc implant. *A*, T1-weighted sagittal spin echo MR image of the temporomandibular joint in a patient with a thin, Proplast-Teflon disc implant of low signal intensity *(arrow)*. The condyle is not seen in the fossa, but a mass of granulation tissue of intermediate signal intensity surrounds the implant *(arrowheads)*. *B*, In the adjacent image, the implant is fragmented *(arrows)*, and the fossa is filled with a mass of granulation tissue *(arrowheads)* that has eroded the condyle. The remnant of the mandible is of low signal intensity where marrow fat (of high signal intensity) is normally seen.

## FURTHER READING

Abrahams JJ, Berger SB: Inflammatory disease of the jaw: Appearance on reformatted CT scans. AJR Am J Roentgenol 170:1085, 1998.

Conway WF, Hayes CW, Campbell RL, et al: Temporomandibular joint after meniscoplasty: Appearance at MR imaging. Radiology 180:749, 1991.

Helms CA, Morrish RB Jr, Kircos LT, et al: Computed tomography of the meniscus of the temporomandibular joint: Preliminary observations. Radiology 145:719, 1982.

Helms CA, Vogler JB III, Morrish RB Jr, et al: Temporomandibular joint internal derangements: CT diagnosis. Radiology 152:459, 1984.

Kaplan PA, Tu HK, Sleder PR, et al: Inferior joint space arthrography of normal temporomandibular joints: Reassessment of diagnostic criteria. Radiology 159:585, 1986.

Katzberg RW, Bessette RW, Tallents RH, et al: Normal and abnormal temporomandibular joint: MR imaging with surface coil. Radiology 158:183, 1986.

Katzberg RW, Keith DA, Guralnick WC, et al: Internal derangements and arthritis of the temporomandibular joint. Radiology 146:107, 1983.

Larheim TA, Westesson P-L, Sano T: Temporomandibular joint disk displacement: Comparison in asymptomatic volunteers and patients. Radiology 218:428, 2001.

Manco LG, Messing SG, Busino LJ, et al: Internal derangements of the temporomandibular joint evaluated with direct sagittal CT: A prospective study. Radiology 157:407, 1985.

Murphy WA: Arthrography of the temporomandibular joint. Radiol Clin North Am 19:365, 1981.

Murphy WA, Adams RJ, Gilula LA, et al: Magnification radiography of the temporomandibular joint: Technical considerations. Radiology 133:524, 1979.

Scholl RJ, Kellett HM, Neumann DP, et al: Cysts and cystic lesions of the mandible: Clinical and radiologic-histopathologic review. Radiographics 19:1107, 1999.

Suenaga S, Hamamoto S, Kawano K, et al: Dynamic MR imaging of the temporomandibular joint in patients with arthrosis: Relationship between contrast enhancement of the posterior disk attachment and joint pain. AJR Am J Roentgenol 166:1475, 1996.

Tasaki MM, Westesson PL: Temporomandibular joint: Diagnostic accuracy with sagittal and coronal MR imaging. Radiology 186:723, 1993.

Thompson JR, Christiansen E, Sauser D, et al: Dislocation of the temporomandibular joint meniscus: Contrast arthrography vs computed tomography. AJR Am J Roentgenol 144:171, 1985.

Updegrave WJ: Radiography of the temporomandibular joints. Semin Roentgenol 6:381, 1971.

Yune HY, Hall JR, Hutton CE, et al: Roentgenologic diagnosis in chronic temporomandibular joint dysfunction syndrome. AJR Am J Roentgenol 118:401, 1973.

# Target Approach to Articular Disease

# CHAPTER 40

## Target Area Approach to Articular Disorders: A Synopsis

### SUMMARY OF KEY FEATURES

The target area approach is a useful concept in the radiographic evaluation of articular diseases. The pattern of distribution of the lesions in each of the diseases is remarkably constant. Further, because this pattern varies from one disorder to the next, it may be used for accurate differential diagnosis in many cases.

### INTRODUCTION

An accurate radiographic diagnosis of joint disease is based on evaluation of two fundamental parameters: the morphology of the articular lesions and their distribution in the body. Morphologic characteristics vary among the disorders in response to the underlying pathologic aberrations. Equally important in the interpretation of the radiographs is an evaluation of the distribution of articular lesions. Certain disorders have a remarkable proclivity to affect specific joints (and regions of those joints), which is largely unexplained. Radiographic analysis of the distribution of articular lesions is termed the target area approach. The target area approach dictates locations that are predominantly involved in a disease process, not those that are involved exclusively. The pattern of distribution, when coupled with the morphology of the lesions, ensures a confident diagnosis in most patients with articular disease.

### HAND

The joints of the hand consist of the distal interphalangeal, proximal interphalangeal, and metacarpophalangeal joints of the second to fifth digits and the metacarpophalangeal and interphalangeal joints of the thumb.

### Rheumatoid Arthritis (Fig. 40–1)

Both hands are affected in a relatively symmetrical fashion. Major alterations appear in all five metacarpophalangeal joints, the proximal interphalangeal joints, and the interphalangeal joint of the thumb. Abnormalities in the distal interphalangeal joints are less frequent, are mild, and rarely occur in the absence of changes in more proximal locations. The earliest changes most frequently are apparent in the second and third metacarpophalangeal joints and the third proximal interphalangeal joint. Fusiform soft tissue swelling, regional osteoporosis, diffuse loss of interosseous space, and marginal and central bony erosions are the observed findings.

### Juvenile Chronic Arthritis (Fig. 40–2)

A symmetrical or asymmetrical distribution may be evident. Juvenile chronic arthritis can affect any joint of the hand, including the distal interphalangeal joints. The degree of osteoporosis, joint space narrowing, and osseous erosion is variable, and bony proliferation (periostitis and intra-articular fusion) may be a prominent finding.

### Ankylosing Spondylitis (Fig. 40–3)

Bilateral and asymmetrical findings predominate. Distal interphalangeal, proximal interphalangeal, and metacarpophalangeal joints as well as the interphalangeal joint of the thumb can be affected. Osteoporosis, joint space diminution, osseous erosions, and deformities are less striking in this disease than in rheumatoid arthritis. Osseous proliferation can be exuberant.

### Psoriatic Arthritis (see Fig. 40–3)

The distribution of this disease varies widely. Bilateral asymmetrical polyarticular changes are most characteristic, with a predilection for the interphalangeal joints.

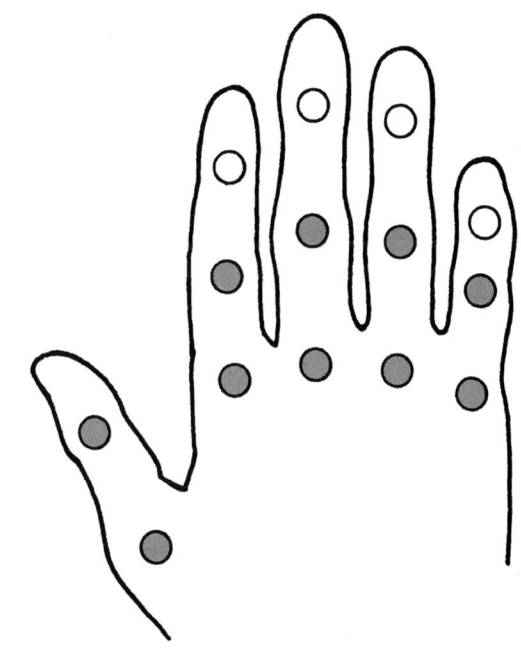

**Figure 40–1.** Rheumatoid arthritis.

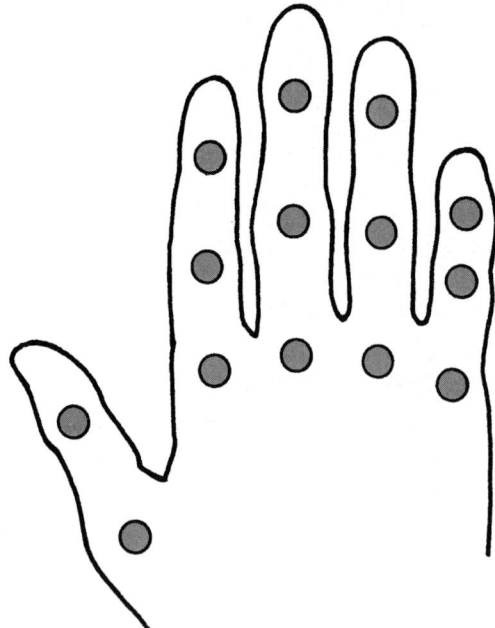

**Figure 40–2.** Juvenile chronic arthritis.

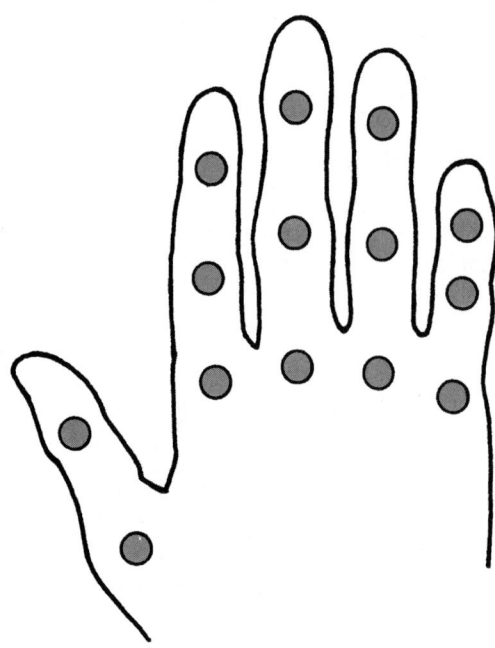

**Figure 40–3.** Ankylosing spondylitis, psoriatic arthritis, and Reiter's syndrome.

In many patients, the extent of distal interphalangeal joint abnormalities is striking. Osteoporosis may be absent and intra-articular osseous fusion and periarticular osseous excrescences can be evident, allowing differentiation from rheumatoid arthritis. Psoriatic arthritis may be accompanied by a raylike distribution in which one or two digits are involved extensively.

### Reiter's Syndrome (see Fig. 40–3)

Asymmetrical changes are most typical. Monoarticular or pauciarticular disease can affect any joint of the hand. Its features are virtually identical to those of psoriatic arthritis.

### Degenerative Joint Disease (Osteoarthritis) (Fig. 40–4)

Bilateral, symmetrical, or asymmetrical findings can be observed. Distal interphalangeal and proximal interphalangeal joints generally are affected to a greater degree than are metacarpophalangeal joints. Further, changes are rarely isolated to the metacarpophalangeal joints. In interphalangeal joints, loss of interosseous space, subchondral eburnation, marginal osteophytes, and small ossicles appear. Findings suggesting a disease other than osteoarthritis are marginal erosions in distal or proximal interphalangeal joints, or in both, and prominent osteophytes or erosions in metacarpophalangeal joints.

### Inflammatory (Erosive) Osteoarthritis (Fig. 40–5)

A bilateral, symmetrical, or asymmetrical distribution is encountered. Distal interphalangeal and proximal interphalangeal joint abnormalities predominate over metacarpophalangeal joint changes. The morphologic aspects of the alterations can be indistinguishable from those of noninflammatory osteoarthritis, although the presence of centrally located osseous defects in combination with osteophytosis allows this specific diagnosis to be made.

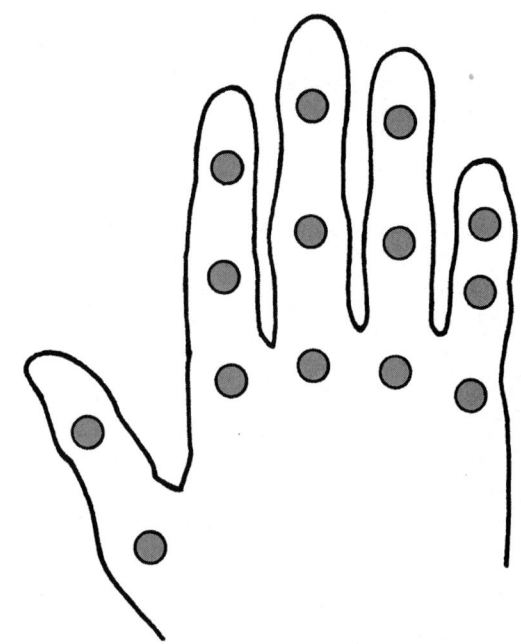

**Figure 40–4.** Degenerative joint disease (osteoarthritis).

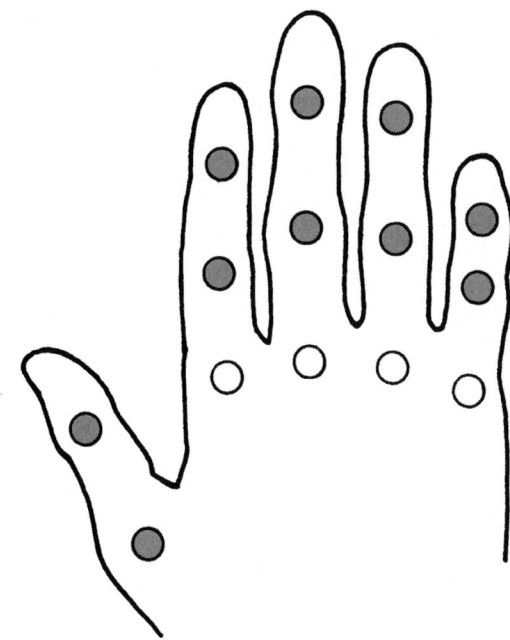

**Figure 40–5.** Inflammatory (erosive) osteoarthritis.

## Systemic Lupus Erythematosus (Fig. 40–6)

A deforming, nonerosive arthropathy with a bilateral and symmetrical distribution affecting metacarpophalangeal and interphalangeal joints of all of the digits, including the thumb, characterizes one type of joint abnormality in this disease. Osteonecrosis at one or more metacarpophalangeal joints is a second pattern of articular disease.

## Scleroderma and Polymyositis (Fig. 40–7)

A bilateral erosive arthritis showing a predilection for the distal interphalangeal and, to a lesser extent, the proximal interphalangeal joints has been observed in some patients with scleroderma. A similar pattern of joint disease rarely is encountered in patients with polymyositis. In both of these diseases, more characteristic findings, such as soft tissue calcification and tuftal resorption, usually are evident.

## Gouty Arthritis (Fig. 40–8)

A bilateral and asymmetrical process predominates. Changes may appear in distal interphalangeal, proximal interphalangeal, or metacarpophalangeal joints, consisting of lobulated soft tissue masses, eccentric intra- and extra-articular osseous erosions, preservation of joint space, proliferation of bone (overhanging edges), and lack of osteoporosis.

## Calcium Pyrophosphate Dihydrate Crystal Deposition Disease (Fig. 40–9)

Idiopathic calcium pyrophosphate dihydrate (CPPD) crystal deposition disease or that associated with hemochromatosis produces bilateral, relatively symmetrical changes that predominate at the metacarpophalangeal joints. In both disorders, changes are most frequent in the second and third metacarpophalangeal joints; in hemochromatosis, the fourth and fifth digits are involved more commonly than in idiopathic CPPD crystal deposition disease. Further, in hemochromatosis, beaklike osseous excrescences arising from the radial aspect of the metacarpal heads are distinctive.

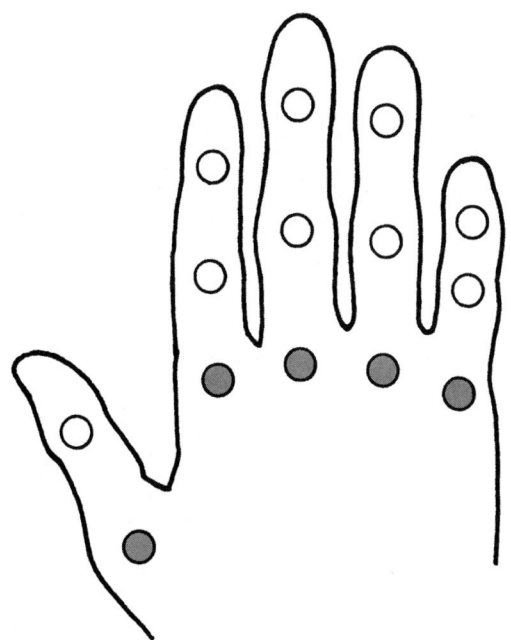

**Figure 40–6.** Systemic lupus erythematosus.

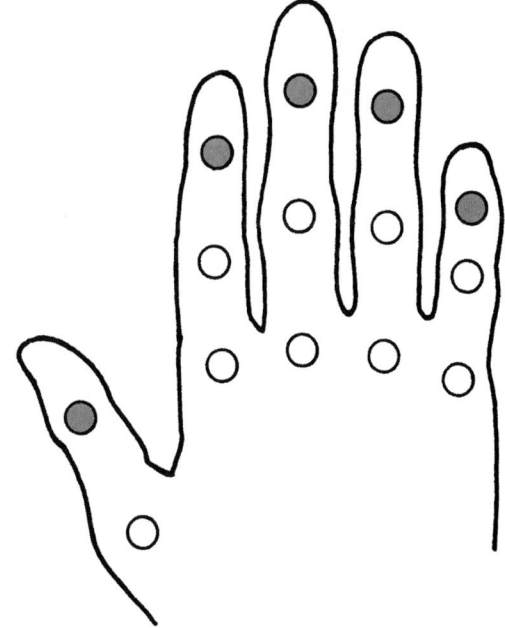

**Figure 40–7.** Scleroderma and polymyositis.

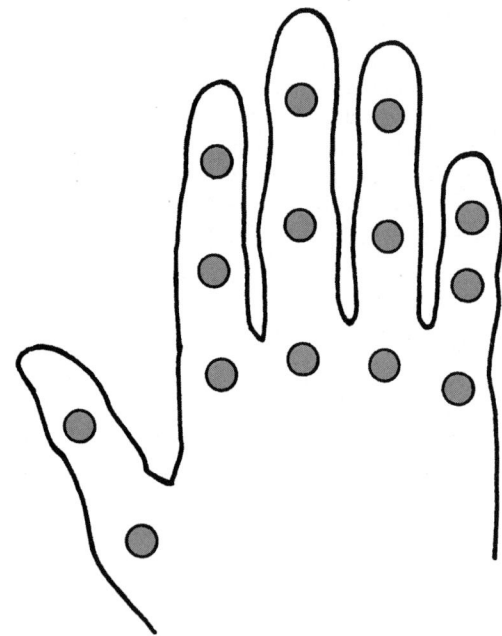

**Figure 40–8.** Gouty arthritis.

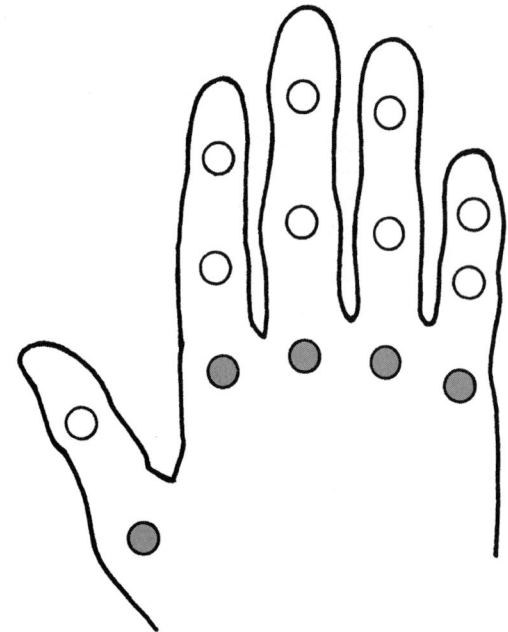

**Figure 40–9.** Calcium pyrophosphate dihydrate crystal deposition disease.

## Other Diseases

*Multicentric reticulohistiocytosis* can lead to significant abnormalities of both hands, which usually are most striking in the distal interphalangeal and, to a lesser extent, the proximal interphalangeal joints. *Thermal injuries*, including frostbite and burns, may produce alterations that also predominate in distal locations. In some cases, the joints of the thumb are spared in frostbite. *Hyperparathyroidism*

(and renal osteodystrophy) can lead to a peculiar "erosive" arthritis of the digits that affects distal interphalangeal, proximal interphalangeal, or metacarpophalangeal joints of both hands. In most cases, the changes are combined with subperiosteal resorption in the phalanges. In *rheumatic fever*, a deforming, nonerosive arthropathy (Jaccoud's arthropathy) predominates in the fourth and fifth digits. *Septic arthritis* of the metacarpophalangeal joints may follow a fistfight in which the fist is cut when it strikes the opponent's teeth. *Hydroxyapatite crystal deposition disease* leads to intra-articular and periarticular calcification in interphalangeal locations. *Wilson's disease* produces indistinct and irregular subchondral bone in the metacarpophalangeal and interphalangeal joints.

## WRIST

The major joints or compartments of the wrist are summarized in Table 40–1 and Figure 40–10.

### Rheumatoid Arthritis (Fig. 40–11)

A bilateral and symmetrical process usually is evident. Although initial abnormalities predominate in the radiocarpal, inferior radioulnar, and pisiform-triquetral compartments, all the compartments of the wrist become involved. Above all, this pancompartmental distribution is an important characteristic of the wrist involvement in rheumatoid arthritis.

### Juvenile Chronic Arthritis (Fig. 40–12)

The pattern of wrist involvement is variable. In some forms of juvenile chronic arthritis, all the carpal bones migrate toward the bases of the metacarpals, reflecting

### TABLE 40–1

**Major Compartments of the Wrist**

| Compartment | Location |
| --- | --- |
| Radiocarpal | Between the distal end of the radius and the proximal carpal row |
| Midcarpal | Between the distal and the proximal carpal rows |
| Common carpometacarpal | Between the distal carpal row and the bases of the four ulnar metacarpals |
| First carpometacarpal | Between the trapezium and the base of the first metacarpal |
| Inferior radioulnar | Between the distal ends of the radius and ulna, separated from the radiocarpal compartment by the triangular fibrocartilage of the wrist |
| Pisiform-triquetral | Between the pisiform and triquetrum |

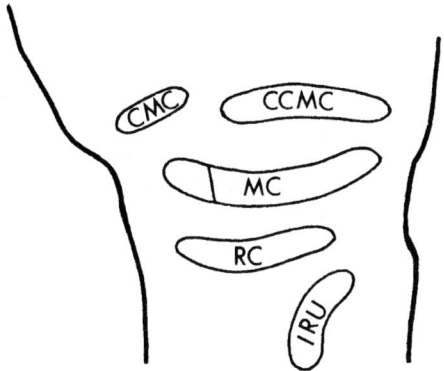

**Figure 40–10.** Joints of the wrist. The pisiform-triquetral compartment is not shown. The trapezioscaphoid region of the midcarpal joint is separated by a vertical line from the remainder of this joint. CCMC, common carpometacarpal compartment; CMC, first carpometacarpal compartment; IRU, inferior radioulnar compartment; MC, midcarpal compartment; RC, radiocarpal compartment.

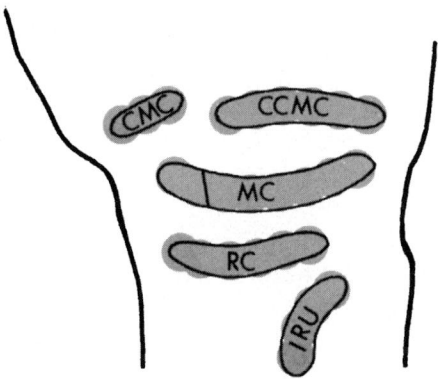

**Figure 40–11.** Rheumatoid arthritis. CCMC, common carpometacarpal compartment; CMC, first carpometacarpal compartment; IRU, inferior radioulnar compartment; MC, midcarpal compartment; RC, radiocarpal compartment.

joint space loss in the midcarpal and common carpometacarpal compartments. In fact, eventual osseous fusion of the proximal and distal carpal rows and bases of the four ulnar metacarpals may be seen, with relative sparing of the first carpometacarpal and radiocarpal compartments. A similar pattern of disease may be apparent in some patients with adult-onset Still's disease.

### Ankylosing Spondylitis, Psoriatic Arthritis, and Reiter's Syndrome (Fig. 40–13)

Asymmetrical findings in the wrist can appear during the course of any of these three disorders. Pancompartmental changes may be seen. Although similar to rheumatoid arthritis, these disorders are associated with less frequent and extensive wrist disease, the absence of osteoporosis, and the presence of poorly defined osseous excrescences or "whiskers."

### Degenerative Joint Disease (Osteoarthritis) (Fig. 40–14)

In the absence of significant accidental or occupational trauma, degenerative joint disease of the wrist is virtually limited to the first carpometacarpal and trapezioscaphoid areas. At the first carpometacarpal joint, radial subluxation of the metacarpal base may be evident, whereas at the trapezioscaphoid area of the midcarpal compartment, joint space narrowing and eburnation may be the only findings.

In the presence of occupational or accidental trauma, more widespread alterations of the wrist may be detected. Post-traumatic abnormalities eventually may become severe and widespread, leading to a pattern that is designated scapholunate advanced collapse (SLAC).

### Inflammatory (Erosive) Osteoarthritis (see Fig. 40–14)

Changes predominate at the first carpometacarpal and trapezioscaphoid areas, a distribution identical to that in

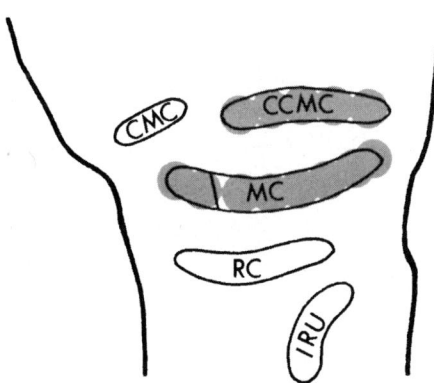

**Figure 40–12.** Juvenile chronic arthritis. CCMC, common carpometacarpal compartment; CMC, first carpometacarpal compartment; IRU, inferior radioulnar compartment; MC, midcarpal compartment; RC, radiocarpal compartment.

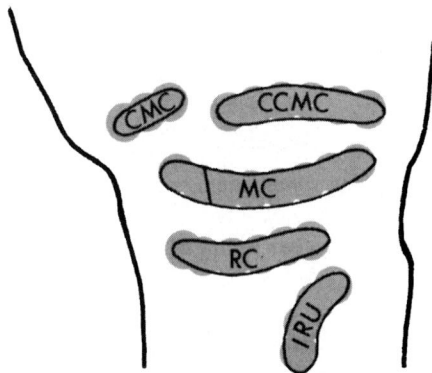

**Figure 40–13.** Ankylosing spondylitis, psoriatic arthritis, and Reiter's syndrome. CCMC, common carpometacarpal compartment; CMC, first carpometacarpal compartment; IRU, inferior radioulnar compartment; MC, midcarpal compartment; RC, radiocarpal compartment.

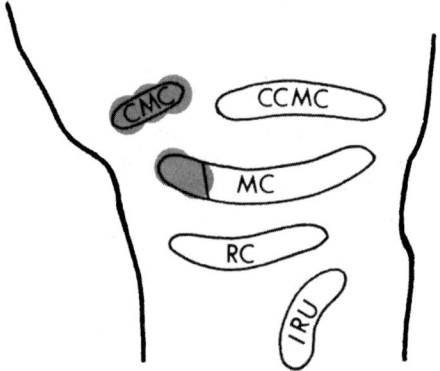

**Figure 40–14.** Degenerative joint disease (osteoarthritis) and inflammatory (erosive) osteoarthritis. CCMC, common carpometacarpal compartment; CMC, first carpometacarpal compartment; IRU, inferior radioulnar compartment; MC, midcarpal compartment; RC, radiocarpal compartment.

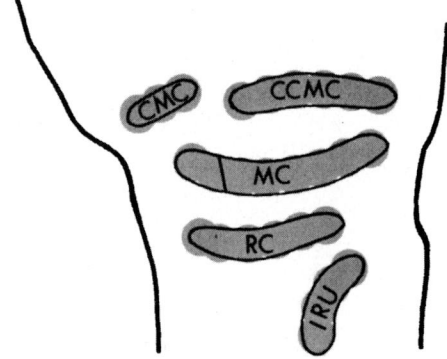

**Figure 40–16.** Gouty arthritis. CCMC, common carpometacarpal compartment; CMC, first carpometacarpal compartment; IRU, inferior radioulnar compartment; MC, midcarpal compartment; RC, radiocarpal compartment.

noninflammatory osteoarthritis. At these sites, joint space narrowing and eburnation predominate, although rarely, erosive abnormalities may be detected.

## Scleroderma (Fig. 40–15)

Selective involvement of one or both first carpometacarpal compartments may be noted in some patients with scleroderma. The changes consist of scalloped erosions of the base of the metacarpal and adjacent trapezium. Similar alterations of the first carpometacarpal joint may be encountered in systemic lupus erythematosus, polymyositis, and Ehlers-Danlos syndrome. In scleroderma, intraarticular and periarticular calcification frequently can be observed about the altered joint.

## Gouty Arthritis (Fig. 40–16)

In long-standing gouty arthritis, bilateral symmetrical or asymmetrical changes can be observed in the wrist. A pan-

compartmental distribution, similar to that in rheumatoid arthritis, may be apparent. Of diagnostic significance, the common carpometacarpal compartment may be the site of the most extensive abnormality in this disease. At this site, scalloped erosions of the bases of one or more of the four ulnar metacarpals are seen. Additional findings, such as the absence of osteoporosis and the presence of eccentric erosions with sclerotic margins, lobulated soft tissue masses, and preservation of joint space, also aid in the differentiation of gouty arthritis from rheumatoid arthritis.

## Calcium Pyrophosphate Dihydrate Crystal Deposition Disease (Fig. 40–17)

CPPD crystal deposition disease leads to bilateral symmetrical or asymmetrical changes that reveal a distinct predilection for the radiocarpal compartment of the wrist. At this site, extensive narrowing of the space between the distal portion of the radius and scaphoid may be seen. Elsewhere in the wrist, the trapezioscaphoid or lunate-

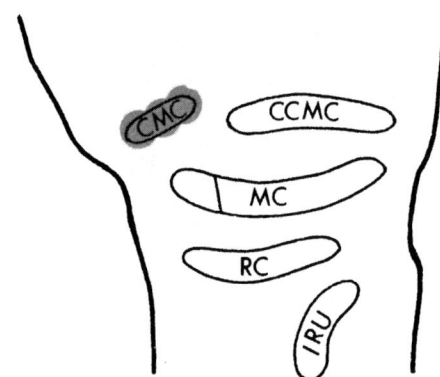

**Figure 40–15.** Scleroderma. CCMC, common carpometacarpal compartment; CMC, first carpometacarpal compartment; IRU, inferior radioulnar compartment; MC, midcarpal compartment; RC radiocarpal compartment.

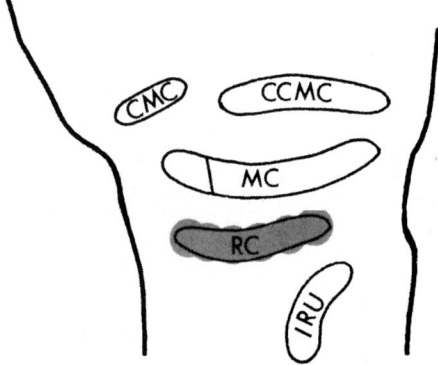

**Figure 40–17.** Calcium pyrophosphate dihydrate crystal deposition disease. CCMC, common carpometacarpal compartment; CMC, first carpometacarpal compartment; IRU, inferior radioulnar compartment; MC, midcarpal compartment; RC, radiocarpal compartment.

capitate area of the midcarpal compartment and the first carpometacarpal compartment may show severe involvement, and calcification about the distal portion of the ulna may be apparent.

## Other Diseases

*Septic arthritis* of the wrist leads to monoarticular disease. Although initially one compartment may be involved, pancompartmental disease is the rule in neglected infection. *Amyloidosis* also can affect one or both wrists. In this disease, localization to the inferior radioulnar compartment is not unusual. *Calcium hydroxyapatite crystal deposition disease* is associated with curvilinear calcification in the flexor carpi ulnaris tendon, adjacent to the pisiform.

## FOREFOOT

The joints of the forefoot include the distal interphalangeal, proximal interphalangeal, and metatarsophalangeal joints of the second to fifth digits and the interphalangeal and metatarsophalangeal joints of the great toe.

## Rheumatoid Arthritis (Fig. 40–18)

A bilateral and symmetrical process of the forefoot represents one of the earliest and most frequent radiographic findings in rheumatoid arthritis. Typically, the predominant changes occur at one or more metatarsophalangeal joints and the interphalangeal joint of the great toe. Significant involvement of the proximal interphalangeal and distal interphalangeal joints of the second to fifth toes is infrequent. At the metatarsophalangeal joints, abnormalities are most commonly encountered on the medial aspect of the metatarsal heads of the second to fourth digits and on the medial and lateral aspects of the metatarsal head of the fifth digit. At the interphalangeal joint of the great toe, a typical erosion appears on the medial aspect of the distal portion of the proximal phalanx.

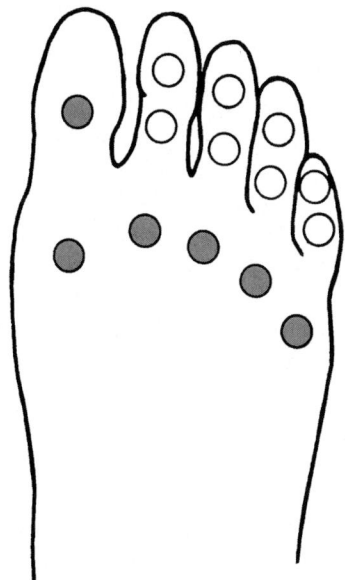

**Figure 40–18.** Rheumatoid arthritis.

## Ankylosing Spondylitis, Psoriatic Arthritis, and Reiter's Syndrome

(Figs. 40–19 and 40–20)

In ankylosing spondylitis, symmetrical or asymmetrical abnormalities may appear at the metatarsophalangeal joints and the interphalangeal joint of the great toe.

Psoriatic arthritis can be associated with a bilateral symmetrical or asymmetrical or unilateral process, with or without a raylike pattern, leading to considerable abnormalities of the forefoot. The most severe changes are commonly seen at the metatarsophalangeal joints and the interphalangeal joint of the great toe. At the latter site,

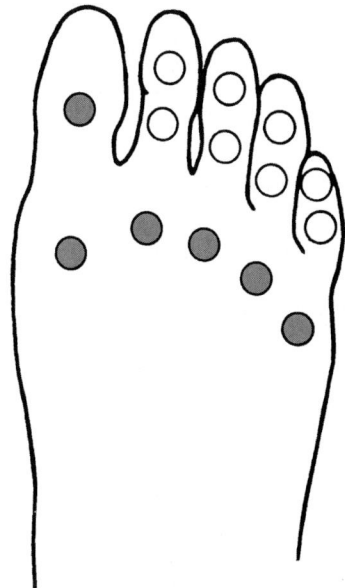

**Figure 40–19.** Ankylosing spondylitis.

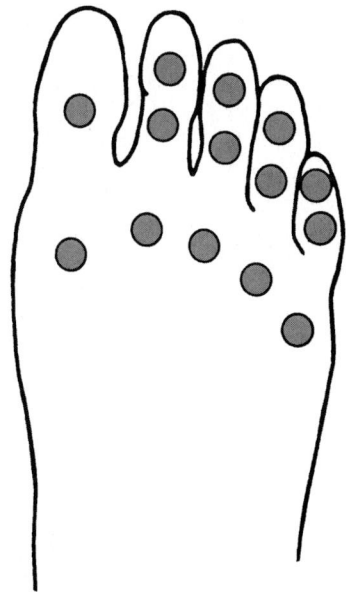

**Figure 40–20.** Psoriatic arthritis and Reiter's syndrome.

the degree of osseous destruction is greater in this disease than in any other articular disorder. Prominent erosions and intra-articular osseous fusion can be evident at other interphalangeal joints as well. In this fashion, the distribution of changes in psoriatic arthritis differs from that in rheumatoid arthritis.

Asymmetrical or unilateral abnormalities of the forefoot are frequent in Reiter's syndrome. Fewer joints are affected in this disorder than in rheumatoid arthritis or psoriatic arthritis. Any joint of the forefoot is a potential site of abnormality, however. Selective involvement of the interphalangeal joint of the great toe can be encountered, similar to that seen in psoriatic arthritis.

### Degenerative Joint Disease (Osteoarthritis)
(Fig. 40–21)

The first metatarsophalangeal joint is affected most frequently in degenerative joint disease. A unilateral or bilateral distribution may be evident, and changes include loss of interosseous space, eburnation, osteophytosis, and even hallux valgus deformity.

### Gouty Arthritis (Fig. 40–22)

Bilateral symmetrical or asymmetrical changes in gouty arthritis can appear in any joint of the forefoot. The characteristic distribution includes the first metatarsophalangeal joint and, to a lesser degree, the interphalangeal joint of the great toe. Prominent changes about other metatarsophalangeal and interphalangeal joints are not infrequent, however. At any involved site, a large soft tissue mass commonly indicates the presence of a tophus.

### Neuropathic Osteoarthropathy (Fig. 40–23)

Neuropathic joint disease, particularly in diabetic patients, frequently affects the forefoot in a bilateral distribution.

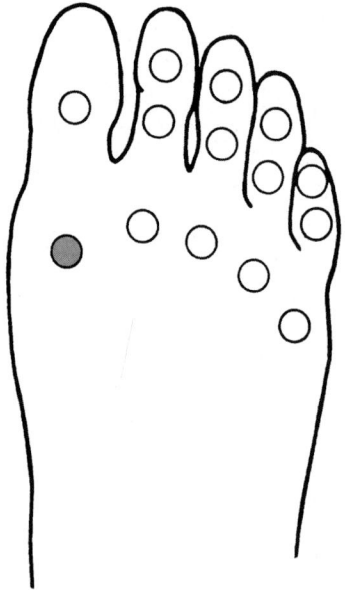

**Figure 40–21.** Degenerative joint disease (osteoarthritis).

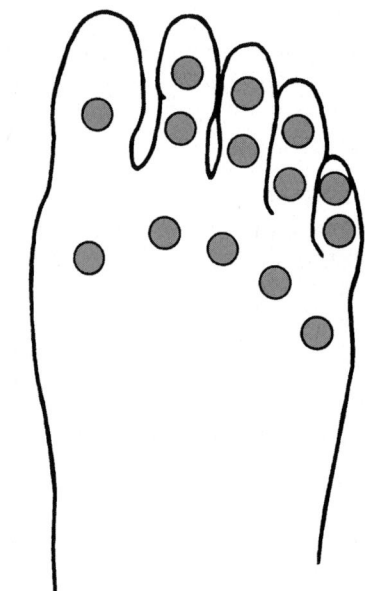

**Figure 40–22.** Gouty arthritis.

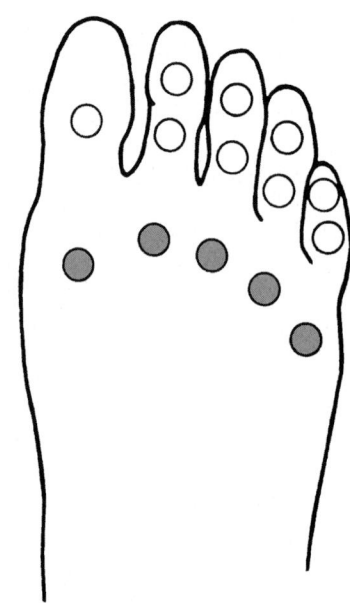

**Figure 40–23.** Neuropathic osteoarthropathy.

Metatarsophalangeal joint abnormalities predominate, although with progressive disease, a great degree of phalangeal resorption may be evident. Other causes of neuropathic osteoarthropathy, such as leprosy and alcoholism, occasionally produce a similar pattern of disease.

### Other Diseases

Infrequently, metatarsophalangeal joint abnormalities may be seen in *CPPD crystal deposition disease, scleroderma, systemic lupus erythematosus,* and *Jaccoud's arthropathy.* Other findings usually ensure an accurate diagnosis in these cases. Similarly, *infectious processes* of the foot may follow diabetes mellitus and local puncture wounds.

## MIDFOOT AND HINDFOOT

The major joints of the midfoot and hindfoot are shown in Figure 40–24.

### Rheumatoid Arthritis (Fig. 40–25)

Rheumatoid arthritis frequently affects all the joints of the midfoot, commonly in association with changes at the metatarsophalangeal joints. Bilateral and symmetrical abnormalities predominate. The most typical sites of involvement are the talonavicular portion of the talocalcaneonavicular joint, the tarsometatarsal joints, and the "posterior" subtalar joint.

### Juvenile Chronic Arthritis (see Fig. 40–25)

Any of the joints of the midfoot can be affected in juvenile chronic arthritis. Bony ankylosis of the tarsal bones and bases of the metatarsal bones of both feet may eventually occur.

### Degenerative Joint Disease (Osteoarthritis) (Fig. 40–26)

Abnormalities of the first tarsometatarsal joint in one or both feet represent the most typical pattern of degenerative joint disease in the midfoot. The findings, consisting of joint space narrowing, sclerosis, and osteophytosis, can simulate those of gout.

### Gouty Arthritis (Fig. 40–27)

Although any of the compartments of the midfoot can be affected, gouty arthritis shows a predilection for the tar-sometatarsal joints. A bilateral symmetrical or asymmetrical process is most frequent. Prominent osseous erosions of the bases of one or more metatarsal bones are especially characteristic.

### Calcium Pyrophosphate Dihydrate Crystal Deposition Disease (Fig. 40–28)

Considerable osseous fragmentation in a bilateral distribution about the talonavicular aspect of the talocalcaneonavicular joint represents an infrequent but distinctive pattern in this disorder. The appearance and distribution are difficult to distinguish from those accompanying the neuropathic osteoarthropathy of diabetes mellitus.

### Neuropathic Osteoarthropathy

The midfoot or hindfoot is not an infrequent site of involvement in diabetes mellitus. Tarsal disintegration with extension to the bases of the metatarsal bones may be combined with changes at one or more metatarsophalangeal joints. In some cases, fragmentation and subluxation at the tarsometatarsal joints simulate the appearance of a Lisfranc's fracture-dislocation.

## CALCANEUS

Five potential target areas exist on the calcaneus: (1) superior surface; (2) posterior surface above the attachment of the Achilles tendon; (3) posterior surface at the site of attachment of the Achilles tendon; (4) plantar surface at the site of attachment of the plantar aponeurosis; and (5) plantar surface anterior to the attachment of the aponeu-

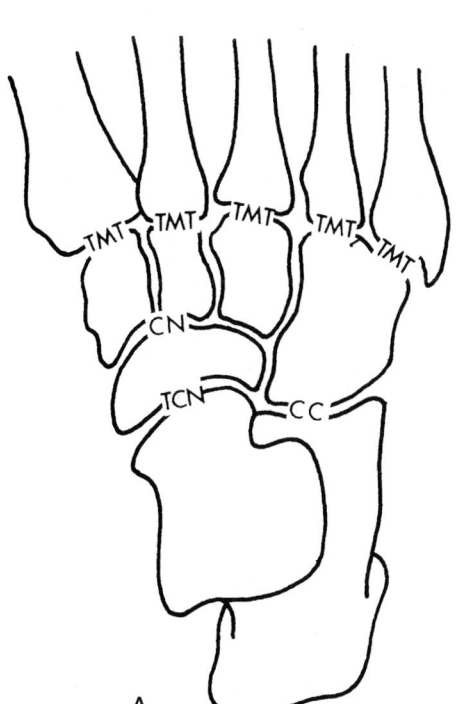

A

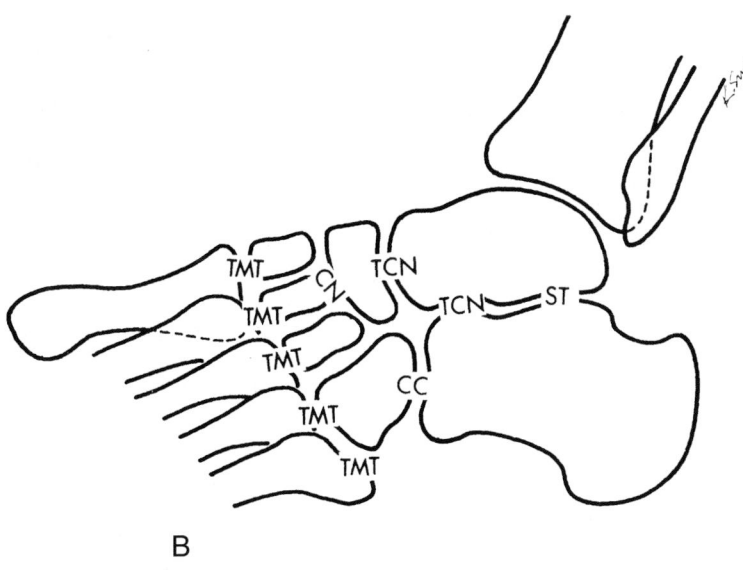

B

**Figure 40–24.** Joints of the midfoot and hindfoot. CC, calcaneocuboid; CN, cuneonavicular; ST, posterior subtalar; TCN, talocalcaneonavicular; TMT, tarsometatarsal.

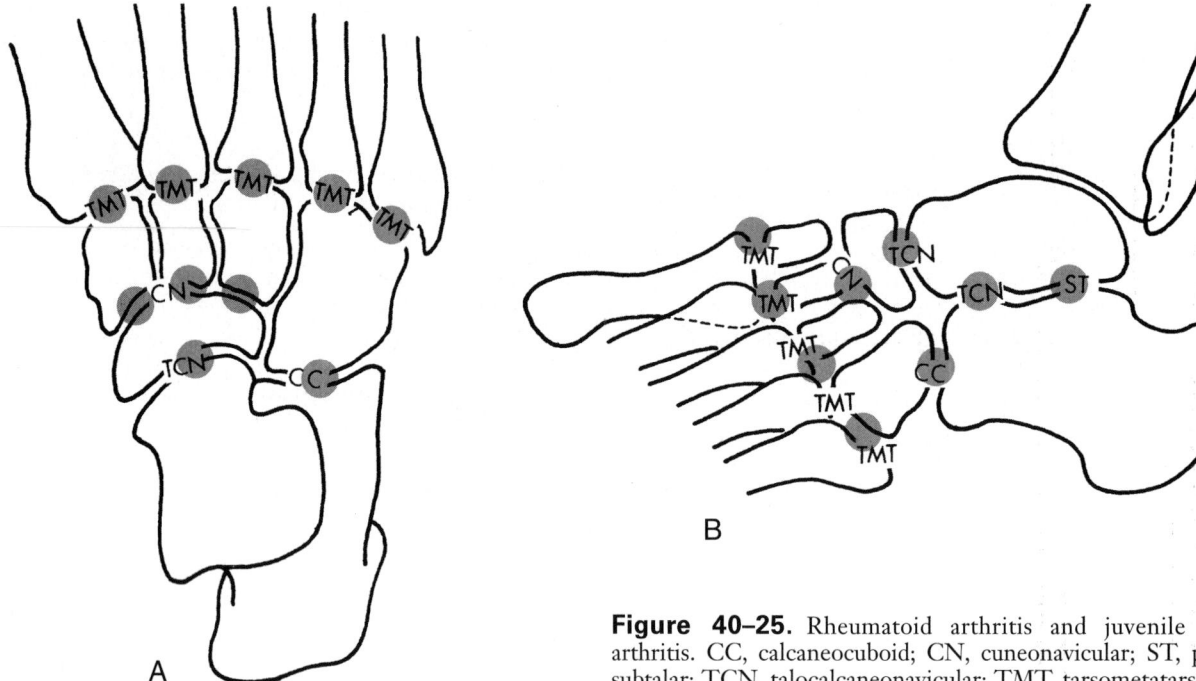

**Figure 40–25.** Rheumatoid arthritis and juvenile chronic arthritis. CC, calcaneocuboid; CN, cuneonavicular; ST, posterior subtalar; TCN, talocalcaneonavicular; TMT, tarsometatarsal.

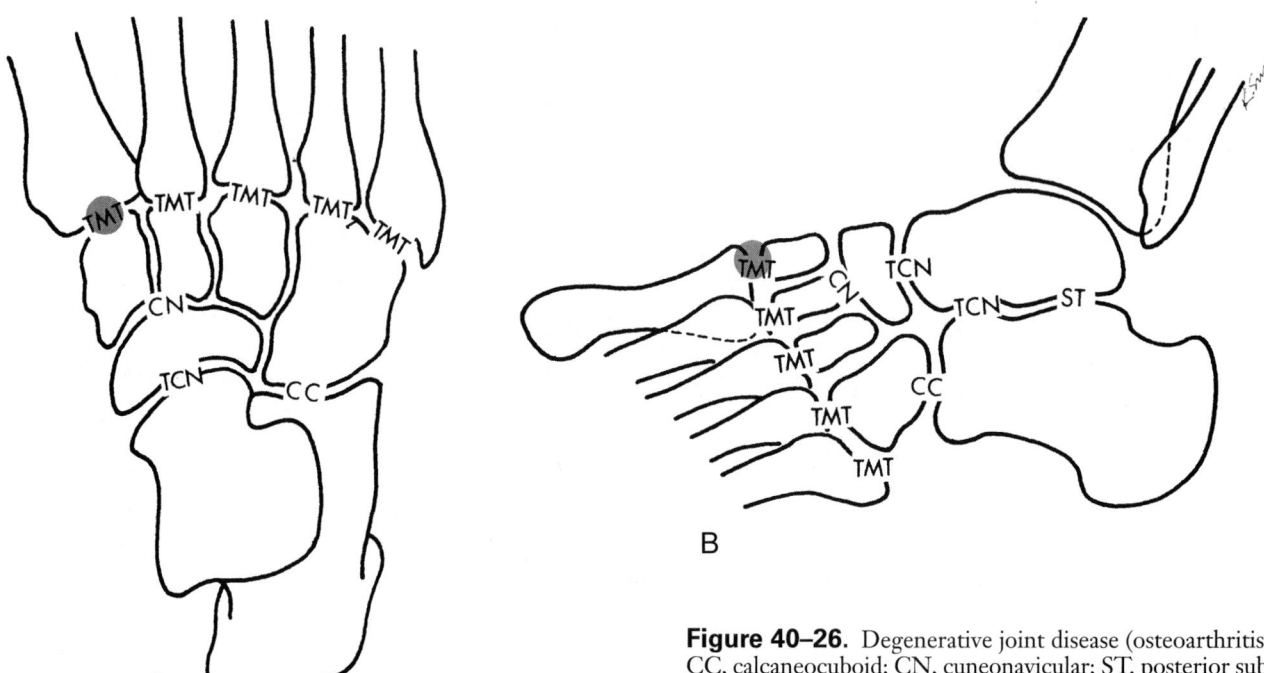

**Figure 40–26.** Degenerative joint disease (osteoarthritis). CC, calcaneocuboid; CN, cuneonavicular; ST, posterior subtalar; TCN, talocalcaneonavicular; TMT, tarsometatarsal.

rosis (Fig. 40–29). Of fundamental importance is the intimate relationship of a synovium-lined sac, the retrocalcaneal bursa, to the posterosuperior aspect of the calcaneus as it lies between the Achilles tendon and the osseous surface.

### Rheumatoid Arthritis (Fig. 40–30)

Retrocalcaneal bursitis leads to unilateral or bilateral calcaneal erosions in both site 1 and site 2. An adjacent soft tissue mass projecting into the pre-Achilles fat pad is frequently evident. Well-defined posterior (site 3) and

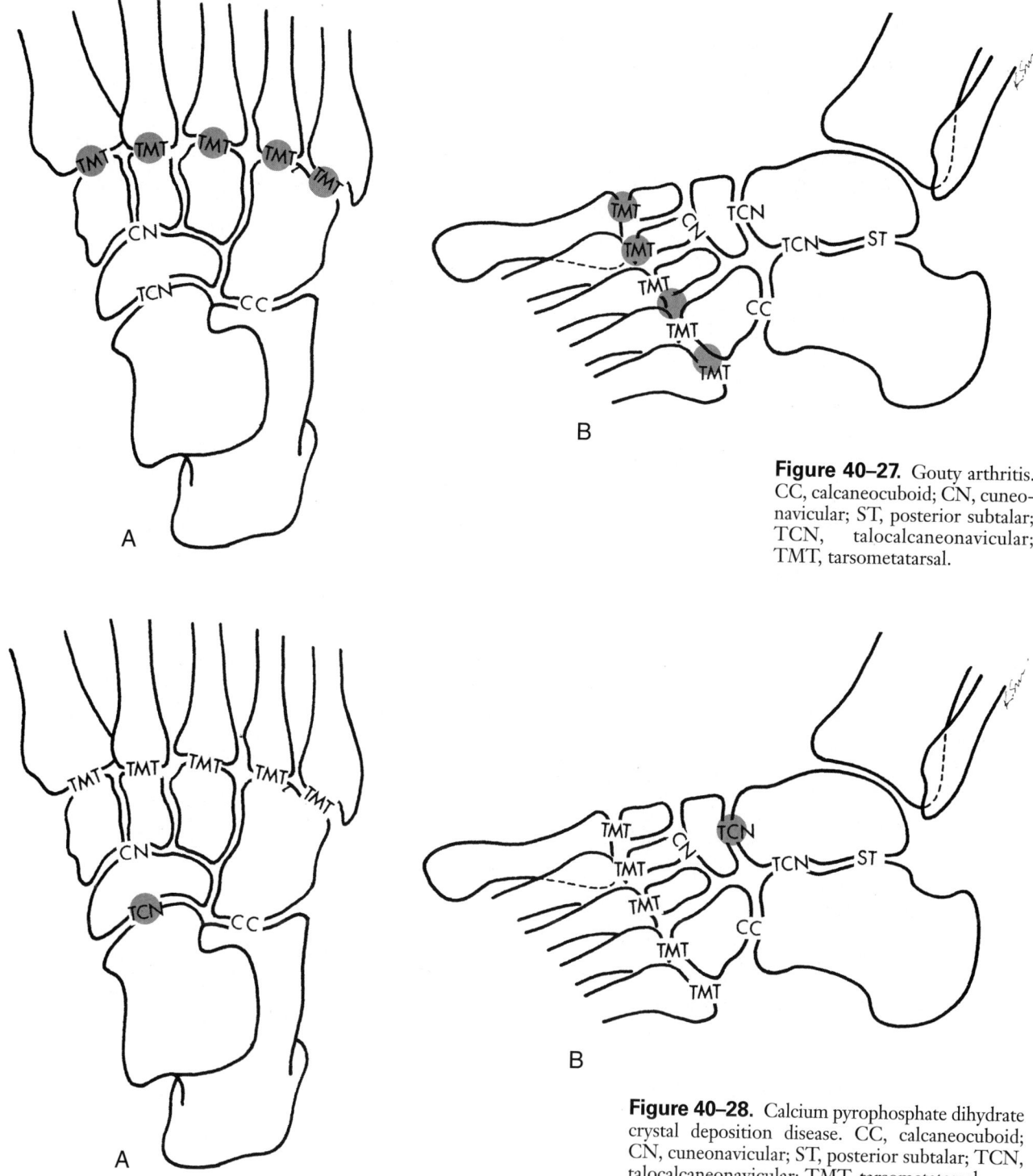

**Figure 40–27.** Gouty arthritis. CC, calcaneocuboid; CN, cuneonavicular; ST, posterior subtalar; TCN, talocalcaneonavicular; TMT, tarsometatarsal.

**Figure 40–28.** Calcium pyrophosphate dihydrate crystal deposition disease. CC, calcaneocuboid; CN, cuneonavicular; ST, posterior subtalar; TCN, talocalcaneonavicular; TMT, tarsometatarsal.

plantar (site 4) calcaneal enthesophytes also are typical. Plantar osseous erosions of considerable size are distinctly unusual. Achilles tendinitis producing an enlarged or poorly defined tendinous outline can be seen.

## Ankylosing Spondylitis and Psoriatic Arthritis (Fig. 40–31)

Similar abnormalities occur in both ankylosing spondylitis and psoriatic arthritis, frequently in a bilateral distribution.

Retrocalcaneal bursitis leads to osseous erosions that predominate at site 2. The changes, which occasionally may be combined with alterations at site 1, resemble the findings in rheumatoid arthritis, although reactive bone formation may be more prominent. Well-defined calcaneal enthesophytes at the site of attachment of the Achilles tendon (site 3) may be observed, a nonspecific finding. On the plantar aspect of the bone, at sites 4 and 5, poorly marginated erosions, reactive sclerosis, and poorly defined enthesophytes may be detected. The outgrowths are more

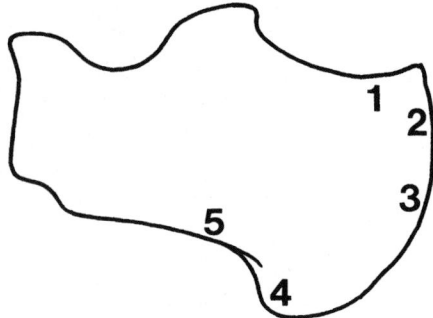

**Figure 40–29.** Target areas of the calcaneus (see text for identification of numbered areas).

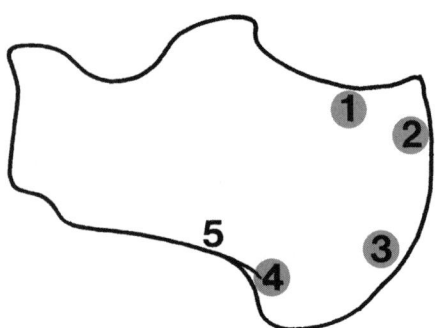

**Figure 40–30.** Rheumatoid arthritis.

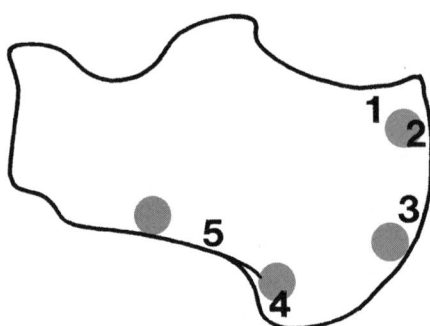

**Figure 40–31.** Ankylosing spondylitis and psoriatic arthritis.

irregular and fuzzy, and the degree of sclerosis is more prominent in these disorders than in rheumatoid arthritis. Achilles tendon thickening can be seen.

### Reiter's Syndrome (Fig. 40–32)

In Reiter's syndrome, unilateral or bilateral alterations can be encountered. Retrocalcaneal bursitis produces erosions at sites 1 and 2 that resemble the findings in rheumatoid arthritis. Abnormalities at site 3, including well-defined calcaneal excrescences, are less frequent than in psoriatic arthritis, ankylosing spondylitis, and rheumatoid arthritis, probably reflecting the younger age of the patients. On the plantar aspect of the bone, osseous erosions and poorly defined bone formation predominate at site 4. The irregular enthesophytes that develop may become better defined over an extended period.

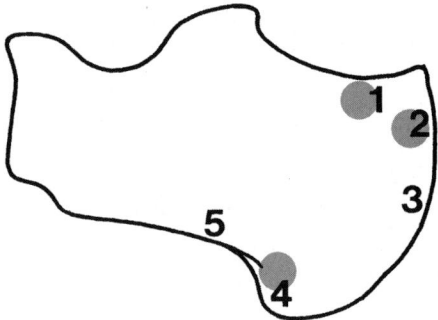

**Figure 40–32.** Reiter's syndrome.

### Gouty Arthritis (Fig. 40–33)

Tophaceous nodules in and about the Achilles tendon can lead to erosions at sites 2 and 3. The findings are combined with other, more typical changes at the metatarsophalangeal and interphalangeal joints.

### Calcium Pyrophosphate Dihydrate Crystal Deposition Disease (Fig. 40–34)

Calcific collections consisting of CPPD crystals can be deposited in the Achilles tendon and plantar aponeurosis of one or both feet in this disorder. The deposits are linear and may be of considerable length. Similar abnormalities may be seen in calcium hydroxyapatite crystal deposition disease.

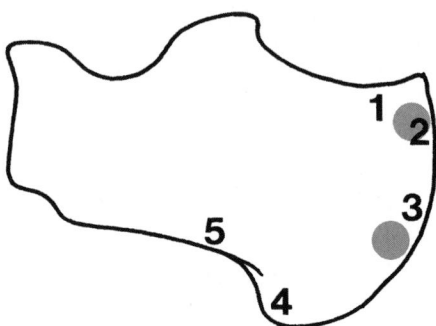

**Figure 40–33.** Gouty arthritis.

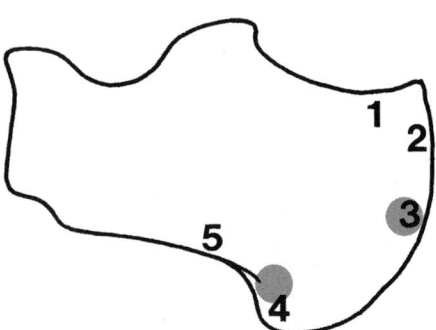

**Figure 40–34.** Calcium pyrophosphate dihydrate crystal deposition disease, xanthomatosis, and diffuse idiopathic skeletal hyperostosis.

### Xanthomatosis (see Fig. 40–34)

Tendinous xanthomas can appear in the Achilles tendon and the plantar aponeurosis in a unilateral or bilateral distribution. They produce eccentric soft tissue masses that do not calcify. On rare occasions, they may erode subjacent bone.

### Diffuse Idiopathic Skeletal Hyperostosis (see Fig. 40–34)

Well-defined outgrowths of variable size occur at the sites of bony attachment of the Achilles tendon and plantar aponeurosis (sites 3 and 4).

### Other Diseases

*Hyperparathyroidism* can lead to subligamentous erosion at site 4, as well as subtle defects elsewhere in the calcaneus, including site 1 (Fig. 40–35). *Haglund's syndrome* is characterized by retrocalcaneal bursitis with a soft tissue mass at sites 1 and 2.

### KNEE

It is useful to analyze separately three major areas or spaces of the knee: the medial femorotibial space, the lateral femorotibial space, and the patellofemoral space. Anteroposterior radiographs allow analysis of the medial and lateral femorotibial compartments, analysis that can be improved by obtaining radiographs with the patient standing. Lateral and axial radiographs allow evaluation of the patellofemoral compartment.

### Rheumatoid Arthritis (Fig. 40–36)

Rheumatoid arthritis usually leads to alterations that are bilateral and symmetrical and affect both medial and lateral femorotibial compartments to an equal degree. Diffuse loss of interosseous space in the medial and lateral compartments may be combined with osteoporosis, marginal or central osseous erosions, and subchondral sclerosis. Crumbling of the osteoporotic bone of the tibia in combination with ligamentous abnormalities may create varus or, more characteristically, valgus angulation of the knee.

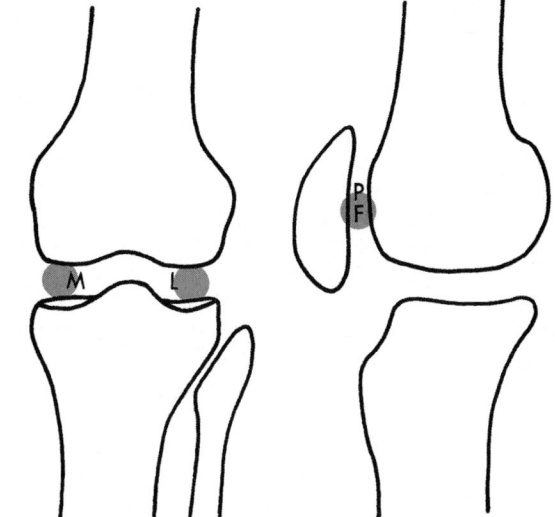

**Figure 40–36.** Rheumatoid arthritis. L, lateral; M, medial; PF, patellofemoral.

Involvement of the patellofemoral space is often combined with involvement of the other two compartments in the knee in rheumatoid arthritis. Although not invariably present, tricompartmental abnormalities that are of equal severity are most suggestive of rheumatoid arthritis.

### Ankylosing Spondylitis, Psoriatic Arthritis, and Reiter's Syndrome (Fig. 40–37)

Any of these three disorders can affect one or both knees. A tricompartmental distribution may be encountered, although the degree of joint space narrowing, osteoporosis, and osseous erosion is less than in rheumatoid arthritis, and the extent of periosteal proliferation or "whiskering" may be pronounced.

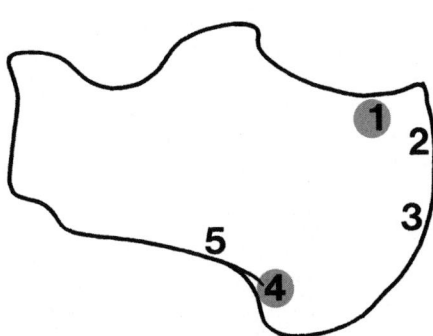

**Figure 40–35.** Hyperparathyroidism.

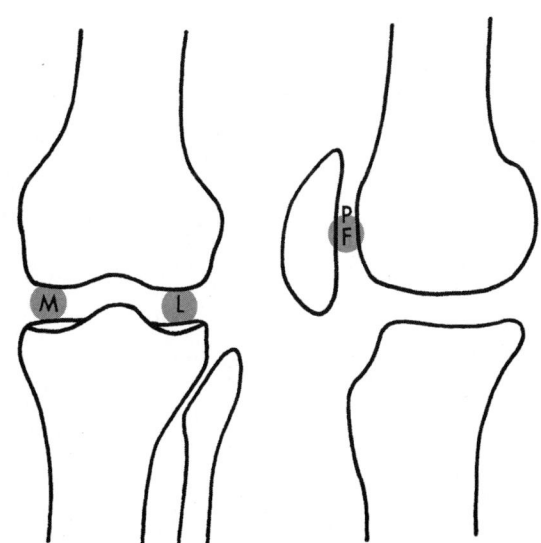

**Figure 40–37.** Ankylosing spondylitis, psoriatic arthritis, and Reiter's syndrome. L, lateral; M, medial; PF, patellofemoral.

## Degenerative Joint Disease (Osteoarthritis)
(Fig. 40–38)

A unilateral or bilateral distribution can be seen. Asymmetrical involvement of the medial and lateral femorotibial compartments predominates, frequently in combination with significant patellofemoral compartment disease. Thus, bicompartmental rather than tricompartmental findings are evident on radiographs. In most instances, it is the medial femorotibial compartment that is more severely affected, and the asymmetrical nature of the process may lead to varus deformity. Severe alterations in the lateral femorotibial compartment and valgus deformity are less common on radiographs of the osteoarthritic knee and, when present, are usually seen in women.

Isolated abnormalities of the patellofemoral compartment are relatively unusual in degenerative joint disease of the knee. The detection of joint space narrowing, sclerosis, and osteophytosis in this location in the absence of similar changes in either the medial or lateral femorotibial space should initiate a search for CPPD crystal deposition disease.

## Calcium Pyrophosphate Dihydrate Crystal Deposition Disease (Fig. 40–39)

The distribution of abnormalities of the knee in patients with CPPD crystal deposition disease is somewhat variable. Usually both knees are affected. The medial femorotibial and patellofemoral compartments are commonly affected simultaneously, a distribution that is identical to that in osteoarthritis. In these cases, the greater extent of osseous destruction and fragmentation may allow accurate differentiation of CPPD crystal deposition disease from osteoarthritis. Lateral femorotibial compartment changes, with or without medial femorotibial compartment abnor-

malities, also can be encountered in this disease and, in some instances, may lead to valgus deformity of the knee. Further, findings isolated to the patellofemoral compartment are observed in some patients. In fact, a "degenerative"-like arthropathy of the patellofemoral compartment, appearing in the absence of significant medial or lateral femorotibial space alterations, raises the possibility that this disease is present.

## Other Diseases

In addition to subperiosteal resorption of bone along the medial aspect of the tibia, *hyperparathyroidism* can produce distinctive types of articular abnormality on knee radiographs. Subchondral resorption of bone may be evident in any compartment. The changes, consisting of poorly defined "erosion" and sclerosis, may be especially marked in the patellofemoral areas (Fig. 40–40).

*Septic arthritis* affecting the knee can become evident initially in any compartment. As in rheumatoid arthritis, the alterations can spread to all areas of the joint, producing tricompartmental disease. A unilateral distribution is most frequent.

*Neuropathic osteoarthropathy* accompanying tabes dorsalis or, more rarely, other diseases with neurologic deficit can lead to involvement of one or both knees with sclerosis, fragmentation, subluxation, and disorganization of the joint.

*Hydroxyapatite crystal deposition disease* or *mixed calcium phosphate crystal deposition disease* has a distinctive appearance in the knee. Involvement predominates in the lateral femorotibial compartment, leading to osseous collapse and fragmentation, and may be combined with changes in the shoulder.

*Ischemic necrosis* commonly involves the distal portion of the femur or, to a lesser extent, the proximal part of the tibia. It may relate to an underlying condition, such as corticosteroid medication, or occur on an idiopathic basis. The medial compartment is typically affected in spontaneous osteonecrosis about the knee.

*Wilson's disease* is associated with abnormality of the patellofemoral compartment (see Fig. 40–40). In *alkaptonuria*, changes resemble those of osteoarthritis, although isolated involvement of the lateral femorotibial compartment and considerable bony collapse and fragmentation are encountered.

## HIP

In evaluating articular disorders that affect the hip, it is useful to define the nature or location of any accompanying joint space loss. With diminution of the articular space, the femoral head migrates in one of three basic directions with respect to the acetabulum. If the loss is confined to the superior aspect of the joint, the femoral head moves in an upward or superior direction; if the loss is confined to the inner third of the joint, the femoral head migrates in a medial direction; and if the joint space loss involves the entire joint, the femoral head migrates in an axial direction along the axis of the femoral neck (Fig. 40–41). Certain disorders are associated with characteristic patterns of femoral head migration.

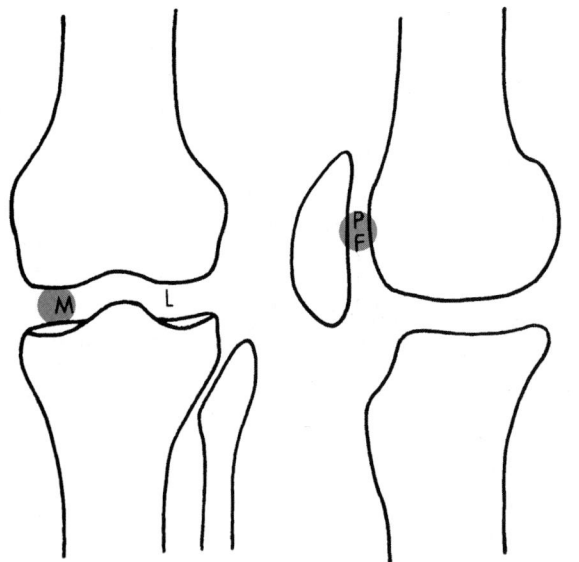

**Figure 40–38.** Degenerative joint disease (osteoarthritis). L, lateral; M, medial; PF, patellofemoral.

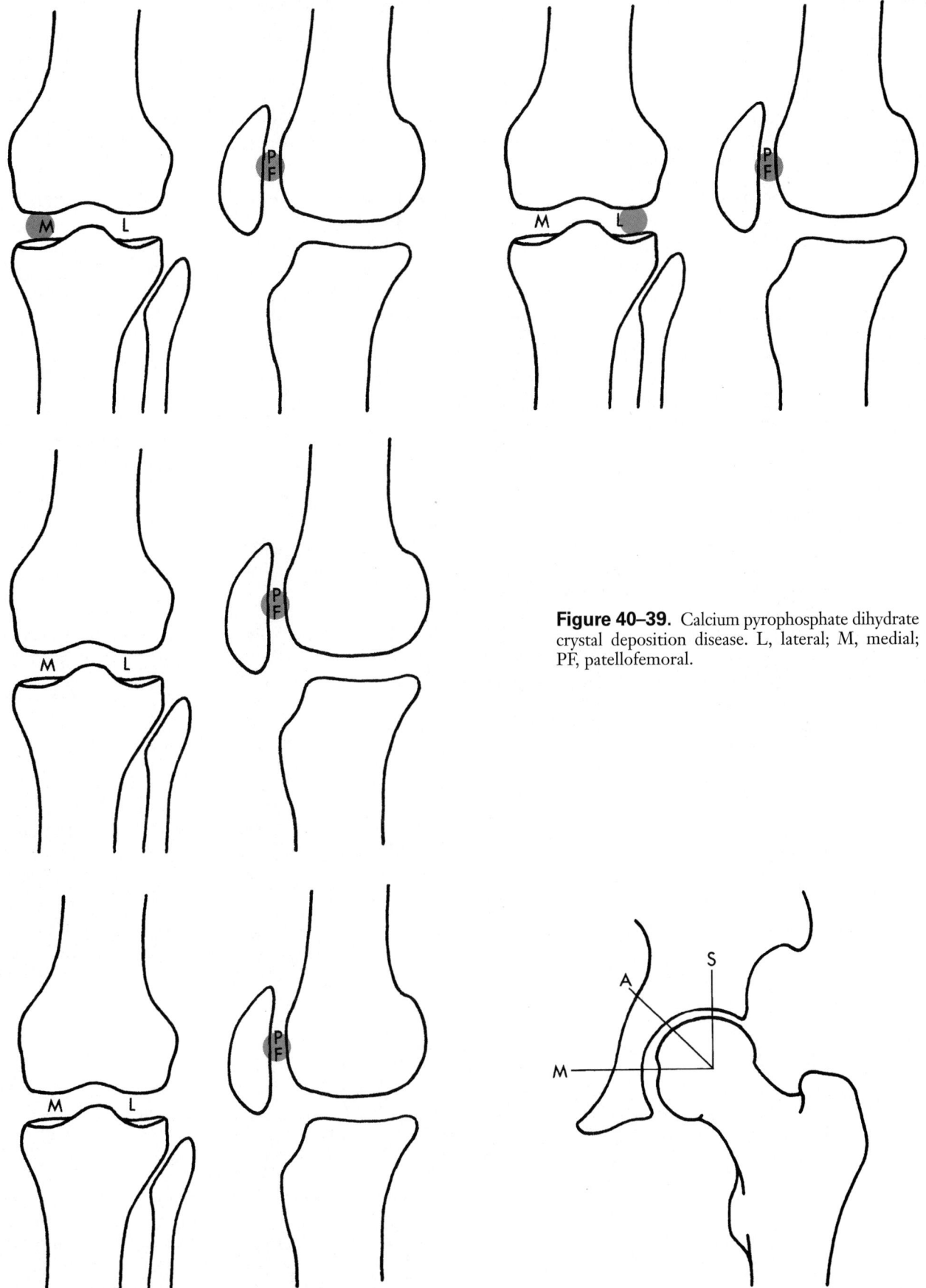

**Figure 40–39.** Calcium pyrophosphate dihydrate crystal deposition disease. L, lateral; M, medial; PF, patellofemoral.

**Figure 40–40.** Hyperparathyroidism and Wilson's disease. L, lateral; M, medial; PF, patellofemoral.

**Figure 40–41.** Patterns of migration of the femoral head. A, axial migration; M, medial migration; S, superior migration.

## Rheumatoid Arthritis (Fig. 40–42)

In rheumatoid arthritis, the entire articular cartilaginous coat of the femoral head and acetabulum is typically affected in a bilateral and symmetrical fashion. Thus, symmetrical loss of the interosseous space occurs with axial migration of the femoral head with respect to the acetabulum. This finding is usually accompanied by marginal and central osseous erosions and cysts and even localized sclerosis. Osteophytosis is not a prominent feature.

## Juvenile Chronic Arthritis

The prevalence and type of hip involvement in juvenile chronic arthritis are influenced by the specific variety of disease that is present. In some patients, diffuse loss of joint space with concentric narrowing of the joint results in axial migration of the femoral head and a radiographic picture that resembles that in adult-onset rheumatoid arthritis. In others, osseous erosions may be unaccompanied by loss of interosseous space. In patients with juvenile-onset ankylosing spondylitis, the radiographic findings are similar to those in adult-onset ankylosing spondylitis.

## Ankylosing Spondylitis (see Fig. 40–42)

A bilateral and symmetrical pattern consisting of axial migration of the femoral head due to diffuse loss of joint space is seen. Although this pattern is identical to that occurring in rheumatoid arthritis, the presence of osteophytosis, commencing on the superolateral aspect of the femoral head and progressing as a collar about the femoral head–neck junction, is distinctive of ankylosing spondylitis. The combination of axial migration of the femoral head and osteophyte formation is most characteristic of ankylosing spondylitis and CPPD crystal deposition disease. Rarely, patients with degenerative joint disease may reveal symmetrical loss of interosseous space. In ankylosing spondylitis, acetabular and femoral cysts, mild acetabular protrusion, and partial or complete intra-articular bony ankylosis can be observed.

## Psoriatic Arthritis and Reiter's Syndrome

Hip involvement is unusual in both psoriatic arthritis and Reiter's syndrome. Occasionally a patient with either disease may reveal concentric loss of joint space resembling that in rheumatoid arthritis, and, rarely, patients with psoriatic arthritis have more extensive osseous destruction, leading to a blunted and eroded femoral head.

## Degenerative Joint Disease (Osteoarthritis) (Fig. 40–43)

Unilateral or bilateral alterations can be delineated. Most commonly, loss of interosseous space is maximal on the upper aspect of the joint, resulting in superior migration of the femoral head with respect to the acetabulum. Less

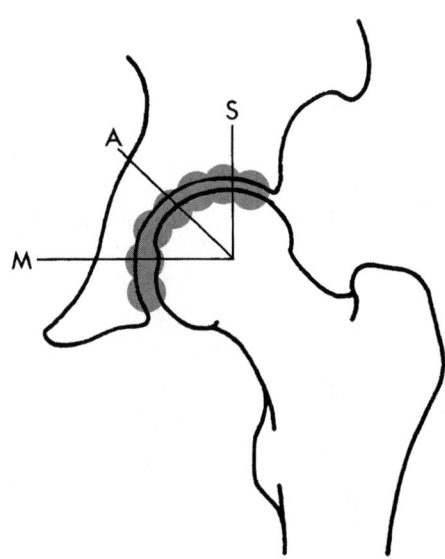

**Figure 40–42.** Rheumatoid arthritis and ankylosing spondylitis. A, axial migration; M, medial migration; S, superior migration.

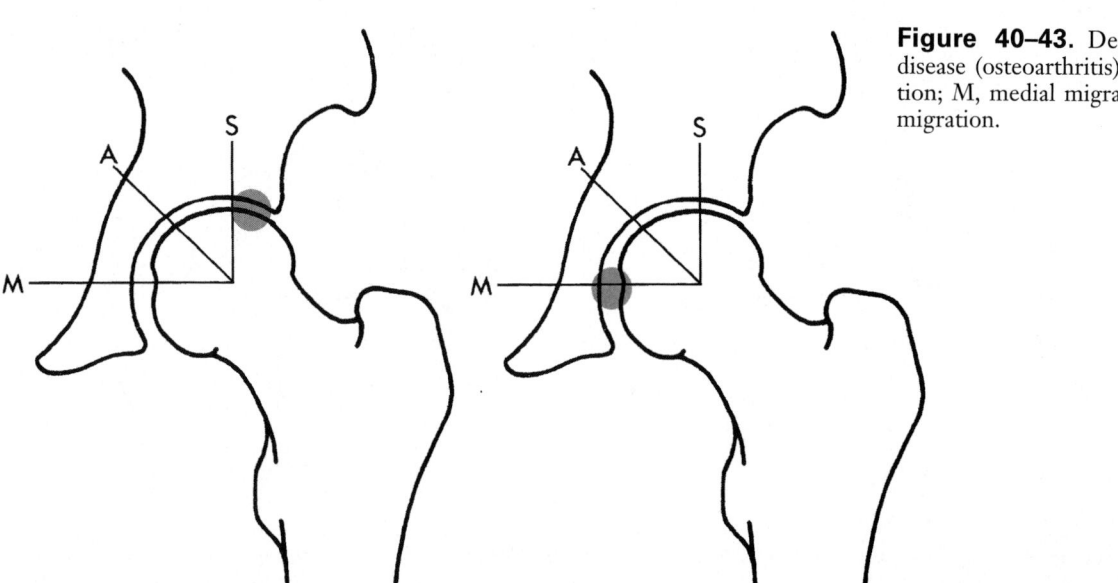

**Figure 40–43.** Degenerative joint disease (osteoarthritis). A, axial migration; M, medial migration; S, superior migration.

frequently, medial loss of joint space is seen, which may be associated with mild protrusio acetabuli deformity. Rarely, axial migration of the femoral head indicates diffuse loss of the cartilaginous surfaces of the femur and acetabulum. In all cases of degenerative joint disease, femoral and acetabular osteophytes, sclerosis, and cyst formation are common, and thickening or buttressing of the medial femoral cortex is apparent.

### Gouty Arthritis

Hip involvement is unusual in gouty arthritis. Rarely, osseous erosion or osteonecrosis can be seen

### Calcium Pyrophosphate Dihydrate Crystal Deposition Disease (Fig. 40–44)

The arthropathy of CPPD crystal deposition disease may involve one or both hips. It is characterized by symmetrical loss of joint space with axial migration, sclerosis, cyst formation, and osteophytosis. The degree of osseous collapse and fragmentation may be extreme, and the resulting radiographic features may be misinterpreted as neuropathic osteoarthropathy or osteonecrosis. Additional findings, such as chondrocalcinosis of the acetabular labrum and symphysis pubis detectable on pelvic radiographs, provide helpful clues to the correct diagnosis.

### Osteonecrosis

Although osteonecrosis of one or both femoral heads can accompany a vast number of diseases, the joint space is remarkably preserved in most cases, even in the presence of significant bony collapse and fragmentation. In longstanding cases, secondary degenerative joint disease can result, owing to the incongruity of the apposing articular surfaces. In these instances, loss of joint space usually

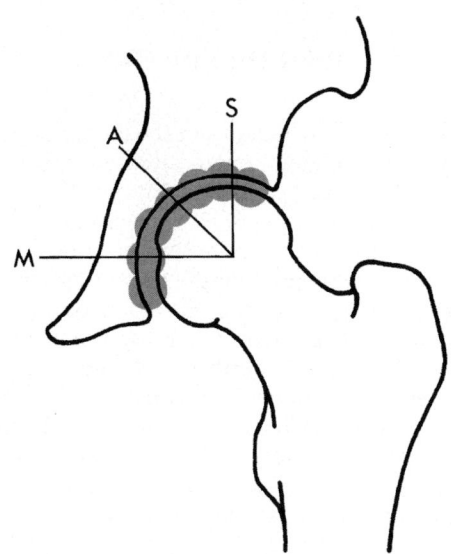

**Figure 40–44.** Calcium pyrophosphate dihydrate crystal deposition disease. A, axial migration; M, medial migration; S, superior migration.

predominates in the superior aspect of the joint, leading to superior migration of the femoral head with respect to the acetabulum. Occasionally, loss of joint space is more diffuse.

### Neuropathic Osteoarthropathy

Disintegration of osseous and cartilaginous tissue in one or both hips can be a manifestation of neuropathic osteoarthropathy. In these cases, tabes is the most typical underlying disorder.

### Other Diseases

In *Paget's disease*, involvement of para-articular osseous tissue can lead to secondary degenerative joint disease. The radiographic findings are influenced by the distribution of pagetic changes; the pattern of joint space loss may differ when the acetabulum is affected alone, when both the acetabulum and femur are affected, and when the femur is the only site of involvement. Because of these variations, any pattern of femoral head migration can appear in Paget's disease.

*Idiopathic chondrolysis* of the hip is rare, but it is associated with diffuse loss of joint space and axial migration of the femoral head with respect to the acetabulum. The appearance may closely resemble that of infection.

*Regional migratory osteoporosis* and *transient osteoporosis of the hip* are self-limited conditions that can produce periarticular osteoporosis that improves spontaneously over several months. A unilateral distribution is typical, and when transient osteoporosis affects a woman in the third trimester of pregnancy, almost invariably the left hip is involved. Preservation of joint space and the absence of significant defects in the subchondral bone plate are features of regional osteoporosis that allow its differentiation from infection.

*Infections* of the hip can have a bacterial, mycobacterial, or fungal cause. The radiographic features and prognosis are influenced by the age of onset. In infants, pyogenic arthritis of the hip requires immediate attention to prevent permanent epiphyseal damage. Joint space loss, which is generally diffuse in nature, is a fundamental finding in all infectious disorders. Other findings include osteoporosis and marginal and central osseous erosions.

*Pigmented villonodular synovitis* and *idiopathic synovial osteochondromatosis* are two disorders that can produce monoarticular disease of the hip. In both conditions, soft tissue swelling and osseous erosions may appear in the absence of joint space narrowing and osteoporosis, although the last two findings are evident in some cases. The presence of cystic erosions of the femoral neck in both conditions and the detection of calcific or ossific foci in idiopathic synovial osteochondromatosis are important diagnostic clues.

*Familial acetabular protrusion* (Otto pelvis) leads to bilateral abnormalities, especially in women, characterized by protrusio acetabuli deformity and, eventually, joint space loss.

*Cartilage atrophy*, secondary to disuse, immobilization, or paralysis, produces diffuse loss of joint space and axial migration of the femoral head. Osteoporosis is evident.

*Irradiation* can lead to collapse of the femoral head, fragmentation of the acetabulum, acetabular protrusion, and concentric joint space loss.

## SHOULDER

In the shoulder region, three potential target areas can be affected in various articular disorders: the glenohumeral joint, the acromioclavicular joint, and the undersurface of the distal end of the clavicle at the site of attachment of the coracoclavicular ligament (Fig. 40–45).

### Rheumatoid Arthritis (Fig. 40–46)

All three target areas on both sides of the body can be involved in rheumatoid arthritis. Glenohumeral joint alterations consist of osteoporosis, symmetrical loss of joint space, and marginal osseous erosions, predominantly on the superolateral aspect of the humeral head. Associated atrophy or tear of the rotator cuff may lead to slow or rapid elevation of the humeral head with respect to the glenoid cavity and narrowing of the acromion–humeral head distance.

Acromioclavicular joint erosion with widening of the articular space is a recognized manifestation of this disease. The margins of the distal end of the clavicle may assume a tapered appearance. Similarly, scalloped erosion on the undersurface of the distal end of the clavicle opposite the coracoid process is an additional manifestation of rheumatoid arthritis.

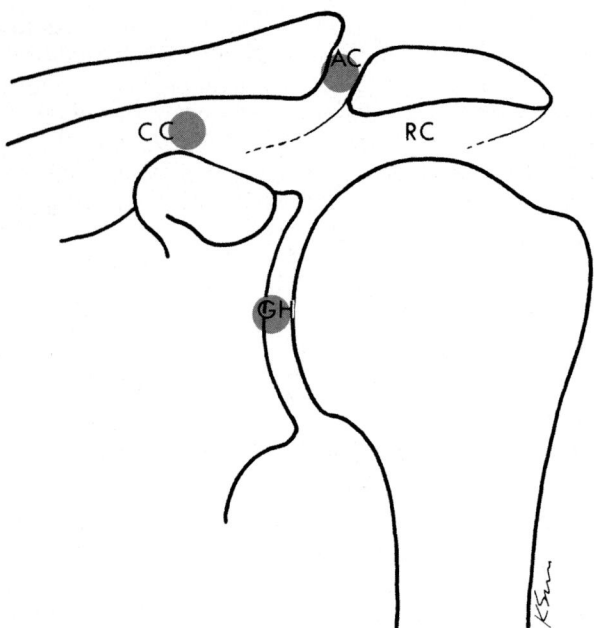

**Figure 40–46.** Rheumatoid arthritis and ankylosing spondylitis. AC, acromioclavicular joint; CC, coracoclavicular ligament; GH, glenohumeral joint; RC, rotator cuff.

### Ankylosing Spondylitis (see Fig. 40–46)

The changes about the shoulder in ankylosing spondylitis resemble those in rheumatoid arthritis. Glenohumeral joint involvement leads to joint space narrowing and osseous erosion. A large bony defect, the "hatchet" deformity, can appear on the superolateral aspect of the humeral head, which is distinctive. The absence of osteoporosis and the presence of bony proliferation about the osseous erosions are additional characteristics of ankylosing spondylitis that are helpful in diagnosis.

### Degenerative Joint Disease (Osteoarthritis) (Fig. 40–47)

Although severe abnormalities in the glenohumeral joint are not typical of uncomplicated osteoarthritis unless significant accidental or occupational trauma has occurred, mild alterations consisting of joint space narrowing, sclerosis, and osteophytosis can be seen even in the absence of such trauma. Disruption of the rotator cuff is frequent in elderly persons, producing elevation of the humeral head. Although the appearance may simulate that of rotator cuff injury in rheumatoid arthritis, the initial absence of significant glenohumeral joint involvement in association with degeneration of the cuff is noteworthy. Further, the appearance of an osseous excrescence on the anteroinferior surface of the acromion is a degenerative alteration responsible for or accompanying the shoulder impingement syndrome.

Acromioclavicular joint degeneration is frequent in middle-aged and elderly persons. Changes consist of articular space narrowing and eburnation.

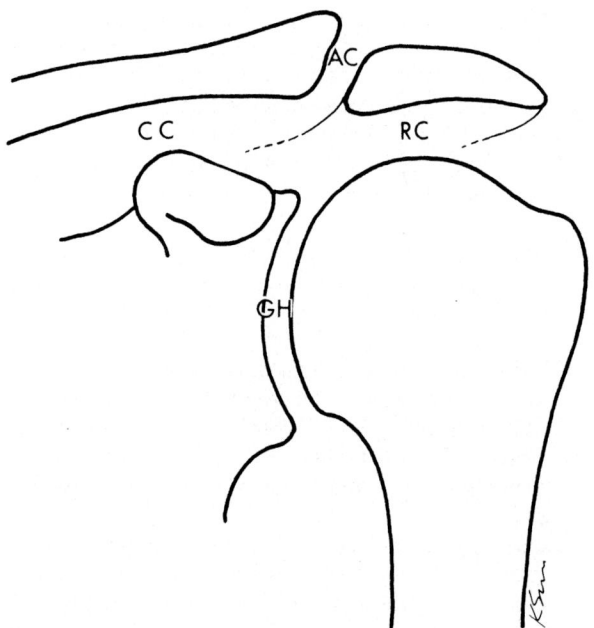

**Figure 40–45.** Target areas of the shoulder. AC, acromioclavicular joint; CC, coracoclavicular ligament; GH, glenohumeral joint; RC, rotator cuff.

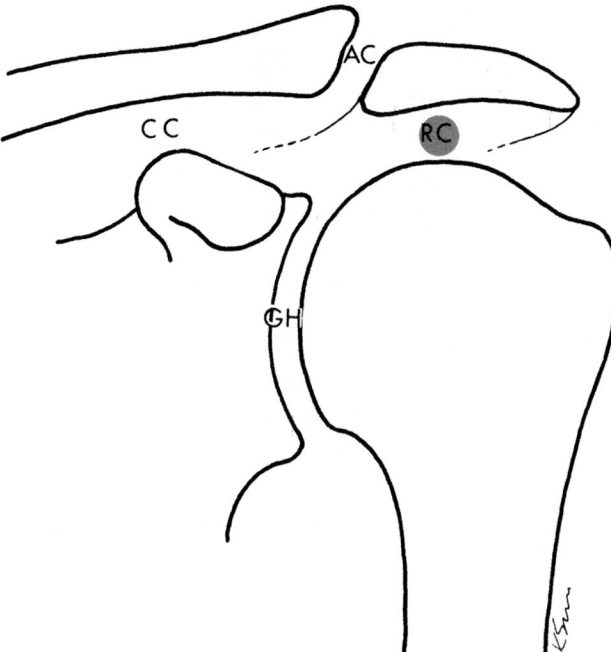

**Figure 40–47.** Rotator cuff degeneration. AC, acromioclavicular joint; CC, coracoclavicular ligament; GH, glenohumeral joint; RC, rotator cuff.

## Calcium Pyrophosphate Dihydrate Crystal Deposition Disease (Fig. 40–48)

Both the glenohumeral and the acromioclavicular joints can be affected in this disease. Fibrocartilage or hyaline cartilage calcification, joint space narrowing, sclerosis, and osteophytosis can appear at either shoulder location.

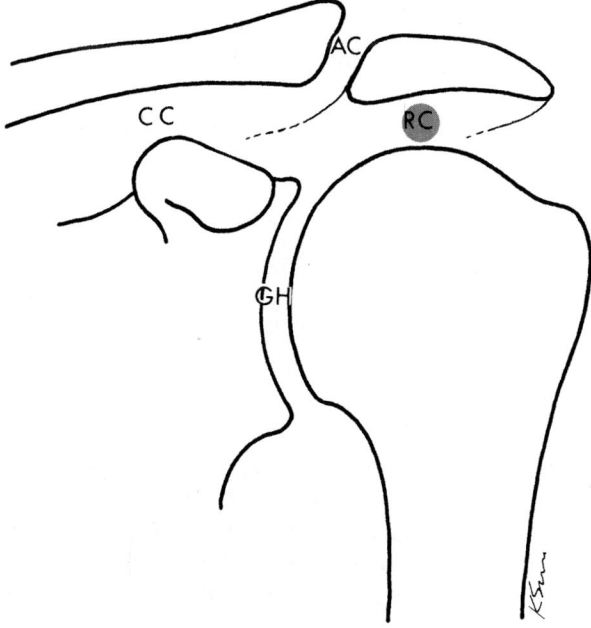

**Figure 40–48.** Calcium pyrophosphate dihydrate crystal deposition disease. AC, acromioclavicular joint; CC, coracoclavicular ligament; GH, glenohumeral joint; RC, rotator cuff.

## Calcium Hydroxyapatite Crystal Deposition Disease

The deposition of calcium hydroxyapatite crystals in the shoulder is responsible for periarticular cloudlike calcification in the rotator cuff or subacromial (subdeltoid) bursa. Such deposition may also be instrumental in a distinctive arthropathy, the Milwaukee shoulder syndrome, that is characterized by destruction of bone and cartilage and deterioration of the rotator cuff.

## Other Diseases

*Alkaptonuria* (ochronosis) can lead to an arthropathy resembling degenerative joint disease of the glenohumeral joint in one or both shoulders. Similar, in *acromegaly*, osteophytosis may be evident in this site, especially on the inferior aspect of the humeral head. *Hyperparathyroidism* leads to osseous resorption of the distal end of the clavicle and adjacent acromion, as well as of the inferior aspect of the clavicle at the site of attachment of the coracoclavicular ligament. *Post-traumatic changes* include osteolysis of the distal end of the clavicle, and degenerative joint disease may be seen in association with recurrent posterior dislocation of the glenohumeral joint.

## SACROILIAC JOINT

The most important aspect in the differential diagnosis of diseases that affect the sacroiliac joint is the distribution of the abnormalities. Findings can be bilateral and symmetrical, bilateral and asymmetrical, or unilateral (Fig. 40–49). In nearly every instance, the synovial portion of the joint (the lower one half or two thirds of the interosseous space between sacrum and ilium) is affected to a greater degree than is the ligamentous portion (the area above the synovium-lined space).

## Rheumatoid Arthritis (see Fig. 40–49B, C)

Abnormalities of the sacroiliac joint in rheumatoid arthritis are generally a minor feature of the disease. Bilateral asymmetrical or unilateral changes predominate, consisting of joint space narrowing, superficial osseous erosions, minor sclerosis, and absence of widespread bony ankylosis.

## Juvenile Chronic Arthritis

The prevalence and appearance of sacroiliac joint changes in juvenile chronic arthritis depend on the subgroup of disease present. Changes usually are not prominent unless juvenile-onset ankylosing spondylitis is evident. In this case, a bilateral and symmetrical distribution is encountered.

## Ankylosing Spondylitis (see Fig. 40–49A)

The classic findings in this disease are bilateral and symmetrical. Erosions, sclerosis, and bony ankylosis of the synovial joint are frequently combined with poorly defined osseous margins in the ligamentous aspect of the joint. Iliac abnormalities predominate.

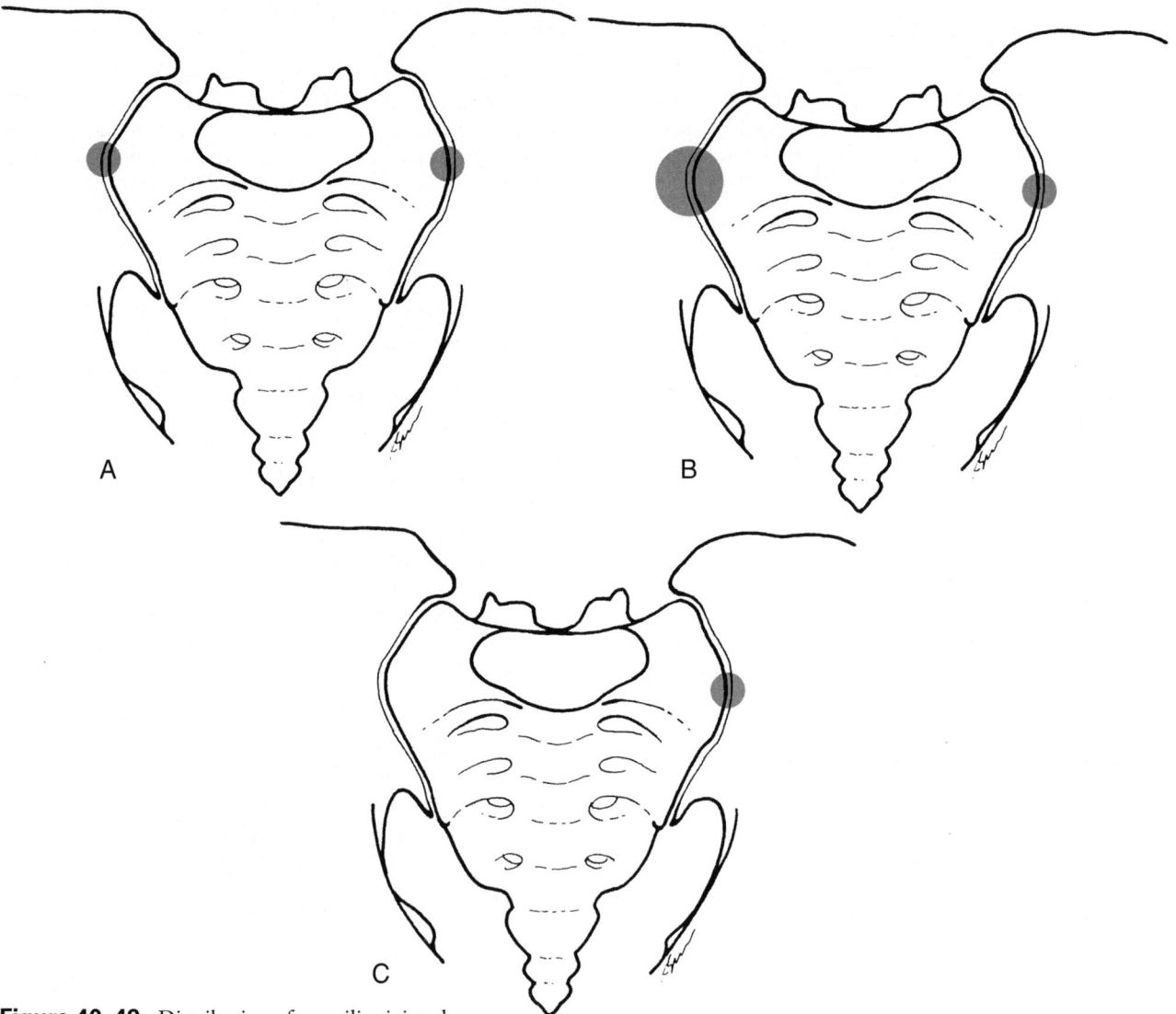

**Figure 40–49.** Distribution of sacroiliac joint changes. *A*, Symmetrical; *B*, Asymmetrical; *C*, Unilateral.

### Psoriatic Arthritis and Reiter's Syndrome
(see Fig. 40–49*A–C*)

The distribution of abnormalities is variable in psoriatic arthritis and Reiter's syndrome. Changes may be bilateral and symmetrical, bilateral and asymmetrical, or unilateral. Osseous erosion and bony sclerosis are similar to the findings in ankylosing spondylitis, although joint space narrowing and bony ankylosis occur with decreased frequency. Proliferation of bone in the ilium and sacrum above the synovial aspect of the joint may be prominent, particularly in Reiter's syndrome.

### Degenerative Joint Disease (Osteoarthritis)
(see Fig. 40–49*A–C*)

Osteoarthritis of the sacroiliac joint can be unilateral or bilateral. Unilateral abnormalities of this joint in con-

junction with osteoarthritis of the contralateral hip may be encountered. Findings include joint space narrowing, sclerosis, and osteophytosis. Erosions are not prominent, and para-articular rather than intra-articular ankylosis predominates.

### Gouty Arthritis (see Fig. 40–49*A–C*)

Abnormalities of the sacroiliac joint can be seen in patients with long-standing tophaceous gout. Bilateral symmetrical, bilateral asymmetrical, or unilateral alterations consisting of large erosions and reactive sclerosis are found.

### Other Diseases

Sacroiliitis accompanying *inflammatory bowel diseases* is bilateral and symmetrical and cannot be differentiated from that seen in ankylosing spondylitis (see Fig. 40–49*A*). In *hyperparathyroidism*, subchondral resorption of bone, especially in the ilium, produces bilateral and symmetrical changes consisting of joint space widening and reactive sclerosis (see Fig. 40–49*A*). Unilateral abnormalities are typical of sacroiliac joint *infection* (see Fig. 40–49*C*). Such infection can be related to bacterial, mycobacterial, or fungal agents and is not infrequent in drug abusers.

*Osteitis condensans ilii* produces bilateral and symmetrical alterations in young women consisting of well-defined triangular sclerosis of the inferior aspect of the ilium (see Fig. 40–49*A*). Sacroiliac joint involvement also may accompany *familial Mediterranean fever, relapsing polychondritis, Behçet's syndrome, alkaptonuria, immobilization,* and *disuse.*

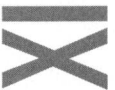

# Metabolic Diseases

# CHAPTER 41

## Osteoporosis

## SUMMARY OF KEY FEATURES

Osteoporosis is an extremely common metabolic disorder that can accompany a variety of disease processes. It can be conveniently divided into generalized, regional, and localized types. Localized osteoporosis is commonly associated with focal skeletal lesions, such as neoplasm and infection. Generalized osteoporosis accompanies senile and postmenopausal states; endocrine disorders such as acromegaly, hyperthyroidism, hyperparathyroidism, and Cushing's disease; pregnancy; heparin administration; and alcoholism. This type of osteoporosis, which must be distinguished from other metabolic disorders such as osteomalacia and osteitis fibrosa cystica, predominates in the axial skeleton, with major effects on the vertebrae; abnormalities of the appendicular skeleton are mild and consist of uniform loss of osseous density (osteopenia). In the vertebral bodies, characteristic changes in radiolucency, trabecular pattern, and osseous contour are encountered.

Regional osteoporosis accompanies disuse or immobilization, reflex sympathetic dystrophy, and transient regional osteoporosis. Changes predominate in the appendicular skeleton. A more aggressive type of bone resorption in these conditions can lead to cortical bone changes at the endosteal, intracortical, and subperiosteal bony envelopes and to spongy bone changes at subchondral and metaphyseal locations.

Additional manifestations of osteoporosis include acute and insufficiency stress fractures and bone bars (reinforcement lines). Magnetic resonance (MR) imaging shows promise in the assessment of some forms of regional osteoporosis and in the detection or further evaluation of complications associated with generalized osteoporosis.

## INTRODUCTION

Osteoporosis is the most frequent metabolic bone disease. It relates to a generalized decrease in bone mass. The remaining bone is structurally normal, as determined by histologic and chemical analysis. Routine radiographic procedures are not very helpful in the early detection of this metabolic condition. It has been estimated that 30% to 50% of skeletal calcium must be lost before a change appears on radiographs. Because of this inadequacy, newer diagnostic techniques have been used for the earlier detection and quantitation of osteoporosis, including photon absorptiometry, transaxial (quantitative)

computed tomography (CT) scanning, dual energy radiographic absorptiometry (DEXA), and ultrasonography, which are discussed elsewhere in this book.

## TERMINOLOGY

Osteoporosis is characterized by qualitatively normal (i.e., a normal mineral-to-matrix ratio) but quantitatively deficient bone. Radiographs in patients with osteoporosis reveal increased radiolucency of bone, a finding that is best termed osteopenia, meaning "poverty of bone." Osteopenia is a generic term, and it can have multiple causes. Other terms, such as demineralization and undermineralization, are not accurate descriptions of this radiographic finding. Demineralization implies a specific loss of mineral without a concomitant loss of the organic component of bone, a phenomenon called halisteresis, which is not prominent in osseous tissue. Undermineralization might be more accurately applied to osteomalacia, a condition characterized by inadequate secretion of mineral into osteoid matrix. The term deossification implies abnormal loss of bone occurring as a result of accelerated bone resorption. In fact, some types of osteoporosis are associated with increased rates of resorption; others are characterized by normal rates of resorption. Thus, osteoporosis and deossification are not equivalent terms.

The World Health Organization has used bone density measurements to classify categories of osteoporosis. These categories include terms such as osteopenia, osteoporosis, and established osteoporosis, which are dependent on the severity of bone loss and the presence or absence of fractures. At present, however, osteopenia is the most suitable term to describe increased radiolucency of bone. Osteopenia occurs when bone resorption exceeds bone formation, no matter what the specific pathogenesis (Table 41–1). Diffuse osteopenia is found in osteoporosis, osteomalacia, hyperparathyroidism, neoplasm, and a variety of other conditions. Accurate diagnosis of osteoporosis rests on the radiographic findings of osteopenia, coupled with typical clinical and histologic features.

Osteoporosis is established when the decrease in bone mass is greater than that expected for a person of a given age, sex, and race and when it results in structural bone failure manifested by fractures. These fractures are most

### TABLE 41–1

**Major Causes of Diffuse Osteopenia**

| | |
|---|---|
| Osteoporosis | Hyperparathyroidism |
| Osteomalacia | Neoplasm |

typical in the spine, proximal portion of the femur, and distal portion of the radius; they are produced by trabecular or cortical bone loss, or both, depending on the site of involvement.

## CAUSE

Osteoporosis can be classified as generalized (involving the major portion of the skeleton, particularly its axial component), regional (involving one segment of the skeleton), or localized (single or multiple focal areas of osteoporosis). The generalized, regional, and localized forms of osteoporosis have many causes. Some of the diseases associated with generalized or regional osteoporosis are discussed here. Localized osteoporosis may accompany focal skeletal lesions such as arthritis, infection, and neoplasm, and it is often overshadowed by the radiographic features of the primary process itself.

### Generalized Osteoporosis

The osseous manifestations of conditions leading to generalized osteoporosis predominate in the axial skeleton and proximal portions of the long bones of the appendicular skeleton. Abnormalities of the spine are particularly prominent and lead not only to osteopenia but also to changes in vertebral contour, characterized by biconcave vertebral bodies ("fish vertebrae") and collapse. Changes in the pelvis include osteopenia and a coarsened trabecular pattern. Trabecular resorption occurs in certain areas of the appendicular skeleton, such as the femoral necks. In both the axial and the appendicular skeleton, the decrease in radiodensity is usually uniform, particularly in conditions with slowly progressive and long-standing osteoporosis. Although some differences are apparent in the distribution and appearance of osteopenia among the various diseases that produce generalized osteoporosis (Table 41–2), the previously mentioned characteristics are most typical.

### Senile and Postmenopausal Osteoporosis

Senescent osteoporosis and postmenopausal osteoporosis (Fig. 41–1) are the most common causes of generalized

**TABLE 41–2**

**Major Causes of Generalized Osteoporosis**

| | |
|---|---|
| Senile and postmenopausal states | Deficiency states |
| Medication | Scurvy |
| Steroids | Malnutrition |
| Heparin | Calcium deficiency |
| Endocrine states | Alcoholism |
| Hyperthyroidism | Chronic liver disease |
| Hyperparathyroidism | Anemic states |
| Cushing's disease | Osteogenesis imperfecta |
| Acromegaly | Idiopathic condition |
| Pregnancy | |
| Diabetes mellitus | |
| Hypogonadism | |

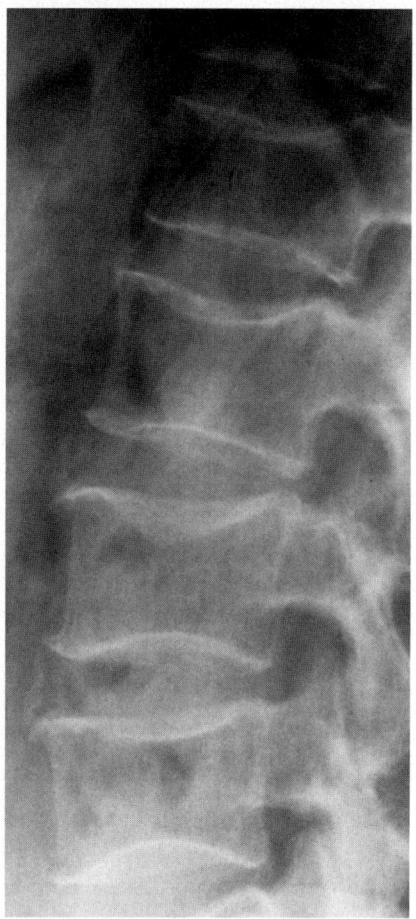

**Figure 41–1.** Senile and postmenopausal osteoporosis. In this elderly woman, a lateral radiograph of the lumbar spine outlines increased lucency and biconcave deformity (fish vertebrae) of multiple vertebral bodies.

osteoporosis. The reported frequency of osteoporosis and vertebral body compression fractures is as high as 20% of men and 29% of women between the ages of 63 and 95 years. Bone mass peaks in the second decade of life. Peak bone mass is approximately 20% greater in men than in women and is greater in black than in white persons. In general, gradual loss of skeletal mass begins to occur in the fifth or sixth decade of life in men and in the fourth decade in women. Although loss of both compact and trabecular bone occurs in older men and women, the magnitude of the loss of compact bone in women after menopause is much greater than the loss in men. Over a lifetime, women lose about 50% of their trabecular bone and 30% of their cortical bone; corresponding figures in men are about two thirds of these values. The endosteal diameter of bone increases more rapidly than the periosteal diameter, which leads to expansion of the medullary cavity at the expense of the cortex. A concomitant reduction in trabecular bone is evident, and the resulting diminution in bone mass produces a decrease in strength and a propensity for fracture.

Patients with senile or postmenopausal osteoporosis may be entirely asymptomatic, although significant loss of bone mass may be accompanied by various clinical findings. Bone pain, particularly in the back, may be associated with loss of height as a result of vertebral compression. Increased thoracic kyphosis is apparent, but neurologic complications are unusual. Patients with osteoporosis in the vertebral column have a high frequency of femoral fracture. The prevalence of osteoporosis in older patients with such fractures has been estimated at 75% to 85%. These fractures occur spontaneously or after minor trauma and may be accompanied by fractures of the ribs, humerus, or radius. Laboratory analysis generally yields unremarkable results.

The pathogenesis of osteoporosis is not clear. Whatever the precise mechanism, the apparent relationship between loss of ovarian function and escalation of osteoporosis after menopause—a relationship supported by the occurrence of osteoporosis in young oophorectomized women, in female athletes with secondary amenorrhea, in women with hyperprolactinemia, and in patients with Turner's syndrome—has led to the preventive and therapeutic use of estrogen.

### Hyperparathyroidism

Osteoporosis may occur during the course of hyperparathyroidism. The characteristic skeletal changes in this disease relate to increased rates of both bone resorption and bone formation. Superimposed on osteoporosis are the typical findings of osteitis fibrosa cystica.

### Steroid-Induced Osteoporosis

Osteoporosis occurring during the course of either Cushing's syndrome or exogenous (iatrogenic) hypercortisolism (Fig. 41–2) is well known. Histologic studies have revealed decreased bone formation and increased bone resorption. Radiographic evaluation discloses the usual findings of osteoporosis, although peculiar condensation of bone at the margins of the vertebral bodies and involvement of extraspinal sites may be encountered. Acute fractures may be evident, especially at sites that contain predominantly trabecular bone (such as the ribs and spine). Insufficiency fractures in the axial (pelvis) and appendicular skeleton are characteristic and easily overlooked.

### Hyperthyroidism

Osteoporosis in hyperthyroidism is associated with an increase in both bone resorption and bone formation. Radiographic findings are typical of osteoporosis, although rapid progression before treatment and rapid improvement after therapy may be evident.

### Acromegaly

Osteoporosis can occur in acromegaly in association with other forms of endocrine dysfunction or in acromegaly unaccompanied by such dysfunction.

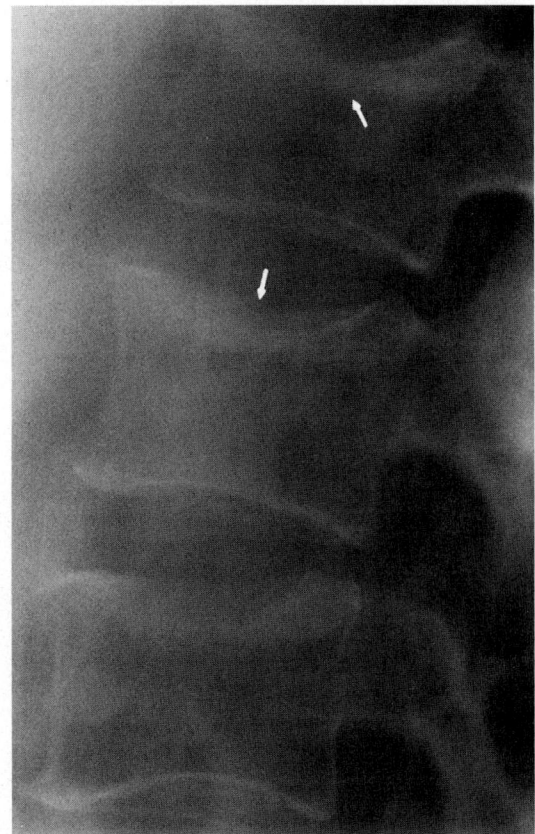

**Figure 41–2.** Steroid-induced osteoporosis. Lateral radiograph of the lumbar spine outlines osteoporosis and compressed vertebral bodies with peripheral condensation of bone (*arrows*). This latter feature, which leads to radiodense superior and inferior vertebral margins, is characteristic of exogenous or endogenous hypercortisolism.

### Pregnancy and Related Conditions

Though uncommon, osteoporosis may be observed in childbearing women. Its cause in this clinical setting has not been documented. Osteoporosis appearing in association with pregnancy or lactation is accompanied by normal results on histologic examination and serum and urinary laboratory analysis.

### Heparin-Induced Osteoporosis

The development of osteoporosis has been documented in patients receiving large doses of heparin (>15,000 units/day). The changes may be reversible with cessation of therapy, but the mechanism of osteoporosis in these patients is not known. Typical radiographic findings in the spine include osteopenia and vertebral compression.

### Alcoholism

Alcoholic patients have reduced bone mass in comparison to controls and increased bone fragility, manifested as a high rate of occurrence of fractures. The cause of this loss in bone mineral is not known.

## Idiopathic Juvenile Osteoporosis

Idiopathic juvenile osteoporosis (Fig. 41–3) is an uncommon, self-limited disease of childhood. Clinically affected children come to medical attention about 2 years before puberty because of spinal and extraspinal symptoms, which may simulate those of arthritis. Difficulty or inability to walk may be an initial manifestation. On radiographic examination, osteoporosis of the spine, particularly in the thoracic and lumbar regions, may be combined with vertebral collapse. Kyphosis is the characteristic spinal

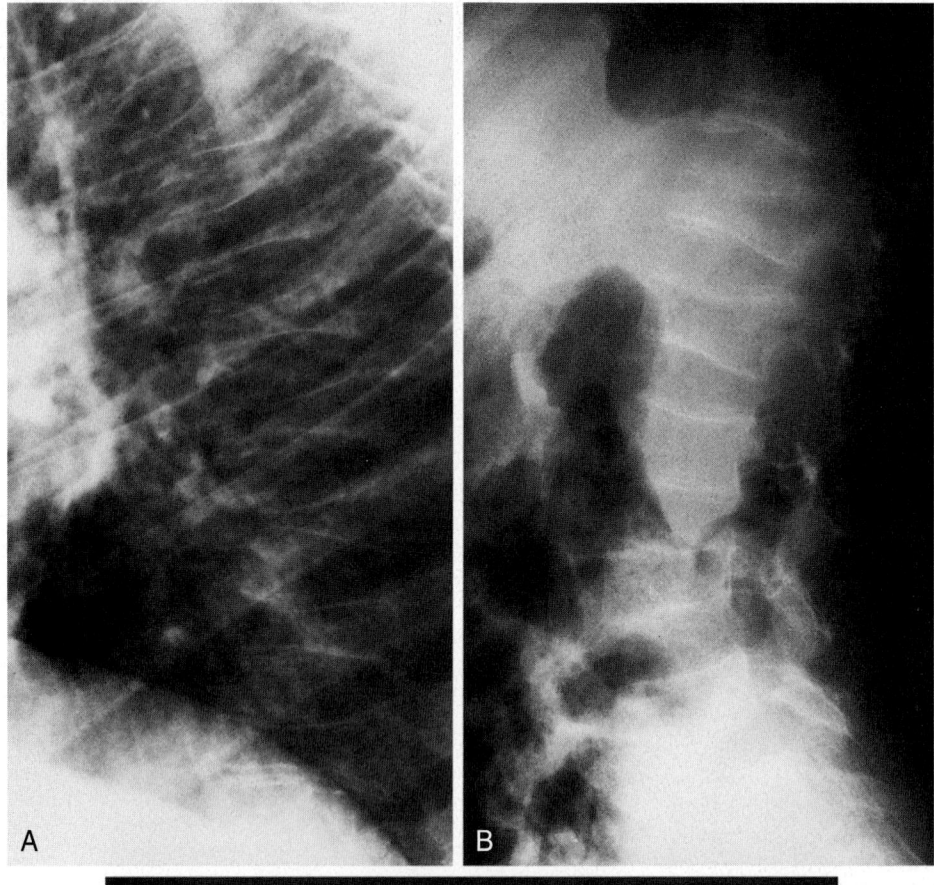

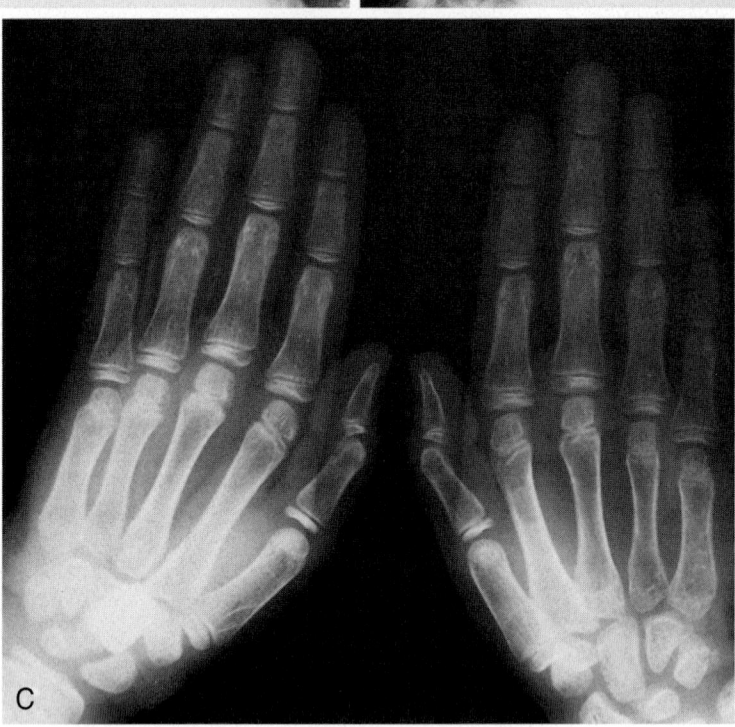

**Figure 41–3.** Idiopathic juvenile osteoporosis. This 11-year-old girl has progressive osteoporosis in the appendicular and axial skeletons. There is no clinical evidence of blue sclerae or deafness. The laboratory evaluation is unremarkable, and the family history is noncontributory. *A*, Lateral radiograph of the thoracic spine reveals severe compression and collapse of multiple radiolucent vertebral bodies. The disc spaces appear ballooned. *B*, In the lumbar spine, similar alterations are evident. Observe the severe osteoporosis of the vertebral bodies. Biconcave deformities and anterior wedging are evident. *C*, Radiograph of the hands outlines osteopenic bones with thinned cortices.

complication. Although transverse and oblique fractures may occur in the bones of the peripheral skeleton, a more typical feature appears to be metaphyseal injury, especially about the knees and ankles. This finding is less common in osteogenesis imperfecta, the disease most likely to be confused with idiopathic juvenile osteoporosis.

The major problem in the differential diagnosis is distinguishing idiopathic juvenile osteoporosis from osteogenesis imperfecta (Fig. 41–4). Osteogenesis imperfecta congenita appears in early infancy and has distinctive features. Osteogenesis imperfecta tarda may not produce abnormalities until late childhood or adolescence. Osteogenesis imperfecta may be associated with blue sclerae and progressive cranial, facial, and pelvic deformities, findings not evident in idiopathic juvenile osteoporosis. In osteogenesis imperfecta, thin diaphyseal cortices lead to characteristic fractures of the shaft. Other childhood disorders, such as leukemia, homocystinuria, Cushing's disease, and juvenile chronic arthritis, are usually easily differentiated from idiopathic juvenile osteoporosis.

## Other Disorders

Generalized osteoporosis may accompany plasma cell myeloma, Gaucher's disease, glycogen storage disease, anemia, nutritional deficiency, diabetes mellitus, immuno-

deficiency states, and chronic liver disease. In some of these disorders (plasma cell myeloma, storage diseases), the primary disease process involves the bone directly; in others (sickle cell anemia, neoplasm), the bone is altered as a complication of the primary disease.

## Differential Diagnosis

Differentiation between generalized osteoporosis and osteomalacia, especially in adults, may be extremely difficult on the basis of radiographic abnormalities and may require histologic evaluation. In infants and children, the presence of rickets, with its characteristic metaphyseal changes, is a valuable diagnostic clue. An accurate diagnosis is especially important in infants, particularly those receiving long-term intravenous hyperalimentation; in these patients, the development of rickets may lead to multiple fractures that contribute to an erroneous diagnosis of osteogenesis imperfecta, the child abuse syndrome, or copper deficiency (Fig. 41–5).

In adults with osteomalacia, diffuse osteopenia simulates generalized osteoporosis. In osteomalacia, however, trabeculae may appear indistinct, and the interface of cortical and medullary bone may be obscured. Osseous deformity (such as acetabular protrusion and a bell-shaped thorax) and insufficiency fractures and pseudofractures (which are most frequent in the pubic rami, medial portion of the femoral neck, axillary margins of the ribs, scapula, and, occasionally, tubular bones) may also be seen (Fig. 41–6). In some forms of osteomalacia and rickets, additional distinctive alterations are apparent. X-linked hypophosphatemic osteomalacia (or rickets) is associated with a generalized enthesopathy in which bone proliferation at sites of tendon and ligament attachment and tendi-

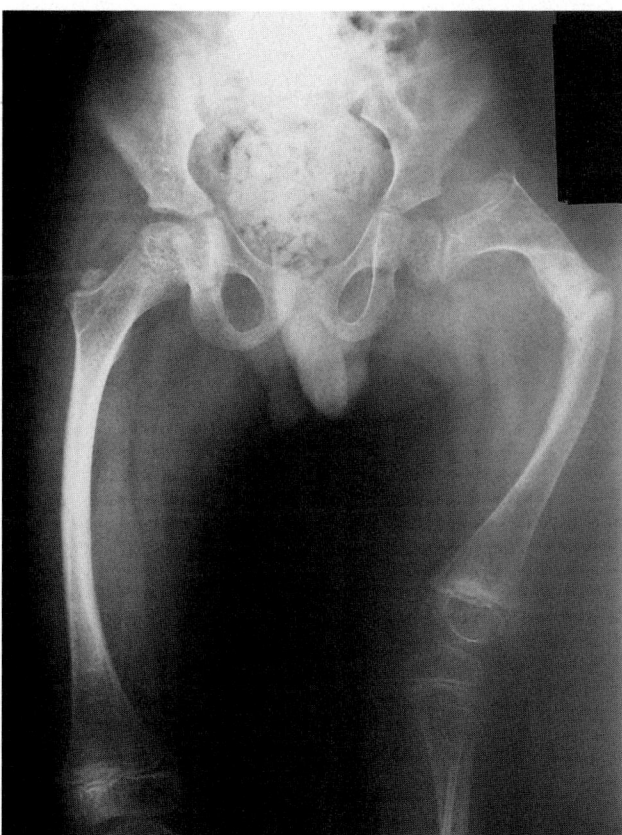

**Figure 41–4.** Osteogenesis imperfecta. In this child, observe the generalized osteoporosis, cortical diminution, and osseous deformity and fracture.

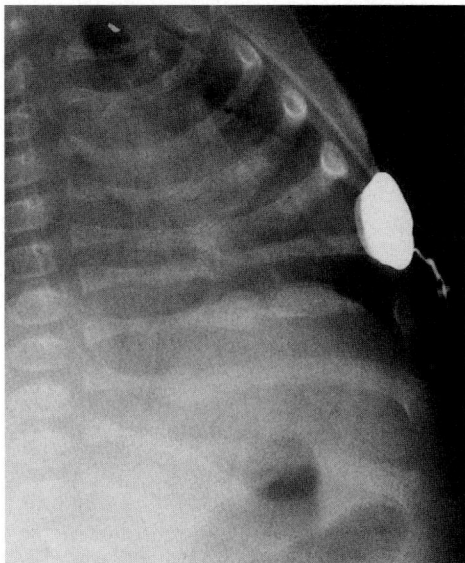

**Figure 41–5.** Rickets secondary to intravenous hyperalimentation. In this infant, multiple fractures of the ribs simulate those seen in the child abuse syndrome. (Courtesy of M. Dalinka, MD, Philadelphia, Pa.)

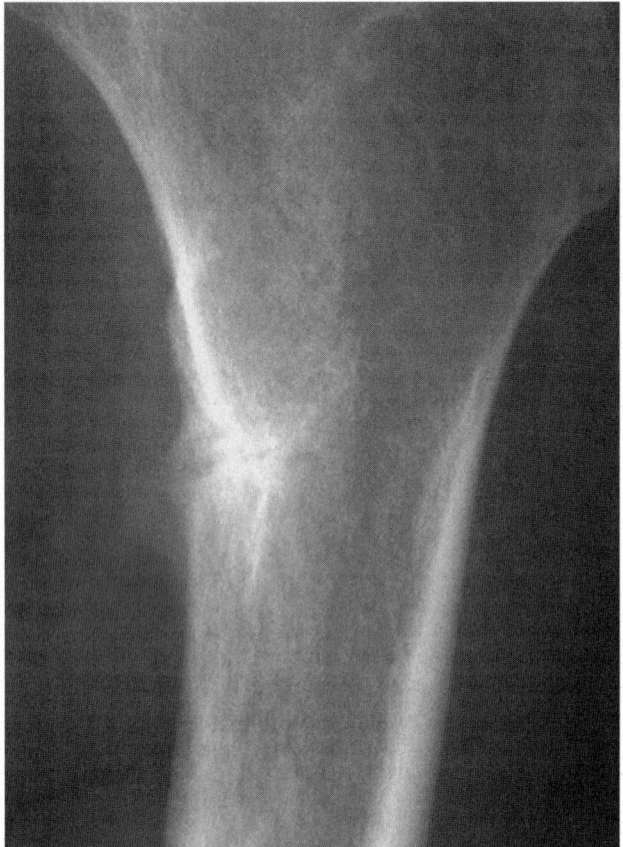

**Figure 41–6.** Osteomalacia. Note pseudofractures in the medial aspect of the femoral neck.

nous, ligamentous, and capsular calcification become evident; calcification of cartilage and small ossicles may also be seen. In addition to osteopenia, hyperparathyroidism produces aggressive bone resorption in subperiosteal, intracortical, endosteal, subligamentous, and subchondral locations. In patients with renal osteodystrophy, these changes are accompanied by osteosclerosis, osteomalacia, and vascular, soft tissue, and periarticular calcification.

## Regional Osteoporosis

Osteoporosis confined to a region or segment of the body is associated with disorders of the appendicular skeleton. The classic example is osteoporosis associated with disuse or immobilization. Other examples include reflex sympathetic dystrophy (RSD) and transient regional osteoporosis (Table 41–3).

The radiographic patterns of regional osteoporosis are variable. Uniform osteopenia may accompany regional osteoporosis of long duration, whereas bandlike osteopenia (in the subchondral or metaphyseal regions) and patchy osteopenia (particularly in the epiphyses) may indicate a more acutely developing osteoporosis. In acute osteoporosis, both cortical and spongy bone can show dramatic alterations. The cortical abnormalities include subperiosteal, intracortical, and endosteal erosion.

**TABLE 41–3**

**Major Causes of Regional Osteoporosis**

Immobilization and disuse
Reflex sympathetic dystrophy
Transient regional osteoporosis
  Transient osteoporosis of the hip
  Regional migratory osteoporosis

## Osteoporosis of Immobilization and Disuse

This type of osteoporosis characteristically occurs in the immobilized regions in patients with fractures, motor paralysis caused by central nervous system disease or trauma, and bone and joint inflammation (Fig. 41–7).

The radiographic appearance of osteoporosis depends on many factors, including the age of the patient (osteoporosis appears sooner in younger persons) and the extent and duration of the negative calcium balance (osteoporosis is more severe when calcium loss is more prominent). After paralysis, osteoporosis generally occurs within 2 or 3 months; the findings initially appear in the appendicular skeleton, although the pelvis may subsequently become abnormal. Spinal abnormalities are not prominent. The radiographic features of osteoporosis occurring after immobilization for fractures are generally similar to those seen after paralysis.

The radiographic patterns associated with osteoporosis of immobilization are uniform osteoporosis (most common type), speckled or spotty osteoporosis (characterized by small, spheroid lucent areas, most frequently in the periarticular regions and in the carpal and tarsal areas), bandlike osteoporosis (in the subchondral or metaphyseal regions), and cortical lamellation or scalloping (translucency of the outer or inner aspects of the cortex). These radiographic appearances may simulate those of malignancy. Finally, it should be recognized that although a regional distribution is the hallmark of disuse osteoporosis, generalized or scattered patterns may be observed in unusual circumstances.

## Reflex Sympathetic Dystrophy

RSD is the most commonly accepted name for a distinct entity that is also known as Sudeck's atrophy or osteodystrophy, reflex dystrophy of the extremities, causalgia, shoulder-hand syndrome, reflex neurovascular dystrophy, and the RSD syndrome. A recently introduced term—complex regional pain syndrome—may eventually prove to be a more appropriate designation. Any neurally related visceral, musculoskeletal, neurologic, or vascular condition is a potential source of RSD, although an incipient cause is frequently not identifiable. The most common initiating event appears to be trauma; RSD is estimated to occur in as many as 5% of patients with traumatic injuries. Other associated conditions include cerebrovascular disorders, degenerative disease of the cervical spine, disc extrusion, postsurgical and post-

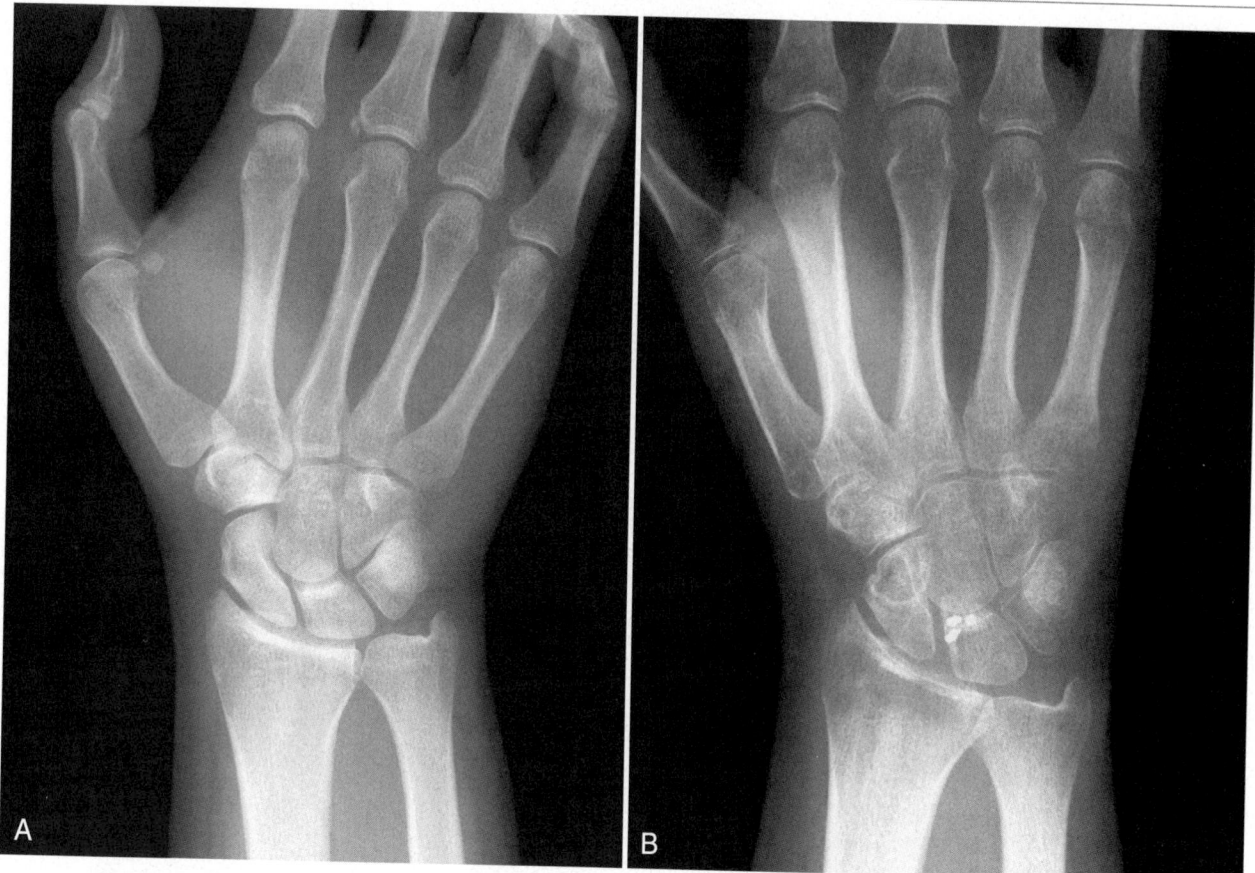

**Figure 41–7.** Osteoporosis of immobilization and disuse. Radiographs obtained immediately before wrist ligament reconstruction (A) and 2 months later (B) are shown. Observe in (B) the extent of the osteopenia.

infectious states, calcific tendinosis, vasculitis, electrical injuries, and neoplasm.

The pathogenesis of RSD is not entirely clear. The most widely held theory is that of the "internuncial pool," in which it is assumed that an injury or lesion produces painful impulses that travel via afferent pathways to the spinal cord, where a series of reflexes are initiated that spread by means of the interconnecting pool of neurons. These latter reflexes stimulate the lateral and anterior tracts and thereby provoke efferent pathways that travel to the peripheral nerves and produce the local findings of RSD.

Clinical symptoms and signs are variable. They may be evident in any involved site, although the characteristic distribution is the shoulder and hand. Rarely, multiple extremities are affected. Initially, stiffness, pain, tenderness, and weakness may be associated with swelling, vasomotor changes, hyperesthesia, and disability. The duration of RSD varies, and in some cases, findings may persist for years and become irreversible.

Soft tissue swelling and regional osteoporosis are the most important radiographic findings (Fig. 41–8). Five types of bone resorption can be detected: (1) resorption in the metaphyseal region, which leads to bandlike, patchy, or periarticular osteoporosis; (2) subperiosteal bone resorption, which is similar to that occurring in cases of hyperparathyroidism; (3) intracortical bone resorption,

which produces excessive striation or tunneling in cortices; (4) endosteal bone resorption, which causes scalloping of the endosteal surface, with subsequent uniform remodeling of the endosteum and widening of the medullary canal; and (5) subchondral and juxta-articular erosion, which may lead to small periarticular erosions and intra-articular gaps in the subchondral bone. Because of the widespread nature and severity of the bone resorption in RSD, radiographs may reveal rapid and severe osteopenia, particularly in the periarticular regions, that simulates the appearance of primary articular disorders. The absence of significant intra-articular erosions and joint space loss usually allows the accurate differentiation of RSD from these various arthritides. The preservation of joint space cannot be overemphasized as a characteristic finding in this syndrome.

Bone and joint scintigraphy demonstrates typical abnormalities in RSD, which may antedate the clinical and radiographic changes. It also reveals increased technetium-99m pertechnetate radionuclide accumulation in the articular regions. This finding appears to be related to increased vascularity of the synovial membrane, and bone-seeking agents likewise reveal increased accumulation in the involved bones in RSD, also related to increased blood flow. With three-phase bone scanning, the delayed images delineate this pattern most frequently, although scintigraphic abnormalities also occur

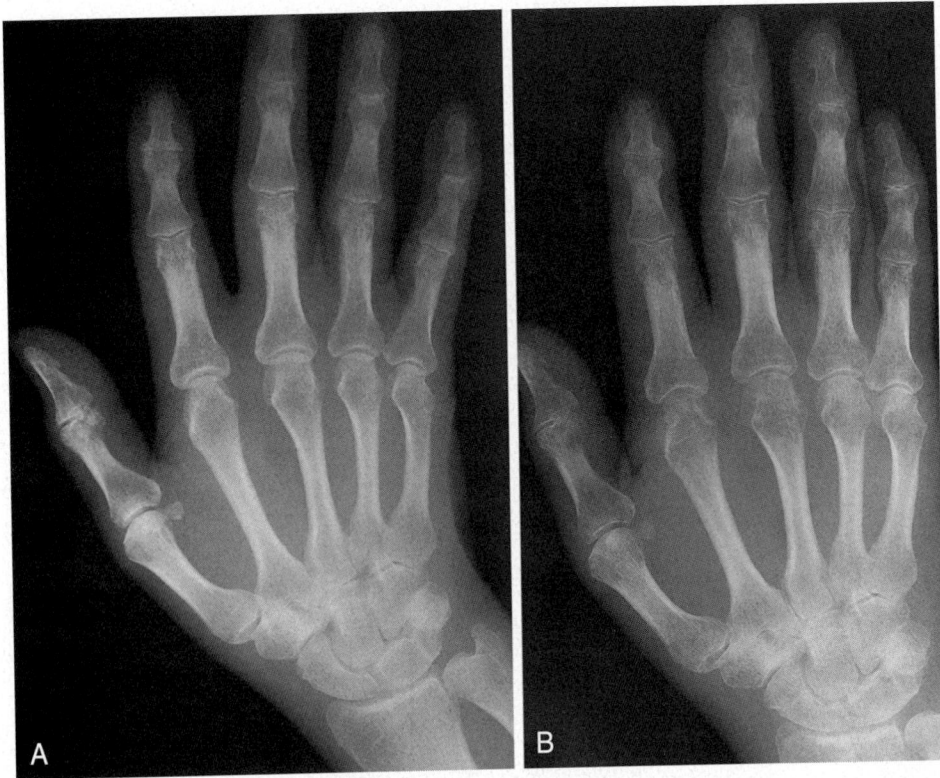

**Figure 41–8.** Reflex sympathetic dystrophy: radiographic abnormalities. Pain and swelling developed in a 65-year-old man after a minor injury to the hand. *A*, The initial film outlines mild periarticular osteoporosis and soft tissue swelling. *B*, Six weeks later, the osteoporosis is much more exaggerated. The periarticular osteoporosis simulates the appearance of rheumatoid arthritis.

during the angiographic and blood pool stages of the study. In these earlier stages of the study, soft tissue uptake may be prominent. Bone scans obtained at different times in a single patient may reveal migration of the scintigraphic abnormality from one side of a joint to another. Rarely, decreased or normal accumulation of the radionuclide is observed on bone scans, a finding that may be more frequent in children.

Radiographic, scintigraphic, and quantitative bone mineral analyses all reveal that RSD is often a bilateral process; the abnormalities are much more marked on one side than the other, however. Almost universally, an entire extremity distal to an affected site is altered. Rarely, a segmental pattern affecting only a portion of an extremity may be encountered. This localized form of RSD may lead to the involvement of one joint in an extremity, one or several digits of the hand or foot, or a portion of an articular surface (e.g., patella, femoral condyle).

### Transient Regional Osteoporosis

Transient regional osteoporosis is a term applied to conditions that share certain features: rapidly developing osteoporosis affecting periarticular bone, self-limited and reversible nature, and the absence of clear-cut evidence of inciting events such as trauma and immobilization. Two important diseases (which are probably related) fall into this category: transient osteoporosis of the hip and regional migratory osteoporosis.

**Transient Osteoporosis of the Hip.** Originally described in the third trimester of pregnancy, transient osteoporosis is now known to typically occur in young and middle-aged adults, particularly men. In male patients, either hip may be involved, whereas in female patients, the left hip is affected almost exclusively. Hip pain begins spontaneously and usually progresses within a few weeks and becomes severe enough to produce a limp. The clinical findings regress in 2 to 6 months without permanent sequelae.

Radiographic findings are characteristic. Progressive and marked osteoporosis of the femoral head, which begins several weeks after the onset of clinical abnormalities, is associated with less extensive involvement of the femoral neck and acetabulum (Fig. 41–9). The joint space is not diminished in size. Incomplete or complete fractures of the femoral neck may occur. This complication has been emphasized in pregnancy or in the immediate postpartum period. Restoration of normal radiographic density of the bone takes place rapidly. Radionuclide studies using bone-seeking agents reveal abnormal accumulation of isotope before radiographically demonstrable osteoporosis. MR imaging may show altered signal intensity of the bone marrow in affected sites and joint effusions.

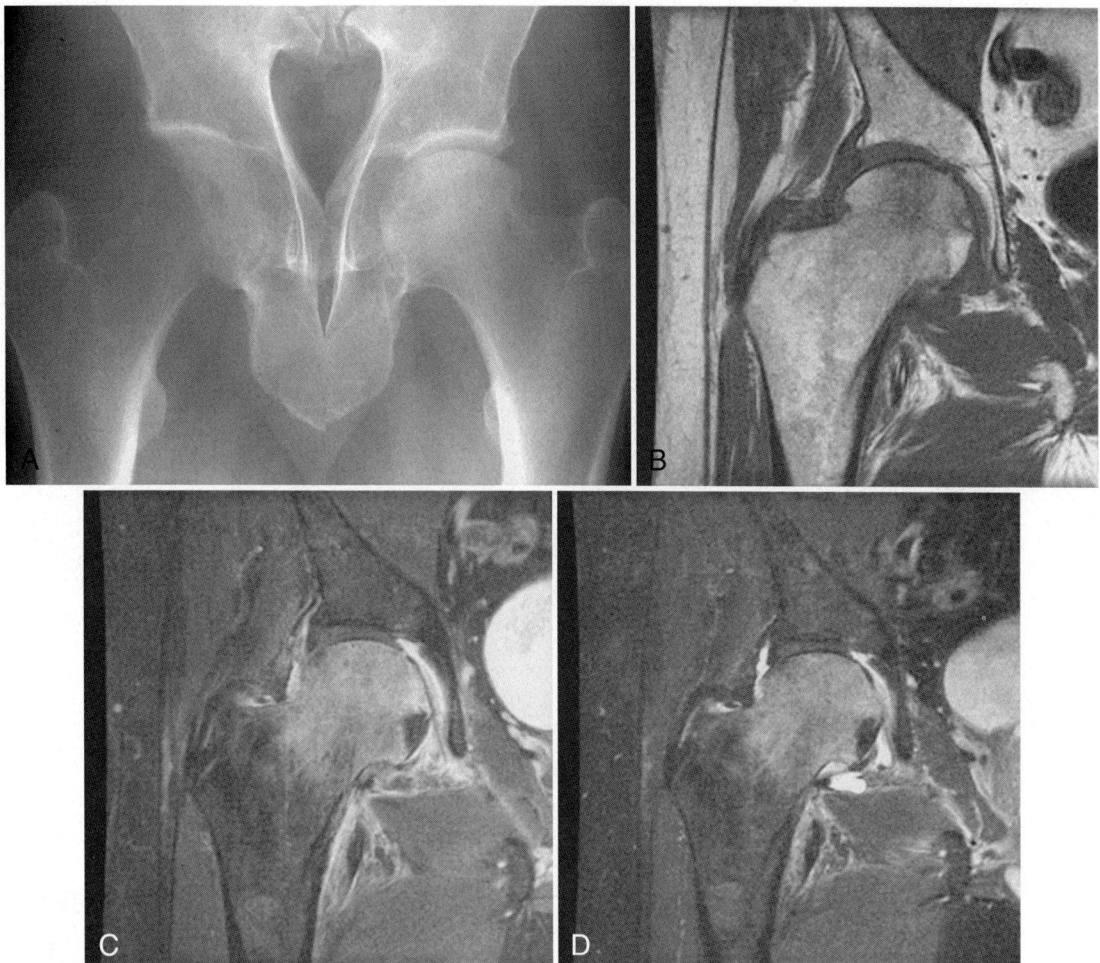

**Figure 41–9.** Transient osteoporosis of the hip in a 66-year-old man. *A*, Radiograph, collimated for comparison of both hip joints, shows dramatic osteopenia of the right femoral head and neck. *B* and *C*, Coronal T1-weighted (TR/TE, 800/15) spin echo *(B)* and STIR (TR/TE, 4000/15; inversion time, 150 msec) *(C)* MR images show the typical features of marrow edema. Note the sparing of the medial aspect of the femoral head and joint effusion. *D*, Corresponding fat-suppressed T1-weighted (TR/TE, 467/15) spin echo MR image following intravenous gadolinium contrast administration shows extensive enhancement of the edema, as well as synovial enhancement.

The cause of this condition is unknown. Although it has been regarded as a self-limited ischemic necrosis of bone, its similarity to RSD suggests a related neurogenic pathogenesis. Because transient osteoporosis of the hip is occasionally bilateral in distribution or may involve other joints, a relationship with regional migratory osteoporosis is possible.

**Regional Migratory Osteoporosis.** The second form of transient osteoporosis is migratory in nature. Abnormalities of the hip are less frequent than abnormalities in other areas, particularly the knee, ankle, and foot. It occurs in men more frequently than women and usually becomes evident in the fourth or fifth decade of life. The disorder is characterized by local pain and swelling, particularly in the lower extremity, that develop rapidly, last up to 9 months, and then diminish and disappear. Subsequent involvement occurs in other regions of the same or opposite extremity, although this migratory

pattern is not invariable. Radiographic evidence of osteoporosis becomes apparent within weeks or months of the onset of clinical findings (Fig. 41–10). It also progresses rapidly, subsequently diminishes, and appears at other sites. In extreme cases, periarticular osteoporosis extends for a considerable distance into the adjacent bone. The joint space is not narrowed, nor can evidence of intra-articular erosion be found. MR imaging shows signal intensity alterations in the bone marrow (see subsequent discussion).

The migratory nature of the syndrome is the major feature that differentiates this condition from transient osteoporosis of the hip. Usually, the joint nearest the diseased one is the next to be involved. The clinical features may overlap, so more than one joint can be symptomatic at a given time. The pathogenesis of this condition is not known, although regional migratory osteoporosis may be closely related to RSD and transient osteoporosis of the hip.

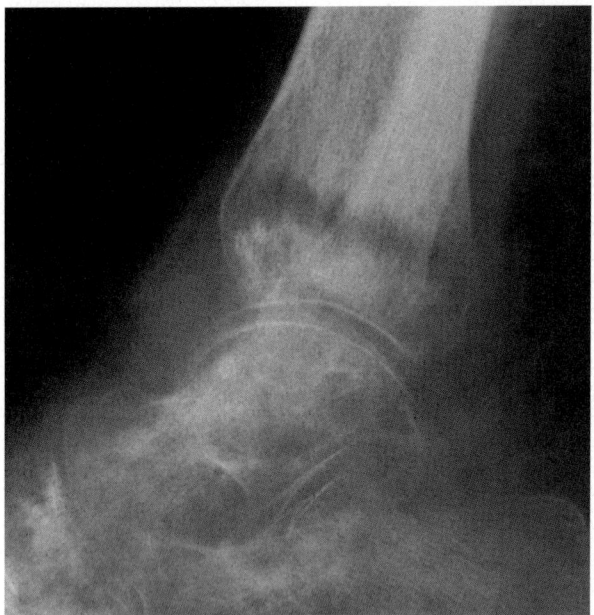

**Figure 41–10.** Regional migratory osteoporosis. Typical in this condition are transient pain and swelling of one joint associated with periarticular osteoporosis, followed by spontaneous improvement and involvement of an adjacent joint. Observe the soft tissue swelling and bandlike osteopenia of the tibia and talus.

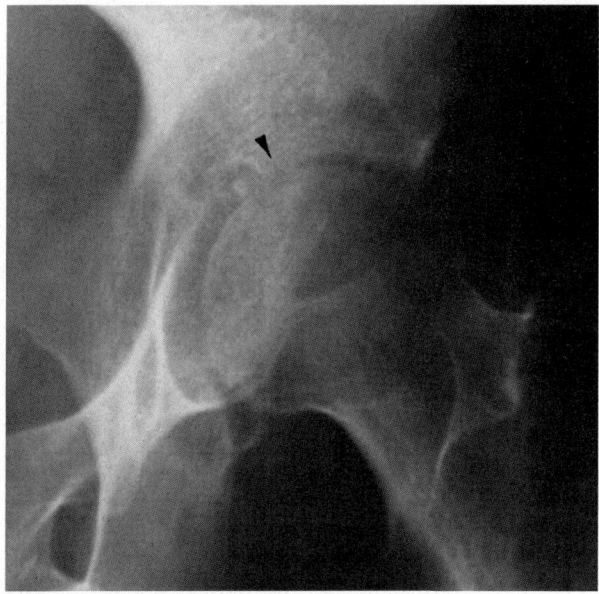

**Figure 41–11.** Osteomyelitis and septic arthritis. Progressive hip pain developed in this 23-year-old Mexican woman over a 1-year period. The appearance of osteoporosis in the femoral head and acetabulum resembles transient osteoporosis of the hip. The presence of joint space narrowing *(arrowhead)*, however, signifies cartilaginous destruction, in this case related to tuberculosis.

### Differential Diagnosis

Accurate diagnosis of regional osteoporosis associated with disuse is not difficult. The osteoporosis associated with RSD, transient osteoporosis of the hip, and regional migratory osteoporosis may simulate other conditions. Septic arthritis can lead to regional osteoporosis (Fig. 41–11); however, joint space narrowing and osseous erosion are eventually observed in infection, whereas in regional osteoporosis, these findings are not apparent. Similarly, in rheumatoid arthritis, intense synovial inflammation can produce significant cartilaginous and osseous destruction. In addition, symmetrical involvement of multiple joints is characteristic of rheumatoid arthritis.

In monoarticular processes such as pigmented villonodular synovitis and idiopathic synovial osteochondromatosis, osteoporosis is not a dominant feature and, when present, occurs late in the course of the articular disease. Monoarticular involvement of the hip or other joints is not infrequent in osteonecrosis (Fig. 41–12). In osteonecrosis, the presence of osteoporosis on radiographic examination, the presence of increased radionuclide accumulation on scintigraphic examination, and the absence of articular space narrowing are findings that are identical to those in regional osteoporosis. Further, the MR imaging features of certain types of regional osteoporosis overlap with those of ischemic necrosis of bone. Although one condition can certainly occur without the other, a meaningful association of the two may exist (see discussion later in this chapter).

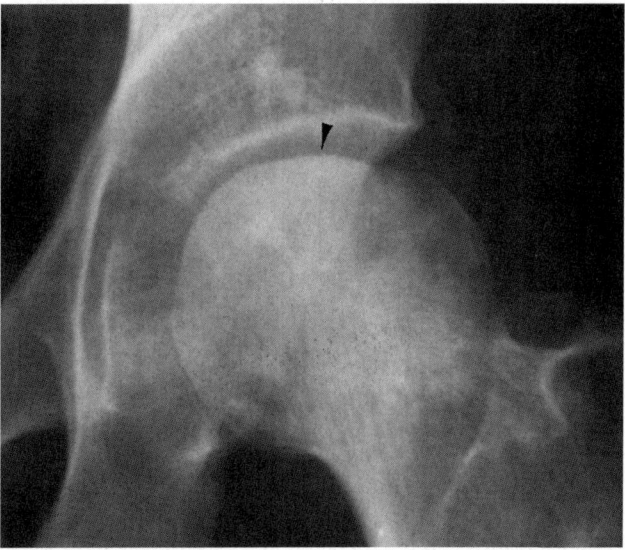

**Figure 41–12.** Osteonecrosis. The diagnosis is established by detecting a depression in the articular surface of the femoral head *(arrowhead)*; this finding is associated with patchy lucent areas and sclerosis.

## RADIOGRAPHIC-PATHOLOGIC CORRELATION
### General Distribution of Abnormalities

Generalized osteoporosis is most prominent in the axial skeleton, particularly the vertebral column, pelvis, ribs, and sternum (Fig. 41–13). Eventually, less extensive changes

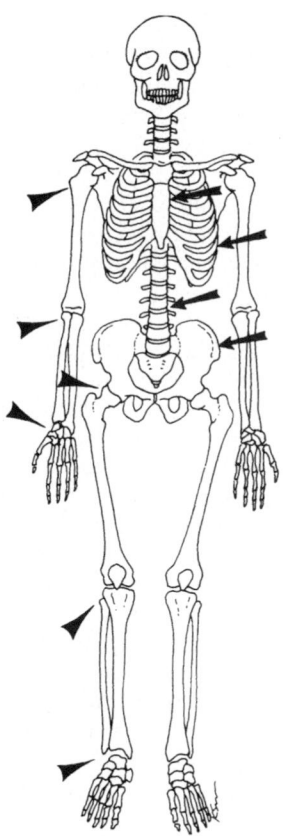

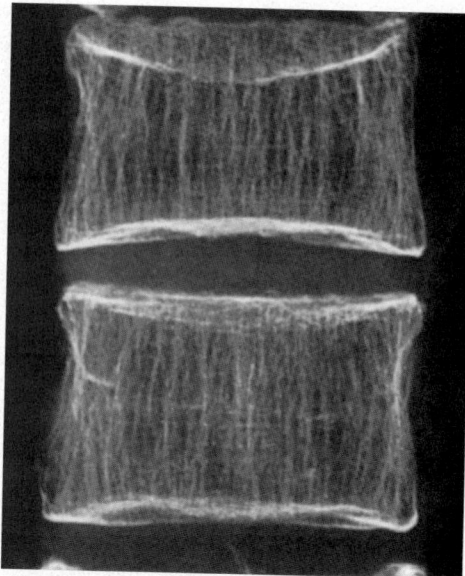

**Figure 41–14.** Osteoporosis: changes in radiolucency and trabecular pattern in the spine. Observe the accentuation of the vertical trabeculae, with preferential resorption of the horizontal trabeculae. Additional findings characteristic of osteoporosis are depression of the superior margin of the vertebral body and a distinct but thinned bone plate at the superior and inferior surfaces of the vertebral bodies.

**Figure 41–13.** Osteoporosis: distribution of abnormalities— generalized versus regional. In generalized osteoporosis (*arrows*, right half of diagram), the spine, pelvis, ribs, and sternum are affected most commonly. In regional osteoporosis (*arrowheads*, left half), the appendicular skeleton is the predominant site of alterations, particularly in periarticular regions.

may become evident in the long and short tubular bones of the appendicular skeleton. Cranial vault alterations are usually mild. In regional osteoporosis, alterations in the appendicular skeleton predominate over those in the axial skeleton.

## Spine

The diagnosis of osteoporosis of the spine is made on the basis of changes in the radiolucency of bone, trabecular pattern, and shape of vertebral bodies.

### Change in Radiolucency

Osteoporosis produces increased radiolucency of vertebral bone (Fig. 41–14). It must be realized, however, that approximately 30% to 80% of bone tissue must be lost before a recognizable abnormality can be detected on spinal radiographs, and the radiographic diagnosis of mild to moderate osteoporosis remains difficult. Associated vertebral compression can lead to an increase in bone density as a result of compaction of trabeculae and callus formation.

### Change in Trabecular Pattern

In osteoporosis, individual trabeculae are thinned, and some are lost. Relative accentuation of the vertical trabeculae leads to vertical radiodense striations (bars) that simulate the appearance of a hemangioma (Fig. 41–15). In osteoporosis, a distinct but thinned subchondral bone plate becomes evident in the superior and inferior portions of the vertebral body. These typical changes in trabecular structure in osteoporosis are different from those in osteomalacia, in which individual trabeculae appear indistinct or fuzzy and produce a coarsened or spongy pattern. In some instances of osteomalacia, the density of the bone is actually increased. The endplate sclerosis seen in renal osteodystrophy, which leads to rugger-jersey spine, is likewise not a feature of osteoporosis.

### Change in Shape of Vertebral Bodies

Characteristic abnormalities in vertebral shape are observed in osteoporosis (Table 41–4) and must be distinguished from normal variations in vertebral contour, as well as from artifacts produced by improper radiographic examination (Fig. 41–16). The posterior heights of the thoracic vertebrae often measure 1 to 3 mm more than the anterior heights. If the normal prominence of the posterior surface of the vertebral body is taken into account, a difference in vertical height of 4 mm or more between the anterior and posterior surfaces should be considered true vertebral compression; if this normal prominence is not used in the measurement, a difference of 2 mm or more in vertical height is in-

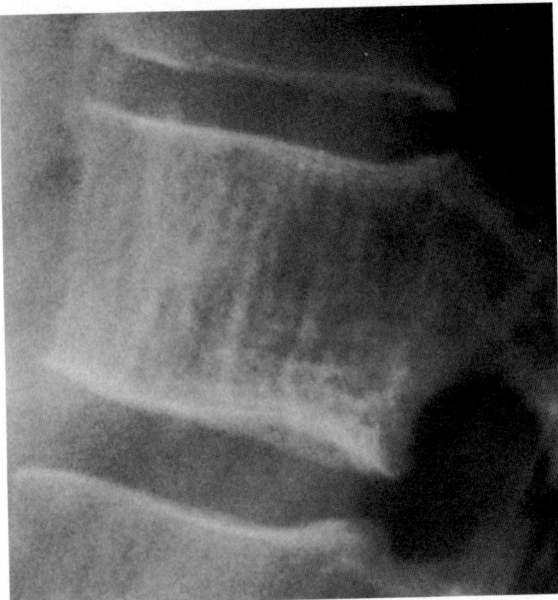

**Figure 41–15.** Hemangioma. Lateral radiograph demonstrates the typical characteristics of a vertebral body hemangioma: increased radiolucency and coarse vertical trabeculae producing a spongy appearance.

dicative of abnormality. The same criteria used to measure thoracic vertebrae can be applied to the measurement of lumbar vertebrae.

Alterations in vertebral shape include wedge-shaped vertebrae, with a reduced anterior border but a normal posterior border, and compression, in which the central portion of the vertebral body alone, both the anterior and central portions of the vertebral body, or the anterior, central, and posterior portions of the vertebral body are decreased. If the degree of compression is severe and uniform, a pancake vertebral body is present.

**Wedged-Shaped and Compressed Vertebrae.** Both wedging and compression (Fig. 41–17) in osteoporosis indicate a fracture of the vertebral body. The particular pattern of altered vertebral shape is influenced by the specific spinal segment affected, the type and amount of stress placed on the spine, and the degree of osteoporosis.

The different patterns of vertebral compression have led to problems in terminology. A compression fracture of the vertebral body is typically thought of as one in which the posterior portion of the vertebral body (the middle column of the spine) is not affected; a burst fracture of the vertebral body is commonly defined as one that affects both the anterior and the posterior portions of the vertebral body (the anterior and middle columns). In line with these definitions, both compression and burst fractures of the vertebral bodies can occur spontaneously in patients with osteoporosis. Burst fractures can be stable, without neurologic compromise (the designation compression fractures with middle column involvement could be used in such cases), or unstable, with neurologic compromise (a more typical burst fracture). Unstable burst fractures in osteoporosis generally occur in the lower thoracic and lumbar spine; stable burst fractures (compression fractures with middle column involvement) have a similar distribution. Typical compression fractures (with an intact middle column) occur predominantly in the lumbar spine, and vertebral wedge fractures (anterior column involvement) are most common in the mid-thoracic region and thoracolumbar junction. Any of these fractures are uncommon cephalad to the seventh thoracic vertebra and rare cephalad to the fourth thoracic vertebra, so fractures above these spinal levels, even in patients with severe osteoporosis, should raise the suspicion of another underlying disease process. Further, although exaggerated thoracic kyphosis may accompany multiple wedged vertebral bodies in an osteoporotic thoracic spine, such kyphosis may occur in the absence of wedge fractures and reflect the presence of another condition, such as senile kyphosis.

---

**TABLE 41–4**

**Abnormalities in Vertebral Body Shape**

| Abnormality | Common Cause | Characteristics |
|---|---|---|
| Biconcave (fish) vertebrae | Osteoporosis<br>Osteomalacia<br>Paget's disease<br>Hyperparathyroidism | Archlike contour defects of the superior and inferior vertebral surfaces, particularly in the lower thoracic and lumbar areas |
| Cupid's bow vertebrae | Normal | Parasagittal concavities on the inferior surface of the lower lumbar vertebrae |
| Butterfly vertebrae | Congenital | Funnel-like defect through a vertebra dividing it into right and left halves |
| Cartilaginous nodes | Scheuermann's disease<br>Trauma<br>Hyperparathyroidism<br>Intervertebral osteochondrosis | Depression and discontinuity of the vertebral endplate with an intraosseous lucent area and surrounding sclerosis |
| H vertebrae | Sickle cell anemia<br>Gaucher's disease | Steplike central depression of the vertebral endplates |

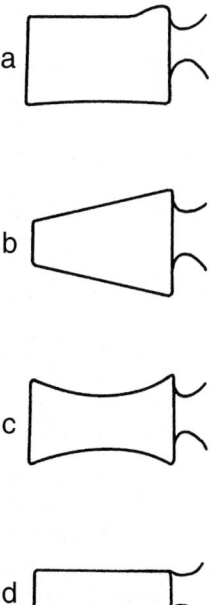

**Figure 41–16.** Osteoporosis: changes in vertebral body shape. a, In a normal situation, the superior and inferior vertebral outlines are relatively parallel, although a slight elevation or protuberance can be seen at the posterosuperior aspect of the vertebral bodies. b, Wedge-shaped vertebrae relate to collapse of the anterior aspect of the vertebral body. c, Biconcave, or fish, vertebrae are characterized by biconcave deformity of the superior and inferior surfaces of the vertebral body. d, Flattened, or pancake, vertebrae are associated with compression of the entire vertebral surface.

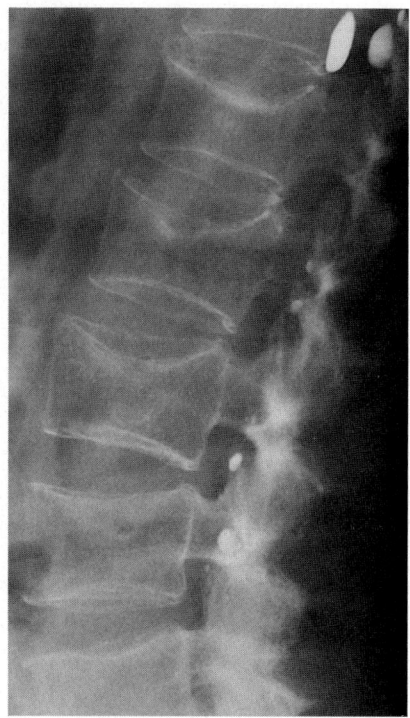

**Figure 41–17.** Osteoporosis: vertebral compression. Lateral radiograph of the lumbar spine in this 68-year-old woman shows multiple compression fractures of the vertebral bodies. Note that the osseous depressions involve mainly the central portion of the superior bone plate and are accompanied by an increase in radiodensity at the fracture site in the first and second lumbar vertebral bodies. Acutely, such radiodense areas may represent compression of trabeculae; subacutely or chronically, they may indicate new bone formation at the site of fracture. In this case, the posterior surface of the vertebral body (the middle column) is not affected. Slight loss of height of the anterior vertebral surface is seen in the first lumbar vertebral body.

Compression fractures of the vertebral bodies may occur as a complication of a single traumatic event, a few separate traumatic events, or slow structural remodeling from chronic microfractures. In the last of these complications, particularly when the compression is confined to the central portion of the vertebral body with an intact anterior margin, the designation "fish vertebrae" is commonly used.

**Fish Vertebrae.** Increased concavity of the vertebral bodies in osteoporosis produces typical fish vertebrae (presumably named for their likeness to the vertebrae of a normal fish). Gradually developing biconcave deformities of the vertebral bodies (fish vertebrae) are characteristic of disorders resulting in diffuse weakening of the bone (Fig. 41–18), including osteoporosis, osteomalacia, Paget's disease, hyperparathyroidism, and neoplasm. Fish vertebrae are particularly common in the lower thoracic and upper lumbar spine.

Fish vertebrae complicating osteoporosis must be differentiated from fish vertebrae in other disorders. In osteomalacia, biconcave vertebral deformities have been reported to be smoother than those in osteoporosis and to involve the superior and inferior margins of the vertebral body with equal severity; adjacent vertebrae are affected to the same extent. Fish vertebrae in Paget's disease, hyperparathyroidism, renal osteodystrophy, and

neoplasm also resemble those in osteoporosis, although additional characteristics of the underlying disease process are usually discernible.

Cupid's bow contour, a name applied to a normal concavity that is seen most commonly on the inferior aspect of the third, fourth, and fifth lumbar vertebral bodies, may resemble the biconcave changes of fish vertebrae (Fig. 41–19). When viewed from the front, parasagittal concavities on the undersurface of the vertebral bodies resemble a bow pointing cephalad, with the spinous processes representing the arrows. On lateral views, these vertebral depressions are located posteriorly.

**Cartilaginous (Schmorl's) Nodes.** This defect can be attributed to displacement of a portion of the intervertebral disc into the vertebral body (Fig. 41–20). These disc displacements are termed cartilaginous, or Schmorl's, nodes. Metabolic disorders produce cartilaginous nodes by diffusely weakening the osseous structure of the vertebral body. With subchondral bone loss, a portion of the cartilaginous endplate becomes depressed into the subjacent bone. The radiographic evidence of cartilaginous node

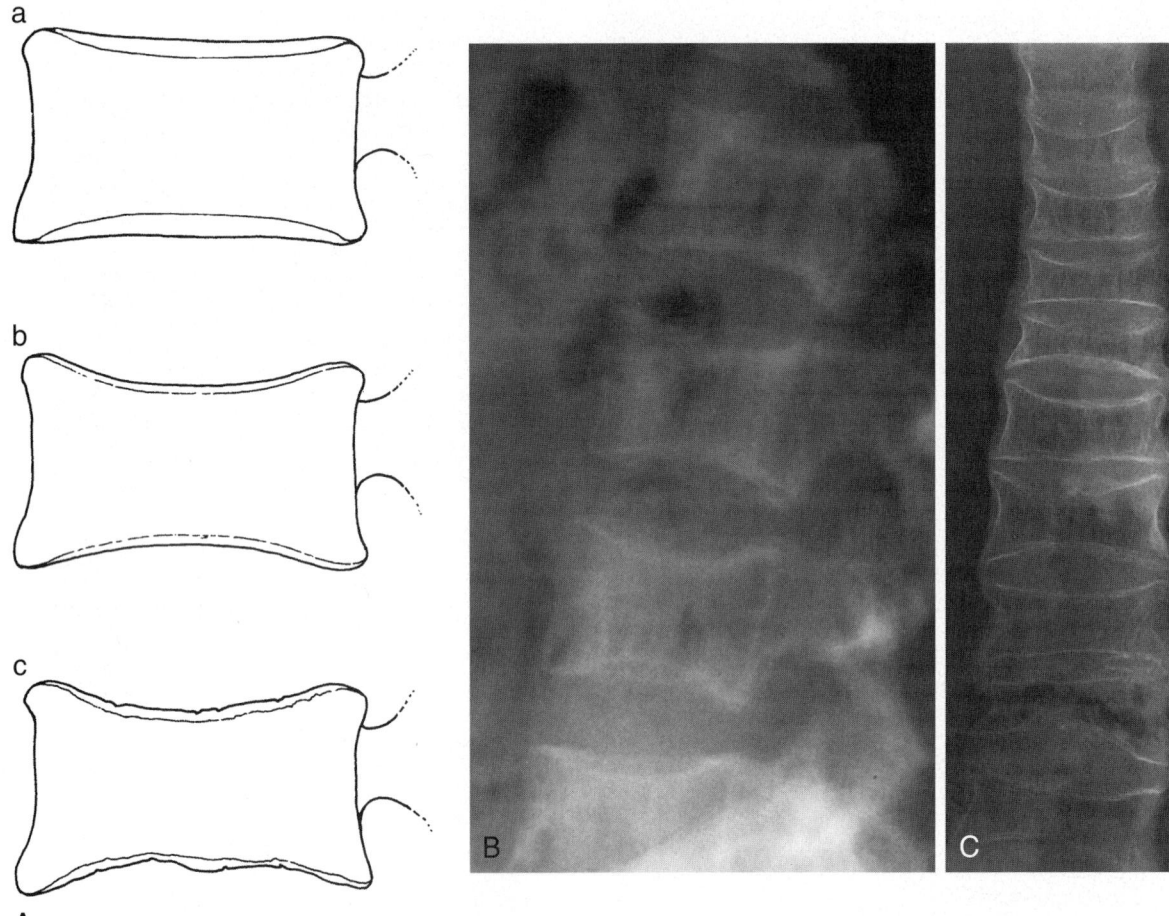

**Figure 41–18.** Fish vertebrae: differential diagnosis of osteoporosis and osteomalacia. *A*, Normal vertebra (a) becomes biconcave in outline in both osteomalacia (b) and osteoporosis (c). In osteomalacia, however, the indentation of the osseous surface is smooth, and both the superior and inferior borders are involved to approximately the same degree. In osteoporosis, the depression is more angular or irregular, and the superior and inferior surfaces of the vertebral body are frequently involved to different degrees. *B*, Osteomalacia. On a lateral radiograph of the lumbar spine, observe the smooth biconcave deformities (fish vertebrae) of the vertebral bodies and the poorly defined trabeculae. Vertical trabeculae are not accentuated. *C*, Osteoporosis. On a radiograph of a coronal section of an involved spine, osteopenia and biconcave deformities are evident in most of the vertebrae. The subchondral bone plates are distinct, and the superior and inferior surfaces of the vertebral bodies are not involved to the same extent.

formation is based on the presence of a break in the subchondral bone plate (corresponding to the site of disc displacement), a lucent area of varying size bordering on the intervertebral disc (corresponding to the site and variable amount of displaced disc material), and a small degree of surrounding bone sclerosis (corresponding to trabecular condensation and thickening).

## Proximal Portion of the Femur

Analysis of the trabecular pattern of the upper end of the femur has been used as an index of osteoporosis (Fig. 41–21). In this region, four major anatomic groups of trabeculae can be identified:

1. *Principal compressive group.* This group comprises the uppermost compression trabeculae, which extend from the medial cortex of the femoral neck to the upper portion of the femoral head in slightly curved radial lines. It contains the thickest and most densely packed trabeculae in the region.

2. *Secondary compressive group.* Trabeculae that arise from the medial cortex of the shaft below the principal compressive group form this group. They curve upward and slightly laterally toward the greater trochanter and the upper portion of the femoral neck. These trabeculae are thin and widely spaced.

3. *Principal tensile group.* Trabeculae that arise from the lateral cortex below the greater trochanter and extend in a curvilinear fashion superiorly and medially across the femoral neck, ending in the inferior portion of the femoral head, form the thickest tensile trabeculae.

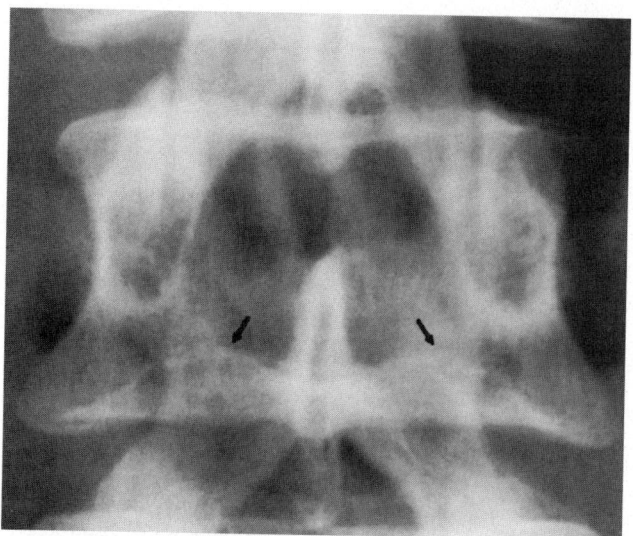

**Figure 41–19.** Cupid's bow contour. Frontal radiograph of a lower lumbar vertebral body reveals a normal variation in vertebral outline, the Cupid's bow contour. Observe the smooth parasagittal concavities on the inferior surface of the vertebral body *(arrows)*.

4. *Secondary tensile group.* These trabeculae arise from the lateral cortex below the principal tensile group. They extend superiorly and medially and terminate after crossing the middle of the femoral neck.

In the femoral neck, a triangular area—Ward's triangle—contains thin and loosely arranged trabeculae. This area is enclosed by trabeculae from the principal compressive, secondary compressive, and principal tensile groups.

Patterns of trabecular loss may correlate with increasing severity of osteoporosis (see Fig. 41–21). With early trabecular resorption, accentuation of the principal compressive and principal tensile groups is seen, and Ward's triangle is more prominent. With an increased degree of trabecular resorption, tensile trabeculae are reduced in number. With a further increase in trabecular resorption, the outer portion of the principal tensile trabeculae opposite the greater trochanter disappears. As the osteoporosis increases in severity, all trabecular groups are resorbed, with the exception of bony trabeculae in the principal compressive group. With severe osteoporosis, even these latter trabeculae may be partially or completely obliterated. The value of this trabecular analysis (termed the Singh index) is debated and has fallen into disuse with the advent of more quantitative methods for assessing bone mineral content.

## Cortex of the Tubular Bones

Osseous resorption of bone cortices may become apparent in three specific sites (Table 41–5; Fig. 41–22): (1) a cellular, vascularized membrane covering the endosteal surface of the cortex, designated the endosteal envelope; (2) an intracortical (haversian) envelope that constitutes the surfaces within the cortical bone (haversian and Volkmann's canals); and (3) a periosteal envelope that covers the surface of the cortex. The response to stimuli induced by various endocrine and metabolic disorders is not always identical in these three bone envelopes.

Endosteal resorption produces scalloped concavities on the inner margin of the cortex that enlarge the marrow cavity. Intracortical resorption is characterized by the appearance of prominent longitudinal striations within

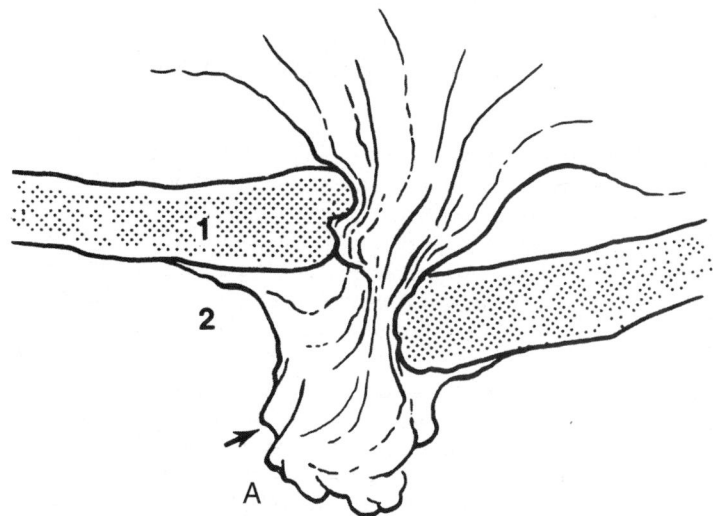

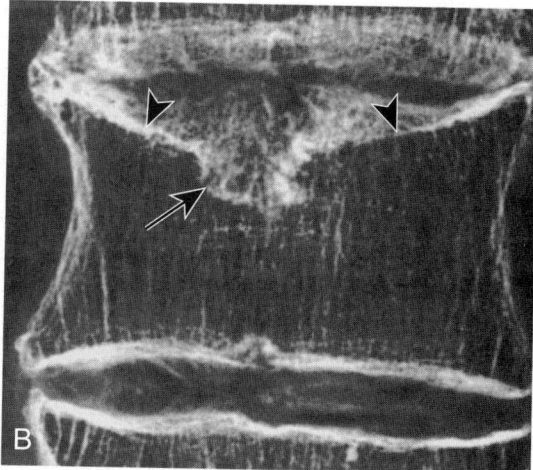

**Figure 41–20.** Osteoporosis: cartilaginous (Schmorl's) nodes. *A,* Schmorl's nodes occur when a portion of the intervertebral disc protrudes into the vertebral body *(arrow)* through a gap in the cartilaginous endplate (1) and subchondral bone plate (2). *B,* Radiograph of a coronal section reveals depression of the subchondral bone *(arrowheads)*. A cartilaginous node *(arrow)* has resulted from disruption of the cartilaginous and bony plates, creating a radiolucent defect within the bones with a small rim of sclerosis. A small cartilaginous node is noted on the opposite side of the vertebral body.

*(B,* From Resnick D, Niwayama G: Intravertebral disk herniations: Cartilaginous [Schmorl's] nodes. Radiology 126:57, 1978.)

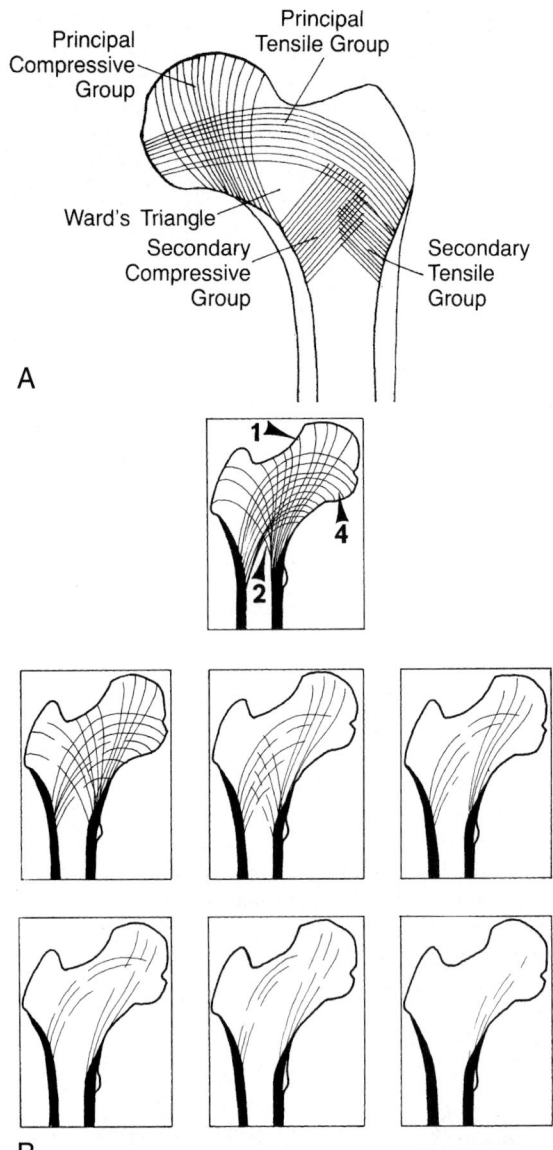

A

B

**Figure 41–21.** Proximal portion of the femur: normal tra-becular pattern and osteoporosis (Singh index). *A,* Four anatomic groups of trabeculae are indicated in this diagram. Ward's triangle lies within the neutral axis, wherein compressive and tensile forces balance each other; this triangle contains thin, widely spaced trabeculae. *B,* In the normal situation, it is often difficult to identify all these groups, but with increasing osteoporosis, they may initially be identifiable and subsequently be resorbed. In the top drawing, three groups can be well seen: principal compressive group (1), secondary compressive group (2), and principal tensile group (4). In the subsequent drawings, increasing degrees of osteoporosis lead to trabecular resorption. The principal compressive group is the last to be obliterated.

the cortex. Abnormal linear radiolucent areas within the cortex can be detected in such disorders as hyperpara-thyroidism, hyperthyroidism, acromegaly, osteomalacia, renal osteodystrophy, disuse osteoporosis, and RSD. Subperiosteal resorption produces irregularity and poor definition of the outer surface of the cortex. It becomes prominent in diseases associated with rapid bone turn-over, particularly hyperparathyroidism.

**TABLE 41–5**

**Patterns of Osseous Resorption in Tubular Bones**

| Site | Pattern |
|---|---|
| Cortex | |
| Endosteal | Diffuse cortical thinning or scalloped erosions |
| Intracortical | Cortical radiolucent areas or striations |
| Periosteal | Subperiosteal erosions |
| Spongiosa | |
| Subchondral | Linear, bandlike, or spotty radiolucent areas |
| Metaphyseal | Bandlike radiolucent areas |
| Diffuse | Homogeneous or spotty radiolucent areas |

## Spongiosa in the Appendicular Skeleton

Spongy bone undergoes early and significant changes in osteoporosis and related metabolic conditions (see Table 41–5). Several radiographic patterns can be distinguished: diffuse or homogeneous osteoporosis; speckled or spotty osteoporosis, which is particularly prominent in peri-articular areas; and linear and bandlike osteoporosis in subchondral and metaphyseal areas (Fig. 41–23).

In subchondral locations, linear radiolucent bands produce thinning of the overlying bone plate, linear or curvilinear radiolucent regions within the bone plate, and small areas of osseous disruption. These last-mentioned bony defects can simulate the erosions of rheumatoid arthritis and related diseases. The degree of periarticular bone resorption in osteoporosis can become striking and produce an alarming radiographic picture that suggests an erroneous diagnosis of arthritis, infection, or even neoplastic disease.

## Additional Skeletal Manifestations

### Fractures

Acute fractures are an important complication of osteo-porosis, with the most common sites being the vertebral bodies, the neck and intertrochanteric region of the femur, the distal portion of the radius, and the humeral neck. Although attempts have been made to define the importance of trabecular bone loss, cortical bone loss, or both, as factors contributing to such fractures, no uniform agreement has been reached. In general, it appears that trabecular bone loss is more significant than cortical bone loss in the pathogenesis of fractures in the spine and distal portion of the radius. Loss of cortical bone must be considered, however, especially in the femur.

The insufficiency type of stress fracture may occur in patients with osteoporosis. Typical sites of involvement are the symphysis pubis (Fig. 41–24), pubic rami, and sacrum (Fig. 41–25). Other areas of involvement include the supra-acetabular area, other regions of the bony pelvis, the femoral neck, proximal and distal portions of the tibia, and the sternum.

Insufficiency fractures of the pubic rami may be accom-panied by considerable osteolysis and fragmentation of

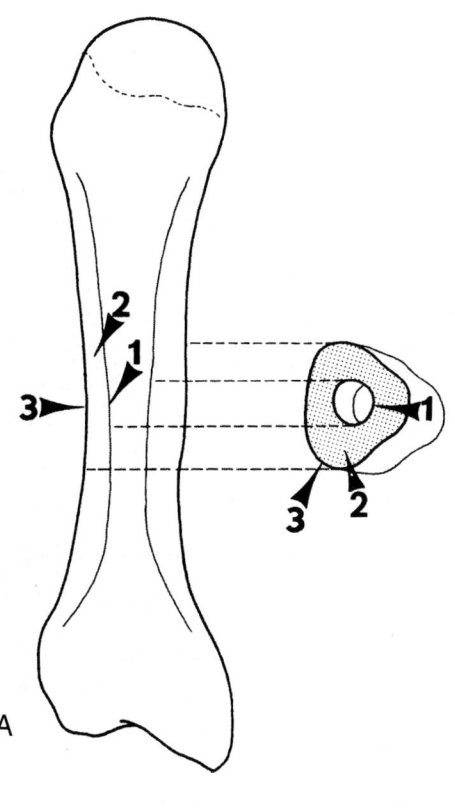

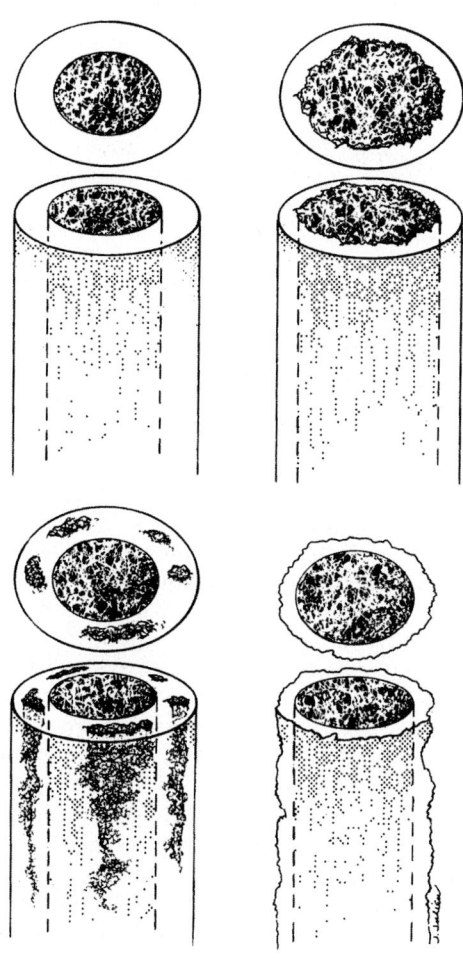

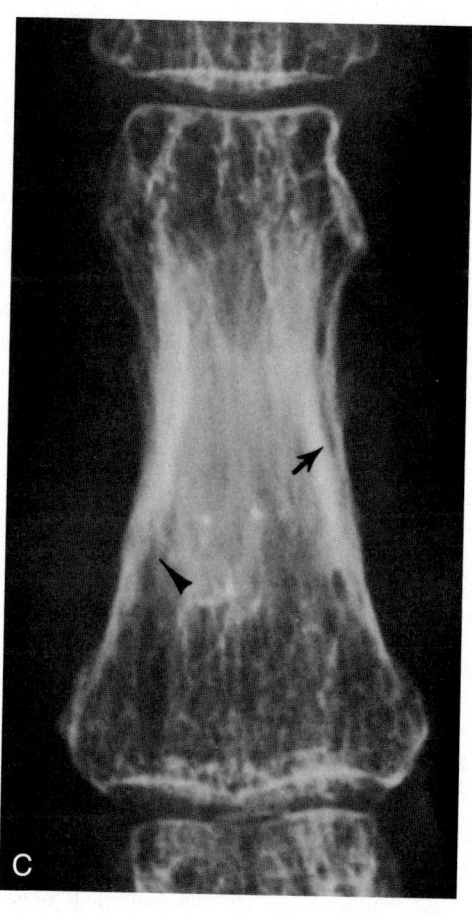

**Figure 41–22.** Cortex of tubular bones: sites of osseous resorption. *A,* Three envelopes exist at which cortical resorption may occur: endosteal envelope (1), intracortical (haversian) envelope (2), and periosteal envelope (3). *B,* Diagram indicates the normal situation (top left), endosteal resorption (top right), intracortical resorption (bottom left), and subperiosteal resorption (bottom right). *C,* Magnification radiograph of a phalanx in a patient with reflex sympathetic dystrophy reveals endosteal *(arrowhead)* and intracortical *(arrow)* resorption.

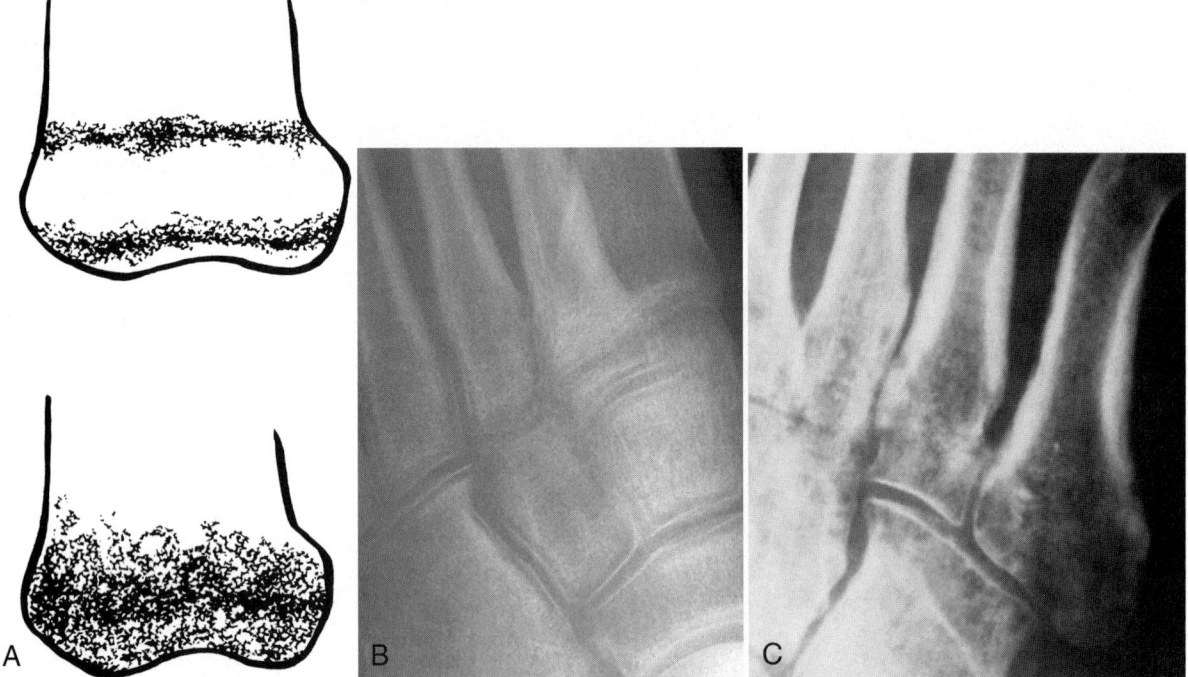

**Figure 41–23.** Spongiosa of tubular bones: sites of osseous resorption. *A*, Patterns of bone loss include bandlike radiolucent areas in the metaphysis or subchondral bone (top drawing) and homogeneous periarticular radiolucent areas (bottom drawing). *B*, Bandlike resorption. Metaphyseal and subchondral linear radiolucent areas are evident. *C*, Spotty resorption. A cystic pattern is apparent.

bone, findings that simulate a malignant tumor. Those of the sacrum are associated with hip, back, or buttock pain and with a characteristic scintigraphic pattern in which vertical and horizontal regions of increased accumulation of the bone-seeking radiopharmaceutical agent produce a configuration referred to as the H pattern. Typical MR imaging abnormalities also occur (see later discussion). Insufficiency fractures of the supra-acetabular bone produce poorly defined linear or punctate zones of increased radiodensity of variable size.

### Reinforcement Lines (Bone Bars)

In patients with chronic osteopenia, radiographs of the tubular bones, particularly the femur and tibia, commonly reveal strands of trabeculae of variable thickness that extend partially or completely across the marrow cavity (Fig. 41–26). These strands, which are referred to as reinforcement lines or bone bars, are evident in both adults and children. The precise pathogenesis of bone bars is not clear.

## MAGNETIC RESONANCE IMAGING ABNORMALITIES

### Generalized Osteoporosis

Potential applications of MR imaging in patients with generalized osteoporosis include assessment of vertebral body fractures, analysis of extraspinal sites of insufficiency fractures, and evaluation of bone mass and strength.

### Vertebral Body Fractures

The common occurrence of both osteoporosis and fractures of the vertebral body in elderly patients presents an immediate diagnostic challenge, particularly in those with known extraosseous malignant neoplasms. Is the vertebral collapse related to osteoporosis alone, or does it indicate that the vertebral body contains metastatic foci? Although routine radiography may be helpful in certain cases, MR imaging is especially useful in this clinical setting. The potential value of this technique relies on alterations in the signal intensity of bone marrow in the involved vertebral body that allow the differentiation of a tumorous process from one accompanying osteoporosis alone. In theory, this method seems attractive, but in practice, difficulties arise because of variations in the signal intensity of normal bone marrow, as well as of bone marrow that has been injured.

The signal intensity of normal vertebral marrow is generally dominated by its fatty content. Therefore, with a standard spin echo technique, high signal intensity is expected on T1-weighted images and intermediate signal intensity is expected on T2-weighted images in the normal marrow of the vertebral body. In the presence of tumor or any other condition in which replacement of marrow fat has occurred, decreased signal intensity is seen in the marrow on T1-weighted images, and T2-weighted images show either low or high signal, depending on the specific pathologic process present. With most tumors, foci of increased signal intensity are noted on T2-weighted spin echo images.

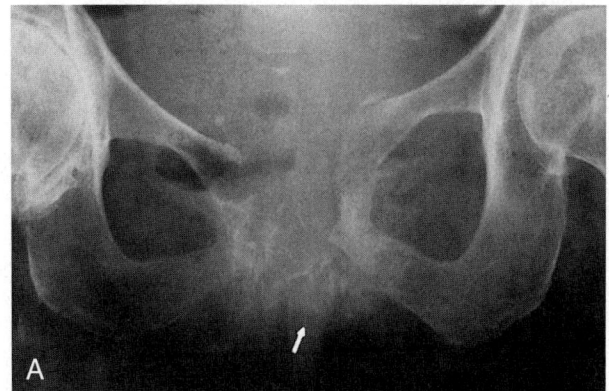

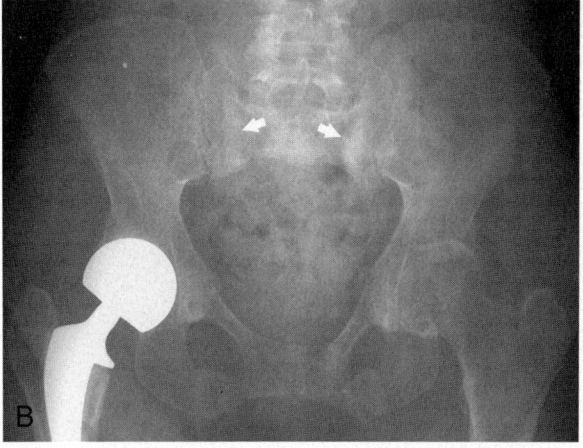

**Figure 41–24.** Osteoporosis: insufficiency fracture of the symphysis pubis. *A*, This 72-year-old woman with rheumatoid arthritis received corticosteroid therapy. Radiograph of the pubis shows considerable bone fragmentation and subluxation *(arrow)*. The findings are diagnostic of an insufficiency fracture, although they are easily misinterpreted as evidence of a malignant neoplasm. *B*, This 79-year-old woman has bilateral insufficiency fractures of the ischium, pubis, and sacrum. The distribution is quite characteristic and suggests the diagnosis. Sacral fractures *(arrows)* are subtle.

In general, pathologic fractures of the vertebral body (defined as fractures related to skeletal metastasis) result in homogeneous replacement of vertebral marrow, with low signal intensity demonstrated on T1-weighted spin echo images and high signal intensity on T2-weighted sequences. The MR imaging findings of a so-called benign fracture, in common with scintigraphic abnormalities, are dependent in part on the age of the fracture. In persons with long-standing or chronic benign fractures, isointense marrow signal comparable with that of normal vertebral bodies is evident on all the MR sequences used. In those with more acute benign fractures, high signal intensity in the bone marrow of the affected vertebral body is evident on fluid-sensitive sequences and is typically characterized by abnormal signal bands that parallel the endplates; these may return to normal on non–fat-suppressed T1-weighted images following contrast enhancement. The MR imaging characteristics of the bone marrow in cases of acute compression fractures usually revert to a normal pattern in 1 to 3 months.

Recent reports have emphasized that most vertebral fractures resulting from metastatic involvement are associated with bone marrow replacement on T1-weighted images (seen as foci of decreased signal intensity), and replacement is total in the vast majority of cases. It is postulated that in cases of tumor, vertebral compression occurs only when the entire bone marrow in the vertebral body is replaced. Other features suggesting tumor include an associated soft tissue or epidural mass and extension of marrow abnormalities into the posterior elements. Concavity to the posterior vertebral body cortex and focal increased or heterogeneous signal on fluid-sensitive or non–fat-suppressed T1-weighted images following contrast enhancement also suggest tumor involvement. MR imaging may also identify other lesions in noncompressed vertebrae.

Although the initial experience with the use of MR imaging to assess vertebral compression fractures has been encouraging, a number of diagnostic difficulties can be predicted. The effects of irradiation and chemotherapy on the signal intensity of vertebral marrow in cases of tumor may complicate the differential diagnosis. The possibility also exists that tumorous involvement of a vertebral body in a patient with preexisting osteoporosis could lead to vertebral collapse before the entire vertebral body is infiltrated with neoplasm. The presence of plasma cell myeloma rather than carcinoma in the collapsed vertebral body produces patterns on MR imaging that closely simulate those of osteoporotic collapse. Heterogeneous (rather than homogeneous) signal intensity of marrow may be encountered in myeloma. Further, the signal intensity of marrow during the treatment of myeloma is somewhat variable.

### Insufficiency Fractures of Extraspinal Sites

In comparison to conventional radiographs, MR imaging has superior sensitivity and specificity in the analysis of insufficiency fractures of the pelvic bones. The sensitivity of MR examination in this situation relates to the occurrence of bone marrow edema as an early manifestation of the fracture. In common with edema from other causes and in other processes in which bone marrow is replaced or modified, the MR imaging characteristics of traumatic edema include decreased signal intensity on T1-weighted spin echo images and increased signal intensity on T2-weighted spin echo and other fluid-sensitive sequences. The specificity of the MR examination relies, in large part, on the morphology and distribution of the abnormal foci. Involvement of the portion of the sacrum located just medial to the sacroiliac joint in a unilateral or bilateral distribution, the portion of the symphysis pubis that abuts on the fibrocartilaginous disc, the inner contour of the ilium, and the supra-acetabular bone is most characteristic of insufficiency fractures of the pelvis (Fig. 41–27). Some diagnostic pitfalls are encountered when MR imaging is used for the analysis of pelvic insufficiency fractures. First, the pelvis is also a frequent site of skeletal metastasis, and the resulting altered signal intensity is similar to that seen in cases of fracture. Second, the cortical disruption and fragmentation accompanying insufficiency fractures may resemble the findings of an aggressive

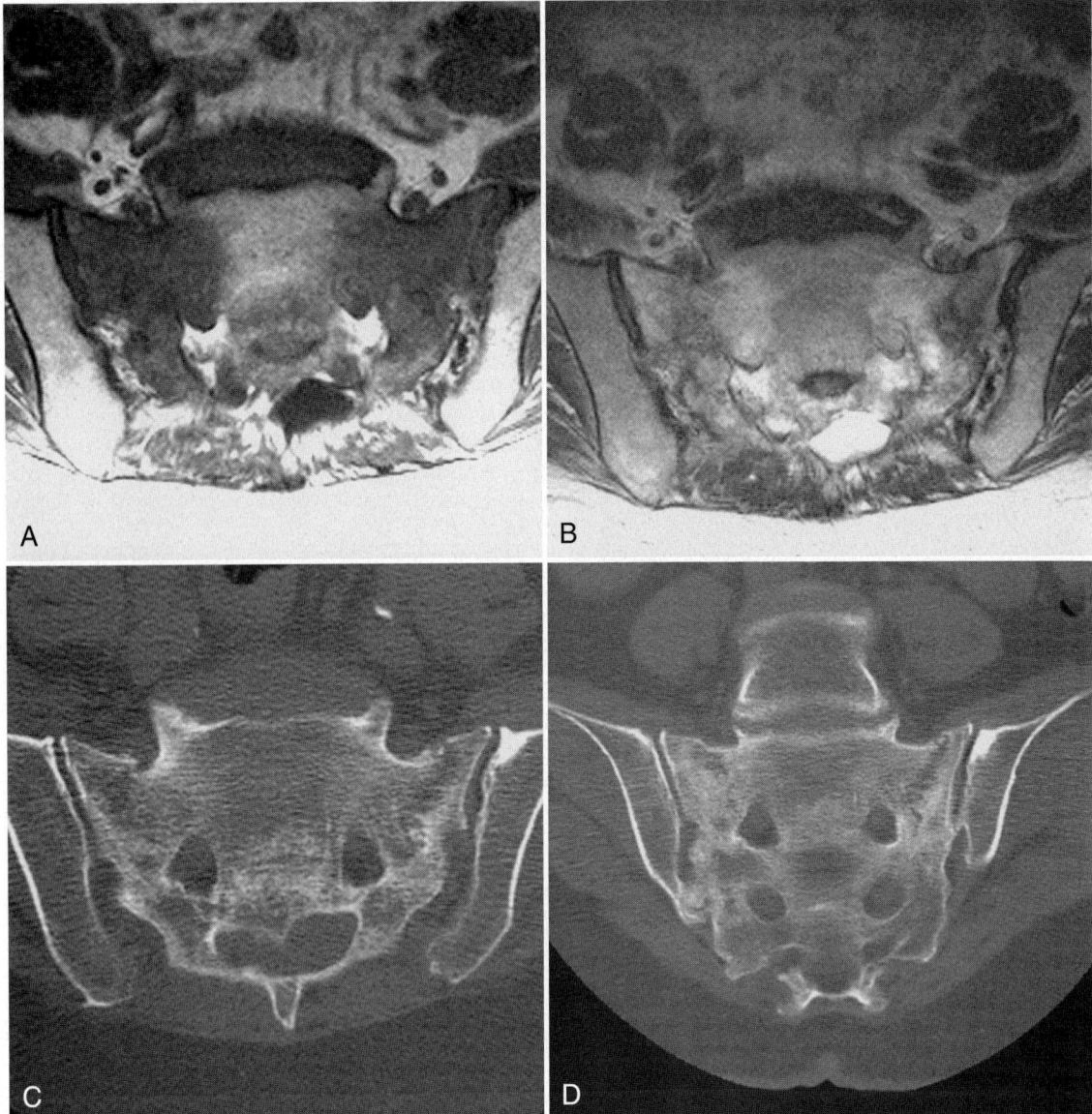

**Figure 41–25.** Osteoporosis: bilateral sacral insufficiency fracture. This 81-year-old woman presented with low back pain. Axial T1-weighted (TR/TE, 600/12) *(A)* and fast T2-weighted (TR/TE, 4000/102) *(B)* spin echo MR images show extensive edema through the sacral ala bilaterally. The fracture line on the left is vaguely seen. Axial *(C)* and reformatted oblique coronal *(D)* noncontrast CT scans show sacral fractures and subtle bone sclerosis. Fractures are seen to better advantage on the reformatted oblique coronal image *(D)*.

tumor. Discrete soft tissue masses, however, do not generally occur in cases of insufficiency fracture. Third, the conversion of hematopoietic marrow to fatty marrow in normal persons is not as complete in the pelvis as it is in other extraspinal locations.

MR imaging can also be useful in the diagnosis of insufficiency fractures of the femoral neck and intertrochanteric region. Insufficiency fractures tend to course horizontally, across the femoral neck, at angles almost perpendicular to those of some of the trabecular groups (Fig. 41–28).

## Regional Osteoporosis

### Transient Bone Marrow Edema

Transient bone marrow edema is the term used to describe the abnormality in patients with clinical manifestations identical to those of transient osteoporosis of the hip but with normal radiographs. The abnormalities in the process relate to the presence of edema in the femoral head and neck. Decreased signal intensity in this area on T1-weighted sequences and increased signal intensity in the corresponding region on T2-weighted sequences are typically observed (Fig. 41–29). Associated joint effusions

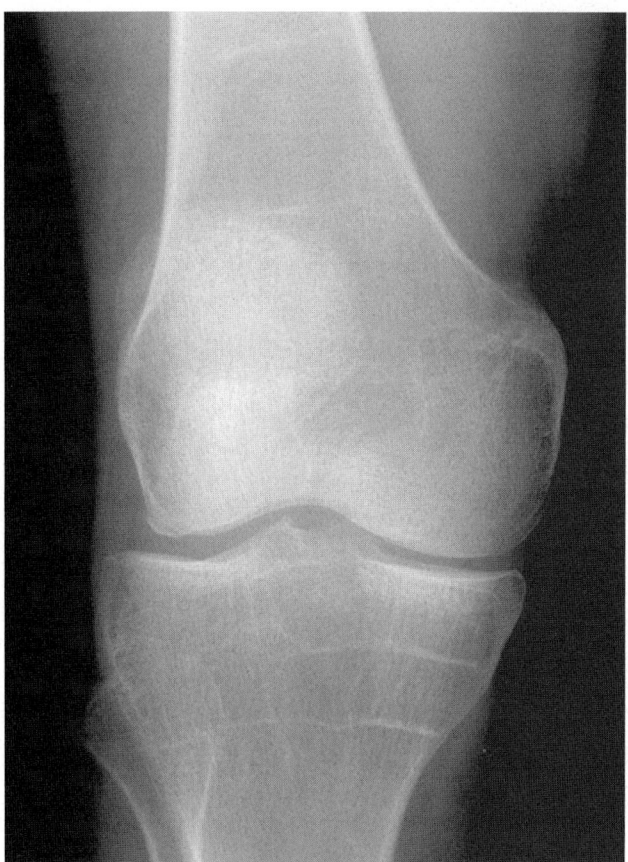

**Figure 41–26.** Reinforcement lines (bone bars): radiographic abnormalities associated with chronic osteoporosis. Observe the numerous thick bone bars in the metaphysis and metadiaphysis of the femur and tibia in association with diffuse osteopenia.

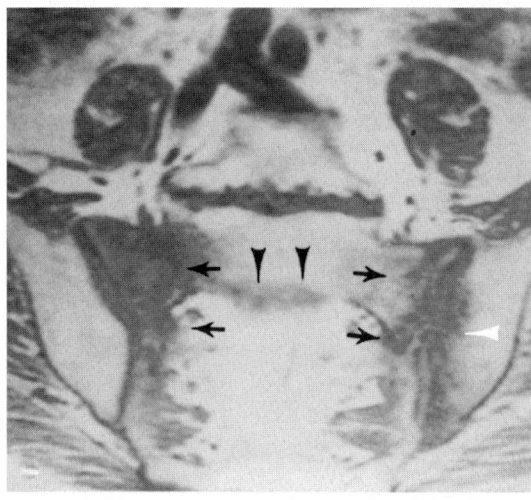

**Figure 41–27.** Insufficiency fractures of the pelvis: sacrum. This 70-year-old woman with low back pain had no history of previous injury to the area. Coronal T1-weighted (TR/TE, 650/20) spin echo MR image shows bands of decreased signal intensity paralleling both sacroiliac joints *(arrows)* and extending across the body of the sacrum *(black arrowheads)*. Decreased signal intensity is also seen along the iliac side of the joint *(white arrowhead)*.

(From Brahme SK, Cervilla V, Vint V, et al: Skeletal Radiol 19:489, 1990.)

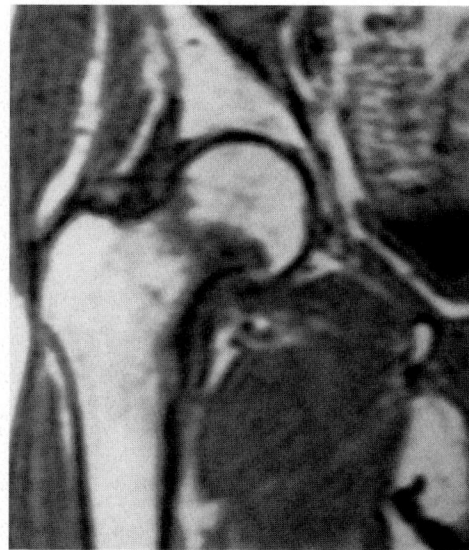

**Figure 41–28.** Insufficiency fracture of the femoral neck. In this 75-year-old woman, a fracture of the right femoral neck occurred spontaneously. A routine radiograph (not shown) was interpreted as negative. Coronal T1-weighted (TR/TE, 600/20) spin echo MR image reveals the characteristic serpentine-like region of low signal intensity in the subcapital region of the right femoral neck.

in the affected hip are common. The MR imaging findings, along with the clinical manifestations, regress partially or completely over a period of months. The use of chemical shift, fat-suppression imaging, and short tau inversion recovery (STIR) imaging can be effective in the detection of transient bone marrow edema.

Three questions regarding transient bone marrow edema require clarification. First, what is its relationship to transient osteoporosis of the hip? Certainly, on the basis of observed clinical manifestations, these disorders are closely related or identical. Documentation that transient bone marrow edema can involve both hips and other joints, with abnormalities moving from one location to another, suggests that this disorder is related to regional migratory osteoporosis as well. Further, partial types of bone marrow edema, with distribution patterns similar to those seen in regional osteoporosis, may be observed.

A second question relates to the specificity of the MR imaging findings in transient bone marrow edema. The most common imaging pattern observed in this condition indicates involvement of both the femoral head and the femoral neck. A similar distribution may characterize the MR imaging appearance of femoral involvement in a number of processes, including transient osteoporosis, but this distribution differs from that typically seen in cases of osteonecrosis of the femoral head.

The final and perhaps most important question regarding transient bone marrow edema concerns its relationship to ischemic necrosis of bone. Recent reports indicate that a subgroup of patients with bone marrow edema in the femoral head will subsequently develop osteonecrosis at this site. This complication is not entirely

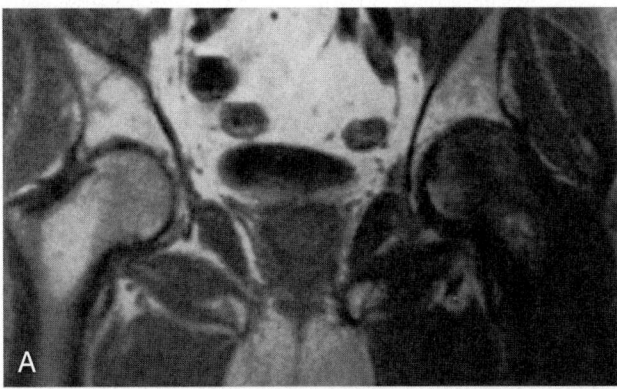

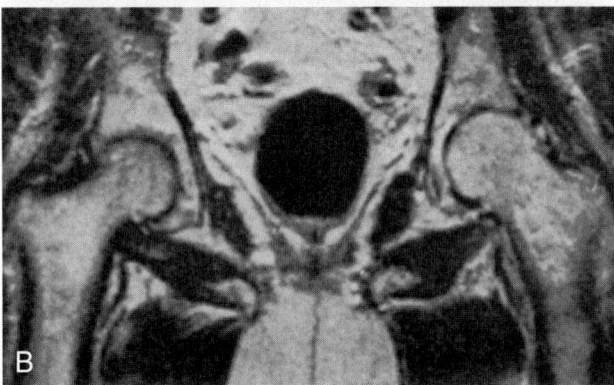

**Figure 41–29.** Transient bone marrow edema. This patient complained of left hip pain of several months' duration. Routine radiographs were normal, and bone scintigraphy was not performed. *A*, Coronal T1-weighted (TR/TE, 930/26) spin echo MR image reveals low signal intensity replacing the normal signal of the bone marrow in the left femoral head and neck. The acetabulum appears normal, as does the opposite hip. *B*, Coronal T2-weighted (TR/TE, 2000/80) spin echo MR image reveals increased signal intensity in the left femoral head and neck. The signal intensity is slightly greater than that on the opposite side. A very small joint effusion is present. The pain and MR imaging abnormalities diminished over 3 months.

surprising, because vascular congestion and edema of the bone marrow are thought to occur early in the course of ischemic necrosis of bone. What is not clear, however, is the percentage of patients with transient bone marrow edema in whom osteonecrosis will develop, the factors responsible for this occurrence in some patients and not in others, and how this complication can be predicted on the basis of an initial MR imaging pattern that indicates only bone marrow edema.

### Reflex Sympathetic Dystrophy

Few data have accumulated with regard to the MR imaging findings in RSD. Preliminary reports indicate that MR imaging is normal in the majority of patients but may show nonspecific soft tissue changes or, uncommonly, bone marrow edema or muscle atrophy.

## FURTHER READING

Arnstein AR: Regional osteoporosis. Orthop Clin North Am 3:585, 1972.

Baker LL, Goodman SB, Perkash I, et al: Benign versus pathologic compression fractures of vertebral bodies: Assessment with conventional spin-echo, chemical-shift, and STIR MR imaging. Radiology 174:495, 1990.

Chen C, Chandnani V, Kang HS, et al: Insufficiency fracture of the sternum caused by osteopenia: Plain film findings in seven patients. AJR Am J Roentgenol 154:1025, 1990.

Cooper KL: Insufficiency fractures of the sternum: A consequence of thoracic kyphosis? Radiology 167:471, 1988.

Cooper KL, Beabout JW, Swee RG: Insufficiency fractures of the sacrum. Radiology 156:15, 1985.

Cummings SR: Are patients with hip fractures more osteoporotic? Review of the evidence. Am J Med 78:487, 1985.

Daniel WW, Sanders PC, Alarcón GS: The early diagnosis of transient osteoporosis by magnetic resonance incoherent motions: Application to diffusion and perfusion in neurologic disorders. Radiology 161:401, 1986.

De Smet AA, Neff JR: Pubic and sacral insufficiency fractures: Clinical course and radiologic findings. AJR Am J Roentgenol 145:601, 1985.

Dietz GW, Christensen EE: Normal "Cupid's bow" contour of the lower lumbar vertebrae. Radiology 121:577, 1976.

Genant HK, Kozin F, Bekerman C, et al: The reflex sympathetic dystrophy syndrome: A comprehensive analysis using fine-detail radiography, photon absorptiometry and bone and joint scintigraphy. Radiology 117:21, 1975.

Houang MTW, Brenton DP, Renton P, et al: Idiopathic juvenile osteoporosis. Skeletal Radiol 3:17, 1978.

Kozin F, McCarty DJ, Simms J, et al: The reflex sympathetic dystrophy syndrome. I. Clinical and histologic studies: Evidence for bilaterality, response to corticosteroids and articular involvement. Am J Med 60:321, 1976.

Lequesne M, Kerboull M, Bensasson M, et al: Partial transient osteoporosis. Skeletal Radiol 2:1, 1977.

McCord WC, Nies KM, Campion DS, et al: Regional migratory osteoporosis: A denervation disease. Arthritis Rheum 21:834, 1978.

Naides S, Resnick D, Zvaifler N: Idiopathic regional osteoporosis. J Rheumatol 12:763, 1985.

Resnick D, Niwayama G: Intravertebral disk herniations: Cartilaginous (Schmorl's) nodes. Radiology 126:57, 1978.

Rosen RA: Transitory demineralization of the femoral head. Radiology 94:509, 1970.

Singh M, Nagrath AR, Maini PS: Changes in trabecular pattern of the upper end of the femur as an index of osteoporosis. J Bone Joint Surg Am 52:457, 1970.

Turner DA, Templeton AC, Selzer PM, et al: Femoral capital osteonecrosis: MR findings of diffuse marrow abnormalities without focal lesions. Radiology 171:135, 1989.

Vande Berg BE, Malghem JJ, Labaisse MA, et al: MR imaging of avascular necrosis and transient marrow edema of the femoral head. Radiographics 13:501, 1993.

Wambeek N, Munk PL, Lee MJ, et al: Intra-articular regional migratory osteoporosis of the hip. Skeletal Radiol 29:97, 2000.

Wilson AJ, Murphy WA, Hardy DC, et al: Transient osteoporosis: Transient bone marrow edema? Radiology 167:757, 1988.

# CHAPTER 42

## Rickets and Osteomalacia

### Michael J. Pitt

## SUMMARY OF KEY FEATURES

The terms *rickets* and *osteomalacia* encompass a group of disorders with similar gross pathologic, histologic, and radiographic findings. Causative factors include abnormalities of vitamin D metabolism and syndromes resulting primarily from renal tubular phosphate loss. Significant advances in the understanding of vitamin D metabolism have yielded new insights into these syndromes.

## INTRODUCTION

The terms *rickets* and *osteomalacia* describe a group of diseases demonstrating similar gross pathologic, radiographic, and histologic abnormalities. The pathologic changes result from inadequate or delayed mineralization of osteoid in mature cortical and spongy bone (osteomalacia) and an interruption in the orderly development and mineralization of the growth plate (rickets). Therefore, before growth plate fusion, rickets and osteomalacia coexist.

The radiographic findings in affected bones and cartilage reflect the gross pathologic and histologic abnormalities. Although the general radiographic findings are similar in all the rachitic and osteomalacic syndromes, some distinctive features may be of help in sorting out the various disease entities.

## BIOCHEMISTRY OF VITAMIN D

Progress in the understanding of vitamin D metabolism has occurred at an exponentially rapid pace in the past 3 decades, resulting in basic modifications of long-standing views. Until recently, the general assumption was that vitamin D was a vitamin and was unaltered metabolically before discharging its physiologic function. It has now been established that what is termed vitamin D (Fig. 42–1) is a prohormone that requires two sequential hydroxylations before the active hormonal form 1,25-dihydroxyvitamin $D_3$ $(1,25[OH]_2D_3)$ is produced. Two prohormonal forms of $1,25(OH)_2D$ are found in humans: vitamin $D_3$ and vitamin $D_2$. Vitamin $D_3$ is the natural, endogenously produced compound resulting from interaction of ultraviolet light with a cholesterol derivative, 7-dehydrocholesterol, in the deeper layers of the skin. Vitamin $D_2$ is prepared artificially by irradiation of ergosterol obtained from yeast or fungi and is the compound used for food supplementation and pharmaceutical preparations.

Both vitamin $D_3$ and Vitamin $D_2$ are hydroxylated at the carbon 25 position to form 25-OH-$D_3$ and 25-OH-$D_2$, respectively. This occurs predominantly in the liver but has also been noted in extrahepatic sites, such as the intestine and kidney. When both vitamin $D_3$ and vitamin $D_2$ are available in adequate amounts, the major portion of the circulating 25-hydroxylated form is 25-OH-$D_3$, which circulates bound to a specific binding protein. 25-Hydroxyvitamin D is hydroxylated further at the $1\alpha$ position, producing the active form of the hormone, $1,25(OH)_2D_3$. The $1\alpha$ hydroxylating enzyme (25-OH-D-$1\alpha$ hydroxylase) is found exclusively in renal tissue. The production of $1,25(OH)_2D_3$ is related directly to body requirements and is closely regulated by multiple factors, which may be integrated into classic hormonal feedback loops. In comparison to 25-OH-D, the serum levels of $1,25(OH)_2D_3$ are relatively low. The latter is produced and metabolized rapidly and, unlike 25-OH-D, has no significant tissue stores.

## Action of Vitamin D

The long-recognized functions of vitamin D are the homeostatic maintenance of serum calcium and phosphorus levels and the mineralization of bone. The physiologic form of the vitamin, $1,25(OH)_2D_3$, acts on two main target organs—the intestine and bone. The kidney and the parathyroid glands also have been identified as sites of action.

**Intestines.** The effect of $1,25(OH)_2D$ on the intestine is to increase the absorption of calcium and phosphorus. Although it is well established that $1,25(OH)_2D$ increases intestinal calcium transport, its influence on phosphate absorption from the intestine was defined only recently. In addition to passive absorption of phosphorus in conjunction with the active intestinal transport of calcium, active phosphate transporting mechanisms reflecting vitamin D activity have been demonstrated.

**Bone.** In the skeleton, $1,25(OH)_2D$ has two actions, which initially appear to be diametrically opposed: mobilization of calcium and phosphorus from previously formed bone, and promotion of maturation and mineralization of organic matrix.

$1,25(OH)_2D$ mobilizes calcium and phosphorus from previously formed bone by stimulating osteocytic osteolysis and, in this way, participates in the breakdown process occurring as part of skeletal homeostasis. The process requires the presence of both $1,25(OH)_2D$ and parathyroid hormone.

The presence of vitamin D is clearly essential for adequate deposition of bone mineral. Two hormonal roles are possible: the maintenance of adequate serum calcium and phosphorus levels, or a direct effect on skeletal tissue (or both). The role of vitamin D in the preservation of normal serum levels of calcium and phosphorus has been firmly established. Undoubtedly, levels of serum calcium or phosphorus (or both), regardless of cause (e.g., defi-

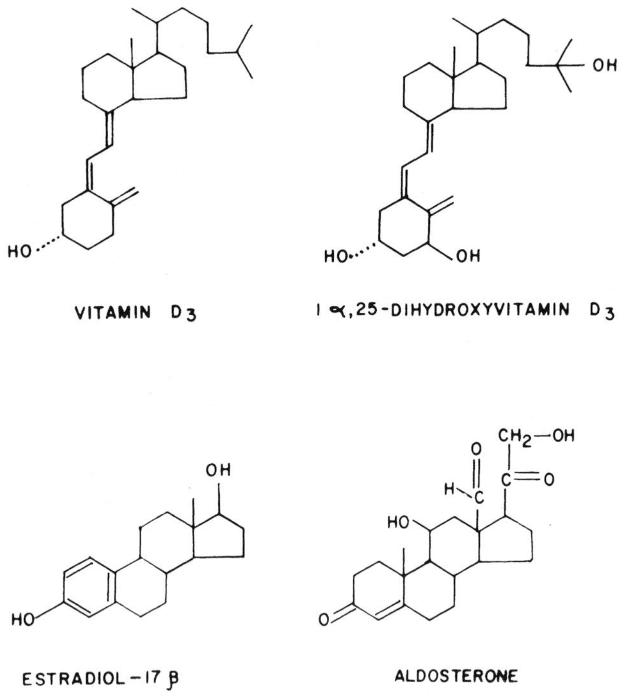

**Figure 42–1.** Chemical structures of vitamin $D_3$ and the active hormonal form, $1,25(OH)_2D_3$. Note the structural similarities to other steroid hormones. (From Pitt MJ, Haussler MR: Biochemistry and clinical applications. Skeletal Radiol 1:191, 1977.)

ciency of $1,25[OH]_2D$, diet, renal loss) are important factors in the development of rickets and osteomalacia; however, clinical experience shows a poor correlation between serum calcium and phosphorus concentrations and the severity of rachitic and osteomalacic states. Administration of vitamin D in these conditions can result in a positive bone mineralization response, which precedes correction of the serum calcium and phosphorus levels. Therefore, there is a distinct possibility that vitamin D metabolites have a direct effect on bone cells and matrix during the process of mineralization.

**Kidneys and Parathyroid Glands.** Although the intestine and skeleton are the major targets of $1,25(OH)_2D_3$ action, the kidney and parathyroid glands also are target organs affected by vitamin D. Vitamin D appears to have a direct suppressive effect on proximal renal tubular function. Further, direct action of $1,25(OH)_2D_3$ on the parathyroid glands has been demonstrated, with resulting suppression of parathyroid hormone secretion.

## Regulators of $1,25(OH)_2D_3$ Production

Considerable evidence exists to justify the designation of vitamin D as a hormone. As with other hormones, only one specific organ, the kidney, produces the substance using the substrates formed in extrarenal sites. $1,25(OH)_2D_3$ is secreted and transported to target organs, where it has an intranuclear mechanism of action resembling that of other steroid hormones. The renal production of $1,25(OH)_2D_3$ is closely regulated by several factors that may be integrated into classic endocrine loops with typical feedback features. The established

regulators are the levels of serum calcium, parathyroid hormone, and serum phosphate. Less certain are the roles of $1,25(OH)D$ itself, calcitonin, corticosteroids, sex hormones, thyroid hormone, and growth hormones.

**Calcium and Parathyroid Hormone.** Although calcium and parathyroid hormone exert a significant regulatory influence on $1,25(OH)_2D$ formation, the issues of how this is accomplished and the importance of parathyroid hormone control must be defined more completely. Available data suggest that the increase in $1,25(OH)_2D_3$ production elicited by hypocalcemia is mediated by the parathyroid glands, although the need for and importance of parathyroid hormone in this loop have been questioned. It is generally believed that under acute conditions, stimulation of $1,25(OH)_2D$ production by signals stemming from low calcium levels is mediated primarily by parathyroid hormone. Physiologically, in the absence of parathyroid hormone–deficient or –resistant states, this is most likely the important operative mechanism. In situations in which chronic parathyroid hormone deficiency or resistance exists, the body apparently has the adaptive capacity to produce $1,25(OH)_2D_3$ in response to low serum calcium levels.

**Phosphate.** Dietary and serum inorganic phosphorus levels have a significant influence on the regulation of $1,25(OH)_2D_3$ formation. Hypophosphatemia is frequently noted in the deficiency rachitic states, however, and is probably the primary factor in the development of rickets and osteomalacia in the syndromes associated with renal tubular phosphate loss (e.g., X-linked hypophosphatemia and Fanconi's syndromes). Indeed, depression of serum phosphate levels may be of more importance than low calcium levels in the development of rickets and osteomalacia. Low dietary phosphate is associated with increased levels of 25-OH-D-1$\alpha$ hydroxylase activity and increased serum levels of $1,25(OH)_2D_3$. Hypophosphatemia stimulates $1,25(OH)_2D_3$ production directly; in contrast to the acute hypocalcemic signal, this effect is independent of parathyroid hormone.

**$1,25(OH)_2D_3$ (a Self-Regulator).** $1,25(OH)_2D_3$ affects its own production by both direct and indirect means. The indirect influence occurs through suppression of parathyroid hormone secretion. A direct negative feedback effect of $1,25(OH)_2D_3$ on its own production also has been demonstrated. Suppression of enzymatic conversion of 25-OH-D$_3$ to $1,25(OH)_2D_3$ in isolated renal tubules occurs in the presence of $1,25(OH)_2D_3$.

**Summary of Regulatory Controls.** Two main regulatory loops initiated by low serum calcium and low serum phosphate levels, respectively, may be postulated (Fig. 42-2). Acute depressions of serum calcium level signal the production of parathyroid hormone, which in turn stimulates $1,25(OH)_2D_3$ production. Serum calcium and phosphate levels rise owing to the subsequent action of $1,25(OH)_2D_3$ on the intestine and to the combined effects of parathyroid hormone and $1,25(OH)_2D_3$ on bone, causing calcium and phosphate mobilization. The elevation of serum phosphate concentration is negated by

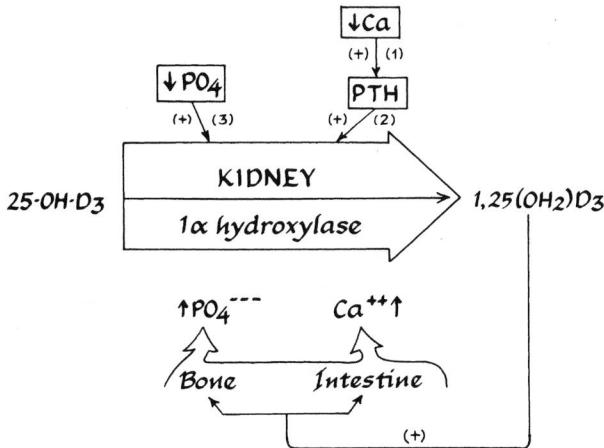

**Figure 42–2.** 25-OH-D is converted in the kidney to $1,25(OH)_2D$ by the action of the renal enzyme $1\alpha$-hydroxylase. This reaction is regulated by serum phosphate (3) and parathyroid hormone (2). Serum calcium (1) influences the reaction indirectly through its effect on the parathyroid glands. The two main target organs of $1,25(OH)_2D$ action, bone and intestine, are depicted. A plus (+) indicates a stimulatory effect. (From Pitt MJ, Haussler MR, Davis J, et al: Current concepts of vitamin D metabolism: Correlation with clinical syndromes. Crit Rev Radiol Sci 10:135,1977.)

increased renal excretion of phosphate from parathyroid action on the renal tubules. The net result is an increase in serum calcium levels.

The hypophosphatemic signal stimulates $1,25(OH)_2D$ production directly. Elevation of serum phosphate and calcium results from $1,25(OH)_2D$ action on the intestine, bone, and kidney. Subsequent suppression of parathyroid hormone secretion, resulting from the $1,25(OH)_2D$-induced elevation of serum calcium level and the direct suppressive effect of $1,25(OH)_2D$ on the parathyroid glands, together with the hypercalcemia, leads to an increase in urinary calcium excretion but a decrease in urinary phosphate excretion. In addition, $1,25(OH)_2D$ may increase serum phosphate concentration by the mobilization of phosphate from soft tissue stores. The total sequence accounts for a net increase in serum phosphate level.

$1,25(OH)_2D$ acts to close each of these controlling loops by (directly and indirectly) depressing its own formation. The role of calcitonin and other hormones awaits further investigation.

## STRUCTURAL PATHOANATOMY OF RICKETS AND OSTEOMALACIA

### Gross Pathology and Histology

Regardless of their causes, the rachitic and osteomalacic syndromes display remarkably similar histologic and radiographic features. The characteristic changes of rickets are identified in the growth plates before closure; abnormalities of osteomalacia are seen in mature areas of trabecular and cortical bone.

The structure of the normal growth plate must be understood before the changes of rickets can be appreciated (Fig. 42-3). The typical growth plate, a complex structure composed of fibrous, cartilaginous, and osseous

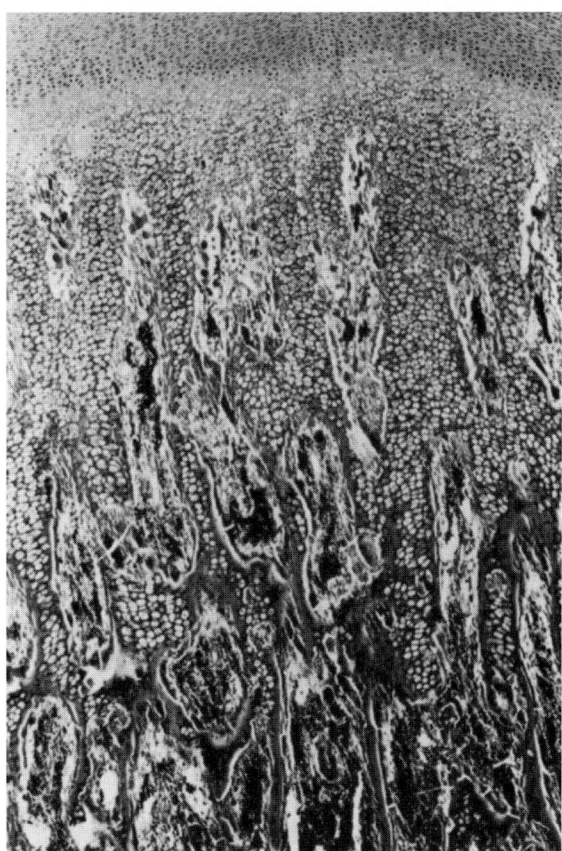

**Figure 42–3.** Normal chick growth plate with zone of proliferation at top. Observe orderly cartilaginous cell columns with zone of primary spongiosa at bottom. (Hematoxylin and eosin stain, 200×.) (From Pitt MJ, Haussler MR, Davis J, et al: Current concepts of vitamin D metabolism: Correlation with clinical syndromes. Crit Rev Radiol Sci 10:140, 1977.)

tissues, is located at the ends of long bones and situated between the epiphysis and the metaphysis. Histologically, the cellular arrangement of the normal growth plate is characterized by *order*. From epiphyseal to metaphyseal side, a progressive increase occurs in the number and size of cartilage cells and in the development of cell columns aligned with the long axis of the shaft. Zones of development may be identified.

1. The *reserve zone* (also termed the resting or germinal zone) is subjacent to the epiphysis. The cartilage cells are few in number, spherical, and randomly situated either singly or in pairs. They are not resting, are not germinal cells, and are not small in comparison to cells in the proliferative zone. Their function may be nutritional.

2. The *proliferating zone* is where the chondrocytes become flattened and arranged into longitudinal, parallel columns. These are the only cells in the cartilaginous portion of the growth plate that actively divide. The function of this zone is matrix production and cellular proliferation.

3. The *hypertrophic zone* is a region that may be subdivided further into zones of *maturation, degeneration,* and *provisional calcification.* The change in cell morphology from the proliferative to the hypertrophic zones is

usually abrupt and marked by sphericity and progressive enlargement. Cells nearing the metaphyseal side of the growth plate become quite large and vacuolated, with the last cells in the column becoming nonviable. The upper portions of this zone are active metabolically, and calcification of intervening cartilage matrix occurs.

4. The *zones of primary* and *secondary spongiosa* are located in the metaphysis immediately subjacent to the growth plate. Cartilage bars are partially or completely calcified and become ensheathed with osteoblasts, which produce layers of osteoid. Bone is produced by endochondral ossification.

The rachitic lesion displays disorganization in the growth plate and subjacent metaphysis (Fig. 42-4). The resting and proliferative zones of the cartilaginous growth plate appear normal. The zone of maturation reveals a disorganized increase in the number of cells and a loss of normal columnar pattern. This cell mass results in an increase in length and width of the growth plate. Concomitantly, vascular intrusion from the metaphysis and subsequent calcification of the intervening cartilaginous bars are decreased and grossly disordered. Defective mineralization in the zone of primary spongiosa and a lack of proper formation of bone lamellae and haversian systems occur.

Osteomalacia (Fig. 42-5) is characterized by abnormal quantities of osteoid (inadequately mineralized bone matrix) coating the surfaces of trabeculae and lining the haversian canals in the cortex ("osteoid seams"). Trabeculae become thin and decrease in number. In the cortex, the haversian systems become irregular, and large channels develop. Osteoid seams are not pathognomonic for osteomalacia and may be found in other states of high bone turnover. In osteomalacia, however, these osteoid seams increase in both number and width. Looser's lines or Milkman's pseudofractures, which strongly suggest the radiographic diagnosis of osteomalacia, are composed of focal accumulations of osteoid. Osteitis fibrosa cystica frequently is superimposed on the lesions of rickets and osteomalacia, reflecting hyperparathyroidism. This feature is particularly prominent in renal osteodystrophy.

## Radiographic Diagnosis of Rickets and Osteomalacia

**Rickets.** Rachitic changes are more obvious in regions of the most active growth; the sites of highest radiographic yield are the costochondral junctions of the middle ribs, the distal part of the femur, the proximal portion of the humerus, both ends of the tibia, and the distal ends of ulna and radius.

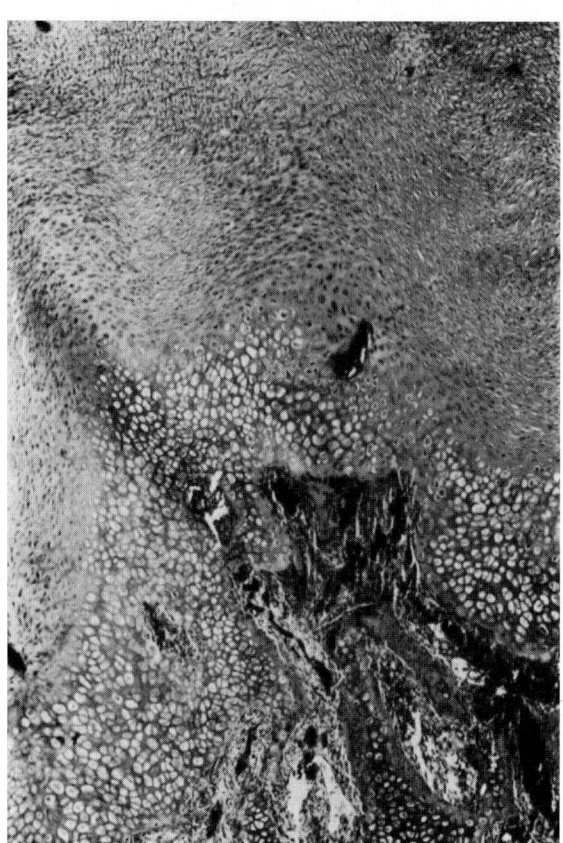

**Figure 42–4.** Rachitic chick growth plate with thick disordered hypertrophic zone virtually filling the field. Epiphyseal side appears at top. (Hematoxylin and eosin stain, 200×.) (From Pitt MJ, Haussler MR, Davis J, et al: Current concepts of vitamin D metabolism: Correlation with clinical syndromes. Crit Rev Radiol Sci 10:140, 1977.)

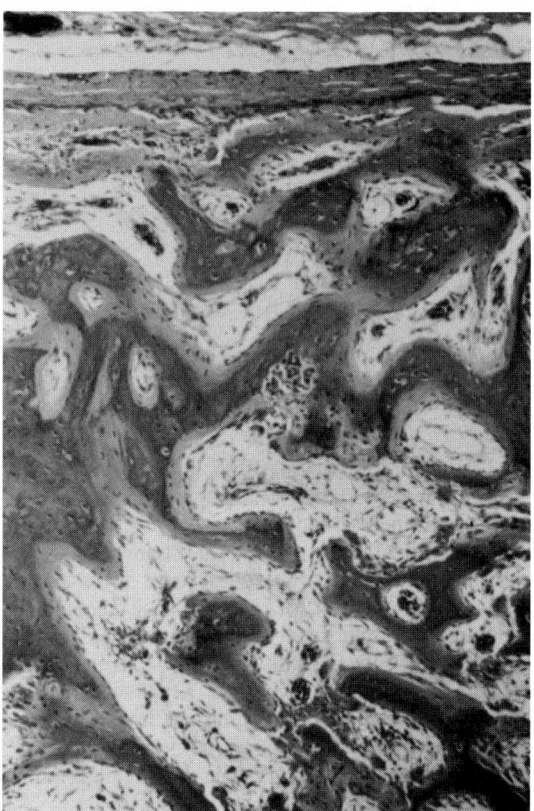

**Figure 42–5.** Osteomalacic cortex and subcortical spongy bone from metaphyseal region of a vitamin D–deficient chick. Trabeculae are thinned and irregular in shape and distribution. Sheaths of lightly stained osteoid almost equal the girth of bone in the trabeculae. Interspicular tissue is loosely fibrocartilaginous. (Hematoxylin and eosin stain, 500×.) (From Pitt MJ, Haussler MR, Davis J, et al: Current concepts of vitamin D metabolism: Correlation with clinical syndromes. Crit Rev Radiol Sci 10: 141, 1977.)

Nonspecific radiographic features include a general retardation in body growth and osteopenia. Characteristic changes appear at the growth plate. These reflect the disordered increase in cell growth in the zone of hypertrophy, coupled with the deficient mineralization of the zone of provisional calcification. Slight axial widening at the growth plate represents the earliest specific radiographic change. This is followed by a decrease in density at the zone of provisional calcification (on the metaphyseal side of the growth plate). As the disease progresses, further widening of the growth plate occurs, and the zone of provisional calcification becomes irregular. Disorganization and "fraying" of the spongy bone occur in the metaphyseal region. Widening and cupping of the metaphysis can be explained by the chaotic cartilage cell growth in the zone of maturation. On occasion, a thin bony margin is seen extending from the peripheral portions of the metaphysis surrounding the uncalcified cartilage mass (Fig. 42-6).

The ossified center of the epiphysis is surrounded by cartilage cells, which are organized in a similar fashion to the growth plate. The peripheral rim of the ossified epiphyseal nucleus is analogous to the zone of provisional calcification. Changes similar to those seen in the growth plate are present, consisting of deossification and unsharpness of the ossified periphery.

The bulky growth plates at the shaft bone-cartilage junctions of long bones and ribs explain some of the characteristic physical findings of rickets. Swelling about joints is typical, and a "rachitic rosary" develops at the costochondral junctions of the middle ribs. An additional semicoronal impression may be found at the costal attachment of the diaphragm (Harrison's groove).

The deformities caused by rickets exhibit different patterns, depending on the child's age when the disease develops. The head is particularly affected during the first months of life. During this period, the skull must accommodate to the most rapidly growing organ, the brain. The rapid accommodation by the skull is associated with excess osteoid formation, particularly at the central margins and outer table. Resorption at the inner table continues. The thin calvaria is subject to supine postural influences, resulting in posterior flattening. Continued accumulation of osteoid in the frontal and parietal regions results in the squared configuration known as craniotabes.

During infancy and early childhood, the long bones show the greatest deformity, both at the cartilage-shaft junctions and in the diaphyses. The characteristic bowing deformities of the arms and legs can be related to the sitting position assumed by infants and children. Bowing also is a result of displacement of the growth centers owing to asymmetrical musculotendinous pulls on the weakened growth plate. For example, the saber shin deformity of the tibia results from the strong posterior pull of the Achilles tendon on the calcaneus.

With increasing age, the effects of weight bearing become prominent. Scoliosis frequently develops and, coupled with bending deformities of long bones, results in an overall decrease in height. The intervertebral discs expand, producing concave impressions on the vertebral endplates. The skull shows basilar invagination, and intrusion of the hip and spine into the soft pelvis produces a triradiate configuration.

**Osteomalacia.** The radiographic confirmation of osteomalacia is difficult. Many changes, such as osteopenia, are nonspecific. Areas of spongy bone show a decrease in the total number of trabeculae; remaining trabeculae appear prominent but indistinct and project a "coarsened" pattern. Lucent sites in the cortex reflect accumulations of osteoid and widened, irregular haversian canals.

Looser's zones or pseudofractures are lucent areas that are oriented at right angles to the cortex and span the diameter of the bone incompletely. They tend to occur in characteristic sites, such as the axillary margins of the scapula, ribs, pubic rami, inner margins of the proximal ends of the femora, and ulnae (Fig. 42-7). Pseudofractures typically are bilateral and symmetrical. Sclerosis often demarcates the intraosseous margins; new bone on the periosteal aspect suggests callus.

Looser's zones are considered an insufficiency type of stress fracture. Radiolucent areas similar to those of pseudofractures may be found in bones affected by Paget's disease and fibrous dysplasia.

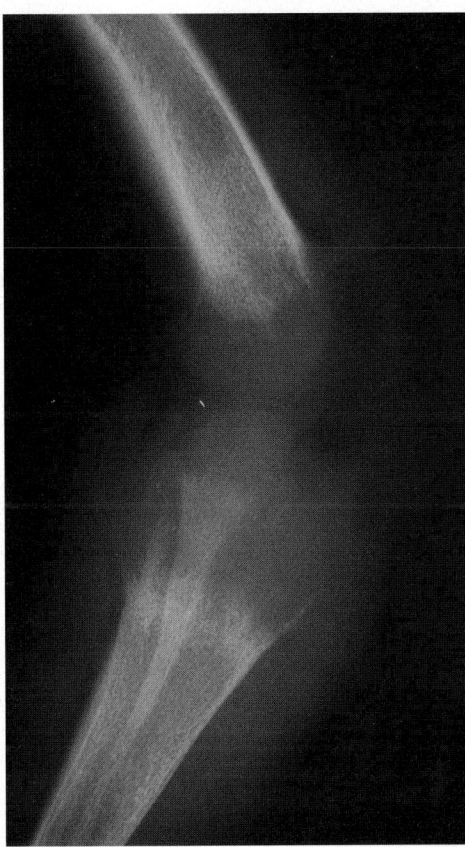

**Figure 42–6.** Knee radiograph of 6-week-old chick showing advanced dietary-deficiency rickets. Observe the advanced demineralization and disorganization in the metaphysis subjacent to the enlarged (unmineralized) growth plates. In the proximal part of the tibia in this specimen, a thin rim of circumferential new bone may be seen surrounding the rachitic growth plate. Also note the thickened, blunted posterior femoral cortex, representing an increase in inadequately mineralized osteoid. (From Pitt MJ, Haussler MR, Davis J, et al: Current concepts of vitamin D metabolism: Correlation with clinical syndromes. Crit Rev Radiol Sci 10:144, 1977.)

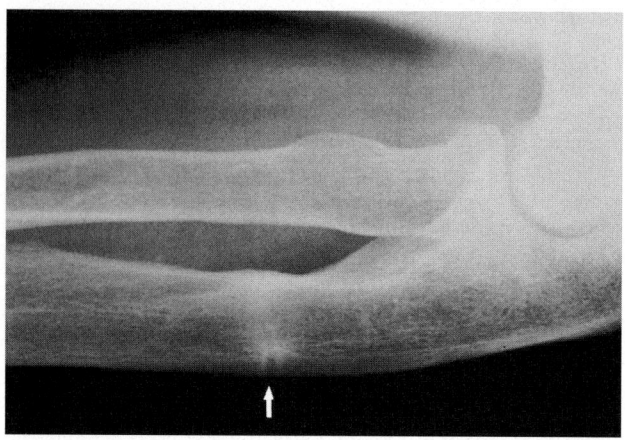

**Figure 42–7.** Pseudofracture *(arrow)* in adult patient with X-linked hypophosphatemic osteomalacia occurring in a characteristic location in the proximal portion of the ulna. Note bowing of the ulna. (From Pitt MJ, Haussler MR, Davis J, et al: Current concepts of vitamin D metabolism: Correlation with clinical syndromes. Crit Rev Radiol Sci 10:145, 1977.)

## CLINICAL SYNDROMES

An etiologic approach to the rachitic and osteomalacic disorders, as shown in Figure 42-8, includes the following:

1. Abnormalities of vitamin D metabolism: prohormone vitamin D, 25-OH-D, or 1,25(OH)$_2$D.

2. Rachitic and osteomalacic syndromes resulting primarily from renal tubular phosphate loss.

3. Rachitic and osteomalacic syndromes that do not show abnormalities of vitamin D metabolism or aberrations of calcium or phosphorus metabolism.

Table 42-1 lists useful points in diagnosing specific syndromes.

## Vitamin D Deficiency

Classic vitamin D–deficiency rickets is encountered uncommonly in the United States today, owing to the widespread addition of synthetic vitamin D$_2$ to foods, notably dairy products and bread. The natural source of vitamin D for humans is not dietary, however. Rather, humans depend mainly on the ultraviolet rays of the sun for endogenous conversion of 7-dehydrocholesterol in the skin to the prohormone vitamin D$_3$ (cholecalciferol). A reasonable degree of exposure to the sun should prevent the development of rickets and osteomalacia in a normal person whose diet contains adequate amounts of calcium and phosphorus.

From a worldwide perspective, deficiency rickets and osteomalacia are still health problems. Although decreased exposure to the sun appears to be important, deficiency rickets and osteomalacia have been reported even in sun-rich areas. Further, in developed countries, osteomalacia occurs in the elderly. The elderly segment of the population may constitute the largest group subject to the development of osteomalacia, particularly those patients who are house-bound or institutionalized for long periods. Although decreased exposure to the sun is a prime cause, other postulated factors include deficient intake of oral vitamin D$_2$, intestinal malabsorption in the elderly, and lower vitamin D hydroxylase activity in the liver and kidney. Although "deficiency" rickets (and osteomalacia) usually connotes a lack of vitamin D, insufficiencies of calcium, phosphorus, or both, should also be considered. Rickets secondary to phosphorus deficiency is usually a result of congenital or acquired renal disease. Proximal renal tubular dysfunction with defective absorption of phosphorus is seen in X-linked hypophosphatemia and Fanconi's syndromes. Phosphate loss also may complicate hemodialysis, cadaveric renal transplantation, or excessive ingestion of aluminum hydroxide, which binds phosphate in the gut. Rickets secondary to insufficient calcium in the diet is rare.

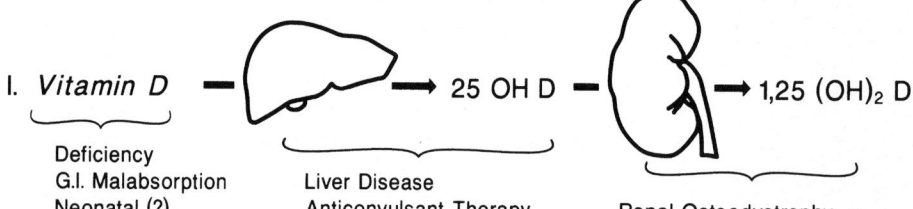

**I. Vitamin D** — 25 OH D — 1,25 (OH)$_2$ D

Deficiency
G.I. Malabsorption
Neonatal (?)

Liver Disease
Anticonvulsant Therapy

Renal Osteodystrophy
Vitamin D Dependent Rickets
Tumor Associated
Parathyroid Disorders
   Hypoparathyroidism
   Pseudohypoparathyroidism
   Hyperparathyroidism

**II. Phosphate loss**
   Renal Tubular Disorders
      X-linked Hypophosphatemia
      Fanconi Syndromes
      Tumor Associated

**III. NORMAL Vitamin D, P, Ca**
   Axial Osteomalacia
   Hypophosphatasia
   Metaphyseal Chondrodysplasia

**Figure 42–8.** Etiologic approach to the rachitic and osteomalacic syndromes organized in a framework of (I) abnormalities of vitamin D, (II) syndromes secondary to renal tubular loss of phosphate, and (III) syndromes in which no known abnormality of vitamin D metabolism or calcium-phosphorus homeostasis exists.

**TABLE 42–1**

### Radiographic Features of Specific Rachitic and Osteomalacic States

1. Nonspecific radiographic changes of rickets and osteomalacia
   a. Patients less than 6 months of age: Consider biliary atresia, vitamin D–dependent rickets, hypophosphatasia, and rickets associated with prematurity.
   b. If resistance to usual doses of vitamin D occurs (in the absence of chronic glomerular renal disease): Consider a renal tubular disorder, tumor association, hypophosphatasia, or metaphyseal chondrodysplasia, type Schmid. Note: Mild changes of secondary hyperparathyroidism may be present.
2. Renal osteodystrophy (uremic osteopathy): Radiographic changes of secondary hyperparathyroidism are usually present and predominate over the pattern of deossification. Osteosclerotic foci, particularly in the spine adjacent to the cartilaginous endplates (rugger-jersey spine), are characteristic. Vascular calcification of the Mönckeberg type and, less commonly, large "tumoral" deposits of amorphous calcification may be identified, particularly around joints.
3. X-linked hypophosphatemia
   a. Children: Rachitic changes at the growth plates are usually only mild to moderate in degree. General osteoporosis is uncommon, and the bones, although bowed, are "strong" in appearance.
   b. Adults: Generalized increase in bone density may be present, particularly in the axial skeleton. Changes may suggest ankylosing spondylitis. Characteristic is paravertebral calcification, multiple small ossified dense areas near joints, and new bone formation at ligamentous and tendinous attachments in the extremities. Biochemical tests reveal hyperphosphaturia with low serum phosphate concentration.
4. Axial osteomalacia: Radiographic abnormalities are confined to the axial skeleton. Dense, coarse trabecular pattern is most marked in the cervical region. Lumbar spine, pelvis, and ribs are also involved. The skull is normal. This disorder affects men, symptoms are minimal, and biochemical values are within normal limits.
5. Primary biliary cirrhosis: Mild to moderate generalized deossification. Hands show small, asymmetrical, intracapsular marginal erosions. Symptoms are mild; the arthritis is nondeforming.
6. Hypophosphatasia: Varies in severity. Newborn infants may show advanced demineralization. Rachitic growth plates show characteristic multiple lucent extensions into the metaphyses. Wormian bones and craniosynostosis may be present.
7. Metaphyseal chondrodysplasia, type Schmid: Multiple small bone projections extend from metaphyses into rachitic growth plates. Long bones maintain normal density. Skull is within normal limits. Spontaneous healing occurs.

### Gastrointestinal Malabsorption

Disorders of the small bowel, hepatobiliary system, and pancreas associated with intestinal malabsorption are the most common causes of vitamin D deficiency in the United States. Rickets and osteomalacia may develop in many small bowel malabsorptive states, including sprue, gluten-sensitive enteropathy (celiac disease) (Fig. 42-9), regional enteritis, scleroderma, and even unusual conditions such as multiple jejunal diverticula or stagnant (blind) loop syndromes. Decreased absorption and excessive fecal loss of both vitamin D and (probably) calcium are contributory. Small intestinal bypass surgery, performed for intractable morbid obesity, and partial gastrectomy have also been associated with osteomalacia.

Malabsorption associated with pancreatic insufficiency, even when pronounced, is infrequently associated with osteomalacia. Children with cystic fibrosis, in contrast to those with other malabsorptive diseases, seldom develop rickets.

### Rickets Associated with Prematurity (Neonatal Rickets; Metabolic Bone Disease of Prematurity)

Abnormal mineral homeostasis with low serum levels of calcium and phosphorus is a well-recognized complication in low-birth-weight premature infants. Radiographs may reveal evidence of rickets and osteomalacia. Affected infants usually weigh less than 1000 g at birth or were less than 28 weeks' gestation at birth. Although bone disease usually appears at about 12 weeks of age, it may develop later, particularly when prolonged parenteral nutrition is required.

The pathogenesis of the bone disease in prematurity can be related to a combination of nutritional, metabolic, and sometimes iatrogenic factors. A premature infant's

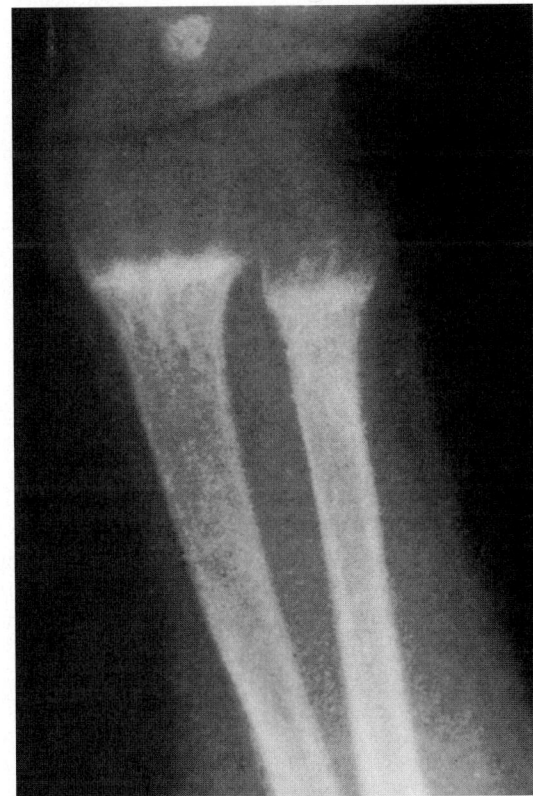

**Figure 42–9.** Rickets in a 4-month-old Mexican infant with celiac disease. The metaphysis is demineralized and disorganized. Metaphyseal widening reflects the enlarged growth plate.

requirements for calcium, phosphorus, and vitamin D are greater than those of an infant born at term. This increased need may not be provided for in the diet. Human milk and standard infant formulas, which are adequate for term babies, have insufficient amounts of vitamin D, phosphorus, and probably calcium for premature infants. Rickets and osteomalacia in these premature infants lead to significant morbidity from fractures, respiratory distress, and skeletal deformity.

## Liver Disease

Metabolic bone disease, termed hepatic osteodystrophy, is a well-recognized complication of chronic biliary ductal and hepatocellular disorders. Both osteoporosis and osteomalacia are found histologically. Although many patients are asymptomatic, morbidity relating to bone pain, tenderness, and fractures may be significant. When present, radiographic changes are usually those of nonspecific osteopenia. Pseudofractures indicate the presence of osteomalacia. Hypertrophic osteoarthropathy has been reported but is not common.

As in renal osteodystrophy, the cause of hepatic osteodystrophy is multifactorial. Because the liver is the major site for the initial hydroxylation of vitamin D, abnormalities in vitamin D metabolism might be expected. 25-Hydroxylation activity of the liver appears to be almost normal, however, and 25-OH-D levels usually can be corrected with vitamin D supplementation. The low serum levels of 25-OH-D are more likely a reflection of inadequate amounts of prohormone resulting from decreased exposure to ultraviolet light, decreased vitamin D supplementation, and—particularly if steatorrhea is present—malabsorption of vitamin D.

Because bile salts are necessary for the absorption of vitamin D, biliary duct obstruction, such as that which occurs in congenital biliary atresia (usually extrahepatic duct involvement), may be associated with typical rachitic changes, which may appear before 6 months of age.

## Anticonvulsant Drug–Related Rickets and Osteomalacia

Rickets and osteomalacia may be seen both histologically and radiographically in patients receiving anticonvulsant drug therapy, particularly phenobarbital and phenytoin (Dilantin). The reported prevalence of clinical bone disease and abnormal radiographic changes in these patients varies, but it is probably low. The mechanisms responsible for the production of rickets and osteomalacia are incompletely understood. When present, radiographic changes are nonspecific and cannot be differentiated from those of rickets or osteomalacia resulting from other causes.

## Renal Osteodystrophy (Uremic Osteopathy)

The bone disease associated with chronic renal failure results from multiple complex factors. Although the pathogenesis remains incompletely explained, two main mechanisms (probably acting in concert) are responsible: secondary hyperparathyroidism and abnormal vitamin D metabolism.

**Secondary Hyperparathyroidism.** Secondary hyperparathyroidism is noted consistently in untreated uremia occurring early in the course of the disease. Parathyroid hormone levels may be increased significantly and frequently are higher than the levels reached in primary hyperparathyroidism. The secondary hyperparathyroidism is provoked by hypocalcemia, which results from several different mechanisms; phosphate retention is the major factor.

**Abnormal Vitamin D Metabolism.** The singular importance of the kidney as the only organ capable of producing the physiologically active form of vitamin D, $1,25(OH)_2D$, was emphasized earlier in this chapter. Loss of renal tissue in acquired renal disease therefore would be expected to be associated with low levels of $1,25(OH)_2D$. The hyperphosphatemia of renal failure also inhibits $1,25(OH)_2D$ production.

**Histology and Radiology.** The histologic and radiographic findings in chronic renal failure reflect hyperparathyroidism and deficiency of $1,25(OH)_2D$. The major abnormalities are osteitis fibrosa cystica, osteomalacia or rickets (or both), osteosclerosis, and osteoporosis (see also Chapter 41).

Histologic evidence of secondary hyperparathyroidism is invariably present and is usually the dominant finding. The extent of bone resorption depends on the duration and degree of parathyroid hormone elevation. Osteomalacia or rickets, or both, is present in variable degrees and in several patterns. An increase in the number of osteoid borders or seams surrounding trabecular bone frequently is present but may result from either parathyroid hormone excess or vitamin D deficiency. An increase in the thickness of the seams indicates vitamin D deficiency. In addition, focal accumulations of osteoid are often found.

Radiographic abnormalities in chronic renal disease are observed in both the bones and the soft tissues. Bone changes reflect the abnormal histologic pattern and display secondary hyperparathyroidism, rickets or osteomalacia (or both), and osteosclerosis (Fig. 42-10). A combination of these abnormalities is frequently present.

Rickets may be the presenting feature and the first indication of chronic renal disease in children. Although rickets is usually the predominant feature, osteitis fibrosa cystica also may be conspicuous. General retardation of growth is noted as the disease progresses. In adults, the earliest radiographic changes are usually found in the hands. Subperiosteal resorption of bone on the radial aspects of the middle phalanges of the index and long fingers is identified radiographically by an unsharp, "lacy" outline of the cortex. A similar lack of definition may be seen in the cortex of the distal phalangeal tufts. With more advanced disease, other bones show evidence of subperiosteal resorption in concave areas ("cutback zones"), such as the medial margin of the femoral neck and inner aspect of the proximal end of the tibia. Widening of various joints, such as the acromioclavicular and sacroiliac joints and symphysis pubis, may occur secondary to subchondral resorption of bone and replacement fibrosis. Brown tumors, previously thought to be unusual

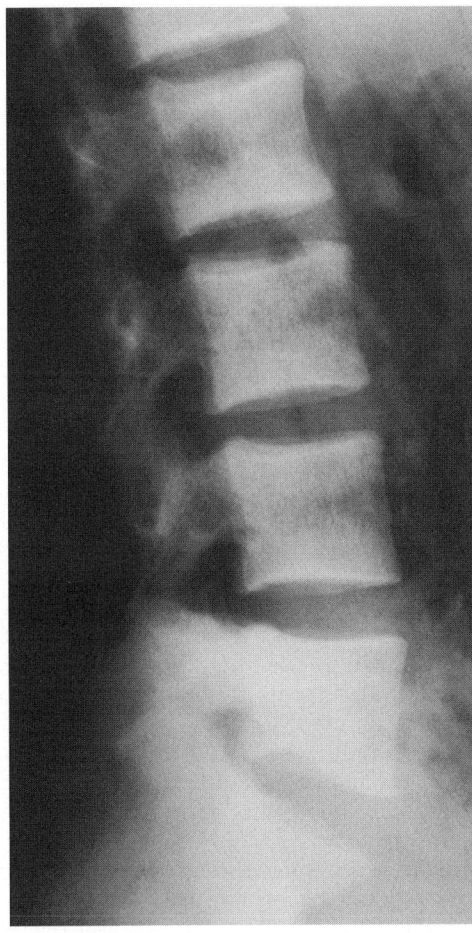

**Figure 42–10.** Areas of increased sclerosis subjacent to the cartilaginous plates (rugger-jersey spine) are demonstrated in a patient with chronic renal failure.

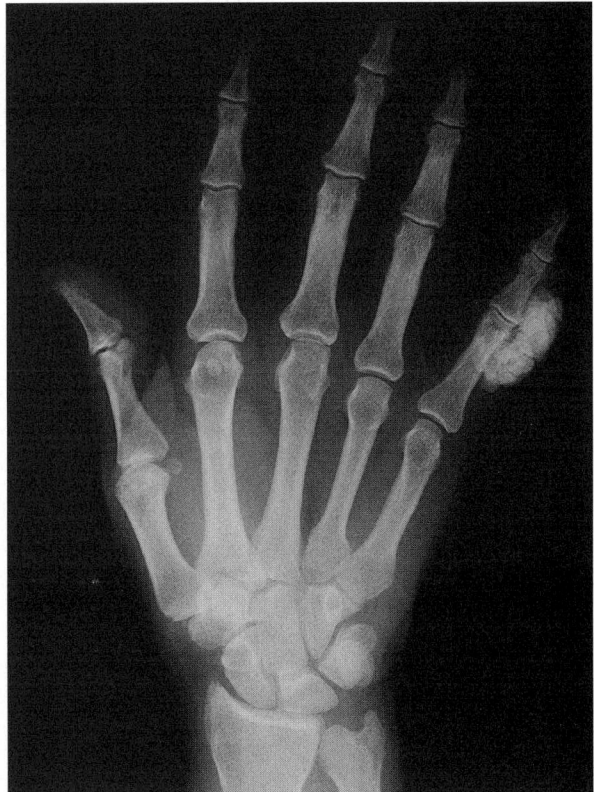

**Figure 42–11.** Tumoral calcinosis adjacent to the proximal interphalangeal joint of the little finger in a patient with chronic renal failure. Note the septated appearance of the calcium deposits. This patient had received large doses of vitamin D. Secondary hyperparathyroidism is reflected by the unsharpness of the phalangeal tufts and subperiosteal bone resorption on the radial aspects of the middle phalanges of the index and long fingers.

in uremic osteopathy, are being reported with increasing frequency.

Areas of increased density (osteosclerosis) are noted frequently in uremic osteopathy, and histologically they represent accumulations of excessive osteoid. These areas are characteristic in the spine, subjacent to the cartilaginous plates, and account for the characteristic rugger-jersey appearance (see Fig. 42-10). Areas of increased sclerosis are also noted in the pelvis and metaphyses of long bones. Subperiosteal new bone in the pelvis and paralleling the shafts of long bones (i.e., periosteal neostosis) likewise has been reported.

Soft tissue calcifications in uremia may be visceral or nonvisceral. Visceral calcifications occur in the heart, lungs, skeletal muscle, stomach, and kidneys. With the exception of the kidneys and lungs, these changes rarely are detected radiographically. Nonvisceral calcification occurs in the eyes, skin, periarticular areas, and arteries. Vascular calcification is of the Mönckeberg type and probably is a reflection of hyperphosphatemia. Accumulations of amorphous calcium in periarticular regions also are a reflection of increased serum phosphate levels. These deposits can become quite large (Fig. 42-11). Periarticular calcification in the capsule and tendons of both large and small joints is not uncommon. Chondro-

calcinosis, a feature of primary hyperparathyroidism, is less common in advanced renal failure.

## Aluminum Toxicity

Patients with chronic renal disease may develop aluminum toxicity, resulting in a low-turnover osteomalacia, termed dialysis osteomalacia or aluminum osteomalacia. Rickets may develop in children. This problem has been associated with significant morbidity and even death. Aluminum toxicity in uremia was first described as a complication of excess amounts of aluminum in the dialysate, due to either excess aluminum in the local water supply or aluminum sulfate added to the dialysate as a flocculating agent to remove particulate matter. Aluminum from oral phosphate binders such as aluminum hydroxide, which lower serum phosphate levels by binding with phosphate in the intestine, is now implicated as the main source.

Although the exact mechanism for the production of bone disease is unknown, aluminum accumulation at the bone-osteoid junction (calcification front) appears to inhibit mineralization. Because skeletal uptake of calcium is blocked, patients reveal a tendency toward hypercalcemia and relative *hypoparathyroidism*. Early symptoms and signs of aluminum toxicity include bone pain, muscle weakness, dementia, microcytic anemia, and hypercalcemia. Advanced complications may include pathologic fractures, seizures, encephalopathy, and death.

Radiographs may be helpful in predicting aluminum toxicity without resorting to biopsy. Diagnostic findings include the following: (1) an increased frequency of fractures, (2) a *lack* of osteosclerosis, (3) a relative *decrease* in subperiosteal resorption (hyperparathyroidism) compared with patients without aluminum toxicity, and (4) a significant increase in osteonecrosis after transplantation.

## Hereditary Vitamin D–Dependent Rickets

Hereditary vitamin D–dependent rickets, also termed pseudovitamin D–deficiency rickets, is a rare autosomal recessive disorder characterized by the clinical, radiographic, and biochemical features of vitamin D deficiency. Vitamin D intake is normal, however, and no evidence exists of other disease states, such as intestinal malabsorption and liver or kidney disorders, that would account for derangement in vitamin D metabolism. Symptoms may be present as early as 3 months of age (in contrast to the later onset of nutritional rickets), with most patients being symptomatic by the age of 1 year. Rachitic bone changes may be severe and rapidly progressive, with pathologic fractures. Although hypophosphatemia is present, the primary rachitogenic factor is hypocalcemia, which results from a decrease in intestinal calcium absorption. This condition is often apparent soon after birth, and secondary hyperparathyroidism follows.

## Rickets and Osteomalacia Secondary to Phosphate Loss

A number of rachitic and osteomalacic syndromes have been identified that, although differing in genetic and clinical features, share one or several renal tubular abnormalities: renal phosphate loss with secondary hypophosphatemia, glycosuria, aminoaciduria, renal tubular acidosis, hypokalemia, and vasopressin-resistant polyuria. These diseases are collectively designated Fanconi's syndrome. The most common is cystinosis; tyrosinemia and the oculocerebrorenal syndrome (Lowe's syndrome) are other, less common examples. In addition to congenital diseases, acquired renal tubular disorders with similar clinical and biochemical features may be secondary to drug toxicity, heavy metal poisoning, paraproteinemias, and tumors.

**X-Linked Hypophosphatemia.** X-linked hypophosphatemia (also known as familial vitamin D–resistant rickets) is the most common form of renal tubular rickets and osteomalacia. The classic syndrome is transmitted genetically as an X-linked dominant trait. Men are affected to a greater degree than women. The syndrome is characterized by lifelong hypophosphatemia that is secondary to renal tubular phosphate loss, decreased intestinal absorption of calcium, and normal serum levels of calcium. Rickets generally appears between 12 and 18 months of age. Remission usually follows growth plate closure, but recurrence of symptoms is common later in life. Patients typically are short, bowlegged, and stocky. The development and severity of rickets may differ among patients with the classic syndrome.

Radiographic features may allow for the specific diagnosis of this syndrome. In children, rachitic changes at the growth plates, in themselves nonspecific, may be only mild in degree. Osteopenia is not prominent. Bowing of long bones, particularly of the lower extremities, may occur, but deformity frequently is minimal. With increasing age, the trabecular pattern becomes coarsened. Looser's zones are more prevalent and can be complicated by complete fractures. By adulthood, a generalized increase in bone density, especially in the axial skeleton, is characteristic. Enthesopathic calcification and ossification develop in the paravertebral ligaments, anulus fibrosus, and capsules of apophyseal and appendicular joints (Figs. 42-12 and 42-13). The spinal changes may resemble those of ankylosing spondylitis or diffuse idiopathic skeletal hyperostosis. In contrast to ankylosing spondylitis, however, the sacroiliac joints in X-linked hypophosphatemia show no bone erosions. Narrowing of the spinal canal, which may relate to ossification of the ligamentum flavum, is common. In the pelvis, multiple sites of calcification may involve the acetabulum, iliolumbar ligaments, and sacroiliac ligaments (see Fig. 42-12B). The appendicular skeleton shows multiple sites of new bone formation at various muscle and ligament attachments. Separate small ossicles may develop around various joints, particularly those in the carpus (see Fig. 42-13).

X-linked hypophosphatemia and the various Fanconi's syndromes produce rickets and osteomalacia principally by renal tubular phosphate loss. Two separate renal tubular mechanisms for phosphate resorption have been identified: a parathyroid hormone–sensitive component, which is responsible for about two thirds of the total net resorption, and an additional system, which is responsive to the serum calcium level. The parathyroid hormone–sensitive component is completely absent in male patients with X-linked hypophosphatemia and is partially absent in female patients. Abnormalities in vitamin D metabolism also have been demonstrated in both X-linked hypophosphatemia and Fanconi's syndromes.

## Tumor-Associated Rickets and Osteomalacia

Hypophosphatemic vitamin D–refractory rickets and osteomalacia in association with various neoplasms are being recognized with increasing frequency. The associated neoplasms occur in children and adults, are located in soft tissues or bone, and vary in size. The lesions typically are vascular and often show foci of new bone formation; the most frequent histologic diagnosis is hemangiopericytoma. Bone lesions include nonossifying fibroma, giant cell tumor, osteoblastoma, and non-neoplastic diseases such as fibrous dysplasia and neurofibromatosis. Radiographic changes of rickets and osteomalacia may be advanced. Hypophosphatemia is the predominant biochemical feature, related to failure of renal tubular reabsorption of phosphate. Circumstantial evidence suggests the existence of a tumor-elaborated humoral substance that affects renal phosphate absorption in the proximal tubule directly.

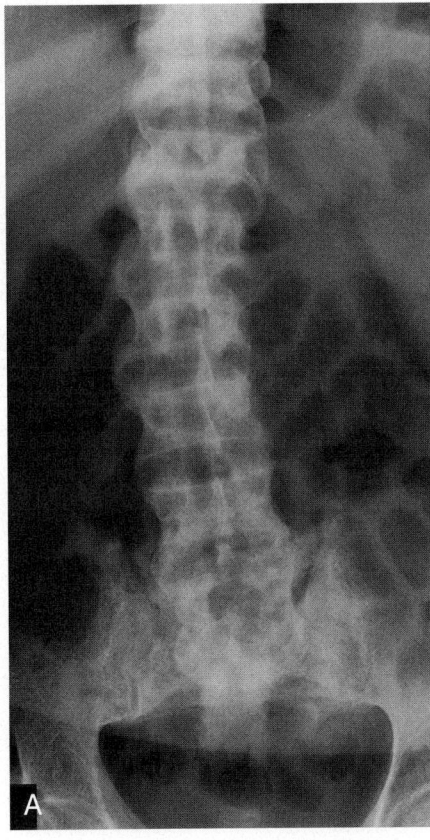

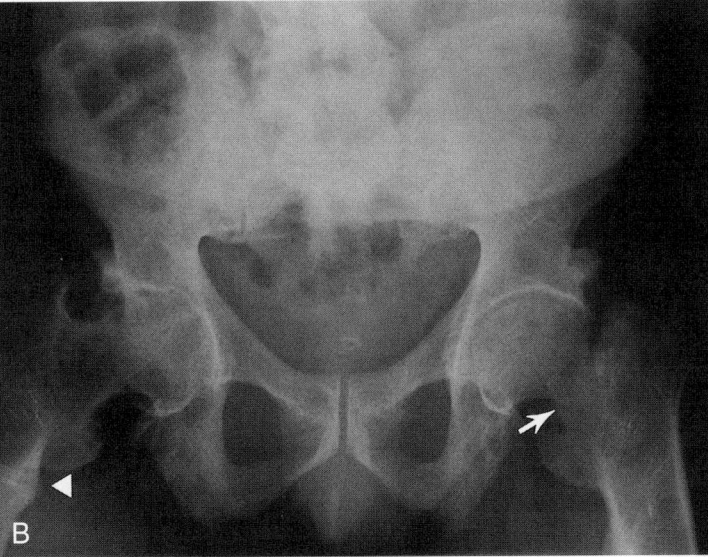

**Figure 42–12.** X-linked hypophosphatemia in a man. *A*, Multifocal areas of paravertebral ossification are similar to those in diffuse idiopathic skeletal hyperostosis or ankylosing spondylitis. Abnormalities of both sacroiliac joints result from ossification of the anterior sacroiliac ligaments. *B*, In the same patient, enthesopathic new bone is seen bilaterally at the supra-acetabular attachments of the rectus femoris muscles and at the adductor muscle attachments to the ischia. A Looser's zone is present in the right proximal portion of the femur *(arrowhead)*. The patient had an intracapsular fracture of the left hip *(arrow)*.

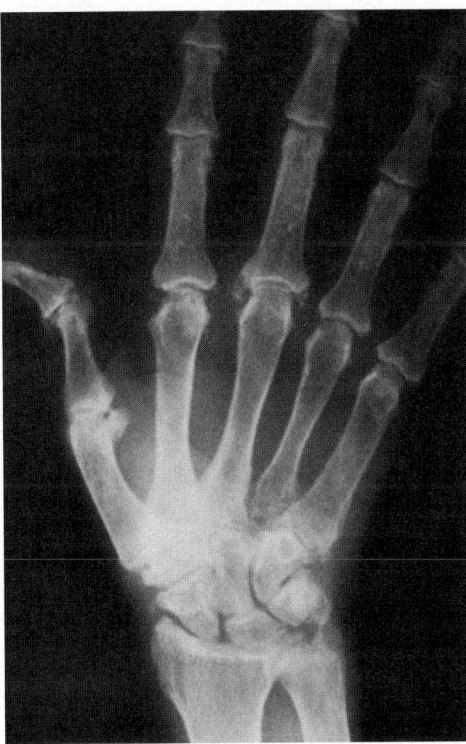

**Figure 42–13.** X-linked hypophosphatemia. Small ossicles are noted at the radial aspect of the wrist, and ossification of the triangular fibrocartilage complex is present. Capsular ossification is noted at multiple interphalangeal and metacarpophalangeal joints.

It is important for the radiologist to be aware of the association between various neoplasms and the development of rickets and osteomalacia. A careful search for these lesions should be made in patients with hypophosphatemic vitamin D–refractory states for which the more common causes have not been identified.

## Atypical Axial Osteomalacia

Atypical axial osteomalacia is a rare condition in which the radiographic changes are characteristic. Skeletal involvement is axial, with sparing of appendicular sites (Fig. 42-14). A dense, coarse trabecular pattern involves primarily the cervical spine but also is present in the lumbar spine, pelvis, and ribs. Looser's zones have not been identified.

All reported patients have been men. Their general health is good, symptoms are minimal, and the biochemical findings are within normal limits. Biopsy of the involved areas demonstrates typical osteomalacia. Patients do not respond to vitamin D therapy.

## Hypophosphatasia

Hypophosphatasia is a rare disorder transmitted genetically in an autosomal recessive pattern. It is characterized by defective skeletal mineralization resembling that of rickets and osteomalacia, low serum alkaline phosphatase levels, and abnormal amounts of phosphoethanolamine in the urine and blood. Although most cases are diag-

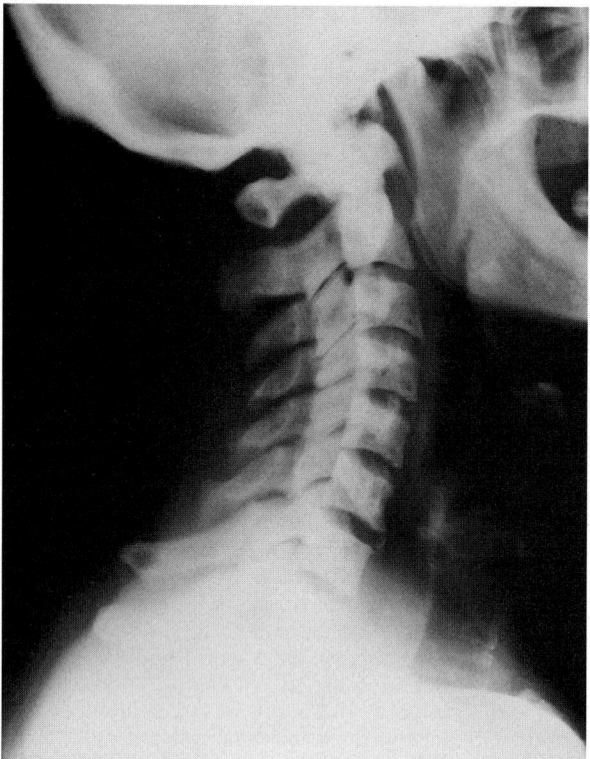

**Figure 42–14.** Atypical axial osteomalacia. A dense, coarse trabecular pattern involves the cervical spine. The appendicular skeleton was normal.

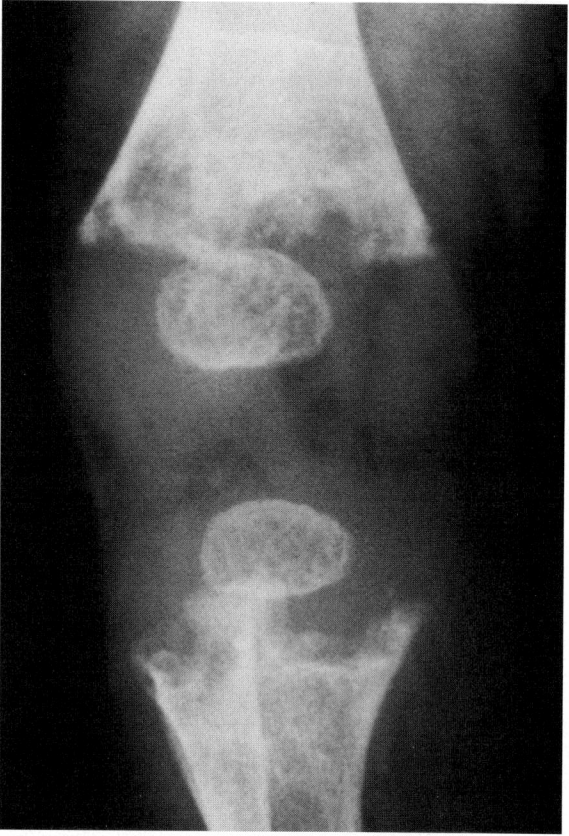

**Figure 42–15.** Hypophosphatasia. Deossification is present adjacent to the growth plates. Characteristic radiolucent areas extend from the growth plates into the metaphysis.

nosed during infancy or childhood, in some patients the condition may not be recognized until adult life. The most severely affected neonates usually die soon after birth. Generalized deficient or absent mineralization is noted radiologically. Fractures with deformity and shortening of the extremities may suggest a dwarfing syndrome.

Patients surviving infancy display varying degrees of skeletal involvement. Radiographic changes at the growth plates may be identified soon after birth. These abnormalities are similar to those of rickets but characteristically demonstrate irregular, often prominent lucent extensions into the metaphysis representing uncalcified bone matrix (Fig. 42-15). Generalized deossification with a coarse trabecular pattern, bowing deformities with or without healing fractures, and subperiosteal new bone accumulation may be present. Craniosynostosis involving all sutures is common, and wormian (intersutural) bones may be identified.

## Metaphyseal Chondrodysplasia (Type Schmid)

Metaphyseal chondrodysplasias encompass a variety of disorders that have in common generalized symmetrical disturbance of endochondral bone formation, primarily at the metaphyses. The type described by Schmid is the most common and has radiographic features very similar to those of X-linked hypophosphatemic rickets (vitamin D–resistant rickets). Normal levels of serum phosphorus, alkaline phosphatase, and calcium differentiate these dis-

orders from other rachitic syndromes.

The disease manifests in childhood with short stature, bowing of long bones, and an accentuated lumbar lordosis with a waddling gait. The clinical course is benign. The disease is transmitted in an autosomal dominant pattern, but spontaneous mutations occur.

In a child, radiographs reveal widening of the growth plates. In contrast to usual rickets, the metaphysis is well mineralized and actually may show increased density. Fine, spurlike projections of organized bone may extend into the growth plate from the metaphysis. The long bones are bowed. The absence of Looser's zones or signs of secondary hyperparathyroidism is notable. The lesions tend to heal spontaneously.

## Parathyroid Gland Abnormalities

Because parathyroid hormone is a major stimulus to $1,25(OH)_2D$ production, the clinical syndromes of hypoparathyroidism, pseudohypoparathyroidism, and pseudopseudohypoparathyroidism are associated with abnormalities of vitamin D metabolism.

**Pseudohypoparathyroidism and Pseudo-pseudohypoparathyroidism.** The term *pseudohypoparathyroidism* was introduced by Albright and associates to describe patients who had a characteristic phenotype consisting of short stature, round face, short neck, and shortening of metacarpal bones (particularly the first, fifth, and fourth) (Fig. 42-16), accompanied by low serum calcium and high serum phosphorus levels consistent with hypoparathyroidism. Administration of parathyroid hormone in these patients did not result in the normally expected increase in urinary phosphate levels, leading investigators to postulate the existing of an end-organ (kidney) unresponsiveness to parathyroid hormone. Subsequently, patients were described who had the characteristic phenotype of pseudo-hypoparathyroidism with normal blood chemistry values, and the term pseudo-pseudohypoparathyroidism was applied to this condition. The renal response to parathyroid hormone in this latter group of patients is normal.

Both pseudohypoparathyroidism (the classic syndrome is termed type I) and pseudo-pseudohypoparathyroidism have the same phenotype. The parathyroid glands are intrinsically normal. Parathyroid hormone levels are normal in pseudo-pseudohypoparathyroidism and elevated in pseudohypoparathyroidism; the latter is a consequence of the ineffective hormone action at the kidney, with secondary hyperphosphatemia and hypocalcemia. Patients have been reported who exhibit this same phenotype but who have true hypoparathyroidism. Parathyroid hormone levels are low, and they have a proper target-organ response to the administration of parathyroid hormone. These patients would be classified as having pseudo-pseudohypoparathyroidism. To clarify the distinctions between these disorders, it has been proposed that the condition with the phenotypic changes originally described by Albright be termed Albright's hereditary osteodystrophy (distinct from Albright's syndrome, which consists of fibrous dysplasia, precocious puberty, and café au lait spots). Hypoparathyroid states should be classified as either true hormone-deficient or hormone-resistant forms. Patients with Albright's hereditary osteodystrophy may exhibit target-organ (kidney and bone) unresponsiveness to parathyroid hormone (pseudohypoparathyroidism) or may exhibit a normal target-organ responsiveness (pseudo-pseudohypoparathyroidism with normal parathyroid hormone levels or pseudo-pseudohypoparathyroidism with true deficiency of parathyroid hormone) (see Chapter 46)

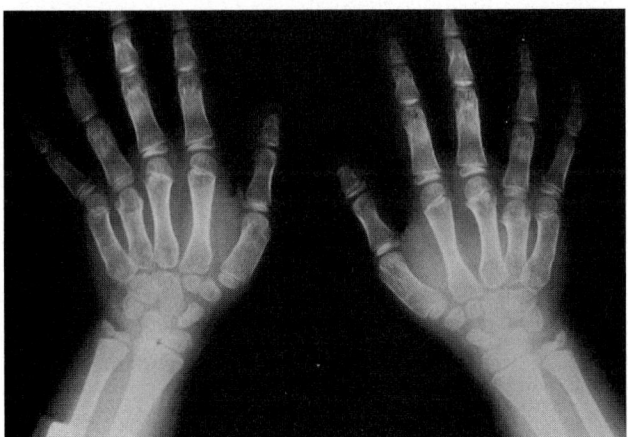

**Figure 42–16.** Pseudohypoparathyroidism (Albright's hereditary osteodystrophy) in a 9-year-old boy, demonstrating shortening of all metacarpal bones, particularly the fourth.

## FURTHER READING

Albright F, Burnett CH, Smith PH, et al: Pseudohypoparathyroidism—an example of Seabright-Bantam syndrome (report of 3 cases). Endocrinology 30:922, 1942.

Brighton CT: Structure and function of the growth plate. Clin Orthop 136:22, 1978.

Burnstein MI, Kottamasu SR, Petitifor JM, et al: Metabolic bone disease in pseudohypoparathyroidism: Radiologic features. Radiology 155:351, 1985.

Burnstein MI, Lawson JP, Kottamasu SR, et al: The enthesopathic changes of hypophosphatemic osteomalacia in adults: Radiologic findings. AJR Am J Roentgenol 153:785, 1989.

Dent CE: Rickets (and osteomalacia), nutritional and metabolic (1919–1969). Proc R Soc Med 63:401, 1970.

Dent CE, Normand ECS: Metaphysial dysostosis, type Schmid. Arch Dis Child 39:444, 1964.

Frame B, Frost HM, Ormond RS, et al: Atypical osteomalacia involving the axial skeleton. Ann Intern Med 55:632, 1961.

Frymoyer JW, Hodgkin W: Adult-onset vitamin D–resistant hypophosphatemic osteomalacia. J Bone Joint Surg Am 59:101, 1977.

Kidd GS, Schaaf M, Adler RA, et al: Skeletal responsiveness in pseudohypoparathyroidism: A spectrum of clinical disease. Am J Med 68:772, 1980.

Kolb FO, Steinbach HL: Pseudohypoparathyroidism with secondary hyperparathyroidism and osteitis fibrosa. J Clin Endocrinol Metab 22:59, 1962.

Linovitz RJ, Resnick D, Keissling P, et al: Tumor-induced osteomalacia and rickets: A surgically curable syndrome, report of two cases. J Bone Joint Surg Am 58:419, 1976.

Lyles KW, Berry WR, Haussler M, et al: Hypophosphatemic osteomalacia: Association with prostatic carcinoma. Ann Intern Med 93:275, 1980.

Mankin HJ: Rickets, osteomalacia, and renal osteodystrophy–Part I. J Bone Joint Surg Am 56:101, 1974.

Mankin HJ: Rickets, osteomalacia, and renal osteodystrophy—Part II. J Bone Joint Surg Am 56:352, 1974.

Mankin HJ: Rickets, osteomalacia, and renal osteodystrophy. Orthop Clin North Am 21:81, 1990.

Nelson AM, Riggs BL, Jowsey JO: Atypical axial osteomalacia: Report of four cases with two having features of ankylosing spondylitis. Arthritis Rheum 21:715, 1978.

Pitt MJ: Rickets and osteomalacia are still around. Radiol Clin North Am 29:97, 1991.

Polisson RP, Martinez S, Khoury M, et al: Calcification of entheses associated with X-linked hypophosphatemic osteomalacia. N Engl J Med 313:1, 1985.

Renton P, Shaw DG: Hypophosphatemic osteomalacia secondary to vascular tumors of bone and soft tissue. Skeletal Radiol 1:21, 1976.

Reynolds WA, Karo JJ: Radiologic diagnosis of metabolic bone disease. Orthop Clin North Am 3:521, 1972.

Shapiro R: Radiologic aspects of renal osteodystrophy. Radiol Clin North Am 10:557, 1972.

Spiegel AM, Levine MA, Marx SJ, et al: Pseudohypoparathyroidism: The molecular basis for hormone resistance—a restrospective. N Engl J Med 307:679, 1982.

Steinbach HL, Kolb FO, Gilfillan R: A mechanism of the production of pseudofractures in osteomalacia (Milkman's syndrome). Radiology 62:388, 1954.

Steinbach HL, Noetzli M: Roentgen appearance of the skeleton in osteomalacia and rickets. AJR Am J Roentgenol 91:955, 1964.

Turner ML, Dalinka MK: Osteomalacia: Uncommon causes. AJR Am J Roentgenol 133:539, 1979.

# CHAPTER 43

## Paget's Disease

## SUMMARY OF KEY FEATURES

Paget's disease is a common disorder of middle-aged and elderly patients that is characterized by excessive and abnormal remodeling of bone. Its radiographic features are virtually diagnostic and include an initial osteolytic phase, most common in the skull and tubular bones, and a subsequent osteosclerotic phase, particularly in the axial skeleton. An enlarged bone with increased radiodensity and an accentuated trabecular pattern is typical. Involvement of specific sites leads to characteristic radiographic signs, including the "cotton-wool" cranial vault and the "picture-frame" vertebral body. Complications associated with Paget's disease are insufficiency fractures, neurologic symptoms and signs, skeletal deformities, neoplasms, and articular alterations. The most important articular abnormality associated with this disorder is degenerative joint disease, particularly in the hip and knee.

## INTRODUCTION

Paget's disease (osteitis deformans) is a condition of unknown cause that affects approximately 3% of the population older than 40 years. Initially described by Paget in 1877, the disease varies considerably in severity. Commonly, it is a process localized to one or several regions of the skeleton without significant clinical findings; occasionally, it is widespread and severe and produces extensive osseous abnormality and deformity. Paget's disease has certain geographic and racial characteristics. It appears to be particularly common in inhabitants of Australia, Great Britain, and certain areas of continental Europe; it is not uncommon in the United States; and it is extremely rare in China and most areas of Africa.

The disease is characterized by excessive and abnormal remodeling of bone. Its active phase is associated with aggressive bone resorption and formation, whereas its quiescent phase is associated with a diminished rate of bone turnover. The combination of osseous resorption and apposition produces a diagnostic pathologic and radiographic appearance. Irregular bony fragments with a thickened and disorganized trabecular (mosaic) pattern are visualized as coarsened and enlarged osseous trabeculae on radiographs.

## CLINICAL FEATURES

Paget's disease is common, particularly in middle-aged and elderly persons. It is unusual in persons younger than 40 years, uncommon between the ages of 40 and 55 years, common (3% to 4%) after the age of 55 years, and frequent (10%) in patients older than 80 years. Paget's disease is slightly more common in men than in women.

In many patients, the disorder is first diagnosed as an incidental finding on radiographs obtained for unrelated purposes. In patients with symptoms, clinical findings vary with the distribution of the disease. Sometimes, Paget's disease affects just one bone and remains limited in distribution throughout its course. At other times, after first being localized to one or two sites, the disorder progresses to involve much of the skeleton. Paget's disease has a predilection for the axial skeleton and may be widespread at the time of initial diagnosis. Local pain and tenderness are frequently present at an affected skeletal site. Pain is often worse at night and unrelated to exercise. Increasing size of bone may produce such clinical findings as head enlargement or prominence of the shins. Skeletal deformities include kyphosis and bowing of the long bones of the extremities. Neuromuscular complications are not infrequent. Neurologic deficits result from impingement on the spinal cord causing muscle weakness, paralysis, and rectal and vesical incontinence. Platybasia is a result of involvement of the base of the skull. Obstructive hydrocephalus may result in ataxia, gait disturbances, incontinence, and dementia. Compression of cranial nerves in their foramina is not common, although deafness may be apparent.

Congestive heart failure has been noted in patients with Paget's disease, which may be related to the presence of arteriovenous shunts in the involved bone.

Laboratory analysis in Paget's disease generally reveals elevated alkaline phosphatase levels in serum and elevated hydroxyproline levels in serum and urine. These chemical abnormalities vary with the distribution and activity of the disease. Generally, serum alkaline phosphatase is thought to be a less sensitive parameter of pagetic activity than urinary hydroxyproline. Serum acid phosphatase values are normal in this disease, whereas serum uric acid levels are commonly elevated.

## CAUSE

The precise cause of Paget's disease remains unknown, although a viral cause has gained support in recent years. Active pagetic bone is characterized by the presence of giant osteoclasts containing large numbers of nuclei. Intranuclear inclusion bodies have been identified in these cells that are not observed in the osteoblasts or osteocytes of pagetic bone or in osseous tissue derived from patients with a variety of other skeletal disorders, even those characterized by osteoclastic proliferation. Ultrastructural characteristics of pagetic osteoclasts suggest that the inclusions are viral in nature. Similar cellular characteristics are observed in disorders produced by certain viruses, specifically, subacute sclerosing panencephalitis related to a paramyxovirus of the measles group. The identification of similar intranuclear inclusions within giant cell tumors in patients with Paget's disease is further evidence of a viral cause of the disorder, and certain immunocytologic data have reinforced this viral hypothesis. In addition, significant and sustained viral antibody titers against the measles virus have been detected in a few patients with Paget's disease.

## PATHOPHYSIOLOGY

Paget's disease is a remarkable disorder of bone that evolves through various stages, or phases, of activity, followed by an inactive or quiescent stage (Table 43–1). Its initial characteristic is an intense wave of osteoclastic activity with resorption of normal bone by giant multinucleated cells. Subsequently, excessive and disorganized new bone formation induced by a vigorous osteoblastic response leads to the appearance of architecturally abnormal osseous tissue that consists of primitive or woven bone with increased vascularity and a pronounced connective tissue reaction. After a variable period of time, osteoblastic activity also declines, and the condition becomes quiescent or inactive. Microscopic evaluation reveals distortion of the normal trabecular appearance, with a mosaic pattern of irregular cement lines joining areas of lamellar bone.

## RADIOGRAPHIC-PATHOLOGIC CORRELATION

### General Stages of the Disease

An initial phase of intense osteoclastic activity with resorption of bone trabeculae may be detected on radiographs as an "osteolytic" form of the disease (Fig. 43–1). This imaging appearance is particularly common in the skull, where it is termed osteoporosis circumscripta. Osteolysis in the cranial vault is observed most frequently in the frontal or occipital region and may progress to involve the entire skull. The advancing radiolucent lesion may be sharply delineated from the adjacent normal bone. The osteolytic phase of Paget's disease may be apparent elsewhere in the skeleton, particularly in the long bones and, less commonly, the pelvis, spine, and small bones of the hands and feet.

Osteolysis begins almost invariably in the subchondral regions of the epiphysis and subsequently extends into the metaphysis and diaphysis; occasionally, the disease may appear at both ends of an involved bone, but only exceptionally is Paget's disease apparent in the diaphysis without involvement of the epiphysis. When present, this latter feature typically occurs in the tibia. As the disease progresses, osteolysis may advance into the diaphysis as a V- or wedge-shaped radiolucent area, clearly demarcated from adjacent bone. This appearance has been likened to a blade of grass or a flame. Within the area of radiolucency, the remaining trabeculae may appear thickened, although they are frequently obliterated, and a hazy "ground-glass" or "washed-out" pattern is observed. The involved bone is commonly enlarged or widened, and pathologic fractures may be evident.

Radiographic evidence of increased density, or sclerosis, of bone may be seen in the active or inactive stages of the disease (Figs. 43–2 and 43–3). In the cranium, bone sclerosis may produce circular radiodense lesions in one

### TABLE 43–1

**Stages of Paget's Disease**

| Stage | Most Common Sites | Appearances |
|---|---|---|
| Active Osteolytic | Cranial vault | Osteoporosis circumscripta |
| | Long tubular bones | Subchondral location, advancing wedge of radiolucency |
| Osteolytic, osteosclerotic, or both | Cranial vault | Osteoporosis circumscripta, focal radiodense areas |
| | Pelvis | Patchy radiolucency and radiodensity |
| | Long tubular bones | Diaphyseal radiolucency, epiphyseal and metaphyseal radiodensity |
| Inactive Osteosclerotic | Cranial vault | "Cotton-wool" appearance, thickened cranial vault, basilar invagination |
| | Spine | "Picture frame" vertebral body, ivory vertebral body |
| | Pelvis | Thickening of pelvic ring, focal or diffuse radiodensity |
| | Long tubular bones | Epiphyseal predilection, coarse trabeculae, widened and deformed bone |

area, whereas osteoporosis circumscripta is noted elsewhere. Similarly, in the long bones, as the flame-shaped advancing edge of osteolysis proceeds toward the shaft, focal radiodensity may become evident in the epiphysis and metaphysis. Cortical thickening, enlargement of bone, and coarsened trabeculae are prominent. Eventually, radiographic evidence of osteolysis may disappear, and the imaging picture is that of osteosclerosis.

### General Distribution of the Disease

When discovered, Paget's disease is generally polyostotic in distribution (Fig. 43–4). Symmetry is not typical of bone involvement, with the exception of the innominate bones. Paget's disease predominates in the axial skeleton. Particularly characteristic is involvement of the pelvis (30% to 75%); sacrum (30% to 60%); spine (30% to 75%), especially the lumbar segment; and skull (25% to 65%). In addition, the proximal portions of the long bones are commonly affected, particularly the femur (25% to 35%). Abnormalities of the axial skeleton or proximal part of the femur are present in approximately 75% to 80% of cases. No bone is exempt, although changes in the ribs, fibula, and small bones in the hand and foot are infrequent. In some patients, the disease is initially or totally monostotic, a pattern that is evident in 10% to 35% of cases.

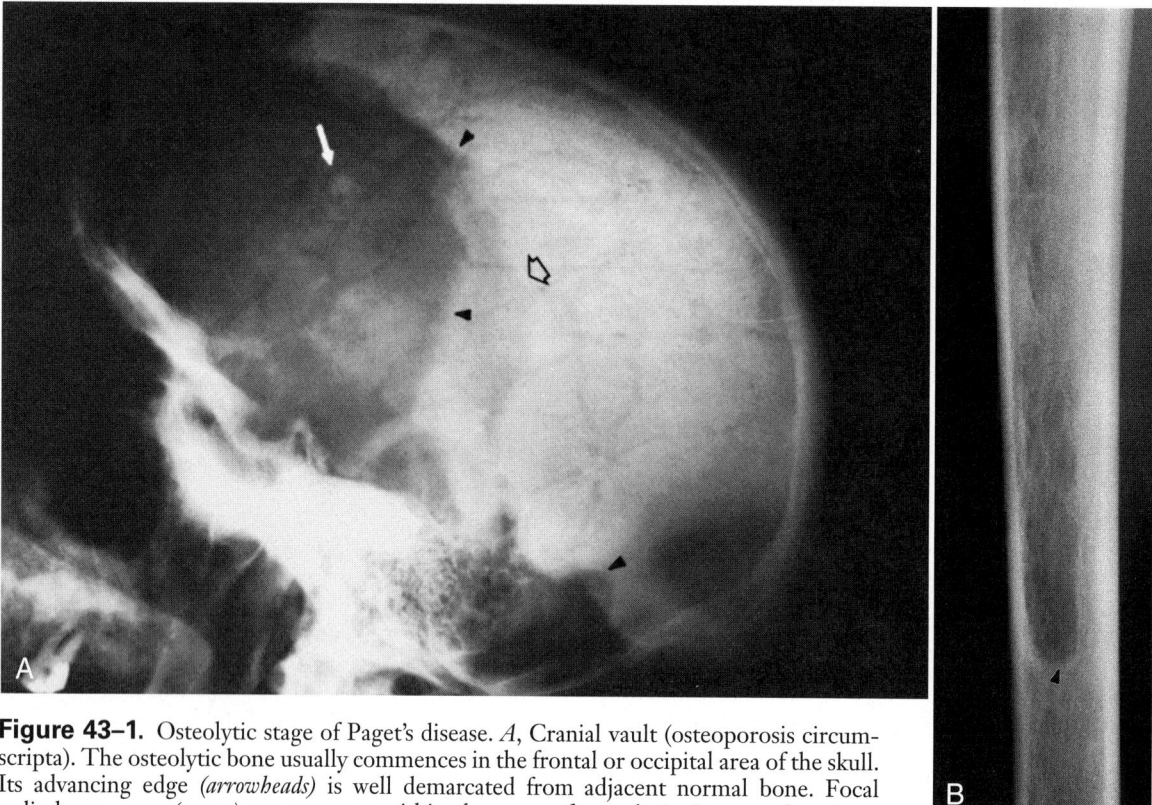

**Figure 43–1.** Osteolytic stage of Paget's disease. *A*, Cranial vault (osteoporosis circumscripta). The osteolytic bone usually commences in the frontal or occipital area of the skull. Its advancing edge *(arrowheads)* is well demarcated from adjacent normal bone. Focal radiodense areas *(arrow)* are apparent within the areas of osteolysis. In some locations, involvement of a portion of the cranial vault creates beveled margins *(open arrow)*. *B*, Tubular bones. An advancing wedge-shaped radiolucent edge *(arrowhead)* is observed in the femur.

## Involvement of Specific Sites

**Cranium**. Pagetic alterations of the skull (see Figs. 43–1 and 43–2) vary from typical osteoporosis circumscripta to widespread sclerosis. Focal radiodense areas exhibiting

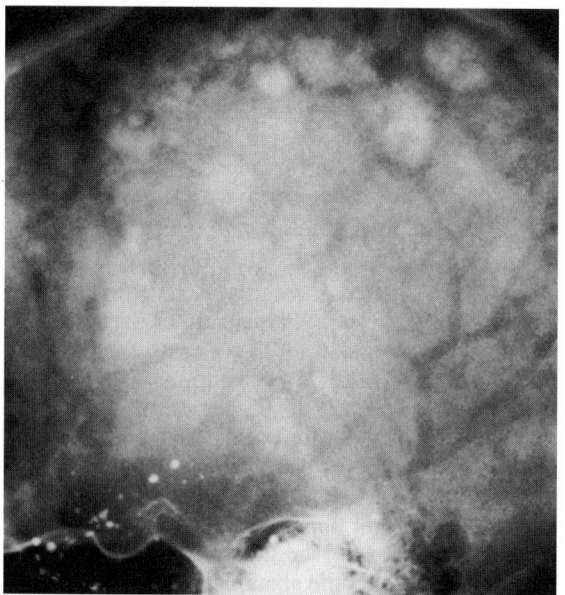

**Figure 43–2.** General stages of Paget's disease: osteolytic and osteosclerotic stage. Cranial involvement showing extensive osteosclerosis is producing the "cotton-wool" appearance.

the "cotton-wool" appearance may be observed. Cranial thickening is occasionally extensive, particularly in the frontal regions, and both bone sclerosis and thickening may be distributed asymmetrically. In contrast to the exuberant facial changes that may be seen in fibrous dysplasia, extensive alterations of the facial bones are infrequent in Paget's disease.

Basilar invagination is seen in about one third of patients with Paget's disease of the skull, and it increases in frequency with progressive severity of the disease. Basilar invagination is characterized by upward protrusion of the foramen magnum and surrounding bone as a result of the effect of gravity and muscle pull. It may be associated with neurologic symptoms and signs. Additional clinical findings are related to impingement on other cranial nerves by the enlarging pagetic bone.

**Vertebral Column**. Paget's disease frequently involves the vertebral column (Fig. 43–5), particularly the lumbar spine and the sacrum. Thoracic and cervical involvement and monostotic disease of the spine may be observed. Five mechanisms have been emphasized in the pathogenesis of the neurologic complications of such involvement: collapse of affected vertebral bodies; increased vascularity of pagetic bone, which "steals" blood from the spinal cord; mechanical interference with the spinal cord blood supply; narrowing of the spinal canal because of new bone formation or soft tissue and ligament ossification; and stenosis of neural foramina resulting from involve-

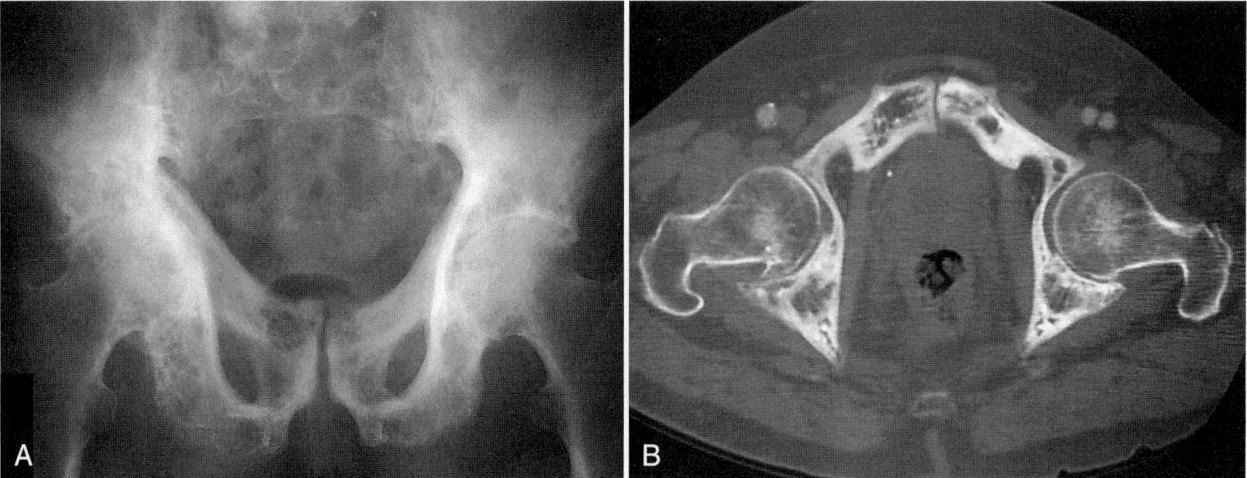

**Figure 43–3.** General stages of Paget's disease: osteosclerotic stage. *A,* Long-standing Paget's disease of the pelvis with diffuse osteosclerosis is evident. Note the degenerative joint disease in both hips. *B,* Axial CT scan at the level of the femoral heads shows dramatic involvement of the pelvis with sparing of the femora. Note the extensive osteosclerosis, coarse trabeculae, and cortical thickening. It is difficult to appreciate the increased size of the involved bone owing to the bilateral involvement.

ment of the vertebral posterior elements. In the lumbar spine, Paget's disease can lead to compression of the cauda equina and encroachment on the foramina. In the thoracic spine, cord compression and intervertebral foraminal impingement may be seen. With cervical involvement, Paget's disease can lead to cord compression and even spastic quadriplegia. Pagetic abnormalities of the vertebral bodies at any level can result in collapse.

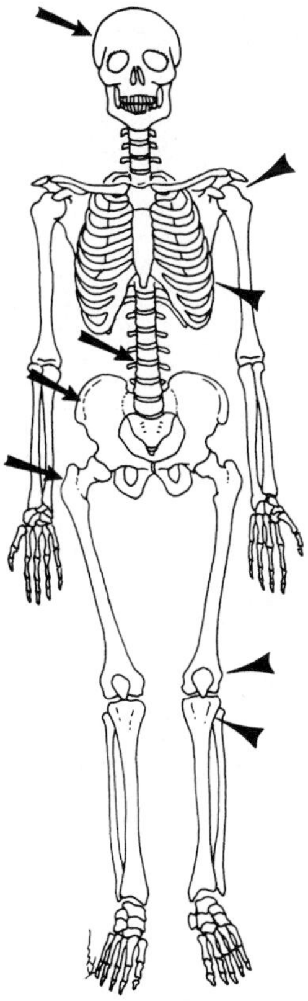

The vertebral bodies and posterior elements may be altered, with the changes being more apparent in the vertebral bodies. Enlarged, coarsened trabeculae are observed, and condensation of bone may be especially prominent along the contours of the vertebral body. In this situation, the highlighted contour of the involved vertebra resembles a picture frame. In some patients, a uniform increase in osseous density produces an ivory vertebra, and differentiation of Paget's disease from other causes of ivory vertebra, such as metastasis and lymphoma, may be difficult. In this situation, if the vertebra is enlarged, the diagnosis of Paget's disease is usually ensured.

Biconcave deformities termed "fish vertebrae" are identical to those occurring in metabolic disorders such as osteoporosis, osteomalacia, and hyperparathyroidism.

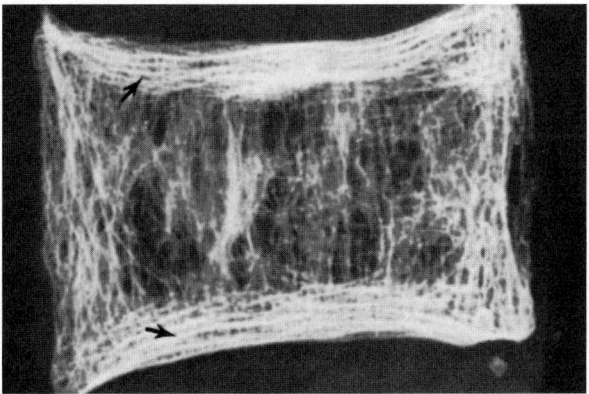

**Figure 43–5.** Radiographic abnormalities in Paget's disease: "picture-frame" vertebral body. In a cadaver, a sectional radiograph reveals the increased thickness of the marginal trabeculae in the vertebral body. Observe the linear, horizontal direction of the trabeculae *(arrows).*

**Figure 43–4.** General distribution of Paget's disease. Very common *(arrows)* and common *(arrowheads)* sites are indicated.

These deformities are related to compression of affected vertebrae by the adjacent intervertebral disc. Pagetic changes in the posterior elements may occur in conjunction with vertebral body abnormalities or as an isolated spinal manifestation of the disease. With pediculate involvement, increased radiodensity may simulate osteoblastic metastasis. Sacral alterations are usually associated with involvement of additional areas of the pelvis. Osteolytic features commonly predominate in the sacrum, and in such instances, a missed diagnosis is not infrequent (Fig. 43–6).

**Pelvis.** Manifestations of Paget's disease in the pelvis (see Fig. 43–3) usually include both bone resorption and bone formation. Trabecular thickening may initially be evident along the inner contour of the pelvis. The iliopubic and ilioischial lines may be prominent, with little other osseous abnormality of the pelvis. Thickening in these areas must be distinguished from irregularity of the iliopubic contour, which is frequent in normal elderly persons, and from calcification of Cooper's ligament. The periphery of the iliac bone may appear radiodense, with a relatively lucent central portion. Iliac sclerosis adjacent to the sacroiliac joint can simulate the changes of osteitis condensans ilii. Involvement of the pubis and ischium is often associated with enlarged osseous contours. Para-acetabular alterations can lead to acetabular protrusion. Diffuse abnormalities of the pelvis are not infrequent and are commonly asymmetrical.

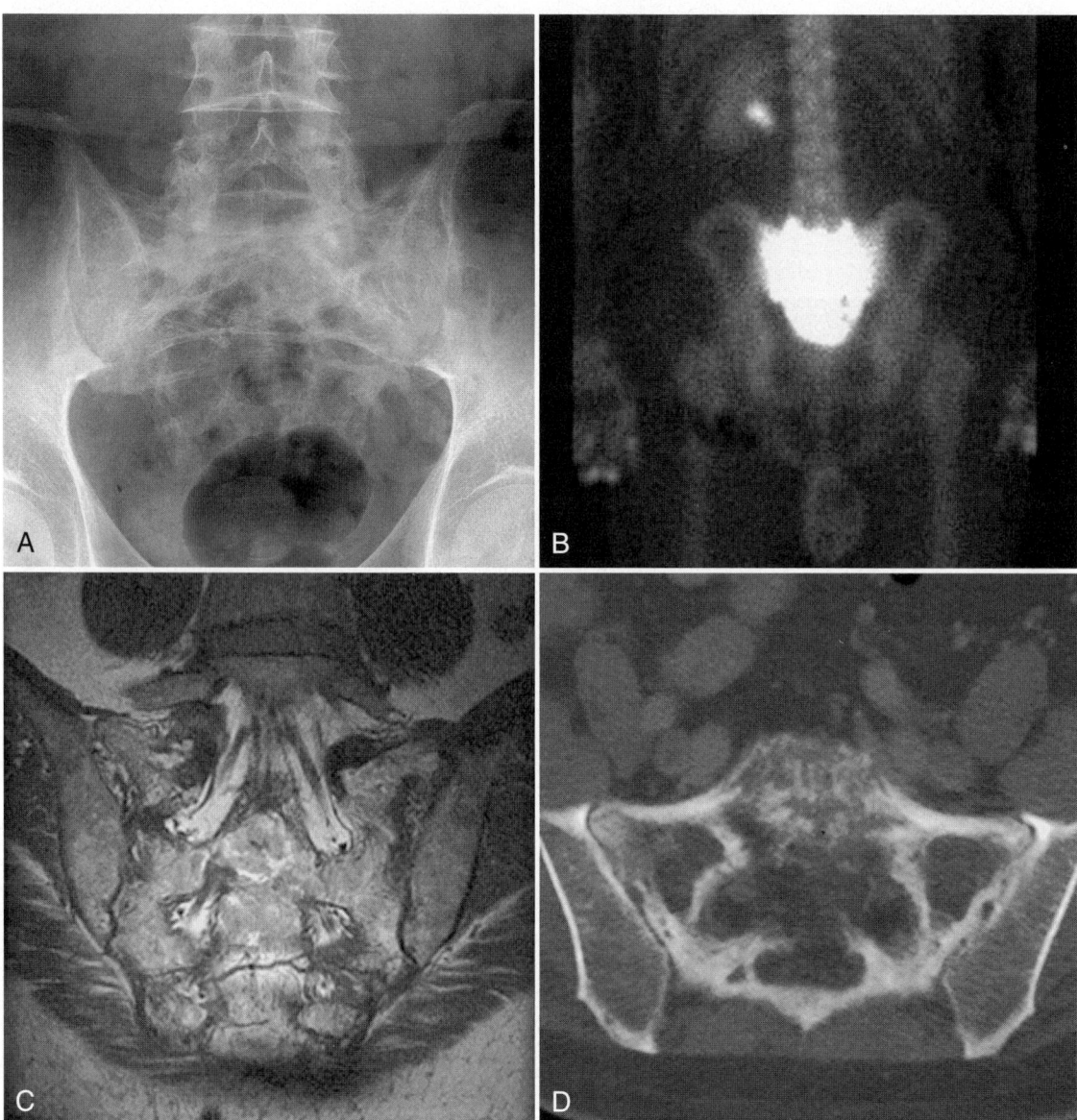

**Figure 43–6.** Radiographic abnormalities in Paget's disease: sacrum in a 76-year-old man. *A,* Radiograph shows few trabeculae, and the entire bone is osteopenic. The remaining trabecular pattern is coarsened, diagnostic of Paget's disease. *B,* Marked focal accumulation is seen throughout the entire sacrum, a pattern virtually diagnostic of Paget's disease. *C,* Oblique coronal T1-weighted (TR/TE, 500/20) spin echo MR image shows preservation of normal fatty marrow. The coarse trabeculae are not well appreciated. *D,* Axial CT scan viewed at a bone window demonstrates increased fatty marrow, with coarse trabeculae and thickened cortex.

**Additional Sites.** Paget's disease can affect any part of the skeleton (Fig. 43–7). Involvement of the tubular bones of the extremities is most common in the femur, tibia, and humerus. As noted previously, such involvement is characterized by an epiphyseal predilection, an advancing wedge of radiolucency, periosteal apposition of new bone leading to widening of the osseous surface, and deformity and fracture. Cortical thickening with encroachment on the medullary canal is evident. In rare instances, the involved bone reveals narrowing or contraction. Diaphyseal changes without epiphyseal abnormality are extremely unusual but may be observed, particularly in the tibia, where pagetic involvement may begin in the mid-diaphysis. A more characteristic site of initial tibial involvement in cases of "diaphyseal" Paget's disease is the anterior tibial tubercle. Peculiarities in the distribution of stress in the lower extremity lead to typical patterns of deformity; most characteristically, exaggerated lateral curvature of the femur and anterior curvature of the tibia become apparent. Lateral bowing of the humerus is also seen. The fibula is frequently spared. Paget's disease of the bones of the feet and hands is less common. In the foot, changes show a predilection for the calcaneus.

## OTHER DIAGNOSTIC METHODS
### Scintigraphy

Bone scintigraphy has been used in the evaluation of patients with Paget's disease (Fig. 43–8). As would be expected, areas of skeletal disease are depicted as sites of increased uptake of bone-seeking radiotracers and, in appropriate locations, as sites of marrow replacement. Scintigraphic abnormalities may precede radiographically detectable changes and can document the extent of the initial lytic phase of Paget's disease. In this phase, increased radionuclide activity may be particularly prominent at the advancing edge of bone. Serial bone scintigraphs may provide objective evidence of the effect of various therapeutic agents.

### Computed Tomography

Computed tomography (CT) scanning is generally not required in the evaluation of uncomplicated Paget's disease. When used, this technique reveals the coarsened trabecular pattern, thickened cortex, increased size of the bone, and decreased size of the medullary cavity that are

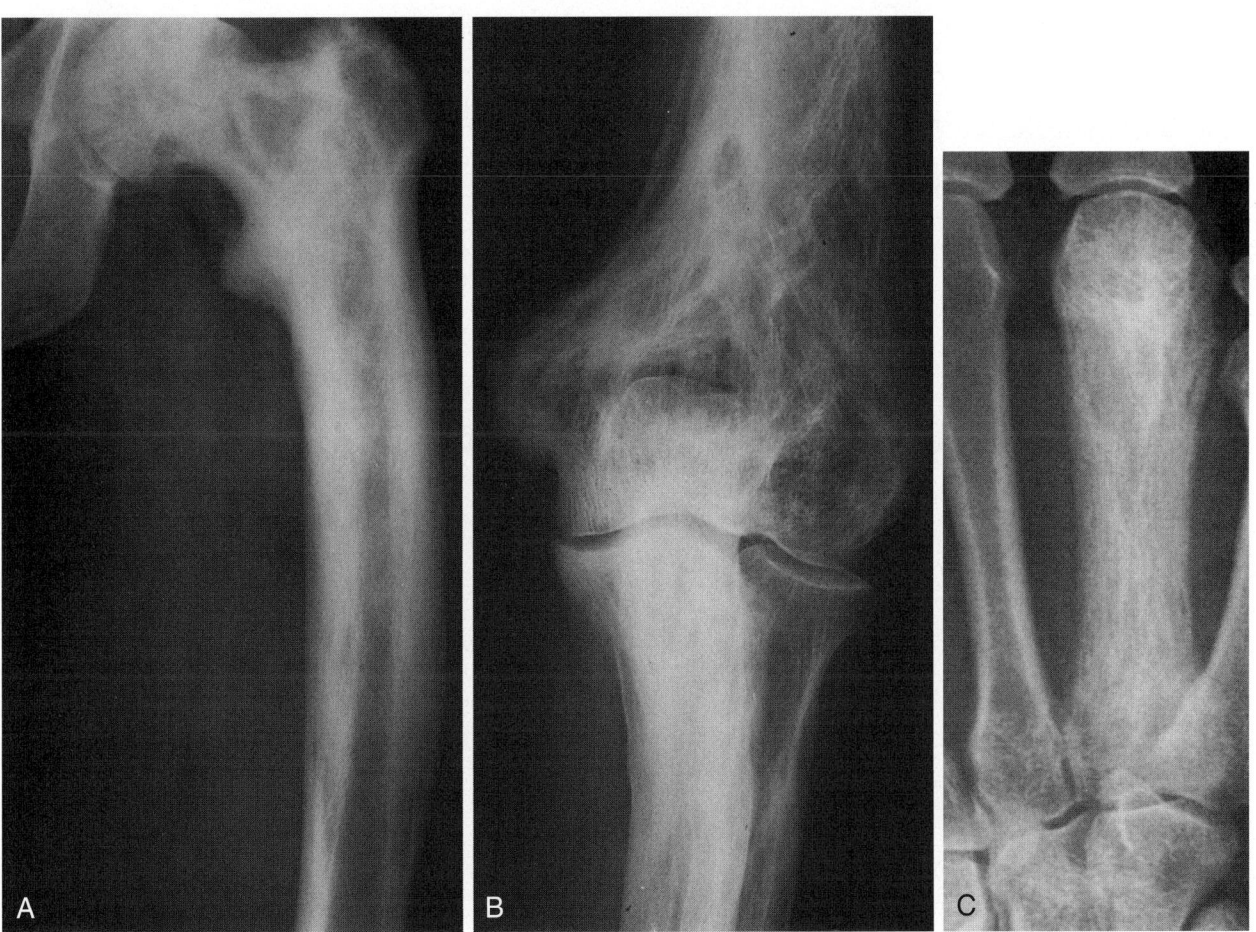

**Figure 43–7.** Radiographic abnormalities in Paget's disease: additional sites. *A,* Femur. Alterations extend from the femoral head to the mid-diaphyseal region. The cortex is thickened, with cortical encroachment on the medullary canal. Observe the coarse trabecular pattern. *B,* Humerus and ulna. Coarsely trabeculated bone is associated with radiolucent regions of varying size. The osseous outlines are enlarged. *C,* Hand. The characteristic findings of Paget's disease are observed throughout an entire metacarpal bone.

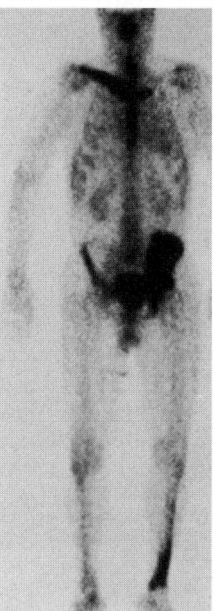

**Figure 43–8.** Scintigraphic abnormalities in Paget's disease: osteosclerotic phase. Note the marked focal accumulation of radionuclide (technetium polyphosphate) in the left hemipelvis, distal portion of the left tibia, and right clavicle. The scintigraphic pattern is virtually diagnostic of Paget's disease.

typical of the disorder (see Figs. 43–3*B* and 43–6*D*). CT is useful in the further delineation of a number of complications of Paget's disease, including articular abnormalities, especially in the hip, neoplastic degeneration, and vertebral involvement with neurologic compromise.

## Magnetic Resonance Imaging

Magnetic resonance (MR) imaging alterations are most characteristic in patients who have long-standing inactive phases of Paget's disease (see Figs. 43–6*C* and 43–9). These changes include cortical thickening, coarse trabeculation, enlargement of bone, reduction in size of the medullary cavity, and, in tubular bones, bowing. Typically, but not invariably, the cortex remains devoid of signal on all imaging sequences. Thickened trabeculae in the medullary cavity also reveal a signal void. The persistence of signal from normal marrow fat is a potential way of differentiating osteosclerotic Paget's disease alone from that associated with fracture or tumor in symptomatic patients. Obliteration of areas of normal fatty marrow would be expected in the presence of edematous or neoplastic tissue.

The active stage of Paget's disease leads to variability in the MR findings. The hematopoietic marrow is replaced by fibrous connective tissue with numerous large vascular channels. These histologic characteristics account for the nonspecific MR features that may resemble the findings in tumor or infection. In common with CT, MR imaging may be effective for evaluating some of the complications of Paget's disease.

## COMPLICATIONS

Numerous complications can be observed in patients with Paget's disease (Table 43–2).

### Fracture

Partial or complete insufficiency (stress) fractures and acute true fractures can complicate Paget's disease (Fig. 43–10). Cortical stress fractures are prominent in the

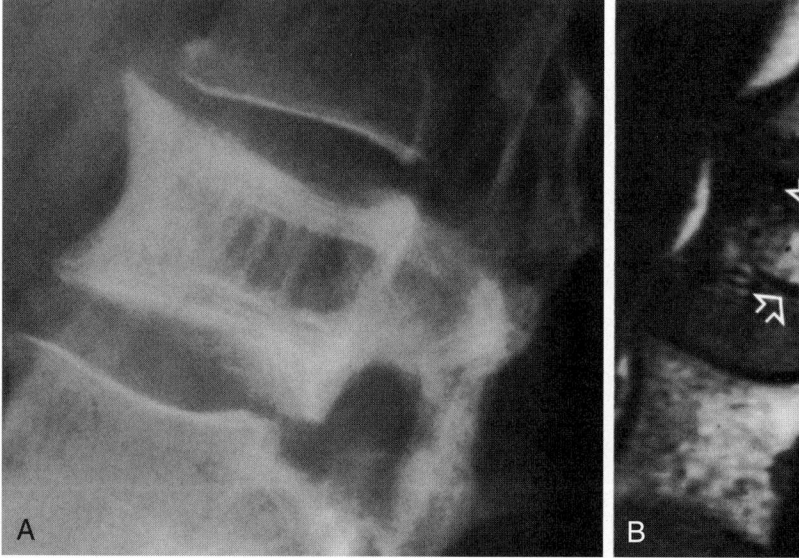
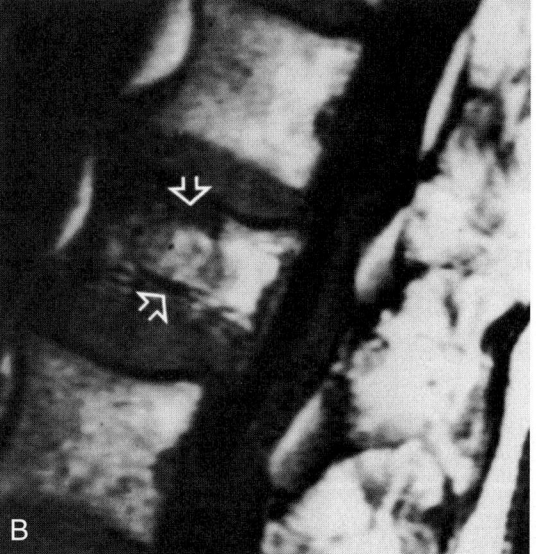

**Figure 43–9.** MR imaging abnormalities in Paget's disease: inactive disease in the spine. *A*, Routine radiograph shows classic pagetic abnormalities with a "picture-frame" appearance. The vertebral body is mildly compressed, and osteophytes are seen. Note the involvement of the posterior osseous elements. *B*, On a sagittal T1-weighted (TR/TE, 600/20) spin echo MR image, coarse trabeculation appears as regions of low signal intensity *(arrows)*.

**TABLE 43–2**

**Musculoskeletal Complications of Paget's Disease**

Neurologic abnormalities
Osseous deformities
Fractures
Neoplasms
Soft tissue masses
Osteomyelitis
Extramedullary hematopoiesis
Crystal deposition
 Monosodium urate
 Calcium pyrophosphate dihydrate*
 Calcific periarthritis
Degenerative joint disease
Rheumatoid arthritis and its variants*

*Questionable association.

lower extremity, particularly in the femur and tibia. They appear as single or multiple horizontal radiolucent areas, with a predilection for the convex aspect of the bone (lateral aspect of the femoral neck and shaft, anterior aspect of the tibia). Although these linear radiolucent areas that partially traverse the bone resemble Looser's zones, which are apparent in osteomalacia, the involvement of convex rather than concave surfaces is distinctive. These stress fractures appear most frequently in patients with long-standing (inactive) disease and have a variable course, healing or remaining unchanged

indefinitely in some patients, or progressing and extending across the entire bone in others. Pathologic fractures in Paget's disease are the most common orthopedic complication and are typically seen in the femur, humerus, tibia, spine, and pelvis. Because the risk of sarcoma is substantial in cases of pathologic fracture in Paget's disease, some authors recommend a biopsy whenever such a fracture develops.

### Neoplasm

Neoplastic involvement in Paget's disease includes sarcomatous degeneration, giant cell tumor, and superimposition of another tumorous condition such as metastatic disease, plasma cell myeloma, and lymphoma. It is generally believed that malignant changes develop in approximately 1% of patients with Paget's disease. The tumor is apparent in areas of pagetic involvement (Figs. 43–11 and 43–12).

Patients with sarcomatous degeneration in Paget's disease are usually between 55 and 80 years of age. Men are affected slightly more frequently than women, and at a younger age. Clinical findings include pain and swelling. The bones most commonly affected are the femur, pelvis, and humerus. Except for the higher frequency of neoplastic changes in the humerus and the lower frequency in the skull and vertebrae, the distribution of sarcomas in Paget's disease is similar to that of the disorder itself. Predominance of certain cells most commonly leads to a diagnosis of osteosarcoma (50% to 60%) or fibrosarcoma (20% to 25%), although additional diagnoses such as chondrosarcoma (10%) may be entertained. No matter which cell type predominates, the

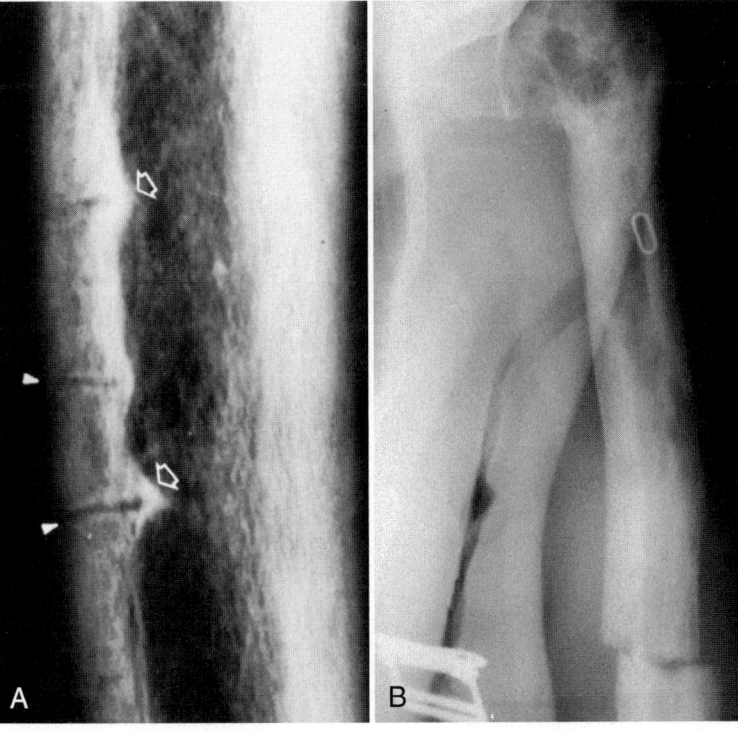

**Figure 43–10.** Complications of Paget's disease: insufficiency (stress) fractures. *A,* Radiograph of the proximal femur demonstrates multiple linear radiolucent areas *(arrowheads)* traversing the thickened femoral cortex. Some of the fractures traverse the entire cortex, whereas others do not. Endosteal callus is evident *(open arrows). B,* In another patient, progression to a completed fracture in the humerus. Note the transverse orientation of the fracture line. (*A,* Courtesy of Y. Dirheimer, MD, Strasbourg, France.)

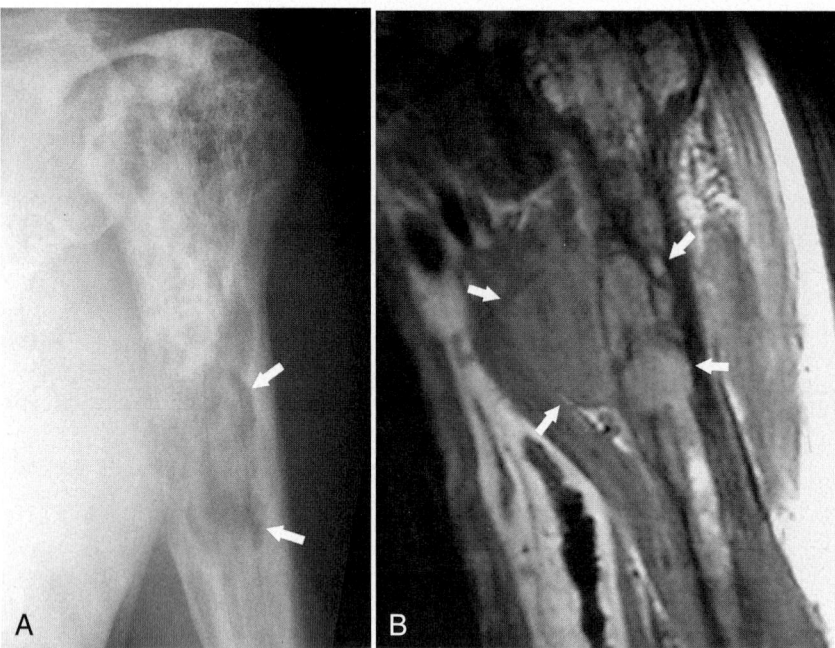

**Figure 43–11.** Paget's disease: sarcomatous degeneration in a 62-year-old man. *A*, Radiograph demonstrates pagetic involvement of the humerus with a focal osteolytic lesion *(arrows)*. *B*, Sagittal T1-weighted (TR/TE, 617/20) spin echo MR image shows osseous destruction with a large soft tissue mass *(arrows)*. The final diagnosis was osteosarcoma in Paget's disease.

prognosis for the patient is ominous. Osteolysis rather than osteosclerosis is the major radiographic characteristic of the sarcoma. In addition to bone destruction, findings include a soft tissue mass, cortical disruption, bony spiculation, and a persistent fracture without evidence of healing.

Giant cell tumors associated with Paget's disease are uncommon but well described; they often occur in the skull, facial bones, pelvis, and clavicle. The tumors invariably affect regions of the skeleton involved in the pagetic process; however, the pagetic involvement may be inconspicuous radiographically. A lytic lesion causing a remodeled, expansile osseous contour without radiologic matrix is observed. The prognosis is usually good. In some cases of giant cell tumor complicating Paget's disease, familial and geographic clustering is evident.

Metastatic disease and Paget's disease may coexist, and it is interesting to speculate that increased local blood flow in the latter disorder may make the bone more susceptible to metastasis. Typical sites of the primary tumor are the breast, lung, kidney, prostate, and colon. Of interest, metastasis to uninvolved skeletal sites has been recorded in patients with Paget's disease.

The diagnosis of neoplasm complicating Paget's disease is usually not difficult. Clinically, increased pain and a soft tissue mass are observed. On radiographs, soft tissue swelling and a lytic lesion may be seen, and in some tumors, the initial sign may be a pathologic fracture. Any enlarging lytic lesion within pagetic bone should be carefully evaluated. These lytic neoplasms must be differentiated from the osteolytic phase of Paget's disease and from lucent areas representing fat-filled marrow spaces (Fig. 43–13). Periosteal bone proliferation in uncomplicated Paget's disease can produce a radiodense soft tissue lesion that may contain new bone (Fig. 43–14) and may also simulate neoplastic degeneration.

## ARTICULAR ABNORMALITIES
### Crystal Deposition

Hyperuricemia has been reported in 40% of patients with symptomatic Paget's disease, related to overproduction of urate, and patients may have typical clinical and radiographic features of gout. Coexistence of calcium pyrophosphate dihydrate crystal deposition and Paget's disease has also been noted, although the frequency of crystal deposition in patients with Paget's disease may not differ significantly from that in controls.

### Degenerative Joint Disease

Clinical and radiographic features of degenerative joint disease may be apparent in patients with Paget's disease. This complication is reported most frequently in the hip and knee. In the hip, the pattern of narrowing of the articular space depends on whether the acetabulum or the femur is involved. The pattern of narrowing in Paget's disease can generally be differentiated from that seen in primary osteoarthritis (Fig. 43–15). Acetabular protrusion may complicate Paget's disease of the acetabulum. Osteophyte formation is usually a mild feature of the disease.

The pathogenesis of the arthritic changes associated with Paget's disease is not clear. Hypervascularity and rapid bone turnover in pagetic subchondral bone may lead to accelerated endochondral bone formation at the expense of articular cartilage. Superimposed on this interference with dynamics at the chondro-osseous junction are mechanical abnormalities about the articulation.

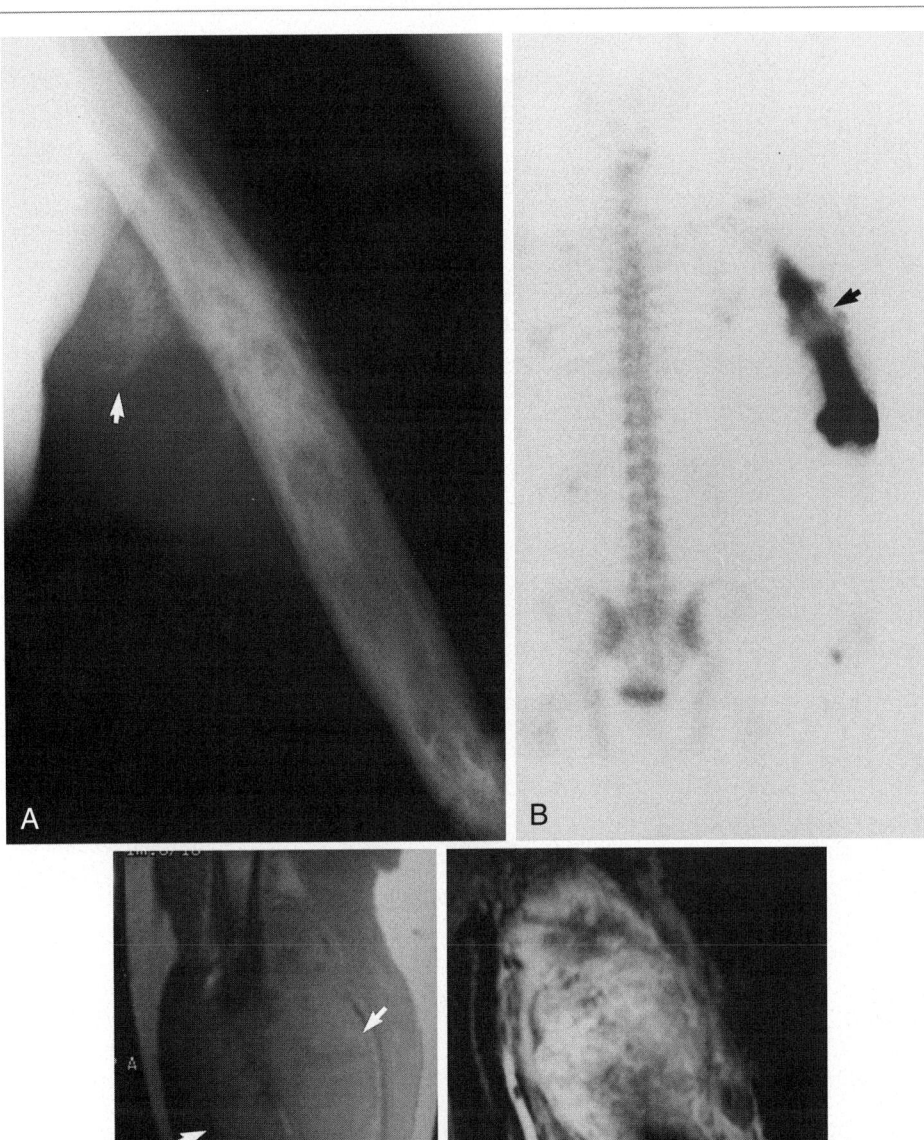

**Figure 43–12.** Complications of Paget's disease: osteosarcoma. *A*, Radiograph of the humerus in a 60-year-old man shows pagetic involvement of the distal portion of the bone and a bone-forming malignant tumor in the diaphysis, along with soft tissue ossification *(arrow)*. *B*, Bone scan shows intense uptake of radionuclide in the distal two thirds of the humerus and a relative photopenic region in the diaphysis *(arrow)* that corresponds to the site of the tumor. This illustration is oriented to correspond to that of the radiograph. *C*, Sagittal T1-weighted (TR/TE, 700/12) spin echo MR image shows that the tumor has low signal intensity in the shaft of the humerus, along with a soft tissue mass *(arrows)*. *D*, Coronal STIR (TR/TE, 4000/39; inversion time, 150 msec) MR image demonstrates high signal intensity in the tumor.

## IMAGING ASPECTS OF THERAPY

Since the 1950s, effective therapeutic agents have been used in Paget's disease. One such agent is calcitonin, a potent inhibitor of bone resorption that acts by inhibiting osteoclasts; it can lead to relief of pain within weeks of its administration and to a decline in serum alkaline phosphatase and urinary hydroxyproline levels. A second agent used in the treatment of Paget's disease is etidronate disodium (EHDP), a diphosphonate. Diphosphonates inhibit bone resorption and mineralization by binding to hydroxyapatite crystals and inhibiting their growth and

dissolution. Radiographic improvement, however, has not been a consistent feature of therapy (Fig. 43–16). Several reports have indicated an increased frequency of fractures in patients with Paget's disease treated with EHDP. Mithramycin is an antibiotic with cytotoxic activity that has been used successfully in the treatment of Paget's disease.

Scintigraphy has advantages over radiography in monitoring the response of pagetic bone to any of these therapeutic agents. A distinct decrease in radionuclide accumulation in diseased areas is characteristic of the pagetic response to treatment. In general, good corre-

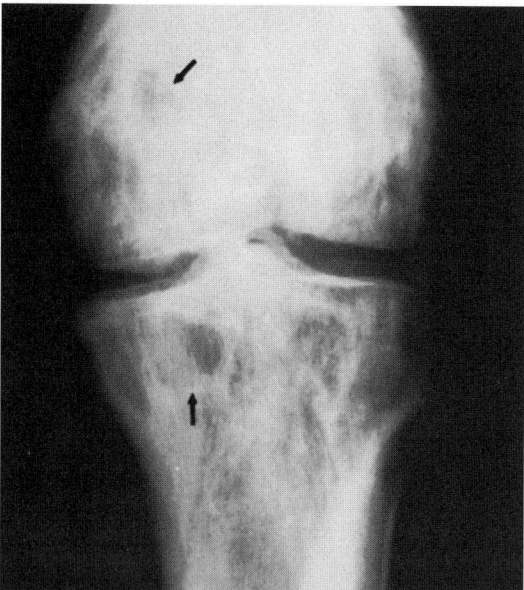

**Figure 43–13.** Pseudoneoplastic osteolytic lesions of varying size *(arrows)* in Paget's disease represent degeneration and necrosis of proliferating fibrous tissue. They should not be mistaken for neoplasm.

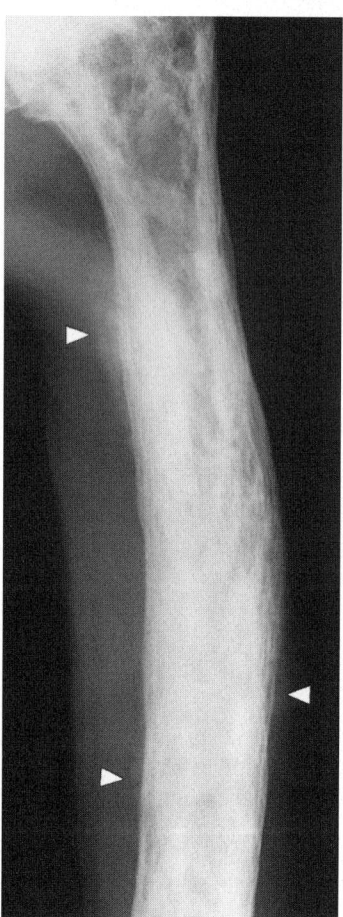

**Figure 43–14.** Paget's disease: soft tissue extension. Note the extraosseous extension of Paget's disease at three sites *(arrowheads)* in the humerus characterized by ill-defined periosteal new bone formation.

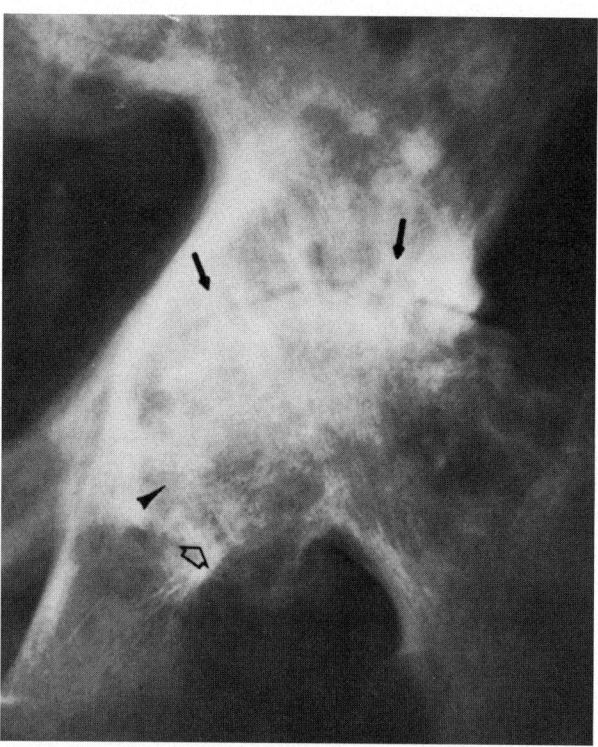

**Figure 43–15.** Paget's disease with secondary degenerative joint disease: acetabular involvement alone. Radiograph demonstrates Paget's disease isolated to the acetabulum, with loss of both superior and axial joint space *(arrows)*. The medial joint space is narrowed only slightly *(arrowhead)*. A medial femoral osteophyte is evident *(open arrow)*.

lation is noted between scintigraphic and biochemical parameters of disease activity. Recurrence of the disorder is typically accompanied scintigraphically by a rise in activity in one or more bones in a diffuse or circumscribed pattern or by the spread of disease into adjacent normal bone.

## DIFFERENTIAL DIAGNOSIS

### General Features

Although the initial lytic phase of Paget's disease may be difficult for an inexperienced observer to identify, its radiographic features are diagnostic. Involvement of the end of a long bone, sharply demarcated bone lysis, and an advancing wedge of radiolucency allow an accurate diagnosis. Widespread sclerosis, which can be apparent in Paget's disease of long duration, also has specific characteristics, such as bony enlargement and a coarsened trabecular pattern, which can be distinguished from findings associated with other diseases. Diffuse increased skeletal radiodensity may be observed in bony metastasis (particularly from prostatic carcinoma; Fig. 43–17), myelofibrosis, fluorosis, mastocytosis (urticaria pigmentosa), renal osteodystrophy, fibrous dysplasia, and tuberous sclerosis. Additional findings in these other disorders ensure their recognition. For example, hepatosplenomegaly (myelofibrosis, mastocytosis), ligamentous ossification (fluorosis), focal radiodensity (mastocytosis and tuberous

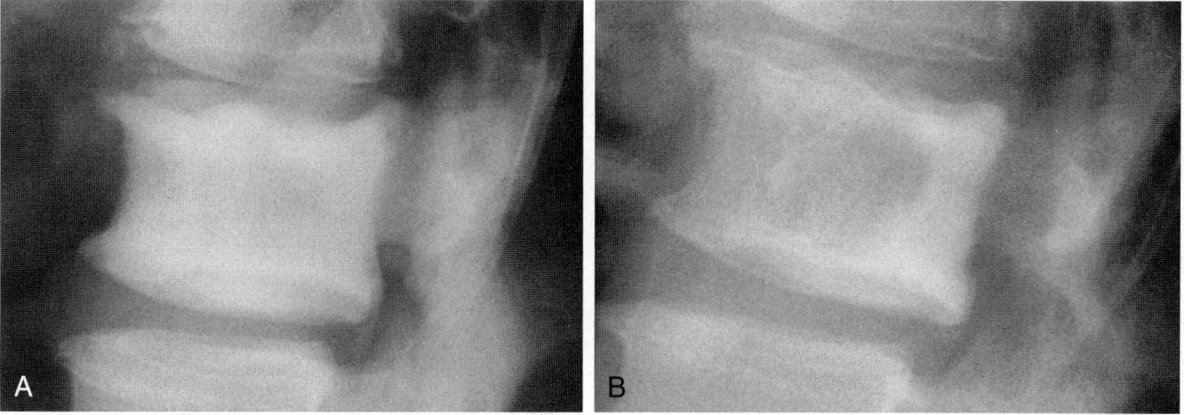

**Figure 43–16.** Treatment of Paget's disease: etidronate disodium (EHDP). Radiographs obtained 1 year after initial manifestation of the disease *(A)* and 4 years 6 months after discontinuation of treatment with EHDP *(B)* reveal improvement in the abnormalities of the second lumbar vertebra on the later examination. (From Nicholas JJ, Helfrich DJ, Cooperstein L, Goodman L: Clinical and radiographic improvement of bone of the second lumbar vertebra in Paget's disease following therapy with etidronate disodium: A case report. Arthritis Rheum 32:776, 1989.)

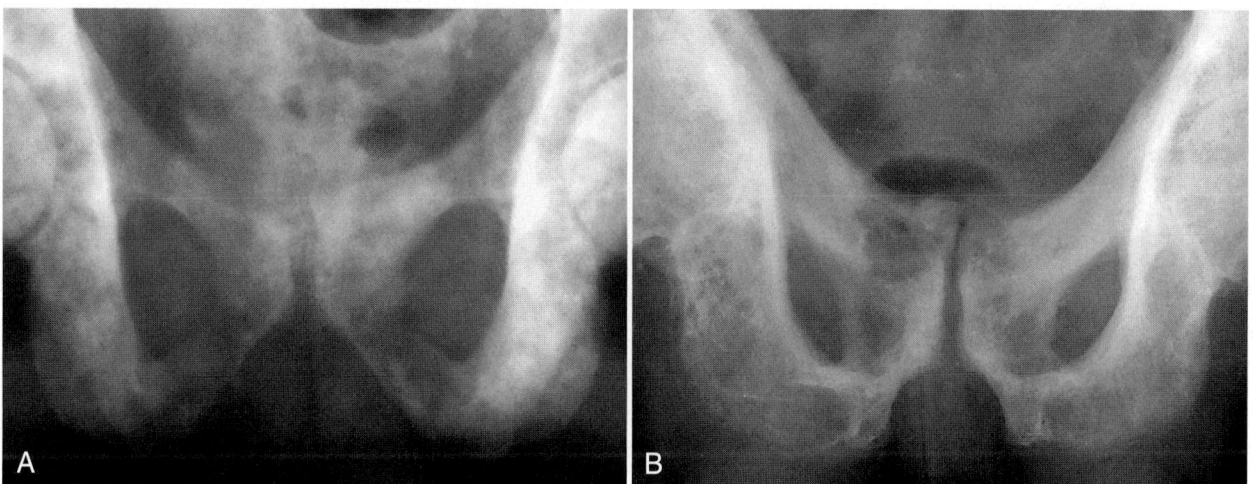

**Figure 43–17.** Skeletal metastasis from prostate carcinoma compared with Paget's disease *A*, Patient with metastatic prostate carcinoma demonstrates patchy osteosclerosis. *B*, Corresponding image from a patient with Paget's disease shows a coarsened trabecular pattern, cortical thickening, and osseous enlargement.

sclerosis), characteristic bowing deformities and a ground-glass appearance (fibrous dysplasia), and subperiosteal and subchondral bone resorption (renal osteodystrophy) are abnormalities associated with these other diseases.

Familial idiopathic hyperphosphatasia (osteitis deformans in children, "juvenile" Paget's disease, hyperostosis corticalis) is a rare disorder of bone occurring in children that is associated with progressive skeletal deformities, coarsely trabeculated and widened bone, and elevation of serum levels of alkaline phosphatase and urinary levels of hydroxyproline. Although some characteristics of this disorder resemble those of Paget's disease, familial idiopathic hyperphosphatasia occurs in younger patients, and the epiphyses may not be involved.

## Calvarial Hyperostosis

Paget's disease of the skull can be confused with other disorders associated with calvarial hyperostosis, including hyperostosis frontalis interna, fibrous dysplasia, anemia, and skeletal metastasis. Hyperostosis frontalis interna predominates in women and produces thickening of the inner table of the frontal squama. Fibrous dysplasia may cause gross enlargement of the skull, although facial involvement is particularly characteristic. In addition, fibrous dysplasia leads to focal involvement of the cranial vault (Fig. 43–18), whereas Paget's disease is often diffuse in distribution. Both disorders produce diploic widening and can extend across suture lines. Certain anemias, such as sickle cell anemia and thalassemia, produce thickening

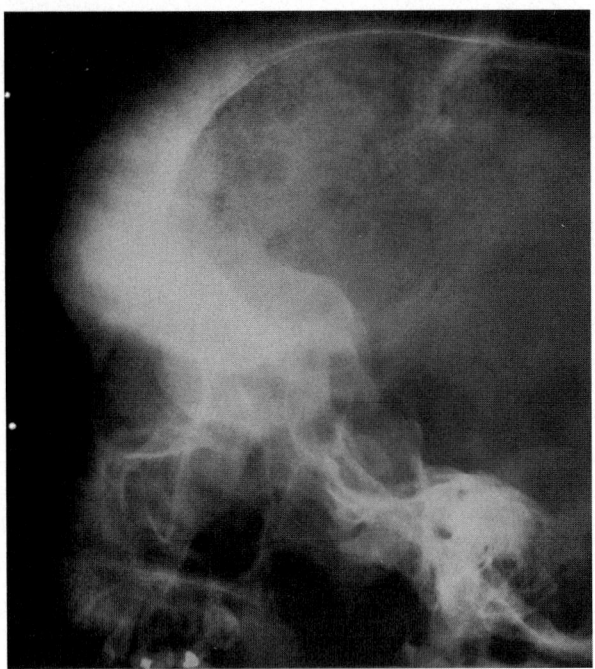

**Figure 43–18.** Fibrous dysplasia. Characteristic hyperostosis and calvarial thickening can be seen in the frontal region. The facial bones are also affected.

of the cranial vault and a radiating trabecular pattern (hair-on-end appearance). The base of the skull is generally spared. Osteoblastic metastasis can simulate the cotton-wool radiodense lesions of Paget's disease.

## Vertebral Sclerosis

Condensation of the periphery of a vertebral body—the "picture-frame" vertebra—is almost diagnostic of Paget's disease. It differs from the accentuated vertical trabeculae of hemangiomas and the rugger-jersey spine of renal osteodystrophy. Some patients with Paget's disease have diffuse sclerosis of an entire vertebral body—the ivory vertebra—which can simulate skeletal metastasis and lymphoma.

## Pelvic Abnormalities

Although pelvic sclerosis in Paget's disease can mimic the findings of osteoblastic metastasis, an asymmetrical or unilateral distribution, accentuated trabecular pattern, and enlargement of the involved bone are typical of Paget's disease. In elderly patients, thickening of the iliopubic line and Cooper's ligament calcification should not be interpreted as early radiographic signs of Paget's disease.

## FURTHER READING

Altman RD, Collins B: Musculoskeletal manifestations of Paget's disease of bone. Arthritis Rheum 23:1121, 1980.

Barry HC: Paget's Disease of Bone. Edinburgh, E&S Livingstone, 1969, p 16.

Bowerman JW, Altman J, Hughes JL, et al: Pseudo-malignant lesions in Paget's disease of bone. AJR Am J Roentgenol 124:57, 1975.

Fenton P, Resnick D: Metastases to bone affected by Paget's disease: A report of three cases. Int Orthop 15:397, 1991.

Goldman AB, Bullough P, Kammermans S, et al: Osteitis deformans of the hip joint. AJR Am J Roentgenol 128:601, 1977.

Greditzer HG III, McLeod RA, Unni KK, et al: Bone sarcomas in Paget disease. Radiology 146:327, 1983.

Hamdy RC: Paget's Disease of Bone: Assessment and Management. New York, Praeger, 1981.

Jacobs P: Osteolytic Paget's disease. Clin Radiol 25:137, 1974.

Kaufmann GA, Sundaram M, McDonald DJ: Magnetic resonance imaging in symptomatic Paget's disease. Skeletal Radiol 20:413, 1991.

McNairn JDK, Damron TA, Landas SK, et al: Benign tumefactive soft tissue extension from Paget's disease of bone simulating malignancy. Skeletal Radiol 30:157, 2001.

Mills BG, Singer FR: Nuclear inclusions in Paget's disease of bone. Science 194:201, 1976.

Murphy WA, Whyte MP, Haddad JG Jr: Paget bone disease: Radiologic documentation of healing with human calcitonin therapy. Radiology 136:1, 1980.

Paget J: On a form of chronic inflammation of bones (osteitis deformans). Med Chir Tr 60:37, 1877.

Pathak HJ, Nardi PM, Thornhill B: Multiple giant cell tumors complicating Paget's disease. AJR Am J Roentgenol 172:1696, 1999.

Resnick D: Paget's disease of bone: Current status and a look back to 1943 and earlier. AJR Am J Roentgenol 150:249, 1988.

Singer FR, Mills BG: Evidence for a viral etiology of Paget's disease of bone. Clin Orthop 178:245, 1983.

Smith J, Botet JF, Yeh SDJ: Bone sarcomas in Paget's disease: A study of 85 patients. Radiology 152:583, 1984.

Steinbach HL: Some roentgen features of Paget's disease. AJR Am J Roentgenol 86:950, 1961.

Tehranzadeh J, Fung Y, Donohue M, et al: Computed tomography of Paget disease of the skull versus fibrous dysplasia. Skeletal Radiol 27:664, 1998.

Tins BJ, Davies AM, Mangham DC: MR imaging of pseudo-sarcoma in Paget's disease of bone: A report of two cases. Skeletal Radiol 30:161, 2001.

Wick MR, McLeod RA, Siegal GP, et al: Sarcomas of bone complicating osteitis deformans (Paget's disease): Fifty years' experience. Am J Surg Pathol 5:47, 1981.

Wilner D, Sherman RS: Roentgen diagnosis of Paget's disease (osteitis deformans). Med Radiogr Photogr 42:35, 1966.

Zlatkin MB, Lander PH, Hadjipavlou AG, et al: Paget's disease of the spine: CT with clinical correlation. Radiology 160:155, 1986.

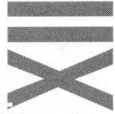
# Endocrine Diseases

# CHAPTER 44

## Pituitary Disorders

### SUMMARY OF KEY FEATURES

The osseous manifestations of acromegaly are the result of the effects of elevated levels of serum growth hormone on the adult skeleton. Reactivation of endochondral bone formation and stimulation of periosteal bone formation in association with connective tissue proliferation are apparent, leading to characteristic radiographic findings, including increased soft tissue thickness and bony overgrowth. Joint abnormalities result from chondrocyte proliferation in articular cartilage. The excessively stimulated cartilage is vulnerable to fissuring, fragmentation, and ulceration, which are followed by a brisk reparative response. These histologic alterations have their radiographic counterparts. Initial joint space widening is followed by joint space narrowing, bony sclerosis, cyst formation, and osteophytosis. The latter radiographic abnormalities simulate those of osteoarthritis. In contradistinction, articular abnormalities in hypopituitarism are infrequent; the dominant osseous abnormalities related to skeletal development are manifested by a delay in the appearance and growth of ossification centers and a similar delay in their fusion and disappearance

### ACROMEGALY AND GIGANTISM

Growth hormone (somatotropin) hypersecretion can be associated with acidophilic or chromophobic adenomas of the anterior lobe of the pituitary gland. Less frequently, such hypersecretion is associated with diffuse hyperplasia of the acidophilic cells or no histologic abnormality at all. In the immature skeleton, in which the growth plates are still open, growth hormone hypersecretion leads to excessive proportional growth of bone (i.e., in both length and width). This results from direct hormonal stimulation of endochondral bone formation at the physeal growth plates. The resulting syndrome is termed hyperpituitary gigantism and is characterized by extreme height. In the mature skeleton, in which the growth plates have closed and endochondral bone formation has ceased, growth hormone hypersecretion may reactivate endochondral bone formation at various existing cartilage-bone junctions (such as the costochondral junctions) and induce periosteal bone formation, leading to widening of osseous structures. This overgrowth of bone in association with enlargement of soft tissue is particularly prominent in the acral parts (hands, feet, lower jaw) of the skeleton, leading to use of the term acromegaly for this condition.

Patients with acromegaly demonstrate distinctive symptoms and signs that relate to the morphologic, biochemical, and metabolic effects of growth hormone excess (Table 44–1).

### General Clinical Features

Typically, the symptoms and signs of acromegaly begin in the third or fourth decade of life; however, older and younger patients can be affected, and acromegaly (as distinct from gigantism) has been recorded in children. Although the physical appearance of a patient with hyperpituitary gigantism is essentially that of a tall, normally proportioned person, the features of a patient with acromegaly may be dramatic. Facial characteristics include a large mandible, producing a "lantern jaw" appearance; poor dental occlusion, with separation of the teeth; coarsening of facial features related to overgrowth of bone and soft tissue; prominence of the forehead, produced by calvarial thickening and enlargement of the frontal sinuses; deepening of the voice; and prominence of the tongue. The hands appear broad and spadelike, and the fingers are separated and blunted. The entire frame enlarges as a result of overgrowth of bone. Hypersecretion of growth hormone also affects other organ systems, producing thickening and coarsening of the skin and enlargement of the kidneys, liver, pancreas, spleen, thyroid gland, and heart. Associated endocrine alterations may be observed, including diabetes mellitus (12% to 25%), persistent lactation (4%), increased secretion of cortisol by the adrenal cortex, and increased frequency of parathyroid and pancreatic islet cell adenomas.

The clinical manifestations of acromegaly may stabilize after the disease has progressed to a certain degree. This fact, in addition to the insidious nature of the disease, may lead to considerable delay before an acromegalic patient seeks medical attention. Headaches and visual disturbances, which are related to the pressure exerted by the enlarging pituitary gland, may eventually lead the patient to a physician.

Rheumatic complaints are common in patients with acromegaly. The fundamental morphologic abnormality

**TABLE 44–1**

**Rheumatic Complaints in Acromegaly**

Backache
Limb arthropathy
Compression neuropathy
Neuromuscular symptoms
Raynaud's phenomenon

leading to articular symptoms and signs appears to be overstimulation of cartilaginous tissue. Rheumatic manifestations generally begin after 20 years of age and are equally frequent in men and women. These clinical findings may be observed at either early or late stages of the disease, and they may persist even after the hyperpituitarism has been treated successfully. Five types of rheumatic complaints may be encountered (see Table 44–1).

**Backache.** Approximately 50% of acromegalic patients have backache, particularly in the lower back. This symptom, which is usually insidious in onset, may be associated with local tenderness and a normal or increased range of spinal and hip motion. Painful kyphosis of the thoracic spine may be observed.

**Limb Arthropathy.** Arthropathy is most common in the large joints, such as the knee, glenohumeral joint, and hip. Symptoms and signs, which are often mild, include soft tissue swelling and minimal pain and tenderness. Infrequently, crystal-induced synovitis attributable to calcium pyrophosphate dihydrate crystal deposition may be seen. In later stages of the articular disease, secondary degenerative changes, particularly in the hip and knee, may produce pain, limitation of motion, deformity, and angulation.

**Compression Neuropathy.** Compression neuropathies are due to overgrowth of connective tissue and bone. The carpal tunnel syndrome is particularly characteristic, occurring in 30% of patients, often with a bilateral distribution. Spinal cord compression with long tract signs has been noted in some patients with acromegaly.

**Neuromuscular Symptoms.** Fatigue and lethargy are two common clinical findings in acromegaly. Muscle wasting generally is not a prominent feature. Neurologic changes are also encountered.

**Raynaud's Phenomenon.** Raynaud's phenomenon is a relatively uncommon manifestation of the disease, more marked in the hands than in the feet.

## Pathologic Features of Skeletal Involvement

Characteristic pathologic aberrations accompany acromegaly, and these pathologic changes correlate well with radiographic abnormalities (Table 44–2).

**Stimulation of Endochondral Ossification.** In patients whose growth plates are not yet closed, excessive growth hormone results in exaggerated longitudinal growth of the skeleton. In the young, true gigantism may result; in persons in whom the cartilaginous growth plates are near fusion, some increase in longitudinal growth is observed, but gigantism is relatively mild. After closure of the growth plates, excessive secretion of growth hormone can result in reactivation of endochondral bone formation at certain chondro-osseous junctions. One such site is the costochondral area of the rib. Thickening of the costal cartilage results from deposition of new cartilage on preexisting cartilage; enlargement of the costochondral junctions is termed the acromegalic rosary.

### TABLE 44–2

**Radiographic-Pathologic Correlation in Acromegaly**

| Pathologic | Radiographic |
| --- | --- |
| Stimulation of endochondral bone formation | Enlargement of costochondral junctions |
|  | Thickening of intervertebral discs |
| Stimulation of periosteal bone formation | Mandibular enlargement |
|  | Thickening of the cranial vault |
|  | Prominence of the supraorbital ridges and facial structures |
|  | Cortical thickening of tubular bones |
|  | Enlargement of phalangeal tufts |
|  | Increase in sagittal and transverse diameters of vertebral bodies |
| Stimulation of subligamentous bone formation | Calcaneal enthesophytes |
|  | Excrescences on patella, tuberosities, trochanters |
| Stimulation of bone resorption | Overtubulation of phalanges, metacarpals, metatarsals |
|  | Intracortical striations |
|  | Medullary widening |
|  | Vertebral scalloping |
| Proliferation of articular cartilage | Widening of articular spaces |
| Cartilaginous degeneration and regeneration | Narrowing of articular spaces |
|  | Periarticular calcifications and ossifications |
|  | Osteophytosis |
| Connective tissue hyperplasia | Increased thickness of skin (e.g., heel pad) |
| Pituitary neoplasm | Sella turcica abnormalities |

**Stimulation of Periosteal Bone Formation.** In acromegaly, subperiosteal bone formation is observed at specific sites. In the skull, this form of bone proliferation is apparent on the alveolar margins of the maxilla and mandible, with resultant deepening of the alveolar sockets and separation of the teeth. Enlargement and forward protrusion of the entire mandible are observed. Bony deposition is also characteristic in the supraorbital ridges, facial bones, and calvarial vault. Subperiosteal and subligamentous bone formation may result in thickening and irregularity of the cortices of the bony shafts, prominence of various tuberosities, and osteophytosis. These alterations account for the enlargement of the phalanges, metacarpals, and metatarsals. Proliferation of the phalangeal tufts is particularly characteristic.

In the vertebral column, there is an increase in both the transverse and the sagittal diameters of the vertebral bodies, owing to prominent subperiosteal bone deposition. This produces an altered vertebral shape, in which the vertebral bodies appear short in height and elongated in sagittal and transverse planes. These vertebral abnormalities are associated with an increase in the size of the intervertebral disc. Osteophytes of the vertebral column may be a prominent feature, perhaps related to excessive spinal mobility, with laxity of paraspinal ligaments and thickening of intervertebral discs.

**Bone Formation and Bone Resorption.** It appears that in acromegaly, subperiosteal and endosteal bone proliferation occurs simultaneously with increased bone resorption. Radiographic and pathologic evidence that cortical bone formation and resorption are occurring simultaneously is the finding of overtubulation of the phalanges and metatarsals, with normal or increased cortical thickness, and periosteal apposition of bone on the anterolateral aspect of the vertebral bodies, with concomitant increased concavity along their posterior margins. In most sites, bony apposition exceeds bony resorption.

**Articular Cartilage Alterations.** Increased growth hormone secretion can lead to proliferation of articular cartilage. Progressive cartilaginous fragmentation and denudation, disordered joint mechanics, and tissue repair with remodeling cause exuberant regenerative changes that lead to joint enlargement with thickened ulcerative cartilage, hypertrophied periarticular tissue, calcinosis, osteophytosis, and periosteal bone formation at insertion sites of tendons, ligaments, and capsule.

## Radiographic Features of Skeletal Involvement

**Changes in Skin Thickness.** Collagen tissue demonstrates a marked response to excessive amounts of growth hormone (Fig. 44–1). Manifestations of this response cause thickening of the skin. Despite some variations in heelpad thickness related to body weight and even race, values greater than 23 mm in men and 21.5 mm in women are suggestive of acromegaly; values greater than 25 mm in men and 23 mm in women are even more diagnostic of this disease if local causes of skin thickening are excluded.

**Abnormalities of the Skull.** Radiographic manifestations of the skull abnormalities in patients with acromegaly include sella turcica alterations; prominence and enlargement of the frontal and maxillary sinuses; excessive pneumatization of the mastoids; prominence of the occipital protuberance; thickening or, less commonly, thinning of the cranial vault; prominence of the supraorbital ridges and zygomatic arches; enlargement and elongation of the mandible; widening of the mandibular angle; and anterior tilting, separation, and hypercementosis of the teeth (Fig. 44–2).

**Abnormalities of the Hand and Wrist.** Initial reports of the radiographic features of acromegaly stressed characteristic findings in the hand (Fig. 44–3). Abnormalities include soft tissue thickening of the fingers, thickening and squaring of the phalanges and metacarpals, tubulation or overconstriction of the shafts of the phalanges, abnormally wide articular spaces, bony excrescences at sites of tendon and ligament attachment to bone, and prominence

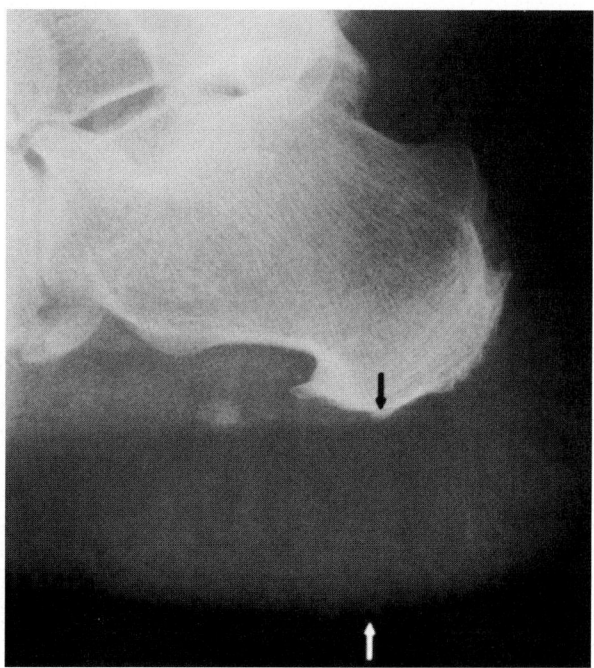

**Figure 44–1.** Acromegaly: increase in skin thickness. Observe the prominence of the soft tissues of the heel, with associated hyperostosis and enthesophytosis of the calcaneus. One technique of measuring these soft tissues evaluates the shortest distance between the calcaneus and the plantar skin surface *(between arrows)*.

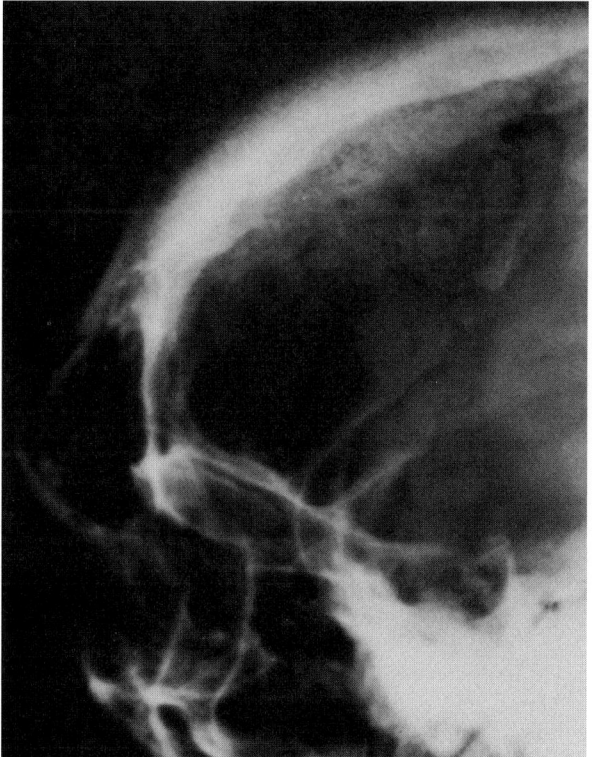

**Figure 44–2.** Acromegaly: skull abnormalities. Findings include increased thickness of the cranial vault, prominent sinuses and supraorbital ridges, and enlarged sella turcica.

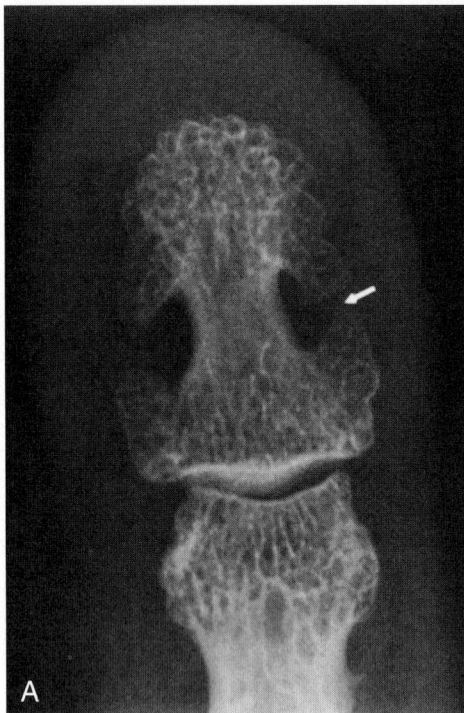

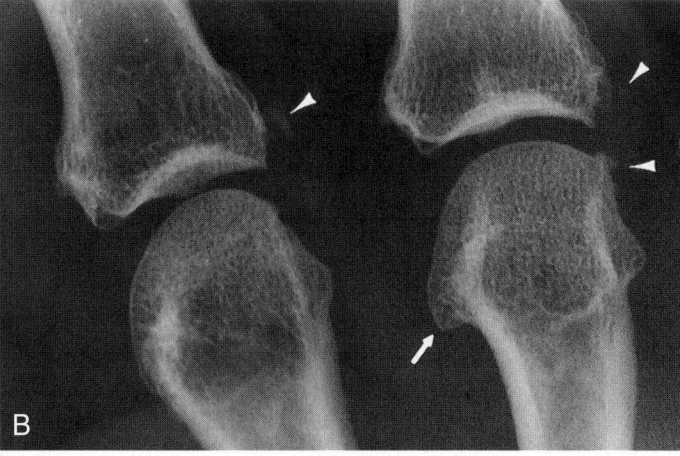

**Figure 44–3.** Acromegaly: abnormalities of the hand. *A,* Terminal phalanx demonstrates typical findings, including soft tissue prominence and enlargement of the tuft and base. Note the formation of pseudoforamina *(arrow)*. *B,* Metacarpophalangeal joints demonstrate widening of articular spaces, beaklike osteophytes on the medial aspect of the metacarpal heads *(arrow)*, and periarticular calcific deposits *(arrowheads)*.

of the ungual tufts. Bone enlargement can be observed about the wrist as well.

To determine the sesamoid index, the size of the medial sesamoid is measured at the first metacarpophalangeal joint. On a nonmagnified radiograph of the hand exposed at a 36-inch focus-film distance, the greatest diameter of this bone is multiplied by the greatest diameter of the same sesamoid image that is perpendicular to the first measurement. Although the reliability of this index has been challenged, a sesamoid index greater than 40 in men and greater than 32 in women is suggestive of acromegaly, whereas a sesamoid index below 30 militates against but does not exclude the diagnosis of acromegaly. Other measurements used in the diagnosis of acromegaly are listed in Table 44–3.

**Abnormalities of the Foot.** Radiographic changes in the foot resemble those in the hand (Fig. 44–4). Thickening of the soft tissues of the toes, enlargement of the sesamoid bones and articular spaces (particularly at the metatarsophalangeal joints), and prominence of the metatarsal

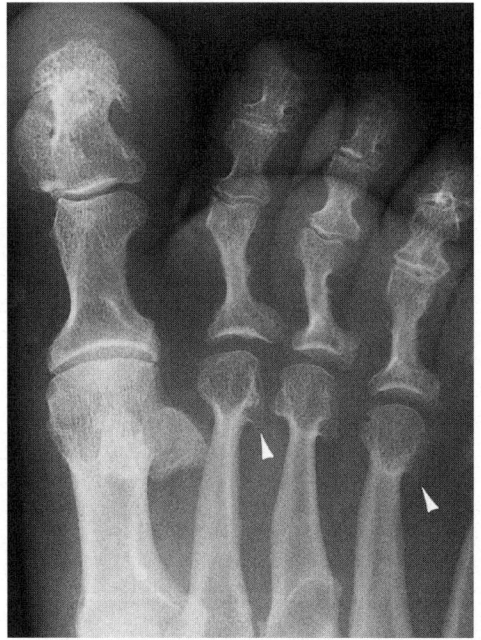

**Figure 44–4.** Acromegaly: abnormalities of the foot. Findings are soft tissue enlargement, prominence of the tufts and bases of the terminal phalanges, pseudoforamina, widening of some of the metatarsophalangeal joints, and beaklike outgrowths of the metatarsal heads *(arrowheads)*. A cystic lesion is seen in the proximal aspect of the third metatarsal.

**TABLE 44–3**

**Bone and Soft Tissue Measurements Suggestive of Acromegaly**

| | |
|---|---|
| Heel-pad thickness | >23 mm (men) |
| | >21.5 mm (women) |
| Sesamoid index (first MCP joint) | >40 (men) |
| | >32 (women) |
| Tuftal width (third finger) | ≥12 mm (men) |
| | ≥ 10 mm (women) |
| Joint space thickness (second MCP joint) | >2.5 mm (men and women) |
| Phalangeal soft tissue thickness (proximal midphalanges) | ≥27 mm (men) |
| | ≥26 mm (women) |

MCP, metacarpophalangeal.

heads are seen. The terminal tufts become prominent, and bony outgrowths arise from the terminal phalangeal base, extending distally. Proliferation at sites of tendon and ligament attachments, such as the calcaneus; thickening of the metatarsal shafts; and constriction of the shafts of the proximal phalanges may be observed.

**Abnormalities of the Vertebral Column.** Elongation and widening of the vertebral bodies are noted in some patients with acromegaly (Fig. 44–5). These findings are more frequent in the thoracic and lumbar spinal regions and less common in the cervical region. Osteophytes of the thoracic and lumbar vertebrae may be extensive, resembling the findings of spondylosis deformans and diffuse idiopathic skeletal hyperostosis. Increased height of the intervertebral disc space, particularly in the lumbar region; hypertrophic changes about apophyseal joints; increased thoracic kyphosis; and increased lumbar lordosis are additional manifestations of acromegaly.

Exaggeration of the normal concavity on the posterior aspect of the vertebral bodies is a recognized abnormality in this disease. The cause of scalloping of the posterior margins of the vertebral bodies in acromegaly is not clear. Scalloping of vertebral bodies is not diagnostic of this condition, as it is found in a variety of disease processes.

**Abnormalities of the Thoracic Cage.** The thorax may appear enlarged owing to elongation of the ribs. Elevation of the lower portion of the sternum and an increased sternal angle have been observed.

**Abnormalities of the Pelvis.** In addition to articular alterations at the sacroiliac joint and hip, enlargement and beaking of the symphysis pubis can be recognized in some patients with acromegaly (Fig. 44–6).

**Abnormalities of the Long Bones.** The simultaneous occurrence of osseous proliferation and resorption is evident in the tubular bones of the extremities. In some of these bones, resorption is predominant, producing a narrow diaphysis with apparent flaring of the metaphysis and epiphysis.

**Miscellaneous Osseous Abnormalities.** Bone proliferation occurs at sites of tendon and ligament attachment to bone (see Fig. 44–1). Particularly characteristic are excrescences on the undersurface of the calcaneus, the anterior margin of the patella, the trochanters of the femur, the tuberosities of the humerus, and the undersurface of the distal end of the clavicle. Localized and generalized osteoporosis has been described in acromegaly.

**Articular Abnormalities.** Radiographic abnormalities of the peripheral joints in acromegaly are seen most frequently in the knee, hip, and glenohumeral joint, although they may be apparent at more distant sites, including the elbow, ankle, hand, wrist, and foot. These abnormalities can be divided into two types: cartilage hypertrophy and cartilaginous and osseous degeneration.

1. Cartilage hypertrophy: Gross thickening of the cartilage is associated with radiographically evident widening of the articular space (Fig. 44–7). Widening of the

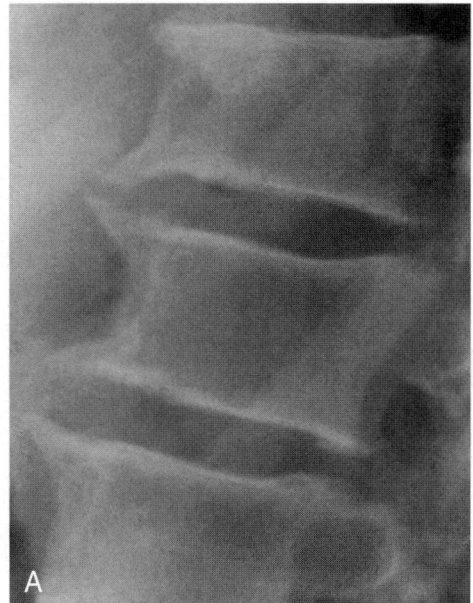

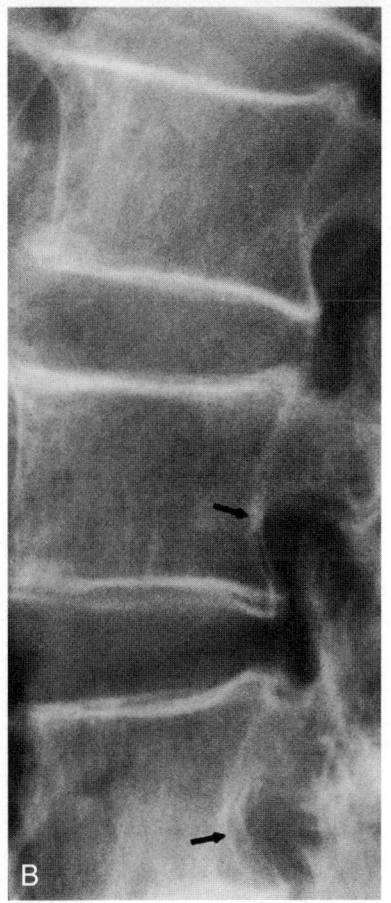

**Figure 44–5.** Acromegaly: abnormalities of the spine. *A*, In the lumbar spine, note bone formation on the anterior aspect of the vertebrae, producing an increase in the anteroposterior diameter of the vertebral bodies. *B*, In a different patient, observe exaggerated concavity on the posterior aspect of multiple lumbar vertebral bodies *(arrows).*

joint space may be apparent in any joint, although it is observed most frequently in the metacarpophalangeal, metatarsophalangeal, and interphalangeal joints.

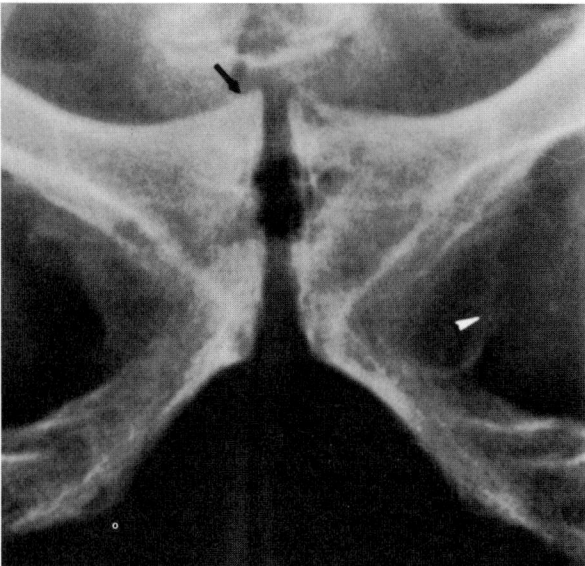

**Figure 44–6.** Acromegaly: abnormalities of the pubis. Findings include "beaking" of the superior aspect of the symphysis *(arrow)* and hyperostosis at sites of ligament attachment to bone *(arrowhead)*.

2. Cartilaginous and osseous degeneration: In later stages of the disease, cartilage fibrillation and erosion lead to secondary degenerative alterations (Fig. 44–8). Initially, osteophytes are seen, and the combination of osteophyte formation and a normal or widened joint space is suggestive of acromegaly. With continued cartilage and bone degeneration, articular space narrowing, cyst formation, sclerosis, and progressive osteophytosis are seen. The eventual appearance resembles that of primary degenerative disease. Involvement of articular

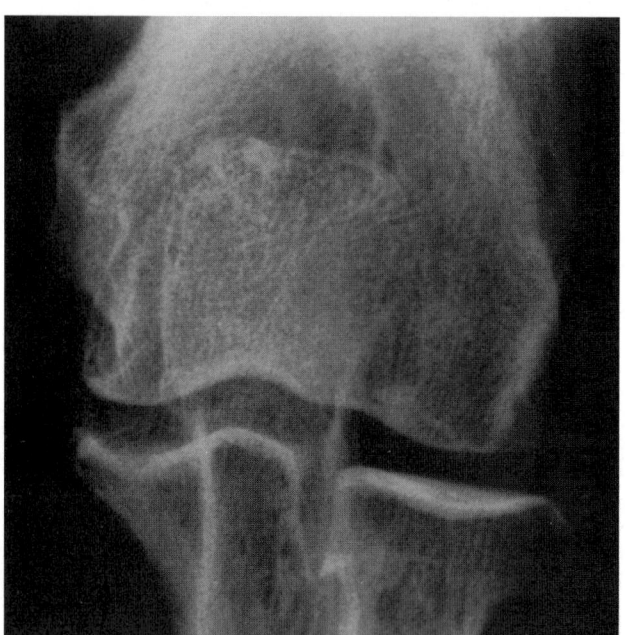

**Figure 44–7.** Acromegaly: cartilage hypertrophy. Joint space widening is apparent in the elbow.

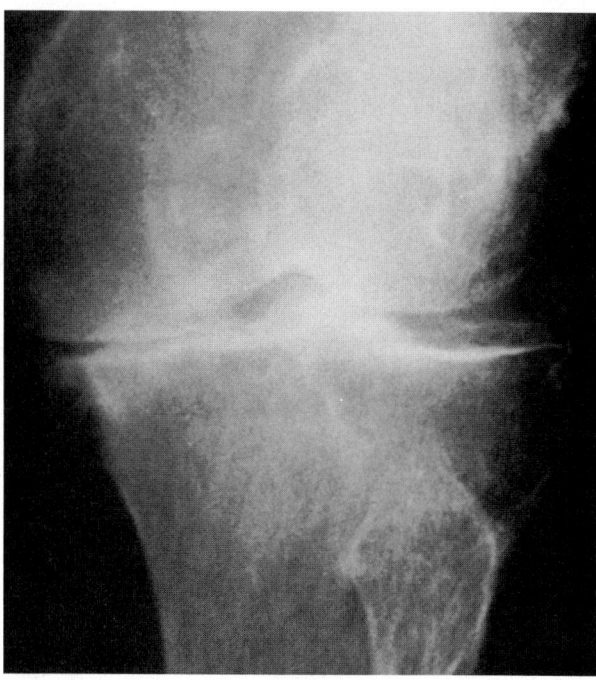

**Figure 44–8.** Acromegaly: cartilaginous and osseous degeneration. In the knee, narrowing of both the medial and lateral femorotibial compartments is seen, with sclerosis and osteophytosis.

sites that are not commonly affected in degenerative joint disease, such as the glenohumeral joint and elbow; the presence of prominent osteophytes and bony excrescences; and the documentation of typical findings of acromegaly elsewhere in the skeleton usually allow an accurate diagnosis of this disease.

## Differential Diagnosis

The combination of radiographic findings in acromegaly is sufficiently characteristic that accurate diagnosis is not difficult, particularly in advanced cases. Individual radiographic signs that are apparent in this disease, such as increased soft tissue width, tuft prominence, and vertebral scalloping, may also be noted in other disorders, however. The early radiographic diagnosis of acromegaly relies on a variety of measurements, especially in the hands and feet.

**General Radiographic Features.** An acromegaly-like syndrome has been associated with pachydermoperiostosis. The characteristic features of this forme fruste familial syndrome are digital clubbing, coarsening of facial features, furrowing and oiliness of the skin, and periosteal new bone formation. Radiographic findings are similar to those of acromegaly, with enlarged sinuses, prominent supraorbital ridges, and thickening of the phalanges (Fig. 44–9). The sella turcica is not enlarged, and severe prominence of the phalangeal tufts and enlargement of the articular space are not observed.

**Enlargement of Phalangeal Tufts.** Widening and prominence of the tufts of the distal phalanges of the hand (and

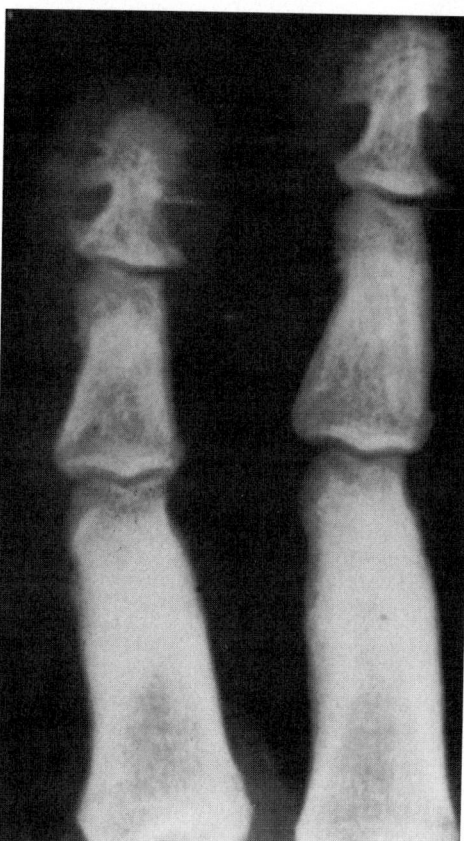

**Figure 44–9.** Pachydermoperiostosis. Findings include soft tissue prominence, thickening of all the phalanges, and enlargement of phalangeal tufts.

**TABLE 44–4**

**Causes of Scalloped Vertebral Bodies**

1. Increased intraspinal pressure
   a. Intradural neoplasms
   b. Intraspinal cysts
   c. Syringomyelia and hydromyelia
   d. Communicating hydrocephalus
2. Dural "ectasia"
   a. Marfan's syndrome
   b. Ehlers-Danlos syndrome
   c. Neurofibromatosis
3. Bone resorption
   a. Acromegaly
4. Congenital disorders
   a. Achondroplasia
   b. Morquio's disease
   c. Hurler's syndrome
5. Physiologic scalloping

From Mitchell GE, Lourie H, Berne AS: The various causes of scalloped vertebrae with notes on their pathogenesis. Radiology 89:67, 1967.

foot) are well-recognized signs of acromegaly. Phalangeal tufts are more prominent in men than in women and in persons who perform heavy manual labor; irregular excrescences on the tuft are occasionally apparent in elderly persons.

**Thickening of Soft Tissues.** Although soft tissue thickening at certain sites, such as the phalanges and heel, can be reliable indicators of acromegaly, similar thickening can occur in other diseases, related to edema, hemorrhage, exudation, or fatty tissue infiltration. Long-term phenytoin therapy may be accompanied by thickening of the heel pad.

**Scalloped Vertebrae.** Exaggerated concavity of the posterior surface of the vertebral bodies is recognized in acromegaly. It is also seen in a variety of other disease processes (Table 44–4).

**Articular Abnormalities.** The initial phase of acromegalic joint disease manifests as increased articular space and enlargement of the osseous surfaces. These radiographic findings are easily differentiated from those accompanying other disease processes. In later stages of acromegalic joint disease, findings include joint space narrowing, cyst formation, sclerosis, and osteophytosis, which are similar to the abnormalities of osteoarthritis. Differentiation between these two disorders may be difficult.

Prominent osteophytes and beaklike excrescences of articular bony surfaces are characteristic in acromegaly. The distribution of degenerative alterations in acromegaly may be similar to that in alkaptonuria and calcium pyrophosphate dihydrate crystal deposition disease. In the former disorder, vertebral osteoporosis, disc calcification, and widespread loss of disc height ensure a proper diagnosis; in the latter disorder, articular and periarticular calcification and more severe and progressive joint destruction are important diagnostic clues, although both acromegaly and calcium pyrophosphate dihydrate crystal deposition disease may occur in the same person.

## HYPOPITUITARISM

Damage to the anterior lobe of the pituitary gland during the period of skeletal growth leads to abnormal osseous development. The cause of damage is variable and includes neoplasm (adenoma, craniopharyngioma, pituitary carcinoma, metastasis), infection (pyogenic, tuberculous, fungal), granuloma (histiocytosis, sarcoidosis), injury, and vascular insult. In approximately 10% of cases, hypopituitarism is familial. The effect on the skeleton is a delay in the appearance and growth of ossification centers and a similar delay in their fusion and disappearance (Fig. 44–10). Eventually, the growth plate may disappear, although osseous fusion occurs at an advanced age.

Clinically, growth failure is usually recognized when the child is 1 to 3 years of age. If the condition is untreated, continued slow growth at the rate of 50% to 60% of normal occurs throughout childhood. Findings include immature body proportions and facial features, abnormal distribution of fat, and delay in eruption of secondary teeth. Mental development generally parallels the chronologic age.

Radiographic abnormalities are reported in association with hypopituitarism, but articular manifestations are infrequent. In rare instances, slipping of the femoral

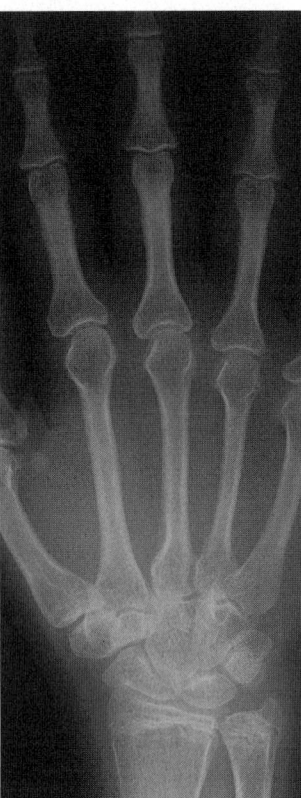

**Figure 44–10.** Hypopituitarism: delayed skeletal maturation. In this 23-year-old woman, a marked reduction in the rate of skeletal maturation is confirmed by the absence of closure of the physes of the distal portions of the radius and ulna. Osteopenia is evident.

capital epiphysis may occur before or during growth hormone therapy in patients with pituitary dysfunction. The differential diagnosis of pituitary dwarfism includes a number of other causes of short stature (Table 44–5). Most of these conditions are easily differentiated from pituitary dwarfism; this is important, because the latter disease probably accounts for fewer than 10% of cases of short stature in children.

## FURTHER READING

Anton HC: Hand measurements in acromegaly. Clin Radiol 23:445, 1972.

Bluestone R, Bywaters EGL, Hartog M, et al: Acromegalic arthropathy. Ann Rheum Dis 30:243, 1971.

Doppman JL, Sharon M, Gorden P: Metatarsal pencilling in acromegaly: A proposed mechanism based on CT findings. J Comput Assist Tomogr 12:708, 1988.

Hernandez RJ, Poznanski AW, Hopwood NJ: Size and skeletal maturation of the hand in children with hypothyroidism and hypopituitarism. AJR Am J Roentgenol 133:405, 1979.

---

### TABLE 44–5

**Causes of Short Stature**

**Endocrine Disorders**
  Hypopituitarism
  Hypothyroidism
  Diabetes mellitus
  Hypercortisolism
  Congenital adrenal hyperplasia
  Deficient somatomedin production (Laron dwarfism)

**Chronic Disorders of Major Organ Systems**
  Chronic renal disease
  Congenital heart disease
  Juvenile chronic arthritis
  Sickle cell anemia
  Malabsorption syndromes

**Skeletal Disorders**
  Achondroplasia
  Osteochondrodysplasias
  Pseudohypoparathyroidism and pseudo-
    pseudo-hypoparathyroidism
  Rickets

**Chromosomal Aberrations**
  Gonadal dysgenesis
  Trisomy conditions

**Miscellaneous Disorders**
  Malnutrition
  Familial short stature
  Inborn errors of metabolism
  Intrauterine infections
  Systemic inflammatory diseases
  Renal tubular disorders
  Psychosocial dwarfism
  Neurologic disorders

Jaffe HL: Metabolic, Degenerative and Inflammatory Diseases of Bones and Joints. Philadelphia, Lea & Febiger, 1972, p 332.

Lang EK, Bessler WT: The roentgenologic features of acromegaly. AJR Am J Roentgenol 86:321, 1961.

Layton MW, Fudman EJ, Barkan A, et al: Acromegalic arthropathy: Characteristics and response to therapy. Arthritis Rheum 31:1022, 1988.

Lin SR, Lee KF: Relative value of some radiographic measurements of the hand in the diagnosis of acromegaly. Invest Radiol 6:426, 1971.

Mitchell GE, Lourie H, Berne AS: The various causes of scalloped vertebrae with notes on their pathogenesis. Radiology 89:67, 1967.

Shimizu C, Kubo M, Kijima H, et al: A rare case of acromegaly associated with pachydermoperiostosis. J Endocrinol Invest 22:386, 1999.

Steinbach HL, Feldman R, Goldberg MB: Acromegaly. Radiology 72:535, 1959.

# CHAPTER 45

## Thyroid Disorders

### SUMMARY OF KEY FEATURES

Distinctive osseous, articular, and soft tissue alterations may accompany hyperthyroid and hypothyroid states. These alterations underscore the importance of thyroid hormone in regulating normal growth, development, and maturation of tissue. Radiographs may provide an important clue to the proper diagnosis when clinical findings are not specific and may serve as a useful parameter for assessing the adequacy of therapy.

### INTRODUCTION

Thyroxine and triiodothyronine are active thyroid hormones that increase the turnover of protein, carbohydrates, fat, and minerals. They circulate in the blood, largely bound to serum proteins, although small quantities are in an active free form. Excessive thyroid hormone produces catabolism of protein and loss of connective tissue; deficiency of thyroid hormone has a dramatic effect on the body, causing defects in bone growth and development.

### HYPERTHYROIDISM

#### General Characteristics

Thyrotoxicosis is a general term indicating biochemical and physiologic abnormalities that result from excessive quantities of thyroid hormones; the term hyperthyroidism is used to describe this syndrome when it is the result of overproduction of these hormones by the thyroid gland itself rather than of abnormalities originating outside the gland. Of the many forms of thyrotoxicosis, toxic diffuse goiter (Graves' disease or Basedow's disease) and toxic nodular goiter produced by single or multiple adenomas are most common. Clinical manifestations of thyrotoxicosis that generally allow an accurate diagnosis include symptoms such as fatigue, weakness, nervousness, hypersensitivity to heat, hyperhidrosis, weight loss, tachycardia, palpitations, eye complaints, and diarrhea; physical signs may include enlargement of the neck, rapid heartbeat, tremor, thyroid bruit, and abnormalities of the eye. Musculoskeletal abnormalities of hyperthyroidism are also well known (Table 45–1).

#### Bone Resorption

In patients with hyperthyroidism, elevation of the serum calcium concentration is apparent, although hypercalcemia generally is not severe or sustained. Additional laboratory findings are elevated levels of serum phosphorus and

---

### TABLE 45–1

**Musculoskeletal Abnormalities of Hyperthyroidism**

Hyperthyroid osteopathy
Accelerated skeletal maturation
Myopathy

---

alkaline phosphatase and hypercalciuria. These features underscore the presence of excessive bone turnover with a negative calcium balance.

The reported frequency of radiographically detectable bone disease in patients with hyperthyroidism varies from 3.5% to 50%. The changes are more common in men than in women; in women, such changes predominate after menopause. Most persons with bone abnormalities have had hyperthyroidism for longer than 5 years, and these abnormalities may be associated with pain, fracture, and deformity. Osseous deformities include reduction in height and exaggerated dorsal kyphosis. Spontaneous fractures in patients with hyperthyroidism are frequent. Clinical as well as radiographic findings may appear quickly, progress rapidly, and stabilize or improve with appropriate treatment of thyrotoxicosis.

The radiographic features of bone loss in hyperthyroidism simulate those associated with other varieties of osteoporosis, although hyperthyroid osteopathy may lead to bone loss not only in the vertebral column but also in the pelvis, cranium, hands, and feet. In the spine, osteoporosis, vertebral compression, and kyphosis (or kyphoscoliosis) are seen (Fig. 45–1). Osteoporosis produces typical rarefaction of the midportion of the vertebral body and fish vertebrae, with exaggerated biconcave deformity of the vertebral body. These changes are more pronounced in the thoracic and lumbar vertebrae but may be observed in the cervical region as well.

In the skull, focal rarefaction of bone, particularly in the frontal region, may produce a radiographic picture reminiscent of multiple myeloma. Increased radiolucency and cystic lesions may also be apparent in long bones, clavicles, hands, feet, and ribs. Both bone resorption and bone formation are increased, but in the presence of reduced skeletal mass, bone resorption is the more dominant abnormality.

#### Additional Abnormalities

Hyperthyroidism in children is associated with acceleration of skeletal maturation and may reach severe proportions. Premature craniosynostosis may be evident. Myopathy is frequent in hyperthyroidism, and its symptoms and signs may simulate arthritis. Weakness, cramps, and muscle tenderness are observed. Neurologic manifestations of hyperthyroidism include peripheral neuropathy, corticospinal tract disease, chorea, seizures, and psychiatric disorders.

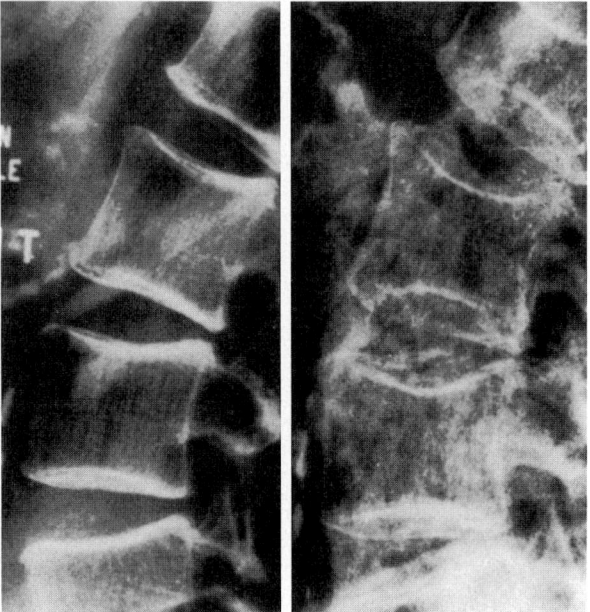

**Figure 45–1.** Hyperthyroidism: spinal abnormalities. Radiographs obtained 5 months apart reveal the rapid course of vertebral osteoporosis that may accompany thyrotoxicosis. On the later film (right), increased radiolucency of the vertebral bodies and biconcave deformities are apparent. (From Meunier PJ, Bianchi GG, Edouard CM, et al: Bony manifestations of thyrotoxicosis. Orthop Clin North Am 3:745, 1972.)

# THYROID ACROPACHY

## General Characteristics

Thyroid acropachy is an unusual manifestation of thyroid disease that may be seen in approximately 0.5% to 1% of patients with thyrotoxicosis. Although the cause is unknown, this condition is usually observed after treatment of hyperthyroidism, at which time the patient may be euthyroid or hypothyroid. Men and women are affected equally. Clinical findings in thyroid acropachy include exophthalmos, which may be severe and progressive; painless symmetrical or asymmetrical soft tissue swelling of the fingers and toes, which may be erythematous and fluctuant; pretibial myxedema; and clubbing of the fingers (Table 45–2).

## Radiographic and Pathologic Findings

Radiographic abnormalities are virtually diagnostic (Fig. 45–2). Periosteal bone formation is seen in the diaphyses

---

**TABLE 45–2**

**Clinical and Radiographic Features of Thyroid Acropachy**

Exophthalmos
Soft tissue swelling
Pretibial myxedema
Clubbing
Periostitis

---

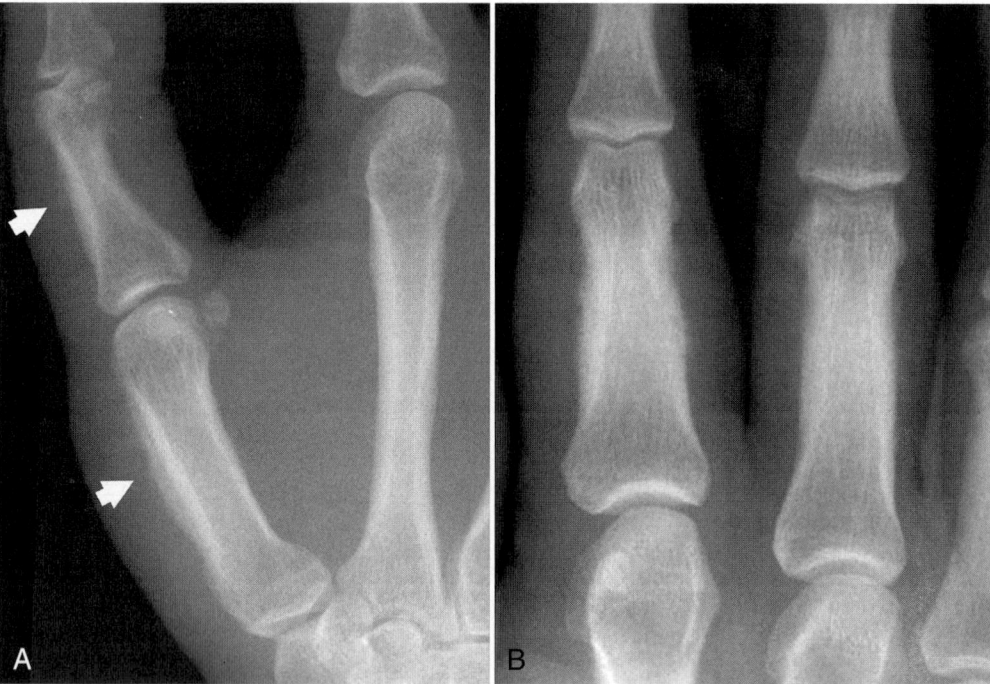

**Figure 45–2.** Thyroid acropachy. *A,* Thick, shaggy periostitis, asymmetrical in distribution, has a predilection for the radial aspect of the proximal phalanx and metacarpal of the thumb *(arrows). B,* In a different patient, observe soft tissue swelling and spiculated or feathery periostitis in the proximal phalanx of the index finger. There are less extensive changes in the middle finger.

of the metacarpals, metatarsals, and proximal and middle phalanges, although this change may be visualized occasionally at other sites, including the long bones. Periostitis is asymmetrical in distribution and more prominent on the radial aspect of the bone; it tends to be dense and solid in appearance, with a feathery contour. Soft tissue swelling in the hands and feet, phalangeal tufts, and anterior tibial region is observed. The osseous abnormalities generally are not progressive, and correcting thyroid function has little or no effect on the acropachy. Increased radionuclide activity in areas of bony alteration has been observed.

## Differential Diagnosis

Thyroid acropachy must be differentiated from other disorders associated with periosteal bone formation (Table 45–3). Hypertrophic osteoarthropathy, which is commonly associated with thoracic neoplasm, is characterized by bony proliferation and soft tissue swelling of the hands and tufts, but the distribution of osseous abnormality differs from that of thyroid acropachy. In hypertrophic osteoarthropathy, periosteal bone formation is observed most commonly in the tibia, fibula, radius, and ulna. Changes limited to the hands and feet are unusual in this condition. Further, the feathery pattern of bony proliferation seen in thyroid acropachy is not typical of hypertrophic osteoarthropathy.

Pachydermoperiostosis is associated with typical facies, soft tissue prominence of the hands, and periostitis. Periosteal bone formation generally is apparent in a symmetrical pattern in the tibia, fibula, radius, and ulna, although the hands may also be affected. Periostitis in this disorder is not limited to the diaphysis but may be exuberant at the metaphyseal and epiphyseal areas.

Hypervitaminosis A and venous stasis may produce periosteal bone proliferation, but clinical and radiographic features allow an accurate diagnosis of these conditions. Fluorosis is associated with more extensive abnormality of the axial skeleton and long bones. Leukemic acropachy is particularly prominent in the terminal phalanges. Periosteal bone formation in acromegaly and vasculitides such as periarteritis nodosa is readily distinguished from the changes of thyroid acropachy. Infectious and traumatic disorders cause alterations in addition to periostitis.

---

**TABLE 45–3**

**Conditions Associated with Periostitis of Multiple Bones**

Hypertrophic osteoarthropathy
Pachydermoperiostosis
Thyroid acropachy
Hypervitaminosis A
Venous stasis
Fluorosis
Leukemia
Vascular insufficiency
Infection
Trauma

---

# HYPOTHYROIDISM
## General Characteristics

Hypothyroidism and myxedema are terms describing a clinical state of thyroxine and triiodothyronine deficiency. The deficiency can be divided into a primary form, in which the thyroid gland itself is involved, and a secondary form, characterized by a deficiency in thyroid-stimulating hormone. Hypothyroidism can have many causes, including atrophy; thyroid gland destruction after radioactive iodine therapy or surgery; thyroiditis, which may be acute or chronic (Hashimoto's disease); infiltrative disorders such as lymphoma, cystinosis, amyloidosis, and metastasis; deficiency in iodine or iodine metabolism; use of certain medications; and a variety of pituitary disorders.

In infants, thyroid deficiency results in cretinism; in children, it produces juvenile myxedema, with mental retardation and developmental abnormalities. Symptoms and signs include lethargy, constipation, enlarged tongue, abdominal distention, hypotonia, dry hair and skin, and delayed dentition. In adults, the disease is more frequent in women and can be associated with dry, coarse skin and hair, fatigue, lethargy, edema, hoarseness, constipation, paresthesias, and bradycardia, as well as other symptoms and signs (Table 45–4).

In adult-onset hypothyroidism, there are altered kinetics in bone but no diagnostic radiographic abnormalities. In cretinism and juvenile myxedema, skeletal manifestations are more marked. Delayed bony maturation is most characteristic, and in infants, absence of the distal femoral and proximal tibial epiphyses is an important radiographic clue. In older children, abnormal epiphyseal maturation leads to distinctive radiographic findings,

---

**TABLE 45–4**

**Symptoms and Signs of Hypothyroidism**

| | Percentage of Cases |
|---|---|
| Dry, coarse skin and hair | 70–97 |
| Fatigue, lethargy, mental or physical slowness | 70–91 |
| Edema; puffy hands, face, or eyes | 67–95 |
| Pallor | 50–59 |
| Cold intolerance | 58–95 |
| Decreased sweating | 68–89 |
| Hoarseness | 48–74 |
| Constipation | 36–61 |
| Weight gain | 48–76 |
| Loss or thinning of hair | 32–57 |
| Paresthesias | 56 |
| Enlarged tongue | 19 |
| Bradycardia | 14 |
| Menstrual disturbance | 16–30 |
| Decreased hearing | 6 |

From Robbins J, et al: The thyroid and iodine metabolism. In Bondy PK, Rosenberg LE (eds): Metabolic Control and Disease, 8th ed. Philadelphia, WB Saunders, 1980, p 1390.

with fragmented, irregular epiphyseal contours, termed epiphyseal dysgenesis. Delayed dental development is a concomitant feature of the disease. Growth retardation in these persons may simulate that associated with growth hormone deficiency.

## Altered Development of Bone

Retardation of skeletal maturation is a fundamental radiographic feature of hypothyroidism, and although this finding can be seen in other disorders, it is more severe in hypothyroidism (Fig. 45–3). The diagnosis of hypothyroidism is suspect if a child has normal maturation. The radiographic confirmation of delayed skeletal maturation relies on a delay in appearance and growth of epiphyseal ossification centers and is facilitated in infants by examination of the knees. This abnormality of epiphyseal development is accompanied by alterations in the development of synchondroses (e.g., between segments of sternum and sacrum) and sutures; physeal growth plates and sutures may persist well beyond the age at which they normally should have disappeared.

In the skull, growth retardation is particularly striking at the base of the cranium. Decreased growth of the spheno-occipital synchondrosis produces brachycephaly. Enlargement of the sella turcica is observed (Fig. 45–4). Additional cranial findings in hypothyroidism include prominent sutures with accessory (wormian) bones (which can also be seen in osteogenesis imperfecta, cleidocranial dysostosis, and other conditions), underdevelopment of the paranasal sinuses and mastoid air cells, and a prognathous lower jaw (Fig. 45–5).

In affected epiphyses, ossification proceeds from multiple centers rather than from a single site, and the resulting irregular appearance is termed epiphyseal dysgenesis (Fig. 45–6). Epiphyseal dysgenesis is particularly frequent in the femoral and humeral heads. The fragmented epiphysis can simulate the appearance of osteonecrosis. With involvement of the femoral head, this leads to a mistaken diagnosis of Legg-Calvé-Perthes disease. Epi-

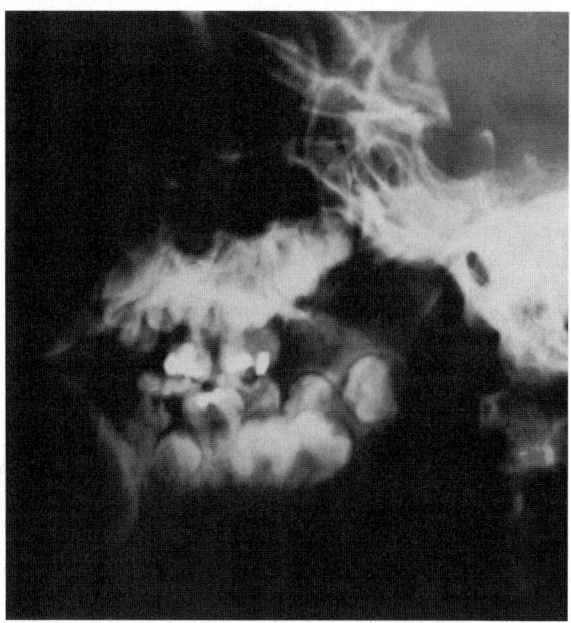

**Figure 45–4.** Hypothyroidism: cranial and facial abnormalities. In a 21-year-old man with cretinism, findings include an enlarged sella turcica, prominent lower jaw, and delayed dental development. (Courtesy of S. Hilton, MD, San Diego, Calif.)

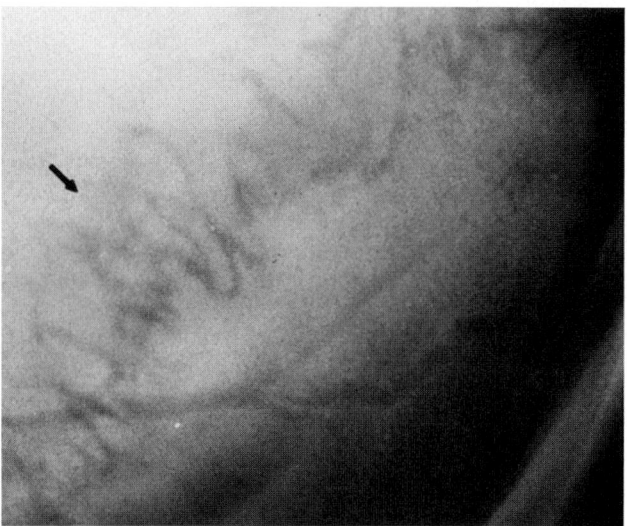

**Figure 45–5.** Hypothyroidism: prominent sutures with accessory (wormian) bones. Examples are shown of intrasutural bones (*arrow*), which are characteristic of hypothyroidism.

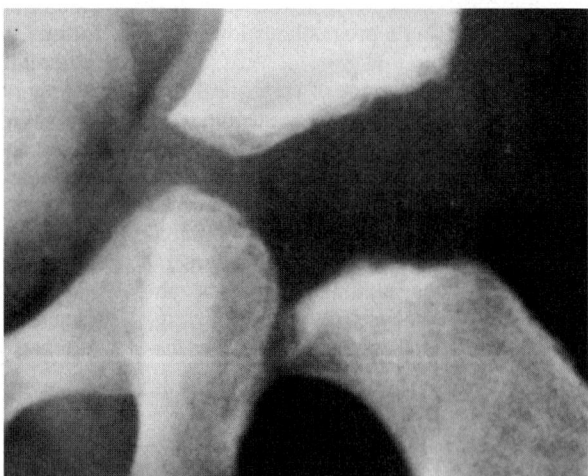

**Figure 45–3.** Hypothyroidism: delayed ossification of epiphyses. In a 3-year-old child with hypothyroidism, the capital femoral epiphysis has not yet ossified.

physeal dysgenesis is not due to vascular insufficiency but relates to an aberration of the ossification pattern in the involved epiphysis. When the patient is treated, coalescence of the fragments may lead to disappearance of epiphyseal dysgenesis within a year or two. With delayed or inadequate therapy, epiphyseal abnormalities may result in secondary articular degeneration, intra-articular osseous and cartilaginous bodies, and angular deformities. In the hip, coxa plana, coxa magna, and coxa vara have been described.

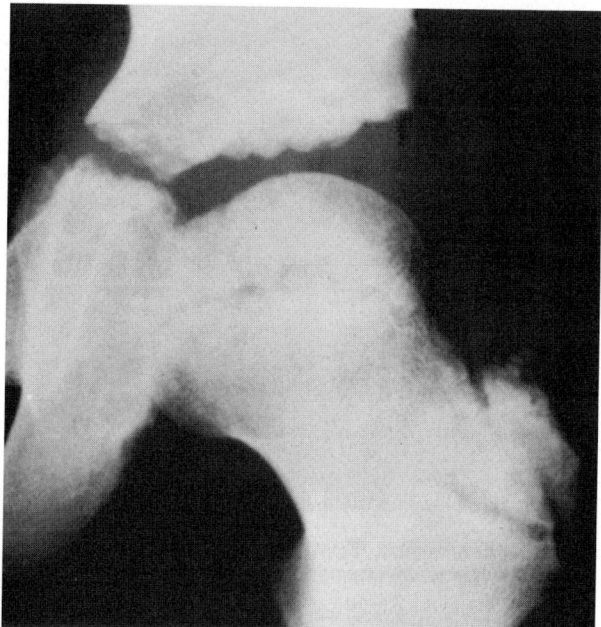

**Figure 45–6.** Hypothyroidism: epiphyseal dysgenesis. Irregularity of the apophysis of the greater trochanter and acetabular margin is associated with flattening and deformity of the proximal capital femoral epiphysis.

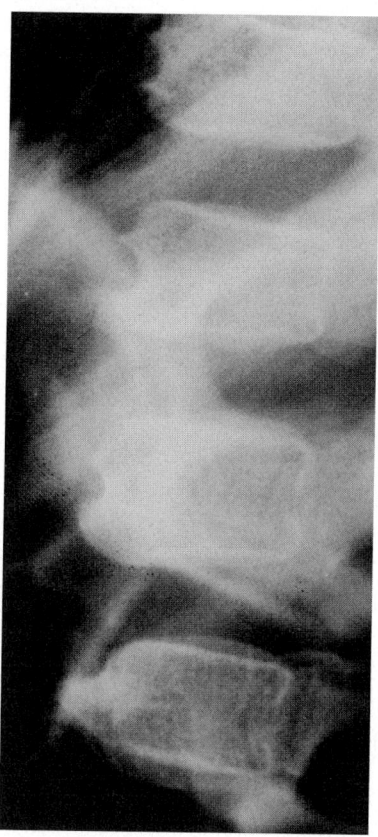

**Figure 45–7.** Hypothyroidism: spinal abnormalities. Note bullet-shaped vertebrae and beaklike anterior surfaces of the vertebral bodies.

Vertebral abnormalities are also common in hypothyroidism and are particularly prominent at the thoracolumbar junction, where short, bullet-shaped 12th thoracic and 1st lumbar vertebral bodies may be visualized (Fig. 45–7). A gibbous deformity may result.

## Abnormal Calcification

In hypothyroidism, abnormal calcium metabolism and excretion are present. Retention of calcium with increased bone sclerosis may be seen in association with soft tissue calcific deposits. Increased bony eburnation in the periorbital region is termed the lunette sign. Parotid calcification and premature atherosclerosis are two examples of abnormal calcific deposition in hypothyroidism.

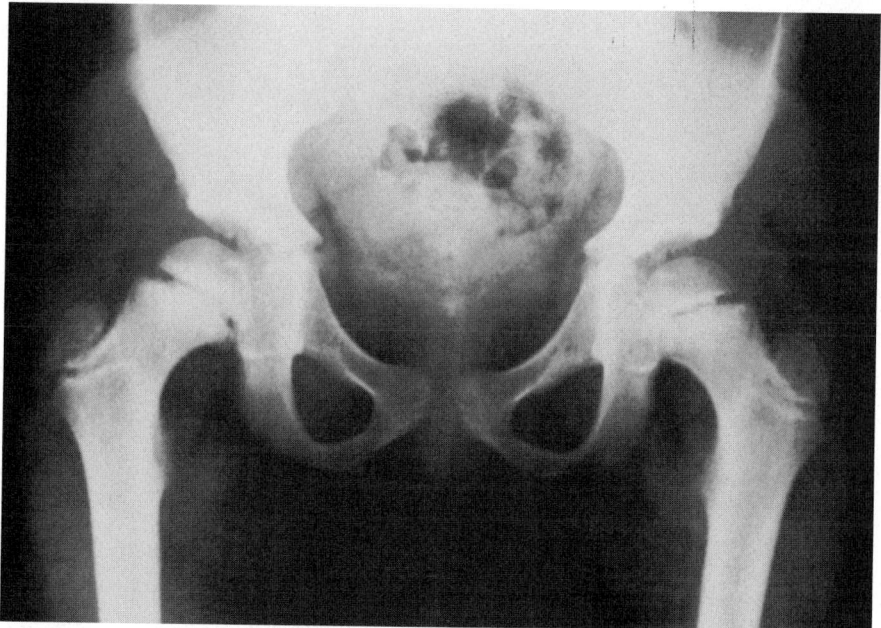

**Figure 45–8.** Hypothyroidism: slipped capital femoral epiphyses. In a 13-year-old girl, bilateral hip pain developed over a 1-year period. Frontal radiograph of the pelvis shows bilateral slipped capital femoral epiphyses, more prominent on the right. Evaluation revealed decreased bone age, and the diagnosis of hypothyroidism was subsequently verified. (Courtesy of G. Greenway, MD, Dallas, Tex.)

## Additional Rheumatologic Manifestations

An entrapment neuropathy, including the carpal tunnel syndrome, is seen in approximately 7% of patients with hypothyroidism. The carpal tunnel syndrome, which is produced by nerve impingement by the myxedematous tissue and accompanying tenosynovitis, may be persistent, showing little response to hydrocortisone injections, although it may improve rapidly after thyroid hormone replacement.

Muscle cramps and stiffness are common in hypothyroidism, with a predilection for the calves, thighs, and shoulders. Symptoms and signs include pain and tenderness that increase after exercise. Prominent soft tissues are due to myxomatous infiltration of soft tissues, and tendon reflexes are characteristically slow, with delayed relaxation.

## Slipped Capital Femoral Epiphysis

Slipped capital femoral epiphyses may occur in either treated or untreated patients with hypothyroidism. Although usually seen in prepubescent subjects, the complication is occasionally apparent in more mature patients. A bilateral or unilateral distribution is evident (Fig. 45–8). The cause of this complication of hypothyroidism is not known. Whatever the cause, slipped capital femoral epiphyses are an important manifestation of hypothyroidism and may be the presenting feature of the disease.

## FURTHER READING ─────────────

Bonakdarpour A, Kirkpatric JA, Renzi A, et al: Skeletal changes in neonatal thyrotoxicosis. Radiology 102:149, 1972.

Borg SA, Fitzer PM, Young LW: Roentgenologic aspects of adult cretinism: Two case reports and review of the literature. AJR Am J Roentgenol 123:820, 1975.

Hernandez RJ, Poznanski AK: Distinctive appearance of the distal phalanges in children with primary hypothyroidism. Radiology 132:83, 1979.

Hernandez RJ, Poznanski AW, Hopwood NJ: Size and skeletal maturation of the hand in children with hypothyroidism and hypopituitarism. AJR Am J Roentgenol 133:405, 1979.

Jaffe HL: Metabolic, Degenerative and Inflammatory Diseases of Bones and Joints. Philadelphia, Lea & Febiger, 1972, p 346.

Lauwers A, Alexandre C: Bone manifestations of untreated hypothyroidism in adults. Rev Rhum Engl Ed 63:612, 1996.

Lintermans JP, Seyhnaeve V: Hypothyroidism and vertebral anomalies: A new syndrome? AJR Am J Roentgenol 109:294, 1970.

McLean RM, Podell DN: Bone and joint manifestations of hypothyroidism. Semin Arthritis Rheum 24:282, 1995.

Meunier PJ, Bianchi GG, Edouard CM, et al: Bony manifestations of thyrotoxicosis. Orthop Clin North Am 3:745, 1972.

Moorefield WG, Urbaniak JR, Ogden WS, et al: Acquired hypothyroidism and slipped capital femoral epiphysis: Report of three cases. J Bone Joint Surg Am 58:705, 1976.

Scanlon GT, Clemett AR: Thyroid acropachy. Radiology 83:1039, 1964.

Vanhoenacker FM, Pelckmans MC, De Beuckeleer LH, et al: Thyroid acropachy: Correlation of imaging and pathology. Eur Radiol 11:1058, 2001.

Wietersen FK, Balow RM: The radiologic aspects of thyroid disease. Radiol Clin North Am 5:255, 1967.

# CHAPTER 46

## Parathyroid Disorders and Renal Osteodystrophy

## SUMMARY OF KEY FEATURES

Elevated levels of parathyroid hormone occurring in primary and secondary hyperparathyroidism produce considerable osseous erosion involving subperiosteal, intracortical, endosteal, trabecular, subchondral, subphyseal, and subtendinous and subligamentous foci. In renal osteodystrophy, the changes of secondary hyperparathyroidism are combined with additional radiographic and histologic features, including osteomalacia, osteoporosis, and soft tissue and vascular calcification, findings that may become exaggerated or arrested after hemodialysis and renal transplantation. A peculiar variety of amyloidosis occurs in dialyzed patients, whereas osteonecrosis is an important complication of renal transplantation. Depressed levels of parathyroid hormone may be associated with osteosclerosis, subcutaneous and basal ganglion calcification, and spinal abnormalities simulating diffuse idiopathic skeletal hyperostosis or ankylosing spondylitis. Pseudohypoparathyroidism and pseudo-pseudohypoparathyroidism may be associated with abnormalities in skeletal maturation and development, peculiar exostoses, and soft tissue calcification and ossification.

## INTRODUCTION

Parathyroid hormone is essential for the proper transport of calcium and other ions in bone, intestine, and kidney. Parathyroid hormone has dramatic, albeit complex, effects on the bone. Its initial effect is to promote the release of calcium into the blood from bone; a second action is to stimulate extensive bone remodeling. Alterations of parathyroid function cause a breakdown in calcium homeostasis, leading to characteristic pathologic and radiographic abnormalities.

## HYPERPARATHYROIDISM

### Background and General Features

Hyperparathyroidism is a general term indicating an increased level of parathyroid hormone in the blood. The condition traditionally is divided into three types: primary, secondary, and tertiary.

Primary hyperparathyroidism is characterized by increased parathyroid hormone secretion as a result of an abnormality in one or more of the parathyroid glands. Autonomous hyperfunction of these glands results from a variety of causes, including diffuse hyperplasia (10% to 40% of cases), single (50% to 80%) or multiple (10%) adenomas, and, rarely, carcinoma (<1%). The fundamental (although not invariable) biochemical parameter of hyperparathyroidism is persistent hypercalcemia.

Secondary hyperparathyroidism is associated with abnormalities in parathyroid gland function induced by a sustained hypocalcemic stimulus, usually resulting from chronic renal failure or, occasionally, from malabsorption states. Pathologic examination generally reveals hyperplasia of all four parathyroid glands; plasma calcium levels are normal or low, and serum inorganic phosphate levels are high (chronic renal disease) or low (intestinal malabsorption). Renal abnormality is associated with additional soft tissue and skeletal changes, and the entire complex is termed renal osteodystrophy.

Tertiary hyperparathyroidism occurs in patients with chronic renal failure or malabsorption and long-standing secondary hyperparathyroidism who develop relatively autonomous parathyroid function and hypercalcemia.

Elevated serum levels of parathyroid hormone provide the most important clue in establishing the diagnosis of hyperparathyroidism. Because of variations in the amount of circulating parathyroid hormone at any given time, multiple measurements of serum calcium are often recommended. Further, hypercalcemia is a known complication of other disease states (Table 46–1), such as neoplasms; 10% to 20% of patients with malignancy have elevated serum calcium levels. The majority of these patients have direct involvement of the skeleton by a malignant lesion. The syndrome consisting of hypercalcemia of malignancy in the absence of demonstrable skeletal metastasis or primary hyperparathyroidism is termed pseudohyperparathyroidism.

In general, clinical findings are most commonly attributable to renal, skeletal, and gastrointestinal changes. The patient's initial complaints are frequently related to the presence of urinary tract calculi and nephrolithiasis, peptic ulcer disease, or pancreatitis. Symptomatic bone disease is observed in 10% to 25% of patients and may consist of tenderness and aching of the peripheral joints and the vertebral column; this may eventually progress to severe pain, swelling, and deformity. Alterations in the central nervous system, skin, and cardiovascular system may also contribute to the initial clinical picture, producing personality disturbance, coma, muscular weakness, fatigue, dry skin, itching, hypertension, and congestive heart failure.

### Fundamental Characteristics of Bone Involvement

In experimental or clinical situations, hyperparathyroidism is accompanied by an increase in the ratio of osteoclasts to osteoblasts. The skeletal effects of parathyroid hormone are mediated through the osteoblast, because osteoclasts do not express the parathyroid hormone receptor. Osteoblasts are able to communicate in some fashion with

## TABLE 46–1

### Differential Diagnosis of Hypercalcemia

**Artifactual Disorders**
  Hyperproteinemia
    Venous stasis during blood collection
    Hyperalbuminemia (e.g., hyperalimentation)
    Hypergammaglobulinemia (e.g., myeloma, sarcoidosis)

**Malignancy**
  Solid tumors (primarily breast cancer)
  Hematologic disorders
    Myeloma
    Lymphoma
    Leukemia

**Endocrinologic Disorders**
  Primary hyperparathyroidism
  Multiple endocrine adenomatoses, types I and II
  Ectopic hyperparathyroidism (malignancy, predominantly
    lung cancer)
  Secondary hyperparathyroidism (e.g., renal failure)
  Hyperthyroidism
  Hypoadrenalism (usually following acute steroid withdrawal)

**Drugs**
  Vitamin A intoxication
  Vitamin D intoxication
  Thiazides
  Calcium
    Milk-alkali syndrome (ingestion of absorbable antacid
      calcium-containing preparations—e.g., calcium
      carbonate)
    Dialysis (with dialysate calcium concentration >7.0 mg/dL)

**Granulomatous Disorders**
  Sarcoidosis
  Tuberculosis
  Histoplasmosis
  Berylliosis
  Rheumatoid arthritis (primary during immobilization)

**Pediatric Disorders**
  Infantile hypercalcemia
  Hypophosphatasia

**Immobilization**
  Paget's disease
  Growth

**Miscellaneous Disorders**
  Pheochromocytoma
  Idiopathic periostitis
  Post–renal transplant surgery
  Benign familial hypercalcemia
  Diuretic phase of acute renal failure

From Aviolo LV, Raisz LG: Bone metabolism and disease. In Bondy PK, Rosenberg LE (eds): Metabolic Control and Disease, 8th ed. Philadelphia, WB Saunders, 1980, p 1734.

osteoclasts to mediate the effects of parathyroid hormone. Mobilization of calcium from the bone has been attributed to the process of osteocytic osteolysis, as evidenced by an apparent increase in the extracellular space of bone lacunae. Extensive bone remodeling may be due to alterations of both osteoblasts and osteoclasts. The stimulation of bone formation by parathyroid hormone is consistent with the occurrence of osteosclerosis in some cases of hyperparathyroidism.

Histologic examination of osseous tissue in hyperparathyroidism demonstrates great variation in the pathologic findings. Abnormalities include those of osteitis fibrosa cystica, with replacement of marrow elements by highly vascular fibrous tissue, as well as the changes of osteoporosis and osteomalacia. In hyperparathyroidism, initial bone changes may be so slight as to be imperceptible on radiographic or gross pathologic examination. More severe skeletal involvement may lead to localized cysts or brown tumors, rarefied and thinned cortices, distorted and blurred cancellous trabeculae, infarctions, fractures, and deformities.

## Bone Resorption

Resorption of osseous tissue is evident on histologic and radiographic examination in patients with primary (or secondary) hyperparathyroidism. Although many skeletal sites are involved, the sensitivity of bone resorption in the hands in the early stages of the disease has been documented repeatedly, indicating that high-quality radiography (with macroradiography or digitized radiography) of this region is adequate for detecting and monitoring the course of skeletal changes in primary and secondary hyperparathyroidism. Bone resorption can be categorized as subperiosteal, intracortical, endosteal, subchondral, subphyseal, trabecular, or subligamentous and subtendinous. Localized lesions or brown tumors may also be seen.

**Subperiosteal Bone Resorption.** Subperiosteal resorption of cortical bone, particularly when prominent, is virtually diagnostic of hyperparathyroid bone disease (Figs. 46–1 and 46–2). Although this change may be visualized in various skeletal locations, it is most frequent along the radial aspect of the phalanges of the hand, particularly in the middle phalanges of the index and middle fingers. The ulnar aspect is affected less significantly. A lacelike appearance of the phalangeal bone may progress to a spiculated contour and, eventually, to complete resorption of the entire cortex. Additional sites of subperiosteal resorption include the phalangeal tufts; medial aspect of the proximal ends of the tibia, humerus, and femur; superior and inferior margins of the ribs; and lamina dura. A distinctive pattern of acro-osteolysis may be seen in the terminal phalanges of the hands (and, less commonly, the feet), consisting of bandlike radiolucent areas that may separate the tuft and the base of the phalanx completely.

Subperiosteal resorption of bone also may be apparent at the margins of certain joints, accounting for one "articular" manifestation of hyperparathyroidism (Table 46–2; Fig. 46–3). Although this may be noted about the acromioclavicular, sternoclavicular, and sacroiliac joints and symphysis pubis, periarticular subperiosteal resorption may be especially prominent in the hand, wrist, and foot. The erosions that are created can simulate the appearance of rheumatoid arthritis, although they may be located slightly farther from the joint margin and are almost always associated with typical subperiosteal resorption of the adjacent phalangeal shafts. Although other forms of bone resorption are frequent in hyperparathyroidism, subperiosteal resorption is the most

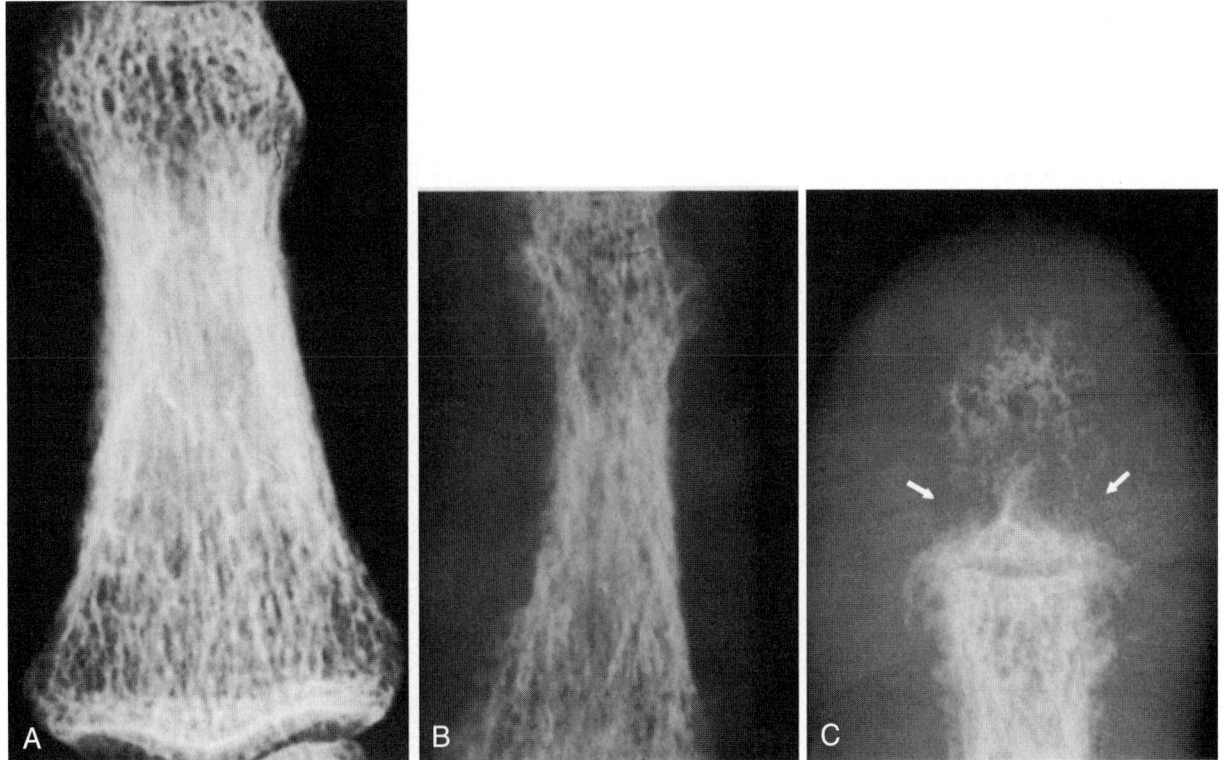

**Figure 46–1.** Hyperparathyroidism: subperiosteal bone resorption in the phalanges and phalangeal tufts. *A* and *B*, Phalanges. Mild *(A)* and severe *(B)* subperiosteal resorption. Early findings include lacelike bone resorption, particularly on the radial aspect of the middle phalanges. This pattern may progress to severe cortical destruction, with loss of definition between cortex and spongiosa. *C*, Phalangeal tufts. Severe tuftal resorption and osteolysis of the phalangeal waist *(arrows)* are seen.

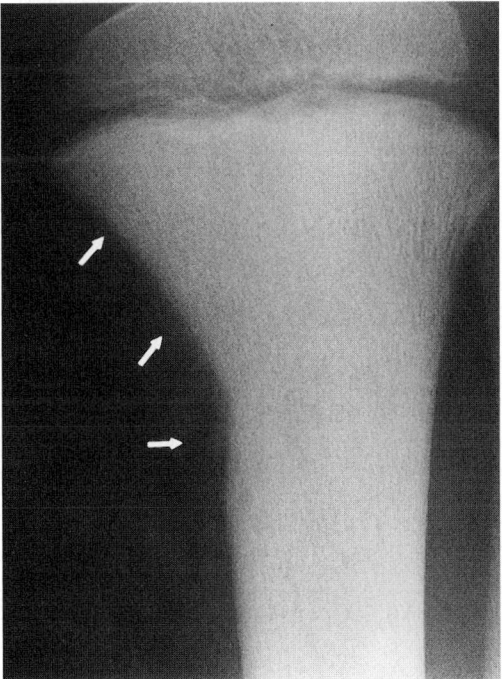

**Figure 46–2.** Hyperparathyroidism: subperiosteal bone resorption in the proximal portion of the tibia. Resorption is particularly prominent on the medial aspect of this bone *(arrows)*.

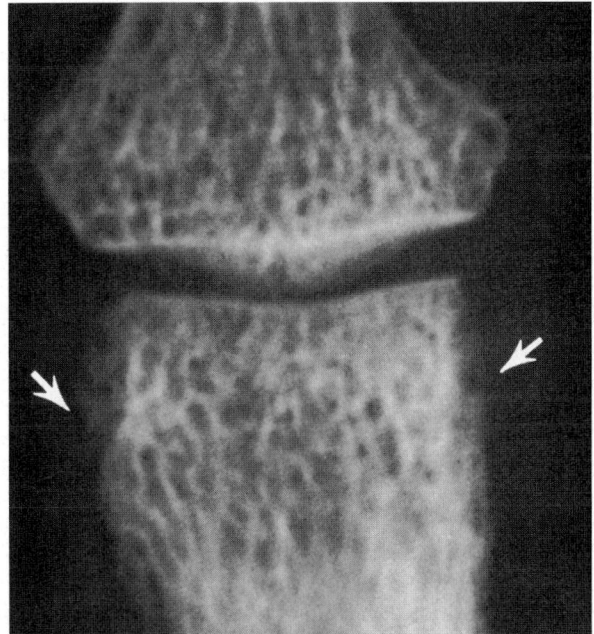

**Figure 46–3.** Hyperparathyroidism: subperiosteal bone resorption and juxta-articular erosions. At the distal interphalangeal joints, subperiosteal resorption at the corners of the joints *(arrows)* is continuous with intra-articular erosions, producing a squared appearance of the phalangeal bone.

**TABLE 46-2**

### Articular Manifestations of Hyperparathyroidism

| Mechanism | Characteristic Sites | Characteristic Appearance |
| --- | --- | --- |
| Subperiosteal bone resorption | Hands, wrists, feet | Marginal erosions with adjacent bone resorption and proliferation |
| Subchondral bone resorption | Sacroiliac, sternoclavicular, and acromioclavicular joints; symphysis pubis; discovertebral junction; large and small joint of the appendicular skeleton | Subchondral erosions, weakening, and collapse |
| Subligamentous and subtendinous bone resorption | Trochanters, ischial tuberosities, humeral tuberosities, calcanei, distal clavicles | Osseous erosion with reactive bone formation |
| CPPD crystal deposition | Knees, wrists, symphysis pubis | Chondrocalcinosis; pyrophosphate arthropathy (rare) |
| Urate crystal deposition | Various sites | Soft tissue swelling, osseous erosions |
| Tendon and ligament laxity | Sacroiliac and acromioclavicular joints, spine | Joint instability, soft tissue swelling, osseous erosion, dislocation, subluxation |
| Tendon avulsion and rupture | Quadriceps, patellar, triceps, flexor and extensor finger tendons | Subluxation and dislocation |

CPPD, calcium pyrophosphate dihydrate.

useful diagnostic sign, and changes in the phalanges are among the initial bony manifestations of the disease.

**Intracortical Bone Resorption.** Osteoclastic resorption of bone within cortical haversian canals can produce radiographically detectable intracortical linear striations (Fig. 46–4). These are best observed in the cortex of the second metacarpal bone. These findings can occur in other disorders with rapid bone turnover, such as acromegaly and hyperthyroidism. Intracortical resorption of bone is almost always associated with subperiosteal resorption.

**Endosteal Bone Resorption.** Osteoclastic resorption occurs along the endosteal surface of bone, particularly in the hands. Radiographic features include localized pocket-like or scalloped defects along the inner margin of the cortex, which are reminiscent of abnormalities occurring in multiple myeloma, and more generalized thinning of the cortex, which can simulate the appearance of osteoporosis.

**Subchondral Bone Resorption.** Subchondral resorption of bone is a common manifestation of hyperparathyroidism (Figs. 46–5 and 46–6). This type of resorption is most frequent in the joints of the axial skeleton at the sacroiliac, sternoclavicular, and acromioclavicular joints; symphysis pubis; and discovertebral junctions. Weakening and collapse of the osseous surface are apparent. Subchondral resorption in hyperparathyroidism at the sacroiliac joints leads to radiographic abnormalities that simulate those of ankylosing spondylitis, with osseous erosion and reactive new bone formation producing a poorly defined and sclerotic articular margin and "pseudo-widening" of the joint space. Subchondral resorption is also common at the acromioclavicular and sternoclavicular joints. The changes are usually symmetrical. Although resorption of the distal end of the clavicle is not a specific sign of hyperparathyroidism, it is helpful in making the diagnosis.

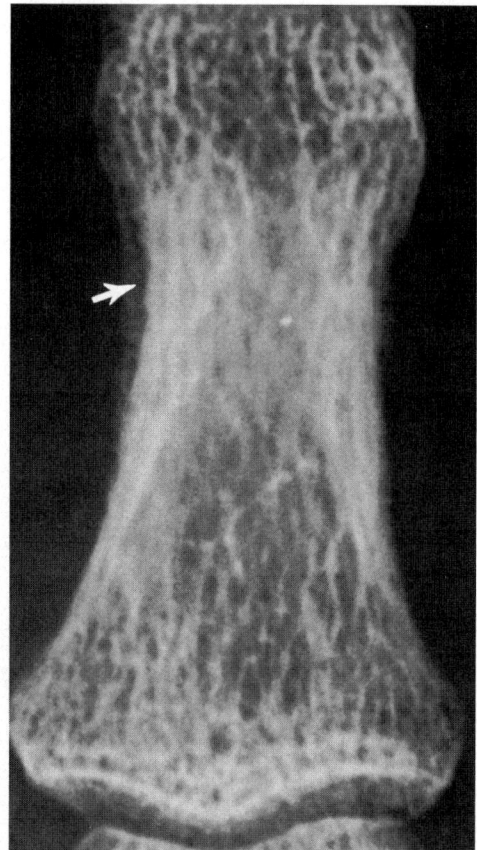

**Figure 46–4.** Hyperparathyroidism: intracortical bone resorption. Slightly exaggerated linear radiolucency of the phalangeal cortices can be observed (arrow).

**Subphyseal Bone Resorption.** In children with primary or secondary hyperparathyroidism, irregular radiolucent areas may appear in the metaphysis adjacent to the growth plate. This finding is reminiscent of the abnormalities accompanying rickets.

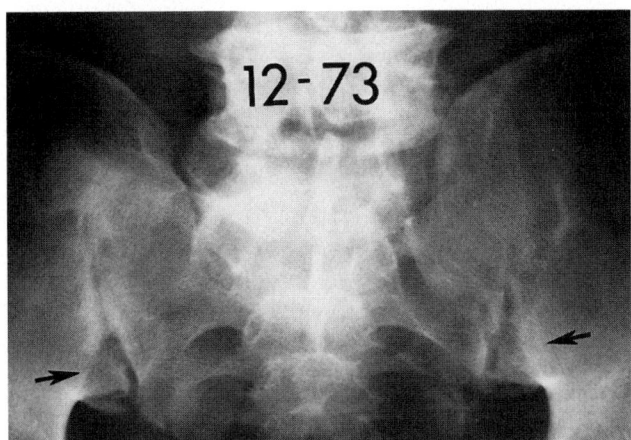

**Figure 46–5.** Hyperparathyroidism: subchondral bone resorption *(arrows)* about both sacroiliac joints. Observe the irregular osseous surface on the ilium and adjacent reactive sclerosis.

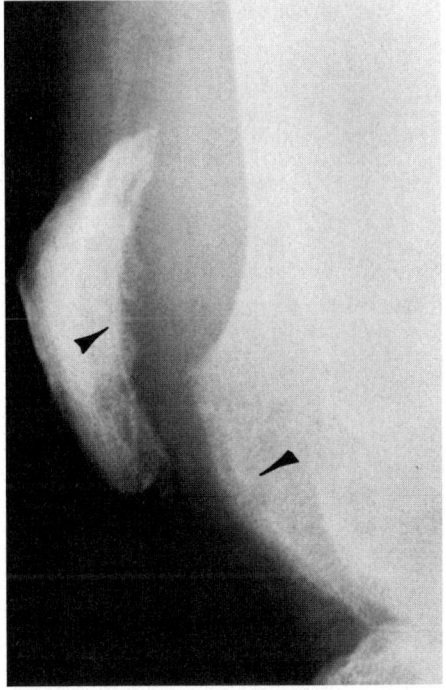

**Figure 46–6.** Hyperparathyroidism: subchondral bone resorption at the patellofemoral joint. There is considerable erosion, with deformity of the posterior surface of the patella and resorption on the anterior surface of the femur *(arrowheads)*. An effusion is present. (Courtesy of R. Shapiro, MD, and K. Weisner, MD, Sacramento, Calif.)

**Trabecular Bone Resorption.** Trabecular resorption within medullary bone occurs throughout the skeleton in hyperparathyroidism, particularly in advanced stages of the disease (Fig. 46–7). Within the cranium it can be especially striking, giving the diploë a speckled appearance, which is termed the "salt and pepper" skull.

**Subligamentous and Subtendinous Bone Resorption.** Osseous resorption occurs at sites of tendon and ligament attachment to bone (Fig. 46–8). This is particularly

frequent at the femoral trochanters, ischial and humeral tuberosities, elbow, inferior surface of the calcaneus, and inferior aspect of the distal end of the clavicle.

**Brown Tumors.** Brown tumors were initially described as being characteristic of primary hyperparathyroidism, but more recently they have been noted with increasing frequency in secondary hyperparathyroidism as well (Fig. 46–9). Brown tumors represent localized accumulations of fibrous tissue and giant cells, which can replace bone and may even produce osseous expansion. They may subsequently undergo necrosis and liquefaction, producing cysts. Brown tumors appear as single or multiple

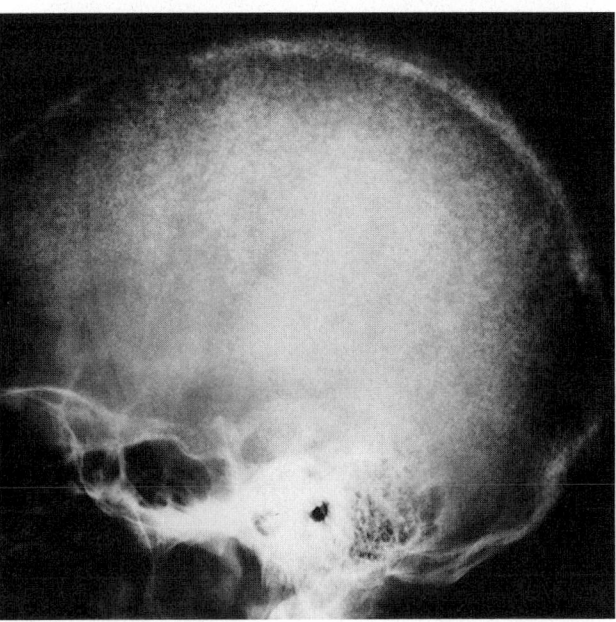

**Figure 46–7.** Hyperparathyroidism: trabecular bone resorption in the cranial vault. Lateral radiograph outlines the characteristic mottling of the vault. Alternating areas of lucency and sclerosis produce the "salt and pepper" appearance.

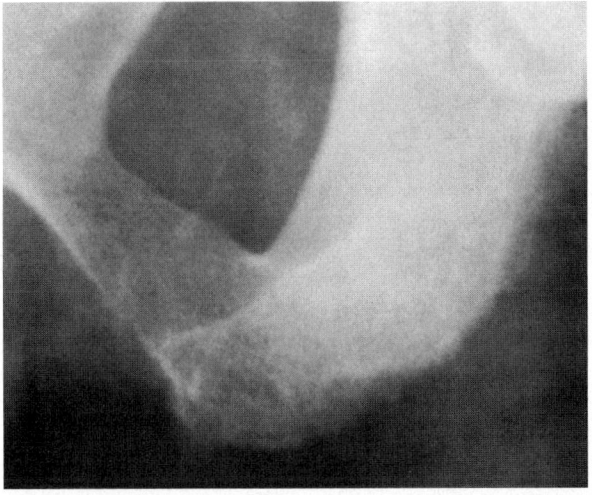

**Figure 46–8.** Hyperparathyroidism: subligamentous and subtendinous bone resorption in the ischial tuberosity. Erosion of bone has produced a poorly defined, irregular osseous surface.

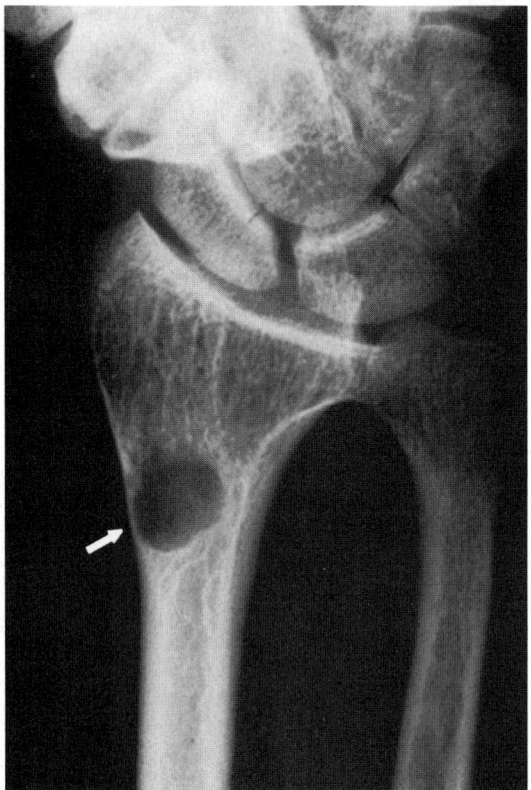

**Figure 46–9.** Hyperparathyroidism: brown tumor *(arrow)* in the distal portion of the radius. Brown tumors can be single or multiple, well demarcated or poorly defined, and eccentric or central in location.

well-defined lesions of the axial or appendicular skeleton, frequently eccentric or cortical in location. Common sites of involvement are the facial bones, pelvis, ribs, and femora. Other manifestations of hyperparathyroidism are generally apparent.

## Bone Sclerosis

Bone sclerosis is observed far more frequently in patients with renal osteodystrophy and secondary hyperparathyroidism, although it may be apparent in primary hyperparathyroidism as well. In patients with primary hyperparathyroidism, bone sclerosis may be localized or patchy, apparent in the metaphyseal regions of the long bones, the skull, or the vertebral endplates. In the spine, bone deposition in the subchondral areas of the vertebral bodies results in the appearance of radiodense bands across the superior and inferior margins (rugger-jersey spine). This manifestation, too, is much more frequent in secondary than in primary hyperparathyroidism. Diffuse bone sclerosis is rarely noted in primary hyperparathyroidism. The mechanism of bone sclerosis in hyperparathyroidism has not been clearly defined.

## Chondrocalcinosis (Calcium Pyrophosphate Dihydrate Crystal Deposition)

The association of primary hyperparathyroidism and calcium pyrophosphate dihydrate (CPPD) crystal deposi-

tion is well known. CPPD crystal deposition may also occur in chronic renal disease, although its frequency is much lower than in primary hyperparathyroidism. Radiographic evidence of such crystal deposition has been reported in 18% to 40% of patients with hyperparathyroidism.

## Additional Rheumatic Manifestations

In addition to subchondral osseous resorption leading to collapse and fragmentation of bone, subperiosteal osseous resorption leading to periarticular erosions, subligamentous and subtendinous osseous resorption, and CPPD crystal deposition, other rheumatic manifestations of hyperparathyroidism may be encountered (Fig. 46–10). Parathyroid hormone may affect ligaments and tendons themselves, with resultant capsular and ligamentous laxity, as well as rupture. It may contribute to joint instability, traumatic synovitis, and cartilaginous and osseous destruction. The acromioclavicular and sacroiliac joints may be particularly vulnerable because of their dependence on soft tissues for support.

Monosodium urate crystals and clinical gout have been described in patients with hyperparathyroidism.

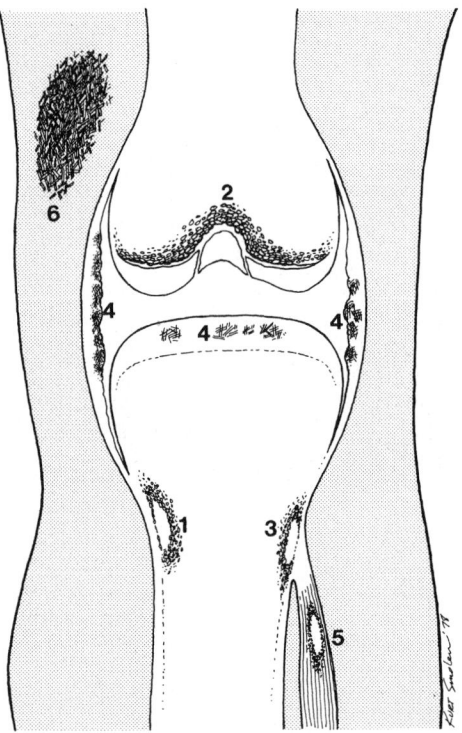

**Figure 46–10.** Rheumatic manifestations of hyperparathyroidism (and renal osteodystrophy). Findings may be related to subperiosteal resorption at the margins of the joint (1); subchondral resorption leading to cartilage and bone disintegration and fragmentation (2); subligamentous and subtendinous resorption (3); intra-articular crystal (calcium pyrophosphate dihydrate, monosodium urate) deposition in cartilage, synovium, and capsule (4); tendinous and ligamentous injury and rupture (5); and periarticular crystal (monosodium urate, calcium hydroxyapatite) deposition in soft tissues (6).

## Hyperparathyroidism in Infants and Children

Primary hyperparathyroidism may be evident in infants and children. Congenital primary hyperparathyroidism is a rare disorder that occurs in infants and demonstrates autosomal recessive inheritance. Symptoms and signs include hypotonicity, respiratory distress, fever, dehydration, constipation, anorexia, lethargy, vomiting, dysphagia, craniotabes, and hepatosplenomegaly. Hypercalcemia is generally but not universally present. Radiographs may reveal severe bone disease with extensive bone resorption. The degree of periostitis may be so severe as to simulate the findings of syphilis. Unless parathyroidectomy is performed, the infants usually die.

A second disorder, transient hyperparathyroidism of the neonate, occurs secondary to hypoparathyroidism in the mother. The radiographic changes are similar to those of congenital primary hyperparathyroidism, although they resolve rapidly.

In older children, skeletal involvement in hyperparathyroidism is characterized by osteopenia, genu valgum, fractures, cystic lesions of bone, and clubbing of the fingers. Renal involvement and rickets-like changes with metaphyseal irregularity may be observed.

## Familial Hypercalcemia

Specific and distinct syndromes of familial hypercalcemia have been identified, including several types of disorders accompanied by tumors of multiple endocrine glands and familial hypocalciuric hypercalcemia (Table 46–3).

Familial multiple endocrine neoplasia (MEN) syndrome type I, which is also referred to as multiple endocrine adenomatosis and Wermer's syndrome, is an autosomal dominant disease associated with primary hyperparathyroidism (95% of cases) and, less frequently, with excessive secretion of gastrin (20% to 40% of cases), insulin (2% to 10% of cases), other pancreatic islet peptides (rare), and anterior pituitary peptides (rare). Nonsecretory neoplastic masses, including lipomas, pituitary chromophobe adenomas (30% to 65% of cases), carcinoid tumors, and adrenal and thyroid adenomas, also occur but rarely metastasize. MEN syndrome type I generally manifests in the third, fourth, or fifth decade

of life. Clinical manifestations are variable but include those related to renal calculi. Hypercalcemia usually is not severe.

Familial MEN type IIA, also called Sipple's syndrome, is inherited as an autosomal dominant trait with very high penetrance for medullary thyroid carcinoma in adults. Abnormalities of other endocrine glands, particularly primary parathyroid hyperplasia and pheochromocytoma, occur in approximately one third of cases, but malignant change related to these other endocrine aberrations is rare.

Familial hypocalciuric hypercalcemia, also called familial benign hypercalcemia, is a rare disorder of unknown cause characterized by autosomal dominant inheritance with high penetrance for expression of hypercalcemia at all ages. The syndrome is associated with lifelong hypercalcemia, low urinary calcium excretion, the absence of prominent symptoms and signs, and the failure of subtotal parathyroidectomy to decrease plasma calcium levels. Superficially, familial hypocalciuric hypercalcemia resembles asymptomatic primary hyperparathyroidism; in the former condition, however, there is no significant reduction of bone mass in the axial or appendicular skeleton, and the prevalence of fractures is not increased.

## Differential Diagnosis

Subperiosteal bone resorption is the most helpful diagnostic clue of hyperparathyroidism on radiographs. Widespread subperiosteal resorption is confined to hyperparathyroid bone disease. Focal areas of subperiosteal bone resorption may be seen in cases of tumor, infection, and even articular disorders, but the resulting contour defects in these cases are much better defined than the defects in hyperparathyroidism. Intracortical bone resorption may be noted in disease states characterized by rapid bone turnover, such as hyperthyroidism and acromegaly, whereas endosteal bone resorption can be produced by osteoporosis or marrow-containing disorders, such as multiple myeloma. The severely depressed and fragmented subchondral bone surface that may accompany hyperparathyroidism can simulate the find-

---

**TABLE 46–3**

### Major Features in Syndromes of Familial Hypercalcemia

| Feature | Multiple Endocrine Neoplasia Type I | Multiple Endocrine Neoplasia Type II* | Hypocalciuric Hypercalcemia |
|---|---|---|---|
| Inheritance | Autosomal dominant | Autosomal dominant | Autosomal dominant |
| Penetrance of hypercalcemia, first decade | Low | Low | High |
| Associated endocrinopathy | Islet cell; anterior pituitary | Medullary thyroid cancer; pheochromocytoma | None |
| Unique biochemical features | Hypergastrinemia | Hypercalcitoninemia | Relative hypocalciuria |
| Subtotal parathyroidectomy | Useful | Useful | Usually no benefit |

*Multiple endocrine neoplasia type IIB rarely has hypercalcemia or hyperparathyroidism.

From Aurbach GD, Marx SJ, Spiegel AM: Parathyroid hormone, calcitonin, and the calciferols. In Williams RH (ed): Textbook of Endocrinology; 7th edn. Philadelphia, WB Saunders, 1985, p 1176.

ings of septic arthritis, osteonecrosis, or crystal-induced arthropathy.

In the interphalangeal joints of the hand, the findings may resemble inflammatory osteoarthritis, psoriasis, or even rheumatoid arthritis; in the sacroiliac articulations and symphysis pubis, the differential diagnosis includes ankylosing spondylitis and other seronegative spondyloarthropathies; in the acromioclavicular and sternoclavicular joints, hyperparathyroid subchondral bone resorption may simulate the changes of rheumatoid arthritis or ankylosing spondylitis; in the patellofemoral joints, the appearance is almost identical to that in Wilson's disease and CPPD crystal deposition disease; and at the discovertebral junction, hyperparathyroidism with subchondral resorption resembles infection, neuropathic osteoarthropathy, or degenerative disc disease. Subligamentous bone resorption in hyperparathyroidism may produce a radiographic appearance that simulates the changes seen in ankylosing spondylitis and other seronegative spondyloarthropathies. Localized areas of osseous resorption (brown tumors) in hyperparathyroidism resemble a variety of neoplastic or neoplastic-like diseases, particularly giant cell tumor and fibrous dysplasia.

The rugger-jersey spine is a relatively specific finding of secondary hyperparathyroidism, although a similar vertebral sclerosis may occur in Paget's disease (leading to the "picture frame" vertebral body), osteopetrosis, osteomesopyknosis, and osteoporosis. Diffuse bone sclerosis, which is also more frequent in secondary hyperparathyroidism, is seen in many other conditions, including myelofibrosis, fluorosis, mastocytosis, anemia (particularly sickle cell anemia), neoplasm (especially metastasis), irradiation, hypoparathyroidism, sarcoidosis, and Paget's disease.

The CPPD crystal deposition in primary and (less commonly) secondary hyperparathyroidism is identical to that occurring in idiopathic CPPD crystal deposition disease and hemochromatosis. Any patient with chondrocalcinosis should be evaluated for the presence of hyperparathyroidism. Monosodium urate crystal deposition in hyperparathyroidism leads to secondary gout, which resembles primary gout.

In infants and children, periostitis and extensive bone resorption in hyperparathyroidism may simulate the findings of syphilis or leukemia, whereas metaphyseal destruction in the long bones in hyperparathyroidism produces a radiographic picture identical to that of rickets.

## RENAL OSTEODYSTROPHY

### Background and General Features

In the presence of chronic renal insufficiency, the parathyroid glands undergo hyperplasia. This effect is generally attributable to phosphate retention and consequent lowering of the serum calcium level. Secondary hyperparathyroidism, which is a complication of chronic renal disease, is also seen in other conditions, such as malabsorption states, osteomalacia, and pseudohypoparathyroidism. It is merely one of the skeletal changes that occur in patients with chronic renal disease. Because normal kidney function is fundamental to the proper metabolism of vitamin D, renal diseases can lead to rickets and osteomalacia.

Renal osteodystrophy is a term applied to the bone disease that is apparent in patients with chronic renal failure. Osseous abnormalities of renal osteodystrophy have been well outlined and can be divided into hyperparathyroidism, rickets and osteomalacia, osteoporosis, fractures, soft tissue and vascular calcification, and miscellaneous alterations.

## Hyperparathyroidism

The abnormalities associated with hyperparathyroidism may become manifest in patients with renal osteodystrophy, including subperiosteal, intracortical, endosteal, trabecular, subchondral, and subligamentous and subtendinous bone resorption; brown tumors; bone sclerosis; and chondrocalcinosis. The frequency of some of these findings is different in renal osteodystrophy with secondary hyperparathyroidism than in primary hyperparathyroidism (Table 46-4). Modern techniques allow the diagnosis of primary hyperparathyroidism at an early stage, when bone abnormalities are not extensive; therefore, many of the osseous changes originally believed to be more frequent in primary than in secondary hyperparathyroidism are now found to be more typical of the latter.

The reported frequency of brown tumors in association with renal osteodystrophy and secondary hyperparathyroidism is lower than that in primary hyperparathyroidism. Osteosclerosis is a well-known feature of renal osteodystrophy (Fig. 46-11). It predominates in the axial skeleton, with involvement of the pelvis, ribs, and superior and inferior portions of the vertebral bodies (rugger-jersey spine), although the appendicular skeleton (Fig. 46-12) may also be involved, particularly the metaphyseal regions of long bones. Chondrocalcinosis due to CPPD crystal deposition is much more frequent in primary hyperparathyroidism than in renal osteodystrophy.

Periosteal neostosis is a term applied to periosteal bone formation in patients with renal osteodystrophy (Fig. 46-13). Its frequency is estimated to be 8% to 25% in such patients, and it is more frequent in those with severe skeletal abnormalities. Periosteal neostosis is

---

**TABLE 46-4**

**Primary versus Secondary Hyperparathyroidism**

| Findings | Primary Hyperparathyroidism | Secondary Hyperparathyroidism* |
|---|---|---|
| Brown tumors | Common | Less common |
| Osteosclerosis | Rare | Common |
| Chrondrocalcinosis | Not infrequent | Rare |
| Periostitis | Rare | Not infrequent |

*Additional findings of renal osteodystrophy are observed in association with secondary hyperparathyroidism, including rickets, osteomalacia, and soft tissue and vascular calcification.

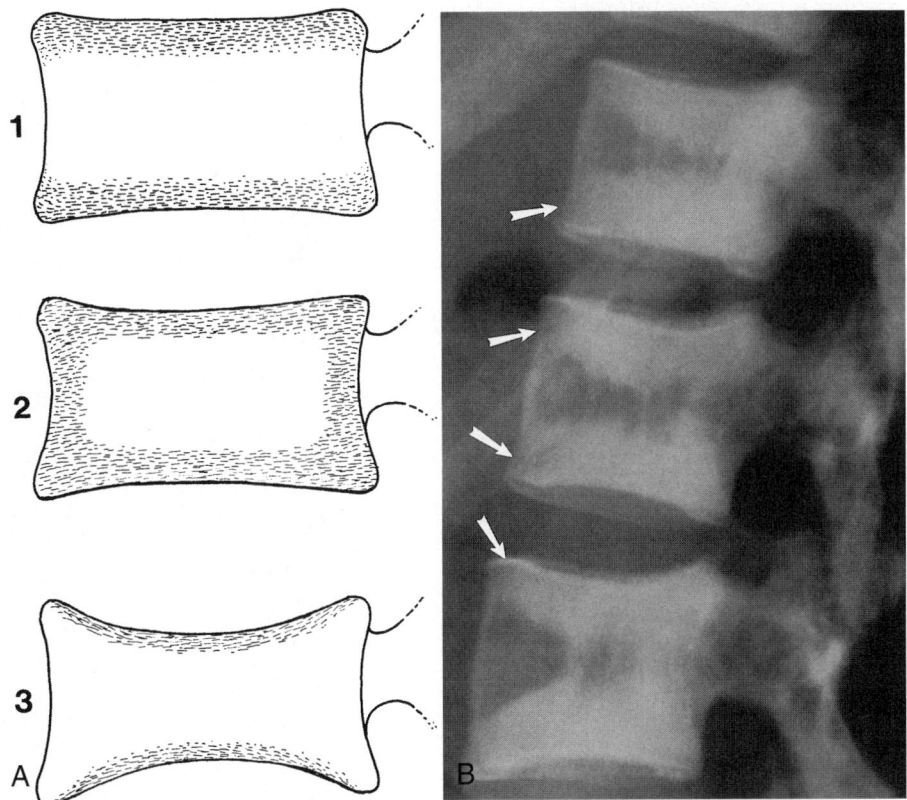

**Figure 46–11.** Renal osteodystrophy: osteosclerosis of vertebral bodies. *A*, Vertebral osteosclerosis in renal osteodystrophy is characterized by bandlike sclerosis on the superior and inferior surfaces of the vertebral body (1), an appearance that is termed the rugger-jersey spine. In Paget's disease (2), sclerosis around the entire vertebral body resembles a picture frame. In osteoporosis (3), particularly that associated with steroid excess, biconcave vertebral bodies (fish vertebrae) may be associated with condensation of bone. *B*, Rugger-jersey spine. Condensation of bone in the superior and inferior margins of the vertebral bodies *(arrows)* is not associated with osseous collapse.

observed most commonly in the metatarsals, femur, and pelvis, particularly the pubic rami, although it may be visualized elsewhere.

## Rickets and Osteomalacia

The cause of the osteomalacia seen in chronic renal disease before dialysis treatment is probably complex. The kidney is essential in the further hydroxylation of 25-hydroxycholecalciferol to 1,25-dihydroxycholecalciferol, which is an active metabolite of vitamin D, and the absence of this metabolite in patients with chronic renal disease can lead to abnormality of bone. Further, patients with renal failure have malabsorption of calcium from the gut, which can also contribute to bone disease. Osteomalacia may also be related to vitamin D deficiency as well as resistance, with the deficiency occurring as a result of anorexia and inadequate diet, the increased requirement of hyperparathyroid bone, and abnormality of the hepatic enzyme system.

The radiographic features of osteomalacia in chronic renal disease include osteopenia, bone deformities, and Looser's zones. The latter abnormalities are narrow radiolucent bands, frequently symmetrical and oriented perpendicular to the osseous surface (Fig. 46–14).

Looser's zones are most common in the pubic rami, ilia, ribs, femoral necks, scapulae, and long bones and are observed in 1% of patients with chronic renal disease. Radiographic features consistent with rickets include osteopenia, irregularity and widening of the growth plate, and poor definition of the epiphysis (Fig. 46–15).

Slipped epiphyses have been described in approximately 10% of children with chronic renal disease. The capital femoral epiphysis is the most common site of involvement by far, although similar changes may be seen at other skeletal locations, including the proximal end of the humerus; the distal portion of the radius, ulna, or femur; and, rarely, the small bones of the hands and feet. Bilateral involvement is frequent. Three radiographic signs may precede slipping of the capital femoral epiphysis in renal osteodystrophy: bilateral subperiosteal erosion on the medial aspect of the femoral neck, increase in width of the cartilaginous growth plate, and bilateral coxa vara (see Fig. 46–15).

## Osteoporosis

A diminution of bone volume occurs in renal osteodystrophy. On radiographs, decreased bone density, or osteopenia, is evident, although the diminished radio-

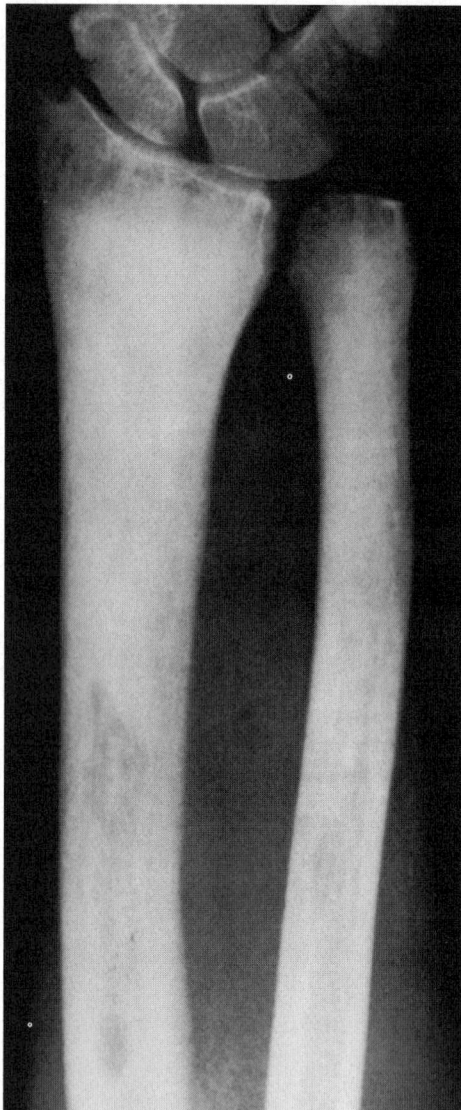

**Figure 46–12.** Renal osteodystrophy: osteosclerosis in the appendicular skeleton. Note osteosclerosis of the diaphyses and metaphyses of the radius and ulna. (Courtesy of L. Cooperstein, MD, Pittsburgh, Pa.)

density is due not only to osteoporosis but also to osteitis fibrosa cystica and osteomalacia.

## Fractures

Pathologic fractures are a recognized complication of renal osteodystrophy. Potential causes of such fractures include hyperparathyroidism itself, osteomalacia, osteoporosis, and aluminum intoxication. In the spine, vertebral compression in association with a rugger-jersey appearance is commonly encountered. Fractures in regions of brown tumors are also characteristic. Insufficiency fractures, which in some cases represent Looser's zones of osteomalacia, are seen in patients with renal osteodystrophy. The medial aspect of the femoral neck is an important and common site of such insufficiency fractures, with bilateral involvement reported in as many as 50% of patients.

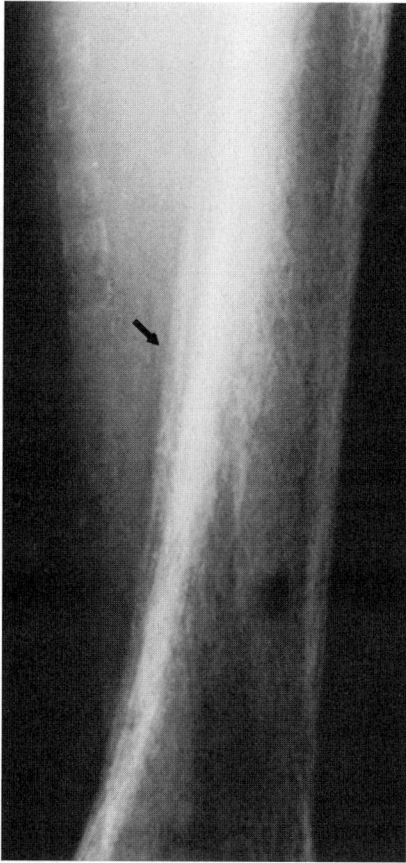

**Figure 46–13.** Renal osteodystrophy: periosteal neostosis. Frontal radiograph of the femur in a patient with renal osteodystrophy outlines laminated periosteal new bone formation (*arrow*). Vascular calcification and bony abnormalities are present.

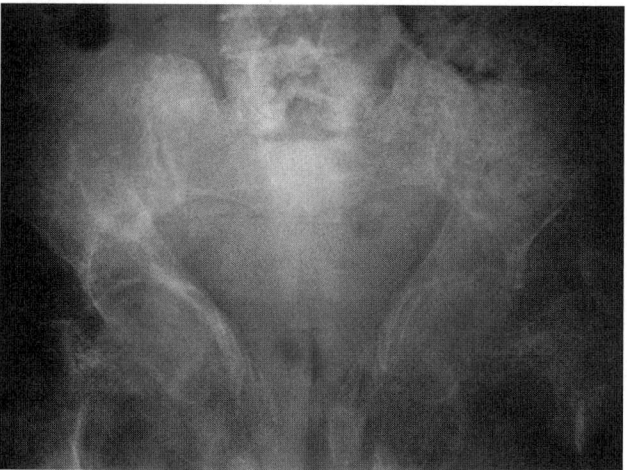

**Figure 46–14.** Renal osteodystrophy: osteomalacia. Observe the bony deformities of the pelvis. Acetabular protrusion, coxa vara, and bowing of the radius, ulna, tibia, and fibula are seen. Trabecular detail is virtually absent.

## Soft Tissue and Vascular Calcification

Although calcification may be observed in the soft tissues and vessels of patients with primary hyperparathyroidism, it is much more frequent in patients with renal osteodystrophy. In patients with chronic renal failure,

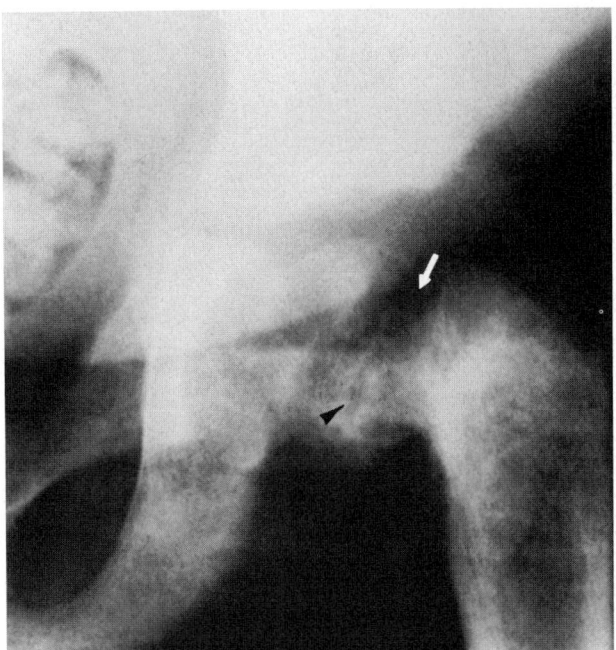

**Figure 46–15.** Renal osteodystrophy: rickets. Note metaphyseal irregularity and resorption *(arrow)*, with surrounding sclerosis and severe coxa vara. The growth plate *(arrowhead)* is oriented in a vertical position, which may predispose to epiphyseal slipping.

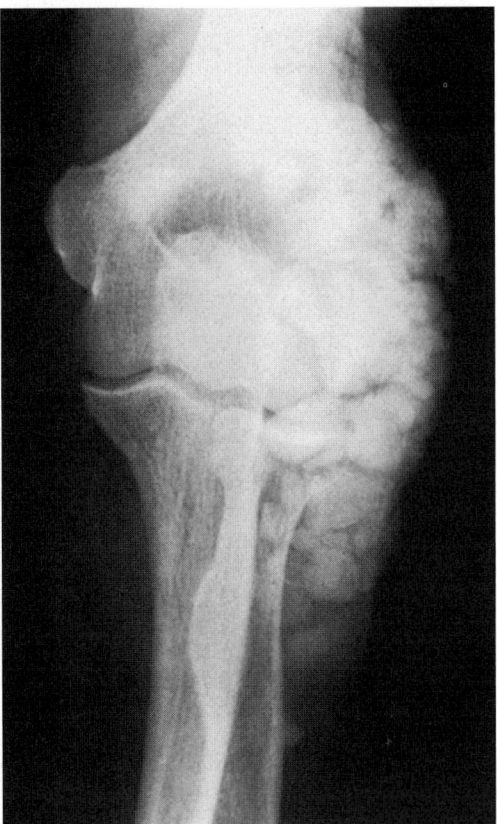

**Figure 46–16.** Renal osteodystrophy: soft tissue calcification. Extensive "tumoral" calcification is apparent in the periarticular regions of the elbow.

soft tissue calcification occurs when multiplication of the respective concentrations (in mg/dL) of plasma calcium and plasma phosphorus produces a value greater than 70. Soft tissue deposits can occur in multiple sites, including corneal and conjunctival tissue, viscera, vasculature, and subcutaneous and periarticular tissue (Fig. 46–16). The deposits may occur in patients with chronic uremia who have not been treated, although they appear to be more frequent and extensive in uremic patients who have undergone hemodialysis or renal transplantation. Periarticular deposits may reach considerable size and produce striking patchy or tumoral radiodense areas, particularly in the hips, knees, shoulders, and wrists. Bilateral symmetrical deposits about multiple joints are not uncommon.

Vascular collections involve not only the heart and great vessels but also the peripheral arteries, especially the dorsalis pedis artery of the foot.

## Miscellaneous Abnormalities

Patients with chronic renal insufficiency have hyperuricemia and may develop secondary gout. Radiographic features resemble those of primary gout, although in secondary gout, atypical articular sites may be affected. Oxalosis of bone may develop as a rare secondary manifestation of chronic renal failure.

## Musculoskeletal Abnormalities after Hemodialysis

In the vast majority of patients with chronic renal failure who are placed on maintenance hemodialysis, many of the bone changes of renal osteodystrophy resolve, provided that the hemodialysis is of adequate quality and duration (Table 46–5; Fig. 46–17). In poorly managed patients on dialysis, increasing osteopenia may be observed in association with spontaneous fractures. These fractures are most frequent in the ribs, although they may occur at other sites, including the femoral necks, vertebrae, pubic rami, tibias, and metatarsals.

**Aluminum Intoxication.** It is generally believed that the primary cause of the progression of skeletal abnormalities in patients on chronic hemodialysis is osteomalacia due to aluminum intoxication (Fig. 46–18). Clinical characteristics of this syndrome include bone pain, myopathy, fracture, and dialysis encephalopathy accompanied by dementia, speech disorders, seizures, and dyspraxia. Fractures of the ribs and proximal portion of the femora are characteristic, although the spine and other tubular bones are also affected. High aluminum levels in tissues, including the brain and bone as well as various articular structures, support the speculation that aluminum toxicity is involved in this syndrome. The source of the aluminum is related to the contents of phosphate-binding gels or the ambient water or dialysate. Aluminum-induced changes, however, have been documented in patients with chronic renal disease who have not undergone dialysis, and in such cases, considerable evidence exists that aluminum is absorbed from the orally administered aluminum-containing phosphate-binding

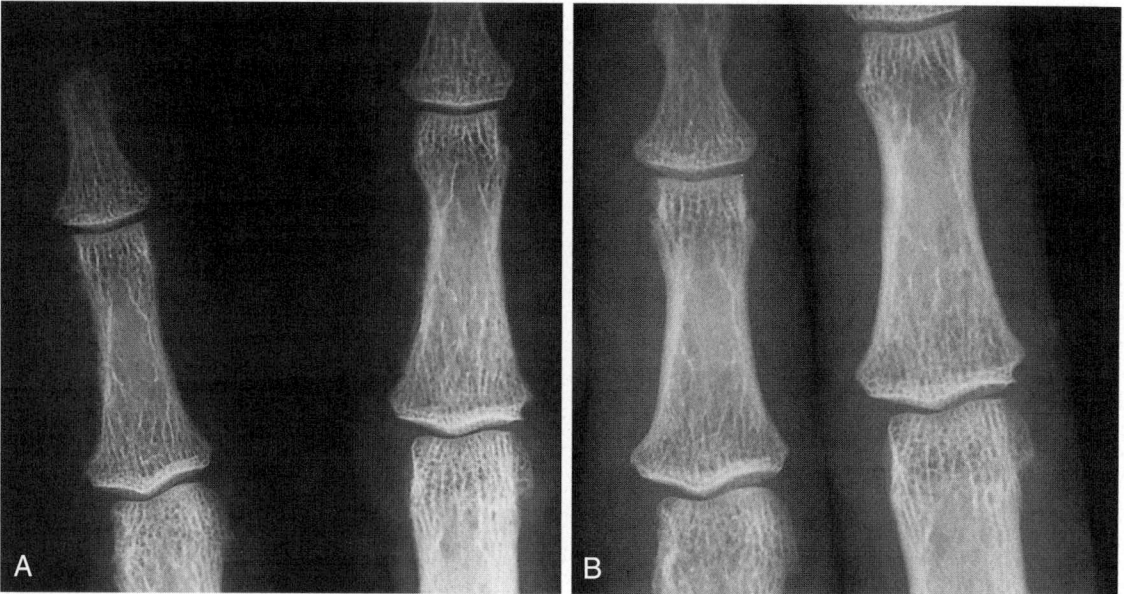

**Figure 46–17.** Renal osteodystrophy: resolution of skeletal abnormalities during hemodialysis. In this 38-year-old man on maintenance hemodialysis, radiographs obtained at presentation (*A*) and after 4 years (*B*) show significant improvement in osseous abnormalities following treatment.

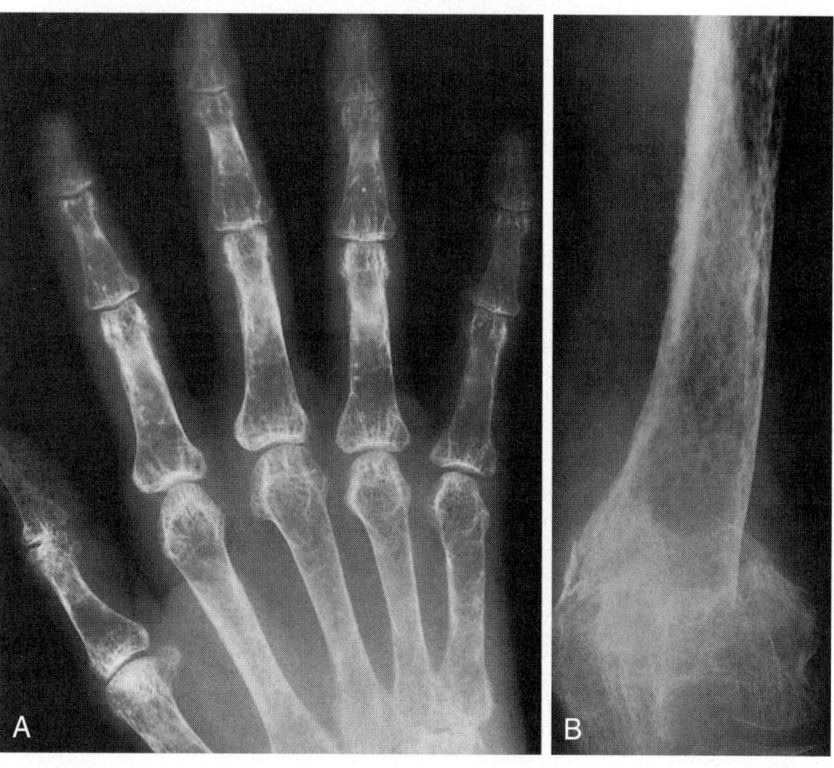

**Figure 46–18.** Renal osteodystrophy: aluminum intoxication during hemodialysis. *A*, Radiograph of the hand reveals marked osteopenia, with indistinctness of the cortical margins and trabeculae. *B*, Radiograph of the lower femur shows osteopenia, cortical tunneling, and a supracondylar fracture with insignificant callus formation 1 year after injury. (From Llewellyn CH, Resnick CS, Brower AC: Case report 288: Osteomalacia and secondary hyperparathyroidism (dialysis-induced), with aluminum deposition. Skeletal Radiol 12:223, 1984.)

medications prescribed for patients with renal failure. Reversal of the findings follows removal of the source of aluminum contamination.

**Soft Tissue and Vascular Calcification.** Soft tissue and vascular calcification is frequent in patients undergoing hemodialysis. Reversal of periarticular and, less commonly, vascular calcification may be seen during dialysis.

Progression of such calcification, however, is a more typical finding.

**Musculoskeletal Infection.** Septicemia, osteomyelitis, and septic arthritis are well-recognized complications of hemodialysis. External or internal arteriovenous fistulas provide an ideal site of entry for infectious organisms. In addition, impaired host resistance related to the presence of a chronic debilitating illness and the use of immuno-suppressive agents and adrenal steroids increase the risk of infection in these persons. Osteomyelitis and septic arthritis may occur at any site.

**Osteonecrosis.** Ischemic necrosis of bone may complicate the administration of steroids in patients with chronic renal disease undergoing dialysis. This same complication is well recognized after renal transplantation. Affected sites include the femoral and humeral heads and the talus.

**Destructive Spondyloarthropathy.** A peculiar pattern of spondyloarthropathy has been identified in 5% to 23% of patients with chronic renal disease who are undergoing hemodialysis. Middle-aged or elderly patients who have been hemodialyzed for several years are affected; it is extremely rare in persons whose dialysis treatment has been ongoing for less than 2 or 3 years. The most common site of involvement is the cervical spine (approximately 70% of cases), followed by the lumbar spine (20%) and thoracic spine (10%). Single or multiple spinal levels reveal rapidly progressive radiographic abnormalities characterized by loss of intervertebral disc space, erosion of subchondral bone in the neighboring vertebral bodies, and new bone formation (Fig. 46–19). The findings resemble infection, neuropathic osteoarthropathy, severe intervertebral (osteo)chondrosis, or CPPD crystal deposition disease. Although the precise cause of the

spinal abnormalities has been debated, accumulating data underscore the importance of amyloid deposition in regions of spinal destruction. Amyloid masses, composed of beta$_2$-microglobulins, have been documented repeatedly, not only in the vertebral column but also in other skeletal and extraskeletal sites in patients undergoing chronic hemodialysis.

**Carpal Tunnel Syndrome.** Carpal tunnel syndrome is well recognized in patients receiving hemodialysis and is usually attributed to alterations in vascular hemodynamics at the access site, resulting in edema, venous distention, and secondary compression of the median nerve within the carpal canal. The rate of occurrence of these abnormalities is directly related to the length of dialysis. Currently, amyloid is also considered an important cause of carpal tunnel syndrome in hemodialyzed patients. Amyloid accumulation also occurs in the accompanying small cystic lesions in the carpal bones (Fig. 46–20).

**Amyloid Deposition.** Amyloid accumulation in osseous and articular structures is a prominent feature of hemodialysis in patients with chronic renal disease. Periarticular soft tissue prominence, intraosseous and subchondral bone destruction, pathologic fracture, and carpal tunnel syndrome are characteristic clinical and radiographic features of amyloid accumulation. The variety of amyloid in this clinical setting is a beta$_2$-microglobulin. Such amyloid deposition must be considered one important factor, in addition to hyperparathyroidism, aluminum intoxication, and crystalline and iron accumulation, in the pathogenesis of the musculoskeletal manifestations of hemodialysis.

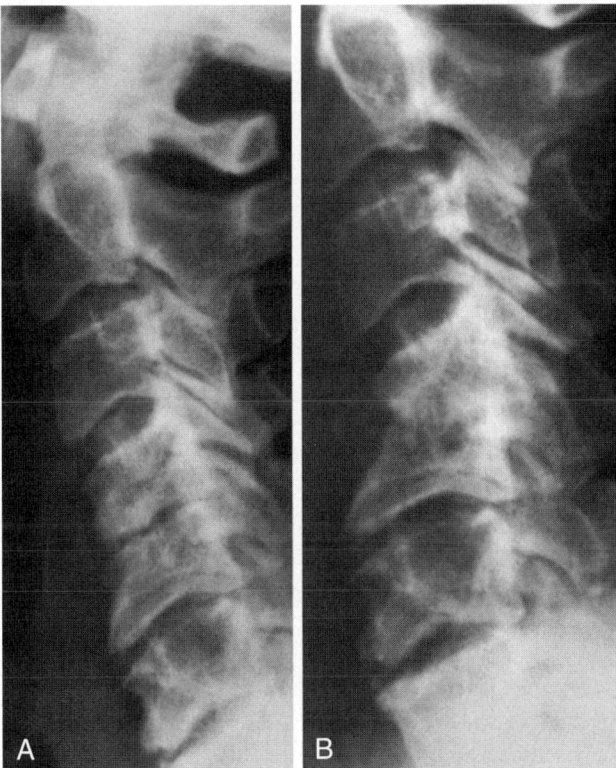

**Figure 46–19.** Renal osteodystrophy: spondyloarthropathy during hemodialysis. *A* and *B*, Radiographs obtained 7 months apart show progressive destruction of the C4–C5 intervertebral disc and both adjacent vertebral bodies. An osteolytic lesion in C6 is also evident.

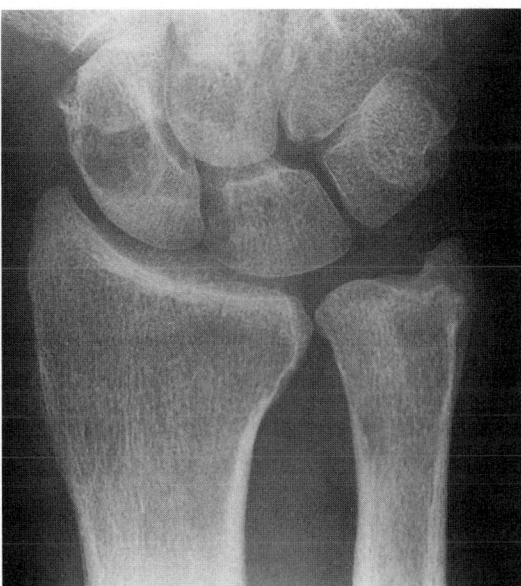

**Figure 46–20.** Renal osteodystrophy: carpal tunnel syndrome and amyloid deposition during hemodialysis. Observe soft tissue swelling and cystic lesions in the scaphoid, lunate, capitate, and ulna. During carpal tunnel release, a biopsy of the synovium and distal portion of the ulna revealed tissue that demonstrated chronic synovitis with amyloid deposition in both the synovium and the bone.

The accumulation of beta$_2$-microglobulin in patients undergoing hemodialysis appears to affect predominantly the musculoskeletal system, and the prevalence of such amyloid deposition increases progressively with the duration of dialysis therapy. Amyloid deposition may lead to arthralgias and arthropathies, especially in the shoulder, but also in the hip, wrist, and other joints; amyloidomas in periarticular bone may produce radiolucent lesions of variable size that may fracture, particularly in the femoral neck and vertebra, but in additional sites as well; amyloid accumulation in soft tissues may produce neurovascular compromise, most evident about the wrist; and masses of amyloid may extend from affected vertebral bodies and intervertebral discs into the spinal canal, leading to significant neurologic compromise. Amyloid deposition in soft tissue, joint capsule, and synovium may lead to prominent periarticular masses about the shoulder, sternoclavicular joint, knee, hip, wrist, and other sites (Fig. 46–21).

Magnetic resonance (MR) imaging has been used to investigate dialysis-related arthropathy and generally reveals that subchondral intraosseous collections of amyloid communicate with the articular surface. Reported signal characteristics of dialysis-related arthropathy are not uniform; however, regions of low signal intensity corresponding to sites of amyloid accumulation on both T1- and T2-weighted spin echo MR images are most typical.

## Musculoskeletal Abnormalities after Peritoneal Dialysis

Bone disease and soft tissue calcification have also been observed in uremic patients undergoing peritoneal dialysis. Some investigators suggest that the osseous and soft tissue changes are less frequent and less severe with this therapeutic technique than with hemodialysis, but others have not found this to be true. Deposition of beta$_2$-microglobulin amyloid has been documented in patients with chronic renal disease receiving long-term peritoneal dialysis. Although there are theoretical reasons why this form of dialysis might lead to such deposition less frequently than hemodialysis does, the known occurrence of arthralgias, destructive arthropathy and spondyloarthropathy, intraosseous lytic lesions, and carpal tunnel syndrome in association with chronic peritoneal dialysis appears to underscore the importance of amyloidosis as a complication of this form of therapy as well.

## Musculoskeletal Abnormalities after Renal Transplantation

After transplantation, normal renal function is restored; the nature and progress of bone disease depend on the state of the bones at the time of transplantation. The occurrence of osteonecrosis after renal transplantation is well known (Fig. 46–22). Osteonecrosis generally becomes evident 4 to 36 months after surgery. It is generally assumed that osteonecrosis in the post-transplant period is due to steroid medications; the reported frequency is 1.4% to 40%. The occurrence of clinically occult ischemic bone necrosis, detected only by MR imaging, in renal transplant patients makes analysis of the prevalence of osteonecrosis difficult. The most common site of osteonecrosis after renal transplantation is the femoral head; additional sites are the distal end of the femur, humeral head, talus, humeral condyles, cuboid, and carpal bones.

Radiographic manifestations of osteonecrosis are characteristic but are seen late in the disease process. A linear subchondral radiolucent shadow represents a fracture beneath the cartilaginous surface. Focal areas of sclerosis are observed about this lucent area, as well as

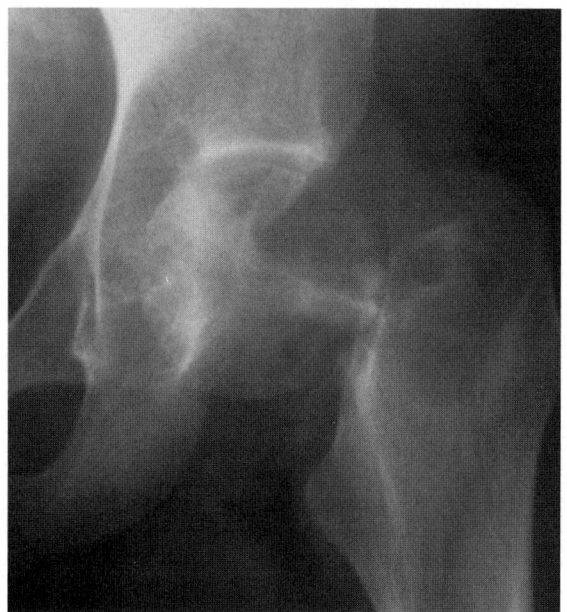

**Figure 46–21.** Renal osteodystrophy: amyloid deposition during hemodialysis leading to pathologic fracture. Note the displaced fracture of the femoral neck, with osteolytic destruction of the femoral head and neck. Additional destructive lesions of the acetabulum and pubic ramus are present. (Courtesy of A. Newberg, MD, Boston, Mass.)

| TABLE 46–5 |
| --- |
| **Musculoskeletal Abnormalities Following Dialysis and Renal Transplantation** |

Hyperparathyroidism
Osteomalacia and rickets
Osteosclerosis
Fractures
Soft tissue and vascular calcification
Osteomyelitis and septic arthritis
Osteonecrosis
Crystal deposition
Destructive spondyloarthropathy
Amyloidosis
Carpal tunnel syndrome
Digital clubbing
Aluminium toxicity
Dialysis cysts
Olecranon bursitis

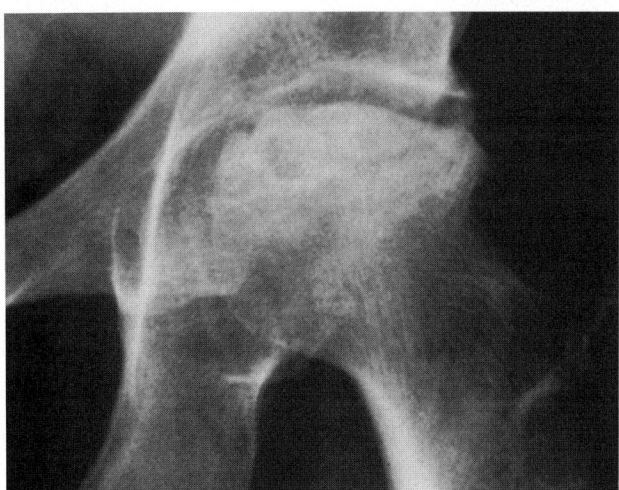

**Figure 46–22.** Renal osteodystrophy: complications of renal transplantation. The radiographic features of osteonecrosis are characteristic, including patchy radiolucency and sclerosis and collapse of the femoral head.

bony eburnation. Spontaneous fractures are not infrequent after renal transplantation and have been observed in 5% to 25% of patients. Although the cause is not known, a reduction in bone mass clearly contributes to spontaneous complete fractures, as well as insufficiency-type stress fractures. Bone and joint infection may also be noted.

Tendinosis and spontaneous tendon ruptures have been identified in some patients who have had renal transplants. An increased rate of malignant change may be evident in patients with renal transplants. Possible explanations for this increased risk of neoplasm are the presence of an underlying autoimmune renal disease, transplantation of malignancy, and immunosuppressive therapy.

### Differential Diagnosis

In renal osteodystrophy, the radiographic features of hyperparathyroidism must be distinguished from those accompanying primary hyperparathyroidism. In secondary hyperparathyroidism, diagnostic features include an increased frequency of vascular and soft tissue calcification, more common and widespread bone sclerosis, and a decreased frequency of chondrocalcinosis. Diffuse osteosclerosis in this condition may be particularly prominent and, although usually accompanied by other radiographic changes of renal osteodystrophy, must be differentiated from the increased radiodensity associated with various other endocrine, metabolic, and neoplastic diseases. Periosteal neostosis in renal osteodystrophy produces diffuse periosteal bone formation, a finding that can also occur with hypertrophic osteoarthropathy, neoplasm, and infection.

Osteomalacia in chronic renal disease produces decreased radiodensity of bone, a finding that lacks specificity. Occasionally, Looser's zones appear identical to those accompanying other types of osteomalacia. Rachitic changes of renal osteodystrophy are almost identical to those accompanying rickets related to dietary deficiencies and chronic renal tubular disorders. The presence of slipped epiphyses and genu valgum deformities may be more common in the rickets of renal osteodystrophy.

Periarticular calcification is found not only in renal osteodystrophy but also in various collagen vascular diseases, hypervitaminosis D, milk-alkali syndrome, idiopathic tumoral calcinosis, and idiopathic calcium hydroxyapatite crystal deposition disease. The periarticular, soft tissue, and vascular calcifications of renal osteodystrophy are usually accompanied by other radiographic changes of the disorder.

## HYPOPARATHYROIDISM

### Background and General Features

Hypoparathyroidism is characterized by hypocalcemia and its neuromuscular symptoms and signs. The disease may result from a deficiency in parathyroid hormone production or an end-organ resistance to the action of the hormone. Deficiency of parathyroid hormone most commonly results from excision of or trauma to the parathyroid glands during thyroid surgery, although it can also occur as idiopathic hypoparathyroidism, in which the parathyroid glands are usually absent or atrophied. End-organ unresponsiveness to parathyroid hormone is seen in pseudohypoparathyroidism and pseudo-pseudohypoparathyroidism.

Postsurgical hypoparathyroidism occurs in less than 13% of thyroidectomies, may be unrecognized for years, and becomes evident clinically during pregnancy and lactation. Idiopathic hypoparathyroidism usually occurs in childhood, with girls being affected more commonly than boys. The disease is rare in blacks. A familial occurrence is noted. The disorder may be characterized by the presence of circulating antibodies to the parathyroid, adrenal, and thyroid glands, supporting the concept that idiopathic hypoparathyroidism may be part of a generalized autoimmune disease.

General radiographic abnormalities of this condition include thickening of the cranial vault and facial bones; increased intracranial pressure with sutural diastasis; calcification of the basal ganglia and, rarely, the choroid plexus and cerebellum; ventricular dilatation; dental abnormalities such as hypoplasia of enamel and dentin, delay or failure of eruption, blunting of the roots, and thickening of the lamina dura; and gastrointestinal hypersecretion and spasm.

### Skeletal Abnormalities

Osteosclerosis, which may be generalized or localized, is the most common skeletal abnormality of hypoparathyroidism (Table 46–6). Localized osteosclerosis is more common, reported in 23% of patients; generalized osteosclerosis is seen in 9%. In addition to osteosclerosis, typical radiographic findings of hypoparathyroidism (and pseudohypoparathyroidism) include calvarial thickening and hypoplastic dentition (Fig. 46–23). Also noteworthy are peculiar bandlike areas of increased radiodensity in

**TABLE 46–6**

**Radiographic Features of the Skeleton in Hypoparathyroidism**

Osteosclerosis
Calvarial thickening
Hypoplastic dentition
Subcutaneous calcification
Basal ganglion calcification
Premature physeal fusion
Spinal ossification

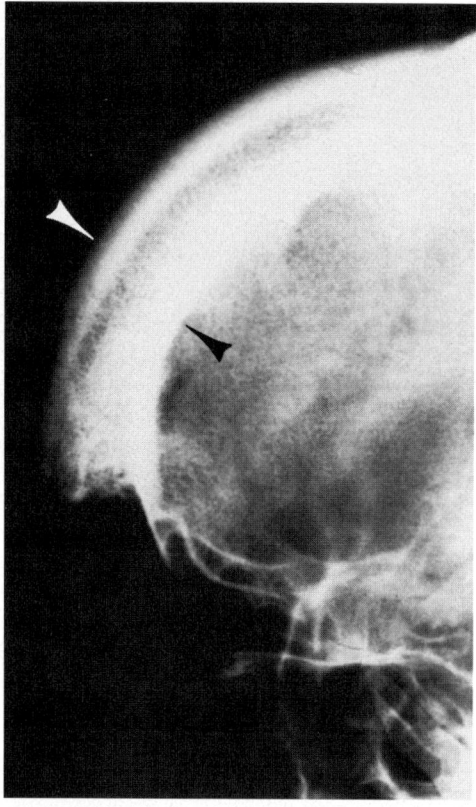

**Figure 46–23.** Hypoparathyroidism: calvarial thickening. Lateral radiograph of the anterior aspect of the skull shows thickening of the cranial vault (*arrowheads*) with narrowing of the diploic space.

the metaphyses of long bones, associated with increased density of the iliac crest and marginal sclerosis of the vertebral bodies. Subcutaneous calcification may be seen, especially about the hips and shoulders. The deposits are generally asymptomatic.

In rare situations, distinctive abnormalities of the spine resembling those of ankylosing spondylitis or diffuse idiopathic skeletal hyperostosis have been reported in patients with hypoparathyroidism. Radiographic evaluation outlines calcification of the anterior longitudinal ligament and posterior paraspinal ligaments with spinal osteophytes (Fig. 46–24). In some cases, these spinal changes are associated with bony proliferation about the pelvis, hip, and long bones and calcification of soft tissue and tendon.

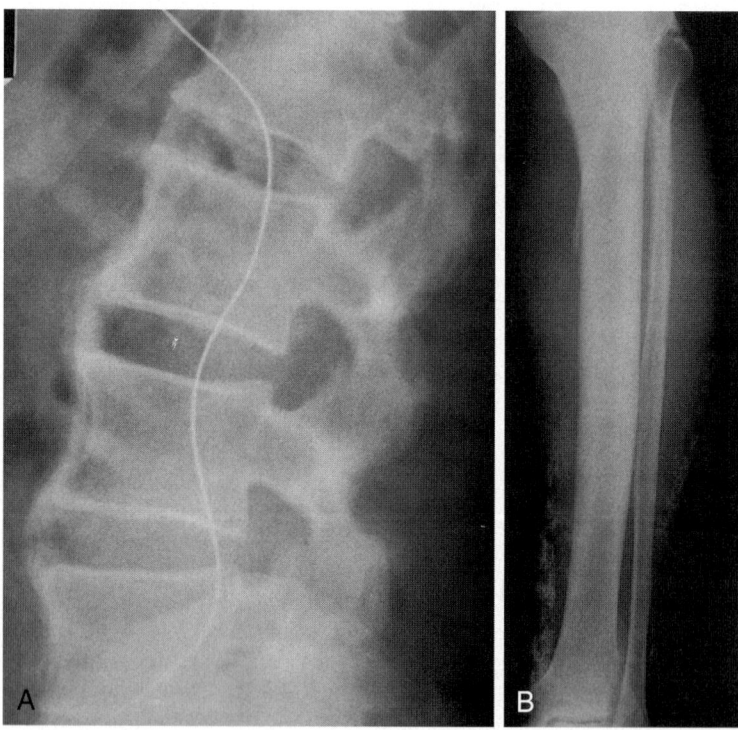

**Figure 46–24.** Hypoparathyroidism: enthesopathy and soft tissue calcification. *A,* Changes resemble those of diffuse idiopathic skeletal hyperostosis, including flowing anterior vertebral ossification. *B,* Soft tissue calcification in the calf and bone excrescences arising from the proximal portion of the tibia are evident. (Courtesy of P. Cockshott, MD, Hamilton, Ontario, Canada.)

## Differential Diagnosis

Widespread osteosclerosis, particularly of the axial skeleton, may be identified in hypoparathyroidism, but it is also seen in certain other disorders, including osteoblastic metastasis, myelofibrosis, Paget's disease, fluorosis, renal osteodystrophy, sickle cell anemia, and mastocytosis. In these diseases, other radiographic features are usually apparent, allowing an accurate diagnosis. In hypoparathyroidism (and pseudohypoparathyroidism), additional findings such as calvarial thickening and hypoplastic dentition are helpful clues, although other causes of generalized sclerosis, such as Paget's disease, sickle cell anemia, and even metastasis, may produce increased thickness and sclerosis of the cranial vault. Hypoplastic dentition is also seen in a variety of congenital syndromes, including cleidocranial dysostosis and pyknodysostosis, and in a number of other endocrine disorders, such as hypopituitarism and hypothyroidism. Sclerosis of the metaphyseal region of the long bones, which is seen in some patients with hypoparathyroidism, is not specific. A similar finding may be noted in systemic illnesses in infancy and childhood, leading to growth recovery lines, leukemia during treatment, heavy metal poisoning, hypothyroidism, healing scurvy, and hypervitaminoses, although additional radiographic and clinical features usually allow easy differentiation among these disorders.

Basal ganglion calcification is particularly characteristic of hypoparathyroidism and pseudohypoparathyroidism. It is also seen in infectious disorders such as toxoplasmosis and cytomegalic inclusion disease, in Fahr's syndrome (ferrocalcinosis), after radiation therapy and exposure to toxic substances such as carbon monoxide, and rarely in certain other diseases. Also, subcutaneous calcification, seen in hypoparathyroidism and pseudohypoparathyroidism, is not a specific finding, being observed in collagen vascular disease, hypervitaminosis D, milk-alkali syndrome, and renal osteodystrophy.

The "pseudospondylitic" manifestations of hypoparathyroidism are of particular interest. Descriptions of these manifestations bear a striking resemblance to those of diffuse idiopathic skeletal hyperostosis, including the tendency toward spinal and extraspinal ligament ossification, osteophytosis, and bony excrescences at sites of tendon and ligament attachment to bone. Similar spinal alterations may be seen in fluorosis and ankylosing spondylitis, although, unlike in the latter disorder, thin vertical syndesmophytes, erosion, and intra-articular ankylosis of the sacroiliac joints are not characteristic of hypoparathyroidism.

# PSEUDOHYPOPARATHYROIDISM AND PSEUDO-PSEUDOHYPOPARATHYROIDISM

## Background and General Features

Pseudohypoparathyroidism (PHP) is a heritable disorder that shares many features with idiopathic hypoparathyroidism, including hypocalcemia, hyperphosphatemia, and basal ganglion and soft tissue calcification. PHP differs from idiopathic hypoparathyroidism in several respects; it involves end-organ resistance to the action of parathyroid hormone and is associated with a charac-

teristic somatotype, which includes short stature, obesity, round face, and brachydactyly. Additional clinical findings of this disease are abnormal dentition, mental retardation, strabismus, dermatoglyphic abnormalities, and impaired taste and olfaction. Typical radiographic features of PHP are short metacarpals, metatarsals, and phalanges; exostoses; cone epiphyses; and wide bones. In some cases, changes of secondary hyperparathyroidism are seen.

PHP is more frequent in women than in men and appears to be transmitted as an X-linked dominant trait. PHP is usually diagnosed in the second decade of life. Affected persons reveal increased levels of serum phosphorus, decreased levels of serum calcium, and diminished phosphaturia. In addition, because of similarities in somatotypic findings, some investigators suggest that PHP may be related to other hereditary syndromes, such as multiple epiphyseal dysplasia, basal cell nevus syndrome, and Turner's syndrome.

PHP results from end organs' inability to respond to parathyroid hormone rather than from deficient secretion of the hormone or the presence of a biologically ineffective hormone. Excessive secretion of parathyroid hormone has been demonstrated in patients with PHP. In fact, reports indicate an apparently rare variation of PHP characterized by renal unresponsiveness to parathyroid hormone but a normal osseous response to the hormone. This condition, termed pseudohypohyperparathyroidism, is associated with histologic findings similar to those of renal osteodystrophy. Abnormal somatic features may or may not be present. Radiographic abnormalities are those of hyperparathyroidism, including subperiosteal bone resorption, brown tumors, osteosclerosis, periosteal neostosis, and slipped capital femoral epiphyses.

Pseudo-pseudohypoparathyroidism (PPHP) is the normocalcemic form of PHP. Patients with PPHP possess the same somatic abnormalities as those with PHP. Both PHP and PPHP may occur in the same family, suggesting a close association of these disorders. Both conditions have been grouped under the term Albright's hereditary osteodystrophy. Patients with PHP frequently come to medical attention with tetany and occasionally with convulsions in late childhood or adolescence. Additionally, they reveal hyperexcitability, cramping of the extremities, and stridor.

## Skeletal Abnormalities

Skeletal abnormalities are an integral part of PHP and PPHP (Table 46–7). Radiographic findings include shortening of all the metacarpals, with premature fusion of the growth plates; broad and short phalanges, with pseudoepiphyses; and soft tissue calcification. The calcification is plaquelike in appearance, asymmetrically distributed, and located beneath the skin surface (Fig. 46–25). Metacarpal shortening shows a predilection for the first and fourth digits (Fig. 46–26), and it is rare to observe metatarsal shortening as an isolated skeletal abnormality. The first metacarpal bone may reveal excessive width and curvature, and the phalanges are short and wide, with cone-shaped epiphyses. Additional findings include basal ganglion calcification, calvarial thickening,

**TABLE 46–7**

**Radiographic Features of the Skeleton in PHP and PPHP**

Soft tissue calcification and ossification
Basal ganglion calcification
Premature physeal fusion
Metacarpal and metatarsal shortening
Calvarial thickening
Exostoses
Abnormalities of bone density
Bowing deformities

PHP, pseudohypoparathyroidism; PPHP, pseudo-pseudohypoparathyroidism.

bowing of the extremities, and exostoses. The exostoses are often located centrally and project at right angles to the bone, differing from the appearance of multiple hereditary exostoses, in which outgrowths are usually directed away from joints. Bone density may be increased, normal, or decreased in PHP and PPHP. The carpal angle may be reduced, and spinal stenosis may occur.

Shortening of the metacarpal bones may lead to a positive metacarpal sign (Fig. 46–27). This sign is not specific; it is also positive in other congenital conditions,

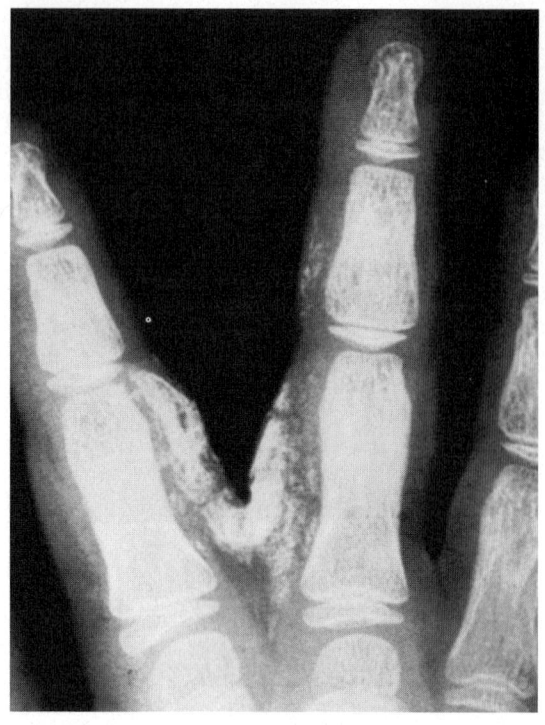

**Figure 46–25.** Pseudohypoparathyroidism: soft tissue calcification. Plaquelike calcification of the subcutaneous tissue of the second and third digits is observed.

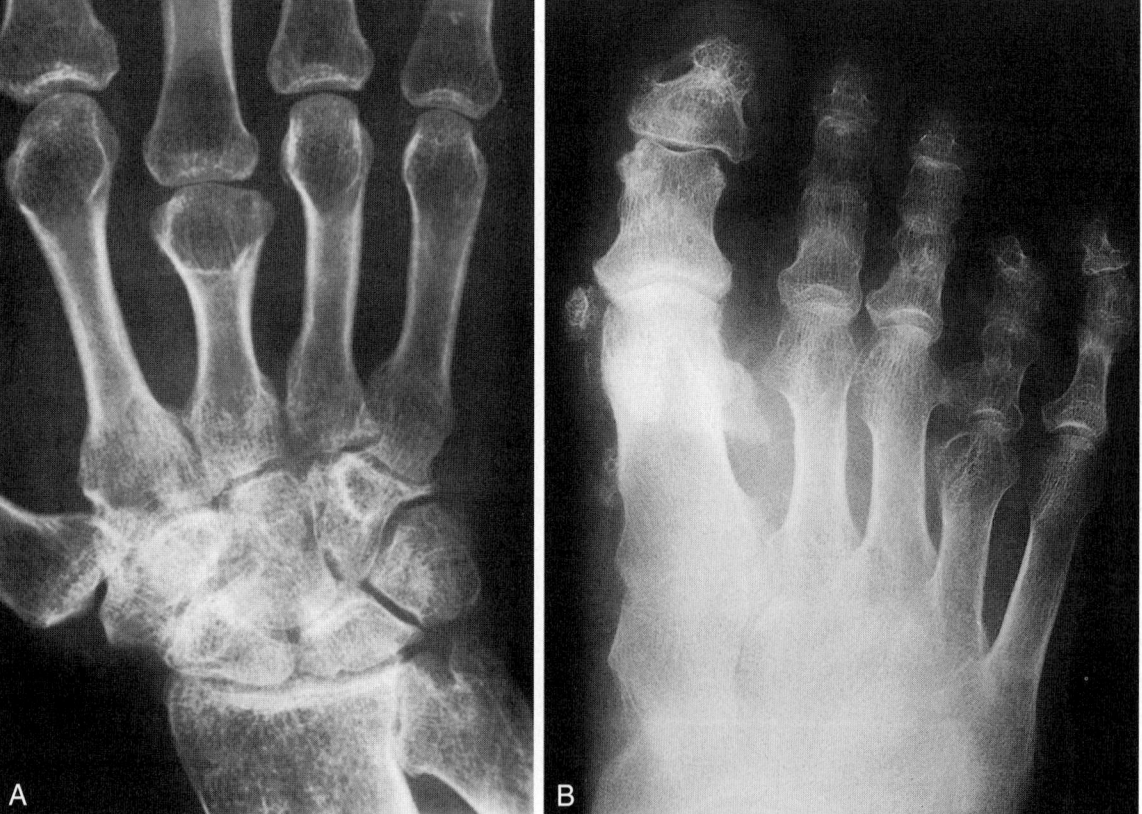

**Figure 46–26.** Pseudohypoparathyroidism: metacarpal and metatarsal shortening. *A*, Shortening of all the metacarpal bones is evident, although the most severe abnormality is in the third digit. Note irregularity of the distal end of the ulna and carpal bones, with joint space narrowing and sclerosis. *B*, Shortening of all the metatarsal bones, particularly the fourth, is associated with soft tissue ossification on the medial aspect of the first digit.

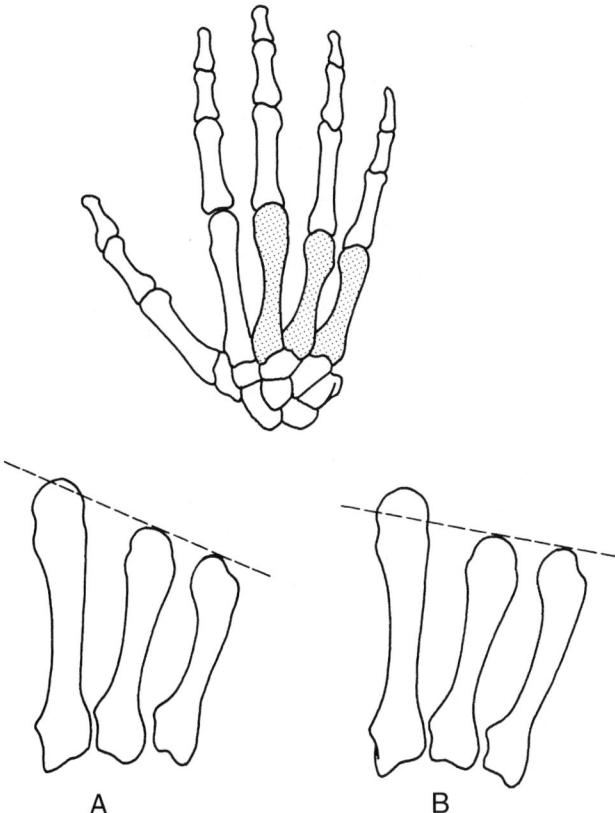

**Figure 46–27.** Pseudohypoparathyroidism and pseudo-pseudohypoparathyroidism: positive metacarpal sign. Normally, a line drawn tangential to the heads of the fourth and fifth metacarpal bones does not intersect the end of the third metacarpal bone or just contacts its articular surface (*A*). A positive metacarpal sign is present when such a line intersects the third metacarpal bone (*B*).

such as basal cell nevus syndrome, multiple epiphyseal dysplasia, and Beckwith-Wiedemann syndrome, as well as in acquired conditions, such as juvenile chronic arthritis, sickle cell anemia with infarction, trauma, and neonatal hyperthyroidism. Further, this sign may be unreliable in diagnosing PHP and PPHP because the third metacarpal bone may also be short in these conditions. Radiographic findings of hyperparathyroidism may be seen in some patients with PHP and PPHP.

## Differential Diagnosis

Radiographic abnormalities of the hand in PHP and PPHP are almost identical. These hand abnormalities resemble the findings in acrodysostosis (except for the much smaller size of the bones in the latter condition), Turner's syndrome (except that the changes in Turner's syndrome may be less severe than those in PHP and PPHP, and drumstick phalanges and thin bones may be apparent in Turner's syndrome), and brachydactyly E and D. Some radiographic features of PHP and PPHP resemble the findings of myositis (fibrodysplasia) ossificans progressiva and multiple hereditary exostoses.

## FURTHER READING

Bywaters EGL, Dixon ASJ, Scott JT: Joint lesions of hyperparathyroidism. Ann Rheum Dis 22:171, 1963.

Cardinal E, Buckwalter KA, Braunstein EM, et al: Amyloidosis of the shoulder in patients on chronic hemodialysis: Sonographic findings. AJR Am J Roentgenol 166:153, 1996.

Chary-Valckenaere I, Kessler M, Mainard D, et al: Amyloid and non-amyloid carpal tunnel syndrome in patients receiving chronic renal dialysis. J Rheumatol 25:1164, 1998.

Dodds WJ, Steinbach HL: Primary hyperparathyroidism and articular cartilage calcification. AJR Am J Roentgenol 104:884, 1968.

Doppman JL: Multiple endocrine syndromes—a nightmare for the endocrinologic radiologist. Semin Roentgenol 20:7, 1985.

Elmstedt E: Avascular bone necrosis in the renal transplant patient: A discriminant analysis of 144 cases. Clin Orthop 158:149, 1981.

Falbo SE, Sundaram M, Ballal S, et al: Clinical significance of erosive azotemic osteodystrophy: A prospective masked study. Skeletal Radiol 28:86, 1999.

Fenves AZ, Emmett M, White MG, et al: Carpal tunnel syndrome with cystic bone lesions secondary to amyloidosis in chronic hemodialysis patients. Am J Kidney Dis 7:130, 1986.

Flipo RM, Cotton A, Chastanet P, et al: Evaluation of destructive spondyloarthropathies in hemodialysis by computerized tomographic scan and magnetic resonance imaging. J Rheumatol 23:869, 1996.

Franco M, Van Elslande L, Passeron C, et al: Tumoral calcinosis in hemodialysis patients: A review of three cases. Rev Rhum Engl Ed 64:59, 1997.

Garrett P, McWade M, O'Callaghan J: Radiological assessment of aluminum-related bone disease. Clin Radiol 37:63, 1986.

Genant HK, Baron JM, Strauss FH II, et al: Osteosclerosis in primary hyperparathyroidism. Am J Med 59:104, 1975.

Genant HK, Heck LL, Lanzl LH, et al: Primary hyperparathyroidism: A comprehensive study of clinical, biochemical, and radiographic manifestations. Radiology 109:513, 1973.

Goldman AB, Lane JM, Salvati E: Slipped capital femoral epiphyses complicating renal osteodystrophy: A report of three cases. Radiology 126:333, 1978.

Greenfield GB: Roentgen appearance of bone and soft tissue changes in chronic renal disease. AJR Am J Roentgenol 116:749, 1972.

Griffiths HJ, Ennis JT, Bailey G: Skeletal changes following renal transplantation. Radiology 113:621, 1974.

Kaplan P, Resnick D, Murphey M, et al: Destructive non-infectious spondyloarthropathy in hemodialysis patients: A report of four cases. Radiology 162:241, 1986.

Kriegshauser JS, Swee RG, McCarthy JT, et al: Aluminum toxicity in patients undergoing dialysis: Radiographic findings and prediction of bone biopsy results. Radiology 164:399, 1987.

Kuntz D, Naveau B, Bardin T, et al: Destructive spondyloarthropathy in hemodialyzed patients: A new syndrome. Arthritis Rheum 27:369, 1984.

Mankin HJ: Metabolic bone disease. J Bone Joint Surg Am 76:760, 1994.

Meema HE, Oreopoulos DG, Rabinovich S, et al: Periosteal new bone formation (periosteal neostosis) in renal osteodystrophy: Relationship to osteosclerosis, osteitis fibrosa, and osteoid excess. Radiology 110:513, 1974.

Milgram JW, Salyer WR: Secondary oxalosis of bone in chronic renal failure. J Bone Joint Surg Am 56:387, 1974.

Orzincolo C, Bedani PL, Scutellari PN, et al: Destructive spondyloarthropathy and radiographic follow-up in hemodialysis patients. Skeletal Radiol 19:483, 1990.

Poznanski AK, Werder EA, Giedion A, et al: The pattern of shortening of the bones of the hand in PHP and PPHP—a comparison with brachydactyly E, Turner syndrome, and acrodysostosis. Radiology 123:707, 1977.

Pugh DG: Subperiosteal resorption of bone: A roentgenologic manifestation of primary hyperparathyroidism and renal osteodystrophy. AJR Am J Roentgenol 66:577, 1951.

Resnick D: Abnormalities of bone and soft tissue following renal transplantation. Semin Roentgenol 13:329, 1978.

Resnick D, Niwayama G: Subchondral resorption of bone in renal osteodystrophy. Radiology 118:315, 1976.

Ross LV, Ross GJ, Mesgarzadeh M, et al: Hemodialysis-related amyloidomas of bone. Radiology 178:263, 1991.

Slavotinek JP, Coates PTH, McDonald SP, et al: Shoulder appearances at MR imaging in long-term dialysis recipients. Radiology 217:539, 2000.

Steinbach HL, Gordan GS, Eisenberg E, et al: Primary hyperparathyroidism: A correlation of roentgen, clinical and pathologic features. AJR Am J Roentgenol 86:329, 1961.

Steinbach HL, Rudhe U, Jonsson M, et al: Evolution of skeletal lesions in pseudohypoparathyroidism. Radiology 85:670, 1965.

Steinbach HL, Young DA: The roentgen appearance of pseudohypoparathyroidism (PH) and pseudo-pseudohypoparathyroidism (PPH): Differentiation from other syndromes associated with short metacarpals, metatarsals and phalanges. AJR Am J Roentgenol 97:49, 1966.

Steinberg H, Waldron BR: Idiopathic hypoparathyroidism: Analysis of 52 cases, including report of new case. Medicine 31:133, 1952.

Sundaram M, Phillipp SR, Wolverson MK, et al: Ungual tufts in the follow-up of patients on maintenance dialysis. Skeletal Radiol 5:247, 1980.

Tervonen O, Mueller DM, Matteson EL, et al: Clinically occult avascular necrosis of the hip: Prevalence in an asymptomatic population at risk. Radiology 182:845, 1992.

Weller M, Edeiken J, Hodes PJ: Renal osteodystrophy. AJR Am J Roentgenol 104:354, 1968.

# CHAPTER 47

## Disorders of Other Endocrine Glands and of Pregnancy

## SUMMARY OF KEY FEATURES

Various musculoskeletal manifestations may accompany endocrine disorders. Further, certain complications are apparent in women during and after pregnancy.

In Cushing's disease, osteoporosis is most typical, and although osteonecrosis is seen occasionally, it is not as frequent as in cases of exogenous hypercortisolism. The list of disorders that may be associated with diabetes mellitus includes crystal-induced arthropathy (gout and calcium pyrophosphate dihydrate crystal deposition disease), osteoarthritis, diffuse idiopathic skeletal hyperostosis, soft tissue contractures, osteomyelitis, septic arthritis, and neuropathic osteoarthropathy. Musculoskeletal anomalies are identified in some infants born to diabetic mothers. After a normal pregnancy, osteitis condensans ilii and osteitis pubis may be apparent, and a similar-appearing abnormality of the clavicle has been described. Other conditions associated with pregnancy include osteonecrosis, transient osteoporosis of the hip, disseminated intravascular coagulation, symphyseal diastasis and rupture, and stress fractures.

## INTRODUCTION

Several endocrine disorders, other than those covered in the preceding chapters, may be associated with significant abnormalities of the skeleton. In addition, musculoskeletal manifestations accompanying or occurring after pregnancy and one miscellaneous disease, osteitis condensans of the clavicle, are discussed.

## CUSHING'S DISEASE

### General Features

Cushing's syndrome is caused by the presence of excessive amounts of adrenocortical glucocorticoid steroids in the body. This excess may be induced by hyperplasia or hyperfunctioning tumors of the adrenal cortex (endogenous Cushing's disease) or by excessive administration of corticosteroid medication (exogenous Cushing's disease). Endogenous Cushing's disease usually results from adrenal hyperplasia (approximately 75% of cases), less commonly from adenoma or carcinoma of the adrenal gland, and rarely from hormone-producing tumors. The disease is most frequent in women between the ages of 20 and 60 years. Its onset is variable. Easy bruising and the development of purpura, especially on the hands and forearms, may be early manifestations. In women, men-strual abnormalities may herald the onset of the disease. Generalized obesity, muscle weakness, emotional disturbance, and backache are common symptoms. On physical examination, patients may demonstrate moon face (increased fullness of the face and cheeks), buffalo hump (fatty deposition over the dorsal spine), increased transparency of the skin, abdominal and axillary purple striae, abnormal distribution of hair with hirsutism, hypertension, and bone tenderness. In children, growth arrest and short stature are observed.

### Osteoporosis

Reduced bone substance in Cushing's syndrome is frequently severe, reflecting decreased bony deposition associated with increased bony resorption. Radiographic examination of patients with Cushing's syndrome reveals typical findings of osteoporosis. The changes predominate in the spine, where diminished bone density, biconcave deformities of vertebral bodies (fish vertebrae), compression fractures, and exaggerated kyphosis are apparent (Fig. 47–1). The appearance is not unlike that in other disorders associated with osteoporosis, although

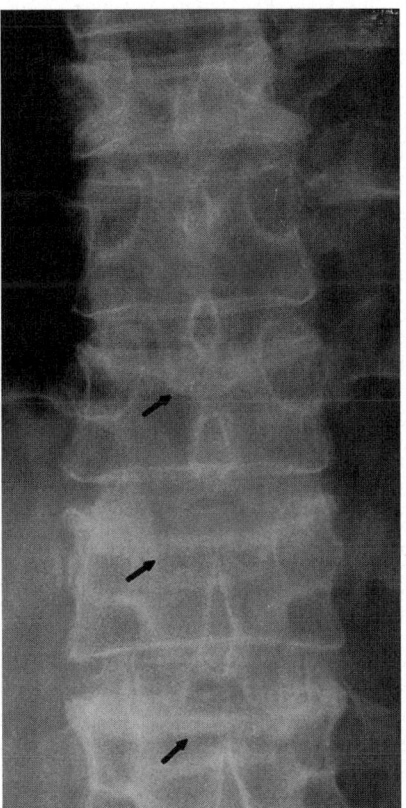

**Figure 47–1.** Endogenous and exogenous Cushing's disease: vertebral osteoporosis. Anteroposterior radiograph outlines osteoporosis of the vertebrae, collapse of multiple vertebral bodies, and condensation of bone (*arrows*) at the vertebral margins.

increased radiodensity of the superior and inferior margins of compressed or collapsed vertebral bodies allows a specific diagnosis in some patients with Cushing's disease. Further, as opposed to the characteristics of postmenopausal and senile osteoporosis, the osteoporosis of Cushing's syndrome may involve the skull, creating peculiar patchy radiolucent areas in the cranial vault. The ribs are also involved, and rib fractures, which are frequent in Cushing's syndrome, may heal with abundant callus formation. Osteoporosis of the pelvis may be associated with protrusio acetabuli. Osteopenia in the appendicular skeleton generally is not attributed to Cushing's syndrome. Osteoporosis, vertebral compression, and kyphosis may also occur with exogenous corticosteroid therapy.

## Osteonecrosis

Osteonecrosis is a well-recognized complication of exogenous hypercortisolism. In endogenous hypercortisolism, osteonecrosis is less well reported and most frequently involves the femoral head, although changes in the humeral head have also been noted. Considering that similar factors may be operational in both exogenous and endogenous steroid excess, it is surprising that osteonecrosis is not reported more frequently during the course of endogenous Cushing's syndrome. When osteonecrosis occurs in this syndrome, typical radiographic features are evident, with subchondral curvilinear radiolucent shadows, osteoporosis, osteosclerosis, bony collapse and fragmentation, and a relatively normal articular space.

## Other Musculoskeletal Abnormalities

Although systemically or locally administered steroid medication may lead to a variety of abnormalities, including a peculiar destructive arthropathy that simulates neuropathic osteoarthropathy, articular infection, and tendon injury and rupture, these features are rarely if ever reported in endogenous Cushing's disease. Delayed skeletal maturation, growth recovery lines, decreased osteophyte formation about abnormal articulations, and loss of the lamina dura are observed rarely in this disease. Soft tissue changes are related to the redistribution of fat, leading to an accumulation of fatty tissue in the trunks of adults and in the trunks and extremities of children. Muscle atrophy and mediastinal and retroperitoneal fat deposition may be noted.

## CONGENITAL ADRENAL HYPERPLASIA AND ADRENOCORTICAL NEOPLASMS IN CHILDREN

The condition of congenital adrenal hyperplasia and adrenocortical neoplasms, originally called the adrenogenital syndrome, is related to a relative or absolute loss of one of the various enzymes involved in the conversion of cholesterol to normal hormonal steroids. This defect results in excessive amounts of adrenocorticotropic hormone, with resultant adrenal hyperplasia. The clinical picture varies according to the precise enzymatic defect, but the most frequent type of intersex problem is female pseudohermaphroditism. Accelerated growth occurs

initially, but premature physeal closure may eventually lead to short stature. Additional musculoskeletal manifestations include accelerated dental maturation, prominent musculature, and premature calcification of the costal cartilage.

Tumors arising from the adrenal cortex are rare in infants and children. These may be benign (adenomas) or malignant (carcinomas). Because histologic differentiation of the benignancy or malignancy of the tumor is often difficult, these tumors are considered together as adrenocortical neoplasms. Such adrenocortical neoplasms are far less common than neuroblastomas but more common than pheochromocytomas. Adrenocortical neoplasms typically occur before the age of 5 years and are more common in girls than in boys. Clinical findings involve endocrine abnormalities, including those of Cushing's syndrome (often manifested as generalized obesity) and virilization. A characteristic finding is precocious puberty, in which secondary sex characteristics appear before the age of 8 years in girls and before the age of 9 years in boys.

Adrenocortical neoplasms may be associated with hemihypertrophy ipsilateral or contralateral to the side of the tumor. They also may be part of the Beckwith-Wiedemann syndrome. This syndrome, which is sometimes referred to as exomphalos-macroglossia-gigantism syndrome, is accompanied by benign and malignant tumors of multiple organs. The most common associated neoplasm is nephroblastoma (Wilms' tumor), followed in frequency by adrenocortical carcinoma and hepatoblastoma.

## ADDISON'S DISEASE

Destruction of the adrenal cortex leading to Addison's disease can be attributed to a variety of processes, including infections, such as tuberculosis or fungal diseases, and infiltrating neoplasms; most commonly, however, idiopathic atrophy of the adrenal glands is observed. The clinical manifestations are usually insidious and related to deficiencies of aldosterone and cortisol. Musculoskeletal manifestations are not frequent or prominent; findings include migratory myalgias, back pain, and sciatica. Radiographs in patients with Addison's disease may reveal calcification in the adrenal glands, external ear, periarticular areas, and costal cartilage, and skeletal maturation may be delayed.

## PHEOCHROMOCYTOMA

A pheochromocytoma arises from chromaffin elements, typically in the adrenal medulla but also in the para-aortic and thoracic sympathetic chains, the organs of Zuckerkandl, the carotid body, and the urinary bladder. Adults between the ages of 30 and 50 years are usually affected. Clinical abnormalities can result from the physical presence of the neoplasm itself but are more often related to the increased production of catecholamines, leading to hypertension, flushing or blanching, palpitations, excessive sweating, headache, anorexia, weight loss, decreased gastrointestinal motility, and psychosis. Osteolytic and osteosclerotic regions in the metaphyses of the tubular bones of children, presumably related to ischemia and infarction, have been reported (Fig. 47–2). The lesions regress after surgical treatment of the tumor. Single or multiple osteolytic metastases, which predominate in the axial skeleton, may be seen.

## NEUROBLASTOMA

Tumors of the sympathetic nervous system are generally classified as neuroblastoma, ganglioneuroblastoma, and ganglioneuroma. Of these, neuroblastoma is most frequent and usually arises in the adrenal medulla. In common with pheochromocytoma, the tumor may be accompanied by excessive production of catecholamines and catecholamine metabolites; however, neuroblastoma is a very aggressive tumor characterized by rapid growth and widespread metastases. Approximately 80% of patients are children younger than 5 years, and most of these are younger than 2 years. Boys and girls are affected in equal numbers. Skeletal metastases are frequent, often demonstrating bilateral and symmetrical osseous lesions, especially in the metaphyseal segments (Fig. 47–3). Osteolytic lesions with permeative bone destruction predominate, particularly in the femur and tibia; sclerosis is less common and is a late manifestation of the disease, but it may become extensive. In the skull, increased intracranial pressure (due to leptomeningeal involvement and leading to sutural diastasis), vertical osseous striations extending from the outer table, and soft tissue swelling are seen. Additional manifestations of the skeletal metastases include "floating" teeth related to mandibular involvement, vertebral collapse, rib alterations with extrapleural extension, and pelvic bone destruction with soft tissue masses compressing nearby viscera, such as the bladder. The differential diagnosis includes Ewing's sarcoma, lymphomas, leukemias, and metastases from other tumors, such as rhabdomyosarcoma, medulloblastoma, retinoblastoma, and Wilms' tumor.

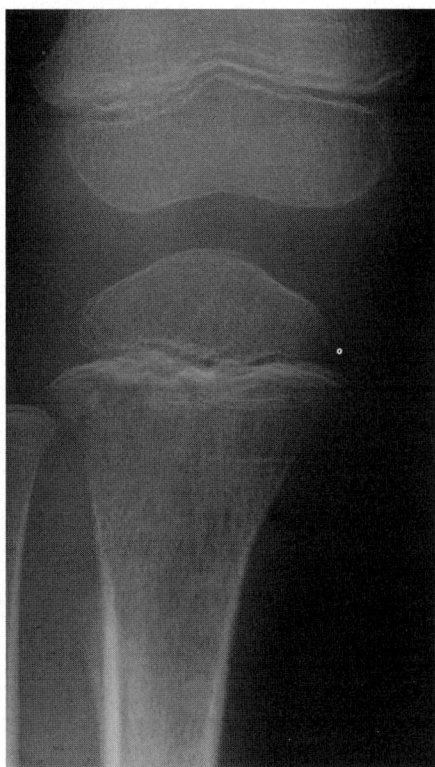

**Figure 47–3.** Neuroblastoma: skeletal metastasis. Note permeative bone destruction and periostitis in the metaphysis of the tibia. Growth recovery lines are also evident.

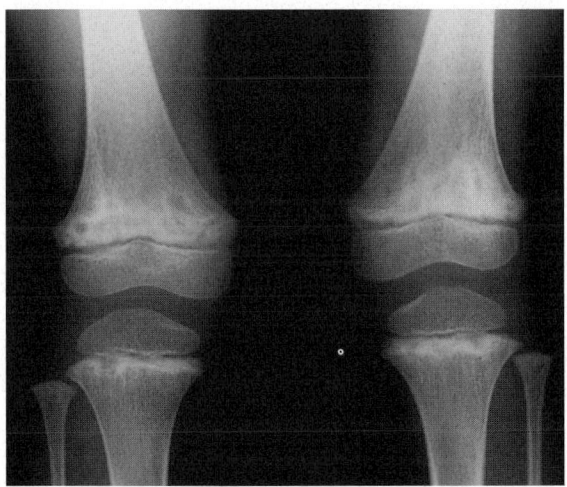

**Figure 47–2.** Pheochromocytoma: metaphyseal abnormalities. Metaphyseal alterations in children with pheochromocytoma regress after surgical treatment of the tumor. (Courtesy of J. C. Hoeffel, MD, Nancy, France.)

## DIABETES MELLITUS

### General Features

Although numerous musculoskeletal disorders have been described in conjunction with diabetes mellitus (Table 47–1), the association between them has not been well documented. Much of the difficulty in associating diabetes and additional rheumatic conditions is related to its extreme frequency; thus, the occurrence of diabetes in combination with another disease process may be no more than the coincidental appearance of two diseases in the same patient.

### Gouty Arthritis

The relationship between diabetes mellitus and gouty arthritis is not well defined. When patients with gout are compared with age- and weight-matched control subjects, no significant difference in glucose metabolism is found between the two groups. This evidence suggests that the prevalence of diabetes in patients with gout is related to the high frequency of obesity in hyperuricemic subjects.

### Calcium Pyrophosphate Dihydrate Crystal Deposition Disease

The frequency of diabetes mellitus in patients with calcium pyrophosphate dihydrate (CPPD) crystal deposition disease may be quite high, as may the frequency of CPPD crystal accumulation in persons with diabetes mellitus. Thus,

**Musculoskeletal Manifestations of Diabetes Mellitus**

Gout*
Calcium pyrophosphate dihydrate crystal deposition disease*
Degenerative joint disease*
Diffuse idiopathic skeletal hyperostosis
Soft tissue and muscle syndromes
  Periarthritis
  Diabetic cheiroarthropathy
  Dupuytren's contracture
  Flexor tenosynovitis
  Carpal tunnel syndrome
  Skeletal muscle infarction
Osteomyelitis
Septic arthritis
Neuropathic osteoarthropathy
Forefoot osteolysis

*Possible association

the true association of diabetes mellitus and CPPD crystal deposition disease is not clear.

## Osteoarthritis

A possible association between diabetes mellitus and degenerative joint disease (osteoarthritis) has been suggested in some reports, although this association is not well documented.

## Diffuse Idiopathic Skeletal Hyperostosis

Diffuse idiopathic skeletal hyperostosis (DISH) is particularly frequent in diabetic and obese patients and is seen with greater frequency in diabetic than in nondiabetic patients. In general, diabetes mellitus is mild in patients with DISH, and the severity of the disease does not correspond to the extent of DISH.

## Soft Tissue and Muscle Syndromes

Several syndromes involving soft tissues or skeletal muscle may be observed in patients with diabetes mellitus. Not included here is the increased frequency of soft tissue (as well as visceral) arterial calcification, as well as the rare occurrence of dystrophic calcification of subcutaneous soft tissues at sites of chronic insulin injection.

**Periarthritis.** Periarthritis produces a painful stiff shoulder (adhesive capsulitis) characterized by loss of joint motion, particularly internal rotation and abduction, without evidence of intra-articular disease. The condition is more common in women and in persons older than 40 years. It may be bilateral or unilateral in distribution. Periarthritis of the shoulder may be four or five times more common in diabetic patients than in nondiabetic patients. Radiographic examination occasionally reveals calcific bursitis or calcific tendinitis. Magnetic resonance (MR)

imaging reveals thickening of the capsule and enhancement of its signal intensity following intravenous gadolinium administration (Fig. 47–4).

**Diabetic Cheiroarthropathy.** This syndrome has been described in as many as 40% of patients with insulin-dependent (type I) juvenile diabetes. Characteristic findings of this syndrome, which is variously termed diabetic cheiroarthropathy and diabetic hand syndrome, are mild to moderately severe joint contractures of the fingers, particularly at the proximal interphalangeal joints and in the fourth and fifth digits; thickening and a waxy appearance of the skin on the dorsum of the hand; and short stature. There is no evidence of palmar fascial thickening or Dupuytren's contracture.

**Dupuytren's Contracture.** A high frequency (3% to 40%) of Dupuytren's contracture has been reported in patients with either type I or type II diabetes. In diabetic patients, the frequency of Dupuytren's contracture increases with long-standing disease. It is generally mild, rarely requiring surgery. This condition develops insidiously as nodular or plaquelike thickening of the palmar fascia, initially over the ulnar side of the hand. Extension of the fibrous process to the metacarpophalangeal and proximal interphalangeal joints may result in finger contracture. The cause of this condition is unknown.

**Flexor Tenosynovitis.** Flexor tenosynovitis (trigger finger, stenosing tenovaginitis) refers to a condition of one or

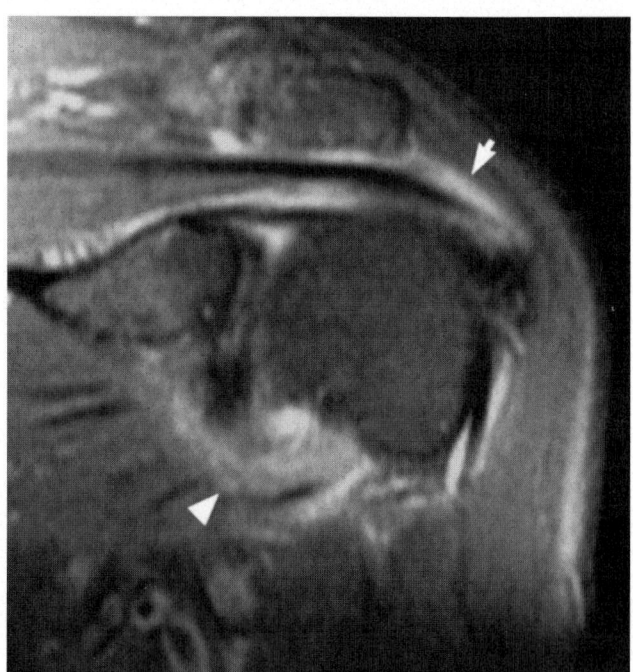

**Figure 47–4.** Diabetes mellitus and adhesive capsulitis. Oblique coronal, fat-suppressed, T1-weighted (TR/TE, 650/14) spin echo MR image, obtained after the intravenous administration of a gadolinium-containing contrast agent, shows enhancement of signal intensity in the subacromial-subdeltoid bursa (*arrow*), axillary recess of the glenohumeral joint (*arrowhead*), and tendon sheath about the biceps tendon.

more fingers associated with snapping, pain, locking, and limited motion of the interphalangeal joint due to obstruction of the flexor tendon in a constricted tendon sheath. The sheath is thickened, with local inflammatory changes, fibrous proliferation, and collagenous degeneration. Some reports suggest that diabetes mellitus may coexist in 10% to 30% of patients with flexor tenosynovitis.

**Carpal Tunnel Syndrome.** Carpal tunnel syndrome results from entrapment of the median nerve within the carpal tunnel on the volar aspect of the wrist. Tissue infiltration in leukemia, sarcoidosis, amyloidosis, and neoplasm; tissue edema in acromegaly and hypothyroidism; tissue hemorrhage occurring after trauma; and tissue inflammation in rheumatoid arthritis, systemic lupus erythematosus, dermatomyositis, gout, and CPPD crystal deposition disease are potential causes. The frequency of diabetes mellitus in patients with carpal tunnel syndrome is reportedly 5% to 17%. It has been suggested that an increased occurrence of this syndrome in association with diabetes may be due to ischemic changes related to microvascular disease.

**Skeletal Muscle Infarction.** This complication is typically seen in patients with poorly controlled disease and results in excruciating pain and tender swelling or a mass in the involved muscle. The muscles in the lower extremity, especially in the thigh and calf, are involved most commonly, and multiple sites in one or both legs may be affected. Involvement of the quadriceps musculature and adductor muscles of the hip is characteristic. Clinical manifestations may simulate those of myositis, abscess, neoplasm, deep venous thrombosis, or ruptured synovial cyst. MR imaging reveals diffuse enlargement of affected muscles (without a focal mass) and partial loss of normal fatty intermuscular septa. Subcutaneous edema and subfascial fluid may be evident. T1-weighted spin echo images show normal or low signal intensity in the involved muscles. High intramuscular signal intensity is apparent in fluid-sensitive sequences (Fig. 47–5). The diagnosis of muscle infarction should be considered in a diabetic patient presenting with an acute painful thigh or leg swelling.

## Osteomyelitis and Septic Arthritis

Soft tissue ulceration and infection, which are frequent in diabetes, may lead to contamination of contiguous bones and joints. This sequence is particularly frequent in the diabetic foot. Initial soft tissue lesions are especially frequent beneath the first and fifth metatarsophalangeal joints and the calcaneus at pressure points. The initial radiographic findings include defects in soft tissue contour, loss of tissue planes, and swelling. As the infection reaches the bone, the radiographic findings of osteomyelitis and septic arthritis become evident. It should be noted that periosteal new bone formation and osteopenia may not be prominent in the diabetic foot, because bony proliferation and diffuse, patchy, or periarticular osteoporosis require an adequate vascular supply. Spontaneous fracture, subluxation, and dislocation may be seen, frequently in association with neuropathic osteoarthropathy.

## Neuropathic Osteoarthropathy

Diabetes mellitus is by far the leading cause of neuropathic osteoarthropathy (see Chapter 66). Diabetic neuropathic osteoarthropathy has a unique distribution, frequently involving the tarsometatarsal, intertarsal, and metatarsophalangeal joints (Fig. 47–6). Abnormalities of the ankle and interphalangeal joints are less frequent. Occasionally, changes occur at other sites, including the knee, spine, and joints of the upper extremity. Spontaneous fractures and dislocations are not infrequent. In this regard, diabetic neuropathic osteoarthropathy with findings resembling Lisfranc's fracture-dislocation at the tarsometatarsal joints is well recognized.

## Forefoot Osteolysis

A distinct osteolysis of the forefoot has been described in patients with diabetes mellitus, characterized by patchy or generalized osteoporosis of the distal metatarsals and proximal phalanges, accompanied by a variable degree of pain. The articular surfaces are spared initially, although progressive osteolysis may become apparent with the disappearance of adjacent bone. The process may terminate at any stage, and resolution may commence with partial or complete restoration of bony architecture. The cause of this condition is not clear.

## Osteopenia

Osteopenia is a well-recognized manifestation of insulin-treated diabetes mellitus in patients of all ages; in many series, its frequency in insulin-dependent disease is reported to be approximately 50%. Although correlation of bone loss with the severity of the disorder is poor, bone loss is particularly marked initially and in younger age groups. The pathogenesis of diabetic osteopenia is not clear.

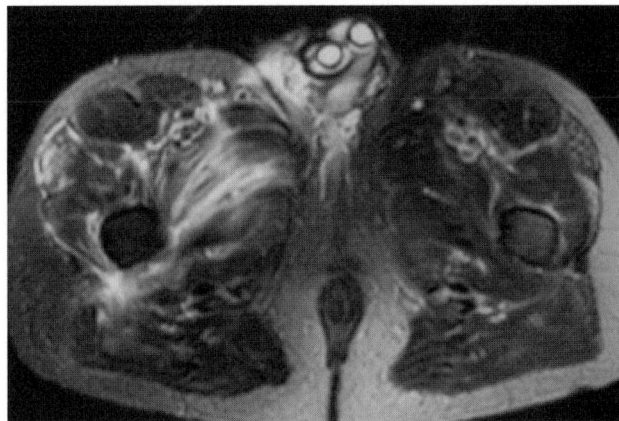

**Figure 47–5.** Diabetes mellitus and muscle infarction. Fat-suppressed transverse (TR/TE, 3000/102) fast spin echo MR images show slight enlargement and high signal intensity in multiple muscles (including the adductors, vastus lateralis, and tensor fasciae latae muscles) in the right thigh. No discrete mass is evident.

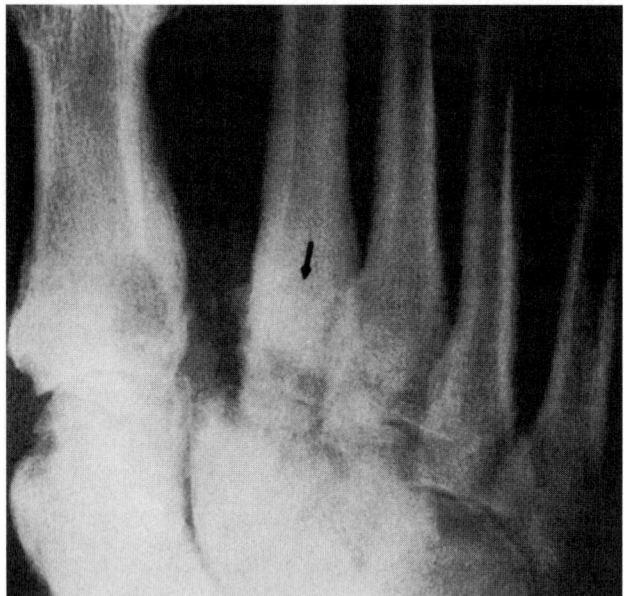

**Figure 47–6.** Diabetes mellitus: association with neuropathic osteoarthropathy. In a patient with diabetes, neurologic deficit, and soft tissue infection, note the degree of sclerosis and fragmentation of the tarsometatarsal joint (*arrow*), a common site of occurrence of neuropathic osteoarthropathy in diabetic patients. Lateral displacement of the metatarsal bases is also seen.

## Vascular Calcification

Arterial calcifications, especially of the internal carotid and renal arteries, the aorta, and the arteries of the lower extremities and pelvis, are commonly observed during radiography in patients with diabetes mellitus. In the leg, arterial calcifications of the media, rather than the intima, are the typical lesions of diabetes mellitus and lead to regular, diffuse, and fine-grained collections that generally affect the whole circumference of the vessel and accumulate in rings. Although common in diabetes mellitus, arterial calcifications generally do not impinge on the lumen of the vessel; however, such calcifications are more frequent in diabetic patients with gangrene than in those without gangrene, suggesting that arterial calcific deposits can lead to impaired circulation owing to the increased rigidity of the vessel wall. The cause of the angiopathy is not clear.

## LIPOATROPHIC DIABETES
### General Features

Lipoatrophic diabetes is characterized by insulin-resistant diabetes, hepatosplenomegaly, hyperlipidemia, hypermetabolism, accelerated growth and maturation, muscular overdevelopment, hirsutism, hyperpigmentation, and progressive loss of adipose tissue without ketosis. Additional clinical features are cutaneous xanthomas, protuberant abdomen, corneal opacities, and mental retardation. Lipoatrophic diabetes may be congenital or acquired. In the

congenital form, there is a paucity of fat at the time of birth, and affected children are frequently the product of consanguineous marriages. Diabetes commonly appears in the second decade of life. Acquired lipodystrophy may be related to a previous infection, such as pertussis or mumps. This form of the disease is more common in women than in men and may have its onset after a difficult labor and delivery. The cause of this disorder is unknown.

### Radiographic Findings

The most striking radiographic finding is a decrease or absence of body fat, manifested as loss of soft tissue planes. A markedly advanced bone age may be seen in children with this syndrome. Thickening of the diaphyseal cortices, metaphyseal sclerosis, and hypertrophy of the epiphyses have been described in the long bones. Small cystic lesions may appear in the metaphysis. Changes in the skull may include dolichocephaly, brachycephaly, calcification of the falx cerebri, thickening of the calvaria, and advanced dentition. Evidence of organomegaly may be seen in the chest and abdomen.

Cystic and sclerotic foci are particularly common in periarticular regions, and the findings may resemble those of osteonecrosis or osteopoikilosis (Fig. 47–7). The regions of increased density may extend into the metaphysis and involve the margins of the vertebral bodies. It has been suggested that the radiodense foci represent an osteoblastic reaction to loss of fat in the bone marrow. Because there are wide variations in the radiographic appearance of lipoatrophic diabetes, its differential diagnosis depends on the distribution and severity of imaging findings in the particular patient. This condition should be differentiated from partial lipodystrophy, in which loss of facial, trunk, and upper extremity fat is apparent in children between the ages of 5 and 15 years. A decrease in subcutaneous fat may also be seen in hyperthyroidism, anorexia nervosa, progeria, and various other congenital and acquired disorders. The gigantism of lipoatrophic diabetes must be distinguished from pituitary and cerebral gigantism. In pituitary gigantism, increased subcu-

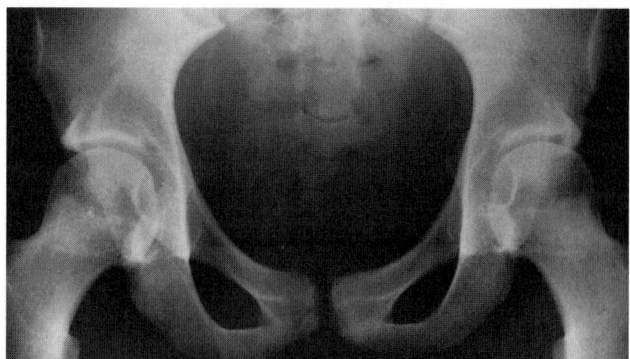

**Figure 47–7.** Lipoatrophic diabetes. Note the increased radiodensity in the femoral necks. (From Gold RH, Steinbach HL: Lipoatrophic diabetes mellitus (generalized lipodystrophy): Roentgen findings in two brothers with congenital disease. AJR Am J Roentgenol 101:884, 1967.)

taneous fat and typical osseous changes are apparent, whereas in cerebral gigantism, there is excessive body fat and an absence of hepatosplenomegaly.

## ANOMALIES IN INFANTS OF DIABETIC MOTHERS

Hyperinsulinemia in the fetus of a diabetic mother is presumed to be the result of maternal hyperglycemia, because insulin does not traverse the placental barrier. Elevated levels of insulin can promote abnormal growth, which is manifested in the newborn as visceromegaly and increased body fat. The frequency of congenital anomalies in the offspring of diabetic mothers may be as high as 20% but is probably far less. These include respiratory anomalies (respiratory distress syndrome, wet lung syndrome, persistence of fetal circulation); cardiomyopathy and congenital heart disease; hyperviscosity, thrombosis, and hemorrhage; renal anomalies (hydronephrosis, duplication, cystic kidneys, renal agenesis, pseudohermaphroditism, renal vein thrombosis); small left colon syndrome; and alterations in the musculoskeletal system.

Sacrococcygeal agenesis, or the caudal regression syndrome, is one of the most specific anomalies in these infants. Approximately 20% of patients with this syndrome are the children of diabetic mothers, and approximately 16% of children born to diabetic mothers have sacral anomalies. Agenesis varies in severity; in some cases, only minor coccygeal changes are present, whereas in others, aplasia of the lower thoracic and entire lumbar spine is combined with absence of one or more segments of the sacrum (Fig. 47–8). Associated abnormalities include meningocele, arthrogryposis, hip dislocation, flexion contractures of the knee and hip, foot deformities, and urinary tract anomalies.

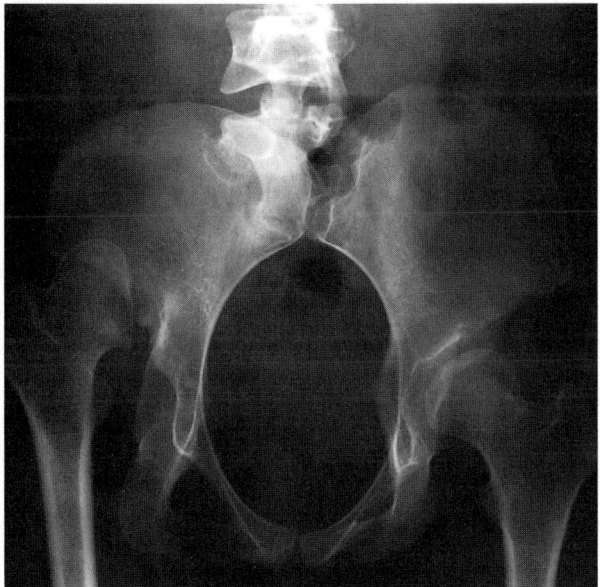

**Figure 47–8.** Anomalies in children of diabetic mothers: caudal regression syndrome. In this 27-year-old daughter of a diabetic mother, aplasia of the lower lumbar spine and sacrum is associated with pelvic and acetabular deformity and dislocation of the right hip. (Courtesy of S. Hilton, MD, San Diego, Calif.)

## DISORDERS AND COMPLICATIONS OF PREGNANCY

In women, there is an increase in lumbar lordosis and angulation at the lumbosacral junction, as well as an increase in obliquity of the pelvic bones themselves. During pregnancy, certain biomechanical changes occur that produce increased stress on the pelvic joints. As a result of increased weight during pregnancy, the degree of lumbar lordosis increases, and the center of mass is displaced. Sliding movement at the sacroiliac joint, which is evident in normal persons, becomes accentuated owing to softening and relaxation of adjacent ligaments and diastasis. It is generally assumed that relaxation of the joints of the pelvis is an essential and normal accompaniment of pregnancy, which ensures the accommodation of the growing fetus and facilitates vaginal delivery. The major radiographic findings associated with physiologic and pathologic changes during pregnancy occur at the sacroiliac joints and symphysis pubis. Bony eburnation about the sacroiliac joint is termed osteitis condensans ilii, whereas that at the symphysis pubis is termed osteitis pubis. Although either condition may be apparent in nulliparous women or even men, both are observed most frequently in multiparous women.

### Osteitis Condensans Ilii

Osteitis condensans ilii is a condition of the pelvis that involves predominantly the ilium adjacent to the sacroiliac joint. Usually, though not invariably, it is a bilateral and relatively symmetrical process in women; rarely, men are affected, and asymmetrical or unilateral changes may be observed. Osteitis condensans ilii is associated with well-defined triangular sclerosis on the iliac aspect of the sacroiliac joint (Fig. 47–9). The bony eburnation involves the inferior portion of the bone, and the apex of the sclerosis extends into the articular portion of the ilium. The subchondral bone is generally well defined, highlighted by the radiodensity of the involved osseous surface. Significant narrowing of the sacroiliac joint and extensive involvement of the sacrum are distinctly unusual.

The cause of osteitis condensans ilii is not clear. The predominant theory suggests that the condition is secondary to mechanical stress across the sacroiliac joint coupled with increased vascularity during pregnancy. Its occurrence in nulliparous women and in men is inconsistent with this theory, although mechanical stress of a different cause may be operational in these people. Generally, this disorder is easily differentiated from ankylosing spondylitis (Table 47–2).

### Osteitis Pubis

Osteitis pubis is a painful condition of the symphysis pubis that may become apparent within 1 month or longer after delivery or other pelvic procedures or operations. In men, osteitis pubis is particularly frequent after prostate (or bladder) surgery. Clinical findings are characterized by local pain and tenderness, muscle spasm, and unstable gait. The disorder should be distinguished from the normal symphyseal separation and hypermobility that may occur

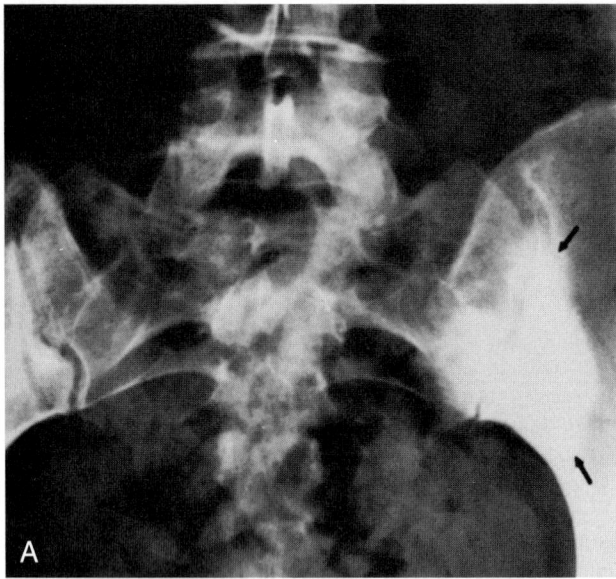
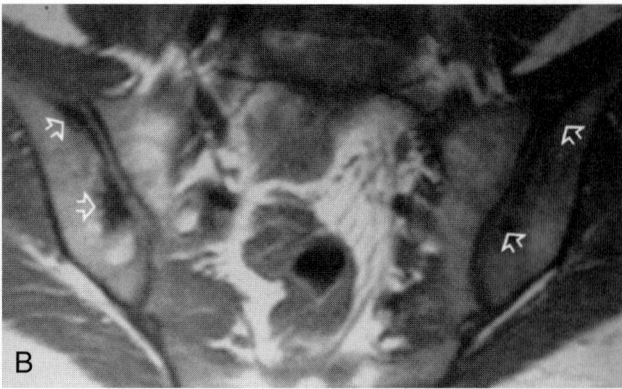

**Figure 47–9.** Osteitis condensans ilii. *A*, Typical radiographic features include well-defined triangular sclerosis on the iliac aspect of the joint (arrows). The joint space is relatively well preserved. *B*, In a different patient, transverse T1-weighted (TR/TE, 550/20) spin echo MR image shows low signal intensity *(arrows)* in both ilia. The joints are normal. Similar findings were seen on a corresponding T2-weighted image.

during pregnancy. In this normal situation, widening of the symphysis can be detected radiographically and is accentuated by the patient's standing on one leg at a time. The width of the articulation is usually less than 7 mm, and the symphyseal changes regress within a few months post partum. In the unusual case in which the pubic changes do not regress and are associated with bony erosion, resorption, and eburnation, osteitis pubis may be diagnosed.

The radiographic appearance of osteitis pubis includes mild to severe subchondral bony irregularity of the symphysis pubis with resorption (Fig. 47–10). The condition usually involves both pubic bones in a symmetrical

fashion, although asymmetrical or unilateral findings are occasionally encountered. The degree of resorption or sclerosis may rarely become striking, with osteolysis of a large segment of the pubic bones. Restoration of the osseous surface with disappearance of the sclerosis may be associated with bony ankylosis of the joint.

In most cases, the cause of osteitis pubis remains speculative. The differential diagnosis of osteitis pubis includes not only trauma and infection but also a variety of articular disorders characterized, in part, by inflammation of the symphysis pubis. Subchondral resorption of bone in primary and secondary hyperparathyroidism

---

**TABLE 47–2**

**Osteitis Condensans Ilii (OCI) versus Ankylosing Spondylitis (AS)**

|  | OCI | AS |
|---|---|---|
| **Age** | Young adults | Young adults |
| **Sex** | Women > men | Men > women |
| **Clinical symptoms, signs** | Absent or mild | Mild to severe |
| **HLA-B27** | Present in 8% (same as controls) | Present in 90% |
| **Sacroliliac joint abnormalities** | | |
| **Distribution** | Bilateral, symmetrical; iliac | Bilateral, symmetrical; iliac > sacral |
| **Sclerosis** | Well defined | Poorly defined |
| **Joint space** | Normal | Narrowed |
| **Erosion** | Absent | Common |
| **Bony ankylosis** | Absent | Common |
| **Spinal abnormalities** | Absent | Common |
| **Symphysis pubis abnormalities** | Less common | More common |

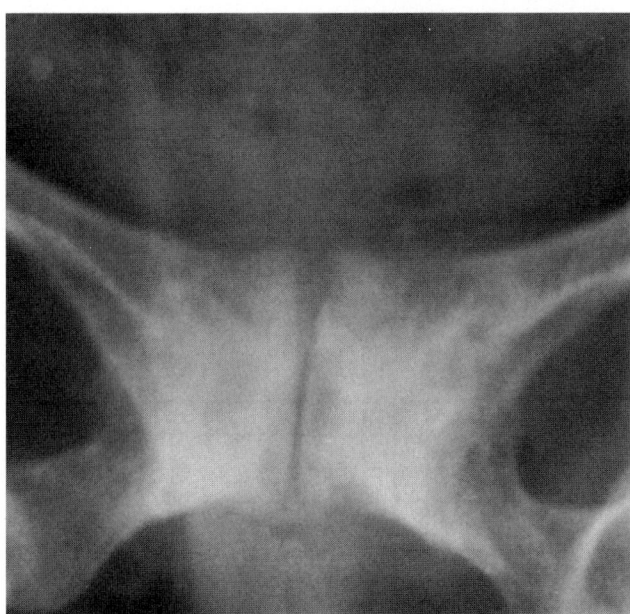

**Figure 47–10.** Osteitis pubis. Radiograph reveals considerable bone sclerosis on both sides of the symphysis, with narrowing of the joint space. (Courtesy of M. Austin, MD, Newport Beach, Calif.)

and stress or insufficiency fractures in this condition, as well as in osteomalacia and osteoporosis and following radiation therapy, can produce abnormalities that simulate osteitis pubis.

### Symphyseal Diastasis and Rupture

Symphyseal separation is a known complication of pregnancy. It is generally asymptomatic and appears to be related to an increased elasticity of the pubic ligaments in response to the hormones progesterone and relaxin. The frequency of this finding in pregnant women is variable but has been estimated to be as high as 30%. The width of the symphysis pubis may change progressively throughout the course of pregnancy, without a marked increase

during labor or delivery. The width of the symphysis pubis in this physiologic condition is usually less than 7 mm. In rare circumstances, rupture of the symphysis pubis occurs during the final stages of pregnancy, particularly during labor and delivery. Radiographs reveal symphyseal separations varying from 1 to 12 cm (Fig. 47–11). Nonoperative treatment is generally sufficient, and functional recovery should be complete.

### Ischemic Necrosis of Bone

Although it occurs infrequently, well-documented instances of ischemic necrosis of bone related to pregnancy have been reported. Ischemic necrosis of bone is usually identified in close association with childbirth, and the femoral head or, less commonly, the humeral head is the principal target. Most reports of pregnancy-related ischemic necrosis of bone have been anecdotal, so a meaningful association between the two has yet to be proved.

### Transient Osteoporosis of the Hip

As discussed in Chapter 41, periarticular osteoporosis of the hip has been identified in women during the third trimester of pregnancy and has occasionally been inaccurately described as ischemic necrosis. Affected women have joint pain, an antalgic limp, and restricted hip motion. The left side is involved almost exclusively, although changes in the right hip, both hips, and other joints have been noted.

### Generalized Osteopenia

Osteopenia associated with pregnancy and lactation is infrequent, because most pregnant women adjust well to the large placental transfer of calcium and phosphorus to the developing fetus and to the calcium demands during lactation. Certain changes in maternal levels of serum calcium, parathyroid hormone, thyrocalcitonin, and vitamin D metabolites are considered physiologic and are not accompanied by a propensity to fracture. Why things go wrong in some women, leading to significant osteopenia during pregnancy and lactation, is not clear,

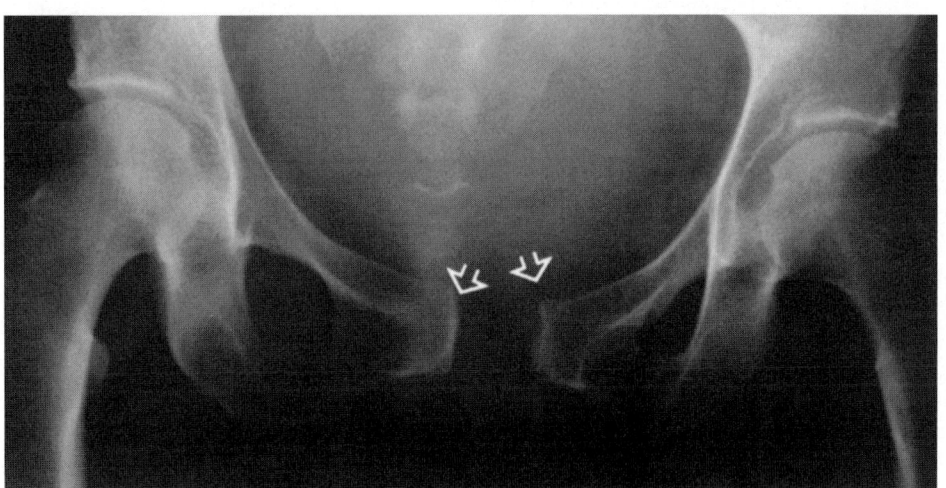

**Figure 47–11.** Symphyseal diastasis after pregnancy. In this 38-year-old woman, continued symphyseal pain and tenderness occurred in the postpartum period. Radiograph reveals abnormal widening (>10 mm) of the symphysis pubis (*arrows*).

although histologic data suggest that the decrease in bone mass is related principally to low-turnover osteoporosis.

## Stress Fractures

Stress fractures have been observed in the later stages of pregnancy and in the postpartum period. Pelvic sites such as the parasymphyseal bone and sacrum are typically involved. A potential cause of such fractures in the pubic rami in the final stages of pregnancy is the forceful descent of the fetal head against a pelvic ring that contains lax ligaments. Stress fractures in the postpartum period may be related to increased body weight and increased levels of physical activity.

## Other Complications

Carpal tunnel syndrome is a frequent finding during pregnancy, often occurring bilaterally in the second or third trimester. It is probably related to soft tissue swelling in and around the carpal tunnel, as the syndrome is associated with swelling of the fingers, generalized edema, preeclampsia, and hypertension. Tenosynovitis, especially De Quervain's, is also encountered during pregnancy, generally attributed to fluid retention.

## OSTEITIS CONDENSANS OF THE CLAVICLE

Although this relatively newly described condition is not a complication of pregnancy, osteitis condensans of the clavicle shares morphologic and radiographic features with osteitis condensans ilii and osteitis pubis. Patients are women with an average age of 40 years (range, 20 to 50 years). A history of stress to the region of the sternoclavicular joint, usually associated with heavy lifting or sports activity, is typical. Pain is most commonly referred to the ipsilateral shoulder and is accentuated with abduction of the arm. No definite association with osteitis pubis or osteitis condensans ilii has been reported.

Radiographs reveal bone sclerosis and mild enlargement of the inferomedial aspect of the clavicle, as well as osteophytes in the inferior margin of the clavicular head

(Fig. 47–12). The sternoclavicular joint space is not narrowed, and adjacent soft tissue and osseous structures are not affected. Scintigraphy demonstrates increased accumulation of bone-seeking radiopharmaceutical agents. Computed tomography scanning and MR imaging can be used to document the extent of bone involvement. The cause of condensing osteitis of the clavicle is unknown. Its occurrence in women of childbearing age suggests a common causative agent with osteitis condensans ilii, and stress-induced changes are most likely.

The differential diagnosis of this clavicular lesion is limited. The most difficult entity to exclude is ischemic necrosis of the medial clavicular epiphysis (Friedreich's disease). This rare disorder typically occurs in children and adolescents and is believed to be related to direct trauma or to an embolic event that results in obliteration of the vascular supply to the medial clavicular epiphysis. Sternocostoclavicular hyperostosis is a second disease that affects the medial end of the clavicle. Hyperostosis of the clavicle, sternum, and upper anterior ribs, with ossification of intervening soft tissues, is observed. In contrast to condensing osteitis of the clavicle, this condition is more common in older patients and in men, is usually bilateral, and is often accompanied by pustular lesions of the palms and soles (pustulosis palmaris et plantaris). Pyarthrosis of the sternoclavicular joint, especially the type seen in intravenous drug abusers, may mimic condensing osteitis of the clavicle, although laboratory values and radiographic evidence of narrowing of the sternoclavicular joint and osseous destruction assist in the differential diagnosis. Osteoarthritis of the sternoclavicular joint may also resemble condensing osteitis; however, joint space narrowing, osteophytosis, and subchondral cysts are seen on both sides of the articulation.

Chronic recurrent multifocal osteomyelitis, also referred to as cleidometaphyseal or plasma cell osteomyelitis, is an unusual syndrome seen in children and adolescents that leads to symmetrical lesions of the tubular bones and clavicles. Hyperostosis is a prominent feature of clavicular involvement, producing bone enlargement that resembles the findings in sternocostoclavicular hyperostosis. Chronic recurrent multifocal osteomyelitis and

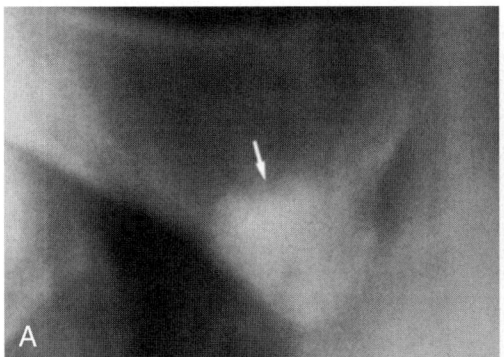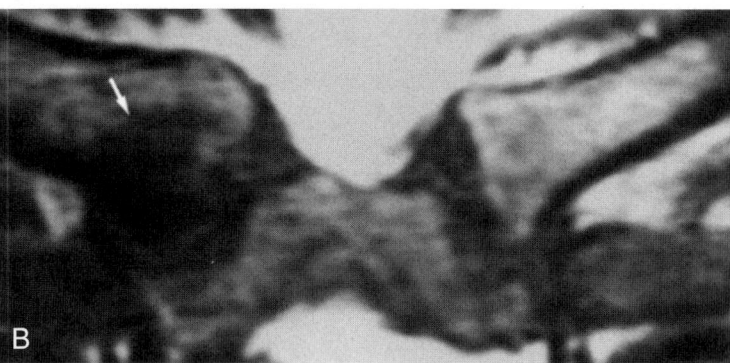

**Figure 47–12.** Condensing osteitis of the clavicle. This 40-year-old woman developed pain and tenderness over the medial end of the right clavicle. *A,* Conventional tomography reveals bone sclerosis involving the inferomedial aspect of the bone *(arrow). B,* Coronal T1-weighted (TR/TE, 300/11) spin echo MR image shows low signal intensity in this area *(arrow).* The diminished signal intensity persisted on T2-weighted spin echo and gradient echo images (not shown). (Courtesy of G. Greenway, MD, Dallas, Tex.)

potentially related disorders such as sternocostoclavicular hyperostosis and the synovitis-acne-pustulosis-hyperostosis-osteitis (SAPHO) syndrome are discussed in Chapters 53 and 82.

## FURTHER READING

Agrons GA, Lonergen GJ, Dickey GE, et al: Adrenocortical neoplasms in children: Radiologic-pathologic correlation. Radiographics 19:989, 1999.

Barnes WC, Malament M: Osteitis pubis. Surg Gynaecol Obstet 117:277, 1963.

Brower AC, Sweet DE, Keats TE: Condensing osteitis of the clavicle: A new entity. AJR Am J Roentgenol 121:17, 1974.

Cone RO, Resnick D, Goergen TG, et al: Condensing osteitis of the clavicle. AJR Am J Roentgenol 141:387, 1983.

Dhar S, Anderton JM: Rupture of the symphysis pubis during labor. Clin Orthop 283:252, 1992.

Dunn V, Nixon GW, Jaffe RB, et al: Infants of diabetic mothers: Radiographic manifestations. AJR Am J Roentgenol 137:123, 1981.

Gold RH, Steinbach HL: Lipoatrophic diabetes mellitus (generalized lipodystrophy): Roentgen findings in two brothers with congenital disease. AJR Am J Roentgenol 101:884, 1967.

Gray RG, Gottlieb NL: Rheumatic disorders associated with diabetes mellitus: Literature review. Semin Arthritis Rheum 6:19, 1976.

Greenspan A, Gerscovich E, Szabo RM, et al: Condensing osteitis of the clavicle: A rare but frequently misdiagnosed condition. AJR Am J Roentgenol 156:1011, 1991.

James RE, Baker HL, Scanlon PW: The roentgenologic aspects of metastatic pheochromocytoma. AJR Am J Roentgenol 115:783, 1972.

Jelinek JS, Murphey MD, Aboulafia AJ, et al: Muscle infarction in patients with diabetes mellitus: MR imaging findings. Radiology 211:241, 1999.

Johnson JP, Carey JC, Gooch WM III, et al: Femoral hypoplasia—unusual facies syndrome in infants of diabetic mothers. J Pediatr 102:866, 1983.

Kincaid OW, Hodgson JR, Dockerty MB: Neuroblastoma: A roentgenographic and pathologic study. AJR Am J Roentgenol 78:420, 1957.

Madell SH, Freeman LM: Avascular necrosis of bone in Cushing's syndrome. Radiology 83:1068, 1969.

Mendelson EB, Fisher MR, Deschler TW, et al: Osteomyelitis in the diabetic foot: A difficult diagnostic challenge. Radiographics 3:248, 1983.

Numaguchi Y: Osteitis condensans ilii, including its resolution. Radiology 98:1, 1971.

Nunez-Hoyo M, Gardner CL, Motta AO, et al: Skeletal muscle infarction in diabetes: MR findings. J Comput Assist Tomogr 17:986, 1993.

Pognowska MJ, Collins LC, Dobson HL: Diabetic osteopathy. Radiology 89:265, 1967.

Rand T, Schweitzer M, Rafii M, et al: Condensing osteitis of the clavicle: MRI. J Comput Assist Tomogr 27:291, 1998.

Segal G, Kellogg DS: Osteitis condensans ilii. AJR Am J Roentgenol 71:643, 1954.

Sinha S, Munichoodappa CS, Kozak GP: Neuro-arthropathy (Charcot joints) in diabetes mellitus (clinical study of 101 cases). Medicine 51:191, 1972.

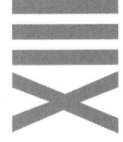

# Diseases of the Hematopoietic System

# CHAPTER 48

## Hemoglobinopathies and Other Anemias

### SUMMARY OF KEY FEATURES

The hemoglobinopathies are associated with characteristic abnormalities of the skeleton. In general, the abnormalities are related to marrow hyperplasia, vascular occlusion, and several additional problems, including fracture and infection. Although these features are apparent in almost all the hemoglobin disorders, their severity varies, which in some cases allows differentiation among these disorders. The articular manifestations in the hemoglobinopathies can be attributed to epiphyseal osteonecrosis, growth disturbances, osseous weakening, infection, crystal deposition, hemarthrosis, and synovial membrane microvascular obstruction. In some patients, these articular abnormalities overshadow other clinical manifestations of the disease.

### INTRODUCTION

Anemia should be regarded as a clinical finding rather than a specific disease. It is characterized by a reduction in the blood's capacity to transport oxygen. Oxygen combined with hemoglobin is transported by the red cell; therefore, anemia occurs when the circulating red cell mass is abnormally low. Because the red cell mass is generally correlated with the concentration of hemoglobin or the hematocrit value, anemia is usually accompanied by a decrease in hemoglobin concentration (below 13.5 g/dL in men and 12.0 g/dL in women) and a fall in hematocrit.

Hemoglobin represents approximately 33% of the wet weight of the red blood cell and 95% of its dry weight. Ninety-seven percent of the molecule consists of the polypeptide chains of globin, and 3% consists of the heme groups. The structure of 97% of the hemoglobin in a normal adult, which consists of two pairs of coiled polypeptide chains (two alpha chains composed of 141 amino acids, and two beta chains composed of 146 amino acids) is termed Hb A. A smaller fraction of hemoglobin (approximately 2%), termed Hb A2, may also be found; this fraction contains a different set of polypeptide chains. In the fetus, another type of hemoglobin is found, termed Hb F. This hemoglobin is present in infants at birth and varies in concentration from 60% to 90%. It generally decreases in concentration during the neonatal period and, in most infants, has almost disappeared by 4 months of age, by which time Hb A becomes predominant. In an adult, Hb F makes up the remaining 1% of hemoglobin.

The clinical manifestations of anemia are variable and influenced by its rate of development and the status or function of the cardiovascular, cerebrovascular, and renal systems. Characteristic abnormalities include exertional dyspnea, tachycardia, claudication, vertigo, and angina, conditions indicating an inadequate supply of oxygen to the body's tissues. Specific types of anemia (of which there are many) are sometimes associated with typical clinical clues, including the cholelithiasis seen in chronic hemolytic states and the bone pain and tenderness accompanying osseous metastasis with compromise of the bone marrow.

The hypoxia of anemia is a stimulus for increased erythropoiesis through the action of the hormone erythropoietin, formed principally in the kidneys. This hormone is responsible for increased cellular activity, leading to an augmented rate of formation of red blood cells from precursor cells. In the presence of bone marrow compromise, which may be related to marrow infiltration by tumor or myelofibrosis, extramedullary sites such as the liver and spleen become actively involved in hematopoiesis. Hepatosplenomegaly and even paravertebral masses are radiographic findings consistent with such hematopoiesis.

### SICKLE CELL ANEMIA

#### General Features

Sickle cell disease is a term that describes all conditions characterized by the presence of Hb S. These conditions include sickle cell anemia (Hb SS), sickle cell trait (Hb AS), and diseases in which Hb S is combined with another abnormal hemoglobin. Hb S is characterized by a normal alpha chain and an abnormal beta chain in which valine has replaced glutamic acid. It has been estimated that the sickle cell trait exists in approximately 7% of North American blacks and that sickle cell anemia occurs in approximately 0.3% to 1.3% of North American blacks.

#### Clinical Features

Symptomatic, painful crises affecting the bones and joints of the extremities usually commence during the second or third year of life. These crises are characterized by gradual or rapid worsening of anemia as a result of erythrocyte destruction and are associated with fever, icterus, nausea, vomiting, abdominal pain, and prostration. The basic pathogenesis of the sickle crisis appears to be deformation of red blood cells, which produces vaso-occlusion and tissue death. Osseous and articular pain and tenderness are frequently related to infarction of bone marrow. Indeed, such pain and tenderness appear to be the only clinical findings that can consistently and specifically be related to bone marrow necrosis; other associated abnormalities, which may include malaise, weight loss, and fever, are more likely manifestations of the underlying disease. In patients with sickle cell trait, painful crises are not usually apparent unless the patient is exposed to an atmosphere low in oxygen.

Sickle cell anemia rarely has its clinical onset in infants younger than 6 months because of the persistence of Hb F, which reduces the sickling properties of the red blood cell. Fever, pallor, and swelling of the hands are observed in children with this disease, apparently related in part to infarction of the small tubular bones. This "hand-foot" syndrome, or dactylitis, is most frequent between the ages of 6 months and 2 years. It is the initial manifestation of the disease in approximately 30% of cases. The clinical features are self-limited, with a duration that varies from a few days to several weeks.

Other clinical manifestations that may be apparent in sickle cell anemia are hepatosplenomegaly; cardiac enlargement; chronic leg ulcers, particularly over the malleoli; osteomyelitis; septic arthritis; pulmonary abnormalities, including pneumonia and infarction; abdominal pain; cholelithiasis; jaundice; peptic ulcer disease; hematuria; priapism; neurologic and muscular findings; and lymphadenopathy. Death may result from infection, cardiac decompensation related to severe anemia, or thrombosis and infarction of various organs. In recent years there has been increased longevity, and many affected persons live past the age of 50 years.

## Radiographic and Pathologic Features

### Marrow Hyperplasia

Hypercellularity of the bone marrow in this disease is a response to anemia of long duration. In infants with sickle cell anemia, red marrow extends into all the bones, including those of the hands and feet; in older children and adults, red marrow recedes from some of these small bones but persists in the ankles, wrists, and shafts of the long bones. Marrow hyperplasia produces widening of the medullary cavities and intertrabecular spaces and rarefaction of the remaining trabeculae in the spongiosa and cortex. These pathologic findings are associated with radiographic abnormalities, including increased radiolucency of osseous tissue, fewer and more accentuated bony trabeculae, and cortical thinning.

In the skull, diffuse widening of the diploic space is associated with thinning of both the outer and inner tables. The appearance is that of a coarse, granular osteoporosis involving the entire cranial vault except for the base of the occiput, which is relatively spared (Fig. 48–1). Localized areas of hyperplastic marrow (or infarcts) lead to focal radiolucent areas simulating metastasis or myeloma. In rare instances, focal or diffuse osteosclerosis of the cranium is observed, perhaps related to myelofibrosis. The facial bones, with the exception of the mandible, are not generally involved in sickle cell anemia. Prominence of the lamina dura may be observed.

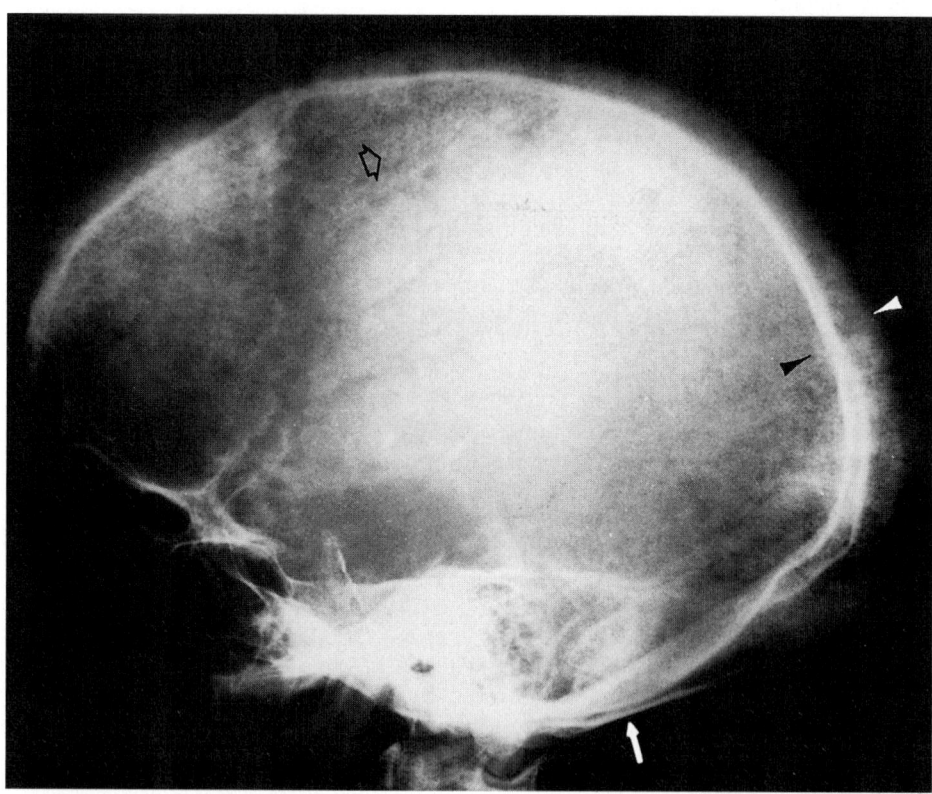

**Figure 48–1.** Sickle cell anemia: marrow hyperplasia. Lateral view of the skull demonstrates widening of the diploic space *(arrowheads)*. The base of the occiput is spared *(arrow)*. Focal areas of increased radiodensity *(open arrow)* may represent myelofibrosis or healing infarcts.

Osteoporosis of the vertebrae is commonly noted in patients with sickle cell anemia. Radiographically, osteoporosis is manifested as increased radiolucency of the vertebral bodies, prominence of vertical trabeculae, and smooth deformity of the contour of the vertebral bodies (fish vertebrae) as a result of compression by the adjacent intervertebral discs. Another vertebral sign—squared-off indentations of the vertebral bodies—is virtually diagnostic of sickle cell anemia or related disorders. This abnormality in vertebral contour apparently relates to bone infarction and arrested growth and is discussed later in this chapter. Marrow hyperplasia in bones of the thorax and extremities may also lead to osteoporosis and cortical thinning. The findings in the appendicular skeleton are not as prominent in adults as in children because of the normal fatty conversion of the marrow of the extremities that occurs with advancing age.

## Vascular Occlusion

Osteonecrosis is a well-recognized and significant complication of sickle cell anemia and its variants. Clinically, patients with osteonecrosis have fever, soft tissue swelling, bone pain and tenderness, and leukocytosis. Other clinical manifestations depend on the site of osteonecrosis.

**Sickle Cell Dactylitis.** In children between the ages of 6 months and 2 years, osteonecrosis may involve the small tubular bones of the hands and feet (Fig. 48–2). Osteonecrosis in this clinical setting is termed the hand-foot syndrome, or dactylitis. The syndrome may be present in as many as 20% to 50% of children with sickle cell anemia. Clinical manifestations include soft tissue swelling of the hands and feet, pain, tenderness, elevated temperature, and limitation of motion. These findings in a black child should arouse suspicion of this diagnosis.

In the early stages of sickle cell dactylitis, soft tissue swelling is frequently seen. Within 1 to 2 weeks, patchy radiolucency of the shaft with surrounding periostitis is observed in the metacarpals, metatarsals, and phalanges. The findings are relatively symmetrical in distribution in most persons and may affect the hands and feet simultaneously (Fig. 48–3). Focal osteosclerosis is also seen, and the osseous outline may be lost. The findings resemble those of osteomyelitis, and differentiation of these two conditions is extremely difficult. During a period of several months, bone reconstitution may lead to a completely normal osseous shadow. The hand-foot syndrome is rare after the age of 6 years because the red marrow recedes from the distal bones of the extremities and is replaced by fibrous tissue, which has less rigid oxygen demands.

The differential diagnosis of the clinical and radiographic manifestations of this syndrome includes tuberculosis, syphilis, yaws, smallpox, other types of infection, leukemia, and fat necrosis.

**Diaphyseal Infarction of Larger Tubular Bones.** The long tubular bones are common sites of such infarction (Fig. 48–4), and involvement of the diaphysis or one or both epiphyses can occur. The most frequent site of infarction is the proximal aspect of the femur, although the proximal humerus, distal femur, proximal tibia, and other locations may be affected.

Extensive infarction of the shaft is associated with patchy radiolucency and sclerosis of the medullary bone. Infarction of a large segment of cortical bone is followed by subperiosteal bone proliferation, periosteal inflammatory reaction, edema, exudation, and bone formation. On radiographic examination, such periosteal new bone initially appears as a linear radiodense area adjacent to

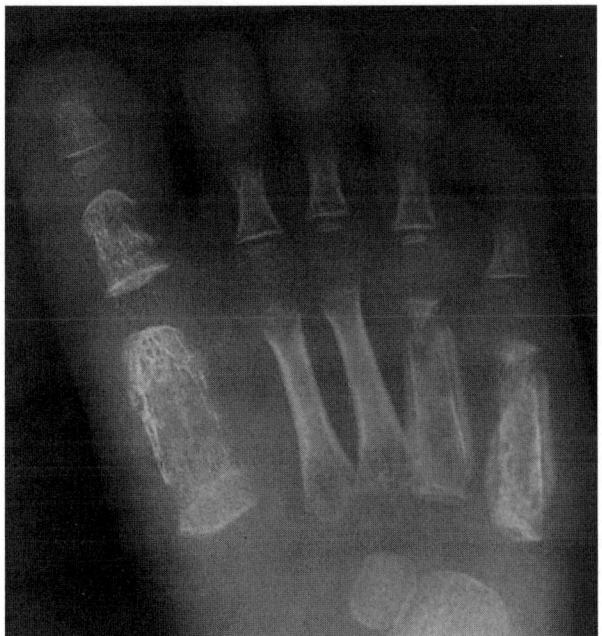

**Figure 48–2.** Sickle cell anemia: vascular occlusion in sickle cell dactylitis. Observe the soft tissue swelling, small osteolytic lesions (especially in the proximal phalanx of the great toe and the first, fourth, and fifth metatarsal bones), areas of more prominent osteolysis (including the distal portions of the fourth and fifth metatarsals), focal osteosclerosis, and periostitis. (Courtesy of P. Kaplan, MD, Boston, Mass.)

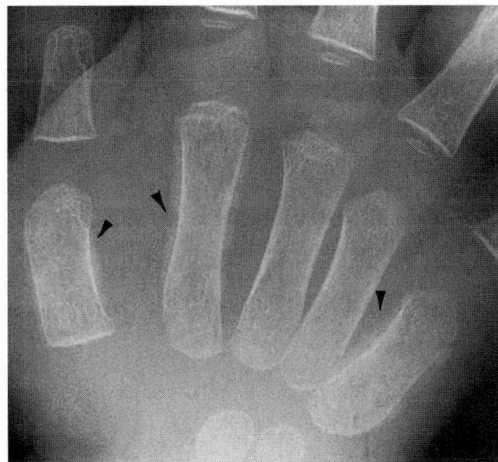

**Figure 48–3.** Sickle cell anemia: vascular occlusion in sickle cell dactylitis. Radiograph of the hand at 18 months of age (8 weeks after the onset of symptoms) delineates medullary lytic defects with periostitis (*arrowheads*) of multiple metacarpal bones.

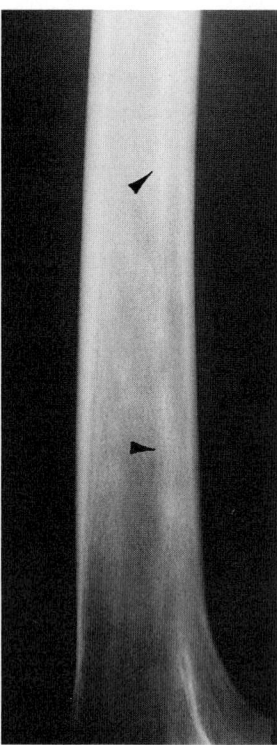

**Figure 48–4.** Sickle cell anemia: vascular occlusion and diaphyseal infarction of large tubular bones. The typical bone-within-bone appearance is caused by diaphyseal infarction. Observe the linear sclerosis beneath the cortex *(arrowheads)* on this lateral view of the femur.

the cortex that may extend along the entire shaft. Subsequently, the bone is incorporated into the cortex, and cortical thickening results. Within the bone along the inner surface of the cortex, laminated new bone formation in response to infarction can produce concentric cylinders of bone paralleling the cortical surface. On radiographs, discrete linear bands beneath the cortical bone produce a bone-within-bone appearance, which is diagnostic of osteonecrosis.

**Infarction of Other Bones.** Osteosclerosis in association with medullary infarction of bone (Fig. 48–5) can reach extreme proportions in sickle cell anemia and simulate the appearance of osteoblastic metastasis or Paget's disease. These sclerotic findings are particularly common in the pelvis, spine, thorax, tibia, and fibula and produce increased radiodensity of bone and a coarsened trabecular pattern. Ischemic necrosis in the small bones of the wrist and hindfoot is observed in sickle cell anemia but is less common than osteonecrosis in the tubular bones. Sclerosis in the terminal phalanges of the hand, similar to that described in patients with various collagen vascular diseases, has been observed to occur with increased frequency in patients with sickle cell anemia.

**Epiphyseal Infarction.** Epiphyseal infarcts in sickle cell anemia (Fig. 48–6) are frequent, although they are more prevalent in adults than in children. In older children, infarction of the capital femoral epiphysis occasionally leads to an appearance simulating that of Legg-Calvé-

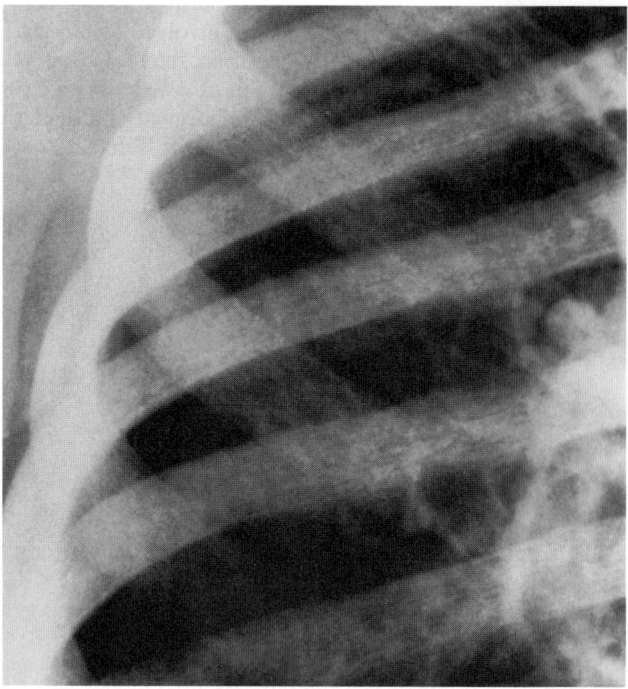

**Figure 48–5.** Sickle cell anemia: vascular occlusion and infarction of other bones. In the ribs, diffuse sclerosis has resulted in a coarsened trabecular pattern.

Perthes disease. Children with sickle cell anemia and necrosis of the proximal part of the femur are older than those with Legg-Calvé-Perthes disease, however. In addition, bilateral femoral involvement and occurrence in blacks are two features suggestive of sickle cell anemia or its variants. Epiphyseal infarction has a predilection for the capital femoral and proximal humeral epiphyses.

Osteonecrosis of the epiphysis in an adult with sickle cell anemia mimics the necrosis and collapse of epiphyses that accompany other processes, including steroid-induced and fracture-related conditions. Focal radiolucency and sclerosis, subchondral linear or curvilinear radiolucent shadows, collapse, and fragmentation are evident in involved epiphyses. Although collapse and disintegration of epiphyses, followed by the development of osteoarthritis, may be observed in weight-bearing areas such as the hip, epiphyseal necrosis in non–weight-bearing sites may lead to osteosclerosis without significant loss of epiphyseal contour. This finding is frequent in the proximal part of the humerus, where alternating areas of radiolucency and sclerosis produce a "snow-capped" appearance.

**Growth Disturbances.** Numerous growth disturbances occur in sickle cell anemia, presumably related to bone infarction. Damage to the epiphyseal circulation may produce arrested or decreased cartilage proliferation in the growth plate, which leads to shortening of the bone. Ingrowth of blood vessels from the metaphysis may cause osseous fusion, particularly in the central portion of the growth plate. This localization appears to be related to the fact that the central aspect of the plate is supplied by diaphyseal vessels, whereas the peripheral aspects are nourished by periosteal vessels. A variety of epiphyseal-

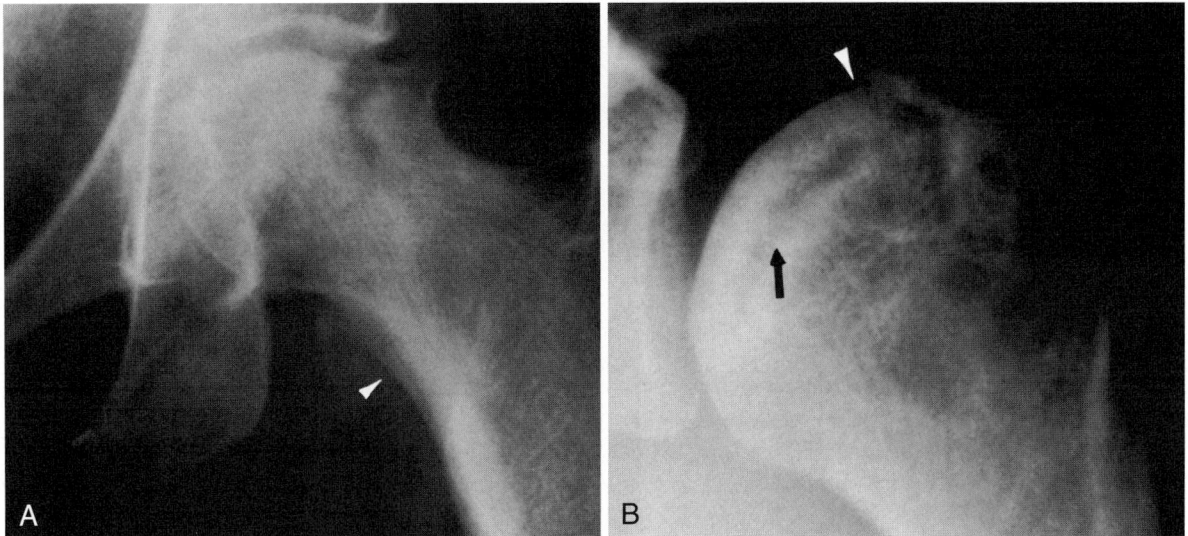

**Figure 48–6.** Sickle cell anemia: vascular occlusion and epiphyseal infarction. *A*, Osteonecrosis of the femoral head is characterized by focal areas of sclerosis and subsequent collapse, with irregularity of the articular surface. Observe the lateral femoral osteophytes and buttressing *(arrowhead)* of the femoral neck. *B*, The "snow-capped" appearance of the humeral head is related to patchy sclerosis. Collapse of the articular surface *(arrowhead)* and subchondral fractures *(arrow)* are evident.

metaphyseal growth disturbances have also been emphasized in this disease and are particularly frequent in the hands and feet, although they may occur elsewhere, including the long tubular bones. Cone-shaped epiphyses and inverted V, "cup," or "channel" deformities of the adjacent metaphyses are observed in sickle cell anemia, but similar changes occur in many other disorders.

Tibiotalar deformity consists of slanting of the articular surfaces of the distal portion of the tibia and the talus. It is an infrequent sign of sickle cell anemia and may also be seen in hemophilia, juvenile-onset rheumatoid arthritis, and multiple epiphyseal dysplasia.

Central depression of the vertebral bodies may be an additional growth disturbance of sickle cell anemia. The resulting deformity of the vertebra consists of squared-off endplate depressions, the H vertebra (Fig. 48–7). This deformity has been postulated to result from ischemia of the central portion of the vertebral growth plate, a vulnerability paralleling that of the central aspect of the growth plate in the peripheral skeleton.

## Miscellaneous Findings

**Fractures.** Fractures in the appendicular and axial skeletons in patients with sickle cell anemia can occur spontaneously or after minor trauma. In the long tubular bones, marrow hyperplasia produces cortical thinning, which predisposes to this complication. In the spine, marrow hyperplasia results in diffuse weakening of the entire vertebral body. Typical deformities result from compression of the bone by the adjacent intervertebral discs (fish vertebrae) or from intraosseous displacement of portions of the intervertebral disc (cartilaginous, or Schmorl's, nodes).

**Osteomyelitis and Septic Arthritis.** The frequency of osteomyelitis related to a variety of organisms in patients with sickle cell anemia is reported to be more than 100 times that seen in normal persons. Bone and joint infections in sickle cell anemia are caused by salmonellae in

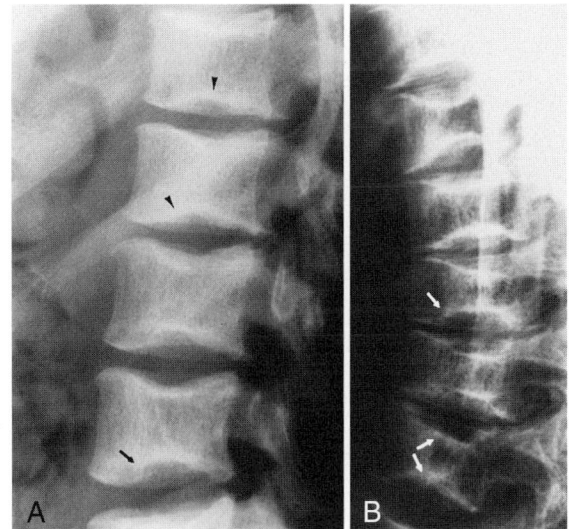

**Figure 48–7.** Sickle cell anemia: growth disturbance and H vertebrae. *A* and *B*, Two examples of H vertebrae, which are characterized by central indentations of the vertebral bodies. Initially, the abnormalities may simulate cartilaginous nodes or fish vertebrae *(arrowheads)*, although eventually, typical squared-off indentations *(arrows)* are observed.

over 50% of cases. It is suggested that these organisms gain entry to the bloodstream as a result of intestinal infarction produced by sickling within mesenteric vessels; typically, *Salmonella* bacteremia precedes osteomyelitis, and the organisms then lodge in the bone marrow. Staphylococci are a second common cause of osteomyelitis in sickle cell anemia and, in some series, are implicated more frequently than salmonellae. Osteomyelitis is most frequent in the long tubular bones. Infection may produce symmetrical involvement with diaphyseal localization (Fig. 48–8). Osteomyelitis in these patients may be related not only to hematogenous dissemination of infection to bone but also to direct spread from a contiguous soft tissue infection. Septic arthritis complicating sickle cell anemia is less frequent than osteomyelitis. Radiographic findings are typical of septic arthritis: soft tissue swelling, joint space narrowing, variable osteoporosis, and osseous destruction.

**Crystal Deposition.** Hyperuricemia occurs in some patients with sickle cell anemia. The reported frequency of this laboratory finding in adults with the disease varies from 20% to 40%. The frequency of clinical attacks of gout and successful recovery of urate crystals from inflamed joints in patients with sickle cell anemia is lower.

**Joint Effusions.** Joint effusions in sickle cell anemia that are not associated with infection, crystal deposition, or hemarthrosis are relatively common. Fluid production is

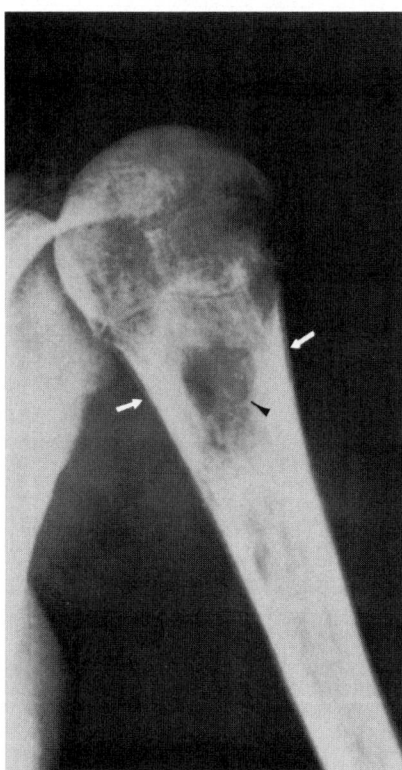

**Figure 48–8.** Sickle cell anemia: osteomyelitis and septic arthritis. *Salmonella* infection of the humerus has led to lytic lesions *(arrowhead)*, with surrounding periostitis *(arrows)*. This organism may produce symmetrical diaphyseal osteomyelitis of the long tubular bones in patients with sickle cell anemia.

generally confined to one or two joints and subsides in 2 to 14 days. Radiographic examination may demonstrate osteonecrosis of adjacent bones.

## Radionuclide Findings

In normal adults, bone marrow is located predominantly in the axial skeleton and proximal portions of the femora and humeri; in patients with various anemias, the marrow expands symmetrically to occupy the long bones and skull. During asymptomatic periods, patients with sickle cell anemia and related disorders may reveal focal areas of decreased uptake, which can probably be attributed to sites of previous infarction. During a crisis, additional areas are found that are without radionuclide activity, surrounded by active marrow. After a crisis, the infarcted marrow may return to normal in 1 to 12 months or progress to permanent fibrosis, with corresponding changes in radionuclide activity.

Bone scanning agents such as technetium-99m ($^{99m}$Tc) polyphosphate demonstrate uptake related to the integrity of blood flow and the presence of new bone formation. In patients with sickle cell anemia and related diseases, marrow expansion is associated with increased blood flow and an increased accumulation of radionuclide in the skeleton, particularly in the lower extremities. Immediately after a crisis, an area of infarction may demonstrate decreased or absent radionuclide activity (Fig. 48–9). The size of this defect in activity is generally smaller on bone scans than on bone marrow scans. One to 2 weeks after the crisis, increased activity on bone scanning is due to reactive bone formation about the area of infarction. This abnormal activity may persist for several months.

It has been suggested that scanning with both bone- and bone marrow–seeking radionuclides allows differentiation of osteomyelitis and osteonecrosis in patients with sickle cell anemia. The combination of a large defect on the bone marrow scan and a smaller defect on the bone scan is typical of osteonecrosis. Marrow scans with $^{99m}$Tc sulfur colloid may also outline sites of extramedullary hematopoiesis in sickle cell anemia or related disorders.

## Magnetic Resonance Imaging Findings

**Normal Findings.** From a functional viewpoint, bone marrow is often divided into red marrow and yellow marrow, although components of both types of marrow are frequently encountered at any particular anatomic site. Red marrow is considered hematopoietically active and involved in the production of red cells, white cells, and platelets; yellow marrow is considered hematopoietically inactive and is composed predominantly of fat cells. The chemical composition of red marrow is approximately 40% water, 40% fat, and 20% protein; yellow marrow consists of approximately 15% water, 80% fat, and 5% protein. The precise amount of red and yellow marrow is dependent on a number of factors, including the anatomic site, age of the person, and hematopoietic demands of the body. Under normal circumstances, a well-documented, orderly, and predictable transition, or conversion, of red to yellow marrow takes place. Transition begins in the immediate postnatal period

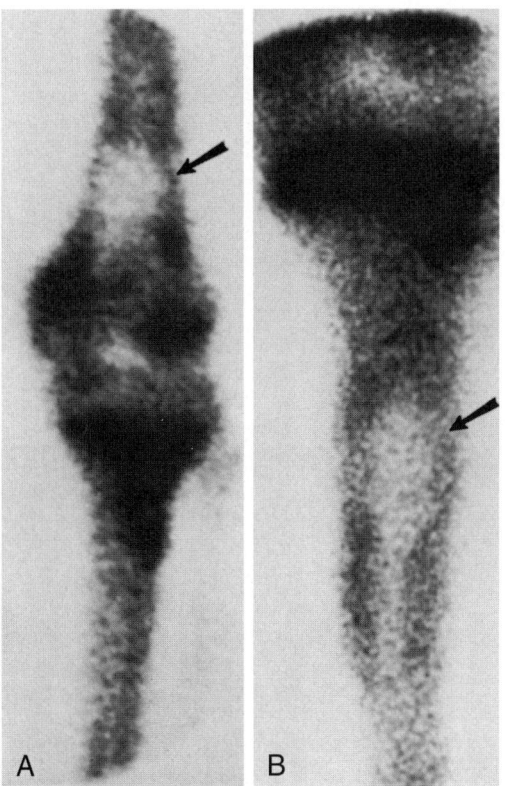

**Figure 48–9.** Sickle cell anemia: radionuclide abnormalities shown by technetium-labeled polyphosphate bone scanning. Diaphyseal infarctions of the distal portion of the femur *(A)* and proximal end of the tibia *(B)* are associated with focally decreased accumulation of radionuclide *(arrows)*. Increased metaphyseal activity is apparent.

and generally progresses from appendicular to axial sites and, in the tubular bones, from diaphyseal to metaphyseal locations. The most dramatic changes occur in the tubular bones and in the first 2 decades of life. Conversion begins in the bones of the hands and feet, progresses to the distal and then the proximal ends of the long tubular bones, and finally occurs in the flat bones and vertebral bodies; the adult pattern is generally achieved by age 25 years. At any age, the apophyses and epiphyses of the skeleton contain predominantly yellow marrow.

In regions of yellow marrow, fat is the tissue that contributes most heavily to the magnetic resonance (MR) imaging signal. The short T1 relaxation time and the long T2 relaxation time of adipose tissue are the factors most responsible for the MR imaging characteristics of yellow marrow. The contribution of fat to the MR imaging signal pattern of red marrow is also significant, although the increased cellularity and water and protein content in hematopoietic tissue lead to longer T1 and T2 relaxation times. With spin echo imaging, yellow marrow appears as areas of high signal intensity on T1-weighted sequences; because of the variability of the T1 value of hematopoietic marrow, however, its appearance on T1-weighted spin echo MR images is more variable. Such marrow may have a signal intensity ranging from less than that of muscle to greater than that of muscle but less than that of

fat (in hematopoietic marrow that contains a greater proportion of fat). With more heavily T2-weighted spin echo MR images, differences in T2 relaxation times dictate the resulting appearance of the bone marrow. Discrimination between red and yellow marrow, which may be characterized by relatively small differences in T2 relaxation times, is generally poorer on T1-weighted images.

Short tau inversion recovery (STIR) imaging provides a method whereby the MR imaging signal derived from fat can be eliminated. Thus, the signal intensity of yellow marrow is nullified, and it appears black, allowing its differentiation from red marrow. STIR imaging is also an effective technique in accentuating pathologic processes that replace yellow marrow, although discrimination between these and hematopoietic marrow may be difficult. Chemical shift imaging can also be used to produce selective elimination of the fat signal; it shares with STIR imaging the benefit of accentuating differences between red and yellow marrow.

**Marrow Reconversion.** Reversal of the normal sequence of conversion from red to yellow marrow, a process termed reconversion, may occur when an increased demand for hematopoiesis exists, as in patients with various types of anemia and in those with diseases that infiltrate or replace normal bone marrow, such as plasma cell myeloma, myelofibrosis, or skeletal metastasis. Marrow reconversion commences in the spine and flat bones, after which the tubular bones in the extremities are affected in a proximal to distal sequence that is the reverse of marrow conversion. In patients with sickle cell anemia, an expanded distribution of hematopoietic bone marrow is indicated by diffuse or focal areas of diminished signal intensity seen with T1-weighted spin echo sequences (Fig. 48–10). The signal characteristics on T2-weighted sequences are more variable and depend on the amount of cellularity and tissue water, and abnormal regions of marrow may reveal signal intensity that is less than, equal to, or slightly greater than that of subcutaneous fat on such sequences. The extent of reconversion of marrow is proportional to the severity of the process. In some patients with chronic disorders of erythropoiesis, iron overload from recurrent hemolysis and frequent blood transfusions leads to iron deposition in the liver, spleen, and bone marrow. This deposition results in regions of low signal intensity on both T1- and T2-weighted images (Fig. 48–11). Reconversion of bone marrow that accompanies anemic states leads to signal changes on MR imaging that lack specificity, and similar findings may be seen in patients with lymphoma, leukemia, plasma cell myeloma, myelofibrosis, or (less commonly) skeletal metastasis.

Even in healthy persons, foci of marrow reconversion may occur, simulating the appearance of such tumors. This clinically insignificant process appears to be more frequent and extensive in obese women of menstruating age and in athletes involved in sports demanding long endurance. Sparing or minimal involvement of the epiphysis has also been emphasized as an MR imaging finding that occurs in this benign condition, whereas epiphyseal involvement may be seen in more significant bone marrow disorders.

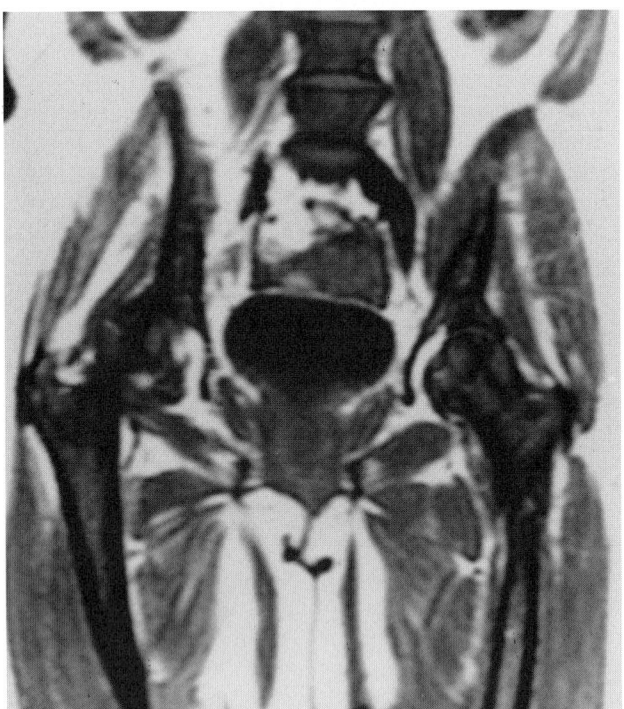

**Figure 48–10.** Sickle cell anemia: marrow ischemia and reconversion. In this 26-year-old woman, a T1-weighted (TR/TE, 600/20) spin echo MR image reveals an expanded distribution of hematopoietic marrow, resulting in low signal intensity in all visualized bone marrow, including the diaphyses of the femora. The irregularity and collapse of both femoral heads are consistent with osteonecrosis.

**Marrow Ischemia.** In sickle cell anemia, ischemia with infarction may occur in diametaphyseal or subchondral locations, or both (Fig. 48–12). The MR imaging features of osteonecrosis are detailed in Chapter 67.

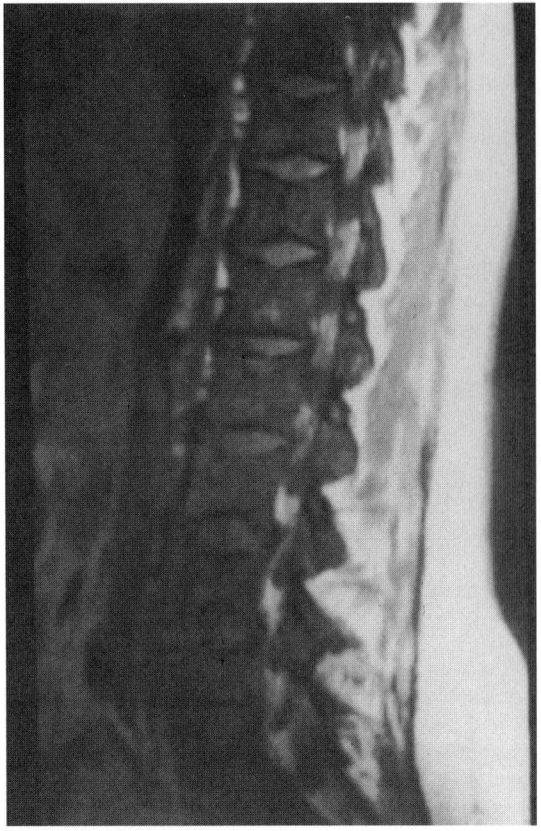

**Figure 48–11.** Sickle cell anemia: iron overload. In this adolescent patient, a T1-weighted spin echo MR image of the spine shows diffuse decreased signal intensity in the bone marrow of the vertebrae. The signal intensity of the marrow remained low on T2-weighted images (not shown). (From Moore SG, Bisset GS 3rd, Siegel MJ, Donaldson JS: Pediatric musculoskeletal MR imaging. Radiology 179:345, 1991.)

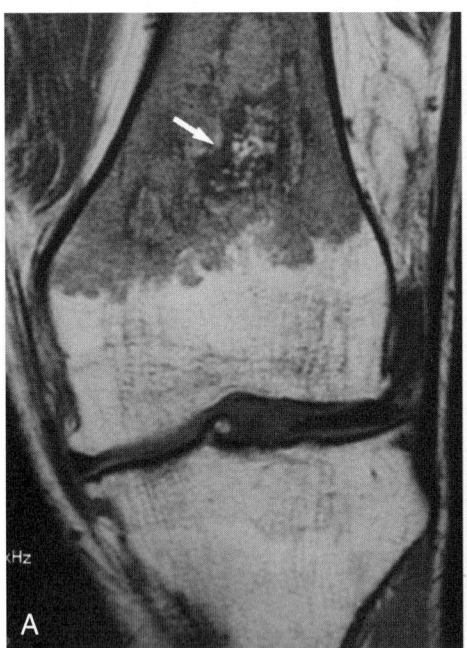

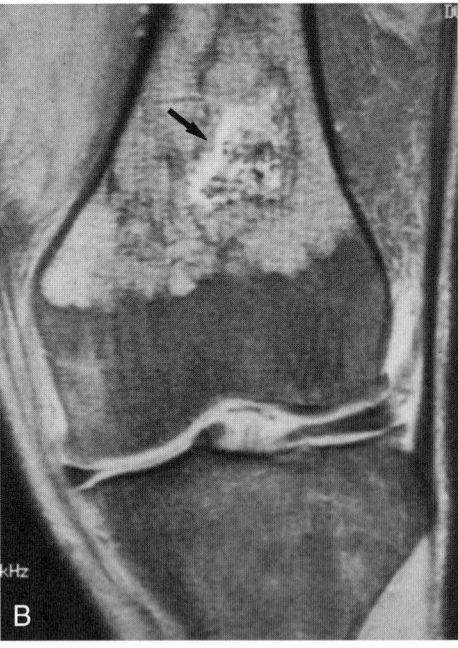

**Figure 48–12.** Sickle cell anemia: marrow ischemia and reconversion. In this 50-year-old woman with hemoglobinopathy (sickle cell–thalassemia disease), coronal T1-weighted (TR/TE, 516/13) spin echo (A) and fat-suppressed (TR/TE, 3000/12) fast spin echo (B) MR images show evidence of marrow reconversion and infarction in the distal metaphyseal portion of the femur. In A, note that the reconverted marrow is of low signal intensity, and an area of bone infarction in the metaphysis is characterized by inhomogeneous signal intensity (arrow). In B, the hematopoietic marrow in the femur has a signal intensity similar to that of muscle, and the infarct (arrow) has inhomogeneous but mainly higher signal intensity.

**Osteomyelitis.** The MR imaging characteristics of osteomyelitis relate to replacement or infiltration of the normal (or ischemic) marrow by inflammatory cells. As a result of the increased water content and cellularity, the affected region demonstrates decreased signal intensity on T1-weighted spin echo MR images and increased signal intensity on T2-weighted spin echo MR images. In patients with sickle cell anemia, it may be impossible to differentiate osteomyelitis and acute marrow ischemia and infarction by means of MR imaging.

**Marrow Heterotopia.** Extramedullary hematopoiesis may be encountered in patients with chronic hemolytic anemias, especially thalassemia (see later discussion), but also sickle cell and other anemias. The resulting masses of hematopoietic tissue may be detected with MR imaging. On T1-weighted images, low signal intensity similar to that of hematopoietic marrow characterizes the masses, although a rim of higher signal intensity similar to that of fat has been emphasized as an MR imaging finding of paraspinal sites of extramedullary hematopoiesis.

**Muscle and Soft Tissue Abnormalities.** Alterations in skeletal muscle occurring during sickle crises relate to hemorrhagic or ischemic changes that lead to inflammation and edema. Single or multiple foci occur in one or more extremities, especially the legs, with resultant soft tissue swelling and pain. Involvement of the intrinsic musculature of the foot is also characteristic. Early diagnosis may be provided by MR imaging, particularly T2-weighted spin echo sequences, in which increased signal intensity can be detected in the involved musculature. Healing of infarcts in skeletal muscle may be accompanied by fibrosis, with regions of low signal intensity on T1- and T2-weighted spin echo images. In general, MR imaging abnormalities confined to the soft tissues exclude the presence of marrow infarction or osteomyelitis in patients with sickle cell anemia, and they raise the possibility of muscle infarction.

## SICKLE CELL TRAIT

Sickle cell trait is characterized by the presence of Hb AS. It can be associated with sickling if the blood is exposed to low oxygen tension. Patients with sickle cell trait are not jaundiced or anemic. Hyperplasia of bone marrow is not present. The frequency of musculoskeletal findings related to sickle cell trait is low.

## SICKLE CELL–HEMOGLOBIN C DISEASE

Sickle cell–hemoglobin C disease is the second most frequent sickling disorder. The clinical disability is less severe than in homozygous sickle cell disease (sickle cell anemia) because Hb S accounts for approximately 50% of the total hemoglobin; therefore, the diagnosis is often not established until adulthood. A typical complaint is musculoskeletal pain, which may localize in the joints. Marrow hyperplasia in sickle cell–hemoglobin C disease may result in calvarial alterations in 25% of patients. Reported changes in the skull include granular osteoporosis, diploic widening, and thinning of the outer table.

Spinal abnormalities consisting of biconcavity of the vertebral bodies and narrowing of the intervertebral discs may be seen. Osteonecrosis of the femoral and humeral heads may be apparent. Some investigators have suggested that the frequency of bone necrosis is higher in this disease than in sickle cell anemia, perhaps related to greater blood viscosity in SC hemoglobinopathy than in SS hemoglobinopathy (Fig. 48–13).

## SICKLE CELL–THALASSEMIA DISEASE

Sickle cell–thalassemia disease is caused by the inheritance of one gene for Hb S and one gene for thalassemia. The clinical and radiographic features of this disease vary: some patients have manifestations that are almost identical to those associated with sickle cell anemia, whereas other patients are entirely asymptomatic. The clinical manifestations generally parallel the amount of Hb A present. Ischemic changes in the skeleton are common in sickle cell–thalassemia disease. Diaphyseal and epiphyseal infarcts are seen (Fig. 48–14). The former leads to patchy sclerosis and radiolucency and a bone-within-bone appearance, whereas the latter is most common in the proximal epiphyses of the femora and humeri and consists of radiolucency, sclerosis, collapse, and fragmentation. Osteomyelitis and septic arthritis may occur in sickle cell–thalassemia disease. *Salmonella* is frequently the causative agent, and infection may occur in the appendicular or axial skeleton.

## THALASSEMIA
### General Features

In 1925, Cooley and Lee described a form of severe anemia associated with splenomegaly and bone abnormalities that they designated thalassemia, from the Greek word

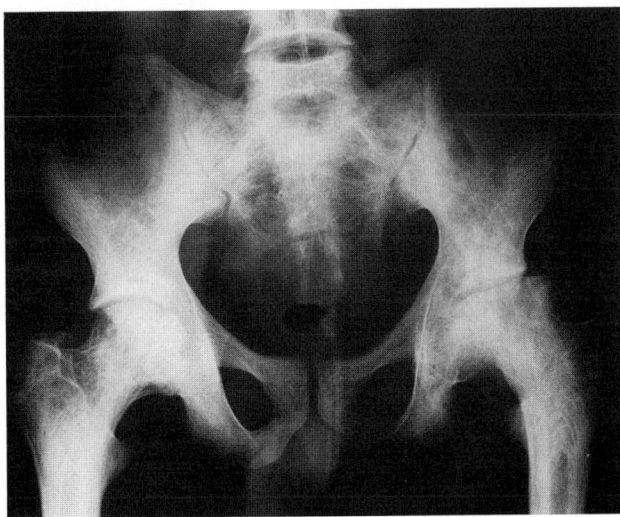

**Figure 48–13.** Sickle cell–hemoglobin C disease: vascular occlusion. Diffuse osteosclerosis of the pelvis and proximal long bones is associated with osteonecrosis of the femoral heads. Significant collapse of the left femoral head is apparent.

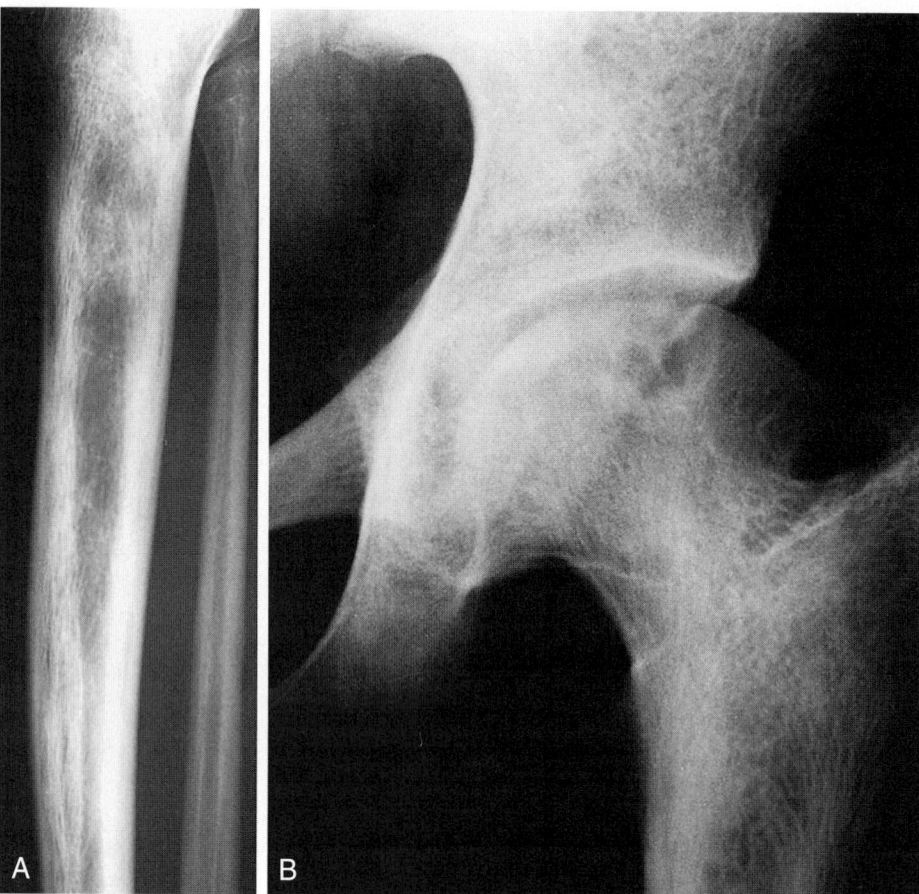

**Figure 48–14.** Sickle cell–thalassemia disease: vascular occlusion. *A,* In the tibia, extensive bone infarction has resulted in a bone-within-bone appearance. *B,* Osteonecrosis of the femoral head is evident.

for "sea," because their patients were of Mediterranean origin. It is now known that thalassemia is not a single disease but a group of disorders related to an inherited abnormality in globin production. These disorders differ from sickle cell anemia, which results from an inherited structural abnormality in one of the constituent globin chains; the thalassemias result from inherited defects in the rate of synthesis of one of the globin chains. This abnormality leads to an imbalance in globin chain production, which contributes to ineffective erythropoiesis, hemolysis, and a variable degree of anemia.

Thalassemia is divided into two main groups: alpha-thalassemia is characterized by a deficiency in alpha-globin chain synthesis, and beta-thalassemia is characterized by a deficiency in beta-globin chain synthesis. Because Hb F contains alpha chains, the fetus is affected by alpha-thalassemia; beta-thalassemia becomes apparent after the newborn period, when Hb A replaces Hb F. Thalassemia may exist in a homozygous form, called thalassemia major, or a heterozygous form, termed thalassemia minor or minima.

## Clinical Features

Homozygous beta-thalassemia (thalassemia major), typically seen in persons of Mediterranean ancestry, is characterized by severe anemia, prominent hepatosplenomegaly, and early death, often in childhood. Heterozygous beta-

thalassemia (thalassemia minor) is generally associated with mild clinical findings, including slight to moderate anemia, splenomegaly, and jaundice. It is observed throughout the world, most commonly in Mediterranean populations, and occurs in approximately 1% of American blacks, most of whom are entirely asymptomatic.

## Radiographic and Pathologic Features

**Marrow Hyperplasia.** The radiographic and pathologic features of beta-thalassemia are due in large part to marrow hyperplasia. Initially, both the axial and the appendicular skeletons are altered, but as the patient reaches puberty, the appendicular skeletal changes diminish because of normal regression of the hematopoietic marrow. The changes in thalassemia major are much more severe than those in thalassemia minor.

In the skull, the frontal bones reveal the earliest and most severe changes, and the inferior aspect of the occiput is usually unaltered. Findings include granular osteoporosis, widening of the diploic space, and thinning of the outer table. Bony proliferation on the outer table of the vault leads to a hair-on-end appearance. Marrow hyperplasia of the skull is not confined to the cranial vault but involves the facial bones as well (Fig. 48–15). In infancy and early childhood, osseous expansion of the nasal and temporal bones leads to obliteration of the air spaces of the paranasal sinuses. Maxillary alterations can produce lateral displacement of the orbits, leading to hypertelorism, malocclusion of the jaws, and displacement of dental structures, with a resultant "rodent" facies. The extent and severity of the cranial vault changes, including the hair-on-end appearance, are much greater in thalassemia than in other anemic disorders.

Osteoporosis of the vertebrae is most evident in the vertebral bodies. In the spine, reduction in the number of trabeculae, thinning of the subchondral bone plates,

accentuation of vertical trabeculation, and biconcave deformities (fish vertebrae) are evident. Medullary hyperplasia is also evident in other bones of the axial skeleton, including the ribs, pelvis, and clavicles, as well as the bones of the appendicular skeleton (Figs. 48–16 and 48–17). Similarly, the tubular bones reveal a widened marrow cavity, cortical thinning, and a coarse, trabeculated appearance. The contour of some of the long bones is altered; normal concavity is lost, and the bones may

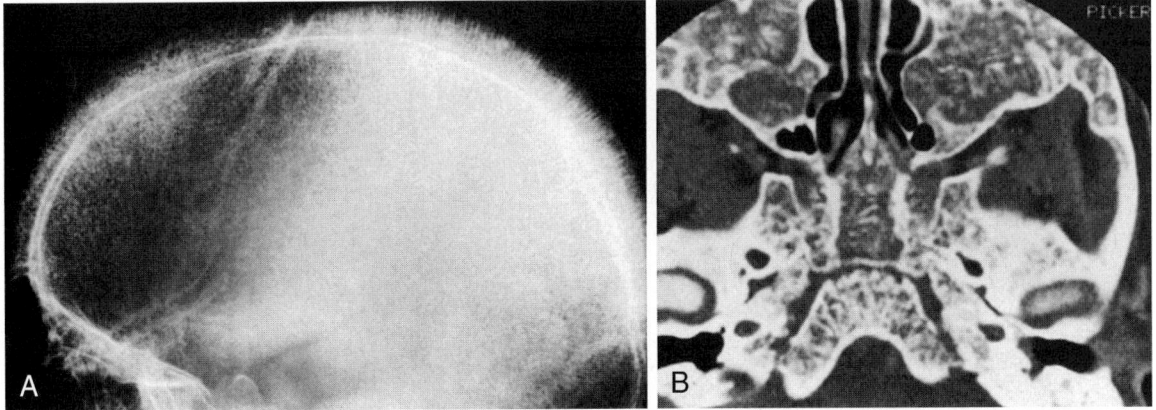

**Figure 48–15.** Marrow hyperplasia in the skull and face. In this example, a hair-on-end appearance is well shown on a routine radiograph *(A)*, and overgrowth of the facial bones is delineated with transaxial CT scanning *(B)*. (Courtesy of S. K. Brahme, MD, San Diego, Calif.)

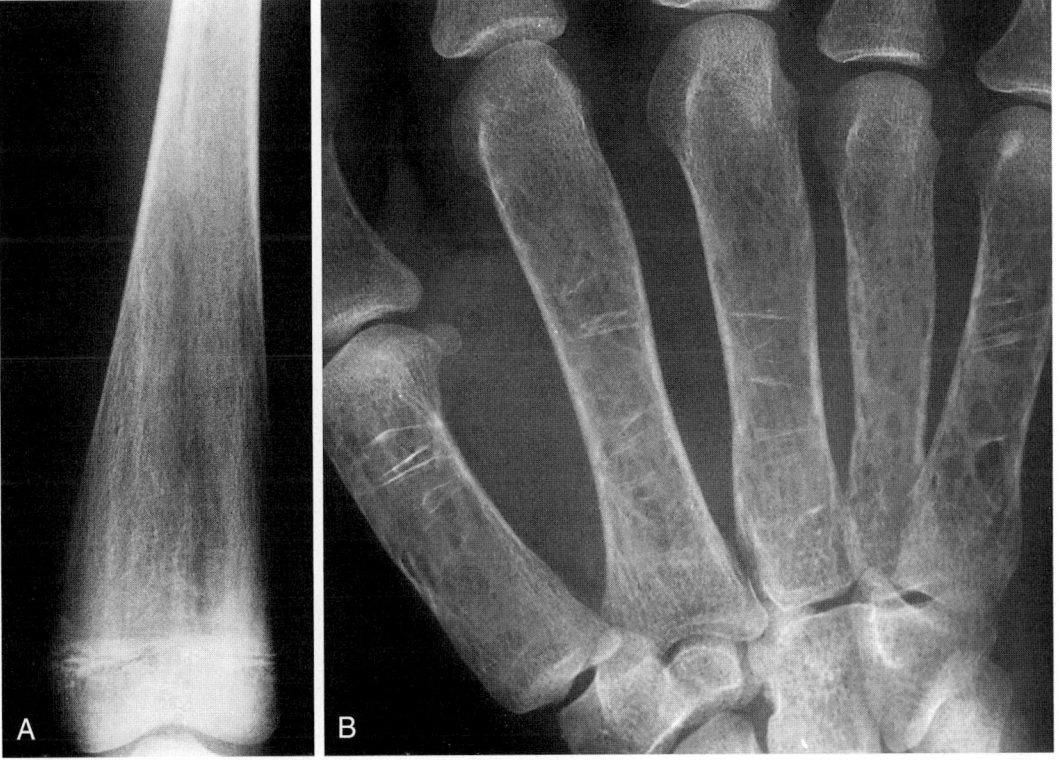

**Figure 48–16.** Thalassemia major: marrow hyperplasia in the axial and appendicular skeletons. *A,* Femur. An Erlenmeyer flask deformity is apparent, with loss of normal concavity and straightening or convexity of the osseous contour, particularly along the medial aspect of the bone. *B,* Hands. Osteopenia, small cystic lesions, and bone reinforcement lines are apparent. (*B,* Courtesy of S. K. Brahme, MD, San Diego, Calif.)

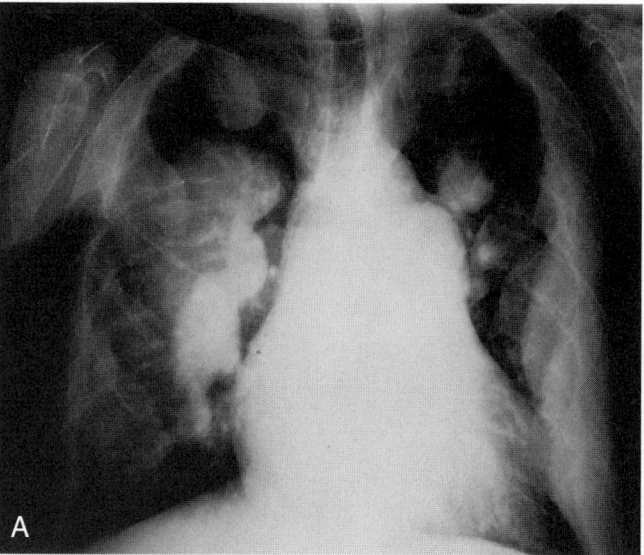

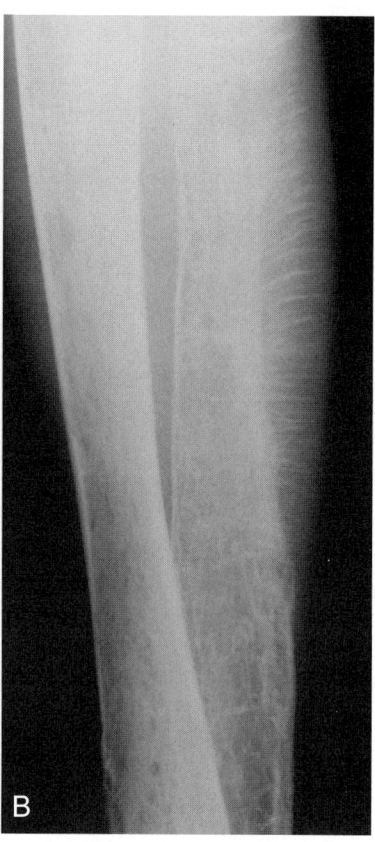

**Figure 48–17.** Thalassemia major: marrow hyperplasia in the axial and appendicular skeletons Widespread and marked involvement of the ribs is associated with osteopenia, cortical thinning, and bone expansion. The entire thorax and the humeri are affected. (Courtesy of A. Brower, MD, Norfolk, Va.)

have a straight or convex appearance. The widening of the metaphyses and epiphyses resembles an Erlenmeyer flask. Radionuclide studies in patients with thalassemia and diffuse marrow hyperplasia may reveal a generalized decrease in the skeletal uptake of bone-seeking pharmaceutical agents.

**Growth Disturbances.** The modeling (Erlenmeyer flask) deformity is only one of the tubular bone growth disturbances that may be encountered in patients with thalassemia. Premature fusion of the physes (growth plates) in the tubular bones of the extremities is a common finding in children with thalassemia major, noted in 10% to 15% of patients. It generally occurs after the age of 10 years and is most frequent in the proximal portion of the humerus and distal end of the femur. Shortening and deformity of the extremity may be apparent.

**Fractures.** Infarctions or spontaneous fractures (Fig. 48–18) are not uncommon in patients with thalassemia. They are most frequent in the long bones of the lower extremity, particularly the femur; in the bones of the forearm; and in the vertebrae.

**Crystal Deposition.** Secondary hemochromatosis resulting from repeated transfusions can be seen in patients with thalassemia. The arthropathy in these patients resembles that of primary hemochromatosis, with joint space narrowing and sclerosis in the metacarpophalangeal joints, knees, and hips. Calcium pyrophosphate dihydrate crystal deposition may lead to chondrocalcinosis. Hyper-

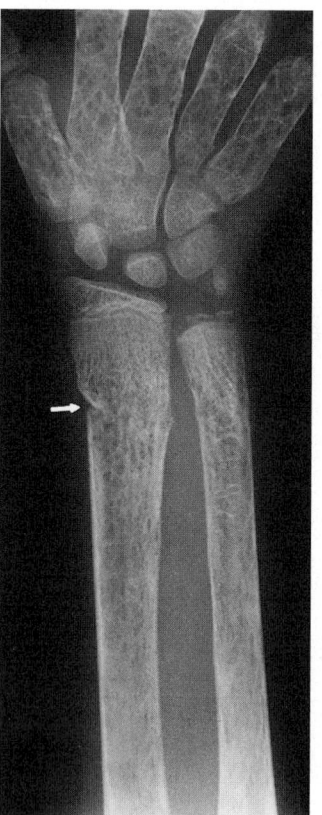

**Figure 48–18.** Thalassemia major: fracture. Note the extreme osteoporosis. The cortices are extensively thinned or absent, and a fracture can be observed (*arrow*).

uricemia and acute gouty arthritis may appear during the clinical course of thalassemia.

**Extramedullary Hematopoiesis.** In thalassemia, posterior paravertebral mediastinal masses (Fig. 48–19), representing sites of extramedullary hematopoiesis, result from extraosseous extensions of medullary tissue derived from vertebral bodies and ribs. Radiographs of the ribs in such cases document expanded and thinned cortices and cortical perforations with lobulated soft tissue masses; these findings are particularly well shown with computed tomography (CT) or MR imaging. In beta-thalassemia, this complication is almost universally seen in the thoracic region, a localization that is also noted in other hematologic diseases such as sickle cell anemia and hereditary spherocytosis. Extramedullary hematopoiesis in thalassemia, as well as in other anemias, can involve the retroperitoneal space and pelvis (Fig. 48–20).

**Miscellaneous Abnormalities.** Enlargement of nutrient foramina in the phalanges of the hand has been identified in beta-thalassemia. This finding is presumably related to hyperactive and hyperemic bone marrow.

## Other Diagnostic Techniques

The iron overload resulting from repeated blood transfusions in thalassemia is associated with a reduction in skeletal uptake of phosphorus-containing bone-seeking radiopharmaceutical agents and an increase in renal and soft tissue radioactivity. Similarly, analysis of sites of extramedullary hematopoiesis by radionuclide techniques can be accomplished if appropriate caution is exercised.

CT scanning can document the abnormal deposition of iron that follows multiple blood transfusions in patients with thalassemia (or other anemias). This technique can also be used to document sites of extramedullary hematopoiesis, particularly in the posterior mediastinum, spinal canal, and pelvis.

MR imaging has been used as an additional diagnostic method in some patients with thalassemia. The intensity of the MR image provides a means of assessing the amount of iron deposited in the tissues of the body. Depression of spin echo intensities in the liver and bone marrow and elevation of these intensities in the kidneys and muscles correlate with changes in iron concentration and iron content per ferritin molecule. In addition, MR imaging is useful in documenting the bone marrow's response to therapeutic manipulation of various anemias. MR imaging may also be used effectively in the assessment of marrow heterotopia, and it allows documentation of the effect of sites of extramedullary hematopoiesis on surrounding tissues and organs (see Fig. 48–19).

## Effects of Therapeutic Modalities

Therapeutic methods that have been used in patients with thalassemia include repeated blood transfusions to

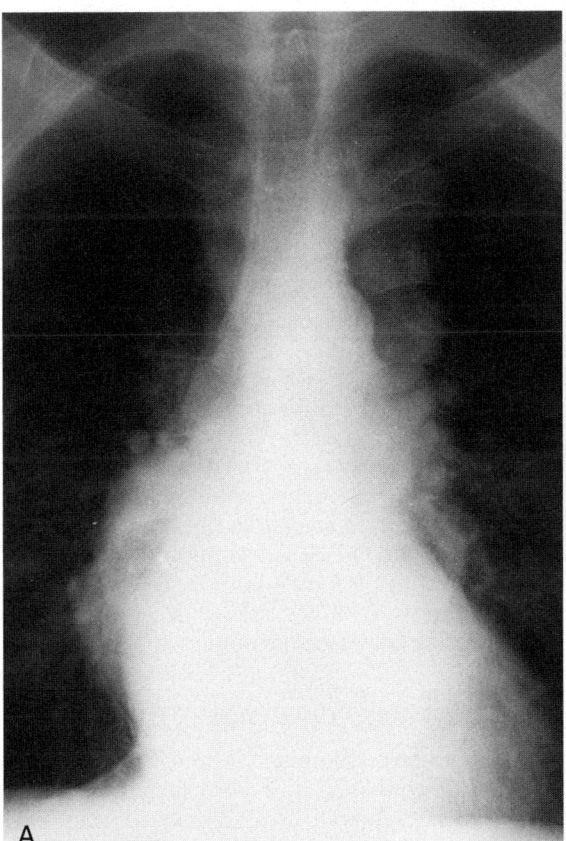

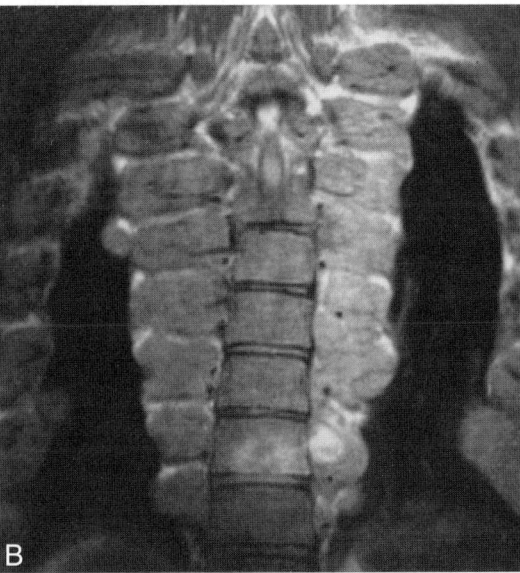

**Figure 48–19.** Thalassemia major: extramedullary hematopoiesis. *A*, Bilateral lobulated posterior mediastinal masses can be seen. The heart is enlarged. *B*, In a different patient, a coronal T1-weighted (TR/TE, 700/20) spin echo MR image of the thorax reveals evidence of marrow reconversion and heterotopia. Note the presence of hematopoietic marrow in the vertebral bodies and ribs. The posterior portions of the ribs are expanded dramatically.

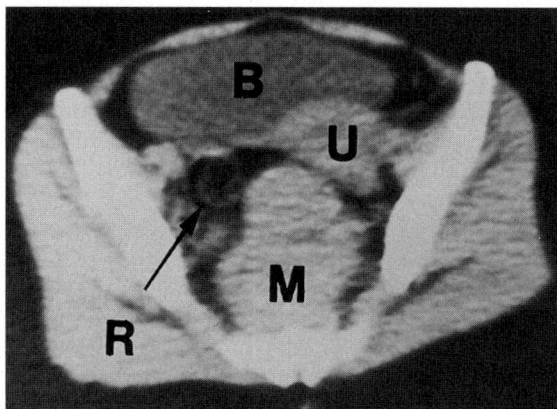

**Figure 48–20.** Thalassemia major: extramedullary hematopoiesis. Transaxial CT image of the pelvis demonstrates the posterior mass (M), representing extramedullary hematopoiesis. Note the anterior displacement of the rectum (R) and the position of the bladder (B) and uterus (U). (Courtesy of J. Sebes, MD, Memphis, Tenn.)

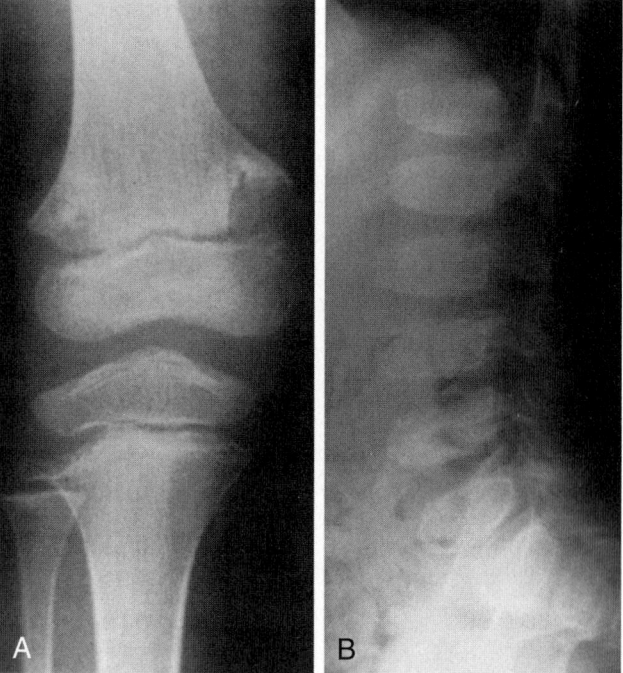

**Figure 48–21.** Thalassemia major: deferoxamine-induced bone changes. *A*, In an anteroposterior radiograph of the knee, the metaphyses of the distal portion of the femur and proximal end of the tibia are deficient circumferentially. Note the irregularity of the femoral metaphysis and, to a lesser extent, the tibial and fibular metaphyses. *B*, In the lumbar spine, flattened vertebral bodies are evident. (From Brill PW, Winchester P, Giardina PJ, Cunningham-Rundles S: Deferoxamine-induced bone dysplasia in patients with thalassemia major. AJR Am J Roentgenol 156:561, 1991.)

maintain acceptable levels of hemoglobin and chelation to remove the excessive amounts of iron that result from such transfusions. Although these methods have succeeded in prolonging the life span of some patients with various types of thalassemia, complications related to chelation therapy have been identified.

One of the chelation agents, deferoxamine, may lead to significant skeletal abnormalities. Clinically, affected patients have short trunks with moderate sternal protrusion, genu valgum, generalized joint stiffness, and periarticular bone deformities. Irregular flattening of the vertebral bodies in the thoracic and lumbar spine may be observed. More dramatic alterations affect the metaphyses of the tubular bones of the extremities (Fig. 48–21). The bone changes are typically bilateral, and common sites of involvement include the distal femoral, proximal tibial, and distal ulnar areas. Although the skeletal abnormalities resemble those encountered in spondylometaphyseal dysplasia, the findings do not precisely correspond to any of the recognized genetic dysplasias. The precise relationship among the dose of deferoxamine, the age of the patient, and the severity of the skeletal alterations remains to be established.

## IRON DEFICIENCY ANEMIA

In children, iron deficiency anemia results from insufficient intake or excessive loss of iron during the first 6 months of life, which depletes the iron that was stored during late prenatal life. This type of anemia is most frequent between 9 months and 2 years of age. Skeletal abnormalities are generally mild. Marrow hyperplasia may result in changes in the cranial vault, with thinning of the outer table and diploic widening observed in the frontal, parietal, or occipital bone. Radial striations extending from the outer table are rare and usually mild in iron deficiency anemia, allowing its distinction from thalassemia.

## HEREDITARY SPHEROCYTOSIS

This hemolytic anemia, which is inherited as an autosomal dominant disorder, is worldwide in distribution but most common in northern Europeans. It is characterized by abnormally shaped red blood cells, or spherocytes, in the peripheral blood that are hemolyzed in the spleen. Clinical features include anemia, jaundice, and splenomegaly. Gallstones and chronic leg ulcerations are two other potential manifestations of this disorder. Coincident syndromes have been described, including unconjugated hyperbilirubinemia, familial myocardiopathy, and spinal cord dysfunction.

As in other hemolytic diseases, compensatory hyperplasia of the bone marrow occurs, with extension of red marrow into the diaphyses of long bones. In the cranial vault, diploic widening and thinning of the outer table are evident. Because anemia in this condition may not manifest until late childhood or adolescence, significant long bone changes are unusual. Occasionally, extramedullary hematopoiesis may result in paravertebral masses simulating infection or tumor.

## HEREDITARY ELLIPTOCYTOSIS

In hereditary elliptocytosis, red blood cells are oval or elliptic in shape. The disorder is closely linked to hereditary spherocytosis. Hemolysis occurs in the spleen. The bone abnormalities are largely undescribed.

# NONSPHEROCYTIC HEMOLYTIC ANEMIA

Nonspherocytic hemolytic anemia is a designation that can be used for hereditary hemolytic processes not attributable to thalassemia, spherocytosis, elliptocytosis, or one of the hemoglobinopathies. The two most important disorders in this category are pyruvate kinase deficiency and glucose-6-phosphate dehydrogenase deficiency anemias. Radiographic changes have been documented in association with pyruvate kinase deficiency, including marrow hyperplasia producing osteoporosis, diploic widening, and thinning of the cranial vault. Unlike with thalassemia, the facial bones and sinuses are unaffected.

# APLASTIC ANEMIA

An uncommon condition, aplastic anemia is characterized by acellular or hypocellular bone marrow and is accompanied by pancytopenia, including anemia, neutropenia, and thrombocytopenia. Its causes are diverse, including drugs (chloramphenicol, phenytoin, gold, benzene), radiation, paroxysmal nocturnal hemoglobinuria, Fanconi's anemia, viral hepatitis, pregnancy, and thymoma, although many cases are idiopathic. Patients with aplastic anemia have an impaired ability to incorporate iron into marrow erythroid precursors. Various types of therapy, including repeated blood transfusions or marrow transplantation, can effect partial or complete recovery of the bone marrow.

MR imaging may be useful in the initial diagnosis of aplastic anemia and as a method of monitoring the therapeutic response. MR imaging in untreated patients with aplastic anemia emphasizes an augmentation of marrow signal intensity because of the presence of fat. During therapy, focal areas of low signal intensity, representing islands of active hematopoietic cells scattered in otherwise fatty marrow, may be evident.

# DIFFERENTIAL DIAGNOSIS

## Differentiation among the Anemias
(Table 48–1)

Extensive thickening of the cranial vault associated with marked diploic expansion and a hair-on-end appearance is most characteristic of thalassemia. Its occurrence in patients with sickle cell anemia has been overemphasized, as this finding is evident in less than 5% of patients with the disease. Some thickening of the cranial vault may be apparent in sickle cell–hemoglobin C disease, sickle cell–thalassemia disease, iron deficiency anemia, hereditary spherocytosis, and pyruvate kinase deficiency, but widespread and severe skull alterations are rare.

Changes of marrow hyperplasia in the peripheral skeleton are most common and marked in thalassemia. In iron deficiency anemia and sickle cell–thalassemia disease, changes of marrow hyperplasia in the tubular bones are absent or mild. Bone infarction is particularly common in sickle cell anemia and sickle cell–hemoglobin C disease. Ischemic skeletal changes are less frequent in sickle cell–thalassemia disease and sickle cell trait and are not characteristic of thalassemia or iron deficiency anemia. Osteonecrosis of the epiphyses may be more frequent in

sickle cell–hemoglobin C disease than in sickle cell anemia, although this point is debated. Diaphyseal infarction with surrounding sclerosis producing a bone-within-bone appearance is suggestive of sickle cell anemia or sickle cell–hemoglobin C disease because it is rare in other anemias. Infarction of the small bones of the hands and feet in children with subsequent dactylitis and the hand-foot syndrome is almost diagnostic of sickle cell anemia.

Abnormalities in vertebral body contour consisting of squared-off compressions of the vertebrae (H vertebrae) occur in sickle cell anemia, sickle cell–hemoglobin C disease, and sickle cell–thalassemia disease, although such abnormalities may be seen in thalassemia and in other conditions such as Gaucher's disease. Flaring of the ends of the tubular bones, the Erlenmeyer flask appearance, is most suggestive of thalassemia. Premature fusion of the growth plate has been described in both sickle cell anemia and thalassemia. Osteopenia, which may be found in many of the anemic disorders, leads to osseous weakening and thereby predisposes to skeletal fractures. Pathologic fractures have been noted in sickle cell anemia and thalassemia, although they are to be expected in the other anemias as well. Osteomyelitis, particularly that associated with *Salmonella* infection, is a known complication of sickle cell anemia, although infections of bones and joints can be observed in thalassemia and other hemoglobinopathies.

## Differentiation of Anemia from Other Conditions

In anemic disorders, diffuse skeletal abnormality characterized by decreased radiographic density (osteopenia) is an indication of marrow hyperplasia. This finding may be simulated by changes in other disorders. Other primary marrow diseases, such as Gaucher's disease and Niemann-Pick disease, are associated with similar findings. Osteopenia may also accompany osteogenesis imperfecta, idiopathic juvenile osteoporosis, hyperparathyroidism, and leukemia.

Thickening of the cranial vault is a radiographic finding that is apparent in many disorders. In anemias, this thickening frequently involves the entire cranium, with the exception of the inferior aspect of the occipital bone and base of the skull. Fibrous dysplasia and leontiasis ossea can lead to excessive hyperostosis of the skull, but changes usually predominate in the frontal regions and face. The hair-on-end appearance is characteristic of thalassemia.

Epiphyseal and diaphyseal bone infarction occurs not only in anemia but also in other diseases. Epiphyseal ischemia, particularly of the femoral head, is noted in endogenous and exogenous corticosteroid excess, caisson disease, Gaucher's disease, Legg-Calvé-Perthes disease, collagen vascular disorders, alcoholism with pancreatitis, and radiation therapy, as well as after trauma and in many other processes. Diametaphyseal ischemia is seen in association with steroid administration, caisson disease, pancreatitis, and Gaucher's disease.

Abnormality in vertebral body contour characterized by steplike depressions of the osseous surface, the H vertebra, is a relatively specific radiographic sign of anemia. It has been noted rarely in other conditions. An

**TABLE 48-1**

## Characteristic Skeletal Findings in the Anemias

| Disease | Marrow Hyperplasia | | | Bone Infarction | | Growth Disturbances | | Fractures | Osteomyelitis and Septic Arthritis | Crystal Deposition | |
|---|---|---|---|---|---|---|---|---|---|---|---|
| | Cranial Vault | Facial Bones | Tubular Bones | Long Tubular Bones | Hands, Feet | H Vertebrae | Flaring of Tubular Bones | | | Calcium Pyrophosphate Dihydrate | Monosodium Urate |
| Sickle cell anemia | + | | + | + | + | + | | + | + | | + |
| Sickle cell trait | | | | + | | + | | | + | | |
| Sickle cell-hemoglobin C disease | + | | | + | | | | | | | |
| Sickle cell-thalassemia disease | + | | + | + | | + | | | + | | |
| Thalassemia | + | + | + | | | + | + | + | + | + | + |
| Iron deficiency anemia | + | + | + | | | | | | | | |
| Spherocytosis | + | | | | | | | | | + | |
| Nonspherocytic hemolytic anemia | + | | | | | | | | | | |

H vertebra with its abrupt endplate indentations can be distinguished from a fish vertebra, which has a smooth biconcave appearance. Fish vertebrae may be observed in anemias, but the changes are not specific because they appear in all forms of osteoporosis and in other conditions producing diffuse weakening of bone.

Sickle cell dactylitis may simulate the changes of other disorders associated with destruction and periostitis of the small tubular bones of the hands and feet. Tuberculous dactylitis, termed spina ventosa, is characterized by soft tissue swelling, bone destruction, periostitis, and bone expansion. The findings of infarction of the long and short tubular bones in sickle cell anemia can simulate osteomyelitis.

The extramedullary hematopoiesis accompanying thalassemia and, less commonly, other anemias leads to enlargement of the posterior portions of the ribs, a finding simulating that of fibrous dysplasia; it also leads to lobulated posterior mediastinal masses resembling neoplasm. With regard to the rib lesions, multiplicity, bilaterality, and the known presence of an anemia generally allow sites of extramedullary hematopoiesis to be differentiated from other causes of rib expansion.

## FURTHER READING

Agarwal KN, Dhar N, Shar MM, et al: Roentgenologic changes in iron deficiency anemia. AJR Am J Roentgenol 110:635, 1970.

Barton CJ, Cockshott WP: Bone changes in hemoglobin SC disease. AJR Am J Roentgenol 88:523, 1962.

Bohrer SP: Growth disturbances of the distal femur following sickle cell bone infarcts and/or osteomyelitis. Clin Radiol 25:221, 1974.

Brasch RC, Wesbey GE, Gooding CA, et al: Magnetic resonance imaging of transfusional hemosiderosis complicating thalassemia major. Radiology 150:767, 1984.

Caffey J: Cooley's anemia: A review of the roentgenographic findings in the skeleton. AJR Am J Roentgenol 78:381, 1957.

Chan Y, Li C, Chu WC, et al: Deferoxamine-induced bone dysplasia in the distal femur and patella of pediatric patients and young adults: MR imaging appearance AJR Am J Roentgenol 175:1561, 2000.

Cooley TB, Lee P: A series of cases of splenomegaly in children with anemia and peculiar bone changes. Trans Am Pediatr Soc 37:29, 1925.

Coskun E, Keskin A, Suzer T, et al: Spinal cord compression secondary to extramedullary hematopoiesis in thalassemia intermedia. Eur Spine J 7:501, 1998.

Currarino G, Erlandson ME: Premature fusion of epiphyses in Cooley's anemia. Radiology 83:656, 1964.

Fink IJ, Pastakia B, Barranger JA: Enlarged phalangeal foramina in Gaucher disease and B-thalassemia major. AJR Am J Roentgenol 143:647, 1984.

Janus WL, Dietz MW: Osseous changes in erythroblastosis fetalis (21 cases). Radiology 53:39, 1949.

Juhl JH, Wesenberg RL, Gwinn JL: Roentgenographic findings in Fanconi's anemia. Radiology 89:646, 1967.

Kaneko K, Humbert JH, Kogutt MS, et al: Iron deposition in cranial bone marrow with sickle cell disease: MR assessment using a fat suppression technique. Pediatr Radiol 23:435, 1993.

Kaplan PA, Asleson RJ, Klassen LW, et al: Bone marrow patterns in aplastic anemia: Observations with 1.5-T MR imaging. Radiology 164:441, 1987.

Lawson JP, Ablow RC, Pearson HA: The ribs in thalassemia. I. The relationship to therapy. Radiology 140:663, 1981.

Lawson JP, Ablow RC, Pearson HA: The ribs in thalassemia. II. The pathogenesis of the changes. Radiology 140:673, 1981.

Lutzker LG, Alavi A: Bone and marrow imaging in sickle cell disease: Diagnosis of infarction. Semin Nucl Med 6:83, 1976.

Mirowitz SA, Apicella P, Reinus WR, et al: MR imaging of bone marrow lesions: Relative conspicuousness on T1-weighted, fat-suppressed T2-weighted, and STIR images. AJR Am J Roentgenol 162:215, 1994.

O'Hara AE: Roentgenographic osseous manifestations of the anemias and the leukemias. Clin Orthop 52:63, 1967.

Pauling L, Itano HA, Singer SJ, et al: Sickle cell anemia, a molecular disease. Science 110:543, 1949.

Reynolds J: A re-evaluation of the "fish vertebra" sign in sickle cell hemoglobinopathy. AJR Am J Roentgenol 97:693, 1966.

Reynolds J: The Roentgenological Features of Sickle Cell Disease and Related Hemoglobinopathies. Springfield, Ill, Charles C Thomas, 1965.

Sebes JI, Brown DL: Terminal phalangeal sclerosis in sickle cell disease. AJR Am J Roentgenol 140:763, 1983.

Tunaci M, Tunaci A, Engin G, et al: Imaging features of thalassemia. Eur Radiol 9:1804, 1999.

# CHAPTER 49

## Plasma Cell Dyscrasias and Dysgammaglobulinemias

### SUMMARY OF KEY FEATURES

Musculoskeletal findings occur in various plasma cell dyscrasias and dysgammaglobulinemias. In plasma cell myeloma, such findings are a predominant manifestation of the disease and lead to characteristic pathologic and radiographic abnormalities. Widespread or localized osteolysis can be attributed, in large part, to plasma cell infiltration in the bone marrow. Accompanying amyloid deposition in some patients may manifest as articular and periarticular alterations. The skeletal and articular manifestations of Waldenström's macroglobulinemia, though less frequent and less well known, resemble those of plasma cell myeloma. Amyloidosis, which can occur in both plasma cell myeloma and Waldenström's macroglobulinemia, can also appear in a primary form without antecedent cause or in a secondary form in various other conditions. In both primary and secondary types, amyloid deposition can lead to significant bone and joint changes, including osteoporosis, osseous lytic lesions, and tumorous foci in both articular and extra-articular locations.

### INTRODUCTION

Plasma cells are the functional unit of the immune defense system. They are found in various areas of the human body, particularly the lymph nodes, spleen, bone marrow, and submucosa of the gastrointestinal tract, and they are responsible for antibody synthesis. Plasma cells are derived from B lymphocytes and are the principal source of immunoglobulins, proteins of high molecular weight that function as antibodies. In the presence of infectious disease, the number of plasma cells in the bone marrow increases, with a similar increase in the production of immunoglobulins. This response is termed plasmacytosis and is a normal consequence of infection or other processes that result in antigenic stimulation. When plasma cell proliferation appears as an inappropriate or uncontrolled event, a plasma cell dyscrasia exists (e.g., multiple myeloma, Waldenström's macroglobulinemia, amyloidosis).

Plasma cell dyscrasias are characterized by the uncontrolled proliferation of plasma cells in the absence of an identifiable antigenic stimulus; the elaboration of electrophoretically and structurally homogeneous monoclonal, M-type (plasma cell myeloma, macroglobulinemia) gamma globulins or excessive quantities of homogeneous polypeptide subunits of these proteins (Bence Jones proteins, H chains), or both; and a commonly associated deficiency in the synthesis of normal immunoglobulins. Some of these dyscrasias, such as plasma cell myeloma, macroglobulinemia, amyloidosis, and heavy chain diseases, have a typical constellation of clinical manifestations that permits a specific diagnosis, whereas others initially or ultimately defy precise classification. Disease states in the latter category include premyeloma, essential hypergammaglobulinemia, essential cryoglobulinemia, dysgammaglobulinemia, and idiopathic monoclonal gammopathy.

Plasma cell dyscrasias result in the synthesis of large quantities of a single protein related to one of the five major classes of immunoglobulins: IgG, IgM, IgA, IgD, IgE. All of them consist of two identical heavy (H) chains linked to two identical light (L) chains. The type of immunoglobulin that is being abnormally elaborated can be identified by its electrophoretic pattern and varies among the plasma cell dyscrasias. For example, in patients with multiple myeloma, IgG predominates (approximately 55% of cases), followed, in order of decreasing frequency, by IgA, IgD, IgM, and IgE. In Waldenström's macroglobulinemia, the elaboration of large amounts of IgM is apparent. Further, a subunit of one of these proteins may be identified in some of these dyscrasias; in multiple myeloma, large quantities of Bence Jones proteins (representing free light chains) are common and may be identified in the urine in approximately 50% of cases.

### PLASMA CELL MYELOMA

Plasma cell myeloma is a malignant disease of plasma cells that usually originates in the bone marrow but may involve other tissues as well.

#### Clinical Features

Plasma cell myeloma is a common disease, representing approximately 1% of all malignancies and 10% to 15% of malignancies of the hematologic system. The disease can occur between the ages of 25 and 80 years but is more predominant in older patients; the average age of involved patients is 60 to 70 years. It appears to be slightly more common in men than in women. An even more striking male predilection may be seen in cases of solitary myeloma (single lesion). Myeloma is particularly common in blacks. In large part, the clinical manifestations are a consequence of excessive proliferation of abnormal plasma cells, which creates a mechanical burden that compromises the skeleton by displacing and eroding bony trabeculae. Symptoms include bone pain, particularly of the back and chest, that is sudden in onset and aggravated by movement; weakness; fatigue; and the presence of deformities, such as exaggerated kyphosis and loss of height. Additionally, fever, weight loss, bleeding, and neurologic signs may be seen. With coexistent amyloidosis, additional clinical manifestations may be the result of macroglossia or cardiac and renal failure.

Laboratory investigation reveals moderate or severe anemia, an elevated erythrocyte sedimentation rate, a normal or slightly elevated leukocyte count, thrombocytopenia, hypercalcemia, and hyperuricemia. Renal insufficiency may lead to an elevated serum creatinine concentration. Most patients with plasma cell myeloma have an increase in total serum protein, usually attributable to an increase in the globulin fraction. Serum electrophoresis confirms the abnormality of the globulin fraction in 80% to 90% of patients with multiple lesions. When patients with plasma cell myeloma are grouped according to the type of protein produced by the tumor, approximately 55% to 60% have IgG myeloma, 20% have IgA myeloma, and 1% to 2% have IgD myeloma; IgE and IgM myelomas are rare. On rare occasions (approximately 1% of cases), no abnormal protein is observed, a phenomenon called nonsecretory myeloma. Nonsecretory myeloma, which is often accompanied by hypogammaglobulinemia, is characterized by sepsis, widespread osteolytic lesions, and the absence of renal complications. In patients with myeloma, the major causes of death are infection and renal failure. Urinary electrophoresis is an important laboratory examination in patients with myeloma because it may demonstrate abnormalities even when the serum electrophoretic pattern is entirely normal. Bence Jones proteinuria is apparent in 40% to 60% of patients with this disease. Excretion of these proteins (light chains) can lead to damage to the proximal renal tubules, which may be due to the proteins' toxic effect on the renal tubular epithelium. Increased serum viscosity is a common feature in plasma cell myeloma. In general, this manifestation can be attributed to the large molecular size of certain immunoglobulins, such as IgG and IgM.

## Pathogenesis

Whatever the cause of the plasmacytosis in this disease, abnormal accumulation of plasma cells in myeloma is associated with single or multiple areas of bone lysis. It is now known that plasma cells can produce an osteoclast-stimulating factor that may be responsible for the osteolytic lesions that are characteristic of myeloma. This factor also leads to inhibition of osteoblasts.

## Radiographic Features

**General Abnormalities.** In almost all patients, the predominant radiographic pattern in plasma cell myeloma is osteolysis. Rarely, focal or diffuse sclerotic lesions are seen. Although multiple sites of involvement are characteristic, solitary lesions, or plasmacytomas, may exist for prolonged periods.

Typically, the axial skeleton is the predominant site of abnormality (Fig. 49–1). Multiple lesions are most commonly apparent in the vertebral column, ribs, skull, pelvis, and femur, in descending order of frequency. Solitary plasmacytomas have a similar distribution, although well over 50% of these lesions are localized in the vertebrae, followed by the pelvis, skull, sternum, and ribs. Diffuse lesions of the appendicular skeleton have been described in plasma cell myeloma, usually accompanying extensive involvement of the axial skeleton. Mandibular abnormalities are observed in approximately one third of patients.

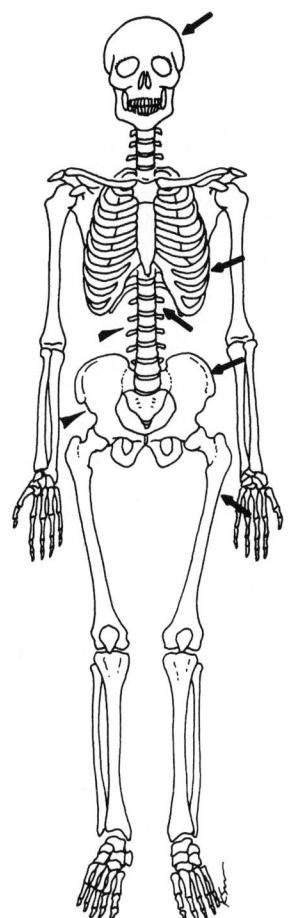

**Figure 49–1.** Plasma cell myeloma: distribution of abnormalities. The most common sites of multiple lesions of myeloma are indicated on the right half of the diagram *(arrows)*. These sites include the spine, pelvis, ribs, and skull. The most common sites of solitary plasmacytoma are indicated on the left *(arrowheads)* and include the spine and pelvis.

Differentiation between myeloma and metastatic skeletal disease may be difficult. Classically, multiple myeloma first manifests as widespread osteolytic lesions with discrete margins that appear uniform in size (Fig. 49–2). These characteristic morphologic features are seen much less frequently in bone metastasis. Although smaller myelomatous areas may coalesce into larger segments of destruction, such large foci are more commonly seen in skeletal metastasis.

Particularly distinctive in plasma cell myeloma is a subcortical circular or elliptic radiolucent shadow, most often observed in the long tubular bones. An associated mild periosteal proliferation may act as a buttress that prevents or resists fracture. The subcortical defects cause erosion of the inner margins of the cortex and, when extensive, create a scalloped and wavy contour throughout the endosteal bone. This appearance is highly suggestive of plasma cell myeloma, is occasionally seen in cases of rapid and aggressive osteoporosis, and is unusual in skeletal metastasis.

Diffuse skeletal osteopenia without well-defined areas of lysis can also be observed in plasma cell myeloma, a

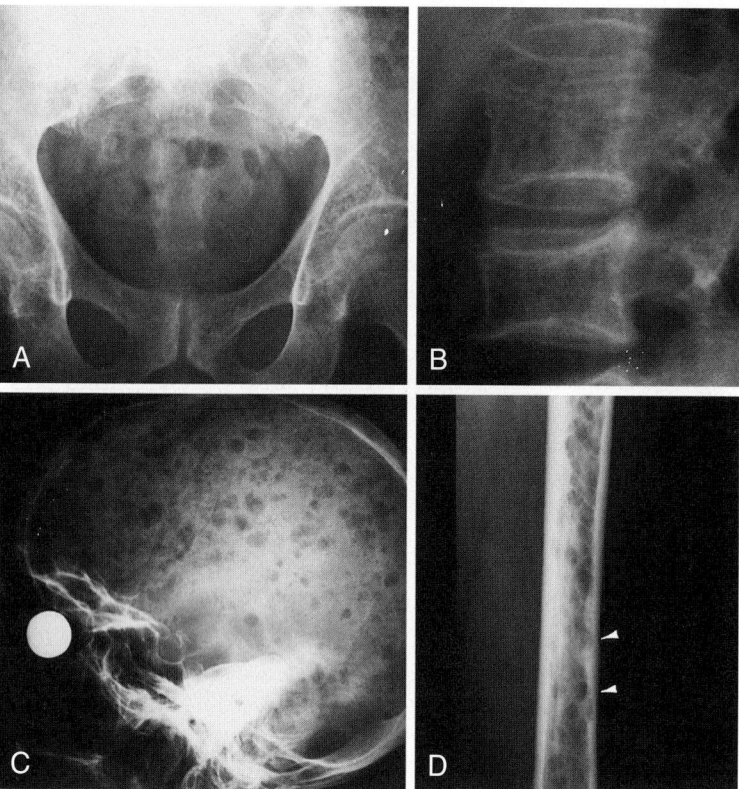

**Figure 49–2.** Plasma cell myeloma: multiple lytic lesions. *A*, Pelvis. Although the major radiographic pattern is one of diffuse osteopenia, some lytic lesions can be identified, particularly in the ilium, ischium, and pubis. *B*, Spine. On a lateral radiograph of the lumbar spine, observe the lytic lesions of multiple vertebral bodies, with evidence of vertebral compression. Pediculate involvement is mild. *C*, Skull. Well-circumscribed radiolucent lesions without surrounding sclerosis are obvious. They are relatively uniform in size, a feature that is more suggestive of myeloma than of skeletal metastasis. The radiodense area overlying the orbit represents an eye prosthesis. *D*, Femur. On this frontal radiograph, striking radiolucent lesions are seen throughout the diaphysis and are producing scalloping of the endosteal margin of the cortex *(arrowheads)*. This latter feature is particularly characteristic of plasma cell myeloma.

pattern of involvement that is infrequent with metastasis but can simulate the appearance of osteoporosis (Fig. 49–3). Sclerosis in plasma cell myeloma is generally seen after pathologic fracture, irradiation, or chemotherapy for lytic lesions, although it is occasionally noted in conjunction with intact and untreated lesions. Bone sclerosis may occur as a solitary focus or as multiple foci. Diffuse sclerosis is apparent in less than 3% of patients with plasma cell myeloma (Fig. 49–4). It can simulate the appearance of osteoblastic metastasis, lymphoma, mastocytosis, renal osteodystrophy, and myelofibrosis. Sclerotic myeloma has been reported to occur in younger persons and is known to be associated with peripheral neuropathy. The cause of the osteosclerosis in plasma cell myeloma is unknown.

**Specific Sites of Involvement.** In the skull, numerous discrete lytic areas of uniform size are more common in plasma cell myeloma than in skeletal metastasis. Myeloma may demonstrate a predilection for mandibular involvement, an uncommon site for skeletal metastasis. Sternal involvement in myeloma is not infrequent and may lead to pathologic fracture. In the spine, preferential destruction of the vertebral bodies, with sparing of the posterior elements, has been emphasized. Paraspinal and extradural extension of tumor is quite characteristic of myeloma. Preferential involvement of the distal end of the clavicle, acromion, glenoid, and ulnar olecranon is seen, whereas this distribution is less common in metastatic disease involving the skeleton.

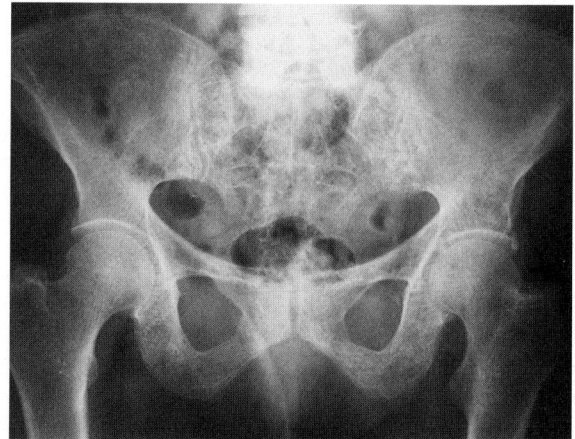

**Figure 49–3.** Plasma cell myeloma: diffuse osteopenia. Radiograph of the pelvis reveals increased radiolucency of the skeleton and a coarsened trabecular pattern. No evidence of discrete lytic lesions can be seen. The pattern resembles that in osteoporosis or osteomalacia.

## Pathologic Features

Myelomatous involvement of the skeleton is variable in extent and predominates in regions of red marrow. Extraosseous involvement is most common in the spleen, liver, and lymph nodes. Pathologic fractures are frequent,

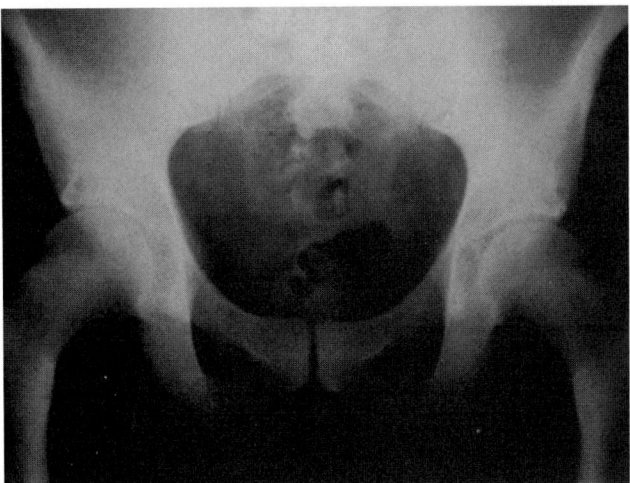

**Figure 49–4.** Plasma cell myeloma: osteosclerosis. In this 70-year-old man, diffuse osteosclerosis is seen in the pelvis and proximal portions of the femora.

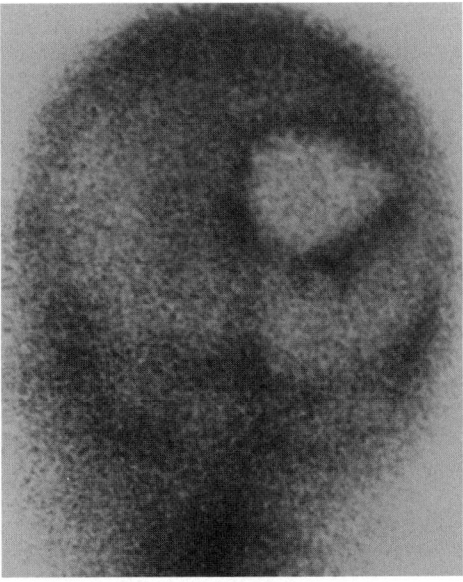

**Figure 49–5.** Plasma cell myeloma: scintigraphic abnormalities. The center of this large lesion of the cranial vault shows a relative lack of accumulation of the bone-seeking radiopharmaceutical agent ("cold" lesion), with a peripheral rim of augmented radionuclide activity. This appearance is termed the doughnut sign.

especially in the vertebrae and ribs; other sites, such as the pelvis, sternum, clavicle, and tubular bones, are fractured less commonly.

Histologically, myeloma is characterized by closely packed plasma cells ranging from undifferentiated to well differentiated. Accompanying amyloid deposits are histologically apparent in approximately 10% of patients. Calcification within these amyloid deposits may be evident.

## Radionuclide Examination

Although radionuclide bone scanning is valuable in the early detection of most neoplastic processes of the skeleton, the results of this examination are less predictable in patients with myeloma (Fig. 49–5). False-negative scans are not uncommon. The current belief is that radionuclide examination in patients with myeloma does not reveal all lesions and that radiography is a more valuable technique for assessing the distribution of lesions, with the possible exception of rib abnormalities, which may be seen more easily with scintigraphy. Further, areas of increased uptake in some persons may indicate the presence not of tumor but of amyloid deposition. In fact, fractures account for augmented radionuclide uptake in a large percentage of patients with myeloma.

Although radiographic examination appears to be more sensitive than scintigraphy in detecting the osseous alterations of plasma cell myeloma, it is far from ideal for monitoring the course of the disease. Clinical and laboratory evidence of patient improvement is commonly associated with a lack of change on serial radiographic studies. Reports indicate that scintigraphy is a potential aid in monitoring patients with myeloma who are receiving chemotherapy; remission is characterized by significant regression or disappearance of the scintigraphic abnormalities in many of these patients.

## Computed Tomography

In contrast to plain film radiography, in which extensive osseous destruction is required before abnormalities

become apparent, computed tomography (CT) may indicate minor alterations in radiodensity that reflect the presence of intramedullary myelomatous foci (Fig. 49–6). CT is well suited to assess the degree of osseous destruction. In general, however, magnetic resonance (MR) imaging is used to document the presence and extent of myelomatous involvement of the skeleton.

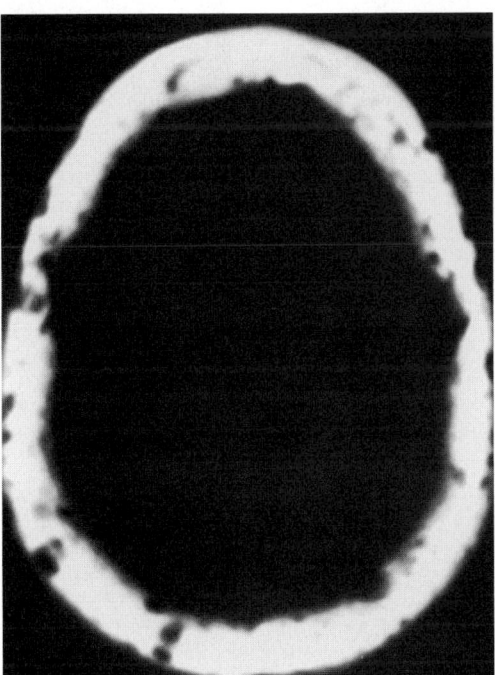

**Figure 49–6.** Plasma cell myeloma: CT abnormalities in the skull. Observe the well-defined radiolucent lesions involving the diploic portion and both tables of the skull.

## Magnetic Resonance Imaging

With MR imaging, normal or abnormal marrow has an appearance that is directly related to the specific sequence or method being used. Spin echo techniques are not ideal for the assessment of some marrow alterations because they are relatively insensitive to subtle changes in free water content, with signal intensities that are most dependent on the presence or absence of fat. Irrespective of which MR imaging sequence is chosen, detection of myelomatous involvement of the vertebral bodies (or elsewhere) is dependent on contrast differences between regions of tumor infiltration and background tissue composed of areas of either hematopoietic or fatty marrow, or both (Fig. 49–7).

The results of three early reports in which standard spin echo methods were applied to the analysis of vertebral abnormalities in plasma cell myeloma underscore some of the diagnostic difficulties encountered using T1- and T2-weighted spin echo sequences. These reports noted variable patterns of marrow replacement on T1-weighted spin echo images that varied from total to focal to normal (Fig. 49–8). Variable signal intensities may also include high signal intensity on T1-weighted images, perhaps related to hemorrhagic areas.

These reported observations led to efforts to improve diagnostic accuracy through the use of additional MR imaging methods and sequences. Gadolinium-supplemented T1-weighted images are characterized by widely disseminated or inhomogeneous enhancement of diffuse

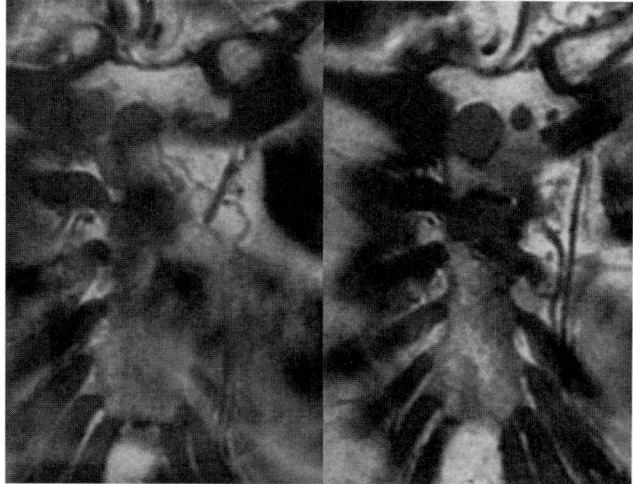

**Figure 49–7.** Plasma cell myeloma: MR imaging abnormalities in the sternum. These sequential coronal T1-weighted (TR/TE, 600/20) spin echo MR images reveal multiple well-defined foci of tumor that appear as regions of diminished signal intensity, highlighted by the bright signal of the predominantly fatty bone marrow.

or variegated marrow involvement. The pattern of enhancement of myelomatous foci differs from that typically encountered in regions of hematopoietic bone marrow. Although normal marrow may enhance

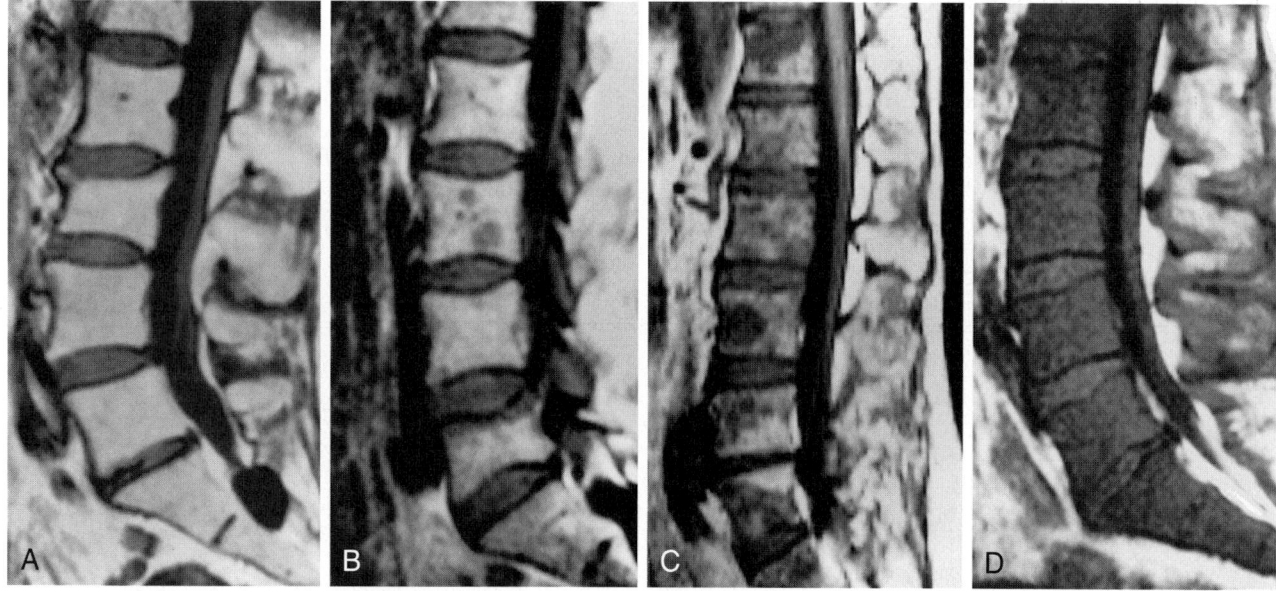

**Figure 49–8.** Plasma cell myeloma: MR imaging abnormalities in the spine. Sagittal T1-weighted (TR/TE, 350/20) spin echo MR images show four patterns of marrow involvement seen in patients with monoclonal gammopathies. *A*, Normal-appearing marrow (62-year-old woman). Note the absence of diffuse or focal abnormalities of signal intensity. One possible lesion is seen in the second lumbar vertebral body, and loss of height of the third lumbar vertebral body is evident. *B*, Focal lesions (54-year-old woman). Several foci of low signal intensity are seen in the second and third lumbar vertebral bodies, and collapse of the superior endplate of the fifth lumbar vertebral body is evident. *C*, Focal lesions (45-year-old man). Numerous foci of low signal intensity are seen in every visualized vertebral body. *D*, Diffuse infiltration (50-year-old man). The signal intensity of the vertebral bodies is lower than that of the intervertebral discs. (From Lecouvet FE, Malghem J, Michaux L, et al: Vertebral compression fractures in multiple myeloma. Part II. Assessment of fracture risk with MR imaging of spinal bone marrow. Radiology 204:201, 1997.)

markedly when a gadolinium-based contrast agent is administered intravenously to young children, such enhancement has been reported to be subtle or absent in adults. In plasma cell myeloma, especially in cases of more aggressive disease, the degree of enhancement of signal intensity in involved marrow tends to be greater than that of normal marrow (Fig. 49–9). Further, gadolinium-related diffuse enhancement of marrow in vertebral bodies occurs not only in myeloma but also in lymphomas, leukemias, and myelofibrosis.

Short tau inversion recovery (STIR) sequences may allow the detection of small focal collections of tumor that escape visualization with standard spin echo MR imaging methods. Other fat-suppression techniques, such as chemical shift imaging, can also be used in patients with plasma cell myeloma and may be combined with the use of intravenous gadolinium-based contrast agents, although the value of these modified MR imaging methods has yet to be proved in patients with this disease.

**Clinical and Prognostic Value.** Although MR imaging findings in cases of plasma cell myeloma lack specificity, their potential role in providing information about the stage and prognosis of the disease has been emphasized. Whereas conventional radiography was used in the past to determine tumor mass in myeloma patients, comparative studies of MR imaging, routine radiography, and scintigraphy in this clinical setting clearly indicate that MR imaging results in the highest detection rate. In general, the frequency of abnormal MR imaging findings in patients with plasma cell myeloma increases with advancing stages of the disease. In reports of patients with stage III myeloma, MR imaging indicated the presence of marrow abnormalities in approximately 80% of cases.

**Vertebral Collapse.** Collapse of one or more vertebral bodies is a common and well-recognized complication of plasma cell myeloma. Although MR imaging criteria have been developed with regard to the differentiation of

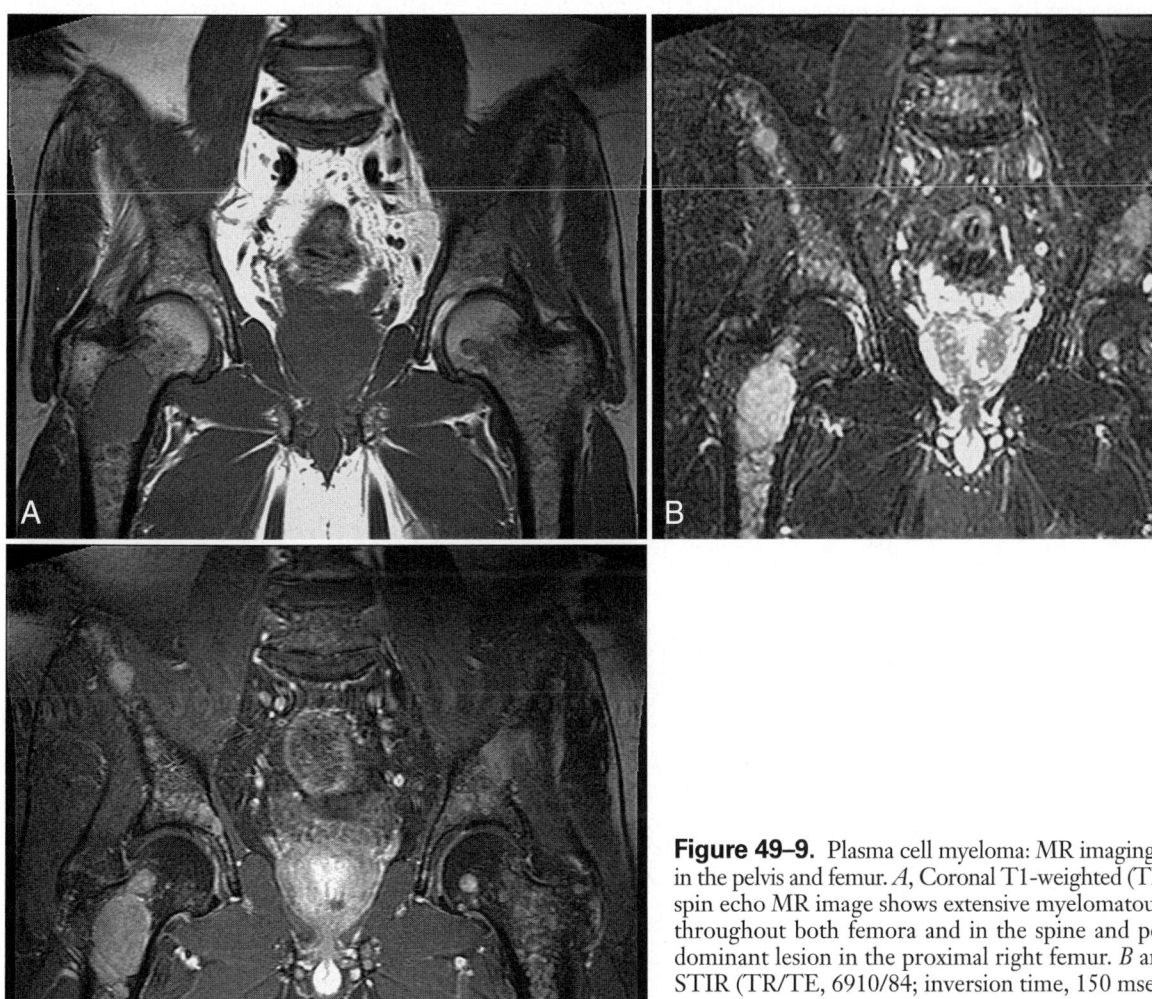

**Figure 49–9.** Plasma cell myeloma: MR imaging abnormalities in the pelvis and femur. *A,* Coronal T1-weighted (TR/TE, 690/16) spin echo MR image shows extensive myelomatous involvement throughout both femora and in the spine and pelvis, with the dominant lesion in the proximal right femur. *B* and *C,* Coronal STIR (TR/TE, 6910/84; inversion time, 150 msec) *(B)* and fat-suppressed gadolinium-enhanced T1-weighted (TR/TE, 584/16) *(C)* spin echo MR images reveal the myelomatous lesions to have high signal intensity and prominent enhancement.

nontumorous and tumorous collapse of vertebral bodies (see Chapters 41 and 72), these criteria may be less valuable in cases of myeloma. Specifically, the preservation of signal intensity typical of fat in collapsed vertebral bodies, generally believed to indicate a nontumorous pathogenesis, has been noted in cases of myelomatous infiltration. Whether specific MR imaging patterns of vertebral involvement in plasma cell myeloma are predictive of fracture risk is not clear.

**Extraspinal Sites of Involvement.** Even though existing data relate mainly to the assessment of spinal involvement in plasma cell myeloma, MR imaging can also be applied to the evaluation of disease presence and extent in extraspinal sites and to the analysis of solitary or multifocal plasmacytomas.

## Plasmacytoma

Myeloma can occur as a solitary lesion of bone. Although laboratory analysis may reveal the same abnormalities that occur in disseminated myelomatosis, this is not always the case. In some patients with solitary plasmacytoma, serologic tests are negative, or abnormal patterns of serum electrophoresis disappear after excision of the tumor. In many cases of apparently solitary plasmacytoma, multiple lesions eventually appear if the patient is monitored long enough; in fact, some investigators believe that all patients with plasmacytoma will eventually demonstrate multiple lesions.

Compared with multiple myeloma, solitary plasmacytoma is rare (representing <5% of plasma cell dyscrasias), affects younger patients (average age, about 50 years), is commonly accompanied by neurologic manifestations, and can simulate giant cell tumor on radiographic examination. Plasmacytoma is most common in the spine (especially the thoracic and lumbar segments) and pelvis, although it may occur at many other axial and extra-axial sites. The radiographic features are variable. A multi-

cystic expansile lesion with thickened trabeculae or a purely osteolytic focus without expansion may be observed (Figs. 49–10 and 49–11). Sclerotic lesions have also been identified; in fact, solitary plasmacytoma may appear as a radiodense vertebral body, the ivory vertebra (Fig. 49–12). Calcification or even ossification in plasmacytomas may indicate amyloid deposition, and the resulting radiographic appearance can simulate that of osteosarcoma or chondrosarcoma.

Solitary plasmacytoma of the spine deserves special emphasis. This diagnosis must be considered in any middle-aged or elderly patient with a single osteolytic lesion of a vertebral body or, less commonly, a vertebral arch. An involved vertebral body may collapse and disappear completely, or the lesion may extend into the spinal canal or across the intervertebral disc and invade the adjacent vertebral body.

## Rheumatologic Manifestations

**Neurologic Findings.** Sciatica and brachial neuralgia related to nerve root pressure are encountered in patients with spinal disease. In addition, patients with sclerotic plasma cell myeloma (or, rarely, osteolytic myeloma) may have an associated peripheral neuropathy. It has been suggested that peripheral neuropathy may be related to dysglobulinemia. It occurs in less than 1% of plasma cell neoplasms.

**POEMS Syndrome.** A syndrome of plasma cell dyscrasia, chronic progressive polyneuropathy, and endocrine disturbances, including diabetes mellitus, has been recognized (Fig. 49–13). To facilitate recognition of the most constant features of this syndrome—polyneuropathy (P), organomegaly (O), endocrinopathy (E), M proteins (M), and skin changes (S)—the acronym POEMS has been suggested. M protein abnormalities, if present, are lambda light chains, unlike the kappa light chains evident

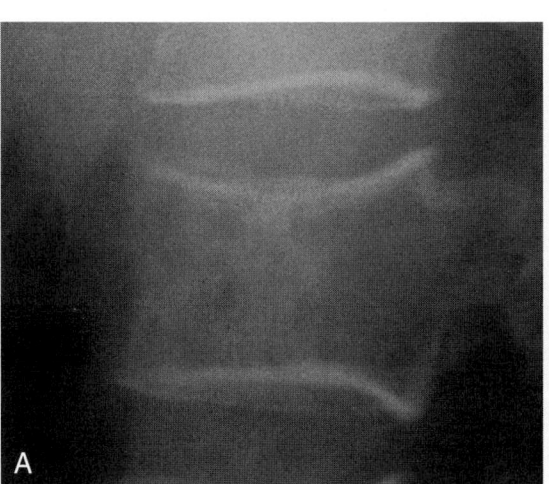
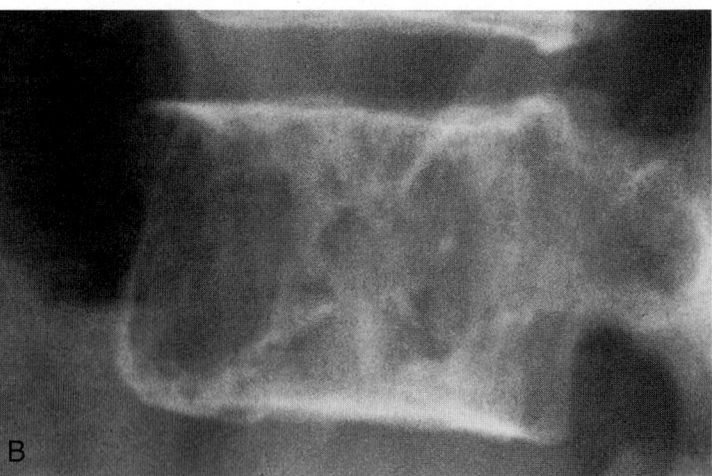

**Figure 49–10.** Plasmacytoma: spine. Progressive changes in the spine in a 37-year-old man with low back pain. *A*, The initial radiograph demonstrates increased radiolucency of the third lumbar vertebral body, with slight compression of its superior surface. *B*, Two years later, the lesion has progressed and appears "bubbly" or septated.

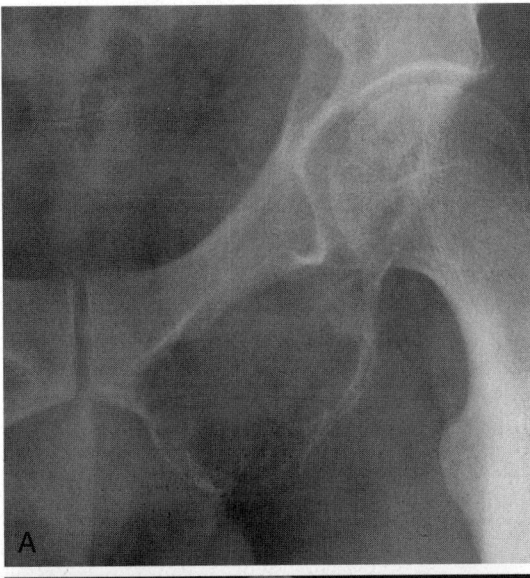

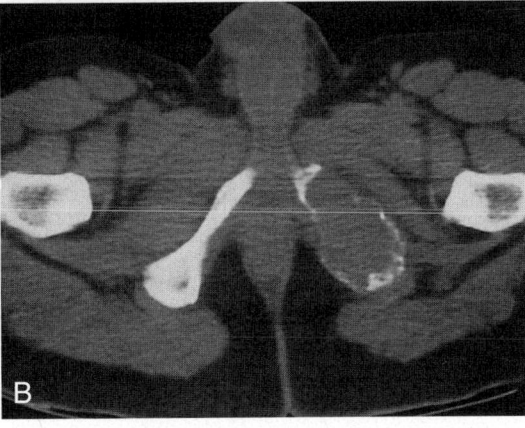

**Figure 49–11.** Plasmacytoma: pelvis. This 34-year-old man had left hip pain that progressed over a 2-year period. *A,* Radiograph reveals an expansile trabeculated lesion of the ischium. *B,* Transaxial CT image at the level of the ischial tuberosity, obtained at the same time as *(A),* reveals the expansile lesion, cortical thinning and perforation, and absence of a soft tissue mass. Open biopsy confirmed the diagnosis of plasmacytoma. (Courtesy of G. Greenway, MD, Dallas, Tex.)

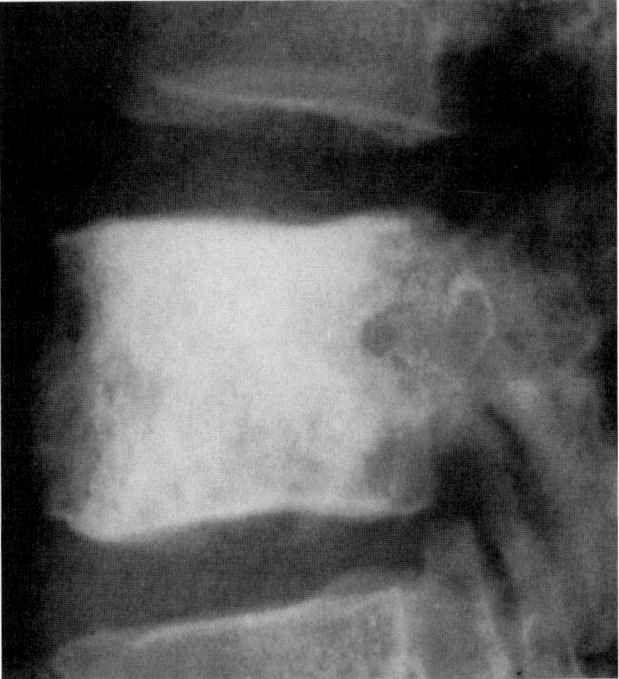

**Figure 49–12.** Plasmacytoma: ivory vertebra. In this 33-year-old man with a 1-month history of low back pain, laboratory evaluation revealed normal serum and urine electrophoresis. Osteosclerosis of the entire third lumbar vertebral body is observed, with areas of permeative bone destruction. The intervertebral disc spaces are normal. Open biopsy documented the presence of a plasmacytoma.

in classic myeloma. Additional characteristics of this syndrome are thickening and pigmentation of the skin (sometimes resembling scleroderma), cutaneous angiomas, edema, excess perspiration, hirsutism, impotence, gynecomastia or amenorrhea, thrombocytosis, and hepatosplenomegaly. Affected patients do not have associated amyloidosis and rarely exhibit Bence Jones proteinuria. The syndrome is more frequent in men and usually has its onset at a young age. Sclerotic plasmacytomas are evident in most cases, particularly in the spine and pelvis. The lesions may be uniformly sclerotic or appear target-like, with a peripheral margin of bone sclerosis. Ivory vertebral bodies may be evident, and areas with features similar to those of bone islands may be seen. Bone proliferation is apparent at sites of tendon and ligament attachment to bone. Particularly characteristic are irregular bony excrescences involving the posterior

elements of the spine, including the articular, transverse, and spinous processes. Similar findings are observed about the sacroiliac and costovertebral joints. The cause of this syndrome is not known.

**Polyarthritis and Amyloid Deposition.** Plasma cell myeloma may manifest as a polyarthritis that superficially resembles rheumatoid arthritis. These articular manifestations can precede any overt manifestation of myelomatosis or develop after the onset of the latter disease.

Amyloidosis occurs in approximately 15% of patients with plasma cell myeloma. The distribution of amyloid in these patients resembles that in primary amyloidosis. In fact, differentiation of myeloma with coexistent amyloidosis from primary amyloidosis may be extremely difficult. It appears that most patients with plasma cell myeloma and polyarthritis have coexistent amyloidosis. These patients must be distinguished, however, from those with plasma cell myeloma and coincidental rheumatoid arthritis, from patients with primary amyloidosis and joint manifestations, and from those with rheumatoid arthritis and serum M components without myeloma or amyloidosis.

Rarely, a circumscribed mass of amyloid may be identified within a plasmacytoma in the skeleton. Its presence can be suspected when areas of calcification or ossification are evident in the lesion. The resulting radiographic abnormalities resemble those of osteosarcoma or chondrosarcoma (Fig. 49–14).

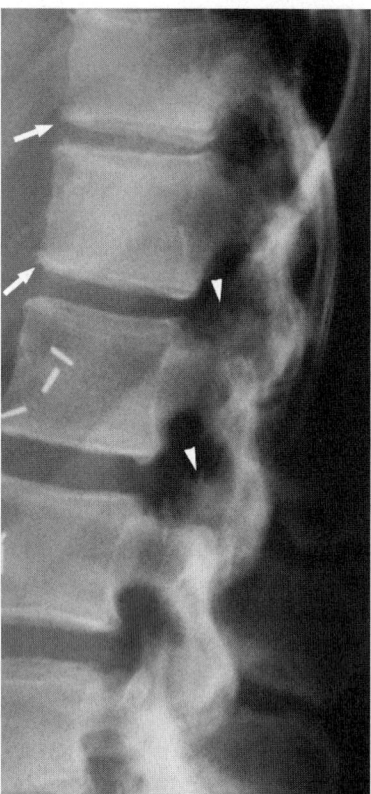

**Figure 49–13.** Syndrome of plasma cell dyscrasia, polyneuropathy, and endocrine disturbances (POEMS syndrome). On a lateral radiograph of the lumbar spine, observe the peculiar proliferative changes about the apophyseal joints *(arrowheads)* and, to a lesser extent, the discovertebral junctions *(arrows)*. The bones appear radiodense.

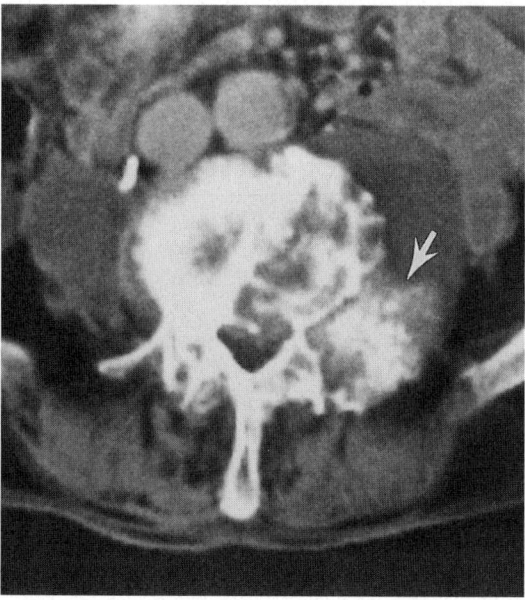

**Figure 49–14.** Plasmacytoma with amyloid deposition. Biopsy of solitary lesion of the skeleton documented the presence of a plasmacytoma with amyloid deposition. Transaxial CT image shows the extent of bone destruction and the presence of calcification *(arrow)*. (Courtesy of J. Castello, MD, Madrid, Spain.)

**Gouty Arthritis.** Several reports have noted the association of plasma cell myeloma and gout. Joint symptoms may precede the recognition of myeloma by a prolonged period.

**Infection.** Hypogammaglobulinemia in myeloma results in impairment in humoral immunity and an increased susceptibility to infection. The most frequent sites of infection are the lung and the urinary tract, but soft tissue involvement is also common. Osteomyelitis and septic arthritis may be seen.

## Percutaneous Vertebroplasty

Percutaneous vertebroplasty is a recently introduced technique for reducing pain and strengthening bone in patients with plasma cell myeloma (or skeletal metastasis) involving the spine, as well as in patients with osteoporotic vertebral collapse. This method entails the injection, usually with fluoroscopic or CT guidance, of a polymer of methylmethacrylate through a large needle into the weakened vertebral body. The pain relief provided by percutaneous vertebroplasty is frequent and often dramatic; it may be related to tumor necrosis, destruction of sensory nerve endings, stabilization of microfractures, or a combination of these mechanisms. The degree of pain relief is independent of the percentage of the lesion that is filled with methylmethacrylate during the injection procedure. Certain patterns of extraosseous leakage of methylmethacrylate, such as foraminal or spinal canal leakage, may require decompressive surgery because of the occurrence of neurologic symptoms and signs.

## Differential Diagnosis

Widespread osteolytic lesions in a middle-aged or elderly patient should arouse suspicion of myeloma or skeletal metastasis, and differentiation of the radiographic features of these two disorders causes some difficulty (Table 49–1). Certain features favor the diagnosis of myeloma, including symmetrically distributed lesions of equal size without adjacent sclerosis; subcortical lucent areas with endosteal scalloping; involvement of the mandible, shoulder girdle, and elbow region; and spinal lesions with preservation of the pediculate shadow. None of these characteristics is pathognomonic of myeloma, however. Other disorders may also be associated with widespread osteolysis, including macroglobulinemia, leukemia, histiocytosis, Gaucher's disease, vascular tumor, infection, fibrous dysplasia, hyperparathyroidism, pancreatitis with fat necrosis, and Weber-Christian disease.

Diffuse osteosclerosis is unusual in plasma cell myeloma. When present, the pattern simulates that associated with myelofibrosis, osteoblastic metastasis, sickle cell anemia, Paget's disease, fibrous dysplasia, lymphoma, mastocytosis, tuberous sclerosis, renal osteodystrophy, and sarcoidosis. Single (or several) lytic foci in myeloma are difficult to distinguish from many other primary and secondary skeletal neoplasms and infections. Expansile myelomatous lesions can simulate skeletal metastasis (particularly from thyroid and renal carcinoma), brown tumors of hyperparathyroidism, fibrous dysplasia, angiomatous lesions, hemophilic pseudotumors, and several primary bone tumors.

**TABLE 49-1**

**Plasma Cell Myeloma versus Skeletal Metastasis**

| | Plasma Cell Myeloma | Skeletal Metastasis |
|---|---|---|
| Disribution and common sites | Symmetrical<br>Axial skeleton, proximal portions of long bones, shoulder and elbow region | Asymmetrical<br>Axial skeleton, proximal portions of long bones |
| Predominant pattern | Osteolytic lesions > osteosclerotic lesions<br>Diffuse osteopenia (common)<br>Diffuse osteosclerosis (rare) | Osteolytic or osteosclerotic lesions<br>Diffuse osteopenia (rare)<br>Diffuse osteoclerosis (common with prostatic carcinoma) |
| Morphology of lesions | Well-circumscribed lesions of uniform size<br>Medullary or subcortical lucent lesions with cortical scalloping<br>Expansile lesions, soft tissue mass, or both (common in ribs, spine) | Poorly circumscribed lesions of varying size<br>Medullary, subcortical, or cortical lucent lesions with cortical destruction<br>Expansile lesions, soft tissue mass, or both (common in thyroid and renal carcinoma) |

## WALDENSTRÖM'S MACROGLOBULINEMIA

Macroglobulinemia is a disorder of middle-aged and elderly persons. It is a disease of differentiating B lymphocytes that is associated with the production of monoclonal macroglobulins. Symptoms include weakness, weight loss, bleeding diathesis, dyspnea, and personality changes; physical findings include retinal hemorrhage, hepatosplenomegaly, and lymphadenopathy. Laboratory analysis reveals anemia, an elevated sedimentation rate, increased serum viscosity, hyperglobulinemia, and increased cerebrospinal fluid protein. Cellular infiltration (lymphocytes, plasma cells, histiocytes, and mast cells) into various organs accounts for the clinical and radiographic manifestations of this disease.

### Skeletal Manifestations

Skeletal findings in Waldenström's macroglobulinemia are similar to those of multiple myeloma. Osteopenia, widening of the marrow spaces, and endosteal erosion are evident. The remaining trabeculae may be coarsened and result in focal osteosclerosis. Vertebral collapse is encountered. Osteolytic lesions may also be observed, with a reported frequency of 10% to 15% (Fig. 49–15). Involvement of the pelvis, perhaps with a predilection for the para-acetabular regions, is not uncommon. Large lesions in periarticular locations may result in joint destruction. MR imaging of spinal lesions in Waldenström's macroglobulinemia shows diffuse or patchy patterns of marrow involvement, similar to those of plasma cell myeloma. Ischemic necrosis of the femoral or humeral heads, which could be related to the hyperviscosity of blood, may be an additional manifestation of Waldenström's macroglobulinemia.

### Rheumatologic Manifestations

As in myeloma with secondary amyloidosis, the resulting arthropathy may simulate rheumatoid arthritis because of the presence of subcutaneous nodules, symmetrical

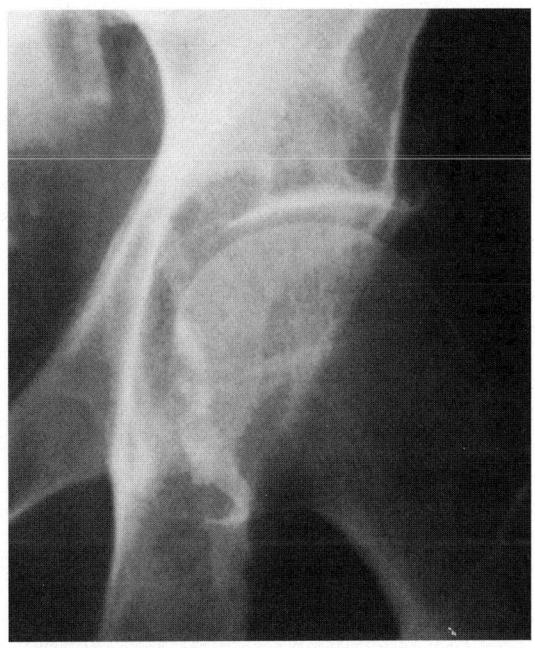

**Figure 49–15.** Waldenström's macroglobulinemia. Observe the osteolytic lesions of the para-acetabular region.

synovial thickening, and osseous erosions. Secondary gouty arthritis can be observed in patients with Waldenström's macroglobulinemia.

## AMYLOIDOSIS

Amyloidosis can be classified as primary, secondary, heredofamilial, senile, or localized amyloid tumors, based primarily on clinical parameters. In addition, in patients undergoing chronic hemodialysis, amyloid deposition consists of beta$_2$-microglobulin, which in rare circumstances can accumulate in the tissues of patients without a history of renal disease or hemodialysis. This last type of amyloidosis is discussed in detail in Chapter 46.

**Primary Amyloidosis.** The primary form of amyloidosis occurs without coexistent or antecedent disease. Most frequently it involves certain mesenchymal structures such as the heart, muscle, tongue, synovial membrane, and perivascular connective tissue. In many patients, primary amyloidosis is associated with multiple myeloma, which is generally nearly simultaneous in onset.

**Secondary Amyloidosis.** The secondary form is associated with various chronic diseases, including rheumatoid arthritis, sepsis, neoplasm, inflammatory disorders, and familial Mediterranean fever. It is an important complication of Crohn's disease and cystic fibrosis, as well as of chronic drug abuse. Amyloid deposition of the secondary type shows a predilection for the liver, spleen, kidneys, and adrenals.

**Heredofamilial Amyloidosis.** An increasing number of heredofamilial amyloid syndromes have been described. These syndromes can be classified by the site of predominant organ involvement. Thus, heredofamilial amyloidoses include neuropathies, nephropathies, cardiomyopathies, and miscellaneous types.

**Senile Amyloidosis.** Senile amyloidosis refers to a type whose incidence increases with age.

**Localized Amyloid Tumors.** In this type of amyloidosis, focal growths occur in the larynx, trachea, bronchi, and, rarely, skin (lichen amyloidosus).

## General Clinical Features

Primary amyloidosis is more frequent in men than in women, and its onset is generally between the ages of 40 and 80 years. Cardiac deposition of amyloid results in decompensation with dyspnea, edema, and pleural effusion. Macroglossia produces dysphagia and dysarthria. If amyloid is deposited in the liver, spleen, and kidney, hepatosplenomegaly and renal abnormality become evident, although these organs are more frequently involved in secondary amyloidosis.

Secondary amyloidosis can develop at any age, depending on the underlying disease process. Amyloid deposition in the kidneys leads to the nephrotic syndrome with albuminuria, cylindruria, edema, hypoalbuminemia, and hypercholesterolemia. Hepatosplenomegaly and adrenal insufficiency may become apparent. Amyloidosis of the gastrointestinal tract may manifest as obstruction, malabsorption, hemorrhage, protein loss, and diarrhea.

Amyloidosis occurring in association with plasma cell myeloma may be difficult to detect because of the presence of significant clinical findings related to the latter disease. Renal involvement and hepatosplenomegaly may be apparent.

Heredofamilial amyloidoses are associated with neurologic (including sensory neuropathies, autonomic nervous system symptoms and signs, and cranial nerve alterations), cardiac, and renal abnormalities.

Localized amyloid tumors of the respiratory tract may cause hoarseness, dyspnea, epistaxis, dysphagia, and hemoptysis.

Although no laboratory findings are pathognomonic of amyloidosis, the diagnosis can be substantiated by performance of the Congo red test. The gingiva, rectum, liver, spleen, kidney, small intestine, and skin have been used for diagnostic biopsy, although aspiration biopsy of the subcutaneous abdominal fat pad has become the method of choice.

## Musculoskeletal Features

Osseous and articular abnormalities can appear during the course of amyloidosis. In many instances, the abnormalities are the result of amyloid deposition in bone, synovium, and soft tissue. In some varieties of amyloidosis, the musculoskeletal features are indicative of an underlying disease process.

**Amyloidosis Complicating Rheumatologic Disorders.** The association of rheumatoid arthritis and secondary amyloidosis is well established, with an occurrence rate of 5% to 25%. Amyloidosis rarely develops in patients with rheumatoid arthritis who have had that disease for less than 2 years. The clinical diagnosis of secondary amyloidosis in patients with rheumatoid arthritis is supported by the presence of proteinuria, although hepatosplenomegaly and gastrointestinal bleeding are other important diagnostic findings. Amyloidosis in children is most frequently secondary to juvenile-onset rheumatoid arthritis, but it may also complicate chronic suppurative diseases and familial Mediterranean fever in this age group. Amyloidosis may occur during the course of ankylosing spondylitis, as well as other spondyloarthropathies and collagen vascular disorders.

**Bone Lesions.** Osteoporosis, lytic lesions of bone, and pathologic fractures may be observed (Fig. 49–16). Radiolucent areas of variable size are detected within medullary and cortical bone, particularly in the proximal portion of the femur and proximal end of the humerus. These lesions produce scalloping along the endosteal margin of the cortex, a finding simulating the appearance of plasma cell myeloma (see Table 49–1). They are produced by focal deposits of amyloid, some of which may localize in subchondral bone. In this latter location, secondary occlusion of blood vessels related to perivascular amyloidosis can lead to osteonecrosis of the epiphyses, with collapse. Amyloidosis of bone marrow can produce vertebral osteoporosis and collapse.

Tumorous lesions of bone containing amyloid (amyloidomas) have occasionally been reported. These lesions predominate in patients with plasma cell myeloma and coexistent amyloidosis and are usually associated with plasma cell infiltration as well. Calcification or ossification within these lesions may be evident.

**Articular and Periarticular Lesions.** The articular manifestations of amyloidosis are characterized by the accumulation of this substance in synovial tissue, other intra-articular structures, peritendinous areas, and surrounding soft tissue (Fig. 49–17). Soft tissue amyloid deposition produces nodules resembling those of rheumatoid arthritis. Amyloid nodules may become large and simulate

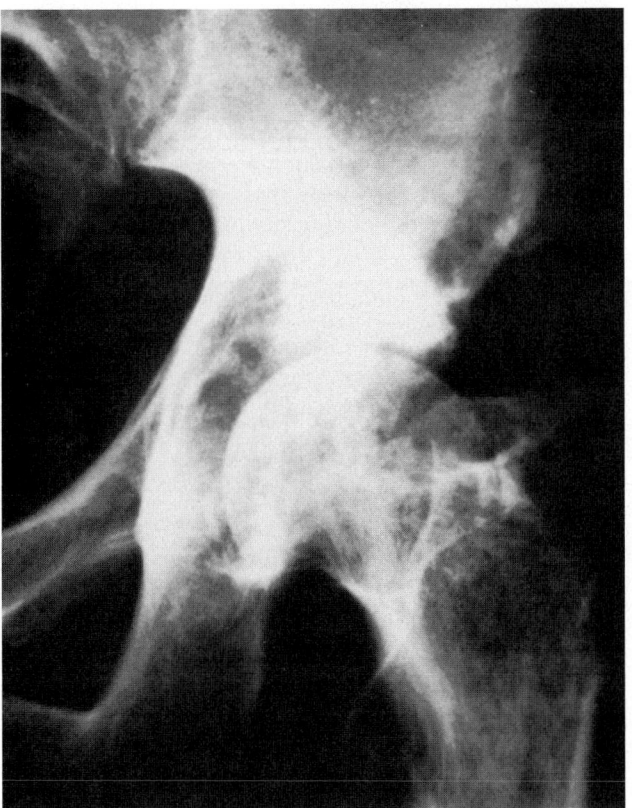

**Figure 49–16.** Amyloidosis: lytic lesions and osteoporosis. Osteolytic lesions with reactive sclerosis can be seen in the ilium and proximal portion of the femur.

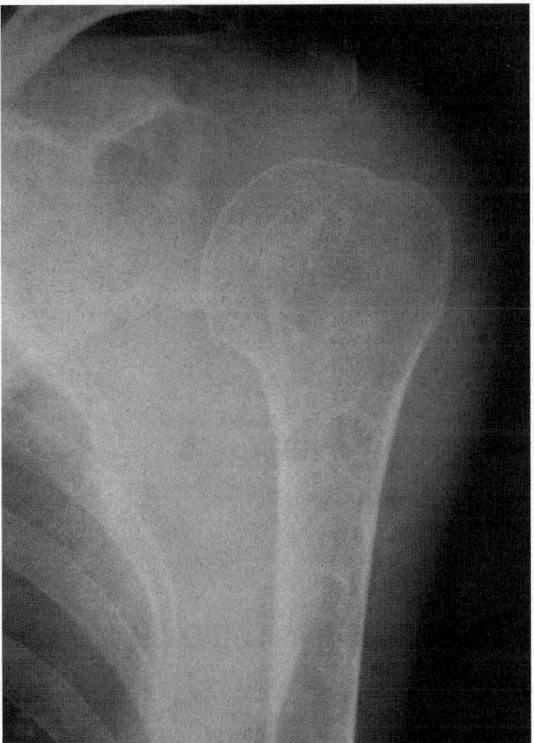

**Figure 49–17.** Amyloidosis: soft tissue abnormalities. Radiograph shows soft tissue swelling and associated osteoporosis of underlying bones.

tumors, and they are particularly prominent in the olecranon region and about the joints of the hand and wrist. Extensive infiltration about the shoulders produces rubbery, hard masses that are accentuated by surrounding muscle atrophy; the appearance resembles that of shoulder pads worn by football players. Similar deposits in the carpal canal can lead to carpal tunnel syndrome. In fact, 5% to 10% of patients with this syndrome may have amyloid infiltration in the adjacent soft tissues, and 10% to 30% of patients with primary amyloidosis have carpal tunnel syndrome.

The clinical findings of amyloid joint disease resemble the manifestations of rheumatoid arthritis. Bilateral, symmetrical arthritis of the large and small joints characterized by pain, stiffness, swelling, and palpable nodules is seen in both disorders. Amyloidosis may lead to joint contractures, which are usually the result of muscle and nerve involvement.

The radiographic findings of joint involvement in amyloidosis reflect this intra-articular and periarticular distribution of amyloid (Table 49–2). Asymmetrical soft tissue masses, periarticular osteoporosis, widening of the articular space, subchondral cysts, and erosions are seen. Subluxation, lytic lesions of bone, and pathologic fractures are additional manifestations. Involvement is frequently bilateral in distribution. Although the radiographic appearance is reminiscent of that in rheumatoid arthritis, extensive soft tissue nodular masses, well-defined cystic lesions with or without surrounding sclerosis, and preservation of the joint space are more characteristic of amyloid joint disease. Extensive joint destruction is occasionally encountered in amyloidosis.

## Magnetic Resonance Imaging

MR imaging of amyloid arthropathy demonstrates a homogeneous intermediate signal intensity of amyloid deposition on both T1- and T2-weighted spin echo sequences. The persistence of areas of low signal intensity within deposits of amyloid in T2-weighted images represents a key element in accurate diagnosis, although gouty tophi reveal similar areas. In amyloidosis, enhancement of signal intensity may occur after intravenous gadolinium administration, but the degree of enhancement is often mild, and portions of the amyloid deposits may fail to show any enhancement. Significant enhance-

---

**TABLE 49–2**

**Radiographic Manifestations of Musculoskeletal Involvement in Amyloidosis**

Osteoporosis
Lytic lesions
Pathologic fractures
Osteonecrosis
Soft tissue nodules and swelling
Subchondral cysts and erosions
Joint subluxations and contractures
Neuropathic osteoarthropathy

ment of leptomeningeal deposits of amyloid with the use of gadolinium-containing contrast agents has been noted, however (Fig. 49–18).

## Differential Diagnosis

**Bone Lesions.** Diffuse lytic lesions in amyloidosis are indistinguishable from those accompanying more com-mon disorders, particularly skeletal metastasis and plasma cell myeloma. Bone lysis in Waldenström's macroglobu-linemia is also virtually identical to that accompanying amyloidosis.

Localized destructive lesions of the skeleton in amyloidosis resemble sites of metastasis or a primary bone neoplasm. A soft tissue mass (which may contain calcifications) is common, but periostitis is rare.

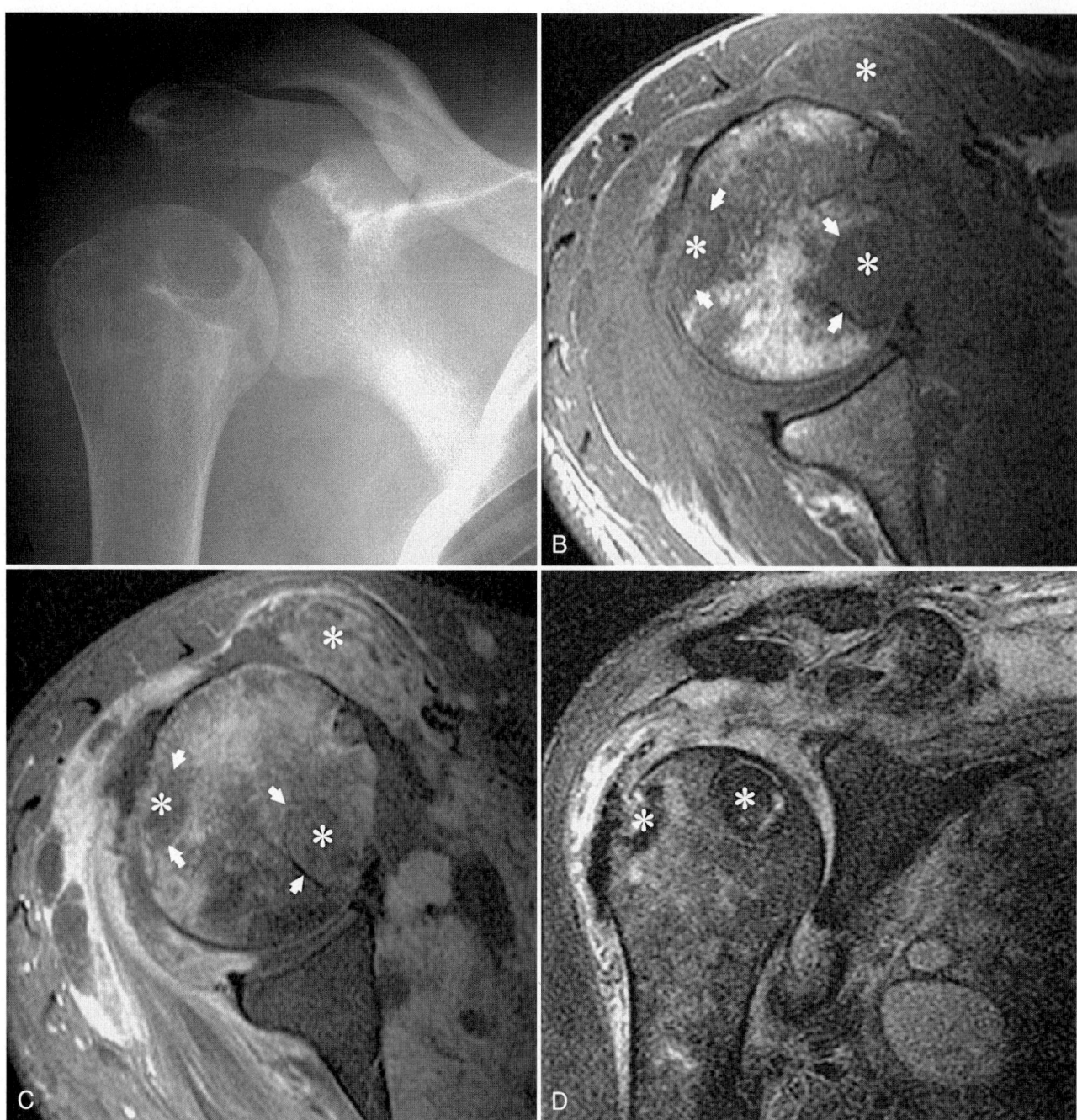

**Figure 49–18.** Dialysis-related amyloidosis: soft tissue masses and joint destruction. In this patient with renal disease who was receiving long-term hemodialysis, pain and swelling developed about multiple joints, and a gradually enlarging soft tissue mass appeared around the shoulder. *A*, Anteroposterior radiograph of the shoulder shows multiple well-defined erosions in the humeral head and acromion. *B* and *C*, Transverse T1-weighted (TR/TE, 650/14) *(B)* and fat-suppressed gadolinium-enhanced T1-weighted (TR/TE,600/14) *(C)* spin echo MR images show multiple enhancing soft tissue masses *(asterisks)*. Note the associated osseous erosions *(arrows)* and enhancing synovitis. *D*, Coronal conventional T2-weighted (TR/TE, 2000/80) spin echo MR image shows the masses *(asterisks)* to have an inhomogeneous but mainly low signal intensity. Note the massive rotator cuff tear with associated synovitis and fluid.

**Articular Lesions.** Articular lesions in amyloidosis are characterized by bulky soft tissue masses, well-defined erosions and cysts, and preservation of the joint space. These features can usually be distinguished from those of rheumatoid arthritis, which is associated with diffuse or fusiform soft tissue swelling, early joint space loss, and marginal erosions of bone. Amyloid joint disease shares many radiographic characteristics with gouty arthritis and xanthomatosis, but the clinical and laboratory manifestations of these latter disorders usually ensure an accurate diagnosis. The arthropathy of amyloidosis also resembles pigmented villonodular synovitis; some distinguishing features of the former include multiple sites of involvement, juxta-articular osteoporosis, and older patient age.

## FURTHER READING

Abdelwahab IF, Miller TT, Hermann G, et al: Transarticular invasion of joints by bone tumors: Hypothesis. Skeletal Radiol 20:279, 1991.

Bardwick PA, Zvaifler NJ, Gill GN, et al: Plasma cell dyscrasia with polyneuropathy, organomegaly, endocrinopathy, M protein, and skin changes: The POEMS syndrome. Medicine 59:311, 1980.

Barnett EV, Winkelstein A, Weinberger HJ: Agammaglobulinemia with polyarthritis and subcutaneous nodules. Am J Med 48:40, 1970.

Bataille R, Chevalier J, Rossi M, et al: Bone scintigraphy in plasma cell myeloma: A prospective study of 70 patients. Radiology 145:801, 1982.

Buckley RH: Specific immunodeficiency diseases, excluding acquired immunodeficiency syndrome. In Kelly WN, Harris ED Jr, Ruddy S, Sledge CB (eds): Textbook of Rheumatology, 5th ed. Philadelphia, WB Saunders, 1997, p 1282.

Clarisse PDT, Staple TW: Diffuse bone sclerosis in multiple myeloma. Radiology 99:327, 1971.

Fahey JL, Barth WF, Solomon A: Serum hyperviscosity syndrome. JAMA 192:464, 1965.

Flores M, Nadarajan P, Mangham DC: Soft-tissue amyloidoma: A case report. J Bone Joint Surg Br 80:654, 1998.

Gootnick LT: Solitary myeloma: Review of sixty-one cases. Radiology 45:385, 1945.

Grayzel AI, Marcus R, Stern R, et al: Chronic polyarthritis associated with hypogammaglobulinemia: A study of two patients. Arthritis Rheum 20:887, 1977.

Grossman RE, Hensley GT: Bone lesions in primary amyloidosis. AJR Am J Roentgenol 101:872, 1967.

Grover SB, Dhar A: Imaging spectrum in sclerotic myelomas: An experience of three cases. Eur Radiol 10:1828, 2000.

Heiser S, Schwartzman JJ: Variation in the roentgen appearance of the skeletal system in myeloma. Radiology 58:178, 1952.

Jacobson HG, Poppel MH, Shapiro JH, et al: The vertebral pedicle sign: A roentgen finding to differentiate metastatic carcinoma from multiple myeloma. AJR Am J Roentgenol 80:817, 1958.

Katz GA, Peter JB, Pearson CM, et al: The shoulder-pad sign—a diagnostic feature of amyloid arthropathy. N Engl J Med 288:354, 1973.

Lecouvet FE, Malghem J, Michaux L, et al: Vertebral compression fractures in multiple myeloma. Part II. Assessment of fracture risk with MR imaging of spinal bone marrow. Radiology 204:201, 1997.

Libshitz HI, Malthouse SR, Cunningham D, et al: Multiple myeloma: Appearance at MR imaging. Radiology 182:833, 1992.

Meszaros WT: The many facets of multiple myeloma. Semin Roentgenol 9:219, 1974.

Murata H, Kusazaki K, Hashiguchi S, et al: Bilateral metachronous periosteal tibial amyloid tumors. Skeletal Radiol 29:346, 2000.

Narvaez JA, Majos C, Narvaez J, et al: POEMS syndrome: Unusual radiographic, scintigraphic and CT features. Eur Radiol 8:134, 1998.

Reinus WR, Kyriakos M, Gilula LA, et al: Plasma cell tumors with calcified amyloid deposition mistaken for chondrosarcoma. Radiology 189:505, 1993.

Renner RR, Nelson DA, Lozner EL: Roentgenologic manifestations of primary macroglobulinemia (Waldenström). AJR Am J Roentgenol 113:499, 1971.

Renner RR, Smith JR: Plasma cell dyscrasias (except myeloma). Semin Roentgenol 9:209, 1974.

Resnick D, Greenway GD, Bardwick PA, et al: Plasma-cell dyscrasia with polyneuropathy, organomegaly, endocrinopathy, M-protein, and skin changes: The POEMS syndrome. Radiology 140:17, 1981.

Subbarao K, Jacobson HG: Amyloidosis and plasma cell dyscrasias of the musculoskeletal system. Semin Roentgenol 21:139, 1986.

Tong D, Griffin TW, Laramore GE, et al: Solitary plasmacytoma of bone and soft tissues. Radiology 135:195, 1980.

Vermess M, Pearson KD, Einstein AB, et al: Osseous manifestations of Waldenström's macroglobulinemia. Radiology 102:497, 1972.

Weinfeld A, Stern MH, Marx LH: Amyloid lesions of bone. AJR Am J Roentgenol 108:799, 1970.

# CHAPTER 50

## Lipidoses, Histiocytoses, and Hyperlipoproteinemias

## SUMMARY OF KEY FEATURES

Musculoskeletal findings are a significant part of the lipidoses, histiocytoses, and hyperlipoproteinemias. In Gaucher's disease, cellular accumulation in the bone marrow leads to replacement of trabeculae, endosteal erosion of the cortex, cortical thinning, lytic defects, and fractures. Osteonecrosis and modeling deformities of the long bones are characteristic. The findings in Niemann-Pick disease may resemble those of Gaucher's disease, although osteonecrosis is not encountered. This latter abnormality is detected in Fabry's disease.

Multicentric reticulohistiocytosis is characterized by the proliferation of histiocytes in various tissues. Skeletal involvement can lead to a symmetrical destructive polyarthritis with a predilection for the interphalangeal joints of the hands and feet, early and severe abnormalities of the atlantoaxial joints, and changes in other articulations of the appendicular skeleton.

The Langerhans cell histiocytoses consist of three disorders: eosinophilic granuloma, Hand-Schüller-Christian disease, and Letterer-Siwe disease. Although these disorders share numerous radiographic and pathologic features, their classic clinical characteristics allow their separation into discrete entities.

Erdheim-Chester disease is an unusual lipidosis leading to characteristic skeletal abnormalities. Its relationship to the histiocytoses is not clear. Sinus histiocytosis with massive lymphadenopathy is a self-limited disease associated with osteolytic lesions.

The hyperlipoproteinemias are divided into five types, according to the predominant lipoprotein pattern. Similar clinical and radiographic manifestations are observed in these disorders, including xanthomatous collections in soft tissue, tendon, subperiosteal, and intraosseous locations, as well as gout, arthralgias, and arthritis.

## INTRODUCTION

No agreement has been reached regarding the classification of lipid storage and histiocytic disorders, in part because of the lack of a clear understanding of their cause and pathogenesis. A classification system of lipid storage and histiocytic diseases based on a composite of several systems is presented in Table 50–1. This chapter covers some of these diseases, particularly those with prominent musculoskeletal involvement.

**TABLE 50–1**

### Lipid Storage and Histiocyctic Disorders

**Lipid Storage Diseases**
Gaucher's disease (glycosylceramide lipidosis)
Niemann-Pick disease (sphingomyelin lipidosis)
Fabry's disease (glycolipidosis)
Refsum's disease (phytanic acid storage disease)
Krabbe's disease (galactosylceramide lipidosis)
Metachromatic leukodystrophy (sulfatide lipidosis)
Farber's lipogranulomatosis (ceramidase deficiency)
Gangliosidoses
Sea-blue histiocytosis
Tay-Sachs disease
Fucosidosis

**Reactive Histiocytoses**
Multicentric reticulohistiocytosis
Langerhans cell histiocytosis
Lipid granulomatosis (Erdheim-Chester disease)
Sinus histiocytosis with lymphadenopathy
Erythrophagocytic lymphohistiocytosis

**Neoplastic Histiocytoses**
Acute monocytic leukemia
Chronic myelomonocytic leukemia
Histiocytic lymphoma
Malignant histiocytosis (histiocytic medullary reticulosis)

**Disorders of Lipoprotein Metabolism**
Hyperlipoproteinemias
Hypolipoproteinemias

**Miscellaneous Disorders**
Membranous lipodystrophy

## GAUCHER'S DISEASE

### General Features

Gaucher's disease is a rare familial, autosomal recessive disorder of cerebroside metabolism caused by the deficit of a specific enzyme (glucocerebroside hydrolase or beta-glucosidase) that leads to abnormal accumulation of lipid material in the reticuloendothelial cells of the body. The disease affects both men and women and may develop at any age, although it is particularly frequent in childhood and early adulthood. Many patients are Ashkenazic Jews; however, others may be affected, including white, black, and Asian groups.

The manifestations of Gaucher's disease can be attributed to the accumulation of Gaucher cells in various tissues of the body; however, the pathogenesis of cerebroside infiltration within these cells is not known. Proliferation of Gaucher cells in the liver and spleen in Gaucher's disease leads to hepatosplenomegaly. Similarly, accumulation of these cells in the lymph nodes produces lymphadenopathy, and accumulation in the brain produces glial cell proliferation and degenerative changes in the pyramidal cells of the cerebral cortex. The bone marrow is not immune. Accumulation of Gaucher cells in this location may cause osseous destruction, hematologic abnormalities, and articular manifestations.

## Clinical Features

Gaucher's disease has been divided into three clinical forms: types 1, 2, and 3. Common to all three types are recessive inheritance, hepatosplenomegaly, deficient acid beta-glucosidase activity, elevated non–tartrate-inhibitable acid phosphatase activity, and characteristic Gaucher cells in the bone marrow.

Type 1 disease, termed chronic non-neuronopathic or "adult" Gaucher's disease, is the most frequent; it occurs in Ashkenazic Jews and leads to clinical manifestations that may initially appear in childhood but subsequently worsen as the patient enters the second and third decades of life. Such manifestations include a protuberant abdomen and episodic pain, often severe, in the arms, legs, and back. Laboratory findings include microcytic anemia, leukopenia, and a decreased number of platelets in association with easy bruising and a bleeding diathesis. Bone involvement is common.

Type 2, or acute neuronopathic, Gaucher's disease is a rare, fatal neurodegenerative disorder with no particular ethnic predilection; it manifests clinically shortly after birth or in the first few months of life. Bone abnormalities are limited. The average time of survival is approximately 1 year.

Type 3, or subacute neuronopathic (juvenile), Gaucher's disease is uncommon and characterized by hepatosplenomegaly appearing in the first few years of life. Neurologic

and skeletal manifestations appear during childhood or adolescence.

The presence of enlarged, lipid-laden histiocytes—the Gaucher cells—represents the hallmark of all types of this disease. Gaucher cells are particularly prominent in the red pulp of the spleen, the bone marrow, and the sinusoids and medullary portions of the lymph nodes.

## Musculoskeletal Abnormalities

Osteoarticular findings may be minimal in young infants with the acute, fulminant disease. These findings are more pronounced in older infants, children, and adults who suffer from the more chronic form of Gaucher's disease. In some patients, skeletal disease is the earliest and most prominent feature and can occur before the onset of splenomegaly.

**Marrow Infiltration.** Accumulation of Gaucher cells within the bone marrow is associated with cellular necrosis, fibrous proliferation, and resorption of spongy trabeculae (Fig. 50–1). Erosion of the endosteal surface of the cortex is also apparent, causing increased radiolucency of bone and cortical scalloping and thinning. Abnormalities predominate in the axial skeleton and proximal portions of the long bones, although they may be detected at other skeletal sites. Abnormalities of the long bones are usually bilateral and frequently symmetrical.

In the spine, cellular infiltration results in loss of trabeculae, with increased radiolucency of the vertebral bodies, accentuation of vertical trabeculae, and multiple compression fractures with kyphosis and gibbous defor-

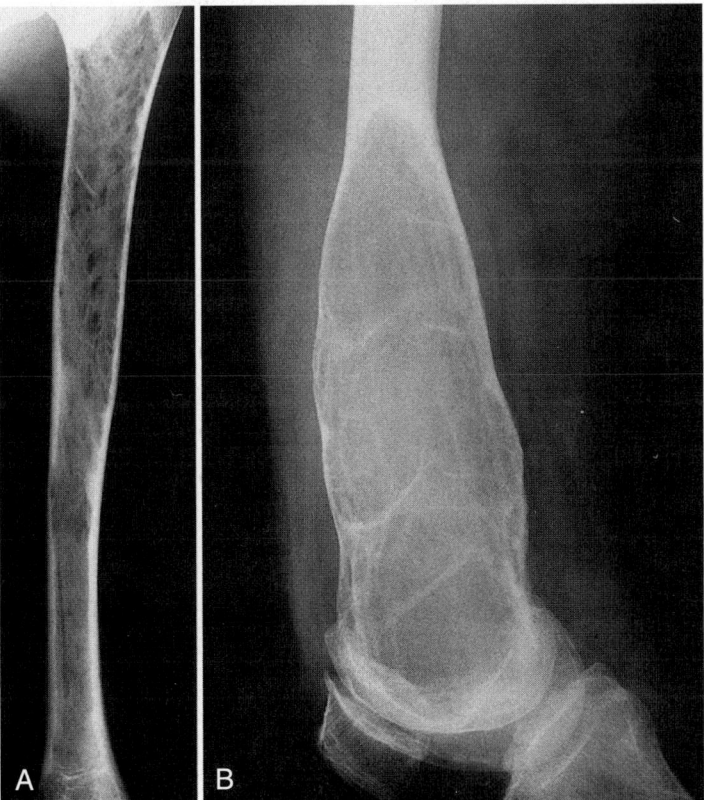

**Figure 50–1.** Gaucher's disease: marrow infiltration in the appendicular skeleton. *A*, Radiographic abnormalities of Gaucher's disease include osteopenia, osteolytic lesions, medullary widening, and cortical diminution. The resemblance to features of plasma cell myeloma is obvious. *B*, Observe the long expansile lesion of the distal end of the femur with a "ground-glass" appearance, crossing trabeculae, and cortical diminution.

mity. Spinal cord compression is rare. In the calvaria, trabecular destruction and thinning of both the outer and inner tables can be seen. Mandibular involvement is not unusual.

**Fractures.** Infiltration of the marrow spaces with Gaucher cells and trabecular resorption produce osseous weakening, which may result in pathologic fractures (Fig. 50–2). Most frequently, fractures appear in the vertebral column. Intraosseous disc displacement (cartilaginous or Schmorl's nodes) and compression of the vertebral bodies are seen. The involved vertebral body may become completely flattened (vertebra plana). This appearance, which is identical to that accompanying the histiocytoses, may be evident at multiple levels and is associated with paravertebral soft tissue swelling. Fractures are also observed in the ribs and in the long and short tubular bones of the appendicular skeleton, particularly the femur, tibia, and humerus. These fractures may appear in the diaphyses or the epiphyses, although in the latter location, their occurrence may reflect underlying osteonecrosis.

**Modeling Deformities.** One of the most characteristic osseous manifestations of chronic Gaucher's disease is modeling deformities. Expansion of the contour of the long tubular bones is most frequent in the lower ends of both femoral shafts, particularly medially. It results in cortical thinning and loss of the normal concavity of the bony outline. This appearance has been termed an Erlenmeyer flask deformity (Fig. 50–3); it is very suggestive of the diagnosis of Gaucher's disease, particularly when associated with epiphyseal osteonecrosis.

Peculiar steplike depressions of the superior and inferior margins of the vertebral bodies (Fig. 50–4) have been described in Gaucher's disease and are identical to the depressions typical of sickle cell anemia and other hemoglobinopathies. This deformity, which is called the H vertebra, has been attributed to ischemic growth disturbance at the chondro-osseous junction.

**Osteonecrosis.** Osteonecrosis of the epiphyses and diaphyses is well recognized in Gaucher's disease (Fig. 50–5). Risk factors may include previous splenectomy and male gender. In the shafts of long bones, alternating radiolucency and sclerosis are seen, with associated periostitis; this bone-within-bone appearance is identical to that seen in sickle cell anemia.

Epiphyseal bone necrosis can be visualized in the femoral head, humeral head, and tibial plateau. The resulting radiographic picture of osteonecrosis is identical to that accompanying many other diseases.

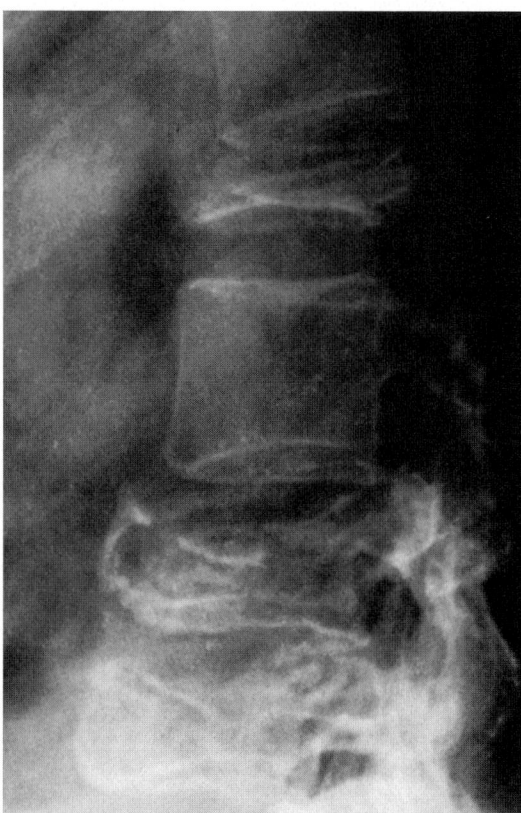

**Figure 50–2.** Gaucher's disease: fractures. Vertebral fracture and collapse are particularly frequent. In this case, marrow replacement has led to the dramatic collapse of multiple vertebral bodies, some of which have been reduced to a flattened structure (vertebra plana).

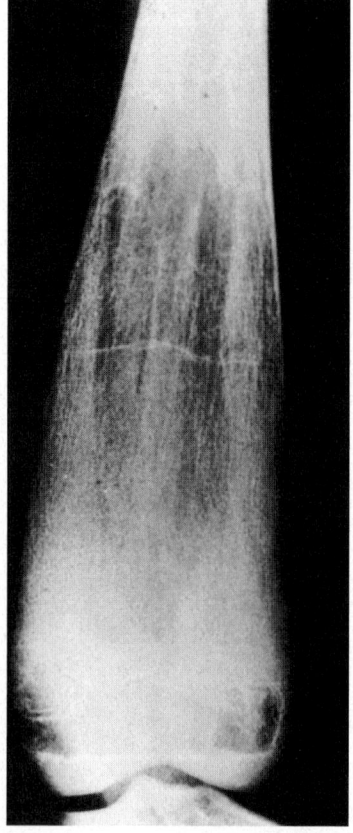

**Figure 50–3.** Gaucher's disease: modeling deformities. Erlenmeyer flask deformity of the distal end of the femur is observed. Note the expansion of the contour of the long tubular bone, with straightening and convexity of the osseous margin, particularly along the medial aspect of the metaphysis.

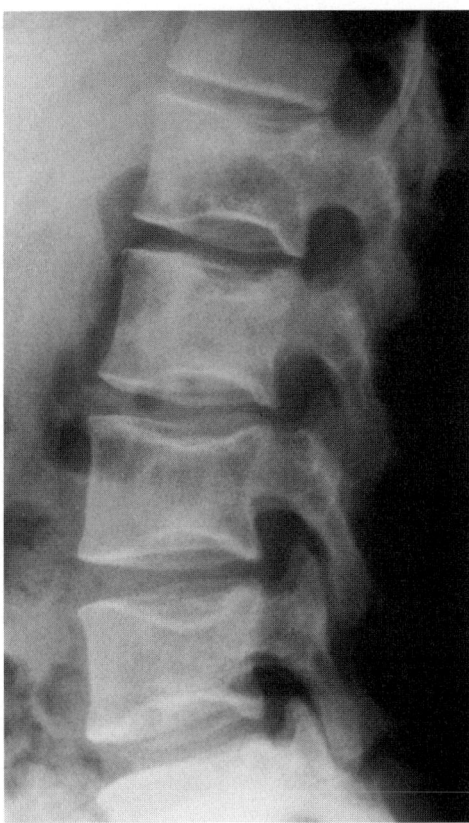

**Figure 50–4.** Gaucher's disease: modeling deformities. Observe the central depressions of the superior and inferior surfaces of multiple lumbar vertebral bodies in this 35-year-old woman.

**Infection.** Patients with Gaucher's disease have an increased susceptibility to the development of bone infection. Infection may involve any skeletal site and can be caused by various organisms, including salmonellae.

### Advanced Imaging Methods

Radionuclide techniques, including bone scintigraphy (i.e., technetium-labeled diphosphonates) and bone marrow scintigraphy (i.e., technetium-labeled sulfur colloid), have been used to determine the extent and severity of skeletal involvement in patients with Gaucher's disease (Fig. 50–6). At the onset of a crisis, the bone scan typically shows decreased uptake or, rarely, no uptake ("cold" bone scan) of the radionuclide at the involved site; several weeks later, a margin of increased uptake surrounding a region of decreased uptake may be evident, and months later, the radionuclide scan may appear normal.

The expanding role of magnetic resonance (MR) imaging in the analysis of bone marrow disorders extends to Gaucher's disease. The T1-weighted signal characteristics of affected bone marrow are identical to those in other disorders characterized by marrow infiltration, such as metastatic disease, leukemia, lymphoma, and plasma cell myeloma, although the distribution and morphology of the process vary, to some extent, among these disorders. More helpful in terms of diagnosing Gaucher's disease is persistent low signal intensity on T2-weighted spin echo

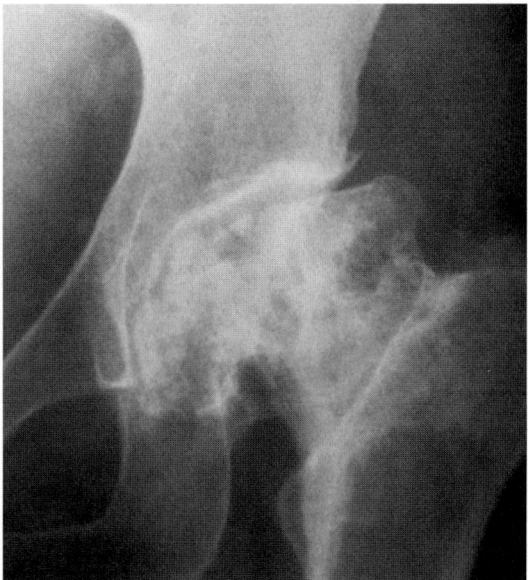

**Figure 50–5.** Gaucher's disease: osteonecrosis. Radiograph delineates ischemic necrosis of the femoral head, with collapse of bone and secondary osteoarthritis. (Courtesy of G. Greenway, MD, Dallas, Tex.)

MR images (Fig. 50–7), which differs from the higher signal intensity that may accompany skeletal metastasis, certain other tumors, and infection. The signal pattern, however, is not specific, because the T2 values of tumors

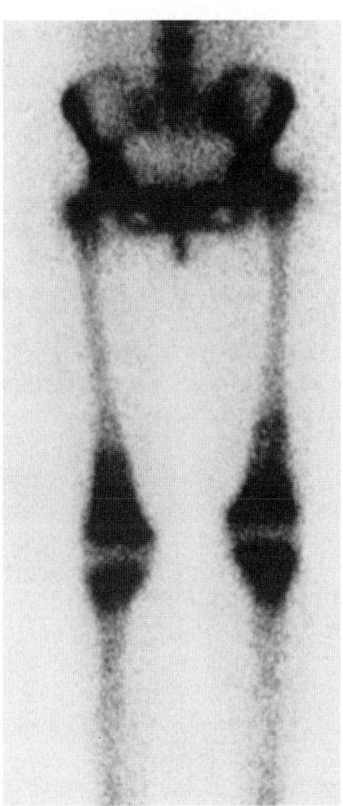

**Figure 50–6.** Gaucher's disease: radionuclide abnormalities. Bone scintigraphy shows intense accumulation of radionuclide in the periarticular and metaphyseal regions, particularly about the knee. Note the Erlenmeyer flask deformities of the femora.

show considerable variability, the T2 values of hyperplastic normal marrow are also variable, and high signal intensity on T2-weighted spin echo MR sequences in the bone marrow of patients with Gaucher's disease has been encountered.

MR imaging can also be used effectively to study the skeletal complications that occur in Gaucher's disease. Bone marrow ischemia and necrosis, osteomyelitis, and vertebral collapse are among the complications that may be assessed with MR imaging (Fig. 50–8).

## Differential Diagnosis

The generalized increased radiolucency (osteopenia) seen in Gaucher's disease is also apparent in a variety of metabolic (osteoporosis, osteomalacia, hyperparathyroidism), hematologic (sickle cell anemia, thalassemia), and neoplastic (plasma cell myeloma, leukemia) disorders. In Gaucher's disease, localized lucent areas and cystic lesions producing a honeycomb appearance may simulate the findings of plasma cell myeloma, amyloidosis, and skeletal metastasis.

Generalized or localized osteosclerosis is likewise not specific for Gaucher's disease and may be seen in skeletal metastasis, tuberous sclerosis, mastocytosis, myelofibrosis, and Hodgkin's disease. In Gaucher's disease, the sclerosis includes a coarsened trabecular pattern and a bone-

within-bone appearance, a finding that is not apparent in these other disorders. Similar changes, however, can be seen in sickle cell anemia and its variants; this similarity is related to the occurrence of bone infarction and necrosis in these anemias and in Gaucher's disease. Epiphyseal osteonecrosis, particularly of the femoral head, which is seen in both Gaucher's disease and hemoglobinopathies, is also apparent in Cushing's syndrome and exogenous hypercortisolism, pancreatitis, caisson disease, collagen vascular disorders, and numerous other diseases.

An Erlenmeyer flask appearance is seen in Gaucher's disease and other disorders (Table 50–2), including certain anemias, fibrous dysplasia, Niemann-Pick disease, (cranio)metaphyseal dysplasia (Pyle's disease), heavy metal poisoning, and osteopetrosis. In many of these diseases, other findings allow an accurate diagnosis. The diagnosis of Gaucher's disease should be considered in any patient with hepatosplenomegaly who has widespread osteopenia with a coarsened trabecular pattern, focal osteosclerosis, ischemic necrosis, and flaring or Erlenmeyer flask deformities of the distal portions of the femora.

## NIEMANN-PICK DISEASE

### General Features

Niemann-Pick disease is a rare, genetically determined disorder characterized by the widespread accumulation

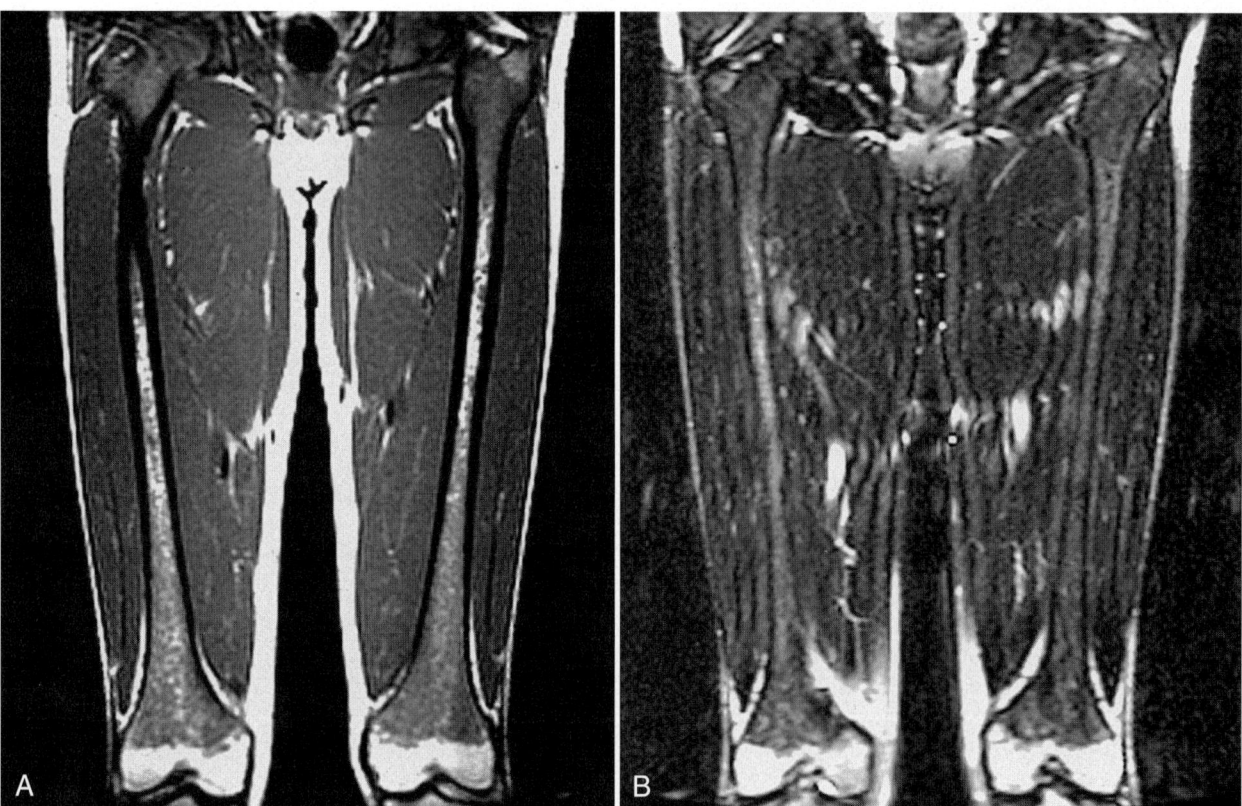

**Figure 50–7.** Gaucher's disease: MR imaging abnormalities. Marrow infiltration has occurred in this 30-year-old man with type 1 disease. Corresponding coronal T1-weighted (TR/TE, 566/11) *(A)* and fast T2-weighted (TR/TE, 5000/108) *(B)* spin echo MR images show replacement of the normal marrow with a signal intensity similar to that of muscle on both pulse sequences.

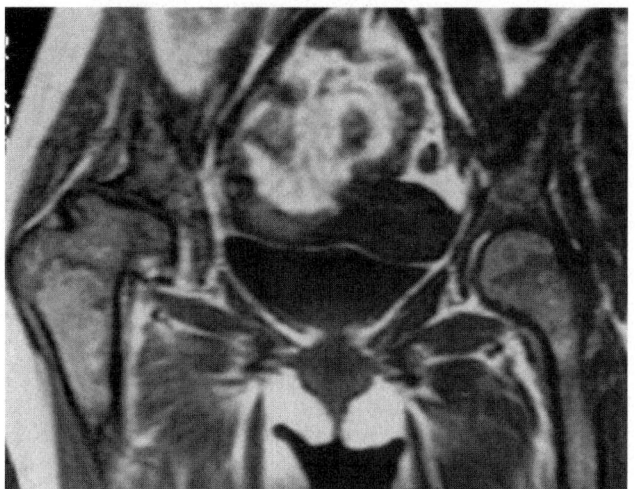

**Figure 50–8.** Gaucher's disease: MR imaging abnormalities. Marrow infiltration and osteonecrosis are evident in this 31-year-old woman. Coronal T1-weighted (TR/TE, 600/20) spin echo MR image shows abnormally low signal intensity in the marrow of the femora and innominate bones. Note the deformity of the right femoral head, indicative of osteonecrosis.

of lipid, particularly sphingomyelin, in the body. Niemann-Pick disease is not a single entity; five types have been reported.

**Type A.** This acute neuronopathic form, often observed in Ashkenazic Jews, is characterized by a rapidly fatal disease of infancy, with involvement of viscera and the nervous system.

**Type B.** This chronic form, without nervous system involvement, is often seen in non-Jewish persons and is characterized by visceral involvement in infants and a moderate to severe deficiency of sphingomyelinase.

**Type C.** This is a subacute (juvenile) form causing neurologic abnormalities in childhood and usually leading to death by adolescence. There is questionable sphingomyelinase deficiency.

**Type D.** This is also called the Nova Scotia form, in which patients with Nova Scotian ancestry otherwise resemble those with type C disease.

---

**TABLE 50–2**

**Conditions Characterized by Erlenmeyer Flask Deformity**

Gaucher's disease
Niemann-Pick disease
Anemias
Fibrous dysplasia
Metaphyseal dysplasia (Pyle's disease)
Osteopetrosis
Heavy metal poisoning

---

**Type E.** This is an indeterminate form that occurs in adults. There is visceral involvement and questionable sphingomyelinase deficiency.

## Clinical Features

The clinical manifestations vary with the specific disease type. In general, symptoms and signs become apparent during infancy, progress rapidly, and lead to the patient's demise. Findings in these infants may include jaundice, hepatosplenomegaly, abdominal enlargement, lymphadenopathy, emaciation, and decreased visual acuity or blindness. In some patients, clinical manifestations may not be detected until later in childhood, and affected children may live into adolescence.

## Musculoskeletal Abnormalities

Lipid-containing foam cells accumulate in the bone marrow and produce abnormalities in the adjacent bony trabeculae (Fig. 50–9). These changes are particularly frequent in children who have a type of Niemann-Pick disease that is compatible with longer life (type B). On radiographs, this combination of spongiosa and cortical abnormalities results in increased osseous radiolucency and medullary widening with cortical diminution, findings similar to those of Gaucher's disease. Modeling deformities in Niemann-Pick disease are also similar to those of Gaucher's disease and consist of straightening and convexity of the distal femoral contour. As in Gaucher's disease, MR imaging is effective in documenting marrow infiltration in the long tubular bones.

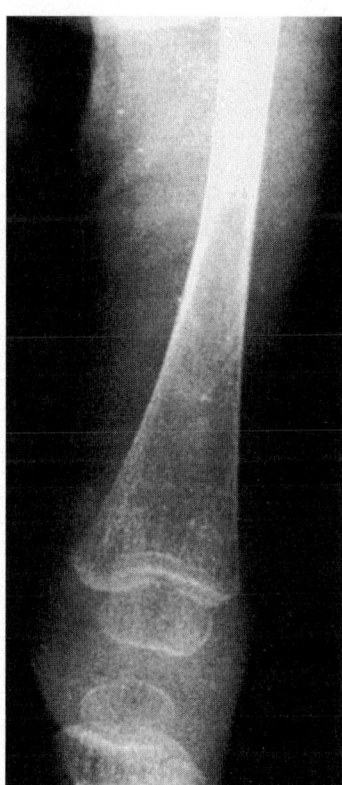

**Figure 50–9.** Niemann-Pick disease: marrow infiltration. The distal femoral shaft is both osteopenic and expanded.

## Differential Diagnosis

The skeletal manifestations of Niemann-Pick disease are similar to those of Gaucher's disease, which is not surprising, in view of their nearly identical pathogenesis (Table 50–3). Medullary widening, cortical thinning, and modeling deformities are seen in both disorders. Unlike Gaucher's disease, Niemann-Pick disease has not been associated with epiphyseal osteonecrosis or with a high frequency of well-circumscribed radiolucent lesions. These differences facilitate the radiographic diagnosis of Niemann-Pick disease.

## FABRY'S DISEASE

### General Features

Fabry's disease, or glycosphingolipidosis, is a hereditary, X-linked systemic disorder characterized by the accumulation of ceramide trihexoside in various tissues because of the absence of an enzyme (ceramide trihexosidase) required for its catabolism. The initial clinical manifestations may involve multiple organ systems and vary in men and women and in hemizygous and heterozygous patients. The characteristic skin lesion of this disease is bilaterally distributed in the lower part of the abdomen and the legs, with involvement of the back, thighs, buttocks, hips, pelvis, and scrotum. The patient may die in the fifth or sixth decade of life because of renal failure and hypertension. The diagnosis is established by the detection of a characteristic skin lesion, corneal epithelial dystrophy, and abnormal levels of birefringent lipid material in the skin or kidney.

### Musculoskeletal Abnormalities

Periarticular swelling may be seen in the knees, elbows, and small joints of the fingers. Osteonecrosis is observed at many sites, including the femoral head and talus. Presumably, the pathogenesis of the bone necrosis is similar to that in Gaucher's disease, with lipid infiltration in marrow and vessel walls.

## MULTICENTRIC RETICULOHISTIOCYTOSIS

### General Features

Multicentric reticulohistiocytosis is an uncommon systemic disease of unknown cause that usually becomes apparent

**TABLE 50–3**

**Musculoskeletal Manifestations of Gaucher's Disease and Niemann-Pick Disease**

| | Gaucher's Disease | Niemann-Pick Disease |
|---|---|---|
| Osteopenia | + | + |
| Cortical thinning or erosion | + | + |
| Coarsened trabecular pattern | + | + |
| Lytic lesions | + | – |
| Modeling deformity | + | + |
| Osteonecrosis | + | – |

in adulthood and is characterized by the proliferation of histiocytes in the skin, mucosa, subcutaneous tissue, synovium, and, on occasion, bone and periosteum. Other names for this disease are lipoid dermatoarthritis, reticulohistiocytoma, and giant cell reticulohistiocytosis.

### Clinical Features

Multicentric reticulohistiocytosis demonstrates no particular geographic predilection. Its onset is most frequently in middle age (40 to 50 years). Women are affected more frequently than men. In approximately 60% to 70% of patients, polyarthritis is the first manifestation of the disease, followed months to years later by a nodular eruption of the skin. In the remainder of patients, skin nodules are present when the disorder initially develops. These nodules are pruritic, firm, yellow to red in color, and common in the ears, nose, scalp, face, dorsum of the hands, forearms, and elbows. Small tumefactions about the nail folds are characteristic and may lead to alterations in nail growth.

Polyarticular manifestations are symmetrical and involve, in descending order of frequency, the interphalangeal joints of the fingers, knees, shoulders, wrists, hips, ankles, feet, and elbows. Clinical findings are soft tissue swelling, stiffness, and tenderness; these abnormalities resemble the findings of rheumatoid arthritis, although there is a greater frequency of distal interphalangeal joint changes in multicentric reticulohistiocytosis, and joint involvement may be more severe. In fact, arthritis mutilans develops in almost 50% of patients with multicentric reticulohistiocytosis.

In addition to skin lesions and polyarthritis, patients may have xanthelasmas. Xanthomas are related to the presence of hypercholesterolemia and involve predominantly the eyelids. Tendon sheath swelling, hypertension, lymphadenopathy, ganglia, erythema, joint hypermobility, and pathologic fractures (in descending order of frequency) are other clinical manifestations.

### Radiographic Abnormalities

The musculoskeletal radiographic features of multicentric reticulohistiocytosis are bilateral symmetrical involvement; predilection for the interphalangeal joints of the hand and foot; early and severe involvement of the atlanto-axial articulation; erosive arthritis beginning at the margins of the joint, spreading centrally, and producing separation of osseous surfaces; lack of significant periarticular osteoporosis or periosteal bone formation; and uncalcified nodules of the skin, subcutaneous tissues, and tendon sheaths (Table 50–4).

The most characteristic site of involvement is the interphalangeal joints of the hands, which may be altered in as many as 75% of patients with this disease (Fig. 50–10). Soft tissue swelling and marginal erosions, distributed symmetrically, are the initial features in this location. The erosions are well circumscribed and resemble the defects of gouty arthritis. The articular space may be widened or narrowed. Abnormalities of the feet resemble those of the hands.

Changes may be evident in other joints of the appendicular skeleton, including the glenohumeral and acromio-

**TABLE 50–4**

### Radiographic Characteristics of Multicentric Reticulohistiocytosis

Bilateral symmetrical involvement
Predilection for interphalangeal joints of the hand, foot
Atlantoaxial subluxation
Marginal erosions
Absence of osteoporosis
Soft tissue nodules

clavicular joints, as well as the hip, knee, elbow, and ankle. In each location, the severity of the process may vary. Changes in the sacroiliac joint include erosion and obliteration, with bony ankylosis of the articular space. Severe destructive abnormalities in the cervical spine, including subluxation at the atlantoaxial joint, may be seen.

## Differential Diagnosis

The articular manifestations of multicentric reticulohistiocytosis must be distinguished from those of other conditions (Table 50–5). The early erosive changes at the margins of joints resemble the erosions in a variety of synovial diseases, such as rheumatoid arthritis, psoriatic arthritis, ankylosing spondylitis, and Reiter's syndrome.

Although symmetrical involvement and absence of new bone formation are seen in both multicentric reticulohistiocytosis and rheumatoid arthritis, periarticular osteoporosis and early joint space loss are characteristic of rheumatoid arthritis but may be absent in multicentric reticulohistiocytosis. In addition, significant destructive changes of the distal interphalangeal joints are not common in rheumatoid arthritis but represent an important finding in multicentric reticulohistiocytosis. Atlantoaxial subluxation may be seen in both conditions.

Certain findings in psoriatic arthritis resemble the changes in multicentric reticulohistiocytosis, including a predilection for the interphalangeal joints, marginal and central erosions with separation of osseous surfaces, and lack of osteoporosis. Distinguishing features in psoriasis are asymmetrical involvement, new bone formation and proliferation with poorly defined erosive alterations, and intra-articular bony ankylosis. The character of the erosions in Reiter's syndrome and ankylosing spondylitis resembles that of psoriatic arthritis (poorly defined erosive changes with proliferation) and differs from that of multicentric reticulohistiocytosis. In addition, the distribution of articular involvement in both Reiter's syndrome and ankylosing spondylitis is characteristic.

Inflammatory (erosive) osteoarthritis and scleroderma are two other diseases that may be associated with osseous erosion of the interphalangeal joints. In the former disease, erosive changes may predominate in the central portion of the joint—a distinctive characteristic—and may be

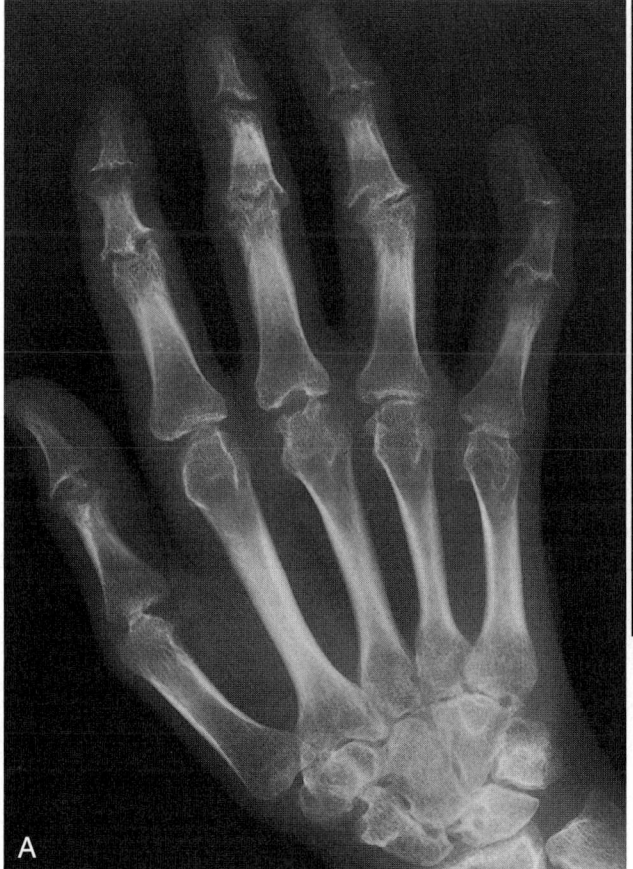

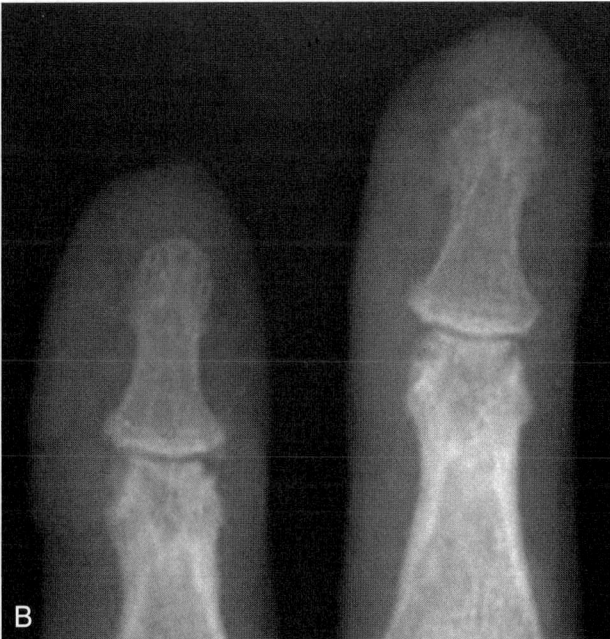

**Figure 50–10.** Multicentric reticulohistiocytosis: hand and wrist involvement. *A*, Radiograph reveals well-defined erosions of the interphalangeal and metacarpophalangeal joints, as well as throughout the wrist. *B*, In a different patient with mild involvement, note characteristic interphalangeal joint involvement, with erosive changes at the margins of the joints. Soft tissue nodules are readily apparent. (*A*, Courtesy of A. Brower, MD, Norfolk, Va.)

**TABLE 50–5**

Differential Diagnosis of Multicentric Reticulohistiocytosis

| | Symmetrical Involvement | Involvement of DIP Joints | Marginal Erosions | Osteo-porosis | Intra-articular Bony Ankylosis | Atlantoaxial Subluxation | Soft Tissue Nodules |
|---|---|---|---|---|---|---|---|
| Multicentric reticulohistiocytosis | + | + | + | − | − | + | + |
| Rheumatoid arthritis | + | − | + | + | − | + | + |
| Psoriatic arthritis | ± | + | + | − | + | + | − |
| Inflammatory (erosive) osteoarthritis | + | + | ± | − | + | − | − |
| Gouty arthritis | ± | + | + | − | − | − | + |

DIP, distal interphalangeal.

associated with osteophytosis and intra-articular bony ankylosis. These latter features are not part of the radiographic picture of multicentric reticulohistiocytosis. Distal interphalangeal joint erosions are unusual in scleroderma and, when present, are associated with more typical findings, such as tuftal resorption and soft tissue calcification.

Gouty arthritis is characterized by soft tissue nodular masses, sharply marginated erosions, and lack of osteoporosis, radiographic findings identical to those of multicentric reticulohistiocytosis. Preservation of articular space is noted in gout and may be apparent in multicentric reticulohistiocytosis, particularly in the early phases of the disease. An asymmetrical distribution, partially calcified soft tissue masses, and bone production with overhanging edges are findings of gout that are not apparent in multicentric reticulohistiocytosis.

## LANGERHANS CELL HISTIOCYTOSIS (HISTIOCYTOSIS X)

### General Features

The three major conditions in the category of Langerhans cell histiocytosis are eosinophilic granuloma, Hand-Schüller-Christian disease, and Letterer-Siwe disease. The term histiocytosis X has been used as a comprehensive designation for these three conditions, as an expression of the same basic pathologic process underlying them. Eosinophilic granuloma, the mildest form of histiocytosis, manifests as single or multiple lesions of bone. Hand-Schüller-Christian disease, the most varied form, involves chronic dissemination of osseous lesions. Letterer-Siwe disease, the acute form, is characterized by rapid dissemination and a poor clinical prognosis.

Clear distinction among these entities on the basis of clinical and radiographic manifestations is not always possible. Some patients initially have solitary bone lesions consistent with eosinophilic granuloma and subsequently develop more widespread skeletal and extraskeletal involvement, consistent with Hand-Schüller-Christian disease. Other patients have a fulminant onset consistent with Letterer-Siwe disease that progresses to a more chronic form. Clear separation among these three forms of

histiocytosis is also difficult on the basis of histologic manifestations. Additionally, in all three entities, specific histiocytic cells (Langerhans cells) containing cytoplasmic inclusion bodies (Langerhans granules, or X bodies) are found. Langerhans cells are believed to be virtually diagnostic of the histiocytoses.

Despite the presence of Langerhans cells in the three classic forms of histiocytosis, many observers maintain that the three disorders are unrelated and emphasize their differing clinical manifestations. Early and diffuse organ involvement and rapid patient demise, characteristics of Letterer-Siwe disease, support its classification as a malignant lymphoma, although the Langerhans cells, which are unreactive with antilymphocytes, appear to be of other than lymphatic or myelocytic origin. On the other side of the spectrum, eosinophilic granuloma is certainly benign in its clinical characteristics and resembles an inflammatory process more than a neoplasm. Hand-Schüller-Christian disease is believed by some investigators to be a multifocal variety of eosinophilic granuloma. The precise cause and pathogenesis of Langerhans cell histiocytosis remain unclear, however. Evidence exists that the disorder is a manifestation of or is associated with immunologic aberrations.

### Eosinophilic Granuloma

Eosinophilic granuloma is characterized by single or multiple skeletal lesions occurring predominantly in children, adolescents, or young adults, but occasionally in older persons. It represents approximately 70% of the total number of cases of Langerhans cell histiocytosis; it is more common in men than in women and in whites than in blacks. Clinical manifestations include local pain, tenderness, and swelling related to adjacent skeletal lesions. Fever and leukocytosis may also be apparent.

Solitary lesions are more common than multiple lesions, although it has been estimated that multifocal osseous (and extraosseous) disease eventually develops in about 10% of patients with solitary lesions. In general, new skeletal lesions occur within 1 or 2 years after the initial solitary lesion is identified. The most common sites of involvement are the skull, mandible, spine, ribs, pelvis, and long bones, particularly the femur and humerus. In older patients, changes in the flat bones are more common than changes in the tubular bones. Spinal involvement predominates in the thoracic and lumbar regions. Vertebral body localization is most typical. Involvement of the sternum and clavicles is also encountered. Epiphyseal lesions may occur in children, and these lesions may cross the open physeal plate.

The radiographic characteristics of eosinophilic granuloma vary with its skeletal location. In long and short tubular bones, the lesions appear as relatively well defined radiolucent areas, particularly in the medullary cavity (Fig. 50–11). With further growth, they encroach on the cortical bone, with endosteal erosion of the cortex and periosteal new bone formation. The appearance can simulate that of osteomyelitis or malignant neoplasm,

such as Ewing's sarcoma and lymphoma. In the ribs, single or multiple lesions can lead to pathologic fractures (Fig. 50–12). In the skull and pelvis, the lytic areas may be particularly well defined, with or without surrounding sclerosis. A radiodense focus within a lytic cranial lesion (or, rarely, in another location) has been termed a "button" sequestrum (Fig. 50–13). Skull lesions are especially prevalent in the frontal and parietal bones. Nonuniform growth of the lesion leads to beveled bone margins and unequal destruction of the inner and outer tables of the vault (Fig. 50–14). Flat bone lesions may demonstrate a "hole within a hole" appearance (Fig. 50–15). In the mandible, radiolucent lesions about the teeth may lead to loss of supporting bone and a "floating teeth" appearance.

Vertebral destruction can lead to a flattened vertebral body, termed vertebra plana, a finding that is much more frequent in children than in adults (Fig. 50–16). Thoracic and lumbar spine involvement predominates. The height of the intervening intervertebral disc is usually normal. A paraspinal mass may be evident, simulating a soft tissue abscess related to vertebral osteomyelitis. Rarely, neurologic manifestations ensue.

### Hand-Schüller-Christian Disease

The classic triad of Hand-Schüller-Christian disease is diabetes insipidus, unilateral or bilateral exophthalmos, and single or multiple areas of bone destruction. The finding of diabetes insipidus is attributable to extensive

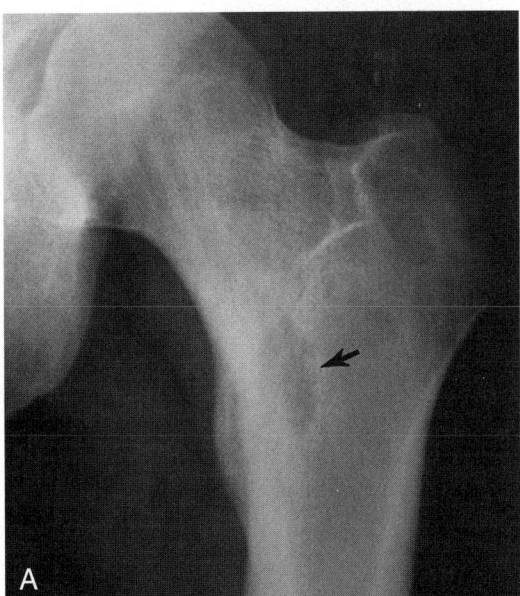
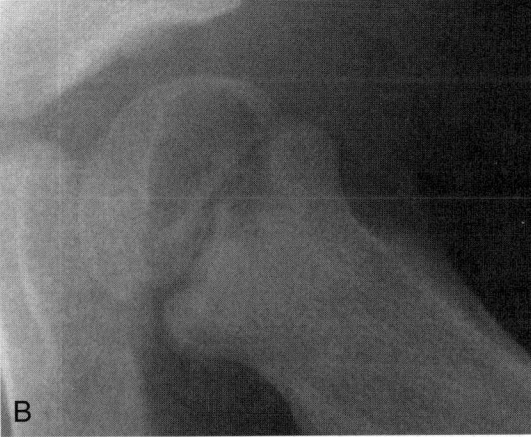

**Figure 50–11.** Eosinophilic granuloma: radiographic abnormalities in the tubular bones of the appendicular skeleton. *A,* In this 33-year-old man, thigh pain developed that was worse at night and relieved by aspirin. Radiograph reveals an eccentric osteolytic lesion *(arrow)* with a sharp zone of transition between the abnormal and normal bone. Biopsy confirmed the presence of an eosinophilic granuloma. *B,* In another patient, a lesion has violated the growth plate, with involvement of both the epiphysis and the metaphysis. (*A,* Courtesy of P. Ellenbogen, MD, Dallas, Tex. *B,* Courtesy of M. Murphey, MD, Washington, D.C.)

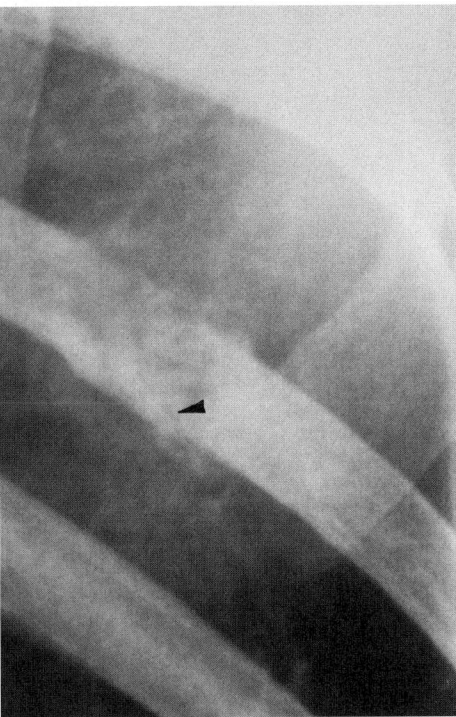

**Figure 50–12.** Eosinophilic granuloma: radiographic abnormalities in the ribs. This 44-year-old woman had pleuritic chest pain of 1 month's duration. Radiograph reveals a poorly defined osteolytic lesion. A pathologic fracture *(arrowhead)* extends across the lesion. An eosinophilic granuloma was found on examination of the resected rib. (Courtesy of G. Greenway, MD, Dallas, Tex.)

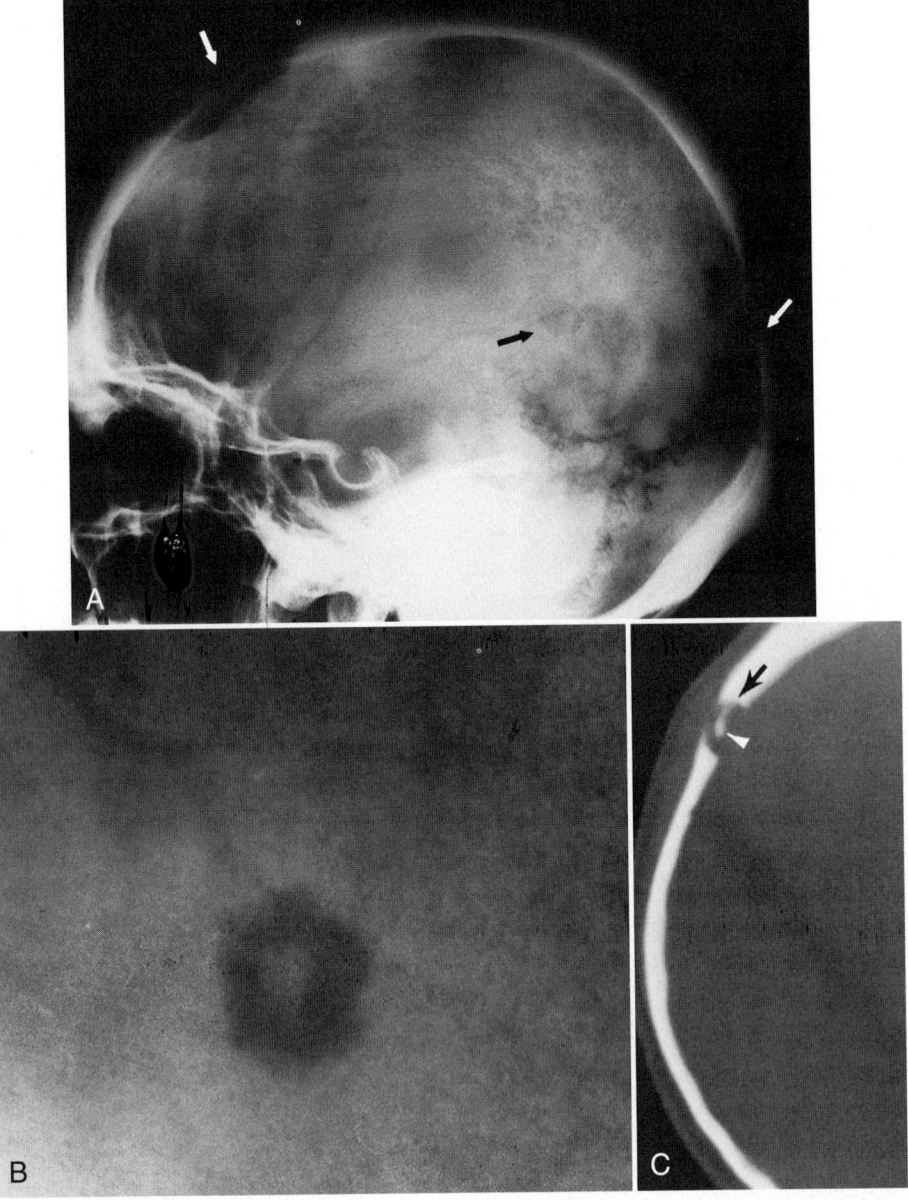

**Figure 50–13.** Eosinophilic granuloma: radiographic abnormalities in the skull. *A*, Widespread lytic lesions of variable size are observed *(arrows)*. Most of them are sharply defined. *B*, Lytic lesion with a central radiodense area, the "button" sequestrum. *C*, Computed tomography scan of the skull in a different patient shows an osteolytic lesion *(arrow)* with a radiodense center representing the "button" sequestrum *(arrowhead)*. Note adjacent soft tissue prominence.

destruction of bone at the base of the skull and is not universally present in this disease. In fact, the classic triad may be apparent in less than 10% of patients. Hand-Schüller-Christian disease predominates in children (approximately two thirds of patients are younger than 5 years at the initial clinical examination).

Clinical characteristics are otitis media; cutaneous involvement consisting of eczema, xanthomatosis, and soft tissue nodules; ulceration of the gums; lymphadenopathy; and hepatosplenomegaly. Visceral involvement of the lungs, kidneys, brain, liver, and spleen is observed. Anemia, when present, is a grave prognostic sign. In

general, the disease runs a protracted course, sometimes extending over a period of 10 to 20 years.

The skeletal lesions of Hand-Schüller-Christian disease may be widely disseminated (Fig. 50–17). The radiographic manifestations of individual lesions are similar to those of eosinophilic granuloma. In the skull, which is involved in more than 90% of patients, confluent areas of destruction may isolate islands of bone and create a geographic, or maplike, skull. With mandibular involvement, osteolytic lesions can surround the teeth, giving a "floating teeth" appearance. A diagnosis of Hand-Schüller-Christian disease or a related

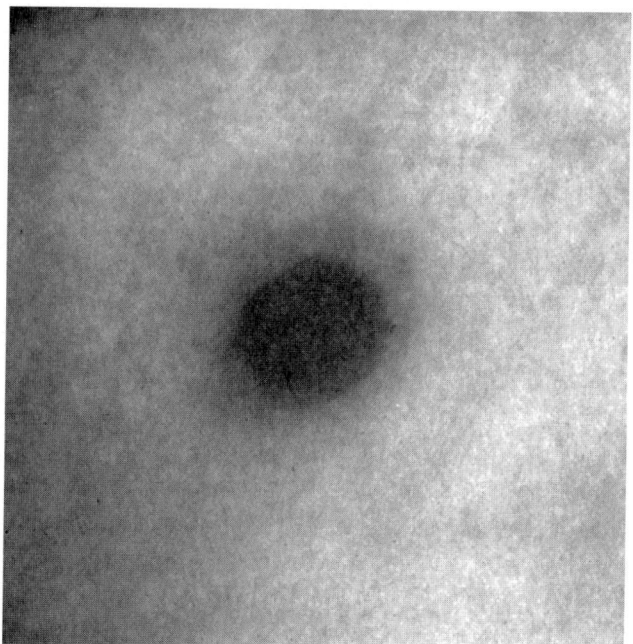

**Figure 50–14.** Eosinophilic granuloma: radiographic abnormalities. Unequal involvement of the tables of the skull gives the margins of the lesion a "beveled edge" appearance.

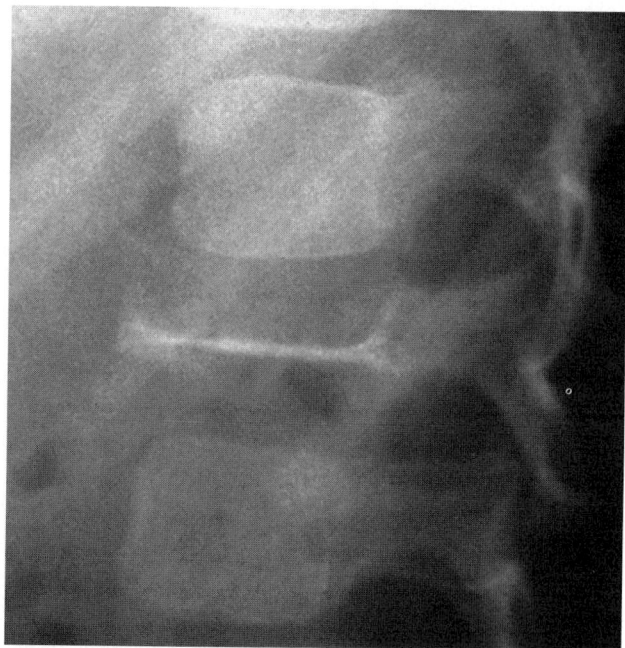

**Figure 50–16.** Eosinophilic granuloma: vertebra plana. Observe the flattened vertebral body with preserved adjacent disc spaces.

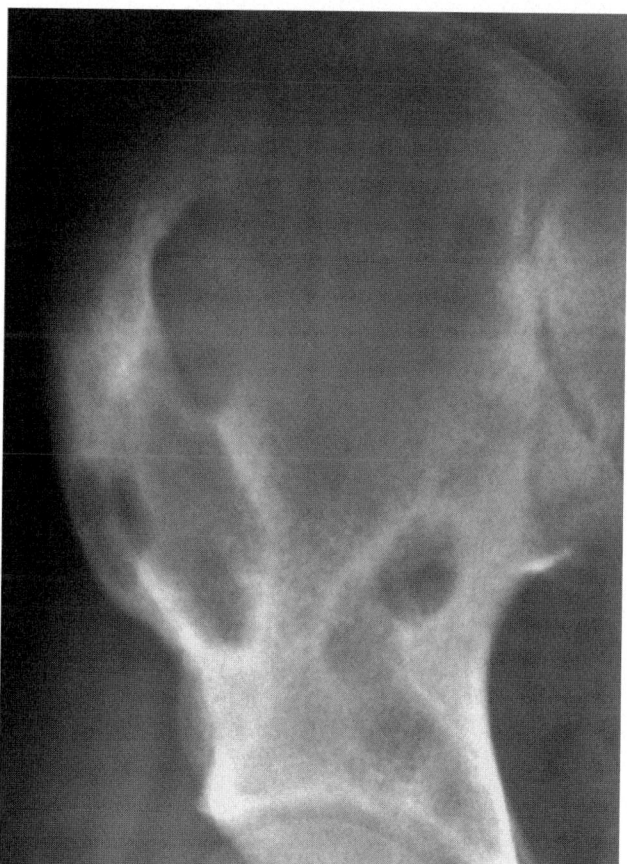

**Figure 50–15.** Eosinophilic granuloma: radiographic abnormalities. Confluence of flat bone lesions gives a characteristic "hole within a hole" appearance.

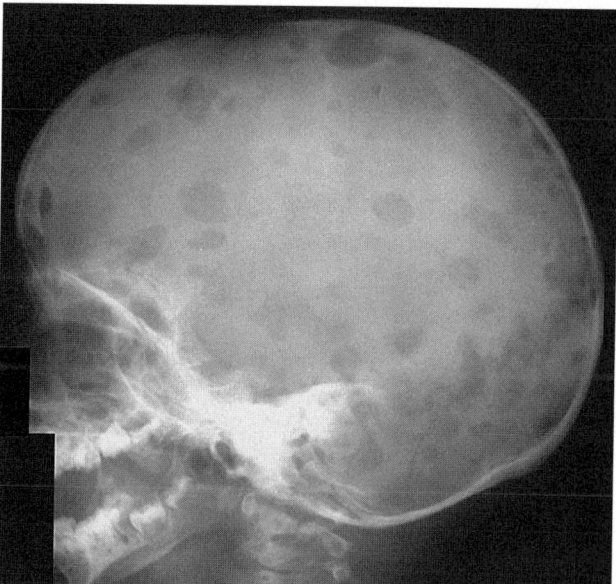

**Figure 50–17.** Hand-Schüller-Christian disease: radiographic abnormalities in the skull. Multiple well-defined lytic lesions are apparent, some of which have beveled margins.

histiocytosis should be considered in any infant or child with osteolytic lesions of the pelvis or skull.

The outcome in cases of Hand-Schüller-Christian disease is variable. In some instances, the bone lesions resolve gradually. In other instances, the bone lesions progress; in fact, cases with initial involvement identical to that of eosinophilic granuloma may be associated with increased osseous dissemination and visceral complications. The prognosis worsens with involvement of multiple organ systems, and the disease is fatal in 10% to 30% of cases.

## Letterer-Siwe Disease

Letterer-Siwe disease is a relatively acute syndrome that is most frequent in children younger than 3 years, although occasional cases are encountered in late childhood or young adulthood. This disorder is characterized by histiocytic proliferation in multiple visceral organs. It accounts for approximately 10% of all cases of Langerhans cell histiocytosis.

Clinical manifestations include febrile episodes, cachexia, hepatosplenomegaly, lymphadenopathy, purpuric skin eruption, hyperplasia of the gums, and progressive anemia. The course is generally rapidly progressive; most patients die within 1 or 2 years, although occasionally a more prolonged clinical course, with features of Hand-Schüller-Christian disease, develops.

Single or multiple areas of bone destruction are observed, particularly in the calvaria, base of the skull, and mandible. More diffuse skeletal involvement can be encountered, although the hands and feet are usually spared. During treatment, extensive bone sclerosis may be observed. Histologically and radiographically, the bone lesions simulate those in eosinophilic granuloma. Osteolytic lesions, which are relatively well defined and lack significant surrounding bony eburnation, represent sites of histiocytic proliferation.

## Disease Prognosis and Evolution of Osseous Abnormalities

In general, the prognosis of any of the types of histiocytosis is related to the location and extent of organ involvement, so the clinical, radiographic, and laboratory evaluation must include an examination of all potential target areas of disease. The greater the number of tissues or systems affected, the poorer the prognosis. Patients with polyostotic disease tend to fare worse than those with monostotic disease and are more likely to have visceral involvement. The prognosis of the histiocytoses is also related to the age of the patient at the onset of clinical abnormalities; generally, the younger the patient, the poorer the prognosis.

Healing of skeletal lesions, whether initiated through aggressive intervention or complete neglect, is accompanied by characteristic radiographic changes. Bone sclerosis typically develops in osteolytic lesions in extraspinal locations during resolution, and the lesions may divide into smaller isolated areas as a result of septation. Additional findings at these sites during the healing process include periosteal reaction, cortical thickening, and pathologic fracture, and the changes may resemble those of Paget's disease. Because sclerosis appears to represent the hallmark of the healing response, its appearance in the form of a partial or complete rim of increased radiodensity or patchy or diffuse bone reaction in untreated lesions may indicate spontaneous resolution and should be regarded as a favorable prognostic sign. Conversely, enlargement of foci of osseous destruction or the appearance of new areas of lysis is indicative of an unfavorable prognosis. The typical healing response of spinal lesions that have produced vertebra plana is partial reconstitution of vertebral height. The degree of recovery of vertebral body height is potentially greater when the patient is young.

Intralesional injection of methylprednisolone sodium succinate after bone biopsy has become a popular method of treatment of the histiocytoses. Progressive healing of the osseous lesions generally becomes detectable radiographically after 2 to 4 months, as evidenced by a decrease in size, sclerosis of marginal bone, and increasing trabeculation. Clinical improvement, manifested as diminution of pain, accompanies the radiographic changes. The mechanism of action of the corticosteroid preparation after intralesional administration is not clear, and the possibility that the lesions will resolve spontaneously or after biopsy alone complicates the interpretation of the benefits of such a therapeutic procedure.

## Scintigraphy

In general, in the evaluation of patients with Langerhans cell histiocytosis, bone scintigraphy has proved to be less sensitive than radiography in the detection of osseous lesions, with falsely negative radionuclide studies commonly reported. The purely lytic nature of the lesions is cited by some investigators as the reason for the disappointing results of bone scintigraphy. When bone scan findings are present, osseous lesions in histiocytosis demonstrate a spectrum of radionuclide abnormalities, ranging from "cold" areas with decreased or absent accumulation of the radionuclide to areas of augmented activity.

## Magnetic Resonance Imaging

Spin echo imaging of the skeleton in patients with histiocytosis reveals one or more foci of decreased signal intensity on T1-weighted images and increased signal intensity on T2-weighted images (Fig. 50–18). Lesion enhancement after the intravenous injection of a gadolinium contrast agent may be seen. The MR imaging abnormalities of the musculoskeletal system in Langerhans cell histiocytosis include features that simulate those of aggressive tumors and infection. Cortical perforation, periostitis, and soft tissue extension are known radiographic manifestations of eosinophilic granuloma and the other histiocytoses. The large size, poor definition, and signal inhomogeneity of the soft tissue component accompanying skeletal involvement in the histiocytoses must be emphasized.

The value of MR imaging of the musculoskeletal system in patients with Langerhans cell histiocytosis lies in its sensitivity rather than specificity. Although MR imaging is not a practical screening method for skeletal involvement in these diseases, its usefulness in defining the extent of involvement at one or a few skeletal sites, such as the spine, has been established. Problems exist, however, even in this regard, because it is difficult to determine the degree of cortical violation (a task better accomplished with computed tomography) and to distinguish between histiocytic tissue and surrounding edema.

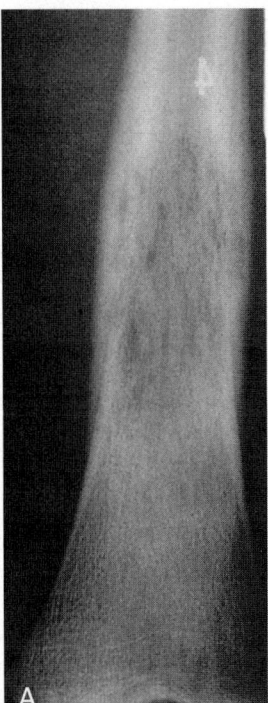

**Figure 50–18.** Eosinophilic granuloma: MR imaging abnormalities in the femur. This 4-year-old girl experienced pain and swelling in the thigh. *A*, Routine radiograph shows an osteolytic lesion with moth-eaten bone destruction and thick periosteal reaction in the diaphysis of the femur. *B*, Coronal T1-weighted (TR/TE, 500/20) spin echo MR image reveals low signal intensity in the diaphyseal and distal metaphyseal portions of the femur. Periosteal new bone also exhibits low signal intensity. *C*, With T2 weighting (TR/TE, 2000/90), the femoral lesion is inhomogeneous but generally of high signal intensity. Note the elevated periosteum with new bone formation and the irregular and extensive soft tissue component with very high signal intensity. Differentiation of the lesion itself and adjacent edema is impossible. (Courtesy of M. Pathria, MD, San Diego, Calif.)

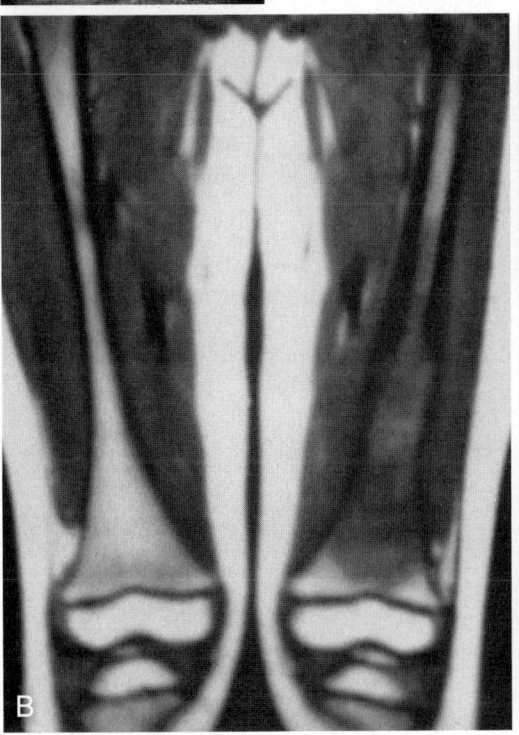

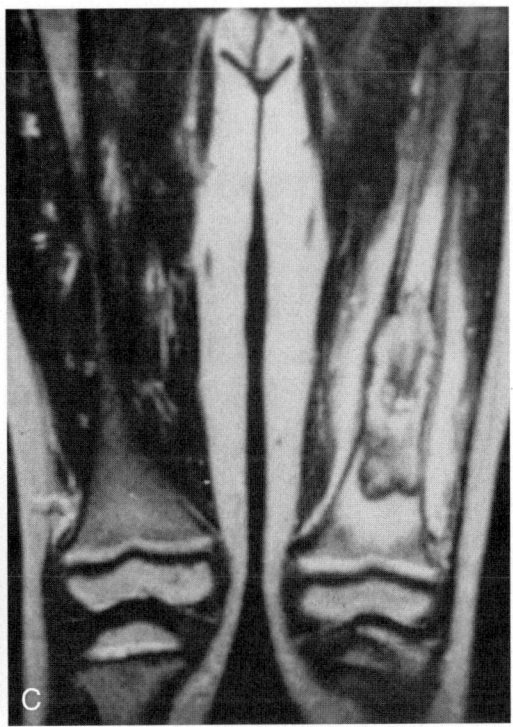

## Differential Diagnosis

The predominant pattern of the histiocytoses is osteolysis. Osteolytic lesions may be single or multiple. Single lytic defects must be differentiated from neoplastic and inflammatory lesions, as well as fibrous dysplasia. Multiple lytic lesions may simulate infection, skeletal metastasis, leukemia, lymphoma, hyperparathyroidism with brown tumors, and Gaucher's disease.

## LIPID GRANULOMATOSIS (ERDHEIM-CHESTER DISEASE)

Lipid granulomatosis is a distinctive and unusual lipidosis. The clinical manifestations are not well defined, although men and women in the fifth through seventh decades of life appear to be affected. Cardiac and pulmonary manifestations are caused by liberation of cholesterol from foam cells, and xanthomatous patches in the eyelids may

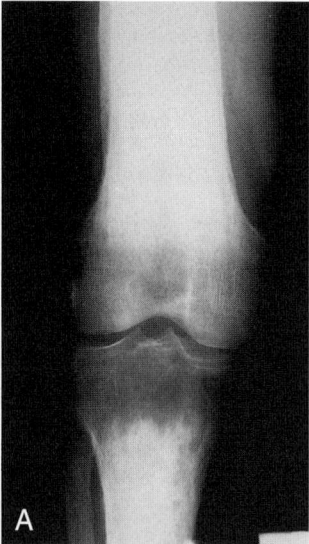

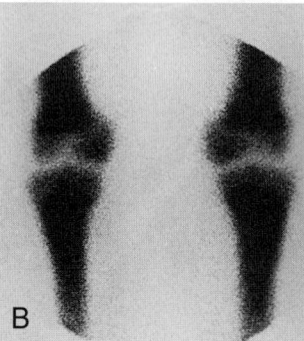

**Figure 50–19.** Erdheim-Chester disease. *A,* Sclerotic lesions of the distal femur and proximal tibia. The epiphyses are spared, and the opposite side was similarly involved. *B,* Radionuclide studies reveal increased uptake of bone-seeking agents. (Courtesy of G. Greenway, MD, Dallas, Tex.)

be seen. Mild local pain and tenderness over areas of skeletal abnormality are noted, although patients may be entirely asymptomatic.

Radiographic abnormalities are distinctive (Fig. 50–19). The major long bones of the limbs are invariably affected, whereas axial skeletal involvement, which has been documented in the skull, ribs, and innominate bone, is unusual. A patchy or diffuse increase in density, a coarsened trabecular pattern, medullary sclerosis, and cortical thickening appear in the diaphysis and metaphysis, with minor changes or sparing of the epiphysis. Symmetry is the rule. Radionuclide studies using bone-seeking radiopharmaceutical agents demonstrate increased accumulation of isotope in areas of radiographic abnormality. Although data regarding the MR imaging findings in this disease are limited, replacement of normal marrow fat by lipid infiltration has been accompanied by a decrease in signal intensity on T1-weighted spin echo MR images and regions of low and high signal intensity on T2-weighted images. Inhomogeneous enhancement of areas of marrow involvement, with nonenhancing cystic components, is seen following intravenous gadolinium administration. Periosseous soft tissue masses are also detected with MR imaging.

Pathologic findings show that spongiosa is replaced by sclerotic bone, especially in the metaphyseal regions. The pathologic aberrations in bone most resemble those of Hand-Schüller-Christian disease. The precise relationship of Erdheim-Chester disease to the histiocytoses is not known.

## SINUS HISTIOCYTOSIS WITH LYMPHADENOPATHY

Sinus histiocytosis with massive lymphadenopathy, or Rosai-Dorfman disease, is a non-neoplastic, self-limited disease occurring predominantly in the first 3 decades of life, especially in black patients. It is characterized by painless bilateral cervical adenopathy, adenopathy in other lymph node chains, fever, an elevated erythrocyte sedimentation rate, neutrophilic leukocytosis, occasional eosinophilia, and hypergammaglobulinemia. Involved lymph nodes reveal distinctive microscopic abnormalities, including a marked proliferation of sinus histiocytes, which often contain phagocytized lymphocytes. Extranodal sites of involvement include the upper respiratory tract, salivary glands, orbits, eyelids, testes, and bone.

Osseous manifestations of this disease, which may rarely occur without lymphadenopathy, are generally restricted to multiple or, less frequently, solitary osteolytic lesions (Fig. 50–20) principally involving the long tubular bones but also the skull, pelvis, sternum, vertebral bodies, phalanges, metacarpals, and ribs. The lesions are usually asymptomatic, although spinal involvement may be associated with paresis. The epiphysis, diaphysis, and metaphysis are affected singly or in any combination. Of variable size, the lesions are usually medullary in location, but an occasional cortical focus is encountered. Intralesional calcification and periostitis are absent. Surrounding sclerosis is sometimes apparent. Radionuclide and MR imaging features are not specific. Serial radiographs may reveal a continual decrease in the size of the lytic defects, with eventual complete disappearance.

## HYPERLIPOPROTEINEMIAS

### General Features

The primary familial hyperlipoproteinemias are a group of heritable diseases associated with an increase in the plasma concentration of cholesterol or triglycerides. These disorders result from defects that occur in the various regulatory steps of lipoprotein metabolism. Currently, these diseases are divided into five major types, according to the plasma lipoprotein (Table 50–6).

**Type I.** Primary type I hyperlipoproteinemia is related to a hereditary (autosomal recessive) abnormality in chylomicron removal characterized by deficient plasma postheparin lipoprotein lipase activity. Massive amounts of chylomicrons are apparent while the patient is ingesting a normal diet and disappear within a few days after commencing a fat-free diet. Type I hyperlipoproteinemia may occur in a secondary form in diabetes mellitus, pancreatitis, and alcoholism. Primary type I hyperlipoproteinemia is diagnosed in most patients in the first or second decade of life. Clinical findings include lipemia retinalis, hepatosplenomegaly, abdominal pain, and pancreatitis.

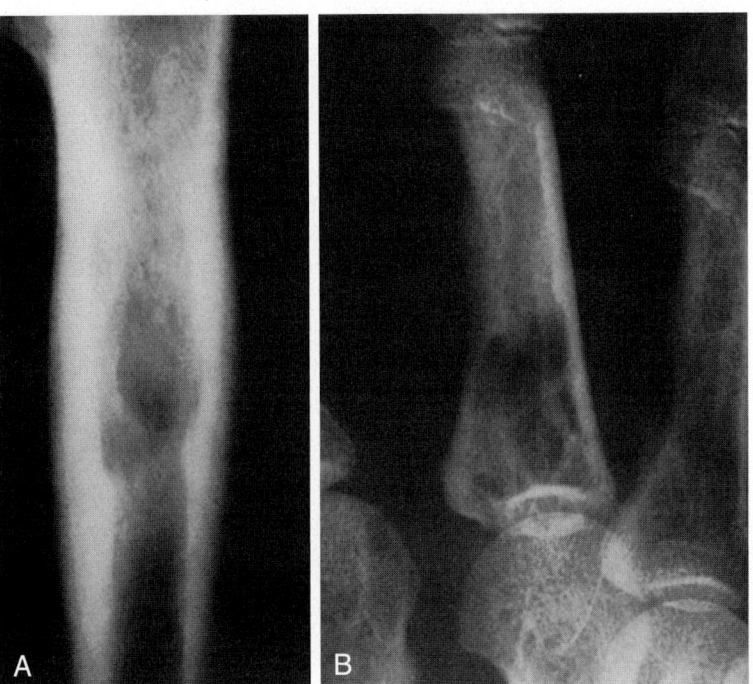

**Figure 50–20.** Sinus histiocytosis with lymphadenopathy. Osteolytic foci are apparent in the femur *(A)* and small tubular bones of the hand *(B)*. (Courtesy of D. Sartoris, MD, San Diego, Calif.)

**TABLE 50–6**

**Hyperlipoproteinemias**

| Type | Lipoprotein Abnormality | Primary Form | Secondary Forms | Xanthomas | Arthralgia or Arthritis | Hyper-uricemia |
|------|------------------------|--------------|-----------------|-----------|------------------------|----------------|
| I | Chylomicrons | Autosomal recessive | Diabetes mellitus<br>Pancreatitis<br>Alcoholism | Skin | | |
| II | Beta lipoprotein | Autosomal dominant | Hypothyroidism<br>Myeloma<br>Macroglobulinemia<br>Obstructive hepatic disease | Skin<br>Tendinous<br>Tuberous<br>Subperiosteal | + | |
| III | Beta or pre-beta lipoprotein | Autosomal recessive (?) | Diabetes mellitus<br>Hypothyroidism | Skin<br>Tendinous<br>Tuberous<br>Subperiosteal | | + |
| IV | Pre-beta lipoprotein | Autosomal recessive | Diabetes mellitus<br>Pancreatitis<br>Alcoholism<br>Hypothyroidism<br>Glycogen storage disease<br>Gaucher's disease<br>Gout<br>Hypercalcemia | Skin<br>Tuberous<br>Intraosseous | + | + |
| V | Pre-beta lipoprotein, chylomicrons | Autosomal dominant (?) | | Skin | | + |

**Type II (Familial Hypercholesterolemia).** Type II, the most common type, is related to an increase in the plasma concentration of low-density lipoproteins or beta lipoproteins. Type II is further divided into two subgroups: types IIA and IIB. The former is characterized by an excess of beta lipoproteins, and the latter by an excess of both beta and pre-beta lipoproteins. In its primary form, type II hyperlipoproteinemia is an autosomal dominant hereditary abnormality. It may also be secondary to many disorders, including hypothyroidism, plasma cell myeloma, macroglobulinemia, and obstructive liver disease. The diagnosis of primary type II hyperlipoproteinemia is usually established in early childhood. Findings include xanthomas and premature coronary, cerebral, and peripheral vascular disease.

**Type III ("Broad-Beta" Disease).** Type III, an uncommon type, is associated with beta or pre-beta lipoprotein abnormality. In its primary form, type III hyperlipoproteinemia may be an autosomal recessive disorder. Rarely, it is secondary to severe insulinopenic diabetes and hypothyroidism. Primary type III hyperlipoproteinemia may not be detected until the third, fourth, or fifth decade of life, or even later. It is rarely observed in patients younger than 25 years. Xanthomas and premature peripheral vascular disease are apparent.

**Type IV.** Type IV is characterized by the presence of increased low-density lipoproteins or pre-beta lipoproteins without chylomicronemia. In its primary form, the disease appears to be an autosomal recessive disorder. Type IV hyperlipoproteinemia may be secondary to many diseases, including diabetes mellitus, pancreatitis, alcoholism, hypothyroidism, glycogen storage disease, Gaucher's disease, gout, and hypercalcemia. In its primary form, the disease is rarely detected in those younger than 20 years. Xanthomas, hyperuricemia, and coronary vascular disease may be evident.

**Type V.** Type V is similar to type IV, with an increase in low-density lipoproteins and chylomicrons. In its primary form, it is probably an autosomal dominant hereditary disease that is rarely clinically manifested in childhood. Xanthomas, hyperuricemia, abdominal pain, hepatosplenomegaly, paresthesias, and lipemia retinalis may be detected.

## Musculoskeletal Abnormalities

### Xanthoma

Xanthomas may be apparent in all five types of hyperlipoproteinemia and in primary and secondary forms of the disease. Xanthomas can be classified as eruptive, tendinous, tuberous, or subperiosteal and osseous.

**Eruptive Xanthomas.** Yellow papules containing triglycerides, with surrounding erythema, occur on the knees, buttocks, back, and shoulders.

**Tendinous Xanthomas.** Localized deposits occur in the tendons of the palm and dorsum of the hand, patellar tendon, Achilles tendon, plantar aponeurosis, and peroneal tendons; deposits may also appear around the elbow and in the fascia and periosteum overlying the lower part of the tibia. These deposits are situated within the tendon fibers and not on the tendon sheath.

**Tuberous Xanthomas.** Soft subcutaneous masses occur over extensor surfaces, including the elbows, knees, and hands, as well as the buttocks.

**Subperiosteal and Osseous Xanthomas.** Lipid deposits occur beneath the periosteum or replace trabeculae within the spongiosa and lead to osteolytic defects, periosteal or

endosteal erosion of the cortex, and even pathologic fracture or osteonecrosis from vascular occlusion.

In type I hyperlipoproteinemia, xanthomas are of the eruptive type; they may appear at times of severe hyperlipidemia and disappear when the triglyceride level is reduced with a low-fat intake.

In type II hyperlipoproteinemia, xanthomas may occur in as many as 80% of patients before death. In persons who are homozygous with respect to the abnormal gene, xanthomatosis occurs in childhood and may be extensive. In heterozygotes, tendinous xanthomas do not usually appear until age 30 years. In type III hyperlipoproteinemia, tuberous, tendinous, and subperiosteal xanthomas may occur. In addition, lipid deposition (planar xanthoma) may produce yellowish elevation on the palmar surface of the hands and fingers, a distinctive clinical manifestation that may also be seen in homozygous type II and possibly type IV hyperlipoproteinemia. The frequency of planar xanthomas in type III patients may reach 65% to 70%.

Tuberous and tendinous xanthomas produce nodular masses in soft tissue and tendons (Fig. 50–21). These rarely calcify. Subtle thickening of the tendon may be the only radiographic abnormality. Subperiosteal xanthomas are associated with scalloping of the external cortical surface. Intramedullary lipid deposition leads to lytic defects, endosteal erosion, subchondral collapse, juxta-articular erosive changes, and pathologic fractures (Fig. 50–22). In general, the osseous defects are well defined, with a sharp zone of transition between abnormal and normal bone.

The diagnosis of soft tissue xanthomas, particularly those of the Achilles tendon, can be accomplished with ultrasonography and MR imaging. With ultrasonography, xanthomas appear as focal or confluent hypoechoic regions.

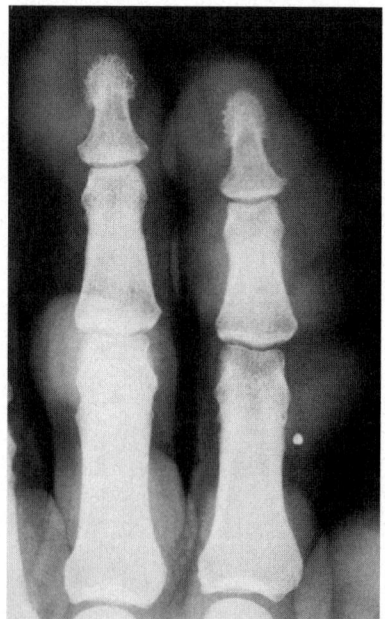

**Figure 50–21.** Hyperlipoproteinemia: xanthomas without osseous abnormalities. Radiograph reveals asymmetrical soft tissue masses in periarticular and periosseous locations. Neither soft tissue calcification nor significant osseous erosions are present.

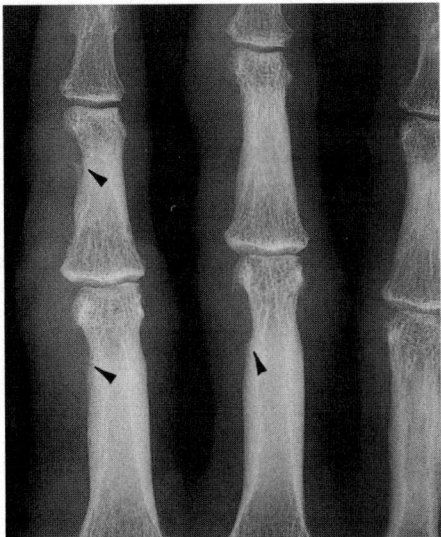

**Figure 50–22.** Hyperlipoproteinemia: xanthomas with bony abnormalities. Observe the nodular soft tissue masses with subjacent osseous erosion *(arrowheads)*. The osseous defects are eccentric and well defined. Osteoporosis and joint space narrowing are not apparent.

The signal intensity of xanthomas on MR images is variable, depending in part on the chemical constituents of the lesions. In vitro studies have documented that triglycerides may lead to high signal intensity on some MR imaging sequences, whereas cholesterols do not. Most reports of the MR imaging features of such lesions have documented persistently low to intermediate signal intensity on T1- and T2-weighted spin echo MR images and signal inhomogeneity (Fig. 50–23).

## Gout

Hyperuricemia and clinical gout have been reported in association with types III, IV, and V hyperlipoproteinemia, but not with type I or II.

## Arthralgias and Arthritis

In type II hyperlipoproteinemia, a migratory polyarthritis affecting large and small peripheral joints may be detected. Involved sites include the ankles, knees, hips, elbows, wrists, and, rarely, hands. Tendinous xanthomas are commonly apparent, and these tumors may produce concomitant mechanical defects or tendinosis. Symptoms and signs may migrate from one joint to another, similar to the findings in rheumatic fever. Soft tissue swelling may be observed on radiographs of involved joints. Arthralgias may occur in patients with type IV hyperlipoproteinemia. Joint pain, tenderness, and stiffness may be evident, but synovitis is not detectable.

## Cerebrotendinous Xanthomatosis

Cerebrotendinous xanthomatosis, a xanthomatous disorders without hyperlipidemia, is a rare disease characterized by xanthomas, cataracts, progressive cerebellar ataxia, and dementia. Accumulation of cholesterol and

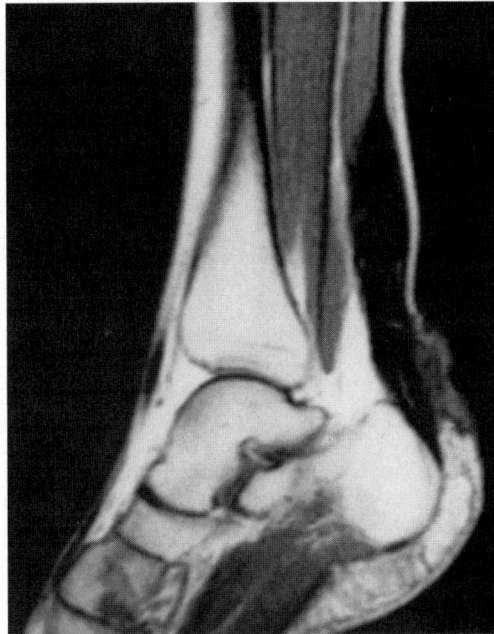

**Figure 50–23.** Hyperlipoproteinemia: xanthomas. Sagittal T1-weighted (TR/TE, 550/30) spin echo MR image shows a thickened and irregular Achilles tendon of low signal intensity. (From Liem MSL, Leuven JAG, Bloem JL, et al: Magnetic resonance imaging of Achilles tendon xanthomas in familial hypercholesterolemia. Skeletal Radiol 21:453, 1992.)

cholesterol-like crystals occurs in the white matter of the brain and in xanthomas. Cerebrotendinous xanthomatosis is an autosomal recessive disorder whose biochemical basis is not entirely known. Disability is progressive, although patients may survive until the sixth or seventh decade of life. Tendinous xanthomas are most frequent in the Achilles tendon but may also involve the triceps tendon, extensor tendons of the fingers, and tibial tuberosities.

## Differential Diagnosis

One radiographic characteristic of the hyperlipoproteinemias, consisting of eccentric masses without calcification, can be simulated by changes in other diseases, particularly gouty arthritis. This similarity is accentuated by localization of the masses to periarticular soft tissues, tendons, and subperiosteal and osseous areas; by the adjacent bone lysis; and by the simultaneous occurrence of both hyperlipidemia and hyperuricemia. Secondary gout may complicate hyperlipidemia and may be accentuated by lipid-lowering agents. The osseous erosions in both disorders share common features, including well-defined margins, eccentricity, and intra- and extra-articular distribution. Similar joints are involved. The soft tissue swelling of gout may contain radiographically evident calcification, a finding that is not characteristic of xanthoma. The erosions in hyperlipoproteinemia may also resemble the defects in multicentric reticulohistiocytosis, although large soft tissue masses are not characteristic of the latter disorder.

The subperiosteal xanthomas in the hyperlipoproteinemias produce subjacent bone erosion.

# FURTHER READING

Barrow MV, Holubar K: Multicentric reticulohistiocytosis: A review of 33 patients. Medicine 48:287, 1969.

Carranza-Bencano A, Fernadez-Centeno M, Leal-Cerro A, et al: Xanthomas of the Achilles tendon: Report of a bilateral case and review of the literature. Foot Ankle 20:314, 1999.

Cohen M, Zornoza J, Cangir A, et al: Direct injection of methylprednisolone sodium succinate in the treatment of solitary eosinophilic granuloma of bone: Report of 9 cases. Radiology 136:289, 1980.

David R, Oria RA, Kumar R, et al: Radiologic features of eosinophilic granuloma of bone. AJR Am J Roentgenol 153:1021, 1989.

Dee P, Westgaard T, Langholm R: Erdheim-Chester disease: Case with chronic discharging sinus from bone. AJR Am J Roentgenol 134:837, 1980.

Dunnick NR, Parker BR, Warnke RA, et al: Radiographic manifestations of malignant histiocytosis. AJR Am J Roentgenol 127:611, 1976.

Gold RH, Metzger AL, Mirra JM, et al: Multicentric reticulohistiocytosis (lipoid dermatoarthritis): An erosive polyarthritis with distinctive clinical, roentgenographic, and pathologic features. AJR Am J Roentgenol 124:610, 1975.

Greenfield GB: Bone changes in chronic adult Gaucher's disease. AJR Am J Roentgenol 110:800, 1970.

Hasegawa Y, Inagaki Y: Membranous lipodystrophy (lipomembranous polycystic osteodysplasia): Two case reports. Clin Orthop 181:229, 1983.

Jaffe HL: Metabolic, Degenerative and Inflammatory Diseases of Bones and Joints. Philadelphia, Lea & Febiger, 1972, p 506.

Jaffe HL, Lichtenstein L: Eosinophilic granuloma of bone: A condition affecting one, several or many bones, but apparently limited to the skeleton and representing the mildest clinical expression of the peculiar inflammatory histiocytosis also underlying Letterer-Siwe disease and Schüller-Christian disease. Arch Pathol 37:99, 1944.

Kaye JJ, Freiberger RH: Eosinophilic granuloma of the spine without vertebra plana: A report of two unusual cases. Radiology 92:1188, 1969.

Kushihashi T, Munechika H, Sekimuzu M, et al: Erdheim-Chester disease involving bilateral lower extremities: MR features. AJR Am J Roentgenol 174:875, 2000.

Lachman R, Crocker A, Schulman J, et al: Radiological findings in Niemann-Pick disease. Radiology 108:659, 1973.

Levin B: Gaucher's disease. Clinical and roentgenologic manifestations. AJR Am J Roentgenol 85:685, 1961.

Lichtenstein L: Histiocytosis X: Integration of eosinophilic granuloma of bone, "Letterer-Siwe disease" and "Schüller-Christian" disease as related manifestations of a single nosologic entity. Arch Pathol 56:84, 1953.

Liem MSL, Leuven JAG, Bloem JL, et al: Magnetic resonance imaging of Achilles tendon xanthomas in familial hypercholesterolemia. Skeletal Radiol 21:453, 1992.

Owman T, Sjoblad ST, Gothlin J: Radiographic skeletal changes in juvenile GM$_1$-gangliosidosis. ROFO Fortschr Geb Rontgenstr Nuklearmed 132:682, 1980.

Pastershank SP, Yip S, Sodhi HS: Cerebrotendinous xanthomatosis. J Can Assoc Radiol 25:282, 1974.

Ponseti I: Bone lesions in eosinophilic granuloma, Hand-Schüller-Christian disease, and Letterer-Siwe disease. J Bone Joint Surg Am 30:811, 1948.

Puczynski MS, Demos TC, Suarez CR: Sinus histiocytosis with massive lymphadenopathy: Skeletal involvement. Pediatr Radiol 15:259, 1985.

Resnick D, Greenway G, Genant H, et al: Erdheim-Chester disease. Radiology 142:289, 1982.

Rosai J, Dorfman RF: Sinus histiocytosis with massive lymphadenopathy: A newly recognized benign clinicopathological entity. Arch Pathol 87:63, 1969.

Rosenthal DI, Mayo-Smith W, Goodsitt MM, et al: Bone and bone marrow changes in Gaucher disease: Evaluation with quantitative CT. Radiology 170:143, 1989.

Siegelman SS, Schlossberg I, Becker NH, et al: Hyperlipoproteinemia with skeletal lesions. Clin Orthop 87:228, 1972.

Sistermann R, Katthagen B-D: Erdheim Chester disease: A rare cause of knee and leg pain. Arch Orthop Trauma Surg 120:112, 2000.

Sundaram M, deMello D, Falbo S, et al: Sinus histiocytosis with massive lymphadenopathy (Rosai-Dorfman disease) presenting with skeletal lesions. Skeletal Radiol 27:115, 1998.

Waite RJ, Doherty PW, Liepman M, et al: Langerhans cell histiocytosis with the radiographic findings of Erdheim-Chester disease. AJR Am J Roentgenol 150:869, 1988.

Warnke RA, Kim H, Dorfman RF: Malignant histiocytosis (histiocytic medullary reticulosis). I. Clinicopathologic study of 29 cases. Cancer 35:215, 1975.

# CHAPTER 51

## Lymphoproliferative and Myeloproliferative Disorders

### Donald Resnick and Parviz Haghighi

## SUMMARY OF KEY FEATURES

Musculoskeletal abnormalities accompany a variety of myeloproliferative disorders. In leukemias, such abnormalities are particularly frequent in children. Osseous involvement from the primary disease leads to local symptoms and signs. Synovial involvement from leukemic infiltration and hemorrhage can result in articular findings. Hyperuricemia and secondary gout can complicate this disease. Bone destruction and secondary gout may also be observed in the lymphomas. Sjögren's syndrome is associated with an arthritis that usually appears identical to rheumatoid arthritis. In systemic mastocytosis, characteristic skeletal abnormalities include focal or diffuse lytic or sclerotic lesions. In polycythemia vera, osteonecrosis, osteopenia, and hyperuricemia may appear. Myelofibrosis may be accompanied by osteosclerosis, particularly in the axial skeleton. In addition, hyperuricemia and secondary gout are relatively common in this disorder.

## INTRODUCTION

Certain lymphoproliferative and myeloproliferative (i.e., hematoproliferative) disorders are associated with definite skeletal manifestations, which may be an initial or dominant part of the entire clinical picture. In some instances, musculoskeletal symptoms and signs related to the primary disease process are responsible for these clinical findings; in other instances, metabolic consequences of the primary disease are responsible.

## LEUKEMIAS

### General Features

It is convenient to divide the leukemias into acute and chronic forms (Table 51–1). Acute leukemias are accompanied by the accumulation of immature, or blast, cells as a result of a defect in the production of mature hemic cells; chronic leukemias are accompanied by massive overgrowth of mature cells. Determination of the phenotypes of lymphoid and myeloid cells can be accomplished by using monoclonal antibodies that are generally directed against surface membrane proteins. Two broad populations of lymphocytes involved in the immune response can be identified: thymus-derived lymphocytes (T cells), which require the thymus for normal differentiation, and bone marrow–derived lymphocytes (B cells), which

**TABLE 51–1**

**Skeletal Alterations in the Leukemias**

| | Acute Childhood Leukemia | Acute Adult Leukemia | Chronic Leukemia |
|---|---|---|---|
| Osteopenia | ++ | ++ | + |
| Metaphyseal abnormalities | ++ | + | − |
| Osteolysis | ++ | ++ | + |
| Periostitis | ++ | + | + |
| Osteosclerosis | + | + | + |
| Articular abnormalities | ++ | + | + |

++, common; +, uncommon; −, absent.

undergo initial differentiation in the bone marrow. Thus, leukemias can be classified not only on the basis of their acute or chronic nature but also according to their predominant cellular morphology and their T-cell or B-cell constituency.

Acute leukemia can affect both children and adults. In children, acute leukemia is almost always lymphoblastic in cell origin, and the survival time is limited to approximately 1 year; in adults, acute leukemia is frequently myeloid in cell origin. Chronic leukemia may be granulocytic or lymphocytic. The chronic types of leukemia have a peak age of onset of 35 to 55 years and an average survival time of approximately 3 years. The general clinical manifestations of the leukemias are a consequence of the distribution of abnormal cells in the various organs and tissues of the body.

### Acute Childhood Leukemia

Acute leukemia, the most common form of childhood malignancy, is a disease of the first few years of life, with the peak prevalence occurring between 2 and 5 years of age. In some children, acute leukemia has a paucity of clinical signs, but this lack of signs is more typical of acute myeloblastic leukemia than acute lymphoblastic leukemia, in which numerous clinical findings may be encountered, including lymphadenopathy and splenomegaly. Bone and joint pain, tenderness, and swelling, which are common findings in children with leukemia, may be confused with rheumatic fever, juvenile chronic polyarthritis, or osteomyelitis. Arthralgias and arthritis are attributable to hemorrhage or to leukemic masses in the metaphyseal periosteum, subarticular bone, and synovium. Several radiographic findings may be observed.

**Diffuse Osteopenia (15% to 100%).** Osteopenia, with medullary widening and cortical thinning in tubular bones, and vertebral compression are encountered. Osteopenia may progress slowly without treatment or improve with therapy. The occurrence of unexplained generalized osteopenia in a child should initiate a search for clinical and laboratory manifestations of leukemia.

**Radiolucent and Radiodense Metaphyseal Bands (10% to 55%).** Symmetrical metaphyseal bandlike radiolucent areas are observed in leukemia and other chronic childhood illnesses (Fig. 51–1). This nonspecific finding probably reflects a nutritional deficit that interferes with proper osteogenesis. It is most commonly seen at sites of rapid bone growth, including the distal femoral, proximal tibial, proximal humeral, and distal radial metaphyses. After the age of 2 years, radiolucent metaphyseal bands are more characteristic of leukemia than of other conditions. Radiodense metaphyseal bands may be noted adjacent to the areas of increased radiolucency. Parallel radiodense growth recovery lines (of Harris) are presumably related to alternating periods of arrest and acceleration of bone growth. They may be observed in 50% of children with leukemia. Transverse radiolucent bands may also be observed under the vertebral endplates.

**Osteolytic Lesions (30% to 50%).** Multiple (or solitary) radiolucent lesions related to bone destruction are encountered in tubular and flat bones (Figs. 51–1 and 51–2). In the long bones of the extremities, the radiolucent lesions of a metaphysis can extend into the diaphysis. Similar lesions are seen in the cranial vault, pelvis, ribs, and shoulder girdle. The medial cortex of the proximal portion of the humerus is a characteristic site of involvement.

**Periostitis (10% to 35%).** Periosteal bone formation can be associated with lytic lesions (see Fig. 51–2). Proliferating leukemic cells in the marrow invade the cortex via haversian canals and extend to subperiosteal locations, where they cause elevation of the periosteal membrane. Subperiosteal hemorrhage may be an associated finding. Periostitis is particularly prominent in the long bones.

Prominent symmetrical periosteal new bone deposition in the tubular bones simulates the appearance of secondary hypertrophic osteoarthropathy, syphilis, and prostaglandin-induced periostitis.

**Osteosclerosis (5% to 10%).** Osteosclerosis is a relatively infrequent finding in leukemia. When apparent, it is particularly prominent in the metaphyses of long bones.

**Other Skeletal Abnormalities.** Sutural diastasis is common in infants and children with leukemia (Fig. 51–3). It is produced by an increase in intracranial pressure resulting from leukemic cell infiltration of the meninges or cerebrum or from intracerebral hemorrhage.

**Course of the Skeletal Lesions.** The extent of the bone lesions correlates poorly with the progress of leukemia. During treatment, resolution of the lytic defects is observed. The disappearance of lucent metaphyseal bands during remission has also been noted and may be associated with transient metaphyseal sclerosis. Skeletal lesions may or may not reappear during relapse.

**Articular Abnormalities.** The joint manifestations of acute leukemia that can lead to significant clinical findings are due to intra-articular leukemic cell infiltration and hemorrhage and, more commonly, to periarticular bone lesions. Pauciarticular and asymmetrical involvement appears to be most characteristic. Severe pain is a common clinical finding. Soft tissue swelling, effusion, and juxta-articular osteoporosis are occasionally seen.

Epiphyseal osteonecrosis may occur in some patients, particularly those treated with steroid medications. It has also been documented in leukemic patients before such therapy and has led to the early onset of symptoms. In such cases, potential mechanisms include leukemic infiltration in the bone marrow or walls of the blood vessels and hyperviscosity of the blood. Osteonecrosis occurring in association with leukemia typically affects the femoral

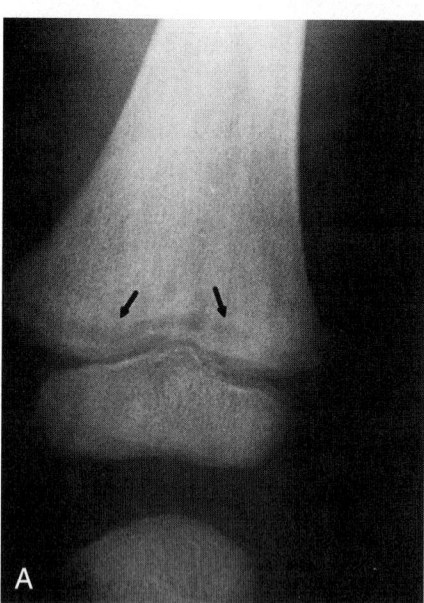
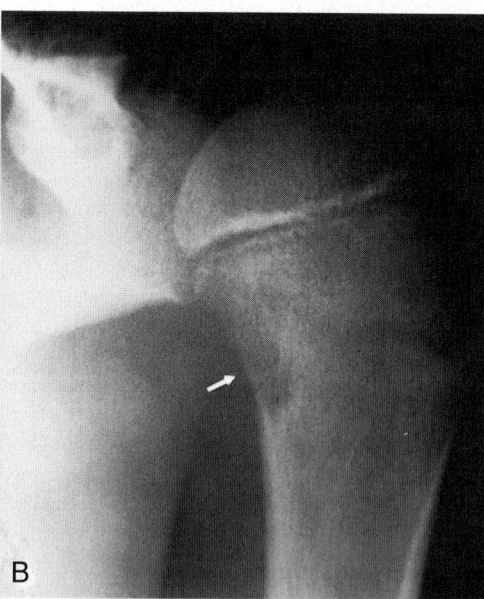

**Figure 51–1.** Acute childhood leukemia: metaphyseal abnormalities. *A,* Transverse band of radiolucency *(arrows)* in the metaphysis of the distal end of the femur. Adjacent minimal sclerosis and epiphyseal radiolucency are evident. *B,* Lytic lesion in the medial metaphysis of the proximal portion of the humerus *(arrow).* Note the metaphyseal transverse lucent band.

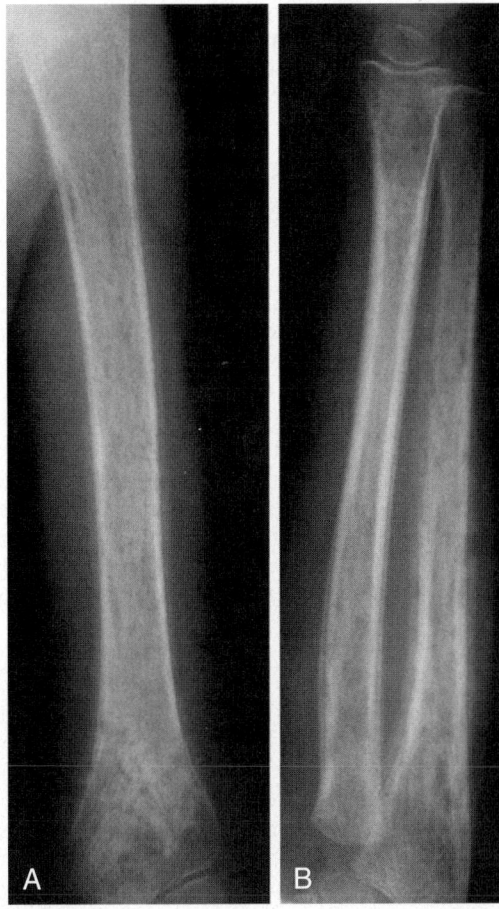

**Figure 51–2.** Acute childhood leukemia: osteolysis and periostitis. Observe the diffuse, small osteolytic lesions in the humerus, radius, and ulna. Periostitis is apparent.

epiphyses and condyles and the proximal portion of the humerus. Septic arthritis and osteomyelitis can complicate the acute leukemias in both children and adults.

**Differential Diagnosis.** The skeletal lesions of acute leukemia are similar to those in other disease processes. Metaphyseal radiolucency is a nonspecific finding that may also be encountered in systemic childhood illnesses, including transplacental infections (toxoplasmosis, rubella, cytomegalic inclusion disease, herpes, syphilis), scurvy, juvenile chronic polyarthritis, healing rickets, and neuroblastoma. The last-mentioned disorder is associated with many of the radiographic findings seen in acute leukemia, including widespread osteolytic lesions and periostitis. Similar findings are also observed in sickle cell anemia, skeletal metastasis (especially from retinoblastoma and embryonal rhabdomyosarcoma), infection, and syphilis.

### Acute Adult Leukemia

Clinical and radiographic evidence of skeletal involvement in leukemia is less common in adults than in children. Acute leukemia in adults may be associated with bone pain and tenderness. Articular symptoms and signs are less frequent than in children with acute leukemia. Adults with acute leukemia, however, may initially have articular findings simulating those of rheumatoid arthritis, and proliferative synovitis may be documented on histologic analysis.

The radiographic features in the skeleton in acute adult leukemia are diffuse osteopenia, discrete osteolytic lesions, and metaphyseal radiolucency. Diffuse osteopenia is a nonspecific finding simulating osteoporosis and other metabolic disorders. Lytic lesions may be evident in the skull, pelvis, and proximal ends of the long bones.

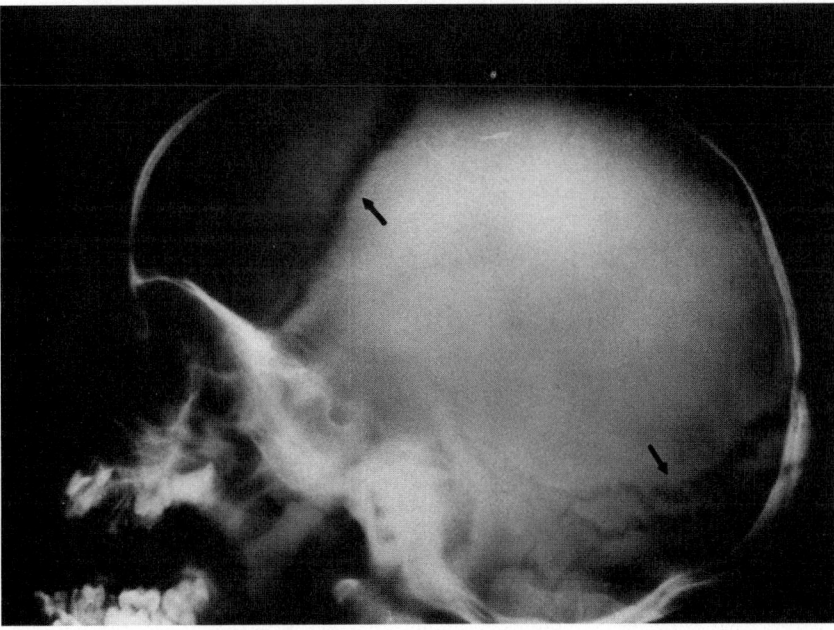

**Figure 51–3.** Acute childhood leukemia: sutural diastasis. In an infant with leukemia, the sutures in both the frontal and occipital regions are widened (*arrows*).

Metaphyseal radiolucent bands are not as frequent as in children with acute leukemia. Rare radiographic findings are large destructive lesions, periostitis, acro-osteolysis, discrete subperiosteal erosions, and focal or diffuse osteosclerosis.

## Chronic Leukemia

The osseous and articular manifestations of chronic leukemia are less common and less severe than those of acute leukemia. Marrow hyperplasia in some patients may become evident as nonspecific diffuse osteopenia, particularly in the axial skeleton. Discrete osteolytic lesions are observed in less than 3% of persons, particularly in the femur and humerus (Fig. 51–4). Occasionally, larger and more aggressive lesions may be encountered. Rarely, widespread or multifocal bone sclerosis is evident, perhaps related to diffuse marrow fibrosis. Soft tissue accumulation of masses of leukemic cells (chloromas) can produce subjacent osseous erosion.

In adults (and in children), leukemic involvement of the small bones of the hand may be associated with soft tissue edema, clubbing, and bone destruction. This combination of findings is termed leukemic acropachy. Clinical findings are usually a late manifestation of the disease and show a predilection for the knees, shoulders, and ankles. Radiographic findings are limited; osteopenia and soft tissue swelling may be evident, however. Epiphyseal osteonecrosis has been described and is usually, but not

invariably, related to steroid administration. Secondary gout is a well-known complication of chronic leukemia. Septic arthritis and osteomyelitis may also be evident (Fig. 51–5).

## Special Types of Leukemia

**Hairy Cell Leukemia.** Hairy cell leukemia, which is also termed leukemic reticuloendotheliosis, is responsible for approximately 2% of all cases of leukemia. Its name originates from the numerous short villi, resembling hairs, about the membranes of lymphocytes. The major clinical consequences of the disease are related to depressed bone marrow function and hypersplenism.

Hairy cell leukemia typically develops in adults. Its insidious onset is characterized by fatigue, weakness, infectious episodes, abdominal pain (or, more rarely, hemorrhage), splenic rupture, and pathologic fracture of bone. Splenomegaly, hepatomegaly, and lymphadenopathy are present, in order of decreasing frequency. The disease is slowly progressive, but most patients die in the

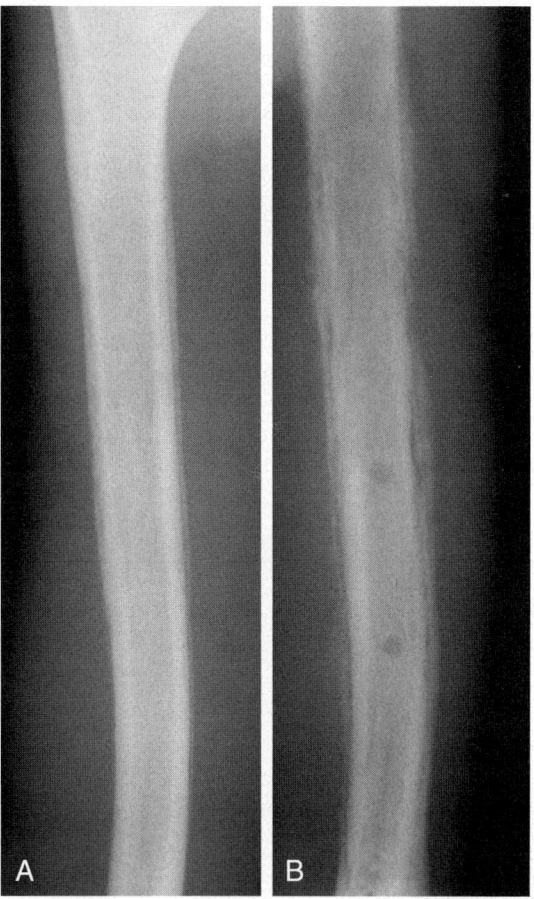

**Figure 51–5.** Chronic leukemia: osteomyelitis. In this 34-year-old woman, osteomyelitis from *Salmonella* infection occurred in the humerus. As depicted in these radiographs obtained 2 weeks apart, findings include poorly defined osteolysis in the diaphysis associated with periostitis, abnormalities seen in uncomplicated leukemia as well. A biopsy of bone undertaken in the interval between the two studies (*A*, initial radiograph; *B*, 2 week follow-up) explains the circular osteolytic defects in the later radiograph. *Salmonella* organisms were recovered from the biopsy material.

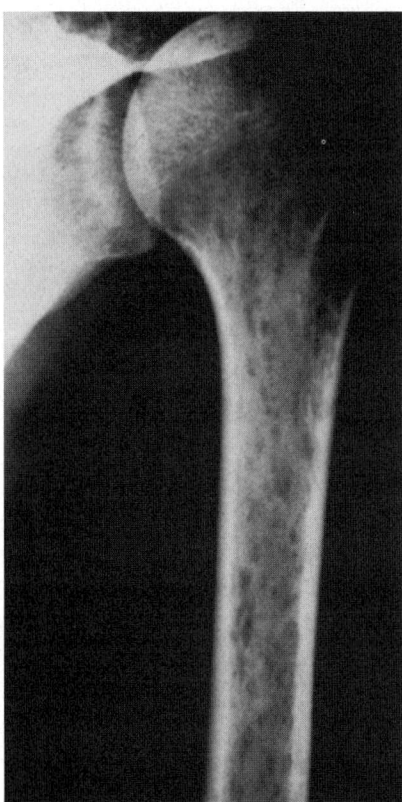

**Figure 51–4.** Chronic leukemia: osteolytic lesions. A 27-year-old woman with chronic leukemia demonstrates small, focal radiolucent lesions in the proximal portions of the humerus and femur.

first 5 years. Bone involvement is an infrequent feature of hairy cell leukemia. When present, such involvement can lead to solitary or, less commonly, multiple (usually two) osteolytic lesions, with a predilection for the spine and proximal portions of the femora (head and neck). Bone sclerosis is rare. Spontaneous fracture is a recognized complication of such lesions. Radiation therapy and chemotherapy can lead to a decrease in symptoms and regression of the osteolytic process.

**Acute Megakaryoblastic Leukemia.** This rare disorder, also termed malignant myelofibrosis, affects children and adults and demonstrates a progressive course characterized by anemia, pancytopenia, and diffuse marrow fibrosis. Splenomegaly is absent or mild. The proliferating cells in the bone marrow are variable in type, immature, and dominated by megakaryocytes.

In children, radiolucency in the metaphyseal regions of tubular bones and osteolytic lesions are seen. The degree of periosteal bone formation can be profound. In adults, focal or diffuse bone sclerosis is observed.

**Granulocytic Sarcoma (Chloroma).** Granulocytic sarcoma is a localized tumor mass composed of immature cells of the granulocyte series (Fig 51–6). Its designation as chloroma stems from the greenish color of the tumor. Granulocytic sarcoma is most commonly associated with acute leukemia of the myeloid type, especially in children, although it is also observed in adults and in patients with other varieties of leukemia, with other myeloproliferative disorders, or without obvious bone marrow dysfunction.

Granulocytic sarcomas are more common in children than in adults and may be single or multiple. Frequent sites of involvement are bone, periosteum, soft tissue, orbits, lymph nodes, and skin. Lytic lesions characterize intraosseous involvement and are especially prominent in the skull, spine, ribs, long tubular bones, and sternum. Soft tissue tumors can lead to masses, as in a paraspinal location, that may subsequently erode the neighboring bone.

## Magnetic Resonance Imaging

Broad applications of magnetic resonance (MR) imaging to the analysis of musculoskeletal involvement in patients with leukemia include determination of the extent of bone marrow alterations before the initiation of therapy, assessment of the response of the disease to such therapy, detection of some of the skeletal complications of the disease or the therapeutic regimen, and investigation of some special forms of leukemia, such as hairy cell leukemia and granulocytic sarcoma.

The MR imaging abnormalities accompanying leukemic infiltration of bone marrow are similar or identical to those in a number of other infiltrative processes (e.g., plasma cell myeloma, lymphoma, metastasis) (Fig. 51–7). Most commonly, leukemic marrow demonstrates prolongation of the T1 relaxation value, which leads to diminution of marrow signal intensity on T1-weighted spin echo MR images. Diffuse or focal abnormalities are evident, with the latter pattern being especially evident in acute myelogenous leukemia. Because many of the leukemias affect children, the resulting decrease in signal intensity is sometimes difficult to differentiate from the signal intensity of normal hematopoietic marrow. T2 changes are more variable and less dramatic. Quantitative chemical shift MR imaging has been used in patients with leukemia to determine the stage of the disease. This technique can help distinguish the individual contributions of fat and water to the total signal intensity, thus rendering a more quantitative assessment of the bone marrow than can be accomplished with conventional MR imaging techniques.

The role of other MR imaging techniques, such as gadolinium enhancement and short tau inversion recovery (STIR) and in-phase and out-of-phase gradient echo imaging, in the evaluation of the therapeutic response of patients with leukemia (and other disseminated malignant disorders of bone marrow) is still to be determined. Although the value of MR imaging as a technique for monitoring disease activity requires further study, its value in defining local complications of musculoskeletal involvement is well established. Soft tissue extension of intraosseous lesions and compromise of the spinal cord accompanying vertebral involvement, especially in focal lesions associated with hairy cell leukemia and granulocytic sarcoma, are well shown with standard MR imaging techniques. Further, assessment of complications resulting from chemotherapy, such as ischemic necrosis of bone, can be accomplished with these techniques.

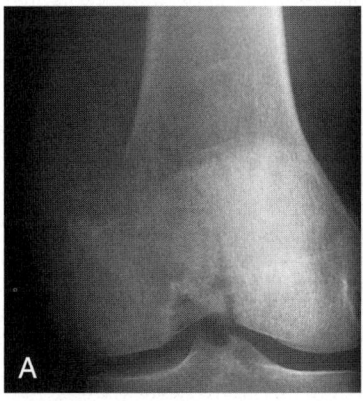
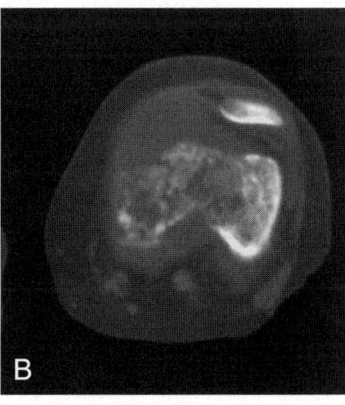

**Figure 51–6.** Granulocytic sarcoma (chloroma). Routine radiograph *(A)* and transaxial computed tomography scan *(B)* show an osteolytic lesion with a soft tissue mass that, on biopsy, was found to be a granulocytic sarcoma. (Courtesy of G. Greenway, MD, Dallas, Tex.)

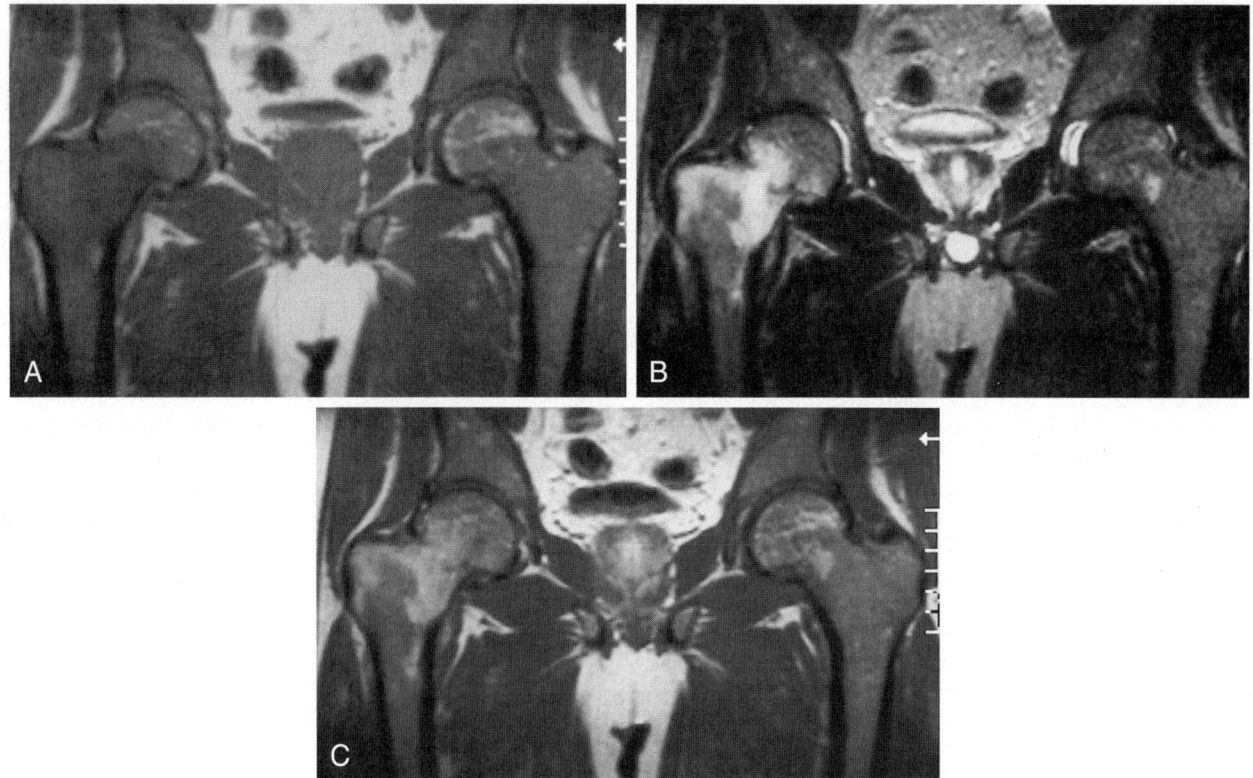

**Figure 51–7.** Leukemia: MR imaging abnormalities—spin echo and gadolinium-enhanced techniques. This adult patient has a pathologic fracture of the femur. *A*, Standard coronal T1-weighted (TR/TE, 525/25) spin echo MR image reveals diffuse low signal intensity in the marrow of the diaphyses and metaphyses of the femora and the innominate bones. The distribution of this signal intensity is too widespread to represent normal sites of hematopoietic marrow in an adult patient. Some fatty marrow with high signal intensity is seen in the femoral epiphyses and, on the left side, in the femoral metaphysis and diaphysis. *B*, With T2 weighting (TR/TE, 2200/90), regions of very high signal intensity are evident in the femoral necks, especially on the right side, and joint effusions are apparent in both hips. The remaining portions of the bone marrow are of moderately low signal intensity. *C*, Coronal T1-weighted (TR/TE, 525/25) spin echo MR image obtained after the intravenous administration of a gadolinium contrast agent shows enhancement of signal intensity in the marrow, particularly in both femoral necks. The distribution of the abnormal signal changes in the femora is similar to that in *(B)*. (Courtesy of J. Kramer, MD, Vienna, Austria.)

## LYMPHOMAS

### General Features

A variety of diseases are grouped together as lympho-reticular neoplasms, including non-Hodgkin's lymphoma, Hodgkin's lymphoma, Burkitt's lymphoma, and mycosis fungoides. The classification of such diseases is complicated and debated, and it is made even more difficult because the terminology is continually undergoing modification.

Lymphomas are generally divided into two broad categories—Hodgkin's disease and malignant lymphomas. Malignant lymphomas occur about three times more commonly than Hodgkin's disease. Non-Hodgkin's lymphomas have been classified, based on histologic characteristics, into low-grade, intermediate-grade, and high-grade categories, each of which can be further divided according to specific cellular characteristics (Table 51–2). Common to all types of lymphoma are lymphadenopathy, mediastinal and abdominal masses, hepatomegaly or splenomegaly (or both), and, not uncom-

monly, constitutional symptoms that include fever, night sweats, and weight loss. Some of these neoplasms arise in extraskeletal sites and appear as single or multiple tumors in the lymph nodes, spleen, or gastrointestinal tract. From these locations, abnormal cells may circulate in the blood and lodge in distant sites, such as the bone marrow, where they may flourish. Alternatively, lymphoreticular neoplasms may arise as a primary process of bone, an occurrence that accounts for approximately 5% of all primary malignant osseous tumors. Most of these cases result from the histiocytic type of lymphoma. Such lymphomas originating in bone are observed in older patients and in men more commonly than women.

Skeletal changes are common in all the lymphomas. Abnormalities may be identified in 5% to 50% of cases, depending on the specific disease being investigated and the method of detection. Because the prognosis of lymphoreticular neoplasms is intimately related to the extent of disease, the initial evaluation must include a search for sites of involvement, a process called staging. Lower stages of disease are characterized by localization

**Proposed WHO Classification of Lymphoid Neoplasms***

B-cell neoplasms
  Precursor B-cell neoplasm
    Precursor B-lymphoblastic leukemia/lymphoma (precursor
      B-cell acute lymphoblastic leukemia)
  Mature (peripheral) B cell neoplasms[†]
    B-cell chronic lymphocytic leukemia/small lymphocytic
      lymphoma
    B-cell prolymphocytic leukemia
    Lymphoplasmacytic lymphoma
    Splenic marginal zone B-cell lymphoma (± villous
      lymphocytes)
    Hairy cell leukemia
    Plasma cell myeloma/plasmacytoma
    Extranodal marginal zone B-cell lymphoma of MALT type
    Nodal marginal zone B-cell lymphoma (± monocytoid B
      cells)
    Follicular lymphoma
    Mantle-cell lymphoma
    Diffuse large B-cell lymphoma
      Mediastinal large B-cell lymphoma
      Primary effusion lymphoma
    Burkitt's lymphoma/Burkitt cell leukemia

T-cell and NK-cell neoplasms
  Precursor T-cell neoplasm
    Precursor T-lymphoblastic lymphoma/leukemia (precursor
      T-cell acute lymphoblastic leukemia)
  Mature (peripheral) T-cell neoplasms[†]
    T-cell prolymphocytic leukemia
    T-cell granular lymphocytic leukemia
    Aggressive NK-cell leukemia
    Adult T-cell lymphoma/leukemia (HTLV1 +)
    Extranodal NK/T-cell lymphoma, nasal type
    Enteropathy-type T-cell lymphoma
    Hepatosplenic gamma-delta T-cell lymphoma
    Subcutaneous panniculitis-like T-cell lymphoma
    Mycosis fungoides/Sézary's syndrome
    Anaplastic large-cell lymphoma, T/null cell, primary
      cutaneous type
    Peripheral T-cell lymphoma, not otherwise characterized
    Angioimmunoblastic T-cell lymphoma
    Anaplastic large-cell lymphoma, T/null cell, primary
      systemic type

Hodgkin's lymphoma (Hodgkin's disease)
  Nodular lymphocyte-predominant Hodgkin's lymphoma
  Classic Hodgkin's lymphoma
    Nodular sclerosis Hodgkin's lymphoma (grades 1 and 2)
    Lymphocyte-rich classic Hodgkin's lymphoma
    Mixed cellularity Hodgkin's lymphoma
    Lymphocyte depletion Hodgkin's lymphoma

*Only major categories are included.

[†]B- and T-/NK-cell neoplasms are grouped according to major clinical
presentations (predominantly disseminated/leukemic, primary extranodal,
predominantly nodal).

HTLV1 +, human T-cell leukemia virus; MALT, mucosa-associated lymphoid
tissue; NK, natural killer; WHO, World Health Organization.

From Harris NL, Jaffe ES, Diebold J, et al: World Health Organization
classification of neoplastic diseases of the hematopoietic and lymphoid tissues:
Report of the clinical advisory committee meeting–Airlie House, Virginia,
November 1997. J Clin Oncol 17:3835, 1999.

in a single lymph node or in a single extralymphatic site or by involvement of lymph nodes, spleen, or extralymphatic sites confined to one side of the diaphragm. Higher stages of disease are characterized by transdiaphragmatic spread or by diffuse or disseminated involvement of extralymphatic sites (e.g., liver, lung, bone marrow), with or without lymph node involvement. A truly primary bone lesion is considered stage I non-Hodgkin's lymphoma, whereas a bone lesion associated with disease in other sites is considered stage IV.

## Skeletal Abnormalities

**Non-Hodgkin's Lymphoma.** Involvement of bone in non-Hodgkin's lymphoma is more commonly a manifestation of diffuse disease than of a primary lesion. Estimates of the prevalence of skeletal alterations in widespread non-Hodgkin's lymphoma are 10% to 20% in adults and 20% to 30% in children. Such alterations generally appear after the initial manifestation of the disease. Abnormalities of the axial skeleton predominate, with frequent involvement of the spine, pelvis, skull, ribs, and facial bones. Hematogenous spread of tumor is responsible for most of these lesions, but alterations can also develop as a result of osseous invasion from surrounding soft tissues and lymph nodes. Multiple osteolytic lesions with moth-eaten or permeative bone destruction predominate (Fig. 51–8). Periostitis occurs but is less frequent and severe than in Hodgkin's disease.

Primary non-Hodgkin's lymphoma of bone occurs at any age and affects men more frequently than women. Systemic symptoms and signs are characteristically absent, but localized pain and swelling may be evident. The lesions predominate in the bones of the appendicular skeleton, especially those in the lower extremities (Fig. 51–9). An osteolytic lesion with poorly defined margins in the metaphyseal (or, rarely, epiphyseal or diaphyseal) region of a long tubular bone is most typical. Pathologic fractures and soft tissue masses are common. The presence of soft tissue masses without extensive cortical destruction has been emphasized in cases of primary lymphoma of bone. Detached pieces of bone, or sequestra, are reported to occur in approximately 10% of cases.

**Hodgkin's Disease.** Skeletal involvement in Hodgkin's disease is quite common, detectable on radiographs in 10% to 25% of cases. Such involvement is infrequent at the initial clinical examination. Bone abnormalities are more common in adults than in children. Tumor may reach osseous tissue through either hematogenous dissemination or direct spread from contiguous involved lymph nodes. The most common sites of involvement in Hodgkin's disease are the spine, pelvis, ribs, femora, and sternum. Multiple lesions occur with a slightly greater frequency than solitary lesions.

Osteosclerosis alone, osteolysis alone, or osteosclerosis combined with osteolysis may be evident. The reported frequency of sclerotic lesions varies from 14% to 45%. Diffuse sclerosis of the vertebral body (ivory vertebra) is similar to that observed in other lymphomas, skeletal

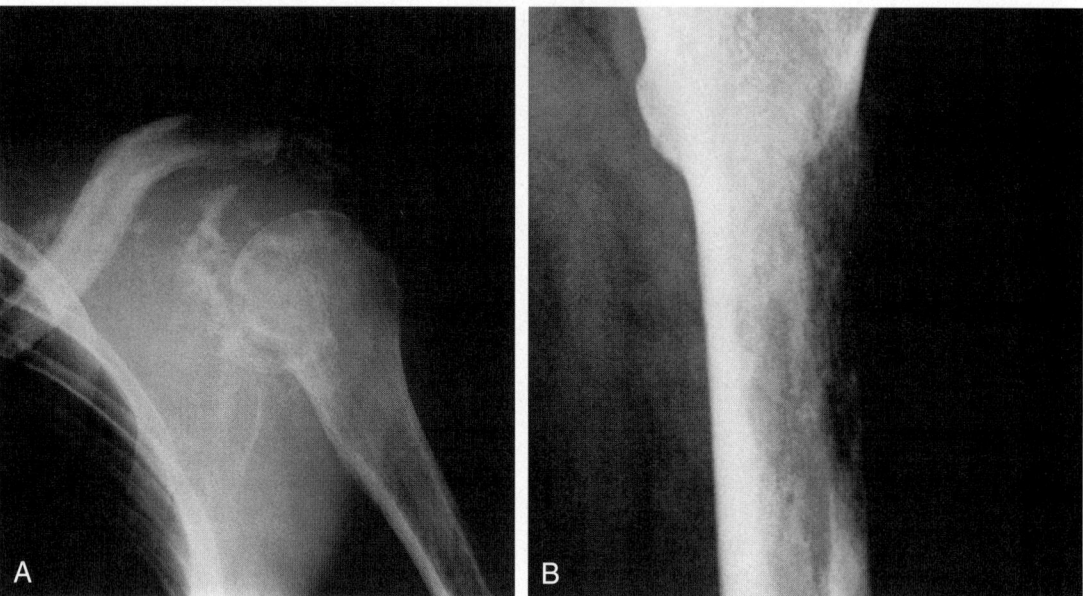

**Figure 51–8.** Non-Hodgkin's lymphoma: histocytic type with disseminated disease. *A,* Extensive destructive lesion of the scapula in a 58-year-old man is characterized by a soft tissue mass, osteolysis of the glenoid process and adjacent bone, and osteosclerosis. The humeral head appears to be involved, and the shaft reveals osteoporosis. *B,* In this 47-year-old man, multiple organ systems are affected. Observe an eccentric diaphyseal lesion of the femur, with moth-eaten bone destruction and cortical violation.

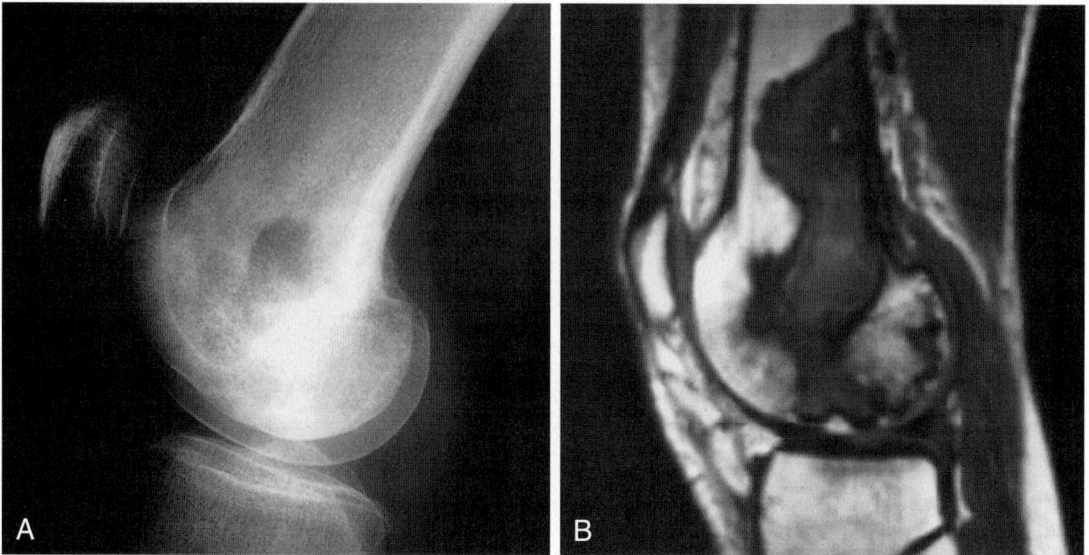

**Figure 51–9.** Non-Hodgkin's lymphoma: histocytic type with primary bone involvement. *A,* Patchy osteolysis in the distal end of the femur is evident on the radiograph. *B,* Sagittal T1-weighted (TR/TE, 700/15) spin echo MR image reveals the extent of the tumor, which is of low signal intensity. No enhancement of the lesion was evident on MR images obtained after the intravenous administration of a gadolinium contrast agent (not shown). (Courtesy of J. Kramer, MD, Vienna, Austria.)

metastasis, and Paget's disease (Fig. 51–10). Widespread osteosclerosis may result from an osseous response to extensive bone marrow involvement or bone marrow fibrosis rather than from frank involvement of the bone itself. Osteolytic lesions are poorly defined and associated with periostitis in approximately one third of cases. Similar periosteal bone formation may indicate associated hypertrophic osteoarthropathy.

**Burkitt's Lymphoma.** Burkitt's lymphoma is a stem cell lymphoma that is seen predominantly in children. This type of lymphoma is strongly associated with the Epstein-Barr virus. It is the most common malignant disease of children in tropical Africa. Involvement of the facial bones is particularly characteristic. Early radiographic changes include loss of the lamina dura, particularly around the molar teeth, and diminution and obscuration

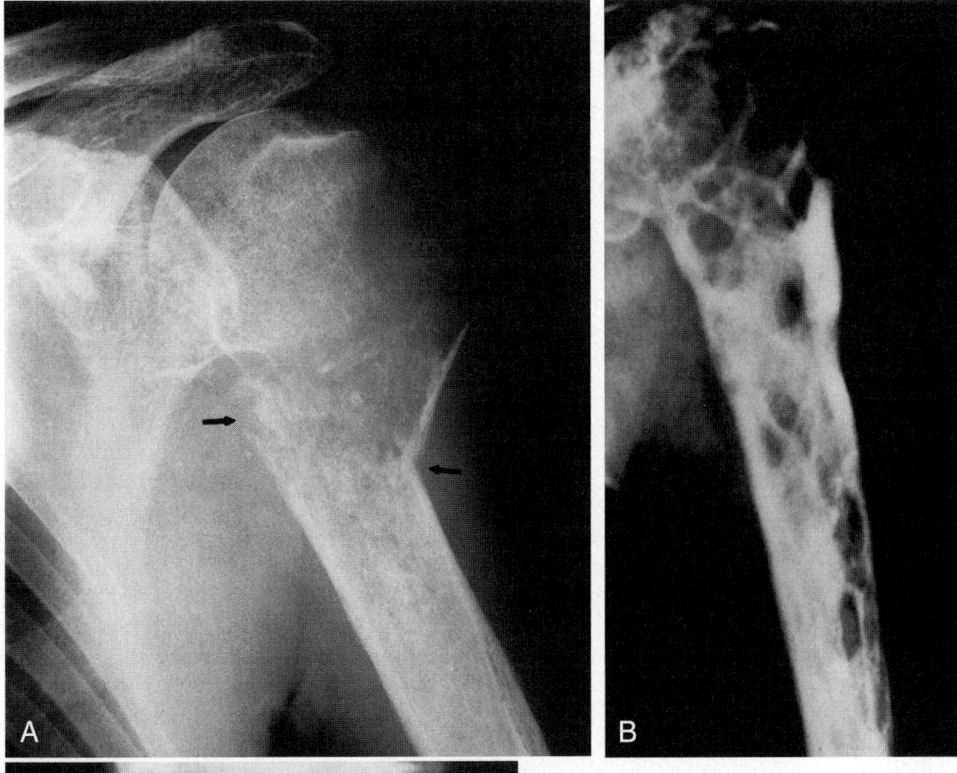

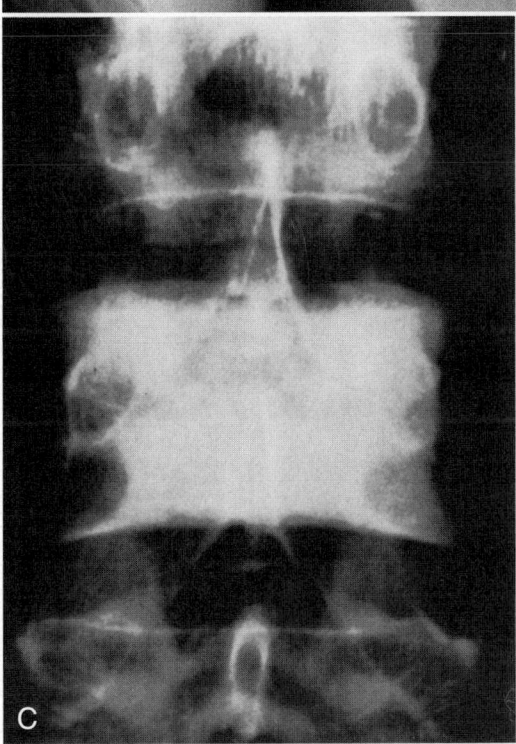

**Figure 51–10.** Hodgkin's disease: skeletal manifestations. *A*, Large osteolytic lesion of the proximal end of the humerus has resulted in a pathologic fracture *(arrows)*. *B*, Multiple large "cystic" osteolytic lesions of the proximal end of the humerus are associated with adjacent bony eburnation. *C*, In a different patient, frontal radiograph reveals an ivory vertebra. Note the homogeneous increase in radiodensity of the vertebral body, without osseous enlargement.

of trabeculae in cancellous bone. With disruption of the cortex, a soft tissue mass may extend into the buccal cavity or maxillary antrum.

Lesions in the tubular bones and pelvis have been described but are less frequent. The femur and tibia are especially vulnerable. Osteolytic foci develop in the medullary portion of the bone, coalesce, penetrate the cortex, produce periostitis, and lead to a soft tissue mass.

**Mycosis Fungoides.** Mycosis fungoides is considered an unusual form of malignant (T-cell) lymphoma with primary involvement of the skin. It is uncommon but not rare. Its onset is in the fourth or fifth decade of life. Initially, mycosis fungoides may appear as nonspecific skin ulcerations. Cutaneous lesions may be associated with localized or generalized lymphadenopathy. In the tumor stage, extracutaneous manifestations with visceral involvement are evident. After the tumor stage, death commonly occurs within a few years, frequently as a result of septicemia.

Bone marrow involvement is rare. When present, bone lesions occur in the appendicular skeleton, with discrete or poorly defined medullary defects, cortical destruction, periostitis, and soft tissue swelling. Although the skeletal abnormalities are similar to those accompanying other aggressive lesions, such as metastasis and plasma cell myeloma, involvement of the peripheral skeleton, including the hand, may be a helpful clue in the diagnosis of mycosis fungoides.

## Muscle Abnormalities

Enlargement of one or more muscles is a recognized manifestation of the lymphomas. Such enlargement can be painful and may affect the musculature of the axial or the appendicular skeleton, or both. Lymphomatous infiltration of the muscle related to either contiguous tumor mass or lymph node represents one mechanism for enlargement of the muscle. Similar enlargement, however, can occur without histologic evidence of lymphomatous infiltration, although the pathogenesis of the finding in this situation is not clear.

With ultrasonography, muscle involvement is characterized by an ill-defined hypoechoic mass. With com-

puted tomography, a mass effect is often seen, although the involved tissue may have attenuation values similar to those of normal muscle. On MR images, signal intensity similar to that of normal muscle is typical on T1-weighted sequences, with relatively high signal intensity on T2-weighted sequences (Fig. 51–11). The adjacent fat is often infiltrated, and multiple muscle compartments and a long segment of an extremity may be involved. The differential diagnosis of muscle involvement in lymphoma includes various types of myositis, muscle infarction, denervation changes in muscle, and sarcoidosis.

## Effects of Therapy

The association between ischemic necrosis of bone and treatment of lymphoma with combination chemotherapy regimens that include intermittent corticosteroids has been reported. The frequency of this complication in treated patients is approximately 1% to 3% in Hodgkin's disease and somewhat lower in non-Hodgkin's lymphoma, typically occurring 1 to 3 years after the initiation of therapy. The femoral head and, less commonly, the humeral head are preferred sites of involvement.

A second complication of therapy in leukemia and, less typically, lymphoma is related to the administration of methotrexate. Skeletal changes, termed methotrexate osteopathy, usually occur 6 to 18 months after institution

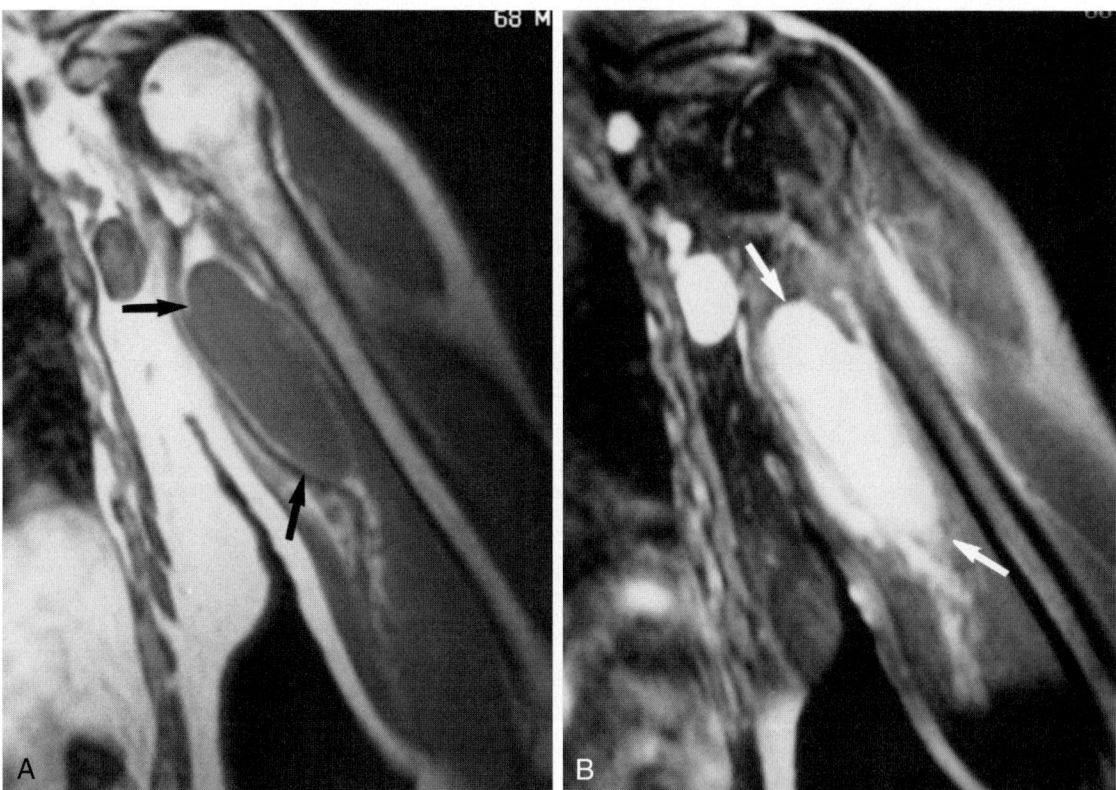

**Figure 51–11.** Non-Hodgkin's lymphoma: muscle involvement. In a 68-year-old man, oblique coronal T1-weighted (TR/TE, 400/16) spin echo *(A)* and fat-suppressed fast spin echo (TR/TE, 3500/39) *(B)* MR images show fusiform enlargement of a long segment of the involved muscle *(arrows)*, characterized by signal intensity identical to that of normal muscle in *(A)* and high signal intensity in *(B)*. Note the associated lymphadenopathy. (Courtesy of C. Chen, MD, Kaohsiung, Taiwan.)

of the therapy and are characterized by pain, osteopenia, growth recovery lines, dense metaphyseal bands, and insufficiency or complete fractures. Periostitis is either absent or localized. The cause of methotrexate osteopathy is not known.

## Magnetic Resonance Imaging

MR imaging shows lymphomatous infiltration of the marrow as focal or diffuse regions of low signal intensity on T1-weighted spin echo images (Fig. 51–12). Most descriptions of such infiltration have emphasized regions of high signal intensity on T2-weighted spin echo images, but this observation has not been entirely consistent. Periosseous invasion of tissue such as muscle in lymphoma can be shown with standard MR imaging. MR imaging is particularly useful for determining the extent of bone and soft tissue involvement in patients who have spinal lymphoma. The use of gradient echo sequences in the analysis of marrow involvement in lymphoma (as well as in other infiltrative processes) may lead to diagnostic difficulty. Normal marrow exhibits a shortened effective transverse relaxation time on gradient echo sequences because of local magnetic field inhomogeneity and, therefore, low signal intensity on these sequences.

## Other Lymphoproliferative Disorders

**Angioimmunoblastic Lymphadenopathy.** Angioimmunoblastic lymphadenopathy is a systemic lymphoproliferative disease characterized by lymphadenopathy, hepatosplenomegaly, skin rash, anemia, lymphocytopenia, and polyclonal hypergammaglobulinemia. Corticosteroid therapy or the administration of cytotoxic agents may lead to remission, although median survival is only 3 years. The disease may be transformed into a malignant lymphoblastic lymphoma. Articular involvement occurs in approximately 10% of cases. Joint effusions, soft tissue swelling, and, rarely, periarticular osteoporosis, joint space narrowing, and osseous erosions have been encountered.

**Angiofollicular Lymphoid Hyperplasia.** Angiofollicular lymphoid hyperplasia, or Castleman's disease, has variable clinical features that depend on the precise histologic aberrations. Two distinct histologic subtypes of disease have been identified: the hyaline vascular form (90% of cases) and the plasma cell form (10% of cases). Patients with the first subtype of disease are generally asymptomatic, whereas those with the plasma cell form may exhibit fever, anemia, and hypergammaglobulinemia. Widespread abnormalities and an aggressive clinical course may result in hepatosplenomegaly, lymphadenopathy, sepsis, and, in some instances, death. Masses of abnormal lymphoid tissue may be found in the thorax, mediastinum, retroperitoneum, axilla, or abdominal or pelvic cavities. An additional association of Castleman's disease is neoplasia, including lymphoma, Kaposi's sarcoma, plasmacytoma, and colon carcinoma.

## SJÖGREN'S SYNDROME

### General Features

The classic triad of Sjögren's syndrome consists of keratoconjunctivitis sicca (dry eyes), xerostomia (dry mouth), and rheumatoid arthritis. In some patients, however, rheumatoid arthritis is replaced by another disorder such as systemic lupus erythematosus, periarteritis nodosa, progressive systemic sclerosis, or polymyositis. The diagnosis is established by the presence of two of the three major components.

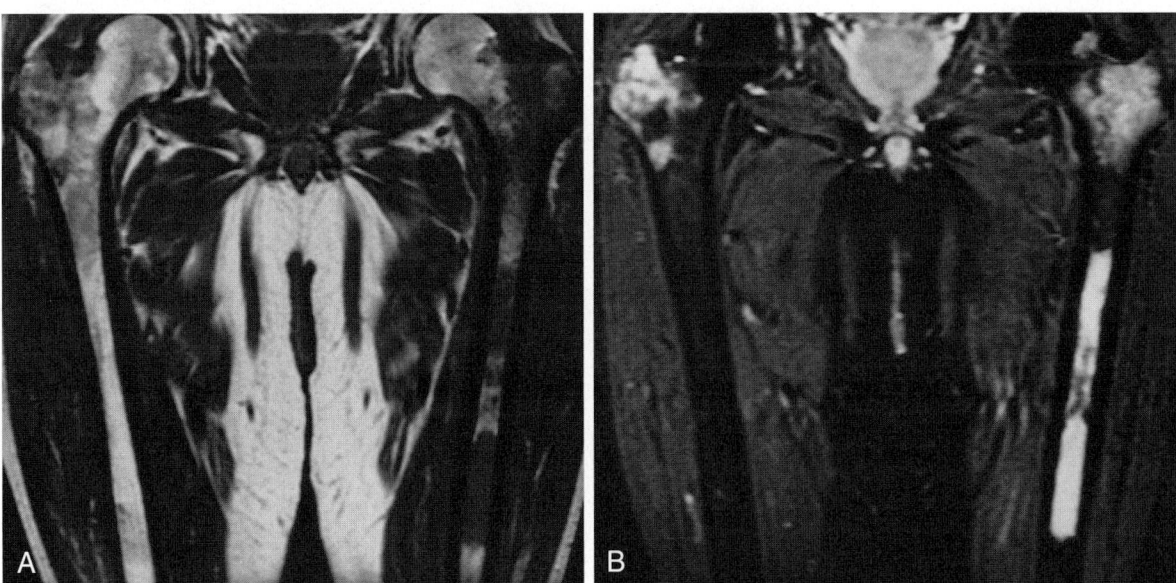

**Figure 51–12.** Non-Hodgkin's lymphoma: disseminated disease. Spin echo and STIR MR imaging techniques. *A*, Coronal T1-weighted (TR/TE, 800/20) spin echo MR image reveals bilateral femoral involvement, greater on the left side. Focal areas of low signal intensity are evident in the bone marrow. *B*, With STIR imaging (TR/TE, 2000/30; inversion time, 160 msec), the lesions are of high signal intensity.

## Clinical Abnormalities

Sjögren's syndrome is a common disorder, affecting about 500,000 to 2 million persons in the United States. It is far more frequent in women than in men, and the average age at the time of diagnosis is 40 to 50 years. The two most common clinical patterns are (1) slowly progressive development of the sicca complex in a patient with chronic rheumatoid arthritis and (2) a more rapid development of oral and ocular dryness accompanied by episodic parotitis in an otherwise healthy person. Parotid gland enlargement is evident in approximately 50% of patients.

Articular symptoms and signs may or may not be present. Clinical manifestations are almost invariably those of rheumatoid arthritis. In 10% to 15% of patients with rheumatoid arthritis, keratoconjunctivitis sicca develops after an average duration of arthritis of 9 years. Subcutaneous nodules are apparent in approximately 60% of patients with arthritis and are histologically typical of rheumatoid nodules. The eventual outcome of the joint disease is similar to that in uncomplicated rheumatoid arthritis. Additional manifestations of Sjögren's syndrome include Raynaud's phenomenon (20%), splenomegaly and leukopenia suggestive of Felty's syndrome, infections, vasculitis, peripheral neuropathy, glomerulonephritis, and purpura.

## Radiographic Abnormalities

The major articular findings are those of rheumatoid arthritis and consist of soft tissue swelling, periarticular osteoporosis, marginal erosions, joint space narrowing, and intra-articular cystic lesions. Typical target sites are the same as those of rheumatoid arthritis.

## Relationship to Lymphoma and Other Malignancies

It is well known that lymphoma and leukemia can affect the lacrimal and salivary glands and produce abnormalities resembling those of Sjögren's syndrome. In addition, follow-up studies in patients with Sjögren's syndrome reveal that malignant lymphoma, including mucosa-associated lymphoid tissue (MALT lymphoma), or another lymphoproliferative disease develops in some persons.

## SYSTEMIC MASTOCYTOSIS

### General Features

Systemic mastocytosis is a rare proliferative disorder affecting both men and women that begins in adulthood. It is a systemic process whose clinical manifestations resemble those of lymphoma or leukemia. Multiple organ systems may be altered, including the liver, spleen, lymph nodes, and skeleton, although cutaneous involvement is most common and characteristic. The skin or mucous membrane lesions resemble urticaria pigmentosa of childhood.

Typically, patients with systemic mastocytosis are in the fifth to eighth decades of life. Men and women are affected equally. The clinical features relate, in part, to histamine release and consist of local urticaria, flushing, shocklike episodes, diarrhea, and vomiting. In more severe cases, weight loss, weakness, malaise, hepatosplenomegaly, lymphadenopathy, and peptic ulcer disease are encountered. Hematologic abnormalities include anemia, leukopenia, thrombocytopenia, and eosinophilia. Hepatic dysfunction occurs as a result of mast cell proliferation and periportal fibrosis. The prognosis is variable, depending on the extent of systemic involvement. When the disease is confined to the skin and skeleton, it may run a mild, protracted course.

### Skeletal Abnormalities

Mast cell proliferation in skeletal tissue may cause tenderness, soft tissue mass, and deformity secondary to pathologic fracture. Such fractures are especially common in the spine. Mast cell infiltration into the bone marrow stimulates fibroblastic activity and a granulomatous reaction, which lead to trabecular destruction and replacement with adjacent new bone formation. These abnormalities, which occur in 70% of patients, can be classified into two types: (1) osteopenia and bone destruction and (2) osteosclerosis (Fig. 51–13). In either type, a focal or diffuse distribution may be seen. Diffuse lesions predominate in the axial skeleton, whereas focal lesions occur in both the axial and the appendicular skeletons. Progression of skeletal lesions is not uncommon, and the initial focal lesions may become diffuse. Scintigraphy has been used to identify skeletal involvement in mastocytosis. Radionuclide patterns vary according to the distribution of the osseous lesions.

**Osteopenia and Bone Destruction.** Diffuse osteopenia or multiple lytic lesions may be observed in systemic mastocytosis. Generalized rarefaction simulates the appearance of osteoporosis and is most frequent in the skull, pelvis, spine, and ribs. It may relate to the effects of heparin or prostaglandins, by-products of mast cell metabolism. The lesions can simulate the findings of cystic osteoporosis, Gaucher's disease, or thalassemia.

**Osteosclerosis.** Focal or diffuse bone sclerosis is another radiographic pattern in systemic mastocytosis that may appear in combination with osteolysis. Focal sclerotic lesions correspond to areas of prominent trabeculae, with cortical thickening and narrowing of the marrow spaces, and may be misinterpreted as skeletal metastases. In the axial skeleton, loss of delineation of bony trabeculae and the resulting homogeneous radiodense appearance resemble the abnormalities associated with myelofibrosis, fluorosis, sickle cell anemia, Paget's disease, and skeletal metastasis. In systemic mastocytosis, the cause of the osteosclerosis is not known.

### Magnetic Resonance Imaging

MR imaging is sensitive in detecting marrow abnormalities in patients with mastocytosis. Although findings are nonspecific, several patterns of altered signal intensity are encountered, including both diffuse and focal abnormalities paralleling the pathologic findings that charac-

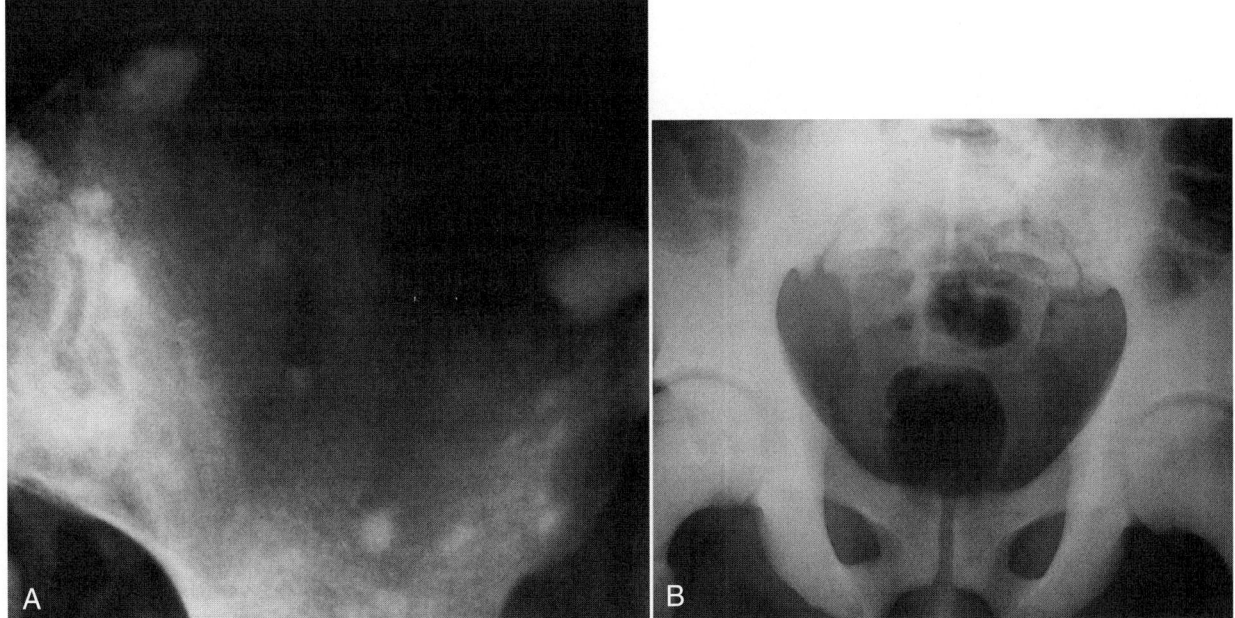

**Figure 51–13.** Mastocytosis: radiographic abnormalities in extraspinal sites. *A*, Observe the multiple focal, well-defined osteosclerotic lesions in the hemipelvis. *B*, In a different patient, diffuse osteosclerosis of the entire pelvis and proximal ends of the femora is evident.

terize marrow involvement in this disease. The high signal intensity of affected sites in T2-weighted spin echo and STIR images may be more profound than that seen in lymphomas, leukemias, plasma cell myeloma, and myelofibrosis, although such altered signal intensity is not uniformly seen (Fig. 51–14).

## Differential Diagnosis

The skeletal manifestations of systemic mastocytosis are nonspecific (Table 51–3). The diffuse osteopenia in this disease is nearly identical to that in osteoporosis, osteomalacia, hyperparathyroidism, and plasma cell myeloma. The diffuse lesions in systemic mastocytosis can simulate

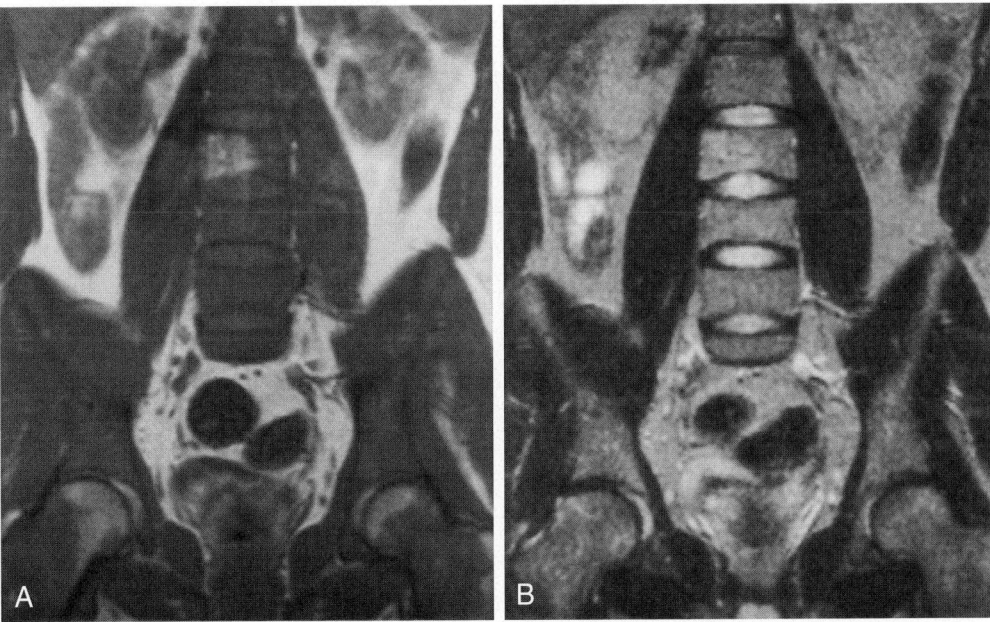

**Figure 51–14.** Mastocytosis: MR imaging abnormalities. Coronal T1-weighted (TR/TE, 550/25) *(A)* and T2-weighted (TR/TE, 2200/90) *(B)* spin echo MR images show marrow infiltration in the spine and osseous pelvis, as well as the proximal portions of the femora, manifested as low signal intensity in *(A)* and intermediate signal intensity (similar to that of fat) in *(B)*. (Courtesy of J. Kramer, MD, Vienna, Austria.)

**TABLE 51–3**

**Differential Diagnosis of Osteosclerosis**

| | Skeletal Metastasis | Mastocytosis | Myelofibrosis | Lymphomas | Paget's Disease | Fluorosis | Renal Osteodystrophy | Axial Osteomalacia |
|---|---|---|---|---|---|---|---|---|
| Distribution | Axial > appendicular | Axial > appendicular | Axial > appendicular | Axial > appendicular | Axial > appendicular | Axial > appendicular | Axial > appendicular | Axial |
| Diffuse sclerosis | + | + | + | + | + | + | + | + |
| Focal sclerosis | + | + | – | + | + | – | – | – |
| Osteopenia or bone lysis | + | + | + | + | + | – | + | – |
| Bony enlargement | – | – | – | – | + | – | – | – |
| Osteophytosis, ligament ossification | – | – | – | – | – | + | – | – |
| Splenomegaly | – | + | + | + | – | – | – | – |

+, common; – uncommon or rare.

the appearance of osteoporosis, sickle cell anemia, Gaucher's disease, and plasma cell myeloma. Diffuse osteosclerosis is observed not only in systemic mastocytosis but also in myelofibrosis, skeletal metastasis, fluorosis, Paget's disease, renal osteodystrophy, and numerous other conditions. The multiple focal osteosclerotic lesions in systemic mastocytosis resemble the findings in skeletal metastasis and tuberous sclerosis.

## POLYCYTHEMIA VERA

### General Features

Polycythemia vera (primary polycythemia), a disease of unknown cause characterized by hyperplasia of all the cellular elements in the bone marrow (primarily erythrocytes), results in an elevated red blood cell count, leukocytosis, and thrombocytosis. Polycythemia vera occurs in middle-aged or elderly patients. Clinical complaints include headache, dizziness, weakness, fatigue, paresthesias, dyspnea, and visual disturbances. On physical examination, a ruddy complexion, hepatosplenomegaly, and systolic hypertension are seen. Vascular thrombosis is a recognized complication of the disease that is related to thrombocytosis and increased blood viscosity. Occlusion of hepatic veins (Budd-Chiari syndrome) and cirrhosis of the liver may be evident. In the later stages of the disease, myelofibrosis, progressive myeloid metaplasia, and anemia are encountered.

### Musculoskeletal Abnormalities

Vascular thrombosis can lead to osteonecrosis, particularly of the femoral head, and generalized marrow hyperplasia can produce patchy radiolucent lesions throughout the bone. The cranial abnormalities may resemble those of thalassemia major. Myelofibrosis is associated with generalized increased radiodensity of the skeleton. Extramedullary hematopoiesis is seen in later stages of the disease. Hyperuricemia is not infrequent in (primary) polycythemia vera or secondary polycythemia. Gouty arthritis has been estimated to occur in 5% to 8% of all cases.

## MYELOFIBROSIS

### General Features

Myelofibrosis is an uncommon disease associated with fibrotic or sclerotic bone marrow and extramedullary hematopoiesis. Its cause has not been precisely determined. Myelofibrosis is usually divided into two forms: primary (or idiopathic) and secondary. The basic pathologic finding is fibrosis of the bone marrow, which in some instances may replace almost the entire marrow tissue. Focal or diffuse areas of hypercellular marrow may be combined with trabecular thickening and overgrowth. The degree of bone marrow fibrosis is generally thought to indicate the severity of the disease process.

### Clinical Abnormalities

Myelofibrosis is usually a disease of middle-aged and elderly men and women. Most affected patients are in the sixth or seventh decade of life. The disease is generally insidious in onset. Symptoms include weakness, fatigue, weight loss, abdominal pain, anorexia, nausea, vomiting, and dyspnea. Physical signs may include abdominal swelling, hepatosplenomegaly, and purpura. Hematologic evaluation frequently reveals moderate to severe anemia, an increased number of nucleated red blood cells, leukocytosis, or leukopenia. The diagnosis is established by bone marrow biopsy. The prognosis of the disease is variable. Some patients die within a few months of the initial diagnosis, whereas others survive for a prolonged time.

### Musculoskeletal Abnormalities

The radiographic picture reflects the pathologic changes. In some instances, normal or osteopenic bone and osteolytic lesions are observed, but in general, osteosclerosis is the predominant radiographic pattern and is observed in 40% to 50% of patients in both the axial skeleton and the proximal ends of the long bones (Fig. 51–15). The bones altered most commonly are the spine, pelvis, skull, ribs, proximal end of the humerus, and proximal portion of the femur. The osseous structures may be uniformly dense or demonstrate small areas of relative radiolucency. In the long bones, cortical thickening may be observed and is predominantly due to endosteal sclerosis. This abnormality results in obliteration of the normal demarcation between cortical and medullary bone. In the spine, increased radiodensity or condensation of bone at the superior and inferior margins of the vertebral body (sandwich vertebrae) may be encountered. Extramedullary hematopoiesis in this condition can create lobulated, paravertebral intrathoracic masses.

### Articular Abnormalities

Hemarthrosis has been described in association with myeloproliferative disease and can be its initial manifestation. Impaired platelet function presumably contributes to the bleeding episodes. Fifty percent to 80% of patients have elevated serum or urinary uric acid levels. Secondary gout, which may antedate the diagnosis of myelofibrosis, occurs in 5% to 20% of patients and may be associated with tophi and renal uric acid stones. The polyarthralgias and polyarthritis in myelofibrosis may resemble rheumatoid arthritis.

### Magnetic Resonance Imaging

Fibrotic replacement of the marrow, when examined with standard spin echo MR sequences, is characterized by decreased signal intensity on both T1- and T2-weighted images. Regions of intermediate to high signal intensity at sites of marrow involvement have been described with STIR imaging and after intravenous gadolinium administration. A focal or diffuse pattern of alteration in signal intensity may be encountered. MR imaging abnormalities are evident in the vertebrae, pelvis, and ribs (Fig. 51–16). Subsequent pathologic events, such as reconversion from fatty to hematopoietic marrow and marrow fibrosis, occur in the tubular bones, especially the femur, humerus, and

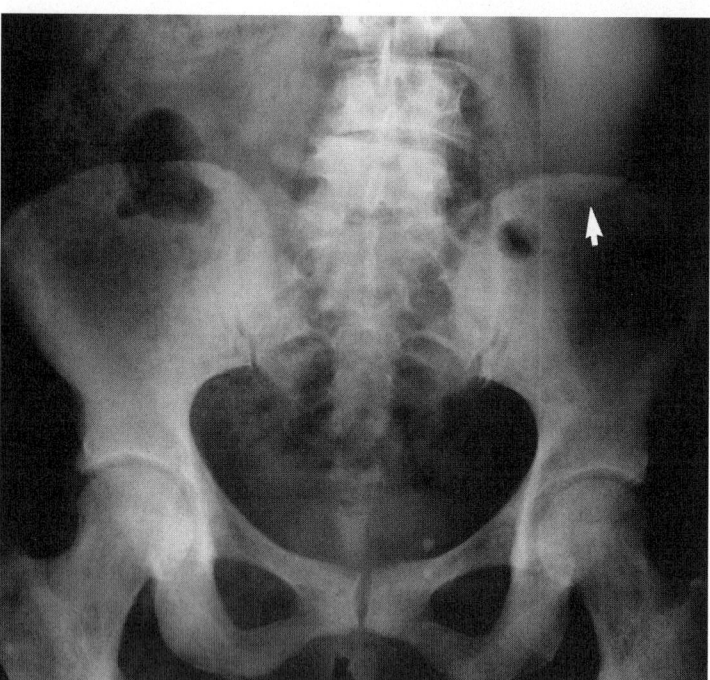

**Figure 51–15.** Myelofibrosis: radiographic abnormalities. Patchy osteosclerosis of the entire pelvis is associated with small radiolucent areas. The spleen is enlarged (*arrow*).

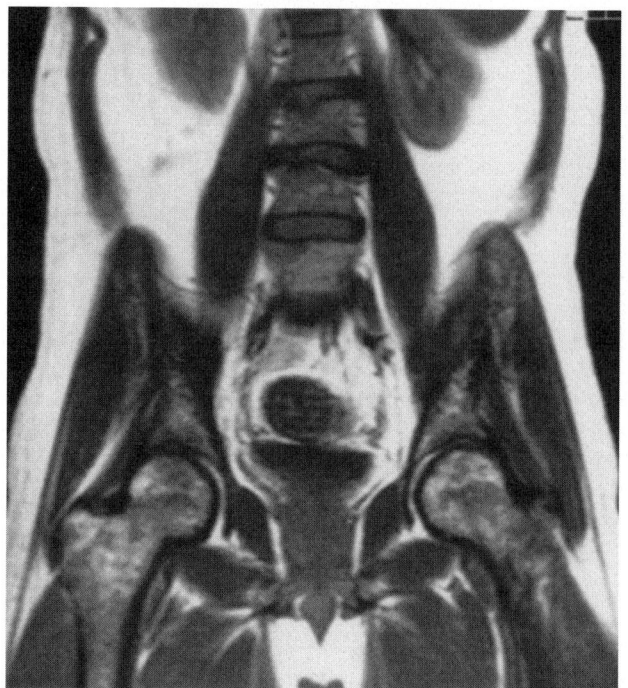

**Figure 51–16.** Myelofibrosis: MR imaging abnormalities in the axial skeleton. On a coronal T1-weighted (TR/TE, 650/30) spin echo MR image of the pelvis, the marrow of the vertebral bodies, pelvic bones, and proximal ends of the femora is predominantly low in signal intensity. This pattern is consistent with the presence of hematopoietic marrow or fibrosis. Schmorl's nodes are evident, and the spleen is enlarged. (Courtesy of T. Mattsson, MD, Riyadh, Saudi Arabia.)

tibia, and they account for the same pattern of signal abnormality encountered in the axial skeleton. In-phase and chemical shift opposed-phase spin echo MR sequences may be a useful adjunct in evaluating the presence of non-fatty marrow in the femoral neck and intertrochanteric region, findings considered abnormal in middle-aged and elderly individuals.

## Differential Diagnosis

The radiographic diagnosis of myelofibrosis should be suggested when axial skeleton osteosclerosis is combined with splenomegaly in a middle-aged or elderly patient (see Table 51–3). Although lymphoma and leukemia can lead to splenomegaly, the extent of the bone sclerosis is less in these conditions than in myelofibrosis. Systemic mastocytosis can produce diffuse or focal osteosclerosis and hepatosplenomegaly, and it may be difficult to distinguish this condition from myelofibrosis.

Increased radiodensity of bone without splenic enlargement may be seen in some patients with myelofibrosis and is apparent in patients with this disorder who have had splenectomies. This combination of findings may be evident in other processes as well, including skeletal metastasis, fluorosis, Paget's disease, axial osteomalacia, and renal osteodystrophy. Differentiation of myelofibrosis and skeletal metastasis can be difficult. In most cases, the sclerosis observed in metastatic disease of the bone is less generalized, less symmetrical, and more frequently associated with osteolytic lesions. In fluorosis, spinal osteophytosis, ligament calcification and ossification, and periostitis may be noted. In renal osteodystrophy, other changes are evident, including those of hyperparathyroidism. In Paget's disease, a characteristic coarsened trabecular pattern is present.

# BONE MARROW TRANSPLANTATION

Bone marrow transplantation is a technique for replenishing the bone marrow with normal pluripotential stem cells. Normal marrow cells from a histocompatible allogeneic donor are used to repopulate the diseased marrow, and such transplantation is frequently combined with intensive chemotherapy or immunosuppressive therapy. The marrow is usually obtained from the donor's iliac crest.

Infections developing immediately before or soon after bone marrow transplantation relate to the effects of chemotherapy and radiation therapy, as well as the transplantation itself. Bacterial and fungal infections dominate in the pretransplantation period, and viral infections may also be encountered. During the first 2 or 3 weeks after transplantation, severe granulocytopenia, fever, and, in about 50% of patients, at least one episode of bacteremia are seen. Neutropenia at this time predisposes to infections caused by opportunistic organisms. Delayed post-transplantation infections are usually related to varicella-zoster virus or recurrent bacterial or fungal infections.

Graft-versus-host disease, which is discussed in detail in Chapter 24, is believed to be the result of allogeneic T cells that were transfused with the graft or that developed from its reaction to targets of the genetically different host. An immunologic attack on the recipient's tissues develops. Acute graft-versus host disease occurs within the first 3 months after transplantation and is associated with lesions of the skin, liver, and gastrointestinal tract. Specific clinical findings include an erythematous maculopapular skin rash on the face, trunk, and extremities, as well as abdominal pain, diarrhea, nausea, and vomiting. Chronic graft-versus-host disease affects 20% to 40% of patients who survive more than 6 months after transplantation. It involves the skin, oral mucosa, serosal surfaces, skeletal muscle, gastrointestinal tract, liver, and lung, and its manifestations resemble those of a collagen vascular disorder, particularly scleroderma.

Chemotherapy and radiotherapy administered in the pretransplantation period are designed not only to induce immunologic suppression in the recipient but also to eliminate any residual malignant cell populations. The initial response of the bone marrow to such therapy is congestion and edema. Subsequently, hematopoietic tissue disappears, and the marrow becomes predominantly fatty. High signal intensity is observed on T1-weighted spin echo MR images, and intermediate signal intensity is seen on T2-weighted spin echo images, signal characteristics that are typical of adipose tissue. During transplantation, bone marrow cells are infused intravenously. After transient residence in the lungs and spleen, the infused stem cells migrate to the bone marrow. Hematologic engrafting typically takes 3 to 4 weeks and is heralded by a peripheral rise in granulocytes. Repopulation of the bone marrow in the spine after transplantation can be studied with MR imaging. On T1-weighted spin echo MR images, the superior and inferior margins of the vertebral bodies reveal low signal intensity, whereas the central portion of the vertebral bodies show high signal intensity, consistent with fat. With STIR sequences, the opposite situation is apparent, with high signal intensity at the superior and inferior vertebral margins and low signal intensity centrally. At histologic examination, the marginal, or peripheral, regions of the vertebral body are found to contain a concentrated collection of repopulating cells, and the central region contains predominantly marrow fat.

# FURTHER READING

Amano Y, Onda M, Amano M, et al: Magnetic resonance imaging of myelofibrosis: STIR and gadolinium-enhanced MR images. Clin Imaging 21:264, 1997.

Avila NA, Ling A, Metcalfe D, et al: Mastocytosis: Magnetic resonance imaging pattern of marrow disease. Skeletal Radiol 27:119, 1998.

Bloch KJ, Buchanan WW, Whol MJ, et al: Sjögren's syndrome: A clinical, pathological and serological study of sixty-two cases. Medicine 44:187, 1965.

Braunstein EM, White SJ: Non-Hodgkin's lymphoma of bone. Radiology 135:59, 1980.

Chew FS, Schellingerhout D, Keel SB: Primary lymphoma of skeletal muscle. AJR Am J Roentgenol 172:1370, 1999.

Coles WC, Schulz MD: Bone involvement in malignant lymphoma. Radiology 50:458, 1948.

Dalinka MK: Primary lymphoma of bone: Radiographic appearance and prognosis. Radiology 147:288, 1983.

Demanes DJ, Lane N, Beckstead JH: Bone involvement in hairy-cell leukemia. Cancer 49:1697, 1982.

Ferris RA, Hakkai HG, Cigtay OS: Radiologic manifestations of North American Burkitt's lymphoma. AJR Am J Roentgenol 123:614, 1975.

Glatt W, Weinstein A: Acropachy in lymphatic leukemia. Radiology 92:125, 1969.

Harris NL, Jaffe ES, Diebold J, et al: World Health Organization classification of neoplastic diseases of the hematopoietic and lymphoid tissues: Report of the clinical advisory committee meeting–Airlie House, Virginia, November 1997. J Clin Oncol 17:3835, 1999.

Kaplan KR, Mitchell DG, Steiner RM, et al: Polycythemia vera and myelofibrosis: Correlation of MR imaging, clinical, and laboratory findings. Radiology 183:329, 1992.

Lecouvet FE, Dechambre S, Malghem J, et al: Bone marrow transplantation in patients with multiple myeloma: Prognostic significance of MR imaging. AJR Am J Roentgenol 176:91, 2001.

Leigh TF, Corley CC Jr, Huguley CM Jr, et al: Myelofibrosis: The general and radiologic findings in 25 proven cases. AJR Am J Roentgenol 82:183, 1959.

McKenna MJ, Frame B: The mast cell and bone. Clin Orthop 200:226, 1985.

Metzler JP, Fleckenstein JL, Vuitch F, et al: Skeletal muscle lymphoma: MRI evaluation. Magn Reson Imaging 10:491, 1992.

Neiman RS, Barcos M, Berard C, et al: Granulocytic sarcoma: A clinicopathologic study of 61 biopsied cases. Cancer 48:1426, 1981.

Nixon GW, Gwinn JL: The roentgen manifestations of leukemia in infancy. Radiology 107:603, 1973.

Olson DO, Schields AF, Scheurich CJ, et al: Magnetic resonance imaging of the bone marrow in patients with leukemia, aplastic anemia, and lymphoma. Invest Radiol 21:540, 1986.

O'Reilly GV, Clark TM, Crum CP: Skeletal involvement in mycosis fungoides. AJR Am J Roentgenol 129:741, 1977.

Parker BR, Marglin S, Castellino RA: Skeletal manifestations of leukemia, Hodgkin disease and non-Hodgkin lymphoma. Semin Roentgenol 15:302, 1980.

Patzik SB, Smith C, Kubicka RA, et al: Bone marrow transplantation: Clinical and radiologic aspects. Radiographics 11:601, 1991.

Pettigrew JD, Ward HP: Correlation of radiologic, histologic and clinical findings in agnogenic myeloid metaplasia. Radiology 93:541, 1969.

Phillips WC, Kattapuram SV, Doseretz DE, et al: Primary lymphoma of bone: Relationship of radiographic appearance and prognosis. Radiology 144:285, 1982.

Poppel MH, Gruber WF, Silber R, et al: The roentgen manifestations of urticaria pigmentosa (mastocytosis). AJR Am J Roentgenol 82:239, 1959.

Rafii M, Firooznia H, Golimbu C, et al: Pathologic fracture in systemic mastocytosis: Radiographic spectrum and review of the literature. Clin Orthop 180:260, 1983.

Schabel SI, Tyminski L, Holland RD, et al: The skeletal manifestations of chronic myelogenous leukemia. Skeletal Radiol 5:145, 1980.

Schwartz AM, Leonidas JC: Methotrexate osteopathy. Skeletal Radiol 11:13, 1984.

Silbiger ML, Peterson CC Jr: Sjögren's syndrome: Its roentgenographic features. AJR Am J Roentgenol 100:554, 1967.

Simmons CR, Harle TS, Singleton EB: The osseous manifestations of leukemia in children. Radiol Clin North Am 6:115, 1968.

Talbott JH: Gout and blood dyscrasias. Medicine 38:173, 1959.

Vogler JB III, Murphy WA: Bone marrow imaging. Radiology 168:679, 1988.

White LM, Schweitzer ME, Khalili K, et al: MR imaging of primary lymphoma of bone: Variability of T2-weighted signal intensity. AJR Am J Roentgenol 170:1243, 1998.

# CHAPTER 52

## Bleeding Disorders

## SUMMARY OF KEY FEATURES

The skeletal abnormalities associated with hemophilia and other bleeding diatheses are characteristic. They result from hemorrhage in soft tissue, muscle, and subperiosteal, intraosseous, and intra-articular locations. In involved joints, typical findings are radiodense effusions, regional or periarticular osteoporosis, subchondral bony erosions and cysts, and joint space narrowing. Hyperemia may lead to epiphyseal overgrowth in a child affected by these disorders. Tumor-like lesions are occasionally encountered that are due to massive subperiosteal, osseous, or soft tissue hemorrhage, with erosion and distortion of adjacent bone. Hemosiderin deposition in any of these disorders leads to characteristic findings on magnetic resonance imaging. The differential diagnosis is usually not difficult when both clinical and imaging features are studied.

## INTRODUCTION

Hemophilia is a term applied to a group of disorders characterized by an anomaly of blood coagulation caused by a deficiency in a specific plasma clotting factor. This anomaly leads to easy bruising and prolonged and excessive bleeding. Of these disorders, two are associated most commonly with intraosseous and intra-articular bleeding: classic hemophilia (hemophilia A), characterized by a functional deficiency of antihemophilic factor (factor VIII), and Christmas disease (hemophilia B), marked by a functional deficiency of plasma thromboplastin component (factor IX). These two types of hemophilia are X-linked recessive disorders that are clinically manifested in men and carried by women. Rarely, other disorders of blood coagulation may manifest as bone and joint abnormalities. One such disorder is von Willebrand's disease, a rare familial disease of both men and women that apparently is attributable to a dominant autosomal mutant gene; in this disease, both factor VIII and functional platelet abnormalities occur.

## HEMOPHILIA

### Clinical Abnormalities

Classic hemophilia occurs in approximately 1 of every 10,000 men and boys in the United States. Christmas disease occurs about one tenth as often as classic hemophilia. Although both forms are confined almost exclusively to male subjects, reports exist of significant clinical and radiographic abnormalities in female patients. The severity of the clinical manifestations in either form of hemophilia varies. In mild forms of disease, excessive bleeding may be apparent only during surgery. With moderate or severe forms, bleeding episodes may also occur spontaneously or after minor or significant trauma. The diagnosis is established by performing appropriate laboratory tests to detect defects in blood coagulation.

Hemarthrosis is a particularly characteristic abnormality, occurring in approximately 75% to 90% of patients. It may begin in the early years of life, and young children and adolescents demonstrate more frequent episodes of joint bleeding than adults do. The joints altered most commonly are the knee, elbow, ankle, hip, and glenohumeral joint, in descending order of frequency. Joints such as the knee, whose stability depends on adjacent soft tissue structures rather than intrinsic factors, are particularly vulnerable. Usually a single joint is involved in each episode, although eventually multiple joints are affected. Joint involvement may be markedly asymmetrical or even unilateral.

Clinical manifestations of hemophilic arthropathy can be divided into three types, although they are not rigidly defined:

1. *Acute hemarthrosis.* Joint bleeding may occur rapidly, producing a tense, swollen, red, and tender articulation that is painful and stiff. Associated muscle spasm leads to flexion of the extremity and restricted motion. Symptoms decrease quickly after administration of the appropriate clotting factor.

2. *Subacute hemarthrosis.* After multiple acute episodes, complete recovery of the joint is not evident. Joint motion is restricted, a finding that appears to best correlate with the degree of cartilaginous destruction, and contractures and muscle atrophy become evident.

3. *Chronic hemarthrosis.* After 6 months to 1 year, a chronic stage may develop. More severe and persistent contractures are found, particularly in the elbow and knee. The final stage is a fibrotic, contracted, and destroyed joint. Approximately 50% of hemophilic patients develop permanent changes in the peripheral joints.

Articular bleeding may be accompanied by hemorrhage into muscles, fascial planes, and bones. Soft tissue bleeding can lead to fixed joint deformities and soft tissue necrosis. Compartment syndromes may complicate intramuscular bleeding in the upper or lower extremities. The most common of these in hemophilia are Volkmann's contractures, related to massive hemorrhage into the volar muscles of the forearm. Hemorrhage in and around the spinal cord can lead to neurologic abnormalities. Subperiosteal and intraosseous bleeding can induce trabecular distortion and destruction, and large expansile lesions, particularly of the femur and ilium (hemophilic pseudotumors), may simulate neoplasm.

### Pathologic Abnormalities

After an acute episode of intra-articular bleeding, blackish fluid containing clots is apparent. With each recurring episode of bleeding, resorption of blood is less complete and more permanent findings are apparent, particularly in the synovial membrane, with brownish discoloration caused by the absorption of blood pigment. Synovial villi become more numerous and enlarged, and the entire membrane thickens. The subsynovial tissue undergoes dense fibrous proliferation. Marginal cartilaginous erosion appears adjacent to synovial pannus, and eventually numerous small or large serrated erosions are scattered throughout the cartilaginous surface. Loss of the subchondral bone plate occurs, so that the calcified layer of cartilage rests on the cancellous bone. Trabecular thinning and resorption lead to enlarging subchondral cysts. Osseous cystic lesions are particularly prominent in this disease. Productive changes may appear, with sclerotic trabeculae and osteophytes (Table 52–1; Fig. 52–1).

Massive periosteal or intraosseous hemorrhage creates neoplastic-like lesions called hemophilic pseudotumors (Fig. 52–2). In subperiosteal locations, the periosteal membrane is lifted from the parent bone, and hemorrhage may extend into the adjacent soft tissues. Periosteal bone formation follows, creating expanded and irregular osseous contours. In intraosseous locations, large defects with geographic (relatively well-defined) bone destruction may be seen. In the immature skeleton, chronic hyperemia of the epiphyseal cartilage can produce accelerated maturation and enlargement of epiphyses.

## Radiographic Abnormalities

### General Features

The findings of hemophilia have been divided into five stages on the basis of a variety of radiographic abnormalities: (1) soft tissue swelling, (2) osteoporosis, (3) osseous subchondral cystic lesions, (4) narrowing of the interosseous space with cartilage destruction, and (5) joint disorganization with severe cartilaginous and osseous abnormalities. The division of the radiographic changes into stages

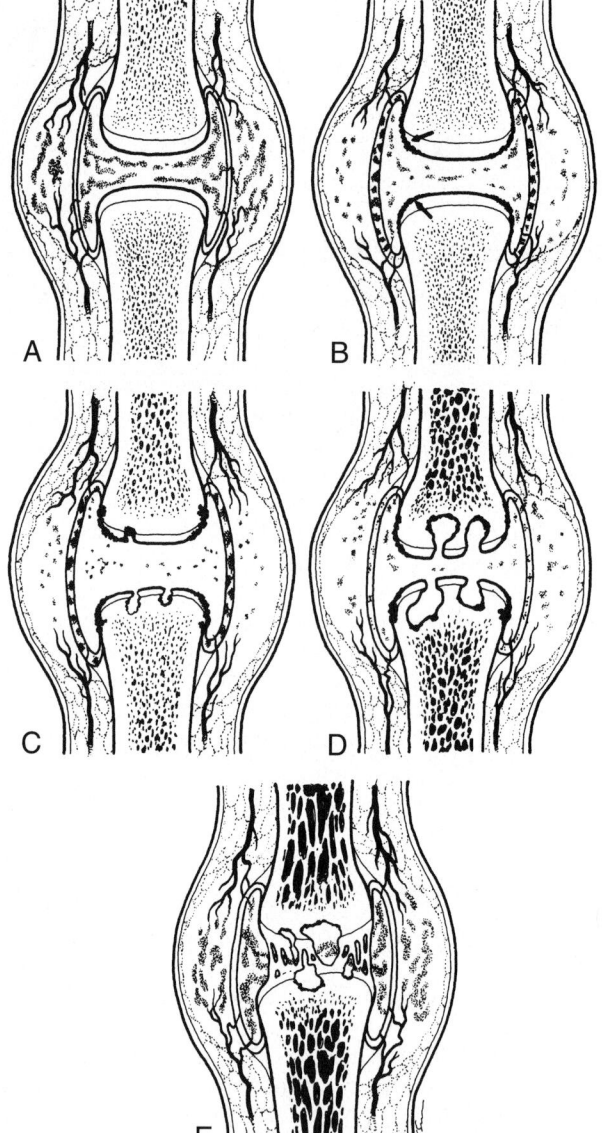

**Figure 52–1.** Hemophilia: pathologic abnormalities—intra-articular findings. *A,* Acute episodes of bleeding lead to accumulation of blood in the articular cavity and periarticular soft tissues. *B,* After numerous bleeding episodes, absorption of blood is incomplete from the articular cavity and soft tissues. Brownish discoloration of the synovial membrane is associated with hypertrophy and hyperemia. Synovial inflammatory tissue, or pannus, appears at the margins of the articular cartilage *(arrows). C,* At a later stage, periarticular osteoporosis and focal areas of cartilage and osseous destruction become apparent. Cystic lesions are evident, which generally communicate with the joint cavity. Note areas of relatively normal cartilage and bone. *D,* Continued destruction of cartilage and bone leads to enlarging cystic lesions, surface irregularities, osteoporosis, and joint space narrowing. *E,* In late stages of the disease, fibrous adhesions extend across the articular space. New episodes of bleeding occur.

---

**TABLE 52–1**

**Hemophilia: Radiographic-Pathologic Correlation**

| Pathology | Radiology |
| --- | --- |
| Recurrent intra-articular hemorrhage with hemosiderin-laden hypertrophied synovial membrane | Radiodense joint effusions |
| Synovial inflammation and pannus formation; hyperemia | Osteoporosis; epiphyseal overgrowth; accelerated skeletal maturation |
| Cartilaginous erosion; subchondral trabecular resorption and collapse | Bony erosions and cysts |
| Cartilaginous denudation | Joint space narrowing |
| Bony proliferation | Sclerosis and osteophytosis |
| Soft tissue, superiosteal, and intraosseous hemorrhage | Pseudotumors |

(see Fig. 52–1) does not imply that all cases follow this sequence of events. Further, radiographic abnormalities do not always develop in a systematic fashion. Although bone change usually precedes cartilage loss, this is not

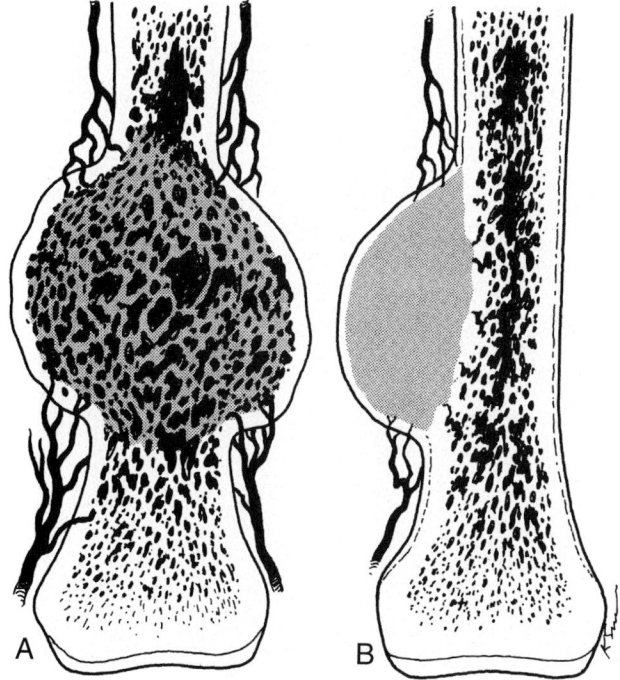

**Figure 52–2.** Hemophilia: pathologic abnormalities—intraosseous (A) and subperiosteal (B) hemorrhage. These types of hemorrhage can lead to hemophilic pseudotumors, with destruction and deformity of bone.

always the case. In some patients, articular involvement never progresses beyond the first or second stage; in other patients, despite appropriate medical or surgical therapy, severe arthropathy develops.

## Distribution of Abnormalities

The knee, ankle, and elbow are the joints involved most frequently. Bilateral involvement is common, but the changes need not be symmetrical.

**Knee.** The knee is affected most often (Fig. 52–3). Dense joint effusions are common. Periarticular osteoporosis creates lucent epiphyses of both the distal end of the femur and the proximal part of the tibia. Irregularity of the articular surface of the femoral condyles, the tibial plateaus, and the posterior surface of the patella may become apparent. Multiple subchondral cysts are frequent and sometimes grow to a large size.

Overgrowth of the distal femoral and proximal tibial epiphyses may result. The distal condylar surface may appear flattened, and the intercondylar notch of the femur is commonly widened. Squaring of the inferior pole of the patella has been detected in as many as 20% to 30% of patients with hemophilia. However, squaring of the patella is not specific for hemophilia, being a recognized manifestation of juvenile chronic arthritis. Differentiation between these two disorders on the basis of knee radiographs is very difficult.

**Ankle.** The radiographic findings in the ankle are similar to those in other involved joints, including soft tissue swelling, osteoporosis, marginal and central osseous erosions, and joint space narrowing (Fig. 52–4). Tibiotalar slanting may be observed, creating an angular joint surface, a finding observed in epiphyseal dysplasias, juvenile chronic arthritis, and perhaps sickle cell anemia. Bony ankylosis of the subtalar joints has also been described in hemophilia. Osteonecrosis of the talus may be observed.

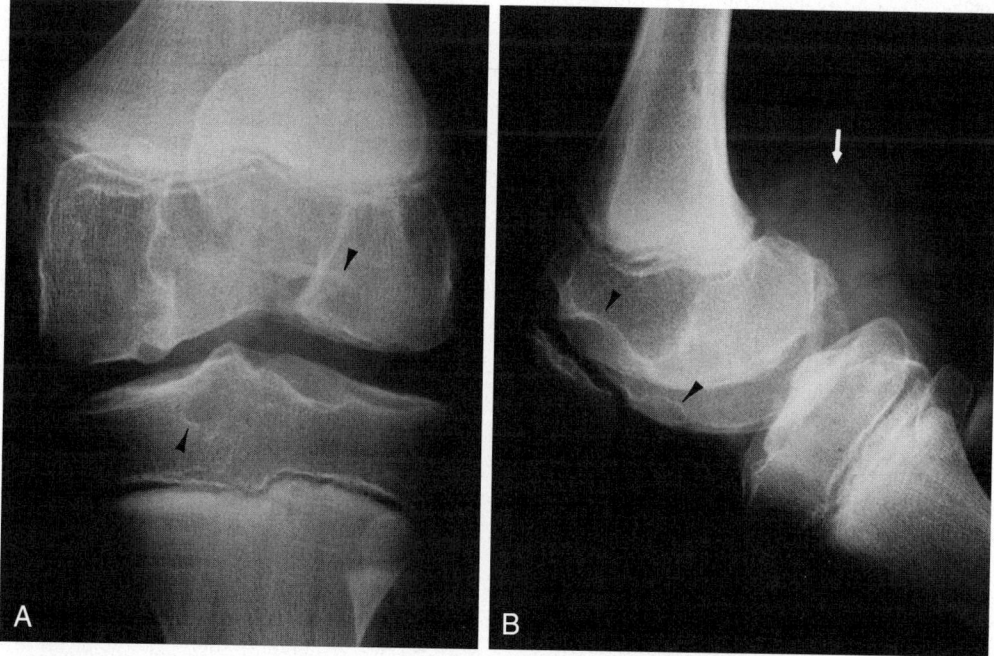

**Figure 52–3.** Hemophilia: knee joint abnormalities. Frontal (A) and lateral (B) radiographs demonstrate characteristic findings of hemophilia. The bones are mildly osteoporotic, and the epiphyses are enlarged. Note the well-defined or "etched" erosions of subchondral bone (arrowheads), the radiodense joint effusion (arrow), and the widened intercondylar notch of the femur.

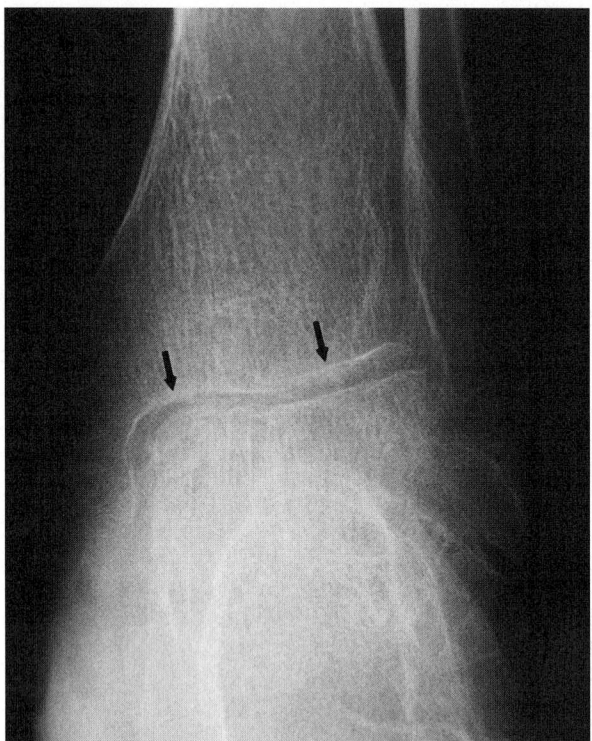

**Figure 52–4.** Hemophilia: ankle joint abnormalities. Extensive abnormalities in the ankle include osteoporosis and joint space narrowing. Note the tibiotalar slant with an angular joint surface *(arrows)*.

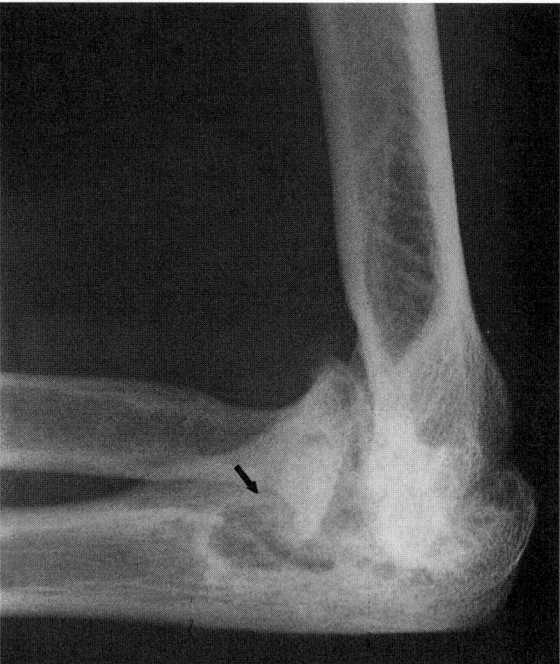

**Figure 52–5.** Hemophilia: elbow joint abnormalities. Observe sclerosis, flattening, and deformity of the bones. The radial head is widened. Note the enlargement of the radial fossa *(arrow)*.

**Elbow.** Radiodense effusion, osteoporosis, and cartilaginous and osseous destruction are evident in the elbow in hemophilia (Fig. 52–5). The trochlear and radial notches of the ulna are frequently widened, and the radial head may be enlarged.

**Other Joints.** Typical hemophilic abnormalities may be apparent in other joints, including the hip, glenohumeral joint, and small articulations of the hand and foot.

### Additional Abnormalities

Several other abnormalities may be associated with hemophilia.

**Osteonecrosis.** Epiphyseal fragmentation and collapse may be apparent in hemophilia. These findings appear to be related to intraosseous bleeding, with subsequent collapse of bone, or to intracapsular bleeding, with elevation of intra-articular pressure, vascular occlusion, and subsequent osteonecrosis. These changes are particularly common in the femoral head and talus (Fig. 52–6).

**Ectopic Ossification.** Ossification may appear in periarticular soft tissue (Fig. 52–7). This complication is most frequently apparent in the lower half of the body, particularly in the pelvis, where ossification extending from the lateral aspect of the ilium or ischium to the proximal end of the femur may be observed.

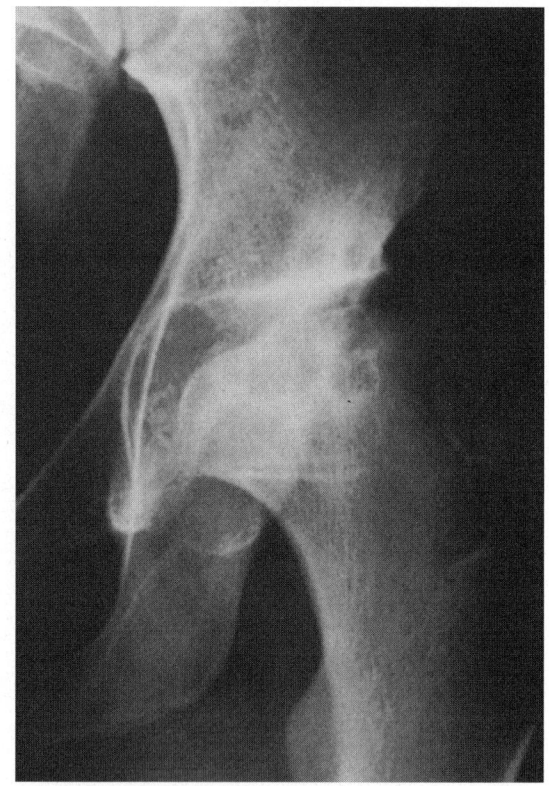

**Figure 52–6.** Hemophilia: osteonecrosis of the hip. Intra-articular bleeding can produce osteonecrosis of the femoral head. Findings include considerable flattening of the femoral head, subchondral cysts, mild joint space narrowing, and acetabular deformity.

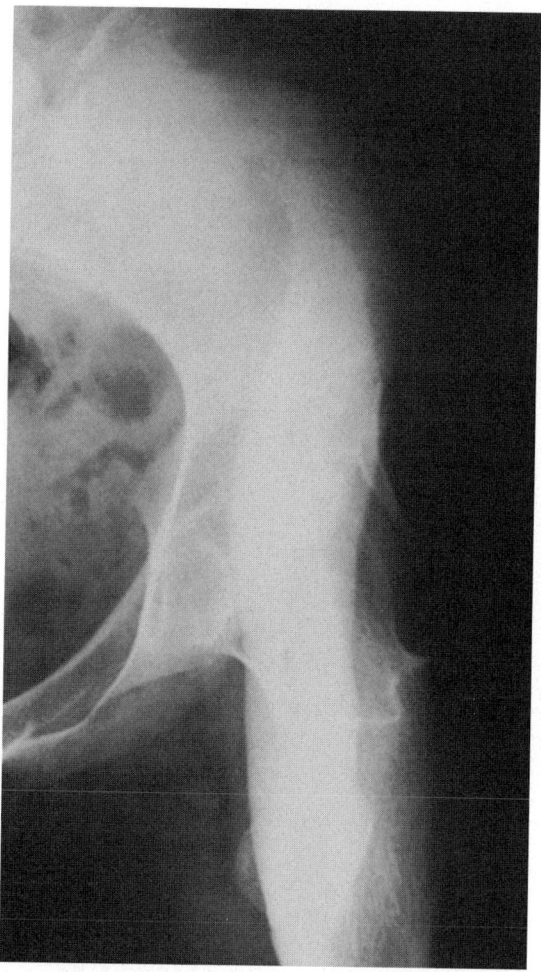

**Figure 52–7.** Hemophilia: ectopic ossification. A large band of ossification extends from the lateral aspect of the ilium to the proximal portion of the femur. (Courtesy of M. Dalinka, MD, Philadelphia, Pa.)

**Fractures.** In hemophilia, fractures may occur spontaneously or after minor trauma. Fracture healing in hemophilic patients proceeds normally, although pseudotumors may develop at the site of fracture.

**Hemophilic Pseudotumor.** Hemophilic pseudotumor is a relatively uncommon manifestation of the disease, probably occurring in less than 2% of cases. The bones that are implicated most frequently, in descending order of frequency, are the femur, the components of the osseous pelvis, the tibia, and the small bones of the hands. Pseudotumors may be intraosseous or subperiosteal, or they may occur within the soft tissues. It is probable that pseudotumors arise from hemorrhage.

Medullary bone destruction may produce small or large central or eccentric radiolucent lesions that are fairly well demarcated. Trabeculae can extend across the lesions, and the surrounding bone is frequently sclerotic. Cortical violation and periosteal bone formation may reach considerable proportions. A large soft tissue mass may be encountered. Mild, moderate, or massive bleeding may occur in subperiosteal locations. In the immature skeleton, the periosteum is lifted easily by the accumulation of blood.

Cortical atrophy due to abnormal pressure, subperiosteal bone formation, and soft tissue extension are evident (Fig. 52–8). Tumors arising in the soft tissue enlarge slowly, develop a fibrous capsule, and distort the subjacent osseous tissue by pressure erosion. Soft tissue hemophilic pseudotumors are most common in the thigh and the gluteal region. Infrequently, the soft tissue masses calcify.

Initially, a subperiosteal hematoma in hemophilia produces periostitis that can simulate malignancy (Ewing's sarcoma, skeletal metastases) or infection. An intraosseous hematoma leading to osteolytic lesions of varying size simulates primary and secondary neoplasms, tumor-like lesions, and infection. In many patients, accurate diagnosis relies on knowledge of the patient's underlying disease.

**Other Articular Manifestations.** In hemophilia, joint contractures may complicate intra-articular destruction or soft tissue hemorrhage, with impingement on vessels and nerves.

### Scintigraphy

Increased sensitivity of the isotopic examination compared with clinical and radiographic evaluation is not unexpected, particularly at sites of acute arthropathy. The radionuclide examination lacks specificity, however, and it is less effective in evaluating joints with chronic arthropathy.

### Computed Tomography

Because hemophilic pseudotumors commonly arise in or extend to periosseous soft tissues, they are often well characterized by computed tomography. Soft tissue ossification in hemophilia is also well shown with this technique (Fig. 52–9).

### Magnetic Resonance Imaging

Spin echo magnetic resonance (MR) imaging sequences typically reveal regions in the joint with low to intermediate signal intensity on T1- and T2-weighted images, with foci of increased signal intensity on T2-weighted images. Persistent low signal intensity in both types of images is consistent with the presence of synovial fibrosis, hemosiderin deposition, or both (Fig. 52–10). The foci of high signal intensity on T2-weighted images are consistent with areas of synovial inflammation or fluid. Owing to the changing signal characteristics of resolving hemorrhage, it may be difficult to distinguish between viscous joint fluid and fresh blood with MR imaging in this disease. The intravenous administration of paramagnetic contrast agents, such as those containing gadolinium, may be useful in distinguishing among synovial inflammation, hemorrhage, and joint effusion. The MR imaging characteristics of hemosiderin deposition in this disease are similar to those seen in other disorders accompanied by recurrent episodes of intra-articular bleeding. Such processes include pigmented villonodular synovitis, neoplasms such as synovial hemangiomas, neuropathic osteoarthropathy, and chronic renal disease. Hemosiderin collections lead to low signal intensity on all spin echo

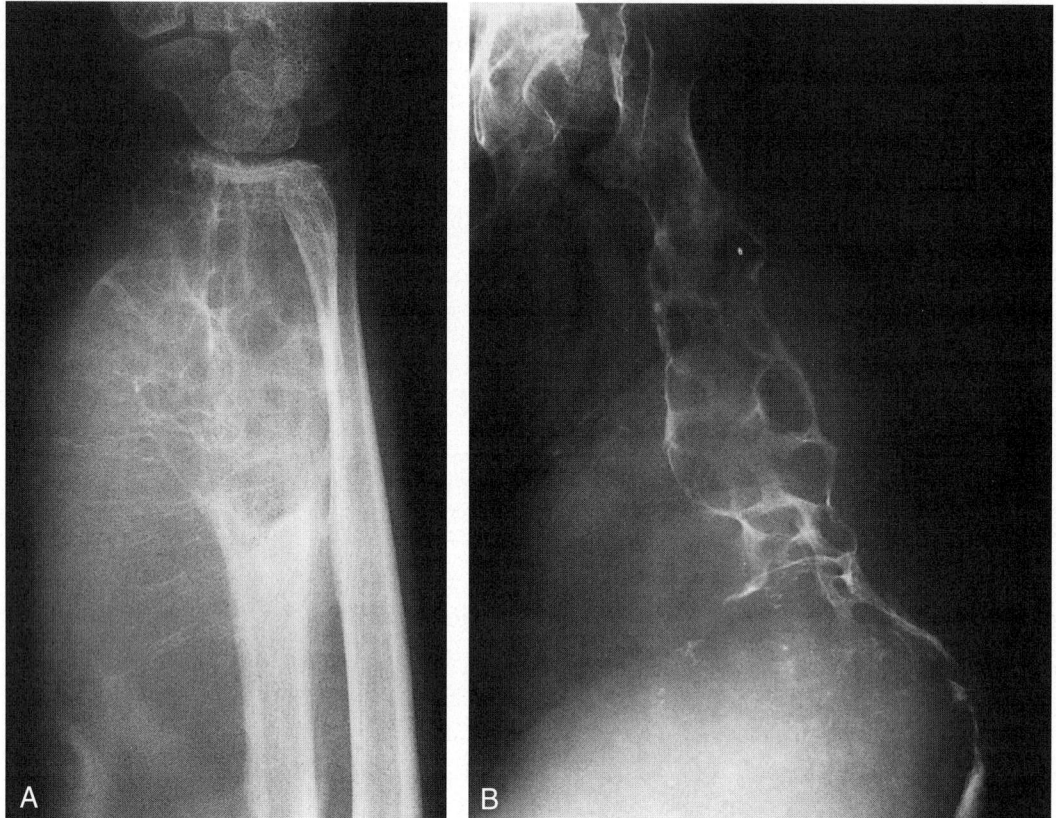

**Figure 52–8.** Hemophilia: pseudotumors. *A*, Radiograph of the forearm reveal a pseudotumor involving the distal portion of the radius. Note new bone formation extending into the soft tissues, with destruction and deformity of the underlying bone. *B*, Striking bone and soft tissue abnormalities may accompany bleeding in hemophilia. The deformed femur has a "cystic" appearance, and in places, its contour has been obliterated completely. The hip is also abnormal. (*A*, Courtesy of A. Brower, MD, Norfolk, Va.)

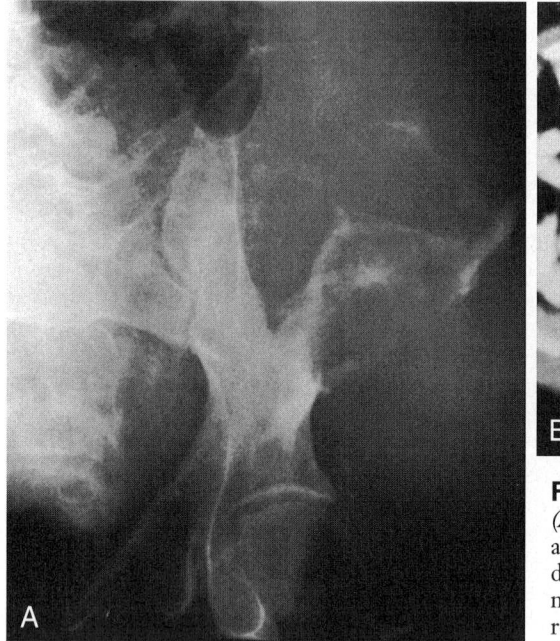

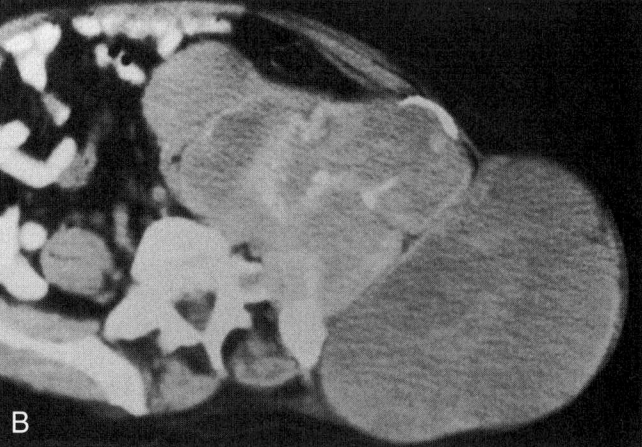

**Figure 52–9.** Hemophilia: pseudotumors. Routine radiography *(A)* and transaxial computed tomography *(B)* reveal both bone and soft tissue abnormalities. The extent of the process is better delineated with computed tomography, which shows a lobulated mass of low attenuation, a partial rim of higher attenuation, and residual and distorted trabeculae. (Courtesy of R. Cone, MD, San Antonio, Tex.)

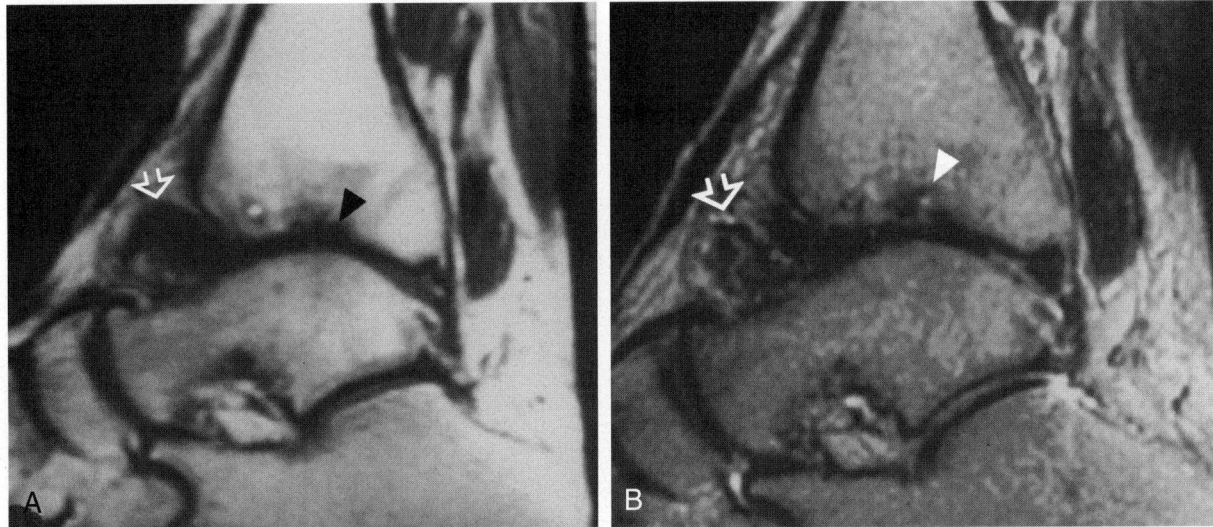

**Figure 52–10.** Hemophilia: MR imaging. *A*, Sagittal T1-weighted (TR/TE, 500/16) spin echo MR image shows anterior extension of the joint *(arrow)*. The intra-articular contents are of low signal intensity. Irregularity of the subchondral bone of the tibia is evident *(arrowhead)*. *B*, Sagittal T2-weighted (TR/TE, 2000/80) spin echo MR image shows persistent low signal intensity anteriorly, with peripheral regions of higher signal intensity *(arrow)*. Abnormal signal intensity is also seen in the tibia *(arrowhead)*. The articular findings indicate synovial fibrosis or hemosiderin deposition (low signal intensity) and inflammation (high signal intensity).

sequences and, to a greater degree, on all gradient echo sequences (Fig. 52–11).

Subchondral cystic lesions, a prominent feature of hemophilic arthropathy, can be evaluated with MR imaging. The signal characteristics of these cysts, however, are dependent on the precise imaging sequence used and the contents of the lesions. Fluid, fibrotic material, hemorrhage, or hemosiderin, in various combinations, may be present in the subchondral cysts, leading to inhomogeneity in signal intensity in some cases. Cysts with high signal intensity on both T1- and T2-weighted spin echo MR images are related to recent hemorrhage; those with low signal intensity on T1-weighted and high signal intensity on T2-weighted spin echo MR images contain nonhemorrhagic fluid; and those with low signal intensity in both types of MR images relate to the presence of fibrous tissue and hemosiderin (see Fig. 52–11).

The signal behavior of these pseudotumors is complex, reflecting the effects of remote and recurrent bleeding and clot organization. A peripheral margin of low signal intensity on T1- and T2-weighted spin echo MR sequences is consistent with the presence of fibrous tissue or hemosiderin, or both, in the wall of the pseudotumor. Less uniform, however, are the signal characteristics of the interior portions of the pseudotumor, which may reveal regions of either high or low signal intensity on one or both of these sequences. Intramuscular pseudotumors (as well as those in other locations) may reveal mural nodules (Fig. 52–12).

## Pathogenesis of Hemophilic Arthropathy

Generally, it is assumed that arthropathy in hemophilia results from intra-articular and periarticular hemorrhage.

In the synovial membrane, hypertrophy and inflammation, subsynovial fibrosis, and hemosiderin deposition are known responses to experimental hemarthrosis and resemble the findings in other articular disorders, particularly pigmented villonodular synovitis. Cartilaginous abnormalities occurring after hemarthrosis are less constant. The role of intra-articular iron deposits in the pathogenesis of hemophilic arthropathy is not clear. The osseous abnormalities in hemophilic joints may result from certain toxic and chemical effects on bone and elevation of intra-articular pressure (due to hemarthrosis) and intramarrow pressure (due to focal destruction of weight-bearing surfaces). Hyperemia may be responsible for epiphyseal overgrowth in hemophilia. Osteoporosis may relate to increased blood flow in capsular and epiphyseal blood vessels, as well as to disuse and immobilization.

## Differential Diagnosis

Hemarthrosis is not confined to hemophilic arthropathy. It is frequent after trauma, in other articular and nonarticular disorders such as scurvy or myeloproliferative disease, and after excessive administration of anticoagulant medication. In these other conditions, permanent cartilaginous and osseous findings resembling those of hemophilia are not encountered.

Articular abnormalities of hemophilia most resemble the changes of juvenile chronic arthritis (Table 52–2). It is often impossible to distinguish between these two disorders on the basis of radiographic abnormalities in a single joint. Rather, it is the distribution of articular abnormalities in hemophilia and juvenile-onset rheumatoid arthritis (and other forms of juvenile chronic arthritis) that permits an accurate radiographic diagnosis. In

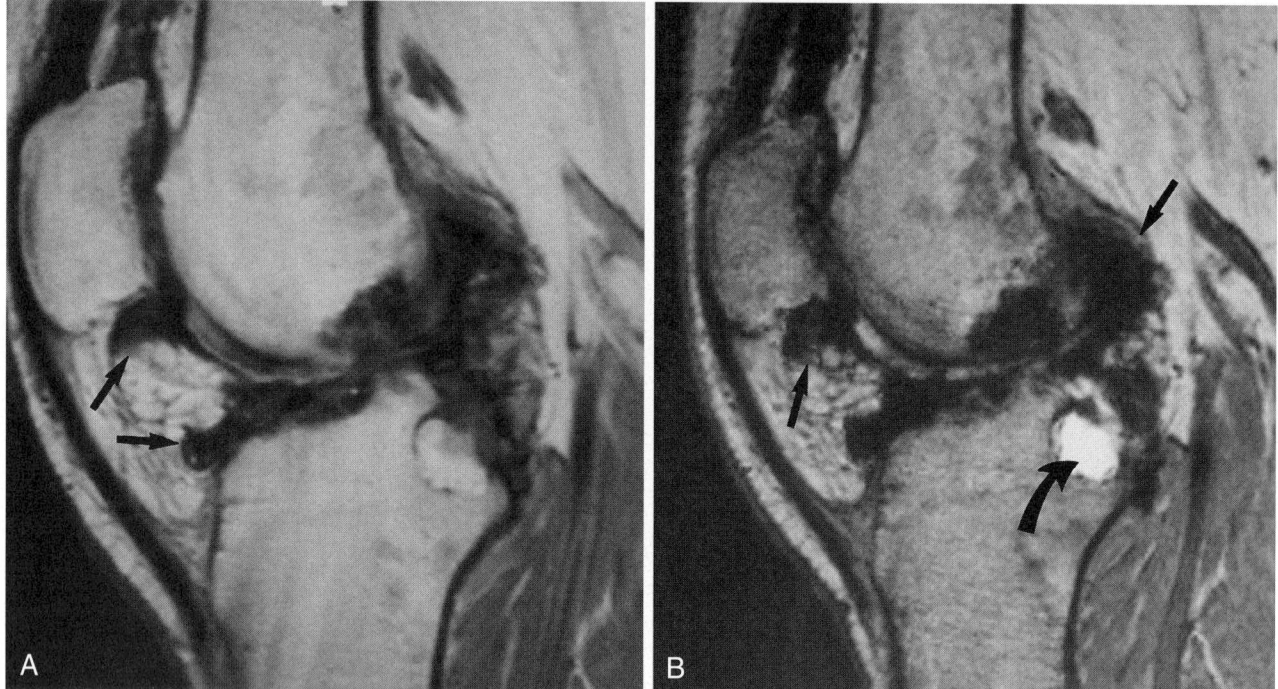

**Figure 52–11.** Hemophilia: MR imaging—hemosiderin deposition. *A*, Sagittal intermediate-weighted (TR/TE, 2100/20) spin echo MR image demonstrates synovial proliferation of low signal intensity extending into and distorting Hoffa's fat pad *(arrows)*. *B*, Sagittal T2-weighted three-dimensional (TR/TE, 30/10; flip angle, 40 degrees) gradient echo MR image demonstrates "blooming" of the hemosiderin within the synovium *(arrows)* and a posterior tibial cyst containing fluid or hemorrhage *(curved arrow)*.

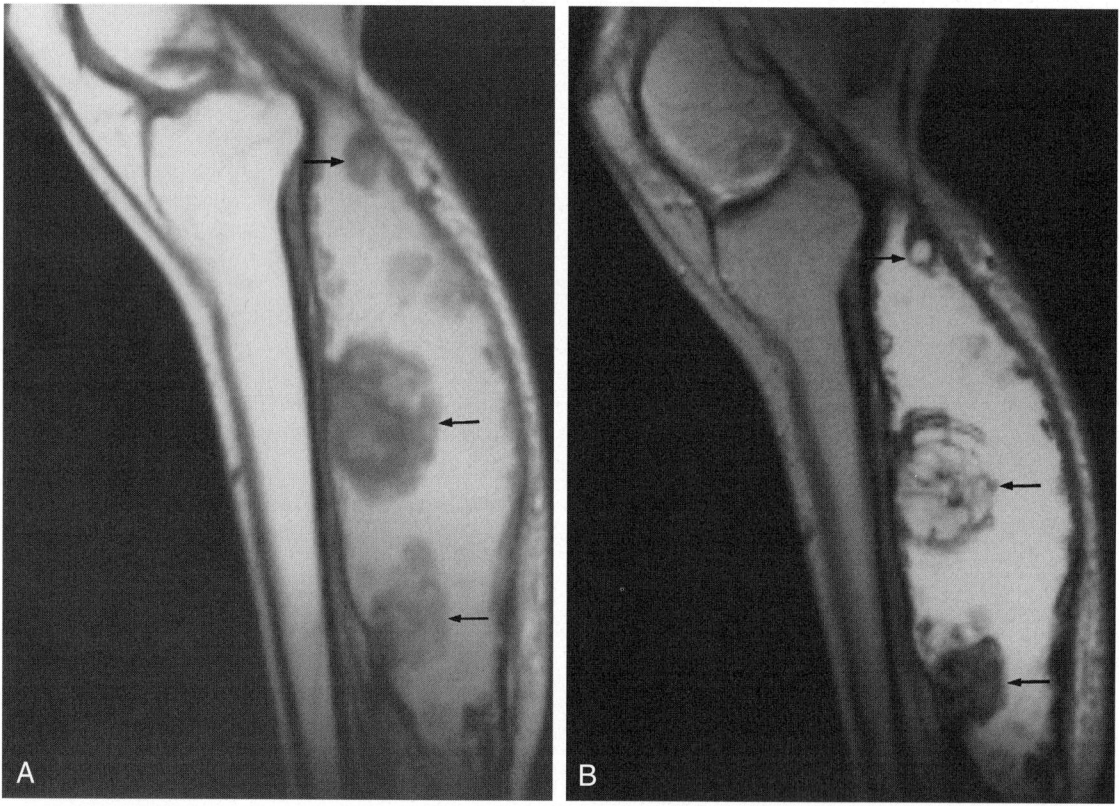

**Figure 52–12.** Hemophilia: MR imaging—pseudotumors. Sagittal T1-weighted (TR/TE, 600/20) *(A)* and T2-weighted (TR/TE, 1500/80) *(B)* spin echo MR images reveal a pseudotumor in the gastrocnemius muscle with an elliptic shape. Multiple various-sized lobulated nodules are seen attached to the capsule *(arrows)*, exhibiting heterogeneous signal intensity compatible with blood clots in various stages of organization. (From Jaovisidha S, Ryu KN, Hodler J, et al: Hemophilic pseudotumor: Spectrum of MR findings. Skeletal Radiol 26:468, 1997.)

**TABLE 52–2**

**Hemophilia versus Juvenile-Onset Rheumatoid Arthritis (JRA)**

|  | Hemophilia | JRA |
|---|---|---|
| Common articular sites | Knee, wrist, elbow | Knee, ankle, wrist, hand |
| Soft tissue swelling | + | + |
| Osteoporosis | + | + |
| Joint space narrowing | ± | ± |
| Bony ankylosis | − | + |
| Epiphyseal overgrowth | + | + |
| Growth inhibition | − | + |
| Epiphyseal collapse or osteonecrosis | + | + |
| Periostitis | ± | + |
| Pseudotumors | + | − |
| Spondylitis | − | + |

+, present; −, absent.

hemophilia, the knee, ankle, and elbow are altered most commonly; in juvenile-onset rheumatoid arthritis, the articulations of the hands and wrists, as well as the larger joints and the spine, may be affected.

In some joints, the findings of hemophilia may simulate those of pigmented villonodular synovitis or infection. These latter disorders are characteristically monoarticular, whereas joint involvement in hemophilia is usually polyarticular. Articular and skeletal alterations accompanying neuromuscular diseases such as cerebral palsy, muscular dystrophy, and poliomyelitis may also resemble those of hemophilia. On rare occasions, intra-articular bleeding in association with certain hemorrhagic diatheses may lead to an arthropathy identical to that of hemophilia (Table 52–3).

## BLEEDING DIATHESES AND HEMANGIOMAS

### General Features

Hemangiomas are vascular tumors, most often located in the skin, that appear in the early postnatal period. Hemangiomas may be associated with unusual syndromes, some of which produce hematologic abnormalities.

The association of varicose veins, soft tissue and bony hypertrophy, and cutaneous hemangiomas is known as Klippel-Trénaunay syndrome. An underlying vascular abnormality consisting of atresia and hypoplasia or obstruction of the deep venous system is noted. When these findings are associated with an arteriovenous fistula, the condition is commonly called Parke-Weber syndrome. Additional variations of Klippel-Trénaunay syndrome include cutaneous lymphangiomas and facial hemihypertrophy. Klippel-Trénaunay syndrome affects both sexes. The nevus is usually present at birth, and varices appear, sometimes at birth but typically in the first few years of life. Osseous and soft tissue hypertrophy is also evident in early life but becomes more obvious during the adolescent growth spurt. Usually only one lower limb is involved. The natural history of Klippel-Trénaunay syndrome is variable, although worsening of venous insufficiency is the rule.

**TABLE 52–3**

**Heritable Disorders of Blood Coagulation**

| Disorder | Hereditary | Hemorrhagic Tendency | Hemarthrosis |
|---|---|---|---|
| Classic hemophilia (factor VIII deficiency) | X-linked | Mild to severe | Common |
| Christmas disease (factor IX deficiency) | X-linked | Mild to severe | Common |
| von Willebrand's disease (factor VIII deficiency, platelet abnormalities) | Autosomal dominant | Mild to severe | Uncommon |
| Plasma thromboplastin antecedent (PTA, factor IX) deficiency | Autosomal recessive | Mild | Rare |
| Hageman trait (deficiency of Hageman factor, factor XII) | Autosomal recessive | None to mild | Usually absent |
| Fletcher trait (deficiency of plasma prekallikrein) | Autosomal recessive | None | Absent |
| Fitzgerald trait (deficiency of high-molecular-weight kininogen) | Autosomal recessive | None | Absent |
| Parahemophilia (factor V deficiency) | Autosomal recessive | Moderate | Rare |
| Stuart factor deficiency (factor X deficiency) | Autosomal recessive | Severe | Variable |
| Factor VII deficiency | Autosomal recessive | Mild to moderate | Variable |
| Hereditary hypoprothrombinemia (prothrombin deficiency) | Autosomal recessive | Mild to severe | Variable |
| Congenital deficiency of fibrinogen | Autosomal recessive | Severe | Variable |
| Congenital dysfibrinogenemia (structural abnormality of fibrinogen) | Autosomal dominant | None to mild | Variable |
| Congenital deficiency of fibrin-stabilizing factor (factor XIII deficiency) | Unknown | Severe | Rare |

Kasabach-Merritt syndrome consists of papillary hemangiomas and extensive purpura. Hematologic abnormalities associated with Kasabach-Merritt syndrome include thrombocytopenia; deficiencies of factors V, VII, VIII, and IX; prothrombin depression; hypofibrinogenemia; and microangiopathic hemolytic anemia. A consumption coagulopathy caused by intravascular coagulation within the hemangioma makes these patients (usually infants) susceptible to hemorrhage.

## Articular Abnormalities

Arthropathies are not commonly reported in either Klippel-Trénaunay syndrome or Kasabach-Merritt syndrome, although, in the latter condition, patients may

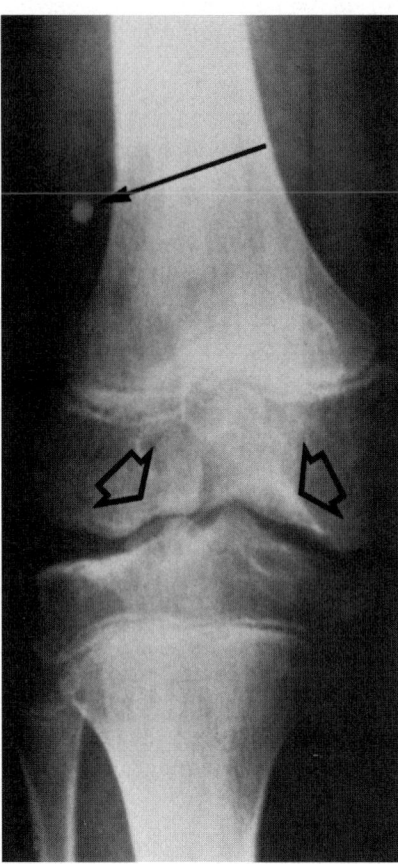

**Figure 52–13.** Arthropathy in association with hemangiomas and bleeding diatheses. This 11-year-old had recurrent bilateral knee pain and abdominal discomfort. At the age of 6 weeks, multiple hemangiomas of the lower extremities and abdomen were noted. Extensive clinical and laboratory evaluation confirmed the diagnosis of multiple giant hemangiomas and varicosities (Klippel-Trénaunay syndrome), Kasabach-Merritt syndrome, and a consumption coagulopathy. On this radiograph of the knee, a soft tissue phlebolith *(arrow)* is apparent. The distal femoral and proximal tibial epiphyses are enlarged, with irregularities of the subchondral bone and a widened intercondylar notch *(open arrows)*. (From Resnick D, Oliphant M: Hemophilia-like arthropathy of the knee associated with cutaneous and synovial hemangiomas: Report of 3 cases and review of the literature. Radiology 114:323, 1975.)

suffer joint stiffness and "degenerative" changes. Rarely, an arthropathy of the knee resembling hemophilia may be evident (Fig. 52–13).

## FURTHER READING

Arnold WD, Hilgartner MW: Hemophilic arthropathy: Current concepts of pathogenesis and management. J Bone Joint Surg Am 59:287, 1977.

Brant EE, Jordan HH: Radiologic aspects of hemophilic pseudotumors in bone. AJR Am J Roentgenol 115:525, 1972.

deValderrama JAF, Matthews JM: The haemophilic pseudotumor or haemophilic subperiosteal haematoma. J Bone Joint Surg Br 47:256, 1965.

Gaary E, Gorlin JB, Jaramillo D: Pseudotumor and arthropathy in the knees of a hemophiliac. Skeletal Radiol 25:85, 1996.

Greene WB, Yankaskas BC, Guilford WB: Roentgenographic classifications of hemophilic arthropathy. J Bone Joint Surg Am 71:237, 1989.

Hermann G, Gilbert MS, Abdelwahab IF: Hemophilia: Evaluation of musculoskeletal involvement with CT, sonography, and MR imaging. AJR Am J Roentgenol 158:119, 1992.

Johnson JB, Davis TW, Bullock WH: Bone and joint changes in hemophilia. Radiology 63:64, 1954.

Jordan HH: Hemophilic Arthropathies. Springfield, Ill, Charles C Thomas, 1958.

Kasabach HH, Merritt KK: Capillary hemangioma with extensive purpura: Report of a case. Am J Dis Child 59:1063, 1940.

Kontras SB: The Klippel-Trenaunay-Weber syndrome. Birth Defects 10:177, 1974.

Pettersson H, Ahlberg S, Nilsson IM: A radiologic classification of hemophilic arthropathy. Clin Orthop 149:153, 1980.

Pettersson H, Gilbert MS: Diagnostic Imaging in Hemophilia. Berlin, Springer-Verlag, 1985.

Phillips GN, Gordon DH, Martin EC, et al: The Klippel-Trenaunay syndrome: Clinical and radiological aspects. Radiology 128:429, 1978.

Plazanet FR, du Boullay CH, De Faux F, et al: Open synovectomy for the prevention of recurrent hemarthrosis of the ankle in patients with hemophilia: A report of five cases with magnetic resonance imaging documentation. Rev Rhum Engl Ed 64:166, 1997.

Resnick D, Oliphant M: Hemophilia-like arthropathy of the knee associated with cutaneous and synovial hemangiomas: Report of 3 cases and review of the literature. Radiology 114:323, 1975.

Richardson ML, Helms CA, Vogler JB III, et al: Skeletal changes in neuromuscular disorders mimicking juvenile rheumatoid arthritis and hemophilia. AJR Am J Roentgenol 143:893, 1984.

Roebuck DJ: Klippel-Trenaunay and Parke-Weber syndromes. AJR Am J Roentgenol 169:311, 1997.

Roosendaal G, Vianen ME, Wenting MJG, et al: Iron deposits and catabolic properties of synovial tissue from patients with haemophilia. J Bone Joint Surg Br 80:540, 1998.

Vaz W, Cockshott WP, Martin RF, et al: Myositis ossificans in hemophilia. Skeletal Radiol 7:27, 1981.

Weber FP: Hemangiectatic hypertrophy of limbs—congenital phlebacteriectasis and so-called congenital varicose veins. Br J Child Dis 15:13, 1918.

Wilson DA, Prince JR: MR imaging of hemophilic pseudotumors. AJR Am J Roentgenol 150:349, 1988.

# Infectious Diseases

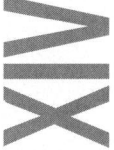

# CHAPTER 53

## Osteomyelitis, Septic Arthritis, and Soft Tissue Infection: Mechanisms and Situations

## SUMMARY OF KEY FEATURES

A thorough understanding of regional anatomy is fundamental to the accurate interpretation of clinical, radiographic, and pathologic characteristics of infections of bone, joint, and soft tissue. In most persons with such infections, a specific mechanism of contamination can be recognized; infection may be derived from hematogenous seeding, spread from a contiguous source, direct implantation, or operative contamination. The radiographic findings of osteomyelitis (including abscess, involucrum, and sequestration), septic arthritis (including joint space loss and marginal and central osseous erosions), and soft tissue suppuration (including swelling, radiolucent streaks, and periostitis) are generally delayed for a variable period after the clinical onset of infection. Other diagnostic techniques, including scintigraphy and magnetic resonance imaging, allow an accurate diagnosis at an earlier stage of the process.

## INTRODUCTION

Infection of bone, joint, and soft tissue is a common and disturbing problem that often represents a diagnostic and therapeutic challenge. Early diagnosis is imperative because it allows prompt treatment, which can prevent many of the dreaded complications.

## TERMINOLOGY

*Ostemyelitis* implies an infection of bone and marrow. It most commonly results from bacterial infections, although fungi, parasites, and viruses can infect the bone and the marrow.

*Infective (suppurative) osteitis* indicates contamination of the bone cortex. Infective osteitis can occur as an isolated phenomenon or, more frequently, as a concomitant to osteomyelitis.

*Infective (suppurative) periostitis* implies contamination of the periosteal cloak that surrounds the bone. In this situation, a subperiosteal accumulation of organisms frequently leads to infective osteitis and osteomyelitis.

*Soft tissue infection* indicates contamination of cutaneous, subcutaneous, muscular, fascial, tendinous, ligamentous, or bursal structures. This may be seen as an isolated condition or as a complication of periosteal, osseous, marrow, or articular infection.

*Articular infection* implies a septic process of the joint itself. Septic arthritis can occur as an isolated condition that may soon spread to the neighboring bone or as a complication of adjacent osteomyelitis or soft tissue infection.

A *sequestrum* represents a segment of necrotic bone that is separated from living bone by granulation tissue. Sequestra may reside in the marrow for protracted periods, harboring living organisms that have the capability of evoking an acute flare-up of the infection.

An *involucrum* denotes a layer of living bone that has formed about the dead bone. It can surround and eventually merge with the parent bone.

*Cloaca* is an opening in the involucrum through which granulation tissue and sequestra can be discharged.

*Sinuses* are tracts leading to the skin surface from the bone.

A *bone abscess (Brodie's abscess)* is a sharply delineated focus of infection. It is of variable size, can occur at single or multiple locations, and represents a site of active infection. It is lined by granulation tissue and frequently is surrounded by eburnated bone.

*Garré's sclerosing osteomyelitis* is a sclerotic, nonpurulent form of osteomyelitis. Although this term is applied carelessly to any form of osteomyelitis with severe osseous eburnation, it should be reserved for those cases in which intense proliferation of the periosteum leads to bony deposition and in which no necrosis or purulent exudate and little granulation tissue are present.

The clinical stages of osteomyelitis are frequently designated acute, subacute, and chronic. This does not imply that definitive divisions exist between one stage and another, nor does it signify that all cases of osteomyelitis progress through each of these phases. The relatively abrupt onset of clinical symptoms and signs during the initial stage of infection is a clear indication of the acute osteomyelitic phase; if this acute phase passes without complete elimination of infection, subacute or chronic osteomyelitis can become apparent. The transition from acute to subacute and chronic osteomyelitis may indicate that therapeutic measures have been inadequate.

## OSTEOMYELITIS

### Routes of Contamination

Osseous (and articular) structures can be contaminated by four principal routes:

1. *Hematogenous spread of infection.* Infection can reach the bone (or joint) via the bloodstream.

2. *Spread from a contiguous source of infection.* Infection can extend into the bone (or joint) from an adjacent contaminated site. Cutaneous, sinus, and dental infections are three important sources of extraskeletal infective foci.

3. *Direct implantation*. Direct implantation of infectious material into the bone (or joint) may occur following puncture or penetrating injuries.

4. *Postoperative infection*. Postoperative infection may occur via direct implantation, spread from a contiguous septic focus, or hematogenous contamination of the bone (or joint).

## Hematogenous Infection

### Bacteremia

Bacteria usually enter the blood vessels (or the lymphatics and then the blood vessels) by direct extension from extravascular sites of infection, which include the genitourinary, gastrointestinal, biliary, and respiratory systems; the skin and soft tissue; and other structures. In some instances, no primary source of infection is identifiable. Bacteremia is often transient and totally asymptomatic; however, in some cases, prominent clinical manifestations may occur.

A single pathogenic organism is usually responsible for hematogenous osteomyelitis. In neonates and infants, *Staphylococcus aureus*, group B streptococcus, and *Escherichia coli* are the bone isolates recovered most frequently. In children older than 1 year of age, *S. aureus*, *Streptococcus pyogenes*, and *Haemophilus influenzae* are responsible for most cases of hematogenous osteomyelitis. In those older than 4 years, staphylococci are the major pathogens in this disease, as the prevalence of osteomyelitis related to *H. influenzae* decreases. Gram-negative organisms assume importance as pathogens in bone and joint infections in adults and in intravenous drug abusers. A recent surgical procedure or concurrent soft tissue infection is frequently associated with staphylococcal septicemia and osteomyelitis; disorders of the gastrointestinal or genitourinary tract may initiate a gram-negative septicemia; and an acute or chronic respiratory infection is important in the pathogenesis of tuberculous, fungal, and pneumococcal osteomyelitis. Blood cultures are positive in approximately 50% of patients with acute hematogenous osteomyelitis.

### General Clinical Features

Childhood osteomyelitis can be associated with a sudden onset of high fever, a toxic state, and local signs of inflammation, although this presentation is not uniform. Indeed, as many as 50% of children have vague complaints, including local pain of 1 to 3 months' duration with minimal if any temperature elevation. In infants, hematogenous osteomyelitis often leads to less dramatic findings, including pain, swelling, and an unwillingness to move the affected bones.

The adult form of hematogenous osteomyelitis may have a more insidious onset, with a relatively longer period between the appearance of symptoms and signs and accurate diagnosis. In all age groups, the prior administration of antibiotics for treatment of the febrile state can attenuate or alter the clinical (and imaging) manifestations of the bone infection. Single or multiple bones can be infected; involvement of multiple osseous sites appears to be particularly common in infants. In the younger age group, the long tubular bones of the extremities are especially vulnerable; in adults, hematogenous osteomyelitis is encountered more frequently in the axial skeleton.

### Vascular Anatomy

The vascular supply of a tubular bone is derived from several points of arterial inflow, which become complicated sinusoidal networks within the bone (Fig. 53–1). One or two diaphyseal nutrient arteries pierce the cortex and divide into ascending and descending branches. As they extend to the ends of the bones, they branch repeatedly, becoming finer channels, and are joined by the terminals of metaphyseal and epiphyseal arteries. The metaphyseal arteries originate from neighboring systemic vessels, whereas the epiphyseal arteries arise from periarticular vascular arcades. The arteries within the bone marrow form a series of cortical branches that connect with the fenestrated capillaries of the haversian systems. At the bony surface, the cortical capillaries form connections with overlying periosteal plexuses, which themselves are derived from the arteries of the neighboring muscles and soft tissues. The cortices of the tubular bones derive nutrition from both the periosteal and the medullary circulatory systems. The central arterioles drain into a thin-walled venous sinus, which subsequently unites with veins that retrace the course of the nutrient arteries, piercing the cortex at various points and joining larger and larger venous channels.

Joints receive blood vessels from periarterial plexuses that pierce the capsule to form a vascular plexus in the deeper part of the synovial membrane. The blood vessels of the synovial membrane terminate at the articular margins as looped anastomoses (circulus articularis vasculosus). The epiphysis and the adjacent synovium share a common blood supply.

The radiographic and pathologic features of osteomyelitis differ in children, infants, and adults, related in large part to peculiarities of the vascular anatomy of the tubular bones in each age group (Fig. 53–2; Table 53–1).

**Childhood Pattern.** Between the age of approximately 1 year and the time when the open cartilaginous growth plates fuse, a childhood vascular pattern can be recognized in the ends of the tubular bones (see Fig. 53–2*A*). In the metaphysis, the vessels turn in acute loops to join large sinusoidal veins, which occupy the intramedullary portion of the metaphysis; here, the blood flow is slow and turbulent. The epiphyseal blood supply is distinct from that on the metaphyseal aspect of the plate. This anatomic characteristic explains the peculiar predilection of hematogenous osteomyelitis to affect metaphyses and equivalent locations in children.

**Infantile Pattern.** A fetal vascular arrangement may persist in some tubular bones up to the age of 1 year (see Fig. 53–2*B*). Some vessels at the surface of the metaphysis penetrate the preexisting growth plate, ramifying in the epiphysis. This arrangement affords a vascular connection between the metaphysis and epiphysis and explains the frequency of epiphyseal and articular infection in infants.

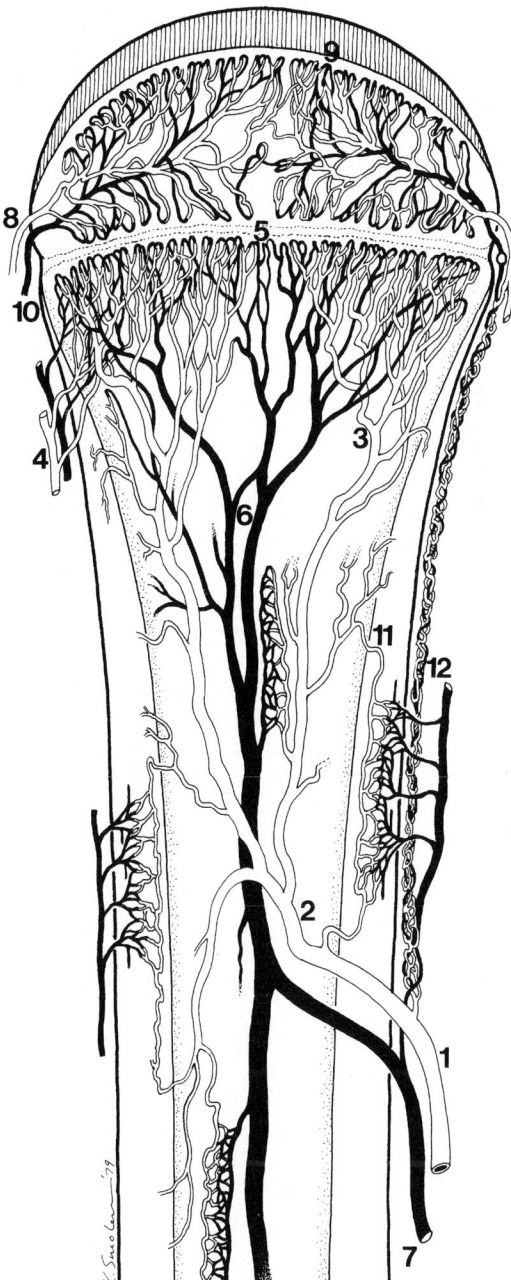

**Figure 53–1.** Normal osseous circulation to a growing tubular bone. Nutrient arteries (1) pierce the diaphyseal cortex and divide into descending and ascending (2) branches. These latter vessels continue to divide, becoming fine channels (3) as they approach the end of the bone. They are joined by metaphyseal vessels (4) and, in the subepiphyseal (growth) plate region, form a series of end-arterial loops (5). The venous sinuses extend from the metaphyseal region toward the diaphysis, uniting with other venous structures (6) and eventually piercing the cortex as a large venous channel (7). At the ends of the bone, nutrient arteries of the epiphysis (8) branch into finer structures, passing into the subchondral region. At this site, arterial loops (9) are again evident, some of which pierce the subchondral bone plate before turning to enter the venous sinusoid and venous channels of the epiphysis (10). At the bony surface, cortical capillaries (11) form connections with overlying periosteal plexuses (12). Note that in the growing child, distinct epiphyseal and metaphyseal arteries can be distinguished on either side of the cartilaginous growth plate. Anastomoses between these vessels either do not occur or are infrequent.

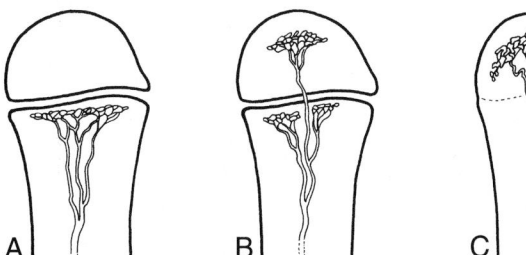

**Figure 53–2.** Normal vascular patterns of tubular bone, based on age. *A*, In the child, the capillaries of the metaphysis turn sharply, without violating the open growth plate. *B*, In the infant, some metaphyseal vessels may penetrate or extend around the open growth plate, ramifying in the epiphysis. *C*, In the adult, with closure of the growth plate, a vascular connection between the metaphysis and epiphysis can be recognized.

**Adult Pattern.** With narrowing and closing of the physeal growth plate, metaphyseal vessels progressively reestablish a vascular connection between the metaphysis and the epiphysis (see Fig. 53–2*C*). Blood within the nutrient vessels can then reach the surface of the epiphysis through large anastomosing channels.

### Age-Related Patterns

The development of hematogenous osteomyelitis varies according to age-related characteristics of the bones (Fig. 53–3; Table 53–2).

**Childhood.** In childhood hematogenous osteomyelitis, the metaphyseal location is related to (1) the peculiar anatomy of the vascular tree, (2) the inability of vessels to penetrate the open physeal plate, (3) the slow rate of blood flow in this region, (4) a decrease in phagocytic ability of neighboring macrophages, or (5) secondary thrombosis of the nutrient artery. Primary involvement of an epiphysis or secondary extension across the physis to an epiphysis is encountered rarely.

Inflammation in the adjacent bone of the metaphysis is characterized by vascular engorgement, edema, cellular response, and abscess formation. Transudates extend from

---

**TABLE 53–1**

**Vascular Patterns of Tubular Bones**

| Pattern | Age (yr) | Characteristics |
|---|---|---|
| Infantile | 0–1* | Diaphyseal and metaphyseal vessels may perforate open growth plate |
| Childhood | 1–16† | Diaphyseal and metaphyseal vessels do not penetrate open growth plate |
| Adult | >16 | Diaphyseal and metaphyseal vessels penetrate closed growth plate |

*Upper age limit depends on specific local anatomic variation in the appearance and growth of the ossification center.

†Upper age limit is related to the time at which the open growth plate closes.

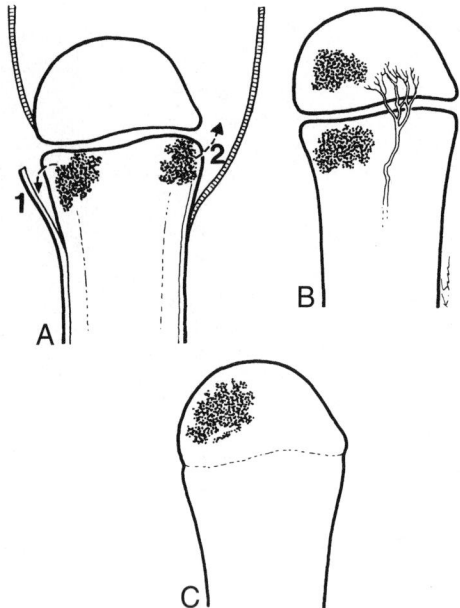

**Figure 53–3.** Sites of hematogenous osteomyelitis of tubular bone, based on age. *A*, In the child, a metaphyseal focus is frequent. From this site, cortical penetration can result in a subperiosteal abscess in locations where the growth plate is extra-articular (1) or in a septic joint in locations where the growth plate is intra-articular (2). *B*, In the infant, a metaphyseal focus may be complicated by epiphyseal extension, owing to the vascular anatomy in this age group. *C*, In the adult, a subchondral focus in an epiphysis is not unusual, owing to the vascular anatomy in this age group.

the marrow to the adjacent cortex. A rise in intramedullary pressure, caused by the presence of inflammatory and edematous tissue confined by the rigid cortical columns of bone, encourages the extension of infected fluid by way of haversian and Volkmann's canals. The inflammatory process soon reaches the outer surface of the cortex and abscesses develop, lifting the periosteum and disrupting the periosteal blood supply to the external cortical surface. Elevation of the periosteum is prominent in the immature skeleton because of its relatively loose attachment to the subjacent bone. The elevated

periosteum produces single or multiple layers of bone (i.e., periostitis) and eventually lays down bone in the form of an involucrum. Infection may penetrate the periosteal membrane, producing cloacae (Fig. 53–4).

Childhood hematogenous osteomyelitis is not confined to tubular bones. In flat or irregular bones such as the calcaneus, clavicle, and bones of the pelvis, childhood osteomyelitis may show a predilection for metaphyseal-equivalent osseous locations adjacent to an apophyseal cartilaginous plate and epiphyseal-equivalent locations adjacent to articular cartilage.

**Infancy.** In infants, because some of the vessels in the metaphysis penetrate the growth plate, a suppurative process of the metaphysis may extend into the epiphysis (Fig. 53–5). Epiphyseal infection can then result in articular contamination and damage to the cells on the epiphyseal side of the growth cartilage, leading to arrest or disorganization of growth and maturation. Articular involvement is also facilitated by the frequent localization of infantile osteomyelitis to the ends of bones in which the growth plate is intra-articular (e.g., hip).

**Adulthood.** Unique manifestations of hematogenous osteomyelitis are seen in adults (see Table 53–2). The disease in the mature skeleton does not commonly localize in the tubular bones; hematogenous osteomyelitis of the spine, pelvis, and small bones is more common in adult patients. In cases in which involvement of tubular bones is evident, the free communication of the metaphyseal and epiphyseal vessels through the closed growth plate allows infection to localize in the subchondral (beneath the articular cartilage) regions of the bone (Fig. 53–6). Joint contamination can complicate this epiphyseal location.

The firm attachment of the periosteum to the cortex in adults resists displacement; therefore, subperiosteal abscess formation, extensive periostitis, and involucrum formation are relatively unusual in this age group. Extensive sequestration is not a common feature. In adults, infection violates and disrupts the cortex itself, producing atrophy and osseous weakening, and predisposes the bone to pathologic fracture.

| **TABLE 53–2** | | | |
| --- | --- | --- | --- |
| **Hematogenous Osteomyelitis of Tubular Bones** | | | |
| **Aspect** | **Infant** | **Child** | **Adult** |
| Localization | Metaphyseal with epiphyseal extension | Metaphyseal | Epiphyseal |
| Involucrum | Common | Common | Not common |
| Sequestrum | Common | Common | Not common |
| Joint involvement | Common | Not common | Common |
| Soft tissue abscess | Common | Common | Not common |
| Pathologic fracture | Not common | Not common | Common* |
| Sinus tracts | Not common | Variable | Common |

*In neglected cases.

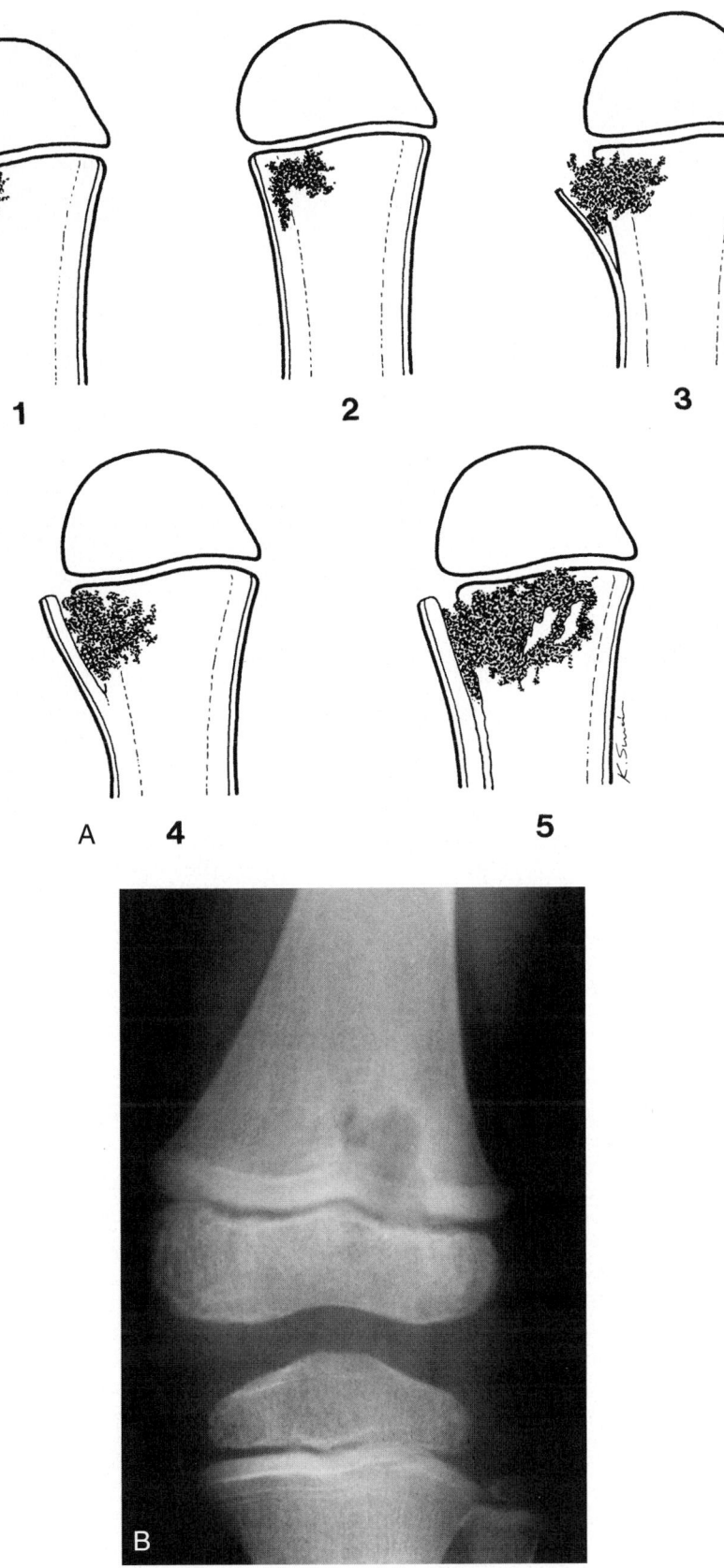

**Figure 53–4.** Hematogenous osteomyelitis of tubular bone in a child. *A*, Sequential steps in the initiation and progression of infection: 1, a metaphyseal focus is common; 2, the infection spreads laterally, reaching and invading the cortical bone; 3, cortical penetration is associated with subperiosteal extension and elevation of the periosteal membrane; 4, subperiosteal bone formation leads to an involucrum or shell of new bone; 5, the involucrum may become massive with continued infection. *B*, Lytic metaphyseal focus in the femur is readily apparent. It extends to the growth cartilage (causative organism is *Staphylococcus*).

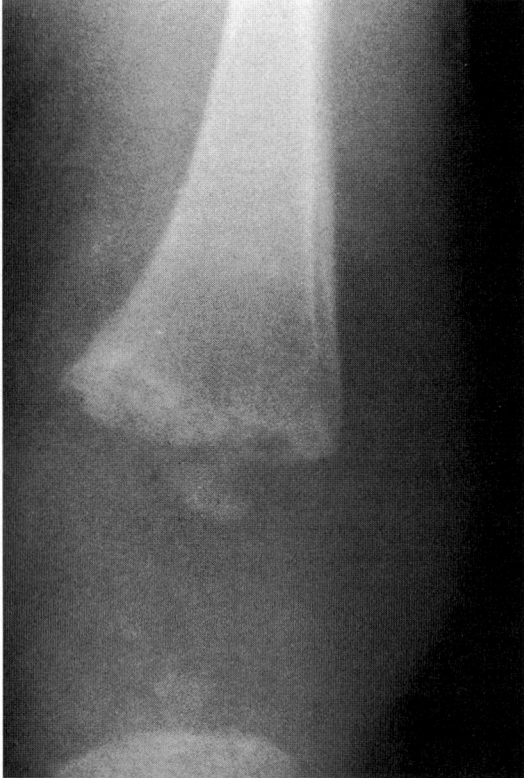

**Figure 53–5.** Hematogenous osteomyelitis of tubular bone in an infant. In this infant with acute staphylococcal osteomyelitis, metaphyseal and epiphyseal involvement of the distal end of the femur is associated with periostitis and articular involvement.

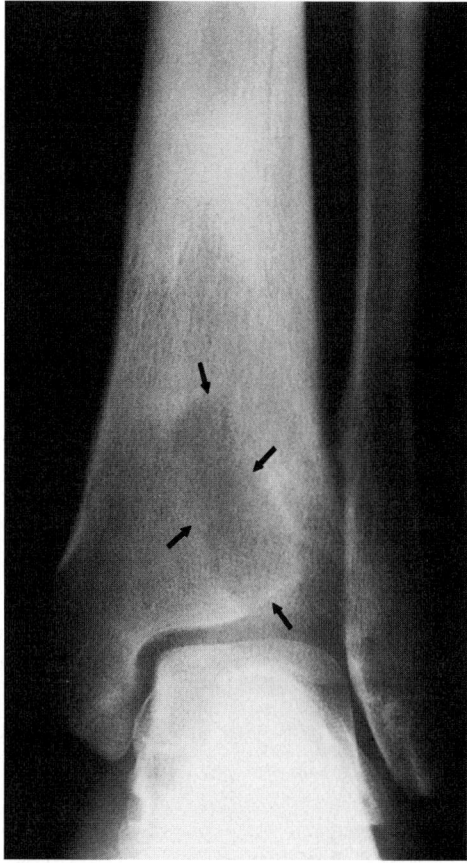

**Figure 53–6.** Hematogenous osteomyelitis of tubular bone in an adult. Epiphyseal localization is not infrequent in this age group. Observe the lytic lesion (abscess), with surrounding sclerosis extending to the subchondral bone plate *(arrows)*. Metaphyseal and diaphyseal sclerosis is evident. The elongated shape of the lesion is typical of infection (causative organism is *Staphylococcus*).

## Radiographic and Pathologic Abnormalities

### Acute Hematogenous Osteomyelitis

The pathologic changes associated with acute hematogenous pyogenic osteomyelitis are described in Table 53–3. Radiographic evidence of significant osseous destruction is delayed for a period of days to weeks. Nevertheless, initial and subtle radiographic changes in the soft tissues may appear within 3 days after bacterial contamination of bone, although radiographically evident bone destruction and periostitis can be delayed for 1 to 2 weeks. Eventually, large destructive lesions become evident on the radiograph. In children, these lesions appear as enlarging, poorly defined lucent shadows of the metaphysis, surrounded by varying amounts of eburnation; the lucent lesions extend to the growth plate and, on rare occasions, may violate it. In addition, destruction progresses horizontally, reaching the cortex, and periostitis follows. In infants, the epiphyses are unossified or only partially ossified, making radiographic recognition of epiphyseal destruction extremely difficult. Metaphyseal lucent lesions, periostitis, and joint effusion are helpful radiographic clues. In adults, soft tissue alterations are more difficult to detect on radiographic examination. Epiphyseal, metaphyseal, and diaphyseal osseous destruction creates radiolucent areas of varying size, which are associated with mild periostitis. Cortical resorption can be identified as

endosteal scalloping, intracortical lucent regions or tunneling, and poorly defined subperiosteal bony defects.

### Subacute and Chronic Hematogenous Osteomyelitis

**Brodie's Abscess.** Single or multiple radiolucent abscesses may be evident during subacute or chronic stages of osteomyelitis. These abscesses are now defined as circumscribed lesions showing a predilection for (but not confined to) the ends of tubular bones; they are found characteristically in subacute pyogenic osteomyelitis and are usually of staphylococcal origin. It has been suggested that bone abscesses develop when an infective organism has a reduced virulence or when the host demonstrates increased resistance to infection. Brodie's abscesses are especially common in children, more typically in boys. In this age group, they appear in the metaphysis, particularly that of the distal or proximal portion of the tibia. In young children and infants, Brodie's abscesses may occur in epiphyses.

Radiographs outline radiolucent areas with adjacent sclerosis (Fig. 53–7). This lucent region is commonly located in the metaphysis, where it may connect with the

---

**TABLE 53-3**

### Hematogenous Osteomyelitis: Radiographic-Pathologic Correlation

| Pathologic Abnormality | Radiographic Abnormality |
|---|---|
| Vascular changes and edema of soft tissues | Soft tissue swelling with obliteration of tissue planes |
| Infection in medullary space with hyperemia, edema, abscess formation, and trabecular destruction | Osteoporosis, bone lysis |
| Infection in haversian and Volkmann's canals of cortex | Increasing lysis, cortical lucency |
| Subperiosteal abscess formation with lifting of the periosteum and bone formation | Periostitis, involucrum formation |
| Infectious penetration of periosteum with soft tissue abscess formation | Soft tissue swelling, mass formation, obliteration of tissue planes |
| Localized cortical and medullary abscesses | Single or multiple radiolucent cortical or medullary lesions with surrounding sclerosis |
| Deprivation of blood supply to cortex due to thrombosis of metaphyseal vessels and interruption of periosteal vessels, cortical necrosis | Sequestration |
| External migration of dead pieces of cortex with breakdown of skin and subcutaneous tissue | Sinus tracts |

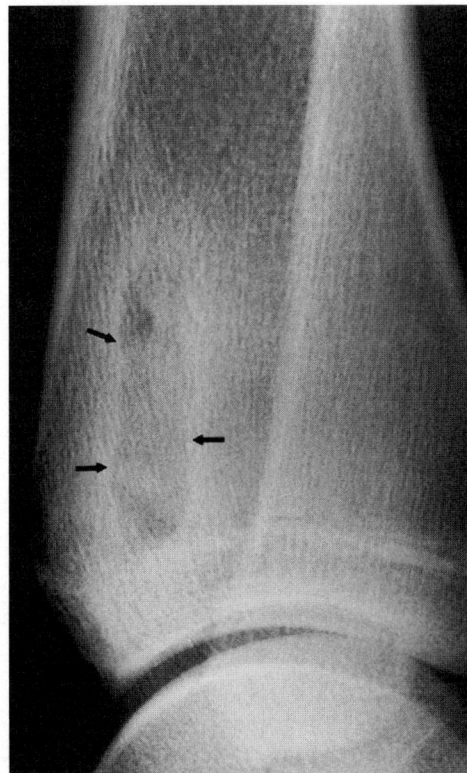

**Figure 53-7.** Brodie's abscess: radiographic abnormalities. Lateral radiograph outlines a typical appearance of an abscess of the distal end of the tibia caused by staphylococci. Observe the elongated radiolucent lesion, with surrounding sclerosis extending to the closing growth plate (*arrows*). The channel-like shape of the lesion is important in the accurate diagnosis of this condition.

---

growth plate by a tortuous channel. Radiographic detection of this channel is important; identification of a metaphyseal defect connected to the growth plate by such a tract ensures the diagnosis of osteomyelitis. In the diaphysis, the radiolucent abscess cavity may be located in central or subcortical areas of the spongiosa or in the cortex itself and may contain a central sequestrum. In an epiphysis, a circular, well-defined osteolytic lesion is seen, which, in the immature skeleton, may border on the chondro-osseous junction or on the physis, where it may extend into the metaphysis. When an abscess is located in the cortex, its radiographic appearance, consisting of a lucent lesion with surrounding sclerosis and periostitis, simulates that of an osteoid osteoma or stress fracture. A rounded radiolucent lesion without calcification is characteristic of a cortical abscess; a circular lucent area with or without calcification that is smaller than 2 cm is more typical of an osteoid osteoma; and a linear lucent shadow without calcification is characteristic of a stress fracture. In any skeletal location, computed tomography (CT) or magnetic resonance (MR) imaging can be used to better assess the extent of the abscess and any signs of its reactivation (Fig. 53–8).

**Sequestration.** During the course of hematogenous osteomyelitis, cortical sequestration may become evident.

One or more areas of osseous necrosis are commonly situated in the medullary aspect of a tubular bone (sequestration is less prominent in flat bones), where they create radiodense bony spicules (Fig. 53–9). The sequestrum frequently is marginated sharply, surrounded by granulation tissue. Sequestra may extrude through cortical breaks, extending into the adjacent soft tissues, where they eventually may be discharged through draining sinuses.

**Sclerosing Osteomyelitis.** In the subacute and chronic stages of osteomyelitis, considerable periosteal bone formation can surround the altered cortex, and an increased number and size of spongy trabeculae can reappear in the affected marrow, leading to considerable radiodensity and contour irregularity of the affected bone (Fig. 53–10). Cystic changes may occur within the sclerotic area, but sequestra are uncommon. At any site, the radiographic findings of sclerosing osteomyelitis resemble those of osteoid osteoma, fibrous dysplasia, and Ewing's sarcoma.

### Infection from a Contiguous Source

#### General Clinical Features

In most cases of osteomyelitis and septic arthritis arising from such a contiguous source, soft tissue infections are

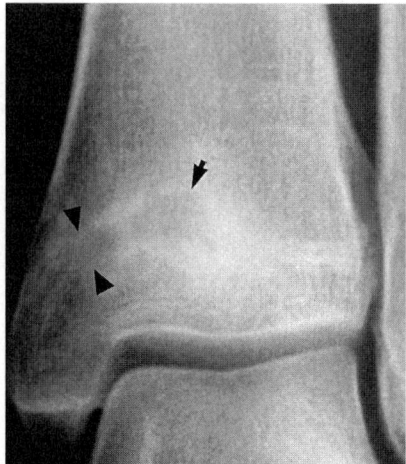

**Figure 53–8.** Brodie's abscess: radiographic abnormalities. Tibial metaphyseal involvement in a 19-year-old woman. Routine radiograph shows a metaphyseal radiolucent lesion *(arrow)* with a medial channel *(arrowheads)*. (Courtesy of M. Mitchell, MD, Halifax, Nova Scotia, Canada.)

implicated. The importance of osteomyelitis of the mandible and maxilla in persons with poor dental hygiene and of the frontal portion of the skull and face in persons with chronic sinusitis is undeniable. Soft tissue infections that lead to bone and joint contamination are frequent after trauma, animal and human bites, puncture wounds, irradiation, burns, and decubitus or pressure ulcers in paralyzed or immobilized patients.

### General Radiographic and Pathologic Features

Whereas the direction of contamination in hematogenous osteomyelitis is from the bone outward into the soft tissue, the direction of contamination in osteomyelitis resulting from adjacent sepsis is from the soft tissues inward into the bone (or joint) (Table 53–4; Fig. 53–11). Periosteal bone formation is commonly the initial radiographic manifestation of osteomyelitis. After traumatic initiation of soft tissue infection, periostitis may appear early in response to injury and may not reflect actual bone infection. With further accumulation of pus, subperiosteal resorption of bone and cortical disruption ensue. As infection gains access to the spongiosa, it may spread in the marrow, producing lytic osseous defects on the radiograph.

### Specific Locations

**Hand.** Three distinct routes are available to organisms that become lodged in the soft tissues of the hand; infection may disseminate via tendon sheaths, fascial planes, or lymphatics (Fig. 53–12). Infective digital tenosynovitis can result from a puncture wound, particularly in a flexor crease of the finger, where skin and sheath are intimately related. A sheath infection may perforate into an adjacent bone or joint in the finger; the most characteristic site of such extension is the proximal interphalangeal articulations and adjacent middle phalanx (Fig. 53–13). The

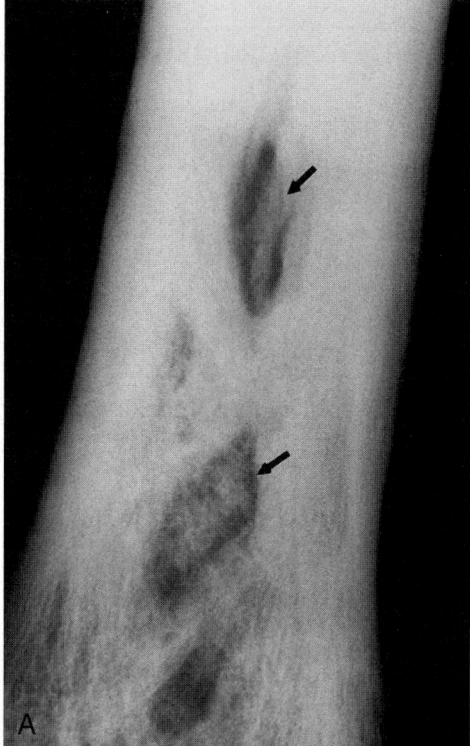

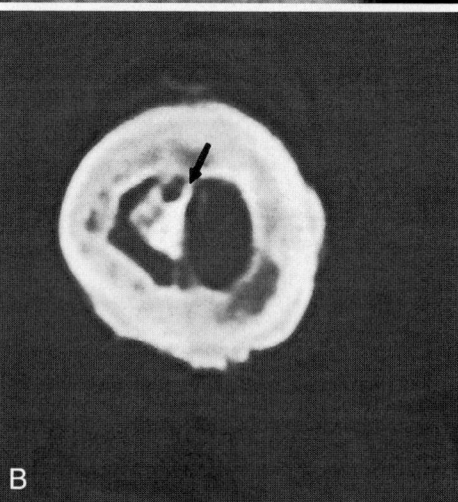

**Figure 53–9.** Chronic osteomyelitis: sequestration. *A,* In this radiograph of a femur, chronic osteomyelitis is associated with several radiodense, sharply marginated foci *(arrows)* within lucent cavities that contain granulation tissue. *B,* CT scanning identifies sequestered bone *(arrow).*

metacarpophalangeal joints are altered less commonly. Such tenosynovitis causes exquisite tenderness over the course of the sheath, a semiflexed position of the finger, severe pain on extension of the finger, and fusiform swelling of the digit.

Infections in the fascial planes of the hand are numerous but result in joint or bone alterations less frequently than do those in the synovial sheaths. Lymphangitis may result from superficial injuries. In intense cases, complications may include tenosynovitis, septicemia, osteomyelitis, and septic arthritis.

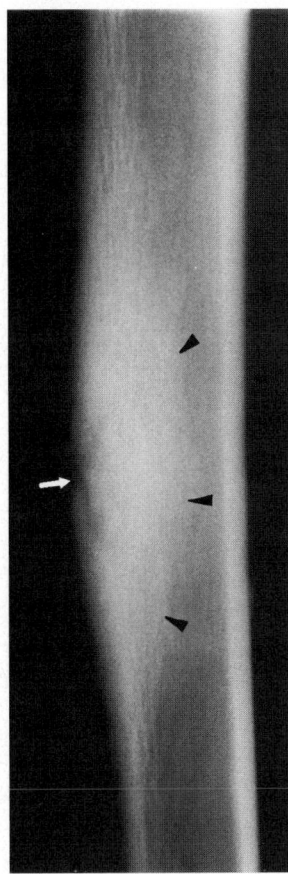

**Figure 53–10.** Chronic sclerosing osteomyelitis. Chronic osteomyelitis can be associated with considerable new bone formation. In this patient, a cortical abscess contains a sequestrum *(arrow)* and is surrounded by sclerosis *(arrowheads)*. The appearance is reminiscent of that of an osteoid osteoma.

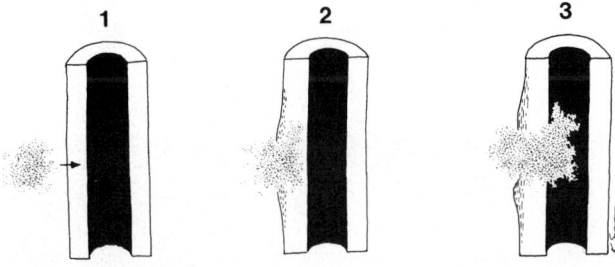

**Figure 53–11.** Diagrammatic representation of the sequential steps of osteomyelitis resulting from a contiguous contaminated source. 1, Initially, a soft tissue focus of infection is apparent. Occasionally, such a focus can irritate the underlying bone, producing periostitis without definite invasion of the cortex. 2, The infection subsequently invades the cortex, spreading via haversian and Volkmann's canals. 3, Finally, the medullary bone and marrow spaces are affected.

A felon results from infection in the terminal pulp space. Bone involvement is not infrequent in neglected cases because of the close proximity of the terminal phalanx (Fig. 53–14). Subcuticular abscesses of the nail fold are termed paronychia. On rare occasions, osseous destruction of a terminal phalanx may be evident (Fig. 53–15).

**Foot**. The plantar aspect of the foot is especially vulnerable to soft tissue infection. Foreign bodies, puncture wounds, or skin ulceration from weight bearing can represent the portal of entry for various organisms. In a diabetic patient, soft tissue breakdown over certain pressure points (e.g., metatarsal heads, calcaneus) leads to infection that is combined with vascular and neurologic abnormalities.

Puncture wounds of the plantar aspect of the foot can lead to osteomyelitis and septic arthritis (Fig. 53–16). The infective organisms can vary, but gram-negative agents such as *Pseudomonas aeruginosa* are frequently implicated; this is not surprising, because these organisms are usually found in the soil and may be normal inhabitants of skin. Typically, local pain and swelling appear within days after a puncture wound, although radiographs usually are normal at this time. After a delay of 1 to 3 weeks, the radiographs reveal typical abnormalities of osteomyelitis or septic arthritis. Osteomyelitis of the os calcis is a recognized complication of repeated heel punctures in neonates.

The clinical, radiographic, and pathologic characteristics of osteomyelitis (and septic arthritis) complicating foot infections in diabetic patients are modified by the associated problems of these persons, including vascular insufficiency and neurologic deficit. The radiographic picture usually reveals significant soft tissue swelling and mottled osteolysis (Fig. 53–17). Osteosclerosis, fragmentation, periostitis, and soft tissue gas may be seen. In some diabetic patients with foot infections complicated by osteomyelitis, findings can simulate those of diabetic neuropathic osteoarthropathy, and differentiation of neurologic and infectious processes can be difficult. In fact, both infection and neuropathic osteoarthropathy of the midfoot and forefoot frequently coexist in diabetic patients.

**Pelvis**. Soft tissue breakdown that occurs in debilitated persons who maintain a single position for long periods is referred to as a pressure sore, decubitus ulcer, or bedsore. Although other sites (e.g., heels) may be affected, most pressure sores develop about the pelvis,

**TABLE 53–4**

**Osteomyelitis Due to Spread from a Contiguous Source of Infection: Radiographic-Pathologic Correlation**

| Pathologic Abnormality | Radiographic Abnormality |
| --- | --- |
| Soft tissue contamination and abscess formation | Soft tissue swelling, mass formation, obliteration of tissue planes |
| Infectious invasion of the periosteum with lifting of the membrane and bone formation | Periostitis |
| Subperiosteal abscess formation and cortical invasion | Cortical erosion |
| Infection in haversian and Volkmann's canals of cortex | Cortical lucency and destruction |
| Contamination and spread in marrow | Bone lysis |

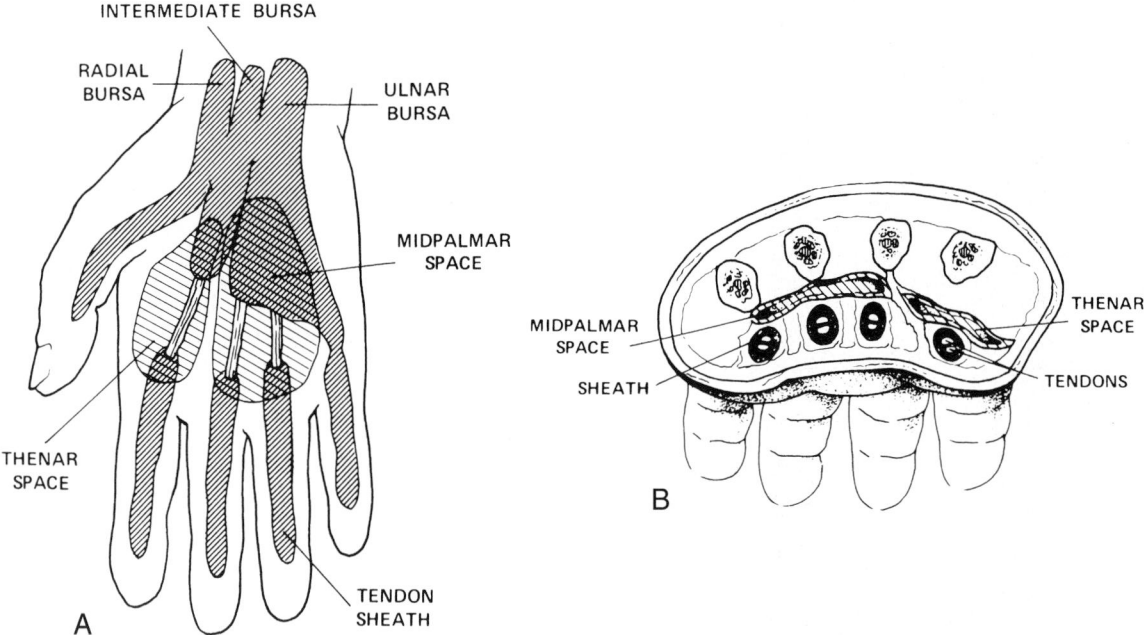

**Figure 53–12.** Spread of infection in the hand: available anatomic pathways *A*, Drawing demonstrates the relationships of the tendon sheaths, bursae, and fascial planes (thenar space, midpalmar space). *B*, Drawing of a section through the metacarpal bones outlines two spaces—the midpalmar and thenar spaces—separated by a septum and located above the digital flexor tendon sheaths. Note the close relationship between the sheath of the index finger and the thenar space and between the sheaths of the third, fourth, and fifth fingers and the midpalmar space. (From Resnick D: Osteomyelitis and septic arthritis complicating hand injuries and infections: Pathogenesis of roentgenographic abnormalities. J Can Assoc Radiol 27:21, 1976.)

especially near the sacrum, ischial tuberosities, trochanteric regions, and buttocks. Local soft tissue infection and bacteremia are commonly associated with decubitus ulcers. Osteomyelitis is observed most commonly in the innominate bones and proximal portions of the femora, areas subjacent to sites of skin breakdown, and is related to spread from a contiguous contaminated source.

The accurate diagnosis of osteomyelitis complicating pressure sores is difficult, owing to a number of other conditions that may become evident in immobilized or paralyzed patients. Pressure-related changes in bone are not infrequent, leading to flattening and sclerosis of bony

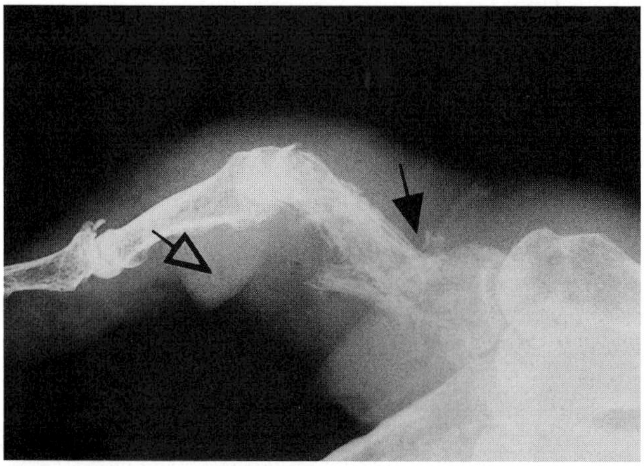

**Figure 53–13.** Spread of infection in the hand: digital flexor tenosynovitis. After a neglected puncture wound, a 45-year-old woman developed tenosynovitis and osteomyelitis. Note the soft tissue swelling, particularly along the volar surface of the proximal phalanx *(open arrow)*; the semiflexed position of the finger; and extensive permeative osseous destruction, with pathologic fracture *(solid arrow)* of the proximal phalanx. (From Resnick D: Osteomyelitis and septic arthritis complicating hand injuries and infections: Pathogenesis of roentgenographic abnormalities. J Can Assoc Radiol 27:21, 1976.)

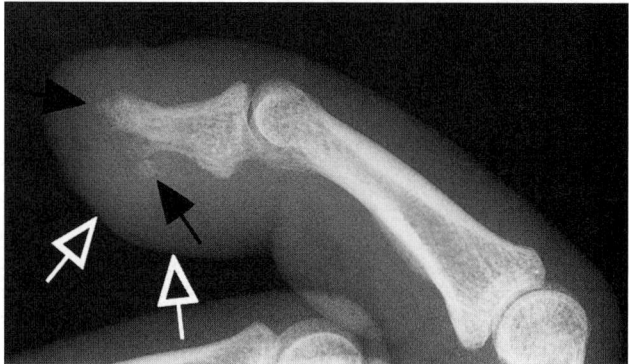

**Figure 53–14.** Spread of infection in the hand: felon. An infection in the pulp space has produced considerable soft tissue swelling *(open arrows)*. Extension into the tuft and diaphysis of the terminal phalanx is apparent *(solid arrows)*. Shrapnel from a previous injury can be seen. (From Resnick D: Osteomyelitis and septic arthritis complicating hand injuries and infections: Pathogenesis of roentgenographic abnormalities. J Can Assoc Radiol 27:21, 1976.)

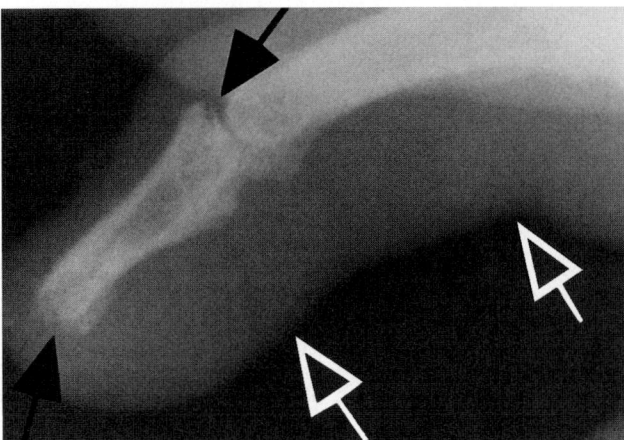

**Figure 53–15.** Spread of infection in the hand: paronychia. Widespread infection of the pulp space, digital flexor tendon sheath, terminal tuft, and distal interphalangeal joint *(solid arrows)* resulted from an initial subcuticular abscess. Soft tissue swelling along the tendon sheath can be noted *(open arrows)*. (From Resnick D: Osteomyelitis and septic arthritis complicating hand injuries and infections: Pathogenesis of roentgenographic abnormalities. J Can Assoc Radiol 27:21, 1976.)

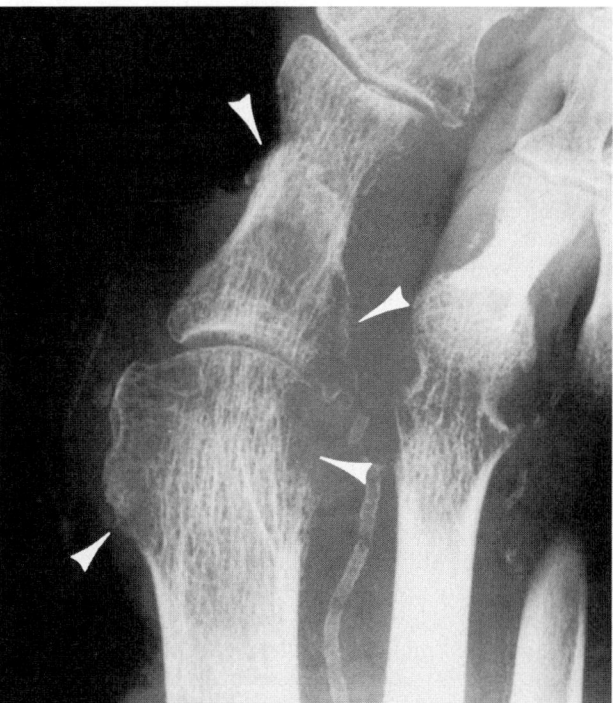

**Figure 53–17.** Spread of infection in the foot: diabetes mellitus. Radiograph reveals a soft tissue infection about the first metatarsophalangeal joint, with ulcerations and erosion of bone *(arrowheads)*. Observe vascular calcification and alterations at the second metatarsophalangeal joint.

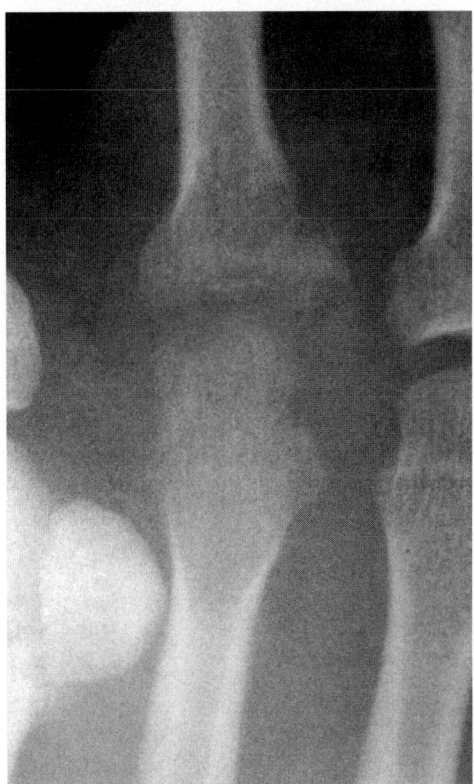

**Figure 53–16.** Spread of infection in the foot: puncture wounds. After a puncture wound from a nail, this patient developed a plantar soft tissue infection that led to osteomyelitis and septic arthritis. Observe osseous destruction of the metatarsal head and proximal phalanx, joint space narrowing, and soft tissue swelling.

prominences such as the femoral trochanters and ischial tuberosities. Heterotopic ossification, a well-recognized accompaniment of neurologic injury, further complicates the early diagnosis of osteomyelitis. Routine radiography is reported to be insensitive and nonspecific in the diagnosis of bone infection in patients with pressure sores, related in part to the difficulty of differentiating changes caused by abnormal pressure from those of osteomyelitis. CT and MR imaging are helpful, although precise diagnosis frequently requires histologic examination of the bone.

## Direct Implantation of Infection

### General Clinical Features

Puncture wounds of the hand and foot can lead to osteomyelitis (and septic arthritis) by contamination of adjacent soft tissues or by direct inoculation of the bone or joint. This latter complication is especially prevalent in the foot, where nails, splinters, or glass can lead to deep puncture wounds; in the hand, where a human bite received during a fistfight can directly injure osseous and articular structures; and in any site after an animal bite.

### General Radiographic Features

The features of bone (and joint) involvement after direct implantation of an infectious process are virtually identical to those occurring after spread of infection from a contiguous contaminated source. Commonly, osseous destruction and proliferation lead to focal areas of lysis, sclerosis, and periostitis. Soft tissue swelling is common, related not to infection but to edema resulting from the injury itself.

## Human Bites

The most common cause of human bite injury is a fist blow to the mouth that results in laceration of the dorsum of the metacarpophalangeal joint. Joint infection is more common than bone infection in these cases. *S. aureus* or *Streptococcus* species are the usual implicated organisms. The radiographic findings, which are particularly well shown on steep oblique and lateral radiographs, include peculiar bony defects and fractures, tooth fragments, and osseous and articular destruction (Fig. 53–18).

## Animal Bites

Superficial animal bites or scratches can inoculate local soft tissues, leading to infection of underlying bones and joints. Deep animal bites can introduce organisms directly into osseous and articular structures. Dog bites account for approximately 90% of these injuries and cat bites for about 10%. Approximately 5% of dog bites and 20% to 50% of cat bites become infected significantly. The infecting organisms vary, but *Pasteurella multocida* is commonly implicated, especially in cat bites. Any anatomic site can be affected, although animal bites are seen predominantly in the hand, arm, and leg (Fig. 53–19).

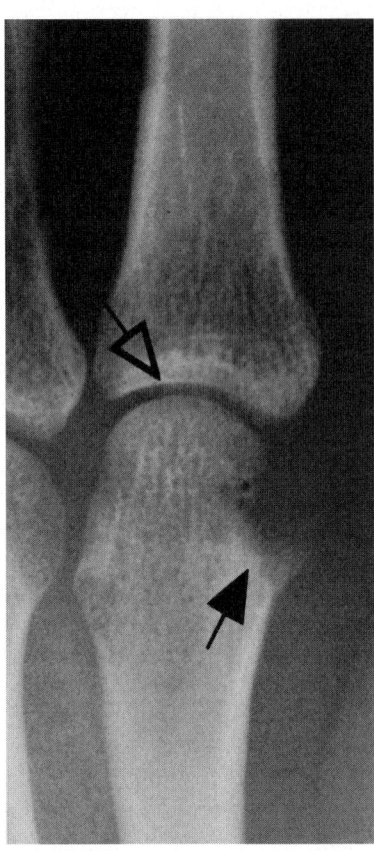

**Figure 53–18.** Infection due to direct implantation: human bites. Destruction of the third metacarpal head (*solid arrow*) and a narrowed metacarpophalangeal joint (*open arrow*) resulted from infection after a fistfight in which the patient's fist struck the opponent's teeth. (From Resnick D: Osteomyelitis and septic arthritis complicating hand injuries and infections: Pathogenesis of roentgenographic abnormalities. J Can Assoc Radiol 27:21, 1976.)

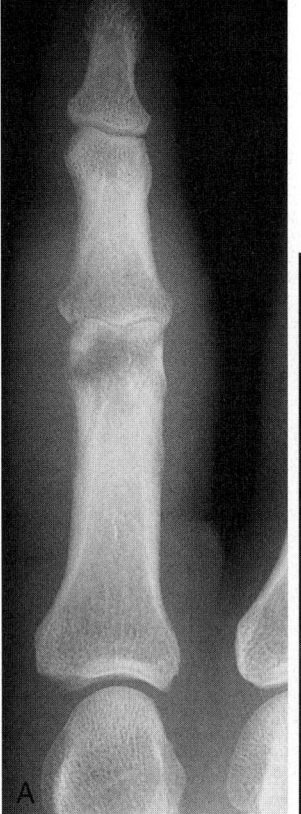
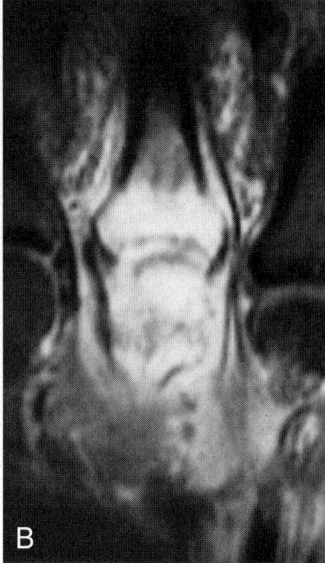

**Figure 53–19.** Infection due to direct implantation: animal bites. *A,* After a cat bite, this patient developed *Pasteurella* osteomyelitis and septic arthritis. Observe soft tissue swelling, osseous destruction of the proximal and middle phalanges, and joint space narrowing and flexion at the proximal interphalangeal joint. *B,* In a different patient who developed *Pasteurella* osteomyelitis and septic arthritis after a cat bite, a coronal T1-weighted (TR/TE, 800/20) spin echo MR image obtained with fat saturation technique and intravenous gadolinium enhancement shows high signal intensity in the third metacarpophalangeal joint and adjacent bone and soft tissue.

## Open Fractures and Dislocations

Whenever a fracture or dislocation is complicated by disruption of the overlying skin, direct inoculation of bones and joints can occur. This problem is especially relevant to injuries of the tibia. Despite the early administration of antibiotics, chronic osteomyelitis is frequent in this setting.

## Postoperative Infection

Postoperative infections occur as a result of contamination of bones and joints from adjacent infected soft tissues, direct inoculation of osseous and articular tissue at the time of surgery, or, less frequently, hematogenous spread to an operative site from a distant location. Particularly troublesome are instances of infection that occur after internal fixation of fractures, intervertebral disc surgery, median sternotomy, and various types of reconstructive procedures and arthroplasty. One or more organisms may be implicated; *S. aureus* is the most common pathogen.

One special type of postoperative infection relates to the transcutaneous insertion of pins into bone. The causative organisms vary, but infections caused by gram-negative bacteria are common. The mechanisms of contamination are also variable; in some cases, the pins are inserted into bones that are already the site of osteomyelitis, whereas in others, osseous infection occurs at the time of or after pin insertion. Radiographs reveal progressive osteolysis about the metal or, after removal of the pin, a ring sequestrum (Fig. 53–20). In the latter instance, the central circular radiolucent area created by the pin itself is surrounded by a ring of bone, which, in turn, is surrounded by an area of osteolysis.

## Complications

**Severe Osteolysis.** If osteomyelitis is not treated adequately or early enough, severe osteolysis may ensue. Large foci of destruction eventually can lead to disappearance of long segments of tubular or flat bones.

**Epiphyseal Growth Disturbance.** Injury to the cartilage cells on the epiphyseal side of the growth plate is irreparable, and subsequent growth disturbances are to be expected. Even with severe epiphyseal disintegration, however, some regeneration of the epiphysis can occur after eradication of the infection (Fig. 53–21). It is difficult to predict the occurrence and extent of epiphyseal recovery after injury.

**Neoplasm.** Epidermoid carcinoma arising in a focus of chronic osteomyelitis is not uncommon. The latent period between the onset of osteomyelitis and the appearance of neoplasm is variable, although a time span of 20 to 30 years is typical. Neoplasm most frequently arises adjacent to the femur and the tibia and is clinically evident as pain, increasing drainage, hemorrhage, onset of a foul odor from the sinus tract, a mass, and lymphadenopathy. Radiographically, there is progressive destruction of bone (Fig. 53–22). The prognosis is guarded.

**Amyloidosis.** Secondary amyloidosis can complicate chronic osteomyelitis. This complication has become less frequent, however, owing to improvement in the chemotherapy of infection. It is seen in less than 5% of cases of chronic osteomyelitis.

## Modifications and Diagnostic Difficulties

**Antibiotic-Modified Osteomyelitis.** The previous discussion was concerned with the radiographic and pathologic findings of untreated osteomyelitis. During the early healing phase of osteomyelitis, bone resorption continues as damaged osseous tissue is removed. Therefore, radiographically evident increased destruction can occur at a time when the clinical picture is improving.

**Active and Inactive Chronic Osteomyelitis.** Differentiation of active and inactive chronic osteomyelitis by imaging techniques can be extremely difficult, but certain indications on the radiograph may be helpful (Table 53–5).

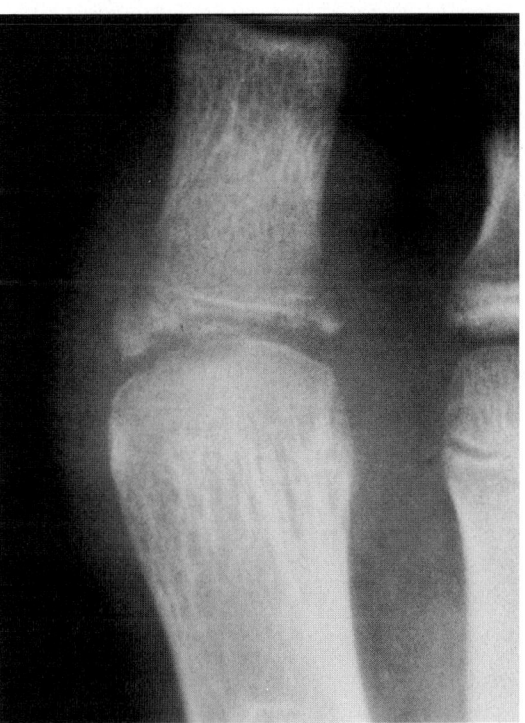

**Figure 53–21.** Complications of osteomyelitis: epiphyseal destruction. This 11-year-old boy developed osteomyelitis and septic arthritis of the first metatarsophalangeal joint. One week after initial presentation, the epiphysis has fragmented and largely disappeared, and osteolysis of both the metatarsal bone and the phalanx can be noted. Joint space narrowing is seen. (Courtesy of T. Goergen, MD, Escondido, Calif.)

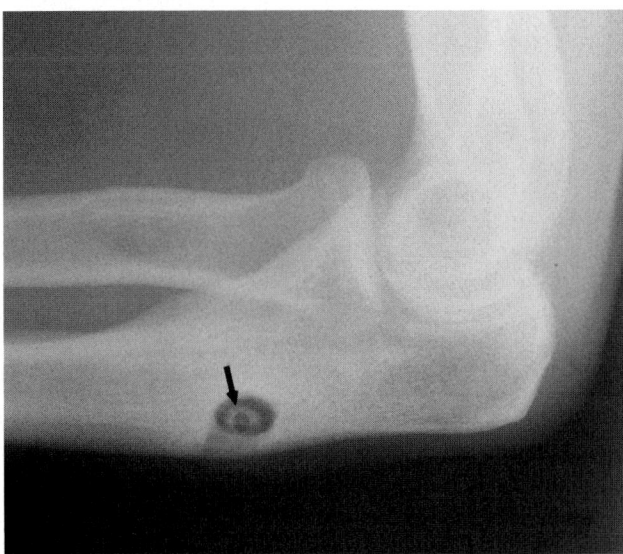

**Figure 53–20.** Postoperative infection: pinhole ring sequestrum. Percutaneous pins were used to treat a fracture about the wrist in this 27-year-old man. Purulent drainage occurred, requiring removal of the pins. Note the classic radiographic findings of a ring sequestrum (*arrow*).

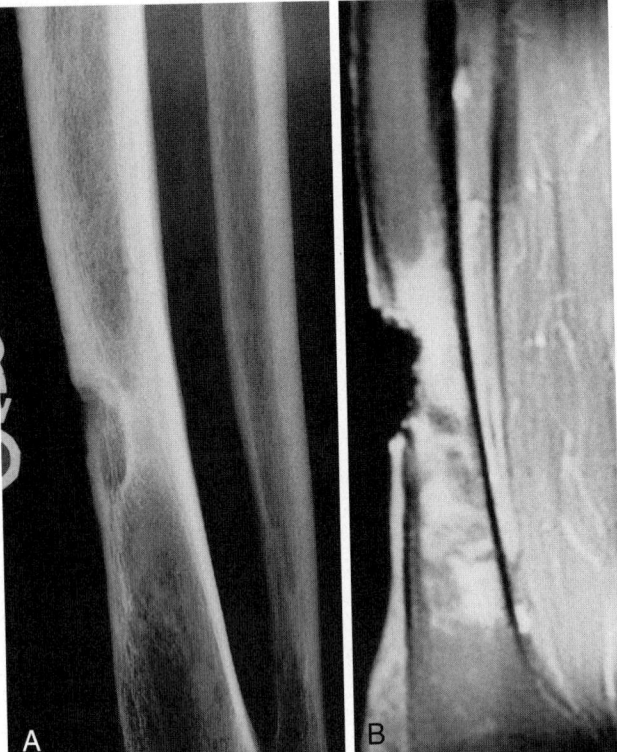

**Figure 53–22.** Complications of osteomyelitis: neoplasm. This 69-year-old man developed a squamous cell carcinoma of a sinus tract after years of osteomyelitis of the tibia with drainage. *A*, Lateral radiograph shows osteolysis of the tibia, which was related to tumorous involvement of the bone. A soft tissue mass at this site cannot be seen in this image. The soft tissue mass and involved bone were excised. *B*, In the immediate postoperative period, a sagittal fat-suppressed T1-weighted (TR/TE, 550/20) spin echo MR image obtained after intravenous gadolinium contrast agent administration shows edema of high signal intensity in the tibia, presumably related to the surgery, although the presence of residual intraosseous tumor could not be excluded.

Periostitis that is thin and linear in quality and separated from the subjacent bone suggests activity. Poorly defined or fluffy periosteal excrescences extending into the adjacent soft tissues also suggest active infection. Finally, documentation of an abscess or sequestration on routine radiography, conventional tomography, CT, or MR imaging implies activity, because necrotic osseous fragments or abscesses commonly harbor viable organisms.

## Differential Diagnosis

**General Features.** The combination of clinical and imaging characteristics in osteomyelitis usually ensures the correct diagnosis. Occasionally, aggressive bone destruction combined with periostitis and soft tissue swelling simulates the changes in malignant neoplasms, especially Ewing's sarcoma or osteosarcoma in children, histiocytic lymphoma in young adults, and skeletal metastasis in older persons. The imaging features of osteomyelitis may resemble those of bone infarction, especially in the diaphysis of a long

| **TABLE 53–5** |
| --- |
| **Radiographic Signs of Activity in Chronic Osteomyelitis** |

Change from previous radiograph
Poorly defined areas of osteolysis
Thin, linear periostitis
Sequestration

bone. Further, patients who have sickle cell anemia or Gaucher's disease, and those who have lymphoproliferative disorders or are receiving steroid medications, are predisposed to the development of either osteomyelitis or bone infarction (or both), compounding the diagnostic difficulty.

**Periostitis.** The nature of the periosteal proliferation accompanying osteomyelitis is varied. In some patients, single or multiple osseous shells appear. This "onion-skinning" is not specific for osteomyelitis, because it may also be evident in malignant neoplasm (e.g., Ewing's sarcoma). A triangular area (Codman's triangle) of periostitis, similar to that seen in osteosarcoma, may be evident in osteomyelitis. In cases of osteomyelitis in which a single thick layer of periosteal bone is seen, the changes are reminiscent of eosinophilic granuloma or traumatic periostitis.

**Osteolytic Foci.** In a child, identification of a metaphyseal radiolucent lesion abutting the growth plate or connected to it by a channel suggests the presence of an abscess. Although osteosarcoma is typically metaphyseal in location, and Ewing's sarcoma may be metaphyseal, the osteolytic foci in these tumors are more poorly marginated, and considerable neoplastic bone production may be evident in osteosarcoma. In a child, epiphyseal infection with abscess formation leads to radiographic features similar to those of chondroblastoma, enchondroma, or eosinophilic granuloma.

**Osteosclerosis.** In some cases of osteomyelitis, exuberant bone formation produces widespread sclerosis. This may be uniform or combined with mottled radiolucent shadows. The resulting radiographic picture can simulate malignant bone tumors (e.g., osteosarcoma, Ewing's sarcoma, histiocytic lymphoma, chondrosarcoma), osteonecrosis, fibrous dysplasia, or Paget's disease.

**Sequestration.** Radiodense foci representing sequestra are reliable indicators of infection. Their occasional appearance in tumors (e.g., fibrosarcoma) does not significantly diminish the diagnostic nature of the finding.

**Soft Tissue Masses and Swelling.** In general, tumors are associated with circumscribed soft tissue masses that displace surrounding soft tissue planes and frequently contain visible tumor matrix. Infections lead to infiltration and obscureness of soft tissue planes. This differentiation is not uniformly reliable, however.

# SEPTIC ARTHRITIS

## Articular Manifestations of Infection

Septic arthritis is but one of several processes that can cause or perpetuate articular disease in patients with infection. An infectious agent may trigger a sterile synovitis at a site distant from the primary infective focus. A classic example is the reactive arthritis of acute rheumatic fever occurring as a complication of streptococcal throat infection. Clinical characteristics common to reactive arthritides include a symptom-free interval, a self-limited course in which cartilage or bone destruction is rare, a characteristic clinical presentation that includes acute migratory polyarthritis, a tendency in some patients toward involvement of the heart, and a negative serologic test for rheumatoid factor. Inciting infections commonly reach the body through one of three portals of entry: the oronasopharynx and respiratory tract, the urogenital tract, and the intestinal tract. The existence of reactive arthritis in patients with infection underscores the importance of performing joint aspiration and attempting to isolate the causative organisms in all cases of suspected septic arthritis.

## Routes of Contamination

The potential routes of contamination of joints can be divided into the same categories used in the previous discussion of osteomyelitis (Fig. 53–23).

1. *Hematogenous spread of infection.* Hematogenous seeding of the synovial membrane results from either direct transport of organisms within the synovial vessels or spread from an adjacent epiphyseal focus of osteomyelitis by means of vascular continuity between the epiphysis and the synovial membrane.

2. *Spread from a contiguous source of infection.* A joint may become contaminated by intra-articular extension of osteomyelitis from an epiphyseal or metaphyseal focus or of neighboring suppurative soft tissue processes.

3. *Direct implantation.* Inoculation of a joint can occur during aspiration or arthrography or after a penetrating wound.

4. *Postoperative infection.* An intra-articular suppurative process can occur after arthroscopy or any other type of joint surgery.

## Hematogenous Infection

### Pathogenesis

Hematogenous spread of infection to a joint indicates that organisms are transported within the vasculature of the synovial membrane directly from a distant infected source or indirectly from an adjacent bone infection. In either case, infection of the synovial membrane precedes contamination of the synovial fluid. Therefore, initial arthrocentesis may suggest bland inflammation of the joint. The reaction of the synovial tissue to the contained organisms varies according to the local and general resistance of the patient and the number, type, and virulence of the infecting agents.

## General Clinical Features

Monoarticular involvement is the major pattern of presentation, especially in younger age groups. The specific site or sites of infection depend on the age of the patient, the organism, and the existence of an underlying disease or problem. The knee, particularly in children, infants, and adults, and the hip, especially in children and infants, are frequently affected. With pyogenic infection, an acute onset with fever and chills is typical, although a prodromal phase of several days' duration with malaise, arthralgia, and low-grade fever can be encountered. Pain, tenderness, redness, heat, and soft tissue swelling of the involved joint are common. Leukocytosis and positive blood and joint cultures are important laboratory parameters of pyogenic arthritis. Elevated erythrocyte sedimentation rates and C-reactive protein levels are also encountered. The organism most commonly implicated is *S. aureus. H. influenzae* represents an important and common cause of septic arthritis in children younger than 5 years.

## Radiographic-Pathologic Correlation

In response to bacterial infection, the synovial membrane becomes edematous, swollen, and hypertrophied. Increased amounts of synovial fluid are produced; the fluid may be thin and cloudy, contain large numbers of leukocytes, and reveal a lowered sugar level and an elevated protein count. After a few days, frank pus accumulates in the articular cavity, and destruction of cartilage begins (Table 53–6; Fig. 53–24). Prominent abnormality may appear at the margins or in central portions of joints, accompanied by growth of the inflamed synovium across the surface of the cartilage or between cartilage and bone. Cartilaginous erosion (from superficially located pannus) and disruption of the chondral surface (from subchondral pannus) can develop. With further fluid, the capsule becomes distended, surrounding soft tissue edema is evident, and osseous abnormalities ensue. Superficial marginal and central bony erosions may progress to extensive destruction of large segments of the articular surface. Fibrous or bony ankylosis can eventually occur.

Radiographic abnormalities parallel the pathologic changes in pyogenic arthritis (Fig. 53–25). Interosseous space narrowing, which is frequently diffuse, reflects damage and disruption of the chondral surface. Osseous erosions at the edges of the joint, related to the effects of diseased synovium on bone, lead to marginal defects. Subchondral extension of pannus destroys the bone plate and adjacent trabeculae, leading to poorly defined gaps in the subchondral "white" line on the radiograph. Further destruction of bone becomes evident, and in late stages, bony ankylosis of the joint may be seen.

Rapid destruction of bone and cartilage is characteristic of bacterial arthritis, whereas in tuberculosis and fungal diseases articular changes occur more slowly. In tuberculosis, marginal osseous erosions with preservation of joint space and periarticular osteoporosis may be prominent. Infrequently, gas formation within a joint complicates septic arthritis. Much more frequently, the appearance of radiolucent collections in an infected joint indicates that a prior arthrocentesis has been performed.

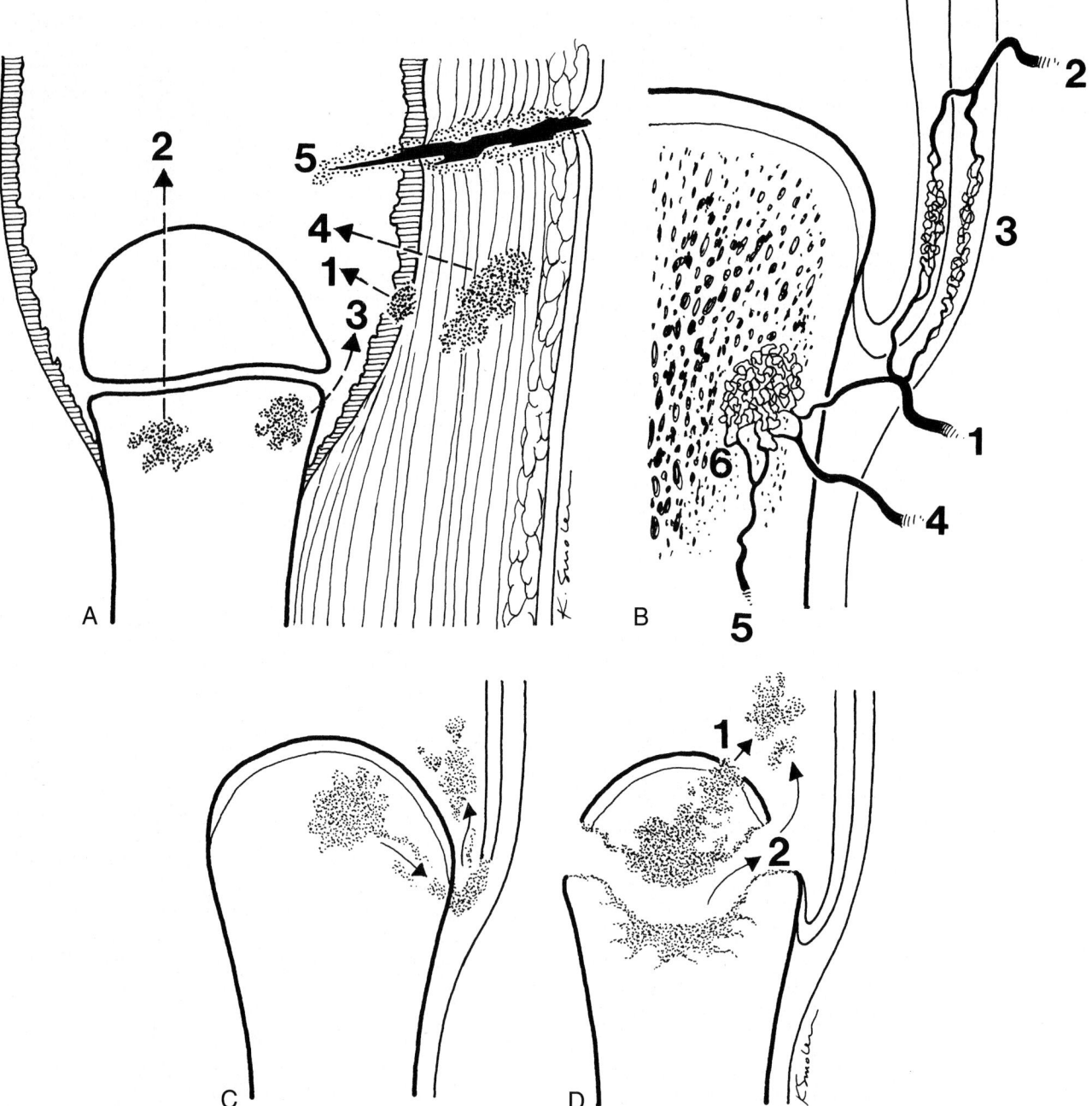

**Figure 53–23.**  Septic arthritis: potential routes of contamination. *A,* Hematogenous spread of infection to a joint can result from direct lodgment of organisms in the synovial membrane (1). Spread into the joint from a contiguous source can occur from a metaphyseal focus that extends into the epiphysis and from there into the joint (2), from a metaphyseal focus with extension into the joint when the growth plate is intra-articular (3), or from a contiguous soft tissue infection (4). Direct implantation after a penetrating wound (5) can also lead to septic arthritis. *B,* Hematogenous spread of infection to a joint can occur owing to vascular continuity between the epiphysis and the synovial membrane. The vessels shown include arterioles (1), venules (2), and capillaries (3) of the capsule; periosteal vessels (4); the nutrient artery (5); and metaphyseal-epiphyseal anastomoses (6). *C,* Sequence of events by which the synovial membrane can become infected from an osseous focus before the joint fluid is contaminated. *D,* Spread from a contiguous osseous surface can result from penetration of the cartilage (1) or pathologic fracture with articular contamination (2). In this situation, synovial fluid may become infected before the synovial membrane.

**TABLE 53–6**

### Septic Arthritis: Radiographic-Pathologic Correlation

| Pathologic Abnormality | Radiographic Abnormality |
| --- | --- |
| Edema and hypertrophy of synovial membrane with fluid production | Joint effusion, soft tissue swelling |
| Hyperemia | Osteoporosis |
| Inflammatory pannus with chondral destruction | Joint space loss |
| Pannus destruction of bone | Marginal and central osseous erosion |
| Fibrous or bony ankylosis | Bony ankylosis |

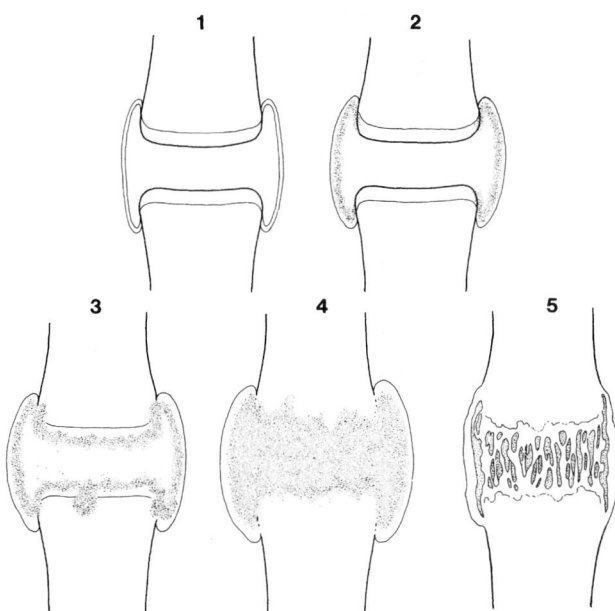

**Figure 53–24.** Septic arthritis: pathologic abnormalities. 1, Normal synovial joint. 2, An edematous, swollen, and hypertrophic synovial membrane becomes evident. 3 and 4, Accumulating inflammatory pannus leads to chondral destruction and to marginal and central osseous erosions. 5, Bony ankylosis may eventually result.

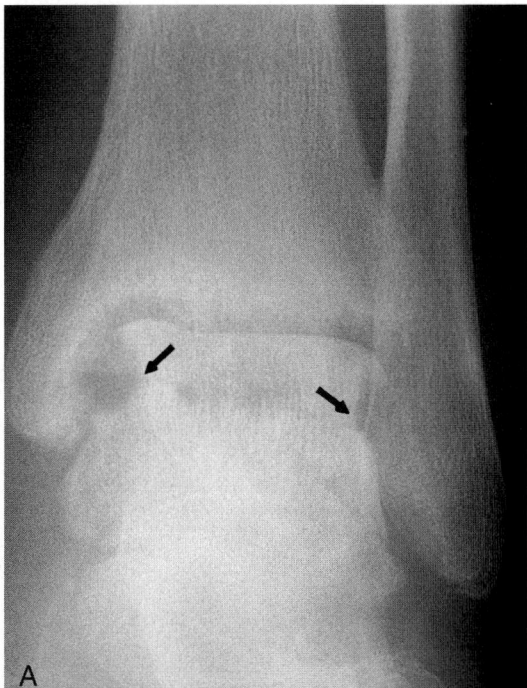

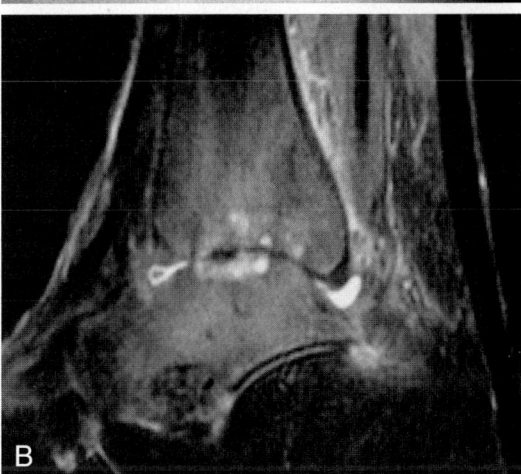

**Figure 53–25.** Septic arthritis: hematogenous spread of infection. *A*, Radiograph reveals joint space narrowing and osseous erosions, which predominate at the margins of the talus *(arrows)*. *B*, In this patient with acquired immunodeficiency syndrome, a sagittal STIR (TR/TE, 3200/18; inversion time, 150 msec) MR image show classic features of septic arthritis of the ankle, with cartilage and bone erosion and marrow edema in the tibia and talus.

## Infection from a Contiguous Source

### Pathogenesis

In certain age groups, osteomyelitis can be complicated by contamination of the adjacent articulation. Septic arthritis complicating osteomyelitis occurs in as many as one third of patients and is seen most commonly in the hip and knee. In infants, the presence of vascular communication between metaphyseal and epiphyseal segments of tubular bones allows organisms within nutrient vessels to localize in the epiphysis and subsequently extend into the joint. In adults, vascular connections between the epiphysis and metaphysis are reestablished as the growth plate closes. Hematogenous osteomyelitis thus can affect the epiphysis in this age group.

A second situation in which septic arthritis can occur as a result of contamination from a contiguous source is related to adjacent soft tissue infection or, more infrequently, nearby visceral infection (e.g., vesicoacetabular or enteroacetabular fistulas). Predisposing factors include pelvic trauma, surgical manipulation, and diverticulitis.

Joint infection may also develop as a result of extension from a surrounding suppurative process in sites where the growth plate has an intra-articular location; the most important such sites are the hip and the glenohumeral joint. Because of this anatomic arrangement, osteomyelitis localized to the metaphysis can enter the joint by extending laterally without violating the growth plate.

### Radiographic-Pathologic Correlation

Usually, radiographic evidence exists that the infective process originates outside the articulation. This evidence may include soft tissue deficit, swelling, or gas formation; osteomyelitis with typical epiphyseal or metaphyseal destruction; and diverticulitis or cystitis with fistulization. In certain situations, however, joint effusion and cartilaginous and subchondral osseous destruction are the first radiographic clues to infection. Once the articulation has been violated, the radiographic and pathologic abnormalities of the infection are virtually identical to those associated with hematogenously derived suppurative joint disease.

### Specific Entities

Neonatal septic arthritis affects the hip joint most frequently, and *S. aureus* is the organism most commonly implicated. In this age group, infection can reach the hip via spread from a metaphyseal focus of osteomyelitis either directly into the joint (the growth plate is intra-articular) or to the epiphysis by way of vascular channels that cross the growth plate. Clinically, infants with septic arthritis of the hip may manifest irritability, loss of appetite, and fever. Initial radiographs of the hip are frequently unremarkable. With accumulation of intra-articular fluid, pathologic subluxation or dislocation of the femoral head can occur, although the lack of ossification in most of the proximal capital femoral epiphysis makes this sign difficult to apply (Fig. 53–26). A helpful finding, however, is radiographically detectable osteomyelitis of the femoral metaphysis manifested as osteolysis, osteosclerosis, or periostitis.

The radiographic findings of hip infection in infants can simulate those of other conditions; therefore, aspiration of the joint is mandatory to firmly establish the diagnosis of septic arthritis and to provide guidelines for adequate therapy. Only as the child develops and ossification of the immature skeleton proceeds will the degree of residual deformity from destruction of the cartilaginous femoral head and acetabulum become apparent (Fig. 53–27).

Septic arthritis of the hip is also frequent in children, although the overall frequency of this problem and the extent of its devastating effects on local cartilage and bone are less than in infants. It may be associated with the acute onset of fever, pain, swelling, and limping, as well as a dramatic leukocytosis. On radiographs, accumulation of intra-articular fluid may produce soft tissue swelling, capsular distention, and subtle lateral displacement of the ossified epiphysis. The prognosis of septic arthritis of the hip for a child is far better than that for an infant. Osteonecrosis of the femoral head occurring after metaphyseal or epiphyseal infection in a

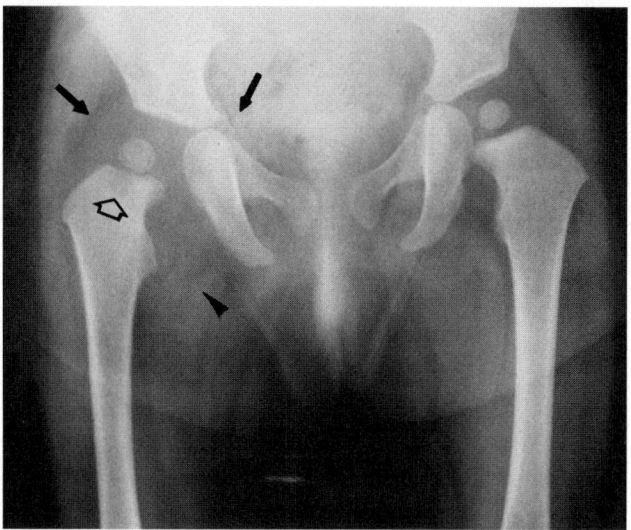

**Figure 53–26.**  Septic arthritis of the hip: infancy. This infant developed septic arthritis of the right hip and osteomyelitis. Note displacement of the "capsular" and obturator fat planes *(solid arrows)*, obliteration of the iliopsoas fat plane *(arrowhead)*, and a metaphyseal focus of infection *(open arrow)*. The femoral head is displaced laterally and is slightly enlarged. The soft tissue findings indicative of intra-articular fluid may be of more diagnostic help in this age group than in adults. (Courtesy of J. Weston, MD, Lower Hutt, New Zealand.)

child (or infant) is an important complication of the disease (Fig. 53–28). Osteonecrosis of the epiphysis is usually not recognized until 6 to 8 weeks after the onset of infection. The epiphysis can reveal a generalized increase in radiodensity, followed by fragmentation and, less commonly, collapse.

### Direct Implantation of Infection

Arthrocentesis for the evaluation of synovial contents or for arthrography can introduce gram-positive or gram-negative bacteria. Similarly, penetrating injuries, such as those that occur in a fistfight or from a bullet, knife, nail, or other sharp object, can lead to septic arthritis.

### Postoperative Infection

Articular surgery in the form of arthroscopy, arthrotomy, arthrodesis, arthroplasty, or another procedure can be complicated by joint infection in the postoperative period. Infections occurring soon after such procedures are usually related to direct inoculation of the joint during the operation or to intra-articular spread from an adjacent contaminated focus (e.g., soft tissue abscess). Joint infection occurring long after surgery is frequently associated with obvious preceding sepsis elsewhere in the body and may relate to hematogenous spread to the joint from this distant process.

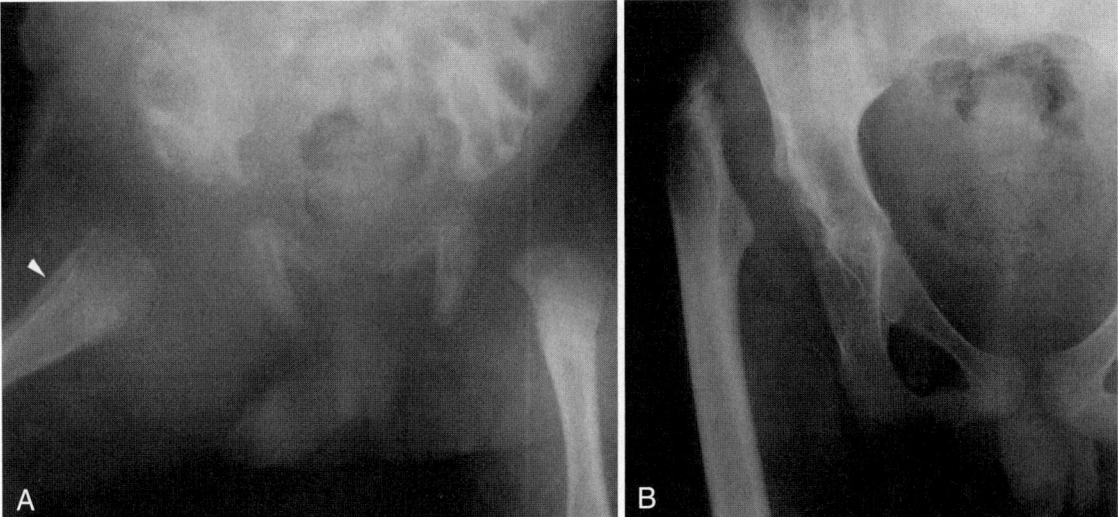

**Figure 53–27.** Septic arthritis of the hip: infancy. *A,* This neonate developed septic arthritis of the right hip. The initial radiograph reveals soft tissue swelling and periosteal reaction along the femur *(arrowhead).* *B,* At age 13 years, the ossification centers of the greater and lesser trochanters are apparent. Femoral dislocation, acetabular shallowness, and absence of epiphyseal ossification are evident. (From Freiberger RH, Ghelman B, Kaye JJ, and Spragge JW: Hip disease of infancy and childhood. In Moseley RD Jr, et al [eds]: Current Problems in Radiology. Chicago, Year Book Medical Publishers, 1973.)

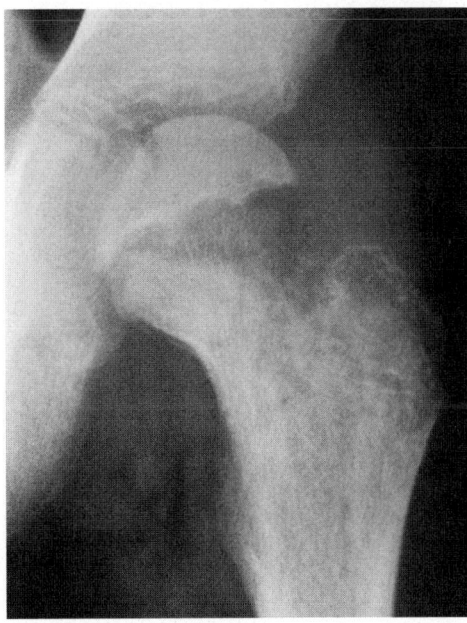

**Figure 53–28.** Septic arthritis of the hip: childhood. The complication of osteonecrosis in a child with septic arthritis of the hip is well demonstrated in this patient. Subsequently, progressive osteomyelitis and septic arthritis produced increased intra-articular fluid and osteonecrosis of the femoral head, manifested as increased radiodensity. Eventually, disintegration of the femoral head occurred.

## Complications

Several potential complications of septic arthritis deserve emphasis. The frequency of synovial cyst formation in septic arthritis appears to be low. Infrequently, synovial rupture of the cyst, with or without sinus tract formation, is observed. Septic arthritis can lead to disruption of adjacent capsular, tendinous, and soft tissue structures. This complication has been well documented in the glenohumeral joint.

Radiographic and pathologic evidence of osteomyelitis is associated with septic arthritis. Bony abnormalities can antedate and be the source of the suppurative joint process, or they can indicate the contamination of adjacent bony surfaces from a primary joint infection. Partial or complete osseous fusion may represent the residual findings of septic arthritis. This complication is not frequent; however, bone ankylosis is occasionally encountered after pyogenic processes. Significant destruction of articular cartilage from joint sepsis can lead to incongruity of apposing articular surfaces and, later, to changes of secondary osteoarthritis. The resulting radiographic findings, consisting of joint space narrowing, sclerosis, and osteophytosis, may be difficult to differentiate from primary osteoarthritis.

## Modifications and Diagnostic Difficulties

Inadequate or inappropriate administration of antibiotics can modify articular infection. Clinical manifestations may be masked, appearing relatively late in the course of the disease, and radiographic changes may be less dramatic, less extensive, and much delayed. When infection is superimposed on a previous articular disorder such as rheumatoid arthritis, calcium pyrophosphate dihydrate crystal deposition disease, or osteoarthritis, the clinical and radiographic abnormalities can be hidden or changed by the underlying disease process.

## Differential Diagnosis

Although numerous disorders such as pigmented villonodular synovitis, idiopathic synovial osteochondromatosis, juvenile chronic arthritis, and even adult-onset rheumatoid arthritis can be associated with mono-articular changes, infection must be considered the prime diagnostic possibility until proved otherwise. This is particularly true when the joint process is associated with loss of interosseous space, poorly defined or "fuzzy" osseous margins, and a sizable effusion. In patients with pyogenic infection, the articular destruction can be rapid. Diagnostic difficulty arises when the septic process involves more than one joint or when septic arthritis appears during the course of another articular disorder.

Of all the radiographic features of infection, it is the poorly defined nature of the bony destruction that is most characteristic. Osseous erosions or cysts in gout, rheumatoid arthritis, seronegative spondyloarthropathies, osteoarthritis, pigmented villonodular synovitis, idiopathic synovial osteochondromatosis, hemophilia, and calcium pyrophosphate dihydrate crystal deposition disease are more sharply marginated. Further, concentric loss of interosseous space is typical in infection, but focal diminution of the articular space (as noted in osteo-arthritis) and relative preservation of articular space (as seen in gout, pigmented villonodular synovitis, idiopathic synovial osteochondromatosis, and hemophilia) are rare in pyogenic infection.

Marginal erosions are frequent in processes associated with significant synovial inflammation, such as sepsis, rheumatoid arthritis, and the seronegative spondylo-arthropathies. They may also be observed in gout and, less commonly, in pigmented villonodular synovitis and idiopathic synovial osteochondromatosis. Similarly, peri-articular osteoporosis can be encountered in rheumatoid arthritis, Reiter's syndrome, juvenile chronic arthritis, hemophilia, and nonpyogenic suppurative processes, such as tuberculosis or fungal disease. Intra-articular bony ankylosis can represent the end stage of septic arthritis, the seronegative spondyloarthropathies, and, in some locations, rheumatoid arthritis and juvenile chronic arthritis.

## SOFT TISSUE INFECTION

### Routes of Contamination

Infection of soft tissue structures commonly results from direct contamination after trauma. Any process that disrupts the skin surface can lead to secondary infection. Hematogenous spread is less important as a mechanism in soft tissue contamination than it is in osteomyelitis and septic arthritis.

### Radiographic-Pathologic Correlation

Swelling with obliteration of adjacent tissue planes is characteristic of soft tissue infection. Radiolucent streaks within the contaminated area can relate to collections of air derived from the adjacent skin surface or to gas formation by various bacteria (Fig. 53–29). Erosion of bone due to pressure from an adjacent soft tissue mass is much more frequent when the mass is neoplastic rather than infectious in origin. When osseous abnormalities appear after soft tissue contamination, infective perios-

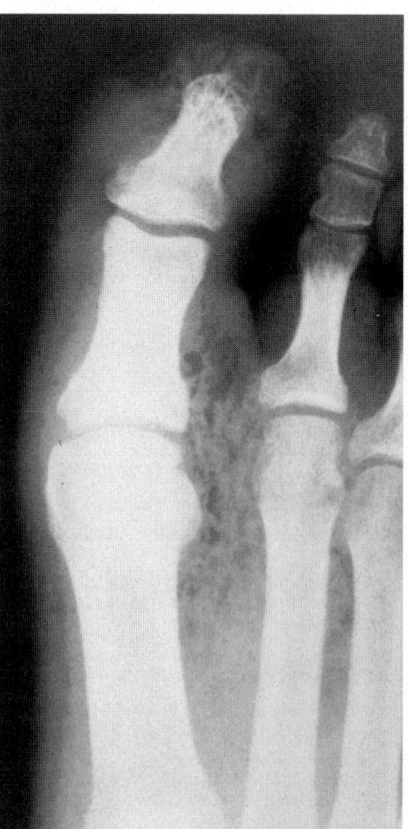

**Figure 53–29.** Soft tissue infection: gas formation. *Escherichia coli* infection in diabetes mellitus. Note the "bubbly" radiolucent collections in the foot.

titis, osteitis, or osteomyelitis is usually present (Fig. 53–30). A well-defined soft tissue mass is less typical of infection than of neoplasm. The edema of an infectious process usually leads to infiltration of surrounding soft tissues rather than displacement.

### Specific Entities

**Septic Subcutaneous Bursitis.** Septic bursitis most frequently localizes to the olecranon and the prepatellar and, less frequently, the subdeltoid regions. A history of recent injury, occupational trauma, or puncture is frequently, though not invariably, present. Clinical manifestations include painful swelling localized to the involved bursa, subcutaneous edema, a normal range of joint motion, and fever. Routine radiography, bursography, or MR imaging (Fig. 53–31) may be used to define the extent of the soft tissue infection. Septic bursitis is usually not associated with infectious arthritis.

**Septic Tenosynovitis.** Septic processes originating from a distant or local focus or occurring after trauma can also lead to tenosynovitis. Soft tissue swelling and surface resorption and erosion of underlying bony structures may be evident. MR imaging (Fig. 53–32) and ultrasonography are appropriate diagnostic methods applied to the assessment of suppurative tenosynovitis.

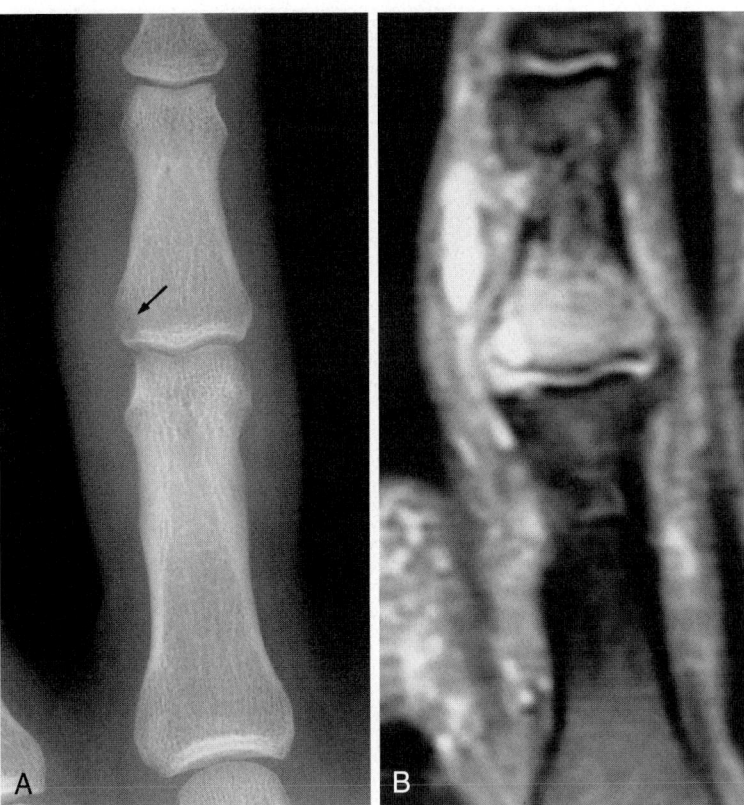

**Figure 53–30.** Soft tissue infection: osteomyelitis. This 30-year-old man developed a soft tissue infection after an injury. *A,* Radiograph shows soft tissue swelling and bone erosion in the middle phalanx *(arrow)*. *B,* Coronal fat-suppressed fast spin echo (TR/TE, 2000/21) MR image confirms the presence of osteomyelitis with bone erosion and edema and a soft tissue infective focus manifested as a region of high signal intensity.

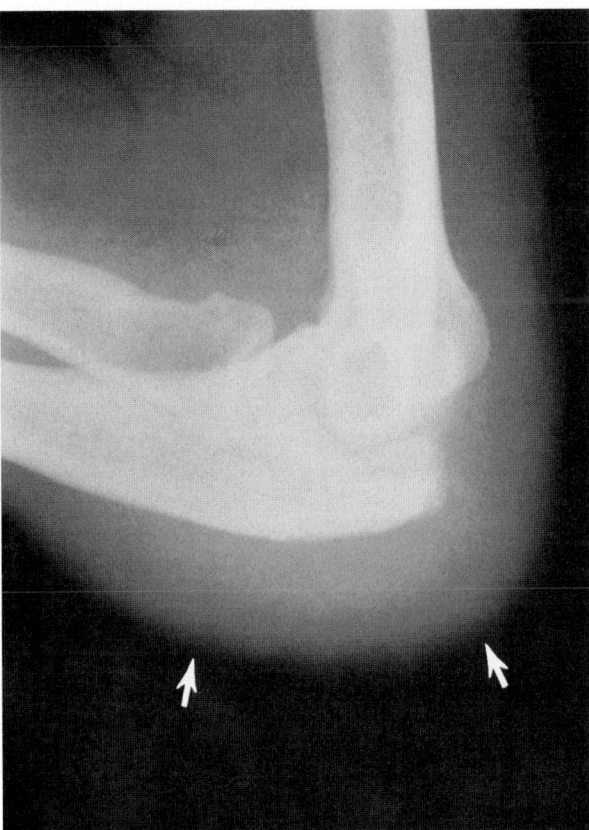

**Figure 53–31.** Septic olecranon bursitis. Note olecranon swelling *(arrows)* and soft tissue edema due to *Staphylococcus aureus*. Previous surgery and trauma are the causes of the adjacent bony abnormalities.

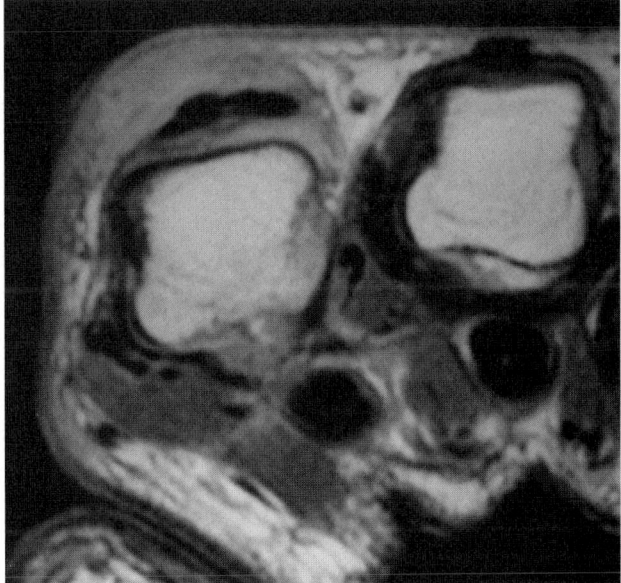

**Figure 53–32.** Infective tenosynovitis and cellulitis: extensor tendons of wrist and fingers. In this 50-year-old man with a puncture wound on the dorsum of the hand, a transverse intermediate-weighted (TR/TE, 2000/43) spin echo MR image shows infection involving the subcutaneous soft tissues and peritendinous tissue of the second finger.

**Lymphadenitis.** Lymphadenitis, usually with an accompanying cellulitis, can complicate streptococcal or staphylococcal infections. Nodular or diffuse soft tissue swelling and underlying periostitis may be encountered. Cat-scratch disease often manifests in this fashion.

**Cellulitis.** Cellulitis represents an acute inflammatory process of the deeper subcutaneous tissue; involvement of deep fasciae and muscles is unusual in cases of uncomplicated cellulitis. Clinical findings include pain or tenderness, redness, swelling, warmth, and mild to moderate fever. Cellulitis generally results from a streptococcal or, less commonly, a staphylococcal infection. Radiographic findings are nonspecific and are usually confined to the soft tissues. With T2-weighted spin echo MR imaging, cellulitis is characterized by subcutaneous thickening and hyperintense streaks or fluid collections in the subcutaneous fat and superficial fascial tissues. Enhancement of signal intensity in these regions is evident when gadolinium-containing contrast agents are administered intravenously (see Fig. 53–32).

**Necrotizing Fasciitis.** Necrotizing fasciitis represents a rare type of soft tissue infection that is accompanied by widespread fascial necrosis in the absence of muscular or cutaneous infection. It is a serious condition associated with systemic toxicity and, if untreated, death. Routine radiography may reveal evidence of soft tissue gas, although the clinical findings of fever, pain, swelling, and bullae usually allow an accurate diagnosis. MR imaging shows involvement of both superficial and deep soft tissue structures; the demonstration of deep fasciae with fluid collections, thickening, and enhancement of signal intensity with intravenous gadolinium-containing contrast agents generally distinguishes this condition from cellulitis (Fig. 53–33).

**Infectious Myositis.** Inflammation of muscle may occur in a variety of infectious disorders caused by viruses, bacteria, protozoa, and parasites. Pyogenic myositis (pyomyositis) is a well-recognized and serious infection affecting children and young adults in tropical regions (tropical pyomyositis) and, less frequently, in other locations. Although the disease, as described classically, occurs in otherwise healthy persons, it is being recognized with increasing frequency in malnourished and immunodeficient patients. Pyomyositis is related to *S. aureus* infection in about 90% of cases (streptococci account for most of the remaining cases). Sonographically guided percutaneous drainage may be helpful in the diagnosis and management of the condition, and MR imaging may further delineate the location and extent of the disease process. MR imaging findings (Fig. 53–34) include muscle enlargement; abscesses characterized by a peripheral rim of increased signal intensity on T1-weighted spin echo MR images, a central region (representing fluid) of intense signal on T2-weighted images, and peripheral enhancement after intravenous administration of gadolinium-based contrast medium; and associated abnormalities of subcutaneous edema in some cases.

## SPECIFIC SITUATIONS

### Chronic Granulomatous Disease

This heterogeneous disorder is a hereditary condition, usually transmitted as an X-linked recessive trait, that occurs in male children, although a similar syndrome has

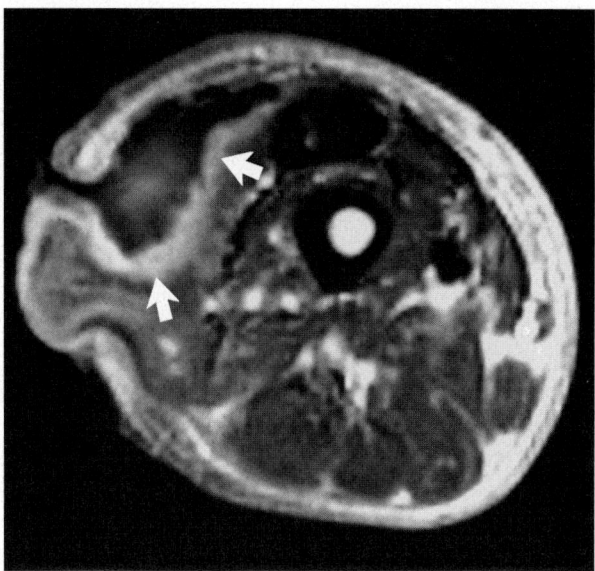

**Figure 53–33.** Necrotizing fasciitis and myositis with abscess formation and fistula: thigh. After the intravenous administration of a gadolinium-containing contrast agent, a transverse T1-weighted (TR/TE, 400/15) spin echo MR image reveals peripheral enhancement *(arrows)*, consistent with an abscess. Note the presence of the fistula. (From Rahmouni A, Chosidow O, Mathieu D, et al: MR imaging in acute infectious cellulitis. Radiology 192:493, 1994.)

been identified in female and male children without a family history of disease. The syndrome is characterized by purulent granulomatous and eczematoid skin lesions, granulomatous lymphadenitis with suppuration, hepatosplenomegaly, recurrent and persistent pneumonias, and chronic osteomyelitis (25% to 35%). It is frequently fatal (40%), and death before adolescence is common. Virtually every organ or tissue is vulnerable to infection in this disorder. Histologically, granulomas composed primarily of plasma cells, lymphocytes, macrophages, and multinucleated giant cells, with or without central caseation, are seen. A defect has been noted in the ability of the polymorphonuclear leukocytes and monocytes to destroy certain pathogenetic organisms adequately. Certain clinical and radiographic peculiarities characterize the osteomyelitis of chronic granulomatous disease of childhood:

1. The disease lacks the usual early clinical signs and symptoms of osteomyelitis, so that initial radiographs frequently reveal considerable bony involvement.

2. The causative organisms are usually of low virulence.

3. The most frequent site of involvement is the small bones of the hands and feet.

4. Osteomyelitis may result either from contamination related to an adjacent focus of infection, especially in the thoracic region, or from hematogenous dissemination.

5. The radiographic abnormalities are characterized by extensive osseous destruction with minimal reactive sclerosis.

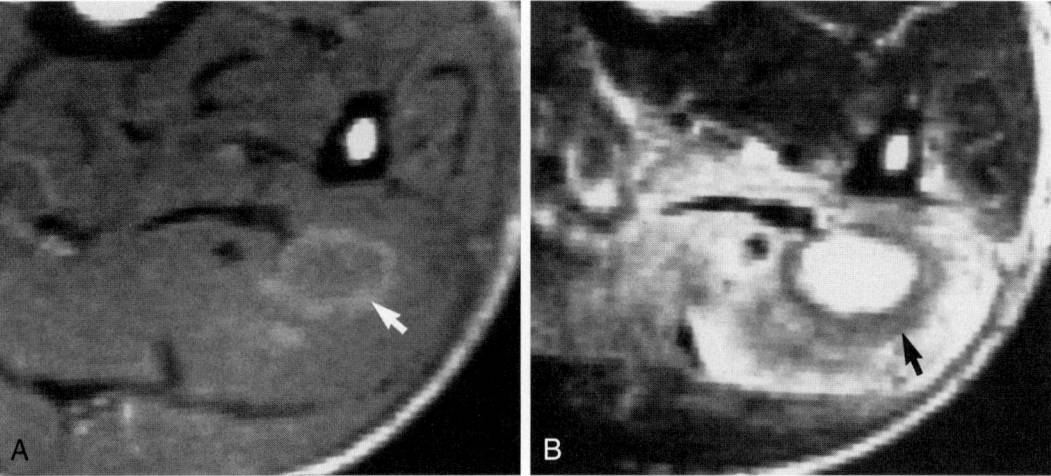

**Figure 53–34.** Infective myositis: soleus muscle. *Staphylococcus aureus* infection in a 34-year-old patient with acquired immunodeficiency syndrome. *A,* On a transaxial T1-weighted (TR/TE, 500/30) spin echo MR image, a rim of increased signal intensity *(arrow)* is evident. *B,* With T2 weighting (TR/TE, 2000/90), a similar transaxial image shows a central area of marked hyperintensity surrounded by a hypointense band *(arrow)*, which is itself surrounded by a more diffuse region of hyperintensity. The MR imaging findings are those of an abscess. (From Fleckenstein JL, Burn DK, Murphy FK, et al: Differential diagnosis of bacterial myositis in AIDS: Evaluation with MR imaging. Radiology 179:653, 1991.)

6. Osteomyelitis may develop in new areas despite continuous therapy.

7. Osteomyelitis eventually responds to long-term antibiotic therapy, so operative intervention is seldom necessary.

## Chronic Recurrent Multifocal Osteomyelitis

Chronic recurrent multifocal osteomyelitis (CRMO), which is also discussed as part of the SAPHO (synovitis, acne, pustulosis, hyperostosis, osteitis) syndrome in Chapter 82, is a variety of subacute and chronic osteomyelitis of unknown cause that occurs in childhood and frequently causes multiple and symmetrical alterations. It has also been referred to as condensing osteitis of the clavicle in childhood, chronic symmetrical plasma cell osteomyelitis, chronic sclerosing osteomyelitis, and multifocal chronic osteomyelitis. The usual age of onset of the disease is 5 to 10 years, although infants and adults may be affected. Skin lesions, including pustulosis palmaris et plantaris, acne fulminans, and psoriasis, are observed in some patients. CRMO has also been associated with Wegener's granulomatosis, inflammatory bowel disease, and leukemia. The metaphyses of the bones of the lower extremity and the medial ends of the clavicles are particularly vulnerable. Osteolysis with intense sclerosis may be noted. In certain locations, such as the clavicle, the bone may become massive (Fig. 53–35). The dominant radiographic feature at any skeletal site is bone sclerosis (Fig. 53–36). This feature is similar or identical to that described in cases of Garré's sclerosing osteomyelitis.

Both bone scintigraphy and MR imaging can be used to detect skeletal lesions in CRMO. With the former method, diagnostic difficulty is sometimes encountered owing to the normal uptake of radionuclide in the meta-

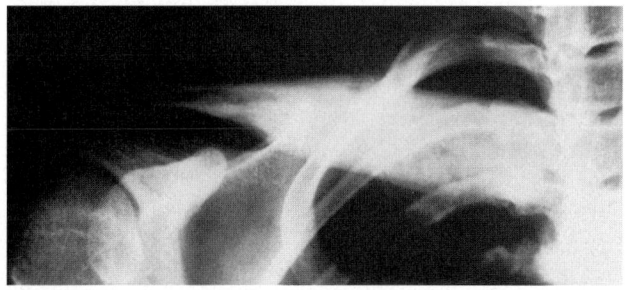

**Figure 53–35.** Chronic recurrent multifocal osteomyelitis: clavicle. Note massive enlargement of the clavicle. Biopsy and histologic evaluation indicated only chronic osteitis. Cultures were negative. (Courtesy of G. Greenway, MD, Dallas, Tex.)

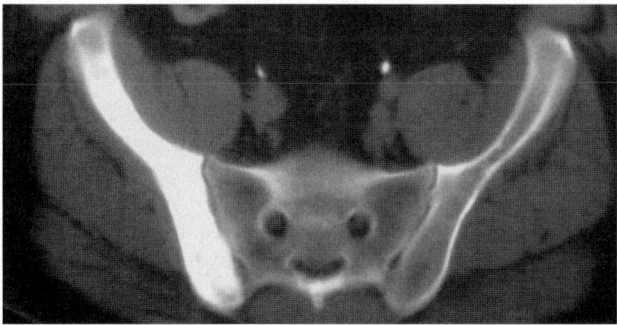

**Figure 53–36.** Chronic recurrent multifocal osteomyelitis: pelvis. Transaxial CT scan shows diffuse sclerosis of the ilium. Note that the sacrum is unaffected. (Courtesy of M. Pathria, MD, San Diego, Calif.)

physeal region of tubular bones. With MR imaging, low signal intensity in affected regions is seen on T1-weighted spin echo images, and variable signal intensity is noted on T2-weighted images. Laboratory analysis is usually nonspecific, and cultures of blood or bone after biopsy may be nonrewarding. Although the long-term prognosis is good, the condition may run a protracted course with resultant skeletal deformities.

Of considerable interest, the selective hyperostosis of the clavicle in this condition may also be seen in two other disorders. Osteitis condensans (condensing osteitis) of the medial end of the bone has been reported, especially in young women (see Chapter 47). Sternocostoclavicular hyperostosis of unknown cause, with painful swelling of the sternum, clavicles, and upper ribs, has also been described. Men and women are both affected, and the usual age at onset is in the fifth or sixth decade of life. Sternocostoclavicular hyperostosis is discussed further in Chapter 82. The relationship of CRMO to these other conditions is not clear, although the common involvement of the clavicle, as well as several other features, suggests an association.

## Osteomyelitis and Septic Arthritis in Intravenous Drug Abusers

An increased frequency of infectious disease has been noted in intravenous drug abusers. The mechanisms for this association are not entirely known. Use of contaminated narcotics or needles, colonization of the skin during previous hospitalizations, and alterations of the bacterial flora by pretreatment with antibiotics are three potential mechanisms that may explain an increased frequency of infection in intravenous drug abusers.

Hematogenous osteomyelitis and septic arthritis in intravenous drug users are characterized by unusual localization and unusual organisms. Although staphylococcal infection may be seen, *Pseudomonas*, *Klebsiella*, and *Serratia* are commonly implicated. The axial skeleton is frequently affected, especially the spine, sacroiliac joint, and sternoclavicular joint, with less common involvement of the manubriosternal joint (Fig. 53–37). The precise cause of axial skeletal involvement in intravenous drug abusers is not clear.

The occurrence of systemic candidiasis in heroin addicts deserves emphasis. Contamination of the lemon used to dissolve "brown" heroin by strains of *Candida albicans* previously colonizing the oropharynx and skin of heroin addicts is probably the source of the infection. Musculoskeletal sites of involvement include, foremost, the costochondral joints and, less commonly, the spine, sacroiliac joints, knees, and wrists. Additional musculoskeletal manifestations in intravenous drug abusers include lymphedema, thrombophlebitis, subcutaneous fat necrosis, atrophy and calcification, pyomyositis, myonecrosis, tenosynovitis, and chemical inflammation of the synovium due to direct intra-articular administration of the drug.

## OTHER DIAGNOSTIC TECHNIQUES
### Computed Tomography

The primary applications of CT to the evaluation of musculoskeletal infections are the delineation of the

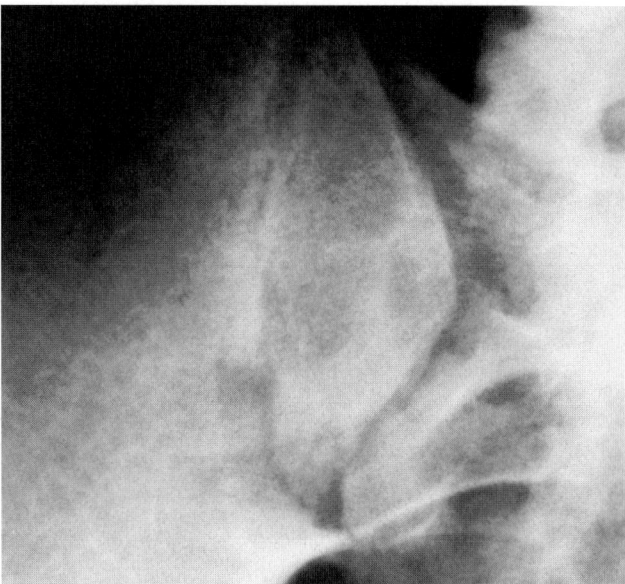

**Figure 53–37.** Hematogenous osteomyelitis and septic arthritis in an intravenous drug abuser: sacroiliac joint. Note indistinct margins about a narrowed sacroiliac joint.

osseous and soft tissue extent of the disease process, especially in areas of complex anatomy such as the vertebral column, and the monitoring of percutaneous aspiration and biopsy procedures, particularly of the spine, retroperitoneal tissues, and sacroiliac joints.

Many of the CT abnormalities in osteomyelitis are shared by primary and secondary malignant neoplasms affecting the skeleton, including an increased attenuation value in the medullary canal, destruction of cortical bone, new bone formation, and a soft tissue mass. With CT scanning, the detection of gas within the medullary canal is an infrequent but reliable diagnostic sign of osteomyelitis that may not be as evident on radiographs or MR imaging. (Fig. 53–38); it is analogous to the presence of gas within soft tissue abscesses. Fat-fluid levels within the

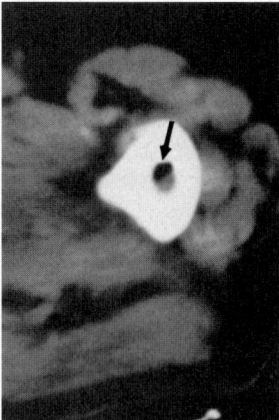

**Figure 53–38.** Acute osteomyelitis: CT. In this 54-year-old man with *Enterobacter* osteomyelitis of the hip and femur, transaxial CT scan at the level of the proximal portion of the femur reveals intramedullary gas collections *(arrow).* (Courtesy of V. Vint, MD, San Diego, Calif.)

medullary canal or in the adjacent joint are also reported in osteomyelitis and septic arthritis. CT evaluation in patients with subacute or chronic osteomyelitis may reveal cortical sequestration, cloacae, and bone and soft tissue abscesses (Fig. 53–39).

## Sinography

Retrograde injection of contrast material defines the course and extent of the sinus tract and its possible communication with an underlying bone or joint. Sinography may be combined with CT scanning or MR imaging for better delineation of the sinus tracts.

## Arthrography

The principal reason for performing a joint puncture in the clinical setting of infection is to obtain fluid for bacteriologic examination. After removal of the joint contents, however, contrast opacification of the joint can be used to outline the extent of the synovial inflammation and the presence of capsular, tendinous, and soft tissue injury.

## Ultrasonography

Ultrasonography is a useful technique for detecting effusions in the hip in children with transient synovitis, septic arthritis, or Legg-Calvé-Perthes disease. The absence of joint fluid in this joint on sonographic examination excludes the diagnosis of septic arthritis, though it does not eliminate the possibility of osteomyelitis. Further, sonography can be used to monitor aspiration of the effusion. Ultrasonography can also be employed in the detection of joint fluid in adults with septic arthritis of the hip and, in a similar fashion, to assess the presence and extent of infected fluid in superficially located joints, synovial cysts, bursae, and tendon sheaths in both children and adults.

## Radionuclide Examination

Although the use of scintigraphy in the evaluation of musculoskeletal infections is discussed in Chapter 7, a few comments are appropriate here. Technetium phosphate bone scans become abnormal within hours to days after the onset of bone infection and days to weeks before the disease becomes manifest on conventional radiographs. The scintigraphic abnormality initially may be evident as

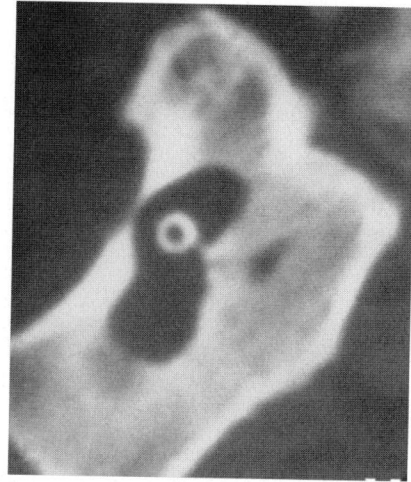

**Figure 53–39.** Chronic osteomyelitis: CT. Transverse CT scan reveals bone destruction and a sequestrum in the calcaneus that resulted from a pin tract infection.

a photo-deficient area ("cold" spot), a finding that is related to fulminant infection with thrombosis or vascular compression; within a few days, however, increased accumulation of the radioisotope ("hot" spot) is typical (Fig. 53–40). The bone scan can also be used to monitor the disease course and response to treatment, although several weeks may be required before the scan returns to normal, and the correlation between clinical and scintigraphic improvement is not uniformly good. Occasional difficulty in interpreting the bone scan in younger patients arises from an inability to differentiate between normal and abnormal activity in the metaphyseal region.

A gallium scan can be performed in conjunction with a technetium scan in the same patient, and the resulting information may be more useful than that obtained by either examination alone (Table 53–7; see Fig. 53–40). Gallium scans may reveal abnormal accumulation in patients with active osteomyelitis when technetium scans reveal decreased activity (cold lesions) or perhaps normal activity (transition period between cold and hot lesions). It should be remembered that gallium is a bone scanning agent that accumulates in regions of increased bone remodeling, such as occur in osteomyelitis. Therefore, its accumulation in osseous sites that are also positive on technetium phosphate scans is not unexpected, and such accumulation by itself does not increase the specificity of the radionuclide examination. Rather, when both tech-

## TABLE 53–7

### Radionuclide Evaluation of Osseous and Soft Tissue Infection

| Agent | Cellulitis | Acute Osteomyelitis | Chronic Osteomyelitis |
|---|---|---|---|
| Technetium phosphates | Early scans show increased uptake; later scans are normal | Early and late scans show increased uptake (scans in early acute osteomyelitis may reveal "cold" spots) | Scans may remain positive, even in inactive disease |
| Gallium | Increased uptake | Increased uptake | Increased uptake in areas of active disease |

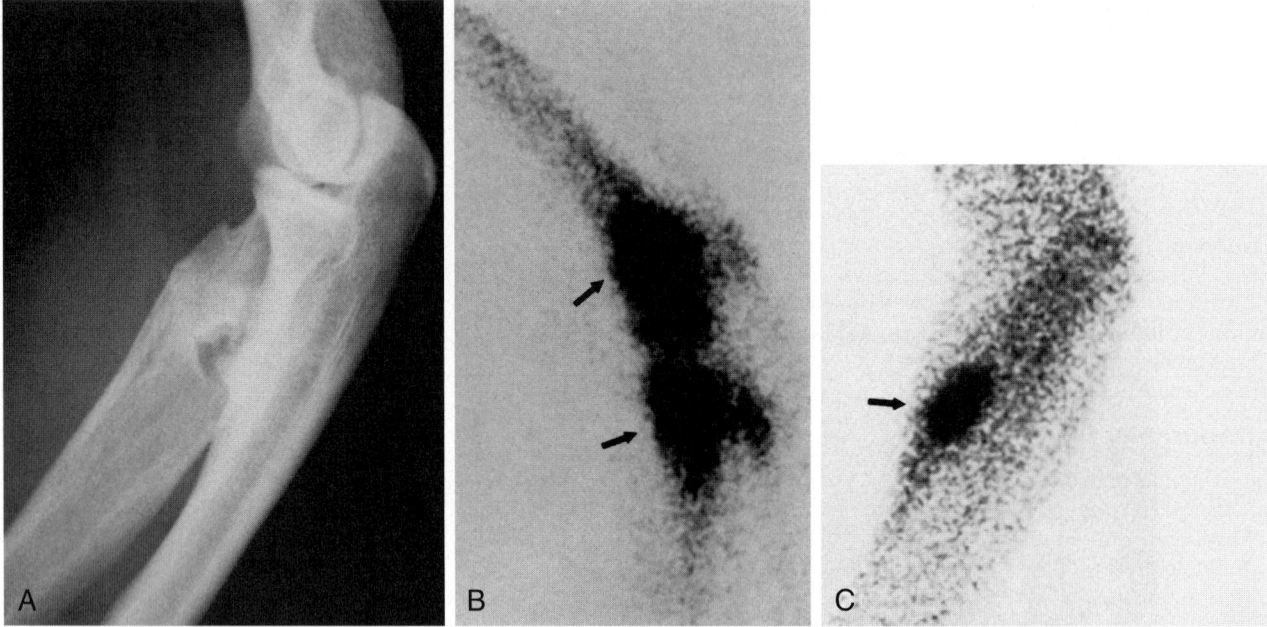

**Figure 53–40.** Soft tissue infection: imaging findings. This 37-year-old man, with a history of chronic inactive osteomyelitis of the proximal portion of the radius, developed a staphylococcal soft tissue infection. *A*, Radiograph shows soft tissue swelling and osseous deformity of the proximal portion of the radius and ulna. *B*, Technetium phosphate bone scan reveals accentuated uptake of the radiopharmaceutical agent *(arrows)* in the humerus, radius, and ulna about the elbow. *C*, Gallium scan indicates abnormality of soft tissue alone *(arrow)*. (Courtesy of V. Vint, MD, San Diego, Calif.)

netium phosphate and gallium scanning are used, it is important to compare the degree and extent of radionuclide uptake on the two examinations. Disparate distribution of uptake or increased intensity of uptake on the gallium study is an important sign of osteomyelitis. Such infection is unlikely when both technetium phosphate and gallium scanning are negative or when the distribution of both tracers is spatially congruent and the relative intensity of gallium uptake is less than that of the bone tracer.

Although a negative delayed bone image appears to be specific in excluding infection, a positive finding during the delayed static phase of the examination lacks specificity for infection and has stimulated considerable interest in "three-phase" examinations in patients with musculoskeletal infection. This encompasses serial images obtained during the first minute after a bolus injection of a technetium compound (angiographic phase), a postinjection image obtained at the end of the first minute or after several minutes (blood pool phase), and additional images obtained 2 or 3 hours later (delayed phase). If increased accumulation of radionuclide within bone is observed in all three phases, the diagnosis of osteomyelitis is highly likely. Conversely, if such an increase is present only on the delayed image, an alternative diagnosis should be considered. Soft tissue infections are characterized by delayed images that either are normal or reveal minimally increased tracer accumulation within the bone, presumably because of regional hyperemia. Septic arthritis is usually accompanied by increased uptake of the radiopharmaceutical agent in juxta-articular bone in the delayed images, moderate and diffuse blood pool hyperemia, and, on the radionuclide angiogram, increased flow to the joint space (Fig. 53–41). The addition of a fourth

phase to the scintigraphic examination, representing a static image obtained 24 hours after injection of the bone-seeking radiopharmaceutical agent, may help in this differentiation. Advantages of the 24-hour image relate to continued accumulation of the technetium phosphate

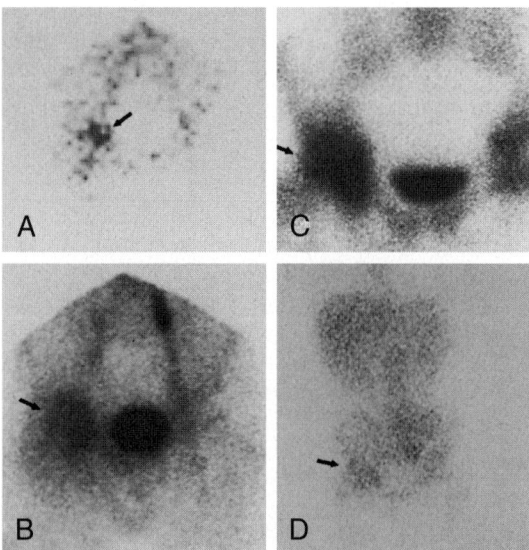

**Figure 53–41.** Septic arthritis: bone scanning. *A* to *C*, Three-phase technetium phosphate study documents increased flow *(arrow)* in the angiographic phase *(A)*, diffuse hyperemia about the hip *(arrow)* in the blood pool stage *(B)*, and increased uptake of the radiopharmaceutical agent *(arrow)* in the delayed image *(C)*. These findings indicate septic arthritis. *D*, Gallium scan is also abnormal, with increased scintigraphic activity about the hip *(arrow)*. (Courtesy of G. Greenway, MD, Dallas, Tex.)

radionuclide in the abnormal woven bone about foci of infection.

The accumulation of leukocytes at sites of abscess formation has led to the use of indium-labeled autologous leukocytes for the evaluation of inflammatory processes. In general, [111]In-labeled leukocyte scintigraphy is less sensitive in detecting bone infections than soft tissue infections and leads to difficulty in differentiating osteomyelitis and septic arthritis. It can demonstrate soft tissue extension from an area of bone infection. Positive leukocyte images are encountered in musculoskeletal conditions other than infection. Rheumatoid arthritis and other synovial inflammatory disorders can lead to findings simulating those of septic arthritis, and primary or secondary tumors in the soft tissue or bone can produce positive leukocyte images similar to those accompanying infection. Compared with bone imaging with [99mTc] compounds, [111]In scintigraphy has increased sensitivity in the detection of early osteomyelitis.

## Magnetic Resonance Imaging

Acute osteomyelitis typically appears as an area of low signal intensity on T1-weighted spin echo MR images and high signal intensity on T2-weighted images, its conspicuity being influenced by the hematopoietic or fatty nature of the adjacent marrow (Fig. 53–42). The process of subacute and chronic osteomyelitis has a more variable MR imaging appearance, although in cases of chronic active infection, similar characteristics of signal intensity are observed. Additional MR imaging abnormalities in either acute or chronic osteomyelitis include cortical erosion or perforation, periosteal bone formation, soft tissue involvement, and, in chronic osteomyelitis, abscesses, bone sequestration, and sinus tracts. With short tau inversion recovery (STIR) imaging, osteomyelitis and soft tissue infection appear as areas of markedly increased signal intensity that are reportedly more conspicuous than on routine spin echo MR images (Fig. 53–43).

After intravenous administration of a gadolinium contrast agent, areas of vascularized inflammatory tissue reveal enhancement of signal intensity, but nonvascularized abscess collections show either no enhancement or enhancement at the margin of the lesion. Brodie's abscesses (Fig. 53–44) typically appear as well-defined intraosseous regions of low signal intensity on T1-weighted spin echo MR images (with a rim of intermediate signal intensity related to a layer of highly vascularized granulation tissue, termed the penumbra sign, surrounded by a variable amount of low signal intensity related to marrow edema) and as areas of high signal intensity on T2-weighted spin echo MR images (with a rim of low signal intensity due to sclerotic bone surrounded by a variable amount of high signal intensity related to marrow edema); they may be better delineated with gadolinium-enhanced MR imaging.

Sequestra, although better seen on CT scans, appear as regions of low to intermediate signal intensity on both T1- and T2-weighted images and do not show enhancement of signal intensity after intravenous administration of a gadolinium-based contrast agent. The inflamed

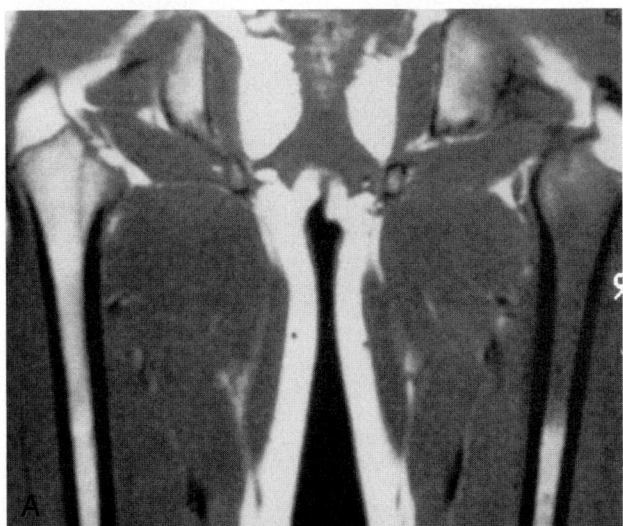
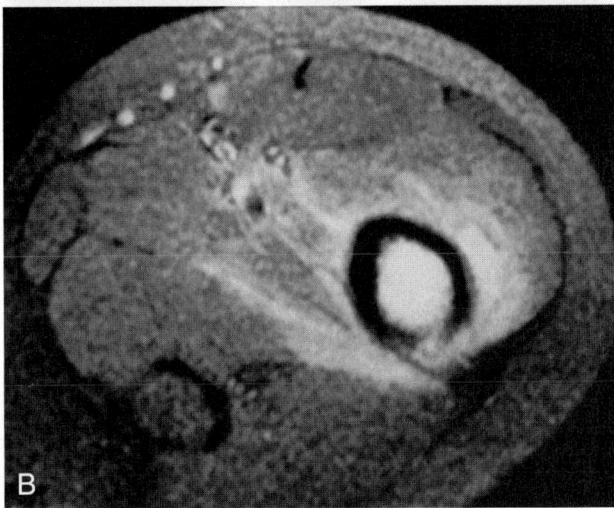

**Figure 53–42.** Acute osteomyelitis: MR imaging. *A,* Coronal T1-weighted (TR/TE, 650/20) spin echo MR image shows a long segment of abnormal bone marrow manifested as a region of low signal intensity. *B,* Transaxial T2-weighted (TR/TE, 2000/80) spin echo MR image shows that the infection, demonstrating high signal intensity, has extended from the marrow through the posterior cortex into the soft tissues. Documentation of the extent of the soft tissue infection, which requires its differentiation from edema, is difficult. (Courtesy of G. Greenway, MD, Dallas, Tex.)

synovial membrane in cases of septic arthritis, as in rheumatoid arthritis, is enhanced after the intravenous injection of a gadolinium agent.

Although numerous reviews have emphasized the sensitivity of MR imaging in the diagnosis of musculoskeletal infections, it is this very sensitivity that can lead to diagnostic problems, particularly in defining the extent of the process. Several specific problem areas can be defined:

1. In acute osteomyelitis, differentiating soft tissue extension of infection from soft tissue edema or differentiating osteomyelitis from surrounding intraosseous reactive edema.

2. In septic arthritis, differentiating secondary osteomyelitis from bone marrow edema; or in acute osteomyelitis

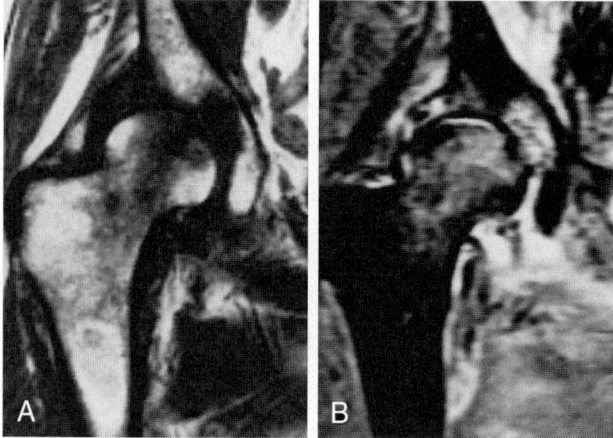

**Figure 53–43.** Septic arthritis and osteomyelitis: MR imaging. *A*, Coronal T1-weighted (TR/TE, 350/20) spin echo MR image displays the infectious process in this 75-year-old woman as areas of low signal intensity in the proximal end of the right femur and adjacent acetabulum. A joint effusion of low signal intensity is evident. *B*, Coronal STIR (TR/TE, 2700/30; inversion time, 160 msec) image better delineates the bone and soft tissue abnormalities, which are of high signal intensity. Although extremely sensitive in the documentation of inflammation, STIR imaging can lead to an overestimation of the extent of the process. (Courtesy of M. Pathria, MD, and D. Bates, MD, San Diego, Calif.)

affecting epiphyses, differentiating secondary septic arthritis from sympathetic effusions.

3. In chronic osteomyelitis, differentiating active and inactive disease.

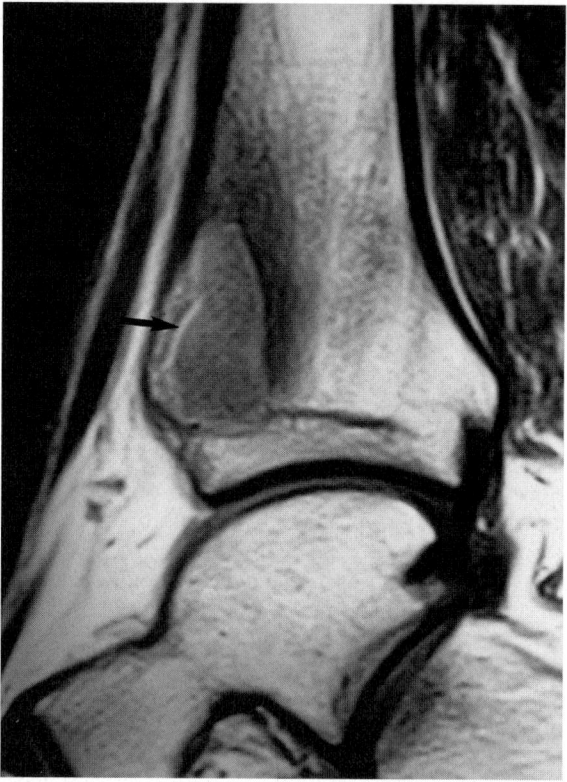

**Figure 53–44.** Brodie's abscess: MR imaging. In a sagittal T1-weighted (TR/TE, 567/20) spin echo MR image, the wall of the abscess in the distal metaphysis of the tibia has intermediate signal intensity *(arrow)*, the penumbra sign. Note surrounding marrow edema of low signal intensity. (Courtesy of D. Goodwin, MD, Hanover, N.H.)

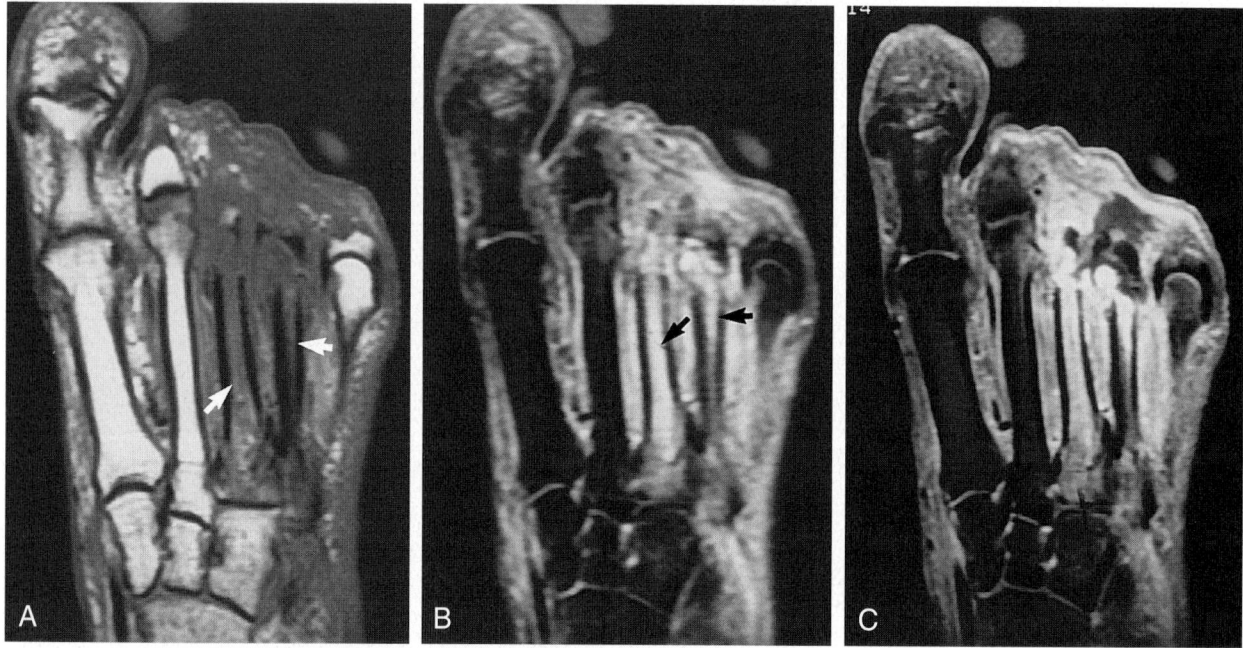

**Figure 53–45.** Diabetic foot infection: MR imaging. This 63-year-old man required amputation of the third toe at the level of the metatarsophalangeal joint for control of infection. He later developed clinical manifestations of recurrent infection. *A*, Transverse T1-weighted (TR/TE, 700/15) spin echo MR image shows abnormally low signal intensity in the third and fourth metatarsal bones *(arrows)* and in the adjacent soft tissues. The head of the second metatarsal bone also appears to be involved. *B*, Transverse STIR (TR/TE, 1800/25; inversion time, 160 msec) image reveals high signal intensity in these metatarsal bones *(arrows)* and soft tissues. *C*, Transverse T1-weighted (TR/TE, 900/13) fat-suppressed image obtained in conjunction with intravenous administration of gadolinium contrast agent provides information similar to that in *(B)*. A third and fourth ray resection confirmed the presence of osteomyelitis.

4. In soft tissue infections, differentiating infective periostitis, osteitis, or osteomyelitis from bone marrow edema.

The assessment of infection in the feet of diabetic patients provides unique challenges (Fig. 53–45). Although reported data indicate the value of scintigraphic methods, particularly [111]In-labeled leukocyte imaging with or without bone scintigraphy, the day-to-day clinical experience of many physicians suggests otherwise. A normal bone scan virtually excludes the presence of osteomyelitis, neuropathic osteoarthropathy, or both. The hyperemia associated with either process can lead to positive results with three-phase bone scintigraphy. Decreased blood flow and possible impaired leukocyte responsiveness limit the sensitivity achievable with [111]In-labeled leukocyte scintigraphy in diabetic foot infections; however, reports indicate that the finding of definite increased uptake on leukocyte scans has a high positive predictive value, and the absence of increased leukocyte uptake in or near bone makes the diagnosis of osteomyelitis very unlikely. Although high signal intensity in the bone marrow on T2-weighted spin echo and STIR images and on T1-weighted spin echo MR images (with or without fat saturation) after the intravenous administration of gadolinium contrast agent is compatible with the diagnosis of osteomyelitis, it is not a specific finding (see Fig. 53–43). Neuropathic osteoarthropathy in the absence of coexistent infection is accompanied by persistent low signal intensity in the bone marrow on T2-weighted spin echo MR images, although this is not a constant finding. In rapidly developing neuropathic osteoarthropathy, acute fragmentation of bone is associated with marrow edema, resulting in high signal intensity on T2-weighted spin echo and STIR images and those images obtained after the intravenous administration of a gadolinium-containing contrast agent (Fig. 53–46). With application of the last of these methods, the presence of soft tissue or osseous abscesses suggests that the accompanying marrow altera-

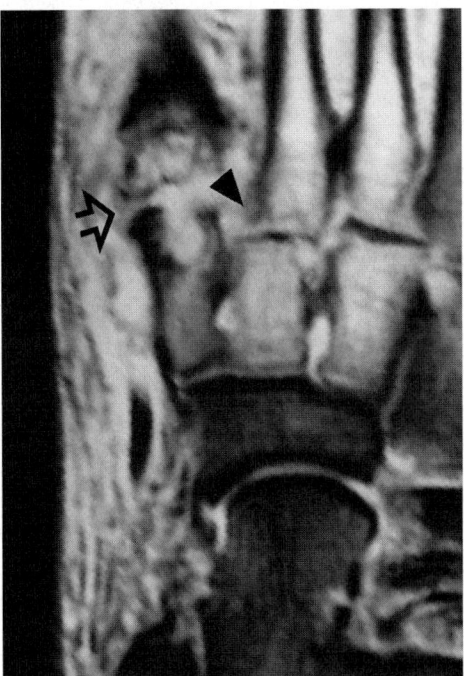

**Figure 53–46.** Diabetic neuropathic osteoarthropathy and osteomyelitis: MR imaging. Transverse STIR (TR/TE, 1800/20; inversion time, 125 msec) MR image shows high signal intensity in the marrow of the second and third metatarsal bones, in the intermediate and lateral cuneiform bones, and in the soft tissues. Note the neuropathic changes about the first tarsometatarsal joint (*arrow*) and a Lisfranc pattern of subluxation (*arrowhead*). In such cases, it is difficult to differentiate sites of osteomyelitis from neuropathic disease with marrow edema.

tions are related to osteomyelitis rather than to neuropathic osteoarthropathy. Some guidelines for this choice in cases of osteomyelitis, septic arthritis, and soft tissue infections are provided in Table 53–8.

### TABLE 53–8

**Some Useful MR Imaging Protocols in Assessment of Musculoskeletal Infections**

| Condition | Suggested Protocols |
|---|---|
| Osteomyelitis in red marrow | T2-weighted spin echo<br>T1-weighted spin echo with gadolinium contrast enhancement<br>STIR |
| Osteomyelitis in yellow marrow | T1-weighted spin echo<br>T1-weighted spin echo with gadolinium contrast enhancement and fat suppression<br>STIR |
| Septic arthritis | T1-weighted spin echo with gadolinium contrast enhancement with or without fat suppression |
| Soft tissue infection | T1-weighted spin echo with gadolinium contrast enhancement with or without fat suppression |

STIR, short tau inversion recovery.

### FURTHER READING

Azouz EM: Computed tomography in bone and joint infections. J Can Assoc Radiol 32:102, 1981.
Bonakdar-pour A, Gaines VD: The radiology of osteomyelitis. Orthop Clin North Am 14:21, 1983.
Boutin RD, Resnick D: The SAPHO syndrome: An evolving concept for unifying several idiopathic disorders of bone and skin. AJR Am J Roentgenol 170:585, 1998.
Bressler EL, Conway JJ, Weiss SC: Neonatal osteomyelitis examined by bone scintigraphy. Radiology 152:685, 1984.
Butt WP: The radiology of infection. Clin Orthop 96:20, 1973.
Butt WP: Radiology of the infected joint. Clin Orthop 96:136, 1973.
Capitanio MA, Kirkpatrick JA: Early roentgen observations in acute osteomyelitis. AJR Am J Roentgenol 108:488, 1970.
Curtiss PH Jr: The pathophysiology of joint infections. Clin Orthop 96:129, 1973.
Davis LA: Antibiotic modified osteomyelitis. AJR Am J Roentgenol 103:608, 1968.
Erdman WA, Tamburro F, Jayson HT, et al: Osteomyelitis: Characteristics and pitfalls of diagnosis with MR imaging. Radiology 180:533, 1991.

Fitzgerald RH, Brewer NS, Dahlin DC: Squamous-cell carcinoma complicating chronic osteomyelitis. J Bone Joint Surg Am 58:1146, 1976.

Fletcher BD, Scoles PV, Nelson AD: Osteomyelitis in children: Detection by magnetic resonance. Work in progress. Radiology 150:57, 1984.

Gilday DL, Paul DJ, Paterson J: Diagnosis of osteomyelitis in children by combined blood pool and bone imaging. Radiology 117:331, 1975.

Goldberg JS, London WL, Nagel DM: Tropical pyomyositis: A case report and review. Pediatrics 63:298, 1979.

Graif M, Schweitzer ME, Deely D, et al: The septic versus nonseptic inflamed joint: MRI characteristics. Skeletal Radiol 28:616, 1999.

Green NE, Beauchamp RD, Griffin PP: Primary subacute epiphyseal osteomyelitis. J Bone Joint Surg Am 63:107, 1981.

Grey AC, Davies AM, Mangham DC, et al: The "penumbra sign" on T1-weighted MR imaging in subacute osteomyelitis: Frequency, cause and significance. Clin Radiol 53:587, 1998.

Handmaker H, Leonards R: The bone scan in inflammatory osseous disease. Semin Nucl Med 6:95, 1976.

Hofer P: Gallium and infection. J Nucl Med 21:484, 1980.

Kahn M-F, Chamot A-M: SAPHO syndrome. Rheum Dis Clin North Am 18:225, 1992.

Kaye JJ: Bacterial infections of the hips in infancy and childhood. Curr Probl Radiol 3:17, 1973.

Kemp HBS, Lloyd-Roberts GC: Avascular necrosis of the capital epiphysis following osteomyelitis of the proximal femoral metaphysis. J Bone Joint Surg Br 56:688, 1974.

Kido D, Bryan D, Halpern M: Hematogenous osteomyelitis in drug addicts. AJR Am J Roentgenol 118:356, 1973.

McAfee JG, Subramanian G, Gagne G: Technique of leukocyte harvesting and labeling: Problems and perspective. Semin Nucl Med 14:83, 1984.

Mendelson EB, Fisher MR, Deschler TW, et al: Osteomyelitis in the diabetic foot: A difficult diagnostic challenge. Radiographics 3:248, 1983.

Miller TT, Randolph DA Jr, Staron RB, et al: Fat-suppressed MRI of musculoskeletal infection: Fast T2-weighted techniques versus gadolinium-enhanced T1-weighted images. Skeletal Radiol 26:654, 1997.

Miller WB, Murphy WA, Gilula LA: Brodie abscess: Reappraisal. Radiology 132:15, 1979.

Mok PM, Reilly BJ, Ash JM: Osteomyelitis in the neonate: Clinical aspects and the role of radiography and scintigraphy in diagnosis and management. Radiology 145:677, 1982.

Murray SD, Kehl DK: Chronic recurrent multifocal osteomyelitis: A case report. J Bone Joint Surg Am 66:1110, 1984.

Pennington WT, Mott MP, Thometz JG, et al: Photopenic bone scan osteomyelitis: A clinical perspective. J Pediatr Orthop 19:695, 1999.

Rasool MN: Primary subacute haematogenous osteomyelitis in children. J Bone Joint Surg Br 83:93, 2001.

Resnick D: Osteomyelitis and septic arthritis complicating hand injuries and infections: Pathogenesis of roentgenographic abnormalities. J Can Assoc Radiol 27:21, 1976.

Resnick D, Pineda CJ, Weisman MH, et al: Osteomyelitis and septic arthritis of the hand following human bites. Skeletal Radiol 14:263, 1985.

Rosenbaum DM, Blumhagen JD: Acute epiphyseal osteomyelitis in children. Radiology 156:89, 1985.

Solheim LF, Paus B, Liverud K, et al: Chronic recurrent multifocal osteomyelitis. Acta Orthop Scand 51:37, 1980.

Tehranzadeh J, Wang F, Mesqarzadeh M: Magnetic resonance imaging of osteomyelitis. CRC Crit Rev Diagn Imaging 33:495, 1992.

Trueta J: Studies of the Development and Decay of the Human Frame. Philadelphia, WB Saunders, 1968, p 254.

Unger E, Moldofsky P, Gatenby R, et al: Diagnosis of osteomyelitis by MR imaging. AJR Am J Roentgenol 150:605, 1988.

Waldvogel FA, Vasey H: Osteomyelitis: The past decade. N Engl J Med 303:360, 1980.

Wolfson JJ, Kane WJ, Laxdal SD, et al: Bone findings in chronic granulomatous disease of childhood: A genetic abnormality of leukocyte function. J Bone Joint Surg Am 51:1573, 1969.

Wood BP: The vanishing epiphyseal ossification center: A sequel to septic arthritis of childhood. Radiology 134:387, 1980.

# CHAPTER 54

## Osteomyelitis, Septic Arthritis, and Soft Tissue Infection: Axial Skeleton

## SUMMARY OF KEY FEATURES

The routes of contamination of the spine, the sacroiliac joint, and other axial skeletal sites are identical to those of the appendicular skeleton. In the spine, early loss of intervertebral disc space is characteristic of pyogenic infection and is associated with lysis and sclerosis of neighboring bone. These findings can simulate those of other disorders, such as rheumatoid arthritis, intervertebral (osteo)chondrosis, and conditions complicated by cartilaginous node formation. Sacroiliac joint infection is typically unilateral in distribution, a feature that allows its differentiation from many other articular processes. Additional locations in the axial skeleton are not uncommonly infected in intravenous drug abusers and in patients after trauma, surgery, or diagnostic and therapeutic procedures.

## INTRODUCTION

The distribution of osteomyelitis and septic arthritis is dramatically influenced by the age of the patient, the specific causative organism, and the presence or absence of any underlying disorder or situation. In children and infants, frequent involvement of the bones and joints of the appendicular skeleton is evident, whereas in adults, localization of infection to the osseous and articular structures of the vertebral column is common. Spinal infection is also frequent in intravenous drug abusers and in patients with tuberculosis.

## SPINAL INFECTIONS

### Routes of Contamination

**Hematogenous Spread of Infection.** Hematogenous spread through arterial and venous routes (Batson's paravertebral venous system) can result in lodgment of organisms in the bone marrow of the vertebrae. This vascular arrangement allows two direct routes for the hematogenous spread of infection: via the nutrient arteries and via the paravertebral venous system. Although the contribution of each system to cases of spinal osteomyelitis is a matter of debate, it is attractive to implicate the valveless venous plexus—whose direction and extent of flow are dramatically influenced by changes in abdominal pressure—in the frequent spread of infection (and neoplasm) to the spine from pelvic sources (Fig. 54–1). Urinary tract infections or surgery, rectosigmoid disease and enteric fistulas, and septic abortion or postpartum infection are well-

recognized pelvic precursors of vertebral osteomyelitis. The common localization of early foci of osteomyelitis in the subchondral region of the vertebral body, an area richly supplied by nutrient arterioles, emphasizes that arterial rather than venous pathways may be more important in hematogenous osteomyelitis of the spine.

The role of hematogenous spread of infection directly into the intervertebral disc has stimulated great interest. It has been suggested that in children and adolescents younger than 19 or 20 years, vascular channels perforate the vertebral endplate and allow organisms in the bloodstream to have direct access to the intervertebral disc. This concept has led to the application of such popular terms as "discitis." A similar occurrence in adults has been attributed to a persistent disc blood supply or to a supply that has been reinstated by vascular invasion of degenerating disc tissue.

**Spread from a Contiguous Source of Infection.** Vertebral or intervertebral disc infection can result from contamination by an adjacent soft tissue suppurative focus. Even in cases in which bone or cartilage involvement follows soft tissue infection, it is extremely difficult to eliminate the possibility that osteomyelitis or disc infection is a result of hematogenous or lymphatic seeding. Tuberculous and fungal infection, however, can extend from the spine to the neighboring tissue, dissect along the subligamentous areas for a considerable distance, and then reenter the vertebral body or intervertebral disc. Further, cases of osteomyelitis and infective discitis have been reported as a complication of colonic, hypopharyngeal, and esophageal perforation or instrumentation. In all these examples, however, the role of bacteremia with subsequent hematogenous seeding of the spine must be considered.

A specific entity that may be related to this mechanism of infection is Grisel's syndrome, in which spontaneous atlantoaxial subluxation accompanies inflammation of neighboring soft tissues, mainly in children (Fig. 54–2). Proposed causes of this phenomenon include muscle spasm, ligamentous laxity, and synovial effusion; the direct continuity of the periodontoidal venous plexus and the suboccipital epidural sinuses with the pharyngovertebral veins suggests the existence of a hematogenous route for the transport of peripharyngeal septic exudates to the upper cervical spine structures.

**Direct Implantation.** Organisms can be directly implanted into the intervertebral disc (and, far less commonly, the vertebra) during attempted puncture of the spinal canal, intervertebral disc, paravertebral and peridural tissues, or aorta, or in penetrating injuries. Usually, the intervertebral disc is the initial site of infection, especially in cases of misguided puncture, and the vertebra becomes contaminated as a secondary event.

**Postoperative Infection.** The more frequent and aggressive spinal operations that are currently being undertaken

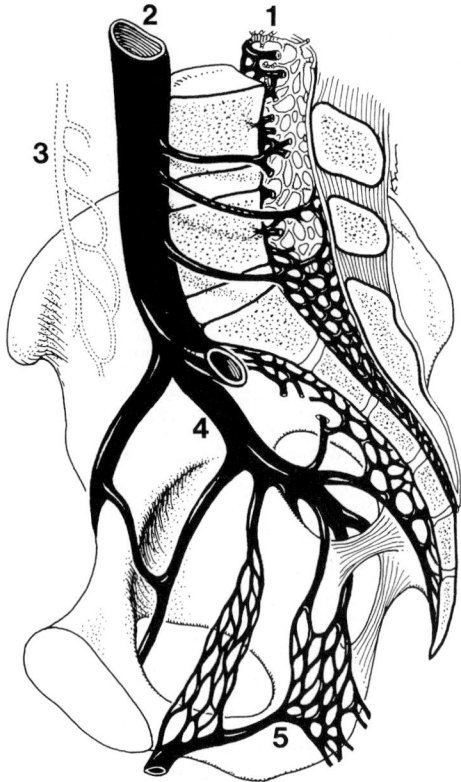

**Figure 54–1.** Anatomic considerations: Batson's paravertebral venous system. This valveless, plexiform set of veins lies outside the thoracoabdominal cavity and anastomoses with the cavitary veins at each segmental level. Thus, communication exists between the pelvic and vertebral venous system, femoral and iliac veins, inferior and superior venae cavae, and other important venous structures. 1, paravertebral venous plexus; 2, inferior vena cava; 3, inferior mesenteric vein; 4, internal iliac vein; 5, pelvic plexus. (Modified from Vider M, Maruyama Y, Narvaez R: Significance of the vertebral venous (Batson's) plexus in metastatic spread in colorectal carcinoma. Cancer 40:67, 1977.)

have led to an increase in postoperative infection of the spinal column. Laminectomy, discectomy, instrumentation, and fusion can each be complicated by osteomyelitis or disc infection. The localization of osseous or articular contamination depends on the precipitating surgical event.

## Clinical Abnormalities

The reported frequency of osteomyelitis and disc space infection (together termed infective spondylitis) has risen dramatically. Initially, infective spondylitis was thought to represent less than 1% of all cases of osteomyelitis; now it appears that 2% to 4% is a more accurate estimate. Men are affected more commonly than women. The highest frequency of septic spondylitis occurs in the fifth and sixth decades of life. The lumbar spine is the most typical site of involvement, followed by the thoracic spine; sacral and cervical abnormalities occur with about equal frequency. The usual location of infection in the vertebra is the vertebral body.

A history of recent primary infection, instrumentation, or a diagnostic, therapeutic, or surgical procedure is common. The most frequently encountered (55% to 90%) pyogenic organism is *Staphylococcus aureus* or, less commonly, *Staphylococcus epidermidis*, although other grampositive and, less typically, gram-negative agents may be implicated. Clinical manifestations vary with the virulence of the organism and the nature of the host's resistance. General findings include fever, malaise, anorexia, and weight loss. Back pain is a common initial local manifestation and may be intermittent or constant, exacerbated by motion, and throbbing at rest. With accompanying soft tissue abscess formation, hip contracture can occur (psoas muscle irritation). Appropriate culture of the blood can identify the causative organism in some cases, although more drastic methods, such as needle biopsy or aspiration, may be necessary.

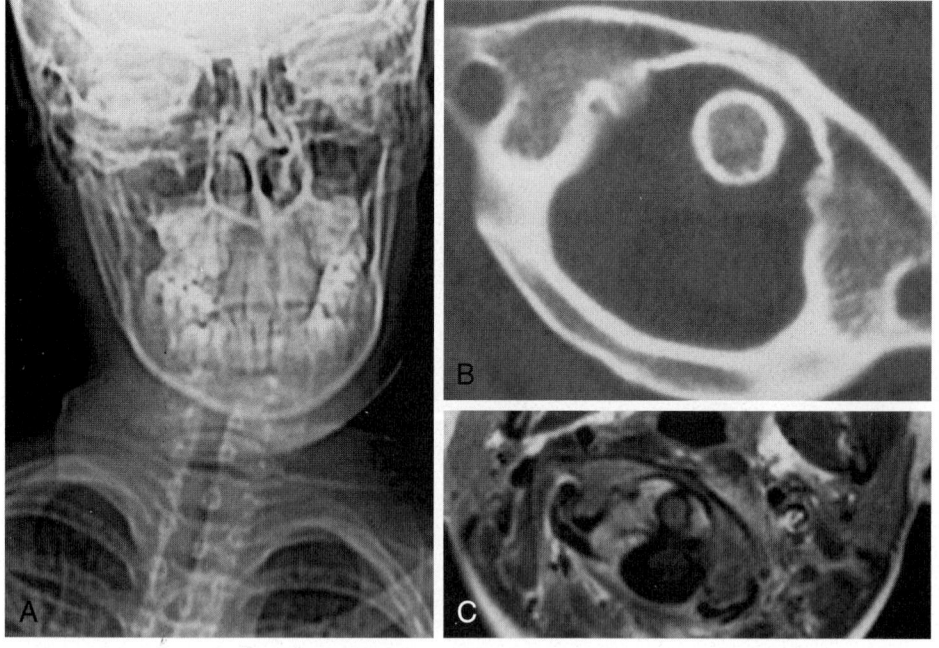

**Figure 54–2.** Grisel's syndrome. A head tilt developed in this 11-year-old boy after an ear infection. *A*, Scout view from a CT study reveals deviation of the head to the left side. *B*, Transaxial CT scan at the level of the atlas shows that it is rotated about the odontoid process, with the right side of the atlas located anterior to the left side. *C*, Transaxial T1-weighted (TR/TE, 300/15) spin echo MR image obtained after the intravenous injection of a gadolinium contrast agent reveals a similar position of the atlas, which is rotated with respect to the axis. The adjacent soft tissues show some degree of hyperintensity because of gadolinium enhancement. The rotational abnormality resolved slowly over a period of months. (Courtesy of S. Wall, MD, San Francisco, Calif.)

## Radiographic-Pathologic Correlation

**Early Abnormalities.** Hematogenous spread of infection frequently leads to a focus in the anterior subchondral regions of the vertebral body adjacent to the intervertebral disc (Fig. 54–3). Disc perforation soon ensues. At this stage, radiographs may be entirely normal. Soon (1 to 3 weeks), however, decrease in intervertebral disc height is accompanied by loss of normal definition of the subchondral bone plate and enlarging destructive foci within the neighboring vertebral body (Fig. 54–4). The combination of rapid loss of intervertebral disc height and adjacent lysis of bone is most suggestive of an infectious process. Such involvement of two contiguous vertebral bodies is almost uniformly associated with transdiscal infection and is rarely the result of multicentric involvement.

**Later Abnormalities.** After a variable period (10 to 12 weeks), regenerative changes manifesting as sclerosis or eburnation appear in the bone. The osteosclerotic response is

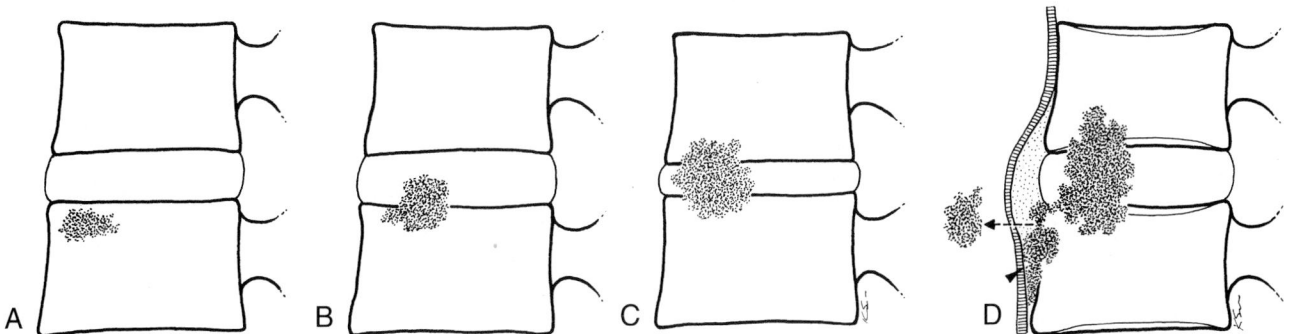

**Figure 54–3.** Spinal infection: sequential stages. *A,* An anterior subchondral focus in the vertebral body is typical. *B,* Infection may then perforate the vertebral surface and reach the intervertebral disc space. *C,* With further spread of infection, contamination of the adjacent vertebral body and narrowing of the intervertebral disc space are recognizable. *D,* With continued dissemination, infection may spread in a subligamentous fashion and erode the anterior surface of the vertebral body *(arrowhead)* or perforate the anterior ligamentous structures *(arrow).*

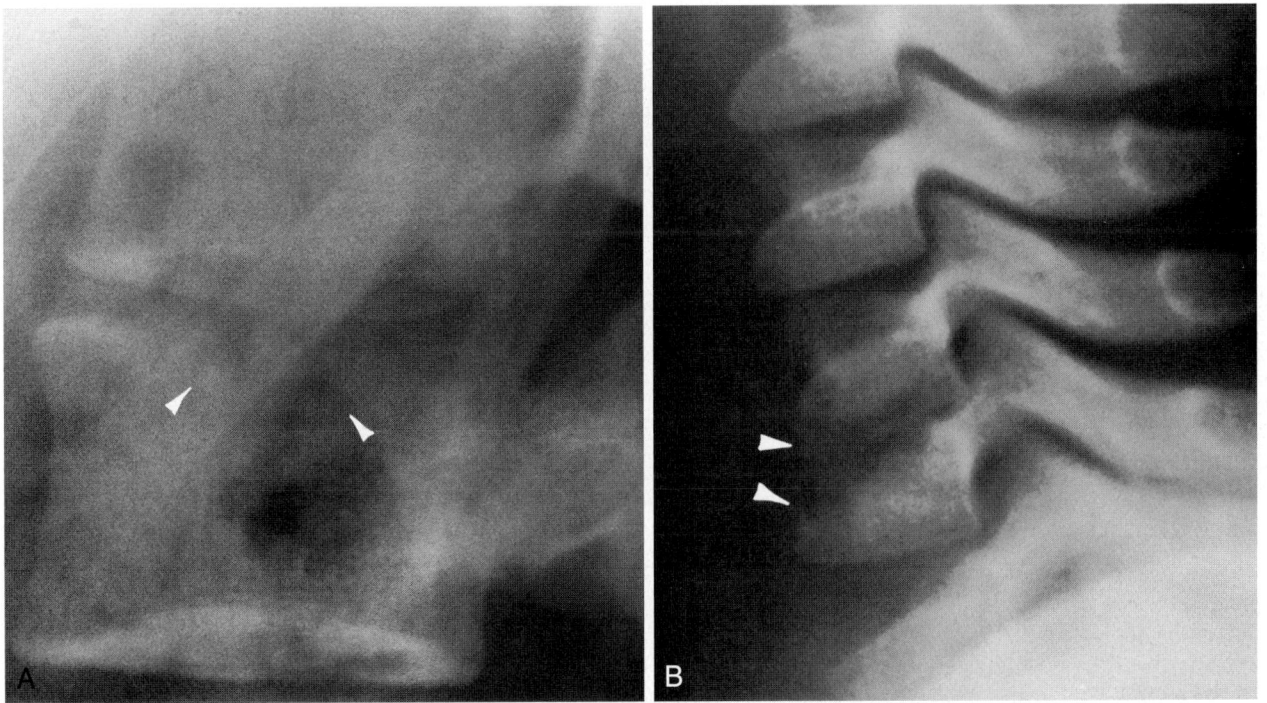

**Figure 54–4.** Spinal infection: early and later radiographic abnormalities. *A,* Observe the loss of definition of the superior aspect of a lumbar vertebral body *(arrowheads),* with narrowing of the adjacent intervertebral disc space. This appearance (in a middle-aged man with pyogenic infection) conforms to the stage in Figure 54–3*B. B,* In this young child, a staphylococcal infection has led to destruction of two adjacent vertebral bodies *(arrowheads)* and narrowing of the intervening intervertebral disc. A soft tissue mass is apparent. This appearance corresponds to the stage in Figure 54–3*D.*

variable in severity and has been used in the past as a helpful sign in differentiating pyogenic from tuberculous infection. Although such sclerosis is indeed common in pyogenic (nontuberculous) spondylitis, it may also be evident in tuberculosis. More helpful in this differentiation is a combination of findings that strongly indicates tuberculous spondylitis, including the presence of a slowly progressive vertebral process with preservation of intervertebral discs, subligamentous spread of infection with erosion of the anterior vertebral margins, large and calcified soft tissue abscesses, and the absence of severe bony eburnation (Fig. 54–5).

In the lumbar spine, such extension can lead to obliteration or displacement of the psoas margin; in the thoracic spine, a paraspinal mass can be encountered; and in the cervical spine, retropharyngeal swelling can lead to displacement and obliteration of adjacent prevertebral fat planes. With early and proper treatment, reconstitution can result, with production of a radiodense (ivory) vertebra, a relatively intact or ankylosed intervertebral disc, and surrounding osteophytosis (Fig. 54–6).

## Special Types of Spinal Infection

Most infections of the intervertebral disc occur as an extension of vertebral osteomyelitis or direct inoculation during diagnostic or surgical procedures. In children, however, a hematogenous route to the disc still exists, and hematogenous contamination of disc tissue is possible. Clinical symptoms and signs may become evident between 1 and 16 years of age (average age, approximately 5 years), and a preexisting infectious condition

(upper respiratory tract, urinary tract, or ear infection) is usually apparent. Manifestations are generally mild and include back pain, abdominal pain, hip irritability, and altered gait. Low-grade fever, irritability, malaise, elevation of the erythrocyte sedimentation rate, and, on occasion, leukocytosis are noted in many cases. When positive, blood or bone biopsy culture most typically reveals *S. aureus*. Negative culture results are reported in 50% to 90% of cases.

Scintigraphy may reveal increased accumulation of bone-seeking pharmaceuticals at a relatively early stage. Intervertebral disc space narrowing is later accompanied by erosion of the subchondral bone plate and osseous eburnation (Fig. 54–7). Magnetic resonance (MR) imaging in cases of childhood discitis reveals findings similar to those in adults with infective spondylitis.

## Other Diagnostic Techniques

The role of radionuclide studies in establishing the presence of spinal infection at a stage when radiographs are entirely normal is well documented. Technetium-, gallium-, and indium-labeled radiopharmaceutical agents can be used in this regard. The application of pinhole scintigraphy and single photon emission computed tomography (SPECT) has further increased the sensitivity of bone scanning in the diagnosis of infective spondylitis.

Computed tomography (CT) scanning allows definition of the extent of osseous and disc destruction and paravertebral and intraspinal involvement (Fig. 54–8). The intravenous injection of contrast material aids in the

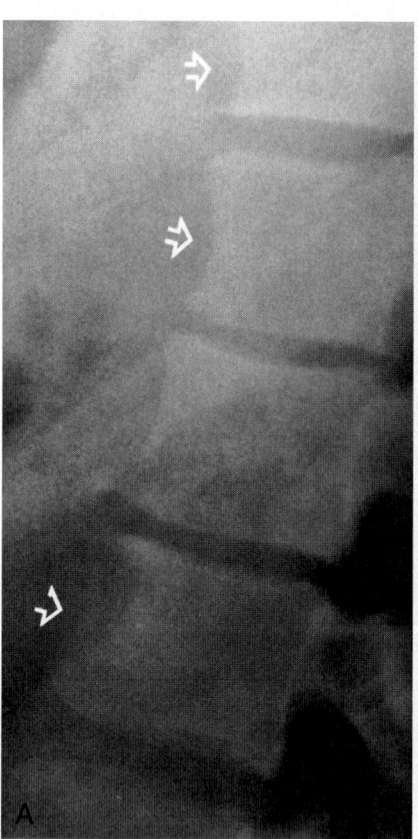
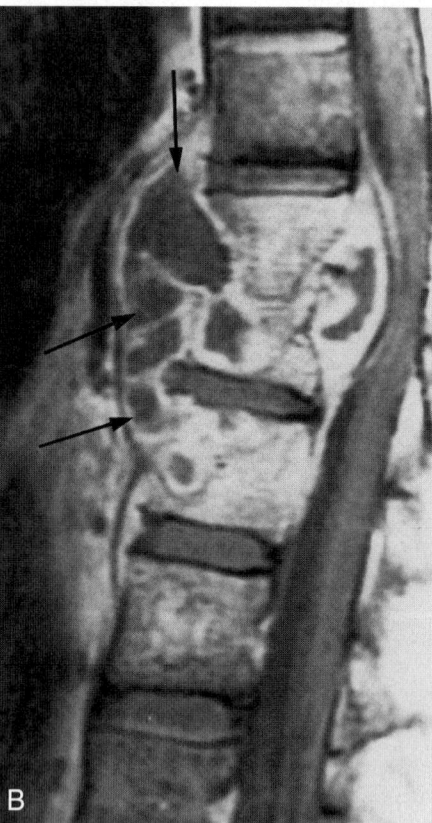

**Figure 54–5.** Spinal infection: tuberculosis with subligamentous spread. *A,* Note the erosion of the anterior surface *(arrows)* of multiple vertebral bodies. *B,* In a different patient, a sagittal T1-weighted spin echo MR image obtained after intravenous gadolinium administration shows involvement of multiple contiguous vertebral bodies (manifest as high signal intensity) and anterior abscess formation *(arrows),* with elevation of the anterior longitudinal ligament. Intraosseous and posterior abscesses are also seen. (*A,* Courtesy of A. Nemcek, MD, Chicago, Ill. *B,* Courtesy of A. D'Abreu, MD, Porto Alegre, Brazil.)

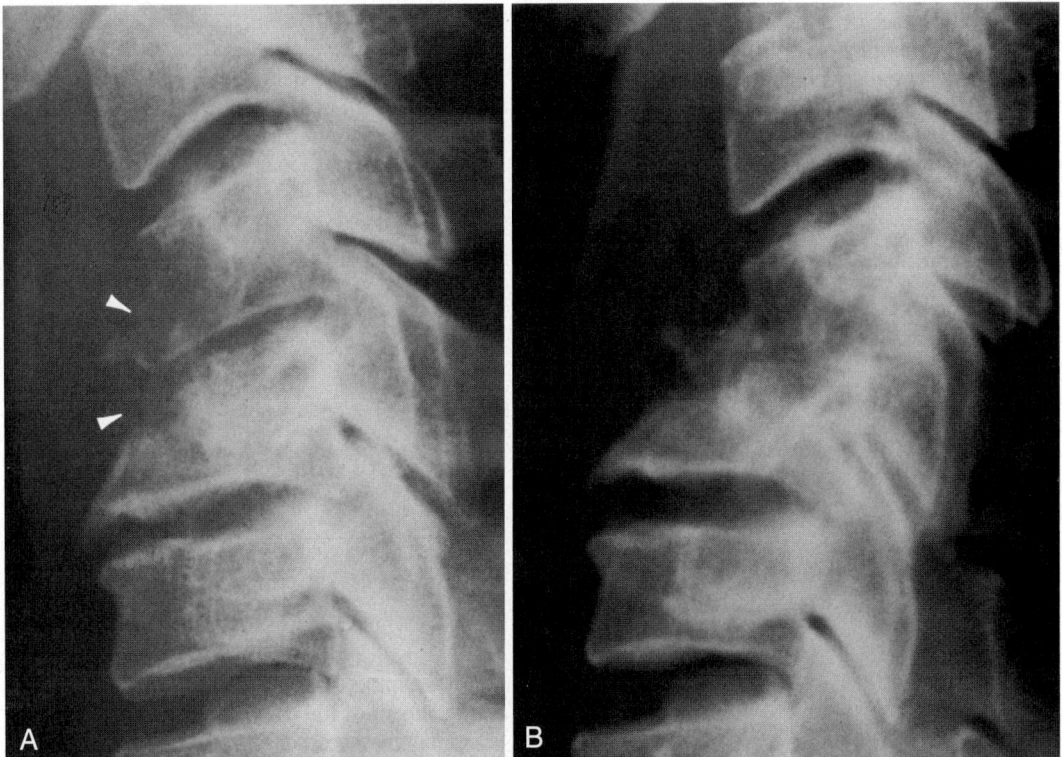

**Figure 54–6.** Spinal infection: residual deformity. *Klebsiella* spondylitis developed in the cervical region in this 41-year-old man. *A,* Three weeks after the onset of infectious spondylitis, note the collapse and fragmentation of the superior aspect of the fifth cervical vertebral body and lysis of the interior aspect of the fourth cervical vertebral body *(arrowheads).* Soft tissue swelling is evident. *B,* Two weeks later, angulation and subluxation are apparent. Soft tissue swelling is again seen.

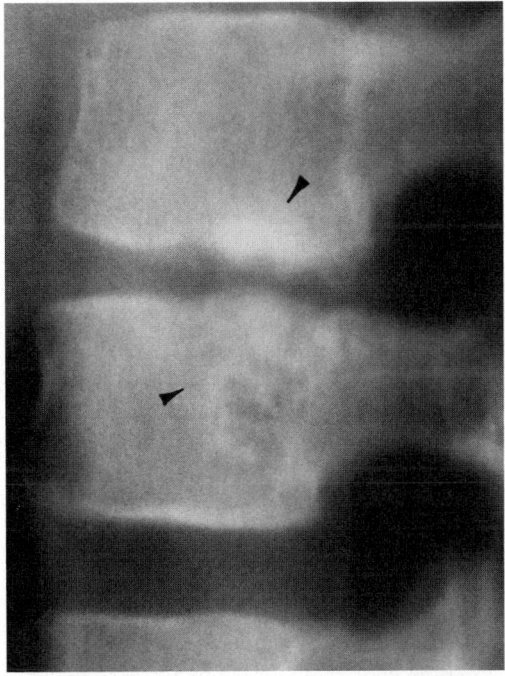

**Figure 54–7.** Intervertebral disc infection: discitis. This 6-year-old girl had symptoms and signs consistent with spinal infection. Bacteriologic studies were not helpful. Observe the narrowing of the intervertebral disc between the second and third lumbar vertebral bodies, with osseous radiolucency and sclerosis *(arrowheads).* The appearance is consistent with infection. (Courtesy of L. Lurie, MD, Chula Vista, Calif.)

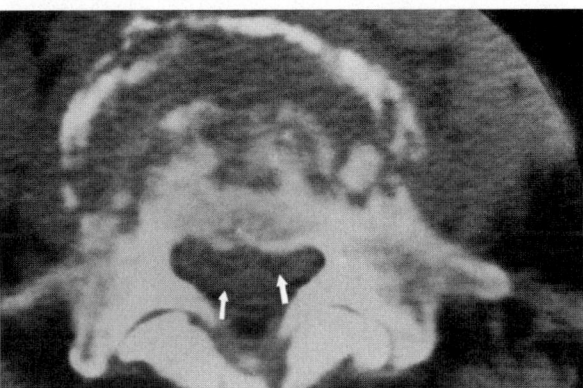

**Figure 54–8.** Spinal infection: role of CT scanning. Transaxial CT scan at the L4–L5 level documents the extent of spinal destruction and a soft tissue mass in paraspinal and intraspinal locations *(arrows).* This mass explained the patient's prominent neurologic manifestations.

separation of abnormal and normal soft tissue. Gas may be identified in the infected soft tissue or, rarely, in the intervertebral disc itself.

The MR imaging characteristics of infective spondylitis are influenced by the specific nature and extent of the process and the precise imaging protocols used. Further, the age of the patient affects these characteristics because of the changing constituency of the bone marrow (i.e., red versus yellow marrow). In acute pyogenic osteomyelitis, affected regions typically show decreased signal intensity on T1-weighted spin echo MR images and increased signal intensity on T2-weighted spin echo images (Fig. 54–9). The conspicuity of the bone marrow infection on these MR images depends on the extent of red and yellow marrow in the vertebral body and is more variable on T2-weighted spin echo MR images. Imaging with long repetition and echo times (as well as fat suppression) is beneficial in demonstrating high signal intensity within the marrow.

With MR imaging, irregularity of the vertebral endplates and narrowing of the intervertebral disc may be evident. On T2-weighted spin echo MR sequences, the infected disc reveals increased signal intensity with absence of the normal nuclear cleft (i.e., the normal anatomic structure that, on T2-weighted images, appears as an area of signal void in the center of lumbar discs in subjects 30 years or older). The high signal intensity of the intervertebral disc in cases of pyogenic spondylitis is an important diagnostic sign. Additional MR imaging findings of pyogenic spondylitis are less frequent but include epidural and paraspinal extension, posterior disc protrusion, vertebral collapse, and spinal deformity.

Infected marrow usually enhances diffusely after the administration of gadolinium. In some instances, however, this technique may produce a decrease rather than an increase in the contrast between normal and infected vertebral bodies (Fig. 54–10). The combination of contrast enhancement and fat suppression in cases of pyogenic spondylitis may eliminate this problem. Vertebral marrow involvement in cases of infection (or tumor) may also be effectively demonstrated by using short tau inversion recovery (STIR) sequences.

### Differential Diagnosis

The radiographic hallmark of infective spondylitis is intervertebral disc space narrowing, frequently accompanied by lysis or sclerosis of adjacent vertebrae (Table 54–1). A similar radiographic pattern can be encountered in various articular disorders, such as rheumatoid arthritis,

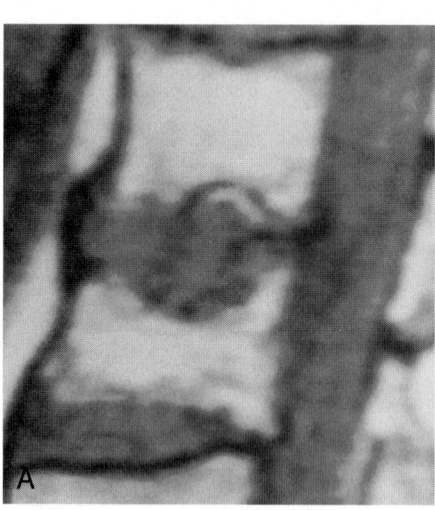 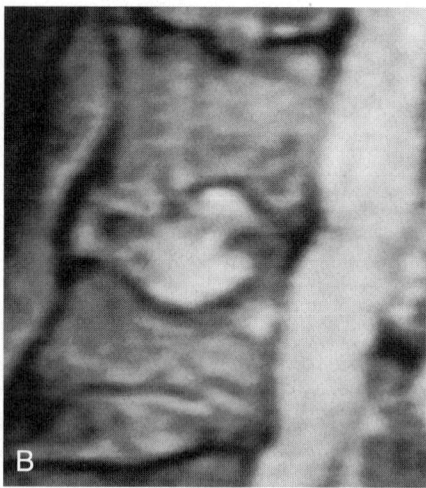

**Figure 54–9.** Spinal infection: MR imaging in pyogenic spondylitis. Sagittal T1-weighted (TR/TE, 600/25) *(A)* and T2-weighted (TR/TE, 2000/60) *(B)* spin echo MR images reveal characteristic findings of infective spondylitis. Abnormal morphology of the endplates of the first and second lumbar vertebral bodies and the L1–L2 intervertebral disc is evident on both images. In *(B)*, note the increased signal intensity in the infected disc. (Courtesy of D. Belovich, MD, Mechanicsburg, Pa.)

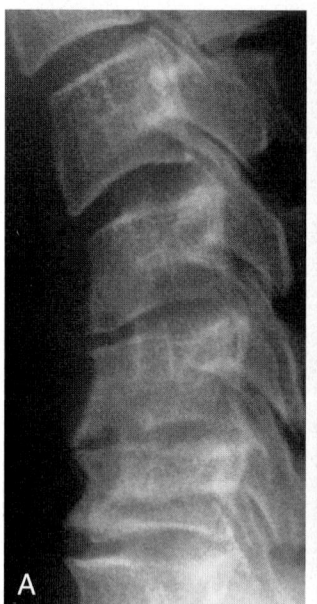 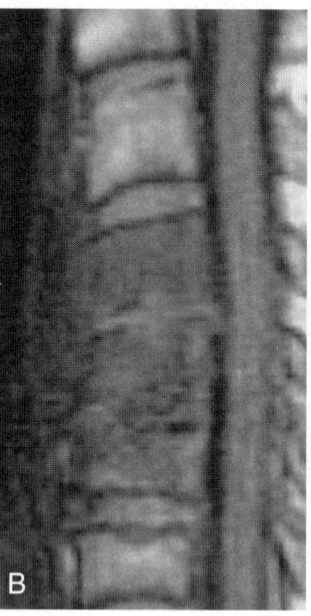 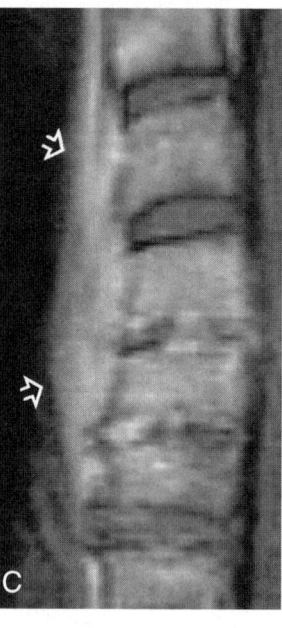

**Figure 54–10.** Spinal infection: MR imaging in pyogenic spondylitis. Infective spondylitis developed in this 40-year-old man after multilevel cervical discography. *A,* Routine radiography shows narrowing of the intervertebral discs at the C4–C5 and C5–C6 levels. Prevertebral soft tissue swelling is also evident. *B,* Sagittal T1-weighted (TR/TE, 500/12) spin echo MR image reveals low signal intensity of the marrow of the fourth, fifth, and sixth cervical vertebral bodies. *C,* After intravenous administration of a gadolinium contrast agent, sagittal T1-weighted (TR/TE, 500/12) spin echo MR image shows hyperintensity in the prevertebral soft tissues *(arrows)*. In comparison with the findings in *(B)*, the marrow involvement is less apparent.

**TABLE 54-1**

**Differential Diagnosis of Disorders Producing Disc Space Narrowing**

| Disorder | Discovertebral Margin | Sclerosis | Vacuum Phenomena | Osteophytosis | Other Findings |
|---|---|---|---|---|---|
| Infection | Poorly defined | Variable* | Rare† | Absent | Vertebral lysis, soft tissue mass |
| Intervertebral osteochondrosis | Well defined | Prominent | Present | Variable | Cartilaginous nodes |
| Rheumatoid arthritis | Poorly or well defined with "erosions" | Variable | Absent | Absent or mild | Apophyseal joint abnormalities, subluxation |
| Calcium pyrophosphate dihydrate crystal deposition disease | Poorly or well defined | Prominent | Variable | Variable | Fragmentation, subluxation |
| Neuropathic osteoarthropathy | Well defined | Prominent | Variable | Prominent | Fragmentation, subluxation, disorganization |
| Trauma | Well defined | Prominent | Variable | Variable | Fracture, soft tissue mass |
| Sarcoidosis | Poorly or well defined | Variable, may be prominent | Absent | Absent | Soft tissue mass |

*Usually evident in pyogenic infections and in tuberculosis in black patients.

†Vacuum phenomena may initially be evident when intervertebral osteochondrosis is also present or, rarely, when a gas-forming microorganism is responsible for the infection.

the seronegative spondyloarthropathies, calcium pyrophosphate dihydrate crystal deposition disease, alkaptonuria, and neuropathic osteoarthropathy; in each of these disorders, however, clinical and additional radiographic features usually ensure an accurate differential diagnosis.

Sarcoidosis can occasionally be associated with disc space narrowing and bone eburnation at one or more levels of the spine. Diminution of intervertebral disc height and bony sclerosis are associated with cartilaginous node formation (Schmorl's nodes). In general, the poor definition of the subchondral bone plate is less in cases of cartilaginous nodes than in cases of infection. MR imaging can also be applied to the differentiation of cartilage node formation and infection, although diagnostic difficulties are encountered. The widespread cartilaginous nodes detected in Scheuermann's disease (juvenile kyphosis) create an appearance that is not generally confused with that of infection.

Intervertebral (osteo)chondrosis also produces intervertebral disc space narrowing and reactive sclerosis of the neighboring bone (see Chapter 30). The resulting radiographic picture can resemble that of infective spondylitis. In intervertebral (osteo)chondrosis, the vertebral endplates are usually smooth and well defined, although focal defects can represent sites of intervertebral disc displacement (cartilaginous nodes). Of particular diagnostic significance is the presence of one or more radiolucent collections overlying the intervertebral disc in intervertebral (osteo)chondrosis. These vacuum phenomena represent gaseous collections (nitrogen) within the nucleus pulposus and are a reliable sign of disc degeneration. They are exceedingly rare in cases of disc infection, and their detection makes the diagnosis of infection very unlikely. Similarly, the presence of gas in the vertebral body virtually eliminates the diagnosis of

infection. Rarely, infections by gas-forming bacteria may lead to a vacuum phenomenon–like appearance.

In general, primary or metastatic tumor in the spine does not lead to significant loss of intervertebral disc space; the combination of widespread lysis or sclerosis of a vertebral body and an intact adjacent intervertebral disc is much more characteristic of tumor than of infection. Certain neoplasms such as plasma cell myeloma, chordoma, and even skeletal metastasis can extend across or around the intervertebral disc to involve the neighboring vertebra, however. Paraspinal masses occur in infective spondylitis and traumatic and neoplastic disorders. Infection is likely if such masses contain gas.

Accurate radiographic differentiation of pyogenic infective spondylitis from granulomatous infections (tuberculosis and fungal disorders) can be difficult. Rapid loss of intervertebral disc height, extensive sclerosis, and the absence of calcified paraspinal masses are findings that are more typical of pyogenic infection.

## SACROILIAC JOINT INFECTIONS

### Routes of Contamination

The sacroiliac joint may become infected by the hematogenous route, by contamination from a contiguous suppurative focus, by direct implantation, or after surgery. Hematogenous involvement of this joint likely begins in the subchondral bone of the ilium.

Contamination of the sacroiliac joint or neighboring bone can occur from an adjacent infection. Pelvic abscesses can disrupt the anterior articular capsule or the periosteum and cortex of the ilium or sacrum. Thus, vaginal, uterine, ovarian, bladder, and intestinal processes can lead to iliac or sacral osteomyelitis and sacroiliac joint suppuration by contiguous contamination (as well as by hematogenous spread via Batson's plexus). Pressure sores related to prolonged immobilization are not infrequent in the sacral region and can lead to subsequent articular and osseous infection. Direct implantation of organisms after diagnostic, therapeutic, or surgical procedures represents another, though uncommon, source of sacroiliac joint infection.

## Clinical Abnormalities

Pyogenic infection of the sacroiliac joint may develop in patients of all ages. Unilateral alterations predominate. Fever, local pain and tenderness, and a limp may be evident. Accurate diagnosis is often delayed in cases of septic sacroiliitis, which increases the frequency of such extra-articular contamination. Elevation of the erythrocyte sedimentation rate and leukocytosis are common but variable laboratory findings. Identification of the causative organisms from blood culture or joint aspiration can be difficult. Gram-negative bacterial agents are especially common in pyogenic arthritis of the sacroiliac joint in intravenous drug abusers.

## Radiographic-Pathologic Correlation

In almost all cases of sacroiliac joint infection, a unilateral distribution is encountered. In pyogenic arthritis, radiographic findings generally occur in 2 or 3 weeks and are characterized by blurring and indistinctness of the subchondral osseous line and narrowing or widening of the interosseous space. Although these two alterations frequently coexist, their time of appearance is dictated by the initial site of contamination: if osteomyelitis precedes septic arthritis, bony abnormalities may antedate the articular changes; if the joint is affected initially, cartilaginous and osseous alterations may coexist. In both situations, the most extensive findings are commonly evident about the inferoanterior aspect of the joint (Fig. 54–11). Surrounding condensation of bone is variable in frequency and degree, and it is influenced by the type and virulence of the infecting microorganism.

## Other Diagnostic Techniques

Scintigraphy, with the use of technetium phosphate, gallium, or both, may outline increased accumulation of radionuclide when findings on routine radiographs and conventional tomograms are unimpressive Abnormal unilateral uptake of isotope in the sacroiliac joint indicates infection until proved otherwise.

CT scanning is valuable in the early diagnosis of septic sacroiliitis, because it reveals cartilaginous and osseous destruction as well as intraosseous gas, and as an aid to aspiration and biopsy techniques. The latter procedures can be difficult without CT guidance (Fig. 54–12).

MR imaging shows marrow edema in the sacrum and ilium, irregularity of the subchondral bone on either side of the joint space, joint fluid, muscle edema, fluid-filled channels, sinus tracts, and fistulas. Intravenous administration of a gadolinium contrast agent can be used to accentuate the MR imaging abnormalities and to delineate adjacent soft tissue involvement (Fig. 54–13).

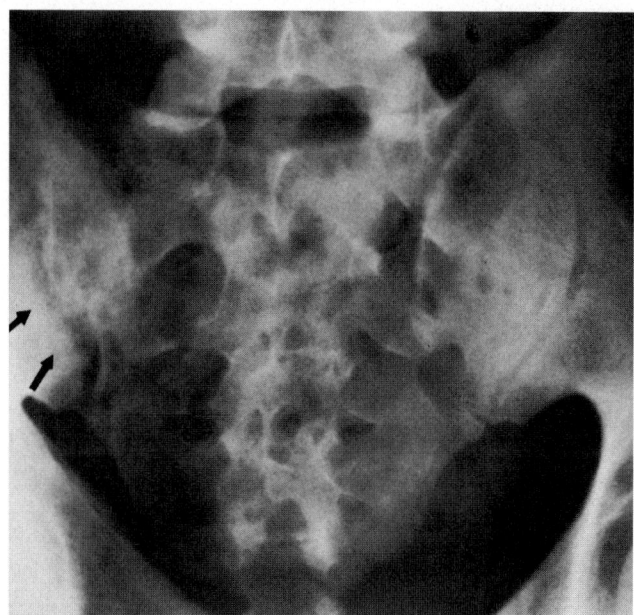

**Figure 54–11.** Sacroiliac joint infection: early abnormalities. *Pseudomonas* osteomyelitis and septic arthritis developed in a 35-year-old male heroin addict. Radiograph reveals changes in the right sacroiliac joint consisting of subchondral osseous erosion, poorly defined articular margins, and widening of the joint space (*arrows*).

## Differential Diagnosis

The unilateral nature of infective sacroiliac joint disease

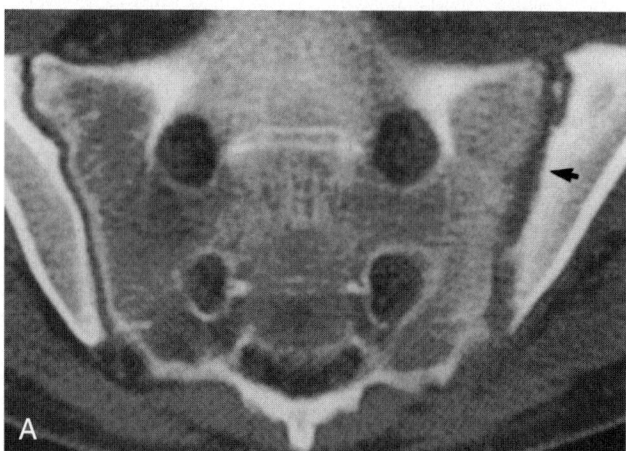
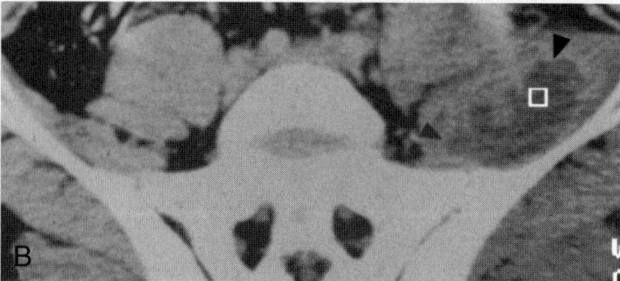

**Figure 54–12.** Sacroiliac joint infection: CT scanning. In this 20-year-old intravenous drug abuser, CT scans with bone (*A*) and soft tissue (*B*) windows show involvement of the left sacroiliac joint (*arrow*) and an abscess (*arrowheads*) in the iliac muscle. (Courtesy of J. Hodler, MD, Zurich, Switzerland.)

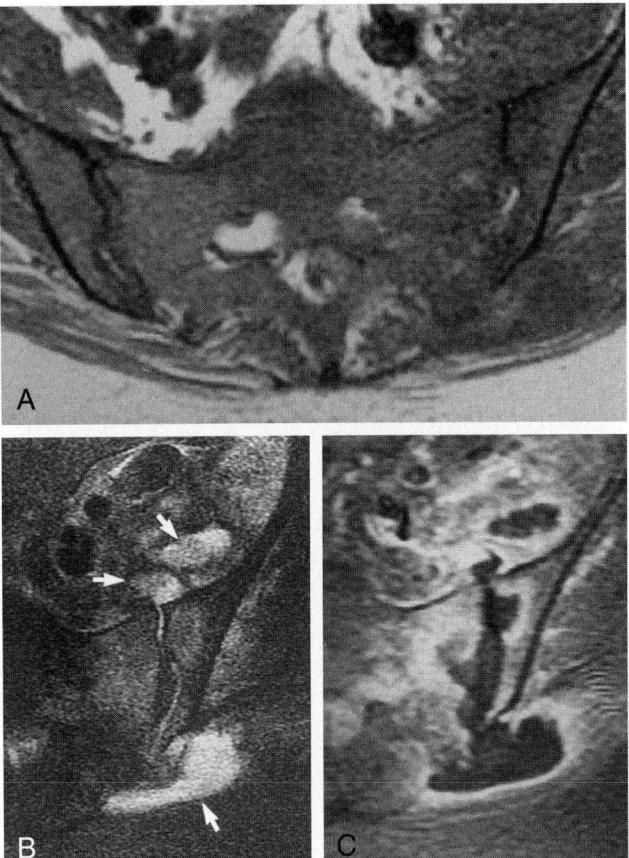

**Figure 54–13.** Sacroiliac joint infection: MR imaging. Staphylococcal infection of the left sacroiliac joint developed in this 48-year-old woman. *A*, The infectious process in the sacrum and ilium is not well visualized on this transaxial T1-weighted (TR/TE, 650/11) spin echo MR image because of the similar signal intensity of the inflammatory response and the hematopoietic bone marrow. The soft tissue extension of infection is not evident either. *B*, Transaxial fat-suppressed T2-weighted (TR/TE, 6000/102) fast spin echo MR image reveals high signal intensity in the sacrum and ilium, as well as in the anterior and posterior soft tissues and musculature *(arrows)*. *C*, Transaxial T1-weighted (TR/TE, 500/11) spin echo MR image obtained with fat saturation technique after the intravenous injection of a gadolinium contrast agent reveals the inflammatory reaction, with high signal intensity in the bone and about the anterior and posterior abscesses. Note the low signal intensity of the fluid in the joint and in the soft tissues and musculature. (Courtesy of M. Schweitzer, MD, Philadelphia, Pa.)

is its most useful diagnostic feature. Bilateral symmetrical or asymmetrical articular changes are characteristic of ankylosing spondylitis, psoriasis, Reiter's syndrome, osteitis condensans ilii, and hyperparathyroidism. Unilateral changes can be encountered in rheumatoid arthritis, gout, Reiter's syndrome, psoriasis, and paralysis (because of chondral atrophy).

## INFECTION AT OTHER AXIAL SITES

In intravenous drug abusers, osteomyelitis and septic arthritis of the sternoclavicular and acromioclavicular joints, in addition to the spine and sacroiliac joint, may be

evident. After urologic procedures or athletic endeavors, osteomyelitis of the symphysis pubis may be difficult to differentiate from osteitis pubis. Infection of the sternum and the manubriosternal and sternoclavicular joints can result from direct hematogenous inoculation (Fig. 54–14) or secondary contamination resulting from local injury, surgery, or diagnostic or therapeutic procedures. In some sites, such as the sternoclavicular joint, abscess formation and inflammation in nearby tissues are common, and these complications are well studied by CT scanning or MR imaging.

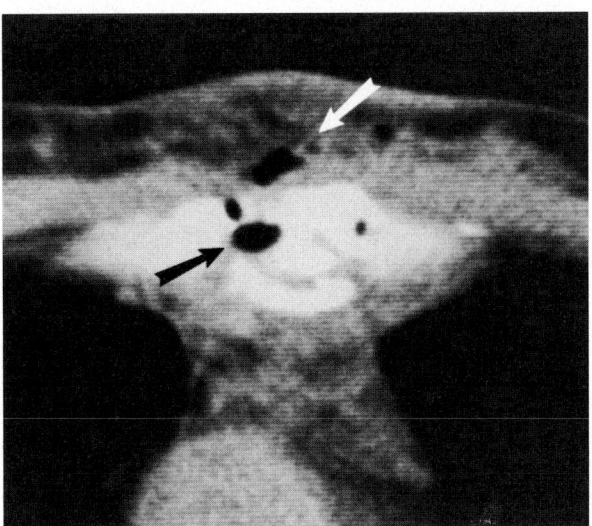

**Figure 54–14.** Sternal infection. Group B streptococcal septicemia resulting in infections in the hip, spine, and sternum developed in this 47-year-old man. Transaxial CT scan shows a destroyed sternum and an anterior soft tissue mass, both containing gas *(arrows)*, and mediastinal adenopathy. Mediastinitis was confirmed at surgery.

## FURTHER READING

Allen EH, Cosgrove D, Millard FJC: The radiological changes in infections of the spine and their diagnostic value. Clin Radiol 29:31, 1978.

Batson OV: The vertebral vein system. AJR Am J Roentgenol 78:195, 1957.

Brant-Zawadzki M, Burke VD, Jeffrey RB: CT in the evaluation of spine infection. Spine 8:358, 1983.

Dagirmanjian A, Schils J, McHenry M, et al: MR imaging of vertebral osteomyelitis revisited. AJR Am J Roentgenol 167:1539, 1996.

Fernandez-Ulloa M, Vasavada PJ, Hanslits ML, et al: Diagnosis of vertebral osteomyelitis: Clinical radiological and scintigraphic features. Orthopedics 8:1141, 1985.

Goldin RH, Chow A, Edwards JE Jr, et al: Sternoarticular septic arthritis in heroin users. N Engl J Med 289:616, 1973.

Jamison RC, Heimlich EM, Miethke JC, et al: Non-specific spondylitis of infants and children. Radiology 77:355, 1961.

Larde D, Mathieu D, Frija J, et al: Vertebral osteomyelitis: Disk hypodensity on CT. AJR Am J Roentgenol 139:963, 1982.

Lewkonia RM, Kinsella TD: Pyogenic sacroiliitis: Diagnosis and significance. J Rheumatol 8:153, 1981.

Modic MT, Weinstein MA, Pavlicek W, et al: Magnetic resonance imaging of the cervical spine: Technical and clinical observations. AJR Am J Roentgenol 141:1129, 1983.

Murphy KJ, Brunberg JA, Quint DJ, et al: Spinal cord infection: Myelitis and abscess formation. AJNR Am J Neuroradiol 19:341, 1998.

Numaguchi Y, Rigamonti D, Rothman MI, et al: Spinal epidural abscess: Evaluation with gadolinium-enhanced MR imaging. Radiographics 13:545, 1993.

Pinckney LE, Currarino G, Higgenboten CL: Osteomyelitis of the cervical spine following dental extraction. Radiology 135:335, 1980.

Rosenberg D, Baskies AM, Deckers PJ, et al: Pyogenic sacroiliitis: An absolute indication for computerized tomographic scanning. Clin Orthop 184:128, 1984.

Sandrasegaran K, Saifuddin A, Coral A, et al: Magnetic resonance imaging of septic sacroiliitis. Skeletal Radiol 23:289, 1994.

Sartoris DJ, Moskowitz PS, Kaufman RA, et al: Childhood diskitis: Computed tomographic findings. Radiology 149:701, 1983.

Sharif HS: Role of MR imaging in the management of spinal infections. AJR Am J Roentgenol 158:1333, 1992.

Wiley AM, Trueta J: The vascular anatomy of the spine and its relationship to pyogenic vertebral osteomyelitis. J Bone Joint Surg Br 41:796, 1959.

# CHAPTER 55

# Osteomyelitis, Septic Arthritis, and Soft Tissue Infection: Organisms

## SUMMARY OF KEY FEATURES

Osseous, articular, and soft tissue structures may become involved in many infectious disorders. Bacteria, mycobacteria, spirochetes, fungi, viruses, rickettsiae, protozoa, and worms are all capable of affecting the musculoskeletal system. In many instances, imaging features, though typical of an infection, do not allow the diagnosis of a specific causative agent; in some cases, the distribution and morphology of the lesions are sufficiently characteristic to suggest a single infectious process. In all cases, the imaging studies must be interpreted in conjunction with the clinical and pathologic manifestations.

## INTRODUCTION

Although the skeleton can react in only a limited number of ways, certain characteristics of its response to a particular infectious agent may differ, at least subtly, from the changes encountered in the presence of another agent. Thus, certain organisms produce rapid and destructive osseous or articular disease, whereas others are associated with a more indolent process. Further, some agents show a predilection for certain anatomic regions of the skeleton.

## BACTERIAL INFECTION
### Gram-Positive Cocci

#### Staphylococcal Infection

Staphylococci are responsible for most cases of acute osteomyelitis and nongonococcal infectious arthritis. The two major pathogens are *Staphylococcus aureus* (coagulase positive) and *Staphylococcus epidermidis* (coagulase negative). *S. aureus* is most typical in pyogenic osteomyelitis. Localization of the infection to the metaphysis of the tubular bones in children is typical, and Brodie's abscesses may be seen (Fig. 55–1). Staphylococci are also responsible for many of the deep infections that occur after bone or joint surgery; the foot infections in diabetic patients; cases of osteomyelitis and septic arthritis in hemodialysis patients with infected shunts, intravenous drug addicts, and patients with rheumatoid arthritis; and the osseous, articular, and soft tissue suppurative processes that follow penetrating or open wounds. *S. aureus* is implicated in most cases of pyomyositis.

#### Streptococcal Infection

Streptococci are gram-positive cocci that can be classified on the basis of the type of hemolysis they produce on sheep blood agar plates (e.g., beta-hemolytic streptococci). In infants, hemolytic streptococcal agents are an important causative factor in neonatal or infantile osteomyelitis. The clinical manifestations of streptococcal bone infection may be mild, even in the presence of significant radiographic alterations. Infection of a single bone is most frequent, and a predilection for the humerus has been noted (Fig. 55–2). Lytic lesions with mild or absent sclerosis and periostitis may be seen. The joints may be infected by streptococcal organisms either by extension from a neighboring site of osteomyelitis or cellulitis or directly.

#### Pneumococcal Infection

Formerly termed *Diplococcus pneumoniae*, the pneumococcus is now referred to as *Streptococcus pneumoniae*. Pulmonary infections and those of the upper respiratory tract predominate. Pneumococcal arthritis is not frequent. Pneumococcal osteomyelitis is rare and generally confined to periarticular bone or the spine. Sickle cell anemia may be an underlying problem.

### Gram-Negative Cocci
#### Meningococcal Infection

Meningococcal infection caused by *Neisseria meningitidis* occurs almost exclusively in persons who have no measurable antimeningococcal antibody. It varies remarkably in severity, from benign and asymptomatic to a fulminant and fatal disorder. Septicemia may lead to contamination of many sites, but the microorganisms commonly lodge in the central nervous system, skin, adrenal glands, and serosal surfaces. Meningococcemia leads to the rapid development of fever, shaking chills, skin eruption, petechiae, myalgias, and a variety of neurologic manifestations. In fulminant cases (Waterhouse-Friderichsen syndrome), hypotension, confusion, tachypnea, peripheral cyanosis, and consumptive coagulopathy develop. In children, characteristic skeletal abnormalities have been described in which localized premature fusion of part of several physes is seen, usually in a bilateral and relatively symmetrical distribution (Fig. 55–3). Commonly, the central aspect of the physis is affected, and a cupped or cone-shaped metaphysis results. Subsequently, epiphyseal disintegration and bowing and angular deformities appear, especially in the legs, and lead to limb shortening.

#### Gonococcal Infection

Gonorrhea is produced by the microorganism *Neisseria gonorrhoeae*, which infects the mucous membranes of the urethra, cervix, rectum, and pharynx. The frequency of

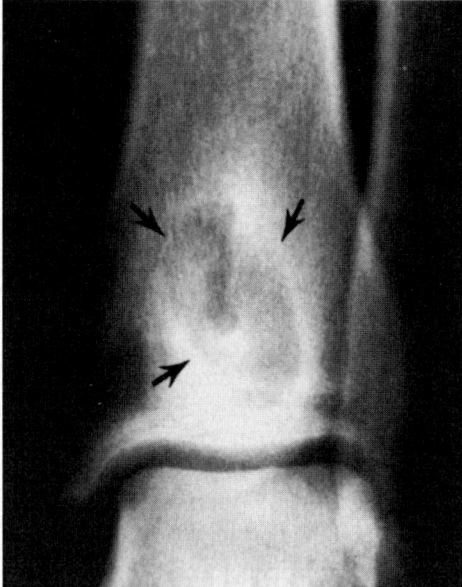

**Figure 55–1.** Staphylococcal osteomyelitis. Well-defined lucent lesion surrounded by a sclerotic margin at the end of the tubular bone *(arrows)* is typical of Brodie's abscess.

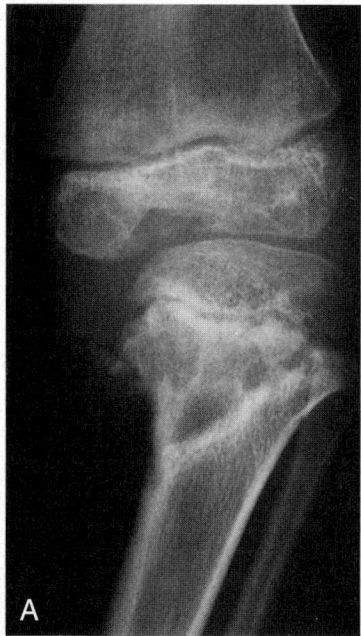

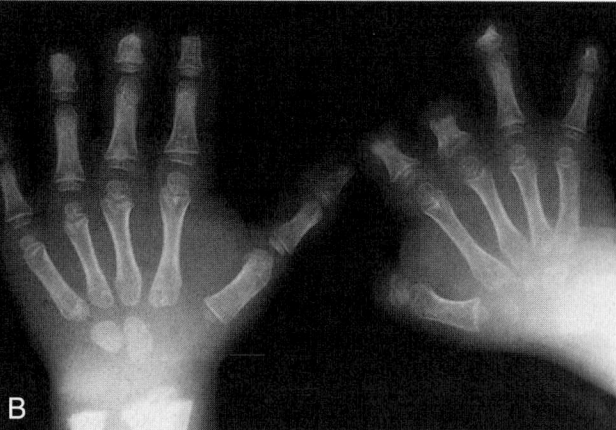

**Figure 55–3.** Meningococcemia with skeletal deformities. This 5 year-old-boy demonstrates the skeletal deformities that can follow meningococcemia with intravascular coagulation. *A*, Findings in the knee include metaphyseal sclerosis, epiphyseal irregularity and deformity, subluxation, and, in one tibia, a previous fracture. *B*, Observe the metaphyseal cupping and irregularity in the phalanges, metacarpal bones, and radii, with amputation of some of the digits. (Courtesy of M. Dalinka, MD, Philadelphia, Pa.)

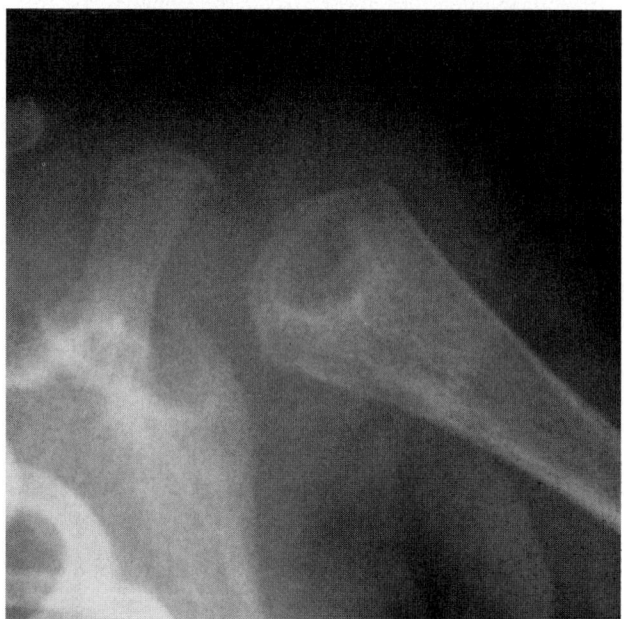

**Figure 55–2.** Streptococcal osteomyelitis and septic arthritis. In this infant, radiography shows an osteolytic lesion of the metaphysis of the humerus. The proximal epiphysis is not ossified. (Courtesy of J. Tomanek, MD, Johnson City, Tenn.)

gonococcal arthritis is rising, possibly owing to an increasing resistance to antibiotics. The disease is transmitted almost exclusively through sexual contact with persons who have asymptomatic or ignored symptomatic infection. It is also encountered during pregnancy and after gonococcal vulvovaginitis in children and neonates. Only a minority of gonococcal infections eventually disseminate. Gonococcemia leads to skin rash, fever, and arthritis, the

last occurring in approximately 75% of disseminated cases. The articular disease may have an insidious onset with fleeting arthralgias or a sudden onset with fever and red, hot, swollen, and tender joints. Polyarticular findings are frequent, but the infection tends to localize in one or two joints. The affected articulations, in decreasing order of frequency, are the knee, ankle, wrist, and joints of the shoulder, foot, and spine. In approximately 50% to 70% of cases, acute asymmetrical tenosynovitis or periarthritis is evident, particularly in the dorsal aspect of the fingers, hand, or wrist or in the ankle.

If appropriate treatment is delayed, more prominent radiographic findings are encountered, including joint space narrowing, marginal and central osseous erosions, lytic destruction of adjacent metaphyses and epiphyses, and periostitis (Fig. 55–4). These features are identical to those accompanying other pyogenic infections, although abnormalities at multiple joints and tenosynovitis are helpful clues to a specific diagnosis of gonococcal infection. Differentiating the radiographic features of gonococcal pyarthrosis and Reiter's syndrome can be extremely difficult; clinical differentiation is complicated by the presence of skin rash, urethral discharge, and articular abnormalities in both conditions.

## Enteric Gram-Negative Bacilli

Although the terminology related to this group of bacteria is not constant, two major families of microorganisms are identified: Enterobacteriaceae and Pseudomonadaceae. In general, these gram-negative bacilli are responsible for as many as 25% of skeletal infections.

### Coliform Bacterial Infection

The coliform bacteria are gram-negative bacilli that normally inhabit the human intestinal tract. The best-known organisms in this group are *Escherichia coli* and *Enterobacter (Aerobacter) aerogenes*. Articular and osseous infections with these agents are rare except in intravenous drug abusers, those with preexisting joint disease, and patients with chronic debilitating disorders. No specific radiographic features are evident.

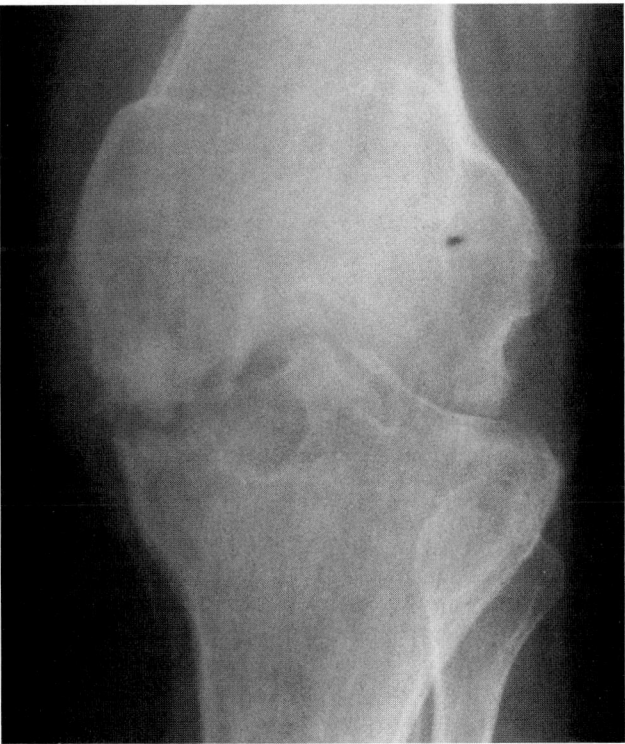

**Figure 55–4.** Gonococcal arthritis: knee. Observe the joint space loss, poorly defined marginal and central osseous erosions, and soft tissue swelling. The lack of osteoporosis is impressive. Bone proliferation is evident along the distal medial portion of the femur.

### *Proteus* Infection

*Proteus mirabilis* infection of a joint is rarely observed. Monoarticular involvement of the knee or another joint is typical. Osteomyelitis related to this microorganism is also rare.

### *Pseudomonas* Infection

Premature infants, children with congenital anomalies, intravenous drug abusers, patients with myeloproliferative disorders or those receiving immunosuppressive agents, and geriatric patients with debilitating diseases are susceptible to osteomyelitis or septic arthritis from *Pseudomonas aeruginosa*. Hematogenous spread of infection is common in intravenous drug abusers; *Pseudomonas* infection commonly localizes in the axial skeleton and affects the spine and the sacroiliac, sternoclavicular, and acromioclavicular joints. *Pseudomonas* osteomyelitis is a recognized complication of puncture wounds. No specific radiographic features characterize skeletal involvement with this organism.

### *Klebsiella* Infection

Rarely, *Klebsiella pneumoniae* results in osteomyelitis and septic arthritis in a host with diminished resistance. Emphysematous septic arthritis may also be seen.

### *Salmonella* Infection

*Salmonella typhi* produces a systemic infection, typhoid fever. Bone infection in such cases is rare. Involvement can occur in spinal locations, with a radiographic picture resembling that of tuberculosis. An association exists between *Salmonella* infection and sickle cell anemia and other hemoglobinopathies, as well as leukemia, lymphoma, bartonellosis, cirrhosis of the liver, and systemic lupus erythematosus. It has been postulated that multiple bowel infarcts allow the organisms to leave the colon and enter the bloodstream and that *Salmonella* organisms are well suited for survival in areas of medullary bone infarction. In fact, *Salmonella* osteomyelitis frequently originates in the medullary cavity of a tubular bone. *Salmonella* infection may be characterized by a symmetrical distribution, a combination of lysis and sclerosis, and periostitis, findings that are difficult to differentiate from those of infarction alone.

### *Shigella* Infection

Two to 3 weeks after an episode of acute bacillary dysentery, a noninfectious polyarthritis showing a predilection for the knees, elbows, wrists, or fingers may be evident. It simulates rheumatic fever.

### *Yersinia* Infection

Two types of bone or joint affliction can occur in association with infection caused by *Yersinia enterocolitica*. A nonsuppurative, self-limited polyarthritis, especially of the knees and ankles, can appear approximately 3 weeks after the onset of illness. This articular manifestation may be complicated by sacroiliitis and presence of the HLA-B27 antigen. The second type of affliction relates to the presence of *Y. enterocolitica* septicemia, particularly in patients with underlying abnormalities. Septic arthritis or osteomyelitis may appear in this setting.

### *Serratia* Infection

*Serratia marcescens* can cause infection of the musculoskeletal system, especially in persons with underlying disorders such as diabetes mellitus, systemic lupus erythematosus, neutrophil dysfunction syndromes, and rheumatoid arthritis. It can also occur after trauma; placement of intravenous, arterial, or urinary catheters; ischemic necrosis of bone; or intravenous drug abuse. The usual pathway for articular and osseous infection with this organism is the bloodstream. Radiographic features are entirely nonspecific.

## Other Gram-Negative Bacilli

### *Haemophilus* Infection

Acute septic arthritis caused by *Haemophilus influenzae* is more frequent in children, particularly those between the ages of 7 months and 4 years, than in adults (Fig. 55–5).

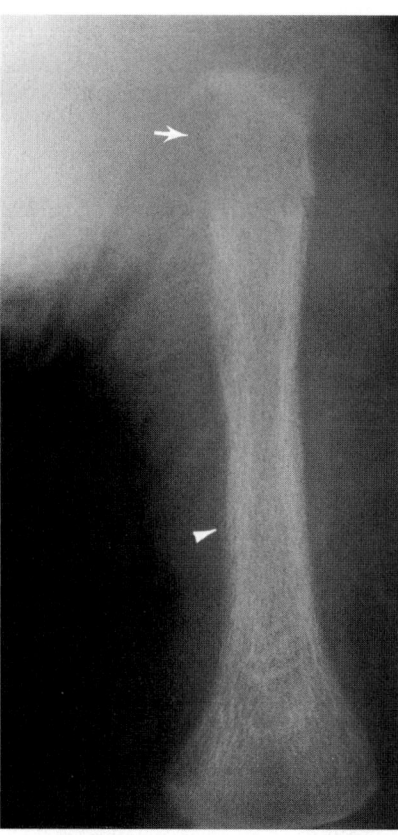

**Figure 55–5.** *Haemophilus* osteomyelitis and septic arthritis. Osteomyelitis of the proximal metaphysis and diaphysis of the humerus, with glenohumeral joint involvement, developed in this infant secondary to *Haemophilus* infection. Observe the metaphyseal erosion *(arrow)*, permeative bone destruction, and periostitis *(arrowhead)*.

In fact, this microorganism appears to be the leading cause of pyarthrosis in the first 2 years of life. Hematogenous spread is the usual mechanism of joint infection. Single or, less commonly, multiple joints may be affected, with the knee and ankle being the most frequent sites of involvement.

### *Brucella* Infection

Brucellosis (undulant fever) is endemic in Saudi Arabia, South America, Spain, Italy, and the midwestern United States. It is transmitted to humans from animals such as goats, cows, and hogs through the ingestion of milk or milk products containing viable bacteria or through skin contact with infected tissues or secretions. The disease is rarely transmitted from one human to another. The invading organisms localize in tissues of the reticuloendothelial system, such as the liver, spleen, lymph nodes, and bone marrow.

Involvement of joints, bones, and bursae is relatively uncommon, although an inflammatory process in any one of these sites in a farmer or meat handler should arouse suspicion of brucellosis. The arthritis is usually monoarticular or pauciarticular, with the hip and knee being involved most frequently. Alterations in bursae may be especially characteristic, with inflammation common in the prepatellar region.

Osteomyelitis of long, short, or flat bones may be encountered. Brucellar spondylitis, which appears to be the most common form of musculoskeletal disease, typically affects the lumbar spine and is associated with an acute clinical onset and rapid progression of radiographic findings (Fig. 55–6). Abnormalities include destruction of vertebrae and intervertebral discs, sclerosis, paravertebral abscess formation, and healing with intraosseous fusion and osteophytosis. A large, parrot beak–like osteophyte has been reported as a characteristic feature of spinal brucellosis, although this radiographic abnormality resembles that in other types of pyogenic or tuberculous spondylitis.

### *Aeromonas* Infection

*Aeromonas hydrophila* is an aerobic gram-negative rod found in fresh water, tap water, swimming pools, and soil, as well as in the stools of some persons. Although rarely a pathogen, it can cause infection in patients with neoplasm or chronic liver disease. A history of exposure to water in a pool or lake, especially when combined with trauma, is characteristic. Necrotizing lesions can lead to gas formation. After initiation of septic arthritis resulting from hematogenous spread of infection, patients respond poorly to therapy.

### *Pasteurella* Infection

Typical pathogens in animals, *Pasteurella* organisms can also produce human infection. Cutaneous and subcutaneous abscesses, cellulitis, and lymphangitis are local and regional manifestations of *Pasteurella* infection and can be followed by septicemia and involvement of distant sites. Localization of infection in the knee is common,

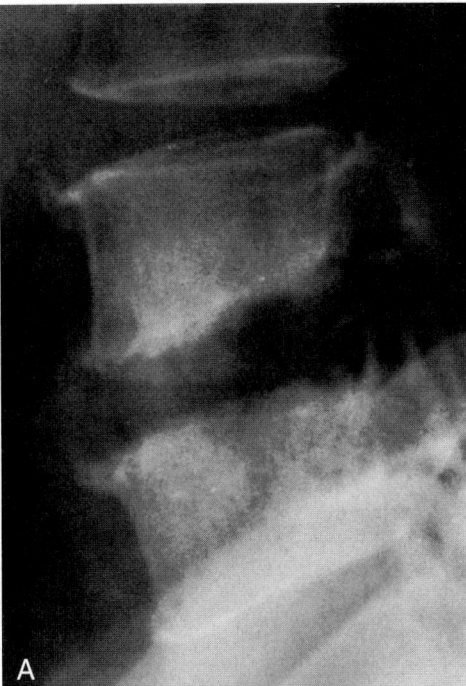

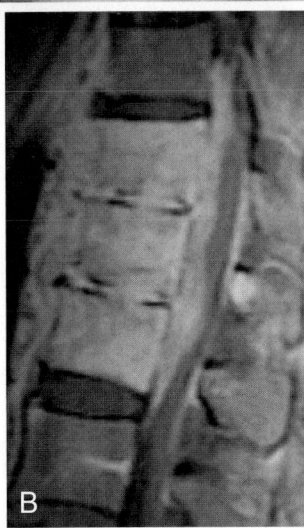

**Figure 55–6.** Brucellar spondylitis: lumbar spine. *A*, Involvement in this case is characterized by irregular destruction of the osseous surfaces of two adjacent vertebrae with reactive sclerosis. Note the parrot beak–like osteophytes. *B*, In another patient, findings include disc space loss at two levels (T12–L1, L1–L2) with osteophyte formation. A sagittal fat-suppressed T1-weighted (TR/TE, 600/20) spin echo MR image obtained after the intravenous administration of a gadolinium contrast agent reveals high signal intensity in the affected vertebral bodies and intervertebral discs, as well as in the anterior soft tissues and intraspinal regions. The spinal cord is displaced and encased by the infection.

although any joint can be affected. Bone and joint contamination in the hand or foot is commonly related to direct inoculation of organisms or spread of infection from involved soft tissues as a result of injury (animal bite or scratch).

## Other Bacteria

### Clostridial Infection

Wounds that are contaminated by gas gangrene may contain a mixture of clostridial organisms. These organisms are anaerobic and are capable of producing extensive tissue destruction with gas formation at the site of invasion. Soft tissue contamination with gas gangrene develops in devitalized tissues in which the arterial blood supply has been compromised. War wounds, vehicular trauma, surgery, burns, and decubitus ulcers are some predisposing factors. Clinical manifestations of clostridial myonecrosis may become evident within 6 to 8 hours of injury and include severe pain and an edematous, pulseless, and gangrenous limb. Crepitation with detection of gas in the soft tissues is apparent in later stages. The clinical manifestations of clostridial cellulitis are less striking.

On radiographs, radiolucent collections may appear within subcutaneous or muscular tissue (Fig. 55–7). In the former location, they produce linear or netlike lucent areas. Gas in muscular tissue may produce circular collections of varying size. It should be emphasized, however, that soft tissue gas is not specific for clostridial infection, because it is evident in some cases of infection with *E. coli*, other coliform bacteria, streptococci, and *Bacteroides* species. Clostridial organisms can be introduced into a joint by contamination from a penetrating injury or, rarely, by hematogenous spread from its normal site of residence in the gastrointestinal tract. Monoarticular disease, particularly of the knee, is typical. Synovial edema and inflammation and cartilaginous destruction may be evident, perhaps related to the effect of the highly toxic enzymes produced by these bacteria. In addition to joint space narrowing and osseous defects, radiographs may delineate gas in the adjacent soft tissues or in the articulation itself.

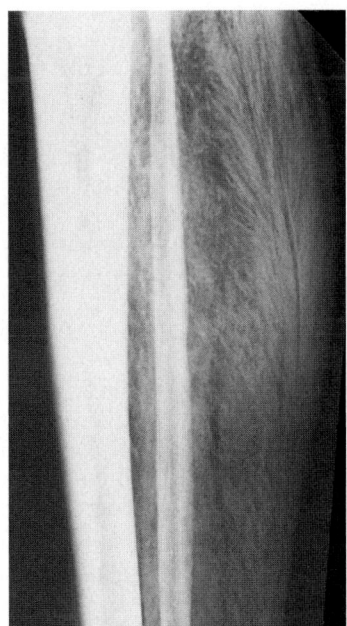

**Figure 55–7.** Clostridial soft tissue infection. Linear collections of gas in subcutaneous and muscular tissue reflect the presence of clostridial myositis and cellulitis.

### *Bacteroides* and Related Anaerobic Infection

In comparison to clostridia, which are spore-forming obligate anaerobic bacteria, *Bacteroides* and several other anaerobic bacteria are non–spore-forming obligate anaerobes. Many of these organisms exist as part of the normal microflora on the skin and adjacent mucous membranes, and clinically evident infections result when breaks in the mucosa or skin allow the microflora to become displaced into deeper tissues and reach the bloodstream. Characteristics of such infections include localization to a site normally inhabited by anaerobic bacteria, traumatic disruption of the skin or mucous membrane, and a history of diabetes mellitus or other chronic debilitating disease. In the musculoskeletal system, crepitant cellulitis, necrotizing fasciitis, and myonecrosis are typical expressions. Septic arthritis, infective spondylitis, and osteomyelitis are rare and may be manifestations of hematogenous dissemination. Gas formation in the soft tissues or, rarely, the articular cavity or intervertebral disc aids in the precise radiographic diagnosis.

## Mycobacteria

### Tuberculous Infection

The frequency of tuberculosis has changed dramatically since the advent of appropriate chemotherapy for this disease; however, even when pulmonary tuberculosis was common, musculoskeletal involvement was not frequent. Currently, the rate of pulmonary tuberculosis is on the rise, and the frequency of musculoskeletal tuberculosis has also increased. Contributing factors to this increase in tuberculosis cases include a greater number of people who have suppressed immune systems, the development of drug-resistant strains of mycobacteria, an aging population, and an increase in the number of health care workers exposed to the disease. Further, the use of modern therapeutic techniques, including bacille Calmette-Guérin (BCG) vaccination, has produced examples of iatrogenic infection (see the discussion later in this chapter).

Additionally, the pattern of osteoarticular tuberculosis has changed over the years. Initially, the disease was usually encountered in children and young adults; currently, patients of all ages are affected. Persons with underlying disorders, those receiving corticosteroid medication, alcoholic patients, intravenous drug abusers, persons who harbor human immunodeficiency virus (HIV), and immigrants may be hosts for this disease. Tuberculous spondylitis is the most typical form of the disease, with the spine being involved in 25% to 50% of cases of skeletal tuberculosis. In recent years, however, articular changes in extraspinal sites, such as the hip, knee, wrist, and elbow, have become more prominent. Tuberculous dactylitis, multiple sites of involvement, and tendon sheath abnormalities are also commonly encountered.

### *Clinical Abnormalities*

Skeletal tuberculosis can affect persons of all ages. Extrapulmonary tuberculosis is more common in children than in adults. The vertebral column, pelvis and hip, and knee are the most frequent sites of involvement. Tuber-

culous arthritis can lead to pain, swelling, weakness, muscle wasting, a draining sinus, and other manifestations, which may be present for 1 to 2 years before diagnosis. Tuberculous spondylitis first manifests clinically as an insidious onset of back pain, stiffness, local tenderness, and possibly fever. Tuberculous dactylitis usually appears as painless swelling of the hand or foot. Tuberculous tenosynovitis and bursitis can produce soft tissue swelling and tenderness in the ulnar or radial bursa, fingers, and toes.

A positive skin test for tuberculosis is of little help in diagnosing this disease (older patients who have never exhibited any clinical manifestations of tuberculosis have a high frequency of positive skin tests), although a negative skin test usually (but not invariably) excludes the diagnosis. A negative chest radiograph in an adult patient does not exclude the possibility of skeletal tuberculosis. In a child, such a radiograph makes tuberculosis an unlikely cause of bony abnormalities.

### *Pathogenesis*

It is generally accepted that skeletal involvement in tuberculosis occurs mainly by the hematogenous route. Hematogenous seeding of the skeleton may arise from a primary infection of the lung, particularly in children, or, at a later date, from a quiescent primary site or an extraosseous focus. Pulmonary involvement may be evident in 50% of cases, is more frequent in children, and on radiographs may appear either active or inactive. Urogenital lesions may coexist with skeletal involvement in 20% to 45% of cases.

### *General Pathologic Considerations*

The typical response of tissue is the formation of tubercles that are sharply demarcated from surrounding tissue. Around a central zone are clusters of epithelioid cells. In the central part of the tubercle are multinucleated giant cells, whereas at the periphery of the tubercle is a mantle of lymphocytes. Central caseating necrosis is characteristic of these tubercles and is incited by the tuberculin produced by the bacilli.

It should be emphasized that granulomatous disease, including that of the bone marrow, is a nonspecific response to a persistent antigenic stimulus and has been identified in a wide range of illnesses (Table 55–1).

### *Tuberculous Spondylitis*

The vertebral column is affected in 25% to 60% of cases of skeletal tuberculosis. The first lumbar vertebra is most commonly affected, and the frequency of involvement decreases equally as one proceeds in either direction from this level. Tuberculous infection of the upper cervical and sacroiliac joint is not rare. More than one vertebra is typically affected, and the vertebral body is involved more commonly than the posterior elements (Fig. 55–8). In the vertebral body, an anterior predilection is striking. Tuberculous spondylitis is generally thought to result from hematogenous spread of infection. Whether the primary vascular pathway is supplied by the

**TABLE 55–1**

### Diseases Associated with Bone Marrow Granuloma

**Infectious Diseases**
Bacterial infection and exposures
  Mycobacterial disease
    Tuberculosis
    BCG vaccination
    Leprosy
  Brucellosis
  Tularemia
  Glanders
Fungal infection (disseminated)
  Histoplasmosis
  Cryptococcosis
  Paracoccidioidomycosis
  *Saccharomyces cerevisiae* infection
Viral infection
  Infectious mononuclesosis
  Cytomegalovirus infection
  Viral hepatitis
Parasitic infection
  Toxoplasmosis
  Leishmaniasis
Other
  Rocky Mountain spotted fever
  Q fever
  *Mycoplasma pneumoniae* infection

**Malignant Diseases**
Hodgkin's disease
Non-Hodgkin's lymphoma
Metastatic carcinoma
Acute lymphocytic leukemia

**Drugs**
Chlorpropamide
Phenylbutazone (oxyphenbutazone)
Allopurinol
Procainamide
Ibuprofen
Phenytoin

**Autoimmune or Allergic Diseases**
Rheumatoid arthritis (Felty's syndrome)
Systemic lupus erythematosus
Primary biliary cirrhosis
Farmer's lung

**Miscellaneous**
Syndrome of marrow and lymph node granuloma, uveitis, and
  reversible renal failure
Berylliosis
Sarcoidosis

BCG, bacille Calmette-Guérin.

From Bodem CR, Hamory BH, Taylor HM, et al: Granulomatous bone marrow
disease: A review of the literature and clinicopathologic analysis of 58 cases.
Medicine (Baltimore). 62:372, 1983.

chondral bone plate (Fig. 55–9). Infection may spread to the adjacent intervertebral discs. Such spread may occur if the bacilli extend beneath the anterior or posterior longitudinal ligament to violate the peripheral disc tissue

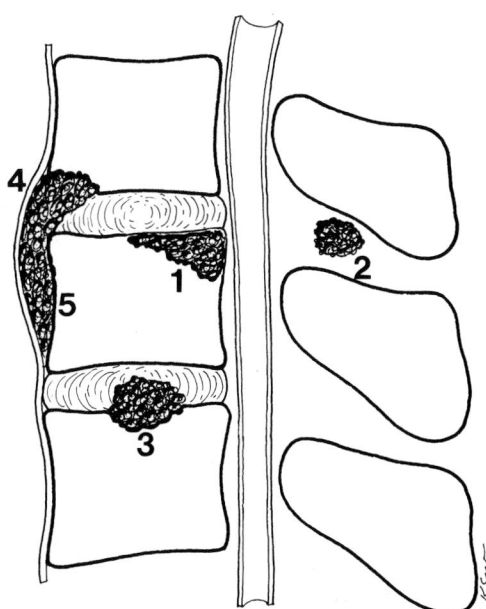

**Figure 55–8.** Tuberculous spondylitis: sites of involvement. Tuberculous lesions can localize in the vertebral body (1) or, more rarely, the posterior osseous or ligamentous structures (2). Extension to the intervertebral disc (3) or prevertebral tissues (4) is not infrequent. Subligamentous spread (5) can lead to erosion of the anterior vertebral surface.

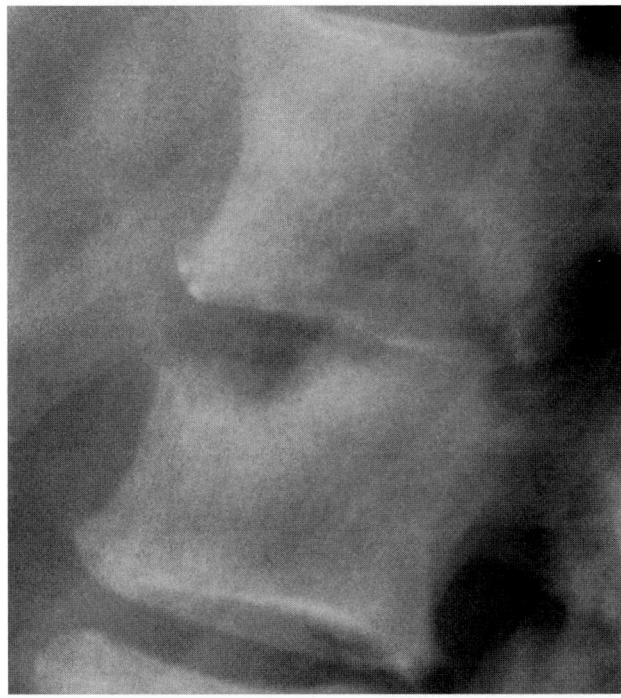

**Figure 55–9.** Tuberculous spondylitis: discovertebral lesion. Radiograph reveals subchondral destruction of two vertebral bodies, with mild surrounding eburnation and loss of intervertebral disc height. The appearance is identical to that in pyogenic spondylitis.

arterial route or the paravertebral venous plexus of Batson is debated, however.

**Radiographic-Pathologic Correlation.** In most cases, tuberculous spondylitis begins as an infectious focus in the anterior aspect of the vertebral body adjacent to the sub-

(Fig. 55–10); if the organisms penetrate the subchondral bone plate and overlying cartilaginous endplate to enter the intervertebral disc; or if an intraosseous lesion weakens the vertebral body to such a degree that it produces disc displacement (cartilaginous node), contamination of invading disc tissue, and subsequent spread through the defect into the intervertebral disc. The combination of vertebral body and disc destruction in tuberculosis is similar to that occurring in pyogenic spondylitis, although the tuberculous process is not usually rapidly progressive. Only rarely does vertebral body tuberculosis extend into the pedicles, laminae, or transverse or spinous processes.

**Paraspinal Extension.** Extension of tuberculosis from vertebral and disc sites to the adjacent ligaments and soft tissue is frequent, usually occurring anterolaterally. Subligamentous extension of a tuberculous abscess can allow osseous and disc invasion at distant sites (Fig. 55–11). Burrowing abscesses can extend for extraordinary distances before perforating an internal viscus or the body surface. Abscess formation in tuberculosis can produce soft tissue swelling on radiographs that appears out of proportion to the degree of osseous and disc destruction. Psoas abscesses are usually easy to identify and may contain calcification (Fig. 55–12); nontuberculous psoas abscesses rarely calcify. Tuberculous abscesses of the psoas muscle calcify in two distinct patterns: faint amorphous deposits, which may become quite dense with progressive healing, and teardrop-shaped calcification. Psoas abscess formation can complicate 5% of cases of tuberculous spondylitis. Magnetic resonance (MR) imaging of tuberculous spondylitis, in common with computed tomography (CT), provides an accurate display of paraspinal and intraspinal extension of

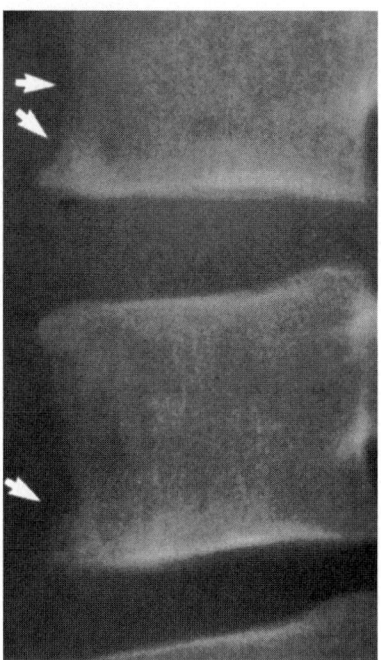

**Figure 55–11.** Tuberculous spondylitis: subligamentous extension. The findings, though subtle, include erosion of the anterior surface of the vertebral bodies *(arrows)*. (Courtesy of C. Resnik, MD, Baltimore, Md.)

disease, as well as the extent of bone and disc involvement (Fig. 55–13).

**Posterior Element Lesions.** Occasionally, the posterior elements may be the initial spinal site of tuberculosis. In these instances, radiographic findings include pediculate or laminal destruction, erosion of the posterior cortex of the vertebral body and adjacent ribs, a large paraspinal mass, and relative sparing of the intervertebral discs.

**Solitary Vertebral Involvement.** Rarely, tuberculosis leads to isolated involvement of a single vertebral body. In children or adults, vertebra plana can appear and simulate eosinophilic granuloma.

**Kyphosis, Scoliosis, and Ankylosis.** Collapse of partially destroyed vertebral bodies during the course of tuberculous spondylitis can lead to severe tuberculous kyphosis or a gibbous deformity. Despite the striking nature of the deformity, the diameter of the spinal canal may not be significantly altered (Fig. 55–14). Although not as frequent as kyphosis, lateral deviation of the spine can occur in tuberculous spondylitis. This abnormality accompanies asymmetrical or unilateral destruction of the vertebral bodies and intervertebral discs and is virtually confined to the lower thoracic and lumbar vertebrae. Healing in tuberculous spondylitis can be associated with osseous fusion of the vertebral bodies.

**Atlantoaxial Destruction.** Involvement of the upper cervical spine is rare, occurring in less than 2% of cases of tuberculous spondylitis. Quadriparesis may be observed in as many as 40% of patients with cervical tuberculosis.

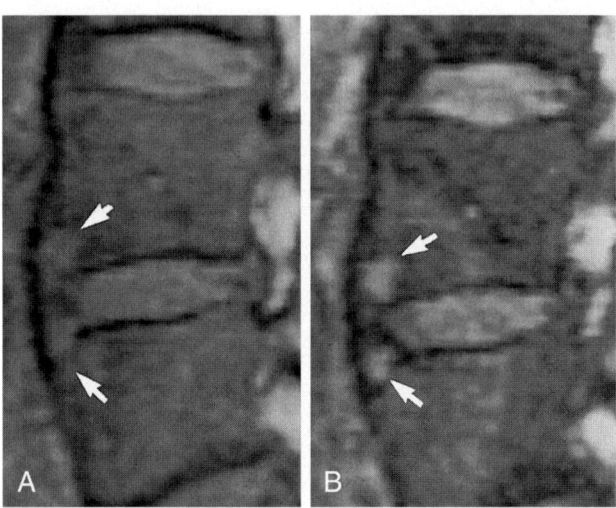

**Figure 55–10.** Tuberculous spondylitis: discovertebral lesion. In this 55-year-old man who had low back pain for 2 months, sagittal intermediate-weighted (TR/TE, 2000/30) *(A)* and T2-weighted (TR/TE, 2000/70) *(B)* spin echo MR images show tuberculous changes at the L3–L4 spinal level. Note the anterior lesions of the vertebral bodies *(arrows)*, with bowing of the adjacent anterior longitudinal ligament and contamination of the anterior portion of the L3–L4 intervertebral disc. The lesions are of higher signal intensity in *(B)*. (Courtesy of P. VanderStoep, MD, St. Cloud, Minn.)

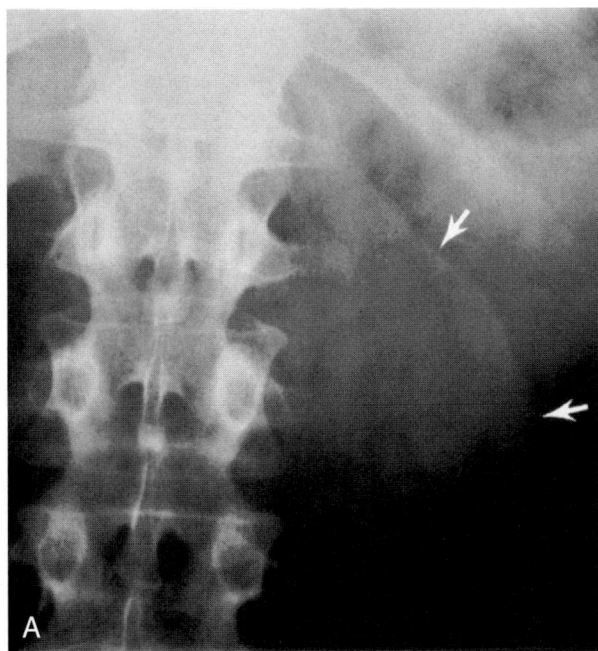

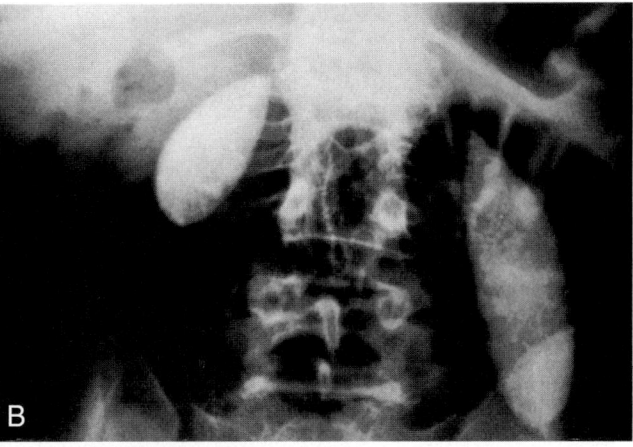

**Figure 55–12.** Tuberculous spondylitis: psoas abscess. *A*, Large, noncalcified left psoas abscess *(arrows)*. *B*, Diffusely calcified psoas abscesses are noted in association with spinal abnormalities.

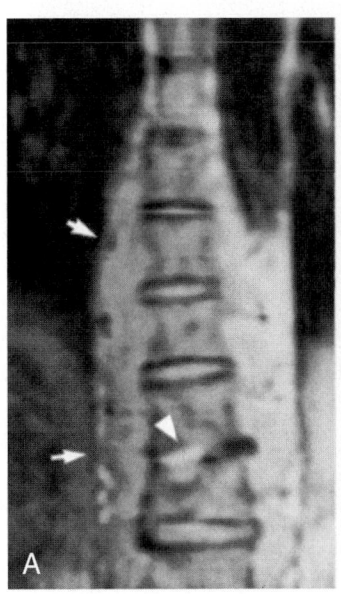

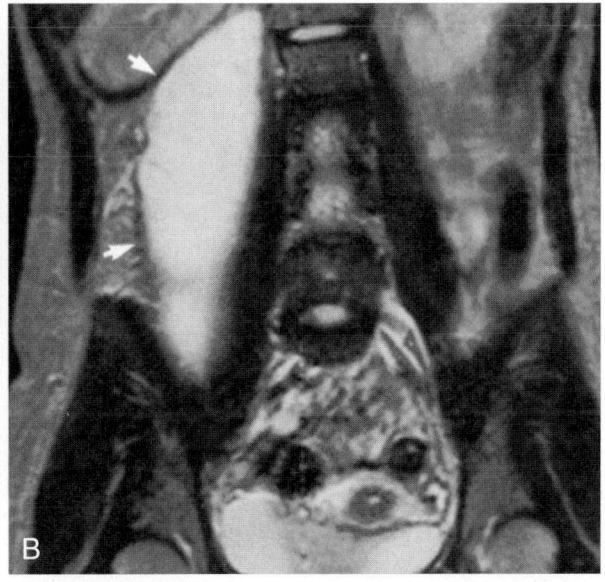

**Figure 55–13.** Tuberculous spondylitis: paraspinal and intraspinal extension. *A*, Coronal intermediate-weighted (TR/TE, 2800/19) spin echo MR image shows paraspinal extension of disease, which is more evident on the right side *(arrows)*, originating from a discovertebral lesion *(arrowhead)*. *B*, Coronal T2-weighted (TR/TE, 1800/80) spin echo MR image confirms the psoas extension *(arrows)*. (Courtesy of R. Kerr, MD, Los Angeles, Calif.)

Radiographic abnormalities include occipitoatlantoaxial subluxation, bone erosion, and a prevertebral soft tissue mass (Fig. 55–15).

**Differential Diagnosis.** Differentiation of tuberculous and pyogenic vertebral osteomyelitis can be extremely difficult. Radiographic features favoring tuberculosis are involvement of one or more segments of the spine, a delay in destruction of the intervertebral discs, a large and calcified paravertebral mass, and absence of sclerosis. None of the radiographic findings is pathognomonic. Intervertebral disc space destruction is more characteristic of infectious lesions of the spine.

### Tuberculous Osteomyelitis

Tuberculous osteomyelitis is relatively infrequent and is almost uniformly related to hematogenous dissemination. Most often, it arises from septic arthritis. Virtually any bone can be affected, including the pelvis, phalanges and metacarpals (tuberculous dactylitis), and long bones. In the long tubular bones, tuberculosis usually originates in one of the epiphyses and soon spreads into the neighboring joint (Fig. 55–16). This feature deserves emphasis, because pyogenic infections arising in the metaphyseal segment of a child's tubular bone generally do not extend across the physis, and detection of a transphyseal spread of infection favors the diagnosis of a granulomatous infec-

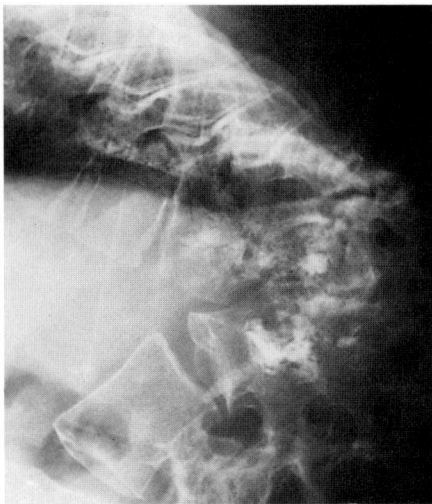

**Figure 55–14.** Tuberculous spondylitis: kyphosis. Severe thoracolumbar kyphosis, associated with calcification and an increased superoinferior dimension of a lumbar vertebral body, is evident. (Courtesy of T. Yochum, DC, Denver, Colo.)

tious process. On radiographs, foci of osteolysis are accompanied by varying amounts of eburnation and periostitis. Sequestrum formation may be encountered as a spicule of increased radiodensity within the zone of destruction.

### Cystic Tuberculosis

A rare variety of tuberculosis is associated with disseminated lesions. Cystic lesions of one or multiple bones are encountered much more frequently in children than in adults (Fig. 55–17). In children, these lesions usually but not invariably affect the peripheral skeleton, favor the metaphyseal regions of tubular bones, may be symmetrical, are of variable size, and are generally unaccompanied by sclerosis. The prognosis in this variety of

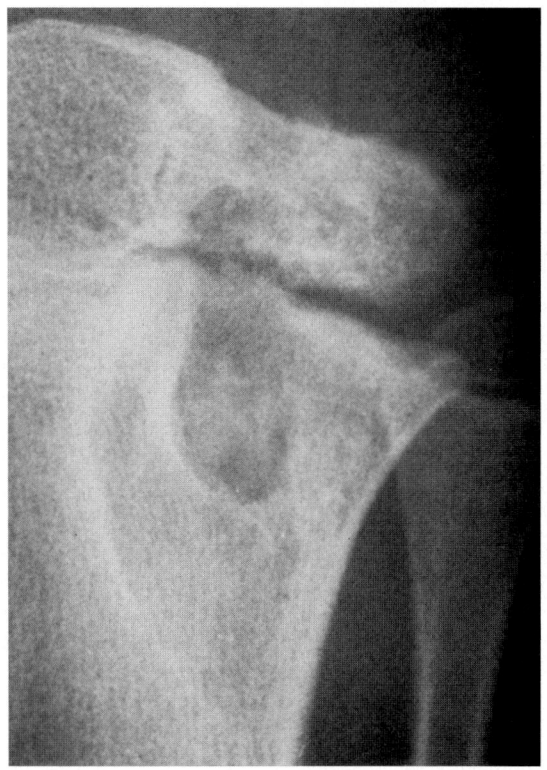

**Figure 55–16.** Tuberculous osteomyelitis: tubular bones. Transphyseal spread of a metaphyseal lesion into the epiphysis is evident.

tuberculosis is good. The radiographic characteristics of cystic tuberculosis resemble those of eosinophilic granuloma, sarcoidosis, cystic angiomatosis, plasma cell myeloma, fungal infection, metastasis, and other conditions.

### Tuberculous Dactylitis

Tuberculous involvement of the short tubular bones of the hands and feet is termed tuberculous dactylitis. It is

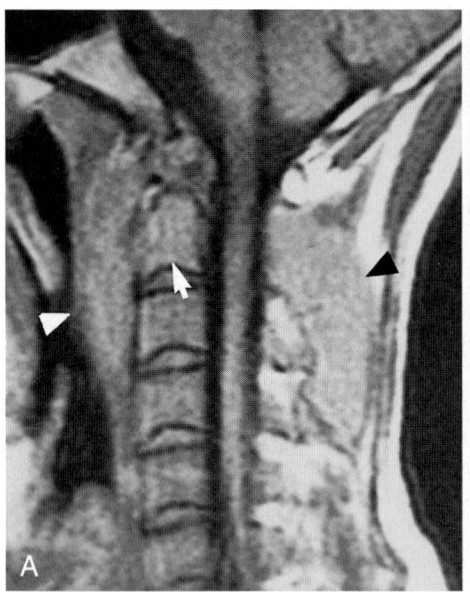

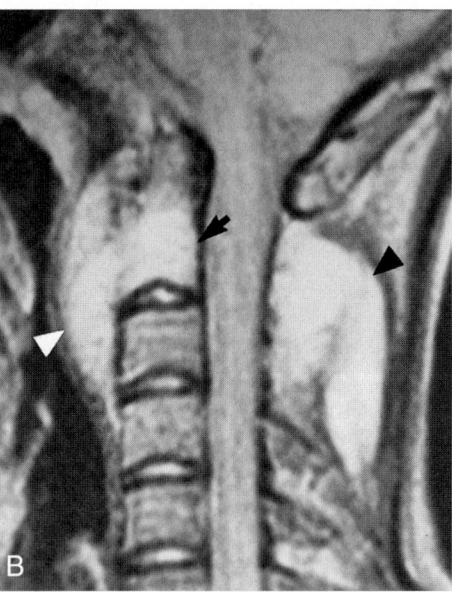

**Figure 55–15.** Tuberculous spondylitis: atlantoaxial destruction. A and B, In this 23-year-old man, sagittal T1-weighted (TR/TE, 450/30) (A) and T2-weighted (TR/TE, 1800/50) (B) spin echo MR images reveal tuberculous involvement of the upper cervical spine. Findings include abnormalities of the axis (arrows), with anterior and posterior extension of the process (arrowheads). (Courtesy of T. Mattsson, MD, Riyadh, Saudia Arabia.)

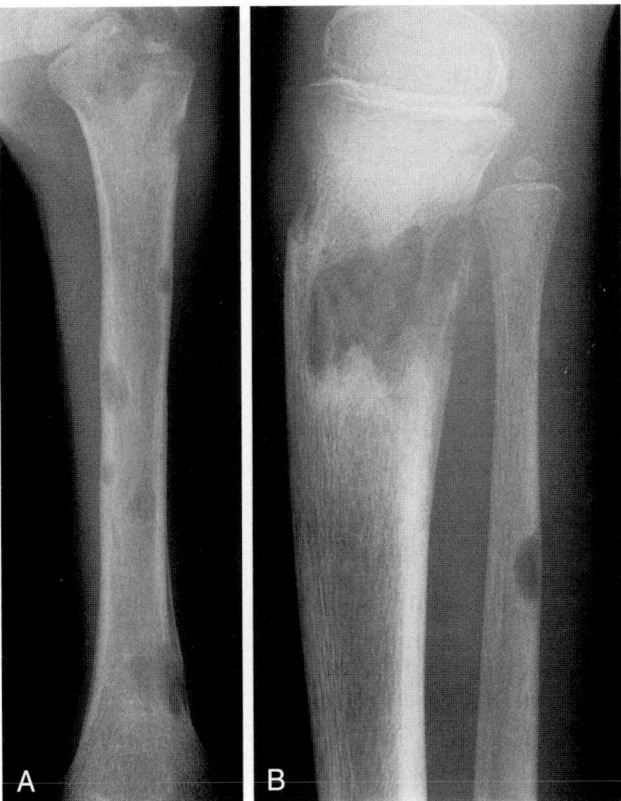

**Figure 55–17.** Cystic tuberculosis. *A*, Note the well-defined lytic lesions of the medullary and cortical areas of the metaphysis and diaphysis of the humerus. The proximal epiphysis is also affected. Sclerosis is absent, although periostitis can be seen. *B*, Similar lesions are present in the tibia and fibula. Some of these lesions are central, whereas others are eccentric or peripheral.

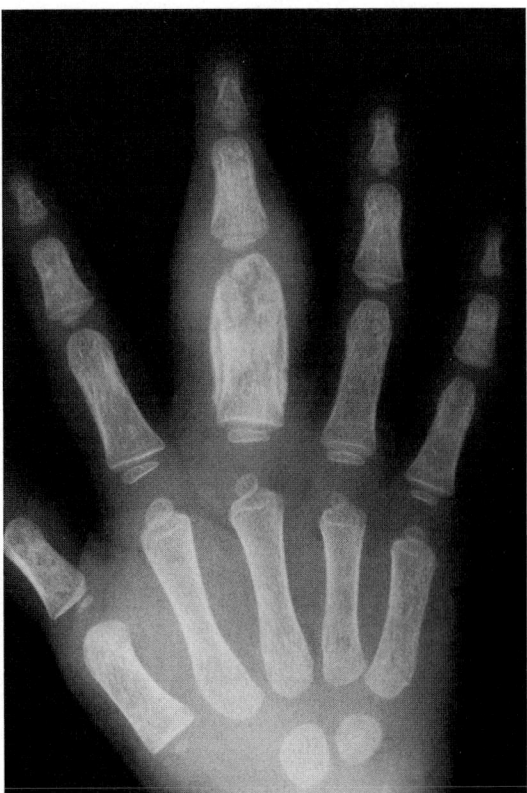

**Figure 55–18.** Tuberculous dactylitis. Radiographic findings in this child include soft tissue swelling of multiple digits, lytic lesions of several middle and proximal phalanges and metacarpals, and exuberant periostitis and enlargement of the proximal phalanx of the third finger.

especially frequent in young children, uncommon after the age of 5 years, and rare after the age of 10 years. Although involvement of one bone of the hand or foot is common, multiple osseous foci can be identified in 25% to 35% of cases and are especially characteristic of childhood dactylitis. Soft tissue swelling is usually the initial manifestation. Mild or exuberant periostitis of the phalanges, metacarpals, or metatarsals may be evident (Fig. 55–18). Cystlike expansion of the bone is termed spina ventosa. Infection with a pyogenic or fungal origin may have similar radiographic manifestations. Syphilitic dactylitis in infants and children produces bilateral and symmetrical involvement; in that disease, periostitis is more exuberant and soft tissue swelling is less prominent than in tuberculous dactylitis. Fibrous dysplasia, hyperparathyroidism, leukemia, sarcoidosis, and sickle cell anemia may produce phalangeal, metacarpal, and metatarsal changes, although characteristic radiographic alterations at other sites allow an accurate diagnosis in many cases.

### Tuberculous Arthritis

Tuberculous arthritis typically affects large joints such as the knee and hip, although any articular site can be involved. Monoarticular disease is the rule. Most joint lesions occur secondary to adjacent osteomyelitis. Most patients are middle-aged or elderly, and many have underlying disorders or have received intra-articular injections of steroids. Tuberculous joint disease may persist and cause chronic pain and only minimal signs of inflammation. Delay in diagnosis is frequent, and correct diagnosis requires the use of synovial fluid and tissue for culture and histologic studies.

A triad of radiographic findings (Phemister's triad) is characteristic of tuberculous arthritis: juxta-articular osteoporosis, peripherally located osseous erosions, and gradual narrowing of the interosseous space (Fig. 55–19). Marginal erosions are especially characteristic of tuberculosis in "tight" or weight-bearing articulations such as the hip, knee, and ankle. They produce corner defects simulating the erosions of other synovial processes, such as rheumatoid arthritis. The combination of regional osteoporosis, marginal erosions, and relative preservation of joint space is highly suggestive of tuberculous arthritis. In rheumatoid arthritis, early loss of articular space is more typical. The rapidity of joint space loss in tuberculosis is highly variable. Bony proliferation is generally not as exuberant in tuberculous arthritis as it is in pyogenic arthritis. The eventual result in tuberculous arthritis is usually fibrous ankylosis of the joint. Bony ankylosis is occasionally seen, but this sequela is more frequent in pyogenic arthritis.

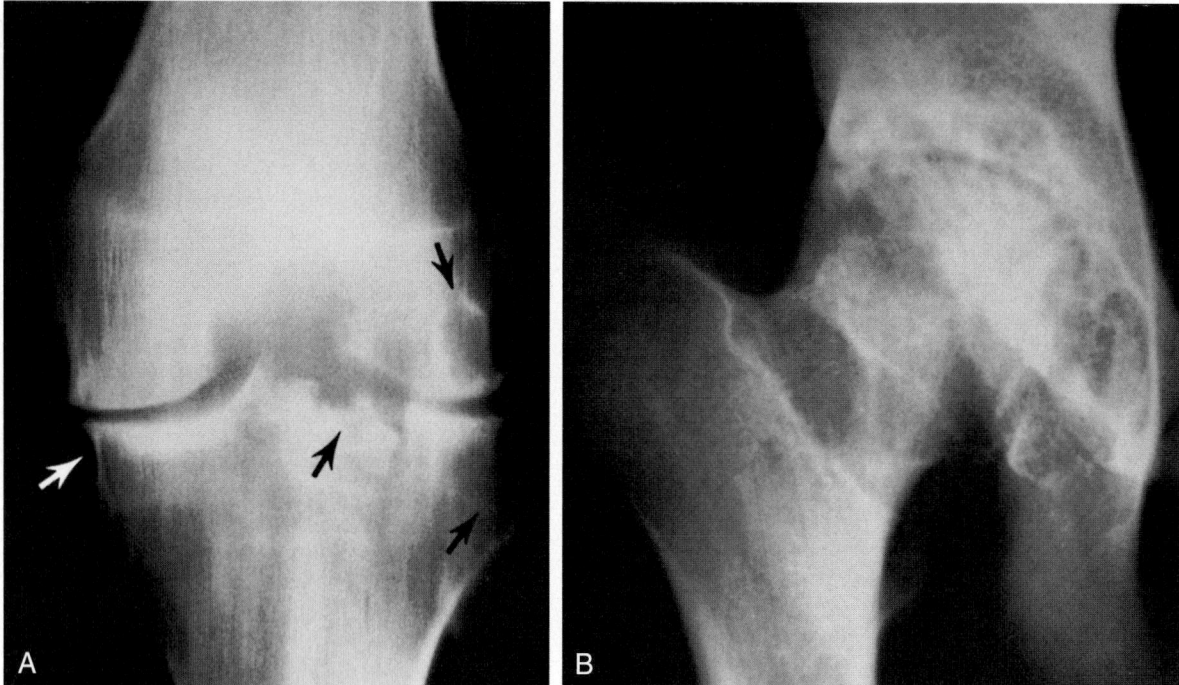

**Figure 55–19.** Tuberculous arthritis. *A*, Knee. On a conventional tomogram, typical marginal and central osseous erosions *(arrows)* accompany tuberculous arthritis. Osteoporosis is not prominent. *B*, Hip. In a different patient, osseous erosions on both sides of the joint, diffuse loss of interosseous space, and osteoporosis are evident. (*B*, Courtesy of J. Kaye, MD, Nashville, Tenn.)

The diagnosis of tuberculous arthritis is not difficult when classic radiographic features appear in typical locations, such as the knee, hip, wrist, or elbow. The appearance of periarticular osteoporosis, marginal erosions, and absent or mild joint space narrowing is most helpful in the accurate diagnosis of this disease (Table 55–2). In rheumatoid arthritis, osteoporosis and marginal erosions are accompanied by early and significant loss of articular space. In gout, osteoporosis is mild or absent, although marginal erosions and preservation of interosseous space can be observed. In regional osteoporosis, marginal osseous defects are not apparent, and the joint space is maintained. In idiopathic chondrolysis, osteoporosis and early joint space loss are evident, especially in the hip, although they occasionally occur in other locations as well.

### Tuberculous Bursitis and Tenosynovitis

The synovial membrane of bursae and tendon sheaths and the tendons themselves may be involved in tuberculosis (Fig. 55–20). Typical sites include the radial and ulnar bursae of the hand, the flexor tendon sheaths of the fingers, the bursae about the ischial tuberosities, and the subacromial (subdeltoid) and subgluteal bursae. Rarely, other tendon sheaths are affected. Osseous destruction can be encountered in the region of the greater trochanter, and the hip joint may become infected secondarily. In any bursal location, dystrophic calcification may appear, a finding that is especially characteristic about the hip and elbow.

### BCG Vaccination–Induced Infection

BCG is a vaccine of an attenuated bovine tubercle bacillus that has been used for immunization against tuberculosis. Although complications are unusual, generalized BCG infection and bone and joint infection have been identified after vaccination. The former complication is almost invariably fatal and is especially common in patients with immunologic deficiency. The latter complication results from hematogenous spread of BCG infection to the skeleton, is not usually associated with immunologic disorders, and has a favorable prognosis. The interval between

---

**TABLE 55–2**

**Comparison of Tuberculous and Pyogenic Arthritis**

|  | Tuberculous Arthritis | Pyogenic Arthritis |
|---|---|---|
| Soft tissue swelling | + | + |
| Osteoporosis | + | ± |
| Joint space loss | Late | Early |
| Marginal erosions | + | + |
| Bony proliferation (sclerosis, periostitis) | ± | + |
| Bony ankylosis | ± | + |
| Slow progression | + | − |

+, common; ±, infrequent; −, rare or absent.

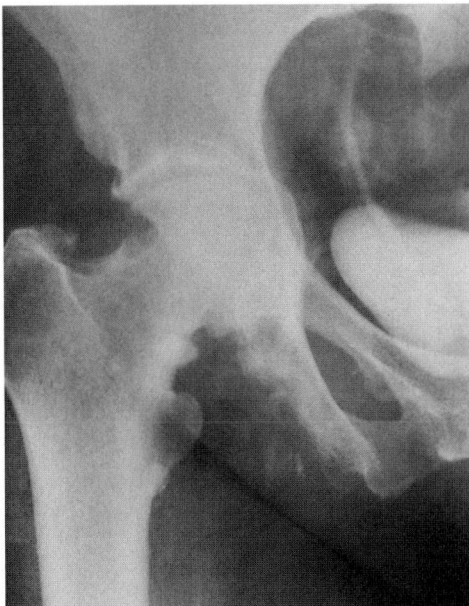

**Figure 55–20.** Tuberculous bursitis: ischial tuberosity. Observe the erosion of the ischial tuberosity and soft tissue calcification. The latter finding is typical of tuberculous bursitis. (Courtesy of J. Jimenez, MD, Oviedo, Spain.)

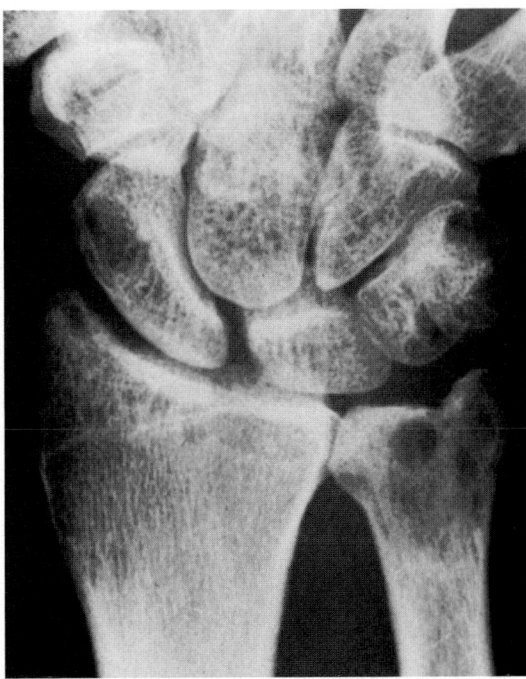

**Figure 55–21.** Atypical mycobacterial infection: septic arthritis caused by *Mycobacterium avium*. Radiograph shows cystic areas in the ulna, radius, scaphoid, triquetrum, and pisiform bones. The joint spaces are preserved. Synovial biopsy indicated hypertrophy of the synovial membrane with chronic granulomatous inflammation. *M. avium* was recovered from the tissue. (Courtesy of J. Scavulli, MD, San Diego, Calif.)

the time of vaccination and the diagnosis of osteomyelitis is widely variable but is commonly within 6 to 12 months after vaccination.

BCG osteomyelitis involves boys and girls between the ages of 5 months and 6 years. It usually affects the metaphyses and the epiphyses of the tubular bones. Lesions in tubular bones are more frequent on the side of the body where the vaccine was given. Solitary lesions predominate and are characterized by well-defined lytic foci with only minor degrees of sclerosis or periostitis.

## Atypical Mycobacterial Infection

Acid-fast bacteria that are morphologically similar to tubercle bacilli are commonly associated with skin and pulmonary disease, although they can be associated with bone and joint alterations as well. Mycobacterial osteomyelitis and arthritis can complicate connective tissue disorders and may be evident in patients with impaired resistance, those who have received renal transplants, patients with acquired immunodeficiency syndrome (AIDS), or those receiving corticosteroids. They may also occur in an otherwise normal host. Mechanisms of the musculoskeletal alterations include hematogenous spread and contamination after injury or surgery.

Radiographic characteristics include the following: multiple lesions predominate over solitary lesions, the metaphyses and diaphyses of long bones are commonly affected, discrete lytic areas may contain sclerotic margins, osteoporosis may not be as striking as in tuberculous infection, a tendency for the development of abscesses and sinus tracts is present, and articular disease can simulate tuberculosis or rheumatoid arthritis (Fig. 55–21). Accurate diagnosis remains difficult, although clinical findings such as tenosynovitis and carpal tunnel syndrome are characteristic. Information regarding a specific occupational history or recreational activities is important. For example, gardening may allow the introduction of *Mycobacterium terrae* organisms, which can be found in soil and vegetables. Fishermen or aquarium workers may acquire infections from *Mycobacterium marinum*, because these organisms grow in fresh or salt water.

## Leprosy (Hansen's Disease)

Leprosy is an infectious disease caused by *Mycobacterium leprae*. Despite its infrequent occurrence in the United States, it is not uncommon in areas of Africa, South America, and Asia. Leprosy is characterized by a lengthy incubation period and a chronic course, with involvement of the skin, mucous membranes, and peripheral nervous system. Involvement of peripheral nerves is especially characteristic. The lesions of leprosy have been divided into four principal types, according to their microscopic appearance: lepromatous, tuberculoid, dimorphous, and indeterminate. The clinical manifestations vary among these types.

### Clinical Abnormalities

Organisms enter the body through the skin or mucous membranes, especially the nasal mucosa, and are disseminated via the bloodstream and the lymphatics and localize in the skin, the nerves, and, in advanced cases, many of the viscera. The incubation period has been estimated to be 3 to 6 years. The disease may begin at any age, although leprosy commonly manifests before 20 years of age. Prodromal symptoms and signs include malaise, fever, drowsiness, rhinitis, and profuse sweating. Lymphadenopathy is seen in all types of leprosy, although it is most striking in the lepromatous variety.

Laboratory abnormalities may include a positive lepromin skin test (in tuberculoid leprosy), an elevated erythrocyte sedimentation rate, and a positive serologic test for syphilis (20% to 40% of cases). The diagnosis is established by demonstration of the bacilli in typical histologic lesions.

### Musculoskeletal Abnormalities

Musculoskeletal abnormalities include (1) those directly related to the presence of the bacilli, in which granulomatous lesions appear in the osseous tissue, and (2) those that involve the skeleton indirectly as a result of neural abnormalities.

**Leprous Periostitis, Osteitis, and Osteomyelitis.** The frequency of direct involvement of the skeleton in leprosy is low and varies from 3% to 5% in hospitalized patients. The changes are usually confined to the small bones of the face, the hands, and the feet. In these cases, osseous involvement is usually due to extension of the infection from overlying dermal or mucosal areas; initially, the periosteum is contaminated (leprous periostitis), and subsequently, the subjacent cortex, spongiosa, and marrow (leprous osteitis and osteomyelitis) become involved (Fig. 55–22). Less commonly, hematogenous spread of infection to bone can occur. In the face, nasal destruction is most characteristic. Destruction of the alveolar process and anterior nasal spine of the maxilla appears to be related to direct lepromatous contamination of the bone, as well as secondary infection. In the tubular bones, symmetrical periostitis of the tibia, fibula, and distal portion of the ulna may be noted. Intractable pain and tenderness may develop. The constellation of erythematous skin lesions, pain, and periostitis involving the lower extremity has been called red leg.

**Neuropathic Musculoskeletal Lesions.** The skeletal abnormalities occurring on a neurologic basis are much more frequent and severe than those produced by direct leprous infiltration of bone. These changes may be evident in 20% to 70% of hospitalized patients. They result from denervation and produce sensory or motor impairment, or both. Repeated injuries and secondary infections subsequently lead to considerable osseous and articular destruction. The bones of the hands, wrists, ankles, and feet are especially susceptible. Denervation can be associated with the absorption of cancellous bone and the development of concentric bone atrophy. The result is a tapered appearance of the end of the bone, termed the licked candy stick (Fig. 55–23). In the foot, progressive resorption of the metatarsals and proximal phalanges occurs. In the hand and the foot, distal phalangeal resorption is also encountered. Although all insensitive digits can be altered, the index and long fingers are usually the

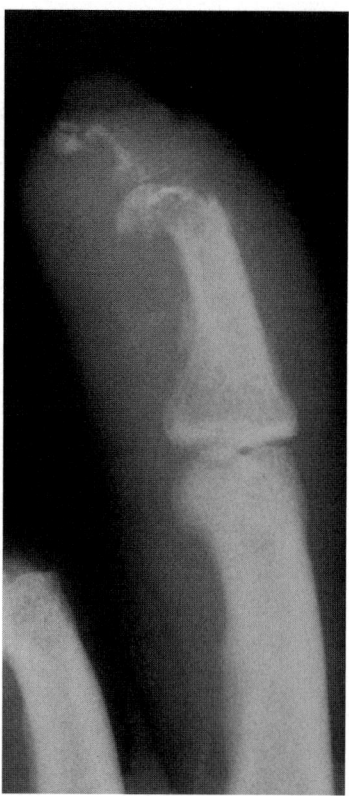

**Figure 55–22.** Leprous tenosynovitis, periostitis, osteitis, and osteomyelitis. Contamination of the soft tissues, tendon sheath, tendon, and phalanges occurred secondary to skin involvement.

first affected. Tarsal disintegration alone or in combination with ankle involvement is not infrequent and is attributable to sensory and motor dysfunction, trauma, and secondary infection. The radiographic appearance of neuropathic osteoarthropathy in leprosy resembles that in syphilis, diabetes mellitus, congenital insensitivity to pain, and syringomyelia.

**Secondary Infection.** Ulceration followed by secondary infection and pyogenic osteomyelitis is common in anesthetic feet. Differentiating the effects of pyogenic osteomyelitis and arthritis from leprous osteomyelitis or neuropathic osteoarthropathy is extremely difficult.

**Soft Tissue Calcification and Neoplasm.** Rarely, linear calcification of involved nerves can be seen on radiographs (Fig. 55–24). Similarly, abscess formation within the nerve, especially the ulnar nerve, can be associated with calcification. Leprosy with cutaneous ulcerations may be complicated by the development of secondary neoplasia, specifically, squamous cell carcinoma of the skin.

## Spirochetes and Related Organisms

### Syphilis

Syphilis is a chronic systemic infectious disease caused by *Treponema pallidum*, a slender spirochete. Syphilis is transmitted by direct and intimate contact with moist infectious lesions of the skin and mucous membranes.

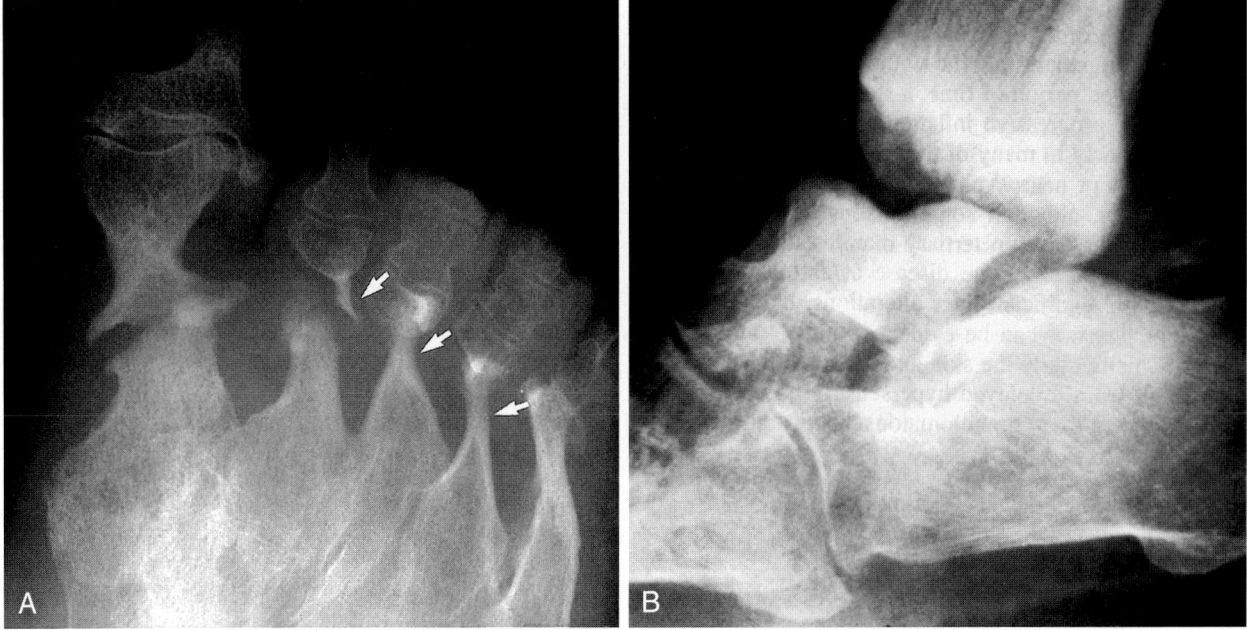

**Figure 55–23.** Leprosy: neuropathic lesions. *A*, Examples of concentric bone atrophy in the foot illustrate the tapered osseous surfaces *(arrows)* and phalangeal osteolysis. *B*, Fragmentation and collapse of the talar, tibial, and calcaneal surfaces can be seen. The appearance is similar to that in tabes dorsalis. (*A*, Courtesy of W. Coleman, MD, Carville, La.)

Infection is usually spread during sexual contact. Children may acquire the disease by sharing a bed with an infected person. Such cases are termed acquired syphilis. In addition, the fetus may be infected by transmission of the organism through the placenta, termed congenital syphilis.

Approximately 3 to 6 weeks after the organism has entered the body, a primary lesion, called a chancre, develops at the site of inoculation. This skin ulceration heals spontaneously. About 6 weeks later, a generalized skin eruption known as secondary syphilis develops. After healing of both primary and secondary manifestations, the patient may be without symptoms and signs for a protracted period—a stage termed latent syphilis—although progressive inflammatory alterations may be slowly occurring in many of the organ systems. Cardiovascular syphilis or neurosyphilis may manifest 10 to 30 years later; however, tertiary manifestations of syphilis never develop in approximately 50% of cases. In patients with significant later alterations, large destructive lesions, or gummas, may be evident in almost any organ of the body, particularly the skin and the bones.

*Congenital Syphilis*

The disorder originates from transplacental migration of the treponema and invasion of the perichondrium, periosteum, cartilage, bone marrow, and sites of active endochondral ossification, especially in the metaphyseal regions of tubular bones. The spirochetes inhibit osteogenesis. A fetus that is heavily infiltrated with spirochetes may be aborted or die shortly after birth. Others survive and develop the stigmata of congenital syphilis. Approximately 75% of cases of congenital syphilis are diagnosed

in children older than 10 years. Such children may have the hutchinsonian triad, which consists of Hutchinson's teeth, interstitial keratitis, and nerve deafness. Additional manifestations include fissuring about the mouth and

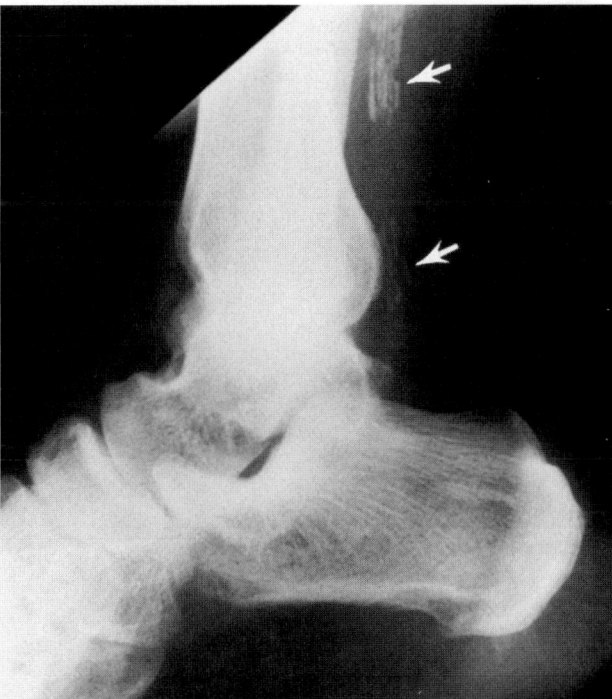

**Figure 55–24.** Leprosy: calcification of nerves. The linear radiodense regions *(arrows)* represent calcification of nerves. This finding, though rare, suggests the diagnosis of leprosy but must be distinguished from vascular calcification. (Courtesy of M. Dalinka, MD, Philadelphia, Pa.)

anus (rhagades), anterior bowing of the lower part of the leg (saber shin), collapse of the nasal bones (saddle nose), and perforation of the palate.

**Early Osseous Lesions.** In fetuses, neonates, and very young infants, bony abnormalities include osteochondritis, diaphyseal osteomyelitis (osteitis), periostitis, and miscellaneous changes.

Syphilitic osteochondritis usually results in symmetrical involvement of sites of endochondral ossification. The epiphyseal-metaphyseal junction of tubular bones, the costochondral regions, and, in severe cases, the flat and short tubular bones and the centers of ossification of the sternum and vertebrae are affected. In the growing metaphyses of the long bones, particularly about the knee, widening of the provisional calcification zone, serrations, and adjacent osseous irregularity are seen, which on histologic evaluation are found to result from a disturbance in endochondral ossification. Radiographs outline broad horizontal radiolucent bands reminiscent of those identified in leukemia or metastasis from neuroblastoma. If the process continues, metaphyseal irregularities appear (Fig. 55–25). On radiographs, irregular erosive lesions appear along the contour of the bone at the metaphyseal–growth plate junction. Epiphyseal separation may result. The medial surface of the proximal tibial shaft is a particularly characteristic site of erosion, a finding termed Wimberger's sign. The lesions of osteo-chondritis generally heal quickly with specific therapy; healing is evident within 2 weeks and may be complete within 2 months.

Diaphyseal osteomyelitis (osteitis) can appear in infants with congenital syphilis who have not received therapy or in whom treatment has been inadequate. Granulation tissue in the metaphysis may extend into the diaphysis and induce infective foci of variable size (Fig. 55–26). Osteolytic lesions with surrounding bony eburnation and overlying periostitis may be seen on radiographs of involved tubular bones.

Periostitis is a less frequent manifestation of congenital syphilis than is osteochondritis. The long tubular bones and, less commonly, the flat bones are affected. Reparative (reactive) periostitis is a second type of periosteal response that may be noted about healing foci of osteochondritis or after epiphyseal slipping.

**Late Osseous Lesions.** The early manifestations of congenital syphilis generally regress or disappear in the first few years of life, even in the absence of adequate therapy. Exacerbation of disease may appear in a young child or adolescent (5 to 20 years of age), however. Although the evolving skeletal lesions that occur late in the course of congenital syphilis may rarely resemble those of early congenital syphilis (osteochondritis, osteomyelitis, periostitis), they more typically resemble the changes observed in acquired syphilis (see later discussion). Osteomyelitis

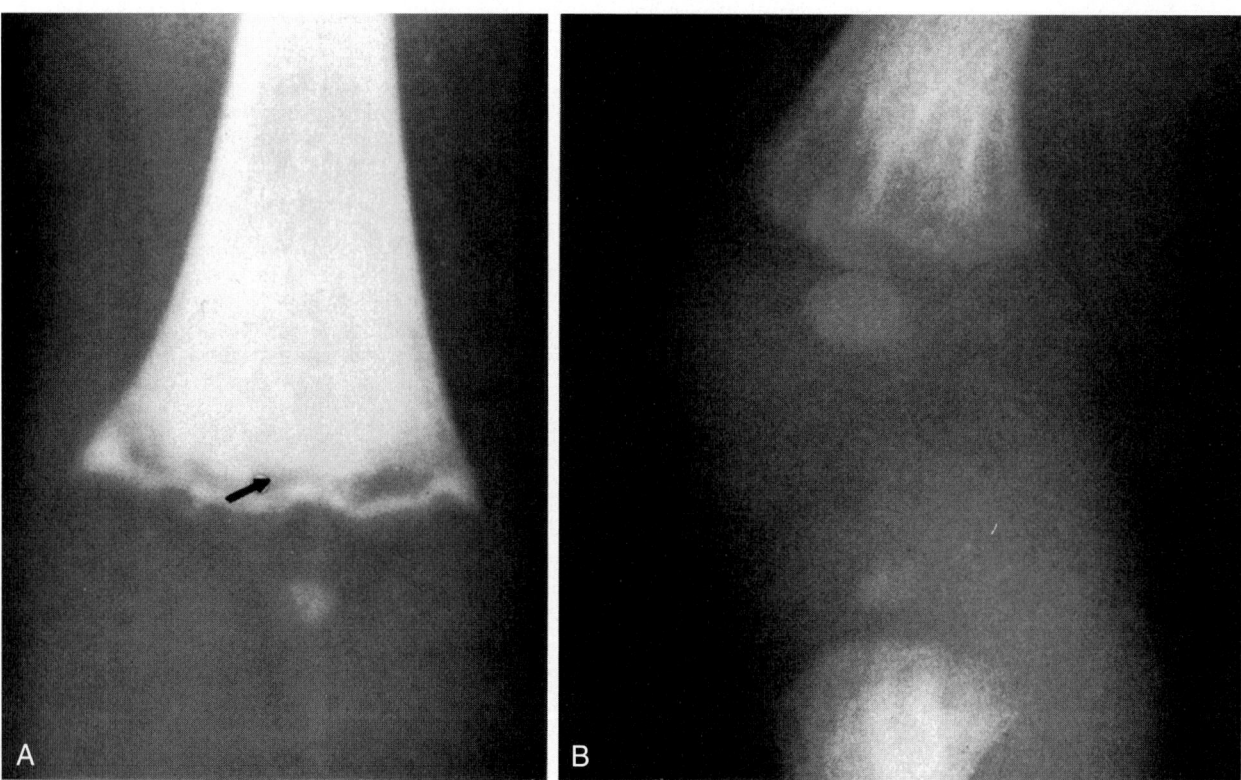

**Figure 55–25.** Congenital syphilis: osteochondritis. *A,* In this 3-week-old infant, the lucent band in the metaphysis *(arrow)* is caused by a disturbance in endochondral ossification. The appearance is similar to that in leukemia or neuroblastoma. *B,* In another infant with syphilis, a "celery stalk" appearance, with alternating longitudinal lucent and sclerotic bands caused by an abnormality in endochondral ossification, resembles the changes seen in rubella. *(B,* Courtesy of D. Edwards, MD, San Diego, Calif.)

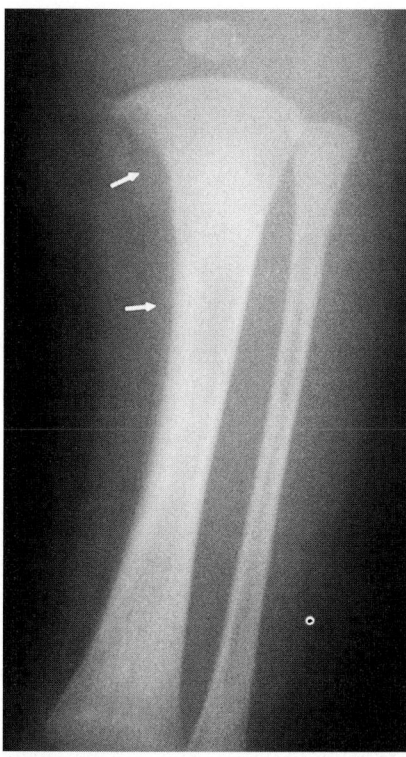

**Figure 55–26.** Congenital syphilis: osteochondritis and osteomyelitis. Note tibial erosion with periostitis *(arrows)*. The predilection for the medial tibial metaphysis is noteworthy.

and periostitis can involve the tubular bones, the flat bones, and even the cranium.

Gummatous or nongummatous osteomyelitis or periostitis results in diffuse hyperostosis of the involved bone. Endosteal bony proliferation produces encroachment on the medullary cavity, whereas periosteal bony proliferation creates an enlarged, undulating, and dense osseous contour. In the tibia, a typical saber shin may be encountered, with anterior bending of the bone. Its radiographic appearance may resemble that of Paget's disease, although the syphilitic hyperostosis may not extend to the epiphysis (Fig. 55–27). Lucent defects within areas of hyperostosis may represent gummas. Abnormalities of the skull and mandible include destruction of the nasal bones, calvarial gumma, and Hutchinson's teeth (characterized by peg-shaped, notched, and hypoplastic dental structures). Bilateral painless effusions, especially of the knee, have been termed Clutton's joints.

### Acquired Syphilis

The osseus and articular manifestations of acquired syphilis usually appear in the latent or tertiary phase of the disease. The frequency of osseous lesions varies from rare to as high as 8% to 20%.

**Early Acquired Syphilis.** Spirochetemia appearing 1 to 3 months after documentation of a primary lesion can lead to dissemination of organisms throughout the body.

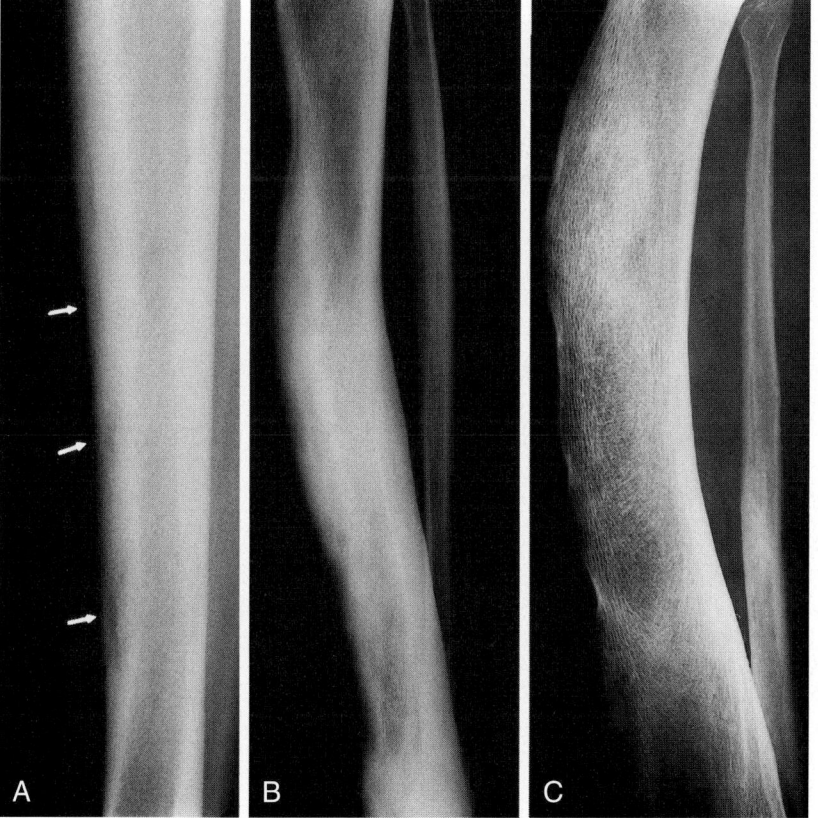

**Figure 55–27.** Congenital syphilis: late osseous changes. *A*, Observe the radiolucent foci within the anterior cortex of the tibia *(arrows)*, along with periostitis and endosteal proliferation. *B*, In a different patient, more exuberant hyperostosis of both the tibia and the fibula has resulted in bowed and prominent osseous surfaces. The changes are somewhat reminiscent of those in Paget's disease. *C*, A typical saber shin deformity of the tibia is associated with anterior bowing of the bone. The fibula is also involved.

The spirochetes can reach the bone, with development of osteochondritis, periostitis, osteitis, or osteomyelitis. Proliferative periostitis is the most common osseous lesion in early acquired syphilis. It may be especially prominent in the tibia, skull, ribs, and sternum, although other bones, such as the clavicle, femur, fibula, and osseous structures of the hand and foot, can also be affected. Destructive bone lesions occur much less commonly than periostitis in early syphilis. These lesions are attributable to osteomyelitis and infective osteitis (as well as septic arthritis) (Fig. 55–28). Involvement of the skull is particularly characteristic and has been noted in nearly 9% of patients with secondary syphilis.

**Late Acquired Syphilis.** Osseous lesions occurring during the later stages of acquired syphilis can be related to gummatous or nongummatous inflammation. A gumma is a discrete or confluent area of variable size that contains caseous necrotic material and is related to the effects of the toxic products of spirochete degeneration, although the organisms themselves are not usually demonstrable within the lesions.

The radiographic features are characterized by lytic and sclerotic areas of bone, which may reach considerable size. Involvement of the cranial vault, nasal bones, maxilla, mandible, tubular bones of the appendicular skeleton, spine, and pelvis has been noted. The degree of periosteal proliferation can become extreme and, in tubular bones, can lead to gross enlargement of osseous tissue. The resultant radiographic and pathologic features resemble those in the late stages of congenital syphilis, including the saber shin deformity. Dactylitis, which is not infrequent in congenital syphilis, is less typical of acquired disease.

## Articular Involvement

The frequency of articular involvement in syphilis is low. Joint abnormalities may occur in either the congenital or the acquired form of the disease. In congenital syphilis, articular changes predominate in the late phases of the disorder; in acquired syphilis, joint manifestations appear in the tertiary or, less frequently, the secondary stage. Joint effusions associated with pain and tenderness, which may be infectious or noninfectious in origin, are commonly bilateral and most typically affect the knee. Infectious syphilitic arthritis can occur in any axial or extra-axial site. Syphilitic infectious arthritis is associated with an effusion and capsular distention. The synovial membrane may become hypertrophied, with cellular infiltration. Synovial inflammation with pannus can lead to cartilaginous and osseous destruction. On radiographs, osteoporosis, joint space narrowing, bony destruction, sclerosis, and intra-articular osseous fusion may be seen, findings similar to those occurring in other infectious arthritides.

## Yaws

Yaws is an infectious disorder caused by *Treponema pertenue*. Yaws occurs in tropical climates and is prevalent in Africa, South America, the South Pacific islands, and the West Indies. It is generally acquired before puberty during contact with open lesions containing the spirochetes. Transmission of the disease is rarely associated with sexual contact. Within a period of weeks after inoculation, a granulomatous primary lesion appears, referred to as the mother yaw. Approximately 1 to 3 months later, a generalized papular skin eruption occurs on the extremities, buttocks, neck, and face. Involvement of the soles, called

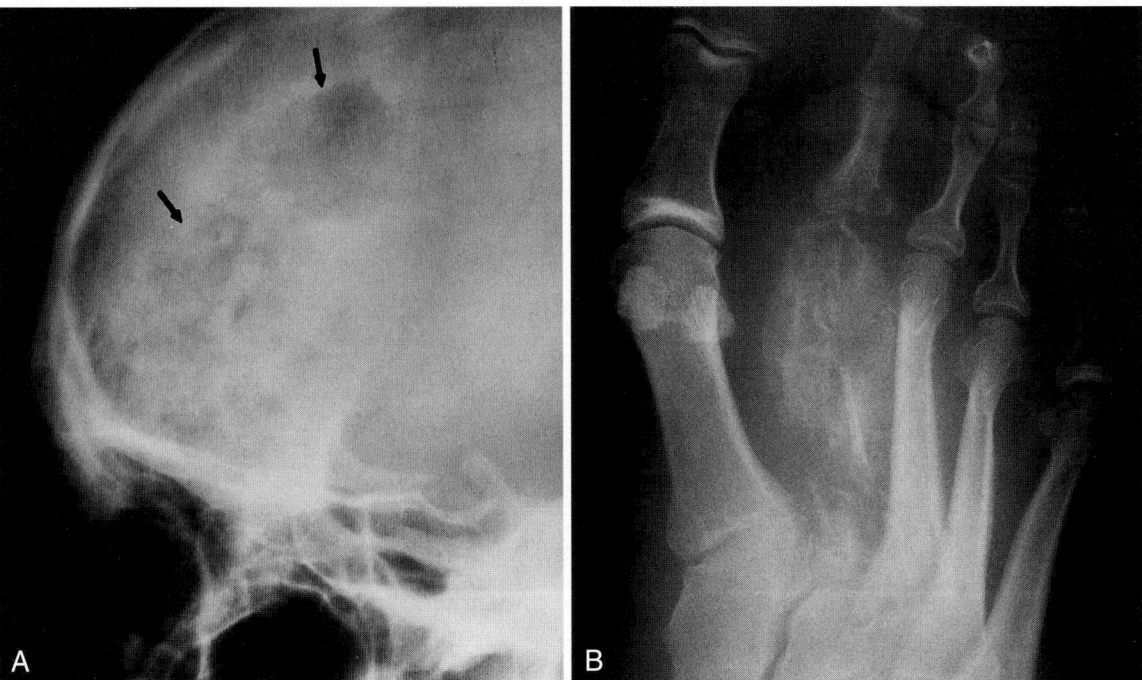

**Figure 55–28.**  Acquired syphilis: osteitis, osteomyelitis, and periostitis. *A*, Lytic lesions of the frontal region of the skull (*arrows*) are accompanied by reactive sclerosis. *B*, Note the osteolysis of the metatarsal bones and phalanges, associated with soft tissue swelling, periostitis, pathologic fracture, and articular involvement.

crab yaws, may make walking painful. After several years, late destructive lesions may become evident in cutaneous and osseous tissue.

The tubular bones of the extremities, including those of the hands and feet, the pelvis, the skull, and the facial bones may become the sites of periostitis or osteitis. Lucent lesions in the cortex or spongiosa are accompanied by florid periosteal bone formation (Fig. 55–29). Saber shin deformities (as in syphilis), dactylitis, and nasal destruction may be encountered. Localized expansile lesions in the epiphyses of tubular bones may simulate neoplasms, and destructive changes in the fingers and toes can resemble leprosy or psoriatic arthritis. In yaws, however, the distal phalanges are usually spared. The radiographic changes in the skeleton in patients with yaws are similar to those of syphilis.

## Tropical Ulcer

Tropical ulcers are seen in patients of all ages from Central and East Africa. The initial lesions are painful, tense swellings with a serosanguineous discharge that appear on the anterolateral aspect of the distal portions of the lower limbs and spread rapidly. Because the ulcer erodes muscles and tendons, it may reach the underlying bone. The favorite target area is the middle third of the tibia; fibular involvement is less frequent and, when present, is most common in the distal third of the shaft. Periostitis leads to broad-based excrescences resembling

osteomas (Fig. 55–30). Approximately 25% of cases show malignant degeneration leading to epidermoid carcinomas of the involved skin, which can cause destruction of subjacent cortical and medullary tissue. The cause of tropical ulcer appears to be multifactorial. Trauma is common, and cultures of the lesion frequently isolate Vincent's types of fusiform bacilli and spirochetes.

## Lyme Disease

First observed in 1975, Lyme disease is an inflammatory articular condition named for the Connecticut town where it was initially encountered. In the United States, most cases of Lyme disease have occurred in the Northeast, Upper Midwest, and Far West. Both children and adults are affected. Clinical manifestations generally appear within 7 days of a tick bite. The illness characteristically begins in the summer in the form of a distinctive skin lesion, erythema chronicum migrans, in the area of a previous tick bite. The rash disappears over a period of weeks. Although the cutaneous manifestations are an important clue to the correct diagnosis, they are not constant. Approximately 2 to 6 months later, joint manifestations appear and are characterized by a monoarticu-

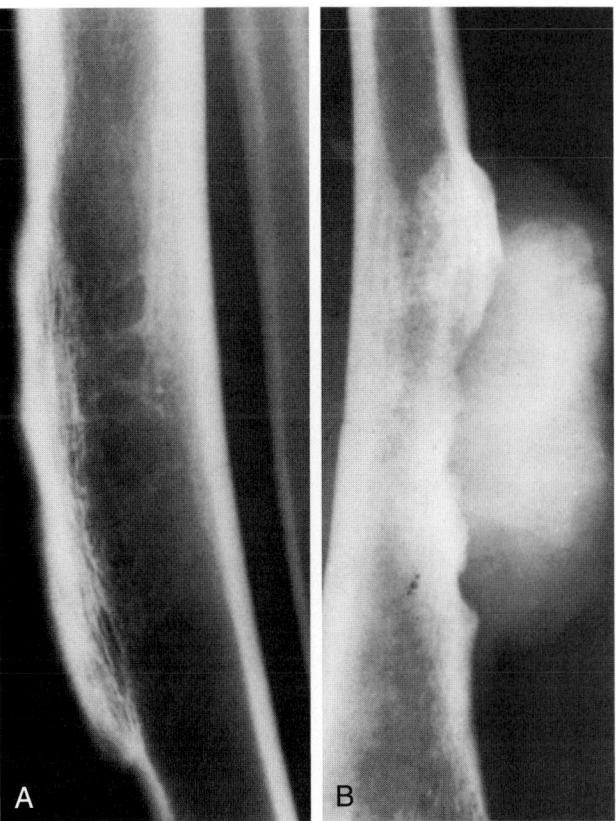

**Figure 55–30.** Tropical ulcer. *A*, The anterior surface of the tibia reveals a broad-based excrescence and an ivory osteoma. The bone is bowed, and the thickened trabeculae in the medullary bone indicate a response to altered stress. *B*, In a different patient, malignant degeneration at the site of skin ulceration has led to destruction of the underlying bone. Note the irregularity of the involved soft tissues. (Courtesy of S. Bohrer, MD, Winston-Salem, N.C.)

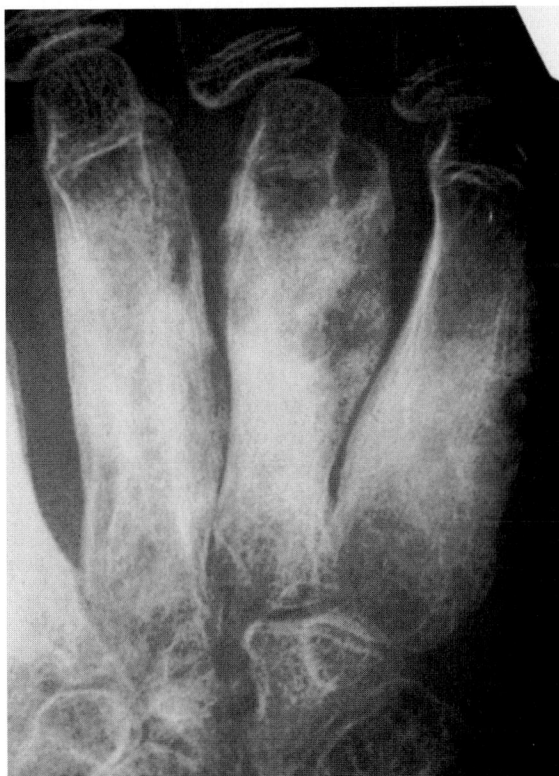

**Figure 55–29.** Yaws. Dactylitis is characterized by lytic lesions surrounded by florid periosteal proliferation. Note the enlarged and sclerotic osseous contours. (Courtesy of W. P. Cockshott, MD, Hamilton, Ontario, Canada.)

lar, oligoarticular, or polyarticular process that is sudden in onset, short in duration, and associated with recurrence and, sometimes, migration from one location to another. Sites of involvement, in order of decreasing frequency, are the knee, shoulder, and elbow.

The radiographic characteristics of joint involvement are soft tissue swelling and effusions. Infrequently, a chronic oligoarthritis develops, especially in the knees, that is associated with persistent and prominent joint swelling. This finding may occur in as many as 10% of untreated patients. In such cases, juxta-articular osteoporosis, cartilage loss, and marginal bone erosions may appear (Fig. 55–31). Lyme disease is transmitted by *Ixodes dammini* or related ixodid ticks. The disease itself is caused by a recently recognized spirochete. The clinical and radiographic features of Lyme disease resemble those of juvenile chronic arthritis, Reiter's syndrome, and granulomatous infections such as tuberculosis.

## FUNGAL AND HIGHER BACTERIAL INFECTION

A variety of pathogenic fungi can produce human disease. Although healthy persons may become hosts for fungal diseases, these pathogens become more virulent in subjects with depressed immunologic function, in whom widespread and sometimes fatal abnormalities may occur.

### Actinomycosis

Actinomycosis is a noncontagious suppurative infection caused by anaerobic organisms that are normally found in the mouth. These organisms are higher bacteria that resemble mycobacteria and are frequently misclassified as fungi. The infections are especially frequent in the face and neck, which is probably explained by the prevalence of these organisms within the oral and nasal cavities. Trauma is important in the introduction of organisms into tissues. From infective foci in the face, lung, or bowel, hematogenous dissemination of organisms can lead to contamination of subcutaneous tissue, liver, spleen, kidneys, brain, bones, and joints.

Typically, the skeleton becomes contaminated from an adjacent infected soft tissue focus; less commonly, hematogenous seeding of osseous or articular tissue occurs. The mandible, the flat bones of the axial skeleton (pelvis, ribs, spine), and the major joints of the appendicular skeleton are most commonly affected. Mandibular and maxillary bone involvement may follow trauma or extraction of a tooth. Osseous involvement is characterized by a combination of lysis and sclerosis (Fig. 55–32). In the ribs, the degree of bony proliferation may be extensive, and the combination of severe osseous eburnation, cutaneous sinus tracts, and pleuritis is suggestive of actinomycosis. In the vertebral column, infection can originate from adjacent mediastinal or retroperitoneal foci. Several vertebrae are commonly affected and demonstrate lytic defects with surrounding sclerosis, and the intervening intervertebral discs may be spared. Paravertebral abscesses may appear, but they are usually smaller than the abscesses in tuberculosis and do not calcify.

### Cryptococcosis (Torulosis)

Cryptococcosis, a serious disease of worldwide distribution, is caused by *Cryptococcus neoformans*, an organism that demonstrates an unusual predilection for the central nervous system. The disease is generally acquired by the respiratory route through the inhalation of aerosolized spores. Once they reach the body and proliferate, cryptococci can be detected in the brain, meninges, lungs, other viscera, and bones and joints. Neurologic manifestations of the disease predominate, and many patients die within

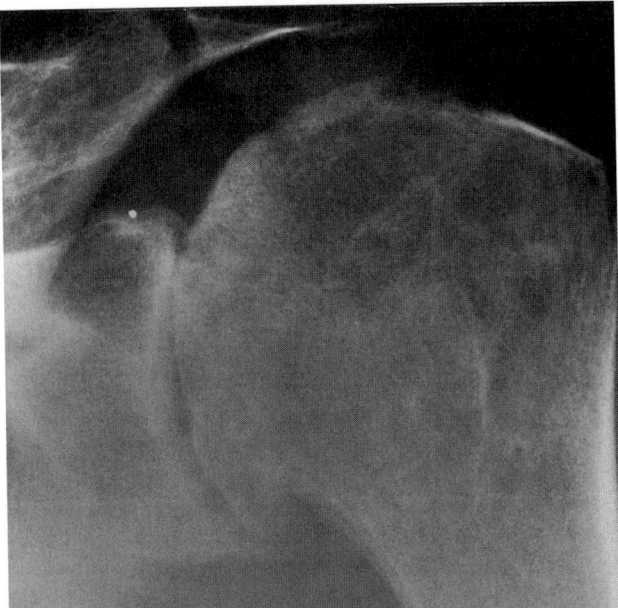

**Figure 55–31.** Lyme disease. The glenohumeral joint space is narrowed, and erosions and osteophytes in the humeral head are seen. (Courtesy of J. Lawson, MD, New Haven, Conn.)

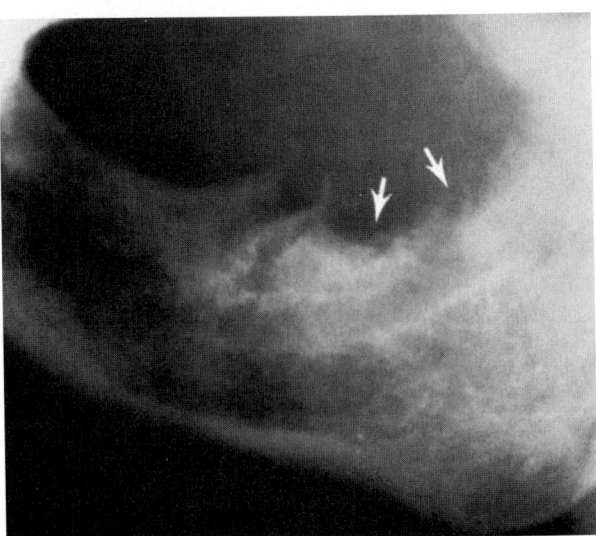

**Figure 55–32.** Actinomycosis has led to erosion and sclerosis of a segment of the mandible *(arrows)*. (Courtesy of R. Taketa, MD, Long Beach, Calif.)

a few months. *Cryptococcus* infection may be seen in association with leukemia, lymphoma, Hodgkin's disease, sarcoidosis, tuberculosis, and diabetes mellitus, as well as in persons with AIDS, those receiving steroid medications, and those who have undergone renal transplantation.

Osseous involvement is a manifestation of disseminated cryptococcosis and appears in 5% to 10% of such cases. Adults are affected far more frequently than children. The most commonly involved skeletal sites are the spine, pelvis, ribs, skull, tibia, and bones about the knees, in descending order of frequency. Bony prominences may be affected, a peculiarity that is also evident in other fungal disorders such as coccidioidomycosis. Single or multiple osseous foci are associated with soft tissue swelling and pain. The radiographic features of bony involvement are not specific. Osteolytic lesions predominate, with discrete margins, mild surrounding sclerosis, and little or no periosteal reaction (Fig. 55–33). Arthritis related to cryptococcosis is very uncommon and almost invariably is the result of intra-articular extension of organisms from an adjacent osseous focus.

## North American Blastomycosis

This fungal disease is produced by *Blastomyces dermatitidis*. In the United States, its frequency is highest in the Ohio and Mississippi River valleys and in the Middle Atlantic states. The skin appears to be the portal of entry in some cases, with infection commonly following cutaneous injuries. The respiratory tract may be a second site of entry. In the skin, cutaneous abscesses develop beneath the epidermis and are surrounded by a granulomatous reaction. Similar lesions may be encountered in the lungs.

The bones may be altered in as many as 50% of patients with disseminated disease. Skeletal changes can occur from hematogenous seeding or by direct extension from overlying cutaneous lesions. One or several osseous sites can be affected, especially the vertebra, rib, tibia, and carpus and tarsus (Fig. 55–34). No portion of the skeleton is immune. The radiographic features of blastomycotic osteomyelitis are not specific. Moth-eaten bony destruction may be seen in association with osteoporosis and periostitis. In the tubular bones of the extremities, eccentric saucer-shaped erosions may be detected beneath cutaneous abscesses, or areas of focal or diffuse osteomyelitis may be encountered in the subchondral regions of the epiphysis or in the metaphysis. The lesions frequently possess sclerotic margins and are surrounded by periostitis. Extension from the infected foci to soft tissues or joints is not unusual. Draining sinuses and cortical sequestration may appear in neglected cases. In the spine, blastomycosis resembles tuberculosis. Articular involvement is usually related to extension from an adjacent site of osteomyelitis.

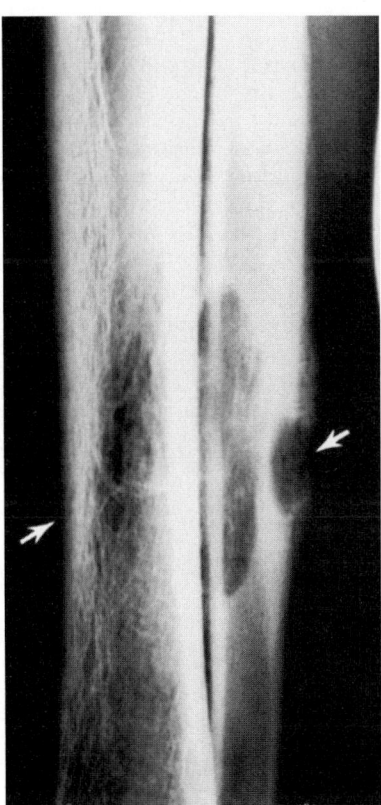

**Figure 55–33.** Cryptococcosis (torulosis). Discrete osteolytic foci with surrounding sclerosis and, in some places, periosteal reaction are seen *(arrows)*.

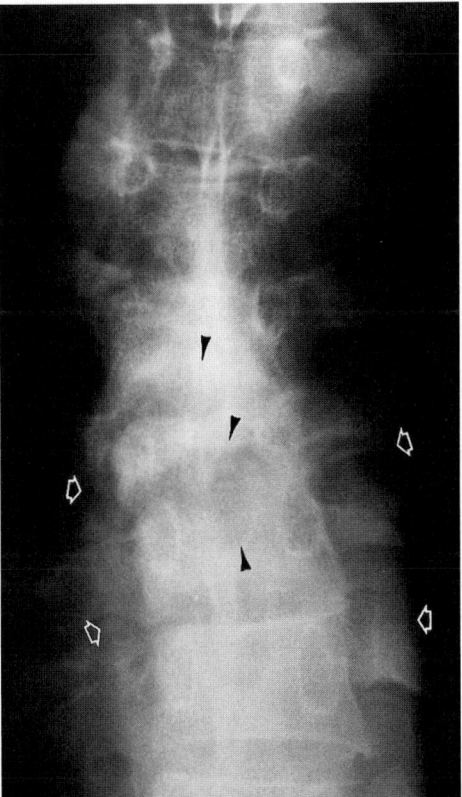

**Figure 55–34.** North American blastomycosis. In this patient, blastomycosis involves the lung and bone. Note vertebral body and intervertebral disc destruction *(arrowheads)*, accompanied by a paravertebral mass *(open arrows)*. (Courtesy of A. Brower, MD, Norfolk, Va.)

## South American Blastomycosis (Paracoccidioidomycosis)

The fungal disorder called South American blastomycosis, caused by the organism *Blastomyces (Paracoccidioides) brasiliensis*, occurs only in South America and in areas of Mexico and Central America. The infective agents invade the pharynx, presumably after inhalation, and from there spread locally or are disseminated throughout the body. Nasopharyngeal ulceration and local lymphadenopathy may antedate the clinical findings in other locations. Hematogenous spread of infection to the lungs, spleen, other abdominal viscera, and bones can occur. In general, the features of musculoskeletal involvement are similar to those in North American blastomycosis. Solitary or multiple lytic lesions, geographic or well-defined bone destruction, marginal sclerosis, and periostitis are observed radiographic findings.

## Coccidioidomycosis

Coccidioidomycosis results from inhalation of the fungus *Coccidioides immitis* in endemic areas in the southwestern United States, Mexico, and some regions of South America. After inhalation, the organisms lodge in the terminal bronchioles and alveoli of the lungs, where an inflammatory reaction may ensue. In some persons, disseminated disease may develop, with spread of infection to the liver, spleen, lymph nodes, skin, kidneys, meninges, pericardium, and bones. Clinical manifestations vary in accordance with the distribution of the lesions, and in cases of wide dissemination, the mortality rate is high.

Although an acute, self-limited arthritis (desert rheumatism) may develop in approximately 33% of cases of coccidioidomycosis, granulomatous lesions in the bones and joints develop in only 10% to 20% of patients. Bone alterations relate to hematogenous spread, although cutaneous infection can lead to contamination of subjacent bones (and joints). Osseous involvement can be confined to a single bone, but multiple, symmetrical osseous lesions may be seen. Radiographs frequently reveal multiple osseous lesions in the metaphyses of long tubular bones and in bony prominences (patella, tibial tuberosity, calcaneus, ulnar olecranon) (Fig. 55–35). Well-demarcated lytic foci of the spongiosa are typical. Periostitis may be seen, but bone sclerosis and sequestration are unusual. Lesions involving the ribs are typically marginal in location and can be associated with prominent extrapleural masses (Fig. 55–36). In the spine, abnormalities of one or more vertebral bodies, with paraspinal masses and contiguous rib changes, are typical (Fig. 55–37). Joint involvement is most common in the ankle and knee (Fig. 55–38). In general, articular changes result from extension of an osteomyelitic focus. Monoarticular involvement is most typical, with radiographs showing osteoporosis, effusion, joint space narrowing, and bony destruction.

## Histoplasmosis

Histoplasmosis is caused by the dimorphic fungus *Histoplasma capsulatum*, which is present in many areas of the United States, particularly the Mississippi River valley in the central portion of the country. Histoplasmosis, which is the most common systemic fungal infection in the United States, results from exposure to soil containing the spores of this fungus. The portal of entry is usually the respiratory tract, although the gastrointestinal system may be an additional portal in some persons. Diffuse disease can result, and the fungus proliferates most exten-

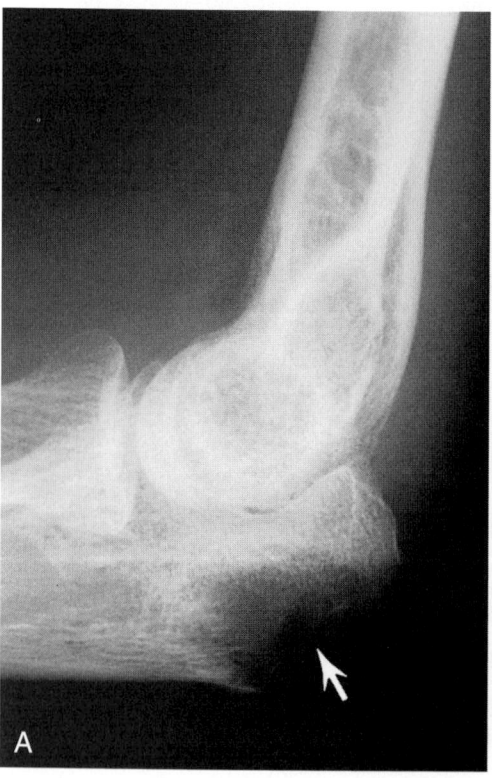
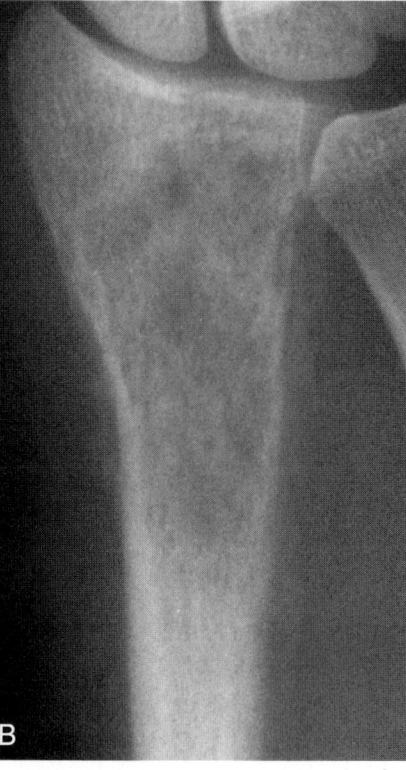

**Figure 55–35.** Coccidioidomycosis: osteomyelitis (appendicular skeleton). *A*, Note the involvement of bony protuberances such as the ulnar olecranon *(arrow)*. Discrete lesions with surrounding sclerosis are evident. *B*, In another patient, the radiograph shows an osteolytic lesion with moth-eaten bone destruction and periostitis of the radius.

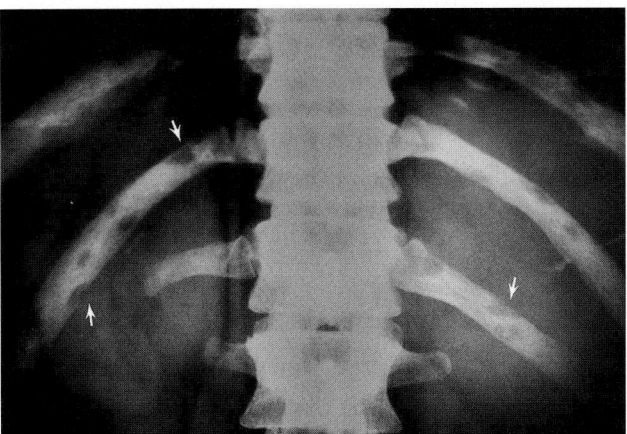

**Figure 55–36.** Coccidioidomycosis: osteomyelitis (axial skeleton). The diagnosis of disseminated coccidioidomycosis was established by skin biopsy, bone marrow and cerebrospinal fluid examination, and positive serologic test results. Radiography outlines lytic lesions with surrounding sclerosis *(arrows)* involving the ribs.

sively in cells of the reticuloendothelial system. Involvement of the brain, lymph nodes, spleen, adrenal gland, lungs, bowel, and bone marrow is most typical.

Skeletal involvement is usually associated with *H. capsulatum* and typically involves the pelvis, skull, ribs, and small tubular bones; children are affected more commonly than adults. Joint alterations have been noted, especially in the knees, ankles, wrists, and joints of the hands, and lead to clinical (pain, swelling), radiographic (osteoporosis, joint space narrowing, erosion), and pathologic (granulation tissue with phagocytic cells) findings. These abnormalities are similar to those of sarcoidosis and tuberculosis. In histoplasmosis caused by *Histoplasma duboisii*, a related organism, granulomatous ulcerating and papular lesions of the skin can be associated with osseous and articular changes in as many as 80% of patients (Fig. 55–39).

## Sporotrichosis

Sporotrichosis, a chronic fungal disease caused by *Sporothrix schenckii*, is characterized by suppurating nodular lesions of the skin and subcutaneous tissue. The fungus resides as a saprophyte on vegetation and can invade the human body through a skin wound; the disease is not uncommon after cutaneous puncture with thorns. After inoculation, a painless, ulcerating cutaneous lesion develops, and the organisms spread locally and produce nodular lesions of the lymphatic channels. Rarely, disseminated disease can evolve, commonly in patients with an underlying disorder such as a malignant lesion or myeloproliferative disease. In the disseminated form of sporotrichosis, bone and joint changes may appear in 80% of cases, and death can occur rapidly.

Localization in one or more joints is especially characteristic, with a predilection for the knee, wrist and hand, ankle, elbow, and metacarpophalangeal joints. Soft tissue swelling, effusion, and joint space loss are seen, as well as irregularity, poor definition, and destruction of subchon-

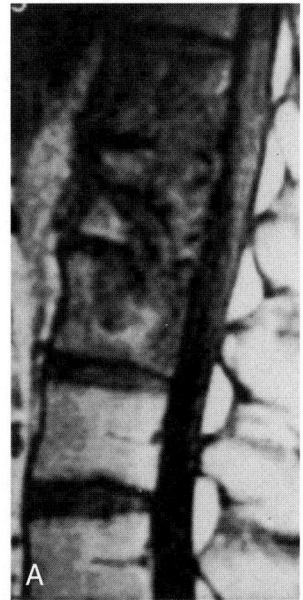

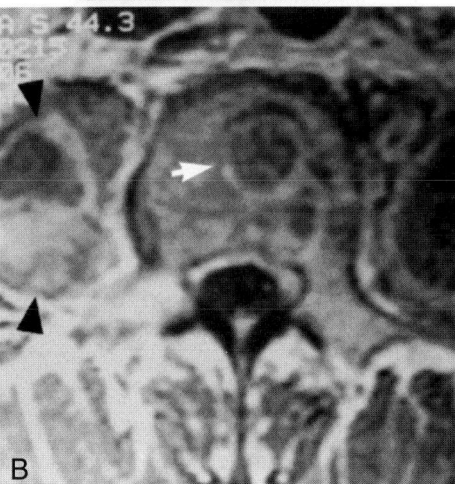

**Figure 55–37.** Coccidioidomycosis: spondylitis. *A,* Sagittal T1-weighted (TR/TE, 400/20) spin echo MR image shows foci of low signal intensity in the 12th thoracic and 1st and 2nd lumbar vertebral bodies, as well as in the intervening intervertebral discs. *B,* Transaxial T1-weighted (TR/TE, 800/20) spin echo image obtained immediately after the intravenous injection of a gadolinium contrast agent reveals enhancing vertebral *(arrow)* and psoas muscle *(arrowheads)* lesions. (Courtesy of D. Witte, MD, Memphis, Tenn.)

dral bony margins (Fig. 55–40). Osteophytes may or may not be evident. Bone changes may take several forms. Eccentric erosions beneath subcutaneous lesions (especially in the tibia) may be encountered but are more typical of blastomycosis. Single or multiple lytic areas in bone can appear as a result of hematogenous spread directly to osseous tissue or to synovium, with extension into neighboring bone. The tibia, fibula, femur, humerus, and short tubular bones of the hand (Fig. 55–41) and foot are involved most commonly. Osteolysis predominates, whereas periostitis is usually absent. The radiographic features of osseous and articular involvement in sporotrichosis simulate those of tuberculosis, other fungal dis-

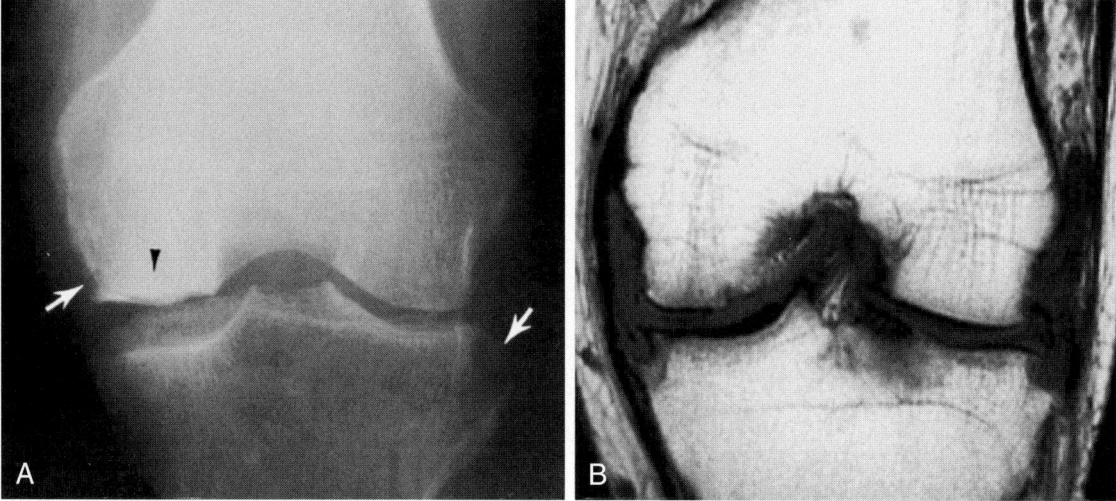

**Figure 55–38.** Coccidioidomycosis: septic arthritis. *A*, Radiograph reveals soft tissue swelling, marginal osseous erosions *(arrows)*, and flattening with sclerosis of the medial femoral condyle *(arrowhead)*. The last-mentioned findings resemble those in spontaneous osteonecrosis of the knee. *B*, In a different patient, a coronal T1-weighted (TR/TE, 500/16) spin echo MR image shows similar marginal erosions, especially in the tibia, along with marrow edema and a joint effusion.

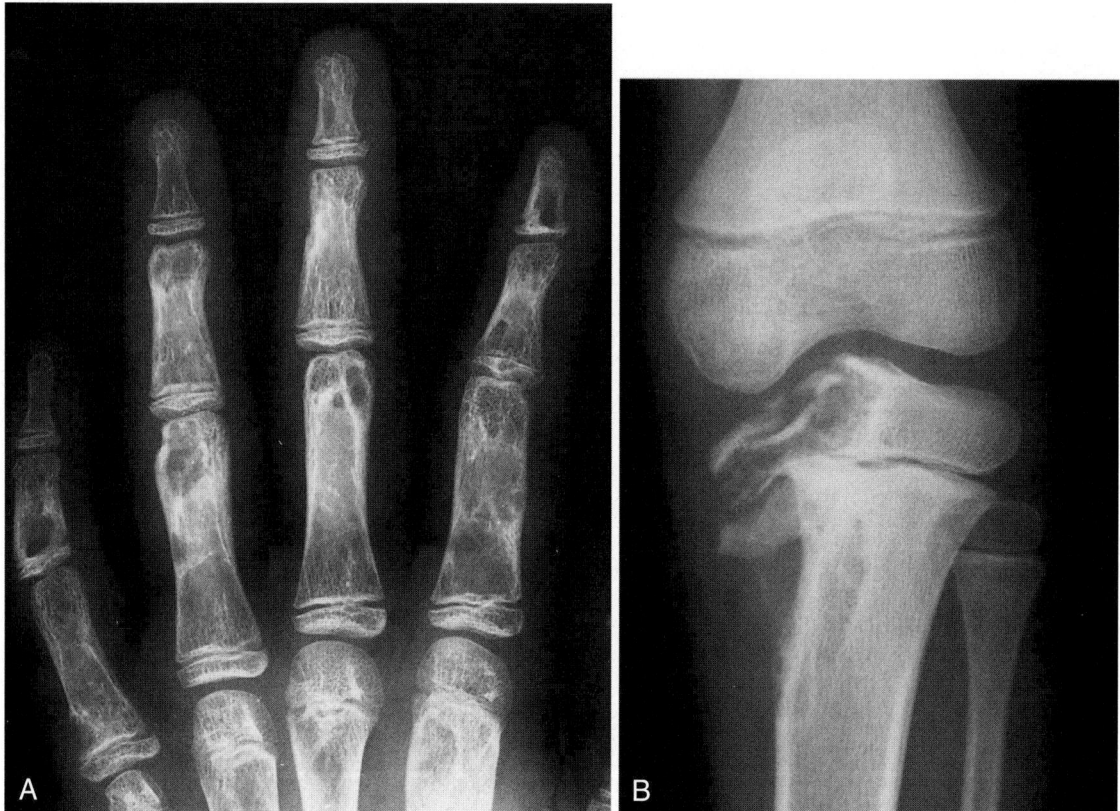

**Figure 55–39.** *Histoplasma capsulatum* var. *duboisii* osteomyelitis. *A*, Radiograph of the hand reveals cystic lesions of the metacarpal bones and phalanges. In many areas, they are well marginated and surrounded by reactive bone formation and mature periostitis. *B*, Extensive lesions of the tibial epiphysis and metaphysis have produced collapse of the articular surface, with sclerosis and mild periostitis. Extension across the growth cartilage is not unusual in fungal infections. (*A*, From Cockshott WP, Lucas AO: *Histoplasmosis duboisii*. Q J Med 33:223, 1964.)

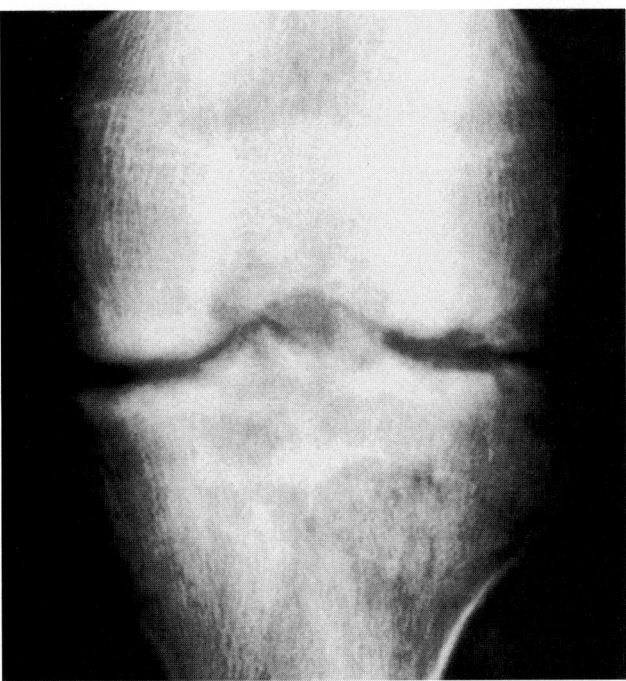

**Figure 55–40.** Sporotrichosis: septic arthritis. Note soft tissue swelling, joint space loss, and irregularity and poor definition of subchondral bone, with marginal and central osseous erosions. The changes are identical to those in other forms of septic arthritis. Joint involvement is not infrequent in this disorder, and osteoporosis may or may not be present. (Courtesy of A. Brower, MD, Norfolk, Va.)

orders, or pigmented villonodular synovitis. Involvement of the small joints of the hands and feet appears to be more characteristic of this fungal disease than the others.

## Candidiasis (Moniliasis)

Of the various *Candida* species, *Candida albicans* is most commonly associated with human disease. *Candida* organisms normally reside on the mucous membranes. Abnormal proliferation on these membranes may occur in otherwise normal persons but is especially characteristic in debilitated children or adults, in patients receiving broad-spectrum antibiotics, in those with diabetes mellitus, and in patients with intravenous or Foley catheters. In the mouth, a mucocutaneous infection can be found, consisting of white patches (thrush) with subjacent inflammation of the buccal mucosa. Rarely, widespread infection may develop.

*Candida* infection of the musculoskeletal system occurs when host resistance is depressed. Intravenous drug addicts may be affected, and a distinctive syndrome leading to systemic candidiasis with costochondral involvement has been recognized in approximately one third of heroin addicts. Bone involvement in cases of disseminated candidiasis is relatively rare, evident in less than 1% to 2% of cases. When present, such osseous involvement can result from direct hematogenous seeding or extension from an overlying soft tissue abscess. Osteomyelitis in any age group can occur in one or more sites, including the tubular bones of the extremities, flat bones, and spine. Common patterns of distribution are involvement of a single long bone, involvement of the sternum, and involvement of two consecutive vertebral bodies (Fig. 55–42). Septic arthritis is also observed in candidiasis. Typically, infection predominates in large weight-bearing joints; the knee is the most common site of involvement. The pathogenesis of the articular infection can relate to

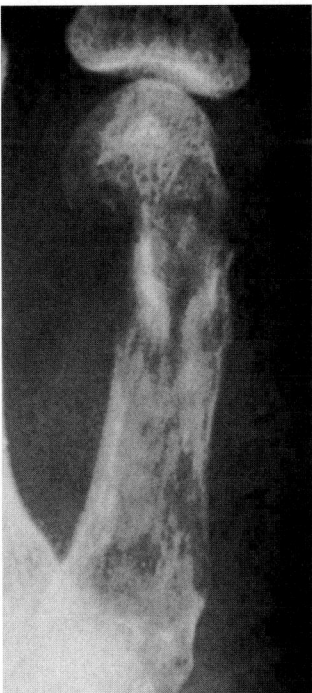

**Figure 55–41.** Sporotrichosis: osteomyelitis. Note osteolysis of the fifth metacarpal bone, along with a pathologic fracture. (Courtesy of A. G. Bergman, MD, Stanford, Calif.)

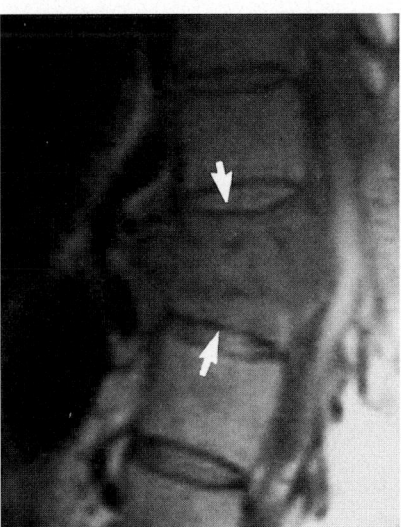

**Figure 55–42.** Candidiasis: spondylitis. Sagittal T1-weighted (TR/TE, 600/26) spin echo MR image shows involvement of two contiguous vertebral bodies (*arrows*) and the intervening intervertebral disc. The process is of low signal intensity with both anterior and posterior extension.

hematogenous contamination or extension from an adjacent infected osseous or soft tissue structure. Radiographic findings include soft tissue swelling, joint space narrowing, irregularity of subchondral bone, and more widespread changes of osteomyelitis (Fig. 55–43).

## Aspergillosis

*Aspergillus* is normally a harmless inhabitant of the upper respiratory tract. Uncommonly, in patients with low resistance or in those who have received an overwhelming inoculum, a chronic localized pulmonary infection may result. The usual organism is *Aspergillus fumigatus*. The musculoskeletal system is rarely involved in aspergillosis. Two potential mechanisms of infection have been emphasized: hematogenous infection, which reportedly predominates in adults, and spread from a pulmonary or cutaneous infective site, a mechanism that may predominate in children. Indeed, pulmonary aspergillosis leading to chest wall involvement has been emphasized as a finding of chronic granulomatous disease in children (Fig. 55–44).

## Maduromycosis (Mycetoma)

Maduromycosis, a chronic granulomatous fungal disease, affects the feet (Madura foot). It can be observed throughout the world but is especially prevalent in India; in fact, the town of Madura in India is the source of its name. In the United States, a variety of organisms may cause Madura foot.

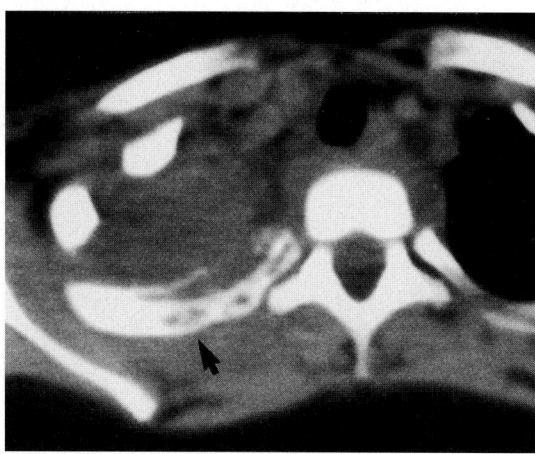

**Figure 55–44.** Aspergillosis: osteomyelitis. Transaxial CT scan of the thorax in a 5-year-old boy with X-linked chronic granulomatous disease shows consolidation in the right apical portion of the lung, soft tissue swelling, loss of fat planes, and osteolytic lesions *(arrow)* in the posteromedial aspect of the right third rib. (From Kawashima A, Kuhlman JE, Fishman EK, et al: Pulmonary *Aspergillus* chest wall involvement in chronic granulomatous disease: CT and MRI findings. Skeletal Radiol 20:487, 1991.)

Infection of the foot (and, less commonly, other sites) results from post-traumatic soft tissue invasion by organisms that are normal inhabitants of soil. After soft tissue contamination, the organisms may penetrate the underlying structures. Sinus tracts arising from the infected osseous tissues are common. The course of maduromycosis is usually progressive. Initially, soft tissue swelling is seen. Over a period of months to years, the foot becomes swollen, deformed, and necrotic. The radiographic findings vary with the virulence of the invading organism. In some cases, single or multiple localized osseous defects are evident; in others, extensive soft tissue and bony disruption occurs, with associated periostitis and sclerosis. Intra-articular osseous fusion may occur and lead to an appearance that is termed "melting snow" (Fig. 55–45).

## VIRAL INFECTION

### Rubella (German Measles)

Rubella is a contagious viral disease. Although it is generally a benign disorder in adults, maternal infection in the first half of pregnancy can lead to serious skeletal and nonskeletal alterations in the fetus.

**Postnatal Rubella.** In adult patients (especially women), rubella arthritis may occur within a few days to 1 week of the skin rash. Persistent or migratory articular findings are most common in the small joints of the hands and wrists.

After live, attenuated rubella virus became available for active immunization, episodes of acute arthritis were noted in children injected with the virus. A chronic arthropathy in children and adults has also been associated with rubella vaccination. In this arthropathy, recurrent episodes of knee stiffness (catcher's crouch syndrome) are evident. Oligoarthritis and polyarthritis are the clinical patterns observed.

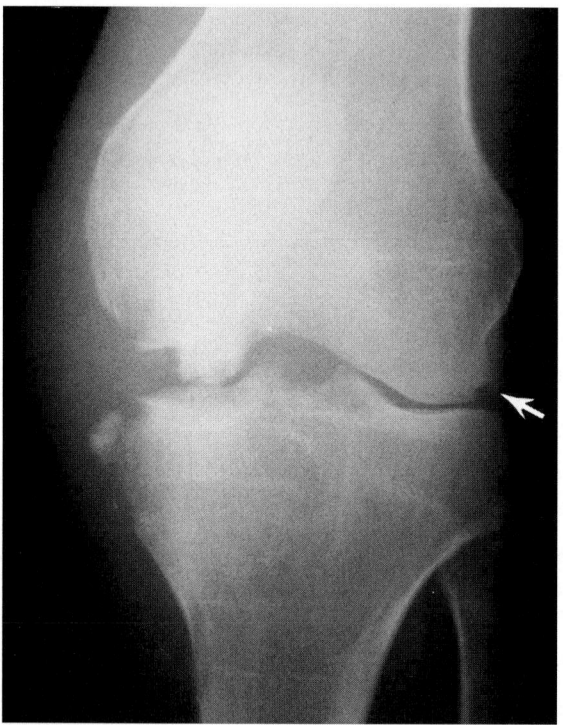

**Figure 55–43.** Candidiasis: septic arthritis. Observe the massive soft tissue swelling, marginal osseous erosions *(arrow)*, bone collapse and fragmentation, and joint space narrowing.

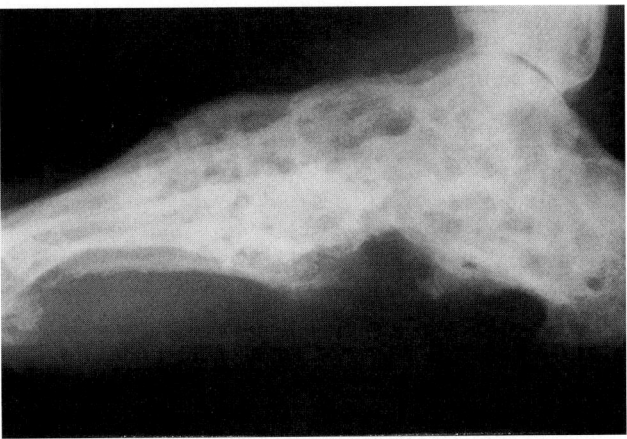

**Figure 55–45.** Maduromycosis: Madura foot. Lateral radiographs delineate the osseous and articular effects of chronic involvement of the foot. Bony destruction and widespread intra-articular osseous fusion can be noted.

Radiographic findings are variable but include intra-articular bone erosions. The arthropathy resembles juvenile chronic arthritis, and reports indicate that rubella antibody levels are elevated not only in rubella vaccine–induced arthritis but also in a significant proportion of children (approximately 33%) with juvenile chronic arthritis, suggesting a possible role of rubella infection in this disease.

**Intrauterine Rubella.** The radiographic features consist of metaphyseal lesions in long bones characterized by symmetry, linear areas of radiolucency, and increased bone density producing a longitudinally oriented striated pattern ("celery stalk" appearance), as well as the absence of periostitis. These features can either disappear completely if the child recovers from the intrauterine viral infection or persist with increasing density of the juxtaepiphyseal region if the infection continues (Fig. 55–46). With healing, beaklike exostoses can be noted at the metaphyses. It is generally believed that the metaphyseal and diaphyseal lesions of rubella are related to alterations in bone formation. These osseous alterations may occur in as many as 45% of cases of intrauterine rubella.

## Cytomegalic Inclusion Disease

Intrauterine infection related to cytomegalic inclusion disease can lead to intracranial calcifications and rubella-like abnormalities of the skeleton (Fig. 55–47). Metaphyseal osteopenia, irregularity of the growth plate, and a striated pattern parallel to the long axis of the bone characterized by alternating lucent and sclerotic bands are noted. The metaphyseal changes are usually evident in the first few days of life and then disappear completely within a period of days to weeks. They are generally attributed to a disturbance in endochondral bone formation rather than osteomyelitis.

## Variola (Smallpox)

Osteomyelitis and septic arthritis are well-known complications of smallpox. No apparent relationship has been

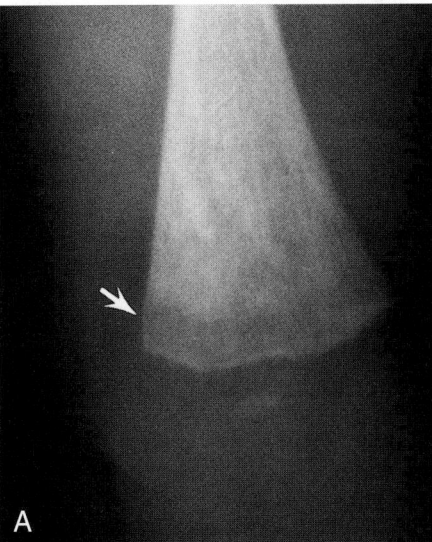

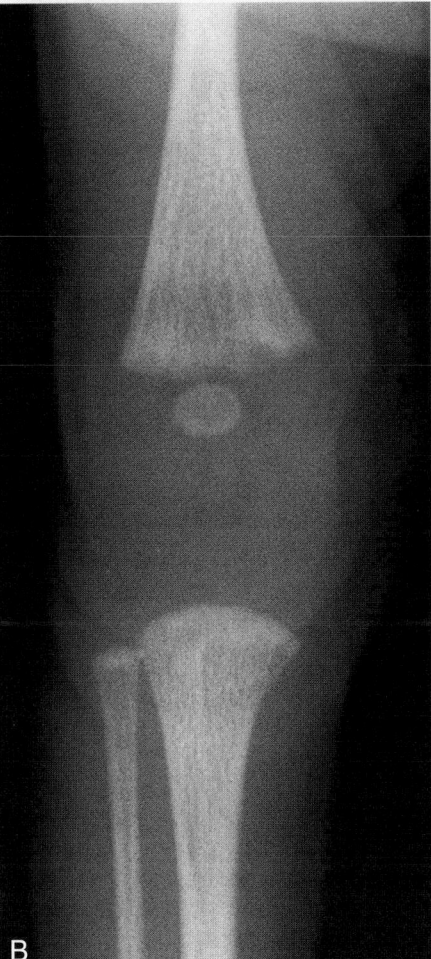

**Figure 55–46.** Intrauterine rubella infection. *A,* Radiolucent metaphyseal bands *(arrow)* in the distal ends of the femora of this infant are associated with relative sclerosis of the diaphyses. *B,* In a different infant, longitudinal striations have produced the characteristic "celery stalk" appearance. Periostitis is absent.

found between the severity of the infection and the frequency or severity of osteomyelitis or septic arthritis. Infection may originate in the bone, joint, or both; most typically, osseous and articular changes occur together.

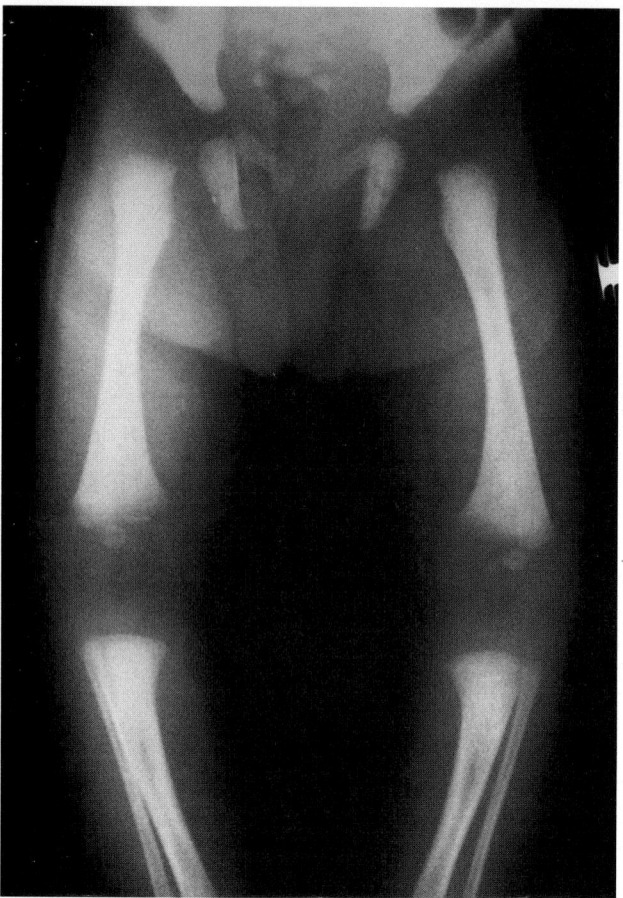

**Figure 55–47.** Cytomegalic inclusion disease. Metaphyseal changes consist of irregularity of the growth plate and osseous fragmentation, most evident in the distal ends of the femora. (Courtesy of F. N. Silverman, MD, Palo Alto, Calif.)

Symmetrical involvement is frequent, and articular infection reveals an unusual affinity for the elbow (80% of patients).

Three types of bone and joint lesions have been described: (1) a necrotic, nonsuppurative osteomyelitis, probably caused by the smallpox virus itself; (2) a suppurative arthritis related to contamination of the joint, probably due to secondary infection of a pustule; and (3) a nonsuppurative arthritis that appears 1 to 4 weeks after the initial infection. Polyarticular and symmetrical abnormalities are common and are characterized by pain, swelling, and restriction of motion. During the acute stage of osteomyelitis variolosa, findings simulate those of pyogenic osteomyelitis. Juxtametaphyseal osteoporosis and destruction, epiphyseal extension, periostitis, involucrum formation, and articular contamination are seen. The elbow is commonly affected (Fig. 55–48).

## Human Immunodeficiency Virus Infection

HIV infection leads to compromise of the body's defense mechanisms, which in turn predisposes infected persons to a variety of opportunistic infections, anemia, arthritis, myositis, and immune-related neoplasms. Musculoskeletal alterations in such persons are not infrequent.

### Rheumatologic Disorders

Many of the rheumatologic manifestations of HIV infection fall within the spectrum of differentiated and undifferentiated forms of spondyloarthropathy. In patients with HIV infection, the classic triad of clinical abnormalities in Reiter's syndrome is commonly lacking because of the infrequent occurrence of conjunctivitis. Fasciitis and enthesopathy occur, especially in the feet (Fig. 55–49),

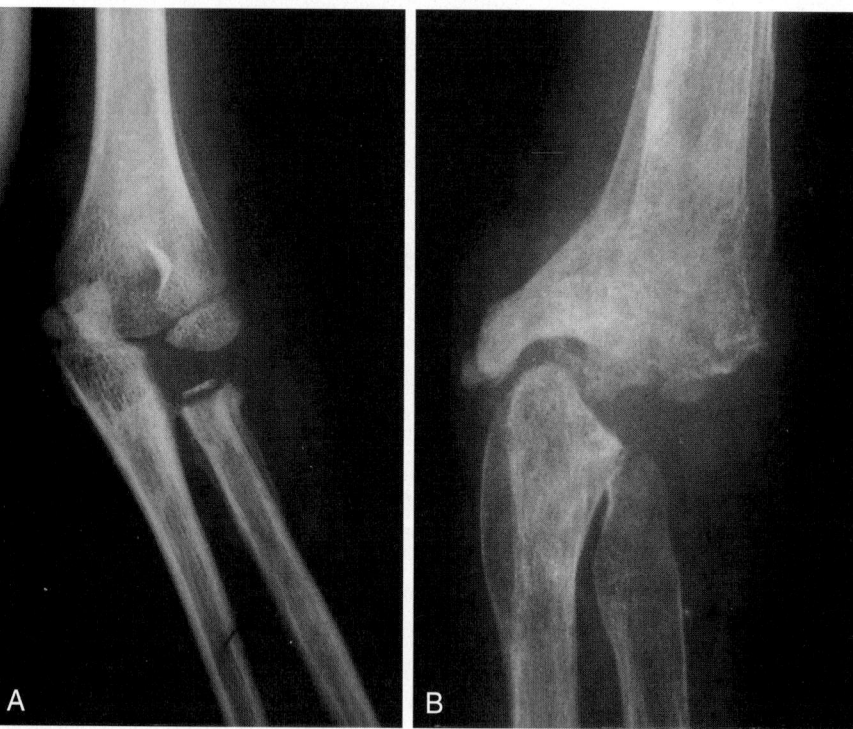

**Figure 55–48.** Variola osteomyelitis and septic arthritis: elbow involvement. Stages in the process of bone and joint disease are illustrated in two different patients. *A,* Initial findings include destructive foci with periostitis. *B,* Subsequently, irregularity of the articular surfaces can be seen. (Courtesy of W. P. Cockshott, MD, Hamilton, Ontario, Canada.)

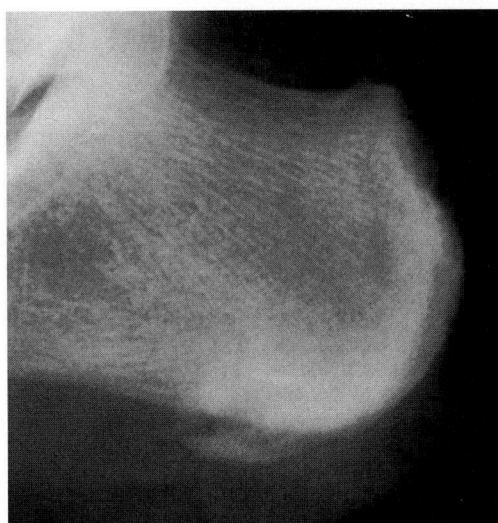

**Figure 55–49.** Human immunodeficiency virus infection: reactive arthritis with enthesopathy and bursitis. Note enthesitis, with bone proliferation in the plantar aspect of the calcaneus, and retrocalcaneal bursitis, with erosion of the posterosuperior portion of the calcaneus.

and are accompanied by marked muscle wasting. These characteristics, which are nearly diagnostic, have been referred to as the AIDS foot. As with Reiter's syndrome, psoriasis-like joint involvement may be seen in patients with HIV infection.

## Infectious Disorders

Osteomyelitis, septic arthritis, pyomyositis, and septic bursitis are among the most frequent complications associated with HIV infection. Although the knee is the most common site of involvement, joints of the upper extremity and the acromioclavicular, sternoclavicular, and sacroiliac joints may also be affected. *S. aureus* or *S. pneumoniae* is implicated most often, but opportunistic pathogens represent additional potential causative agents.

Pyomyositis is a bacterial infection of muscle that is generally, but not exclusively, caused by *S. aureus* and is endemic in tropical regions of Africa, Southeast Asia, and South America. It commonly affects patients who are immunologically compromised or who have underlying chronic disorders such as HIV infection. Almost 95% of reported cases of pyomyositis associated with HIV infection involve localization in the lower extremity. Multiple abscesses are identified in about 50% of cases. The most typical pattern of disease, however, appears to be a solitary abscess in the quadriceps musculature. Clinical findings include fever and local muscle pain, redness, and swelling; if untreated, this may be accompanied by marked edema and septicemia.

## Kaposi's Sarcoma

Among the malignant tumors encountered with increased frequency in patients with HIV infection are lymphomas, Hodgkin's disease, and Kaposi's sarcoma. The last of these tumors arises from lymphatic endothelial cells, and it has

been reported to be present in 15% to 20% of patients with HIV infection. In these patients, Kaposi's sarcoma is aggressive in behavior, with multiorgan involvement.

## Bacillary Angiomatosis

Bacillary angiomatosis is a disorder characterized by histologic evidence of vascular proliferation in affected tissues such as the skin, bone, lymph nodes, and brain and by the presence of numerous bacillary organisms. Recent biologic and microbiologic investigations have confirmed that at least two organisms, *Rochalimaea henselae* and *Rochalimaea quintana*, can cause this disease. Bacillary angiomatosis can occur in patients infected with HIV, but it is not restricted to such patients; it has also been observed in immunocompetent patients and in recipients of organ transplants. The typical clinical manifestation is that of a cutaneous disorder with multiple friable angiomatous papules closely resembling pyogenic granulomas, as well as the skin lesions of Kaposi's sarcoma. Fever, chills, weight loss, night sweats, cellulitis, and subcutaneous nodules are additional clinical features. Bone lesions may also be seen, sometimes as an initial manifestation of the disease. Tubular bones of the extremities are typically affected (Fig. 55–50), with the flat and irregular bones affected less commonly. Osteolysis is the dominant radiographic feature, and the osteolytic focus or foci may

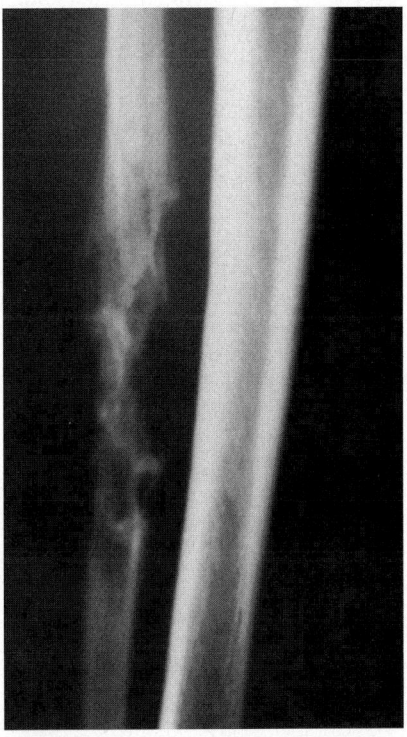

**Figure 55–50.** Human immunodeficiency virus infection: bacillary angiomatosis. This 34-year-old homosexual man had pain and swelling in the calf for 6 weeks. A poorly defined osteolytic lesion of the fibula is evident. (From Conrad SE, Jacobs D, Gee J, et al: Pseudoneoplastic infection of bone in acquired immunodeficiency syndrome. A case report involving the cat-scratch disease bacillus. J Bone Joint Surg Am 73:774, 1991.)

be either well or poorly defined. Cortical or medullary destruction, or both, is seen, and an adjacent soft tissue mass is an associated feature. Periostitis is often identified, and this finding combined with skin lesions in a patient with AIDS is considered strong evidence of bacillary angiomatosis.

## RICKETTSIAL INFECTION

### Cat-Scratch Disease

Cat-scratch disease (CSD) has been linked to two soil-borne proteobacteria, *Bartonella henselae* and, occasionally, *Afipia felia*. CSD is often manifested as a local lymphadenitis with lymphadenopathy occurring within 1 or 2 weeks after being scratched by a cat. Such lymphadenopathy is generally preceded by an erythematous pustule or papule at the site of inoculation that resolves spontaneously within several weeks to months. Involvement of the central nervous system, lung, liver, spleen, bone, and skin may complicate CSD in as many as 2% of cases. A serologic test (indirect fluorescent antibody) for *R. henselae* is currently considered a useful adjunct for obtaining the correct diagnosis. Affected persons are between the ages of 5 and 21 years, and CSD is probably the leading cause of chronic benign lymphadenopathy. More than 90% of patients with CSD have a history of exposure to cats.

The initial clinical manifestations are cutaneous and consist of skin eruptions at the site of inoculation. Because the hands and forearms are the most frequent sites of inoculation, adenopathy often develops around the elbow, axilla, and head and neck; specific areas of adenopathy, in decreasing order of frequency, are the axillary and epitrochlear nodes, the cervical and submandibular nodes, the groin, and the preauricular, postauricular, and supraclavicular chains. Conventional radiographs reveal soft tissue edema, masses, or both. Although ultrasonography can also be used to study the soft tissue and systemic manifestations of CSD, MR imaging may be more sensitive and is often diagnostic. An ill-defined mass with heterogeneous low signal intensity on T1-weighted spin echo MR images and intermediate to high signal intensity on T2-weighted spin echo MR images in the region of the epitrochlear nodes about the elbow should suggest

the diagnosis of CSD (Fig. 55–51). Surrounding edema is common, and enhancement of signal intensity in the peripheral portion of the mass may be noted after intravenous gadolinium administration. Osseous lesions, probably related to hematogenous dissemination and spread from a contiguous contaminated source, such as a lymph node, are encountered uncommonly. These lesions are not specific when studied by conventional radiography because they resemble other processes such as eosinophilic granuloma.

## PROTOZOAN INFECTION

### Toxoplasmosis

Toxoplasmosis is an infectious disorder caused by an intracellular protozoan parasite, *Toxoplasma gondii*. Human infections with *Toxoplasma* may be either congenital or acquired. The congenital variety of toxoplasmosis can be severe. An infant may be stillborn at term or be born prematurely with active infection characterized by fever, rash, hepatosplenomegaly, mental retardation, chorioretinitis, and convulsions, which may lead to death in 10% to 20% of cases. Osseous lesions are unusual, although metaphyseal alterations in tubular bones may simulate those of rubella, cytomegalic inclusion disease, or syphilis. Cerebral calcification may be evident. The acquired variety of the disease can occur at any age and may display variable manifestations, including rash, lymphadenopathy, ocular changes, and widespread vascular alterations. Myalgias and myositis can accompany acquired toxoplasmosis. Radiographically evident osteoporosis, soft tissue swelling, and osseous cystic lesions have been described.

## HELMINTHIC INFECTION

A variety of helminths (worms) can cause infection (Table 55–3).

### Hookworm Disease

Hookworm disease is produced by *Ancylostoma duodenale* or *Necator americanus*. Anemia and its complications are

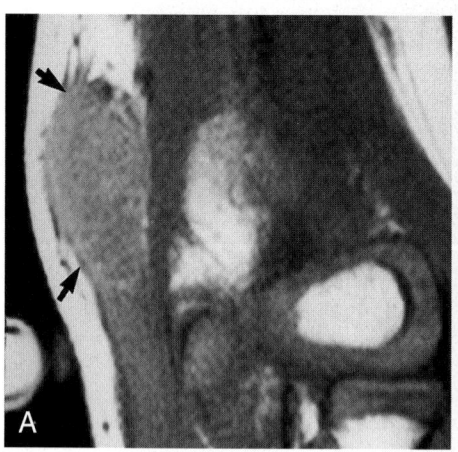
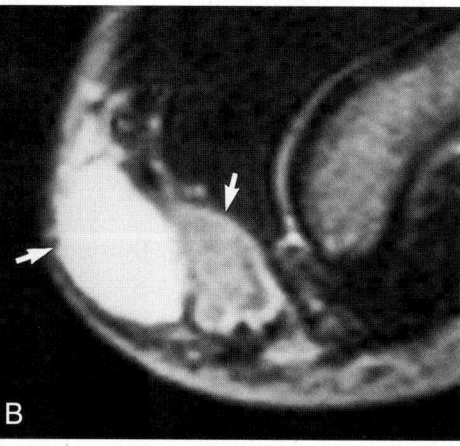

**Figure 55–51.** Cat-scratch disease. This young boy was bitten and scratched by a cat while trying to put the animal in a clothes dryer several weeks earlier. A soft tissue mass developed on the medial aspect of the elbow. The granulomatous process *(arrows)* is well shown on coronal intermediate-weighted (TR/TE, 1600/40) *(A)* and transaxial T2-weighted (TR/TE, 2000/100) *(B)* spin echo MR images. (Courtesy of A. Motta, MD, Cleveland, Ohio.)

**TABLE 55–3**

**Major Helminthic Infections of Humans**

| Nematodes (Roundworms) | | Trematodes (Flatworms) | | Cestodes (Tapeworms) | |
|---|---|---|---|---|---|
| *Intestinal* | *Tissue* | *Tissue* | *Intravascular* | *Pathogenic Form: Adult* | *Pathogenic Form: Larva* |
| Ancylostoma duodenale | Wuchereria bancrofti | Clonorchis sinensis | Schistosoma mansoni | Diphyllobothrium latum | Echinococcus granulosus |
| Necator americanus | Brugia malayi | Fasciola hepatica | Schistosoma japonicum | Taenia saginata | Echinococcus multilocularis |
| Ascaris lubricoides | Onchocerca volvulus | Fasciolopsis buski | Schistosoma haematobium | Taenia solium | Taenia solium |
| Enterobius vermicularis | Loa loa | Paragonimus westermani | Hymenolepsis nana | Hymenolepsis nana | Hymenolepsis nana |
| Trichuris trichiura | Trichinella spiralis Toxocara canis Dracunculus medinensis | | | | |

From Korzeniowdki OM: Diseases due to helminths. In Stein JH (ed): Internal Medicine. Boston, Little, Brown, 1983, p 1455.

the major clinical manifestations of this disorder. Musculoskeletal abnormalities are rare.

## Loiasis

Loiasis is prevalent in West and Central Africa and is produced by the filaria *Loa loa* (African eyeworm). Infective larvae are deposited in the victim's skin after a bite of the mango fly. The larvae burrow into the deeper subcutaneous tissue, where they mature to adult worms over a period of 6 months or longer. The dead worms cause abscesses or undergo calcification, or both. Calcific deposits in subcutaneous tissue may be fine, coiled, lacelike, and filamentous (calcification of the worm), or they may be thicker, beadlike, and lobulated (calcification of the fibrous capsule surrounding the worm) (Fig. 55–52; Table 55–4). Polyarthritis has been associated with loiasis.

## Onchocerciasis

Onchocerciasis is a form of filariasis produced by *Onchocerca volvulus* and transmitted by flies. It is prevalent in Africa and Central and South America. Soft tissue calcifications, similar to those in loiasis, may be detected, although radiographic demonstration of the calcified areas is extremely difficult because of their small size.

## Filariasis

Filariasis is produced by adult worms of the species *Wuchereria bancrofti* or *Brugia malayi*, which localize in the lymphatic and soft tissues of the human body. The disease is predominant in tropical areas of Asia, Africa, South America, Australia, and the South Pacific islands. After prolonged and repeated attacks, filariasis can lead to massive lymphedema or elephantiasis, especially of the legs and scrotum. Radiographs show an affected limb to

be greatly enlarged, with soft tissue thickening, blurring of subcutaneous fat planes, and a linear striated pattern. Soft tissue calcification has been noted in *W. bancrofti* infestation; elongated radiodense shadows in the subcutaneous tissue represent calcified, dead, encysted filariae.

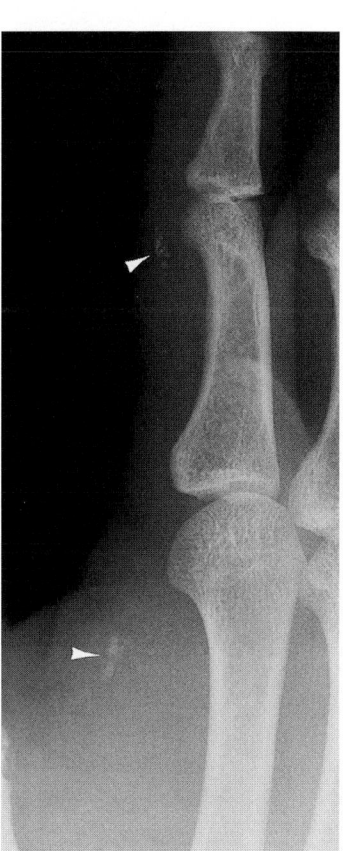

**Figure 55–52.** Loiasis (African eyeworm disease). Soft tissue calcifications *(arrowheads)* are evident in the hand of this 29-year-old man. (Courtesy of M. Dalinka, MD, Philadelphia, Pa.)

### TABLE 55–4

**Helminths (Worms) Associated with Calcification**

| Helminth (Disease) | Frequency of Radiographic Calcification | Typical Location of Calcification | Typical Appearance of Calcification |
|---|---|---|---|
| *Loa loa* (loiasis) | Common | Widespread; subcutaneous tissues | Extended or coiled, linear or beaded, variable in size |
| *Onchocerca volvulus* (river blindness) | Rare | Legs, trunk, head; subcutaneous nodules | Extended or coiled, linear or beaded, small |
| *Wuchereria bancrofti, Brugia malayi* (filariasis) | Rare | Thighs, legs, scrotum; subcutaneous tissues | Straight or coiled, small |
| *Dracunculus medinensis* (guinea worm disease) | Common | Extremities | Extended or coiled, long |
| *Taenia solium* (cysticercosis) | Common | Widespread; muscular tissues | Numerous, linear or oval, variable in size, lie in plane of muscle |
| *Echinococcus granulosus* (echinococcosis) | Common | Liver, lungs, other organs | Curvilinear, cystic, eggshell |
| *Sarcocystis lindemanni* (sarcosporidiosis) | Common | Extremities; muscular and subcutaneous tissues | Numerous, linear or oval, variable in size and orientation |
| *Armillifer armillatus*, Porocephalida, Pentastomida (porocephaliasis) | Variable | Abdomen, thorax | Multiple, crescent shaped or oval |
| *Schistosoma haematobium* (schistosomiasis) | Variable | Bladder, urinary tract | Linear, nodular |

The calcifications are smaller than those in loiasis and occur predominantly in the lymphatic channels of the scrotum, thighs, and legs.

## Dracunculiasis (Guinea Worm Disease)

The guinea worm, *Dracunculus medinensis*, can cause human disease, particularly in parts of Africa, the Middle East, South America, India, and Pakistan. The disorder is contracted when larvae in contaminated water are ingested by a water flea (*Cyclops*), which in turn is swallowed in the drinking water by humans. The larvae eventually enter the circulation and mature within human subcutaneous tissue. When the female parasites die, they may calcify and produce long, curled radiodense shadows in the lower extremities (Fig. 55–53) and hands or, less commonly, in the perineum and abdominal and chest walls. The deposits are usually multiple and may become fragmented because of the action of adjacent musculature.

## Trichinosis

After ingestion of infected pork, humans may contract trichinosis from the intestinal nematode *Trichinella spiralis*. Calcification of the cysts of the parasite is commonly detected on microscopic examination but is rarely, if ever, noted on radiographic evaluation. Clinical features resemble those of dermatomyositis.

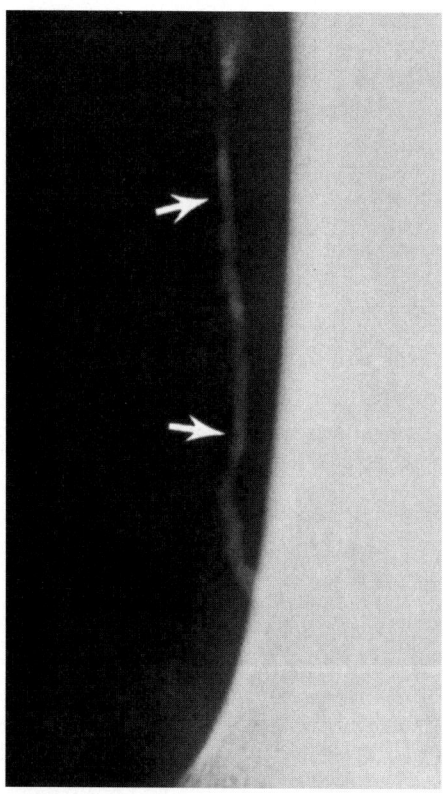

**Figure 55–53.** Dracunculiasis (guinea worm disease). Observe the long linear calcification (*arrows*) adjacent to the lower part of the tibia caused by the presence of a dying female worm.

## Cysticercosis

The relationship between humans and the pork tapeworm *Taenia solium* is twofold: humans are the only definitive host of the adult tapeworm (the parasite inhabits the intestine), and humans may serve as an intermediate host (the usual intermediate host is the hog) and harbor the larval stage, *Cysticercus cellulosae*. In the latter case, deposits of the larval form of the tapeworm may appear in subcutaneous and muscular tissue and in a variety of viscera, including the heart, brain, lung, liver, and eye. When the larvae die, a foreign body reaction may ensue, followed over a period of years by caseation and calcification. On radiographs, linear or oval elongated calcifications appear in the soft tissues and musculature and may reach 23 mm in length. The long axis of the calcified cysts lies in the plane of the surrounding muscle bundles (Fig. 55–54).

## Echinococcosis

Echinococcosis is produced principally by the larval stage of *Echinococcus granulosus* and is most prevalent in sheep- and cattle-raising areas of North and South Africa, South America, Central Europe, Australia, and Canada; less commonly, *Echinococcus multilocularis* is the causative agent, especially in Alaska and Eurasia. In humans, *E. granulosus* is contracted by ingestion of the eggs, which are contained in the feces of dogs (sheep or cattle dogs). After ingestion, the embryos escape from the eggs, traverse the intestinal mucosa, and are disseminated via venous and lymphatic channels. Cysts may develop in various viscera, particularly the liver and the lungs. They may calcify and produce irregular curvilinear radiodense areas.

Bone lesions are reported in 1% to 2% of cases of echinococcosis. Osseous involvement is almost invariably related to primary infection and is not the result of extension from a neighboring soft tissue lesion. Although hematogenous seeding of the skeleton can conceivably occur at any site, one bone, a few adjacent bones, or one skeletal region is usually affected. The vertebral column, pelvis, long bones, and skull are most commonly involved. The spine is involved in about 50% of cases.

Radiographs can reveal single or multiple expansile, cystic, osteolytic lesions containing trabeculae (Fig. 55–55). These lesions may be associated with cortical violation and soft tissue mass formation, with subsequent calcification. The radiographic characteristics are similar to those of fibrous dysplasia, plasmacytoma, giant cell tumor, cartilaginous neoplasm, skeletal metastasis (especially from a tumor of the kidney or thyroid), brown tumor of hyperparathyroidism, angiosarcoma, or hemophilic pseudotumor. CT features of echinococcosis include a soft tissue mass adjacent to sites of bone involvement; the center of the mass contains fluid with water attenuation values. Cystic lesions within the bone and adjacent soft tissue are also identified with MR imaging; the signal characteristics of the cyst are variable (dependent on the type of cyst present and whether it is intact, ruptured, infected,

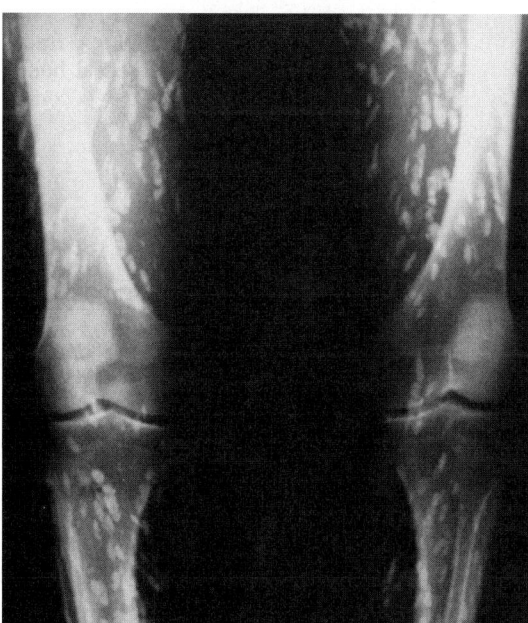

**Figure 55–54.** Cysticercosis. The typical appearance of soft tissue calcification in this disorder consists of dense, elongated, linear or oval lesions oriented in the plane of the surrounding muscle bundles. (Courtesy of B. Howard, MD, Charlotte, N.C.)

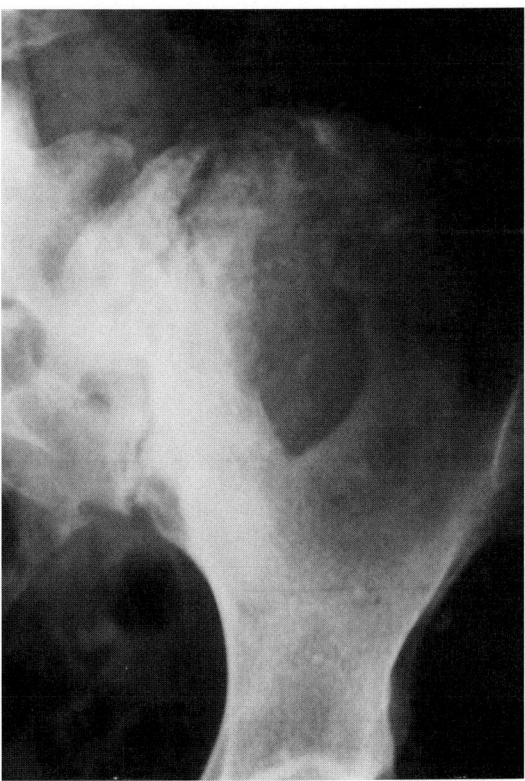

**Figure 55–55.** Echinococcosis. An osteolytic lesion in the ilium is accompanied by sclerosis extending to the sacroiliac joint. (Courtesy of A. D'Abreu, MD, Porto Alegre, Brazil.)

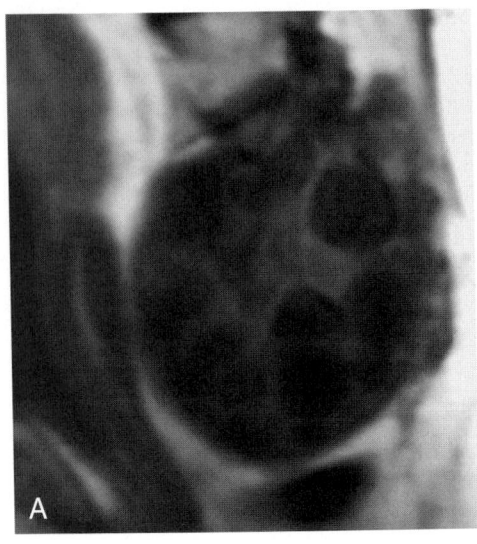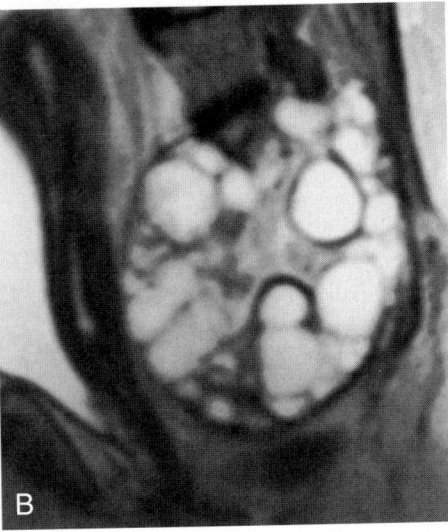

**Figure 55–56.** Echinococcosis. *A,* Sagittal T1-weighted (TR/TE, 650/20) spin echo MR image reveals a large mass involving predominantly the sacrum, with anterior extension leading to displacement of pelvic viscera. Note the circular regions of low signal intensity within the mass, consistent with fluid-filled cysts. *B,* Sagittal T2-weighted (TR/TE, 4348/150) spin echo MR image reveals the cysts as regions of high signal intensity. (Courtesy of J. Kramer, MD, Vienna, Austria.)

or dead) and may not be diagnostic (Fig. 55–56). The presence of numerous cystic lesions of high signal intensity on T2-weighted spin echo MR images appears to be characteristic.

## ADDITIONAL DISORDERS WITH A POSSIBLE INFECTIOUS CAUSE

### Ainhum

Ainhum (dactylolysis spontanea) is a self-limited dermatologic disorder that is characteristically found in African blacks or their descendants. Most typically, the fifth toe on one or both feet is affected, although other toes (especially the fourth) and even the fingers can be involved. A deep soft tissue groove corresponding to a hyperkeratotic band within the epidermis appears and is associated with dermal fibrosis. The groove is initially evident along the medial aspect of the fifth toe and progressively deepens and encircles the toe. Bony resorption begins on the medial aspect of the distal portion of the proximal phalanx or the middle phalanx of the fifth toe (Fig. 55–57). The cause of ainhum is not clear. Traumatic and infectious factors appear most likely.

### Tietze's Syndrome

Tietze's syndrome and costochondritis are terms used to describe pain, tenderness, and swelling at the costosternal joints. This condition is common and may occur in as many as 10% of patients with chest pain. Tietze's syndrome is benign and self-limited. Typically, painful swelling and tenderness to local palpation of one or more costosternal junctions are observed. Radiographs are seldom revealing, although rarely, soft tissue swelling, calcification, osteophytosis, and periostitis are encountered. Increased activity may be demonstrated on bone scans. CT scanning may reveal sclerosis of the sternal manubrium, partial calcification of costal cartilage, and soft tissue swelling. The cause is unknown.

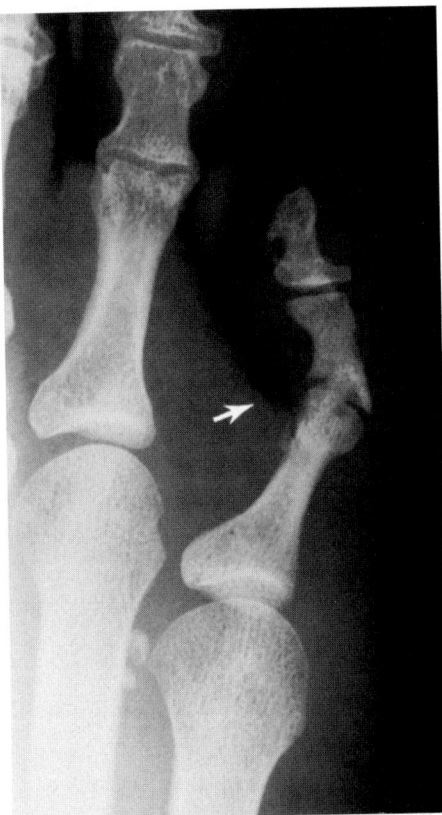

**Figure 55–57.** Ainhum. Note the soft tissue groove (*arrow*) and osseous resorption, especially on the medial aspect of the proximal and middle phalanges of the fifth toe. Periostitis is absent.

## FURTHER READING

Alexander GH, Mansuy MM: Disseminated bone tuberculosis (so-called multiple cystic tuberculosis). Radiology 55:839, 1950.

Allen JH Jr: Bone involvement with disseminated histoplasmosis. AJR Am J Roentgenol 82:250, 1959.

Baron AL, Steinbach LS, LeBoit PE, et al: Osteolytic lesions and bacillary angiomatosis in HIV infection: Radiographic differentiation from AIDS-related Kaposi sarcoma. Radiology 177:77, 1990.

Barre PS, Thompson GH, Morrison SC: Late skeletal deformities following meningococcal sepsis and disseminated intravascular coagulation. J Pediatr Orthop 5:584, 1985.

Beggs I: The radiology of hydatid disease. AJR Am J Roentgenol 145:639, 1985.

Bertcher RW: Osteomyelitis variolosa. AJR Am J Roentgenol 76:1149, 1956.

Bonakdarpour A, Zadeh YFA, Maghssoudi H, et al: Costal echinococcosis: Report of six cases and review of the literature. AJR Am J Roentgenol 118:371, 1973.

Braithwaite PA, Lees RF: Vertebral hydatid disease: Radiological assessment. Radiology 140:763, 1981.

Brown JS, Middlemiss JH: Bone changes in tropical ulcer. Br J Radiol 29:213, 1956.

Casado E, Olivé A, Holgado S, et al: Musculoskeletal manifestations in patients positive for human immunodeficiency virus: Correlation with CD4 count. J Rheumatol 28:802, 2001.

Chang AC, Destouet JM, Murphy WA: Musculoskeletal sporotrichosis. Skeletal Radiol 12:23, 1984.

Chapman M, Murray RO, Stoker DJ: Tuberculosis of the bones and joints. Semin Roentgenol 14:266, 1979.

Chilton SJ, Aftimos SF, White PR: Diffuse skeletal involvement of streptococcal osteomyelitis in a neonate. Radiology 134:390, 1980.

Comstock C, Wolson AH: Roentgenology of sporotrichosis. AJR Am J Roentgenol 125:651, 1975.

Cremin BJ, Fisher RM: The lesions of congenital syphilis. Br J Radiol 43:333, 1970.

Dalinka MK, Dinnenberg S, Greendyke WH, et al: Roentgenographic features of osseous coccidioidomycosis and differential diagnosis. J Bone Joint Surg Am 53:1157, 1971.

de Roos A, van Meerten ELVP, Bloem JL, et al: MRI of tuberculous spondylitis. AJR Am J Roentgenol 146:79, 1986.

Dong PR, Seeger LL, Yao L, et al: Uncomplicated cat-scratch disease: Findings at CT, MR imaging, and radiography. Radiology 195:837, 1995.

Duran H, Ferrandez L, Gomez-Castresana F, et al: Osseous hydatidosis. J Bone Joint Surg Am 60:685, 1978.

Ehrlich I, Kricun ME: Radiographic findings in early acquired syphilis: Case report and critical review. AJR Am J Roentgenol 127:789, 1976.

Enna CD, Jacobson RR, Rausch RO: Bone changes in leprosy: A correlation of clinical and radiographic features. Radiology 100:295, 1971.

Faget GH, Mayoral A: Bone changes in leprosy: A clinical and roentgenological study of 505 cases. Radiology 42:1, 1944.

Fang D, Leong JCY, Fang HSY: Tuberculosis of the upper cervical spine. J Bone Joint Surg Br 65:47, 1983.

Feldman F, Auerbach R, Johnston A: Tuberculous dactylitis in the adult. AJR Am J Roentgenol 112:460, 1971.

Fetterman LE, Hardy R, Lehrer H: The clinico-roentgenologic features of ainhum. AJR Am J Roentgenol 100:512, 1967.

Gelman MI, Everts CS: Blastomycotic dactylitis. Radiology 107:331, 1973.

Goldblatt M, Cremin BJ: Osteo-articular tuberculosis: Its presentation in coloured races. Clin Radiol 29:669, 1978.

Goldenberg DL: "Postinfectious" arthritis: New look at an old concept with particular attention to disseminated gonococcal infection. Am J Med 74:925, 1983.

Green WH, Goldberg HI, Wohl GT: Mucormycosis infection of the craniofacial structures. AJR Am J Roentgenol 101:802, 1967.

Harisinghani MG, McLoud TG, Shepard JO, et al: Tuberculosis from head to toe. Radiographics 20:449, 2000.

Harverson G, Warren AG: Tarsal bone disintegration in leprosy. Clin Radiol 30:317, 1979.

Haygood TM, Williamson SL: Radiographic findings of extremity tuberculosis in childhood: Back to the future? Radiographics 14:561, 1994.

Hong SH, Kim SM, Ahn JM, et al: Tuberculous versus pyogenic arthritis: MR imaging evaluation. Radiology 218:848, 2001.

Hook EW, Campbell CG, Weens HS, et al: *Salmonella* osteomyelitis in patients with sickle cell anemia. N Engl J Med 257:403, 1957.

Jacobs P: Osteo-articular tuberculosis in coloured immigrants: A radiological study. Clin Radiol 15:59, 1964.

Jaffe HL: Metabolic, Degenerative and Inflammatory Diseases of Bones and Joints. Philadelphia, Lea & Febiger, 1972.

Keats TE: Cysticercosis: A demonstration of its roentgen manifestations. Mo Med 58:457, 1961.

Kelly PJ, Martin WJ, Schirger A, et al: Brucellosis of the bones and joints: Experience with 36 patients. JAMA 174:347, 1960.

Kumar R, Gulati MS, Nag HL: MR appearances in a case of femoral echinococcosis. Skeletal Radiol 29:235, 2000.

Lawson JP, Rahn DW: Lyme disease and radiographic findings in Lyme arthritis. AJR Am J Roentgenol 158:1065, 1992.

Lawson JP, Steele AC: Lyme arthritis: Radiologic findings. Radiology 154:37, 1985.

Lewall DB, Ofole S, Bendl B: Mycetoma. Skeletal Radiol 14:257, 1985.

Lewis R, Gorbach S, Altner P: Spinal *Pseudomonas* chondro-osteomyelitis in heroin users. N Engl J Med 286:1303, 1972.

Lifeso RM, Harder E, McCorkell SJ: Spinal brucellosis. J Bone Joint Surg Br 67:345, 1985.

Martinoli C, Derchi LE, Bertolotto M, et al: US and MR imaging of peripheral nerves in leprosy. Skeletal Radiol 29:142, 2000.

McGahan JP, Graves DS, Palmer PES, et al: Classic and contemporary imaging of coccidioidomycosis. AJR Am J Roentgenol 136:393, 1981.

McLaughlin GE, Utsinger PD, Trackat WF, et al: Rheumatic syndromes secondary to guinea worm infestation. Arthritis Rheum 27:694, 1974.

Merten DF, Gooding CA: Skeletal manifestations of congenital cytomegalic inclusion disease. Radiology 95:333, 1970.

Mertz LE, Wobig GH, Duffy J, et al: Ticks, spirochetes, and new diagnostic tests for Lyme disease. Mayo Clin Proc 60:402, 1985.

Mortensson W, Eklöf O, Jorulf H: Radiologic aspects of BCG-osteomyelitis in infants and children. Acta Radiol (Diagn) 17:845, 1976.

Patriquin HB, Trias A, Jeoquier S, et al: Late sequelae of infantile meningococcemia in growing bones of children. Radiology 141:77, 1981.

Rabinowitz JG, Wolf BS, Greenberg EI, et al: Osseous changes in rubella embryopathy (congenital rubella syndrome). Radiology 85:494, 1965.

Reeder MM: Tropical diseases of the foot. Semin Roentgenol 5:378, 1970.

Rehm-Graves S, Weinstein AJ, Calabrese LH, et al: Tuberculosis of the greater trochanter bursa. Arthritis Rheum 26:77, 1983.

Sachdev M, Bery K, Chawla S: Osseous manifestations in congenital syphilis: A study of 55 cases. Clin Radiol 33:319, 1982.

Samuel E: Roentgenology of parasitic calcification. AJR Am J Roentgenol 63:512, 1950.

Sengupta S: Musculoskeletal lesions in yaws. Clin Orthop 192:193, 1985.

Sharif HS, Aideyan OA, Clark DC, et al: Brucellar and tuberculous spondylitis: Comparative imaging features. Radiology 171:419, 1989.

Silverman FN: Virus diseases of bone: Do they exist? AJR Am J Roentgenol 126:677, 1976.

Steinbach HL: Infections of bone. Semin Roentgenol 1:337, 1966.

Steinbach LS, Tehranzadeh J, Fleckenstein JL, et al: Human immunodeficiency virus infection: Musculoskeletal manifestations. Radiology 186:833, 1993.

Weaver P, Lifeso RM: The radiological diagnosis of tuberculosis of the adult spine. Skeletal Radiol 12:178, 1984.

Woolfitt R, Park H-M, Greene M: Localized cryptococcal osteomyelitis. Radiology 120:290, 1976.

Yousefzadeh DK, Jackson JH: Neonatal and infantile candidal arthritis with or without osteomyelitis: A clinical and radiographical review of 21 cases. Skeletal Radiol 5:77, 1980.

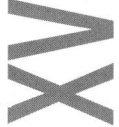
# CHAPTER 56

## Physical Injury: Concepts and Terminology

Donald Resnick and Thomas G. Goergen

## SUMMARY OF KEY FEATURES

In addition to such complications as reflex sympathetic dystrophy, osteolysis, osteonecrosis, many of the osteochondroses, neuropathic osteoarthropathy, heterotopic bone formation, and infection, physical trauma may lead to a variety of radiographic abnormalities. The radiographic characteristics of fractures in the various skeletal sites are explained on the basis of biomechanical principles. Special types of injuries include pathologic, stress, greenstick, torus, bowing, and transchondral fractures; trabecular microfractures; and osseous infractions accompanying subluxations and dislocations. The precise cause of osteochondritis dissecans is not clear, but trauma is suspected. Trauma to synovial joints may lead to synovitis, hemarthrosis, and lipohemarthrosis; trauma to symphyses may result in intraosseous cartilaginous displacement (cartilaginous nodes); trauma to synchondroses may cause variable patterns of acute or chronic growth plate injury; and trauma to supporting structures, syndesmoses, and entheses may lead to tendinous and ligamentous laceration and disruption, avulsion, and diastasis. A variety of skeletal muscle alterations are related to physiologic stress and acute or chronic injury. Characteristic skeletal abnormalities also appear in abused children.

## INTRODUCTION

Physical injury contributes to a wide variety of alterations in bones, joints, and soft tissues. In addition to fractures, dislocations, subluxations, and capsular, tendinous, muscular, and ligamentous tears, trauma can affect the growth plate of immature skeletons, as well as the hyaline cartilaginous and fibrocartilaginous joint structures. Further complications of trauma, covered in other chapters, include reflex sympathetic dystrophy, osteolysis, osteonecrosis, many of the osteochondroses, neuropathic osteoarthropathy, infection, and heterotopic bone formation. Trauma has also been implicated in the development of certain neoplasms, such as aneurysmal bone cysts. Nonmechanical trauma to the musculoskeletal system can result from thermal and electrical injury, irradiation, and chemical substances.

## DIAGNOSTIC TECHNIQUES

The sensitivity as well as the availability of conventional radiography has led to its routine use in the delineation of skeletal injuries. In the evaluation of trauma in children, comparison views provide important information in less than 5% of cases and should be obtained selectively. They are most useful in the evaluation of Salter-Harris type I growth plate injuries and in the assessment of bowing fractures and injuries about the elbow. In certain situations, radiographs obtained during the application of manual stress (i.e., stress radiography) can be effective in uncovering an articular injury that is not apparent on initial radiographs (Fig. 56–1). This technique is used most commonly for injuries to the acromioclavicular joint, knee, and ankle.

The role of computed tomography (CT) in the diagnosis of skeletal trauma is prominent. In general, this technique is able to define the presence and extent of certain fractures or dislocations; detect intra-articular abnormalities, including cartilage damage and osteocartilaginous bodies; and assess nearby soft tissues. Its application to traumatic abnormalities in regions of complicated anatomy, such as the spine, the bones in the face and pelvis, the glenohumeral and sternoclavicular joints, and the midfoot and hindfoot, is especially noteworthy (Fig. 56–2). Recent advances in CT scanning, such as helical scanning and three-dimensional reconstruction of image data, ensure rapid examination and vivid display of abnormalities, respectively.

After trauma to the musculoskeletal system, arteriography may be useful for the identification and possible treatment of vascular abnormalities, including disruption and occlusion of major vessels, arteriovenous fistulas, and aneurysms. Peripheral pulses may be palpable even with complete transection of an artery, however, and absent distal pulses may occur secondary to hypovolemia, pre-existing atherosclerosis, or vasospasm. The vessels that are injured most commonly are in close proximity to a bone and held in a relatively fixed position by fascial or muscular attachment; for example, the subclavian artery may be injured by the distal fragment of a clavicular fracture, or the axillary artery may be damaged in glenohumeral joint dislocations. Mechanisms leading to vascular injury include a tear from the presence of a sharp bone fragment, compression related to hematoma or swelling within a tight fascial compartment, a shearing type of injury, and entrapment in the fracture fragments with angulation and occlusion. Magnetic resonance (MR) angiography can be used as a substitute for arteriography in some patients.

Scintigraphy is useful in the evaluation of patients with skeletal trauma, particularly in the diagnosis of stress fractures. It also may be helpful in detecting subtle acute fractures when radiographs are normal or in excluding

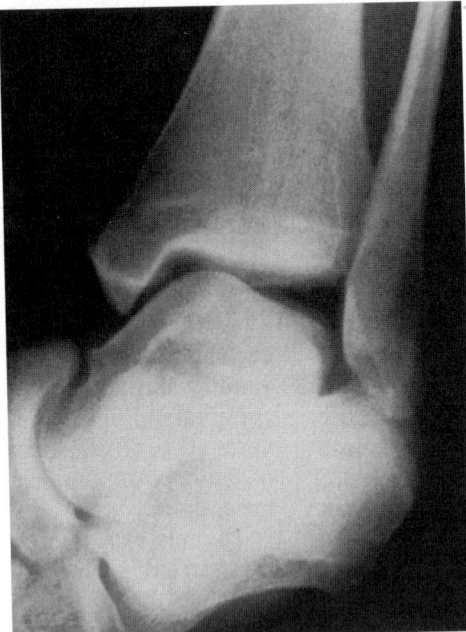

**Figure 56–1.** Physical injury: stress radiography. Injuries involving the ligaments about the ankle may not be detected on routine radiographs, but the application of manual stress may allow their detection. In this case, radiographs obtained during varus stress of the plantar-flexed foot clearly demonstrate displacement of the talus with respect to the tibia, indicative of an injury to the anterior talofibular ligament.

fractures in the presence of significant clinical findings. In addition, scintigraphy can be used to evaluate the healing response. The vast majority of fractures are detected by bone scintigraphy within hours of the injury, with some delay in the identification of scintigraphic abnormalities in older patients, particularly those with osteoporosis. The radionuclide alterations are not specific for fracture because they also occur in soft tissue, synovial, and ligamentous injuries. The minimal time required

for the bone scan to return to normal after fracture is about 5 to 7 months, and in 90% of cases, the scan is normal by 2 years after the injury.

The extreme sensitivity of MR imaging to bone (and cartilage) injury makes it an indispensable supplementary technique in trauma patients whose initial radiographs are either negative or have equivocal findings (Fig. 56–3). In this regard, MR imaging competes favorably with bone scintigraphy and single photon emission computed tomography (SPECT). The MR imaging examination is also well suited to the assessment of osteochondral and stress fractures. MR imaging is far better when used to evaluate a single region of the body, whereas bone scintigraphy is more effective as a general skeletal survey, which is important in cases of multiple injuries or child abuse.

## FRACTURES

### Epidemiology

The likelihood, location, and configuration of a fracture after an injury depend on a number of factors, including the age and sex of the person, the type and mechanism of the injury, and the presence of any predisposing factors that might alter the bones or soft tissues of the musculoskeletal system. Birth-related trauma in a newborn, sports-related activities in an adolescent or young adult, occupation-related stresses in a mature adult, and normal activities in the elderly are typical situations leading to skeletal injury.

### Terminology

Basically, a *fracture* is a break in the continuity of bone, cartilage, or both. Each fracture is associated with soft tissue injury, the character and degree of which have additional therapeutic implications. Alternatively, in an attempt to emphasize the soft tissue component, a fracture might be defined as a soft tissue injury with a break in bone or cartilage. A *transchondral fracture* is one that

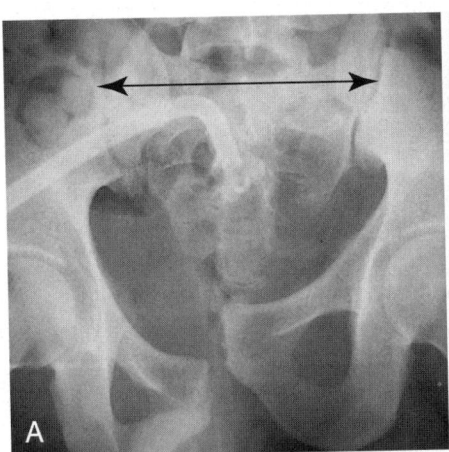
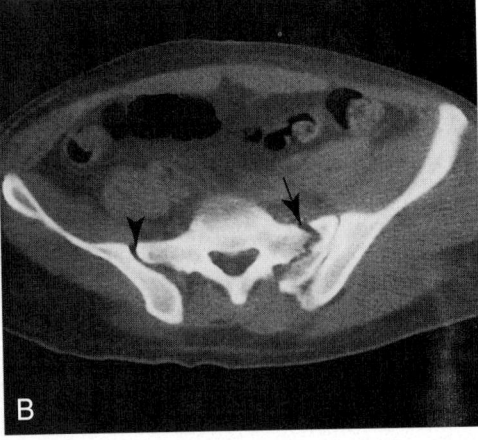

**Figure 56–2.** Physical injury: osseous pelvis. *Double-headed arrow* indicates the approximate level of the transaxial CT scan. Although the initial radiograph *(A)* shows symphyseal diastasis and a fracture of the sacrum *(arrow)*, the latter is better demonstrated with CT *(B)*, which also reveals diastasis of the contralateral sacroiliac joint with a vacuum phenomenon *(arrowhead)*.

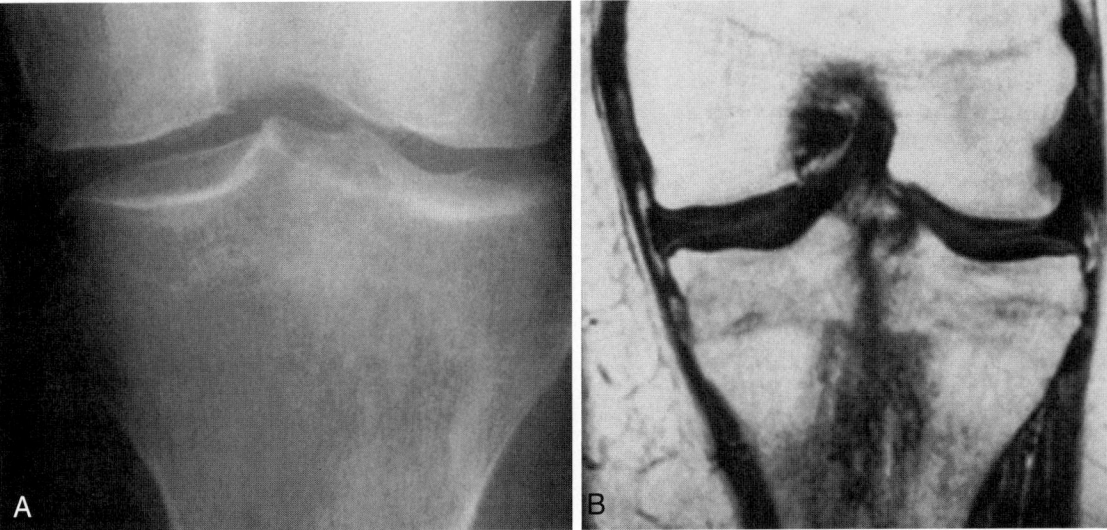

**Figure 56–3.** Physical injury: proximal portion of the tibia. *A*, Initial radiograph reveals minimal sclerosis beneath the tibial eminences but was interpreted as normal. *B*, Coronal T1-weighted (TR/TE, 750/20) spin echo MR image vividly displays the fracture.

involves a cartilaginous surface. If the cartilage alone is involved, the term *chondral fracture* is used; a fracture involving cartilage and subjacent bone is termed an *osteochondral fracture*.

In a *closed (simple) fracture*, the skin is intact and thus prevents communication between the fracture and the outside environment. An *open fracture* allows communication between the fracture and the outside environment because of the disruption of skin. Bone fragments may or may not protrude through the cutaneous defect. Although closed and open fractures are clinically distinguishable, specific findings accompanying an open fracture may be apparent on radiographs (Table 56–1). Open fractures have a higher rate of disturbances in healing, in part related to an increased frequency of infection.

A *complete fracture* occurs when the entire circumference of a tubular bone or both cortical surfaces of a flat bone have been disrupted. In an *incomplete fracture*, a break in the cortex does not extend completely through the bone. When angular deformity is present, the intact cortex may prevent satisfactory realignment. Incomplete fractures occur in the resilient elastic bones of children and young adults. They may be further classified into various types, including bowing, greenstick, and torus fractures. The descriptive nomenclature of fractures can be amplified by the use of terms denoting the direction of the fracture line with reference to the shaft (long bones) or cortex (irregular bones). Four basic types of linear fractures involving the shaft of a tubular bone are recognized: *transverse*, *oblique*, *oblique-transverse*, and *spiral*.

A *comminuted fracture* is one with more than two fracture fragments, regardless of the total number of such fragments. Comminuted fractures may result from a variety of different mechanisms, but in general, the greater the applied force and the more rapid its application, the greater the energy absorption by the bone and the more severe the comminution. *Crush fractures* result in severe comminution and associated soft tissue injury.

Certain distinctive subtypes of comminuted fractures exist. A *butterfly fragment* (Fig. 56–4) is a wedge-shaped fragment arising from the shaft of a long bone at the apex of the force input. A *segmental fracture* (Fig. 56–5) is one in which the fracture lines isolate a segment of the shaft of a tubular bone. Segmental fractures have special implications in terms of the adequacy of the blood supply and the healing rate.

The *alignment* of a fracture refers to the longitudinal relationship of one fragment to another. If no significant angulation is seen, the fracture is said to be in anatomic or near anatomic alignment. By convention, angulation of the distal fragment is described in relation to the proximal one. Such angulation may be medial or lateral, dorsal or ventral, or, in the forearm, radial or ulnar. *Varus* refers to angulation of the distal fracture fragment toward the midline of the body, and *valgus* refers to its angulation away from the midline (Fig. 56–6). Anterior angulation at the fracture site means that the apex of the fracture is directed anteriorly (ventrally). Conversely, posterior angulation at the fracture site indicates that the apex of the fracture site is directed posteriorly (dorsally).

Fracture *position* describes the relationship of the fracture fragments, exclusive of angulation, to the normal anatomic situation. Deviation from anatomic position is

---

**TABLE 56–1**

**Radiographic Signs of Open Fractures**

Soft tissue defect
Bone protruding beyond soft tissues
Subcutaneous or intra-articular gas
Foreign material beneath skin
Absent pieces of bone

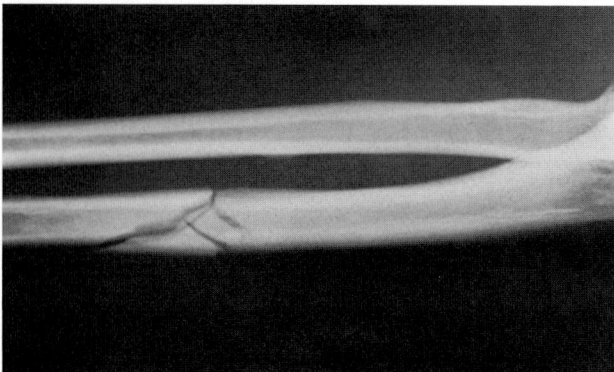

**Figure 56–4.** Butterfly fracture fragment. A comminuted fracture of the midportion of the shaft of the ulna contains a wedge-shaped butterfly fragment.

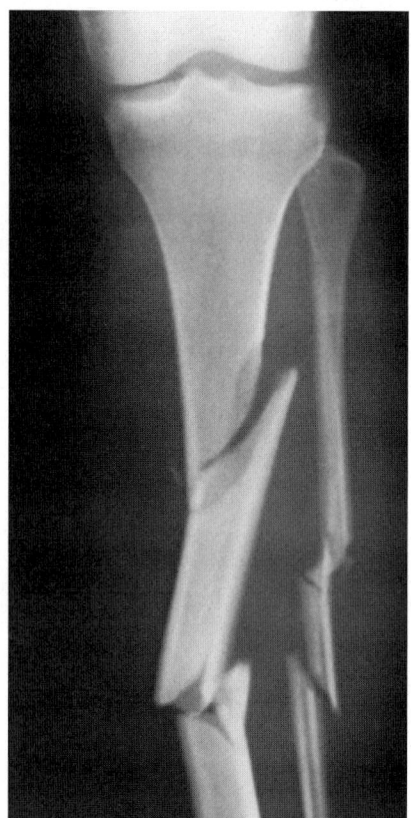

**Figure 56–5.** Segmental fracture. A segment of the shaft of the tibia and a portion of the fibula have been isolated in this injury.

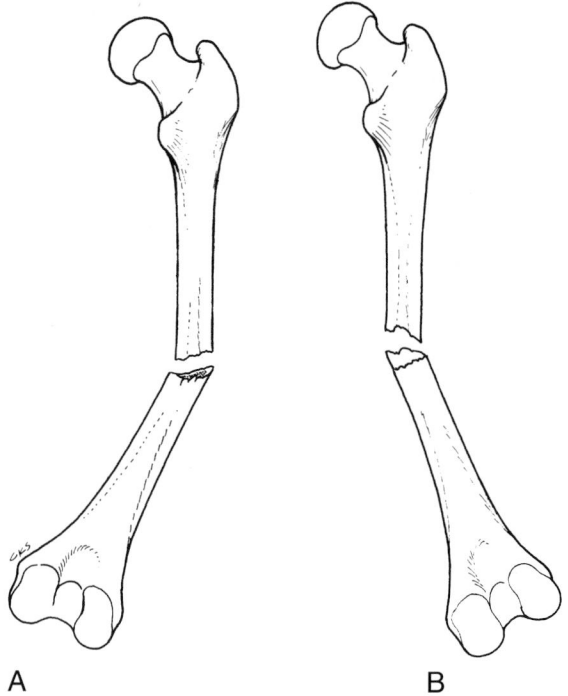

A                                                    B

**Figure 56–6.** Varus and valgus angulation. *A*, Varus angulation. The distal fragment is angulated toward the midline. *B*, Valgus angulation. The distal fragment is angulated away from the midline.

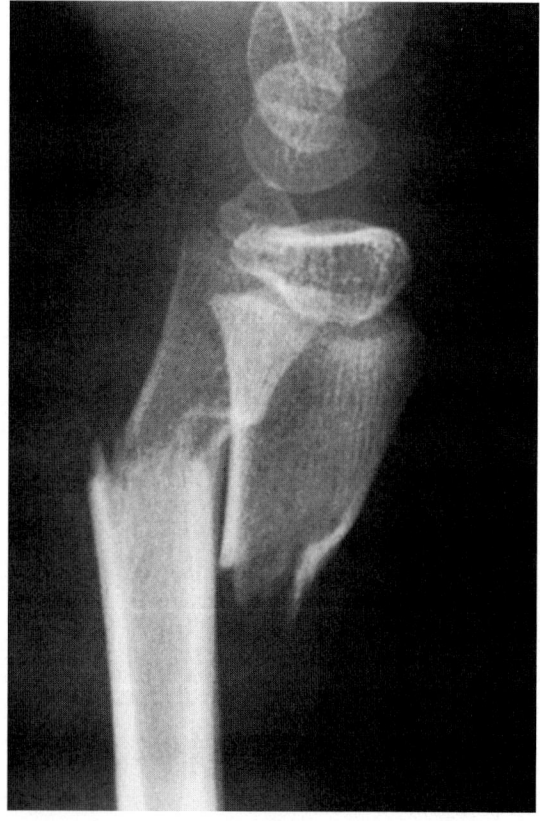

**Figure 56–7.** Bayonet deformity. Observe the fractures of the distal portions of the radius and ulna. The radial fragment is displaced dorsally with overriding—a bayonet deformity.

called *displacement*, which is described in terms of apposition and rotation. *Apposition* considers the degree of bone contact at the fracture site. A fracture with complete, or 100%, apposition is usually called undisplaced. Partial degrees of surface contact can be roughly quantitated by using percentages (e.g., 25%, 50%, or 75% apposition). If the fracture surfaces are separated, the amount of distraction can be measured. Overlapping fracture surfaces with resultant shortening are described as a bayonet deformity (Fig. 56–7). Visualization of *rotatory* displacement of a fracture (i.e., rotation about the long axis of a bone) is facilitated by including the joints both proximal and distal to the fracture on the film (Fig. 56–8).

An *avulsion fracture* occurs when an osseous fragment is pulled from the parent bone by a tendon or ligament (Fig. 56–9). An *impaction fracture* results when one fragment of bone is driven into an apposing fragment (Fig. 56–10). Two specific types of impaction fractures are recognized. A *depression fracture* results when the impacting forces occur between one hard (i.e., stronger) bone surface and an apposing softer (i.e., weaker) surface. A *compression fracture* is a type of impaction fracture characteristically involving the vertebral bodies (Fig. 56–11).

## Fracture Healing

After a fracture, a remarkable series of events takes place that leads to osseous healing in most cases (Fig. 56–12). Three indistinctly separated phases of healing are recognized: an inflammatory phase (representing approximately 10% of the entire healing time), a reparative phase (about 40%), and a remodeling phase (the longest phase, accounting for 50% to as much as 70% of healing time). Initially, bleeding takes place from the damaged ends of the bones and from the neighboring soft tissues. Formation of a hematoma within the medullary canal, between the frac-

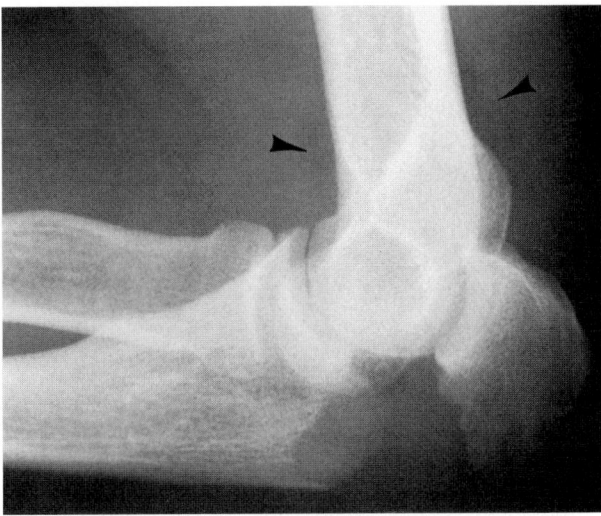

**Figure 56–9.** Avulsion fracture. The triceps tendon is attached to the large fracture fragment. A joint effusion is noted *(arrowheads)*.

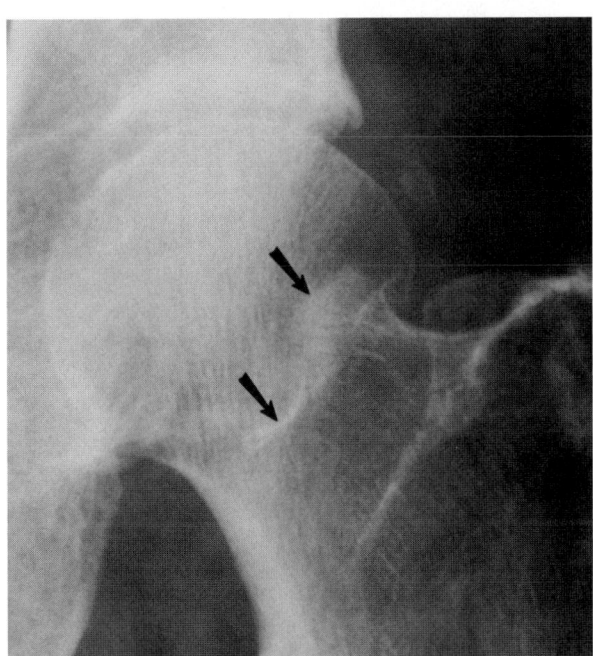

**Figure 56–10.** Impaction fracture. A sclerotic line extends across the lateral aspect of the subcapital region *(arrows)*.

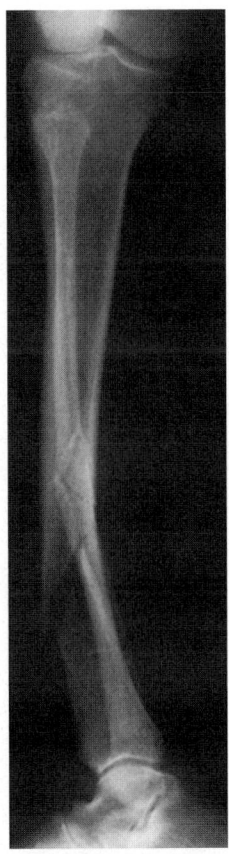

**Figure 56–8.** Rotatory displacement. Radiograph of the lower portion of the leg reveals that the knee is in an oblique position and the ankle is in a lateral attitude. Fractures of the shafts of the tibia and fibula are observed, with marked lateral rotation of the distal fragments.

ture ends, and beneath the elevated periosteum is followed by clot formation. This leads to an intense, acute inflammatory response. The reparative phase begins with organization of the fracture hematoma and invasion by fibrovascular tissue, which replaces the clot and lays down the collagen fibers and matrix that will later become mineralized to form the woven bone of the provisional or primary callus. Callus envelops the bone ends rapidly and thereby produces increasing stability at the fracture site. During the process of repair, a remodeling phase can also be identified; this phase is associated with resorption of unnecessary segments of callus and proliferation of trabeculae along lines of stress.

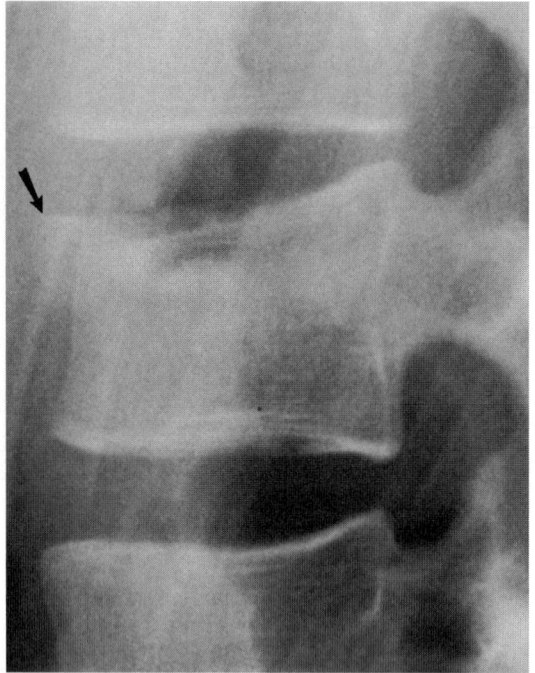

**Figure 56–11.** Compression fracture. A compression fracture of the superior surface of the second lumbar vertebral body is present, with a small comminuted corner fragment (*arrow*).

Many local factors can modify the healing process: degree of trauma, degree of bone loss, type of bone involved, extent of immobilization, presence of infection, presence of an underlying pathologic process, use of radiation therapy, presence of extensive osteonecrosis, and occurrence of intra-articular extension. Systemic factors such as the age of the patient and the presence of abnormal serum levels of certain hormones can also be influential in fracture repair.

In some instances, the healing process is markedly slowed (*delayed union*) or arrested altogether (*nonunion*). Because the rate of fracture healing depends on many local and systemic factors, no definition of delayed union has been uniformly accepted, although clinical application of the term implies that the healing attempt is proceeding. Nonunion generally indicates that the fracture site has failed to heal completely during a period of approximately 6 to 9 months after the injury and that a typical *pseudarthrosis* (consisting of a synovium-lined cavity and synovial fluid, typically related to persistent motion at the nonunion site) or fibrous union has developed. Nonunion of fractures may occur with or without the formation of a pseudarthrosis. Nonunion of scaphoid, tibial, and femoral fractures is encountered most commonly (Fig. 56–13). Nonunion of a type 2 odontoid fracture leads to an os odontoideum. Delayed union and nonunion of fractures should be distinguished from *malunion*. A malunited fracture is one that has healed in an improper position (e.g., excessive angular or rotational deformity). Malunion of a fracture in a child may be a temporary phenomenon that spontaneously disappears with further skeletal growth.

## Special Types of Fractures

### Pathologic Fractures

A pathologic fracture is one in which the bone is disrupted at a site of preexisting abnormality, frequently by a stress that would not have fractured a normal bone. Any

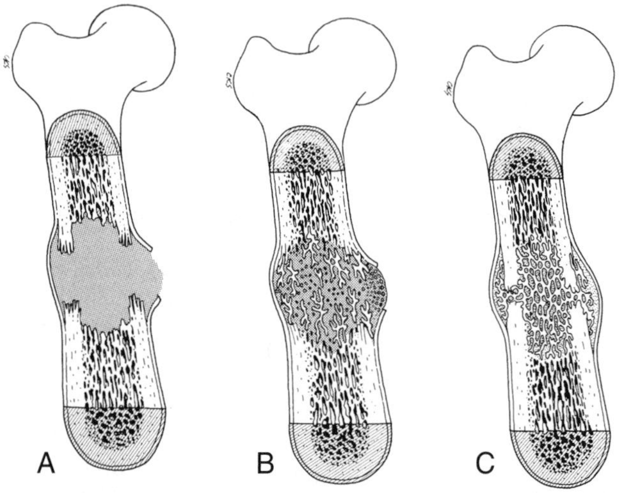

**Figure 56–12.** Normal fracture healing. *A*, After the injury, bleeding is related to osseous and soft tissue damage. A hematoma, followed by clot formation, develops within the medullary canal between the fracture ends and beneath the periosteal membrane, which may have been torn. *B*, Callus formation takes place and consists of external bridging callus at the periosteal surface, intramedullary callus, and primary callus at the ends of the fracture fragments. *C*, Callus envelops the bone ends rapidly and produces increasing stability at the fracture site.

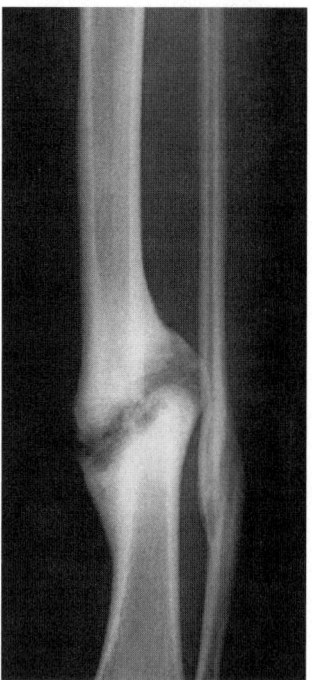

**Figure 56–13.** Abnormal fracture healing: nonunion in the tibia. Classic hypertrophic nonunion is evident. Prominent external callus and irregular bone ends are seen. The adjacent fibular fracture has healed.

process that weakens the osseous tissue structurally can result in a pathologic fracture. Of the tumorous causes of pathologic fracture, skeletal metastasis predominates. Radiographic distinction between a pathologic and a nonpathologic fracture is not always easy. Such differentiation is not difficult, however, when a fracture line traverses a large area of osseous destruction or when the adjacent or distant bones are riddled with additional lesions (Fig. 56–14). When a smaller lesion is present, the fracture itself may obscure the area of lysis or sclerosis, especially in the presence of displacement at the fracture site. The absence of a history of trauma or fracture pain and the presence of symptoms and signs of a preexisting abnormality, such as angular deformity, painless swelling, or generalized bone pain, are clinical aids to the diagnosis of a pathologic fracture. Diagnostic difficulty may be encountered in a patient who has a nonpathologic fracture that is days to weeks old, because resorption, osteolysis, or rotation about the fracture site may create the illusion of an underlying lesion.

## Trabecular Microfractures (Bone Bruises)

The use of MR imaging to evaluate musculoskeletal injuries has led to the identification of intraosseous regions of altered signal intensity, which have been designated occult intraosseous fractures or bone bruises. These injuries, which are typically located close to a joint surface, are believed to result from compression or impaction forces. It appears likely that the trabecular alterations that characterize a bone bruise are very similar, if not identical, to those associated with stress fractures. Resolution of the MR imaging abnormalities associated with bone bruises generally occurs over one to several months and may coincide with a decrease in or disappearance of the patient's symptoms.

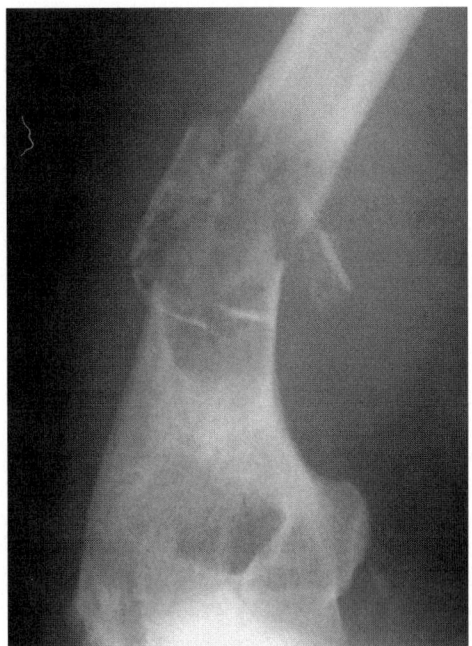

**Figure 56–14.** Pathologic fracture. Transverse fracture line through a metastatic focus from renal cell carcinoma can be detected in the distal portion of the humerus. Note the osteolysis and cortical irregularity.

The characteristics of these trabecular microfractures on MR images are remarkably constant and are those of marrow fluid, with regions of low signal intensity on T1-weighted spin echo MR images and regions of high signal intensity on T2-weighted spin echo and short tau inversion recovery (STIR) images. Bone bruises are displayed most prominently on STIR images (Fig. 56–15), which may lead to overestimation of their size, and they may be

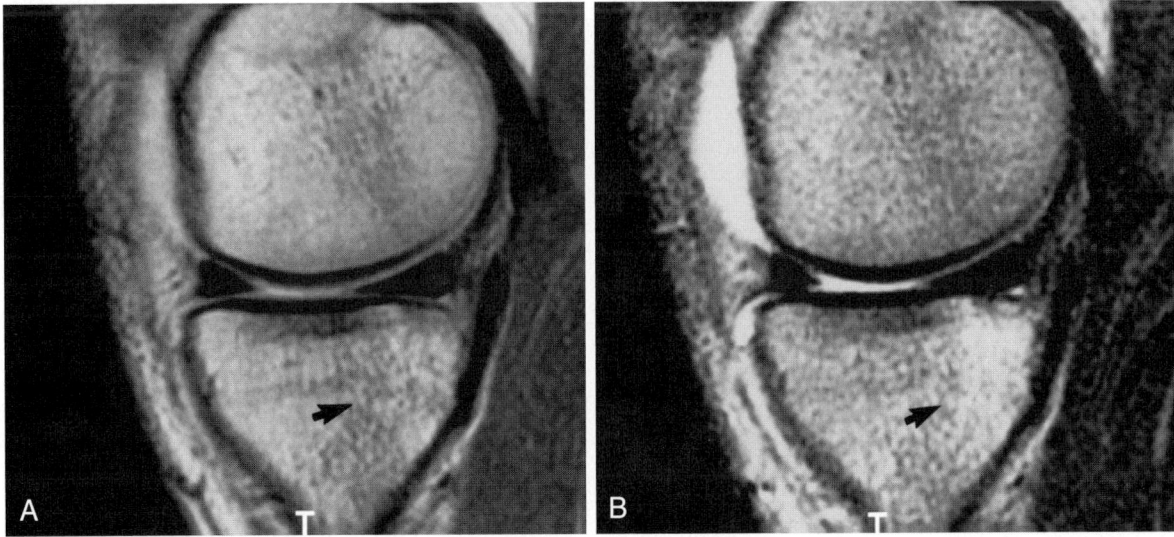

**Figure 56–15.** Trabecular microfracture (bone bruise). Sagittal intermediate-weighted (TR/TE, 2200/30) *(A)* and T2-weighted (TR/TE, 2200/80) *(B)* spin echo MR images show the characteristic finding of a bone bruise *(arrows)*, which in this case involves mainly the posterior portion of the medial tibial plateau. The lesion is of high signal intensity in *(B)*. Note the joint effusion.

vividly apparent when fat-suppression techniques are used with or without the intravenous administration of a gadolinium contrast agent. The detection of bone bruises at specific anatomic sites provides secondary evidence that other injuries may be present; examples include the occurrence of bone bruises in the lateral femoral condyle and posterolateral portion of the tibia in patients with injuries to the anterior cruciate ligament, bone bruises in the lateral femoral condyle in persons with injuries to the medial collateral ligament of the knee, and bone bruises in the lateral femoral condyle and medial portion of the patella in patients with lateral patellar dislocation.

## Stress Fractures

Stress fractures can occur in normal or abnormal bone that is subjected to repeated cyclic loading with a load less than that which causes acute fracture of bone. Two types of stress fracture are recognized: *fatigue fracture*, which results from the application of abnormal stress or torque on a bone with normal elastic resistance, and *insufficiency fracture*, which occurs when normal stress is placed on a bone with deficient elastic resistance.

Fatigue fractures frequently share the following features: the activity is new or different for the person, the activity is strenuous, and the activity is repeated with a frequency that ultimately produces symptoms and signs. Fatigue fractures are relatively common in athletes and military recruits undergoing basic training; they are especially frequent in runners and ballet dancers, and their sites of involvement can often be predicted by an analysis of the specific sporting activity. Typical examples are the fatigue fractures that occur in the metatarsal bones of military recruits ("march" fractures) and in the lower extremities in athletes, joggers, and dancers.

The causes of insufficiency fractures are diverse and include rheumatoid arthritis, osteoporosis, Paget's disease, osteomalacia or rickets, hyperparathyroidism, renal osteodystrophy, osteogenesis imperfecta, osteopetrosis, fibrous dysplasia, and irradiation. Of these causes, rheumatoid arthritis and osteoporosis are most common (Fig. 56–16). Fatigue and insufficiency fractures are not infrequent after certain surgical procedures that result in altered stress or an imbalance of muscular force on normal or abnormal bones. Common examples are noted in the metatarsal bones after bunion surgery and in the lower extremities after arthrodesis or arthroplasty.

Although routine radiography plays an essential role in the diagnosis of stress fractures, radionuclide examination is one means of early detection (Fig. 56–17). The finding of abnormal scintigraphic patterns in athletic individuals in whom stress fractures do not subsequently develop has led to a redefinition of some osseous stress injuries. A shin splint is one of these conditions. In patients with shin splints, radionuclide angiograms and blood pool images are normal, whereas on delayed images, a longitudinally oriented area of increased radionuclide accumulation is seen in the posteromedial cortex of the tibia (Fig. 56–18). This pattern of abnormality differs from that typically seen in an acute stress fracture (in which all phases of the radionuclide examination are abnormal and a more fusiform area of augmented activity

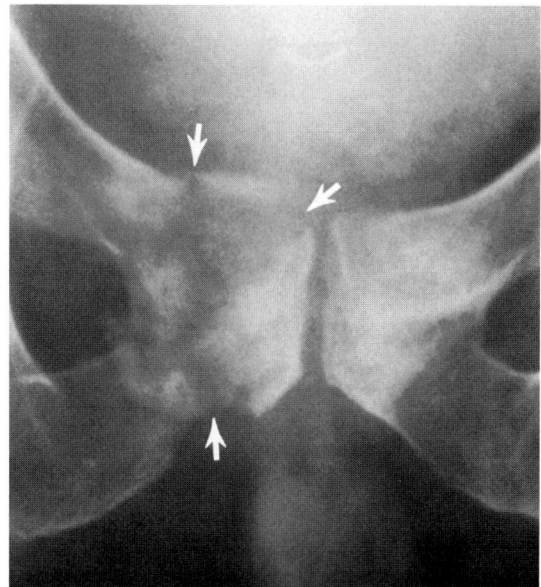

**Figure 56–16.** Insufficiency fracture: rheumatoid arthritis and osteoporosis. In parasymphyseal bone, such fractures *(arrows)* are accompanied by osteolysis, osteosclerosis, and bone fragmentation.

is apparent) and is consistent with the belief that shin splints represent periosteal disruptions of varying length, possibly caused by the rupture of Sharpey's fibers that extend from the muscle through the periosteum into the cortical structure of bone.

MR imaging has comparable sensitivity and superior specificity with respect to bone scintigraphy in the assessment of stress fractures. Stress fractures typically appear as a linear zone of low signal intensity surrounded by a broader, poorly defined area of slightly higher (though still low) signal intensity on T1-weighted spin echo MR images and as a linear area of low signal intensity surrounded by a broader region of high signal intensity on T2-weighted spin echo images (Fig. 56–19). High signal intensity on STIR images and after the intravenous administration of a gadolinium contrast agent may also be observed. The fracture line may or may not be evident. Soft tissue edema may be an associated feature.

The clinical findings of stress fractures are characteristic. Activity-related pain that is relieved by rest is typical. Localized tenderness and soft tissue swelling may also be observed. The specific site of involvement is influenced by the type of physical activity engaged in. The bones in the lower extremity are affected more frequently than those in the upper extremity. More than one site can be involved simultaneously, more than one stress fracture can occur in a single bone, and symmetrical changes are not unusual. The radiographic abnormalities are influenced by the location of the fracture and the interval between the time of injury and the radiographic examination. In a diaphysis, a linear cortical radiolucent area is frequently associated with periosteal and endosteal cortical thickening (Fig. 56–20). In some cases, multiple radiolucent striations that extend partially or completely across the cortex are seen. In an epiphyseal or metaphyseal location or in a cancellous area, focal sclerosis repre-

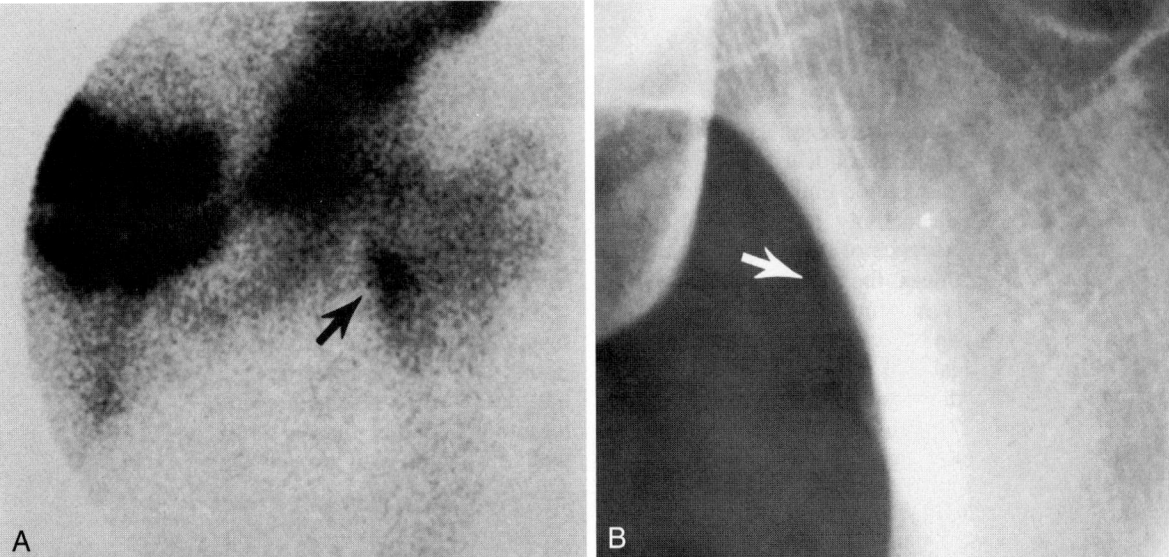

**Figure 56–17.** Stress fracture. This athletic young woman complained of persistent hip pain aggravated by activity. *A*, Radionuclide examination reveals a focal, sharply marginated area of increased activity in the femoral neck *(arrow)*. *B*, Radiograph of the hip delineates a minimal amount of indistinct new bone formation along the medial aspect of the femoral neck *(arrow)*.

senting condensation of trabeculae is the typical finding, and periostitis is not prominent (Fig. 56–21). With healing at either site, the sclerosis may become more diffuse, and eventually, it and the fracture line can disappear.

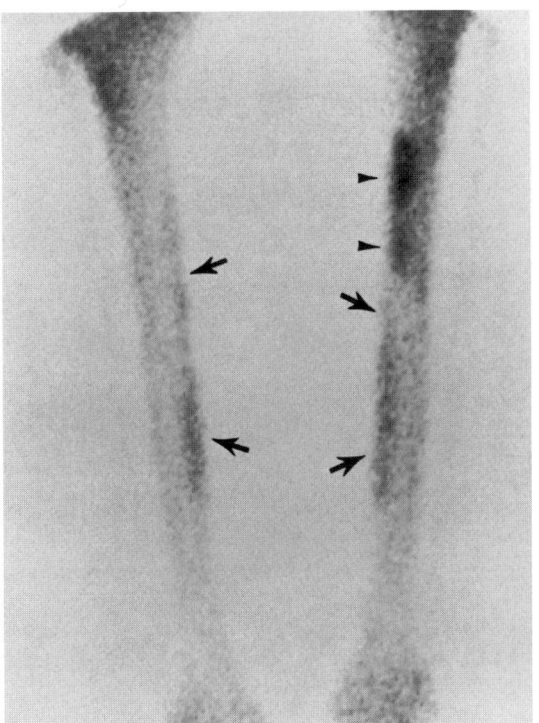

**Figure 56–18.** Stress changes: shin splints. On a frontal view of the lower legs during the delayed portion of a bone scan, longitudinally oriented areas of increased tracer accumulation are apparent in the medial cortex of the midportion of the tibias *(arrows)*. Two localized areas of increased radionuclide activity in the left tibia *(arrowheads)* may represent stress fractures.

Specific examples of activities that cause stress fractures are listed in Table 56–2.

**Calcaneal or Other Tarsal Stress Fracture.** Fatigue fractures of the calcaneus are not uncommon in military recruits, and insufficiency fractures in this site can accompany rheumatoid arthritis, neurologic disorders, and other diseases (Fig. 56–22). Stress fractures in other tarsal bones are less common. Those in the tarsal navicular bone have been observed in physically active persons, especially basketball players and runners (Fig. 56–23).

**Fibular Stress Fracture.** Changing muscular stress can result in a "runner's fracture." Jumping can also produce fibular stress fractures; classically, the proximal portion of the bone is affected in jumping, whereas the distal portion may be altered in running.

**Tibial Stress Fracture.** Stress fractures of the proximal diaphysis of the tibia can occur during running, particularly in children (Fig. 56–24), and stress fractures of the middle and distal tibial diaphysis can occur during long-distance running, marching, and ballet dancing. The posteromedial portion of the cortex is affected more frequently than the anterolateral portion. Shin splints are one cause of the medial tibial stress syndrome, and the resulting pain is more diffuse than that of a stress fracture. Bone scintigraphy and MR imaging allow an accurate differential diagnosis.

**Femoral Stress Fracture.** Stress fractures of the shaft or neck of the femur can result from numerous activities, including long-distance running, ballet dancing, and marching. Two types of stress fracture of the femoral neck are described: the transverse (or tensile) type is more frequent in older patients, appears as a small radiolucent area in the superior aspect of the femoral neck,

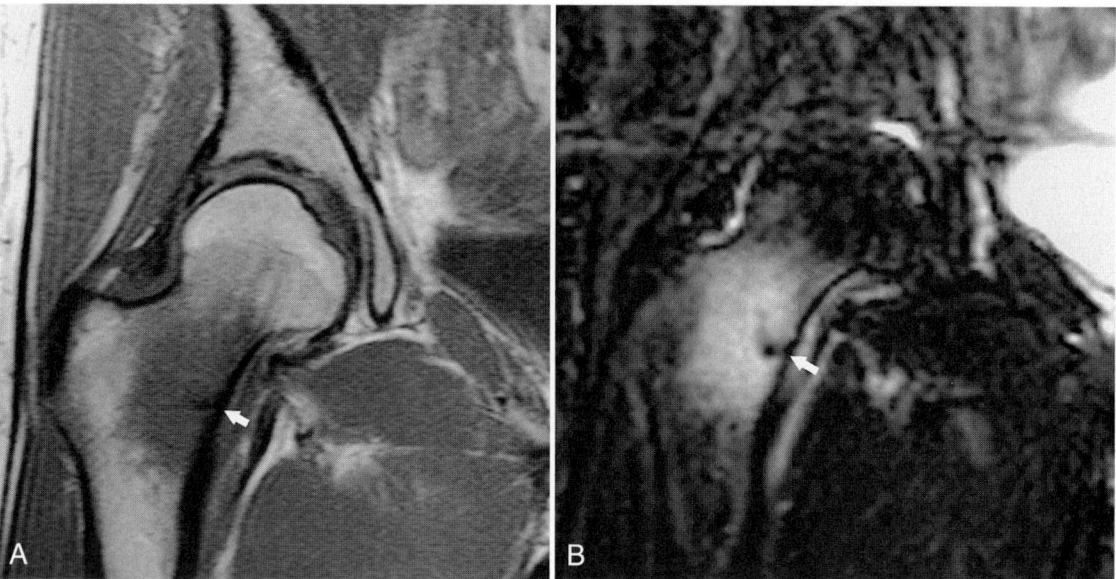

**Figure 56–19.** Stress fracture: fatigue fracture of the femur in a runner. Coronal T1-weighted (TR/TE, 634/16) spin echo *(A)* and STIR (TR/TE, 3940/72; inversion time, 150 msec) *(B)* images show a linear focus of decreased signal *(arrows)*, representing sclerosis, with surrounding edema.

and becomes displaced in some situations; the compression type is more common in younger patients, appears as a haze of callus in the inferior aspect of the neck, and is stable in most cases (Fig. 56–25).

**Metatarsal Stress Fracture.** The metatarsal bones are frequent sites of stress fracture, which may be caused by marching, ballet dancing, prolonged standing, foot deformities, and surgical resection of adjacent metatarsal bones. The middle and distal portions of the shafts of the second and third metatarsal bones are affected most often, but any metatarsal bone can be involved. In the first metatarsal, the base of the bone is altered, and periostitis, a frequent finding at other metatarsal sites, is relatively uncommon (Fig. 56–26). Occasionally, stress fractures involve the metatarsal heads and lead to sclerosis and flattening of subchondral bone, findings resemble those of Freiberg's infraction.

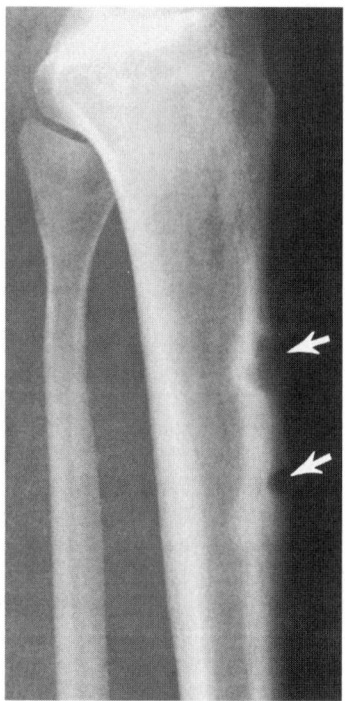

**Figure 56–20.** Stress fracture: radiographic abnormalities in diaphyses. Note the irregular radiolucent areas *(arrows)* in the anterior cortex of the proximal portion of the tibia. Periosteal and endosteal new bone formation about the fractures is evident. (Courtesy of M. Dalinka, MD, Philadelphia, Pa.)

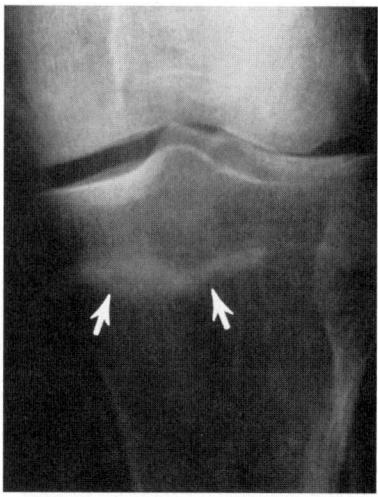

**Figure 56–21.** Stress fracture: radiographic abnormalities in metaphyses and epiphyses. Bandlike focal sclerosis *(arrows)* is typical of a stress fracture in the proximal portion of the tibia.

### TABLE 56-2

#### Activities That Lead to Stress Fractures at Specific Locations

| Location | Activity or Event |
|---|---|
| Sesamoids of metatarsal bones | Prolonged standing |
| Metatarsal shaft | Marching, stamping on ground, prolonged standing, ballet, sequelae of bunionectomy |
| Navicular | Stamping on ground, marching, long-distance running |
| Calcaneus | Jumping, parachuting, prolonged standing, recent immobilization |
| Tibia: Midshaft and distal shaft | Long-distance running |
| Proximal shaft (children) | Running |
| Fibula: Distal shaft | Long-distance running |
| Proximal shaft | Jumping, parachuting |
| Patella | Hurdling |
| Femur: Shaft | Ballet, long-distance running |
| Neck | Ballet, marching, long-distance running, gymnastics |
| Pelvis: Obturator ring | Stooping, bowling, gymnastics |
| Lumbar vertebra (pars interarticularis) | Ballet, lifting heavy objects scrubbing floors |
| Lower cervical, upper thoracic spinous process | Clay shoveling |
| Ribs | Carrying a heavy pack, golfing, rowing, coughing, sequelae of radical neck surgery |
| Clavicle | Sequelae of radical neck surgery |
| Coracoid of scapula | Trapshooting |
| Humerus: Distal shaft | Thowing a ball |
| Ulna: Coronoid | Pitching a ball |
| Shaft | Pitchfork work, propelling a wheelchair |
| Hook of hamate | Holding a golf club, tennis racquet, baseball bat |

Modified from Daffner RH: Stress fractures: Current concept. Skeletal Radiol 2:221, 1978.

**Pubic Rami and Symphysis Stress Fracture.** Stress fractures of the pubic arch and parasymphyseal bone are encountered in pregnant women, joggers, long-distance runners, and marathoners. Similar fractures occur in patients with osteoarthritis of the hip, those who have undergone hip arthroplasty, and patients in whom extensive removal of bone graft material about the sacroiliac joint has led to ligamentous disruption, as well as after irradiation and in association with osteoporosis and rheumatoid arthritis (Fig. 56–27). Complications of such stress fractures include osteolysis simulating malignancy (see Fig. 56–16).

**Other Pelvic Stress Fractures.** Although fatigue fractures of the sacrum have been described in children, athletes, and pregnant women, the occurrence of insufficiency fractures of the sacrum and other pelvic sites in patients

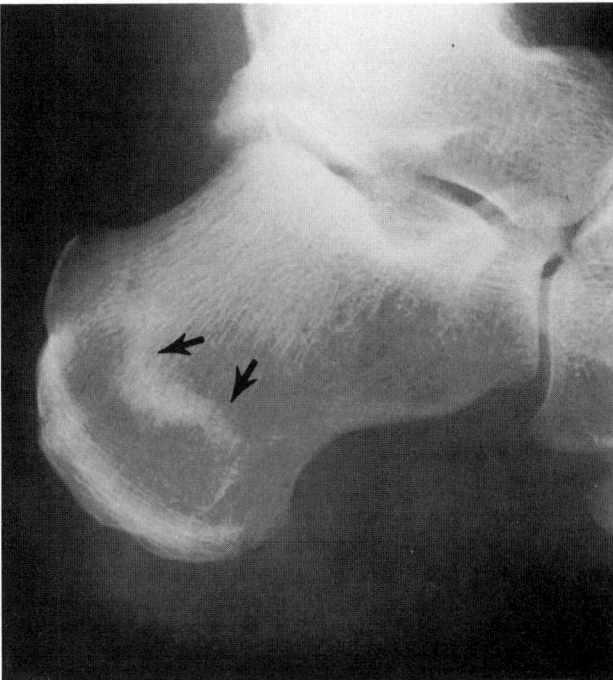

**Figure 56–22.** Calcaneal stress fracture. Note the meandering, vertically oriented sclerotic line *(arrows)*. An examination performed 2 months earlier was normal.

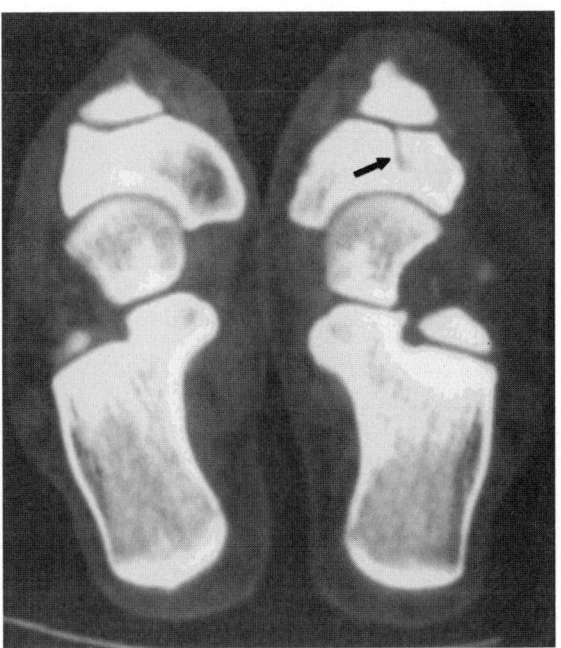

**Figure 56–23.** Tarsal navicular stress fracture. In a professional basketball player, direct transverse CT scan shows a stress fracture in the tarsal navicular bone that has progressed to a complete fracture *(arrows)*. (Courtesy of L. Rogers, MD, Winston-Salem, N.C.)

with postmenopausal or senile osteoporosis or rheumatoid arthritis and in those who have received corticosteroid medications or radiation therapy has been given far more emphasis (Fig. 56–28). Sacral insufficiency fractures may lead to significant clinical manifestations that

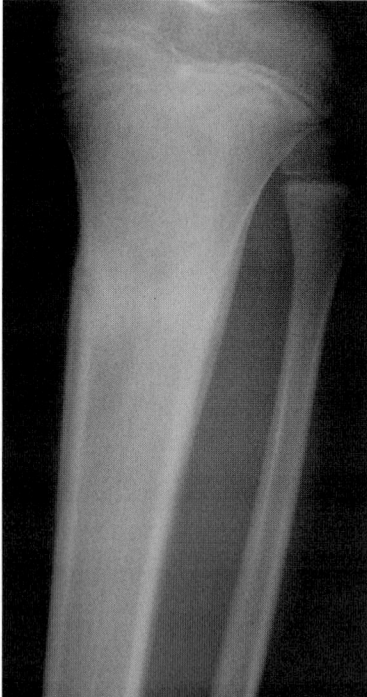

**Figure 56–24.** Tibial stress fracture. In this 12-year-old boy, observe a band of sclerosis across the proximal metadiaphysis of the bone, along with periostitis. (Courtesy of K. Van Lom, MD, San Diego, Calif.)

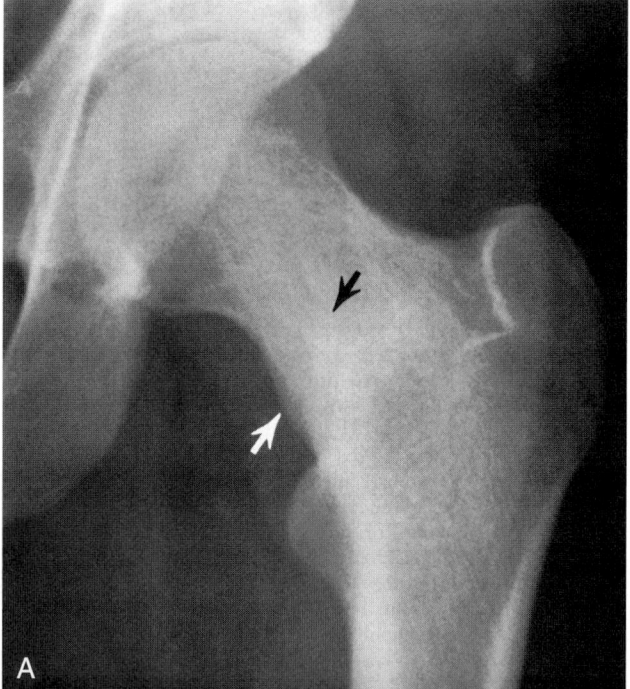

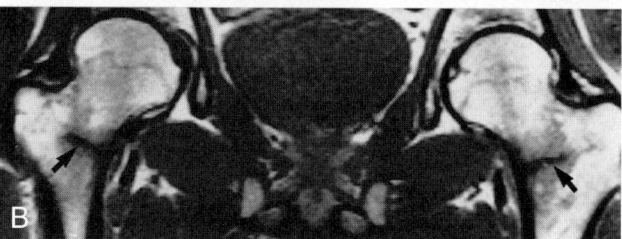

**Figure 56–25.** Femoral neck stress fracture. *A,* In the medial portion of the femoral neck, observe the presence of buttressing and sclerosis *(arrows).* *B,* Coronal intermediate-weighted (TR/TE, 2000/20) spin echo MR image reveals bilateral fatigue fractures *(arrows)* in the medial portion of the femoral neck. The fracture itself and the surrounding marrow edema are of low signal intensity.

simulate the findings associated with skeletal metastasis, including sciatica and severe low back or groin pain. Sacral insufficiency fractures involve one or both sides of the bone, with vertical fracture lines typically located close to the sacroiliac joint or joints. These vertically oriented fractures may lead to subtle interruption of the superior cortical surface or arcuate lines of the sacrum. Horizontal fracture lines may also be evident. Bone scintigraphy reveals the accumulation of radionuclide at the fracture

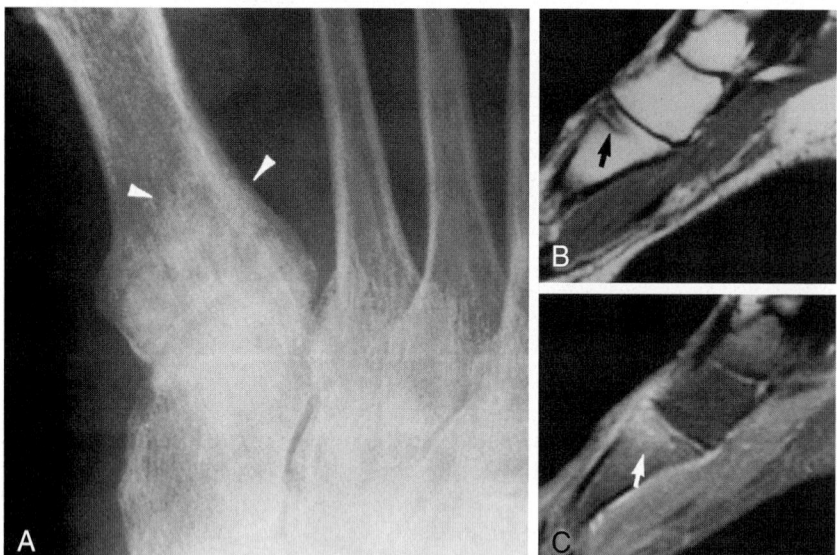

**Figure 56–26.** First metatarsal stress fracture. *A,* Note patchy bone sclerosis *(arrowheads).* The findings are compatible with an insufficiency type of stress fracture. *B,* In a different patient, sagittal T1-weighted (TR/TE, 650/20) spin echo MR image shows a stress fracture *(arrow)* involving the dorsal aspect of the base of the first metatarsal bone. *C,* In the same patient as in *(B),* corresponding fat-saturated T1-weighted (TR/TE, 415/15) spin echo image following contrast reveals enhancement in the bone and soft tissues *(arrow).*

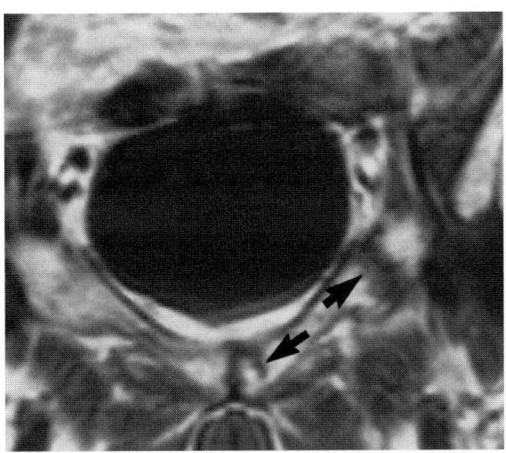

**Figure 56–27.** Pubic rami stress fracture. In this 80-year-old man, coronal T1-weighted (TR/TE, 600/11) spin echo MR image shows two fractures (*arrows*) appearing as linear regions of low signal intensity in the iliopubic bone column of the pelvis. (Courtesy of S. K. Brahme, MD, La Jolla, Calif.)

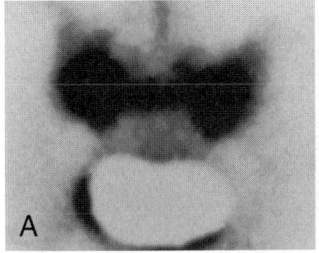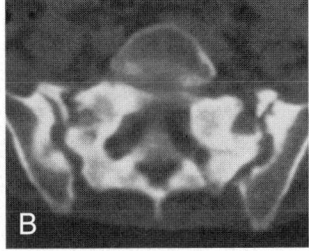

**Figure 56–28.** Sacral stress fracture. The typical imaging features of insufficiency fractures of the sacrum, as shown in this 65-year-old woman, include an "H" pattern of radionuclide uptake on a bone scan (*A*) and comminuted fracture lines with sclerosis on transaxial CT (*B*). In this case, the ilium adjacent to both sacroiliac joints is also involved. (Courtesy of G. Greenway, MD, Dallas, Tex.)

sites, sometimes producing an "H" pattern of increased radiotracer uptake in the sacrum (see Fig. 56–28). The transaxial displays provided by CT and MR imaging are well suited to the detection of sacral insufficiency fractures. MR images usually reveal low signal intensity in the involved marrow on T1-weighted spin echo images and high signal intensity in this marrow on T2-weighted spin echo images. Sacral insufficiency fractures may occur as an isolated finding, although they are frequently associated with other insufficiency fractures of the pelvis, including the ischium, para-acetabular bone, ilium, para-symphyseal locations, and acetabular roof.

**Upper Extremity Stress Fracture.** These fractures are far less frequent than stress fractures in the bones of the lower extremity. Typical sites include the coracoid process of the scapula in trap shooters; the acromion of the scapula in golfers; the ulna in bowlers, tennis players, baseball pitchers, and golfers; the hook of the hamate in

tennis players, golfers, and baseball players; the olecranon process in baseball pitchers and javelin throwers; the phalangeal tufts in guitar players; the phalanges of the hand in bowlers; and the inferior edge of the glenoid fossa in baseball pitchers.

**Stress Fracture of the Neural Arch of the Vertebra (Spondylolysis).** Spondylolysis represents a defect in the pars interarticularis of the vertebra. It may or may not be associated with slippage of one vertebral body onto the adjacent one; this slippage is termed spondylolisthesis. Spondylolysis is observed most frequently in the lumbar region of the spine, with the fifth lumbar vertebra most commonly affected (approximately 67% of cases); the frequency diminishes as one proceeds cephalad. It has been estimated that 3% to 7% of vertebral columns reveal at least one area of spondylolysis. The frequency of spondylolysis appears to be greater in athletes, particularly those involved in gymnastics, diving, weightlifting, pole-vaulting, and American football. Typically, spondylolysis is discovered in childhood or early adulthood. The cause of lumbar spondylolysis has long been debated, although the current consensus strongly supports an acquired traumatic lesion originating sometime between infancy and early adulthood.

Spondylolysis is usually evident on a lateral radiographic projection; however, oblique views are particularly helpful. The spine has a "Scottie dog" appearance on oblique projections (Fig. 56–29). A unilateral or bilateral radiolucent area through the neck of the "Scottie dog" is well demonstrated. Reactive sclerosis about the radiolucent band may be seen, although true callus is unusual. Wedging and hypoplasia of the fifth lumbar vertebra in association with spondylolysis may create a radiographic appearance of spondylolisthesis even when true slippage is not present. In cases of unilateral spondylolysis, hypertrophy and reactive sclerosis, as well as fracture of the contralateral pedicle and lamina, may be detected as a physiologic response to the presence of an unstable neural arch (Fig. 56–30). Scintigraphy (including SPECT) allows the detection of more recently acquired and symptomatic spondylolysis; such defects accumulate the bone-seeking radiotracer, whereas older and nonsymptomatic spondylolysis does not.

CT has been used to delineate areas of spondylolysis. On transaxial scans, it may be difficult to differentiate the defect in the pars interarticularis from the nearby apophyseal joint unless serial images are studied carefully. Multiplanar reconstruction of the image data aids in this differentiation and distinguishing foraminal encroachment and indentation of the neural canal from soft tissue or bone callus formation. CT also allows the detection of other clefts and fractures in the neural arch that are rarer than those in the pars interarticularis (Fig. 56–31). MR imaging is more suited to the assessment of some of the complications of spondylolysis, such as spondylolisthesis, nerve root impingement, and disc degeneration and extrusion. The sagittal plane is more useful than the transaxial plane in demonstrating the entire pars interarticularis. A cortical defect or cortical discontinuity is a reliable MR imaging finding of spondylolysis, but it is shown equally well by CT.

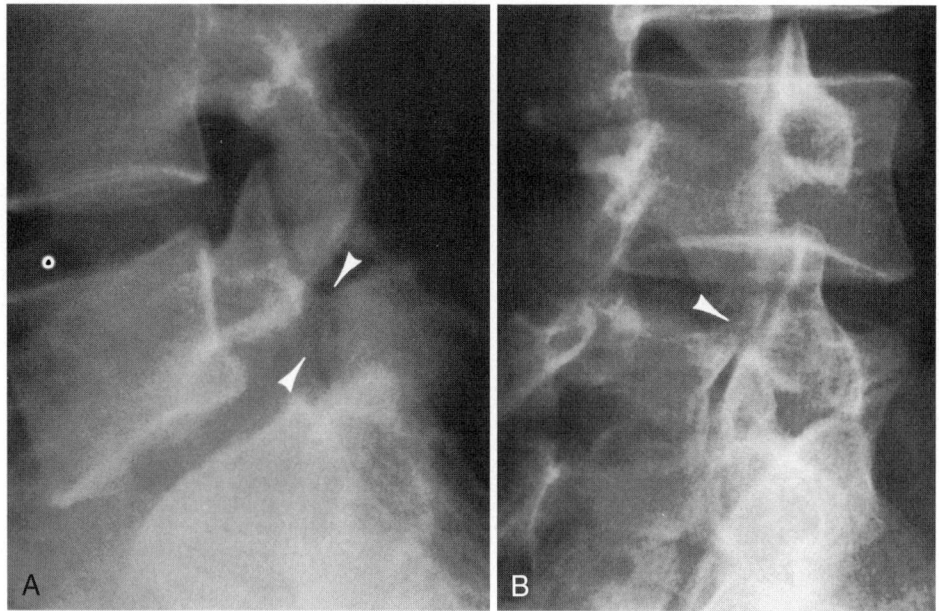

**Figure 56–29.** Spondylolysis in the lumbar spine: L5. Lateral *(A)* and left posterior oblique *(B)* projections reveal a defect through the pars interarticularis *(arrowheads)*. The spine has a "Scottie dog" appearance on oblique views. The resulting lucent lesion has produced a break in the "neck" of the "Scottie dog" in the oblique projection. Grade I spondylolisthesis of L5 on S1 can be noted on the lateral radiograph.

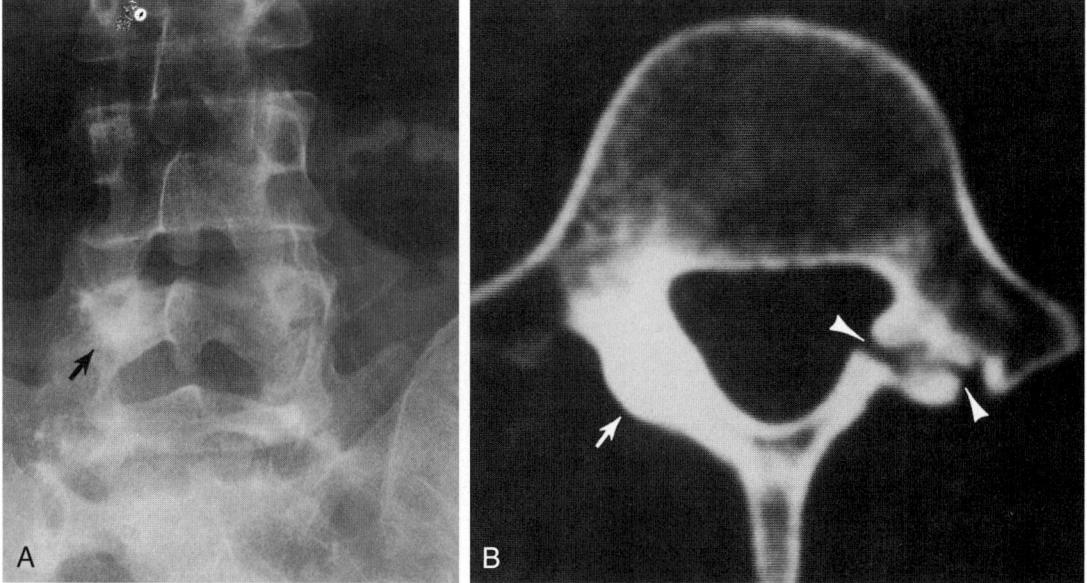

**Figure 56–30.** Unilateral spondylolysis with contralateral bony hypertrophy and reactive sclerosis. The predominant abnormality on a frontal radiograph of the lumbar spine *(A)* is osteosclerosis in the region of the right pedicle of the fifth lumbar vertebra *(arrow)*. The left transverse process of this vertebra is smaller than that on the right. A transaxial CT scan *(B)* of this vertebra reveals spondylolysis *(arrowheads)* and contralateral bone hypertrophy *(arrow)*. (Courtesy of J. A. Amberg, MD, San Diego, Calif.)

## Greenstick, Torus, and Bowing Fractures

In an immature skeleton, fractures that do not completely penetrate the entire shaft of a bone are not infrequent. A *greenstick fracture* is one that perforates one cortex and ramifies within the medullary bone (Fig. 56–32). The name is derived from this fracture's resemblance to a young tree branch that, when broken, is disrupted on its outer surface but remains intact on its inner surface. Typical locations of greenstick fractures are the proximal metaphysis or diaphysis of the tibia and the middle third of the radius and ulna. A *torus (buckling) fracture* results from an injury insufficient in force to create a complete

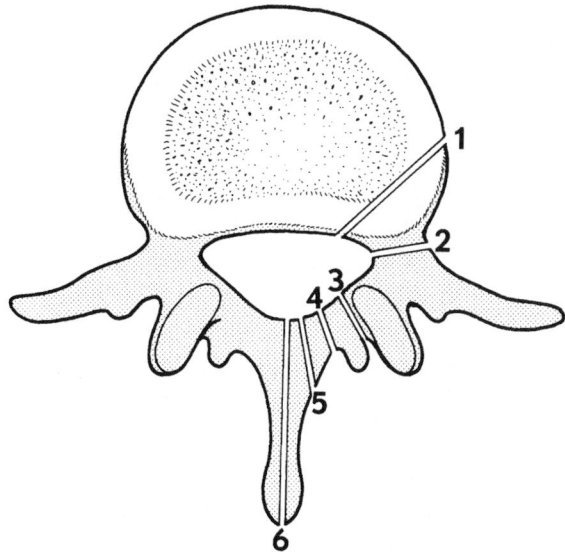

**Figure 56–31.** Clefts in the neural arch. 1, Persistent neuro-central synchondrosis; 2, pediculate, or retrosomatic, cleft; 3, pars interarticularis cleft, or spondylolysis; 4, retroisthmic cleft; 5, paraspinous cleft; 6, spinous cleft. (From Johansen JG, McCarty DJ, Haughton VM: Retrosomatic clefts: Computed tomographic appearance. Radiology 148:447, 1983.)

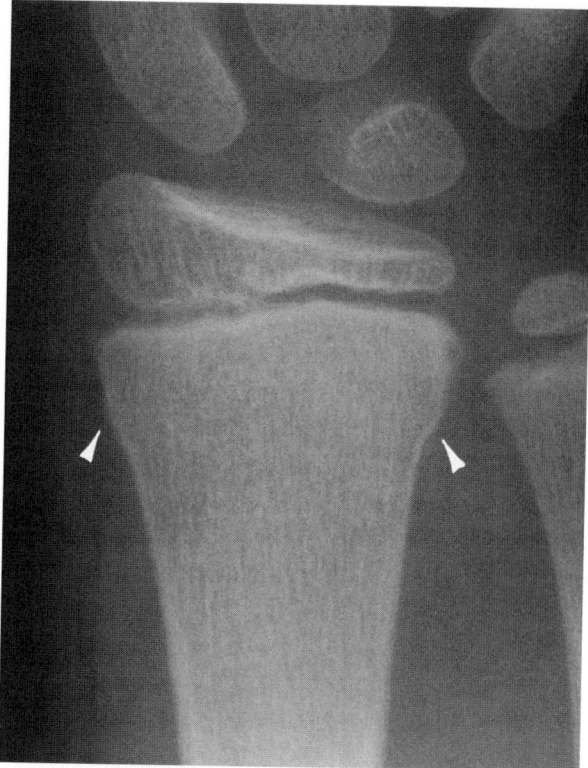

**Figure 56–33.** Torus fracture. Note the buckling of the cortex *(arrowheads)*.

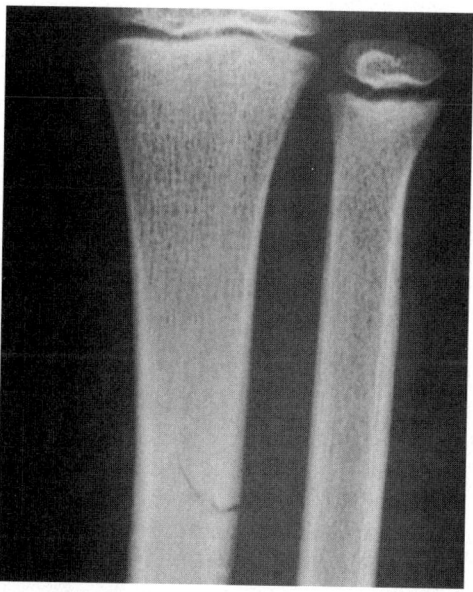

**Figure 56–32.** Greenstick fracture. Observe that the fracture involves one side of the radius and extends incompletely through the bone.

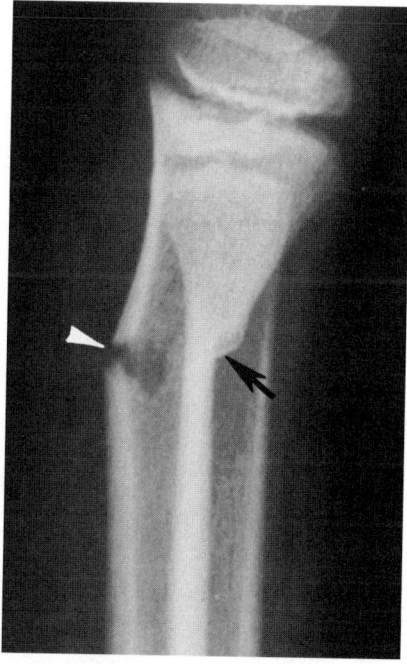

**Figure 56–34.** "Lead pipe" fracture. Note a torus fracture of the dorsal surface of the radius *(arrow)* and a greenstick fracture of the volar surface *(arrowhead)*.

discontinuity of bone but sufficient to produce buckling of the cortex (Fig. 56–33). Torus fractures are common in metaphyseal regions of long bones. Radiographs may be interpreted as normal unless subtle bulging of the cortex is identified. With the application of both compressive and angular forces, a combination of greenstick and torus fractures may result; this is termed a *lead pipe fracture* (Fig. 56–34).

*Bowing fractures* are a plastic response, usually to longitudinal stress in a bone. They occur virtually exclusively in children, typically in the radius and ulna. In bowing fractures, plastic deformation occurs and results in permanent bowing of the bone. Further increases in stress lead to fracture. Radiographic analysis of bowing deformities reveals lateral or anteroposterior bending of the affected bone (Fig. 56–35). The abnormality may be subtle and necessitate comparison radiographs of the opposite side for correct diagnosis. Sequential radiographs of a plastic bowing deformity usually reveal no evidence of periostitis, although thickening of the involved cortex may be detected. Scintigraphy may identify increased uptake of bone-seeking pharmaceutical agents, even when the radiographic findings are only equivocal. MR imaging may reveal marrow edema in the involved bone. A bowed bone generally remains bowed, resists attempts at reduction, holds an adjacent fracture in angulation, and prevents relocation of an adjacent dislocation.

## Toddler's Fractures

Infants and toddlers frequently develop an acute-onset limp without a clear history of specific injury. The classic toddler's fracture is a nondisplaced, oblique fracture of the distal diaphysis of the tibia (Fig. 56–36). Although this fracture is the most common pattern of injury, other causes of these clinical manifestations are occult fractures of the fibula, femur, metatarsal bones (particularly the first), and, less commonly, calcaneus. Most toddlers' fractures occur between the ages of 1 and 3 years; the remainder occur before the age of 1 year.

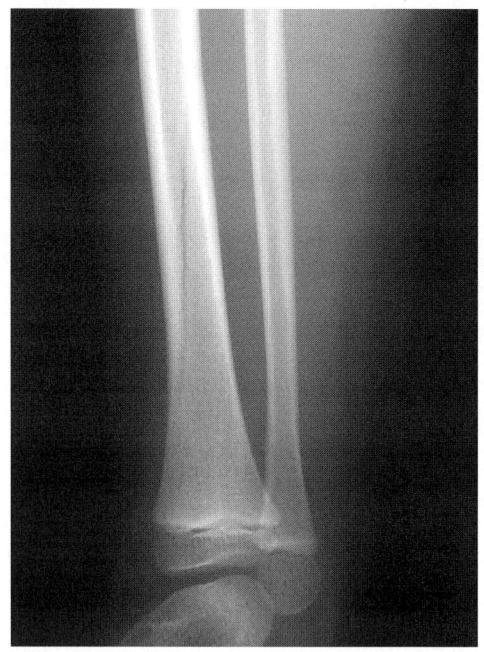

**Figure 56–36.** Toddler's fracture: tibia. Radiograph reveals a nondisplaced oblique fracture of the distal tibia.

## Acute Chondral and Osteochondral Fractures

Shearing, rotational, or tangentially aligned impaction forces generated by abnormal joint motion may produce fractures of one or both of the two apposing joint surfaces. Acute injuries can produce fragments consisting of cartilage alone (chondral fractures) or cartilage and underlying bone (osteochondral fractures). A purely cartilaginous fragment creates no direct radiographic abnormalities, whereas one containing calcified cartilage and bone becomes apparent because of a varying degree of radiodensity (Fig. 56–37). Secondary radiographic signs consisting of soft tissue swelling and joint effusion can be apparent with either chondral or chondro-osseous fragments. After the injury, the detached portion of the articular surface can remain in situ, be slightly displaced, or become loose, or free, within the joint cavity (Fig. 56–38).

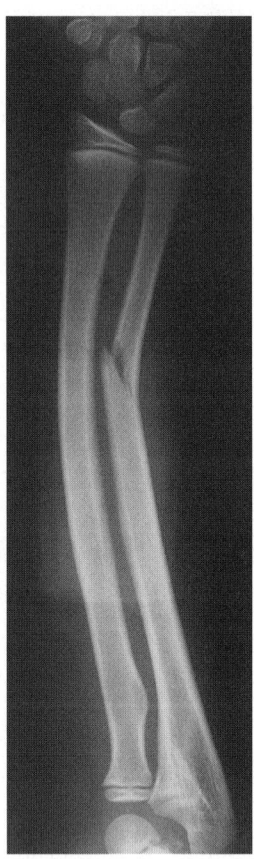

**Figure 56–35.** Bowing deformities of bone. Note the bowing of the radius associated with a fracture of the adjacent ulna.

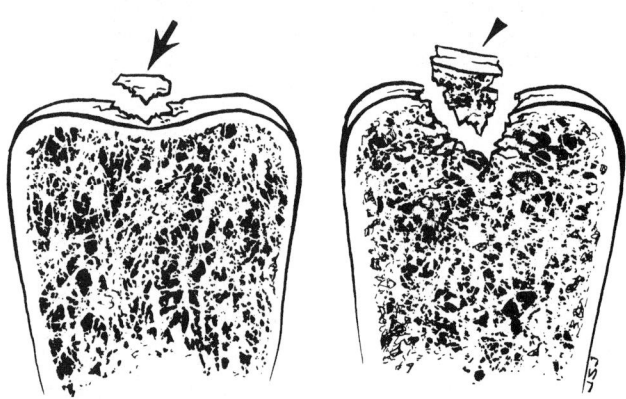

**Figure 56–37.** Acute chondral and osteochondral fractures: fragment components. Fragments can consist of cartilage alone *(arrow)* or both cartilage and bone *(arrowhead)*.

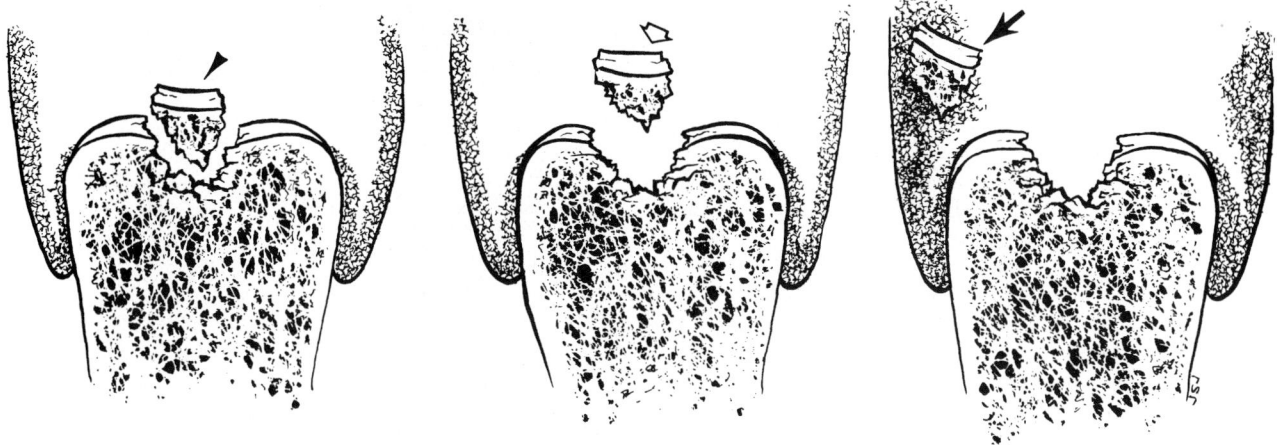

**Figure 56–38.** Acute chondral and osteochondral fractures: fate of fragments. Chondral or osteochondral fragments can remain in situ *(arrowhead)*, be slightly displaced or loose in the articular cavity *(open arrow)*, or become embedded at a distant synovial site and evoke a local inflammatory reaction *(solid arrow)*.

Radiographic identification of loose osteocartilaginous bodies or those attached to the synovial lining requires a careful search of the recesses and dependent portions of the joint. Such bodies are common in the olecranon, coronoid, and radial fossae in the elbow; the axillary and subscapular recesses in the glenohumeral joint; the acetabular fossa and recesses about the zona orbicularis of the hip; and the posterior regions and recesses in the knee. Detection of osteocartilaginous bodies should stimulate a search for their site of origin. Osteochondral injuries are a well-recognized component of a variety of momentary or persistent subluxations and dislocations. Classic examples include injuries to the glenoid region of the scapula and humeral head with dislocation of the glenohumeral joint, injuries to the patella and lateral femoral condyle with dislocation of the patella, and injuries to the femoral head with dislocation of the hip (Fig. 56–39).

### Osteochondritis Dissecans

Osteochondritis dissecans is characterized by fragmentation and possible separation of a portion of the articular surface. The age at onset varies from childhood to middle age, but an onset in adolescence is most common. Patients may be entirely asymptomatic; however, pain aggravated by movement, limitation of motion, clicking, locking, and swelling may be apparent. Single or multiple sites can be affected. The condition is generally believed to be the eventual result of an osteochondral fracture that was initially caused by shearing, rotatory, or tangentially aligned impaction forces.

Considerable interest has developed in determining the stability of the osteochondral fragment. MR imaging is most useful in this regard, with high signal intensity on T2-weighted images adjacent to the osteochondral fragment indicative of fluid or granulation tissue, which is strong but not infallible evidence of an unstable lesion; the presence of fluid encircling the fragment or focal cystic areas beneath the fragment are the best indicators of instability (Fig. 56–40). Similarly, the absence of a

zone of high signal intensity at the interface of the fragment and the parent bone is a reliable sign of lesion stability. Unstable lesions are characterized by (1) the presence of a line of high signal intensity at the interface between the osseous fragment and the adjacent bone, (2) an articular fracture indicated by joint fluid of high signal intensity passing through the subchondral bone plate, (3) a focal osteochondral defect filled with joint fluid, and (4) a 5 mm or larger fluid-filled cyst deep to the lesion. MR arthrography may also be useful in the evaluation osteochondritis dissecans and in establishing fragment stability.

**Femoral Condyle.** One of the most common locations of osteochondritis dissecans is the condylar surfaces of the distal portion of the femur, accounting for as many as 75% of cases. With regard to femoral involvement, men are affected more frequently than women, and the average age at the onset of symptoms and signs is 15 to 20 years, although the age range is highly variable. Unilateral changes predominate over bilateral changes by a ratio of

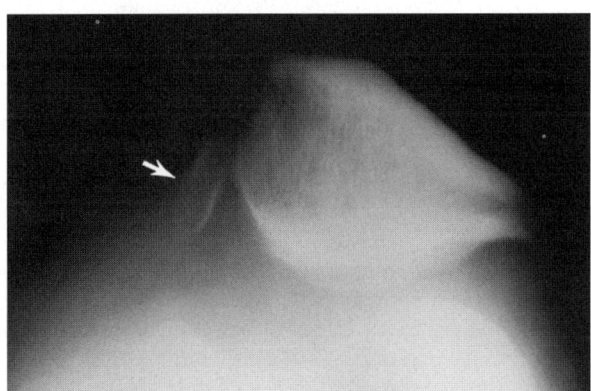

**Figure 56–39.** Acute chondral and osteochondral fractures: lateral patellar dislocation. Note the fracture of the medial margin of the patella *(arrow)* and lateral subluxation of the patella on the axial radiograph.

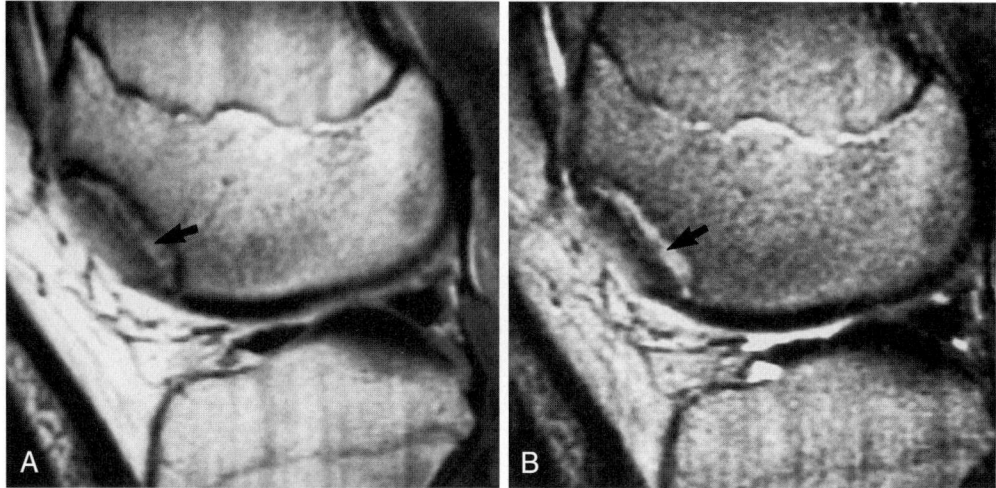

**Figure 56–40.** Osteochondritis dissecans of the lateral femoral condyle. Sagittal intermediate-weighted (TR/TE, 2200/30) *(A)* and T2-weighted (TR/TE, 2200/80) *(B)* spin echo MR images reveal the lesion involving the anterior surface of the lateral condyle. The fragment is ossified, and the junction between it and the parent bone *(arrows)* demonstrates intermediate signal intensity in *(A)* and high signal intensity in *(B)*. The abnormalities are consistent with granulation tissue or fluid in this junctional area. Although the overlying cartilage is not seen well, the MR imaging findings suggest the presence of an unstable lesion. (Courtesy of J. Blassinghame, MD, San Diego, Calif.)

approximately 3:1. The medial condyle is affected most frequently, with the defect occurring in the non–weight-bearing surface, although other sites may be involved (Fig. 56–41). The classic location is the lateral aspect of the medial femoral condyle. The osseous component of an osteochondral lesion is detectable with routine radiography or standard CT (Fig. 56–42). Purely chondral lesions require arthrography (conventional, CT, or MR) for identification.

The major differential diagnosis of the radiographic features of condylar osteochondritis dissecans is spontaneous osteonecrosis of the knee. This latter lesion occurs in older persons, is associated with a sudden onset of clinical manifestations, and almost invariably involves the weight-bearing portion of the medial femoral condyle.

**Patella.** Compared with osteochondritis dissecans of the femoral condyle, involvement of the patella is rare. The typical site of the lesion is the medial facet of the patella. The lateral facet is affected in approximately 30% of cases, and the most medial, or "odd," facet is generally spared. The middle or lower portion of the bone is affected almost universally, whereas the superior portion is uninvolved. The cause of the lesion appears to be traumatic. The lesions are optimally identified on lateral and axial radiographs, where they appear as osseous defects near the convexity between the condylar articular surfaces of the patella (Fig. 56–43).

The major differential diagnoses are chondromalacia patellae, a dorsal defect of the patella, and osteochondral fractures related to direct injury or recurrent dislocation. Chondromalacia patellae is usually confined to the cartilaginous layer of the bone. A dorsal defect of the patella, which likely represents an anomaly of ossification and may be part of the spectrum of a bipartite or multipartite patella, is associated with a round and lytic defect with well-defined margins in the superolateral aspect of the

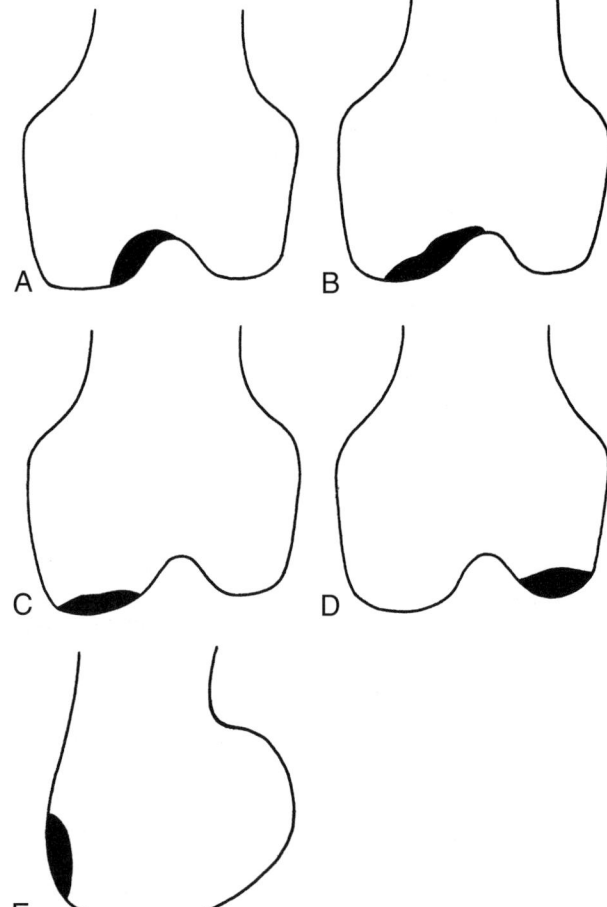

**Figure 56–41.** Osteochondritis dissecans of the femoral condyles: sites of occurrence. *A,* Classic (medial condyle). *B,* Extended classic (medial condyle). *C,* Inferocentral (medial condyle). *D,* Inferocentral (lateral condyle). *E,* Anterior (lateral condyle).

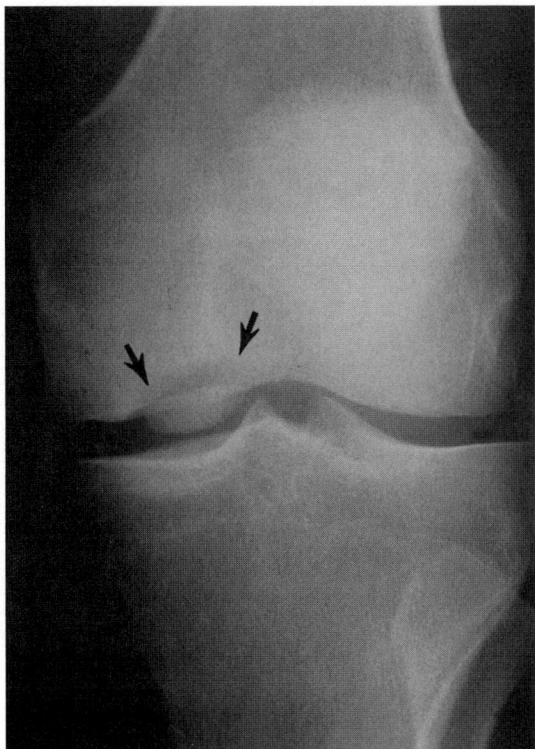

**Figure 56–42.** Osteochondritis dissecans of the femoral condyles. Classic defect of the medial condyle *(arrows)*.

bone. This defect occurs in both sexes, may be bilateral, and is not associated with symptoms and signs; it demonstrates intact cartilage on arthrography. Dislocation of the patella is associated with an osteochondral fracture on the medial side of the patella and, less frequently, at the lateral margin of the lateral femoral condyle.

**Talus.** Osteochondritis dissecans is common in the talar dome. The middle third of the lateral border of the talus and the posterior third of the medial border of the talus are the two most common sites of injury, and they are involved with approximately equal frequency. Centrolateral (or anterolateral) lesions are commonly encountered in patients who have had previous episodes of ankle injury. Patients are usually in the second to fourth decades of life. Carefully obtained radiographs can usually delineate the site of injury. These views may be supplemented by radiographs taken with the ankle in stress or by CT scanning. The osseous defects may be quite subtle and consist of slight irregularity of the articular surface, shallow excavations with or without adjacent sclerosis, and small "flake" fracture fragments (Fig. 56–44). Arthrography or computed arthrotomography is indicated in some cases to better delineate the fracture site, define the condition of the overlying chondral coat, and detect intra-articular osseous and cartilaginous bodies. MR imaging has also been used to detect the abnormality, although its precise role is not yet clear.

**Capitulum of the Humerus.** Osteochondritis dissecans about the elbow usually involves the capitulum. Radiographic abnormalities include flattening, cystic and

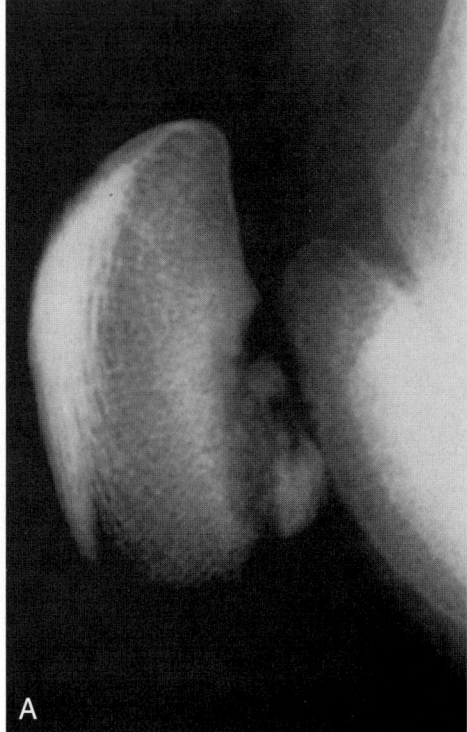

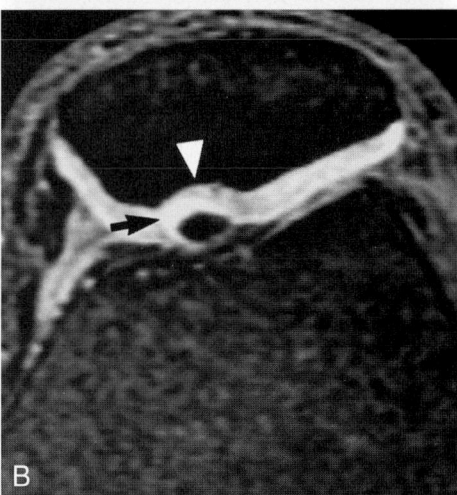

**Figure 56–43.** Osteochondritis dissecans of the patella. *A,* Lateral radiograph reveals bone fragmentation in the lower surface of the patella. *B,* In another patient, transaxial spoiled gradient recalled acquisition in the steady state (TR/TE, 58/10; flip angle, 60 degrees) MR image, obtained with volumetric acquisition and fat suppression, shows the bone fragment, adjacent high signal intensity *(arrow)* in the junctional zone, and the osseous bed *(arrowhead)* in the patella. The articular cartilage of the patella is thinned or absent at the site of the bone fragment. (*A,* Courtesy of J. Schills, MD, Cleveland, Ohio.)

sclerotic changes, and fragmentation of the capitulum (Fig. 56–45). The resulting bone fragments may remain at their site of origin or become partially or completely detached. Free intra-articular bodies may migrate to any region of the elbow, although they often lodge in the fossa of the distal end of the humerus. CT scanning, CT arthrography, ultrasonography, MR imaging (Fig. 56–46), and MR arthrography have all been used to assess this lesion.

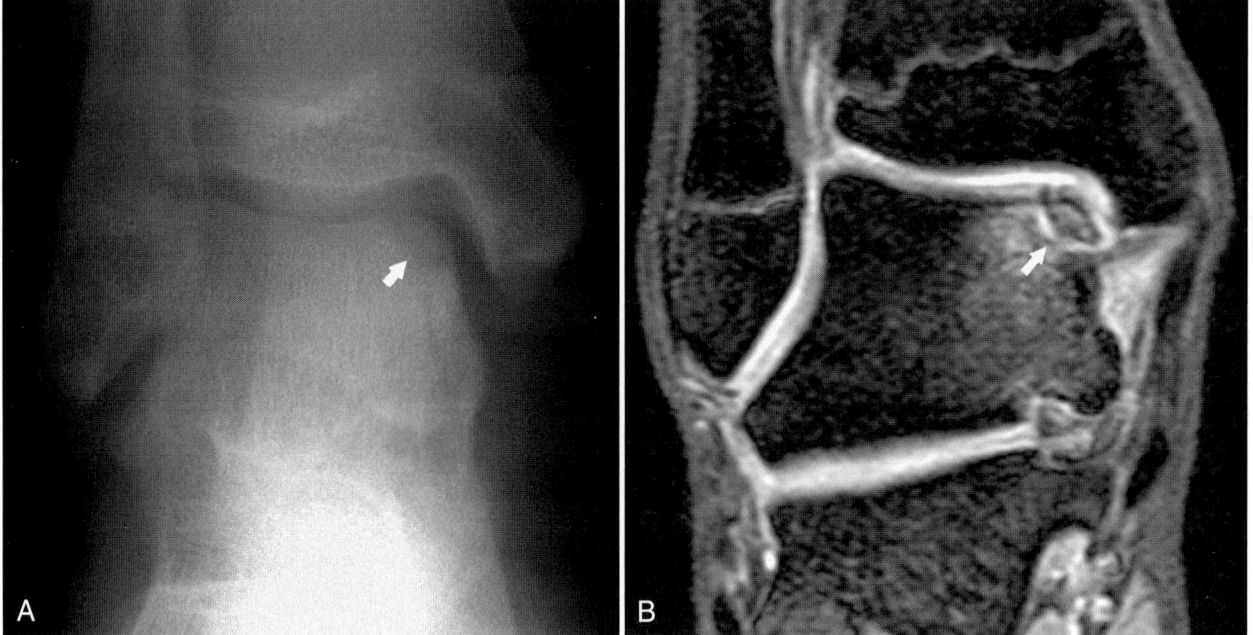

**Figure 56–44.** Osteochondritis dissecans of the talus: medial lesion. *A,* Note the lucent lesion of the medial talar dome *(arrow)*, the site of an osteochondral fragment. *B,* Corresponding coronal, volume gradient (TR/TE, 28/7; flip angle, 25 degrees) MR image shows the nondisplaced fragment.

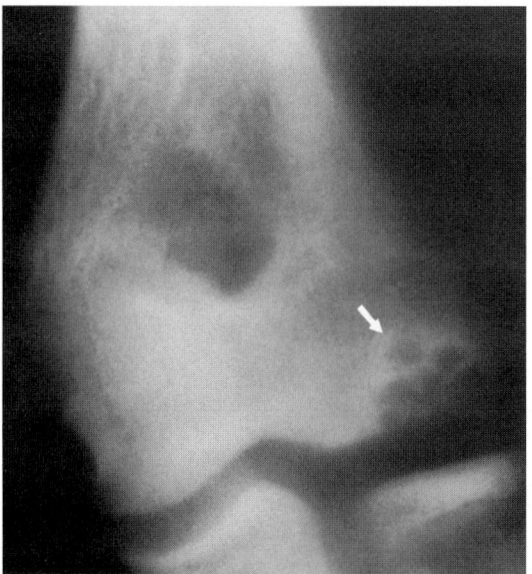

**Figure 56–45.** Osteochondritis dissecans lesion *(arrow)* of the capitulum of the humerus. (Courtesy of G. Greenway, MD, Dallas, Tex.)

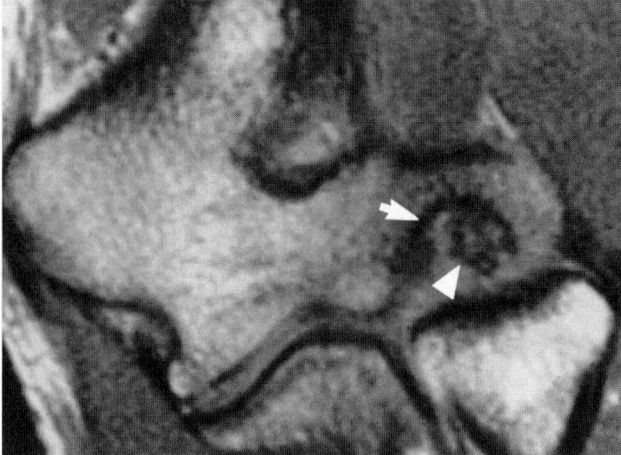

**Figure 56–46.** Osteochondritis dissecans of the capitulum of the humerus. Coronal intermediate-weighted (TR/TE, 2000/20) spin echo MR image reveals the capitular lesion *(arrow)* containing a bone fragment *(arrowhead)*. The overlying articular cartilage is not well seen. (Courtesy of M. Schweitzer, MD, Philadelphia, Pa.)

With regard to the differential diagnosis, Panner's disease, related to irregular ossification of the capitulum, is seen in a younger age group.

**Other Sites.** Post-traumatic osteochondral fractures, osteochondritis dissecans, and necrosis can be identified at other sites, including other tarsal bones, tibia, humeral head, acetabulum, and glenoid cavity.

## Fractures of the Shafts of Long Tubular Bones

It is the application of an abnormal force to a bone, a process termed loading, that results in an injury. The ability of bone to absorb energy varies with the person's age, sex, and metabolic status; the integrity of surrounding tissue; and the specific bone involved. The bones of children are more plastic (ductile) than the comparatively brittle bones of adults; this fact contributes to the occurrence of incomplete and bowing fractures in children, whereas these injuries are almost never seen in adults. Additional factors that contribute to the production of a fracture are the presence of a preexisting lesion and a previous surgical procedure.

Four basic types of load can be applied to an object such as a long tubular bone: *tension* (or *traction*) forces act perpendicular to the cross section of the bone and pull trabeculae apart, *compression* forces act in a similar perpendicular direction and press trabeculae together, *torsion* (or *rotational*) forces are twisting in nature, and *bending* forces lead to angulation (Fig. 56–47). Of these types of force, compression, torsion, and bending forces working independently or in combination are common causes of bone injury. The fracture configuration or pattern depends on the interaction of a particular load and a specific bone. Several types are recognized (Fig. 56–48; Table 56–3).

*Transverse fracture* (mechanism: bending, or angular, forces in long bones; tensile, or traction, forces in short bones). A transverse fracture line, which occurs at a right angle to the shaft, is usually the result of a bending force. Tensile failure of the bone takes place on its convex side (opposite the input force), with subsequent compressive failure on its concave side. Often, the cortex on the compressive side fails before the transverse fracture is complete, resulting in cortical splintering. Transverse fractures (i.e., avulsion fractures) can also be caused by traction forces at sites of tendon or ligament insertion into bone.

*Oblique fracture* (mechanism: combination of compression, bending, and torsion forces). Combined forces consisting of compression, torsion, and, to a lesser extent, bending typically lead to an oblique fracture. Such a fracture resembles a spiral fracture superfi-

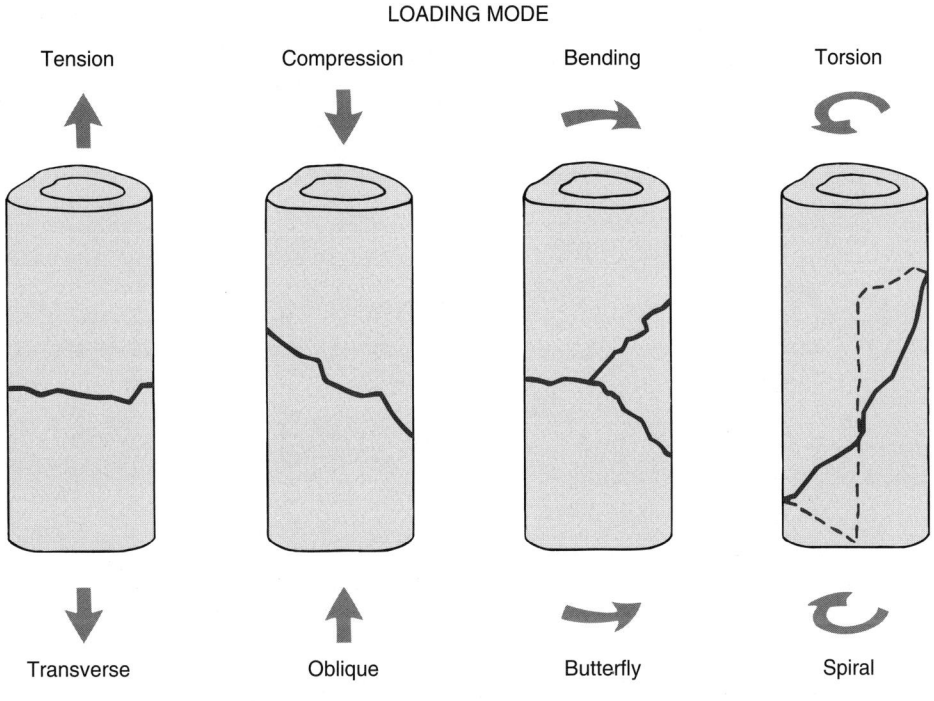

**Figure 56–47.** Biomechanics of fractures in long tubular bones: basic types of load. (From Browner BD, Jupiter JB, Levine AM, Trafton PG [eds]: Skeletal Trauma: Fractures, Dislocations, Ligamentous Injuries. Philadelphia, WB Saunders, 1992, p 101.)

LOADING MODE

Tension — Compression — Bending — Torsion

Transverse — Oblique — Butterfly — Spiral

FRACTURE TYPE

**TABLE 56–3**

**Biomechanics of Fractures in Long Tubular Bones**

| Fracture Pattern | Mechanism of Injury | Location of Soft Tissue Hinge | Energy Load | Common Sites |
|---|---|---|---|---|
| Transverse | Bending | Concavity | Low | Diaphyses |
| Oblique | Compression, bending, and torsion | Concavity (often destroyed) | Moderate | Radius, ulna, tibia, fibula |
| Oblique-transverse | Compression and bending | Concavity or side of butterfly fragment | Moderate | Femur, tibia, humerus |
| Spiral | Torsion | Vertical segment | Low | Tibia, humerus |
| Diaphyseal impaction | Compression | Variable | Variable | Humerus, femur, tibia |
| Comminuted | Variable | Destroyed | High | Variable |

From Gonza ER, Harrington IJ: Biomechanics of Musculoskeletal Injury. Baltimore, Williams & Wilkins, 1982, p 2.

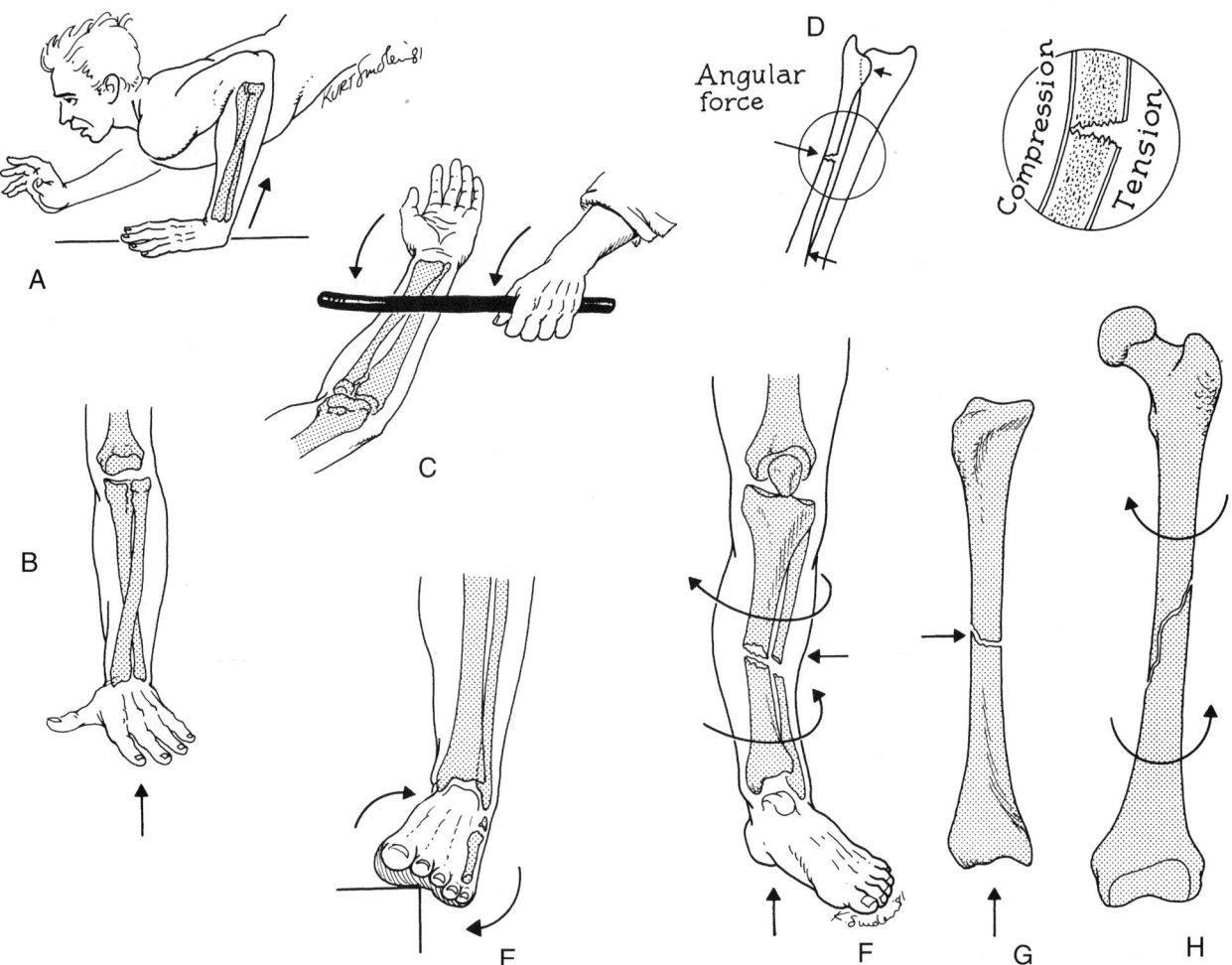

**Figure 56–48.** Biomechanics of fractures in long tubular bones. *A* and *B*, Application of longitudinal compression force (axial compression). Loading of a long bone in this manner may cause an incomplete (bowing or torus) fracture in a child or impaction of the diaphysis into the metaphysis in an adult (e.g., intercondylar fracture of the distal portion of the humerus or femur). *C* and *D*, Application of angular force (bending). Angular force may result in a greenstick fracture in a child or a transverse fracture in an adult. Cortical bone is stronger in compression than in tension, so the bone fails initially on the tension side (opposite the input force) and the fracture propagates transversely to the long axis of the bone. The periosteum may be preserved on the side of the input force. *E*, Traction force (tension) at the site of a tendon or ligament insertion may result in a transverse (avulsion) fracture. *F*, An oblique fracture configuration results from a combination of multiple forces, including longitudinal compression and angular and rotational forces. *G*, An oblique-transverse fracture results from a combination of angular and axial compression forces. The direction of the fracture line is determined by the relative magnitude of the two forces: when axial compression force predominates, the oblique component is larger; conversely, a predominantly angular force results in a more transverse fracture configuration. The oblique fragment may separate in a butterfly configuration. *H*, A spiral fracture results from rotational forces. The fracture line approximates an angle of 40 to 45 degrees, and the direction of the spiral denotes the direction of the rotational forces.

cially; differentiation between the two is important, however, because oblique fractures have a higher frequency of nonunion, whereas spiral fractures usually heal uneventfully. In an oblique fracture, the ends of the bones are short and blunt, a vertical segment is not identified, and a clear space may be seen; in a spiral fracture, long, sharp, pointed ends and a vertical segment are characteristic, and unless the fracture is distracted, no clear space is evident (Fig. 56–49).

*Oblique-transverse fracture* (mechanism: combination of axial compression and bending forces). This combina-

tion of forces can lead to several different types of fracture: if the compression forces are larger than the bending forces, an oblique fracture is produced; if the bending forces are sufficiently large, a purely transverse fracture is seen; and if both the compression and the bending forces are of sufficient magnitude, an oblique-transverse fracture results (see Fig. 56–49). A butterfly fragment may be an added component of the oblique-transverse fracture pattern.

*Spiral fracture* (mechanism: torsion force). Spiral fractures are relatively uncommon and result from twisting or rotational forces, perhaps combined with axial compression. They are usually observed in the humerus and the tibia (see Fig. 56–49).

*Diaphyseal impaction fracture* (mechanism: axial compression force). In certain locations, such as the humerus, femur, and tibia, an axially applied load drives the diaphyseal bone, with its thick and rigid cortex, into the thin metaphyseal bone. Examples of this injury are a supracondylar fracture of the femur and a comminuted fracture of the tibial plateaus.

*Comminuted fracture* (mechanism: variable). Indirect or direct application of force, usually of high energy, leads to multiple osseous fragments of varying size.

## DISLOCATIONS

### Terminology

*Dislocation* is complete loss of contact between two osseous surfaces that normally articulate. *Subluxation* is a partial loss of this contact. Closed subluxation or dislocation exists when the skin and soft tissues remain intact over the injured joint; open dislocation or subluxation exists if associated soft tissue injury exposes the joint to the outside environment (Fig. 56–50). Subluxations and dislocations are usually caused by physical trauma, although they can also occur when congenital or acquired conditions produce muscle imbalance. Many dislocations and subluxations related to trauma are associated with fracture of a neighboring bone. Typical examples of such fractures are the Hill-Sachs lesion of the humeral head

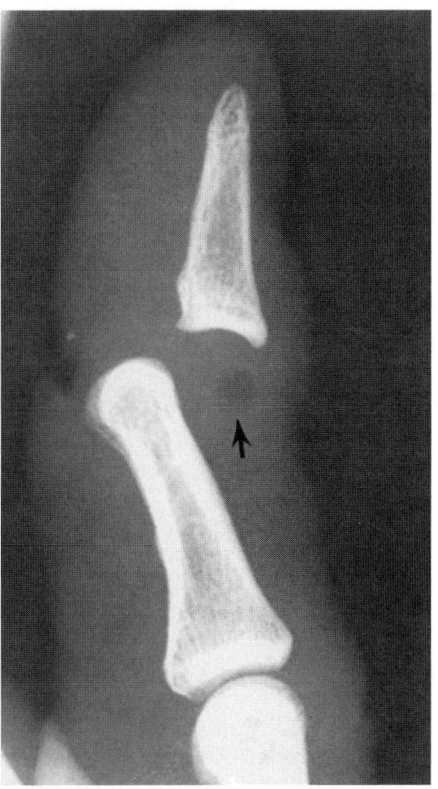

**Figure 56–50.** Open dislocation. Dorsal dislocation of the terminal phalanx at the interphalangeal joint of the thumb is associated with a soft tissue defect in the volar surface of the finger and soft tissue air *(arrow)*.

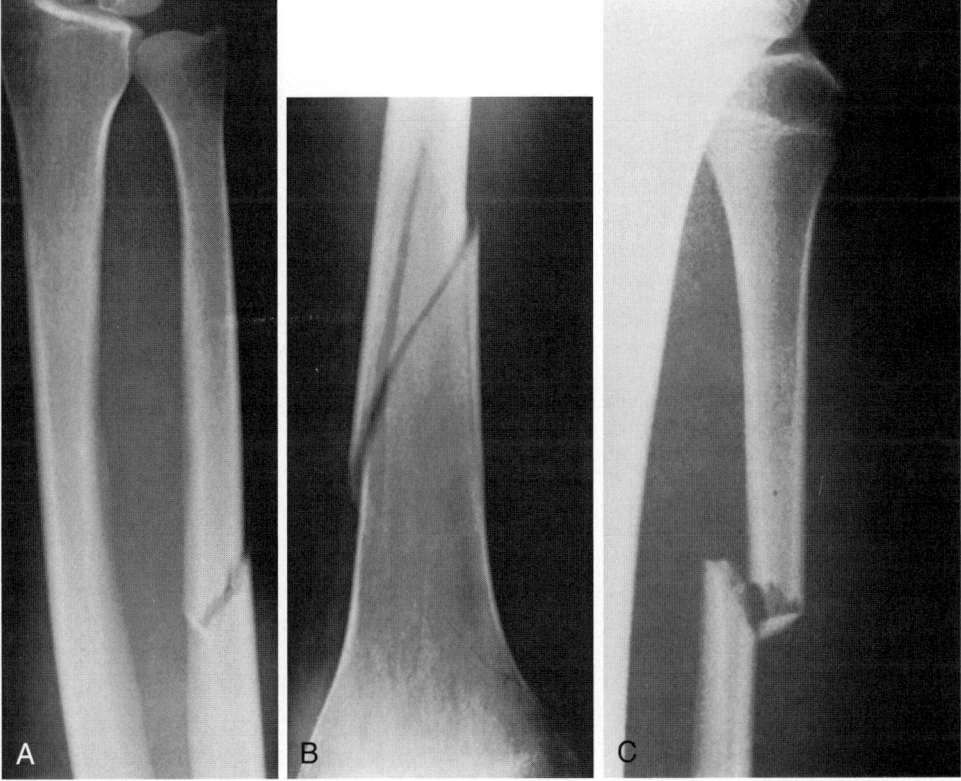

**Figure 56–49.** Long bone fracture. *A,* Oblique (tapping) fracture of the midshaft of the ulna resulting from a direct blow. *B,* Spiral fracture of the femoral diaphysis. *C,* Oblique-transverse fracture with mild comminution.

after anterior dislocation of the glenohumeral joint and fractures of the femoral head that accompany either anterior or posterior dislocation of the hip.

The terminology used to describe a dislocation or subluxation varies with the anatomic complexity of the involved joint. When the joint is composed of two bones, the joint injury derives its name from that joint (e.g., dislocation of the hip). When the joint comprises more than two bones, the dislocation is still named after the involved articulation if it affects the two major bones. If the smallest of the three bones is dislocated, the injury is named after that bone (e.g., dislocation of the patella). The term *diastasis* refers to abnormal separation of a joint that is normally only slightly movable (e.g., the symphysis pubis) (Fig. 56–51).

## Biomechanics

Conventional classification schemes define four types of joint motion: gliding and angular movements, circumduction, and rotation. They may occur independently or, far more frequently, in various combinations. In any location, the precise characteristics of joint movement are governed principally by the shape of the articular surfaces (Table 56–4). In general, increasing freedom of movement is achieved at the expense of joint stability.

Traumatic dislocation of a joint implies that the joint capsule and protective ligaments have been damaged. Alternatively, the capsule may be stripped from one of its osseous sites of attachment, or a stretched ligament may lead to avulsion of a bone fragment. Although trauma can produce dislocation of any articulation, the most commonly involved sites are the glenohumeral joint, elbow, ankle, hip, and interphalangeal joints.

## TRAUMA TO SYNOVIAL JOINTS

### Traumatic Synovitis and Hemarthrosis

A joint effusion appearing within the first few hours after trauma is usually related to a hemarthrosis; nonbloody effusions generally appear 12 to 24 hours after injury. Bloody or nonbloody effusions occurring after trauma

**TABLE 56–4**

**Morphologic Classification of Synovial Joints**

| Type of Joint | Motion | Examples |
|---|---|---|
| Plane | Uniaxial | Intermetatarsal, intercarpal |
| Hinge | Uniaxial | Humeroulnar, interphalangeal |
| Pivot | Uniaxial | Proximal radioulnar, median atlantoaxial |
| Bicondylar | Uniaxial (minimal movement also in a second axis) | Knee, temporomandibular |
| Ellipsoid | Biaxial | Radiocarpal, metacarpophalangeal |
| Sellar | Biaxial | First carpometacarpal, ankle, calcaneocuboid |
| Spheroidal | Triaxial | Hip, glenohumeral |

Adapted from Williams PL, Warwick R: Gray's Anatomy, 36th Br ed. Philadelphia, WB Saunders, 1980, p 430.

are associated with radiographic findings related to displacement of intra-articular fat pads and edema of extra-articular fat planes. Typical examples of these findings are widening of the suprapatellar pouch in cases of knee trauma, and ventral and posterior displacement of the fat pads about the distal end of the humerus (Fig. 56–52).

In general, the displacement and distortion of many of these fat planes indicate only the presence of fluid or a mass in the joint; however, in the clinical setting of trauma,

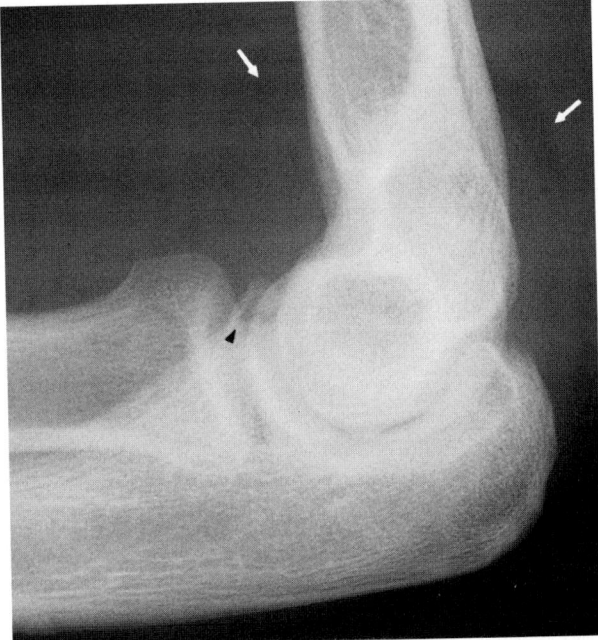

**Figure 56–52.**  Traumatic synovitis, hemarthrosis, and soft tissue edema. Displacement of the anterior and posterior fat pads (*arrows*) about the elbow after trauma usually indicates intra-articular fluid or blood. Note the fracture of the coronoid process of the ulna (*arrowhead*).

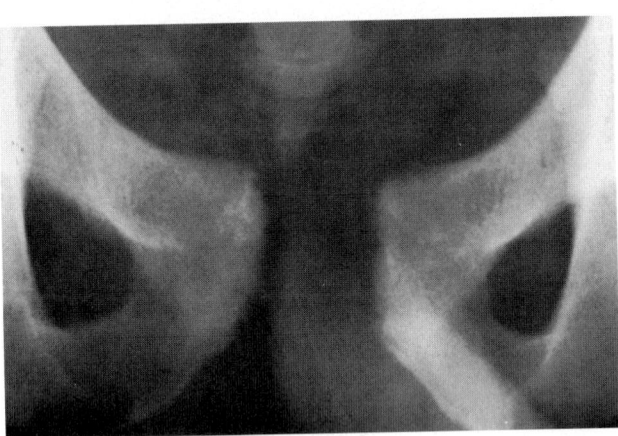

**Figure 56–51.**  Diastasis. Abnormal widening of the symphysis pubis is apparent.

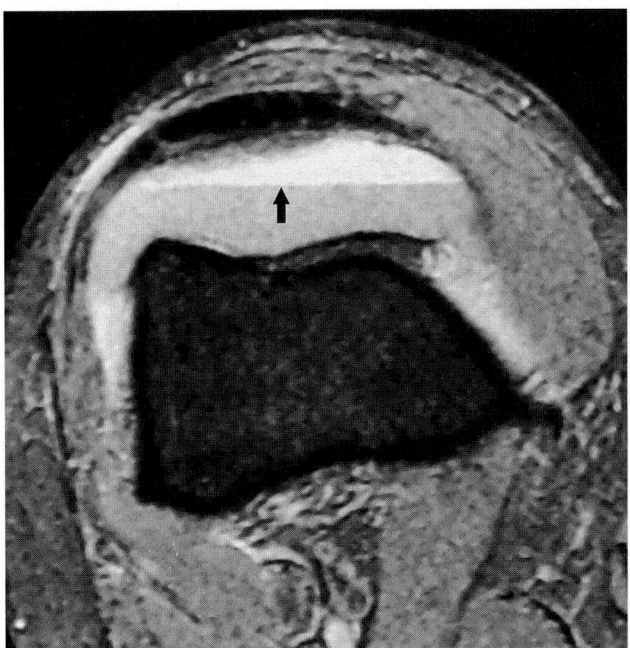

**Figure 56–53.** Hemarthrosis. Coronal gradient (TR/TE, 634/16; flip angle, 25 degrees) MR image in a patient with a lower pole patellar fracture shows a hemarthrosis characterized by a fluid level *(arrow)* separating serum above from the cellular components of blood below.

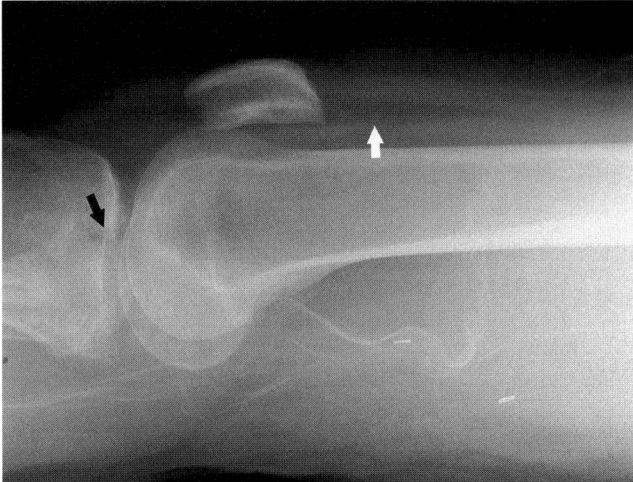

**Figure 56–54.** Lipohemarthrosis. On a cross-table lateral radiograph, a straight radiodense fluid line *(white arrow)* at a fat-blood interface can be a helpful clue to the underlying but subtle tibial plateau fracture *(black arrow)*.

detection of these changes should encourage a thorough search for a subtle fracture or subluxation, although such a search may not be successful. CT scanning and MR imaging in cases of acute hemarthrosis document characteristic findings. A fluid level, or interface, is often noted between two components of the bloody joint effusion (Fig. 56–53). The upper component is serum, and the lower component relates to the cellular components of blood; each component has different CT and MR imaging findings.

## Lipohemarthrosis

Bloody synovial fluid containing fat droplets and bone marrow spicules is reliable evidence of an intra-articular fracture. Frequently, however, a hemorrhagic effusion containing fat may be observed in patients without fracture, probably related to significant cartilaginous or ligamentous injury.

Radiographic examination using a horizontal beam technique may demonstrate a fat-blood fluid level after injury to the joint (Fig. 56–54). Most commonly, this finding is seen in a knee or shoulder, although it may also be noted in other joints. In the knee, subtle tibial plateau fractures may be the source of the fat. Lipohemarthroses can also be detected with CT or MR imaging (Fig. 56–55). With MR imaging, the appearance of a lipohemarthrosis is more complex. The most superior zone contains floating fat, a central zone contains serum, and an inferior zone contains dependent red blood cells. A signal void, representing a chemical shift artifact, may be visible at the interface of fat and serum.

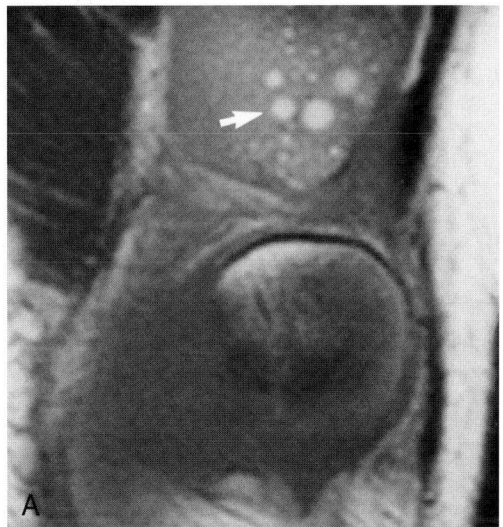

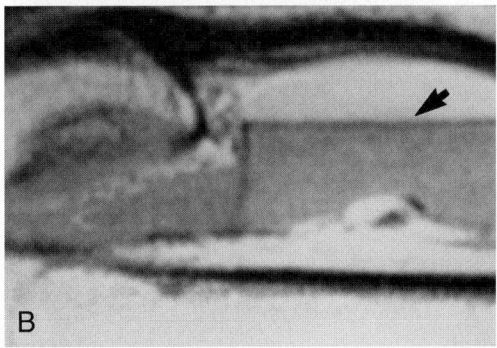

**Figure 56–55.** Lipohemarthrosis. *A,* On a coronal T1-weighted (TR/TE, 500/20) spin echo MR image of the knee, globules of fat *(arrow)* in the suprapatellar pouch, above the patella, are of high signal intensity. The bloody joint effusion is of intermediate signal intensity. *B,* Sagittal T1-weighted (TR/TE, 900/30) spin echo MR image shows a dominant fluid level *(arrow)* at the interface of fat (above) and serum (below). The image has been rotated 90 degrees to simulate the orientation of a cross-table radiograph. (*A,* Courtesy of R. Reinke, MD, Long Beach, Calif. *B,* Courtesy of R. Stiles, MD, Atlanta, Ga.)

## TRAUMA TO SYMPHYSES

Traumatic insult to symphyses, including the symphysis pubis, manubriosternal joint, and intervertebral disc, is not infrequent. Subluxation (i.e., diastasis) or dislocation of the symphysis pubis leads to a single break in the pelvic ring and is commonly combined with a second injury causing pelvic disruption, such as fracture of the ilium or sacrum or diastasis of the sacroiliac joint. Subluxation or dislocation of the manubriosternal joint usually indicates significant trauma and may be seen after automobile accidents in which the chest strikes the steering wheel. Similar displacement at this site occasionally occurs spontaneously owing to the exaggerated thoracic kyphosis associated with generalized osteoporosis, osteomalacia, renal osteodystrophy, or plasma cell myeloma. Violation of the intervertebral disc may be combined with fractures of the vertebral bodies and posterior elements, leading to spinal instability. One injury that can lead to disruption of both the intervertebral disc (plus surrounding bone) and the posterior spinal structures is the seatbelt fracture (Fig. 56–56). During an automobile accident, the trunk flexes over the seat belt. A horizontal fracture of the vertebral body (Chance fracture) or tearing of the intervertebral disc may be combined with laminar and spinous process fractures or ligamentous tear.

Trauma to the discovertebral junction can result from obvious or occult injury. In either situation, violation of the cartilaginous endplate and subchondral bone plate of the vertebral body may allow intraosseous displacement of disc material (cartilaginous or Schmorl's nodes). These nodes can result in an obvious compression fracture of the vertebral body or subtle injury at the discovertebral junction. Fracture of the cancellous bone of the vertebral body and disruption of the cartilaginous endplate allow disc material to enter the vertebral body. Typically, the cranial disc protrudes into the vertebra, although both

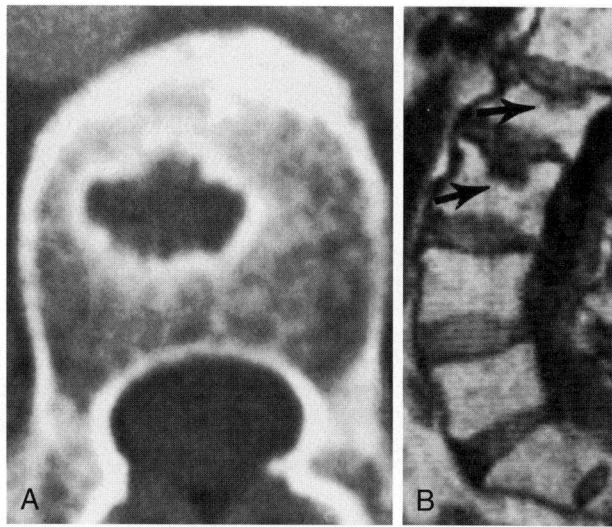

**Figure 56–57.** Cartilaginous nodes. *A*, Transaxial CT scan reveals the typical appearance of a cartilaginous node. It is generally well defined, circular or lobulated, close to the discovertebral junction, and accompanied by a rim of bone sclerosis. *B*, Sagittal T1-weighted (TR/TE, 600/20) spin echo MR image shows the location and appearance of cartilaginous nodes in the lumbar spine *(arrows)*. (*B*, Courtesy of M. Solomon, MD, San Jose, Calif.)

cranial and caudal discs may be involved. The intravertebral disc material may be associated with surrounding osseous compression and reactive bone formation. Radiographs reveal one or more radiolucent areas, with bony sclerosis in the vertebral body that may be combined with intervertebral disc space loss. CT and MR imaging may clarify the nature of the abnormalities (Fig. 56–57).

Another type of injury of the discovertebral junction occurs at the site of attachment of the anulus fibrosus to the rim of the vertebral body. In a developing skeleton, this union is far more solid than that between the cartilage in the vertebral rim and the ossified portion of the vertebral body. Thus, in a young patient, injury with prolapse of the contiguous intervertebral disc can lead to displacement of the ossified portion of the vertebral rim as a result of separation of the osteocartilaginous junction between the rim and the remaining vertebral body. This injury may occur either anteriorly or posteriorly; the latter is associated with displacement of a bony ridge into the spinal canal (Fig. 56–58).

## TRAUMA TO SYNCHONDROSES (GROWTH PLATES)

### Mechanism and Classification

The growth plate of an immature skeleton is especially vulnerable to injury; approximately 6% to 15% of fractures of the tubular bones of children younger than 16 years involve the growth plate and neighboring bone. Forces that produce ligamentous tear or joint dislocation in adults may lead to growth plate injury in children and adolescents because the joint capsule and ligamentous

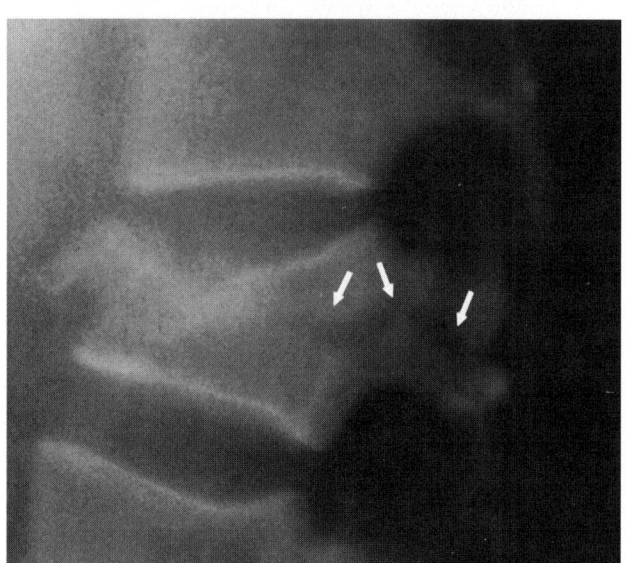

**Figure 56–56.** Seat-belt injury. After an automobile accident, a transverse fracture of an upper lumbar vertebra is sometimes associated with a transverse fracture through the pedicles and laminae *(arrows)*.

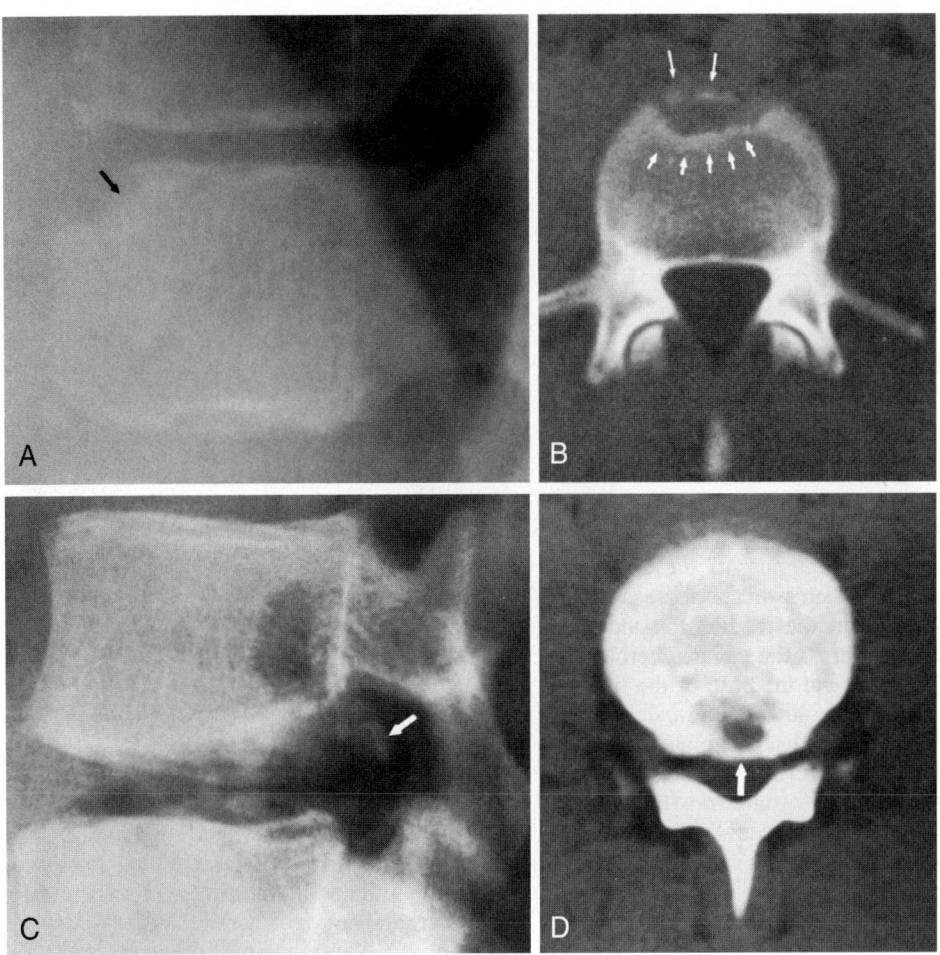

**Figure 56–58.** Cartilaginous nodes: anterior and posterior prolapse. *A*, In this young child, the radiograph shows a radiolucent area in the vertebral body *(arrow)* resulting from a cartilaginous node. This finding, in combination with loss of height of the intervertebral disc, simulates infection. *B*, In a different patient, transaxial CT shows the characteristics of a limbus vertebra. A radiolucent area is accompanied by bone spicules anteriorly, which represent a portion of the ossified vertebral rim, as well as bone sclerosis posteriorly *(arrows)*. *C* and *D*, Posterior prolapse leading to intraspinal bone displacement in an 18-year-old weight-lifter with an acute onset of back and leg pain. Lateral radiograph *(C)* shows displacement of a portion of the ring apophysis *(arrow)* into the spinal canal. Transaxial CT *(D)* reveals the location of the displaced bone *(arrow)*. *(A*, Courtesy of A. D'Abreu, MD, Porto Alegre, Brazil. *B*, Courtesy of R. Yagan, MD, Cleveland, Ohio. *C* and *D*, Courtesy of G. Greenway, MD, Dallas, Tex.)

structures are approximately two to five times stronger than the cartilaginous plate. Four types of stress may produce growth plate injury: shearing or avulsive forces account for approximately 80% of injuries, and splitting or compressive stresses account for the remainder. Sites most typically affected are the phalanges; the distal tibial, fibular, ulnar, and radial growth plates; and the proximal humeral growth plate. Growth plate injuries may occur acutely as a result of a single episode of trauma or chronically as a consequence of prolonged stress, particularly that associated with athletics (e.g., gymnastics).

Metaphyseal failure is more common in sites where the metaphysis is not protected from compression stress; one example is the vertebral endplate, where a compression fracture can produce a cartilaginous node. Metaphyseal fragility is also accentuated by any condition associated with osseous weakening, whether related to the osteoclastosis of hyperparathyroidism or the hypervascularity of the normal growth spurt. Avulsion injury to the growth plate is commonly observed at sites of apophyses. Examples include the lesser trochanter and the medial epicondyle of the distal portion of the humerus. The vulnerability of any specific apophysis to avulsion injury is governed by its development and maturation and depends on the time of appearance and fusion of the apophysis. Radiographically evident residua of growth disturbances related to previous physeal injury may be observed. Such residua include transphyseal linear ossific

striations and growth recovery lines that are modified in appearance according to the sites of arrested physeal growth. Large physeal bars, or bridges, may also be detected (Fig. 56–59).

Although several classification systems of growth plate injuries have been proposed, that of Salter and Harris is accepted most widely. This original system separated the

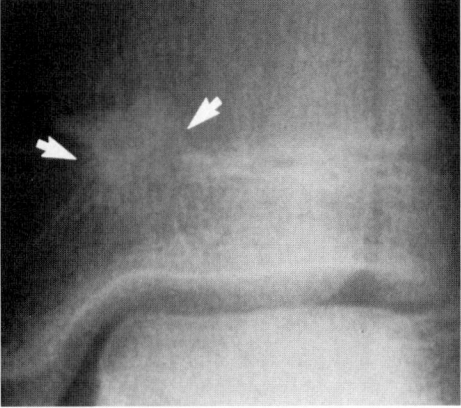

**Figure 56–59.** Growth plate injury: physeal bar. An ossific bridge *(arrows)* involving the medial aspect of the distal tibial physis resulted from a previous Salter-Harris type II injury to this physis (which was associated with a displaced distal fibular fracture).

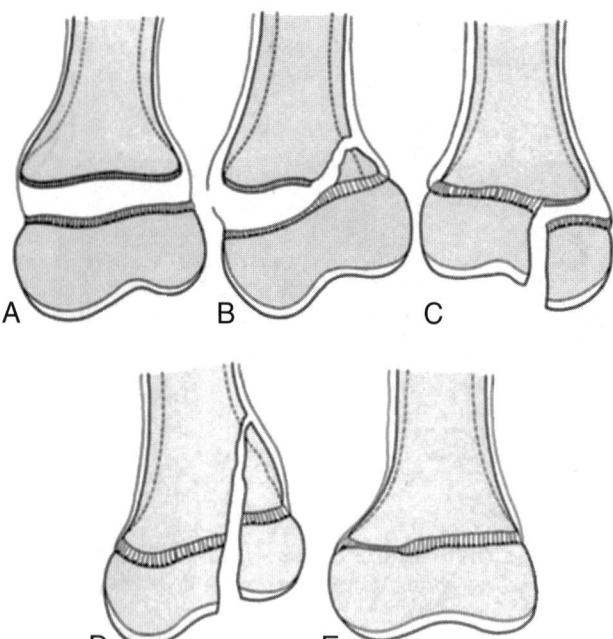

**Figure 56–60.** Growth plate injury: classification system. *A,* Type I. A split in the growth plate occurs through the zone of hypertrophic cells. The periosteum is intact. *B,* Type II. The growth plate is split, and the fracture enters the metaphyseal bone and creates a triangular fragment. The periosteum about the fragment is intact, whereas that on the opposite side may be torn. *C,* Type III. A vertical fracture line extends through the epiphysis to enter the growth plate. It then extends transversely across the hypertrophic zone of the plate. *D,* Type IV. A fracture extends across the epiphysis, growth plate, and metaphysis. Note the incongruity of the articular surface and violation of the germinal cells of the growth plate. *E,* Type V. Compression of a portion of the growth plate may not be associated with immediate radiographic abnormalities.

lesions into five types, according to their radiographic appearance (Fig. 56–60); in recent years, however, the Salter-Harris classification scheme has been modified and expanded.

*Type I* (6%). A type I injury represents pure epiphyseal separation, with the fracture isolated to the growth plate itself (Fig. 56–61A). This type of injury has a favorable prognosis and becomes apparent at a relatively young age, at a time when the growth plate is wide; it is especially frequent in children younger than 5 years. The proximal portions of the humerus and femur and distal portion of the humerus are the sites affected most commonly. Radiographic recognition of this injury is not difficult when the growth plate is wide and the epiphysis remains displaced. If spontaneous reduction of the separation takes place, the radiographic diagnosis is more difficult. Helpful signs are soft tissue swelling, particularly when centered at the physeal level, and minimal widening or irregularity of the growth plate. Comparison radiographs of the opposite (uninvolved) side are of further diagnostic help.

*Type II* (75%). A type II injury, the most common type of growth plate injury, results from a shearing or avulsion force that splits the growth plate for a variable distance before entering the metaphyseal bone and separating a small fragment of the bone—the *Thurston Holland* or *corner sign* (see Fig. 56–61B). The periosteum on the side of the metaphyseal fracture remains intact, but that on the opposite side is disrupted in conjunction with growth plate separation. Because of the intact periosteum, the fracture fragment is usually easily reduced. The usual age at injury is 10 to 16 years, and common sites of involvement are the distal ends of the radius, tibia, fibula, femur, and ulna, in order of decreasing frequency. The prognosis after this injury is generally good because of the absence of subsequent growth disturbance.

*Type III* (8%). In a type III injury, the fracture line extends vertically through the epiphysis and growth plate and then horizontally across the growth plate itself, usually on one side or the other (see Fig. 56–61C). Type III injuries are especially common in children between the ages of 10 and 15 years and in the medial or lateral portion of the distal part of the tibia, with less frequent involvement of the proximal end of the tibia and distal part of the femur. Radiography usually allows prompt recognition of the fracture, although multiple projections and stress views are sometimes necessary. Displacement is generally minimal, and growth arrest and deformities are rare.

*Type IV* (10%). A vertically oriented splitting force can produce a fracture that extends across the epiphysis, the growth plate, and the metaphysis to create a fragment that consists of a portion of both the epiphysis and the metaphysis (see Fig. 56–61D). This injury is most frequently encountered in the distal portions of the humerus and tibia. The radiographic diagnosis is facilitated by the presence of considerable metaphyseal and epiphyseal bone within the fragment; however, in younger children in whom the epiphysis is unossified or only partially ossified, the injury may be mistaken for a type II growth plate fracture. A type II injury is easily reduced and is associated with a good prognosis, whereas a type IV injury may require open reduction and careful realignment so that growth arrest and joint deformity are not encountered later.

*Type V* (1%). A crushing or compressive injury to the end of a tubular bone can lead to a rare type V growth plate fracture. Injury to the vascular supply of the plate occurs without any immediate radiographic signs; no irregularity or widening of the growth plate is seen. Subsequent radiographic examination may indicate focal areas of diminished or absent bony growth, which, in the presence of normal development in adjacent areas, can lead to angular deformity. Premature osseous fusion of the injured portion of the plate may be identified, particularly when tomographic techniques or MR imaging is used (see later discussion). This injury is more prominent in older children and adolescents, particularly those 12 to 16 years old. The physes of the distal portions of the femur and tibia and proximal portion of the tibia are usually affected.

*Type VI.* An injury (e.g., physical trauma, burn, infection) to the perichondrium can produce reactive bone for-

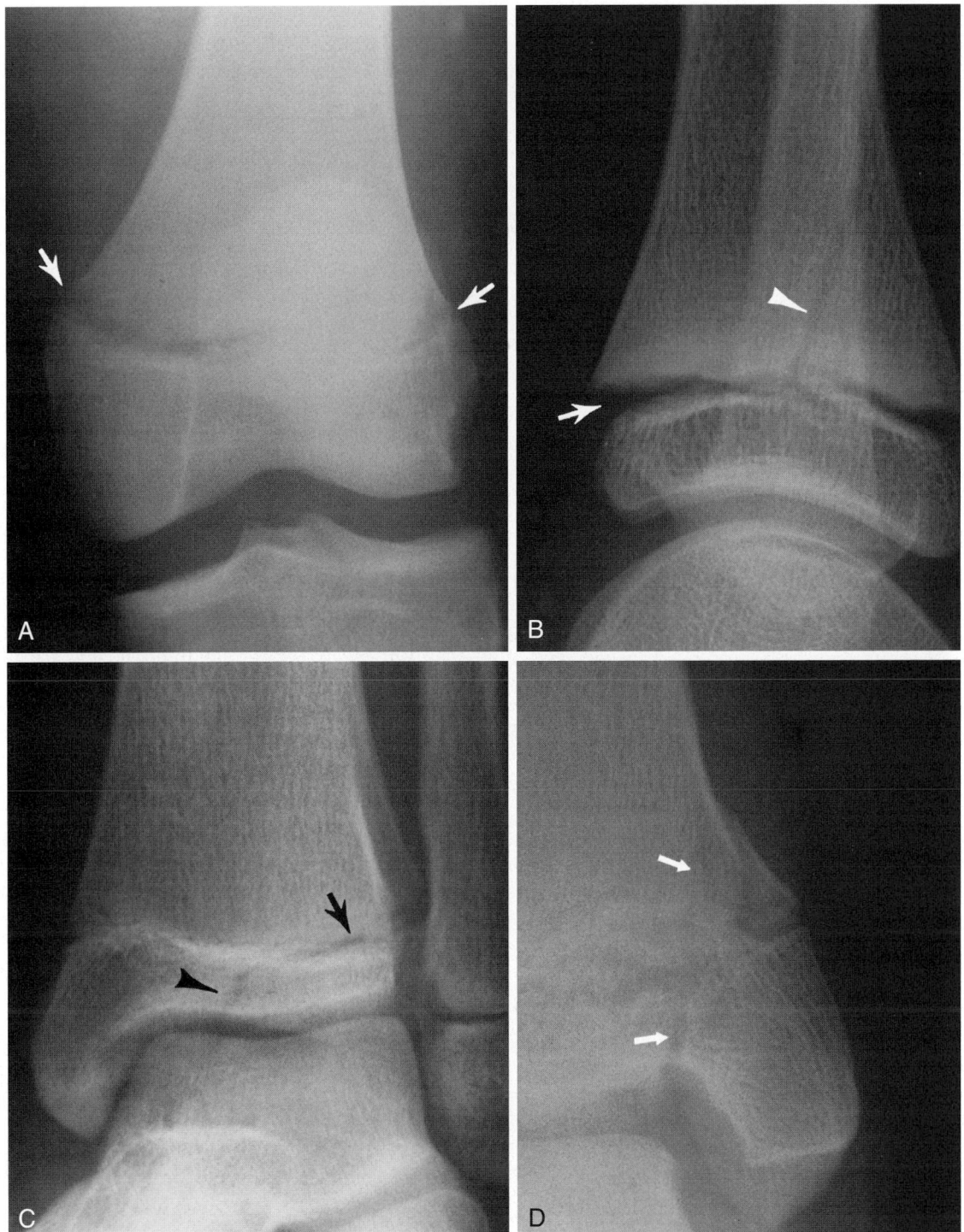

**Figure 56–61.** Growth plate injury: fracture types. *A*, Type I. Note the widening *(arrows)* of the growth plate of the distal end of the femur. *B*, Type II. Observe the widening of the growth plate *(arrow)* and the metaphyseal fracture *(arrowhead)*. *C*, Type III. The epiphyseal fracture line *(arrowhead)* and growth plate violation *(arrow)* can be recognized. *D*, Type IV. Observe the fracture line extending vertically through the epiphysis and metaphysis *(arrows)*.

mation external to the growth plate. The resultant osseous bridge may act as a barrier to growth of the adjacent portion of the plate, and progressive osseous angulation may occur.

*Type VII.* This relatively common type of injury is associated with epiphyseal alterations in the absence of involvement of the growth plate or metaphysis. Transchondral fractures and osteochondritis dissecans are examples of type VII injuries.

*Type VIII.* This injury affects metaphyseal growth and remodeling mechanisms in an immature skeleton, primarily as a result of effects on the blood supply.

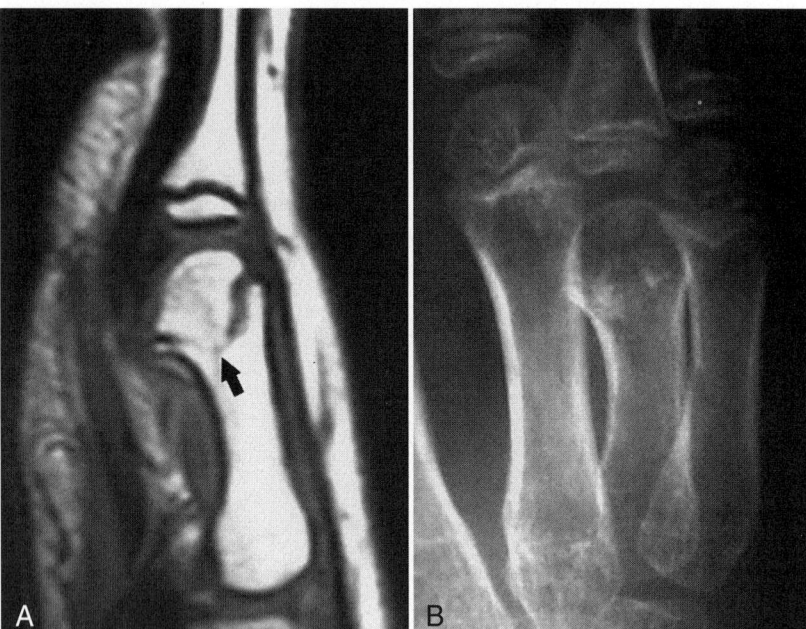

**Figure 56–62.** Growth plate injury: premature partial arrest of growth from previous fracture. *A*, Sagittal T1-weighted (TR/TE, 415/16) spin echo MR image shows partial arrest of the growth plate with a physeal bar *(arrow)*. *B*, Corresponding radiograph shows growth deformity.

*Type IX.* An injury to the periosteum of the diaphysis may, in rare circumstances, result in disruption of normal diaphyseal growth and remodeling. Segmental comminuted fractures, wringer injuries, and severe burns are examples of the type of trauma that can lead to this kind of injury.

Some degree of growth deformity develops in approximately 25% to 30% of patients with growth plate injuries, and in 10% of patients, this deformity is significant. The prognosis is related to the age of the patient, the anatomy of the vascular supply to the region, the type of injury, and the immediacy and adequacy of the reduction. In general, the younger the patient at the time of injury, the poorer the prognosis for residual deformity. Type I, II, and III injuries have a relatively good prognosis, whereas type IV injuries carry a guarded prognosis and type V and VI injuries have a poor prognosis. Late sequelae include growth impairment, premature growth plate fusion, epiphyseal malposition and rotation, and osteonecrosis.

Premature partial arrest of growth is produced by a bridge of bone, or bone bar, that extends from the metaphysis to the epiphysis across a portion of the physis. Continued growth of the remaining portion of the physis results in increasing angular deformity. Type IV injuries characteristically lead to closure of a portion of the physis; type V injuries may result in premature closure of the entire growth plate. MR imaging allows accurate assessment of the extent of the initial injury (Fig. 56–62), as well as the extent of physeal arrest (Fig. 56–63).

## Specific Injuries

### Slipped Capital Femoral Epiphysis

Slippage of the capital femoral epiphysis is typically observed between the ages of 10 and 17 years in boys and 8 and 15 years in girls. Boys are affected more frequently than girls, and black patients are affected more frequently than whites; overweight children have an especially high occurrence. About 20% to 35% of patients with slipped capital femoral epiphysis have bilateral involvement, which is more frequent in girls. A variety of contributing factors have been emphasized in the pathogenesis of this injury:

- *Trauma.* Although trauma is an important precipitating event in infants and young children, it appears to be only a minor factor in older persons. Less than 50% of patients have a history of significant injury.

- *Adolescent growth spurt.* The association between slipped capital femoral epiphysis and the adolescent growth spurt involves the relatively wide physis during this period and its change in configuration from a horizontal to an oblique plane, with increased shearing stress.

- *Hormonal influences.* The list of endocrine diseases associated with this femoral disorder includes hypothyroidism, hypoestrogenic states, acromegaly, gigantism, cryptorchidism, and pituitary and parathyroid tumors. Despite these observations, no clear evidence exists that levels of growth hormone are abnormal in patients with slipped capital femoral epiphysis.

- *Weight and activity.* One of the most striking characteristics of patients with slipped capital femoral epiphysis is a tendency to be overweight. Obesity increases the shearing stress on the growth plate and can lead to slippage even during usual activity. The propensity for epiphyseal slippage appears to be greater in physically active adolescents than in those who are less active.

The femoral head seated in the acetabulum is located in a posterior and medial direction with respect to the remainder of the femur. By convention, reference is made to the movement of the femoral head with respect to the shaft in cases of slipped capital femoral epiphysis.

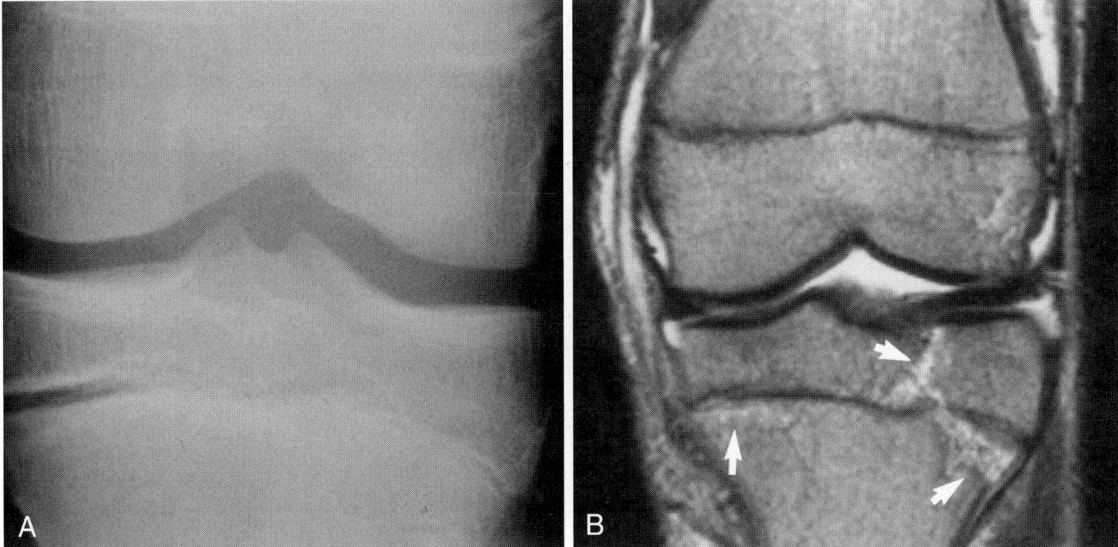

**Figure 56–63.** Growth plate injury. *A*, Routine radiograph shows widening of the medial portion of the proximal tibial physis, suggestive of a Salter-Harris type I injury. *B*, Coronal T2-weighted (TR/TE, 2000/80) spin echo MR image reveals high signal intensity *(arrows)* in the tibia, consistent with a Salter-Harris type IV injury; in a bone bruise in the lateral portion of the distal femoral epiphysis; and in and about the medial collateral ligament, indicative of ligamentous disruption and soft tissue edema. An effusion is present. (Courtesy of A. Newberg, MD, Boston, Mass.)

Although posteromedioinferior slippage of the capital femoral epiphysis is typical, other directions can be seen.

Radiographic analysis remains essential to the diagnosis of slipped capital femoral epiphysis. Both anteroposterior and frog-leg or lateral projections are mandatory; abnormalities on the frontal projection alone may be subtle, even in the presence of significant epiphyseal displacement. Comparison radiographs of the opposite side can be very useful. On the anteroposterior view, osteoporosis of both the femoral head and the femoral neck is common (Fig. 56–64). The margin of the metaphysis may seem blurred or indistinct, and the growth plate may appear widened. A tangential line along the lateral border of the femoral neck may fail to intersect any part of the epiphysis or may cross only a small portion of it. CT scanning and MR imaging appear to be more sensitive for the early diagnosis of this condition at a time when routine (and specialized) radiographs are normal. In chronic stages of slipped capital femoral epiphysis, routine radiography shows reactive bone formation along the medial and posterior portions of the femoral neck, a buttressing phenomenon similar to that which occurs in degenerative joint disease.

Sequelae of slipped capital femoral epiphysis include severe varus deformity, shortening and broadening of the femoral neck, osteonecrosis, chondrolysis, and degenerative joint disease. Osteonecrosis has been described in 6% to 15% of patients with this disorder. Chondrolysis may be observed in as many as 40% of patients with epiphyseal slippage and is more frequent in black than white patients, in women than men, and in persons with severe slippage. It usually occurs within 1 year of the slippage and may be evident in untreated or treated persons. Radiographs outline osteoporosis, concentric narrowing of the interosseous space, and eburnation and osteophy-

tosis of apposing osseous margins. Some joint space recovery may be seen after a period of months in approximately one third of patients. Its cause is unknown.

### Growth Plate Injuries about the Knee

Growth plate trauma in the distal portion of the femur may be related, in many cases, to birth or to athletic or automobile injuries. Examples include the wagon-wheel fracture resulting when children catch their legs between the spokes of wagon or bicycle wheels and the clipping injury of adolescent football players. Salter-Harris type II and III injuries are especially common. Injury to the proximal tibial physis is relatively rare.

### Growth Plate Injuries about the Ankle

Injuries to the growth plate in the distal portion of the tibia are common. Type II injury is most frequent, followed in order of decreasing frequency by type III, IV, and I lesions. Ten percent to 12% of physeal injuries at this site are followed by growth disturbance.

Triplane fractures of the distal portion of the tibia represent approximately 5% to 10% of all injuries in this location. The primary mechanism of injury appears to be external rotation of the foot, although plantar flexion has also been suggested. The resulting injury has several variations, including a two-plane fracture pattern (Tillaux or Kleiger fracture) that involves only the epiphysis, and a three-plane fracture pattern in which an additional metaphyseal fracture is present (Fig. 56–65). Radiographically, a triplane fracture resembles two different types of Salter-Harris injury (a type III lesion on the anteroposterior radiograph and a type II lesion on the lateral radiograph), although in reality, it is a variation of a type

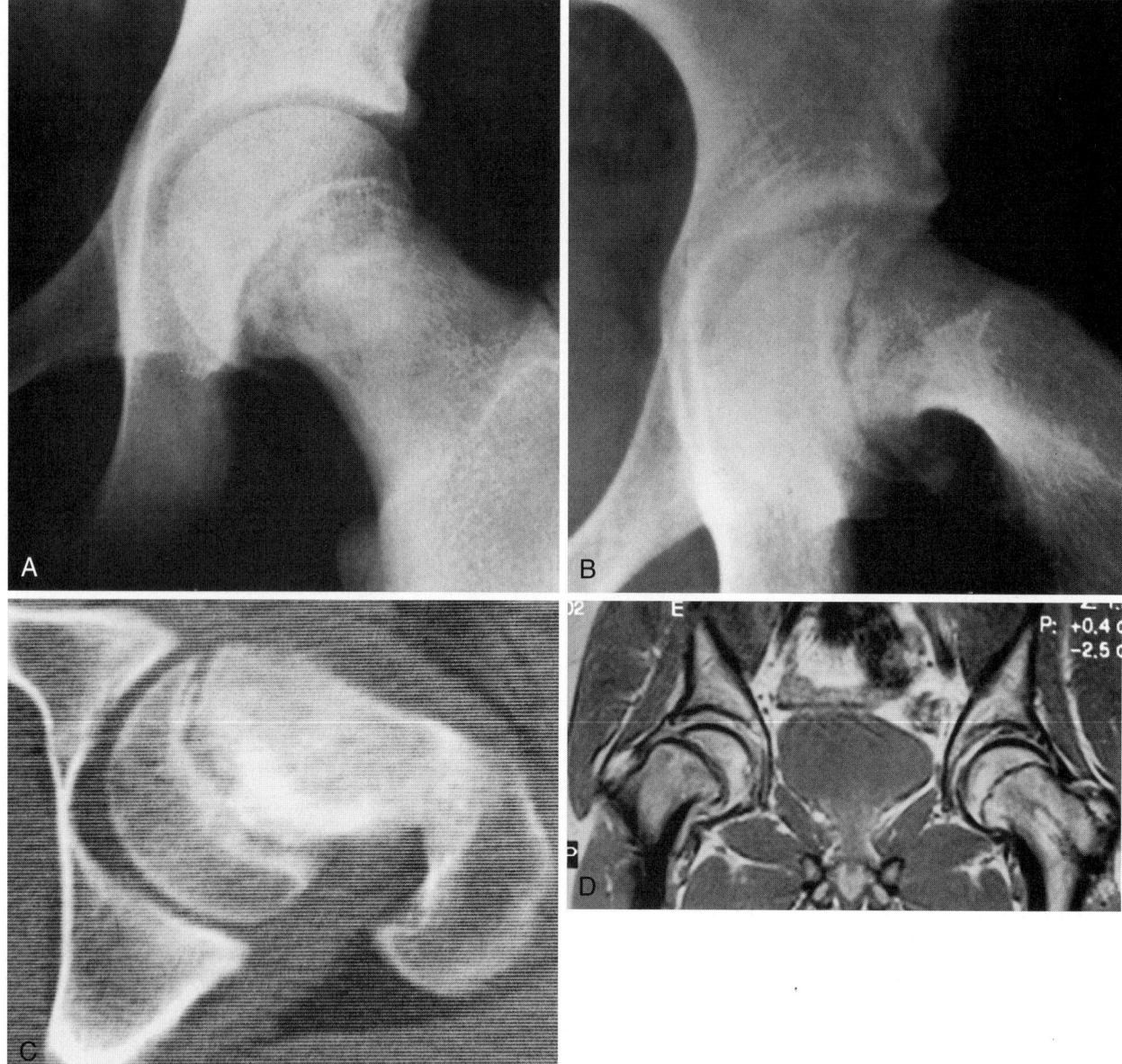

**Figure 56–64.**  Slipped capital femoral epiphysis: radiographic abnormalities. *A*, Anteroposterior radiograph shows subtle findings, including mild osteoporosis of the proximal portion of the femur and an indistinct metaphyseal margin. *B*, In the frog-leg view, the degree of posterior slippage is readily apparent. Note the widened growth plate. *C*, Transaxial CT scan in a different patient reveals that the femoral head is displaced posteriorly with respect to the femoral neck. *D*, In a third patient, coronal intermediate-weighted (TR/TE, 2000/20) spin echo MR images reveal posteromedial displacement of the right proximal femoral epiphysis. A T2-weighted image confirmed the presence of a joint effusion and periphyseal marrow edema. (*C*, From Busch MT, Morrissy RT: Slipped capital femoral epiphysis. Orthop Clin North Am 18:637, 1987. *D*, Courtesy of A. Vieira, MD, Porto, Portugal.)

IV injury pattern (Fig. 56–66). Two, three, or four fragments may result, with two fragments being most common. Because of the complexity of the injury, CT is an excellent technique for delineating the site and extent of involvement.

An isolated vertical fracture of the distal tibial epiphysis occurs in the adolescent age group. This injury, often designated the juvenile fracture of Tillaux, classically involves the lateral portion of the distal tibial epiphysis and conforms to a Salter-Harris type III injury because of lateral extension of the fracture through the open physis (Fig. 56–67).

### Growth Plate Injuries about the Shoulder

Disruption of the epiphysis and physis in the proximal portion of the humerus is relatively infrequent. Its occurrence in adolescent baseball pitchers as an epiphysiolysis is termed the Little League shoulder syndrome. Separation of the proximal humeral epiphysis may result

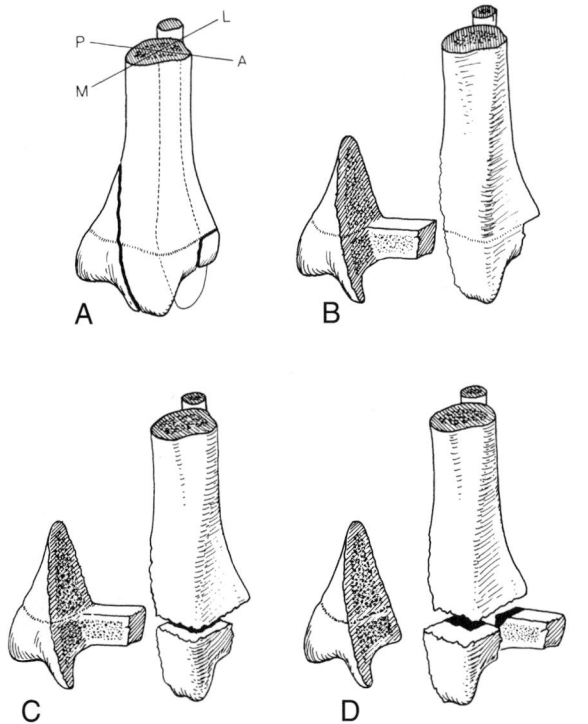

**Figure 56–65.** Growth plate injury: triplane ankle fracture. *A* and *B*, Two-part triplane fracture in place *(A)* and separated *(B)*, as viewed from the medial side. *C*, Three-part triplane fracture. *D*, Four-part triplane fracture. A, anterior; L, lateral; M, medial; P, posterior.

from an injury at birth, particularly during a difficult delivery.

The epiphysis of the inner margin of the clavicle ossifies at approximately 18 to 20 years of age and, with closure of the growth plate, merges with the shaft of the clavicle at approximately 25 years of age. Injury to the medial end of the clavicle in an immature skeleton can produce an epiphyseal separation that may be misdiagnosed as sternoclavicular joint dislocation. Physeal injuries about the shoulder may account for pseudodislocations of the acromioclavicular joint in children. Such injuries include displacement of the distal portion of the clavicle from its periosteal sleeve and avulsion of the epiphysis of the coracoid process.

## Growth Plate Injuries about the Elbow

Accurate diagnosis of elbow injury in an immature skeleton is complicated by the presence of multiple ossification centers. A mnemonic that can be used to remember the sequence of appearance of some of these ossification centers is CRIT: C, capitulum (1 year); R, radial head (3 to 6 years); I, internal or medial epicondyle (5 to 7 years); and T, trochlea (9 to 10 years). The olecranon center of the ulna appears at 6 to 10 years, and the final center to appear is the lateral epicondyle at 9 to 13 years.

Normally, the metaphysis of the distal portion of the humerus and the capitulum are anteverted about 140 degrees relative to the shaft of the humerus. A line drawn along the anterior cortex of the humerus on a lateral radiograph—the anterior humeral line—should intersect

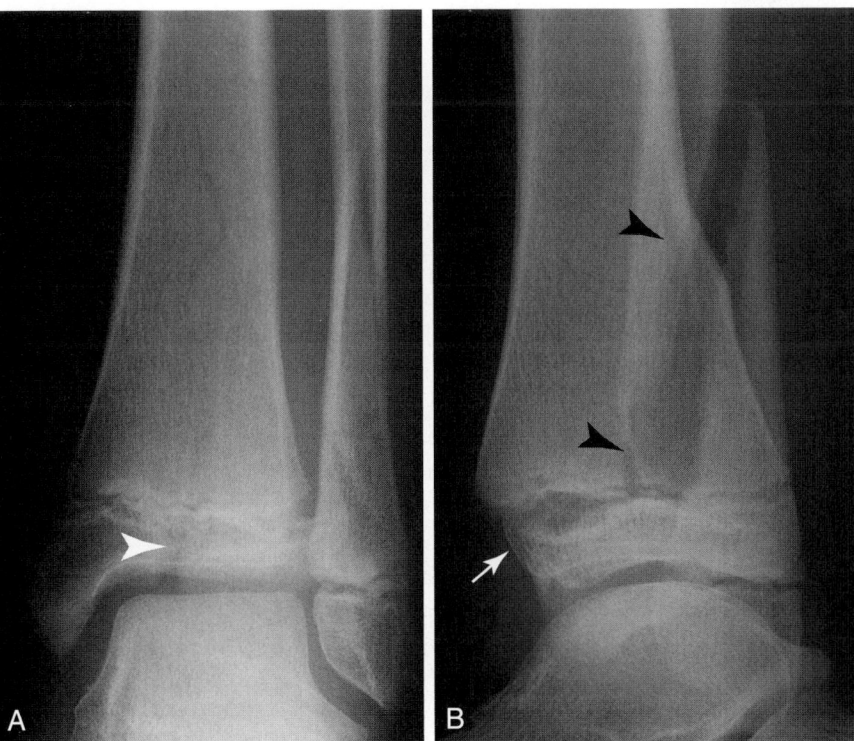

**Figure 56–66.** Growth plate injury: triplane ankle fracture. *A*, Anteroposterior radiograph shows an injury that has the appearance of a type III lesion *(arrowhead)*. *B*, On a lateral radiograph, a type II lesion is apparent *(arrowheads)*. Note the posterior displacement of the distal tibial epiphysis *(arrow)* and an oblique fibular fracture.

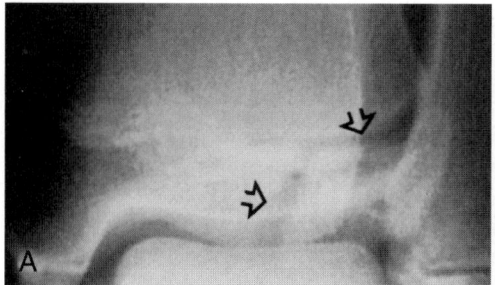
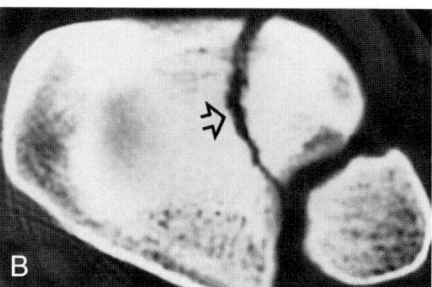

**Figure 56–67.** Growth plate injury: ankle—juvenile fracture of Tillaux. Frontal radiograph *(A)* and transaxial CT image *(B)* show the injury *(open arrows)* involving the anterolateral portion of the epiphysis. It represents a Salter-Harris type III injury.

the middle third of the capitular ossification center. In the presence of supracondylar fractures of the humerus (the most common fracture about the elbow in children), posterior displacement or angulation of the distal fragment allows the anterior humeral line to pass through the anterior third of the ossification center or even anterior to the capitulum (Fig. 56–68). Because of absent or incomplete ossification of the developing centers about the elbow in infants and children, complete assessment of injuries may not be possible with conventional radiography.

Fracture of the lateral condyle is frequent and represents a Salter-Harris type IV injury. The fracture line splits the epiphysis and separates a portion of the adjacent metaphysis and the capitulum. Separation of the medial epicondyle ossification center is a result of stress placed on the flexor pronator tendon that attaches to this site; this represents approximately 10% of all elbow injuries. In some instances, the epicondyle may become entrapped within the joint (Fig. 56–69). In this situation, the displaced epicondylar ossification center can simulate a normal trochlear center; however, the appearance of a trochlear center without a medial epicondylar center is inconsistent with the normal sequence of ossification about the distal portion of the humerus.

Separation, with or without fracture, of the entire distal humeral epiphysis may be mistaken for fracture of the lateral humeral condyle or dislocation of the elbow (Fig. 56–70). In most cases, a Salter-Harris type I or II injury is present. Radiographs usually reveal normal alignment of the radial shaft and capitellar ossification center, normal alignment of the radius and ulna, and malalignment of these bones with the humerus.

### Other Growth Plate Injuries

The relative frequency of some physeal injuries is indicated in Table 56–5.

**Figure 56–68.** Elbow injury: supracondylar fracture of the humerus. On a lateral radiograph, elevation of the intracapsular fat pads and a subtle supracondylar fracture line *(arrow)* are seen. A line drawn along the anterior cortex of the humerus intersects the anterior third of the capitular ossification center, indicative of minimal posterior displacement at the fracture site.

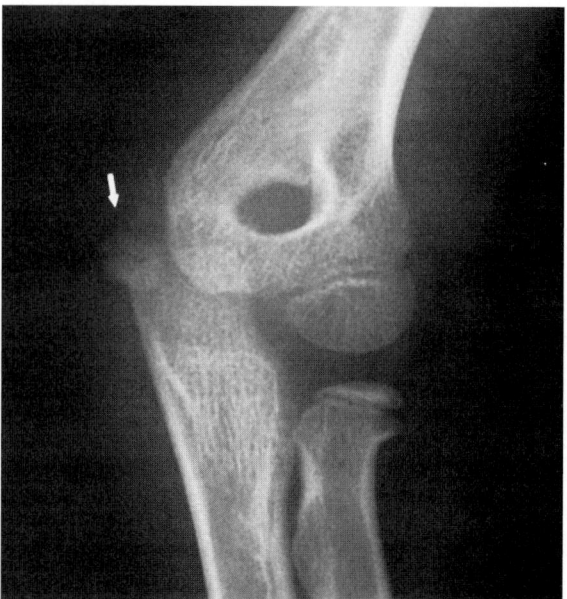

**Figure 56–69.** Injury of the medial epicondyle of the humerus. Note the position of the avulsed epicondyle *(arrow)*.

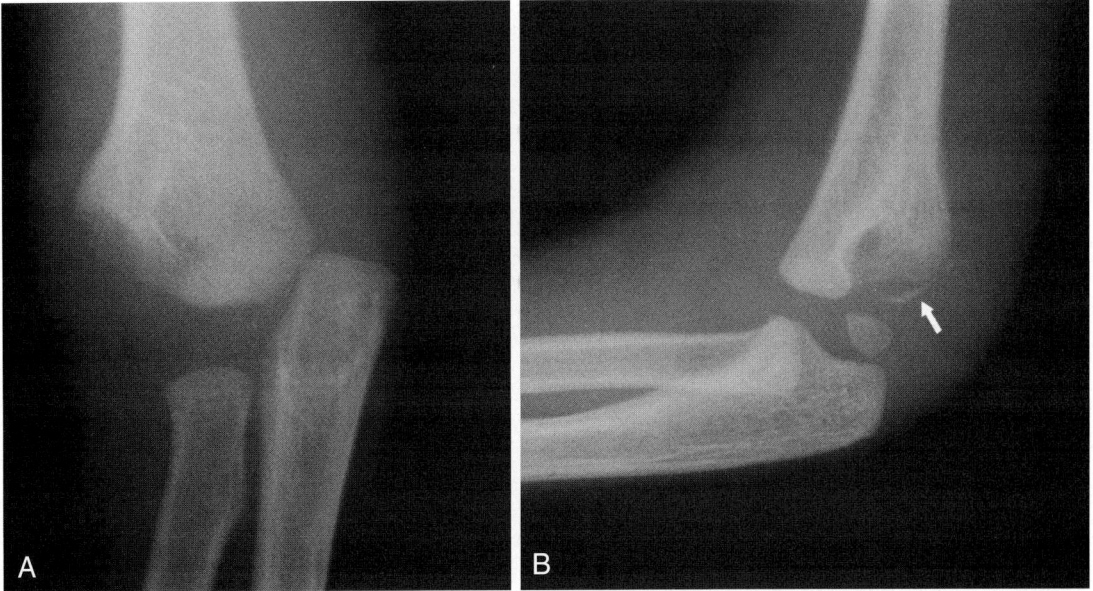

**Figure 56–70.** Growth plate injury of the distal portion of the humerus. Although an anteroposterior radiograph *(A)* appears to delineate dislocation of the elbow, with medial displacement of the ulna and radius, a lateral radiograph *(B)* identifies the metaphyseal ossific flake *(arrow)* and normal alignment of the radius and capitulum, findings indicating that separation of the distal humeral growth plate has occurred.

**TABLE 56–5**

**Relative Frequency of Physeal Injuries**

| | Frequency (%) | Typical Age* (Yr) | Age Range (Yr) |
|---|---|---|---|
| Distal portion of radius | 49.9 | 9–14 | |
| Distal portion of humerus† | 16.7 | Birth–5‡ | |
| | | 6§ | 3–10 |
| Distal portion of tibia | 11.0 | 12 | 8–13 |
| Distal portion of fibula | 9.1 | | |
| Distal portion of ulna | 5.7 | | |
| Proximal portion of radius | 4.2 | 9–10 | 8–13 |
| Proximal portion of humerus | 3.1 | 14–15 | 10–16 |
| Distal portion of femur | 1.2 | 11–12 | 10–15 |
| Proximal portion of ulna | 0.7 | | |
| Proximal portion of tibia | 0.5 | 13–15 | |
| Proximal portion of femur | 0.1 | 2–6 | |
| | | 12–15 | |
| Other | 0.8 | | |

*Girls, because of earlier skeletal maturity and advanced skeletal age relative to boys, have injuries at an average age 1 to 2 years younger than boys.

†The majority of these fractures are lateral condyle lesions.

‡Distal humeral fracture-separations.

§Lateral humeral condyle fracture-separations.

From Shapiro F: Epiphyseal growth plate fracture-separations: A pathophysiologic approach. Orthopedics 5:720, 1982.

## Chronic Stress Injuries

A variety of musculoskeletal manifestations related to the chronic application of stress can occur in professional and recreational athletes. Growth plates in the distal portions of the radius and ulna, proximal portion of the humerus, distal aspect of the femur, and distal end of the tibia are affected most commonly. The general radiographic abnormalities accompanying the chronic stress are similar in each of these locations. Part or all of the physis appears widened and irregular, with varying degrees of accompanying sclerosis in the adjacent metaphysis (Fig. 56–71). Superficially, these radiographic abnormalities resemble those occurring in rickets, hypophosphatasia, or metaphyseal dysplasia. In some cases, a unilateral or asymmetrical distribution of changes provides an important diagnostic clue.

## TRAUMA TO SUPPORTING STRUCTURES, SYNDESMOSES, AND ENTHESES

### Tendon and Ligament Injury and Healing

In most regions of the body, tendons are subjected to axial loading. Acute failure of a musculotendinous system may occur at the junction between muscle and tendon or at the osseous site of tendinous attachment; the latter sometimes results in an avulsion fracture (e.g., mallet finger). Failure within the tendon itself is rare unless preexisting tendon degeneration is present. Tendon tears or ruptures can appear at virtually any site in the body. Typical examples are injuries to the tendons in the hands and feet and to the patellar, triceps, peroneal, quadriceps, rotator cuff, and Achilles tendons. In many cases, a significant traumatic event initiates the tendon injury, although spontaneous rupture has been documented, especially in patients with rheumatoid arthritis and systemic lupus erythematosus and in those receiving local corticosteroid injections. The gold standard for the evaluation of tendons is MR imaging, and its role is discussed in detail in Chapter 59.

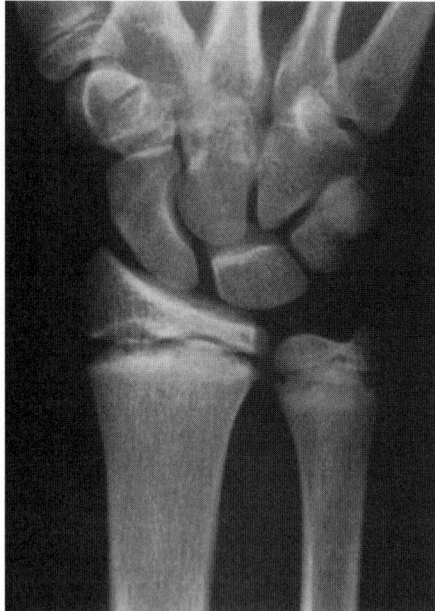

**Figure 56–71.** Growth plate injury: chronic stress involving the wrist in a gymnast. Note the subtle physeal widening and irregularity in the radius and ulna. (Courtesy of R. Dussault, MD, Boston, Mass.)

Ligament tears or ruptures are also widely distributed and are particularly noteworthy about the wrist, ankle, elbow, and knee. In these cases, radiography may require supplementation with stress radiography; however, MR imaging is becoming the modality of choice for ligament evaluation.

## Avulsion Injuries

Abnormal tensile stress on ligaments and tendons caused by a single violent injury or repetitive injuries may lead to characteristic avulsions at their sites of attachment to bone. For example, avulsion of a portion of the calcaneus, patella, or ulnar olecranon may accompany exaggerated pull of the Achilles, quadriceps, or triceps tendon, respectively. Avulsion injuries of the proximal portion of the humerus, which generally occur during dislocation of the glenohumeral joint, may involve either of the tuberosities and are related to tendinous traction provided by the various components of the rotator cuff. Avulsion may also accompany ligamentous, tendinous, and other injuries about the knee (Fig. 56–72) and spinal trauma. The size of the avulsed fragment is quite variable; in adults, only small osseous flecks may be pulled from the parent bone, whereas in children or adolescents, an entire apophysis may undergo avulsion.

Because tendinous, ligamentous, and capsular tissue is much stronger than physeal cartilage, forces that might produce a ligamentous or tendinous injury or dislocation in an adult may lead to physeal avulsion in a child. Such injuries commonly involve the apophyses of the skeleton. In an older child or adolescent with more extensive ossification of the skeleton, the size of the displaced bone fragment may be larger and thus facilitate the proper diagnosis and interpretation of the injury. Apophyseal avulsions can occur at many different skeletal sites, although those of the pelvis and hip are encountered most frequently.

Several avulsion injuries about the pelvis and hip in young athletes have characteristic radiographic features, including avulsion injuries of the anterior superior iliac spine, which occur in sprinters as a result of stress at the origin of the tensor fasciae or the sartorius muscle; avulsion injuries of the anterior inferior iliac spine, which relate to stress at the origins of the straight and reflected heads of the rectus femoris muscle (Fig. 56–73*A*); avulsion injuries of the apophysis of the lesser trochanter caused by stress on the psoas major muscle during strenuous hip flexion; avulsion injuries of the apophysis of the ischial tuberosity resulting from violent contraction of the hamstring muscles, often occurring in soccer players and hurdlers; avulsion injuries of the greater trochanter of the femur produced by gluteal muscle contraction; avulsion of the apophysis of the iliac crest secondary to severe contraction of the abdominal muscles associated

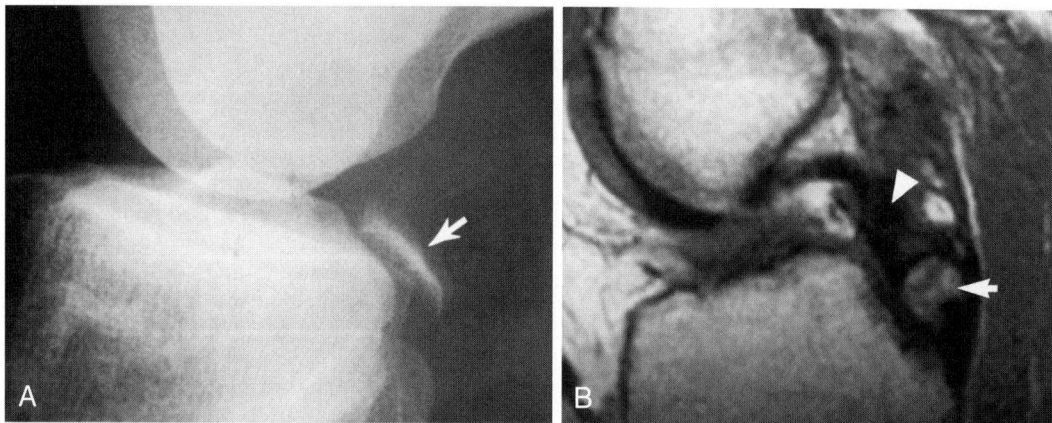

**Figure 56–72.** Avulsion injury: cruciate ligament avulsion. *A,* Observe the posterior bony fragment *(arrow)* from an old posterior cruciate ligament injury. *B,* Sagittal intermediate-weighted (TR/TE, 1000/40) spin echo MR image shows a tibial avulsion fracture *(arrow)* related to the site of attachment of the posterior cruciate ligament *(arrowhead)*.

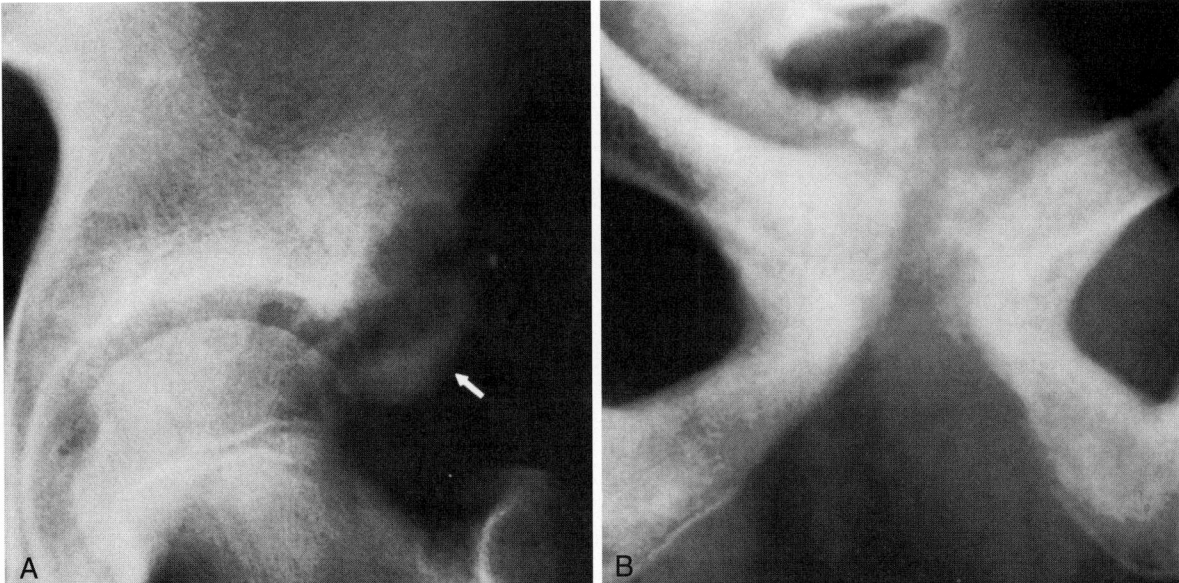

**Figure 56–73.** Avulsion injury: pelvis. *A*, Anterior inferior iliac spine. The avulsed fragment *(arrow)* is related to stress at the origin of the rectus femoris muscle. *B*, Symphysis pubis and inferior pubic ramus. The osseous irregularity may result from avulsion injuries caused by stress in the adductor brevis, adductor longus, and gracilis muscles. (*B*, From Schneider R, Kaye JJ, Ghelman B: Adductor avulsive injuries near the symphysis pubis. Radiology 120:567, 1976.)

with abrupt directional change during running; and avulsion injuries near the symphysis pubis related to adductor muscle (adductor longus, adductor brevis, gracilis) insertion sites (see Fig. 56–73*B*). Follow-up radiographs may show considerable new bone formation or healing with incorporation of the fragment into the parent bone, which in some cases is associated with bizarre skeletal overgrowth.

### Diastasis

The term diastasis implies a separation of normally joined bony elements; it is frequently applied to syndesmoses and, specifically, to injuries of the ligaments that extend between the lower portions of the tibia and fibula. Complete or partial diastasis can occur, depending on the extent of damage to the tibiofibular and interosseous ligaments. Radiographs may reveal abnormal separation of the tibia and fibula in which the space (la ligne claire) between the medial cortex of the fibula and the posterior edge of the peroneal groove is greater than 5 to 5.5 mm on an anteroposterior radiograph. Soft tissue ossification and even ankylosis between the tibia and the fibula may subsequently occur. The term diastasis is likewise applied to separation of apposing bone surfaces about symphyses (e.g., symphysis pubis).

### TRAUMA TO SKELETAL MUSCLE

Trauma to skeletal muscle may result from any type of accidental injury, but it is encountered most often in the setting of physical exertion, particularly athletic endeavors. Intense and prolonged exercise can produce a muscle strain or pull related to rapid and violent contraction of the muscle, but this mechanism is only one of a spectrum

of injuries that can affect skeletal muscle. Skeletal muscles do not act independently. Rather, they transmit their contractile forces to adjacent structures through tendinous attachments. The junctional region between muscle fibers and the tendinous attachment is termed the myotendinous, or musculotendinous, junction. Many, if not most, of the injuries to muscle occur at the myotendinous junction.

### Muscle Anatomy and Physiology

Most muscles show a mixture of two types of fibers: type I, or slow, fibers, and type II, or fast, fibers. Histochemical differences are used to distinguish between these types of fibers. Type I fibers are better suited to a relatively slow but repetitive type of contraction, such as the tonic forces characteristic of postural muscles, and are more resistant to fatigue than type II fibers are. Hence, type I fibers are involved more in endurance activities than in those requiring speed and strength of short duration. Type II fibers, in contrast, are adapted to produce rapid phasic forces that are operational in large-scale movements of the human body. Type I fibers have been designated slow-twitch fibers and type II as fast-twitch fibers.

### Muscle Injury and Repair

Skeletal muscle contracts in response to injury. The sheath that encloses the muscle, the epimysium, and the overlying fascia act as a relatively rigid tissue. As a consequence, large intracompartmental hematomas can develop within the muscle. The anatomic arrangement of muscle tissue within the surrounding sheath contributes to the frequent development of compartment syndromes after trauma. Skeletal muscle is capable of limited regeneration. With extensive muscle damage, however, such regeneration is not possible, and connective tissue is formed to replace the injured muscle, with resultant loss of function. In certain situations, such as after laceration, healing of skeletal muscle is associated with extensive scarring and ossification.

## Direct Muscle Injury

**Muscle Laceration.** Muscle lacerations result from penetrating injuries. The typical healing response results in the formation of a scar composed of dense connective tissue. MR imaging in cases of lacerated muscle is characterized by a defect, often transverse, with interruption of the continuity of the muscle and changes in signal intensity reflecting the presence of blood and edema.

**Muscle Contusion.** Compression of a muscle from direct trauma leads to a contusion. The term *charley horse* is sometimes used to describe the injury. The gastrocnemius and quadriceps muscles are typical sites of involvement. Injury results in capillary rupture and interstitial hemorrhage (bleeding between the fibers of the damaged connective tissue), followed by edema and an inflammatory mass. Contusions vary in severity, and the muscle is still able to function, even in severe cases.

There are four basic MR imaging characteristics of a muscle contusion: (1) the affected muscle is usually slightly increased in girth; (2) edema leads to an increase in signal intensity on T2-weighted spin echo and STIR images; (3) a feathery, interstitial pattern is evident that relates to the dispersion of inflammatory fluid within and between the muscle fibers; and (4) no evidence of disruption of muscle fibers is present (Fig. 56–74).

## Indirect Muscle Injury

Indirect injuries to muscle occur from overzealous use during physical exercise. Certain muscles are prone to exercise-related, or exertional, muscle injury and show several typical characteristics. First, such muscles commonly perform eccentric actions (e.g., hamstring muscles). Second, the muscles commonly act across two joints (e.g., biceps brachii and gastrocnemius muscles). Such muscles often limit the range of joint motion because of their intrinsic tightness. For example, when the knee is extended, the gastrocnemius muscle restricts dorsiflexion of the ankle, and when the hip is flexed, the hamstring muscles limit extension of the knee. Third, muscles that have type II, or fast, fibers and are involved in activities requiring sudden acceleration or deceleration are typically affected (e.g., hip flexors and adductors, rectus femoris muscle).

The precise MR imaging findings are influenced by the severity of the strain and its duration. Minor, or grade 1, strains produce MR imaging findings similar to those of a muscle contusion. With moderate, or grade 2, muscle strains, a focal masslike lesion or a stellate defect, or both, may be observed. The signal intensity of the involved muscle reflects the presence of edema or blood. With severe, or grade 3, muscle strains, discontinuity of the muscle is evident, and blood collects between the torn edges (Fig. 56–75).

Delayed-onset muscle soreness represents another response to physical exertion. Clinical findings consisting of muscle soreness and tenderness to palpation occur within 1 to several days after muscle exertion. The soreness is initially most evident at the musculotendinous junction and later becomes more diffuse. MR imaging findings resemble those of grade 1 muscle strains.

## Muscle Herniation

Focal herniation of muscle through a defect in its enclosing fascia may occur as a complication of local blunt trauma or as a result of muscle hypertrophy. Typically, the lower part of the leg, especially the anterior tibial compartment, is involved, and the tibialis anterior muscle is affected most frequently. MR imaging is an effective diagnostic technique when such herniation is suspected.

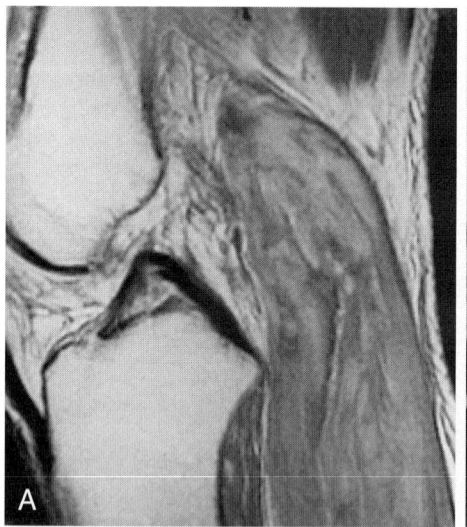 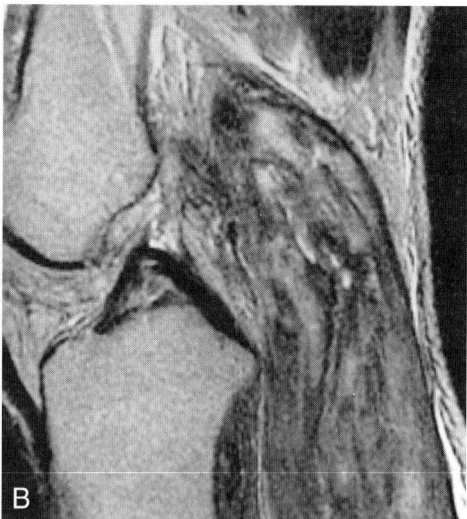

**Figure 56–74.** Skeletal muscle injury: contusion. Sagittal intermediate-weighted (TR/TE, 2000/30) *(A)* and T2-weighted (TR/TE, 2000/80) *(B)* spin echo MR images show enlargement of the medial head of the gastrocnemius muscle. The muscle is inhomogeneous in signal intensity on both images and is generally of higher signal intensity than normal.

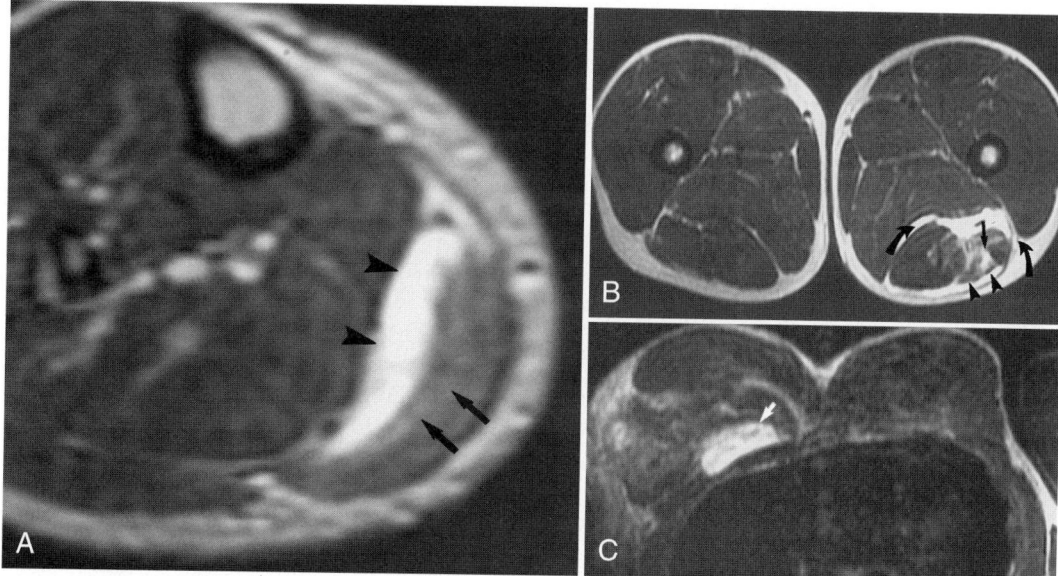

**Figure 56–75.** Skeletal muscle injury in three different patients. *A*, Grade 1 strain. Transaxial T2-weighted (TR/TE, 2000/80) spin echo MR image reveals increased signal intensity of the gastrocnemius muscle *(arrows)* and a perifascial fluid collection *(arrowheads)*. *B*, Grade 2 strain. On a transaxial T2-weighted (TR/TE, 2000/80) spin echo MR image, note that the biceps femoris muscle demonstrates edema throughout its substance *(arrowheads)*, with several small focal areas that may represent limited interruption of muscle fibers *(small arrow)*. The perifascial edema *(large arrows)* is striking. *C*, Grade 3 strain—ruptured right pectoralis muscle. Transaxial T2-weighted (TR/TE, 2000/80) spin echo MR image shows the distortion of muscle anatomy, with localized edema and a focal hematoma *(arrow)* of high signal intensity. (*B*, From Deutsch AL, Mink JH, Kerr R: MRI of the Foot and Ankle. New York, Raven, 1992. *C*, From Fleckenstein JL, Shellock FG: Exertional muscle injuries: Magnetic resonance imaging evaluation. Top Magn Reson Imaging 3:50, 1991.)

## Rhabdomyolysis

Rhabdomyolysis is a relatively common syndrome of muscle injury that alters the integrity of the cell membrane and allows cellular contents to escape into the general circulation. Causative factors include burns, crush injuries, prolonged muscle compression, drug overdose, and extremely intense exercise, especially in hot climates. Although multiple intracellular enzymes may be released, creatine kinase is the most sensitive to muscle injury. Myoglobulin can be detected in the urine. Clinical findings include fever and intense pain and weakness. Ultrasonography, CT, scintigraphy, and MR imaging can be used to investigate this condition and its complications. Swelling and regions of low attenuation in muscles are typical CT findings of rhabdomyolysis. Muscle calcification may also be detected. MR imaging reveals increased intramuscular signal intensity on T2-weighted spin echo and STIR images.

## Compartment Syndrome and Myonecrosis

Compartment syndrome is a condition characterized by elevated pressure within an anatomically confined space that leads to irreversible damage to its contents (i.e., muscle and neurovascular components). Any condition that increases the contents of a compartment or reduces the volume of a compartment may lead to a compartment syndrome. Common causes are trauma with hemorrhage, fractures, increased capillary permeability after thermal burns, and intense physical activity.

The clinical manifestations of a compartment syndrome may be acute or chronic. Typical acute findings are pain out of proportion to the extent of the injury, weakness and pain on passive stretching of the extremity, hypoesthesia in the distribution of the nerves traversing the compartment, and the presence of a tense, swollen compartment. Pulses are always palpable in cases of acute compartment syndrome. If not diagnosed and treated early, an acute compartment syndrome may be associated with muscle necrosis and permanent neurologic damage with fibrous contracture (e.g., Volkmann's contracture).

MR imaging findings in patients with an acute compartment syndrome include swelling of the affected extremity and abnormalities in signal intensity in the muscles of the involved compartment and, less commonly, other compartments. Similar and often transient MR imaging abnormalities may accompany chronic compartment syndromes. Complications such as myonecrosis can be delineated with MR imaging, and radiography may reveal diagnostic findings in cases of long-standing compartment syndrome (Fig. 56–76). One such finding is sheetlike calcification involving the anterolateral portion of the lower part of the leg, commonly associated with dysfunction of the peroneal nerve.

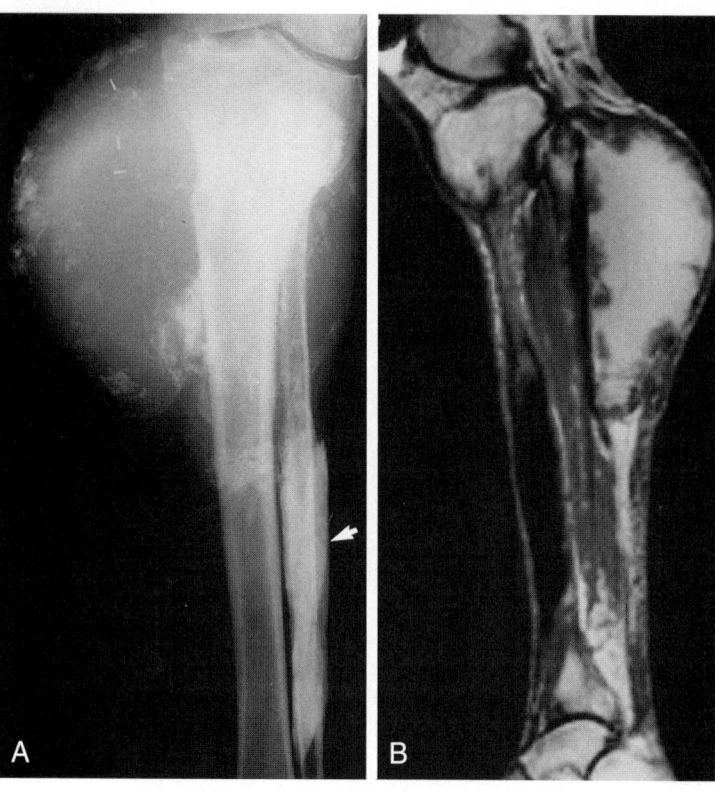

**Figure 56–76.** Skeletal muscle injury: compartment syndrome and myonecrosis. *A,* Chronic compartment syndrome in the lower leg after a tibial fracture led to enlargement and calcification of the gastrocnemius muscle, evident with routine radiography. Also note the sheetlike calcification *(arrow)* in the anterolateral compartment of the leg. *B,* Sagittal intermediate-weighted (TR/TE, 2000/15) spin echo MR image shows the enlarged muscle with central high signal intensity. Cystic degeneration of the gastrocnemius muscle produced these findings. Calcification, with its signal void, is seen in the anterior soft tissues and periphery of the gastrocnemius muscle. (Courtesy of J. Spaeth, MD, Minneapolis, Minn.)

## TRAUMATIC ABUSE OF CHILDREN (ABUSED CHILD SYNDROME)

It has been estimated that as many as 200,000 incidents of child abuse are reported each year in the United States. Radiographic abnormalities can be detected in 50% to 70% of cases.

Traumatic insult to the child's skeleton can produce elevation of the periosteal membrane, which is loosely attached to the diaphysis of tubular bones. Although the resultant periostitis is a delayed radiographic finding (Fig. 56–77A), it should be emphasized that firm attachment of the periosteal membrane to the metaphyses of the tubular bones can lead to an immediate radiographic abnormality—single or multiple metaphyseal bone fragments (see Fig. 56–77B). The resultant fragments consist of a disc of bone and calcified cartilage. Reactive bone formation with sclerosis can be a prominent change associated with periostitis and metaphyseal fracture. Physeal injuries also occur.

The proper workup of a child suspected of having been physically abused includes a radiographic survey of all the long bones, the pelvis, the spine, the ribs, and the skull. A single radiograph of the entire skeleton is diagnostically inadequate. Scintigraphy with bone-seeking pharmaceutical agents may also be a useful adjunct. Radiographic findings include single or multiple fractures, especially in the ribs (see Fig. 56–77C); other sites, in order of decreasing frequency, include the humerus, femur, tibia, small bones of the hand and foot, and skull.

Multiple skull fractures and those that are bilateral and cross sutures are suggestive of child abuse. Diaphyseal or metaphyseal fractures, most commonly transverse, can be seen in various stages of healing. The metaphyseal infractions may be quite subtle and require multiple projections for adequate visualization. "Unusual" fractures, such as those of the sternum, lateral aspect of the clavicle, scapula, and vertebral bodies (especially the anterior portions) and posterior osseous elements, as well as complex physeal injuries of the distal portion of the humerus, should arouse suspicion of abuse. Other clues to a correct diagnosis include overabundant callus formation, bilateral acute fractures, and fractures in the lower extremities in infants and young children who are not walking.

Subperiosteal bone formation may be apparent between 7 and 14 days after the injury. Late skeletal findings include metaphyseal cupping, growth disturbances, subluxation, and diaphyseal widening caused by subperiosteal apposition. Extensive extraosseous alterations may also be present, including myositis, pancreatitis, hepatic and renal injuries, ocular lesions such as retinal detachment, and intracranial and subdural hematomas.

Disorders or conditions that must be differentiated from this syndrome are the normal periostitis of infancy, metaphyseal changes of normal growth, osteogenesis imperfecta, types of congenital insensitivity to pain, spondylometaphyseal and metaphyseal dysplasias, and infantile cortical hyperostosis. Metaphyseal avulsion fractures may similarly accompany abnormal copper metabolism in the kinky-hair syndrome (Menkes' syndrome).

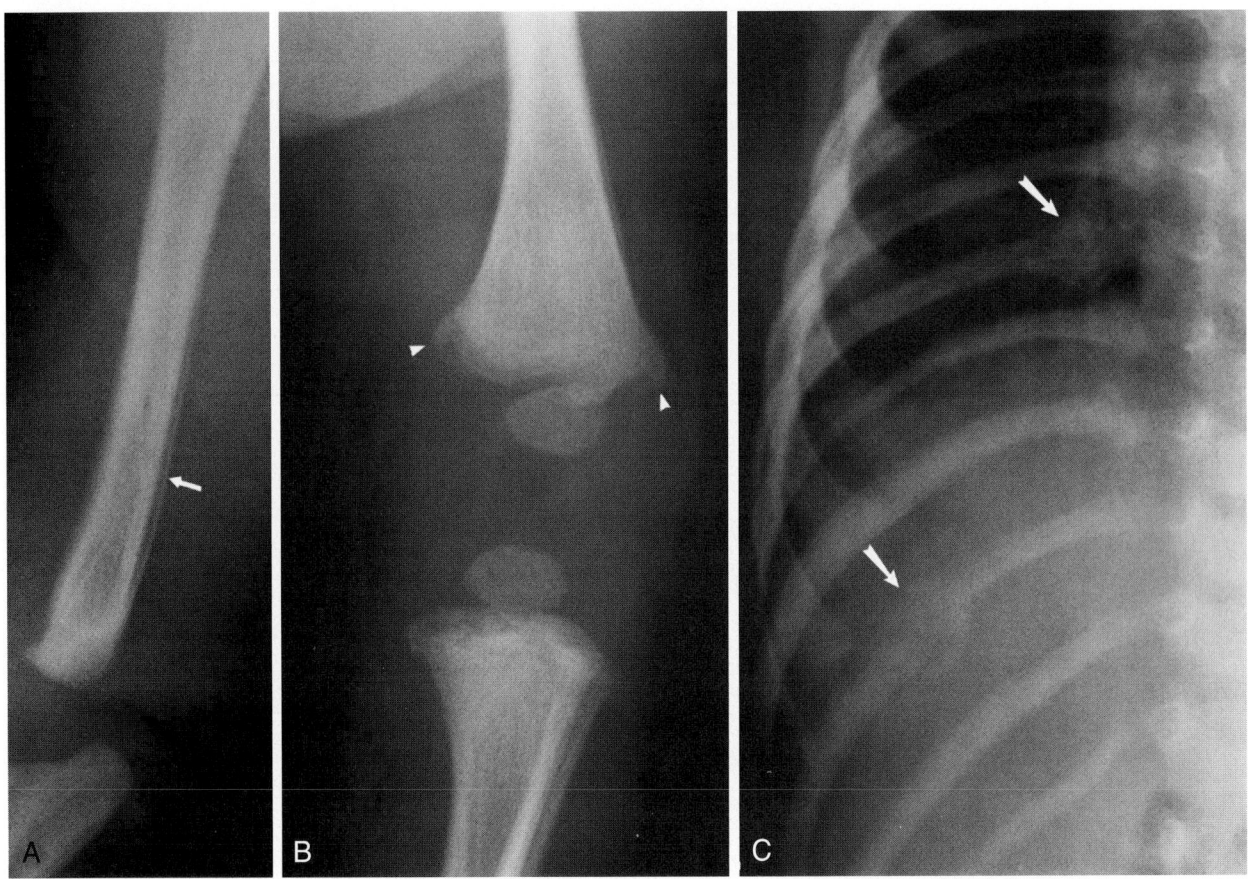

**Figure 56–77.** Abused child syndrome: radiographic abnormalities. *A,* Periostitis *(arrow)* is a delayed radiographic sign of trauma. *B,* Metaphyseal irregularity and corner fractures *(arrowheads)* are more immediate radiographic clues to child abuse. *C,* Rib fractures *(arrows)* are frequent in an abused child. (Courtesy of D. Edwards, MD, San Diego, Calif.)

## FURTHER READING

Berquist TH: Imaging of Orthopedic Trauma, 2nd ed. New York, Raven, 1991.

Cone RO III, Nguyen V, Flournoy JG, et al: Triplane fracture of the distal tibial epiphysis: Radiographic and CT studies. Radiology 153:763, 1984.

De Smet AA, Fisher DR, Graf BK, et al: Osteochondritis dissecans of the knee: Value of MR imaging in determining lesion stability and the presence of articular cartilage defects. AJR 155:549, 1990.

Deutsch AL, Mink JH: Magnetic resonance imaging of musculoskeletal injuries. Radiol Clin North Am 27:983, 1989.

Evans GFF, Haller RG, Wyrick PS, et al: Submaximal delayed-onset muscle soreness: Correlations between MR imaging findings and clinical measures. Radiology 208:815, 1998.

Fleckenstein JL, Weatherall PT, Parkey RW, et al: Sports-related muscle injuries: Evaluation with MR imaging. Radiology 172:793, 1989.

Hagglund G, Hansson LI, Ordeberg G: Epidemiology of slipped capital femoral epiphysis in southern Sweden. Clin Orthop 191:82, 1984.

Harrington IJ: Biomechanics of joint injuries. In ER Gozna, IJ, Harrington (eds): Biomechanics of Musculoskeletal Injury. Baltimore, Williams & Wilkins, 1982, p 31.

Harris JH, Harris WH: The Radiology of Emergency Medicine. Baltimore, Williams & Wilkins, 1975.

John SD, Moorthy CS, Swischuk LE: Expanding the concept of the toddler's fracture. Radiographics 17:367, 1997.

Kleinman PK, Raptopoulos VD, Brill PW: Occult nonskeletal trauma in the battered-child syndrome. Radiology 141:393, 1981.

Mammone JF, Schweitzer ME: MRI of occult sacral insufficiency fractures following radiotherapy. Skeletal Radiol 24:101, 1995.

Milgram JW: The development of loose bodies in human joints. Clin Orthop 124:292, 1977.

Mink JH, Deutsch AL: Occult cartilage and bone injuries of the knee: Detection, classification, and assessment with MR imaging. Radiology 170:823, 1989.

Murray RO, Duncan C: Athletic activity in adolescence as an etiological factor in degenerative hip disease. J Bone Joint Surg Br 53:406, 1971.

Neer CS II: Displaced proximal humeral fractures. Part 1. Classification and evaluation. J Bone Joint Surg Am 52:1077, 1970.

Pfirrmann CWA, Resnick D: Schmorl nodes of the thoracic and lumbar spine: Radiographic-pathologic study of prevalence, characterization, and correlation with degenerative changes of 1,650 spinal levels in 100 cadavers. Radiology 219:368, 2001.

Quinn SF, McCarthy JL: Prospective evaluation of patients with suspected hip fracture and indeterminate radiographs: Use of T1-weighted MR images. Radiology 187:469, 1993.

Resnick D, Niwayama G: Intravertebral disk herniations: Cartilaginous (Schmorl's) nodes. Radiology 126:57, 1978.

Rockwood CA, Green DP: Fractures in Adults, 2nd ed. Philadelphia, JB Lippincott, 1984.

Rogers LF, Poznanski AK: Imaging of epiphyseal injuries. Radiology 191:297, 1994.

Rogers LF: Radiology of Skeletal Trauma, 2nd ed. New York, Churchill Livingstone, 1992.

Rorabeck CH: Compartment syndromes. In BD Browner, JB Jupiter, AM Levine, et al (eds): Skeletal Trauma. Fractures, Dislocations, Ligamentous Injuries. Philadelphia, WB Saunders, 1992, p 285.

Salter RB, Harris WR: Injuries involving the epiphyseal plate. J Bone Joint Surg Am 45:587, 1963.

Salter RB, Harris WR: Injuries of the growth plate. In M Rang (Ed): The Growth Plate and Its Disorders. London, E & S Livingstone, 1969, p 132.

Salter RB: Injuries of the ankle in children. Orthop Clin North Am 5:147, 1974.

Shapiro F: Epiphyseal growth plate fracture-separations: A pathophysiologic approach. Orthopedics 5:720, 1982.

Stevens MA, El-Khoury GY, Kathol MH, et al: Imaging features of avulsion injuries. Radiographics 19:655, 1999.

Steinbach LS, Fleckenstein JL, Mink JH: MR imaging of muscle injuries. Semin Musculoskel Radiol 1:127, 1997.

White PG, Mah JY, Friedman L: Magnetic resonance imaging in acute physeal injuries. Skeletal Radiol 23:627, 1994.

# CHAPTER 57

## Physical Injury: Extraspinal Sites

## SUMMARY OF KEY FEATURES

Routine radiographic findings are emphasized in this chapter, although reference is made to the assessment of such injuries with other methods such as computed tomography and magnetic resonance imaging. Both these techniques are fundamental to the evaluation of internal derangements of joints.

## INTRODUCTION

This survey of physical injuries at extraspinal sites begins in the upper extremity, proceeding in a proximal to distal direction; then considers the lower extremity, again in a proximal to distal direction; and finally extends to the bony pelvis and thoracic cage. It is not meant to compete with standard references but rather to provide an overview of the more important physical injuries occurring in extraspinal sites. A discussion of injuries to the cranium and facial bones is beyond the scope of this chapter.

## UPPER EXTREMITY

### Shoulder

Injuries about the shoulder are among the most commonly encountered traumatic abnormalities, although their precise patterns vary according to the person's age.

### Glenohumeral Joint Dislocation

Even under normal circumstances, the glenohumeral joint is relatively unstable, and this instabilty results in a spectrum of abnormalities. Anterior dislocation accounts for more than 95% of such injuries. Anterior dislocations are further classified as subcoracoid (the most common type), subglenoid (second in frequency), and subclavicular and intrathoracic (rare) (Fig. 57–1). Intrathoracic dislocations are generally accompanied by fractures of the proximal portion of the humerus. Anterior dislocations are best evaluated radiographically by the inclusion of a lateral scapular projection, an axillary projection, or both, in addition to standard frontal views of the shoulder (Fig. 57–2).

Anterior dislocations are associated with a compression fracture on the posterolateral aspect of the humeral head that is produced by impaction of the humerus against the anterior rim of the glenoid fossa. This osseous defect of the humerus is called a *Hill-Sachs lesion* (see Fig. 57–2). This lesion is observed in many cases of anterior dislocation of the glenohumeral joint. Films obtained in various degrees of internal rotation are mandatory because such rotation of the humerus produces a tangential view of the osseous lesion (Fig. 57–3).

A second type of injury accompanying anterior dislocation of the humeral head involves the glenoid fossa and is called a *Bankart lesion* (Fig. 57–4). Although large osseous fractures of the glenoid are occasionally apparent, the fracture may include only the cartilaginous surface of the bone. Conventional magnetic resonance (MR) imaging or MR arthrography are the methods of choice for detecting alterations in the glenoid labrum (see Chapter 59).

A number of other osseous and nonosseous injuries can accompany anterior dislocations of the glenohumeral joint. An avulsion fracture of the greater tuberosity of the humerus occurs in 10% to 15% of cases. Disruption of the rotator cuff may complicate anterior dislocation of the glenohumeral joint, particularly in patients who are older than 40 years. Injuries to the brachial plexus occur in 7% to 45% of anterior glenohumeral joint dislocations; such injuries are more common in older patients and those with large hematomas. Approximately 40% of anterior glenohumeral joint dislocations are recurrent. Recurrent dislocations are more likely in cases of subcoracoid and subglenoid dislocations and in younger persons. Many types of surgical procedures have been advocated for the treatment of patients with recurrent anterior glenohumeral joint dislocations, some of which are listed in Table 57–1.

Posterior dislocation of the glenohumeral joint is rare and accounts for approximately 2% to 4% of all shoulder dislocations. More than 50% of these cases are unrecognized on initial evaluation, despite the presence of a history of trauma, pain, swelling, and limitation of motion. Many cases of posterior dislocation result from convulsions, and in these instances, bilateral dislocations may be evident. Physical examination reveals a posteriorly displaced humeral head that is held in internal rotation. Absence of external rotation and limitation of abduction are present in virtually all cases. Associated injuries include stretching of the posterior capsule, fracture of the posterior aspect of the glenoid rim, avulsion fracture of the lesser tuberosity of the humerus, and stretched or detached subscapularis tendon.

On an anteroposterior radiograph, posterior dislocation of the humeral head distorts the normal elliptic radiodense area created by overlapping of the head and the glenoid fossa (Fig. 57–5). An empty, or vacant, glenoid cavity is a second radiographic sign of dislocation in this projection; posterior displacement of the humeral head may create a space between the anterior rim of the glenoid and the humeral head that is frequently greater than 6 mm. In addition, the normal parallel pattern of the articular surfaces of the glenoid concavity and the humeral head convexity is lost. Other radiographic signs of posterior dislocation on frontal radiographs include a fixed position of internal rotation of the humerus and a second cortical line, the trough line, parallel and lateral to the subchondral articular surface of the humeral head. This line represents the margin of a troughlike impaction frac-

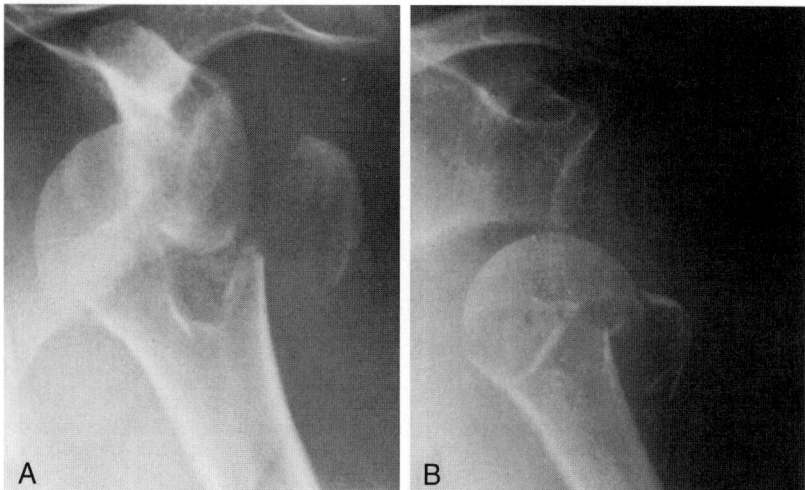

**Figure 57–1.** Glenohumeral joint: anterior dislocation. *A,* Subcoracoid type. Note the anterior and medial displacement of the humeral head and fracture of the greater tuberosity. *B,* Subglenoid type. The humeral head is displaced anteriorly and inferiorly, and the greater tuberosity is fractured.

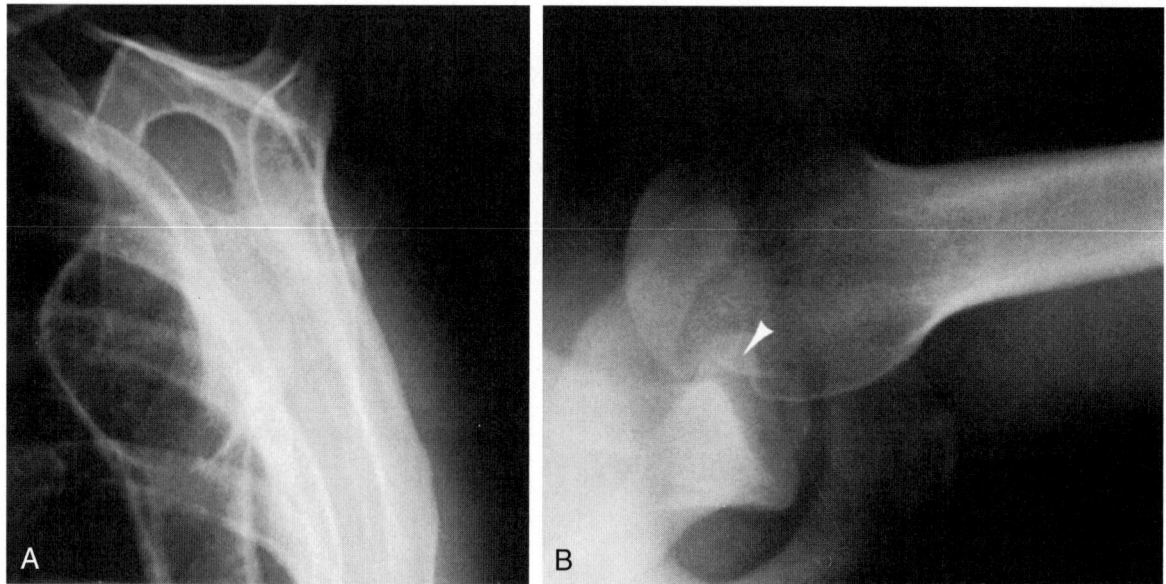

**Figure 57–2.** Glenohumeral joint: anterior dislocation. *A,* Tangential scapular projection reveals the abnormal position of the humeral head, which is located in front of the glenoid cavity. *B,* In a different patient, axillary radiograph reveals an anterior dislocation of the humeral head. Impaction of the anterior glenoid process and the posterolateral aspect of the humeral head has produced a Hill-Sachs lesion *(arrowhead).* Although the dislocation is well shown on this radiograph, axillary projections are difficult to obtain while the humeral head is still displaced.

ture of the humeral head that is created when this structure contacts the posterior glenoid rim during dislocation (Fig. 57–6). As such, it is analogous to the Hill-Sachs lesion seen in association with anterior glenohumeral joint dislocation and is diagnostic of a posterior dislocation. Computed tomography (CT) is an additional imaging technique that can be used to evaluate patients with acute (or chronic) posterior dislocations of the glenohumeral joint (Fig. 57–7).

Superior dislocation of the glenohumeral joint is rare (Fig. 57–8). An extreme forward and upward force on an adducted arm can produce extensive damage to the rotator cuff, capsule, biceps tendon, and surrounding muscu-

lature, as well as fracture of the acromion, clavicle, coracoid process, or humeral tuberosities. Inferior dislocation of the glenohumeral joint (luxatio erecta) is also rare (Fig. 57–9). A direct axial force on a fully abducted arm or a hyperabduction force leading to leverage of the humeral head across the acromion is responsible for this type of dislocation. After this injury, the superior aspect of the articular surface of the humeral head is directed inferiorly and does not contact the inferior glenoid rim; as a result, the arm is held over the patient's head.

A special type of inferior displacement of the humeral head is termed the *drooping shoulder* (Fig. 57–10). It can be associated with uncomplicated fractures of the surgical

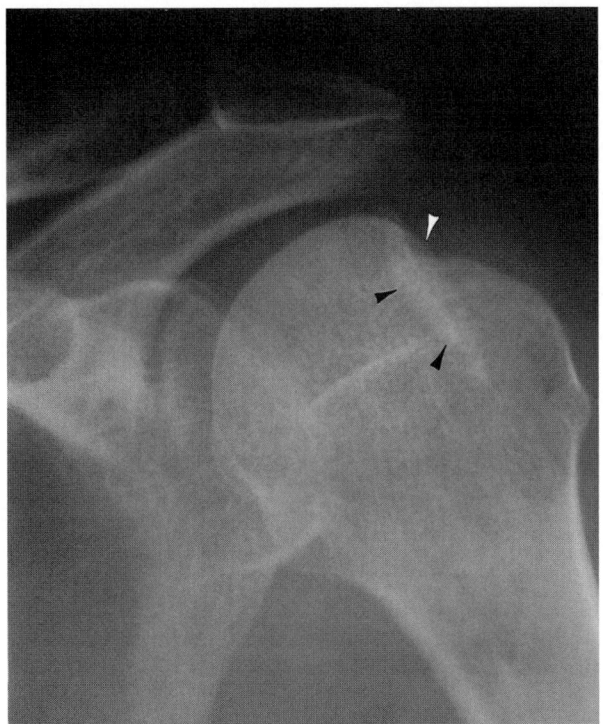

**Figure 57–3.** Glenohumeral joint: Hill-Sachs lesion. In a patient with a previous anterior dislocation, an internal rotation view reveals the extent of the Hill-Sachs lesion *(arrowheads)*.

neck of the humerus. The frequency of inferior humeral displacement in such cases is about 40%, although the cause is not clear. Recognition of this condition eliminates the possibility of an erroneous diagnosis of fracture-dislocation of the proximal humerus, and conservative

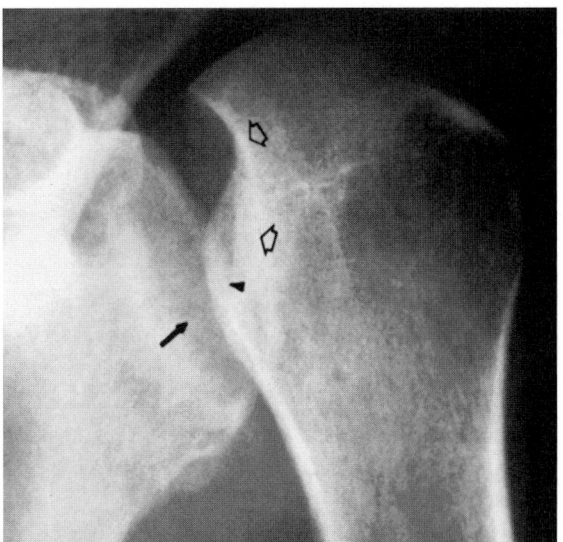

**Figure 57–5.** Glenohumeral joint: posterior dislocation. Findings on the anteroposterior radiograph include distortion of the normal elliptic radiodense region created by the overlying humeral head and glenoid fossa *(arrowhead)*, a "vacant" glenoid cavity *(solid arrow)*, loss of parallelism between the articular surfaces of the glenoid cavity and humeral head, internal rotation of the humerus, and an impaction fracture *(open arrows)*.

therapy leads to disappearance of the drooping shoulder over a period of weeks.

### Acromioclavicular Joint Dislocation

Subluxation or dislocation of the acromioclavicular joint is a common injury that accounts for approximately 10%

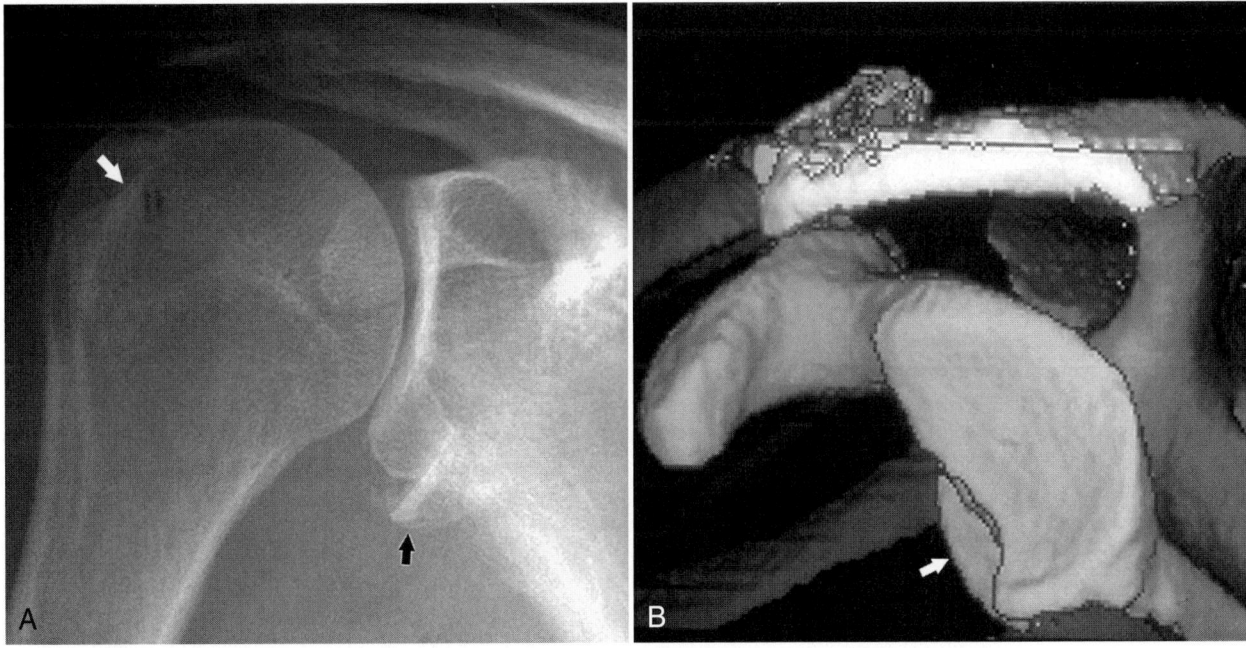

**Figure 57–4.** Glenohumeral joint: Bankart lesion. *A,* In addition to a Hill-Sachs lesion *(white arrow)*, note the fragmentation of the glenoid rim *(black arrow)*, representing an osseous Bankart lesion. *B,* Three-dimensional CT of the shoulder with the humerus electronically removed shows the osseous Bankart lesion *(arrow)*; the fragment is displaced medially from the anterior inferior glenoid.

**TABLE 57–1**

**Surgical Procedures Used for Recurrent Anterior Glenohumeral Joint Dislocation**

| Procedure | Technique |
|---|---|
| Bankart | Repair of anterior capsular mechanism with drill holes and sutures |
| Putti-Platt | Shortening of anterior capsule and subscapularis muscle |
| Magnuson-Stack | Transfer of subscapularis tendon from lesser tuberosity to greater tuberosity |
| Eden-Hybbinette | Bone graft to anterior glenoid region |
| Oudard | Bone graft to coracoid process |
| Trillat | Osteotomy with displacement of coracoid process |
| Bristow-Helfet | Transfer of coracoid process with its attached tendons to neck of scapula |

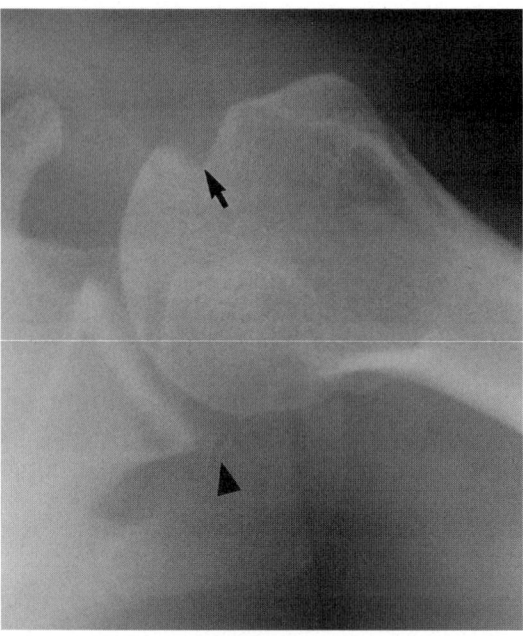

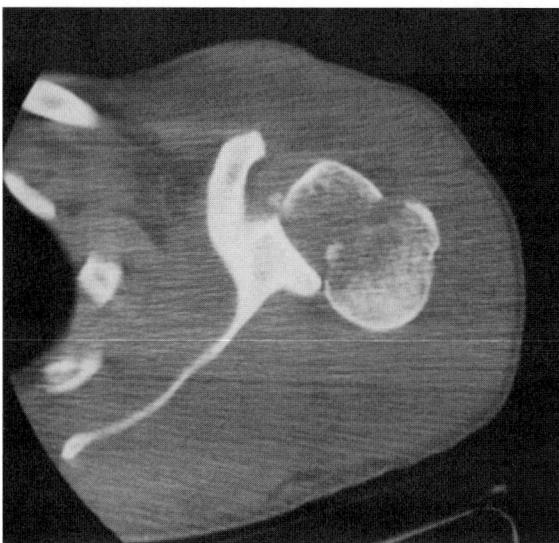

**Figure 57–7.** Glenohumeral joint: posterior dislocation. Transaxial CT scan shows posterior dislocation of the glenohumeral joint and the avulsed tuberosity.

**Figure 57–6.** Glenohumeral joint: posterior dislocation and trough fracture. Axillary radiograph reveals a fracture *(arrow)* involving the anteromedial portion of the humeral head, indicative of a previous posterior dislocation of the glenohumeral joint. Note the fragmentation *(arrowhead)* of the posterior aspect of the glenoid rim.

of all shoulder dislocations. Injury to the acromioclavicular joint can result from indirect or, more commonly, direct forces. Injuries to the acromioclavicular joint are classified in several ways, according to the extent of ligament damage. The initial classification systems used three grades of injury (Fig. 57–11). A type I injury, indicative of a mild sprain, is associated with stretching or tearing of the fibers of the acromioclavicular ligaments. A type II injury, indicative of a moderate sprain, is associated with disruption of the acromioclavicular ligaments and the aponeurosis of the deltoid and trapezius muscle attachments to the distal portion of the clavicle. The coracoclavicular ligament may be sprained but is otherwise intact, and the distal aspect of the clavicle may sublux in a posterior or superior direction. A type III injury, which

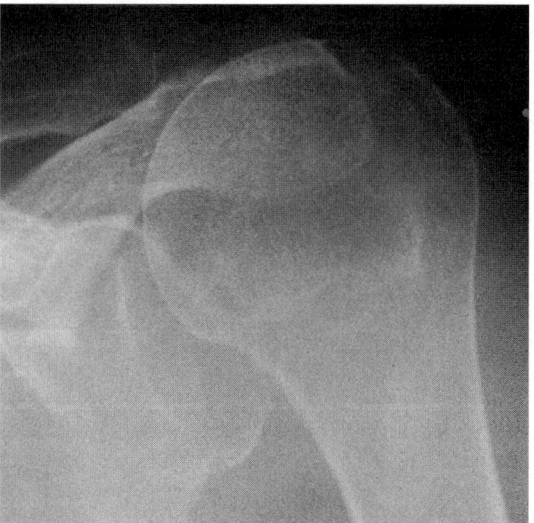

**Figure 57–8.** Glenohumeral joint: superior dislocation. Note the elevation of the humeral head with respect to the glenoid cavity.

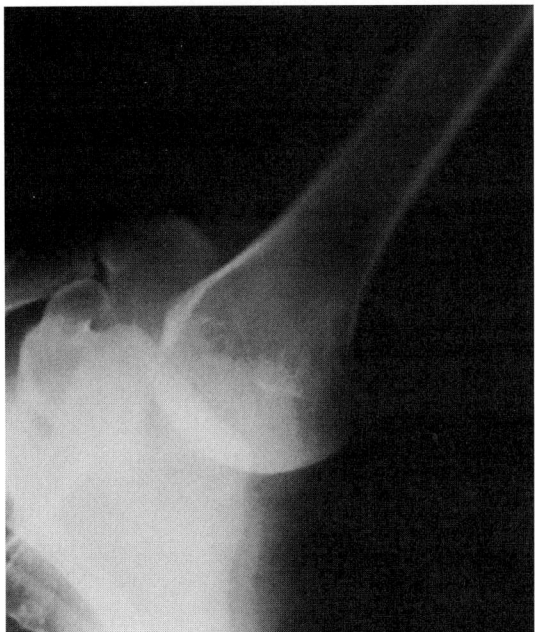

**Figure 57–9.** Glenohumeral joint: inferior dislocation. With acute inferior dislocation of the glenohumeral joint, the arm is held over the head.

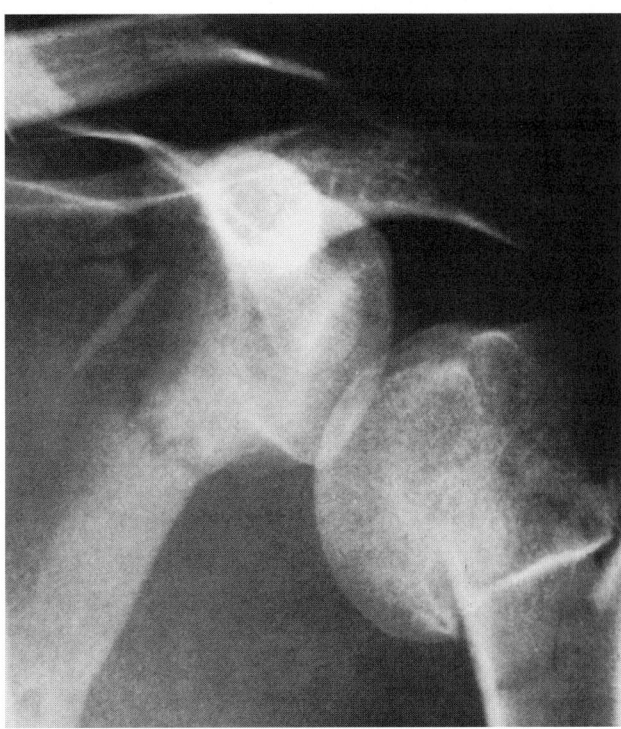

**Figure 57–10.** Glenohumeral joint: drooping shoulder. Fracture of the surgical neck of the humerus is associated with inferior subluxation of the head with respect to the glenoid cavity. Observe an associated scapular fracture.

represents a severe sprain, is characterized by disruption of both the acromioclavicular and the coracoclavicular ligaments, along with the muscle aponeurosis; on radiographs, elevation of the distal aspect of the clavicle with

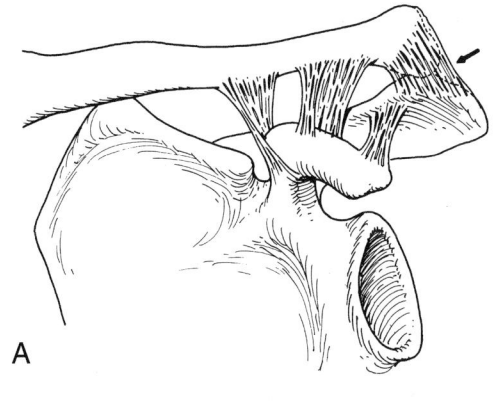

A

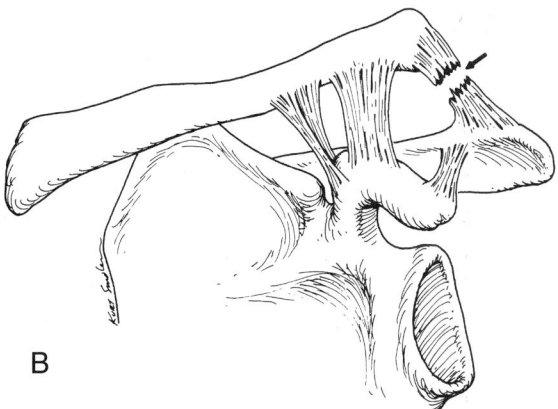

B

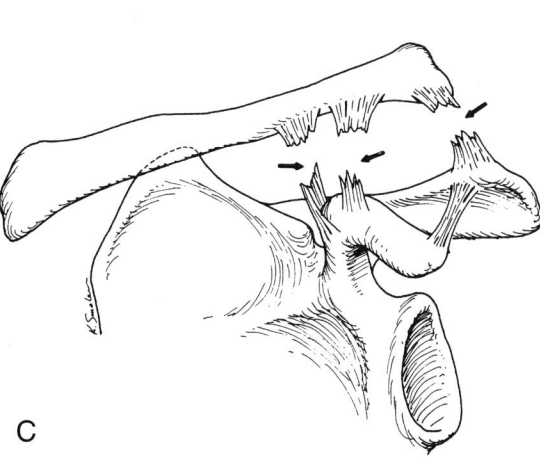

C

**Figure 57–11.** Acromioclavicular joint: classification of injuries (original method). *A*, Type I injury. Stretching or tearing of the fibers of the acromioclavicular ligaments *(arrow)* constitutes a mild sprain. The relationship between the distal portion of the clavicle and the acromion remains normal. *B*, Type II injury. Disruption of the acromioclavicular ligaments *(arrow)* constitutes a part of this injury, which is classified as a moderate sprain. The coracoclavicular ligament may be mildly sprained but is otherwise intact. Minor elevation of the distal portion of the clavicle or widening of the acromioclavicular joint, or both, is the anticipated radiographic abnormality. *C*, Type III injury. This severe sprain is characterized by disruption of both the acromioclavicular and coracoclavicular ligaments *(arrows)* and dislocation of the acromioclavicular joint.

respect to the acromion is detected. This injury produces an unstable clavicle. Subsequently, a more detailed classification system consisting of six types of injury was introduced (Figs. 57–12 and 57–13; Table 57–2).

Fractures of the coracoid process are associated with acromioclavicular joint dislocations. Coracoclavicular ligamentous calcification or ossification can appear after the injury, regardless of the type of treatment initiated. Post-traumatic osteolysis of the distal portion of the clavicle is another complication of acute or repetitive injury to the acromioclavicular joint. The natural course of the osteolytic process is variable but typically continues for 12 to 18 months. Osteoarthritis is an additional complication of dislocation or subluxation.

## Sternoclavicular Joint Dislocation

Sternoclavicular joint injuries are rare and account for only about 2% to 3% of all shoulder dislocations. Traumatic dislocation of the sternoclavicular joint requires a direct or indirect force of great magnitude. Anterior, or presternal, dislocations are caused by forces that move the shoulder backward and outward or downward. Serious complications are rare after this type of dislocation, although a "cosmetic bump" may remain indefinitely. Posterior, or retrosternal, dislocations of the sternoclavicular joint may be accompanied by signs related to clavicular impingement on adjacent neurovascular structures and airways. A pneumothorax or hemothorax may be an associated finding (Fig. 57–14).

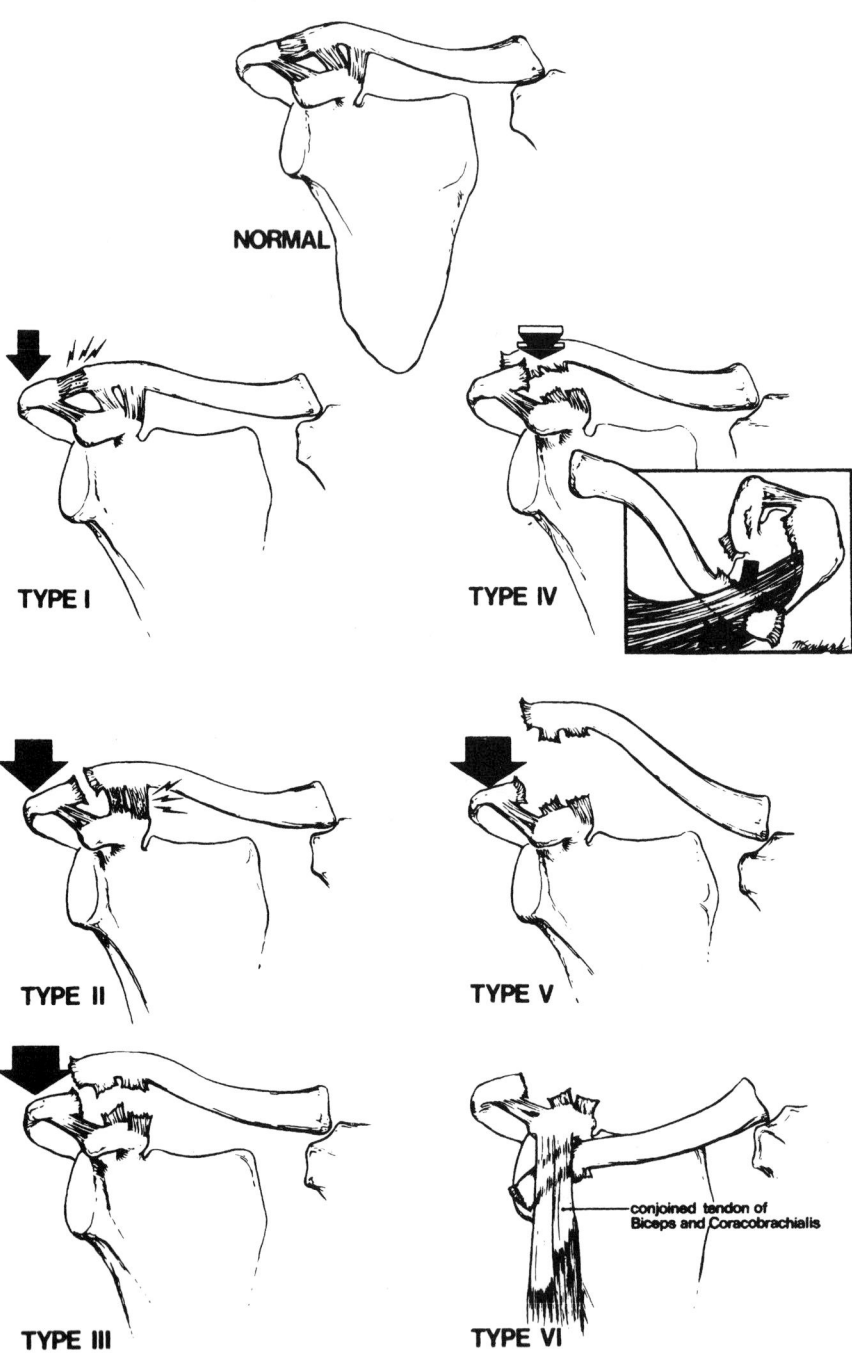

**Figure 57–12.** Acromioclavicular joint: classification of injuries (new method). Type I: A mild force applied to the point of the shoulder does not disrupt either the acromioclavicular or the coracoclavicular ligaments. Type II: A moderate to heavy force applied to the point of the shoulder disrupts the acromioclavicular ligaments, but the coracoclavicular ligaments remain intact. Type III: When a severe force is applied to the point of the shoulder, both the acromioclavicular and the coracoclavicular ligaments are disrupted. Type IV: In this major injury, the acromioclavicular and coracoclavicular ligaments are disrupted, and the distal end of the clavicle is displaced posteriorly into or through the trapezius muscle. Type V: A violent force has been applied to the point of the shoulder that not only ruptures the acromioclavicular and coracoclavicular ligaments but also disrupts the deltoid and trapezius muscle attachments and creates a major separation between the clavicle and the acromion. Type VI: Another major injury is inferior dislocation of the distal end of the clavicle to the subcoracoid position. The acromioclavicular and coracoclavicular ligaments are disrupted. (From Rockwood CA, Jr, Matsen FA III [eds]: The Shoulder, 2nd ed. Philadelphia, WB Saunders, 1998, p 495.)

NORMAL

TYPE I

TYPE IV

TYPE II

TYPE V

TYPE III

TYPE VI

conjoined tendon of Biceps and Coracobrachialis

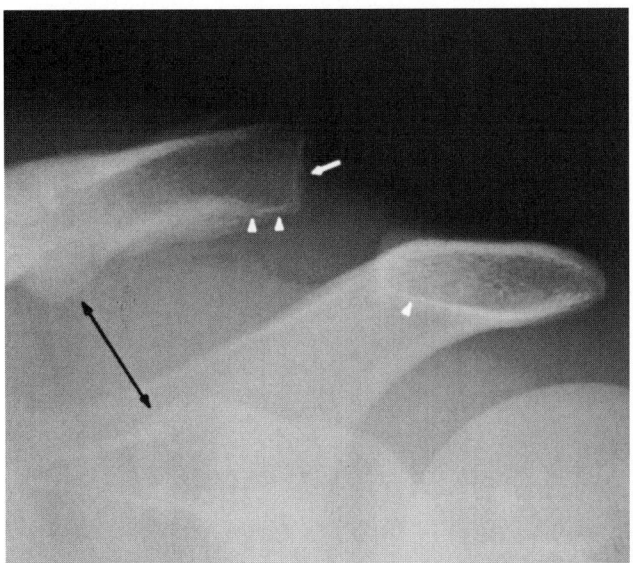

**Figure 57–13.** Acromioclavicular joint dislocation: type V injury. Observe the superior displacement of the clavicle *(arrow)* with respect to the acromion. The inferior margin of the clavicle is no longer aligned with the inferior margin of the acromion *(arrowheads)*. Widening of the acromioclavicular joint and an increased distance between the clavicle and the coracoid process *(double-ended arrow)* are apparent.

## Fracture of the Proximal Portion of the Humerus

The type of injury is dependent, to a large extent, on the age of the person. In the immature skeletons of children or adolescents, physeal separation with or without associated fracture is encountered; in young adults, glenohumeral joint dislocation or subluxation predominates. It is in middle-aged adults (older than 45 years) and in the elderly that fractures of the proximal portion of the humerus are typically seen (Table 57–3).

Classification of fractures of the proximal humerus (Neer's system) emphasizes the presence or absence of significant displacement of one or more of the four major osseous segments (Fig. 57–15): the articular segment containing the anatomic neck, the greater tuberosity, the lesser tuberosity, and the shaft and surgical neck. Approximately 80% of fractures of the proximal portion of the humerus are undisplaced because of the protection afforded by the periosteum, joint capsule, and rotator cuff. A displaced fracture exists if any of the four segments is separated by more than 1 cm from its neighbor or is angulated more than 45 degrees. Nondisplaced fractures or fractures with minimal displacement that do not meet these criteria are considered one-part fractures. A two-part fracture is one in which only a single segment is displaced; two-part fractures represent approximately 15% of all fractures of the proximal humerus. A three-part fracture, which accounts for approximately 3% to 4% of all humeral fractures, occurs when two segments are displaced, and a four-part fracture, which occurs in approximately 3% to 4% of cases, exists when all the humeral segments are displaced (Fig. 57–16). The term *fracture-dislocation* is used to indicate that the articular segment of the humerus is displaced beyond the joint space (Fig. 57–17). CT can be used to more accurately determine the fracture pattern.

Several patterns of intra-articular fracture of the humeral head may be encountered. Impaction of the articular surface against the anterior or posterior rim of the glenoid cavity in cases of anterior or posterior glenohumeral joint dislocation was considered earlier in this chapter. More severe fragmentation or comminution can accompany central impaction of the humeral head against the glenoid cavity. Complications of fractures of the articular head of the humerus include lipohemarthrosis, production of intra-articular osteocartilaginous fragments, inferior displacement of the humeral head (drooping shoulder), and osteoarthritis.

---

**TABLE 57–2**

**Acromioclavicular Injuries**

| Type | Radiographic Findings | Structural Findings |
|------|----------------------|---------------------|
| I | Normal | Acromioclavicular ligament sprain, intact coracoclavicular ligaments and deltoid and trapezius muscles |
| II | Minimal superior subluxation of the clavicle | Acromioclavicular ligament disruption, coracoclavicular ligament sprain, intact deltoid and trapezius muscles |
| III | 25–100% superior subluxation or dislocation of the clavicle | Acromioclavicular ligament disruption, coracoclavicular ligament disruption, clavicular detachment of the deltoid and trapezius muscles |
| IV | Posterior displacement of the clavicle | Acromioclavicular ligament disruption, coracoclavicular ligament disruption, clavicular detachment of the deltoid and trapezius muscles, clavicle displaced posteriorly into or through the trapezius muscle |
| V | >100% superior dislocation of the clavicle | Acromioclavicular ligament disruption, coracoclavicular ligament disruption, more extensive clavicular detachment of the deltoid and trapezius muscles |
| VI | Displacement of the clavicle below the acromion or coracoid process | Acromioclavicular ligament disruption, coracoclavicular ligament disruption, clavicular detachment of the deltoid and trapezius muscles |

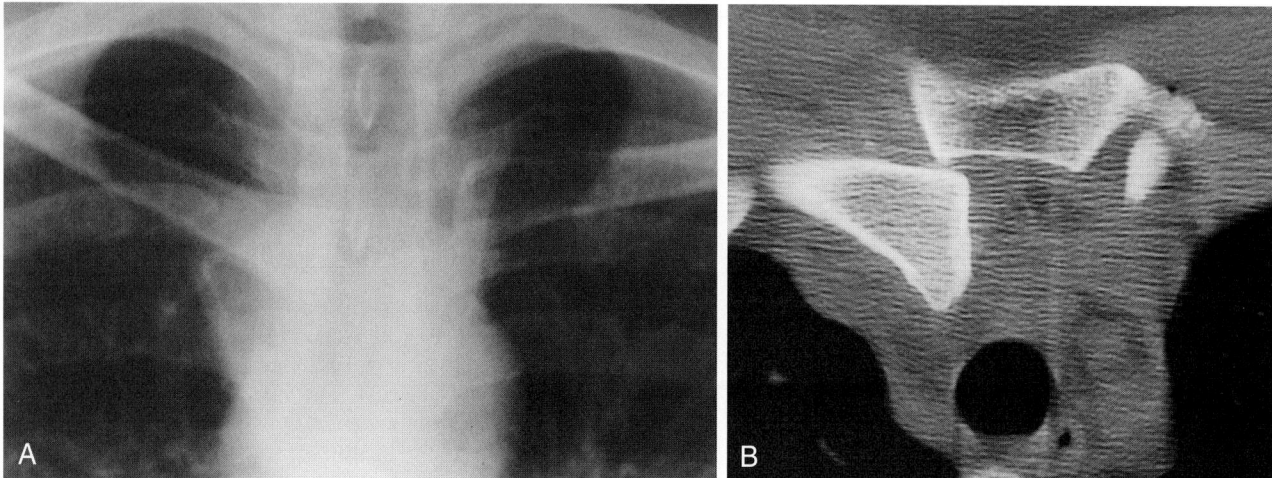

**Figure 57–14.** Sternoclavicular joint: posterior dislocation. *A,* Frontal chest radiograph shows asymmetry in the position of the medial margins of the clavicle, with the right clavicle (on the injured side) being located inferior to the left clavicle. *B,* Transverse CT scan confirms posterior dislocation of the right sternoclavicular joint.

Delayed union or nonunion can occur with any type of fracture of the proximal portion of the humerus and may be accompanied by significant angulation at the fracture site. Osteonecrosis is reported in 7% to 50% of cases and is most typical with displaced fractures and severe fractures or fracture-dislocations of the bone (four-part fractures) (Fig. 57–18). Less commonly, injury to the nearby brachial plexus and the axillary artery may be seen. A brachial plexus injury, which results from contusion or mild traction, may be self-limited.

## Fracture of the Clavicle

It is convenient to divide the clavicle into three functional segments: a distal, or interligamentous, segment consisting of the outer 25% to 30% of the bone—the region about and distal to the coracoclavicular ligament; an intermediate segment consisting of the middle 40% to 50% of the bone; and an inner segment consisting of the medial 25% of the bone. Approximately 75% to 80% of clavicular fractures involve the middle segment of the bone, 15% to 20% involve the distal segment, and 5% affect the inner segment. The prognosis of clavicular fractures depends on the precise site of involvement; for example, nonunion is frequent in fractures distal to the coracoclavicular ligament, whereas this complication is rare in fractures of the medial segment.

The middle segment, located at the junction of the two curvatures of the clavicle, is the most common site of fracture. In adults and children, the mechanism of injury is usually a fall onto an outstretched hand or a fall on the shoulder. In most cases, the radiographic findings permit a prompt and accurate diagnosis (Fig. 57–19). Fractures of the distal portion of the clavicle, related to a force applied to the shoulder that drives the humerus and scapula downward, are divided into two types: type I fractures, in which the coracoclavicular ligaments are intact, and type II fractures, in which a portion (conoid

portion) of the coracoclavicular ligaments is severed (Fig. 57–20). A characteristic medial flange of bone extending from the distal clavicular fragment may be evident in type II fractures. Type II fractures have a poorer prognosis related to more significant displacement at the fracture site and to nonunion. Associated fractures of the coracoid process and ribs may be evident.

Direct trauma accounts for most fractures of the medial end of the clavicle. They have been divided into transverse fractures, which do not become displaced because of ligamentous and musculature attachments, and intra-articular fractures. Intra-articular fractures may be overlooked unless conventional tomography or CT scanning is used.

In children, clavicular fractures heal rapidly without significant sequelae. In adults, exuberant callus affecting the middle segment of the clavicle can be associated with persistent neurologic defects and circulatory disturbances because of compression of the adjacent structures. Nonunion of a clavicular fracture is uncommon and, when present, is associated with lack of immobilization. Posttraumatic pseudarthrosis of the clavicle must be differentiated from congenital pseudarthrosis. Congenital pseudarthrosis of the clavicle usually manifests as a painless swelling overlying the middle third of the bone, more frequently on the right side. These patients are infants, and callus and periosteal bone formation are absent.

## Fracture of the Scapula

Scapular fractures are infrequent. Although they may occur as an isolated phenomenon, as many as 95% of cases are associated with additional injuries. Scapular fractures may involve one or more of the following anatomic regions: glenoid fossa and articular surface, neck, body, spinous process, acromion process, and coracoid process (Fig. 57–21). They are found most frequently in the scapular body, followed by the neck and other regions of the bone.

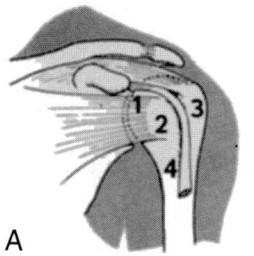

A

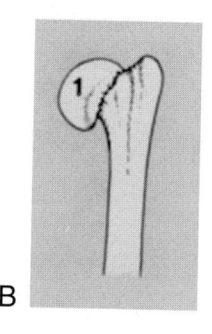

B

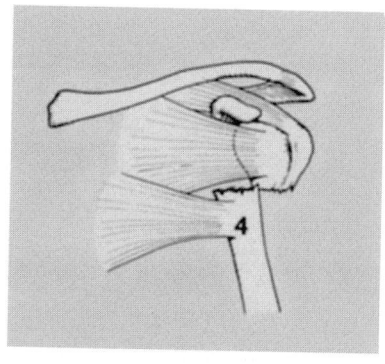

C

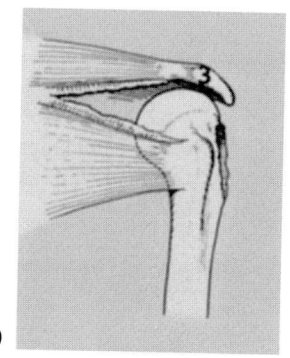

D

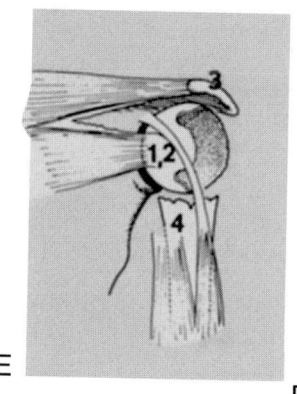

E

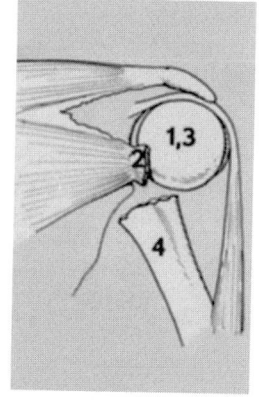

F

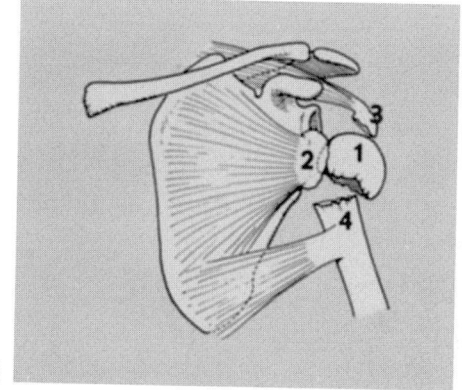

G

**Figure 57–15.** Fractures of the proximal end of the humerus: classification system. *A*, Normal situation. Four major segments of the proximal portion of the humerus are identified: 1, humeral head; 2, lesser tuberosity; 3, greater tuberosity; 4, humeral shaft. *B*, Two-part fracture. In this example, a fracture of the anatomic neck has led to displacement of the humeral head (1). Ischemic necrosis may complicate this rare injury. *C*, Two-part fracture. In this example, displacement of the humeral shaft (4) relates to the pull of the pectoralis major muscle. The rotator cuff is intact and holds the humeral head in a neutral position. Variations of this fracture pattern relate to the extent of impaction, angulation, and comminution. *D*, Two-part fracture. In this example, displacement of the greater tuberosity (3) occurs in response to the forces generated by a portion of the rotator cuff musculature. Retraction of the entire greater tuberosity or one of its facets of more than 1 cm is pathognomonic of a longitudinal tear of the rotator cuff. The fragment tends to be large in younger patients and small in older patients. A complication of this injury is impaired motion of the shoulder. *E*, Three-part fracture. In this injury, the greater tuberosity (3) is displaced and the subscapularis muscle rotates the humeral head (1 and 2) so that its articular surface faces posteriorly. The diaphysis (4) is displaced relative to the rotated head because of the action of the pectoralis major muscle. *F*, Three-part fracture. In this type of injury, the lesser tuberosity (2) is detached and displaced by the action of the subscapularis muscle, and the supraspinatus and external rotators cause the articular surface of the humeral head (1 and 3) to face anteriorly. 4, Humeral shaft. *G*, Four-part fracture. The articular segment (1) is detached from the tuberosities (2 and 3) and from its circulation; is displaced laterally (as shown), anteriorly, or posteriorly; and loses contact with the glenoid cavity. The tuberosities are usually retracted by the attached musculature. (From Neer CS II, Rockwood CA Jr: Fractures and dislocations of the shoulder. In Rockwood CA Jr, Green DP [eds]: Fractures in Adults, 2nd ed. Philadelphia, JB Lippincott, 1984, p 675.)

A fracture of the rim of the glenoid cavity occurs in approximately 20% of traumatic glenohumeral joint dislocations. The fracture fragment may be cartilaginous or osteocartilaginous in nature. Either the anterior glenoid rim (in anterior dislocations) or the posterior glenoid rim (in posterior dislocations) may be affected. Larger portions of the glenoid fossa may be fractured when the humeral head is driven against the glenoid cavity by a direct force.

A fracture in the neck of the scapula characteristically occurs after a direct blow to the shoulder. The fracture

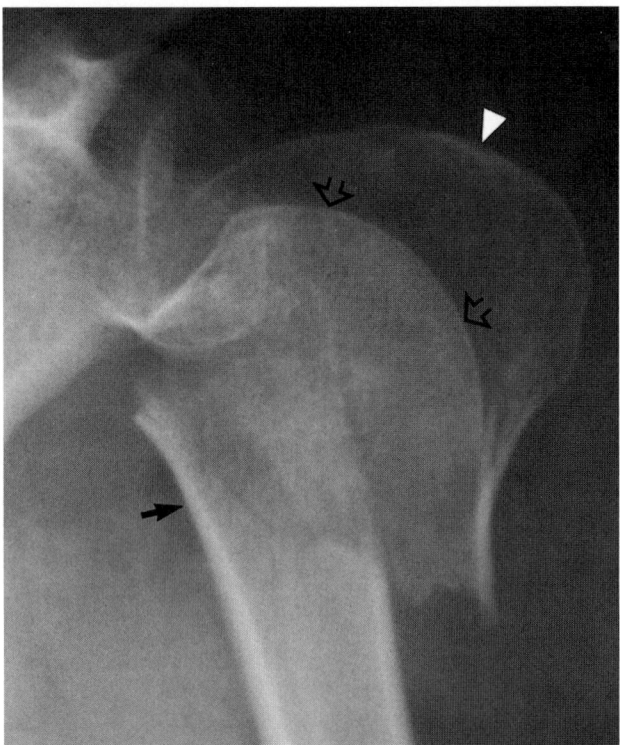

**Figure 57–16.** Fractures of the proximal humerus: three-part fractures. Fractures involve the surgical neck and greater tuberosity of the humerus. Medial displacement of the humeral shaft *(closed arrow)*, superior displacement of the greater tuberosity *(arrowhead)*, and rotation of the humeral head with its articular surface facing posteriorly *(open arrows)* can be seen. CT confirmed that the lesser tuberosity was intact.

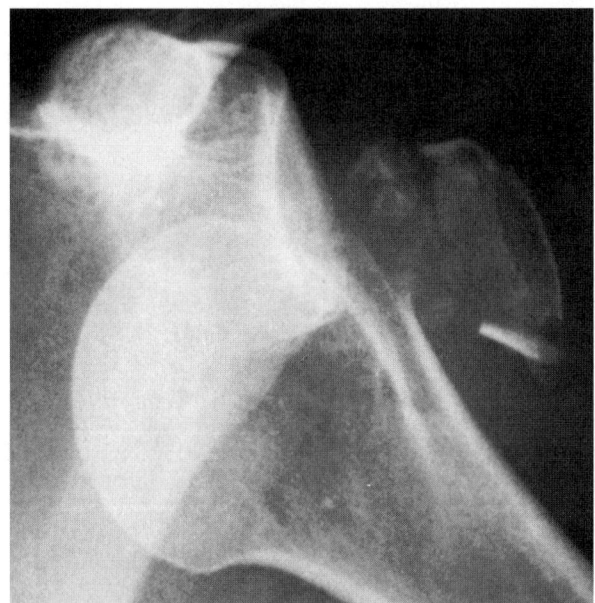

**Figure 57–17.** Fracture-dislocation of the glenohumeral joint. Anterior (subcoracoid) dislocation of the glenohumeral joint is associated with a displaced and comminuted fracture of the greater tuberosity of the humerus.

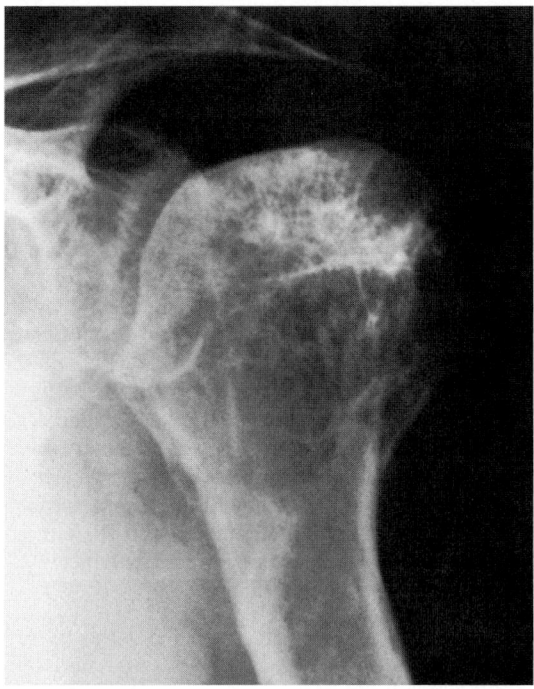

**Figure 57–18.** Osteonecrosis: humeral head. After a fracture of the proximal portion of the humerus, ischemic necrosis of the humeral head occurred and was radiographically manifested as patchy bone sclerosis and irregularity of the articular surface.

line, which may be impacted, extends from the supra-clavicular notch above to the coracoid process below (Fig. 57–22). CT scanning or MR imaging can be used to document the presence or absence of intra-articular extension of the fracture.

Approximately 50% to 70% of scapular fractures involve the body of the bone (see Fig. 57–22). The typical mechanism of injury is a direct force of considerable magnitude, which may also result in fractures of neigh-

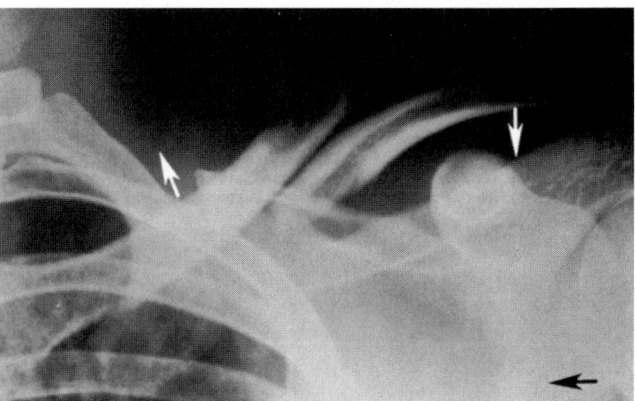

**Figure 57–19.** Clavicular fracture: intermediate segment. The typical fracture configuration is illustrated. Note that the medial portion of the clavicle is pulled upward by the sternocleidomastoid muscle; the lateral portion is pulled downward by the weight of the arm and inward by the pectoralis major and latissimus dorsi muscles. Arrows indicate the direction of these forces. The result is a bayonet deformity at the fracture site.

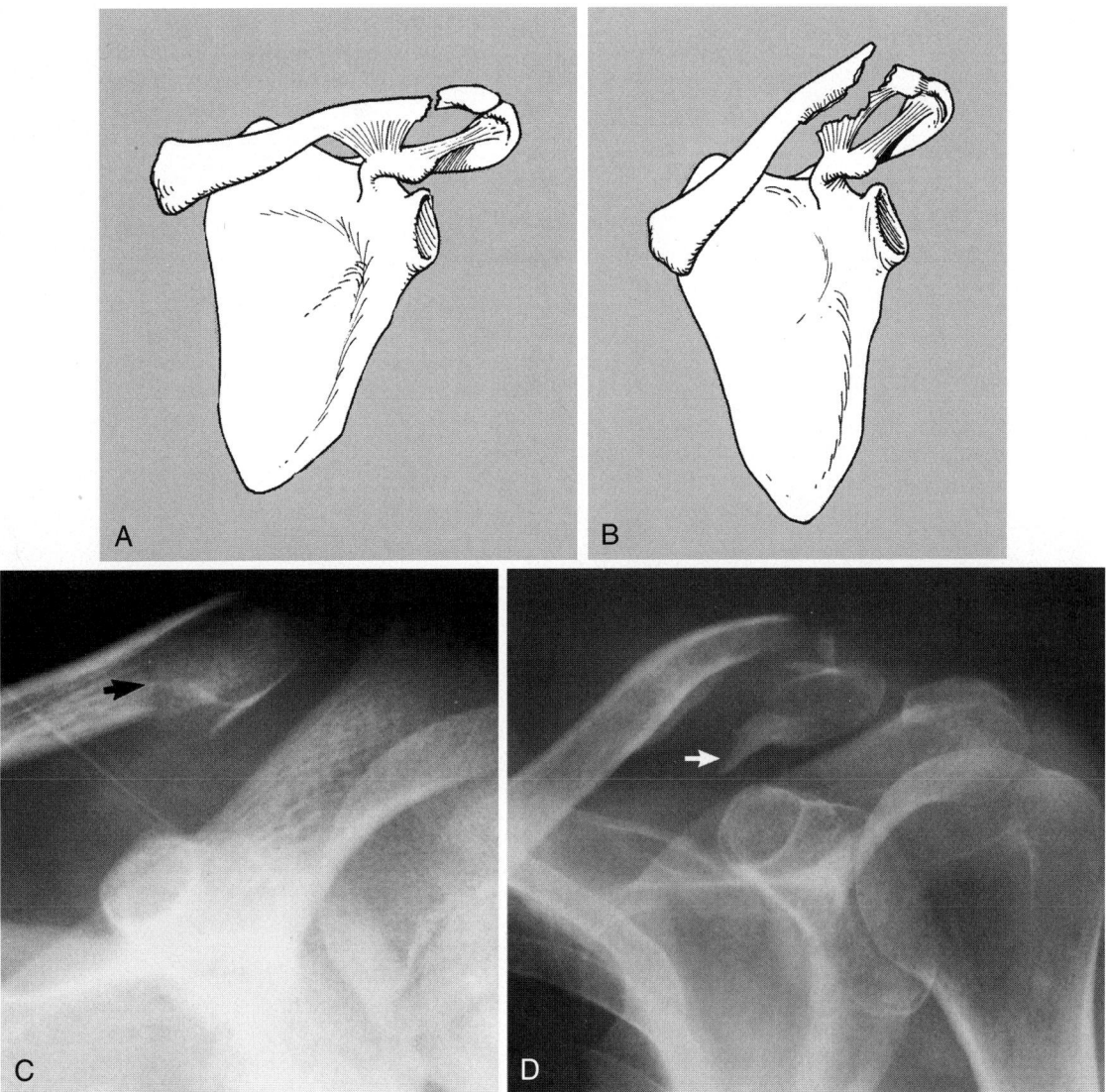

**Figure 57–20.** Clavicular fracture: distal segment. *A*, Type I injury. The coracoclavicular ligaments remain intact. *B*, Type II injury. The conoid portion of the coracoclavicular ligaments is severed. *C*, Type I injury. A subtle fracture *(arrow)* of the distal end of the clavicle in a child is unassociated with clavicular displacement. *D*, Type II injury. Disruption of the conoid portion of the coracoclavicular ligament has allowed superior migration of the proximal segment of the clavicle. Note the bone flange *(arrow)* extending from the distal clavicular segment to which the trapezoid portion of the coracoclavicular ligament inserts.

boring ribs and pneumothorax. Isolated fractures of the spinous process of the scapula are infrequent and, when present, are a result of direct trauma. Fractures of the acromion process generally follow direct trauma, although muscular traction can rarely produce a similar lesion. On radiographs, a fracture line is evident, usually adjacent to the acromioclavicular joint, though occasionally at the base of the acromion process. Significant neurologic injury, although rare, is a recognized complication.

Fractures of the coracoid process are caused by a direct injury from a dislocating humeral head; a direct force on the tip of the coracoid itself; or an avulsion resulting from traction on the coracoclavicular ligament, the short head of the biceps brachii muscle, or the coracobrachialis muscle. Fractures of the anterior aspect

of the coracoid process do not disrupt the coracoclavicular ligaments. Anteroposterior radiographs may not demonstrate the coracoid process adequately and must be supplemented with a lateral scapular view, axillary projection, or both (Fig. 57–23). The tip of this process may be displaced in an inferior and medial direction, similar to the appearance of a normal accessory ossification center (infracoracoid bone).

## Fracture of the First and Second Ribs

Fractures of the first or second rib indicate major trauma to the thorax or shoulder. Associated abnormalities are frequent and potentially serious; they include rupture of the apex of the lung or the subclavian artery, aneurysm

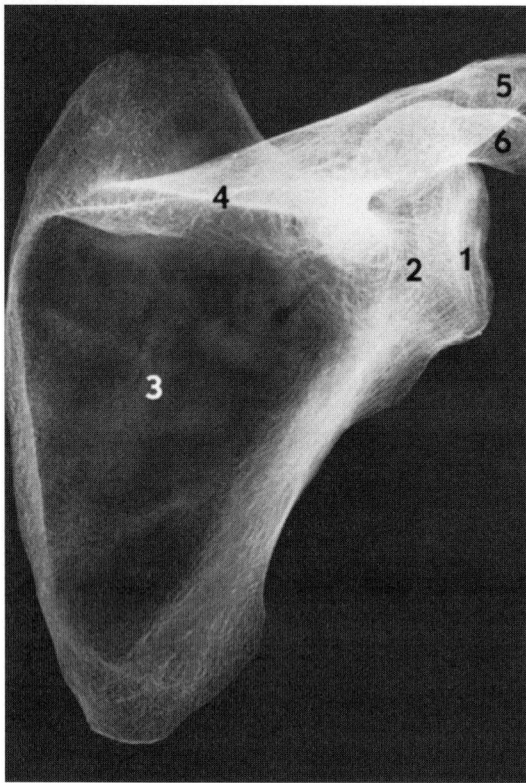

**Figure 57–21.** Scapular fracture: sites of injury. Fractures of the scapula may involve the glenoid fossa and articular surface (1), the neck (2) or body (3) of the bone, or the spinous (4), acromion (5), or coracoid (6) process. They are most common in the scapular body and neck.

of the aortic arch, tracheoesophageal fistula, pleurisy, hemothorax, cardiac alterations, neurologic injury, and additional fractures. Because of the serious implications of these accompanying abnormalities, detection of a fracture of the first rib requires careful evaluation of the intrathoracic structures to exclude the presence of additional injuries.

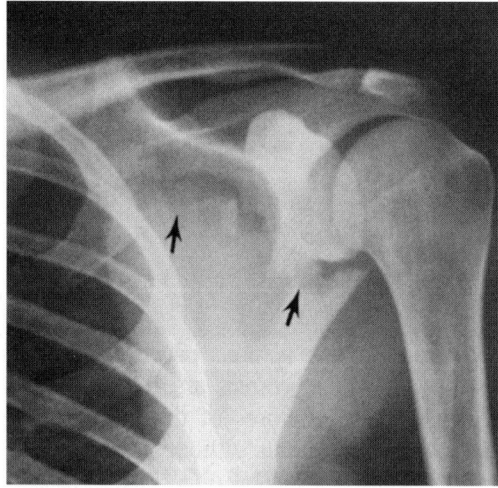

**Figure 57–22.** Scapular fracture: injuries of the scapular body and neck. Horizontal fracture involving the body and neck of the bone *(arrows)*.

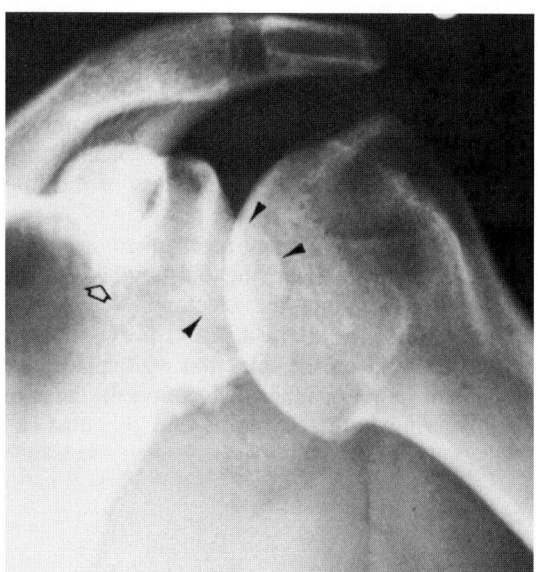

**Figure 57–23.** Scapular fracture: injuries of the coracoid process. Frontal radiograph demonstrates fracture of the coracoid process *(arrowheads)*. Note incidental infracoracoid bone *(open arrow)*.

## Humeral Diaphysis

Fractures of the humeral diaphysis account for about 3% to 5% of all fractures (see Table 57–3). These humeral fractures may occur as a result of either direct trauma (e.g., motor vehicle accidents, blows received during a physical assault, gunshot wounds) or indirect forces, including torsional forces that occur during athletic endeavors. In fractures occurring above the insertion of the tendon of the pectoralis major muscle (Fig. 57–24), the proximal fragment is displaced into abduction and external rotation as a result of the action of the rotator cuff musculature; fractures occurring in the interval between the insertion of the pectoralis major tendon proximally and the deltoid insertion distally result in adduction of the proximal fragment and lateral displacement of the distal fragment; and fractures occurring distal to the insertion of the deltoid muscle result in abduction of the proximal fragment and proximal displacement of the distal fragment.

Transverse fractures of the humeral shaft are most frequent and represent 50% to 70% of all diaphyseal fractures of the humerus; oblique or spiral fractures, each representing about 20% of all humeral diaphyseal fractures, result from torsional forces; and segmental and comminuted fractures constitute the other patterns of humeral shaft fracture (Fig. 57–25). Approximately three fourths of all such fractures involve the middle third of the bone.

Among the complications of fracture of the humeral diaphysis, neurologic injury is most common. Radial nerve palsy occurs in as many as 18% of closed fractures of the humeral shaft and is associated most often with transverse fractures of the diaphysis, particularly those occurring in the junction of the middle and distal thirds of the bone. Injury to the median or ulnar nerve is rare in cases of humeral diaphyseal fracture. Vascular compromise occurs in less than 5% of patients with fracture of the humeral

**TABLE 57–3**

**Fractures of the Humeral Metaphyses and Shaft**

| Site | Characteristics | Complications |
|------|-----------------|---------------|
| Proximal | Middle-aged and elderly adults<br>Classified as one-part to four-part, based on the degree and location of displacement | Lipohemarthrosis<br>Drooping shoulder related to hemarthrosis, capsular tear, muscle or nerve injury<br>Osteonecrosis, especially with displaced fractures of the humeral neck and four-part fractures<br>Osteoarthritis<br>Heterotopic ossification<br>Rotator cuff tear<br>Brachial plexus and, less commonly, axillary artery injury<br>Painful arc of motion |
| Middle | Adults > children<br>Most common at the junction of the distal and middle thirds<br>Associated fractures in 25% of cases (ulna, clavicle, or humerus)<br>Characteristic displacements related to sites of muscular attachment | Delayed union or nonunion when the fracture is transverse or distracted<br>Radial nerve injury in 5–15% of cases<br>Brachial artery injury |
| Supracondylar | Children >> adults<br>Extension (95%) and flexion (5%) types<br>Paradoxical posterior fat pad sign<br>Supracondylar process may fracture | Brachial artery injury<br>Median, ulnar, or radial nerve injury<br>Alignment abnormalities<br>Heterotopic ossification<br>Volkmann's ischemic contracture |

shaft. Delayed union or nonunion of humeral shaft fractures is encountered. In general, transverse, segmental, long oblique, or open fractures unite more slowly than do spiral or short oblique fractures or comminuted fractures.

## Elbow

Fractures and dislocations about the elbow represent 5% to 8% of all such injuries. Either direct injury, such as impact on the radius and ulna, or indirect injury, such as

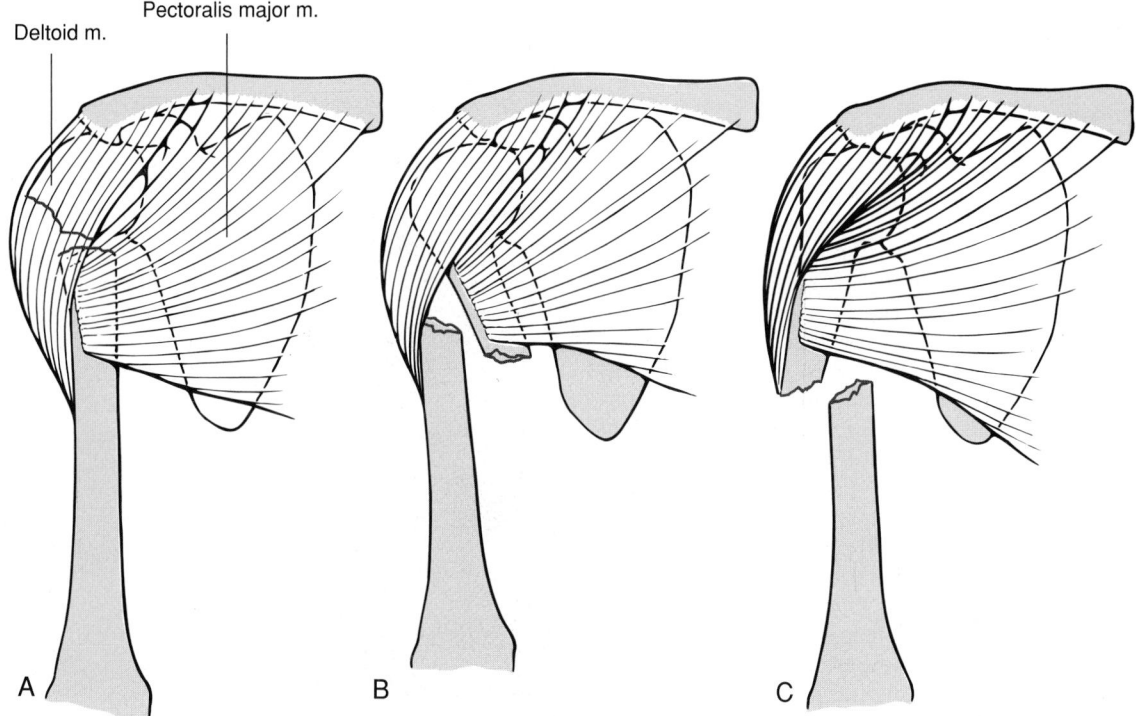

**Figure 57–24.** Humeral diaphysis: muscular anatomy. Effects of muscular forces in cases of humeral shaft fractures are illustrated. (From Browner BD, Levine AM, Jupiter JB, Trafton PG [eds]: Skeletal Trauma, vol 2, 2nd ed. Philadelphia, WB Saunders, 1998, p 1526.)

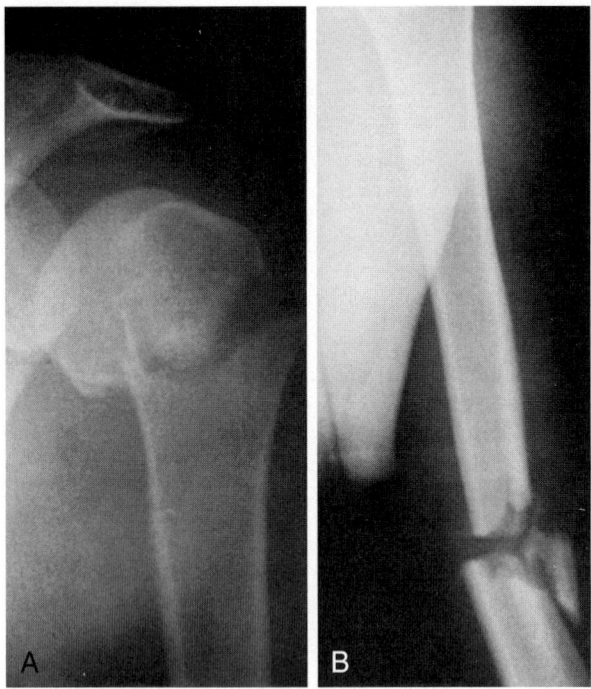

**Figure 57–25.** Humerus: segmental fracture. A fracture of the surgical neck of the bone *(A)* may be entirely overlooked if attention is directed solely at the diaphyseal fracture *(B)*. A fracture of the scapula was also present in this patient.

that transmitted through the bones of the forearm, lead to elbow fractures and dislocations.

### Elbow Dislocation

The elbow joint is the third most common site of dislocation (after the glenohumeral joint and interphalangeal joints of the fingers), and it is the most common site of dislocation in children. The most commonly reported mechanism of injury is hyperextension (e.g., a fall on an outstretched hand). In cases of dislocation involving both the radius and the ulna, posterior dislocation (Fig. 57–26) is most frequent (approximately 80% to 90% of all elbow dislocations). In adults, this injury may be complicated by fracture of the coronoid process of the ulna, the capitulum of the humerus, or the radial head; in children and adolescents, the medial epicondylar ossification center is frequently avulsed and may become entrapped during reduction. Medial, lateral, and anterior dislocations of the elbow are not common.

Isolated dislocation of the ulna at the elbow is unusual. Similarly, isolated radial head dislocation without an associated fracture in the ulna is rare in adults. In children, subluxation of the radial head, which is usually but not invariably transient, is termed *nursemaid's elbow* or pulled elbow. Routine radiographs are therefore normal. Rarely, the annular ligament becomes entrapped in the joint, and surgical reduction is required.

The combination of an ulnar fracture and radial head dislocation is termed Monteggia's fracture-dislocation (Fig. 57–27). Various types of Monteggia's fracture-dislocations

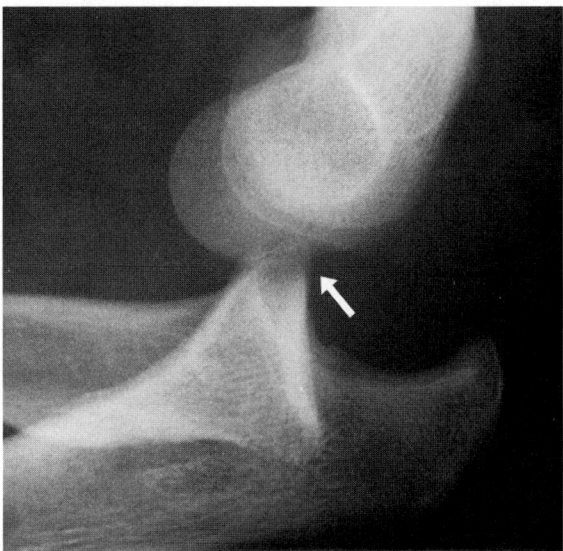

**Figure 57–26.** Elbow: posterior dislocation of both the radius and the ulna. Lateral radiograph shows posterolateral displacement of the radius and ulna with respect to the humerus. Note contact between the trochlea of the humerus and the coronoid process of the ulna *(arrow)*.

are recognized (Table 57–4). These patterns emphasize the typical occurrence of injuries to more than one structure in the forearm. Monteggia's fracture-dislocation is a common injury in adults (but rare in children) and is easily overlooked.

In infants and young children, separation of the entire distal humeral epiphysis may be confused with elbow dislocation. Correct diagnosis of this injury rests on two observations: a normal relationship between the capitulum and radius, and medial displacement of the radius and ulna with respect to the humerus. Complications of elbow dislocation include heterotopic calcification and ossification and neural and vascular injury.

### Intra-articular Fracture of the Distal Portion of the Humerus

Intra-articular fractures of the distal portion of the humerus in a mature skeleton are usually classified as transcondylar, intercondylar, condylar, epicondylar, transchondral, or

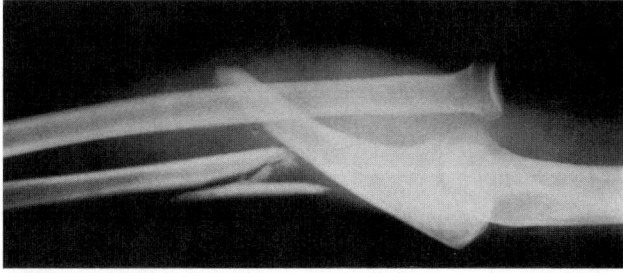

**Figure 57–27.** Monteggia's fracture-dislocation. In a type I Monteggia's fracture-dislocation, note the fracture of the upper third of the ulna, with anterior angulation at the fracture site and anterior dislocation of the radial head.

**TABLE 57–4**

**Fractures of the Radial and Ulnar Shafts**

| Site | Characteristics | Complications |
|------|-----------------|---------------|
| Ulna (alone) | "Nightstick" fracture: direct blow to the forearm, distal >middle> proximal segments of the ulna | Displacement at the fracture site (uncommon) |
| | Monteggia's injury: | Injury to branches of the radial nerve (approximately 20% of cases) |
| | Type I: fracture of the middle or upper third of the ulna with anterior dislocation of the radial head (65%) | |
| | Type II: fracture of the middle or upper third of the ulna with posterior dislocation of the radial head (18%) | |
| | Type III: fracture of the ulna just distal to the coronoid process with lateral dislocation of the radial head (16%) | |
| | Type IV: fracture of the upper or middle third of the ulna with anterior dislocation of the radial head and proximal radial fracture (1%) | |
| Radius (alone) | Proximal and middle segments: uncommon because usually associated with an ulnar fracture | |
| | Galeazzi's injury: fracture of the radial shaft with dislocation or subluxation of the inferior radioulnar joint caused by a direct blow or a fall on the outstretched hand with pronation of the forearm, variable degrees of displacement at the fracture site | Angulation<br>Entrapment of the extensor carpi ulnaris tendon (rare)<br>Delayed union or nonunion |
| Radius and ulna | Closed or open<br>Nondisplaced or displaced (displacement more common in adults than children) | Delayed union or nonunion (especially of ulna)<br>Infection, especially in open fractures<br>Nerve and vascular injuries, especially in open fractures and those with severe displacement<br>Compartment syndromes<br>Synostosis between the radius and ulna (rare) |

miscellaneous. Transcondylar fractures resemble supracondylar fractures (Fig. 57–28) but are intra-articular in location. The fracture line traverses both condylar surfaces in a horizontal direction. Intercondylar fractures of the distal portion of the humerus (Fig. 57–29) result in comminuted and complex fracture lines that generally include one component that traverses the supracondylar region of the humerus in a transverse or oblique fashion and a second component, vertical or oblique in nature, that enters the articular lumen. The resulting configuration of the fracture is thus T- or Y-shaped. These fractures should be distinguished from those involving only an epicondyle (medial or lateral epicondylar fracture) and those affecting the capitulum or the trochlea.

Condylar fractures are relatively uncommon and occur predominantly in children. Fractures of the lateral condyle are more frequent than those of the medial condyle (Fig. 57–30). Each can be associated with significant instability and restriction of motion, especially if the fracture fragment is large. In this regard, a classification system has been devised on the basis of the size of the fragment and the presence or absence of disruption of the lateral trochlear ridge. This structure, which separates the trochlea and capitulum, is important in providing medial and lateral stability to the elbow. In type I fractures of the condyles, the lateral trochlear ridge is not disrupted, whereas in type II fractures, the larger fracture fragment contains the separated condyle and a portion of this ridge. This latter pattern of injury allows translocation of the radius

and ulna in a mediolateral direction and is termed a fracture-dislocation.

The epicondyles, as well as other osseous structures throughout the elbow, are injured more frequently in children or adolescents than in adults (Fig. 57–31). In a mature skeleton, the medial epicondyle is fractured more commonly than the lateral epicondyle, and the injury is related in most cases to a direct force applied to the epicondyle. Injury to the adjacent ulnar nerve may also be apparent. Isolated fractures of the lateral epicondyle are very rare in adults.

### Fracture of the Olecranon and Coronoid Processes of the Ulna

Fractures of the olecranon process, which represent approximately 20% of all elbow injuries in adults, result from direct injury, indirect injury, or a combination of the two (Fig. 57–32). The pull of the triceps muscle accounts for displacement of the fragment or fragments. Significant posterior displacement of the olecranon fragment, combined with anterior movement of the remaining portion of the ulna and the radial head, is a serious injury that is termed a fracture-dislocation of the elbow. Complications of olecranon fractures include a decreased range of elbow motion, osteoarthritis, and nonunion and ulnar nerve damage. Isolated fractures of the coronoid process of the ulna are rare and are commonly associated with posterior dislocation of the elbow.

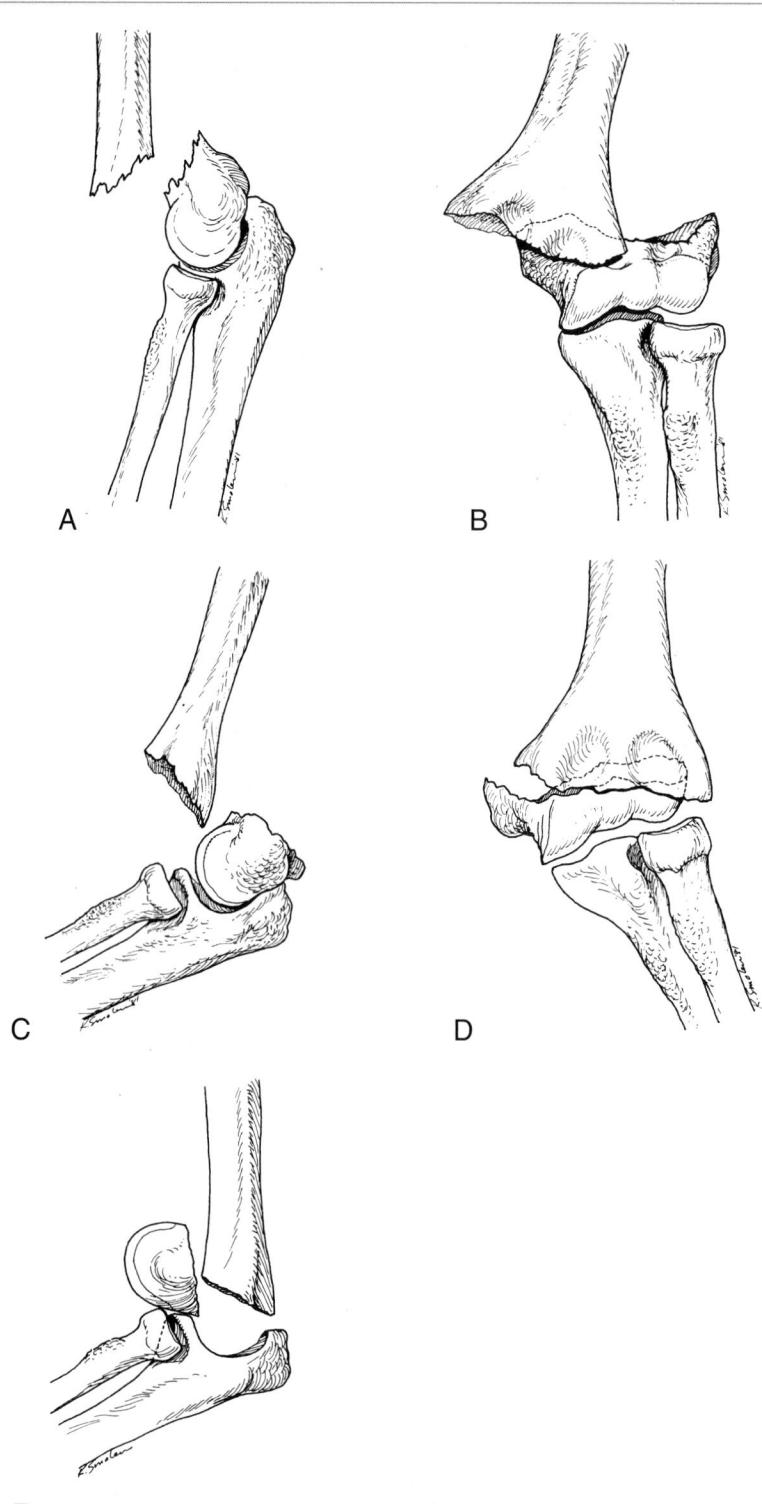

**Figure 57–28.** Humeral fracture: supracondylar and transcondylar. *A* and *B*, Supracondylar fracture (extension type) probably caused by a fall on an outstretched hand with the elbow in extension. On a lateral view *(A)*, the fracture line extends obliquely upward from a more distal point anteriorly to a more proximal point posteriorly. Posterior and proximal displacement of the distal fragment results, in part, from the force of the triceps muscle attaching to the ulna. Observe the sharp margin of the proximal fragment, which projects into the antecubital fossa; this accounts for the associated injuries to the brachial artery and median nerve. On an anteroposterior view *(B)*, the fracture line is generally transverse in configuration. Displacement and angulation at the fracture site are of variable degree. *C* and *D*, Transcondylar fracture (extension type). The fracture line passes through the condyles of the humerus and is intracapsular in location. On a lateral view *(C)*, posterior displacement of the distal fragment predominates. On a frontal view *(D)*, the fracture line is commonly transverse and inferior to that of a supracondylar fracture. *E*, Transcondylar fracture (Posadas type). Note the anterior displacement of the condylar fragment and dislocation of the radius and ulna posteriorly, with the coronoid process wedged between the condyles and the humeral shaft. (*E*, From DeLee JC, Green DP, Wilkins KE: Fractures and dislocations of the elbow. In Rockwood CA Jr, Green DP [eds]: Fractures in Adults, 2nd ed. Philadelphia, JB Lippincott, 1984, p 573.)

## Fracture of the Head and Neck of the Radius

Radial head fractures are common injuries in adults and result principally from indirect trauma. Such fractures are classified as undisplaced fractures (Mason type I), marginal fractures with displacement (e.g., angulation, depression, impaction; Mason type II), comminuted fractures (Mason type III), and, in recognition of their poorer prognosis, fractures associated with elbow dislocation. In addition, an impaction fracture of the radial neck, without involvement of the radial head, is encountered frequently. The diagnostic importance of a positive fat pad sign, as well as of oblique and specialized radiographic projections, is well recognized, and identification of an associated capitulum fracture or intra-articular osseous fragments has been emphasized (Fig. 57–33).

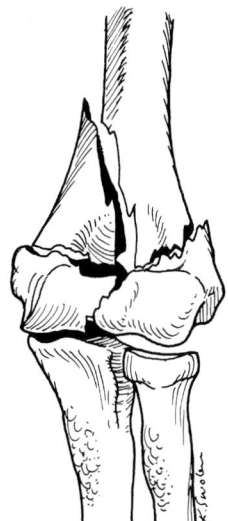

**Figure 57–29.** Humeral fracture: intercondylar. In this example, a comminuted fracture has led to separation of the trochlear and capitular fragments. Rotation at the fracture site and incongruity of the articular surface are potential complications.

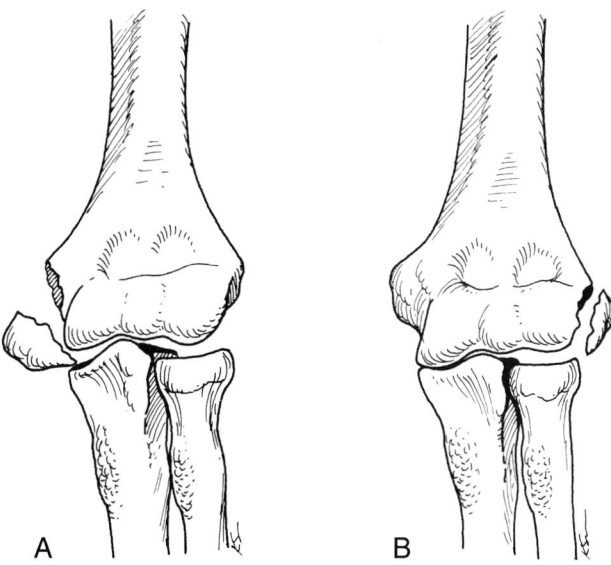

A　　　　　　　　　　　　　　　　B

**Figure 57–31.** Humeral fracture: epicondylar. *A*, Fracture of the medial epicondyle. *B*, Fracture of the lateral epicondyle.

Complications after radial head fractures are infrequent and consist of limited range of motion, osteoarthritis, and, in more severe injuries, heterotopic ossification. Such fractures, however, may be part of a more complex or widespread injury such as elbow dislocation, fracture of the capitulum, subluxation of the distal radioulnar joint (Essex-Lopresti injury), or other carpal bones. The Essex-Lopresti injury consists of a comminuted and displaced radial head fracture and disruption of the distal radioulnar joint.

### Radial and Ulnar Diaphyses

When a fracture occurs in one or both bones of the forearm, the muscles that join these bones—pronator quadratus, pronator teres, and supinator—serve to decrease the interosseous space. The final resting position of the radius after fracture depends on the action of these muscles and others, such as the biceps brachii muscle, and is influenced by the level of the fracture itself. These patterns of rotation of the proximal portion of the radius are important to orthopedic surgeons, who, when reducing the radial fracture, must attempt to eliminate any rotational malalignment. Routine radiography, often supplemented with specialized projections, can be used to judge the degree of supination and pronation of the proximal portion of the radius by analysis of the appearance of the bicipital tuberosity. The bicipital tuberosity

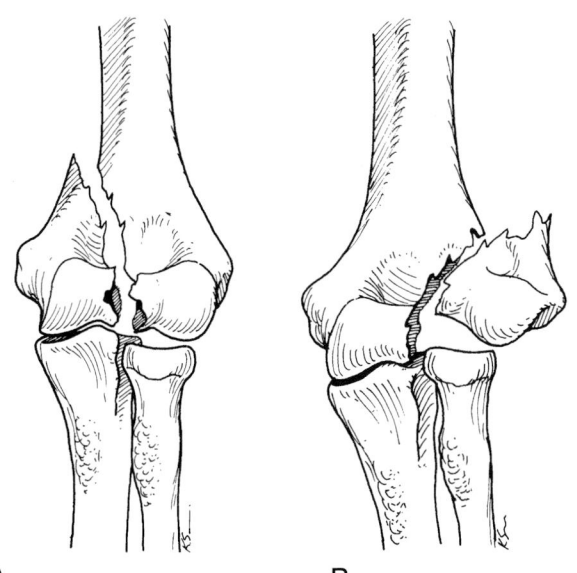

A　　　　　　　　　　B

**Figure 57–30.** Humeral fracture: condylar. *A*, Fracture of the medial condyle. *B*, Fracture of the lateral condyle.

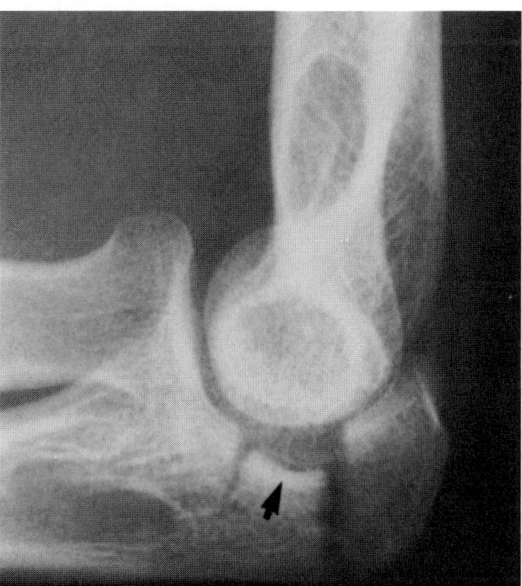

**Figure 57–32.** Ulnar fracture: olecranon process. A comminuted fracture has led to depression of the articular surface *(arrow)*. A joint effusion is present.

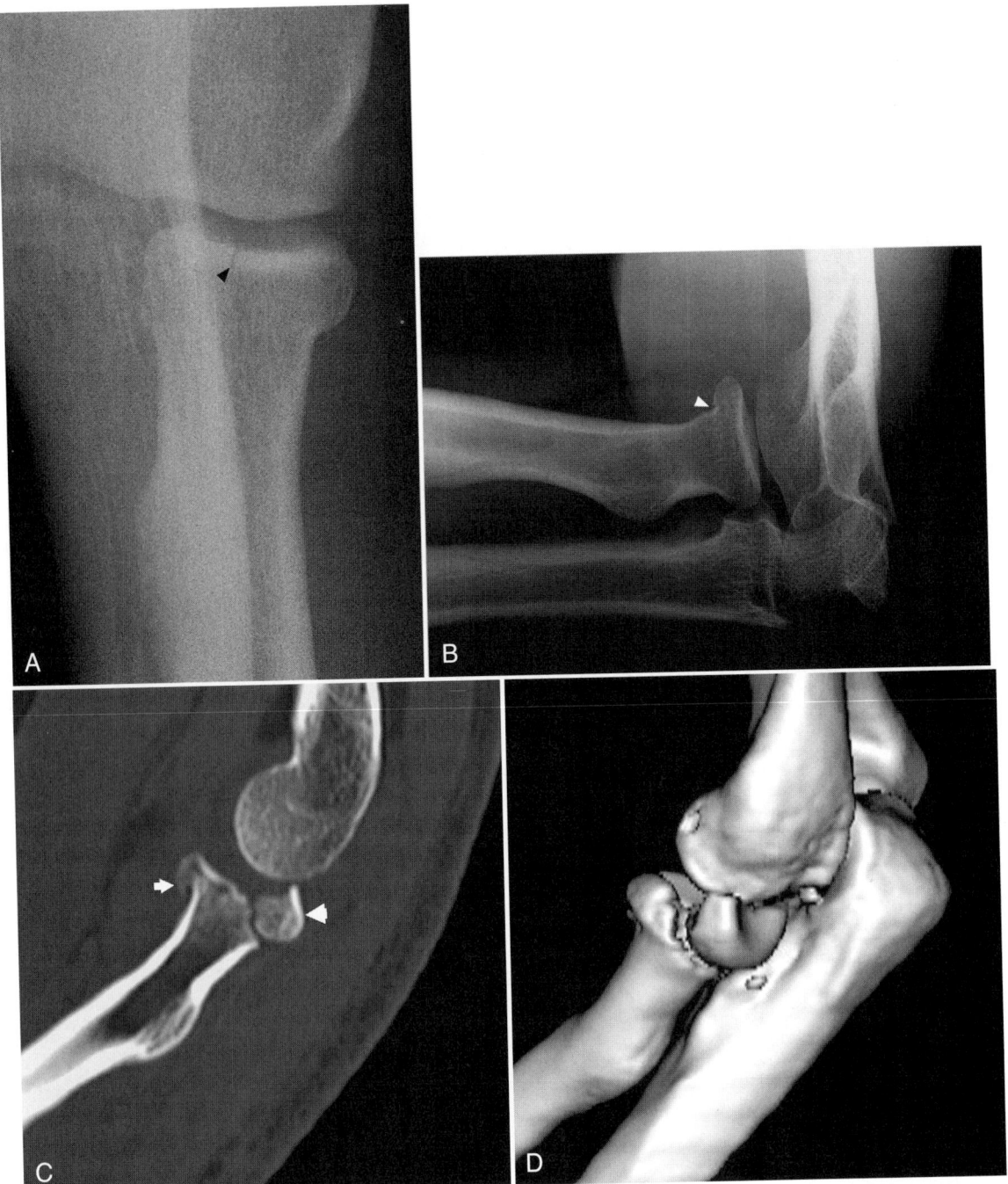

**Figure 57–33.** Radial fracture: head of the radius. *A,* Magnification radiography is used to illustrate a subtle radial head fracture *(arrowhead). B,* Specialized radiographic projection is used to demonstrate a radial head fracture *(arrowhead). C* and *D,* In a different patient, reformatted CT *(C)* shows an impacted fracture of the radial head *(arrow),* with a displaced posterior fragment *(arrowhead).* Surface-rendering three-dimensional CT *(D)* shows to better advantage the displaced and rotated articular surface.

of the radius is located medially when the arm is positioned in full supination, laterally when the arm is positioned in full pronation, and posteriorly when the arm is positioned in midpronation. Radiographs of the forearm generally include a frontal anteroposterior projection with the arm supinated. In such a position, the ulnar styloid process is not a border-forming structure on the outer aspect of the distal end of the ulna; on a frontal (posteroanterior) pro-

jection of the forearm with the arm pronated, the styloid process is located on the outer margin of the distal part of the ulna.

Injuries involving a single anatomic structure in the forearm are rare (see Table 57–4). In common with the pelvis, mandible, and ankle, the forearm can be considered a ring structure because of the ligamentous and articular connections of the radius and ulna. Disruption of the ring at one site is usually accompanied by disruption at a second (or even third) site. When both injuries are fractures, accurate diagnosis with routine radiography is not difficult. When a fracture and dislocation are components of the two injuries (e.g., Monteggia's and Galeazzi's fracture-dislocations, Essex-Lopresti injury), routine radiographic diagnosis is straightforward as long as the entire forearm (i.e., elbow to wrist) is surveyed. When subluxation is a component of the injury pattern, however, the initial radiographic examination may be interpreted as showing only a single lesion, particularly if the subluxation is transient or appears only in certain positions of the forearm. In such cases, scintigraphy, CT, or MR imaging may provide diagnostic assistance.

## Fracture of Both the Radius and the Ulna

Fractures involving both bones of the forearm are common and usually result from direct injury. The middle segment of the diaphyseal portion of the bones is typically involved, although the peripheral segments may also be affected. The fractures in the radius and ulna may occur at approximately the same level or at different levels. Considerable displacement, angulation, and rotation at the fracture sites are common and lead to deformity and loss of function. In children, the distal third of the diaphyses of the radius and ulna is involved most commonly; the site of a radial fracture is generally more distal than that of an ulnar fracture. Complications of these fractures include delayed union or nonunion, neurologic and vascular injury, compartment syndrome, and synostoses.

## Fracture of the Ulna

Fractures involving the diaphysis of the ulna may occur as part of Monteggia's fracture-dislocation (see previous discussion) or as an isolated phenomenon. Isolated fractures of the ulnar shaft are common; typically, they result from a direct injury and are designated *nightstick fractures* (Fig. 57–34). Significantly displaced fractures of the ulnar diaphysis are usually associated with dislocations of the proximal or distal radioulnar joint.

## Fracture of the Radius

Fractures of the diaphysis of the radius occur most commonly as part of Galeazzi's fracture-dislocation (see later discussion) and rarely as an isolated phenomenon. Isolated fractures of the proximal portion of the radial shaft result from a direct blow and are less common than those of the ulna.

## Wrist

### Fracture of the Distal Portions of the Radius and Ulna

The most common mechanism of injury to the wrist is a fall on an outstretched hand. Fractures of the distal regions of the radius and ulna are approximately 10 times more frequent than those of the carpal bones; the latter

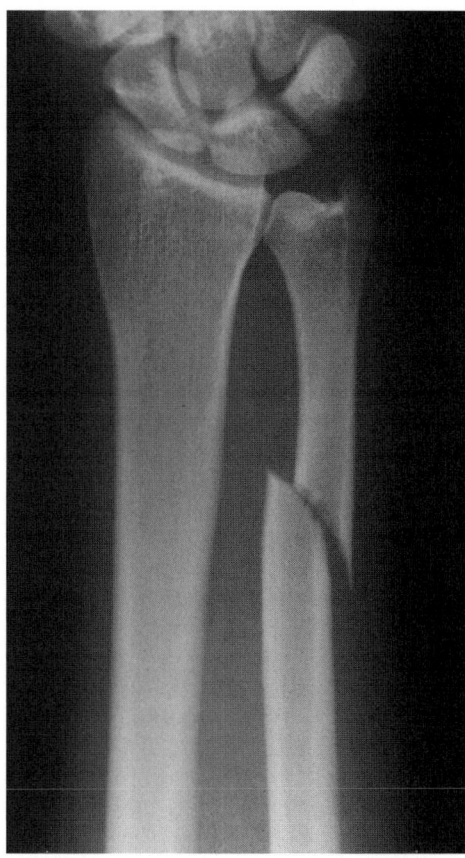

**Figure 57–34.** Fractures of the diaphyses of the radius and ulna: isolated fracture of the ulna (nightstick fracture). Note the oblique, slightly displaced fracture of the distal portion of the ulna.

are especially infrequent in children. Many eponyms have been used to describe fractures of the distal ends of the radius and ulna, and major characteristics of these fractures are described in Table 57–5. Although these designations are still used, descriptions related to the intra-articular or extra-articular nature of the fracture, the number of fracture fragments, and the presence and degree of displacement or angulation are becoming more common. CT scanning and MR imaging may serve as useful supplements to standard radiography in assessing fracture comminution, depression and incongruity of articular surfaces, and associated soft tissue abnormalities (Fig. 57–35).

The classic Colles' fracture is a transverse fracture, with or without comminution, that extends from the volar to the dorsal surface of the distal part of the radius and is accompanied by impaction and displacement of the dorsal surface of the radius (Fig. 57–36). The typical mechanism is a fall on an outstretched hand. Fracture of the ulnar styloid process occurs in approximately 50% to 60% of cases, and violation of one or both of these articulations occurs in most cases. Radial shortening and dorsal inclination of the articular surface of the radius (which normally has a volar inclination of 5 to 15 degrees) are important sequelae of Colles' fractures that, if not corrected, may influence subsequent wrist function. Complications are diverse and common, including unstable

**TABLE 57–5**

**Fractures of the Distal Portions of the Radius and Ulna**

| Fracture | Mechanism | Characteristics | Complications |
|---|---|---|---|
| Colles' (Pouteau's) | Dorsiflexion | Fracture of the distal portion with dorsal displacement<br>Classification system based on extra-articular versus intra-articular location, presence or absence of an ulnar fracture<br>Varying amounts of radial displacement, angulation, and shortening<br>Ulnar styloid fracture in about 50–60% of cases<br>Associated injuries to the carpus, elbow, humerus, femur (in osteoporotic patients), inferior radioulnar joint | Deformity related to radial shortening and angulation<br>Subluxation or dislocation of the inferior radioulnar joint<br>Reflex sympathetic dystrophy syndrome<br>Injury to the median or, less commonly, radial or ulnar nerve<br>Osteoarthritis<br>Tendon rupture |
| Barton's | Dorsiflexion and pronation | Fracture of the dorsal rim of the radius with intra-articular extension | Similar to those of Colles' fracture |
| Radiocarpal fracture dislocation | Dorsiflexion | Uncommon and severe injury<br>Associated fractures of the dorsal rim and styloid process of the radius, ulnar styloid process<br>May be irreducible | Entrapment of the ulnar nerve and artery, tendons |
| Hutchinson's (chauffeur's) | Avulsion by the radial collateral ligament | Fracture of the styloid process of the radius<br>Usually nondisplaced | Scapholunate dissociation<br>Osteoarthritis<br>Ligament damage |
| Smith's (reverse Colles') | Variable | Fracture of the distal portion of the radius with palmar displacement<br>Less common than Colles' fracture<br>Varying amounts of radial comminution, articular involvement<br>Associated fracture of the ulnar styloid process | Similar to those of Colles' fracture |
| Ulnar styloid process | Dorsiflexion or avulsion by the ulnar collateral ligament or triangular fibrocartilage complex | Usually associated with radial fractures, rarely isolated<br>Usually nondisplaced | Nonunion |

reduction, articular incongruity, subluxation or dislocation of the distal radioulnar joint, median nerve compression, ulnar nerve injury, entrapment of flexor tendons, reflex sympathetic dystrophy, carpal malalignment, delayed union, or nonunion.

A distal radial fracture similar in position to Colles' fracture but associated with volar (or palmar) angulation or displacement of the distal fragment is known as Smith's fracture (Fig. 57–37). Smith's fracture is much less common than Colles' fracture. Complications of Smith's fractures are similar to those of Colles' fractures and may include injury to the extensor tendons.

Barton's fracture involves an injury to the dorsal rim of the distal portion of the radius, generally related to dorsiflexion and pronation of the forearm on a fixed wrist (Fig. 57–38). Differentiation from Colles' fracture can be accomplished based on findings on a lateral radiograph of the wrist. Barton's fracture extends in an oblique fashion from the dorsal surface of the radius proximally to the articular surface of the radius distally. It does not violate the volar surface of the radius and is accompanied by dorsal displacement of the carpus. A variant of Barton's fracture affects the volar rim of the distal end of the radius and is sometimes referred to as a reverse Barton's fracture or a type of Smith's fracture.

A fracture of the styloid process of the radius (see Fig. 57–35) is often referred to as Hutchinson's fracture or, because of its original occurrence when the starting crank of a car engine suddenly reversed during a backfire, chauffeur's fracture.

## Dislocation of the Inferior Radioulnar Joint

Dislocations of the inferior radioulnar joint may occur in association with a fracture of the radius. This combination of findings is termed Galeazzi's fracture-dislocation (Fig. 57–39). Classically, the shaft of the radius is fractured. Fractures of the distal end of the radius may be associated with dislocation of the ulnar head. Fractures of the radial neck and head, which may be associated with dislocation of the inferior radioulnar joint, are not regarded as Galeazzi's fracture-dislocations unless the radial shaft is also fractured. Dislocation of the ulna usually occurs in a distal, dorsal, and medial direction; volar dislocation is less frequent.

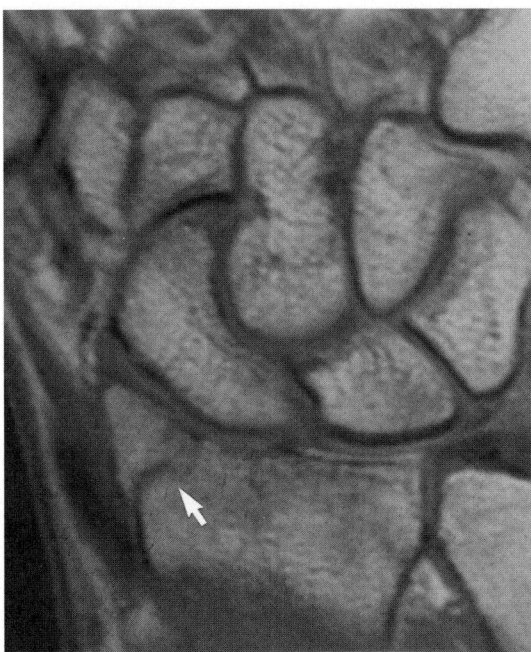

**Figure 57–35.** Wrist fracture: radial styloid process. Coronal T1-weighted (TR/TE, 733/20) spin echo MR image reveals an occult fracture *(arrows)* of the radial styloid process (Hutchinson's fracture). (Courtesy of S. Eilenberg, MD, San Diego, Calif.)

## Carpal Instability

Two important concepts regarding the radiographic anatomy of the wrist should be emphasized. First, on a posteroanterior view, three smooth carpal arcs define the normal intercarpal relationships. Arc 1 follows the proximal surfaces of the scaphoid, lunate, and triquetrum; arc 2 is located along the distal surfaces of these same carpal bones; and arc 3 defines the curvature of the proximal surfaces of the capitate and hamate. In the normal situa-

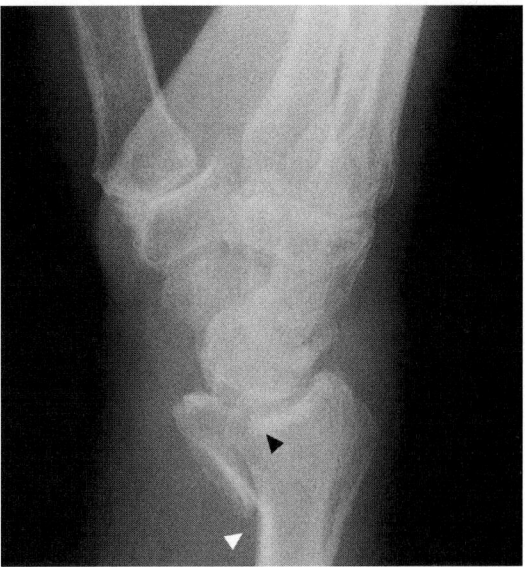

**Figure 57–37.** Wrist fracture: Smith's fracture. A fracture of the distal portion of the radius *(arrowheads)* involves the volar surface. Note the mild volar and proximal displacement of the fracture fragment of the carpus.

tion, with the wrist in neutral position, these curvilinear arcs are roughly parallel, without disruption, and the interosseous spaces are approximately equal in size. Second, a lateral radiograph of a normal wrist (in neutral position) is characterized by a specific relationship of the longitudinal axes of the radius, scaphoid, lunate, capitate, and third metacarpal. A continuous line can be drawn through the axes of the radius, lunate, and capitate, and this line intersects a second line through the longitudinal axis of the scaphoid and creates an angle of 30 to 60 degrees. Alterations in these relationships (as well as others) indicate carpal instability, which in most instances is related to trauma.

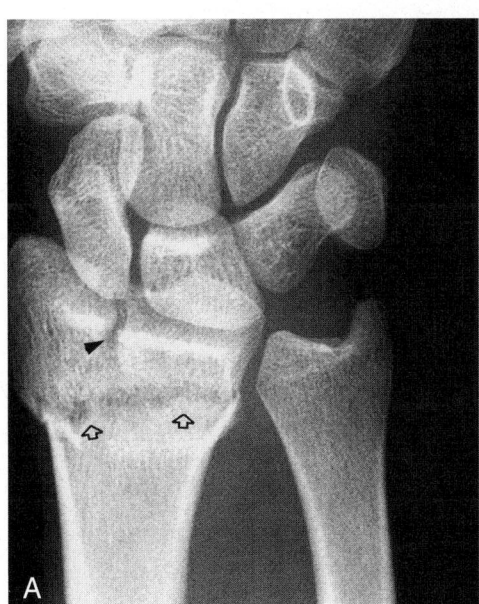
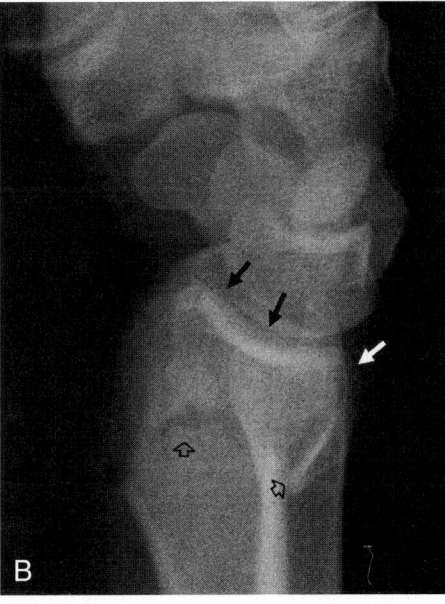

**Figure 57–36.** Wrist fracture: Colles' fracture. *A*, Observe the transverse fracture of the distal portion of the radius *(open arrows)*, with extension into the radiocarpal joint *(arrowhead)*. *B*, In the lateral projection, dorsal angulation of the articular surface of the radius *(solid arrows)* is apparent and caused by compaction of bone dorsally. This injury is a three-part fracture. The ulnar styloid process is intact, and no evidence of subluxation of the distal portion of the ulna can be seen.

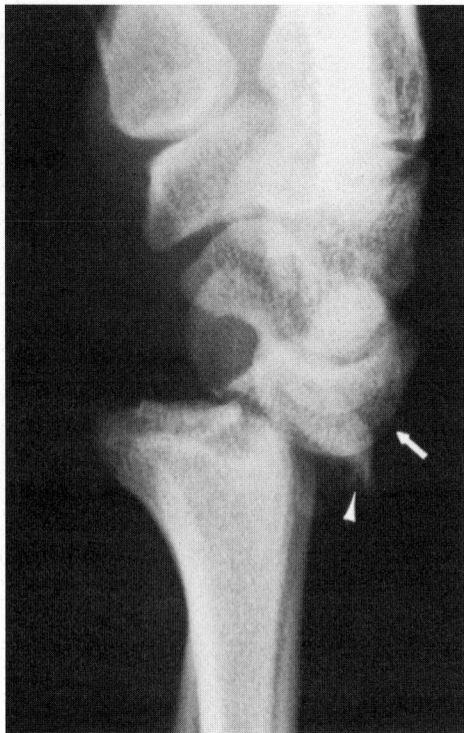

**Figure 57–38.** Wrist fracture: Barton's fracture. The dorsal rim of the distal portion of the radius is fractured *(arrowhead)*. It is displaced proximally and posteriorly, and dorsal subluxation of the carpus *(arrow)* is present.

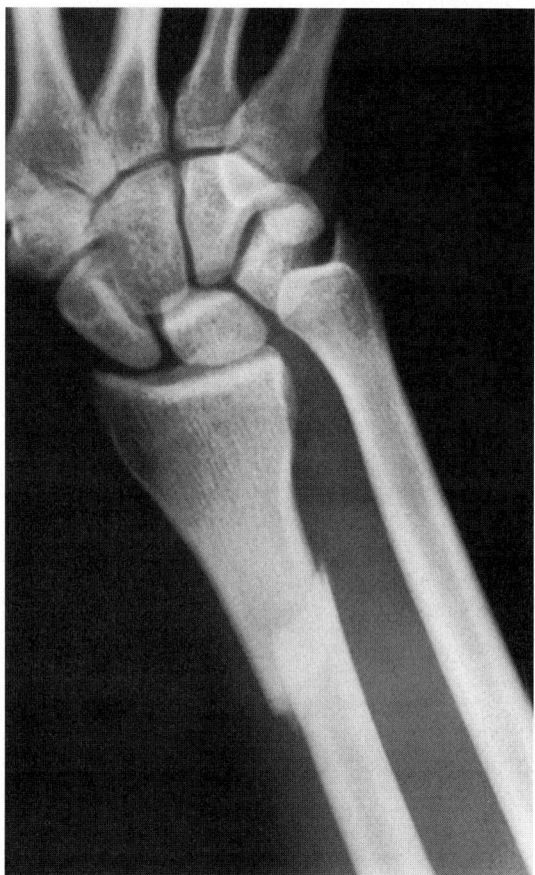

**Figure 57–39.** Galeazzi's fracture-dislocation. Transverse radial fracture is associated with significant overlapping, shortening, and angulation, as well as volar dislocation of the distal end of the ulna.

Carpal instability is considered to be present when symptomatic malalignment exists and the normal kinematics are disrupted during any portion of the arc of motion of the wrist. Several characteristic and distinct patterns of carpal instability are recognized. Such patterns may be defined as either static, when malalignment among the carpal bones is evident on routine radiographs, or dynamic, when such malalignment requires manipulation. Two patterns of instability require emphasis. Dorsal intercalary segment carpal instability is the more common of the two; in this pattern, the lunate is tilted dorsally, the scaphoid is flexed, and the scapholunate angle is greater than 70 degrees. The second pattern, volar intercalary segment carpal instability, occurs when the lunate is tilted in a palmar direction and the scapholunate angle is decreased below the normal value of approximately 47 degrees (Fig. 57–40). Dorsiflexion instability commonly occurs after scaphoid fractures with scapholunate separation or dissociation, as well as after fractures of the proximal portion of the radius; palmar flexion instability may be seen after disruption of the lunotriquetral interosseous ligament, excision of the triquetrum, and sprains of the midcarpal joint that attenuate the extrinsic ligaments.

Scapholunate dissociation (rotatory subluxation of the scaphoid) is suggested when the distance between the scaphoid and lunate is 2 mm or wider and can be diagnosed almost unequivocally when this distance is 4 mm or more (Fig. 57–41). In addition to widening of the scapholunate space (Terry Thomas sign) and palmar tilt-

ing of the scaphoid, rotatory subluxation of the scaphoid is associated with other radiographic findings; these include, on a posteroanterior view, a ring produced by the cortex of the distal pole of the scaphoid and a foreshortened scaphoid.

A common pattern of carpal injury is a perilunate dislocation or transscaphoid perilunate fracture-dislocation. In perilunate dislocation, the lunate remains aligned with the distal end of the radius, and the other carpal bones dislocate, usually dorsally (Fig. 57–42). When the wrist is hyperextended, the dorsal cortex of the distal radial articular surface fixes the lunate in place and apposes the scaphoid waist. A fall on a hyperextended hand, which creates abnormal force through the radius, can produce a fracture of the scaphoid and, with sufficient stress, dislocation of the carpus. The distal fragment of the scaphoid may move with the distal carpal row, and the proximal fragment may move with the proximal carpal row. With continued hyperextension force, the capitate may force the lunate ventrally, thus converting the perilunate dislocation into a lunate dislocation in which the lunate is displaced in a palmar direction and the capitate appears to be aligned with the distal end of the radius (Fig. 57–43).

Close inspection of the functional anatomy of the wrist and the patterns of injury indicates that a predictable

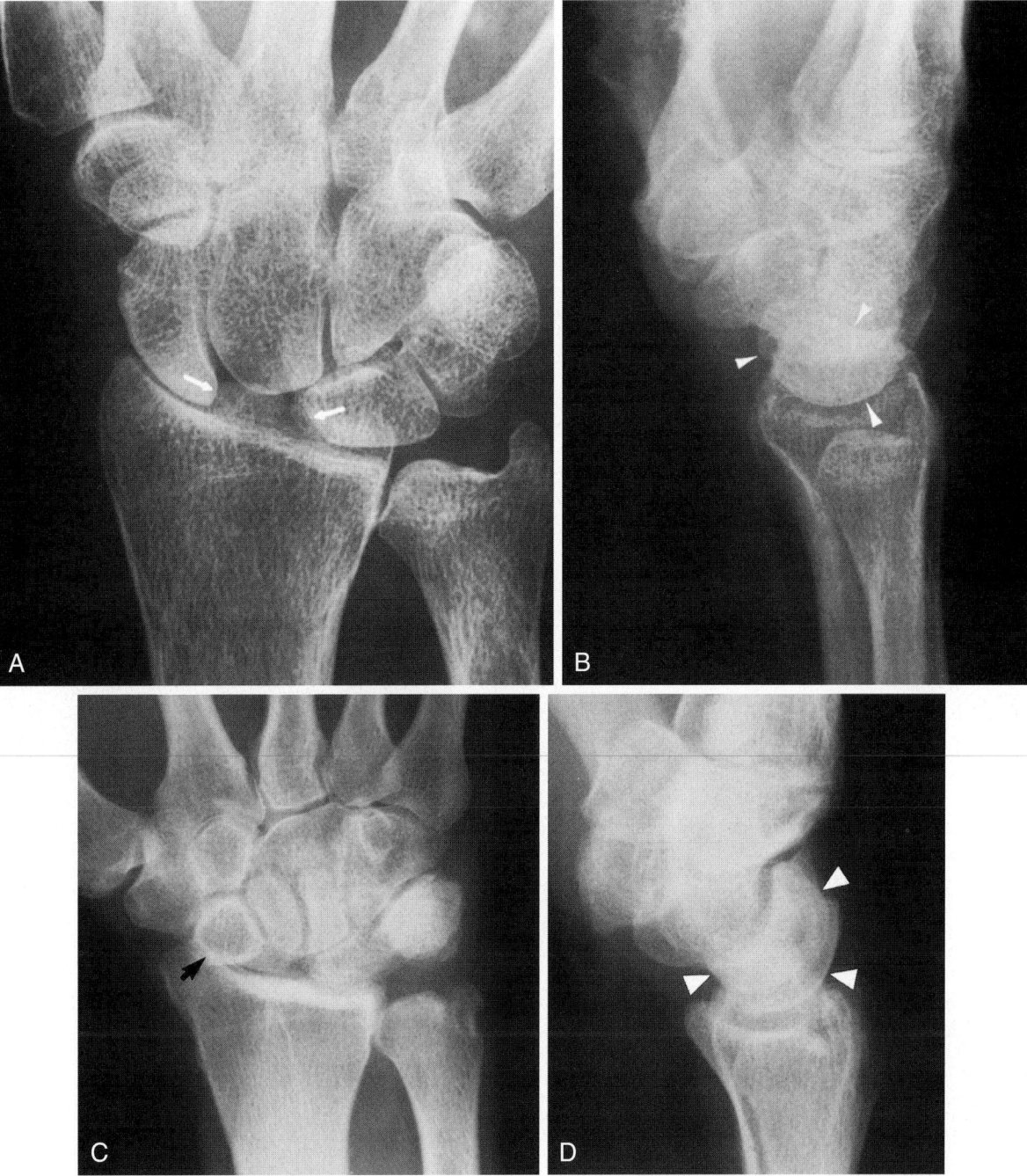

**Figure 57–40.** Lateral (static) carpal instability. *A* and *B*, Dorsal intercalary segment instability. Observe the gap or widening in the scapholunate space *(arrows)* on the posteroanterior radiograph *(A)* and dorsiflexion of the lunate *(arrowheads)* on the lateral radiograph *(B)*. The radiocarpal and midcarpal joints are narrowed. A small fracture of the volar surface of the lunate is seen. *C* and *D*, Volar intercalary segment instability. Findings include palmar displacement of the distal pole of the scaphoid, resulting in a ringlike shadow *(arrow)* and volar tilting of the lunate *(arrowheads)*.

sequence of events generally occurs after trauma (Fig. 57–44). Lesser arc injuries occur in four stages, with each successive stage indicating increased carpal instability. A stage I injury represents scapholunate dissociation with rotatory subluxation of the scaphoid; a stage II injury is characterized by perilunate dislocation; a stage III injury creates ligamentous disruption at the triquetrolunate; and a stage IV injury is associated with lunate dislocation.

Greater arc injuries represent fracture-dislocation patterns as this arc passes through the scaphoid, capitate, hamate, and triquetrum.

## Fracture of the Carpal Bones

Approximately 65% of all carpal bone fractures involve the scaphoid bone. Fractures of the scaphoid are classi-

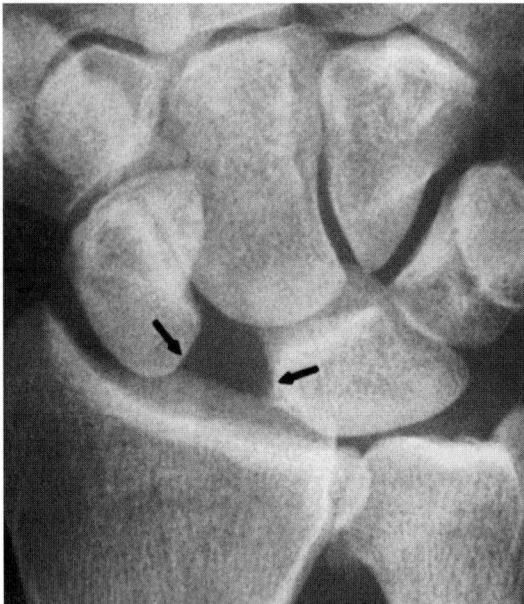

**Figure 57–41.** Scapholunate dissociation (rotatory subluxation of the scaphoid). Findings include widening of the scapholunate distance *(arrows)* and a foreshortened scaphoid.

fied principally according to their location (proximal pole, waist, distal body, tuberosity, distal articular), because the site of involvement affects the likelihood of ischemic necrosis and the rate of healing. In general, the prognosis of distal fractures is better than that of proximal fractures. The most frequent scaphoid fractures occur in the waist (approximately 70%) or proximal pole (approximately 20%). The frequency of delayed union or nonunion is greatest in fractures of the proximal pole and in those associated with displaced fragments. Radiographic

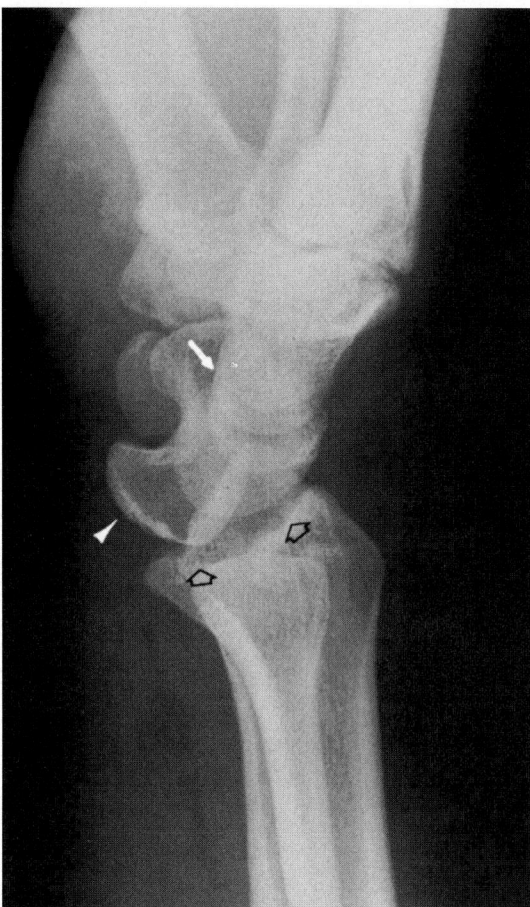

**Figure 57–43.** Lunate dislocation. Note the volar displacement of the lunate *(arrowhead)*, with the capitate *(solid arrow)* resting on the dorsal surface of the bone. Neither the lunate nor the capitate is truly aligned with the distal surface of the radius *(open arrows)*, illustrating the difficulty of classifying such lesions as lunate or perilunate dislocations. (Courtesy of G. Greenway, MD, Dallas, Tex.)

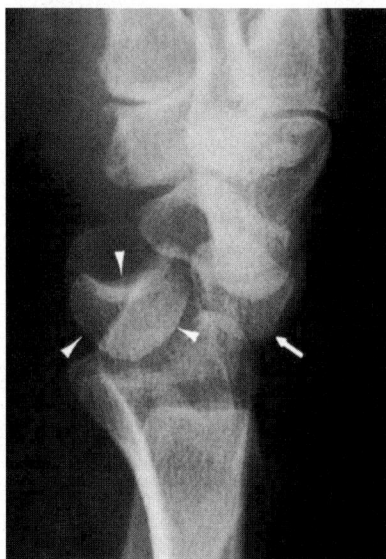

**Figure 57–42.** Perilunate dislocation. Observe the alignment of the lunate *(arrowheads)* with the distal end of the radius and dorsal displacement of the capitate *(arrow)* and the rest of the carpal bones.

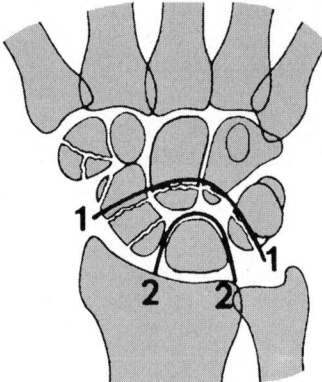

**Figure 57–44.** Wrist injuries: greater and lesser arcs. The locations of the greater (1) and lesser (2) arcs are shown, as are the common sites of carpal fractures that can be produced experimentally. A pure greater arc injury consists of a transscaphoid, transcapitate, transhamate, transtriquetral fracture-dislocation; a pure lesser arc injury is a perilunate or lunate dislocation. Various combinations of these injury patterns are seen clinically. (From Johnson RP: The acutely injured wrist and its residuals. Clin Orthop 149:33, 1980.)

abnormalities of scaphoid nonunion (Fig. 57–45), which occurs in approximately 5% to 15% of cases, include bone sclerosis, cyst formation, widening of the scapholunate space, bone resorption, and, subsequently, osteoarthritis. The frequency of ischemic necrosis after scaphoid fractures is approximately 10% to 15%; this frequency rises to 30% to 40% in the case of nonunion.

Isolated fractures of the other carpal bones are less frequent. Triquetral fractures represent 3% to 4% of all carpal fractures. The dorsal surface of the triquetrum is typically fractured, related either to contact with the hamate or ulnar styloid process or to avulsion by the dorsal radiotriquetral ligaments (Fig. 57–46). Isolated fractures of the lunate constitute 2% to 7% of all carpal fractures.

Hamate fractures account for 2% to 4% of all carpal fractures and may involve any portion of the bone. Fractures of the hook of the hamate deserve emphasis. These injuries may result from a fall on a dorsiflexed wrist, with force transmitted through the transverse carpal and pisohamate ligaments, or from a direct force, such as occurs in athletes who use rackets, bats, or clubs. Accurate clinical and radiographic diagnosis is difficult, and specialized radiographic projections and techniques, particularly conventional tomography or CT, may be required. Complications of fractures of the hook of the hamate include nonunion, osteonecrosis, injuries to the ulnar or median nerve, and tendon rupture (Fig. 57–47).

## Hand

### Metacarpophalangeal and Interphalangeal Joint Dislocation

Dislocation of a metacarpophalangeal joint (excluding the thumb) occurs considerably less frequently than dislocation of a proximal interphalangeal joint of a finger, and it results from a fall on an outstretched hand that forces the joint into hyperextension. The index finger is most commonly involved. In cases of complex dislocation, radiographs may reveal a widened joint space, indicative of interposition of the volar plate within the joint. An adja-

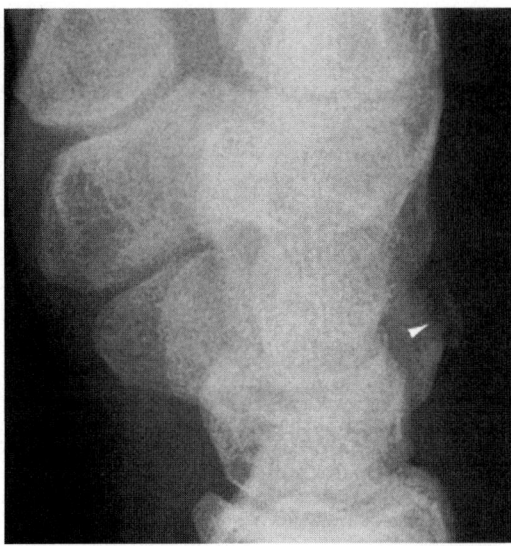

**Figure 57–46.** Carpal fracture: dorsal surface of the triquetrum (*arrowhead*).

cent sesamoid can also become displaced into the joint space.

Dislocations of the proximal interphalangeal joints are very common and may occur with or without a major adjacent phalangeal fracture. These dislocations can occur in a posterior or, more rarely, anterior direction (Fig. 57–48). Posterior dislocation results from a hyperextension injury, and ligamentous and volar plate disruption is a frequent associated finding.

Bennett's fracture-dislocation is a relatively common intra-articular injury that occurs at the base of the first metacarpal. The base of the metacarpal is pulled dorsally and radially. A second intra-articular fracture, Rolando's fracture, results in a Y- or T-shaped comminuted fracture line (Fig. 57–49).

Dislocations and collateral ligament injuries of the first metacarpophalangeal joint are important complications of trauma. Gamekeeper's thumb, related to a sudden valgus stress applied to the metacarpophalangeal joint of the thumb, has received the most attention. Initially described as an occupational hazard in English game wardens, the injury is now recognized to occur in various settings, including skiing. Attenuation or disruption of the ligamentous apparatus along the ulnar aspect of the thumb is seen. Initial radiographs may be negative, although small avulsed fragments from the base of the proximal phalanx can be delineated in some instances (Fig. 57–50). An abnormal folded position of the ulnar collateral ligament, called the Stener lesion, can be identified by MR imaging.

### Fracture of the Metacarpal Bones and Phalanges

Fractures of the metacarpal bones, which predominate in the first and fifth digits, are generally classified according to anatomic location: metacarpal head, metacarpal neck, metacarpal shaft, and metacarpal base. Typical locations of fractures include the shaft and neck of the fifth metacarpal (boxer's fracture); the shaft of the third or

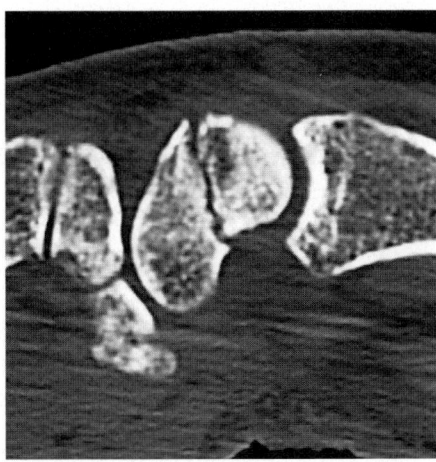

**Figure 57–45.** Carpal scaphoid fracture: nonunion and osteonecrosis. Direct sagittal CT scan shows a fracture gap, with increased density of the proximal portion of the scaphoid bone.

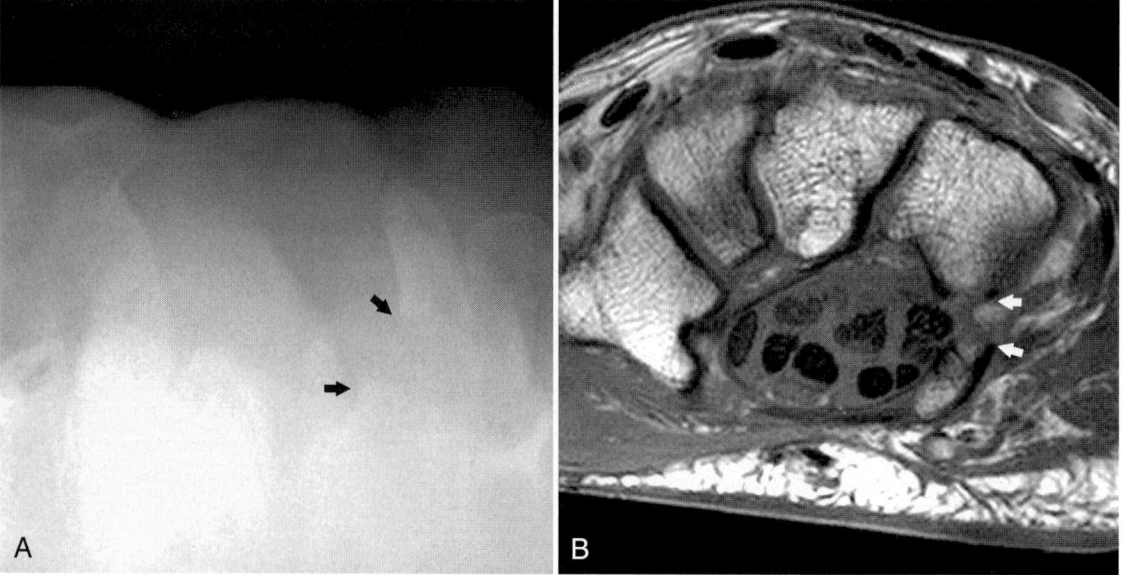

**Figure 57–47.**  Carpal fracture: hamate. *A,* Carpal tunnel view shows occult fracture of the hook of the hamate. Arrows identify the radial aspect of the base and a displaced fragment. *B,* Axial T1-weighted (TR/TE, 564/16) spin echo MR image shows the flexor tendon of the little finger entrapped between fracture fragments (arrows mark the ulnar aspect of the hamate hook base and the displaced fragment).

fourth metacarpal, or both; and the articular surface of the second metacarpal (Fig. 57–51).

Phalangeal fractures are more frequent than metacarpal fractures and typically involve the distal phalanges,

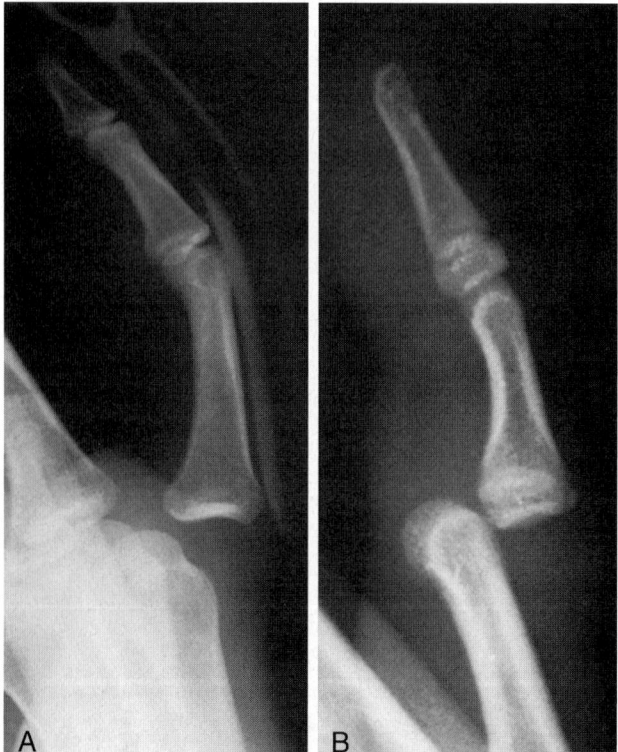

**Figure 57–48.**  Metacarpophalangeal and interphalangeal joint dislocation. *A,* Dorsal dislocation of the second metacarpophalangeal joint. *B,* Dorsal dislocation of the fifth proximal interphalangeal joint with a small dorsal phalangeal fracture.

followed in order of frequency by the proximal phalanges and the middle phalanges. Important varieties include a mallet fracture (in which an avulsion injury at the base of the dorsal surface of the terminal phalanx is produced by damage to the extensor mechanism); a volar plate fracture (in which dorsal dislocation of a proximal interphalangeal joint may be associated with an avulsion fracture in the middle phalanx at the site of attachment of the volar plate); a central slip attachment fracture (in which an intra-articular fracture of the dorsal part of the middle phalanx at the proximal interphalangeal joint accompanies palmar dislocation of this articulation); and, in an immature skeleton, physeal separation at the base of the distal phalanx (the nail-bed injury, in which an open skin surface leads to secondary infection) (Fig. 57–52).

## LOWER EXTREMITY

### Hip

#### Hip Dislocation

Dislocation of the femoral head with or without an acetabular fracture usually follows considerable trauma and represents approximately 5% of all dislocations. Hip dislocations are generally classified as anterior, posterior, or central.

Anterior dislocation of the hip represents 5% to 10% of all hip dislocations, and it is caused by forced abduction and external rotation of the leg. On radiographs, the abnormal position of the femoral head is readily apparent; on frontal radiographs, an anteriorly displaced femoral head typically moves inferomedially (i.e., obturator dislocation) with the femur abducted and externally rotated, and a posteriorly displaced femoral head is usually located superolaterally with the femur adducted and internally rotated. In anterior hip dislocations, associated fractures

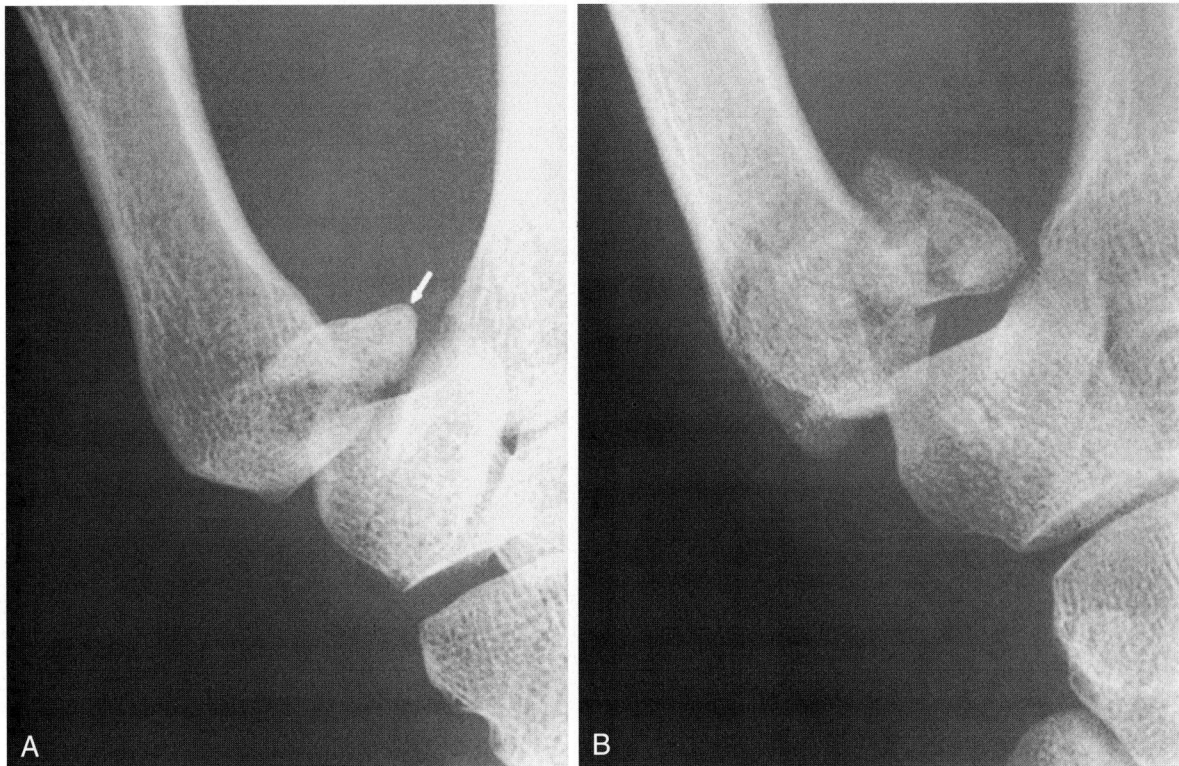

**Figure 57–49.** Fracture and dislocation of the base of the first metacarpal bone. *A*, Bennett's fracture-dislocation. Observe the typical oblique fracture of the volar lip of the first metacarpal bone *(arrow)*. *B*, Rolando's fracture. A comminuted fracture of the metacarpal base is evident.

of the acetabular rim, greater trochanter, femoral neck, or femoral head may be observed (Fig. 57–53).

Posterior dislocation of the hip represents approximately 80% to 85% of all hip dislocations and may result from a "dashboard injury," in which the flexed knee strikes the dashboard during a head-on automobile collision. The leg is shortened, internally rotated, and adducted. A persistently widened hip joint may indicate abnormally placed fragments or significant acetabular injury. CT can be used to identify small osseous fragments (Fig. 57–54).

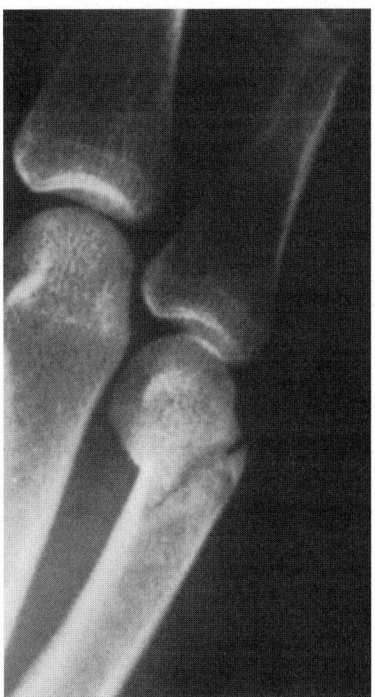

**Figure 57–51.** Metacarpal fracture: neck of the fifth metacarpal.

**Figure 57–50.** Gamekeeper's thumb. Note the slight displacement of a small fragment *(open arrow)* arising from the ulnar aspect of the proximal phalanx of the thumb.

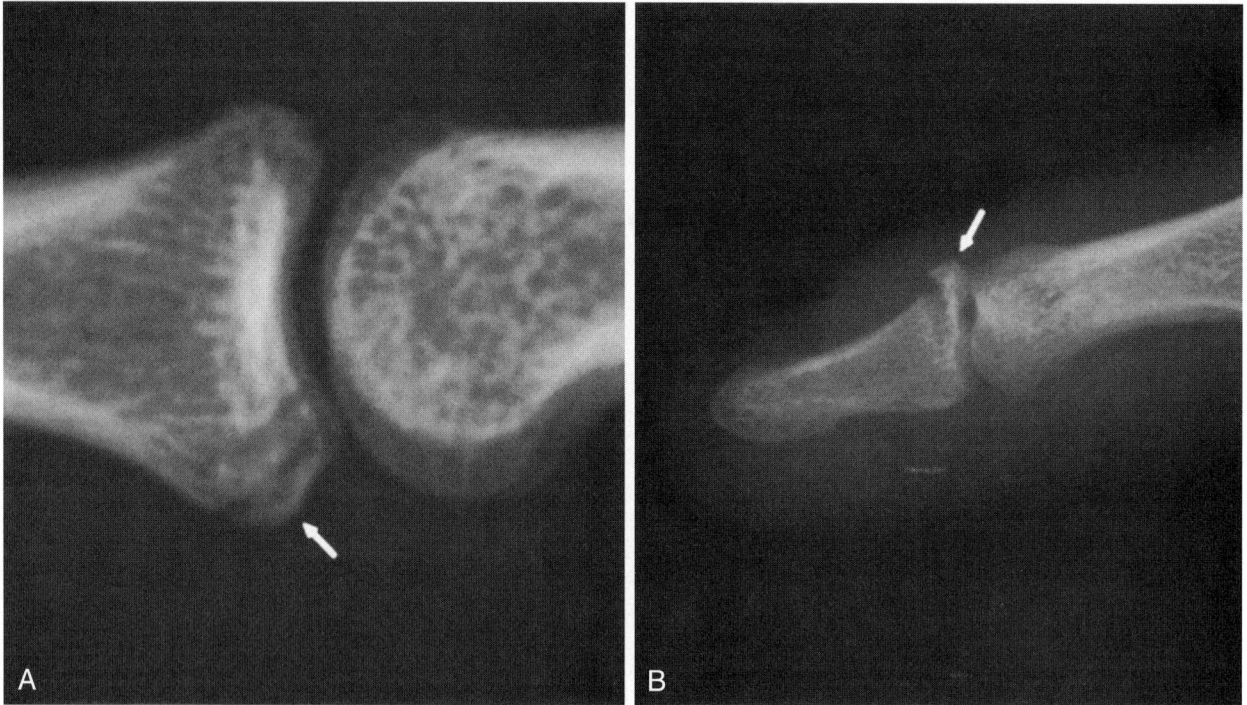

**Figure 57–52.** Phalangeal fracture. *A* and *B,* Avulsion fractures. Small avulsion fractures *(arrows)* near the proximal interphalangeal or distal interphalangeal joint can result from traction on the volar plate *(A)* or extensor tendons *(B).* Dislocations may also be evident.

Central acetabular fracture-dislocation usually results from a force applied to the lateral side of the trochanter and pelvis, with the stress applied through the femoral head. Various patterns of acetabular fracture complicate this injury, and hemorrhage into the pelvis may be observed. Secondary degenerative joint disease is not infrequent. In general, CT scanning is the preferred imaging method (Fig. 57–55).

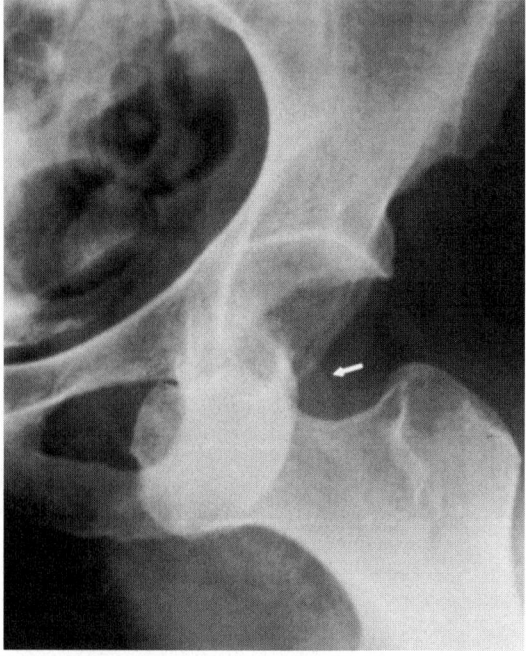

**Figure 57–53.** Hip dislocation: anterior dislocation. Radiograph reveals an inferomedial position of the femoral head and a fracture fragment of the lateral portion of the head *(arrow).*

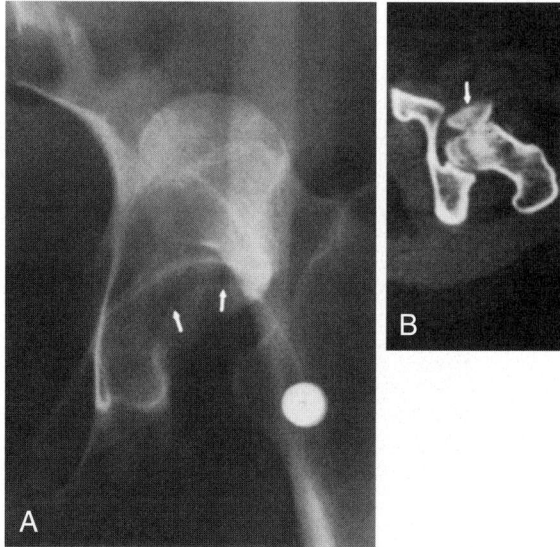

**Figure 57–54.** Hip dislocation: posterior dislocation. *A,* Radiograph shows posterosuperior displacement of the femoral head and a curvilinear bone fragment *(arrows)* in the joint. *B,* Transaxial CT scan reveals the fragment *(arrow),* which represents a portion of the femoral head. This fragment has rotated approximately 180 degrees.

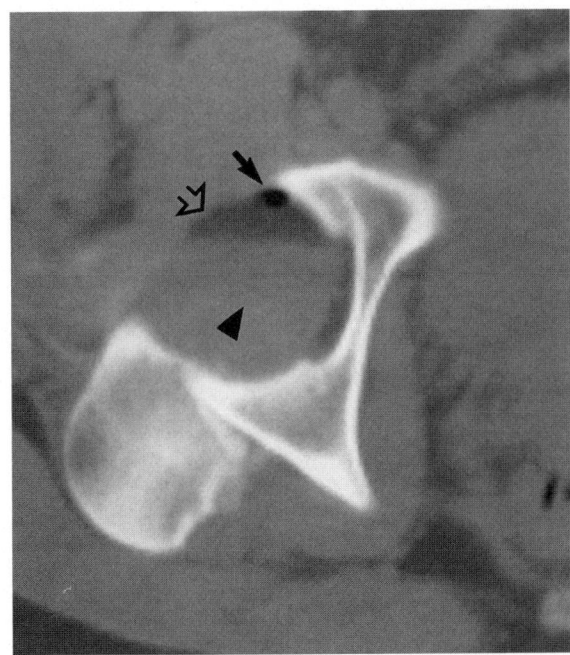

**Figure 57–55.** Hip dislocation. In association with posterior dislocation of the hip, a transverse CT scan shows gas *(solid arrow)*, fat *(open arrow)*, and a fluid level *(arrowhead)* between the serum above and the cellular components of blood below.

## Fracture of the Proximal Portion of the Femur

Fractures of the proximal portion of the femur in elderly persons with osteopenia, particularly women with osteoporosis, have received great attention. In this situation, the injuries are similar to insufficiency stress fractures, although a history of minor trauma is usually evident. Nondisplaced fractures of the proximal portion of the femur may escape detection on initial routine radiographic examination. Diagnostic help is provided by MR imaging (Fig. 57–56).

No classification system for fractures of the proximal femur is uniformly accepted. Anatomic designations, including subcapital, transcervical, basicervical, intertrochanteric, and subtrochanteric, are frequently used to define the location of the fracture and can be modified to include intracapsular fractures (those in the subcapital and transcervical regions) and extracapsular fractures (those in the basicervical and trochanteric regions). Subcapital fractures occur immediately beneath the articular surface of the femoral head, transcervical fractures pass across the middle of the femoral neck, basicervical fractures occur at the base of the femoral neck, intertrochanteric fractures are located in a line between the greater and lesser trochanters, and subtrochanteric fractures occur subjacent to this position.

Intracapsular fractures are approximately twice as frequent as those in the trochanteric region. Classification of intracapsular fractures according to the degree of displacement on prereduction radiographs is commonly referred to as the Garden system. Four types of fractures are identified: type I, incomplete or impacted; type II, complete without osseous displacement; type III, complete but with partial displacement of fracture fragments; and type IV, complete with total displacement of fracture fragments (Fig. 57–57). Type III and IV fractures are associated with significant complications and technical failure.

Under normal circumstances, femoral neck fractures reveal evidence of healing in the first 6 to 12 months. Complications are not uncommon, and nonunion occurs in approximately 5% to 25% of cases; ischemic necrosis of the femoral head occurs in 10% to 30% of cases. MR imaging and bone scintigraphy have been used not only for the initial diagnosis of the fracture but also as a means of detecting osteonecrosis and other complications.

Intertrochanteric fractures predominate in elderly patients, with a somewhat higher frequency in women (unlike the overwhelming female predilection observed in intracapsular femoral neck fractures). Fracture comminution is common and leads to multiple fragments of bone, which may include the greater trochanter, lesser trochanter, or both (Fig. 57–58). Radiographic analysis is complicated by this comminution, as well as by the

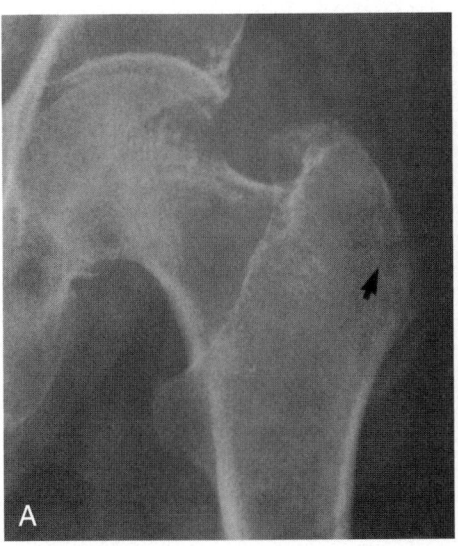
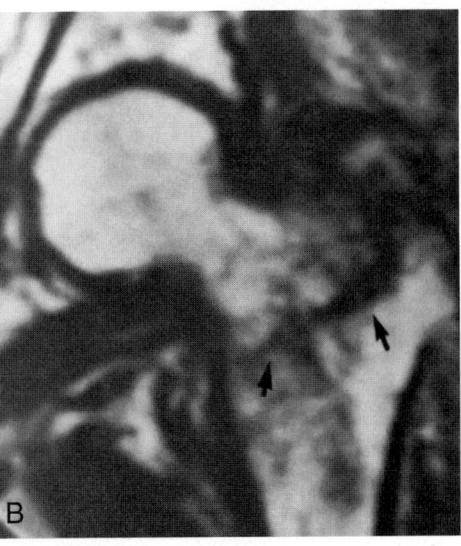

**Figure 57–56.** Fracture of the femoral neck: intertrochanteric fracture. *A* and *B*, Although a subtle fracture is evident on the initial radiograph *(arrow, A)*, it is identified more optimally on a coronal T1-weighted (TR/TE, 600/20) spin echo MR image *(arrows, B)*.

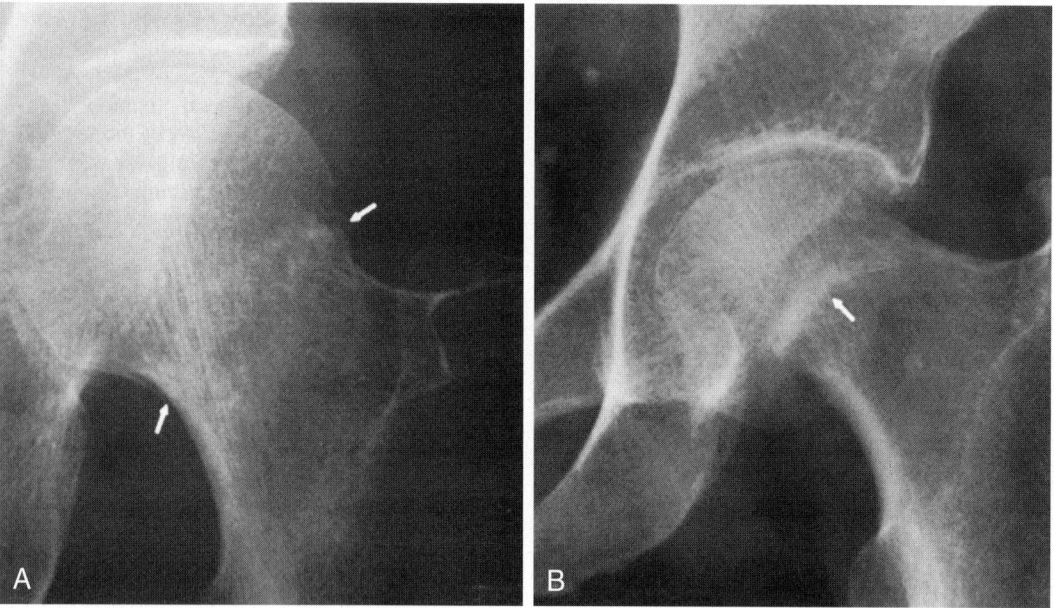

**Figure 57–57.** Fracture of the femoral neck: intracapsular fracture. *A* and *B*, Observe the bands of increased radiodensity in each case *(arrows)*. According to the Garden classification system, these injuries represent a type II fracture *(A)* and a type III fracture *(B)*, but accurate classification requires analysis of lateral radiographs as well. With regard to anatomic location, these fractures are predominantly subcapital.

typical displacement and rotation that occur. No uniform classification system exists for intertrochanteric fractures. MR imaging is a sensitive and specific method for the diagnosis of intertrochanteric fractures. Incomplete rather than complete fractures are seen in some cases and appear to be associated with a better prognosis (Fig. 57–59).

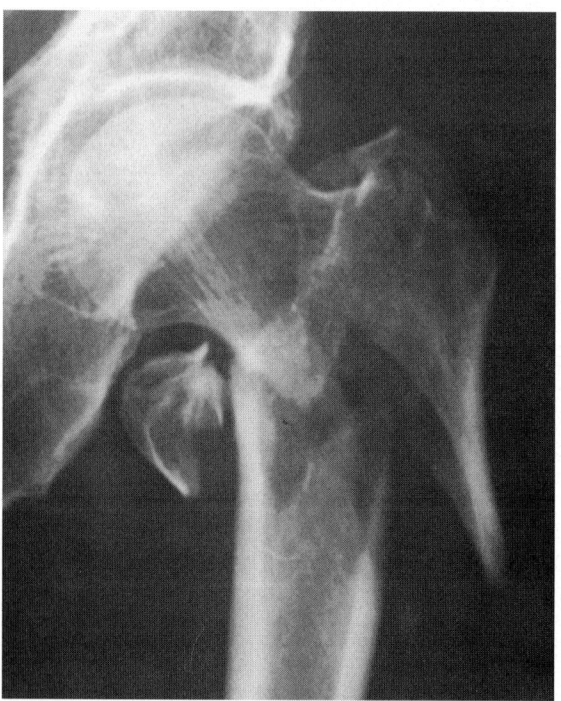

**Figure 57–58.** Fracture of the femoral neck: intertrochanteric fracture. A comminuted fracture is evident, with displacement of both trochanters.

In adults, isolated fractures of the greater trochanter are infrequent and are generally related to injury from a fall, particularly in elderly persons. Differentiation of a fracture of the greater trochanter from one that also involves the proximal portion of the femur may require advanced imaging techniques. Greater trochanter fractures are not usually significantly displaced, and their detection may be difficult. Fractures of the femur that commence immediately below the trochanter are considered subtrochanteric in location. Approximately 5% to 30% of fractures of the proximal portion of the femur occur in the subtrochanteric region. These fractures occur in older patients with relatively minor injuries and in younger patients with major trauma. Pathologic fractures also occur in this region of the femur and are typical of Paget's disease.

### Fracture of the Acetabulum

Although the radiographic examination is an important step in the initial evaluation of acetabular fractures, CT plays an important and expanding role. With any imaging system, delineation of four bony landmarks—anterior acetabular rim, posterior acetabular rim, iliopubic (anterior) column, and ilioischial (posterior) column—remains fundamental to a proper assessment of the extent of injury. With CT, additional features can be readily determined, including the integrity of the acetabular dome and quadrilateral surface, as well as the presence of intra-articular osseous fragments and associated fractures of the bony pelvis (Fig. 57–60).

Acetabular fractures result from the impact of the femoral head against the central regions of the acetabulum or its rims, especially the posterior rim in association with posterior dislocation of the hip. Isolated fractures of

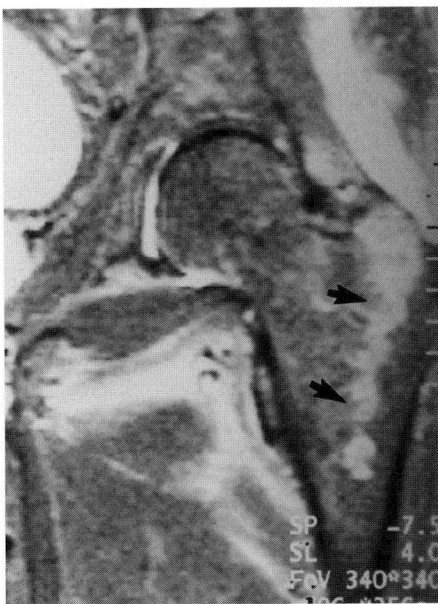

**Figure 57–59.** Fracture of the femoral neck: intertrochanteric fracture. A coronal short tau inversion recovery (STIR; TR/TE, 4000/30; inversion time, 140 msec) MR image shows an incomplete fracture *(arrows)* that extends downward and medially from the greater trochanter. Note the intramuscular and soft tissue bleeding superiorly and medially.

the anterior or superior portion of the acetabular rim are unusual. Fractures may involve the anterior or posterior column alone, or a transverse fracture may involve both columns. The designation *elementary fractures* has been used to describe injuries to one structural component of the acetabulum or its supporting structures; such fractures involve the posterior wall, are transverse, involve the anterior or posterior column, or affect the anterior wall, in decreasing order of frequency. A second designation, *associated fractures*, refers to various combinations of elementary fractures, including fractures of the posterior wall combined with transverse fractures, fractures of both columns, T-shaped fractures, and other fracture patterns, again in decreasing order of frequency. Complications of acetabular fractures include osteoarthritis of the hip, ischemic necrosis of the femoral head, heterotopic ossification, and hemorrhage, as well as urinary tract, bowel, and peripheral nerve injury.

### Femoral Diaphysis

Because the femoral shaft is the strongest portion of the longest and most resilient bone in the human body, fracture requires violent force. Strong muscle attachments to the greater and lesser trochanters lead to abduction, flexion, and external rotation of the proximal femoral fragment, and insertion of the adductor muscles on the medial portion of the distal femoral fragment leads to its medial angulation. All these factors contribute to the varus deformity that typifies fractures involving the middle segment of the femoral diaphysis.

Femoral shaft fractures can be classified in a number of ways, including on the basis of whether they are open

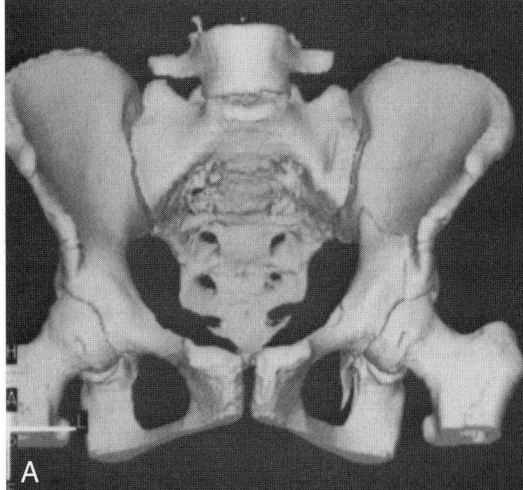

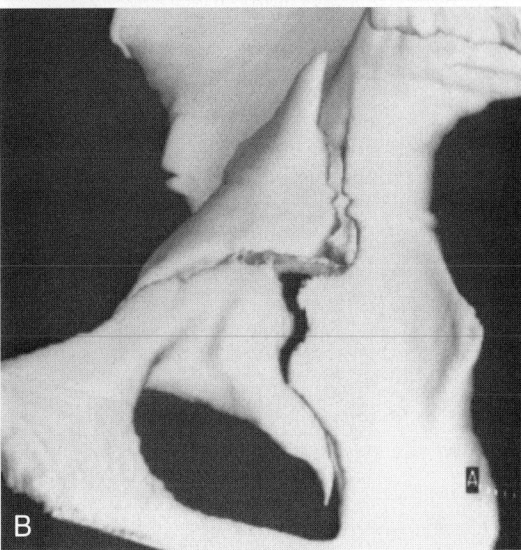

**Figure 57–60.** Acetabular fracture. Three-dimensional images derived from transaxial CT data show, in vivid fashion, a comminuted fracture of the acetabulum, with involvement primarily of the iliopubic column.

or closed, fracture morphology, or what portion of the shaft is involved (Table 57–6). Femoral shaft fractures may be classified as simple (with transverse, oblique, or spiral components), segmental, or comminuted. Although transverse or oblique fractures of the femoral diaphysis are very common, comminuted fractures with one or more butterfly fragments are also encountered regularly. Occult injuries of the knee occur in 5% to 15% of femoral shaft fractures and, in adolescents, may include physeal injuries in the distal end of the femur. Complications of femoral shaft fractures include arterial injuries, malunion, refracture, and fat embolization.

### Knee

#### Fracture of the Distal Portion of the Femur

These fractures can be classified as supracondylar, intercondylar, or condylar. Most of these injuries result from axial loading combined with varus or valgus stress and

**TABLE 57-6**

**Fractures of the Femoral Shaft**

| Site | Characteristics | Complications |
| --- | --- | --- |
| Any level | Major violence with associated injuries to the femur, tibia, patella, acetabulum, hip, and knee<br>Open or closed<br>Spiral, oblique, or transverse fracture with a possible butterfly fragment and comminution | Refracture<br>Peroneal nerve injury from skeletal traction<br>Vascular injury (femoral artery)<br>Thrombophlebitis<br>Nonunion (1% of cases), malunion, or delayed union<br>Infection<br>Fat embolization (approximately 10% of cases) |
| Proximal | Associated with osteoporosis and Paget's disease<br>Less common than midshaft fractures<br>Commonly extend into the subtrochanteric region | Malalignment<br>Nonunion |
| Middle | Most common site<br>Transverse fracture is most typical | |
| Distal and supracondylar | Less common than midshaft fractures | Malalignment<br>Arterial injury |

rotation. Supracondylar fractures (without intra-articular extension) are commonly transverse or slightly oblique in configuration, with varying degrees of displacement and comminution of the fracture fragments. Supracondylar fractures may be accompanied by a vertical fracture line extending into the knee that leads to intercondylar fractures. In condylar fractures, sagittal or coronal fracture lines are isolated to the region of a single condyle (Fig. 57–61).

### Fracture of the Patella

These fractures result from direct or indirect forces, the latter related to contraction of the quadriceps muscles. Transverse fractures are typical and account for approximately 50% to 80% of all patellar fractures, and they are generally the product of indirect force (Fig. 57–62). Longitudinal (25%) and stellate or comminuted (20% to 35%) fractures are less frequent and usually result from direct injury.

Fracture should be differentiated from bipartite patella, in which separate ossification centers develop in the superolateral aspect of the bone. Fragmentation and separation of the lower pole of the patella, referred to as Sinding-Larsen-Johansson disease, are stress-related phenomena that may also mimic a fracture.

### Fracture of the Proximal Portion of the Tibia

These fractures may be extra-articular or intra-articular. Oblique and horizontal beam projections and CT or MR imaging are frequently required for the accurate assessment and diagnosis of occult fractures. Tibial plateau fractures predominate in middle-aged and elderly persons when the relatively stronger condylar portion of the femur impacts against the plateau. Valgus stress is far more common than varus stress, such that isolated lateral plateau fractures (75% to 80% of all fractures of the tibial plateau) and combined lateral and medial plateau fractures (10% to 15%) are more frequent than isolated medial

plateau fractures (5% to 10%). Important imaging considerations related to tibial fractures include the detection of lipohemarthrosis, avulsion fractures and sites of ligamentous detachment (femoral condyle, fibular head, intercondylar eminence), meniscal injuries, abnormal widening of the joint space during the application of stress, and disruption of the articular surface (Fig. 57–63).

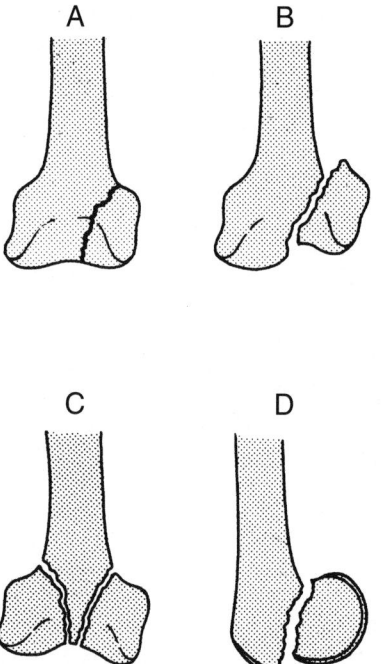

**Figure 57–61.** Fracture of the distal portion of the femur: classification of condylar fractures. Such fractures may be undisplaced (*A*) or displaced (*B* to *D*), involve one (*A* and *B*) or both (*C* and *D*) condyles, and be oriented principally in the sagittal (*A* to *C*) or coronal (*D*) plane. (From Hohl M, Larson RL, Jones DC: Fractures and dislocations of the knee. In Rockwood CA Jr, Green DP [eds]: Fractures in Adults, 2nd ed. Philadelphia, JB Lippincott, 1984, p 1444.)

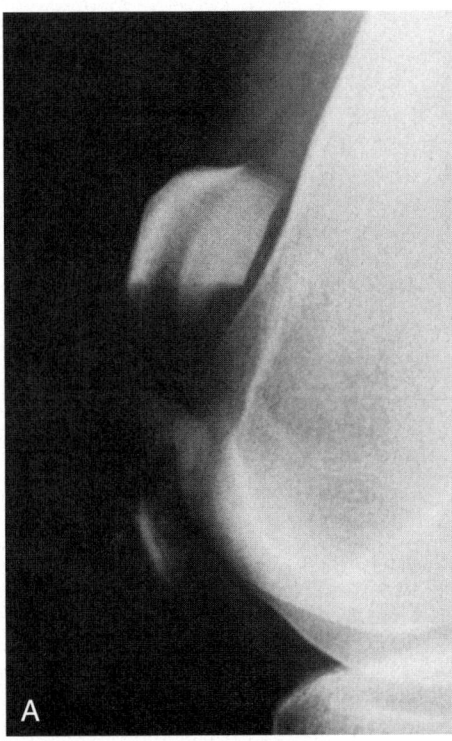

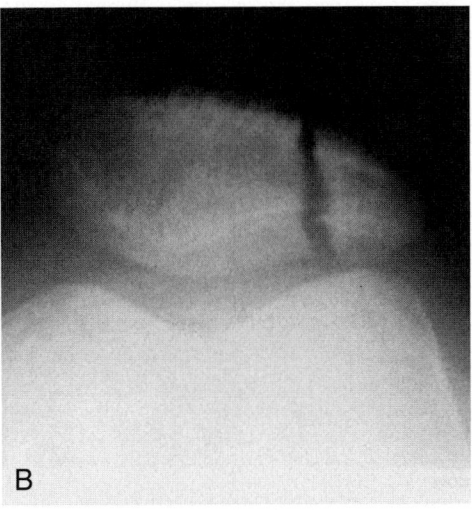

**Figure 57–62.** Patellar fracture. *A,* Transverse patellar fracture with comminution and displacement on a lateral radiograph. *B,* Longitudinal patellar fracture. The lateral radiograph reveals an effusion, but an axial or tangential projection is required for accurate diagnosis.

Fractures of the tibial spine or intercondylar eminence are indicative of possible damage to the cruciate ligaments of the knee. Varying degrees of osseous displacement are seen. Either the anterior tibial spine or, less commonly, the posterior tibial spine is affected; rarely, both are involved. Avulsion injuries of the anterior tibial spine occur more commonly in children and adolescents than in adults. Such fractures in adults are typically accompanied by ligamentous and meniscal injury, whereas in children they may be an isolated phenomenon. Routine radiography supplemented with tunnel projections, radiographs obtained during the application of stress, arthrography, and MR imaging are important in the assessment of these injuries (Fig. 57–64).

An avulsion fracture at the site of insertion of the lateral capsular ligament, termed a Segond fracture, occurs with the knee in flexion because of internal rotation of the tibia. Disruption of the anterior cruciate ligament occurs in 75% to almost 100% of patients with a Segond fracture; medial ligamentous damage may also be present, and anterolateral rotatory instability of the knee is evident on clinical examination (Fig. 57–65).

### Fracture of the Proximal Portion of the Fibula

Fibular head or neck fractures can result from a direct blow, a varus force (in which an avulsion fracture of the proximal pole or styloid process of the fibula occurs), a valgus force (which is accompanied by a fracture of the lateral tibial plateau and injury to the medial collateral ligament), and a twisting force at the ankle (in which pronation and external rotation may lead to a fracture in the fibular neck). The combination of adduction stress on the knee, rupture of the lateral capsular and ligamentous structures, peroneal nerve injury, and, possibly, avulsion fracture of the fibula is termed the ligamentous peroneal nerve syndrome.

### Knee Dislocation

Knee dislocation is a rare but serious injury because of the neurovascular insult that may result from popliteal artery and peroneal nerve damage. Anterior, posterior,

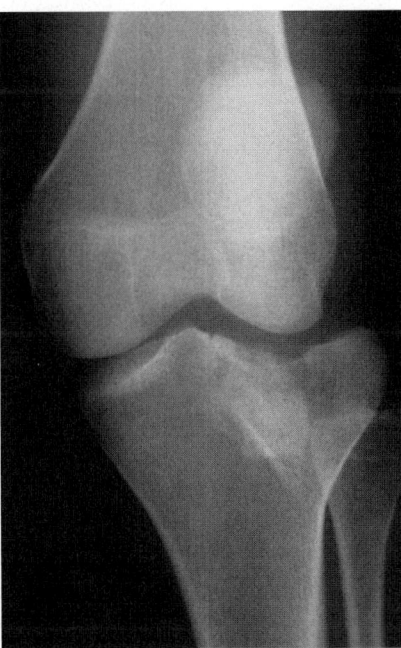

**Figure 57–63.** Fracture of the proximal portion of the tibia: lateral plateau fracture. Valgus stress has led to a markedly displaced fracture, as shown on a frontal radiograph.

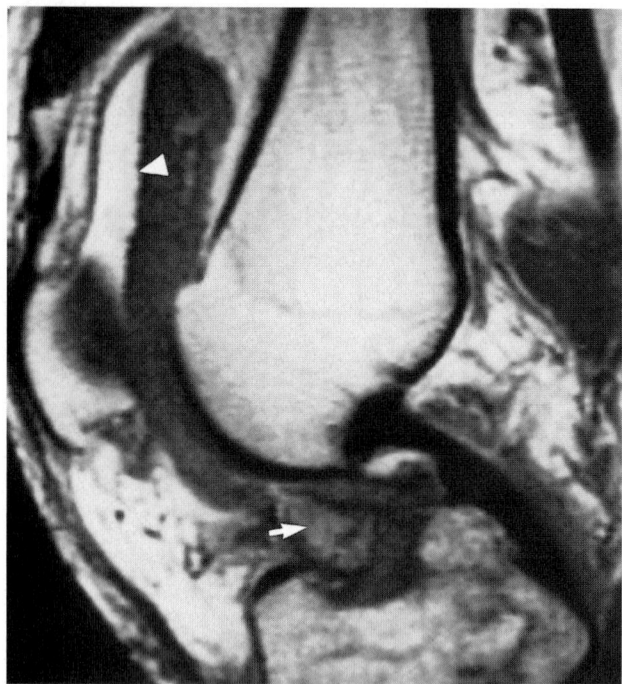

**Figure 57–64.** Fracture of the proximal portion of the tibia: intercondylar eminence fracture. Sagittal T1-weighted (TR/TE, 886/15) spin echo MR image reveals an avulsion fracture *(arrow)* of the proximal portion of the tibia and a lipohemarthrosis *(arrowhead)*. In this image, the anterior cruciate ligament cannot be evaluated.

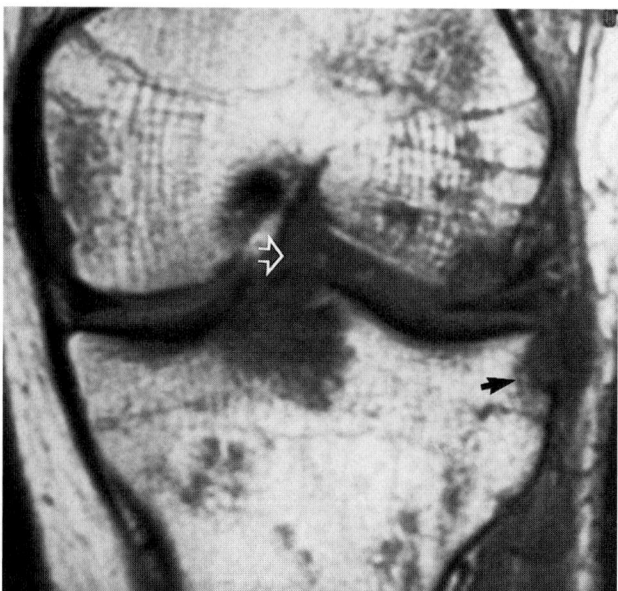

**Figure 57–65.** Fracture of the proximal portion of the tibia: Segond fracture. Coronal T1-weighted (TR/TE, 800/16) spin echo MR image shows a marginal defect *(solid arrow)* in the lateral margin of the tibia—the Segond fracture—and disruption of the anterior cruciate ligament *(open arrow)*. An osteochondral fracture of the lateral femoral condyle and bone bruises are also evident.

lateral, medial, and rotatory types of dislocation are recognized. Anterior dislocation is the most common type (30% to 50% of all knee dislocations) and apparently results from hyperextension of the knee with tearing of the posterior capsule and posterior cruciate ligament. Posterior dislocations are next in frequency. As a general rule, detection of disruption of four major ligaments of the knee (cruciate ligaments and collateral ligaments) implies that dislocation of the joint has occurred. The presence of injuries to both cruciate ligaments also suggests that such a dislocation has occurred (Fig. 57–66), even when the knee is not dislocated at the time of clinical assessment.

Radiographic diagnosis is not difficult in most knee dislocations. Arteriography or MR angiography should be used to delineate the status of the popliteal artery injury that occurs in 25% to 50% of knee dislocations. Nerve injury occurs in approximately 25% of knee dislocations.

### Patellar Dislocation

Traumatic dislocation of the patella can be produced by a direct blow or an exaggerated contraction of the quadriceps mechanism. Abnormalities predisposing to displacement may include an abnormally high patella (patella

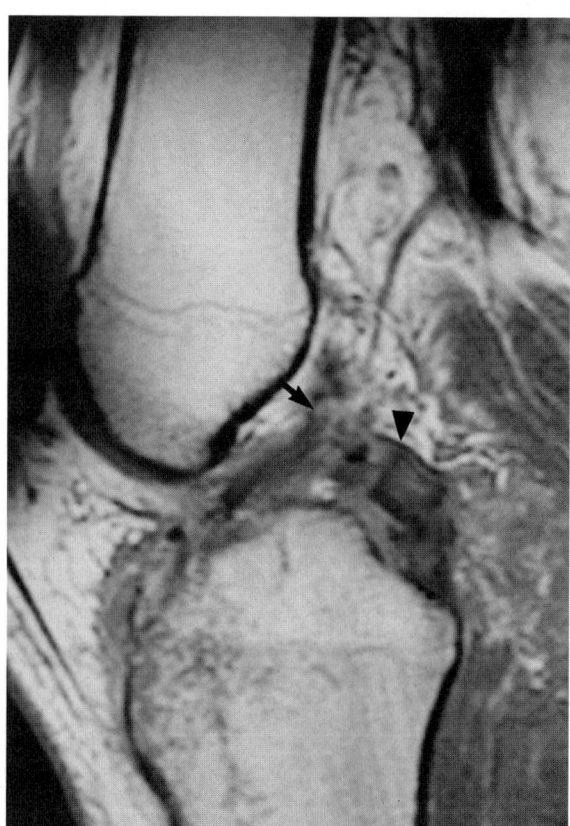

**Figure 57–66.** Knee dislocation. Sagittal T1-weighted (TR/TE, 600/14) spin echo MR image in a patient with a recent knee dislocation shows disruption of both the anterior *(arrow)* and posterior *(arrowhead)* cruciate ligaments. A fracture of the anterior aspect of the tibia is also present. An artifact obscures visualization of the patella. (Courtesy of Naval Hospital, San Diego, Calif.)

alta), deficient height of the lateral femoral condyle, shallowness of the patellofemoral groove, genu valgum or recurvatum, lateral insertion of the patellar tendon, muscle weakness, and excessive tibial torsion. Lateral dislocation, which may be transient, predominates; consequently, the patella may no longer be dislocated on initial radiographs. Identification of characteristic associated fractures therefore assumes diagnostic importance. In particular, osteochondral fractures of the medial patellar facet and lateral femoral condyle are common. Axial radiographs are most useful in detecting these fractures. The MR imaging features of patellar dislocation include hemarthrosis, intra-articular chondral or osteochondral bodies, osteochondral fractures or marrow edema of the medial aspect of the patella and the anterior aspect of the lateral femoral condyle, and disruption of the medial patellar retinaculum (Fig. 57–67).

## Proximal Tibiofibular Joint Dislocation

Though rare, proximal tibiofibular joint dislocation may be seen in parachuting, hang-gliding, skydiving, and horseback riding injuries. Anterior or, less frequently, posterior dislocation of the fibular head may be noted. Peroneal nerve injury may appear after posterior dislocation of this joint. As the fibular head is displaced anteriorly, it also moves laterally. In cases of posterior dislocation, the fibular head is displaced medially.

## Tibial and Fibular Diaphyses

Of all the long tubular bones, the tibia is fractured most commonly (Table 57–7). In general, the more severe the force, the more likely it is that both bones will fracture. Isolated fractures of the shaft of the fibula are uncommon and result from a direct blow. More typically, an apparently isolated fibular fracture is actually one component of a more complicated injury involving the ankle as well (see later discussion). Tibial and fibular fractures occurring together may appear at the same level, although it is common for them to occur at different levels. Additional injuries are not uncommon and may be clinically occult. Survey radiographs of the pelvis and ipsilateral femur may be appropriate when a severe injury of the tibia and fibula has occurred.

Tibial shaft fractures generally heal more quickly in children than in adults. The diagnosis of delayed union or nonunion of a tibial shaft fracture is made on the basis of both clinical and radiographic parameters. Additional complications of tibial (and fibular) shaft fractures include malunion, infection, neurovascular injury, and compartment syndromes. In children, distinctive fractures of the tibial shaft include a spiral fracture in the first 3 years of life, designated a toddler's fracture, and a fracture involving the proximal metaphysis of the bone. Fractures of the proximal metaphyseal region of the tibia may be associated with a subsequent valgus deformity at the fracture site.

## Ankle

### Fractures about the Ankle

Stability of the ankle joint depends on the integrity of a ring formed by the tibia, fibula, and talus, united by the surrounding ligaments (Fig. 57–68). A single break in the ring does not allow subluxation of the talus in the mortise, whereas two or more breaks in the ring, whether frac-

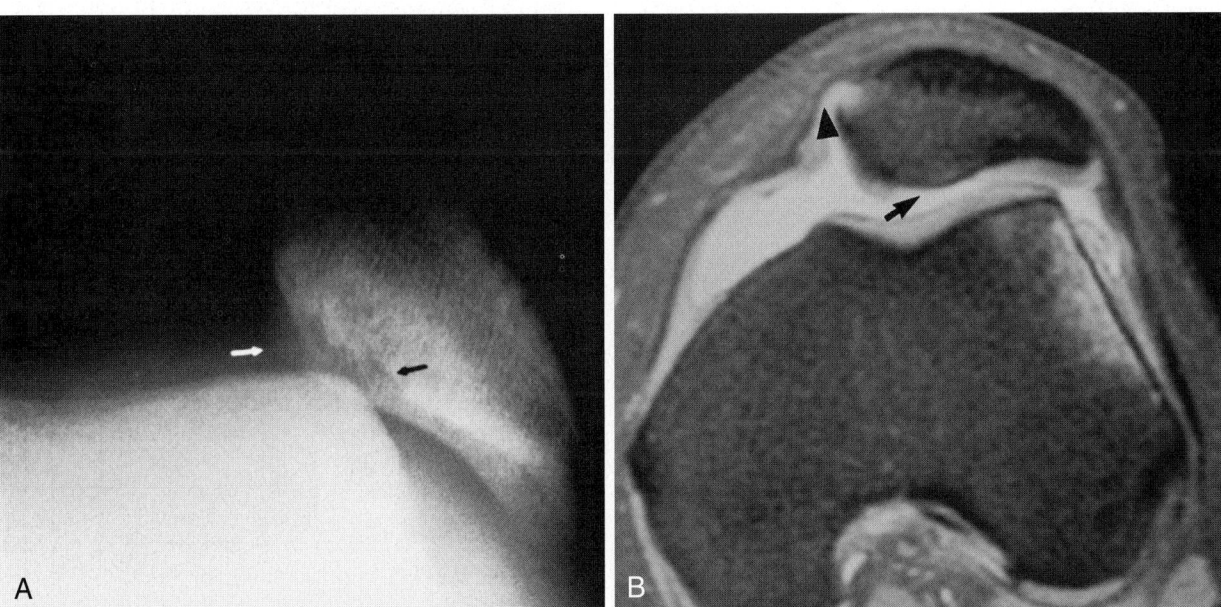

**Figure 57–67.** Patellar dislocation. *A*, Axial radiograph reveals lateral dislocation of the patella, with fragmentation and erosion of a portion of the patellar articular surface *(arrows)*. *B*, In a different patient, transverse fat-suppressed fast spin echo (TR/TE, 2000/19) MR image shows a joint effusion, marrow edema (representing a bone bruise) in the anterior aspect of the lateral femoral condyle, irregularity of the medial margin of the patella, partial disruption of the medial retinaculum *(arrowhead)*, and a chondral defect *(arrow)* in the patella.

**TABLE 57–7**

**Fractures of the Tibial and Fibular Shafts**

| Site | Characteristics | Complications |
|---|---|---|
| Tibia | Direct or indirect trauma | Delayed union (no osseous union at 20 wk) in 5–15% of cases |
| | Associated fractures of the fibula, especially in direct and severe trauma | Nonunion (no osseous union at 6 mo to 1 yr) is most common in the distal third of the tibia |
| | Transverse or comminuted fracture in direct trauma, oblique or spiral fracture in indirect trauma, sometimes segmental fractures | Infection with or without nonunion |
| | Middle and distal thirds > proximal third | Vascular injury (to the anterior tibial artery or, less commonly, the posterior tibial artery) |
| | Minor, moderate, or major categories of injury, the last associated with comminuted and open fractures | Compartment syndrome (anterior > posterior or lateral compartment) |
| | Prognosis related to the amount of displacement, degree of comminution, open or closed fracture, and infection | Nerve injury (uncommon, peroneal and posterior tibial nerves) |
| | Childhood fractures: | Refracture (especially in athletes) |
| |    Toddler fracture—spiral fracture, undisplaced | Leg shortening |
| |    Proximal metaphyseal fracture—associated with genu valgum deformity | Osteoarthritis (if fracture extends into the joint) |
| | | Reflex sympathetic dystrophy syndrome |
| Fibula | Isolated fractures are rare and related to direct injury | Related to those of the associated tibial or ankle injury |
| | Associated fractures of tibia and ankle injuries | |

tures or a fracture in combination with a ruptured ligament, allow abnormal talar motion. Displacement of the talus in the ankle joint may be evident on routine radiographs, including the mortise view (Fig. 57–69), although application of stress to the ankle during radiographic examination can be of considerable diagnostic help.

Ankle fractures are classified, according to the mechanism of injury, into five major fracture complexes. Within each group are stages of injury designated by Roman numerals; the higher the number, the greater the applied force and resultant damage. Each group is designated by two terms. The first term is either pronation or supination, which refers to the position of the foot at the time of injury. The foot is pronated when the forefoot is outwardly rotated and everted and the hindfoot is abducted. Supination represents inward rotation and inversion of the forefoot with adduction of the hindfoot. The second term reflects the direction in which the talus is displaced or rotated relative to the mortise formed by the distal regions of the tibia and fibula. Five directions of talar displacement are possible: external rotation (in which the talus is displaced externally, or laterally), internal rotation (in which the talus is displaced internally, or medially), abduction (in which the talus is displaced laterally without significant rotation), adduction (in which the talus

is displaced medially without significant rotation), and dorsiflexion (in which the talus is dorsiflexed on the tibia). Thus, with the foot in either pronation or supination, the talus may be subjected to one of these five vectors of force.

1. *Supination–external rotation (SER) injury* (stages I to IV). The SER category constitutes almost 60% of all ankle injuries (Fig. 57–70). The fracture complex is caused by external rotation of the supinated foot. External rotation of the foot forces the talus against the fibula, commonly rupturing the anterior tibiofibular ligament (stage I). As the mechanism of injury continues, a short oblique fracture of the distal portion of the fibula occurs (stage II). Stage III is a fracture of the posterior aspect of the tibia of varying size. Stage IV is characterized by fracture of the medial malleolus or rupture of the deltoid ligament (Fig. 57–71).

2. *Supination-adduction (SAD) injury* (stages I and II). The SAD category constitutes about 20% of all ankle injuries (Fig. 57–72). These injuries are produced by a medially directed force acting on a supinated foot. Supination causes tension on the lateral ligaments, and with adduction, either a lateral ligament rupture or a transverse fracture of the distal portion of the fibula occurs (stage I). The characteristic transverse fibular

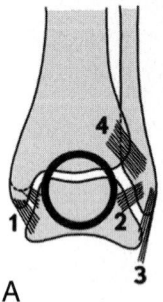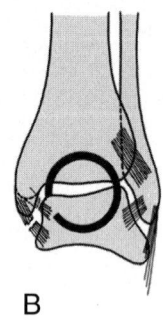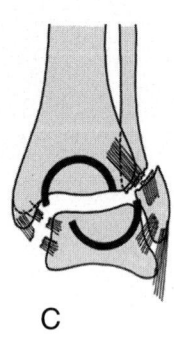

A    B    C

**Figure 57–68.** Ankle: stable and unstable characteristics. *A*, The stability of the ankle joint is determined by the status of a ring comprising the mortise and surrounding ligaments. The latter include the deep and superficial deltoid ligaments (1), the anterior (2) and posterior (not shown) talofibular ligaments, the calcaneofibular ligament (3), the anterior (4) and posterior (not shown) tibiofibular ligaments, the inferior transverse ligament (not shown), and the interosseous membrane and ligament (not shown). *B*, A single break in this ring does not allow displacement of the mortise. *C*, Two or more breaks in the ring allow displacement of the mortise.

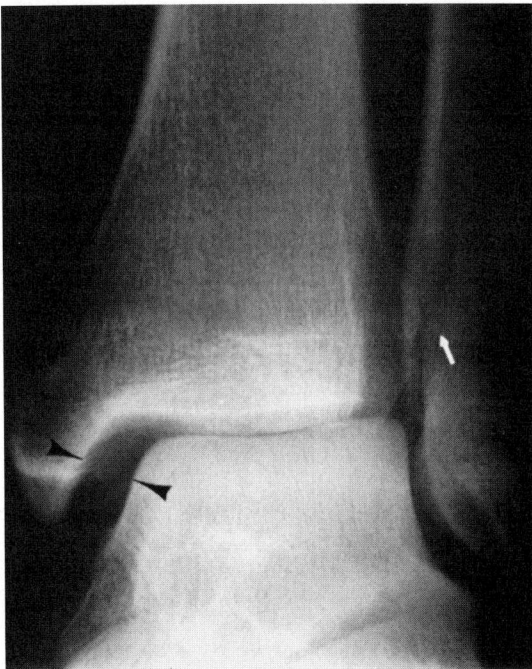

**Figure 57–69.** Ankle instability: routine radiography. Direct lateral displacement of the talus with respect to the tibia results in widening of the medial "clear" space *(arrowheads)*, indicative of rupture of the deep deltoid ligament. The superficial deltoid ligament may also be torn. A fibular fracture *(arrow)* is allowing the talus to move laterally.

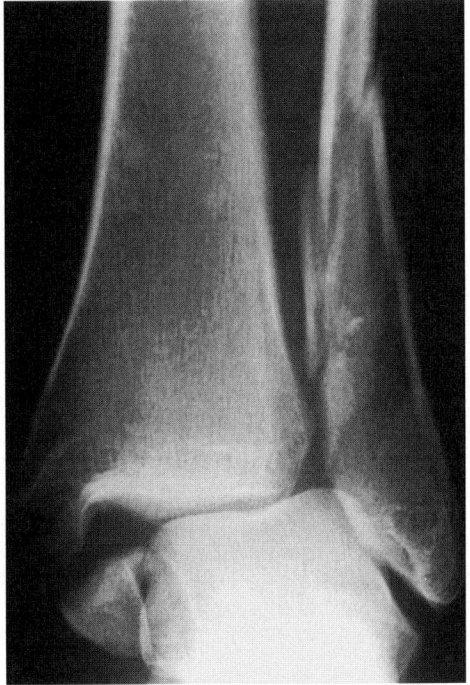

**Figure 57–71.** Ankle injuries: supination–external rotation injury, stage IV. Anteroposterior radiograph reveals an oblique fibular fracture and fracture of the medial malleolus.

fracture usually arises just distal to the tibiotalar articulation. Continued pressure from the medially directed talus results in fracture of the medial malleolus or rupture of the deltoid ligament (stage II). The malleolar fracture is often oblique or nearly vertical (Fig. 57–73).

3. *Pronation–external rotation (PER) injury* (stages I to IV). These injuries are described, along with pronation–abduction injuries, in the following paragraph.

4. *Pronation–abduction (PAB) injury* (stages I to III). PER (Fig. 57–74) and PAB (Fig. 57–75) injuries constitute about 20% of all injuries occurring about the ankle. The two groups are commonly considered together because PER stage I and II injuries and PAB stage I and II injuries cannot be distinguished radiographically. Forceful external rotation or abduction of the talus results in either deltoid ligament rupture (60%) or fracture of the medial malleolus (40%) (PER or PAB stage I). In a PER or PAB stage II lesion, rupture

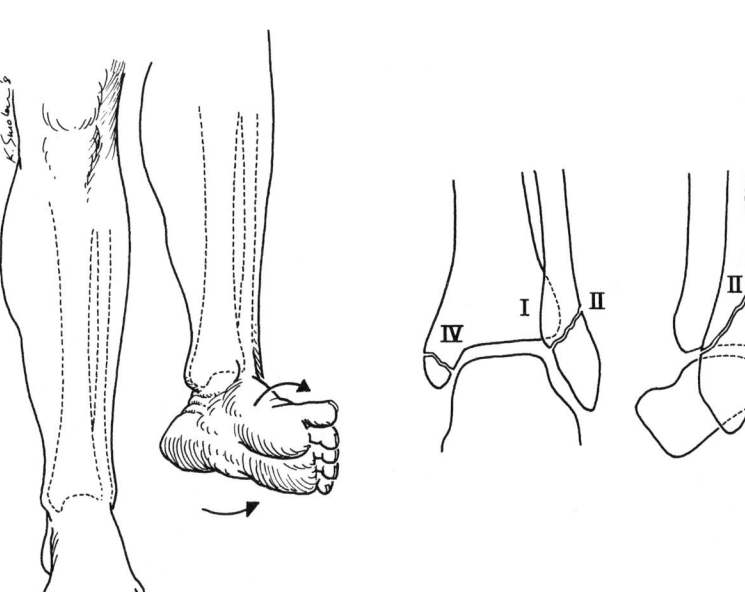

**Figure 57–70.** Ankle injuries: supination–external rotation injury. External rotation forces applied to a supinated foot initially result in rupture of the anterior tibiofibular ligament (stage I). As the forces continue, a short oblique fracture of the distal portion of the fibula occurs (stage II). Stage III involves a fracture of the posterior aspect of the tibia. Stage IV is a fracture of the medial malleolus.

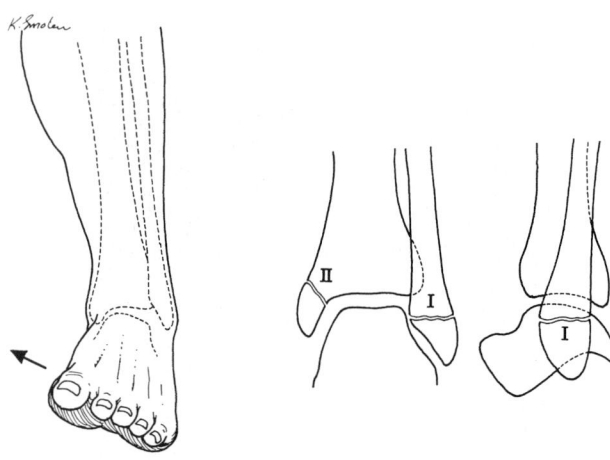

**Figure 57–72.** Ankle injuries: supination-adduction injury. Adduction forces applied to a supinated foot initially result in a traction or avulsion fracture of the distal portion of the fibula or rupture of the lateral ligaments (stage I). As forces continue, fracture of the medial malleolus or rupture of the deltoid ligament occurs (stage II). The fibular fracture is typically transverse, and that of the medial malleolus is oblique or nearly vertical.

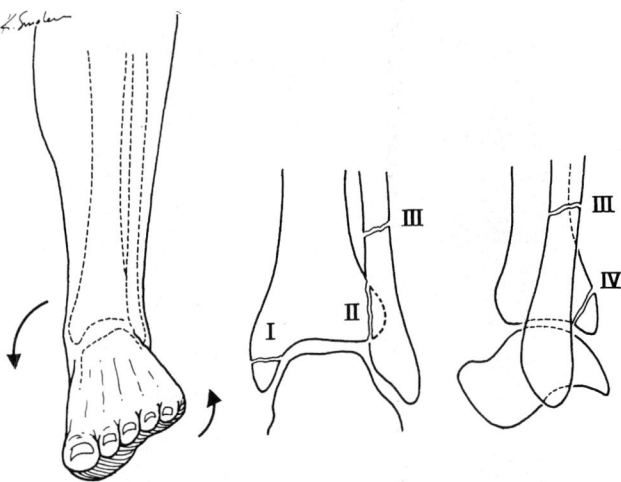

**Figure 57–74.** Ankle injuries: pronation–external rotation injury. Forces of external rotation applied to a pronated foot initially result in rupture of the deltoid ligament or fracture of the medial malleolus (stage I). As forces continue, the anterior tibiofibular ligament is ruptured (stage II). A high fibular fracture (stage III) and fracture of the posterior tibial margin (stage IV) are the final stages in this mechanism of injury.

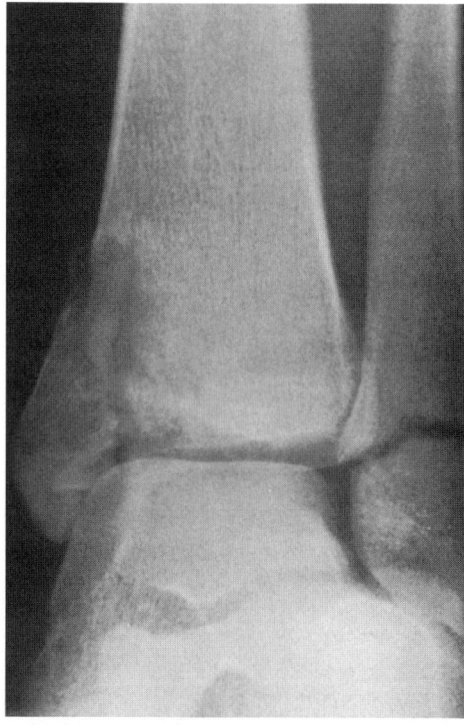

**Figure 57–73.** Ankle injuries: supination-adduction injury, stage II. Note the transversely oriented fibular fracture and the nearly vertical fracture of the medial malleolus.

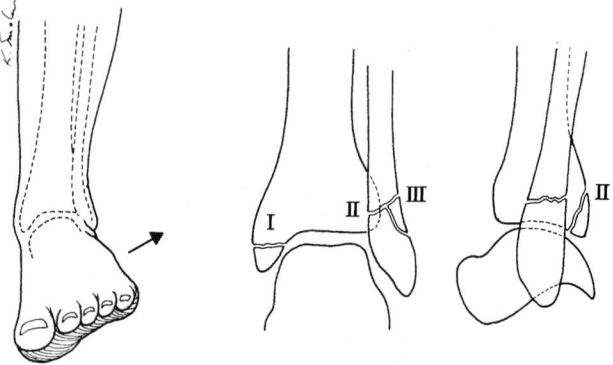

**Figure 57–75.** Ankle injuries: pronation-abduction injury. The first two stages of this injury are identical to those of the pronation–external rotation fracture complex. Stage III is a transverse supramalleolar fibular fracture that may be comminuted laterally.

of the distal tibiofibular syndesmosis also occurs. This latter injury may be purely ligamentous or may be an avulsion. PAB stage III injuries are stage I and II injuries combined with a transverse supramalleolar fibular fracture (Fig. 57–76). PER stage III injuries consist of stage I and II abnormalities plus a short spiral fracture of the fibula more than 2.5 cm above

the tibiotalar joint (Fig. 57–77). This fibular fracture is usually 6 to 8 cm above the ankle and may be even more proximal in location. PER stage IV injuries are stage III injuries in combination with a fracture of the posterior tibial margin.

A fibular fracture occurring above the joint line and proximal to the distal tibiofibular synostosis may be an important manifestation of an ankle injury. Dupuytren's fracture is one type that occurs in this position and involves the lower portion of the fibular shaft. When it results from a PER injury, the fracture extends from the anterior edge of the fibula in a posteroinferior direction; in a PAB injury, the fracture is oblique and extends from the lateral surface of the bone in an inferomedial direction; and in an SER injury, the fibular fracture is oblique, located approximately 4 cm from the distal tip of the fibula, and

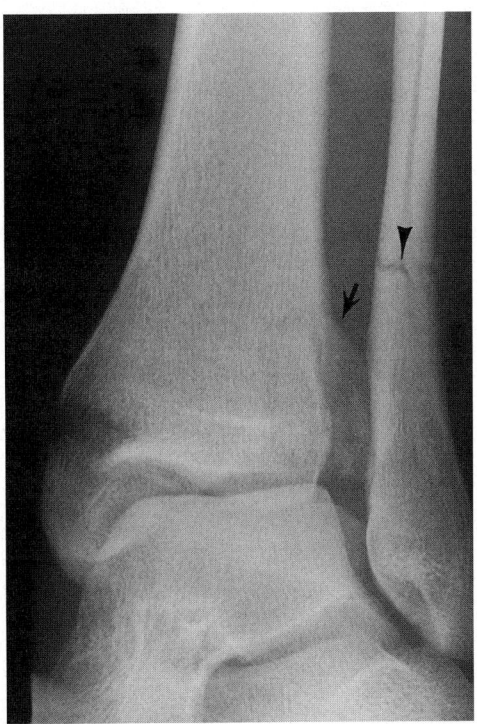

**Figure 57–76.** Ankle injuries: pronation-abduction injury, stage III. Findings include a transverse supramalleolar fibular fracture *(arrowhead)* and fractures of the medial malleolus and anterior tibial tubercle *(arrow)*.

extends from the anterior edge of the bone in a postero-superior direction. Maisonneuve's fracture is a second type and involves the proximal portion of the fibular shaft.

5. *Pronation-dorsiflexion (PDF) injury* (stages I to IV). The PDF category includes the group of lesions produced by axial loading; they are also designated pilon (pestle) fractures because the talus is driven into the tibial plafond. Pilon fractures of the tibia constitute less than 0.5% of all ankle fractures. Their mechanism is forced dorsiflexion of the pronated foot (Fig. 57–78). In stage I, a fracture of the medial malleolus is seen. In stage II, a second fracture arises from the anterior tibial margin. A supramalleolar fracture of the fibula characterizes stage III, and in stage IV, this is accompanied by a relatively transverse fracture of the posterior aspect of the tibia that connects with the anterior tibial fracture.

## Ankle Dislocation

Subluxations and dislocations of the ankle, particularly those in a medial or lateral direction, are commonly asso-

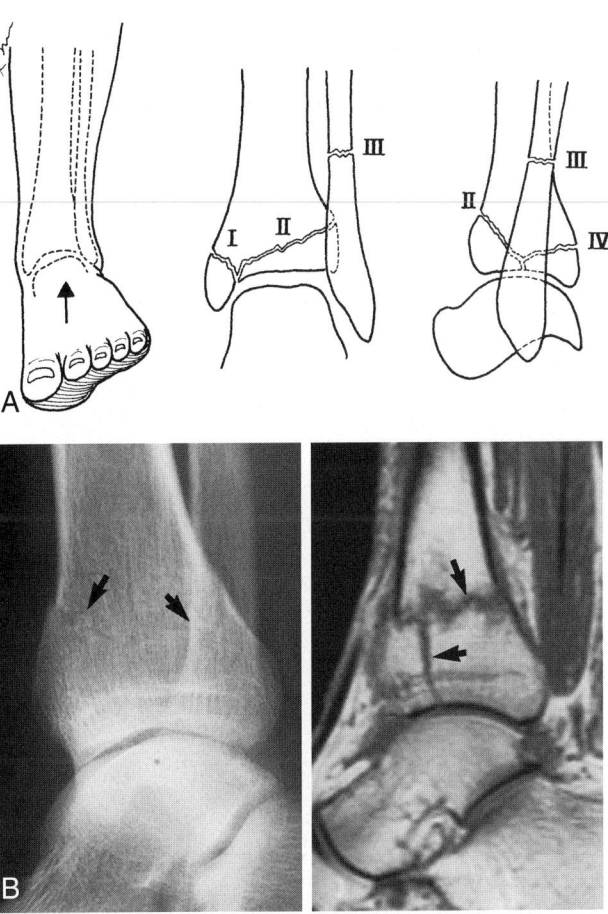

**Figure 57–78.** Ankle injuries: pronation-dorsiflexion injury. *A,* Initially, a fracture of the medial malleolus occurs (stage I). Subsequent injuries include a fracture of the anterior tibial margin (stage II), a supramalleolar fracture of the fibula (stage III), and a transverse fracture of the posterior aspect of the tibia that connects with the anterior tibial fracture (stage IV). *B* and *C,* Stage IV injury. Routine radiograph *(B)* and sagittal T1-weighted (TR/TE, 500/12) spin echo MR image *(C)* show the characteristics of the distal tibial fracture *(arrows)*.

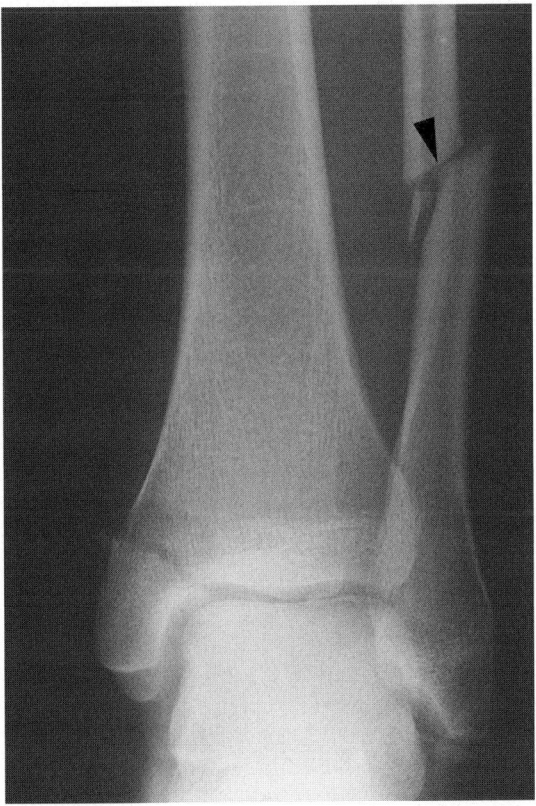

**Figure 57–77.** Ankle injuries: pronation–external rotation injury, stage III. Findings include fracture of the medial malleolus and an oblique fracture of the fibula *(arrowhead)*, well above the level of the ankle joint.

ciated with fracture of the adjacent malleolar surfaces. Medial dislocation of the talus appears to be the most common type, although any type may be associated with a fracture of the tibial surface. A peculiar type of ankle injury resulting from severe external rotation of the foot may lead to posterior displacement of the fibula, which becomes locked behind the tibia. This injury is sometimes referred to as a Bosworth fracture-dislocation of the ankle.

## Foot

### Fracture and Dislocation of the Talus

The talus is second only to the calcaneus as a site of fracture in the tarsal bones. Such fractures occur after sudden hyperextension of the forefoot (e.g., sudden application of the brakes in an automobile to avoid an accident). Avulsion fractures predominate and occur in the superior surface of the talar neck and the lateral, medial, and posterior aspects of the body; major injuries to the talus are also seen. CT scanning is generally regarded as the best of the advanced imaging methods for detecting and fully assessing these injuries.

Avulsion fractures are typically the result of a twisting or rotational force combined with flexion or extension stresses (Fig. 57–79). A longitudinal compression force in combination with acute plantar flexion presumably accounts for the avulsion fracture of the anterosuperior surface of the talar neck. Eversion stress may lead to osseous avulsion at the site of attachment of the deep fibers of the deltoid ligament to the body of the talus. The posterior process may be fractured during severe plantar flexion of the foot because of compression between the posterior surface of the tibia and the calcaneus. Disruption of the talar body where the bone projects beneath the tip of the lateral malleolus may result from severe dorsiflexion and external rotation. Fractures involving the posterior process of the talus may be difficult to differentiate from the os trigonum.

Fractures of the talar neck are second in frequency to avulsion injuries of the bone (Fig. 57–80). Dorsiflexion related to a force from below or, more rarely, a direct blow to the talus produces this fracture. Complications of talar neck fractures include delayed union or nonunion, infection, osteoarthritis of adjacent articulations, and ischemic necrosis, the last occurring in a minority of nondisplaced fractures but in as many as 80% to 90% of displaced fractures, particularly those with dislocations. The appearance of a linear subchondral lucent area (Hawkins' sign) in the talar dome on radiographs obtained 1 to 3 months after a talar neck fracture relates to hyperemia and continuity of the blood supply and should not be misinterpreted as a crescent sign of osteonecrosis.

Fractures of the body of the talus are infrequent; they may involve the posterior or lateral process, the articular surface, or all regions, especially in instances of fracture comminution. Fractures of the lateral process of the talus are believed to result from inversion of the ankle with the foot in dorsiflexion. They are considered intra-articular in nature, are related most often to a fall from a height, and are a recognized injury of snowboarders.

Subluxations or dislocations of the talus are generally accompanied by fractures of the bone, although they may occur as an isolated phenomenon. Medial subtalar dislocations are most frequent and represent approximately 55% to 80% of all such dislocations. Lateral subtalar dislocations are second in frequency, followed by anterior and posterior subtalar dislocations, which are rare. Total dislocation of the talus is an extremely infrequent and serious injury.

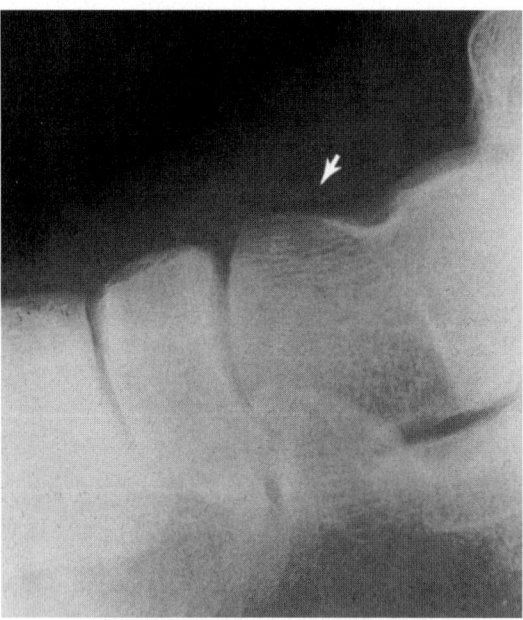

**Figure 57–79.** Talar injuries: avulsion fracture of the talar neck. An example of this relatively common injury is shown (*arrow*).

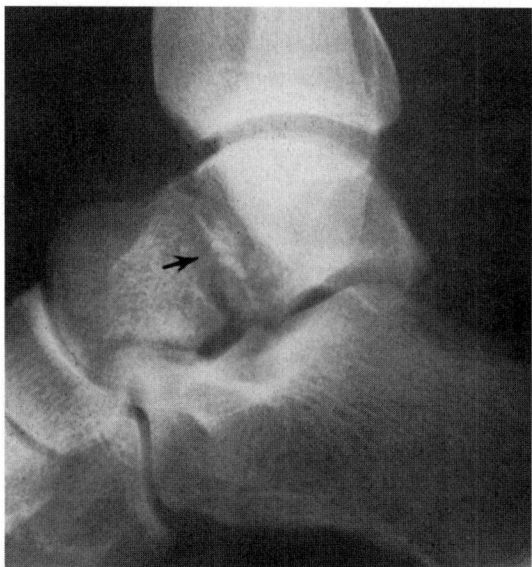

**Figure 57–80.** Talar injuries: fracture of the talar neck. Observe the vertical fracture line (*arrow*) with slight subluxation, leading to widening of the talocalcaneal space in the region of the sustentaculum tali. An acute fracture of the posterior tubercle of the talus also occurred.

## Fracture of the Calcaneus

The calcaneus is the most common site of tarsal fracture. Although an accurate diagnosis is commonly provided by routine and specialized radiographs—especially if attention is directed at Bohler's angle, as depicted on the lateral projection (Fig. 57–81)—the complexity of calcaneal anatomy has prompted the use of CT, which better displays the extent of injury. Fractures of the calcaneus can be broadly classified into those that are intra-articular (approximately 75%) and those that are extra-articular (approximately 25%); the former are associated with a poorer prognosis because of displacement of fragments.

Intra-articular fractures generally occur as a result of a vertical fall in which the talus is driven into the cancellous bone of the calcaneus; this mechanism of injury explains the frequency (10%) of bilateral calcaneal fractures, as well as the simultaneous occurrence of spinal injuries. The precise orientation of the fracture lines is debated, however. CT is a useful technique for the delineation of complex intra-articular fractures (Fig. 57–82). Intra-articular calcaneal fractures may be accompanied by lateral dislocation of the peroneal tendons, and such dislocation is often associated with a fibular avulsion fracture at the site of attachment of the superior peroneal retinaculum.

Extra-articular calcaneal fractures result from several different mechanisms, the most important of which are twisting forces. They may localize to the anterior or medial processes, the sustentaculum tali, the body, or the tuberosity. Certain avulsion injuries, such as those affecting the calcaneal tuberosity, are relatively easy to detect on radiographic examination; others, including those that apparently arise at the origin of the extensor digitorum brevis muscle on the lateral surface of the bone, may be more subtle (Fig. 57–83).

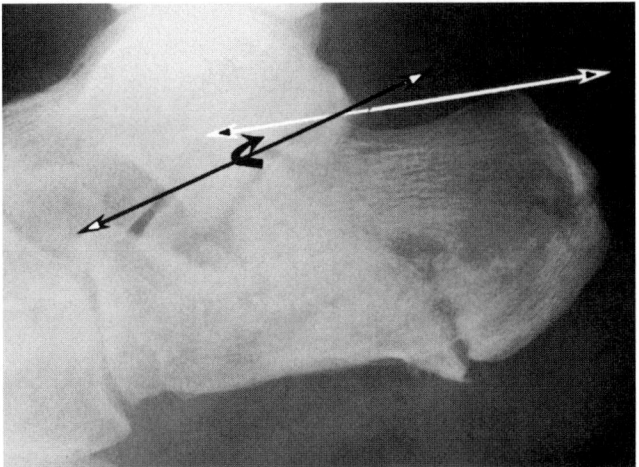

**Figure 57–81.** Calcaneal injuries: measurement of Bohler's angle. This angle (*curved arrow*) is formed by the intersection of two lines: the first line is drawn from the highest part of the anterior process of the calcaneus and the highest point of the posterior articular surface; the second line is drawn between the latter point and the most superior part of the calcaneal tuberosity. Bohler's angle normally measures between 25 and 40 degrees. In this example, it is decreased because of a complex intra-articular calcaneal fracture.

## Fracture of Other Tarsal Bones

Fractures elsewhere in the tarsus are infrequent. Typical sites of injury in the tarsal navicular bone are its dorsal surface near the talonavicular space and the tuberosity and body of the bone. Fractures of the navicular tuberosity may be combined with injuries of the calcaneus and cuboid, whereas isolated fractures of the cuboid and the cuneiforms are rare.

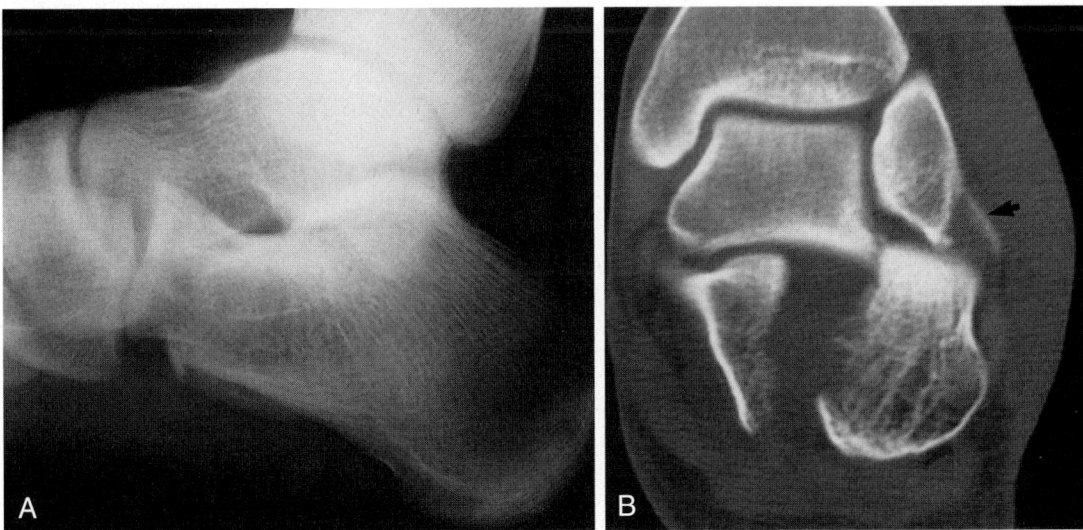

**Figure 57–82.** Calcaneal injuries: intra-articular fracture. *A*, Although routine radiography reveals an intra-articular fracture of the calcaneus, the status of the posterior subtalar joint is difficult to determine. *B*, Direct coronal CT scan shows marked lateral displacement of the lateral portion of the calcaneus, abutment of this region of the calcaneus and the distal end of the fibula, displacement of the peroneal tendons with a fibular avulsion fracture (*arrow*), and uncovering of the posterior facet of the talus.

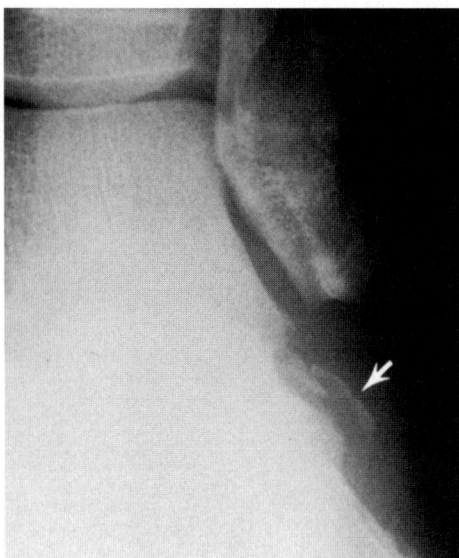

**Figure 57–83.** Calcaneal injuries: extra-articular fracture. Fracture at the origin of the extensor digitorum brevis muscle *(arrow)*.

## Tarsal Dislocation

Lisfranc's fracture-dislocation of the tarsometatarsal joints is an important injury (Fig. 57–84). Normally, the heads of the metatarsal bones are joined by transverse ligaments. Similarly, the bases of the metatarsal bones reveal ligamentous connections, except between the bases of the first and second metatarsal bones. An oblique ligament extending between the medial cuneiform and the second metatarsal base anchors the base of this metatarsal bone, which is also stabilized because of its recessed position between the cuneiforms.

Injuries to the tarsometatarsal joints can result from direct or, more commonly, indirect trauma. In the latter situation, violent abduction of the forefoot can lead to lateral displacement of the four lateral metatarsal bones, with or without a fracture at the base of the second metatarsal and the cuboid (see Fig. 57–84). Associated dorsal displacement is more frequent than plantar displacement. The first metatarsal bone may dislocate in the same direction as the other metatarsal bones (i.e., homolateral dislocation) or in the opposite direction (i.e., divergent dislocation), depending on the precise vectors of the force.

A consistent relationship in a normal foot is alignment of the medial edge of the base of the second metatarsal bone with the medial edge of the second cuneiform on frontal and oblique views. A small space or gap between the bases of the first and second metatarsal bones does not, by itself, represent a definite sign of dislocation; rather, disruption of the alignment of the second metatarsal bone and second cuneiform, with a step-off between the bones, is more diagnostic of an injury. The normal alignment of the bases of the fourth and fifth metatarsal bones with the cuboid and the alignment of the base of the first metatarsal bone with the medial cuneiform are more variable.

## Metatarsophalangeal and Interphalangeal Joint Dislocation

Dislocations at the metatarsophalangeal joints can occur in any direction. The first metatarsophalangeal joint is commonly affected. Similarly, patterns of dislocation of the interphalangeal joints in the foot are variable, but the interphalangeal joint of the hallux is typically affected.

## Fracture of the Metatarsal Bones and Phalanges

Metatarsal fractures, which may result from direct or indirect forces or occur in response to chronic stress or neuropathic osteoarthropathy, may be transverse, oblique, spiral, or comminuted. Those of the shaft and neck of the bone commonly result from a heavy object falling on the foot. Fractures of the metatarsal head are uncommon, result from direct injury, and are usually accompanied by fractures of adjacent metatarsal necks or shafts.

Fractures of the base of the fifth metatarsal bone are of two types: an avulsion fracture of the tuberosity, and a transverse fracture of the proximal portion of the diaphysis. The latter injury is termed a Jones fracture. Avulsion of a portion of the tuberosity of the fifth metatarsal bone results from an indirect injury associated with sudden inversion of the foot. The osseous fragment varies considerably in size, and the fracture line is usually transverse and may enter the cuboid-metatarsal joint space. Differentiating a fracture from a normal-appearing apophysis of the fifth metatarsal bone can be difficult in children; the latter is oriented in a longitudinal direction, and the radiolucent line that exists between it and the parent bone does not enter the cuboid-metatarsal space (Fig. 57–85).

A fracture in the proximal diaphyseal region of the fifth metatarsal bone, a true Jones fracture, results from either direct or indirect forces and is associated with delayed union or nonunion and refracture. Of particular importance are displaced intra-articular fractures (which may require surgical reduction) and, in children, physeal injuries of the distal phalanx.

# AXIAL SKELETON
## Pelvis
### Fracture and Dislocation of the Pelvis

The bony pelvis is intimate with vital internal organs, and the evaluation of these organs is mandatory in cases in which osseous or ligamentous disruption is apparent. Hemorrhage caused by vascular injury to arteries, urinary tract injury, compression of peripheral nerves, and disruption of viscera are among the significant complications of pelvic fractures and dislocations. Radiographic examinations directed at the detection of such complications are as fundamental to the proper analysis of pelvic fractures and dislocations as are radiographs of the bones themselves.

Fractures of the pelvis, which account for approximately 3% of all fractures, have been classified in a number of ways, based on such factors as the site of involvement, direction of force, and mechanism of injury. The major forces acting on the pelvic ring are external rotation, lateral compression (internal rotation), vertical shear, and

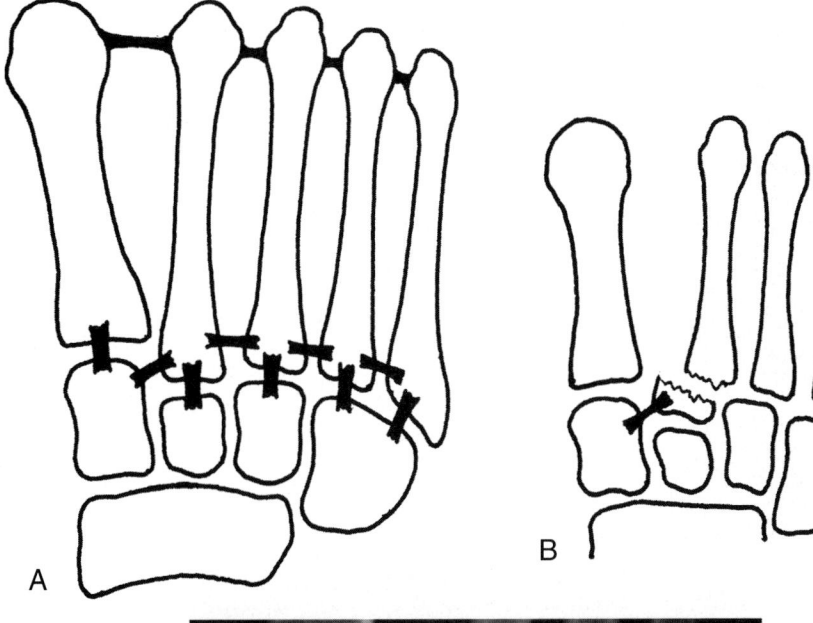

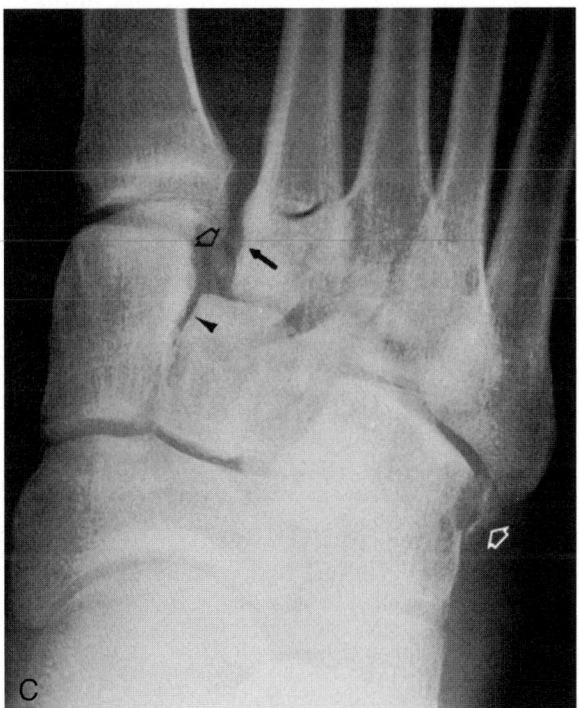

**Figure 57–84.** Lisfranc's fracture-dislocation of the tarsometatarsal joints. *A,* Normal ligamentous anatomy. *B,* Lateral dislocation of the second through fifth metatarsal bones may be associated with fractures of the base of the second metatarsal bone and cuboid. *C,* In this patient, note the subtle displacement of the second through fifth metatarsal bases. The medial edge of the second metatarsal base *(solid arrow)* is not aligned with the medial edge of the second cuneiform *(arrowhead).* Fractures of the base of the second metatarsal bone and cuboid are evident *(open arrows).* (*A* and *B,* From Wiley JJ: The mechanism of tarso-metatarsal joint injuries. J Bone Joint Surg Br 53:474, 1971.)

complex forces, as detailed in Figure 57–86. In this scheme, stability of the pelvic ring is considered to depend primarily on the integrity of its ligamentous structures, especially those located posteriorly. Instability is most characteristic of injuries resulting from vertical shear and complex forces. In other classification systems, stable fractures are generally considered to be those that either do not disrupt the osseous ring or disrupt it in only one place, and unstable fractures are those that disrupt the ring in two or more places (Table 57–8; Fig. 57–87).

**Type I Injuries.** Type I injuries, which do not lead to disruption of the pelvic ring, represent approximately 30% of all injuries that involve the bony pelvis. Avulsion fractures occur at sites of muscular and tendinous inser-

tions, such as the anterior superior iliac spine, anterior inferior iliac spine, and ischial tuberosity. Unilateral fractures of a single ramus are common, occur in elderly patients after a fall or in the form of stress fractures in athletes and after hip surgery, and are somewhat more frequent in the superior ramus than the inferior ramus. These fractures are extremely stable but may be associated with subsequent osteolysis simulating that of a malignant tumor.

A fracture of the iliac wing, Duverney's fracture, follows a direct injury and is rarely displaced. An isolated transverse fracture of the sacrum is rare and can be easily overlooked on radiographic examination. Neurologic compromise, related to disruption of higher or lower sacral nerve roots, is a recognized complication of these frac-

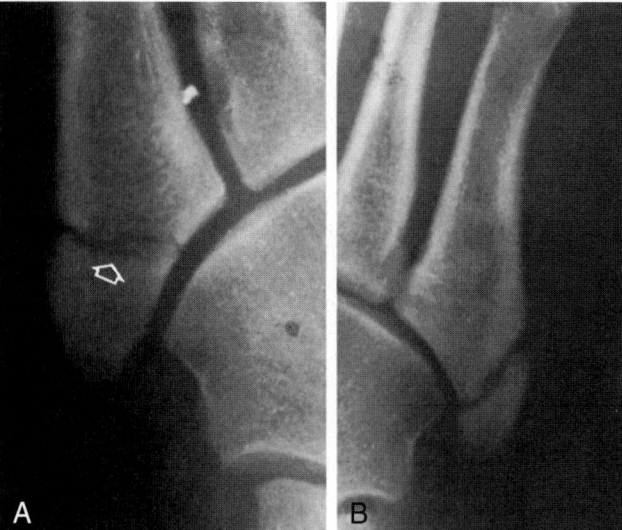

**Figure 57–85.** Metatarsal bone fracture: base of the fifth metatarsal. *A*, The fracture line *(open arrow)* is identified entering the space between the metatarsal base and the cuboid. *B*, On the opposite side, a normal apophysis is present. The radiolucent line between it and the metatarsal bone does not enter the joint.

| **TABLE 57–8** |
| --- |
| **Injuries of the Bony Pelvis** |

**Injuries without Disruption of the Pelvic Ring**
Avulsion fracture
Fracture of the pubis or ischium
Fracture of the iliac wing
Fracture of the sacrum
Fracture or dislocation of the coccyx

**Injuries with a Single Break in the Pelvic Ring**
Fractures of two ipsilateral rami
Fracture near or subluxation of the symphysis pubis
Fracture near or subluxation of the sacroiliac joint

**Injuries with Double Breaks in the Pelvic Ring**
Double vertical fractures or dislocations of the pubis (straddle fracture)
Double vertical fractures or dislocations of the pelvis (Malgaigne's fracture)
Multiple fractures

**Injuries to the Acetabulum**
Undisplaced fractures
Displaced fractures

From Kane WJ: Fractures of the pelvis. In Rockwood CA Jr, Green DP (eds): Fractures in Adult, 2nd ed. Philadelphia, JB Lippincott, 1984, p 1112.

tures. Transverse fractures of the upper or lower portion of the sacrum should be distinguished from vertical fractures of the sacrum (Fig. 57–88), which may be associated with additional osseous and ligamentous injuries, and from insufficiency stress fractures, which occur in an osteopenic skeleton and have both a vertical and a horizontal configuration. In all instances of sacral fracture, careful radiographic analysis of the foramina and arcuate lines is required.

**Type II Injuries.** Ipsilateral fractures of both pubic rami, a fracture of the symphysis itself, subluxation of the sacroiliac joint or symphysis pubis, and a fracture near the sacroiliac articulation are examples of type II pelvic injuries. The greater the degree of joint diastasis or the more extensive the displacement at the fracture site, the more likely the occurrence of a second break in the pelvic ring (type III pattern). Diastasis of the symphysis pubis greater than 15 mm and symphyseal disruption with overlapping of the pubis represent anterior injuries that should raise the strong possibility of disruption of the posterior aspect of the pelvic ring as well.

**Type III Injuries.** Examples of these injuries, which represent double breaks in the pelvic ring (Fig. 57–89), include straddle fractures (characterized by vertical fractures of the rami or dislocation of the symphysis pubis) and Malgaigne's fractures (characterized by simultaneous disruption of both the anterior and posterior aspects of the pelvic ring).

Straddle injuries are typified by disruption of the anterior portion of the pelvis in two places; bilateral vertical fractures involving both pubic rami or a unilateral fracture of both rami combined with symphyseal diastasis fulfills this criterion. These injuries represent 20% of all

pelvic fracture patterns and are accompanied by urethral or visceral damage in about 30% to 40% of cases.

The term Malgaigne's fracture is generally applied to a variety of injuries that have in common disruption of the anterior and posterior regions of the pelvic ring. Forms of this injury include (1) a vertical fracture of both pubic rami combined with either dislocation of the sacroiliac joint or fracture of the ilium or sacrum and (2) symphyseal dislocation combined with either dislocation of the sacroiliac joint or fracture of the ilium or sacrum. Malgaigne's fractures represent approximately 15% of all injuries to the bony pelvis. More extensive disruptions of the pelvis result from massive crushing injuries in which the osseous ring is disrupted in multiple locations or completely shattered (Fig. 57–90).

**Type IV Injuries.** Fractures of the acetabulum were considered earlier in this chapter.

With regard to the complications of pelvic fractures and dislocations, excessive bleeding may accompany many of these fractures, particularly type III injuries. Injuries to the urinary tract are typically associated with symphyseal diastasis, fractures of the pubic rami, or both; urethral damage is somewhat more frequent than injury to the bladder. Damage to the peripheral nerves occurs in approximately 10% of patients after injuries to the bony pelvis, and this frequency increases in those with sacral fractures.

## Thoracic Cage

### Fracture and Dislocation of the Sternum

The usual mechanism leading to fracture or dislocation of the sternum is direct trauma, and associated injuries of the anterior portion of the ribs and costocartilage are common. Aortic, other arterial, tracheal, cardiac, and

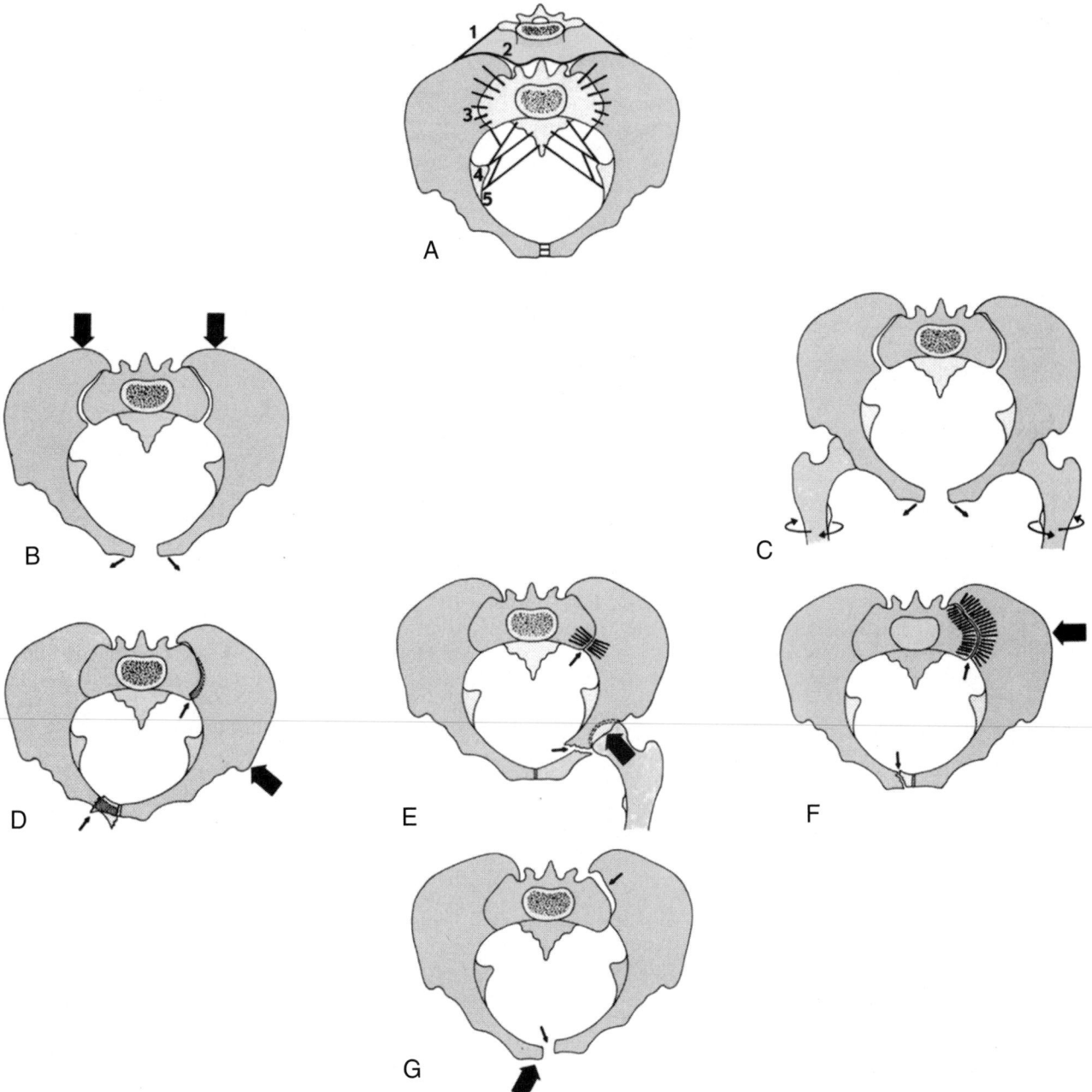

**Figure 57–86.** Fracture and dislocation of the pelvis: biomechanical principles. *A*, Normal situation, illustrating the major ligamentous structures. These structures include the iliolumbar ligaments (1), posterior (2) and anterior (3) sacroiliac ligaments, sacrospinous ligaments (4), and sacrotuberous ligaments (5). *B*, External rotation forces. A direct blow to the posterior superior iliac spines *(large arrows)* leads to opening of the symphysis pubis *(small arrows)*. Without the addition of a shearing force, the posterior ligamentous complex remains intact. *C*, External rotation forces. External rotation of the femora *(curved arrows)* or direct compression against the anterior superior iliac spines also produces springing of the symphysis pubis *(small arrows)*. Without the addition of a shearing force, the posterior ligamentous complex remains intact. *D*, Lateral compression forces. A lateral compression force against the iliac crest *(large arrow)* causes the hemipelvis to rotate internally. The anterior portions of the sacrum and pubic rami *(small arrows)* are injured. *E*, Lateral compression forces. A direct force against the greater trochanter *(large arrow)* leads to similar injuries to the pubic rami and ipsilateral sacroiliac joint ligamentous complex *(small arrows)*. *F*, Lateral compression forces. A force *(large arrow)* directed parallel to the trabeculae about the sacroiliac joint may produce impaction of bone posteriorly and disruption of the pubic rami *(small arrows)*. *G*, Vertical shearing forces. A shearing force *(large arrow)* crosses perpendicular to the main trabecular pattern and causes both anterior and posterior injuries *(small arrows)*. (From Tile M: Fractures of the Pelvis and Acetabulum. Baltimore, Williams & Wilkins, 1984, p 22.)

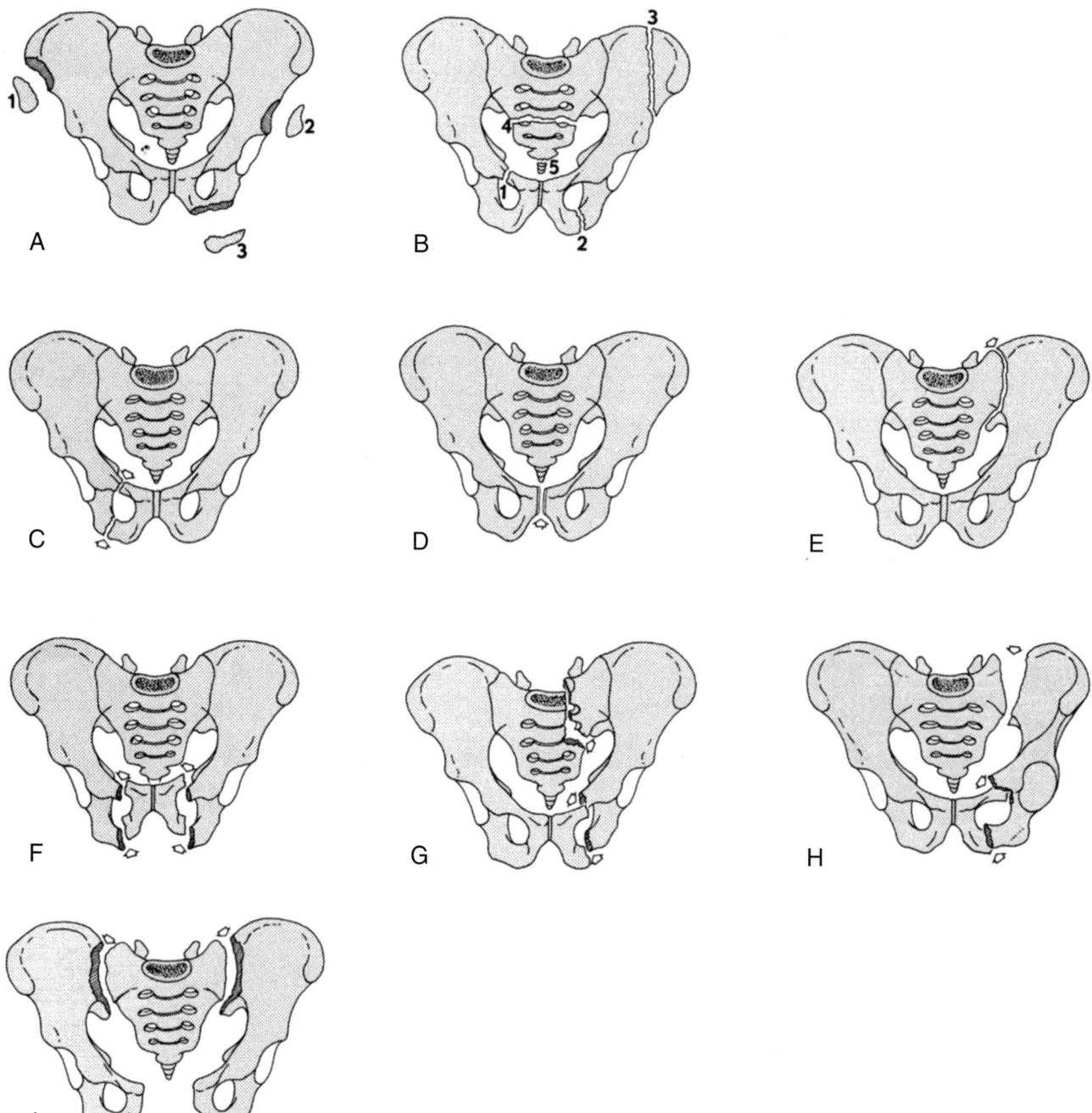

**Figure 57–87.** Fracture and dislocation of the pelvis: classification system. *A*, Type I injury: avulsion fracture. This injury may involve the anterior superior iliac spine (1), anterior inferior iliac spine (2), or ischial tuberosity (3). *B*, Type I injury: fracture of a single pubic ramus or iliac wing (Duverney's fracture). A single break in the superior or inferior pubic ramus (1 and 2), certain fractures of the ilium (3), and some types of fractures of the sacrum (4) or coccyx (5) do not lead to disruption of the pelvic ring. *C*, Type II injury: ipsilateral fractures of the pubic rami. Such fractures *(open arrows)* lead to a single break in the pelvic ring. *D*, Type II injury: diastasis of the symphysis pubis. This injury *(open arrow)*, or an isolated fracture of parasymphyseal bone, also leads to a single break in the pelvic ring. *E*, Type II injury: subluxation of the sacroiliac joint. This subluxation *(open arrow)*, or an isolated fracture near the sacroiliac joint, is an additional example of a single break in the pelvic ring. *F*, Type III injury: straddle fracture. Note the disruption of the pelvis in two places as a result of bilateral vertical fractures involving both pubic rami *(open arrows)*. *G*, Type III injury: Malgaigne's fracture. Vertical fractures of both pubic rami on one side combined with a sacral fracture *(open arrows)* lead to disruption of the pelvic ring in two places. *H*, Type III injury: Malgaigne's fracture. Similar vertical fractures of both pubic rami on one side combined with dislocation of the sacroiliac joint *(open arrows)* produce disruption of the pelvic ring in two places. *I*, Complex injury: "sprung" pelvis. Disruptions of the pelvic ring relate to bilateral dislocations of the sacroiliac joint and diastasis of the symphysis pubis *(open arrows)*.

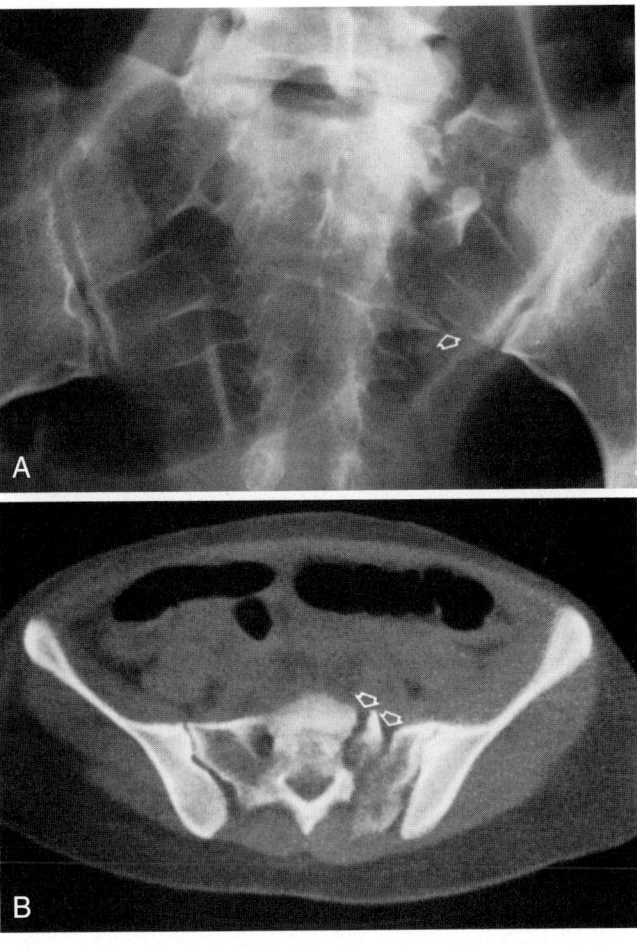

**Figure 57–88.** Fracture and dislocation of the pelvis: type II and III fractures of the sacrum. *A,* Vertical fractures of the sacrum disrupt the arcuate lines *(open arrow),* as depicted on a frontal radiograph. *B,* CT is better able to define the extent of injury *(open arrows).*

pulmonary injuries represent serious complications of direct sternal trauma.

Indirect mechanisms resulting in sternal fracture or dislocation include a blow to the upper thoracic or cervical segment of the spine (which may be fractured), with transmission of the force through the upper ribs or clavicle to the sternum, and stress fractures or collapse (i.e., buckling) of the sternum (Fig. 57–91).

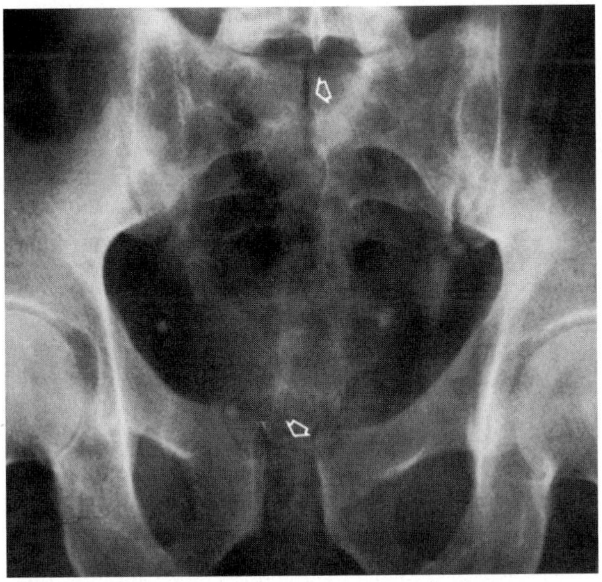

**Figure 57–89.** Fracture and dislocation of the pelvis: type III injury. Symphyseal diastasis and a vertical fracture of the sacrum *(open arrows)* have led to disruption of the pelvic ring in two locations.

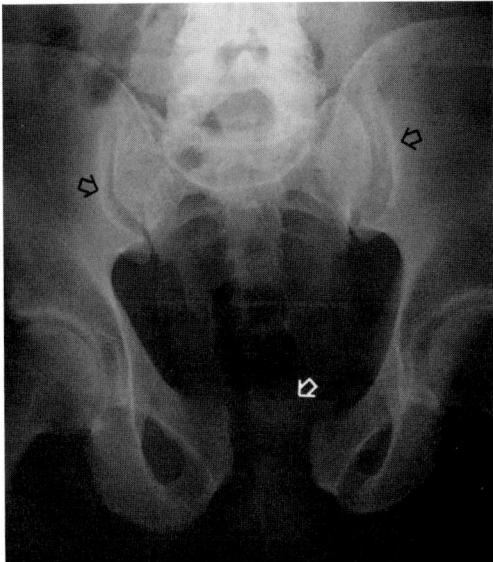

**Figure 57–90.** Fracture and dislocation of the pelvis: Complex injury. "Sprung" pelvis is characterized by subluxations or dislocations of both sacroiliac joints and symphyseal diastasis *(open arrows).*

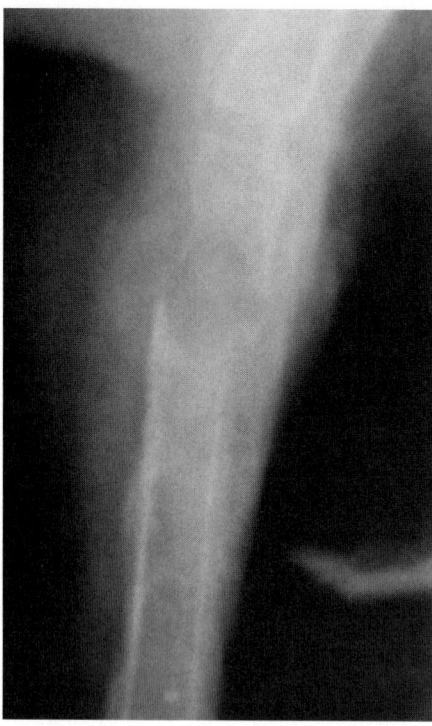

**Figure 57–91.** Fracture of the sternum: insufficiency fracture in osteomalacia. Note the resorption about the fracture site and soft tissue prominence. Biopsy documented the presence of a healing fracture. (Courtesy of J. Schills, MD, Cleveland, Ohio.)

## Fracture of the Ribs

Rib fractures result from direct injuries caused by blows to the chest or falls and are generally less significant than simultaneous injuries in the nearby lung. Commonly, adjacent areas of multiple ribs are affected. Soft tissue emphysema implies that the lung has been violated and should prompt a careful search for a pneumothorax. Fractures of the first and second ribs generally imply severe trauma and may be associated with vascular disruption.

## FURTHER READING

Ayella RJ: Radiologic Management of the Massively Traumatized Patient. Baltimore, Williams & Wilkins, 1978.

Cisternino SJ, Rogers LF, Stufflebam BC, Kruglik GD: The trough line: A radiographic sign of posterior shoulder dislocation. AJR Am J Roentgenol 130:951, 1978.

DePalma AF: The Management of Fractures and Dislocations, 2nd ed. Philadelphia, WB Saunders, 1970.

Deutsch AL, Resnick D, Mink JH: Computed tomography of

the glenohumeral and sternoclavicular joints. Orthop Clin North Am 16:497, 1985.

Goldfarb CA, Yin Y, Gilula LA, et al: Wrist fractures: What the clinician wants to know. Radiology 219:11, 2001.

Harris JH, Harris WH: The Radiology of Emergency Medicine. Baltimore, Williams & Wilkins, 1975.

Higgins TF, Baumgaertner MR: Diagnosis and treatment of fractures of the talus: A comprehensive review of the literature. Foot Ankle 20:595, 1999.

Hill HA, Sachs MD: The grooved defect of the humeral head: A frequently unrecognized complication of dislocations of the shoulder joint. Radiology 35:690, 1940.

Hougaard K, Lindequist S, Nielsen LB: Computerised tomography after posterior dislocation of the hip. J Bone Joint Surg Br 69:556, 1987.

Judet R, Judet J, Letournel E: Fracture of the acetabulum: Classification and surgical approaches for open reduction. J Bone Joint Surg Am 46:1615, 1964.

Kane WJ: Fractures of the pelvis. In Rockwood CA Jr, Green DP (eds): Fractures in Adults, 2nd ed. Philadelphia, JB Lippincott, 1984, p 1093.

Kilcoyne RF, Shuman WP, Matsen FA III, et al: The Neer classification of displaced proximal humeral fractures: Spectrum of findings on plain radiographs and CT scans. AJR Am J Roentgenol 154:1029, 1990.

Kristiansen B, Anderson ULS, Olsen CA, et al: The Neer classification of fractures of the proximal humerus: An assessment of interobserver variation. Skeletal Radiol 17:420, 1988.

Lauge-Hansen N: Fractures of the ankle: Genetic roentgenologic diagnosis of fractures of the ankle. AJR Am J Roentgenol 71:456, 1954.

Lauge-Hansen N: Fractures of the ankle. V. Pronation-dorsiflexion fracture. Arch Surg 67:813, 1953.

Letournel E: Acetabulum fractures: Classification and management. Clin Orthop 151:81, 1980.

Neer CS II, Rockwood CA Jr: Fractures and dislocations of the shoulder. In Rockwood CA Jr, Green DP (eds): Fractures in Adults, 2nd ed. Philadelphia, JB Lippincott, 1984, p 675.

Newberg AH, Greenstein R: Radiographic evaluation of tibial plateau fractures. Radiology 126:319, 1978.

Rizzo PF, Gould ES, Lyden JP, et al: Diagnosis of occult fractures about the hip: Magnetic resonance imaging compared with bone-scanning. J Bone Joint Surg Am 75:395, 1993.

Rockwood CA Jr, Green DP (eds): Fractures in Adults, 2nd ed. Philadelphia, JB Lippincott, 1984.

Rogers LF: Fractures and dislocations of the elbow. Semin Roentgenol 13:97, 1978.

Rogers LF: Radiology of Skeletal Trauma, 2nd ed. New York, Churchill Livingstone, 1992.

Rogers LF, Campbell RE: Fractures and dislocations of the foot. Semin Roentgenol 13:157, 1978.

Tachdjian MO: Pediatric Orthopedics. Philadelphia, WB Saunders, 1972.

Taylor AR, Arden GP, Rainey HA: Traumatic dislocation of the knee: A report of forty-three cases with special reference to conservative treatment. J Bone Joint Surg Br 54:96, 1972.

Young JWR, Resnick CS: Fracture of the pelvis: Current concepts of classification. AJR Am J Roentgenol 155:1169, 1990.

# CHAPTER 58

## Physical Injury: Spine

### Mini N. Pathria

## SUMMARY OF KEY FEATURES

Spinal trauma is complex, involving a wide range of soft tissue and osseous injuries in a variety of spinal regions. Knowledge of the anatomic and functional characteristics of the different spinal regions allows the physician to understand the injuries that are unique to each area. This chapter emphasizes the role of diagnostic imaging in evaluating patients with acute spinal injury.

## INTRODUCTION

Fractures, dislocations, and soft tissue injuries can affect the spine at any level. In most cases, prominent clinical manifestations and radiographic abnormalities allow a prompt and accurate diagnosis. The advent of computed tomography (CT) scanning and magnetic resonance (MR) imaging has had a significant impact on the ability to detect and categorize traumatic lesions of the spine.

## BASIC PRINCIPLES

Injuries to the spine can be categorized according to anatomic location, presumed mechanism of injury, and presence or absence of instability. When discussing spinal injuries, it is convenient to divide the spine into five distinct anatomic and functional segments: occipitoatlantoaxial, lower cervical, upper thoracic, thoracolumbar, and lower lumbar.

Most spinal injuries occur in the lower cervical and thoracolumbar regions, areas of the spine that are capable of voluntary straightening and normally have a large range of motion. The cervicocranium and upper thoracic region also have significant but lower rates of injury; the risk of neurologic damage is particularly high in these regions, however. Multilevel noncontiguous injuries occur in approximately 7% of patients. Spinal injuries can also be classified on the basis of their presumed mechanism (Table 58–1).

The basic spinal unit consists of two adjacent vertebrae, their anterior articulation via the intervertebral disc, their posterior facet articulations, and their ligamentous attachments. The intervertebral disc and spinal ligaments are highly resistant to compression, distraction, flexion, and extension but are vulnerable to rotary and horizontal shear forces. The disc and ligaments are largely incompressible, whereas bone is less able to resist vertically applied loads. The osseous endplates, rather than the intervertebral soft tissues, fail when pure compressive or tensile forces are applied to the spine. Axial compression results in vertebral endplate failure, followed by protrusion of nuclear material into cancellous bone. Hence, pure compression or distraction produces fractures, whereas rotary or shear forces result in intervertebral dislocations.

Spinal injuries can be subdivided further into stable and unstable categories. Fractures in which the interspinous ligaments are intact are considered stable, whereas injuries associated with disruption of the interspinous ligaments are unstable. Biomechanical analysis of the spine has shown that it can be divided into three columns. This three-column classification system is widely used in the assessment of spinal trauma.

1. *The anterior column* consists of the anterior longitudinal ligament, anterior portion of the anulus fibrosus, and anterior half of the vertebral body.
2. *The middle column* consists of the posterior longitudinal ligament, posterior portion of the anulus fibrosus, and posterior half of the vertebral body.
3. *The posterior column* is formed by the posterior osseous arch and the posterior ligaments, consisting of the capsular ligaments, ligamenta flava, interspinous ligaments, and supraspinous ligaments.

Spinal fractures can be divided into minor and major types as a guide to the likelihood of instability. Minor fractures include isolated fractures of the transverse process, articular facet, pars interarticularis (i.e., spondylolysis), or spinous process. These injuries all involve the posterior column, are limited to that column, and do not lead to acute instability. Major injuries involve more than one column or result in sufficient deformity to be considered a separate group of injuries. Major spinal injuries are classified into four categories: compression fractures (48%), burst fractures (14%), fracture-dislocations (16%), and seat-belt–type injuries (5%).

The middle column is most important in determining the potential for instability. Five radiographic signs that indicate the presence of instability as defined by middle column disruption are (1) vertebral displacement greater than 2 mm, (2) widened interlaminar space, (3) widened facet joints, (4) disruption of the posterior margin of the vertebral body, and (5) widened interpediculate distance.

Three types of spinal instability are described. Instability of the first degree (mechanical instability) refers to cases in which the spine is insufficiently constrained against buckling and angulation. This type of instability places the patient at risk for progressive chronic kyphosis. Instability of the second degree (neurologic instability) applies to those patients at risk for delayed neurologic compromise even if no deficit exists at presentation. Instability of the third degree (mechanical and neurologic instability) includes those cases in which both progressive osseous displacement and progressive neurologic injury may develop.

**TABLE 58–1**

**Classification of Injuries of the Cervical Spine**

**Hyperflexion Injuries**
Disruptive hyperflexion
  Hyperflexion sprain (momentary dislocation)
  Hyperflexion-dislocation (locked facets)
    Bilateral
    Unilateral (with associated rotational force)
  Spinous process fracture
Compressive hyperflexion
  Wedgelike compression of vertebral body
  Comminuted (teardrop) fracture of vertebral body
  Hyperflexion fracture-dislocation (type IV)
Hyperflexion or shearing forces
  Anterior atlanto-occipital dislocation (?)
  "Pure" anterior atlantoaxial dislocation (without
    associated fracture)
  Anterior fracture-dislocation of the dens

**Hyperextension Injuries**
Disruptive hyperextension
  Horizontal fracture of the anterior arch of C1
  Hangman's fracture (traumatic spondylolisthesis of C2)
  Anteroinferior margin of the body of the axis (C2)
  Hyperextension sprain (momentary dislocation)
  Spinous process fracture

Compressive hyperextension
  Posterior arch of the atlas fracture
  Vertebral arch fracture (articular pillar, pedicle, lamina)
  Hyperextension fracture-dislocation (types IV, V)
Hyperextension or shearing forces
  Posterior fracture-dislocation of the dens
  "Pure" posterior atlantoaxial dislocation (without associated fracture)

**Hyperrotation Injuries**
Rotary atlantoaxial dislocation
Anterior and posterior ligament disruption

**Lateral Hyperflexion Injuries**
Fracture of transverse process
Uncinate process fracture
Lateral fracture-dislocation of the dens
Brachial plexus avulsion association with cervical fractures or
  dislocations, or both
Lateral wedgelike compression of vertebral body

**Axial Compressive Injuries**
Isolated fracture of the lateral mass of the atlas
Jefferson's burst fracture (C1)
Vertical and oblique fractures of the axis body
Burst fracture of a vertebral body

From Gehweiler JA Jr, Osborne RL Jr, Becker RF: The Radiology of Vertebral Trauma. Philadelphia, WB Saunder, 1980, p 107.

## IMAGING METHODS

### Radiography

The initial screening examination for the injured spine consists of radiographs. The goal of radiography in injured patients is to obtain high-quality diagnostic images without moving the patient inappropriately or placing the patient at any neurologic risk.

### Computed Tomography

Multislice CT with reformations has become an essential modality in the evaluation of spinal trauma. Osseous anatomy is seen best on CT scans obtained with thin (1.5 to 2 mm) sections, using small body calibration to obtain high spatial resolution. Spinal immobilization or traction must be maintained throughout the study, and dislodgment of any traction equipment as the CT table moves must be avoided. Multislice CT, which provides volumetric data acquisition simultaneous with patient movement through the gantry, significantly shortens the time necessary for assessment of the spine, allowing the entire spine to be evaluated quickly and efficiently (Fig. 58–1).

CT has higher sensitivity than conventional radiography in the detection of vertebral fractures, particularly those involving the posterior osseous elements. Although CT allows the detection of numerous fractures not seen on radiographs, most (but not all) of these are second fractures occurring in vertebrae that have already been identified as abnormal. CT also appears to be the optimal method for detecting pneumorachis (gas within the spinal canal). Pneumorachis is most often iatrogenic, caused by a lumbar or cervical puncture, or it may be due to penetrating wounds to the spinal canal.

### Magnetic Resonance Imaging

MR imaging is emerging as the examination of choice for injuries with a high likelihood of spinal cord involvement or vascular occlusion.

The bone marrow changes associated with acute fractures are most obvious on inversion recovery sequences, but the exact plane of the fracture line is best assessed on T1-weighted images. The integrity of the cortex and alterations in the vertebral configuration are well evaluated on T1-weighted or intermediate-weighted spin echo MR sequences. Vertebral body fractures are detected readily, although a greater number of fractures and fragments and their sites of origin can be seen with CT, particularly in the case of comminuted fractures.

Ligamentous injury can be identified by noting alterations in both the morphology and the signal intensity of the spinal ligaments and paraspinal soft tissues. Ligament tears can be seen directly by observing the presence of ligamentous discontinuity or associated soft tissue hemorrhage, or they can be diagnosed by noting indirect criteria, such as kyphosis and malalignment. Supraspinous ligament rupture typically occurs in the midportion, between the osseous elements. Rupture of the anterior longitudinal ligament and posterior longitudinal ligament is easiest to detect in the region at the periphery of the disc, where the ligaments blend with the outermost fibers of the anulus fibrosus.

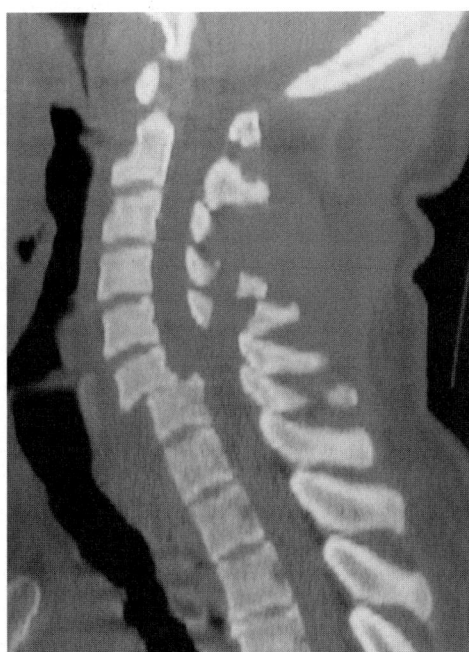

**Figure 58–1.** Fracture-dislocation: helical CT scanning. Sagittal reconstructed CT image shows anterior listhesis of C6 relative to C7 in a patient with a facet lock on the right side at C6–C7, as well as bilateral fractures of the C6 laminae. The entire cervical spine and the cervicothoracic junction can be scanned with the helical technique.

## SPINAL CORD TRAUMA

### General Considerations

The prevalence of spinal cord injury in patients with vertebral trauma is difficult to estimate. Many patients with minor vertebral injuries do not come to medical attention or are not hospitalized, leading to overestimation of the risk of spinal cord injury when only hospitalized patients are included in a survey. The risk of spinal cord injury in a patient with vertebral injury has been estimated to be as high as 14%. The risk is highest in patients with displaced fractures involving both the vertebral body and the posterior osseous elements in the cervical region.

### Classification of Injuries

Acute spinal cord injury may result from irreversible structural lesions, such as laceration, transection, or severe contusion; intrinsic reversible lesions, such as concussion or mild contusion; or extrinsic reversible lesions, such as cord compression. Spinal cord concussion (spinal shock) produces a transient neurologic deficit without any recognizable morphologic or microscopic alterations in the cord. The initial neurologic deficit may be profound and is thought to be due to alterations at a neurochemical or neuroendocrine level. Spinal cord concussion is typically the result of injuries producing a rapid change in cord velocity after trauma and, by definition, resolves completely within 24 to 48 hours. The cervical cord is affected most frequently, perhaps related to preexisting lesions producing spinal canal narrowing or hypermobility.

Transection and laceration are irreversible lesions of the spinal cord produced by anatomic discontinuity of the spinal cord nerve tracts. The spinal cord is surprisingly tough and is rarely torn, lacerated, or transected, even in the presence of massive fracture-dislocations. It may be difficult to distinguish transection from massive contusion if the cord is examined more than a few days after the injury. Spinal cord dissolution owing to autodestruction after severe contusive injuries typically develops 24 to 48 hours after the injury and can simulate the appearance of complete cord rupture. Unlike transection, there is a potential for neurologic improvement in patients with contusion.

## CERVICAL SPINE: GENERAL CONSIDERATIONS

It is generally accepted that early radiographs should be obtained in all injured patients with pain or neurologic deficit referable to the cervical spine, as well as in injured patients who are not fully alert and cooperative at the time of the initial evaluation. Virtually all patients with cervical spine injuries and a normal level of consciousness have symptoms or signs referable to the cervical spine.

### Screening Radiographic Examination

The goals of initial radiographic screening of the cervical spine include detection of all injuries, assessment of neural canal or foraminal encroachment, and determination of spinal stability. Considerable controversy exists regarding how many and which radiographic views constitute an adequate examination of the cervical spine. Increasingly, high-speed helical CT scanning is being used to screen high-risk patients, as well as to evaluate patients with incomplete or inadequate radiographic evaluations. In patients at high risk for cervical injury owing to the force of the initial trauma, altered mental status, abnormal neurologic examination, or prominent cervical symptoms, CT scanning can be cost-effective and is certainly easier to perform than conventional radiography. The role of helical CT for the screening of moderate- and low-risk patients remains to be established.

### Soft Tissue Swelling

Retropharyngeal and retrotracheal soft tissue swelling is an important indirect indicator of cervical trauma. Other indirect signs suggestive of cervical injury include displacement or obliteration of the prevertebral fat stripe, tracheal displacement or contour abnormalities, laryngeal dislocation, and tracheal laceration with retropharyngeal gas and elevation of the hyoid bone.

Examination of the cervical radiographs should include a careful evaluation of the width and contour of the prevertebral soft tissues. Prevertebral soft tissue swelling may not be present acutely, and its absence should not be relied on to exclude significant injury. Swelling due to edema and hemorrhage is maximal within the first 3 days after injury. Traditionally, 4 to 5 mm, or 0.3 times the anteroposterior dimension of the vertebral body width, is considered the normal maximum width of the prevertebral soft tissues at the level of the retropharynx, anterior to the upper four cervical vertebrae. Unfortunately, there is significant overlap in the measurements obtained in injured and noninjured patients. No significant difference in the width of the retropharyngeal soft tissues is seen with flexion and extension of the cervical spine in adults. Dramatic changes in the retropharyngeal measurement can take place with axial rotation, lateral bending, and swallowing, however. The largest increase in the prevertebral tissues is due to screaming. Soft tissue thickness also increases with body weight and age in normal persons.

The cervical prevertebral fat stripe is a thin radiolucent line located immediately anterior to the vertebrae and represents alveolar tissue in the retropharyngeal and retroesophageal spaces. A thin collection of air in the esophagus, a frequent normal finding, should not be confused with this structure. Widening of the prevertebral fat stripe due to obesity may result in an abnormal retropharyngeal and retrotracheal soft tissue thickness.

## OCCIPITOATLANTOAXIAL REGION

### General Considerations

The occipitoatlantoaxial region, also known as the cervicocranial junction, differs both anatomically and functionally from the remainder of the cervical spine and serves as the transition between the cranium and the cervical spine. Injuries to the occipitoatlantoaxial region are typically the result of direct trauma to the head rather than to the spine.

The osseous anatomy of both the C1 vertebra (atlas) and the C2 vertebra (axis) differs considerably from that of the remaining spinal vertebrae. The occipitoatlantal joint is reinforced by a unique ligamentous arrangement that allows moderate flexion and extension and minimal lateral flexion but restricts other movements markedly. In contradistinction, the primary motion at the C1–C2 joint is rotation rather than flexion and extension, which are the dominant motions in the lower cervical segment.

### Atlanto-occipital Dislocation

Atlanto-occipital dislocation, subluxation, and instability may be secondary to acute trauma or a variety of nontraumatic conditions, including rheumatoid arthritis, congenital skeletal anomalies, Down's syndrome, infection, and calcium pyrophosphate dihydrate crystal deposition at the craniovertebral junction. Although the large majority of cases of atlanto-occipital dislocation result in death, the injury is not invariably fatal or neurologically catastrophic. Most survivors have some neurologic injury, but up to 20% have no deficit at the time of presentation. Cranial nerve dysfunction, most commonly involving the sixth and more caudal cranial nerves, is the most common neurologic abnormality, presumably resulting from avulsion of the nerve roots from the brain stem. This injury is more common in children than in adults and typically results from motor vehicle accidents to pedestrians. Traumatic atlanto-occipital dislocation has also been documented in postmortem studies of abused children.

The lateral radiograph is the initial examination that suggests the presence of this unusual injury. Radiographically, however, the diagnosis of atlanto-occipital dislocation may be difficult to establish, with up to 40% of cases not being appreciated on the initial examination. The most apparent finding is retropharyngeal soft tissue swelling. Typically, the cranium is subluxed anteriorly relative to the cervical spine; however, superior displacement or, rarely, posterior subluxation occurs in other cases. Specific signs of anterior or posterior atlanto-occipital dislocation include displacement of the basion (midsagittal point of the anterior lip of the foramen magnum at the lower tip of the clivus) from its normal position superior to the odontoid process, malalignment between the spinolaminar line of C1 and the posterior margin of the foramen magnum, and failure of the clival line to intersect the odontoid process.

A quantitative technique for evaluating anterior cranial subluxation is based on the ratio between two lines rather than on absolute measurements. This technique, known as the Powers ratio, is unaffected by variations in patient size or film magnification (Fig. 58–2). The first line (BC) is the distance between the basion (B) and the posterior arch of C1 (C) at the spinolaminar line. The second line (AO) is the measurement between the posterior margin of the anterior arch (A) of C1 and the posterior lip of the foramen magnum, known as the opisthion (O). These anatomic landmarks are not affected significantly during flexion, extension, or rotation of the neck and can usually be identified on the lateral view, although the opisthion is often difficult to delineate.

In normal persons, the ratio of BC/AO is 0.77 ± 0.09. In patients with atlanto-occipital dislocation, the ratio is 1.15 or greater. This method is valid only when atlanto-occipital dislocation results in anterior translation of the cranium; it is insensitive for longitudinal or posterior displacement (Fig. 58–3).

CT allows assessment of the osseous alignment in this region without moving the patient. Both coronal and sagittal image reconstructions are necessary to comprehend the pattern of displacement fully. Sagittal reconstruction can be used to derive the Powers ratio, because all the necessary anatomic landmarks are well visualized in this plane. Associated findings observed in the upper cervical region with CT scanning include hemorrhage

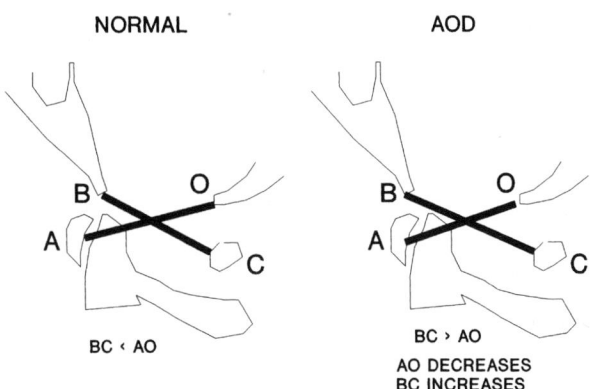

**Figure 58–2.** Powers ratio. This ratio can be used to identify atlanto-occipital dislocation.

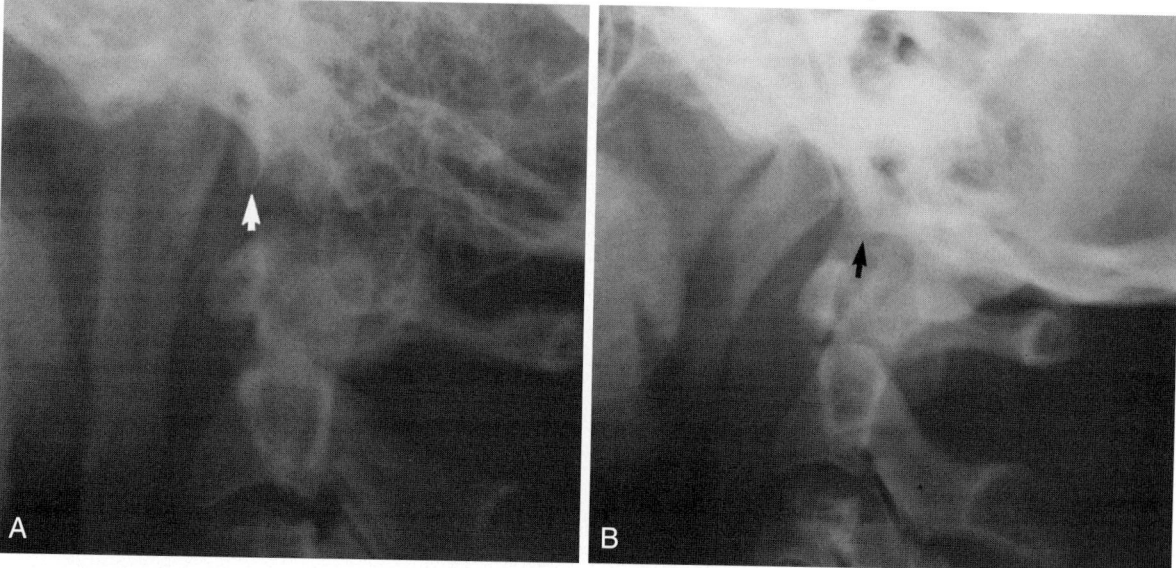

**Figure 58–3.** Atlanto-occipital dislocation: horizontal translation type. *A,* The basion *(arrow)* is displaced anteriorly relative to its normal position above the tip of the odontoid process. *B,* Similar malalignment of the basion *(arrow)* is seen in a different patient with atlanto-occipital dislocation. Note the extensive soft tissue swelling in both examples. The Powers ratio is abnormal in both cases.

around the foramen magnum, thickening of the anterior tectorial membrane, and extradural hemorrhage. MR imaging has also been used to establish the diagnosis of atlanto-occipital dislocation, and some investigators have suggested that MR imaging is the best method for such evaluation, owing to the ability to visualize the ligamentous structures directly.

## Atlantoaxial Subluxation

Isolated post-traumatic atlantoaxial subluxation is a rare injury. Nontraumatic atlantoaxial subluxation is far more frequent, and rheumatoid arthritis is probably the most common cause of transverse ligament incompetence. Numerous other arthritides and connective tissue disorders, including the seronegative spondyloarthropathies, have an association with atlantoaxial subluxation. Five percent to 30% of patients with Down's syndrome have laxity of the transverse ligament.

Traumatic tears of the transverse ligament or avulsion fractures at its site of insertion are sufficient to allow displacement of C1 relative to C2 (Fig. 58–4). Almost all cases of atlantoaxial displacement manifest anterior dislocation of the atlas relative to the axis. Displacements of up to 5 or even 10 mm can develop after isolated transverse ligament rupture; further displacement requires insufficiency of the alar and other secondary ligaments. The normal distance between the dens and the posterior margin of the anterior arch of C1 is less than 3 mm in adults and 5 mm in children. Measurements of the atlantoaxial distance are reliable only when the odontoid process is intact and attached to the C2 body. In many normal persons, the width of the atlantoaxial interval is uneven, with superior widening resulting in a V-shaped predens space. Nine percent of adults show this configuration. A normal atlantoaxial distance is seen in these patients when

it is measured at the lower aspect of the anterior arch of C1.

The distance between the anterior arch of C1 and the dens can be assessed with CT, but the CT examination is typically performed in the neutral or extended position, limiting its sensitivity for atlantoaxial subluxation. In transaxial CT scans, the normal atlantoaxial space appears to be less than 1 mm wide. Normal findings on a CT examination, however, do not exclude atlantoaxial subluxation unless the study is obtained with cervical flexion. MR imaging affords a more sensitive method for the detection of atlantoaxial instability and allows concomitant assessment of the degree of cord compression.

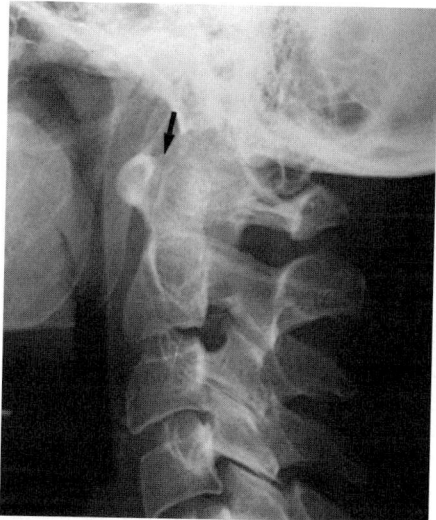

**Figure 58–4.** Atlantoaxial subluxation. Flexion view shows abnormal widening of the atlantoaxial space *(arrow),* which measures 4 mm.

## Atlantoaxial Rotatory Fixation

Atlantoaxial rotatory fixation can be defined as persistent pathologic fixation of the atlantoaxial joints in a rotated position, such that the atlas and axis move as a unit rather than independently. This form of C1–C2 malalignment often occurs after minor or moderate trauma, but it may develop spontaneously or after an inflammatory condition involving the pharynx or upper respiratory tract.

The primary function of the C1–C2 joint is rotation. Normally, the atlas rotates 30 to 50 degrees in either direction relative to the axis. Only after a minimum of 20 to 30 degrees of rotation at this level does rotation of the lower cervical spine develop. When the head is rotated to the right, the left articular mass of C1 slides anteriorly while the right articular mass rotates posteromedially. With continued rotation, the left articular mass continues to move anteriorly but also rotates in a medial direction. The movement of the right articular mass is always greater, causing the left alar ligament to become taut and restrict any further motion. Lateral tilting of the head to the left in this situation relaxes the alar ligament, allowing rotation to continue. This relationship explains why rotation is facilitated by a slight tilt of the head to the opposite direction. In atlantoaxial rotatory fixation, the relationship is generally fixed within the range of motion attainable during normal rotation.

Atlantoaxial rotatory fixation can be classified into four types, based on the direction and degree of displacement:

*Type 1* atlantoaxial rotatory fixation is the most common and consists of fixed rotation within the physiologic range of motion, with an intact transverse ligament and a normal atlantoaxial distance.

*Type 2* lesions are characterized by deficiency of the transverse ligament with atlantoaxial displacement of 3 to 5 mm.

*Type 3* atlantoaxial rotatory fixation consists of atlantoaxial subluxation of more than 5 mm, owing to deficiency of both the transverse and the secondary (predominantly the alar) ligaments.

*Type 4* lesions are extremely rare and occur when both lateral masses of C2 are displaced posteriorly relative to those of C1.

The patient has a persistent, painful torticollis and the typical "Cock Robin" position of the head, consisting of slight flexion, cranial rotation, and tilting of the head contralateral to the direction of rotation. Vertebral artery compromise may occur with severe rotation, particularly when combined with anterior subluxation of C1 and C2. Despite the dramatic clinical and radiographic findings, neurologic deficit is seen in only a minority of patients.

The most characteristic radiographic abnormality in rotatory fixation is a persistent abnormality in the relationship of the odontoid process to the lateral masses of C2. This abnormal relationship of C1 and C2 is best demonstrated in the anteroposterior open-mouth odontoid view (Fig. 58–5). In this view, the dens is positioned eccentrically between the lateral masses of C1, and the anteriorly displaced lateral mass appears wider, more rectangular, and closer to the midline. This appearance occurs because the long axis of the lateral mass is almost

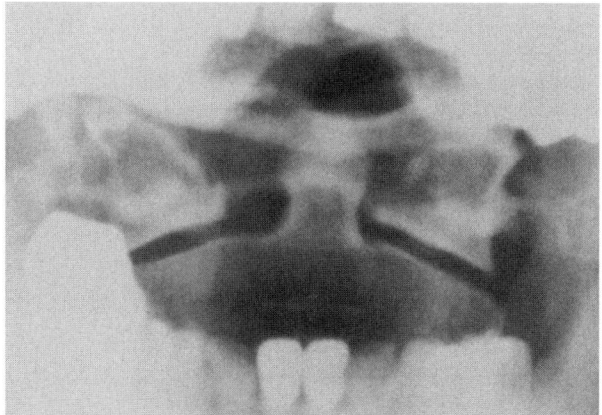

**Figure 58–5.** Atlantoaxial rotatory fixation. In this patient, persistent rotation of the C1–C2 vertebrae was present. Note the asymmetry in the shape of the C1 lateral masses and the asymmetrical distance between the dens and the lateral masses of the atlas.

45 degrees oblique; with rotation, the anterior mass is seen en face, whereas the posterior mass appears foreshortened (Fig. 58–6). Spinous process deviation is not a prominent feature clinically or radiographically, unless an associated lateral tilting of the head is present.

Rotatory fixation can be diagnosed only when the abnormal relationship between the lateral masses of the atlas and axis is shown to be irreducible. Serial exposures taken with different amounts of rotation can be used to

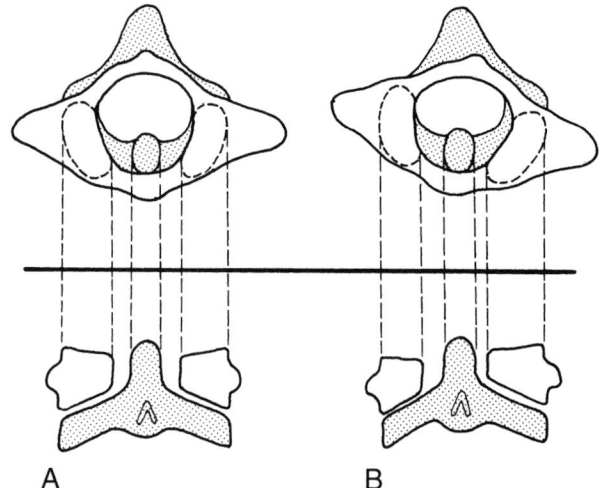

**Figure 58–6.** Atlantoaxial rotatory fixation. The atlantoaxial joint is seen in the neutral position *(A)* and on rotation to the right side *(B)*, viewed from above (top) and from the frontal plane (bottom). *A,* In the neutral position, the odontoid process is located midway between the lateral masses of the atlas. The lateral atlantoaxial joints are symmetrical. *B,* With rotation, anteromedial rotation and upward shift of the left atlantal articular mass are associated with medial approximation to the odontoid process. The right atlantal articular mass moves inferiorly and posteromedially, and it possesses a narrow profile. The left lateral atlantoaxial joint is widened, and the right is narrowed. Persistence of the findings is consistent with atlantoaxial rotatory fixation.

evaluate the C1–C2 relationship. Anteroposterior views of the odontoid process obtained with 15 degrees of rotation of the head to both sides and similar views with lateral tilting of the head to both sides have been advocated. CT scanning both in the resting position and with maximal rotation of the head to the contralateral side is now considered the optimal method for evaluation. Thick slices are actually easier to assess because the axis of a tilted vertebra can be determined from a single slice. In patients with rotatory fixation, no change in the relationship of C1 and C2 is evident when the resting and contralateral rotation studies are compared (Fig. 58–7).

Grisel's syndrome is the term applied to unilateral or bilateral atlantoaxial subluxation in association with an inflammatory condition of the head or neck. Unilateral anterior subluxation, producing rotatory malalignment, is most common. Typically, patients are between 5 and 12 years of age; there is no sex predominance. Rotatory displacement is the most typical deformity; the term displacement, rather than fixation, is preferred, because many patients have some residual motion in the upper cervical region. Infection of the C1–C2 joint itself usually is not present in Grisel's syndrome, and the exact pathogenesis is not well understood.

## Fracture of the Atlas

Atlantal fractures constitute 2% to 13% of cervical fractures and account for 1% to 2% of all vertebral fractures. In general, fractures of C1 are not associated with neurologic deficit. A variety of fractures of the osseous ring of C1 have been described, but only a few occur with significant frequency. Fractures of C1 are classified into five types: (1) Jefferson's burst fractures, (2) posterior arch fractures, (3) horizontal fractures of the anterior arch, (4) lateral mass fractures, and (5) transverse process fractures. The last two types are extremely rare.

The most common fracture of C1 is disruption of its posterior arch as it is compressed between the basiocciput and the posterior arch of C2 during hyperextension of the neck. Fractures of the posterior arch can be unilateral or bilateral. Isolated fractures of the posterior arch are stable. They are usually readily apparent on the lateral view of the cervical spine, particularly when they are bilateral (Fig. 58–8). Transaxial CT scans obtained along

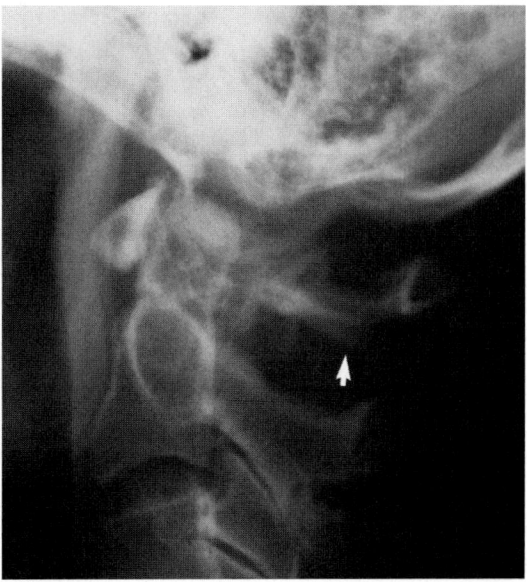

**Figure 58–8.** Fracture of the posterior arch of the atlas. Fracture *(arrow)* occurred after a hyperextension injury. Note the absence of soft tissue swelling with this isolated posterior injury.

the plane of the posterior arch are recommended when the radiographic findings are equivocal or when there is strong clinical suspicion of an atlas fracture. Fractures must be differentiated from congenital clefts of the posterior arch, which are present in 4% of persons.

Axial compressive loading of C1 results in Jefferson's fracture, which occurs when the lateral masses of C1 are compressed between the occipital condyles and the articular facets of C2. The wedge-shaped articular masses are driven apart by the compressive force, resulting in fractures of both the anterior and the posterior arches. The classic Jefferson's fracture consists of bilateral disruption of both anterior and posterior arches with lateral displacement of both lateral masses. The classic four-part fracture as described by Jefferson appears to be relatively rare, however, and most cases studied with CT scanning manifest fewer than four fracture lines. It is now recognized that this injury can be unilateral or bilateral and can manifest two, three, or four fracture lines. Marked prever-

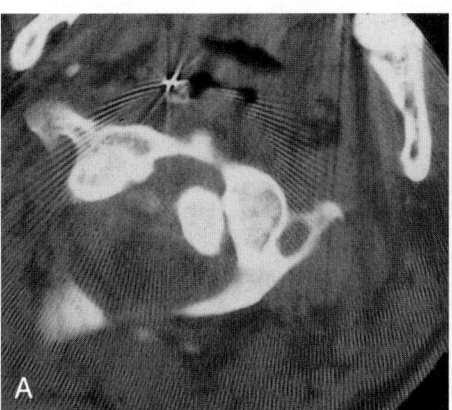
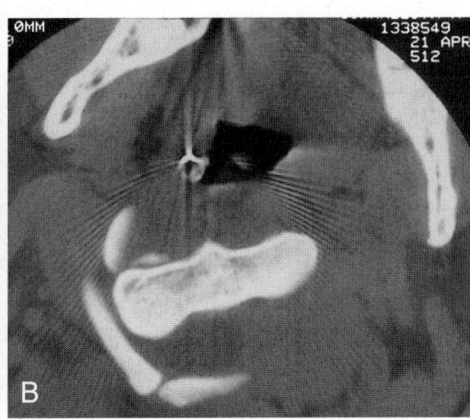

**Figure 58–7.** Atlantoaxial rotatory fixation. Transaxial CT scans through ring of C1 *(A)* and upper body of C2 *(B)* show rotatory malalignment between C1 and C2. This abnormal relationship did not change with cranial rotation.

tebral edema is suggestive of Jefferson's fracture. The fracture is characterized more readily on the open-mouth odontoid view, owing to the presence of lateral displacement of the lateral masses of the atlas relative to those of the axis. Unilateral offset of the lateral masses or bilateral offset, particularly when the combined displacement is 3 mm or greater, is highly specific for injuries to the atlantoaxial region (Fig. 58–9). True offset of the lateral masses must be differentiated from malalignment produced by uneven skeletal maturation of C1 and C2, head positioning, and normal variations in the size of the lateral masses. Minimal degrees of displacement of the lateral masses of the atlas and axis may be seen in healthy persons, and offsets of 1 mm are within the normal range and can be safely discounted. Currently, CT is used most widely to evaluate the integrity of the anterior arch of the atlas.

## Fracture of the Axis

The axis serves as the transitional vertebra between the cervicocranium above and the remaining portion of the cervical spine below. The dens, in conjunction with the anterior arch of C1 and the transverse ligament, prevents anterior and posterior subluxation of C1 on C2.

**Fracture of the Odontoid Process.** Fractures of the odontoid process make up 7% to 13% of all cervical spine injuries. They represent the most common fracture of the axis in most series, accounting for up to 55% of C2 fractures. The mechanism of injury is complex, and the fracture is a result of a combination of extreme flexion, extension, or rotation, along with a shearing force. Most fractures of the dens are the result of a major force. The majority of patients with odontoid fractures have no neurologic deficit and manifest posterior upper cervical pain, which often radiates to the occiput, and paravertebral spasm. The most common neurologic deficits are transient mild upper extremity weakness, lower extremity hyperreflexia, and diminished occipital sensation.

The classification of odontoid fractures is based on fracture location and has both therapeutic and prognostic implications:

*Type 1* odontoid fractures are rare, and some authorities doubt their existence. They are unilateral oblique fractures occurring through the tip of the dens and are probably secondary to alar ligament avulsion. The fracture can be differentiated easily from the round, corticated os terminale, a normal ossicle located at the superior tip of the odontoid process.

*Type 2* fractures are probably the most common type of odontoid fracture, representing 31% to 65% of dens fractures. This injury occurs at the junction of the dens and the body of C2 and disrupts the blood supply to the odontoid process, which enters adjacent to its base (Fig. 58–10). Approximately 50% of type 2 fractures are displaced more than 2 mm at the time of presentation. Displacement of more than 4 mm is generally considered evidence of instability. The rate of nonunion for type 2 fractures is high (26% to 36%). Most authors believe that an os odontoideum is an acquired post-traumatic abnormality in the majority of cases. The mechanism is believed to be post-traumatic disruption of the bone, followed by interruption of the blood supply to the base of the dens, leading to osteonecrosis and resorption of bone. This ossicle can be distinguished from an acute odontoid fracture radiographically by noting the presence of a rounded or oval ossified mass with smooth, thin cortical borders and its smaller size than expected for a complete odontoid process.

*Type 3* fractures are also relatively common injuries. In these cases, horizontal or oblique fractures adjacent to the base of the dens extend into the cancellous bone of the C2 vertebral body. The fracture line usually extends into the joints between the lateral masses of C1 and C2. Although the fractures frequently are displaced, fracture nonunion is unusual. Lateral tilting of the dens greater than 5 degrees may be seen.

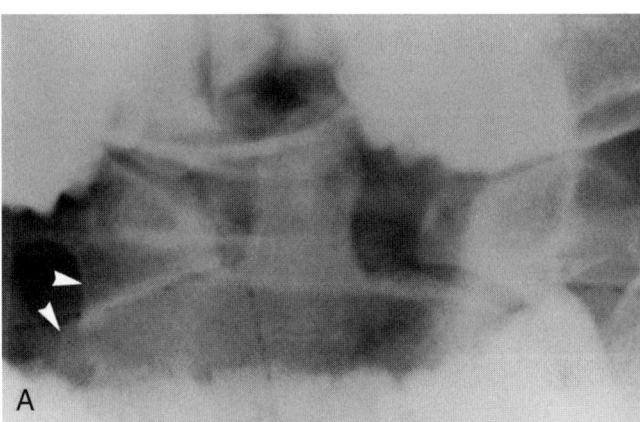
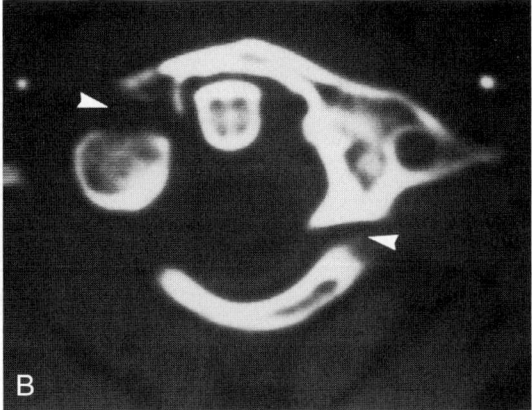

**Figure 58–9.** Jefferson's fracture. *A,* Initial open-mouth radiograph shows an asymmetrical position of the odontoid process between the lateral masses of the atlas. The right lateral atlantoaxial joint is obliterated, and the position of the lateral borders of the right lateral masses of the atlas and axis is offset *(arrowheads).* *B,* CT scanning reveals two fractures of the atlas *(arrowheads).* Identification of such fractures requires analysis of multiple contiguous transaxial scans.

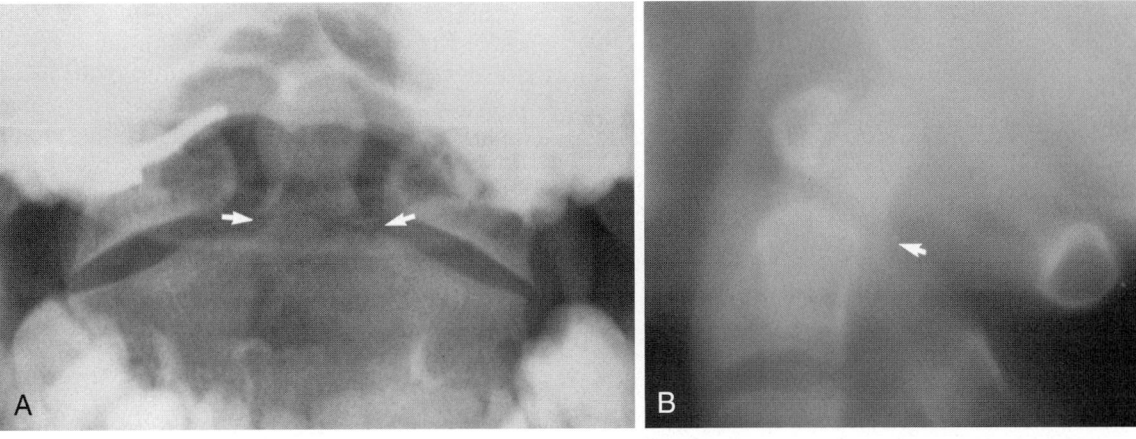

**Figure 58–10.** Type 2 odontoid fracture. *A*, Anteroposterior open-mouth view shows a transverse fracture *(arrows)* across the base of the dens at the same level as the articulation of the C1–C2 lateral masses. *B*, Lateral conventional tomogram confirms the presence of a fracture *(arrow)* at the base of the dens.

The lateral and anteroposterior open-mouth odontoid views are most useful in the assessment of the dens. Flexion and extension views should be avoided in a patient with a dens fracture, because the resultant bone displacement may be fatal. Because many odontoid fractures are horizontal, reformatted thin-section CT scans are preferable to routine transaxial CT images. Transaxial CT scans may fail to detect fractures at the base of the odontoid process. Fractures of the odontoid process are best demonstrated on the anteroposterior open-mouth view. Type 1 fractures are seen only on this projection, provided there is adequate visualization of the tip of the odontoid process. In type 2 and 3 fractures, the fracture line at the base of the odontoid process or within the C2 centrum can be identified, even if the upper part of the odontoid process is obscured. The fracture line may be very subtle in cases of undisplaced fractures. Lateral tilting of the odontoid process more than 5 degrees likewise has been emphasized as an important indicator of a type 3 odontoid fracture. Displaced or angulated odontoid fractures are usually apparent on the lateral view. Even if the odontoid step-off is not visualized, malalignment between the spinolaminar lines of C1 and C2 may be apparent. The lateral view may not demonstrate the odontoid fracture in the absence of displacement or angulation, although prevertebral soft tissue swelling typically is present. Type 3 fractures can be distinguished from type 2 fractures by noting disruption of the "ring shadow" of the axis, a feature seen only in type 3 injuries (Fig. 58–11). The ring shadow is a composite of structures, including the junction of the body of the axis with its lateral masses, the cortex of the facet joints, and the vertebral margin; the dens itself does not form any of the borders of the ring.

**Fracture of the Body and Posterior Arch of the Axis.** With the exception of odontoid fractures, the most common injury of the axis vertebra is traumatic spondylolisthesis of the pars interarticularis, accounting for 4% to 23% of all cervical spine fractures. Typically resulting from a motor vehicle accident or a fall, this fracture is termed

the hangman's fracture because of its similarity to the osseous injury produced by hanging.

This injury is defined as bilateral avulsion of the neural arches from the vertebral body, with or without subluxation, with the odontoid process remaining intact. The fractures occur through the pars interarticularis of C2 or through the adjacent portion of the articulating facet (Fig. 58–12). Extension into the posterior vertebral cortex is seen in up to 18% of cases and is considered a variant or part of the spectrum of this injury. Extension into one or both vertebral artery foramina is also common. The incidence of vertebral artery injury following fracture extension into the vascular foramen is unknown.

The lateral view of the cervical spine demonstrates the fracture in more than 90% of patients. Prevertebral hematoma is found in patients with associated disc disruption. The fracture lines run obliquely in a superopos-

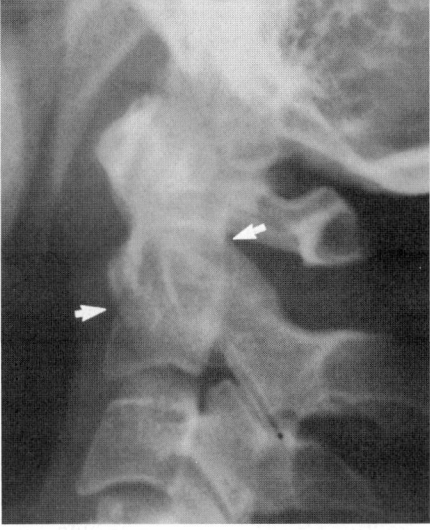

**Figure 58–11.** Type 3 odontoid fracture. Disruption of the "ring shadow" of the axis is seen on the lateral view *(arrows)*, owing to extension of the fracture lines into the C2 vertebral body.

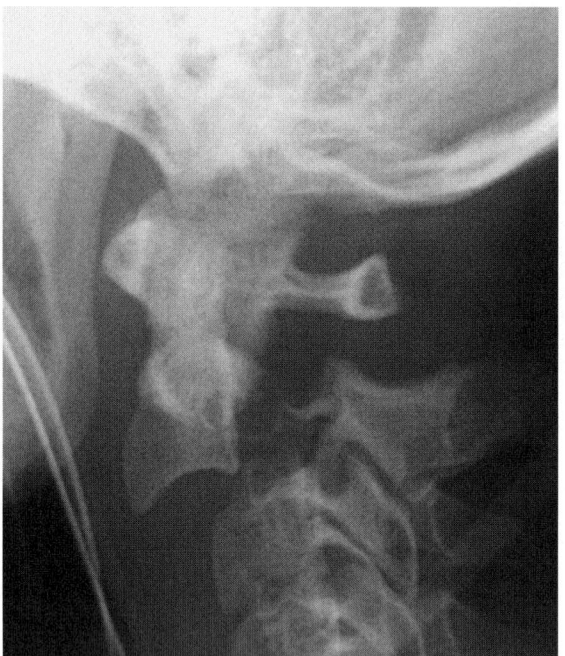

**Figure 58–12.** Hangman's fracture. Fractures through the pars interarticularis on both sides of the axis are present, with marked anterior displacement of the C2 vertebral body. Note the lack of concomitant anterior displacement of the spinolaminar line.

terior to anteroinferior direction and are located immediately anterior to the inferior articular facet. Anterior subluxation of the C2 vertebral body relative to the body of C3 typically is present. In addition, retrolisthesis of the posterior elements of C2 relative to those of C3 may be present. Retrolisthesis can be recognized by noting posterior displacement of the spinolaminar line of C2 relative to C3. Displacement of this line by 2 to 3 mm is a normal variant seen in both children and adults. CT scanning may be necessary for the detection of undisplaced fractures of the pars interarticularis. CT scans demonstrate the fracture lines, their extension into the vertebral foramina, and displaced bony fragments to better advantage than does routine radiography.

Although this injury is generally considered unstable, usually little neurologic damage occurs, owing to decompression of the spinal canal by the separated fragments (Fig. 58–13). The paucity of neurologic injury contrasts with the immediate death produced by hanging with the use of a "long drop" and a submental knot. In hanging, the hyperextension force is sustained and associated with tensile injury to the bone, soft tissues, and spinal cord owing to the gravitational pull of the body across the injury site.

Other fractures that frequently involve C2 are the extension teardrop fracture (Fig. 58–14) and avulsion fractures seen in association with hyperextension dislocation. These two injuries account for 19% of all C2 injuries. The extension teardrop fracture characteristically does not produce any neurologic impairment, whereas the avulsion fracture associated with extension dislocation is accompanied by an acute cervical central cord syndrome. Extension teardrop fractures can occur at any cervical level but are most common at C2. The extension teardrop fracture of C2 is more common in older patients with osteoporosis or underlying cervical spondylosis.

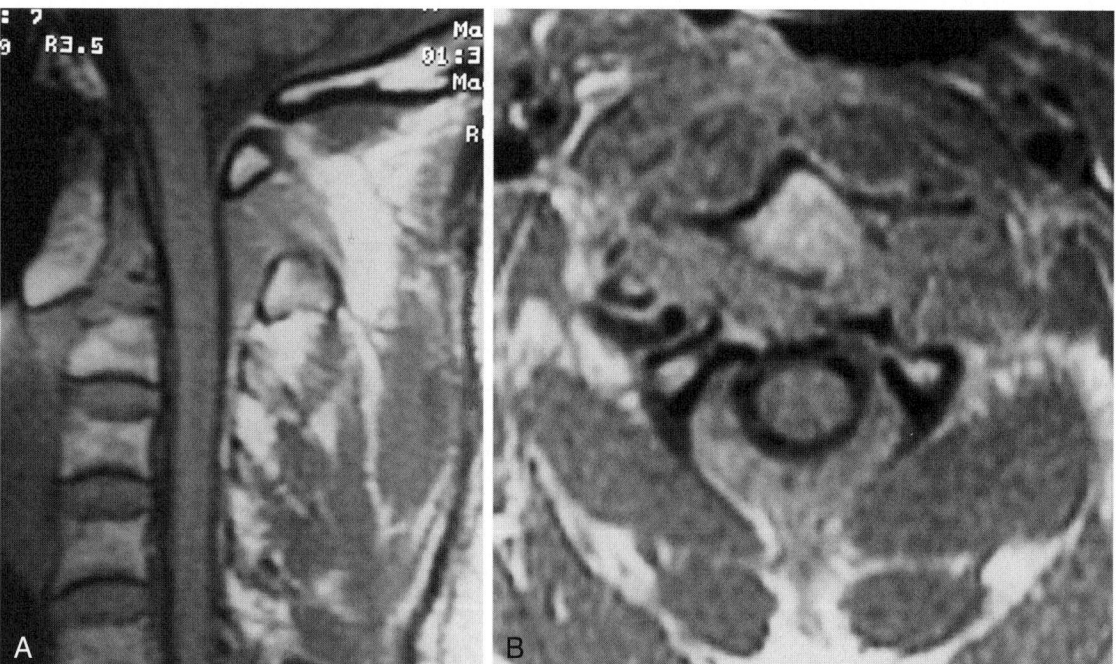

**Figure 58–13.** Hangman's fracture. Sagittal *(A)* and transverse *(B)* T1-weighted (TR/TE, 600/20) spin echo MR images of a patient with a type 2 hangman's fracture. *A,* Hangman's fracture extends into the C2 vertebral body at its posteroinferior corner. The C2 vertebral body is displaced anteriorly. *B,* The left vertebral artery canal is involved in the fracture, and the normal flow void of the vertebral artery is absent. The patient had no clinical evidence of vascular compromise.

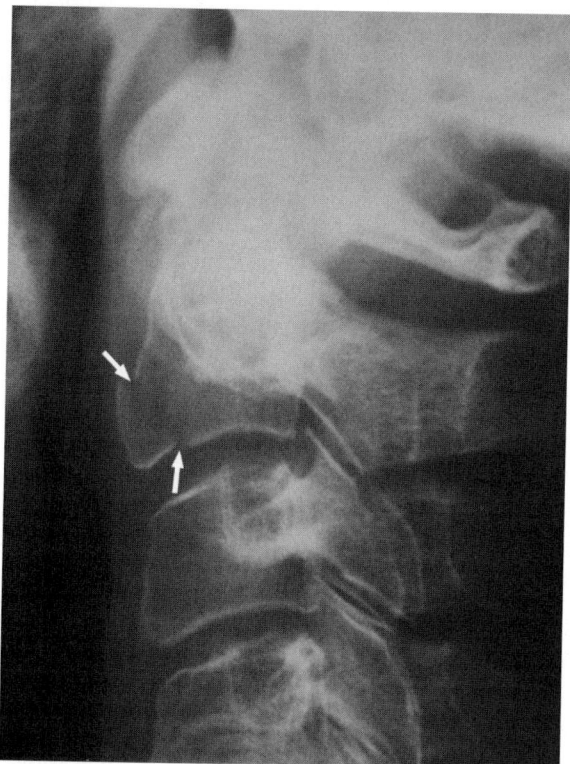

**Figure 58–14.** C2 extension teardrop fracture. A triangular fracture *(arrows)* is present at the anteroinferior margin of the axis. Note that the height of the fragment exceeds its width.

## LOWER CERVICAL REGION

### General Considerations

Fractures of the lower cervical spine are extremely common. It is estimated that 65% to 81% of nonfatal vertebral injuries in adults involve this region. Unlike the situation with fractures of the cervicocranium, radiographic evaluation of injuries in the lower cervical spine is often used to predict the mechanism of injury. Most injuries are due to hyperextension or hyperflexion, either alone or combined with rotation. Axial loading, lateral bending, and shearing account for a much smaller proportion of lower cervical injuries.

### Hyperextension Injuries

Hyperextension of the lower cervical spine is a common mechanism of injury, accounting for 25% to 50% of all cervical injuries. Hyperextension injuries occur as a result of abrupt deceleration, most commonly during motor vehicle accidents involving rear-end collisions and deceleration hyperextension or whiplash injury. The force in hyperextension is maximal in the lower cervical region, at C5 and C6. Many hyperextension injuries in the lower cervical region reveal few or no radiographic abnormalities, even when the injury is unstable or results in severe neurologic damage. Lower cervical injuries associated with hyperextension include avulsion of the ring apophysis, extension teardrop fracture, hyperextension dislocation, and hyperextension sprain.

**Avulsion of the Ring Apophysis.** In the immature spine, hyperextension may produce an avulsion fracture of the inferior ring apophysis. Its appearance is similar to that of the avulsion fracture that occurs with hyperextension in the adult spine. However, unlike its adult counterpart, the apophyseal avulsion fracture characteristically is not associated with soft tissue swelling or other osseous injury. Follow-up examinations show that healing occurs with the formation of a pronounced bone excrescence in the inferior vertebral margin, related to fusion of the avulsed apophysis with the underlying vertebral body.

**Extension Teardrop Fracture.** The extension teardrop fracture is an avulsion fracture that arises from the antero-inferior corner of a vertebral body. The axis is involved most commonly, and the fracture usually is not associated with any neurologic deficit. Unlike the flexion teardrop fracture, the triangular fracture produced by hyperextension is small; its size does not exceed one quarter of the sagittal diameter of the vertebral body. It is not associated with vertebral body displacement, a feature that is typically present in flexion teardrop injuries. The most characteristic feature is that the vertical height of this fracture fragment exceeds its horizontal dimension.

**Hyperextension Dislocation.** This injury occurs when the spine is hyperextended without any associated axial compression. The C5–C6 level is affected most frequently, followed by C4–C5. Hyperextension dislocation injuries occur when a traumatic force causes injury to the anterior longitudinal ligament and then either ruptures the disc or produces an avulsion fracture at the site of insertion of the anulus fibrosus.

This injury may produce no or very subtle radiographic alterations. In up to 30% of cases, prevertebral hematoma is the only radiographic finding. Thus, the diagnosis of hyperextension dislocation is based on the clinical findings and nonspecific radiographic indicators, such as soft tissue swelling. A hyperextension dislocation injury is often suspected because of the profound neurologic deficit produced, despite the paucity of radiographic findings.

Retrolisthesis of the vertebra above the discal injury is often present but may be of minimal degree. Retrolisthesis is seen in 20% of patients with hyperextension-induced cord damage (Fig. 58–15). The characteristic avulsion fracture seen in hyperextension dislocation appears as a thin, linear shadow arising from the inferior vertebral endplate. This fracture is produced by avulsion at the site of attachment of Sharpey's fibers and is typically wider than it is tall. Because no fracture occurs in a large number of cases, this injury is often difficult to recognize radiographically and is probably underreported.

**Hyperextension Sprain.** In a spondylitic spine, hyperextension dislocation can cause neurologic deficit, even in the absence of ligament damage or frank vertebral displacement, and radiographs may be normal. This injury, often referred to as a hyperextension sprain, does not result in significant disruption of the spinal ligaments, osseous structures, or discs. In a hyperextension sprain, neurologic damage is sustained during the injury, but

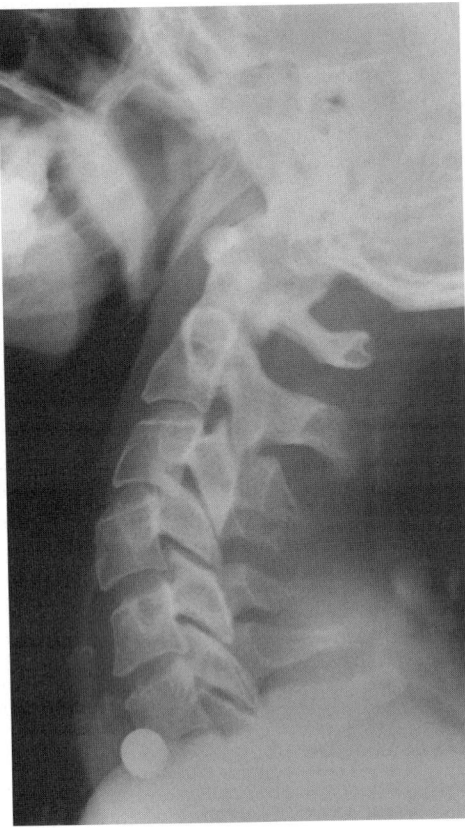

**Figure 58–15.** Hyperextension injury: retrolisthesis and focal hyperlordosis. This woman injured her spine 2 weeks before this radiograph was taken. The initial radiograph (not shown) appeared normal. This view was obtained in active supervised extension of the neck. There is focal increased lordosis at the C3–C4 level, and there is more than 5 mm of retrolisthesis of the C3 vertebral body relative to C4.

spinal stability is maintained. Distinction between a sprain and a reduced dislocation may be impossible on the basis of conventional radiographic findings. In both hyperextension sprain and hyperextension dislocation, severe neurologic damage is thought to occur when the spinal cord is caught between the posterior margin of the vertebral body or posterior osteophytes and the infolded ligamenta flava, particularly in a spondylitic spine. The characteristic neurologic defect in hyperextension sprain is the central cord syndrome, related to hemorrhage in the central gray matter. MR imaging is the optimal method for evaluating patients with neurologic injuries whose radiographic findings are equivocal.

## Extension-Rotation Injuries

A combination of extension, compression, and rotation produces unilateral pillar or facet fractures, which represent 3% to 11% of all cervical spine fractures. Fractures of the lateral masses are more common than is generally appreciated because they are difficult to detect on conventional radiographs, and their true prevalence is underestimated. Facet fractures occur most commonly at C6 and C7 and result in radiculopathy in 6% to 39% of patients.

Fractures of the articular mass (pillar) are often difficult to visualize on frontal and lateral projections unless they are displaced or severely comminuted. The oblique projection is most useful for detecting fractures of the pillar region. Pillar views can also be used to evaluate the lateral masses. The pillar view is oriented tangentially to the facet joints and shows the lateral masses along their short axis. This view is obtained in the anteroposterior supine position with the head rotated maximally away from the facet joints that are being evaluated. The central ray is directed caudally at an angle of 35 degrees, entering at the inferior border of the thyroid cartilage. A single pillar view can be obtained by hyperextending the non-rotated head with the central ray directed 20 to 30 degrees caudally. Conventional tomography and CT scanning are more sensitive for detecting fractures of the articular process than are conventional radiographic projections. Because of the small size of the facets, fractures are best detected with CT using thin overlapping acquisitions with reformatted images.

## Hyperflexion Injuries

One of the most common, if not the most common, mechanisms resulting in cervical spine injury is hyperflexion of the cervical region. Indeed, 46% to 79% of all cervical injuries are due to hyperflexion. Hyperflexion injuries are usually caused by a blow to the posterior aspect of the cranium, forcing the face toward the chest.

**Hyperflexion Sprain.** Hyperflexion sprain is predominantly a ligamentous injury consisting of disruption of the ligaments of the posterior column and, in severe cases, the posterior longitudinal ligament and posterior portion of the anulus fibrosus in the middle column. The injury typically occurs in the absence of any fracture, although minor wedgelike compressions of the anterior portion of the vertebral body occasionally coexist. The injured ligaments, in order of disruption, are the supraspinous ligament, interspinous ligament, ligamenta flava, and capsule of the facet joint. Neurologic defect is usually mild and reversible. Approximately 20% to 33% of patients with posterior ligamentous disruption who are treated conservatively develop progressive kyphosis and delayed spinal instability.

Radiographs of the cervical spine frequently are normal despite the presence of a clinically evident cord injury. When radiographs are positive, widening of the interspinous distance or the posterior aspect of the apophyseal joints is evident. Interspinous widening that is more than 2 mm greater than the width at both adjacent levels has been suggested as a sensitive criterion of spinal instability. An interspinous distance that is more than 1.5 times the distance at both adjacent levels is definitely abnormal and indicates the presence of anterior cervical dislocation. Localized kyphotic angulation of the cervical spine is highly suggestive of this injury. Focally exaggerated kyphosis is required for diagnosis of the injury, because diffuse kyphosis of the cervical spine may result from voluntary flexion or muscle spasm. Another radiographic feature in patients with hyperflexion injury of the cervical spine is kyphosis at a single spinal level with persistent lordosis in the remaining portions of the cervical spine. If this injury is suspected, it has been suggested that supervised flexion and extension views of the cervical spine may help demonstrate these radiographic findings (Fig. 58–16).

**Hyperflexion Injury.** A pure hyperflexion injury of the spine may spare the posterior ligaments and result only in osseous disruption limited to the anterior vertebral column. In the immature cervical spine, flexion may produce an avulsion of the anterior portion of the superior vertebral ring apophysis. This injury characteristically is associated with other vertebral abnormalities, particularly compression fractures of the superior endplate. In adults, simple compression fractures of one or more vertebrae are encountered. The wedge compression fracture consists of comminution of the anterosuperior aspect of the endplate of that vertebral body, without concomitant injury to the posterior portion of the vertebral body, posterior bony elements, or spinal ligaments. These simple compression fractures are relatively benign injuries because they do not compromise the neural canal and generally heal uneventfully. The fracture is best seen on the lateral view and is manifested as loss of anterior vertebral height, buckling or step-off of the anterior or superior endplate (or both), and soft tissue swelling.

**Clay-Shoveler's Fracture.** The clay-shoveler's fracture is an oblique fracture of the spinous process of the sixth cervical through third thoracic vertebrae that results from avulsion by the supraspinous ligament. The injury derives its name from its common occurrence in Australian clay miners. The fracture may involve a single spinous process or multiple spinous processes (Fig. 58–17). The most commonly fractured level is C6 or C7, although the T1 and T2 vertebrae are also injured frequently. Isolated fractures of the spinous process are due to hyperflexion in most cases. These fractures are best seen on the lateral view, unless the spinous processes are obscured by overlying soft tissues. The anteroposterior view may show malalignment and displacement of the inferior tip of the involved spinous process. Occasionally, a "double spinous process" shadow, related to simultaneous visualization of the fractured base and the caudally displaced tip of the spinous process, is evident in this view.

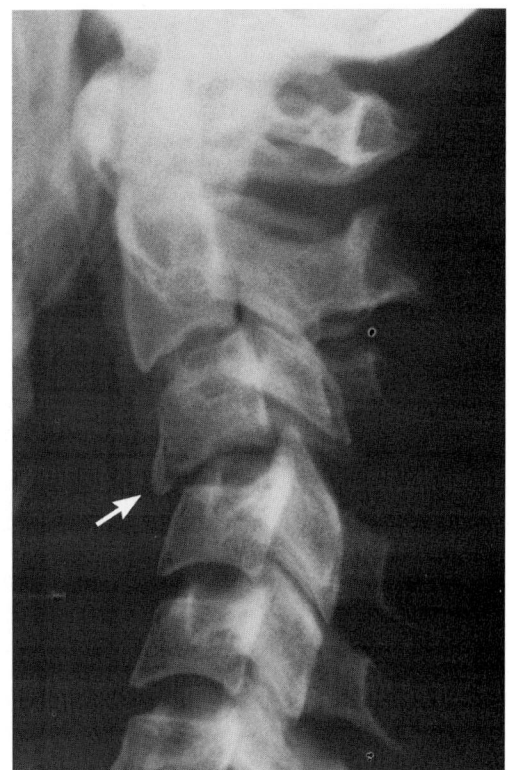

**Figure 58–16.** Hyperflexion injury. Lateral radiograph of the cervical spine obtained with flexion shows a subtle fracture of the third vertebral body *(arrow)*. Anterior displacement of the C3 vertebral body with respect to C4 is obvious. Note the narrowing of the anterior aspect of the intervening intervertebral disc and widening of the apophyseal joints and interspinous distance at this level. Vertebral alignment was normal in extension.

**Bilateral Facet Lock.** Bilateral facet lock represents an unstable injury resulting from severe flexion forces that cause complete ligamentous disruption of the posterior and middle spinal columns and variable disruption of the anterior spinal column. The horizontal orientation of the cervical facet joints allows dislocation to occur in the absence of bony disruption. Rupture of the posterior portion of the anulus fibrosus, the posterior longitudinal

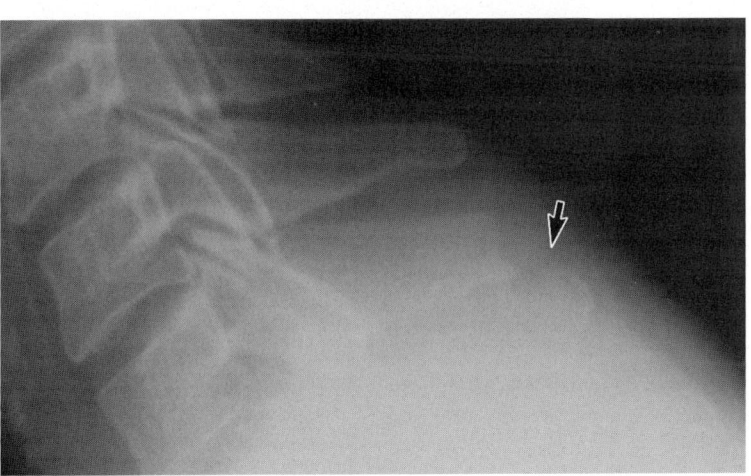

**Figure 58–17.** Fracture of the spinous process. Lateral view shows an isolated fracture of the tip of the spinous process of C6 *(arrow)* due to hyperflexion (clay-shoveler's fracture).

ligament, and the capsular, interspinous, and supraspinous ligaments invariably is present. As the facet joints lock, marked narrowing of the spinal canal and intervertebral neural foramen results. Such narrowing leads to a neurologic deficit in up to 75% of patients with this injury. Vascular injury to the vertebral artery has been shown to be a common complication of facet joint dislocation, although the vascular lesion is typically asymptomatic or associated with nonspecific findings.

Bilateral facet lock is recognized easily on lateral radiographs, owing to the severe spinal malalignment. Anterior displacement of the superior vertebra invariably is present and typically is greater than half the width of the vertebral body (Fig. 58–18). On transverse CT scans and MR images, this injury produces the naked facet sign bilaterally, whereby the articular surfaces of both apophyseal joints at one spinal level are no longer in apposition.

**Flexion Teardrop Fracture.** Flexion teardrop fractures, like bilateral facet locks, are highly unstable injuries that characteristically result in severe neurologic deficit. Complete quadriplegia, paraplegia, Brown-Séquard syndrome, or the anterior cord syndrome develops in 87% of patients with this injury. The characteristic neurologic deficit is the anterior cord syndrome, consisting of complete motor paralysis and partial sensory dysfunction, with loss of pain, touch, and temperature sensations but preservation of posterior column function. This injury is the result of combined flexion and axial loading, with the most common inciting events being diving and motor vehicle accidents. The flexion teardrop injury typically

involves the lower cervical spine, with C5 being the most common level of involvement. The vertebral body is divided into a smaller anteroinferior fragment and a larger posterior fragment (Fig. 58–19). The anteroinferior teardrop fragment may be large and often involves one third to one half of the vertebral body. The teardrop fragment typically remains aligned with the vertebral body below or shows minimal anterior and downward displacement. The most specific finding in this injury is posterior displacement of the inferior aspect of the larger posterior fragment of the fractured vertebral body relative to the vertebra below. The most commonly associated fracture is a sagittal vertebral body fracture.

## Flexion-Rotation Injuries

Unilateral facet lock is the only common cervical injury produced by the combination of flexion and rotation and represents between 4% and 16% of all cervical spine injuries. Rupture of the interspinous ligament and the capsule of the apophyseal joint allows the ipsilateral inferior facet of one vertebra to pivot, dislocate, and come to rest in the neural foramen anterior to the superior facet of the vertebra below. The spinal cord is impinged on by the posterosuperior aspect of the body below and by the lamina above. The most common levels of involvement are C4–C5 and C5–C6. Although this injury is considered mechanically stable, the presence of neurologic damage or an associated facet fracture should suggest potential mechanical and neurologic instability.

Unilateral facet lock produces alterations of spinal alignment on the lateral and anteroposterior projections but is easiest to recognize on oblique views. Anterior subluxation of the superior vertebra is typically present, but the degree of subluxation is less than that seen with bilateral facet lock, averaging one quarter of the sagittal

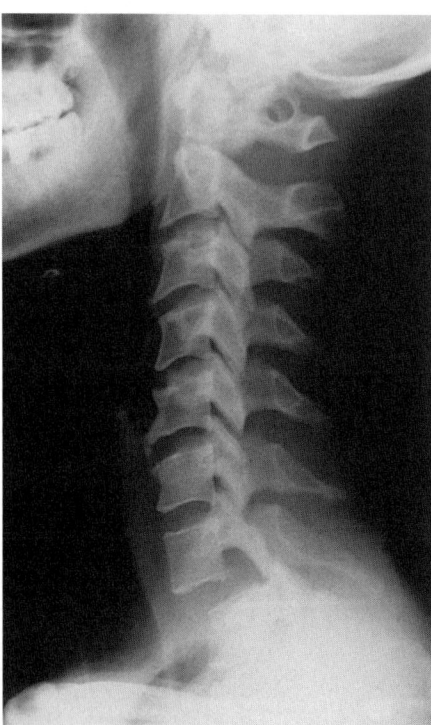

**Figure 58–18.** Bilateral facet lock: radiographic findings. Bilateral facet locks at the C7–T1 vertebral level show marked anterolisthesis and lack of rotation at the injured level.

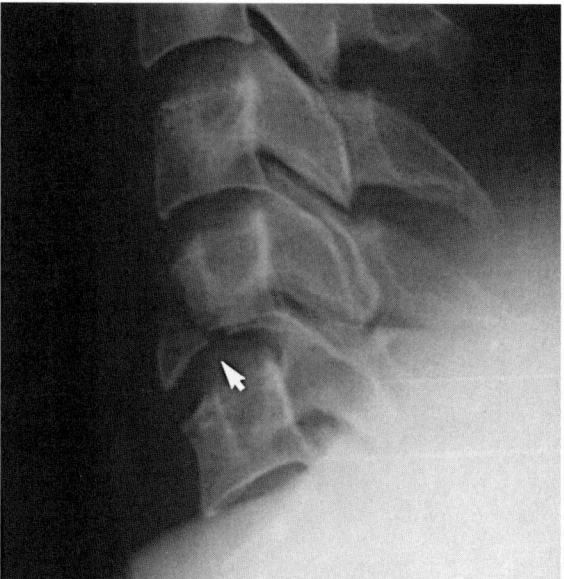

**Figure 58–19.** Flexion teardrop fracture. Triangular fracture *(arrow)* of the anteroinferior margin of the C5 vertebral body is present. Posterior displacement of this vertebral body is minimal.

diameter of the vertebral body. The magnitude of the anterolisthesis is never greater than half this sagittal diameter. The lateral view demonstrates abrupt rotation of the facet joints at the level of the dislocation, with loss of normal superimposition of the paired facets at and superior to the level of injury (Fig. 58–20). The vertebrae above the lock are seen in the oblique rather than the lateral projection, as are the caudal vertebrae. Displacement and rotation of the articular facets produce the classic "bow-tie" appearance, formed by the anteriorly displaced facet above and the normally positioned facet below.

The anteroposterior view demonstrates rotation of the spinous processes at the site of the lock, with lateral step-off of the spinous processes above the site of injury. Associated fractures typically involve the vertebral bodies and spinous processes. On CT scans, facet subluxation can be recognized by noting the malalignment of the articular processes. With facet subluxation and perched facets, the "naked" facet sign is seen, in which a bare articular surface is visualized without its corresponding articular facet. With a frank lock, the convex portions of the joints, rather than the straight portions, are in contact; the flat articular portions of the facets form the anterior and posterior margins of the joint on the side of the lock (Fig. 58–21). Associated uncovertebral joint subluxation at the level of the injury, due to rotation of one vertebral body relative to the other, is often present.

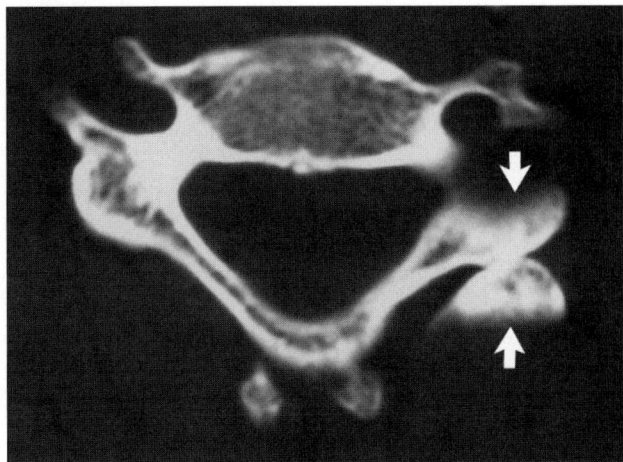

**Figure 58–21.** Unilateral facet lock. Transaxial CT scan of a unilateral left-sided facet lock shows that the straight articular surfaces (*arrows*) no longer are in contact. The curved, nonarticular bony margins are in abnormal contact, denoting a facet lock.

## Lateral Hyperflexion Injuries

Lateral hyperflexion injuries are caused by a force delivered directly to the lateral aspect of the skull or cervical spine. The most well known fracture produced by this mechanism is unilateral lateral wedging of the vertebral body and its associated lateral mass. However, a variety of other osseous injuries can result from lateral bending, including transverse process fracture, uncinate process fracture, laterally displaced odontoid fracture, brachial plexopathy in association with a cervical fracture or dislocation, and lateral wedge-type fracture of a vertebral body. Associated fractures of the neural arches, similar to those occurring in extension, are present in the majority of patients. These injuries are uncommon and represent only 6% of all injuries to the cervical spine. The degree of neurologic deficit varies, depending on the level of injury and its severity; death, complete quadriplegia, and minor transient deficits have all been documented.

## Axial Loading Injuries

Burst fractures of the cervical vertebrae are typically the result of combined flexion and axial loading. This type of fracture is seen predominantly in areas of the spine capable of voluntary straightening, such as the occipitocervical junction, lower portion of the cervical spine, and thoracolumbar spine. Of these three sites, burst fractures of the lower cervical spine are the least common. Neurologic deficit is common.

Burst fractures of the cervical spine characteristically result in retropulsion of the posterosuperior vertebral margin into the spinal canal (Fig. 58–22). Sagittal vertebral widening and the presence of retropulsed bone may lead to confusion with a flexion teardrop injury, but the burst fracture lacks the characteristic anteroinferior triangular fragment, is more comminuted, exhibits more loss of vertebral height, and is not associated with cervical kyphosis, interspinous fanning, or subluxation of the facet

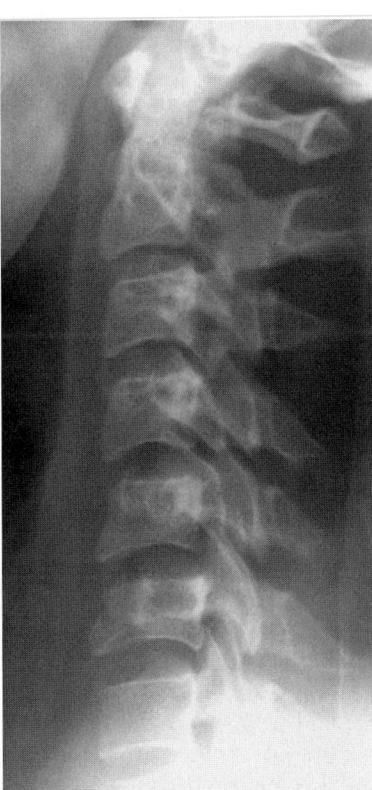

**Figure 58–20.** Unilateral facet dislocation. A unilateral facet lock is present at the C5–C6 spinal level, with a fracture of the anteroinferior margin of the C6 vertebral body. Note the minimal anterolisthesis in this patient. The facet joints at the C6 and C7 levels are superimposed normally, whereas all the facet joints above the level of the unilateral lock are rotated.

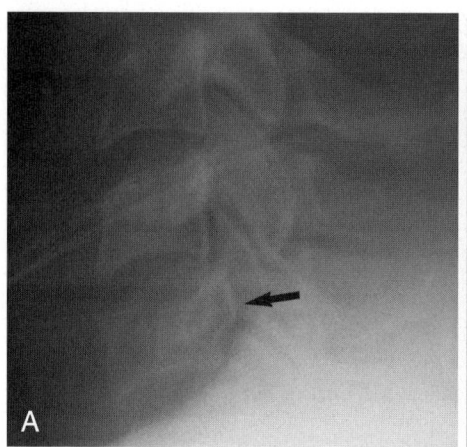
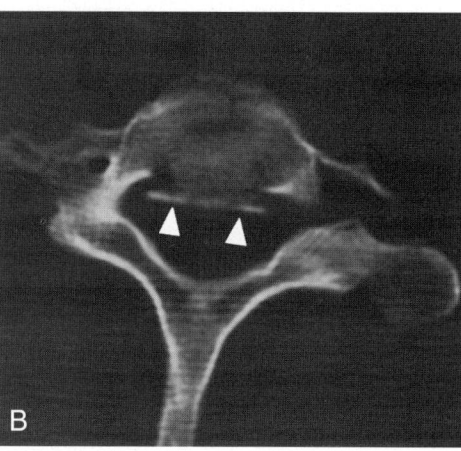

**Figure 58–22.** Cervical burst fracture. *A,* Lateral radiograph demonstrates loss of height of the C7 vertebral body with retropulsed bone *(arrow)* within the spinal canal. *B,* Transaxial CT scan shows the displaced bone *(arrowheads)* narrowing the spinal canal.

joints. The flexion teardrop fracture is grossly unstable, whereas burst fractures typically maintain the integrity of the ligaments of the posterior spinal column. On the anteroposterior view, burst fractures characteristically are associated with a sagittal fracture line that extends across the entire height of the involved vertebral body. This sagittal fracture line is difficult to appreciate on conventional radiographs but may be recognized on a well-penetrated anteroposterior view.

## UPPER THORACIC SPINE

### General Considerations

If compression deformities secondary to osteoporosis are excluded, fractures of the thoracic spine above the thoracolumbar junction are uncommon. It has been estimated that only 30% of all traumatic thoracic fractures occur above the T10 level. The majority of significant upper thoracic spine injuries are due to motor vehicle accidents or falls. The magnitude of force necessary to overcome the inherent stability of the upper thoracic spine is greater than that required for the remainder of the spine. The relatively small cross-sectional area of the spinal canal in the upper thoracic region, combined with the high force necessary to create an unstable injury in this region, leads to a high rate of neurologic damage when such injury occurs.

### Imaging Studies

The initial radiographic examination of the traumatized upper thoracic spine consists of supine anteroposterior and lateral radiographs. The upper four thoracic vertebrae are particularly difficult to see on lateral radiographs. A modified swimmer's view can be helpful for evaluating the upper vertebral bodies, but this projection requires arm movement. In some patients, conventional tomography or CT scanning is necessary to assess a suspected injury of the upper thoracic region.

The majority of acute fractures are associated with the development of a focal paraspinal hematoma that is centered at the level of injury. A hemothorax is also common in association with severe spinal injury. Mediastinal widening, paraspinal hematoma, and left apical capping are features that can be seen in both vertebral and vascular injuries.

## Compression Fracture

Compression fractures of the midthoracic spine are common in patients with osteoporosis. Eighteen percent of white women older than 50 years demonstrate at least one compression fracture, and prevalence rates approach 78% among women older than 90 years. These fractures typically result from flexion or axial forces, or both, producing compression loading of the vertebral body. The cancellous bone of the vertebral body is weaker in compression than in tension. The force required to fracture the vertebral body in an osteoporotic person can be trivial. The distribution of acute compression fractures is bimodal, with one peak at the T6–T7 level and the second, larger peak at the thoracolumbar junction. Typical compression fractures cause localized pain and kyphosis but generally do not manifest any acute neurologic deficit. Paraspinal swelling, loss of vertebral height, and cortical disruption are apparent (Fig. 58–23). By definition, the middle column is intact in compression fractures, so there is no loss of height of the posterior margin of the vertebral body and no vertebral subluxation. The anteroposterior view may show interspinous widening in geometric proportion to the degree of anterior vertebral wedging.

Typical compression fractures result in failure confined to the anterior column. Because the middle column is normal, this injury is generally considered stable. The major risk factor for early kyphosis after traumatic compression fractures in nonosteoporotic patients is the presence of multiple fractures in the upper thoracic region. Conversely, progressive kyphosis is rare with fractures at the thoracolumbar region. Anterior wedging that is greater than 50% of the height of the vertebral body allows the middle column to act as a fulcrum, potentially leading to damage to the posterior ligamentous complex. Less commonly, nontraumatic compression fractures manifest both anterior and middle column failure, resulting in fractures with a configuration similar to that of burst fractures, with retropulsed fragments of bone and potential neurologic compromise.

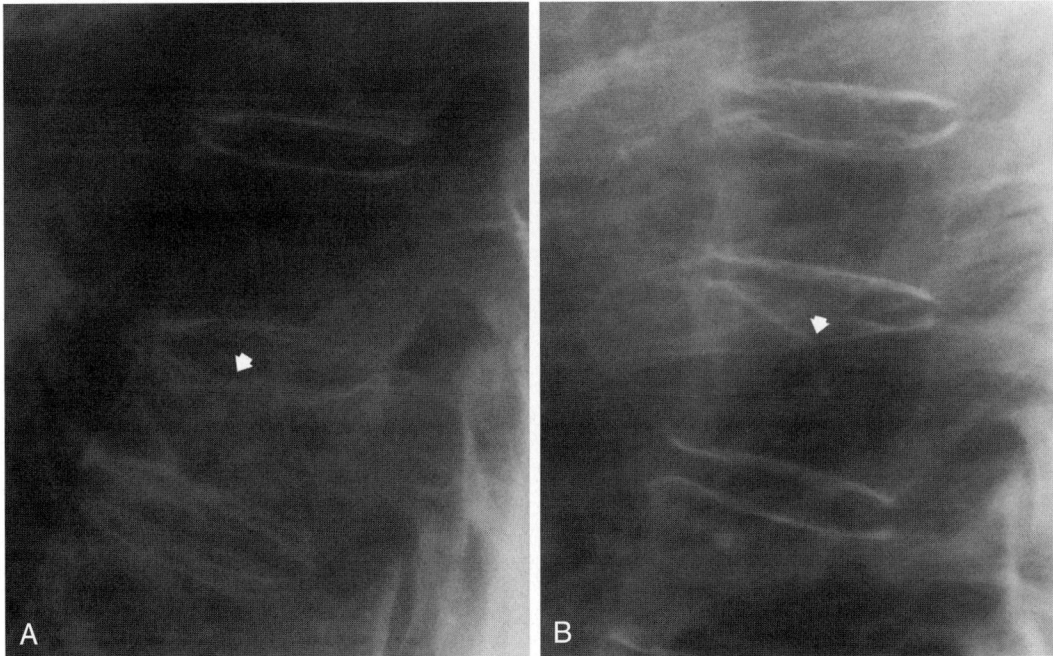

**Figure 58–23.** Compression fracture. *A,* Lateral radiograph reveals compression of the anterior and middle portions of the superior endplate *(arrow),* with loss of height of the vertebral body anteriorly. *B,* Central compression fracture of the seventh thoracic vertebral body produces a central deformity *(arrow)* of the superior endplate, with preservation of height of the vertebral body anteriorly and posteriorly.

Middle and lower thoracic compression deformities are encountered in elderly patients. Solitary compression fractures related to osteoporosis are uncommon above the seventh thoracic vertebra. Identification of an isolated compression fracture in the high thoracic region suggests a cause other than simple osteoporosis. Distinguishing benign compression fractures from pathologic fractures can be very difficult. Radiographs, CT scans, and MR images can all be used to determine the cause of nontraumatic fractures. The typical deformity of the vertebral endplates in osteoporotic compression fractures consists of anterior wedging, diffuse compression, or central compression with smooth, diffuse concavity of the upper or lower endplate. Biconcavity caused by depression of both the upper and lower endplates has been termed "fish vertebra." Fish vertebrae typically are seen at the thoracolumbar or lower lumbar level; the characteristic deformity created by osteoporotic compression fractures in the upper thoracic spine is kyphosis, with anterior collapse or wedging of the vertebral body.

The signal intensity characteristics of an acutely fractured vertebra on MR images are nonspecific. With MR imaging, preservation of normal fatty marrow within the compressed vertebral body is a reliable indicator of a benign fracture that is probably chronic (Fig. 58–24). Incomplete replacement of the bone marrow adjacent to the fracture can be seen in about 25% of vertebral compression fractures, particularly acute fractures. Complete replacement of the bone marrow generally occurs when vertebral compression is related to the presence of skeletal metastasis. The presence of posterior retropulsed bone is more common with benign fractures, whereas convexity

and bulging of the posterior vertebral cortex suggest that the vertebral body has been replaced by tumor. Both acute benign and pathologic fractures show low signal intensity on T1-weighted MR images and high signal intensity on T2-weighted and short tau inversion recovery (STIR) MR images, but the pattern of increased signal intensity is less homogeneous and less intense in cases of benign fracture. Marrow replacement is often partial and bandlike in the presence of a benign fracture, whereas the entire body is more likely to show signal abnormalities if the fracture is pathologic. Benign fractures tend to show a return to normal marrow signal intensity following the intravenous administration of a gadolinium-containing contrast agent, whereas pathologic fractures show increased signal intensity within the affected vertebra on both T1- and T2-weighted images.

### Fracture in Children and Adolescents

Upper thoracic fractures in very young children must be evaluated carefully. This region is rarely traumatized in this age group, so underlying neoplasm, seizures, or child abuse must be considered. Compression fractures of the vertebral bodies, vertebral subluxation, and avulsion fractures of the spinous processes in the thoracic spine are known to occur in abused infants. The most common spinal abnormality in an abused child consists of a superior endplate compression fracture, producing notching of the anterior aspect of the vertebral body, associated with mild disc space narrowing. Forceful shaking, resulting in repetitive flexion and extension of the infant's trunk, is the presumed mechanism for the injuries to the verte-

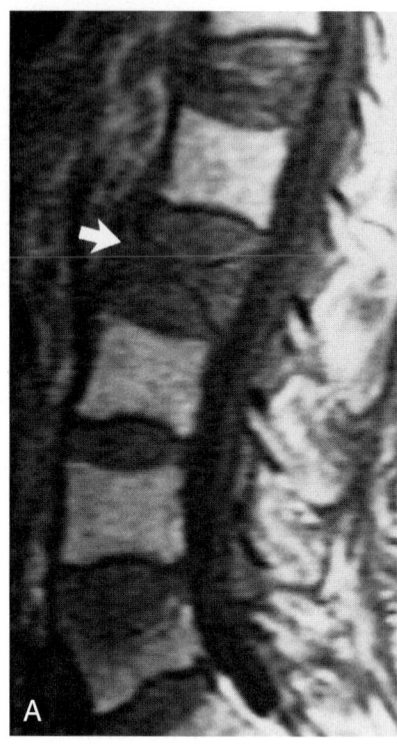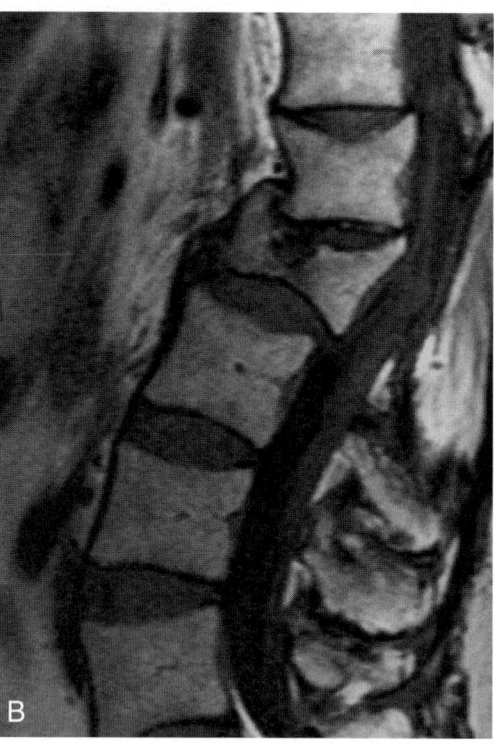

**Figure 58–24.** Compression fracture. *A*, Sagittal T1-weighted (TR/TE, 600/20) spin echo MR image shows diffuse loss of marrow signal intensity at the collapsed T12 and L2 levels *(arrow)*. The collapsed L5 vertebral body shows normal fat signal intensity at its inferior aspect. Biopsy of the L2 vertebral body revealed a healing fracture, and the patient had no evidence of malignancy at long-term follow-up. *B*, Sagittal T1-weighted (TR/TE, 600/20) spin echo MR image in a patient with chronic osteoporotic fractures shows deformity of the vertebral bodies but preservation of normal fat signal within the marrow space.

bral body and spinous process. Other manifestations of child abuse, such as skull and rib fractures, as well as the characteristic metaphyseal fractures, are typically present.

In older children and adolescents, exaggerated vertebral wedging, vertebral endplate irregularities, Schmorl's nodes, and disc space narrowing are characteristic of Scheuermann's disease. Although numerous theories have been advanced to explain this common condition, the most likely cause of Scheuermann's disease is repetitive traumatic stress to the growing spine. Although Schmorl's nodes are a constant finding in Scheuermann's disease, such lesions are more often seen as an isolated finding on lateral spinal radiographs. A Schmorl's node represents a site of displacement of the nucleus pulposus into the vertebral body via a defect in the vertebral endplate. It appears as a well-defined rounded or hemispheric lucent lesion with a thin sclerotic margin abutting a vertebral endplate. These intraosseous extensions of the disc are very common, found in 36% to 79% of cadaveric studies. MR imaging obtained after the intravenous administration of a gadolinium-containing contrast agent shows enhancement surrounding the Schmorl's node, as well as adjacent bone marrow edema, in up to 19% of such lesions.

## Kümmell's Disease

Kümmell's disease is a form of delayed, post-traumatic collapse of the vertebral body that occurs weeks or even months after an injury. The most widely accepted mechanism for Kümmell's disease is osteonecrosis. The presence of gas within the vertebral body, also known as the intravertebral vacuum cleft, suggest that the basis

for Kümmell's disease may be ischemia associated with trauma, which leads to osteonecrosis and delayed collapse of the vertebral body. Almost all reported cases of intravertebral vacuum clefts occur in noninfectious and non-neoplastic conditions.

The typical vacuum cleft appears as a transverse radiolucent line seen in the centrum of the collapsed vertebral body or adjacent to one of its endplates. This linear intraosseous gas collection must be differentiated from the common finding of gas within a degenerated disc. The vacuum cleft is exaggerated by spinal extension, particularly in the lateral decubitus position, and diminishes with spinal flexion and prolonged supine positioning. On CT scans, the gas collection may appear more inhomogeneous and irregular than it does on plain films. On MR images, gas is of low signal intensity on all sequences, with magnetic inhomogeneity effects evident on gradient echo images (Fig. 58–25). This thin, linear, horizontal collection of high signal intensity located centrally within the vertebral body is suggestive of vertebral osteonecrosis.

## Fracture-Dislocation

Fracture-dislocation is an unstable injury usually resulting from a combination of hyperflexion and axial loading of the vertebrae, combined with ligamentous disruption by rotatory and shear forces. These severe injuries are associated with a very high rate of neurologic injury. Most injuries resulting in complete paraplegia occur in the mid-dorsal spine, with the majority located at the T3 to T8 levels (Fig. 58–26). The combination of the severe force necessary to cause vertebral injury and the relatively small cross-sectional area of the spinal canal in the upper thoracic spine makes this area particularly vulnerable to spinal cord damage. Rarely, thoracic spine translocation occurs without the development of a neurologic deficit.

Unfortunately, most patients with an upper thoracic fracture-dislocation develop an intrinsic cord lesion or severe cord compression. The typical injury produced by this combination is a fracture-dislocation involving two adjacent vertebrae and all the intervening soft tissues. A predominantly osseous injury or a mixture of osseous and soft tissue injuries may be evident; pure soft tissue injury disrupting all three columns is rare. The more superior vertebral body may show a variety of fractures, with avulsion fractures of its inferior margin being most common. The superior vertebra is subluxed anteriorly with respect to the inferior vertebra. The intervening disc and interspinous ligaments are disrupted, and the disc may be herniated. Rotational deformity, manifested by rotatory malalignment of the pedicles and spinous processes above and below the injury, may also be seen.

CT scanning and MR imaging can be used to evaluate these complex injuries. Typically, the malalignment and degree of displacement are assessed more readily using MR imaging. CT scanning is superior for identifying fractures of the posterior elements and determining the extent of encroachment on the spinal canal by displaced bone fragments. MR imaging is the method of choice for evaluation of the spinal cord, which is often injured in association with upper thoracic injuries.

## THORACOLUMBAR SPINE

### General Considerations

The thoracolumbar junction is one of the most commonly injured areas of the spine. This region is particularly vulnerable because of its wide range of motion, a facet joint orientation that changes from a sagittal to a coronal plane, and the absence of significant adjacent supporting structures, such as the rib cage or psoas muscles. Most injuries in this region are secondary to pure flexion or to flexion combined with compression, rotatory, or distraction forces. Spinal flexion results in distraction forces posteriorly and compression forces anteriorly.

Major injuries of the thoracolumbar region can be divided into four types (Table 58–2). The first type is the compression fracture resulting from hyperflexion, with compression of only the anterior column and an intact middle column; the majority of these fractures are associated with a normal posterior column as well. In severe anterior compressive injuries, partial failure of the posterior column related to tension may be present. The second category of major injury is the burst fracture, characterized by failure of both the anterior and middle columns in compression. The posterior column remains intact functionally, although fractures of the lamina and splaying of the facet joints are often present. The third major

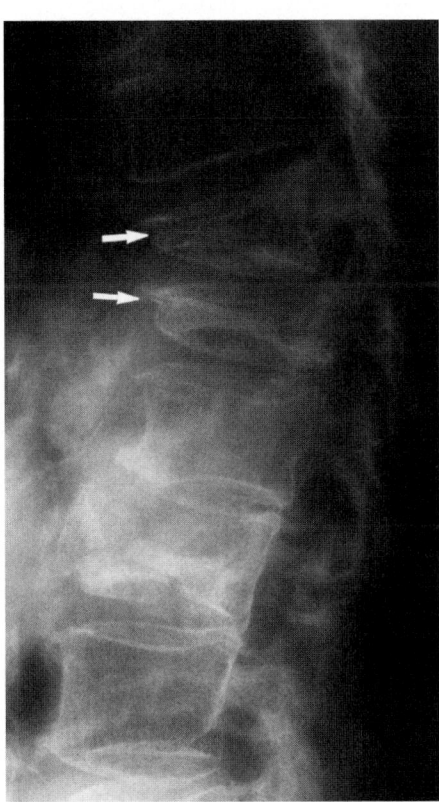

**Figure 58–25.** Kümmell's disease. Lateral radiograph illustrates multiple thoracic and lumbar compression fractures. Horizontal collections of gas are present within the T12 and L1 vertebral bodies (*arrows*), indicating osteonecrosis.

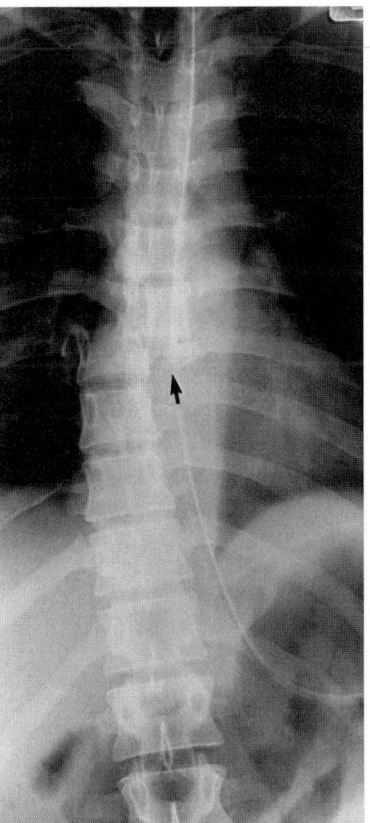

**Figure 58–26.** Thoracic fracture-dislocation. Dislocation is present at the T7–T8 spinal level, with lateral displacement and telescoping of the spine at the injured level. The T8 vertebral body has an oblique fracture within its substance. A small portion of the left T8 vertebral centrum (*arrow*) remains aligned with T7.

**TABLE 58–2**

### Major Fractures and Dislocations of the Thoracolumbar Spine

| | Site of Injury | | |
| --- | --- | --- | --- |
| Type of Injury | *Anterior Column* | *Middle Column* | *Posterior Column* |
| Compression fracture | Compression | None | None or distraction |
| Burst fracture | Compression | Compression | None |
| Seat-belt injury | None or compression | Distraction | Distraction |
| Fracture-dislocation | Compression, rotation, shear | Distraction, rotation, shear | Distraction, rotation, shear |

From Denis F: The three column spine and its significance in the classification of acute thoracolumbar spinal injuries. Spine 8:817, 1983.

category, the seat-belt–type injury, represents failure in tension of both the middle and posterior columns as a result of spinal flexion and, in some cases, additional distraction. The anterior column may fail partially due to compression, but the anterior longitudinal ligament maintains its ability to act as a "hinge." The last major category is the fracture-dislocation. In this injury, all three columns are disrupted owing to a combination of compression, tension, rotation, and shear. The spine is free to subluxate or dislocate, although radiographs may show little malalignment in the resting position. Most patients with this injury demonstrate vertebral subluxation or dislocation at the time of initial presentation. Malalignment in the sagittal, coronal, or transaxial plane may be translational or rotatory.

Supine anteroposterior and cross-table lateral radiographs constitute an adequate screening examination for the thoracolumbar region in the setting of trauma. Collimated coned views centered on the thoracolumbar region can be very helpful, because this area is not well seen in the conventional thoracic and lumbar projections. Most injuries to the thoracolumbar region produce kyphosis, which is often reduced in the supine position. Soft tissue alterations due to thoracolumbar injuries, unlike injuries of the upper thoracic spine, are absent on conventional radiographs.

### Compression Fracture

The thoracolumbar region is the most common site of traumatic compression fractures, and it is also a major site of fractures resulting from trivial injury in persons with osteoporosis. The most common sites of involvement are L1 and L2, followed in frequency by T12, T7, and L3. Most traumatic compression fractures occur between T12 and L2. Among osteoporotic compression fractures, a large proportion involve the thoracolumbar region, although the midthoracic region shows a slightly higher prevalence of compression deformities.

The typical thoracolumbar compression fracture results in loss of height of the anterior vertebral body, with preservation of the middle and posterior spinal columns. In severe compression fractures, partial or complete posterior ligamentous injury may be present. The usual treatment for these injuries is conservative. Progressive kyphosis is unusual after thoracolumbar compression

fracture in a nonosteoporotic person. Vertebral compression that leads to loss of more than 40% of the height of the anterior portion of the vertebral body often requires posterior stabilization, even in the absence of neurologic deficit, to prevent progressive spinal deformity.

In uncomplicated vertebral body fractures, the intervertebral disc remains intact, and no disc space loss is apparent. On CT scans, compression fractures of the thoracolumbar region can be recognized by the presence of an arc of irregular bony fragments displaced circumferentially from the vertebral body. The posterior vertebral wall remains intact, and no retropulsed fragments of bone are present. Fracture lines involving the vertebral body typically involve only its superior aspect, with normal bone seen below the level of the pedicles.

### Burst Fracture

Axial loading, or compression, of the vertebral body, usually combined with flexion, produces the commonly seen burst fracture. Burst fractures represent 1.5% of all spinal fractures and 14% of thoracolumbar injuries. The peak site of spinal burst fractures is the thoracolumbar junction, with T12, L1, and L2 being the most common levels involved. The majority of such fractures are associated with neurologic deficit. Burst fractures can occur only in the spinal segments with the ability to straighten—the cervical and thoracolumbar regions.

Characteristic components of this injury are centripetal disruption, increased sagittal diameter, and moderate to marked anterior wedging of the vertebral body; unilateral or bilateral laminar fractures; an increased interpediculate distance; involvement of the inferior endplate; and narrowing of the spinal canal related to retropulsion of the posterosuperior portion of the vertebral body. It is essential to differentiate the burst fracture from the more common simple compression fracture because of the potential for spinal instability and compromise of the neural canal in the former. Anterior vertebral wedging can be pronounced in either injury. In burst fractures, the average degree of wedging of the anterior portion of the vertebral body does not differ significantly from that seen with compression fractures. Careful evaluation of the posterior margin of the vertebral body usually allows accurate differentiation of these two injuries. The posterior aspect of the normal vertebral body is seen clearly on a well-penetrated, nonrotated lateral view. The posterior cortical line is continuous except in the center of the vertebral body, where it is interrupted by the entry of the nutrient vessels. Disruption, displacement, or rotation of this line indicates disruption of the middle spinal column (Fig. 58–27).

The retropulsed bone fragment in burst fractures characteristically arises from the posterosuperior corner of the fractured vertebral body superior to the basivertebral foramen. On lateral views, the fragment is often triangular, with its sides formed by the posterior part of the superior endplate, the superior part of the posterior vertebral margin, and the fracture line itself. The retropulsed fragment frequently is comminuted. Posterior element fractures are seen in 50% to 100% of patients with burst fractures. Typical fractures of the posterior elements associated with burst fractures include vertical fractures of one or both laminae and the spinous process. Posterior element fractures may be difficult to identify on conventional radiographs, and a higher rate of posterior element fractures is reported in studies using CT scanning.

Normally, the interpediculate distance increases gradually from the T6 spinal level caudally. In the thoracic region, comparison of measurements made at the injured level with those obtained at both adjacent levels is recommended. The mean value for the interpediculate distance in cases of burst fracture is increased by 25%; however, such widening is not present in all cases. CT scanning is the optimal method for identifying the presence of posterior element fractures and retropulsed bone fragments, features not present in simple compression fractures (Fig. 58–28). The failure of the posterior vertebral wall is usually readily apparent. With CT, the degree of narrowing of the spinal canal produced by retropulsed bone fragments can be quantitated in the preoperative and immediate postoperative periods.

### Seat-Belt Injury

The term seat-belt or lap-belt injury refers to a variety of osseous and ligamentous injuries caused by hyperflexion

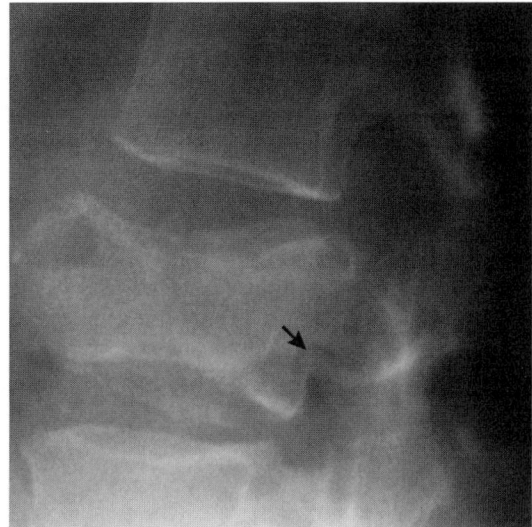

**Figure 58–27.** Thoracolumbar burst fracture. Lateral radiograph reveals loss of height of the vertebral body, with involvement of the cortex both anteriorly and posteriorly (*arrow*).

and, in some cases, superimposed distraction of the spinal column. Not all patients sustaining injuries of this type are wearing seat belts at the time of injury. Such injuries occur most frequently at the thoracolumbar and upper lumbar levels, particularly L1 or L2; these levels are involved in the majority of adults. In children restrained by lap belts, the midlumbar level is injured more frequently than the thoracolumbar region.

The fulcrum of flexion in lap-belt injuries is located anterior to the vertebral body, at the level of the anterior abdominal wall where it abuts on the seat belt. Hyperflexion in this setting subjects the middle and posterior vertebral columns, or all three columns, to distraction forces. The resulting tensile force can lead to purely osseous, purely ligamentous, or combined bony and soft tissue injuries. Because, in general, ligaments withstand tension better than bone does, fractures are typically

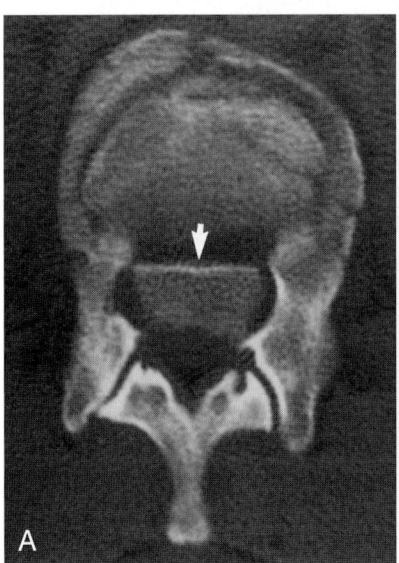
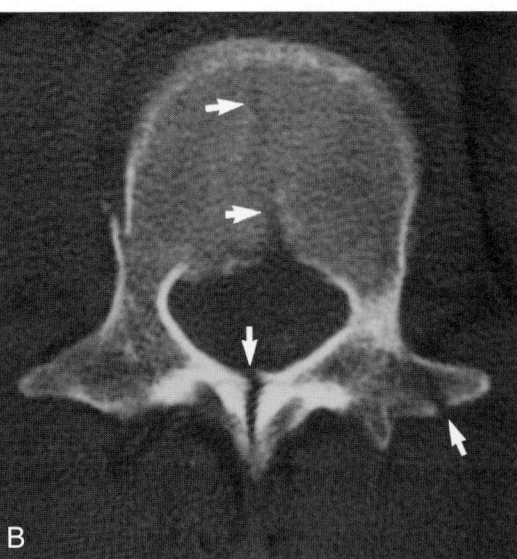

**Figure 58–28.** Thoracolumbar burst fracture. *A,* Transaxial CT scan through the superior aspect of the L3 vertebral body shows comminution of the superior endplate and a large fragment of retropulsed bone within the spinal canal. Note the rotation of the fragment, with the superior cortex (*arrow*) directed anteriorly. *B,* A more caudal image shows sagittal fracture lines involving the left transverse process, spinous process, and inferior aspect of the vertebral body (*arrows*).

present, particularly in the posterior elements. These injuries, of which the horizontal Chance fracture is the best-known subtype, begin posteriorly and propagate anteriorly.

The radiographic findings of a seat-belt injury depend on whether the injury is predominantly osseous or soft tissue. In general, distraction at the level of the posterior fracture or sites of ligament disruption, relative preservation of or increase in the height of the vertebral body, and mild focal kyphosis are seen (Fig. 58–29). Posterior ligamentous damage results in interspinous widening; increased height of the intervertebral foramina; and widening, superior subluxation, perching, or locking of the facet joints. Interspinous widening is often difficult to assess in this region, owing to the changing orientation of the spinous processes. Sufficient angulation may be present to give rise to an "empty" or "vacant" appearance of the vertebral body as a result of cephalad displacement of the posterior elements of the cranial vertebra. If the posterior fibers of the anulus fibrosus are disrupted, widening of the posterior portion of the disc space may be apparent. The characteristic injury seen with this mode of failure is a horizontal fracture extending transversely through the vertebral body, pedicles, and other posterior elements. Careful scrutiny of these structures on the anteroposterior view is recommended, because the posterior elements are often obscured on the lateral radiograph. CT scanning is helpful in elucidating the nature of the posterior injury and is essential for excluding posterior element fractures and facet disruption.

## Fracture-Dislocation

The main characteristic of this severe injury is complete disruption of all three spinal columns, allowing vertebral subluxation and dislocation. The spinal distribution of fracture-dislocations is bimodal, as with compression fractures, with one peak at the T6–T7 level and a second peak at the thoracolumbar junction. The vast majority of these injuries are caused by a combination of spinal flexion and rotation. The posterior and middle columns fail in tension and rotation, whereas the anterior column fails in compression and rotation. Fracture-dislocations are associated with a very high rate of neurologic deficit, with 53% to 93% of patients developing a permanent neurologic deficit, typically complete paraplegia, after their injury.

The major hallmark of these severe injuries is the presence of intervertebral subluxation or dislocation; loss of height of a vertebral body is not a characteristic feature in these injuries. In one series, anterior subluxation averaged one third the width of the vertebral body. Such subluxation is better seen on the lateral view, whereas rotation and lateral translation are seen to better advantage on the anteroposterior projection. Radiographic signs suggestive of rotation injury include slice fractures of the vertebral body, multiple fractures of the ribs or transverse processes, dislocation of the costotransverse joints, unilateral displaced fractures of the articular facets, and rotatory malalignment between the pedicles and spinous processes of vertebrae located above and below the injury (Fig. 58–30). The rotational slice fracture is a horizontal fracture involving the superior endplate and a horizontal, sliver-like fracture of the vertebral body below the dislocation; the upper vertebra, intervertebral disc, and slice fracture fragment are displaced as a unit, which pivots relative to the caudal vertebra. The interpediculate distance is normal, and the posterior cortex of the vertebral body characteristically remains intact. Radiographic signs suggestive of shear injury include lateral vertebral translation, severely comminuted fractures of the articular processes, multiple fractures of the spinous processes, and free-floating laminae.

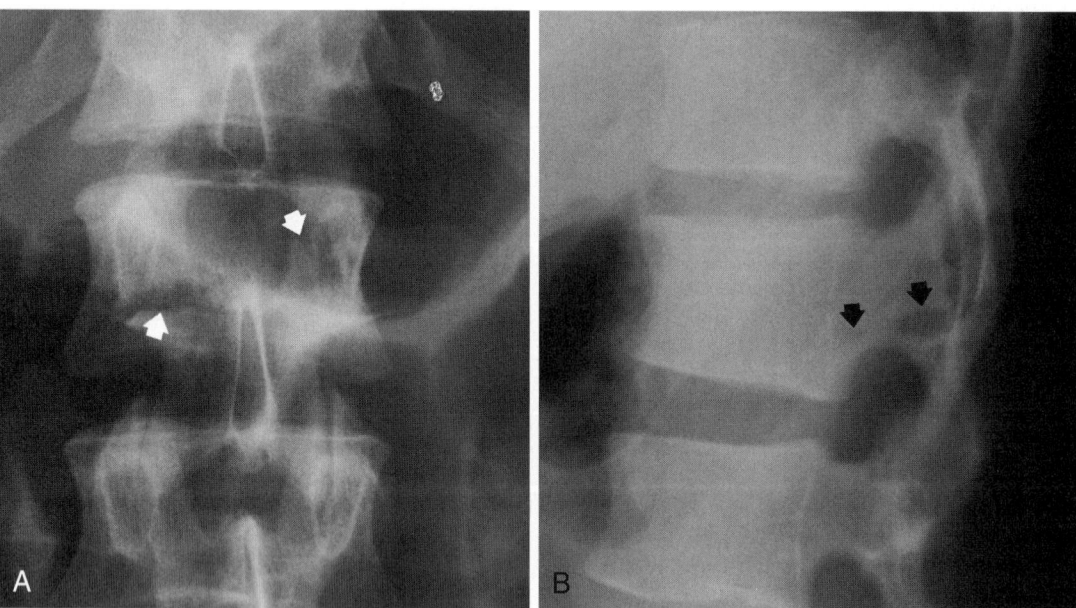

**Figure 58–29.** Thoracolumbar seat-belt injury. Frontal *(A)* and lateral *(B)* radiographs reveal a horizontal fracture *(arrows)* involving the laminae, articular processes, pedicles, and posterior portion of the first lumbar vertebral body. Note the widening of the distance between the spinous processes of the T12 and L1 vertebrae.

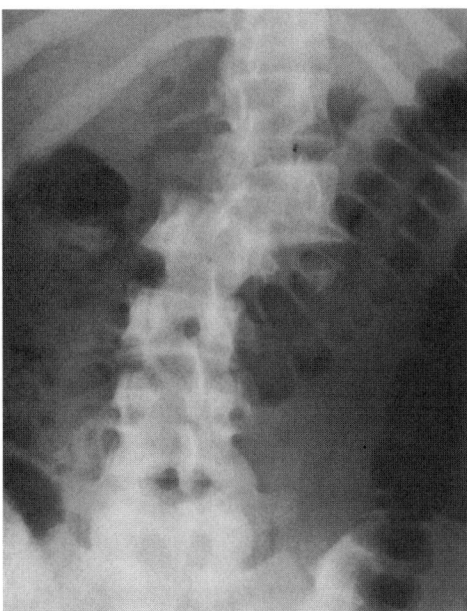

**Figure 58–30.** Thoracolumbar fracture-dislocation. Antero-posterior radiograph demonstrates a fracture-dislocation at the L1-L2 vertebral level. Multiple fractures are present. Severe comminution of the L2 vertebral body and posterior elements on the left is seen. Note the rotational deformity at the level of the dislocation, with a change in orientation of the spinous process and pedicle.

## LOWER LUMBAR SPINE

### General Considerations

Fractures and dislocations of the lumbar spine below L2 are relatively uncommon. The lower lumbar region is well protected by overlying soft tissues and is relatively immobile. The lumbar vertebrae are bulky and have thicker cortices than the vertebrae in other regions of the spine. Although injuries of the lower lumbar region are less common than those in more mobile spinal regions, fractures, subluxations, and dislocations of the lower lumbar region are not uncommon in the setting of severe multisystem trauma.

### Fracture and Dislocation

Compression fractures of the lower lumbar spine in patients with osteoporosis are uncommon. When they develop, central endplate compression resembling Schmorl's nodes, rather than anterior vertebral wedging, is seen. Mechanical testing has shown that resistance to collapse is greatest in the lumbar vertebrae, owing to the presence of a thick anterior vertebral cortex that resists compression. Preferential central depression of the superior and inferior endplates occurs. Compression fractures involving the anterior column of the lower lumbar spine are also uncommon. Burst fractures of the lower lumbar vertebrae are far less common than the same injuries at the thoracolumbar junction. Vertebral dislocation is also much less common in the lower lumbar spine than in the thoracic region or at the thoracolumbar junction.

Fractures of the transverse processes of the vertebrae result from lateral flexion-extension or, less commonly, from a direct blow, or they may be seen in association with Malgaigne's fracture of the pelvis. These fractures tend to occur in the absence of other vertebral fractures, although multiple transverse processes may be involved. The most commonly involved levels are L3 and L4. These fractures are stable injuries, although they may be associated with abdominal, thoracic, and genitourinary injuries. The fractures are most evident on the antero-posterior radiograph, in which disruption of the cortex and displacement of the fractured tip of the transverse process can be seen. Isolated fractures of the transverse processes may be difficult to identify, however, owing to the relatively thin bone in this region and overlying bowel gas. Isolated fractures of the pedicles may be related to trauma or may represent fatigue fractures caused by repetitive stress.

### Spondylolisthesis and Spondylolysis

Spondylolisthesis, with anterior slippage of the superior vertebra on the inferior one, may be due to a variety of osseous lesions, the most common being osteoarthritis of the facet joints and defects of the pars interarticularis. Bilateral pars interarticularis defects effectively divide the vertebra into two segments. The anterosuperior segment consists of the vertebral body, pedicles, transverse processes, and superior facets. The posteroinferior segment consists of the inferior facet, laminae, and spinous process. Acute fractures of the pars interarticularis are far less common than chronic spondylolysis as a cause of traumatic anterior vertebral displacement. Distinction from a chronic spondylolysis is based on a history of severe trauma, the acute appearance of a fracture line, evidence of subsequent callus formation during healing, and increased accumulation of radionuclide on bone scintigraphy.

Spondylolisthesis can be divided into five types: (1) dysplastic, related to congenital anomalies of the upper portion of the sacrum or neural arch of L5; (2) isthmic, caused by fatigue fractures, elongation, or acute fractures of the pars interarticularis; (3) degenerative, related to intersegmental instability; (4) traumatic, secondary to fractures of the neural arch in regions other than the isthmus; and (5) pathologic, resulting from generalized or localized bone disease. The most common types are isthmic and degenerative.

The prevalence of pars interarticularis defects has been reported to be between 2.3% and 10%. The majority of these defects appear to be asymptomatic. An increased prevalence is seen in males, and a strong hereditary component appears to exist. Definite racial differences in the prevalence of these defects are seen: only 1.95% of blacks have pars interarticularis defects, whereas in certain Eskimo communities, the prevalence may be as high as 60%. Virtually all defects of the pars interarticularis develop by the age of 18 years (Fig. 58–31). Patients with such defects have been noted to have a higher frequency of spina bifida occulta at the level of the defect.

Radiographic abnormalities of the pars interarticularis parallel those seen with stress fractures in other locations.

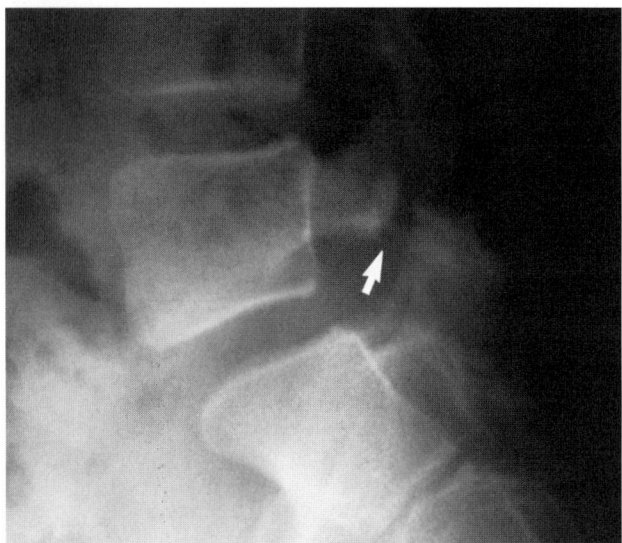

**Figure 58–31.** Spondylolysis of the L5 vertebra. Radiolucent defects *(arrow)* are seen in the pars interarticularis of the L5 vertebra in this 10-year-old child. Spondylolisthesis is minimal, but the vertebral body is normal in morphology.

The earliest radiographic change is osteopenia, followed by the development of endosteal callus. The fracture line itself may not be apparent at this phase. When no discrete fracture line is seen, sclerosis is the dominant finding. With healing, sclerosis, narrowing, and elongation of the pars interarticularis can be seen. The lateral view usually demonstrates the defect, particularly in the presence of spondylolisthesis. The fracture line courses from a posterosuperior to an anteroinferior direction through the pars interarticularis (see Fig. 58–31).

The anteroposterior view demonstrates the pars interarticularis defect in only a small proportion of cases, although secondary signs such as laminar thickening, laminar fragmentation, and vertebral malalignment may be recognized. Oblique radiographs usually are not necessary but occasionally may be helpful. On oblique radiographs, the isthmic defect appears as a collar around the neck of the so-called Scottie dog of Lachapèle. Oblique views do not always show pars interarticularis defects, partly because of the changing obliquity of the isthmic region from a cranial to caudal direction in the spine.

Approximately one fifth of patients with spondylolysis have a unilateral defect. Whether the defect is truly unilateral or whether the patient had bilateral defects with healing on only one side is not known. Unilateral spondylolysis is associated with reactive sclerosis and hypertrophy of the contralateral pedicle and lamina. This appearance can lead to an erroneous diagnosis of osteoid osteoma, although the absence of a nidus and the presence of dense homogeneous sclerosis favor reactive hypertrophy.

Spondylolisthesis associated with bilateral defects of the pars interarticularis occurs most frequently at the L5–S1 level. More than 90% of pars interarticularis defects that allow slippage occur at this level, with the remainder occurring mainly at L4–L5. By contrast, degenerative spondylolisthesis secondary to facet osteoarthritis occurs at L4–L5 in 90% of cases and is four times more frequent in women. Degenerative spondylolisthesis can be distinguished from isthmic spondylolisthesis by noting the presence of defects in the pars interarticularis and elongation of the anteroposterior dimension of the spinal canal in the latter condition.

Vertebral slippage can be categorized as tangential or angular. Tangential slipping at the L5–S1 level can be further classified into five grades, according to the resulting relationship between the fifth lumbar vertebral body and the superior surface of the sacrum. Grade 1 slippage is present when there is anterior migration of the L5 vertebral body by 25% of the anteroposterior dimension of the superior sacral endplate. The grade increases with each quarter of the anteroposterior dimension that is uncovered by the anterior displacement of the L5 vertebral body. Grade 5, or complete spondyloptosis, is the most severe form of listhesis, consisting of complete displacement of the L5 vertebral body, such that it rests entirely anterior to the sacrum. Angular slipping results in an increase in lumbar lordosis related to diminished contact between the posterior surfaces of the fifth lumbar and first sacral vertebrae as the body of L5 tilts anteriorly on the sacrum. This grading system can be applied to spondylolisthesis at other levels, although it was originally developed for quantifying slippage at the lumbosacral junction.

On transaxial images, the CT slice cephalad to the neural foramen is at the top, or above the superior aspect of the apophyseal joints. At this level, a normal appearance is that of an intact ring, consisting of the posterior wall of the vertebral body, the medial walls of the pedicles, the anteromedial pars interarticularis, the laminae, and the anterior margin of the spinous process. In all cases of spondylolysis, a defect, or incomplete ring, is apparent on the slice above the neural foramen. The plane of this level usually corresponds to the defect in the posterior vertebral margin where the basivertebral vein exits the vertebral body. The presence of a complete ring on CT scans at this level excludes the presence of a pars interarticularis defect. Pars interarticularis defects can be differentiated from facet joints by noting the absence of dense subarticular margins, the presence of irregularity or fragmentation at the edges of the spondylolytic defect, and the absence of normal notches about the facet joint that serve as insertion sites for the joint capsule. A pars interarticularis defect also appears more horizontal than the typical facet joint, which has a smooth, oblique orientation (Fig. 58–32).

Anterior displacement of the vertebral body, combined with posterior displacement of the posterior arch, produces widening of the anteroposterior diameter of the spinal canal. With severe spondylolisthesis, there may be a double canal appearance. In addition, in spondylolisthesis, CT scans may reveal pseudobulging of the intervertebral disc caused by soft tissue projecting posteriorly into the spinal canal. This artifactual appearance is related to projection of a portion of the anulus fibrosus posterior to the slipped vertebra. On MR images, pars interarticularis defects are typically of intermediate signal intensity on all pulse sequences, although their signal intensity is somewhat variable, depending on the exact composition of the tissues within the defect. In the sagittal plane,

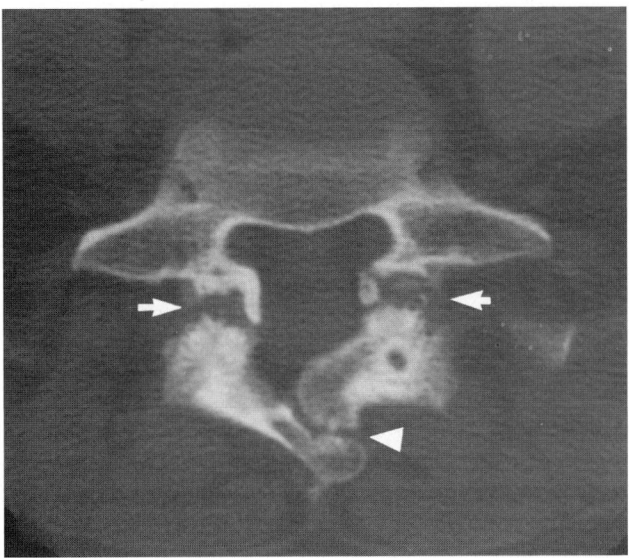

**Figure 58–32.** Spondylolisthesis. Transaxial CT scan through the bilateral defects of the pars interarticularis shows irregularity and fragmentation at the margins of the defects *(arrows)*. Note the horizontal inclination of the spondylolytic regions. Spina bifida is also present *(arrowhead)*.

Bone scintigraphy allows a functional assessment of metabolic activity in the region of the isthmus. Discordance between radiographic and scintigraphic finding in pars interarticularis defects is well recognized. Acute stress injuries of the pars interarticularis may not be apparent radiographically, and long-standing spondylolysis may not be active metabolically. The scintigraphic appearance of spondylolysis is not specific, and a final diagnosis depends on clinical and radiographic evaluation. Single photon emission computed tomography (SPECT) is more sensitive for the detection of stress injuries to the pars interarticularis than is conventional planar imaging.

## Avulsion of the Ring Apophysis

The ring apophyses are narrow cartilaginous mounds present at both the superior and inferior vertebral endplates, from which they are separated by a thin layer of cartilage. The ring apophyses normally begin to calcify at the age of 6 years; ossification occurs at the beginning of adolescence. The apophyses fuse with the vertebral body at the end of skeletal growth by age 18 to 25 years. Avulsions of the posterior apophyseal ring of the lumbar vertebrae, like spondylolysis, are traumatic lesions that develop in children and adolescents. Patients typically first come to medical attention in adolescence or young adulthood with back and leg pain, paraspinal spasm, mechanical findings of nerve entrapment, and a relative paucity of focal neurologic findings. Associated disc herniation is present in up to 90% of patients. Whether the disc herniation produces the avulsion fracture or whether the fracture results in annular disruption is unclear. Disc herniation in patients younger than 21 years is associated with vertebral endplate avulsions in as many as 19% of cases.

normal variations in marrow signal intensity of the pars interarticularis are common and may make detection of pars interarticularis defects difficult when spondylolisthesis is not present. The pars interarticularis is best evaluated in a sagittal imaging plane that passes through the medial pedicle. The central and foraminal stenosis associated with spondylolisthesis is also well depicted on MR images.

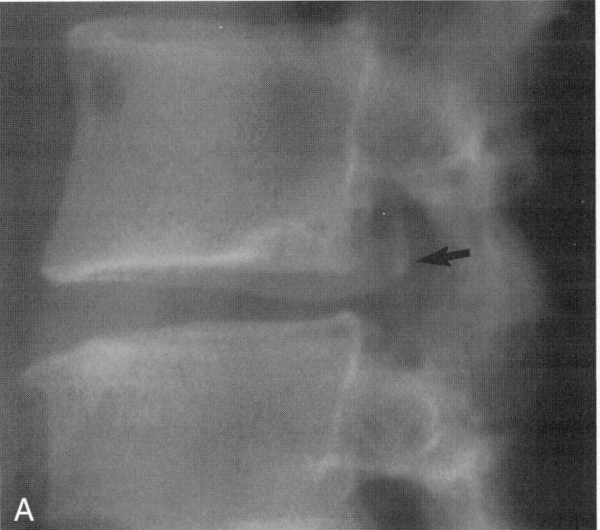
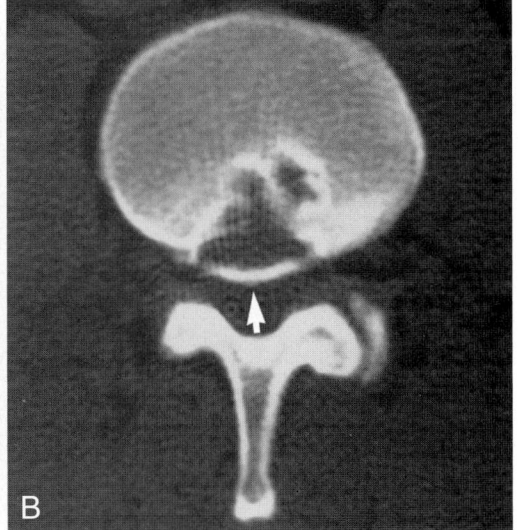

**Figure 58–33.** Avulsion of the posterior ring apophysis. *A*, Lateral radiograph shows a bone fragment *(arrow)* located posterior to the L3–L4 intervertebral disc. Note the narrowing of the intervertebral disc space and the irregularity of the posteroinferior margin of the L3 vertebral body, the source of the displaced bone fragment. *B*, CT scan demonstrates the characteristic arcuate configuration of the displaced apophyseal fragment *(arrow)* and the Schmorl's node at the posteroinferior margin of the vertebral body.

Apophyseal fractures can occur throughout the spine, but the most common levels of involvement are the inferior ring apophyses of the lower lumbar vertebrae, particularly the posteroinferior margin of L4. Alternatively, some authors have suggested that the posterior cephalad rim of the sacrum is affected most frequently. This discrepancy can be explained by the imaging method used; rim avulsions of the sacrum are extremely difficult to visualize on conventional radiographs and are diagnosed by CT scanning or MR imaging in most cases.

Conventional radiographs must be examined carefully, because these lesions are difficult to see. Findings on the lateral view include mild disc space narrowing, irregularity of the posterior vertebral corner, and an irregular wedge-shaped ossific defect displaced into the spinal canal. On CT scans, the osseous fracture fragment has a characteristic arcuate or semilunar configuration that parallels the border of the posterior vertebral body (Fig. 58–33). The fragment may appear irregular rather than arcuate if it contains a large fragment of the vertebral body. This fragment must be differentiated from osteophytes, calcified disc fragments, and calcification or ossification of the posterior longitudinal ligament. The fragment is more difficult to characterize on MR images because it may be hard to distinguish the osseous rim from the low signal intensity of the posterior longitudinal ligament.

## FURTHER READING

Acheson MB, Livingston RR, Richardson ML, et al: High-resolution CT scanning in the evaluation of cervical spine fractures: Comparison with plain film examinations. AJR Am J Roentgenol 148:1179, 1987.

Anderson LD, D'Alonzo RT: Fractures of the odontoid process of the axis. J Bone Joint Surg Am 56:1663, 1974.

Bundschuh CV, Alley JB, Ross M, et al: Magnetic resonance imaging of suspected atlanto-occipital dislocation: Two case reports. Spine 17:245, 1992.

Daffner RH, Deeb ZL, Goldberg AL, et al: The radiologic assessment of post-traumatic vertebral stability. Skeletal Radiol 19:103, 1990.

Denis F: The three column spine and its significance in the classification of acute thoracolumbar spinal injuries. Spine 8:817, 1983.

El-Khoury GY, Kathol MH, Daniel WW: Imaging of acute injuries of the cervical spine: Value of plain radiography, CT, and MR imaging. AJR Am J Roentgenol 164:43, 1995.

Flanders AE, Schaefer DM, Doan HY, et al: Acute cervical spine trauma: Correlation of MR imaging findings with degree of neurologic deficit. Radiology 177:25, 1990.

Frankel HL, Hancock DO, Hyslop G, et al: The value of postural reduction in the initial management of closed injuries of the spine with paraplegia and tetraplegia. Paraplegia 7:179, 1969.

Gehweiler JA, Duff DE, Martinez S, et al: Fractures of the atlas vertebra. Skeletal Radiol 1:97, 1976.

Kliewer MA, Gray L, Paver J, et al: Acute spinal ligament disruption: MR imaging with anatomic correlation. J Magn Reson Imaging 3:855, 1993.

McArdle CB, Crofford MJ, Mirfakhraee M, et al: Surface coil MR of spinal trauma: Preliminary experience. AJNR Am J Neuroradiol 7:885, 1986.

Mirvis SE, Young JWR, Lim C, et al: Hangman's fracture: Radiologic assessment in 27 cases. Radiology 163:713, 1987.

Orrison WW, Johansen JG, Eldevik OP, et al: Optimal computed-tomographic techniques for cervical spine imaging. Radiology 144:180, 1982.

Penecot GF, Couraud D, Hardy JR, et al: Roentgenographical study of the stability of the cervical spine in children. J Pediatr Orthop 4:346, 1984.

Pennell RG, Maurer AH, Bonakdarpour A: Stress injuries of the pars interarticularis: Radiologic classification and indications for scintigraphy. AJR Am J Roentgenol 145:763, 1985.

Powers B, Miller MD, Kramer RS, et al: Traumatic anterior atlanto-occipital dislocation. Neurosurgery 4:12, 1979.

Sherk HH, Nicholson JT: Fractures of the atlas. J Bone Joint Surg Am 52:1017, 1970.

Tarr RW, Drolshagen LF, Kerner TC, et al: MR imaging of recent spinal trauma. J Comput Assist Tomogr 11:412, 1987.

Traughber PD, Havlina JM Jr: Bilateral pedicle stress fractures: SPECT and CT features. J Comput Assist Tomogr 15:338, 1991.

Wiltse LL, Newman PH, Macnab I: Classification of spondylolisis and spondylolisthesis. Clin Orthop 117:23, 1976.

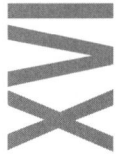
# CHAPTER 59

## Internal Derangements of Joints

### SUMMARY OF KEY FEATURES

This chapter summarizes some of the important internal derangements and related conditions occurring in six anatomic regions. Abnormalities of articular cartilage, subchondral bone, synovial membrane, joint capsule, ligament, tendon, muscle, and nerve are emphasized, with particular attention to anatomy and concepts of pathology and pathophysiology.

These abnormalities can be delineated with a variety of imaging methods, including routine radiography, arthrography, tenography, bursography, ultrasonography, bone scintigraphy, computed tomography, computed arthrotomography, and magnetic resonance imaging. Although clinical assessment is the key to correctly diagnosing many of these conditions, the contributions of these imaging methods are significant.

### INTRODUCTION

This chapter reviews the diagnostic imaging methods for internal derangements of joints in six anatomic regions: wrist, elbow, shoulder, hip, knee, and ankle and foot. Although ancillary techniques such as arthrography and computed arthrotomography are addressed, their coverage is brief because of the prominent role of magnetic resonance (MR) imaging. A number of conditions occurring around these anatomic regions are included, even though they do not precisely fall into the category of internal derangement of joints.

### WRIST

#### Anatomy

The osseous and articular anatomy of the wrist is shown in Figure 59–1. The radiocarpal compartment is formed proximally by the distal surface of the radius and the triangular fibrocartilage (TFC) and distally by the proximal row of carpal bones, exclusive of the pisiform. In the coronal plane, the radiocarpal compartment is a C-shaped cavity with a smooth, shallow curve that is concave distally. The distal radioulnar joint is stabilized primarily by the triangular fibrocartilage complex (TFCC) of the wrist. The components of the TFCC are not agreed on but include the TFC itself, the dorsal and volar radioulnar ligaments, the ulnomeniscal homologue, the ulnar collateral ligament, and the sheath of the extensor carpi ulnaris tendon.

The flexor tendons of the fingers, the sublimis digitorum and profundus digitorum, are enveloped by digital sheaths from the line of insertion of the flexor profundus to a line 1 cm proximal to the proximal border of the deep transverse ligament (Fig. 59–2). This arrangement, which is not constant, is most frequent in the index, middle, and

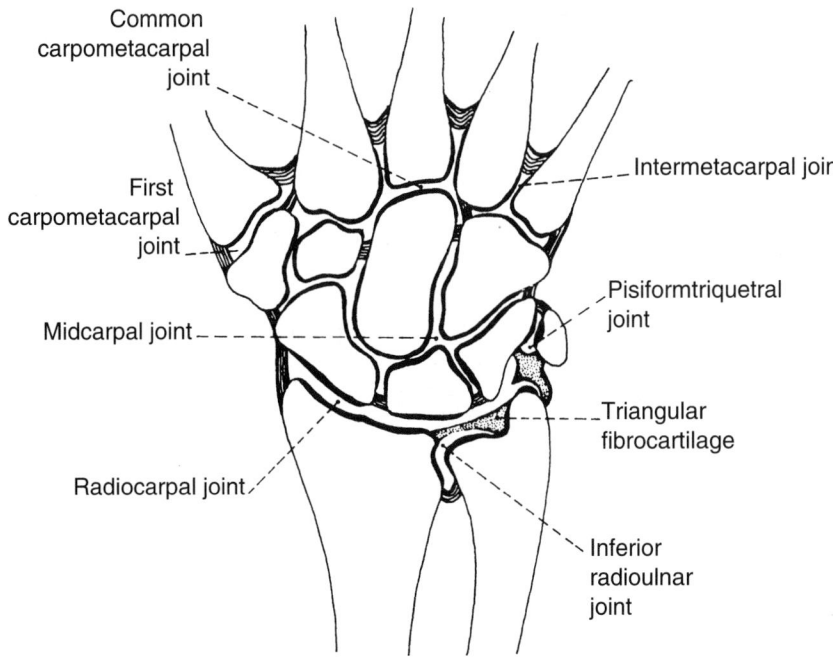

Common carpometacarpal joint

First carpometacarpal joint

Midcarpal joint

Radiocarpal joint

Intermetacarpal joint

Pisiformtriquetral joint

Triangular fibrocartilage

Inferior radioulnar joint

**Figure 59–1.** Articulations of the wrist: general anatomy. The various wrist compartments are illustrated on a schematic drawing of a coronal section.

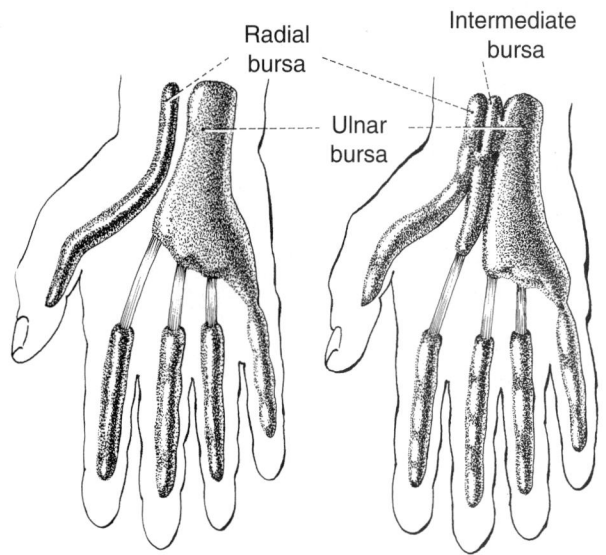

**Figure 59–2.** Digital flexor tendon sheaths and synovial sacs of the palm. The radial and ulnar bursae may be separate, distinct cavities or may communicate via an intermediate bursa. Note the flexor tendon sheaths, which in the second, third, and fourth fingers usually terminate just proximal to the metacarpophalangeal joints. The tendon sheaths in the first and fifth fingers generally communicate with the bursae in the wrist. (From Resnick D: AJR Am J Roentgenol 124:44, 1975.)

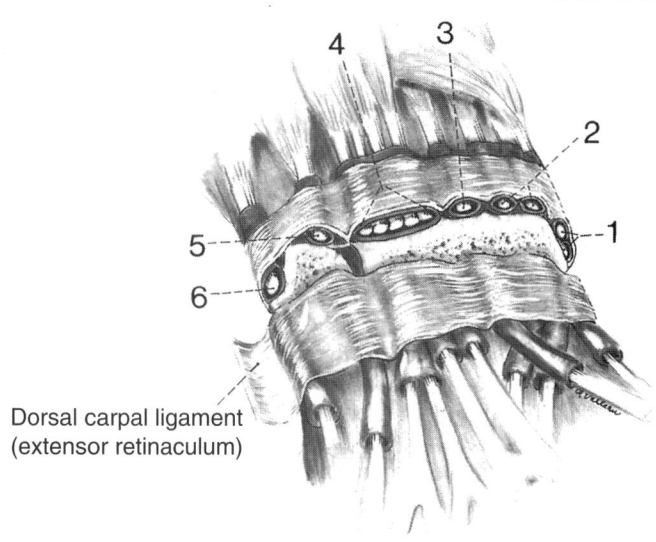

**Figure 59–3.** Extensor tendons and tendon sheaths. Illustration of the dorsal carpal ligament and extensor tendons surrounded by synovial sheaths traversing the dorsum of the wrist within six separate compartments. These compartments are created by the insular attachment of the dorsal carpal ligament on the posterior and lateral surfaces of the radius and ulna. The extensor carpi ulnaris tendon and its sheath are in the medial compartment (6) and are closely applied to the posterior surface of the ulna. (From Resnick D: Rheumatoid arthritis of the wrist: The compartmental approach. Med Radiogr Photogr 52:50, 1976.)

ring fingers. may be found enveloping the index flexor tendons. Additionally, a small synovial sac may enclose the tendon of the flexor carpi radialis muscle as it passes under the crest of the trapezium.

Several synovial sheaths are located in the dorsum of the wrist beneath the dorsal carpal ligament; they extend for a short distance proximal and distal to that ligament (Fig. 59–3). Six distinct avenues are created for transport of the ligamentous structures (Table 59–1).

## Distal Radioulnar Joint Abnormalities

**Functional Anatomy.** Features that are fundamental to the optimal function of the distal radioulnar joint include the following:

1. The articulating surface between the ulnar head and the sigmoid notch of the radius must be intact. As the forearm moves from supination to pronation, the ulnar head rotates up to 150 degrees and also glides several millimeters in a proximal to distal direction within the sigmoid notch.

2. The soft tissue and ligamentous support system of the distal radioulnar joint must be intact. This includes the various components of the TFCC (consisting of the TFC or articular disc, dorsal and volar radioulnar ligaments, ulnar collateral ligament, meniscus homologue, and sheath of the extensor carpi ulnaris tendon).

3. A proper relationship must exist between the lengths of the radius and ulna (Fig. 59–4). Changes in the length of the ulna relative to the length of the radius, designated positive and negative ulnar variance, alter

---

**TABLE 59–1**

**Extensor Tendon Compartments of the Wrist**

1. Abductor pollicis longus
   Extensor pollicis brevis
2. Extensor carpi radialis longus
   Extensor carpi radialis brevis
3. Extensor pollicis longus
4. Extensor digitorum communis
   Extensor indicis proprius
5. Extensor digiti quinti proprius
6. Extensor carpi ulnaris

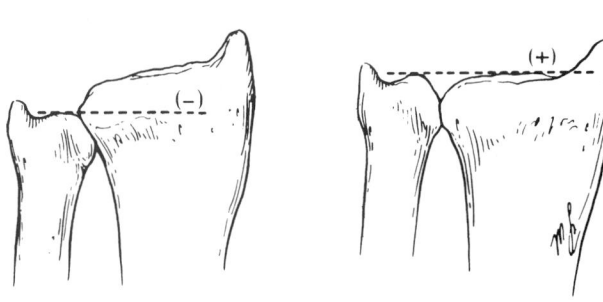

**Figure 59–4.** Ulnar variance. Negative and positive ulnar variance are illustrated.

the distribution of compressive forces across the wrist. The consequences of a short ulna, or negative ulnar variance, include increased force applied to the radial side of the wrist and to the lunate bone, which may explain the association of negative ulnar variance and Kienböck's disease. A consequence of a long ulna, or positive ulnar variance, is the ulnar impaction or ulnar abutment syndrome.

## Lesions of the Triangular Fibrocartilage Complex

Lesions of the TFCC are variable in extent; they may be confined to the horizontal, or flat, portion of the TFCC (referred to as the TFC or articular disc) or involve one or more components of the TFCC with or without instability of the distal radioulnar joint.

Degenerative lesions of the TFC are more common than traumatic lesions. Either type may result in full-thickness defects, as can be documented with arthrography and MR imaging. In young persons, a normal TFC is characterized by homogeneously low signal intensity on virtually all MR pulse sequences in the coronal, sagittal, and transverse planes. In the coronal plane, a normal TFC usually appears as an elongated triangle with its apex attaching to the articular cartilage of the radius (Fig. 59–5). The triangle may be thinner in persons with positive ulnar variance and thicker in those with negative ulnar variance. The ulnar attachment of the TFC may appear bifurcated, with two bands of low signal intensity separated by a region of higher

signal intensity. Although MR images of a normal TFC generally show low signal intensity, regions of higher signal intensity within the TFC are regularly encountered on T1-weighted spin echo MR images in older individuals, related to degenerative change.

The increased signal intensity in a degenerative TFC on T1-weighted spin echo MR images can simulate the appearance of traumatic lesions. Detection of a less high signal intensity in the TFC on T2-weighted spin echo MR images is useful in differentiating TFC degeneration from TFC perforation, in which high signal intensity on T2-weighted spin echo MR images is evident. Although differentiating between a traumatically induced communicating defect of the TFC and one related to degeneration is difficult with the use of MR imaging (or standard arthrography), characteristic MR imaging features frequently allow an accurate diagnosis of some type of communicating defect or perforation of the structure. Linear regions of high signal intensity, identical to that of fluid, that traverse the entire thickness of the TFC on T1- and T2-weighted spin echo MR images (or gradient echo images) are strong evidence that a communicating defect is present (Fig. 59–6). Similar regions of high signal intensity extending partially through the thickness of the TFC are compatible with the diagnosis of a noncommunicating defect.

Most previous investigations of the value of MR imaging in the assessment of the TFC relied on findings derived from spin echo sequences. Gradient echo imaging sequences may also be valuable, however. On multiplanar gradient recalled (MPGR) MR images in which a low flip angle is used, fluid accumulating within communicating defects in the TFC is of high signal intensity. When

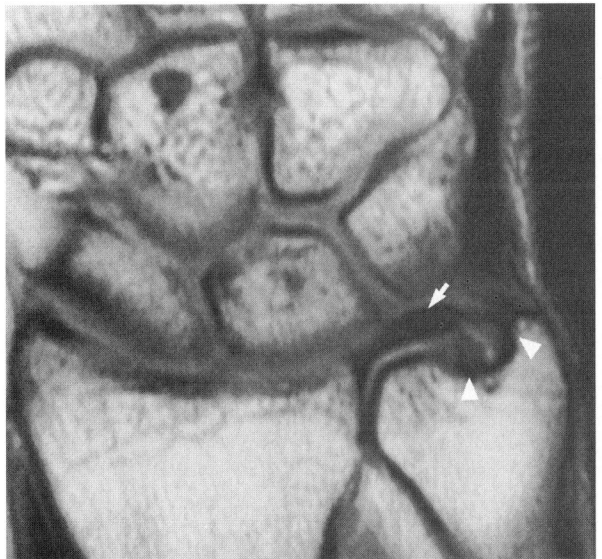

**Figure 59–5.** Triangular fibrocartilage complex: normal appearance. On a coronal intermediate-weighted (TR/TE, 2000/20) spin echo MR image, observe the low signal intensity of the triangular fibrocartilage *(arrow)*, with bifurcated bands of low signal intensity *(arrowheads)* attaching to or near the styloid process of the ulna. The scapholunate and lunotriquetral interosseous ligaments are not well seen on this image. Note the two bone islands, which appear as foci of low signal intensity, in the lunate and capitate. (Courtesy of A. G. Bergman, MD, Stanford, Calif.)

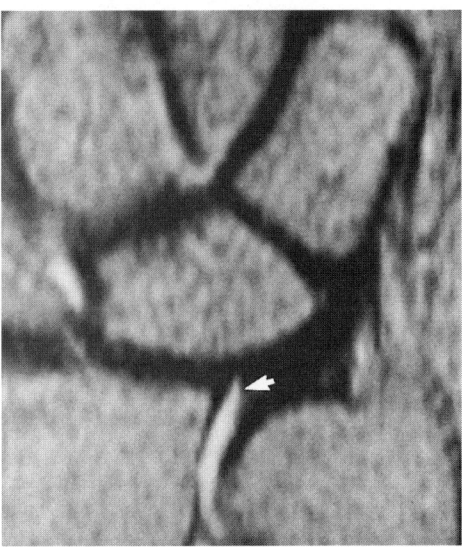

**Figure 59–6.** Triangular fibrocartilage complex: communicating defect. T2-weighted (TR/TE, 2500/80) spin echo MR image shows fluid of high signal intensity in the defect *(arrow)* within the triangular fibrocartilage and in the distal radioulnar joint. Fluid is also present in the midcarpal joint. (Courtesy of M. Zlatkin, MD, Hollywood, Fla.)

gradient recalled imaging is combined with volumetric acquisition, thin sections of the TFC can be obtained and might accentuate the abnormalities associated with such defects. The results of MR imaging and arthrography in the assessment of defects of the TFC appear to agree closely. At this time, state-of-the-art MR imaging and arthrography can be considered equally accurate in this assessment.

## Ulnar Impaction Syndrome

The ulnar impaction syndrome, also termed ulnar abutment syndrome, is defined as a degenerative condition characterized by ulnar-sided wrist pain, swelling, and limitation of motion related to excessive load bearing across the ulnar aspect of the wrist. Chronic impaction of the ulnar head against the TFCC and ulnar-sided carpal bones results in progressive deterioration of the TFCC, chondromalacia of the lunate and head of the ulna, and attrition of the lunotriquetral interosseous ligament. The ulnar impaction syndrome is almost always associated with a positive ulnar variance.

Routine radiographs in patients with the ulnar impaction syndrome may reveal alterations in the lunate, triquetrum, and ulnar head. Findings include bone sclerosis, cysts, and osteophytes. Arthrography often demonstrates communicating defects of the TFC and disruption of the lunotriquetral interosseous ligament. MR imaging also documents these abnormalities of the TFC and lunotriquetral interosseous ligament, as well as chondromalacia and alterations in the subchondral bone of the proximal surfaces of the lunate and triquetrum (Fig. 59–7).

## Ulnar Impingement Syndrome

The ulnar impingement syndrome is associated with clinical manifestations that are similar to but often more disabling than those accompanying the ulnar impaction syndrome. Pain may be aggravated during pronation and supination of the forearm. Three radiographic features are characteristic of the ulnar impingement syndrome: negative ulnar variance, scalloped concavity of the distal radius, and convergence of the ulna with the distal portion of the radius.

## Instability of the Distal Radioulnar Joint

The distal radioulnar joint is involved in pronation and supination of the forearm, during which the radius moves with respect to a relatively fixed ulna. Clinical manifestations include pain, weakness, loss of forearm rotation, and snapping. Dorsal instability predominates, and physical examination confirms a dorsal prominence of the ulnar head, especially in a position of forearm pronation.

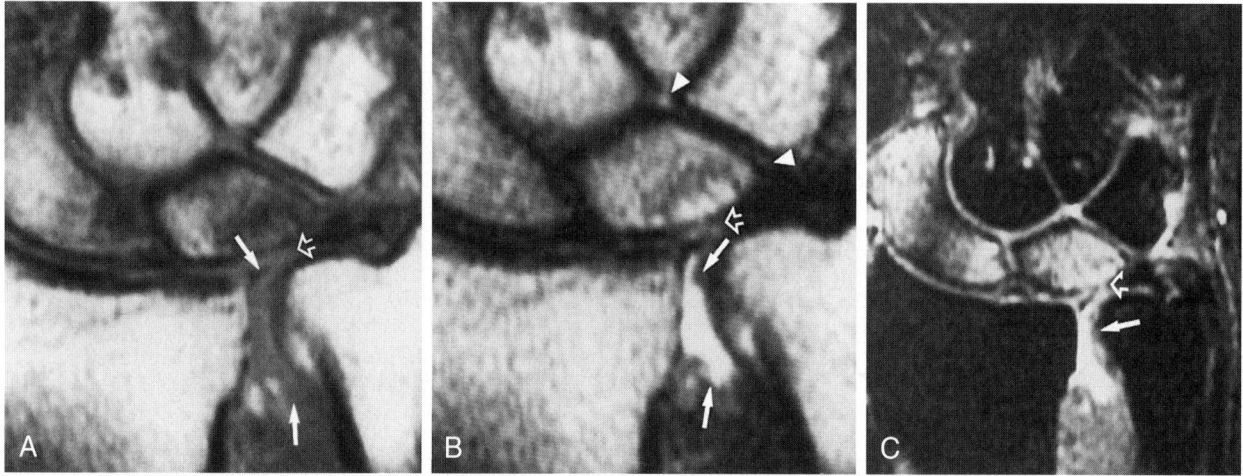

**Figure 59–7.** Ulnar impaction syndrome. *A*, Coronal intermediate-weighted (TR/TE, 1700/20) spin echo MR image shows a large communicating defect *(open arrow)* in the triangular fibrocartilage. Fluid *(solid arrows)* is apparent in the distal radioulnar joint. The lunotriquetral interosseous ligament is not well seen. Note the abnormal regions of low signal intensity in the lunate and scaphoid, consistent with marrow edema. The lunate changes occurred as a consequence of the ulnar impaction syndrome. *B*, Coronal T2-weighted (TR/TE, 1700/70) spin echo MR image also shows the communicating defect *(open arrow)* in the triangular fibrocartilage. Fluid fills the distal radioulnar joint *(solid arrows)* and is seen in the midcarpal joint *(arrowheads)*, including the space between the lunate and triquetrum. High signal intensity in the proximal portion of the lunate is indicative of marrow edema. *C*, Coronal STIR MR image (TR/TE, 1650/25; inversion time, 160 msec) shows defects in the triangular fibrocartilage *(open arrow)* and lunotriquetral interosseous ligament. Fluid fills the distal radioulnar joint *(solid arrow)* and portions of the radiocarpal and midcarpal joints. Marrow edema in the scaphoid and lunate is manifested as regions of increased signal intensity. (From Schweitzer ME, Brahme SK, Hodler J, et al: Radiology 182:205, 1992.)

Detection of subluxation of the distal portion of the ulna is best evaluated with computed tomography (CT). Accurate appraisal of the relative position of the ulna with respect to the radius requires imaging of the wrist in supination, neutral, and pronation and the construction of a number of lines, as shown in Figure 59–8. When the wrist is pronated, the ulna moves dorsally, and when the wrist is supinated, the head moves in a volar direction.

## Carpal Abnormalities

### Carpal Instability

Anatomically, three types of carpal instability are recognized: lateral instability, which usually occurs between the scaphoid and the lunate; medial instability, which occurs between the triquetrum and the lunate or between the triquetrum and the hamate; and proximal instability, which occurs when the abnormal carpal alignment is secondary to an injury to the radius or massive radiocarpal disruption. The patterns of instability that result from ligamentous disruption in the proximal carpal row (i.e., between the scaphoid and lunate or between the lunate and triquetrum) include scapholunate dissociation, which

produces dorsal intercalated segmental instability , and lunotriquetral dissociation, which leads to volar intercalated segmental instability (Fig. 59–9).

Diagnosis of many of the static patterns of carpal instability can be established on the basis of routine radiographic findings. Arthrography can be used for the diagnosis of communicating defects of the scapholunate and lunotriquetral interosseous ligaments. Such defects, however, may relate not to injury but to progressive deterioration, a process that increases in frequency with advancing age.

MR imaging is useful for the identification of defects of the scapholunate and lunotriquetral interosseous ligaments. The coronal plane is most useful for delineating

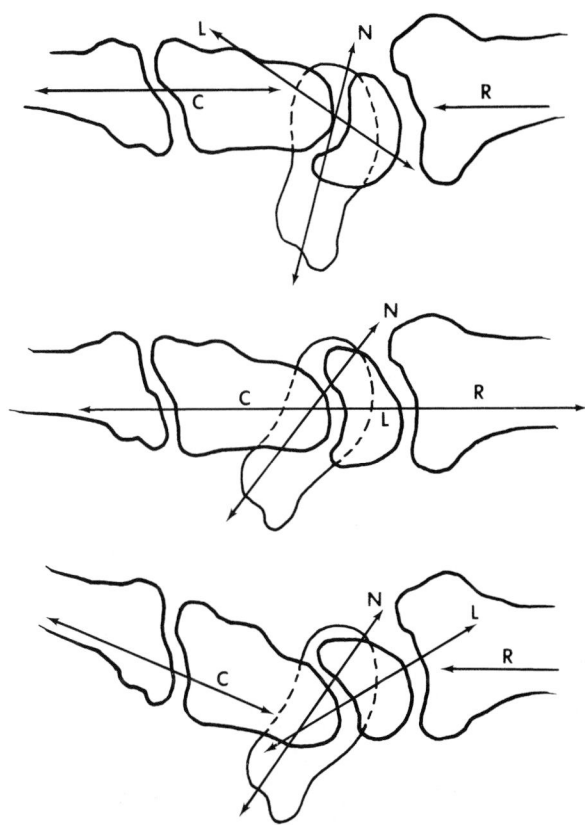

**Figure 59–9.** Dorsal and volar intercalated segmental instability: lateral projection. The upper drawing depicts the longitudinal axes of the third metacarpal, navicular (N) or scaphoid, lunate (L), capitate (C), and radius (R) in dorsal intercalated segmental instability (DISI). The middle drawing depicts the normal situation, and the lower drawing depicts volar intercalated segmental instability (VISI). When the wrist is normal, a continuous line can be drawn through the longitudinal axes of the capitate, lunate, and radius; this line intersects a second line through the longitudinal axis of the scaphoid and creates an angle of 30 to 60 degrees. In DISI, the lunate is flexed toward the back of the hand, and the scaphoid is displaced vertically. The angle of intersection between the two longitudinal axes is greater than 60 degrees. In VISI, the lunate is flexed toward the palm, and the angle between the two longitudinal axes is less than 30 degrees. (From Linscheid RL, Dobyns JH, Beabout JW, et al: Traumatic instability of the wrist: Diagnosis, classification, and pathomechanics. J Bone Joint Surg Am 54:1612, 1972.)

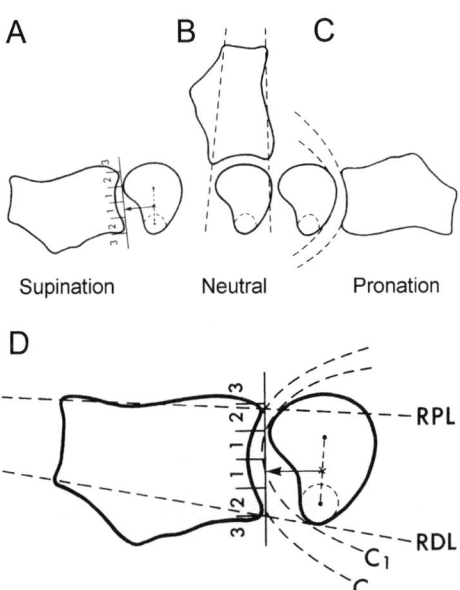

**Figure 59–8.** Methods for assessing radioulnar subluxation. *A* and *D*, Supination—epicenter method. A perpendicular line is drawn from the center of rotation of the distal radioulnar joint (a point halfway between the ulnar styloid process and center of the ulnar head) to a cord of the sigmoid notch. The joint is considered normal if this line is in the middle of the sigmoid notch. The dashed lines represent the location of the styloid process. *B*, Neutral—radioulnar line method. Articulation of the ulnar head with the radius is normal if the head falls between the two pictured lines. *C*, Pronation—congruity method. Note congruity of the arc of the ulnar head with that of the sigmoid notch. (From Wechsler RJ, Wehbe MA, Rifkin MD, et al: Computed tomography diagnosis of distal radioulnar subluxation. Skeletal Radiol 16:1,1987.)

the interosseous ligaments. Of the two interosseous ligaments, the scapholunate is visualized more consistently, although some investigators have indicated that the lunotriquetral ligament can also be identified regularly. On coronal spin echo or gradient echo images, a normal scapholunate interosseous ligament is typically seen as a thin or triangular (delta shaped) structure of low signal intensity traversing the space between the scaphoid and the lunate (Fig. 59–10). When visualized, a normal lunotriquetral interosseous ligament has a similar appearance and extends between the lunate and the triquetrum. Variations in the normal appearance of these ligaments include a linear shape and circular or linear regions of intermediate signal intensity within them.

An abnormality of the scapholunate interosseous ligament is suggested when it is elongated, appears incomplete, courses other than in a horizontal direction, or is not seen at all (Fig. 59–11). An abnormality of the lunotriquetral interosseous ligament is suggested when it is elongated, is incomplete, or extends in a direction other than horizontal. Although successful visualization of a lunotriquetral interosseous ligament is dependent on the specific imaging parameters used, its nonvisualization on MR images is not a reliable indicator of abnormality. Volumetric gradient echo imaging provides thin contiguous sections of the wrist (see Fig. 59–10). With this method, the scapholunate and lunotriquetral interosseous ligaments are generally well delineated. Nonvisualization of either ligament, particularly the scapholunate interosseous ligament, with volumetric imaging is strong evidence that an abnormality exists.

### Osteonecrosis

Osteonecrosis of the carpal bones affects three principal sites: the lunate bone (i.e., Kienböck's disease), the scaphoid bone (particularly its proximal portion after fracture of the waist of the bone), and, less commonly, the capitate bone (typically its proximal portion, either idiopathically or after injury). The features of osteonecrosis at these sites are discussed in Chapter 67. MR imaging is currently regarded as the most sensitive and specific imaging method for the detection of osteonecrosis (Fig. 59–12).

### Improper Fracture Healing

Although fractures may involve any of the carpal bones, fracture of the scaphoid is most common and may be followed by improper fracture healing (i.e., delayed union and nonunion). Causes of improper fracture healing of the scaphoid bone include a delay in the initial diagnosis of the fracture, rotation or displacement at the fracture site, inadequate immobilization, interposition of soft tissue in the fracture gap, and a tenuous blood supply. Routine radiography provides some diagnostic information regarding delayed union or nonunion, although CT provides more definitive evidence of a persistent fracture line, especially if direct or reformatted coronal or sagittal images are included.

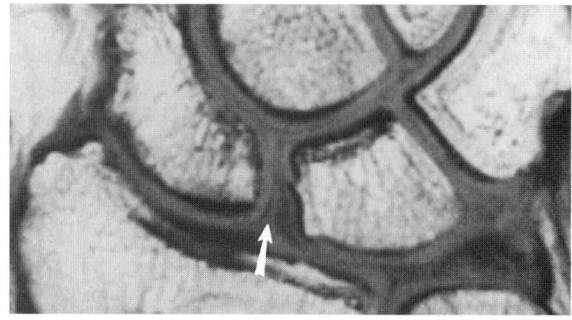

**Figure 59–11.** Intercarpal ligaments: communicating defect of the scapholunate interosseous ligament. Coronal T1-weighted (TR/TE, 800/20) spin echo MR image shows discontinuity of the scapholunate interosseous ligament *(arrow)*. The lunotriquetral interosseous ligament is not seen.

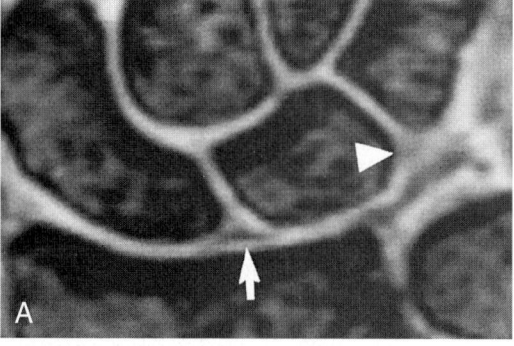 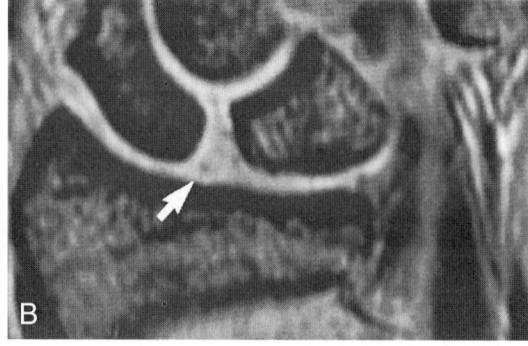

**Figure 59–10.** Intercarpal ligaments: three-dimensional Fourier transform (3DFT) gradient recalled MR imaging. *A,* Normal scapholunate interosseous ligament. Coronal 3DFT (TR/TE, 60/11; flip angle, 10 degrees) MR image shows the low signal intensity and linear morphology that characterize normal scapholunate *(arrow)* and lunotriquetral *(arrowhead)* interosseous ligaments. The triangular fibrocartilage is also normal. *B,* Communicating defect of the scapholunate interosseous ligament. Coronal oblique 3DFT (TR/TE, 60/10; flip angle, 30 degrees) MR image shows altered morphology *(arrow)* of the scapholunate interosseous ligament. *(A,* Courtesy of S. K. Brahme, MD, La Jolla, Calif.)

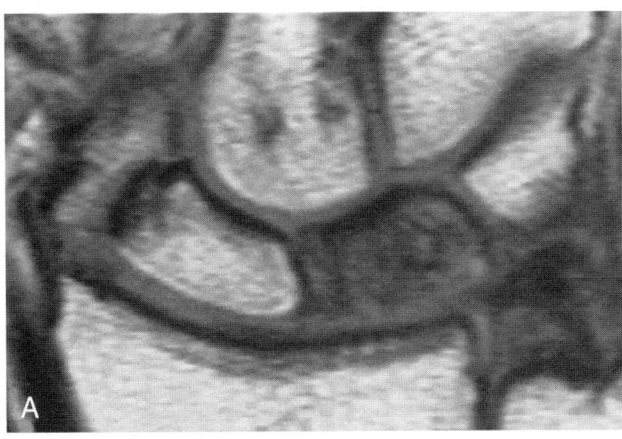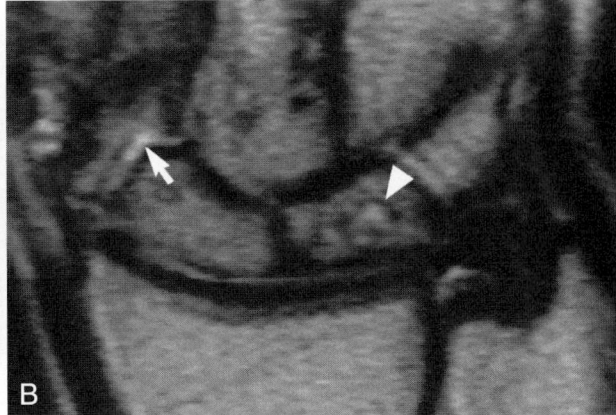

**Figure 59–12.** Kienböck's disease and nonunion of a scaphoid fracture. *A*, Coronal T1-weighted (TR/TE, 800/20) spin echo MR image reveals low signal intensity throughout the lunate bone and in the fracture gap of the scaphoid bone. *B*, Coronal T2-weighted (TR/TE, 2500/60) spin echo MR image shows foci of high signal intensity *(arrowhead)* in the lunate bone. Fluid of high signal intensity *(arrow)* is evident in a portion of the fracture gap in the scaphoid bone.

MR imaging shares many of the advantages of CT in the diagnosis of fracture complications. High signal intensity in the fracture defect on T2-weighted spin echo and certain gradient echo MR images is consistent with the presence of fluid, a sure sign of fracture nonunion (see Fig. 59–12). Persistent low signal intensity on T1- and T2-weighted spin echo MR images may indicate the presence of fibrosis at the fracture site. Marrow continuity across the fracture line is strong evidence that fracture healing has occurred.

## Carpal Tunnel Abnormalities

### Carpal Tunnel Syndrome

As indicated in Chapter 65, carpal tunnel syndrome is a relatively common entrapment neuropathy that affects the median nerve within the carpal tunnel in the palmar aspect of the wrist. Clinical findings include paresthesias of the fingers in the distribution of the median nerve and weakness and atrophy of the thenar muscles. Diagnostic imaging plays a minor role in the assessment of carpal tunnel syndrome. Ultrasonography, CT, and MR imaging have been used for this purpose. There are four consistent MR imaging findings in carpal tunnel syndrome: (1) swelling of the median nerve, best evaluated at the level of the pisiform bone; (2) flattening of the median nerve, best evaluated at the level of the hamate bone; (3) palmar bowing of the flexor retinaculum, best evaluated at the level of the hamate bone; and (4) increased signal intensity of the median nerve on T2-weighted spin echo images (Fig. 59–13). The pattern of enlargement of the median nerve is variable; the nerve may be diffusely enlarged or focally enlarged, especially at the level of the pisiform bone.

Inflammation of the flexor tendon sheaths is considered an important and perhaps the most common cause of carpal tunnel syndrome. The MR imaging abnormalities of such tenosynovitis include enlargement of individual tendon sheaths, as a result of effusion and increased sepa-ration between adjacent tendons in the carpal tunnel; increased signal intensity, resulting from fluid in the enlarged tendon sheaths; and volar bowing, or convexity, of the flexor retinaculum.

### Ulnar Tunnel Syndrome

Compression of the ulnar nerve as it traverses through the ulnar tunnel, or Guyon's canal, in the volar aspect of the wrist is well recognized (see Chapter 65). Causes of such entrapment include masses, vascular injury, anatomic variations, muscle hypertrophy, fracture, and hypertrophy of the transverse carpal ligament. Although the MR imaging abnormalities associated with ulnar tunnel syndrome are not well documented, findings similar to those of carpal tunnel syndrome are likely.

## Abnormalities of the Extensor and Flexor Tendons and Tendon Sheaths

### Tendinosis and Tenosynovitis

The MR imaging abnormalities of tendinosis and tenosynovitis include enlargement and increased signal intensity of the affected tendon and enlargement of its sheath as a result of the accumulation of fluid or synovitis. De Quervain's syndrome consists of tendinosis and tenosynovitis of the abductor pollicis longus and extensor brevis tendons and sheaths in the first extensor compartment. Involvement occurs at the level of or just proximal to the styloid process of the radius. Inflammation in the second extensor compartment (which contains the extensor carpi radialis longus and brevis tendons and sheaths) leads to the intersection syndrome, which is related to friction where the tendons in the first and second compartments cross, or intersect. Similarly, involvement of the extensor carpi ulnaris tendon and sheath in the sixth extensor compartment at the level of the distal portion and styloid process of the ulna may be evident (Fig. 59–14).

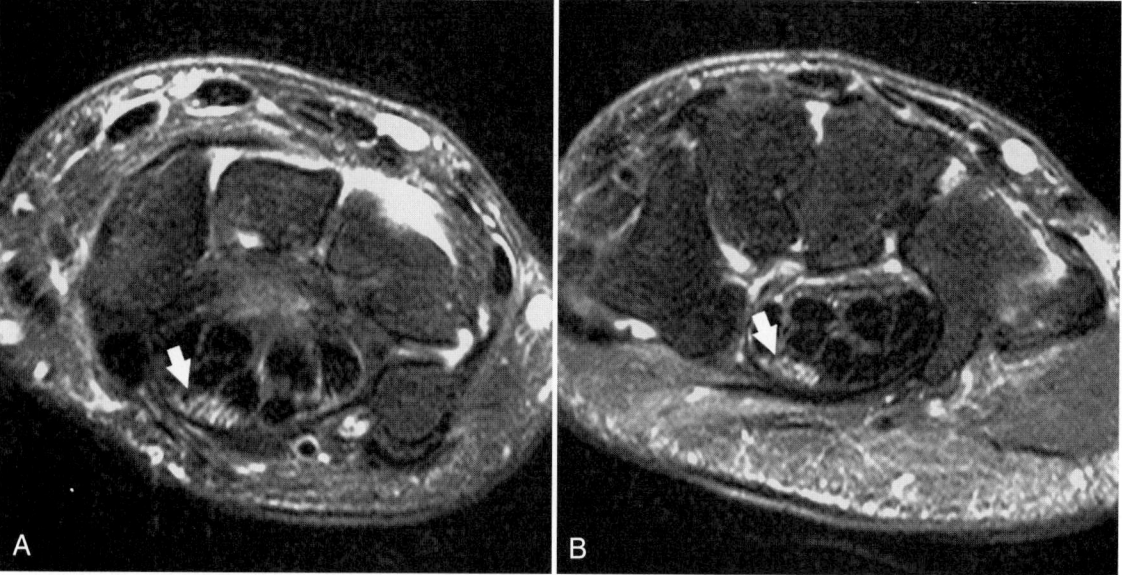

**Figure 59–13.** Carpal tunnel syndrome. *A,* Transaxial T2-weighted (TR/TE, 3000/66) fat-suppressed fast spin echo MR image of the wrist at the level of the pisiform bone. Note the enlargement and increased signal intensity in the median nerve *(arrow)*. *B,* Transaxial image distal to *(A)* at the level of the hook of the hamate bone. Although the signal intensity in the median nerve *(arrow)* is increased, the nerve is smaller at this level than at the level of the pisiform bone.

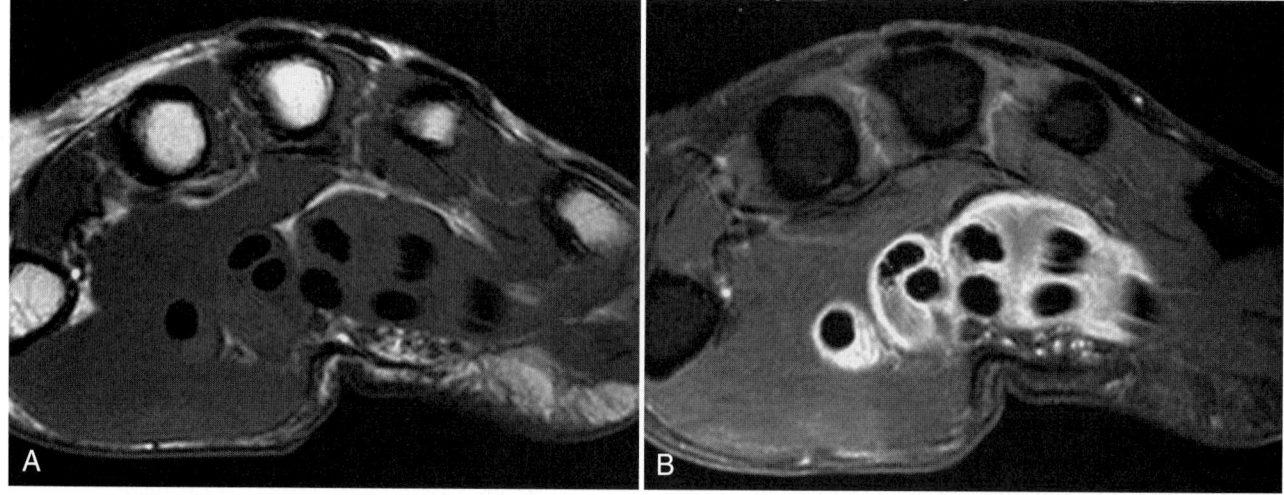

**Figure 59–14.** Tenosynovitis. Transaxial T1-weighted (TR/TE, 500/16) *(A)* and fat-suppressed, contrast-enhanced T1-weighted (TR/TE, 550/16) *(B)* spin echo MR images of the wrist at the midmetacarpal level show marked thickening and enhancement of the flexor tendons.

## Tendon Rupture

Any of the extensor or flexor tendons of the wrist, as well as those of the fingers, can rupture in response to an acute injury or chronic inflammation, such as occurs with infection or rheumatoid arthritis. Interruption of the tendon and the presence of surrounding fluid or inflammatory tissue are the findings noted on MR images. The degree of tendon retraction and the distance between the torn ends of the tendon can be determined (Fig. 59–15).

## Giant Cell Tumor of the Tendon Sheath

As indicated in Chapter 71, giant cell tumors of soft tissue may arise from tendon sheaths (as well as joint capsules and ligamentous tissue). Even though they may be observed about the wrist, they are far more frequent in the fingers. Soft tissue swelling or a mass, with or without erosion of the subjacent bone and without calcification, is evident. The presence of hemosiderin deposition or dense acellular fibrous tissue typically gives the lesion a low to intermediate signal intensity on both T1- and T2-weighted spin echo MR images.

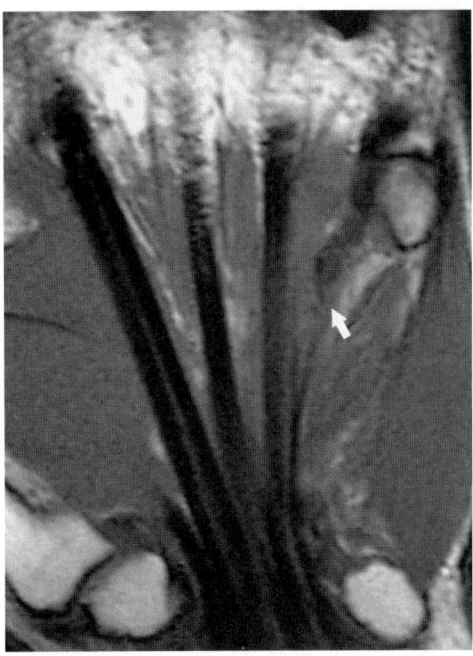

**Figure 59–15.** Tendon rupture. Coronal T1-weighted (TR/TE, 500/14) spin echo MR image of the hand shows rupture of the flexor tendon of the little finger. The free edge of the thickened, retracted, ruptured tendon (*arrow*) is well seen.

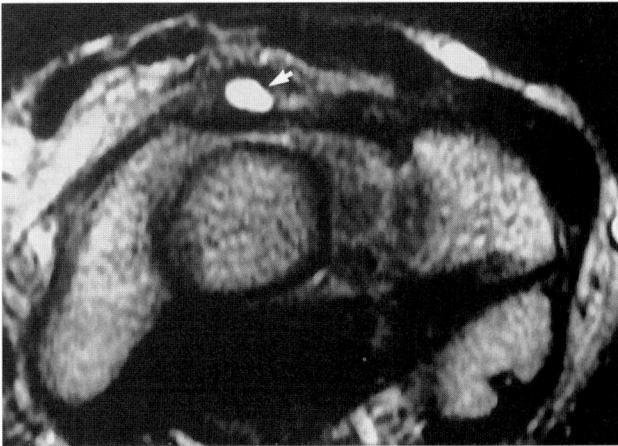

**Figure 59–16.** Ganglion cyst. Transaxial T2-weighted (TR/TE, 2000/80) spin echo MR image of the wrist at the level of the midcarpal joint shows a small ganglion cyst (*arrow*) just superficial to the dorsal intercarpal ligament and deep to the extensor tendons. (Courtesy of A. G. Bergman, MD, Stanford, Calif.)

## Abnormalities of the Joint Synovium and Capsule

### Ganglion Cyst

Ganglion cysts about the wrist are common, although their precise cause is debated (see Chapter 71). Most commonly, ganglion cysts appear on the dorsum of the wrist, but they also occur volarly and in other locations. The site of origin may be the joint capsule, tendon, or tendon sheath. A higher frequency of abnormalities of the TFCC and interosseous ligaments has been noted in patients with such ganglion cysts. Ganglion cysts contain fluid that may be slightly more viscous than joint fluid. They rarely calcify. Anechoic oval, round, or lobulated cystic masses are seen with ultrasonography. Low to intermediate signal intensity on T1-weighted spin echo MR images and high signal intensity on T2-weighted spin echo MR images within the ganglion cyst are typical (Fig. 59–16).

### Adhesive Capsulitis

Adhesive capsulitis is encountered most frequently in the shoulder, although involvement of the ankle, hip, and wrist is also seen. Physical and neurologic injuries are two potential causes of this condition. Restricted joint capacity with extravasation of contrast material is evident during arthrography. MR imaging of adhesive capsulitis is generally not rewarding.

### Articular Diseases

MR imaging has been used to assess the extent of rheumatoid arthritis and other synovial inflammatory diseases in the wrist. Its advantages compared with routine radiography include more accurate assessment of cartilage and bone destruction, extent of synovial inflammation, and activity of the disease process. Marginal and central bone erosions and subchondral cystic lesions can be identified because of the tomographic nature of the study and the high signal intensity of synovial fluid and inflammatory tissue on T2-weighted spin echo and gradient echo MR images. The diagnosis of pigmented villonodular synovitis and idiopathic synovial (osteo)chondromatosis can also be established with MR imaging (see Chapter 71).

## Other Abnormalities

**Occult Bone Injuries.** The use of MR imaging to evaluate occult bone injuries is discussed in Chapter 56. Such injuries include acute infractions and chronic stress fractures. Although most reports on this use of MR imaging are based on studies of occult bone injuries about the knee and hip, a similar role exists for MR imaging in cases of wrist and hand fractures. Occult fractures of the distal portion of the radius in elderly persons and occult scaphoid fractures in young adults are two examples of injuries that can be detected with MR imaging.

**Gamekeeper's Thumb.** Classically described in English game wardens, and thus known as gamekeeper's thumb, tears of the ulnar collateral ligament of the first metacarpophalangeal joint are common, usually the result of violent abduction of the thumb. When disrupted, the torn end of the ulnar collateral ligament can become displaced superficial to the adductor pollicis aponeurosis, a finding known as the Stener lesion. The interposed aponeurosis interferes with healing, and surgery has been advocated for the treatment of displaced tears of the ulnar collateral ligament.

MR imaging can be used to identify a Stener lesion. On coronal MR images of the first metacarpophalangeal joint, a normal ulnar collateral ligament appears as a band of low signal intensity medial to the joint. The adductor aponeurosis is often visible as a paper-thin band of low signal intensity superficial to the ulnar collateral ligament and extending from the distal half of that ligament over the base of the proximal phalanx. A nondisplaced tear of the ulnar collateral ligament appears as a discontinuity of the ligament distally, without ligamentous retraction and with the adductor aponeurosis covering the distal end of the ligament. Displacement of the ulnar collateral ligament, or the Stener lesion, is associated with proximal retraction or folding of the ligament. The proximal margin of the adductor aponeurosis may be seen to abut the folded ulnar collateral ligament, thereby creating a rounded region of low signal intensity that has been designated a "yo-yo on a string" appearance (Fig. 59–17).

## ELBOW

### Anatomy

The articulation about the elbow has three constituents: (1) humeroradial, the area between the capitulum of the humerus and the facet on the radial head; (2) humero-ulnar, the area between the trochlea of the humerus and the trochlear notch of the ulna; and (3) superior (proximal) radioulnar, the area between the head of the radius and the radial notch of the ulna and the annular ligament.

A fibrous capsule completely invests the elbow. Lateral and medial collateral ligamentous complexes reinforce the fibrous capsule of the elbow (Fig. 59–18).

The annular ligament is a thick band of fibrous tissue that attaches to the anterior and posterior margins of the radial notch of the ulna. It serves as a restraining ligament that prevents withdrawal or inferior displacement of the head of the radius from its socket.

It is convenient to divide the many muscles about the elbow into four groups: posterior, anterior, lateral, and medial. The muscles of the posterior group are the triceps and the anconeus; those of the anterior group are the biceps brachii and brachialis; the lateral group of muscles includes the supinator and brachioradialis muscles and the extensor muscles of the wrist and hand; and the medial group of muscles includes the pronator teres, palmaris longus, and flexors of the hand and wrist.

Three major nerves are located in the elbow region. The median nerve parallels the course of the brachial artery, courses anterior to it in the cubital area, and descends farther between the superficial and deep heads of the pronator teres muscle. The ulnar nerve is present on the posteromedial side of the elbow and passes in a groove between the olecranon process of the ulna and the medial epicondyle of the humerus. The radial nerve descends above the elbow between the brachialis and brachioradialis muscles and divides near the elbow into deep and superficial branches.

### Tendon and Muscle Abnormalities

Although uncommon, avulsions (and tears) of tendons about the elbow are encountered. The tendons of the biceps brachii and the triceps are involved most commonly. Routine radiographic features of such avulsions include joint effusion and bone fragmentation and displacement.

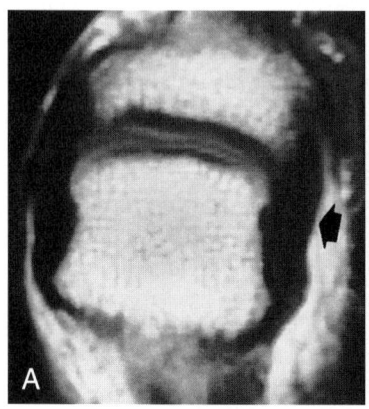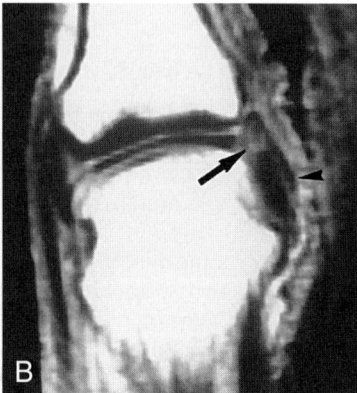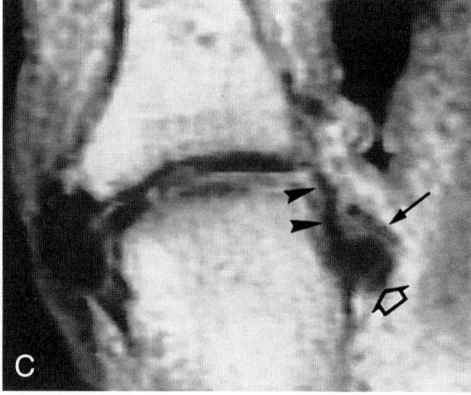

**Figure 59–17.** Gamekeeper's thumb. *A,* Normal ulnar collateral ligament. Coronal T1-weighted (TR/TE, 500/20) spin echo MR image of the first metacarpophalangeal joint shows the normal ulnar collateral ligament *(arrow)* as a band of low signal intensity. The adductor aponeurosis is not visible. *B,* Nondisplaced tear of the ulnar collateral ligament. Coronal T1-weighted (TR/TE, 500/20) spin echo MR image of the first metacarpophalangeal joint shows disruption of the ulnar collateral ligament *(arrow)* and a superficial curvilinear structure of low signal intensity *(arrowhead)* representing the adductor aponeurosis. *C,* Displaced tear of the ulnar collateral ligament (Stener lesion). Coronal T1-weighted (TR/TE, 500/20) spin echo MR image of the first metacarpophalangeal joint reveals a yo-yo appearance. The adductor pollicis aponeurosis *(arrowheads)* looks like a string holding a yo-yo—the balled-up, displaced ulnar collateral ligament *(open arrow).* The thin region of low signal intensity *(solid arrow)* represents an avulsed bone fragment. (From Spaeth HJ, Abrams RA, Bock GW, et al: Gamekeeper thumb: Differentiation of nondisplaced and displaced tears of the ulnar collateral ligament with MR imaging. Work in progress. Radiology 188:553, 1993.)

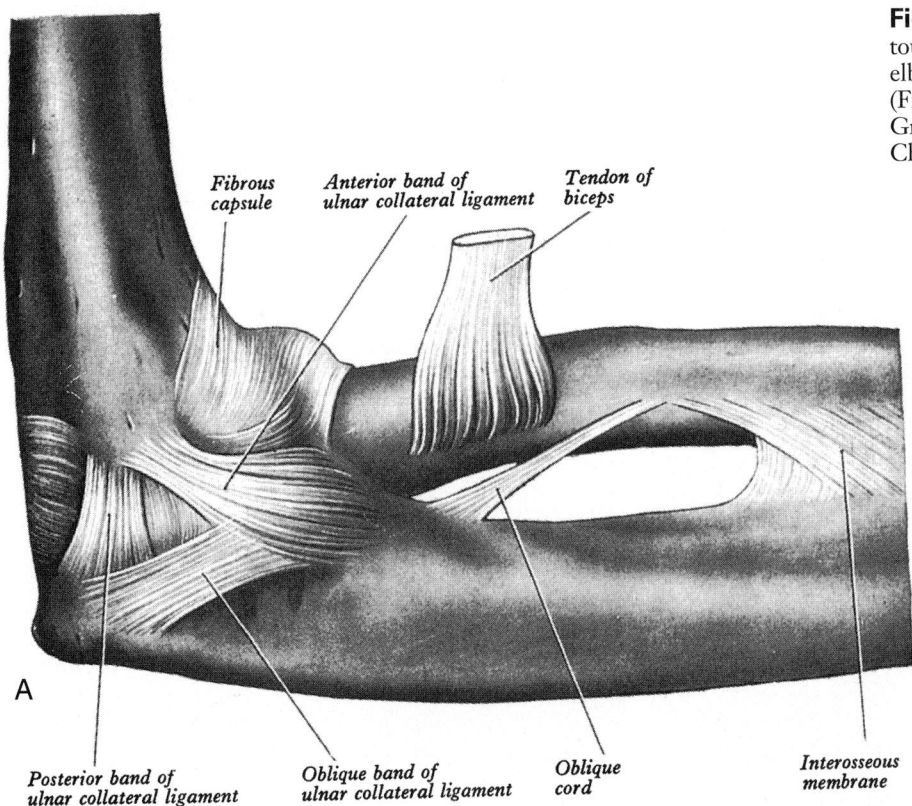

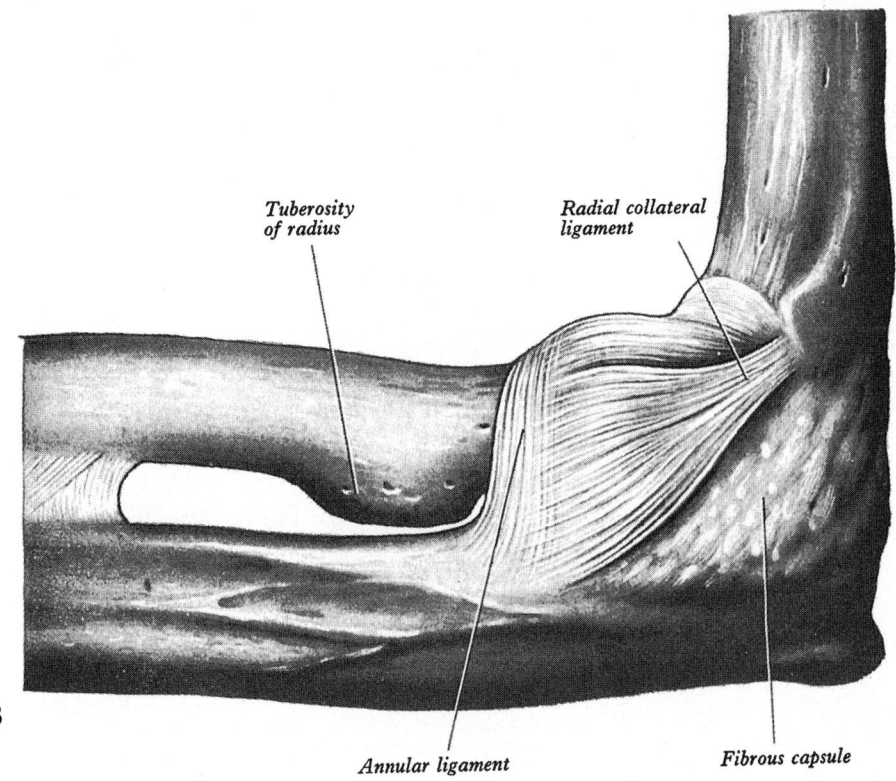

**Figure 59–18.** Elbow joint: ligamentous anatomy. *A*, Medial aspect of the elbow. *B*, Lateral aspect of the elbow. (From Williams PL, Warwick R [eds]: Gray's Anatomy, 36th Br ed. Edinburgh, Churchill Livingstone, 1980, p 431.)

Although other imaging methods, such as CT and ultrasonography, may be used to delineate tendinous injuries, MR imaging is most suited to this task.

Normal tendons about the elbow (and elsewhere) appear as smooth, linear structures of low signal intensity on MR imaging sequences. A magic angle phenomenon, however, occasionally leads to regions of intermediate signal intensity within the tendons when MR sequences with short TE are used. Tendinous tears and avulsion are associated with irregular and frayed contours and altered signal intensity of the tendons (Fig. 59–19). Complete tears are accompanied by discontinuity and retraction of the tendon, and partial tears are accompanied by some remaining intact tendinous fibers. Alterations in signal intensity depend on the age of the injury, although high signal intensity within the tendon itself and the adjacent soft tissues and bone is commonly present on T2-weighted spin echo MR images. Tears of the tendon of the triceps brachii muscle are uncommon, with complete tears dominating over partial tears. Rupture of the distal portion of the tendon of the biceps brachii muscle constitutes less than 5% of all biceps tendon injuries.

Chronic overuse syndromes can also lead to tendinous alterations. Clinical and imaging abnormalities predominate on the lateral side of the joint, in the region of the humeral epicondyle and capitulum. This condition is often described as tennis elbow. Although the type of pathologic lesion associated with chronic overuse syndromes of the elbow varies, partial tearing of fibers within the extensor tendons (and, less commonly, the flexor tendons) from their epicondylar attachments is typical. Regions of high signal intensity on T2-weighted spin echo images in the tendon, the soft tissue, and the bone may be evident (Fig. 59–20).

## Ligament Abnormalities

Ligamentous disruptions about the elbow can accompany severe physical trauma (e.g., elbow dislocation) or can occur as a response to less extensive acute trauma (e.g., valgus injury) or chronic stress (e.g., baseball pitching). Clinical findings include pain and tenderness in the medial aspect of the elbow, symptoms of ulnar nerve compression,

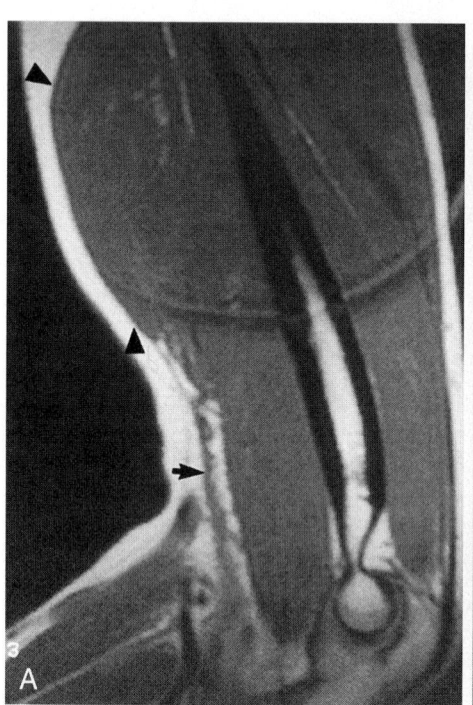
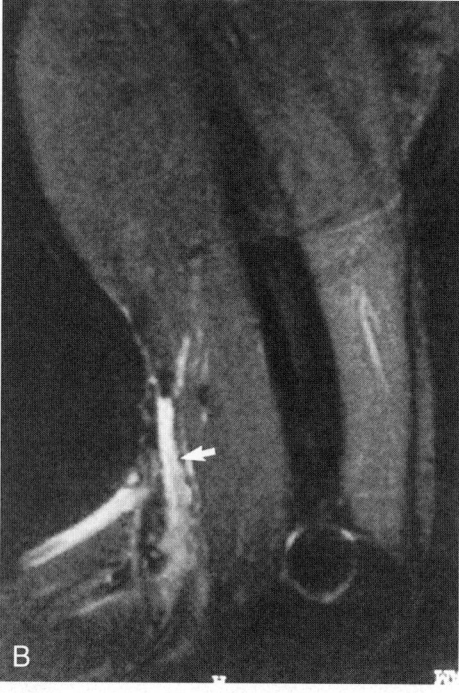

**Figure 59–19.** Biceps brachii tendon tear. Complete rupture in a 41-year-old man who noted a popping sensation while lifting a heavy weight. *A,* Sagittal T1-weighted (TR/TE, 570/15) spin echo MR image shows a corkscrew-like appearance of the biceps brachii tendon *(arrow).* Note the retracted muscle *(arrowheads).* A wraparound artifact relates to patient positioning for the MR imaging examination. *B,* Sagittal STIR (TR/TE, 6200/22; inversion time, 150 msec) MR image shows the abnormal biceps brachii tendon *(arrow).* (Courtesy of C. Wakeley, MD, Bristol, England.)

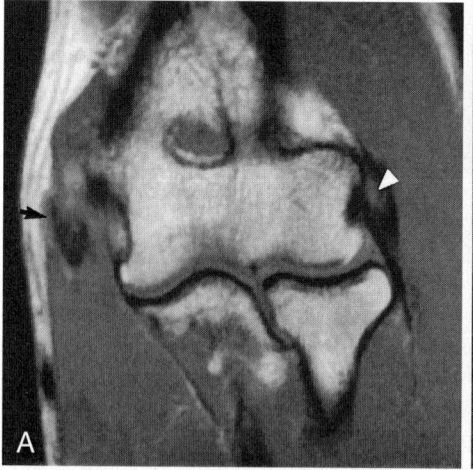
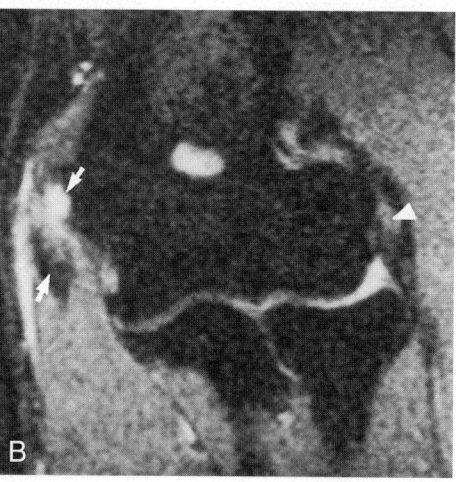

**Figure 59–20.** Flexor tendon tear: acute avulsive injury of the common flexor tendons. *A,* Coronal T1-weighted (TR/TE, 600/30) spin echo MR image shows avulsion of the flexor tendons *(arrow)* from the medial epicondyle of the humerus. Abnormal signal intensity is also evident in the common extensor tendons *(arrowhead).* *B,* Coronal STIR MR image reveals high signal intensity at the site of flexor tendon avulsion *(arrows),* altered signal intensity in the common extensor tendons *(arrowhead),* and a joint effusion. (Courtesy of C. Ho, MD, Palo Alto, Calif.)

and increased valgus stress exerted on a partially flexed joint. MR imaging can be used to assess acutely or chronically injured ligaments about the elbow. Normally, the collateral ligaments, especially the medial collateral ligament, are seen on coronal images of the elbow as thin linear bands of low signal intensity. Coronal oblique MR imaging planes directed along the longitudinal axes of the most important components of the collateral ligaments may improve visualization. With injury to these ligaments, MR imaging findings are laxity, irregularity, poor definition, and increased signal intensity within and around the affected ligament (Fig. 59–21).

## Nerve Abnormalities

Entrapment and compression neuropathies about the elbow may involve the ulnar, radial, or median nerve, with those involving the ulnar nerve most common. Entrapment of the ulnar nerve in the fibro-osseous tunnel posterior to the medial epicondyle of the humerus results in the cubital tunnel syndrome. Typical causes of this syndrome are injury and progressive cubitus valgus deformity (tardy ulnar nerve palsy); other causes include osteoarthritis, rheumatoid arthritis, nerve subluxation, prolonged bed rest, anomalous muscles, and masses. Clinical manifestations include weakness of the flexor carpi ulnaris muscle, flexor digitorum profundus muscle of the fourth and fifth fingers, and intrinsic hand muscles. MR imaging is the preferred diagnostic modality, showing displacement or shift of the ulnar nerve, soft tissue mass, and enlargement and increased signal intensity in the compressed nerve (Fig. 59–22).

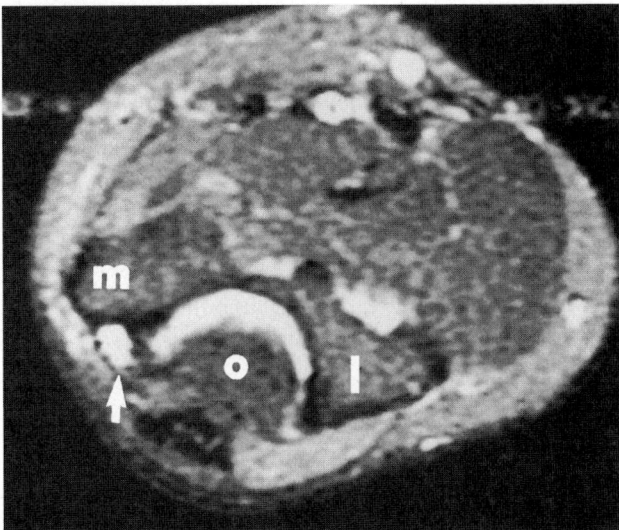

**Figure 59–22.** Entrapment neuropathy: cubital tunnel syndrome. Transaxial T2-weighted (TR/TE, 2000/70) spin echo MR image, accomplished with fat suppression, shows increased signal intensity in the ulnar nerve *(arrow)* within the cubital tunnel. The medial (m) and lateral (l) epicondyles of the humerus and the olecranon process (o) of the ulna are indicated. A joint effusion is present. (Courtesy of S. K. Brahme, MD, La Jolla, Calif.)

## Bone Abnormalities

### Osteochondral Fracture and Osteochondritis Dissecans

Osteochondritis dissecans about the elbow usually affects the capitulum. This disorder differs from a developmental alteration of the capitular ossification center known as Panner's disease. MR imaging of osteochondritis dissecans of the capitulum may be used to gain information regarding the integrity of the adjacent articular cartilage, the viability of the separated fragment, and the presence or absence of associated intra-articular osseous and cartilaginous bodies. The presence of joint fluid or granulation tissue at the interface between the fragment and the parent bone, manifested as increased signal intensity on T2-weighted spin echo MR images, generally indicates an unstable lesion (Fig. 59–23). MR arthrography performed after the intra-articular injection of gadolinium compounds may be advantageous. Computed arthrotomography provides similar information.

### Chondroepiphyseal Injuries

Accurate radiographic diagnosis of elbow injuries in young children is difficult because of the large number of developing ossification centers, the normal irregularities of bone in these centers, and the cartilaginous component of these centers, which is not visible on routine radiographs. Differentiation among the many Salter-Harris lesions of the growth plate may be impossible when standard radiography alone is performed. Because such differentiation has prognostic implications, a diagnostic role may exist for imaging methods such as arthrography and MR imaging.

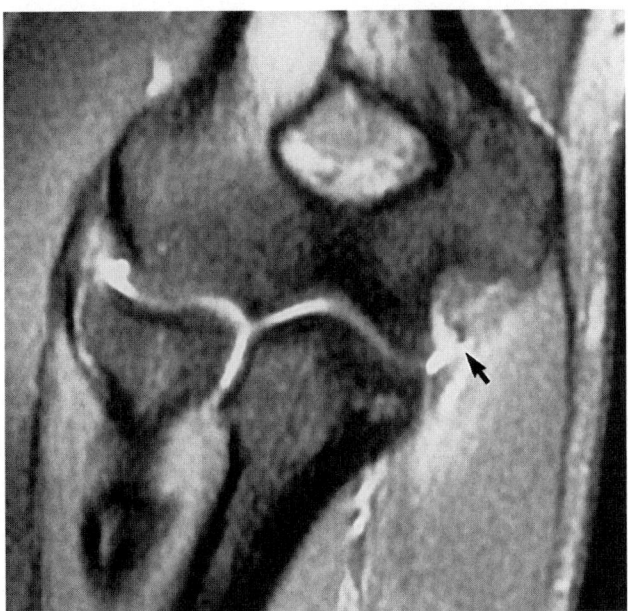

**Figure 59–21.** Medial (ulnar) collateral ligament tear. Coronal fat-suppressed, fast spin echo (TR/TE, 4000/18) MR image in a baseball pitcher shows disruption *(arrow)* of the anterior band of the medial collateral ligament, with surrounding edema and hemorrhage.

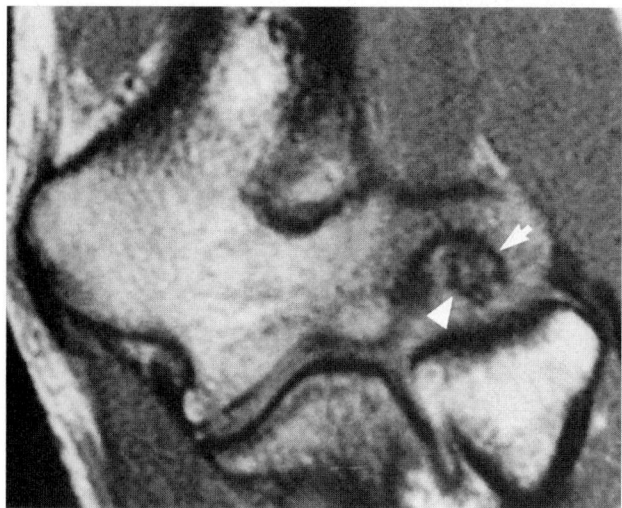

**Figure 59–23.** Osteochondritis dissecans: capitulum of the humerus. Coronal intermediate-weighted (TR/TE, 2000/20) spin echo MR image shows the osseous defect *(arrow)* containing an ossified body *(arrowhead)*. The integrity of the adjacent articular cartilage cannot be determined. (Courtesy of M. Schweitzer, MD, Philadelphia, Pa.)

Spin echo or gradient echo MR images provide direct visualization of the cartilaginous and osseous components of the chondroepiphyses about the elbow. Physeal separation and violation, fractures, and edema are readily detectable on such images.

## Synovial Abnormalities

### Synovial Proliferation

Synovial proliferation in the elbow may accompany a variety of disease processes, including rheumatoid arthritis, septic arthritis, crystal deposition disorders, pigmented villonodular synovitis, and idiopathic synovial osteochondromatosis. Accumulation of joint fluid leads to a characteristic displacement of the extrasynovial fat pads of the elbow, which can be recognized with routine radiography, CT, and MR imaging. The finding lacks specificity and indicates only the presence of an effusion.

Rheumatoid arthritis and other synovial inflammatory disorders affecting the elbow lead to proliferation of the synovial membrane and accumulation of joint fluid. The signal intensity characteristics of the abnormal synovium and fluid are similar on standard MR imaging sequences. Intravenous administration of gadolinium compounds leads to enhancement of the signal intensity of the inflammatory tissue; it does not affect the signal intensity of fluid on MR images obtained immediately after the injection. Pigmented villonodular synovitis may involve the elbow, and the diagnosis may be suggested by an appropriate clinical history and typical radiographic abnormalities. The deposition of hemosiderin in the affected synovial tissue produces regions of persistently low signal intensity on spin echo and, especially, gradient echo MR images. This finding may also be observed in cases of

chronic hemarthrosis, hemophilia, synovial hemangioma, and other conditions.

Idiopathic synovial osteochondromatosis, related to metaplasia of the synovial lining, is accompanied by synovial proliferation and the formation of intrasynovial nodules of cartilage. The fate of these nodules is variable; they may calcify or ossify or may become free within the joint cavity and later become embedded in a distant synovial site. Routine radiography is sensitive to the detection of calcified and ossified intra-articular bodies but insensitive to the detection of nonossified bodies. Arthrography, in which the bodies appear as multiple filling defects within the opacified joint, and MR imaging can be helpful diagnostically (Fig. 59–24).

### Synovial Cyst

Para-articular synovial cysts that communicate with the elbow joint are a recognized manifestation of rheumatoid arthritis, but theoretically they can occur with any process leading to elevated intra-articular pressure in the elbow. Arthrography, cystography, ultrasonography, CT, and MR imaging are all effective in establishing the diagnosis and determining whether the contents of the cyst have ruptured.

### Intra-articular Osteocartilaginous Body

Any process leading to disintegration of the articular surface of the elbow joint may be responsible for intra-articular osteocartilaginous bodies, although trauma is the most important cause. In common with intra-articular bodies in other locations, bodies originating from the joint

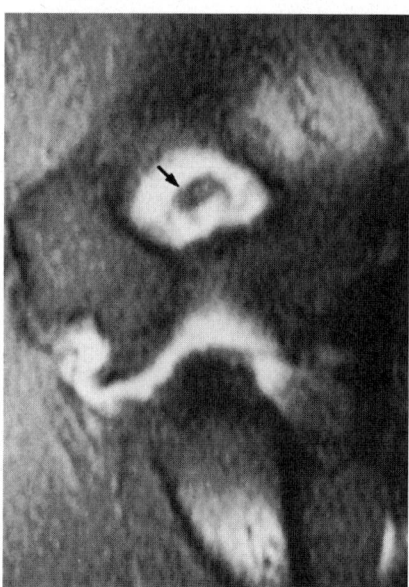

**Figure 59–24.** Intra-articular osteocartilaginous bodies: MR arthrography. Coronal T1-weighted (TR/TE, 950/13) spin echo MR image obtained after the intra-articular injection of a gadolinium compound and with fat suppression shows a body *(arrow)* in the olecranon fossa.

surface may be composed of cartilage alone or cartilage and bone together. Free bodies in the elbow joint commonly migrate to dependent portions of the joint and to sites of normal depressions in bone, particularly the olecranon fossa.

Calcified bodies in the elbow joint can be detected by routine radiography; however, those that lodge in the olecranon fossa may be overlooked unless conventional tomography or CT is used. Noncalcified bodies are more difficult to detect, requiring arthrography, computed arthrotomography, or MR imaging. Of these techniques, computed arthrotomography is often preferred. Conventional MR imaging is relatively insensitive to the diagnosis of small calcified bodies because the signal void of these bodies is easily overlooked. Further, small noncalcified cartilaginous bodies are characterized by high signal intensity on T2-weighted spin echo images, similar to the signal intensity of joint fluid. MR arthrography (see Fig. 59–24) may be useful in the detection of small calcified or noncalcified bodies.

## SHOULDER

### Anatomy

**Articular.** In the glenohumeral joint, the articular surfaces of the glenoid and humerus are covered with hyaline cartilage (Fig. 59–25). The cartilage on the humeral head is thickest at its center and thinner peripherally, whereas the reverse is true on the glenoid portion of the joint. A fibrocartilaginous structure, the labrum, attaches to the

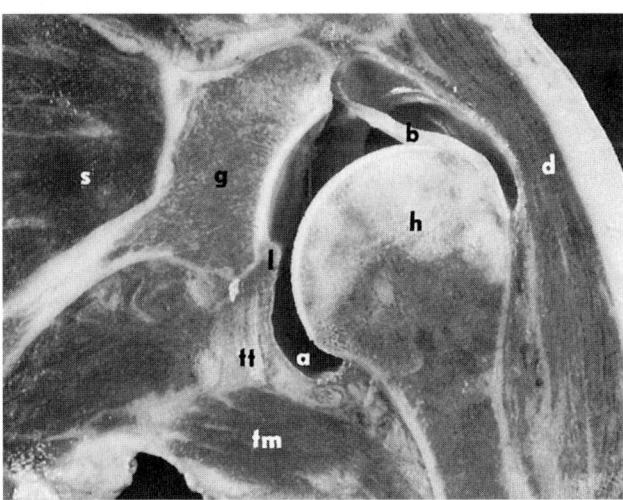

**Figure 59–25.** Glenohumeral joint: articular anatomy. Coronal section of an air-distended articular cavity reveals the glenoid region of the scapula (g); humeral head (h); axillary pouch (a); inferior portion of the labrum (l); tendon of the long head of the biceps brachii muscle (b); portions of the subscapularis (s), deltoid (d), and teres major (tm) muscles; and tendon of the long head of the triceps muscle (tt). Note the hyaline cartilage covering both the glenoid cavity and the humeral head. The size of the articular surface of the humerus is much larger than that of the glenoid cavity.

glenoid rim and adds an element of stability to the glenohumeral articulation. A loose fibrous capsule arises from the circumference of the glenoid labrum or from the neck of the scapula and inserts distally into the humerus. In certain areas, the fibrous capsule is strengthened by its intimate association with the surrounding ligaments and tendons; with regard to tendons, the capsule is reinforced above by the supraspinatus, below by the long head of the triceps, anteriorly by the subscapularis, and posteriorly by the infraspinatus and teres minor. The tendons of the supraspinatus, infraspinatus, teres minor, and subscapularis form a cuff (the rotator cuff) that blends with and reinforces the fibrous capsule.

The coracohumeral ligament strengthens the upper part of the capsule. It arises from the lateral edge of the coracoid process, extends over the humeral head, and attaches to the greater tuberosity. Anteriorly, the capsule may thicken to form the superior, middle, and inferior glenohumeral ligaments. These ligaments and the recesses formed between them are variable in configuration. Several openings may be found in the fibrous capsule, although they are variable in number and location. One or two anterior perforations, or foramina, below the coracoid process establish joint communication with the bursa behind the subscapularis tendon, the subscapular "recess." Although another opening between the greater and lesser tuberosities has been described, allowing passage of the tendon and synovial sheath of the long head of the biceps brachii muscle, this tendon typically invaginates the synovial membrane rather than piercing it. Another inconstant perforation may exist posteriorly and allow communication of the articular cavity and a bursa under the infraspinatus tendon.

Several bursae are located about the glenohumeral joint; the most important of these is the subacromial (subdeltoid) bursa, which lies between the deltoid muscle and joint capsule (Fig. 59–26). It extends underneath the acromion and the coracoacromial ligament. The subacromial (subdeltoid) bursa is separated from the articular cavity by the rotator cuff and does not communicate with the joint unless the cuff has been perforated. The acromioclavicular joint also has a surrounding fibrous capsule. Surrounding ligaments include the acromioclavicular and coracoclavicular ligaments (Fig. 59–27).

**Glenohumeral Ligaments.** The glenohumeral ligaments represent thickenings, or reinforcements, of the joint capsule (Fig. 59–28). The three glenohumeral ligaments are the superior, middle, and inferior glenohumeral ligaments. In any person, the number of ligaments present is variable, and they can vary considerably in size. The superior glenohumeral ligament is present in 90% to 97% of cases, the middle glenohumeral ligament is present in 73% to 92% of cases, and the inferior glenohumeral ligament is present in almost 100% of cases. Each extends from the anterior aspect of the glenoid cavity, near the glenoid labrum, to the proximal portion of the humerus (i.e., anatomic neck). The middle glenohumeral ligament shows the most variability in size. The inferior glenohumeral ligament is the main stabilizer of an abducted glenohumeral joint. The inferior glenohumeral ligament complex consists of an anterior band, a posterior band, and an intervening axillary pouch.

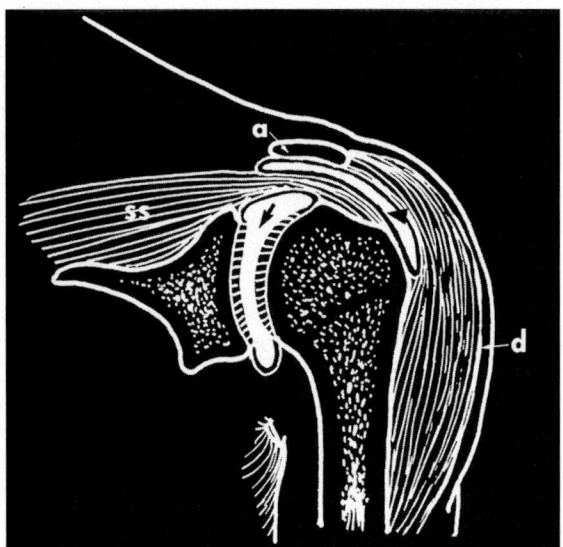

**Figure 59–26.** Subacromial (subdeltoid) bursa: normal anatomy. Diagram of a coronal section of the shoulder shows the glenohumeral joint *(arrow)* and subacromial (subdeltoid) bursa *(arrowhead)*, separated by a portion of the rotator cuff (i.e., supraspinatus tendon). The supraspinatus (ss) and deltoid (d) muscles and the acromion (a) are indicated.

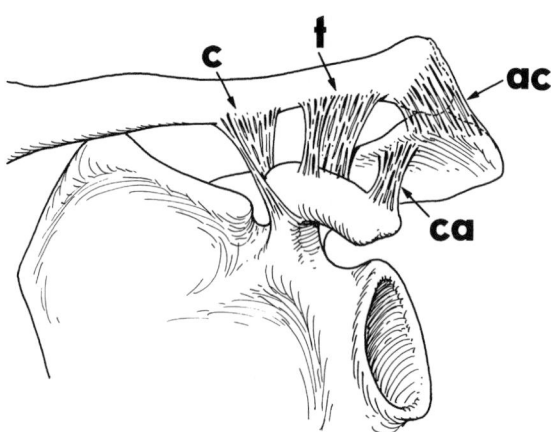

**Figure 59–27.** Acromioclavicular joint: normal ligamentous anatomy. Important structures include the fibrous capsule of the joint, which is strengthened by the acromioclavicular ligament (ac), coracoacromial ligament (ca), and conoid (c) and trapezoid (t) portions of the coracoclavicular ligament.

**Glenoid Labrum.** The glenoid labrum is a cuff of fibrous and fibrocartilaginous tissue surrounding the glenoid cavity that serves to deepen the glenoid fossa and allow attachment of the tendon of the long head of the biceps brachii muscle and the glenohumeral ligaments (see Fig. 59–28). It is often described in terms of the face of a clock; its superior portion is designated 12 o'clock. The superior part of the labrum tends to be meniscal in appearance and is normally loosely attached. This normal laxity leads to difficulty in diagnosing superior labral, anterior and posterior (SLAP) lesions (see later discussion). The

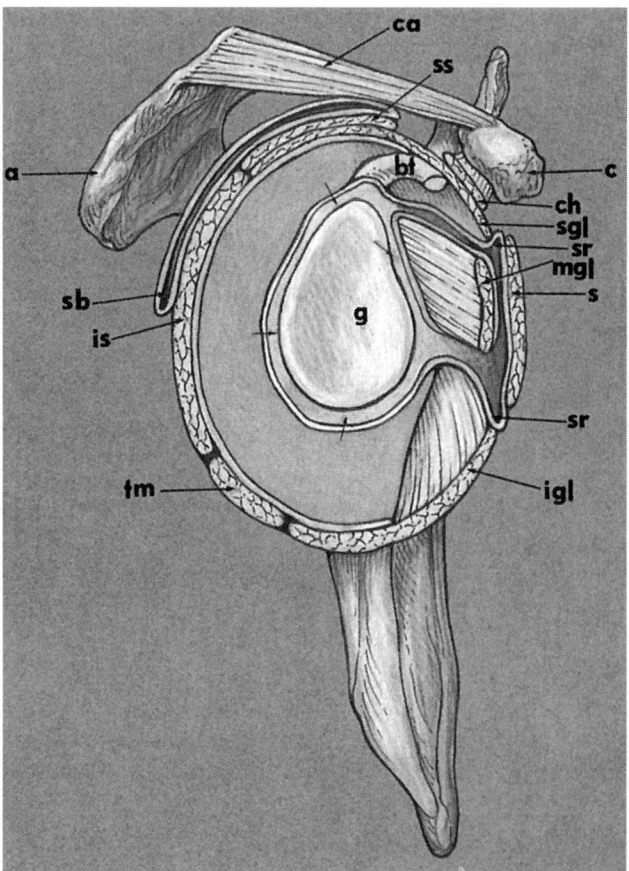

**Figure 59–28.** Glenohumeral joint: ligamentous and capsular anatomy. Lateral view of an opened glenohumeral joint in which the humeral head has been removed. Identified structures (beginning superiorly and continuing in a clockwise direction) are the coracoacromial ligament (ca), supraspinatus tendon (ss), tendon of the long head of the biceps brachii muscle (bt), coracoid process (c), coracohumeral ligament (ch), superior glenohumeral ligament (sgl), an opening into the subscapular recess (sr), middle glenohumeral ligament (mgl), subscapularis tendon (s), a second opening into the subscapular recess (sr), inferior glenohumeral ligament (igl), teres minor tendon (tm), infraspinatus tendon (is), subacromial (subdeltoid) bursa (sb), and acromion (a). Also identified is the cartilage-covered glenoid cavity (g) surrounded by the glenoid labrum *(arrows)*.

anterior capsular insertions have been divided into two or three types, based on the proximity of the insertion site to the anterior portion of the labrum. In the three-part classification system, which is used throughout this chapter, a type I capsular insertion occurs close to or in the labrum, a type II capsular insertion occurs more medially, and a type III capsular insertion occurs in the scapular neck.

**Rotator Cuff.** The tendons of four muscles contribute to the rotator cuff of the shoulder: supraspinatus, infraspinatus, teres minor, and subscapularis (Fig. 59–29). The supraspinatus muscle extends laterally over the humeral head and inserts into the uppermost and middle facets in the greater tuberosity, in close proximity to the infraspinatus tendon posteriorly and the coracohumeral ligament anteriorly. The triangular infraspinatus muscle originates

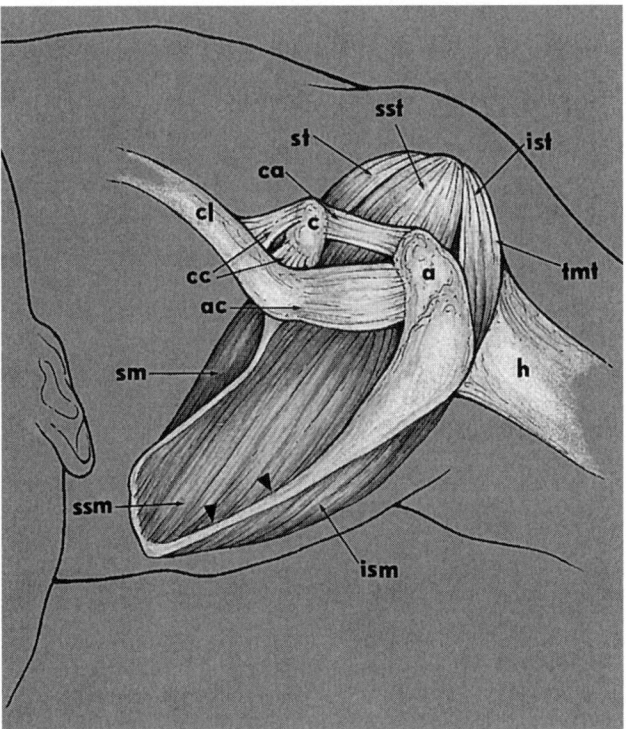

**Figure 59–29.** Rotator cuff: normal anatomy. Superior view of the rotator cuff and related structures. Identified structures (beginning at the top and continuing in a clockwise direction) are the supraspinatus tendon (sst), infraspinatus tendon (ist), teres minor tendon (tmt), infraspinatus muscle (ism), supraspinatus muscle (ssm), subscapularis muscles (sm), acromioclavicular ligament (ac), coracoclavicular ligament (cc), coracoacromial ligament (ca), and subscapularis tendon (st). Also identified are the clavicle (cl), coracoid process (c), acromion (a), humerus (h), and spine of the scapula *(arrowheads)*.

from the infraspinatus fossa to form a single tendon or multiple tendons that insert in the middle facet in the greater tuberosity of the humerus. The teres minor muscle is narrow and inserts into the lowest of the three facets in the greater tuberosity. The subscapularis muscle is large, arises on the anterior surface of the scapula, and attaches to the lesser tuberosity of the humerus. These four components of the rotator cuff are important dynamic stabilizers of the glenohumeral joint.

**Coracoacromial Arch.** The coracoacromial arch is intimate with portions of the rotator cuff, the tendon of the long head of the biceps brachii muscle, and the subacromial bursa. It consists of the coracoacromial ligament, the coracoid process, and the acromion (see Fig. 59–29). Abnormalities of any of the structures of the arch and the acromioclavicular joint can lead to impingement on the adjacent soft tissue structures, particularly the rotator cuff, a situation designated the external subacromial impingement syndrome. Variations in the morphology of the acromion have received a great deal of attention because of their possible association with rotator cuff pathology. The profile shape of the acromion is divided into three types, based on the undersurface of the bone: flat (type I),

curved (type II), or hooked (type III) (Fig. 59–30). A type I acromion appears to have the lowest association with the external subacromial impingement syndrome, and a type III acromion appears to have the highest association with this syndrome.

## Shoulder Impingement Syndromes

### External Impingement

The basis of the external subacromial impingement syndrome is the restricted space between the coracohumeral arch above and the humeral head and tuberosities below. Through this space pass the tendons of the rotator cuff and, within the rotator interval, the tendon of the long head of the biceps brachii muscle and the coracohumeral ligament. Compression of these structures leads to impingement syndrome. Among its causes are structural factors and functional factors. Structural factors relate to the acromioclavicular joint (congenital anomalies or osteophytes), acromion (alterations in shape, fractures with malunion or nonunion, os acromiale, or osteophytes), coracoid process (congenital anomalies or post-traumatic or post-surgical changes), subacromial (subdeltoid) bursa (inflammation, thickening, or surgical or nonsurgical foreign bodies), rotator cuff (calcification, thickening, or irregularity related to tendon tears or postoperative or post-traumatic scars), or humerus (congenital anomalies, fractures with malunion, or altered position of a humeral head prosthesis).

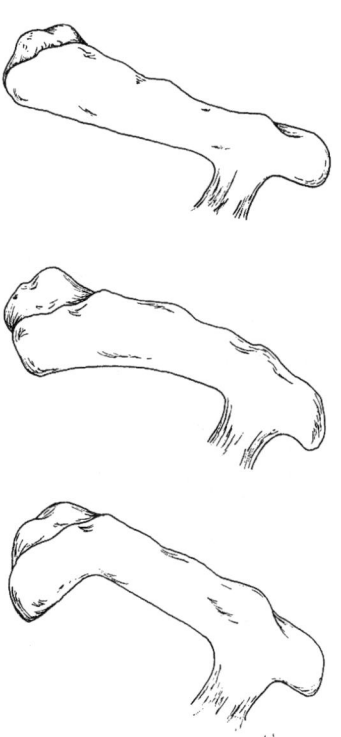

**Figure 59–30.** Acromion: variations in morphology in the sagittal plane. Three variations in acromial shape are illustrated. The upper drawing depicts a flat undersurface of the acromion, the middle drawing depicts a curved undersurface, and the lower drawing depicts a hooked undersurface.

Impingement syndromes are divided into two major categories: primary impingement, which is related to alterations in the coracoacromial arch and occurs mainly in nonathletic persons, and secondary impingement, which is related to either glenohumeral or scapular instability and occurs mainly in athletes involved in sports requiring overhead movement of the arm. The clinical manifestations of this syndrome are well documented and include chronic shoulder pain, stiffness, and weakness— findings that may be accentuated when the arm is flexed or internally rotated.

Routine radiography plays a minor diagnostic role in the evaluation of patients with early clinical stages of external subacromial impingement. Nonspecific sclerosis and cyst formation in the greater tuberosity or osteoarthritis of the acromioclavicular joint may be seen. A rather specific but late radiographic manifestation of the external subacromial impingement syndrome is an anterior acromial enthesophyte (Fig. 59–31). More advanced imaging methods, such as arthrography, computed arthrotomography, ultrasonography, and MR imaging, may be used to define the extent and the precise cause of the impingement syndrome. The only MR imaging finding that is relatively specific for this syndrome is a subacromial enthesophyte (Fig. 59–32).

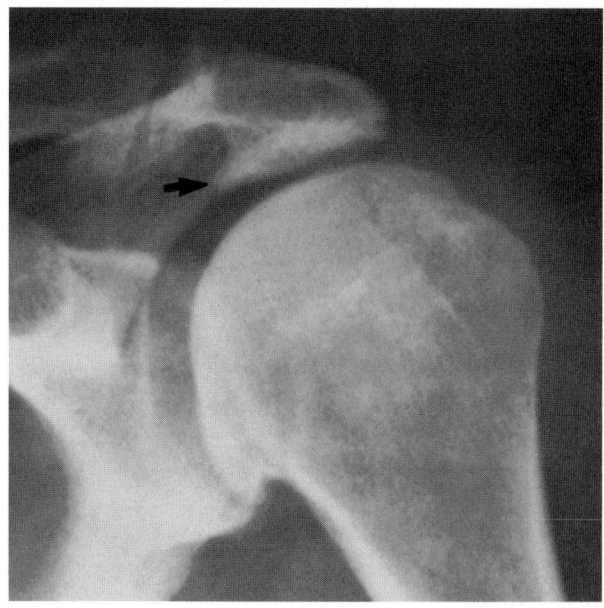

**Figure 59–31.** External subacromial impingement syndrome: routine radiographic abnormalities. Frontal radiograph of the shoulder shows a large enthesophyte *(arrow)* extending from the anteroinferior portion of the acromion and associated with osteophytes at the acromioclavicular joint and in the inferior portion of the humeral head.

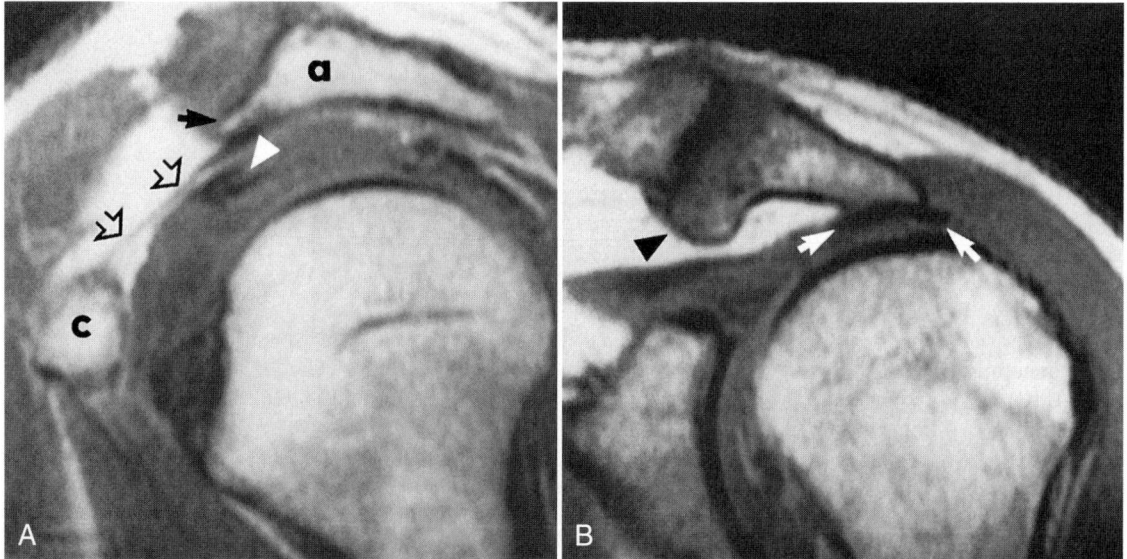

**Figure 59–32.** External subacromial impingement syndrome: MR imaging abnormalities. *A,* On a sagittal oblique T1-weighted (TR/TE, 800/20) spin echo MR image, a subacromial enthesophyte *(solid arrow)* containing marrow projects from the anterior surface of the acromion (a) toward the coracoid process (c). Note its relationship to the coracoacromial ligament *(open arrows)* and supraspinatus tendon *(arrowhead).* *B,* In a second patient, a coronal oblique intermediate-weighted (TR/TE, 2000/30) spin echo MR image reveals the flattened contour and low signal intensity characteristic of a subacromial enthesophyte *(arrows).* Also observe osteoarthritis of the acromioclavicular joint manifested as osteophytosis *(arrowhead)* and an elevated position of the humeral head, indicative of a rotator cuff tear. The tear was demonstrated better on other MR images (not shown).

## Internal Impingement

Impingement related to coracoacromial arch and glenohumeral joint instability has been recognized for many years. More recently, attention has been given to another form of impingement that is seen especially in athletes whose sports require overhead arm motion. In these patients, when the arm is placed in abduction and external rotation (i.e., the throwing position), impingement is found between the posterosuperior margin of the glenoid cavity and the undersurface of the tendinous insertions of the supraspinatus and infraspinatus muscles. There are five characteristic sites of injury: (1) superior portion of the labrum, (2) tendons of the rotator cuff, (3) greater tuberosity of the humerus, (4) inferior glenohumeral ligament complex or adjacent labrum, and (5) superior glenoid bone. All five sites must be surveyed when such patients are evaluated. Although standard arthrography and CT allow analysis of some of these sites, MR imaging and MR arthrography are preferred.

## Rotator Cuff Tear

**Classification and Prevalence.** A variety of methods can be used to classify failure of the rotator cuff. One simple method is to divide tears of the rotator cuff into acute and chronic tears. A second method of classification relates to the depth of the rotator cuff tear. Full-thickness (or complete) tears extend from the articular surface to the bursal surface of the cuff, and partial-thickness (or incomplete) tears involve only the articular surface or the bursal surface of the cuff. A tear within the substance of the rotator cuff (intrasubstance tear) represents a special type of incomplete tear. Massive tears are full-thickness tears involving multiple tendons of the rotator cuff. Lesions of the rotator cuff generally begin in the supraspinatus tendon, and their extension into other components of the rotator cuff is well established.

Partial-thickness tears of the rotator cuff are more common than full-thickness tears, and those on the articular side are probably slightly more common than those on the bursal side. Intratendinous tears appear to be less frequent than tears involving the articular or bursal portion of the rotator cuff. Because no existing method allows the detection of all intrasubstance tears, their true prevalence is difficult to ascertain. The prevalence of rotator cuff disruption increases in the later decades of life. The incidental discovery of chronic tears of the rotator cuff on chest radiographs obtained for unrelated reasons is common.

**Cause and Pathogenesis.** Proposed causes of rotator cuff failure include trauma, attrition, ischemia, and impingement. There is a well-known association between rotator cuff tears and acute traumatic episodes; however, most rotator cuff tears are unrelated to an acute injury. Rather, rupture of the rotator cuff occurs during movements and activities that should not (and usually do not) damage the involved musculotendinous units. This occurrence can be designated a spontaneous rupture. Normal tendons do not rupture spontaneously. Most full-thickness tears of the rotator cuff appear to occur in tendons that have been weakened by some combination of age, repetitive stress, corticosteroid injection, hypovascularity, or damage produced by impingement.

**Clinical Abnormalities.** Tears of the rotator cuff predominate in patients older than 40 years, in men, and in the dominant arm. Shoulder pain, stiffness, and weakness are common clinical manifestations, although patients may be entirely asymptomatic. Weakness of flexion, abduction, and external rotation of the arm may be apparent. The clinical manifestations of rotator cuff disease may allow an accurate diagnosis; however, in some cases, they simulate the findings of other disorders of the shoulder, such as adhesive capsulitis and calcific or noncalcific tendinosis.

**Radiographic Abnormalities.** No radiographic findings are diagnostic of an acute rotator cuff tear that has occurred in the absence of glenohumeral joint dislocation. Radiographs obtained during active abduction of the shoulder to 90 degrees from the horizontal or to the maximum extent possible may reveal narrowing of the coracoacromial distance in patients with rotator cuff disruption. With chronic tears of the rotator cuff, a number of radiographic abnormalities may become apparent (Fig. 59–33):

1. Narrowing of the acromiohumeral space. This interosseous space may measure less than the lower limit of normal, 0.6 to 0.7 cm.

2. Reversal of the normal inferior acromial convexity. Elevation of the humeral head leads to closer apposition

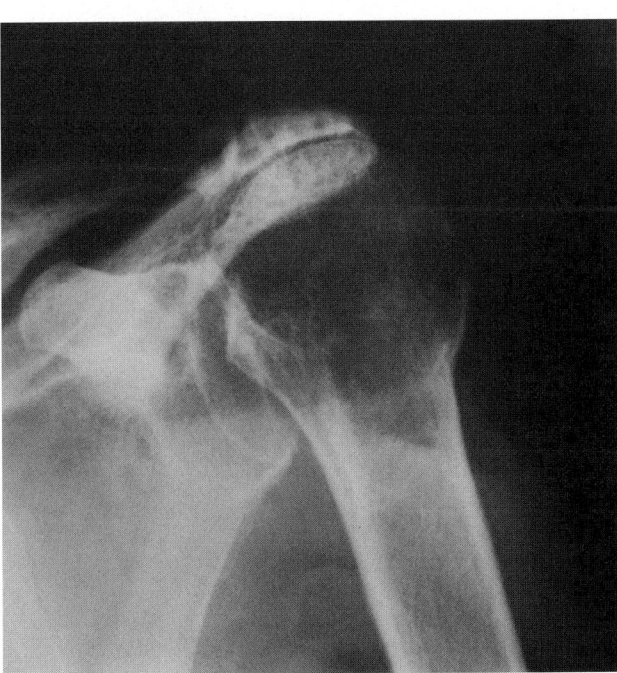

**Figure 59–33.** Rotator cuff tear: routine radiographic abnormalities. In this patient with a chronic rotator cuff tear, note the elevation of the humeral head with respect to the glenoid, contact of the humeral head and the acromion, concavity of the inferior surface of the acromion, and sclerosis and cyst formation on apposing surfaces of the acromion and humeral head.

of the humerus and the acromion and repeated traumatic insult to the acromion. Straightening and concavity of the undersurface of the acromion may then become evident.

3. Cystic lesions and sclerosis of the acromion and humeral head. Small cystic lesions surrounded by a thin rim of sclerosis can be noted along the inferior aspect of the acromion and within the greater tuberosity.

**Arthrographic Abnormalities.** Standard arthrography remains a popular technique for the diagnosis of some tears of the rotator cuff. Complete tears of the rotator cuff are associated with abnormal communication between the glenohumeral joint cavity and the subacromial (subdeltoid) bursa (Fig. 59–34). Contrast material can be identified within the bursa as a large collection superior and lateral to the greater tuberosity and adjacent to the undersurface of the acromion. Tears within the substance of the cuff generally escape arthrographic detection. Tears involving the superior surface of the cuff are not demonstrated on glenohumeral joint arthrography; rarely, they may be seen with direct subacromial bursography. Tears of the inferior surface of the rotator cuff can be diagnosed with arthrography. In these cases, an irregular

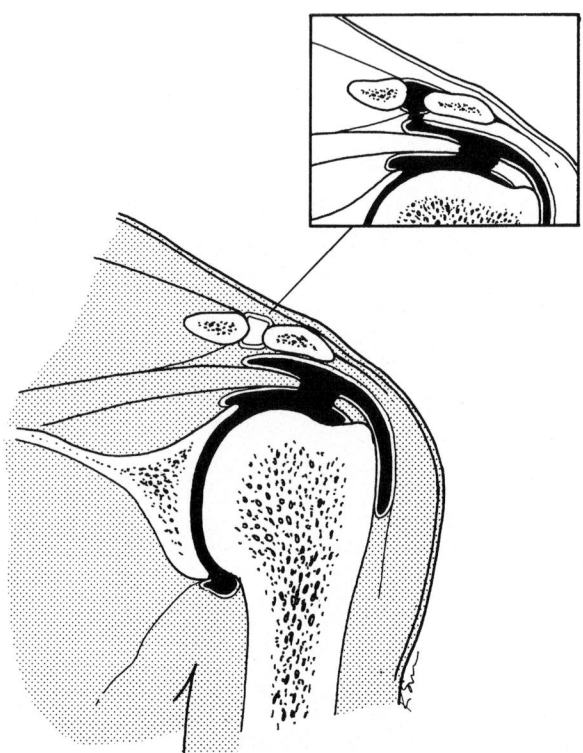

**Figure 59–34.** Full-thickness rotator cuff tear: glenohumeral joint arthrography. Contrast material extends from the glenohumeral joint through the rotator cuff into the subacromial (subdeltoid) bursa. The inset reveals contrast material extending from the glenohumeral joint through the rotator cuff into the subacromial bursa and from there into the acromioclavicular joint.

circular or linear collection of contrast material may be identified above the opacified joint cavity. The intact superficial fibers of the rotator cuff prevent opacification of the subacromial bursa. A false-negative arthrogram in the presence of a partial tear of the rotator cuff may indicate that the tear is too small for recognition or that a fibrous nodule has occluded the defect.

**Ultrasonographic Abnormalities.** The value of ultrasonography in the assessment of the rotator cuff is discussed in Chapter 6.

**Magnetic Resonance Imaging Abnormalities.** The normal tendons of the supraspinatus, infraspinatus, teres minor, and subscapularis muscles usually appear as regions of low signal intensity on all MR imaging sequences, in contrast to the areas of high signal intensity on some MR imaging sequences that are characteristic of tears. Although these differences in signal intensity in normal and torn tendons of the rotator cuff are fundamental to the diagnosis of cuff disruption, regions of intermediate signal intensity and inhomogeneity of signal intensity in intact tendons of the rotator cuff are regularly encountered and create some diagnostic difficulty. Specifically, regions of intermediate and sometimes high signal intensity within the outer portion of the supraspinatus tendon on T1- and intermediate-weighted spin echo MR images have been encountered. These areas relate to the magic angle phenomenon, partial volume averaging, variations in normal anatomy, and histologic findings of myxoid degeneration.

As a general rule, on T2-weighted spin echo MR images, the signal intensity of nondisrupted tendons of the rotator cuff, including the supraspinatus tendon, is equal to or less than that on T1- and intermediate-weighted spin echo MR images. When the signal intensity of the rotator cuff tendons is higher on T2-weighted than on T1- and intermediate-weighted spin echo MR images, tendon disruption is usually present. Unfortunately, there are exceptions to this rule. Further, when fast spin echo sequences are combined with fat suppression, a surprisingly high signal intensity may be seen in tendons that are not torn.

The most definite feature of such tears is a tendinous defect that is filled with fluid, granulation tissue, or both (Fig. 59–35). These tears show high signal intensity on short tau inversion recovery (STIR), T2-weighted spin echo, and other fluid-sensitive MR sequences. A second feature is retraction of the musculotendinous junction beyond the limits of normal. When the first of these two signs is present alone, or when both are present together, the diagnosis of a full-thickness tear of the rotator cuff can be made confidently. A number of other signs of a full-thickness tear of the rotator cuff have been described (Fig. 59–36), but none of them occurring in isolation is diagnostic of such a tear. These signs include fluid in the subacromial (subdeltoid) bursa or in the subcoracoid bursa, fluid in the glenohumeral joint, loss of the peribursal fat plane, and muscle atrophy.

Analysis of coronal oblique and sagittal oblique images provides information regarding the extent of a full-thickness rotator cuff tear. Initial tears in the supraspinatus tendon may extend anteriorly to involve the coracohumeral ligament and subscapularis tendon and extend posteriorly

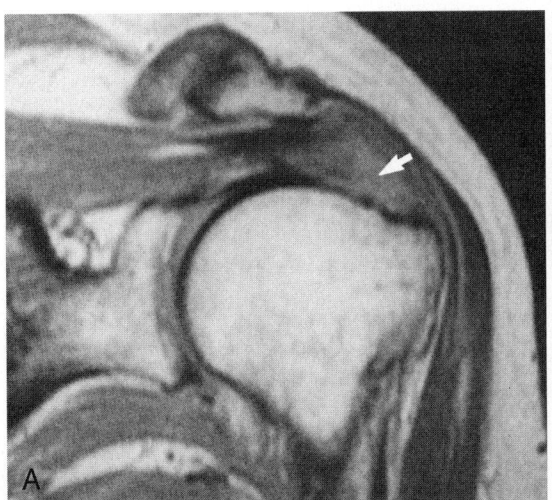
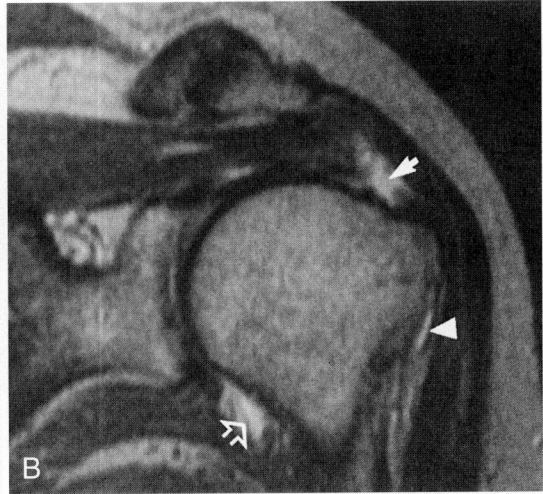
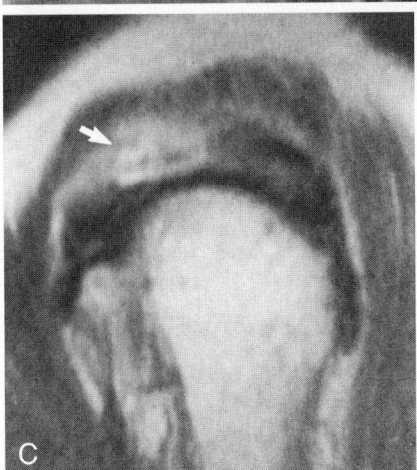

**Figure 59–35.** Full-thickness rotator cuff tear: MR imaging. *A* and *B*, In the coronal oblique plane, intermediate-weighted (TR/TE, 2000/20) *(A)* and T2-weighted (TR/TE, 2000/80) *(B)* spin echo MR images show fluid in a gap *(solid arrows)* in the supraspinatus tendon; the fluid is of increased signal intensity in *B*. Also in *B*, note the increased signal intensity related to fluid in the glenohumeral joint *(open arrow)* and subdeltoid bursa *(arrowhead)*. Osteoarthritis of the acromioclavicular joint is evident. *C*, In the same patient, sagittal oblique T2-weighted (TR/TE, 2000/60) spin echo MR images show the site *(arrow)* of disruption of the supraspinatus tendon, which is of high signal intensity.

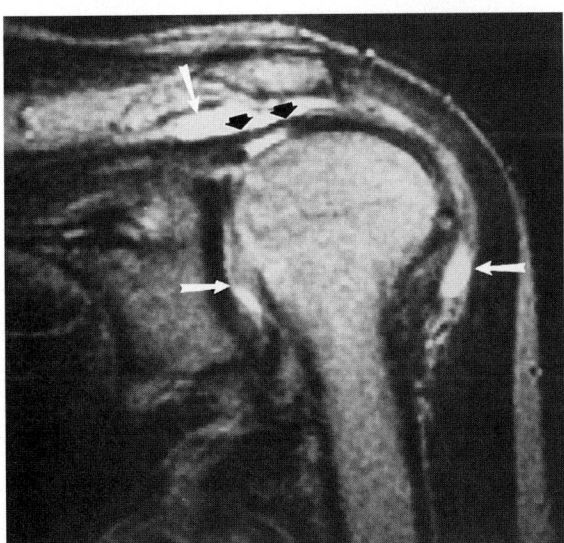

**Figure 59–36.** Full-thickness rotator cuff tear: MR imaging. Coronal oblique T2-weighted (TR/TE, 2000/70) spin echo MR image confirms the presence of an attenuated supraspinatus tendon *(small arrows)* and reveals fluid of increased signal intensity in the glenohumeral joint and subacromial (subdeltoid) bursa *(large arrows)*. (From Kursunoglu-Brahme S, Resnick D: Magnetic resonance imaging of the shoulder. Radiol Clin North Am 28:941, 1990.)

to involve the infraspinatus tendon and, rarely, the teres minor tendon or both. Fatty degeneration and atrophy of the torn and nearby tendons of the rotator cuff progress over time and decrease the likelihood of successful surgical repair (Fig. 59–37).

Partial-thickness tears of the rotator cuff are incomplete tears that extend into or exist within the substance of the cuff. Among partial-thickness tears, deep (articular-sided) tears appear to be most frequent, followed by superficial (bursal-sided) tears and those occurring within the substance of the tendon. Incomplete tears of the rotator cuff may be twice as common as full-thickness tears. MR imaging in cases of partial-thickness tears of the rotator cuff requires careful analysis of patterns of signal intensity and morphologic alterations in the distal portion of the tendons, particularly the supraspinatus tendon. Even with such analysis, MR imaging is not as good diagnostically for partial-thickness tears as it is for full-thickness tears. A region of increased signal intensity in the superficial portion of the tendon, perpendicular to the long axis of the tendon, on coronal oblique T2-weighted spin echo (or other fluid-sensitive) images is most consistent with the diagnosis of a partial-thickness tear involving the bursal side of the tendon; a similar region in the deep portion of the tendon, again perpendicular to the long axis of the tendon, on these images is most consistent with the

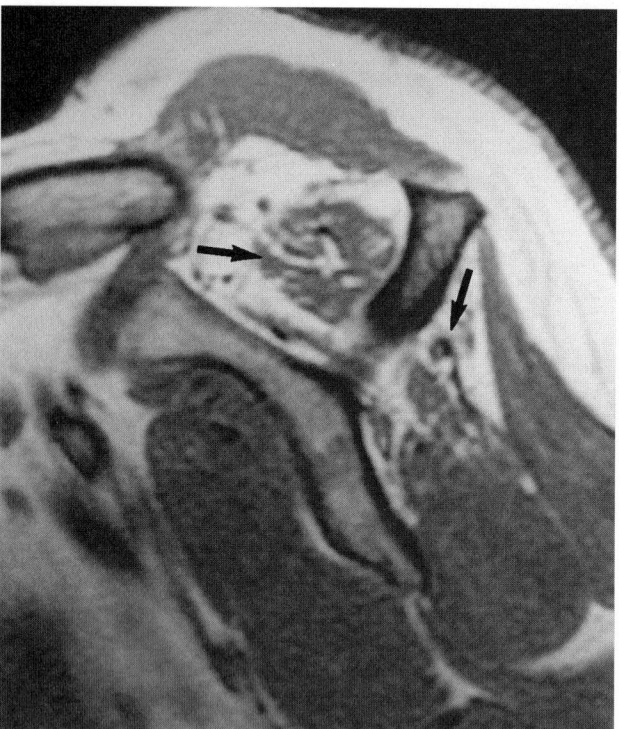

**Figure 59–37.** Full-thickness rotator cuff tear: muscle atrophy. In a 55-year-old woman with chronic tears of the supraspinatus and infraspinatus tendons, atrophy *(arrows)* of the corresponding muscles is seen on an oblique sagittal T1-weighted (TR/TE, 320/10) spin echo MR image.

diagnosis of a partial-thickness tear involving the articular side of the tendon; a region of increased signal intensity on T2-weighted spin echo (or other fluid-sensitive) MR images that extends in a linear fashion through the entire cuff, without retraction of the tendon, is most consistent with the diagnosis of a small full-thickness tear of the tendon; and a region of increased signal intensity on these images that is parallel to the long axis of the tendon is most consistent with the diagnosis of an intrasubstance tear of the tendon (Fig. 59–38). With standard MR imaging or MR arthrography, some partial-thickness articular-sided tendon tears (and, occasionally, small full-thickness tears) are associated with intramuscular fluid-filled (or contrast-filled) cysts.

## Rotator Cuff Tendinosis or Tendinopathy

The designation "tendinitis" is often loosely applied to a variety of shoulder problems that lead to focal pain and tenderness and subacromial crepitation. Histologic findings in such cases are more compatible with an ischemic or degenerative process than an inflammatory one, and a more appropriate term for this process is tendinosis or tendinopathy.

The reported MR imaging characteristics of rotator cuff tendinosis or tendinopathy include increased signal intensity in a tendon with normal or abnormal morphology and an intact peribursal fat plane. The increase in signal intensity is generally moderate and not extreme and creates an inhomogeneous appearance of the tendon. It is

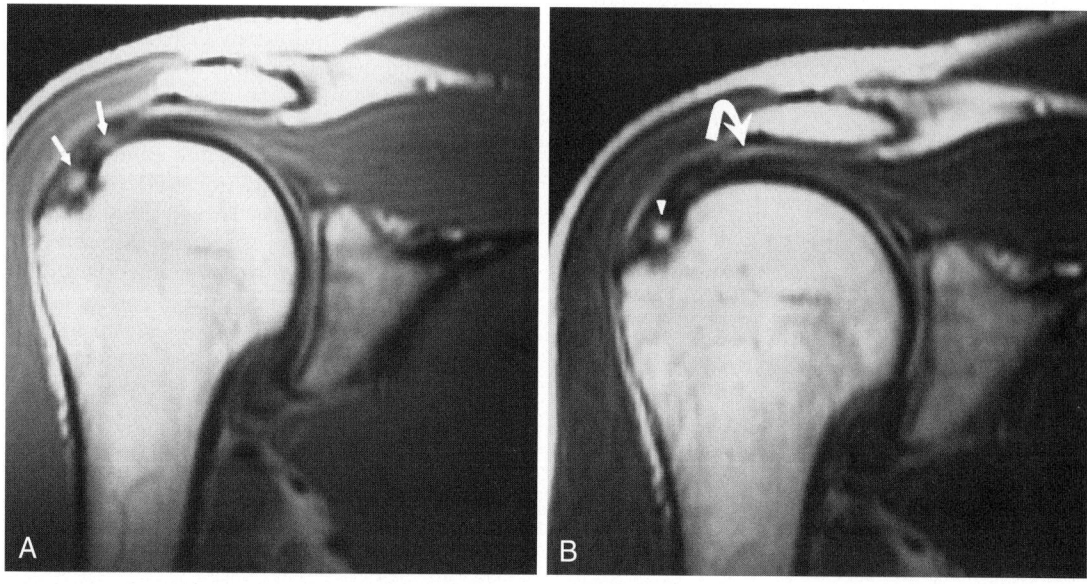

**Figure 59–38.** Partial-thickness rotator cuff tear: articular side of the supraspinatus tendon. Coronal oblique intermediate-weighted (TR/TE, 2000/20) *(A)* and T2-weighted (TR/TE, 2000/70) *(B)* spin echo MR images show two small regions of altered signal intensity *(arrows in A)* in the distal portion of the supraspinatus tendon. One of these regions shows a further increase in signal intensity *(arrowhead in B)*. No fluid is present in the subacromial (subdeltoid) bursa *(curved arrow in B)*. (From Kursunoglu-Brahme S, Resnick D: Magnetic resonance imaging of the shoulder. Radiol Clin North Am 28:941, 1990.)

apparent on T1- and intermediate-weighted spin echo MR images and less evident on T2-weighted spin echo MR images (Fig. 59–39). Regions of intense signal intensity within the cuff tendons on T2-weighted spin echo MR images, similar to the signal intensity of fluid, are not compatible with the diagnosis of tendinosis or tendinopathy and suggest the presence of a full-thickness or partial-thickness tear.

## Adhesive Capsulitis

Adhesive capsulitis is one of several terms applied to a clinical condition characterized by severe restriction of active and passive motion of the glenohumeral joint for which no other cause can be documented.

Glenohumeral joint arthrography is the modality most frequently used in the diagnosis and treatment of adhesive capsulitis (Fig. 59–40). The diagnostic role of MR imaging is not yet clear. Thickening of the joint capsule adjacent to the medial cortex of the humerus has been described as a finding of adhesive capsulitis. More specific, however, is the presence of increased signal intensity in pericapsular tissue on fluid-sensitive images and, in particular, after intravenous gadolinium administration (Fig. 59–41).

## Glenohumeral Joint Instability

**Classification.** Glenohumeral joint instability is generally considered a symptomatic clinical situation characterized by altered movement of the humeral head with respect to the glenoid cavity. Methods of classification of glenohumeral joint instability are based on the degree and direction of instability, its chronology, and its pathogenesis.

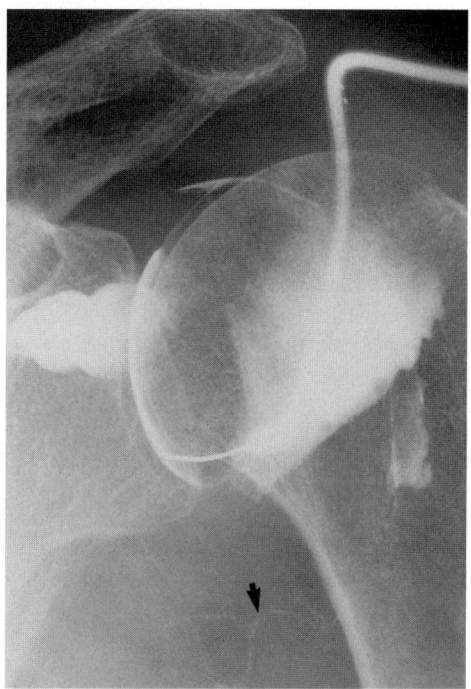

**Figure 59–40.** Adhesive capsulitis: arthrography. Frontal radiograph obtained after the injection of 5 mL of radiopaque contrast material into the glenohumeral joint reveals a tight-appearing articulation with lymphatic filling *(arrow)*. No axillary pouch is seen.

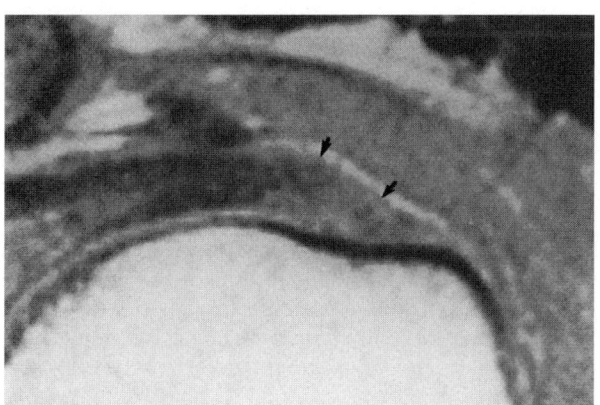

**Figure 59–39.** Tendinosis or tendinopathy of the rotator cuff: MR imaging and histopathology. Coronal oblique intermediate-weighted (TR/TE, 2000/25) spin echo MR image reveals increased signal intensity in the distal part of the supraspinatus tendon *(arrows)*. No further increase in signal intensity was seen on T2-weighted spin echo MR images. The peribursal fat plane is intact. (From Kjellin I, Ho CP, Cervilla V, et al: Alterations in the supraspinatus tendon at MR imaging: Correlation with histopathologic findings in cadavers. Radiology 181:837, 1991.)

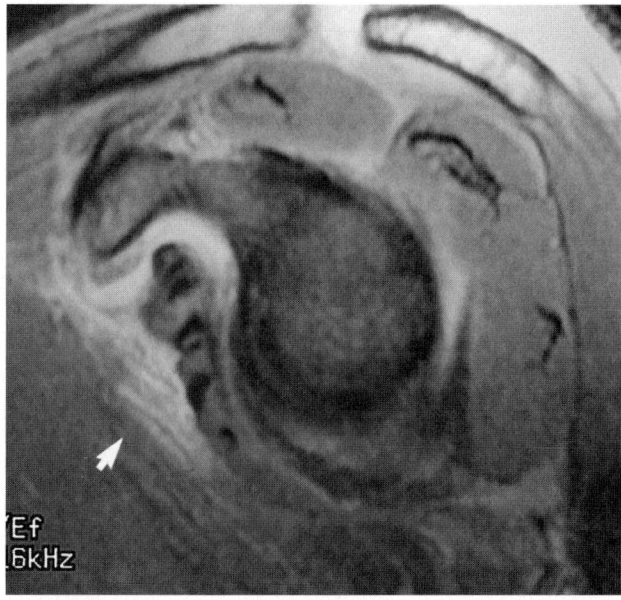

**Figure 59–41.** Adhesive capsulitis: MR imaging. On an oblique sagittal fast spin echo (TR/TE, 2200/42) MR image obtained with fat suppression, note the high signal intensity about the joint capsule and, in particular, superficial to the subscapularis tendon *(arrow)*.

With regard to the degree of instability, dislocations or subluxations of the joint may be encountered. In dislocation, no contact remains between the apposing surfaces of the glenoid cavity and the humeral head. With subluxation, abnormal translation of the humeral head in relation to the glenoid cavity is evident; it is not accompanied by complete separation of the apposing articular surfaces, and it is usually greater than the small amount of translation of the humeral head that represents normal range of motion. Subluxation of the glenohumeral joint is transient and often momentary. Dislocation and subluxation of the glenohumeral joint may occur in several different directions: anterior, posterior, superior, and inferior.

With regard to the chronology of instability, acute dislocations are defined as those seen within the first 24 to 48 hours, and chronic dislocations are defined as those evaluated after this time. Dislocations and subluxations of the glenohumeral joint may also be categorized according to their pathogenesis. They may be traumatic or atraumatic, congenital or acquired, and voluntary or involuntary. The acronym TUBS describes patients with traumatic instability who usually have unilateral involvement, typically have a Bankart lesion, and often require surgery; AMBRI refers to patients with atraumatic instability who have multidirectional instability, often with bilateral involvement, and may respond to a rehabilitation program or require inferior capsular shift (Table 59–2).

**Cause and Pathogenesis.** Although developmental factors may lead to congenital instability of the glenohumeral joint, trauma is the leading cause of subluxation and dislocation of the glenohumeral joint. Indirect forces are more common than direct forces as causes of glenohumeral joint instability. Many structures, such as the components of the rotator cuff, the glenoid labrum, the glenohumeral ligaments, the joint capsule and supporting musculature, and the coracoacromial arch, contribute to glenohumeral joint stability (Fig. 59–42). Both static (passive) and dynamic (active) constraints are believed to contribute to shoulder stability. Static constraints include the bone configuration of the glenohumeral joint and the capsule and ligamentous complex that surrounds the shoulder; dynamic constraints include the muscle and tendon units that surround the glenohumeral joint, particularly the muscles and tendons of the rotator cuff.

The capsule of the glenohumeral joint is large, loose, and redundant, thereby allowing great range of motion.

Reinforcing the capsule of this joint are the coracohumeral ligament and the three glenohumeral ligaments (Fig. 59–43). Although the glenohumeral ligaments are inconstant and variable in size, their importance in providing stability to the glenohumeral joint is undisputed. Of the three glenohumeral ligaments, emphasis has been given to the inferior glenohumeral ligament complex, particularly its anterior band, which is understood to be the primary static restraint against anterior instability when the arm is in an abducted and externally rotated position.

No single or essential lesion appears to be the basis of anterior or posterior instability of the joint. Identification of a detached portion of the glenoid labrum (Bankart lesion), a compression fracture of the posterolateral surface of the humeral head (Hill-Sachs lesion), a deficiency of one or more of the glenohumeral ligaments, capsular laxity, disruption of one or more tendons of the rotator cuff, or detachment or lengthening of the subscapularis muscle as the primary cause of shoulder instability is an oversimplification of a complex process.

**Clinical Abnormalities.** The clinical abnormalities related to instability of the glenohumeral joint are variable and influenced by its atraumatic or traumatic pathogenesis and by its acute or chronic nature. Many patients recall an experience in which the humeral head felt displaced, whether initiated by trauma or not. Fixed dislocations of the glenohumeral joint are usually identifiable during physical examination, particularly in a patient with anterior dislocation of the glenohumeral joint. Posterior dislocations of this joint are associated with more subtle but definite clinical manifestations, including fixed internal rotation of the affected arm with limited external rotation and elevation. Complications of anterior or posterior dislocations, such as neurovascular injury, may provide additional clinical findings. Although provocative tests may be used during physical examination to establish the occurrence of subluxation of the glenohumeral joint, imaging examinations are fundamental to an accurate diagnosis.

**Radiographic and Arthrographic Abnormalities.** The routine radiographic abnormalities associated with dislocation of the glenohumeral joint are discussed in Chapter 57. In addition to confirming an abnormal position of the humeral head with respect to the glenoid cavity, conventional radiographs are useful in the identification of bone injuries that may occur during dislocation. Foremost among these injuries are Hill-Sachs lesions of the humerus and Bankart-type lesions of the anterior portion of the glenoid rim. Standard arthrography also has a limited role in the assessment of glenohumeral joint instability and is discussed in Chapter 5.

**Computed Arthrotomographic Abnormalities.** Computed arthrotomography is especially useful for assessing the shoulder in patients who are unable to undergo MR imaging. Abnormalities of the glenoid labrum depicted on computed arthrotomography include foreshortening or thinning or contrast imbibition along its free margin (Fig. 59–44). The labrum may also be completely detached (a true Bankart lesion). An osseous Bankart-type lesion is

---

| **TABLE 59–2** | | |
| --- | --- | --- |
| **Clinical Categories of Glenohumeral Joint Instability** | | |
| **AMBRI** | **TUBS** | **AIOS** |
| Atraumatic | Traumatic | Acquired |
| Multidirectional | Unilateral | Instability |
| Bilateral | Bankart lesion | Overstress |
| Rehabilitation | Surgery | Surgery |
| Inferior capsular shift | | |

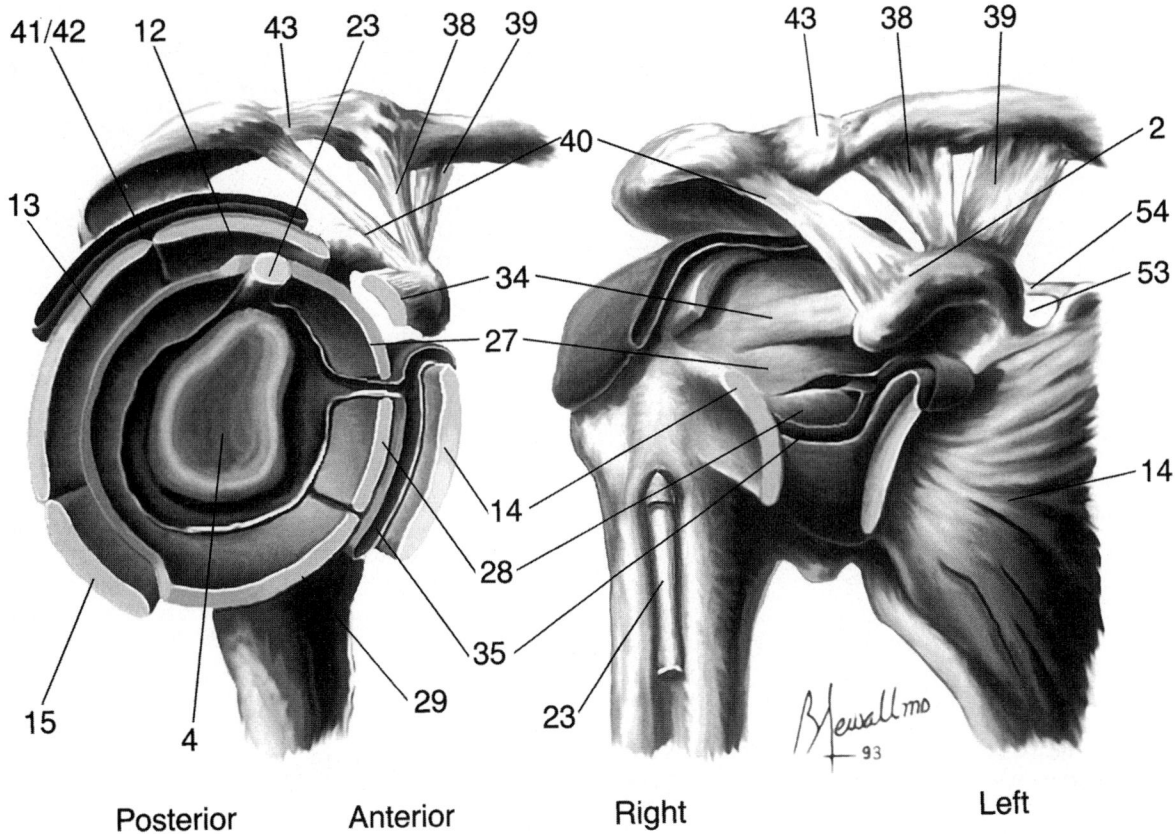

**Figure 59–42.** Capsular complex of the glenohumeral joint, rotator cuff, and supraspinatus outlet: normal anatomy. *Right*, A right shoulder is sketched as though all the muscles have been dissected away to reveal the glenohumeral, coracohumeral, coracoacromial, and coracoclavicular ligaments. The tendons of the long head of the biceps brachii muscle, the subacromial (subdeltoid) bursa, and the subscapularis bursa are also depicted. *Left*, The relationships of these structures in the sagittal plane are emphasized. In numerical order, the structures are the following:

2. Coracoid process
4. Glenoid cavity
12. Supraspinatus muscle and tendon
13. Infraspinatus muscle and tendon
14. Subscapularis muscle and tendon
15. Teres minor muscle
23. Tendon of the long head of the biceps brachii muscle
27. Superior glenohumeral ligament
28. Middle glenohumeral ligament
29. Inferior glenohumeral ligament
34. Coracohumeral ligament
35. Subscapularis bursa
38. Trapezoid ligament
39. Conoid ligament
40. Coracoacromial ligament
41. Subacromial bursa
42. Subdeltoid bursa
43. Acromioclavicular joint and ligaments
53. Suprascapular notch
54. Superior transverse scapular ligament

(Courtesy of B. O. Sewell, MD, San Diego, Calif.; from Petersilge CA, Witte DH, Sewell BO, et al: Normal regional anatomy of the shoulder. Magn Reson Imaging Clin N Am 1:1, 1993.)

typically visualized as elevation of a small sliver of bone and irregularity of the adjacent glenoid rim. A depression along the posterolateral aspect of the humeral head is indicative of a Hill-Sachs lesion.

Distention of the glenohumeral joint accomplished during computed arthrotomography (and during MR arthrography) allows visualization of the anterior and posterior capsular insertions of the glenohumeral ligaments, as well as the coracohumeral ligament. In cases of anterior glenohumeral joint instability, the capsular reflections may appear lax or distorted, with either loss or thickening of the anterior subscapular soft tissues (Fig. 59–45). With

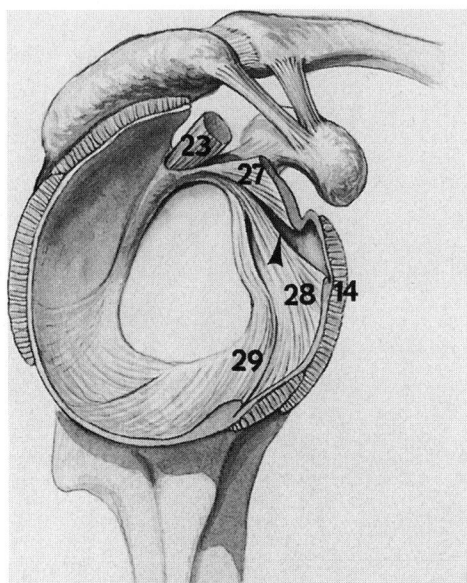

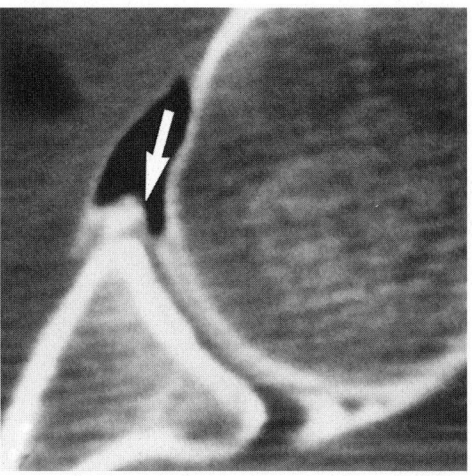

**Figure 59–44.** Glenoid labrum: computed arthrotomography—abnormal appearance. Anterior portion of the labrum is foreshortened and imbibes contrast material *(arrow)*. (From Deutsch AL, Resnick D, Mink JL, et al: Computed and conventional arthrotomography of the glenohumeral joint: normal anatomy and clinical experience. Radiology 153:603, 1984.)

**Figure 59–43.** Capsular complex of the glenohumeral joint: normal anatomy. Simplified depiction of the anterior capsular complex of the glenohumeral joint. The following structures are indicated:

14. Subscapularis muscle and tendon
23. Tendon of the long head of the biceps brachii muscle
27. Superior glenohumeral ligament
28. Middle glenohumeral ligament
29. Inferior glenohumeral ligament
Arrowhead. Opening into the subscapularis bursa
(From Zlatkin M, Bjorkengren AG, Gylys-Morin V, et al: Cross-sectional imaging of the capsular mechanism of the glenohumeral joint. AJR Am J Roentgenol 150:151, 1988.)

**Magnetic Resonance Imaging Abnormalities.** With MR imaging, the normal anterior and posterior portions of the glenoid labrum show low signal intensity and a smooth, wedge-shaped appearance. Irregularity in contour and intermediate or high signal intensity are indicative of a torn labrum (Fig. 59–46). As with computed arthrotomography, MR imaging displays the many variations of labral shape that occur in asymptomatic persons. The presence of a smooth triangular structure generally allows the most confident diagnosis of a normal labrum. The attachment sites of the glenohumeral ligaments and, superiorly, the attachment site of the tendon of the long head of the biceps brachii muscle may also alter the apparent shape of a normal labrum. Most of the normal variations in the labroligamentous complex occur at the 11 to 3 o'clock positions, whereas most of the pathologic findings asso-

posterior instability of the glenohumeral joint, the posterior portion of the glenoid labrum may be torn, shredded, or detached, and capsular laxity may be apparent. Both anterior and posterior abnormalities may be seen with computed arthrotomography in patients with multidirectional instability.

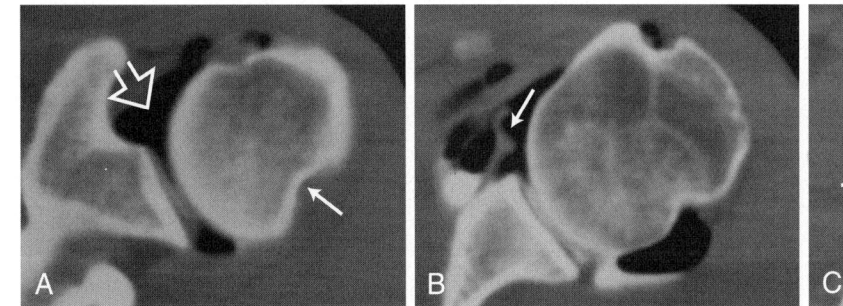
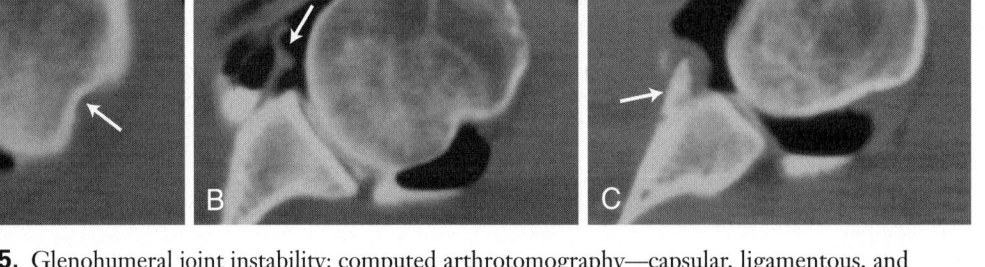

**Figure 59–45.** Glenohumeral joint instability: computed arthrotomography—capsular, ligamentous, and labral abnormalities. Three transaxial CT arthrographic images obtained at the level of the superior aspect of the joint (level 1) *(A)*, the midglenoid level (level 3) *(B)*, and the inferior glenoid level (level 4) *(C)* show a number of abnormalities indicative of previous anterior glenohumeral joint dislocation. In *A*, observe a Hill-Sachs lesion *(arrow)*, irregularity of the superior glenohumeral ligament *(open arrow)*, and nonvisualization of the superoanterior portion of the labrum. In *B*, findings include avulsion of the anterior portion of the labrum at the site of attachment of the middle glenohumeral ligament *(arrow)* and a redundant anterior capsule. In *C*, observe a fracture *(arrow)* of the anterior surface of the glenoid rim.

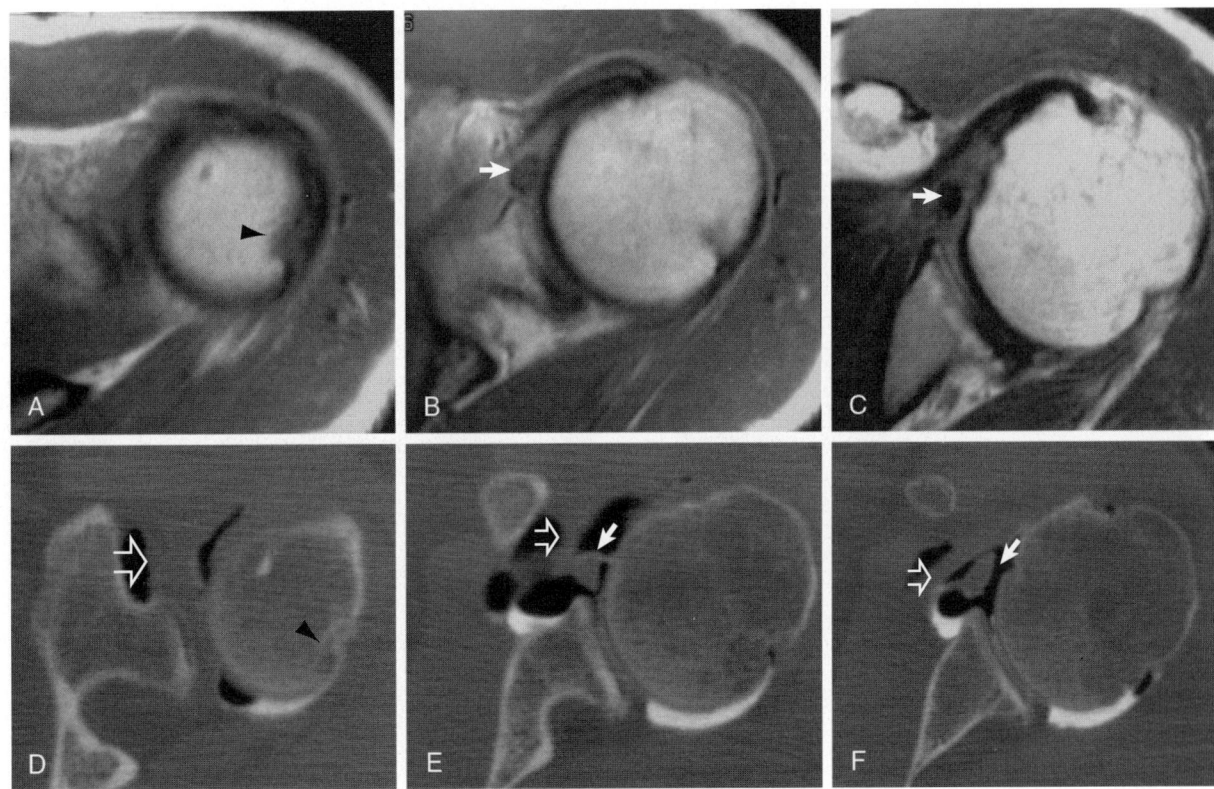

**Figure 59–46.** Glenoid labrum: MR imaging and CT-arthrography—abnormal appearance. Three transaxial intermediate-weighted (TR/TE, 2000/19) spin echo MR images (*A* to *C*) and three transaxial CT-arthrographic scans (*D* to *F*) demonstrate an abnormal anterior portion of the labrum, including a glenoid labrum ovoid mass (GLOM). *A,* At the level of the base of the coracoid process, note a Hill-Sachs lesion (*arrowhead*) of the humeral head. *B,* Slightly below the level of (*A*), observe a GLOM (*arrow*) of low signal intensity, diagnostic of a labral tear and detachment. *C,* Slightly below the level of *B*, in the midglenoid region, the GLOM (*arrow*) is again evident. *D,* At the level of the base of the coracoid process, note the Hill-Sachs lesion (*arrowhead*) and a thick superior glenohumeral ligament (*open arrow*). *E,* Slightly below the level of *D*, note the GLOM (*solid arrow*) adjacent to the inferior portion of the superior glenohumeral ligament (*open arrow*). *F,* Slightly below the level of *E*, in the midglenoid region, the GLOM (*solid arrow*) is contiguous with the middle glenohumeral ligament (*open arrow*). (Courtesy of J. Quale, MD, Englewood, Colo.)

ciated with anterior glenohumeral joint instability occur at the 3 to 6 o'clock positions.

*Labral Variations.* The superior portion of the labrum may normally have a tight (i.e., slablike) or loose (i.e., meniscus-like) attachment to the glenoid margin. If the attachment is loose, a potential space or recess exists between it and the glenoid bone. This space is designated the sublabral recess, or sulcus, and it may fill with contrast agent during MR arthrography. This opacification simulates the appearance of a detached labrum, a type of SLAP lesion. This normal variant is encountered in about 10% of normal persons. This foramen is considered a nonsignificant finding, although its imaging appearance may simulate that of pathologic labral conditions. It extends inferiorly no lower than the 3 o'clock position (Fig. 59–47). Almost invariably, a sublabral recess is also present. A relatively uncommon variation of capsulolabral anatomy designated the Buford complex is characterized by a cordlike middle glenohumeral ligament that originates directly from the superior portion of the labrum at the base of the biceps tendon and crosses the subscapularis tendon to insert on the humerus. No anterosuperior labral tissue is present between this attachment site and the midglenoid notch. This anomaly, which may be present in 2% to 5% of persons, may simulate labral detachment (Fig. 59–48).

*Osseous Abnormalities.* A variety of osseous injuries accompany glenohumeral joint instability and may be detected with MR imaging. These injuries include fractures of the anterior or posterior portion of the glenoid rim, Hill-Sachs and trough lesions, and avulsion fractures of the lesser or greater tuberosity of the humerus (Fig. 59–49). The presence of a normal groove in the posterolateral aspect of the proximal humeral metaphysis can lead to difficulty in the diagnosis of a Hill-Sachs lesion on transaxial CT scans and MR images. This groove, however, is located lower than a Hill-Sachs lesion. The latter is almost universally apparent on the first two or three transaxial images through the superior portion of the humeral head (with a 3- or 5-mm slice thickness).

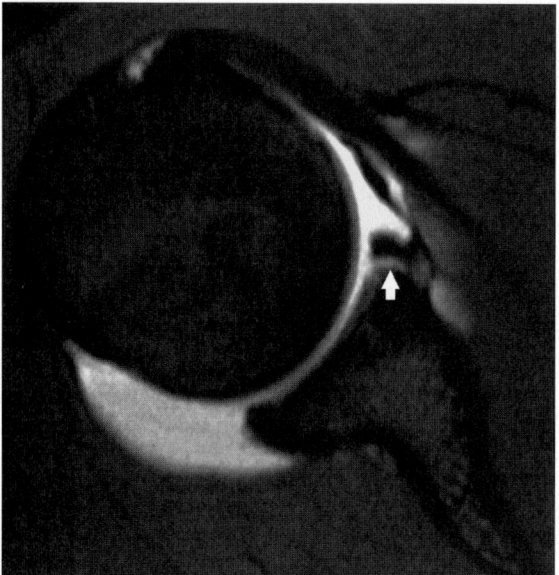

**Figure 59–47.** Normal variations: sublabral foramen (hole). Transverse fat-suppressed T1-weighted (TR/TE, 550/17) MR arthrographic image shows contrast agent between the anterosuperior portion of the labrum and the glenoid margin *(arrow)*.

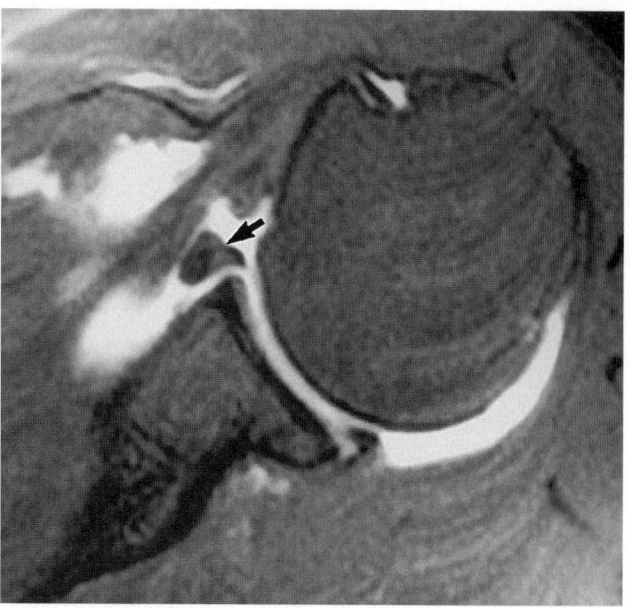

**Figure 59–48.** Normal variations: Buford's complex. This complex consists of a cordlike middle glenohumeral ligament *(arrows)*, with absence of the anterosuperior portion of the labrum. This is well shown on a fat-suppressed transverse T1-weighted (TR/TE, 666/14) MR arthrographic image.

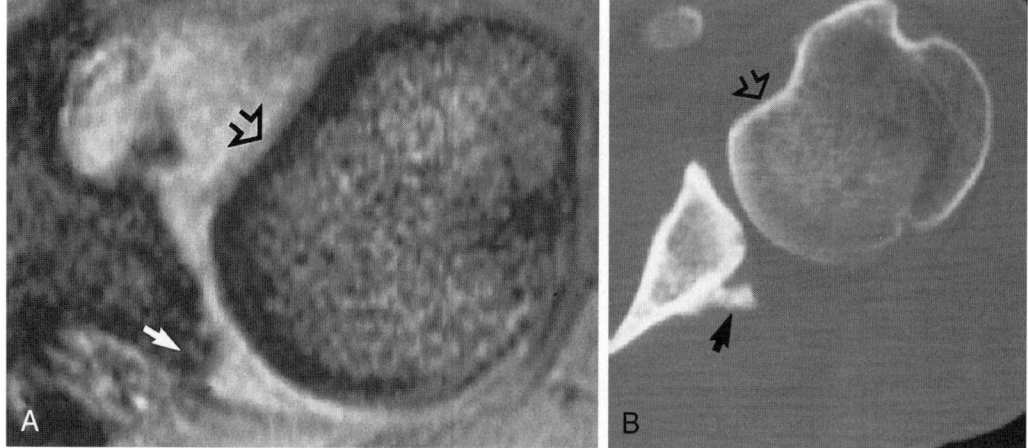

**Figure 59–49.** Posterior glenohumeral joint instability. *A,* Transaxial SPGR (TR/TE, 45/15; flip angle, 20 degrees) MR image shows posterior subluxation of the humeral head, irregularity of the posterior glenoid rim *(solid arrow)*, and a trough fracture *(open arrow)* involving the anterior surface of the humeral head. *B,* Transaxial CT scan at a slightly lower level in the same patient confirms posterior displacement of the humeral head, a fracture of the posterior glenoid region *(solid arrow)*, and a trough fracture of the humeral head *(open arrow)*. (Courtesy of M. Schweitzer, MD, Philadelphia, Pa.)

*Labroligamentous Abnormalities.* Numerous labroligamentous abnormalities have been described, most often in association with glenohumeral joint instability (Table 59–3). These abnormalities can be broadly divided into two categories: those that are associated with such instability, and those that are generally not. In cases of anterior glenohumeral joint instability, abnormalities are usually related to the anterior band of the inferior glenohumeral ligament complex. Failure of this complex may occur at its glenoid insertion site (approximately 70% to 75% of cases), at its humeral insertion site (5% to 10% of cases), or within its substance (15% to 20% of cases). Lesions associated with glenoid-sided failure are the Bankart lesion (cartilaginous or both bony and cartilaginous), anterior labroligamentous periosteal sleeve avulsion, and Perthes' lesion (Fig. 59–50). Lesions associated with humeral

**TABLE 59–3**

**Labroligamentous Lesions**

| Unstable | Stable |
|---|---|
| Glenoid failure (70–75%) | Labral |
| Bankart lesion | Flap/bucket-handle tear |
| ALPSA lesion | Labral—cartilage |
| Perthes' lesion | GLAD lesion |
| Capsular failure (15–20%) | Labral—tendon |
| Tear/laxity | SLAP lesion |
| Humeral failure (5–10%) | |
| HAGL lesion | |
| BHAGL lesion | |
| Humeral and glenoid failure | |
| (floating AIGHL) | |

*AIGHL*, alvulsion of the inferior glenohumeral ligament complex; *ALPSA*, anterior labroligamentous periosteal sleeve avulsion; *BHAGL*, bony humeral avulsion of the glenohumeral ligament; *GLAD*, glenolabral articular disruption; *HAGL*, humeral avulsion of the glenohumeral ligament; *SLAP*, superior labral, anterior and posterior lesion.

failure are humeral avulsion of the glenohumeral ligament lesion and its bony counterpart. Failure of this ligament at both its glenoid and humeral insertion destabilizes both ends of the anterior band of the inferior glenohumeral complex (floating avulsion of the inferior glenohumeral ligament complex). Similar lesions related to the posterior band of this ligament complex have been associated with posterior glenohumeral joint instability.

The Bankart lesion represents an avulsion of the labroligamentous complex from the anteroinferior portion of the glenoid bone. The periosteum of the scapula is lifted and disrupted (Fig. 59–51). The Bankart lesion is located at the 3 to 6 o'clock positions. In some cases, failure results in avulsion of a piece of bone, producing the bony Bankart-like lesion. This piece arises from the anteroinferior aspect of the glenoid rim. CT may be effective in showing this lesion. Recurrent unidirectional anterior instability of the glenohumeral joint may be associated not only with a classic Bankart lesion (avulsion of the anterior labroligamentous structures from the

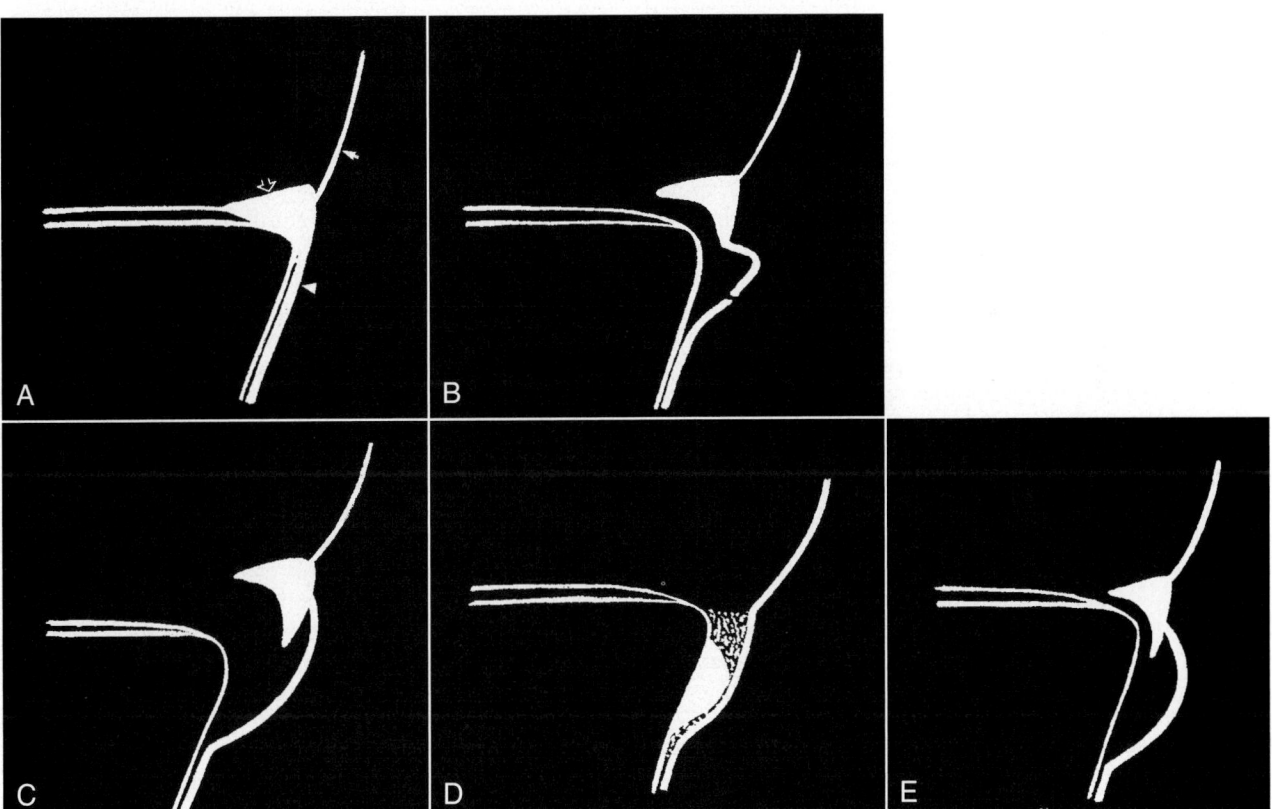

**Figure 59–50.** Anterior glenohumeral joint instability: lesions associated with failure of the anterior band of the inferior glenohumeral ligament complex at its glenoid attachment. *A,* Normal. Structures depicted are the anterior band of the inferior glenohumeral complex *(solid arrow)*, labrum *(open arrow)*, and scapular periosteum *(arrowhead)*. *B,* Bankart lesion. This lesion represents an avulsion of the labroligamentous complex, with lifting and disruption of the scapular periosteum. *C,* Acute anterior labroligamentous periosteal sleeve avulsion (ALPSA) lesion. This lesion represents an avulsion of the labroligamentous complex, with lifting but not disruption of the scapular periosteum. *D,* Chronic ALPSA lesion. This lesion represents an acute ALPSA lesion that is followed by anteromedial displacement of the labrum and the formation of scar tissue. *E,* Perthes' lesion. This lesion represents a nondisplaced labroligamentous avulsion, with lifting but not disruption of the scapular periosteum. (Courtesy of N. Lektrakul, MD, San Diego, Calif.)

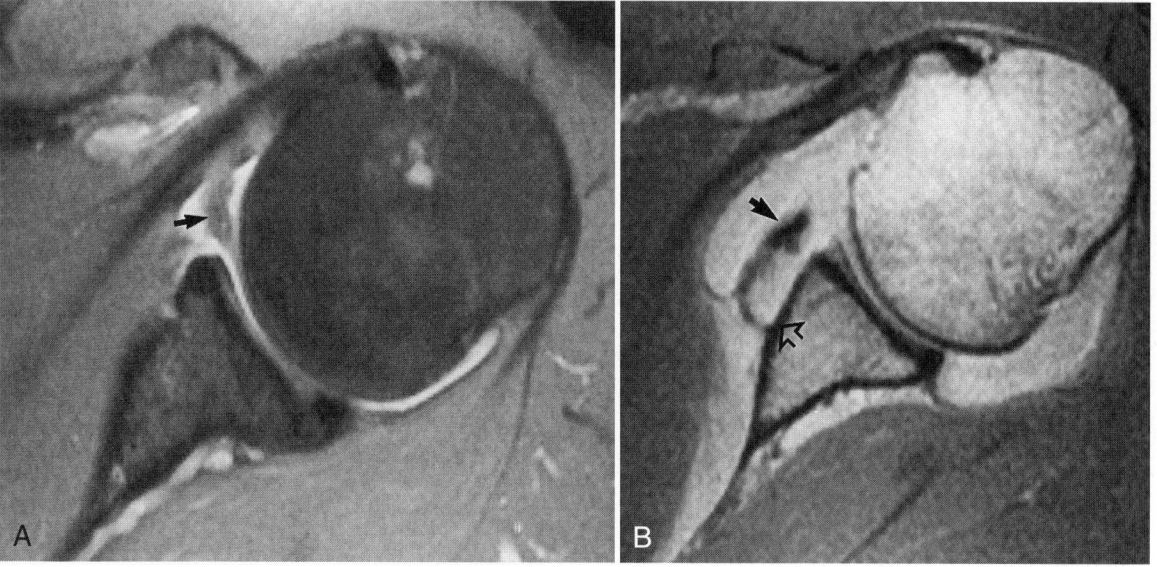

**Figure 59–51.** Anterior glenohumeral joint instability: Bankart and anterior labroligamentous periosteal sleeve avulsion (ALPSA) lesions. *A*, Transaxial fat-suppressed fast spin echo (TR/TE, 2500/15) MR arthrographic image shows the avulsed and displaced labroligamentous complex *(arrow)* characteristic of ALPSA lesion. *B*, In a different patient, transaxial intermediate-weighted (TR/TE, 1800/30) spin echo MR image shows anteromedial displacement of the detached labrum *(solid arrow)*, with lifting *(open arrow)* but not disruption of the scapular periosteum. (Courtesy of C. Ho, MD, Stanford, Calif.)

anterior glenoid rim) but also with avulsion of the periosteal sleeve of the anterior portion of the scapula (see Fig. 59–51). This lesion differs from a Bankart lesion, in that the anterior scapular periosteum does not rupture. Perthes' lesion, another variation of a Bankart lesion, is characterized by a labroligamentous avulsion injury without displacement of the labrum and with stripping but not disruption of the scapular periosteum.

The labroligamentous injuries associated with posterior glenohumeral joint instability have been less well documented than those associated with anterior instability. Posterior labral lesions are less diagnostic of posterior instability than are anterior labral lesions in the setting of anterior instability. Posterior labral tears and detachments, ligamentous injuries, and capsular tears or stripping may occur, and the resulting pathologic variations may resemble those seen in anterior glenohumeral joint instability.

### Superior Labral, Anterior and Posterior Lesion

In athletes subjected to repetitive overhead use of the arm, an injury to the superior portion of the glenoid labrum may result from sudden forced abduction of the arm. This injury may be related to excessive traction caused by a sudden pull of the tendon of the long head of the biceps brachii muscle and is frequently referred to as a SLAP lesion or tear. The lesion begins posteriorly and extends anteriorly, terminates before or at the midglenoid notch, and includes the anchor of the biceps tendon to the glenoid labrum.

The SLAP lesion was initially divided into four types. Type I lesions (approximately 10% of all SLAP lesions) are associated with degenerative fraying of the superior portion of the labrum. Type II lesions (40%) are characterized by separation of the superior portion of the glenoid labrum and the tendon of the long head of the biceps brachii muscle from the glenoid rim. Type III lesions (30%) are bucket-handle tears of the superior portion of the labrum without involvement of the attachment site of the tendon of the long head of the biceps brachii muscle. Type IV lesions (15%) are characterized by bucket-handle tears of the superior portion of the labrum that extend into the biceps tendon. Additional types of SLAP lesions have also been described.

Detection of a SLAP lesion requires analysis of both coronal oblique and transaxial MR images. Type I lesions are characterized by irregularity in labral contour and a slight increase in its signal intensity. Type II lesions are associated with a globular region of high signal intensity interposed between the superior part of the glenoid labrum and the superior portion of the glenoid fossa. Type III lesions are accompanied by superior labral tears, and type IV lesions are associated with diffuse high signal intensity in the superior portion of the labrum and in the proximal part of the biceps tendon. The coronal plane is most sensitive in the diagnosis of SLAP lesions. MR arthrography may be more sensitive and specific (Fig. 59–52).

### Perilabral Ganglion Cyst

Certain tears of the anterior or posterior portion of the labrum are accompanied by the development of perilabral cysts or ganglia. The pathogenesis of these cystic lesions is not certain, although similar lesions have been described in association with meniscal tears of the knee. In the shoulder, such perilabral cysts or ganglia may extend into

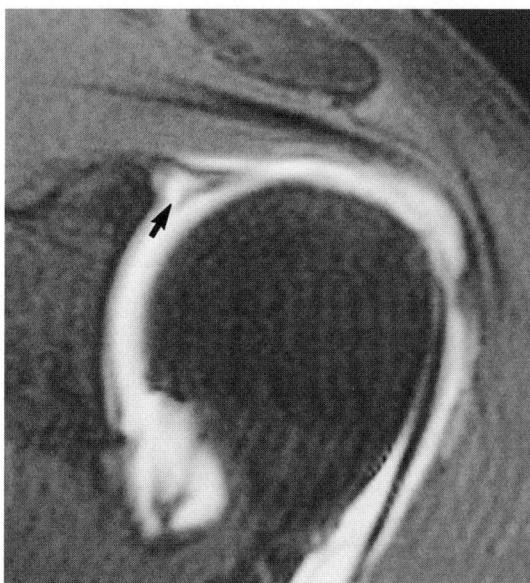

**Figure 59–52.** Superior labral, anterior and posterior (SLAP) lesion: type II. On this oblique coronal T1-weighted (TR/TE, 517/14) fat-suppressed spin echo MR arthrographic image, note the contrast agent *(arrow)* between the biceps-labrum complex and the glenoid margin.

the spinoglenoid notch, the suprascapular notch of the scapula, or both and produce an entrapment neuropathy (see later discussion). During MR arthrography, however, the contrast agent may not reach them, so in addition to the standard T1-weighted sequences, T2-weighted sequences are required (Fig. 59–53). Table 59–4 summarizes the many normal variants and lesions involving the labroligamentous complex and surrounding structures.

## Biceps Tendon Abnormalities

**Anatomic Considerations.** The tendon of the long head of the biceps brachii muscle, with rare exception, arises from the supraglenoid tubercle or the superior portion of the glenoid labrum or from both structures, and it extends obliquely across the top of the humeral head into the intertubercular sulcus or groove. This groove is bounded by the tuberosities of the humerus. The tendon emerges from the joint at the lower portion of the groove, almost surrounded by a sheath that communicates directly with the joint. The subscapularis tendon inserts, in part, into the lesser tuberosity of the humerus. Disruption of the subscapularis tendon leaves the biceps tendon unhindered to slip medially over the lesser tuberosity into the glenohumeral joint.

### Tendinosis and Tenosynovitis

The frequency of bicipital tendinosis and tenosynovitis (with or without tendon subluxation) is unknown. Its association with anterior shoulder pain in athletes required to throw a ball and in golfers and swimmers has been noted. The diagnostic role of MR imaging in cases of bicipital tendinosis and tenosynovitis is not clear. Abnormal signal intensity in the tendon is consistent with tendinosis but may also indicate a tendon tear. Evidence of fluid in the tendon sheath of the long head of the biceps tendon should be considered abnormal only if it completely surrounds the tendon and a sizable joint effusion is not present.

### Tendon Subluxation and Dislocation

Medial subluxation or dislocation of the tendon of the long head of the biceps brachii muscle may occur as an isolated lesion but is generally observed in association

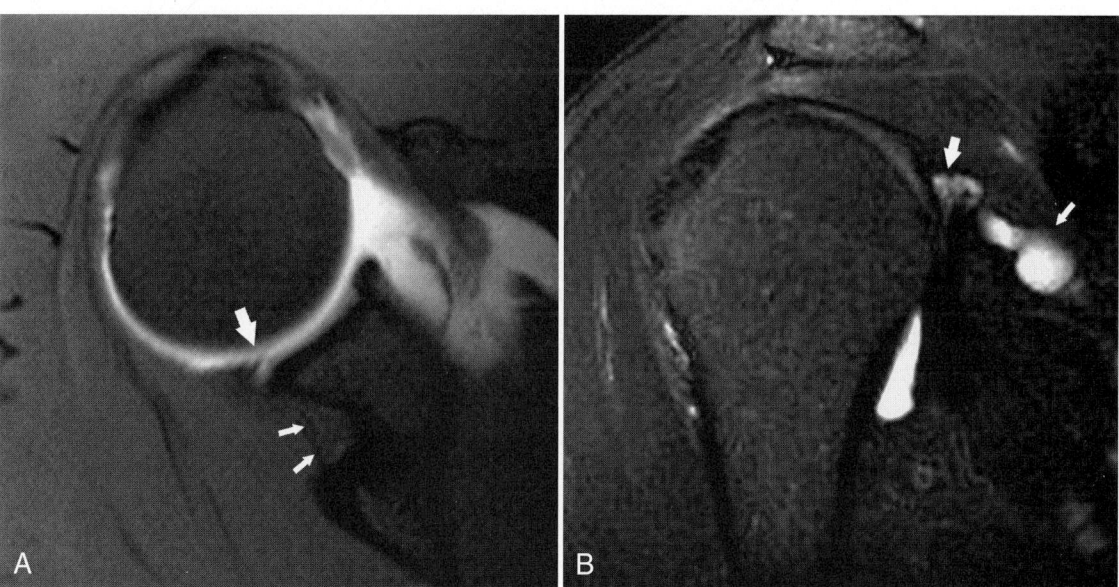

**Figure 59–53.** Perilabral cyst. *A,* Transaxial fast T1-weighted (TR/TE, 500/15) fat-suppressed MR arthrographic image shows a small tear of the posterior superior labrum *(large arrow).* A small perilabral cyst *(small arrows)* is not readily apparent. *B,* Coronal T2-weighted (TR/TE, 3800/105) fat-suppressed MR image shows the perilabral cyst *(small arrow),* as well as its connection to the posterior labrum *(large arrow).*

**TABLE 59–4**

**Terms Applied to Normal Variations or Lesions of the Labroligamentous Complex and Surrounding Structures of the Shoulder**

| Term | Description |
| --- | --- |
| Hill-Sachs lesion | Fracture of the posterior surface of the humeral head, indicative of previous anterior glenohumeral joint dislocation |
| Trough lesion | Fracture of the medial surface of the humeral head, indicative of previous posterior glenohumeral joint dislocation |
| Bankart lesion | Injury of the anteroinferior portion of the glenoid labrum, indicative of previous anterior glenohumeral joint dislocation |
| Sublabral foramen | Normal variation in which a foramen is identified between the anterosuperior portion of the glenoid labrum and the anterior glenoid rim |
| Buford complex | Normal variation in which a cordlike middle glenohumeral ligament is associated with absence of the anterosuperior portion of the glenoid labrum |
| GLOM sign | Designation for a glenoid labral ovoid mass (GLOM), indicative of an injury with avulsion of a portion of the anterior aspect of the glenoid labrum |
| ALPSA lesion | Designation for anterior labroligamentous periosteal sleeve avulsion (ALPSA) associated with recurrent anterior glenohumeral joint dislocation caused by incompetence of the anterior portion of the inferior glenohumeral ligament complex |
| Perthes' lesion | Designation for avulsion of the anteroinferior portion of the glenoid labrum without displacement and with stripping of the periosteal membrane |
| HAGL lesion | Designation for humeral avulsion of the glenohumeral ligament (HAGL); usually seen in older patients and associated with recurrent anterior glenohumeral joint instability and a tear of the subscapularis tendon |
| BHAGL lesion | Designation for a bony HAGL (BHAGL) lesion that is associated with an avulsion fracture of the humerus |
| GLAD lesion | Designation for glenolabral articular disruption (GLAD), which is associated with a tear of the anteroinferior portion of the labrum and erosion of the articular cartilage of the glenoid fossa and not associated with anterior glenohumeral joint instability |
| SLAP lesion | Designation for superior labral, anterior and posterior (SLAP) tear, often seen in athletes involved in sports requiring repetitive overhead use of the arm and varying in severity but involving the superior portion of the glenoid labrum and, sometimes, the biceps anchor |
| Bennett's lesion | Enthesophyte that arises from the posteroinferior portion of the glenoid rim, often seen in baseball pitchers and probably arising at the site of insertion of the posterior band of the inferior glenohumeral ligament complex |
| Osteochondritis dissecans | A lesion of the glenoid cavity related to an impaction force. |
| GARD lesion | Designation for glenoid articular rim divot (GARD) indicative of a lesion involving the posterior glenoid rim, glenoid cavity, or both and related to an impaction injury |
| Perilabral ganglion cyst | Ganglion cyst arising adjacent to the glenoid labrum and often associated with a labral tear |

with massive tears of the rotator cuff. Medial displacement of the biceps tendon may also accompany isolated tears or avulsion of the subscapularis muscle or tendon. Factors predisposing to dislocation of the biceps tendon include anomalies and dysplastic changes of the intertubercular groove, degenerative and attritional changes in the tendon itself, and capsular and ligamentous (i.e., coracohumeral ligament) abnormalities.

Ultrasonography, arthrography, and MR imaging may be used in the assessment of medial dislocation of the biceps tendon. The arthrographic diagnosis of this condition is established by direct visualization of a bicipital tendon within its opacified sheath that is not located in the inter-tubercular groove but is typically located medial to the lesser tuberosity. On MR imaging, the dislocated tendon is seen medial to the bicipital groove, particularly on transaxial images (Fig. 59–54). The tendon may appear thickened and may contain abnormal increased signal intensity, and fluid may be seen in the surrounding tendon sheath. Disruption of one or more components of the rotator cuff and the coracohumeral ligament may also be evident. Intra-articular entrapment of the tendon of the long head of the biceps brachii muscle may be documented; access to the joint is provided by disruption of the subscapularis tendon or by detachment of this tendon from the lesser tuberosity of the humerus (Fig. 59–55).

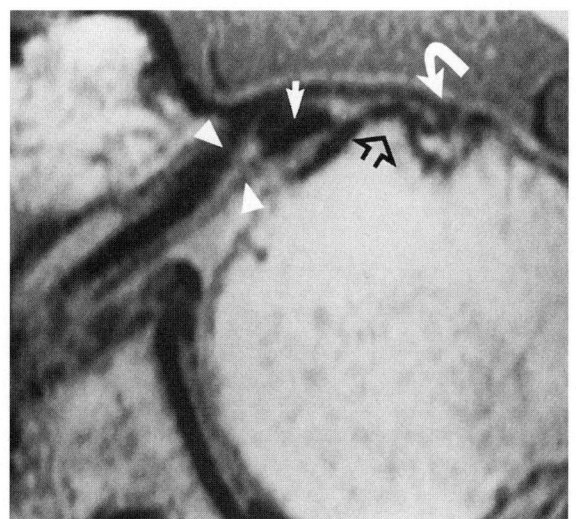

**Figure 59–54.** Tendon of the long head of the biceps brachii muscle: medial displacement. This 54-year-old man fell on his shoulder while skiing and was subsequently unable to abduct his arm. Transaxial intermediate-weighted (TR/TE, 2000/30) spin echo MR image shows that the biceps tendon *(solid straight arrow)* has slipped medially over the lesser tuberosity *(open arrow)* and appears to be lying between the partially displaced fibers *(arrowheads)* of the subscapularis tendon. The transverse humeral ligament *(curved arrow)* appears intact.

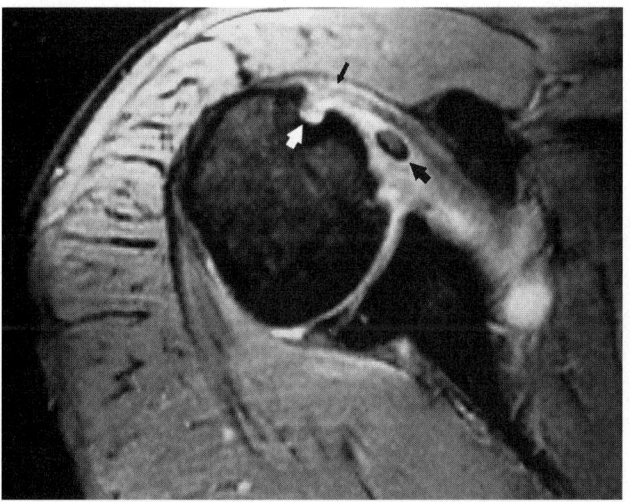

**Figure 59–55.** Tendon of the long head of the biceps brachii muscle: medial displacement with intra-articular entrapment. Axial MPGR (TR/TE, 650/18; flip angle, 20 degrees) MR image at the level of the midglenoid reveals an empty intertubercular sulcus *(white arrow)* and intra-articular displacement of the biceps tendon *(large black arrow)*. Note that the subscapularis tendon is torn *(small black arrow)*.

## Tendon Rupture

Complete rupture of the tendon of the long head of the biceps brachii muscle may occur proximally as a result of impingement or tendon degeneration or, rarely, distally as a result of an injury. The weakest portion of the tendon is the segment just distal to its exit from the joint cavity (extracapsular portion), although intracapsular tears of the bicipital tendon are also encountered. The diagnosis is usually obvious on clinical examination and requires no further diagnostic tests. Partial tears of the biceps tendon, however, may be more subtle, and in these cases, ultrasonography, arthrography, and MR imaging may be useful.

## Entrapment Neuropathies

Several entrapment neuropathies occurring about the shoulder are discussed in Chapter 65, but only three of them are summarized here because of the importance of MR imaging in their diagnosis.

### Suprascapular Nerve Entrapment

The suprascapular nerve passes beneath the superior transverse scapular ligament in the suprascapular notch to enter the supraspinatus fossa; it then runs deep to the supraspinatus muscle beneath the inferior transverse scapular ligament at the lateral margin of the spine of the scapula to enter the infraspinatus fossa through the spinoglenoid notch. Two motor branches supplying the supraspinatus muscle are derived from the portion of the suprascapular nerve in the supraspinatus fossa; similarly, two motor branches supplying the infraspinatus muscle are derived from the portion of the suprascapular nerve in the infraspinatus fossa. Therefore, depending on the precise site of involvement, entrapment of the suprascapular nerve can lead to weakness and atrophy of both the supraspinatus and infraspinatus muscles or to weakness and atrophy of the infraspinatus muscle alone (Fig. 59–56).

The first pattern, that of proximal involvement, is more frequent in the general population, whereas distal entrapment of the nerve leading to isolated involvement of the infraspinatus muscle is often seen in male athletes. Although a variety of causes of suprascapular nerve entrapment have been reported, the documentation of periarticular ganglion cysts with MR imaging has been emphasized (Fig. 59–57). These ganglia may lead to proximal or distal entrapment of the suprascapular nerve and are seen as well-defined, smooth masses with low signal intensity on T1-weighted spin echo MR images and high signal intensity on T2-weighted spin echo MR images. An associated finding is atrophy or edema of the infraspinatus muscle alone or of both the infraspinatus and supraspinatus muscles. Such ganglia may be accompanied by tears in the adjacent portion of the glenoid labrum (see Fig. 59–53).

### Axillary Nerve Entrapment

The quadrilateral space syndrome is an entrapment neuropathy of the axillary nerve that occurs within the quadrilateral space of the shoulder. This space is located posteriorly and is bounded by the teres minor muscle above, the teres major muscle below, the long head of the triceps muscle medially, and the humeral neck laterally (see Fig. 59–56). Passing through this space are the axillary nerve and the posterior humeral circumflex artery. Thus, neurologic manifestations, vascular manifestations, or both may be observed. Clinical findings include skin paresthesias

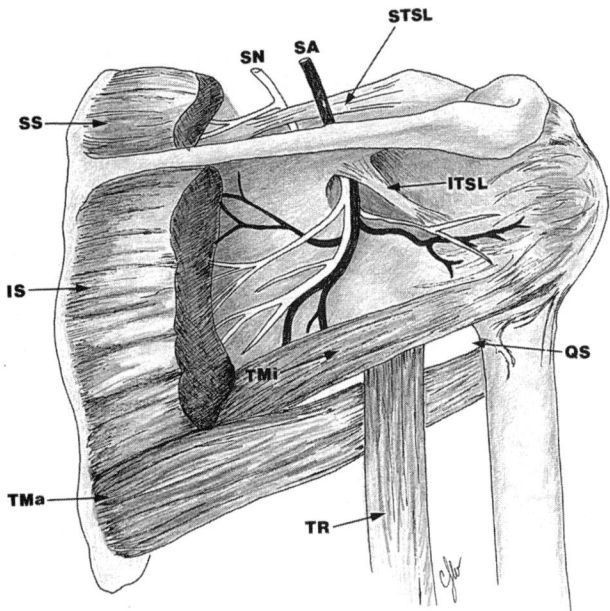

**Figure 59–56.** Suprascapular nerve: normal anatomy. The suprascapular nerve (SN) adjacent to the suprascapular artery (SA) passes beneath the superior transverse scapular ligament (STSL) in the suprascapular notch and then runs deep to the suprascapular muscle (SS) and the inferior transverse scapular ligament (ITSL) to pass through the spinoglenoid notch. The infraspinatus muscle (IS), teres minor muscle (TMi), teres major muscle (TMa), and long head of the triceps muscle (TR) are also indicated. The quadrilateral space (QS) is shown. The axillary nerve and the posterior humeral circumflex artery traverse this space. (Modified from Fritz RC, Helms CA, Steinback LS, et al: Suprascapular nerve entrapment: evaluation with MR imaging. Radiology 182:437, 1992.)

in the distribution of the axillary nerve, weakness of the teres minor or deltoid muscle, and tenderness on palpation of the quadrilateral space. Ganglion cysts are a second well-documented cause of this syndrome. MR imaging reveals atrophy with fatty infiltration of the teres minor or deltoid muscle, or both (Fig. 59–58).

### Brachial Neuritis

Acute brachial neuritis, also known as Parsonage-Turner syndrome, is a painful neuromuscular disorder associated with weakness of the musculature about the shoulder. Its cause is not known, although the syndrome may be related to a viral neuritis. Most commonly, the involved shoulder muscles are those innervated by the suprascapular nerve, but additional muscles may also be affected, such as those innervated by the axillary nerve. Thus, the suprascapular, infraspinatus, deltoid, and teres minor muscles, in various combinations, may be abnormal when studied with MR imaging. Denervation edema and, later, atrophy are observed. The major differential diagnostic considerations are the entrapment neuropathies listed in Table 59–5.

## HIP

### Anatomy

**Articular.** The femoral head is covered with articular cartilage, although a small area on its surface is devoid of cartilage, where the ligament of the head of the femur, or ligamentum teres, attaches (Fig. 59–59). The lunate surface is covered with articular cartilage; the floor of the acetabular fossa within this surface does not contain car-

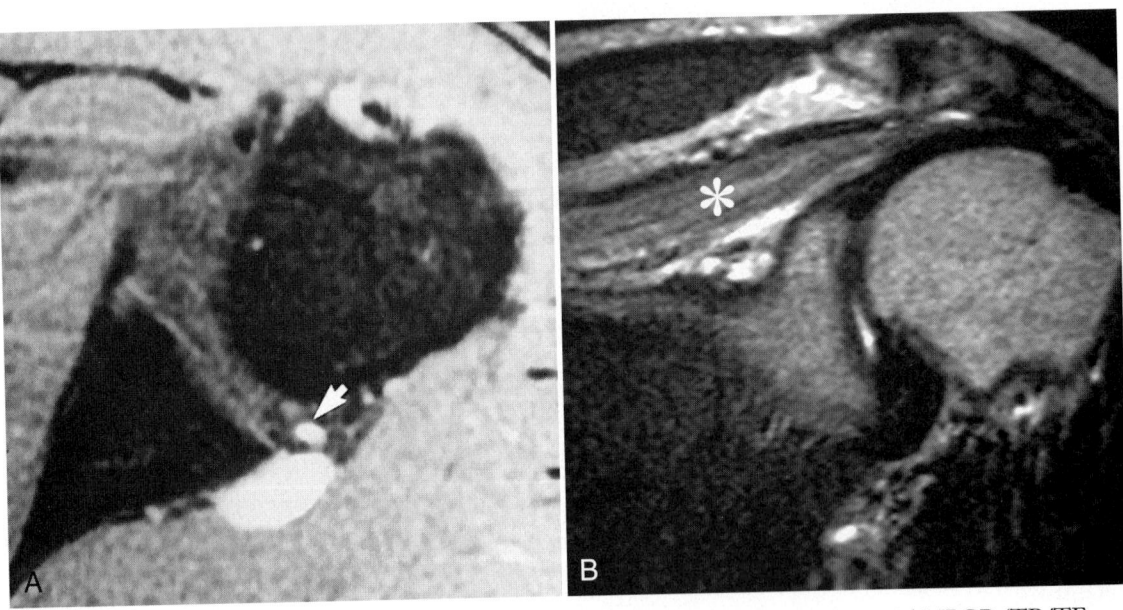

**Figure 59–57.** Suprascapular nerve: entrapment related to ganglion cysts. *A,* Transaxial MPGR (TR/TE, 383/12; flip angle, 15 degrees) MR image reveals a ganglion cyst of high signal intensity adjacent to the posterior margin of the glenoid cavity. Observe a tear in the adjacent labrum *(arrow). B,* In a different patient with documented suprascapular nerve palsy, coronal T2-weighted (TR/TE, 2000/80) spin echo MR image at the level of the suprascapular muscle shows changes of denervation in the suprascapular muscle *(asterisk),* with diffuse increased signal intensity.

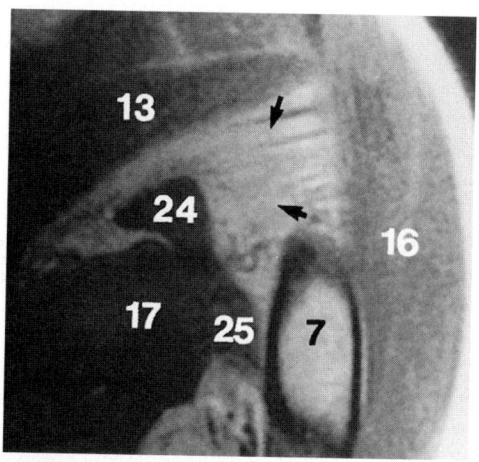

**Figure 59–58.** Quadrilateral space syndrome. Coronal oblique intermediate-weighted (TR/TE, 2000/25) spin echo MR image shows selective atrophy with fatty replacement of the teres minor muscle (*arrows*). The infraspinatus muscle (13), deltoid muscle (16), teres major muscle (17), and long (24) and lateral (25) heads of the triceps muscle are identified and are not involved. The humeral diaphysis (7) is also seen. (Courtesy of W. Glenn, MD, Long Beach, Calif.)

tilage but has a fibroelastic fat pad covered with synovial membrane. A fibrous capsule encircles the joint and much of the femoral neck. The capsule attaches proximally to the acetabulum, labrum, and transverse ligament of the acetabulum. Distally, it surrounds the femoral neck (Fig. 59–60). The fibrous capsule is strengthened by surrounding ligaments, including the iliofemoral, pubofemoral, and ischiofemoral ligaments. The acetabular labrum, the fibrocartilaginous rim about the acetabulum, is firmly attached to the bony rim and transverse ligament, is triangular on cross section, and has a free edge or apex that forms a smaller circle that closely embraces the femoral head.

The iliopsoas bursa is the largest and most important bursa about the hip. It may extend proximally and communicates with the joint space in approximately 15% of normal hips through a gap between the iliofemoral and pubofemoral ligaments.

**Vessels and Nerves.** The major arterial supply of the adult femoral head originates from the medial and lateral femoral circumflex arteries, which are branches of either the femoral artery or the deep femoral artery. The contribution to the blood supply of the femoral head provided by the artery of the ligamentum teres is variable.

## TABLE 59–5

### Muscle Involvement in Neuropathies of the Shoulder

|  | Supraspinatus Muscle | Infraspinatus Muscle | Teres Minor Muscle | Deltoid Muscle |
|---|---|---|---|---|
| Suprascapular nerve entrapment syndrome | + | + | – | – |
| Quadrilateral space syndrome | – | – | + | + |
| Brachial neuritis | + | + | + | + |

+, may be involved.
–, not involved.

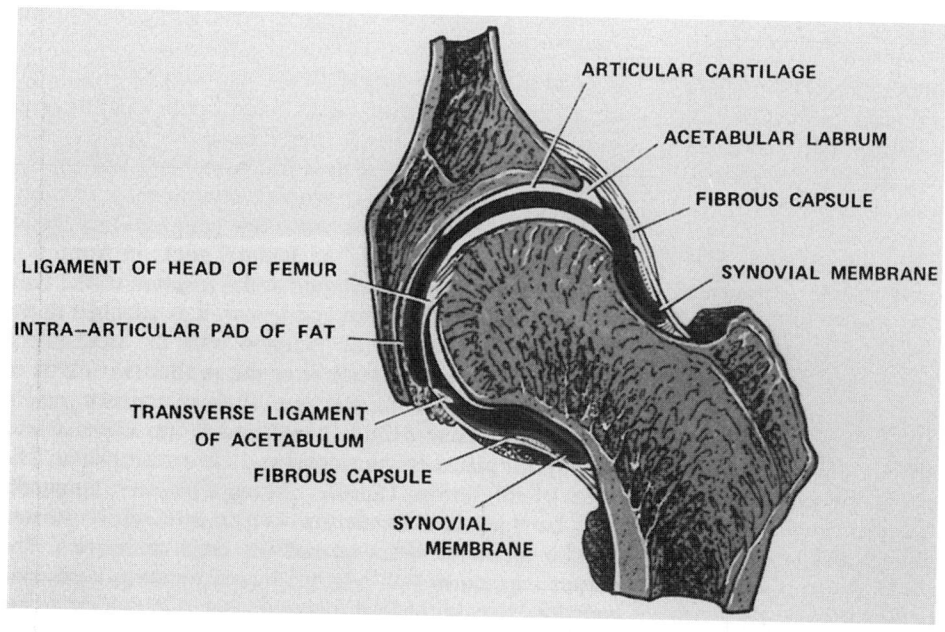

ARTICULAR CARTILAGE

ACETABULAR LABRUM

FIBROUS CAPSULE

SYNOVIAL MEMBRANE

LIGAMENT OF HEAD OF FEMUR

INTRA–ARTICULAR PAD OF FAT

TRANSVERSE LIGAMENT OF ACETABULUM

FIBROUS CAPSULE

SYNOVIAL MEMBRANE

**Figure 59–59.** Hip joint: normal articular anatomy. Drawing of a coronal section through the hip.

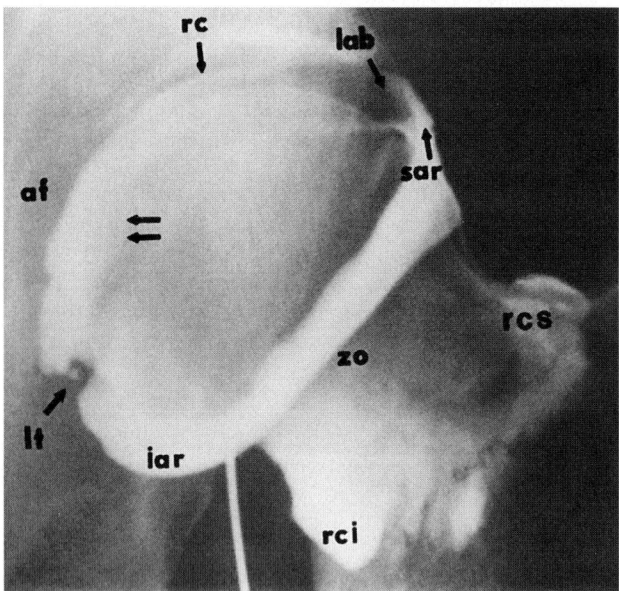

**Figure 59–60.** Hip joint: normal articular anatomy. On a hip arthrogram, the recessus capitis (rc) is a thin, smooth collection of contrast medium between apposing articular surfaces and is interrupted only where the ligamentum teres *(double arrows)* enters the fovea centralis of the femoral head. The ligamentum transversum (lt) is seen as a radiolucent defect adjacent to the inferior rim of the acetabulum. The inferior articular recess (iar) forms a pouch at the inferior base of the femoral head below the acetabular notch and ligamentum transversum. The superior articular recess (sar) extends cephalad around the acetabular labrum (lab). The acetabular labrum is seen as a triangular radiolucent area adjacent to the superolateral lip of the acetabulum. The zona orbicularis (zo) is a circumferential lucent band around the femoral neck that changes configuration with rotation of the femur. The recessus colli superior (rcs) and recessus colli inferior (rci) are poolings of contrast material at the apex and base of the intertrochanteric line and are the most caudal extensions of the synovial membrane. (From Guerra J Jr, Armbruster TG, Resnick D, et al: The adult hip: An anatomic study. Part II: The soft-tissue landmarks. Radiology 128:11, 1978.)

The sciatic nerve exits the pelvis at the right sciatic notch, intimate with the piriformis muscle. Some variation exists, however, in the relationship of these two structures.

## Labral Abnormalities

Abnormalities of the acetabular labrum occur in both children and adults. Those associated with developmental dysplasia of the hip in infants and young children are discussed in Chapter 73.

### Labral Tear

In adults, an association exists between acetabular labral tears and developmental dysplasia of the hip. In these patients, radiographic evidence of acetabular dysplasia is evident. Additional radiographic findings include subchondral cysts in the acetabulum and a relatively rapid appearance of osteoarthritis of the hip (Fig. 59–61). Standard

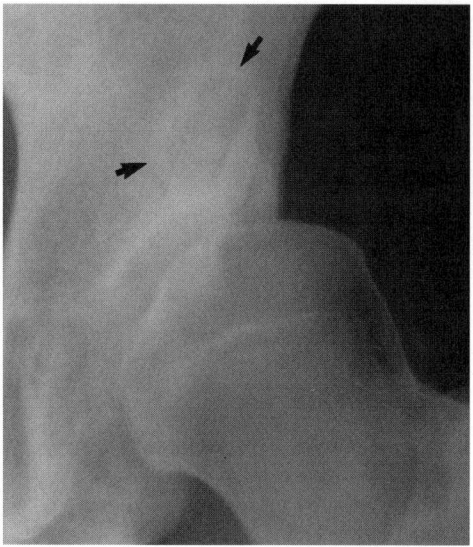

**Figure 59–61.** Acetabulum and acetabular labrum: developmental dysplasia associated with intraosseous ganglion cyst and labral tear. Radiograph reveals developmental dysplasia of the hip (manifested as a steep, flat acetabular roof and lateral displacement of the femoral head) and a ganglion cyst *(arrows)* in the acetabulum.

arthrography reveals evidence of a labral tear, which manifests as an opacified channel extending into the labrum after the introduction of radiopaque contrast material into the hip. Tears of the acetabular labrum may also be seen in patients with no evidence of hip dysplasia. Pain, especially during physical activity and on passive flexion and medial rotation of the hip, is a constant clinical manifestation. Arthrography in some patients may show an abnormal shape of the acetabular labrum characterized by enlargement and a rounded contour, but the actual tear may not be opacified.

### Cystic Degeneration of the Labrum and Ganglion Cyst

A combination of labral tears, acetabular dysplasia, osteoarthritis of the hip, acetabular ganglion cysts, and para-acetabular soft tissue ganglia may be found in the hips of adult patients. Gas adjacent to and within the acetabulum represents a diagnostic clue in some of these patients. MR images show soft tissue ganglion cysts adjacent to the labrum; they appear as well-defined masses of low signal intensity on T1-weighted spin echo MR images and high signal intensity on T2-weighted spin echo images (Fig. 59–62).

The role of standard MR imaging in the assessment of a torn acetabular labrum is not clear. MR arthrography clearly shows labral detachments and most labral tears, although small tears may escape detection. The instillation of pain medication at the time of arthrography can confirm that the articulation itself is the source of the symptoms (Fig. 59–63). Labral detachments are identified at the time of MR arthrography by the presence of contrast material at the acetabular-labral junction, with

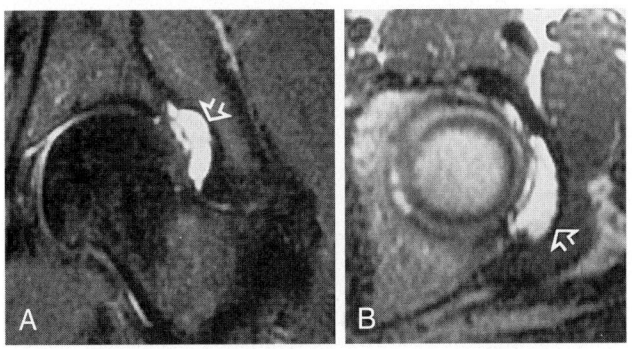

**Figure 59–62.** Acetabular labrum: tear and cystic degeneration. In a 39-year-old woman, a coronal STIR (TR/TE, 4000/17; inversion time, 150 msec) MR image *(A)* shows a cystic collection of high signal intensity *(open arrow)* within the labrum. A transaxial T2-weighted (TR/TE, 2100/70) spin echo MR image *(B)* reveals the posterolateral location of the cystic lesion *(open arrow)*. (Courtesy of S. K. Brahme, MD, La Jolla, Calif.)

or without displacement of the labrum. Criteria for labral tears include contrast material within portions of the labrum and surface irregularity. The identification of perilabral ganglion cysts in the hip is an important sign of labral pathology, with a presumed pathogenesis similar to that of perilabral ganglion cysts in the glenohumeral joint and meniscal cysts. These cysts may not opacify during MR arthrography, although they are clearly visible on T2-weighted MR images.

## Synovial Abnormalities

### Synovitis

Involvement of the hip in a variety of synovial disorders is well known and is covered in appropriate sections of this book. In some cases, routine radiography allows a precise diagnosis, although data provided by clinical assessment, other imaging methods, and, occasionally, joint aspiration or examination of synovial tissue may be required.

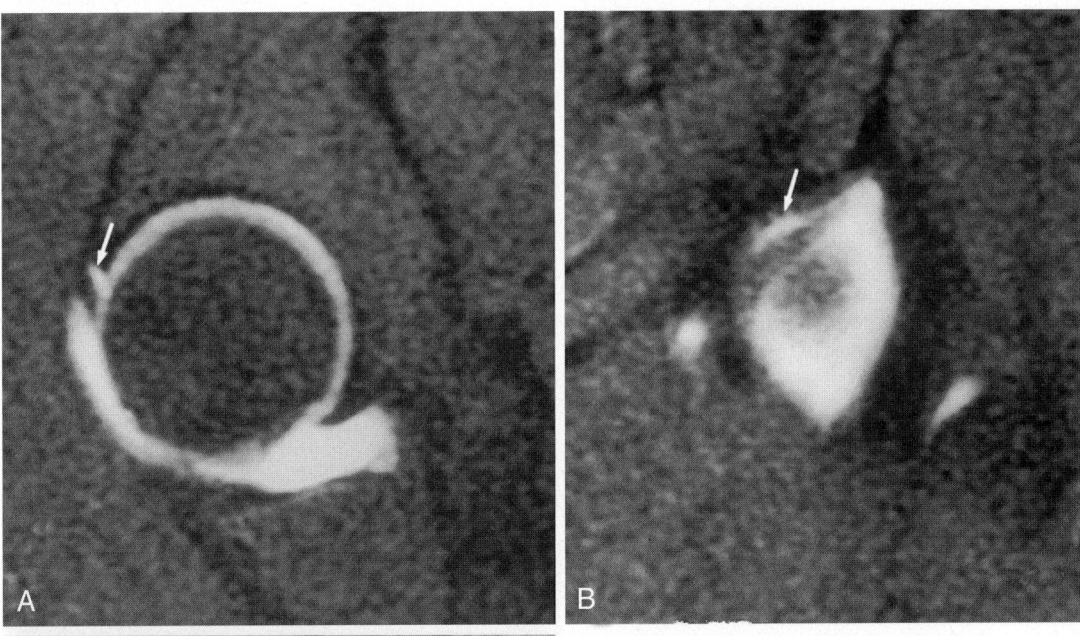

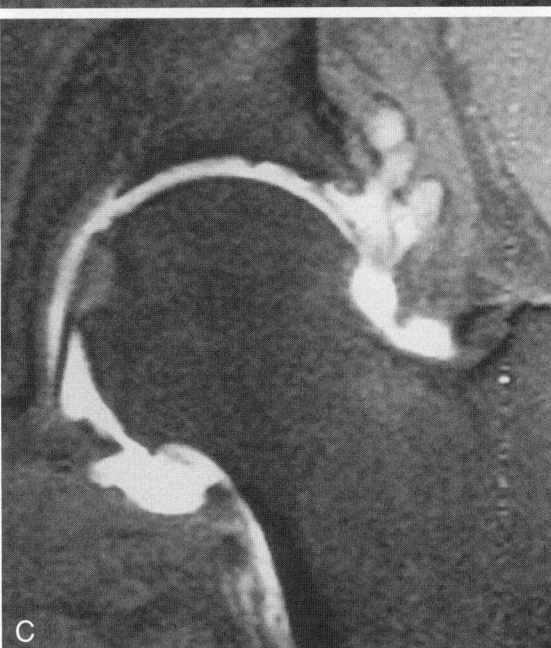

**Figure 59–63.** Acetabular labrum: tear and cystic degeneration. *A* and *B*, Partial detachment of the anterosuperior portion of the labrum *(arrows)* is seen on fat-suppressed sagittal *(A)* and coronal *(B)* T1-weighted (TR/TE, 600/16) spin echo MR arthrographic images. *C*, In a different patient, a fat-suppressed coronal T1-weighted (TR/TE, 700/12) spin echo MR arthrographic image demonstrates a massive superior labral tear with a perilabral ganglion cyst. (*A* and *B*, Courtesy of J. Tomanek, MD, Johnson City, Tenn.)

MR imaging provides information regarding the extent of synovial disease in the hip that is not available on routine radiographs (Fig. 59–64). Abnormal collections of joint fluid may be detected. As in other locations, such as the knee, the differentiation of synovial inflammatory tissue and joint effusion by MR imaging may require the intravenous administration of gadolinium compounds.

## Synovial Cyst

With any process of the hip that leads to an elevation in intra-articular pressure, escape of fluid from the joint through a number of anatomic pathways serves to decompress the articulation. Typically, the fluid passes into a surrounding synovial sac, and its distention can be seen or palpated. These synovial cysts can also be assessed with imaging methods. Of all the potential locations of synovial cysts about the hip, the iliopsoas bursa deserves special emphasis.

**Iliopsoas Bursal Distention.** Communication of the hip and iliopsoas bursa in the presence of intra-articular diseases such as osteoarthritis, rheumatoid arthritis, pigmented villonodular synovitis, infection, calcium pyrophosphate dihydrate crystal deposition disease, and idiopathic synovial (osteo)chondromatosis may lead to bursal enlargement and produce a mass in the ilioinguinal region that simulates a hernia and causes obstruction of the femoral vein. The iliopsoas bursa communicates with the hip joint via an aperture ranging in diameter from 1 mm to 3 cm, and enlargement of this channel in the 15% of normal adults who possess this aperture, or creation of a communicating pathway in adults who do not, is an expected consequence of virtually any disease process of the hip that leads to an elevation in intra-articular pressure (Fig. 59–65).

Suspected iliopsoas bursal distention should be evaluated by ultrasonography. If a nonpulsatile fluid collection without Doppler evidence of flow is demonstrated, this technique can be used for diagnostic aspiration of its contents. Fluid analysis should distinguish a synovial cyst or iliopsoas bursitis from a lymphocele, abscess, or hematoma. Subsequent injection of contrast material into the bursa or cyst may opacify the hip joint and thus confirm the diagnosis; if not, hip arthrography, CT, or MR imaging may be desirable to delineate potential articular communication if surgery is being contemplated.

## Iliopsoas Bursitis

The synovium lining the iliopsoas bursa can be involved in a variety of processes, including rheumatoid arthritis and infection. CT, MR imaging, and ultrasonography are the best techniques for evaluating an inflamed and distended iliopsoas bursa. Afflictions of other bursal cavities about the hip and pelvis can be similarly evaluated (Fig. 59–66).

## Bone Abnormalities

Three conditions are important in any discussion of hip disorders: osteonecrosis of the femoral head, transient bone

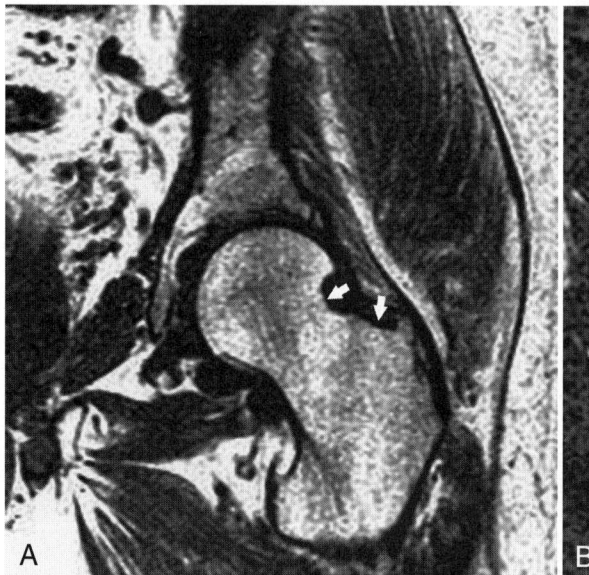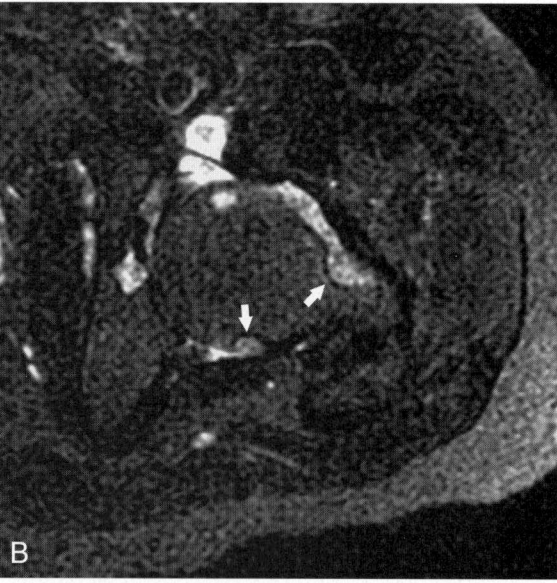

**Figure 59–64.** Synovial disorders: idiopathic synovial (osteo)chondromatosis. Coronal T1-weighted (TR/TE, 633/17) *(A)* and fast T2-weighted (TR/TE, 4000/91) *(B)* spin echo MR images show joint distention with multiple osseous erosions *(arrows)* in this 75-year-old man with chronic hip pain. In *A,* the intra-articular process is of low signal intensity; in *B,* it is of intermediate to high signal intensity. The MR imaging findings simulate those of synovitis with a joint effusion.

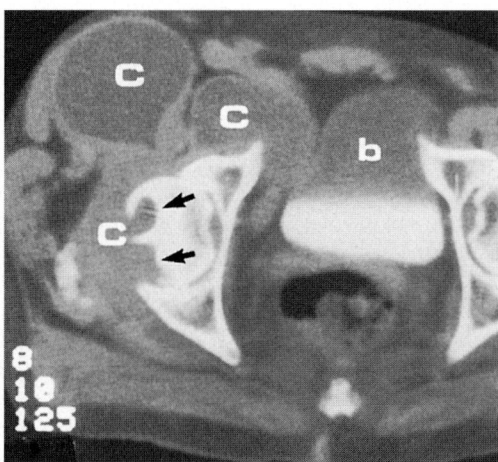

**Figure 59–65.** Iliopsoas bursal distention. CT was performed to evaluate swelling in the right side of the groin of a middle-aged man with rheumatoid arthritis. Transaxial scan reveals several collections of fluid density (C) around and anterior to the right hip joint, one of which extends into the pelvis, with leftward displacement of the urinary bladder (b). Bone erosions are also apparent *(arrows)*. (From Sartoris DJ, Danzig L, Gilula L, et al: Synovial cysts of the hip joint and iliopsoas bursitis: A spectrum of imaging abnormalities. Skeletal Radiol 14:85, 1985.)

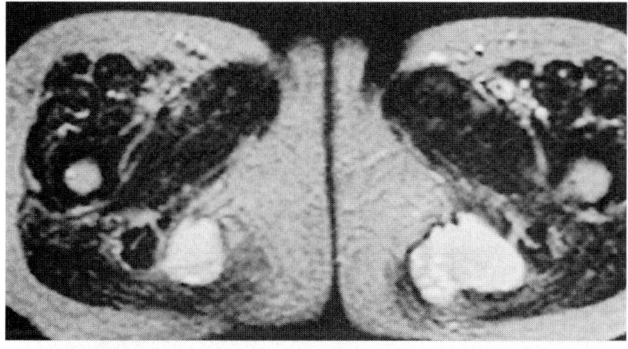

**Figure 59–66.** Ischial bursitis. Transaxial T2-weighted (TR/TE, 1500/90) spin echo MR image shows evidence of bilateral ischial bursitis. (Courtesy of J. Dillard, MD, San Diego, Calif.)

marrow edema (and related disorders), and intracapsular and extracapsular fractures of the femoral neck. Although each of these conditions is considered in detail in other chapters (see Chapters 41, 57, and 67), a few comments are appropriate here.

### Osteonecrosis

The causative factors leading to ischemic necrosis of bone are diverse and include trauma, corticosteroid medications, sickle cell anemia and other hemoglobinopathies, Gaucher's disease, alcoholism, pancreatitis, and radiation; in many cases, a specific causative factor cannot be identified (idiopathic osteonecrosis). The femoral head, femoral condyles, and humeral head are commonly involved.

Routine radiography and CT are not reliable in the diagnosis of early osteonecrosis of the femoral head. Scintigraphy using bone-seeking radiopharmaceutical agents is sensitive to the early changes of osteonecrosis, but the scintigraphic findings lack specificity.

MR imaging characteristics of osteonecrosis of the femoral head are variable and evolve over time. A diffuse pattern of bone marrow edema, identical to that of transient bone marrow edema, may be identified in the early stages of the process. Subsequently, a more focal process within the femoral head allows a more specific diagnosis (Fig. 59–67). The area of ischemic marrow may be surrounded by a reactive interface characterized by low signal intensity on T1-weighted spin echo MR images and an outer margin of low signal intensity and an inner margin of high signal intensity on T2-weighted spin echo MR images. This pattern, often designated a double line sign, is virtually diagnostic of osteonecrosis.

### Transient Bone Marrow Edema

The association of transient pain and limitation of motion in the hip, radiographically evident osteopenia, and an MR imaging pattern consistent with bone marrow edema has been found by many investigators. Also observed is the presence of identical marrow findings on MR imaging in patients with painful hips whose routine radiographs do not reveal osteopenia; this is not surprising, given the relative insensitivity of conventional radiography in the detection of minor to moderate degrees of bone loss. Therefore, the designation of transient bone marrow edema appears to be more comprehensive than that of transient osteoporosis about the hip (Fig. 59–68). The relationship between transient bone marrow edema and osteonecrosis of the femoral head, however, is not clear.

### Occult Femoral Fracture

Fractures of the femoral neck may result from a significant injury, but they also occur spontaneously or after a

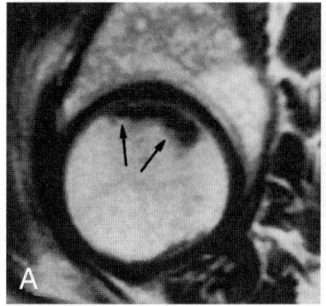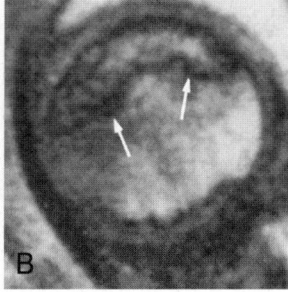

**Figure 59–67.** Osteonecrosis. *A,* Sagittal T1-weighted (TR/TE, 966/12) spin echo MR image shows a curvilinear region of low signal intensity *(arrows)* representing osteonecrosis of the femoral head. *B,* Sagittal T1-weighted (TR/TE, 800/20) spin echo MR image in a different patient reveals a large area of osteonecrosis of the femoral head manifested as a serpentine region of low signal intensity *(arrows)* with a central zone whose signal intensity is similar to that of fat.

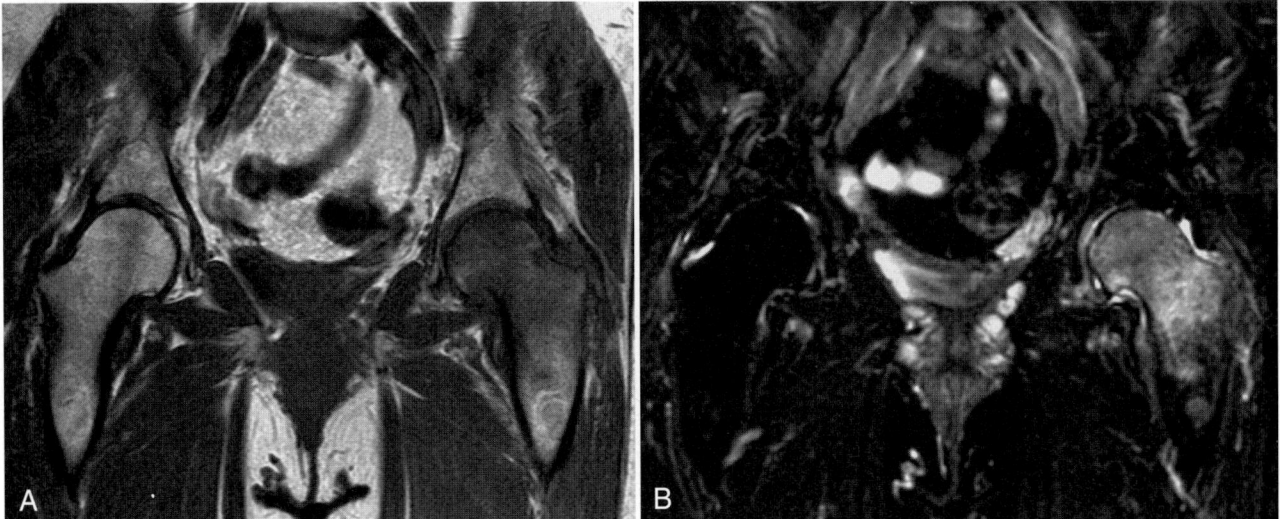

**Figure 59–68.** Transient bone marrow edema. Coronal T1-weighted (TR/TE, 500/15) *(A)* and fat-suppressed fast T2-weighted (TR/TE, 4000/90) *(B)* spin echo MR images reveal characteristic features of transient bone marrow edema. In *(A)*, note the low signal intensity in the marrow of the left femoral head and neck, with normal signal intensity in the adjacent acetabulum. The opposite femur and acetabulum are also normal. In *B*, note the high signal intensity in the involved marrow in the left femur and a joint effusion. The altered signal intensity extends to the base of the femoral neck.

minor injury in elderly patients and as a response to the cumulative effects of prolonged stress (i.e., fatigue or insufficiency fractures). The difficulty of detecting nondisplaced acute fractures of the femoral neck with conventional radiographic techniques has led to the application of other imaging methods. Of these, MR imaging appears to be most specific.

The MR imaging characteristics of a nondisplaced fracture of the femoral neck on T1-weighted spin echo sequences consist of a well-defined linear zone of low signal intensity that may be surrounded by a broader, ill-defined zone of low signal intensity consistent with marrow edema. On T2-weighted spin echo MR images, the fracture line may still be of low signal intensity, but the edematous zone demonstrates high signal intensity. STIR images are very sensitive in the detection of these fractures, which appear as broad bands of high signal intensity within the normal, low-signal-intensity bone marrow; however, these images are less specific because the fracture line itself may not be identifiable. When MR imaging is applied to the analysis of acute trochanteric fractures, some of these fractures are found to extend completely or incompletely across the femoral neck (Fig. 59–69). MR imaging is also highly sensitive and specific for the diagnosis of stress fractures in the femur and pelvic bones.

## Soft Tissue and Muscle Abnormalities

The many soft tissue abnormalities that can lead to significant clinical manifestations in the hip (and elsewhere) are discussed in Chapter 72, and those related to muscle

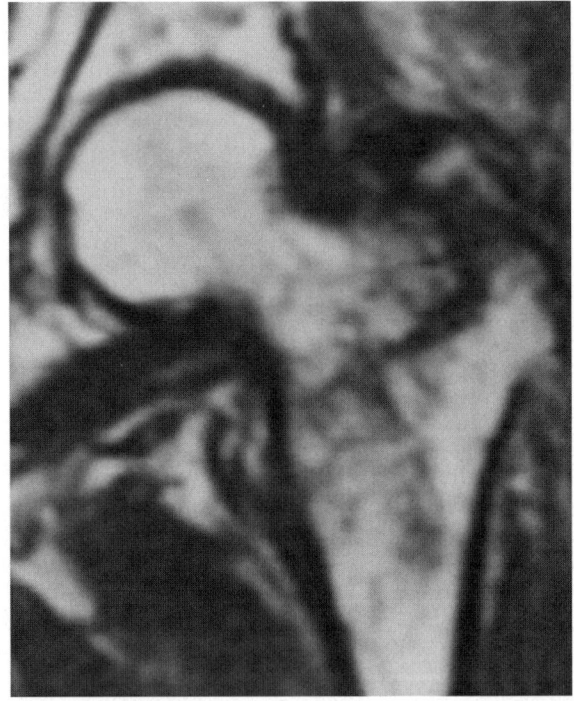

**Figure 59–69.** Femoral neck fracture. Although a routine radiograph was interpreted as normal, a coronal T1-weighted (TR/TE, 600/20) spin echo MR image shows a nondisplaced intertrochanteric fracture of the left femur. The fracture is manifested as an irregular line of low signal intensity surrounded by less well defined regions of low signal intensity. (Courtesy of D. Bates, MD, La Jolla, Calif.)

injury are described in Chapter 79. Only a single entity, snapping hip syndrome, is discussed here.

A variety of causes have been implicated in this syndrome of hip pain associated with audible snapping. Intra-articular abnormalities, including single or multiple osteocartilaginous bodies, typically result in a faint sound associated with true femoral-acetabular motion; extra-articular causes are often characterized by a loud snap and, in some cases, a sudden jump of the fascia lata or gluteus maximus over the greater trochanter as the hip moves in a well-delineated fashion. Other proposed causes include slipping of the iliopsoas tendon over the iliopectineal eminence and slipping of the iliofemoral ligaments over the anterior portion of the hip capsule.

Subluxation of the iliopsoas tendon is one cause of a snapping hip. Iliopsoas bursography, iliopsoas tenography, or hip arthrography in which the iliopsoas bursa is also opacified confirms the changing position of the iliopsoas tendon and its displacement over the iliopectineal line during flexion and extension of the hip. An abrupt change in the position of the tendon coincident with the audible sound and palpable snap is observed.

## Miscellaneous Abnormalities

Although MR imaging is useful in the assessment of many processes involving the hip and adjacent bones and soft tissues, some conditions are better evaluated with other imaging methods. Intra-articular bodies in the hip (and in other joints) may escape detection when MR imaging is used alone. Such bodies, which commonly localize in the region of the acetabular fossa, are detected more easily with routine radiography supplemented with CT or arthrography. Osteoid osteomas are better evaluated with CT (Fig. 59–70).

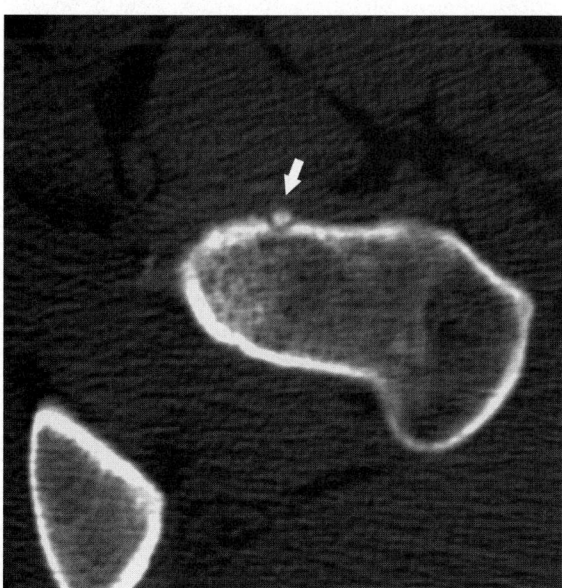

**Figure 59–70.** Osteoid osteoma. Calcified nidus *(arrow)* of a subperiosteal osteoid osteoma is effectively shown on a transaxial CT scan.

## KNEE

The knee joint is the largest and most complicated articulation in the human body. In this articulation, three functional spaces exist: the medial femorotibial space, the lateral femorotibial space, and the patellofemoral space.

### Anatomy

The articular surfaces of the femur, tibia, and patella are not congruent; the adjacent articular surfaces of the tibia and femur are more closely fitted together by the presence of the medial and lateral menisci (Fig. 59–71). The medial meniscus is nearly semicircular in shape, with a broadened or widened posterior horn. The peripheral aspect of the medial meniscus is attached to the fibrous capsule and the medial, or tibial, collateral ligament. The

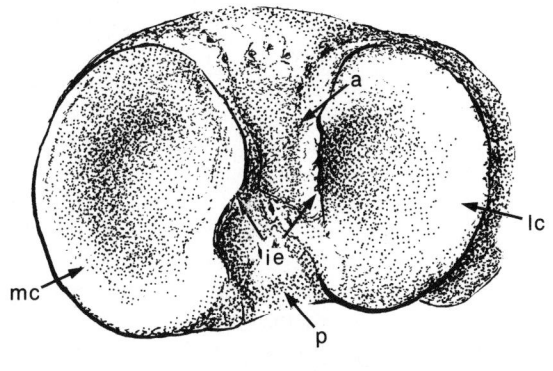

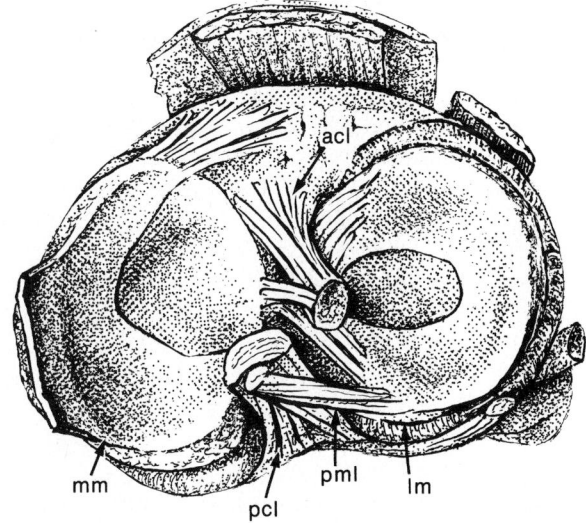

**Figure 59–71.** Knee joint: normal anatomy—menisci and cruciate ligaments. Drawings show the tibial articular surfaces without *(above)* and with *(below)* the addition of soft tissue structures. Note the medial condyle (mc), lateral condyle (lc), intercondylar eminences (ie), anterior intercondylar area (a), and posterior intercondylar area (p). Soft tissue structures are the medial meniscus (mm), lateral meniscus (lm), posterior cruciate ligament (pcl), posterior meniscofemoral ligament (pml), and anterior cruciate ligament (acl).

lateral meniscus, which is of relatively uniform width throughout, resembles a ring. The lateral meniscus is grooved posteriorly by the popliteus tendon and its accompanying tendon sheath. The meniscofemoral ligaments, both anterior and posterior, are attached to or intimate with the posterior horn of the lateral meniscus.

The fibrous capsule of the knee joint is not a complete structure; anteriorly, the fibrous capsule is absent above and over the patellar surface. The ligamentous sheath in this area is composed mainly of a tendinous expansion from the rectus femoris and vastus musculature that descends to attach around the superior half of the bone. Superficial fibers continue to descend onto the strong ligamentum patellae. This structure, which is a continuation of the quadriceps muscle, is attached above to the apex of the patella and below to the tibial tuberosity. Adjacent fibers, the medial and lateral patellar retinacula, pass from the osseous margins of the patella to the tibial condyles. Posteriorly, capsular fibers extend from the femoral surface above the condyles and the intercondylar line to the posterior border of the tibia. Laterally, capsular fibers run from the femoral to the tibial condyles. In this area is found the fibular (i.e., lateral) collateral ligament, which is attached above to the lateral epicondyle of the femur and below to the fibular head. Medially, the capsule is strengthened by tendinous expansions from the sartorius and semimembranosus muscles. These fibers pass upward to the medial collateral ligament, which is attached above to the medial epicondyle of the femur and below to the medial tibial condyle and shaft. The medial and fibular collateral ligaments reinforce the medial and lateral sides of the joint. They are taut in joint extension, and in this position, they prevent rotation of the knee.

The synovial membrane of the knee joint is the most extensive in the body and can be conveniently divided into several parts (Fig. 59–72):

1. *Central portion.* This portion extends between the patella and the patellar surface of the femur to the cruciate ligaments. An infrapatellar fat pad below the patella, located deep to the patellar ligament, presses the synovial membrane posteriorly.

2. *Suprapatellar synovial pouch.* This cavity extends vertically above the patella between the quadriceps muscle anteriorly and the femur posteriorly.

3. *Posterior femoral recesses.* These recesses lie behind the posterior portion of each femoral condyle, deep to the lateral and medial heads of the gastrocnemius muscle.

4. *Subpopliteal recess.* A small synovial cul-de-sac lies between the lateral meniscus and the tendon of the popliteus; this cul-de-sac may communicate with the superior tibiofibular joint in 10% of adults.

Numerous additional bursae may be found about the knee, including the subcutaneous prepatellar and subfascial prepatellar bursae anterior to the patella; the deep infrapatellar bursa between the upper part of the tibia and the ligamentum patellae; the anserine bursa between the medial collateral ligament and tendons of the sartorius, gracilis, and semitendinosus muscles; and bursae between the semimembranosus tendon and medial collateral ligament and between the biceps tendon and fibular collateral ligament.

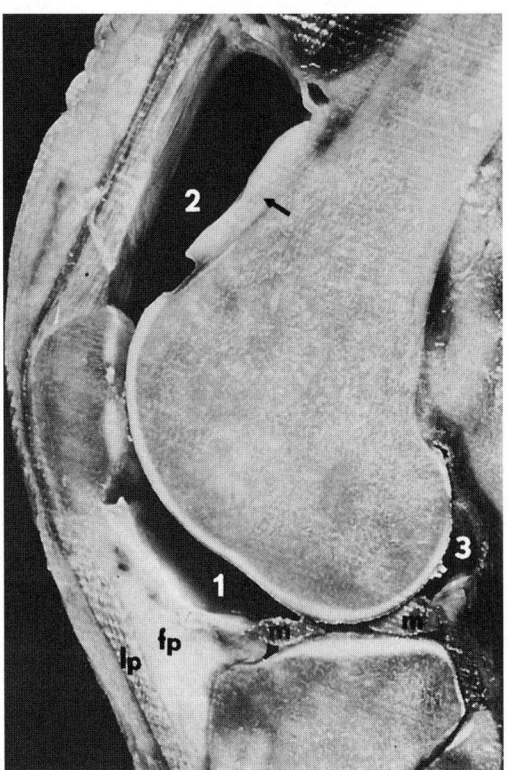

**Figure 59–72.** Knee joint: normal anatomy. Photograph of an air-distended knee joint outlining the ligamentum patellae (lp), infrapatellar fat pad (fp), and menisci (m). The articulation can be divided into a central portion (1), suprapatellar pouch (2), and posterior femoral recesses (3). Note the fatty tissue *(arrow)* pressed against the anterior aspect of the femur.

## Synovial Abnormalities

### Joint Effusion

In normal joints, including the knee, fluid is present in small quantities sufficient to coat the numerous folds of the synovial membrane. The precise amount of fluid that may be present in a normal knee joint is not clear. The lateral radiograph of the knee is the most sensitive of all routine radiographic projections for the detection of a joint effusion. Enlargement of the normally collapsed suprapatellar recess is appreciated radiographically on a lateral projection by abnormal separation between a fat body above the patella and the prefemoral fat body (Fig. 59–73). A measurement of 10 mm between these fat bodies is considered definitely abnormal, and a measurement between 5 and 10 mm is considered possibly abnormal. An abnormal measurement can result not only from joint fluid but also from an intra-articular mass or hypertrophy of the synovial membrane. Approximately 4 to 5 mL of fluid is required in the knee joint before an effusion can be detected with conventional radiography.

MR imaging is extremely sensitive to the presence of intra-articular fluid. Such fluid is of low signal intensity on T1-weighted spin echo MR images and high signal intensity on T2-weighted spin echo and many gradient echo images. Sagittal MR images allow the detection of as little as 1 mL of fluid.

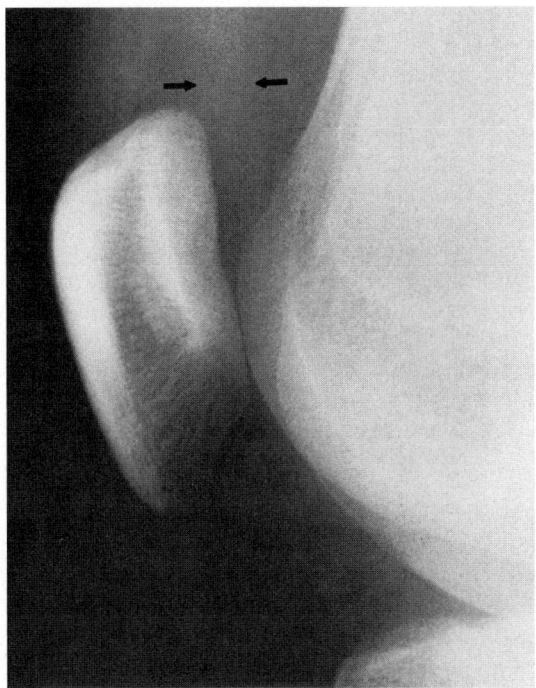

**Figure 59–73.** Knee joint: radiographic anatomy. In the presence of intra-articular fluid, distention of the suprapatellar pouch creates a radiodense region of increased thickness with blurred margins *(arrows)*.

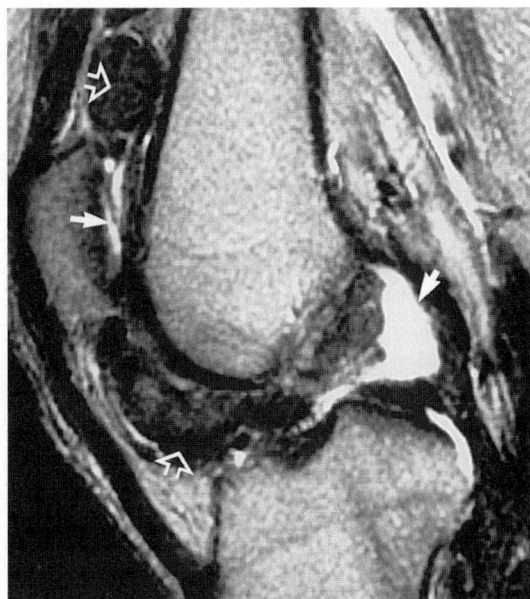

**Figure 59–74.** Chronic hemarthrosis: pigmented villonodular synovitis. Sagittal T2-weighted (TR/TE, 2000/80) spin echo MR image reveals distention of the knee in a patient with pigmented villonodular synovitis. Note the intra-articular fluid of high signal intensity *(solid arrows)* and intrasynovial hemosiderin deposits of low signal intensity *(open arrows)*.

## Hemarthrosis and Lipohemarthrosis

Hemarthrosis may result from an injury or from a number of articular processes, including proliferative disease, tumor, and arthritis. Post-traumatic hemarthrosis of the knee is generally considered a manifestation of serious ligamentous injury, particularly in adults.

MR imaging allows a specific diagnosis in some types of hemarthrosis. Although acute hemorrhagic effusions may have signal intensity characteristics similar to those of normal synovial fluid, subacute and chronic hemarthrosis may demonstrate high signal intensity on both T1- and T2-weighted spin echo MR images. A fluid level representing a layering phenomenon between serum (above) and sediment (below) may also be seen. In cases of chronic hemarthrosis, hemosiderin deposition within the synovial membrane leads to regions of low signal intensity on both T1- and T2-weighted spin echo MR images and, especially, on gradient echo images (Fig. 59–74).

The identification of lipohemarthrosis is a reliable (but not certain) sign that a fracture has occurred. The amount of fat in synovial fluid is directly proportional to the severity of the joint injury. Detection of lipohemarthrosis can be accomplished with several different imaging methods (Fig. 59–75). Routine radiographic examination using the horizontal beam technique allows the demonstration of a fat-blood fluid level after injury to the joint. Transaxial images provided by CT also demonstrate lipohemarthrosis as a fat-blood fluid level. This technique appears to be more sensitive than routine radiography, but MR imaging is probably the most sensitive method for the detection of lipohemarthrosis.

## Synovitis

Differentiating synovial inflammatory tissue and joint fluid is important to physicians treating patients with rheumatoid arthritis and related disorders. With most imaging methods, including routine radiography and CT, such differentiation is not possible. MR imaging holds promise in this area, however (Fig. 59–76).

Intravenous administration of a gadolinium compound allows one to make the distinction between effusion and abnormal synovium, with the effusion remaining of low signal intensity and the synovium demonstrating enhancement and increased signal intensity on T1-weighted spin echo MR images immediately after injection. Standard spin echo MR images (i.e., those obtained without the intravenous administration of gadolinium compounds) can be used for the same purpose, with thickened synovium demonstrating intermediate signal intensity on T1-weighted spin echo MR images (versus the lower signal intensity of joint effusion) and intermediate signal intensity on T2-weighted spin echo MR images (versus the high signal intensity of joint effusion).

## Synovial Plicae

Synovial plicae are remnants of synovial tissue that, in early development, originally divided the joint into three separate compartments; they are normally found in adult knees. Arthrographic evaluation is covered in Chapter 5. The three most commonly encountered plicae are classified according to the partitions from which they took origin: suprapatellar, medial patellar, and infrapatellar

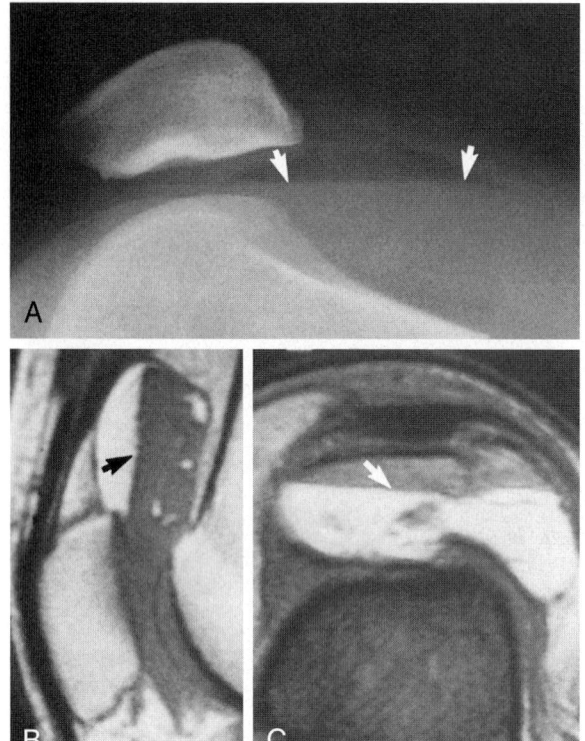

**Figure 59–75.** Lipohemarthrosis. *A*, Routine radiography. In a patient with a tibial plateau fracture, a cross-table radiograph (obtained with horizontal beam technique) shows a fluid level *(arrows)* between fat above and blood below. *B* and *C*, MR imaging. In a patient with an avulsion at the tibial site of attachment of the anterior cruciate ligament, a sagittal T1-weighted (TR/TE, 886/15) spin echo MR image *(B)* and a transaxial MPGR (TR/TE, 424/18; flip angle, 20 degrees) MR image *(C)* show a fluid level *(arrows)*, indicative of a lipohemarthrosis. In *B*, the upper layer, representing fat, is of high signal intensity; the lower layer, representing blood, is of low signal intensity, although it contains regions of high signal intensity indicative of fat. In *C*, the upper layer is of intermediate signal intensity, again representing fat, and the lower layer is of high signal intensity and contains regions of intermediate signal intensity representing fat.

(Fig. 59–77). Of these, infrapatellar plica is most frequent (found in approximately 65% of knees), followed by suprapatellar plica (55% of knees) and medial plica (25% of knees).

Suprapatellar plica is best visualized on a lateral view with the knee in full extension. This position allows for complete distention of the suprapatellar pouch. The plica is seen as a thin, delicate fold obliquely crossing the suprapatellar pouch to insert near the patella. With MR imaging, it is seen more easily when fluid is present in the joint. The medial patellar plica has been referred to variously as a wedge, a band, or a shelf. This synovial remnant has its origin on the medial wall of the knee joint, near the suprapatellar plica, and courses obliquely downward relative

to the patella to insert into the synovium covering the infrapatellar fat pad. The infrapatellar plica, or ligamentum mucosum, is often fan shaped, with a narrow femoral margin in the intercondylar notch that widens as it descends through the inferior joint space to attach distally to the inferior and medial aspects of the patellar articular cartilage. It is also demonstrable on MR images, especially in the sagittal plane (Fig. 59–78).

Symptomatic plicae are most commonly encountered in what has been referred to as the plica syndrome. Most asymptomatic plicae are 1 to 2 mm thick, and most symptomatic plicae are greater than 2 mm thick and may reach 1 cm in size; however, no absolute thickness can be used to distinguish between them (Fig. 59–79).

## Periarticular Synovial and Ganglion Cyst

Minor variations in histologic features and inconsistencies in terminology have led to great confusion regarding the classification of synovial cysts and other periarticular fluid collections. As classically described, synovial cysts about the knee are most frequent in the popliteal region, where communication between the joint and normal posterior bursae can be identified. The most commonly involved bursa is the gastrocnemiosemimembranosus bursa. Swelling of this posterior bursa is termed a Baker's cyst.

MR imaging is effective in the demonstration of intact as well as ruptured popliteal cysts. The typical appearance of a popliteal cyst is a well-defined mass of variable size with the signal intensity characteristics of fluid located between the tendons of the medial head of the gastrocnemius muscle and the semimembranosus muscle (Fig. 59–80). Changes in these signal intensity characteristics may indicate hemorrhage or intrabursal osteocartilaginous bodies. The relationship of the cyst to nearby arteries and veins and documentation of cyst rupture are easily accomplished with MR imaging.

Ganglion cysts classically contain a jelly-like viscous fluid, are loculated or septated, may arise within muscle bundles or be attached to a tendon sheath, and may (but typically do not) communicate with a joint. Those occurring about the knee are usually located close to the proximal tibiofibular joint and fibular head (Fig. 59–81), where they may lead to compression of the common peroneal nerve. As in other sites, ganglion cysts near the pes anserinus tendons can be diagnosed with ultrasonography, cystography, CT, or MR imaging. Usually, but not invariably, the signal intensity characteristics of the lesion on various MR imaging sequences are those of fluid.

### Intra-articular Ganglion Cyst

Ganglion cysts arising within the knee joint are encountered infrequently. These cysts arise most typically at two specific sites: the alar folds that cover the infrapatellar fat body, and the cruciate ligaments. These cysts may manifest as knee pain similar to that of a torn meniscus, joint fullness, or an effusion. They are generally seen as well-defined, smooth masses, and with MR imaging, the signal intensity abnormalities of the lesions are those of fluid (Fig. 59–82).

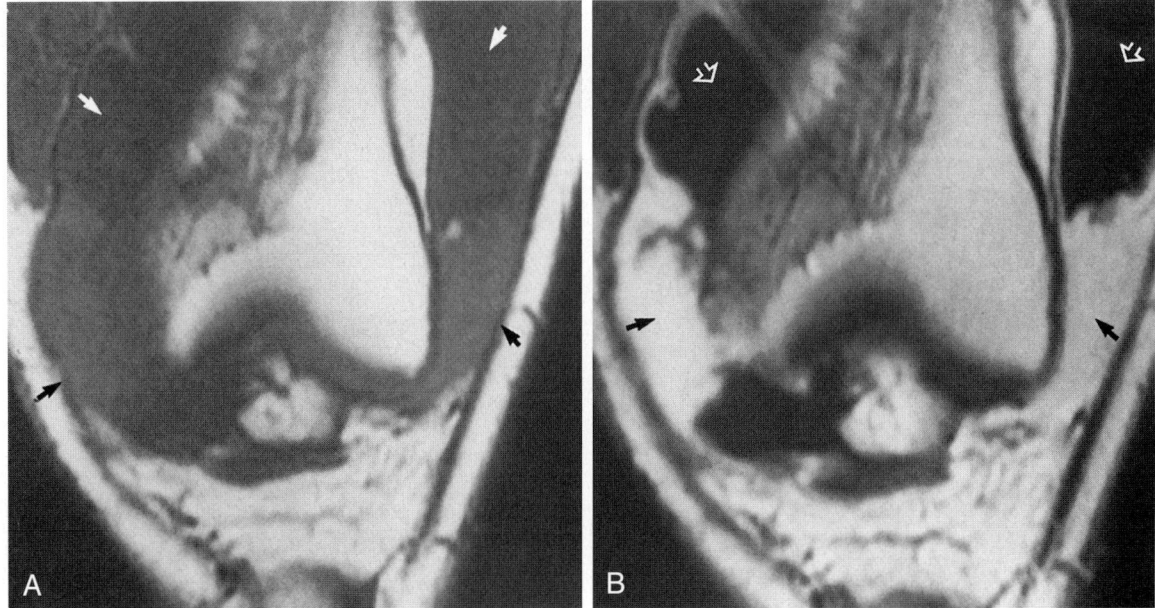

**Figure 59–76.** Synovitis: MR imaging with and without intravenous gadolinium administration in a patient with rheumatoid arthritis. *A,* Coronal T1-weighted (TR/TE, 600/20) spin echo MR image shows distention of the knee with fluid or pannus of inhomogeneous low signal intensity *(arrows)*. *B,* Identical T1-weighted (TR/TE, 600/20) spin echo MR image obtained immediately after the intravenous administration of a gadolinium compound reveals pannus of high signal intensity *(solid arrows)* and joint fluid of low signal intensity *(open arrows)*. (Courtesy of S. K. Brahme, MD, La Jolla, Calif.)

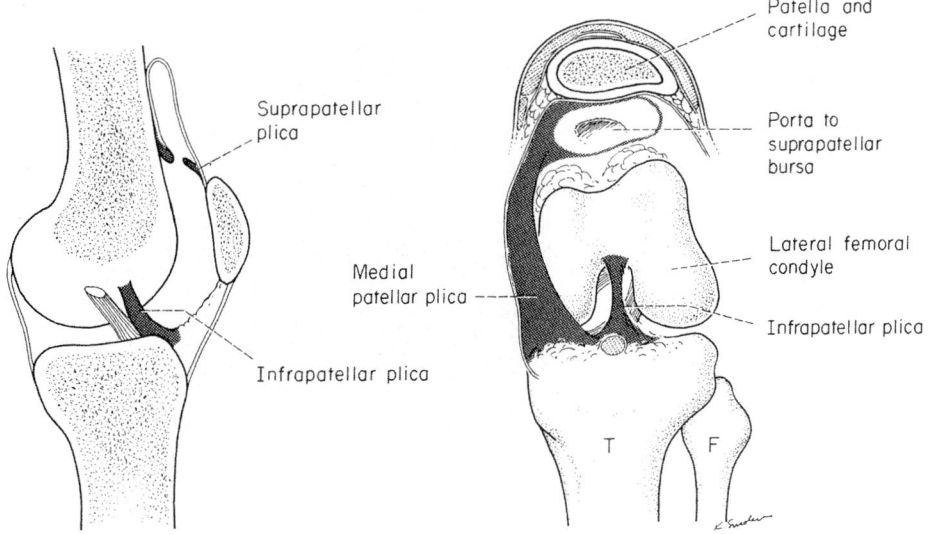

Suprapatellar plica

Infrapatellar plica

Patella and cartilage

Porta to suprapatellar bursa

Medial patellar plica

Lateral femoral condyle

Infrapatellar plica

T    F

**Figure 59–77.** Synovial plicae: classification. Schematic drawing depicts the three most commonly encountered synovial plicae. T, tibia; F, fibula. (From Deutsch AL, Resnick D, Dalinka MK, et al: Synovial plicae of the knee. Radiology 141:627, 1981.)

## Tumors and Tumor-Like Lesions

A number of tumors and tumor-like lesions may arise from the synovium or capsule of the knee joint or nearby intra-articular tissue. These lesions include pigmented villonodular synovitis and localized nodular synovitis, idiopathic synovial (osteo)chondromatosis, synovial hemangioma, intracapsular and capsular chondroma, synovial chondrosarcoma, synovial lipoma, and lipoma arborescens (all covered in Chapter 71).

## Meniscal Abnormalities

**Anatomic Considerations.** The menisci of the knee are composed of fibrocartilage and are located between the articular surfaces of the condyles of the femur and the tibial plateaus (Fig. 59–83). The lateral meniscus appears as a circular structure and, when compared with the medial meniscus, covers more of the articular surface of the tibia. Its width is relatively constant from its anterior to posterior portions. The lateral meniscus has a loose

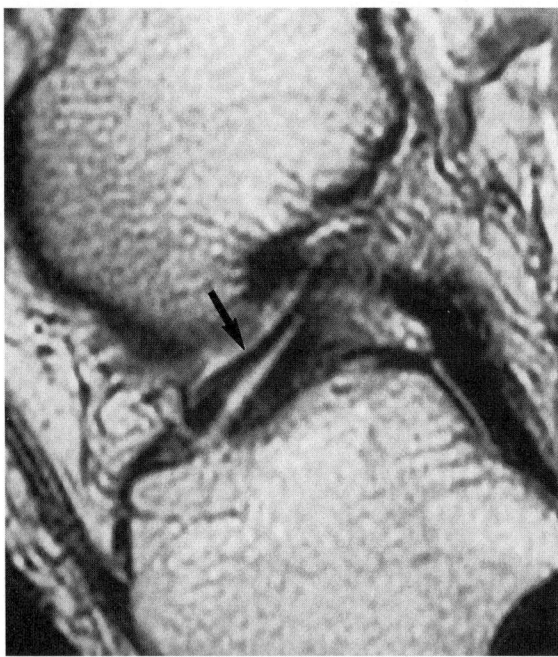

**Figure 59–78.** Synovial plica: infrapatellar. Sagittal T2-weighted (TR/TE, 2000/102) spin echo MR image reveals an infrapatellar plica *(arrow)* in front of the anterior cruciate ligament. (Courtesy of A. D'Abreu, MD, Porto Alegre, Brazil.)

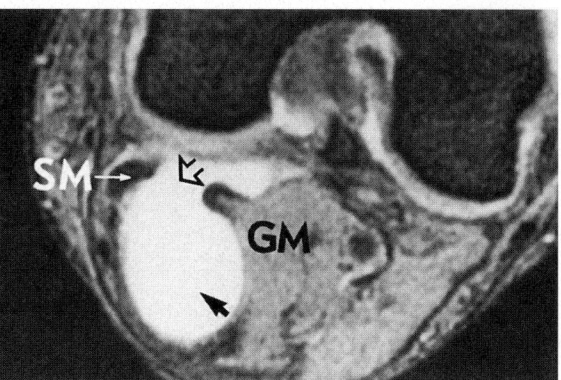

**Figure 59–80.** Synovial cyst. Transaxial MPGR (TR/TE, 500/11; flip angle, 15 degrees) MR image shows the channel *(open arrow)* and the synovial cyst *(solid arrow)* located between the semimembranosus tendon (SM) and the medial head of the gastrocnemius muscle and its tendon (GM). (Courtesy of S. K. Brahme, MD, La Jolla, Calif.)

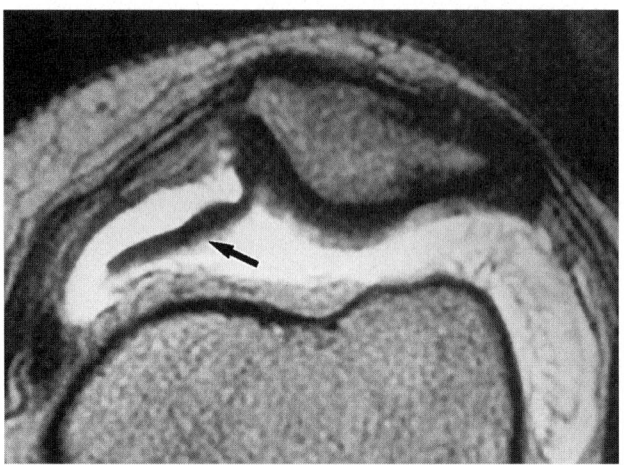

**Figure 59–79.** Synovial plica: plica syndrome. Transverse T2-weighted (TR/TE, 2000/102) spin echo MR image reveals a markedly thickened medial plica *(arrow)* and diffuse abnormality of the patellar cartilage.

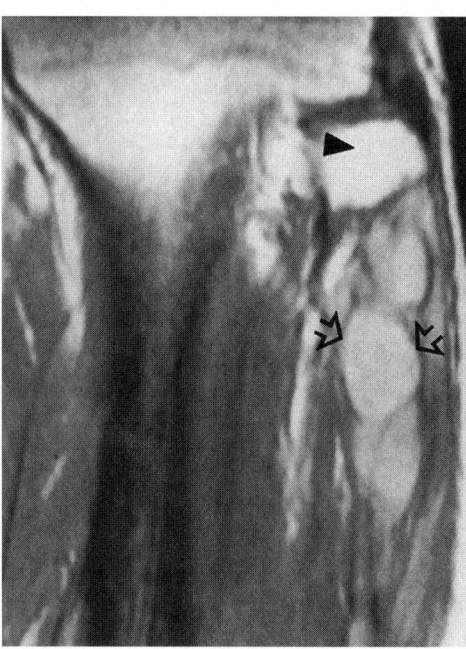

**Figure 59–81.** Periarticular ganglion cyst. Coronal intermediate-weighted (TR/TE, 2000/35) spin echo MR image shows a septated ganglion cyst *(open arrows)* containing fluid of intermediate signal intensity located adjacent to the fibular head *(arrowhead)*. (Courtesy of T. Broderick, MD, Orange, Calif.)

peripheral attachment and, posteriorly, is separated from the capsule by the popliteus tendon and its sheath. The shape of the medial meniscus is semicircular, and its width is greater posteriorly than anteriorly. The width of its central portion is variable. Peripherally, the medial meniscus is firmly attached to the joint capsule, particularly in its midportion, in the region of the medial (tibial) collateral ligament. The tibial attachment of the meniscus is often referred to as the coronary ligament.

The posterior horn of the medial meniscus inserts directly anterior to the tibial insertion of the posterior cruciate ligament, and the insertion site of the anterior horn of the lateral meniscus is adjacent to the tibial insertion of the anterior cruciate ligament. Some of the tibia-inserting fibers of the anterior cruciate ligament are intimate with the insertion site of the anterior horn of the medial meniscus.

The meniscofemoral ligaments are accessory ligaments of the knee that extend from the posterior horn of the

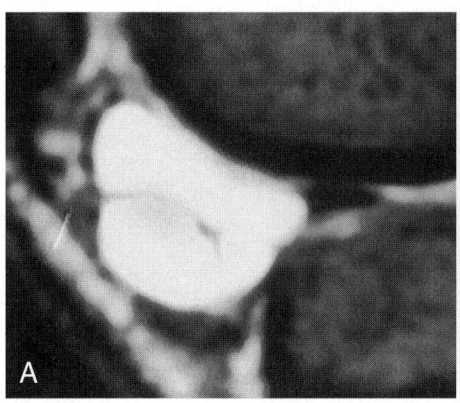 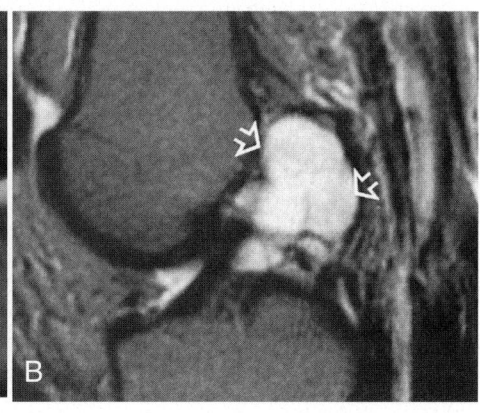

**Figure 59–82.** Intra-articular ganglion cyst. *A*, Alar folds. Sagittal MPGR (TR/TE, 550/25; flip angle, 25 degrees) MR image shows a septated ganglion cyst located anteriorly and extending into the infrapatellar fat body. *B*, Posterior cruciate ligament. Sagittal T2-weighted (TR/TE, 2000/80) spin echo MR image shows a large ganglion cyst *(open arrows)* that arose from the posterior cruciate ligament. (*A*, Courtesy of J. Schils, MD, Cleveland, Ohio.)

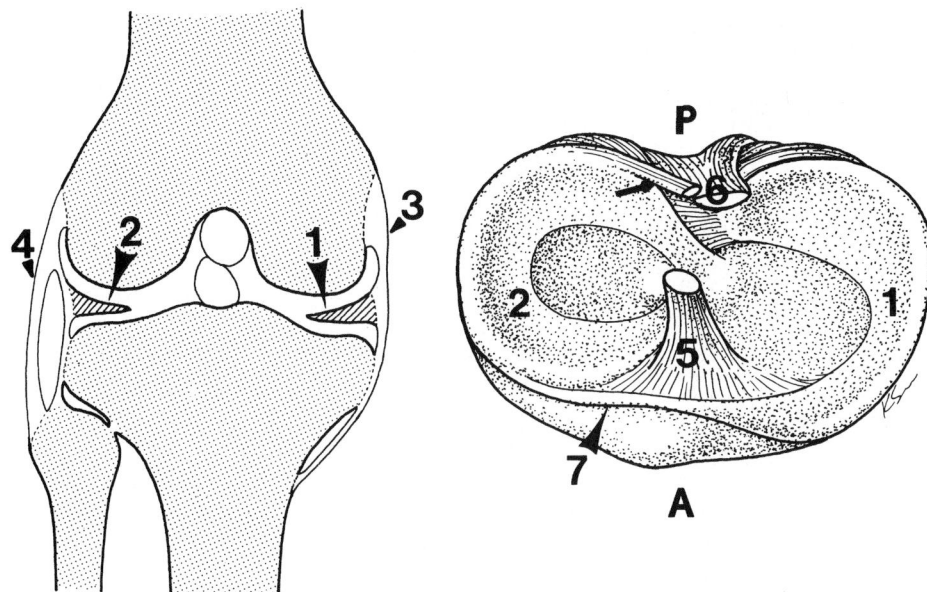

**Figure 59–83.** Menisci of the knee: normal anatomy. Coronal section *(left)* and view of the upper portion of the tibia *(right)*. Visualized structures are the medial meniscus (1), lateral meniscus (2), medial collateral ligament (3), fibular collateral ligament (4), anterior cruciate ligament (5), posterior cruciate ligament (6), transverse ligament of the knee (7), and meniscofemoral ligament of Wrisberg *(arrow)*. Observe the relatively large posterior horn of the medial meniscus and its firm attachment to the medial collateral ligament and the more circular configuration of the lateral meniscus with its relatively uniform size. A, anterior; P, posterior.

lateral meniscus to the lateral aspect of the medial femoral condyle. As they extend across the knee, they are intimate with portions of the posterior cruciate ligament. The anterior meniscofemoral ligament, or Humphry's ligament, passes in front of the posterior cruciate ligament, whereas the posterior meniscofemoral ligament, or Wrisberg's ligament, passes behind the posterior cruciate ligament. The reported incidence of one of the two meniscofemoral ligaments occurring in a single knee is 70% to 100%, and the reported incidence of both ligaments occurring in a single knee is 6% to 80%.

## Meniscal Tear

Two categories of meniscal tears are commonly identified: traumatic and degenerative. Traumatic tears are believed to result from excessive application of force to a normal meniscus; they are usually vertical tears that propagate in a longitudinal direction. Less commonly, longitudinal horizontal or oblique tears may result from this mechanism of injury. Displacement of these latter tears may result in flaps of meniscal tissue (i.e., flap tears). Degenerative tears are believed to result from normal forces acting on a degenerated structure. They are typically horizontal cleavage lesions that occupy the posterior half of the menisci. In young persons, especially athletes, a single traumatic episode is responsible for most meniscal lesions. Degenerative tears occur more commonly in older persons and in association with osteoarthritis of the knee.

No classification system for meniscal tears has been uniformly accepted. Most classification systems emphasize the direction of the tear, describing tears as longitudinal, radial, vertical, or horizontal (or combinations of these) and as complete, incomplete, or complex. With most (but not all) types of tears, the medial meniscus is involved more frequently than the lateral meniscus, and the posterior horn of the medial meniscus and the anterior horn of the lateral meniscus are most commonly affected.

Longitudinal tears are the most common type encountered. Such tears may occur in a vertical direction and divide the meniscus into inner and outer segments, or they may occur in a horizontal direction and divide the meniscus into an upper and lower segment resembling a fish mouth. Vertical longitudinal tears are more common in the medial meniscus than in the lateral meniscus (approximately 3:1). When a large part of the meniscus is affected, the tear is often regarded as unstable and the inner fragment may be displaced into the central part of the joint, a phenomenon termed a bucket-handle tear. Horizontal longitudinal tears are the cleavage lesions common in older persons and in degenerated menisci. A radial tear is a special type of vertical tear that involves the inner margin of the meniscus (Fig. 59–84). Parrot-beak tears generally represent displaced radial tears. Although it would be optimal to differentiate among these various types of tears on the basis of imaging abnormalities, such differentiation may not be possible, and many tears are complex in nature and demonstrate features of more than one type of lesion. Localization of a tear to the peripheral portion of the meniscus has therapeutic importance because of the possibility of spontaneous healing of this tear (see later discussion). Tears in this region may appear hemorrhagic on gross inspection, related to the prominent vascular supply to the peripheral portion of the meniscus.

### Clinical Abnormalities

A history of pain and a slowly developing joint effusion are helpful clues, but neither finding is diagnostic of a meniscal tear. With a bucket-handle tear of the meniscus, the patient may report locking of the knee. Pain and tenderness on palpation of the meniscal margin near the site of the tear may be elicited. A positive McMurray's test, characterized by an audible snap or pop as an abnormal meniscus extends over a bony protuberance, lends support to the clinical diagnosis of a meniscal tear.

### Magnetic Resonance Imaging

Spin echo MR imaging is the most commonly used method for assessing disorders of the knee, including those of the menisci. No agreement has been reached regarding the type of spin echo sequences that should be used in the coronal and sagittal planes. Typically, in one of these planes (usually the sagittal), intermediate- and T2-weighted spin echo MR images are acquired, and in the other plane (usually the coronal), T1-weighted spin echo MR images are obtained. Two aspects of the MR imaging appearance of normal menisci relate to their morphology and internal signal intensity.

**Morphology.** The normal morphology of a meniscus is characterized by a triangular shape and a sharp central tip. This appearance is apparent in both the coronal and sagittal planes (Fig. 59–85). In the sagittal plane, in peripheral sections, the anterior and posterior horns of the menisci unite and form a structure shaped like a bow tie. In central sections, the menisci normally have a rhomboid shape. In the coronal plane, far posterior sections show the menisci as broad and elongated structures extending far into the central portion of the joint.

Although classic morphologic changes (e.g., blunting of the tip, displacement of a portion, interrupted appearance, and abnormal size of a segment) occur in the presence

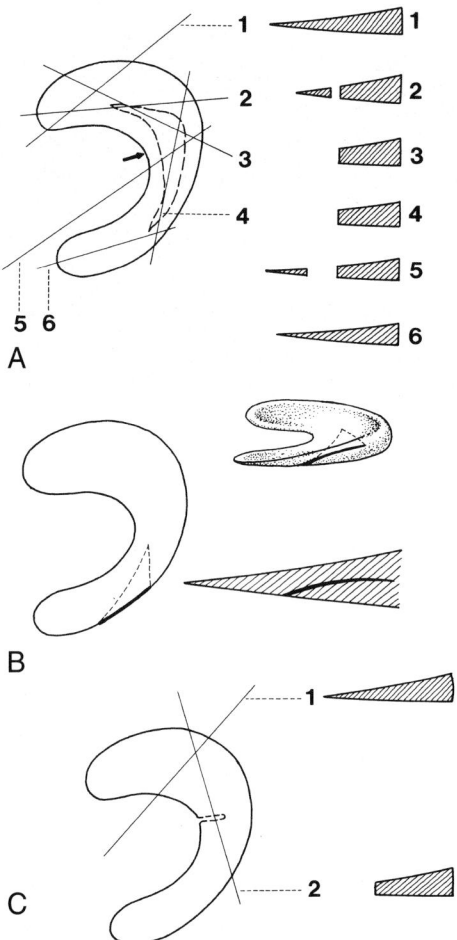

**Figure 59–84.** Meniscal tears: classification. *A*, Longitudinal vertical tears (with displacement). The medial meniscus is viewed from above, with the posterior horn located superiorly. In a longitudinal vertical tear, the inner fragment may be displaced centrally *(arrow)*. The arthrographic appearance, as well as the appearance on radial sections obtained with MR imaging, depends on the specific site of the tear. A view of the posterior aspect of the meniscus (1) is normal. Slightly more anteriorly (2), a vertical tear is apparent, with minimal displacement of the fragment. At positions 3 and 4, an amputated meniscal shadow is apparent. At position 5, significant displacement of the inner fragment is observed. The anterior horn of the meniscus (6) appears normal. *B*, Longitudinal horizontal tears. The medial meniscus is viewed from above *(left)*, in front *(top right)*, and in longitudinal section *(bottom right)*. The extent and appearance of the tear can be appreciated. *C*, Radial tear. The medial meniscus is viewed from above, with its posterior horn located superiorly. A radial tear is evident on the inner contour of the meniscus. Some arthrographic or MR imaging views (with radial sections) appear normal (1), whereas others passing through the tear (2) reveal a blunted, contrast-coated inner meniscal shadow.

of a meniscal tear, certain normal variations in the morphology of the menisci can lead to diagnostic difficulty, including the following:

1. *Anterior transverse meniscal ligament of the knee.* This ligament extends between the convex portions of the anterior horns of the medial and lateral menisci. It is usually identified on sagittal MR images of the knee,

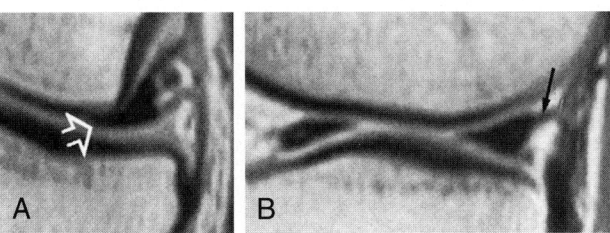

**Figure 59–85.** Lateral meniscus of the knee: normal appearance. *A,* On a coronal intermediate-weighted (TR/TE, 2000/20) spin echo MR image, note the normal lateral meniscus *(open arrow).* It is of uniform low signal intensity. *B,* Sagittal intermediate-weighted (TR/TE, 2000/30) spin echo MR image reveals the anterior and posterior horns of the lateral meniscus. The lateral meniscus is of low signal intensity, and its morphology is normal. Note the superior fascicle *(arrow)* of the lateral meniscus.

and its course can be traced on sequential sagittal MR images of the central portion of the knee (Fig. 59–86).

2. *Popliteus tendon.* The popliteus tendon and its synovial sheath course between the posterior horn of the lateral meniscus and the joint capsule. An area of intermediate signal intensity between the posterior horn of the lateral meniscus and the popliteus tendon on sagittal MR images may be misinterpreted as evidence of a tear (see Fig. 59–86).

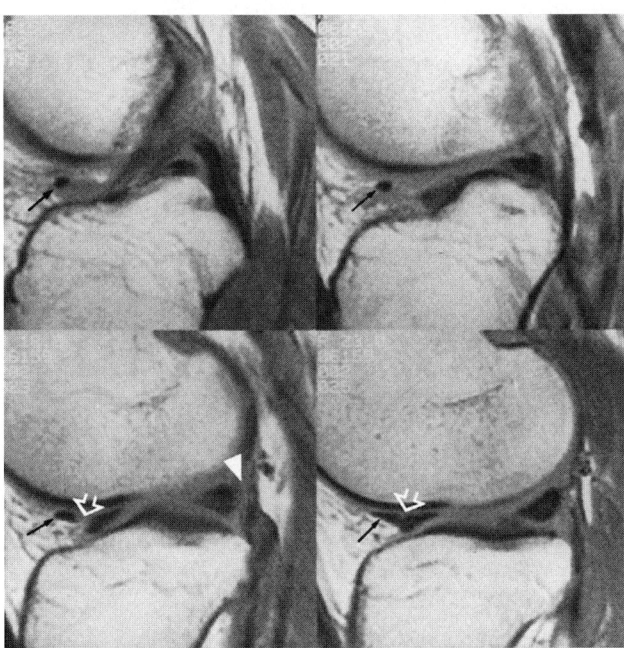

**Figure 59–86.** Pseudotears of the menisci: transverse ligament of the knee and popliteus tendon. Four sagittal intermediate-weighted (TR/TE, 2000/20) spin echo MR images show the course of the transverse ligament of the knee *(solid arrows)* from its most central position *(top left)* to its most lateral position *(bottom right).* As it approaches the anterior horn of the lateral meniscus, a space of intermediate signal intensity *(open arrows)* between it and the meniscus may be misinterpreted as evidence of a meniscal tear. Posteriorly, the popliteus tendon *(arrowhead)* separates the posterior horn of the lateral meniscus and the joint capsule. This region may also be misinterpreted as evidence of a meniscal tear.

3. *Meniscofemoral ligaments.* The meniscofemoral ligaments extend from the posterior horn of the lateral meniscus to the medial condyle of the femur. The relatively high signal intensity of the loose connective tissue between either of these ligaments and the most medial part of the posterior horn of the lateral meniscus may be misinterpreted as evidence of a meniscal tear (Fig. 59–87).

**Internal Signal Intensity.** Although the menisci are commonly described as structures of uniformly low signal intensity, this description is misleading and inaccurate. Regions of intermediate signal intensity are frequently encountered within the menisci of asymptomatic persons. Such regions are also observed in asymptomatic children, perhaps related to normal vascularity of the meniscus, and they predominate in the posterior horn of the medial meniscus.

Three patterns of intrameniscal signal intensity are recognized, as illustrated in Figure 59–88. Correlation

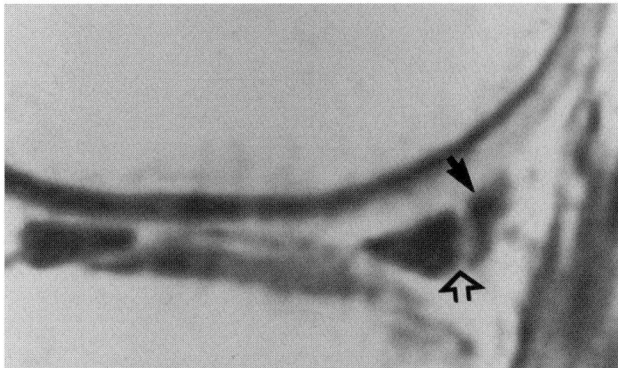

**Figure 59–87.** Pseudotears of the menisci: anterior meniscofemoral ligament (Humphry's ligament). Sagittal intermediate-weighted (TR/TE, 2300/30) spin echo MR image photographed with meniscal windowing reveals the course of the anterior meniscofemoral ligament. Note the ligament *(solid arrow)* adjacent to the posterior horn of the lateral meniscus; the space *(open arrow)* between them may be misinterpreted as evidence of a meniscal tear.

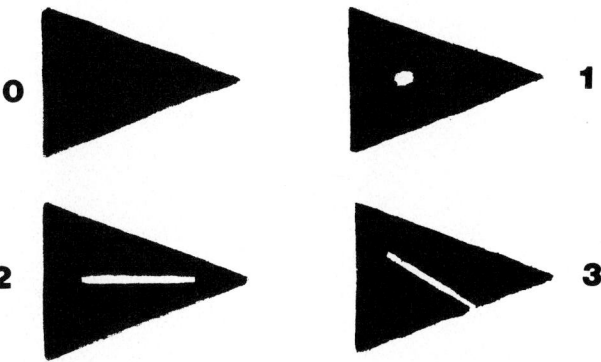

**Figure 59–88.** Grades of intrameniscal signal intensity. The meniscus may appear to be of uniform low signal intensity (grade 0), it may contain one or several circular foci of intermediate signal intensity (grade 1) or a linear region of intermediate signal intensity that does not extend to an articular surface (grade 2), or it may reveal linear or irregular regions of intermediate signal intensity that extend to the articular surface (grade 3).

between grade of signal intensity and histologic findings confirms that there are increasing amounts of degenerative changes in menisci with grade 1 and 2 imaging findings and evidence of fibrocartilaginous tears in menisci with grade 3 imaging findings. Differentiation between grade 2 signal intensity that extends close to the articular surface of the meniscus and grade 3 signal intensity that violates this surface is obviously important, because the first pattern is generally regarded as evidence of degenerative changes that cannot be detected at the time of arthroscopy, and the second pattern is evidence of a meniscal tear that can be found and treated during arthroscopy.

In clinical practice, caution is required to avoid "overcalling" the extent of intrameniscal signal intensity. Studies have shown that a meniscal tear is unlikely when the focus of altered intrameniscal signal intensity does not unequivocally involve the meniscal surface. Similarly, the presence of regions of intermediate signal intensity within the meniscus that contact its surface on only one image should be regarded as a possible tear rather than a definite tear.

Although most patients with altered signal intensity that does not extend to the meniscal surface do not have a torn meniscus, two exceptions deserve emphasis. First, prominent areas of intermediate signal intensity confined to the substance of a discoid meniscus may indicate extensive cavitation of that meniscus, which is often regarded as evidence of an intrameniscal tear at the time of arthroscopy (see later discussion). Second, the presence of extensive intermediate signal intensity confined to the substance of a meniscus, when combined with a meniscal cyst, is often indicative of a meniscal tear.

**Diagnostic Criteria.** The two MR imaging criteria for diagnosis of a meniscal tear are intrameniscal signal intensity that extends to a meniscal surface and abnormal meniscal morphology (Fig. 59–89). The sagittal plane and T1- and intermediate-weighted spin echo MR images are more valuable in this regard than are the coronal and transaxial

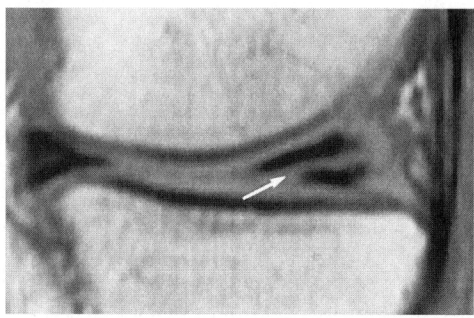

**Figure 59–89.** Meniscal tear: abnormal intrameniscal signal intensity and meniscal morphology. On a sagittal intermediate-weighted (TR/TE, 2000/20) spin echo MR image of the posterior horn of the medial meniscus, a grade 3 pattern of intrameniscal signal intensity (*arrow*) and altered meniscal morphology are evident.

planes and T2-weighted spin echo MR images. Although some meniscal tears fill with fluid and appear as regions of high signal intensity on T2-weighted spin echo images, most do not. When fluid is observed within a meniscal tear and leads to high signal intensity on such images, an unstable meniscal tear is often present.

Alterations in the morphology of torn menisci take several forms. The inner portion of the meniscus may appear blunted on coronal or sagittal MR images. The meniscus may have a normal triangular shape but appear too small. Diagnosis of tears of the free edge of the meniscus often requires careful analysis of both sagittal and coronal MR images so that subtle blunting or poor definition of the involved portion of the meniscus is recognized. An abrupt change in contour or a focal deformity of the meniscus (Fig. 59–90), designated the notch sign, is an important indicator of a meniscal tear, but it can be simulated by the normal meniscal flounce.

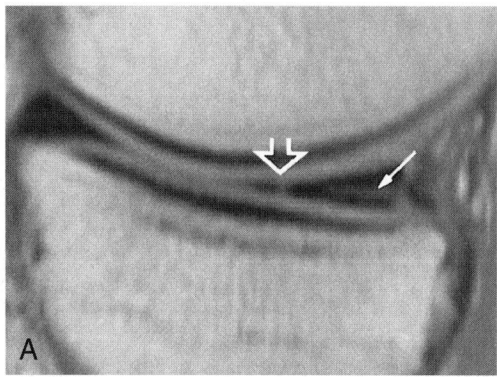
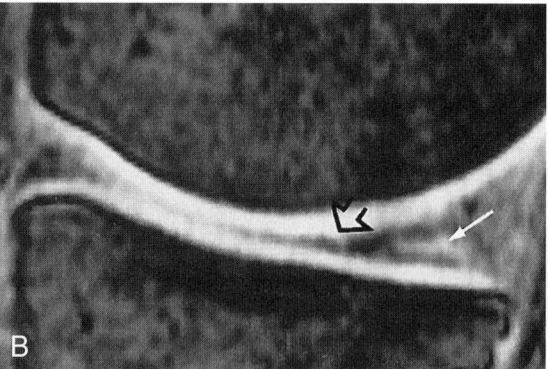

**Figure 59–90.** Meniscal tear: abnormal intrameniscal signal intensity and meniscal morphology—posterior horn of the medial meniscus. Sagittal intermediate-weighted (TR/TE, 2200/20) spin echo MR image (*A*) and sagittal three-dimensional Fourier transform SPGR (TR/TE, 58/10; flip angle, 60 degrees) MR image obtained with fat suppression (*B*) show altered intrameniscal signal intensity (*solid arrows*), with a further increase in signal intensity in (*B*) and an irregular notch (*open arrows*) in the superior surface of the meniscus.

Radial tears of the menisci may be difficult to recognize. Such tears are oriented perpendicular to the long circumferential axis of the meniscus, may be full thickness (extending from the apex to the peripheral portion of the meniscus) or partial thickness, and may be straight (true radial tear) or obliquely oriented (parrot-beak tear). The MR imaging findings vary according to the specific type of tear present, but such findings include complete absence of visualization of the meniscus on at least one image and blunting of the apex of the meniscus (Fig. 59–91).

Displaced meniscal tears are of three classic types: bucket-handle tears (displaced longitudinal tears), parrot-beak tears (displaced radial or oblique tears), and flap tears (displaced horizontal tears). Bucket-handle tears of the meniscus (so named because of their appearance) are associated with characteristic MR imaging abnormalities; the inner displaced meniscal fragment resembles a handle, and the peripheral nondisplaced portion of the meniscus looks like a bucket. Bucket-handle tears are usually observed in the medial meniscus, and they may be associated with a history of locking of the knee joint. MR imaging findings include a foreshortened and blunted meniscus with central displacement of its inner fragment. On sagittal MR images, the displaced fragment of a bucket-handle meniscal tear often lies in front of, below, and parallel to the posterior cruciate ligament (Fig. 59–92).

### Meniscocapsular Separation

Meniscocapsular separation refers to disruption of the meniscal attachment to the joint capsule. The posterior horn of the medial meniscus is involved most frequently. The presence of fluid between the peripheral portion of the posterior horn of the medial meniscus and the joint capsule is the most important finding.

The differential diagnosis of meniscocapsular separation includes normal recesses that may appear above or below the peripheral portion of the meniscus, a large joint effusion displacing the meniscus, a longitudinal vertical tear through the periphery of the meniscus, and bursitis beneath the medial collateral ligament.

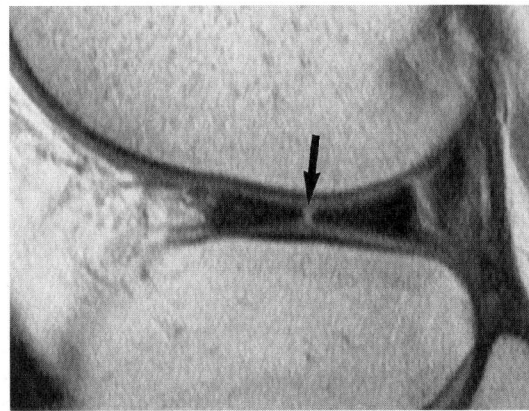

**Figure 59–91.** Meniscal tear: abnormal meniscal contour—radial tear of the body of the lateral meniscus. Note the blunted inner contour (*arrow*) of the body of the lateral meniscus on a sagittal intermediate-weighted spin echo MR image. (Courtesy of J. Edwards, MD, Savannah, Ga.)

### Meniscal Cyst

Meniscal cysts are multiloculated collections of mucinous material of unknown cause that generally occur at the periphery of the meniscus and therefore appear as a focal mass or swelling at the joint line. They are observed in approximately 1% of meniscectomies. Meniscal cysts on the lateral side of the knee are three to seven times more frequent than those on the medial side, and medial meniscal cysts tend to be larger. Most meniscal cysts are associated with myxoid degeneration and horizontal cleavage tears of the adjacent meniscus that extend into the parameniscal region. Fluid from the joint extending into a horizontal tear of the meniscus and subsequently into the cystic lesion is one explanation for their occurrence. On MR images, an ovoid mass of variable size containing fluid is seen (Fig. 59–93). Although high signal intensity of the cyst on T2-weighted spin echo MR images is typical, it is not invariable. Meniscal cysts arising from

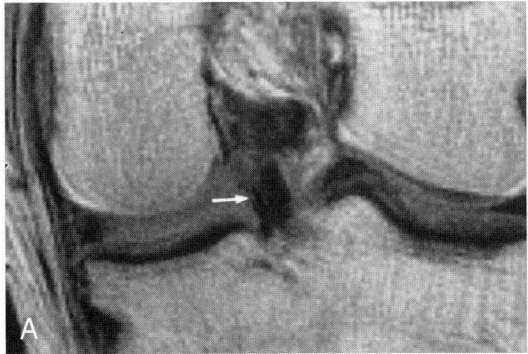 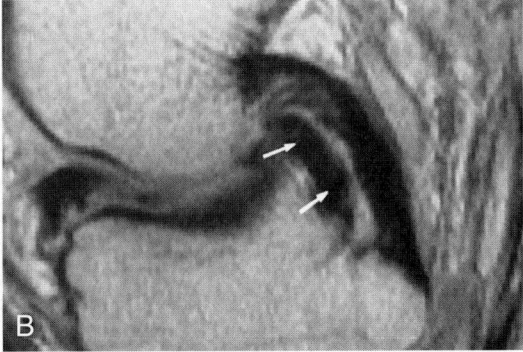

**Figure 59–92.** Meniscal tear: bucket-handle tear—medial meniscus. Coronal intermediate-weighted (TR/TE, 1750/20) (*A*) and sagittal intermediate-weighted (TR/TE, 3000/20) (*B*) spin echo MR images reveal a bucket-handle tear of the medial meniscus, with central displacement (*arrows*) of the inner portion of the meniscus. In *B*, the meniscal fragment is located in front of the posterior cruciate ligament. (Courtesy of R. Stiles, MD, Atlanta, Ga.)

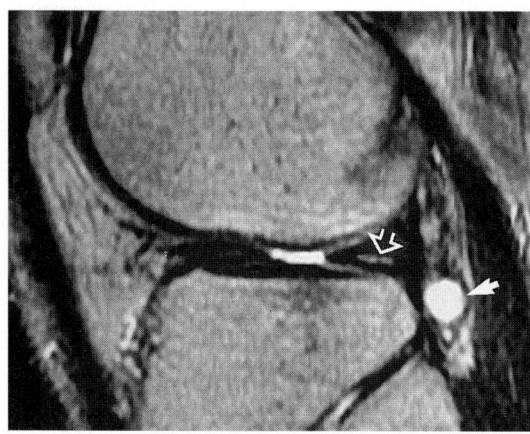

**Figure 59–93.** Meniscal cyst: lateral meniscus. Sagittal T2-weighted (TR/TE, 2200/80) spin echo MR image shows a meniscal cyst *(solid arrow)* associated with a horizontal tear of the lateral meniscus *(open arrow)*. Note that the cyst is displacing the lateral (fibular) collateral ligament.

tears of the posterior horn of the medial meniscus may extend centrally, become intimate with the posterior cruciate ligament, and simulate the appearance of a ganglion cyst of that ligament.

### Discoid Meniscus

A discoid meniscus has an altered shape with a broad and disclike appearance rather than a semilunar configuration, although intermediate varieties of discoid menisci have been described, including the slab type (flat, circular meniscus), biconcave type (biconcave disc, thinner in its central portion), wedge type (large but normally tapered meniscus), anterior type (enlarged anterior horn), ring type (oval meniscus with a hole in the middle), forme fruste (slightly enlarged meniscus), and grossly torn type (too deformed for accurate classification). A discoid lateral meniscus is much more common than a discoid medial meniscus. The reported frequency of discoid lateral menisci varies from 0% to 2.7%. The usual age of patients at the time of the initial clinical examination is between 15 and 35 years.

MR imaging has been used to confirm either an intact or a torn discoid meniscus (Fig. 59–94). Observations based on sagittal images relate to the number of consecutive scans that reveal a bow-tie appearance of the meniscus in which the anterior and posterior horns of the meniscus are still connected, or continuous. This number is directly related to the width of the meniscus; an enlarged meniscus is compatible with the diagnosis of a discoid meniscus, although no precise dimensions are available for normal menisci. The average transverse diameter of the lateral meniscus appears to be approximately 11 or 12 mm; visualization of a bow-tie appearance on three or more contiguous sagittal sections that are 5 mm thick, an abnormally thickened bow tie, or both are evidence of a discoid lateral meniscus.

### Meniscal Ossicle

Meniscal ossicles represent foci of ossification within the menisci. They should be differentiated from meniscal calcifications, which are frequent and relate to calcium pyrophosphate dihydrate crystal deposition in many cases. The origin of meniscal ossicles in humans is not known. There is an association between meniscal ossicles and longitudinal tears of the medial meniscus. Patients with knee ossicles may be asymptomatic or have local pain and swelling.

Initial films reveal ossification of variable shape in the anterior or posterior portion of either the medial or the lateral meniscus. The most common site is the posterior horn of the medial meniscus. MR imaging may also be used to diagnose or confirm a meniscal ossicle. Because the ossicle may contain bone marrow, the signal intensity characteristics of fat may be seen within the ossicle (Fig. 59–95). The ossicle may also have low signal intensity on all MR imaging sequences.

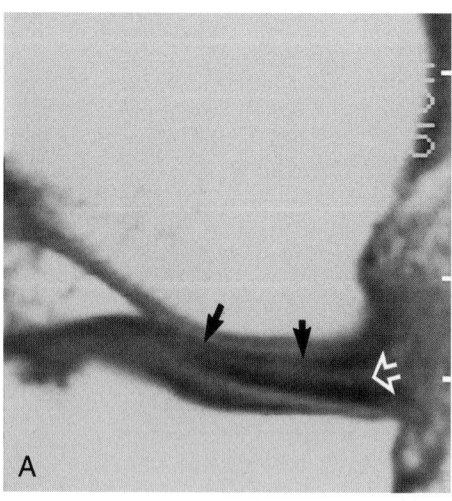

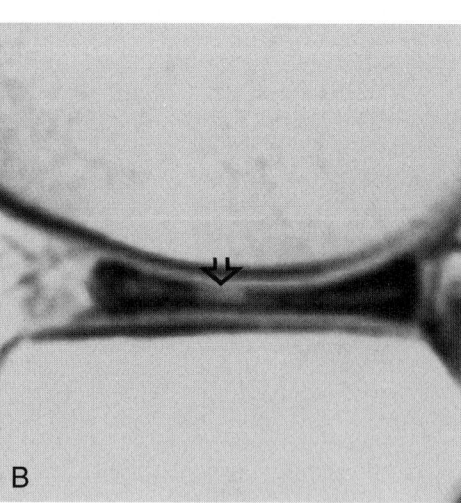

**Figure 59–94.** Discoid meniscus: lateral meniscus. Coronal T1-weighted (TR/TE, 750/20) spin echo MR image *(A)* and sagittal intermediate-weighted (TR/TE, 2300/30) spin echo MR image *(B)*, both photographed with meniscal windowing, show an enlarged meniscus *(solid arrows)* and meniscal tear *(open arrows)*. The presence of large regions of intermediate signal intensity within a discoid meniscus is generally indicative of a tear.

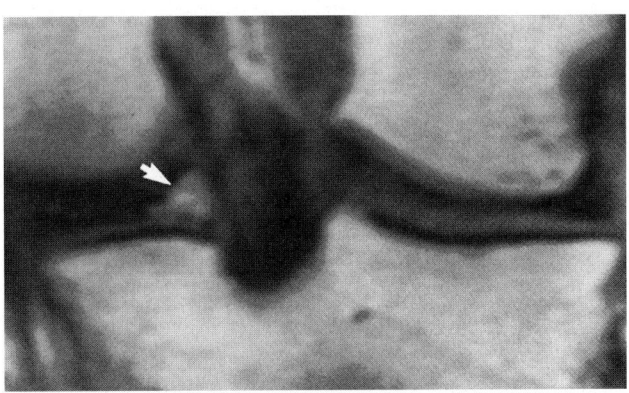

**Figure 59–95.** Meniscal ossicles. Coronal T1-weighted (TR/TE, 600/15) spin echo MR image shows an ossicle containing fat *(arrow)* within the posterior horn of the medial meniscus. (Courtesy of A. Deutsch, MD, Los Angeles, Calif.)

## Postoperative Meniscus

Significant changes in the surgical management of meniscal abnormalities in the knee are a consequence of two major factors: recognition that menisci have a weight-bearing capacity and transmit an important component of the load during daily physical activities, and the current popularity of arthroscopic surgery. The development and refinement of arthroscopic techniques have led to the choice of meniscal repair, meniscal preservation, and even meniscal transplantation rather than meniscal resection as better means of maintaining meniscal function and, ultimately, preserving the integrity of the knee joint.

Despite considerable interest in the role of MR imaging in the assessment of menisci after partial meniscectomy or meniscal repair, the value of this technique is unclear, and its diagnostic superiority over standard arthrography remains unproved. A spectrum of MR imaging findings consisting of altered intrameniscal signal intensity and contour alterations is seen after partial meniscectomy or surgical repair of a torn meniscus, and it is difficult to sort out what is clinically significant from what is not. Caution must be used in applying the classic diagnostic criteria of meniscal tears in the assessment of a postoperative meniscus.

## Abnormalities of the Medial Supporting Structures

**Anatomic Considerations.** The gross anatomy of the supporting structures on the medial side of the knee (Fig. 59–96) is often discussed in terms of layers. The most superficial of the three layers is represented by fascia that covers the quadriceps mechanism, invests the sartorius tendon, and continues on as the deep fascia of the leg. It is rarely torn with injury. The second layer is the superficial portion of the medial collateral ligament (also called the tibial collateral ligament or superficial medial ligament). The superficial portion of the medial collateral ligament is approximately 10 to 11 cm long. It is composed of two bundles of fibers, one vertical and one oblique. The bundle of oblique fibers is often designated the posterior oblique ligament. The superficial portion of the medial collateral ligament has no meniscal attachment and slides posteriorly over the proximal portion of the tibia during flexion of the knee. The third layer is the capsule of the knee joint, which attaches to the margins of the joint. The capsule is thin anteriorly and provides little stability to the joint. It holds the meniscal rim to the tibia (i.e., the coronary ligament) and, to a lesser extent, to the femur (i.e., the meniscofemoral ligament). The superficial and deep portions of the medial collateral ligament are separated by a bursa that allows movement between the two.

The medial supporting structures of the knee are injured more frequently than are the lateral supporting structures. Indeed, the medial collateral ligament is the most commonly injured ligament about the knee. Most of the major injuries to the medial capsuloligamentous complex are the result of a valgus stress. O'Donoghue's triad of injury consists of tears of the anterior cruciate ligament, medial collateral ligament, and medial meniscus.

## Medial Collateral Ligament Injuries

Tears of the medial collateral ligament may be classified as acute, subacute, or chronic, or they may be classified according to their severity, from a ligament sprain (grade I) to partial (grade II) or complete (grade III) rupture. A knee with a grade I sprain is stable on stress testing, although there is microscopic tearing of ligament fibers. With a grade II sprain, stress testing shows an unstable knee with a firm end point, and a macroscopic partial tear of the ligament is present. A knee with a grade III sprain is unstable, with a soft end point on stress testing, and is characterized by a macroscopic complete tear of the ligament.

Routine radiographic abnormalities associated with acute injuries to the medial collateral ligament of the knee include medial soft tissue swelling, with or without joint effusion; rarely, an avulsion fracture at the sites of insertion of the ligament; and evidence of associated injuries, such as fracture of the lateral tibia. Avulsion of the intercondylar eminence of the tibia indicates an accompanying injury to the anterior cruciate ligament. Widening of the medial femorotibial joint space may indicate intra-articular entrapment of a completely torn ligament. In cases of chronic injury to the medial collateral ligament, ligamentous calcification or ossification may occur (Pellegrini-Stieda syndrome). Such ossification may involve the medial collateral ligament alone, the adductor magnus tendon alone, or both structures.

The coronal plane best displays the medial collateral ligament. In the coronal plane, the superficial longitudinal fibers of the medial collateral ligament appear as a smooth structure of low signal intensity that extends from the medial epicondyle of the femur above to the proximal metaphysis of the tibia below (Fig. 59–97). In its lowest portion, the ligament may be separated from the tibial cortex by medial inferior genicular vessels. At the level of the joint line, the medial collateral ligament is separated from the periphery of the medial meniscus by a bursa and surrounding fat. The deep portion of the medial collateral ligament consists of the meniscofemoral and meniscotibial (i.e., coronary) ligaments, which can also be seen optimally on coronal images.

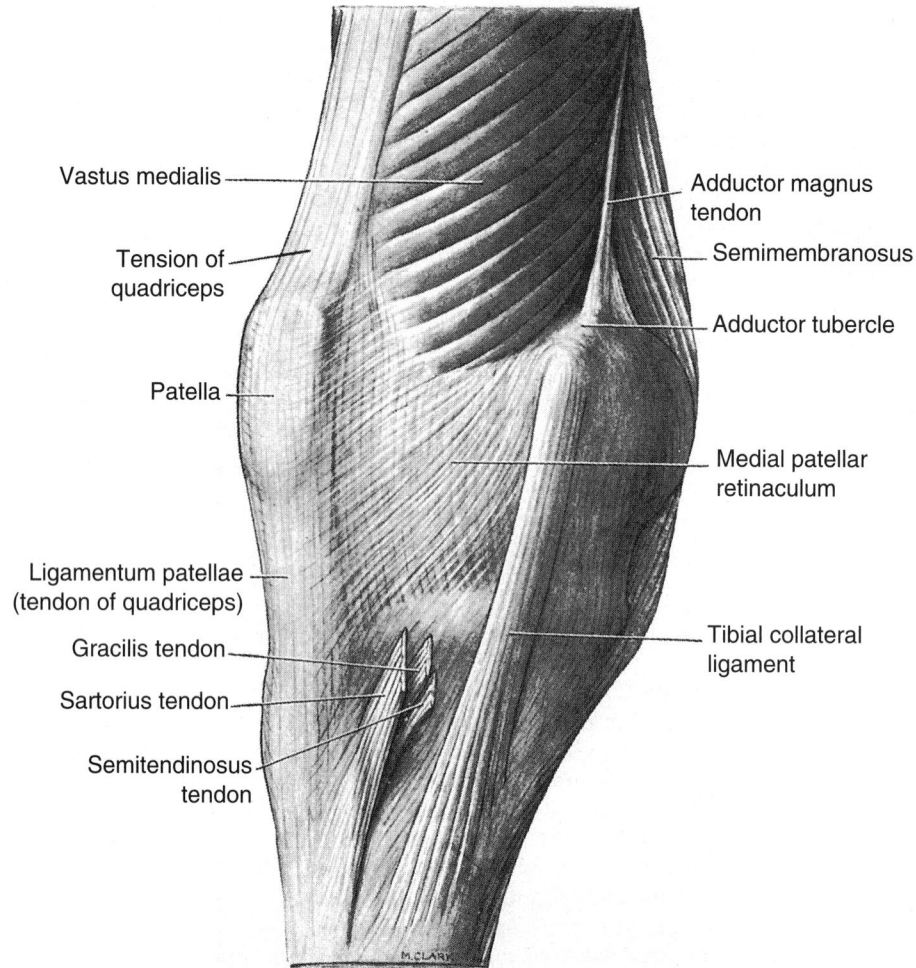

**Figure 59–96.** Medial supporting structures: anatomic considerations. (From Williams PL, Warwick R [eds]: Gray's Anatomy, 35th Br ed. Philadelphia, WB Saunders, 1973, p 453.)

Injuries to the medial collateral ligament vary in severity and include sprains, partial tears, and complete tears. The MR imaging characteristics are dependent on the severity of the injury and its acute or chronic nature. With acute injuries, subcutaneous edema or hemorrhage and, in some cases, a joint effusion are evident; with chronic injuries, such edema and hemorrhage are not apparent. Sprains of the medial collateral ligament may lead to slight contour irregularity or thickening of the ligament, but no discontinuity of its fibers. In acute sprains, subcutaneous edema is an associated finding, but the signal intensity of the ligament is usually normal. Partial tears of the medial collateral ligament lead to discontinuity of some of its fibers, which in acute injuries is associated with increased signal intensity (particularly on T2-weighted spin echo and gradient echo MR images) within the substance of the ligament and in the subcutaneous tissues. Complete tears of the medial collateral ligament are associated with frank discontinuity of all its fibers. In the acute stage, hemorrhage and edema within the ligament and subcutaneous tissues are also evident (Fig. 59–98).

### Semimembranosus Tendon Abnormalities

Many injuries to the posteromedial corner of the knee also involve other medial supporting structures, as well as the medial meniscus, and any peripheral tear of the posterior horn of the medial meniscus usually includes a tear of the posterior oblique ligament. Isolated avulsion injuries involving this corner of the knee are rare.

### Abnormalities of the Lateral Supporting Structures

**Anatomic Considerations.** As on the medial side of the knee, the anatomy of the lateral supporting structures can be considered in terms of layers (according to the depth of the tissues) or in terms of their position in an anteroposterior plane. Three layers of tissue can be defined: superficial, intermediate, and deep. The superficial layer is composed of the deep fascia of the thigh and calf, including the condensed portion known as the iliotibial tract. This tract has functionally important capsular and bone attachments that are sometimes referred to as the anterolateral ligament of the knee; some fibers of the

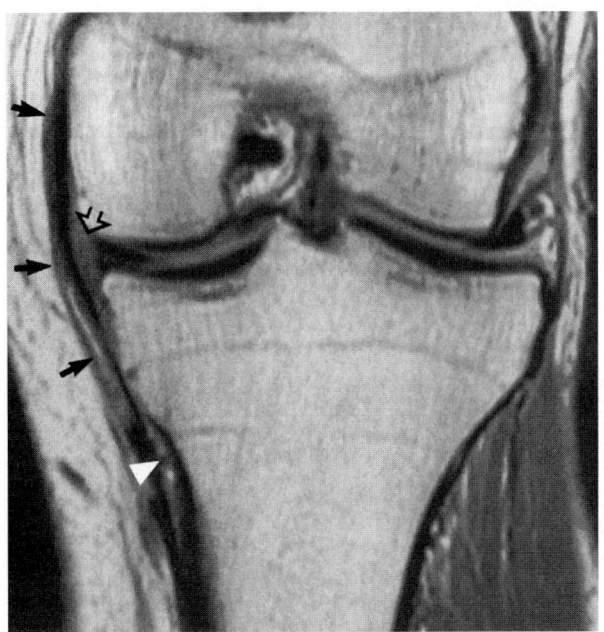

**Figure 59–97.** Medial collateral ligament: normal appearance. Coronal T1-weighted (TR/TE, 800/20) spin echo MR image shows the course of the vertical fibers of the superficial portion of the medial collateral ligament *(solid arrows)*. Note that this portion of the ligament is separated *(open arrow)* from the medial meniscus. The medial inferior genicular vessels are seen *(arrowhead)*.

the capsule of the knee joint and the lateral (fibular) collateral ligament. The lateral collateral ligament extends from the lateral epicondyle of the femur to the proximal lateral surface of the fibular head. The fibular collateral ligament is taut when the knee is extended and loose when the knee is flexed, and it serves as the primary restraint to varus stress at the knee. The popliteus muscle originates in the posterior surface of the proximal portion of the tibia, attaches to the posterior horn of the lateral meniscus and to the arcuate ligament, and terminates in the lateral femoral condyle, distal and posterior to the attachment site of the lateral collateral ligament. The anatomy of the posterolateral corner of the knee (Fig. 59–99) is complex and is not agreed on.

The lateral supporting structures restrain varus angulation at the knee and external rotation of the tibia. Injuries involving both the lateral collateral ligament and these deep posterolateral structures are associated with greater varus instability than are injuries confined to the lateral collateral ligament. Lateral instability patterns are less frequent than those on the medial side of the knee, although they may eventually be more disabling.

### Lateral Collateral Ligament Injuries

With injury to the lateral collateral ligament of the knee, routine radiography generally does not reveal specific findings. Focal soft tissue swelling may be evident in some cases. Further, because the lateral collateral ligament, along with the tendon of the biceps femoris muscle, attaches to the fibular head and styloid process, avulsion fractures of this portion of the fibula may be seen. The fragment is of variable size and may be large, although it is usually displaced only minimally. On MR imaging, the integrity of the lateral collateral ligament and the adjacent tendon of the biceps femoris muscle is well demonstrated (Fig. 59–100).

iliotibial tract are continuous with those of the vastus lateralis tendon and aponeurosis, and together they form the lateral patellar retinaculum. The second layer consists of the retinaculum of the patella and the patellofemoral ligaments. The third and deepest layer is composed of

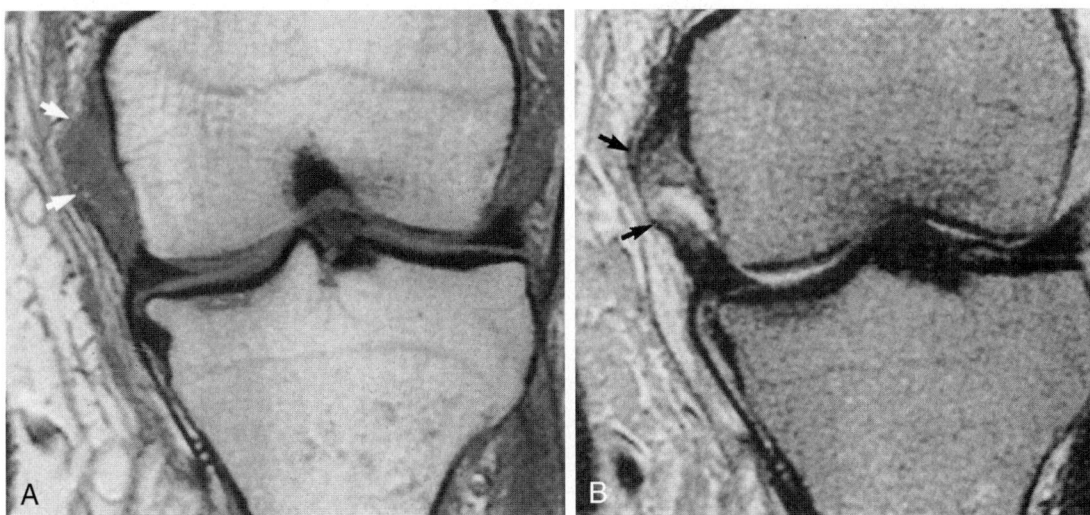

**Figure 59–98.** Injuries of the medial collateral ligament: complete tear. Coronal intermediate-weighted (TR/TE, 1500/12) *(A)* and T2-weighted (TR/TE, 1500/80) *(B)* spin echo MR images show complete disruption *(arrows)* of the fibers of the medial collateral ligament. Note the increase in signal intensity in the ligament and soft tissues in *B*. A joint effusion is present. Additional injuries in this patient included tears of the lateral meniscus and anterior cruciate ligament. (Courtesy of V. Chandnani, MD, Pittsburgh, Pa.)

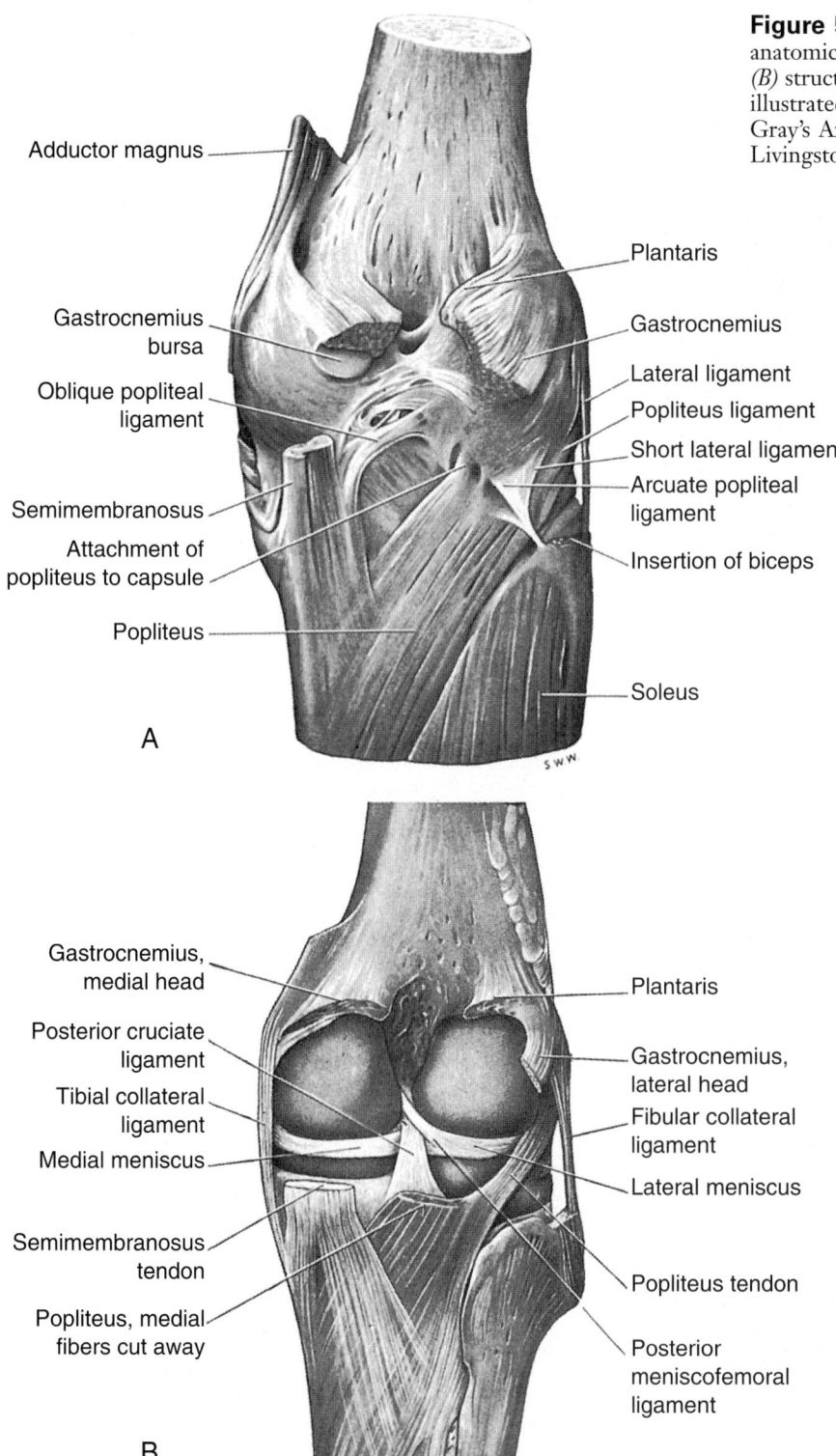

**Figure 59–99.** Posterolateral corner of the knee: anatomic considerations. Superficial *(A)* and deep *(B)* structures in the posterior aspect of the knee are illustrated. (From Williams PL, Warwick R [eds]: Gray's Anatomy, 36th Br ed. Edinburgh, Churchill Livingstone, 1980, pp 452, 453.)

These structures can be identified on sagittal, coronal, and transaxial MR images. Disruption of the lateral collateral ligament, the tendon of the biceps femoris muscle, or both is recognized on MR images as an interruption or waviness of these tendons or regions of high signal inten-sity on T2-weighted spin echo MR images within or adja-cent to these tendons (Fig. 59–101). Associated injuries to other lateral supporting structures or to the cruciate ligaments may also be evident. In dislocations of the knee, injuries to lateral, medial, and cruciate ligaments are encountered.

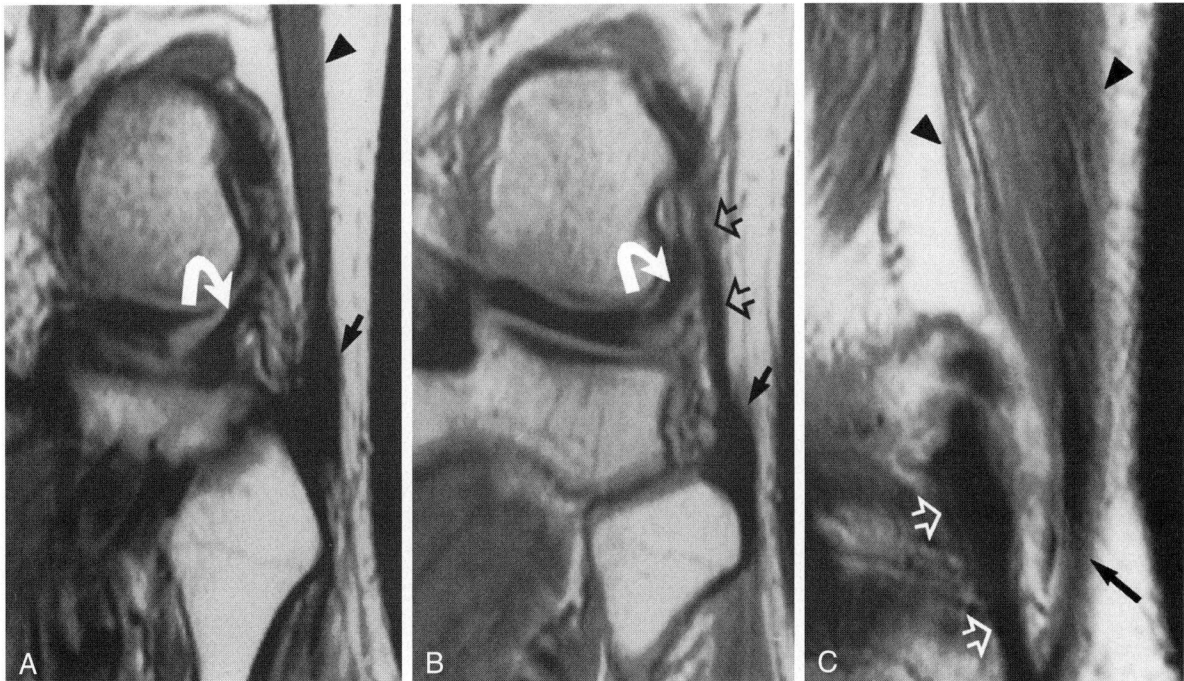

**Figure 59–100.** Lateral collateral ligament and biceps femoris muscle and tendon: normal appearanace. *A* and *B*, Two consecutive coronal intermediate-weighted (TR/TE, 2200/20) spin echo MR images show the normal biceps femoris muscle *(arrowhead)* and its tendon *(solid straight arrows)* and the normal lateral collateral ligament *(open arrows)*. In *A*, the more posterior image, the biceps femoris muscle and tendon are seen extending lateral to the joint and inserting into the proximal portion of the fibula. In *B*, the lateral collateral ligament extends from the fibula superiorly to insert into the femur. The popliteus tendon *(curved arrows)* is identified. *C*, Sagittal intermediate-weighted (TR/TE, 2200/20) spin echo MR image of the lateral aspect of the knee shows the biceps femoris muscle *(arrowheads)* and its tendon *(solid arrow)* and the lateral collateral ligament *(open arrows)*. Note the V-like pattern created at the junction of the biceps femoris tendon and lateral collateral ligament.

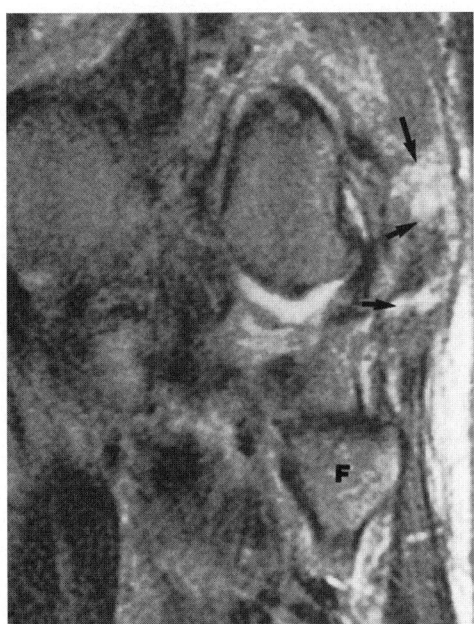

**Figure 59–101.** Injuries of the lateral collateral ligament and biceps femoris muscle and tendon. Coronal T2-weighted (TR/TE, 2500/80) spin echo MR image reveals complete disorganization in the posterolateral region of the knee. Although the fibular head (F) is seen, the tendon of the biceps femoris muscle and the lateral collateral ligament are not identifiable. A joint effusion is present. Note the high signal intensity within the biceps femoris muscle *(arrows)*. This patient also had an injury to the anterior cruciate ligament.

## Popliteus Muscle and Tendon Injuries

Injuries to the popliteus muscle and tendon may occur in association with injuries to other lateral supporting structures of the knee or, rarely, as an isolated phenomenon. Clinical findings include acute hemarthrosis, lateral tenderness, and, rarely, injury to the tibial nerve. Avulsion fracture of the femur may be seen with routine radiography, and an abnormal course or abnormal signal intensity within the popliteus tendon or hemorrhage in the popliteus muscle may be seen with MR imaging.

## Iliotibial Tract Abnormalities

Injuries to the iliotibial tract are usually combined with injuries to other lateral supporting structures of the knee. Rarely, they may occur as an isolated phenomenon. Avulsion injuries may occur at the tibial insertion site of the iliotibial tract (i.e., Gerdy's tubercle). MR imaging can be used to detect traumatic abnormalities involving this structure. A normal iliotibial tract is observed on coronal MR images as a structure of low signal intensity traversing the lateral portion of the thigh, extending across the lateral aspect of the knee, and inserting (in part) in Gerdy's tubercle in the tibia (Fig. 59–102). Discontinuity of this structure and edema in the tibia adjacent to the site of its attachment may be observed when this tract is injured.

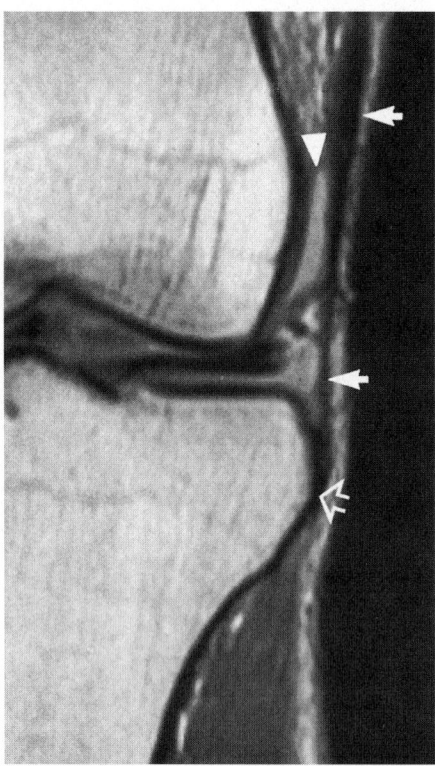

**Figure 59–102.** Iliotibial tract: normal appearance. Coronal intermediate-weighted (TR/TE, 2000/20) spin echo MR image shows the iliotibial tract (*solid arrows*) attaching to Gerdy's tubercle (*open arrow*) in the tibia. A small joint effusion is evident just medial to the iliotibial tract (*arrowhead*).

## Other Lateral Capsular and Ligament Injuries

An important injury is an avulsion fracture of the tibial rim that reportedly occurs at the site of attachment of the lateral capsular ligament of the knee. Termed a Segond fracture, this fracture results from forces of internal rotation and varus stress at the knee. The resulting bone fragment is easily overlooked unless the lateral margin of the tibia is carefully analyzed on anteroposterior and tunnel radiographic views of the knee (Fig. 59–103). An elliptically shaped piece of bone measuring up to 10 mm long occurs at the joint line or just proximal to it, and the donor site in the tibia reveals an irregular surface. The Segond fracture is highly associated with injuries to the anterior cruciate ligament (75% to 100% of cases) and tears of the menisci (60% to 70% of cases). The MR imaging findings of a Segond fracture are also characteristic. Marrow edema, though not extensive, may be evident. The fracture fragment itself is often not visible because of its small size.

## Plantaris Muscle Injuries

The plantaris muscle is thin and small and lies just deep to the lateral head of the gastrocnemius muscle in the proximal portion of the lower part of the leg. It extends obliquely downward and medially to accompany the Achilles tendon. The muscle may be absent in 7% to 10% of persons.

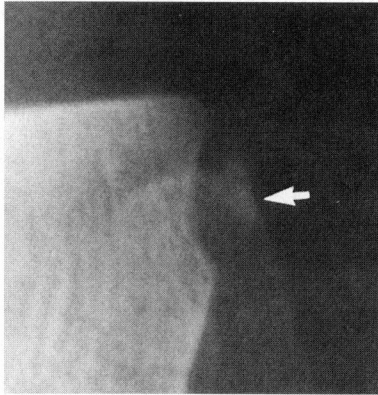

**Figure 59–103.** Injuries of the lateral capsular ligament (Segond fracture): routine radiography and MR imaging. The typical appearance of a Segond fracture fragment (*arrow*) is evident. (Courtesy of G. Bock, MD, Winnipeg, Manitoba, Canada.)

Despite its intimate relationship to the Achilles tendon, it often remains intact when the Achilles tendon ruptures. The proximal aspect of the plantaris tendon may rupture as a result of violent contracture of the muscle. This injury may represent one cause of tennis leg, and it may lead to lower leg pain, especially in athletes. MR imaging and ultrasonography may be helpful in making an accurate diagnosis.

## Abnormalities of the Anterior Supporting Structures

**Anatomic Considerations.** In the anterior aspect of the knee, ligaments, muscles, aponeuroses, and the joint capsule converge to surround the centrally located patella and provide an adequate stabilizing system. These structures lead to forces on the patella that are oriented superiorly (quadriceps muscles), inferiorly (patellar tendon), medially (medial patellar retinaculum and vastus medialis muscle), or laterally (lateral patellar retinaculum, vastus lateralis muscle, and iliotibial tract). Together, they stabilize the patella.

The major passive stabilizer of the patella is the patellar tendon extending from the inferior pole of the patella to the tibial tuberosity. The four components of the quadriceps muscle represent the active elements of the soft tissue stabilizers. These components are the rectus femoris, vastus lateralis, vastus medialis, and vastus intermedius muscles, which terminate as four tendons that merge several centimeters above the patella to form the quadriceps tendon and subsequently attach to the patella. The deep infrapatellar, or pretibial, bursa is situated at the base of the infrapatellar fat body, between the patellar tendon in front and the anterosuperior portion of the tibia behind. Prepatellar bursae are present in front of the patella itself.

Abnormalities of the anterior supporting structures of the knee are related to alterations in the anatomy of the patella and the adjacent patellar articular surface of the femur and the constantly changing compressive and tensile forces generated during complex movement of this joint. Syndromes and disorders related to disuse, overuse, misuse, or injuries to various anterior supporting structures include chondromalacia patellae, patellar tendinosis, disruption of the quadriceps musculature and tendon and the patellar tendon, osteochondritis dissecans of the patella, osteochondral fractures of the patella and femur, patellar instability with subluxation or dislocation, Osgood-Schlatter disease, and deep infrapatellar, superficial infrapatellar, and prepatellar bursitis, many of which are discussed elsewhere in this text.

## Patellar Tendinosis

Patellar tendinosis appears to be an overuse syndrome related to sudden and repetitive extension of the knee that may occur in persons, particularly athletes, involved in such activities as kicking, jumping, and running. This syndrome, often referred to as jumper's knee, leads to local pain, swelling, and tenderness that may ultimately result in disruption of the patellar tendon. The major histologic findings associated with patellar tendinosis are not those of inflammation but rather those of fiber failure, mucoid degeneration, and fibrinoid necrosis, so the term "tendinitis" is inappropriate. Clinical manifestations include activity-related pain below the patella that is initially intermittent but may become persistent.

Routine radiographs do not usually provide diagnostic information in cases of patellar tendinosis. Soft tissue swelling, thickening of the patellar tendon, and obscuration of portions of the infrapatellar fat body may be evident. Bone scintigraphy shows nonspecific accumulation of radionuclide in the infrapatellar soft tissues or patella. Ultrasonography reveals an enlarged and hypoechoic tendon, particularly in its proximal portion. MR images in the sagittal plane display the entire length of the patellar tendon (Fig. 59–104). MR imaging in patients with patellar tendinosis shows an enlarged sagittal diameter of the tendon (Fig. 59–105). The proximal portion of the patellar tendon is usually thickened more than its distal portion.

## Tears of the Patellar and Quadriceps Tendons

Indirect forces applied to the extensor mechanism of the knee can lead to failure of one or more of its components. Failure of the patella resulting in fracture is common, especially in adults. Systemic disorders such as rheumatoid arthritis, chronic renal disease, and systemic lupus erythematosus contribute to failure of the quadriceps and patellar tendons, although such failure, particularly failure of the patellar tendon, may occur in the absence of these causative factors. Patellar tendon ruptures are not uncommon in persons with chronic patellar tendinosis. Failure of the patellar tendon usually occurs at its junction with the inferior pole of the patella or, less commonly, the tibial tuberosity, although intrasubstance disruption of the patellar tendon may also occur. Complete tears of the patellar tendon are associated with a high position of the patella, designated patella alta. Incomplete tears are not associated with this change in patellar position. Although ultrasonography can be used to verify complete

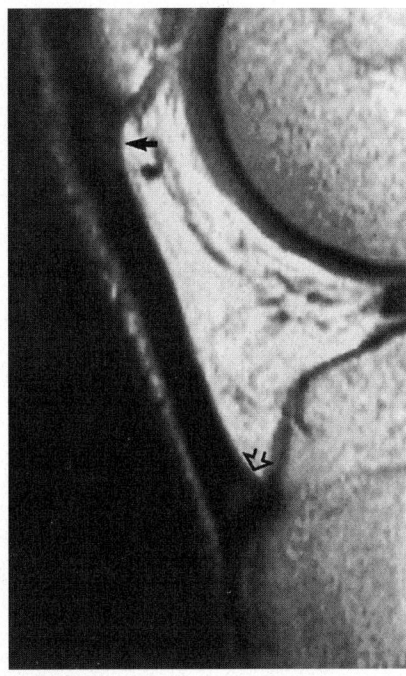

**Figure 59–104.** Patellar tendon: normal appearance. As shown on this sagittal intermediate-weighted (TR/TE, 3000/20) spin echo MR image, the patellar tendon typically has low signal intensity throughout its length, although intermediate signal intensity in the posterior margin of the proximal portion of the tendon *(solid arrow)* and in a triangular area near its distal insertion *(open arrow)* may be evident. (Courtesy of J. Yu, MD, Columbus, Ohio.)

or incomplete tears of the patellar tendon, MR imaging displays these tears more vividly (Fig. 59–106).

Partial or complete tears of the quadriceps tendon may result from an injury involving a direct blow to the tendon or forceful flexion of the knee, or they may occur spontaneously in association with such chronic diseases as systemic lupus erythematosus, rheumatoid arthritis, gout, or renal failure or after corticosteroid therapy. Rarely, spontaneous rupture of the quadriceps tendon occurs in healthy persons. The clinical diagnosis of a complete tear of the quadriceps tendon is usually obvious from the patient's history.

Routine radiographic findings associated with complete tears of the quadriceps tendon include soft tissue swelling, distortion of soft tissue planes above the patella, an inferior position of the patella (patella infra, or baja), calcification or ossification within portions of an avulsed patellar fragment, and an undulating patellar tendon. Similar but less dramatic findings accompany partial tears of the quadriceps tendon. Sagittal MR images display the quadriceps tendon in exquisite detail (Fig. 59–107). A laminated appearance with two, three, or four layers of tissue characterizes the MR imaging appearance of a normal quadriceps tendon. Tears of the quadriceps tendon lead to partial or complete interruption of its fibers (Fig. 59–108).

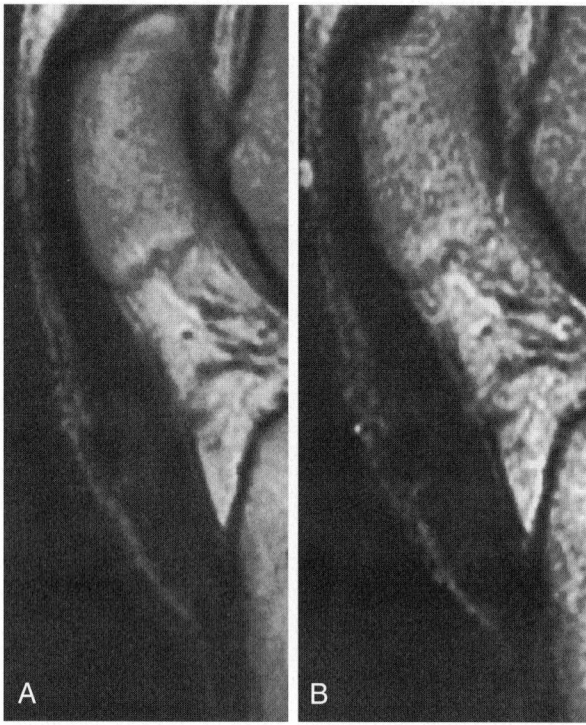

**Figure 59–105.** Chronic patellar tendinosis. Sagittal intermediate-weighted (TR/TE, 2200/30) *(A)* and T2-weighted (TR/TE, 2200/80) *(B)* spin echo MR images show marked thickening of the entire patellar tendon, more pronounced in the middle and distal segments, and indistinctness of the anterior margin of the tendon. No increase in signal intensity within the patellar tendon is seen in *B*. (Courtesy of J. Yu, MD, Columbus, Ohio.)

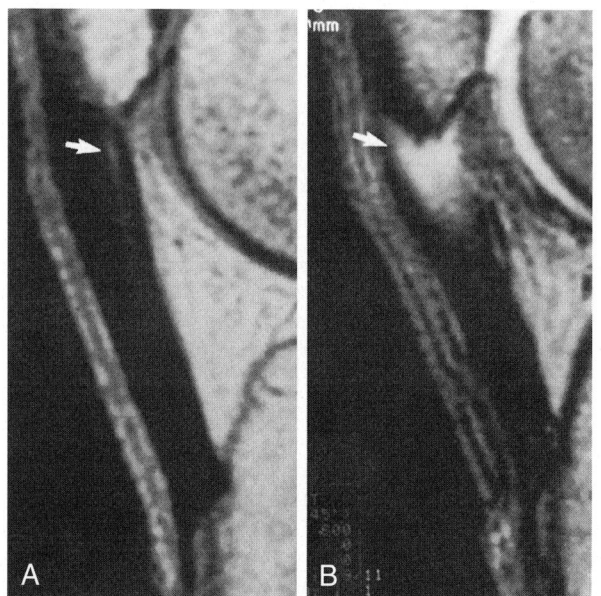

**Figure 59–106.** Patellar tendon: partial tear. Sagittal T1-weighted (TR/TE, 850/25) spin echo MR image *(A)* and sagittal MPGR (TR/TE, 600/20; flip angle, 45 degrees) MR image *(B)* reveal a partial tear *(arrows)* involving the proximal portion of the patellar tendon and thickening of the entire tendon, indicative of chronic patellar tendinosis. The findings of partial patellar tendon rupture are much more pronounced in *B*. (Courtesy of S. Fernandez, MD, Mexico City, Mexico.)

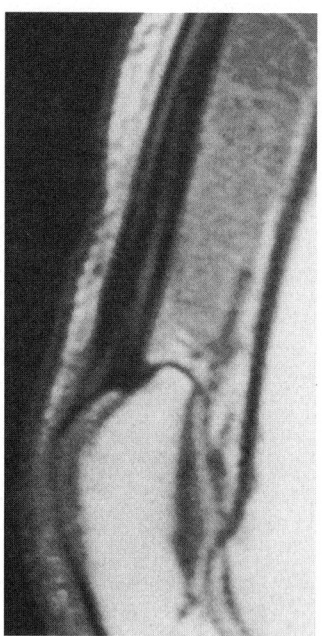

**Figure 59–107.** Quadriceps tendon: normal appearance. Sagittal intermediate-weighted (TR/TE, 3000/20) spin echo MR image shows a trilaminar appearance of the quadriceps tendon. The superficial layer relates to the tendon of the rectus femoris muscle, the middle layer relates to the tendons of the vastus medialis and vastus lateralis muscles, and the deep layer relates to the tendon of the vastus intermedius muscle. (Courtesy of J. Yu, MD, Columbus, Ohio.)

## Patellofemoral Instability

Patellofemoral instability is a frequent and complex problem. Clinical diagnosis of such instability is often difficult because the resulting symptoms and signs may simulate those of other disorders of the knee. A number of different methods based on the position of the patella on the lateral radiograph have been described to confirm the presence of patella alta or baja. The Insall-Salvati ratio (Fig. 59–109) compares the patella tendon length to the longest length of the patella, with a normal ratio of approximately 1. Axial radiographic views to assess the configuration of the trochlea, the shape of the patella, the sulcus angle, and the relationship of the patella to the femur have also been used (Fig. 59–110).

Lateral dislocation (or subluxation) of the patella is often a transient phenomenon with spontaneous reduction. The patella is pulled laterally from the trochlea and across the lateral femoral condyle, with resultant osteochondral injuries to the medial patellar facet, lateral femoral condyle, or both structures. The medial retinaculum is injured as a result of distraction, or a small avulsion fracture occurs at the patellar site of attachment of the medial retinaculum. These pathologic findings can be observed directly on MR images of the knee obtained shortly after the injury. Typical MR imaging features of an acute patellar dislocation include hemarthrosis, chondral and osteochondral fractures, disruption or attenuation of the medial retinaculum, and intra-articular bodies (Fig. 59–111).

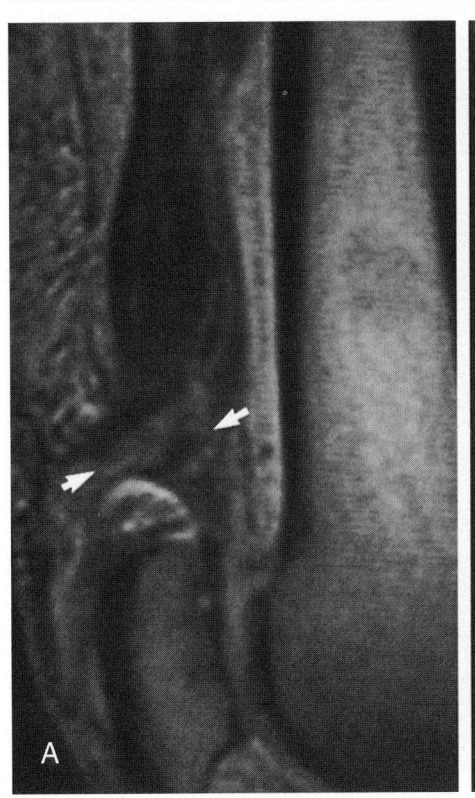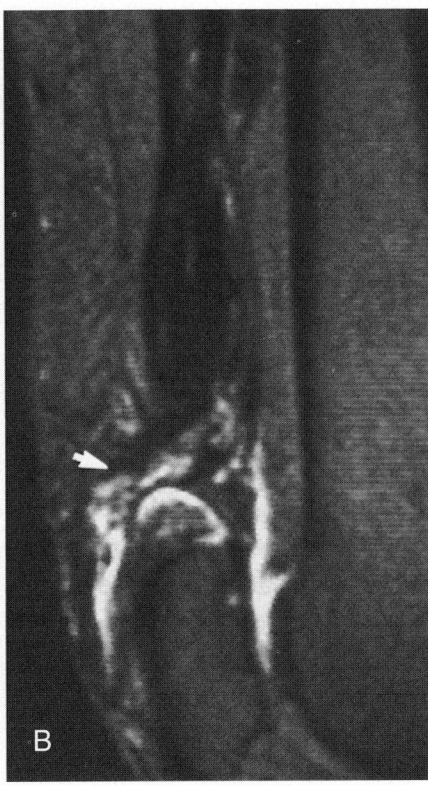

**Figure 59–108.** Quadriceps tendon: complete tear. Sagittal intermediate-weighted (TR/TE, 2500/30) *(A)* and T2-weighted (TR/TE, 2500/80) *(B)* spin echo MR images show a complete tear *(arrows)* of the quadriceps tendon at the tendo-osseous junction. Note the high signal intensity at the site of the tear in *B*. The patella is displaced inferiorly.

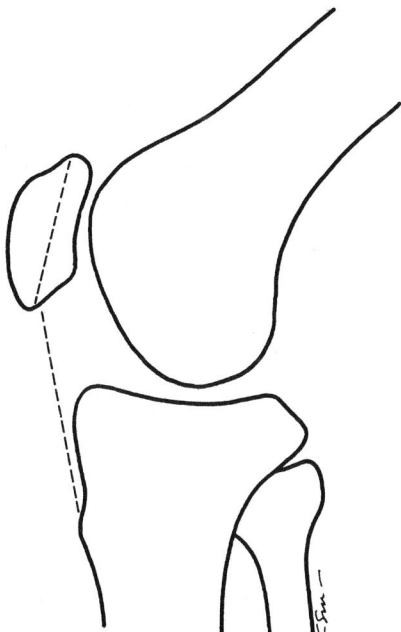

**Figure 59–109.** Patellar position: Insall-Salvati method. The ratio of patellar tendon length to the greatest diagonal length of the patella can be used to diagnose patella alta.

## Chondromalacia Patellae

Chondromalacia patellae is a term applied to cartilage loss involving one or more portions of the patella that leads to patellofemoral pain. Fundamental to the diagnosis of chondromalacia patellae is the presence of histologic abnormalities affecting the articular cartilage of the patella. The use of imaging techniques to assess patellar cartilage loss is an area of great clinical interest. MR imaging appears to be the best noninvasive diagnostic technique for the assessment of patellar cartilage (see later discussion).

## Abnormalities of the Central Supporting Structures

**Anatomic Considerations.** The anterior and posterior cruciate ligaments are intracapsular, extrasynovial structures (Fig. 59–112). The anterior cruciate ligament is proximally attached to a fossa on the posterior aspect of the medial surface of the lateral femoral condyle. Distally, the anterior cruciate ligament is attached to a fossa in front of and lateral to the tibial spines. The posterior cruciate ligament attaches inferiorly to the tibia in a depression just posterior to and below its articular surface. Some fibers of the posterior cruciate ligament extend laterally and blend with the attachment site of the posterior horn of the lateral

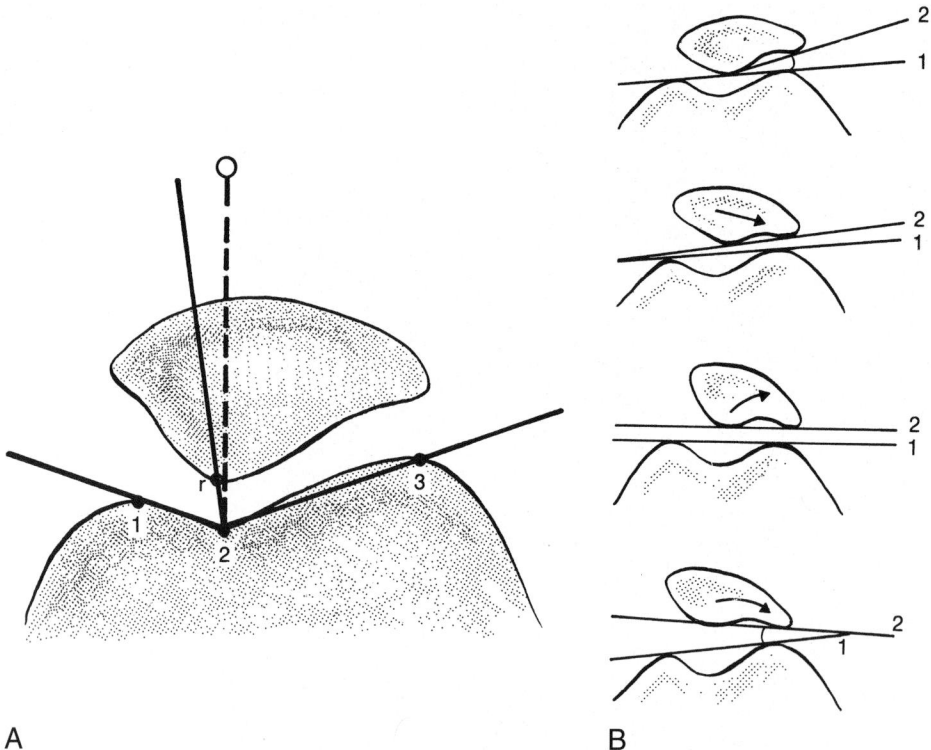

A                                      B

**Figure 59–110.** Patellar position: methods of measuring lateral patellar displacement and patellar tilt. *A*, Merchant and coworkers (J Bone Joint Surg Am 56:1391, 1974) suggested that on an axial radiograph, the line connecting the median ridge of the patella (r) and trochlear depth (2) should fall medial or slightly lateral to a line (O) bisecting angle 1-2-3. Here, the first line lies medial to line O, a normal finding. *B*, Laurin and coworkers indicated other measurements that might be appropriate. The upper two diagrams reveal the normal situation; the lower two diagrams indicate the abnormal situation. On axial radiographs, an angle formed between a line connecting the anterior aspect of the femoral condyles (1) and a second line along the lateral facet of the patella (2) normally opens laterally. In patients with abnormal tilting of the patella, these lines are parallel, or the angle of intersection opens medially. (*B*, From Laurin CA, Levesque HP, Dussault R, et al: The abnormal lateral patellofemoral angle: A diagnostic roentgenographic sign of recurrent patellar subluxation. J Bone Joint Surg Am 60:55, 1978.)

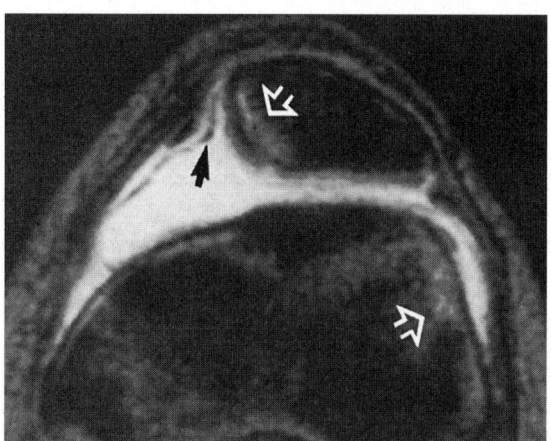

**Figure 59–111.** Patellofemoral instability. Transaxial MPGR (TR/TE, 500/11; flip angle, 15 degrees) MR image shows disruption of the medial patellar retinaculum *(solid arrow)* and marrow edema, with increased signal intensity *(open arrows)* in the medial aspect of the patella and the lateral femoral condyle. A large joint effusion is present.

meniscus. The proximal attachment site of the posterior cruciate ligament is the posterior aspect of the lateral surface of the medial femoral condyle.

The cruciate ligaments attach to the femur and tibia not as a single cord but as a collection of individual fascicles. Two groups of fascicles are evident in the anterior cruciate ligament, and two groups are evident in the posterior cruciate ligament. In the anterior cruciate ligament, these two groups are designated the anteromedial bundle and the larger posterolateral bundle. The anterior cruciate ligament functions as the primary restraint to anterior displacement of the tibia at the knee, but it offers no restraint to posterior displacement of the tibia. The posterior cruciate ligament is the primary restraint to posterior displacement of the tibia at the knee. Disruption of one or both of the cruciate ligaments leads to knee instability.

## Anterior Cruciate Ligament Injuries

Injuries to the anterior cruciate ligament are among the most frequent sequelae of knee trauma. Approximately

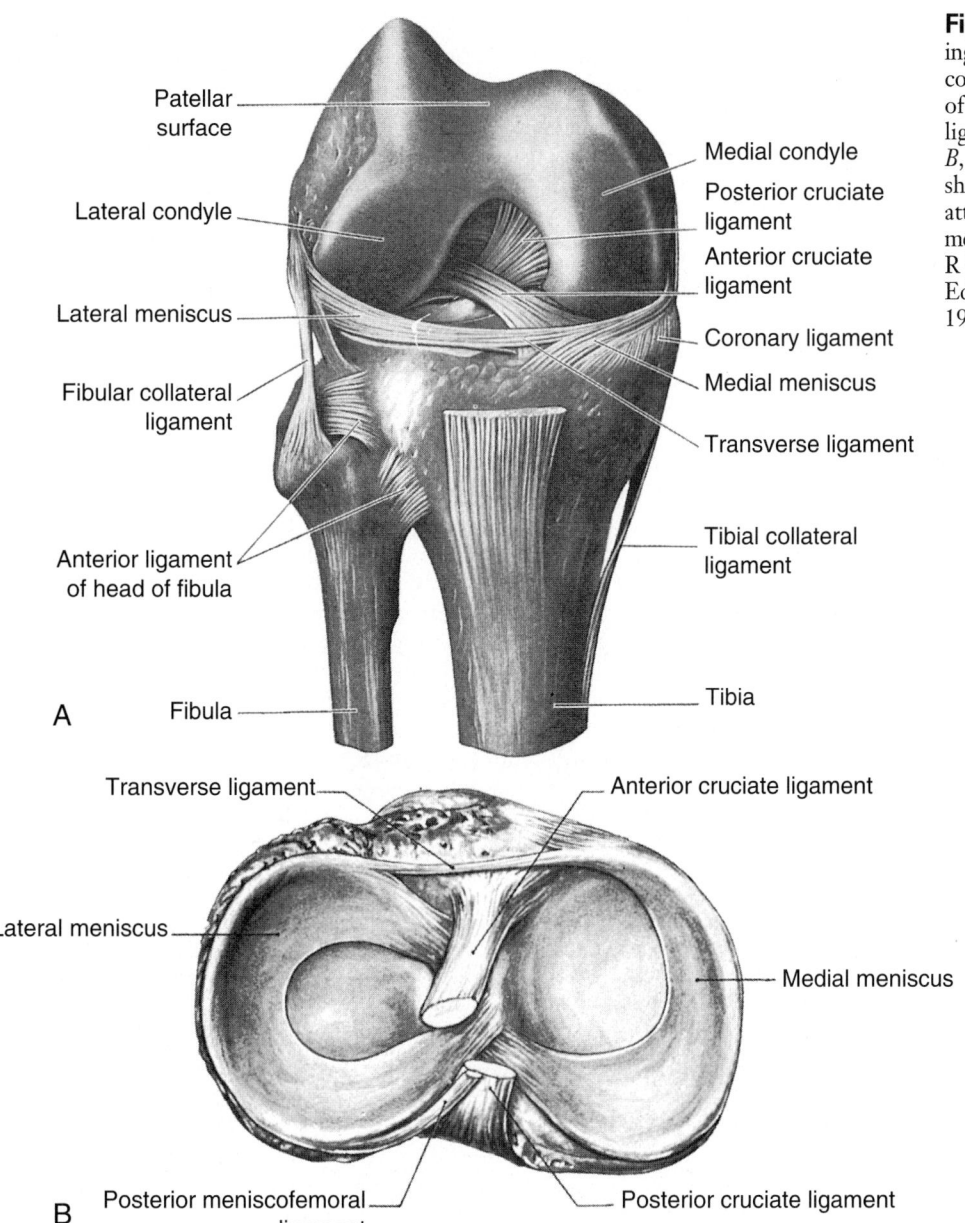

**Figure 59–112.** Central supporting structures of the knee: anatomic considerations. *A*, Anterior aspect of the knee showing the cruciate ligaments and nearby structures. *B*, Superior aspect of the tibia showing the menisci and the tibial attachments of the cruciate ligaments. (From Williams PL, Warwick R [eds]: Gray's Anatomy, 36th Br ed. Edinburgh, Churchill Livingstone, 1980, pp 400, 485, 486.)

60% to 75% of acute traumatic hemarthroses are associated with anterior cruciate ligament injury. The classic mechanism of injury to the anterior cruciate ligament (which is frequently evident in skiers and American football players) is indirect trauma leading to deceleration, hyperextension, or twisting forces, often accompanied by an audible pop and the rapid onset of pain, soft tissue swelling, and disability. The combination of external rotation of the tibia with respect to the femur, knee flexion, and valgus stress may also produce an anterior cruciate ligament injury, often combined with additional injuries to the medial collateral ligament and the medial meniscus. O'Donoghue's triad of injury consists of a tear of the anterior cruciate ligament, complete disruption of the medial collateral ligament, and a tear (or capsular separation) of the peripheral portion of the medial meniscus. The mid-

substance of the anterior cruciate ligament is injured most commonly.

**Associated Osseous Injuries.** In patients with acute tears of the anterior cruciate ligament, nonspecific soft tissue swelling and a joint effusion may be evident. Several types of fracture of the proximal portion of the tibia and distal portion of the femur, however, are specific for or imply the likelihood of an injury to the anterior cruciate ligament:

1. Avulsion fracture of the anterior tibial eminence.
2. Lateral tibial rim fracture (Segond fracture).
3. Posterior fracture of the lateral or medial tibial plateau.
4. Osteochondral fracture of the lateral femoral condyle.

A constant localized chondral or transchondral lesion occurring in the region of the condylopatellar sulcus of the lateral femoral condyle has been observed and is designated the lateral notch sign. The lateral notch sign is considered present when the depth of the sulcus is greater than 1.5 to 2 mm (Fig. 59–113). A depth greater than 2 mm has a specificity and a positive predictive value of 100% for a complete tear of the anterior cruciate ligament.

**Magnetic Resonance Imaging.** The best plane for analysis of either cruciate ligament is the sagittal plane, but the supplementary data supplied by coronal and transaxial MR images are important. The sagittal images are commonly obtained with the leg externally rotated 15 to 30 degrees, or they are obtained by determining the orientation of the anterior cruciate ligament from initial transaxial (or coronal) MR images and using a sagittal oblique imaging plane parallel to this orientation (i.e., a 15- to 30-degree internally rotated imaging plane).

Identification of a normal anterior cruciate ligament begins with analysis of the sagittal MR images (Fig. 59–114). In choosing a proper sagittal section in which a normal anterior cruciate ligament should be visualized, it is often useful to find one that displays the intercondylar roof of the femur as a straight line of low signal intensity. Typically,

in this section (or sections), the anterior cruciate ligament appears as a straight band of low signal intensity whose course parallels or is steeper than that of the intercondylar line. The anterior cruciate ligament may not be seen in its entirety on this image (or images), but the course of the visible portion of the anterior cruciate ligament should still be parallel to this line of low signal intensity. On coronal and transaxial MR images, the normal anterior cruciate ligament can again be identified. The dominant pattern of signal intensity in a normal anterior cruciate ligament is low, although it is not as low as the signal intensity in the posterior cruciate ligament.

### Anterior Cruciate Ligament Tears

MR imaging is a sensitive (90% to 98%), specific (90% to 100%), and accurate (90% to 98%) method for identifying tears of the anterior cruciate ligament. The MR imaging diagnosis of injuries to the anterior cruciate ligament relates to the documentation of (1) abnormalities in the anterior cruciate ligament itself, (2) alterations in the appearance of other structures (e.g., posterior cruciate ligament and patellar tendon) related to the abnormal alignment of the tibia and femur that results from an anterior cruciate ligament tear, and (3) abnormalities that result from bone impaction.

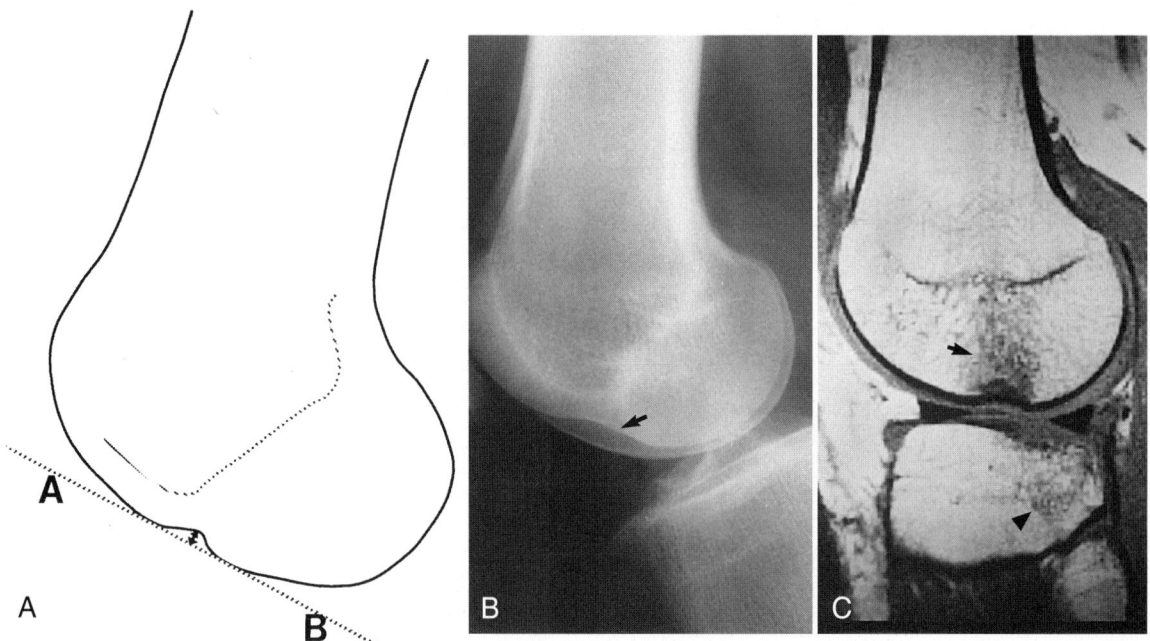

**Figure 59–113.** Injuries of the anterior cruciate ligament. *A,* Method of measuring the depth of the lateral condylopatellar sulcus. A line (AB) drawn tangentially across the lower articular surface of the lateral aspect of the femur forms the reference line. The depth of the sulcus is measured perpendicular to this line at the deepest point *(arrowheads). B,* In a patient with a chronic tear of the anterior cruciate ligament, note the prominent condylopatellar sulcus *(arrow). C,* In a different patient with a torn anterior cruciate ligament and a deep lateral condylopatellar sulcus, a T1-weighted (TR/TE, 800/30) spin echo MR image shows alterations in marrow signal intensity in the midportion of the lateral condyle *(arrow)* and in the posterolateral portion of the tibia *(arrowhead).* These findings are consistent with marrow edema related to impaction fractures. (*A,* From Cobby MJ, Schweitzer ME, Resnick D: The deep lateral femoral notch: An indirect sign of a torn anterior cruciate ligament. Radiology 184:855, 1992. *C,* Courtesy of M. Pathria, MD, San Diego, Calif.)

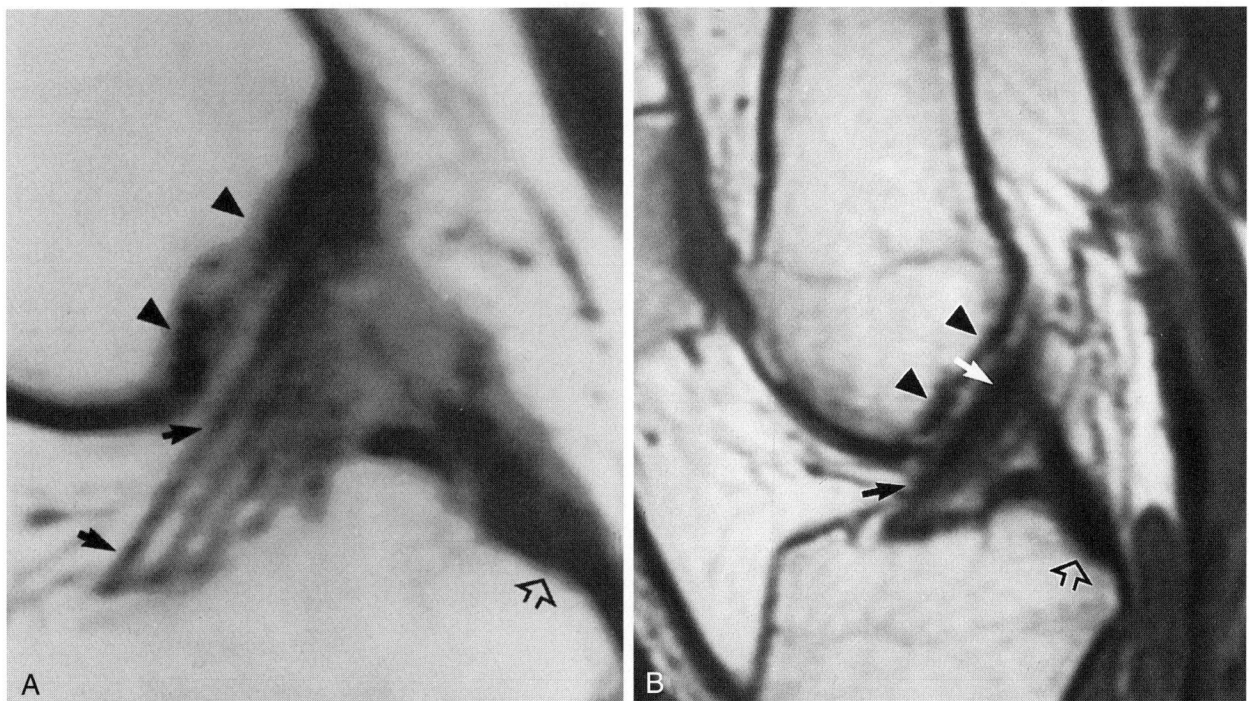

**Figure 59–114.** Anterior cruciate ligament: normal appearance. *A,* Sagittal intermediate-weighted (TR/TE, 2000/20) spin echo MR image depicts the intercondylar roof *(arrowheads)* as a straight line of low signal intensity. The anterior cruciate ligament *(solid arrows)* is seen as individual fibers whose course is straight and parallel to the course of the intercondylar roof. The tibial insertion site of the posterior cruciate ligament *(open arrow)* is also apparent. *B,* In another sagittal intermediate-weighted (TR/TE, 2000/20) spin echo MR image, the intercondylar roof *(arrowheads)* is again visualized as a straight line of low signal intensity. Although individual fibers of the anterior cruciate ligament are not seen, the ligament *(solid arrows)* is of low signal intensity and has a course that is parallel to that of the intercondylar roof. The tibial insertion site of the posterior cruciate ligament *(open arrow)* is evident.

**Abnormalities of the Anterior Cruciate Ligament Itself.** The two major alterations occurring within the ligament itself are changes in its morphology or course and changes in its signal intensity. A complete tear of the anterior cruciate ligament is accompanied by disruption of all its fibers and an irregular or wavy contour. These findings are more evident on sagittal than on coronal MR images. On sagittal MR images, the course of a completely torn anterior cruciate ligament may appear depressed (Fig. 59–115), with a decreased slope of residual fibers extending almost parallel to the tibial surface rather than at an angle to this surface and parallel to the intercondylar roof. In some chronic complete tears of the anterior cruciate ligament, the development of scar tissue leads to attachment of the torn ligament to the posterior cruciate ligament. With acute or chronic tears of some but not all the fibers of the anterior cruciate ligament, the ligament may appear attenuated, or small, and its course may or may not be altered (Fig. 59–116). The presence of increased signal intensity within the anterior cruciate ligament on intermediate- and T2-weighted spin echo or STIR MR images usually indicates an acute or subacute injury (see Fig. 59–116).

**Alterations in Other Structures Related to Abnormal Alignment of the Tibia and Femur.** Anterior cruciate ligament injuries are often associated with anterolateral

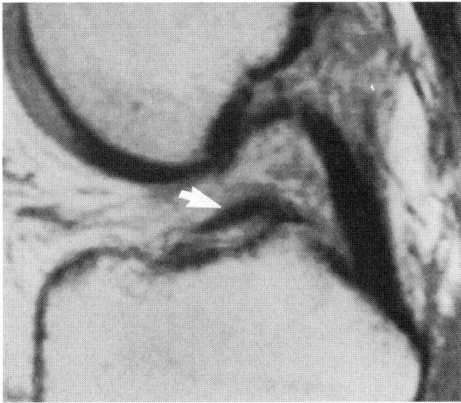

**Figure 59–115.** Injuries of the anterior cruciate ligament: chronic complete anterior cruciate ligament tear. Sagittal intermediate-weighted (TR/TE, 2000/30) spin echo MR image shows alterations in ligament morphology and course *(arrow)* in a patient with a chronically torn anterior cruciate ligament.

instability that may be manifested as a forward shift of the tibia with respect to the femur. This shift, if severe, can be easily recognized from the position of the two bones. A line drawn from the posterior cortex of the medial or lateral femoral condyle fails to pass within 5 mm of the

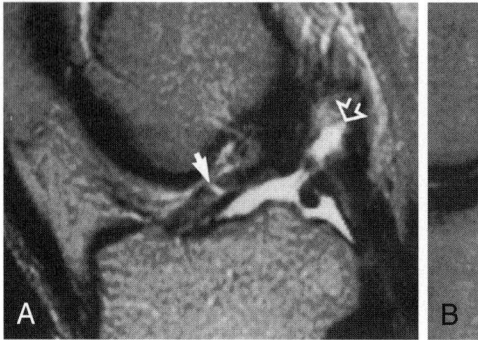
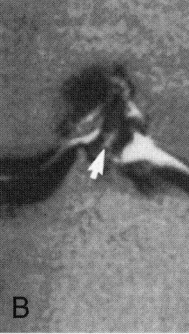

**Figure 59–116.** Injuries of the anterior cruciate ligament: acute partial anterior cruciate ligament tear. Sagittal T2-weighted (TR/TE, 4000/105) *(A)* and coronal T2-weighted (TR/TE, 3200/108) *(B)* fast spin echo MR images show an attenuated appearance of the anterior cruciate ligament, with intraligamentous regions of high signal intensity *(solid arrows)*. Note that joint fluid is collecting between the anterior and posterior cruciate ligaments *(open arrow)*, consistent with a tear in the synovial lining surrounding these ligaments.

posterior cortex of the tibia on sagittal MR images. Additional signs are a relative posterior displacement of the lateral meniscus in comparison to the posterior margin of the lateral tibial plateau ("uncovered lateral meniscus" sign) and a change in the curvature of the posterior cruciate ligament.

The uncovered lateral meniscus sign is positive if a vertical line drawn tangent to the most posterior cortical margin of the lateral tibial plateau on sagittal MR images intersects any part of the posterior horn of the lateral meniscus; this sign is negative if the vertical line does not intersect the lateral meniscus but, rather, is posterior to the meniscus (Fig. 59–117). Changes in the curvature of the posterior cruciate ligament in cases of tears of the anterior cruciate ligament have been emphasized. A forward shift in the position of the tibia with respect to the femur occurs in patients with anterior cruciate ligament–deficient knees, and this shift may alter the appearance of the smooth curve of the posterior cruciate ligament (Fig. 59–118).

**Abnormalities Related to Bone Impaction and Other Forces.** Impaction of portions of the femur and tibia may occur acutely in patients with anterolateral instability of the knee. Subcortical infraction and medullary edema and hemorrhage lead to changes in signal intensity of the affected bone marrow, a finding designated a bone bruise. In patients with acute tears of the anterior cruciate ligament, bone bruises have been observed most often in the midportion of the lateral femoral condyle (near the condylopatellar sulcus) and in the posterior portion of the lateral tibial plateau (Fig. 59–119).

### Incomplete Tears of the Anterior Cruciate Ligament

The designation "partial" tear of the anterior cruciate ligament is used inconsistently in the literature, is rarely defined, and is sometimes replaced by such terms as ligament laxity and incompetence. Partial tear implies that some but not all the ligament fibers are torn. MR imaging

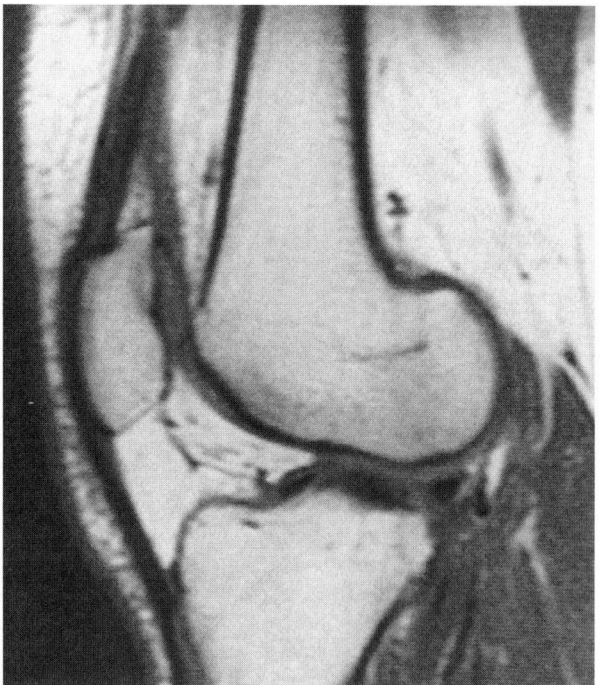

**Figure 59–117.** Injuries of the anterior cruciate ligament: chronic complete anterior cruciate ligament tear with anterior translation of the tibia. Sagittal T1-weighted (TR/TE, 600/20) spin echo MR image shows obvious forward movement of the tibia with respect to the lateral femoral condyle. Note the uncovering of the posterior horn of the lateral meniscus.

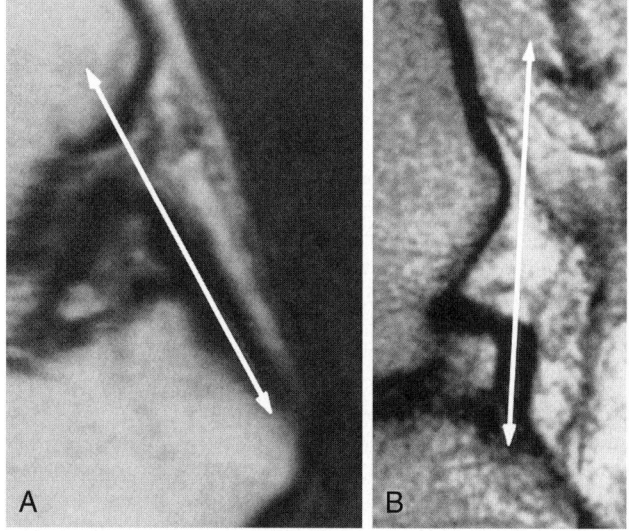

**Figure 59–118.** Injuries of the anterior cruciate ligament: normal and abnormal configuration of the posterior cruciate ligament. *A,* Normal appearance. As shown on this T1-weighted (TR/TE, 600/20) spin echo MR image, a line drawn along the course of the lower portion of the posterior cruciate ligament, when extended superiorly, intersects the femur. *B,* Acute complete anterior cruciate ligament tear. As shown on a sagittal T2-weighted (TR/TE, 2000/70) spin echo MR image, the appearance of the posterior cruciate ligament may be altered in association with a complete tear of the anterior cruciate ligament. In this case, acute angulation of the posterior cruciate ligament is evident. A line drawn along the course of the lower portion of the posterior cruciate ligament, when extended superiorly, does not intersect the femur. (Courtesy of S. K. Brahme, MD, La Jolla, Calif.)

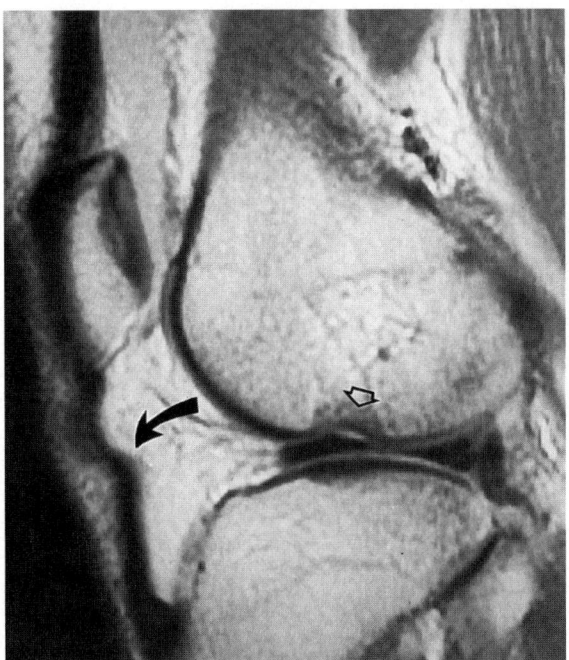

**Figure 59–119.** Injuries of the anterior cruciate ligament: acute complete anterior cruciate ligament tear with redundancy of the patellar tendon and osteochondral impaction fracture. Sagittal intermediate-weighted (TR/TE, 2000/30) spin echo MR image shows buckling of the patellar tendon *(curved solid arrow)* and an alteration in signal intensity *(open arrow)* in the lateral condylopatellar sulcus related to an impaction injury. A large joint effusion is present. (From Cobby MJ, Schweitzer ME, Resnick D: The deep lateral femoral notch: An indirect sign of a torn anterior cruciate ligament. Radiology 184:855, 1992.)

diagnosis of incomplete tears of the anterior cruciate ligament is clearly more difficult than that of complete tears. MR imaging findings of abnormal intraligamentous signal intensity, bowing of the ligament, and inability to identify all the fibers of the ligament are not highly sensitive or specific.

### *Postoperative Anterior Cruciate Ligament*

Operative procedures used for the treatment of a torn anterior cruciate ligament include primary repair of the ligament, ligament repair plus augmentation using various autogenous grafts, and ligament reconstruction with autogenous materials, allografts, or prosthetic devices. Of the autogenous intra-articular reconstructions, the bone–patellar tendon–bone graft has become the anterior cruciate ligament substitute with which all others are compared. The middle third of the patellar tendon is used, along with its accompanying bone plugs or blocks. The femoral insertion site chosen is generally close to or at the normal insertion site of the anterior cruciate ligament. Similarly, the tibial insertion site of the graft usually closely corresponds to that of the anterior cruciate ligament itself.

Radiographs provide indirect information regarding the placement of the graft material, based on the position of the tunnels in the tibia and femur. MR imaging allows direct visualization of the graft itself and is a potentially superior imaging method for establishing the diagnosis of graft impingement.

### Posterior Cruciate Ligament Injuries

Injuries to the posterior cruciate ligament are less frequent than those to the anterior cruciate ligament; they require greater force and may initially be unrecognized, thus leading to a delay in diagnosis. They may occur as an isolated phenomenon (30% of cases) or in association with other capsular, ligamentous, or meniscal injuries (70% of cases). Pain, swelling, and hemarthrosis may be evident. The posterior drawer test, in which stress is applied to the anterior surface of the tibia in an attempt to produce posterior translation of the tibia with respect to the femur, is positive in 30% to 75% of cases.

Routine radiography may reveal avulsion fractures at the tibial insertion site of the ligament. A joint effusion may be present. Routine radiographs rarely contribute to the diagnosis of a posterior cruciate ligament injury. The posterior cruciate ligament normally appears as a band-like structure of low signal intensity on sagittal, coronal, and transaxial MR images (Fig. 59–120). It is seen in its entirety on a single MR image or possibly two contiguous MR images in the sagittal plane. Tears of the posterior cruciate ligament usually occur in its midsubstance. Disruption of all or a portion of its fibers is evident, especially on sagittal MR images (Fig. 59–121). Regions of high signal intensity within the ligament may be evident on T2-weighted spin echo MR images in cases of acute or subacute tears. Regions of altered signal intensity in the bone marrow, compatible with contusions or fractures, are also common.

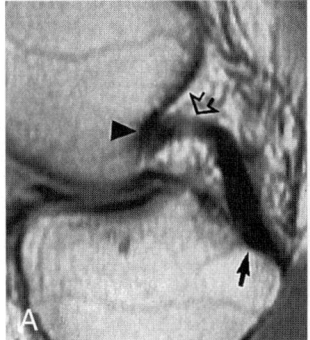
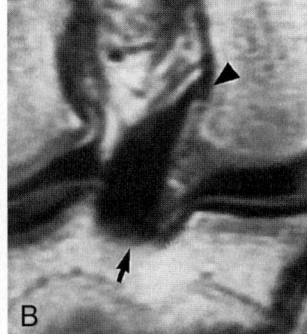

**Figure 59–120.** Posterior cruciate ligament: normal appearance. *A*, Sagittal intermediate-weighted (TR/TE, 2000/20) spin echo MR image. Note the femoral *(arrowhead)* and tibial *(solid arrow)* insertion sites of the posterior cruciate ligament. It has an arcuate course and is of low signal intensity, except for its proximal portion *(open arrow)*, where intermediate signal intensity may relate to the magic angle phenomenon. *B*, Coronal intermediate-weighted (TR/TE, 2000/20) spin echo MR image. The femoral *(arrowhead)* and tibial *(solid arrow)* insertion sites of the posterior cruciate ligament are identified. The ligament is of low signal intensity and has a smooth contour.

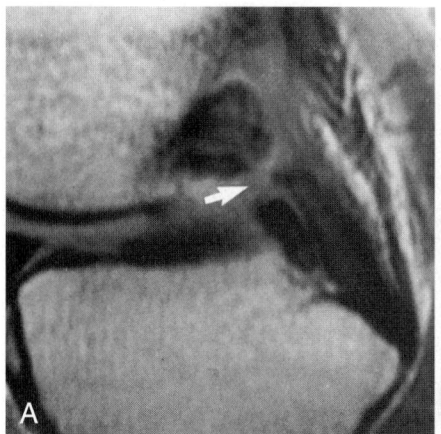
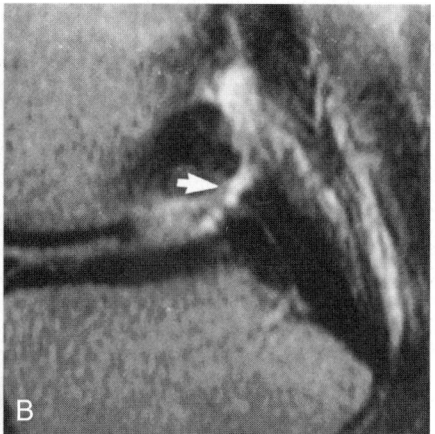

**Figure 59–121.** Injuries of the posterior cruciate ligament: acute complete posterior cruciate ligament tear. Sagittal intermediate-weighted (TR/TE, 2000/30) *(A)* and T2-weighted (TR/TE, 2000/80) *(B)* spin echo MR images reveal complete disruption *(arrows)* of the posterior cruciate ligament, with an increase in signal intensity in *B*.

Tears of the posterior cruciate ligament may be treated by primary repair, which involves suturing of the ligament and, perhaps, graft augmentation. The specific therapeutic strategy, however, is often dictated by the pattern of injury. Acute tears isolated to the posterior cruciate ligament may be treated nonoperatively, whereas those involving multiple ligaments often require surgical reconstruction.

## Abnormalities of Multiple Ligaments

Knee dislocation is the classic cause of multiple ligamentous injuries. Although the precise number of ligaments that are torn, stretched, or avulsed during knee dislocation depends on the magnitude of the force and the specific type of dislocation, injury to both cruciate ligaments is common. When injuries to both cruciate ligaments are documented, even when no other ligaments are torn, knee dislocation is likely even when the knee is reduced at the time of initial evaluation. The most common injury pattern of knee dislocation involves both cruciate ligaments and the medial collateral ligament. Vascular and bone injuries are also important complications of knee dislocation.

## Cartilage Abnormalities

None of the standard imaging methods used to evaluate cartilage degeneration is ideal. Routine radiographic assessment with weight bearing, varus or valgus stress, knee flexion, or combinations of these techniques (e.g., weight bearing and knee flexion) is adequate for the determination of cartilage loss in the more involved weight-bearing compartment. Contrast material injected into the joint cavity allows portions of the articular cartilage to be visualized. The role of ultrasonography in the assessment of articular cartilage is limited by the necessity of positioning the joint in a manner that provides proximity to the articular surface for a probe placed on the skin. MR imaging appears to be unique in its ability to demonstrate not only cartilage loss but the internal structure as well.

Although severe chondral abnormalities, including full-thickness defects and denudation of the articular surface,

are delineated with MR imaging, the detection of more superficial cartilage lesions with this imaging method is far more challenging. A multitude of MR pulse sequences have been advocated, and MR arthrography enhanced with intra-articular administration of gadolinium compounds has been shown to be effective in the detection of cartilage abnormalities. With fat-suppressed gradient echo sequences, cartilage has a trilaminar appearance consisting of a superficial region of high signal intensity, an intermediate region of low signal intensity, and a deep region of high signal intensity (Figs. 59–122 to 59–124).

## Abnormalities of Subchondral Bone

**Occult Injuries.** The detection of occult injuries in the distal portion of the femur and the proximal portion of the tibia with MR imaging has been emphasized. MR imaging may document soft tissue swelling, joint effusions, and alterations in signal intensity in the bone marrow. Such alterations in signal intensity within subchondral marrow after injury to the knee (or other joints) led to the introduction of the term *bone bruise*. The precise histologic correlates of a bone bruise are not clear, although microfractures of trabeculae and hyperemia, edema, and hemorrhage in adjacent marrow appear to contribute to the changes in signal intensity. Reticulated regions of low signal intensity are apparent on T1-weighted spin echo MR images, and similar regions of inhomogeneous high signal intensity are observed on T2-weighted spin echo MR images (Fig. 59–125). STIR imaging sequences dramatically display these lesions as areas of high signal intensity within involved marrow. The MR imaging characteristics of bone bruises are similar to those noted in cases of transient painful bone marrow edema. Additional occult cartilage and bone injuries about the knee include stress fractures (insufficiency and fatigue fractures), osteochondral fractures, and acute fractures of the femoral condyles and tibial plateaus that generally extend into the chondral surfaces.

**Hematopoietic Hyperplasia.** Islands of hypercellular but otherwise normal-appearing hematopoietic marrow may

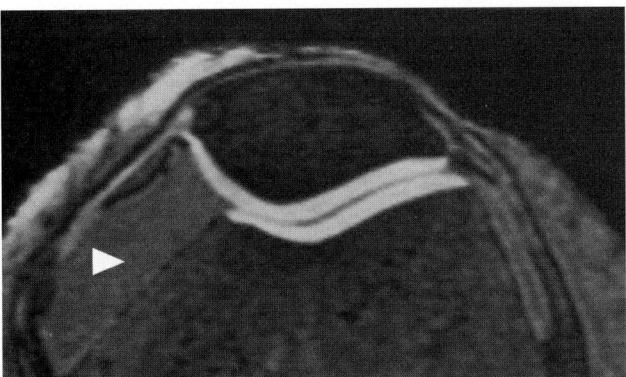

**Figure 59–122.** Patellofemoral articular cartilage: normal appearance. On a transaxial three-dimensional Fourier transform SPGR (TR/TE, 52/10; flip angle, 60 degrees) MR image obtained with fat suppression, the articular cartilage is of high signal intensity, and the bone and synovial fluid (*arrowhead*) are of low signal intensity. The articular cartilage possesses a trilaminar appearance, best appreciated in the lateral patellar facet and the lateral femoral condyle; the superficial portion of articular cartilage is of high signal intensity, a thin intermediate region shows low signal intensity, and the deep portion of the articular cartilage is of high signal intensity.

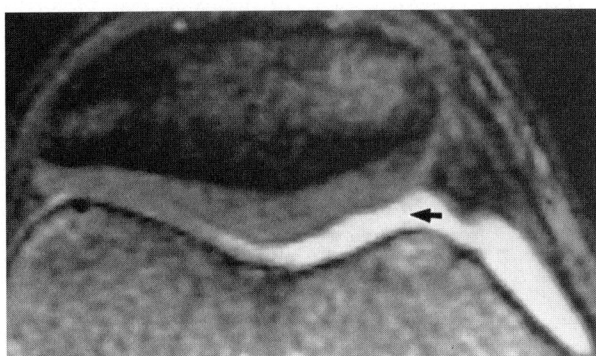

**Figure 59–123.** Patellofemoral articular cartilage: normal appearance. On this transaxial MPGR (TR/TE, 450/20; flip angle, 15 degrees) MR image, the presence of joint fluid (*arrow*) of high signal intensity allows improved visualization of the surface of the articular cartilage.

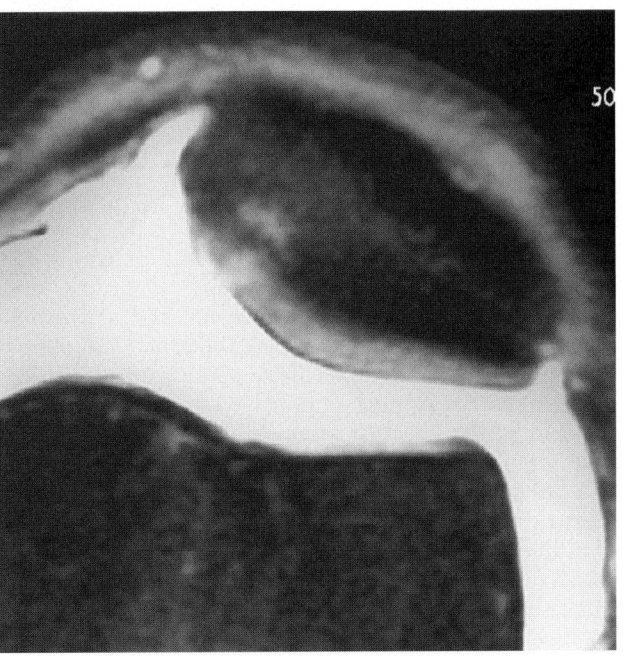

**Figure 59–124.** Patellofemoral articular cartilage abnormalities. On this transverse fast spin echo (TR/TE, 2750/13) fat-suppresssed MR image, note the traumatic defect of the cartilage in the medial facet of the patella, subchondral edema, and a large joint effusion. (Courtesy of D. Goodwin, MD, Hanover, N.H.)

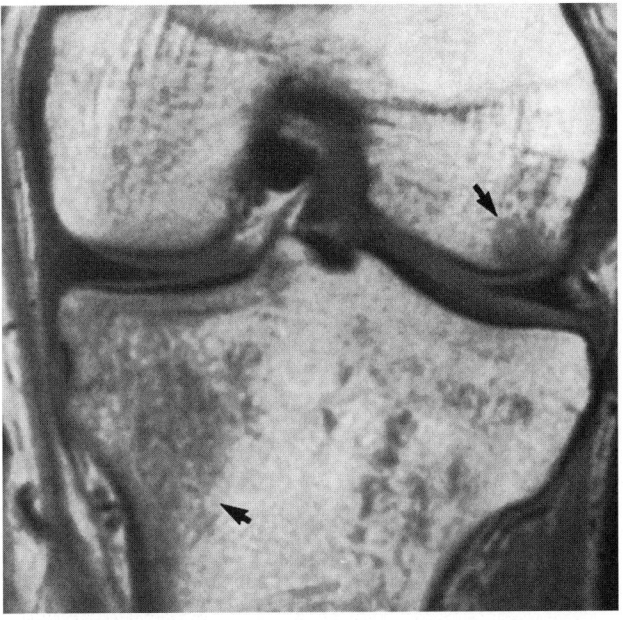

**Figure 59–125.** Bone bruise. In a patient with an anterior cruciate ligament tear, a coronal T1-weighted (TR/TE, 600/20) spin echo MR image shows the typical reticulated regions of low signal intensity (*arrows*) principally involving the medial tibial plateau and the lateral femoral condyle. These regions revealed increased signal intensity on T2-weighted spin echo MR images (not shown). (From Bosch E, Pathria M, Resnick D: Difficult-to-detect osseous injuries—MRI gives greater specificity. Physician Sportsmed 21:116, 1993.)

occur in the distal femoral metaphysis in asymptomatic persons, particularly obese women of menstruating age who are also cigarette smokers. These islands demonstrate low signal intensity on both T1- and T2-weighted spin echo MR images. The major differential diagnostic considerations based on MR imaging findings are lymphoma or other lymphoproliferative or myeloproliferative disorders and sickle cell anemia or other hemoglobinopathies. On fat-suppressed T2-weighted fast spin echo and STIR images, however, hematopoietic hyperplasia appears as foci of increased signal intensity. The resulting signal is similar to that of normal muscle.

**Osteonecrosis.** The frequency of ischemic necrosis involving the bones about the knee is second only to that of the femoral head. Typical sites of involvement are the femoral condyles and proximal portion of the tibia, although involvement of the diaphyseal and metaphyseal regions of the femur and tibia is encountered (see Chapter 67).

## Miscellaneous Abnormalities

**Intra-articular Bodies.** Large calcified free or embedded intra-articular bodies are usually easily identified with routine radiography. Smaller bodies, unless heavily calcified, are more difficult to detect with routine radiography. With any imaging method, the search for intra-articular bodies is more rewarding if normal recesses and dependent portions of the knee (or other joint) are analyzed carefully. Common locations of intra-articular bodies in the knee are the suprapatellar recess, popliteus hiatus or tunnel, recesses beneath the menisci, and intercondylar notch. Free bodies within the knee may pass into an adjacent synovial cyst. Multiple intra-articular bodies in the knee are present in approximately 30% of cases. Detection of small calcified or noncalcified bodies in the knee may require the combination of arthrography and CT (Fig. 59–126). Small calcified or noncalcified bodies in the knee may escape detection with MR imaging, especially if there is no joint effusion present (joint effusion makes their detection easier). In the absence of a knee effusion, MR arthrography may be an effective technique for demonstrating such bodies. In general, however, the diagnosis of free or embedded bodies in the knee is better accomplished with computed arthrotomography than with MR imaging.

**Bursitis.** Any of the bursae about the knee may become inflamed and subsequently accumulate bursal fluid.

Ultrasonography and MR imaging are the two most effective imaging methods for the diagnosis of these conditions. With MR imaging, bursal fluid is of high signal intensity on T2-weighted spin echo images, as well as on STIR images.

**Hoffa's Disease.** Hoffa's disease refers to traumatic and inflammatory changes occurring in the infrapatellar fat body. This rare condition is seen in young athletic persons, in whom pain, swelling, and limitation of joint motion may occur. MR imaging reveals alterations in signal intensity in the infrapatellar fat body (Fig. 59–127) that resemble those related to scarring after knee arthroscopy.

## ANKLE AND FOOT

### Anatomy

**Articular.** The articular surfaces are covered by cartilage, and the bones are connected by a fibrous capsule and by the deltoid, anterior and posterior talofibular, and calcaneofibular ligaments. The capsule is weak both anteriorly and posteriorly, but it is reinforced medially and laterally by various ligaments, including the following:

1. *Deltoid ligament.* This medial ligament is triangular in shape and is attached above to the apex and the posterior and anterior borders of the medial malleolus. It contains superficial, middle, and deep fibers, although classification of the fibers of this ligament is not uniform.

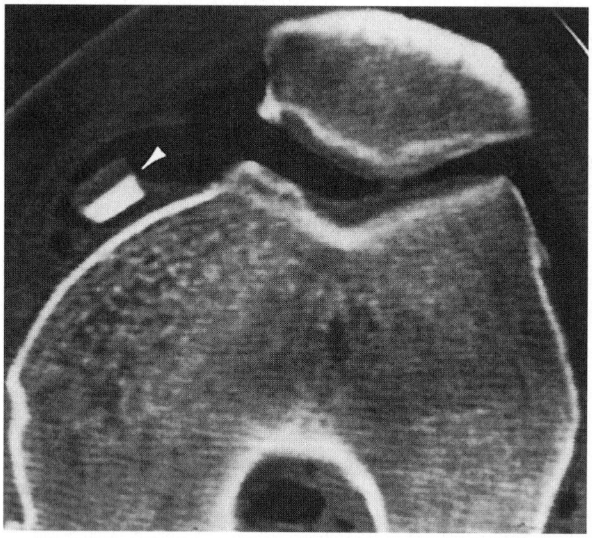

**Figure 59–126.** Intra-articular bodies: CT-arthrography. After the introduction of air into the knee joint, a transaxial CT scan reveals a fragment (*arrowhead*) consisting of cartilage and bone in the medial aspect of the articulation.

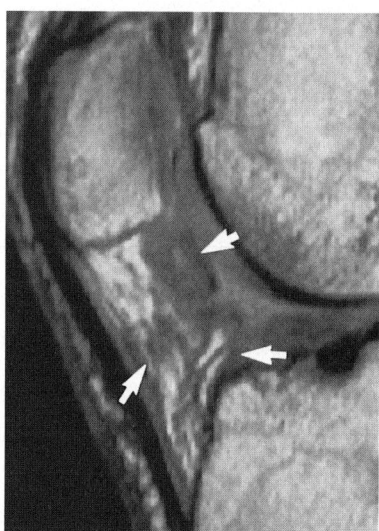

**Figure 59–127.** Hoffa's disease. This male adolescent underwent several arthroscopic procedures in which a medial patellar plica and an enlarged and inflamed infrapatellar fat body were resected. He later sought medical assistance for recurrent anterior knee pain. A sagittal intermediate-weighted (TR/TE, 2700/20) spin echo MR image shows serpentine and irregular areas of low signal intensity (*arrows*) in the deep infrapatellar fat body. Repeat arthroscopy confirmed inflammation of the fat pad and adjacent synovial membrane. (Courtesy of G. Bock, MD, and P. Major, MD, Winnipeg, Manitoba, Canada.)

Superficial fibers run anterior to the tuberosity of the tarsal navicular bone and blend with the plantar calcaneonavicular ligament (or spring ligament). Middle fibers attach to the sustentaculum tali of the calcaneus, and posterior fibers pass to the medial talar surface, including its tubercle.

2. *Anterior talofibular ligament.* This ligament extends from the anterior margin of the lateral malleolus to the lateral articular facet on the neck of the talus.

3. *Posterior talofibular ligament.* This ligament attaches to the lateral malleolar fossa and extends horizontally to the lateral tubercle of the talus and medial malleolus.

4. *Calcaneofibular ligament.* This structure extends from the lateral malleolus to the lateral surface of the calcaneus. It is crossed by the peroneus longus and peroneus brevis tendons.

The soft tissue anatomy of the talocrural joint governs the radiographic manifestations of an articular effusion. On lateral radiographs, an ankle effusion produces a teardrop-shaped dense shadow anterior to the joint that extends along the neck of the talus.

The distal tibiofibular joint consists of a strong interosseous ligament that unites the convex surface of the medial aspect of the distal end of the fibula and the concave surface of the adjacent fibular notch of the tibia. Additionally, the anterior and posterior tibiofibular ligaments reinforce this articulation. Below this ligamentous joint, an upward prolongation of the synovial membrane of the ankle (talocrural joint) can extend 3 to 5 mm. There are two talocalcaneal joints: the subtalar (posterior talocalcaneal or posterior subtalar) joint and the talocalcaneonavicular (anterior subtalar) joint. These articulations are separated by the tarsal canal and sinus and their contents.

**Tendon Sheath and Bursa.** Tendons with accompanying tendon sheaths are intimate with the ankle joint (Fig. 59–128). Anteriorly, sheaths encase the tendons of the tibialis anterior, extensor hallucis longus, extensor digitorum longus, and peroneus tertius muscles. Medially, sheaths are present about the tendons of the tibialis posterior, flexor digitorum longus, and flexor hallucis longus muscles. Laterally, the common sheath of the tendons of the peroneus longus and peroneus brevis muscles is found. The plantar aponeurosis, with its three portions, contains strong fibers that in large part adhere to the posteroinferior surface of the bone. The Achilles tendon, which is the thickest and strongest human tendon, attaches to the posterior surface of the calcaneus approximately 2 cm below the upper surface of the bone. The retrocalcaneal bursa is located between the Achilles tendon and the posterosuperior surface of the calcaneus.

Owing to the tendons' change in orientation from a vertical attitude in the lower leg to a horizontal attitude in the foot, five retinacula act to maintain close approximation of the tendons to the bones about the ankle and thereby prevent bowstringing of these tendons (see Fig. 59–128):

1. *Superior extensor retinaculum.* The superior extensor retinaculum is attached to the anterior surface of the lateral malleolus and to the anterior surface of the medial portion of the tibia, and it is continuous with the deep fascia of the lower part of the leg. This structure serves to reinforce the crural fascia and contain the tendons of the tibialis anterior, extensor hallucis longus, extensor digitorum longus, and peroneus tertius muscles on the dorsal surface of the ankle.

2. *Inferior extensor retinaculum.* The inferior extensor retinaculum is a Y-shaped structure whose base is attached laterally to the calcaneus. This retinaculum serves to prevent bowstringing of the dorsal tendons.

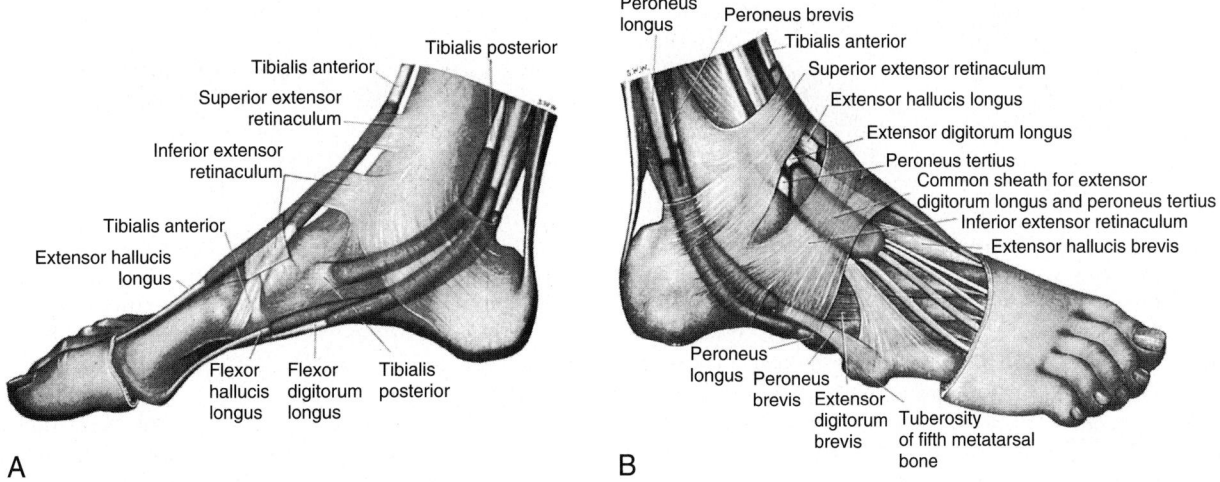

**Figure 59–128.** Tendon sheaths about the ankle: normal anatomy. *A*, Medial aspect of the ankle. *B*, Lateral aspect of the ankle. (From Williams PL, Warwick R [eds]: Gray's Anatomy, 36th Br ed. Edinburgh, Churchill Livingstone, 1980, pp 611, 612.)

3. *Flexor retinaculum.* The flexor retinaculum is located medially and encloses the tarsal tunnel. It extends between the medial malleolus and the calcaneus.

4 and 5. *Superior and inferior peroneal retinacula.* The two peroneal retinacula are laterally located fascial thickenings that extend from the lateral malleolus to the calcaneus. These retinacula serve to hold the tendons of the peroneus longus and brevis muscles firmly in place behind the fibula.

The tendons of the flexor hallucis longus, flexor digitorum longus, and tibialis posterior muscles are intimately related at the levels of the medial malleolus and below. At these levels, the tendon of the tibialis posterior muscle is most anterior, the tendon of the flexor digitorum longus muscle is in the intermediate position, and the tendon of the flexor hallucis longus muscle is located posteriorly. A mnemonic device, "Tom, Dick, and Harry," indicates the anterior to posterior relationships of these three tendons: T for the tibialis posterior tendon, D for the flexor digitorum longus tendon, and H for the flexor hallucis longus tendon.

The tendons of the tibialis anterior, extensor hallucis longus, and extensor digitorum longus muscles lie alongside one another in the anterior portion of the lower part of the leg. The most medial of these structures is the tibialis anterior tendon, the most lateral is the extensor digitorum longus tendon, and the tendon of the extensor hallucis longus muscle lies in an intermediate position. The mnemonic device "Tom, Harry, and Dick" can be used to define the medial to lateral relationships of these three tendons: T for tibialis anterior, H for extensor hallucis longus, and D for extensor digitorum longus.

## Tendon Abnormalities

**Anatomic Considerations.** With the exception of the Achilles tendon, all the foot tendons change from a vertical orientation in the lower leg to a horizontal orientation at or near the level of the ankle, a modification in direction that is accomplished by means of a pulley system consisting of either bone (i.e., the malleoli) or retinacula. Where tendons are applied to the surface of a bone, a groove or sulcus is present to promote the angular deviations in their course that occur about the ankle. The groove behind the fibula, through which pass the tendons of the peroneus brevis and peroneus longus muscles, is the smallest and most shallow, perhaps explaining the occurrence of subluxation of these tendons.

Disorders of the tendons about the ankle and in the foot include the following: tenosynovitis, tethering, tears, dislocations, tumors and pseudotumors, ossification, congenital anomalies, contractures, and iatrogenic injuries. Inflammatory changes about a tendon, often designated tenosynovitis, can be more precisely defined according to the type of tissue affected. If inflammation affects a tendon sheath, the term tenosynovitis is most appropriate. Paratenosynovitis refers to inflammation of tissues about a tendon sheath, and paratendinitis refers to inflammation about a tendon that has no sheath. Peritendinitis is defined as inflammation of a peritenon. Tendinosis (or tendinopathy) indicates degeneration within the substance

of the tendon. Inflammation and degeneration of any or all of these structures may relate to direct or indirect injury, occupational stress and overuse syndromes, misuse syndromes related to anomalies of the foot or other structures, and local or systemic rheumatic diseases. Adhesions may develop between the sheath and the tendon (i.e., stenosing or constrictive tenosynovitis) and lead to altered or restricted movement in a tendon sheath–tendon unit that normally requires smooth, almost frictionless function.

A tethered tendon is one whose range of movement is limited because of its abnormal fixation to an adjacent structure. Causes of such tethering include anatomic anomalies, fractures with resulting deformities that lead to abnormal fixation or displacement of the tendon or its sheath, a hypertrophied os trigonum that leads to constriction and displacement of the flexor hallucis longus tendon within its sheath, fracture-dislocations of the ankle that may lead to tethering or even incarceration of one or more regional tendons, and checkrein deformities resulting from abnormal fixation of the flexor hallucis longus tendon under or just proximal to the flexor retinaculum or under the annular ligament.

Partial or complete tears of the tendons of the foot and ankle may relate to a laceration, especially in the sole of the foot, or more commonly, they may occur spontaneously. Spontaneous rupture of these tendons usually implies some type of intrinsic pathologic process, because normal tendons rarely rupture in this fashion. Tendon degeneration in older persons or chronic tendon overuse in younger persons, particularly athletes, may predispose to spontaneous rupture. Although virtually any tendon of the foot or ankle can be affected, spontaneous disruptions of the tibialis posterior tendon and the Achilles tendon are encountered most frequently.

**Imaging Considerations.** MR imaging is generally considered the best method for the detection of tendinosis, tenosynovitis, and partial and complete tendon rupture. CT is superior to MR imaging in the delineation of tendon calcification and retinacular avulsion of bone, and CT and MR imaging are of approximately equal value when applied to the analysis of tendon dislocation.

Routine radiographic findings associated with abnormalities of the tendons and tendon sheaths of the foot and ankle include soft tissue swelling; change in contour, calcification, or ossification of a tendon; bone proliferation; fracture fragments; and sesamoid displacement. Achilles tendinosis or rupture of the Achilles tendon may be accompanied by edema or hemorrhage, with obscuration of portions of the pre-Achilles fat body. Associated retrocalcaneal bursitis (which may occur in systemic rheumatic disorders and in Haglund's syndrome) leads to obliteration of the normal radiolucent retrocalcaneal recess between the Achilles tendon and the posterosuperior portion of the calcaneus (Fig. 59–129).

MR imaging has been applied to the assessment of tendons and other structures in the ankle and foot. The tibialis posterior tendon and the Achilles tendon have received the greatest attention. The most commonly used MR imaging sequences in the ankle and foot are standard spin echo, fast spin echo, MPGR, and STIR sequences.

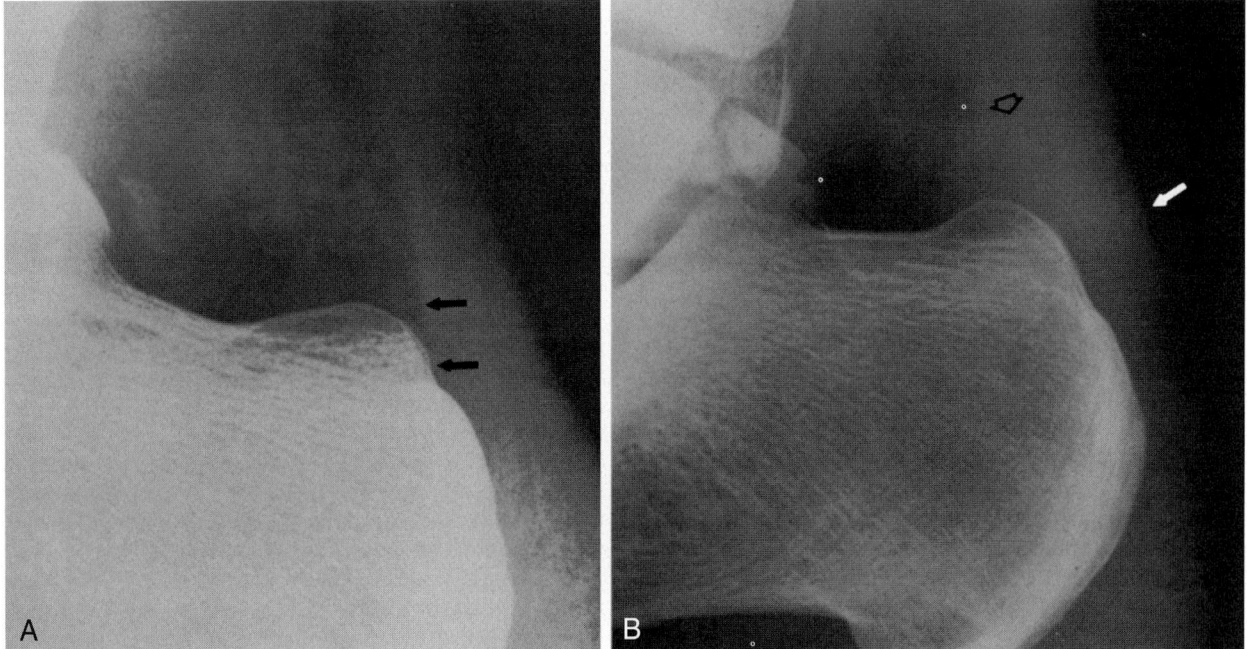

**Figure 59–129.** Retrocalcaneal bursa: normal appearance and retrocalcaneal bursitis. *A*, Normal appearance. Normally, with the foot in neutral position, fat about the retrocalcaneal bursa produces a triangular radiolucent area *(arrows)*, designated the retrocalcaneal recess, between the Achilles tendon and the calcaneus on lateral radiographs of the ankle. *B*, Retrocalcaneal bursitis. Inflammation, synovial hypertrophy, and effusion have resulted in an enlarged, fluid-filled retrocalcaneal bursa that extends above the calcaneus as a radiodense area *(open arrow)*. The Achilles tendon and surrounding tissue are also thickened *(solid arrow)*.

With minor exceptions, the normal tendons in the ankle and foot are homogeneous and of low signal intensity with all MR imaging sequences. They are generally equal in size on the two sides of the body and have a smooth contour. Some exceptions to these general rules may be noted, however:

1. *Magic angle effect.* As indicated earlier, increased signal intensity may be seen in normal tendons oriented obliquely with respect to the main magnetic field, an effect that is greatest when this orientation is at 55 degrees to that of the magnetic field (Fig. 59–130). This effect is greater when the MR imaging examination uses spin echo techniques with short TEs or gradient echo techniques with short TEs and high flip angles.

2. *Tenosynovial fluid.* Differentiation of a thickened tendon from one surrounded by a fluid-filled synovial sheath is difficult on T1-weighted spin echo MR images. Further, the presence of small or even moderate amounts of fluid within a tendon sheath is, by itself, not diagnostic of an abnormality, because such fluid is seen in asymptomatic persons. Tenosynovial fluid is more frequent in flexor tendons than extensor tendons and may be particularly prominent about the flexor hallucis longus tendon.

3. *Bulbous tendon insertion sites.* Insertion sites of tendons may appear bulbous (Fig. 59–131), perhaps related to volume averaging of their signal intensity with that of adjacent cortical bone. This appearance can simulate that of a tendon disruption, particularly disruption of the tibialis posterior tendon.

4. *Tendon striations.* When three-dimensional gradient recalled MR images are obtained, longitudinal lines of intermediate signal intensity in the distal portion of the tibialis posterior tendon may be noted. These lines probably represent branches of the tendon. Similar striations are caused by fat interspersed among the fibers of some of the ankle ligaments.

In common with the findings derived by ultrasonography and CT, the major MR imaging finding of tenosynovitis is abnormal accumulation of fluid within the tendon sheath. This fluid has low signal intensity on T1-weighted spin echo MR images and high signal intensity on T2-weighted spin echo images. Pannus and scar formation about a tendon are characterized by intermediate signal intensity on T1-weighted spin echo MR images and intermediate to high signal intensity on T2-weighted spin echo MR images. Intratendinous tears are accompanied by focal areas of high signal intensity within the substance of the tendon on intermediate- and T2-weighted spin echo MR images. With chronic tendinosis, the tendon is enlarged and of low or intermediate signal intensity on both T1- and T2-weighted spin echo MR images.

Tendon ruptures may be acute or chronic and partial or complete. With MR imaging, recent tendon tears frequently reveal regions of increased signal intensity on T2-weighted spin echo MR images and certain gradient

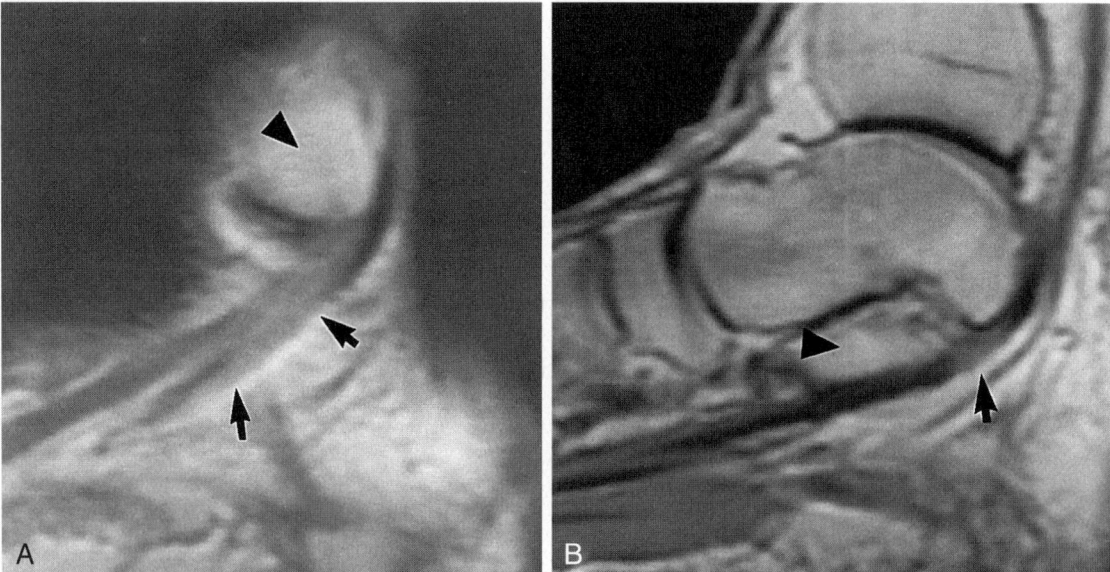

**Figure 59–130.** Tendons about the ankle: normal variations—magic angle phenomenon. *A*, Peroneus longus and brevis tendons. Sagittal T1-weighted (TR/TE, 600/20) spin echo MR image reveals a slight increase in signal intensity *(arrows)* of the peroneus tendons as they course about the distal portion of the fibula *(arrowhead)*. This alteration in signal intensity relates to the magic angle phenomenon. *B*, Flexor hallucis longus tendon. Sagittal T1-weighted (TR/TE, 600/20) spin echo MR image shows a slight increase in signal intensity *(arrow)* in the flexor hallucis longus tendon near the sustentaculum tali *(arrowhead)* related to the magic angle phenomenon. (Courtesy of D. Goodwin, MD, Hanover, N.H., and D. Salonen, MD, Toronto, Ontario, Canada.)

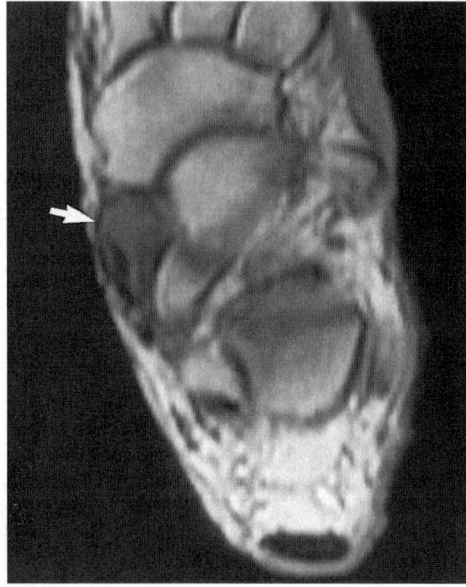

**Figure 59–131.** Tendons about the ankle: normal variations—bulbous tendon insertion sites. As shown on this transaxial T1-weighted (TR/TE, 600/20) spin echo MR image, the navicular insertion site *(arrow)* of the tibialis posterior tendon may normally look bulbous and have increased signal intensity. (Courtesy of D. Goodwin, MD, Hanover, N.H., and D. Salonen, MD, Toronto, Ontario, Canada.)

echo images because of the presence of edema and hemorrhage. Remote tendon tears generally do not have these high-signal-intensity characteristics because of the presence of scar tissue. With regard to the extent of the tendon tear, three MR imaging patterns have been described (Fig. 59–132):

*Type 1.* Partial tendon rupture with tendon hypertrophy. The involved tendon appears hypertrophied and has heterogeneous signal intensity.

*Type 2.* Partial tendon rupture with tendon attenuation. The involved tendon is stretched and attenuated in size.

*Type 3.* Complete tendon rupture with tendon retraction. The involved tendon is discontinuous, and in some cases, a gap filled with fluid, fat, or scar tissue is evident, depending on the age of the tear.

## Abnormalities of the Achilles Tendon

The Achilles tendon, formed by the confluence of the gastrocnemius and soleus tendons, courses along the posterior surface of the ankle and is separated from the ankle joint by the pre-Achilles fat body. Superiorly, the Achilles tendon is a flattened band of tissue. As it descends, it becomes rounded, and close to the point of attachment of the tendinous fibers to the calcaneus, the fibers take a

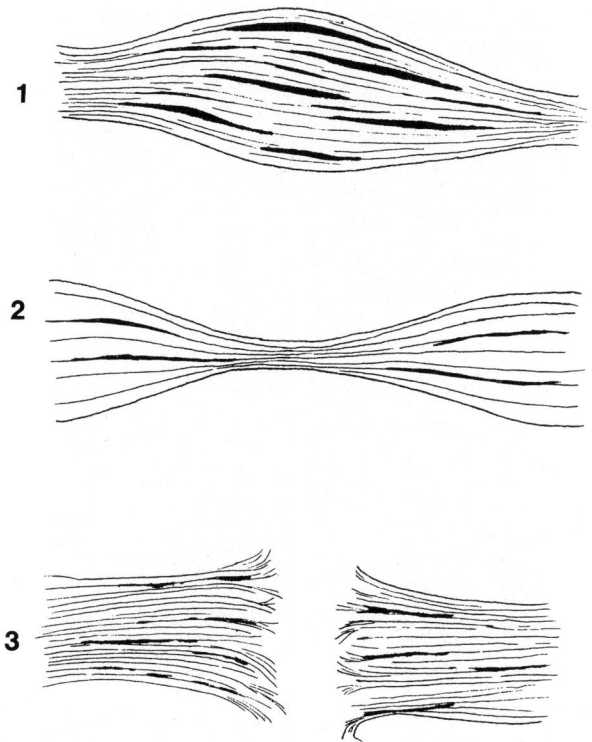

**Figure 59–132.** Tendons about the ankle: types of tendon tears. Type 1 tears are characterized by partial disruption of the tendon, with vertical splits and a bulbous or hypertrophied appearance. Type 2 tears are characterized by partial disruption of the tendon, which appears attenuated. Type 3 tears are characterized by complete disruption of the tendon and retraction of the torn ends. (Modified from Rosenberg ZS, Cheung Y, Jahss MH, et al: Rupture of posterior tibial tendon: CT and MR imaging with surgical correlation. Radiology 169:229, 1988.)

spiral twist. The vulnerable region of the Achilles tendon is just proximal to the inception of this spiral twist and involves a segment between 2 and 6 cm from its insertion into the calcaneus. The normal blood supply in this region is tenuous. The Achilles tendon does not possess a tendon sheath.

The MR imaging features of the Achilles tendon parallel the anatomic features (Fig. 59–133). The average anteroposterior diameter of the Achilles tendon is 5.2 mm. The anterior margin of the tendon is mildly convex in 10% of asymptomatic persons.

Chronic tendinosis leads to thickening of the Achilles tendon. The involved tendon feels thickened, fibrotic, and nodular on physical examination, and it may be tender to palpation. Radiography, CT, and ultrasonography can all document the enlarged Achilles tendon that characterizes chronic tendinosis. The classic MR imaging feature of chronic Achilles tendinosis, with or without surrounding peritendinitis and paratendinitis, is a diffusely or focally enlarged or thickened tendon (Fig. 59–134). The signal intensity in the involved portion of the Achilles tendon is generally low; when intratendinous foci of increased signal intensity are observed on T2-weighted spin echo MR images, an accompanying partial tear of the Achilles tendon is likely.

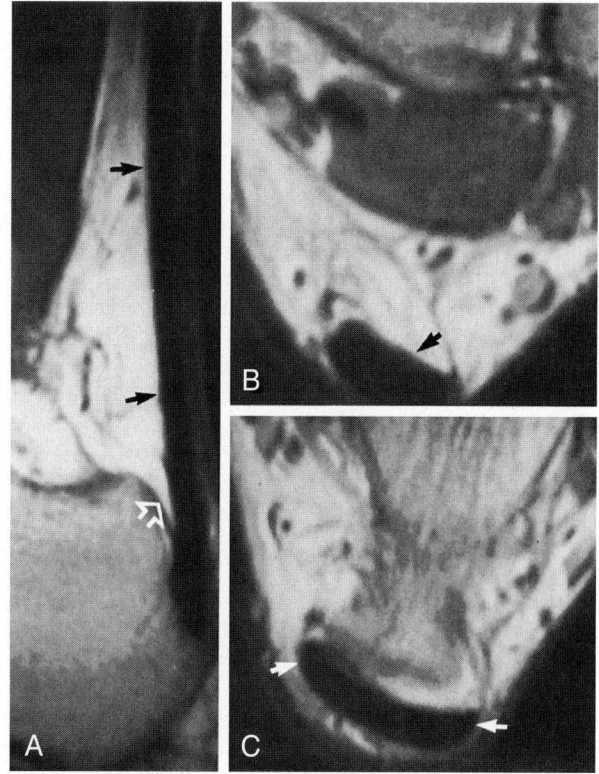

**Figure 59–133.** Achilles tendon: normal appearance. *A,* Sagittal T1-weighted (TR/TE, 650/20) spin echo MR image shows the smooth, straight contour of the Achilles tendon *(solid arrows)* and its sharp interface with the pre-Achilles fat pad. Note the triangular region of fat *(open arrow)* that separates the Achilles tendon and the posterosuperior portion of the calcaneus. *B* and *C,* Transaxial T1-weighted (TR/TE, 650/20) spin echo MR images at the level of the ankle joint *(B)* and just above the calcaneal atttachment of the Achilles tendon *(C)* show the changing shape of the Achilles tendon *(arrows)*. In *B,* the anterior margin of the Achilles tendon is flat or slightly concave; in *C,* a wider structure with a flat anterior margin is evident.

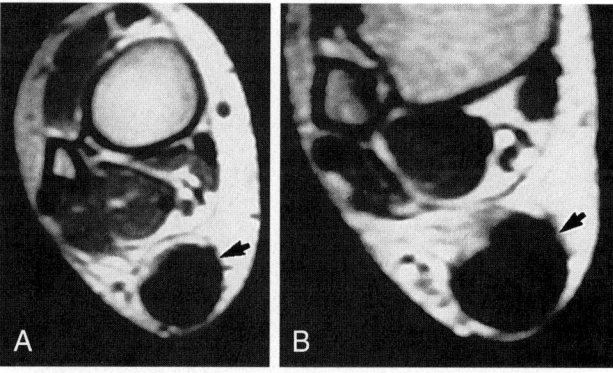

**Figure 59–134.** Chronic Achilles tendinosis. Transaxial intermediate-weighted (TR/TE, 2500/20) spin echo MR image at the level of the distal portions of the tibia and fibula *(A)* and transaxial T2-weighted (TR/TE, 2500/70) spin echo MR image at a slightly lower level *(B)* show a markedly enlarged Achilles tendon *(arrows)* that is of low signal intensity on both images.

Complete disruption of the Achilles tendon by indirect violence is five to six times more common in men than in women. Complete rupture of this tendon usually occurs in persons between the ages of 30 and 50 years. The typical patient is a middle-aged sedentary man who partakes in strenuous activity requiring sudden or forceful dorsiflexion or push-off of the foot. Clinical findings include severe pain, local soft tissue swelling and hemorrhage, and a positive Thompson's test, in which the patient is unable to stand on tiptoe on the affected leg.

MR imaging findings of a partial or complete tear of the Achilles tendon (Fig. 59–135) include discontinuity of some or all of its fibers, intratendinous regions of increased signal intensity on T2-weighted spin echo and STIR MR images, and, in the case of total disruption, a tendinous gap that is filled with blood and edema of increased signal intensity on these images.

## Abnormalities of the Tibialis Posterior Tendon

The tibialis posterior muscle plays a critical role in stabilizing the hindfoot, including the talus and subtalar joints, by preventing valgus deformity of the hindfoot and excessive pronation of the forefoot. As it descends in the lower portion of the leg, the tendon of the tibialis posterior muscle is deep to that of the flexor digitorum longus muscle and lies within a groove behind the medial malleolus of the tibia (Figs. 59–136 and 59–137). From there, the tendon of the tibialis posterior muscle enters the foot by passing deep to the flexor retinaculum and superficial to the deltoid ligament. Distally, the tibialis posterior tendon inserts via a superficial branch into the tuberosity of the navicular

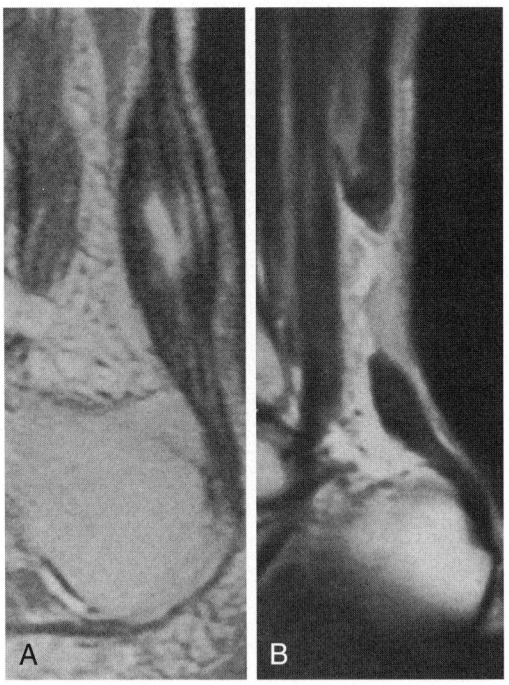

**Figure 59–135.** Chronic Achilles tendinosis with a partial or complete tear. *A*, Partial tear. Sagittal T2-weighted (TR/TE, 2000/70) spin echo MR image shows an enlarged Achilles tendon containing irregular regions of high signal intensity. *B*, Complete tear. Sagittal intermediate-weighted (TR/TE, 3000/30) spin echo MR image shows complete disruption of the Achilles tendon and a proximal segment that is inhomogeneous in signal intensity. Note the edema and hemorrhage of high signal intensity about the acutely torn tendon.

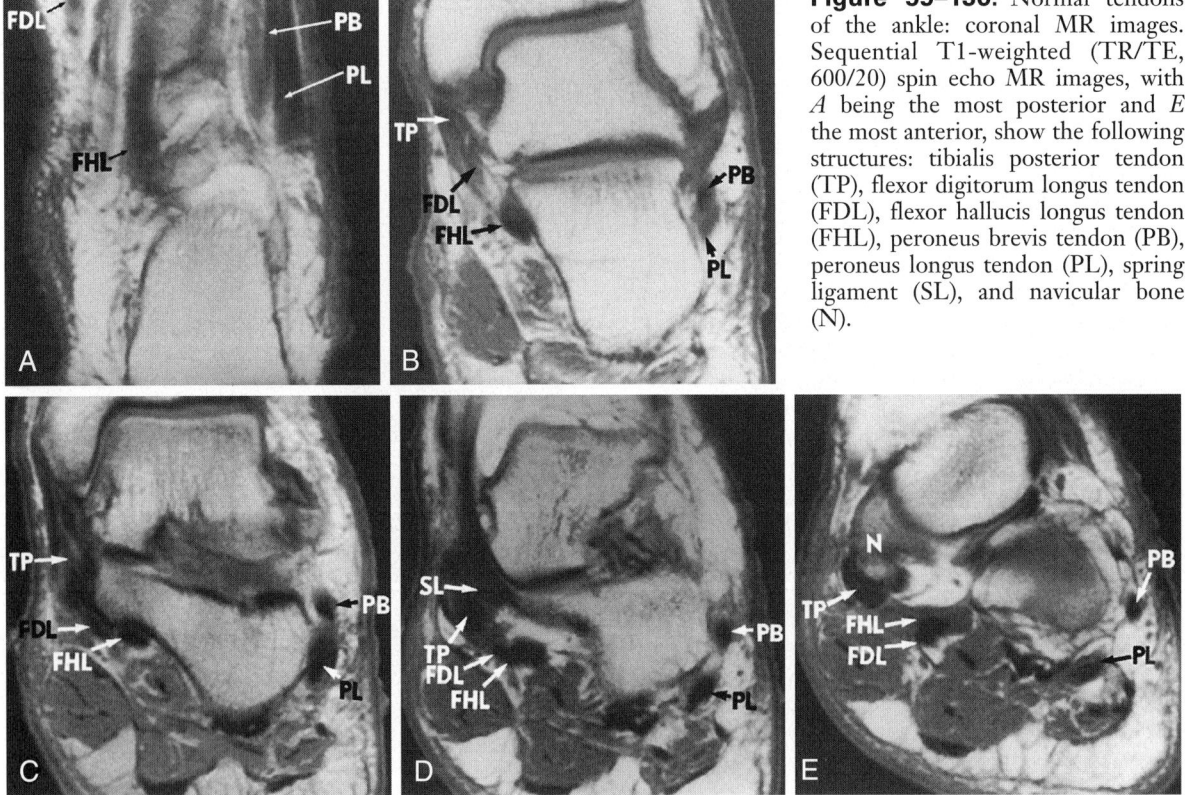

**Figure 59–136.** Normal tendons of the ankle: coronal MR images. Sequential T1-weighted (TR/TE, 600/20) spin echo MR images, with *A* being the most posterior and *E* the most anterior, show the following structures: tibialis posterior tendon (TP), flexor digitorum longus tendon (FDL), flexor hallucis longus tendon (FHL), peroneus brevis tendon (PB), peroneus longus tendon (PL), spring ligament (SL), and navicular bone (N).

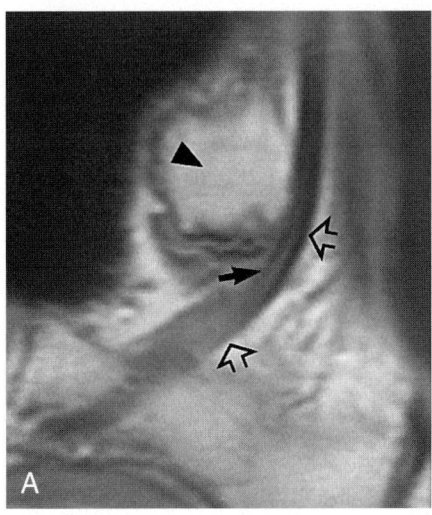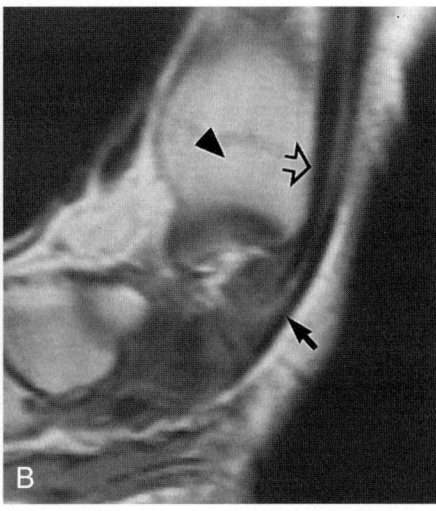

**Figure 59–137.** Normal tendons of the ankle: sagittal MR images. *A*, T1-weighted (TR/TE, 600/20) spin echo MR image through the lateral malleolus *(arrowhead)* shows portions of the peroneus longus *(open arrows)* and peroneus brevis *(solid arrow)* tendons. *B*, T1-weighted (TR/TE, 600/20) spin echo MR image through the medial malleolus *(arrowhead)* reveals the tibialis posterior *(open arrow)* and flexor digitorum longus *(solid arrow)* tendons.

bone, the inferior capsule of the cuneonavicular joint, and the medial cuneiform bone. Disruption of the tibialis posterior tendon, which is being recognized with increasing frequency, is associated with an inability to supinate and invert the foot and, in some cases, with progressive and painful planovalgus deformity of the foot.

Degenerative changes in the tendon and inflammatory changes in the tendon sheath of the tibialis posterior muscle are encountered as a result of altered mechanics of the foot or as a response to a systemic articular disease such as rheumatoid arthritis or a seronegative spondyloarthropathy. Spontaneous rupture of the tibialis posterior tendon is classically seen in patients in the fifth and sixth decades of life, with two thirds of cases occurring in women. Initial manifestations include pain, swelling, and tenderness to palpation of the affected tendon. Progressive involvement results in weakness of inversion of the foot and flattening of the medial longitudinal arch of the foot, with the eventual appearance of severe pes planus deformity. Spontaneous rupture of the tibialis posterior tendon unrelated to a systemic rheumatic disease appears to result from local mechanical factors. Acute angulation of the tendon behind the medial malleolus and, perhaps, a vulnerable blood supply make it susceptible to injury. Further, an accessory ossicle of the navicular bone may provide the site of attachment of some of the fibers of the tibialis posterior tendon, also predisposing to failure of the tendon mechanism.

Although routine radiographs and those obtained during weight bearing allow the diagnosis of long-standing disruption of the tibialis posterior tendon, these methods are less useful in the diagnosis of early disruption because of the presence of a number of deformities (e.g., an increase in the angle between the long axis of the talus and that of the calcaneus, a sag at the calcaneonavicular and naviculocuneiform articulations, and lateral subluxation of the navicular bone with respect to the talus). CT and MR imaging appear to be more valuable than ultrasonography and tenography in the evaluation of degeneration and disruption of the tibialis posterior tendon.

With both CT and MR imaging, type 1 partial tears are associated with tendon hypertrophy and, when longitudinal splitting is prominent, tendon division into two parts. With MR imaging, an abnormal increase in signal intensity may be seen within the enlarged or bifurcated tibialis posterior tendon, especially on intermediate-weighted spin echo MR images, but also occasionally on T2-weighted spin echo and STIR images. Type 2 partial tears lead to a diminution in size of the tibialis posterior tendon, especially its width. Complete tears of the tibialis posterior tendon are associated with tendon retraction and a gap (Fig. 59–138).

### Abnormalities of the Flexor Hallucis Longus Tendon

Abnormalities of the flexor hallucis longus tendon are encountered less commonly than those of the Achilles

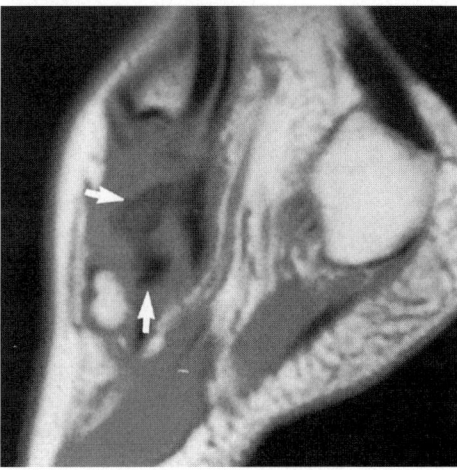

**Figure 59–138.** Injuries of the tibialis posterior tendon: acute complete tear. Sagittal T1-weighted (TR/TE, 800/12) spin echo MR image shows disorganization of the tibialis posterior tendon *(arrows)* near its navicular site of insertion. Note a mass of intermediate signal intensity about the tendon.

and tibialis posterior tendons. Such abnormalities include tendinosis and partial or complete disruption, partial tethering (i.e., os trigonum syndrome), and complete tethering (i.e., checkrein deformity). Flexor hallucis longus tendinosis usually occurs behind the medial malleolus.

MR imaging can be used to assess degeneration or rupture of the flexor hallucis longus tendon (Fig. 59–139), although fluid in the sheath of this tendon may be a normal finding in patients with large ankle effusions because of communication between the sheath and the ankle, which occurs in approximately 20% of normal persons. Partial tethering of the tendon of the flexor hallucis longus muscle may result from hypertrophy of the os trigonum, a condition designated the os trigonum syndrome. The posterior aspect of the talus normally has two tubercles, the medial tubercle and the lateral tubercle, between which is found the fibro-osseous tunnel of the flexor hallucis longus tendon. The os trigonum is the ununited lateral tubercle of the talus, is present in approximately 10% of persons, and is bilateral in 50%. The medial edge of the os trigonum (or trigonal process of the talus) lies under the flexor hallucis longus tendon, on the lateral side of the flexor hallucis longus tunnel, and it may lead to compression of the tendon in this area. CT or MR imaging is useful in defining the relationship between the os trigonum and flexor hallucis longus tendon in some patients with this syndrome.

The checkrein deformity consists of a fixed tethering of the flexor hallucis longus tendon under or just proximal to the flexor retinaculum (internal annular ligament) of the ankle; such tethering leads to unexplained flexion contracture of the interphalangeal joint of the hallux with a mild extension contracture of the first metatarsophalangeal joint (claw hallux). A healing fracture of the lower portion of the tibia may lead to this deformity as a result of post-traumatic adhesions.

### Abnormalities of the Tibialis Anterior Tendon

Spontaneous rupture of the tibialis anterior tendon is rare. Spontaneous ruptures typically appear in patients older than 45 or 50 years, and they may be complete or partial in extent. Rupture of the tibialis anterior tendon may also develop in athletes such as runners, soccer players, and hikers. On clinical examination, a mass related to protrusion of the proximal portion of the torn tendon above the inferior retinaculum may be noted. Retraction of the torn end beneath the superior retinaculum may also be seen. Inflammation of the adjacent tendon sheaths is frequently apparent. MR imaging (Fig. 59–140) and CT allow an accurate diagnosis in most cases.

### Abnormalities of the Peroneal Tendons

The peroneus longus and brevis muscles are important lateral stabilizers of the ankle joint. The peroneus longus muscle serves to evert and dorsiflex the foot, and the brevis muscle contributes to eversion of the foot. During its course, the peroneus longus tendon undergoes an abrupt change in direction at two points: at the tip of the lateral malleolus, and at the distal (lateral) edge of the cuboid bone. In both these locations, the tendon is thickened, and at the point of contact with the smooth surface of the edge of the cuboid bone, a sesamoid composed of fibrocartilage or bone may be found within the tendon. The tendon of the peroneus brevis muscle, after passing behind the fibula, runs forward on the lateral surface of the calcaneus, above the peroneus longus tendon to insert into the tuberosity of the lateral aspect of the base of the fifth metatarsal bone.

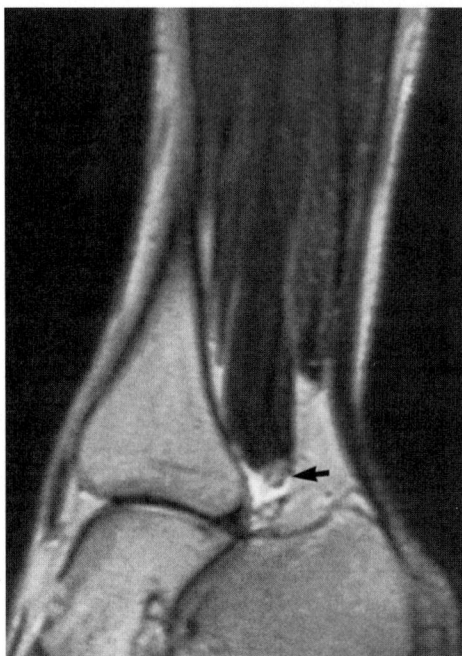

**Figure 59–139.** Injuries of the flexor hallucis longus tendon: acute partial tear. This 43-year-old man heard a pop while running that was immediately followed by severe pain. Sagittal T2-weighted (TR/TE, 3500/102) fast spin echo MR image shows the site of tendon tear *(arrow)*, which is associated with high signal intensity. Other images showed that some of the tendinous fibers were intact.

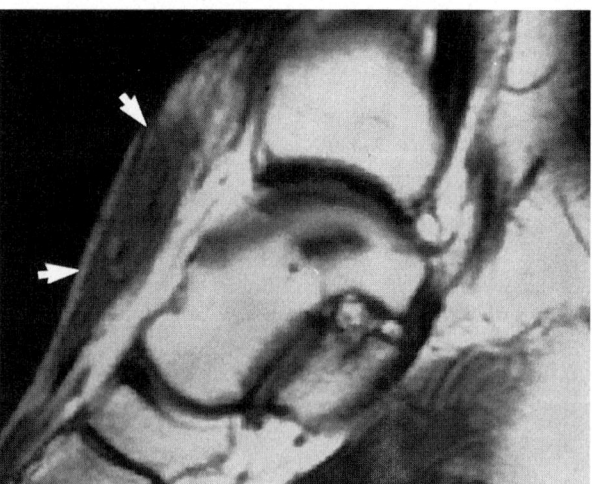

**Figure 59–140.** Injuries of the tibialis anterior tendon: acute complete tear. Sagittal T1-weighted (TR/TE, 450/15) spin echo MR image shows an enlarged tibialis anterior tendon and sheath *(arrows)* containing foci of increased signal intensity.

On MR imaging, the peroneus longus and brevis tendons are approximately equal in size, although the peroneus brevis tendon in the region of the fibular groove is often elongated and flattened in shape. At this level, this tendon is located anterior, medial, or anteromedial to the peroneus longus tendon. Changes in the appearance of these tendons occur with alterations in the position of the foot.

Subluxation and dislocation of the peroneal tendons are often classified as habitual (i.e., voluntary) and traumatic. Habitual subluxations are commonly bilateral and are reproduced by voluntary maneuvers involving the ankle and foot, often leading to a snapping sensation or sound. Traumatic dislocations of the peroneal tendons are associated with disruption of the superior retinaculum or stripping of the periosteal membrane in the distal portion of the fibula at the sites of attachment of this retinaculum. In either situation, the retinaculum becomes functionally deficient, thereby allowing the peroneal tendons to subluxate in a lateral or forward direction.

Routine radiography may disclose a small avulsion fracture adjacent to the lateral surface of the lateral malleolus, an important and often diagnostic observation (Fig. 59–141). The bone fragment is 1 to 1.5 cm long and is best appreciated on the ankle mortise view. Identification of subluxation or dislocation of the peroneal tendons can also be accomplished with peroneal tenography, ultrasonography, CT, and MR imaging.

Fractures of the calcaneus may be associated with lateral displacement of the lateral wall of the bone, with resultant narrowing of the fibulocalcaneal space. Entrapment of the peroneal tendons between the fibula, calcaneus, and talus; subluxation or dislocation of the peroneal tendons; or a combination of the two may result. Clinical manifestations of peroneal tendon entrapment include tenosynovitis, limited subtalar motion, local tenderness, and an antalgic gait. Ultrasonography, tenography, and MR imaging (Fig. 59–142) can be used to diagnose degeneration of the peroneal tendons and inflammation of their sheaths. Differentiation of physiologic and pathologic collections of fluid in the peroneal tendon sheath is difficult. In general, however, tenosynovitis in this location is relatively unusual.

Partial or complete disruption of one or both peroneal tendons can accompany an acute injury or occur spontaneously. Such disruptions are often associated with ligamentous injuries and ankle laxity. Spontaneous ruptures of these tendons are rare. Partial tears are more common than complete disruptions, and complete tears of both tendons are rare. Retraction of the torn tendon is less common in cases of peroneal tendon disruption than in cases of Achilles tendon disruption. In the usual situation, longitudinal splits and hypertrophy of the peroneus brevis tendon are evident pathologically.

In some cases, longitudinal splits divide the peroneus brevis tendon into two parts (peroneal split syndrome). Typically, these longitudinal tears are 2.5 to 5 cm long, begin near the tip of the lateral malleolus, and propagate distally or proximally or in both directions. Longitudinal splitting of the tendon of the peroneus brevis muscle into two halves that are connected proximally and distally is termed a bucket-handle tear. Tears of the peroneus longus tendon are often found distally as the tendon enters the cuboid groove. Complete ruptures may be associated with a change in position of the os peroneum, which may be retracted proximally.

## Ligament Abnormalities

### Anatomic Considerations

Anatomically, the ligaments of the ankle are grouped according to their location into three complexes: tibiofibular, medial, and lateral (Table 59–6). The ligaments in the lateral complex are injured most commonly, usually related

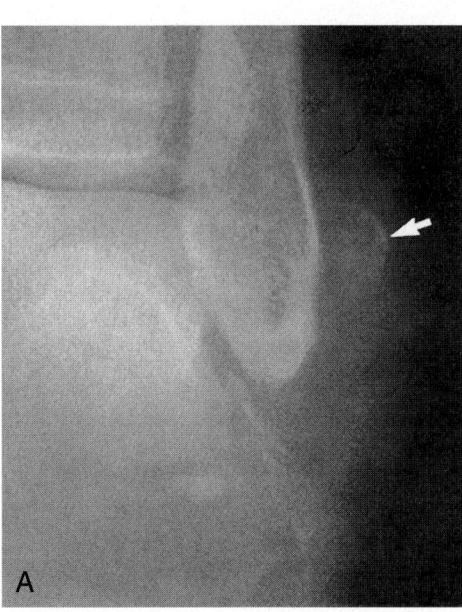
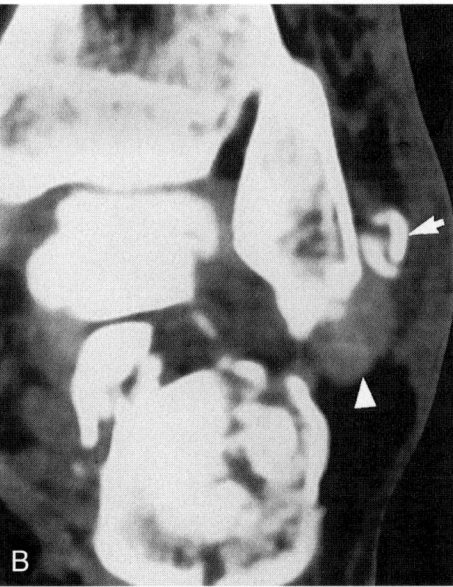

**Figure 59–141.** Injuries of the peroneal tendons and sheath: peroneal tendon dislocation. In this patient with a comminuted calcaneal fracture, a routine radiograph *(A)* reveals the avulsed fibular bone fragment *(arrow)* that is characteristic of peroneal tendon dislocation. Coronal CT scan *(B)* confirms the bone avulsion *(arrow)*. Note its relationship to the peroneal tendons *(arrowhead)* and the fracture of the calcaneus.

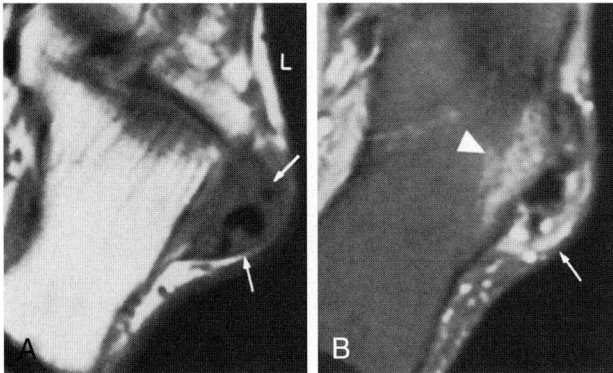

**Figure 59–142.** Injuries of the peroneal tendons and sheath: peroneal tendinosis and tenosynovitis. Transaxial T1-weighted (TR/TE, 400/17) spin echo MR image *(A)* and transaxial T2-weighted (TR/TE, 3300/100) fast spin echo fat-suppressed MR image *(B)* obtained at a slightly more inferior level show a fluid-filled mass *(arrows)* about the peroneus longus and peroneus brevis tendons. Note the reactive edema of the marrow of the calcaneus *(arrowhead in B)*. (Courtesy of S. Eilenberg, MD, San Diego, Calif.)

---

**TABLE 59–6**

**Major Ligaments about the Ankle**

**Lateral Complex**
  Anterior talofibular ligament
  Posterior talofibular ligament
  Calcaneofibular ligament
**Medial Complex**
  Superficial portion
    Tibionavicular ligament
    Tibiospring ligament
    Tibiocalcaneal ligament
    Superficial tibiotalar ligament
  Deep portion
    Deep posterior tibiotalar ligament
    Deep anterior tibiotalar ligament
**Tibiofibular Complex**
  Interosseous ligament
  Anterior tibiofibular ligament
  Posterior tibiofibular ligament
  Transverse tibiofibular ligament

---

to an inversion stress; the ligaments in the medial complex are injured less frequently, generally related to an eversion stress and often in association with a fibular fracture; the ligaments of the tibiofibular complex may be injured as a result of external rotation at the ankle or forced dorsiflexion of the foot, often in combination with a fracture of the fibula.

**Tibiofibular Complex.** Four ligaments, collectively designated the syndesmotic ligaments, bind the apposing portions of the tibia and fibula together (Fig. 59–143). From above downward, they are the interosseous ligament, the anterior tibiofibular ligament, the posterior tibiofibular

ligament, and the transverse tibiofibular ligament. The interosseous ligament represents the lowermost portion of the crural interosseous membrane. The anterior tibiofibular ligament extends between the anterolateral surface of the tibia (including the anterior tubercle) to the adjacent anterior surface of the fibula. As the fibers pass from the tibia to the fibula, they are directed downward and laterally. This ligament is the weakest of the four syndesmotic ligaments. The posterior tibiofibular ligament is the posterior counterpart of the anterior tibiofibular ligament and extends from the posterolateral surface of the tibia (including the posterior tubercle) to the adjacent posterior surface of the fibula. The fibers of this ligament pass upward and medially. External rotation and posterior displacement of the fibula lead to disruption of this ligament. The transverse tibiofibular ligament is the lowermost portion of the posterior tibiofibular ligament and is sometimes designated the deep component of the posterior tibiofibular ligament.

**Medial Complex.** The medial or tibial collateral ligament of the ankle is the strong triangular or fan-shaped deltoid ligament. The deltoid ligament is often (but inconsistently) divided into superficial and deep portions (Fig. 59–144). The superficial portion of the deltoid ligament is further divided into three sets of fibers; in an anterior to posterior direction, they are the tibionavicular, tibiocalcaneal, and superficial tibiotalar fibers. The deep portion of the

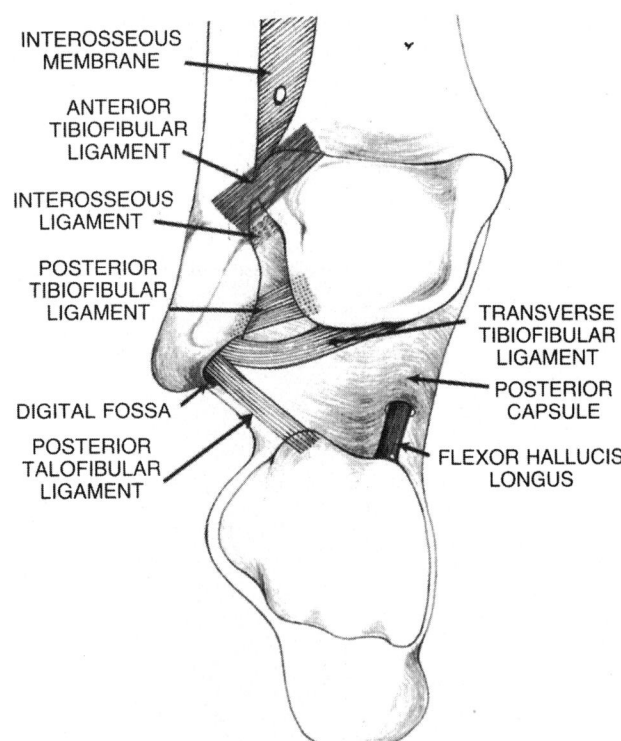

**Figure 59–143.** Syndesmotic ligaments and related structures: normal anatomy. (From Kelikian H, Kelikian AS: Disorders of the Ankle. Philadelphia, WB Saunders, 1985, p 5.)

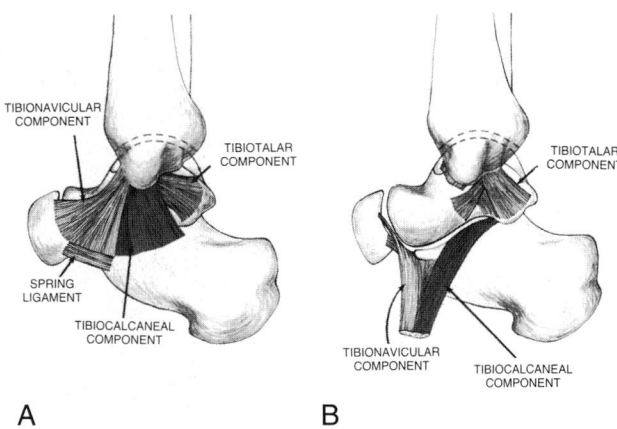

**Figure 59–144.** Medial (tibial) collateral ligament: normal anatomy. (From Kelikian H, Kelikian AS: Disorders of the Ankle. Philadelphia, WB Saunders, 1985, p 20.)

deltoid ligament extends from the tip of the medial malleolus to the entire nonarticular medial surface of the body of the talus. The tendons of the tibialis posterior and flexor digitorum longus muscles are located superficial to the deltoid ligament. The fibers of the deep portion of the deltoid ligament prevent the talus from being displaced laterally.

**Lateral Complex.** The lateral ligamentous complex of the ankle, referred to as the fibular collateral ligament, consists of three components, or fasciculi, all of which attach to the lateral (fibular) malleolus (Fig. 59–145). The anterior talofibular ligament passes from the anterior margin of the fibular malleolus in a forward and medial direction to attach to the lateral articular facet and lateral aspect of the neck of the talus. The anterior talofibular ligament is almost horizontal with the talus in a neutral position, is directed slightly upward as it passes medially with the talus in dorsiflexion, and is directed downward as it passes medially with the talus in plantar flexion. This

component of the lateral ligamentous complex is the weakest and is injured most often. The calcaneofibular ligament extends across two joints (the talocrural and posterior subtalar joints) in an inferior and posterior direction from a depression in front of the apex of the lateral malleolus to attach to a tubercle on the lateral surface of the calcaneus. The tendons of the peroneus longus and peroneus brevis muscles and their sheaths cross over this ligament. This ligament serves to stabilize the posterior subtalar joint. The posterior talofibular ligament is a strong, horizontally oriented structure that passes from the lower part of the fossa of the lateral malleolus to the lateral tubercle of the posterior process of the talus.

### *Pathologic Considerations*

Injuries to the ligaments about the ankle are one of the most frequently encountered consequences of trauma. They are typically seen in young adults, particularly those involved in sports. The lateral ligamentous complex is injured more commonly than the medial or tibiofibular complex. Of the lateral ligaments, the anterior talofibular ligament is affected most frequently, either alone or in combination with an injury to the calcaneofibular ligament.

Classification of ligamentous injuries is based on the specific site or sites of involvement and their severity. Injuries to the collateral ligaments of the ankle are often designated low ankle sprains, and injuries to the syndesmotic ligaments are commonly termed high ankle sprains. The severity of the injury may be categorized as grade I, II, or III. Grade I injuries are the least severe, apparently representing failure of some of the tendinous fibers; grade III injuries are the most severe and are associated with complete ligamentous disruption and instability of the ankle joint; and grade II injuries are intermediate in severity. Instability of the ankle implies abnormal joint motion during the application of varus or valgus stress or positive results during an anterior drawer test.

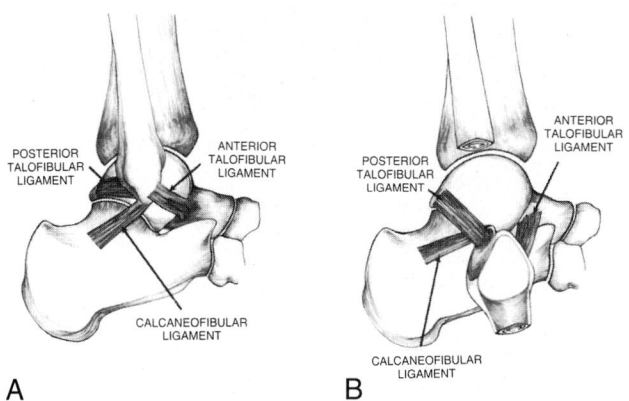

**Figure 59–145.** Lateral ligamentous complex of the ankle: normal anatomy. (From Kelikian H, Kelikian AS: Disorders of the Ankle. Philadelphia, WB Saunders, 1985, p 20.)

## Imaging Considerations

Initial assessment of injuries to the medial, lateral, and syndesmotic ligaments about the ankle requires routine radiography, which allows the detection of any accompanying fractures (see Chapter 57), and radiography obtained during the application of stress. Complementary imaging methods are arthrography and MR imaging; ultrasonography may also be helpful.

MR imaging has been used extensively to evaluate ligamentous injuries about the ankle. Whether the ankle ligaments are evaluated with the foot in a neutral position, plantar-flexed, dorsiflexed, or in some combination of these positions, three MR imaging planes are usually required to fully evaluate all the ligaments of the ankle. Normal ligaments are thin and of low signal intensity. The anterior talofibular ligament is the easiest to identify, particularly on transaxial MR images (Fig. 59–146). It is usually homogeneous in appearance. Similarly, the posterior talofibular ligament is identified most readily in the transaxial plane (although it is also seen on coronal images), and its posterior aspect is intimately related to the peroneal longus tendon and its sheath (see Fig. 59–146). The MR imaging findings associated with disruption of the ligaments about the ankle include interruption of part or all of a ligament, ligament laxity or waviness, thickening and irregularity of the ligament, surrounding hemorrhage and edema (in acute injuries), and accumulation of abnormal amounts of fluid in adjacent joints and tendon sheaths (Fig. 59–147). An inability to visualize a ligament may indicate a tear, but the reliability of this finding depends on the ligament being considered and the technical aspects of the MR imaging examination.

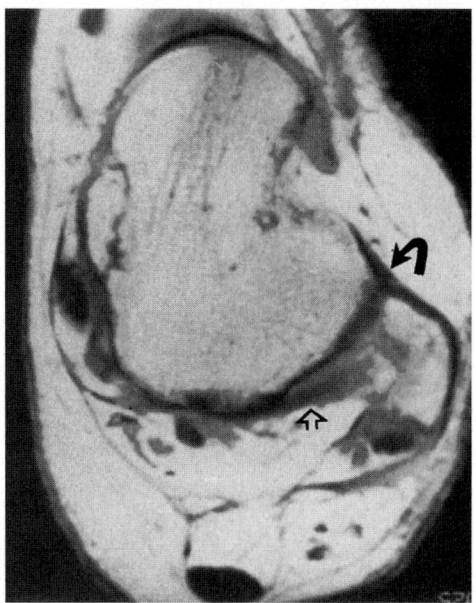

**Figure 59–146.** Normal ligaments of the ankle: anterior and posterior talofibular ligaments. Transaxial T1-weighted (TR/TE, 600/20) spin echo MR image shows the anterior talofibular ligament *(curved arrow)* and posterior talofibular ligament *(open arrow)*.

### Sinus Tarsi Syndrome

Between the two subtalar joints—the posterior subtalar and the talocalcaneonavicular joints—a cone-shaped region designated the tarsal sinus and tarsal canal is found. The apex of the cone is located posteromedially and represents

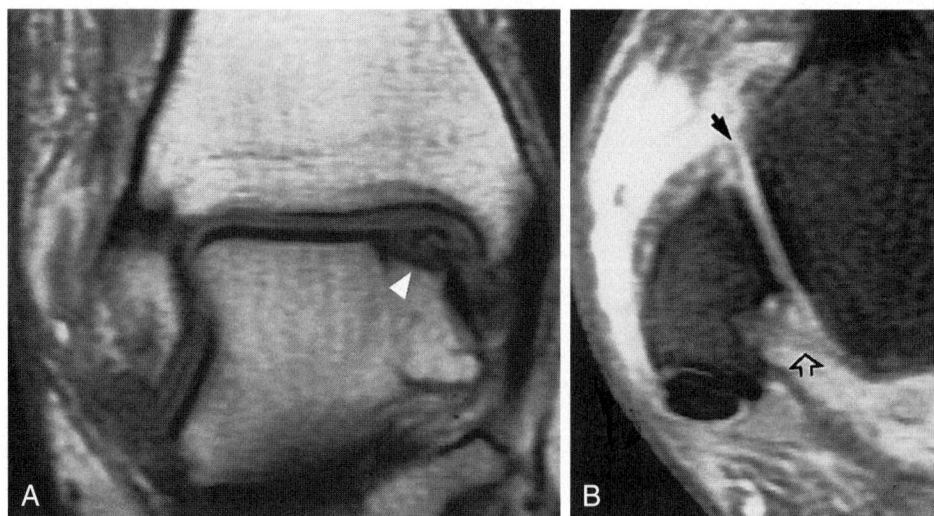

**Figure 59–147.** Injuries of the talofibular ligaments: acute complete tear of the anterior talofibular ligament and acute partial tear of the posterior talofibular ligament. *A,* Coronal T1-weighted (TR/TE, 600/20) spin echo MR image reveals subcutaneous edema laterally and an osteochondral fracture of the talus *(arrowhead).* *B,* Transaxial intermediate-weighted (TR/TE, 2000/20) spin echo MR image obtained with fat suppression at a level just below the ankle shows soft tissue edema and hemorrhage (of high signal intensity), complete disruption of the anterior talofibular ligament *(solid arrow),* and attenuation of the posterior talofibular ligament *(open arrow).* (Courtesy of C. Sebrechts, MD, San Diego, Calif.)

the tarsal canal, and the expanded anterolateral portion of the cone represents the tarsal sinus. The contents of the tarsal canal and sinus include fat, an arterial anastomosis with branches from the posterior tibial and peroneal arteries, joint capsules, nerve endings, and five ligaments. These ligaments are the medial, intermediate, and lateral roots of the inferior extensor retinaculum; the cervical ligament; and the ligament of the tarsal canal (i.e., talocalcaneal interosseous ligament). Injury to these structures leads to the sinus tarsi syndrome, which is associated with lateral foot pain, tenderness, and hindfoot instability. The high association between tarsal sinus and canal injury and injury to the lateral ligaments of the ankle requires careful analysis of the sinus tarsi in all patients with inversion injuries of the ankle.

MR imaging has been used to study the normal contents of the tarsal sinus and canal and to investigate patients with the sinus tarsi syndrome. The cervical ligament and portions of the inferior extensor retinaculum are seen in all normal ankles, and the interosseous ligament is evident in most normal ankles (Fig. 59–148). Fluid collections with increased signal intensity on T2-weighted spin echo MR images are normally evident in the recesses about the talocalcaneal interosseous ligament, although absence of these recesses on MR imaging does not allow a diagnosis of sinus tarsi syndrome. MR imaging findings of this syndrome include poor definition or disruption of soft tissue structures, edema or fibrosis, and abnormal fluid collections (Fig. 59–149). Abnormalities of adjacent structures, such as the anterior talofibular ligament, calcaneofibular ligament, and tibialis posterior tendon, may also be evident.

## Impingement Syndromes

Several impingement syndromes may lead to restricted motion of the ankle joint. These syndromes can be divided into six types: anterior, posterior, posterolateral, anterolateral, syndesmotic, and medial (Table 59–7).

### Anterior Impingement Syndrome

The anterior impingement syndrome results from impingement of the anterior aspect of the tibia against the superior portion of the neck of the talus. It is commonly observed in young athletic persons. Clinical findings include pain and tenderness in the anterior region of the ankle that are accentuated with dorsiflexion of the joint. Routine radiography reveals osteophytes in the anterior surface of the tibia, neck of the talus, or both (Fig. 59–150). Arthroscopic resection of the osteophytes may lead to symptomatic relief and increased ankle motion.

### Posterior Impingement Syndrome

The posterior impingement syndrome may be related to the presence of an os trigonum (Fig. 59–151) or a prominent Stieda's process in the posterior surface of the talus; alternatively, it may result from soft tissue injury. The first of these two types of posterior impingement is often referred to as the os trigonum or talar compression syndrome; the second type is sometimes designated posterior soft tissue impingement. With regard to the talar compression syndrome, symptoms are common because of limitation of plantar flexion at the ankle. For athletes such as professional ballet dancers, the condition

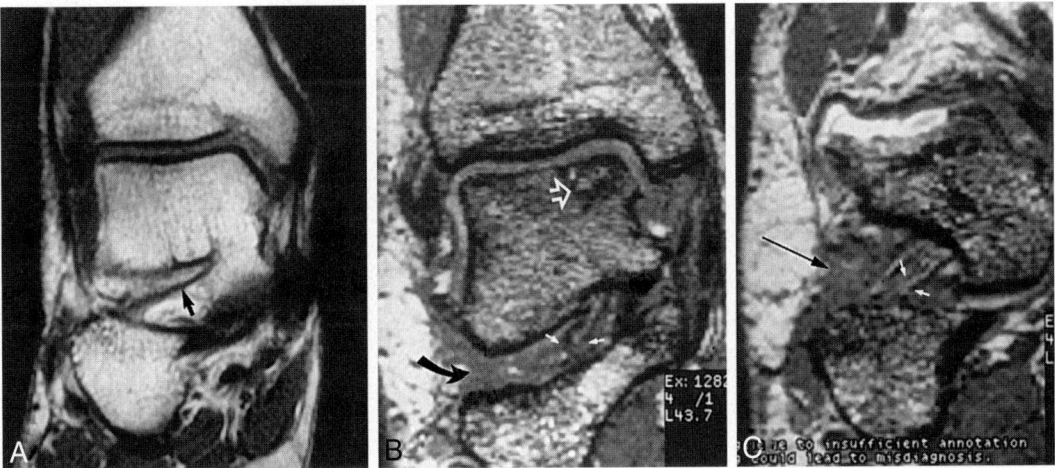

**Figure 59–148.** Sinus tarsi syndrome. *A*, Normal appearance. Coronal T1-weighted (TR/TE, 500/18) spin echo MR image reveals a normal talocalcaneal interosseous ligament *(arrow)*, which is surrounded by fat. *B* and *C*, Sinus tarsi syndrome. Coronal reconstructions from a three-dimensional gradient echo (TR/TE, 30/10; flip angle, 70 degrees) MR image, with *B* being slightly more posterior than *C*, show diffuse infiltration of the tarsal sinus *(black arrow)*. In *B*, partial disruption of the talocalcaneal interosseous ligament has led to a wavy, discontinuous appearance *(solid white arrows)*. A small osteochondral fracture of the medial talar dome *(open white arrow)* is seen. In *C*, partial disruption of the cervical ligament *(white arrows)* is evident. (From Klein MA, Spreitzer AM: MR imaging of the tarsal sinus and canal: normal anatomy, pathologic findings, and features of the sinus tarsi syndrome. Radiology 186:233, 1993.)

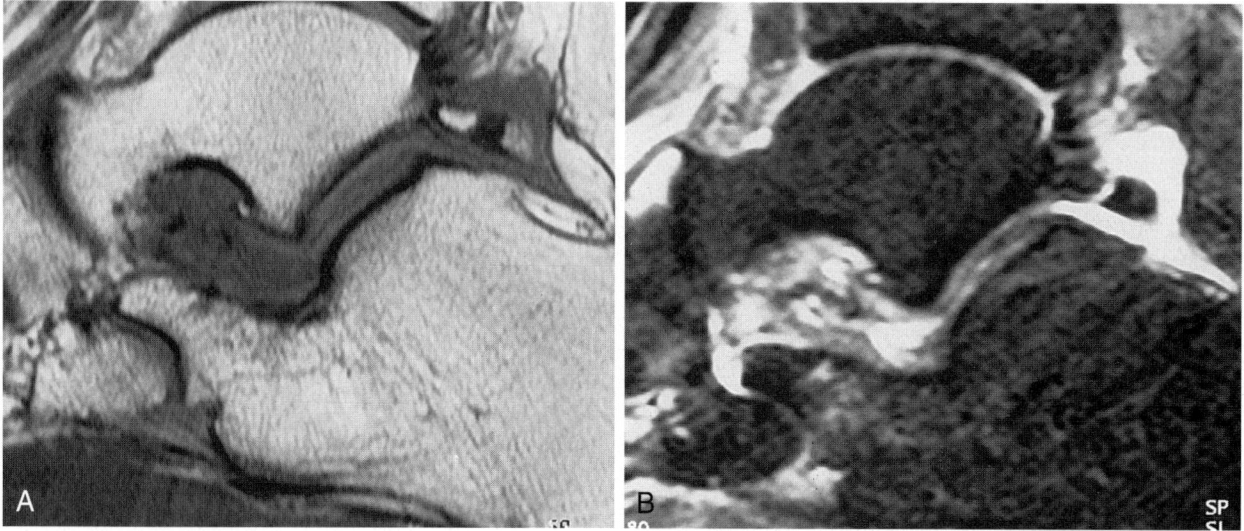

**Figure 59–149.** Sinus tarsi syndrome. Sagittal T1-weighted (TR/TE, 760/20) spin echo *(A)* and STIR (TR/TE, 5300/30; inversion time, 150 msec) *(B)* MR images reveal obliteration of the fat in the tarsal sinus, with high signal intensity in *B*. (Courtesy of J. Edwards, MD, Savannah, Ga.)

---

**TABLE 59–7**

**Impingement Syndromes of the Ankle**

| Location | Pathologic Findings |
|---|---|
| Anterior | Osteoarthritis of the ankle, osteophytes of the anterior portions of the talus and tibia |
| Anterolateral | Injuries to the lateral capsule, anterior tibiofibular ligament, anterior talofibular ligament, or combinations of these structures, with the formation of scar tissue |
| Posterior | Entrapment of the os trigonum or posterior process of the talus |
| Posterolateral | Injuries to the posterior tibiofibular ligament, including the transverse ligament and intermalleolar slip, and the capsule |
| Syndesmotic | Injuries to the anterior tibiofibular ligament and capsule |
| Medial | Cartilage abnormalities at the tip or anterior distal portion of the medial malleolus and the medial facet of the talus |

may be disabling and require excision of the os trigonum. Accompanying inflammation in the sheath about the flexor hallucis longus tendon may be evident.

Posterior (or posterolateral) soft tissue impingement, which may occur alone or in combination with anterolateral impingement, has several causes: hypertrophy or tearing of the inferior portion of the posterior tibiofibular ligament, the transverse tibiofibular ligament, or the posterior intermalleolar ligament, or some combination of these injuries.

## Anterolateral Impingement Syndrome

The anterolateral impingement syndrome generally occurs in young persons who have sustained injuries to the lateral ligaments of the ankle. A complete or partial tear of the anterior talofibular ligament (or other lateral ligaments) is associated with intra-articular hemorrhage and hyperplasia of the part of the synovial membrane that extends into the articular gutter in the lateral aspect of

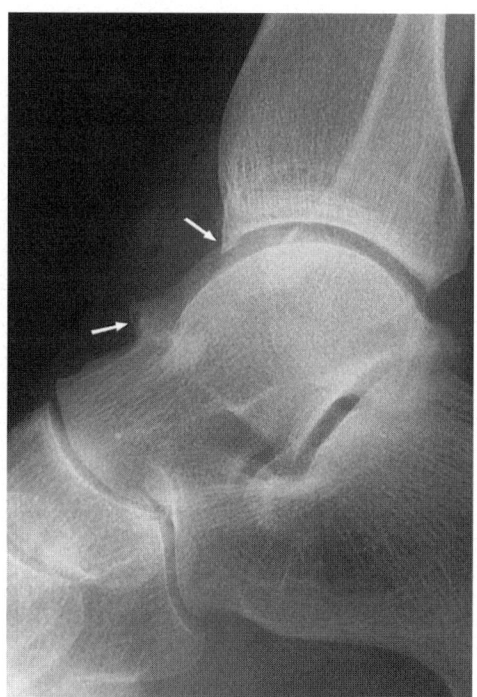

**Figure 59–150.** Anterior impingement syndrome. Observe the osteophytes *(arrows)* involving the anterior surface of the tibia and the talus.

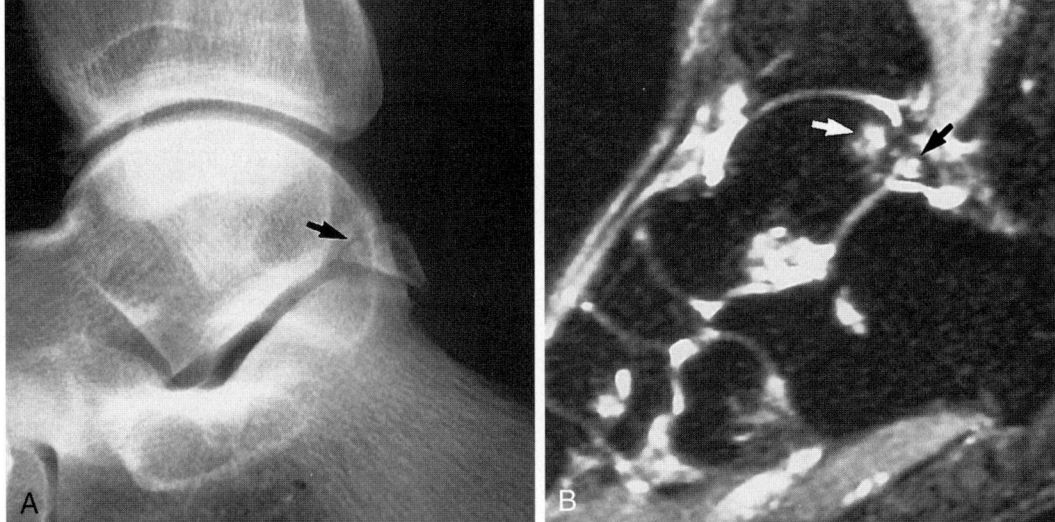

**Figure 59–151.** Posterior impingement syndrome. In this 45-year-old woman, a conventional radiograph *(A)* shows an os trigonum *(arrow)*. A sagittal STIR (TR/TE, 5100/30; inversion time, 150 msec) MR image *(B)* shows high signal intensity *(arrows)* in the os trigonum and adjacent talus, with fluid in the ankle, posterior subtalar joint, and sinus tarsi.

the ankle. CT-arthrography reveals several patterns of abnormal tissue in the anterolateral compartment, including nodular filling defects. MR imaging reveals the mass (Fig. 59–152), which is commonly of low to intermediate signal intensity on both T1- and T2-weighted spin echo MR images.

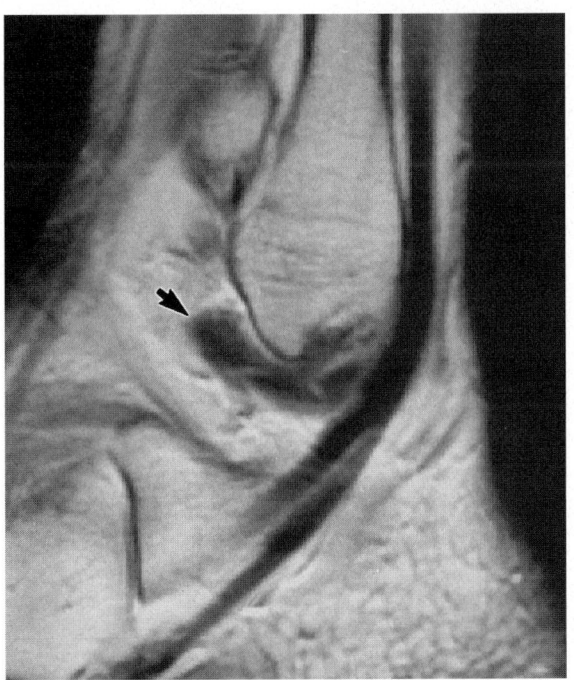

**Figure 59–152.** Anterolateral impingement syndrome. Note a soft tissue mass *(arrow)* anterior to the fibula on a sagittal fast spin echo (TR/TE, 3000/30) MR image. (Courtesy of D. Goodwin, MD, Hanover, N.H.)

### Syndesmotic Impingement Syndrome

Syndesmotic impingement usually results from injuries to the anterior tibiofibular ligament, with or without associated injuries to the interosseous membrane and posterior tibiofibular ligament. Synovitis and scar tissue lead to progressive pain and instability. Excision of the fascicle and débridement of the ankle joint and the anterior tibiofibular ligament may be curative.

### Medial Impingement Syndrome

One cause of this injury is impingement between the medial malleolus and the medial facet of the talus. Chondral abnormalities are detected arthroscopically at these points of abnormal contact, and they differ in location from cartilage lesions of the dome of the talus, which are well recognized after supination injury of the ankle. Other causes of medial ankle pain occurring after inversion injuries of the ankle are partial or complete rupture of the deltoid ligament, chronic synovitis, osteophytes, and scar tissue.

### Synovial and Capsular Abnormalities

#### Adhesive Capsulitis

Although far better known in the glenohumeral joint, post-traumatic adhesive capsulitis is encountered in the ankle. Restriction of ankle motion is detected on clinical examination. Arthrography delineates a decrease in articular capacity, with resistance to injection of contrast material, obliteration of the normal anterior and posterior recesses or the tibiofibular syndesmosis, opacification of lymphatic vessels, and extravasation of contrast material along the needle tract.

## Synovitis

In common with other joints, the ankle may be affected in a variety of systemic rheumatic diseases and local processes. Involvement of surrounding structures such as tendons, tendon sheaths, and bursae and the formation of para-articular synovial cysts may be evident.

## Muscle Abnormalities

### Accessory and Anomalous Muscles

An accessory soleus muscle appears to be a frequent finding, especially on MR imaging examinations. Affected persons are commonly asymptomatic, although soft tissue fullness or a mass and occasionally pain and swelling after exercise may be seen.

The origin and insertion sites of an accessory soleus muscle vary. The muscle may arise from the proximal third of the fibula, the oblique soleal line of the tibia, the aponeurosis of the flexor digitorum longus muscle, the anterior portion of the normal soleus muscle, or some combination of these structures. The insertion sites of an accessory soleus muscle include the Achilles tendon and the superior and medial surfaces of the calcaneus. Diagnosis of this accessory muscle can be accomplished with routine radiography, CT, and MR imaging (Fig. 59–153). Of these techniques, MR imaging appears to be best.

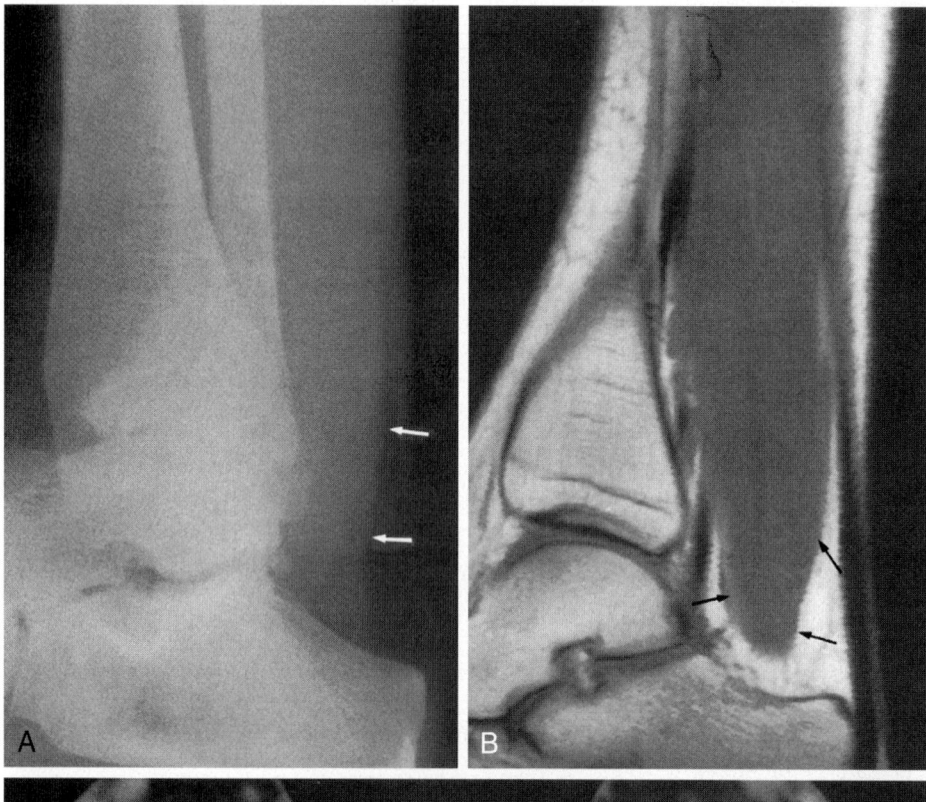

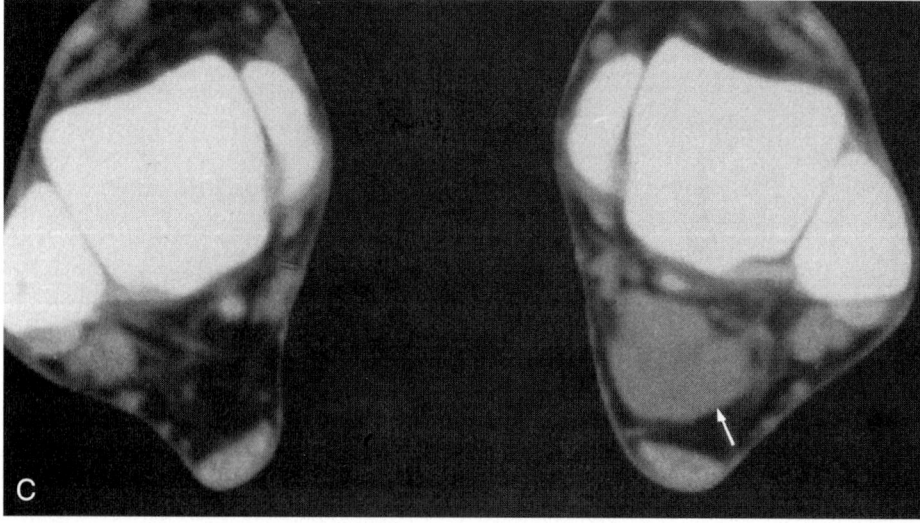

**Figure 59–153.** Accessory soleus muscle. *A* and *B*, Lateral radiograph *(A)* and sagittal T1-weighted (TR/TE, 600/16) spin echo MR image *(B)* show the accessory muscle *(arrows)*. *C*, In a different patient, a transaxial CT scan reveals the accessory soleus muscle *(arrow)*. Compare with the opposite side. (*A* and *B*, Courtesy of G. Greenway, MD, Dallas, Tex. *C*, Courtesy of A. Newberg, MD, Boston, Mass.)

The peroneus quartus muscle, also designated the peroneus accessorius, peroneus externus, and peroneus calcaneus externus muscle, has been associated with chronic pain and swelling about the ankle. Its reported frequency, based on results of cadaveric dissections, varies from approximately 12% to 22%. Its site of origin may include the distal lateral portion of the fibula and the peroneus brevis or longus muscle, and its site of insertion may include the phalanges or metatarsal bone of the fifth toe, the calcaneus, the cuboid bone, and the lateral retinaculum of the ankle. Accurate diagnosis is provided by MR imaging (Fig. 59–154).

## Muscle Hernia

Herniation of a portion of a muscle through its fascial sheath is encountered most often in the leg. Although the tibialis anterior muscle is the typical site of involvement, other muscles can be affected, such as the peroneus longus muscle. Most persons with muscle hernias are asymptomatic, and multiple hernias with bilateral involvement are not uncommon. Accurate diagnosis can be accomplished clinically in many persons. Indeed, the symmetry of bilateral lesions is an important diagnostic clue. MR imaging allows a correct diagnosis in most cases because the subcutaneous masses are seen to be portions of the muscle that extend through defects in the overlying fascia. Ultrasonography is another excellent diagnostic method.

## Abnormalities of the Plantar Soft Tissues

### Plantar Fasciitis

The plantar aponeurosis is a thick, strong band of tissue extending from the calcaneus posteriorly to the region of the metatarsal heads and beyond. It is composed of a prominent central part and lateral and medial parts. Plantar fasciitis represents inflammation of the plantar fascia and perifascial structures. Its causes are divided into three categories: mechanical, degenerative, and systemic. Mechanical factors associated with plantar fasciitis include pes cavus, a pronated foot, and an externally rotated lower extremity. Degenerative causes of plantar fasciitis include atrophy of the heel pad and age-related increases in foot pronation. Systemic causes include a wide variety of rheumatic disorders, especially rheumatoid arthritis and the seronegative spondyloarthropathies.

Clinical findings include pain and tenderness localized to the regions of inflammation. Dorsiflexion of the toes may lead to an exacerbation of the findings as a result of stretching of the fibers of the plantar fascia. Although bone scintigraphy may reveal regions of increased accumulation of the radiopharmaceutical agent at the site of inflammation, the increased scintigraphic activity may be more widespread and produce a nonspecific pattern. With ultrasonography, findings of plantar fasciitis include thickening of the fascia, abnormal echogenicity, and perifascial edema. MR imaging appears to be both sensitive and

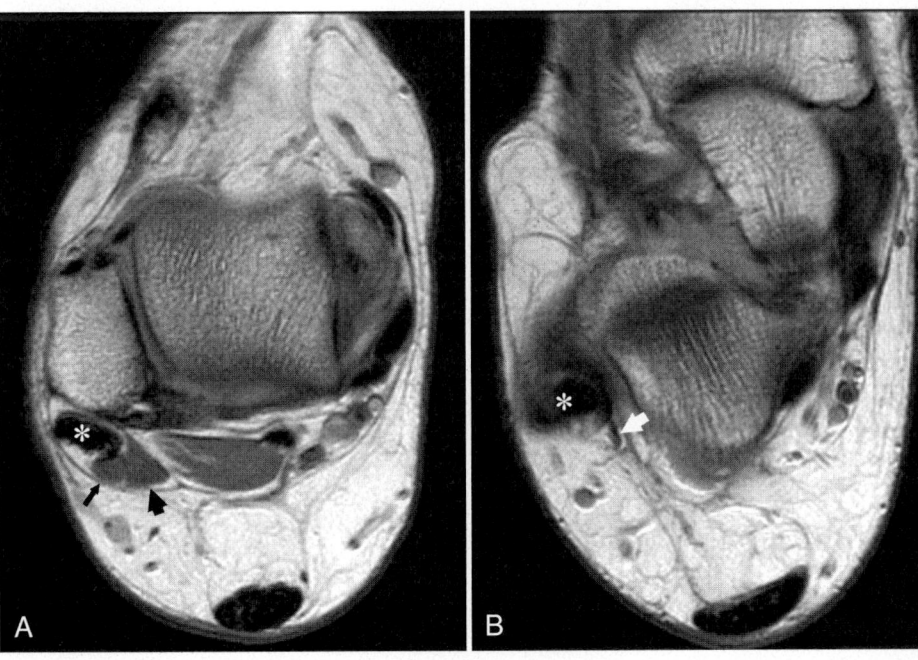

**Figure 59–154.** Accessory peroneus quartus muscle. *A,* Axial fast proton density (TR/TE, 2500/28) spin echo MR image shows the accessory muscle *(large arrow)* medial and adjacent to the peroneal muscle *(small arrow).* The patient was being evaluated for peroneal tendon dysfunction. A longitudinal split tear of the peroneal brevis tendon was found at surgery, as was the peroneal quartus. The peroneal longus tendon *(asterisk)* was intact. *B,* Axial image caudal to *A* shows the peroneal quartus tendon *(arrow)* just proximal to its attachment on the retrotrochlear eminence of the calcaneus. The peroneal longus tendon *(asterisk)* was intact. The split tear of the peroneal brevis tendon is not well seen.

specific in the diagnosis of plantar fasciitis, demonstrating thickening of the plantar fascia (which may grow to 7 or 8 mm from the normal 3 or 4 mm thickness) and intrafascial alterations in signal intensity. On T1-weighted spin echo MR images, foci of intermediate signal intensity may be seen within the plantar fascia, which is normally of uniform low signal intensity. On T2-weighted spin echo and STIR MR images, areas of high signal intensity may be evident in the plantar fascia and subcutaneous tissue (Fig. 59–155). Alterations in signal intensity of the marrow of the calcaneus, reflective of edema, may also be apparent. In some cases, partial fascial tears are seen.

### Plantar Fibromatosis

Plantar fibromatosis is a common condition associated with fibrous proliferation and replacement of portions of the plantar aponeurosis. The disorder is seen in persons of all ages (including children) and is more common in men. Lesions may be solitary or multiple and unilateral or bilateral in distribution. Affected persons are usually asymptomatic, with the nodules being discovered by palpation.

With MR imaging, single or multiple nodules in the plantar fascia and subcutaneous tissue are observed. The medial and central portions of the plantar fascia are typically involved. The lesions are of low signal intensity on T1-weighted spin echo images and low to intermediate signal intensity on T2-weighted spin echo MR images. In some cases, regions of high signal intensity are seen on T2-weighted spin echo or STIR MR images. Enhancement of signal intensity is variable after the intravenous administration of a gadolinium compound.

## Abnormalities of Nerves

### Entrapment Neuropathies

Entrapment neuropathies occurring in the foot and ankle are described in Chapter 65. The most important of these neuropathies relate to compression of the tibial nerve in the medial aspect of the ankle (i.e., the tarsal tunnel syndrome) and entrapment of the deep peroneal nerve.

The tarsal tunnel is located behind and below the medial malleolus; its floor is bony, and its roof is formed by the flexor retinaculum. The resulting fibro-osseous channel allows passage of the tendons of the tibialis posterior, flexor digitorum longus, and flexor hallucis longus muscles; the posterior tibial artery and vein; and the tibial nerve. Causes of compression of the tibial nerve within the tarsal tunnel include tumors of nerves and other structures, tenosynovitis, ganglion cysts (Fig. 59–156), post-traumatic fibrosis, and dilated or tortuous veins. Many of the causes can be defined with CT or MR imaging.

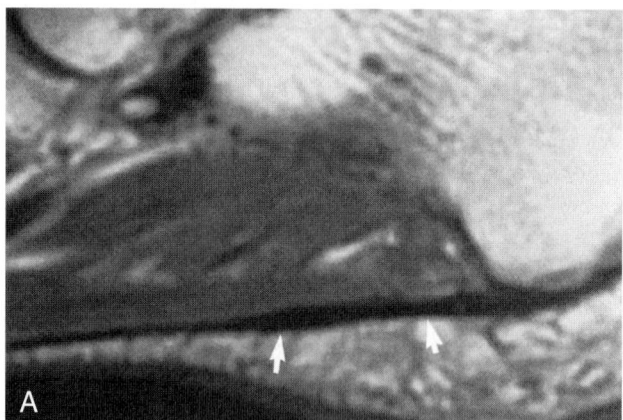

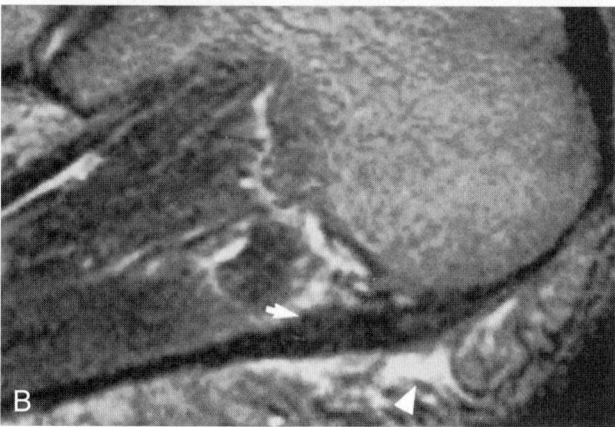

**Figure 59–155.** Plantar fasciitis. *A,* Normal plantar fascia. Sagittal intermediate-weighted (TR/TE, 2000/20) spin echo MR image shows the normal central portion of the plantar fascia *(arrows)* and overlying subcutaneous fibrous septa. *B,* Plantar fasciitis. Sagittal T2-weighted (TR/TE, 2000/80) spin echo MR image reveals subcutaneous edema *(arrowhead)* and focally thickened plantar fascia *(arrow)*. A plantar calcaneal enthesophyte is also present. (From Berkowitz JF, Kier R, Rudicel S: Plantar fasciitis: MR imaging. Radiology 179:665, 1991.)

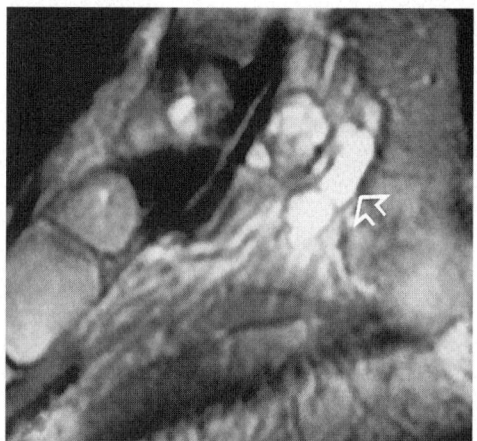

**Figure 59–156.** Entrapment neuropathy. Ganglion cysts in the medial aspect of the ankle led to compression of the tibial nerve. Sagittal T2-weighted (TR/TE, 2000/75) spin echo MR image shows the location of the ganglion cysts *(open arrow)*. (Courtesy of S. Eilenberg, MD, San Diego, Calif.)

Entrapment of the deep peroneal nerve in the ankle and foot may occur in several different locations. The most common site of compression is beneath the inferior extensor retinaculum, a condition referred to as the anterior tarsal tunnel syndrome. Sural nerve entrapment may occur in the ankle and is generally related to fibrosis occurring in response to an ankle sprain, fracture (e.g., calcaneal or fifth metatarsal fracture), Achilles tendon rupture, or ganglion cyst. Entrapment of the superficial peroneal nerve, particularly in the distal portion of the leg and ankle, also occurs, especially as a result of fibrosis secondary to ankle injuries.

### Interdigital Neuroma

Interdigital neuromas, or Morton's neuromas, are not true tumors but represent a fibrotic response that occurs in and about the plantar digital nerves. Interdigital neuromas are encountered most frequently in young and middle-aged persons, especially women. A unilateral distribution predominates but is not universal. The interspace between the third and fourth toes is affected most commonly. The third plantar digital nerve may be most vulnerable because of its large size and relatively fixed position. Clinical findings include pain at the level of the metatarsophalangeal joint that may radiate into the adjacent toes, although these neuromas may be asymptomatic. Because of their persistently low signal intensity on both T1- and T2-weighted spin echo MR images (Fig. 59–157), interdigital neuromas can generally be differentiated from true neuromas, which show high signal intensity on T2-weighted spin echo MR images.

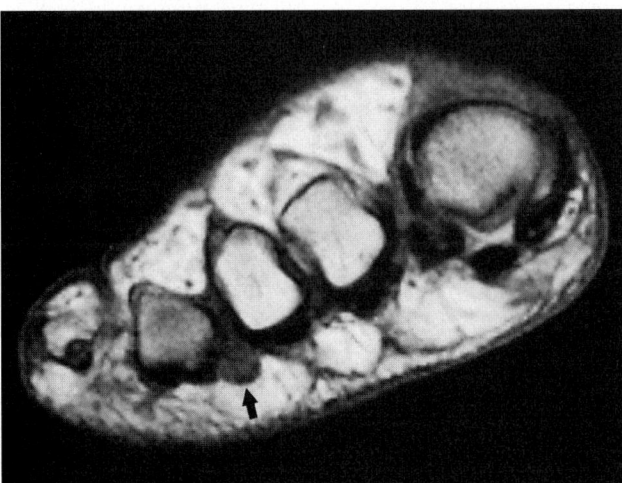

**Figure 59–157.** Morton's neuroma. Coronal T1-weighted (TR/TE, 750/15) spin echo MR image reveals a mass *(arrow)* of low signal intensity between the third and fourth metatarsal bones. Such low signal intensity is characteristic of this lesion.

## FURTHER READING

Berkowitz JF, Kier R, Rudicel S: Plantar fasciitis: MR imaging. Radiology 179:665, 1991.

Bureau NJ, Cardinal E, Hobden R, et al: Posterior ankle impingement syndrome: MR imaging findings in seven patients. Radiology 215:497, 2000.

Campos JC, Chung CB, Lektrakul N, et al: Pathogenesis of the Segond fracture: Anatomic and MR imaging evidence of an iliotibial tract or anterior oblique band avulsion. Radiology 219:381, 2001.

Cervilla V, Schweitzer ME, Ho C, et al: Medial dislocation of the biceps brachii tendon: Appearance at MR imaging. Radiology 180:523, 1991.

Clarke HD, Kitaoka HB, Ehman RL: Peroneal tendon injuries. Foot Ankle 19:280, 1998.

Conway WF, Hayes CW, Loughran T, et al: Cross-sectional imaging of the patellofemoral joint and surrounding structures. Radiographics 11:195, 1991.

De Smet AA, Fisher DR, Graf BK, et al: Osteochondritis dissecans of the knee: Value of MR imaging in determining lesion stability and the presence of articular cartilage defects. AJR Am J Roentgenol 155:549, 1990.

Deutsch AL, Mink JH, Rosenfelt FP, et al: Incidental detection of hematopoietic hyperplasia on routine knee MR imaging. AJR Am J Roentgenol 152:333, 1989.

Deutsch AL, Mink JH, Waxman AD: Occult fractures of the proximal femur: MR imaging. Radiology 170:113, 1989.

El-Khoury GY, Wira RL, Berbaum KS, et al: MR imaging of patellar tendinitis. Radiology 184:849, 1992.

Erickson SJ, Cox IH, Hyde JS, et al: Effect of tendon orientation on MR imaging signal intensity: A manifestation of the "magic angle" phenomenon. Radiology 181:389, 1991.

Erickson SJ, Smith JW, Ruiz ME, et al: MR imaging of the lateral collateral ligament of the ankle. AJR Am J Roentgenol 156:131, 1991.

Haygood TM, Langlotz CP, Kneeland JB, et al: Categorization of acromial shape: Interobserver variability with MR imaging and conventional radiography. AJR Am J Roentgenol 162:1377, 1994.

Hodler J, Kursunoglu-Brahme S, Flannigan B, et al: Injuries of the superior portion of the glenoid labrum involving the insertion of the biceps tendon: MR imaging findings in nine cases. AJR Am J Roentgenol 159:565, 1992.

Hodler J, Resnick D: Current status of imaging of articular cartilage. Skeletal Radiol 25:703, 1996.

Hughston JC, Andrews JR, Cross MJ, et al: Classification of knee ligament instabilities. I. The medial compartment and cruciate ligaments. J Bone Joint Surg Am 58:159, 1976.

Hughston JC, Andrews JR, Cross MJ, et al: Classification of knee ligament instabilities. II. The lateral compartment. J Bone Joint Surg Am 58:173, 1976.

Kaplan PA, Nelson NL, Garvin KL, et al: MR of the knee: The significance of high signal in the meniscus that does not clearly extend to the surface. AJR Am J Roentgenol 156:333, 1991.

Kaplan PA, Walker CW, Kilcoyne RF, et al: Occult fracture patterns of the knee associated with anterior cruciate ligament tears: Assessment with MR imaging. Radiology 183:835, 1992.

Karjalainen PT, Soila K, Aronen HJ, et al: MR imaging of overuse injuries of the Achilles tendon. AJR Am J Roentgenol 175:251, 2000.

Kjellin I, Ho CP, Cervilla V, et al: Alterations in the supraspinatus tendon at MR imaging: Correlation with histopathologic findings in cadavers. Radiology 181:837, 1991.

Kneeland JB, Middleton WD, Carrera WD, et al: MR imaging of the shoulder: Diagnosis of rotator cuff tears. AJR Am J Roentgenol 149:333, 1987.

Kursunoglu-Brahme S, Riccio T, Weisman MH, et al: Rheumatoid knee: Role of gadopentetate-enhanced MR imaging. Radiology 176:831, 1990.

Lektrakul N, Chung CB, Lai Y, et al: Tarsal sinus: Arthrographic, MR imaging, MR arthrographic, and pathologic findings in cadavers and retrospective study data in patients with sinus tarsi syndrome. Radiology 219:802, 2001.

Linscheid RL, Dobyns JH, Beabout JW, et al: Traumatic instability of the wrist: Diagnosis, classification, and pathomechanics. J Bone Joint Surg Am 54:1612, 1972.

Manaster BJ, Remley K, Newman AP, et al: Knee ligament reconstruction: Plain film analysis. AJR Am J Roentgenol 150:337, 1988.

Mesgarzadeh M, Moyer R, Leder DS, et al: MR imaging of the knee: Expanded classification and pitfalls to interpretation of meniscal tears. Radiographics 13:489, 1993.

Mesgarzadeh M, Schneck CD, Bonakdarpour A, et al: Carpal tunnel: MR imaging. II. Carpal tunnel syndrome. Radiology 171:749, 1989.

Mink JH: Ligaments of the ankle. In Deutsch AL, Mink JH, Kerr R (eds): MRI of the Foot and Ankle. New York, Raven Press, 1992, p 173.

Mink JH: Tendons. In Deutsch AL, Mink JH, Kerr R (eds): MRI of the Foot and Ankle. New York, Raven Press, 1992, p 135.

Mink JH, Deutsch AL: Occult cartilage and bone injuries of the knee: Detection, classification, and assessment with MR imaging. Radiology 170:823, 1989.

Mitchell DG, Rao VM, Dalinka MK, et al: Femoral head avascular necrosis: Correlation of MR imaging, radiographic staging, radionuclide imaging, and clinical findings. Radiology 162:709, 1987.

Murphy BJ: MR imaging of the elbow. Radiology 184:525, 1992.

Narváez JA, Narváez J, Ortega R, et al: Painful heel: MR imaging findings. Radiographics 20:333, 2000.

O'Donoghue DH: Surgical treatment of fresh injuries to major ligaments of the knee. J Bone Joint Surg Am 32:721, 1950.

Pao DG: The lateral femoral notch sign. Radiology 219:800, 2001.

Peterfy CG, Majumdar S, Lang P, et al: MR imaging of the arthritic knee: Improved discrimination of cartilage, synovium, and effusion with pulsed saturation transfer and fat-suppressed T1-weighted sequences. Radiology 191:413, 1994.

Quinn SF, Murray WT, Clark RA, et al: Achilles tendon: MR imaging at 1.5T. Radiology 164:767, 1987.

Recht MP, Kramer J, Marcelis S, et al: Abnormalities of articular cartilage in the knee: Analysis of available MR techniques. Radiology 187:473, 1993.

Rockwood CA Jr, Lyons FR: Shoulder impingement syndrome: Diagnosis, radiographic evaluation and treatment with a modified Neer acromioplasty. J Bone Joint Surg Am 75:409, 1993.

Rosenberg ZS, Beltran J, Bencardino JT: MR imaging of the ankle and foot. Radiographics 20(Suppl):153, 2000.

Rosenberg ZS, Cheung Y, Jahss MH, et al: Rupture of posterior tibial tendon: CT and MR imaging with surgical correlation. Radiology 169:229, 1988.

Shellock FG, Mink JH, Fox JM: Patellofemoral joint: Kinematic MR imaging to assess tracking abnormalities. Radiology 168:551, 1988.

Smith DK: Volar carpal ligaments of the wrist: Normal appearance on multiplanar reconstructions of three-dimensional Fourier transform MR imaging. AJR Am J Roentgenol 161:353, 1993.

Vahey TN, Broome DR, Kaye KJ, et al: Acute and chronic tears of the anterior cruciate ligament: Differential features at MR imaging. Radiology 181:251, 1991.

Weinreb JC, Cohen JM, Maravilla KR: Iliopsoas muscles: MR study of normal anatomy and disease. Radiology 156:435, 1985.

Zlatkin MB, Chao PC, Osterman AL, et al: Chronic wrist pain: Evaluation with high-resolution MR imaging. Radiology 173:723, 1989.

Zlatkin MB, Iannotti JP, Roberts MC, et al: Rotator cuff tears: Diagnostic performance of MR imaging. Radiology 172:223, 1989.

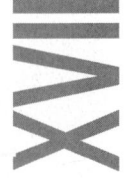
# Thermal, Iatrogenic, Nutritional, and Neurogenic Diseases

# CHAPTER 60

## Thermal and Electrical Injuries

### SUMMARY OF KEY FEATURES

The radiographic features of the skeleton after thermal and electrical injuries are varied. In many cases, they are not specific and must be interpreted with knowledge of the mechanism of injury. Of particular interest are the appearance of epiphyseal abnormalities in frostbite, periarticular calcification and ossification after thermal burns, and pathologic fractures associated with electrocution.

### INTRODUCTION

Exposure of the human body to extremes in temperature or to electricity can lead to significant abnormalities. Osseous and articular structures may participate in the body's response to such insults, and the changes induced may be irreparable. This chapter summarizes musculoskeletal manifestations of thermal and electrical injury (Table 60–1).

### FROSTBITE
#### Terminology and General Abnormalities

Local damage can follow nonfreezing (immersion foot) and freezing (frostbite) injuries. Immersion foot is related to prolonged exposure to low but not freezing temperatures in combination with persistent dampness. Typical examples of immersion foot occur in soldiers (trench foot) and in survivors of shipwrecks. Contributory to the tissue injury in this entity are prolonged exposure to cold and dampness, immobility and dependency of the extremities, semistarvation, dehydration, and exhaustion. Singly or in combination, these factors lead to hypoxic injury in response to decreased blood flow to the affected body part. Plasma escapes through the injured capillary wall, producing edema, which further compromises the integrity of the vascular supply to nerve and muscle tissue. Gangrene and skin necrosis are frequent in the hyperemic stage; induration and fibrosis of subcutaneous tissue, with limitation of joint motion, may be seen for several years after the injury. Nevertheless, complete recovery from immersion foot is common.

Frostbite differs from immersion foot in that blood vessels are injured severely or irreparably, circulation of blood ceases, and the vascular beds within the frozen tissue are occluded by thrombi and cellular aggregation.

**TABLE 60–1**

**Radiographic Findings Associated with Thermal and Electrical Injuries**

Soft tissue swelling, loss, or contracture
Osteoporosis
Acro-osteolysis
Periostitis
Epiphyseal injury and growth disturbance
Articular abnormalities
Periarticular calcification and ossification
Osteolysis, osteosclerosis, and fracture

Once the freezing process has been initiated, it progresses rapidly, and tissue located superficially, such as that in the ears, nose, and digits, is damaged by the formation of tiny ice crystals.

#### Musculoskeletal Abnormalities

During the period of exposure, vascular spasm in the involved extremities is evident. With warming or thawing of the injured parts, vasodilatation leads to increased permeability of the vascular wall, transudation of fluid, perivascular edema, and intravascular stasis, with agglutination of erythrocytes and deposition of fibrin.

Bony and articular manifestations of frostbite apparently are related to cellular injury and necrosis from the freezing process itself or from the vascular insufficiency it produces. Findings are most marked in the hands and the feet, and their severity depends on the length of exposure and the prevailing temperature. Early radiographic manifestations include soft tissue swelling and loss of tissue, especially at the tips of the digits; osteoporosis and periostitis may occur at a slightly later stage. In the hand, the findings predominate in the four medial digits; sparing of the thumb is characteristic but not invariable and can be attributed to clenching of the fist with the thumb clasped in the palm during the exposure to cold.

Late skeletal manifestations are variable. In children, epiphyseal abnormalities are frequent, involving primarily the distal phalanges. Fragmentation, destruction, and disappearance of epiphyseal centers are seen (Fig. 60–1). Premature physeal fusion is also noted, resulting in brachydactyly. Interphalangeal joint abnormalities eventually may simulate those of osteoarthritis (Fig. 60–2). Unilateral or bilateral changes, with joint space narrowing, sclerosis, osteophytosis, and soft tissue hypertrophy, are seen. Deformity and deviation can result from uneven digital involvement. Tuftal resorption of terminal phalanges

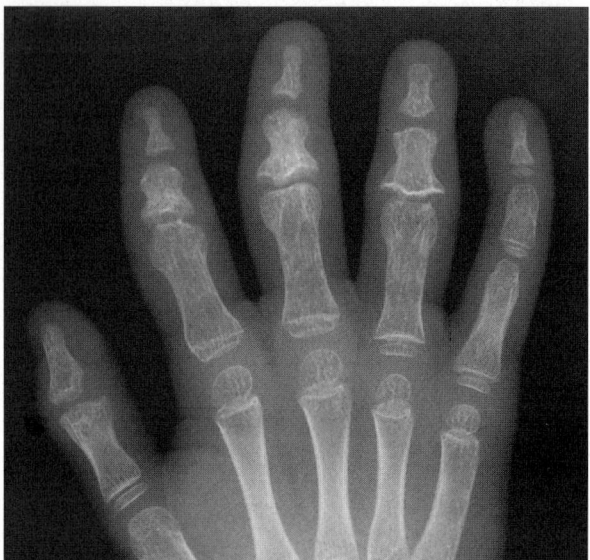

**Figure 60–1.** Frostbite: late changes. Note brachydactyly, irregularity, and contour abnormalities of the proximal, middle, and distal phalanges; epiphyseal destruction; and premature physeal fusion in the proximal phalanges of the second and third fingers. (Courtesy of D. Wilcox, MD, Kansas City, Mo.)

can be traced to loss of overlying soft tissue structures. Unilateral changes and the presence of subchondral cysts may aid in differentiating frostbite arthritis from osteoarthritis.

Frostbite injury of the ears can manifest as calcification and ossification of the pinna. Cartilage calcification at this site after cold injury must be differentiated from that caused by mechanical trauma, hyperparathyroidism, calcium pyrophosphate dihydrate crystal deposition disease, gout, Addison's disease, alkaptonuria, and acromegaly.

Scintigraphy with bone-seeking pharmaceutical agents can be used to assess the viability of involved osseous tissue. The uptake of radionuclide in the region of frostbite depends on the integrity of the vascular tree; absence of such uptake indicates bone that lacks vascular per-

fusion, providing useful information to the surgeon. Persistent perfusion defects indicate nonviable tissue, whereas reperfusion, which may be evident on studies performed weeks after the injury, indicates tissue viability. Triple-phase bone scanning appears to offer advantages over standard techniques (Fig. 60–3). The role of magnetic resonance (MR) imaging in this condition is not known.

### Differential Diagnosis

The normal occurrence of sclerosis of one or more epiphyses (ivory epiphyses) should not be misinterpreted as evidence of epiphyseal necrosis after frostbite. Thiemann's disease (epiphyseal acrodysplasia) is a poorly defined condition occurring predominantly in men in their late teens; in this disease, swelling of the fingers is associated with epiphyseal irregularity, sclerosis, and fragmentation. The distribution of epiphyseal abnormalities, with sparing of the distal phalanges, differs from that of frostbite. Ungual tuftal resorption can occur in a variety of conditions other than frostbite, including collagen vascular disease, epidermolysis bullosa, neuropathic osteoarthropathy, hyperparathyroidism, sarcoidosis, and psoriatic arthritis. In these conditions, the thumb is frequently affected, and other more diagnostic findings are generally present.

### THERMAL BURNS
### General Abnormalities

Thermal injury results in coagulative tissue necrosis with an inflammatory response. A second-degree burn implies that coagulative necrosis involves only the epidermis and part of the dermis and that elements are available for epithelial regeneration; a third-degree burn implies death of tissue to such an extent that epithelial regeneration cannot occur. In both second- and third-degree burns, massive outpouring of protein-rich fluid results from both endothelial capillary damage and interference with normal lymphatic absorption. Secondary bacterial invasion is frequent and may contribute to ischemic necrosis of tissue.

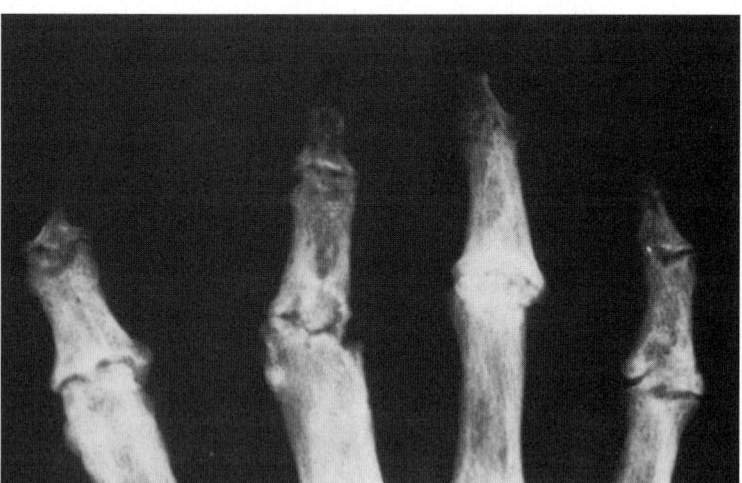

**Figure 60–2.** Frostbite: interphalangeal joint abnormalities. In addition to acro-osteolysis, osseous and cartilaginous destruction is evident in the proximal and distal interphalangeal joints. Subchondral erosion and collapse, sclerosis, osteophytosis, and joint space narrowing with or without intra-articular bony ankylosis simulate the findings of inflammatory (erosive) osteoarthritis. (Courtesy of M. Dalinka, MD, Philadelphia, Pa.)

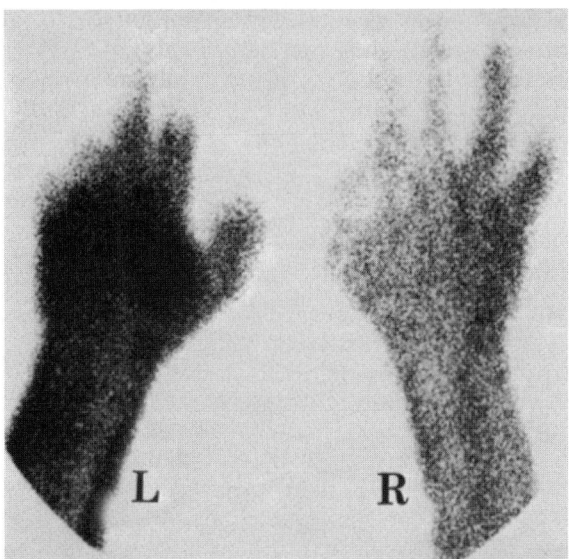

**Figure 60–3.** Frostbite: scintigraphic abnormalities. In this 62-year-old alcoholic man who had been exposed to freezing temperatures with his hands unprotected for 3 hours, a static image shows the following features: in the left (L) hand, marked hyperemia, absent perfusion of the fourth and fifth digits, and diminished perfusion in the middle and distal phalanges of the second digit and the distal phalanx of the first digit; in the right (R) hand, hyperemia in the midpalmar region and the fourth and fifth digits, and diminished perfusion in the distal phalanx of the fifth digit. Eventually, the left fourth and fifth fingers required amputation at the level of the metacarpophalangeal joints, and the right fifth finger and distal parts of the left thumb and index finger required débridement. (From Salimi Z, Vas W, Tang-Burton P, et al: Assessment of tissue viability in frostbite by $^{99m}$Tc pertechnetate scintigraphy. AJR Am J Roentgenol 142:415, 1984.)

## Musculoskeletal Abnormalities

Thermal burns can produce significant skeletal and soft tissue abnormalities that may involve the bone, the joint, or the periarticular tissue. Early radiographic alterations include soft tissue loss, osteoporosis, and periostitis; late alterations include articular and periarticular changes and growth disturbances.

Osteoporosis is the most frequent bony response to thermal burns (Fig. 60–4). The pathogenesis of such osteoporosis probably includes immobilization and disuse, a reflex vasomotor response, or a metabolic reaction to tissue destruction. Osteoporosis can appear within weeks to months after injury, and with increased mobilization of patients during the recovery phase, the finding may diminish or disappear completely. Periostitis appears within months after the injury in those bones that underlie severely burned areas (see Fig. 60–4).

The appearance of irregular periarticular calcification is not infrequent 1 month or longer after thermal injury. The deposits create poorly defined and flocculent radiodense areas that are separate from the underlying bone. They are found most commonly about the elbow. Periarticular ossification is also a well-recognized complication among patients with thermal burns; it is encountered most commonly about the elbow and, less frequently,

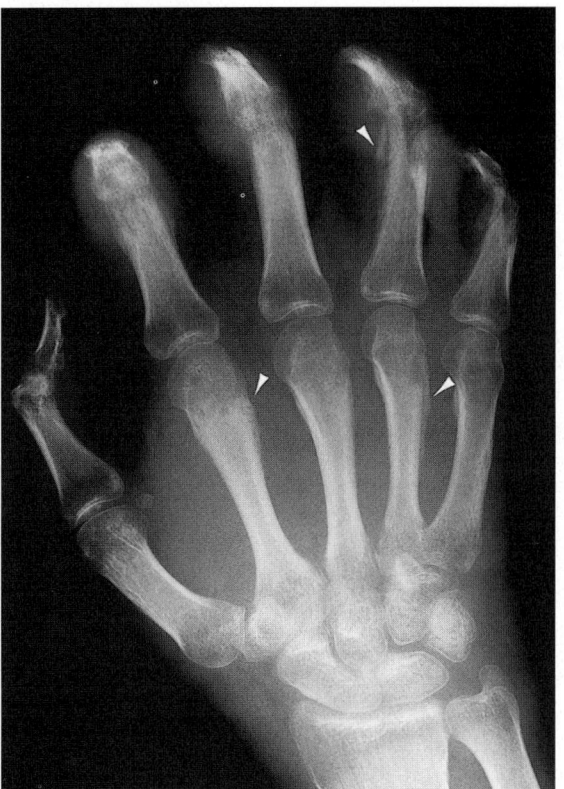

**Figure 60–4.** Thermal burn: early changes. The early radiographic findings in this patient who burned his hand include diffuse soft tissue swelling, soft tissue and bony loss in the digits, severe periarticular osteoporosis, and periostitis, especially of the phalanges and metacarpal bones *(arrowheads)*.

about the hip and shoulder (Fig. 60–5). Such ossification usually becomes evident in the second or third month after injury. Periarticular osseous excrescences that attach to the underlying bone cannot always be differentiated clearly from soft tissue calcification and ossification. These outgrowths may contain recognizable trabeculae and appear to arise from the subjacent bone. They are also most prevalent about the elbow (see Fig. 60–5). The relationships among heterotopic bone formation, periarticular calcification, and osteophytosis are not clear, although all three abnormalities may represent various stages of the same process and frequently occur at the same location.

Heterotopic ossification is intimately associated with the surrounding musculature, although it does not appear to replace the muscle tissue. The bony ridges commonly attach to the adjacent osseous structure. One common pattern of ossification is from the olecranon process to the medial epicondylar ridge of the humerus, along the medial border of the triceps muscle. The pathogenesis of heterotopic calcification and ossification after burns is unknown.

Acromutilation with partial or complete loss of phalanges may be a prominent finding when the hand or foot is burned (Fig. 60–6). Progressive destruction of one or more joints, with eventual fibrous or bony ankylosis, may be evident after thermal burns. Destruction may appear within a few weeks after injury, and ankylosis may

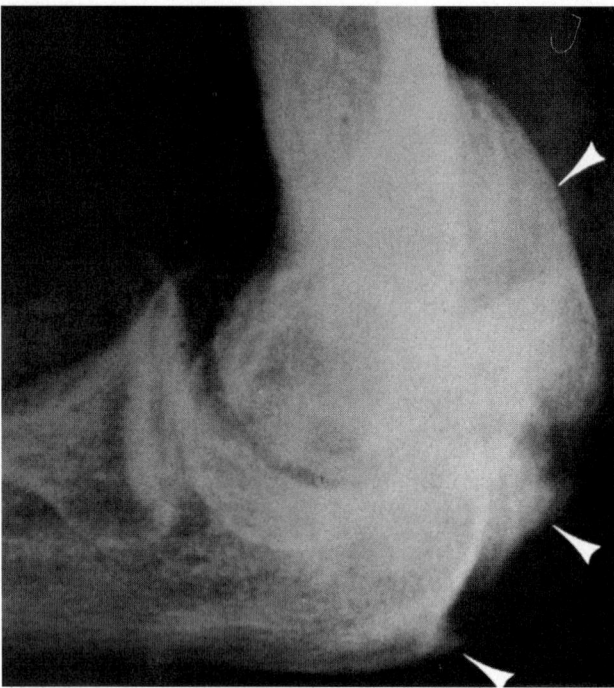

**Figure 60–5.** Thermal burn: osteophytes, soft tissue calcification, and ossification. Several months after a thermal burn, local ossification *(arrowheads)* appears along the posterior surface of the humerus and ulna.

develop within a few months (Fig. 60–7). Initially, fusiform soft tissue swelling and osteoporosis are observed about the involved joint. Progressive loss of interosseous space and subchondral irregularity are seen. Eventually, intra-articular osseous fusion may result. Thermal injury, mechanical trauma, infection, neuropathic osteoarthropathy, and immobilization are all possible factors in the pathogenesis of these articular changes. Contractures caused by soft tissue and muscular changes are also frequently observed in burn patients, especially about the elbow and hand.

## Differential Diagnosis

The radiographic findings of osteoporosis, periarticular calcification and ossification, joint space loss, intra-articular bony ankylosis, and contracture that are encountered in burn patients may also be seen after paralysis (or immobilization). Heterotopic ossification in

these situations is identical. Phalangeal tuftal resorption or destruction occurring after burns must be differentiated from similar changes occurring in association with frostbite, collagen vascular disorders, and articular diseases.

## ELECTRICAL BURNS

### General Abnormalities

Electricity can produce severe injury or death. The extent of bodily harm depends on the type of electricity, the voltage, the water content of tissues, and the points of entry and exit of the charge. Electrical injury associated with a relatively short route—such as a point of entry in the arm to a point of exit in a finger—produces less tissue damage than an injury associated with a longer route—such as entry in the head and exit through a foot. With alternating currents, muscular contraction may prevent a person from releasing the source of electricity, leading to more prolonged and severe tissue damage.

Electrical energy is converted to heat as it traverses the skin. Resulting burns are accentuated by vascular spasm, leading to electrical necrosis. Death from low-voltage electrical injury (<200 volts) usually is caused by ventricular fibrillation; death related to high-voltage electricity (>1000 volts) is caused by inhibition of the respiratory center in the brain.

### Musculoskeletal Abnormalities

The hand, because of its grasping function, is the most commonly affected area. Severe skin burns are encountered at the points of entry and exit of the electrical charge. Osseous and articular changes are related to the effects of heat, mechanical trauma from accompanying uncoordinated muscle spasm, neural and vascular tissue damage, infection, disuse or immobilization, and, perhaps, a specific effect of the electricity itself.

Initial radiographic features include loss of cutaneous, subcutaneous, and osseous tissues owing to tissue charring. Other findings are soft tissue hematomas; compression fractures of the spine, dislocation of joints, and avulsions at tendinous insertions related to muscle spasm; and various fractures resulting from accompanying falls (Fig. 60–8). Small, rounded, dense osseous lesions resembling wax drippings may be attributable to the melting of bone from the intense heat. Focal, tiny disruptions in bony continuity (microfractures) may also be a direct effect of the heat. They may have a zigzag contour with

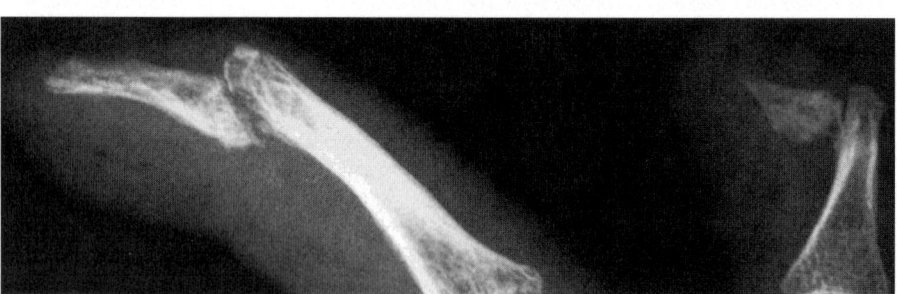

**Figure 60–6.** Thermal burn: acromutilation. Observe the terminal phalangeal destruction of two burned digits. Joint destruction and subluxation are also evident.

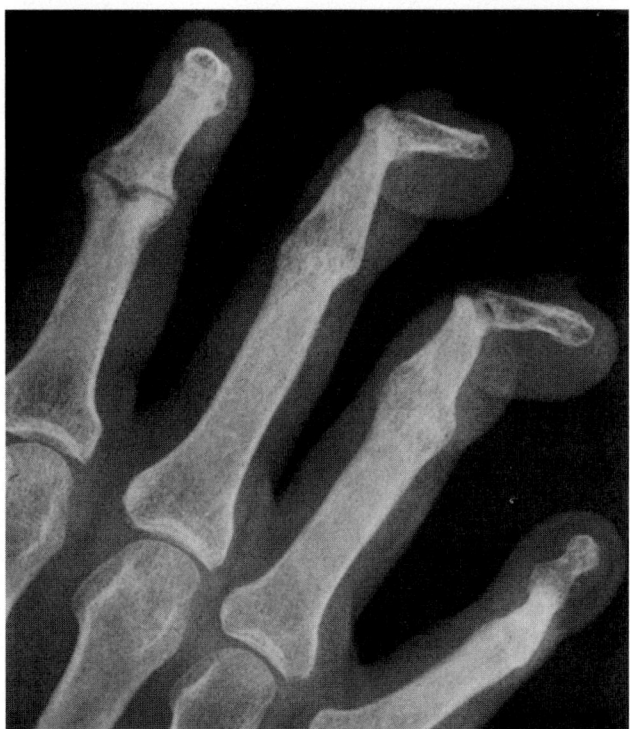

**Figure 60–7.** Thermal burn: articular and osseous changes. In this burned hand, note osteolysis with deformity of phalanges and intra-articular osseous fusion.

discrete margins and can occur anywhere along the route of electricity. Osteolysis and periostitis are also encountered (Fig. 60–9).

Delayed musculoskeletal alterations, which may appear months or years later, are related predominantly to ischemia. Osteonecrosis may develop at sites distal to the entry and exit wounds. Accelerated bone growth and premature fusion of damaged physes may follow electrical injury in children. Secondary infection with osteomyelitis and septic arthritis, nonunion of pathologic fractures, neuropathic osteoarthropathy, and contracture with joint subluxation or dislocation have also been described. Periarticular calcification and ossification and intra-articular bony ankylosis may eliminate joint motion.

A potential role exists for scintigraphic and MR imaging analysis of soft tissue injury occurring as a result of electrical burns. With MR imaging, enhanced signal intensity in areas of injured muscle after the intravenous administration of a gadolinium contrast agent suggests edematous, viable tissue. Lack of such enhancement is indicative of nonviable tissue. However, the presence of normal-appearing muscle on MR images does not eliminate the possibility of electrical injury.

## Differential Diagnosis

The radiographic findings occurring after this type of injury represent a combination of thermal, mechanical,

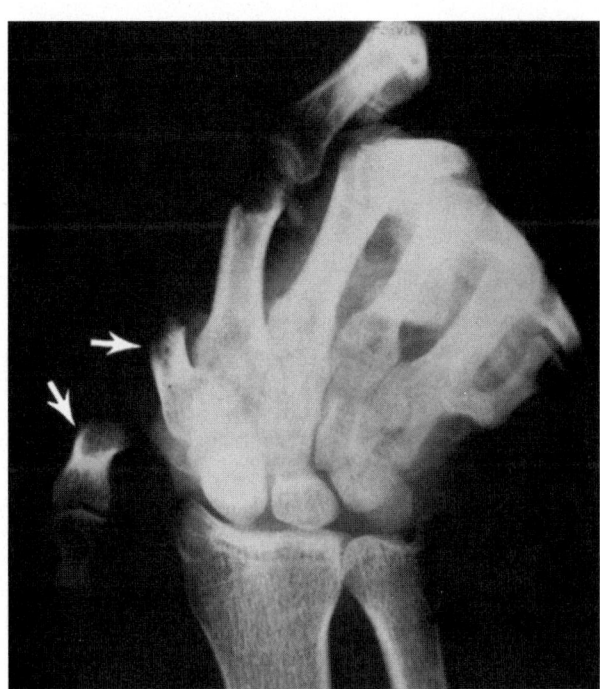

**Figure 60–8.** Electrical burn. This man developed changes in his hands after touching a high-tension wire. The severe alterations in the left hand resulted from sustained grasping of the wire. They include contracture, soft tissue injury, subluxation, dislocation, and fracture *(arrows)*. The right hand was affected similarly.

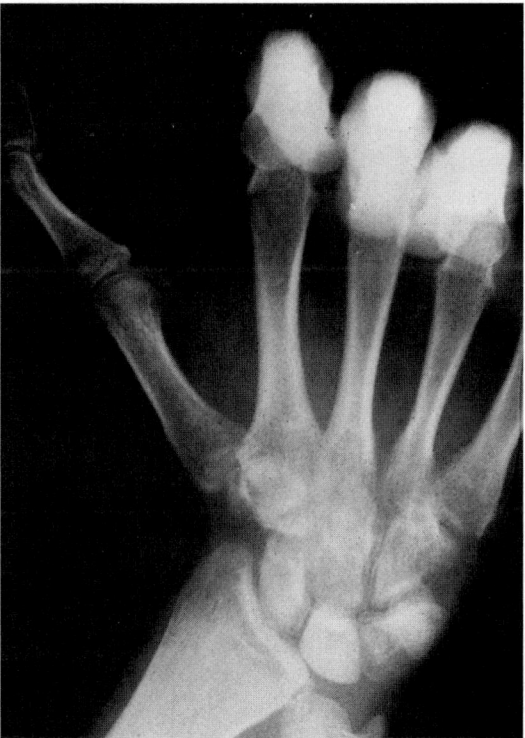

**Figure 60–9.** Electrical burn. This 21-year-old man came into contact with a high-tension wire, resulting in severe injury to both hands (entrance wounds) and to the pretibial regions (exit wounds). Radiograph of a hand reveals contractures of multiple digits and periarticular osteoporosis. (Courtesy of J. Barry, MD, Seattle, Wash.)

and electrical effects on bones and joints. They are complicated by vascular and neurologic damage and secondary infection. Some of the imaging abnormalities are identical to those that occur after trauma from any cause, whereas others resemble those of septic arthritis, neuropathic osteoarthropathy, osteoporosis, thermal burns, frostbite, and neurologic deficit.

## FURTHER READING

Brinn LB, Moseley JE: Bone changes following electrical injury: Case report and review of literature. AJR Am J Roentgenol 97:682, 1966.

Carrera GF, Kozin F, Flaherty L, et al: Radiographic changes in the hands following childhood frostbite injury. Skeletal Radiol 6:33, 1981.

Evans EB, Smith JR: Bone and joint changes following burns: A roentgenographic study—preliminary report. J Bone Joint Surg Am 41:785, 1959.

Fleckenstein JL, Chason DP, Bonte FJ, et al: High-voltage electric injury: Assessment of muscle viability with MR imaging and Tc-99m pyrophosphate scintigraphy. Radiology 195:205, 1995.

Gralino BJ, Porter JM, Rosch J: Angiography in the diagnosis and therapy of frostbite. Radiology 119:301, 1976.

Ogden JA, Southwick WO: Electrical injury involving the immature skeleton. Skeletal Radiol 6:187, 1981.

Reed MH: Growth disturbances in the hands following thermal injuries in children. 2. Frostbite. J Can Assoc Radiol 39:95, 1988.

Salimi Z, Vas W, Tang-Barton P, et al: Assessment of tissue viability in frostbite by $^{99m}$Tc pertechnetate scintigraphy. AJR Am J Roentgenol 142:415, 1984.

Schiele HP, Hubbard RB, Bruck HM: Radiographic changes in burns of the upper extremity. Radiology 104:13, 1972.

Selke AC Jr: Destruction of phalangeal epiphyses by frostbite. Radiology 93:959, 1969.

Tishler J: The soft tissue and bone changes in frostbite injuries. Radiology 102:511, 1972.

# CHAPTER 61

## Radiation Changes

Murray K. Dalinka and Tamara Miner Haygood

## SUMMARY OF KEY FEATURES

The effects of radiation on bone occur as a result of accidental exposure (e.g., radium dial workers) and of diagnostic (e.g., Thorotrast) and therapeutic procedures. Radiation therapy may affect bone growth, cause osseous necrosis, and induce neoplasia. Fortunately, these complications have decreased in frequency owing to advances in the methods of providing such therapy and to the use of both radiation and chemotherapy.

## INTRODUCTION

Within a year after Roentgen published his discovery, the new technique was in clinical use, chiefly for the diagnosis of fractures and the localization of metallic foreign bodies. Deleterious effects of radiation were noted as early as 6 months after Roentgen's initial description, including the development of pigmentation, telangiectasia, fibrosis, alopecia, scarring, ulceration, and dermatitis. More serious was the finding several years later that malignant lesions could be induced by exposure to diagnostic and therapeutic irradiation, as well as to radioactive agents such as radium and thorium.

## RADIUM

Radium was used therapeutically, both orally and intravenously, in the treatment of many ailments between 1910 and 1930. Orally ingested radium is deposited mainly in the outer cortex of bone, and in the 1920s, it was found to cause radium jaw (a type of osteomyelitis), severe aplastic anemia, and osseous neoplasms in radium dial painters.

When large quantities of radium are deposited in bone for more than 20 years, mostly dead osteoid tissue remains. Normal bone physiology becomes erratic, and large resorption cavities are formed. These cavities contain gelatinous material with osteoid-like matrix and appear as sharply defined bone lesions resembling those of multiple myeloma. They occur in the long bones (Fig. 61–1) and skull (Fig. 61–2) and increase in size over time. These areas of cortical resorption are caused by constant alpha particle irradiation.

Metaphyseal sclerosis is frequent, particularly in patients who ingest radium before physeal closure. Areas of increased density probably represent the deposition of new bone on unresorbed trabeculae. These density changes may simulate those of Paget's disease, but the bone is of normal size. Pathologic fractures can occur, and frequently they heal normally. Osteosarcomas and fibrosarcomas,

sometimes multicentric, are seen. The average latent period of these sarcomas is 23 years. Carcinomas of the paranasal sinuses and mastoids have also been reported.

## THORIUM

Thorium dioxide in dextran (Thorotrast) was introduced as a contrast agent in 1928 and was widely used in the United States between 1930 and the early 1950s. Its clinically inert properties and high atomic number made it the agent of choice for hepatolienography, peripheral and cerebral angiography, and the opacification of body cavities.

Extravasation of Thorotrast at the site of injection leads to continuous alpha particle irradiation, resulting in an expanding cicatricial mass (Thorotrastoma) that invades contiguous structures, leading to tissue destruction and vascular compromise. The liver, spleen, and bone marrow are subjected to continuous low-dose alpha radiation. The reticuloendothelial system and adjacent tissues are therefore at risk for radiation-induced neoplasia, particularly hemangioendothelial sarcoma of the liver.

The injection of Thorotrast into growing children may give rise to a "bone-within-bone" or "ghost vertebra" appearance (Fig. 61–3). Thorotrast deposition causes constant alpha radiation and temporary growth arrest. The size of the ghost vertebra corresponds to the vertebral size at the time of injection.

## EFFECTS OF RADIATION THERAPY

### Bone Growth

The effects of radiation on bone growth depend on dosage, quality of the x-ray beam, age of the patient, method of fractionation, length of time after therapy, specific bone or bones involved, and coexistence of trauma or infection. These effects include disruption of normal growth and maturation, scoliosis, osteonecrosis, and neoplasm.

The epiphysis is the area of the bone that is most sensitive to radiation. Decreased growth can occur with as little as 400 cGy. With a low dose of 600 to 1200 cGy, rapid histologic recovery of radiation-induced changes occurs. Secondary changes are limited, but some residua may remain. With 1200 cGy or more, the damage is increased and is maximal to the chondroblasts. Delayed changes take 6 months or longer to appear and are dose related; they include vascular damage, premature cartilage degeneration, and bone marrow atrophy. Growth impairment is related to the age of the patient, with the effect of any given dose being greater at a younger age. The greater the growth potential of a particular bone, the more drastic is the effect. Any skeletal part capable of growth that is exposed to 2000 cGy or more will show growth disturbances. In pediatric patients, irradiation of the growing epiphysis or apophysis may cause shortening of

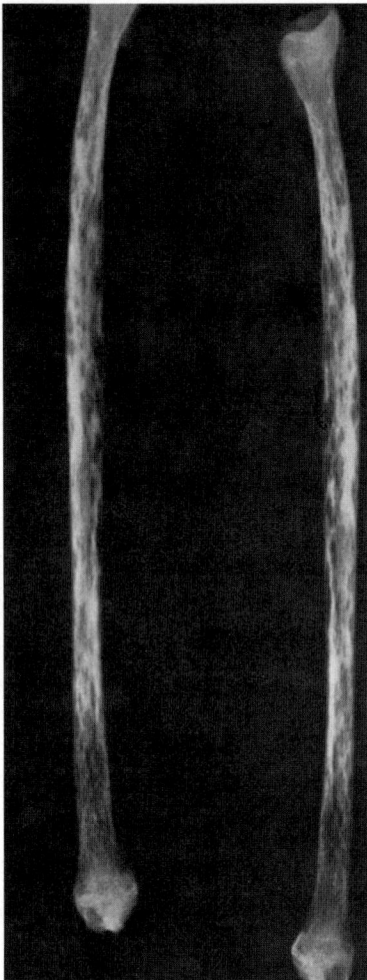

**Figure 61–1.** Radiograph of a specimen from a radium dial worker shows both fibulae with multiple resorption cavities within the shafts. Note the well-defined lucent lesions somewhat resembling those of multiple myeloma.

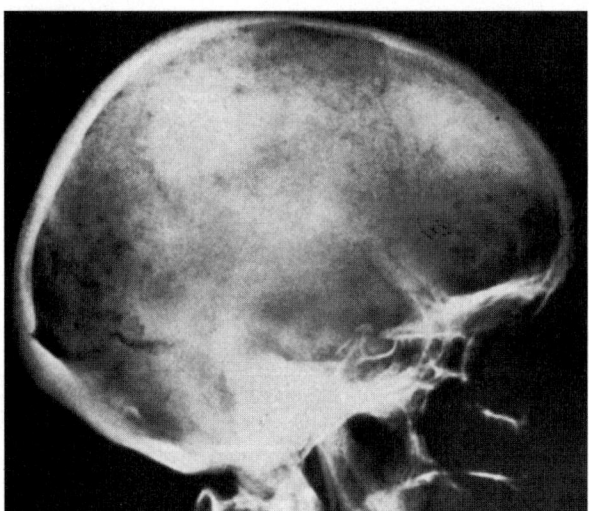

**Figure 61–2.** Skull of a radium dial worker demonstrates multiple small lucent areas within the calvaria, mainly in the parietal region, simulating the lesions of multiple myeloma. (From Dalinka MK, Edeiken J, Finkelstein JB: Complications of radiation therapy: Adult bone. Semin Roentgenol 9:29, 1974.)

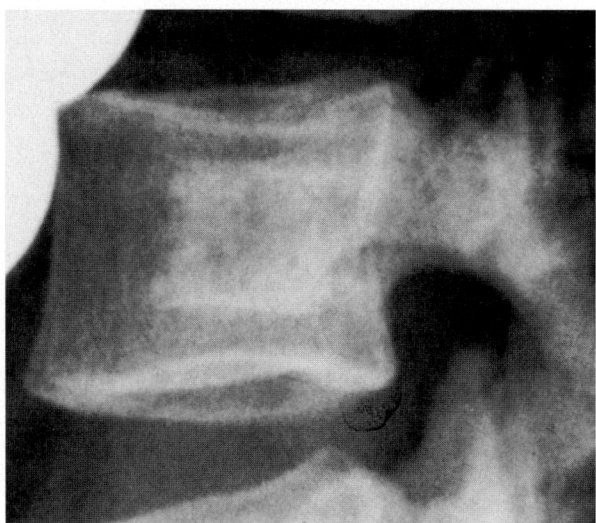

**Figure 61–3.** Coned-down view of lumbar vertebra shows the bone-within-bone appearance in a patient injected with Thorotrast at age 3 years. (From Teplick JG, Head GL, Kricun ME, Haskin ME: Ghost infantile vertebrae and hemipelves within adult skeleton from thorotrast administration in childhood. Radiology 129:657, 1978.)

long bones or hypoplasia of the ilium. Widening of the growth plate has been described as early as 1 to 2 months after treatment. If mild, this returns to normal after approximately 6 months. Joint space widening has also been reported 8 to 10 months after therapy. Metaphyseal changes, including irregularity, fraying, and sclerosis (Fig. 61–4), may superficially resemble those of rickets (Fig. 61–5). Patients with metaphyseal changes may develop a broad band of increased density, which may be a manifestation of repair.

### Slipped Capital Femoral Epiphysis

Slipped capital femoral epiphysis may also develop as a sequel to radiation therapy if the femoral head was included in the field of therapy (Fig. 61–6). The damaged growth plate is unable to withstand the shearing stresses of growth, leading to epiphyseal slippage. Radiation-induced slipped epiphysis usually occurs at an earlier age than the idiopathic variety and may be seen in patients who do not conform to the typical age and body habitus of most children with the idiopathic type. Other changes that may occur when the acetabulum or femoral head, or both, is included in the radiation port are iliac hypoplasia, acetabular dysplasia, coxa vara and coxa valga, and leg shortening.

### Scoliosis

Irradiation to the spine is noted to produce scoliosis. No radiographic abnormality is seen in patients treated with less than 1000 cGy. Children who receive 1000 to 2000 cGy develop changes secondary to growth arrest 9 to 12 months after therapy; these changes consist of horizontal lines of increased density parallel to the vertebral endplates and, on occasion, a bone-within-bone appearance. These abnor-

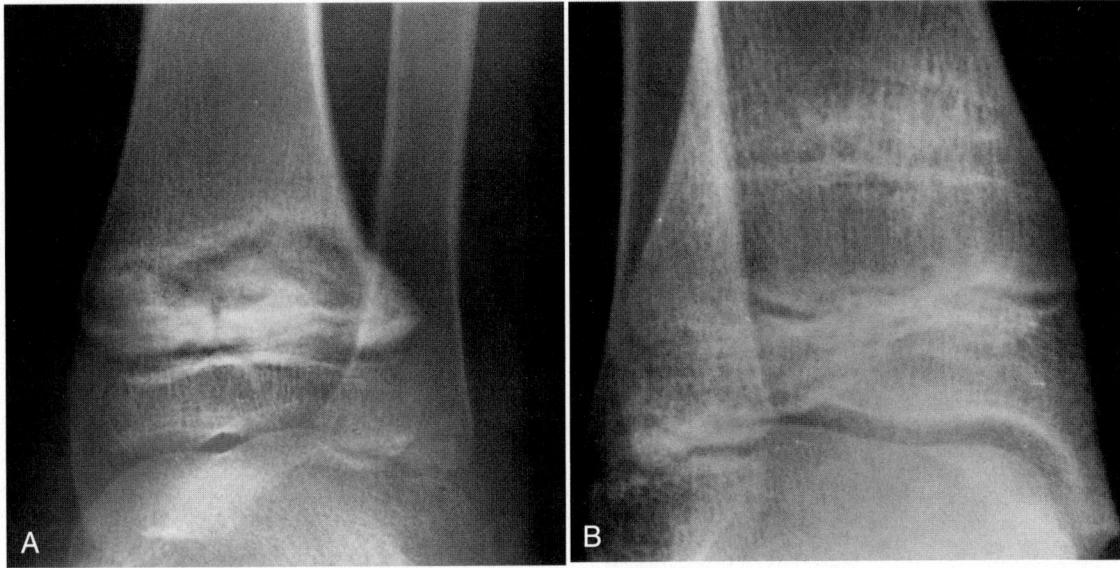

**Figure 61–4.** Radiation-induced lesion of the distal tibial metaphysis after therapy for Ewing's tumor of the proximal end of the tibia. *A*, Six months after the completion of therapy, a lucent lesion is observed in the distal metaphysis; it is well defined and has sclerotic margins. A small fracture is also present. *B*, Six months after *(A)*, the lesion has filled in with normal-appearing bone. A lucent band is present at the proximal extent of the lesion. (From Dalinka MK, Mazzeo VP Jr: CRC Crit Rev Diagn Imaging 23:235, 1985.)

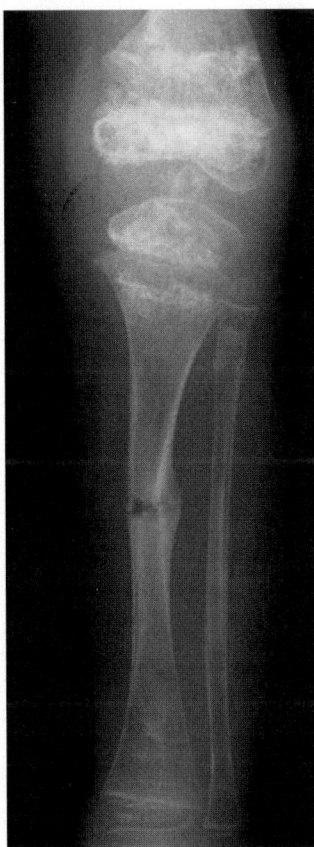

malities are not confined to the treatment field and hence are related to a general effect on bone growth. At doses between 2000 and 3000 cGy, irreversible changes consisting of irregularity and scalloping of the vertebral endplates are confined to the irradiated area and are associated with decreased vertebral height and abnormal bone contour. Changes are more severe in patients treated before the age of 2 years; therefore, the effects of radiation are believed to be both dose and age related.

In many later series, scoliosis occurs despite therapy to the entire vertebral body (Fig. 61–7) and even megavoltage therapy. Nonetheless, scrupulous inclusion of the

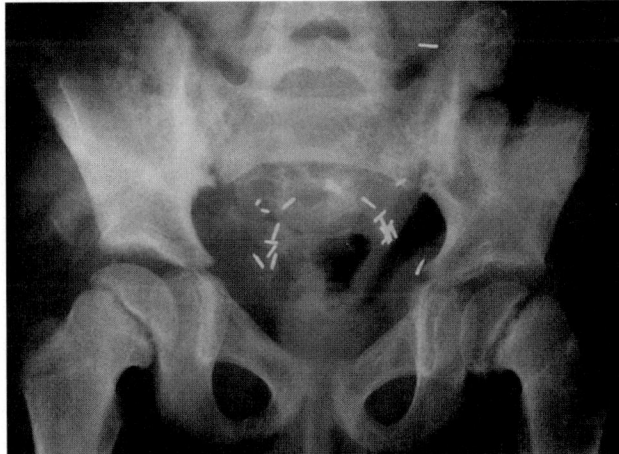

**Figure 61–5.** This patient was irradiated approximately 2 years before this examination for leukemia and knee pain. The treated field included most of the tibia as well as the knee. A fracture through the midshaft of the tibia is seen, with periosteal reaction about it. Periosteal reaction is also noted about the midshaft of the fibula. Metaphyseal irregularity of the distal end of the femur is present, with deformity secondary to radiation therapy. Diffuse osteopenia is also present. (Courtesy of P. Borns, MD, Wilmington, Del.)

**Figure 61–6.** Slipped capital femoral epiphysis after radiation therapy. This 8-year-old child received radiation therapy for an embryonal rhabdomyosarcoma. The pelvis was treated with 5940 cGy, with a femoral shield added at 4500 cGy. In the anteroposterior view of the pelvis, note the slipped epiphysis on the left side. The right sacroiliac joint has sclerotic margins, also secondary to radiation therapy. (Courtesy of A. Newburg, MD, Boston.)

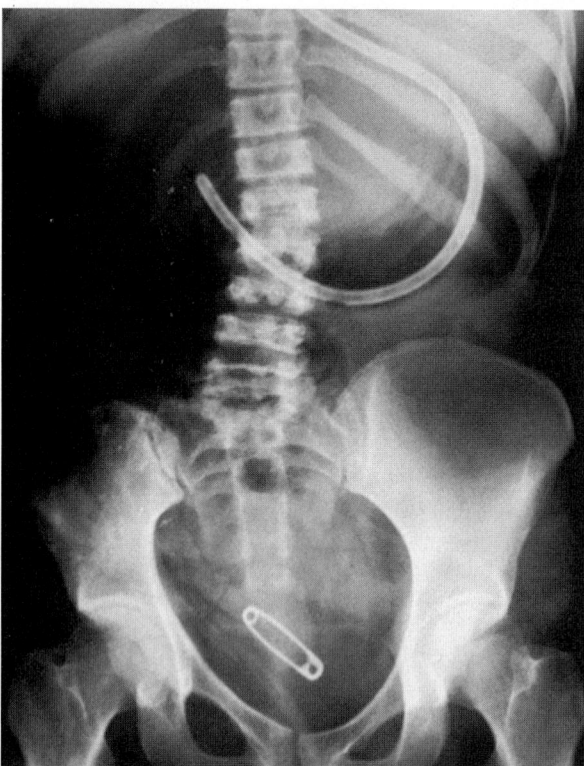

**Figure 61–7.** Spinal changes following radiation. This patient was irradiated for a right-sided Wilms' tumor in childhood. Note the severe decrease in the height of the vertebral bodies and a slight scoliosis convex to the left. The ribs and iliac crest on the right side are also hypoplastic. The long tube is present because of intestinal obstruction, which was later shown to be secondary to radiation enteritis.

entire vertebral body may mitigate the resulting scoliosis. In general, a dose less than 2000 cGy produces no deformity, a dose between 2000 and 3000 cGy is associated with a scoliosis of not more than 20 degrees, and a dose greater than 3000 cGy produces a curvature greater than 20 degrees. It has also become apparent that radiation-induced scoliosis can be progressive, particularly when high doses are given to young patients.

## Radiation Osteitis and Osteonecrosis

The pathologic effects of radiation are independent of their method of production. The effects of radiation in mature bone are mainly on the osteoblasts, with the primary event being decreased matrix production. Immediate or delayed cell death, injury with recovery, arrest of cellular division, abnormal repair, or neoplasia may occur.

Historically, Ewing used the term radiation osteitis to define the effects of radiation on bone. Abnormalities include temporary cessation of growth with recovery, periostitis, bone sclerosis with increased fragility, ischemic necrosis, and infection with osteoradionecrosis. Despite disagreement about the nature of the bone abnormalities that occur after radiation, it has been established that they are dependent on dosage, quality of the x-ray beam, method of fractionation, length of time after therapy,

specific bone or bones involved, and presence of coexistent trauma or infection. The quality of the x-ray beam determines the energy absorption and hence the radiation effect.

Radiation effects in mature bone, like those in growing bone, are dose related: the larger the dose, the greater the effect. Permanent damage to mature bone is very unusual at doses lower than 3000 cGy. Doses between 3000 and 5000 cGy cause permanent damage, and at doses higher than 5000 cGy, cell death and permanent devitalization of bone occur. The vast majority of cases of radiation osteitis occur in the mandible (32%), with the clavicle (18%), humeral head (14%), ribs (9%), and femur (9%) also well represented. The temporal relationships vary according to the bone affected. Mandibular abnormalities frequently manifest within a year after therapy, whereas in most other sites the latent period is longer.

### Regional Effects

**Mandible.** Osteonecrosis is considerably more common in the mandible than in the maxilla because of its compact bone and poor blood supply. The mandible, because of its superficial location, receives a large dose of radiation during the treatment of intraoral cancer. Osteonecrosis is more common when the tumor involves or is adjacent to bone. The necrosis is usually of a mild and temporary nature. Mandibular necrosis may be aseptic or septic; the aseptic or simple type is usually of no consequence.

In children, radiation to the mandible may result in altered patterns of tooth eruption, including malformation of the tooth or its root. These findings, which are well displayed with panoramic radiography, may be more prominent when both radiation and chemotherapy are employed. Mandibular osteonecrosis may be difficult to differentiate from tumor recurrence. Recurrence and osteoradionecrosis usually both occur within 1 year after therapy. Mandibular necrosis frequently manifests as a poorly defined destructive lesion without sequestration (Fig. 61–8). The absence of a soft tissue mass helps in differentiating necrosis from tumor recurrence, but an inflammatory mass may be present with osteonecrosis.

**Skull.** Radiation injury to the calvaria may occur after a maximum absorbed dose of 3600 cGy. The typical finding of radiation change in the calvaria is a mixed region of lysis and sclerosis that starts in the epicenter of the radiation portal and extends outward to the margins of the portal (Fig. 61–9). If soft tissue necrosis is associated with the calvarial changes, secondary infection with osteomyelitis, mastoiditis, or meningitis may occur.

**Shoulder.** Radiation changes in the shoulder girdle after therapy for breast carcinoma have been reported in 1% to 3% of patients. Osteopenia is common after irradiation but also occurs in a substantial number of patients treated by radical mastectomy alone. Osteopenia is commonly associated with a coarse, disorganized trabecular pattern, which may resemble Paget's disease superficially. Rib fractures are also common; they may be subtle and are frequently painless. The early finding is often a sharp change in alignment with or without a fracture line. The

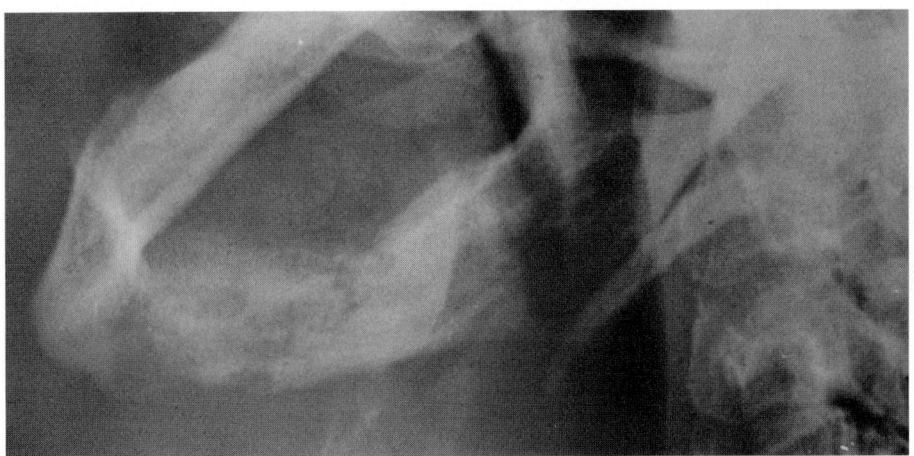

**Figure 61–8.** Oblique view of the mandible in a patient previously treated for carcinoma of the floor of the mouth. There is a poorly defined destructive lesion in the body of the mandible, with a pathologic fracture. No discernible soft tissue mass is present. This represents mandibular necrosis.

lesions commonly occur in the anterior or anterolateral aspects of the ribs and are usually multiple (Fig. 61–10). The edges of the fracture fragments are frequently resorbed, and they may show sclerotic or pointed ends. In some cases, the bone resorption is progressive.

Clavicular fractures are commonly associated with rib fractures and may also be associated with adjacent bone resorption. Radiation necrosis of the humerus (see Fig. 61–10) can be seen 7 to 10 years after therapy, and such necrosis is frequently symptomatic. Associated findings in the ribs, clavicle, and scapula are frequent. Changes in the humerus may include resorption cavities, fractures, and ischemic necrosis of the humeral head.

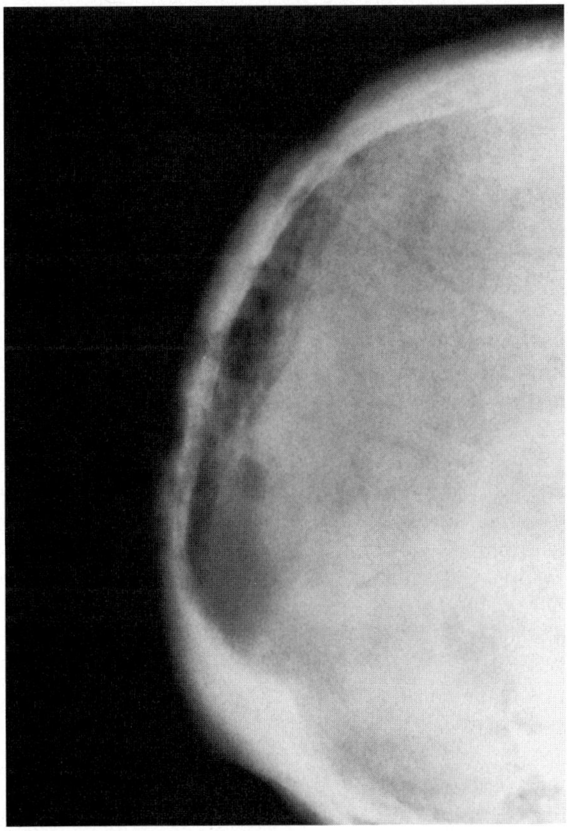

**Pelvis.** Fractures of the femoral neck occurring after radiation therapy to the pelvis (Fig. 61–11) are reported to occur in approximately 2% of patients treated with pelvic radiation. The fractures are usually subcapital in location and typically involve osteopenic bone. Such fractures may be unilateral or bilateral. Fractures of the femoral

**Figure 61–9.** Radiation necrosis of the skull after treatment of basal cell carcinoma. Note that the edges of the lesion are sharp and that the area of necrosis is well defined and relatively superficial. (From Dalinka MK, Mazzeo VP Jr: Complications of radiation therapy. CRC Crit Rev Diagn Imaging 23:235, 1985.)

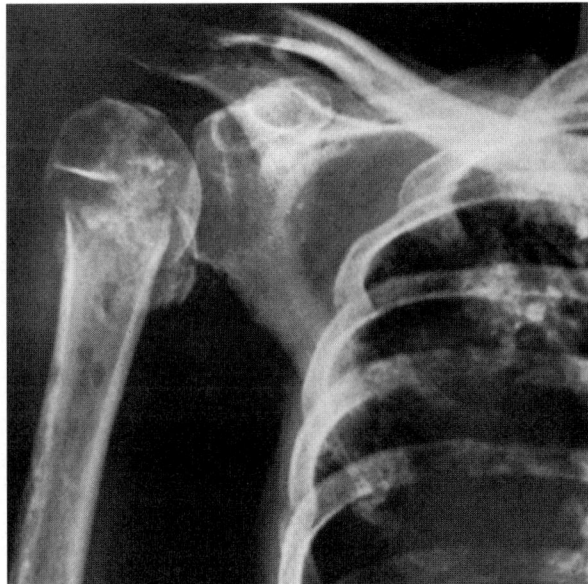

**Figure 61–10.** Radiation necrosis. Examination of the shoulder 10 years after radiation for carcinoma of the breast reveals pathologic fractures of the right humerus and multiple ribs. The lucent lesions in the proximal humeral shaft are also secondary to radiation necrosis. (From Dalinka MK, Edeiken J, Finkelstein JB: Complications of radiation therapy: Adult bone. Semin Roentgenol 9:29, 1974.)

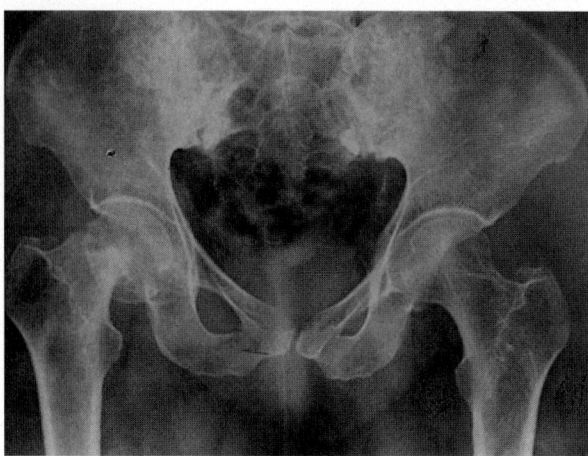

**Figure 61–11.** Fracture of the right femoral neck 4 years after radiation therapy for carcinoma of the cervix. The patient was treated with 2500 cGy external radiation plus two applications of radium. Sclerotic changes are present about both sacroiliac joints, with adjacent calcification.

neck have been reported after as little as 1540 cGy of exposure and as early as 5 months after therapy.

Femoral fractures complicating radiation therapy are believed to begin as insufficiency fractures. Most fractures heal with routine treatment, with adequate callus formation. Osteonecrosis of the femoral head may occur (Fig. 61–12) but is rare after radiation-induced femoral fracture.

Although abnormalities about the sacroiliac joint (simulating those of osteitis condensans ilii and ankylosing spondylitis) are well documented after radiation (Fig. 61–13), fractures represent a more significant complication. These are insufficiency fractures that demonstrate linear sclerosis running vertically in the sacral alae, parallel and adjacent to the sacroiliac joints, although transverse fractures may also develop as a secondary complication from continued stress on the weakened sacrum. Even the iliac side of the articulation may be involved. Bone scintigraphy is a sensitive (and often diagnostic) method for the detection of these fractures. It may demonstrate vertically oriented lines of increased activity running through the sacrum on one or both sides. The lines may be joined by a transverse line to create an H-shaped area of increased activity. Computed tomography scanning may show extensive bone sclerosis about the fracture sites. Although insufficiency fractures about the sacrum are also encountered in patients with osteoporosis, fractures that extend horizontally or obliquely across the ilium are almost specific for radiation injury. Magnetic resonance (MR) imaging can also be used to show radiation-induced fractures of the pelvis (Fig. 61–14). However, marrow edema may obscure the fracture lines when this imaging method is used, so the findings may lack specificity and may simulate those of tumor or infection.

Protrusio acetabuli may also develop, but the mechanism of acetabular protrusion in these patients is unclear. Osteonecrosis of the acetabulum leading to destruction

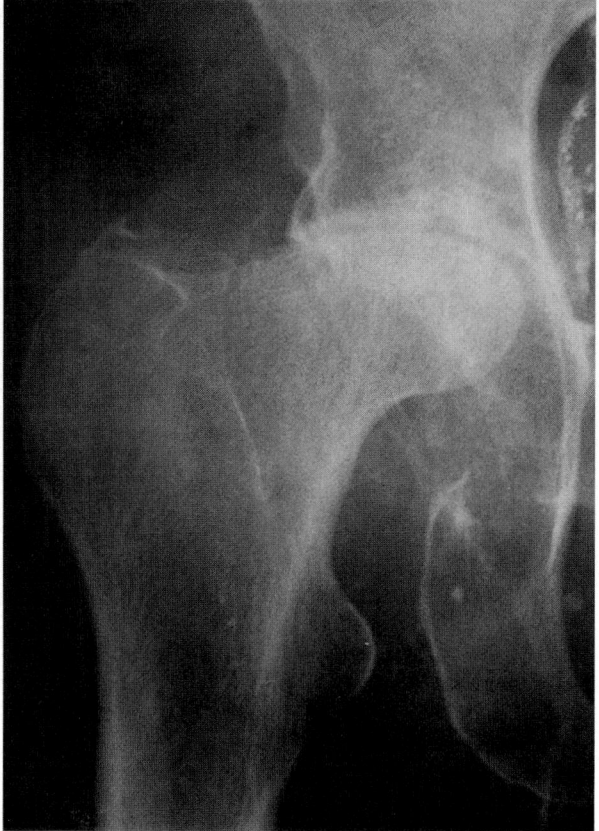

**Figure 61–12.** Radiation necrosis after treatment for carcinoma of the cervix. In this radiograph taken 9 months after therapy, the femoral head has collapsed and there is marked narrowing of the hip joint.

of the hip joint and requiring hip prostheses is also a well-recognized complication of irradiation. Such acetabular changes may be accompanied by fragmentation or resorption of the femoral head and rapid loss of joint space, simulating the appearance of septic arthritis, crystal deposition diseases, neuropathic osteoarthropathy, or idiopathic rapidly destructive hip disease.

**Sternum.** The prevalence and severity of changes in the sternum are directly related to the dose and to the length of follow-up. Mild changes consist of osteoporosis, abnormal bony trabeculae, and localized bone necrosis with sclerosis. Moderate changes include the development of localized pectus excavatum and necrosis involving more than one sternal segment. Severe changes are defined as complete osseous necrosis of one or more sternal segments with deformity.

**Other Sites.** Radiation changes in other areas usually follow a similar pattern. Well-defined lucent shadows are sometimes identified within the field of therapy. These can occur in normal bone after therapy for a soft tissue lesion (Fig. 61–15) or in bone previously treated for an osseous lesion (Fig. 61–16). Small areas of trabecular sclerosis or larger areas of ischemic necrosis may occur, and these may be complicated by superimposed infection.

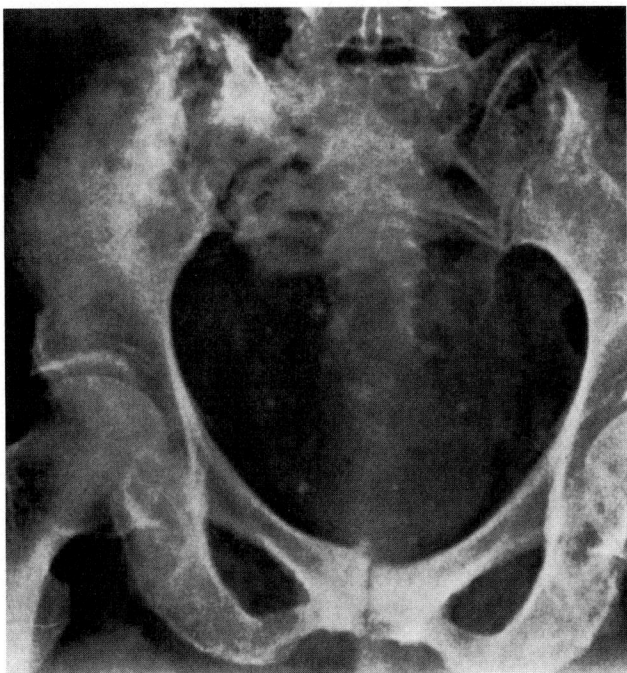

**Figure 61–13.** Radiation necrosis 10 years after treatment for carcinoma of the cervix. The right sacroiliac joint is widened and markedly irregular. Radiation changes in the symphysis pubis simulate osteitis pubis. This patient was treated with 7000 cGy externally using the betatron and 3290 mg-hours of radium. The patient died of a ruptured necrotic bladder and also had radiation necrosis of the bowel. (From Dalinka MK, Edeiken J, Finkelstein JB: Complications of radiation therapy: Adult bone. Semin Roentgenol 9:29, 1974.)

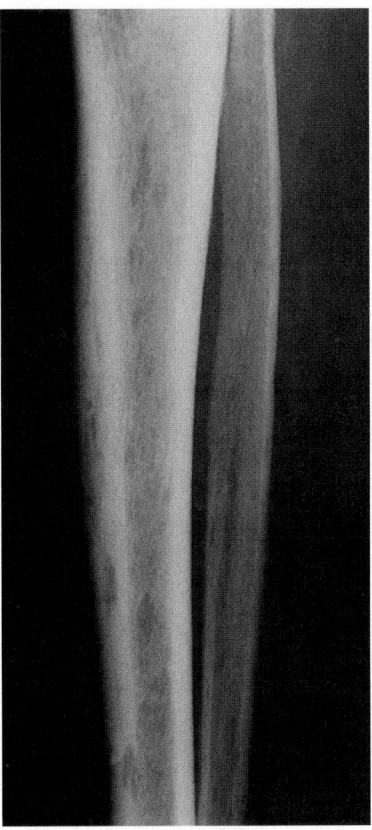

**Figure 61–15.** Radiation changes in the tibia and fibula after treatment for varicose veins. Approximately 50 years after therapy, radiolucent lesions are observed in these long bones. (Courtesy of G. Beauregard, MD, Montreal, Quebec, Canada.)

## Radiation-Induced Neoplasms

**Benign Neoplasms.** Benign radiation-induced neoplasms occur almost exclusively in patients who are treated during childhood, especially those who are younger than 2 years old at treatment. Osteochondromas (exostoses) are the most common benign radiation-induced tumors reported

in humans. They occur exclusively in children and may be seen in any bone in the irradiated field (Fig. 61–17), usually within 5 years after therapy.

Radiation-induced exostoses are identical histologically and radiographically to spontaneously occurring osteochondromas. They typically occur at the periphery of the

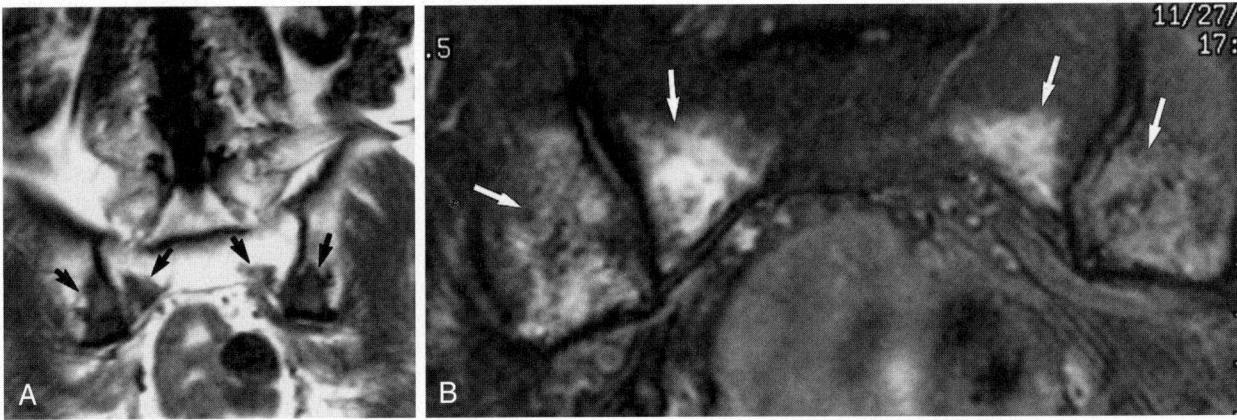

**Figure 61–14.** Radiation changes of the bony pelvis. This 82-year-old man underwent radiation therapy for carcinoma of the prostate. *A*, Coronal T1-weighted (TR/TE, 300/14) spin echo MR image shows regions of low signal intensity *(arrows)* involving the ilium and sacrum about both sacroiliac joints. *B*, Coronal fat-suppressed fast spin echo (TR/TE, 4400/105) MR image reveals edema *(arrows)* at the fracture sites. The fracture lines are poorly seen, but the locations of the lesions are virtually diagnostic of radiation-induced insufficiency fractures. (Courtesy of C. Beaulieu, MD, Palo Alto, Calif.)

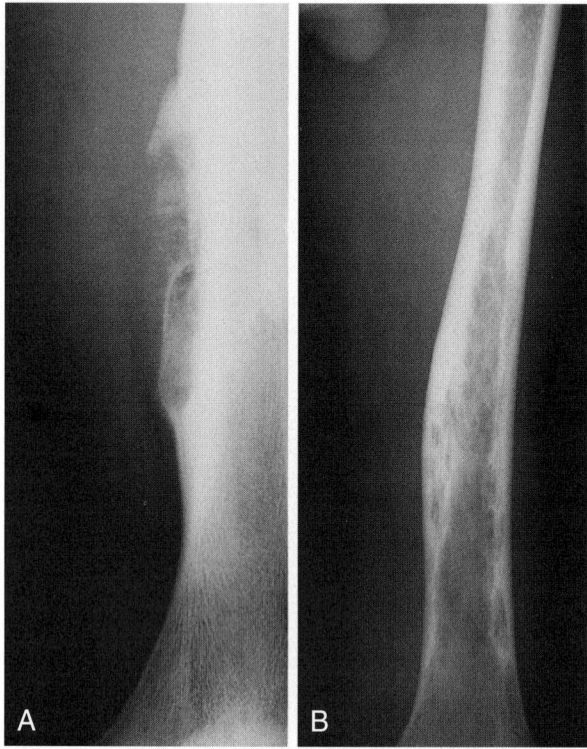

**Figure 61–16.** Ewing's tumor followed by late radiation necrosis. *A,* Oblique view of the femur demonstrates a destructive diaphyseal lesion with saucerization, perpendicular periosteal new bone formation, and a large soft tissue mass. Codman's triangles are present at both edges of the lesion. *B,* In the same patient 31 years later, note the multiple well-defined lucent areas in the shaft of the femur secondary to radiation necrosis.

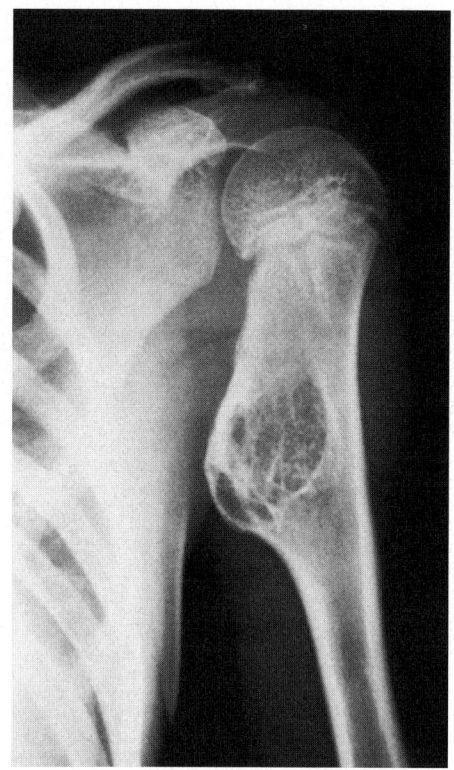

**Figure 61–17.** Radiation-induced exostosis in the proximal portion of the humerus after radiation therapy. This appearance is identical to that of a spontaneously occurring osteochondroma. (Courtesy of W. E. Berdon, MD, New York.)

irradiated field and are reported with doses ranging from 1600 to 6425 cGy. Malignant degeneration of radiation-induced osteochondromas is exceedingly rare but has been reported.

**Malignant Neoplasms.** Radiation-induced malignant neoplasia is a well-recognized complication of radiation therapy. Osseous changes usually precede the development of radiation-induced tumors (Fig. 61–18). Radiation-induced neoplasms form in areas that receive radiation sufficient to induce mutation but not enough to destroy the regenerating capacity of the bone.

The criteria for the diagnosis of radiation-induced sarcoma are as follows:

1. There must be microscopic or radiographic evidence of a nonmalignant condition.

2. Sarcoma must arise within the irradiated field.

3. A long latent period must be present (at least 4 years).

4. Histologic proof of sarcoma must be available.

On the basis of these criteria, radiation-induced sarcomas have been documented in both soft tissue and bone. Before the mid-1980s, osteosarcoma was the most common radiation-induced sarcoma in most series. Since the mid-1980s, malignant fibrous histiocytoma has become estab-

lished as a histologic entity and is the most frequent diagnosis in many series of radiation-induced malignancies. Many soft tissue tumors that would have been considered fibrosarcomas in the past are now being called malignant fibrous histiocytomas.

The evidence that radiation can induce sarcomas is overwhelming. Although sarcomas have been reported with doses as low as 800 cGy for the treatment of bursitis, radiation-induced sarcomas usually require a dose of at least 3000 cGy in 3 weeks, with a threshold appearing at about 1000 cGy. A higher prevalence of radiation-induced tumors would be expected in children because of the longer potential period at risk; however, the latent period does not seem to differ between children and adults. It varies between 4 and 42 years, with an average of 11 years (Fig. 61–19). Radiation-induced bone sarcoma may arise in previously normal or abnormal bone; however, in one series, 70% of patients had preexisting bone disease.

Radiation necrosis can usually be differentiated from sarcoma arising in irradiated bone, although this may be difficult in some cases. It may not be possible to distinguish a new radiation-induced sarcoma from recurrence of the original tumor. Sarcoma, necrosis, and recurrences all occur within the field of radiation and may be seen years after treatment. The presence of pain, a soft tissue mass, or a new focal lucent area favors the diagnosis of

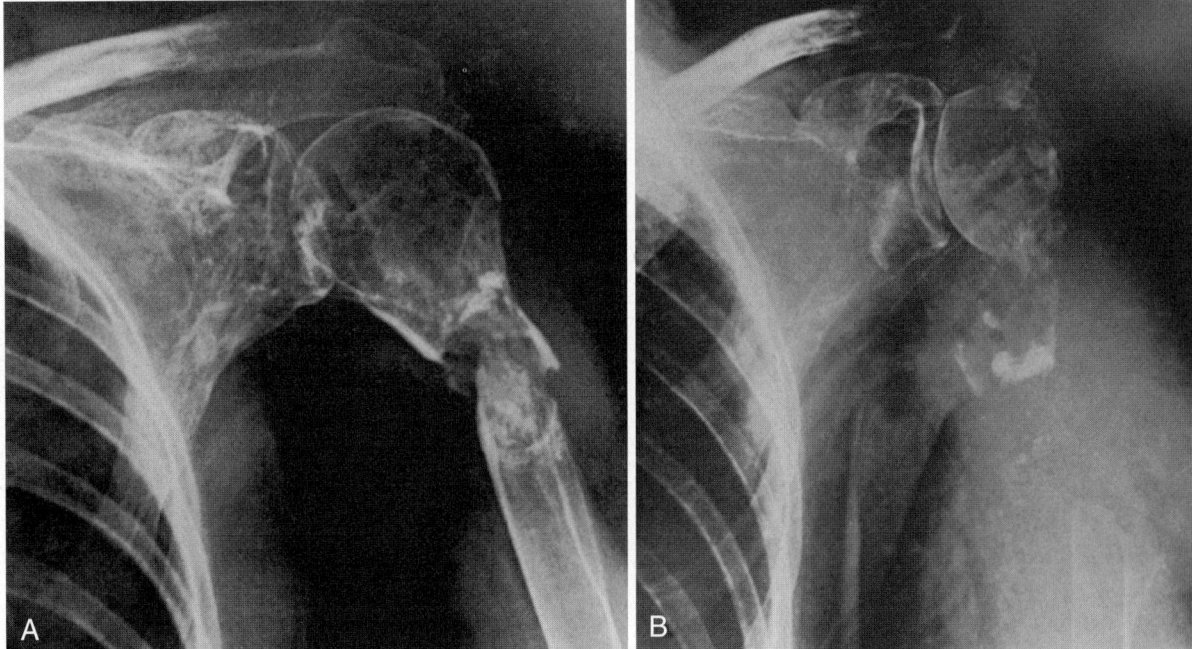

**Figure 61–18.** Sarcoma arising in irradiated bone. *A*, Radiograph 8 years after radiation therapy for breast carcinoma shows a previous pathologic fracture and pseudarthrosis of the humerus, with radiation changes in the scapula and humerus. *B*, In the same patient 6 years later, note an undifferentiated radiation-induced sarcoma of the humerus. (*A*, From Dalinka MK, Edeiken J, Finkelstein JB: Complications of radiation therapy: Adult bone. Semin Roentgenol 9:29, 1974.)

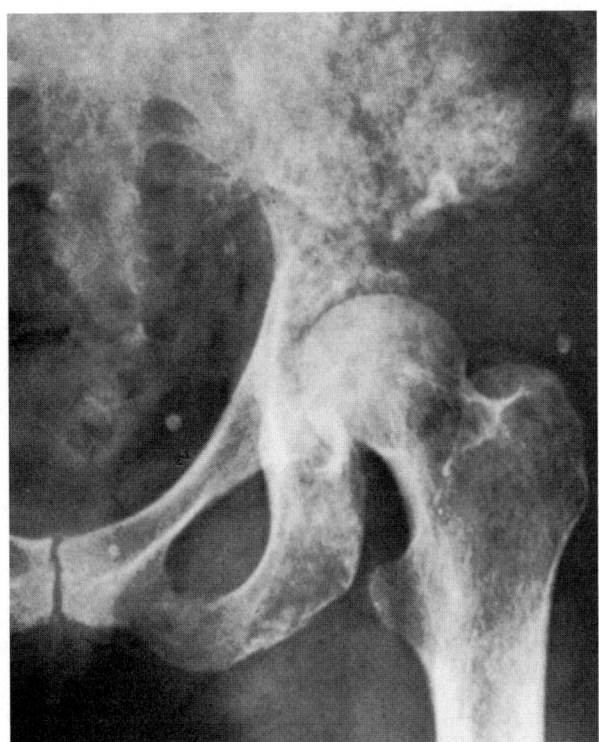

**Figure 61–19.** Anteroposterior view of the pelvis shows osteosarcoma of the left iliac wing 17 years after radiation therapy for cervical carcinoma. (From Dalinka MK, Edeiken J, Finkelstein JB: Complications of radiation therapy: Adult bone. Semin Roentgenol 9:29, 1974.)

recurrent or new neoplasia, whereas their absence favors radiation necrosis. A relative lack of change on serial radiographs favors the diagnosis of radiation necrosis, although healing, remodeling, and development of osteoradionecrosis are dynamic processes that themselves produce radiographic changes (Fig. 61–20).

## Musculoskeletal Applications of Radiation Therapy

Radiation is used extensively in the management of painful myelomatous and metastatic lesions. Patients are treated symptomatically with relatively low doses, frequently with large fractions. A favorable clinical response is often followed by sclerosis in the treated area, with partial or complete healing of the metastatic focus.

Radiation therapy has been used to decrease ectopic bone formation in high-risk patients undergoing total hip arthroplasty. This therapy, sometimes used in conjunction with nonsteroidal anti-inflammatory drugs, prevents heterotopic ossification in approximately 90% of such patients. As yet, there are no definite reported complications of this therapy.

Radiation has been used to sterilize allograft bone before implantation in the recipient. A dose of 2500 cGy is effective against both bacterial and viral pathogens without significant loss of strength. There have been no reported changes in the radiographic appearance of the allograft due to radiation.

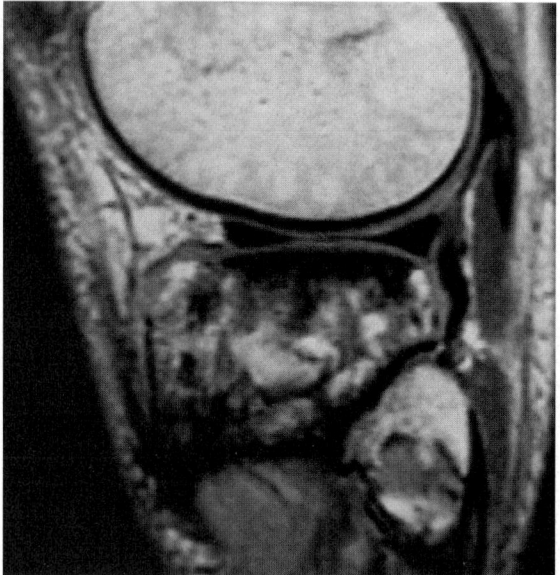

**Figure 61–20.** Radiation changes on MR imaging. This patient underwent radiation therapy for a tibial lymphoma 2 years previously. On this sagittal intermediate-weighted (TR/TE, 1600/16) MR image, areas of signal void probably represent extremely dense sclerotic bone. This appearance was unchanged for more than a year, which, together with involvement of both the tibia and the fibula, suggests radiation change rather than new or recurrent tumor.

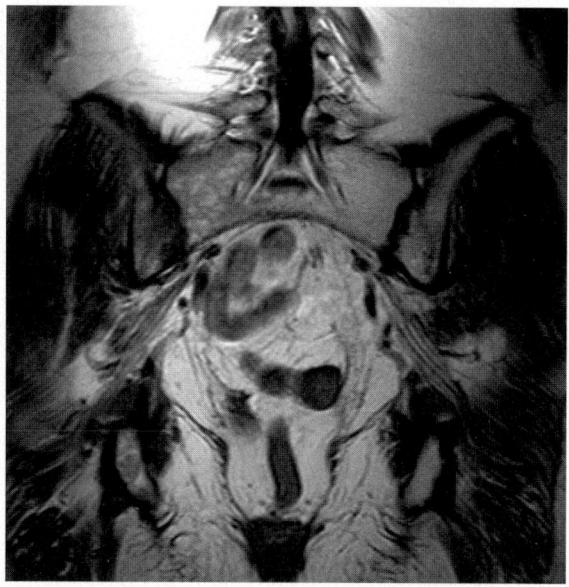

**Figure 61–21.** Radiation changes in the marrow. This patient underwent radiation therapy to the left pelvis. Coronal T1-weighted (TR/TE, 622/17) spin echo MR image shows increased fatty marrow signal from the left sacrum, ilium and ischium.

## MAGNETIC RESONANCE IMAGING

MR imaging is often used to assess the response of malignant bone and soft tissue tumors to radiation therapy. With regard to the marrow, experimental studies indicate that both hemorrhage and fat contribute to the signal intensity characteristics seen on MR images after irradiation. Hemorrhage changes dominate in the early states (i.e., first few days) after radiation therapy. Subsequently, fat accumulates in the marrow. In clinical practice, similar time-dependent changes are observed. For example, as early as 2 months after radiation therapy, T1-weighted spin echo MR images of the spine show increased signal intensity within the bone marrow, probably representing a relative or absolute increase in marrow fat (Fig. 61–21). This change may be permanent, and the presence of tissue in the marrow that does not show the signal intensity characteristics of fat is a strong indicator of recurrent tumor.

With regard to soft tissues, MR imaging may prove useful in the differentiation of radiation fibrosis from recurrent tumor. Radiation fibrosis usually has a low signal intensity similar to that of muscle on both T1- and T2-weighted spin echo MR sequences; in contrast, tumor clearly shows increased signal intensity, especially on T2-weighted spin echo images. However, the presence of increased signal intensity on T2-weighted images does not eliminate the possibility of radiation-induced fibrosis and necrosis. Further, postradiation soft tissue edema can simulate the appearance of recurrent tumor on MR images. The duration and degree of such edema are variable. Edema persists longer in intramuscular septa than in muscle or fat and generally resolves in 2 to 4 years.

## FURTHER READING

Arlen M, Higinbotham NL, Huvos AG, et al: Radiation induced sarcoma of bone. Cancer 28:1087, 1971.

Bonfiglio M: The pathology of fractures of the femoral neck following irradiation. AJR Am J Roentgenol 70:449, 1953.

Brady LW: Radiation induced sarcomas of bone. Skeletal Radiol 41:72, 1979.

Bragg DG, Shidnia H, Chu FCH, et al: The clinical and radiographic aspects of radiation osteitis. Radiology 97:103, 1970.

Chapman JA, Deakin DP, Green JH: Slipped upper femoral epiphysis after radiotherapy. J Bone Joint Surg Br 62:337, 1980.

Cohen J, D'Angio GJ: Unusual bone tumors after roentgen therapy of children. AJR Am J Roentgenol 86:502, 1961.

Cooper KL, Beabout JW, Swee RG: Insufficiency fractures of the sacrum. Radiology 156:15, 1985.

Dalinka MK, Edeiken J, Finkelstein JB: Complications of radiation therapy: Adult bone. Semin Roentgenol 9:29, 1974.

Deleeuw HW, Pottenger LA: Osteonecrosis of the acetabulum following radiation therapy. J Bone Joint Surg Am 70:293, 1988.

DeSmet AA, Kuhns LR, Fayos JV, et al: Effects of radiation therapy on growing long bones. AJR Am J Roentgenol 127:935, 1976.

Glazer HS, Lee JKT, Levitt RG, et al: Radiation fibrosis: Differentiation from recurrent tumor by MR imaging—work in progress. Radiology 156:721, 1985.

Gondos B: Late clinical and roentgen observations following Thorotrast administration. Clin Radiol 24:195, 1973.

Hall FM, Mauch PM, Levene MB, et al: Protrusio acetabuli following pelvic irradiation. AJR Am J Roentgenol 132:291, 1979.

Howland WJ, Loeffler RK, Starchman DE, et al: Post irradiation atrophic changes of bone and related complications. Radiology 117:677, 1975.

Kim JH, Chu FCH, Pope RA, et al: Time dose factors in radiation induced osteitis. AJR Am J Roentgenol 120:684, 1974.

Libshitz HI, Cohen MA: Radiation induced osteochondromas. Radiology 142:643, 1982.

Mitchell MJ, Logan PM: Radiation-induced changes in bone. Radiographics 18:1125, 1998.

Murray EM, Werner D, Greeff EA, et al: Postradiation sarcomas: 20 cases and a literature review. Int J Radiat Oncol Biol Phys 45:951, 1999.

Neuhauser EBD, Wittenborg MH, Berman CZ, et al: Irradiation effects of roentgen therapy on the growing spine. Radiology 59:637, 1952.

Paling MR, Herdt JR: Radiation osteitis: A problem of recognition. Radiology 137:339, 1980.

Phillips TL, Sheline GE: Bone sarcomas following radiation therapy. Radiology 81:992, 1963.

Rubin P, Probhasawat D: Characteristic bone lesions in post irradiated carcinoma of the cervix—metastases versus osteonecrosis. Radiology 76:703, 1961.

# CHAPTER 62

## Disorders Due to Medications and Other Chemical Agents

### *SUMMARY OF KEY FEATURES*

A survey of the musculoskeletal manifestations associated with certain medications and chemical substances indicates that in some cases the therapeutic regimen may be more detrimental than the disease. A variety of teratogenic drugs can lead to significant fetal anomalies. Corticosteroids and other anti-inflammatory agents can produce osteoporosis, osteonecrosis, and neuropathic-like alterations. Osteosclerosis, periostitis, osseous excrescences, ligamentous calcification, and dental abnormalities can accompany fluorosis. Injection of dopamine and related substances may lead to gangrene, requiring amputation, whereas soft tissue calcification may appear after calcium gluconate injection or ingestion of milk and alkali. New bone formation is seen in some patients receiving prostaglandins or isotretinoin. Quinolones may produce tendinosis and tendon rupture.

### INTRODUCTION

Significant musculoskeletal changes can result from medications and other chemical agents. This chapter considers the musculoskeletal alterations that may accompany the administration of certain teratogenic drugs, corticosteroids and other anti-inflammatory agents, fluorine, dopamine, calcium gluconate, milk-alkali, prostaglandins, retinoic acid, and other chemical agents.

### TERATOGENIC DRUGS

It is well recognized that medications administered to a pregnant woman can affect the fetus. Drugs that act on the somatic cells of the developing organism during vulnerable periods of embryogenesis and organogenesis are termed teratogens. Of particular importance with regard to the musculoskeletal system are thalidomide, anticonvulsants, and alcohol.

#### Thalidomide

Thalidomide was previously used to induce sleep in pregnant women, with disastrous results. When it is ingested during the first trimester, thalidomide exposure produces reduction deformities of the limbs of the fetus. The anomalies include dysplasia of the thumb and radial hemimelia, phocomelia, or complete four-limb amelia; these deformities are associated with hypoplasia or aplasia of the external ear and canal, congenital heart defects, gastrointestinal tract atresia or stenosis, and capillary hemangioma of the face. Although abnormalities in the appendicular skeleton predominate in thalidomide embryopathy, peculiar spinal alterations may also be observed. Irregularities of the contour of the vertebral bodies and anterior fusion between adjacent vertebrae are encountered. The resulting radiographic findings simulate those of Scheuermann's disease and idiopathic progressive noninfectious anterior vertebral fusion.

#### Anticonvulsants

When administered to expectant mothers, anticonvulsant medications, especially phenytoin, may lead to congenital anomalies in their infants, including hypoplasia of the distal phalanges, digitate thumb, cleft palate, decreased head circumference, and peculiar facies. The teratogenic potential of anticonvulsants is not accepted by all investigators.

#### Alcohol

Infants born to severely and chronically alcoholic women may exhibit the fetal alcohol syndrome, consisting of prenatal and postnatal growth deficiency and delayed development. Findings may include clinodactyly, camptodactyly, congenital dislocation of the hip, pectus excavatum or carinatum, radioulnar synostosis, scoliosis, and vertebral fusion. The precise cause of fetal alcohol syndrome is unclear. Although ethanol appears to be the principal agent responsible for the findings, a potential role for acetaldehyde, the primary metabolite of ethanol, is possible.

### CORTICOSTEROIDS AND OTHER ANTI-INFLAMMATORY AGENTS

The complications of cortisone therapy can become manifest in almost any system of the body, including the skeleton (Table 62–1).

---

**TABLE 62–1**

**Musculoskeletal Abnormalities Associated with Corticosteroid Medication**

Osteoporosis
Osteonecrosis
Neuropathic-like arthropathy
Osteomyelitis (septic arthritis)
Tendinous injury or rupture
Soft tissue atrophy
Intra-articular calcification
Periarticular calcification
Accumulation of fat

---

## Osteoporosis

The occurrence of generalized osteoporosis in patients receiving systemic corticosteroids has been noted by many observers. Stress (insufficiency) fractures occur and heal with extensive callus formation. Collapse of single or multiple vertebral bodies, with condensation of bone at the superior and inferior surfaces (Fig. 62–1), and infractions of ribs are particularly characteristic. The radiographic diagnosis of insufficiency fractures related to corticosteroid therapy is often difficult, owing to the associated generalized osteopenia. Although bone scintigraphy can be used to enhance the diagnostic accuracy, false-negative results may be encountered. Computed tomography and magnetic resonance (MR) imaging are useful in detecting such fractures in anatomically complex regions. The precise mechanism by which corticosteroids lead to bone loss is not known.

## Osteonecrosis

The true frequency of steroid-induced osteonecrosis is difficult to determine because of the many variables included in different studies. In patients receiving corticosteroids after renal transplantation, the frequency appears to be approximately 5% to 10%. In many reviews of patients with osteonecrosis, steroid medications are implicated in 20% to 35% of cases. The occurrence of steroid-induced bone necrosis appears to be directly related to the dosage level and duration of the medication, and it may become prominent in many persons after prolonged high intake. Single or multiple osseous sites can be affected; the femoral head, humeral head, distal end of the femur, and proximal part of the tibia are altered most commonly, in decreasing order of frequency (Fig. 62–2). Radiographic and pathologic characteristics of osteonecrosis due to corticosteroids are not unique, being evident in cases of bony necrosis from other causes (see Chapter 51). As observed in ischemic necrosis in general, bone scanning and MR imaging are more sensitive than plain film radiography in detecting sites of osseous necrosis in patients receiving corticosteroids (Fig. 62–3). The pathogenesis of steroid-associated osteonecrosis is not clear (Table 62–2).

Changes in the diaphyses and metaphyses of tubular bones are encountered less frequently than epiphyseal alterations in patients being treated with steroids or other anti-inflammatory agents. Osteonecrosis of vertebral bodies in association with steroid medications has been recognized. Radiolucent linear shadows in the subchondral bone reflect fractures of necrotic bone and are reminiscent of the radiolucent areas that appear at other sites of osteonecrosis, such as the femoral and humeral heads (Fig. 62–4). This phenomenon is termed the vacuum vertebral body. Although it is not associated universally with ischemic necrosis of bone, it is most suggestive of that diagnosis.

## Neuropathic-Like Articular Destruction

A neuropathic-like, rapidly progressive joint disease characterized by severe osseous and cartilaginous destruction represents one variety of steroid arthropathy that typically appears after intra-articular injection of the

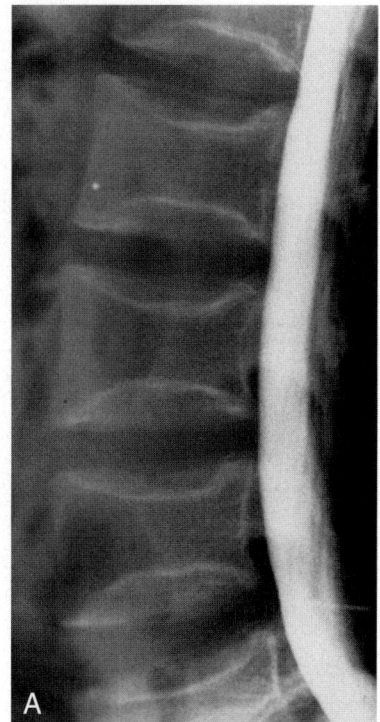
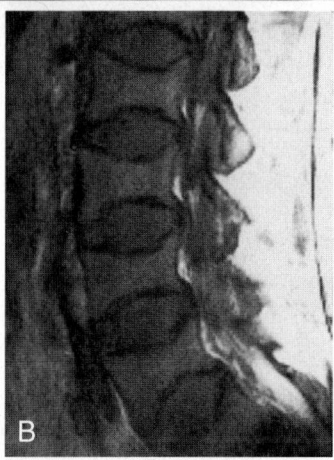

**Figure 62–1.** Steroid-induced osteoporosis. This 22-year-old woman, who had received systemic corticosteroid therapy for many months as a child, developed cushingoid features, with deposition of fat in the shoulders and back and muscle weakness. *A*, Lateral radiograph obtained during a lumbar myelogram (for investigation of low back pain) reveals osteopenia, biconcave deformities of multiple vertebral bodies, and well-defined subchondral bone plates. *B*, Sagittal T1-weighted (TR/TE, 200/26) spin echo MR image of the lumbar spine shows the biconcave deformities to good advantage. The signal intensity of the bone marrow reflects the presence of hematopoietic tissue and is within normal limits. (Courtesy of G. Greenway, MD, Dallas.)

drug (Table 62–3). It may be associated with osteoporosis, osteonecrosis, and an underlying articular disorder, such as rheumatoid arthritis or osteoarthritis (Fig. 62–5). Although any joint can be affected, the hip and knee are involved most frequently. The rapidity of the process can be remarkable. The pathogenesis of the process is not certain.

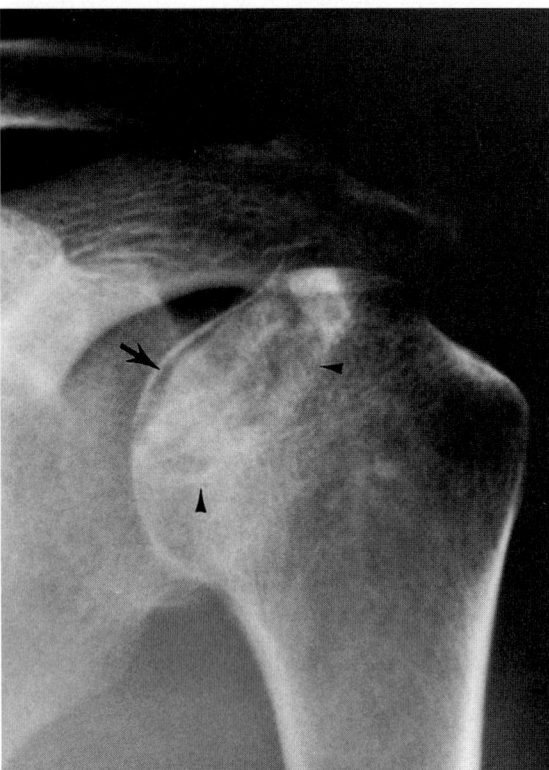

**Figure 62–2.** Steroid-induced osteonecrosis: proximal end of the humerus. Abnormalities consist of flattening of the humeral head with a subchondral radiolucent line—the crescent sign *(arrow)*—surrounding osteolysis and osteosclerosis *(arrowheads)*, and relative preservation of joint space.

## Osteomyelitis and Septic Arthritis

Bone and joint infections can complicate steroid therapy, although such complications are rare. Septic arthritis can appear after oral, intravenous, or intra-articular adminis-

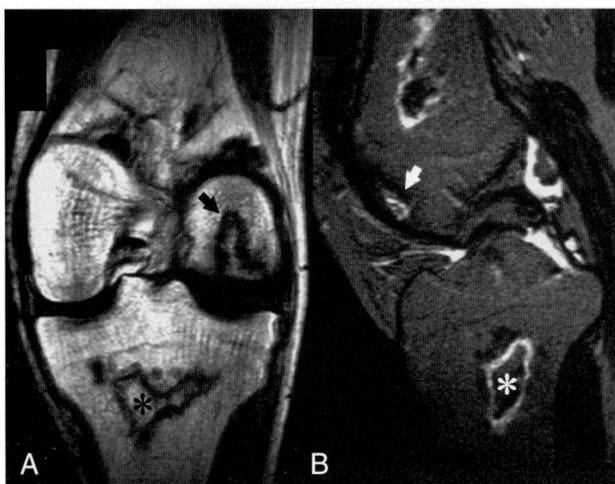

**Figure 62–3.** Steroid-induced osteonecrosis: knee. This 28-year-old woman had received oral corticosteroids for inflammatory bowel disease. Coronal T1-weighted (TR/TE, 550/16) *(A)* and conventional sagittal T2-weighted (TR/TE, 2500/80) *(B)* spin echo MR images reveal osteonecrosis *(arrows)* and bone infarcts *(asterisks)*. Note the "double-line" sign on the T2-weighted image.

**TABLE 62–2**

**Pathogenesis of Steroid-Induced Osteonecrosis**

| Theory | Possible Mechanisms |
|---|---|
| Mechanical | Osteoporosis leading to microfractures and osseous collapse |
| Vascular | Vascular compression from marrow accumulation of fat |
| | Fat embolization following steroid-induced fatty liver |
| | Vasculitis |
| | Hyperviscosity |

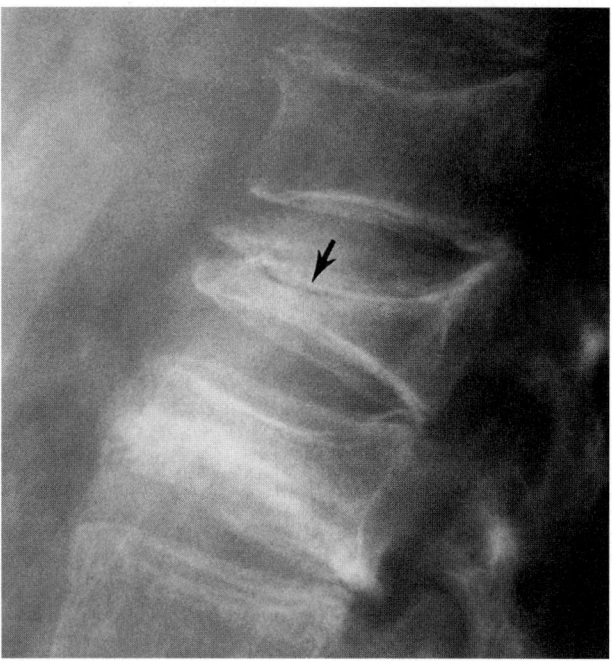

**Figure 62–4.** Steroid-induced osteonecrosis: vertebral bodies. Observe collapse of multiple osteoporotic lumbar vertebral bodies, reactive sclerosis of endplates, and a radiolucent line or crescent within the bone *(arrow)*. The last-mentioned finding differs from a vacuum intervertebral disc, in which the radiolucent collection is located in the disc itself.

**TABLE 62–3**

**Steroid-Induced Neuropathic-Like Alterations**

| Possible Pathogenesis | Characteristics |
|---|---|
| Neuropathic osteoarthropathy due to sensory loss induced by medication | Usually evident after intra-articular administration of drug |
| Osteonecrosis | Predilection for the hip and knee |
| | Rapid onset and progression |
| | Osseous defects ("bites"), collapse, and fragmentation |
| | Cartilaginous destruction |

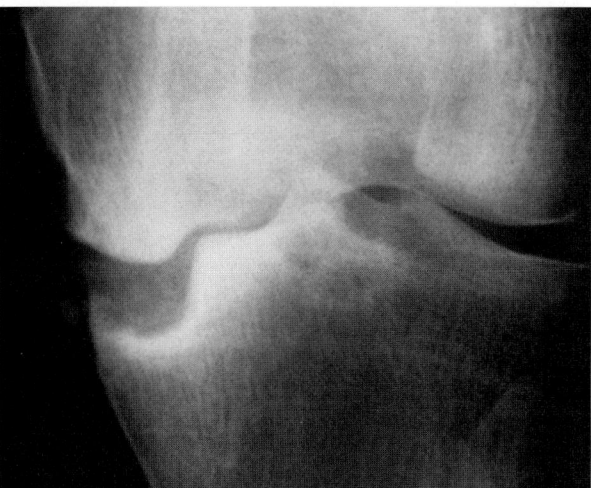

**Figure 62–5.** Steroid-induced neuropathic-like arthropathy. In this 70-year-old woman with rheumatoid arthritis, multiple steroid injections into the knee were associated with significant bone abnormalities. Note the gouged-out area of destruction in the medial tibial plateau.

tration and can affect any joint, particularly the knee. Similarly, osteomyelitis can appear alone or in conjunction with septic arthritis. The initiation and spread of infection are promoted by the medication's interference with normal host defense mechanisms.

## Tendinous and Soft Tissue Injury

Tendinous rupture has been described in association with systemically or locally administered corticosteroids (Fig. 62–6). At this time, it appears likely that steroids, particularly when administered locally, accelerate the degeneration and rupture of a tendon that is already the site of a pathologic process; whether similar complications can occur in healthy tendons after steroid administration is not certain.

## Intra-articular and Periarticular Calcification

The occurrence of calcification in and around joints that have been injected with corticosteroid preparations is well documented. The knee is involved most commonly, and the calcified deposits occur in the infrapatellar fat pad and, less frequently, in the synovial membrane, joint capsule, and adjacent ligaments. The responsible crystal is calcium hydroxyapatite (Fig. 62–7). Periarticular and intra-articular calcification may also be observed after systemic administration of corticosteroids.

## Accumulation of Fat

Endogenous or exogenous corticosteroid excess leads to abnormal accumulations of fat. Mediastinal lipomatosis represents one manifestation of this phenomenon, which may resolve if the steroid dosage is lowered or terminated. Similarly, paraspinal localization may be seen. Although the masses of fat in the thorax and paraspinal regions rarely lead to clinical manifestations, epidural

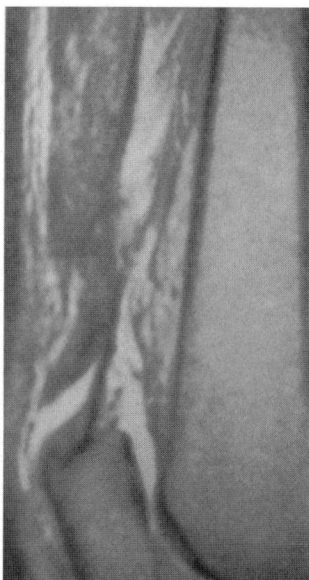

**Figure 62–6.** Steroid-induced tendon injury: quadriceps tendon. In this patient on a long-term systemic steroid regimen, sagittal T2-weighted (TR/TE, 2500/80) spin echo MR image shows rupture of the quadriceps tendon, with peritendinous extravasation of fluid and a joint effusion.

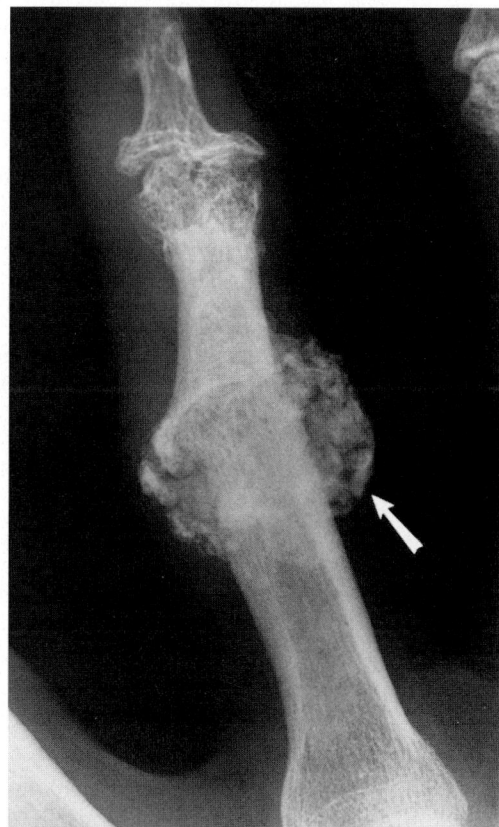

**Figure 62–7.** Steroid-induced intra-articular and periarticular calcification. In this 57-year-old woman with osteoarthritis of the interphalangeal joints of both hands, multiple intra-articular injections of triamcinolone hexacetonide were followed by the development of intra-articular and periarticular calcifications (*arrow*), presumably related to calcium hydroxyapatite crystal deposition. (Courtesy of M. Dalinka, MD, Philadelphia.)

lipomatosis in patients receiving corticosteroid therapy (as well as those with Cushing's disease) may produce neurologic complications, including paraplegia. Cord compression is a far more common complication of epidural lipomatosis in exogenous as opposed to endogenous (i.e., Cushing's disease) steroid excess.

# FLUORINE

Chronic fluorine intoxication (fluorosis) arises when the drinking water contains fluoride in concentrations higher than 4 parts per million (ppm); fluorosis occurs as an endemic problem in certain regions of the world, especially India, where it was first described in the 1930s. The entity may also appear in industrial workers who are exposed to fluorine compounds over a period of years. Bone changes are also recognized in patients with osteoporosis who are treated with sodium fluoride. Investigations have revealed that although a fluoride concentration of 1 ppm can reduce dental caries, a level of 2 ppm or more can lead to mottled enamel, 8 ppm can produce osteosclerosis in 10% of persons, and more than 100 ppm can induce growth disturbances, kidney damage, or death.

Approximately 50% of the absorbed fluoride is excreted, mainly in the urine, and approximately 99% of the fluoride retained in the body is deposited in the calcified tissue. The biologic half-life for bone fluoride is about 8 years, owing to the slow rate of turnover of skeletal tissues. Clinical manifestations of acute fluoride exposure include nausea, vomiting, constipation, loss of appetite, and toxic nephritis; manifestations in cases of more prolonged exposure include joint pain and restriction of motion, back stiffness, restriction of respiratory movements, functional dyspnea, dental alterations, paraplegia, and palpable thickening of the bones, including the clavicle, tibia, and ulna.

## Dental Fluorosis

Mottled enamel is an early dental sign of fluoride intoxication. Progression of the dental changes leads to depressions or pits of variable size and discoloration. Radiographs outline hypoplasia, irregular dental roots, and periapical sclerosis and root resorption.

## Skeletal Fluorosis

**Radiographic Abnormalities.** Involvement of the axial skeleton is characteristic (Table 62–4). Changes are most marked in the spine, pelvis, and ribs. Although osteopenia can appear initially, particularly in children, osteosclerosis usually appears first. Increasing trabecular condensation eventually creates a radiodense or chalky appearance throughout the thorax, vertebral column, and pelvis, with obscuration of bony architecture (Fig. 62–8). The skull and tubular bones of the appendicular skeleton are relatively spared.

Vertebral osteophytosis can lead to encroachment on the spinal canal and intervertebral foramina. In the axial skeleton, hyperostosis and bony excrescences develop at sites of ligamentous attachment, especially in the iliac crests, ischial tuberosities, and inferior margins of the

---

| **TABLE 62–4** |
| --- |
| **Radiographic Abnormalities in Fluorosis** |

Hypoplasia and irregularity of dental structures
Osteosclerosis
Vertebral osteophytosis
Ligamentous calcification
Periostitis

---

ribs. Calcification of paraspinal and intraspinal ligaments, including the posterior longitudinal ligament, and of the sacrotuberous and iliolumbar ligaments can be noted (see Fig. 62–8B).

In the appendicular skeleton, osteopenia with or without growth recovery lines may be an early finding. Periosteal thickening, calcification of ligaments, and excrescences at ligamentous and muscular attachments to bone can also be seen at one or more sites.

**Complications.** Advanced stages of fluorosis can lead to significant and crippling abnormalities, including kyphosis, restricted spinal and chest motion, and contractures and deformities of extraspinal joints such as the hips and knees. Neurologic complications include paresthesias, muscular weakening and wasting, sensory disturbances, and paralysis.

**Reversibility of Skeletal Abnormalities.** The radiographic identification of less striking skeletal abnormalities in retired workers who had been exposed to fluoride while employed is consistent with the concept that such abnormalities are reversible. The resulting radiographic appearance, consisting of a coarsened trabecular pattern without increased radiodensity, resembles that of Paget's disease. The degree of cortical bone thickening and calcification of muscle insertions and ligaments remains unchanged.

**Fluoride Treatment of Osteoporosis.** Sodium fluoride has been used in the treatment of osteoporosis for approximately 25 years. The rationale for its use is fluoride's ability to stimulate new bone formation through increased osteoblastic activity and to depress bone resorption through the deposition of relatively stable fluoroapatite, which is less active in surface exchange reactions. Radiographic changes appear to occur in direct proportion to the duration of treatment, and the first detectable changes are noted at least 1 year after the start of fluoride therapy. Findings include pronounced bone radiodensity, cortical thickening, coarsening of the trabecular pattern, and partial obliteration of the medullary space, and they are observed principally in the axial skeleton, especially the spine and pelvis. Ligamentous calcification, a frequent finding in industrial and endemic fluorosis, is not a feature of iatrogenic fluorosis. The abnormalities simulate those of Paget's disease, myelofibrosis, and renal osteodystrophy. In the appendicular skeleton, periosteal and endosteal bone formation is particularly prominent in areas of high mechanical stress.

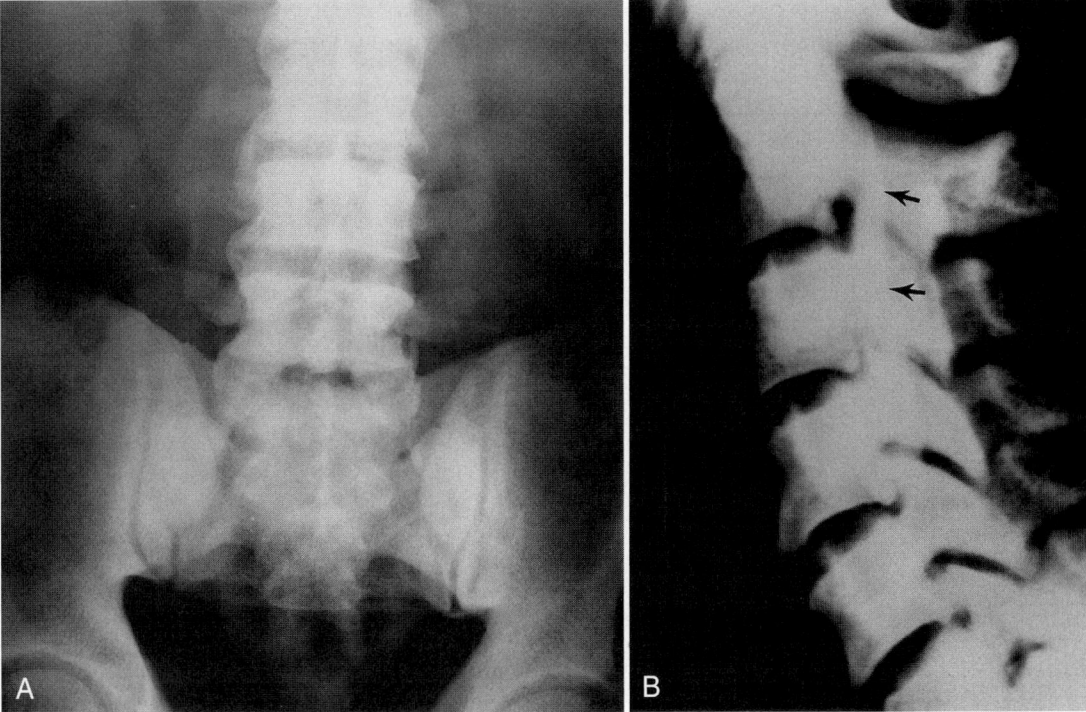

**Figure 62–8.** Fluorosis: axial skeletal abnormalities. *A*, Osteosclerosis and vertebral osteophytosis are evident in a patient with fluorosis. Note the bony eburnation about the sacroiliac joints. *B*, In a different patient, note the extreme increase in radiodensity of the cervical spine, with spinal osteophytes and ossification of the posterior longitudinal ligament *(arrows)*. (*B*, Courtesy of G. Beauregard, MD, Montreal, Quebec, Canada.)

Although the radiographic appearance of osteoporotic bone in patients receiving sodium fluoride is one of progressive osteosclerosis, it is not clear whether a commensurate increase in osseous strength occurs. In fact, fractures of the vertebral bodies and tubular bones during fluoride treatment have been reported.

**Differential Diagnosis.** The combination of findings noted on the radiographs of patients with skeletal fluorosis is virtually diagnostic. Osteosclerosis, osteophytosis, and ligamentous calcification represent a useful triad of abnormalities that are evident on pelvis and spine radiographs. The other alterations that occur in both axial and extra-axial locations, such as periostitis and osseous excrescences at sites of tendinous and ligamentous attachment, provide additional clues to the correct diagnosis.

Osteosclerosis alone is not diagnostic of fluorosis; it is evident in skeletal metastasis, myelofibrosis, mastocytosis, certain hemoglobinopathies, renal osteodystrophy, Paget's disease, congenital disorders, and other conditions as well. Likewise, vertebral osteophytosis or similar outgrowths can accompany many diseases, including fluorosis, spondylosis deformans, diffuse idiopathic skeletal hyperostosis, ankylosing spondylitis, the spondylitis of psoriasis, Reiter's syndrome and inflammatory bowel disorders, acromegaly, neuropathic osteoarthropathy, and alkaptonuria. Proliferative changes at ligamentous and tendinous insertions in bones are apparent not only in fluorosis but also in diffuse idiopathic skeletal hyperostosis, hypoparathyroidism, X-linked hypophosphatemic osteomalacia, and

certain plasma cell dyscrasias. Periostitis similar to that seen in fluorosis can be detected in hypertrophic osteoarthropathy, pachydermoperiostosis, and thyroid acropathy.

## CALCIUM GLUCONATE

Intravenous administration of calcium gluconate has been used in the treatment of neonatal tetany and neonatal asphyxia. Subcutaneous masses of calcification can appear at sites of recent or previous injections. Clinical findings include erythema and bulla formation, which become evident in days and may be followed by skin sloughing and secondary infection. Calcification, which is related to tissue necrosis, can be noted within 4 or 5 days or as late as 3 weeks after injection (Fig. 62–9). It is amorphous and can be localized or distributed along fascial planes. Vascular calcification may also be apparent. With healing, clinical and radiographic manifestations may disappear. The radiographic changes simulate those in subcutaneous fat necrosis and hematomas after trauma.

## MILK-ALKALI

Milk-alkali syndrome was initially observed in patients with chronic peptic ulcer disease and renal insufficiency in whom excessive intake of milk and alkali (over a few to many years) had led to metastatic calcification. These patients exhibit hypercalcemia without hypercalciuria or hypophosphatemia, normal serum alkaline phosphatase levels, azotemia, and mild alkalosis. Soft tissue calcifi-

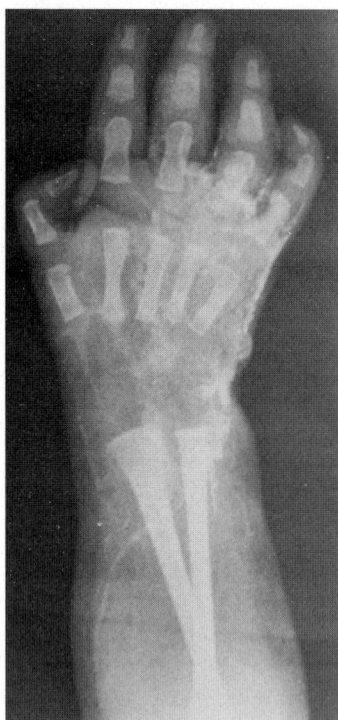

**Figure 62–9.** Calcium gluconate extravasation. This 3-pound, 6-ounce infant received an infusion of calcium gluconate into a vein in the dorsum of the hand that subsequently infiltrated into the soft tissues. Radiograph taken approximately 1 week later reveals extensive linear and platelike subcutaneous deposits, with vascular calcification. (From Berger PE, Heidelberger KP, Poznanski AK: Extravasation of calcium gluconate as a cause of soft tissue calcification in infancy. AJR Am J Roentgenol 121:109, 1974.)

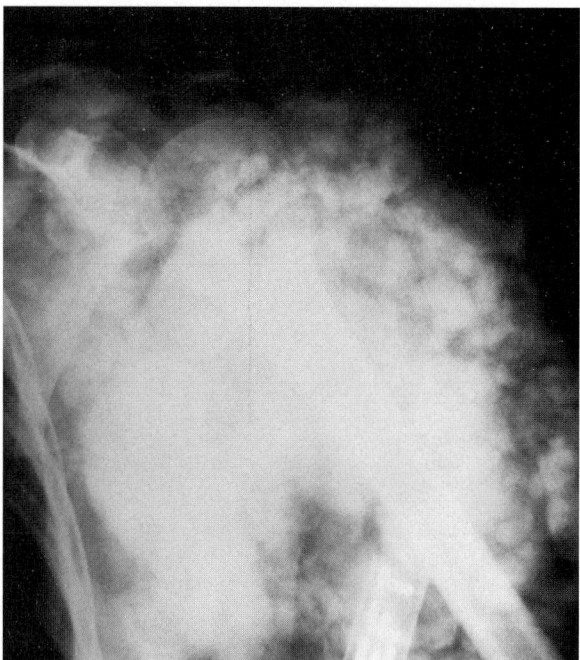

**Figure 62–10.** Milk-alkali syndrome. Extensive calcific collections about the shoulder are seen. (Courtesy of M. K. Dalinka, MD, Philadelphia.)

cation occurs from the following sequence of events: excessive intake of milk and alkali, kidney damage, fixation in urinary calcium excretion, hypercalcemia, supersaturation of calcium phosphate, and calcinosis.

Radiographic manifestations of this syndrome include unilateral or bilateral periarticular calcific deposits, which are amorphous and vary in size from small nodules to bulky tumors (Fig. 62–10). Widespread calcification in blood vessels, kidneys, ligaments, and falx cerebri is also observed, and the osseous tissues are normal.

Milk-alkali syndrome occurs principally in middle-aged men (the male-female ratio is about 4:1) who are ingesting milk and calcium carbonate, or calcium carbonate alone, for abdominal pain or heartburn. Although hypercalcemia, alkalosis, and renal impairment represent the classic triad of the syndrome, the clinical characteristics are variable.

The differential diagnosis of periarticular calcific deposits accompanying milk-alkali syndrome includes collagen vascular disorders, hyperparathyroidism, renal osteodystrophy, hypervitaminosis D, and idiopathic tumoral calcinosis.

## PROSTAGLANDINS

Prostaglandin $E_1$ is commonly used to maintain the patency of the ductus arteriosus in neonates with ductus-dependent congenital heart disease, including interruption or coarctation of the aortic arch, pulmonary atresia complex, and tetralogy of Fallot. Although the duration of prostaglandin $E_1$ administration is usually limited to the time required to stabilize the infant's condition before surgical intervention, longer periods of infusion are occasionally required. A variety of complications have been encountered during and after prostaglandin $E_1$ therapy, including damage of the ductus, hypotension, hyperthermia, diarrhea, apnea, bradycardia, and flushing and edema of the skin.

Periosteal bone formation is characteristic of long-term ( 40 days) prostaglandin $E_1$ infusion, although it may also be seen with short-term therapy (9 to 14 days) and with prostaglandin $E_2$ therapy. Affected sites include the ribs, tubular bones, and, to a lesser extent, mandible, clavicle, scapula, and pelvis. Although multiple areas may be involved, a symmetrical distribution is not uniformly present. Periostitis varies in intensity from subtle and localized osseous deposits to widespread and severe alterations (Fig. 62–11), leading to enlargement of the bone (Fig. 62–12). Generally the process is self-limited, with no apparent effect on subsequent bone growth and development; complete resolution is commonly seen over a period of 6 months to 1 year.

The differential diagnosis of the osseous alterations includes physiologic periostitis, trauma, Caffey's disease, congenital syphilis, hypervitaminosis A, scurvy, hypertrophic osteoarthropathy, leukemia, and skeletal metastasis.

## RETINOIDS

Natural and synthetic forms of vitamin A, known collectively as retinoids, have been employed in the treatment

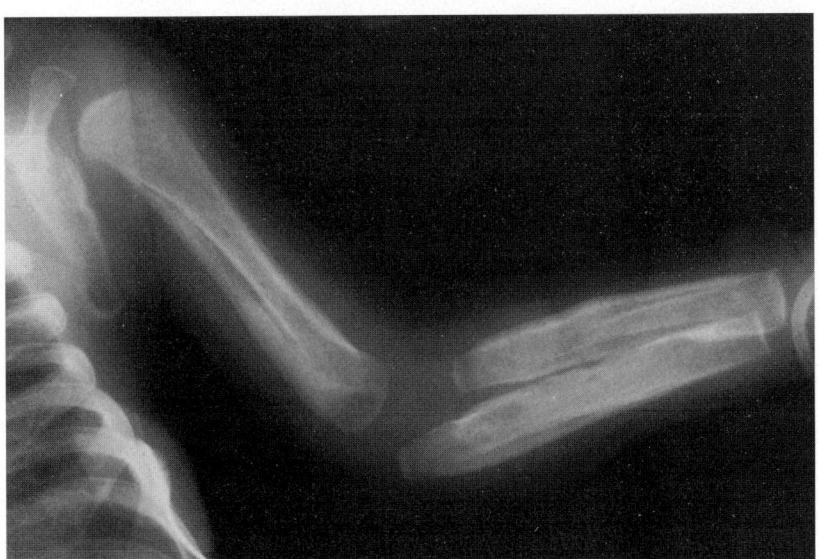

**Figure 62–11.** Prostaglandin periostitis. In this 3-month-old infant receiving prostaglandin E₁ infusions, exuberant periosteal new bone is observed in the ribs, humerus, radius, and ulna. (Courtesy of T. Broderick, MD, Orange, Calif.)

of various dermatologic disorders. Reports indicate that the long-term use of isotretinoin is associated with skeletal hyperostosis resembling that seen in chronic vitamin A intoxication. Both axial and appendicular skeletal sites are affected. Vertebral alterations predominate in the cervical region, although thoracic and lumbar spinal changes may also be evident. The findings, which are usually subtle and require comparison with previous radiographic studies for identification, consist of pointed osseous excrescences arising from the anterior and posterior margins of the vertebral bodies; with time, these excrescences progress to larger osteophytic outgrowths (Fig. 62–13). In the appendicular skeleton, pointlike hyperostosis is seen at the corners and promontories of bones, such as the tarsal navicular and calcaneus. Bilateral and symmetrical changes occur more frequently than unilateral abnormalities. Clinical manifestations are absent or mild.

## QUINOLONES

A number of complications, including arthralgias, arthritis, myalgia, tendinosis, and spontaneous tendon ruptures,

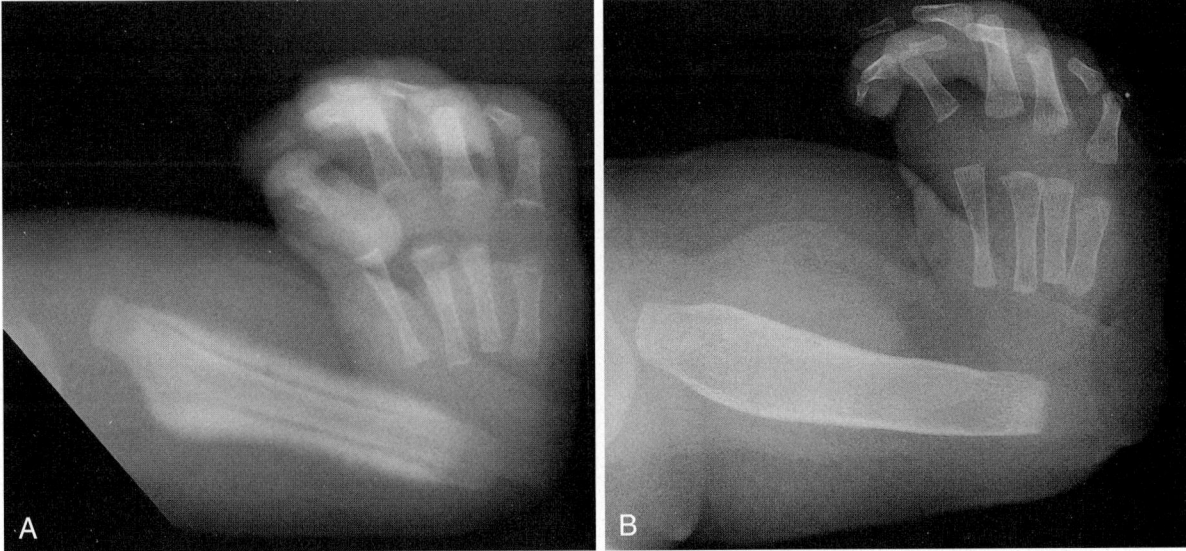

**Figure 62–12.** Prostaglandin periostitis. This male infant was noted to have multiple congenital abnormalities at birth. A cardiac catheterization confirmed the presence of a severe tetralogy of Fallot. An infusion of prostaglandin E was begun when the patient was 3 weeks old and maintained for 7 weeks, after which it was discontinued. Bone changes were observed initially in the ribs and clavicle after 20 days of therapy. *A*, Radiograph of the forearm, obtained when the infant was 43 days old, reveals extensive periosteal elevation in the ulna. Note the absence of the radius, a finding of the VATER syndrome (consisting of vertebral defects, imperforate anus, tracheoesophageal fistula, and radial and renal dyslasia). *B*, At 6 months of age, the periosteal bone has been incorporated into the diaphysis of the ulna. (From Poznanski AK, Fernbach SK, Berry TE: Bone changes from prostaglandin therapy. Skeletal Radiol 14:20, 1985.)

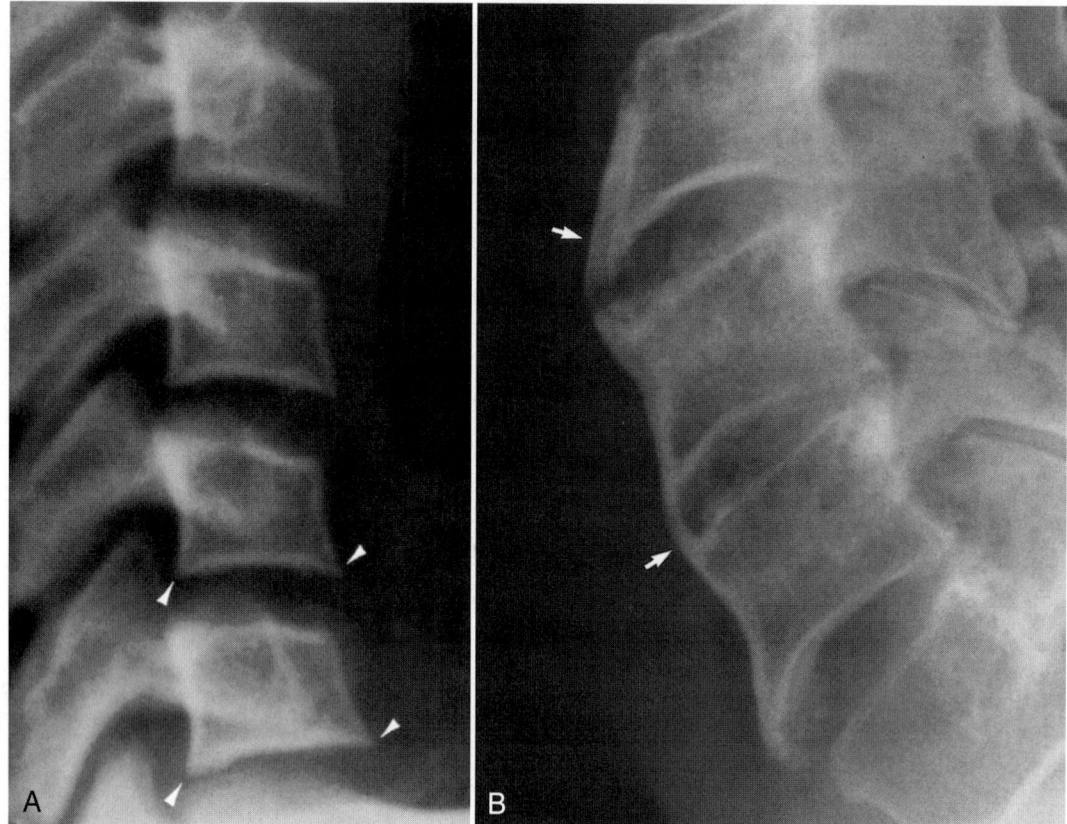

**Figure 62–13.** Isotretinoin hyperostosis. *A*, Lateral radiograph of the cervical spine obtained after 1 year of therapy shows "pointing" of the bone at the anteroinferior and posteroinferior portions of the vertebral bodies *(arrowheads)*. *B*, In a different patient, prominent ligamentous ossification *(arrows)* is apparent in the midcervical spine. (*A*, From Pennes DR, Ellis CN, Madison KC, et al: Early skeletal hyperostoses secondary to 13-cis-retinoic acid. AJR 142:979, 1984.)

have been related to treatment with fluoroquinolones. Although the Achilles tendon is usually involved, other affected structures include the tendons of the rotator cuff, quadriceps tendon, tendons about the elbow, and plantar fascia. Bilateral involvement is common. Risk factors include advanced age, corticosteroid therapy, renal failure (especially with associated dialysis or renal transplantation), and the choice of pefloxacin as the therapeutic agent. The precise pathophysiology of tendon abnormalities related to fluoroquinolone-containing antibiotics is not clear.

## OTHER CHEMICAL AGENTS

Phenytoin (Dilantin) has been associated with calvarial thickening and enlargement of the heel pad, findings resembling those of acromegaly. Phenytoin, as well as heparin, alcohol, and methotrexate, can lead to skeletal osteopenia (Fig. 62–14).

With long-term methotrexate therapy for childhood neoplasms, especially acute lymphocytic leukemia, severe osteopenia and multiple fractures in the tubular bones of the lower extremities (and, to a lesser extent, the upper extremities) are seen; additional findings include growth recovery lines and radiodense areas in the metaphyses and epiphyses, simulating the changes of scurvy (Fig. 62–15). Another chemotherapeutic agent used in the treatment of tumors, ifosfamide, has been associated with hypophosphatemic rickets.

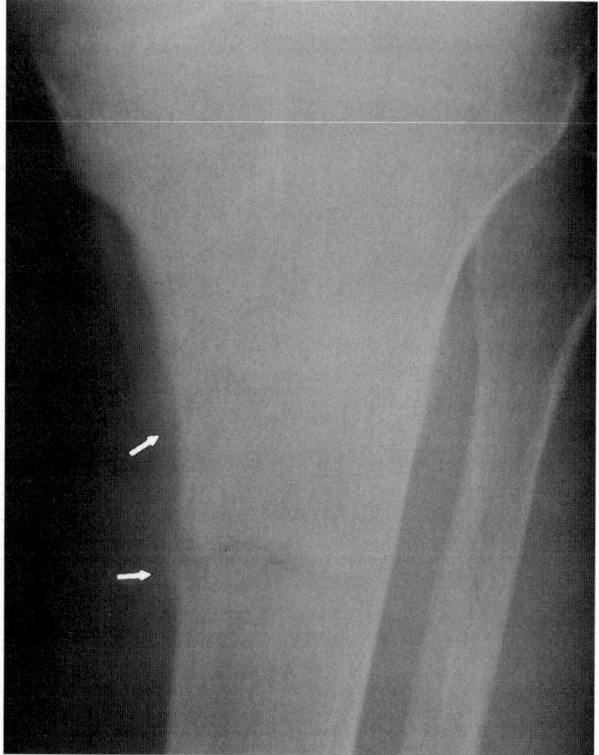

**Figure 62–14.** Phenytoin-induced osteomalacia. In this adult with a seizure disorder, long-term phenytoin therapy has resulted in osteomalacia with Looser's zones, or insufficiency fractures *(arrows)*.

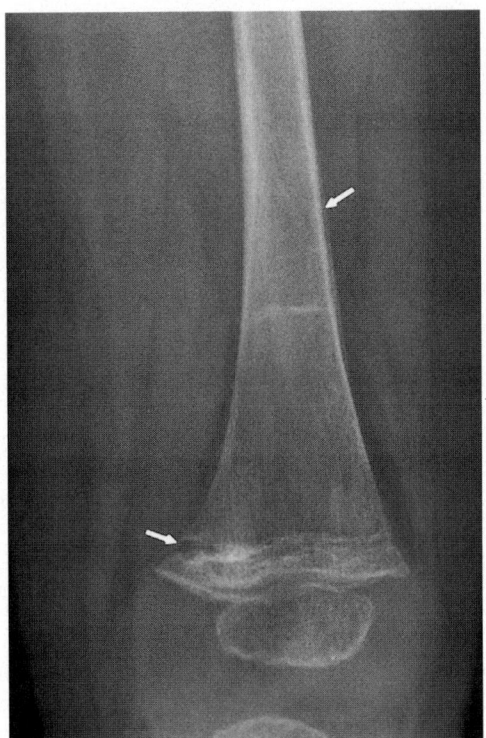

**Figure 62–15.** Methotrexate osteopathy. An 18-month-old boy with acute lymphocytic leukemia was treated with a variety of drugs, including methotrexate. Approximately 2 years later, this radiograph was obtained because the patient had pain and weakness in the legs. Findings include osteopenia, periostitis, and fractures in both the diaphysis and metaphysis of the left femur *(arrows)*. A growth recovery line is seen. (From Schwartz AM, Leonidas JC: Methotrexate osteopathy. Skeletal Radiol 11:13, 1984.)

## FURTHER READING

Abitboul M, Arlet J: Retinol-related hyperostosis. AJR Am J Roentgenol 144:435, 1985.

Berger PE, Heidelberger KP, Poznanski AK: Extravasation of calcium gluconate as a cause of soft tissue calcification in infancy. AJR Am J Roentgenol 121:109, 1974.

Burnett CH, Commons RR, Albright F, et al: Hypercalcemia without hypercalciuria or hypophosphatemia, calcinosis, and renal insufficiency. N Engl J Med 240:787, 1949.

Conklin JJ, Alderson PO, Zizic TM, et al: Comparison of bone scan and radiograph sensitivity in the detection of steroid-induced ischemic necrosis of bone. Radiology 147:221, 1983.

Dalinka MK, Stewart V, Bomalaski JS, et al: Periarticular calcifications in association with intra-articular corticosteroid injections. Radiology 153:615, 1984.

DiGiovanna JJ, Helfgott RK, Gerber LH, et al: Extraspinal tendon and ligament calcification associated with long-term therapy with etretinate. N Engl J Med 315:1177, 1986.

El-Khoury GY, Moore TE, Albright JP, et al: Sodium fluoride treatment of osteoporosis: Radiologic findings. AJR Am J Roentgenol 139:39, 1982.

Grandjean P, Thomsen G: Reversibility of skeletal fluorosis. Br J Indust Med 40:456, 1983.

Halpern AA, Horowitz BG, Nagel DA: Tendon ruptures associated with corticosteroid therapy. West J Med 127:378, 1977.

Harris AA, Ramamurthy RS, Pildes RS: Late onset of subcutaneous calcifications after intravenous injection of calcium gluconate. AJR Am J Roentgenol 123:845, 1975.

Kassner EG: Drug-related complications in infants and children: Imaging features. AJR Am J Roentgenol 157:1039, 1991.

Kattan KR: Calvarial thickening after Dilantin medication. AJR Am J Roentgenol 110:102, 1970.

Kilcoyne RF, Cope R, Cunningham W, et al: Minimal spinal hyperostosis with low-dose isotretinoin therapy. Invest Radiol 21:41, 1986.

Maldague B, Noel H, Malghem J: The intravertebral vacuum cleft: A sign of ischemic vertebral collapse. Radiology 129:23, 1978.

Miller WT, Restifo RA: Steroid arthropathy. Radiology 86:652, 1966.

Murray RO: Iatrogenic lesions of the skeleton. AJR Am J Roentgenol 126:5, 1976.

Murray RO: Radiological bone changes in Cushing's syndrome and steroid therapy. Br J Radiol 33:1, 1960.

Orwoll ES: The milk-alkali syndrome: Current concepts. Ann Intern Med 97:242, 1982.

Pennes DR, Ellis CN, Madison KC, et al: Early skeletal hyperostoses secondary to 13-cis-retinoic acid. AJR Am J Roentgenol 141:979, 1984.

Poppel MH, Zeitel BE: Roentgen manifestations of milk drinker's syndrome. Radiology 67:195, 1956.

Poznanski AK, Fernbach SK, Berry TE: Bone changes from prostaglandin therapy. Skeletal Radiol 14:20, 1985.

Quint DJ, Boulos RS, Sanders WP, et al: Epidural lipomatosis. Radiology 169:485, 1988.

Ringel RE, Brenner JI, Haney PJ, et al: Prostaglandin-induced periostitis: A complication of long-term PGE₁ infusion in an infant with congenital heart disease. Radiology 142:657, 1982.

Sackler JP, Liu L: Heparin-induced osteoporosis. Br J Radiol 46:548, 1973.

Schnitzler CM, Solomon L: Trabecular stress fractures during fluoride therapy for osteoporosis. Skeletal Radiol 14:276, 1985.

Schwartz AM, Leonidas JC: Methotrexate osteopathy. Skeletal Radiol 11:13, 1984.

Silberzweig JE, Haller JO, Miller S: Ifosfamide: A new cause of rickets. AJR Am J Roentgenol 158:823, 1992.

Singh A, Dass R, Hayreh SS, et al: Skeletal changes in endemic fluorosis. J Bone Joint Surg Br 44:806, 1962.

Soriano M, Manchon F: Radiological aspects of a new type of bone fluorosis, periostitis deformans. Radiology 87:1089, 1966.

Stevenson CA, Watson AR: Fluoride osteosclerosis. AJR Am J Roentgenol 78:13, 1957.

Tondreau RL, Hodes PJ, Schmidt ER Jr: Joint infections following steroid therapy: Roentgen manifestations. AJR Am J Roentgenol 82:258, 1959.

Vande Berg BC, Malghem J, Lecouvet FE, et al: Fat conversion of femoral marrow in glucocorticoid-treated patients: A cross-sectional and longitudinal study with magnetic resonance imaging. Arthritis Rheum 42:1405, 1999.

Wang Y, Yin Y, Gilula LA, et al: Endemic fluorosis of the skeleton: Radiographic features in 127 cases. AJR Am J Roentgenol 162:93, 1994.

# CHAPTER 63

## Hypervitaminosis and Hypovitaminosis

## SUMMARY OF KEY FEATURES

Deficiencies and excesses of certain vitamins can have pronounced effects on the musculoskeletal system. In addition to vitamin D deficiency leading to rickets, hypervitaminosis A and D and hypovitaminosis C (scurvy) are examples of vitamin-related disorders that affect the osseous, articular, or soft tissue structures.

## INTRODUCTION

Vitamins are biologically active organic compounds that are not synthesized by the body and are obtained from exogenous sources, mainly the diet. Vitamins, which are essential for normal growth and development, can be classified according to whether they are fat soluble (vitamins A, D, E, and K) or water soluble (vitamins $B_1$, $B_2$, niacin, $B_6$ or pyridoxine, folic acid, cyanocobalamin, C or ascorbic acid, biotin, and pantothenic acid). Musculoskeletal manifestations accompany deficiencies and excesses of certain vitamins. As an example, rickets is caused by a deficiency in vitamin D or its active metabolites (see Chapter 42). In addition, excessive levels of vitamins D and A and depressed levels of the vitamins A and C can produce characteristic changes in the skeleton, which are described in this chapter.

## HYPERVITAMINOSIS A

Vitamin A poisoning appears in both children and adults. Its clinical and radiographic manifestations are influenced by the acute or chronic nature of the vitamin abuse.

### Acute Poisoning

After a massive dose of vitamin A (several hundred thousand units), acute clinical findings can develop, including nausea, vomiting, headache, drowsiness, and irritability. In children, drowsiness, vomiting, and bulging of the fontanelles may develop. Bulging of the fontanelles can appear within 12 hours after vitamin ingestion and usually disappears after 36 to 48 hours. Although skull films can reveal widening of the sutures, this finding is transient.

### Subacute and Chronic Poisoning

In both children and adults, anorexia and itching represent nonspecific early findings of chronic vitamin A poisoning. After a period of weeks or months, hard and tender soft tissue nodules appear in the extremities, particularly in the forearms. Additional manifestations include dry, scaly skin; coarse, sparse hair; hepatosplenomegaly; and digital clubbing. Rapid diminution and disappearance of the symptoms and signs follow withdrawal of vitamin A intake.

Radiographic signs are characteristic and are virtually confined to children. Cortical thickening of the tubular bones is a constant finding and is usually related to the areas in which soft tissue nodules are present. Typically, hyperostosis is observed in the ulna and metatarsal bones, producing a wavy or undulating diaphyseal contour; metaphyseal and epiphyseal segments do not participate in the cortical thickening (Fig. 63–1). Involvement of the clavicle, tibia, and fibula is not uncommon; the femur, humerus, metacarpal bones, and ribs are less commonly affected, and changes in the mandible are rarely observed. Cupping, shortening, and splaying of the metaphyses, irregularity and narrowing of the cartilaginous growth plates, and hypertrophy and premature fusion of the epiphyseal ossification centers may be noted (Fig. 63–2). Although the areas of cortical hyperostosis may gradually disappear after removal of the excess vitamin A, the damage to the epiphyseal cartilage may be irreversible if the poisoning has been protracted. Flexion contractures, short stature, and leg length discrepancies may ensue. As in cases of acute poisoning, increased intracranial pressure has been noted in association with chronic hypervitaminosis A.

The condition that produces skeletal changes most similar to those of chronic hypervitaminosis A is infantile cortical hyperostosis (Caffey's disease) (Table 63–1). In vitamin A intoxication, cortical hyperostosis usually manifests no earlier than the end of the first year of life (whereas infantile cortical hyperostosis may produce changes in the first 6 months of life), mandibular and facial involvement is unusual (whereas these areas are typically affected in infantile cortical hyperostosis), metatarsal alterations are frequent (whereas these bones are generally spared in infantile cortical hyperostosis), and biochemical analysis of the blood reveals marked elevation of vitamin A.

## HYPOVITAMINOSIS A

Chronic vitamin A deficiency in infancy, childhood, or adulthood produces a variety of epithelial alterations, including dry and scaly skin, photophobia, night blindness, and dry conjunctivae; in infancy, additional manifestations include susceptibility to infection, anemia, cranial nerve injury, and growth retardation. Increased intracranial pressure of unknown pathogenesis is observed in this condition, which in infants younger than 6 months of age may lead to widening of the cranial sutures with bulging fontanelles. Vitamin A deficiency may also have a dramatic effect on dental development.

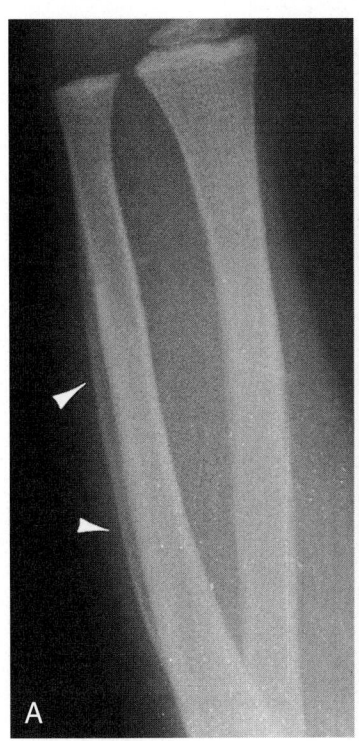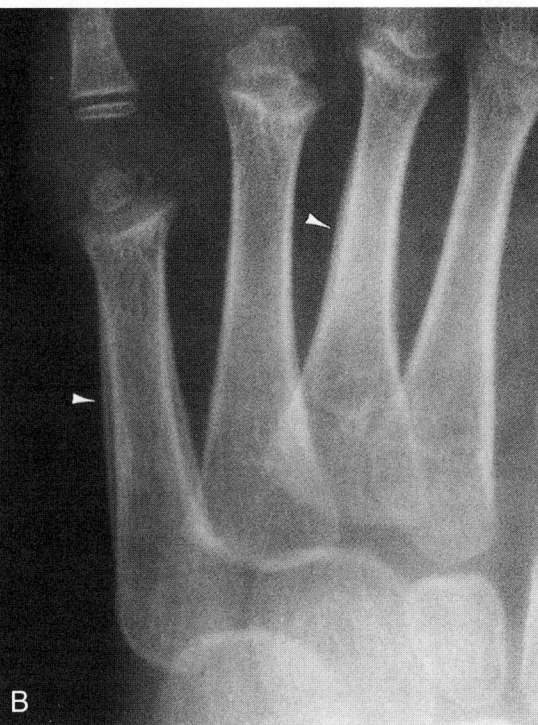

**Figure 63–1.** Hypervitaminosis A: periostitis and cortical hyperostosis. A, Note periosteal bone formation in the diaphysis of the ulna (*arrowheads*). B, In a different child, periosteal proliferation is evident in the diaphyses of multiple metatarsals (*arrowheads*). (A, Courtesy of F. Silverman, MD, Stanford, Calif.)

## HYPOVITAMINOSIS C (SCURVY)

A long-term deficiency of dietary vitamin C (ascorbic acid) results in scurvy. Cases can be divided into those that develop in infancy or childhood (infantile scurvy) and those that occur in adulthood (adult scurvy).

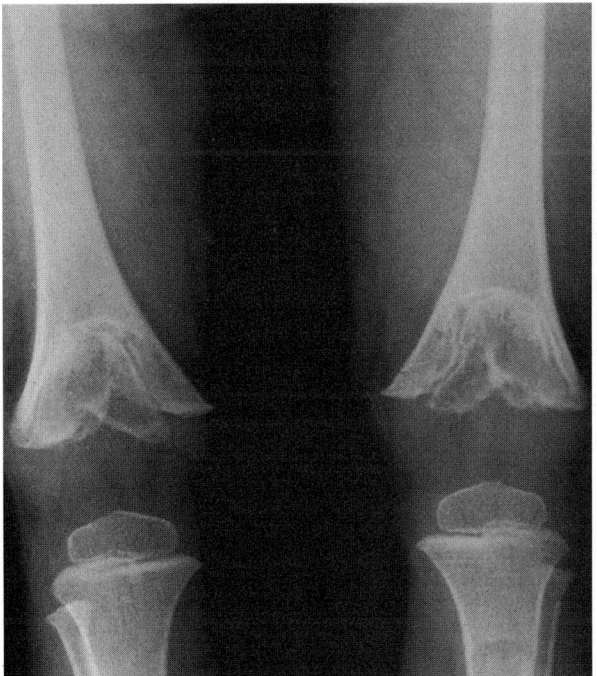

**Figure 63–2.** Hypervitaminosis A: metaphyseal and epiphyseal changes. Observe the striking splaying and cupping of the distal femoral metaphyses, with narrowing of the cartilaginous growth plates and hypertrophy and invagination of the epiphyses.

## Infantile Scurvy

Infantile scurvy occurs in babies who are fed pasteurized or boiled milk; the process of heating the milk leads to disruption of vitamin C and the appearance of the disorder. Clinically apparent disease develops after deficiency of the vitamin has existed for 4 to 10 months; therefore, it is exceedingly unusual to detect this disorder in infants younger than 4 months of age. The manifestations generally becoming apparent at 8 to 14 months. Before the appearance of hemorrhagic tendencies, infants with scurvy can develop nonspecific findings, including failure to thrive and digestive alterations. The onset of pale skin with petechial hemorrhages; swollen, red, and ulcerated gums; palatal petechiae; hematuria; melena; hematemesis; and secondary infections, when combined with characteristic radiographic changes and depressed levels of serum ascorbic acid, ensures an accurate diagnosis.

**Metaphyseal Changes.** Skeletal alterations result from a depression of normal cellular activity, which is most marked in areas of active endochondral bone growth (ends of tubular bones and costochondral junctions). In the region of the cartilaginous growth plate, proliferating cartilage cells are reduced in number, and disorganization of the growth zone is evident (Fig. 63–3). A sparsity of newly formed trabeculae is evident in this junctional region. Brittleness of the trabecular structure contributes to a tendency to fracture through this zone, leading to hemorrhage. The abnormal marrow in the junctional area is termed gerüstmark, and the entire zone consists of detritus (Trümmerfeldzone). Lateral extension of the heavy provisional zones of calcification, in conjunction with elevation and stimulation of the adjacent periosteal membrane, produces small spicules, or excrescences, of the metaphysis.

**TABLE 63–1**

**Hypervitaminosis A versus Infantile Cortical Hyperostosis (Caffey's Disease)**

| Factor | Hypervitaminosis A | Infantile Cortical Hyperostosis |
|---|---|---|
| Age of onset | End of first year of life | First 6 mo of life |
| Findings | Soft tissue nodules | Soft tissue nodules |
| | Periostitis and hyperostosis | Periostitis and hyperostosis |
| | Metaphyseal changes | Growth disturbances |
| | Growth disturbances | |
| | Increased intracranial pressure | |
| Sites of hyperostosis (descending order of frequency) | Ulna | Mandible |
| | Metatarsal | Clavicle |
| | Clavicle | Scapula |
| | Tibia | Rib |
| | Fibula | Tubular bones |
| | Metacarpal | |
| | Other tubular bones | |
| | Rib | |
| Etiology | Vitamin A poisoning | Unknown; possibly a viral disease |

A radiograph of the end of an involved tubular bone reveals several zones (Table 63–2; Fig. 63–4). A radiodense line borders on the growth plate, representing the sclerotic provisional zone. On its metaphyseal side between the provisional zone of calcification and the heavy spongiosa deeper in the shaft is a transverse band of diminished density, the scurvy line. Small, beaklike outgrowths of the metaphysis, incomplete or complete separation of the plate from the shaft due to subepiphyseal marginal clefts and infractions (corner sign or

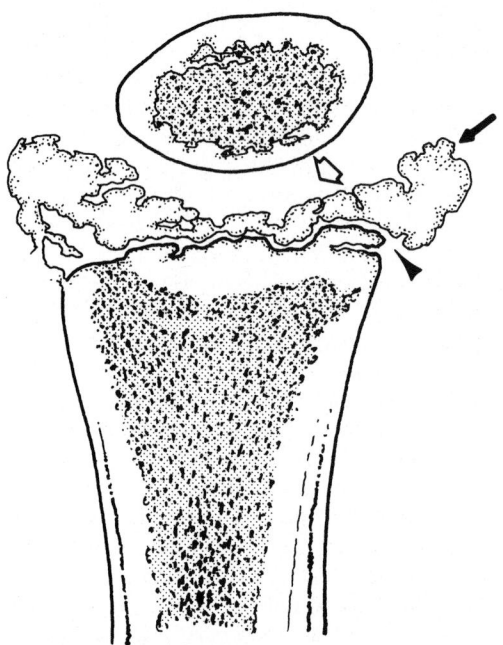

**Figure 63–3.** Hypovitaminosis C (scurvy): pathologic abnormalities. Changes in the ends of tubular bones consist of an irregular arrangement of cartilage cells in the proliferating zone of the growth plate (*open arrow*), a metaphyseal area containing a latticework of calcified cartilage that is free of osseous tissue (*solid arrow*), and a decrease in trabeculae, fracture, and detritus in the junctional area (*arrowhead*). Metaphyseal excrescences can develop.

**TABLE 63–2**

**Hypovitaminosis C (Scurvy): Radiographic-Pathologic Correlation**

| Radiographic Finding | Pathologic Finding |
|---|---|
| Transverse metaphyseal line of increased density | Prominent thickened provisional zone of calcification |
| Transverse metaphyseal line of decreased density ("scurvy line") | Decrease in trabeculae and detritus in junctional area of metaphysis ("Trümmerfeldzone") |
| Metaphyseal excrescences or beaks | Lateral extension of the heavy provisional zone of calcification with periosteal elevation and stimulation |
| Subepiphyseal infractions ("corner sign" or "angle sign") | Decrease and brittleness of trabeculae in junctional area with fracture and hemorrhage |
| Periostitis | Subperiosteal hemorrhage with elevation and stimulation of periosteum |
| Epiphyseal shell of increased density with central lucency (Wimberger's sign of scurvy) | Prominent thickened provisional zone of calcification with atrophy of central spongiosa |

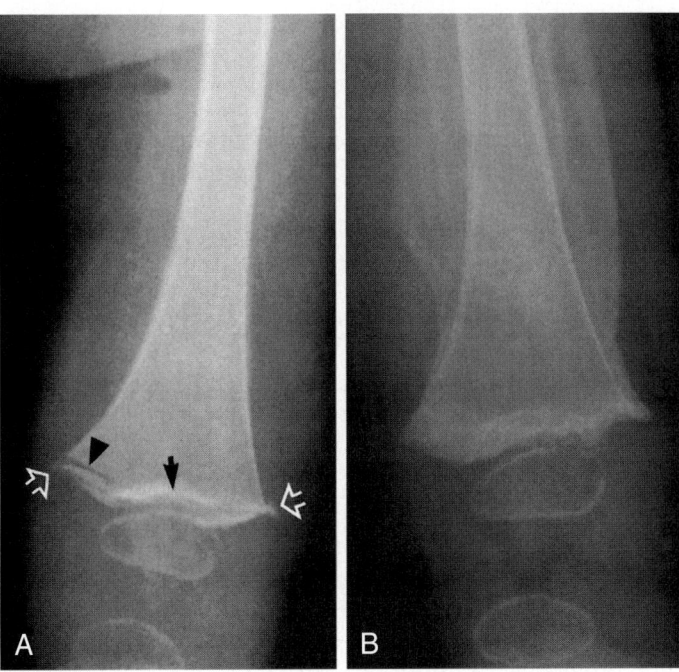

**Figure 63–4.** Hypovitaminosis C (scurvy): radiographic abnormalities. *A* and *B*, Radiographs obtained 1 month apart show, initially *(A)*, a sclerotic metaphyseal line *(arrow)*, beaklike excrescences *(open arrows)*, and a metaphyseal radiolucent line *(arrowhead)*. Subsequently *(B)*, a thicker band of metaphyseal sclerosis and periostitis is seen. A sclerotic line about the epiphysis is also seen in both radiographs.

angle sign), extensive physiolysis with osseous malalignment, and periosteal elevation with new bone formation due to subperiosteal hemorrhage complete the distinctive radiographic picture of the metaepiphyseal regions of tubular bones (and costochondral junctions). These changes are most marked in areas of active endochondral bone formation.

**Epiphyseal Changes.** In the ossification centers of the epiphyses of tubular bones and in the carpus and tarsus, similar but less marked alterations are seen. Persistence and thickening of the provisional zone of calcification produce a radiodense shell around the ossification center that is accentuated by central rarefaction owing to atrophy of the adjacent spongiosa (Wimberger's sign of scurvy).

**Diaphyseal Changes.** Atrophy of spongiosa in the shafts of tubular bones accounts for a nonspecific decreased radiodensity and a "ground-glass" appearance of the diaphyses. Cortical diminution is common and often severe, yet fracture of the shafts is unusual. Subperiosteal hemorrhage is most frequent in the larger tubular bones such as the femur, tibia, and humerus. The degree of hemorrhage is variable and can produce focal or diffuse elevation of the periosteal membrane. Radiographically, soft tissue masses of increased density, displacement of adjacent bones, and small or large shells of periosteal bone, particularly during the healing phase of the disease, are observed.

**Articular Changes.** Hemarthrosis, a rare manifestation of scurvy, demonstrates a predilection for the large weight-bearing joints of the lower extremities.

**Growth Disturbances.** Permanent growth disturbances are unusual after scurvy, despite the frequency and severity of epiphyseal separations. Central segmental metaphyseal

cupping in a bilateral or unilateral distribution can lead to intrusion of the epiphysis into the exaggerated concavity of the metaphysis and apparent early fusion of the growth plate. This complication is not frequent, and the pathogenesis of metaphyseal cupping is not clear.

**Effects of Therapy.** With treatment of the disease, there is thickening of the cortex, increased density of the radiolucent zone of the metaphysis, transverse densities within the shaft caused by burying of the thickened provisional zone of calcification, massive subperiosteal bone formation that later merges with the underlying cortex, spontaneous shifting of the diaphysis to realign with the displaced epiphysis, and increased density of the epiphysis.

**Differential Diagnosis.** The appearance of a radiolucent metaphyseal band in scurvy is not a pathognomonic finding and may be seen in other chronic illnesses, such as leukemia and neuroblastoma. The identification of radiodense lines at the metaphysis and about the epiphysis, metaphyseal fracture, osseous beaks, epiphyseal displacement, and diaphyseal periostitis allows an accurate diagnosis of scurvy. Leukemia can lead to periostitis and diaphyseal destruction in combination with bandlike metaphyseal radiolucency, but fracture and epiphyseal separation are not present. Syphilis produces symmetrical destructive foci in the metaphyses, particularly in the proximal tibia, but the distinctive findings are not confused with those of scurvy. Metaphyseal changes can also accompany rubella, cytomegalic inclusion disease, toxoplasmosis, and a variety of traumatic and dysplastic disorders.

## Adult Scurvy

Currently, scurvy is encountered infrequently in adults, although it may be observed in severely malnourished persons, especially the elderly. A protracted period of vitamin deficiency is required for clinical expression. Nonspecific weakness, anorexia, weight loss, and fatigue usually antedate the more diagnostic hemorrhagic manifestations, such as petechiae and ecchymoses of the skin, subcutaneous tissues, and gums.

Hemarthrosis and bleeding at synchondroses may be observed in adult scurvy. Osteoporosis is prominent in the axial skeleton, especially the spine, and in the tubular bones of the appendicular skeleton.

## HYPERVITAMINOSIS D

Excessive intake of vitamin D can be associated with clinical and radiographic manifestations in both children and adults. Initial reports noted findings of intoxication in infants and young children who had been given excessive levels of vitamin D for the treatment of rickets and other skeletal disorders; similar intoxication was later identified in adult patients who were receiving inordinate amounts of vitamin D for the treatment of Paget's disease.

### Musculoskeletal Abnormalities

Vitamin D poisoning can be acute or chronic. The level of the vitamin required to produce toxic symptoms and signs is extremely variable. Acute clinical manifestations may appear within 3 to 9 days after massive doses of the vitamin and include vomiting, fever, dehydration, abdominal cramps, bone pain and tenderness, convulsions, and coma. With chronic poisoning, lassitude, thirst, anorexia, and polyuria are followed by vomiting, abdominal pain, and diarrhea.

In infants and children, metaphyseal bands of increased density, reflecting heavy calcifications of the matrix of the proliferating cartilage, alternating with areas of increased lucency are evident in the tubular bones. Cortical thickening due to periosteal apposition may be observed at certain sites, and osteoporosis and thinning of the cortices may be evident at other locations. Metastatic calcification of viscera, blood vessels, periarticular structures, muscles, laryngeal and tracheal cartilage, falx cerebri, and tentorium cerebelli may be noted.

In adults, hypervitaminosis D can lead to focal or generalized osteoporosis. The bones of the appendicular skeleton, the spine, the pelvis, and even the skull reveal varying degrees of bone loss. Massive soft tissue calcification can become apparent. Lobulated, smooth, amorphous masses of calcium are evident in periarticular regions, bursae, tendon sheaths, joint capsules, and intra-articular cavities (Fig. 63–5). Pathologic evaluation reveals thick, white, granular calcareous material, usually representing calcium hydroxyapatite, and an inflammatory reaction in the bursal wall or adjacent soft tissues can be seen.

Metastatic soft tissue calcification accompanies a variety of disorders, including hypervitaminosis D, milk-alkali syndrome, hyperparathyroidism, plasma cell myeloma, and skeletal metastasis. Further, soft tissue calcinosis may be evident in various collagen vascular disorders, and dystrophic calcification can occur after tissue injury or devitalization from any cause. Periarticular deposits are most characteristic of hypervitaminosis D, milk-alkali syndrome, hyperparathyroidism, renal osteodystrophy, collagen vascular disorders, and idiopathic tumoral calcinosis.

### Chronic Idiopathic Hypercalcemia

Chronic idiopathic hypercalcemia relates to excessive ingestion of vitamin D over prolonged periods by infants who are slightly sensitive to this vitamin. The major clinical manifestations of this disorder include a peculiar facies, anorexia, hypotonia, mental and physical retardation, and vomiting. Radiographically, a generalized increase in skeletal density is observed.

Infants with Williams' syndrome demonstrate a facies similar to that of patients with idiopathic hypercalcemia; they also have supravalvular aortic stenosis and mental retardation. The detection of hypercalcemia and these variable vascular anomalies suggests that vitamin D excess or hypersensitivity in the expectant mother may be a fundamental cause of congenital malformations of the cardiovascular system of the fetus.

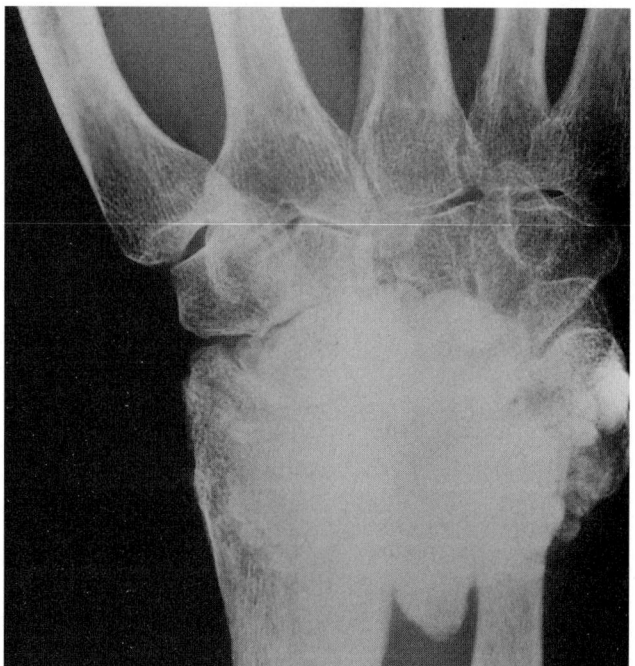

**Figure 63–5.** Hypervitaminosis D: soft tissue abnormalities. In a patient with rheumatoid arthritis who was treated with vitamin D, note massive soft tissue calcification about the wrist.

## FURTHER READING

Caffey J: Chronic poisoning due to excess of vitamin A: Description of the clinical and roentgen manifestations in seven infants and young children. Pediatrics 5:672, 1950.

Caffey J: Traumatic cupping of the metaphyses of growing bones. AJR 108:451, 1970.

Christensen WR, Liebman C, Sosman MC: Skeletal and periarticular manifestations of hypervitaminosis D. AJR 65:27, 1951.

Holman CB: Roentgenologic manifestations of vitamin D intoxication. Radiology 59:805, 1952.

Joffe N: Some radiological aspects of scurvy in the adult. Br J Radiol 34:429, 1961.

Keating JP, Feigin RD: Increased intracranial pressure associated with probable vitamin A deficiency in cystic fibrosis. Pediatrics 46:41, 1970.

Miller JH, Hayon II: Bone scintigraphy in hypervitaminosis A. AJR 144:767, 1985.

Shiers JA, Neuhauser EBD, Bowman JR: Idiopathic hypercalcemia. AJR 78:19, 1957.

Singleton EB: The radiographic features of severe idiopathic hypercalcemia of infancy. Radiology 68:721, 1957.

Sprague PL: Epiphyseo-metaphyseal cupping following infantile scurvy. Pediatr Radiol 4:122, 1976.

# CHAPTER 64

## Heavy Metal Poisoning and Deficiency

## SUMMARY OF KEY FEATURES

In some cases of heavy metal poisoning, radiodense lines or bands may appear in the metaphyses of tubular bones and within flat or irregular bones. The resulting radiographic findings, which are characteristically observed in lead, phosphorus, and bismuth poisoning, must be differentiated from normal variants, stress lines of Park or Harris, and changes in various metabolic, endocrine, and infectious disorders. Significant radiographic abnormalities are also observed in the aluminum accumulation that accompanies dialysis and in nutritional or inherited deficiencies of copper. Finally, metal debris (metallosis) may complicate joint surgery.

## INTRODUCTION

Poisoning with certain heavy metals can produce characteristic musculoskeletal alterations. One of the most well-recognized changes associated with the ingestion, inhalation, or injection of lead or other heavy metals is the appearance of radiodense lines at the ends of tubular bones or along the contours of flat and irregular bones. These lines must be differentiated from the transverse radiodense areas that are commonly observed at some of these locations in persons who have not been poisoned with metals.

## TRANSVERSE OR STRESS LINES

The appearance of opaque transverse lines that extend across the metaphyses of tubular bones is a common radiographic phenomenon that may be observed in children and adults (Fig. 64–1). They are often referred to as Park or Harris lines or as transverse or growth arrest lines. Investigations of these lines have emphasized that they can occur in both healthy and sick persons, that similar lines have been encountered in patients poisoned with a variety of heavy metals, and that the lines may be used as a determinant of growth potential and magnitude. Transverse radiodense lines may be evident at birth or during infancy; they do not appear after growth has ceased, but once formed, they persist into adult life. Similar lines can appear about the margins of the round and the flat bones and in both the appendicular and axial portions of the skeleton (Fig. 64–2).

The close proximity of and similarity between the lines and the growth plate suggest that the bands are related to a disturbance of normal growth patterns. Indeed, the term arrest lines, which is still applied to these dense shadows, underscores the early belief that their appearance signified an arrest in normal growth; however, they are more properly termed recovery lines, indicating periods of renewed or increased growth, presumably after a period of inhibited growth of the bone.

Growth arrest (or recovery) lines are also observed on magnetic resonance (MR) images. They appear as curvilinear regions of low signal intensity, producing a bone-within-bone appearance (Fig. 64–3). The more central aspect often contains fatty marrow of higher signal intensity than that in the periphery.

Transversely or obliquely oriented radiodense lines are regularly encountered in the tubular bones of adults with osteopenia. These lines, which are termed bone bars or reinforcement lines, are discussed more fully in Chapter 41. They are especially frequent in the distal portion of the femur and the tibia in persons with long-term osteoporosis, and they should be regarded as an adaptive response of chronically weakened bone to normal or abnormal stress, not as a manifestation of growth disturbance.

## LEAD POISONING

### General Abnormalities

Lead poisoning results from prolonged ingestion of lead-containing materials such as paint chips, ceramics, and drinking water; inhalation of fumes from burning storage batteries or similar substances; or, infrequently, absorption of the material from bullets or buckshot within a serous cavity after a wound. Lead poisoning may also occur in the fetus of a pregnant woman exposed to lead, because lead can cross the placenta. Delayed dental and skeletal development, lead lines, and osteosclerosis may be evident in infants with congenital lead poisoning.

The onset of symptoms and signs after chronic (subclinical) lead poisoning may be abrupt. Cramping abdominal pain; encephalopathy with convulsions, delirium, coma, or death; peripheral neuritis with muscular paralysis; and mild anemia are recognized clinical manifestations of the chronic disorder. Examining the urine for porphyrin is a useful screening test to establish the diagnosis.

### Musculoskeletal Abnormalities in Infants and Children

Lead poisoning is associated with the appearance of thick, transverse, radiodense lines in the metaphyses of growing tubular bones. Deposition of calcium is the basis of the transverse lines; even though lead is deposited in the metaphysis, the amounts are minute in relation to the content of calcium. Lead lines, which are almost invariable in chronic infantile and juvenile plumbism, are not an early manifestation of the process and, therefore, are of little diagnostic aid. The radiodense zones are especially prominent in the bones about the knee (Fig. 64–4); identification of density in the proximal fibular metaphysis may

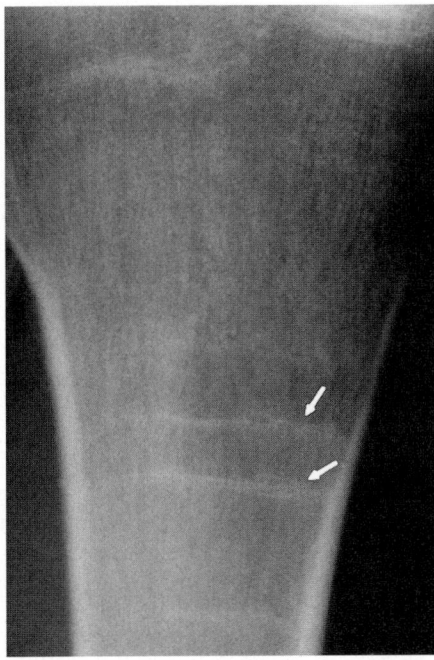

**Figure 64–1.** Transverse or stress lines: appendicular skeleton. In the proximal tibia, multiple transverse radiodense lines extend almost completely across the medullary cavity *(arrows)*.

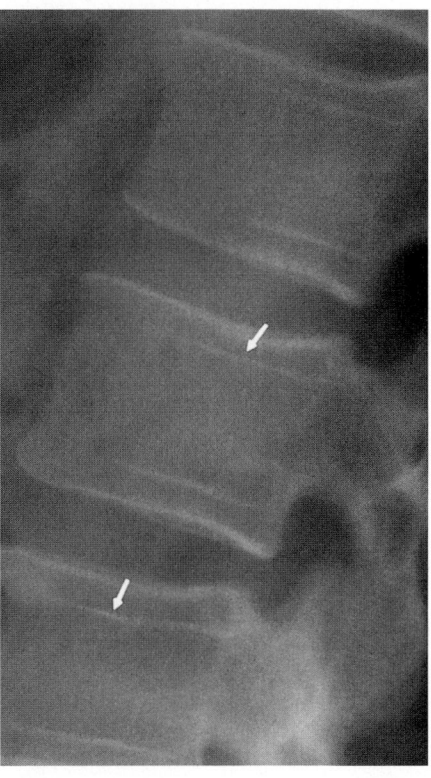

**Figure 64–2.** Transverse or stress lines: axial skeleton. In multiple vertebral bodies, observe radiodense lines paralleling the superior and inferior osseous margins *(arrows)*, creating a bone-within-bone appearance.

be particularly helpful in establishing a radiographic diagnosis of lead poisoning. Radiodense lines can also be evident at other sites, particularly in the wrist (Fig. 64–5). Single transverse bands predominate; however, multiple lines may result from several episodes of lead poisoning. Even the axial skeleton may be affected (Fig. 64–6). In the absence of continued lead poisoning, the migrating lead lines decrease in radiodensity and disappear in approximately 4 years.

An additional manifestation of plumbism is failure of normal modeling of the tubular bones, which is most prominent in the femora. Widening of the metaphyses can resemble the changes in a number of bone dysplasias.

Lead poisoning can be associated with clinical and radiographic signs of increased intracranial pressure. Widening of the cranial sutures may be evident in as many as 10% of cases of chronic lead poisoning.

## Musculoskeletal Abnormalities in Adults

Lead intoxication related to retained lead missiles within the body is commonly overlooked as a diagnostic possibility

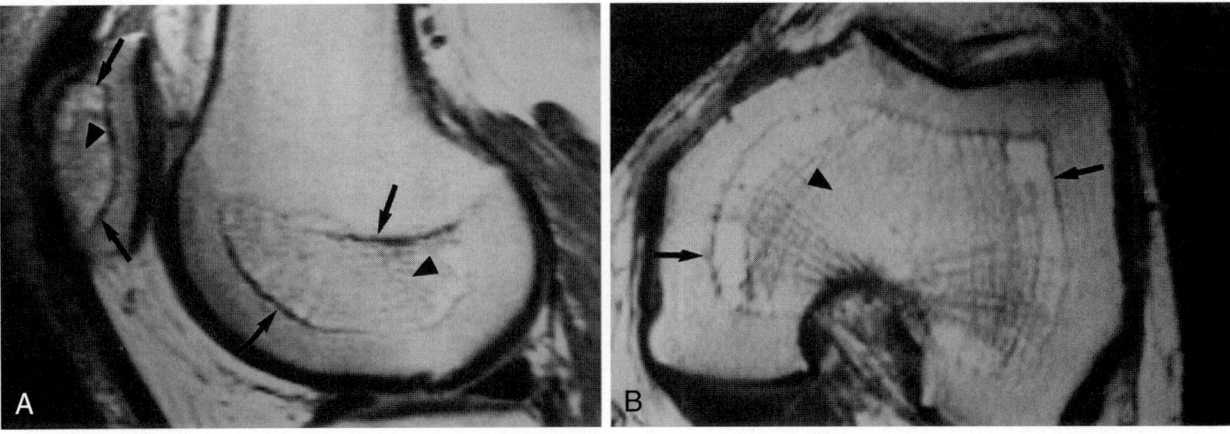

**Figure 64–3.** Transverse growth recovery lines. In sagittal intermediate-weighted (TR/TE, 2500/16) *(A)* and transaxial T1-weighted (TR/TE, 722/20) *(B)* spin echo MR images, note the bone-within-bone appearance *(arrows)*, with the marrow within the central bone having a higher signal intensity *(arrowheads)*.

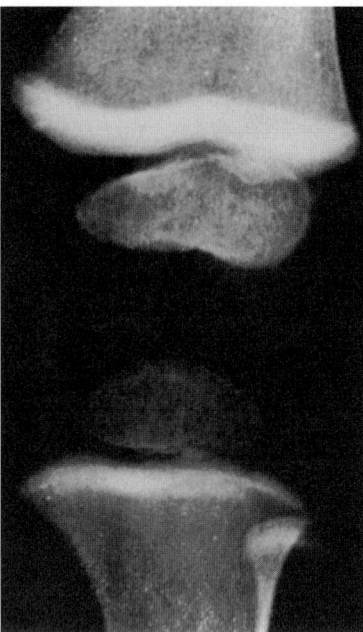

**Figure 64–4.** Lead poisoning: knee. Transverse radiodense bands of the metaphyses of femur, tibia, and fibula.

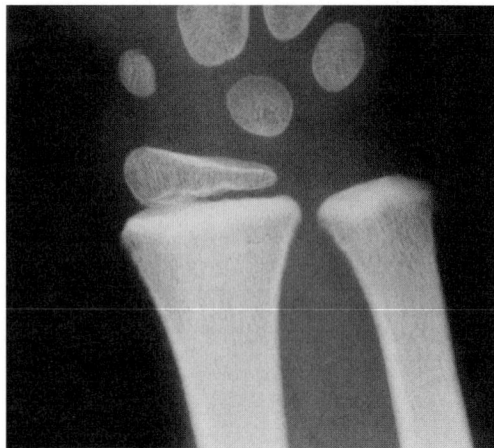

**Figure 64–5.** Lead poisoning: wrist. Transverse radiodense bands of the metaphyses of radius and ulna.

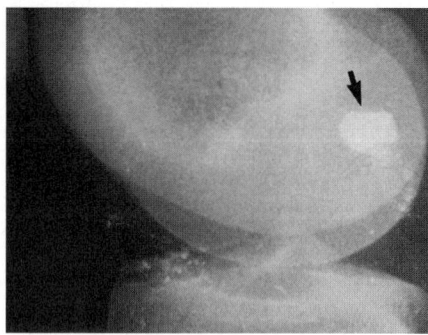

**Figure 64–6.** Lead poisoning: radiographic abnormalities. Observe fragmentation of a missile (*arrow*), with opaque fragments present in the knee joint.

in patients with protean clinical manifestations such as anemia, encephalopathy, nephropathy, neuropathy, and abdominal pain. Bullets, shrapnel, and buckshot are potential sources of the lead, and the resulting clinical findings may be intermittent, delayed for as long as 50 years after the injury. The absorption of lead from the missile generally requires that it be located in a cystic cavity, typically a synovium-lined joint.

Reports have documented lead poisoning in patients with retained missiles in the hip, knee, ankle, elbow, glenohumeral joint, and small joints of the hands and feet. In these cases, localized synovial reaction leading to symptoms and signs of arthritis may occur. It is assumed that some factor in the synovial fluid leads to accelerated solution of the lead. In some cases, systemic manifestations are associated with lead missiles in extra-articular locations.

Radiographic evidence of dissolution of lead missiles is provided by progressive fragmentation, enlargement, and migration of the radiodense foci (see Fig. 64–6). In a joint, this can lead to initial findings resembling a lead arthrogram (plumbogram), which subsequently disappear. In the vertebral column, enlarging radiodense areas in the spinal canal, intervertebral disc, and adjacent connective tissues may be accompanied by osseous and cartilaginous destruction. Saturnine gout is also termed the "moonshine malady" because of its occurrence in moonshiners whose home-brewed liquor contained an appreciable quantity of lead. Saturnine gout appears to be an expression of renal injury from lead in which a tubular defect leading to uric acid retention becomes evident.

### Differential Diagnosis

Radiodense lines in the metaphyses of tubular bones can be seen as a normal variant, as an indication of previous stress, in heavy metal poisoning (including lead poisoning), and in the healing stages of leukemia, rickets, and scurvy (Table 64–1). Similar findings may accompany hypothyroidism, hypervitaminosis D, and transplacental infections (rubella, cytomegalic inclusion disease, herpes simplex, toxoplasmosis, and syphilis). Metaphyseal flaring or widening is seen not only in lead poisoning but also in various anemias (sickle cell anemia, thalassemia), storage disorders (Gaucher's disease, Niemann-Pick disease), and congenital syndromes (Pyle's disease, multiple familial exostoses, osteopetrosis, Ollier's disease) and as a normal variant.

### PHOSPHORUS POISONING

Phosphorus poisoning was previously seen in rachitic and tuberculous children who were being treated with phosphorized cod liver oil, although it is encountered infrequently today. Single or multiple deep bands of increased radiodensity are produced in the ends of growing tubular bones and within flat or irregular bones and persist for many years.

### BISMUTH POISONING

In a pregnant woman with syphilis, injected bismuth may cross the placenta and enter the fetal circulation to be

**TABLE 64–1**

## Historical Summary of Early Published Studies on Lines and Bands

| Date | Author | Summary of Findings | Date | Author | Summary of Findings |
|------|--------|---------------------|------|--------|---------------------|
| 1874 | Wegener | Produced transverse bands of trabeculae by administration of phosphorus to rabbits and chickens | 1941 | Siegling | Used radiopaque lines to determine growth loci in epiphyses of long bones |
| 1877 | Gies | Produced transverse bands by administration of arsenic to rabbits | 1942 | Gill and Abbott | Described shifting proportions of relative growth at both ends of tibia and femur between prenatal and postnatal life in child whose mother had been given bismuth during pregnancy |
| 1903 | Ludloff | Reported transverse striations in radiographs of legs of normal individuals | | | |
| 1904 | Lehndorff | Described transverse striations in scurvy | 1945 | Caffey | Reported lines in sites of accelerated growth, and doubted that growth retardation is essential to development of these lines |
| 1918 | Phemister | Described radiopaque transverse bands in long bones after administration of phosphorus | | | |
| 1921 | Stettner | Interpreted transverse lines as lines of arrested growth | 1952 | Follis and Park | Distinguished between lattice formation, or zones of increased density, and transverse strata, or lines of increased density—the former being primarily a defect in resorptive activity by osteoblasts, whereas in the latter, a cessation of cartilaginous growth is primary |
| 1924 | Asada | Reported experimental production of lines by encasing extremities in plaster | | | |
| 1926 | Harris | Reviewed earlier literature on lines, used lines to demonstrate nonexistence of interstitial growth, explained their presence as manifestations of arrested growth, and discussed their formation with reference to vitamins | 1953 | Park and Richter | Indicated that although initiation of a transverse line is caused by cessation of cartilage growth, thickening is caused by lag of cartilage cell maturation behind resumed osteoblastic activity in recovery phase |
| 1927 | Eliot, Souther, and Park | Concluded from histologic studies that transverse lattice formation might be regarded as temporary halting of cartilage growth but with continuation of osteoblastic activity | | | |
| 1931 | Harris | Presented historical review, case histories, and illustrations of various clinical conditions and experimental evidence indicating that transverse stratum first appears as calcification in proliferative zone of cartilage | 1955 | Hewitt, Westropp, and Acheson | Demonstrated statistically significant association between transverse lines in radiographs of knees and periods of illness in 650 normal children |
| | | | 1956 | Jones and Dean | Reported that more children with kwashiorkor had transverse lines on distal end of radius than normal children and followed development of these lines in serial radiographs |
| 1931 | Park, Jackson, and Kajdi | Reported radiopaque bands following lead poisoning and suggested that lead produced more densely packed trabeculae | 1956 | Dreizen, Currie, Gilley, and Spies | Found transverse lines and nutritive status not to be significantly associated, although relation between resorption of lines and nutritive status was reported |
| 1933 | Park, Jackson, Goodwin, and Kajdi | Discussed transverse formation in lead poisoning and distinguished these "bands" from transverse lines | | | |
| 1933 | Harris | Presented essentially a repetition of his earlier article | 1959 | Acheson | Suggested that in starvation and illness, withdrawal of growth hormone is primary cause of slowing of cartilage growth |
| 1938 | Sontag | Reported striae in tarsal bones of 1-mo-old infants, and attributed their presence to shift from prenatal to postnatal environment | 1960 | Goff | Reviewed previous uses of transverse lines to elucidate relative growth, and gave additional examples of their utility |
| | | | 1962 | Platt and Steward | Produced transverse lines in growing pigs subjected to low-protein diets |
| 1941 | Stammel | Reported two persons with multiple lines and bands on vertebrae, round bones, epiphyses, and phalanges, as well as major long bones and pelvis | 1964 | Dreizen, Spirakis, and Stone | Indicated in longitudinal study of 679 children that frequency of transverse lines on distal end of radius reached a maximum by 5 yr of age and decreased thereafter |

**TABLE 64–1**

**Historical Summary of Early Published Studies on Lines and Bands** *Continued*

| Date | Author | Summary of Findings | Date | Author | Summary of Findings |
|------|--------|---------------------|------|--------|---------------------|
| 1964 | Park | Presented summary and review of work by him and his colleagues on formation and distribution of transverse lines and their distinction from bands produced by phosphorus and heavy metals | 1968 | Gahn, Hempy, and Schwager | Used transverse lines on distal end of tibia in longitudinal series to partition relative contribution of proximal and distal ends of diaphyseal and epiphyseal growth increments |
| 1964 | Wells | Showed prevalence of transverse tibial lines in skeletal remains of children and adults | 1968 | Cornwell and Littleton | Identified radiopaque lines on tibia as subcortical, reaching from endosteal surface to endosteal surface to endosteal surface, as confirmed by transaxial conventional tomograms and bone sections |
| 1965 | Roche | Used transverse lines to demonstrate tibial lines in skeletal remains of children and adults | | | |
| 1966 | Marshall | Found presence of new transverse lines on radius to be associated with illness and inoculation and discussed their use in paleopathology | 1968 | Schwager | Reported statistically significant, low-order associations between episodes of disease and trauma in childhood and appearance of new transverse lines in succeeding period |
| 1967 | Gahn and Schwager | Showed persistent transverse lines on distal end of tibia of adults into ninth decade of life, with decreasing frequency after sixth decade in both sexes | 1968 | McHenry | Showed high frequency of transverse lines on distal end of femur in prehistoric populations and demonstrated such lines to be manifestations of bony lattice within marrow cavity |
| 1967 | Gray | Observed radiopaque lines in 30% of 133 Egyptian mummies, and suggested "a general poor state of health during adolescence in ancient Egypt" | | | |

From Garn SM, Silvermann FN, Hertzog KP, et al: Lines and bands of increased density: Their implication to growth and development. Med Radiogr Photogr 44:60, 1968.

deposited in the skeleton. Single or multiple radiodense bands or lines in the metaphyses of the tubular bones in cases of bismuth poisoning share radiographic and morphologic characteristics with those that appear in cases of lead poisoning.

## ALUMINUM TOXICITY

The oral or parenteral administration of aluminum compounds may lead to its deposition in the body's tissues and, in some sites—such as the brain and bones—to toxic effects. This situation can arise in nonuremic adults, some of whom have peptic ulcer disease, who are ingesting large amounts of aluminum carbonate; in uremic patients who ingest aluminum salts as phosphate binders and whose renal clearance of aluminum is reduced or who are undergoing hemodialysis, and in patients who have lost small bowel function and are maintained on chronic total parenteral nutrition.

The toxic effects of aluminum on the brain and bones have been well studied in patients with chronic renal failure who are maintained on regular hemodialysis or, rarely, on peritoneal dialysis (see Chapter 46). Accumulation of aluminum appears to play a major role in

dialysis encephalopathy. Further, bone toxicity, manifested clinically as pain, tenderness, and deformity, is accompanied by the accumulation of aluminum in osseous tissue.

Osteopenia (related to osteomalacia), Looser's zones (insufficiency fractures), and complete fractures affecting the ribs, spine, and tubular bones are the principal radiographic manifestations of aluminum-induced osteopathy. Periosteal new bone in the shafts of the tibia and fibula and in the pelvis has also been observed. In children, rickets-like metaphyseal abnormalities appear.

## COPPER DEFICIENCY

A disorder associated with hypocupremia has been reported in infants who are malnourished, those receiving long-term parenteral nutrition, or those born prematurely and maintained on diets low in copper. Radiographic findings include osteopenia, metaphyseal radiodense lines and spurs, fractures, and physeal disruptions with malalignment of the epiphysis and metaphysis. Periostitis, which may become profound, is also observed. Reversal of the osseous abnormalities occurs when copper supplementation is employed.

Menkes' syndrome (kinky-hair syndrome) is an inherited disorder with an X-linked pattern of transmission that relates to a defect in copper absorption from the gut. Radiographic findings are similar to those in nutritional copper deficiency, consisting of osteopenia, flaring of the ends of the tubular bones, metaphyseal cupping and irregularity, and osseous spurs. The changes resemble those of rickets and the abused child syndrome.

## METAL DEBRIS (METALLOSIS) ASSOCIATED WITH JOINT IMPLANTS

Although the complications resulting from joint surgery are discussed in Chapter 14, a few comments regarding one of these, metal debris (or metallosis), are appropriate here. Such debris may occur in large amounts in tissues surrounding failed prostheses, especially those containing titanium. Although metallosis is relatively rare, increased serum and urine levels of some metals (e.g., cobalt, chromium, nickel) have been noted in patients with knee and hip prostheses, especially if the prostheses are loose. Dissemination of metal debris to regional lymph nodes has been documented. Concern has been expressed about the effects of particulate metal debris on the immune system, with the potential development of hypersensitivity reactions, infections, and tumors. Within the involved joint, metal debris in the synovial membrane leads to a diagnostic radiographic appearance, with radiodense material observed at the periphery of the joint (Fig. 64–7). Arthrocentesis documents the presence of thick, dark gray or black fluid.

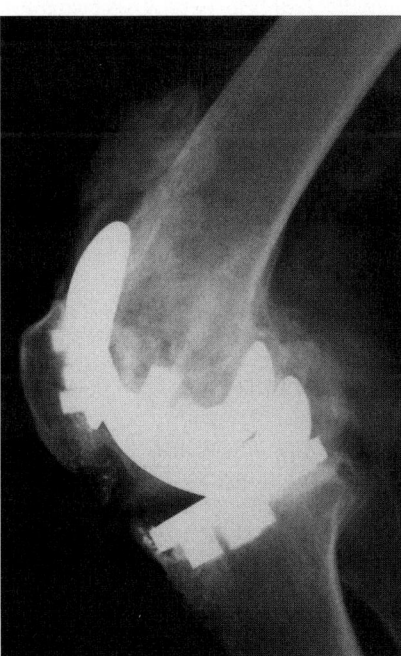

**Figure 64–7.** Metallosis associated with joint implants. Total knee arthroplasty associated with metallosis, with characteristic radiodense shadows within the affected joints. (Courtesy of C. Chen, MD, Kaohsiung, Taiwan.)

## FURTHER READING

Andreoli SP, Smith JA, Bergstein JM: Aluminum bone disease in children: Radiographic features from diagnosis to resolution. Radiology 156:663, 1985.

Ashkenazai A, Levin S, Djaldetti M, et al: The syndrome of neonatal copper deficiency. Pediatrics 52:525, 1971.

Blickman JG, Wilkinson RH, Graef JW: The radiologic "lead band" revisited. AJR Am J Roentgenol 146:245, 1986.

Chew FS, Ramsdell MG, Keel SB: Metallosis after total knee replacement. AJR Am J Roentgenol 170:1556, 1998.

Danks DM, Campbell PE, Stevens BJ, et al: Menkes' kinky hair syndrome: An inherited defect in copper absorption with widespread effects. Pediatrics 50:188, 1972.

DeMartini J, Wilson A, Powell JS, et al: Lead arthropathy and systemic lead poisoning from an intraarticular bullet. AJR Am J Roentgenol 176:1144, 2001.

Edwards DK III: Skeletal growth lines on radiographs of newborn infants: Prevalence and possible association with obstetric abnormalities. AJR Am J Roentgenol 161:141, 1993.

Follis RH Jr, Park EA: Some observations on bone growth with particular respect to zones and transverse lines of increased density in the metaphysis. AJR Am J Roentgenol 68:709, 1952.

Garn SM, Silverman FN, Hertzog KP, et al: Lines and bands of increased density: Their implication to growth and development. Med Radiogr Photogr 44:58, 1968.

Garrett P, McWade M, O'Callaghan J: Radiological assessment of aluminum-related bone disease. Clin Radiol 37:63, 1986.

Klinenberg JR: Saturnine gout—a moonshine malady. N Engl J Med 280:1238, 1969.

Leonard MH: The solution of lead of synovial fluid. Clin Orthop 64:255, 1969.

Leone AJ Jr: On lead lines. AJR Am J Roentgenol 103:165, 1968.

Park EA: The imprinting of nutritional disturbances on the growing bone. Pediatrics 33:815, 1964.

Pearl M, Boxt LM: Radiographic findings in congenital lead poisoning. Radiology 136:83, 1980.

Pease CN, Newton GG: Metaphyseal dysplasia due to lead poisoning in children. Radiology 79:233, 1962.

Sachs HK: The evolution of the radiologic lead line. Radiology 139:81, 1981.

Sclafani SJA, Vuletin JC, Twersky J: Lead arthropathy: Arthritis caused by retained intra-articular bullets. Radiology 156:299, 1985.

Sebes JI, Pinstein ML, Massie JD, et al: Radiographic manifestations of aluminum-induced bone disease. AJR Am J Roentgenol 142:424, 1984.

Wesenberg RL, Gwinn JL, Barnes GR Jr: Radiological findings in the kinky hair syndrome. Radiology 92:500, 1969.

# CHAPTER 65

## Neuromuscular Disorders

### SUMMARY OF KEY FEATURES

The musculoskeletal abnormalities accompanying neuromuscular disorders include osteoporosis, soft tissue atrophy, growth disturbances, deformities, growth plate injuries, infection, heterotopic ossification, cartilage atrophy, synovitis, clubbing, joint capsule alterations, and neuropathic osteoarthropathy. Typical radiographic changes are encountered. Although the pathogenesis of some of the findings is clear, that of heterotopic ossification and sacroiliac joint and spinal alterations is unknown.

Some specific types of neuromuscular disease lead to characteristic clinical and imaging findings. Of particular importance, entrapment neuropathies occur at vulnerable sites along the course of peripheral nerves, as well as in plexuses. Hereditary neuropathies of sensory neurons produce neuropathic osteoarthropathy, which is discussed in Chapter 66.

### INTRODUCTION

Although the specific response of the musculoskeletal system depends to some degree on the nature of the disorder, certain general abnormalities are evident in many of the neuromuscular diseases. These alterations include osteoporosis; fractures; soft tissue atrophy or hypertrophy; growth disturbances and deformities caused by altered muscular forces; growth plate and epiphyseal changes; soft tissue, bone, and joint infections; heterotopic ossification; cartilage and muscle atrophy; spondylopathy; synovitis; and capsular abnormalities.

### GENERAL ABNORMALITIES

#### Osteoporosis and Fractures

Profound osteoporosis accompanies immobilization, disuse, or paralysis. It can affect the entire skeleton or a portion of it, depending on the cause or the circumstances (Fig. 65–1). The pathogenesis of the osteoporosis is not clear. A generalized or localized, uniform or patchy, diffuse or periarticular decrease in spongy bone density is associated with diminution of the cortex and accentuation of stress trabeculae in the peripheral or central skeleton, or in both. In certain bones, such as the humerus and tibia, the resulting radiographic abnormalities, which consist of a permeative pattern of bone destruction, simulate those of plasma cell myeloma or skeletal metastasis (Fig. 65–2).

Several types of fractures are seen. Muscle weakness leads to frequent episodes of falling or stumbling that result in fractures of the tubular bones in the lower extremity. Seizures are associated with direct forces on bone as a result of a fall or with indirect forces on bone secondary to uncontrolled and violent muscle contraction; typical sites of fractures accompanying seizures are the spine, proximal portion of the femur, acetabulum, and shoulder region. "Spontaneous" fractures may be encountered as a result of bone atrophy and weakening aggravated by altered patterns of ambulation, spasticity, contractures, deformities, and, in some instances, vigorous physical therapy; excessive callus formation can appear in the healing phase (Fig. 65–3). Soft tissue ossification and synostosis are seen about fracture sites.

#### Soft Tissue and Muscle Atrophy and Hypertrophy

Soft tissue atrophy with muscle wasting and fatty infiltration accompanies most neuromuscular disorders, particularly denervation. Computed tomography and magnetic resonance (MR) imaging have been used to document the extent of muscle abnormality that occurs in neuromuscular disorders.

Injury to peripheral nerves related to trauma or other causes leads to a spectrum of muscle abnormalities that appear to be time dependent. Such abnormalities can be studied with MR imaging. Subacute denervation reveals prolonged T1 and T2 values, which contribute to conspicuous hyperintensity on short tau inversion recovery (STIR) images. The resulting appearance is similar to that occurring in a variety of other conditions, such as myonecrosis, intramuscular hemorrhage, muscle infarction, polymyositis, muscle edema secondary to tumors, effects of ionizing radiation, and exertional muscle injuries. Subacutely denervated muscles may progress to fatty replacement or may return to normal.

Paradoxically, in rare instances, a muscle's response to denervation is enlargement, not atrophy. Such enlargement may be related to two processes: true hypertrophy, which is enlargement caused by an increase in the size of the remaining innervated muscle fibers, and pseudohypertrophy, which is enlargement related to the accumulation of fat within the muscle (Fig. 65–4).

Myonecrosis (rhabdomyolysis) is associated with compression of musculature as a result of trauma or coma; it can be unifocal or multifocal and unilateral or bilateral. MR imaging supplemented with the intravenous injection of a gadolinium-containing contrast agent shows nonenhancing portions of the muscle, although a similar appearance may be noted in cases of muscle abscess and necrotic tumor and during some stages of hematoma.

#### Growth Disturbances and Deformities Caused by Altered Muscular Forces

Activity is essential to the normal growth and development of bones. With inactivity from any cause, muscle contraction diminishes or is lost, and in an immature skeleton, the growth cartilage is damaged. Neonates with

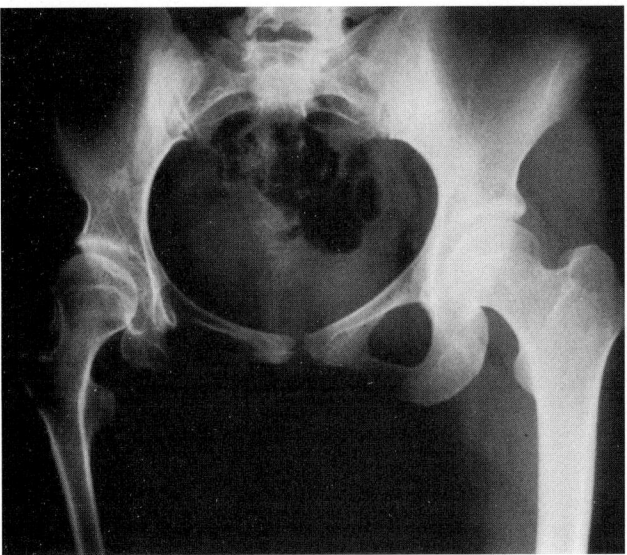

**Figure 65–1.** Osteoporosis, bony underdevelopment, and soft tissue atrophy: poliomyelitis. Note the osteoporosis and underdevelopment of the hemipelvis and femur on the paralyzed right side. Coxa valga, external rotation of the femur, and stress changes in the contralateral sacroiliac joint are also noted.

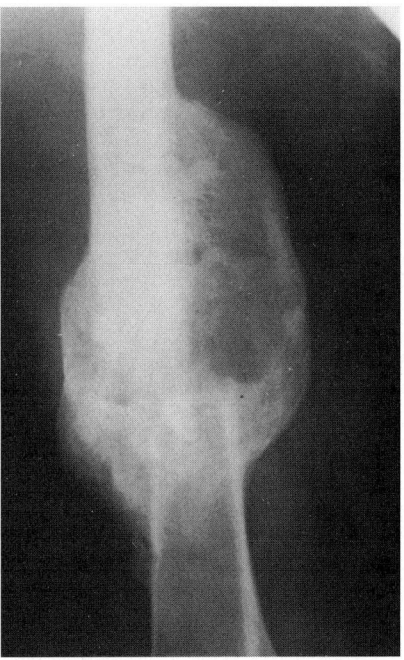

**Figure 65–3.** Osteoporosis and fracture. In this 24-year-old man who became comatose at the time of an automobile accident, subsequent healing of a femoral fracture is associated with exuberant callus and solid bone union.

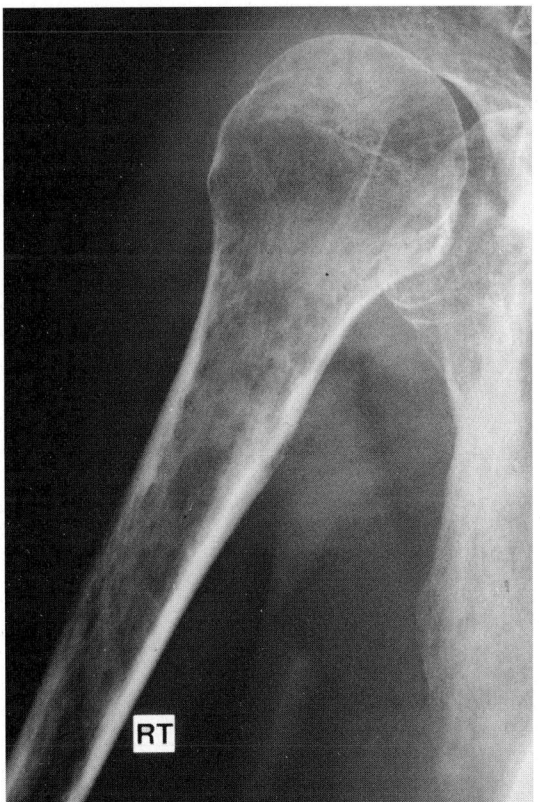

**Figure 65–2.** Osteoporosis. In this patient with hemiplegia, an aggressive pattern of osteoporosis in the humerus simulates the appearance of plasma cell myeloma.

muscle hypotonia or flaccidity and inactive children who spend most of their time in a horizontal position may have vertebral bodies with increased vertical dimensions and narrowed intervertebral discs. Similarly, an increase in the neck-shaft angle of the femur, with the subsequent production of coxa valga (Fig. 65–5), can result from muscular imbalance or a decrease in weight bearing, particularly in very young children. In severe cases, subluxation or dislocation of the hip may occur. The opposite situation, coxa vara, develops when the normal amount of upward muscle pull exceeds the force that can be resisted by weakened bone, such as in osteomalacia and Paget's disease.

Additional effects of altered muscular activity on neighboring bone can be easily identified (Fig. 65–6). In a child with cerebral palsy, for instance, scoliosis, lordosis, and pelvic obliquity may result from unbalanced spine and hip muscle contraction and spasticity; external rotation of the upper portion of the femur, with a prominent lesser trochanter, results from the exaggerated pull of the iliopsoas muscle; and flexion contractures of the hips and knees, with abnormal stress on the quadriceps mechanism, may lead to patella alta, an elongated patellar shape, and fragmentation of the lower pole of the patella and the tibial tuberosity. An exaggerated pull of the flexor muscles of the leg relative to the extensors can produce equinus at the ankle. In a child with poliomyelitis or peroneal muscle atrophy, a pes cavus deformity is attributable to altered muscular function and stress.

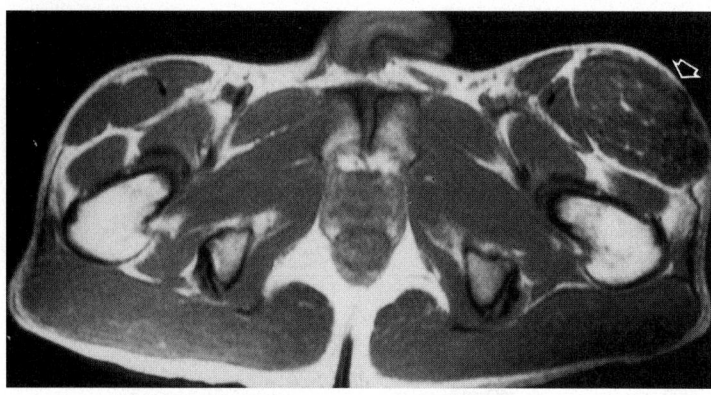

**Figure 65–4.** Denervation with muscle enlargement: true hypertrophy and pseudohypertrophy. Following a stab wound in the left thigh, this 32-year-old man developed a painful mass in the injured area. Transaxial T1-weighted (TR/TE, 770/15) spin echo MR image shows an enlarged left tensor fasciae latae muscle *(arrow)* with signal intensity similar to that of other muscles, although foci of intramuscular fat are seen. (Courtesy of C. A. Petersilge, MD, Cleveland, Ohio.)

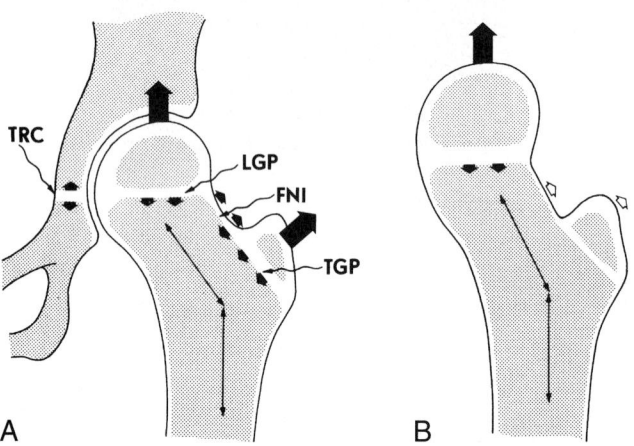

**Figure 65–5.** Pathogenesis of coxa valga. *A*, Normal. The growth zones in this region are the articular cartilage, longitudinal growth plate (LGP), femoral neck isthmus (FNI), and trochanteric growth plate (TGP). The triradiate cartilage (TRC) is present on the acetabular side of the joint. The direction of growth is indicated by small and large bold arrows. The double-headed arrows indicate the normal neck-shaft angle. *B*, Coxa valga. Weakness in the abductor musculature reduces the growth stimulus to the trochanteric growth plate and the femoral neck isthmus *(open arrows)*. The horizontally oriented longitudinal growth plate continues to lengthen the femoral neck in line with the femoral shaft *(small and large bold arrows)*. A valgus angulation results *(double-headed arrows)*. (Modified from Siffert RS: Patterns of deformity in the developing hip. Clin Orthop 160:14, 1981.)

## Growth Plate and Epiphyseal Changes

Premature closure of the growth plate, particularly in the metatarsals and knees, is noted in patients with poliomyelitis (Fig. 65–7). Premature physeal closure can occur in other neuromuscular diseases, and it may be associated with epiphyseal overgrowth (ballooning), findings resembling those of hemophilia or juvenile chronic arthritis.

Epiphyseal and metaphyseal trauma is a recognized manifestation in patients with certain neurologic disorders (meningomyelocele and congenital insensitivity to pain) as a result of their sensory deficiency, osteoporosis, and musculoligamentous laxity (see Chapter 66).

## Osseous, Articular, and Soft Tissue Infection

Generalized or localized infections frequently develop in immobilized and debilitated patients with neuromuscular diseases. Skin breakdown over pressure points is a common and frustrating problem in these patients, and with penetration of the subcutaneous and fascial tissue, infection may reach the underlying bones and joints. The ischial tuberosities, femoral trochanters, hip joints, and other bony protuberances are typically affected, and the characteristic radiographic findings of osteomyelitis or septic arthritis (or both) ensue.

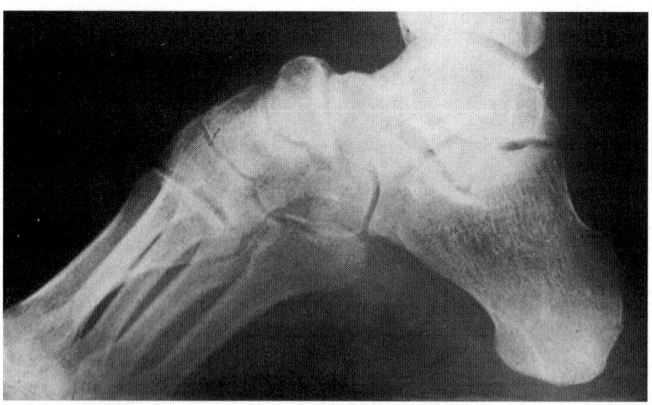

**Figure 65–6.** Osseous effects related to altered muscular activity: pes cavus deformity in poliomyelitis. Observe the exaggerated arch of the foot, soft tissue atrophy, and osteoporosis.

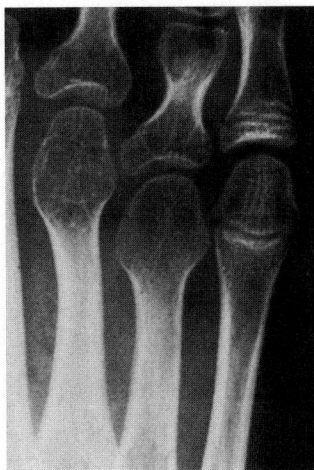

**Figure 65–7.** Premature closure of the growth plate in a patient with poliomyelitis. Closure of the growth plate of the third metatarsal bone has produced shortening of the digit.

## Heterotopic Ossification

Heterotopic new bone formation is a well-documented complication of central nervous system and spinal cord disorders. It is reported most commonly in association with paraplegia secondary to spinal cord trauma. Less frequently, it is evident after acute anoxia, head injury, cerebrovascular accident, encephalomyelitis, poliomyelitis, multiple sclerosis, neoplastic disease, and tetanus. In general, ossification appears 2 to 6 months after injury. Single or multiple and unilateral or bilateral sites may be affected. The areas most typically affected are the hip, knee, and shoulder and, less commonly, the elbow (Fig. 65–8). Although ossification is almost always seen in a paralyzed limb or limbs, this association is not constant.

Radiographic examination initially delineates poorly defined periarticular radiodense areas that do not contain recognizable trabeculae. The collections enlarge, merge with the underlying bone in the form of an irregular excrescence, and demonstrate trabecular architecture. Eventually, complete periarticular osseous bridging may result and lead to significant loss or absence of joint motion. In some instances, ossification develops at a distance from a joint and eventually merges with the subjacent bone.

Scintigraphic examination may be used to determine the evolution of this process and the maturity of the heterotopic ossification. This determination is important, because surgical removal of immature new bone is frequently followed by recurrence of the abnormal deposits. Computed tomography shows ossification progressing from a soft tissue density with lower attenuation than muscle to a calcific density paralleling the radiographic appearance of bone formation. MR imaging patterns of signal intensity are consistent with the presence of ossific shells, marrow fat, hemorrhage and edema of soft tissue, fibrosis, or a combination of these constituents. In the early stages of heterotopic ossification, a region of low signal intensity on T1-weighted spin echo images and a region of high signal intensity on T2-weighted spin echo

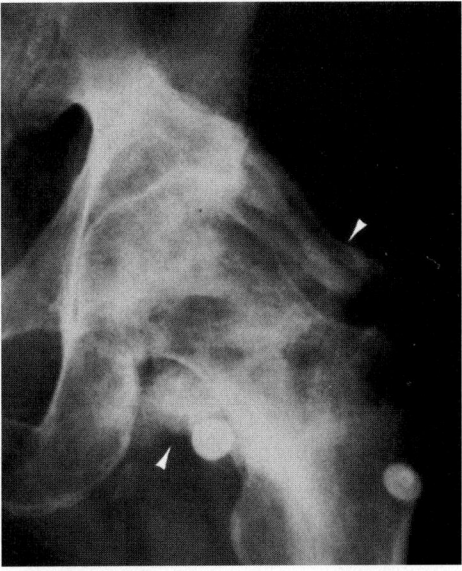

**Figure 65–8.** Soft tissue and bone infection: heterotopic ossification in the hip. The deposit begins as poorly defined opaque areas and progresses to a radiodense lesion of considerable size possessing a trabecular pattern (*arrowheads*).

images are evident. Enhancement of signal intensity in the rim of this region may occur after the intravenous administration of a gadolinium-containing contrast agent, and the resulting appearance simulates that of an abscess or necrotic tumor (Fig. 65–9). Enhancement of signal intensity in adjacent muscles may also be seen on postcontrast images. In the intermediate stages of heterotopic ossification, regions of low signal intensity (corresponding to calcification) at the margins of the lesion and higher signal intensity (corresponding to fat) within the lesion are observed. The chronic stages of heterotopic ossification are characterized by further calcification and ossification, especially at the margin of the lesion, with corresponding MR imaging findings.

The common factor in heterotopic ossification in neurologic disorders is immobilization. Heterotopic ossification of soft tissues is not confined to patients with neuromuscular disease. Burns, mechanical trauma, and venous stasis (varicosities) can lead to similar changes. In addition, a progressive form of ossification of unknown cause, fibrodysplasia (myositis) ossificans progressiva, is recognized.

## Cartilage Atrophy

Articular cartilage is nourished predominantly by diffusion of synovial fluid. Immobilization leads to significant changes in cartilaginous nutrition that are manifested radiographically by chondral changes, with loss of interosseous (joint) space, in patients with neurologic disease (Fig. 65–10). Although this alteration may be observed in any paralyzed body part, such changes are especially characteristic in the hip, knee, and sacroiliac joint.

Reported radiographic changes of the sacroiliac joint consist of periarticular osteoporosis and joint space

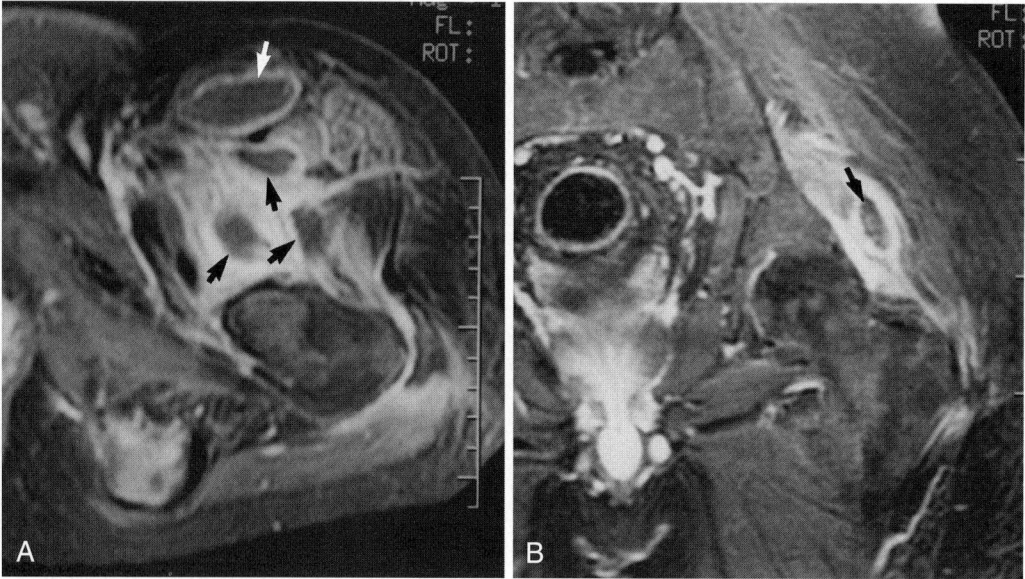

**Figure 65–9.** Heterotopic ossification: MR imaging. In this 37-year-old man with quadriplegia and soft tissue swelling about the hip, axial *(A)* and coronal *(B)* fat-suppressed T1-weighted (TR/TE, 500/14) spin echo MR images obtained after intravenous gadolinium administration show muscle and soft tissue enhancement of signal intensity, with central nonenhancing areas *(arrows)*. Aspiration failed to document infection. Also note the increased signal intensity in the ischial tuberosity in *(A)*, related to chronic stress in this bedridden patient.

narrowing, which may progress to intra-articular bony ankylosis, simulating that of ankylosing spondylitis (Fig. 65–11).

## Spondylopathy

A variety of spinal abnormalities occur in paralyzed persons. Some of them represent neuropathic osteoarthropathy and consist of disc space loss, bone sclerosis, fragmentation, osteophytosis, and subluxation; they are similar to abnormalities appearing in diabetes mellitus, syringomyelia, and syphilis (see Chapter 66). In other instances, bony outgrowths of the spine develop, with characteristics that resemble those of the paravertebral ossification that accompanies psoriatic arthritis or Reiter's syndrome, the flowing ossification of diffuse idiopathic skeletal hyperostosis, or the thin excrescences of ankylosing spondylitis (see Fig. 65–11).

## Joint Capsule Abnormalities

Fibrosis in the joint capsule, especially about the glenohumeral joint, may explain the association between adhesive capsulitis and neurologic injury, particularly hemiparesis. It may also account for the common occurrence of shoulder pain in patients with hemiplegia, although other conditions, such as reflex sympathetic dystrophy and humeral subluxation (see later discussion), as well as osteonecrosis of the humeral head and rotator cuff disruption, may be contributory. With regard to adhesive capsulitis, arthrography documents the restricted capacity of the articular cavity and the irregular accumulation of contrast material consistent with the presence of fibrosis in the joint itself or its normal extensions (such as the bicipital tendon sheath).

Inferior subluxation of the humeral head with respect to the glenoid region of the scapula—the drooping shoulder—is a documented manifestation of paralysis. It is produced by loss of muscular tone, leading to stretching of the supportive musculature and capsule by the weight of the dependent, flaccid upper extremity.

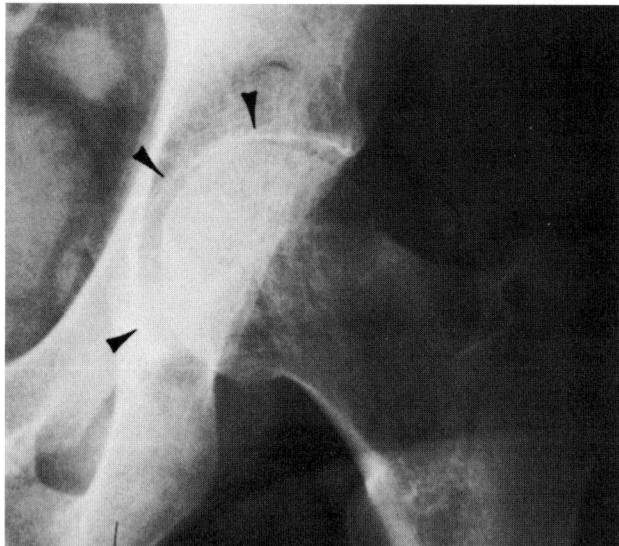

**Figure 65–10.** Cartilage atrophy: radiographic abnormalities. Typical example of symmetrical loss of joint space *(arrowheads)* in the hip secondary to cartilage atrophy resulting from paralysis.

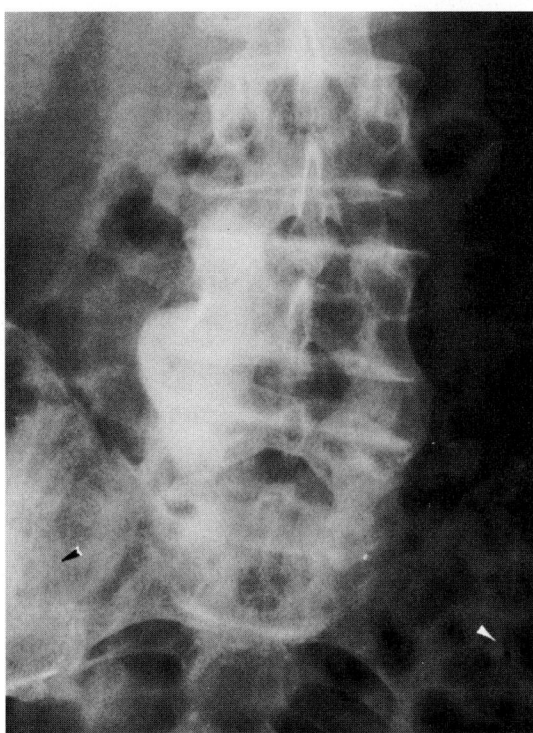

**Figure 65–11.** Sacroiliac joint and spinal abnormalities. In this patient, who had been quadriplegic for more than 5 years, radiograph shows loss of interosseous space in both sacroiliac joints *(arrowheads)* and spinal ossification.

## Miscellaneous Abnormalities

Significant digital clubbing may be encountered in paralyzed patients. This finding is seen in patients who have been paralyzed for more than a year, and it appears to correlate with the presence of decubitus ulcers and persistent subcutaneous edema.

Reflex sympathetic dystrophy has been observed in as many as 25% of hemiplegic patients and is also encountered in quadriplegic patients. Scintigraphy with bone-seeking radiopharmaceutical agents shows increased radionuclide activity in periarticular regions.

## SPECIFIC TYPES OF NEUROMUSCULAR DISEASE

### Peripheral Neuropathies

Peripheral neuropathies represent primary disorders of peripheral motor, sensory, and autonomic neurons and are accompanied by muscle weakness, muscle atrophy, sensory changes, autonomic dysfunction, or any combination of these findings. Classification is commonly accomplished by using the designations mononeuropathy, multiple mononeuropathies, and polyneuropathies (Table 65–1).

### Entrapment Neuropathies

Peripheral nerve entrapment syndromes involve the compression of a short segment of a single nerve at a specific site, frequently as a result of the vulnerability of that nerve as it passes through a fibro-osseous tunnel or an opening in fibrous or muscular tissue. The clinical manifestations vary with the specific site of involvement. In some cases, the manifestations are persistent; in others, they occur only with certain maneuvers of the extremity. The latter situation is often referred to as dynamic compression neuropathy. A variety of provocative clinical tests have been described in which gentle pressure on the nerve at the site of entrapment is accompanied by paresthesias in the distribution of that nerve. These provocative tests, when applied carefully and combined with data derived from the clinical history and routine physical examination, aid in the assessment of entrapment neuropathies. Entrapment neuropathies typically involve the median, ulnar, radial, musculocutaneous, suprascapular, dorsoscapular, or brachial

---

**TABLE 65–1**

**Classification of Peripheral Neuropathies**

| Type | Characteristics | Pathophysiology | Common Cause |
| --- | --- | --- | --- |
| Mononeuropathy | Involves one cranial or peripheral nerve or nerve root | Trauma Compression Entrapment Infarction | Common peroneal palsy Carpal tunnel syndrome Diabetes mellitus |
| Multiple mononeuropathy | Involves several nerves | | |
| | Contiguous nerves | Neoplastic invasion Infarction | Invasion of the brachial plexus by cancer Diabetes mellitus |
| | Noncontiguous nerves | Infarction | Diabetes mellitus Vasculitis |
| Polyneuropathy | Involves the longest nerves first; distal, symmetrical | Toxic-metabolic | Alcoholic-nutritional Diabetes mellitus Uremia Systemic cancer |
| | | Inflammatory or immune (or both) | Guillain-Barré syndrome |

From Sherman DG: Peripheral neuropathies. In Stein JG (ed): Internal Medicine. Boston, Little, Brown, 1983, p 872.

plexus nerve in the upper extremities and the sciatic, common peroneal, tibial, femoral, saphenous, lateral femoral cutaneous, obturator, ilioinguinal, or genitofemoral nerve in the lower extremity (Table 65–2).

### Median Nerve

Entrapment of the median nerve occurs most frequently in the wrist as the carpal tunnel syndrome, but it may also develop in the region of the distal end of the humerus or proximal end of the forearm.

**Ligament of Struthers.** In approximately 1% of limbs, the ligament of Struthers connects an anomalous bony excrescence (the supracondylar process) arising from the anteromedial surface of the distal portion of the humerus to the medial epicondyle of the humerus. Compromise of the median nerve is a possible complication (Fig. 65–12).

**Pronator Syndrome.** An entrapment neuropathy of the median nerve (Fig. 65–13) can occur in the antecubital area where the nerve passes between the two heads of the pronator teres muscle and then under the edge of the flexor digitorum sublimis muscle.

**Anterior Interosseous Nerve Syndrome (Kiloh-Nevin Syndrome).** The anterior interosseous nerve, the largest branch of the median nerve, is purely motor and supplies the flexor pollicis longus, pronator quadratus, and radial part of the flexor digitorum profundus muscles. Its compression leads to weakness of the thumb and index finger and occurs on an idiopathic basis, after radial or supracondylar humeral fractures.

**Carpal Tunnel Syndrome.** The most frequent entrapment syndrome of the median nerve occurs as the nerve passes through the narrow fibro-osseous tunnel that exists between

### TABLE 65–2

**Entrapment Neuropathies**

| Nerve | Syndrome | Site | Muscle Involvement | Some Causes or Findings |
|---|---|---|---|---|
| | | **Neck and Upper Extremity** | | |
| Brachial plexus and its branches (C5, C6, C7, C8, T1) | Thoracic outlet Anterior scalene (scalenus anticus) syndrome | Posterior scalene foramen or interscalene triangle (neurovascular; brachial plexus and subclavian artery) | Variable but neurologic findings dominate | Accessory muscle (scalenus minimus), cervical rib, fibrous band, muscle hypertrophy or insertional variation, asymmetry of thorax, carrying a knapsack (backpack paralysis), work with arms above head, sports activity (e.g., swimming) |
| | Costoclavicular syndrome | Costoclavicular space between clavicle and first rib (neurovascular: brachial plexus and subclavian artery, subclavian vein) | Variable but vascular findings dominate | Fibrous band, clavicular fracture, fracture of first rib, posterior sternoclavicular dislocation, arm elevation, hypertrophy of pectoralis minor muscle, sports activity (e.g., swimming, tennis) |
| | Hyperabduction syndrome | Axilla, in space (coracopectoral tunnel) between pectoralis minor tendon and coracoid process (neurovascular: brachial plexus, subclavian [axillary] artery, subclavian [axillary] vein) | Variable but neurologic findings are infrequent | Abduction of arm during sleep or occupational activity, accessory muscle (chondroepitrochlearis) |
| Cervical and upper thoracic nerve roots | Scapulocostal syndrome | Space between scapula and chest wall | None | Poor posture, muscle spasm, fibromyositis, immobilization, rotator cuff tear, humeral fracture, glenohumeral joint subluxation, stress fracture of upper ribs |
| Suprascapular nerve (C5, C6) | Suprascapular nerve syndrome | Suprascapular or spinoglenoid notch | Supraspinatus, infraspinatus | Scapular fracture, glenohumeral joint dislocation, ganglion, tumor, varices, sports activity |

**TABLE 65–2**

**Entrapment Neuropathies** *Continued*

| Nerve | Syndrome | Site | Muscle Involvement | Some Causes or Findings |
|---|---|---|---|---|
| | | *Neck and Upper Extremity Continued* | | |
| Axillary (circumflex humeral) nerve (C5, C6) | Quadrilateral space syndrome (lateral axillary hiatus syndrome) | Lateral axillary hiatus (neurovascular: axillary nerve, posterior circumflex humeral artery) | Deltoid, teres minor | Humeral fracture, scapular fracture, glenohumeral joint dislocation, tumor, hematoma, sports activity (e.g., baseball pitching), ganglion, fibrous band, neuralgic amyotrophy |
| Dorsal scapular nerve (C5) | Dorsal scapular nerve syndrome | Scalenus medius muscle | Levator scapulae, rhomboids | Muscle hypertrophy |
| Long thoracic nerve (C5, C6, C7) | Long thoracic nerve syndrome | Serratus anterior muscle, between clavicle and first two ribs or in axilla | Serratus anterior | Plaster cast, axillary splint, crutches, tumor, carrying heavy load, sports activity, neuralgic amyotrophy |
| Musculocutaneous nerve (C5, C6, C7) | Musculocutaneous nerve syndrome of upper part of arm | Coracobrachialis muscle | Coracobrachialis, biceps brachii, brachialis | Muscle anomaly (caput tertium, supernumerary head of biceps brachii), muscle hypertrophy, humeral fracture, neuralgic amyotrophy |
| | Musculocutaneous nerve syndrome at elbow | Elbow, near tendon of biceps brachii muscle and lacertus fibrosus | Biceps brachii, brachialis | Elbow injury, sports activity |
| Radial nerve (C5, C6, C7, C9, T1) | Saturday night (sleep or crutch) palsy | Axilla | Triceps, anconeus, extensor muscles of forearm | Abnormal position of arm, anomaly (coracobrachialis, triceps), triceps brachii contraction, crutches, tumor |
| | Radial nerve syndrome | Spiral groove of humerus | Brachioradialis, wrist/finger extensors | Humeral fracture, muscle contraction, tumor, anomaly (triceps) |
| | Radial tunnel syndrome | Elbow (lateral intermuscular septum, arcade of Frohse, multiple other sites) | Extensor muscles of forearm | Elbow fracture and dislocation, rheumatoid arthritis, tumor, fibrous band, vigorous exercise |
| | Supinator syndrome (posterior interosseous nerve syndrome) | Elbow and forearm, beneath supinator muscle in arcade of Frohse | Abductor pollicis longus, extensor pollicis longus, extensor pollicis brevis, extensor indicis | Humeral fracture, Monteggia's fracture, radial head subluxation, tumor, arthritis, fibrous band, sports activity |
| | Distal posterior interosseous nerve syndrome (neuropathy of deep terminal branch of posterior interosseous nerve) | Wrist, dorsal to radius at entrance to joint capsule of wrist | None | Repetitive movement of wrist (gymnasts) |
| | Cheiralgia paresthetica (neuropathy of superficial branch of radial nerve, Waternberg's disease) | Forearm and wrist, beneath tendon of brachioradialis muscle | None | Radial fracture, surgery for de Quervain's tenosynovitis, plaster cast, handcuffs, tight watch strap, sports activity |
| Median nerve (C5, C6, C7, C8, T1) | Supacondylar process syndrome | Distal humerus | All forearm muscle | Ligament of Struthers, supracondylar process fracture, abnormalities of brachial artery, certain elbow and arm positions |

*Table continued on following page*

**TABLE 65–2**

**Entrapment Neuropathies** *Continued*

| Nerve | Syndrome | Site | Muscle Involvement | Some Causes or Findings |
|---|---|---|---|---|
| | | *Neck and Upper Extremity Continued* | | |
| | Pronator syndrome | Cubital fossa (pronator teres, flexor digitorum superficialis muscles) | Thenar muscles, flexors of wrist, fingers (1–3) | Fibrous band, abnormalities of lacertus fibrosus, anomaly of muscle, trauma, myositis, sports activity (e.g., weightlifting, playing baseball) |
| | Anterior interosseous nerve syndrome (Kiloh-Nevin syndrome) | Elbow and forearm, beneath flexor muscles along interosseous membrane | Flexor policis longus, flexor digitorum profundus of second fingers, pronator quadratus | Humeral or forearm fracture, fibrous band, anomaly (muscles, vessels), tumors, sports activity (e.g, weightlifting, throwing) |
| | Carpal tunnel syndrome | Wrist, carpal tunnel | Abductor pollicis brevis, opponens pollicis, all or part of flexor pollicis brevis, adductor pollicis (rare) | Systemic or local factors, idiopathic |
| Ulnar nerve (C7, C8, T1) | Sulcus ulnaris syndrome (cubital tunnel syndrome) | Elbow, behind medial epicondyle | Flexor carpi ulnaris, flexor digitorum profundus (fingers 4, 5) hypothenar, interossei, some lumbricals, adductor pollicis, portion of flexor pollicis brevis | Humeral fracture, elbow dislocation, overuse syndrome, cubitus valgus deformity, arthritis, anomaly (trochlear hypoplasia, epitrochleoanconeus muscle), ulnar nerve subluxation |
| | Flexor carpi ulnaris muscle syndrome (cubital tunnel syndrome) | Elbow, between two heads of flexor carpi ulnaris | Same as above | Idiopathic, trauma, arthritis, tumor, ganglion, anomaly (of muscles) |
| | Ulnar tunnel syndrome (Guyon's canal syndrome) (vascular counterpart is hypothenar hammer syndrome) | Wrist, Guyon's canal | Palmaris brevis, hypothenar, lateral lumbrical, interossei, adductor pollicis, part of flexor profundus brevis, abductor digiti minimi | Ganglion, anomaly (muscles, hamate hook), carpal fracture, edema, tumor, fibrotic band, sports activity (e.g., cycling) |
| | Syndrome of deep branch of ulnar nerve (pisohamate hiatus syndrome) (vascular counterpart is hypothenar hammer syndrome) | Wrist, hypothenar muscles | Same as above, except spares abductor digiti minimi and palmaris brevis | Ganglion, anomaly (muscles, hamate hook), carpal fracture, edema, tumor, fibrotic band, vibrating tools, motorcycle riding |
| | Syndrome of tendinous arch of adductor pollicis muscle (terminal part of deep branch of ulnar nerve) | Volar aspect of hand, transverse and oblique heads of adductor pollicis muscle | Adductor pollicis | Metacarpal (especially third) fracture, tumor, sports activity (sports requiring prolonged gripping, bicycling) |
| | | *Trunk* | | |
| Intercostal nerve (T6–T12) | Syndrome of rectus abdominis muscle (abdominal cutaneous nerve entrapment syndrome) | Abdomen, at point where nerve enters muscle | Abdominal muscles | Pregnancy, physical activity, abdominal surgery, subluxation of interchondral joints (clicking rib syndrome) |

**TABLE 65–2**

**Entrapment Neuropathies** *Continued*

| Nerve | Syndrome | Site | Muscle Involvement | Some Causes or Findings |
|---|---|---|---|---|
| | | *Trunk Continued* | | |
| Iliohypogastric nerve (L1) | Iliohypogastricus syndrome | Posterior part of abdomen, where nerve pierces aponeurosis of transversus abdominis and internal oblique muscles | Transversus abdominis, internal oblique muscles | Trauma, abdominal surgery, bone graft harvesting, pregnancy, tumor (e.g., renal carcinoma) |
| Ilioinguinal nerve (L1) | Ilioinguinal syndrome | Lower part of abdomen, where nerve pierces transversus abdominis muscle | Abdominal muscle | Retroperitoneal or renal tumor, inguinal hernia, hip arthritis |
| Genitofemoral nerve (L1, L2) | Genitofemoral nerve syndrome | Lower part of abdomen, where either nerve passes through psoas major muscle or its branches pass through abdominal wall | Cremaster muscle | Surgery (inguinal hernia repair, cesarean section, appendectomy, laparoscoppy) psoas abscess |
| | | *Lower Extremity* | | |
| L5 nerve | Lumbosacral tunnel syndrome | Tunnel adjacent to lumbosacral ligament | None | Degenerative disc disease (L5–S1), thick lumbosacral ligament, aneurysm, tortuous veins, tumor (spine, sacrum, ilium), pelvic fractures |
| Superior and inferior gluteal nerves (L4, L5, S1, S2) | Gluteal nerve syndrome | Superior gluteal nerve: in suprapiriform foramen; inferior gluteal nerve: in infrapiriform foramen (along with sciatic nerve) | Tensor fasciae latae Gluteal muscles Superior nerve: Gluteus medius Gluteus minimus Tensor fasciae latae Inferior nerve: Gluteus maximus | Pelvic fracture, hip surgery, intramuscular injection, spondylolisthesis, piriformis muscle hypertrophy, trauma |
| Femoral nerve (L2, L3, L4) | Iliacus muscle syndrome (iliacus tunnel syndrome) | Thigh, under inguinal ligament, near iliopectineal arch | Iliacus, psoas, pectineus, sartorius, quadriceps, thigh muscles except tensor fasciae latae | Pelvic surgery (hysterectomy, gynecologic surgery, renal transplantation, anterior spine fusion), hematoma pelvic fracture, retroperitoneal tumor, aneurym, hernia |
| Obturator nerve (L2, L3, L4) | Obturator tunnel syndrome | Obturator tunnel (root— pubic bone; floor— internal and external obturator muscles) | Pectineus, adductor longus, adductor brevis, gracilis, adductor magnus | Pelvic fracture, pelvic tumor, hematoma, retroperitoneal tumor, surgery (total hip arthroplasty, genitourologic surgery), aneurysm, hernia |
| Cutaneous posterior femoral nerve (S1, S2, S3, S4) | Cutaneous posterior femoral nerve syndrome | Thigh, infrapiriform foramen, or under gluteus maximus muscle | None | Hypertrophy or spasm of piriformis muscle, prolonged sitting, trauma |
| Sciatic nerve (L4, L5, S1, S2) | Piriformis muscle syndrome | Infrapiriformis foramen in greater sciatic notch (hilus of gluteus) | Biceps femoris, semitendinosus, semimembranosus, adductor magnus, and all muscles below knee | Piriformis muscle abnormality (spasm, myositis, injury, anomaly), sacroilitis, hematoma, bursitis, anomaly of course of nerve, pelvic fracture tumor, flexion contracture of hip, injection, immobility |

*Table continued on following page*

**TABLE 65–2**

**Entrapment Neuropathies** *Continued*

| Nerve | Syndrome | Site | Muscle Involvement | Some Causes or Findings |
|---|---|---|---|---|
| | | *Lower Extremity Continued* | | |
| Lateral femoral cutaneous nerve (L2, L3) | Meralgia paresthetica | Anterior part of thigh, near inguinal ligament and fascia lata | None | Scoliosis, leg length discrepancy, prolonged standing, seat belt, tight belt, retroperitoneal tumor, aortic aneurysm, abdominal or inguinal surgery, obesity, weight loss, anomaly (nerve passes through sartorius muscle) |
| Saphenous nerve (sensory branch of femoral nerve) | Saphenous nerve syndrome | Medial part of thigh, in adductor canal (Hunter's canal) (nerve along with femoral artery and femoral vein) that is intimate with vastus medialis, sartorius, and adductor longus muscles | None | Trauma, vascular surgery, thrombophlebitis, pes anserinus bursitis, knee surgery |
| Tibial nerve (L4, L5, S1, S2, S3) | Popliteal entrapment syndrome | Popliteal fossa, intimate with popliteal artery and vein | Generally none but rarely gastrocnemius, plantaris, soleus, popliteus, tibialis posterior, flexor digitorum longus, flexor hallucis longus | Anomaly of gastrocnemius, soleus, or plantaris muscle, fibrous band, tumor |
| Common peroneal nerve (L4, L5, S1, S2) | Peroneal tunnel syndrome | Neck of fibula | Anterior tibialis, extensor digitorum longus, extensor hallucis longus, peroneus longus, peroneus brevis | Cast, fibula fracture, dislocation of proximal tibiofibular joint, total knee arthroplasty, ganglion, repetitive activity, popliteal cyst, tumor (e.g., osteochondroma), enlarged fabella, muscle herniation |
| Superficial peroneal nerve (branch of common peroneal nerve) | Superficial peroneal nerve syndrome (or entrapment) | Middle to distal third of leg where nerve pierces crural fascia | Peroneus longus, peroneus brevis (rare) | Muscle hernia, surgery, tight boots, tumor, trauma |
| Sural nerve (sensory branch of tibial nerve) | Sural nerve syndrome | Lower part of leg and behind lateral malleolus | None | Ganglion, tumor, thrombophlebitis, trauma, tight boots, cast, synovial cyst, ankle surgery |
| Deep peroneal nerve (branch of common peroneal nerve) | Anterior tarsal tunnel syndrome | Dorsum of foot at inferior extensor retinaculum or under tendon of extensor hallucis longus muscle | Extensor digitorum brevis, anterior tibialis, extensor digitorum longus, extensor hallucis longus, peroneus tertius | Retinacular abnormality, osteoarthritis of the talonavicular joint, synovial cyst, ganglion, fracture, shoe straps, high-heeled shoes, tenosynovitis, neuroma, aneurysm, sports activity (e.g., running, skiing, ballet dancing) |
| Tibial nerve and its branches, medial and lateral plantar nerves | Tarsal tunnel syndrome | Tarsal tunnel, below medial malleolus | Medial plantar nerve: flexor digitorum brevis, abductor hallucis, flexor hallucis brevis, first lumbrical muscles | Fracture of medial malleolus, talar fracture, ankle dislocation, arthritis, valgus deformity of ankle, pronated foot, muscle hypertrophy of abductor |

**TABLE 65–2**

**Entrapment Neuropathies** *Continued*

| Nerve | Syndrome | Site | Muscle Involvement | Some Causes or Findings |
|---|---|---|---|---|
| | | *Lower Extremity Continued* | | |
| | | | Lateral: digiti quinti, flexor digiti minimi brevis, flexor digitorum accessorius, abductor digiti minimi, interossei, lumbrical, adductor hallucis | hallucis, anomalous muscle, metabolic and endocrine disorder, ganglion, tumor, varicosities, Trevor's disease |
| Medial plantar nerve (branch of tibial nerve) | Jogger's foot | Abductor tunnel, behind navicular tuberosity between navicular bone and abductor hallucis muscle, in region of master knot of Henry | None or flexor digitorum brevis | Trauma, pes cavus deformity, jogging |
| Nerve to abductor digiti quinti muscle (first branch of lateral plantar nerve, which itself is a branch of the tibial nerve) | Jogger's heel | Plantar aspect of foot between fascia of abductor hallucis muscle and medial head of quadratus plantae muscle | Abductor digiti quinti | Sports activity (e.g., running, jogging) |
| Hallucal nerves (branches of plantar nerves) | Hallucal nerve entrapment | Dorsal or plantar aspect of first metatarsal head | None | Bunion, osteoarthritis of first metatarsophalangeal joint, hallux rigidus |
| Digital branch of plantar nerve | Morton's metatarsalgia | Metatarsal heads, especially between third and fourth digits | None | Trauma of metatarsophalangeal joint, Freiberg's infraction, arthritis, ganglion, intermetatarsal bursitis, high-heeled shoes, foot deformity, idiopathic |
| Medical calcaneal nerve (branch of tibial nerve) | Calcaneal nerve entrapment | Ankle or foot, including heel | None | Plantar fasciitis, calcaneal enthesophytes, calcaneal fractures |

the carpal bones and a roof consisting of the inelastic transverse carpal ligament. Although the carpal tunnel view allows analysis of the osseous components of this passageway, delineation of the fibrous roof and the structures within the canal requires ultrasonography or MR imaging (Fig. 65–14).

Causes of carpal tunnel syndrome are numerous (Table 65–3), but many cases occur on an idiopathic basis. Most patients are between the ages of 35 and 65 years. Women are affected more frequently than men, and although bilateral involvement is common, the dominant hand is usually involved first and more severely. Aggravating factors include occupations that require a great deal of repetitive hand and wrist motion, pregnancy, and the use of oral contraceptive agents. Clinical findings include sensory and motor deficits, with numbness and paresthesias of the thumb, index, middle, and half of the ring finger and atrophy and weakness of the thenar mus-

cles. Physical examination documents a positive Tinel's sign (paresthesia after percussion of the nerve in the volar aspect of the wrist).

Four general findings characterize the MR imaging appearance of carpal tunnel syndrome: (1) swelling of the median nerve, best evaluated at the level of the pisiform bone; (2) flattening of the median nerve, judged most reliably at the level of the hamate bone; (3) palmar bowing of the flexor retinaculum, best visualized at the level of the hamate bone; and (4) increased signal intensity of the median nerve on T2-weighted spin echo MR images (Fig. 65–15).

### Ulnar Nerve

Entrapment of the ulnar nerve occurs most commonly near the elbow or wrist and rarely in the forearm.

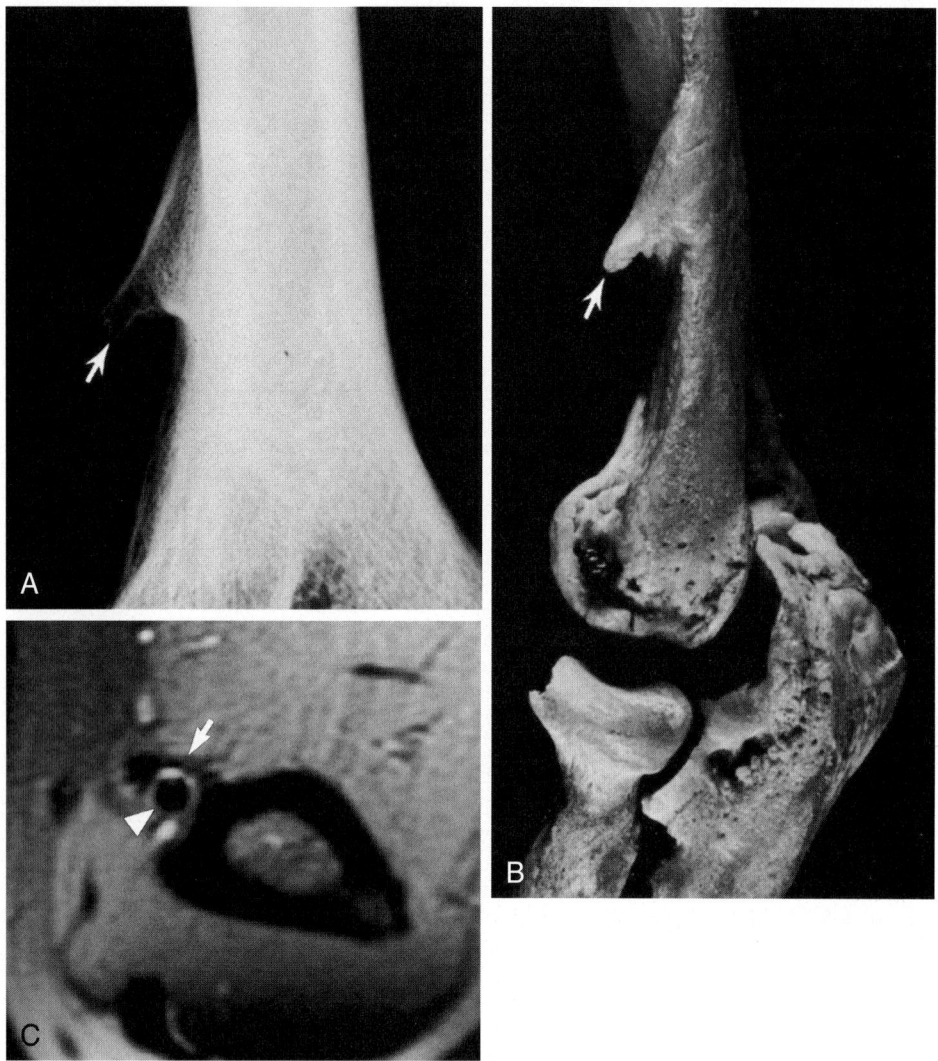

**Figure 65–12.** Entrapment of the median nerve: supracondylar process. *A* and *B*, Radiograph *(A)* and photograph *(B)* show an osseous outgrowth *(arrows)* from the anterior surface of the distal portion of the humerus. The ligament of Struthers may extend from its tip to the medial epicondyle of the humerus and result in compromise of the median nerve. *C*, In a different patient, transverse fat-suppressed T1-weighted (TR/TE, 500/13) spin echo MR image obtained after intravenous gadolinium administration shows a supracondylar process *(arrow)* under which lies the ulnar nerve *(arrowhead)*.

**Cubital Tunnel Syndrome.** Ulnar nerve entrapment is seen most frequently at the level of the cubital tunnel. In this location, the ulnar nerve extends through a fibro-osseous canal formed by the medial epicondyle and an aponeurotic band bridging the dual origin of the flexor carpi ulnaris muscle. Cubital tunnel syndrome is probably the second most common compressive neuropathy of the upper extremity (after carpal tunnel syndrome). Typical causes of compression of the ulnar nerve in the cubital tunnel are trauma, progressive cubitus valgus deformity, and various masses (Fig. 65–16). Clinical findings are sensory deficits and weakness of the flexor carpi ulnaris muscle, flexor digitorum profundus muscle of the fourth and fifth fingers, and intrinsic hand muscles.

**Guyon's Canal Syndrome (Ulnar Tunnel Syndrome).** An entrapment neuropathy of the ulnar nerve may occur in the wrist where the nerve enters the palm through the canal of Guyon (the ulnar tunnel) (Fig. 65–17). The walls of the canal consist of the pisiform bone medially and the hook of the hamate laterally. The floor of the canal is composed of the flexor retinaculum and the origin of the hypothenar muscles, and the roof is composed of the volar carpal ligament, palmaris brevis muscle, and fibers from the palmar fascia. The contents of the canal are the ulnar nerve, ulnar artery, and fatty tissue. The effects of ulnar nerve compression in the ulnar tunnel are dependent on the specific anatomic site affected: with proximal involvement, motor and sensory disturbances are evident; with

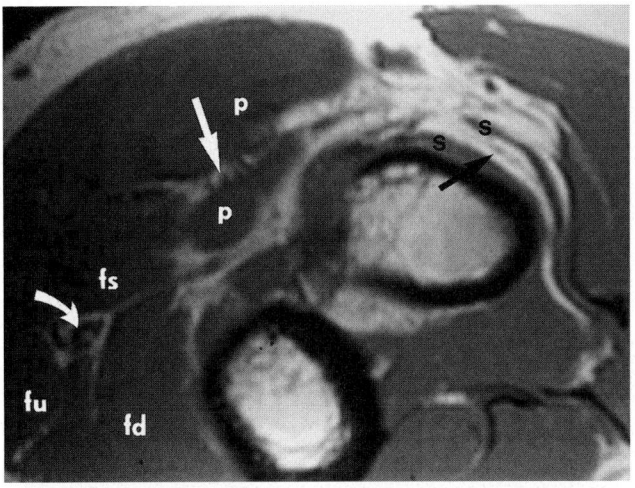

**Figure 65–13.** Median nerve anatomy. Transverse T1-weighted (TR/TE, 500/20) spin echo MR image at the level of the proximal portion of the forearm of an extended elbow shows the median nerve *(straight white arrow)* located between the two heads of the pronator teres (p) muscle; the ulnar nerve *(curved white arrow)* between the flexor digitorum profundus (fd), flexor digitorum superficialis (fs), and flexor carpi ulnaris (fu) muscles; and the radial nerve *(black arrow)* between the two heads of the supinator (s) muscle. (From Kim YS, Yeh LR, Trudell D, et al: Skeletal Radiol 27:419, 1998.)

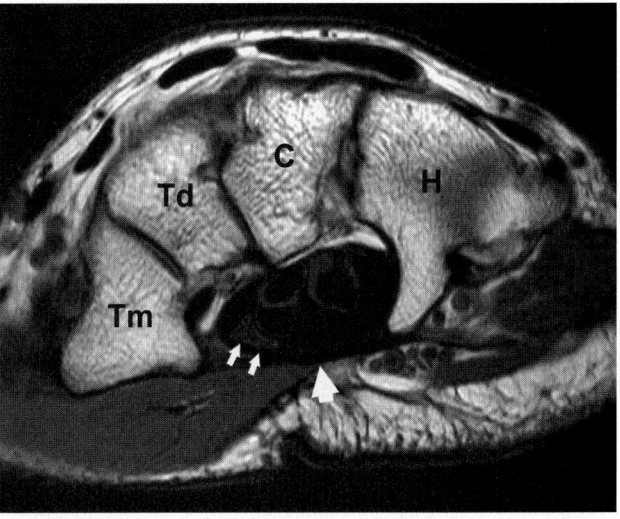

**Figure 65–14.** Entrapment of the median nerve: carpal tunnel syndrome—normal sectional anatomy. On this T1-weighted (TR/TE, 600/20) spin echo MR image at the level of the hook of the hamate, observe the position of the median nerve *(small arrows)* and the flexor retinaculum *(large arrow)*. Also note the capitate (C), hamate (H), trapezoid (Td), and trapezium (Tm).

more distal involvement, either sensory or motor nerve involvement predominates. The most frequent causes of ulnar nerve entrapment in Guyon's canal are ganglia (Fig. 65–18) and accidental, occupational, or recreational (bicycling) trauma.

### Radial Nerve

Entrapment of the radial nerve may occur in the axilla, upper part of the arm, elbow, proximal portion of the forearm, and wrist.

---

**TABLE 65–3**

**Causes of Carpal Tunnel Syndrome**

**Synovitis**
  Rheumatoid arthritis
  Scleroderma
  Systemic lupus erythematosus
  Dermatomyositis
  Seronegative spondyloarthropathies
  Ganulomatous and nongranulomatous infections
  Hemophilia
  Crystal deposition diseases
**Infiltrative Diseases**
  Amyloidosis
  Myxedema
  Acromegaly
  Mucopolysaccharidoses
**Trauma**
  Fractures and dislocations
  Repetitive and prolonged stress
**Tumors and Tumor-Like Lesions**
  Neuromas
  Lipomas
  Synovial cysts
  Ganglia
  Multiple myeloma

**Anatomic Factors**
  Small carpal canal
  Thick transverse carpal ligament
  Anomalous nerves, muscles, bursae
**Medical and Surgical Procedures**
  Arteriovenous fistula
  Artery punctures, catheterizations
**Miscellaneous**
  Diabetes mellitus
  Polymyalgia rheumatica
  Hemorrhage
  Hypoparathyroidism
  Pregnancy
  Use of oral contraceptives
  Gynecologic surgery
  Osteoarthritis
  Pyridoxine deficiency
  Paget's disease
  Idiopathic

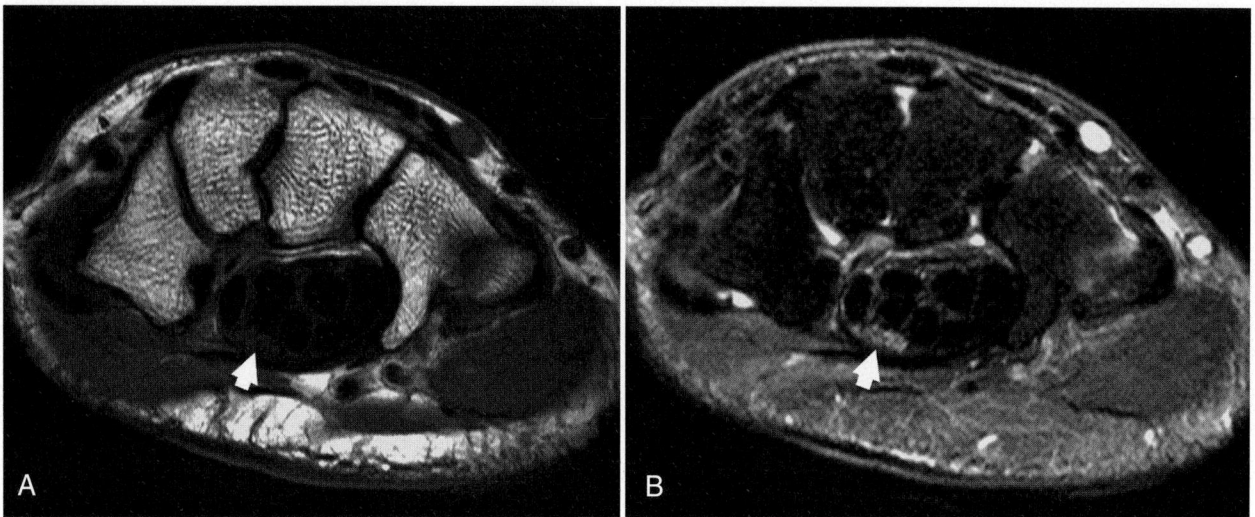

**Figure 65–15.** Entrapment of the median nerve: carpal tunnel syndrome. Transverse T1-weighted (TR/TE, 517/17) *(A)* and fat suppressed fast T2-weighted (TR/TE, 3610/77) *(B)* spin echo MR images at the level of the hook of the hamate show flattening of the median nerve *(arrow)*, mild retinacular bowing, and increased signal from the median nerve in *(B)*.

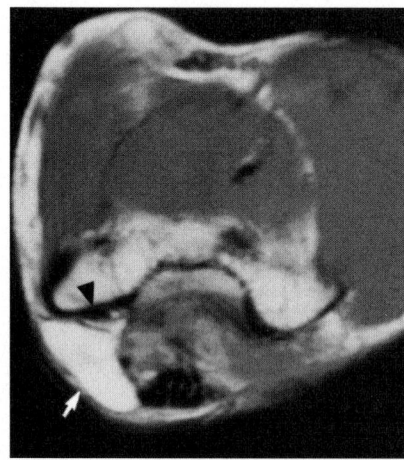

**Figure 65–16.** Entrapment of the ulnar nerve: cubital tunnel syndrome. A lipoma *(arrow)* adjacent to the ulnar nerve *(arrowhead)* is well shown in these transverse intermediate-weighted (TR/TE, 2000/20) spin echo MR images. The lipoma led to clinical findings of ulnar nerve entrapment in this 36-year-old man. (Courtesy of Z. Rosenberg, MD, New York.)

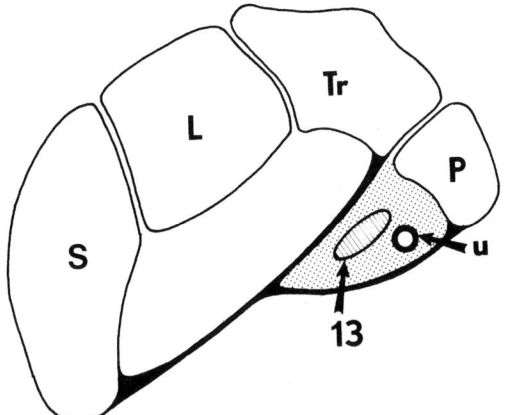

**Figure 65–17.** Entrapment of the ulnar nerve: Guyon's canal syndrome (ulnar tunnel syndrome)—normal sectional anatomy. Observe the ulnar nerve (13) and ulnar artery (u). L, lunate; P, pisiform; S, scaphoid; Tr, triquetrum. (From Grundberg AB Ulnar tunnel syndrome. J Hand Surg [Br] 9:72, 1984.)

**Saturday Night Palsy.** Radial nerve dysfunction may develop because of compression of the radial nerve in the axilla or spiral groove of the humerus in persons who sleep in a position that exerts pressure on the proximal medial aspect of the arm. This type of sleep palsy is particularly common in alcoholics and drug abusers and in patients using crutches.

**Posterior Interosseous Nerve Syndrome.** Compression of the posterior interosseous nerve, a purely motor branch of the radial nerve, occurs just distal to the elbow. Compression of the nerve occurs beneath the proximal edge

of the supinator muscle. Causes of this compression neuropathy include dislocation of the elbow, fracture, rheumatoid arthritis, soft tissue tumor, ganglia, and traumatic or developmental fibrous bands.

**Radial Tunnel Syndrome.** At the elbow, radial nerve compression occurs in the radial tunnel, the most common type of compression of the radial nerve. The motor weakness associated with this entrapment or compressive neuropathy is mild. Causes leading to this syndrome are similar to those producing the posterior interosseous nerve syndrome (some consider both syndromes to be

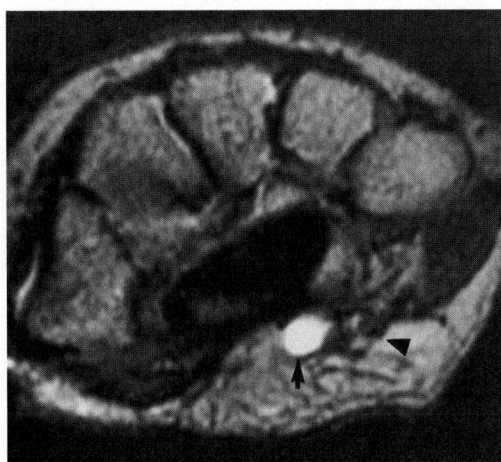

**Figure 65–18.** Entrapment of the ulnar nerve: Guyon's canal syndrome (ulnar tunnel syndrome)—ganglion cyst. Transverse T2-weighted (TR/TE, 2000/80) spin echo MR image shows a ganglion cyst *(arrow)* adjacent to the ulnar nerve and vessels *(arrowhead).*

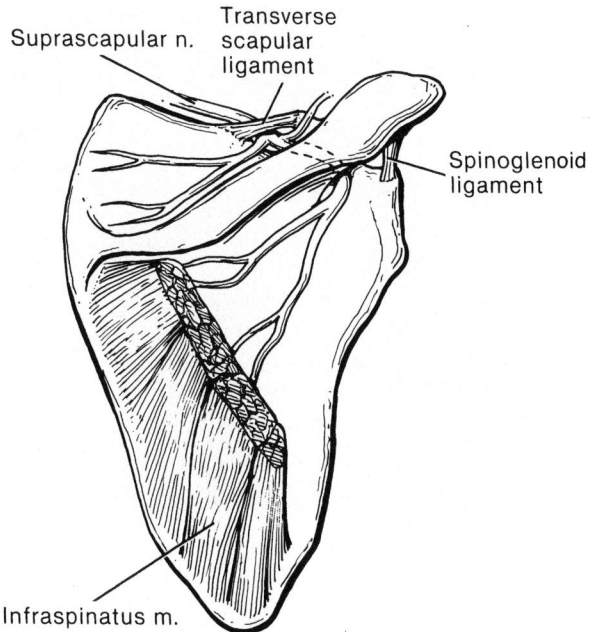

**Figure 65–19.** Suprascapular nerve anatomy. (From Butters KP: Nerve lesions of the shoulder. In DeLee JC, Drez D Jr [eds]: Orthopaedic Sports Medicine: Principles and Practice. Philadelphia, WB Saunders, 1994, p 657.)

variations of a single entity), although tumors are rarely implicated.

### Suprascapular Nerve

Entrapment of the suprascapular nerve occurs most commonly as it passes through the suprascapular notch (Fig. 65–19). This nerve, which contains motor and sensory fibers, arises from the upper trunk of the brachial plexus, runs deep to the trapezius and omohyoid muscles, and enters the supraspinous fossa through the suprascapular notch below the superior transverse scapular ligament. After the suprascapular nerve passes through the notch, it supplies the supraspinatus and infraspinatus muscles. The most frequent site of nerve encroachment is at the point where the suprascapular nerve traverses the suprascapular notch adjacent to the suprascapular ligament. As the nerve continues over the lateral part of the scapular spine and spinoglenoid notch and under the inferior transverse ligament and the spinoglenoid ligament to the infraspinatus fossa, other sites of entrapment are possible, particularly in the spinoglenoid notch. Potential causes of suprascapular nerve entrapment include a scapular fracture or glenohumeral joint dislocation, occupational or recreational injury, ganglia, and tumors. The major clinical findings, which may be unilateral or bilateral, are shoulder pain and weakness and atrophy of the supraspinatus or infraspinatus muscle, or both.

Entrapment neuropathy of the suprascapular nerve by a ganglion deserves special emphasis. Such ganglia arising at the scapular notch compress both motor branches of the suprascapular nerve, with subsequent weakness or atrophy of both the supraspinatus and the infraspinatus muscles; ganglia arising near the spinoglenoid notch affect a more distal segment of the nerve and result in selective involvement of the infraspinatus muscle. On MR images, a fluid-filled mass communicating with the joint, muscle edema or atrophy, and, in some cases, a rotator cuff tear are evident (Fig. 65–20).

### Axillary Nerve

Although rare, a quadrilateral space syndrome is produced by compression of the posterior circumflex humeral artery and the axillary nerve. The syndrome predominates in young men and women, usually in the third or fourth decade of life, and is more common in the dominant upper extremity. The quadrilateral space syndrome may also develop in athletes, especially baseball pitchers. Symptoms include paresthesias in the upper extremity and anterior shoulder pain that may interfere with daily physical activity. MR imaging allows an accurate diagnosis, showing changes in signal intensity (representing regions of edema or fat) within the deltoid and teres minor muscles (Fig. 65–21).

### Digital Branch of the Medial or Lateral Plantar Nerves

Entrapment of a digital branch of the medial or lateral plantar nerves of the foot as a result of injury to these nerves near the transverse intertarsal ligament leads to the development of Morton's neuroma. Ultrasonography and MR imaging can be used to make the diagnosis. The typical sonographic appearance is that of an ovoid, hypoechoic mass oriented parallel to the long axis of the metatarsal bones. MR imaging characteristics include a mass with decreased signal intensity that is well demarcated from adjacent fat tissue on T1-weighted spin echo MR images and is isointense or slightly hypointense to

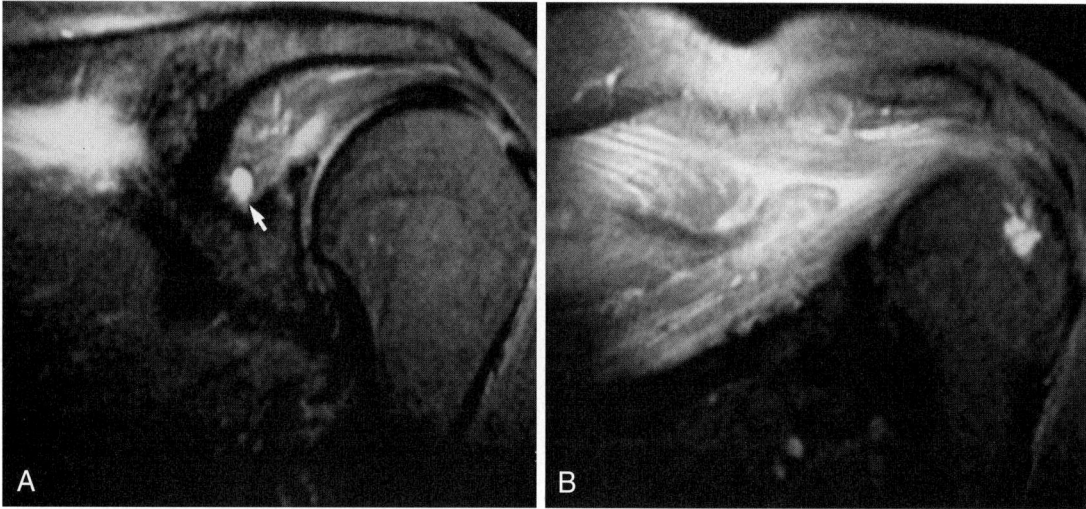

**Figure 65–20.** Entrapment of the suprascapular nerve: ganglia. *A* and *B*, Two oblique coronal fat-suppressed fast spin echo (TR/TE, 2650/48) MR images reveal a ganglion cyst *(arrow)* in the spinoglenoid notch, with intense signal in the infraspinatus muscle related to denervation. Also note an undersurface tear of the infraspinatus tendon and a humeral cyst.

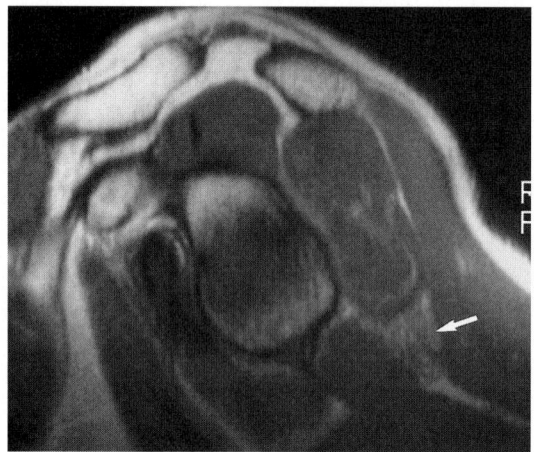

**Figure 65–21.** Quadrilateral space syndrome: neurologic abnormalities. Oblique sagittal fast spin echo (TR/TE, 3000/16) MR image shows selective atrophy of the teres minor muscle *(arrow)*.

fat tissue on T2-weighted spin echo images. MR imaging accomplished with fat-suppression techniques, such as those combined with heavily T2-weighted fast spin echo images and those obtained after the intravenous administration of gadolinium-based contrast agents (Fig. 65–22), may lead to improved detection.

### Distal Tibial Nerve

The proximal tarsal tunnel is a fibro-osseous space located behind the medial malleolus. Its roof is the flexor retinaculum, and its floor is formed by the medial talar surface, sustentaculum tali, and medial calcaneal wall. The posterior tibial artery and vein and the tibial nerve

are found within the proximal tarsal tunnel, and the bifurcation of the tibial nerve into medial and lateral plantar nerves generally occurs within the tarsal tunnel.

The distal tarsal tunnel contains the medial and lateral plantar nerves, which pass through fibrous openings in the origin of the abductor hallucis muscle. The classic tarsal tunnel syndrome refers to compression of nerves within the proximal tarsal tunnel, behind the medial malleolus. A specific cause of this classic syndrome can be identified in about 60% to 80% of cases. Trauma is the leading cause, including such specific injuries as fracture of the distal portion of the tibia. Tumors and tumor-like lesions may also cause the syndrome. An insidious onset of pain and burning sensation aggravated by activity in the plantar aspect of the foot is typical.

Distal tarsal tunnel syndromes relate to entrapment or compression of one or more branches of the tibial nerve. MR imaging is an effective technique for assessing the classic tarsal tunnel syndrome or its variations (Fig. 65–23).

### Peroneal Nerve

Entrapment of the common peroneal nerve, although relatively infrequent, typically occurs as it winds around the neck of the fibula; causes of such entrapment are injury with stretching or traction of the nerve, popliteal cysts, total knee arthroplasty, high tibial osteotomy, arthroscopic surgery of the knee, tight casts, fibular fractures, masses, and ganglia (Fig. 65–24). The deep peroneal nerve arises from the common peroneal nerve and courses distally between the extensor digitorum longus and tibialis anterior muscles in the proximal aspect of the leg. Compression of the superficial peroneal nerve generally occurs where the nerve pierces the crural fascia.

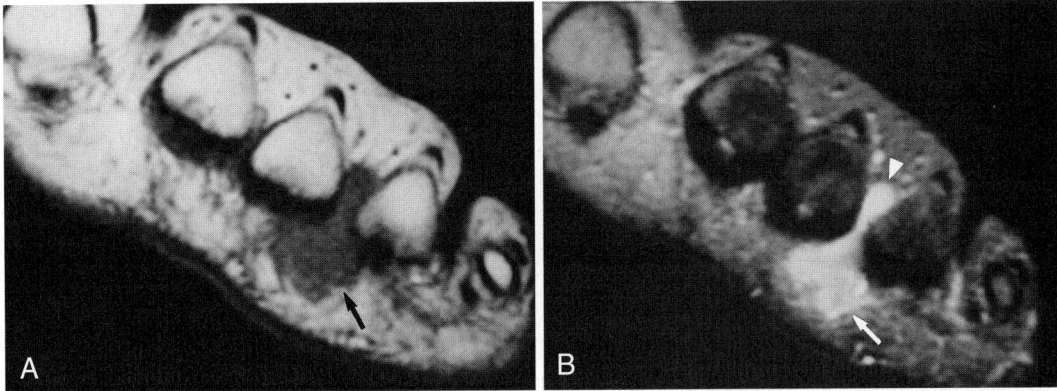

**Figure 65–22.** Morton's neuroma. *A*, Coronal T1-weighted (TR/TE, 600/20) spin echo MR image shows a mass *(arrow)* of low signal intensity between the third and fourth metatarsal heads. *B*, This mass *(arrow)* has high signal intensity on a coronal fat-suppressed fast spin echo (TR/TE, 3500/50) MR image. A small amount of fluid may be present in the intermetatarsal bursa *(arrowhead)*.

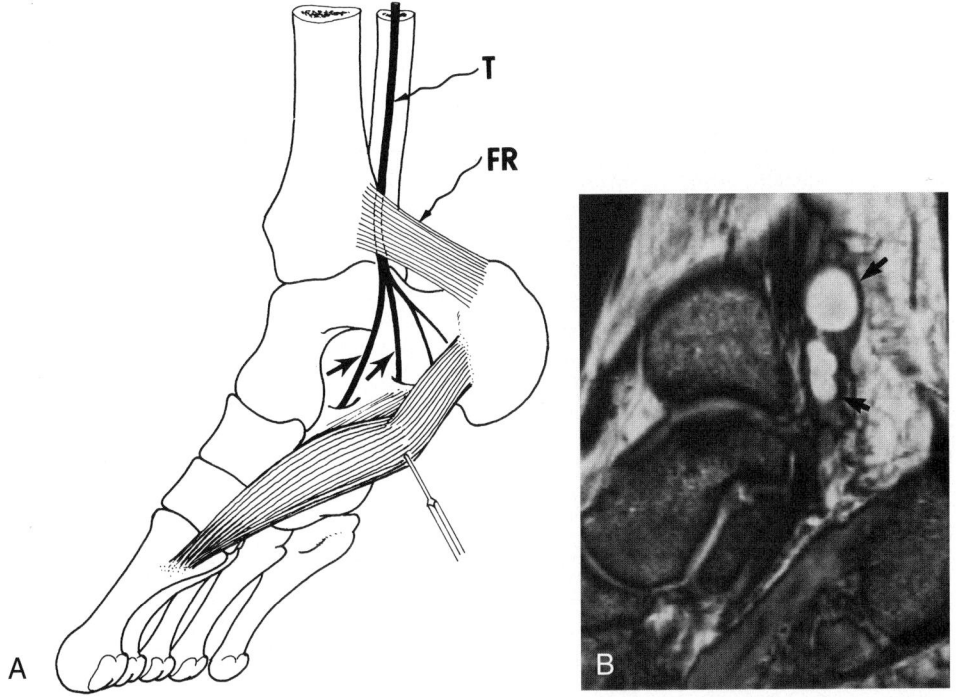

**Figure 65–23.** Entrapment of the tibial nerve: tarsal tunnel syndrome. *A*, Normal anatomy. The tibial nerve (T) passes beneath the flexor retinaculum (FR) and then divides into various nerves, including the medial and lateral plantar nerves *(arrows)*. *B*, Ganglion. Sagittal gradient recalled acquisition in the steady state (GRASS) image obtained with volumetric acquisition (TR/TE, 30/12; flip angle, 40 degrees) show a ganglion *(arrows)* on the medial and posterior portions of the ankle in this 48-year-old man. (*A*, From Kopell HP, Thompson WAL: Peripheral entrapment neuropathies of the lower extremity. N Engl J Med 262:56, 1960. *B*, Courtesy of G. Bock, MD, Winnipeg, Manitoba, Canada.)

## Sciatic Nerve

Most of the important structures connecting the gluteal region with the pelvis pass through the greater sciatic foramen. The piriformis muscle splits the greater sciatic foramen into the suprapiriformis and infrapiriformis regions. The superior gluteal nerve and vessels exit the pelvis through the suprapiriformis region. The sciatic nerve leaves the pelvis through the infrapiriformis region.

Although an extruded intervertebral disc is the most common cause of sciatica, entrapment neuropathies and other processes of the sciatic nerve are also encountered. The proximal portion of the sciatic nerve is infrequently

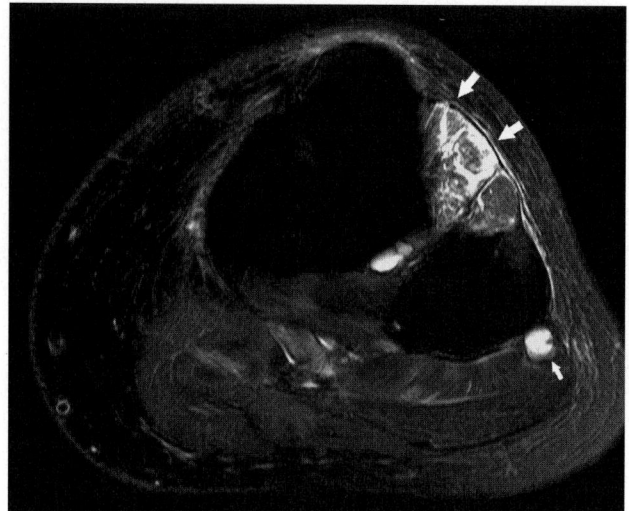

**Figure 65–24.** Peroneal nerve palsy: ganglion. Transverse fat-suppressed fast T2-weighted (TR/TE, 4390/80) MR image shows a small ganglion adjacent to the fibular head, compressing the peroneal nerve *(small arrow)*. The ganglion continued along the course of the nerve and compressed the deep branch of the peroneal nerve, causing denervation changes in the anterior compartment *(arrows)*.

compressed. Slightly more distally, compression neuropathy of the sciatic nerve may be produced by immobility, prolonged squatting, Paget's disease of the ischium, avulsion of the ischial tuberosity, fractures about and dislocations of the hip, post-traumatic ossification in the biceps femoris muscle, intramuscular injections, and hip surgery. Below the sciatic foramen, a piriformis syndrome represents a distinct pattern of nerve compression in which the symptoms and signs resemble those of disc extrusion. It appears to be caused by enlargement, inflammation, or anatomic variations of the piriformis muscle. The relationship of the sciatic nerve and the piriformis muscle is variable (Fig. 65–25). In about 85% of persons, the sciatic nerve exits the pelvis deep (i.e., anterior) to the piriformis muscle. In about 12% of persons, the common peroneal nerve and tibial nerve are split by a portion of the piriformis muscle, with the common peroneal nerve exiting through the substance of the muscle belly. In about 3% of persons, the common peroneal nerve emerges superficial (i.e., posterior) to the piriformis muscle, and the tibial nerve exits deep to the muscle belly. In about 1% of persons, the entire sciatic nerve extends through the piriformis muscle. Some of these variations may predispose to compression of the sciatic nerve or its branches.

## Hereditary Neuropathies

Slowly progressive peripheral neuropathies that are hereditary can be differentiated according to the type of neurons predominantly affected: sensory neurons, motor neurons, or autonomic neurons. Although classification of these disorders on the basis of specific neuron involvement is logical, it is complicated because many of the diseases affect more than one type of neuron. A more useful system may be to divide the disorders into three categories: those that involve sensory and autonomic neurons; those that involve sensory and motor neurons; and those that affect only motor neurons.

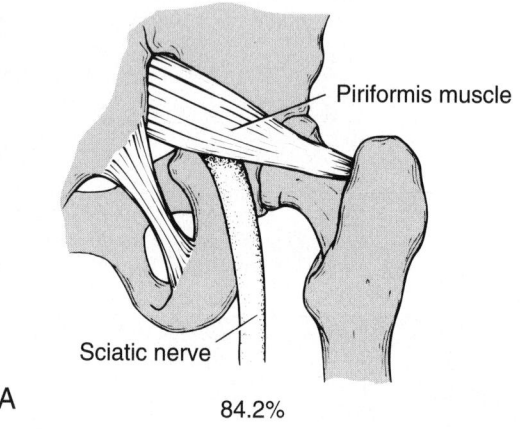

**Figure 65–25.** Sciatic nerve: variations in its relationship with the piriformis muscle. (From Levin P: Hip dislocations. In Browner BD, Jupiter JB, Levine AM, Trafton PG [eds]: Skeletal Trauma. Philadelphia, WB Saunders, 1992, p 1333.)

A   84.2%

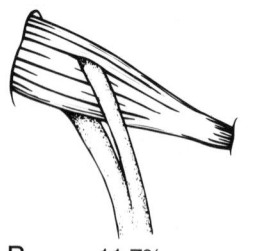

B   11.7%

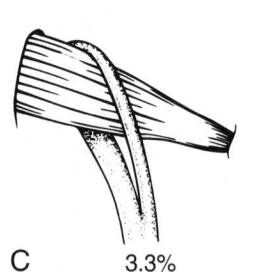

C   3.3%

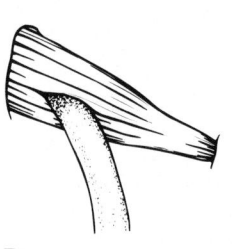

D   0.8%

These disorders also differ in their mode of inheritance, age of onset, natural history and prognosis, distribution of abnormalities, and pathologic alterations. Some disorders, such as those with prominent sensory loss, produce neuropathic osteoarthropathy, which is discussed in Chapter 66.

### Hereditary Sensory and Autonomic Neuropathies

These neuropathies consist of a number of disorders that have in common dysfunction of sensory neurons and, in some cases, autonomic neurons as well. Indifference or insensitivity to pain accounts for the appearance of neuropathic osteoarthropathy (see Chapter 66).

**Type I.** Also termed hereditary sensory radicular neuropathy, mutilating acropathy, and Thévenard's syndrome, this disorder is inherited as a dominant trait. It varies in severity, has a predilection for the lower extremities, and leads to sensory loss complicated by perforating lesions of the soft tissues and foot deformities. Burning feet may be a prominent symptom.

**Type II.** Type II disorder, which is also termed congenital sensory neuropathy, is inherited as a recessive trait, appears in infancy and childhood, predominates in the distal portions of the upper and lower extremities, and leads to soft tissue ulcerations and fractures in the extremities.

**Type III.** Also termed familial dysautonomia of Riley-Day, this inherited disease is seen principally in Jewish infants and children, although non-Jewish persons may be affected. Peripheral sensory, motor, and autonomic neurons are involved. Clinical manifestations include poor feeding, repeated episodes of vomiting and pulmonary infection, autonomic disturbances, areflexia, insensitivity to pain, and early death. Neuropathic osteoarthropathy, abnormalities of spinal curvature, osteomyelitis, and ischemic necrosis of bone are seen.

**Type IV.** This recessive disorder is associated with sensory neuropathy, insensitivity to pain, mental retardation, and anhidrosis and has been attributed to an abnormality of the neural crest. Clinical manifestations generally appear in the first years of life. Neuropathic osteoarthropathy; periostitis; fractures; epiphyseal displacement, disintegration, and necrosis; and osteoporosis may be observed.

### Hereditary Motor and Sensory Neuropathies

Hereditary motor and sensory neuropathies include several distinct progressive disorders.

**Type I.** Type I is a dominantly inherited, hypertrophic form of peroneal muscular atrophy (Charcot-Marie-Tooth disease). It varies in severity but is frequently mild, and some patients have no obvious symptoms or signs.

**Type II.** Type II disorder, which is usually inherited as a dominant trait, represents the neuronal pattern of peroneal muscular atrophy (Charcot-Marie-Tooth disease). Its onset is typically in the second decade of life, although a wide variation in age of onset is reported. Clinical manifestations are symmetrical muscle weakness and atrophy in the feet and ankles and difficulty standing and walking. When compared with patients with type I disease, persons with type II disease may be older at the time of disease onset and have lesser degrees of tremor, ataxia, upper limb involvement, and sensory loss.

### Hereditary Motor Neuropathies

Hereditary motor neuropathies represent a group of chronic neurologic disorders with selective involvement of the anterior horn cells of the spinal cord and lower brain stem and, in some cases, the motor neurons of the corticospinal tract. Sensory deficits and cerebellar dysfunction are absent. These neuropathies are further divided into diseases in which prominent changes in upper neurons are combined with muscle atrophy and weakness (amyotrophic lateral sclerosis) and those in which upper neuron disease is lacking and slowly progressive muscle weakness and wasting occur (progressive muscular atrophy). Two specific types of progressive muscular atrophy deserve emphasis.

**Werdnig-Hoffmann Disease.** This disease exhibits autosomal recessive inheritance or occurs sporadically. It begins in infancy and early childhood and appears clinically as hypotonia, severe weakness, areflexia, tremors and fasciculations, and normal sensation; the proximal muscles are affected more severely than the distal ones, and the lower extremities are weaker than the upper extremities. Orthopedic complications include scoliosis, pelvic tilt, coxa valga, plastic bowing of the ribs, and subluxation or dislocation of the hips.

**Wohlfart-Kugelberg-Welander Disease.** This autosomal recessive disorder differs from Werdnig-Hoffmann disease in its older age of onset (late childhood, adolescence, or adulthood) and slower course; it affects mainly the proximal muscles, especially in the lower extremities. Scoliosis, joint contractures, mild acetabular dysplasia, and coxa valga are apparent.

## Guillain-Barré Syndrome

This syndrome is an acute inflammatory demyelinating polyradiculoneuropathy that is usually preceded by an infectious illness, surgery, or vaccination. Clinical manifestations include ataxia; weakness of the proximal and distal muscles; involvement of the facial, extraocular, and respiratory muscles; and sensory loss. Typically, motor weakness is dominant. The cause of this syndrome is not clear, but an immune-mediated pathogenesis has been emphasized. MR imaging reveals thickening of spinal nerves and the cauda equina, with enhancement of signal intensity after intravenous administration of a gadolinium-containing contrast agent.

## Friedreich's Ataxia

Friedreich's ataxia is one form of spinocerebellar degeneration. It is usually a recessive disorder that begins in childhood or adolescence and manifests as progressive ataxia, dysarthria, and nystagmus, with impairment in vibratory and position sensation and diminished or absent reflexes. Cardiomyopathy may lead to the patient's death in the third or fourth decade of life. Orthopedic complications include severe scoliosis (50% to 75% of cases), coxa valga deformity, subluxation of the hips, instability of the knees and ankles, and pes cavus.

## Muscle Diseases

Diseases of muscle can be classified as congenital or genetic, metabolic, inflammatory or infectious, traumatic, neoplastic, and miscellaneous. Many of these diseases are considered elsewhere in this textbook. Diseases of muscle are better evaluated with computed tomography or MR imaging than with radiography.

**Muscular Dystrophies.** The universal clinical finding in the inherited myopathies is weakness, and the pathologic abnormalities are limited to the skeletal musculature. The muscular dystrophies can be separated into several forms on the basis of their genetic patterns and clinical manifestations such as age of onset, distribution of muscle involvement, and presence or absence of muscle hypertrophy (Table 65–4). Recognized types are Duchenne's (pseudohypertrophic), Becker's (benign pseudohypertrophic), facioscapulohumeral, limb-girdle, ocular or oculopharyngeal, myotonic, and distal dystrophies. Of these patterns, Duchenne's muscular dystrophy is most common and has the greatest relevance to the musculoskeletal system.

Duchenne's muscular dystrophy is characterized by an X-linked recessive inheritance (affecting boys only), disease onset in the first decade of life, weakness in the proximal muscles (especially those in the hips and shoulders), and mild mental retardation. The muscles of the calf are large and firm and have a rubbery consistency. Serum levels of creatine kinase are markedly elevated. Foot deformities, including pes planus and equinovarus, occur relatively early in the course of the disease because of tightening of the Achilles tendon, and progressive contractures appear in the hips and knees. Subsequently, spinal deformities consisting of scoliosis and kyphosis are seen. Respiratory failure, pneumonia, and cardiac decompensation are causes of the patient's demise, commonly by the third decade of life.

## FURTHER READING

Abel MS: Sacroiliac joint changes in traumatic paraplegics. Radiology 55:235, 1950.

Bhate DV, Pizarro AJ, Seitam A, et al: Axial skeletal changes in paraplegics. Radiology 133:55, 1979.

Boerger TO, Limb D: Suprascapular nerve injury at the spinoglenoid notch after glenoid neck fracture. J Shoulder Elbow Surg 9:236, 2000.

Currarino G: Premature closure of epiphyses in the metatarsals and knees: A sequel of poliomyelitis. Radiology 87:424, 1966.

Daher YH, Lonstein JE, Winter RB, et al: Spinal deformities in patients with Friedreich ataxia: A review of 19 patients. J Pediatr Orthop 5:553, 1985.

---

**TABLE 65–4**

**Classification of Human Muscular Dystrophies**

|  | Duchenne's Dystrophy | Facioscapulohumeral Dystrophy | Limb-Girdle Dystrophy | Myotonic Dystrophy |
|---|---|---|---|---|
| Genetic pattern | X-linked recessive | Autosomal dominant | Autosomal recessive | Autosomal dominant |
| Age at onset | Before age 5 yr | Adolescence | Adolescence | Early or late |
| First symptoms | Pelvic | Shoulders | Pelvic | Distal; hands or feet |
| Pseudohypertrophy | + | − | − | − |
| Predominant early weakness | Proximal | Proximal | Proximal | Distal |
| Progression | Relatively rapid; incapacitated in adolescence | Slow | Variable | Slow |
| Facial weakness | − | + | − | Occasional |
| Ocular, oropharyngeal weakness | − | − | − | Occasional |
| Myotonia | − | − | − | + |
| Cardiomyopathy | − or late | − | − | Arrhythmia, conduction block |
| Associated disorders | None (? mental retardation) | None | None | Cataracts; testicular atrophy and baldness in men |
| Serum enzyme levels | Very high | Slight or no increase | Slight or no increase | Slight or no increase |

From Rowland LP: Diseases of muscle and neuromuscular junction. In Beeson PB, McDermott W, Wyngaarden JB (eds): Cecil Textbook of Medicine, 15th ed. Philadelphia, WB Saunders, 1979, p 916.

Dyck PJ, Thomas PK, Lambert EH: Peripheral Neuropathy. Philadelphia, WB Saunders, 1975.

Erickson SJ, Canale PB, Carrera GF, et al: Interdigital (Morton) neuroma: High-resolution MR imaging with a solenoid coil. Radiology 181:833, 1991.

Erickson SJ, Quinn SF, Kneeland JB, et al: MR imaging of the tarsal tunnel and related spaces: Normal and abnormal findings with anatomic correlation. AJR Am J Roentgenol 155:323, 1990.

Fritz RC, Helms CA, Steinbach LS, et al: Suprascapular nerve entrapment: Evaluation with MR imaging. Radiology 182:437, 1992.

Houston CS: The radiologist's opportunity to teach bone dynamics. J Can Assoc Radiol 29:232, 1978.

Houston CS, Zaleski WA: The shape of vertebral bodies and femoral necks in relation to activity. Radiology 89:59, 1967.

Howard CB, Williams LA: A new radiological sign in the hips of cerebral palsy patients. Clin Radiol 35:317, 1984.

Jarvic JG, Kliot M, Maravilla KR: MR nerve imaging of the wrist and hand. Hand Clin 16:13, 2000.

Kaye JJ, Freiberger RH: Fragmentation of the lower pole of the patella in spastic lower extremities. Radiology 101:97, 1971.

Kopell HP, Thompson WAL: Peripheral Entrapment Neuropathies, 2nd ed. Huntington, NY, RE Krieger, 1976.

Lanzieri CF, Hilal SK: Computed tomography of the sacral plexus and sciatic nerve in the greater sciatic foramen. AJR Am J Roentgenol 143:165, 1984.

Lev-Toaff AS, Karasick D, Rao VM: "Drooping shoulder"—nontraumatic causes of glenohumeral subluxation. Skeletal Radiol 12:34, 1984.

Loredo R, Hodler J, Pedowitz R, et al: MRI of the common peroneal nerve: Normal anatomy and evaluation of masses associated with nerve entrapment. J Comput Assist Tomogr 22:925, 1998.

Major P, Resnick D, Greenway G: Heterotopic ossification in paraplegia: A possible disturbance of the paravertebral venous plexus. Radiology 136:797, 1980.

Martinoli C, Bianchi S, Gandolfo N, et al: US of nerve entrapments in osteofibrous tunnels of the upper and lower limbs. Radiographics 20:199, 2000.

McIvor WC, Samilson RL: Fractures in patients with cerebral palsy. J Bone Joint Surg Am 44:858, 1966.

Middleton WD, Kneeland JB, Kellman GM, et al: MR imaging of the carpal tunnel: Normal anatomy and preliminary findings in the carpal tunnel syndrome. AJR Am J Roentgenol 148:307, 1987.

Muheim G, Donath A, Rossier AB: Serial scintigrams in the course of ectopic bone formation in paraplegic patients. AJR Am J Roentgenol 118:865, 1973.

Nakano KK: Entrapment neuropathies. In Kelley WN, Harris ED Jr, Ruddy S, et al (eds): Textbook of Rheumatology, 2nd ed. Philadelphia, WB Saunders, 1985, p 1754.

Pech P, Haughton V: A correlative CT and anatomic study of the sciatic nerve. AJR Am J Roentgenol 144:1037, 1985.

Pool WH Jr: Cartilage atrophy. Radiology 112:47, 1974.

Richardson ML, Helms CA, Vogler JB III, et al: Skeletal changes in neuromuscular disorders mimicking juvenile rheumatoid arthritis and hemophilia. AJR Am J Roentgenol 143:893, 1984.

Rosin AJ: Ectopic calcification around joints of paralysed limbs in hemiplegia, diffuse brain damage, and other neurological diseases. Ann Rheum Dis 34:499, 1975.

Sauser DD, Hewes RC, Root L: Hip changes in spastic cerebral palsy. AJR Am J Roentgenol 146:1219, 1986.

Schwentker EP, Gibson DA: The orthopaedic aspects of spinal muscular atrophy. J Bone Joint Surg Am 58:32, 1976.

Seigel RS: Heterotopic ossification in paraplegia. Radiology 137:259, 1980.

Seybold ME, Sherman DC: Muscle diseases. In Stein JH (ed): Internal Medicine. Boston, Little, Brown, 1983, p 874.

Sugimoto H, Miyaji N, Ohsawa T: Carpal tunnel syndrome: Evaluation of median nerve circulation with dynamic contrast-enhanced MR imaging. Radiology 190:459, 1994.

Termote J-L, Baert A, Crolla D, et al: Computed tomography of the normal and pathologic muscle system. Radiology 137:439, 1980.

Thomas PK: Inherited neuropathies. Mayo Clin Proc 58:476, 1983.

Woodlief RM: Superior marginal rib defects in traumatic quadriplegia. Radiology 126:673, 1978.

# CHAPTER 66

## Neuropathic Osteoarthropathy

### SUMMARY OF KEY FEATURES

The effect of the deprivation of sensory feedback on the musculoskeletal system can be profound. An anesthetized joint or bone that is subject to continuing stress deteriorates progressively, with the appearance of specific radiographic abnormalities. These changes, which include articular space narrowing, bony eburnation, osteophytosis, fragmentation, fracture, and subluxation, can accompany a variety of disorders but are most common in diabetes mellitus, tabes dorsalis, and syringomyelia. When severe, the resulting radiographic picture is diagnostic; in earlier stages, however, the findings may resemble those of osteoarthritis, calcium pyrophosphate dihydrate crystal deposition disease, calcium hydroxyapatite crystal deposition disease, osteonecrosis, or, in the spine, intervertebral (osteo)chondrosis.

### INTRODUCTION

In 1868, Charcot described an apparent cause-and-effect relationship between primary lesions of the central nervous system and certain arthropathies. Charcot continued to study and characterize the disorder for the next 15 years, and although his description was virtually confined to patients with tabes dorsalis, the name "Charcot joint" has become synonymous with all articular abnormalities related to neurologic deficits, regardless of the nature of the primary disease. Other terms applied to this disorder are neuroarthropathy and neurotrophic or neuropathic joint disease. None of these terms is ideal, however, because the initial event in some cases occurs not in the joint itself but in the adjacent bone or even some distance from the articulation. Therefore, the designations neuropathic osteoarthropathy and neuropathic bone and joint disease are more suitable.

### CAUSE AND PATHOGENESIS

Central (upper motor neuron) and peripheral (lower motor neuron) lesions can lead to neuropathic osteoarthropathy. Among the central lesions that may produce neuropathic osteoarthropathy are syphilis, syringomyelia, meningomyelocele, trauma, multiple sclerosis, Charcot-Marie-Tooth disease, congenital vascular anomalies, and other causes of cord compression, injury, or degeneration; peripheral causes include diabetes mellitus, alcoholism, amyloidosis, infection (tuberculosis, yaws, leprosy), pernicious anemia, trauma, and intra-articular or systemic administration of steroids. Additionally, specific syndromes leading to congenital insensitivity to pain and dysautonomia produce similar alterations.

No agreement exists on the pathogenesis of the articular changes. Two fundamental theories of pathogenesis are (1) the "French theory," holding that joint changes are the result of damage to the central nervous system trophic centers, which control nutrition of the bones and joints, and (2) the "German theory," which maintains that unusual mechanical stresses about a weight-bearing joint in an ataxic person lead to recurrent subclinical trauma. Although other theories exist, there is considerable evidence that both mechanical and vascular factors contribute to subsequent disintegration of the joint (Fig. 66–1). What is clear is that loss of normal neurologic function renders a joint (and adjacent bone) susceptible to a sequence of pathologic and radiographic alterations that may ultimately produce its disintegration. Joint instability that precedes neurologic dysfunction may make this sequence more likely.

### GENERAL RADIOGRAPHIC AND PATHOLOGIC ABNORMALITIES

Although the pathologic and radiographic features of advanced neuropathic osteoarthropathy are characteristic, early features may simulate those of osteoarthritis (Fig. 66–2). The presence of an enlarging and persistent effusion, minimal subluxation, fracture, and fragmentation should alert a radiologist to the possibility of neuropathic osteoarthropathy; similarly, the finding of considerable amounts of cartilaginous and osseous debris attached to and incorporated into the synovial membrane (detritic synovitis) in a patient who is presumed to have osteoarthritis should suggest to a pathologist that the changes may represent joint manifestations of neuropathic disease (Table 66–1). These early changes may show rapid progression, and the joint may appear to fall apart in a matter of days or weeks (Fig. 66–3).

More advanced radiographic abnormalities consist of depression, absorption, and shattering of subchondral bone; osseous proliferation in the form of significant sclerosis and osteophytosis; intra-articular osseous fragments; subluxation; massive soft tissue enlargement and effusion; and fracture of neighboring bones (Fig. 66–4). On pathologic examination, the capsule is found to be irregularly thickened by fibrous tissue and ossified; the synovial membrane is indurated, with villous transformation; and considerable fluid and connective tissue adhesions are evident within the joints. In the synovial membrane, diffuse metaplasia of the synovium, with the formation of cartilage and calcification of cartilage within the deeper layers of the membrane, may be noted; this can produce radiographically detectable calcific and ossific dense lesions that may eventually become far removed from the joint itself (Fig. 66–5).

In long-standing neuropathic osteoarthropathy, the radiographic picture is that of a disorganized joint characterized by simultaneous bone resorption and formation. The degree of sclerosis, osteophytosis, and fragmentation

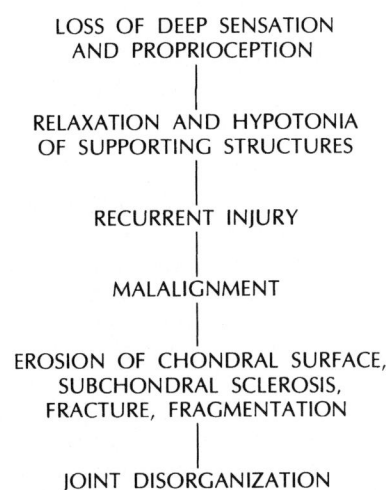

**Figure 66–1.** Pathogenesis of neuropathic osteoarthropathy. Probable sequential steps in the development of the disease are indicated.

in this disorder is greater than that in any other process. Yet the bone shards and irregular articular surfaces produced by the considerable osseous fragmentation and collapse accompanying this disease are generally well defined and sharp. Poorly marginated, "fuzzy" bone contours, as occur in osteomyelitis and septic arthritis, are not usually evident unless infection has become superimposed on the neuropathic process.

## SPECIFIC DISORDERS

Neuropathic osteoarthropathy can accompany many disorders that lead to sensory disturbances. Although some motor function is fundamental in the pathogenesis of the lesions, neuropathic osteoarthropathy can develop in patients with both sensory and motor loss, presumably related to vigorous physical therapy. The radiographic and pathologic features of this condition are generally similar in these various disorders, but certain subtle differences

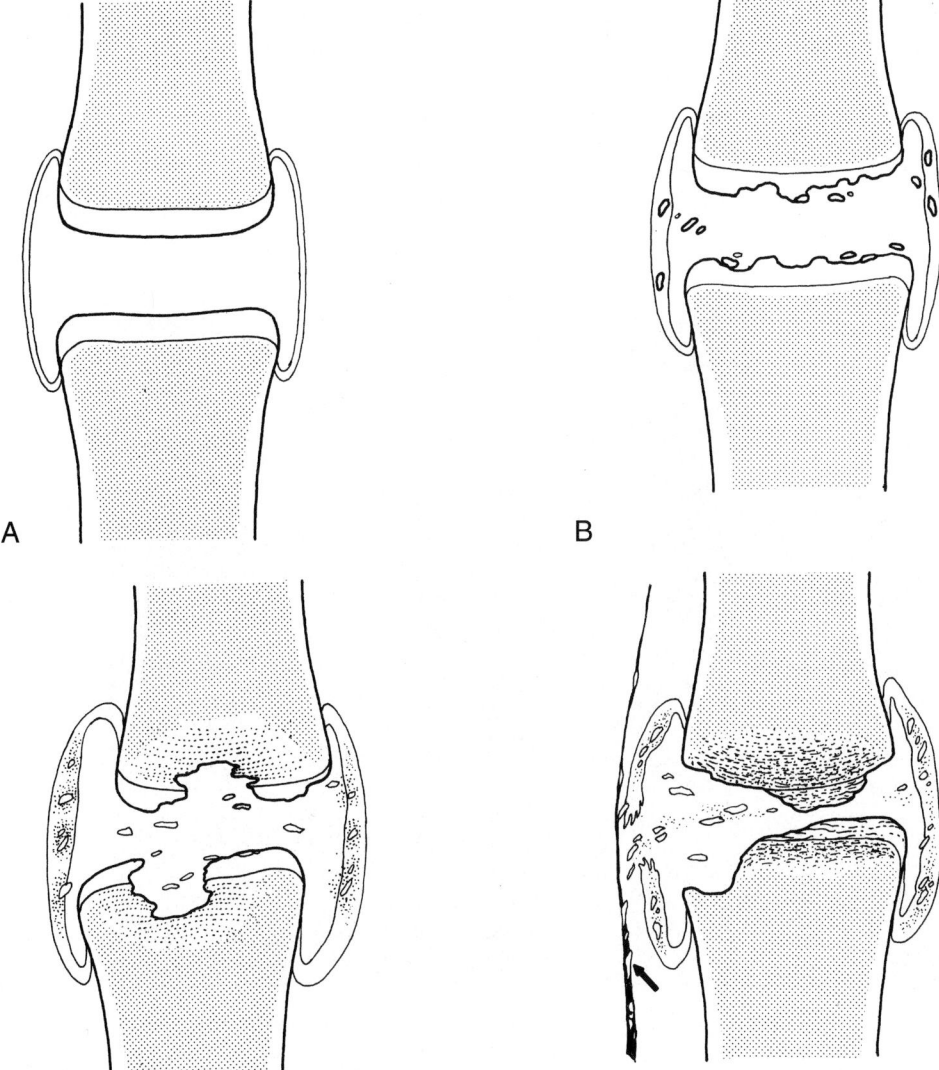

**Figure 66–2.** General radiographic and pathologic abnormalities in the various stages of neuropathic osteoarthropathy. *A*, Normal synovial joint. *B*, Initially, cartilaginous fibrillation and fragmentation can be observed. Some of the cartilaginous debris remains attached to the chondral surface, some is displaced into the articular cavity, and some becomes embedded in the synovial membrane. *C*, Subsequently, osseous and cartilaginous destruction becomes more extensive, and the embedded pieces of cartilage and bone produce local synovial irritation. Bony eburnation and subluxation are also evident. *D*, Eventually, large portions of the chondral coat are lost, sclerosis is extreme, capsular rupture can occur, and shards of bone can dissect along the soft tissue planes *(arrow)*.

## TABLE 66-1

### Causes of Detritic Synovitis

Neuropathic osteoarthropathy
Osteonecrosis
Calcium pyrophoshate dihydrate crystal deposition disease
Psoriatic arthritis
Osteoarthritis
Osteolysis with detritic synovitis

may be evident, and the distribution of abnormalities varies among the disorders (Table 66–2).

## Tabes Dorsalis

It is estimated that 5% to 10% of patients with tabes dorsalis have neuropathic osteoarthropathy. The joints of the lower extremity are affected in 60% to 75% of cases. The knee, hip, ankle, shoulder, and elbow are altered, in descending order of frequency (see Figs. 66–3 to 66–6). Other involved sites include the joints of the forefoot, midfoot, vertebral column, and fingers and the temporomandibular and sternoclavicular joints. Polyarticular alterations are not unusual.

Typically, painless swelling, deformity, weakness, and instability represent the clinical manifestations of tabetic neuropathic osteoarthropathy. In as many as one third of

patients, the affected joints may be painful. Axial neuropathic osteoarthropathy is not uncommon in tabes and may represent 20% of all cases of neuropathic disease encountered in tabetic patients. It is most frequent in the lumbar spine, where one or more vertebrae may be affected. As opposed to the situation in peripheral neuropathic osteoarthropathy, axial involvement is often symptomatic and results in significant pain.

Radiographic features of tabetic axial neuropathic disease may be productive or destructive. In the former group, changes such as intervertebral disc space and apophyseal joint narrowing, sclerosis, and osteophytosis are generally more exaggerated than those of degenerative joint disease and represent "osteoarthritis with a vengeance" (Fig. 66–7). Fracture with osseous fragmentation in spinal and paraspinal locations, as well as malalignment, may also be evident. The resulting radiographic findings, when severe, are unique to this disorder and differ from the spinal manifestations of degenerative joint disease, infection, skeletal metastasis, and Paget's disease (Table 66–3). Less commonly, osteolytic or destructive changes predominate in axial neuropathic osteoarthropathy. These alterations can appear acutely, progress rapidly, and lead to significant bony dissolution in a period of weeks or months. The appearance of this lytic variety of neuropathic disease can resemble that of infection or skeletal metastasis.

## Syringomyelia

It has been estimated that neuropathic osteoarthropathy develops in 20% to 25% of patients with syringomyelia.

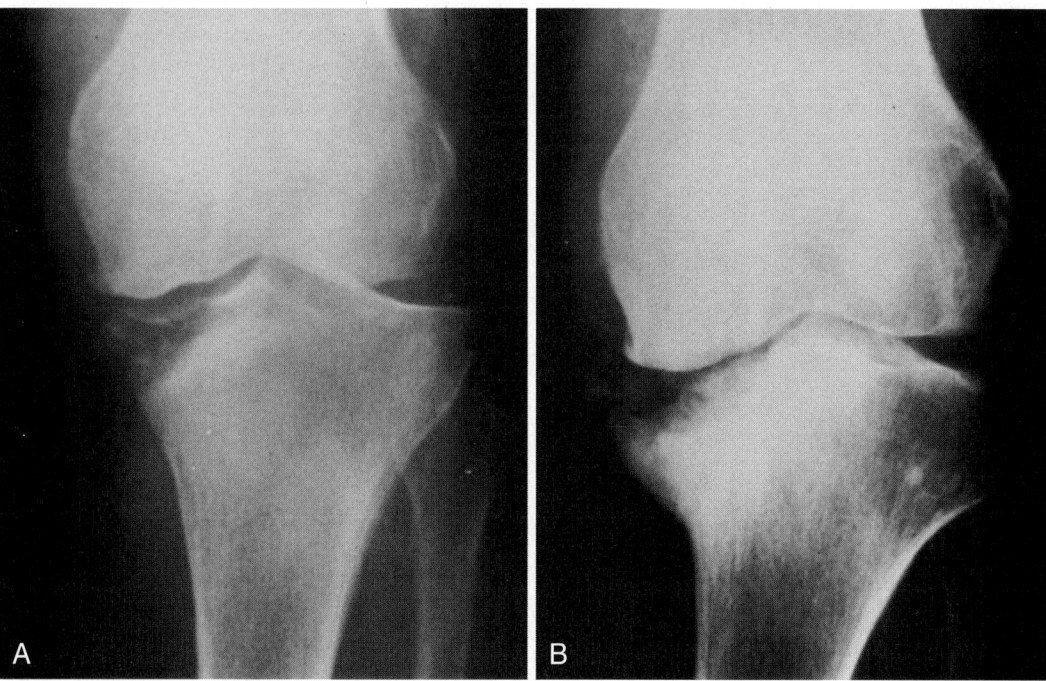

**Figure 66–3.** General radiographic and pathologic abnormalities of neuropathic osteoarthropathy: rapid disease progression. *A* and *B,* The appearance and progression of articular destruction can occur rapidly. Initial foci of chondral and osseous destruction can lead to fragmentation and collapse in a matter of weeks. This patient has tabes dorsalis.

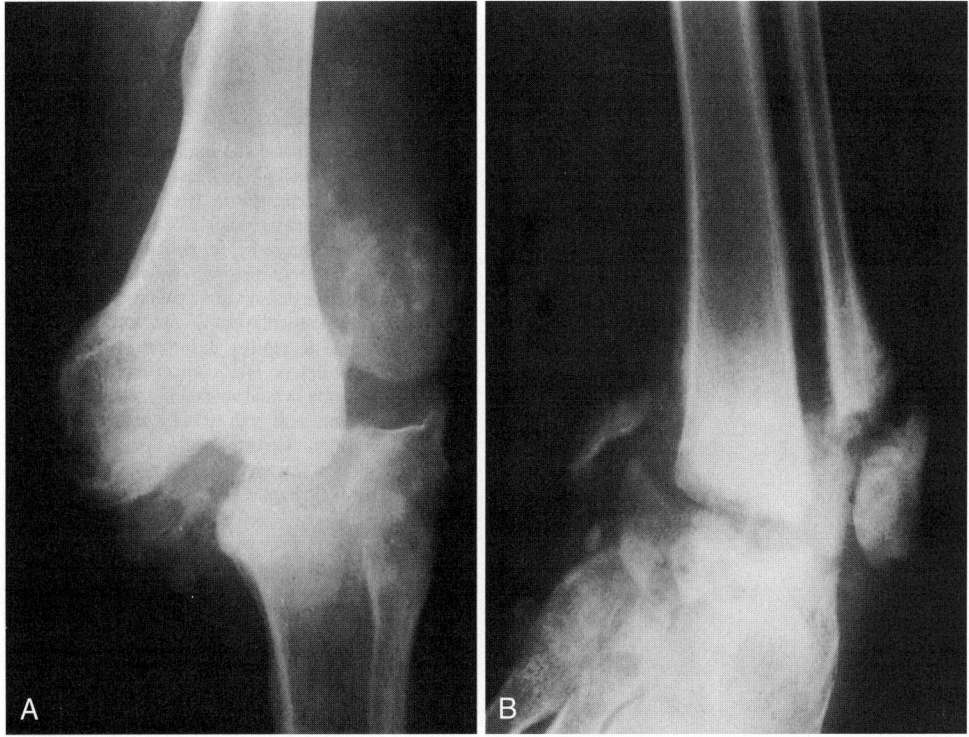

**Figure 66–4.** General radiographic and pathologic abnormalities of neuropathic osteoarthropathy: fractures and subluxations. *A*, Gross disorganization of the joint in a tabetic patient is characterized by lateral subluxation of the tibia on the femur, lateral patellar dislocation, soft tissue swelling, osseous fragmentation and sclerosis, and periostitis. *B*, In a different patient with the same disease, note the angular deformity of the ankle, with fragmentation, sclerosis, and fractures. Periostitis and soft tissue swelling are evident.

Neuropathic changes in syringomyelia are common in the joints of the upper extremity, especially the glenohumeral articulation (Fig. 66–8). In the lower extremity, the knee, ankle, and hip are affected with approximately equal frequency; in both the upper and lower limbs, bilateral symmetrical changes are not as common as in tabes.

Generally, neuropathic osteoarthropathy occurs during the later phases of syringomyelia, but occasionally, joint findings may be the initial or predominant manifestation of the disease. The clinical, radiographic, and pathologic alterations of neuropathic osteoarthropathy in syringomyelia are similar to those in tabes. The degree of fragmentation and sclerosis of the humeral head can be striking, and these changes may be associated with fractures of neighboring bones, including the scapula, clavicle, and ribs. Further, spontaneous dislocation of the glenohumeral joint may be the initial manifestation of neuropathic osteoarthropathy in syringomyelia.

### Diabetes Mellitus

The complexity of diabetic neuropathic osteoarthropathy is well known. Loss of pain and loss of proprioceptive sensation appear to be of major importance in diabetic neuropathic osteoarthropathy and, in the presence of repetitive microtrauma or macrotrauma, promote the changes. Infectious processes are commonly superimposed on neuropathic changes in diabetic patients, especially in superficially located joints. The addition of suppuration can accentuate and accelerate the joint destruction.

Although the exact frequency of neuropathic bone and joint changes in diabetic persons is not clear, this disease has certainly overtaken both syphilis and syringomyelia as the leading cause of neuropathic osteoarthropathy; it represents the underlying disorder in more than 98% of cases. Typically, diabetic neuropathic osteoarthropathy appears in a man or woman with long-standing diabetes mellitus, generally in the fifth to seventh decades of life. The joints of the forefoot and midfoot are altered most commonly. Painless soft tissue swelling, skin ulceration, and joint deformity are encountered. Monoarticular or polyarticular involvement can occur.

Destructive or resorptive bony abnormalities can predominate, depending on the location of the neuropathic changes. In the intertarsal or tarsometatarsal joints, osseous fragmentation, sclerosis, and subluxation or dislocation may be prominent, and complete disintegration of one or more tarsal bones can occur rapidly. Calcaneal fragmentation is typical (Fig. 66–9). Talar disruption and dorsolateral displacement of the metatarsal bones in relation to the cuneiform and cuboid bones are also characteristic, and the resulting radiographic picture may resemble that observed in an acute Lisfranc's fracture-dislocation (Fig. 66–10). At the metatarsophalangeal joints, osseous resorption is frequent and leads to partial or complete

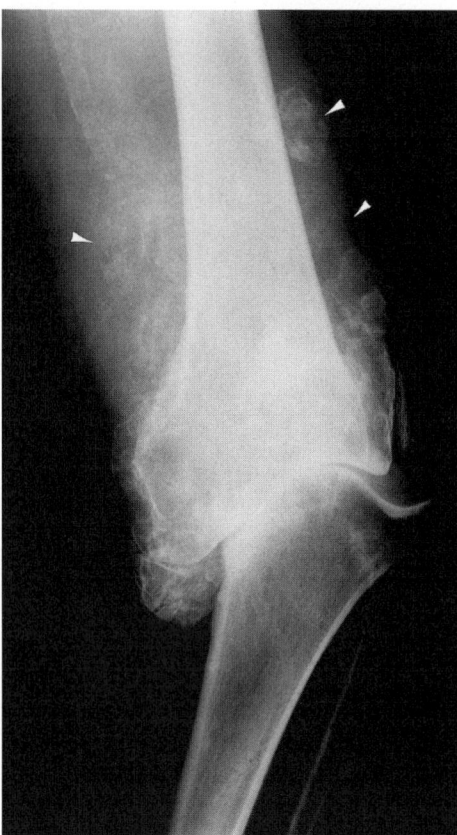

**Figure 66–5.** General radiographic and pathologic abnormalities of neuropathic osteoarthropathy: migration of bony shards. In this patient with syphilis, numerous fragments of bone originating from the destroyed articular surfaces have moved into the far recesses of the joint or migrated along adjacent tissue planes (*arrowheads*).

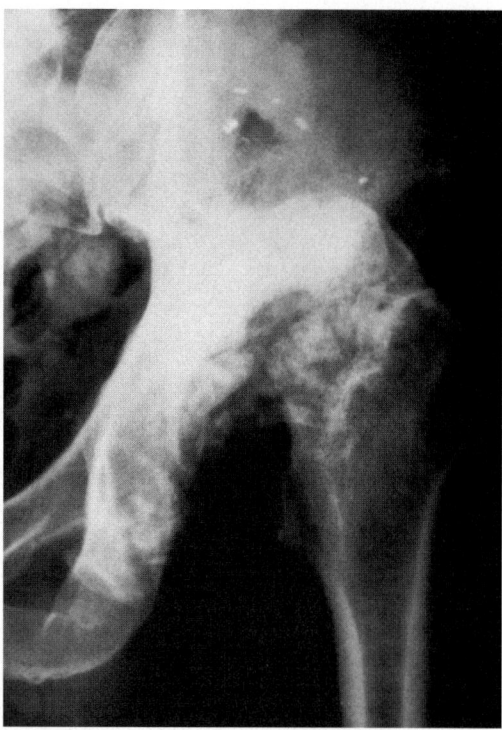

**Figure 66–6.** Tabes dorsalis: neuropathic osteoarthropathy of the appendicular skeleton—hip. Sclerosis and fragmentation are prominent, and deformities, subluxation, and dislocation may be evident.

disappearance of the metatarsal heads and proximal phalanges, with tapering or "pencil-pointing" of the phalangeal and metatarsal shafts (Fig. 66–11). Flattening and fragmentation of the metatarsal heads are particularly characteristic and may resemble the changes of Freiberg's infraction (Fig. 66–12).

Although less frequent than changes in the forefoot or midfoot, ankle involvement may be detected. Knee abnormalities are rare. Diabetic axial neuropathic osteoarthropathy can be generalized or localized. The resulting radiographic changes, which include destruction of vertebral bodies, sclerosis, osteophytosis, fragmentation, bony ankylosis, altered spinal curvature, and spinal angulation, resemble those in tabes or syringomyelia (Fig. 66–13).

### Alcoholism

Although peripheral neuropathy may be evident in as many as 30% of alcoholic patients who are examined at a hospital, reports of neuropathic osteoarthropathy in these persons are infrequent. When present, neuropathic osteoarthropathy is evident in the feet and resembles the changes accompanying diabetic neuropathic disease.

### Amyloidosis

Occasionally, neuropathic bone and joint disease develops in patients with amyloidosis with or without additional plasma cell dyscrasias. The knee and the ankle appear to be the predominant sites of involvement.

**TABLE 66–2**

**Common Sites of Involvement in Neuropathic Osteoarthropathy**

| Disease | Site of Involvement |
| --- | --- |
| Tabes dorsalis | Knee, hip, ankle, spine |
| Syringomyelia | Glenohumeral joint, elbow, wrist, spine |
| Diabetes mellitus | Metatarsophalangeal, tarsometatarsal, interarsal joints |
| Alcoholism | Metatarsophalangeal, interphalangeal joints |
| Amyloidosis | Knee, ankle |
| Meningomyelocele | Ankle, intertarsal joints |
| Congenital sensory neuropathy, hereditary sensory radicular neuropathy | Knee, ankle, intertarsal, metatarsophalangeal, interphalangeal joints |
| Idiopathic | Elbow, shoulder |

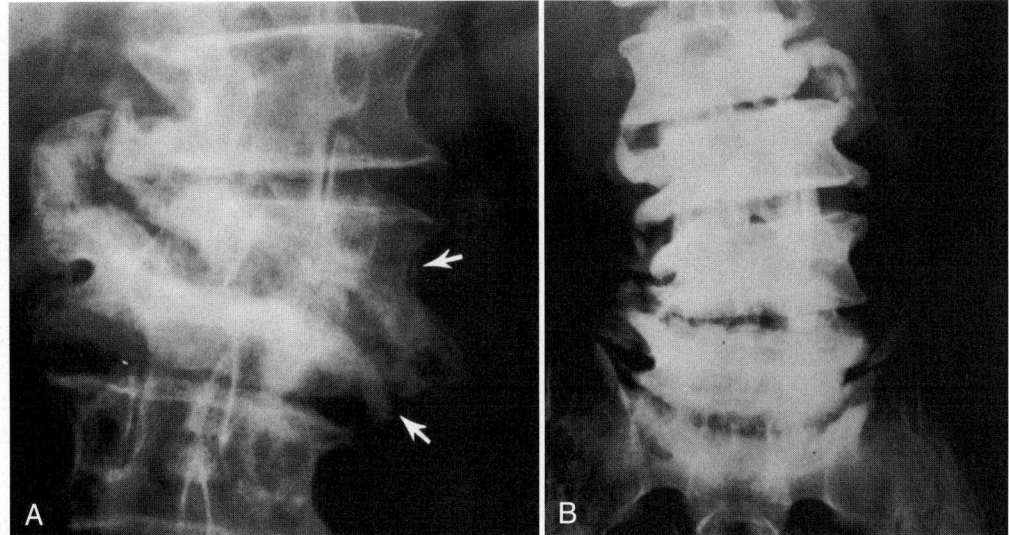

**Figure 66–7.** Tabes dorsalis: neuropathic osteoarthropathy of the axial skeleton—spine. *A,* Localized disease. Frontal and lateral radiographs of the lumbar spine reveal extensive disorganization involving two vertebral bodies *(arrows)* and the intervening intervertebral disc. Note the loss of intervertebral disc space, sclerosis, and osteophytosis. The resulting osseous contours are relatively well defined. *B,* Generalized disease. Widespread abnormalities in the lumbar spine consist of loss of height of multiple intervertebral discs, extreme sclerosis, osteophytes, subluxation, and vertebral angulation.

**TABLE 66–3**

**Axial Neuropathic Osteoarthropathy and Its Differential Diagnosis**

| | Neuropathic Osteoarthropathy | Intervertebral (Osteo)Chondrosis | Infection | CPPD Crystal Deposition Disease |
|---|---|---|---|---|
| Sites of involvement | One or more levels Predominates in thoracolumbar spine* | Frequently widespread Cervical, thoracic, or lumbar spine | Frequently one level Predominates in thoracolumbar spine | Widespread Cervical, thoracic, or lumbar spine |
| Intervertebral disc spaces | Narrowed or obliterated | Narrowed | Narrowed or obliterated | Calcification; narrowed |
| Bony sclerosis | May be extreme | Usually mild to moderate | Variable† | Variable‡ |
| Osteophytosis | May be massive | Absent or moderate in size | Usually absent | Variable |
| Bony fragmentation | May be extreme | Absent or minimal | Usually absent | Variable§ |
| Subluxation, angulation | Common | Rare | Variable‖ | Variable |
| Paravertebral mass | Usually absent | Absent | Common | Absent |

*Influenced by the specific underlying disorder.
†Sclerosis more typical in pyogenic spondylitis and in black patients with tuberculous spondylitis.
‡Disc calcification may appear without sclerosis, or disc space loss may be combined with moderate or severe sclerosis.
§In some patients, fragmentation and deformity may be severe, especially in the cervical spine.
‖In tuberculosis, kyphosis may become prominent.
CPPD, calcium pyrophosphate dihydrate.

## Congenital Indifference to Pain

Indifference or insensitivity to pain is a feature common to several distinct hereditary sensory neuropathies that differ in their patterns of inheritance, precise clinical manifestations, and prognosis. In most of these syndromes, the neurologic deficit can be recognized in infancy or childhood. A decreased or absent reaction to pain, scars on the tongue or fingers related to burns or infections, corneal opacities resulting from unnoticed foreign bodies, and aggressive behavior may be found. Self-mutilation with amputation of fingers and toes is also encountered.

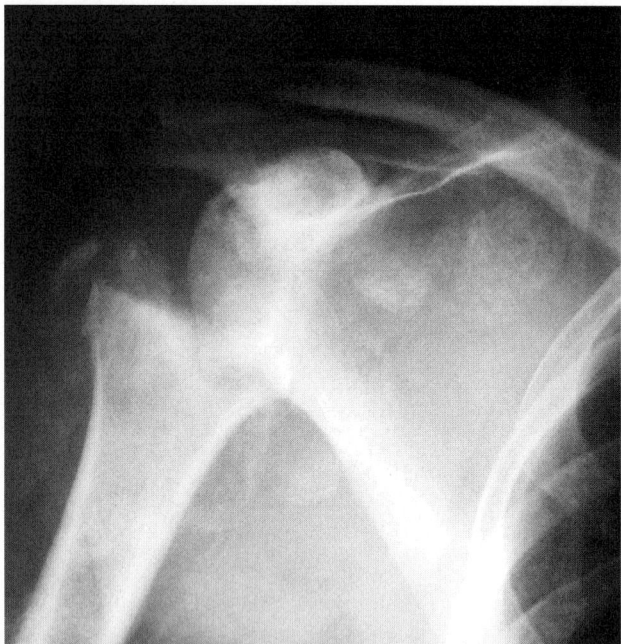

**Figure 66–8.** Syringomyelia. Radiograph of the right shoulder reveals dissolution of the humeral head, with extensive bone fragmentation. The shaft of the humerus is displaced inferiorly.

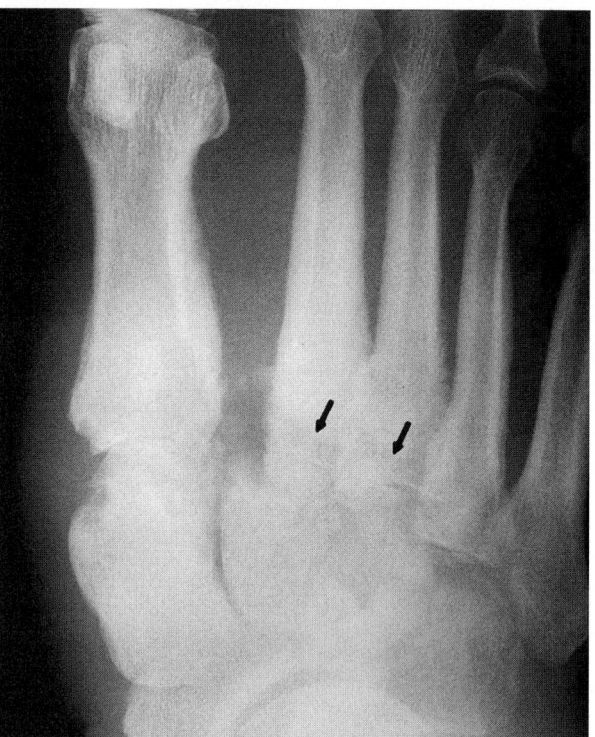

**Figure 66–10.** Diabetes mellitus: tarsometatarsal joints. Note the lateral displacement of the bases of the metatarsals *(arrows)* with respect to the tarsals. This finding, combined with soft tissue swelling and fragmentation, represents a neuropathic Lisfranc's fracture-dislocation.

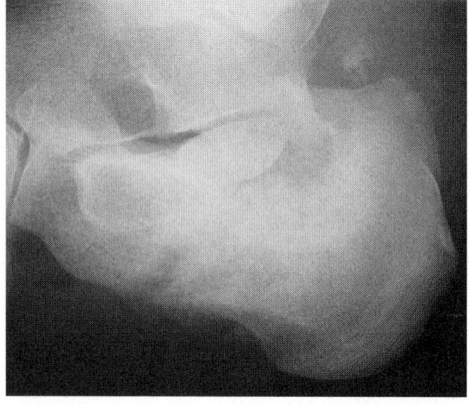

**Figure 66–9.** Diabetes mellitus: calcaneus. Radiograph shows fractures of the posterior aspect of the calcaneus and subtalar region and collapse of the bone.

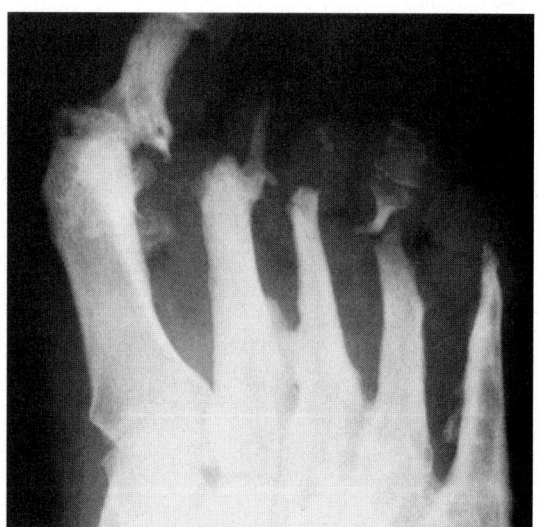

**Figure 66–11.** Diabetes mellitus: metatarsophalangeal and interphalangeal joints. Neuropathic osteoarthropathy and infection in the forefoot of a diabetic patient combine to produce bizarre abnormalities consisting of osteolysis of the distal metatarsals and proximal phalanges, with tapering of the osseous contours.

Skeletal lesions in the syndromes of congenital indifference to pain (and related disorders) demonstrate fractures of the metaphysis and diaphysis of long bones, epiphyseal separations, neuropathic osteoarthropathy, and soft tissue ulcerations (Fig. 66–14). These injuries, which are often unrecognized and untreated, can lead to severe disability and are generally more frequent in the lower extremity than the upper extremity. Epiphyseal separation is the result of chronic trauma or stress, as the growth plate represents the weak link in the child's skeleton;

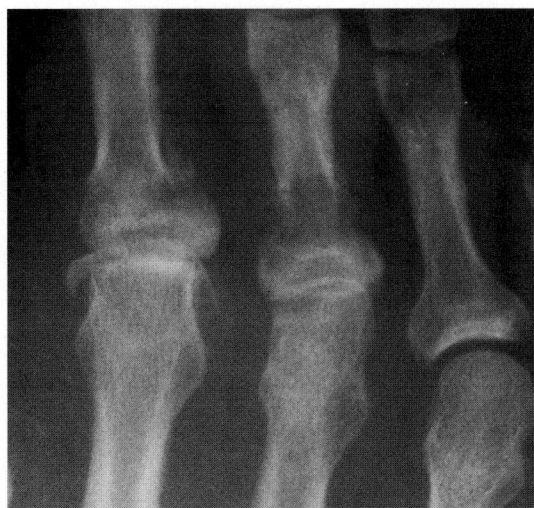

**Figure 66–12.** Diabetes mellitus: metatarsophalangeal joints. Observe the collapse of the second and third metatarsal heads, similar to the findings in Freiberg's infraction. Fractures in the bases of the proximal phalanges are also evident. (Courtesy of A. D'Abreu, MD, Porto Alegre, Brazil.)

widening and irregularity of the growth plate, lysis and sclerosis of the metaphysis, periostitis and callus, and variable degrees of epiphyseal displacement are recognized. Neuropathic osteoarthropathy is especially common in the knee, ankle, and tarsal areas. Overt neurologic symptoms and signs may be absent in children and adolescents with some types of congenital insensitivity to pain.

Therefore, the presence of unusual fractures and physeal abnormalities on radiographs should stimulate a search for a subtle neurologic deficit, especially if the clinical findings appear mild in comparison to the severity of the radiographic alterations. Virtually identical skeletal abnormalities are seen in all the syndromes of congenital insensitivity to pain.

## Meningomyelocele (Spinal Dysraphism)

Sensory impairment resulting from spina bifida and meningomyelocele is the most frequent underlying cause of neuropathic osteoarthropathy in childhood. It affects principally the ankle and the tarsal joints. In active children, radiographic changes may appear in the first 3 years of life. These changes are identical to those in the syndromes of congenital indifference to pain and include osteoporosis, diaphyseal and metaphyseal fractures, injuries to the growth plate, epiphyseal separations, persistent effusions, articular destruction, and soft tissue ulcerations (Fig. 66–15).

## Other Diseases

Numerous other causes of neuropathic skeletal alterations exist, including spinal cord or peripheral nerve injury, myelopathy of pernicious anemia, Charcot-Marie-Tooth disease, Arnold-Chiari malformation, neurofibromatosis, arachnoiditis, intraspinal tumors, degenerative spinal disease, paraplegia, quadriplegia, familial interstitial hypertrophic polyneuropathy of Dejerine and Sottas, chronic inflammatory demyelinating polyradiculoneuropathy, limb replantation, leprosy, paraneoplastic sensory neuropathy,

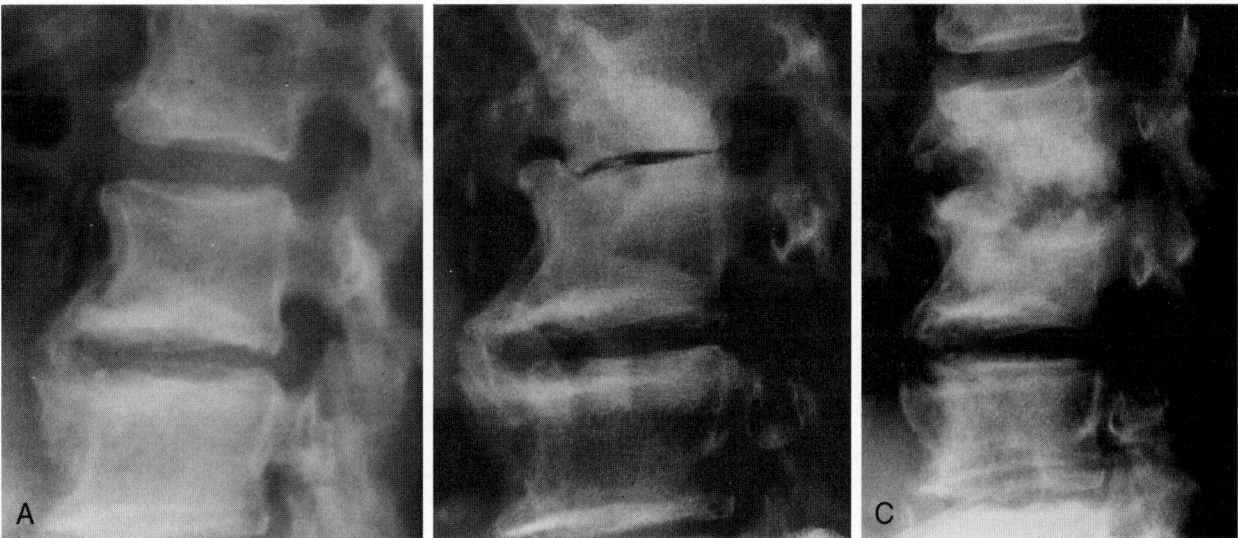

**Figure 66–13.** Diabetes mellitus: spine. Progressive deterioration of the lumbar spine is apparent during a 3-year period of observation. Initially (A), the changes at the lower lumbar level resemble degenerative disc disease. Subsequently (B and C), this level deteriorates slowly; one level above, however, rapid destruction of the intervertebral disc and bone is evident. The vacuum phenomenon in the upper disc, as well as the well-defined and sclerotic bone in (B), makes infection unlikely. In (C), the pattern of disc destruction is identical to that of infection, although the latter was not apparent clinically. (Courtesy of U.S. Naval Hospital, San Diego, Calif.)

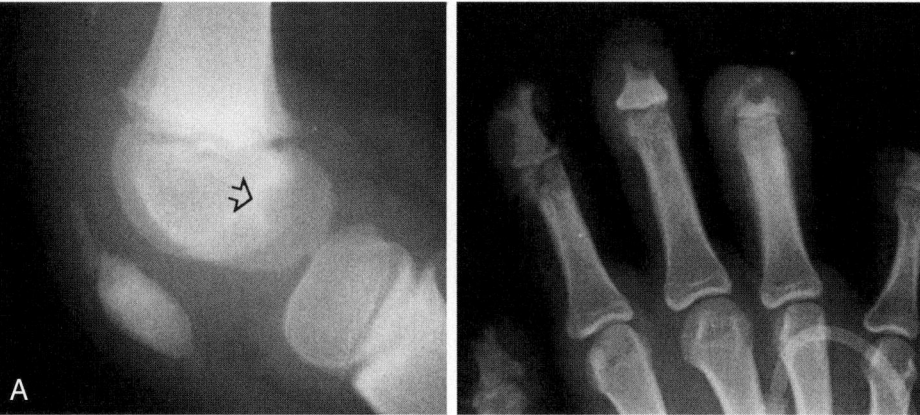

**Figure 66–14.** Syndromes of congenital indifference to pain. *A*, In this 7-year-old boy, fragmentation of the lateral femoral condyle *(arrow)* and patella is associated with a joint effusion and intra-articular osseous bodies. The opposite side (not shown) was similarly affected. *B*, In a 17-year-old patient, osteolysis and autoamputation of multiple phalanges are evident. The opposite hand was similarly involved. (Courtesy of M. Mitchell, MD, Halifax, Nova Scotia, Canada.)

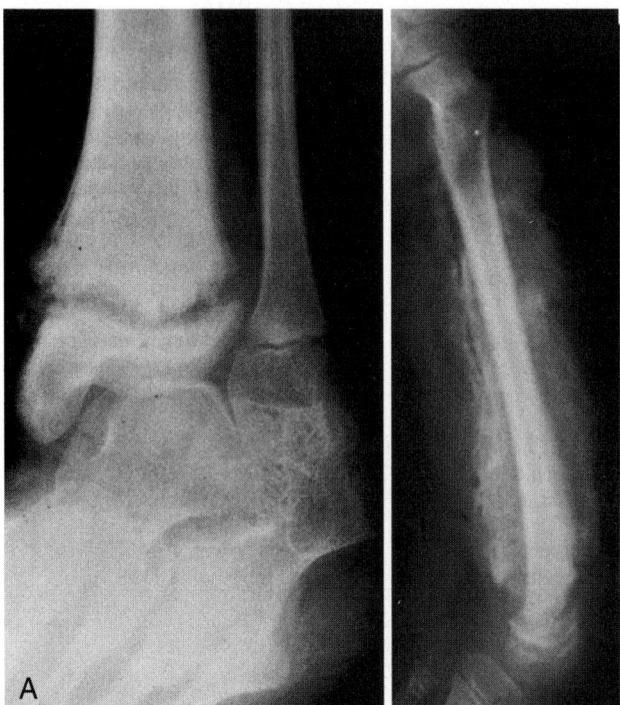

**Figure 66–15.** Meningomyelocele (spinal dysraphism). *A*, In this child with a meningomyelocele, note the epiphyseal separation of the distal end of the tibia, along with a widened and irregular growth plate, sclerosis, and periostitis. *B*, Lateral radiographs of the femora in this child with a meningomyelocele reveal irregular and widened distal femoral growth plates, fracture and fragmentation, and exuberant periostitis. (Courtesy of J. E. L. Desautels, MD, Calgary, Alberta, Canada.)

and yaws. An idiopathic variety of neuropathic osteoarthropathy of the elbow and shoulder has also been identified.

Neuropathic-like changes occur in patients with chronic paraplegia and quadriplegia. Neuropathic osteoarthropathy may be seen in paralyzed patients, initiated by physical therapy and by daily activities such as transferring from a bed to a wheelchair. Most reports of neuropathic osteoarthropathy occurring in paralyzed patients have indicated a predilection for the spine.

## MAGNETIC RESONANCE IMAGING ABNORMALITIES

The general magnetic resonance (MR) imaging findings of neuropathic osteoarthropathy parallel the known pathologic findings and include large joint effusions, capsular distention and rupture, synovial cysts, ligamentous disruption, and intra-articular bodies. In the spine, findings are similar to those of infection (e.g., sclerosis and erosions of the vertebral endplates, decreased height of the intervertebral disc, soft tissue masses), although identification of gas in the affected intervertebral disc, spondylolisthesis, involvement of the facet joints, diffuse abnormalities of signal intensity in the vertebral bodies, and rim enhancement of signal intensity in the intervertebral discs on intravenous gadolinium-enhanced MR images are more suggestive of neuropathic osteoarthropathy than of infection.

Recent attention has been given to the MR imaging findings in diabetic patients with soft tissue and bone infections of the foot and their differentiation from neuropathic abnormalities. Despite the encouraging results of preliminary investigations, diagnostic problems are encountered in the differentiation of osteomyelitis and neuropathic osteoarthropathy in patients with diabetes mellitus. Ongoing neuropathic changes encountered in ambulatory diabetic patients may be associated with edema in both the adjacent bones and the soft tissues. The signal intensity patterns of such edema in neuropathic osteoarthropathy is similar, if not identical, to those encountered in infection (Fig. 66–16). This edema is often prominent in cases of acute neuropathic osteoarthropathy, accompanied by fracture and fragmentation of bone. Additionally, sympathetic joint effusions

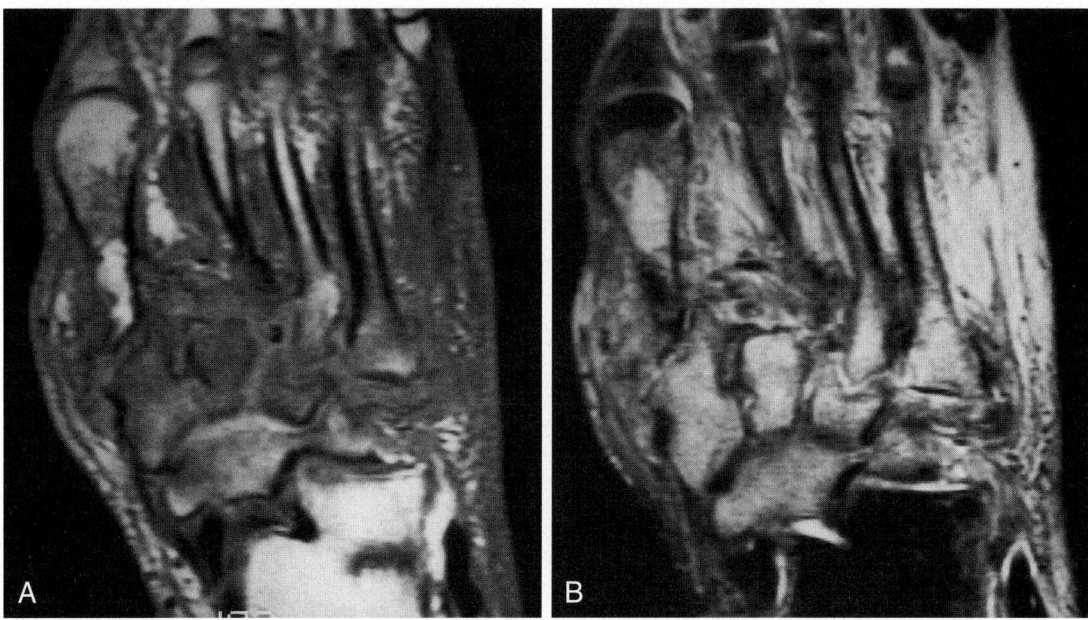

**Figure 66–16.** Neuropathic osteoarthropathy: diabetes mellitus. As shown on these transverse MR images, marrow edema may accompany acute neuropathic changes, which in this case include dislocation and fragmentation at the tarsometatarsal joints. The edema is displayed on a T1-weighted (TR/TE, 600/14) spin echo MR image *(A)* and a short tau inversion recovery (STIR; TR/TE, 4000/20; inversion time, 140 msec) MR image *(B)*.

are consistently observed in the feet of diabetic patients, and this may simulate findings of septic arthritis.

Differences in the MR imaging appearances of infection and neuropathic osteoarthropathy may be seen. In general, pedal osteomyelitis results almost exclusively from contiguous infection and occurs most frequently around the first and fifth metatarsophalangeal joints. Although primary signs of osteomyelitis are not specific, secondary MR imaging signs of osteomyelitis have a high specificity and include adjacent cutaneous ulcer, sinus

tract, and cortical interruption. These are best identified on T1-weighted and gadolinium-enhanced fat-suppressed T1-weighted images. Identification of abscesses is also strong evidence that infection is present (Fig. 66–17).

## DIFFERENTIAL DIAGNOSIS

When severe, neuropathic osteoarthropathy is associated with radiographic changes that are almost pathognomonic. Bony eburnation, fracture, subluxation, and joint

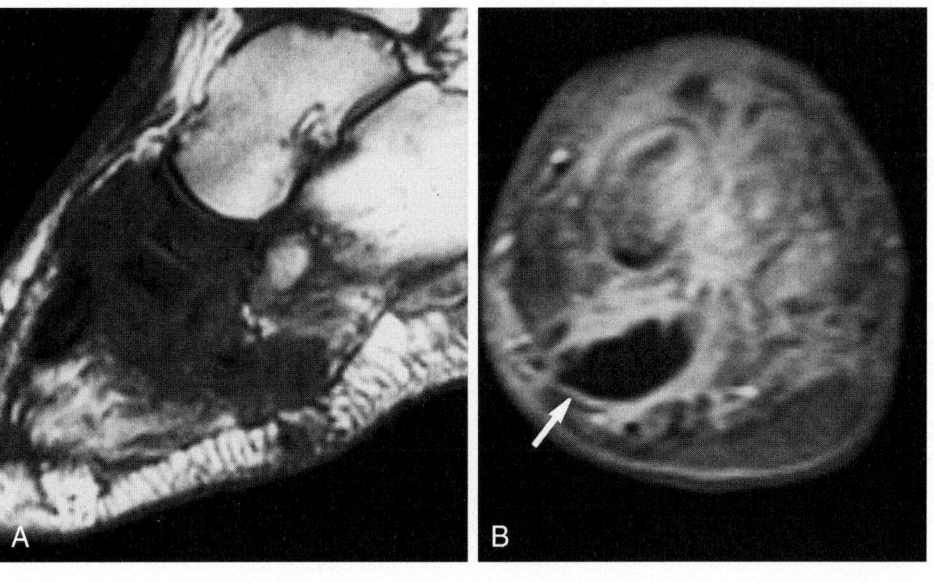

**Figure 66–17.** Osteomyelitis and soft tissue infection: MR imaging. Diabetes mellitus. *A*, sagittal $T_1$-weighted (TR/TE, 450/13) spin echo MR image shows low signal intensity in multiple tarsal bones and adjusted soft tissues. *B*, Axial enhanced fat-suppressed $T_1$-weighted (TR/TE, 500/13) spin-echo MR image reveals an abscess *(arrow)* in the plantar soft tissues, thus suggesting that the bone abnormalities relate to osteomyelitis.

disorganization are more profound in this disorder than in any other condition. In the joints of the appendicular skeleton, joint space loss, sclerosis, and fragmentation in the early stages of neuropathic osteoarthropathy can resemble the changes in osteoarthritis. With progressive flattening and deformity of the articular surfaces, the production of numerous intra-articular osseous dense areas, and the appearance of increasing sclerosis and osteophytosis, the diagnosis of neuropathic osteoarthropathy becomes more obvious.

In calcium pyrophosphate dihydrate crystal deposition disease, a neuropathic-like arthropathy characterized by joint space narrowing, eburnation, and fragmentation can appear, especially in the knee, wrist, and metacarpophalangeal joints. Identification of articular and periarticular calcification, involvement of specific areas of the joint such as the radiocarpal compartment of the wrist and the patellofemoral compartment of the knee, and the variability in osteophyte formation are helpful clues to the accurate diagnosis of pyrophosphate arthropathy. Intra-articular deposition of calcium hydroxyapatite crystals may lead to progressive destruction of a joint, especially in the shoulder, with fracture and dissolution of bone. A similar appearance in the shoulder has been reported as a manifestation of idiopathic "rapid destructive arthropathy."

Bony fragmentation and collapse are also manifestations of osteonecrosis, post-traumatic osteoarthritis, intra-articular steroid arthropathy, neglected infection, and alkaptonuria. In the joints of the axial skeleton, early findings of neuropathic osteoarthropathy, such as intervertebral disc space narrowing and vertebral sclerosis, resemble those of intervertebral osteochondrosis, infection, or alkaptonuria.

Once the radiographic findings are interpreted as those of neuropathic osteoarthropathy, identification of the underlying disorder usually depends on the location of the changes. Tabes typically produces changes in the hip, knee, ankle, and spine; diabetes mellitus leads to alterations in the midfoot and forefoot; syringomyelia affects the articulations of the upper extremity and cervical spine; and the syndromes of congenital indifference to pain and meningomyelocele commonly localize in the joints (including the physes) of the lower extremity. The presence of metaphyseal and growth plate destruction in an immature skeleton is especially characteristic of congenital indifference to pain and meningomyelocele.

## FURTHER READING

Bjorkengren AG, Weisman M, Pathria MN, et al: Neuroarthropathy associated with chronic alcoholism. AJR Am J Roentgenol 151:743, 1988.

Blanford AT, Keane SP, McCarty DJ, et al: Idiopathic Charcot joint of the elbow. Arthritis Rheum 21:723, 1978.

Brower AC, Allman RM: Pathogenesis of the neurotrophic joint: Neurotraumatic versus neurovascular. Radiology 139:349, 1981.

Campbell WL, Feldman F: Bone and soft tissue abnormalities of the upper extremity in diabetes mellitus. AJR Am J Roentgenol 124:7, 1975.

Citron ND, Paterson FWN, Jackson AM: Neuropathic osteonecrosis of the lateral femoral condyle in childhood: A report on four cases. J Bone Joint Surg Br 68:96, 1986.

Clouse ME, Gramm HF, Legg M, et al: Diabetic osteoarthropathy: Clinical and roentgenographic observations in 90 cases. AJR Am J Roentgenol 121:22, 1974.

Eichenholtz SN: Charcot Joints. Springfield, Ill, Charles C Thomas, 1966.

El-Khoury GY, Kathol MH: Neuropathic fractures in patients with diabetes mellitus. Radiology 134:313, 1980.

Feldman F, Johnson AM, Walter JF: Acute axial neuroarthropathy. Radiology 111:1, 1974.

Forrester DM, Magre G: Migrating bone shards in dissecting Charcot joints. AJR Am J Roentgenol 130:1133, 1978.

Giesecke SB, Dalinka MK, Kyle GC: Lisfranc's fracture-dislocation: A manifestation of peripheral neuropathy. AJR Am J Roentgenol 131:139, 1978.

Goldman AB, Freiberger RH: Localized infectious and neuropathic diseases. Semin Roentgenol 14:19, 1979.

Gondos B: The pointed tubular bone: Its significance and pathogenesis. Radiology 105:541, 1972.

Hodgson J, Pugh D, Young H: Roentgenologic aspects of certain lesions of bone: Neurotropic or infectious? Radiology 50:65, 1948.

Jones EA, Manaster BJ, May DA, et al: Neuropathic osteoarthropathy: Diagnostic dilemmas and differential diagnosis. Radiographics 20:279, 2000.

Kathol MH, El-Khoury GY, Moore TE, et al: Calcaneal insufficiency avulsion fractures in patients with diabetes mellitus. Radiology 180:725, 1991.

Katz I, Rabinowitz JG, Dziadiw R: Early changes in Charcot's joints. AJR Am J Roentgenol 86:965, 1961.

Kirkpatrick RH, Riley CR: Roentgenographic findings in familial dysautonomia. Radiology 68:654, 1957.

Ledermann HP, Morrison WB, Schweitzer ME: MR image analysis of pedal osteomyelitis: Distribution, patterns of spread, and frequency of associated ulceration and septic arthritis. Radiology 223:747, 2002.

Meyer GA, Stein J, Poppel MH: Rapid osseous changes in syringomyelia. Radiology 69:415, 1957.

Morrison WB, Schweitzer ME, Batte WG, et al: Osteomyelitis of the foot: Relative importance of primary and secondary MR imaging signs. Radiology 207:625, 1998.

Norman A, Robbins H, Milgram JE: The acute neuropathic arthropathy—a rapid severely disorganizing form of arthritis. Radiology 90:1159, 1968.

Pogonowska MJ, Collins LC, Dobson HL: Diabetic osteopathy. Radiology 89:265, 1971.

Schneider R, Goldman AB, Bohne WH: Neuropathic injuries to the lower extremities in children. Radiology 128:713, 1978.

Siegelman S, Heimann WG, Manin MC: Congenital indifference to pain. AJR Am J Roentgenol 97:242, 1966.

Silverman FN, Gilden JJ: Congenital insensitivity to pain: A neurologic syndrome with bizarre skeletal lesions. Radiology 72:176, 1959.

Westcott MA, Dynes MC, Remer EM, et al: Congenital and acquired orthopedic abnormalities in patients with myelomeningocele. Radiographics 12:1155, 1992.

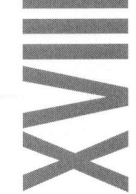
# CHAPTER 67

## Osteonecrosis: Pathogenesis, Diagnostic Techniques, Specific Situations, and Complications

Donald Resnick, Donald E. Sweet, and John E. Madewell

## SUMMARY OF KEY FEATURES

Osteonecrosis can accompany many diverse disease processes, such as trauma, hemoglobinopathy, exogenous or endogenous hypercortisolism, alcoholism, pancreatitis, dysbaric conditions, and Gaucher's disease. It may also become evident without any recognizable disease or event (primary, or spontaneous, osteonecrosis). Post-traumatic osteonecrosis is most frequent in the femoral and humeral heads, scaphoid, and talus, although other sites may be affected. Dysbaric osteonecrosis can produce widespread skeletal alterations of the epiphyseal, metaphyseal, or diaphyseal segments of tubular bones. Spontaneous osteonecrosis is most commonly recognized about the hip and knee. Possible complications of bone necrosis are secondary degenerative joint disease, formation of intra-articular osseous and cartilaginous bodies, septic arthritis, pathologic fracture, and cystic or sarcomatous transformation.

## INTRODUCTION

For most of the 19th century, osteonecrosis was regarded as septic in origin. The identification of well-documented cases with negative bacteriologic studies led to the use of the term aseptic necrosis. Subsequent observations indicated that the necrotic bone foci were not only aseptic but also avascular; hence the terms ischemic necrosis, avascular necrosis, and bone infarction were suggested. As currently used, the term osteonecrosis indicates the occurrence of ischemic death of the cellular constituents of bone and marrow. By convention, the term ischemic necrosis is applied to areas of epiphyseal or subarticular involvement, whereas the term bone infarct is reserved for metaphyseal and diaphyseal involvement. The literature on ischemic bone necrosis indicates, however, considerable overlap and lack of uniformity in applied terminology. A greater consensus exists regarding the many causes of osteonecrosis (Table 67–1).

### TABLE 67–1

**Causes of Osteonecrosis**

Trauma (fracture or dislocation)
Hemoglobinopathies (sickle cell anemia, sickle cell variant states)
Exogenous or endogenous hypercortisolism (corticosteroid medication, Cushing's disease)
Renal transplantation
Alcoholism
Pancreatitis
Dysbaric conditions (caisson disease)
Small vessel disease (collagen disorders)
Gaucher's disease
Gout and hyperuricemia
Irradiation
Synovitis with elevation of intra-articular pressure (infection, hemophilia)

## PRINCIPLES OF INFARCTION

Ischemic necrosis of bone, like infarction in other organ systems, results from a significant reduction or obliteration of the affected area's blood supply. One of the following phenomena can usually be demonstrated or inferred as impeding blood flow: (1) intraluminal obstruction (e.g., thromboembolic disorders, sludging of blood cells, stasis), (2) vascular compression (e.g., external mechanical pressure or vasospasm), or (3) physical disruption of the vessel (e.g., trauma). These factors can act alone or in combination.

Cell death from anoxia is not immediate; rather, it occurs through progressive stages of ischemic injury: stage 1, cessation of intracellular metabolic activity at a chemical level; stage 2, alteration or interruption of intracellular enzyme systems; and stage 3, disruption or dissolution of intracellular nuclear and cytoplasmic ultrastructure. Dissolution of intracellular structural integrity is irreversible and results in cell death.

The production of ischemic injury or necrosis and the rapidity with which cell death occurs depend on the sensitivity of the individual cell type, as well as the degree and duration of anoxia. The sensitivity of the cellular elements of bone and marrow to anoxia varies. The hematopoietic elements are generally acknowledged to be the first to undergo anoxic death, in 6 to 12 hours, followed by bone cells—osteocytes, osteoclasts, and osteoblasts—in 12 to 48 hours and, subsequently, marrow fat cells in 48 hours to 5 days. The variation in sensitivity of the different cellular constituents of bone and the marrow cavity makes it possible for temporary anoxia to result in the death of hematopoietic elements without necessarily being sufficient to cause osteocytic or marrow fat cell death. Once ischemic marrow fat cell death occurs, the involved segment of bone and marrow can clearly be labeled infarcted.

Infarcts, including those in bone, are three dimensional and can be subdivided into four zones: a central zone of cell death surrounded by successive zones of ischemic injury, active hyperemia, and, finally, normal tissue. The ischemic zone reflects a gradation of hypoxic injury ranging from severe cell damage immediately adjacent to the central zone of cell death to marginal cellular alterations adjacent to the hyperemic zone. Once ischemic necrosis is established, the breakdown products of dying and severely damaged cells provoke the initial inflammatory response consisting of vasodilatation, transudation of fluid, fibrin precipitation, and local infiltration of inflammatory cells. This response forms the basis for the development of the hyperemic zone and also represents the initial step of repair, removal, and reconstruction of the infarcted area.

Bone infarcts occurring in the metadiaphyseal intramedullary cavity (Fig. 67–1) have a central core of dead marrow and bone surrounded by zones of ischemically injured marrow and bone, active hyperemia, and viable marrow and bone. Infarcts occurring within an epiphysis or a small, round bone demonstrate a similar three-dimensional pattern, except that one surface is almost always covered by compact subchondral bone and articular cartilage. Because articular cartilage receives the bulk of its nourishment from synovial fluid, its viability is usually not significantly affected at first by the underlying osteonecrosis, except for the cartilage cells below the tidemark, which may die. Because the osteonecrotic segment is by definition avascular, repair begins along its outer perimeter at the junction between the ischemic zone surrounding the dead area and the viable area with an intact circulation (hyperemic zone). This reparative response results in the progressive development of a reactive margin (interface) between the dead zone and adjacent viable tissue.

Because tissue death is essentially a cellular phenomenon, mineralized bone matrix does not appear to be materially altered by ischemic necrosis directly; hence, bone structure is initially unaltered as a direct result of osteocyte death or osteonecrosis. Therefore, any alteration in bone density—either a real increase or a real decrease in radiographic density—is an indication of viability requiring osteoblastic or osteoclastic cell activity, respectively, and will initially be perceived in the viable bone and marrow surrounding the osteonecrotic segment.

## MARROW CAVITY

The medullary cavity is an admixture of cancellous bone, hematopoietic marrow, fatty marrow, and a sinusoidal vascular bed confined by a nonexpandable shell of cortical bone. Radiographically, ischemic necrosis of bone is encountered most commonly within the epiphyseal (especially the femoral and humeral heads) and metadiaphyseal marrow cavities of adult long tubular bones. Occasional involvement occurs in the distal femoral condyles, small bones of the wrist and ankle, and other sites.

The extensive arterial supply to adult long tubular bones—including the nutrient artery, with its ascending and descending diaphyseal branches, and the penetrating metaphyseal and epiphyseal (retinacular) arteries, as well as the superficial periosteal vessels and the diffuse intramedullary sinusoidal vascular bed—provides excellent collateral circulation. Venous outflow is also extensive, as evidenced by numerous perforating channels exiting from the cortex.

Despite the extensive circulation available to the metadiaphyseal cortex and intramedullary cavity, the epiphyseal ends of long bones have limited arterial access and venous outflow because much of their surface is covered by articular cartilage. Arterial access to the epiphysis is further compromised in a growing skeleton because the epiphysis is separated from the metaphysis by the growth plate. Although occasional small arterioles penetrate the physeal growth plate (physis), little or no significant collateral circulation exists between a developing epiphysis and its adjacent metaphysis. In the absence of collateral circulation, the likelihood of a single or dominant artery supplying an entire epiphysis or a significant segment of an epiphysis is increased. The small carpal and tarsal

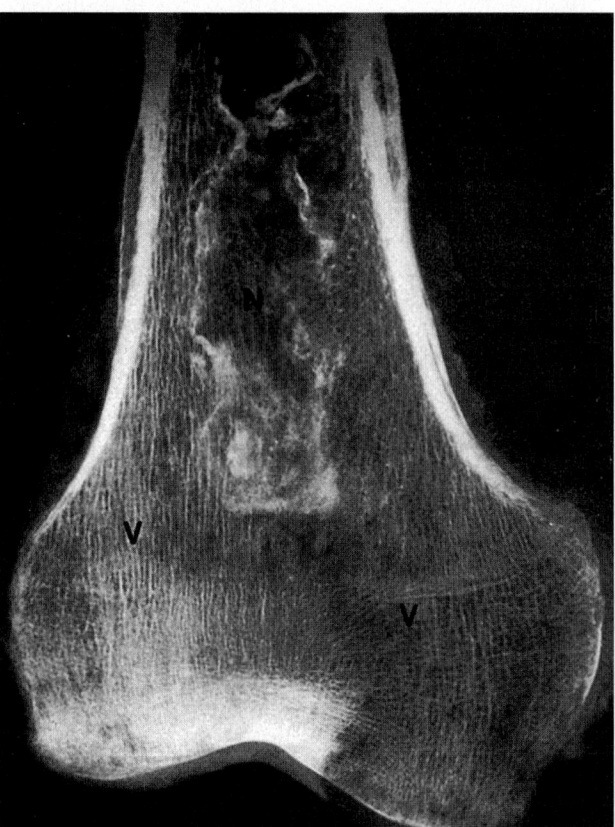

**Figure 67–1.** Intramedullary bone infarct. Specimen radiograph of a coronally sectioned distal end of the femur reveals unaltered density within the central necrotic zone (N), which is separated from the adjacent viable bone and marrow (V) by an irregular linear margin of increased density. Note the localized area of increased density that appears to be within the inferior portion of the infarct.

bones are also covered to a large extent by articular cartilage. In many respects, their ossification centers are analogous to the developing epiphyses of a long bone with regard to blood supply.

Development of a sinusoidal vascular bed appears to be an important prerequisite for the emergence of normal hematopoietic activity. This demand for hematopoiesis is largely a function of age. The marrow cavities of all bones in newborns and young children are actively engaged in hematopoiesis. As the total marrow volume increases with skeletal growth, normal hematopoietic demand can eventually be satisfied by the marrow capacity of the axial skeleton. Therefore, the marrow cavities of the adolescent and adult appendicular skeleton normally contain predominantly fatty marrow, unless some special circumstance requires increased hematopoiesis.

Thus, both radiographic and anatomic observations indicate that ischemic necrosis of bone, either avascular necrosis or bone infarction, occurs almost invariably within areas of predominantly fatty marrow. The converse is equally true; ischemic necrosis in areas of normal active hematopoiesis is distinctly unusual except in sickle cell disease and related hemoglobinopathies or after complete traumatic disruption of the arterial blood supply. Ischemic necrosis of cortical bone is relatively rare and occurs only when the arterial blood supply has been extensively interrupted, as in osteomyelitis.

## HISTOLOGIC-RADIOGRAPHIC CORRELATION

Once osteonecrosis or ischemic injury is an established anatomic fact, the body sets into motion the initial inflammatory host response as the first step toward revival, rehabilitation, or removal and reconstruction (repair).

In the early stages of osteonecrosis, no gross architectural or radiographic alteration is observed. Following this initial phase, there is cell modulation in the zone of ischemic injury and associated hyperemia. The generalized active hyperemia in response to the injured and dying cells results in osteoporosis (mediated through osteoclastic activity) of the adjacent viable bone, the first recognizable radiographic alteration in osteonecrosis; the dead area remains unchanged. As the marrow cells in the ischemic zone undergo morphologic changes, the reactive interface begins to emerge.

The reactive interface demonstrates an increase in vascularity associated with infiltration of inflammatory cells along the outer viable margin and further modulation of ischemic marrow fat toward fibroblastic cells, which may elaborate an atypical-appearing ischemic fiber bone. This ischemic bone may also appear as an appliqué on the surface of preexisting dead bone trabeculae within the ischemic zone. While these changes evolve in the reactive interface, sustained active hyperemia causes progressive osteoporosis in the remaining viable bone. Emergence of the reactive interface within the previously ischemic zone (with focal cancellous bone resorption, minimal trabecular bone reinforcement, and deposition of ischemic fiber bone within the reactive fibrosis) accounts for the earliest alterations in radiographic density between the infarcted and viable zones (Fig. 67–2). With continued repair and remodeling, a reactive interface forms between the viable and osteonecrotic zones, consisting of ischemic fiber bone formation and dystrophic mineralization of dead marrow fat within the necrotic zone adjacent to the fibrous interface. As a result of the continuing hyperemia, the supporting bony architecture may become sufficiently weakened by continued resorption of trabecular bone and subchondral bone plate along the reactive interface that the stress of weight bearing results in subchondral bone plate fracture, with focal articular cartilage buckling and eventual collapse. Fragmentation and compaction of subchondral bony fracture debris lead to the development of a subchondral lucent area along the fracture line, designated the crescent sign (Fig. 67–3). This sign is often best seen radiographically on a frog-leg view. In time, flattening of the articular surface becomes apparent.

## DIAGNOSTIC TECHNIQUES

### Radiography

The radiographic findings of osteonecrosis of an epiphysis, metaphysis, or diaphysis in a tubular bone or a flat or irregular bone are characteristic. Arclike subchondral radiolucent lesions, patchy lucent areas and sclerosis, osseous collapse, and preservation of the joint space in an epiphyseal region (Fig. 67–4); lucent shadows with a peripheral rim of sclerosis and periostitis in a diametaphyseal region (Fig. 67–5); and patchy lucent areas and sclerosis with bony collapse in a flat or irregular bone (Fig. 67–6) are typical radiographic signs of osteonecrosis. Unfortunately, these abnormalities do not appear for several months after the onset of clinical manifestations in many persons and are therefore not a sensitive indication of early disease (Fig. 67–7). Further, the initial radiographic features of osteonecrosis, especially in the diametaphyseal portions of tubular bones, may lack specificity. Subtle, mottled, poorly defined radiolucent lesions may simulate the aggressive pattern of bone destruction that accompanies a variety of malignant tumors, as well as osteomyelitis.

### Computed Tomography

The use of computed tomography (CT) to evaluate ischemic necrosis of bone (especially in the femoral head) has two goals: to allow early diagnosis of the condition, and to identify the presence and extent of bone collapse. Although it appears that CT can delineate subtle alterations in bone when routine radiographs are normal, it is also apparent that scintigraphy and magnetic resonance (MR) imaging are far more sensitive in this respect (see later discussion). CT may also be a useful adjunct in patients unable to undergo MR imaging.

In patients with more advanced changes of osteonecrosis of the femoral head, transaxial CT scans reveal centrally or peripherally located circular areas of decreased attenuation. At this stage, reformation of the CT data in a sagittal or coronal plane is more useful because it delineates areas of subchondral fracture and subtle buckling or collapse of the articular surface (Fig. 67–8). The latter finding has therapeutic significance because the presence of even minimal bone collapse indicates a more advanced

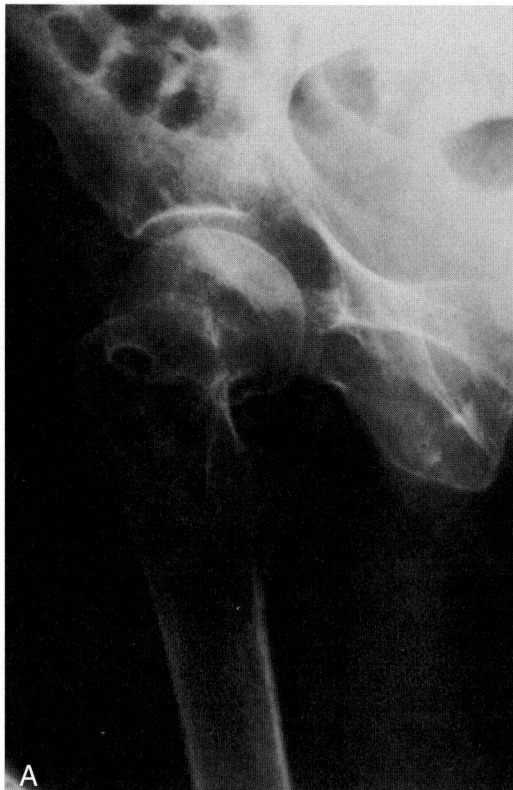

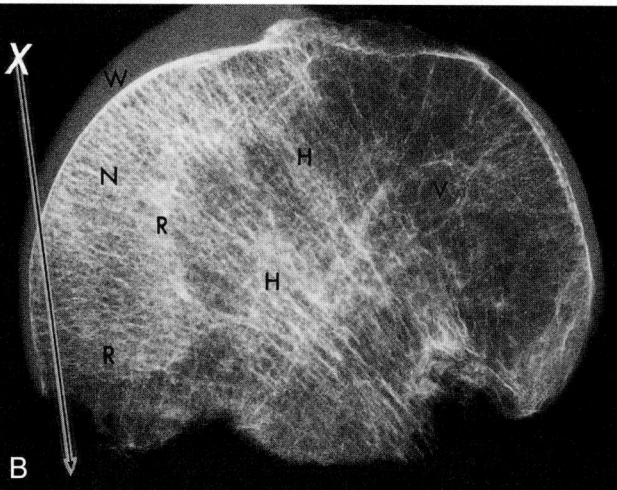

**Figure 67–2.** Reactive interface: fracture of the femoral neck (72 hours old, with ischemic necrosis of 3 to 6 months' duration). *A,* Clinical radiograph of a femoral neck fracture that occurred clinically 3 days before resection. A slight increase in subchondral bone density beneath the weight-bearing area is seen. The degree of relative osteoporosis above the fracture margin indicates an active process older than 3 days. *B,* Specimen radiograph (2.5×) of the sectioned femoral head reveals an area of subchondral radiodensity beneath the weight-bearing area (W) that corresponds to the area of ischemic necrosis (N). The osteonecrotic segment is surrounded by a faintly perceived reactive margin of variable but focally increased density (R). The remaining viable portion of the femoral head is radiolucent (V) in comparison to the ischemic area (N). The articular surface and subchondral plate appear intact.

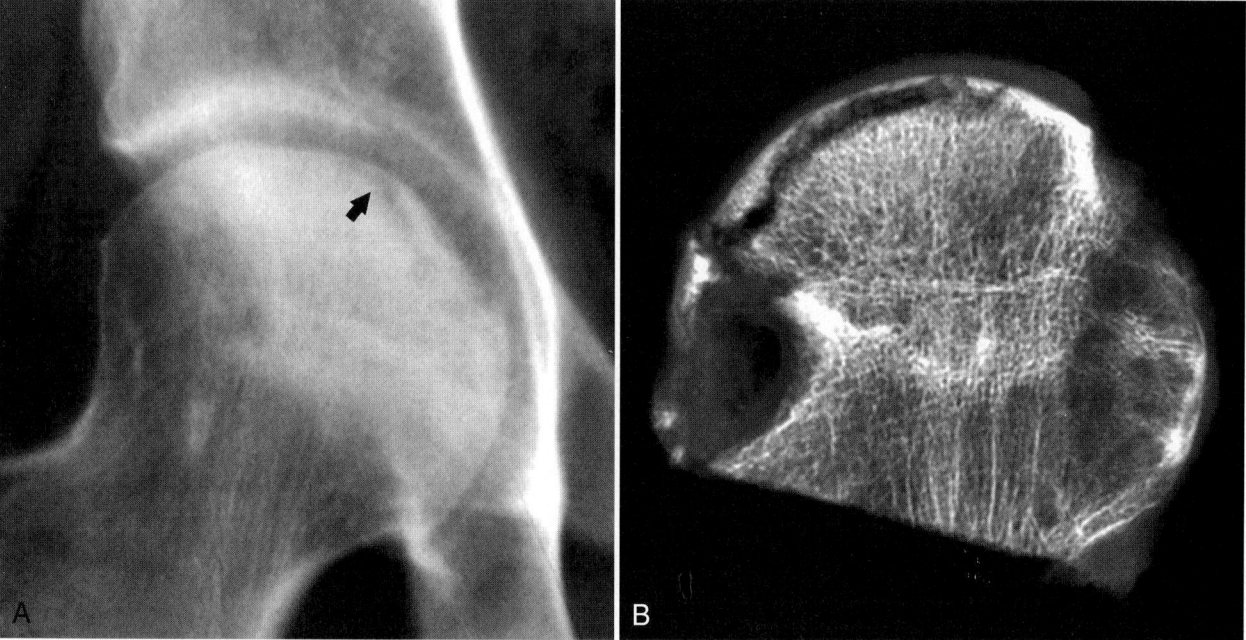

**Figure 67–3.** Ischemic necrosis of the femoral head (nontraumatic). *A,* Radiograph demonstrates flattening of the weight-bearing surface of the femoral head, with a subtle crescent sign *(arrow)* indicating collapse of the articular surface. A serpentine rind of sclerosis surrounding the osteonecrotic region of the femoral head is not well defined. *B,* Specimen radiograph from a different patient shows the crescent sign and fracture to better advantage. The osteonecrotic region of the femoral head has a surrounding rind of sclerosis (reactive interface).

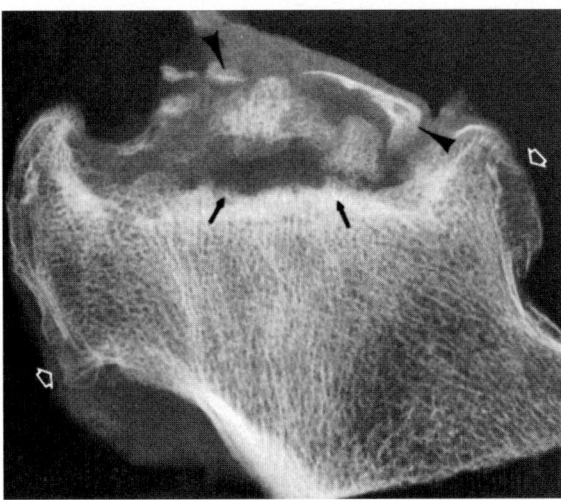

**Figure 67–4.** Osteonecrosis: epiphysis. Sectional radiograph shows displaced cartilage and subchondral bone plate *(arrowheads)*, subjacent osseous resorption *(solid arrows)*, reactive bone formation, and buttressing. Osteophytic lipping is observed *(open arrows)*.

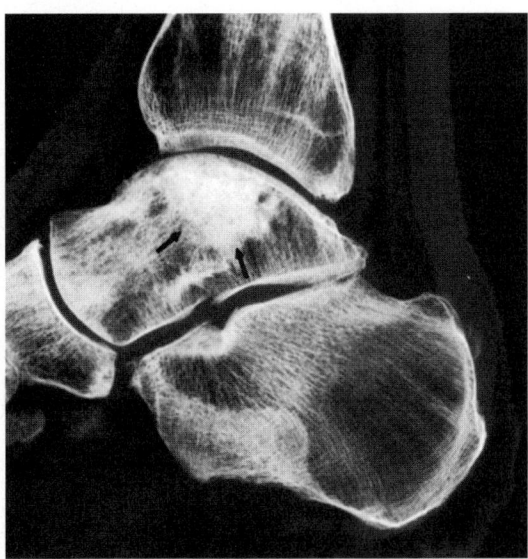

**Figure 67–6.** Osteonecrosis: irregular bone. In this patient with corticosteroid-induced ischemic necrosis of bone, observe the sclerotic zone in the talus (as well as the calcaneus), which corresponds in position to an irregular hemorrhagic area of infarction *(arrows)*.

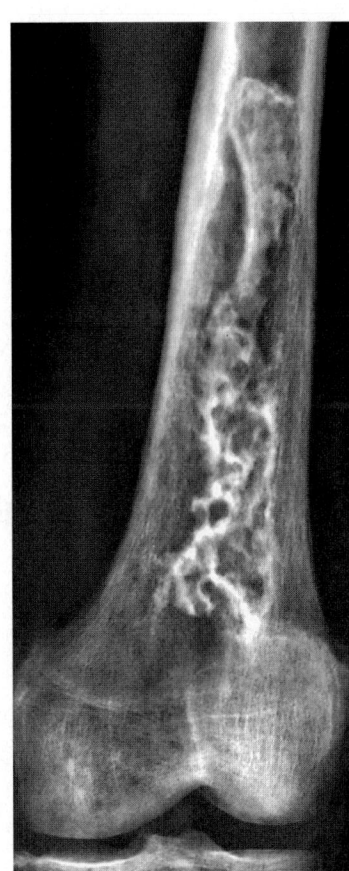

**Figure 67–5.** Osteonecrosis: diametaphysis (bone infarct). Radiograph of the lower half of the left femur of a 69-year-old man with intermittent claudication of 4 years' duration demonstrates a bone infarction. Observe the typical shell-like calcification of the lesion. (From Jaffe HL: Ischemic necrosis of bone. Med Radiogr Photogr 45:57, 1969.)

stage of the disease (Table 67–2) and limits the number of orthopedic procedures that can be used successfully (Table 67–3).

### Scintigraphy

Radionuclide examination is one of the most attractive techniques for the early diagnosis of osteonecrosis. Single photon emission computed tomography (SPECT) may further improve radionuclide sensitivity for this diagnosis. Establishing a correct diagnosis at an early stage is important, because the success of some of the proposed orthopedic procedures requires their application before

**TABLE 67–2**

**Criteria for Staging Osteonecrosis**

| Stage | Characteristics |
|---|---|
| 0 | Normal or nondiagnostic radiograph, bone scan, and MR examination |
| I* | Normal radiograph; abnormal bone scan or MR examination, or both |
| II* | Abnormal radiograph showing cystic and sclerotic changes in the femoral head |
| III* | Subchondral collapse producing a crescent sign |
| IV* | Flattening of the femoral head |
| V* | Joint space narrowing with or without acetabular involvement |
| VI | Advanced degenerative changes |

*The extent or grade of involvement should also be indicated as A, mild; B, moderate; or C, severe.

Modified from Steinberg ME, et al: J Bone Joint Surg Br 77:34, 1995.

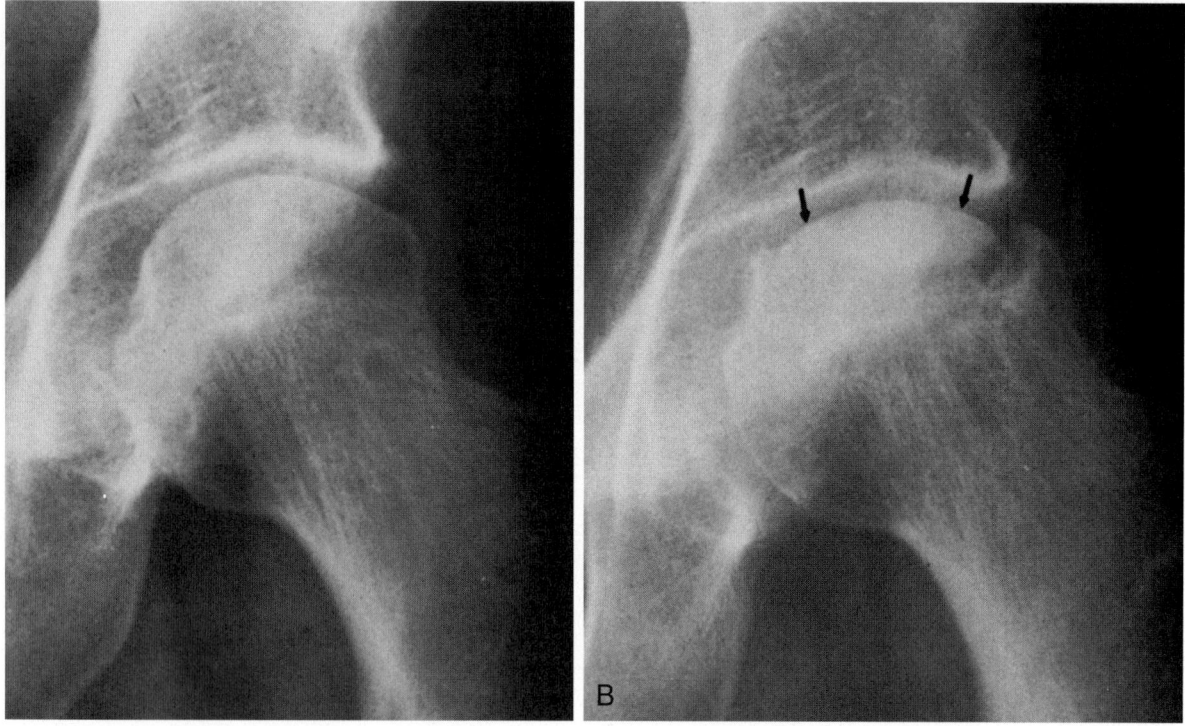

**Figure 67–7.** Osteonecrosis: inadequacy of radiographic examination. This 35-year-old man had hip pain at the time of his initial radiographic examination that progressed over the next 6 to 9 months. *A,* The initial radiograph was interpreted as normal. Neither a bone scan nor MR imaging was performed. *B,* Seven months later, significant collapse of the superolateral aspect of the femoral head is identified *(arrows)*. The joint is not narrowed.

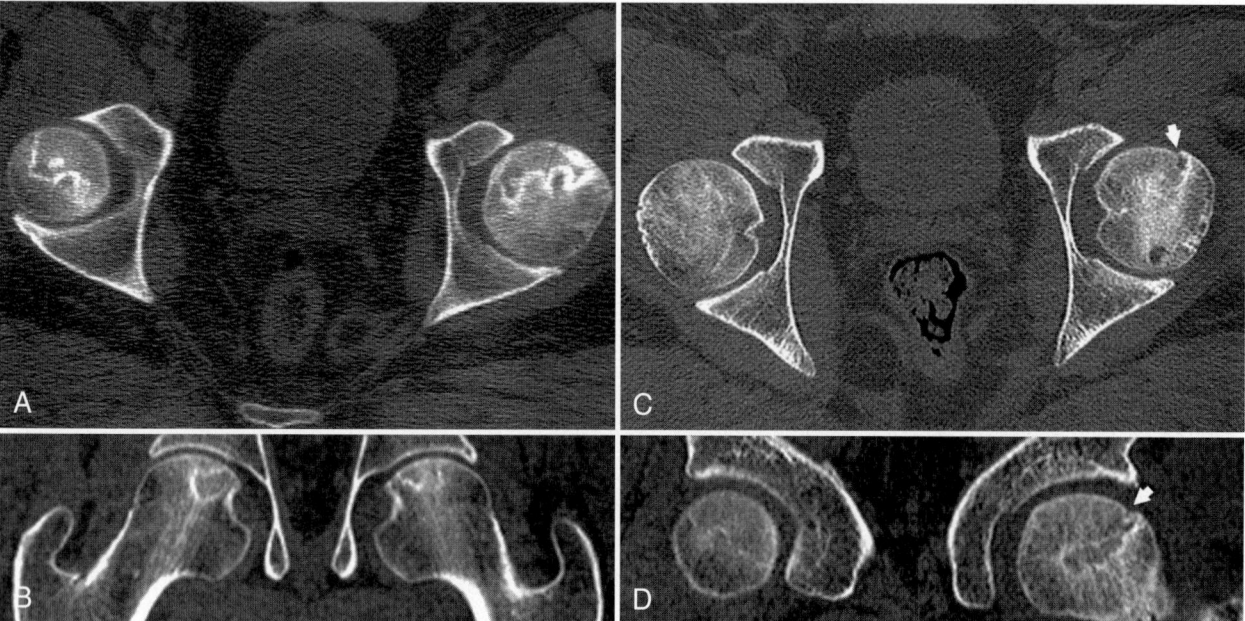

**Figure 67–8.** Osteonecrosis: CT. *A* and *B,* Transaxial CT scan *(A)* and a coronal reconstruction *(B)* illustrates a curvilinear zone of sclerosis, diagnostic of ischemic necrosis of the femoral head. No collapse of the articular surface is evident. *C* and *D,* In similar images from a different patient, observe the degenerative subchondral cysts and articular collapse *(arrows)* of the left femoral head. The joint space is preserved.

**TABLE 67–3**

**Surgical Methods of Treating Ischemic Necrosis of the Femoral Head**

| Method | Rationale |
|---|---|
| Drilling or forage | Multiple drill holes in the femoral head and neck to establish channels for revascularization |
| Core decompression | Coring device to create large and small channels from the trochanteric region to the femoral head to allow decompression of elevated intraosseous pressure |
| Free bone grafts with cancellous or cortical bone | Placement of cortical bone (for mechanical support) or cancellous bone (for rapid incorporation) into channels in the femoral head and neck |
| Vascularized bone grafts with attached muscle pedicle | Same as for free bone grafts, except that living rather than dead bone is used |
| Osteochondral allograft | Replacement of the collapsed portion of the articular surface with an allograft |
| Osteotomy | |
|    Varus or valgus | Shift of the femoral head in the acetabulum to provide a new weight-bearing area |
|    Rotational | Rotation of the femoral head in the acetabulum to provide a new weight-bearing area |
| Electrical stimulation | Use of electrical current to induce bone formation |
| Arthroplasty | Replacement of the abnormal femoral head (and acetabulum) with a prosthesis |

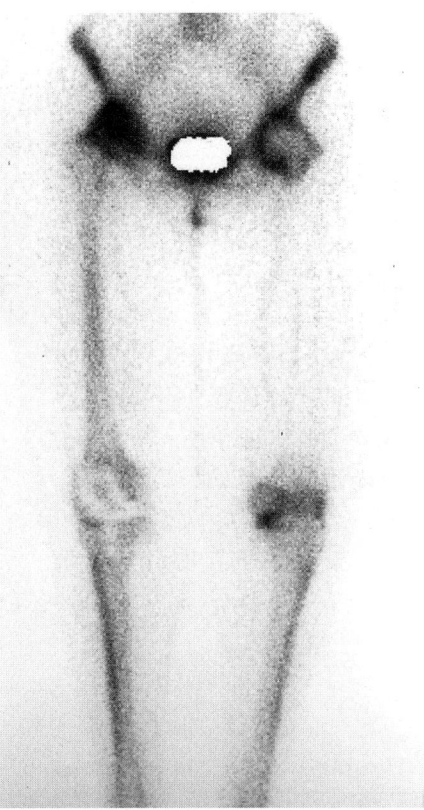

**Figure 67–9.** Osteonecrosis: radionuclide bone scan. In this 75-year-old woman with widespread infarction, a bone scan shows absence of uptake of the radionuclide throughout much of the length of the left femur, consistent with the clinical diagnosis of acute bone infarction. Osteoarthritis in the right hip is associated with increased accumulation of the radiopharmaceutical agent. (Courtesy of K. Nguyen, MD, Wichita, Kans.)

collapse of the articular surface begins. Scintigraphy may be especially useful in studying the contralateral "silent" hip in cases of apparent unilateral osteonecrosis of the femoral head.

Immediately after interruption of the osseous blood supply, scintigraphy with bone-seeking radiopharmaceutical agents can reveal an area of decreased or absent uptake, or a "cold" lesion (Fig. 67–9). After weeks or months, reparative processes in the surrounding bone are associated with revascularization and increased accumulation of the radioisotope, or a "hot" lesion (Fig. 67–10). At some point between these two stages, early in the course of the process, the radionuclide examination may be normal. Even when the study is abnormal, however, it is not specific and must be interpreted with knowledge of the radiographic and clinical findings.

## Magnetic Resonance Imaging

On the basis of a review of the literature, certain observations can be made about the use of MR imaging in the evaluation of osteonecrosis, particularly in the femoral head:

1. MR imaging is a very sensitive method for the early diagnosis of ischemic necrosis of bone and is more sensitive in this regard than bone scintigraphy.

2. A negative MR imaging examination does not eliminate the possibility of osteonecrosis, although it makes this possibility highly unlikely.

3. Although MR imaging abnormalities occur early in the course of osteonecrosis, they are somewhat variable in their time of occurrence and are dependent on alterations of fat cells in the bone marrow. Ischemic changes first become evident in hematopoietic cells 6 to 12 hours after the ischemic event and are then observed in osteocytes, osteoblasts, and osteoclasts within 2 days of the ischemic event. Fat cells are more resistant to ischemia, in that they survive 2 to 5 days after the insult. Further, initial changes in the fat cells may not lead to an alteration in MR imaging signal characteristics. An inflammatory and hyperemic response in viable tissue adjacent to the devascularized regions produces a reactive interface about the osteonecrotic areas that is associated with increased vascularity, inflammation, granulation tissue, and fibrosis. MR imaging is sensitive to the presence of this reactive interface.

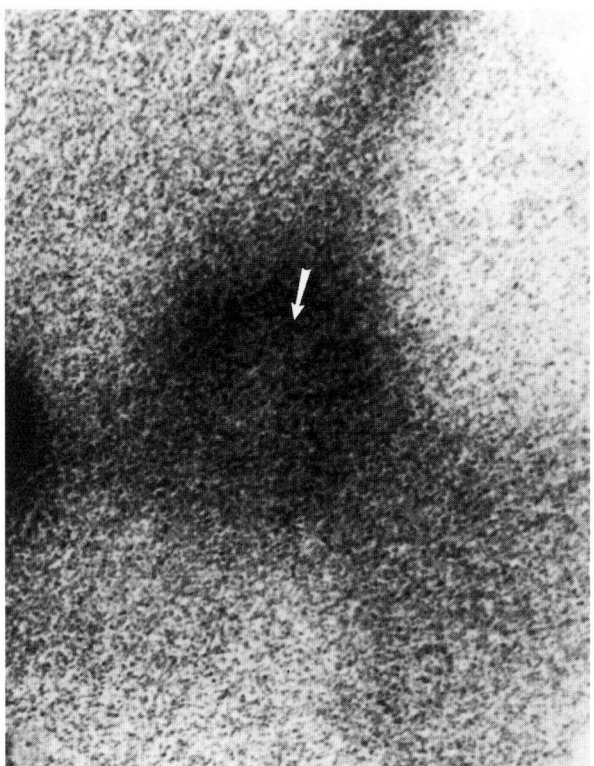

**Figure 67–10.** Osteonecrosis: radionuclide bone scan. Technetium pyrophosphate bone scan depicts a central area of diminished uptake surrounded by a zone of augmented activity *(arrow)*.

4. MR imaging may be able to identify changes that place a femoral head at risk for subsequent osteonecrosis. Two such changes—early conversion of hematopoietic to fatty marrow in the proximal end of the femur, and prominent physeal scars that close off the femoral head—have been identified, but neither appears to be a sensitive or specific predictor of disease.

5. Variations in the pattern of MR imaging abnormalities are indicative of individual differences in the distribution and extent of involvement and in the host response. Focal abnormalities predominate, with some component of diminished signal intensity on T1-weighted spin echo images. The regions of altered signal intensity may be homogeneous or inhomogeneous, however. The most characteristic pattern of involvement is the double line appearance, evident on T2-weighted spin echo MR images at the reactive interface between ischemic and nonischemic bone. On T1-weighted spin echo images, this interface is characterized by a line of low signal intensity reflecting the presence of granulation tissue and, to a lesser extent, sclerotic bone. On T2-weighted spin echo images, a narrower line of low signal intensity, reflecting the presence of bone sclerosis, and an inner zone of high signal intensity, indicating the location of granulation tissue, are apparent. This combination of findings is designated the double line sign. Chemical shift misregistration artifact appears to contribute to the double line sign. On T2-weighted images, the zone of high signal intensity, which represents granulation tissue, is

typically slightly shifted so that it is misregistered with respect to a coexisting area of low signal intensity with the same size and shape (Fig. 67–11). Thus, a double line sign may occur in the absence of bone sclerosis, although its diagnostic significance remains the same. The absence of a double line sign does not eliminate the diagnosis of osteonecrosis.

The crescent sign, which is related to a fracture in the necrotic portion of the femoral head, is often visible with routine radiography. Its appearance on MR images is variable because the fracture gap may be filled with fluid or gas.

Diffusely distributed MR imaging abnormalities in the femoral head and neck may be encountered in cases of osteonecrosis (Fig. 67–12), and the patterns of signal intensity on T1- and T2-weighted spin echo images in such instances may be indistinguishable from those of transient osteoporosis of the hip and, occasionally, infection and tumor. This diffuse pattern has been associated with pain and a tendency for progressive abnormalities, with collapse of bone.

6. Some correlation exists between the MR imaging characteristics of osteonecrosis and histologic parameters. The prognostic significance of the changes in signal intensity within the ischemic zone is not clear, although the presence of fat within this zone appears to correspond to absent or less dramatic radiographic abnormalities, and the presence of fibrous tissue corresponds to more extensive radiographic abnormalities (Fig. 67–13).

7. No agreement exists regarding the choice of imaging plane or specific sequence when using MR imaging to evaluate osteonecrosis of the femoral head. The coronal plane is ideally suited to analysis of the subchondral bone of the femoral head. Sagittal images, particularly when combined with the application of surface coils and small fields of view, appear to increase the sensitivity of MR imaging in the diagnosis of early disease (Fig. 67–14).

8. Although the application of MR imaging to the detection of ischemic necrosis at skeletal sites other than the femoral head has received far less attention, there is little doubt of its efficacy. The basic MR imaging characteristics in these other skeletal locations are similar or identical to those seen in cases of osteonecrosis of the femoral head (Fig. 67–15). The MR imaging changes that occur in association with diametaphyseal infarction vary according to the stage of the process. Early infarcts may have intermediate to high signal intensity on T1-weighted sequences and high signal intensity on T2-weighted sequences; chronic infarcts are typically of low signal intensity on both T1- and T2-weighted images (Fig. 67–16). In both instances, a serpentine zone of low signal intensity that represents bone sclerosis or fibrosis may surround the necrotic region. Diagnostic difficulty may be encountered in cases of acute bone infarction, although islands of entrapped fat within the lesion may be noted.

9. MR imaging may be a useful technique for assessing the response of an osteonecrotic femoral head to

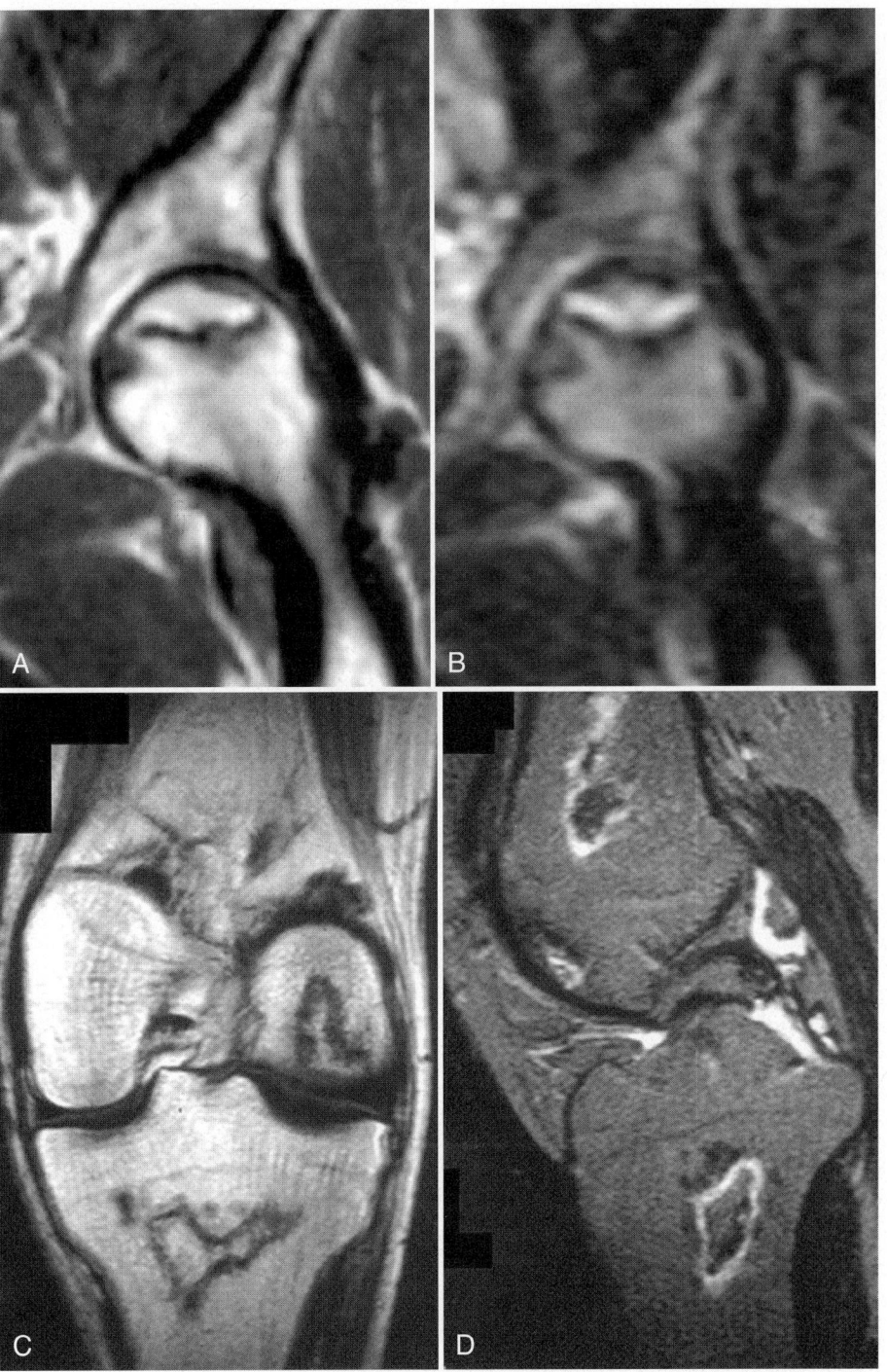

**Figure 67–11.** Osteonecrosis: MR imaging—double line sign. *A* and *B*, On a T1-weighted spin echo MR image *(A)*, a line of decreased signal reflects the presence of granulation tissue and sclerotic bone. On a T2-weighted spin echo MR image *(B)*, an additional line of high signal intensity indicates the location of granulation tissue. This combination of findings is designated the double line sign. *C* and *D*, In a different patient, coronal T1-weighted (TR/TE, 550/16) *(C)* and sagittal T2-weighted (TR/TE, 2800/85) *(D)* spin echo MR images show the double line sign in both areas of osteonecrosis and bone infarct.

operative intervention, especially core decompression. MR imaging performed at variable times after core decompression of osteonecrotic femoral heads may reveal changing patterns of involvement, with ischemic lesions decreasing in size; however, changes are not seen uniformly and are more likely to occur when the initial lesions are small. Patterns of bone marrow edema may also resolve after surgery. Typically, however, there is little change in the MR imaging abnormalities, and the signal intensity characteristics of the necrotic zone remain constant.

## POST-TRAUMATIC OSTEONECROSIS

After a fracture, bone death of variable extent on either side of the fracture line is common. Necrosis of a large segment of bone after fracture or dislocation is generally restricted to sites that possess a vulnerable blood supply, such as the femoral head, body of the talus, and carpal scaphoid. Additional characteristics common to each of these areas are an intra-articular location of necrotic bone and limited attachment of soft tissue. The necrotic portion of bone may appear radiodense as a result of compression of trabeculae, reactive eburnation from the

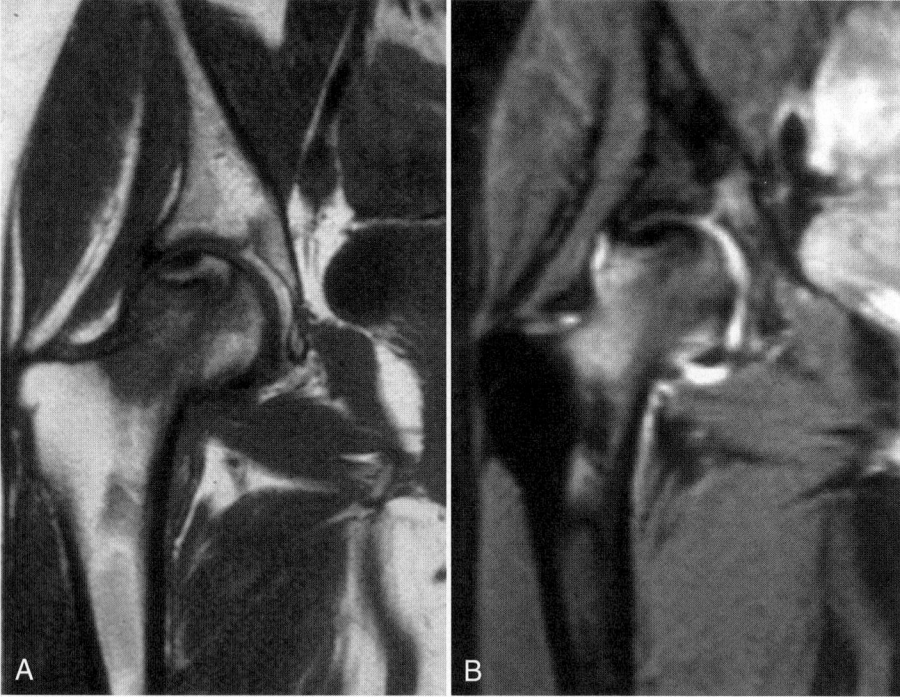

**Figure 67–12.** Osteonecrosis: MR imaging—marrow edema. Corresponding coronal T1-weighted (TR/TE, 600/20) *(A)* and fat-suppressed fast T2-weighted (TR/TE, 4000/70) *(B)* spin echo MR images reveal an area of osteonecrosis in the right femoral head, with associated articular collapse and joint effusion. Note diffusely distributed abnormalities in the femoral head and neck, compatible with marrow edema.

healing process, or lack of participation of the bone in the hyperemia and osteoporosis of neighboring viable bone.

### Femoral Head

Osteonecrosis of the femoral head is a well-recognized complication of femoral neck fractures and hip dislocations. The principal blood supply to the adult femoral head is via the circumflex femoral branches of the profunda femoris artery (Fig. 67–17). A second supply of blood is derived from vessels of the ligamentum teres, which enters the bone of the fovea capitis. It has been established that the superior (lateral) retinacular vessels represent the most important source of blood to the femoral head, and a fracture of the femoral neck that traverses the entry site of the superior retinacular vessels

into the epiphysis can lead to significant disruption of blood supply and subsequent osteonecrosis. The vessels within the ligamentum teres vary in diameter, and their role in the supply of blood to the femoral head is debated.

Fractures of the femoral neck in adults (and in children) can be complicated by osteonecrosis of the femoral head (Fig. 67–18). This complication is more frequent in intracapsular fractures (subcapital, transcervical) than in extracapsular fractures (intertrochanteric); in the latter situation, the blood supply is not compromised by the fracture line. The use of MR imaging to detect acute ischemia of the femoral head, and the use of contrast-enhanced MR imaging in cases of early ischemia, is valuable in patients with acute fractures of the femoral neck.

Other traumatic causes of osteonecrosis of the femoral head include dislocation of the hip and a slipped capital

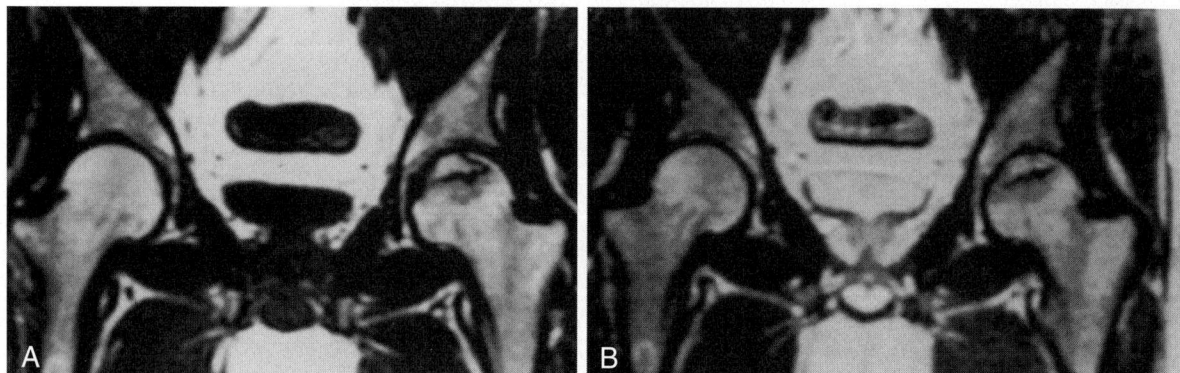

**Figure 67–13.** Osteonecrosis: MR imaging. Coronal T1-weighted (TR/TE, 600/20) *(A)* and T2-weighted (TR/TE, 2500/70) *(B)* spin echo MR images reveal an area of osteonecrosis in the left femoral head, where a serpentine region of low signal intensity surrounds a central region whose signal characteristics are identical to those of fat.

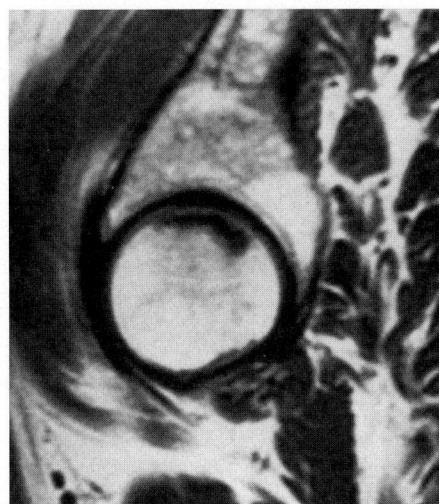

**Figure 67–14.** Osteonecrosis: MR imaging. Sagittal T1-weighted (TR/TE, 966/12) spin echo MR image shows a characteristic serpentine region of low signal intensity, diagnostic of osteonecrosis of the femoral head.

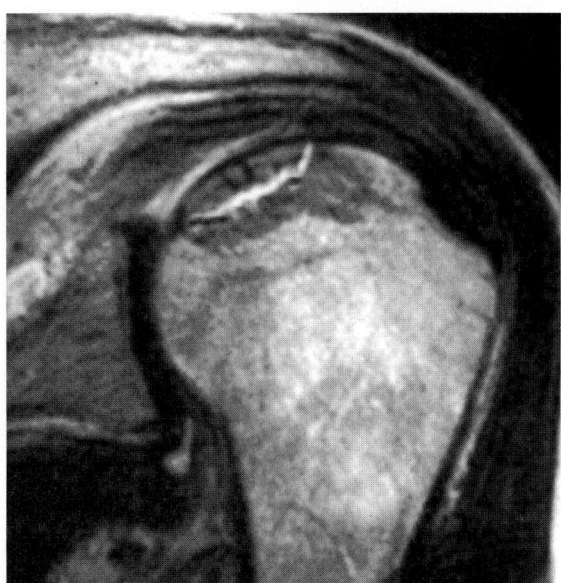

**Figure 67–15.** Osteonecrosis: involvement of the humeral head. Coronal oblique T2-weighted (TR/TE, 3600/96) fast spin echo MR image shows the classic features of osteonecrosis, including a crescent sign. (Courtesy of S. Eilenberg, MD, San Diego, Calif.)

femoral epiphysis. Osteonecrosis of the femoral head has also been recorded in as many as two thirds of patients after developmental dysplasia with dislocation of the hip.

### Talus

Osteonecrosis of the talus is a recognized and disabling complication of various fractures and injuries. The body of the talus is more prone to necrosis than are the talar head and neck. This complication is especially prevalent after fracture of the neck in which dislocation of the subtalar or ankle joint, or both, is also evident. Osteonecrosis of the talus has been reported as a stress injury as well.

Radiographic diagnosis of osteonecrosis of the talus can be difficult, and it is usually delayed until osteoporosis of the surrounding viable bone creates a relatively increased density of the talar body. This finding may be apparent within 1 to 3 months after injury and may be combined with collapse of the articular surface (Fig. 67–19). Conversely, participation of the entire talus in the osteoporosis of immobilization after injury is a good prognostic sign indicating adequate blood supply to the bone. The presence of a subchondral radiolucent band in the proximal part of the talus, Hawkins' sign, represents bony resorption and can be a useful radiographic indication of an intact vascular supply (Fig. 67–20).

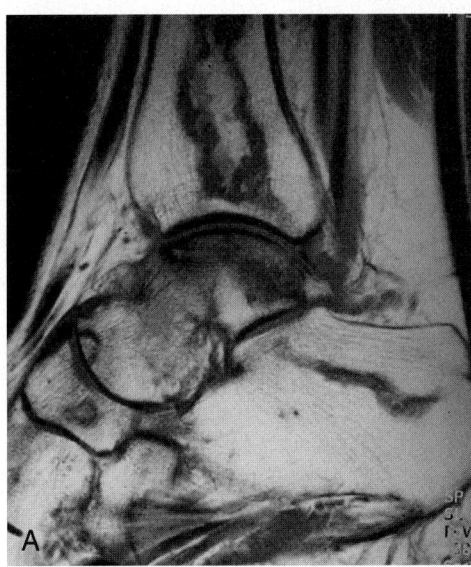
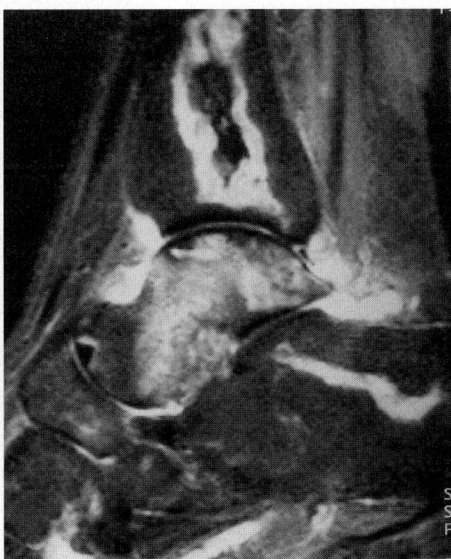

**Figure 67–16.** Osteonecrosis: involvement of the bones about the ankle and foot. Widespread osteonecrosis in the distal portion of the tibia, the talus, the calcaneus, and the navicular bone related to corticosteroid therapy is revealed on sagittal T1-weighted (TR/TE, 650/20) spin echo *(A)* and short tau inversion recovery (STIR; TR/TE, 5830/30; inversion time, 150 msec) *(B)* MR images.

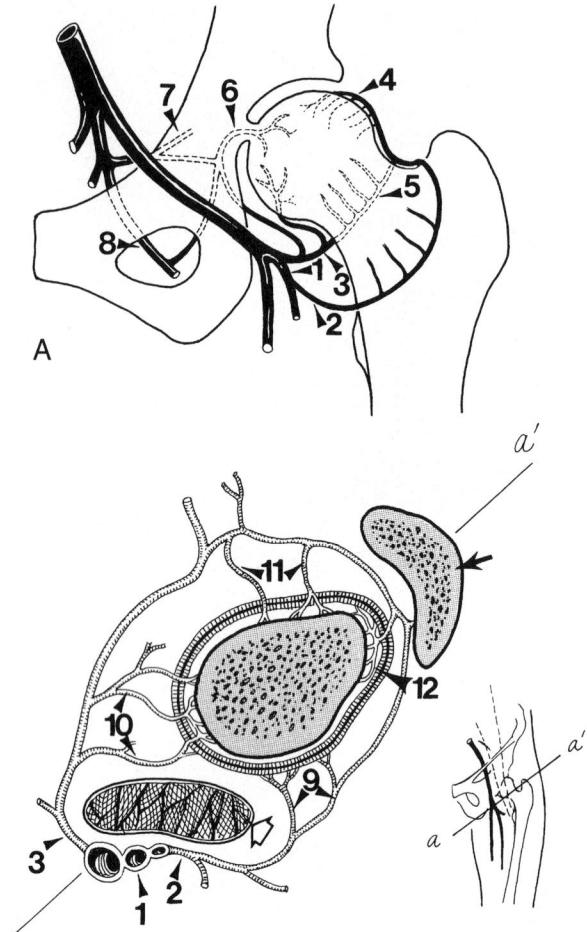

B

**Figure 67–17.** Femoral head: vascular supply in adults. *A,* The major blood supply is derived from the profunda femoris artery (1), from which arise the lateral (2) and medial (3) circumflex arteries. (The medial and lateral circumflex arteries may arise from the femoral artery rather than the profunda femoris artery in some persons.) As these latter vessels pass anterior and posterior to the femur to anastomose at the level of the trochanters, they send off small branches beneath the capsule of the hip joint. These branches, including the superior retinacular (lateral epiphyseal) arteries (4) and the inferior retinacular (inferior metaphyseal) arteries (5), raise the synovial membrane into folds, or retinacula. A second supply of blood is derived from the vessels of the ligamentum teres. Here, the foveal (medial epiphyseal) arteries (6) can be noted. Additional regional vessels are the inferior gluteal artery (7) and the obturator artery (8). *B,* Cross section of the proximal end of the femur at the base of the neck better delineates the nature of the blood supply. The greater trochanter *(arrow)* and iliopsoas muscle *(open arrow)* are indicated. Note the profunda femoris artery (1) and the lateral (2) and medial (3) circumflex arteries. From the lateral circumflex arteries are derived the anterior ascending cervical arteries (9). From the medial circumflex artery are derived the medial (10), posterior (11), and lateral (12) ascending cervical arteries, which, in combination with the anterior ascending cervical arteries, form a subsynovial anastomotic ring on the surface of the femoral neck at the margin of the articular cartilage. The inset shows the plane of section (line *a–a′*). (*A,* After Graham J, Wood S: In Davidson JK [ed]: Aseptic Necrosis of Bone. New York, American Elsevier, 1976, p 101. *B,* After Chung SM: J Bone Joint Surg Am 58:961, 1976.)

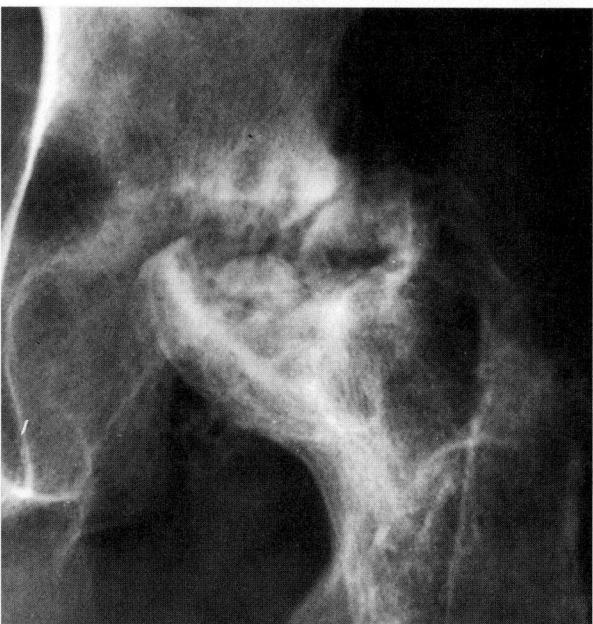

**Figure 67–18.** Post-traumatic osteonecrosis: basicervical fracture of the femoral head. A fracture of the base of the neck led to lateral subluxation of the femur and osteonecrosis of the femoral head associated with massive collapse.

## Humeral Head

The blood supply of the head of the humerus is derived from several major sources (Fig. 67–21). The vascular supply pierces the bony cortex just distal to the anatomic

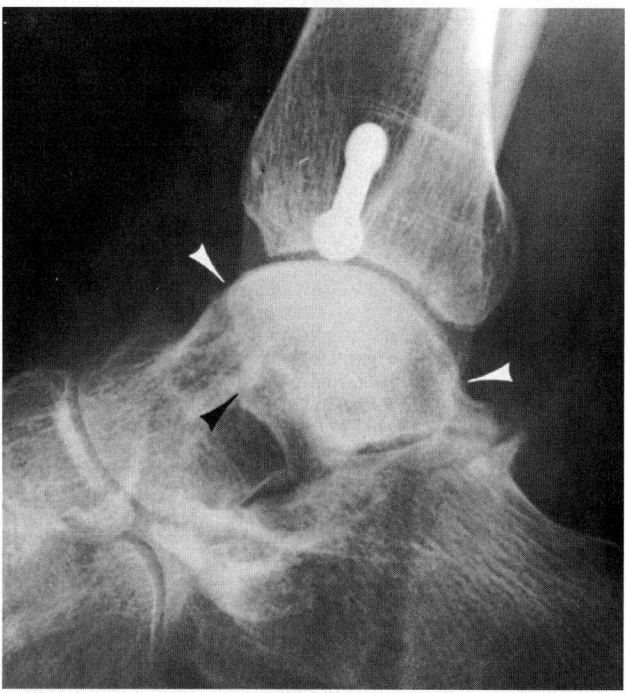

**Figure 67–19.** Post-traumatic osteonecrosis: talus. In this person who sustained a fracture of the body of the talus, as well as a fracture of the medial malleolus (which was transfixed with a screw), note the increased radiodensity of the proximal half of the bone *(arrowheads).*

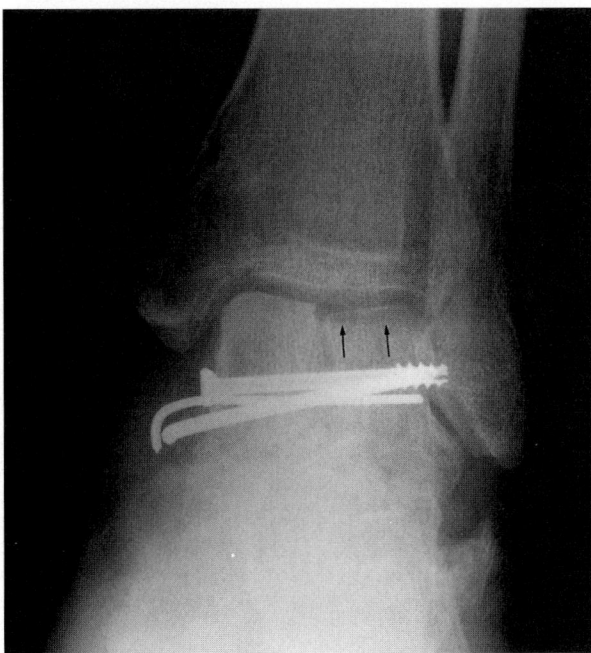

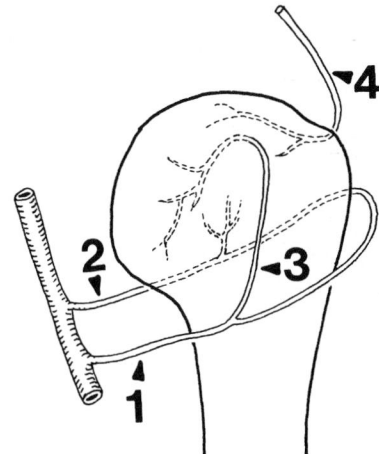

**Figure 67–21.** Humeral head: vascular supply. Vessels include the anterior circumflex humeral artery (1), posterior circumflex humeral artery (2), arcuate artery (3), and vessels of the rotator cuff (4). (After Graham J, Wood S: In Davidson JK [ed]: Aseptic Necrosis of Bone. New York, American Elsevier 1976, p 101.)

**Figure 67–20.** Post-traumatic osteonecrosis: talus. After reduction and internal fixation of a sagittally oriented fracture of the talus, osteopenia with Hawkins' sign (i.e., subchondral lucent line; [*arrows*]) is seen in the lateral portion of the bone, a finding that implies a good prognosis for this osseous segment. The medial portion of the talus is relatively radiodense, however.

neck. Osteonecrosis of the humeral head occurs if a fracture leads to loss of blood supply from both the muscular insertions and the arcuate branch of the anterior circumflex humeral artery; this complication may result after a displaced fracture of the anatomic neck or a severe frac-

ture or fracture-dislocation of the bone. The radiographic findings parallel those in the femoral head (Fig. 67–22).

## Scaphoid

Osteonecrosis of the proximal pole of the carpal scaphoid is a well-documented complication after injury to this bone. Osteonecrosis is most likely to occur when a scaphoid fracture involves the proximal pole of the bone; with more distal infractions, interruption of the blood supply is less constant or less severe. The reported frequency of this complication after scaphoid injuries

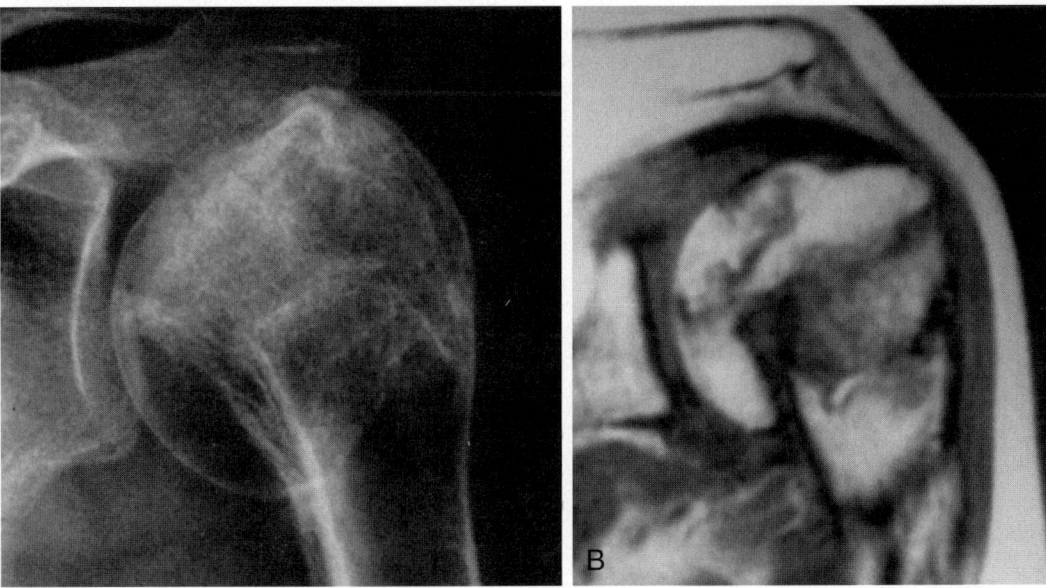

**Figure 67–22.** Post-traumatic osteonecrosis: humeral head. *A,* Although a fracture of the anatomic neck of the humerus has healed, observe the flattened and irregular humeral head, indicative of ischemic necrosis. *B,* In a different patient with a comminuted fracture of the proximal end of the humerus, note a large focus of osteonecrosis in the humeral head on an oblique coronal T1-weighted (TR/TE, 666/20) spin echo MR image. (*A,* Courtesy of J. Schils, MD, Cleveland, Ohio.)

varies with the nature and severity of the fracture or dislocation; a frequency of 11% to 65% has been noted, but 10% to 15% is the most common estimated frequency of this complication. The radiographic diagnosis depends on a relative increase in density of the devitalized portion of the scaphoid in comparison to the osteoporotic viable bone (Fig. 67–23), an appearance that is delayed for 4 to 8 weeks and may be associated with delayed union or nonunion of the fracture, collapse of the necrotic segment, and, eventually, secondary degenerative joint disease of the radiocarpal compartment of the wrist. MR imaging has also been used to diagnose osteonecrosis of the scaphoid (Fig. 67–24). Regions of low signal intensity in the marrow of the proximal pole of the scaphoid on T2-weighted spin echo MR images and, more importantly, the presence of such regions after the intravenous injection of a gadolinium-containing contrast agent are suggestive of osteonecrosis.

## Capitate

Ischemic necrosis of the capitate typically occurs after accidental or occupational trauma or recreational stress, as well as spontaneously in the absence of any type of

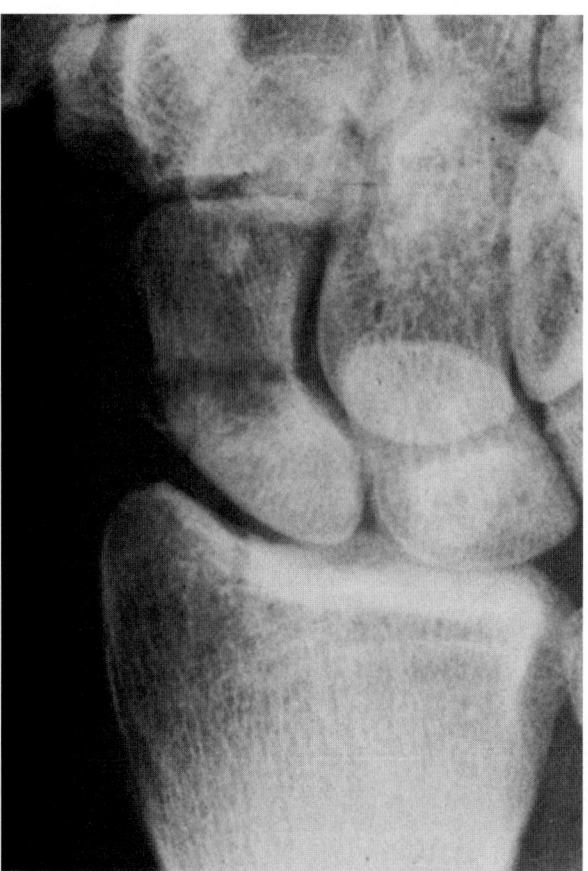

**Figure 67–23.** Post-traumatic osteonecrosis: carpal scaphoid. Radiograph obtained 8 weeks after traumatic scaphoid fracture shows increased radiodensity of the proximal half of the scaphoid, accentuated by osteoporosis of the distal half of the bone, indicative of the presence of osteonecrosis and reparative bone formation.

injury. The proximal pole of the capitate is the site of ischemic necrosis. Osteonecrosis of this bone is a recognized complication of a transscaphoid, transcapitate, perilunate fracture-dislocation (scaphocapitate syndrome).

## Vertebral Body

Delayed post-traumatic collapse of vertebral bodies is termed Kümmell's disease. Current evidence suggests that vertebral collapse occurs as a consequence of a vascular insult leading to secondary bone necrosis. The frequency of Kümmell's disease is not known, but it is probably not uncommon. Affected patients are generally middle-aged or elderly men or women. The interval between the acute traumatic episode and the vertebral collapse varies from days to years, and the lower thoracic and upper lumbar vertebral bodies are principally involved (Fig. 67–25). A gas collection within the collapsed vertebra may be seen (vacuum vertebral body), which may extend into the adjacent psoas musculature.

## Other Sites

After significant injury or prolonged stress, avascular necrosis can appear at other sites, especially when an osseous fragment loses its soft tissue attachments. Areas at risk include the lunate, other carpal bones, tarsal navicular bone, mandibular condyle, patella, femoral condyles, and even metatarsal and metacarpal heads.

## DYSBARIC OSTEONECROSIS

### General Features

Exposure to high-pressure environments occurs as a result of scuba diving, underwater and space exploration, and off-shore oil drilling. One late complication of such exposure is osteonecrosis, which has been designated dysbaric osteonecrosis, caisson disease, pressure-induced osteoarthropathy, and barotraumatic osteoarthropathy.

The term decompression sickness indicates the acute consequences of the liberation of gas bubbles, principally nitrogen, in the blood and tissues of a person who has undergone decompression too rapidly after a period of exposure to a hyperbaric environment. In a high-pressure environment, a person's blood and tissues are saturated with atmospheric gases, and after a rapid return to normal atmospheric pressure, the various gases come out of solution and produce supersaturation of tissues. Ventilation may allow dispersion of the excess oxygen and carbon dioxide, but the released nitrogen may produce bubbles within the vascular tree that act as air emboli. Nitrogen accumulation is greatest in tissues rich in fat, and the fatty marrow does not escape this accumulation.

The association of decompression sickness and dysbaric osteonecrosis is controversial, and in general, there appears to be a lack of correlation between these two conditions. Despite this dissociation of findings, however, it is generally assumed that gas bubbles initiate the manifestations of decompression sickness and that they are probably the cause of osteonecrosis as well. The frequency of dysbaric osteonecrosis appears to be exaggerated in patients with

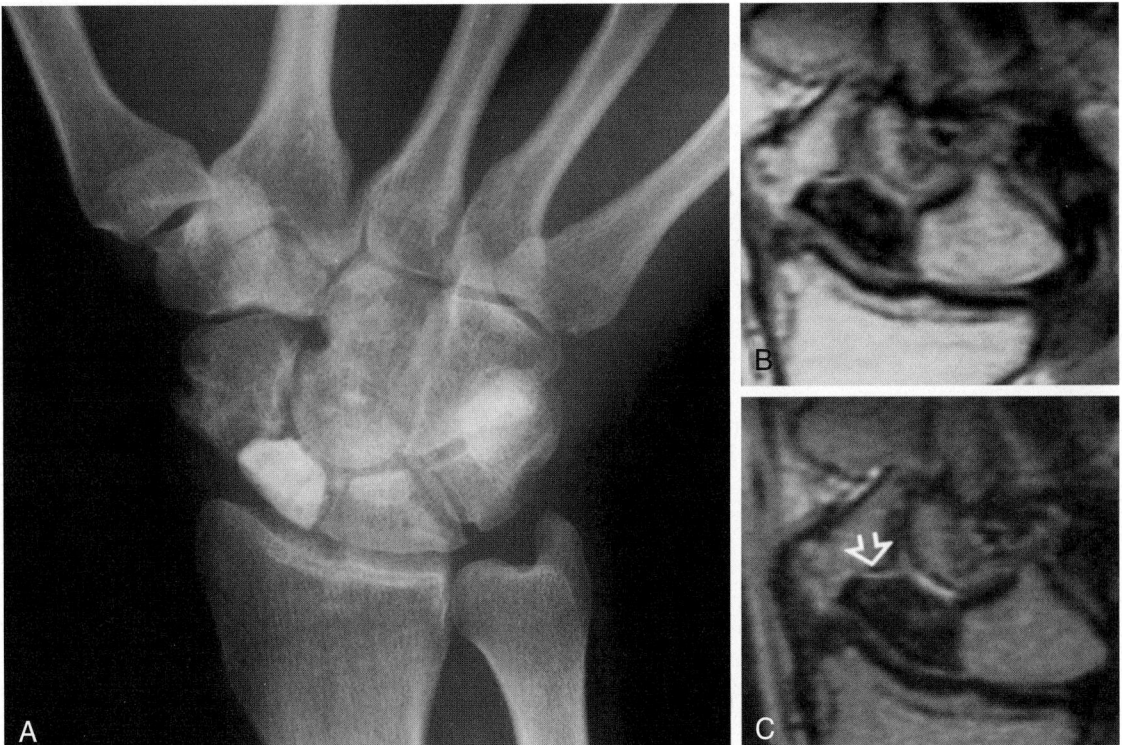

**Figure 67–24.** Post-traumatic osteonecrosis: carpal scaphoid. *A*, Routine radiography reveals typical features of osteonecrosis involving the proximal pole of the bone. No evidence of bone union is apparent at the fracture site in the midportion of the scaphoid bone. *B* and *C*, Coronal intermediate-weighted (TR/TE, 2500/30) *(B)* and T2-weighted (TR/TE, 2500/80) *(C)* spin echo MR images document the abnormally low signal intensity of the marrow in the proximal pole of the bone. In *(C)*, observe fluid in the midcarpal joint, with extension into the fracture gap *(arrow)*.

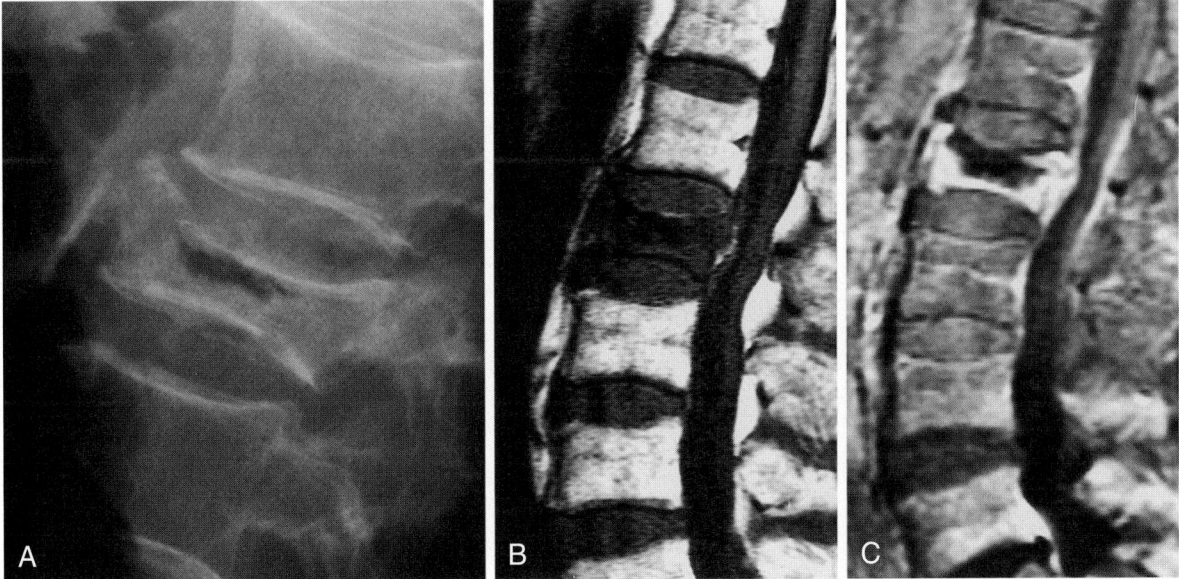

**Figure 67–25.** Post-traumatic osteonecrosis: vertebral body (Kümmell's disease). *A* to *C*, Delayed post-traumatic collapse of the second lumbar vertebral body developed in this 71-year-old man. *A*, Radiograph shows an intraosseous vacuum at this spinal level. *B*, In a sagittal T1-weighted (TR/TE, 300/13) spin echo MR image, low signal intensity is seen in this vertebral body. Narrowing of the spinal canal is evident. *C*, In a sagittal fat-suppressed T1-weighted (TR/TE, 450/11) spin echo MR image obtained after the intravenous administration of a gadolinium compound, low signal intensity persists in the central portion of the vertebral body (consistent with fluid or gas), with enhancement of other portions of the vertebral body. (Courtesy of G. Greenway, MD, Dallas.)

repeated exposure, exposure to greater pressures, a rapid rate of exposure, and obesity.

In compressed-air workers, the reported frequency of osseous lesions varies from almost 0% to 75%, with most estimates being in the range of 10% to 20%. It has been determined that 4 to 12 months usually elapses between the time of exposure and the appearance of any radiographic abnormality. The reported prevalence of osteonecrosis in divers also varies, although the occurrence rate may rise substantially in studies that include long-term follow-up examinations. In divers in the British Royal Navy, a low frequency (4%) has been noted. As in the case of compressed-air workers, a delay of at least 6 to 12 months is typical between divers' first exposure to increased atmospheric pressure and the onset of radiographically evident skeletal alterations.

## Radiographic Abnormalities

Radiographic abnormalities are typically divided into juxta-articular lesions (occurring most frequently in the head of the humerus and femur; Fig. 67–26) and diaphyseal and metaphyseal lesions (situated at a distance from the joint; Fig. 67–27). Juxta-articular alterations consist of radiodense areas between 3 and 20 mm in diameter that are slightly less discrete than bone islands (enostoses); spherical, segmental opaque areas that may eventually produce a "snow-capped" configuration; radiolucent subcortical bands (crescent sign), indicating a fracture of necrotic bone; and osseous collapse and fragmentation. Diaphyseal and metaphyseal abnormalities consist of indistinct, poorly defined radiodense foci; irregular calcified areas with a shell-like configuration; and, rarely, radiolucent lesions, perhaps resulting from sites of necrosis.

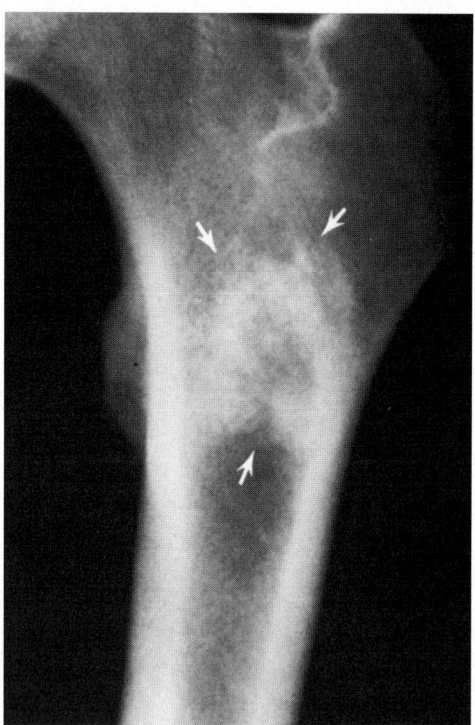

**Figure 67–27.** Dysbaric osteonecrosis: diametaphyseal lesions. In this 28-year-old male scuba diver, a patchy area of increased sclerosis is evident in the proximal femoral shaft *(arrows)*. Note the increased density of the periphery of the lesion. Biopsy with histologic evaluation indicated osseous and marrow necrosis compatible with an infarct.

Multiple or single, bilateral or unilateral alterations can be seen. The distal femoral shaft, humeral head, femoral head, and tibial shaft, in descending order of frequency, are the most typical sites of involvement. An infarct that is limited to the shaft of a tubular bone is not usually associated with clinical complaints; when involvement of an epiphysis leads to collapse of the articular surface, pain and swelling may become apparent.

## Differential Diagnosis

The radiographic findings associated with dysbaric osteonecrosis are generally indistinguishable from those associated with osteonecrosis of other causes such as sickle cell anemia, Gaucher's disease, and steroid medication. Small, dense foci in dysbaric osteonecrosis are virtually identical to bone islands, and only foci that are larger and more numerous may allow an accurate diagnosis of this condition.

## IATROGENIC OSTEONECROSIS

A number of iatrogenic factors can lead to single or multiple sites of osteonecrosis. Certain medications (e.g., corticosteroids) and irradiation are well known in this regard. One additional iatrogenic cause relates to the use of lasers for orthopedic applications such as meniscectomy and discectomy.

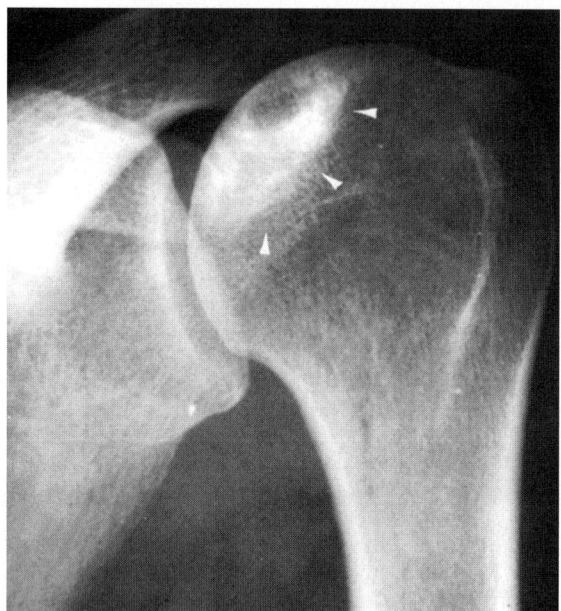

**Figure 67–26.** Dysbaric osteonecrosis: juxta-articular lesions. The sclerosis ("snow-capped" appearance) of the humeral head *(arrowheads)* is typical of dysbaric osteonecrosis but may be evident in other varieties of bone necrosis as well.

# IDIOPATHIC (PRIMARY OR SPONTANEOUS) OSTEONECROSIS

Osteonecrosis may appear in certain locations in the absence of any recognizable underlying disorder or event. Characteristically, the femoral head or femoral condyles are involved, although rarely, spontaneous osteonecrosis can appear at other sites.

## Spontaneous Osteonecrosis of the Femoral Head in Adults

Idiopathic, or spontaneous, osteonecrosis of the femoral head in adults, which is also designated Chandler's disease, affects men more frequently than women and is usually seen between the fourth and seventh decades of life. Unilateral or bilateral involvement may be detected. Despite the frequency of bilateral involvement, the condition usually first manifests as a unilateral symptomatic hip related to osseous collapse on the more severely affected side.

The radiographic features vary with the stage of the disorder. Initially, a femoral head of normal osseous contour may reveal mottled radiodense areas scattered throughout its anterosuperior region, with a faint curvilinear band of diminished density in the anterior subchondral bone (crescent sign). As the disease progresses, a focus of increased radiodensity or a lucent zone with a peripheral rim of increased radiodensity is observed.

A milder form of osteonecrosis of the femoral head, typically found contralateral to a femoral head with the classic features of ischemic necrosis, has been designated minimal or segmental osteonecrosis. This type of involvement is not progressive and affects the superficial zone of the femoral head, producing a wedge-shaped involved area that is related to vascular interruption at the wedge apex and a base situated on the articular surface (Fig. 67–28). The resulting radiographic findings are localized to a small portion of the femoral head but otherwise resemble those seen with more extensive osteonecrosis.

## Spontaneous Osteonecrosis about the Knee in Adults

This disorder, which is sometimes referred to as Ahlbäck's disease, is distinct from osteochondritis dissecans occurring in adolescence (Table 67–4). The cause and pathogenesis of this condition are not clear; however, the dominant opinion implicates vascular insufficiency leading to infarction of bone. It typically affects older patients, more frequently women. Onset occurs with abrupt pain

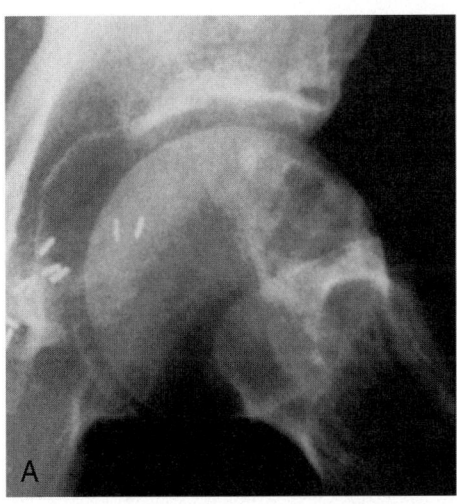 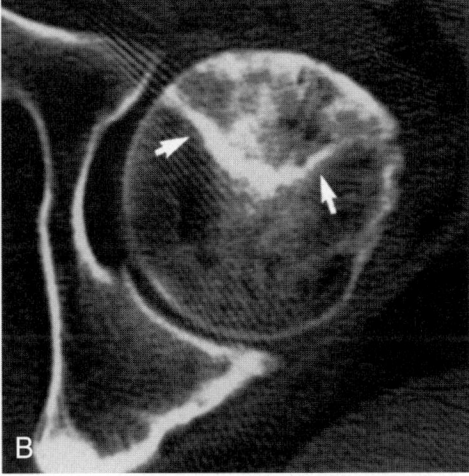

**Figure 67–28.** Spontaneous osteonecrosis of the femoral head: segmental type. *A*, In this 55-year-old man, a lobulated radiolucent lesion involves the anterior portion of the femoral head. No collapse of bone is evident. Surgical clips are seen. *B*, Transaxial CT scan shows a wedge-shaped lesion *(arrows)* with its base situated on the anterior femoral surface. Note the sclerotic margins of this osteonecrotic region.

**TABLE 67–4**

**Spontaneous Osteonecrosis versus Osteochondritis Dissecans (about the Knee)**

|  | Spontaneous Osteonecrosis | Osteochondritis Dissecans |
| --- | --- | --- |
| Age of onset | Middle-aged and elderly | Adolescent |
| Symptoms | Pain, tenderness, swelling, restricted motion | Variable; may be lacking |
| Typical location | Weight-bearing surface of medial femoral condyle | Non–weight-bearing surface of medial femoral condyle |
| Probable pathogenesis | Trauma, perhaps related to meniscal tear or vascular insult | Trauma |
| Sequelae | Degenerative joint disease, intra-articular osteocartilaginous bodies | Intra-articular osteocartilaginous bodies |

in the knee, almost always confined to the medial aspect of the joint. The pain is typically worse at night. Unilateral involvement predominates over bilateral involvement. Initially, radiographs are normal; after weeks or months have passed, a subtle flattening of the weight-bearing articular surface of the medial femoral condyle is seen. A radiolucent lesion in the condyle can be detected over the ensuing weeks; this lesion is initially diffuse and irregular in outline and then becomes more sharply demarcated. Within the lucent area, a radiodense line consisting of cartilage and subchondral bone plate can frequently be identified (Fig. 67–29).

If the affected area is small and weight bearing is avoided, spontaneous healing can occur. If untreated, however, further depression of the bony margin, intra-articular osseous bodies, progressive sclerosis, and periostitis of the distal portion of the femur may be encountered on later examination. Over a period of months or years, joint space narrowing, cyst formation, eburnation, and osteophytosis on apposing margins of the femur and tibia indicate the development of secondary osteoarthritis (Fig. 67–30). It has been speculated that a significant number of cases of degenerative joint disease of the knee have their origin in an ischemic event.

The precise distribution of the lesion about the knee is one of the most important characteristics of spontaneous osteonecrosis. In the vast majority of cases, the weight-bearing surface of the medial femoral condyle is involved. Spontaneous ischemic necrosis is occasionally observed in the medial portion of the tibial plateau or in the lateral femoral condyle, alone or in combination with changes in the medial condyle of the femur.

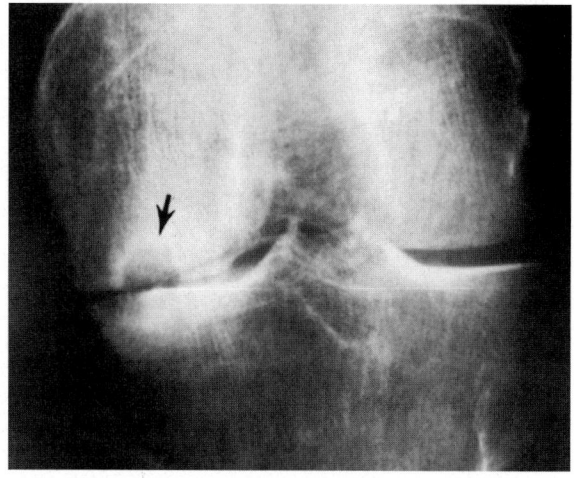

**Figure 67–30.** Spontaneous osteonecrosis about the knee: medial femoral condyle. In this patient, degenerative joint disease is superimposed on spontaneous osteonecrosis. Joint space narrowing and sclerosis are prominent. Although the appearance simulates that of uncomplicated osteoarthritis, the degree of bony flattening and the presence of cystic lesions (*arrow*) in the condyle suggest that osteonecrosis has occurred.

Scintigraphic examination using bone-seeking radio-pharmaceutical agents demonstrates focal accumulation of radionuclide long before radiographic changes appear (Fig. 67–31). MR imaging may also be used as a sensitive method in the diagnosis of spontaneous osteonecrosis about the knee (Fig. 67–32).

The other entities that enter into the differential diagnosis of spontaneous osteonecrosis about the knee are osteonecrosis from other causes, osteochondritis dissecans, calcium pyrophosphate dihydrate crystal deposition disease, transient osteoporosis, stress fracture, and neuropathic osteoarthropathy.

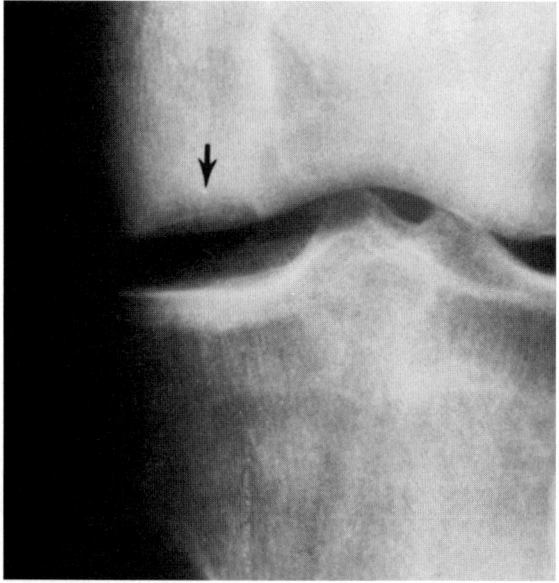

**Figure 67–29.** Spontaneous osteonecrosis about the knee: medial femoral condyle. This 60-year-old man had acute-onset knee pain that was associated with an effusion. No history of trauma could be elicited, and the patient had not received corticosteroids. Two years after the onset of pain, a radiograph reveals flattening of the weight-bearing surface of the medial femoral condyle associated with an osseous excavation (*arrow*) containing a linear radiodense shadow.

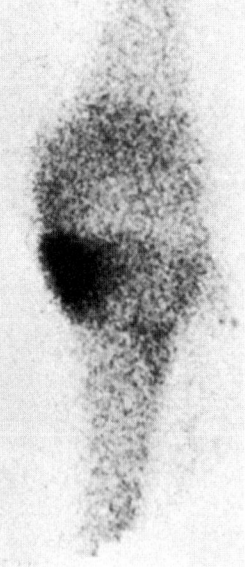

**Figure 67–31.** Spontaneous osteonecrosis about the knee: medial tibial plateau. Although the radiograph (not shown) was essentially normal, the increased accumulation of bone-seeking radionuclide in the medial aspect of the tibia is consistent with spontaneous osteonecrosis.

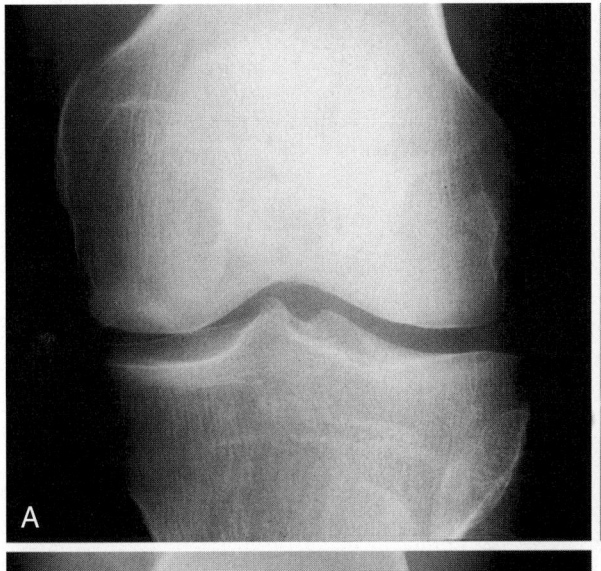

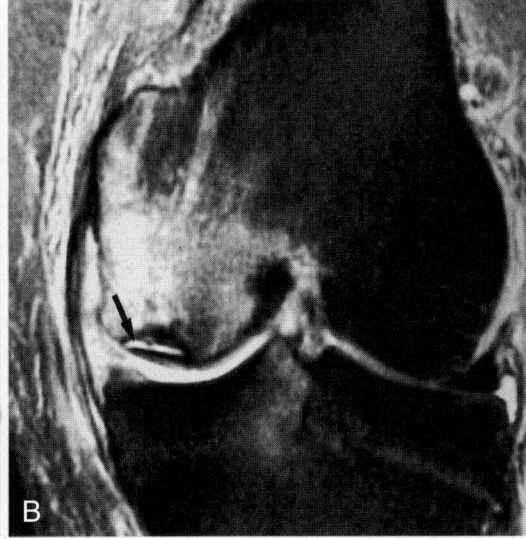

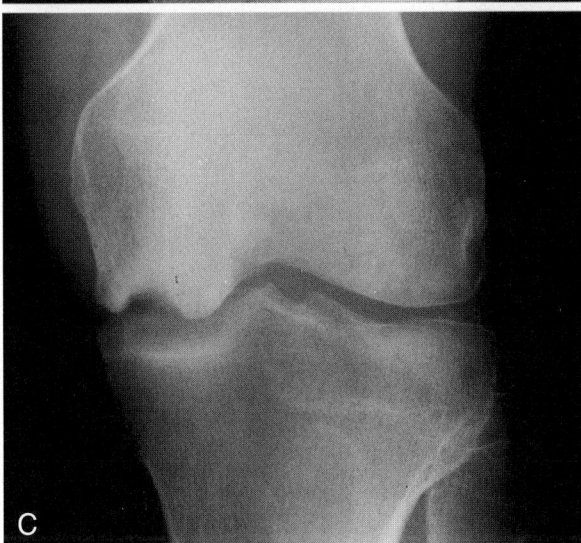

**Figure 67–32.** Spontaneous osteonecrosis about the knee: medial femoral condyle. *A,* Initial frontal radiograph of the knee shows flattening and increased radiodensity in the medial femoral condyle. *B,* One month later, coronal fat-suppressed fast spin echo (TR/TE, 3000/21) MR image shows a subchondral fracture containing fluid *(arrow)* in the medial femoral condyle. Note the surrounding marrow and soft tissue edema, a tear of the medial meniscus, loss of articular cartilage in the medial femorotibial compartment, and edema centrally in the tibia. *C,* Radiograph obtained 3 months after *(A)* shows progressive abnormalities in the medial femoral condyle.

## Spontaneous Osteonecrosis of the Tarsal Navicular Bone in Adults (Mueller-Weiss Syndrome)

Rarely, atraumatic osteonecrosis of the tarsal navicular bone occurs in adults, especially women. Radiographic characteristics include medial or dorsal protrusion of portions of the bone or the entire navicular bone and a comma-shaped deformity caused by collapse of the lateral portion of the bone. Bilateral distribution, asymmetrical involvement, and pathologic fractures represent additional findings in the disease. Also termed Mueller-Weiss syndrome, this form of osteonecrosis is distinct from the well-recognized osteochondrosis of the tarsal navicular bone occurring in children (Köhler's disease). Mueller-Weiss syndrome is a disorder of adults that is characterized by a chronic clinical course, severe and sometimes devastating pain and disability, and progressive deformity.

## COMPLICATIONS

### Cartilaginous Abnormalities

One of the striking pathologic features of osteonecrosis is the intactness of the chondral surface, despite the presence of adjacent severe osseous abnormality. It is also recognized that when osteonecrosis leads to significant collapse of the articular surface, incongruities of apposing bony margins may lead to secondary degenerative joint disease. In this situation, cartilaginous fibrillation and erosion may be revealed on radiographs as diminution of the interosseous space (Fig. 67–33).

### Intra-articular Osseous Bodies

Infrequently, one or more chondral or osteochondral fragments can appear in osteonecrosis. They may exist free in the articular cavity, in situ in the depressed bony area, or embedded in the synovium at a distant site.

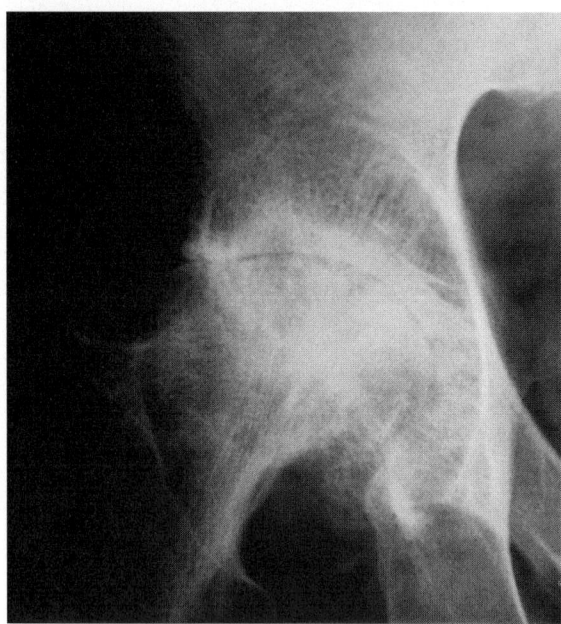

**Figure 67–33.** Osteonecrosis: complications—cartilaginous abnormalities. Radiograph obtained 6 years after collapse of the articular surface shows secondary osteoarthritis, with considerable narrowing of the joint space. In such cases, it is difficult to state with certainty that the changes represent osteoarthritis alone, unless a sequence of radiographs is available for examination.

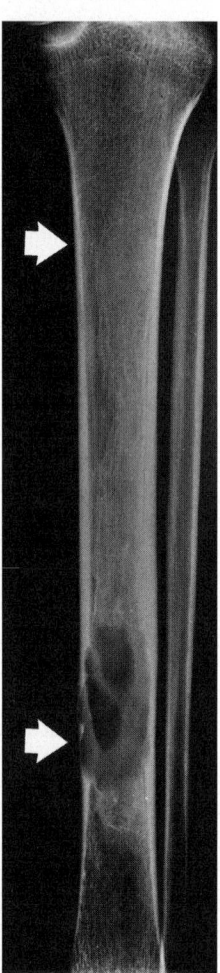

**Figure 67–34.** Osteonecrosis: complications—cyst formation. Observe a bone infarct *(upper arrow)* in the shaft of the tibia. A cystic area *(lower arrow)* has led to erosion of the endosteal margin of the cortex. (From Norman A, Steiner GC: Radiographic and morphological features of cyst formation in idiopathic bone infarction. Radiology 146:335, 1983.)

## Cyst Formation

Cystic degeneration in areas of bone infarction predominates in the diaphyses of tubular bones, especially the tibia (Fig. 67–34) and the humerus. An expanding osteolytic area that erodes the cortex is seen. As it evolves, the cyst becomes sharply marginated. This feature and the absence of cortical disruption suggest the correct diagnosis, although differentiation of a cyst and malignant degeneration of an osseous infarct may be difficult.

## Malignant Degeneration

Sarcoma arising in areas of bone infarction has been documented in both idiopathic cases and those related to caisson disease or other disorders. Men are affected more commonly, and the patient is usually in the fifth to seventh decade of life. Multiple bone infarcts are frequently present. Typically, the distal end of the femur (Fig. 67–35) or the proximal part of the tibia is the site of neoplasm, but other sites may be altered as well. The diametaphyseal portion of the bone is affected almost invariably. The malignant tumor is most often fibrosarcoma or malignant fibrous histiocytoma; more rarely, it is osteosarcoma, angiosarcoma, or pleomorphic sarcoma. It is suggested that these tumors arise from some of the cellular elements involved in the repair process.

There is a long latent period between bone infarction and malignant transformation. Although the prognosis in patients with bone infarction and sarcoma is guarded, and disseminated metastasis and death commonly occur within a short period, the data in no way justify surgical ablation of infarcts because of the apparent rarity of the complication. Radiographic diagnosis is not difficult, inasmuch as a soft tissue mass and osseous destruction appear at a site of obvious infarction. MR imaging may be another useful diagnostic method.

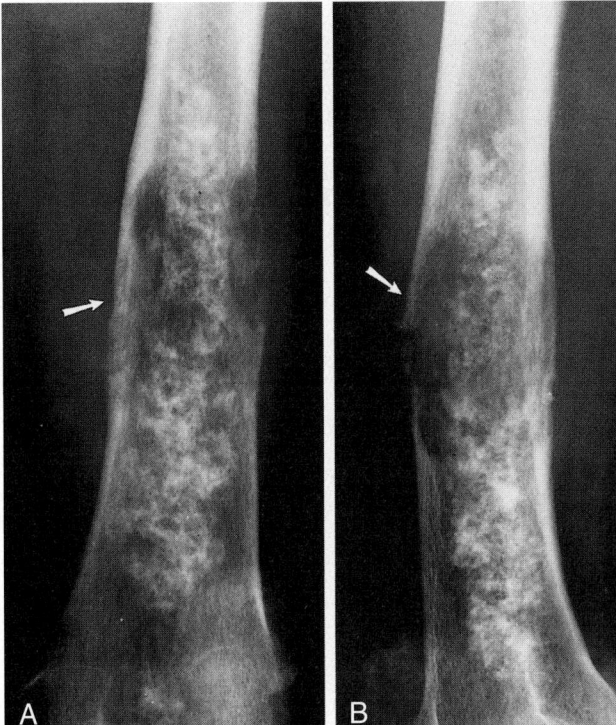

**Figure 67–35.** Osteonecrosis: complications—malignant transformation. In this 76-year-old woman with bone infarction, a fibrosarcoma developed at the site of bone necrosis in the femur. In addition to the typical calcification of a bone infarct, observe the osteolytic destruction *(arrows)*, with a pathologic fracture representing a fibrosarcoma. (Courtesy of V. Vint, MD, La Jolla, Calif.)

## FURTHER READING

Ahlbäck S, Bauer GCH, Bohne WH: Spontaneous osteonecrosis of the knee. Arthritis Rheum 11:705, 1968.

Barquet A: Natural history of avascular necrosis following traumatic hip dislocation in childhood: A review of 145 cases. Acta Orthop Scand 53:815, 1982.

Bell ALL, Edson GN, Hornick N: Characteristic bone and joint changes in compressed air workers: A survey of symptomless cases. Radiology 38:698, 1913.

Bjorkengren AG, AlRowaih A, Lindstrand A, et al: Spontaneous osteonecrosis of the knee: Value of MR imaging in determining prognosis. AJR Am J Roentgenol 154:331, 1990.

Brower AC, Downey EF Jr: Kümmell disease: Report of a case with serial radiographs. Radiology 141:363, 1981.

Burt RW, Matthews TJ: Aseptic necrosis of the knee: Bone scintigraphy. AJR Am J Roentgenol 138:571, 1982.

Catto M: A histological study of avascular necrosis of the femoral head after transcervical fracture. J Bone Joint Surg Br 47:749, 1965.

Davidson JK: Dysbaric osteonecrosis. In Davidson JK (ed): Aseptic Necrosis of Bone. Amsterdam, Excerpta Medica, 1976, p 147.

Davidson JK, Hanison JAB, Jacobs P, et al: The significance of bone islands, cystic areas and sclerotic areas in dysbaric osteonecrosis. Clin Radiol 28:381, 1977.

Dihlmann W: CT analysis of the upper end of the femur: The asterisk knee. Investigation by radionuclide scintimetry and radiography. J Bone Joint Surg Br 53:605, 1970.

Gelberman RH, Menon J: The vascularity of the scaphoid bone. J Hand Surg 5:508, 1980.

Glimcher MJ, Kenzora JE: The biology of osteonecrosis of the human femoral head and its clinical implications. II. The pathological changes in the femoral head as an organ and in the hip joint. Clin Orthop 139:283, 1979.

Gohel VK, Dalinka MK, Edeiken J: Ischemic necrosis of the femoral head simulating chondroblastoma. Radiology 107:545, 1973.

Haller J, Sartoris DJ, Resnick D, et al: Spontaneous osteonecrosis of the tarsal navicular in adults: Imaging findings. AJR Am J Roentgenol 151:355, 1988.

Houpt JB, Alpert B, Lotem M, et al: Spontaneous osteonecrosis of the medial tibial plateau. J Rheumatol 9:81, 1982.

Jaffe HL: Ischemic necrosis of bone. Med Radiogr Photogr 45:57, 1969.

Kim Y-M, Oh HC, Kim HJ: The pattern of bone marrow oedema on MRI in osteonecrosis of the femoral head. J Bone Joint Surg Br 82:837, 2000.

Lecouvet FE, Van de Berg BC, Maldague BE, et al: Early irreversible osteonecrosis versus transient lesions of the femoral condyles: Prognostic value of subchondral bone and marrow changes on MR imaging. AJR Am J Roentgenol 170:71, 1998.

Lotke PA, Ecker ML: Osteonecrosis-like syndrome of the medial tibial plateau. Clin Orthop 176:148, 1983.

Maldague BE, Noel HM, Malghem JJ: The intravertebral vacuum cleft: A sign of ischemic vertebral collapse. Radiology 129:23, 1978.

Mankin HJ, Brower TD: Bilateral idiopathic aseptic necrosis of the femur in adults: "Chandler's disease." Bull Hosp Joint Dis 23:42, 1962.

Martel W, Poznanski AK: The effect of traction on the hip in osteonecrosis: A comment on the "radiolucent crescent line." Radiology 94:505, 1970.

Mirra JM, Bullough PG, Marcove RC, et al: Malignant fibrous histiocytoma and osteosarcoma in association with bone infarcts: Report of four cases, two in caisson workers. J Bone Joint Surg Am 56:932, 1974.

Mitchell DG, Kressel HY, Arger PH, et al: Avascular necrosis of the femoral head: Morphologic assessment by MR imaging with CT correlation. Radiology 161:739, 1986.

Mitchell DG, Rao V, Dalinka M, et al: MRI of joint fluid in the normal and ischemic hip. AJR Am J Roentgenol 146:1215, 1986.

Mont MA, Baumgarten KM, Rifai A, et al: Atraumatic osteonecrosis of the knee. J Bone Joint Surg Am 82:1279, 2000.

Morris HD: Aseptic necrosis of the talus following injury. Orthop Clin North Am 5:177, 1974.

Mulfinger GL, Trueta J: The blood supply of the talus. J Bone Joint Surg Br 52:160, 1970.

Nellen JR, Kindwall EP: Aseptic necrosis of bone secondary to occupational exposure to compressed air: Roentgenologic findings in 59 cases. AJR Am J Roentgenol 115:512, 1972.

Norman A, Baker ND: Spontaneous osteonecrosis of the knee and medial meniscal tears. Radiology 129:653, 1978.

Norman A, Steiner GC: Radiographic and morphological features of cyst formation in idiopathic bone infarction. Radiology 146:335, 1983.

Ohta Y, Matsunaga H: Bone lesions in divers. J Bone Joint Surg Br 56:3, 1974.

Patterson RJ, Bickel WH, Dahlin DC: Idiopathic avascular necrosis of the head of the femur: A study of fifty-two cases. J Bone Joint Surg Am 46:267, 1964.

Saito S, Ohzono K, Ono K: Minimal osteonecrosis as a segmental infarct within the femoral head. Clin Orthop 231:35, 1988.

Shimizu K, Moriya H, Akita T, et al: Prediction of collapse with magnetic resonance imaging of avascular necrosis of the femoral head. J Bone Joint Surg Am 76:215, 1994.

Totty WG, Murphy WA, Ganz WI, et al: Magnetic resonance imaging of the normal and ischemic femoral head. AJR Am J Roentgenol 143:1273, 1984.

Vance RM, Gelberman RH, Evans EF: Scaphocapitate fractures. J Bone Joint Surg Am 62:271, 1980.

Vande Berg B, Malghem J, Labaisse MA, et al: Avascular necrosis of the hip: Comparison of contrast-enhanced and nonenhanced MR imaging with histologic correlation. Radiology 182:445, 1992.

Vogler JB III, Murphy WA: Bone marrow imaging. Radiology 168:679, 1988.

Williams JL, Cliff MM, Bonakdarpour A: Spontaneous osteonecrosis of the knee. Radiology 107:15, 1973.

# CHAPTER 68

## Osteochondroses

## SUMMARY OF KEY FEATURES

The osteochondroses are a heterogeneous group of disorders that are usually characterized by fragmentation and sclerosis of an epiphyseal or apophyseal center in an immature skeleton. Reossification and reconstitution of osseous contour may be evident in some cases. These disorders can be divided into three major categories: (1) conditions characterized by primary or secondary osteonecrosis; (2) conditions related to trauma or abnormal stress, without evidence of osteonecrosis; and (3) conditions that represent variations in normal patterns of ossification. In some cases, a definite pathogenesis cannot be identified.

## INTRODUCTION

The designation osteochondrosis has traditionally been used to describe a group of disorders that share certain features: a predilection for the immature skeleton; involvement of an epiphysis, apophysis, or epiphysioid bone; and a radiographic picture dominated by fragmentation, collapse, sclerosis, and, frequently, reossification with reconstitution of the osseous contour. The radiographic and pathologic features of the osteochondroses were initially interpreted as evidence of a primary impairment in local arterial supply that led to osteonecrosis. With further investigation of these disorders, it became apparent that the dissimilarities among them were considerable and that the osteochondroses were a heterogeneous group of unrelated lesions (Table 68–1). It is now recognized that osteonecrosis is not apparent on histologic examination in some of the osteochondroses, and in others, ischemic necrosis of bone is not a primary event but apparently follows a fracture or other traumatic insult. In fact, some of the osteochondroses are not disorders at all, but appear to represent variations in normal ossification.

Thus, it is important to put to rest the erroneous concept that the osteochondroses are a closely related group of disorders whose basic pathogenesis is vascular insufficiency with osteonecrosis. In this chapter, the osteochondroses are grouped according to their probable pathogenesis rather than their site of involvement.

## GENERAL CHARACTERISTICS

Many of the osteochondroses become apparent in the first decade of life, at a time when the developing bone still contains a cartilaginous model. Almost all these disorders are more frequent in boys than in girls. Although a single and unilateral distribution predominates, involvement of multiple and bilateral sites is not uncommon.

The concept that generalized factors may initiate or aggravate some of the osteochondroses is supported by numerous observations, including their occurrence in several members of a single family, in children who are below average in size and have a delay in skeletal maturation, and in those who have congenital anomalies. The importance of trauma as an initiating event or common pathway in most of these disorders cannot be denied.

Although the radiographic features of the osteochondroses have been well described and documented, interpretation of the changes in some of the syndromes is debated because of the irregularity in endochondral ossification at certain sites, such as the calcaneus and the tarsal navicular bone. Nevertheless, the identification of similar irregularities on radiographs of sites that normally ossify in a uniform fashion and the identification of necrosis, granulation tissue, disorderly ossification, bone absorption, and reparative osteogenesis on histologic inspection support the belief that some of the osteochondroses should not be regarded as variations of normal.

## DISORDERS CHARACTERIZED BY PRIMARY OR SECONDARY OSTEONECROSIS

### Legg-Calvé-Perthes Disease

**Clinical Abnormalities.** Legg-Calvé-Perthes disease affects children, particularly those between the ages of 4 and 8 years. The appearance of Legg-Calvé-Perthes disease in children younger than 4 years is usually associated with a good prognosis. The disorder is more frequent in boys than in girls, with a ratio of approximately 5:1. Either hip can be altered, and bilateral abnormalities are detected in about 10% to 20% of cases, though rarely in girls. When both hips are involved, they are usually affected successively, not simultaneously. Bilateral symmetrical fragmentation of the capital femoral epiphyses should suggest the presence of other diseases, such as hypothyroidism or sickle cell anemia. Legg-Calvé-Perthes disease is rare in blacks. A family history of the condition may be detected in approximately 6% of cases.

The principal clinical signs are limping, pain, and limitation of joint motion. Occasionally, radiographic changes are noted in patients who lack clinical abnormalities. A history of trauma is found in approximately 25% of cases, with an acute onset dating from the time of injury. These variable clinical manifestations represent a diagnostic challenge to a physician examining a child with a painful hip. The possibility of Legg-Calvé-Perthes disease must be considered in any child with acute manifestations in the hip, as well as in those with chronic hip complaints.

**Radiographic Abnormalities.** The radiographic abnormalities of Legg-Calvé-Perthes disease include the following (Fig. 68–1):

1. Soft tissue swelling on the lateral side of the articulation. Capsular bulging with displacement of the capsular fat pad relates to the accumulation of intra-articular fluid.

**TABLE 68–1**

## Osteochondroses

| Disorder | Site | Age (Yr) | Probable Mechanism |
|---|---|---|---|
| Legg-Calvé-Perthes disease | Femoral head | 4–8 | Osteonecrosis, perhaps from trauma |
| Freiberg's infraction | Metatarsal head | 13–18 | Osteonecrosis from trauma |
| Kienböck's disease | Carpal lunate | 20–40 | Osteonecrosis from trauma |
| Köhler's disease | Tarsal navicular | 3–7 | Osteonecrosis or altered sequence of ossification |
| Panner's disease | Capitulum of humerus | 5–10 | Osteonecrosis from trauma |
| Thiemann's disease | Phalanges of hand | 11–19 | Osteonecrosis, perhaps from trauma |
| Osgood-Schlatter disease | Tibial tuberosity | 11–15 | Trauma |
| Blount's disease | Proximal tibial epiphysis | 1–3 (infantile) 8–15 (adolescent) | Trauma |
| Scheuermann's disease | Discovertebral junction | 13–17 | Trauma |
| Sinding-Larsen-Johansson disease | Patella | 10–14 | Trauma |
| Sever's phenomenon | Calcaneus | 9–11 | Normal variation in ossification |
| Van Neck's phenomenon | Ischiopubic synchondrosis | 4–11 | Normal variation in ossification |

2. Smallness of the femoral ossification nucleus. A diminutive ossification center may be apparent in as many as 50% of patients. The pathogenesis of this finding is not clear, but it may represent an actual retardation of bone growth.

3. Lateral displacement of the femoral ossification nucleus. The ossific nucleus may be laterally displaced 2 to 5 mm, producing enlargement of the medial portion of the joint space. This change, which has been reported in as many as 85% of cases, may relate to synovitis with intra-articular fluid accumulation or cartilaginous hypertrophy.

4. Fissuring and fracture of the femoral ossific nucleus. This sign may be detected only on radiographs obtained in the frog-leg position. Linear or curvilinear radiolucent shadows are seen at the margin of the epiphysis, and the fracture fragment may remain in situ or be slightly displaced.

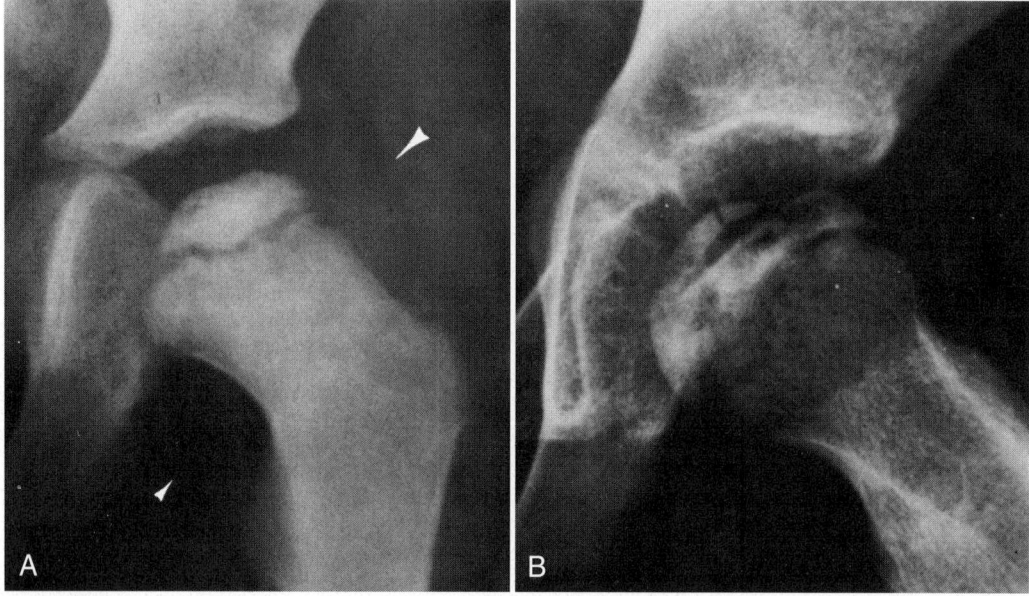

**Figure 68–1.** Legg-Calvé-Perthes disease: radiographic abnormalities. *A,* Early radiographic changes are demonstrated. Note soft tissue distortion *(arrowheads),* a sclerotic femoral ossification center that is laterally displaced and contains radiolucent fissures, and metaphyseal irregularity. *B,* In a different child, a frog-leg projection delineates the fragmented sclerotic femoral ossification center containing several radiolucent fissures.

5. Flattening and sclerosis of the femoral ossific nucleus. Flattening of the epiphyseal nucleus predominates near the fracture lines in the anterolateral superior segment of the femoral head. The frog-leg position is optimal for visualizing the degree of bone flattening. Mild to moderate sclerosis accompanies other radiographic signs of the disease, and on the anteroposterior view, the entire femoral head may appear radiodense.

6. Intraepiphyseal gas. A vacuum phenomenon caused by the release of gas into clefts and gaps in the subchondral trabeculae accentuates the exaggerated radiolucent appearance in this area. In most cases, however, this finding is not present.

7. Metaphyseal "cysts." Although the progression and extent of the disease are highly variable, further compression, disintegration, fragmentation, and sclerosis of the epiphysis may be seen, along with characteristic radiolucent lesions of the metaphysis (Fig. 68–2). The pathogenesis is debated, with some theories supporting osteonecrosis or a disturbance in endochondral bone formation.

8. Widening and shortening of the femoral neck. Widening and irregularity of the growth plate and broadening of the metaphysis are additional manifestations of this disorder. The greater trochanter may appear disproportionately large in comparison to the shortened femoral neck.

**Pathologic Abnormalities.** The fundamental pathologic aberration of the femoral head in this disease is osteonecrosis, accompanied by structural failure of the femoral head with resultant flattening and collapse. As in other varieties of osteonecrosis, the chondral surfaces are remarkably well preserved during the early and intermediate stages of Legg-Calvé-Perthes disease. Healing is characterized by revascularization of the necrotic portion of the femoral head.

**Course of the Disease.** The course of Legg-Calvé-Perthes disease is variable. The degree of reconstitution of the ossific nucleus and the ultimate shape of the femoral head depend on the amount of necrosis, its exact location, and the magnitude of forces across the joint. In some instances, the eventual radiographic appearance of the involved head may be indistinguishable from that of its uninvolved counterpart, whereas in others, coxa plana, shortening and widening of the femoral neck, osteochondroma-like lesions of the femoral neck, degenerative joint disease, and intraarticular osseous bodies may be identified (Fig. 68–3). A radiodense curvilinear shadow at the base of the femoral neck, termed the "sagging rope" sign, probably represents the radiodense shadow cast by the anterior or lateral edge of a severely deformed femoral head (Fig. 68–4).

In most cases of Legg-Calvé-Perthes disease, changes are isolated to or predominantly involve one hip. When bilateral abnormalities are encountered, symmetrical involvement is exceedingly rare, a feature that distinguishes Legg-Calvé-Perthes disease from other disorders that affect the hip. Although the chondral surface is relatively uninvolved in this disease, joint incongruity can lead to secondary osteoarthritis with cartilaginous fibrillation and erosion. A detached osteochondral fragment (osteochondritis dissecans) can be seen in this disease (Fig. 68–5). The reported frequency of this complication is approximately 2% to 4%, and it is observed almost exclusively in male patients.

**Classification and Prognosis.** The variable course of Legg-Calvé-Perthes disease has stimulated investigation into the predictive value of certain radiographic or clinical signs in determining the eventual outcome of the disorder.

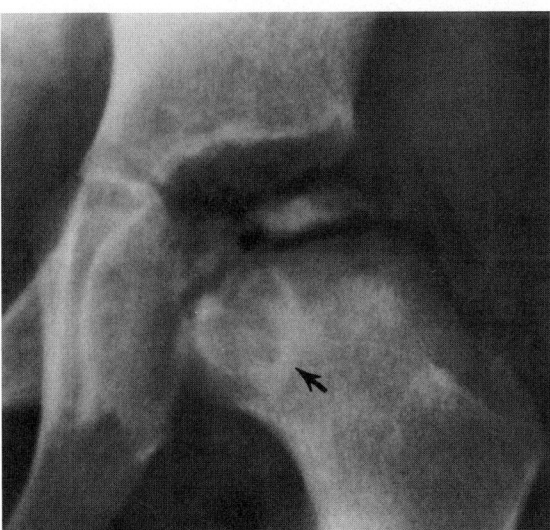

**Figure 68–2.** Legg-Calvé-Perthes disease: metaphyseal "cysts." Observe the large cystic lesion of the medial metaphysis of the femur *(arrow)*, which is associated with a fragmented, sclerotic, and laterally placed ossific nucleus.

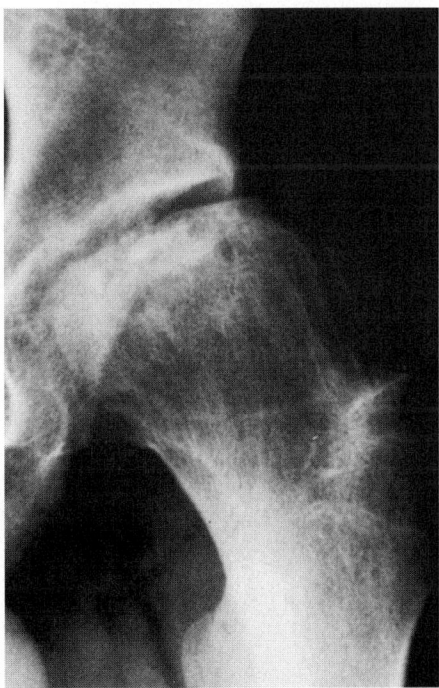

**Figure 68–3.** Legg-Calvé-Perthes disease: coxa plana and coxa magna. Note residual flattening and enlargement of the femoral head, with surface irregularity and widening of the femoral neck. The acetabulum is mildly flattened.

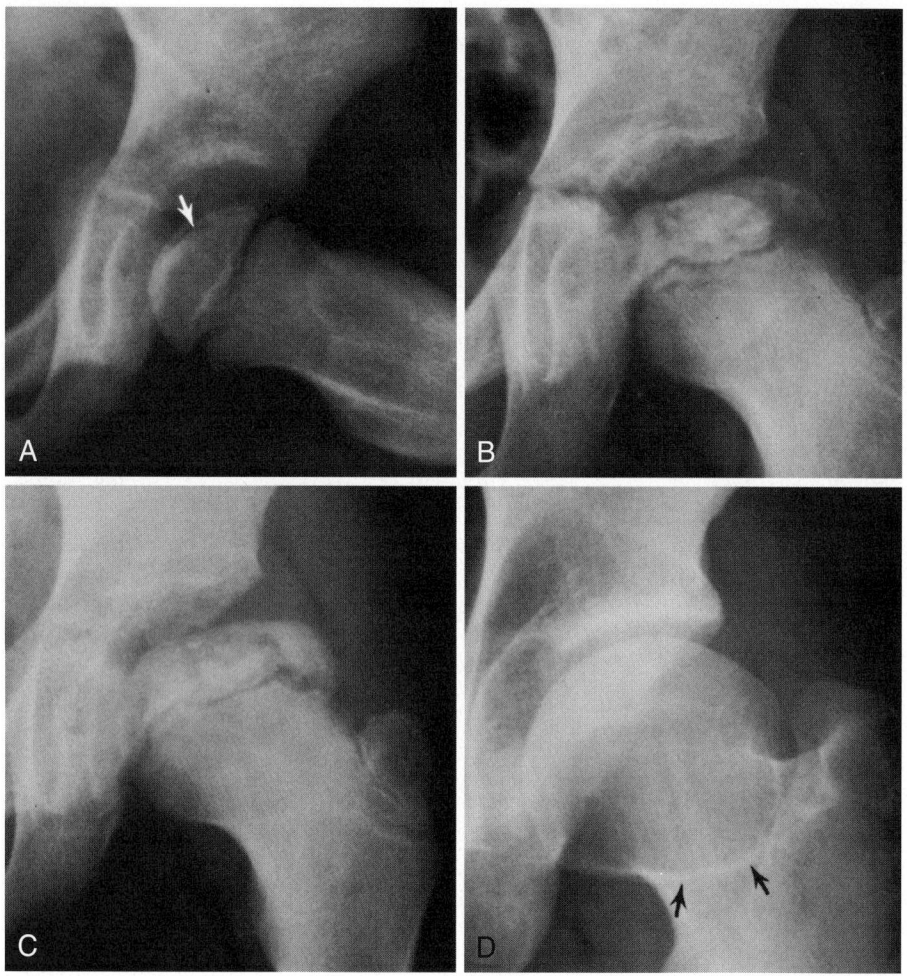

**Figure 68–4.** Legg-Calvé-Perthes disease: "sagging rope" sign. Sequential radiographs of the left hip indicate the course of the disease over a 16-year period. *A*, Age 7 years (phase of disease onset). On this frog-leg view, note the radiolucent crescent sign *(arrow)*. *B*, Age 8 years (phase of fragmentation). The lateral two thirds of the femoral head is collapsed and fragmented, and the lateral portion of the head is not covered by the acetabulum. *C*, Age 9 years (phase of healing). The medial aspect of the epiphysis is larger, and the amount of bone that is present laterally has increased. The femoral head is not completely covered. *D*, Age 22 years (residual phase). The femoral head is slightly flattened and large. Note the radiodense curved line—the sagging rope sign *(arrows)*. (Courtesy of P. VanderStoep, MD, Saint Cloud, Minn.)

In general, a better prognosis is observed in boys and in younger patients (younger than 5 or 6 years), perhaps indicating that a longer elapsed time before skeletal maturity allows more extensive remodeling and healing of the femoral head. Other prognostic signs relate to the extent of epiphyseal involvement, and the disease can be separated into four groups on the basis of this involvement (Table 68–2):

Group I. The anterior part of the epiphysis is the only affected site, and collapse and sequestration are not evident. Metaphyseal changes are unusual but may occur in later stages. Radiographically, the course of the disease is characterized by absorption of the involved segment, followed by regeneration commencing from the periphery.

Group II. Greater involvement is apparent. Collapse and sequestration are followed by absorption and healing.

Group III. Only a small portion of the epiphysis is not sequestered. Anteroposterior radiographs reveal a "head-within-a-head" appearance, and collapse of a centrally placed sequestrum can be identified. Subsequent broadening of the femoral neck is common. The course of the disease is similar to that in group II, although the metaphyseal changes are more generalized.

Group IV. The whole epiphysis is affected. Total collapse may be associated with metaphyseal changes.

The purpose of this classification system is to identify the degree of epiphyseal involvement and to relate this involvement to the prognosis of the disease. In general, patients in groups III and IV have a relatively poor prognosis, whereas those in groups I and II do better. These generalizations are not without exception, however. An additional limitation of this classification system is the difficulty in recognizing which pattern is present in the early phase of the disease; some patients initially placed in one category shift to another group on follow-up radiography.

Early radiographic changes useful to indicate a capital femoral epiphysis at risk for collapse include (1) Gage's sign (a small, osteoporotic segment that forms a transradiant V on the lateral side of the epiphysis), (2) calcification lateral to the epiphysis (reflecting the presence of extruded cartilage), (3) lateral subluxation of the femoral head, and (4) a transverse physeal line.

It is clear that no single radiographic observation is indicative of a good or poor result and that a combination of findings must be used for prognostic accuracy. Most patients are symptom free 30 to 40 years after diagnosis, although persistent radiographic alterations are usually evident. A mild limp, leg shortening, and pain can be seen.

**Other Diagnostic Methods.** Arthrography may be used in the evaluation of Legg-Calvé-Perthes disease. In the early

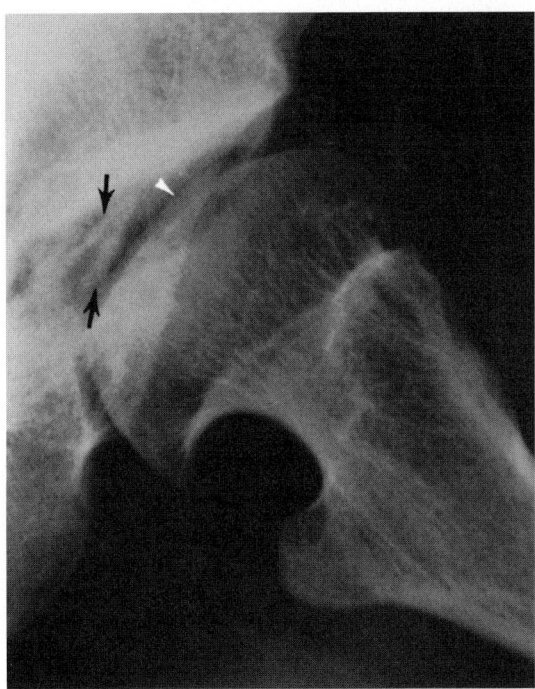

**Figure 68–5.** Legg-Calvé-Perthes disease: osteochondral fragment. Frog-leg view reveals a flattened femoral head, acetabular deformity, and an osseous body *(arrows)* within the joint, highlighted by the spontaneous release of gas into the articulation. The presence of gas also permits the identification of a thinned cartilaginous surface *(arrowhead)*.

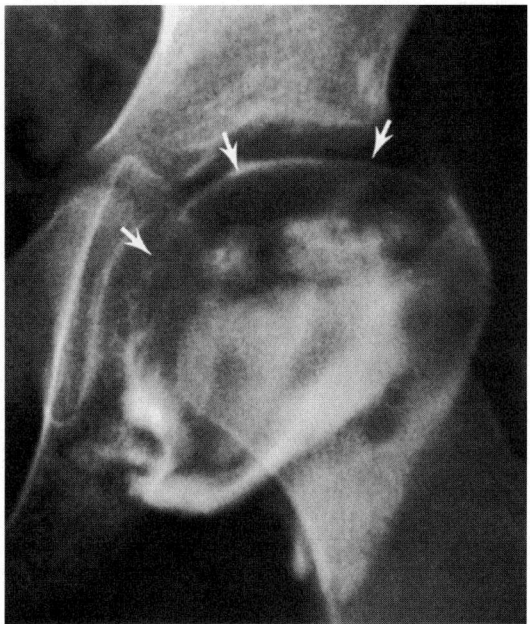

**Figure 68–6.** Legg-Calvé-Perthes disease: arthrographic abnormalities. Arthrogram reveals a relatively smooth cartilaginous surface *(arrows)*, despite the presence of extensive ossific irregularity. Some thickening of the medial chondral surface of the femoral head is apparent. (Courtesy of T. Goergen, MD, Escondido, Calif.)

stages, contrast opacification of the joint can reveal subtle flattening of the chondral surface at the site of osseous fissuring and an increase in width of both the femoral and the acetabular cartilage. In later stages, arthrography frequently indicates a smooth cartilaginous surface, despite the presence of considerable ossific fragmentation (Fig. 68–6).

Radionuclide examination with bone-seeking radiopharmaceutical agents allows the identification of areas of deficient uptake in the early phase of the disease caused by varying degrees of impairment in the blood supply. The scintigraphic abnormality, especially if flow and static images are obtained, antedates the radiographic alterations (Fig. 68–7).

Ultrasonography has been used to define the presence of an effusion and joint space widening in the hips of patients with transient synovitis of the hip or Legg-Calvé-Perthes disease. Ultrasonography has also been used to define the extent of deformity of the femoral head in Legg-Calvé-Perthes disease and may define cartilage thickening in this disease.

Magnetic resonance (MR) imaging has been used to identify infarction of the femoral head in Legg-Calvé-Perthes disease (Fig. 68–8). The MR imaging characteristics of osteonecrosis in this disease, as in other causes of osteonecrosis, are variable and are addressed in Chapter 67. In Legg-Calvé-Perthes disease, information provided by MR imaging, such as the extent of femoral head infarction, the presence or absence of viable regions of the femoral head, and the degree of involvement, if any, of the growth plate, influences the staging of the process and, ultimately, its prognosis. Added benefits of MR imaging include the availability of gadolinium enhancement tech-

**TABLE 68–2**

**Grades of Femoral Involvement in Legg-Calvé-Perthes Disease (Catterall Classification)**

|  | Grade | | | |
|---|---|---|---|---|
|  | *I* | *II* | *III* | *IV* |
| Site of epiphyseal involvement | Anterior part | Anterior part | Almost whole epiphysis | Whole epiphysis |
| Sequestrum | No | Yes | Yes | Yes |
| Crescent sign | No | Anterior | Anterior and extends posteriorly | Anterior and posterior |
| Collapse | No | Yes | Yes | Yes |
| Metaphyseal abnormalities | No | Localized | Diffuse | Diffuse |

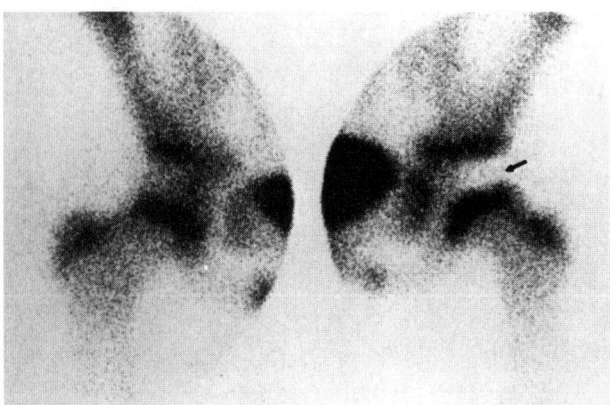

**Figure 68–7.** Legg-Calvé-Perthes disease: radionuclide abnormalities. In this 9-year-old boy, note the characteristic "cold" area *(arrow)* in the left femoral head on the bone scan. The opposite hip is normal. (Courtesy of V. Vint, MD, San Diego, Calif.)

niques for early diagnosis and manual positioning of the hip in an open-magnet configuration for demonstration of articular congruency and femoral head deformity and containment.

**Cause and Pathogenesis.** It is generally held that vascular insufficiency in the femoral head triggers the radiographic and pathologic findings of Legg-Calvé-Perthes disease, although the factors leading to the deficient blood supply have not been precisely identified. Some investigators favor a traumatic cause in which direct compression of the femoral head by the adjacent acetabular roof leads to the characteristic radiographic features of the disease, including fracture, flattening, and sclerosis.

The role of synovitis and raised intra-articular pressure in the pathogenesis of Legg-Calvé-Perthes disease has also been emphasized. Legg-Calvé-Perthes disease has been identified in as many as 12% of patients with transient synovitis of the hip. Obliteration of the blood supply to the femoral head may cause vascular compression from the accumulation of intra-articular fluid. Finally, the delayed skeletal maturation of children with this disease and the reported higher frequency of congenital anomalies in extraskeletal sites suggest to some investigators that genetic and developmental factors are important.

**Differential Diagnosis.** Fragmentation and collapse of the femoral head can be seen in hypothyroidism and in osteonecrosis from other causes (Table 68–3). The appearance of femoral head necrosis in a black patient should lead to hemoglobin analysis before the changes are ascribed to Legg-Calvé-Perthes disease. Similarly, bilateral symmetrical alterations should be interpreted cautiously, because they are uncommon in Legg-Calvé-Perthes disease but may be evident in hypothyroidism, sickle cell anemia, Gaucher's disease, and multiple epiphyseal and spondyloepiphyseal dysplasias.

Meyer's dysplasia of the femoral head (dysplasia epiphysealis capita femoris) is characterized by retarded skeletal maturation, mild or absent clinical signs, and femoral bony nuclei that appear late and are small and granular. The abnormal femoral head epiphyses are usually apparent by age 2 years; they are gradually transformed over the ensuing 2 to 4 years by growth, coalescing into enlarging, normal-appearing ossification centers. Sclerosis and metaphyseal changes are not evident in Meyer's dysplasia, and bilaterality is seen in almost 50% of cases. The earlier age of onset, bilateral nature of the changes, absence of prominent radiographic abnormalities, and lack of progression allow the differentiation of Meyer's dysplasia and Legg-Calvé-Perthes disease.

## Freiberg's Infraction

In 1914, Freiberg described a series of patients with metatarsalgia in whom the metatarsal head appeared to

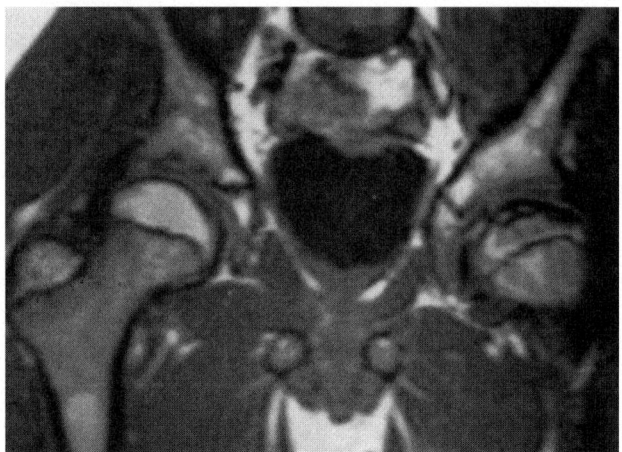

**Figure 68–8.** Legg-Calvé-Perthes disease: MR imaging abnormalities. In this 14-year-old boy, a coronal T1-weighted (TR/TE, 600/20) spin echo MR image reveals evidence of osteonecrosis of the left femoral head. The ossified portion of the capital epiphysis is flattened and contains superior and lateral regions of abnormal signal intensity. The cartilage surface, of intermediate signal intensity, appears more congruent. The acetabulum is slightly flattened. The opposite hip is normal.

### TABLE 68–3

**Causes of Femoral Head Irregularity and Collapse in Infants and Children**

| Disease | Distribution |
| --- | --- |
| Legg-Calvé-Perthes disease | Unilateral or bilateral |
| Meyer's dysplasia | Unilateral or bilateral |
| Hypothyroidism | Bilateral |
| Epiphyseal dysplasia | Bilateral |
| Spondyloepiphyseal dysplasia | Bilateral |
| Sickle cell anemia | Unilateral or bilateral |
| Gaucher's disease | Unilateral or bilateral |
| Infection | Unilateral |
| Eosinophilic granuloma | Unilateral |
| Hemophilia | Unilateral or bilateral |

be crushed or collapsed, and he termed the condition an infraction of bone. The head of the second metatarsal is typically involved, although it is now recognized that the third and fourth metatarsal heads can also be affected. Unilateral changes are characteristic, although bilateral involvement and alterations of more than one digit can be encountered (Fig. 68–9). The disease is usually seen in adolescents (especially girls) between the ages of 13 and 18 years. Clinical features consist of local pain, tenderness, swelling, and limitation of motion of the corresponding metatarsophalangeal joint.

The radiographic features of Freiberg's infraction are virtually pathognomonic. Initial radiographic abnormalities include subtle flattening, increased radiodensity, and cystic lucent lesions of the metatarsal head and widening of the metatarsophalangeal articulation; subsequently, an osteochondral fragment with progressive flattening and sclerosis of the metatarsal head, and periostitis with increased cortical thickening of the adjacent metaphysis and diaphysis of the bone, may be seen (Fig. 68–10). Premature closure of the growth plate, intra-articular osseous bodies, deformity and enlargement of the metatarsal head, and secondary degenerative joint disease are recognized complications of the process. The nearby phalangeal base may enlarge and appear irregular. Increased accumulation of bone-seeking radiopharmaceutical agents is evident in the abnormal sites, and MR imaging reveals abnormalities in osseous contour and alterations of signal intensity in the bone marrow (Fig. 68–11).

The prevailing opinion suggests that single or multiple episodes of trauma represent the primary event in Freiberg's infraction. The high rate of occurrence in women could conceivably be related to the wearing of high-heeled shoes, which creates increased stress on the second metatarsal bone. Repeated injury at this site may lead to disruption of articular cartilage, ischemic necrosis of subchondral bone, compression fracture, collapse, and fragmentation.

## Kienböck's Disease

Also termed lunatomalacia, this peculiar affliction of the carpal lunate was described by Kienböck in 1910. Kienböck's disease is most commonly observed in patients

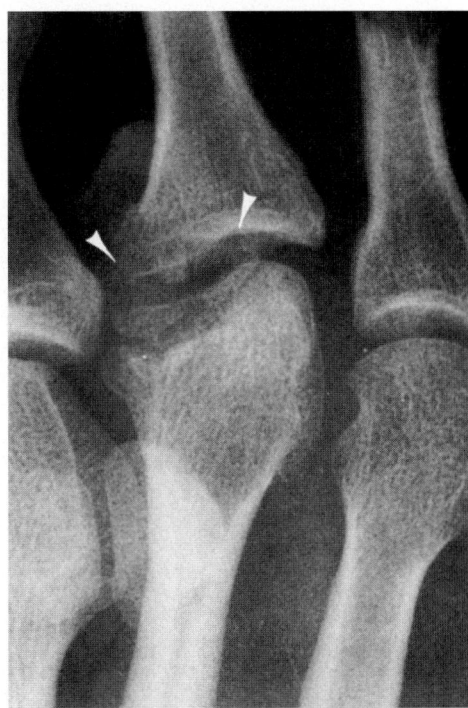

**Figure 68–10.** Freiberg's infraction: late radiographic abnormalities. A loose body had been removed from the second metatarsophalangeal joint 2 years before this evaluation. Note the flattened metatarsal head with two osteochondral fragments *(arrowheads)*, osteophytosis, joint space narrowing, and widening of the phalangeal base.

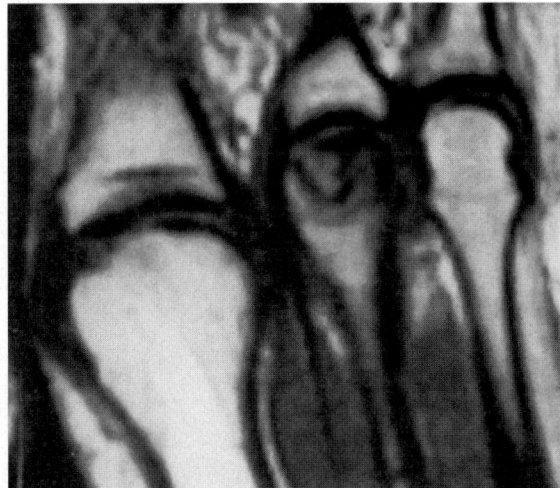

**Figure 68–11.** Freiberg's infraction: MR imaging abnormalities. This 14-year-old girl had pain and tenderness about the second metatarsophalangeal joint of the left foot. On this T1-weighted (TR/TE, 600/20) spin echo MR image obtained in the plantar plane, abnormal signal intensity is observed in the head of the second metatarsal bone. A serpentine region of low signal intensity outlines the area of necrosis, which contains tissue whose signal intensity is identical to that of marrow fat. Surrounding bone marrow edema is characterized by intermediate signal intensity, and an effusion has led to distention of the joint capsule.

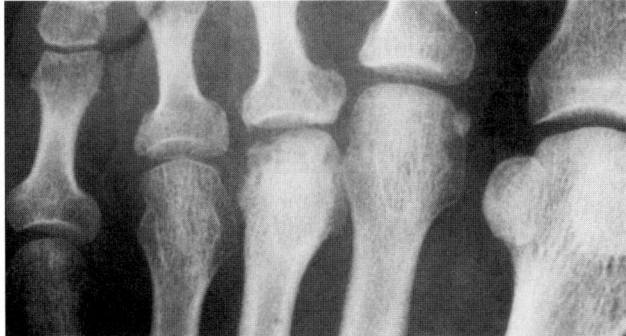

**Figure 68–9.** Freiberg's infraction: radiographic abnormalities. Note the sclerosis and collapse of the third metatarsal head, with narrowing of the adjacent metatarsophalangeal joint. Equivocal increased density of the second metatarsal head is present as well. Adjacent phalangeal new bone formation is seen.

between the ages of 20 and 40 years, and it has a predilection for the right hand. A history of trauma may be elicited but is not a constant feature. Progressive pain, swelling, and disability may be apparent.

Radiographic changes are distinctive. Initially, the lunate may have normal architecture and density, but a linear or compression fracture can be delineated. Subsequently, increased density of the lunate bone relative to the other carpal bones is noted, followed by evidence of altered shape and diminished size of the bone (Fig. 68–12). Eventually, the entire lunate may collapse and fragment. Complications include disruption of carpal architecture, scapholunate dissociation, and secondary degenerative joint disease.

The cause of this condition is not clear. Certain anatomic and biomechanical features of the lunate may predispose this bone to injury and subsequent osteonecrosis. These features include a vulnerable blood supply and a fixed position in the wrist, resulting in substantial forces of various degrees that may be greater than those on neighboring carpal bones. Mechanical forces may be accentuated by the presence of a short ulna (ulnar minus, or negative ulnar, variant), a finding seen in up to 75% of cases (Fig. 68–13).

MR imaging is more sensitive than radiography and, possibly, bone scintigraphy in the detection of Kienböck's disease. MR imaging patterns of abnormality and signal characteristics in Kienböck's disease are variable, as they are in osteonecrosis in other locations (Fig. 68–14). Morphologic evidence of this disease, including fracture, collapse, and fragmentation of the lunate, can be delineated with MR imaging in a manner similar to that permitted by other tomographic methods, including conventional and computed tomography. Equally important, MR imaging appears to be an effective method for eliminating this diagnosis in some patients with wrist symptoms and, in such cases, may provide evidence of an alternative disease process. Osteonecrosis of the lunate may, however, occur

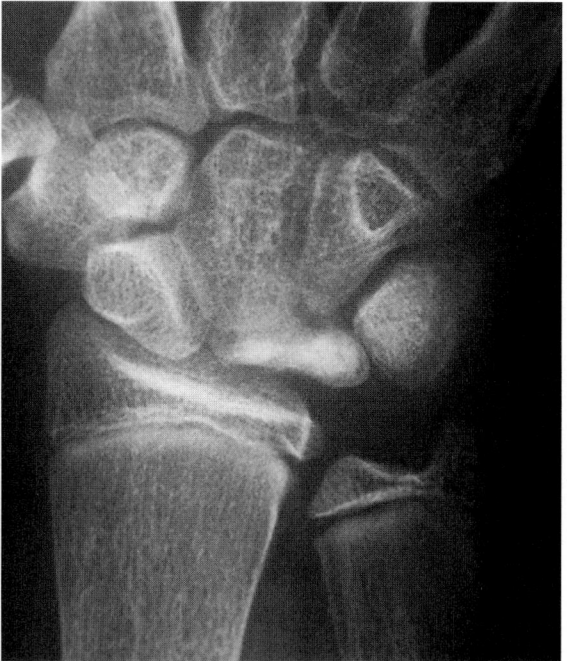

**Figure 68–13.** Kienböck's disease. A collapsed and sclerotic lunate bone is seen in this 12-year-old girl. Although the ulna appears short, determination of ulnar variance in an immature skeleton is difficult.

in association with complex injuries of the wrist, including lunate dislocations, and, rarely, as a consequence of corticosteroid therapy.

## Köhler's Disease

Köhler's disease is a self-limited condition of the tarsal navicular characterized by flattening, sclerosis, and irregular

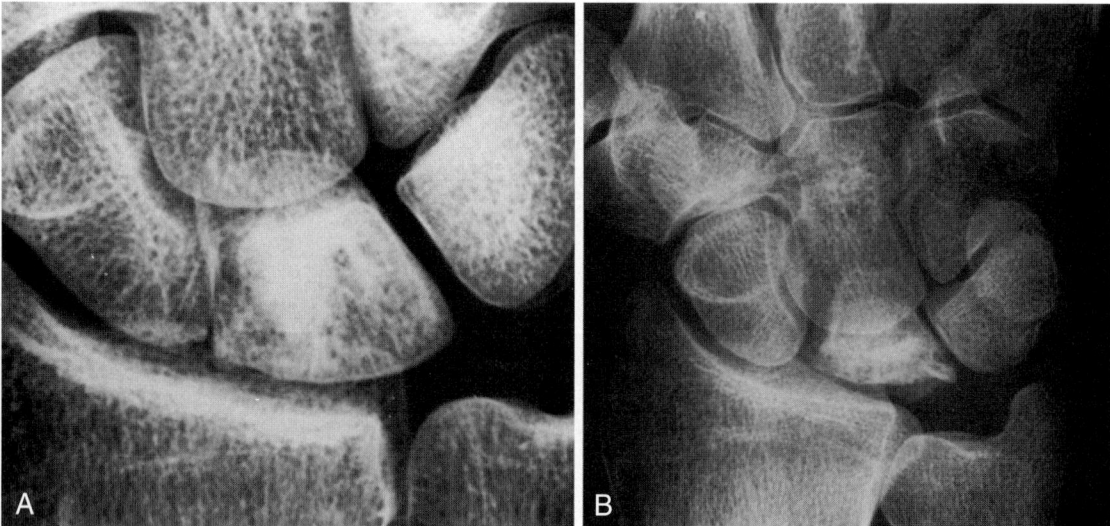

**Figure 68–12.** Kienböck's disease. *A,* Magnification radiograph demonstrates patchy increased density of the lunate, without alterations in the shape of the bone. *B,* In a different patient, observe the collapse of a sclerotic lunate bone. The ulna is shortened (ulna minus variant).

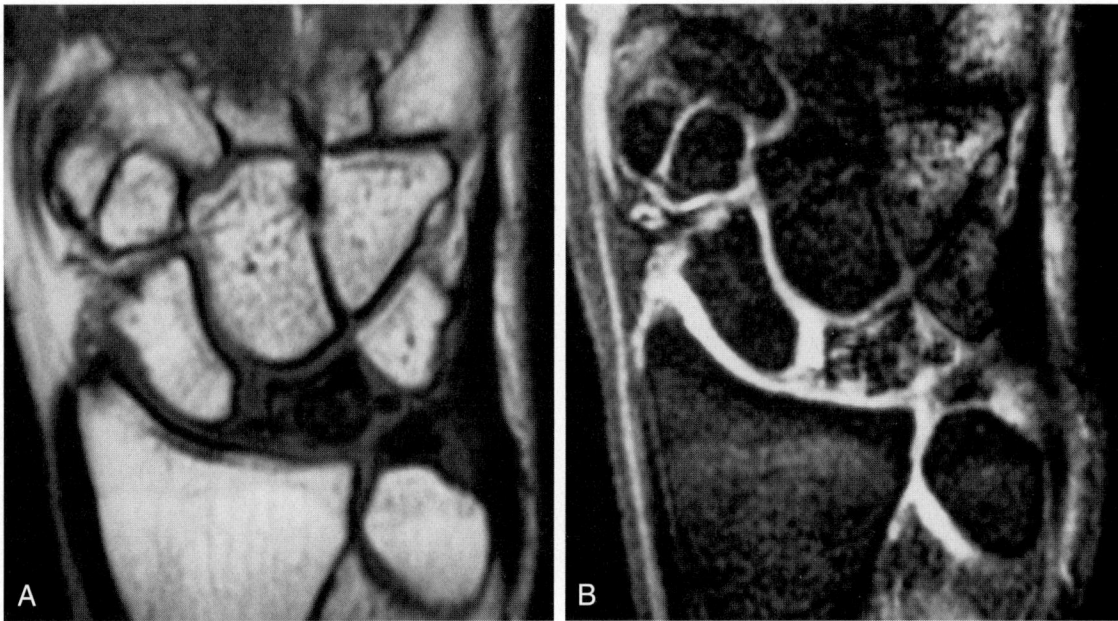

**Figure 68–14.** Kienböck's disease: MR imaging abnormalities. *A*, In this 43-year-old woman, a coronal T1-weighted (TR/TE, 600/15) spin echo MR image shows diffuse low signal intensity in the lunate. Note the scapholunate dissociation. *B*, Coronal gradient echo (TR/TE, 600/15; flip angle, 35 degrees) MR image reveals patchy high signal intensity in the lunate, disruption of the scapholunate interosseous ligament, disruption of the radial aspect of the triangular fibrocartilage, and effusions in the radiocarpal, midcarpal, and inferior radioulnar joints.

rarefaction. It is relatively rare, although its exact frequency is difficult to determine because it is impossible to distinguish its radiographic abnormalities from those that occur as a normal variation of growth. This disorder is discussed here because the predominant theory of its pathogenesis is still one of vascular insufficiency.

The disorder is more frequent in boys, and complaints are most commonly observed between the ages of 3 and 7 years. Unilateral involvement is evident in approximately 75% to 80% of cases. Clinical manifestations may be quite mild and consist of local pain, tenderness, swelling, and decreased range of motion.

Radiographs at an early stage can reveal a patchy increase in density, nodularity, and fragmentation with multiple ossific nuclei. Soft tissue swelling may be evident. The bone may be diminished in size and flattened or wafer-like in appearance, yet the interosseous space between the navicular and neighboring bones may be normal and indicate integrity of the chondral surface (Fig. 68–15). Over a period of 2 to 4 years, the bone may regain its normal size, density, and trabecular structure. Long-term follow-up assessment of adults who had Köhler's disease as children generally reveals an absence of clinical or radiographic sequelae.

The self-limited and reversible nature of the process has led to speculation that the "disease" is actually an altered sequence of tarsal ossification. This apparent overlap with normal patterns of ossification leads to considerable diagnostic difficulty, and two criteria must be used in establishing the presence of Köhler's disease: (1) changes are detected in a previously normal navicular bone, and (2) alterations consisting of resorption and reossification must be compatible with those of osteonecrosis. Further,

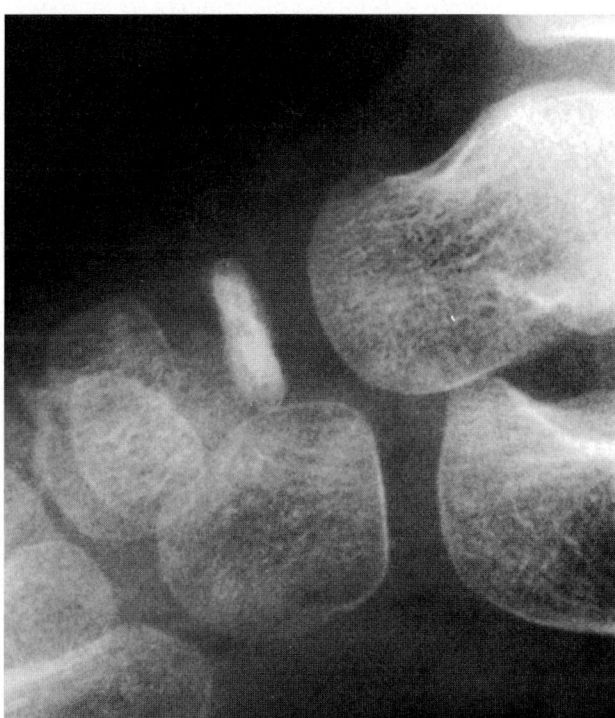

**Figure 68–15.** Köhler's disease. In this 4-year-old boy, a wafer-like radiodense tarsal navicular bone is identified. The neighboring joint spaces are not diminished in width.

clinical manifestations should be present if the diagnosis is to be considered seriously. MR imaging confirms irregular ossification of the developing navicular bone (Fig. 68–16).

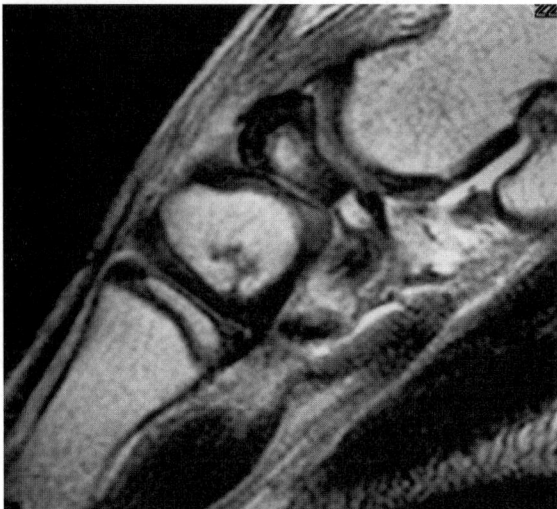

**Figure 68–16.** Köhler's disease: MR imaging abnormalities. Sagittal T2-weighted (TR/TE, 3000/96) spin echo MR image in a 7-year-old boy shows an irregular shape of the navicular bone, which is also inhomogeneous in signal intensity. (Courtesy of A. D'Abreu, MD, Porto Alegre, Brazil.)

## Panner's Disease

Panner's disease, or osteochondrosis of the capitulum of the humerus, is a rare disorder that usually appears between the ages of 5 and 10 years. Boys are affected almost exclusively, and the condition is commonly linked to a history of trauma. It is sometimes termed "Little Leaguer's elbow" because of its frequency in young baseball pitchers. Bilateral involvement is rare. Clinical manifestations are typically mild, and complete recovery is frequent. Pain and stiffness with restricted range of motion of the elbow are seen.

Radiographs reveal fissuring and increased density of the capitulum, decreased size and condensation of bone with an increase in the radiohumeral space, fragmentation, and resorption (Fig. 68–17). Subsequent regeneration and reconstitution of the capitulum are observed, and in most cases, no residual deformity or disability is seen. Hyperemia can lead to abnormal skeletal maturation of the radial head. The disease is differentiated from osteochondritis dissecans of the elbow principally on the basis of the age of the patient. Osteochondritis dissecans typically occurs in adolescents or adults, at a time when ossification of the capitulum is complete.

## Thiemann's Disease

Thiemann's disease is characterized by progressive enlargement of the proximal interphalangeal joints of the fingers, an onset in the second decade of life, and a predilection for boys. Some reports indicate that the principal clinical manifestations of this disease are painless swelling of the proximal interphalangeal articulations, digital shortening, and deformity. Thiemann's disease is familial, probably transmitted as a dominant trait with virtually complete penetrance.

Radiographs reveal irregularity of the epiphyses of the phalanges, especially in the middle fingers. The epiphyses

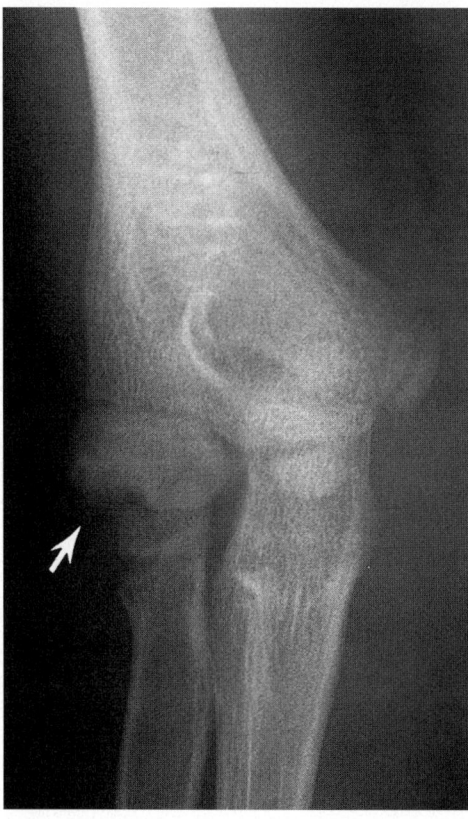

**Figure 68–17.** Panner's disease. Findings include fissuring and fragmentation of the capitulum (*arrow*) and deformity of the adjacent radial head in this child with elbow pain and swelling. (Courtesy of V. Vint, MD, La Jolla, Calif.)

appear sclerotic and fragmented and may contain medial and lateral osseous excrescences (Fig. 68–18). Eventually, the joint space becomes narrowed, the base of the phalanx thickens, and phalangeal shortening is seen (Fig. 68–19).

The differential diagnosis of the phalangeal alterations of Thiemann's disease includes trauma, infection, thermal injury, and juvenile chronic arthritis.

## DISORDERS RELATED TO TRAUMA OR ABNORMAL STRESS WITHOUT EVIDENCE OF OSTEONECROSIS

### Osgood-Schlatter Disease

Osgood-Schlatter disease occurs in adolescents, usually between the ages of 11 and 15 years. Boys are affected more frequently than girls, and a history of participation in sports and a rapid growth spurt before the onset of symptoms and signs are typical. Although the disease is generally unilateral in distribution, bilateral alterations are detected in approximately 25% of cases. Clinically, patients usually have local pain and tenderness of variable severity. Soft tissue swelling and firm masses can be palpated in the involved region, but no synovial effusion is present in the knee.

Initial radiographic abnormalities include soft tissue swelling in front of the tuberosity, resulting from edema of the skin and subcutaneous tissue (Fig. 68–20). The

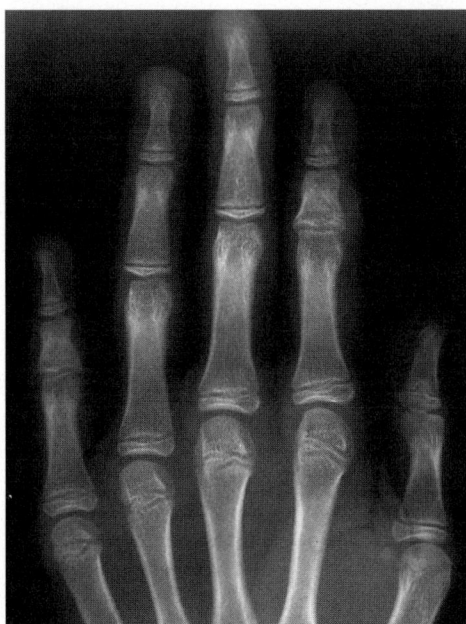

**Figure 68–18.** Thiemann's disease. Radiograph of the hand shows physeal closure and shortened middle phalanges in the second and fifth fingers. The opposite side was similarly affected.

margins of the patellar tendon may be indistinct. Three or 4 weeks later, single or multiple ossific collections in the avulsed fragment become evident (Fig. 68–21). After the acute stage, soft tissue swelling diminishes, and displaced pieces of bone may increase in size or may reunite

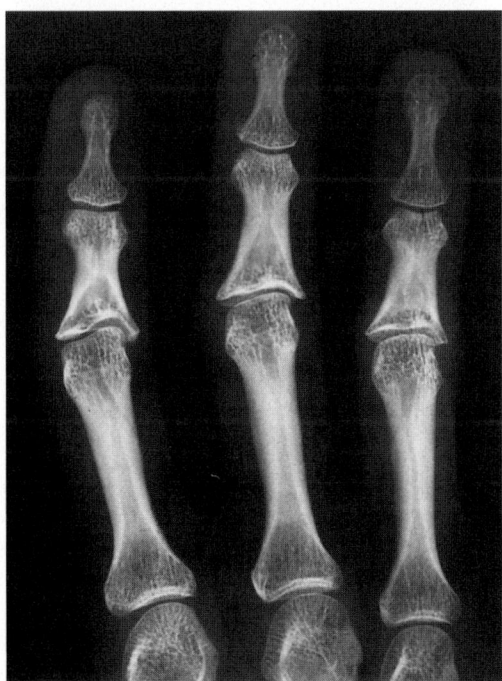

**Figure 68–19.** Thiemann's disease. Residual deformities are seen in this adult. They include shortening of the middle phalanges, broadening of the bases of these phalanges, and narrowing of the interphalangeal joints. The opposite hand was similarly involved. (Courtesy of B. Howard, MD, Charlotte, N.C.)

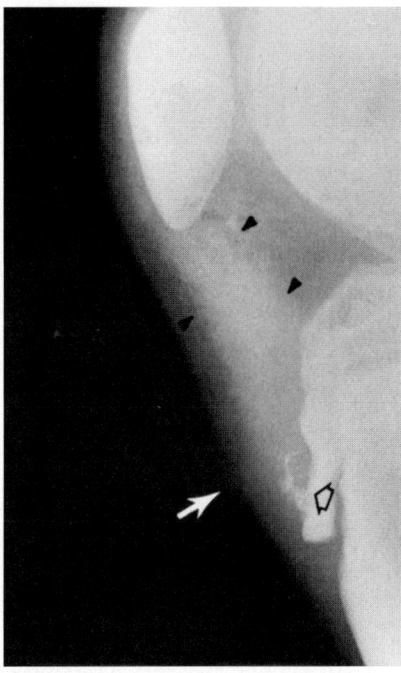

**Figure 68–20.** Osgood-Schlatter disease: soft tissue abnormalities. Low-kilovolt radiography indicates soft tissue edema over the tibial tuberosity *(solid arrow)*. Note the indistinctness of the infrapatellar tendon *(arrowheads)* and osseous irregularity of the tuberosity *(open arrow)*. (Courtesy of J. Weston, MD, Lower Hutt, New Zealand.)

with one another and with the underlying tibial tuberosity. MR imaging may reveal evidence of patellar tendinosis, with an abnormally large tendon demonstrating signal inhomogeneity, as well as evidence of deep infrapatellar bursitis (Fig. 68–22).

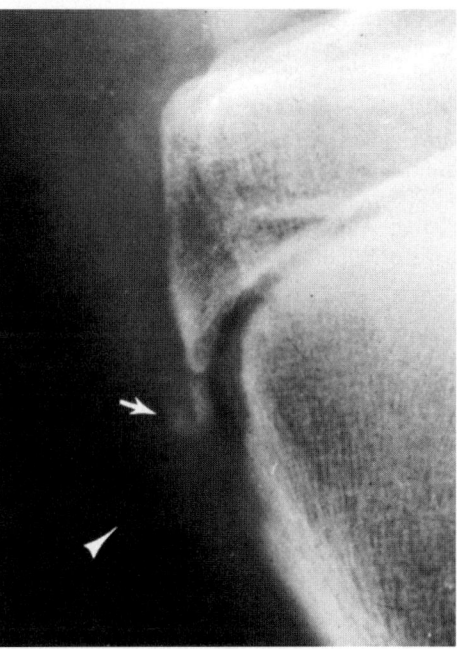

**Figure 68–21.** Osgood-Schlatter disease: osseous abnormalities. Observe the soft tissue swelling *(arrowhead)* and an avulsed osseous fragment of the tibial tuberosity *(arrow)*.

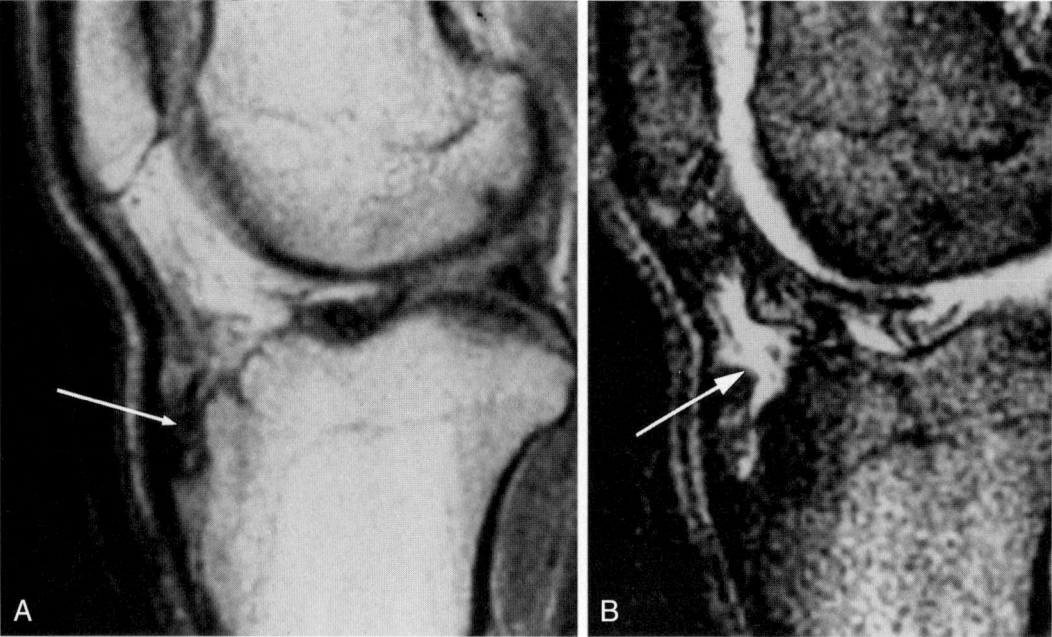

**Figure 68–22.** Osgood-Schlatter disease: MR imaging abnormalities. *A,* Sagittal T1-weighted (TR/TE, 850/25) spin echo MR image demonstrates fragmentation and irregularity of the tibial tuberosity at the insertion site of the patellar tendon *(arrow). B,* On a sagittal gradient echo (TR/TE, 750/20; flip angle, 45 degrees) MR image, note the joint effusion and fluid *(arrow)* in the deep infrapatellar bursa adjacent to the site of fragmentation of the tuberosity.

A fragmented tuberosity can occur in other conditions and, in the absence of current or previous symptoms, may indicate only a normal ossification pattern. Soft tissue swelling is fundamental to the radiographic diagnosis of Osgood-Schlatter disease. In the past, Osgood-Schlatter disease was considered by some investigators to be a type of osteonecrosis. More recent studies, however, indicate that the tibial tuberosity possesses an excellent blood supply and that the pathologic findings in this condition are most consistent with traumatically induced disruption somewhere along the site of attachment of the patellar tendon to the tibial tuberosity. The appearance of fragmentation of the inferior pole of the patella in some patients with Osgood-Schlatter disease supports the concept of a traumatic insult, as does evidence of patellar tendinosis provided by MR imaging.

### Blount's Disease

Blount's disease, also called tibia vara or osteochondrosis deformans tibiae, is a local disturbance in growth of the medial aspect of the proximal tibial epiphysis. The condition is generally classified into two types: an infantile type in which deformity is noted in the first few years of life, and an adolescent type in which deformity appears between the ages of 8 and 15 years (Table 68–4). The infantile type is approximately five to eight times more frequent than the adolescent variety. Recently, the classification of tibia vara has been modified and expanded to include a third and fourth type—late-onset tibia vara, which typically appears in obese black children between the ages of 6 and 13 years, and focal fibrocartilaginous

dysplasia, which leads to abnormalities that may simulate those of classic Blount's disease.

**Infantile Tibia Vara.** Infantile tibia vara appears to develop when normal physiologic bowing persists rather than progressively changes to a straight leg or slight valgus position; it worsens once a growing child becomes heavier and begins to put weight on the knee joint. Additional mechanical factors that may contribute to infantile tibia vara include excessive body weight and abnormal articular laxity, but these factors are not present consistently. Altered mechanical forces in the proximal end of the tibia

**TABLE 68–4**

**Infantile versus Adolescent Tibia Vara**

|  | Infantile | Adolescent |
|---|---|---|
| Age of onset | 1–3 yr | 8–15 yr |
| Distribution | Bilateral: 50–75% | Unilateral: 90% |
| Clinical findings | Obesity | Normal body weight |
|  | Absent pain, tenderness | Pain and tenderness |
|  | Prominent deformity | Mild deformity |
|  | Slight leg shortening | Moderate, severe leg shortening |
| Cause or pathogenesis | Trauma | Trauma |
|  | Growth arrest or dysplasia | Growth arrest |

from various primary causes can increase the mobility of the tibia on the femur and result in a change in direction of weight-bearing forces on the upper tibial epiphysis from perpendicular to oblique. This obliquity tends to displace the tibial epiphysis in a lateral direction, with subsequent overloading of the mediodorsal segment of the bone. Histologic examination confirms the absence of changes attributable to infection or osteonecrosis. The microscopic findings are consistent with the effects of persistent abnormal pressure on the growth plate.

Clinically, progressive bilateral (60%) or unilateral (40%) bowing of the leg during the first year of life is difficult to differentiate from physiologic changes. The tibia may be angulated acutely inward just below the knee. Pain is not evident. Associated findings are obesity, shortening of the leg, tibial torsion, and pronated feet.

Radiographic abnormalities are seldom evident before age 2 years. They simulate those of physiologic bowing but are more severe and can be unilateral or asymmetrical in distribution. Further, altered alignment in Blount's disease occurs in the proximal portion of the tibia, not between the femur and tibia, as occurs in physiologic bowing. In Blount's disease, the tibia is in a varus position because of angulation of the metaphysis, and the tibial shaft is adducted without intrinsic curvature. A depressed medial tibial metaphysis with an osseous excrescence, or outgrowth, is seen. Six stages have been recognized on radiographs (Figs. 68–23 and 68–24):

Stage I (2 to 3 years). A progressive increase in the degree of varus deformity of the tibia is associated with irregularity of the entire growth plate. The medial part of the metaphysis protrudes with a medial and distal beak.

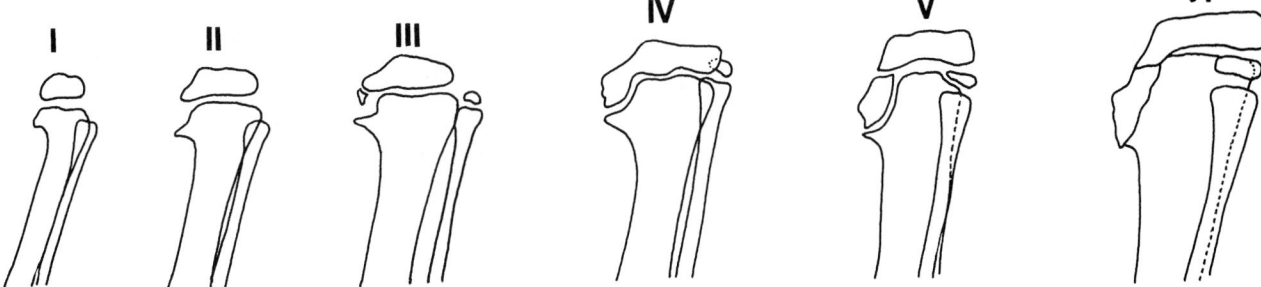

**Figure 68–23.** Blount's disease: infantile tibia vara. Six stages of the disease (see text for details). (After Langenskiöld A: Tibia vara. Osteochondritis deformans tibiae. A survey of 23 cases. Acta Chir Scand 103:1, 1952.)

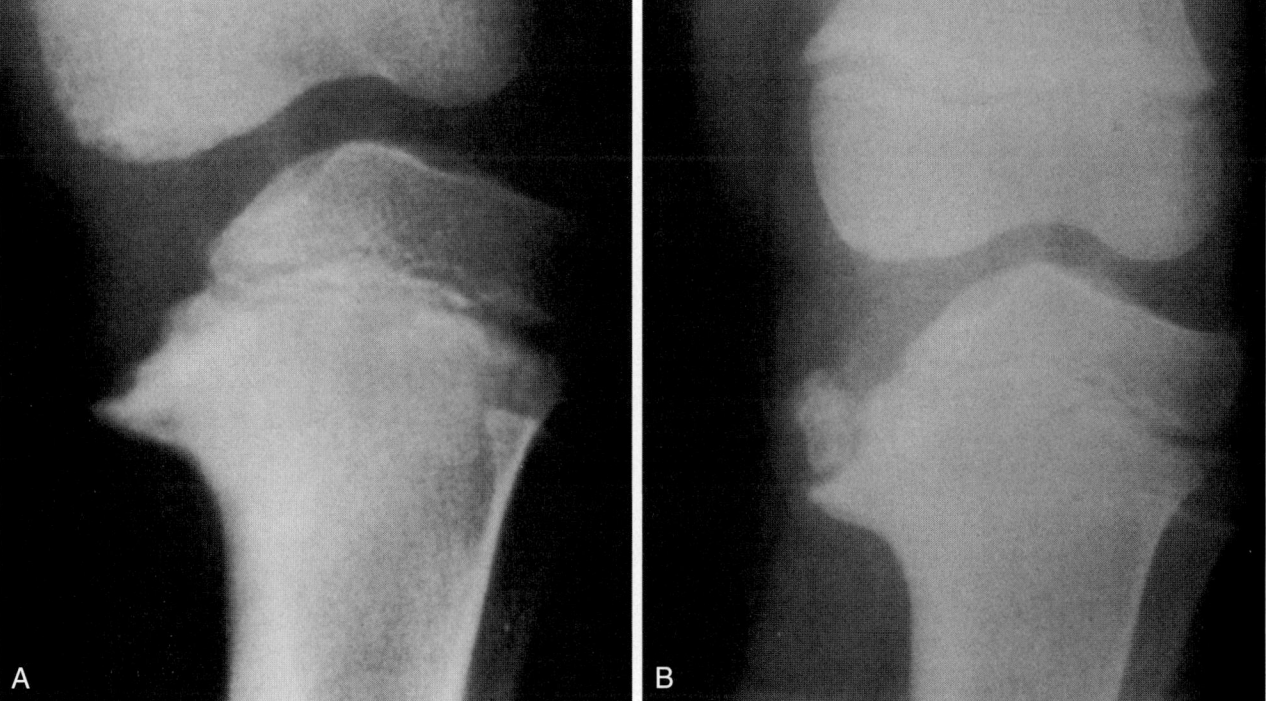

**Figure 68–24.** Blount's disease: infantile tibia vara. The various stages of the disease are well illustrated in this child. *A*, Stage II, at age 4 years. *B*, Stage III–IV, at age 8 years. (Courtesy of L. Danzig, MD, Santa Ana, Calif.)

Stage II (2.5 to 4 years). A lateromedial depression of the ossification line of the medial portion of the metaphysis and a wedge-shaped medial portion of the epiphysis are observed. Complete healing of the lesion is possible at this stage.

Stage III (4 to 6 years). The cartilage-filled depression in the metaphyseal beak deepens. The medial part of the bony epiphysis remains wedge shaped. Small calcific foci may be evident beneath the medial border.

Stage IV (5 to 10 years). With increasing bone maturation, the cartilaginous growth plate is reduced to a narrow plate, and the bony epiphysis occupies an increasing part of the end of the bone. The medial margin of the epiphysis shows definite irregularity. Even at this stage, restoration of a relatively normal epiphysis is possible.

Stage V (9 to 11 years). The epiphysis and articular surface are greatly deformed. A "partial double epiphyseal plate" results as the epiphysis is separated into two portions by a clear band that extends medially from the lateral portion of the growth plate.

Stage VI (10 to 13 years). The branches of the medially located double growth plate ossify, whereas growth continues in the normal lateral part. Stages V and VI represent phases of irreparable structural damage.

Lateral widening of the growth plate of the proximal end of the tibia and, less frequently, the distal end of the femur has been identified in infantile tibia vara. This diastasis may result from the chronic stress of genu varum on the growth plates in the area of the knee.

**Adolescent Tibia Vara.** The adolescent (or juvenile) form, which is much less frequent than infantile tibia vara, develops in children between the ages of 8 and 15 years. As in the infantile variety, black children are affected more frequently than whites. The cause is not clear. A history of trauma or infection is occasionally elicited, and conventional or computed tomography may indicate an osseous bridge between the epiphysis and metaphysis. Unilateral alterations occur in approximately 70% to 90% of cases.

Radiographs outline a proximal tibial profile that is angled about 10 to 20 degrees. The proximal tibial epiphysis reveals medial wedging, and the medial tibial growth plate is diminished in height, but a sharp step-off in the tibial plateau is not usually apparent (Fig. 68–25).

**Late-Onset Tibia Vara.** Late-onset tibia vara occurs between the ages of 6 and 14 years and causes marked knee deformity. Flattening of the medial aspect of the tibial epiphysis, resulting in a wedge-shaped epiphysis, and growth plate irregularity are observed radiographically. The histologic abnormalities of involved portions of the tibia resemble those found in infantile tibia vara, suggesting a relationship between the two conditions. Affected children may have had significant symmetrical physiologic varus in early childhood that corrected spontaneously, though not completely, on the side where tibia vara later develops. Late-onset tibia vara, in common with the adolescent variety, is much less frequent than the infantile type. Because of the overlap in age of onset between the adolescent and late-onset types, the latter is divided into two categories:

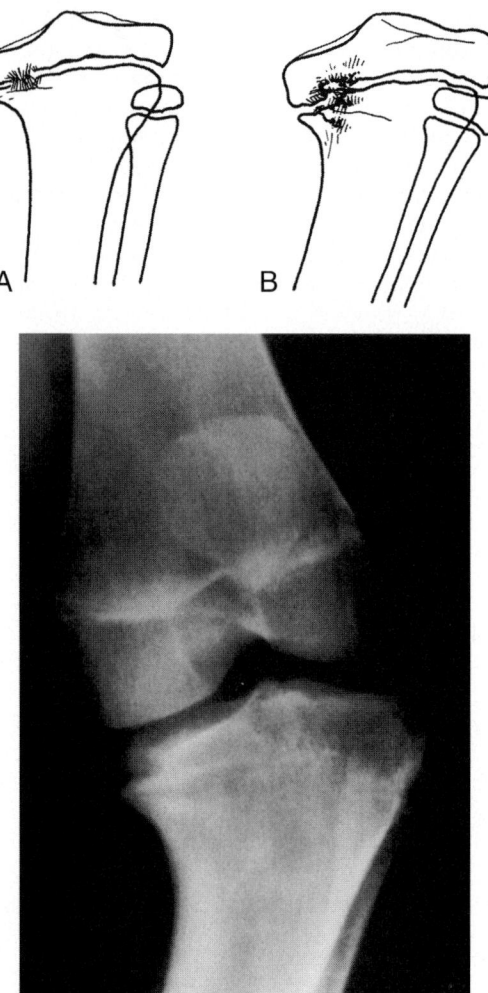

**Figure 68–25.** Blount's disease: adolescent tibia vara. *A* and *B*, Stages of the process. Observe fusion of the medial aspect of the growth plate, with progressive sclerosis and varus deformity. *C*, In this example of adolescent tibia vara, note the varus deformity, depression of the articular surface of the medial tibial plateau, sclerosis, and osteophyte formation. (*A* and *B*, After Langenskiöld A: Acta Chir Scand 103:1, 1952.)

juvenile (previously designated adolescent) and adolescent (the newly described late-onset disease). There is no uniformity in the use of these terms, however.

The preceding observations indicate that a spectrum of abnormalities is encountered in patients with tibia vara and that the disease is best categorized according to age at clinical onset and, thus, amount of remaining growth potential. The infantile type of disease is most likely to lead to the greatest deformity, and the late-onset type is least likely to do so.

**Focal Fibrocartilaginous Dysplasia.** Another condition leading to unilateral tibia vara in early childhood is focal fibrocartilaginous dysplasia. This disorder occurs with equal frequency in boys and girls and is invariably unilateral. The clinical onset occurs between 3 and 18 months of age, and all children with this condition who have not been treated surgically have achieved spontaneous resolution in 1 to 4 years.

Routine radiographs are diagnostic and reveal a well-defined, obliquely positioned radiolucent defect in the metadiaphyseal cortex in the proximal and medial portion of the tibia. Endosteal and periosteal thickening of the cortex is an associated finding (Fig. 68–26). Computed tomography documents the presence of soft tissue medial to the defect that is indistinguishable from the adjacent muscle and tendon. MR imaging reveals cartilage or fibrocartilage within the lesion. The cause of focal fibrocartilaginous dysplasia is unknown.

**Differential Diagnosis.** The radiographic abnormalities in infantile, adolescent, and late-onset tibia vara are usually diagnostic. Some difficulty is occasionally encountered in differentiating the infantile type from physiologic bowed legs, and serial radiographs may be necessary (Fig. 68–27). The sharply angular appearance of infantile tibia vara differs from the gradual curve in physiologic bowed legs.

## Scheuermann's Disease

Originally termed kyphosis dorsalis juvenilis, Scheuermann's disease leads to lower thoracic kyphosis. On the basis of irregularities involving the rims of the vertebral bodies, early investigators concluded that this disorder was related to osteonecrosis. Considerable disagreement now exists, however, regarding the cause and pathogenesis of this disorder. The criteria necessary for a diagnosis of Scheuermann's disease are also debated. Current criteria

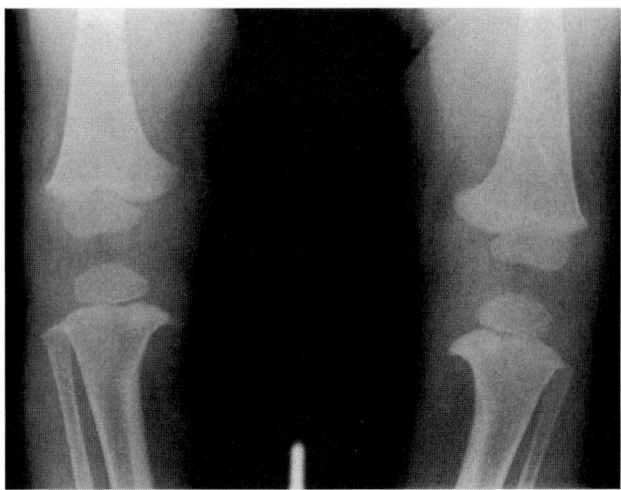

**Figure 68–27.** Physiologic bowed legs. Note the gradual varus curvature of the knees in this child. No evidence of a proximal tibial step-off or varus deformity was apparent.

frequently require the presence of abnormalities in at least three contiguous vertebrae, each with wedging of 5 degrees or more. Such criteria are not ideal, however, because they exclude cases of Scheuermann's disease that are associated predominantly with vertebral irregularity without wedging. The reported frequency during routine examination in military personnel and industrial workers is approximately 4% to 8%. Most affected persons are between the ages of 13 and 17 years.

**Clinical Abnormalities.** Although in some persons the disease is totally asymptomatic, in others, prominent symptoms and signs can be seen. Typically, these findings relate to the middle and lower thoracic spine. Fatigue, defective posture, aching pain aggravated by physical exertion, and tenderness to palpation are encountered. Kyphotic deformity, which may be associated with mild scoliosis, predominates in the thoracic region (75% of patients), although it may be observed in the thoracolumbar (20% to 25%) or lumbar (0% to 5%) segments. Neurologic complaints are not common.

**Radiographic Abnormalities.** On radiographs, an undulant superior and inferior surface of affected vertebral bodies is associated with intraosseous radiolucent zones of variable size (cartilaginous or Schmorl's nodes), along with surrounding sclerosis (Figs. 68–28 and 68–29). Loss of intervertebral disc height and wedging of the anterior portion of the vertebral body may be seen. The degree of thoracic kyphosis is variable.

Prolapse of large foci of intervertebral disc tissue may be observed anteriorly, and the extruded disc material may extend beneath the apophyseal centers of ossification and appear submarginally behind the anterior longitudinal ligament. Under these circumstances, a portion of the proximal or distal ringlike apophyseal centers of ossification may be separated from the vertebral body and produce a limbus vertebra (see Fig. 68–29*B*). Ossification of the anterior portions of the intervertebral disc can lead to synostosis of one vertebral body with its neighbor.

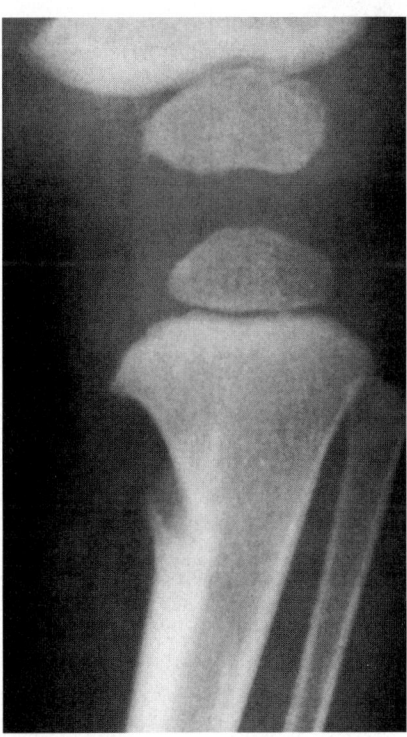

**Figure 68–26.** Focal fibrocartilaginous dysplasia. This 16-month-old girl was first noted to have bowing of the left leg at 14 months of age. A radiograph shows a well-defined defect of the metadiaphyseal portion of the medial cortex of the tibia. Note the thickening of the cortex adjacent to and below the lesion. (From Herman TE, et al: Radiology 177:767, 1990.)

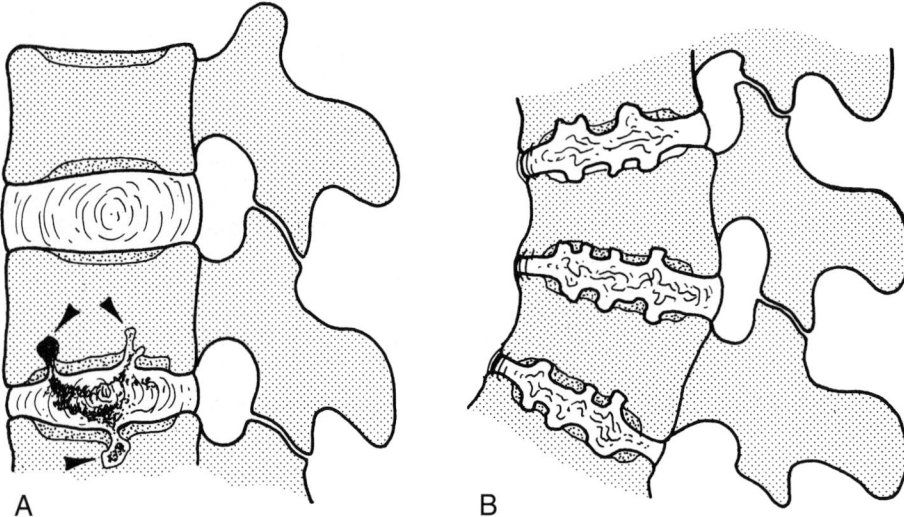

**Figure 68–28.** Scheuermann's disease. The underlying abnormality relates to intraosseous displacement of disc material (cartilaginous nodes) through the cartilaginous endplates *(arrowheads)*. This defect produces radiolucent lesions of the vertebral bodies with surrounding sclerosis, intervertebral disc space narrowing, and irregularity of vertebral contour. Kyphosis may appear.

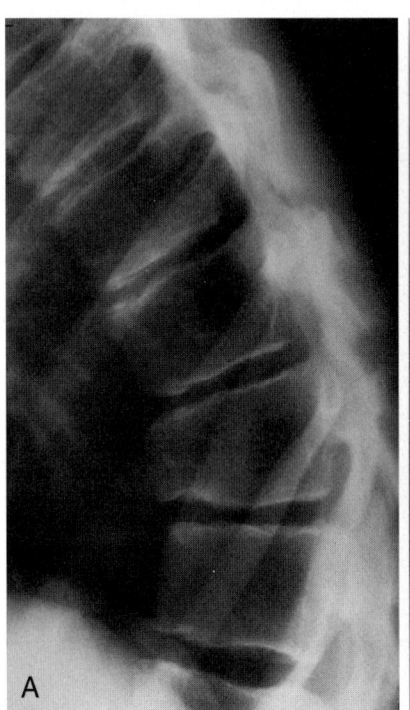
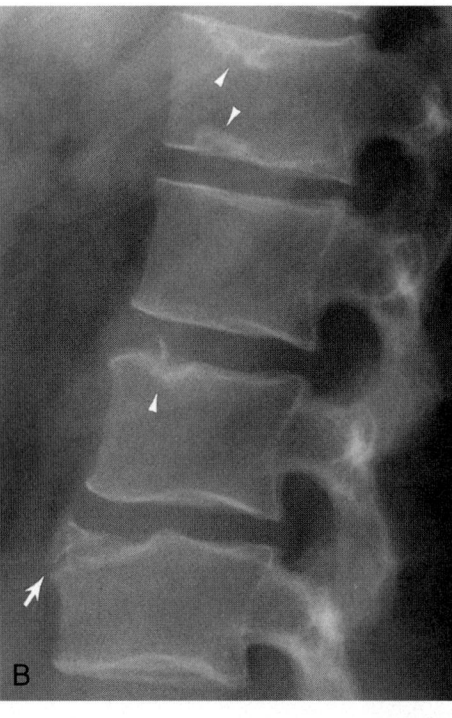

**Figure 68–29.** Scheuermann's disease. *A,* Thoracic spine. Findings include irregularity in vertebral contour, reactive sclerosis, intervertebral disc space narrowing, anterior vertebral wedging, and kyphosis. *B,* Lumbar spine. Observe the cartilaginous nodes *(arrowheads)* creating surface irregularity, lucent areas, and reactive sclerosis. Anterior disc displacement *(arrow)* has produced an irregular anterosuperior corner of a vertebral body—the limbus vertebra.

**Cause and Pathogenesis.** This disorder is most likely a manifestation of cartilaginous node formation. The basis for the nodes is not clear, although stress-induced intraosseous displacement through congenitally or traumatically weakened portions of the cartilaginous endplate appears probable. The radiographic findings reflect the presence of disc material within the vertebral bodies (intraosseous lucent areas) and arrested or abnormal vertebral growth (irregularity in osseous contour), either or both of which can be evident in a patient with the disease.

**Juvenile Lumbar Osteochondrosis.** A condition sharing some features with Scheuermann's disease but localized to the lower thoracic and lumbar spine has been described.

Affected patients have pain, often severe, in the lower part of the back that appears during adolescence. Boys are involved more commonly than girls, and the thoracic deformity seen in Scheuermann's disease is absent.

Radiographs reveal prominent depression of the vertebral endplates, with wedging and an increased anteroposterior dimension of affected vertebral bodies. Decreased height of lumbar intervertebral discs, retrolisthesis of lumbar vertebrae, and findings of spinal stenosis may be apparent. The relationship between this condition and typical Scheuermann's disease is not clear. Of interest in this regard is the occurrence of similar abnormalities of the lumbar spine in patients who have characteristic abnormalities of Scheuermann's disease in the thoracic spine.

Clinical manifestations in patients with isolated alterations in the lumbar spine, however, differ from those of classic Scheuermann's disease, suggesting that it may be a distinct disorder.

**Differential Diagnosis.** Cartilaginous nodes can accompany any disease process that weakens the cartilaginous endplate or subchondral bone of the vertebral body and allows intraosseous disc displacement. A partial list of such processes includes trauma, neoplasm, metabolic disorders (hyperparathyroidism, osteoporosis, Paget's disease), infection, intervertebral osteochondrosis, and articular disorders (rheumatoid arthritis). The combination of kyphosis, cartilaginous nodes, and irregular vertebral outlines is virtually pathognomonic of Scheuermann's disease.

### Sinding-Larsen-Johansson Disease

Sinding-Larsen-Johansson disease occurs most commonly in adolescents between 10 and 14 years of age and consists of tenderness and soft tissue swelling over the lower pole of the patella, accompanied by radiographic evidence of osseous fragmentation. This process is traumatic in origin, and its pathogenesis appears to be similar to that of Osgood-Schlatter disease. It is probably related to a traction phenomenon in which contusion or tendinosis in the proximal attachment of the patellar tendon can be followed by calcification and ossification. The association of fragmentation of the inferior portion of the patella with spastic paralysis is consistent with this traction phenomenon. Similar findings are observed in athletes, in whom the term "jumper's knee" has been applied.

Radiographs reveal small bony fragments adjacent to the distal surface of the patella with overlying soft tissue swelling. The radiodense areas may subsequently coalesce and become incorporated into the patella, eventually yielding a normal radiographic appearance. MR imaging can also be used to substantiate the diagnosis (Fig. 68–30). Patellar fragmentation may also represent a normal variation of ossification or the presence of accessory ossification centers.

## "DISORDERS" CAUSED BY VARIATIONS IN OSSIFICATION

### Sever's Phenomenon

Irregularity of the secondary calcaneal ossification center is a normal variation unrelated to the painful heels of adolescents. It is now generally accepted that fragmentation and sclerosis of the secondary ossification center of the calcaneus may be entirely normal (Fig. 68–31) and, in fact, are the result of proper weight bearing. Such osseous changes may be absent in patients who are immobilized as a result of neurogenic disease or fracture and may appear with resumption of normal levels of activity.

### Ischiopubic Osteochondrosis

Rarefaction and swelling of the ischiopubic synchondrosis is sometimes termed Van Neck's disease or phenomenon. On the basis of clinical, radiographic, scintigraphic, and pathologic observations, this condition is now regarded as a very common, normal pattern of ossification. The

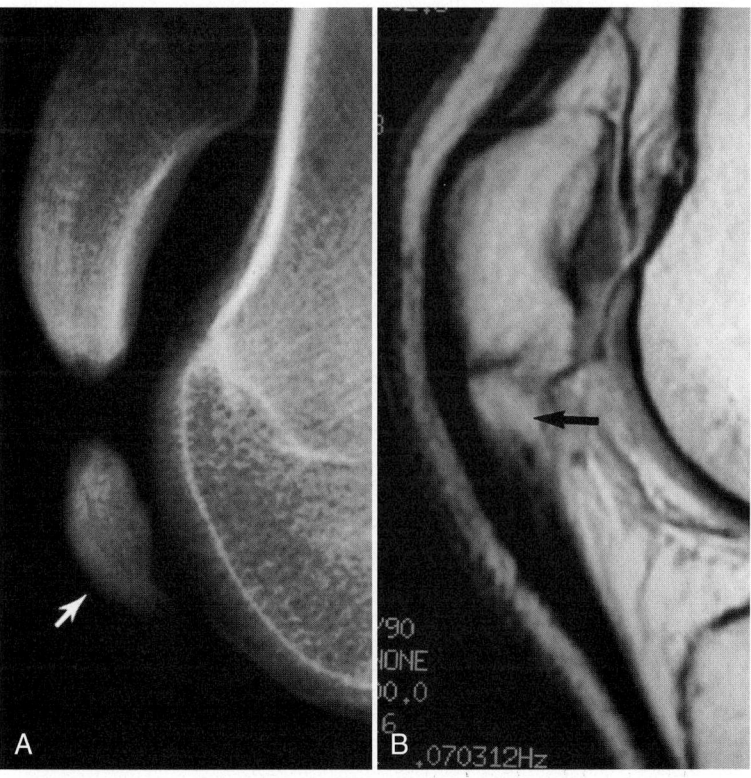

**Figure 68–30.** Sinding-Larsen-Johansson disease. *A,* In this patient with spastic paralysis, observe the fragmentation of the lower pole of the patella *(arrow),* related to abnormal stress. *B,* In a different patient, a sagittal intermediate-weighted (TR/TE, 2500/26) spin echo MR image shows a fragment *(arrow)* of the lower pole of the patella, with thickening of the proximal portion of the patellar tendon.

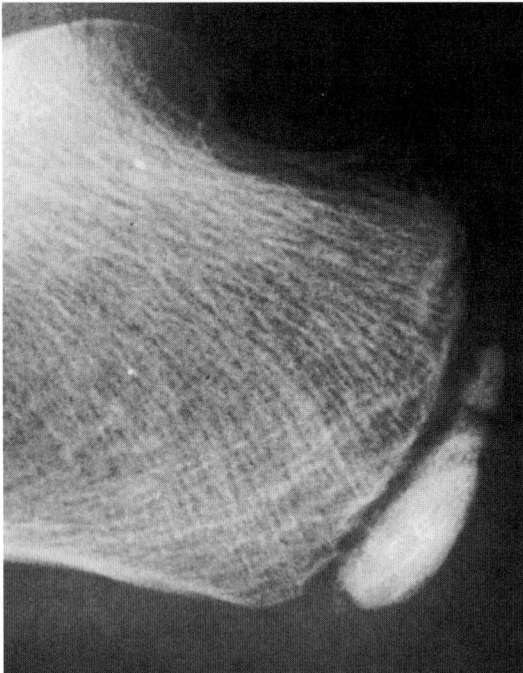

**Figure 68–31.** Sever's phenomenon. Sclerosis and fragmentation of the secondary calcaneal ossification center are illustrated. This finding is a normal consequence of weight bearing.

pattern may be unilateral or bilateral in distribution. The time of closure of the synchondrosis is somewhat variable, but it usually takes place between the ages of 9 and 11 years. Irregular ossification of the synchondrosis is generally most apparent between the ages of 5 and 8 years (Fig. 68–32).

The differential diagnosis of this normal variant includes stress fracture, post-traumatic osteolysis, and infection. Diagnostic difficulty arises because of the accumulation of bone-seeking radionuclides about this normal variant. It has been suggested that if such uptake is equal to or greater than that adjacent to the triradiate cartilage, a pathologic process is present.

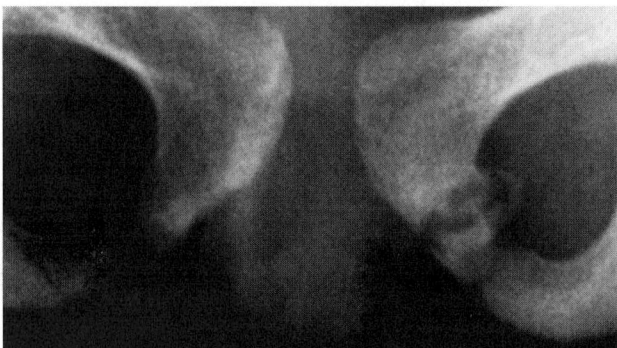

**Figure 68–32.** Ischiopubic osteochondrosis. In this 3-year-old child, the ischiopubic synchondrosis on the right side is open, with adjacent smooth bone margins; on the left side, irregular ossification is evident. This latter pattern of ossification is within normal limits. (Courtesy of J. Goobar, MD, Ostersund, Sweden.)

## MISCELLANEOUS DISORDERS

Osteochondroses have been described in almost every epiphysis and apophysis in the body (Table 68–5). In most cases, boys are affected more frequently than girls, alterations rarely develop before age 3 years or after age 12 years, and developmental irregularities in ossification can be encountered at many of the same skeletal sites.

**TABLE 68–5**

**Some of Osteochondroses**

| Year Reported | Investigator(s) | Location of Lesion |
|---|---|---|
| 1887 | Koenig | Osteochondritis dissecans |
| 1903 | Osgood; Schlatter | Tibial tubercle |
| 1908 | Köhler | Primary patellar center |
| 1908 | Haglund | Os tibiale externum |
| 1908 | Köhler | Tarsal navicular |
| 1909 | Thiemann | Phalangeal bases |
| 1910 | Legg; Calvé; Perthes | Femoral epiphysis |
| 1910 | Kienböck | Carpal lunate |
| 1911 | Preiser | Carpal scaphoid |
| 1912 | Sever | Calcaneal apophysis |
| 1912 | Iselin | Fifth metatarsal base |
| 1914 | Freiberg | Second metatarsal head |
| 1921 | Hass | Head of humerus |
| 1921 | Burns | Lower part of ulna |
| 1921 | Scheuermann | Vertebral apophysis |
| 1921 | Sinding-Larsen | Secondary patellar center |
| 1922 | Mandl | Greater trochanter |
| 1924 | Friedrich | Medial end of clavicle |
| 1924 | Van Neck | Ischiopubic synchondrosis |
| 1925 | Calvé | Vertebral body |
| 1927 | Panner | Capitulum of humerus |
| 1927 | Mauclaire | Heads of metacarpals |
| 1927 | Buchman | Iliac crest |
| 1928 | Diaz | Talus |
| 1929 | Pierson | Symphysis pubis |
| 1932 | Dietrich | Heads of metacarpals |
| 1937 | Blount | Medial proximal tibial shaft |
| 1945 | Caffey | Entire carpus bilaterally |
| 1950 | Liffert and Arkin | Distal tibial center |
| 1953 | Milch | Ischial apophysis |
| 1956 | Caffey | Tibial spines |

After Brower AC: Orthop Clin North Am 14:99, 1983.

## FURTHER READING

Alexander CJ: Scheuermann's disease: A traumatic spondylodystrophy? Skeletal Radiol 1:209, 1977.
Arie E, Johnson F, Harrison MHM, et al: Femoral head shape in Perthes' disease: Is the contralateral hip abnormal? Clin Orthop 209:77, 1986.
Bateson EM: The relationship between Blount's disease and bow legs. Br J Radiol 41:107, 1968.

Bonzar M, Firrell JC, Hainer M, et al: Kienböck disease and negative ulnar variance. J Bone Joint Surg Am 80:1154, 1998.

Braddock GTF: Experimental epiphyseal injury and Freiberg's disease. J Bone Joint Surg Br 41:107, 1968.

Bradish CF, Davies SJ, Malone M: Tibia vara due to focal fibrocartilaginous dysplasia: The natural history. J Bone Joint Surg Br 70:106, 1988.

Caffey J: The early roentgenographic changes in essential coxa plana: Their significance in pathogenesis. AJR Am J Roentgenol 103:620, 1968.

Caffey J, Ross SE: The ischiopubic synchondrosis in healthy children: Some normal roentgenologic findings. AJR Am J Roentgenol 76:488, 1956.

Catterall A: Legg-Calvé-Perthes Disease. Edinburgh, Churchill Livingstone, 1982.

Catterall A: The natural history of Perthes' disease. J Bone Joint Surg Br 53:37, 1971.

Christensen F, Soballe K, Ejsted R, et al: The Catterall classification of Perthes' disease: An assessment of reliability. J Bone Joint Surg Br 68:614, 1986.

Clarke NMP, Harrison MHM, Keret D: The sagging rope sign: A critical appraisal. J Bone Joint Surg Br 65:285, 1983.

Cullen JC: Thiemann's disease: Osteochondrosis juvenilis of the basal epiphyses of the phalanges of the hand. Report of two cases. J Bone Joint Surg Br 52:532, 1970.

Egund N, Wingstrand H: Legg-Calvé-Perthes disease: Imaging with MR. Radiology 179:89, 1991.

Freiberg AH: Infraction òf the second metatarsal bone: A typical injury. Surg Gynecol Obstet 19:191, 1914.

Gelberman RH, Salamon PB, Jurist JM, et al: Ulnar variance in Kienböck's disease. J Bone Joint Surg Am 57:674, 1975.

Goldman AB, Hallel T, Salvati EM, et al: Osteochondritis dissecans complicating Legg-Perthes disease: A report of four cases. Radiology 121:561, 1976.

Herring JA, Lundeen MA, Wenger DR: Minimal Perthes' disease. J Bone Joint Surg Br 62:25, 1980.

Hochbergs P, Eckerwall G, Egund N, et al: Synovitis in Legg-Calvé-Perthes disease: Evaluation with MR imaging in 84 hips. Acta Radiol 39:532, 1998.

Hulting B: Roentgenologic features of fracture of the tibial tuberosity (Osgood-Schlatter's disease). Acta Radiol 48:161, 1957.

Kaye JJ, Freiberger RH: Fragmentation of the lower pole of the patella in spastic lower extremities. Radiology 101:97, 1971.

Klein EW: Osteochondrosis of the capitulum (Panner's disease). Report of a case. AJR Am J Roentgenol 88:466, 1952.

Langenskiöld A, Riska EB: Tibia vara (osteochondrosis deformans tibiae). J Bone Joint Surg Am 46:1405, 1964.

Lowe TG: Scheuermann's disease. Orthop Clin North Am 30:475, 1999.

McCauley RGK, Kahn PC: Osteochondritis of the tarsal navicular: Radioisotopic appearances. Radiology 123:705, 1977.

Melo-Gomes JA, Melo-Gomes E, Viana-Queiros M: Thiemann's disease. J Rheumatol 8:462, 1981.

Murphy RP, Marsh HO: Incidence and natural history of "head at risk" factors in Perthes' disease. Clin Orthop 132:102, 1978.

Ogden JA: Radiology of postnatal skeletal development. X. Patella and tibial tuberosity. Skeletal Radiol 11:246, 1984.

Osgood RB: Lesions of the tibial tubercle occurring during adolescence. Boston Med Surg J 148:114, 1903.

Ozonoff MB: Pediatric Orthopedic Radiology. Philadelphia, WB Saunders, 1979.

Panner HJ: An affection of the capitulum humeri resembling Calvé-Perthes disease of the hip. Acta Radiol 8:617, 1927.

Rosenberg ZS, Kawelblum M, Cheung YY, et al: Osgood-Schlatter lesion: Fracture or tendinitis? Scintigraphic, CT, and MR imaging features. Radiology 185:853, 1992.

Rush BH, Bramson RT, Ogden JA: Legg-Calvé-Perthes disease: Detection of cartilaginous and synovial changes with MR imaging. Radiology 167:473, 1988.

Schmorl G, Junghanns H: The Human Spine in Health and Disease, 2nd ed. Trans EF Besemann. New York, Grune & Stratton, 1971.

Scoles PV, Yoon YS, Makley JT, et al: Nuclear magnetic resonance imaging in Legg-Calvé-Perthes disease. J Bone Joint Surg Am 66:1357, 1984.

Shopfner CE, Coin CG: Effect of weight-bearing on the appearance and development of the secondary calcaneal epiphysis. Radiology 86:201, 1966.

Siffert RS: Classification of the osteochondroses. Clin Orthop 158:10, 1981.

Silverman FN: Lesions of the femoral neck in Legg-Perthes disease. AJR Am J Roentgenol 144:1249, 1985.

Sinding-Larsen MF: A hitherto unknown affection of the patella in children. Acta Radiol 1:171, 1921.

Spragge JW: Legg-Calvé-Perthes disease. In Freiberger RH et al (eds): Hip disease of infancy and childhood. Curr Probl Radiol 3:30, 1973.

Stöhl F: On lunatomalacia (Kienböck's disease): A clinical and roentgenological study, especially on its pathogenesis and the late results of immobilization treatment. Acta Chir Scand Suppl 126:1, 1947.

Swischuk LE, John SD, Allbery S: Disk degenerative disease in childhood: Scheuermann's disease, Schmorl's nodes, and the limbus vertebra: MRI findings in 12 patients. Pediatr Radiol 28:334, 1998.

Tallroth K, Schlenzka D: Spinal stenosis subsequent to juvenile lumbar osteochondrosis. Skeletal Radiol 19:203, 1990.

Wolinski AP, McCall IW, Evans G, et al: Femoral neck growth deformity following the irritable hip syndrome. Br J Radiol 57:773, 1984.

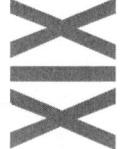
# CHAPTER 69

## Tumors and Tumor-Like Lesions of Bone: Radiographic Principles

### SUMMARY OF KEY FEATURES

Conventional radiographic techniques are of fundamental importance in the analysis of bone tumors and tumor-like lesions. Morphologic characteristics provide important diagnostic information regarding the aggressive or nonaggressive behavior of the lesion. These, when combined with information related to the site or distribution of skeletal involvement, allow the formulation of a single diagnostic choice or several choices that are most likely in any patient. The addition of clinical information, including the age of the patient, information derived from other imaging techniques, and, in some cases, histologic data, is also essential.

### INTRODUCTION

Although the radiographic findings may not allow a simple, precise diagnosis in a patient with a tumor or tumor-like lesion, they do provide reliable information regarding its aggressiveness or rate of growth. This information, coupled with data reflecting the site of the lesion and the age of the patient, allows the formulation of a reasonable diagnosis in most cases. A note of warning regarding this analysis is required. Although aggressive lesions are commonly malignant and benign tumors are commonly nonaggressive, such generalization is not uniformly true. Rapid osseous expansion, an aggressive characteristic, can occur in nonmalignant conditions such as an aneurysmal bone cyst. Similarly, a rim of bone sclerosis about a lesion is a nonaggressive characteristic that, in rare circumstances, may become evident in malignant neoplasms. Further, osteomyelitis is frequently associated with poorly demarcated osteolysis and periostitis, findings resembling those of a malignant tumor.

### MORPHOLOGY

#### Pattern of Bone Destruction

Radiographs are not extremely sensitive in the detection of small amounts of bone destruction, especially if the destructive focus is located in cancellous bone. Cortical lesions are detected more readily than are those in cancellous bone (Fig. 69–1). In fact, detection of a sharply marginated radiolucent area overlying the medullary portion of a tubular bone (especially a large one) in a single radiographic projection almost always implies cortical involvement.

Three radiographic patterns of bone destruction have been identified: geographic, moth-eaten, and permeative.

**Geographic Bone Destruction.** The geographic pattern is the least aggressive pattern of bone destruction, and it is generally indicative of a slowly growing lesion. The margin may be smooth or irregular, but in either case, it is well defined and is easily separated from the surrounding normal bone with a short zone of transition (Fig. 69–2). In some instances, a sclerotic margin of variable thickness surrounds the lesion. The thicker and more complete the sclerotic margin, the less aggressive the process. Benign bone tumors usually demonstrate geographic bone destruction. Malignant diseases such as plasma cell myeloma and metastasis can demonstrate a similar pattern of geographic bone destruction; however, they rarely show a sclerotic margin.

**Moth-eaten Bone Destruction.** The moth-eaten pattern is a more aggressive pattern of bone destruction and is characteristic of a lesion that is growing more rapidly than one that demonstrates geographic bone destruction. The moth-eaten pattern is associated with a less well defined or demarcated lesion margin and with a longer zone of transition from normal to abnormal bone (Fig. 69–3). Malignant bone tumors and osteomyelitis may demonstrate the moth-eaten pattern of bone destruction. Some benign processes, such as eosinophilic granuloma, may be associated with moth-eaten bone destruction, however.

**Permeative Bone Destruction.** The permeative pattern indicates an aggressive bone lesion with rapid growth potential. The lesion is poorly demarcated and may imperceptibly merge with uninvolved osseous segments and create a zone of transition that is very long (Fig. 69–4). Its true size is larger than that evident on radiographs. Certain malignant bone tumors, such as Ewing's sarcoma, may demonstrate permeative bone destruction. Osteomyelitis and rapidly developing osteoporosis, as in reflex sympathetic dystrophy, may reveal permeative bone destruction, however.

#### Size, Shape, and Margin of the Lesion

In general, primary malignant tumors of bone are larger than benign tumors are. The growth rate of a lesion is of great importance in assessing the aggressiveness of any skeletal process. Benign tumors usually grow more slowly than malignant tumors, or they may show no change in size over a long period of observation; however, exceptions to this rule are encountered. Plasma cell myeloma is occasionally associated with slow growth, and histologically low-grade or benign giant cell tumors may enlarge

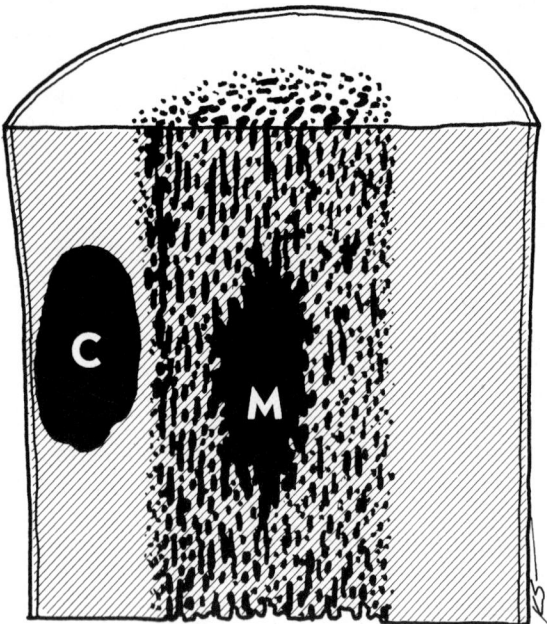

**Figure 69–1.** Cortical versus medullary involvement. A lesion in medullary bone (M) may be more difficult to recognize than one in cortical bone (C). In addition, a nonaggressive cortical lesion produces a sharp interface with the surrounding bone, whereas such a lesion in medullary bone may not.

rapidly. Slowly growing lesions can be associated with reactive sclerosis of the surrounding normal bone. The sclerotic margin can be of variable thickness and may surround the bone lesion partially or completely.

## Presence and Nature of Visible Tumor Matrix

Certain tumors produce matrix that calcifies or ossifies. The resulting radiodense areas must be distinguished from the calcification that may develop in regions of necrotic or degenerative tissue; from callus formation, which may indicate the presence of a pathologic fracture; and from a sclerotic response of non-neoplastic bone to the adjacent tumorous deposit.

Certain cartilage tumors are associated with matrix calcification. These include chondromas, chondroblastomas, chondrosarcomas, and, less frequently, chondromyxoid fibromas. Cartilage matrix calcification is frequently centrally located and may appear as ringlike, flocculent, or flecklike radiodense areas (Fig. 69–5). Similar findings can be apparent within the cartilaginous cap of an osteochondroma.

Visible tumor matrix is also associated with neoplastic bone. Examples of neoplasms producing such tumor matrix are osteosarcomas, parosteal osteosarcomas, ossifying fibromas, osteomas, and osteoblastomas. Certain lesions, such as fibrous dysplasia, can be accompanied by a uniform increase in radiodensity, an appearance designated the "ground-glass" pattern. This pattern is associated with obscuration or obliteration of neighboring trabeculae.

## Internal or External Trabeculation

Within or around the lesion, trabeculated shadows may be identified on the radiograph. In some instances, these shadows reflect the location of residual trabeculae that have been modified or displaced by the neighboring tumor. In other cases, the trabeculation represents new

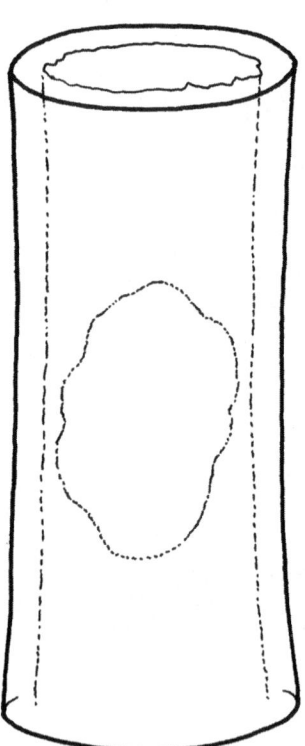

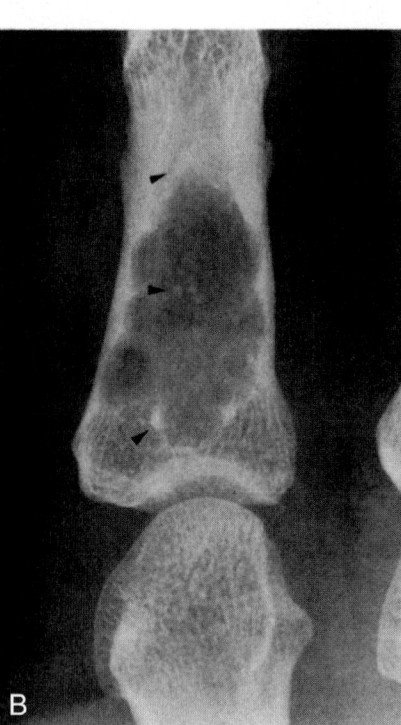

**Figure 69–2.** Geographic bone destruction. *A,* This pattern of bone destruction is characterized by well-defined lesion margins and a short zone of transition from normal to abnormal bone. *B,* The lesion in the proximal phalanx demonstrates geographic bone destruction, a central location, lobulated margins, and small foci of calcification *(arrowheads).* (Final diagnosis, enchondroma.)

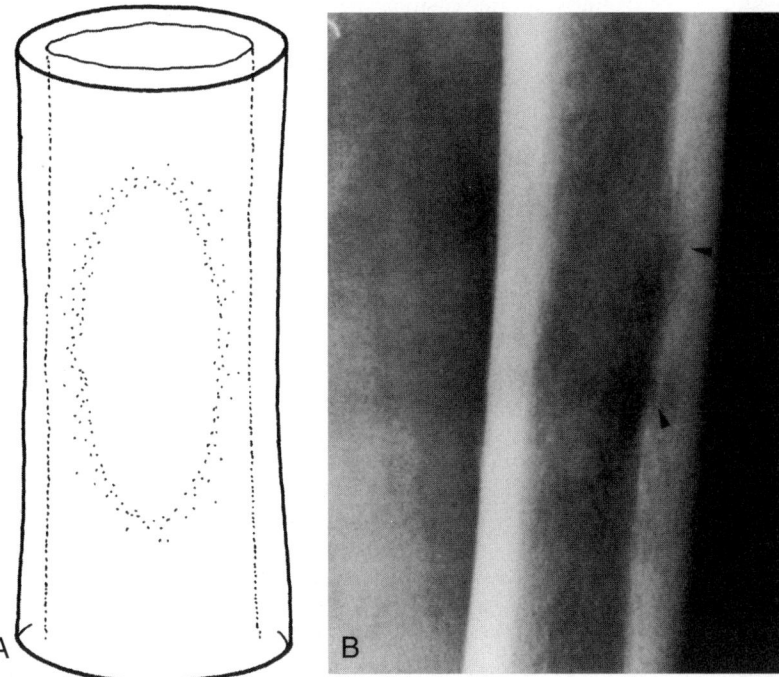

**Figure 69–3.** Moth-eaten bone destruction. *A,* This pattern of bone destruction is associated with lesion margins that are less well defined and a longer zone of transition from normal to abnormal bone. *B,* A lesion with moth-eaten bone destruction is identified in this femur. Note its poorly defined margins and erosion of the endosteal margin of the cortex *(arrowheads).* (Final diagnosis, lymphoma.)

bone formation evoked as a response to the presence of a nearby neoplasm. The location and appearance of the trabeculation provide information regarding the nature of the neoplasm (Table 69–1; Figs. 69–6 and 69–7).

## Cortical Erosion, Penetration, and Expansion

The bony cortex can serve as an effective barrier to the further lateral growth of certain tumors, whereas in other instances, the neoplasm may penetrate the cortex par-

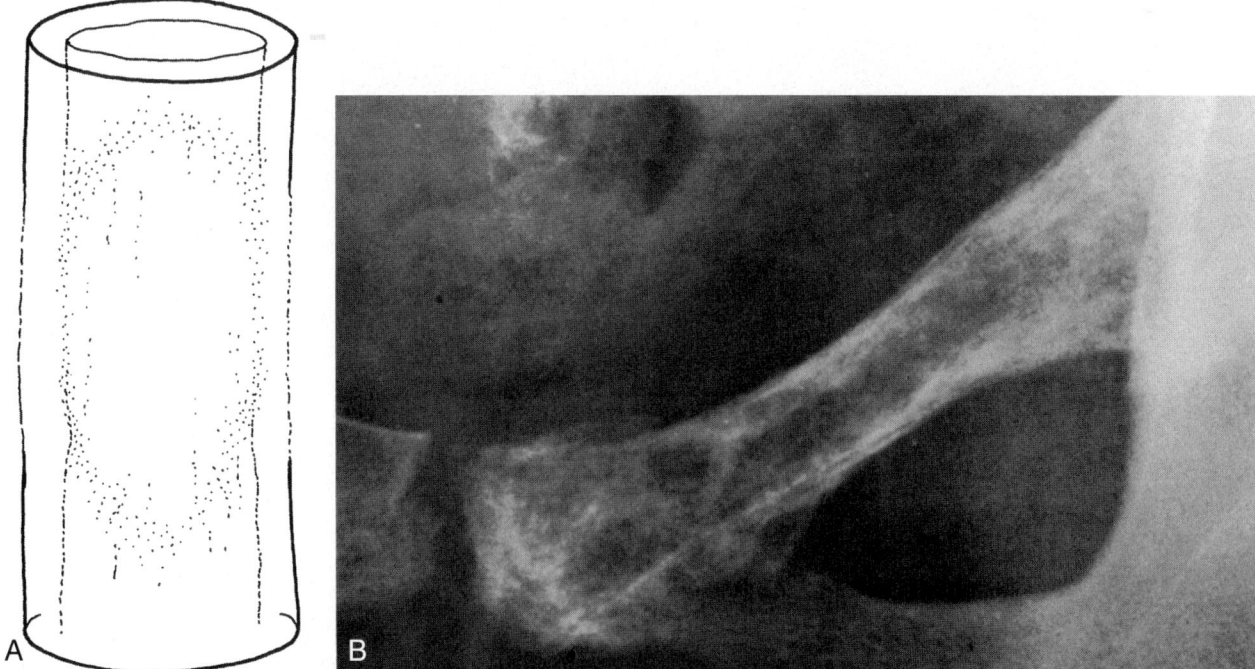

**Figure 69–4.** Permeative bone destruction. *A,* This pattern of bone destruction is associated with very poorly defined lesion margins and a very long zone of transition from normal to abnormal bone. *B,* The lesion in the superior pubic ramus reveals permeative bone destruction with cortical erosion, periostitis, and a soft tissue mass. (Final diagnosis, lymphoma.)

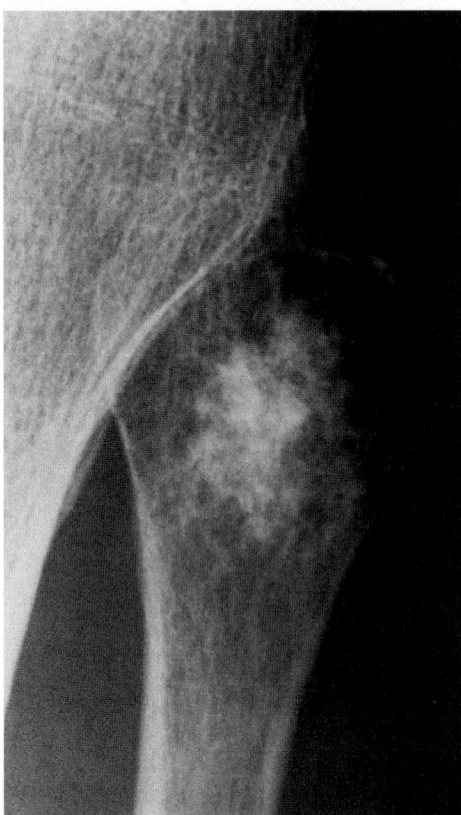

**Figure 69–5.** Matrix calcification. Magnification radiograph shows typical punctate and centrally located calcification of a cartilaginous tumor of the proximal portion of the fibula. (Final diagnosis, enchondroma.) (Courtesy of U. Mayer, MD, Klagenfort, Austria.)

**TABLE 69–1**

**Trabeculated Lesions**

| Lesion | Pattern |
|---|---|
| Giant cell tumor | Delicate, thin |
| Chondromyxoid fibroma | Coarse, thick |
| Desmoplastic fibroma | Coarse, thick |
| Nonossifying fibroma | Lobulated |
| Aneurysmal bone cyst | Delicate, horizontally oriented |
| Hemangioma | Striated, radiating |

tially or completely. Nonaggressive medullary lesions may provoke little change in the endosteal surface of the cortex. Slowly growing lesions, such as enchondromas, can lead to lobulated erosion of the inner margin of the cortex and produce a scalloped endosteal margin. If progressive endosteal erosion is associated with periosteal bone deposition, an expanded osseous contour can be created. The rate of bone expansion is variable. Certain tumors expand bone very slowly, and the accompanying periosteal response may eventually produce a surrounding cortical shell of such thickness that further expansion of the cortex is resisted. Other lesions, such as aneurysmal bone cysts, cause very rapid bone expansion (Fig. 69–8).

## Periosteal Response

A slowly growing tumor that is eroding or penetrating the cortex can evoke a periosteal response in which

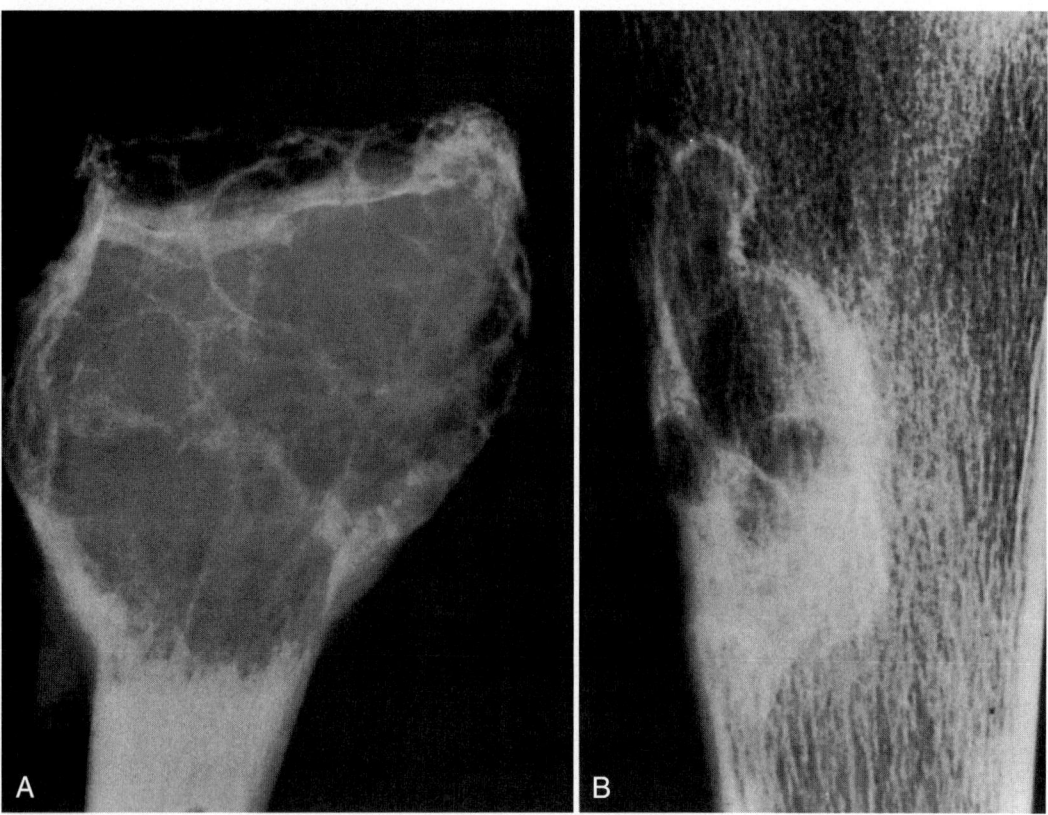

**Figure 69–6.** Trabeculation: specimen radiographs. *A*, Giant cell tumor. Note the delicate trabeculae that extend through and around this lesion of the distal portion of the radius. *B*, Nonossifying fibroma. A lobulated pattern of trabeculation characterizes this lesion of the proximal portion of the tibia.

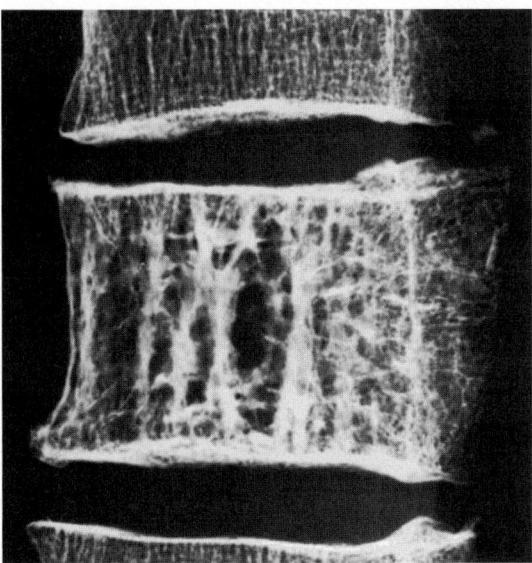

**Figure 69–7.** Trabeculation: hemangioma. Specimen radiograph shows the typical "corduroy" appearance of a vertebral body that contains a hemangioma. Accentuation of the vertical trabecular pattern is present.

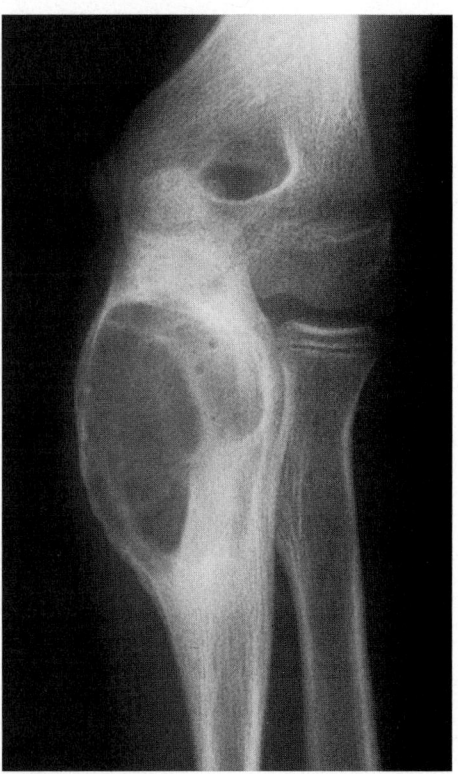

**Figure 69–8.** Bone expansion. This aneurysmal bone cyst of the proximal portion of the ulna is associated with expansion of bone but an intact cortical shell. Chronic periosteal bone formation is noted at the distal portion of the lesion.

additional layers of new bone are added to the exterior and an expanded osseous contour is created (Fig. 69–9). In these instances, the ultimate thickness of the surrounding cortical bone depends on the extent of endosteal erosion and periosteal proliferation. It can be of diminished or "normal" thickness in comparison to the original thickness of the cortex, or the new cortex can be thickened in a uniform or nonuniform fashion. If the interface between the normal and expanded cortex is "filled in" with bone, a buttressed pattern has evolved. With more rapid tumor growth, the periosteal response may be characterized by delicate layers of new bone. Single or multiple laminated bone formation may be identified. Multiple concentric layers of periosteal new bone produce the onion-peel pattern, which can be identified in some cases of Ewing's sarcoma and osteosarcoma.

At the periphery of a neoplasm or an infective focus, a triangular elevation of the periosteum may be identified that is termed Codman's triangle (Fig. 69–10). Usually, the subperiosteal area in the region of Codman's triangle is itself free of tumor. In certain neoplasms, such as osteosarcoma, rays of periosteal bone formation extend away from the bone in a radiating or sunburst pattern and emanate from a single focus in the bone; in other neoplasms, such as Ewing's sarcoma, the rays extend in a direction perpendicular to the underlying bone and create a hair-on-end periosteal pattern.

### Soft Tissue Mass

Soft tissue masses are not infrequently associated with malignant bone neoplasms. Osteomyelitis is also associated with a soft tissue mass or swelling. Although radiographic characteristics that may differentiate an inflammatory mass from a neoplastic mass have been identified, these characteristics are not extremely reliable.

## DISTRIBUTION IN A SINGLE BONE

The distribution of a solitary lesion within a bone provides an important clue to the correct diagnosis.

### Position of Lesions in the Transverse Plane

The center of a lesion can frequently be identified as having a central, eccentric, cortical, juxtacortical (parosteal or periosteal), or soft tissue location (Figs. 69–11 and 69–12). Establishing the position of the center of a lesion is less reliable when a narrow tubular bone, such as the fibula, is the site of involvement.

Some lesions characteristically lie on or close to the central axis of the bone within the medullary canal (i.e., central lesions). These lesions include enchondromas, fibrous dysplasia, some aneurysmal bone cysts, and simple bone cysts. Other lesions arise to one side of the central axis of the bone, still within the medullary canal (i.e., eccentric lesions) or within the cortex (i.e., cortical lesions). It may be difficult to differentiate a lesion arising subcortically from one originating in the cortex. Eccentric lesions include giant cell tumors; mesenchymal sarcomas such as osteosarcoma, chondrosarcoma, and fibrosarcoma; and chondromyxoid fibromas. Cortical lesions include nonossifying fibromas and osteoid osteomas. Lesions arising adjacent to the outer surface of the cortex are generally considered juxtacortical. Juxtacortical lesions can be further divided into those

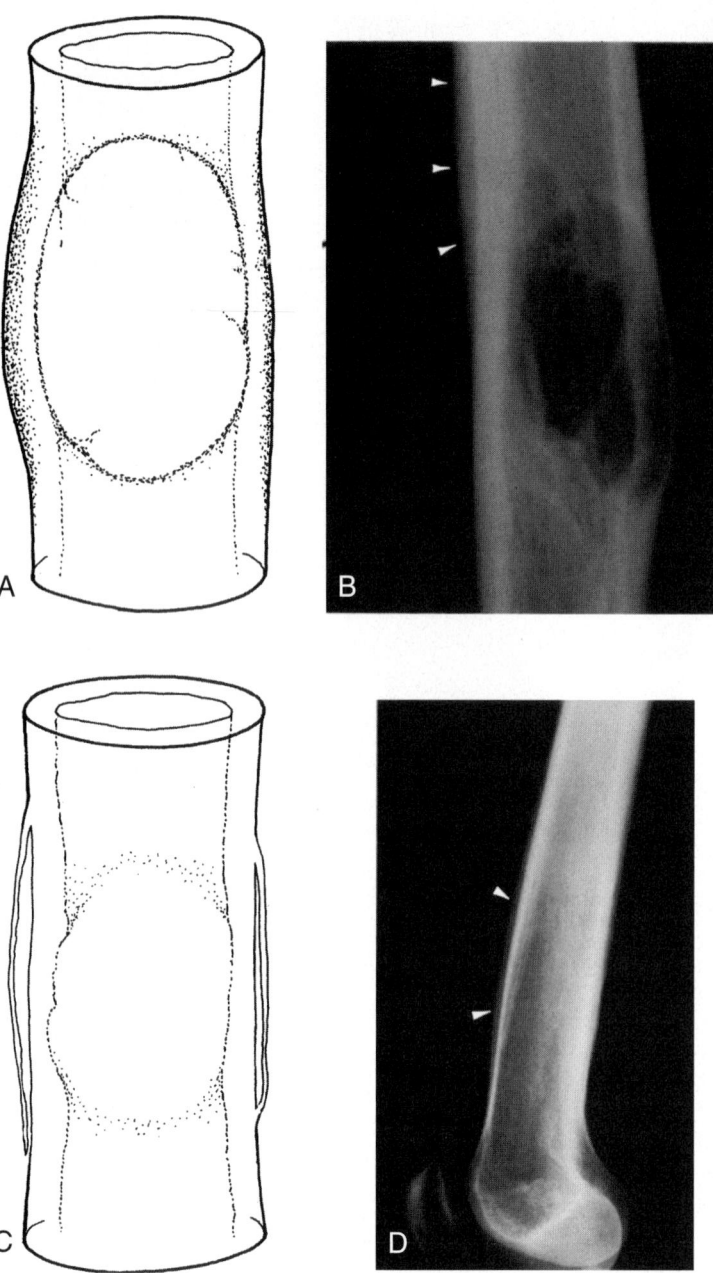

**Figure 69–9.** Periosteal response. *A* and *B*, Periosteal buttressing. The diagram *(A)* indicates that periosteal bone formation in response to a lesion may merge with the underlying cortex and produce a buttressed appearance. On the radiograph *(B)*, a thick single layer of periosteal bone *(arrowheads)* about this femoral lesion is still separated from the underlying cortex. The thickness of the periosteal response indicates a relatively slow-growing lesion. (Final diagnosis, simple bone cyst.) *C* and *D*, Single layer of periosteal bone. The diagram *(C)* demonstrates the appearance of a single thin layer of periosteal bone about a lesion, separated from the underlying bone. The radiograph *(D)* indicates a single layer of periosteal bone on both the anterior and posterior surfaces of the femur. Anteriorly, the periosteal layer is quite thick and still separated from the underlying bone *(arrowheads)*. Posteriorly, the periosteal bone has merged with the femur. (Final diagnosis, hypertrophic osteoarthropathy.)

derived from the deep layer of the periosteum and separating it from the cortex (i.e., periosteal lesions) and those derived from the outer layer of the periosteum and growing in an exophytic pattern (i.e., parosteal lesions). Typical examples of juxtacortical lesions are juxtacortical chondromas, periosteal osteosarcomas, and parosteal osteosarcomas.

## Position of Lesions in the Longitudinal Plane

Certain solitary lesions in the tubular bones show a remarkable propensity to develop in specific anatomic locations, such as the epiphysis, metaphysis, and diaphysis. Examples of lesions that may involve the epiphyses of adults are clear cell chondrosarcoma, metastasis, lipoma

(Fig. 69–13*A*), and intraosseous ganglion. Although originating in the metaphysis, giant cell tumors quickly penetrate the closed growth plate and involve the epiphysis, with extension to the subchondral bone adjacent to the joint (see Fig. 69–13*B*). Examples of epiphyseal lesions in children are chondroblastoma (see Fig. 69–13*C*), osteomyelitis, and, less frequently, osteoid osteoma, enchondroma, and eosinophilic granuloma. Transarticular spread of epiphyseal tumors is encountered most consistently with aggressive lesions, such as bone sarcomas, plasma cell myeloma, and skeletal metastasis, and in joints that lack or have limited mobility, such as the sacroiliac and discovertebral joints.

Metaphyseal lesions include nonossifying fibroma, which characteristically develops a short distance from

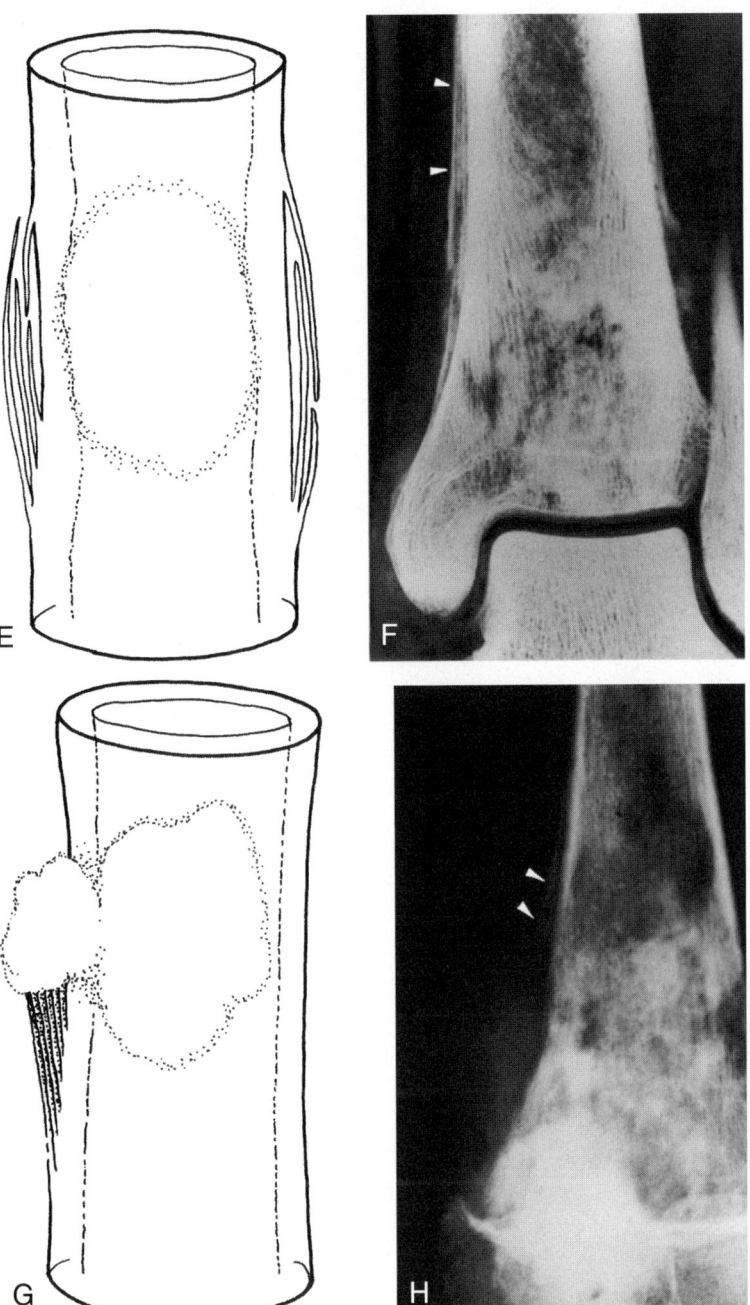

**Figure 69–9.**—*Continued E* and *F,* Multiple layers of periosteal bone: onion-peel pattern. The diagram *(E)* indicates multiple concentric layers of periosteal bone about the lesion. The specimen radiograph *(F)* shows such a pattern along one side of the distal portion of the tibia *(arrowheads).* On the other side of the bone, a more complex pattern of periostitis is seen. The medullary lesion contains radiopaque foci. (Final diagnosis, osteosarcoma.) *G* and *H,* Codman's triangle. The diagram *(G)* reveals triangular elevation of the periosteum beneath an aggressive lesion that is penetrating the cortex. The specimen radiograph *(H)* shows Codman's triangle *(arrowheads).* Note the medullary and cortical bone destruction, soft tissue mass, and radiodense foci within the lesion. (Final diagnosis, osteosarcoma.)

the growth plate; chondromyxoid fibroma, which abuts the growth plate; simple bone cyst; osteochondroma; Brodie's abscess; and mesenchymal sarcomas, such as osteosarcoma and chondrosarcoma (Table 69–2).

Aggressive lesions that may develop in a diaphysis include round cell tumors, such as Ewing's sarcoma. Nonaggressive lesions that may appear in the diaphysis of a tubular bone include nonossifying fibromas, simple bone cysts, aneurysmal bone cysts, enchondromas, osteoblastomas, and fibrous dysplasia.

Although these anatomic divisions are not applied as accurately to lesions in flat bones, epiphyseal-equivalent areas exist beneath the articular cartilage in the bones of

the pelvic and shoulder girdles, such that lesions in these areas are commonly those that show a predilection for the epiphyses in tubular bones. Similar "epiphyseal" lesions may develop in the small bones of the wrist and midfoot and in the patella.

## LOCATION IN THE SKELETON

Certain tumors predominate in areas of red, or hematopoietic, marrow as a result of being derived from cells of the red marrow or being transported to such areas by the vasculature of the marrow. Metastatic disease, plasma cell myeloma, Ewing's sarcoma, and certain types

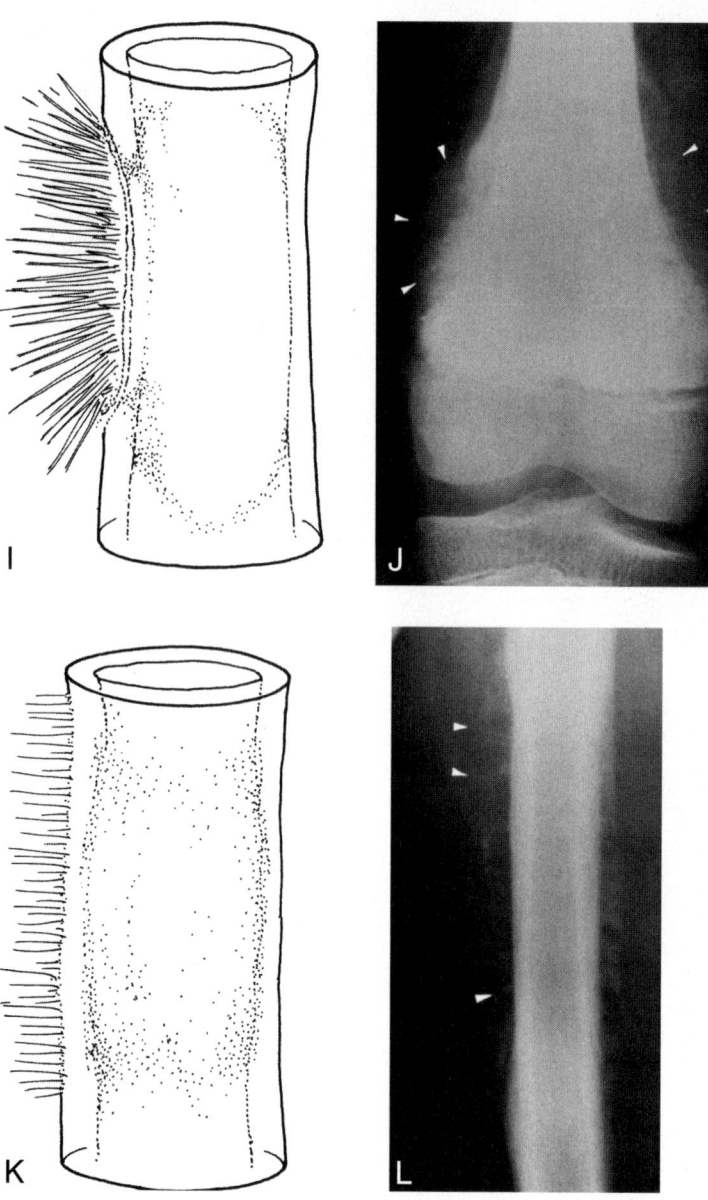

**Figure 69–9.**—*Continued I* and *J*, Radiating spicules of periosteal bone: sunburst pattern. The diagram *(I)* shows radiating spicules that emanate from a single focus within the bone. The radiograph *(J)* indicates such a sunburst pattern of periosteal bone *(arrowheads)* that is intermixed with tumor bone formation. Note the radiodense lesion in the medullary bone and Codman's triangle. (Final diagnosis, osteosarcoma.) *K* and *L*, Radiating spicules of periosteal bone: hair-on-end pattern. The diagram *(K)* demonstrates the parallel horizontal spicules that emanate from the underlying bone. The radiograph *(L)* indicates a femoral lesion characterized by a hair-on-end pattern *(arrowheads)*. The individual striations of periosteal bone have created an inhomogeneous band of radiodensity on the opposite side of the bone. (Final diagnosis, Ewing's sarcoma.)

of lymphoma are among the tumors that localize primarily to hematopoietic marrow. The tendency for these neoplasms to involve both the appendicular and axial skeletons in the young and predominantly the axial skeleton in the aged is consistent with the changing distribution of red marrow that takes place with advancing age.

Many primary osseous neoplasms develop in areas of rapid bone growth, especially the distal portion of the femur and the proximal portions of the tibia and humerus. Further, the vascular anatomy peculiar to this region, which consists of looped vessels and sinusoidal channels, promotes sluggish blood flow and, with it, metastatic seeding of tumor (and infection).

Certain tumors, because of their derivation, predominate in one or more areas of the skeleton. A variety of neoplasms related to dentition are virtually confined to the mandible and maxilla. Chordomas, which develop from remnants of the primitive notochord, are typically seen at the cranial and caudal limits of the vertebral column. Epidermoid cysts, apparently occurring because of implantation of cells from superficial tissue, have a definite predilection for the terminal phalanges and calvaria. Neurilemomas occur most commonly in sites containing extensive intraosseous nerves, such as the mandible and sacrum.

In adults, lesions of the vertebrae relate most frequently to skeletal metastasis, plasma cell myeloma, hemangioma, lymphoma, and osteomyelitis. In children with spinal lesions, important diagnostic considerations are eosinophilic granuloma, aneurysmal bone cyst, osteoblastoma, osteoid osteoma, lymphoma, leukemia, and osteomyelitis. In addition to chordomas, other important lesions of the sacrum include plasmacytomas, metastases, lymphomas, Ewing's sarcoma, giant cell tumors, and a variety of neurogenic cystic lesions. Sternal lesions in adults are

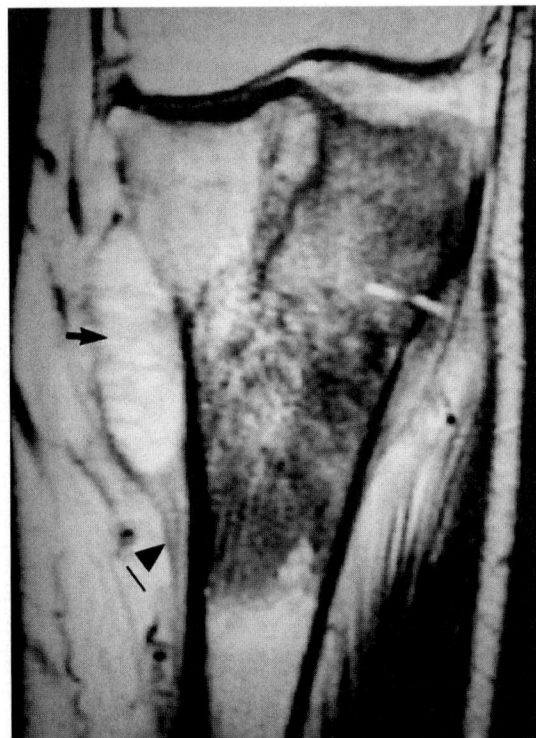

**Figure 69–10.** Periosteal response: Codman's triangle. This coronal fast spin echo (TR/TE, 5400/87) magnetic resonance image reveals a bone-forming tumor that has extended into the adjacent soft tissues *(arrow)*, with triangular elevation of the periosteal membrane (Codman's triangle) at the inferior portion of the lesion *(arrowhead)* in the tibia. (Final diagnosis, osteosarcoma.)

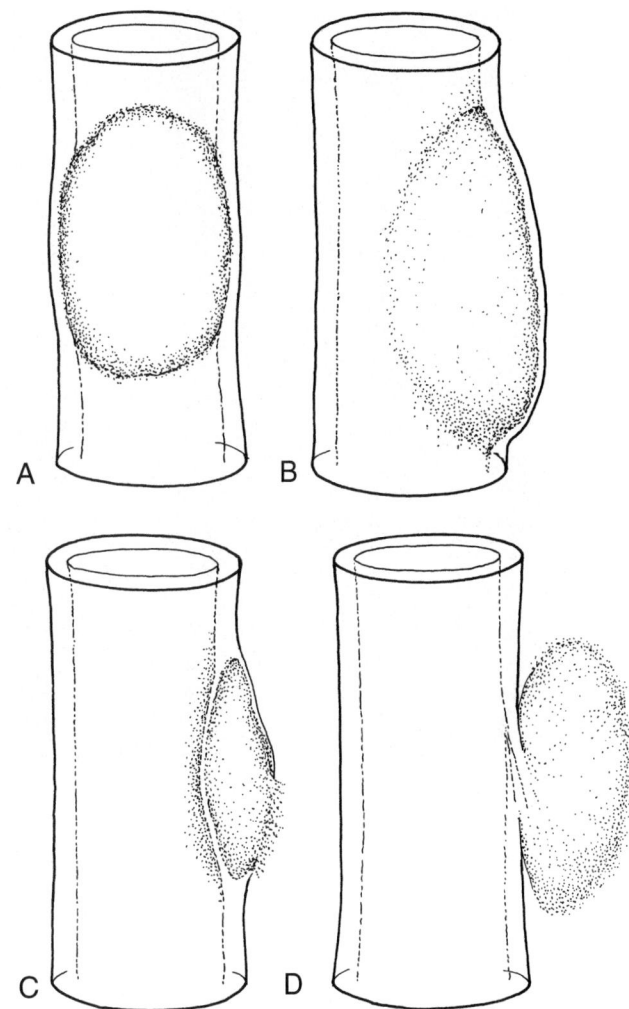

**Figure 69–11.** Position of lesions in the transverse plane. Lesions may be central *(A)*, eccentric *(B)*, cortical *(C)*, or juxtacortical *(D)*. Identification of the precise position of the lesion requires that radiographs be obtained in more than one projection.

typically caused by malignant tumors such as metastasis, plasma cell myeloma, lymphoma, and chondrosarcoma. Similarly, clavicular lesions in adults are usually malignant tumors. Metastasis is the dominant cause of rib lesions in adults, but enchondromas and fibrous dysplasia are other common causes of such lesions. Although enchondroma (Fig. 69–14A) and giant cell tumor should be given serious diagnostic consideration in patients with well-defined lesions of the metacarpal bones and phalanges of the hand, sarcoidosis, giant cell reparative granuloma, fibrous dysplasia, and aneurysmal bone cyst

should also be considered. With regard to the terminal phalanges, additional diagnostic choices include an inclusion cyst (see Fig. 69–14B), glomus tumor, and even metastasis. Patellar lesions are generally benign.

## TABLE 69–2

**Mesenchymal Sarcoma versus Round Cell Sarcoma***

|  | Mesenchymal | Round Cell |
| --- | --- | --- |
| Examples | Osteosarcoma, chondrosarcoma, fibrosarcoma | Ewing's sarcoma, leukemias |
| Location in tubular bones | Metaphyseal | Metadiaphyseal |
| Types of bone destruction | Moth-eaten pattern | Permeative pattern |
| Visible tumor matrix | Common (osteosarcoma, chondrosarcoma) | Rare |
| Periostitis | Sunburst, Codman's triangle | Onion-peel, hair-on-end, Codman's triangle |

*Classic features are indicated for each type of sarcoma, although considerable variability may be evident.

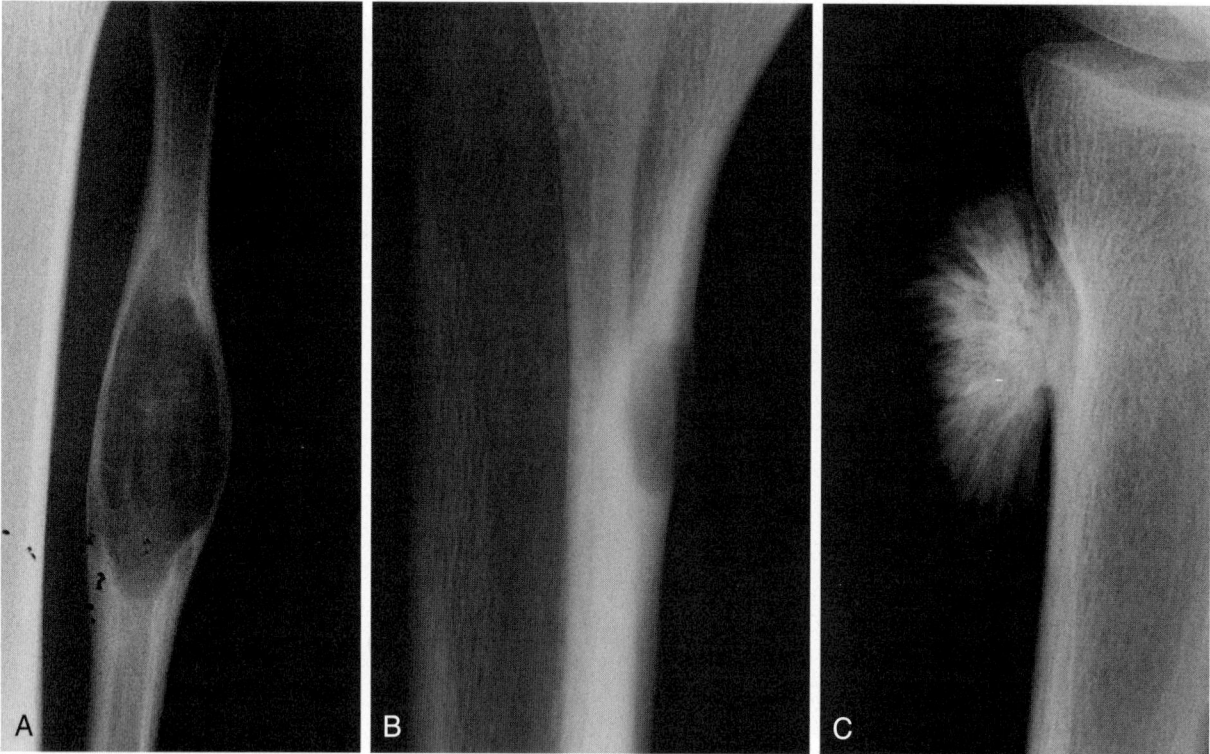

**Figure 69–12.** Position of lesions in the transverse plane. *A*, Central (simple bone cyst). *B*, Cortical (nonossifying fibroma). *C*, Juxtacortical (parosteal osteosarcoma). (*A*, Courtesy of V. Vint, MD, San Diego, Calif. *C*, Courtesy of A. D'Abreu, MD, Porto Alegre, Brazil.)

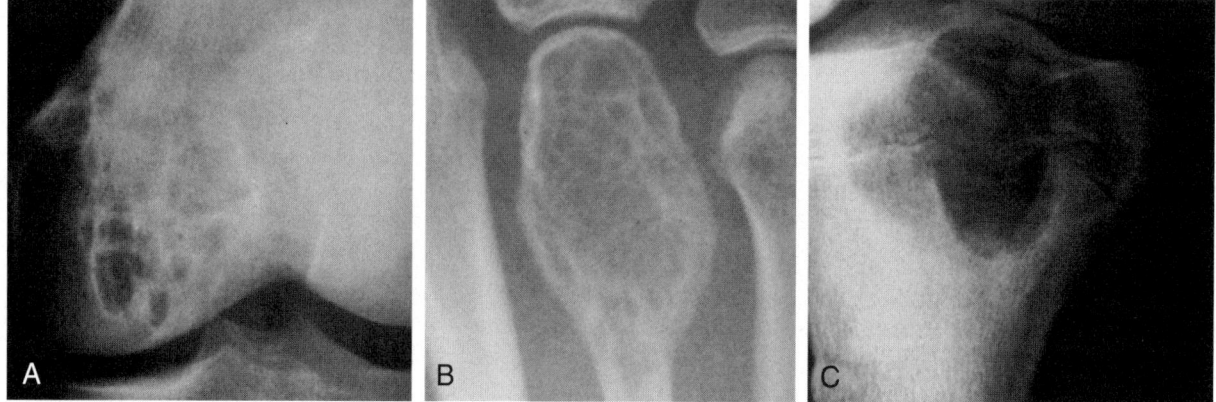

**Figure 69–13.** Position of lesions in the longitudinal plane: lesions involving epiphyses. *A*, Intraosseous lipoma. *B*, Giant cell tumor. *C*, Chondroblastoma. (*A*, Courtesy of A. G. Bergman, MD, Stanford, Calif. *C*, Courtesy of R. Stiles, MD, Atlanta, Ga.)

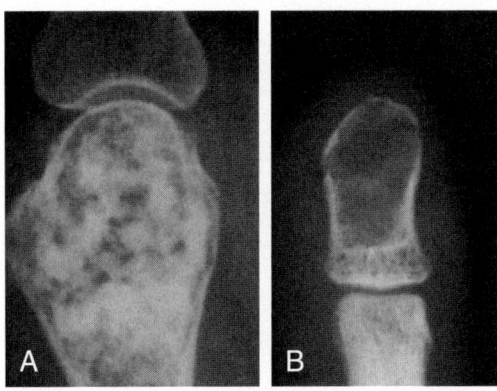

**Figure 69–14.** Lesions of the metacarpal bones and phalanges of the hand. *A*, Enchondroma. *B*, Inclusion cyst. (*A*, Courtesy of S. Kursunoglu-Brahme, MD, San Diego, Calif. *B*, Courtesy of G. Greenway, MD, Dallas, Tex.)

## FURTHER READING

Ehara S, Khurana JS, Kattapuram SV, et al: Osteolytic lesions of the patella. AJR 153:103, 1989.

Jones SN, Stoker DJ: Radiology at your fingertips: Lesions of the terminal phalanx. Clin Radiol 39:478, 1988.

Kricun ME: Radiographic evaluation of solitary bone lesions. Orthop Clin North Am 14:39, 1983.

Kricun ME: Red-yellow marrow conversion: Its effect on the location of some solitary bone lesions. Skel Radiol 14:10, 1985.

Lodwick GS: The bones and joints. In PJ Hodes (Ed): Atlas of Tumor Radiology. Chicago, Year Book Medical Publishers, 1971.

Lodwick GS, Wilson AJ, Farrell C, et al: Determining growth rates of focal lesions of bone from radiographs. Radiology 134:577, 1980.

Lodwick GS, Wilson AJ, Farrell C, et al: Estimating the rate of growth in bone lesions: Observer performance and error. Radiology 134:585, 1980.

Seeger LL, Yao L, Eckardt JJ: Surface lesions of bone. Radiology 206:17, 1998.

Volberg FM Jr, Whalen JP, Krook L, et al: Lamellated periosteal reactions: A radiologic and histologic investigation. AJR 128:85, 1977.

# CHAPTER 70

## Tumors and Tumor-Like Lesions of Bone: Imaging and Pathology of Specific Lesions

### Donald Resnick, Michael Kyriakos, and Guerdon D. Greenway

## SUMMARY OF KEY FEATURES

Many tumors and tumor-like lesions may involve bone. Accurate diagnosis of these lesions requires close cooperation among the orthopedic surgeon, radiologist, and pathologist. The patient's age and the site of skeletal localization are fundamental to the proper interpretation of the abnormalities detected by routine radiography and specialized imaging techniques. In many instances, however, a single diagnosis cannot be offered on the basis of such abnormalities, and careful histologic and, more recently, immunohistochemical analyses are required.

## INTRODUCTION

The number of specific tumors that affect the skeleton is large, and selecting the one that is most likely based on radiographic findings can sorely test the clinical acumen of even the keenest observer. Although additional imaging methods can provide diagnostic help in many cases, the importance of complete and accurate clinical information cannot be overstated. Attempting to interpret imaging studies in the absence of such clinical data significantly increases the likelihood of misdiagnosis. In particular, consideration of the patient's age is fundamental to the correct interpretation of imaging abnormalities. The propensity of a specific tumor to affect infants, children, adolescents, young or middle-aged adults, or the elderly is one of the most characteristic features of many tumors and tumor-like lesions of the skeleton (Table 70–1). Almost equal in diagnostic importance is knowledge of the skeletal sites that are characteristically affected by each of these lesions (Table 70–2).

## BONE-FORMING TUMORS

### Benign Tumors

#### Osteoma

Osteomas, benign lesions composed of dense, compact osseous tissue that usually arise from membranous bones, are discussed in Chapter 82.

### Enostosis (Bone Island)

The common lesions known as enostoses or bone islands are discussed in Chapter 82.

### Osteoid Osteoma

An osteoid osteoma is a benign osteoblastic tumor with distinctive histologic abnormalities consisting of a central core of vascular osteoid tissue and a peripheral zone of sclerotic bone. This lesion has been the focus of intense investigation into its neoplastic or infectious origin and its precise relationship to another lesion of bone, osteoblastoma. In this chapter, osteoid osteoma and osteoblastoma are considered distinct lesions.

#### Clinical Abnormalities

Osteoid osteomas are observed most frequently in patients between the ages of 7 and 25 years, more frequently in males (3:1). With rare exception, pain is the hallmark of the lesion, and without this symptom, the diagnosis is suspect. The pain typically is more intense at night and is ameliorated with small doses of salicylates. Pain may be accompanied by soft tissue swelling and tenderness. In an immature skeleton, significant aberrations in growth, muscle atrophy, and skeletal deformity are recognized complications of osteoid osteomas. Torticollis, spinal stiffness, and scoliosis are among the clinical characteristics of lesions that develop in the vertebral column, whereas joint tenderness, swelling, synovitis, and limitation of motion may be the initial clinical manifestations of intra-articular osteoid osteomas.

Lesions are invariably small; some investigators use 1 cm as the upper limit of the size of an osteoid osteoma, whereas others use 1.5 cm. The femur is the bone involved most frequently, followed by the tibia. These two bones together account for more than half of cases, and the long bones are the site of origin in more than 70% of cases. The bones in the hands and feet are involved in 20% of cases. Within long bones, osteoid osteoma is usually located in the diaphysis, but it may also extend into the metaphysis. Epiphyseal and intra-articular osteoid osteomas are rare.

Vertebral osteoid osteomas usually arise from the posterior elements. The lumbar vertebrae are the sites most typically affected. Additional infrequent sites of localization of osteoid osteoma are the innominate bone, acetabulum, skull, mandible or maxilla, clavicle, scapula, ribs, and radius.

#### Radiographic Abnormalities

When present, the classic radiographic appearance of a centrally located, oval or round radiolucent area measuring less than 1 cm in diameter and surrounded by a zone of uniform bone sclerosis is virtually diagnostic of this lesion.

**TABLE 70–1**

**Tumors and Tumor-Like Lesions: Typical Ages of Patients**

| Tumor | Age (Years) |
|---|---|
| | 0  10  20  30  40  50  60  70  80 |
| *Malignant* | |
| Osteosarcoma | |
| Parosteal osteosarcoma | |
| Chondrosarcoma | |
| Fibrosarcoma | |
| Fibrous histiocytoma | |
| Malignant giant cell tumor | |
| Ewing's sarcoma | |
| Adamantinoma | |
| Angiosarcoma | |
| Histiocytic lymphoma | |
| Chordoma | |
| Plasma cell myeloma | |
| Skeletal metastasis | |
| *Benign* | |
| Osteoma | |
| Osteochondroma | |
| Enchondroma | |
| Chondroblastoma | |
| Chondromyxoid fibroma | |
| Osteoid osteoma | |
| Osteoblastoma | |
| Nonossifying fibroma | |
| Desmoplastic fibroma | |
| Lipoma | |
| Hemangioma | |
| Giant cell tumor | |
| Neurilemoma | |
| Simple bone cyst | |
| Aneurysmal bone cyst | |

Unfortunately, this appearance is not always present; it is modified according to the specific bone affected, as well as the precise site of involvement in that bone. Further, this lesion may occur in the cortex, in medullary or cancellous bone, or in a subperiosteal location, and the resulting radiographic abnormalities are not identical in these three locations.

**Long Tubular Bones.** With regard to the long tubular bones, osteoid osteomas that are diaphyseal in location (and some that are metaphyseal) are typically observed in the cortex and appear as a radiolucent lesion, representing the nidus, that is surrounded by bone sclerosis and cortical thickening caused by endosteal and subperiosteal new bone formation (Fig. 70–1). The nidus itself may be uniformly radiolucent or contain variable amounts of calcification. It is usually small (almost always <1 cm in diameter) and oval or round in configuration; these

characteristics have diagnostic significance and generally allow differentiation between osteoid osteoma and a stress fracture (which is accompanied by a linear, radiolucent cortical area) or osteoblastoma (which is commonly a larger lesion). In rare circumstances, a single osteoid osteoma may contain more than one nidus, or more than one osteoid osteoma, each with its own nidus, may be found. As a general rule, the nidus is located in the center of the sclerotic reaction, but its precise delineation may require additional imaging techniques such as conventional or computed tomography (CT).

Osteoid osteomas that are subperiosteal in location were once thought to be extremely rare. Recent evidence, however, based on analysis of CT scans and magnetic resonance (MR) images, suggests that a subperiosteal origin of this tumor may be common and that the apparent intracortical origin relates mainly to continual remodeling of bone with subperiosteal deposition and endosteal

**TABLE 70–2**

## Tumors and Tumor-Like Lesions: Typical Sites of Skeletal Localization

| Tumor or Tumor-Like Lesion (Number of Cases Evaluated) | Femur | Tibia | Fibula | Foot | Patella | Humerus | Radius | Ulna | Hand, Wrist |
|---|---|---|---|---|---|---|---|---|---|
| Enostosis (371) | 25 | 7 | 1 | 5 | <1 | 9 | 1 | <1 | 9 |
| Osteoid osteoma (661) | 32 | 24 | 4 | 11 | <1 | 7 | 1 | 3 | 9 |
| Osteoblastoma (conventional) (298) | 14 | 10 | 4 | 7 | <1 | 3 | 1 | 2 | 3 |
| Osteoblastoma (aggressive) (47) | 11 | 13 | 6 | 11 | | 2 | | | 2 |
| Osteosarcoma (conventional) (3844) | 46 | 21 | 3 | 1 | <1 | 11 | <1 | <1 | <1 |
| Osteosarcoma (telangiectatic) (191) | 54 | 16 | 5 | <1 | | 14 | <1 | <1 | <1 |
| Osteosarcoma (periosteal) (69) | 44 | 41 | 4 | | | 7 | | | |
| Osteosarcoma (parosteal) (300) | 64 | 11 | 3 | 2 | | 15 | 2 | 1 | <1 |
| Chondroma (enchondroma) (1028) | 11 | 3 | 2 | 7 | <1 | 7 | 2 | <1 | 57 |
| Chondroma (periosteal) (130) | 25 | 8 | 3 | 5 | | 32 | 2 | 2 | 20 |
| Chondroblastoma (642) | 33 | 18 | 1 | 10 | 2 | 22 | 1 | | 2 |
| Chondromyxoid fibroma (231) | 17 | 38 | 8 | 16 | | 1 | 3 | 3 | 2 |
| Osteochondroma (solitary) (1604) | 31 | 18 | 4 | 6 | <1 | 19 | 1 | 1 | 5 |
| Chondrosarcoma (conventional) (1937) | 24 | 7 | 2 | 2 | <1 | 10 | 1 | 1 | 3 |
| Chondrosarcoma (clear cell) (64) | 64 | 5 | | | | 16 | | 2 | 2 |
| Chondrosarcoma (mesenchymal) (92) | 15 | 7 | 1 | 8 | | 7 | | 1 | |
| Chondrosarcoma (dedifferentiated) (107) | 43 | 7 | | | | 17 | | | |
| Nonossifying fibroma (833) | 38 | 43 | 8 | 1 | | 5 | 1 | <1 | 1 |
| Desmoplastic fibroma (121) | 12 | 8 | 2 | 2 | | 10 | 8 | 2 | 1 |
| Fibrosarcoma (621) | 39 | 16 | 3 | 2 | | 11 | 1 | 1 | <1 |
| Giant cell tumor (1949) | 31 | 27 | 4 | 2 | <1 | 6 | 10 | 3 | 4 |
| Fibrous histiocytoma (malignant) (271) | 44 | 21 | 2 | 2 | 1 | 9 | 1 | 1 | |
| Lipoma (66) | 15 | 14 | 20 | 15 | | 9 | | 2 | |
| Hemangioma (solitary) (195) | 4 | 3 | 2 | 5 | 1 | 3 | 1 | 1 | 2 |
| Hemangiopericytoma (48) | 10 | | 6 | 4 | | 15 | 4 | 2 | 2 |
| Angiosarcoma (151) | 18 | 23 | 4 | 6 | 1 | 13 | 2 | | 2 |
| Neurofibroma (42) | | 7 | 5 | | | 2 | | | |
| Neurilemoma (76) | 7 | 4 | 1 | 3 | 3 | 4 | | 5 | 8 |
| Chordoma (503) | | | | | | | | | |
| Simple bone cyst (884) | 27 | 6 | 5 | 1 | | 56 | 1 | 1 | 1 |
| Aneurysmal bone cyst (465) | 14 | 15 | 7 | 8 | <1 | 9 | 3 | 4 | 5 |
| Adamantinoma (189) | 3 | 81 | 3 | 1 | | 6 | 1 | 4 | 1 |
| Ewing's sarcoma (1974) | 22 | 11 | 9 | 3 | | 10 | 2 | 1 | 1 |

*Numbers indicate the percentage of lesions that affect each of the skeletal sites based on analysis of major reports containing the greatest number of cases. Percentages may not always total 100 because numbers were rounded to the nearest whole number.

erosion (Fig. 70–2). Subperiosteal lesions are associated with more limited osseous proliferation immediately adjacent to or at a distance from the lesion.

**Carpus, Tarsus, and Epiphyses.** In the carpal or tarsal bones (Fig. 70–3), as well as in the epiphyses of the long tubular bones, an osteoid osteoma usually arises in the medullary spongiosa and, radiographically, appears as a well-circumscribed lesion that is partially or completely calcified. A radiolucent zone may surround the lesion, and extensive reactive sclerosis is generally absent. In the immature skeletons of children and adolescents, an osteoid osteoma arising in an epiphyseal ossification center can lead to alterations in normal physeal growth.

**Small Bones of the Hand and Foot.** In the metacarpals, metatarsals, and phalanges (Fig. 70–4), osteoid osteomas have a variable radiographic appearance. When located in the cortex, they generally provoke a periosteal response similar to that observed in the diaphysis of long tubular bones. In subperiosteal sites, they produce scalloping of the adjacent cortical surface, and in cancellous bone, a partially or totally calcified lesion with or without a radiolucent margin is identified. In any of these locations, soft tissue swelling may be prominent. Painless osteoid osteomas appear to be more frequent in the phalanges than in other sites.

**Intra-articular Sites.** Osteoid osteomas arising in an intra-articular location are associated with pain, soft tissue

**TABLE 70–2**

## Tumors and Tumor-Like Lesions: Typical Sites of Skeletal Localization *Continued*

| Tumor or Tumor-Like Lesion (Number of Cases Evaluated) | Site* | | | | | | | | |
|---|---|---|---|---|---|---|---|---|---|
| | Scapula | Clavicle | Sternum | Ribs | Vertebrae, Including Sacrum and Coccyx | Innominate Bone | Skull | Face | Mandible, Maxilla |
| Enostosis (371) | 1 | <1 | | 12 | 2 | 25 | | | |
| Osteoid osteoma (661) | 1 | | | <1 | 6 | 2 | <1 | | <1 |
| Osteoblastoma (conventional) (298) | 1 | <1 | | 4 | 30 | 2 | | -4- | 11 |
| Osteoblastoma (aggressive) (47) | 4 | | | 2 | 23 | 13 | 11 | | 2 |
| Osteosarcoma (conventional) (3844) | 1 | <1 | <1 | 1 | 2 | 7 | 1 | <1 | 4 |
| Osteosarcoma (telangiectatic) (191) | 2 | | | 2 | | 3 | 2 | | <1 |
| Osteosarcoma (periosteal) (69) | | | | 1 | | 1 | | | 1 |
| Osteosarcoma (parosteal) (300) | <1 | | | | | 1 | | | |
| Chondroma (enchondroma) (1028) | 1 | <1 | 1 | 5 | 1 | 3 | <1 | | |
| Chondroma (periosteal) (130) | | | | 2 | 1 | 2 | | | |
| Chondroblastoma (642) | 2 | <1 | <1 | 2 | 1 | 4 | 1 | | <1 |
| Chondromyxoid fibroma (231) | 1 | | <1 | 3 | 2 | 6 | <1 | | |
| Osteochondroma (solitary) (1604) | 4 | <1 | <1 | 2 | 2 | 5 | <1 | | |
| Chondrosarcoma (conventional) (1937) | 5 | 1 | 2 | 8 | 6 | 24 | 1 | 1 | 2 |
| Chondrosarcoma (clear cell) (64) | 2 | | | 3 | 3 | 2 | 2 | | 2 |
| Chondrosarcoma (mesenchymal) (92) | 2 | | 1 | 12 | 11 | 12 | 8 | 1 | 14 |
| Chondrosarcoma (differentiated) (107) | 8 | | <1 | 4 | 1 | 22 | | | |
| Nonossifying fibroma (833) | <1 | <1 | | 1 | | 1 | <1 | | <1 |
| Desmoplastic fibroma (121) | 3 | 2 | | 2 | 3 | 11 | 1 | 33 | |
| Fibrosarcoma (621) | 2 | 1 | <1 | 1 | 4 | 10 | 1 | | 7 |
| Giant cell tumor (1949) | <1 | <1 | <1 | 1 | 7 | 4 | 1 | <1 | <1 |
| Fibrous histiocytoma (malignant) (271) | 1 | 1 | <1 | 3 | 2 | 9 | 2 | | 3 |
| Lipoma (66) | | | | 8 | 5 | | 5 | | 9 |
| Hemangioma (solitary) (195) | 2 | 1 | | 9 | 25 | 3 | 29 | 2 | 8 |
| Hemangiopericytoma (48) | 2 | 4 | 4 | 8 | 15 | 11 | 2 | | 10 |
| Angiosarcoma (151) | 3 | | 1 | 5 | 10 | 8 | 3 | | 2 |
| Neurofibroma (42) | | | | | | 7 | | 2 | 76 |
| Neurilemoma (76) | 1 | | | 3 | 16 | 1 | 3 | | 42 |
| Chordoma (503) | | | | | 75 | | 25 | | |
| Simple bone cyst (884) | <1 | <1 | | <1 | | 2 | | | |
| Aneurysmal bone cyst (465) | 2 | 3 | | 3 | 14 | 9 | 2 | <1 | 2 |
| Adamantinoma (189) | | | | 1 | | 1 | | | |
| Ewing's sarcoma (1974) | 5 | 2 | <1 | 8 | 6 | 18 | 1 | <1 | 1 |

*Numbers indicate the percentage of lesions that affect each of the skeletal sites based on analysis of major reports containing the greatest number of cases. Percentages may not always total 100 because numbers were rounded to the nearest whole number.

swelling, and joint effusion (Fig. 70–5). Accurate diagnosis is commonly delayed. A synovial inflammatory response, characterized as lymphofollicular, may lead to irreversible cartilaginous and osseous destruction. Osteopenia, uniform narrowing of the interosseous space, and periarticular subperiosteal bone apposition may be encountered. Eventually, hypertrophic changes similar to those in osteoarthritis may be seen.

**Spine.** Pain, which may be radicular, is commonly prominent with spinal osteoid osteomas. Scoliosis, particularly when combined with pain, has repeatedly been emphasized as an important clinical manifestation of this lesion, although the combination is certainly not specific.

On radiographs, the lesion is characteristically located on the concave aspect of the scoliotic curve, near its apex. Osteosclerosis of a pedicle, lamina, articular process, or, less commonly, transverse or spinous process is observed. A radiolucent nidus may be present, but its identification frequently requires conventional tomography or CT (Fig. 70–6).

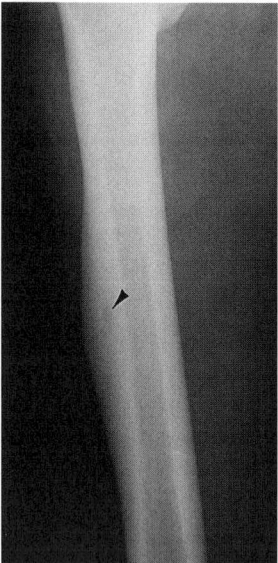

**Figure 70–1.** Osteoid osteoma: femur. Note the radiolucent nidus *(arrowhead)* with surrounding endosteal and periosteal bone formation in the diaphysis of the femur.

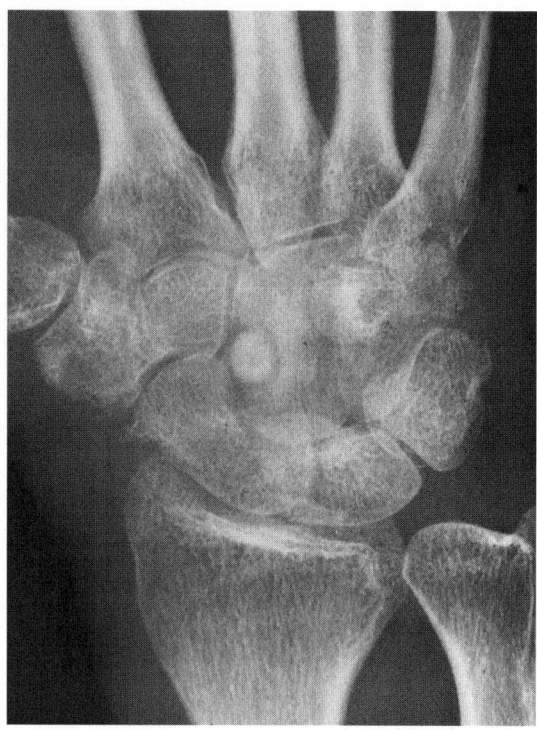

**Figure 70–3.** Osteoid osteoma: carpal bones. This osteoid osteoma in the capitate of a 17-year-old boy manifests as a partially calcified lesion with osteopenia in all the carpal bones.

**Other Skeletal Sites.** In the innominate bones of the pelvis and in the scapula, an osteoid osteoma most typically appears as a radiolucent or partially calcified lesion with limited surrounding bone sclerosis. A para-articular location such as the glenoid or acetabular region is characteristic (Fig. 70–7).

### *Other Imaging Techniques*

On scintigraphy, osteoid osteomas avidly accumulate bone-seeking radiopharmaceutical agents during the vascular, blood pool, and delayed phases of the examination. A distinctive pattern of abnormality, designated the double density sign, has been observed in radionuclide bone scans in patients with osteoid osteoma. This sign is characterized by intense scintigraphic activity centrally in the region of the nidus and less intense accumulation of the radionuclide peripherally in the sclerotic bone (Fig. 70–8).

CT scanning is most valuable in defining osteoid osteomas in the spine, osseous pelvis and femoral neck, and, occasionally, other sites (see Fig. 70–6). The choice of

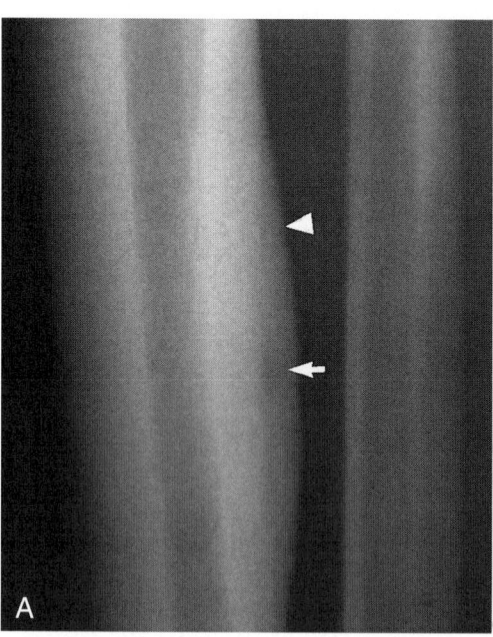

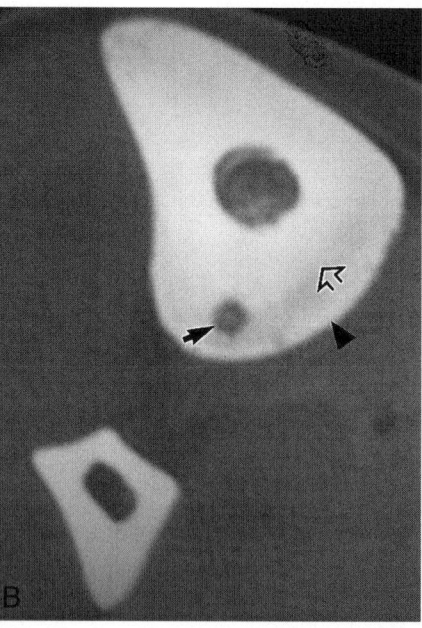

**Figure 70–2.** Osteoid osteoma: subperiosteal lesions. *A,* In this 24-year-old man, a routine radiograph shows periosteal new bone formation *(arrowhead)* in the posterolateral aspect of the midshaft of the tibia. Note the 3-mm radiolucent nidus *(arrow). B,* Transverse CT scan at the level of the tibial lesion shows mature periosteal bone *(arrowhead),* the partially calcified nidus *(solid arrow),* and the location of the original cortex *(open arrow).* The nidus sits on the surface of this original cortex. (From Kayser F, Resnick D, Haghigh P, et al: Evidence of the subperiosteal origin of osteoid osteomas in tubular bones: Analysis by CT and MR imaging. AJR Am J Roentgenol 170:609, 1998.)

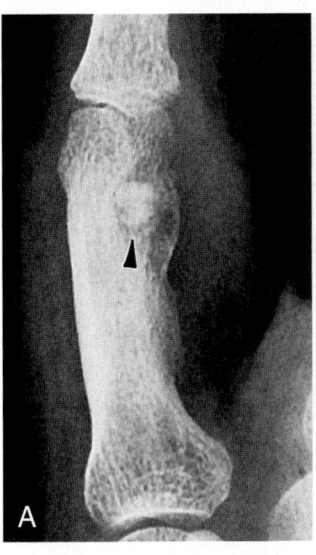
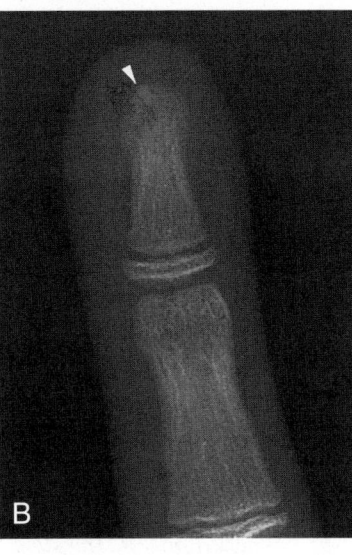

**Figure 70–4.** Osteoid osteoma: phalanges. *A,* In the proximal phalanx of the fifth finger; the nidus *(arrowhead)* is partially calcified, and considerable soft tissue swelling is evident. *B,* Note the radiodense focus *(arrowhead)* in a terminal phalanx, with adjacent soft tissue swelling. (*A,* Courtesy of P. Major, MD, Winnipeg, Manitoba, Canada.)

adequate window settings for visualization of cortical bone is essential for accurate CT documentation of the nidus.

Although MR imaging has been used in the evaluation of osteoid osteomas, it is generally considered less useful than CT scanning for detection of the nidus; further, MR imaging findings in osteoid osteoma may simulate those of a malignant tumor or osteomyelitis as a result of the presence of marrow and soft tissue edema or even a soft tissue mass. MR imaging findings of synovitis and joint effusion (Figs. 70–9 and 70–10) may accompany intra-

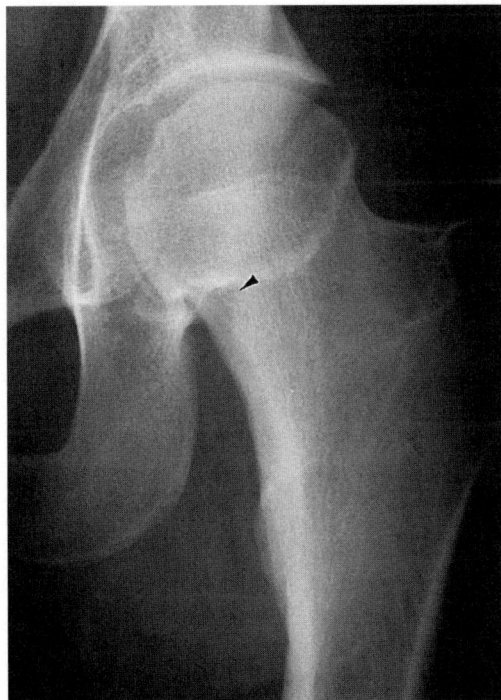

**Figure 70–5.** Osteoid osteoma: hip. An osteoid osteoma with a radiolucent nidus *(arrowhead)* in the femoral neck has produced extensive adjacent new bone formation, osteophytosis, and mild narrowing of the hip joint.

articular osteoid osteomas. When seen on MR images, the nidus of an osteoid osteoma reveals variable patterns of signal intensity, depending on the size of the nidus and the amount of calcification or fibrous tissue present.

### Pathologic Abnormalities

Microscopically, the nidus of an osteoid osteoma consists of bone in various stages of maturity within a highly vascular connective tissue stroma containing numerous dilated capillaries. Seams of osteoid form irregular trabeculae of woven or reticular bone. Histologically, osteoid osteoma and osteoblastoma are similar, although some investigators believe that osteoblastomas may be more vascular and possess more osteoblasts, wider trabeculae, and less organization than osteoid osteomas. Distinction between the two tumors also depends on their size, location, and clinical features.

### Natural History

It is well recognized that surgical resection of the entire nidus is a prerequisite for an optimal clinical response. Recently, percutaneous radiofrequency ablation has been shown to be an effective alternative to open surgery. The method involves placement of a radiofrequency probe using CT guidance and appears to be better suited to removing osteoid osteomas in the long tubular bones (Fig. 70–11) than in small bones or the spine. The natural history of osteoid osteomas that are not removed surgically (or percutaneously) is not clear because precise diagnosis of the lesion requires verification of typical histologic features. In several reported instances, lesions with the clinical and radiographic (and CT or MR imaging) characteristics of osteoid osteoma healed spontaneously over varying time spans.

### Differential Diagnosis

In an intracortical location, a lesion containing a radiolucent center (with or without calcification) and a periph-

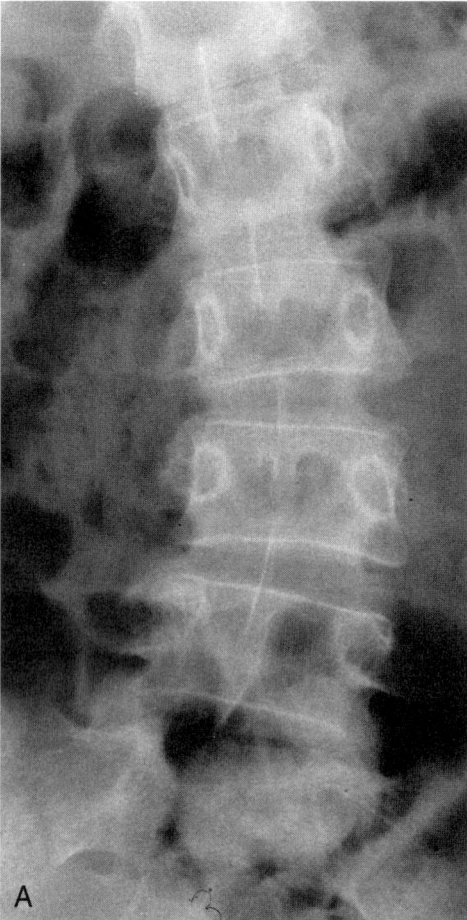

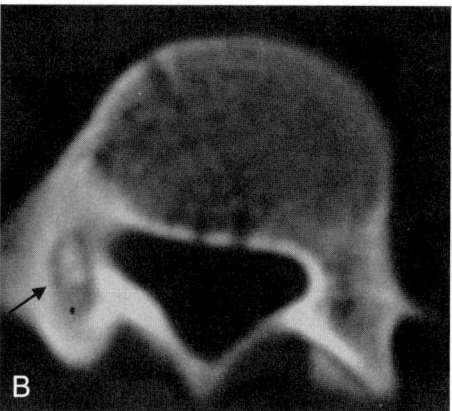

**Figure 70–6.** Osteoid osteoma: spine. *A,* Frontal radiograph of the lumbar spine shows scoliosis but no other significant abnormalities. *B,* Transaxial CT scan at the level of the fifth lumbar vertebra reveals the partially calcified nidus *(arrow)* of an osteoid osteoma. (Courtesy of J. Kirkham, MD, Minneapolis, Minn.)

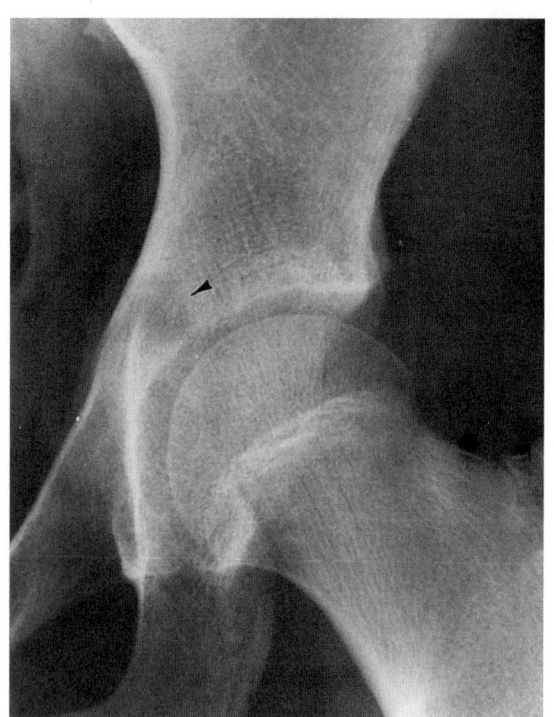

**Figure 70–7.** Osteoid osteoma: innominate bone. Hip pain in this 13-year-old boy resulted from an osteoid osteoma *(arrowhead)* in the acetabular region.

eral zone of bone sclerosis is almost certainly an osteoid osteoma, despite occasional reports of an abscess or a bone tumor (i.e., hemangioma, osteosarcoma). When an osteoid osteoma is in a subperiosteal or intramedullary location or within an articulation, the radiographic diagnosis is more difficult, and in certain sites such as the spine, additional diagnostic methods may be required for precise delineation of the nidus.

## Osteoblastoma

Osteoblastoma can be categorized into conventional and aggressive types.

### Conventional Osteoblastoma

Benign osteoblastoma is a relatively uncommon primary neoplasm of bone that is composed of a well-vascularized connective tissue stroma with active production of osteoid and primitive woven bone.

**Clinical Abnormalities.** Osteoblastoma is observed most frequently in persons younger than 30 years, with approximately 70% of cases appearing in the second or third decade of life. Males are affected more frequently than females, in a ratio of approximately 2:1. Local pain is a common manifestation of osteoblastoma, although it

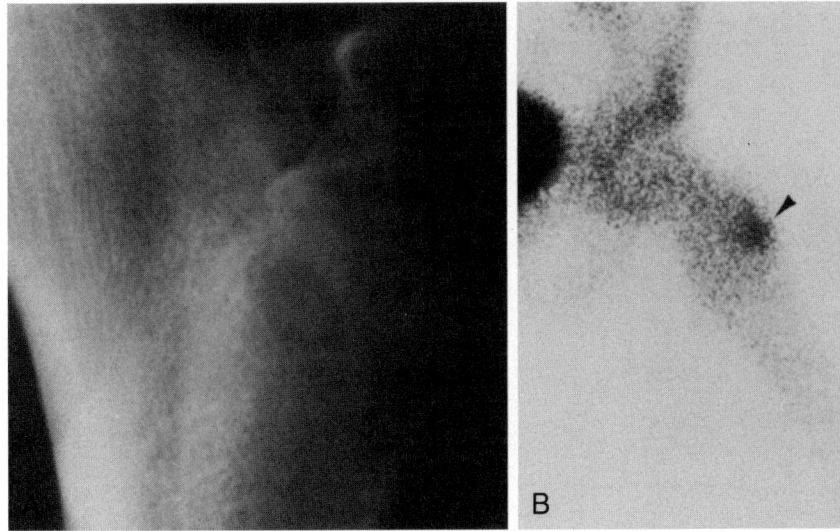

**Figure 70–8.** Osteoid osteoma: scintigraphic abnormalities. *A,* In this 15-year-old boy with a classic osteoid osteoma of the proximal portion of the femur, avid accumulation of bone-seeking radionuclide corresponds to the site of the radiographically evident lesion. *B,* Note that the region of most intense scintigraphic activity *(arrowhead)* is surrounded by a zone of less intense, but abnormal, activity.

is generally mild. Accentuation of pain at night and its amelioration with salicylates are inconstant clinical features of osteoblastoma. Spinal lesions may be accompanied by muscle spasm, scoliosis, and neurologic manifestations.

**Skeletal Location.** Although osteoblastoma can affect virtually any bone, it is most frequently observed in the flat bones or the vertebrae. The vertebrae are the site of origin in 30% of patients, and the long tubular bones are involved in approximately 35% of patients. Fifteen percent of tumors affect the skull, mandible, or maxilla; 5% of tumors occur in the innominate bone; and 10% are localized in the bones of the hands and feet.

In the long tubular bones, approximately 75% of osteoblastomas are situated in the diaphysis, with the remainder in the metaphysis. Epiphyseal involvement is distinctly unusual. Although the femur is the long bone most typically affected by osteoblastoma, the proximal portion of this bone is rarely involved. In the spine, the thoracic and lumbar vertebrae are the most frequent sites of involvement. Vertebral osteoblastomas arise mainly in the pedicles and the laminae. Involvement of the vertebral body is less typical.

**Radiographic Abnormalities.** The radiographic features of osteoblastoma are varied and, in most instances, non-

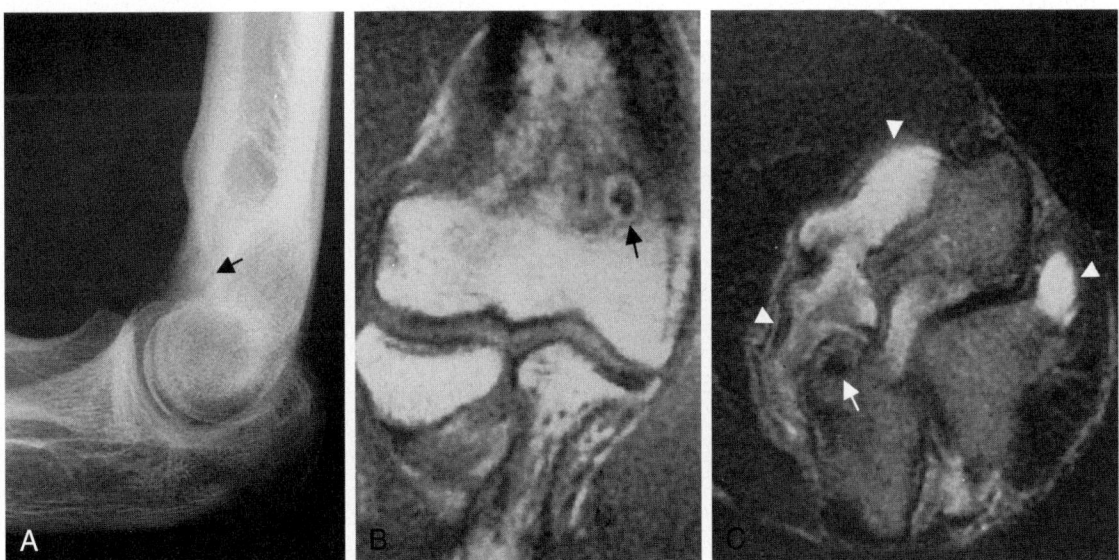

**Figure 70–9.** Osteoid osteoma: radiographic and MR imaging abnormalities. *A,* Lateral radiograph of the elbow shows cortical thickening in the distal portion of the humerus and a partially calcified nidus *(arrow)* of an osteoid osteoma. *B,* On a coronal T1-weighted (TR/TE, 600/20) spin echo MR image, the partially calcified nidus *(arrow)* is identified. *C,* Transaxial T2-weighted (TR/TE, 2500/70) spin echo MR image through the distal portion of the humerus reveals the nidus *(arrow)* and a large joint effusion *(arrowheads).* (Courtesy of P. VanderStoep, MD, St. Cloud, Minn.)

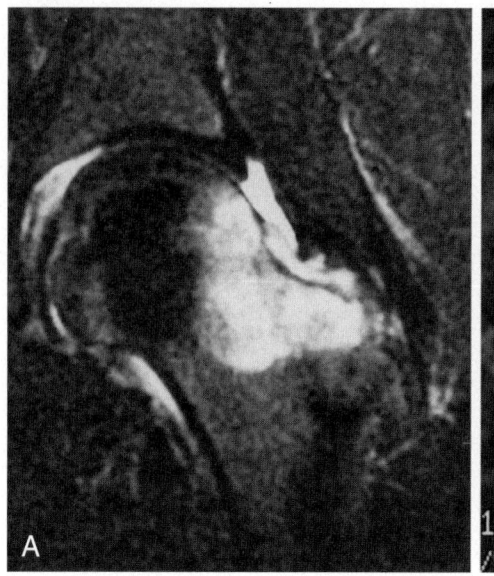
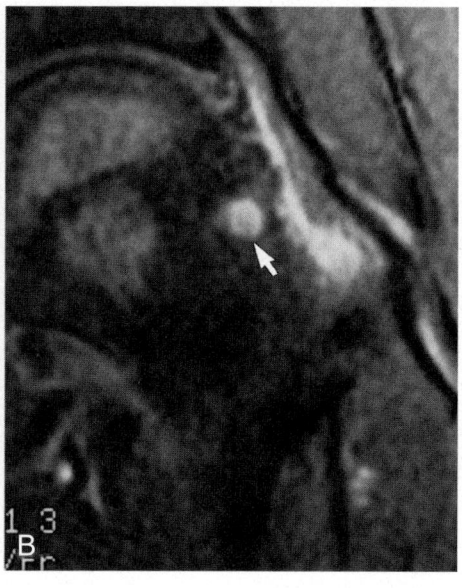

**Figure 70–10.** Osteoid osteoma: MR imaging abnormalities. In this 20-year-old man with hip pain, a coronal fat-suppressed fast spin echo (TR/TE, 5600/102) MR image (A) reveals femoral marrow edema and a joint effusion, but the nidus of an osteoid osteoma is not visible. After intravenous gadolinium administration, a coronal fat-suppressed T1-weighted (TR/TE, 81/3) spin echo MR image (B) shows the enhanced nidus (arrow). (Courtesy of M. Schweitzer, MD, Philadelphia, Pa.)

diagnostic. Osteolysis alone, osteosclerosis alone, or a combination of the two may be observed. Expansion of bone, cortical thinning, and a soft tissue mass may accompany this lesion.

In the long tubular bones, osteoblastomas may originate in medullary or cortical bone (Figs. 70–12 and 70–13) or, rarely, in a subperiosteal location. These lesions are usually round or oval, predominantly osteolytic with areas of calcification or ossification, well margined, and expansile. Bone sclerosis and periostitis may be exuberant. Similar radiographic alterations may accompany osteoblastomas in the small bones of the hands and feet and in the innominate bone (Fig. 70–14).

In the spine, a well-defined, expansile osteolytic lesion that is partially or extensively calcified or ossified and arises from the posterior osseous elements, especially in the thoracic or lumbar segment, should suggest the diagnosis of osteoblastoma (Fig. 70–15). Although not as characteristic as in cases of osteoid osteoma, scoliosis may

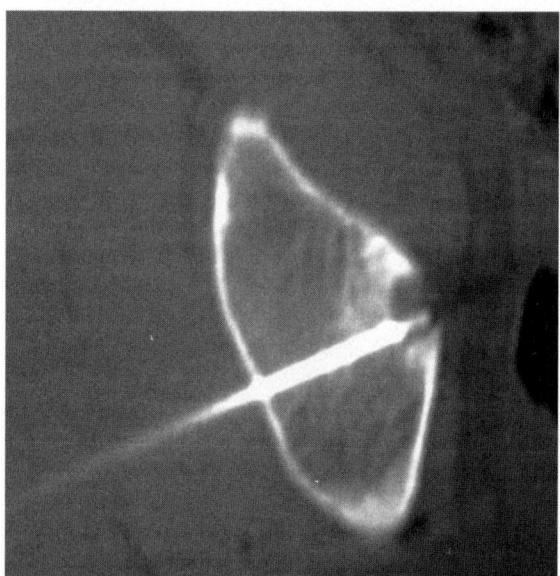

**Figure 70–11.** Osteoid osteoma: radiofrequency ablation. Transaxial CT scan obtained during a percutaneous ablation procedure shows the tip of the radiofrequency probe near the center of the lesion.

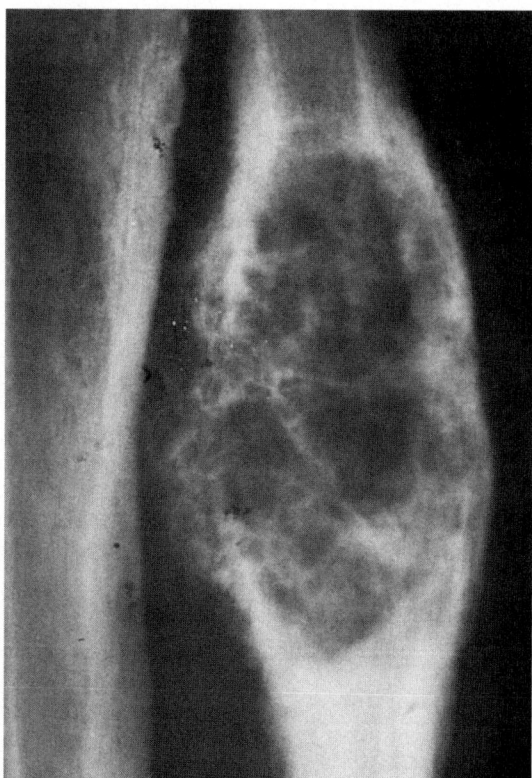

**Figure 70–12.** Osteoblastoma: long tubular bones. This aggressive lesion of the ulnar diaphysis is characterized by irregular osteolysis and osteosclerosis with cortical thickening and osseous expansion. (Courtesy of C. Resnik, MD, Baltimore, Md.)

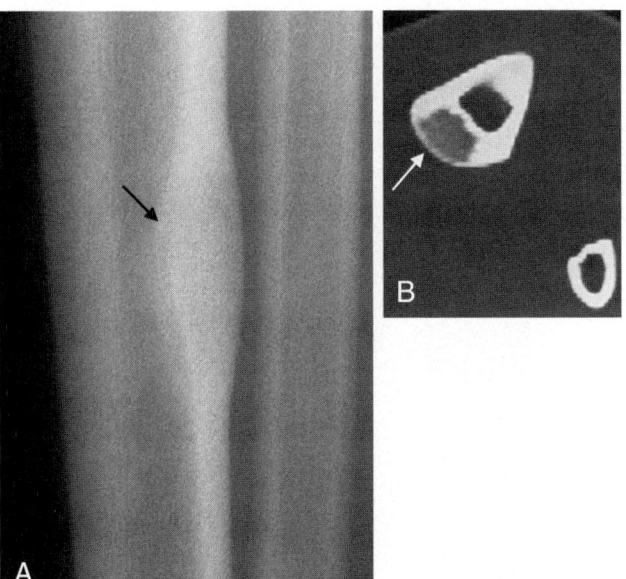

**Figure 70–13.** Osteoblastoma: long tubular bones. This 19-year-old man complained of leg pain. *A,* Routine radiograph shows a region of cortical thickening *(arrow)* containing an elongated radiolucent focus in the posterior aspect of the diaphysis of the tibia. *B,* Transaxial CT scan shows the intracortical tumor *(arrow).* The radiolucent region is larger than a typical osteoid osteoma.

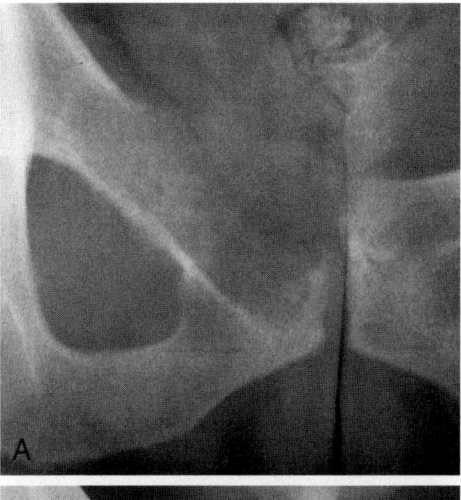

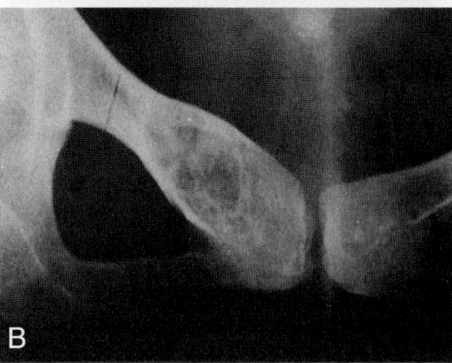

**Figure 70–14.** Osteoblastoma: innominate bone. Two examples show the variability of the radiographic features of this tumor. *A,* An osteolytic, expansile lesion of the parasymphyseal bone is present. *B,* Considerable osteosclerosis and calcification are evident in a lesion in a similar location. (*A,* Courtesy of R. S. Howell, MD, Louisville, Ky. *B,* Courtesy of P. Feldman, MD, Toronto, Ontario, Canada.)

accompany spinal osteoblastomas. Scoliosis may also be associated with osteoblastomas in the ribs. Osteoblastomas are infrequent in the skull.

**Other Imaging Techniques.** Bone scintigraphy reveals increased accumulation of radionuclide at the site of the lesion, and CT and MR imaging allow full delineation of the extent of the process. An inflammatory reaction in the bone about the tumor or in the nearby soft tissues may result in a misleading appearance on MR images that simulates a malignant tumor. Fluid levels may be seen within osteoblastomas.

**Pathologic Abnormalities.** Microscopically, the basic pattern of osteoblastoma is similar to that of osteoid osteoma and consists of a well-vascularized connective tissue stroma with active production of osteoid and primitive woven bone. There is considerable variation in this pattern, however. Some osteoblastomas have large tumor cells with bizarre, atypical hyperchromatic nuclei containing prominent nucleoli, or they may have a cartilaginous matrix, similar to the findings of osteosarcoma; conversely, some cases of osteosarcoma histologically resemble osteoblastoma. Cases are encountered in which foci of osteosarcoma coexist with areas of osteoblastoma, and some osteoblastomas have recurred with "transformation" to osteosarcoma. Whether these phenomena are the result of initial misdiagnosis of an osteosarcoma or true transformation of an osteoblastoma is unclear.

**Differential Diagnosis.** The radiographic abnormalities of osteoblastoma do not commonly allow a precise diagnosis,

although tumors in the posterior osseous elements of the vertebrae (which lead to an expansile, partially calcified area of osteolysis) or in the skull (which produce a sharply marginated radiolucent defect containing central calcification or ossification) may be accurately identified as osteoblastomas. In other sites, this neoplasm has a highly variable radiographic appearance that may include features suggestive of other diagnoses.

### Aggressive and Malignant Osteoblastoma

Although typical osteoblastomas may recur in as many as 10% of cases, particularly after incomplete excision, the documentation of recurrent osteoblastoma with a more aggressive histologic appearance than that of the original tumor serves as a warning that osteoblastomas should not be regarded as uniformly benign. In general, the anatomic distribution of aggressive or malignant osteoblastoma parallels that of conventional osteoblastoma. The vertebrae, tibia, femur, and skull are the most common sites of involvement. In the long tubular bones, a metaphyseal location with extension to the epiphysis may be evident. In all sites, the radiographic and macropathologic features of these lesions resemble the findings of typical

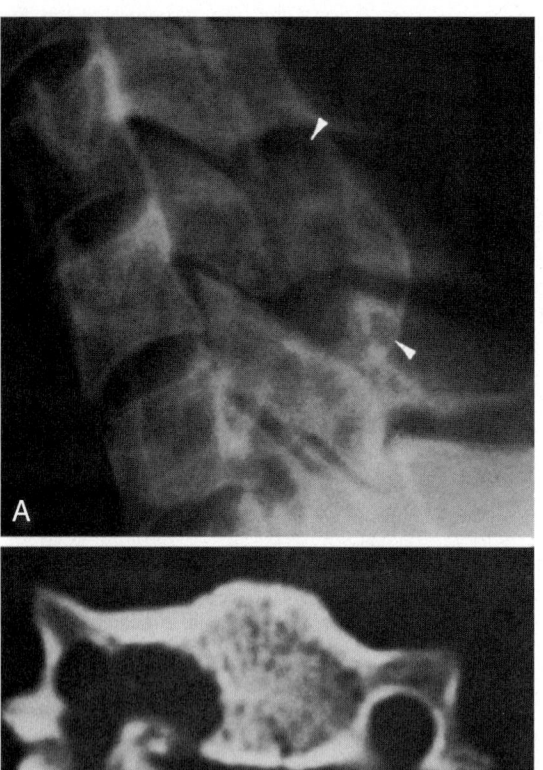

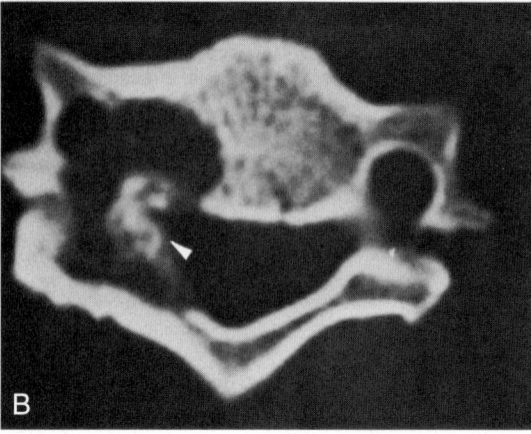

**Figure 70–15.** Osteoblastoma: spine. Two different examples are shown. *A,* An expansile lesion *(arrowheads)* in the lamina of the fifth cervical vertebra is evident. *B,* Note an osteolytic lesion containing calcification or ossification *(arrowhead)* affecting the body, transverse and costal elements, and lamina of a cervical vertebra as depicted on a transaxial CT scan.

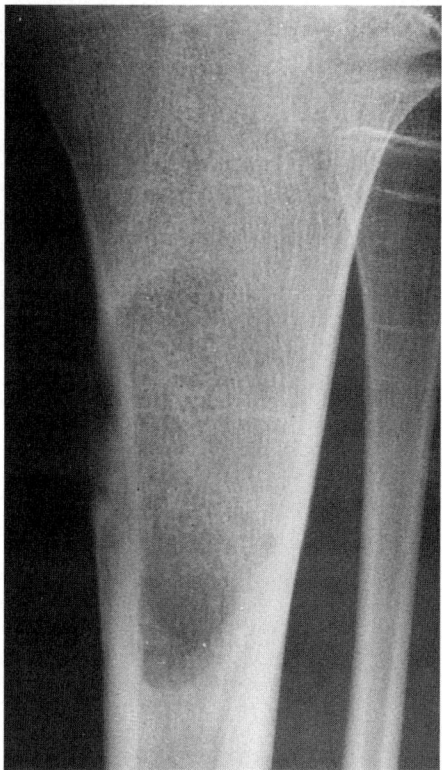

**Figure 70–16.** Aggressive (malignant) osteoblastoma. Radiograph in a 16-year-old girl reveals a well-defined, slightly expansile osteolytic lesion of the tibia. Biopsy confirmed the presence of osteoblastoma. After conservative surgery, the tumor recurred.

osteoblastoma, but with a greater likelihood of soft tissue involvement (Fig. 70–16).

Descriptions of the histologic features of these types of osteoblastoma emphasize the presence of highly cellular tumors containing compact areas of osteoblasts that are larger and have more frequent mitoses than the osteoblasts in conventional osteoblastoma. The major diagnostic problem is differentiating atypical osteoblastoma from osteosarcoma. It is important to differentiate between aggressive osteoblastomas and conventional osteoblastomas, because the former show a far greater likelihood to recur (although some disagree with this distinction). In certain rare instances, aggressive osteoblastoma can lead to the patient's death.

## Ossifying Fibroma

This fibro-osseous lesion is closely related radiographically and pathologically to fibrous dysplasia. Most ossifying fibromas arise in the facial bones. A similar tumor can

appear in a tubular bone, almost exclusively the tibia or fibula, with an earlier age of onset; this tumor is termed ossifying fibroma of long bones, or osteofibrous dysplasia.

**Ossifying Fibroma of Facial Bones.** A variety of fibro-osseous lesions of the craniofacial bones—ossifying fibromas of the jaw—are well-circumscribed, slowly growing expansile lesions. Their similarity to fibrous dysplasia has been emphasized repeatedly. Clinically, a painless expansion of the tooth-bearing portion of the mandible or, less commonly, the maxilla is observed on clinical examination. Radiographically, the lesion is typically 1 to 5 cm in diameter, although larger (and more aggressive) tumors are encountered, especially in children with juvenile aggressive or active ossifying fibromas. Well-defined unilocular or multilocular areas of osteolysis containing varying degrees of calcification are seen (Fig. 70–17).

**Ossifying Fibroma (Osteofibrous Dysplasia) of Tubular Bones.** Ossifying fibromas of the tubular bones are rare. Most cases consist of lesions isolated to the tibia; additional patterns of distribution include involvement of the tibia and ipsilateral fibula, the fibula alone, and both the tibia and fibula. Diaphyseal localization is typical, especially the middle third of the tibia, and the lesion is usually located in the anterior aspect of the bone, apparently beginning as an intracortical tumor that subsequently violates the spongiosa.

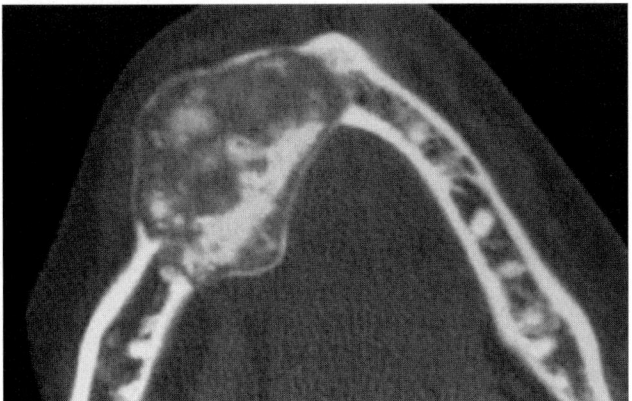

**Figure 70–17.** Ossifying fibroma: mandible. The lesion is well defined, expansile, and partially calcified. (Courtesy of D. Goodwin, MD, Hanover, NH.)

Ossifying fibromas of the tubular bones are generally seen in the first or second decade of life. Neonates may be affected as well. In the tibia, the lesion usually leads to painless enlargement or a mass, and slight or moderate anterior or anterolateral bowing of the bone is the rule. Osseous deformity may be accentuated by pathologic fractures, which may be followed by pseudarthrosis. Intracortical osteolysis clearly marginated by a band of sclerosis may be seen as a single confluent region or as multiple elongated, bubble-like areas. A hazy or "ground-glass" appearance similar to that of osteofibrous dysplasia is commonly evident (Fig. 70–18). Occasionally, the tumor is entirely osteosclerotic. Although ossifying fibroma of the tubular bones is usually stable or may even regress spontaneously on serial radiographic examinations, progression of the lesion is occasionally seen.

Histologically, ossifying fibroma consists of a fairly abundant fibrous stroma in which small trabeculae of metaplastic bone reside. The trabeculae are arranged randomly throughout the stroma in no apparent functional pattern, have the coarse appearance of metaplastic woven bone, and are characteristically rimmed by osteoblasts and occasional osteoclasts (in contrast to the pattern in fibrous dysplasia, in which the metaplastic bone lacks apparent osteoblasts).

Adamantinoma is another lesion sharing many radiographic features with ossifying fibroma, including a propensity to affect the middle region of the tibia. Indeed, a relationship may exist between adamantinoma in young persons and ossifying fibroma.

## Malignant Tumors

### Osteosarcoma

Osteosarcoma is second in frequency only to plasma cell myeloma as a primary malignant neoplasm of bone. It is histologically characterized by malignant tumor cells that directly produce osteoid or immature bone. Classification systems make use of such features as the precise location of the tumor within the bone (intramedullary or central, intracortical, surface, periosteal, or parosteal),

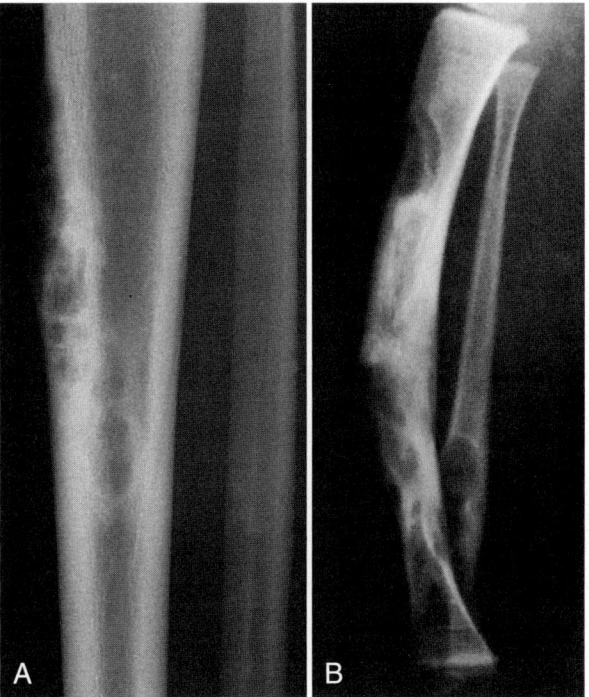

**Figure 70–18.** Ossifying fibroma. *A*, Tibia. In this 16-year-old girl with progressive pain in the anterior portion of the lower leg, a lateral radiograph reveals a sharply marginated, lobulated, eccentric lesion in the diaphysis affecting mainly the anterior cortex. *B*, Tibia and fibula. In this 2-year-old child, note the multiloculated, eccentric cortical lesion of the tibia with an additional lesion of the fibula. Other bones were not affected. Although biopsy indicated only "fibrous" tissue, the appearance is compatible with osteofibrous dysplasia (see text). (*A*, From Goergen TG, Dickman PS, Resnick D, et al: Long bone ossifying fibromas. Cancer 39:2067, 1977. *B*, Courtesy of J. E. L. Desautels, MD, Calgary, Alberta, Canada.)

the degree of cellular differentiation (high grade or low grade), the histologic composition (osteoblastic, chondroblastic, fibroblastic, fibrohistiocytic, telangiectatic, small cell, or clear cell), the number of foci of involvement (single or multicentric), and the status of the underlying bone (normal or the site of disease, such as Paget's disease).

### *Conventional Osteosarcoma*

Conventional osteosarcoma is generally seen in the second and third decades of life, although the neoplasm has been identified in patients of all ages. Men are affected more frequently than women in a ratio of approximately 2:1. Clinical manifestations include pain and swelling, restriction of motion, warmth, and pyrexia.

**Skeletal Location.** The most typical sites of involvement are the tubular bones in the appendicular skeleton (80% of cases), particularly the femur (40%), tibia (16%), and humerus (15%); 50% to 75% of all cases develop in the osseous structures about the knee. With regard to the long tubular bones, a metaphyseal location predominates. Initial involvement of the diaphysis occurs in about 10% of cases.

**Radiographic Abnormalities.** The pattern of osseous involvement is variable, depending to a large extent on the amount of bone produced by the tumor. When bone formation is extensive, a "cumulus cloud" appearance becomes evident. A mixed pattern consisting of both osteolysis and osteosclerosis is most typical, with purely osteolytic or osteosclerotic lesions (Fig. 70–19) being encountered less frequently. Osteolysis is especially characteristic of the telangiectatic variety. With regard to the tubular bones of the appendicular skeleton, conventional osteosarcoma is usually evident as an ill-defined intramedullary, metaphyseal lesion that has extended through the cortex and produced a sizable soft tissue mass. Periosteal reaction in the form of Codman's triangle or a "sunburst" appearance and, rarely, a pathologic fracture are additional radiographic features.

The radiographic features of osteosarcoma in other skeletal sites are similar to those in the tubular bones and include varying degrees of osteolysis and osteosclerosis, cortical violation, periostitis, and a soft tissue mass (Fig. 70–20). Five percent to 10% of osteosarcomas involve the flat bones, including those of the pelvis, and such involvement may be more frequent in older patients.

**Other Imaging Techniques.** Additional imaging methods are useful in defining the extent of the neoplasm and its relationship to surrounding neurovascular structures and in evaluating the response of the tumor to therapy. Radio-

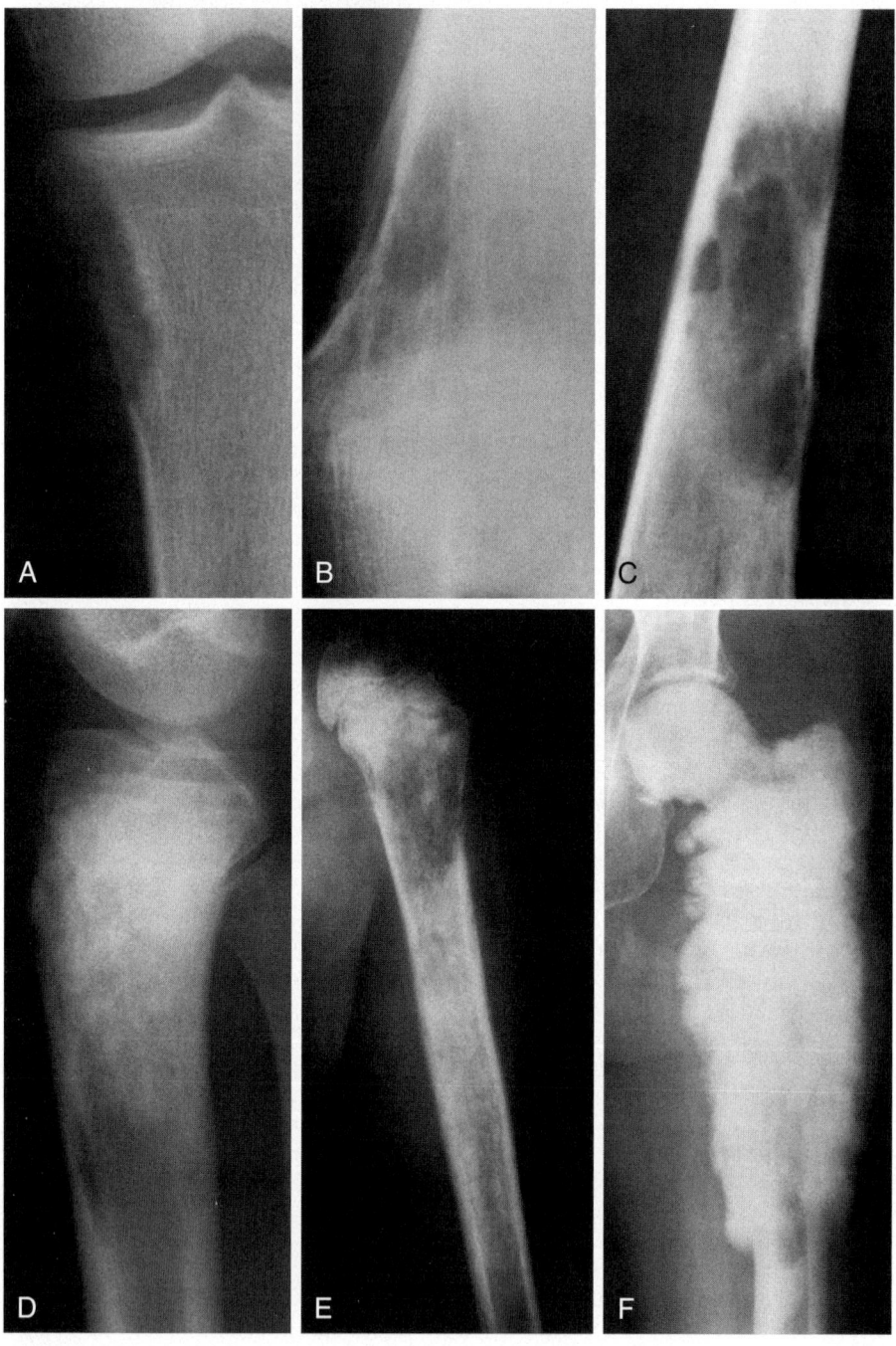

**Figure 70–19.** Conventional osteosarcoma: basic patterns of osseous involvement. *A,* Purely osteolytic pattern (metaphyseal and epiphyseal). *B,* Purely osteolytic pattern (metaphyseal and diaphyseal). *C,* Purely osteolytic pattern (diaphyseal). *D,* Mixed osteolytic and osteosclerotic pattern (metaphyseal and diaphyseal). *E,* Mixed osteolytic and osteosclerotic pattern (metaphyseal and diaphyseal). *F,* Purely osteosclerotic pattern (epiphyseal, metaphyseal, and diaphyseal). (*F,* Courtesy of P. Major, MD, Winnipeg, Manitoba, Canada.)

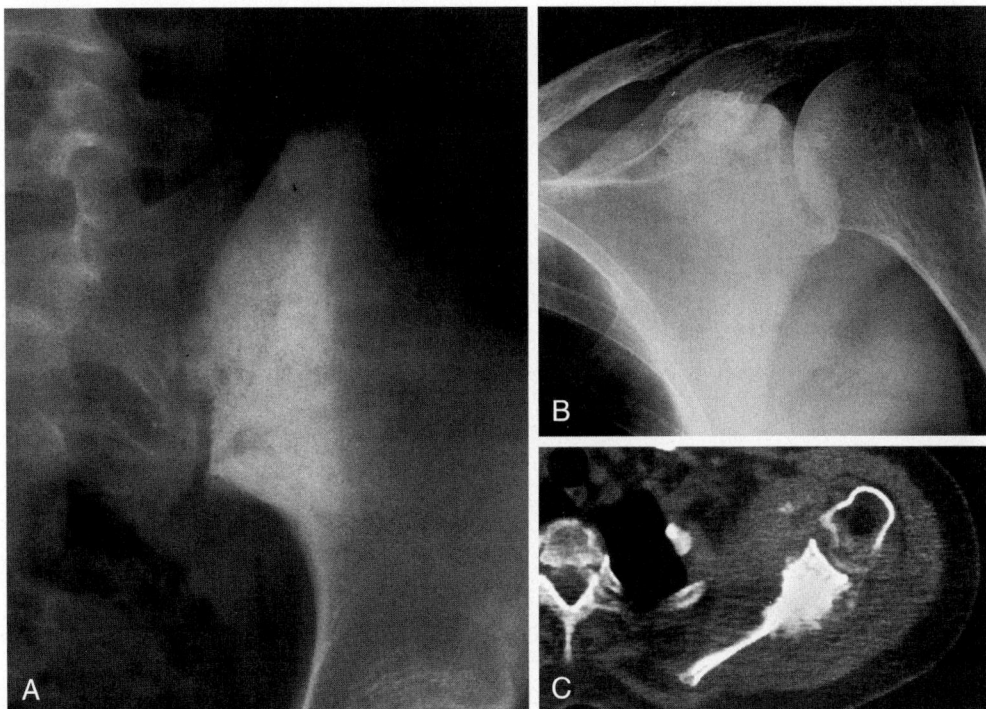

**Figure 70–20.** Conventional osteosarcoma. *A,* Ilium. An osteosclerotic lesion involves the bone about the sacroiliac joint. *B* and *C,* Scapula. Routine radiograph *(B)* and transaxial CT scan *(C)* document an osteosclerotic lesion of the scapula. In *(C)*, observe a soft tissue mass.

nuclide examination uniformly shows increased accumulation of the bone-seeking radiopharmaceutical agent within the primary tumor itself and, less uniformly, at sites of skeletal or extraskeletal metastasis (Fig. 70–21).

MR imaging appears to be superior to CT in defining the intraosseous and extraosseous extent of the tumor. In addition to local staging, large field of view T1-weighted imaging of the entire affected bone is essential to identify additional lesions within the medullary canal, termed "skip" metastases. The neoplasm is typically of low signal intensity on T1-weighted spin echo MR images and can be differentiated from normal fatty marrow (see Fig. 70–18). In some instances, differentiation of soft tissue and intraosseous extension of osteosarcoma and peritumoral edema is difficult. Enhancement of signal intensity in the tumor is evident after the intravenous administration of gadolinium compounds (Fig. 70–22). In general, the absence of joint effusion on MR images has high predictive value for the absence of articular involvement by the tumor; however, the presence of joint effusion is not diagnostic of intra-articular extension of tumor.

**Pathologic Abnormalities.** Because most osteosarcomas occur in young children and adolescents, the neoplasm is usually noted to abut an open physeal plate. It had long been thought that an open physis served as a barrier to prevent extension of the tumor into the epiphysis; however, recent studies indicate that macroscopic or microscopic evidence of transphyseal extension is quite common. Although osteosarcomas do not usually contain areas of tumor that are separate from the main neoplasm, such

"skip" areas have been observed in as many as 25% of cases. Patients with skip lesions and no other evidence of tumor dissemination have a prognosis similar to those presenting with metastatic disease.

The microscopic pathology of conventional osteosarcoma is often pleomorphic. Although osteoblastic, chondroblastic, and fibroblastic differentiation is predominant, other less common histologic types include chondroblastoma-like osteosarcomas, chondromyxoid fibroma–like osteosarcomas, osteoblastoma-like osteosarcomas, and fibrohistiocytic osteosarcomas. In general, all conventional osteosarcomas contain pleomorphic stromal elements that are either plump, spindle-shaped fibroblast-like cells or plump, round to oval osteoblasts with irregular, hyperchromatic nuclei. Abnormal mitotic activity and foci of necrosis, hemorrhage, hemosiderin pigment, and even cystlike vascular spaces similar to those in aneurysmal bone cysts are frequently evident. The form and shape of the malignant osteoid are also highly variable.

**Natural History.** The application of new and innovative chemotherapeutic strategies as a supplement to surgery and irradiation has resulted in a dramatic increase in the number of patients who can be expected to survive for 5 years or more. The response of the neoplasm to intense chemotherapy can be evaluated with serial radiographs; a favorable response is characterized by a decrease in the size of the soft tissue mass and an increase in periostitis, medullary sclerosis, and calcification. Local recurrence and distant skeletal metastasis after such amputation lead to osseous alterations that are similar to those of the

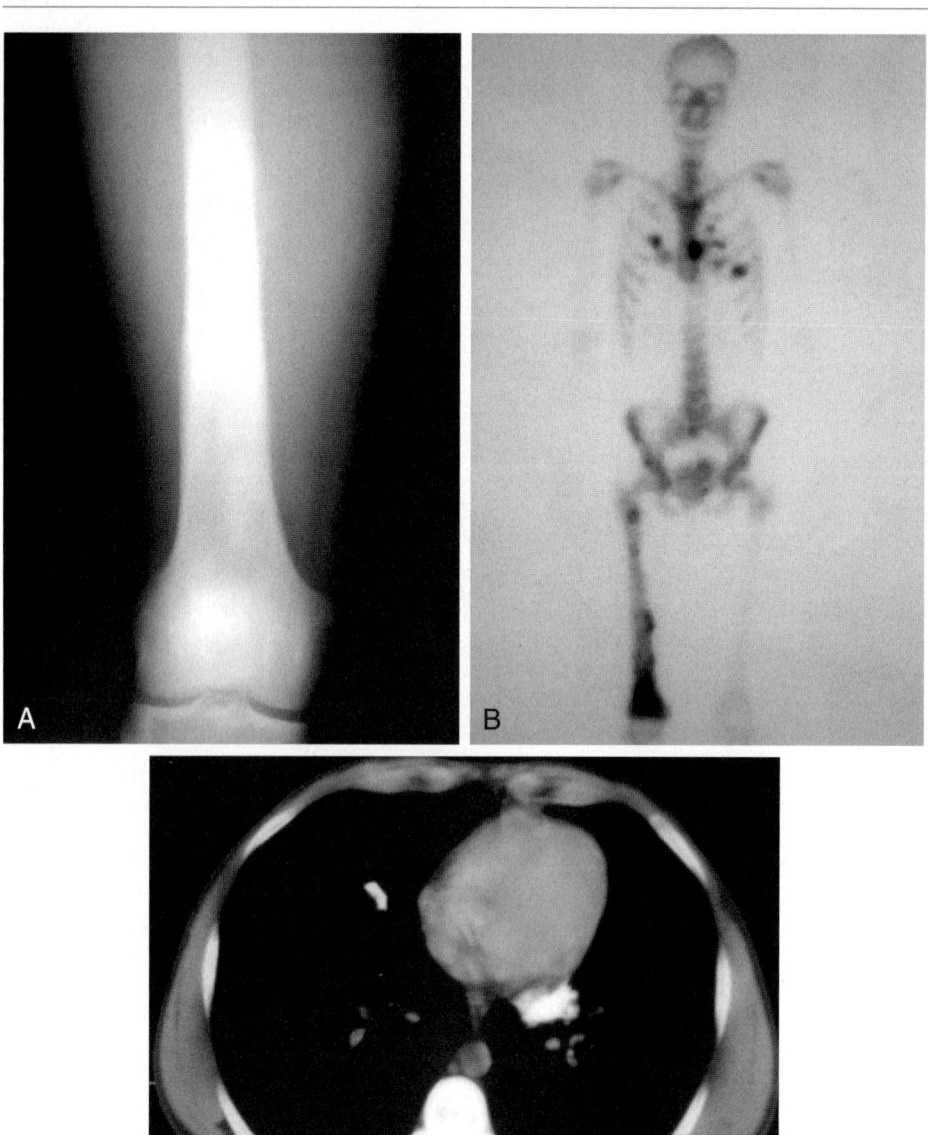

**Figure 70–21.** Conventional osteosarcoma. *A,* Radiograph shows an osteosclerotic lesion in the metaphysis and diaphysis of the femur. *B,* Bone scan reveals an extended pattern of uptake involving the femoral diaphysis and distal epiphysis. Also note "skip" lesions in the proximal femur, as well as pulmonary metastases. *C,* Axial CT scan of the lung bases shows multiple ossified pulmonary metastases.

primary tumor and, in some instances, must be differentiated from multifocal osteosarcomatosis. Of interest, lymph node, soft tissue, or visceral metastases from osteosarcoma may appear as calcified or ossified lesions on radiographs, and pulmonary metastatic foci can be associated with spontaneous pneumothorax.

Although MR imaging has been used to monitor the response of the tumor to chemotherapy, its effectiveness is not entirely clear. An increase in tumor volume during chemotherapy is generally predictive of a poor response. Several different patterns of signal intensity have been observed after preoperative chemotherapy, although detection of decreased signal intensity in the soft tissue mass (compared with the signal intensity before chemotherapy) has been associated with a favorable histologic response in some patients. Dynamic MR imaging studies in which rapid gradient echo imaging is accomplished

after the intravenous injection of a gadolinium compound is another technical modification that has been used to assess tumor viability after chemotherapy.

### Gnathic Osteosarcoma

Osteosarcomas of the mandible or maxilla, which represent about 8% of all osteosarcomas, are considered by some investigators to be distinct from conventional osteosarcomas because of an older age at onset (averaging approximately 30 years) and a decreased tendency for systemic metastases. Tumors arising in the mandible are slightly more frequent than those occurring in the maxilla. Gnathic osteosarcoma may be purely osteolytic or purely osteosclerotic or demonstrate a mixed pattern of osteolysis and osteosclerosis. CT findings of gnathic osteosarcomas include tumor calcification, involvement of the cortex,

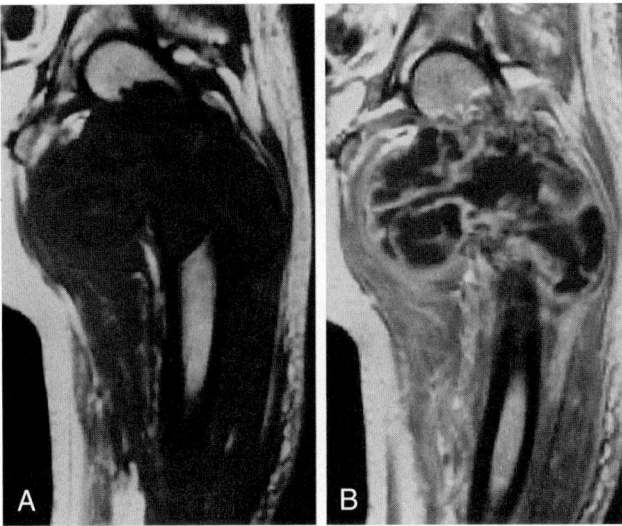

**Figure 70–22.** Conventional osteosarcoma. Coronal T1-weighted (TR/TE, 700/15) spin echo MR images obtained before *(A)* and after *(B)* the intravenous injection of a gadolinium-based contrast agent reveal a tumor of low signal intensity in the femur and adjacent soft tissue, with inhomogeneous enhancement of signal intensity in *(B)*. (Courtesy of J. Kramer, MD, Vienna, Austria.)

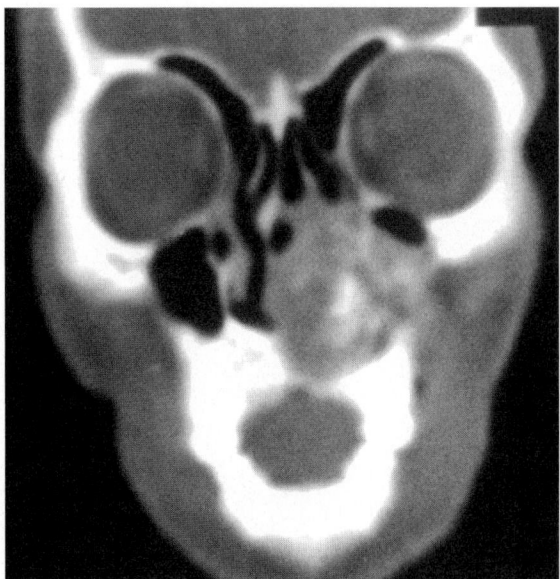

**Figure 70–23.** Gnathic osteosarcoma. Coronal CT scan reveals a predominantly osteolytic lesion in the maxilla.

and soft tissue and intramedullary bone extension (Fig. 70–23). MR imaging reveals similar features, although detection of matrix calcification and bone destruction or reaction is better accomplished with CT.

### Telangiectatic Osteosarcoma

The presence in some osteosarcomas of microscopic features that include large cystic cavities filled with blood has led to the designation telangiectatic (or hemorrhagic) osteosarcoma. Telangiectatic osteosarcoma is primarily a tumor of the long tubular bones; the femur is involved most frequently, followed by the tibia and humerus, a distribution similar to that of conventional osteosarcoma. In these bones, the metaphysis is the usual site of origin, but diaphyseal involvement occurs in approximately 10% of cases.

The radiographic hallmark of telangiectatic osteosarcoma is osteolysis. A large, multilocular or pseudocystic expansile lesion, often lacking periosteal bone production and sometimes possessing a relatively well-defined margin, is characteristic (Fig. 70–24). Pathologic fractures (in approximately 25% to 30% of cases) and soft tissue masses are also encountered. MR imaging may show areas of high signal intensity on T1-weighted spin echo images and fluid levels similar to those seen in aneurysmal bone cysts. Intravenous administration of a gadolinium-containing contrast agent is associated with inhomogeneous enhancement.

### Small Cell Osteosarcoma

Small cell osteosarcomas contain cells that resemble those of Ewing's sarcoma. This neoplasm is usually seen

in the second, third, or fourth decade of life. Pain and swelling of short duration are the typical clinical manifestations. Sites of involvement, in order of decreasing frequency, are the femur, humerus, tibia, and ilium. Lesions in the tubular bones predominate in the epiphysis and metaphysis. The prognosis of the tumor appears to be poorer than that of conventional osteosarcoma.

Radiographically, a large, predominantly osteolytic lesion involving medullary and cortical bone is accompanied by periostitis, a soft tissue mass, or both in approximately 50% of cases. The presence of a tumor with osteoblastic features extending from the metaphysis into the diaphysis and associated with permeative bone destruction is suggestive but not diagnostic of small cell osteosarcoma.

### Intraosseous Low-Grade (Well-Differentiated) Osteosarcoma

Low-grade or well-differentiated osteosarcomas arising within bone are uncommon when compared with the frequency of highly aggressive intraosseous osteosarcomas. These low-grade neoplasms, which appear to be the intramedullary counterpart of the parosteal variety of tumor (see later discussion), lead to clinical, radiographic, and histologic characteristics that may simulate those of benign neoplasms. These tumors typically affect young or middle-aged adults and are located mainly in the tibia or femur. Radiographs usually reveal a relatively large metaphyseal lesion, which may be purely osteosclerotic or both osteolytic and osteosclerotic in appearance (Fig. 70–25). Epiphyseal extension, cortical violation, osseous expansion, and soft tissue extension are encountered inconsistently. Intraosseous low-grade osteosarcoma is associated with a better prognosis than is conventional osteosarcoma.

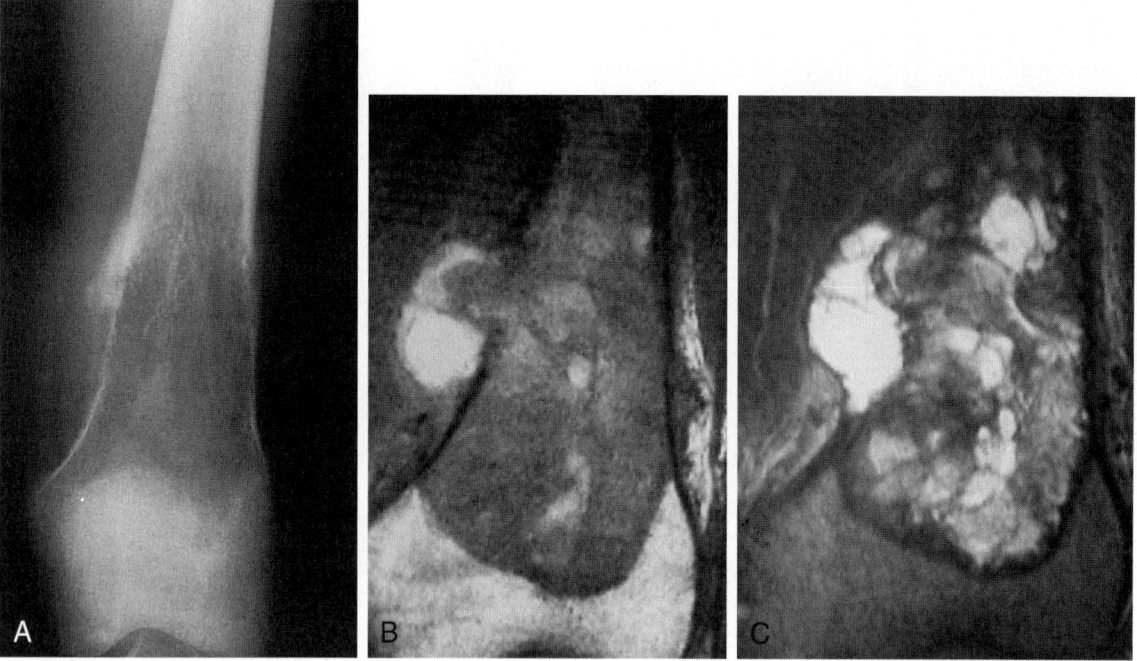

**Figure 70–24.** Telangiectatic osteosarcoma. *A*, Anteroposterior radiograph shows an osteolytic lesion containing small and large areas of bone destruction in the femur. The cortex is thinned or perforated, and Codman's triangle and a large soft tissue mass are evident. *B* and *C*, Coronal T1-weighted (TR/TE, 500/30) *(B)* and T2-weighted (TR/TE, 2000/120) *(C)* spin echo MR images vividly demonstrate the extent of the tumor. In *(B)*, only the soft tissue component of the lesion has high signal intensity; in *(C)*, the overall intensity of the tumor has increased.

### Intracortical Osteosarcoma

This tumor appears to be the rarest form of osteosarcoma, with only a few cases being documented. It arises within the confines of the cortex as an osteolytic lesion with surrounding cortical sclerosis but without radiating osseous spicules. Typically affecting young adults, intracortical osteosarcoma is a diaphyseal lesion of the tibia or femur. A radiolucent focus containing osteoid and surrounded in part by a sclerotic margin is usually seen (Fig. 70–26).

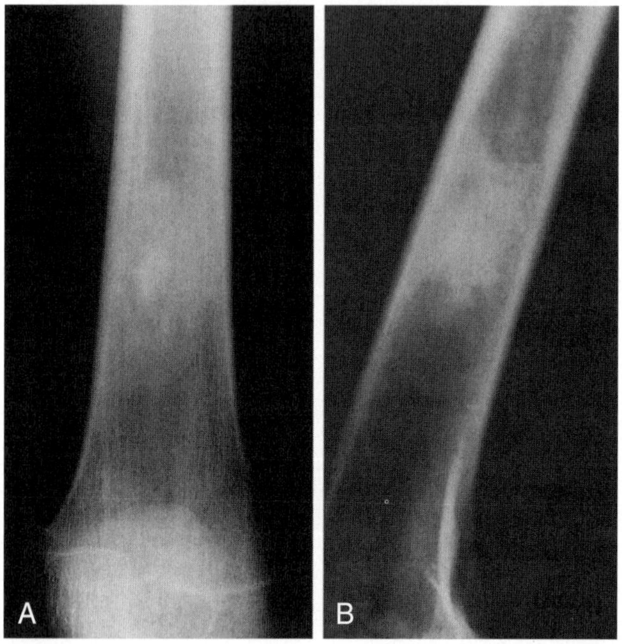

**Figure 70–25.** Intraosseous, low-grade osteosarcoma. Frontal *(A)* and lateral *(B)* radiographs reveal a poorly defined osteosclerotic tumor in the distal portion of the femur. Subtle endosteal erosion is evident.

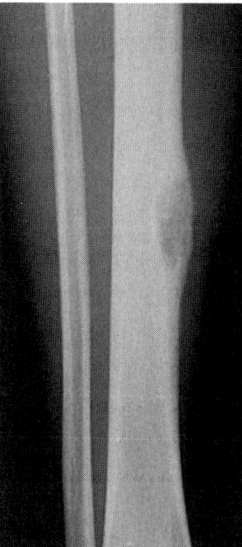

**Figure 70–26.** Intracortical osteosarcoma. Radiolucent lesion of the diaphyseal cortex of the tibia is accompanied by cortical thickening, slight osseous expansion, and narrowing of the medullary canal. (From Kyriakos M: Cancer 46:2525, 1980.)

## Surface (Juxtacortical) Osteosarcoma

With regard to the general nomenclature of surface lesions of bone, periosteal lesions are those processes originating from the deep layer of the periosteum, and parosteal lesions are those originating from the outer fibrous layer of the periosteum. The term *juxtacortical* is flexible and is applied to surface lesions of extracortical origin, regardless of their exact anatomic relationship to the periosteum. Three types of osteosarcoma involve predominantly the surface of bone: high-grade surface osteosarcoma, periosteal osteosarcoma, and parosteal osteosarcoma.

**High-Grade Surface Osteosarcoma.** Most patients with this lesion are in the second or third decade of life. Tubular bones, especially the femur, are involved most frequently, and a diaphyseal location is typical. Histologically, these tumors are identical to conventional osteosarcoma, and their only differentiating feature is localization to the surface of the bone. The radiographic appearance of surface high-grade osteosarcoma is characterized by a broad-based, partially or completely calcified or ossified lesion arising from the external surface of the cortex (Fig. 70–27). The prognosis of this type of tumor appears to be identical to that of conventional high-grade osteosarcoma.

**Periosteal Osteosarcoma.** Periosteal osteosarcoma is an infrequent neoplasm that predominates in the second and third decades of life. Involvement of the diaphysis of a long tubular bone, especially the femur or tibia, is typical. It is significant that when a periosteal osteosarcoma occurs in the distal region of the femur, it is usually located in the anterior, lateral, or medial portion of the bone, in contrast to the posterior femoral involvement that characterizes parosteal osteosarcoma.

Periosteal osteosarcomas are variable in size and on radiographs appear as lesions on the bone surface. The tumor is limited to the cortex, which is thickened and irregular externally; this feature is commonly accompanied by nonhomogeneous, radiating osseous spicules that extend from the superficial region of the cortex into the adjacent soft tissues (Fig. 70–28). It should be emphasized that the medullary cavity, with rare exception, is uninvolved. Histologically, periosteal osteosarcoma is relatively poorly differentiated and predominantly chondroblastic. The prognosis of this tumor is definitely better than that of conventional osteosarcoma and poorer than that of parosteal osteosarcoma.

**Parosteal Osteosarcoma.** This lesion is the most common juxtacortical osteosarcoma, typically affecting patients in the second to fifth decades of life, an age distribution that is significantly older than that of conventional osteosarcoma. Symptoms and signs are typically insidious and consist of pain, swelling, and a palpable mass. Parosteal osteosarcomas occur almost exclusively in the long tubular bones; the femur is the predominant site of involvement (approximately 65% of cases), followed in frequency by the humerus (15%) and tibia (10%). Parosteal osteosarcomas are particularly common on the posterior surface of the distal portion of the femur (50% to 70% of femoral tumors). Involvement of the bones about the knee occurs in approximately 70% of all parosteal osteosarcomas. These tumors characteristically arise in the metaphyseal region of a tubular bone.

The radiographic abnormalities of this tumor are highly characteristic (Figs. 70–29 and 70–30). A large, radiodense, oval or spheroid mass possessing smooth lobulated or irregular margins is evident. Typically, it is attached in a sessile fashion to the external cortex, which itself may be thickened; a thin radiolucent line, or cleavage plane, may separate the remaining portion of the tumor from the underlying bone, although this latter finding is not constant. Ossification within the tumor proceeds from the base of the lesion to its periphery. The pattern of ossification differs from that seen in myositis ossificans, in which the periphery of the lesion is the first to ossify. CT and MR imaging can be used to determine the extent of the neoplasm and, in some cases, the presence of

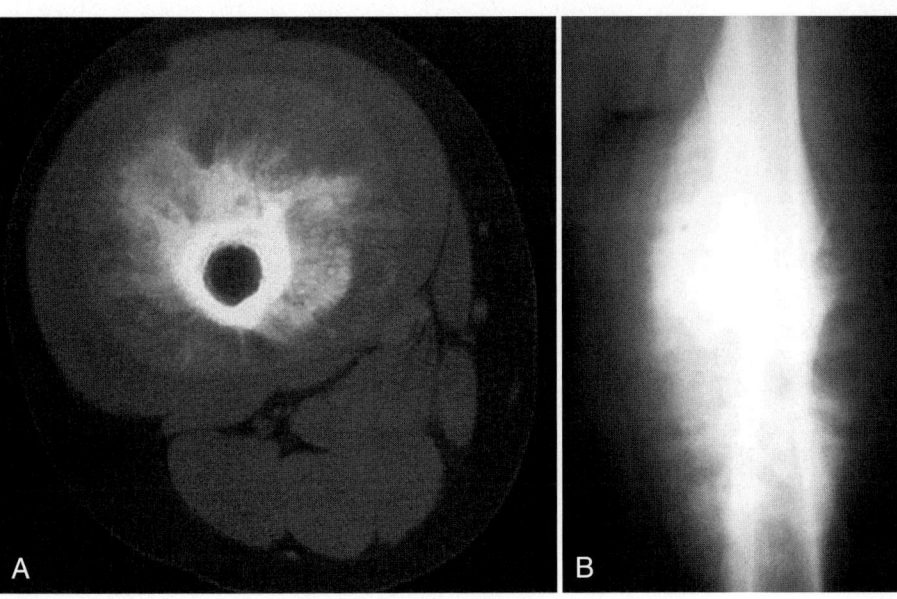

**Figure 70–27.** Surface high-grade osteosarcoma. *A,* Transaxial CT reveals a large ossified mass arising circumferentially from the surface of the femur. Note the normal appearance of the marrow within the medullary canal of the femur. *B,* Anteroposterior radiograph reveals a densely mineralized mass. The juxtacortical origin is difficult to establish based solely on the radiograph.

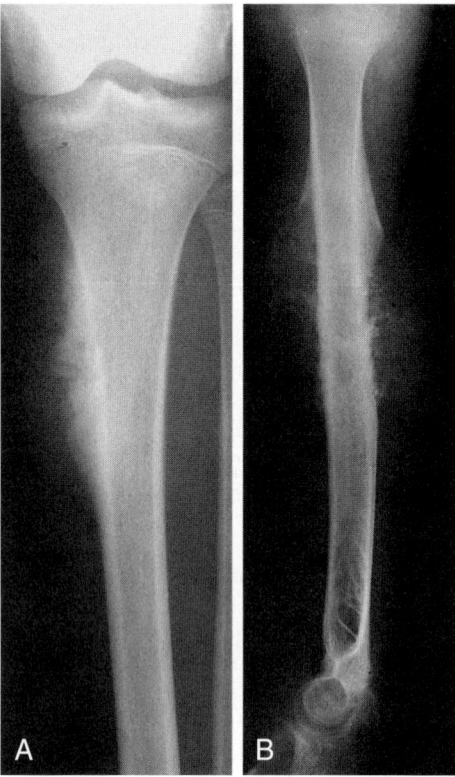

**Figure 70–28.** Periosteal osteosarcoma. *A*, Tibia. The lesion is located in the medial cortex of the tibia, with cortical thickening and radiating, cloudlike osseous proliferation on the external surface of the bone. The medullary portion is uninvolved. *B*, Humerus. This diaphyseal lesion is accompanied by exuberant periostitis, including Codman's triangle; osseous proliferation; and soft tissue prominence.

medullary involvement; however, differentiation between neoplastic invasion of the medullary cavity and reactive non-neoplastic loss of cancellous bone and between tumor bone and thickened adjacent host cortex is not always possible.

Dedifferentiated parosteal osteosarcoma is a term used to describe parosteal osteosarcomas that have developed an additional high-grade mesenchymal component. These lesions appear to evolve from low-grade parosteal osteosarcoma after a long time or a history of local recurrence. Many of the features of parosteal osteosarcoma resemble those of intraosseous low-grade osteosarcoma.

The radiographic and pathologic features of parosteal osteosarcoma must be differentiated from those of post-traumatic heterotopic bone formation (myositis ossificans) and sessile osteochondroma. A clinical history of trauma followed by the rapid appearance of a soft tissue mass—a lesion that initially ossifies at its periphery, with a zonal pattern of maturation in which the periphery of the lesion consists of lamellar bone and the center consists of proliferating mesenchymal cells—is the distinguishing feature of myositis ossificans. An osteochondroma is radiographically characterized by continuity between the cortex and spongiosa of the excrescence and the underlying normal bone. Periosteal osteosarcoma is usually small in comparison to the size of parosteal osteosarcoma; it is accompanied by a distinctive spiculated periosteal reaction and, histologically, is predominantly chondroblastic.

### Multicentric Osteosarcoma

Involvement of more than one skeletal site by osteosarcoma in a single person may be related to several differ-

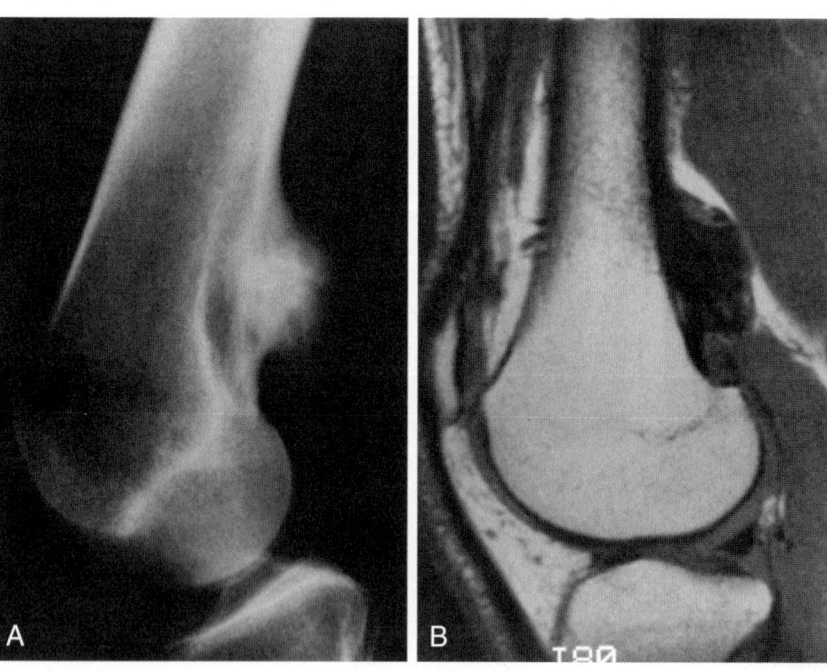

**Figure 70–29.** Parosteal osteosarcoma: femur. *A*, Lateral radiograph shows an irregular ossified lesion involving the posterior aspect of the distal femoral metaphysis. *B*, On a sagittal T1-weighted (TR/TE, 550/20) spin echo MR image, the tumor is of low signal intensity, and the adjacent marrow of the femur is normal.

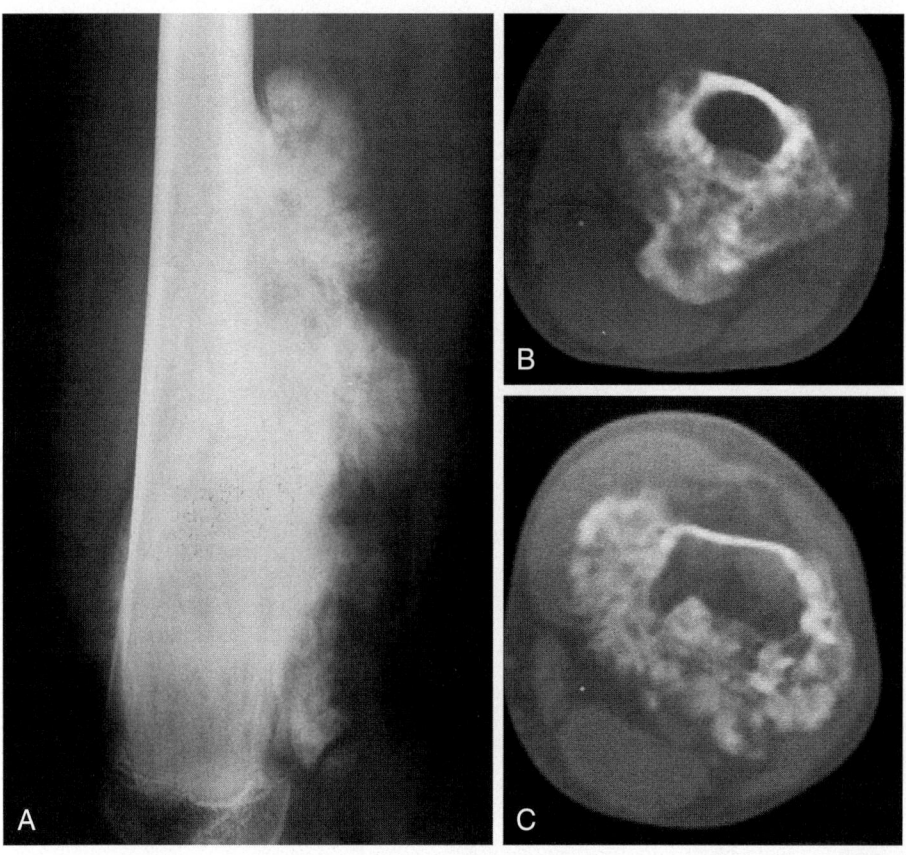

**Figure 70–30.** Parosteal osteosarcoma: femur. *A,* An exuberant, densely ossified lesion involves the posterior metaphyseal and diaphyseal regions of the femur. It has wrapped itself around the femur, accounting for the radiodense shadows seen anterior to the bone. The lesion is lobulated and irregular in outline, and the underlying cortex is thickened. *B* and *C,* Transaxial CT scans at the diaphyseal *(B)* and metaphyseal *(C)* levels show the extent of the ossifying process, which involves not only the posterior surface of the bone but also the medial and lateral surfaces. The cortex is thickened, and the medullary bone appears to be involved. (Courtesy of Regional Naval Medical Center, San Diego, Calif.)

ent mechanisms: multicentric lesions that arise simultaneously (osteosarcomatosis), multicentric lesions that arise metachronously, or a unicentric lesion in which a second neoplastic focus develops in the same bone or in an adjacent bone.

Osteosarcomatosis, which represents the simultaneous occurrence of multiple skeletal osteosarcomas, is regarded by many investigators as a rare, distinct form of disease that predominates in children. There is similarity in the size and radiographic and histologic appearance of the osseous lesions. The identification of a larger (or dominant) lesion in almost all cases supports the contention that osteosarcomatosis represents hematogenous metastatic disease from a single osteosarcoma rather than multiple primary osteosarcomas (Fig. 70–31). Although not all accept this pathogenesis, there is agreement on the uniformly poor prognosis of this form of the disease.

Multiple, metachronous osteosarcomas typically occur in adolescents and young adults. In this situation, one or more new tumors develop after the initial treatment of a primary osteosarcoma. Such metachronous sarcomas may represent late metastases from the original neoplasm or new primary tumors. A unicentric osteosarcoma with subsequent skeletal metastasis represents a definite cause of multicentric lesions. Osseous dissemination in patients with a primary osteosarcoma appears to occur in 10% to 20% of cases. One or more osteosarcomas may also occur in persons with Paget's disease.

## CARTILAGE-FORMING TUMORS

### Benign Tumors

#### Chondroma

A chondroma may arise within a bone (enchondroma) or on the surface of a bone (periosteal chondroma). It may be solitary or multiple (enchondromatosis), and the tumor may be accompanied by soft tissue vascular lesions (Maffucci's syndrome).

##### *Enchondroma*

A solitary enchondroma is a tumor that develops in the medullary cavity and is composed of lobules of hyaline cartilage. The neoplasm is usually discovered in the third or fourth decade of life and is equally frequent in men and women. Lesions, particularly those in the hand, are generally asymptomatic or associated with painless swelling. The appearance of pain should arouse suspicion of malignant transformation, a complication that is infrequent and occurs more commonly in the long tubular bones, especially in bones of the pelvic and shoulder girdles.

**Skeletal Location.** Approximately 40% to 65% of solitary enchondromas occur in the hands or, much less frequently, the feet. Solitary enchondromas occur in the long tubular bones in approximately 25% of cases and are more frequent in the bones of the upper extremity than in those of the lower extremity. Typical sites of involve-

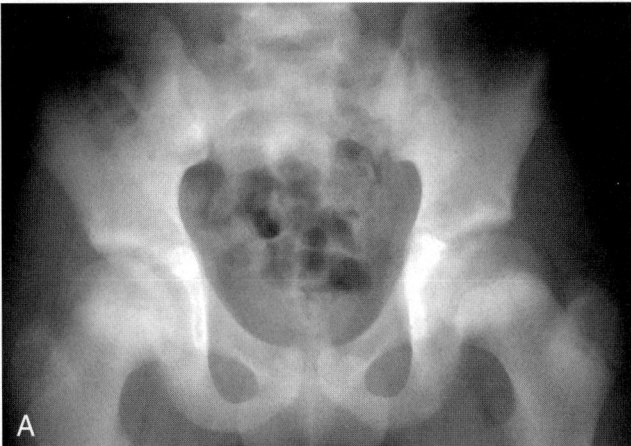

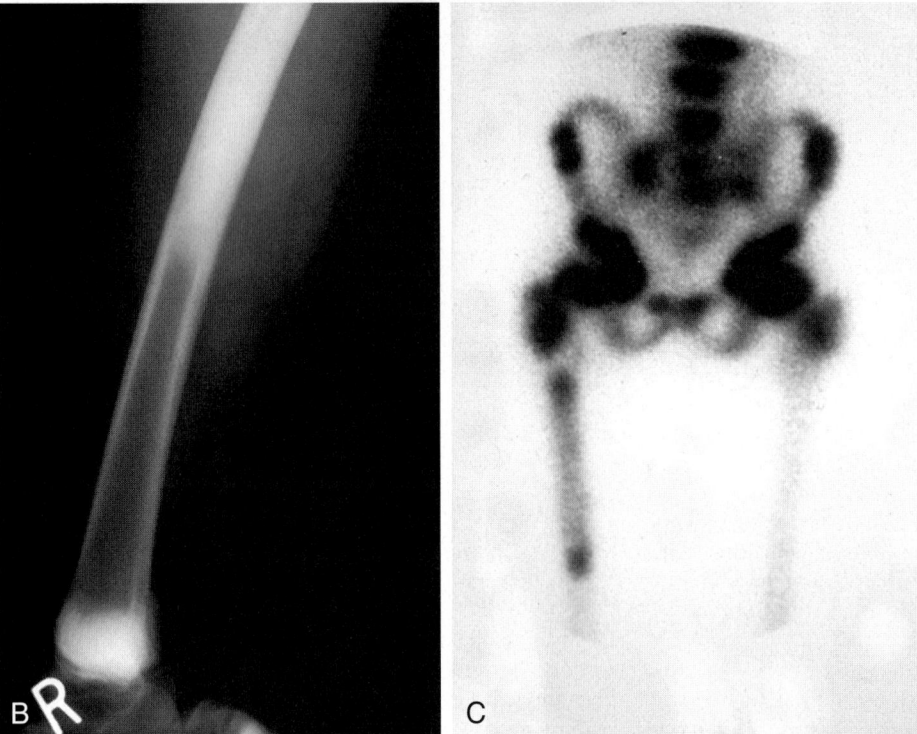

**Figure 70–31.** Multicentric osteosarcoma. *A,* Pelvic radiographs reveal multiple sclerotic foci in metaphyseal-equivalent areas. *B,* Lateral radiograph of the right femur shows a dominant lesion. *C,* Corresponding anteroposterior image of the pelvis from a bone scan shows the dominant femoral lesion, as well as extensive, relatively symmetrical involvement of the pelvis and hips.

ment are the humerus, femur, and tibia. The innominate bones, in which chondrosarcomas are relatively frequent, are the site of less than 3% of all enchondromas. Some enchondromas in the tubular bones may lead to osseous expansion and are designated enchondroma protuberans. Enchondromas are usually central tumors located in the metaphysis of a long tubular bone or in the diaphysis of a short tubular bone in the hand or foot.

**Radiographic Abnormalities.** The radiographic appearance of lesions in the hand (Fig. 70–32) or foot (Fig. 70–33) is usually characteristic. A well-defined, medullary lesion with some degree of calcification, a lobulated contour, and endosteal erosion allows a precise diagnosis in most cases. Cortical expansion or thickening and pathologic fracture are other potential radiographic characteristics. Because enchondroma is the most common benign tumor of the hand, identification of a solitary, well-marginated,

lobulated intraosseous lesion in the bones of the hand should be considered evidence of an enchondroma until proved otherwise. Elsewhere, enchondromas also possess typical radiographic features. In the long tubular bones, a centrally or eccentrically placed medullary, osteolytic tumor of variable size, with or without calcification and leading to lobulated erosion of the endosteal margin of the cortex, is typical (Fig. 70–34). In some cases, channel-like radiolucent areas in the metaphysis are seen (Fig. 70–35). The radiographic abnormalities accompanying an enchondroma in a flat or irregular bone may not be diagnostic.

MR imaging in cases of enchondroma usually shows a well-circumscribed lesion of low signal intensity on T1-weighted spin echo MR images and high signal intensity on T2-weighted spin echo MR images. A lobulated configuration is typical (Fig. 70–36). Calcific foci appear as regions of low signal intensity.

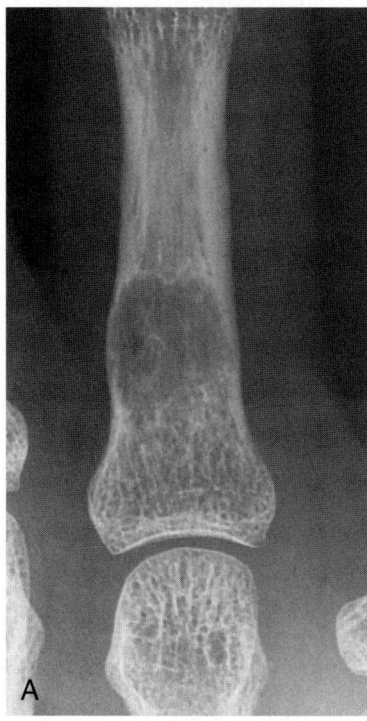
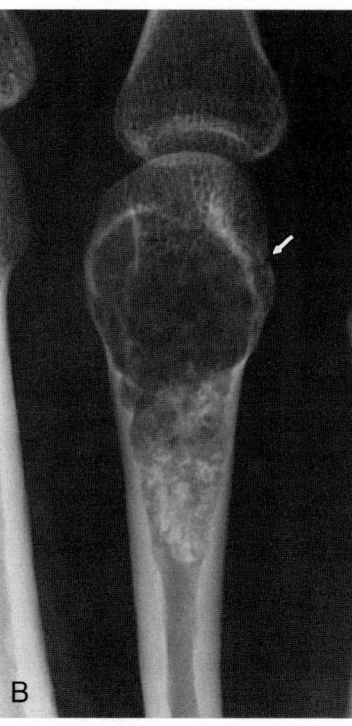

**Figure 70–32.** Enchondroma: tubular bones of the hand. Osteolytic lesions in the metaphyses of the proximal phalanges *(A)* and metacarpal bone *(B)* are well defined, with erosion of the endosteal margin of the cortex. Small foci of calcification are evident in *(A)*; more prominent calcification is demonstrated in *(B)*. Also, in *(B)*, note the lobulated nature of the lesion and a pathologic fracture *(arrow)*.

Differentiation of enchondroma from low-grade chondrosarcoma is a common diagnostic problem. In the tubular bones, extensive endosteal scalloping (more than two thirds of the cortical thickness and along more than two thirds of the lesion), less prominent matrix calcification (calcification located within less than two thirds of the lesion as seen on routine radiographs), periosteal reaction, cortical destruction, and a soft tissue mass are features suggesting chondrosarcoma. An epiphyseal location strongly suggests a chondrosarcoma.

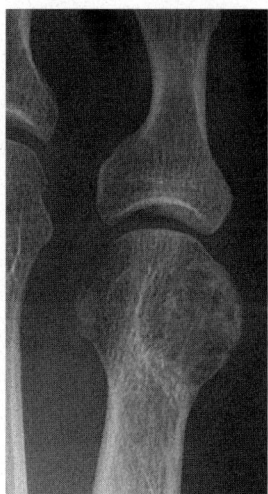

**Figure 70–33.** Enchondroma: tubular bones of the foot. An eccentric lesion in the fifth metatarsal bone contains a sclerotic margin and subtle punctate calcification and has led to osseous expansion.

**Pathologic Abnormalities.** Although most enchondromas are only a few centimeters in size, those in the long tubular bones are often larger. The larger a cartilaginous lesion, the greater the likelihood that it is a chondrosarcoma. Microscopically, most enchondromas consist of lobules of hyaline-type cartilage. The degree of cellularity in enchondromas varies greatly and cannot by itself be used as an indicator of malignancy. Also important is the occurrence of confluence of the cartilage lobules and invasion of the intertrabecular spaces with entrapment of residual normal trabeculae in cases of chondrosarcoma and the lack of these features in enchondroma.

The occurrence of malignant transformation of a solitary, benign enchondroma is exceptional in tumors located in the small bones of the hand or foot and more likely in enchondromas in the long tubular or flat bones. Although chondrosarcoma is the expected result after malignant transformation of an enchondroma, other neoplasms, including malignant fibrous histiocytoma, fibrosarcoma, and osteosarcoma, have been reported in this situation.

### Enchondromatosis (Ollier's Disease)

This disorder is rare and nonhereditary and consists of multiple, asymmetrically distributed intraosseous cartilaginous foci and subperiosteal deposition of cartilage, either exclusively or predominantly involving one side of the body; the affected bones are often shortened and deformed (Fig. 70–37). In childhood, the cartilaginous lesions are subject to pathologic fractures, and in adulthood, they are at risk for malignant transformation. The chondromas in Ollier's disease predominate in the extremities and, less commonly, in the metacarpal and

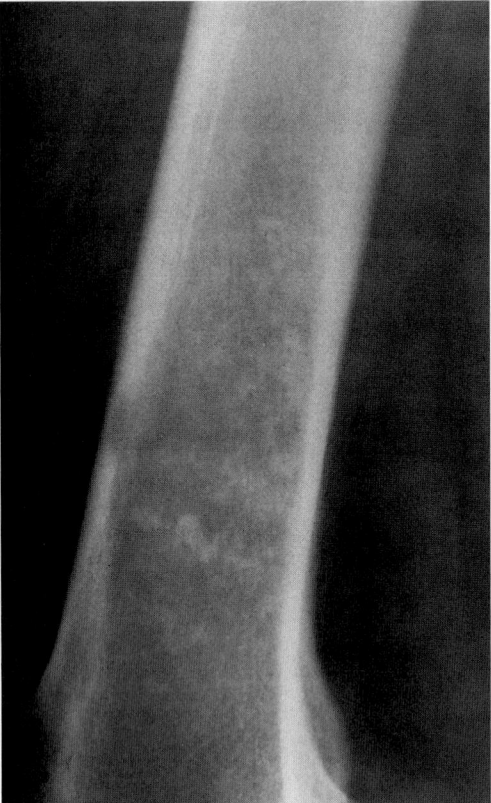

**Figure 70–34.** Enchondroma: long tubular bones. Lateral radiograph shows an elongated, calcified medullary lesion in the diaphysis of the femur, with endosteal erosion of the cortex.

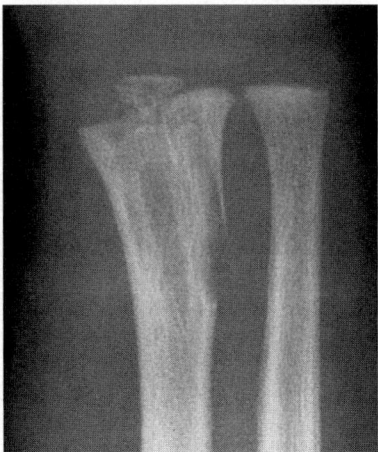

**Figure 70–35.** Enchondroma: long tubular bones. In this child with a solitary lesion, observe the channel-like radiolucent areas extending into the metaphysis of the radius. The appearance is diagnostic of an enchondroma. (Courtesy of E. Bosch, MD, Santiago, Chile.)

metatarsal bones and phalanges. The flat bones, especially those in the pelvis, are also affected.

Clinical manifestations usually appear in the first decade of life and consist of palpable bony masses, asymmetrical shortening of the extremities, and osseous deformities related to fractures. On radiographs, linear or columnar translucencies in the metaphyses, which may reveal calcification, represent sites of persistent cartilaginous tissue. In some instances, erosion and proliferation of the bone

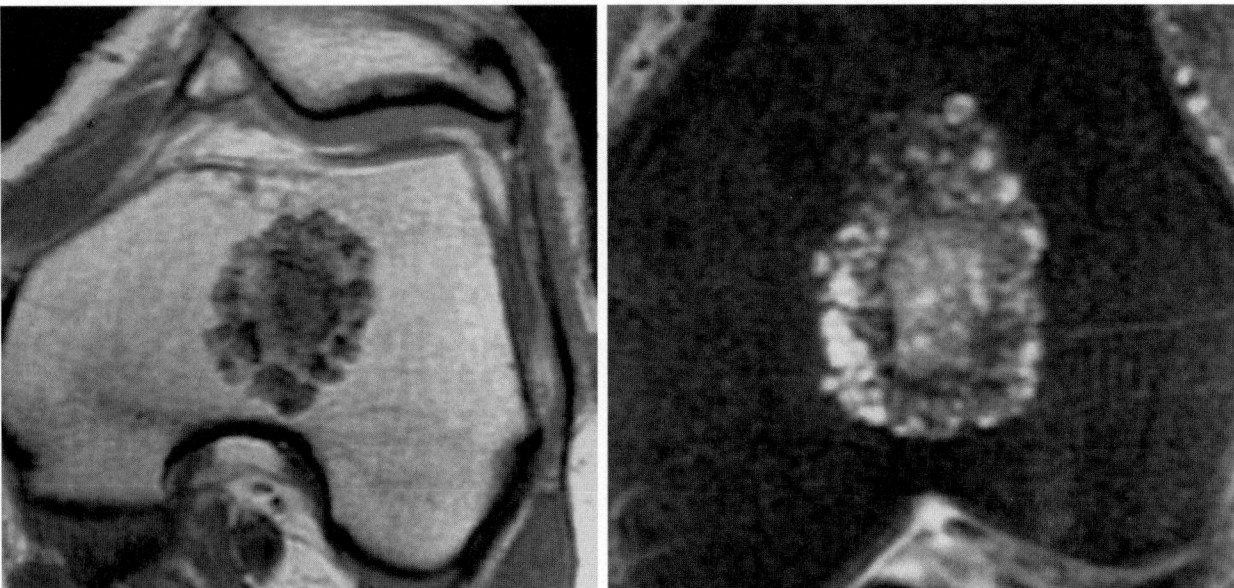

**Figure 70–36.** Enchondroma: long tubular bones. *A,* Transverse T1-weighted (TR/TE, 500/11) spin echo MR image reveals a lobulated lesion of low signal intensity in the medullary cavity of the femur. It is centrally located and well circumscribed. *B,* Coronal STIR (TR/TE, 3266/30; inversion time, 150 msec) MR image shows the lobulated tumor with regions of low signal intensity (representing calcific foci) and high signal intensity (representing cartilage nodules).

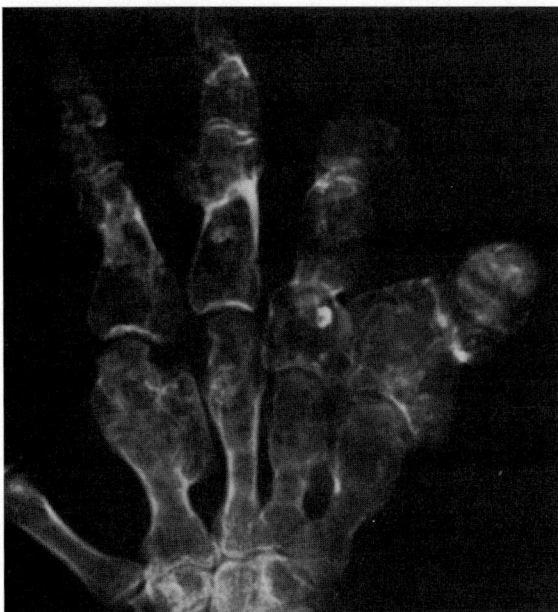

**Figure 70–37.** Enchondromatosis (Ollier's disease). Observe the multiple chondromas involving the metacarpal bones and phalanges. The chondromas have led to calcification and osseous expansion and deformity. (Courtesy of C. Pineda, MD, Mexico City, Mexico.)

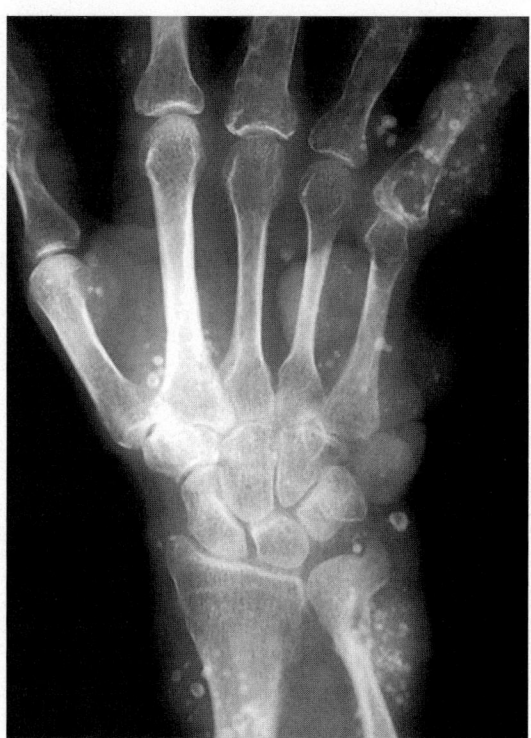

**Figure 70–38.** Maffucci's syndrome. Posteroanterior radiograph of the hand shows enchondromas in multiple phalanges, with phleboliths in the soft tissues.

surface are seen. Some of the lesions may regress during the years of growth. After cessation of normal growth, the lesions do not increase in size unless malignant transformation has occurred, a complication noted in 5% to 30% of cases.

### Maffucci's Syndrome

Maffucci's syndrome is a rare, congenital, nonhereditary mesodermal dysplasia manifested by multiple enchondromas and soft tissue vascular lesions. It causes varying degrees of disability, but malignant transformation within an enchondroma to chondrosarcoma is the most severe complication and occurs in about 20% of patients. Maffucci's syndrome is usually observed in boys and girls in the first decade of life, and the diagnosis is sometimes established at birth. Clinical manifestations are due to osseous deformities and soft tissue abnormalities that include cavernous or capillary hemangiomas and, less commonly, lymphangiomas and epithelioid hemangioendotheliomas.

A unilateral distribution is observed in approximately 50% of cases. Sites of osseous alterations include, most frequently, the metacarpals and phalanges in the hand. The sites of chondromas and soft tissue vascular lesions need not coincide.

Radiographic abnormalities are characteristic and consist of typical central or eccentric radiolucent lesions containing variable amounts of calcification, as well as phleboliths within the affected soft tissues (Fig. 70–38). Additionally, radiographs often reveal sequelae of a dysplasia, including limb length discrepancy and tubulation deformities caused by a lack of normal bone modeling.

The potential for both bone and soft tissue lesions to undergo sarcomatous transformation in this syndrome has been emphasized, although the risk is greater for the skeletal component. Chondrosarcoma is the dominant malignant tumor encountered and is usually seen in adults after age 40 years.

### Periosteal (Juxtacortical) Chondroma

Periosteal chondroma, which is composed of hyaline cartilage, develops adjacent to the cortical surface, beneath the periosteal membrane. This tumor is more frequent in women and predominates in persons younger than 30 years. Clinical manifestations may include initial local swelling and pain. The long tubular bones, particularly the humerus and femur, are affected in approximately 70% of cases, and the bones in the hands or, less commonly, the feet are affected in approximately 25% of cases. Metaphyseal localization predominates.

Radiographically, a soft tissue mass with erosion or saucerization of the adjacent cortex is evident (Fig. 70–39). Medullary sclerosis and periostitis may be seen. Buttressing, or thickening, of the cortex at the distal and proximal margins of the tumor is typical. Calcification within the lesion is evident in approximately 50% of cases and may be extensive in some instances. Periosteal chondromas may also be accompanied by enchondromas, with features resembling those of enchondroma protuberans. With MR imaging, these tumors are generally of high signal intensity on T2-weighted spin echo images. Microscopically, periosteal chondroma is composed of lobules of hyaline cartilage that varies in cellularity.

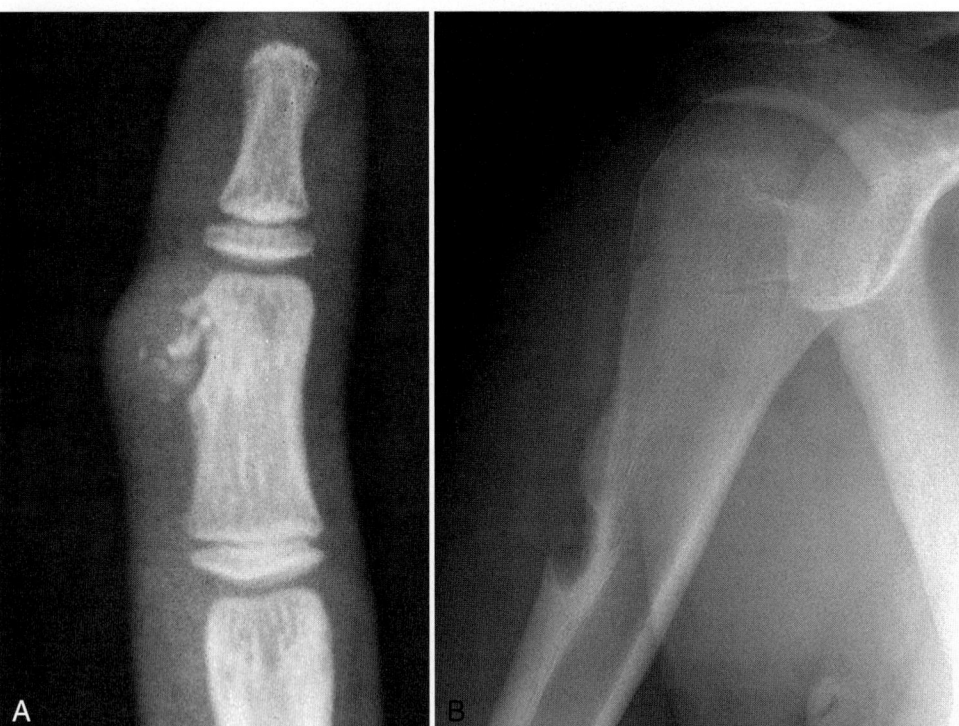

**Figure 70–39.** Periosteal (juxtacortical) chondroma. *A,* Note the calcified soft tissue mass, cortical excavation, and periostitis. *B,* Observe the large, nonmineralized mass scalloping the cortical surface of the humerus.

## Chondroblastoma

Chondroblastoma is a relatively uncommon, benign, cartilaginous neoplasm originating in bone. It is most frequent in the second and third decades of life, and approximately 90% of chondroblastomas occur in persons between 5 and 25 years old. Men are affected more commonly than women, in a ratio of approximately 2:1. The nonspecific symptoms and signs include local pain, swelling, and tenderness. Because the neoplasms are typically located in para-articular bone, joint manifestations are not unexpected, may simulate a primary synovial process, and are accompanied by effusions in as many as 30% of cases.

**Skeletal Location.** Chondroblastomas generally arise in an epiphysis or apophysis of a long tubular bone, although metaphyseal extension of an epiphyseal tumor is not uncommon. The femur (33% of cases), humerus (20% of cases), and tibia (18% of cases) are the most frequent sites of involvement. Approximately 10% of chondroblastomas arise in the bones of the hands and feet, with a particular predilection for the talus and calcaneus.

**Radiographic Abnormalities.** Characteristic radiographic features of this neoplasm consist of an osteolytic lesion that is eccentrically or centrally located in an epiphysis or apophysis, usually less than 5 to 6 cm in size, and well defined and spheroid or oval in shape (Fig. 70–40). A thin sclerotic rim may separate the tumor from adjacent normal bone, and the overlying cartilage may be thinned or eroded. Calcific foci within the lesion are documented in approximately 30% to 50% of patients and are well seen on CT. In sites other than the tubular bones, the radiographic features of chondroblastomas are less specific.

Scintigraphy reveals hypervascularity with avid accumulation of the bone-seeking radiopharmaceutical agent.

Chondroblastomas are of low signal intensity on T1-weighted spin echo MR images and of variable (and often low) signal intensity on T2-weighted spin echo MR images. Chondroblastomas are typically associated with an inflammatory response with high signal intensity on T2-weighted spin echo MR images (Fig. 70–41). This inflammatory response involves the adjacent metadiaphyseal marrow and soft tissues, correlates in extent to the degree of periostitis, and diminishes or disappears after successful surgical intervention. Fluid levels may occasionally be seen and relate to the occurrence of a secondary aneurysmal bone cyst (Fig. 70–42).

**Natural History.** Although intraosseous recurrence of chondroblastoma has been observed after curettage of the neoplasm, the vast majority of these tumors behave in a benign fashion. Occasionally, however, chondroblastomas pursue a more aggressive course, with invasion of joint spaces, soft tissues, or adjacent bones. In fact, metastatic foci of chondroblastoma have been identified in the lungs of patients, usually after some form of surgical therapy for the primary bone tumor. In these instances, removal of the pulmonary lesions has resulted in long-term survival.

**Differential Diagnosis.** The classic radiographic features of chondroblastoma are relatively specific, although other diagnostic considerations may include infection and eosinophilic granuloma. These last two disorders more often lead to metaphyseal or diaphyseal abnormalities, but epiphyseal or apophyseal localization has also been documented. The radiographic features of chondroblas-

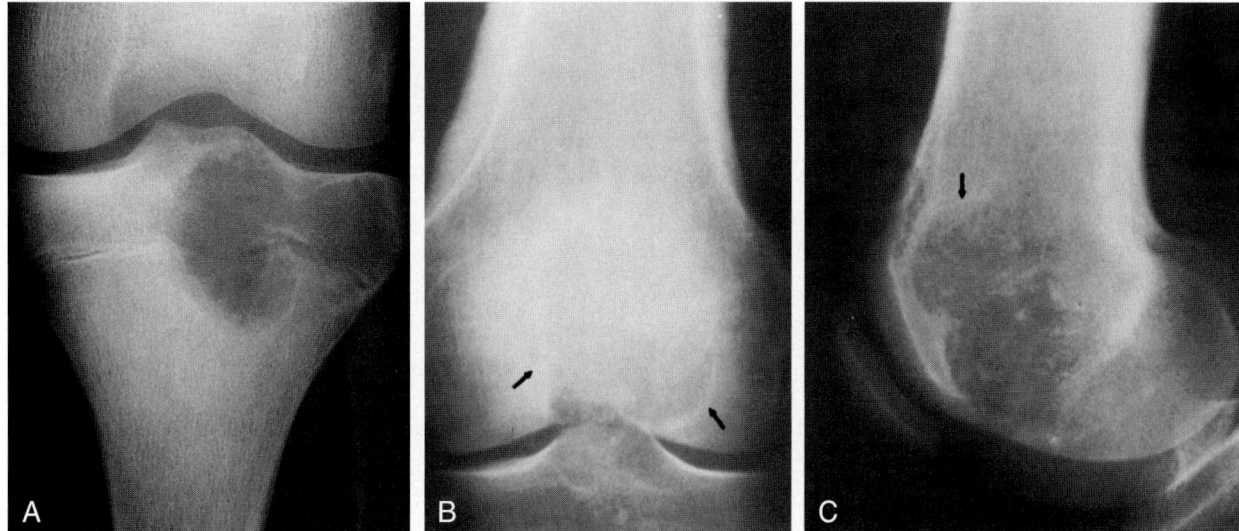

**Figure 70–40.** Chondroblastoma: long tubular bones. *A,* Tibia. Note the radiolucent lesion involving the metaphysis and epiphysis of the proximal portion of the tibia. *B* and *C,* Femur. Frontal *(B)* and lateral *(C)* radiographs in a 22-year-old man show a large epiphyseal and metaphyseal lesion *(arrows)* that contains foci of calcification. An unusual degree of periostitis is apparent in the metaphysis and diaphysis.

toma are generally easily differentiated from those typical of a giant cell tumor (epiphyseal lesion without calcification in a mature skeleton) and chondromyxoid fibroma (metaphyseal lesion with a coarse trabecular pattern); however, in occasional cases, radiographic differentiation among these tumors, as well as others such as enchondroma, osteoblastoma, and chondrosarcoma, may be difficult.

## Chondromyxoid Fibroma

The least common benign neoplasm of cartilage is chondromyxoid fibroma. This tumor is typically identified in persons younger than 30 years and is especially common in the second and third decades of life. Slowly progressive pain, tenderness, swelling, and restriction of motion are observed.

**Skeletal Location.** Chondromyxoid fibroma is observed most frequently in the long tubular bones, especially those in the lower extremity (70% of cases). Involvement of the tibia or femur is evident in approximately 55% of patients. Favored sites of tumor localization are the proximal end of the tibia, proximal and distal ends of the femur and fibula, and, less commonly, innominate bone and small bones of the foot (metatarsal bones, phalanges, calcaneus). In a tubular bone, a metaphyseal focus is favored, with extension into the adjacent epiphysis (in the presence of a closed physeal plate) or diaphysis.

**Radiographic Abnormalities.** When located in a long tubular bone, chondromyxoid fibromas are generally eccentrically situated metaphyseal lesions that are radiolucent, of varying size (2 to 10 cm), and elongated in shape (Fig. 70–43). Cortical expansion, exuberant endosteal sclerosis, and coarse trabeculation are commonly noted. Extensive periostitis and pathologic fractures are unusual,

and calcification is evident in less than 13% of cases. Larger lesions may lead to complete penetration of the cortex; the resulting hemispheric osseous defect, or "bite," when unaccompanied by periostitis, is believed to be highly characteristic of chondromyxoid fibroma.

In the flat and irregular bones, as well as the small bones of the hands and feet (Fig. 70–44), chondromyxoid fibromas lead to osteolysis, scalloped osseous erosions, bone expansion, and a coarse trabecular pattern. CT and MR imaging (see Fig. 70–44) can be used to further define the extent of bone involvement. A multilobulated pattern and high signal intensity on T2-weighted spin echo MR images have been emphasized.

**Natural History.** Although some reports have documented locally aggressive behavior and tumor recurrence, the prevailing view is that chondromyxoid fibroma is a benign cartilaginous neoplasm and that its recurrence, which may take place in as many as 25% of cases, relates to inadequate local excision. Indeed, recurrence of this tumor is most frequent when only curettage of the lesion is accomplished and is least frequent when wide local or block excision of the tumor is performed. Most reported cases of chondromyxoid fibromas that produced metastases are generally viewed as low-grade chondrosarcomas that were histologically misinterpreted as chondromyxoid fibromas. Rare documented cases of malignant transformation of this neoplasm do exist, however.

**Differential Diagnosis.** Accurate diagnosis of chondromyxoid fibroma is least difficult when the osteolytic lesion is localized to the metaphyseal region of a tubular bone and has an eccentric position, endosteal sclerosis, and cortical expansion or violation with a bitelike configuration. The presence of radiographically detectable calcification within this tumor is rare, so this finding

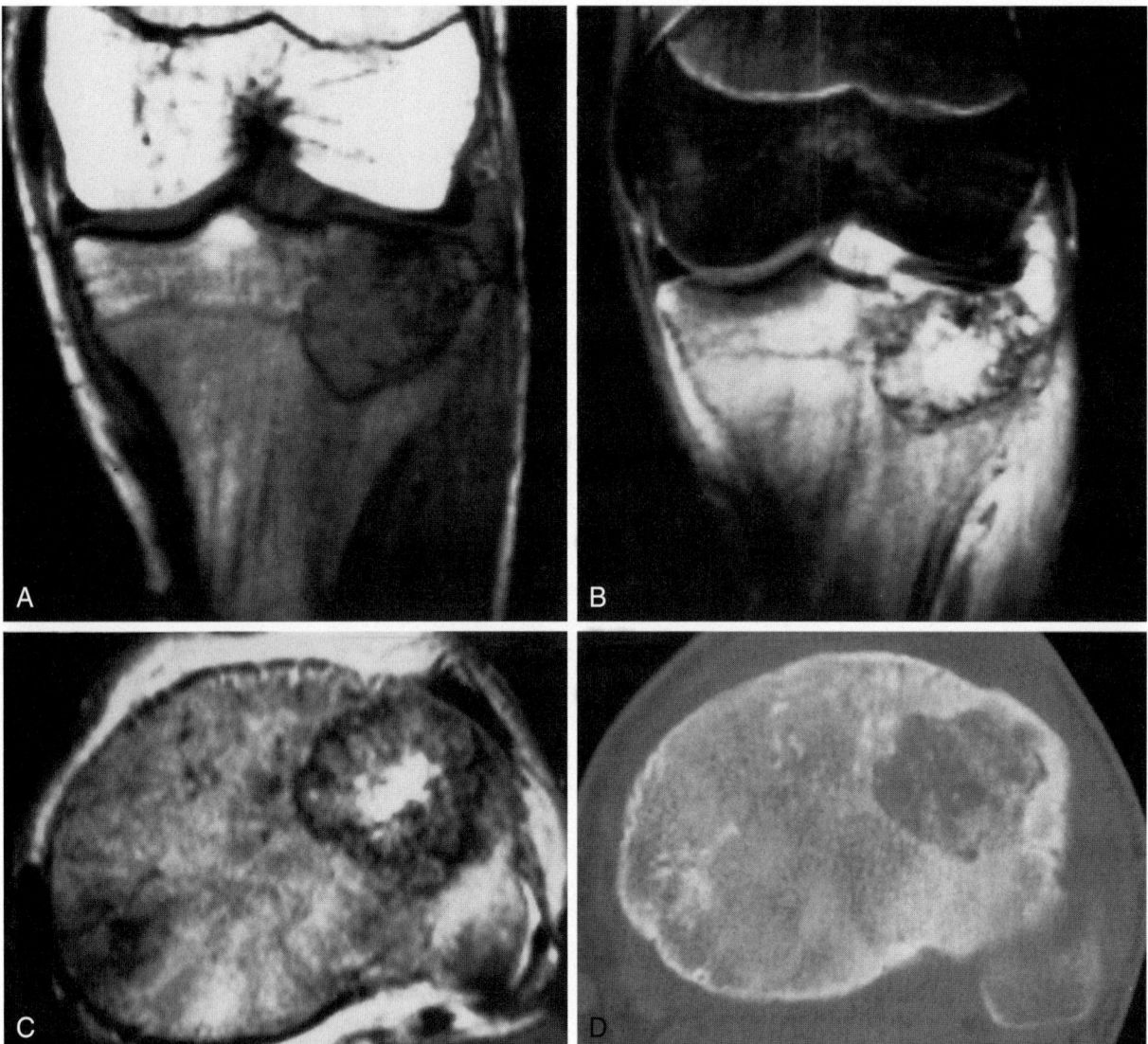

**Figure 70–41.** Chondroblastoma. Coronal T1-weighted (TR/TE, 578/15) spin echo MR image *(A)* and coronal fat-suppressed T1-weighted (TR/TE, 825/15) spin echo MR image obtained after intravenous gadolinium administration *(B)* show the tumor in the lateral epiphyseal and metaphyseal regions of the tibia, with adjacent marrow and muscle edema. Both the tumor and edema are of high signal intensity in *(B)*. These findings are confirmed on a transverse contrast-enhanced, fat-suppressed T1-weighted (TR/TE, 825/15) spin echo MR image *(C)*. The peripheral portion of the tumor remains of low signal intensity. The transverse CT image *(D)* best demonstrates lesion calcification.

should suggest alternative diagnoses such as enchondroma, chondroblastoma, or even fibrous dysplasia. The thick trabeculae commonly found in chondromyxoid fibroma differ from the faint, thin trabeculae of a giant cell tumor or nonossifying fibroma but resemble the trabeculae about a desmoplastic fibroma.

## Osteochondroma

Osteochondromas are cartilage-covered osseous excrescences that arise from the surface of a bone. They may be solitary or multiple (hereditary multiple exostoses) or occur spontaneously or after accidental or iatrogenic injury or irradiation.

### Solitary Osteochondroma

Solitary osteochondroma, or osteocartilaginous exostosis, is a relatively frequent lesion that is regarded as either a true neoplasm or a developmental physeal growth defect. Osteochondromas develop in bones that form through the process of endochondral ossification and are intimately related to the physis.

**Clinical Abnormalities.** Most solitary osteochondromas are discovered in children and adolescents. The vast majority of solitary osteochondromas are asymptomatic and are detected incidentally. Symptomatic lesions usually occur in younger patients. A nontender, painless, slowly growing mass is the most characteristic clinical

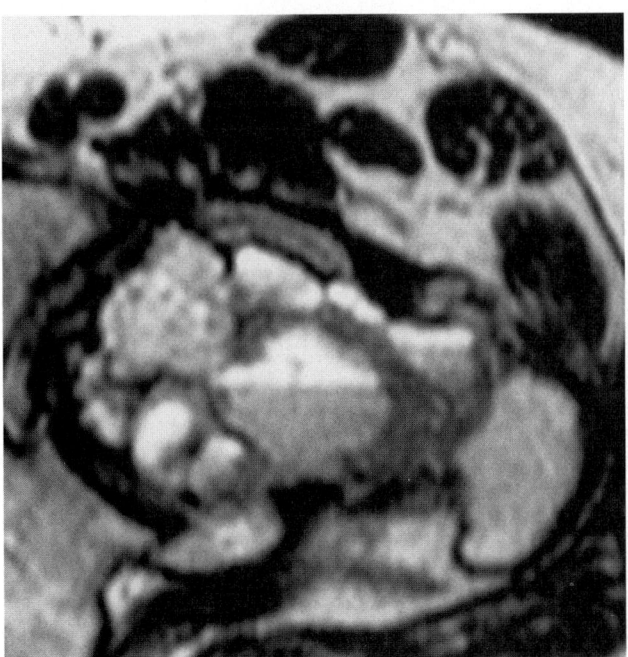

**Figure 70–42.** Chondroblastoma. Transaxial fast spin echo (TR/TE, 4000/91) MR image shows several fluid levels in the tumor. (Courtesy of C. Chen, MD, Kaohsiung, Taiwan.)

manifestation. Large tumors or those occurring at certain anatomic sites may cause symptoms related to fracture, irritation, or damage to adjacent nerves or vessels.

**Skeletal Location.** Any bone that develops by endochondral ossification may be the site of an osteochondroma, although the long tubular bones, especially the femur, humerus, and tibia, are involved most frequently. The bones in the lower extremity are affected more frequently than those in the upper extremity in a ratio of approximately 2:1. In the tubular bones, a metaphyseal location is characteristic. Osteochondromas are rare in the dia-

physis and in the epiphysis; osteochondromas in the latter location are indicative of a separate disorder, Trevor's disease, or dysplasia epiphysealis hemimelica (see later discussion). The small bones of the hand and foot are involved in approximately 10% of cases.

**Radiographic Abnormalities.** An osteocartilaginous exostosis is radiographically characterized by an osseous protuberance arising from the external surface of a long tubular bone and containing spongiosa and cortex that are continuous with those of the parent bone (Fig. 70–45). The outgrowths may be pedunculated (with a narrow stalk and bulbous tip) or sessile (with a broad, flat base) (Fig. 70–46). Typically, lesions point away from the nearby joint and toward the diaphysis. The metaphysis of the tubular bone may be widened as a result of failure of normal tabulation.

The tip of the osteochondroma is covered by a cap composed of hyaline cartilage. The degree of calcification within this cartilage is highly variable. If the cap is small and well defined, with regular, stippled calcification, the appearance is most compatible with a benign outgrowth; if it is large and poorly defined and contains irregular or incomplete calcification, malignant transformation should be given serious consideration.

Osteochondromas arising in the innominate bone (Fig. 70–47) are frequently large and lead to a soft tissue mass and displacement of adjacent structures; the patterns of calcification are variable and commonly irregular. In this instance, differentiation of a benign osteochondroma from one that has undergone malignant transformation is extremely difficult. In the ribs, osteochondromas (as well as enchondromas) are particularly frequent at the costochondral junction.

**Other Imaging Techniques.** CT can be used to evaluate osteochondromas and may be especially useful in demonstrating cortical and medullary continuity where the osseous anatomy is complex. Ultrasonography can be used to analyze the cartilaginous cap of an osteochon-

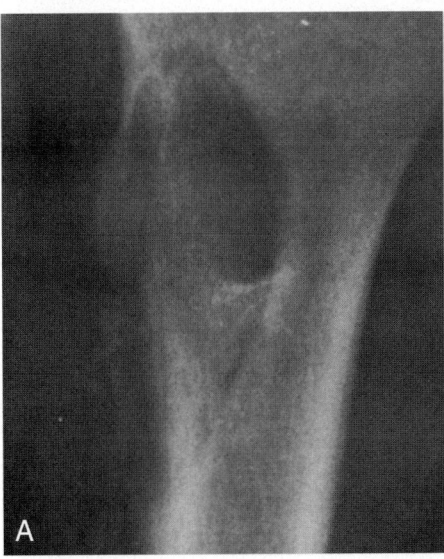

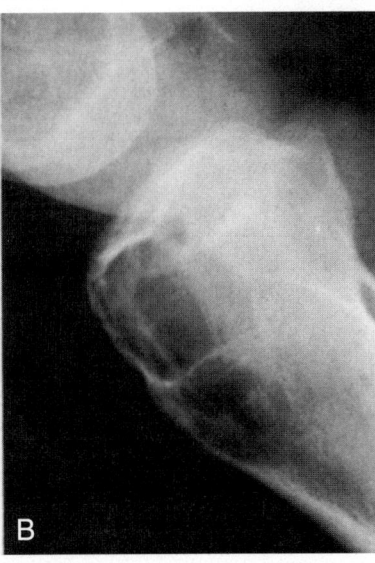

**Figure 70–43.** Chondromyxoid fibroma: long tubular bones. *A*, Femur. An eccentric, osteolytic, slightly expansile lesion of the femoral metadiaphysis is evident. The expanded cortex is thinned and contains small perforations. Calcification and significant periostitis are absent. *B*, Tibia. An eccentric, osteolytic, slightly expansile lesion involves the anterior portion of the metaphysis and epiphysis of the bone and extends to the subchondral region. Slight trabeculation is evident. The lesion is well defined and contains no calcification. Periostitis is absent. (*B*, Courtesy of O. J. Wollenman, MD, Fort Worth, Tex.)

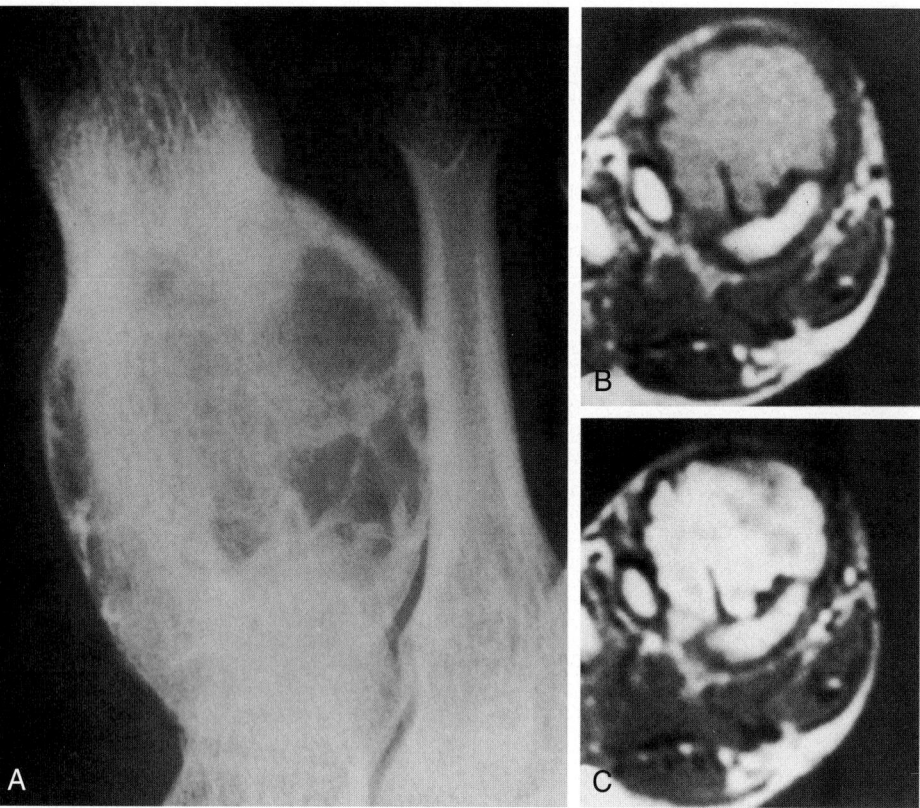

**Figure 70–44.** Chondromyxoid fibroma: small bones of the foot. *A*, An expansile, heavily trabeculated lesion of the first metatarsal bone is evident. *B* and *C*, Coronal T1-weighted (TR/TE, 650/20) spin echo MR images obtained before *(B)* and after *(C)* the intravenous injection of a gadolinium compound reveal the expansile tumor. It is of intermediate signal intensity in *(B)*, and diffuse enhancement of signal intensity is seen in *(C)*. (Courtesy of H. S. Kang, MD, Seoul, Korea.)

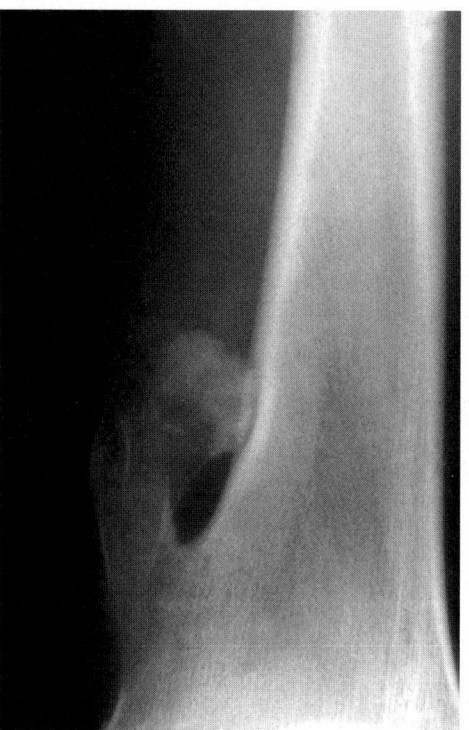

**Figure 70–45.** Solitary osteochondroma: long tubular bones. The pedunculated osteochondroma arising from the distal metaphysis of the femur contains spongiosa and cortex that are continuous with those of the parent bone. The metaphysis itself is slightly widened, a finding that is much more frequent and prominent in cases of multiple osteochondromas.

droma, although lesions that are deeply situated and those oriented inwardly are not well evaluated with this method. Typically, the nonmineralized cartilaginous cap appears as a hypoechoic region that can be differentiated from the hyperechoic surrounding fat and muscle. Acoustic shadowing characterizes areas of mineralization in the cartilaginous cap.

MR imaging is an effective technique for detecting continuity of the cortical and medullary bone. Further, the cartilaginous tissue in the cap of an osteochondroma is of high signal intensity on T2-weighted spin echo MR images, and this tissue is covered with perichondrium that appears to be of low signal intensity on such images. These signal intensity characteristics allow precise identification and even measurement of the cap (Fig. 70–48). MR imaging may therefore provide information regarding the likelihood of malignant change.

**Pathologic Abnormalities.** Osteochondromas vary considerably in size; the average size of lesions arising in the long tubular bones is approximately 4 cm (in maximum dimension), whereas those occurring in the flat or irregular bones are usually larger. When sectioned, the usual osteochondroma is found to contain a cartilaginous cap beneath which is cancellous bone in direct continuity with that of the parent bone. The chondral cap resembles normal cartilage and is generally only a few millimeters thick. The precise thickness of this cap correlates with the age of the patient. In children and adolescents, in whom active bone growth is still occurring, the cap may be as thick as 3 cm; in adults, the cap may be entirely

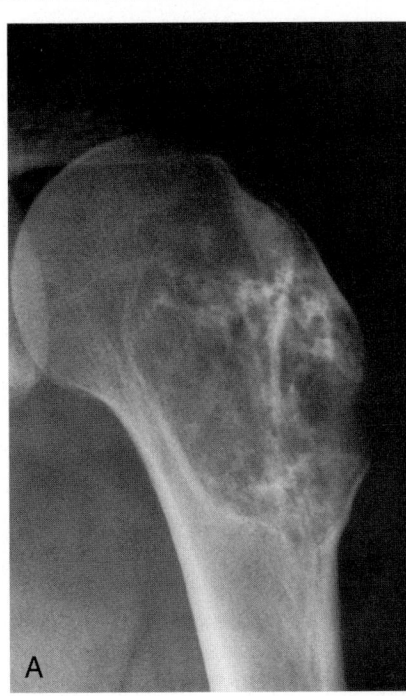

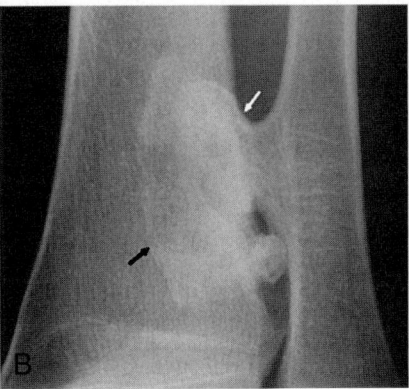

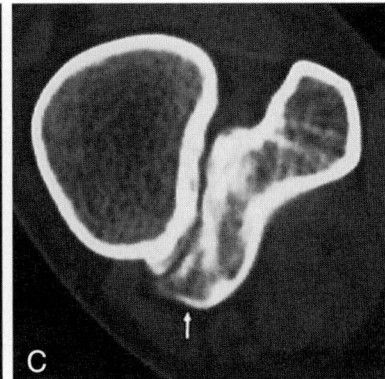

**Figure 70–46.** Solitary osteochondroma: long tubular bones. *A*, Sessile osteochondroma arising from the proximal humerus. The radiographic appearance, which includes calcification, simulates that of an enchondroma. *B* and *C*, Large pedunculated osteochondroma arising from the posteromedial surface of the fibula and wrapping itself about the tibia *(arrows)*, as shown by a routine radiograph *(B)* and transaxial CT scan *(C)*, oriented to allow correlation.

absent. In adults, the occurrence of a cartilage cap that is thicker than 1 cm should raise the possibility of chondrosarcomatous transformation.

**Natural History.** Osteochondromas may continue to increase in size in an immature skeleton. Because such growth usually ceases at puberty, with fusion of the adjacent growth plate, osteochondromas that continue to enlarge after this time must be carefully evaluated for the possibility of malignant transformation; however, growth of benign osteochondromas has been reported in adult patients.

**Complications.** Potential complications of an osteochondroma (or multiple exostoses) include fracture, osseous deformity, vascular injury, neurologic compromise, bursa formation, and malignant transformation.

Fracture is not frequent, but it is not unexpected. Osteochondromas that are large or pedunculated are more likely to result in fracture after an injury. Not unexpectedly, osseous deformity is common (Fig. 70–49) and is more frequently associated with large exostoses and those that arise in one of two anatomically intimate tubular bones. The typical situation is a tibial osteochondroma that produces pressure deformity in the nearby fibula.

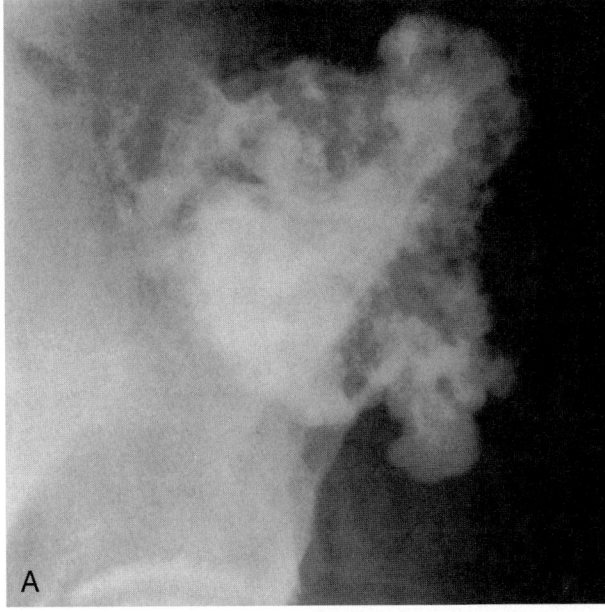

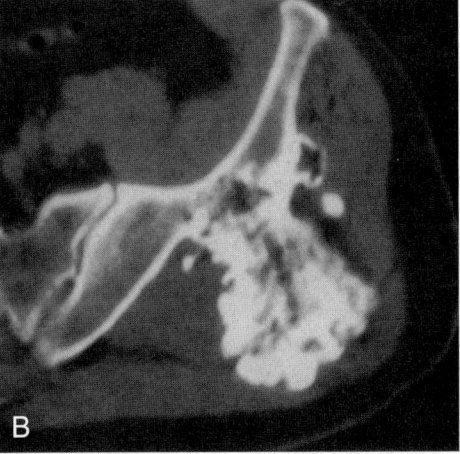

**Figure 70–47.** Solitary osteochondroma: innominate bone. Routine radiograph *(A)* and transaxial CT scan *(B)* show a large pedunculated osteochondroma arising from the posterior surface of the ilium. (Courtesy of R. Sweet, MD, Pomona, Calif.)

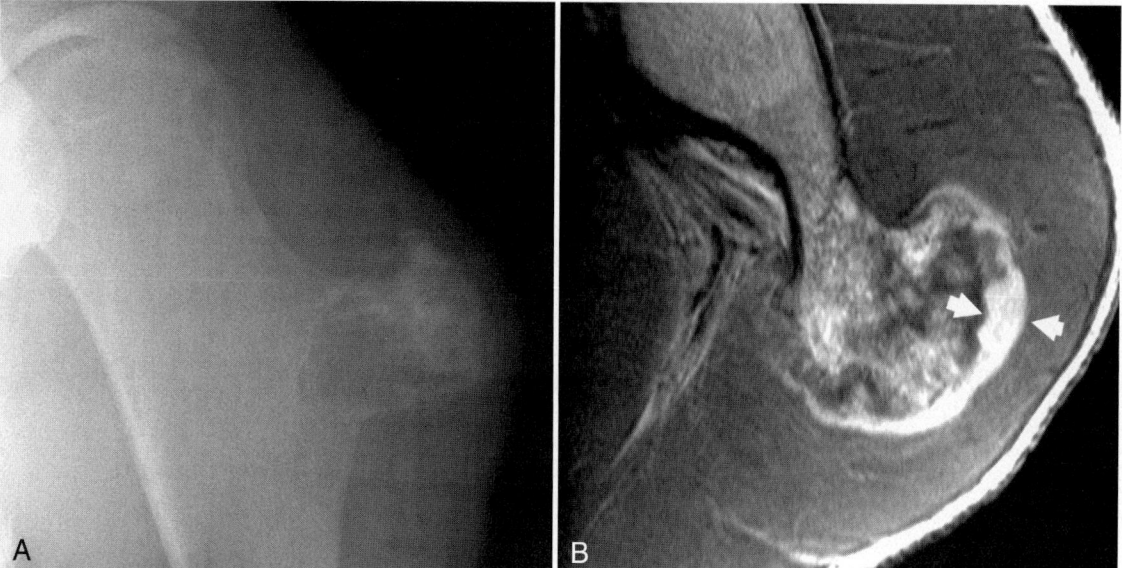

**Figure 70–48.** Solitary osteochondroma. *A*, Radiograph demonstrates a pedunculated osteochondroma in the proximal humerus. *B*, Axial T2-weighted (TR/TE, 2100/90) spin echo MR image demonstrates the cortical and medullary continuity of the pedunculated osteochondroma. Note the high signal intensity from the thin cartilaginous cap *(arrows)*.

The ability of an osteochondroma to displace vessels, particularly those about the knee, is well recognized and relatively common; more severe vascular complications, including arterial or venous stenosis, vessel occlusion or rupture, and pseudoaneurysms, are less frequent but well documented. Almost all the pseudoaneurysms complicating osteochondromas arise in the proximal portion of the popliteal artery. Similarly, osteochondromas may cause neurologic compromise.

An additional complication of an osteochondroma is the formation of a bursal compartment surrounding the tip of the lesion. This finding is particularly frequent when the osteochondroma is large and when it occurs at sites subject to contact and friction with surrounding, unyielding structures such as the scapula and distal portion of the femur (Fig. 70–50). Bursae about any osteochondroma may become inflamed, painful, and distended with fluid, which gives them a firm consistency, especially when they contain fibrin or chondral bodies.

Estimates of the risk of malignant transformation of an osteochondroma vary; however, it appears likely that

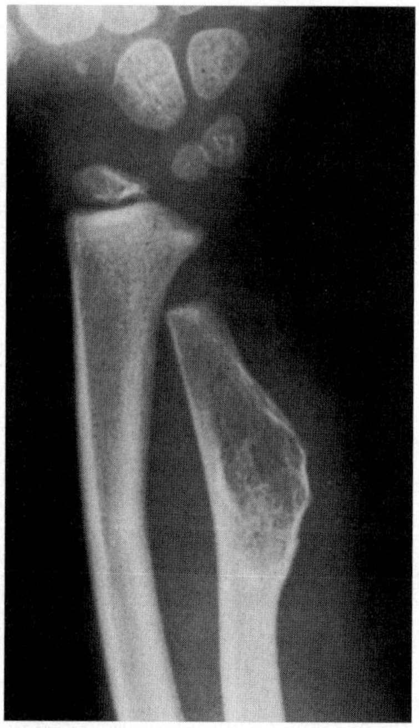

**Figure 70–49.** Solitary osteochondroma: complications—osseous deformity. In this 4-year-old boy, an osteochondroma in the distal portion of the ulna has led to shortening of the bone, with deformity of the wrist.

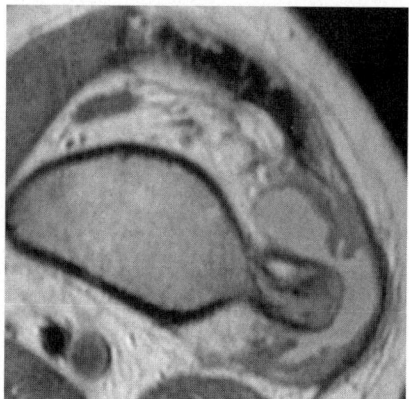

**Figure 70–50.** Solitary osteochondroma: complications—bursa formation. Transverse intermediate-weighted (TR/TE, 1500/11) fast spin echo MR image shows a fractured osteochondroma and adjacent bursitis. (Courtesy of D. Fanney, MD, Virginia Beach, Va.)

the risk of malignant transformation of a solitary osteochondroma is about 1%. The likelihood of malignant transformation is greater in patients with multiple osteochondromas and may reach 25%. Malignant transformation is most commonly to chondrosarcoma. Although certain clinical findings (e.g., pain, swelling, soft tissue mass) and routine radiographic features (e.g., growth of a previously stable osteochondroma, bone erosion, irregular or scattered calcification) aid in the identification of such malignant transformation, they are not entirely reliable.

Scintigraphy accomplished with bone-seeking radionuclides is an effective method for defining osteochondromas that are active metabolically, but it does not allow differentiation of the endochondral ossification occurring in a benign osteochondroma and the hyperemia and osteoblastic reaction occurring in a peripheral chondrosarcoma. A normal bone scan, however, virtually excludes the diagnosis of malignant transformation of an exostosis. CT and MR imaging have met with variable success in differentiating benign from malignant osteochondroma. In general, peripheral chondrosarcomas possess a cartilage cap that is thicker than 1 cm and often greater than 2 cm, whereas in benign exostoses, the thickness is usually less than 1 cm (Fig. 70–51).

**Differential Diagnosis.** The radiographic features of a solitary osteochondroma are usually diagnostic and easily differentiated from other causes of osseous outgrowth, including osteoma, osteophyte, and enthesophyte, and from heterotopic ossification and parosteal osteosarcoma. Osteochondromas or osteochondroma-like lesions are occasionally encountered in systemic disorders, such as pseudohypoparathyroidism, pseudo-pseudohypoparathyroidism, and fibrodysplasia (myositis) ossificans progressiva. The major difficulty arises in distinguishing between a benign osteochondroma and a peripheral chondrosarcoma.

### Hereditary Multiple Exostoses

Hereditary multiple exostoses, an autosomal dominant disorder, leads to clinical abnormalities in the first or second decade of life and characteristic radiographic alterations. Approximately two thirds of affected patients have a positive family history. The specific genetic abnormalities relate to three distinct loci: one each on chromosomes 8, 11, and 19. Palpable osseous protuberances or masses, secondary deformities caused by shortening and bowing of bones, and joint restriction are common and account in part for the early diagnosis of this condition.

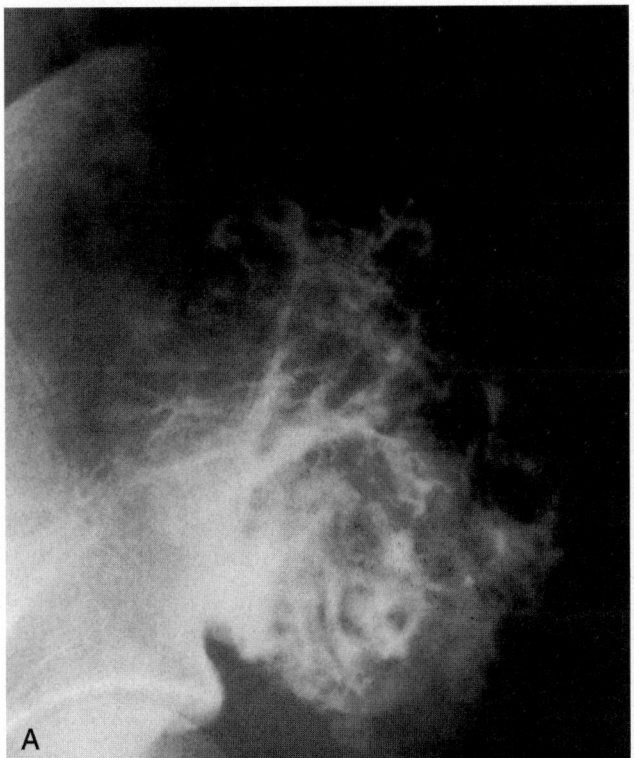

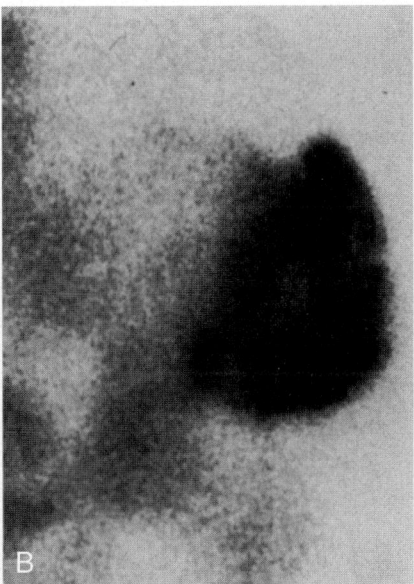

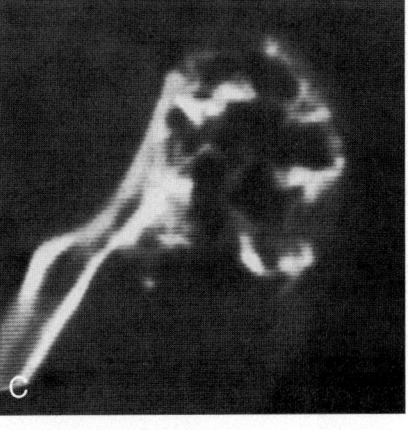

**Figure 70–51.** Solitary osteochondroma: complications—malignant transformation. *A*, Routine radiograph shows a large sessile outgrowth arising from the ilium in a 23-year-old man. *B*, Bone scan reveals nonuniform increased accumulation of radionuclide in the lesion. *C*, Transaxial CT scan shows that the posteriorly located lesion is irregular in outline and contains multiple regions of low attenuation. Biopsy confirmed the presence of a chondrosarcoma.

Typical sites of involvement are the distal and proximal portions of the femur, tibia, and fibula and the proximal portion of the humerus. It is virtually impossible to establish the diagnosis of this disease if exostoses are not present in the bones about the knee. The outgrowths may be bilateral (symmetrical or asymmetrical) or unilateral, depending on the specific genetic type of hereditary multiple exostoses present.

Highly characteristic of this disease is the occurrence of defects in normal modeling of bone and osseous deformities (Fig. 70–52). Of particular note is the presence of bilateral coxa valga and widening of the proximal femoral metaphysis, as well as bilateral and progressive changes about the wrist and shortening of the forearm (Fig. 70–53). An effective radiographic survey designed to delineate some of the more dramatic findings of hereditary multiple exostoses includes frontal radiographs of the knees, pelvis, and wrist.

The complications associated with hereditary exostoses are identical in scope but generally more frequent than those accompanying solitary osteochondromas and include fracture, vascular injury, neurologic compromise, bursa formation, and malignant transformation (Fig. 70–54). The frequency of the last complication has been reported to be between 1% and 27%; it is probably actually about 2% to 5% and is certainly greater than the frequency of malignant transformation in solitary osteochondromas.

### *Dysplasia Epiphysealis Hemimelica (Trevor's Disease)*

Dysplasia epiphysealis hemimelica usually becomes evident in children and young adults and is more common

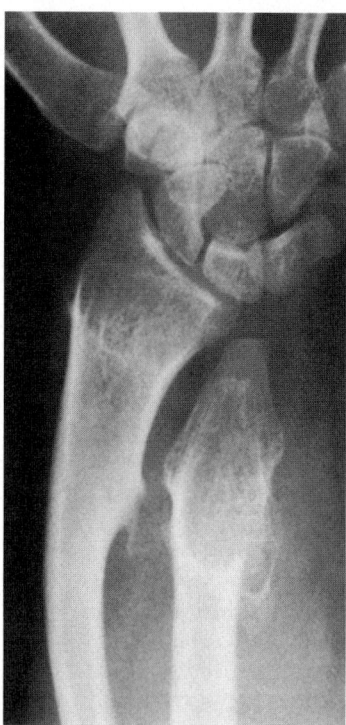

**Figure 70–53.** Hereditary multiple exostoses. The wrist deformity is characterized by osteochondromas of the radius and ulna, with shortening of the ulna, an angular articular surface of the radius, and bowing of the radius. Multiple metacarpal bones were also shortened. (Courtesy of T. Broderick, MD, Orange, Calif.)

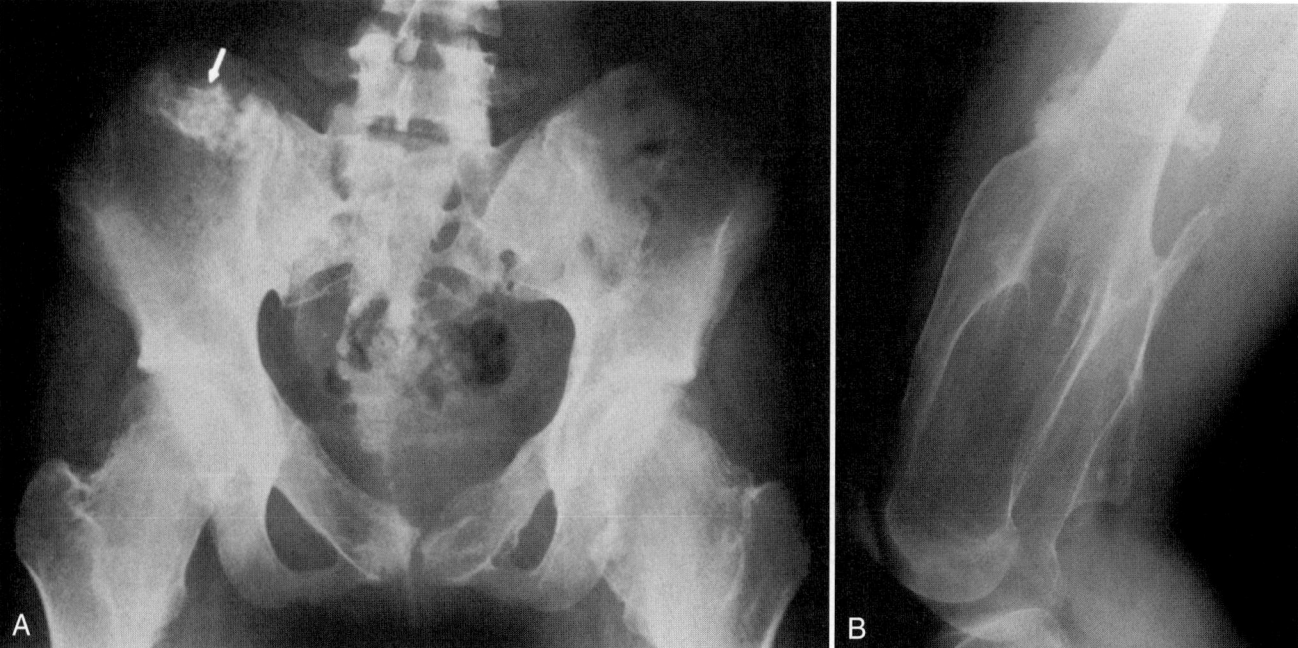

**Figure 70–52.** Hereditary multiple exostoses. *A*, Radiograph reveals bilateral coxa valga deformity, widening of the femoral metaphyses, and multiple osteochondromas in the femora and innominate bones. Observe a large lesion *(arrow)* arising from the ilium. *B*, In a different patient, note the widening and deformity of the distal part of the femur and multiple sessile and pedunculated osteochondromas.

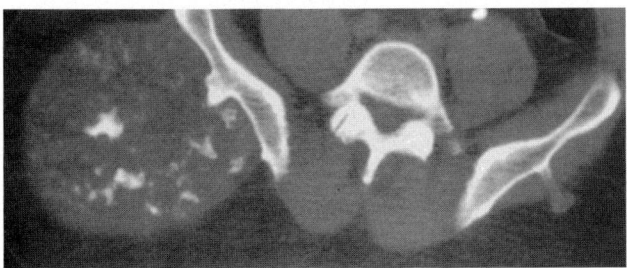

**Figure 70–54.** Hereditary multiple exostoses: complications—malignant transformation. Transaxial CT scan in a 30-year-old man with a buttock mass shows bilateral osteochondromas arising from the posterior surface of the ilii and a calcified mass on the right side representing a chondrosarcoma. (Courtesy of R. Stiles, MD, Atlanta, Ga.)

in males than in females. Typical clinical manifestations include swelling and, less commonly, pain and deformity, which are localized to one side of the body. Lower extremity involvement is far more frequent than upper extremity involvement. The talus, distal portion of the femur, and distal and proximal regions of the tibia are the

principal sites of abnormality. Multiple bones (in a single extremity) are affected in 60% to 70% of cases. This process involves primarily one side of an epiphysis, with the medial side being affected approximately twice as often as the lateral side.

Radiographic findings in an infant or young child include multifocal, irregular ossifications adjacent to one side of an ossifying epiphysis (or carpal or tarsal bone) (Fig. 70–55). The adjacent metaphysis may be widened. Subsequently, the ossifications become confluent with the adjacent bone, eventually appearing as a lobulated osseous mass protruding from the epiphysis. In severe cases, muscle wasting, growth disturbance, and joint deformity are identified.

On macroscopic examination, the lesion is found to be a pedunculated mass with a cartilaginous cap. The histologic features of the lesion are identical to those of an osteochondroma.

### Other Osteochondromas or Osteochondroma-Like Lesions

A subungual exostosis is an uncommon, benign bone tumor arising in the distal phalanx of a digit, beneath or

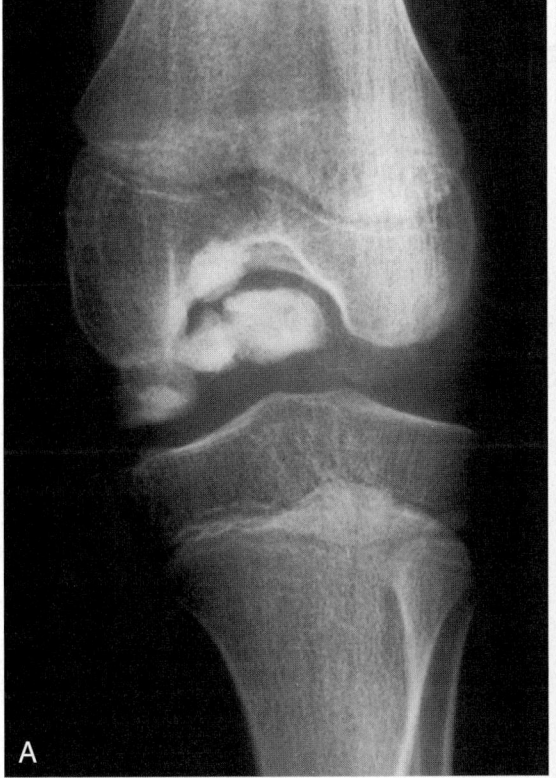

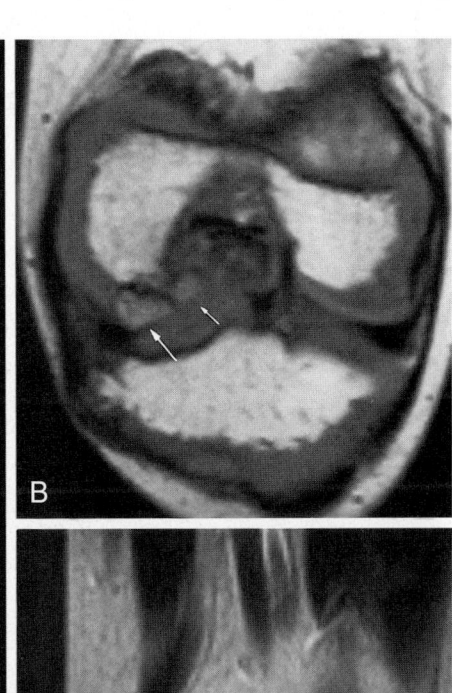

**Figure 70–55.** Dysplasia epiphysealis hemimelica (Trevor's disease): long tubular bones. *A*, In this child, a conventional radiograph shows multiple ossifications about the medial femoral condyle. *B* and *C*, Coronal T1-weighted (TR/TE, 670/25) spin echo *(B)* and fast spin echo (TR/TE, 6445/130) *(C)* MR images document that the ossifications *(arrows)* lie within the epiphyseal cartilage. (Courtesy of T. Hughes, MD, San Diego, Calif.)

adjacent to the nail bed. Clinical manifestations include pain, swelling, and ulcerations of the nail bed or surrounding tissue with secondary infection. The great toe is involved in 70% to 80% of cases. Radiographically, the lesion projects from the dorsal or dorsomedial aspect of the distal portion of a terminal phalanx (Fig. 70–56). Histologically, the lesion consists of a base of trabecular bone with a proliferating fibrocartilaginous cap, features that differ from those of a typical osteochondroma.

A turret exostosis is an infrequent osseous excrescence that typically arises on the dorsal surface of a proximal or middle phalanx in a finger. Clinically, a history of trauma is common. Radiographs show a broad-based bone protuberance on the dorsal surface of the affected phalanx. On the basis of the histologic findings, it is likely that a turret exostosis represents an ossifying, subperiosteal hematoma.

A supracondylar (supracondyloid) process of the humerus represents an outgrowth of bone that occurs on the anteromedial surface of the distal portion of the humerus, approximately 5 to 7 cm above the medial epicondyle. It is believed to represent a phylogenetic vestige of the supracondyloid foramen found in reptiles and some mammals. The supracondylar process is variable in size, and its apex may be roughened or irregular. The process may afford insertion to a persistent part of the coracobrachialis muscle. A band of fibrous tissue, the ligament of Struthers, may join the tip of the supracondylar process and the medial epicondyle. Compression of the median nerve is one complication of this process.

## Malignant Tumors

### Chondrosarcoma

Chondrosarcomas can be categorized according to their location within the bone (central, peripheral, or juxtacortical), their occurrence as an initial (de novo) lesion

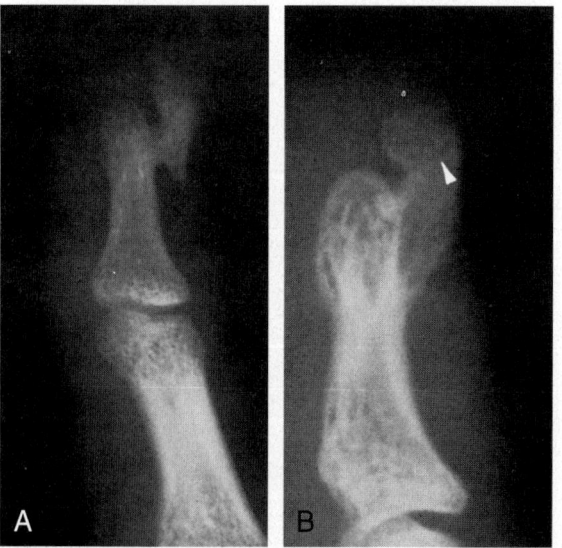

**Figure 70–56.** Subungual exostosis. *A* and *B*, Two examples are shown. In *(B)*, a fracture line *(arrowhead)* extends through the distal portion of the lesion.

(primary chondrosarcoma), or as a lesion superimposed on a preexisting process such as an osteochondroma or enchondroma (secondary chondrosarcoma), their degree of cellular differentiation (low grade, medium grade, or high grade), the presence of unusual histologic characteristics (clear cell or mesenchymal chondrosarcomas), and the occurrence of changes in these histologic characteristics (dedifferentiated chondrosarcoma). Cartilage tumors are designated conventional chondrosarcomas (including central and peripheral types), juxtacortical (periosteal) chondrosarcomas, clear cell chondrosarcomas, mesenchymal chondrosarcomas, and dedifferentiated chondrosarcomas.

### Conventional Chondrosarcoma

In this category are malignant tumors that arise within the medullary cavity either de novo or as a secondary complication of a preexisting enchondroma (central chondrosarcoma) and those that arise near the surface of the bone (peripheral chondrosarcoma). Peripheral chondrosarcomas are sometimes subdivided into two groups: those developing from a preexisting osteochondroma (exostotic chondrosarcoma) and those originating from the periosteal membrane or parosteal tissue (juxtacortical, or periosteal, chondrosarcoma).

**Clinical Abnormalities.** Conventional chondrosarcomas occur more frequently in men than in women. Patients with this tumor are generally between the ages of 30 and 60 years. Patients with peripheral chondrosarcomas tend to be slightly younger than those with central chondrosarcomas. Chondrosarcomas are rare in children. Pain is the most characteristic initial symptom and may occur in association with soft tissue prominence. The average duration of symptoms is 1 to 2 years.

**Skeletal Location.** The long tubular bones are the sites of involvement in approximately 45% of cases, with the femur being the most commonly affected bone (approximately 25% of all cases). Other common locations are the innominate bone (25% of cases) and the ribs (8% of cases). Most chondrosarcomas in the long tubular bones are located in the metaphysis, but with closure of the physis, tumor extension into the epiphysis is encountered. Excluding hematologic tumors, chondrosarcomas are the most frequent malignant neoplasm of the scapula, ribs, sternum, and small bones of the hand. The innominate bone and femur are more characteristic sites of chondrosarcomas than enchondromas, and chondrosarcomas are about twice as frequent in the long bones as enchondromas are.

**Radiographic Abnormalities.** Precise radiographic diagnosis of chondrosarcoma depends on a number of characteristic features, the most important of which is tumoral calcification. Other changes, including the patterns of bone destruction, cortical violation, and periostitis, are more variable. Well-organized calcific rings within cartilage usually signify a low-grade tumor. High-grade chondrosarcomas, which may contain a greater amount of myxoid material, are frequently associated with large areas of noncalcified tumor matrix. Further, when calcification occurs within high-grade chondrosarcomas, it is typically amorphous, punctate, scattered, or irregular. With regard to tumor margins, an ill-defined boundary with a long zone of transition between abnormal and normal portions of bone is usually indicative of an aggressive or high-grade chondrosarcoma.

Central chondrosarcomas occur in both the tubular bones (particularly the femur and humerus) and the flat and irregular bones (especially those in the pelvis). In the tubular bones, radiographs typically reveal an elongated, slightly expansile, multilobulated osteolytic lesion accompanied by periosteal bone formation, cortical thickening, endosteal bone erosion, and scattered stippled or irregular calcification (Fig. 70–57). Such calcification is evident in approximately 60% to 70% of cases, although conventional tomography or CT may be required for its detection. In some cases, obvious features of aggressive behavior are observed, such as poorly defined osteolysis, cortical violation, and a soft tissue mass; more often, however, the radiographic abnormalities are those of a slowly evolving process. In the flat and irregular bones (Fig. 70–58), chondrosarcomas have similar radiographic features, although soft tissue involvement may be more pronounced.

Peripheral chondrosarcomas most commonly arise from a preexisting osteochondroma or, rarely, from the periosteal membrane in the form of a juxtacortical chondrosarcoma (see later discussion); they may occur in flat, irregular, or tubular bones. Distinguishing between a benign osteochondroma and one that has undergone malignant transformation relies on the analysis of data derived from routine radiography. Features suggestive of malignancy are a bulky cartilaginous cap, an irregular or indistinct surface of the calcified tissue beneath the cartilaginous cap, scattered calcifications in the cartilaginous part of the tumor, focal areas of radiolucency in the interior of the osteochondroma, a significant soft tissue mass, and destruction or pressure erosion of the adjacent bone (Fig. 70–59). Rapid growth of an osteochondroma,

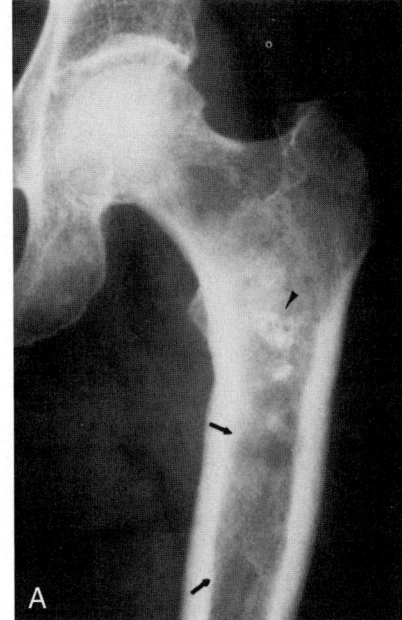
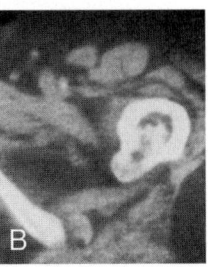

**Figure 70–57.** Conventional chondrosarcoma, central type: long tubular bones. In this 37-year-old man, a routine radiograph *(A)* shows an expansile lesion of the femoral diaphysis. The proximal portion of the lesion is calcified; the distal portion is not. Transaxial CT scan *(B)* reveals internal calcifications and cortical erosion.

though not diagnostic of malignant transformation, is an ominous sign indicating the need to surgically remove the lesion.

**Other Imaging Techniques.** Radionuclide scanning with bone-seeking radiopharmaceutical agents has been used in the evaluation of both central and peripheral chondrosarcomas. In the former, increased accumulation of radionuclide at the site of tumor is uniformly present. In cases of peripheral chondrosarcomas, bone scanning

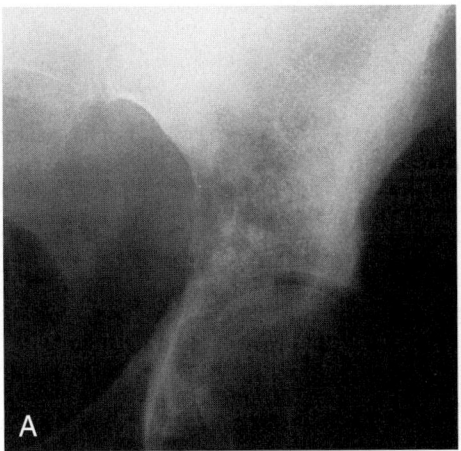
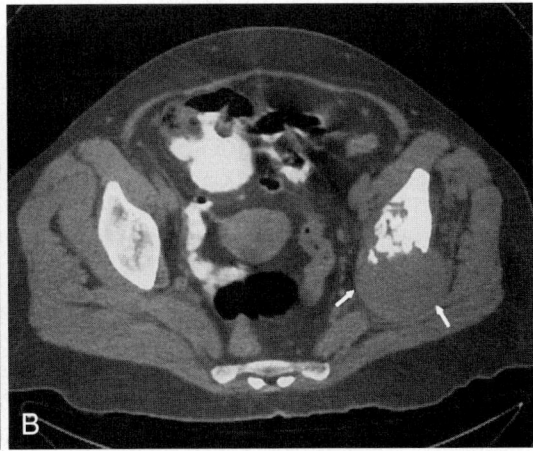

**Figure 70–58.** Conventional chondrosarcoma, central type: innominate bone. In this 50-year-old woman, a routine radiograph *(A)* shows an osteolytic lesion of the para-acetabular bone, with a prominent soft tissue mass. Transaxial CT scan *(B)* documents destruction of the acetabular roof, possible calcification, and a large soft tissue mass *(arrows)*.

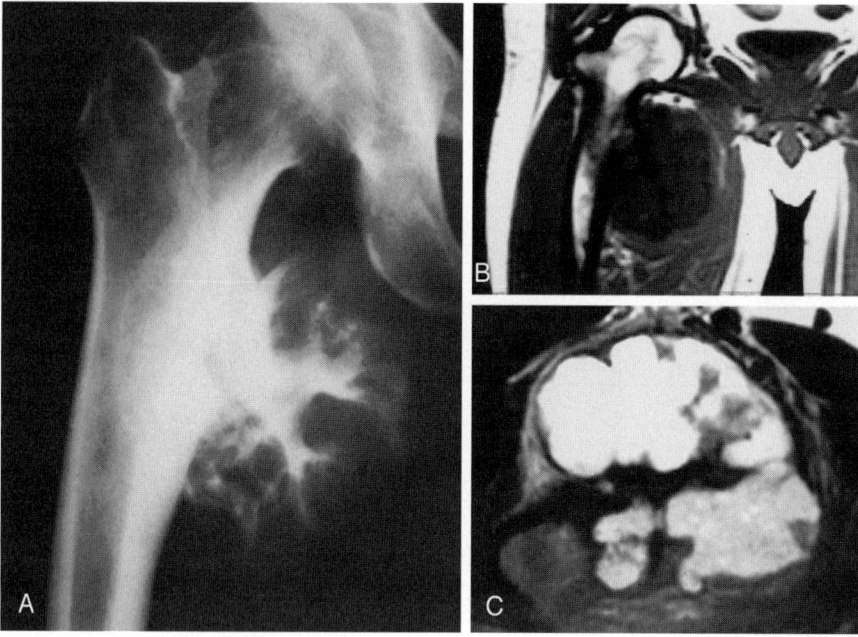

**Figure 70–59.** Conventional chondrosarcoma, peripheral type: long tubular bones. In this 30-year-old man with a firm, nontender mass in the medial aspect of the thigh, a routine radiograph (*A*) shows an irregular excrescence arising from the medial aspect of the femur. Its appearance is not that of a typical osteochondroma. The cortex of the subjacent femur is thickened. Coronal T1-weighted (TR/TE, 500/10) spin echo MR image (*B*) reveals a mass of low signal intensity. On a transaxial T2-weighted (TR/TE, 2000/80) spin echo MR image (*C*), a lobulated tumor of high signal intensity is evident. Vascular displacement and compression are also seen.

allows documentation of osteochondromas that are metabolically active but is unreliable in differentiating between benign and malignant tumors. Absence of uptake of the bone-seeking agent virtually eliminates the possibility of malignant transformation of an osteochondroma.

CT provides important information regarding the intraosseous and soft tissue extent of the neoplasm. It is especially useful in identifying matrix and erosive changes in areas of complex anatomy such as the spine, pelvis, and small bones of the hands and feet. MR imaging has been used to assess both central and peripheral chondrosarcomas (Fig. 70–60). The technique is good for defining the full extent of the tumor. An inhomogeneous or homogeneous lesion of high signal intensity is typical on T2-weighted spin echo MR images. Enhancement of signal intensity in a focal or diffuse fashion within the tumor is evident after the intravenous administration of gadolinium compounds, and the extent of such enhancement may be greater in higher-grade neoplasms. Tumor calcification may be seen with MR imaging but is detected more easily with CT.

**Pathologic Abnormalities.** Central chondrosarcomas frequently erode the cortex and extend into the soft tissue, an important feature that distinguishes them from enchondromas. Peripheral chondrosarcomas that arise from malignant transformation of an osteochondroma are predominantly extraosseous, large, bosselated masses that appear relatively well delineated even though they have invaded the soft tissues. The cartilaginous caps of these tumors are commonly thicker than 2 cm; such caps in benign osteochondromas in adults are usually less than 1 cm thick, whereas in children and adolescents, the cartilaginous caps of benign exostoses may be 2 or 3 cm thick. Chondrosarcomas are usually classified into four grades, I to IV, with the lower grades indicating the better differentiated or less aggressive tumors.

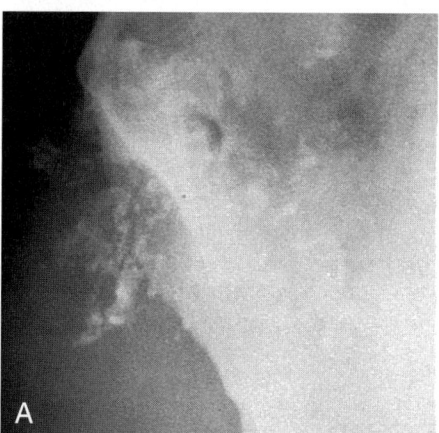

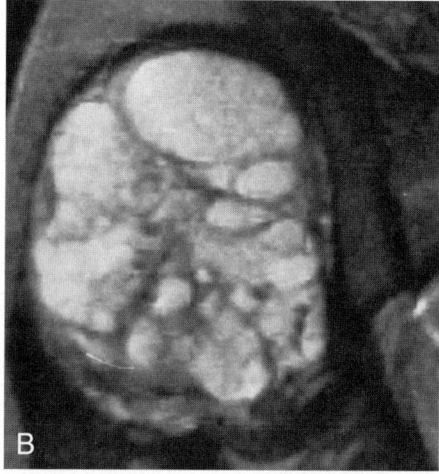

**Figure 70–60.** Conventional chondrosarcoma, peripheral type: innominate bone. *A*, Routine radiograph reveals a calcified lesion extending from the ilium. *B*, On a coronal T2-weighted (TR/TE, 2500/90) spin echo MR image, the tumor is lobulated, is mainly of high signal intensity, and contains septations of low signal intensity. (Courtesy of J. Kramer, MD, Vienna, Austria.)

**Natural History.** The natural history and ultimate prognosis of chondrosarcomas are extremely variable. Chondrosarcomas have the potential to be locally infiltrative and, in some cases, to metastasize through the bloodstream to distant organs. Locally aggressive manifestations of chondrosarcoma include focal or uniform intraosseous extension, transarticular spread, and soft tissue invasion. These manifestations, as well as systemic metastasis, increase in frequency with higher grades of neoplasm. Metastases from well-differentiated (i.e., grade I) chondrosarcomas are rare. Tumor recurrence is also correlated with histologic grade. The reported overall rate of survival for 10 years after treatment varies from 30% to 70%, with the risk of death being greatest for patients with spinal tumors and high-grade chondrosarcomas.

**Differential Diagnosis.** Differentiation of a central chondrosarcoma and an enchondroma may be extremely difficult, although ill-defined osteolysis, a soft tissue mass, and the absence of calcification in part of the lesion are radiographic findings more compatible with a chondrosarcoma. Similarly, differentiation of a peripheral chondrosarcoma and a simple osteochondroma is usually not possible on the basis of conventional radiographic examination, and supplemental imaging techniques are required.

In the flat or irregular bones, a large osteolytic lesion with a soft tissue mass in an adult patient is compatible with a variety of lesions, including chondrosarcoma, plasmacytoma, lymphoma, or a solitary skeletal focus of metastasis. More specific in such cases is the identification of calcification, although its differentiation from ossification, as might be seen in an osteosarcoma, may not be easy.

### *Juxtacortical (Periosteal) Chondrosarcoma*

The clinical and radiographic appearance of juxtacortical chondrosarcoma is similar to that of periosteal osteosarcoma, which has led many investigators to conclude that they are identical neoplasms. Young and middle-aged men or, less commonly, women usually present with pain and a palpable mass. A long tubular bone, especially the femur (often its posterior metadiaphyseal or metaphyseal aspect), is typically affected, and the radiographic alterations include a small lesion on the osseous surface, sometimes accompanied by spotty calcification, radiating bone spicules, and a typical Codman's triangle (Fig. 70–61). In many cases, no periostitis is observed, and the cortical surface is thickened and either irregular or smooth. Macroscopic examination confirms the tumor's origin in the external portion of the cortex.

### *Clear Cell Chondrosarcoma*

Clear cell chondrosarcoma is a low-grade cartilaginous neoplasm that possesses a distinctive histologic appearance based on its constituent tumor cells.

**Clinical Abnormalities.** Clear cell chondrosarcoma occurs more frequently in men and is usually seen in the third, fourth, or fifth decade of life. Symptoms are variable and

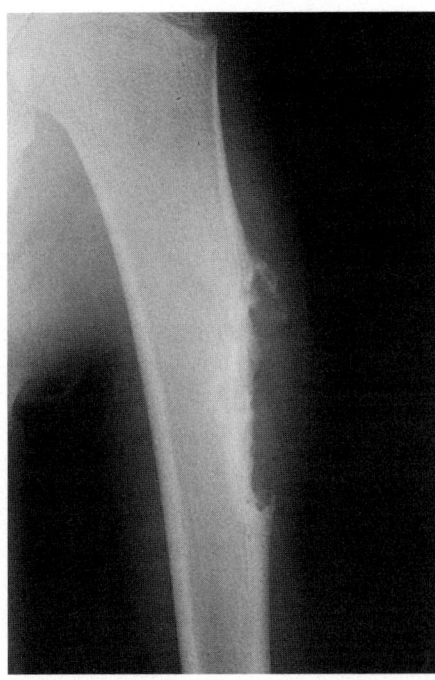

**Figure 70–61.** Juxtacortical (periosteal) chondrosarcoma. Radiograph shows an eccentric osteolytic lesion eroding the external surface of the cortex. The endosteal margin of the cortex is thickened, and mature periosteal elevation is seen at the superior and inferior margins of the tumor.

of long duration and include mild, localized pain and limited range of motion in the adjacent articulation. Pathologic fractures are not infrequent, occurring in approximately 25% of cases.

**Skeletal Location.** Clear cell chondrosarcomas predominate in the long tubular bones (approximately 85% of cases), particularly the femur (approximately 55% of cases) and the humerus (15% to 20% of cases). The bones about the knee are involved in 10% to 15% of cases. Involvement of flat or irregular bones is unusual. In the tubular bones, epiphyseal localization is the rule. The proximal end of the bone is affected in approximately 90% of cases; the most common site of involvement is the proximal portion of the femur, followed in order of decreasing frequency by the proximal portions of the humerus and tibia.

**Radiographic Abnormalities.** Clear cell chondrosarcomas are predominantly osteolytic and slightly expansile. The margin of the tumor may be either poorly defined or well defined, with a sclerotic border. The reported frequency of calcification varies, but it probably occurs in about 35% of cases; in some cases, such calcification is prominent. Endosteal erosion, cortical violation, pathologic fracture, and a soft tissue mass are additional radiographic findings in some cases. The radiographic features, as well as the typical epiphyseal location in a tubular bone (Fig. 70–62), are similar to those of chondroblastoma, and differentiation of these two neoplasms may be difficult. The presence of metaphyseal

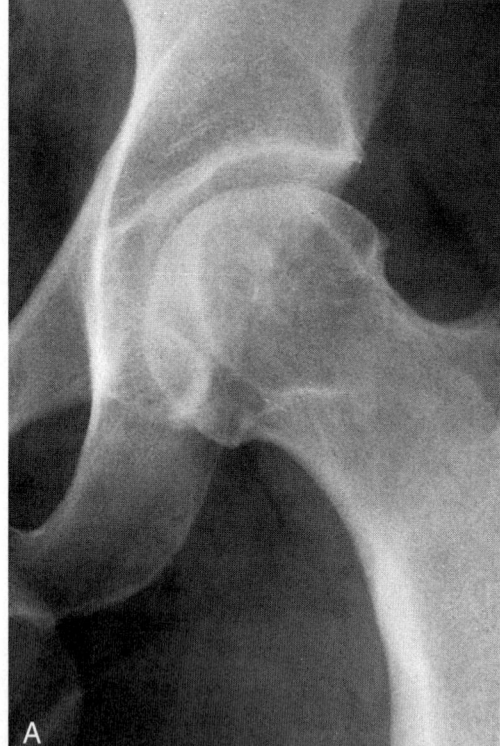

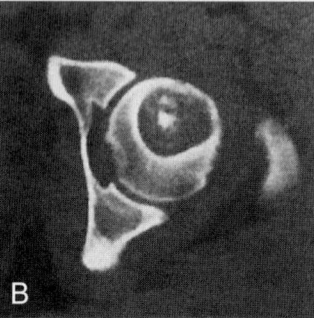

**Figure 70–62.** Clear cell chondrosarcoma. *A*, Routine radiograph shows a large, well-defined osteolytic lesion involving the femoral head and extending into the femoral neck. It contains central calcification and a peripheral sclerotic margin and has led to subtle collapse of the articular surface. *B*, Transaxial CT scan shows the calcified lesion in the femoral head.

involvement and the absence of periostitis are findings that favor the diagnosis of clear cell chondrosarcoma. The absence of associated inflammation on MR imaging also favors the diagnosis of clear cell chondrosarcoma.

**Pathologic Abnormalities.** Clear cell chondrosarcomas are histologically distinctive, with areas of closely compact cells arranged in sheets or separated into faint lobules by thin fibrovascular septa. The tumor cells have an abundant, clear, glycogen-rich cytoplasm with distinct borders. Regions of conventional chondrosarcoma are found in approximately 50% of these tumors.

**Natural History.** Clear cell chondrosarcomas are relatively slow growing, low-grade malignant tumors with a much better prognosis than that associated with conventional

chondrosarcomas. Local extension into the soft tissues and even the adjacent articulation may be encountered. Tumor resection appears to be curative. Disseminated metastases in the lungs, brain, and bones may be seen, however.

**Differential Diagnosis.** Bone lesions that may radiographically resemble clear cell chondrosarcoma are chondroblastoma, aneurysmal bone cyst, osteoblastoma, ossifying lipoma, giant cell tumor, plasmacytoma, skeletal metastasis, and the brown tumor of hyperparathyroidism.

### Mesenchymal Chondrosarcoma

Although relatively rare, mesenchymal chondrosarcomas are one of the few primary malignant tumors of bone that sometimes also arise in the soft tissues (30% to 75% of cases). Mesenchymal chondrosarcomas represent about 13% of all chondrosarcomas arising in bone.

**Clinical Abnormalities.** Men and women are affected in approximately equal numbers; most are in the second, third, and fourth decades of life. Patients with mesenchymal chondrosarcoma are typically younger than those with conventional chondrosarcoma and similar in age to those with conventional osteosarcoma. Pain of several months to years in duration, swelling, a soft tissue mass, and stiffness are the most typical clinical manifestations.

**Skeletal Location.** The most frequent sites of involvement are the femur (15% of skeletal cases), ribs (12%), and spine (11%), followed in order of decreasing frequency by the skull, maxilla, innominate bone, sacrum, humerus, tibia, mandible, calcaneus, and other bones. Mesenchymal chondrosarcomas can arise in any portion of a tubular bone, although a diaphyseal location has been emphasized.

**Radiographic Abnormalities.** Osteolysis, a permeative pattern of bone destruction, an irregular outline, bone sclerosis, periostitis, and intralesional calcification are among the most characteristic of the varied radiographic features of this neoplasm (Fig. 70–63). The pattern of calcification within the osseous or soft tissue component of the lesion is usually stippled. Radiographic abnormalities resemble those of conventional chondrosarcoma; the relatively young age of the patient and the more aggressive pattern of osteolysis may allow a more specific diagnosis of mesenchymal chondrosarcoma.

**Pathologic Abnormalities.** Soft tissue and skeletal mesenchymal chondrosarcomas have an identical histomorphology. Accurate microscopic diagnosis depends on the presence of two components: undifferentiated stromal cells and islands of cartilage.

**Natural History.** Mesenchymal chondrosarcomas represent an aggressive variant of chondrosarcoma and are associated with a poor prognosis. Local recurrence typifies the clinical course, and recurrence may precede the appearance of disseminated metastases. The tendency of this tumor to metastasize to regional and distant lymph

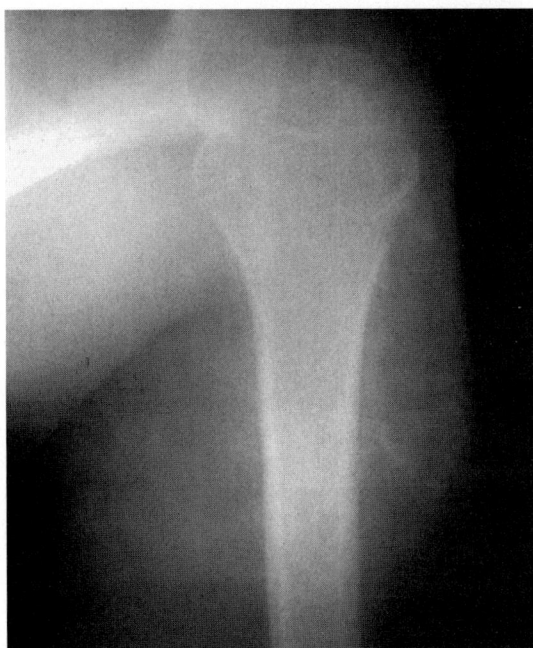

**Figure 70–63.** Mesenchymal chondrosarcoma. Note osteolysis and a permeative pattern of bone destruction, with periostitis and calcification. The pattern of growth suggests an aggressive process.

nodes and to other bones is quite uncharacteristic of an ordinary chondrosarcoma.

**Differential Diagnosis.** Because the radiographic findings of mesenchymal chondrosarcoma are those of an aggressive tumor that contains calcification, it is generally impossible to differentiate this neoplasm from a high-grade conventional chondrosarcoma.

### Dedifferentiated Chondrosarcoma

This variant of conventional chondrosarcoma is a bimorphic neoplasm in which a borderline or low-grade malignant cartilage tumor is in direct association (juxtaposed) with a high-grade sarcoma (of a different cell line). This dedifferentiated neoplasm represents about 10% of all chondrosarcomas. It is locally aggressive and is associated with an extremely poor prognosis.

**Clinical Abnormalities.** Men and women in the fifth, sixth, and seventh decades of life are generally affected. Pain is the most frequent symptom. Soft tissue swelling or a mass and pathologic fractures (10% to 40% of cases) are other common clinical manifestations. Preexisting cartilaginous tumors may or may not be identified.

**Skeletal Location.** Dedifferentiated chondrosarcomas have a distribution similar to that of conventional chondrosarcomas. The femur, humerus, and innominate bone account for most cases. In the long tubular bones, the proximal segments are affected far more frequently.

**Radiographic Abnormalities.** Typically, an osteolytic lesion with moth-eaten bone destruction is observed; the lesion is partially calcified, but in one region such calcification is sparse or entirely absent. These noncalcified areas commonly reveal the most aggressive bone destruction, with erosion and penetration of the cortex, soft tissue swelling, and, in some cases, pathologic fracture. Accurate radiographic diagnosis of a dedifferentiated chondrosarcoma relies on the identification of two characteristic patterns within the lesion. The first is indicative of a low-grade chondrosarcoma, and the second is indicative of the dedifferentiated and more aggressive portion of the tumor (Fig. 70–64).

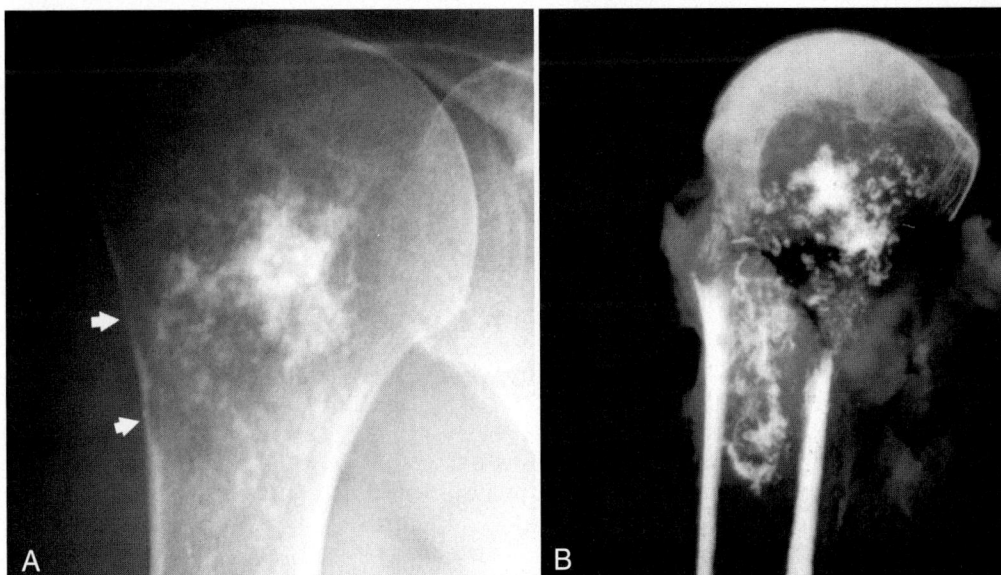

**Figure 70–64.** Dedifferentiated chondrosarcoma. *A,* Radiograph of the proximal humerus shows mineralization, typical of a cartilage tumor. Areas of endosteal scalloping *(arrows)* and lysis have appeared since the previous examination 8 months earlier. *B,* Specimen radiograph shows the cartilage mineralization to better advantage. The pathologic fracture is through the area of the high-grade sarcoma.

**Pathologic Abnormalities.** Histologically, dedifferentiated chondrosarcomas contain foci of a low-grade conventional chondrosarcoma and, in juxtaposition, a pleomorphic or spindle cell sarcoma. The transition between these two components is usually, but not invariably, sharp. The noncartilaginous component may have features of fibrosarcoma, osteosarcoma, or malignant fibrous histiocytoma.

# TUMORS ARISING FROM OR FORMING FIBROUS CONNECTIVE TISSUE

## Benign Tumors

### Fibrous Cortical Defect and Nonossifying Fibroma

Nonossifying fibroma and fibrous cortical defect are common lesions that are composed histologically of whorled bundles of bland connective tissue cells. The two terms are used interchangeably, although it is generally agreed that nonossifying fibroma is more appropriately applied to a larger lesion. The term fibroxanthoma, which is more reflective of the underlying pathology, is sometimes used as a synonym for nonossifying fibroma. The origin and histogenesis of these lesions are still debated, but an unrecognized, local traumatic insult (or insults) to the periosteum resulting in focal hemorrhage and edema is consistent with both the natural history of fibrous cortical defects and their propensity to occur at osseous sites of muscular attachment.

**Clinical Abnormalities.** Small cortical fibrous lesions in the tubular bones are regularly encountered during radiographic examination of healthy children. It has been estimated that one or more cortical defects are apparent in more than 50% of boys and 20% of girls who are older than 2 years. Generally, smaller lesions are clinically silent and are discovered incidentally on radiographs obtained for other reasons. Their rarity in children younger than 2 years is consistent with the belief that muscle pull during weight bearing and walking is important in their pathogenesis, and their infrequency in adults supports the concept that most lesions heal by being replaced by normal bone.

**Skeletal Location.** Small lesions (fibrous cortical defects) occur at either a single site or in multiple locations in one or more bones, whereas large lesions (nonossifying fibromas) are far less commonly multifocal and, when multiple, may or may not be accompanied by other clinical manifestations. Symmetry of involvement is characteristic of bilateral distribution.

The long tubular bones are predominantly affected (approximately 90% of cases). The tibia (43%) and the femur (38%) are the most frequent sites of involvement. Lesions of the upper extremity are uncommon. When evident in sites other than the long bones, these lesions are sometimes designated benign fibrous histiocytomas. In the tubular bones, lesions are predominantly metaphyseal lesions arising close to the physeal plate. With continued growth of the parent bone, these lesions become situated some distance from the physis, and, if they do not involute, they may extend into the diaphysis. Epiphyseal localization or extension is distinctly unusual. Fibrous

cortical defects and nonossifying fibromas usually arise from the posterior wall of the tubular bone and affect the medial (rather than the lateral) osseous surface far more frequently.

**Radiographic Abnormalities.** Fibrous cortical defects and nonossifying fibromas are associated with characteristic radiographic abnormalities that are virtually diagnostic (Fig. 70–65). Smaller lesions produce focal, superficial, shallow radiolucent areas in the cortex with normal or sclerotic adjacent bone. Lesions are circular or oval, well delineated with smooth or lobulated edges, and are not accompanied by significant periostitis. Characteristically, they arise in the metaphysis a short distance from the physis or, less commonly, adjacent to the physeal plate. With growth of the tubular bone, apparent shaftward migration of the lesion may be accompanied by segmental sclerosis within a portion of the osseous defect. Larger lesions are more elongated and have a multiloculated appearance; cortical thinning or slight expansion may be evident.

Other imaging studies are not required due to the specificity of radiographs; however, lesions may be incidentally noted on other modalities. Scintigraphy will show mild accumulation of bone-seeking radiopharmaceutical agents. With MR imaging, these fibrous processes show variability in signal intensity characteristics; although they are typically of low signal intensity on T1-weighted and T2-weighted spin echo MR images, hyperintensity on T2-weighted spin echo MR images may be seen (Fig. 70–66).

**Pathologic Abnormalities.** Both fibrous cortical defects and nonossifying fibromas have an identical histomorphology. They are composed of uniform benign-appearing, spindle-shaped fibroblasts arranged in intersecting bands creating a whorled or storiform pattern. Scattered within this fibrous stroma are multinucleated osteoclast-type giant cells. Foam (xanthoma) cells occur in 30% to 50% of cases and are more common in older lesions.

**Natural History.** The initially small radiolucent lesions arising in the metaphysis, which are generally regarded as fibrous cortical defects, may enlarge, migrate shaftward, shrink, acquire sclerotic borders (beginning in their diaphyseal aspect), and finally disappear, although this sequence is not uniform; nor is the duration of the natural life of these tumors constant. The relative infrequency of fibrous cortical defects in a mature skeleton versus an immature skeleton, however, supports their typically self-limited nature. The behavior of larger lesions, which are generally designated nonossifying fibromas, is less predictable. Although some of these lesions may involute, others continue to grow, become very large, and predispose to fracture.

**Complications.** The occurrence of pathologic fractures through larger nonossifying fibromas is well documented. This complication may be seen after minor trauma and is observed most frequently in the bones of the lower extremity (see Fig. 70–65). Cortical defects rarely fracture.

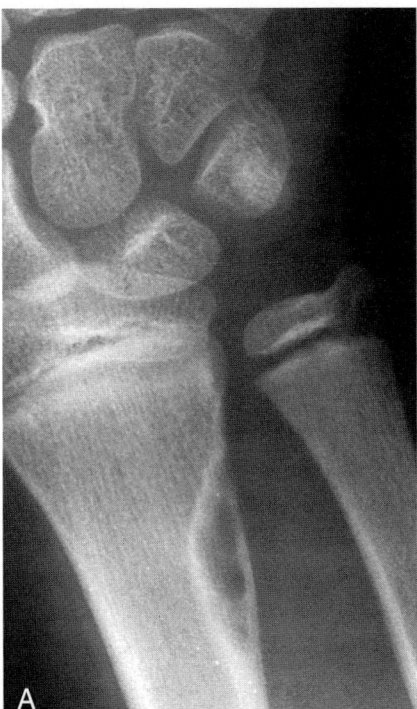

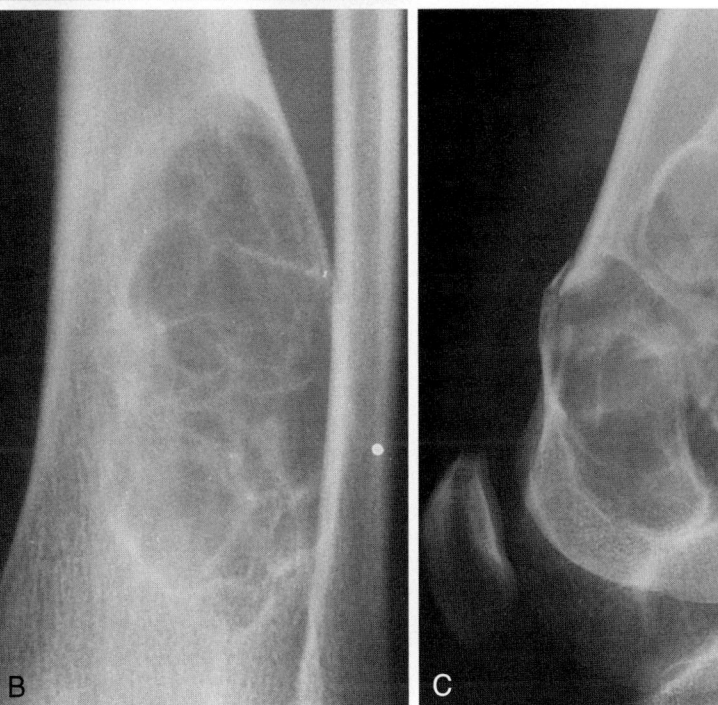

**Figure 70–65.** Nonossifying fibroma and fibrous cortical defect: spectrum of radiographic changes. *A*, This eccentric, radiolucent lesion in the radius has a sclerotic inner margin. It is located a short distance from the physis. *B*, This large nonossifying fibroma of the distal portion of the tibia has produced deformity of the adjacent fibula. Note the eccentric location, geographic bone destruction, radiolucent lesion with lobulated trabeculation, internal sclerotic border, and cortical expansion. This lesion, too, is located a short distance from the neighboring physis. *C*, This large nonossifying fibroma of the distal portion of the femur has led to a spontaneous fracture. Its upper border indicates its eccentric location.

### *Jaffe-Campanacci Syndrome*

Jaffe-Campanacci syndrome is rare and consists of multiple nonossifying fibromas (at least three) and extraskeletal congenital anomalies, including café au lait spots, mental retardation, hypogonadism or cryptorchidism, ocular abnormalities, and cardiovascular malformations. The precise relationship of this condition to neurofibromatosis is not clear. Multiple nonossifying fibromas may occur in the absence of café au lait spots and extraskeletal anomalies. The lesions may be large and distributed symmetrically.

Such cases should be considered distinct from the Jaffe-Campanacci syndrome.

### Periosteal (Juxtacortical) Desmoid

A periosteal desmoid is a tumor-like alteration of the periosteum characterized by fibroblastic proliferation analogous to that occurring in a desmoplastic fibroma (see later discussion). It is usually apparent in patients between the ages of 15 and 20 years and may show a

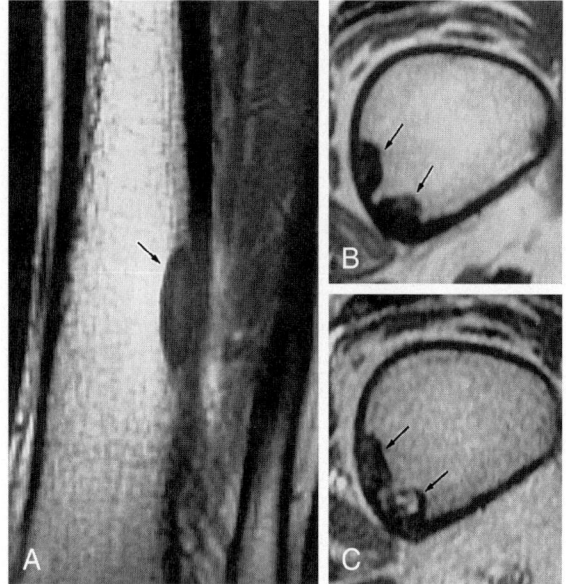

**Figure 70–66.** Nonossifying fibroma (fibrous cortical defect): MR long tubular bones. *A,* Tibia. Coronal T1-weighted (TR/TE, 600/25) spin echo MR image in an 18-year-old man documents an elongated eccentric lesion *(arrow)* in the lateral aspect of the tibia. It is sharply defined and of low signal intensity. Signal intensity remained low on T2-weighted spin echo MR images. *B* and *C,* Femur. Multiple eccentric lesions *(arrows)* in the distal femoral metaphysis are well delineated on transaxial T1-weighted (TR/TE, 400/20) *(B)* and T2-weighted (TR/TE, 2000/80) *(C)* spin echo MR images in this 14-year-old boy. One of the lesions shows an increase in signal intensity in *(C).* (*A,* Courtesy of A. Peck, MD, Portland, Ore. *B* and *C,* Courtesy of P. VanderStoep, MD, St. Cloud, Minn.)

slight male predilection. Almost all cases are localized to the posteromedial cortex of the distal end of the femur, adjacent to the femoral condyle. A history of local trauma or chronic physical activity is frequent. The radiographic characteristics of a periosteal desmoid include soft tissue swelling and a saucer-like defect of the cortex, with adjacent sclerosis and periostitis (Fig. 70–67).

It is unlikely that a periosteal desmoid is a true neoplasm. Rather, it appears to be a reaction to trauma occurring at the musculotendinous insertion site of the adductor magnus muscle or, less commonly, the medial head of the gastrocnemius muscle. As such, it is often designated an avulsive cortical irregularity.

### Desmoplastic Fibroma

This rare benign neoplasm of bone is characterized by abundant collagen formation and the absence of both significant cellularity and pleomorphism.

**Clinical Abnormalities.** Desmoplastic fibromas are most common in the second and third decades of life, with approximately 75% of tumors occurring in patients younger than 30 years. Pain and swelling of weeks' to months' duration are the major clinical manifestations.

**Skeletal Location.** Desmoplastic fibromas typically arise in the mandible, long tubular bones (femur, humerus, tibia, radius), and innominate bone (ilium). In the tubular bones, a central location in the metaphysis is characteristic.

**Radiographic Abnormalities.** Desmoplastic fibromas are osteolytic lesions with a trabeculated, soap bubble, or honeycomb pattern (Fig. 70–68). Endosteal erosion and limited periosteal bone formation may be accompanied by osseous expansion, an appearance that may resemble that of nonossifying fibroma, chondromyxoid fibroma, giant cell tumor, aneurysmal bone cyst, or fibrous dysplasia. Though generally well delineated, desmoplastic fibromas occasionally become large and have a more aggressive appearance.

**Pathologic Abnormalities.** Histologically, desmoplastic fibroma is composed of uniform small, spindle-shaped fibroblasts that have oval or elongated nuclei. The cells lack any significant degree of hyperchromasia, pleomorphism, or atypia, and mitotic figures are either absent or extremely scarce. The histologic characteristics of this lesion resemble those of soft tissue desmoid tumor.

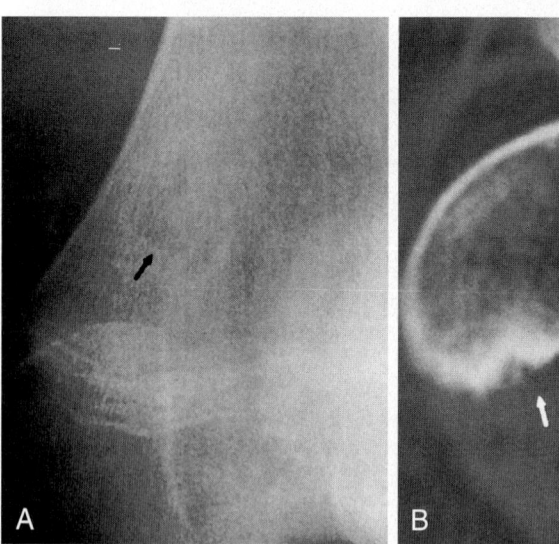

**Figure 70–67.** Periosteal (juxtacortical) desmoid. Routine radiograph *(A)* and transaxial CT scan *(B)* in an athletic patient reveal an area of cortical osteolysis *(arrows),* with endosteal bone formation *(arrowhead).* This lesion occurred at the osseous site of attachment of the medial head of the gastrocnemius muscle and thus supports a traumatic pathogenesis. (Courtesy of T. Goergen, MD, San Diego, Calif.)

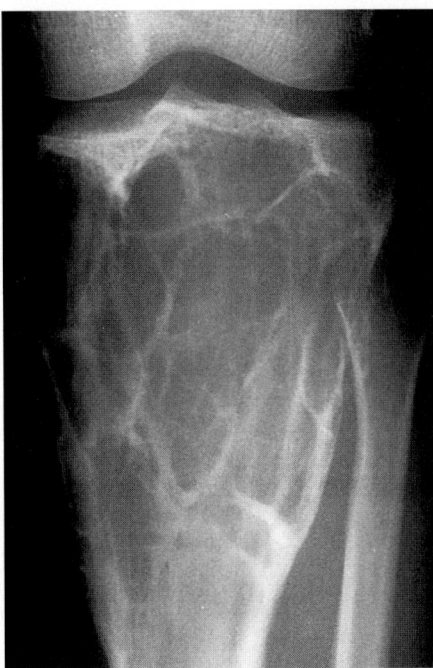

**Figure 70–68.** Desmoplastic fibroma: tibia. This osteolytic lesion involving the metaphyseal and epiphyseal segments of the bone possesses coarse trabeculae. (Courtesy of B. Flanagan, MD, Los Angeles, Calif.)

**Natural History.** Although tumor recurrence may be evident after conservative surgery, wide resection of the lesion is usually curative.

## Malignant Tumors

### Fibrosarcoma

Fibrosarcoma, a rare malignant tumor of bone, is histologically characterized by poorly differentiated to well-differentiated fibrous tissue proliferation that is not associated with the production of cartilage, osteoid, or bone. Fibrosarcomas in bone can occur de novo or as a secondary phenomenon in areas of Paget's disease, osteonecrosis, or chronic osteomyelitis; after irradiation; or related to dedifferentiation of other neoplasms, especially chondrosarcoma.

**Clinical Abnormalities.** Fibrosarcomas of bone are observed in men and women with approximately equal frequency and are most common in the third through sixth decades of life. Clinical manifestations include local pain, swelling, and limitation of motion. Pathologic fractures are present at the time of initial evaluation in approximately 33% of patients.

**Skeletal Location.** The skeletal distribution of fibrosarcoma is similar to that of osteosarcoma and malignant fibrous histiocytoma. The long tubular bones are involved in 70% of cases. The bones about the knee account for 33% to 80% of fibrosarcomas. In the tubular bones, a metaphyseal or metadiaphyseal location is the preferred site. Epiphyseal extension of a metaphyseal tumor is not infrequent.

**Radiographic Abnormalities.** Fibrosarcomas are radiographically characterized by (1) osteolytic foci with a geographic, moth-eaten, or permeative pattern of bone destruction and, generally, a wide zone of transition between normal and abnormal bone and (2) little osteosclerosis or periostitis (Fig. 70–69). Indeed, the degree of bone destruction and the absence of significant osseous reaction can be striking. Cortical destruction and soft tissue masses are seen. Visible tumor matrix is not evident. In the tubular bones, fibrosarcomas may be central or eccentric in position. The radiographic abnormalities of fibrosarcomas generally indicate an aggressive or malignant process. The absence of tumoral calcification or ossification in fibrosarcomas has diagnostic importance.

**Pathologic Abnormalities.** Fibrosarcomas are large, destructive, infiltrating tumors. Histologically, fibrosarcomas may be categorized as well-differentiated, moderately differentiated, or poorly differentiated neoplasms. Most fibrosarcomas are either moderately or poorly differentiated.

**Natural History.** Osseous fibrosarcomas are aggressive tumors with a tendency for one or more recurrence. The rate of such recurrence, as well as the likelihood of patient survival, correlates with the histologic grade of the neoplasm. Fibrosarcomas of bone carry a poorer prognosis than do those of soft tissue.

## HISTIOCYTIC OR FIBROHISTIOCYTIC TUMORS

### Benign Tumors

#### Fibrous Histiocytoma

Fibrous histiocytoma is a term that has been used to describe a benign tumor of bone that is histologically

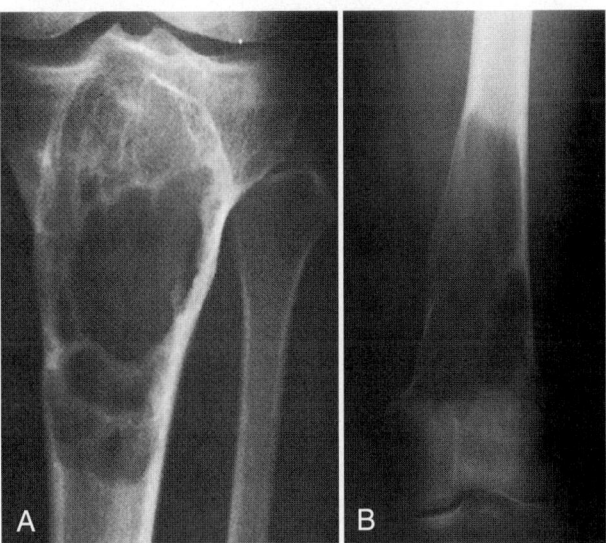

**Figure 70–69.** Fibrosarcoma: long tubular bones. *A*, Tibia. The epiphyseal and metaphyseal segments are affected. The lesion is osteolytic and possesses a pattern of geographic bone destruction. Note the relative absence of periostitis. *B*, Femur. Radiograph shows a long osteolytic lesion of the metadiaphyseal portion of the femur.

identical to nonossifying fibroma (fibroxanthoma). Its existence as a separate lesion is not uniformly accepted, and investigators who distinguish between fibrous histiocytoma and nonossifying fibroma emphasize their different clinical manifestations. Almost all fibrous histiocytomas occur in patients older than 20 years, and many are accompanied by pain; in constrast, nonossifying fibromas are virtually confined to patients younger than 20 years and are painless. Investigators who consider fibrous histiocytoma and nonossifying fibroma to be identical tumors emphasize the histiocytic origin of both lesions.

The radiographic findings are variable and not diagnostic; osteolysis, trabeculation, and bone sclerosis are seen, and the resulting radiographic pattern may resemble that of nonossifying fibroma, fibrous dysplasia, enchondroma, eosinophilic granuloma, osteoblastoma, and chondromyxoid fibroma (Fig. 70–70). Involvement of an epiphysis or diaphysis in cases of benign fibrous histiocytoma appears to have diagnostic importance, although metaphyseal localization (as in cases of nonossifying fibroma) has also been documented.

## Locally Aggressive Tumors

### Giant Cell Tumor

The placement of giant cell tumor in this section is arbitrary, because the precise origin of this lesion is not

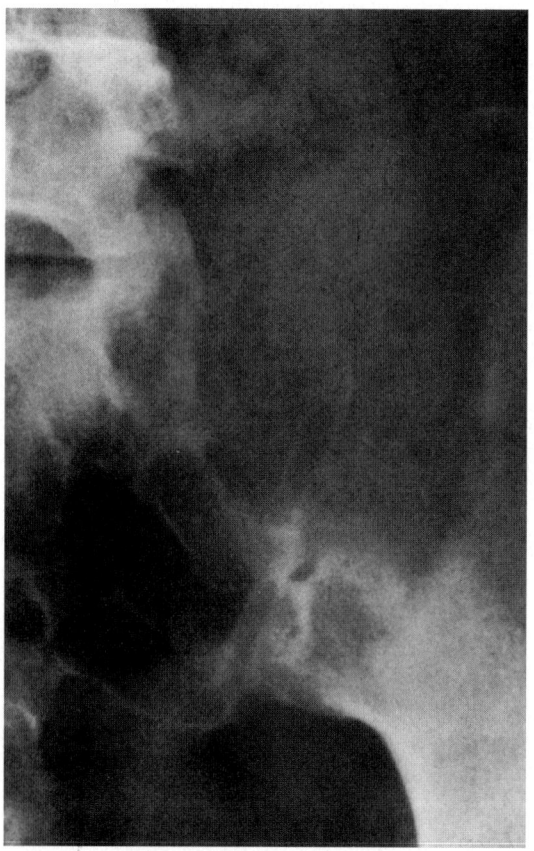

**Figure 70–70.** Fibrous histiocytoma. Large osteolytic lesion of the ilium is associated with sclerosis in the inferior aspect of the bone adjacent to the sacroiliac joint. The radiographic findings are not specific. (Courtesy of H. F. Holman, MD, Maryville, Ill.)

clear. This relatively common and locally aggressive lesion is composed of connective tissue, stromal cells, and giant cells that vary in amount and appearance. Giant cells are not specific for giant cell tumor, however, because they are observed in many neoplastic and non-neoplastic skeletal disorders.

**Clinical Abnormalities.** Giant cell tumors are usually discovered in the third and fourth decades of life. The frequency of giant cell tumors is greater in women than in men. Pain is the most common symptom, followed in order of frequency by local swelling and limitation of motion in the adjacent articulation. A pathologic fracture may be evident at the time of clinical assessment in approximately 10% to 15% of patients. Tenderness to palpation is a consistent physical finding.

**Skeletal Location.** Giant cell tumors predominate in the long tubular bones (75% to 90% of all cases), especially in the femur (approximately 30%), tibia (25%), radius (10%), and humerus (6%). The distal portions of the femur and radius and the proximal portion of the tibia are the most common sites of involvement (approximately 50% of cases). The bones about the knee are affected in 50% to 65% of giant cell tumors. In the vertebral column, the sacrum is the most typical site of localization.

In the skull and the facial bones, giant cell tumors may be accompanied by Paget's disease, and in these locations, identification of giant cell tumor is complicated by the occurrence of a similar lesion, giant cell reparative granuloma. Approximately 5% of giant cell tumors localize in the bones of the hands or, less commonly, the feet.

In the tubular bones, giant cell tumors typically involve the epiphyseal region, although more recently, a metaphyseal origin has been emphasized. Although the lesion is uncommon in the immature bones of children or adolescents, in such cases, metaphyseal localization (with or without subsequent transphyseal spread) has been repeatedly documented.

**Radiographic Abnormalities.** The radiographic appearance of a giant cell tumor is highly characteristic. In a long tubular bone (Fig. 70–71), an eccentric osteolytic lesion extends to the subchondral bone, producing cortical thinning and expansion, and a delicate trabecular pattern is seen. The margins of the lesion may be well or poorly defined, although an extensive sclerotic rim and periostitis are generally not evident. Involvement of a portion of the metaphysis is also characteristic, and, as indicated previously, isolated metaphyseal lesions may be encountered in a child or adolescent (Fig. 70–72).

In the short tubular bones of the hands (Fig. 70–73) and feet, the radiographic features of giant cell tumors are similar to those in the long tubular bones. Epiphyseal involvement, subchondral extension, osteolysis, delicate trabeculae, and osseous expansion are among the characteristics of such neoplasms. Involvement of the head of a metacarpal bone or the base of the proximal phalanx in the hand should be sought.

Less uniformity is seen in the radiographic characteristics of giant cell tumors of flat and irregular bones. Sternal and sacral lesions are osteolytic and, because of

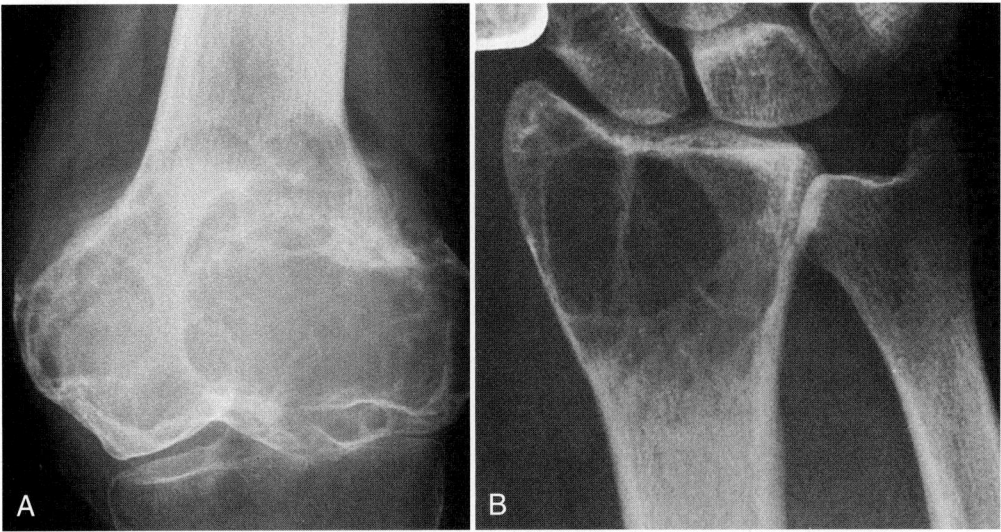

**Figure 70–71.** Giant cell tumor: long tubular bones. *A*, Femur. Note the large, trabeculated, osteolytic lesion involving the metaphysis and epiphysis of the distal portion of the femur. It extends to the subchondral region. The bone is expanded, and collapse of the articular surface has occurred. *B*, Radius. Radiograph shows a geographic, eccentric, osteolytic lesion with trabeculation. The lesion is metaphyseal and epiphyseal in location, with extension to subchondral bone.

their large size and soft tissue component, may simulate the appearance of a malignant neoplasm. In the sacrum (and, occasionally, in other locations), transarticular extension of the tumor may be noted. In the innominate bone, an epiphyseal-equivalent area is commonly affected, such as the bone adjacent to the sacroiliac or hip articulation.

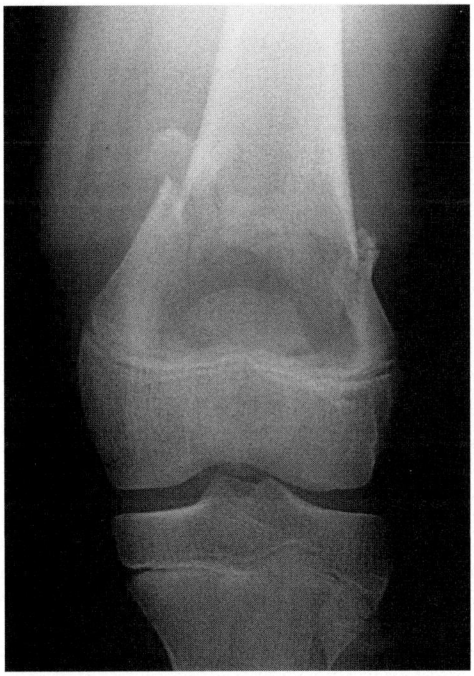

**Other Imaging Techniques.** Scintigraphy shows an extended pattern of activity beyond the true limits of the tumor due to the hyperemia associated with the lesion. Consequently, it cannot reliably define the extent of the tumor. CT and MR imaging allow evaluation of the extraosseous and intraosseous extent of the tumor and its relationship to major vessels and nerves. The identification of one or more fluid levels within a giant cell tumor (Fig. 70–74) is of interest, although neither this finding nor other abnormalities enable a specific diagnosis to be made.

**Figure 70–72.** Giant cell tumor: femur. Note the purely metaphyseal lesion in the distal portion of the femur on a conventional frontal radiograph. The lesion is osteolytic, with a pathologic fracture. (Courtesy of G. Bock, MD, Winnipeg, Manitoba, Canada.)

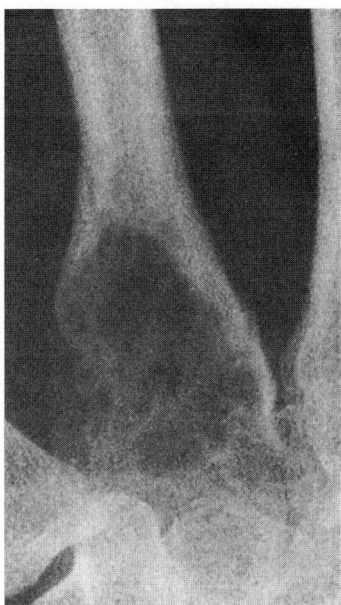

**Figure 70–73.** Giant cell tumor: short tubular bones. In this 15-year-old girl with pain and swelling in the hand, note the slightly expansile, trabeculated, osteolytic lesion of the second metacarpal bone that extends to its base.

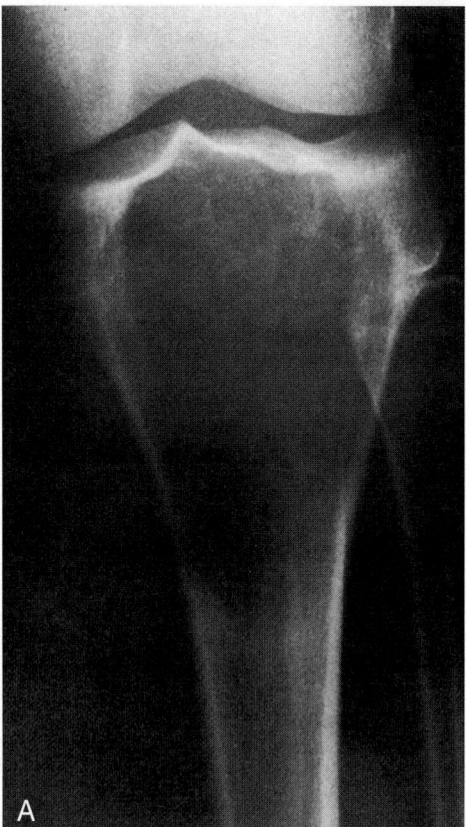

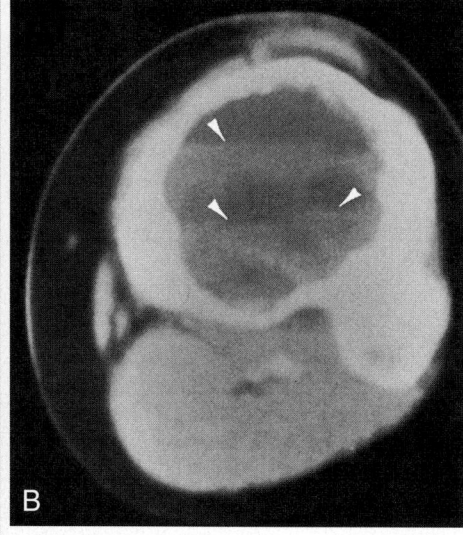

**Figure 70–74.** Giant cell tumor. *A,* Routine radiograph in a 14-year-old girl reveals a large osteolytic lesion of the tibia. *B,* Transaxial CT scan through the lesion with the patient in a supine position shows multiple fluid levels *(arrowheads).* (Courtesy of P. Kaplan, MD, Boston, Mass.)

With MR imaging, the tumor is of low signal intensity on T1-weighted spin echo MR images and of variable but often high signal intensity on T2-weighted spin echo MR images, and it is generally well defined (Fig. 70–75). Inhomogeneity of signal intensity and a poorly delineated tumor margin may be encountered. Hemorrhage within a giant cell tumor is associated with hemosiderin deposition, which may be extensive, thus explaining why foci of very low signal intensity may be apparent in all pulse sequences and may be a dominant finding. Fluid levels are identified on the MR images of some giant cell tumors, representing secondary aneurysmal bone cyst formation.

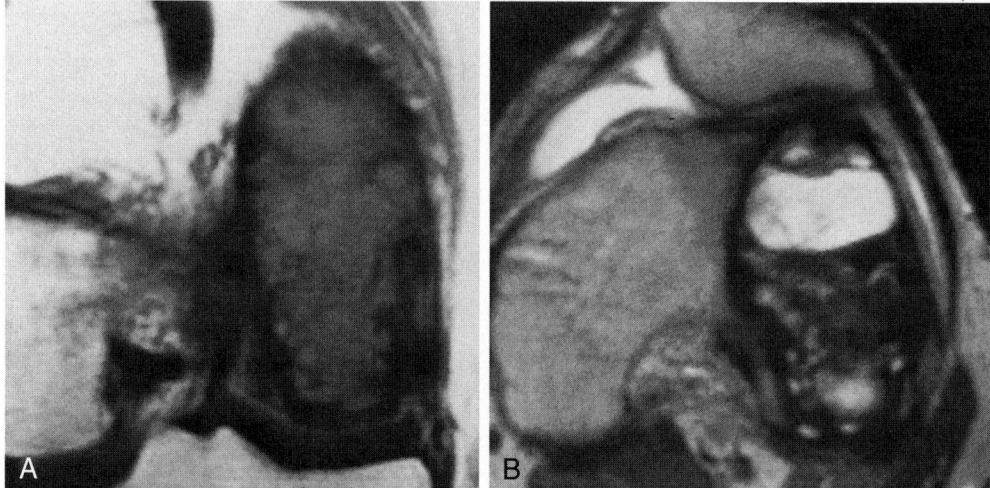

**Figure 70–75.** Giant cell tumor. *A,* In this 26-year-old man, a coronal T1-weighted (TR/TE, 775/20) spin echo MR image reveals a tumor of low signal intensity involving the lateral femoral condyle. *B,* On a transaxial T2-weighted (TR/TE, 2000/70) spin echo MR image, the tumor is of inhomogeneous signal intensity; high signal intensity is observed anteriorly, with mainly low signal intensity posteriorly. The low signal intensity is probably related to hemosiderin deposition. A joint effusion is also present. (Courtesy of M. Mitchell, MD, Halifax, Nova Scotia, Canada.)

**Pathologic Abnormalities.** Giant cell tumors are often fairly large. The tumor itself is commonly soft, fleshy, and friable. Small or large cystic areas filled with fresh or clotted blood or serosanguineous fluid are not uncommon. Cortical erosion with soft tissue extension is detected in 20% to 50% of cases. Areas with features of an aneurysmal bone cyst are not uncommon, especially in larger tumors.

**Natural History.** Local extension, regional and systemic tumor implantation, and malignant transformation with widespread metastases are among the reported manifestations of these neoplasms, indicative of their aggressive and unpredictable nature. Although the histologic appearance of a giant cell tumor is the most important indicator of its behavior, analysis of additional data provided by clinical and radiographic examination and by the gross pathologic features of this neoplasm is essential for the appropriate management of patients.

The rate of recurrence of giant cell tumor is quite high, with estimates generally ranging from 40% to 60%. However, modern therapeutic methods, including wide surgical excision, cryosurgery and bone grafting, and radiotherapy, have reduced the frequency of tumor recurrence, such that estimates of 5% to 10% seem more accurate. Recurrent giant cell tumors are generally observed within the first 2 years after treatment of the neoplasm. The radiographic abnormalities associated with recurrent giant cell tumors are characteristic. With regard to intraosseous recurrence, osteolysis adjacent to the area of surgical resection or delayed resorption of a bone graft may be evident. At the time of surgery, local implantation of giant cell tumor can occur in the adjacent soft tissues (Fig. 70–76). The soft tissue implants may remain radiographically invisible, or they may appear as enlarging masses with peripheral ossification in the form of a radiodense thin shell or thick rind.

The frequency of malignant giant cell tumor (or malignant transformation of benign giant cell tumor) is difficult to ascertain, although an appropriate estimate would be 5% to 10%. To be certain of the diagnosis of malignant giant cell tumor, the pathologist must be able to delineate obviously sarcomatous stroma and zones of typical benign giant cell tumor in the neoplasm under appraisal or in tissue obtained earlier from the same neoplasm. The vast majority (but not all) of malignant giant cell tumors develop after irradiation of the original giant cell tumor. Such neoplasms may best be considered radiation-induced sarcomas rather than malignant giant cell tumors. Approximately 2% to 5% of conventional giant cell tumors metastasize to the lungs. Such lesions are termed benign metastasizing giant cell tumors and are typically, though not invariably, seen following surgery.

**Multicentric Involvement.** The presence of more than one primary giant cell tumor in the same patient is an unusual event, with an estimated frequency of 0.5% to 5%. Multicentric giant cell tumors may appear simultaneously or metachronously. The bones of the hand are affected more frequently in multicentric disease than in solitary giant cell tumors. Additionally, patients with multifocal lesions have an increased propensity for metaphyseal involvement and for pathologic fracture.

**Differential Diagnosis.** Although chondroblastoma, intraosseous ganglion, and a variety of cystic lesions can affect the epiphysis, clinical and radiographic characteristics usually allow differentiation of giant cell tumor from these other entities. Chondroblastoma typically occurs in the immature skeleton of a child or adolescent and may contain calcifications. An intraosseous ganglion is observed most frequently in the medial malleolus of the tibia, in the carpal bones, or in periarticular regions such as the hip. Although a variety of articular processes can lead to subchondral cysts, such cysts are commonly multiple, communicate with the joint, and are associated with additional articular abnormalities. Other differential diagnostic considerations in patients with giant cell tumors include aneurysmal bone cyst, fibrous dysplasia, eosinophilic granuloma, the brown tumor of hyperparathyroidism, and giant cell reparative granuloma. Most of these diagnoses can be eliminated through careful evaluation of the radiographs.

## Giant Cell Reparative Granuloma

A giant cell reparative granuloma is an uncommon bone lesion that has slightly different histologic characteristics and a more benign clinical course than a giant cell tumor. This lesion was initially thought to represent a response to intraosseous hemorrhage rather than being a true neoplasm, although subsequent reports indicate only an

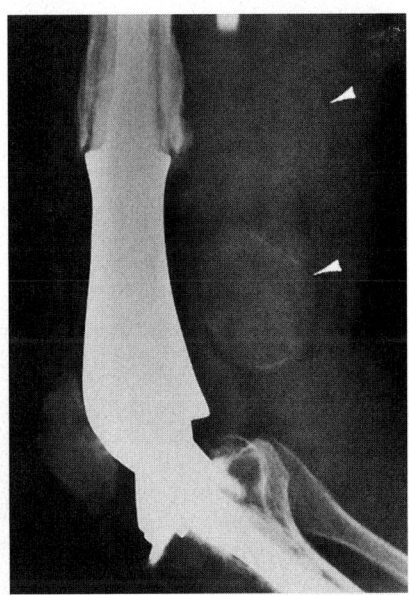

**Figure 70–76.** Giant cell tumor: natural history—intraosseous and extraosseous recurrence. This 36-year-old man had a giant cell tumor of the distal portion of the femur that was treated by curettage and grafting. Five months later, further curettage was required, and the lesion was packed with methylmethacrylate. A pathologic fracture later developed and required resection of bone and a custom total knee arthroplasty. A soft tissue tumor deposit was found in one of the surgical scars at the time of the arthroplasty. Two years after this surgical procedure, as shown on a lateral radiograph, ossified soft tissue masses (*arrowheads*) are present. (From Cooper KL, Beabout JW, Dahlin DC, et al: Giant cell tumor: Ossification in soft-tissue implants. Radiology 153:597, 1984.)

incidental relationship to trauma. It is uniformly agreed, however, that a giant cell reparative granuloma is distinct from a true giant cell tumor and represents less than 10% of all benign tumors of the jaw. Radiographically, a giant cell reparative granuloma in the facial bones appears as a round or oval radiolucent lesion that may be trabeculated and expansile and may contain ossification (Fig. 70–77).

Giant cell reparative granulomas arising in the hands and feet occur more commonly in women than in men. The age range of affected patients is wide (6 to 53 years). A history of trauma is infrequent. Clinical manifestations include pain, discomfort, swelling, and tenderness, and the bone may feel enlarged when palpated. The phalanges of the hand are the most common site of involvement, followed in order of decreasing frequency by the metacarpal, metatarsal, carpal, and tarsal bones and the phalanges of the foot. Radiographically, the lesions are osteolytic, trabeculated, and slightly expansile and involve the metaphysis and diaphysis, but they may also extend to the epiphysis and subchondral bone (Fig. 70–78).

Accurate radiographic diagnosis of giant cell reparative granuloma in the bones of the hands and feet is difficult because similar radiographic features may occur in a variety of processes, including enchondroma, aneurysmal bone cyst, and true giant cell tumor. Giant cell reparative granulomas do not calcify (in contrast to enchondromas) and usually occur after closure of the physeal plate (which is not a typical characteristic of aneurysmal bone cysts). Their differentiation from giant cell tumors may be impossible based solely on radiographic features.

## Malignant Tumors

### Malignant Fibrous Histiocytoma

Malignant fibrous histiocytoma of bone is a rare tumor that can occur de novo or in association with other osseous abnormalities, including bone infarction, intraosseous lipoma, and Paget's disease, and after radiation therapy.

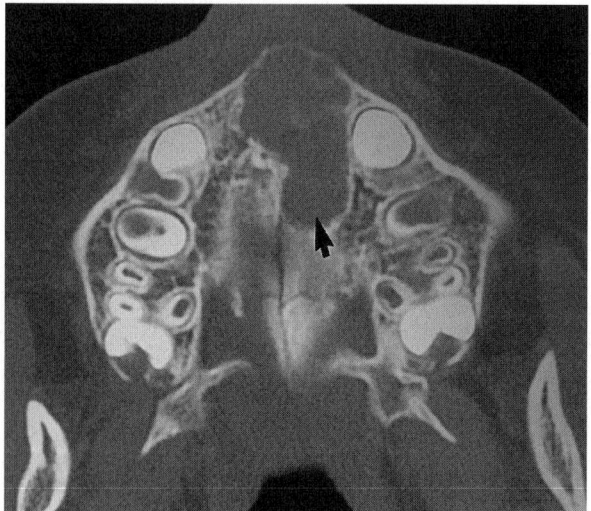

**Figure 70–77.** Giant cell reparative granuloma. Transverse CT scan reveals a slightly trabeculated, radiolucent lesion (*arrow*) in the maxilla. (Courtesy of V. Wing, MD, Walnut Creek, Calif.)

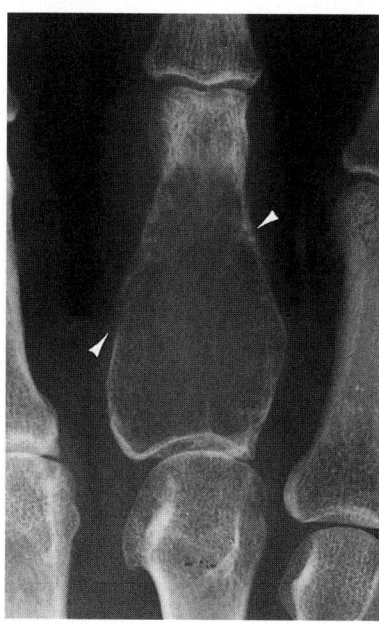

**Figure 70–78.** Giant cell reparative granuloma: differential diagnosis. Radiograph shows an expansile, trabeculated lesion involving the proximal three quarters of the proximal phalanx of a finger. There appears to be a subtle pathologic fracture (*arrowheads*). The radiographic appearance is similar to that of giant cell tumor.

**Clinical Abnormalities.** Malignant fibrous histiocytoma of bone occurs in men more frequently than in women (approximate ratio of 3:2) and in patients of any age, although most affected persons are in the fifth, sixth, and seventh decades of life. Pain, tenderness, and an enlarging mass are the predominant symptoms. Pathologic fracture may eventually occur in 30% to 50% of patients. A palpable and tender mass is the most common physical finding associated with malignant fibrous histiocytoma of bone.

**Skeletal Location.** The skeletal distribution of malignant fibrous histiocytomas is similar to that of osteosarcoma, with the ends of the long tubular bones chiefly affected (approximately 75% of cases). The bones in the lower extremity are involved more frequently than those in the upper extremity; the femur (approximately 45% of cases), tibia (20%), and humerus (9%) are the most common sites of tumor localization. The innominate bone is affected in approximately 10% of cases. Within the long tubular bones, metaphyseal localization is the rule, with frequent extension of the tumor into the epiphysis, diaphysis, or both. The bones about the knee account for approximately 50% of all tumors involving the tubular bones.

**Radiographic Abnormalities.** Osteolysis with a moth-eaten or permeative pattern of bone destruction, cortical erosion, limited periostitis, and a soft tissue mass are the characteristic radiographic abnormalities of malignant fibrous histiocytoma (Fig. 70–79). The lesions are variable in size but may extend from the epiphysis to the diaphysis of a tubular bone, throughout the innominate

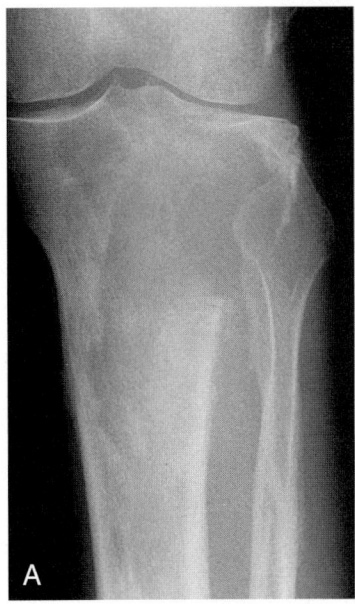
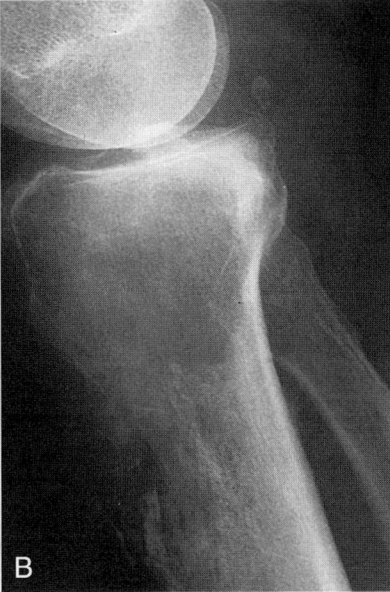

**Figure 70–79.** Malignant fibrous histiocytoma: tibia. Frontal *(A)* and lateral *(B)* radiographs reveal moth-eaten bone destruction in the diaphysis, metaphysis, and epiphysis of the proximal portion of the tibia. The cortex is eroded, and a soft tissue mass and scalloped deformity of the adjacent fibula are seen. Limited periostitis is evident. (Courtesy of I. S. Tolod, MD, Alton, Ill.)

bone, or between the body and posterior osseous elements of the vertebra. Osseous expansion is unusual. Pathologic fractures are relatively frequent.

It should be emphasized that these radiographic features indicate an aggressive skeletal process but are not specific in nature. In addition to malignant fibrous histiocytoma, osseous metastasis, plasmacytoma, lymphoma, osteolytic osteosarcoma, and fibrosarcoma can produce such abnormalities.

**Other Imaging Techniques.** As in the case of most malignant neoplasms of bone, CT and MR imaging can be used to assess the intraosseous or extraosseous extent of the lesion, as well as its relation to the neurovascular structures. MR imaging is probably best for local staging.

**Pathologic Abnormalities.** Macroscopically, malignant fibrous histiocytoma is usually located centrally within the bone and produces little or no osseous expansion. Cortical destruction with tumor extension into soft tissue is found in 80% to 100% of cases. Although malignant fibrous histiocytomas do not have a uniform histologic pattern, they all share common light-microscopic features marked by the presence, in varying amounts, of cells with fibroblastic or histiocyte-like characteristics, or both. The spindle-shaped fibroblasts that are evident in the fibrous regions of a malignant fibrous histiocytoma are not arranged in the classic herringbone pattern of a fibrosarcoma; rather, the cells radiate outward in a spiral array from a central focus and produce a nebula or storiform appearance. Such storiform areas are found in about 80% of these tumors.

**Natural History.** The aggressive nature of malignant fibrous histiocytoma of bone is underscored by the frequency of local recurrence (as many as 80% of tumors) and metastasis to regional lymph nodes and distant sites. Although the reported 5-year survival rate in patients with this neoplasm varies considerably, the malignant nature of this tumor is not questioned, and the ultimate prognosis is guarded.

## TUMORS OF FATTY DIFFERENTIATION

### Benign Tumors

#### Lipoma

Lipomas are among the most common soft tissue lesions but among the more unusual osseous lesions. The infrequency of lipomas of bone may be explained, in part, by their benign radiographic appearance, which may lessen the need for surgical confirmation of the diagnosis, and by the classification of osseous lipomas as other processes, including ischemic necrosis, bone infarct, simple (unicameral) or aneurysmal bone cysts, or fibrous dysplasia, on the basis of their radiographic or histologic characteristics, or both. Lipomas can be categorized according to their location in bone as intraosseous or parosteal lesions.

#### *Intraosseous Lipoma*

**Clinical Abnormalities.** Intraosseous lipomas are observed in men and women with about equal frequency and in patients of all ages, although most are identified in persons in the fourth, fifth, or sixth decade of life. Approximately two thirds of patients with intraosseous lipomas have localized pain, although lesions may be an incidental finding.

**Skeletal Location.** Intraosseous lipomas have been reported most commonly in the long tubular bones, especially the fibula (20% of cases), femur (15%), tibia (13%), and calcaneus (15%). Other reported sites include the ribs, skull, sacrum, ilium, and ischium. In the tubular bones, a metaphyseal localization is characteristic. Multifocal lesions are exceedingly rare, although bilateral involvement of the calcaneus is encountered.

**Radiographic Abnormalities.** Intraosseous lipomas typically appear as osteolytic lesions surrounded by a thin, well-defined sclerotic border. Lobulation or internal osseous ridges are frequently present, and osseous expansion may be evident. Cortical destruction and periosteal reaction are notably absent.

The radiographic abnormalities in intraosseous lipoma vary and correspond to those evident histologically. Stage I lesions, histologically characterized as containing viable non-necrotic fat with trabecular resorption, are seen radiographically as purely radiolucent areas. Histologically, stage II lesions contain viable fat, as well as fat necrosis and dystrophic calcification. Corresponding radiographs reveal radiolucent areas, sometimes expansile, that contain focal radiodense regions. In stage III, involution of the lesions is seen histologically, and with conventional radiography, sclerotic margins about radiolucent areas become apparent. Similar stages of intraosseous lipoma are identified with MR imaging.

The aforementioned radiographic features are not entirely specific, but in two locations—the calcaneus and the proximal portion of the femur—the constellation of radiographic alterations is virtually diagnostic. In the calcaneus, intraosseous lipoma occurs almost invariably in the triangular area between the major trabecular groups, in the same location as simple cysts (Fig. 70–80). An osteolytic area with sclerotic margins and, often, a central calcified or ossified nidus is evident. In the proximal portion of the femur (Fig. 70–81), intraosseous lipoma is characterized by marked ossification involving a large portion of the lesion's margin. In this site, lipomas most commonly occur along the intertrochanteric line or in the femoral neck. In the calcaneus, the major alternative diagnostic possibilities are variations in the normal trabecular pattern and simple bone cyst; in the proximal portion of the femur, intraosseous lipomas must be differentiated from fibrous dysplasia, simple bone cyst, and liposclerosing myxofibrous tumor (see later discussion).

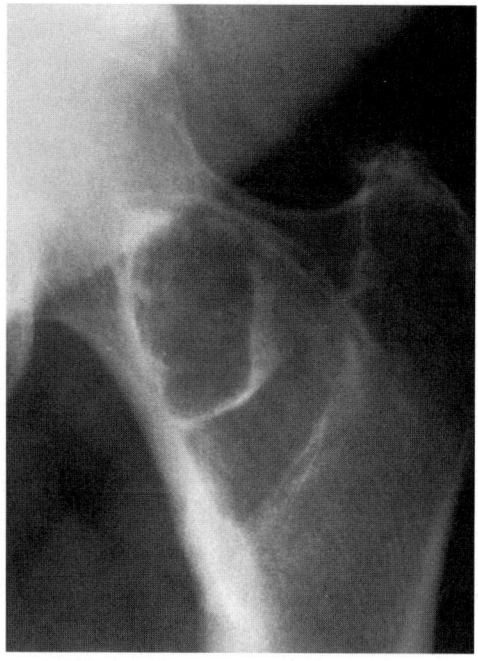

**Figure 70–81.** Intraosseous lipoma: proximal portion of the femur. Note the ossification involving principally the margin of this large osteolytic lesion located in the femoral neck above the intertrochanteric line.

**Other Imaging Techniques.** Although it is not generally necessary, CT allows definitive identification of the fatty component of an intraosseous lipoma, as well as its sclerotic margins and internal calcifications. MR imaging findings vary according to the stage of the process but generally include regions of fat (with relatively high signal intensity on routine spin echo and fast spin echo sequences and low signal intensity on fat-suppressed and short tau inversion recovery [STIR] sequences) that may be combined with internal regions of calcification (low

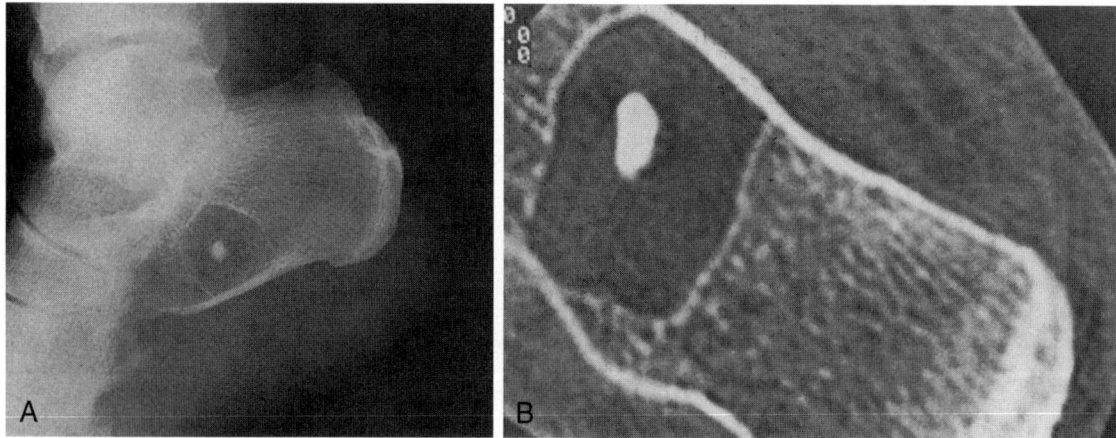

**Figure 70–80.** Intraosseous lipoma: calcaneus. A classic lipoma is shown with radiography *(A)* and transaxial CT *(B)*. The lesion is well defined, radiolucent, and surrounded by a thin sclerotic margin, and it contains a central radiodense focus. Documentation of fat in the lesion can be accomplished with measurements of attenuation derived from CT data. (Courtesy of J. Castello, MD, Madrid, Spain.)

signal intensity) and peripheral thick or thin rims of bone sclerosis (low signal intensity). The distribution and amount of fat are variable, however.

**Pathologic Abnormalities.** Intraosseous lipomas are divided into lobules of various sizes by delicate fibrous septa. Occasionally, central areas of hyalinized fibrous tissue are found, as well as necrotic foci containing dystrophic calcification. These latter areas account for the sclerotic central regions noted on radiographs.

### *Parosteal Lipoma*

Parosteal lipomas are rare lesions that truly arise in the periosteal membrane. It should be noted that a soft tissue lipoma that abuts bone may be difficult to distinguish from a parosteal lipoma. These lesions show no specific age or sex predilection and are generally asymptomatic, although they may rarely lead to a soft tissue mass. Usually, a long tubular bone is affected, most commonly the femur, humerus, or tibia. The diagnosis may be suggested on the basis of radiographic findings when a radiolucent mass (of fat density) is adherent to the external osseous surface, in combination with cortical hyperostosis or periostitis. Such cortical changes may produce an osteochondroma-like configuration (Fig. 70–82).

### Liposclerosing Myxofibrous Tumor of Bone

Liposclerosing myxofibrous tumor of bone is a benign fibro-osseous lesion characterized by a complex mixture of histologic elements that may include lipoma, fibroxanthoma, myxoma, myxofibroma, fibrous dysplasia–like features, cyst formation, fat necrosis, ischemic ossification, and, rarely, cartilage. Other designations for this tumor include polymorphic fibro-osseous lesion of bone and polymorphic fibrocystic disease of bone. The age

range of affected patients is from the second to seventh decades of life, with a mean age of about 40 years and an equal distribution in men and women. The proximal portion of the femur is involved in about 80% of cases. Typical radiographic features include a well-defined and often sclerotic margin, internal mineralization, and mild expansion of the bone in some cases (Fig. 70–83). CT and MR imaging reveal a mixture of internal elements without evidence of fat. Malignant transformation has been noted. The relationship of this lesion to intraosseous lipoma and fibrous dysplasia is not clear.

## Malignant Tumors

### Liposarcoma

Liposarcoma rarely arises in bone. Only a few such occurrences have been reported, and the presence of osteosarcomatous foci in some of these cases would probably lead to their reclassification as osteosarcoma or malignant mesenchymoma on the basis of current diagnostic criteria. Liposarcoma almost invariably occurs in the long tubular bones, including the tibia and femur and, less commonly, the fibula, humerus, and ulna. The diaphysis, metaphysis, or epiphysis may be affected, and large tumors may extend from one of these segments to an adjacent one. Radiographically, a nonspecific, well-defined or poorly defined area of osteolysis is observed. To establish a firm diagnosis of intraosseous liposarcoma, two criteria must be met: the tumor must have the histologic features of liposarcoma, with no evidence of any other tumor type, and a soft tissue origin or metastatic neoplasm must be excluded.

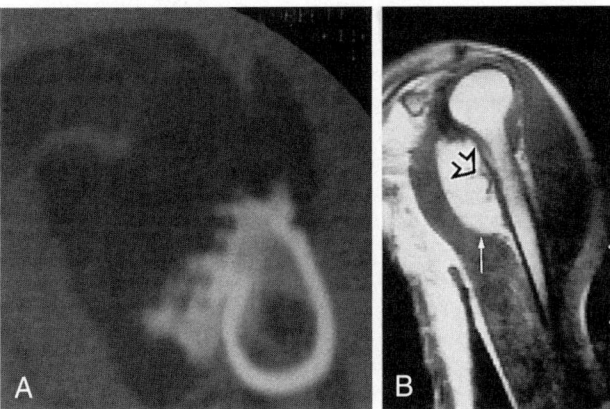

**Figure 70–82.** Parosteal lipoma. In this 32-year-old man with a slowly enlarging mass in the shoulder, transaxial CT scan (*A*) confirms the fatty nature of the mass and subjacent hyperostosis and bone proliferation in the humerus. On a coronal T1-weighted (TR/TE, 500/16) spin echo MR image (*B*), the fatty composition of the mass (*solid arrow*) is confirmed. Irregular bone spicules (*open arrow*) of low signal intensity are evident. (Courtesy of M. Murphey, MD, Washington, D.C.)

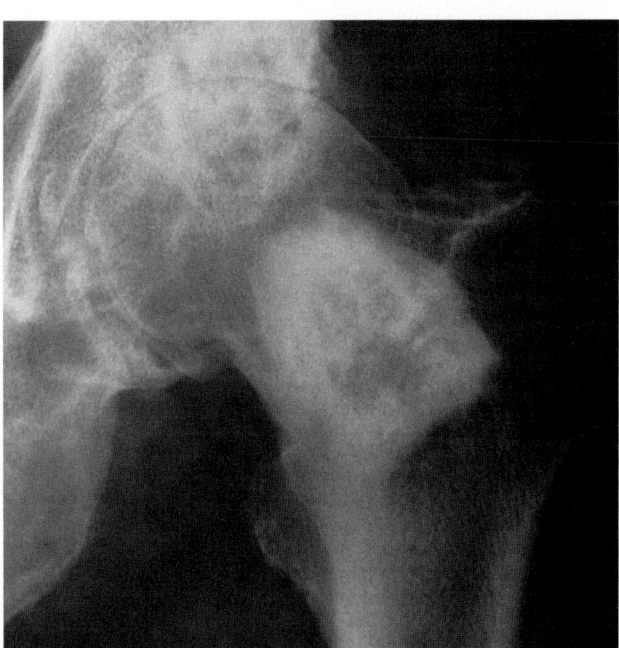

**Figure 70–83.** Liposclerosing myxofibrous tumor of bone. Although clearly not diagnostic, the radiographic appearance is that of a lesion of the femoral neck with a thick sclerotic margin and internal mineralization. Differential diagnostic considerations include fibrous dysplasia and involuting lipoma. Osteoarthritis of the hip is also evident.

## TUMORS OF MUSCLE DIFFERENTIATION

### Benign Tumors

#### Leiomyoma

This neoplasm of smooth muscle is well recognized in extraskeletal sites. It may also occur in the superficial soft tissues of the extremity, in close proximity to blood vessels or hair follicles; on rare occasion, a leiomyoma can apparently arise in the periosteal membrane or in bone.

### Malignant Tumors

#### Leiomyosarcoma

Leiomyosarcoma is a malignant neoplasm of smooth muscle cells that occurs predominantly in the uterus and gastrointestinal tract. Such extraosseous tumors, especially those in the uterus, may metastasize to distant sites, including the lung, liver, kidney, and, less commonly, bone. Leiomyosarcomas originating in bone are exceedingly rare. The diagnosis is established by the exclusion of a primary malignant neoplasm in an extraosseous site, the presence of the bulk of the tumor within the bone, and documentation of characteristic histopathologic features. In these instances, it is generally assumed that the leiomyosarcoma arose from preexisting smooth muscle cells. Only a few cases of primary leiomyosarcoma of bone have been documented.

The lesions predominate in the tubular bones, especially the femur and tibia, and involvement of the bones about the knee is particularly characteristic. Metaphyseal or, less commonly, epiphyseal or diaphyseal abnormalities typically consist of a poorly defined osteolytic lesion (Fig. 70–84) with or without a soft tissue mass and, rarely, periostitis or intralesional calcification. The course of

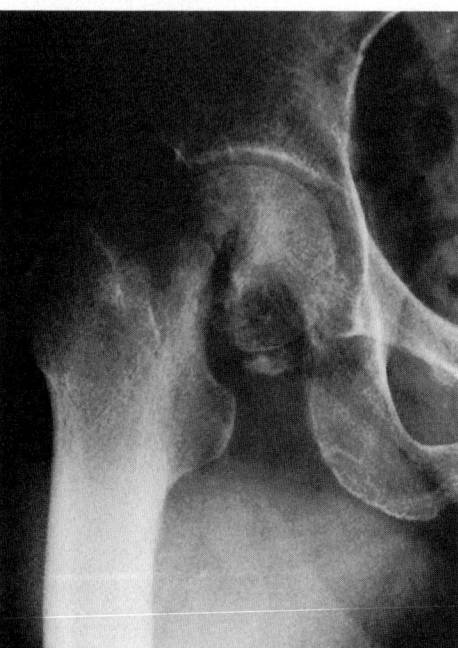

**Figure 70–84.** Leiomyosarcoma. A mass developed in the right hip of this 60-year-old woman after a fall. Two months after the injury, a radiograph shows an osteolytic lesion in the femoral neck and head with a pathologic fracture.

osseous leiomyosarcomas is variable; rapid local extension and widespread metastases are evident in some cases, whereas in others, appropriate therapy leads to long-term patient survival.

#### Rhabdomyosarcoma

Rhabdomyosarcoma is a common malignant tumor in children that arises principally in the soft tissues of the head and neck, the urogenital tract, and the retroperitoneum; its occurrence as a primary neoplasm of bone is exceedingly rare. Primary rhabdomyosarcoma of bone must be differentiated from an extraskeletal rhabdomyosarcoma that has metastasized to bone or one that originates in the periosseous soft tissue and secondarily invades bone.

## TUMORS OF VASCULAR DIFFERENTIATION

### Benign Tumors

#### Hemangioma

Hemangiomas of bone are composed of vascular channels that are cavernous, capillary, or venous in type. Hemangiomas in the spine are common, occurring in perhaps 10% of vertebral columns, whereas extraspinal hemangiomas of bone are infrequent.

**Clinical Abnormalities.** Osseous hemangiomas are identified in middle-aged patients, particularly those in the fourth and fifth decades of life. Women are affected about twice as frequently as men. Many hemangiomas, particularly those in the spine, are clinically insignificant and are discovered incidentally on radiographs or imaging obtained for unrelated reasons. Other hemangiomas, especially those in extraspinal sites, may be associated with soft tissue swelling or pain, particularly in the presence of a pathologic fracture. On rare occasion, vertebral hemangiomas may be accompanied by symptoms and signs of spinal cord compression as a result of extension of the lesion into the epidural space; expansion of the involved vertebrae, leading to narrowing of the spinal canal; epidural hemorrhage arising from the lesion; compression fractures of the involved vertebrae; or some combination of these causes. Hemangiomas of bone and soft tissue may also lead to hemihypertrophy of an extremity.

**Skeletal Location.** Single lesions predominate. The two most common sites of involvement are the vertebrae and the skull or facial bones. It has been estimated that hemangiomas can be found in approximately 10% of spines that are examined carefully at autopsy. In the spine, hemangiomas are most frequent in the thoracic segment and in the vertebral body, but hemangiomas may extend into or localize primarily in the posterior osseous elements of the vertebrae. Most vertebral hemangiomas are small and asymptomatic. Although hemangiomas in the skull are less frequent than those in the spine, they are typically more significant clinically.

Hemangiomas in the long tubular bones are uncommon and are usually observed in the diaphyseal and metaphyseal regions, especially in the femur, tibia, and humerus. Epiphyseal involvement in these tubular bones has been described.

**Radiographic Abnormalities.** Hemangiomas in the spine produce diagnostic radiographic alterations. A coarse, vertical trabecular pattern—the corduroy appearance—is identified in the vertebral body and may extend into the pedicles and laminae (Fig. 70–85). The trabeculae are more prominent than those that accompany osteoporosis, and their vertical orientation differs from the condensation that typifies Paget's disease (picture-frame vertebral body) or renal osteodystrophy (rugger-jersey vertebral body). Hemangiomas may lead to focal radiolucent areas with coarse trabeculae arranged in a honeycomb or cartwheel configuration. Extension of the lesion into the paraspinal soft tissues and spinal canal may be evident and result in radiographic abnormalities that simulate those of a malignant neoplasm.

In extraspinal sites, a radiolucent, slightly expansile, well-defined intraosseous lesion possessing a radiating, lattice-like, or weblike trabecular pattern is highly suggestive of the diagnosis (Fig. 70–86). Cortical thinning and osseous expansion may be seen, but extensive periostitis or a soft tissue mass is rare. In all locations, the distinctive trabecular pattern of hemangiomas is the most helpful diagnostic clue.

Intracortical and periosteal hemangiomas, though less common, predominate in the diaphysis of long tubular bones, especially the tibia or fibula. Radiographically, intracortical hemangiomas are associated with a well-defined osteolytic area, with or without cortical thickening and periostitis, whereas periosteal hemangiomas lead to cortical thickening and periostitis in association with a cup-shaped or saucer-like depression in the outer surface of the cortex.

**Other Imaging Techniques.** On scintigraphy, skeletal hemangiomas may show no or moderate accumulation of bone-seeking radionuclide; a photopenic region at the site of tumor may also be evident. CT is most useful for assessing hemangiomas in the spine and demonstrates the full extent of tumor. Vertebral lesions are often characterized by reinforced trabeculae and fatty stroma, and a polka-dot pattern within the vertebral body is often apparent on transaxial CT scans. MR imaging typically reveals areas of high signal intensity on T1- and T2-weighted spin echo MR images; these areas are related to the presence of fatty marrow intimate with the dilated vascular channels within the tumor (Fig. 70–87). Such signal intensity characteristics are not seen uniformly, however. Enhancement of signal intensity after the intravenous administration of a gadolinium compound is typical of hemangiomas.

**Pathologic Abnormalities.** Hemangiomas of bone do not differ in their histomorphology from those in the skin or soft tissues. Cavernous and capillary hemangiomas are most frequent. The cavernous variety is composed of large, gaping, thin-walled vessels lined by flat endothelial cells and filled with fresh blood. Capillary hemangiomas are composed of similar but smaller vessels with narrow lumina. Cavernous hemangiomas are most common, but mixed hemangiomas containing both cavernous and capillary vessels may be encountered, as well as venous or arteriovenous hemangiomas. Epithelioid hemangioma of bone is a rare variant that is characterized histologically by proliferating blood vessels lined by epithelioid endothelial cells; however, it is not radiographically distinct.

**Natural History.** Solitary or multiple hemangiomas are benign lesions that may grow slowly. Clinical manifes-

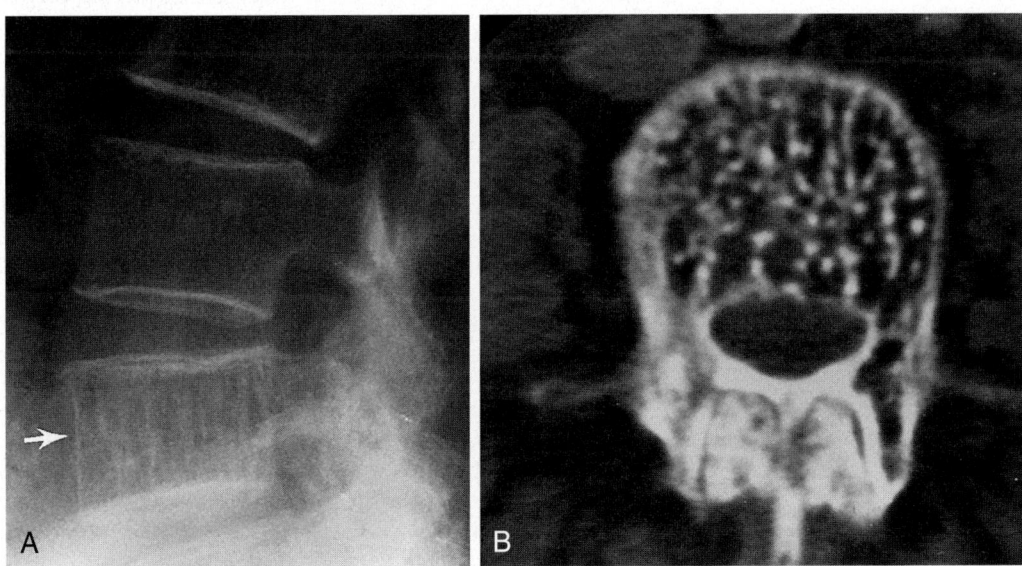

**Figure 70–85.** Hemangioma: lumbar spine. This elderly patient had hemangiomas in multiple vertebral bodies. *A*, Lateral radiograph shows osteopenia of the fifth lumbar vertebral body *(arrow)* and pedicles. *B*, Transaxial CT scan through this vertebra documents hemangiomatous involvement of the vertebral body and at least the left pedicle. (Courtesy of V. Vint, MD, San Diego, Calif.)

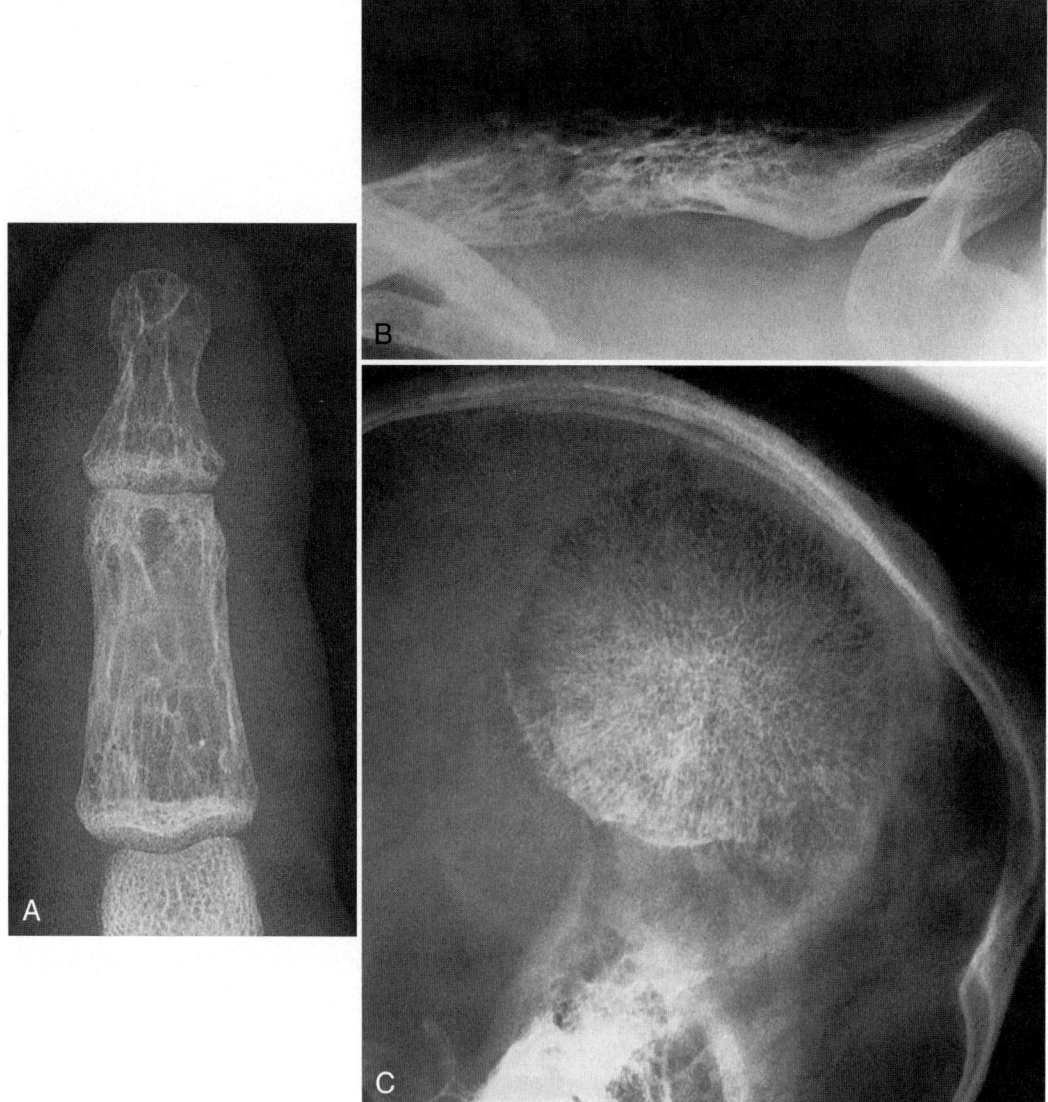

**Figure 70–86.** Hemangioma. *A,* Phalanges of the hand. Note the osteopenia of the middle and distal phalanges of a finger, with a weblike trabecular pattern. Hemangiomas in the adjacent soft tissues have led to swelling. *B,* Clavicle. An elongated lesion in the midportion of the clavicle is associated with osseous expansion and a lattice-like trabecular pattern. *C,* Skull. Note the large, sharply marginated lesion with a honeycomb or cartwheel configuration. (Courtesy of V. Wing, MD, Pasadena, Calif.)

tations, when present, are related to the local effects of the hemangioma, such as osseous expansion, soft tissue extension, or hemorrhage. Malignant degeneration of hemangiomas is not encountered.

### Cystic Angiomatosis

This rare skeletal disorder, which has also been designated diffuse angiomatosis, hemangiomatosis, and hemangiolymphangiomatosis, is characterized by widespread cystic lesions of bone that are frequently combined with visceral involvement. This latter involvement, which occurs in approximately 60% to 70% of cases, is usually responsible for the patient's symptoms and signs, although the skeletal lesions can produce pain and swelling, especially if a pathologic fracture has developed or if neigh-

boring soft tissues are altered. This disease should be distinguished from massive osteolysis, or Gorham's disease, and from single or multiple (but otherwise typical) hemangiomas of bone. The precise relationship of cystic angiomatosis and lymphangiomatosis is not clear.

**Clinical Abnormalities.** Patients are usually in the first, second, or third decade of life, and males are affected about twice as often as females. In patients without visceral lesions, symptoms and signs may be entirely absent. In persons with both visceral and osseous involvement, dramatic clinical abnormalities related to lesions in the soft tissues; spleen; liver; lungs; kidneys; thymus gland; peritoneal, pleural, and pericardial membranes; lymph nodes; larynx; and other organs or tissues may be evident, and such patients may die at an early age.

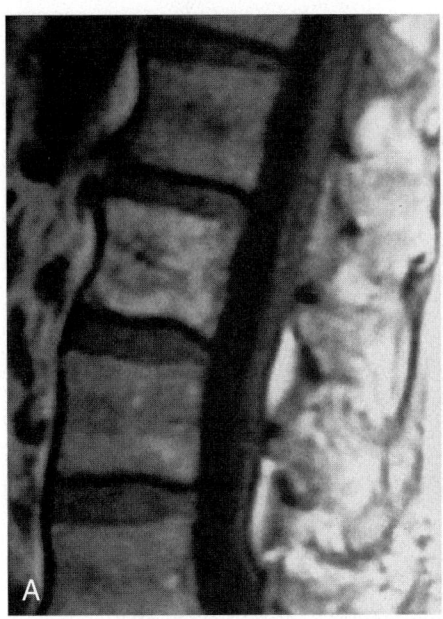
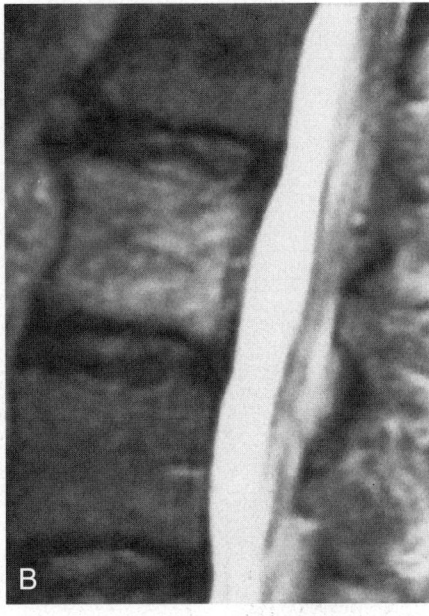

**Figure 70–87.** Hemangioma: spine. Sagittal T1-weighted (TR/TE, 500/11) spin echo MR image *(A)* and sagittal T2-weighted (TR/TE, 3800/144) fast spin echo MR image *(B)* reveal a hemangioma involving the second lumbar vertebral body, which is of high signal intensity in both images. The lesion is more obvious in *(B)*.

**Skeletal Location.** The femur, ribs, vertebrae, skull, innominate bone, humerus, scapula, tibia, radius, fibula, and clavicle, in order of decreasing frequency, are typically involved, but other osseous sites may be affected. Involvement of the axial skeleton is therefore characteristic. The lesions of cystic angiomatosis may be located anywhere within the bone and tend to involve the medullary portion.

**Radiographic Abnormalities.** Well-defined, round or ovoid osteolytic lesions of variable size surrounded by a rim of sclerotic bone are usually seen (Fig. 70–88). Medullary involvement predominates, and cortical invasion, osseous expansion, and periostitis are unusual. In some instances, osteosclerotic lesions simulating skeletal metastases from carcinoma of the prostate are observed. Pathologic fractures are also encountered, especially in the presence of large areas of bone destruction.

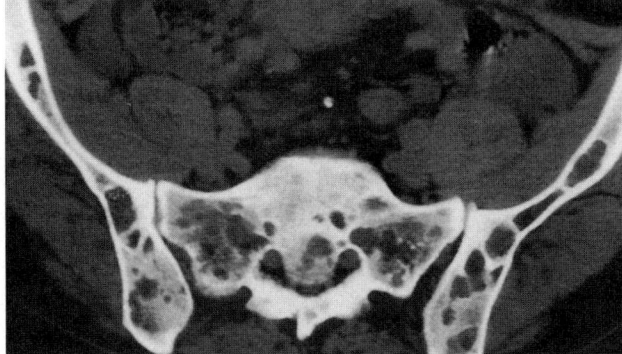

**Figure 70–88.** Cystic angiomatosis. Transaxial CT scan of the pelvis in an adult patient reveals multiple osteolytic lesions of variable size, each well circumscribed and with a sclerotic margin. A symmetrical distribution is apparent. (Courtesy of D. Levey, MD, Corpus Christi, Tex.)

The major differential diagnostic considerations include eosinophilic granuloma and other histiocytoses, hyperparathyroidism, fibrous dysplasia, lipomatosis, lymphangiomatosis, neurofibromatosis, skeletal metastasis, plasma cell myeloma, mastocytosis, sarcoidosis, and lymphoma.

Although other imaging methods have been used to assess the skeletal lesions of cystic angiomatosis, the findings are generally not specific. With bone scanning, the degree of radionuclide uptake in the lesions is variable. Both CT and MR imaging are effective in documenting the location and extent of extraosseous lesions (Fig. 70–89).

**Pathologic Abnormalities.** The lesions of cystic angiomatosis do not differ histologically from cavernous or capillary hemangiomas or even from lymphangiomas. Most contain numerous widely dilated, cavernous, thin-walled vascular channels lined by flat endothelial cells. These channels fill the intertrabecular spaces and rest against the adjacent trabeculae. Some lesions have features of both capillary and cavernous hemangiomas.

### Lymphangioma and Lymphangiomatosis

Lymphangioma of bone can appear as one or more isolated lesions or, in a more diffuse form, as part of the spectrum of either cystic angiomatosis or massive osteolysis (Gorham's disease). Solitary lymphangiomas are extremely rare, with only a few cases documented. Localized intraosseous lymphangiomas are most frequent in children or adolescents, although older patients can also be affected. The typical sites of involvement are the tibia, humerus, ilium, skull, mandible, vertebrae, and small bones in the hand.

Clinical manifestations are variable. Radiographic abnormalities are not specific; an osteolytic lesion arising in the medullary portion of the bone is most characteristic (Fig. 70–90). A multiloculated, septate, or bubble-

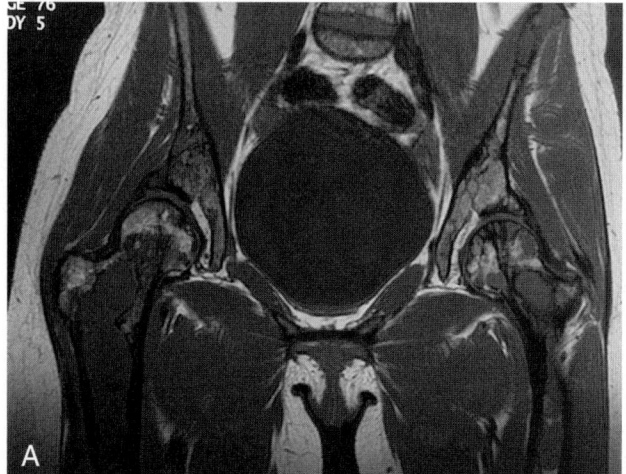

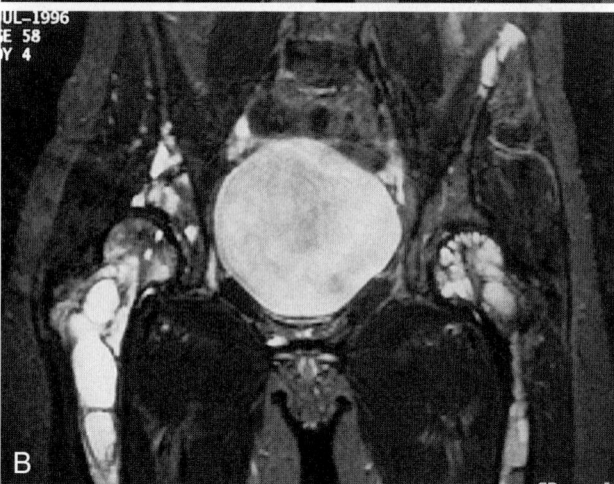

**Figure 70–89.** Cystic angiomatosis. In this relatively asymptomatic 33-year-old man, coronal T1-weighted (TR/TE, 560/15) spin echo *(A)* and STIR (TR/TE, 5000/60; inversion time, 120 msec) *(B)* MR images show widespread skeletal lesions in the femora and ilii. (Courtesy of M. de Maeseneer, MD, Brussels, Belgium.)

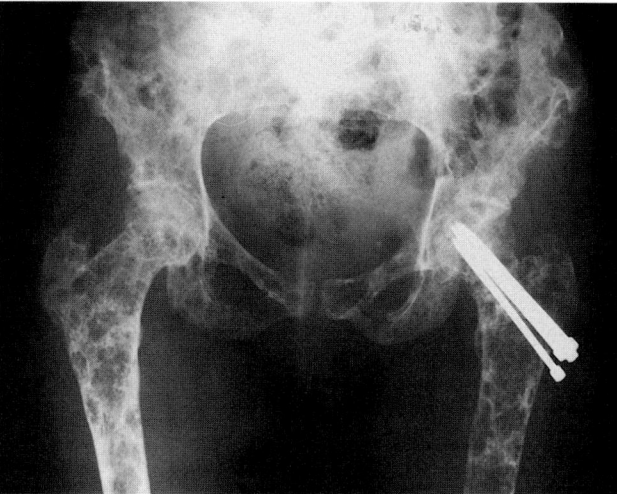

**Figure 70–90.** Lymphangioma and lymphangiomatosis. This adult had lesions scattered throughout the skeleton. A pathologic fracture of the left femoral neck occurred and was treated with multiple orthopedic lag screws. The radiographic appearance, which consists of poorly defined osteolytic lesions, resembles that of plasma cell myeloma or skeletal metastases.

like appearance is encountered, similar to that of hemangioma.

Multiple intraosseous lymphangiomas may occur in several situations: involvement of two or more widely separated bones, involvement of two or more bones in one region of the body (e.g., shoulder girdle or spine), or diffuse involvement of many bones. Additional lymphangiomatous lesions may be evident in the soft tissues or viscera and can lead to a variety of findings, including chylothorax, chylopericardium, hepatosplenomegaly, lymphedema, and cystic hygromas. In these patients, the extraosseous manifestations can lead to considerable morbidity, as well as early demise. The bone lesions are primarily osteolytic and septate but may be associated with involvement of the adjacent soft tissues.

The development of extensive intraosseous gas in cases of lymphangiomatosis has been observed. The precise pathogenesis of this finding, which is not related to osteomyelitis, is not clear. It is possible that resorption of fluid within the lymphangiomatous tissue creates a nega-

tive pressure that allows nitrogen from the blood to accumulate in the tissue. A specific diagnosis can be achieved with lymphangiography because of the accumulation of contrast material in intraosseous lymphangiomas.

Microscopically, the features of a lymphangioma are similar to those of a cavernous hemangioma and consist of widely patent, thin-walled vascular spaces lined by flat endothelial cells. Typically, in a lymphangioma, these spaces are filled with eosinophilic, granular, proteinaceous fluid and do not contain red blood cells.

It should be noted that there can be variations in the microscopic appearance of a lymphangioma, so its differentiation from a hemangioma may be extremely difficult or impossible. It is because of this difficulty that hemangioma, lymphangioma, cystic angiomatosis, hemangiomatosis, and even massive osteolysis (Gorham's disease) are sometimes considered part of the spectrum of a single disease process.

### Glomus Tumor

Glomus tumor (angioglomoid tumor) is a rare lesion that arises from the neuromyoarterial glomus, which is normally located in some of the internal organs of the body, such as the stomach, and in the dermis and superficial subcutaneous tissues in the extremities, particularly the palmar and plantar areas and the fingertips in the region of the nail bed. Glomus tumors are far more often extraosseous than intraosseous. In the extremities, glomus tumors are most common in the region of the fingertips or nail beds, with approximately 75% of such lesions appearing in the upper extremities. Bone involvement is usually a secondary manifestation related to invasion of the bone by a soft tissue glomus tumor. True intraosseous lesions are rare.

**Clinical Abnormalities.** Glomus tumors can be observed in patients of any age, although many persons are in the fourth or fifth decade of life. Lesions are typically solitary, and aching pain and exquisite point tenderness are usually present. Exposure to cold or minimal trauma may induce severe paroxysmal attacks of pain, a finding that is highly suggestive of a glomus tumor.

**Skeletal Location.** Secondary involvement of a bone adjacent to a soft tissue glomus tumor is observed in 15% to 65% of cases, especially in the hand. Tumors are also characteristically observed in the distal phalanx of the hand. Rarely, they occur elsewhere.

**Radiographic Abnormalities.** Soft tissue glomus tumors produce shallow, well-marginated erosions in the subjacent bone, usually the dorsal, medial, or lateral surface in the tuft of a terminal phalanx of a finger. A sclerotic margin may be apparent about the erosion. In some instances, a partial shell of bone extends into the soft tissue, making the distinction between a soft tissue and an intraosseous lesion difficult. The latter appears as a well-defined osteolytic region encased by cortical bone, usually in a terminal phalanx. The resulting radiographic appearance resembles that of an inclusion cyst (Fig. 70–91). The absence of calcification in an intraosseous glomus tumor assumes diagnostic importance, inasmuch as calcific regions may be evident in an enchondroma.

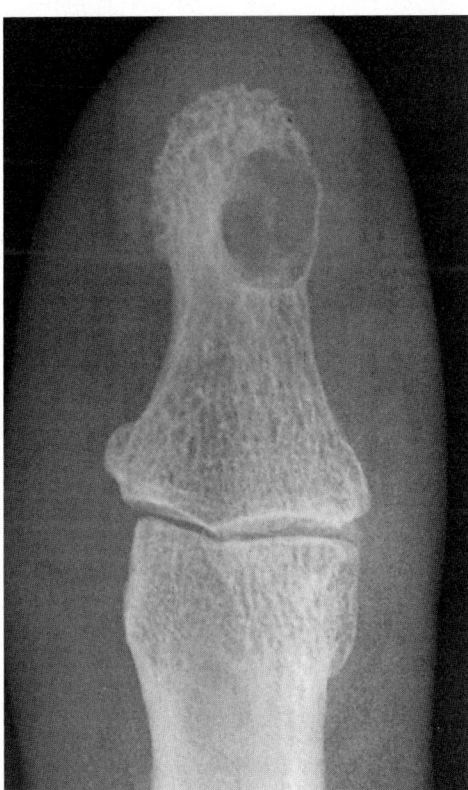

**Figure 70–91.** Glomus tumor: terminal phalanx. An eccentric, osteolytic lesion of the distal phalanx in a finger is characterized by geographic bone destruction. This appearance is typical of a glomus tumor originating in or involving bone.

**Other Imaging Techniques.** With ultrasonography, a hypoechoic mass is typical. With MR imaging, the glomus tumor is of high signal intensity on T2-weighted spin echo images; this technique may be useful for initial detection of the lesion and for identification of tumor recurrence after surgery.

**Pathologic Abnormalities.** Extraosseous and intraosseous glomus tumors are usually only a few millimeters in maximum dimension. The cortex of the involved bone is extremely thin, and beneath it is located a red or violet, soft, friable lesion that may appear jelly-like. Glomus tumors are usually composed of various-sized vascular channels lined by flat or cuboid endothelial cells that are cuffed by masses of polyhedral tumor (glomus) cells.

## Benign or Malignant Tumors

### Hemangiopericytoma

Hemangiopericytoma is an uncommon tumor of pericytes with a propensity to involve soft tissues and behave in an erratic or unpredictable fashion. Hemangiopericytomas arising in bone are rare. Most affected patients are middle-aged or elderly. Nonspecific symptoms and signs are present, including local pain and swelling. Rarely, the findings of hypophosphatemic osteomalacia (oncogenic osteomalacia) are evident.

Involvement of the axial skeleton or proximal ends of long bones is characteristic; the humerus, spine or sacrum, femur, and mandible are the bones affected most frequently. The long tubular bones are involved in approximately 40% of cases, and the innominate bone is involved in approximately 10%. Within the tubular bones, a diaphyseal or metaphyseal location is the preferred site. The nonspecific radiographic appearance of hemangiopericytoma of bone (Fig. 70–92) is characterized by osteolysis; delicate trabeculation with a honeycomb appearance; mild osseous expansion; and, in tumors of the sternum, spine, and calcaneus, significant bone sclerosis. Periostitis is exceedingly rare.

Hemangiopericytoma is characterized by the presence of abundant ramifying, thin-walled blood vessels surrounded by closely packed plump, round to spindle-shaped stromal cells that have relatively scant cytoplasm and indistinct cell borders. Definitive diagnosis of an intraosseous hemangiopericytoma may rest on the identification of pericytes by electron microscopy. Hemangiopericytomas have a broad spectrum of behavioral features. Radiographic abnormalities such as cortical violation or destruction and a soft tissue mass are usually indicative of a more aggressive hemangiopericytoma of bone.

## Malignant Tumors

### Angiosarcoma

Angiosarcoma, a rare malignant tumor of bone, is composed of irregular anastomosing vascular channels lined by one or several layers of atypical endothelial cells. The nomenclature used to describe this tumor is far from consistent. Although the designation hemangioendothelioma has been used most frequently to describe a malignant low-grade vascular tumor and angiosarcoma, the

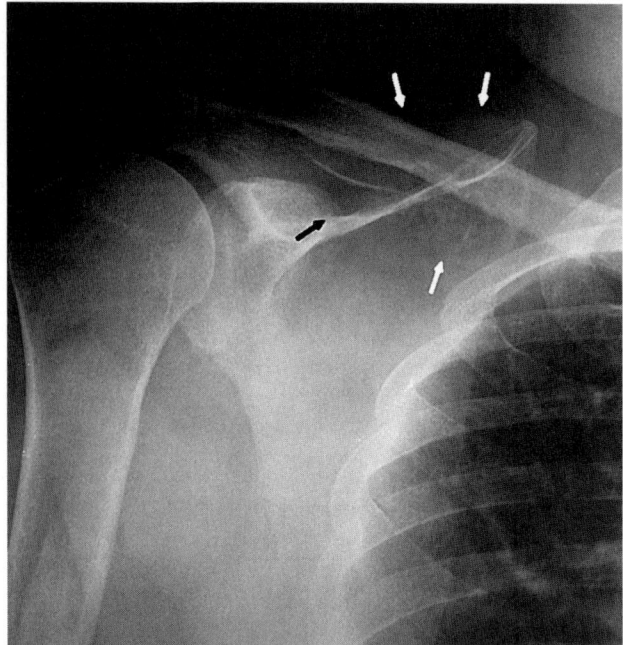

**Figure 70–92.** Hemangiopericytoma. A nonspecific osteolytic lesion with a soft tissue mass *(arrows)* involves the superomedial aspect of the scapula. (Courtesy of J. D. Bauer, MD, St. Louis, Mo.)

term angiosarcoma is used here as the general diagnostic term, with adjectives such as low-grade and high-grade applied appropriately to a given tumor.

**Clinical Abnormalities.** Osseous angiosarcomas are more frequent in men than in women (approximately 2:1). The tumors are observed most frequently in the third through fifth decades of life. Patients with multifocal disease are usually about 10 years younger than those with single lesions. Local pain and, less commonly, swelling are the two most characteristic clinical findings. Pathologic fractures are observed in approximately 10% of patients. Angiosarcomas have been observed at sites of bone infarction, chronic osteomyelitis, Paget's disease, or other neoplasms.

**Skeletal Location.** Angiosarcomas predominate in the long tubular bones, especially those in the lower extremity. The long bones are affected in approximately 60% of cases, with preferential involvement of the tibia (approximately 23% of cases), femur (18%), and humerus (13%). A metaphyseal or diaphyseal location is typical, with rare instances of primary epiphyseal tumors. Of the flat bones, those in the pelvis (7% of cases) and skull (4%) are altered most commonly. The ribs are affected in approximately 5% of cases, and the vertebrae are involved in approximately 10%.

One of the characteristic features of angiosarcoma is synchronous or metachronous multicentric disease, a phenomenon that is observed in 20% to 50% of cases. Multiple lesions may occur in a single bone, or one or more tumor foci may be apparent in multiple bones in a single extremity (especially the lower extremity) or

throughout the skeleton. A regional pattern of involvement of a tubular bone is an important diagnostic sign.

**Radiographic Abnormalities.** The principal radiographic pattern is one of osteolysis; this is uncommonly accompanied by osteosclerosis. Bone sclerosis alone is not evident. The lesions are variable in size, may localize in the cortex or in medullary bone, and possess either well-delineated or poorly defined margins. Cortical thinning and mild or moderate osseous expansion are additional radiographic features of angiosarcomas, and periostitis is infrequent. Extensive periosteal bone formation, cortical violation, and a soft tissue mass are indicative of more aggressive tumors. Multifocal involvement is an important radiographic pattern of this neoplasm. It may manifest as two or more osteolytic lesions involving a long segment of a single bone or as osteolysis in contiguous bones (Fig. 70–93). The radiographic demonstration of multiple neoplastic foci in the cortical bone or spongiosa, or both, leading to a bubble-like appearance and osseous expansion without periostitis in a tubular bone (or bones) of a lower extremity, is highly characteristic. In the flat or irregular bones, a similar osteolytic pattern may be demonstrated.

**Pathologic Abnormalities.** Two fundamental histologic criteria are required: (1) the formation of atypical endothelial cells in greater numbers than would be

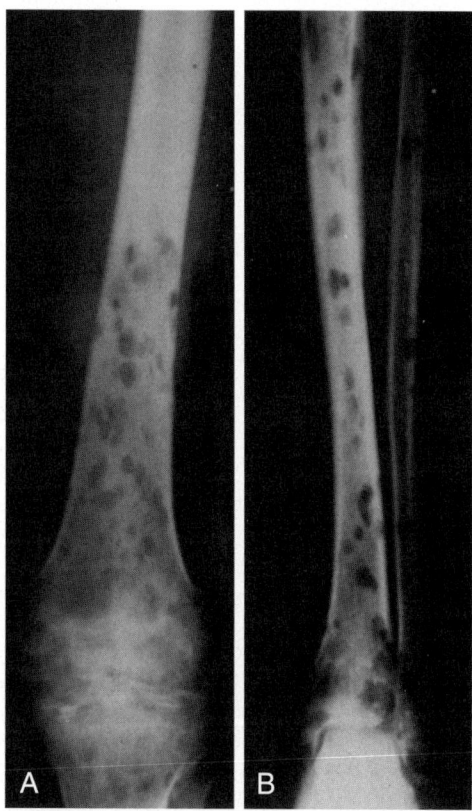

**Figure 70–93.** Angiosarcoma: long tubular bones. *A* and *B*, Note the multiple, well-defined, small osteolytic lesions scattered throughout the tibia, fibula, and femur. This type of regional distribution is one of the characteristic patterns of angiosarcoma. (Courtesy of H. J. Spjut, MD, Houston, Tex.)

required to line vessels with a simple endothelial membrane, and (2) the formation of vascular tubes and channels that possess a delicate framework of reticulin fibers and commonly anastomose. Very well differentiated angiosarcomas usually contain numerous blood vessels whose endothelial cells show only minimal nuclear atypia, such that the lesions are difficult to distinguish from hemangiomas. An important histologic variation is epithelioid hemangioendothelioma; however, this lesion is not radiographically distinct from other low-grade angiosarcomas.

**Natural History.** The ultimate prognosis in patients with angiosarcoma of bone depends largely on the histologic grade of the tumor. Well-differentiated or low-grade neoplasms are associated with a more favorable prognosis. The prognosis for long-term survival in cases of high-grade angiosarcoma of bone remains grave.

## TUMORS OF NEURAL DIFFERENTIATION

Primary osseous tumors of neurogenic origin are rare. Major benign neural tumors are separated into neurofibroma and neurilemoma (schwannoma). The malignant counterpart of these lesions is designated malignant peripheral nerve sheath tumor; older terms include neurogenic sarcoma and malignant schwannoma.

### Benign Tumors

#### Solitary Neurofibroma

Although multiple neurogenic tumors are well recognized as part of neurofibromatosis (see Chapter 81), solitary neurofibromas are uncommon. These lesions generally occur in persons between the ages of 25 and 45 years and originate from the cranial, peripheral, and sympathetic nerves. Neurofibromas arising from peripheral nerves and appearing in the soft tissues are discussed in Chapter 71. When occurring adjacent to a bone, these tumors, as well as those arising in the periosteum or at the outer portion of the osseous neurovascular foramina, may lead to eccentric bone erosion. True intraosseous neurofibromas are rare.

Clinical manifestations are usually mild because of the slow growth of these neoplasms and include local pain, swelling, and tenderness. In certain locations, such as the sacrum, more prominent symptoms may be evident. The mandible is the bone affected most often and is involved in approximately two thirds of cases; other sites of involvement include the maxilla and vertebral column (especially the sacrum). Neurofibromas generally appear in the posterior portion of the mandible. Central or eccentric osteolytic lesions are encountered and may result in cortical destruction and periosteal reaction. Intraosseous neurofibromas can be associated with neurofibromatosis, as well as with congenital bowing of a tubular bone.

#### Neurilemoma

Neurilemomas, which arise from a nerve sheath, rarely originate in bone. Men and women of all ages are affected. Clinical manifestations include pain, swelling, and, less frequently, impairment of sensory and motor function. The most frequent sites of involvement are the mandible, sacrum, maxilla, femur, and humerus, in order of descending frequency. It is of interest that the mandible and sacrum are bones that normally contain lengthy nerve segments, perhaps explaining the predilection of neurilemomas (and neurofibromas) for these sites. Mandibular tumors predominate in the posterior portion of the bone; lesions in the long tubular bones are evident in the diaphysis, metaphysis, or both, with rare involvement of the epiphysis.

The radiographic characteristics of neurilemomas are not specific. Three radiographic presentations are encountered: (1) central involvement characterized by a cystic osteolytic focus with a sclerotic margin; (2) localization to the nutrient canal, with production of a dumbbell lesion; and (3) periosteal involvement leading to cortical erosion or excavation.

### Malignant Tumors

#### Malignant Peripheral Nerve Sheath Tumor

This tumor has been reported to arise in bone only rarely, in some cases in patients with neurofibromatosis. Malignant peripheral nerve sheath tumors usually appear in patients in the third to fifth decades of life. Fewer than 50 cases of such tumors arising in bone have been recorded, most occurring in the mandible or maxilla. Rarely, an identical lesion is documented in the spine, long bones, or small bones in the hand or foot. Typical radiographic features include an osteolytic process with or without soft tissue extension, but such features are not specific.

## TUMORS OF NOTOCHORD ORIGIN

### Locally Aggressive or Malignant Tumors

#### Chordoma

Chordoma is a rare lesion of notochord origin characterized by a lobular arrangement and composed of highly vacuolated (physaliphorous) cells and mucoid intercellular material. It is a locally aggressive tumor that grows slowly, invades surrounding soft tissue structures, and metastasizes infrequently.

#### *Clinical Abnormalities*

Chordomas can become evident in men and women of all ages, although most patients are in the fourth through seventh decades of life. Chordomas occurring in children are rare and appear to be more aggressive. Sacrococcygeal lesions are more common in men than in women (approximately 2:1); spheno-occipital chordomas have an equal sex distribution. Chordomas arising in the sacrococcygeal region produce gradually progressive perineal pain and numbness. Additional manifestations depend on the pressure exerted by the tumor on surrounding structures, including the rectum, bladder, and emerging nerve roots. Spheno-occipital chordomas lead to increased intracranial pressure and encroachment on adjacent structures and manifest as headaches, blurred vision, diplopia, weakness, memory loss, and emotional instability. Dysfunction of the pituitary gland may be accompanied by amenorrhea, sterility, loss of libido, and visual disturbances. Vertebral chordomas progressively involve the adjacent spinal cord and nerve roots and result in pain, numbness, motor weakness, and, eventually, paralysis.

### Skeletal Location

Favored locations of chordomas are the sacrococcygeal region (50% to 60% of cases), spheno-occipital region (25% to 40%), and other portions of the vertebral column (15% to 20%); of the vertebrae above the sacrum, those in the cervical region are affected most commonly, followed by the lumbar and thoracic vertebrae. Spinal chordomas generally arise in the vertebral body, although they may extend into the posterior osseous elements of the vertebra.

### Radiographic and Other Imaging Abnormalities

Osteolysis with or without calcification, cortical violation, and a soft tissue mass are the predominant radiographic findings.

**Sacrococcygeal Tumors.** The fundamental radiographic features of these chordomas are irregular destruction of bone, osseous expansion, and an anterior soft tissue mass. Calcification (50% to 70% of cases) and osteosclerosis are additional abnormalities that are prominent in some cases (Fig. 70–94). CT and MR imaging may define the

extent of the tumor, particularly its soft tissue component, and may detect calcification in as many as 90% of cases. Such calcification is amorphous and predominates in the periphery of the tumor (Fig. 70–95). Myelography, scintigraphy, and angiography are other techniques that can be used to evaluate sacrococcygeal chordomas. Photon-deficient (or "cold") lesions are the typical scintigraphic findings in sacrococcygeal chordomas.

**Spheno-Occipital Tumors.** Destruction of the clivus and sella turcica, osseous expansion, a soft tissue mass, and extension of tumor to the petrous and sphenoid bones and the nasopharynx may be evident. Reticular, nodular, or scattered calcifications within the lesion are detected in 20% to 70% of cases. Of interest in this regard is the identification of a chondroid chordoma, a specific variety that exhibits cartilaginous features, represents approximately one third of all chordomas in this region, and is accompanied by a better prognosis (see later discussion).

CT and MR imaging allow further evaluation of spheno-occipital chordomas. With MR imaging, spheno-occipital chordomas typically have low to intermediate signal intensity on T1-weighted spin echo MR images and lobulated regions of high signal intensity with septations of low signal intensity on T2-weighted spin echo MR images. MR imaging appears to be superior to CT in demonstrating the tumor's relationship to the cavernous internal carotid artery and the vertebral and basilar arteries; CT appears to be superior in defining the presence and extent of tumoral calcification.

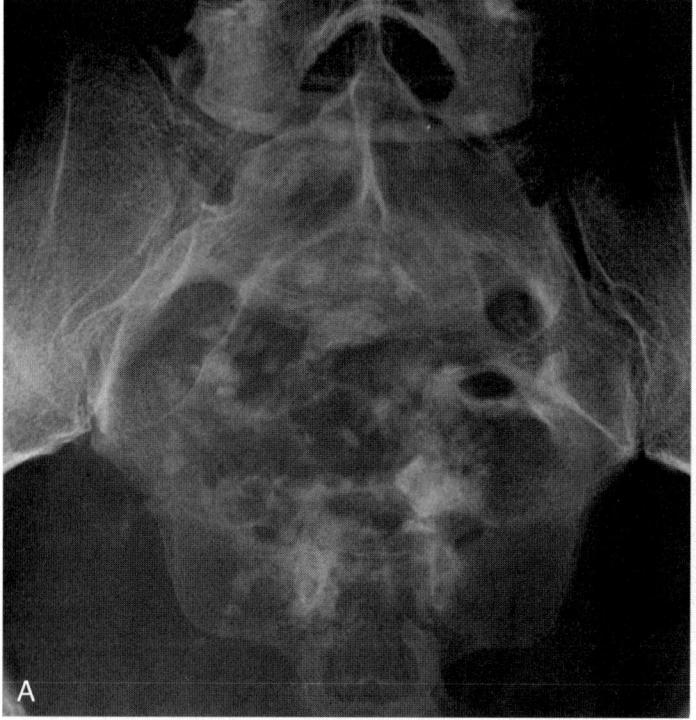

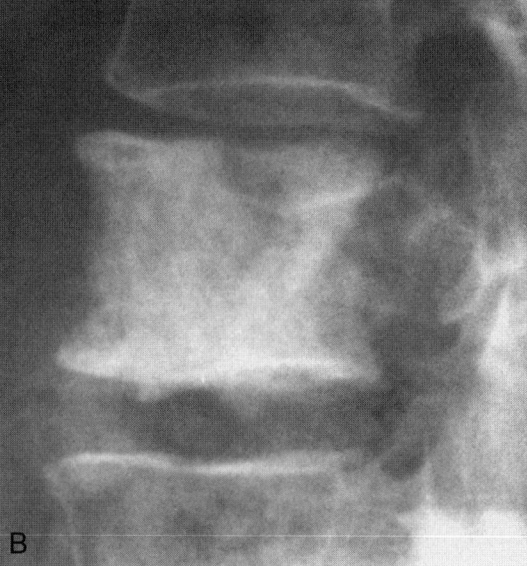

**Figure 70–94.** Chordoma. *A,* Sacrococcygeal tumor. Within the sacrum, this large chordoma has led to osteolysis with prominent calcification. *B,* Vertebral tumor. Osteosclerosis is the predominant abnormality in this chordoma of a vertebral body. Note the erosion of the posterior aspect of the vertebral body and narrowing of the intervertebral disc above the involved vertebra.

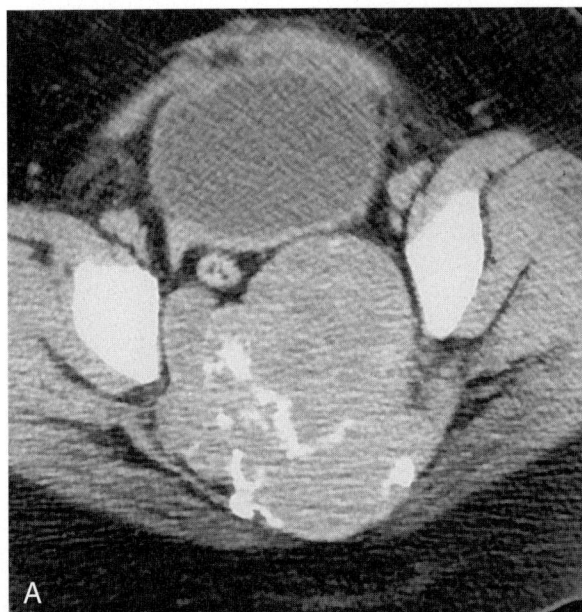

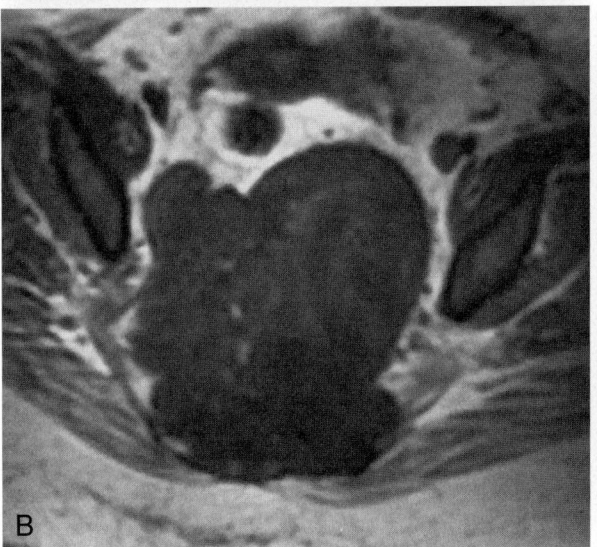

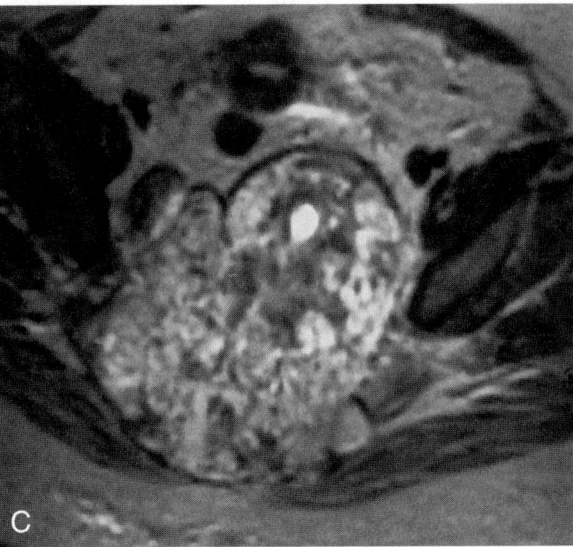

**Figure 70–95.** Chordoma: sacrococcygeal tumor. Contrast-enhanced transaxial CT image *(A)* reveals a large, partially calcified sacral tumor with a large soft tissue mass. Transverse T1-weighted (TR/TE, 600/16) spin echo *(B)* and T2-weighted (TR/TE, 4000/85) fast spin echo *(C)* MR images show the large tumor with inhomogeneous signal intensity.

**Vertebral Tumors.** Initially, destruction of the vertebral body is unaccompanied by loss of height of the adjacent intervertebral disc. Subsequently, osteosclerosis and soft tissue abnormalities may become prominent, and contiguous vertebral bodies may be affected, with involvement of the intervertebral discs. Cervical lesions are most likely to involve contiguous vertebrae. Calcification in an anterior soft tissue mass occurs in approximately 30% of cases. Vertebral collapse, radiodense vertebral bodies (ivory vertebrae), and enlarged neural foramina are additional manifestations of this lesion. CT and MR imaging can also be used to evaluate spinal chordomas. MR imaging combined with the intravenous administration of a gadolinium compound is useful for assessing the epidural extension of the tumor (Fig. 70–96).

### *Pathologic Abnormalities*

The size of chordomas is extremely variable, and those in the sacrococcygeal region may be enormous; spheno-

occipital chordomas tend to be small. The macroscopic features of chordomas include a lobulated configuration. Focal areas of hemorrhage and cyst formation may be evident. The most prominent histologic feature of a chordoma is its abundant production of intracellular and extracellular mucin.

### *Natural History*

The prognosis of a chordoma is variable, depending on its location and its extent at the time of discovery. Unfortunately, many chordomas are massive when initially evaluated and, because of their locally aggressive behavior, have already infiltrated adjacent structures. In these instances, debulking procedures are the only option. In primary or recurrent tumors or in those that have been irradiated, large areas of sarcomatous-appearing cells may develop, similar to those of malignant fibrous histiocytoma, fibrosarcoma, chondrosarcoma, or osteosarcoma. Such lesions are referred to as dedifferentiated chordo-

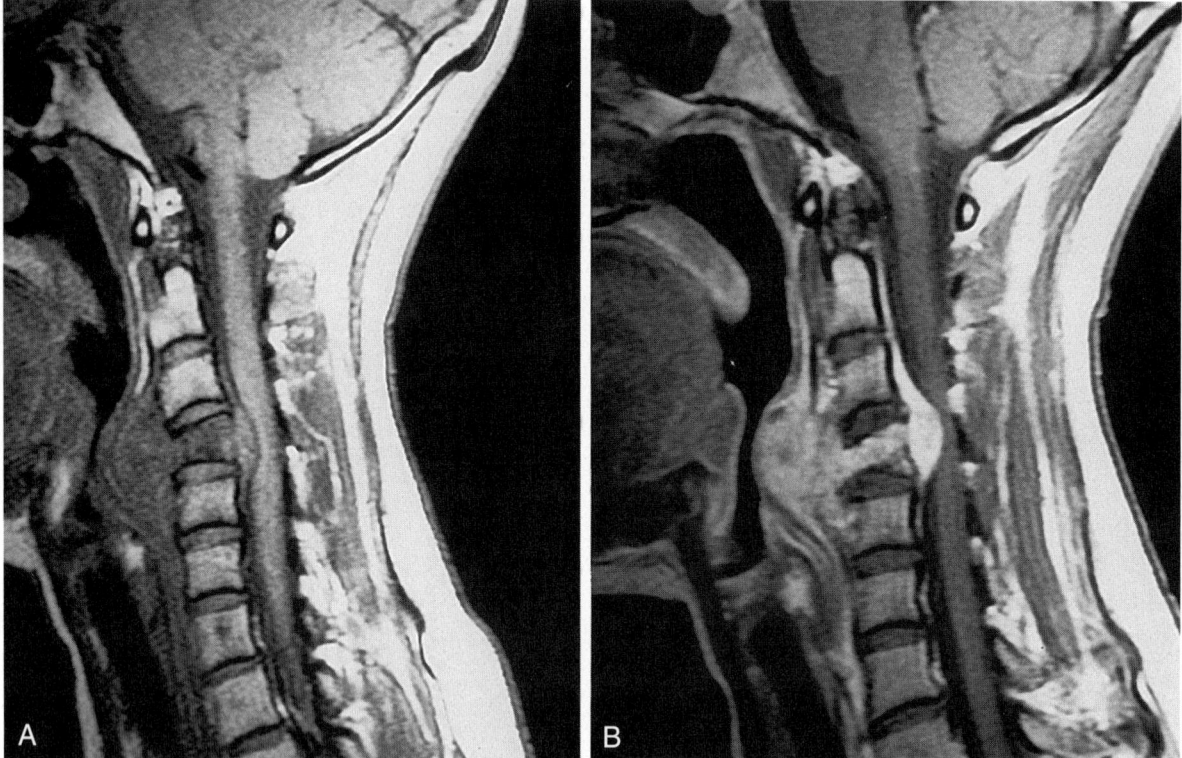

**Figure 70–96.** Chordoma: vertebral tumor. Chordoma arising from the fourth cervical vertebral body extends anteriorly, as shown on sagittal T1-weighted (TR/TE, 600/16) spin echo MR images obtained before *(A)* and after *(B)* intravenous gadolinium administration. Note an anterior epidural mass at this level. (Courtesy of D. Goodwin, MD, Hanover, NH.)

mas. Hematogenous metastases may eventually be evident in 10% to 40% of patients with chordomas. This phenomenon is far more frequent in chordomas of the sacrococcygeal region or spine than in chordomas of the base of the skull.

### Ecchondrosis Physaliphora and Notochordal Hamartoma

Microscopic vestiges of the notochord are detected in as many as 2% of cadavers at the time of autopsy. These vestiges are most common in the region of the spheno-occipital synchondrosis, where they are designated ecchondrosis physaliphora spheno-occipitalis. Ecchondrosis physaliphora is considered to be a gelatinous hamartoma without clinical significance; whether it can occur as a symptomatic lesion is debated.

The prevalence of intraosseous notochord vestiges in adults is uncertain. Recent reports note the occurrence of a proliferation of notochord cells within the vertebral bodies of adult patients, believed to represent a benign hamartomatous process that can be distinguished from a chordoma by the lack of bone destruction or soft tissue extension and by the absence of cellular atypia. Conventional radiographs in such cases either show mild bone sclerosis or are normal.

### Chondroid Chordoma

Chondroid chordomas arise at the base of the skull and rarely at other sites. Approximately 33% of chordomas at the base of the skull are chondroid in type. Chondroid chordomas are associated with distinctive behavioral characteristics, such as a proclivity to invade bone and entwine themselves around vital structures. They are slightly more frequent in women than in men and are usually observed in patients younger than 40 years. Their radiographic and gross morphologic features are similar to those of typical chordomas, although calcification is particularly prominent. Histologically, the cartilaginous foci in chondroid chordomas may resemble those of a chondroma or a low-grade chondrosarcoma.

## TUMORS AND TUMOR-LIKE LESIONS OF MISCELLANEOUS OR UNKNOWN ORIGIN

### Benign Tumors

#### Simple (Solitary or Unicameral) Bone Cyst

The simple bone cyst is a common lesion of unknown cause and pathogenesis. Recent evidence supports the importance of venous obstruction and blocking of interstitial fluid drainage in a rapidly growing and remodeling area of cancellous bone in the pathogenesis of such cysts.

**Clinical Abnormalities.** Lesions are typically discovered in the first and second decades of life and affect boys with greater frequency than girls (ratio of 2:1). In patients younger than 20 years, cysts are generally observed in the tubular bones, particularly the proximal ends of the humerus and femur. Less than 15% of cysts occur in patients older than 20 years, at which time cysts have a predilection for the innominate bone and the calcaneus. At any site, simple bone cysts are rarely symptomatic unless a pathologic fracture has occurred.

**Skeletal Location.** A simple bone cyst is observed most frequently in a long tubular bone (approximately 90% to 95% of cases). The humerus (56% of cases), femur (27%), and tibia (6%) are involved most commonly. With the exception of the calcaneus, which is affected in approximately 3% of cases, simple bone cysts are rare in the small bones of the hand and foot. In the osseous pelvis, the ilium (2%) is usually involved. Rare sites of localization are the ischium, sacrum, pubic bone, ribs, patella, scapula, clavicle, gnathic bones, and spine.

In the long tubular bones, a metaphyseal location is the preferred site. Diaphyseal involvement occurs in 4% to 12% of lesions in the tubular bones. Epiphyseal localization or extension is exceedingly rare. Simple bone cysts located in the metaphysis adjacent to the growth plate are considered active because of their capacity for growth, whereas those that have "migrated" away from the plate toward the diaphysis are considered latent, although this division based on location in the bone is not entirely accurate, and activity appears to correlate better with the age of the patient.

**Radiographic Abnormalities.** A centrally located radiolucent lesion with cortical thinning and mild osseous expansion is the radiographic hallmark of this lesion. Some cysts may possess a multilocular appearance. A thin, sclerotic margin is a frequent finding that produces a classic pattern of geographic bone destruction with a short zone of transition from abnormal to normal bone. In a long tubular bone, additional radiographic features include a lesion confined mainly to the metaphysis and juxtaposed to the physis, as well as an elongated shape, with the longitudinal axis of the lesion parallel to that of the parent bone (Fig. 70–97). In some cases, other diagnoses must be considered, such as an aneurysmal bone cyst, enchondroma, and fibrous dysplasia.

A pathologic fracture through a simple bone cyst is a common associated abnormality and may be accompanied by a vertical fragment within the cyst that migrates to a dependent portion of the lesion because of its fluid content. This finding (Fig. 70–98), which has been designated the "fallen fragment" sign, virtually ensures an accurate analysis of the radiographs.

In some instances, diaphyseal lesions are large, multiloculated, and slightly expansile (Fig. 70–99) and resemble fibrous dysplasia, chondromyxoid fibroma, desmoplastic fibroma, and eosinophilic granuloma. Characteristic features of a simple bone cyst, including a central location, an elongated shape, and prominent radiolucency, usually allow its differentiation from these other processes. With epiphyseal involvement or extension, the cyst may produce radiographic abnormalities simulating those of chondroblastoma; alternatively, because of considerable deformity of the articular surface, the cyst may resemble ischemic necrosis of bone.

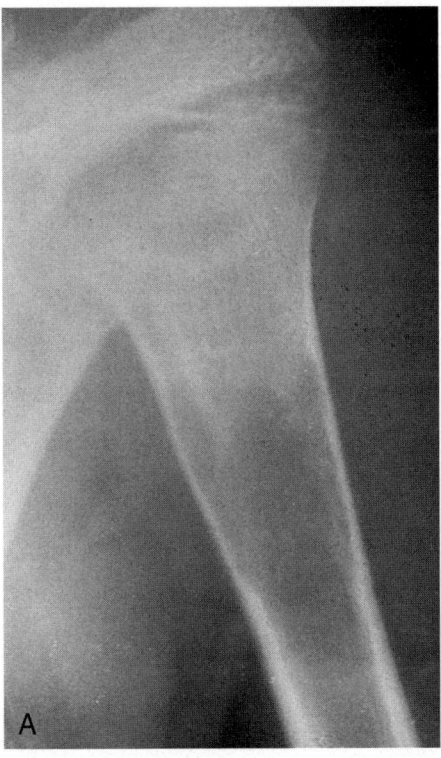

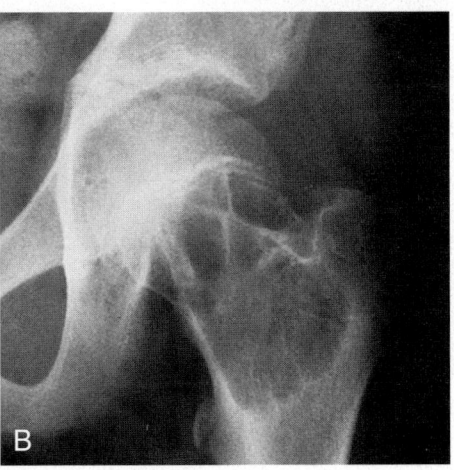

**Figure 70–97.** Simple (solitary or unicameral) bone cyst: long tubular bones. *A*, Humerus. A relatively well-defined, central osteolytic lesion in the proximal metaphysis of the humerus in this 8-year-old boy is virtually diagnostic of a simple bone cyst. Note the elongated shape of the lesion and endosteal bone erosion. *B*, Femur. Radiograph shows a well-marginated, osteolytic metaphyseal lesion juxtaposed to the physis.

A
B

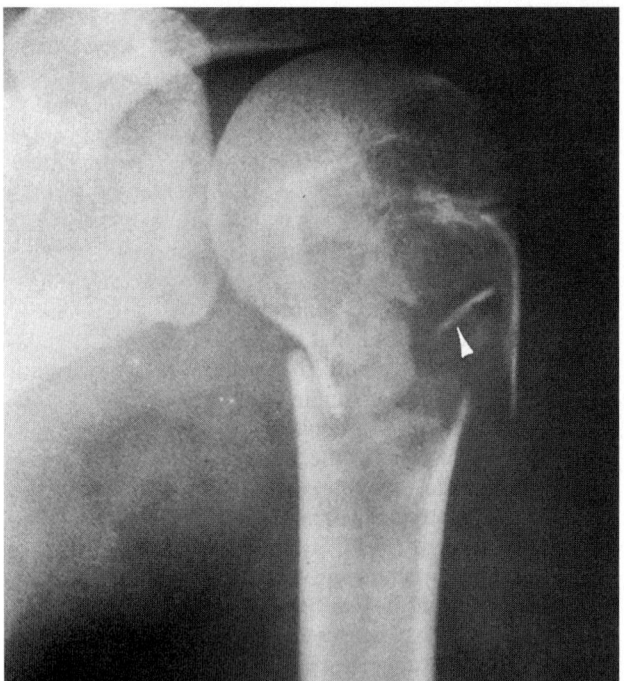

**Figure 70–98.** Simple (solitary or unicameral) bone cyst: pathologic fracture. A transverse pathologic fracture through a cystic lesion of the humerus is evident. Note the piece of cortex *(arrowhead)* that lies within the lesion. (Courtesy of D. Pate, San Diego, Calif.)

In the calcaneus, the cyst is a well-defined radiolucent lesion, almost invariably occurring in the base of the calcaneal neck just inferior to the anterior portion of the posterior facet (Fig. 70–100). The major differential diagnostic considerations are lipoma and thinning of trabeculae, which occurs normally in this portion of the calcaneus. Simple cysts of the ilium may be large. Radiographically, they are well defined and radiolucent, and they commonly possess a sclerotic margin.

**Other Imaging Techniques.** CT can be used to evaluate the extent of lesions in anatomically complex areas such as the spine or osseous pelvis. CT analysis of simple bone cysts and other cystic lesions of bone occasionally demonstrates intralesional gas (pneumatocyst), gas-fluid levels, or fluid-fluid levels. MR imaging can confirm the fluid content of a simple bone cyst by documenting that the lesion has prolonged T1 and T2 relaxation times. Enhancement of signal intensity in the peripheral portion of a simple bone cyst or within internal septations is evident after the intravenous injection of gadolinium-based contrast agents (Fig. 70–101). In cysts that have fractured, however, these enhancement patterns are often more complex and may be characterized by enhancement of focal nodules within the lesion.

**Pathologic Abnormalities.** On macroscopic examination, the affected bone has an expanded cortex, resembling an eggshell, that is covered by intact periosteum. The cyst usually contains fluid that is clear, yellow, orange, red, or brown, depending on whether a previous fracture with hemorrhage has occurred. A membrane generally lines the cystic cavity. Microscopically, the wall of the cyst is thin, and the membrane lining the cyst contains a fibrous stroma.

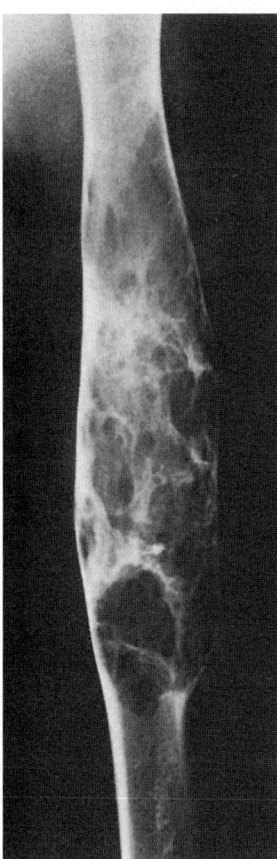

**Figure 70–99.** Multilocular bone cyst. Observe this multiloculated, expansile, osteolytic lesion in the diaphysis of the humerus. (Courtesy of A. D'Abreu, MD, Porto Alegre, Brazil.)

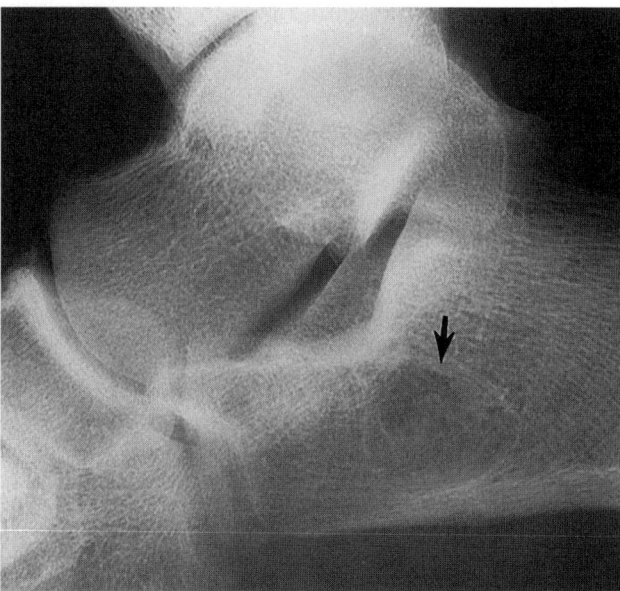

**Figure 70–100.** Simple (solitary or unicameral) bone cyst: calcaneus. Note the typical appearance and location of this simple bone cyst *(arrow)*.

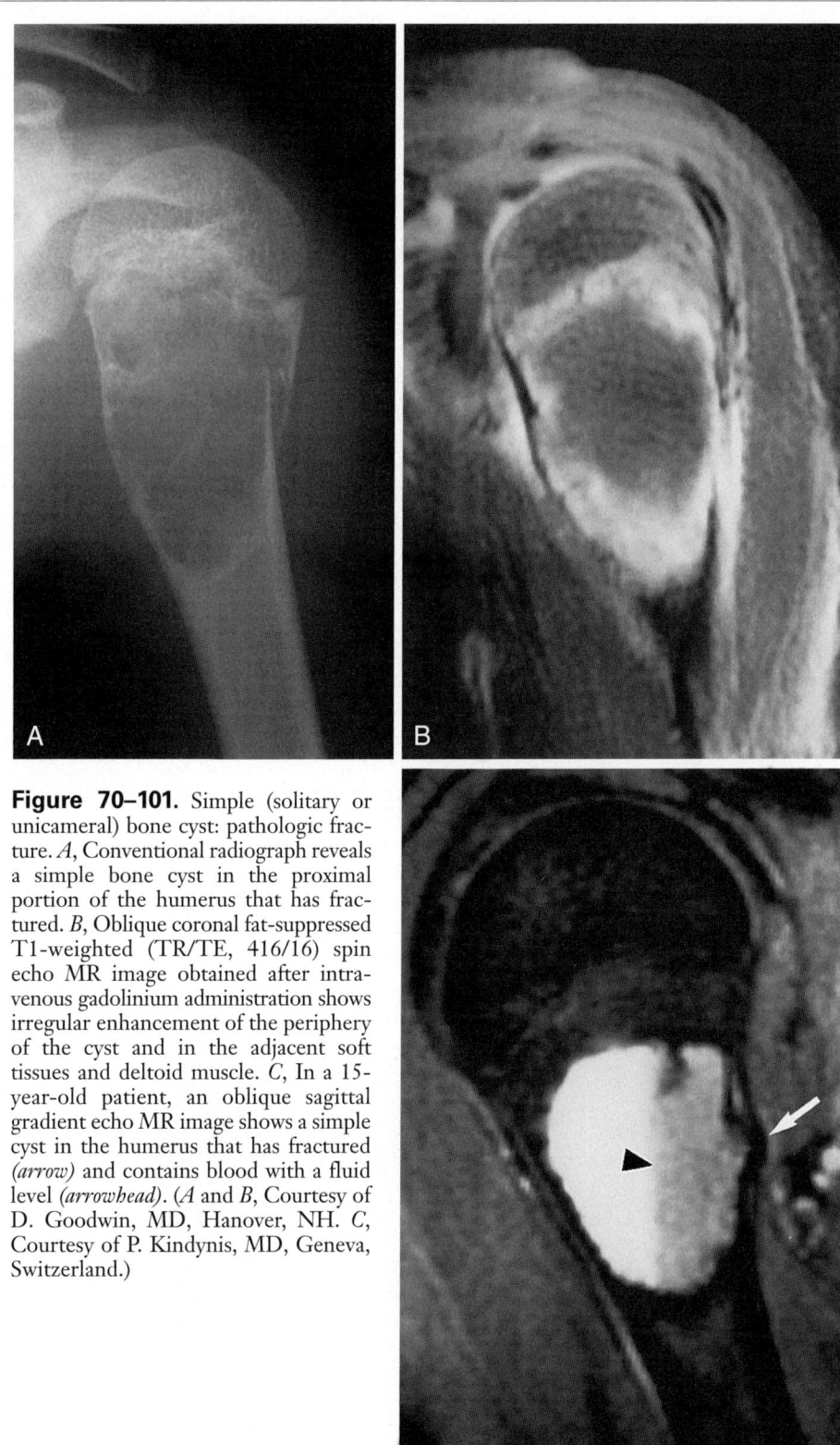

**Figure 70–101.** Simple (solitary or unicameral) bone cyst: pathologic fracture. *A*, Conventional radiograph reveals a simple bone cyst in the proximal portion of the humerus that has fractured. *B*, Oblique coronal fat-suppressed T1-weighted (TR/TE, 416/16) spin echo MR image obtained after intravenous gadolinium administration shows irregular enhancement of the periphery of the cyst and in the adjacent soft tissues and deltoid muscle. *C*, In a 15-year-old patient, an oblique sagittal gradient echo MR image shows a simple cyst in the humerus that has fractured (*arrow*) and contains blood with a fluid level (*arrowhead*). (*A* and *B*, Courtesy of D. Goodwin, MD, Hanover, NH. *C*, Courtesy of P. Kindynis, MD, Geneva, Switzerland.)

**Natural History.** Aggressive growth potential and a high frequency of recurrence after treatment appear to be characteristic of lesions discovered in children or adolescents; these features are not dependent on the precise anatomic location of the bone cyst within the bone. Although bone cysts may rarely undergo spontaneous regression, even after fracture, the usual approach to the management of simple bone cysts is not to wait and watch but rather to intervene.

Depending on the type of surgical procedure performed, as many as 40% of simple bone cysts may recur. An alternative method of treatment that has been advocated in recent years is the injection of steroid preparations (methylprednisolone acetate) directly into the cyst. This injection method has been reported to be effective in 70% to 95% of cases of simple bone cyst, although the lesion still recurs in 10% to 20% of cases and additional steroid injections are required in some patients.

**Complications.** Several potential complications deserve emphasis. Fracture is the most common complication, although its frequency in patients with simple bone cysts is difficult to define because of the probability that many cysts that do not fracture are never discovered. It is unquestioned that fracture is a significant sequela of simple bone cysts and one that generally results in the patient seeking medical attention. In some instances, however, incomplete infractions of bone about the cyst occur and are characterized by minor clinical and radiographic manifestations.

Acellular, amorphous, granular fibrin-like material surrounded by osteoblasts is identified histologically in approximately 10% to 15% of simple bone cysts. The material may undergo calcification and ossification and produce a substance that by ordinary light microscopy superficially resembles odontogenic cementum. In some instances, the term cementoma or cementifying fibroma has been applied to lesions containing this material, which is apparently a unique feature of simple bone cysts.

Rarely, malignant tumors occurring in simple bone cysts have been reported, including chondrosarcoma, liposarcoma, osteosarcoma, fibrosarcoma, and Ewing's sarcoma. In some instances, irradiation was used in the treatment of the cyst, suggesting that the malignancy was a complication not of the cyst itself but of the therapeutic method.

## Epidermoid Cyst

Epidermoid cysts of bone are uncommon. Although their pathogenesis is debated, a history of blunt or penetrating trauma is evident in most affected patients, which suggests that such an injury may lead to intraosseous implantation of ectodermal tissue and the subsequent development of an epidermoid cyst. This concept is consistent with the typical localization of the lesion to superficially situated bones. Men are affected more frequently than women, and patients are usually in the second, third, or fourth decade of life. Clinical manifestations may include pain and swelling.

Intraosseous epidermoid cysts arise almost exclusively in the skull and phalanges of the hand, with the former being the most common site of involvement. In the hands, the terminal phalanx is involved in almost all cases. Rare sites of epidermoid cysts are the metacarpal bones, tibia, ulna, femur, sacrum, and sternum. Any bone of the skull can be affected, with the frontal and parietal bones being the most typical locations. Epidermoid cysts are also observed in the mandible and maxilla.

The radiographic findings are highly characteristic. In the terminal phalanges of the fingers or toes, a well-defined osteolytic lesion possessing a sclerotic margin is observed (Fig. 70–102). A portion of the overlying cortex may be disrupted. Soft tissue swelling may also be evident. The findings are not unlike those of an enchondroma, although the latter tumor rarely localizes in the terminal phalanx. One other differential diagnostic consideration is a glomus tumor. In the skull, a well-marginated radiolucent lesion is typical of an epidermoid cyst. Erosion of both the inner and outer tables occurs in about 50% of cases. The characteristically sharp edge of an epidermoid cyst differs from the pattern of poorly

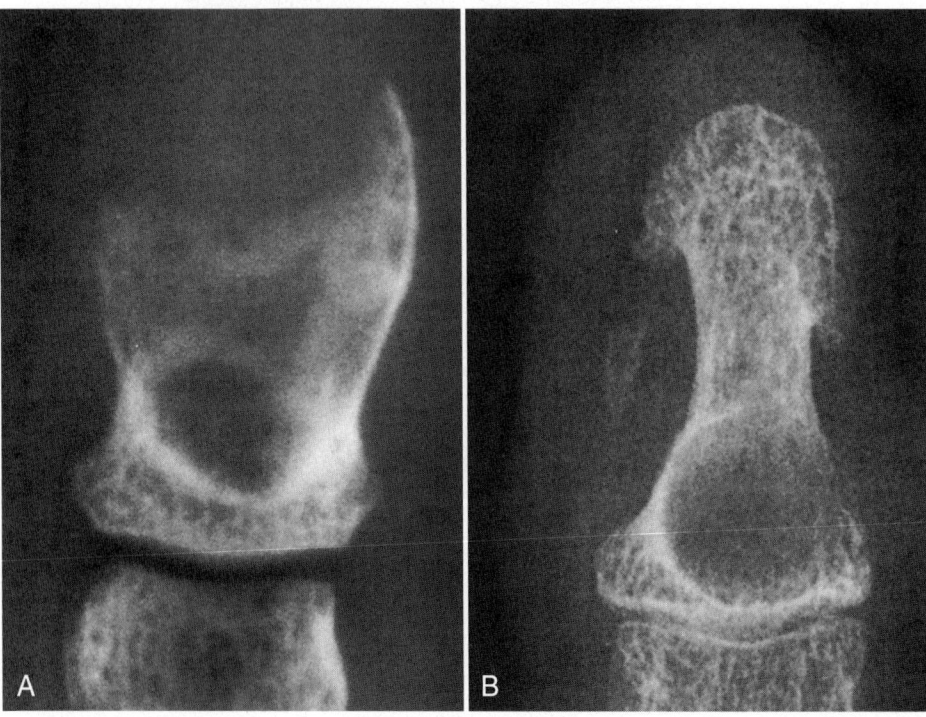

**Figure 70–102.** Epidermoid cyst: terminal phalanx. Two examples of lesions in the hand are shown. *A,* A large, well-defined osteolytic lesion possesses a sclerotic margin. The distal cortex is incomplete. *B,* Frontal radiograph reveals an epidermoid cyst involving the base of a terminal phalanx.

defined osteolysis that accompanies skeletal infection or metastasis.

## Aneurysmal Bone Cyst

An aneurysmal bone cyst is a hemorrhagic lesion containing thin-walled, blood-filled cystic cavities. It is generally regarded as non-neoplastic in nature, and trauma appears to be important in the pathogenesis of some aneurysmal bone cysts, with well-documented examples of this lesion developing subsequent to acute fractures or other injuries. This observation has led to speculation that local postinjury alterations in hemodynamics related to venous obstruction or arteriovenous fistulas are important in the pathogenesis of aneurysmal bone cysts, a concept that is supported by angiographic data.

It is also well documented that aneurysmal bone cysts may accompany a variety of benign processes of the skeleton, including chondroblastoma, chondromyxoid fibroma, nonossifying fibroma, osteoblastoma, giant cell tumor, giant cell reparative granuloma, fibrous histiocytoma, brown tumor, solitary cyst, and fibrous dysplasia, and, less frequently, some malignant tumors such as osteosarcoma, chondrosarcoma, fibrosarcoma, malignant fibrous histiocytoma, and angiosarcoma. The coexistence of an aneurysmal bone cyst and a companion lesion is consistent with the concept that a precursor tumor or event (e.g., trauma) leads to local hemodynamic changes that provide the ideal environment for superimposition of a secondary aneurysmal bone cyst. It is also possible that alterations in osseous hemodynamics resulting from the companion process may give rise to rapid enlargement of an already existing aneurysmal bone cyst. A preexisting lesion can be definitively identified in one third of patients with aneurysmal bone cysts.

### Clinical Abnormalities

Aneurysmal bone cysts are usually observed in the first, second, or third decade of life. Approximately 80% of affected patients are younger than 20 years. There appears to be a slight female preponderance. Local findings include pain and swelling. Other clinical manifestations depend on the specific site of involvement.

### Skeletal Location

Aneurysmal bone cysts are most frequent in the long tubular bones and spine, which together account for approximately 60% to 70% of cases. Specific sites of involvement include the tibia, vertebrae, femur, humerus, and innominate bone. The small bones in the feet and, less frequently, the hands are affected in approximately 10% to 14% of cases. Rare sites of involvement include the patella, sacrum, and acetabular region. Metachronous multiple aneurysmal bone cysts have been described.

Within the long tubular bones, aneurysmal bone cysts are seen almost exclusively in a metaphysis. Diaphyseal involvement occurs in about 8% of cases. Epiphyseal extension of a metaphyseal aneurysmal bone cyst is uncommon and is usually (but not invariably) apparent after closure of the growth plate. Aneurysmal bone cysts

may also arise within the cortex or in a subperiosteal location of a tubular bone.

In the spine, the thoracic, lumbar, cervical, and sacral levels may be affected, in order of decreasing frequency. Vertebral aneurysmal bone cysts generally arise in the posterior osseous elements, including the neural arches, laminae, and transverse and spinous processes; the vertebral bodies are affected less frequently and rarely without concomitant posterior osseous abnormalities.

### Radiographic Abnormalities

Osteolysis and osseous expansion are the dominant radiographic abnormalities of aneurysmal bone cysts (Fig. 70–103).

**Tubular Bones.** An eccentric, osteolytic, occasionally trabeculated process centered in a metaphysis of a long tubular bone is the classic appearance of an aneurysmal bone cyst. The inner margin of the lesion is usually well defined, with or without a rim of bone sclerosis, and the cortical surface of the affected bone is expanded or ballooned. Loss of cortical definition and apparent extension of the lesion into the adjacent soft tissue are alarming features that simulate the appearance of a malignant tumor. More correctly, these abnormalities should be considered indications of an aggressive and rapidly expansile intraosseous cyst. Horizontally oriented trabeculae extending into the soft tissue component of the lesion from the parent bone and a partial or complete osseous shell at the margin of this component are fundamental features in the analysis of radiographs.

Although a more central location of an aneurysmal bone cyst, leading to symmetrical expansion of the entire metaphysis, is occasionally evident in a long tubular

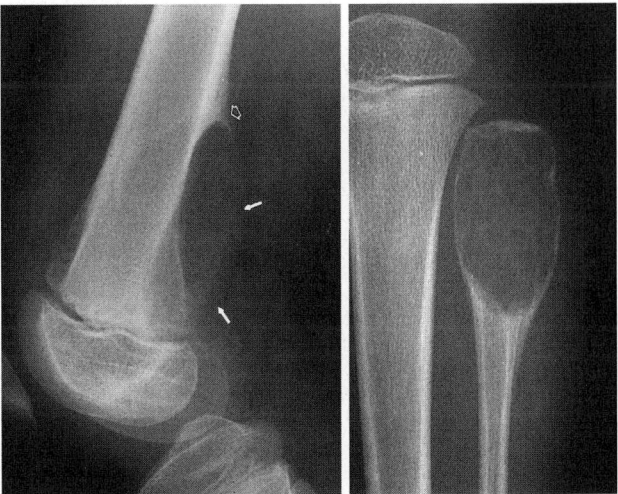

**Figure 70–103.** Aneurysmal bone cyst: tubular bones. *A,* Radiograph shows an aggressive, eccentric, osteolytic lesion. Observe the soft tissue mass *(solid arrows)* and Codman's triangle *(open arrow)*. *B,* In a young child, a centrally located aneurismal bone cyst of the proximal metaphysis of the fibula is osteolytic, expansile, and trabeculated and is accompanied by periostitis and an ossified shell. (*B,* Courtesy of W. Ewing, MD, Pueblo, Colo.)

bone, this pattern is more frequent in the short tubular bones of the hands and feet. The radiographic features may resemble those of a giant cell tumor (which more characteristically involves the epiphysis), enchondroma (which is less expansile and contains calcification), giant cell reparative granuloma, brown tumor of hyperparathyroidism, osteoblastoma, and, rarely, infection.

**Spine.** The typical spinal lesion is osteolytic and expansile and involves either the posterior osseous elements or both the posterior elements and the vertebral body (Fig. 70–104). When an aneurysmal bone cyst is confined to the spinous or transverse process in a child or adolescent, an accurate diagnosis is generally possible based on the radiographic alterations, although osteoblastoma and hemangioma are reasonable alternatives.

**Other Sites.** In the innominate bone (Fig. 70–105), osteolysis and bone expansion occur. Although a sclerotic margin about the lesion may indicate the nonmalignant nature of the process, soft tissue extension with displacement of viscera such as the bladder may make differentiation from sarcoma difficult. Similar difficulties are encountered when interpreting radiographs in patients with aneurysmal bone cysts of the ribs, scapula, and sternum (where malignant neoplasms are more frequent than benign tumors).

### Other Imaging Techniques

Angiography is one alternative imaging technique, with aneurysmal bone cysts usually described as hypovascular lesions with localized regions of hypervascularity. On scintigraphy, the predominant pattern is accumulation of the radiopharmaceutical agent at the periphery of the lesion and little activity in its center, a finding that is evident in approximately 65% of cases. This scintigraphic

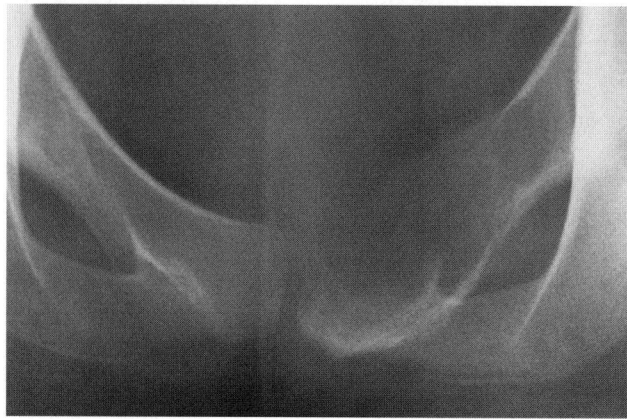

**Figure 70–105.** Aneurysmal bone cyst: pubic bone. An expansile, osteolytic lesion is evident on a routine radiograph.

pattern is not specific, however. CT is most useful in delineating the size and location of the intraosseous and extraosseous components of an aneurysmal bone cyst, especially in anatomically complex areas such as the spine and osseous pelvis. Detection of fluid levels with CT and MR imaging in some aneurysmal bone cysts is of interest (Fig. 70–106). Although such levels are not diagnostic of an aneurysmal bone cyst (occurring in giant cell tumors, simple bone cysts, chondroblastomas, and telangiectatic osteosarcomas as well), they are most compatible with the diagnosis of an aneurysmal bone cyst (Table 70–3). Fluid levels in aneurysmal bone cysts (and, less commonly, other lesions) may be solitary or multiple. An expansile and lobulated or septated lesion is typical. The internal septations create cystic cavities whose walls contain diverticulum-like projections.

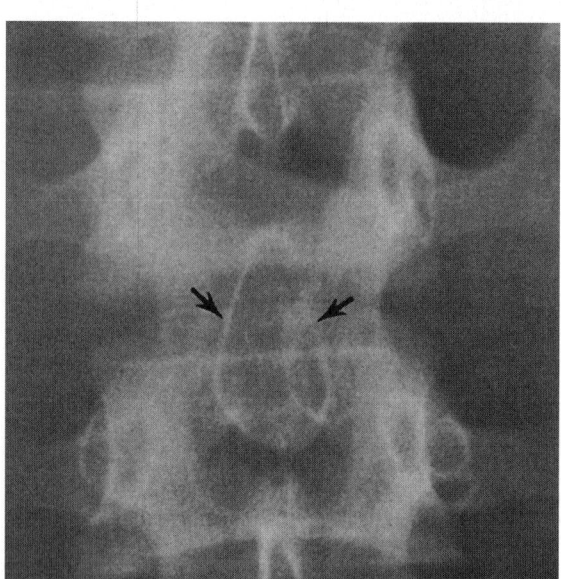

**Figure 70–104.** Aneurysmal bone cyst: spine. Uniform enlargement of the spinous process of a lumbar vertebra is seen (*arrows*). (Courtesy of D. Pate, San Diego, Calif.)

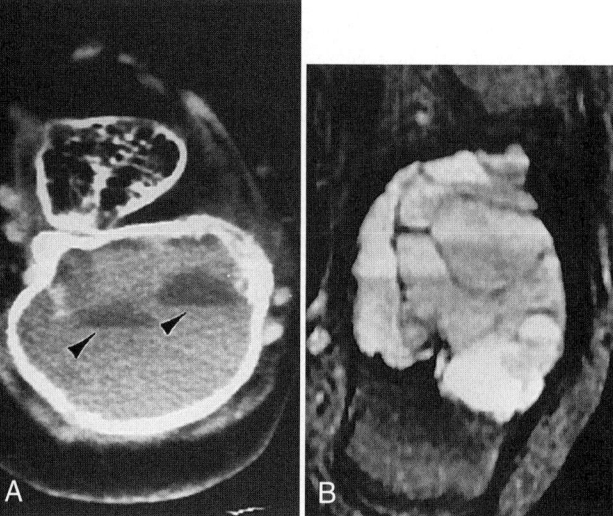

**Figure 70–106.** Aneurysmal bone cyst: fluid levels. *A*, Direct coronal CT scan reveals an expansile lesion of the calcaneus with fluid levels (*arrowheads*). *B*, In a different patient, transverse T2-weighted (TR/TE, 2000/80) spin echo MR image reveals involvement of a large portion of the calcaneus. Note the multiple fluid levels. (*A*, Courtesy of T. Broderick, MD, Orange, Calif.)

**TABLE 70–3**

**Bone Lesions Associated with Fluid Levels Visualized with CT or MR Imaging**

| Benign | Malignant |
|---|---|
| Aneurysmal bone cyst | Telangiectatic osteosarcoma |
| Simple bone cyst | Fibrosarcoma |
| Ganglion cyst | Plasmacytoma |
| Chondroblastoma | Metastases |
| Giant cell tumor | |
| Fibrous dysplasia | |
| Osteomyelitis (abscess) | |
| Osteoblastoma | |
| Brown tumor (hyperparathyroidism) | |

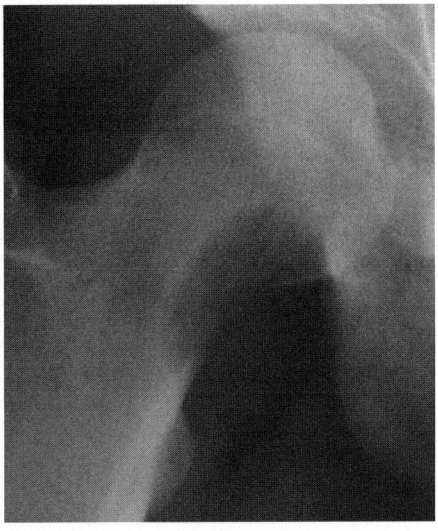

**Figure 70–107.** Aneurysmal bone cyst: solid variant. Hip pain developed in this 13-year-old girl. Routine radiograph shows an eccentric, well-marginated lesion in the medial portion of the femoral neck. (Courtesy of C. Gundry, MD, Minneapolis, Minn.)

### Pathologic Abnormalities

The lesion may contain a single large cystic cavity with a few fragments of friable red tissue on its wall or, more commonly, a meshwork of multiple cysts varying in maximum dimension from a few millimeters to several centimeters. The resulting appearance is that of a blood-filled sponge. Microscopically, the cavernous blood-filled cysts that characterize the gross morphology of an aneurysmal bone cyst do not represent true vascular channels but, rather, are lined by fibroblasts and multinucleated osteoclast-type giant cells. The cysts may be filled with fresh blood or appear empty because of draining during histologic processing. The solid portions of the lesion are composed predominantly of fibrous tissue that frequently contains numerous multinucleated giant cells, not unlike the appearance of a giant cell tumor.

### Natural History

Although an aneurysmal bone cyst is a non-neoplastic condition with no propensity to metastasize, its potential for rapid growth, considerable destruction of bone, and extension into adjacent soft tissue generally necessitates aggressive therapy, despite reports documenting spontaneous regression or regression after simple biopsy of the lesion. Such regression appears to be a rare phenomenon. One or more recurrences of an aneurysmal bone cyst are seen in approximately 10% to 20% of patients.

### Additional Types of Lesions

A solid variant of aneurysmal bone cyst has been identified. Solid aneurysmal bone cysts appear to have a preference for axial involvement (e.g., spine and innominate bone), in contrast to the usual distribution of the classic type of lesion. The long tubular bones, especially the femur, may also be involved. Radiographically, the solid variant of aneurysmal bone cyst is characterized by a spectrum of abnormalities consisting of, at one end, lesions that are indistinguishable from classic aneurysmal bone cysts (Fig. 70–107) and, at the other end, lesions (especially in the axial skeleton) that are highly aggres-

sive, with moth-eaten bone destruction, cortical violation, and soft tissue extension. The typical aneurysmal sinusoids of conventional aneurysmal bone cysts may or may not be present. Intralesional curettage or marginal resection of the lesion is generally curative.

Aneurysmal bone cysts associated with other skeletal lesions have been designated secondary aneurysmal bone cysts. The associated osseous lesions include chondroblastoma, chondromyxoid fibroma, fibrous dysplasia, giant cell tumor, osteoblastoma, simple bone cyst, hemangioma, brown tumor of hyperparathyroidism, telangiectatic osteosarcoma, fibrosarcoma, malignant fibrous histiocytoma, angiosarcoma, giant cell reparative granuloma, eosinophilic granuloma, and nonossifying fibroma. It is difficult to determine the relative frequency of primary aneurysmal bone cysts and those associated with other lesions; estimates of the incidence of a precursor lesion in cases of aneurysmal bone cyst vary, but 30% to 35% is a reasonable estimate.

### Intraosseous Ganglion Cyst

Intraosseous ganglion cysts are common lesions of uncertain pathogenesis that predominate in the subchondral regions of tubular bones, in the acetabulum, and in the carpal bones, especially the lunate. Their true prevalence, however, is difficult to define because of inconsistencies in terminology and, in many instances, the absence of histologic verification of the diagnosis. Most investigators regard intraosseous ganglion cysts as entities separate from post-traumatic and degenerative cysts of bone. The precise pathogenesis of intraosseous ganglion cysts is not clear, however. Although the lesion appears to arise de novo within bone, intraosseous ganglion cysts, cutaneous myxoid cysts, and soft tissue ganglion cysts are histologically identical. Further, the simultaneous occurrence of intraosseous and periosseous ganglion cysts is well recognized and has led to an alternative theory that intraosseous ganglion cysts relate to the extension of an adjacent soft tissue ganglion into bone. Continuity between the soft tissue and osseous lesions is consistent with gradual erosion of the bone surface as a cause of an intraosseous ganglion cyst. Intraosseous ganglia and soft tissue ganglia may occur independently, however.

Intraosseous ganglion cysts occur in persons of all ages, although most are discovered in adults. Intraosseous ganglia are often clinically silent; however, chronic pain, which sometimes increases with physical activity, may be evident. Lesions associated with soft tissue ganglion cysts may be accompanied by swelling or a mass. Nerve compression may also be apparent and is related to either an associated soft tissue ganglion or, more rarely, bone expansion. Although solitary lesions predominate, multiple and bilateral intraosseous ganglion cysts are encountered.

A subchondral lesion in a long tubular bone is most characteristic. Common sites of involvement are the femoral head, distal portions of the radius and ulna, distal portion of the femur, proximal aspect of the tibia, and medial malleolus. The acetabulum is a frequent site of involvement. Carpal involvement is more characteristic than tarsal involvement; of the carpal bones, the lunate and scaphoid bones are most commonly affected, although intraosseous ganglion cysts may occur in any of the carpal bones.

Radiographically, intraosseous ganglia are osteolytic lesions of variable size that are well demarcated and sharply circumscribed (Fig. 70–108). They may be solitary or multiple and, when multiple, may be localized to a single bone or adjacent bones. A sclerotic margin about the lesion is often evident. Pathologic fractures and soft tissue masses (representing ganglion cysts) are additional findings. In a long tubular bone, an intraosseous ganglion is generally eccentric in location, often extending to the subchondral bone plate. Although the bone plate may appear intact, tomographic techniques sometimes reveal that it is violated. Larger lesions may extend into the metaphysis and lead to mild expansion of bone.

Radionuclide examination shows increased accumulation of the bone-seeking agent. With MR imaging, a lesion of low signal intensity on T1-weighted spin echo MR images and high signal intensity on T2-weighted spin echo MR images is evident. Fluid levels have been observed. Adjacent soft tissue lesions may also be noted.

Pathologically, intraosseous ganglia are most often located at the end of the bone, with normal-appearing adjacent articular cartilage. The "cyst" is smooth and round or oval, and it may have a bluish color; typically it is not fluid filled but contains thick, gelatinous material, as opposed to the clearer, less viscid synovial fluid or the serous or serosanguineous contents of a simple or aneurysmal bone cyst. Multiple small or large cavities that communicate or are separated by connective tissue septa are evident. Histologically, the structure of an intraosseous ganglion cyst is identical to that of soft tissue ganglia. Curettage or excision of the bone lesion is usually curative, although recurrent lesions develop in some cases.

The differential diagnosis of the radiographic findings of intraosseous ganglion cysts includes a variety of lesions that lead to epiphyseal and subchondral radiolucent foci,

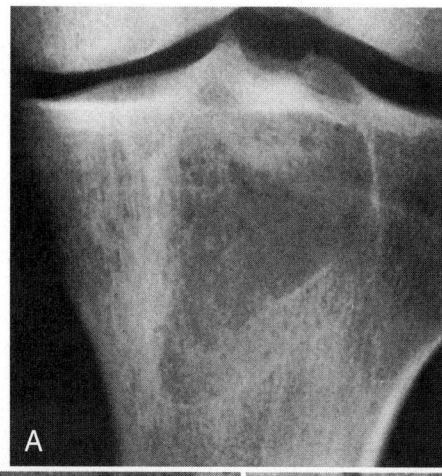
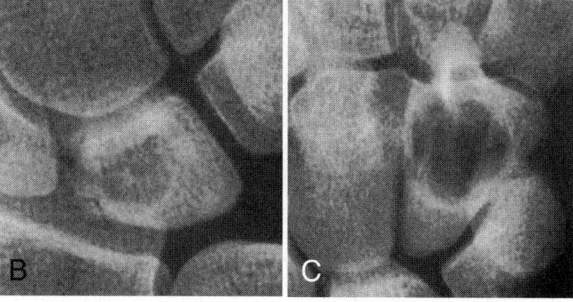

**Figure 70–108.** Intraosseous ganglion cysts. *A,* Tibia. Radiograph reveals a well-marginated osteolytic lesion in the proximal portion of the tibia that extends to subchondral bone. *B,* Lunate bone. A focal radiolucent region is affecting the radial aspect of the lunate bone. *C,* Hamate bone. A similar lesion of the hamate bone is evident.

such as giant cell tumor and chondroblastoma. The sclerotic margin about the ganglion cyst and the absence of calcification generally allow its differentiation from these tumors. Intraosseous ganglion cysts, however, share many radiographic features with the subchondral cysts of osteoarthritis.

## Locally Aggressive or Malignant Tumors

### Adamantinoma

Adamantinoma is an extremely rare, locally aggressive or malignant bone lesion. The lesion is similar to the more common ameloblastoma of the bones of the jaw. Recent studies have found that the cells of an adamantinoma have an epithelial phenotype. A number of investigations have addressed the relationship of adamantinoma to other lesions, particularly fibrous dysplasia and ossifying fibroma of long bone (osteofibrous dysplasia).

**Clinical Abnormalities.** Adamantinomas are slightly more common in men than in women. Although the age of patients with this lesion is variable, most are in the second through fifth decades of life; females are affected at an earlier age.

**Skeletal Location.** Its striking predilection for the long tubular bones (97% of cases) and, specifically, the tibia (80% to 85% of cases) is the most characteristic feature of this tumor. Other bones that are involved include the humerus, ulna, femur, fibula, and radius. An extratibial location, however, is so unusual that alternative diagnoses must be carefully excluded before accepting such cases as examples of adamantinoma. Multifocal lesions may rarely develop in a single bone or in two or more bones. Within a long tubular bone, diaphyseal localization predominates, although metaphyseal extension of lesions within the diaphysis or isolated involvement of a metaphysis is occasionally encountered.

**Radiographic Abnormalities.** In the tibia, adamantinoma is usually localized in the middle third of the bone and appears as a central or eccentric, multilocular, slightly expansile, sharply or poorly delineated osteolytic lesion. Although this osteolytic lesion is similar or identical to that of ossifying fibroma, abnormality of the medullary bone, which occurs with more extensive involvement in adamantinoma, is not characteristic of ossifying fibroma. In adamantinoma, reactive bone sclerosis and small satellite radiolucent foci in direct continuity with the major lesion may be identified. In fact, lesions in the adjacent fibula may be seen (Fig. 70–109). Periostitis is not usually apparent in the absence of a pathologic fracture.

Radiographically, differentiation of adamantinoma, fibrous dysplasia, and osteofibrous dysplasia may be very difficult. The most important findings suggesting a diagnosis of fibrous dysplasia are, in order of decreasing importance, young age; presence of a "ground-glass" appearance, with or without additional opacification; absence of multilayered periosteal reaction and moth-eaten bone destruction; and presence of anterior bowing of the tibia. The presence of infantile or congenital pseudarthrosis of the tibia, although an infrequent find-ing of fibrous dysplasia, excludes the diagnosis of adamantinoma. Similarly, the features of adamantinoma and osteofibrous dysplasia of the tibia may be indistinguishable.

**Pathologic Abnormalities.** The microscopic pattern is generally one in which epithelial-like cells assume a variety of forms and reside within a fibrous stroma. The fibrous stroma commonly consists of benign-appearing fibroblasts arranged in a cartwheel or storiform pattern similar to that found in fibrous histiocytoma, ossifying fibroma, or fibrous dysplasia.

**Relationship to Other Lesions.** The term "differentiated" adamantinoma has been used for purely intracortical locations in the tibia, fibula, or both, with a uniform histologic pattern indistinguishable from what was previously termed ossifying fibroma (osteofibrous dysplasia). The lesion may contain occasional inconspicuous nests of small epithelial cells. This lesion differs from conventional adamantinoma, in which patients are usually young to middle-aged adults, the epithelial component is widespread, and any ossifying fibroma–like component is generally seen only at the periphery of the lesion. This has led some investigators to conclude that at least some examples of ossifying fibroma represent a regressive form of adamantinoma; however, this is not fully accepted. The relationship of fibro-osseous lesions to adamantinoma is unclear: some authors indicate that the fibro-osseous lesions represent regressive changes in underlying adamantinoma, others indicate that they may be precursor lesions to adamantinoma, and still others suggest that they have no relationship to the development of adamantinoma. Resolution of this controversy awaits further reports of these unusual lesions.

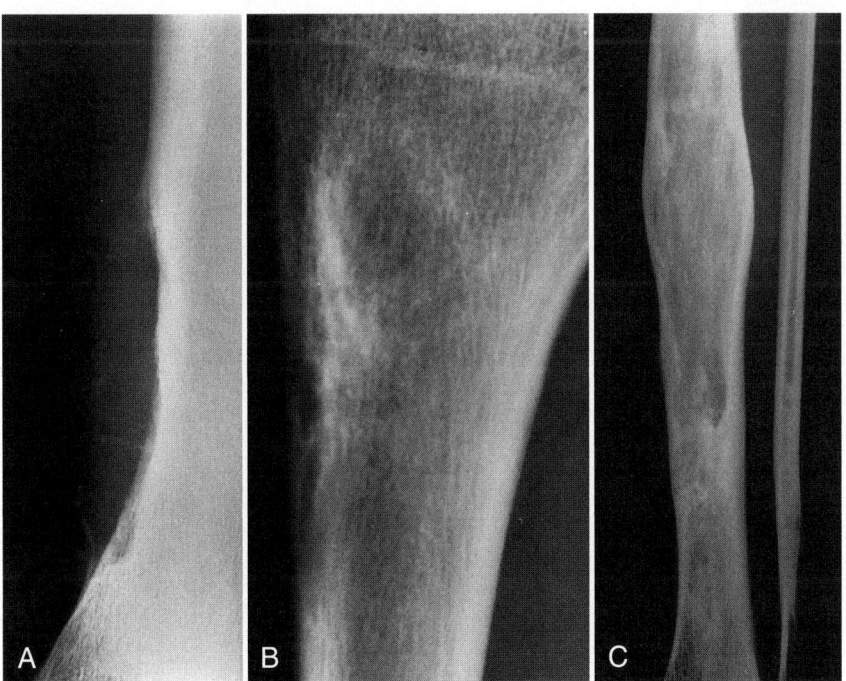

**Figure 70–109.** Adamantinoma. *A,* In this 35-year-old man with an enlarging mass in the medial aspect of the lower leg, a radiograph shows an expansile lesion arising from the distal tibial surface. The external portion of the cortex is eroded, and trabeculae extend into the soft tissue component of the lesion. Minimal periostitis is seen. *B,* In a different patient, an eccentric, predominantly osteolytic lesion involves the proximal metaphysis of the tibia. Bone sclerosis is also apparent, and periostitis is absent. *C,* In this patient, lesions accompanied by both bone sclerosis and lysis are observed in the tibia and fibula. (*B,* Courtesy of R. Freiberger, MD, New York, NY. *C,* Courtesy of R. Kerr, MD, Los Angeles, Calif.)

**Natural History**. Adamantinomas are locally aggressive tumors with the potential to metastasize. Growth of the initial tumor may be slow. Recurrence of tumor is frequent after inadequate therapy. Although the 10-year patient survival rate has been estimated to be as high as 65%, a lower figure is probably more accurate.

## Malignant Tumors

### Ewing's Sarcoma

Ewing's sarcoma is a relatively common malignant tumor of unresolved histogenesis. Recent immunohistochemical and cytogenic studies suggest a neuroectodermal origin of the tumor. Recent descriptions show a close relationship between Ewing's sarcoma and peripheral neuroectodermal tumor (see later discussion), both of which share a common chromosomal translocation.

#### *Clinical Abnormalities*

Ewing's sarcoma is usually identified in patients in the first, second, or third decade of life; approximately 90% of persons with this neoplasm are between 5 and 30 years old at the initial clinical examination. A slight male predilection and an overwhelming preponderance of white patients have been noted. The rarity of Ewing's sarcoma in blacks deserves emphasis. Localized pain and swelling may be combined with fever, weight loss, anemia, and leukocytosis, similar to the clinical findings of infection. Other manifestations depend on the specific site of involvement.

#### *Skeletal Location*

Ewing's sarcoma affects principally the lower segment of the skeleton, with the sacrum, innominate bone, and bones in the lower extremity accounting for approximately two thirds of all cases. The most frequent sites of involvement are the femur, ilium, tibia, humerus, fibula, and ribs; Ewing's sarcoma is relatively uncommon in the vertebrae above the sacrum. In the long tubular bones, Ewing's sarcoma is metadiaphyseal or diaphyseal in location or, less commonly, metaphyseal. Isolated involvement of the epiphysis is rare.

In the vertebral column, sacral involvement dominates, followed in order of decreasing frequency by the lumbar, thoracic, cervical, and coccygeal regions. The vertebral body is primarily affected, although the neoplasm may extend from this region to the posterior osseous elements of the vertebra. With regard to the thoracic cage, Ewing's sarcoma predominates in the ribs, with less common or rare involvement of the scapula, clavicle, and sternum.

#### *Radiographic Abnormalities*

The fundamental radiographic findings in Ewing's sarcoma reflect the aggressive nature of this lesion and include osteolysis, cortical erosion or violation, periostitis, and a soft tissue mass. The bone destruction is generally permeative or moth-eaten in appearance; the periosteal response is often exuberant and may consist of multiple layers of new bone (laminated, onionskin, or onion-peel

pattern) or horizontally oriented, thin osseous strands extending at right angles to the parent bone (hair-on-end pattern). Although Ewing's sarcoma is classically a medullary lesion, changes in the cortex of the bone may be dominant.

Common manifestations include poorly marginated bone destruction (96% of cases), soft tissue involvement (80%), laminated periostitis (57%), and osteosclerosis (40%). The last finding apparently results from reactive bone formation and osteoid deposition on foci of necrotic bone. Less common manifestations include spiculated (hair-on-end or sunburst) periostitis (28%), thickening (21%) or violation (19%) of the cortex, pure osteolysis (19%), pathologic fracture (15%), osseous expansion (13%), and cystic abnormality (12%).

**Tubular Bones**. A poorly defined, osteolytic, metadiaphyseal lesion in a long tubular bone accompanied by cortical erosion, periostitis, and a soft tissue mass is the classic description (Fig. 70–110). The bone sclerosis in some cases resembles that seen in osteosarcoma. Similar abnormalities are observed in Ewing's sarcoma in the metacarpal and metatarsal bones and in the phalanges. The major differential diagnostic considerations in the bones of the peripheral skeleton are osteosarcoma, lymphoma, and infection.

**Vertebral Column**. Ewing's sarcoma in a vertebral body leads to bone destruction, which may be followed by fracture and collapse (Fig. 70–111). Less frequently, osteosclerosis of a vertebral body or even a pedicle or other posterior osseous element is observed. Extension of the process into the paraspinal and intraspinal tissues is well described. In the sacrum, osteolysis, cortical destruction, and a soft tissue mass are encountered. The differential diagnosis of Ewing's sarcoma in the vertebral column includes pyogenic or tuberculous osteomyelitis, lymphoma, leukemia, histiocytosis, and metastatic disease.

**Innominate Bone**. Although the radiographic abnormalities accompanying Ewing's sarcoma in the innominate bone are similar to those in other skeletal sites, a large soft tissue mass containing calcification may be evident (Fig. 70–112). When combined with significant alterations in the bone itself, the resulting radiographic appearance is easily misinterpreted as evidence of osteosarcoma or chondrosarcoma.

**Other Sites**. In the ribs, Ewing's sarcoma produces lesions that are predominantly osteolytic or osteosclerotic or exhibit both osteolysis and osteosclerosis. The large size of the extrapleural mass in comparison to the subtle rib destruction can be striking.

#### *Other Imaging Techniques*

Bone scintigraphy generally shows increased uptake of the radionuclide in foci of Ewing's sarcoma. MR imaging and CT are best used to define the extent of Ewing's sarcoma (Figs. 70–113 and 70–114). Available data regarding the role of MR imaging in evaluating the response of Ewing's sarcoma to chemotherapy are not uniform.

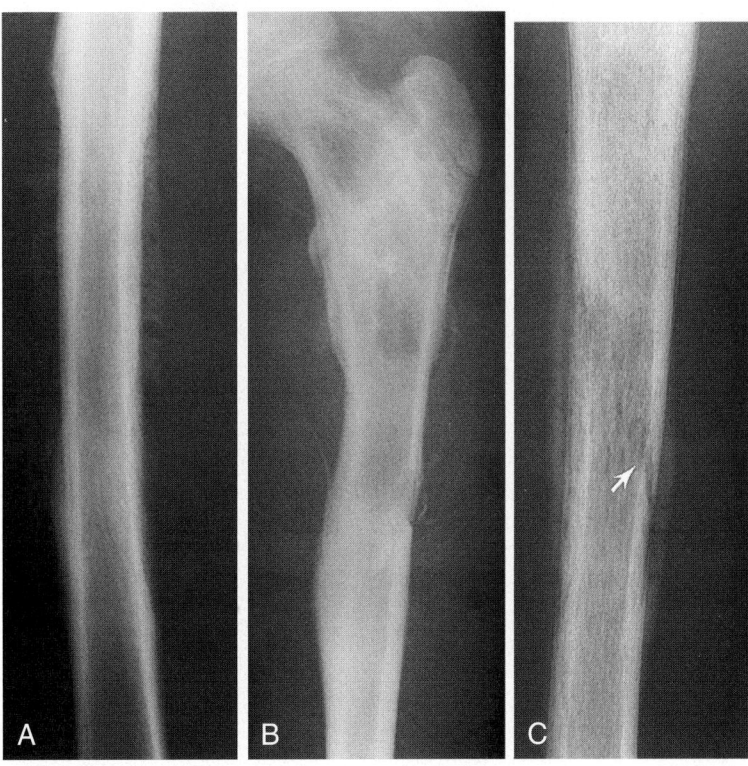

**Figure 70–110.** Ewing's sarcoma: long tubular bones. *A,* Observe a long lesion in the diaphysis of the femur. The predominant abnormalities are evident on the surface of the bone in the form of cortical saucerization and a hair-on-end periosteal reaction. *B,* Ill-defined osteolysis in the metaphysis and diaphysis of the femur is accompanied by various types of periostitis, cortical erosion, and a soft tissue mass. *C,* Permeative bone destruction and periostitis are observed in the humerus. A pathologic fracture *(arrow)* is present.

### Pathologic Abnormalities

Ewing's sarcomas are relatively large at the time of initial clinical evaluation. An associated extraosseous neoplastic component is present in 80% to 100% of cases.

Pathologic fractures are evident in up to 15% of cases. Ewing's sarcoma is composed of essentially small, round, undifferentiated tumor cells. The tumor cells are usually crowded together in sheets or segregated in lobules by fine fibrovascular septa. Ewing's sarcomas are usually vascular, with frequent hemorrhagic areas and extensive necrosis.

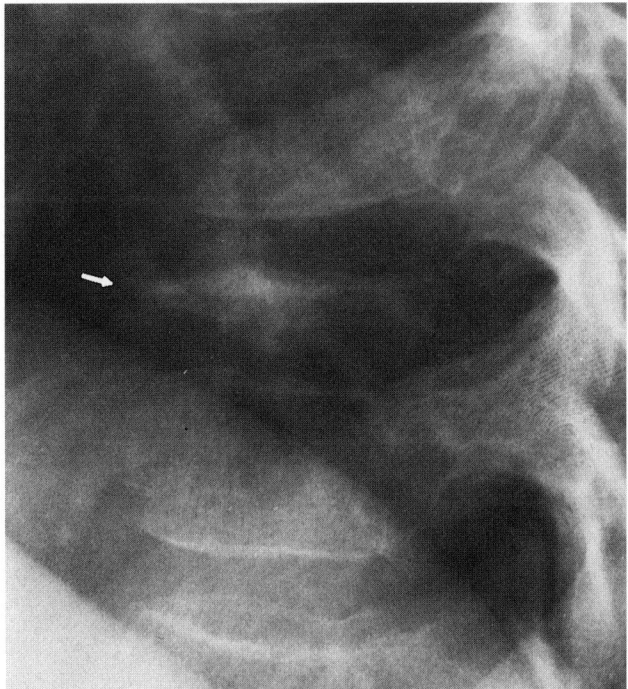

**Figure 70–111.** Ewing's sarcoma: vertebral column. Note the complete collapse of a thoracic vertebral body *(arrow).* Although this abnormality occurred as a result of skeletal metastasis from Ewing's sarcoma, a similar change is observed in primary Ewing's sarcoma.

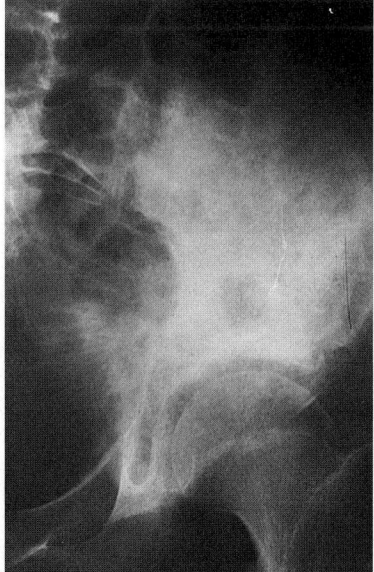

**Figure 70–112.** Ewing's sarcoma: ilium and ischium. Extensive osteosclerosis, periosteal response, and soft tissue radiodense areas are seen.

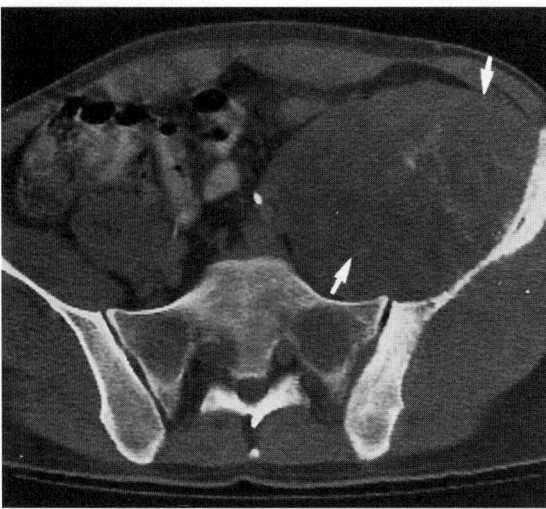
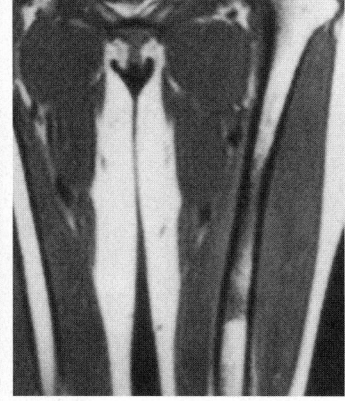
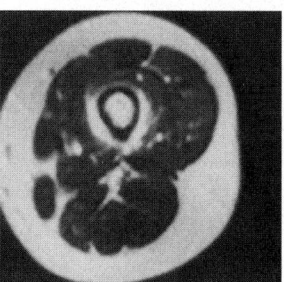

**Figure 70–113.** Ewing's sarcoma. *A*, CT scan depicts Ewing's sarcoma of the pelvis. Note osteolytic and osteosclerotic lesion involving the entire ilium. A soft tissue mass is observed extending into the pelvis. Note the periosteal response and mineralization in the intrapelvic soft tissue mass. *B* and *C*, is a different patient with involvement of the femoral shaft, coronal T₁-weighted (TR/TE, 2200/80) spin-echo MR image shows the marrow replacement as well as extension into the periosseous tissue.

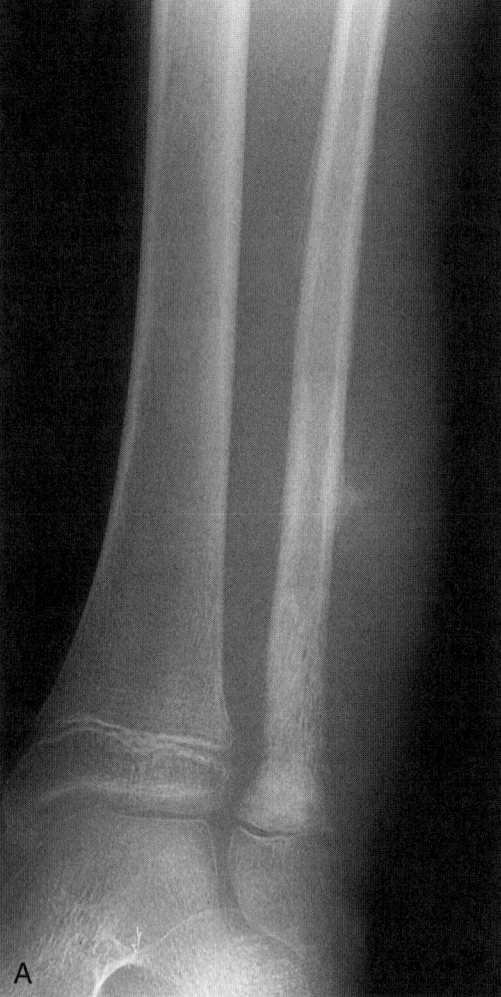
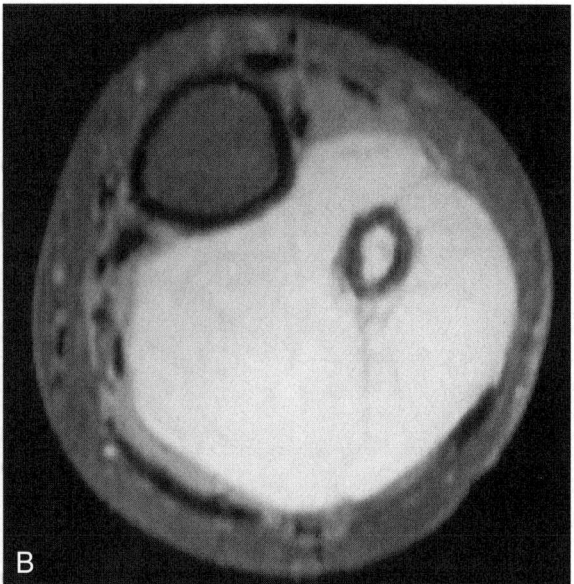

**Figure 70–114.** Ewing's sarcoma: fibula. In this 10-year-old boy, a conventional radiograph *(A)* documents a permeative lesion in the distal portion of the fibula, with a large soft tissue mass containing a small amount of ossification. The size of the soft tissue component is evident on a transverse fat-suppressed fast spin echo (TR/TE, 3800/17) MR image *(B)*.

## Natural History

Ewing's sarcoma is regarded as a highly aggressive tumor with the propensity to invade local tissues and disseminate throughout the body. It has been estimated that between 15% and 30% of patients with Ewing's sarcoma have metastatic disease. The recent use of both radiation therapy and chemotherapy, sometimes in combination with surgery, has had a dramatically favorable impact on the prognosis of patients with this type of cancer.

Routine radiography can be used to evaluate patients who have received therapy for Ewing's sarcoma. Radiographic changes suggesting healing occur within a period of months and include maturation of the periosteal response, reconstitution of the cortex, and increasing bone sclerosis; changes suggesting recurrent or persistent disease also occur within months and include failure of the predicted healing pattern to develop or progression of the initial neoplastic changes.

## Additional Types of Lesions

A large cell (atypical) type of Ewing's sarcoma that represents approximately 5% to 15% of all such sarcomas has been described. The large cell variant is usually observed in patients in the first or second decade of life and is more common in males than in females. Localization in a tubular bone is most frequent, and a permeative pattern of osteolysis is the dominant radiographic abnormality.

A soft tissue neoplasm resembling Ewing's sarcoma (extraskeletal Ewing's sarcoma) has also been described. Both men and women are affected, and the age of involved patients is quite varied. Common sites of involvement are the thigh, paravertebral region, pelvis, and lower extremity. Although a soft tissue mass is the hallmark of the lesion, osseous changes such as bone sclerosis and periosteal reaction may be evident.

Primary (primitive) neuroectodermal tumors (PNETs) of bone resemble Ewing's sarcoma on histologic analysis and relate to the same chromosomal translocation. Hence, many investigators believe that Ewing's sarcoma may constitute a poorly differentiated form of PNET. PNET may also occur in the soft tissues, including the retroperitoneum, pelvis, chest wall, and extremities. Askin's tumor, which typically occurs in the thoracopulmonary soft tissues in children and adolescents, has been shown to be a peripheral neuroectodermal tumor.

## FURTHER READING

Allman RA: RPC of the month from the AFIP. Radiology 93:167, 1969.

Arata MA, Peterson HA, Dahlin DC: Pathological fractures through non-ossifying fibromas: Review of the Mayo Clinic experience. J Bone Joint Surg Am 63:980, 1981.

Azouz EM, Slomic AM, Marton D, et al: The variable manifestations of dysplasia epiphysealis hemimelica. Pediatr Radiol 15:44, 1985.

Baker ND, Greenspan A, Neuwirth M: Symptomatic vertebral hemangiomas: A report of four cases. Skeletal Radiol 15:458, 1986.

Beggs IG, Stoker DJ: Chondromyxoid fibroma of bone. Clin Radiol 33:671, 1982.

Beltran J, Simon DC, Levy M, et al: Aneurysmal bone cysts: MR imaging at 1.5T. Radiology 158:689, 1986.

Bertoni F, Boriani S, Laus M, et al: Periosteal chondrosarcoma and periosteal osteosarcoma: Two distinct entities. J Bone Joint Surg Br 64:370, 1982.

Bertoni F, Calderoni P, Bacchini P, et al: Desmoplastic fibroma of bone: A report of six cases. J Bone Joint Surg Br 66:265, 1984.

Bjorkengren AG, Resnick D, Haghighi P, et al: Intraosseous glomus tumor: Report of a case and review of the literature. AJR Am J Roentgenol 147:739, 1986.

Blumberg ML: CT of iliac unicameral bone cysts. AJR Am J Roentgenol 136:1231, 1981.

Bonakdarpour A, Levy WM, Aegerter E: Primary and secondary aneurysmal bone cyst: A radiological study of 75 cases. Radiology 126:75, 1978.

Boriani S, Bacchini P, Bertoni F, et al: Periosteal chondroma: A review of twenty cases. J Bone Joint Surg Am 65:205, 1983.

Boyko OB, Cory DA, Cohen MD, et al: MR imaging of osteogenic and Ewing's sarcoma. AJR Am J Roentgenol 148:317, 1987.

Boyle WJ: Cystic angiomatosis of bone: A report of three cases and review of the literature. J Bone Joint Surg Br 54:626, 1972.

Broderick TW, Resnick D, Goergen TG, et al: Enostosis of the spine. Spine 3:167, 1978.

Brower AC, Culver JE Jr, Keats TE: Diffuse cystic angiomatosis of bone: Report of two cases. AJR Am J Roentgenol 118:456, 1973.

Bucy PC, Capp CS: Primary hemangioma of bone with special reference to roentgenologic diagnosis. AJR Am J Roentgenol 23:1, 1930.

Buirski G, Ratliff AHC, Watt I: Cartilage-cell-containing tumours of the pelvis: A radiological review of 40 patients. Br J Radiol 59:197, 1986.

Buirski G, Watt I: The radiological features of "solid" aneurysmal bone cysts. Br J Radiol 57:1057, 1984.

Byers P, Mantle J, Salm R: Epidermal cysts of phalanges. J Bone Joint Surg Br 48:577, 1966.

Caffey J: On fibrous defects in cortical walls of growing tubular bones: Their radiologic appearance, structure, prevalence, natural course, and diagnostic significance. Adv Pediatr 7:13, 1955.

Campanacci M, Baldini N, Boriani S, et al: Giant-cell tumor of bone. J Bone Joint Surg Am 69:106, 1987.

Campanacci M, Boriani S, Giunti A: Hemangioendothelioma of bone: A study of 29 cases. Cancer 46:804, 1980.

Campanacci M, Cervellati G: Osteosarcoma: A review of 345 cases. Ital J Orthop Traumatol 1:5, 1975.

Campanacci M, Laus M: Osteofibrous dysplasia of the tibia and fibula. J Bone Joint Surg Am 63:367, 1981.

Campanacci M, Picci P, Gherlinzoni F, et al: Parosteal osteosarcoma. J Bone Joint Surg Br 66:313, 1984.

Capanna R, Albisinni U, Caroli GC, et al: Contrast examination as a prognostic factor in the treatment of solitary bone cyst by cortisone injection. Skeletal Radiol 12:97, 1984.

Capanna R, Dal Monte A, Gitelis S, et al: The natural history of unicameral bone cyst after steroid injection. Clin Orthop 166:204, 1982.

Carlson DH, Wilkinson RH, Bhakkaviziam A: Aneurysmal bone cysts in children. AJR Am J Roentgenol 116:644, 1972.

Cohen EK, Kressel HY, Frank TS, et al: Hyaline cartilage–origin bone and soft-tissue neoplasms: MR appearance and histologic correlation. Radiology 167:477, 1988.

Cooper KL, Beabout JW, Dahlin DC: Giant cell tumor: Ossification in soft-tissue implants. Radiology 153:597, 1984.

Dahlin DC: Giant cell tumor of bone: Highlights of 407 cases. AJR Am J Roentgenol 144:955, 1985.

Dahlin DC, Coventry MB, Scanlon PW: Ewing's sarcoma: A critical analysis of 165 cases. J Bone Joint Surg Am 43:185, 1961.

Dahlin DC, Ivins JC: Benign chondroblastoma: A study of 125 cases. Cancer 30:401, 1972.

Dahlin DC, McLeod RA: Aneurysmal bone cyst and other nonneoplastic conditions. Skeletal Radiol 8:243, 1982.

de Lange EE, Pope TL Jr, Fechner RE: Dedifferentiated chondrosarcoma: Radiographic features. Radiology 160:489, 1986.

Demos TC, Bruno E, Armin A, et al: Parosteal lipoma with enlarging osteochondroma. AJR Am J Roentgenol 143:365, 1984.

de Santos LA, Murray JA, Finklestein JB, et al: The radiographic spectrum of periosteal osteosarcoma. Radiology 127:123, 1978.

de Santos LA, Spjut HJ: Periosteal chondroma: A radiographic spectrum. Skeletal Radiol 6:15, 1981.

Destouet JM, Gilula LA, Murphy WA: Computed tomography of long-bone osteosarcoma. Radiology 131:439, 1979.

Destouet JM, Kyriakos M, Gilula LA: Fibrous histiocytoma (fibroxanthoma) of a cervical vertebra: A report with a review of the literature. Skeletal Radiol 5:241, 1980.

Dwyer AJ, Glaubiger DL, Ecker JG, et al: The radiographic follow-up of patients with Ewing's sarcoma: A demonstration of a general method. Radiology 145:327, 1982.

Edeiken J, Farrell C, Ackerman LV, et al: Parosteal sarcoma. AJR Am J Roentgenol 111:579, 1971.

Edeiken J, Raymond AK, Ayala AG, et al: Small-cell osteosarcoma. Skeletal Radiol 16:621, 1987.

El-Khoury GY, Bassett GS: Symptomatic bursa formation with osteochondromas. AJR Am J Roentgenol 133:895, 1979.

Enneking WF, Springfield DS: Osteosarcoma. Orthop Clin North Am 8:785, 1977.

Eversole LR, Rovin S: Differential radiographic diagnosis of lesions of the jawbones. Radiology 105:277, 1972.

Eyre-Brook AL, Price CHG: Fibrosarcoma of bone: Review of fifty consecutive cases from the Bristol bone tumour registry. J Bone Joint Surg Br 51:20, 1969.

Feldman F, Hecht HL, Johnston AD: Chondromyxoid fibroma of bone. Radiology 94:249, 1970.

Feldman F, Johnston A: Intraosseous ganglion. AJR Am J Roentgenol 118:328, 1973.

Feldman F, Norman D: Intra- and extraosseous malignant histiocytoma (malignant fibrous xanthoma). Radiology 104:497, 1972.

Fernbach SK, Blumenthal DH, Poznanski AK, et al: Radiographic changes in unicameral bone cysts following direct injection of steroids: A report on 14 cases. Radiology 140:689, 1981.

Firooznia H, Pinto RS, Lin JP, et al: Chordoma: Radiologic evaluation of 20 cases. AJR Am J Roentgenol 127:797, 1976.

Freiberger RH, Loitman BS, Helpern M, et al: Osteoid osteoma: A report on 80 cases. AJR Am J Roentgenol 82:194, 1959.

Friedman MM: Neurofibromatosis of bone. AJR Am J Roentgenol 51:623, 1944.

Ginaldi S, de Santos LA: Computed tomography in the evaluation of small round cell tumors of bone. Radiology 134:441, 1980.

Glass TA, Mills SE, Fechner RE, et al: Giant-cell reparative granuloma of the hands and feet. Radiology 149:65, 1983.

Goergen TG, Dickman PS, Resnick D, et al: Long bone ossifying fibromas. Cancer 39:2067, 1977.

Goldenberg RR, Campbell CJ, Bonfiglio M: Giant-cell tumor of bone: An analysis of two hundred and eighteen cases. J Bone Joint Surg Am 52:619, 1970.

Greenway G, Resnick D, Bookstein JJ: Popliteal pseudoaneurysm as a complication of an adjacent osteochondroma: Angiographic diagnosis. AJR Am J Roentgenol 132:294, 1979.

Hart JAL: Intraosseous lipoma. J Bone Joint Surg Br 55:624, 1973.

Healey JH, Ghelman B: Osteoid osteoma and osteoblastoma: Current concepts and recent advances. Clin Orthop 204:76, 1986.

Henderson ED, Dahlin DC: Chondrosarcoma of bone: A study of two hundred and eighty-eight cases. J Bone Joint Surg Am 45:1450, 1963.

Hudson TM: Fluid levels in aneurysmal bone cysts: A CT feature. AJR Am J Roentgenol 141:1001, 1984.

Hudson TM, Chew FS, Manaster BJ: Scintigraphy of benign exostoses and exostotic chondrosarcoma. AJR Am J Roentgenol 140:581, 1983.

Hudson TM, Hamlin DJ, Fitzsimmons JR: Magnetic resonance imaging of fluid levels in an aneurysmal bone cyst and in anticoagulated human blood. Skeletal Radiol 13:267, 1985.

Hudson TM, Schiebler M, Springfield DS, et al: Radiology of giant cell tumors of bone: Computed tomography, arthrotomography, and scintigraphy. Skeletal Radiol 11:85, 1984.

Hudson TM, Springfield DS, Benjamin M, et al: Computed tomography of parosteal osteosarcoma. AJR Am J Roentgenol 144:961, 1985.

Huvos AG: Bone Tumors: Diagnosis, Treatment and Prognosis. Philadelphia, WB Saunders, 1979.

Huvos AG, Marcove RC: Adamantinoma of long bones: A clinicopathological study of fourteen cases with vascular origin suggested. J Bone Joint Surg Am 57:148, 1975.

Jacobs P: The diagnosis of osteoclastoma (giant-cell tumour): A radiological and pathological correlation. Br J Radiol 45:121, 1972.

Jaffe HL: Osteoid-osteoma of bone. Radiology 45:319, 1945.

Jaffe HL: Tumors and Tumorous Conditions of the Bones and Joints. Philadelphia, Lea & Febiger, 1958.

Jaffe HL, Lichtenstein L: Benign chondroblastoma of bone: A reinterpretation of the so-called calcifying or chondromatous giant cell tumor. Am J Pathol 18:969, 1942.

Jaffe HL, Lichtenstein L: Chondromyxoid fibroma of bone: A distinctive benign tumor likely to be mistaken especially for chondrosarcoma. Arch Pathol 45:541, 1948.

Jaffe HL, Lichtenstein L: Solitary unicameral bone cyst: With emphasis on the roentgen picture, the pathologic appearance and the pathogenesis. Arch Surg 44:1004, 1942.

Jaffe HL, Lichtenstein L, Portis RB: Giant cell tumor of bone: Its pathologic appearance, grading, supposed variants and treatment. Arch Pathol 30:993, 1940.

Jones SN, Stoker DJ: Radiology at your fingertips: Lesions of the terminal phalanx. Clin Radiol 39:478, 1988.

Keats T: Dysplasia epiphysealis hemimelica. Radiology 68:558, 1957.

Kenney PJ, Gilula LA, Murphy WA: The use of computed tomography to distinguish osteochondroma and chondrosarcoma. Radiology 139:129, 1981.

Kransdorf MJ, Sweet DE: Aneurysmal bone cyst: Concept, controversy, clinical presentation, and imaging. AJR Am J Roentgenol 164:573, 1995.

Kroon HM, Bloem JL, Holscher HC, et al: MR imaging of edema accompanying benign and malignant bone tumors. Skeletal Radiol 23:261, 1994.

Kumar R, David R, Cierney G: Clear cell chondrosarcoma. Radiology 154:45, 1985.

Kyriakos M, Land VJ, Penning L, et al: Metastatic chondroblastoma: Report of a fatal case with a review of the literature on atypical, aggressive, and malignant chondroblastoma. Cancer 55:1770, 1985.

Landon GC, Johnson KA, Dahlin DC: Subungual exostoses. J Bone Joint Surg Am 61:256, 1979.

Laredo J-D, Assouline E, Gelbert F, et al: Vertebral hemangiomas: Fat content as a sign of aggressiveness. Radiology 177:467, 1990.

Laredo J-D, Reizine D, Bard M, et al: Vertebral hemangiomas: Radiologic evaluation. Radiology 161:183, 1986.

Lavallee G, Lemarbre L, Bouchard R, et al: Ewing's sarcoma in adults. J Can Assoc Radiol 30:223, 1979.

Lee BS, Kaplan R: Turret exostosis of the phalanges. Clin Orthop 100:186, 1974.

Levy WM, Miller AS, Bonakdarpour A, et al: Aneurysmal bone cyst secondary to other osseous lesions: Report of 57 cases. Am J Clin Pathol 63:1, 1975.

Lichtenstein L: Aneurysmal bone cyst: A pathological entity commonly mistaken for giant-cell tumor and occasionally for hemangioma and osteogenic sarcoma. Cancer 3:279, 1950.

Lichtenstein L: Benign osteoblastoma: Category of osteoid- and bone-forming tumors other than classical osteoid osteoma, which may be mistaken for giant-cell tumor or osteogenic sarcoma. Cancer 9:1044, 1956.

Lindell MM Jr, Shirkhoda A, Raymond AK, et al: Parosteal osteosarcoma: Radiologic-pathologic correlation with emphasis on CT. AJR Am J Roentgenol 148:323, 1987.

Lodwick GS: The radiologist's role in the management of chondrosarcoma. Radiology 150:275, 1984.

Lorenzo JC, Dorfman HD: Giant-cell reparative granuloma of short tubular bones of the hands and feet. Am J Surg Pathol 4:551, 1980.

Manizer F, Minagi H, Steinbach HL: The variable manifestations of multiple enchondromatosis. Radiology 99:377, 1971.

Mathis WH Jr, Schulz MD: Roentgen diagnosis of glomus tumors. Radiology 51:71, 1948.

McFarland GB, Morden ML: Benign cartilaginous lesions. Orthop Clin North Am 8:737, 1977.

McInerney DP, Middlemiss JH: Giant-cell tumour of bone. Skeletal Radiol 2:195, 1978.

McIvor J: The radiological features of ameloblastoma. Clin Radiol 25:237, 1974.

McLeod RA, Beabout JW: The roentgenographic features of chondroblastoma. AJR Am J Roentgenol 118:464, 1973.

McLeod RA, Dahlin DC, Beabout JW: The spectrum of osteoblastoma. AJR Am J Roentgenol 126:321, 1976.

Meyer JE, Lepke RA, Lindfors KK, et al: Chordomas: Their CT appearance in the cervical thoracic and lumbar spine. Radiology 153:693, 1984.

Milgran JW: The origins of osteochondromas and enchondromas: A histopathologic study. Clin Orthop 174:264, 1983.

Mindell ER: Chordoma. J Bone Joint Surg Am 63:501, 1981.

Mirra JM, Bernard GW, Bullough PG, et al: Cementum-like bone production in solitary bone cysts (so-called "cementoma" of long bones): Report of three cases. Electron microscopic observations supporting a synovial origin to the simple bone cyst. Clin Orthop 135:295, 1978.

Mirra JM, Brien EW: Giant notochordal hamartoma of intraosseous origin: A newly reported benign entity to be distinguished from chordoma. Report of two cases. Skeletal Radiol 30:698, 2001.

Mirra JM, Gold RH, Rand F: Disseminated nonossifying fibromas in association with café-au-lait spots (Jaffe-Campanacci syndrome). Clin Orthop 168:192, 1982.

Mirra JM, Marcove RC: Fibrosarcomatous dedifferentiation of primary and secondary chondrosarcoma: Review of five cases. J Bone Joint Surg Am 56:285, 1974.

Moseley JE, Starobin SG: Cystic angiomatosis of bone: Manifestation of a hamartomatous disease entity. AJR Am J Roentgenol 91:1114, 1964.

Murphey MD, Nomikos GC, Flemming DJ, et al: Imaging of giant cell tumor and giant cell reparative granuloma of bone: Radiologic-pathologic correlation. Radiographics 21:1283, 2001.

Nakashima Y, Yamamuro T, Fujiwara Y, et al: Osteofibrous dysplasia (ossifying fibroma of long bones): A study of 12 cases. Cancer 52:909, 1983.

Norman A, Schiffman M: Simple bone cysts: Factors of age dependency. Radiology 124:779, 1977.

Norman A, Sissons HA: Radiographic hallmarks of peripheral chondrosarcoma. Radiology 151:589, 1984.

Ohno T, Abe M, Tateishi A, et al: Osteogenic sarcoma: A study of one hundred and thirty cases. J Bone Joint Surg Am 57:397, 1975.

O'Neal LW, Ackerman LV: Chondrosarcoma of bone. Cancer 5:551, 1952.

Onitsuka H: Roentgenologic aspects of bone islands. Radiology 123:607, 1977.

Picci P, Baldini N, Boriani S, et al: Giant cell reparative granuloma and other giant cell lesions of the bones of the hands and feet. Skeletal Radiol 15:415, 1986.

Rambo VB, Davies NE: Giant ameloblastomas. JAMA 238:418, 1977.

Ramos A, Castello J, Sartoris DJ, et al: Osseous lipoma: CT appearance. Radiology 157:615, 1985.

Reinus WR, Gilula LA, IESS Committee: Radiology of Ewing's sarcoma: Intergroup Ewing Sarcoma Study (IESS). Radiographics 4:929, 1984.

Reinus WR, Gilula LA, Shirley SK, et al: Radiographic appearance of Ewing sarcoma of the hands and feet: Report from the Intergroup Ewing Sarcoma Study. AJR Am J Roentgenol 144:331, 1985.

Reiter FB, Ackerman LV, Staple TW: Central chondrosarcoma of the appendicular skeleton. Radiology 105:525, 1972.

Resnick D, Greenway G: Distal femoral cortical defects, irregularities, and excavations: A critical review of the literature with the addition of histologic and paleopathologic data. Radiology 143:345, 1982.

Reynolds J: The "fallen fragment sign" in the diagnosis of unicameral bone cysts. Radiology 92:949, 1969.

Ros PR, Viamonte M Jr, Rywlin AM: Malignant fibrous histiocytoma: Mesenchymal tumor of ubiquitous origin. AJR Am J Roentgenol 142:753, 1984.

Rose JS, Hermann G, Mendelson DC, et al: Extraskeletal Ewing sarcoma with computed tomography correlation. Skeletal Radiol 9:234, 1983.

Rosen RS, Schwinn CP: Adamantinoma of limb bone: Malignant angioblastoma. AJR Am J Roentgenol 97:727, 1966.

Rosenthal DI, Schiller AL, Mankin HJ: Chondrosarcoma: Correlation of radiological and histological grade. Radiology 150:21, 1984.

Rosenthal DI, Scott JA, Mankin HJ, et al: Sacrococcygeal chordoma: Magnetic resonance imaging and computed tomography. AJR Am J Roentgenol 145:143, 1985.

Rousselin B, Vanel D, Terrier-Lacombe MJ, et al: Clinical and radiologic analysis of 13 cases of primary neuroectodermal tumors of bone. Skeletal Radiol 18:115, 1989.

Salvador AH, Beabout JW, Dahlin DC: Mesenchymal chondrosarcoma: Observations on 30 new cases. Cancer 28:605, 1971.

Samter TG, Vellios F, Shafer WG: Neurilemmoma of bone: Report of 3 cases with a review of the literature. Radiology 75:215, 1960.

Schajowicz F: Tumors and Tumorlike Lesions of Bones and Joints. New York, Springer-Verlag, 1981.

Schajowicz F, Aiello CL, Slullitel I: Cystic and pseudocystic lesions of the terminal phalanx with special reference to epidermoid cysts. Clin Orthop 68:84, 1970.

Schajowicz F, Gallardo H: Epiphyseal chondroblastoma of bone: A clinico-pathological study of sixty-nine cases. J Bone Joint Surg Br 52:205, 1970.

Schajowicz F, Lemos C: Osteoid osteoma and osteoblastoma: Closely related entities of osteoblastic derivation. Acta Orthop Scand 41:272, 1970.

Seiss SW, Enzinger FM: Malignant fibrous histiocytoma: An analysis of 200 cases. Cancer 41:2250, 1978.

Sherman RS, Soong KY: Aneurysmal bone cyst: Its roentgen diagnosis. Radiology 68:54, 1957.

Sherman RS, Soong KY: Ewing's sarcoma: Its roentgen classification and diagnosis. Radiology 66:529, 1956.

Sherman RS, Wilner D: The roentgen diagnosis of hemangioma of bone. AJR Am J Roentgenol 86:1146, 1961.

Sim FH, Dahlin DC, Beabout JW: Multicentric giant-cell tumor of bone. J Bone Joint Surg Am 59:1052, 1977.

Smith J, Ahuja SC, Huvos AG, et al: Parosteal (juxtacortical) osteogenic sarcoma: A roentgenological study of 30 patients. J Can Assoc Radiol 29:167, 1978.

Smith J, Heelan RT, Huvos AG, et al: Radiographic changes in primary osteogenic sarcoma following intensive chemotherapy: Radiological-pathological correlation in 63 patients. Radiology 143:355, 1982.

Smith RW, Smith CF: Solitary unicameral bone cyst of the calcaneus: A review of twenty cases. J Bone Joint Surg Am 56:49, 1974.

Snarr JW, Abell MR, Martel W: Lymphofollicular synovitis with osteoid osteoma. Radiology 106:557, 1973.

Spjut HJ, Dorfman HD, Fechner RE, et al: Tumors of bone and cartilage. In Atlas of Tumor Pathology, 2nd ser, fascicle 5. Washington, DC, Armed Forces Institute of Pathology, 1971.

Steiner GM, Farman J, Lawson JP: Lymphangiomatosis of bone. Radiology 93:1093, 1969.

Sundaram M, McGuire MH, Herbold DR: Magnetic resonance imaging of osteosarcoma. Skeletal Radiol 16:23, 1987.

Swee RG, McLeod RA, Beabout JW: Osteoid osteoma: Detection, diagnosis, and localization. Radiology 130:117, 1979.

Taber DS, Libshitz HI, Cohen MA: Treated Ewing sarcoma: Radiographic appearance in response, recurrence, and new primaries. AJR Am J Roentgenol 140:753, 1983.

Thayer C, Rogers LF: Unicentric osteosarcoma of bone with subsequent skeletal metastases. Skeletal Radiol 4:148, 1979.

Unni KK, Dahlin DC, Beabout JW, et al: Chondrosarcoma: Clear-cell variant. J Bone Joint Surg Am 58:676, 1976.

Unni KK, Dahlin DC, McLeod RA, et al: Intraosseous well-differentiated osteosarcoma. Cancer 40:1337, 1977.

Unni KK, Ivins JC, Beabout JW, et al: Hemangioma, hemangiopericytoma, and hemangioendothelioma (angiosarcoma) of bone. Cancer 27:1403, 1971.

Utne JR, Pugh DG: The roentgenologic aspects of chordoma. AJR Am J Roentgenol 74:593, 1955.

Vanel D, De Paolis M, Monti C, et al: Radiologic features of 24 periosteal chondrosarcomas. Skeletal Radiol 30:208, 2001.

Varma DGK, Ayala AG, Carrasco CH, et al: Chondrosarcoma: MR imaging with pathologic correlation. Radiographics 12:687, 1992.

Weiss SW, Dorfman HD: Adamantinoma of long bone: An analysis of nine new cases with emphasis on metastasizing lesions and fibrous dysplasia-like changes. Hum Pathol 8:141, 1977.

Wenger DE, Wold LE: Malignant vascular lesions of bone: Radiologic and pathologic features. Skeletal Radiol 29:619, 2000.

Wilner D: Radiology of Bone Tumors and Allied Disorders. Philadelphia, WB Saunders, 1982.

Wilson AJ, Kyriakos M, Ackerman LV: Chondromyxoid fibroma: Radiographic appearance in 38 cases and in a review of the literature. Radiology 179:513, 1991.

Wold LE, Unni KK, Beabout JW, et al: High-grade surface osteosarcoma. Am J Surg Pathol 8:181, 1984.

Wold LE, Unni KK, Cooper KL, et al: Hemangiopericytoma of bone. Am J Surg Pathol 6:53, 1982.

Woods ER, Martel W, Mandell SH, et al: Reactive soft-tissue mass associated with osteoid osteoma: Correlation of MR imaging features with pathologic findings. Radiology 186:221, 1993.

Zimmer WD, Berquist TH, McLeod RA, et al: Magnetic resonance imaging of osteosarcomas: Comparison with computed tomography. Clin Orthop 208:289, 1986.

# CHAPTER 71

## Tumors and Tumor-Like Lesions of Soft Tissues

### SUMMARY OF KEY FEATURES

The number of tumors and tumor-like lesions of soft tissues is impressive. Routine radiography is relatively insensitive in their detection, and it does not allow a specific diagnosis in most cases. Ultrasonography, computed tomography, scintigraphy, and magnetic resonance imaging are diagnostic methods with greater sensitivity for the detection of soft tissue masses, although in many instances, the specific cause of the mass remains elusive.

### INTRODUCTION

Both localized and generalized processes can affect the soft tissues. In this chapter, a general imaging approach to the correct identification and differential diagnosis of tumors and tumor-like lesions of the soft tissues is presented. Although the choice of an imaging method to assess soft tissue masses was rather limited not so long ago, recent technologic advances have been profound and are presenting both an opportunity and a challenge to physicians. The development of computed imaging techniques, especially magnetic resonance (MR) imaging, has led to the ability to manipulate imaging data and hence identify soft tissue processes. This chapter is not intended as a comprehensive review but as an overview, emphasizing the use of MR imaging in the evaluation of these lesions and highlighting those diagnoses that may be suggested by imaging.

In general, malignant tumors tend to be larger than benign ones. Serial or comparison films allow an assessment of the rate of growth. Very rapid enlargement of a mass can indicate hemorrhage, inflammation, or perhaps a malignant neoplasm, but caution is required because some malignant tumors may present as slowly growing masses. Shape and margin are also variable; however, malignancies tend to grow in a centrifugal fashion, compressing the adjacent normal tissue and forming a pseudocapsule, which may be remarkably well defined on imaging evaluation.

Tumor location is helpful in two ways in establishing a diagnosis. First, certain lesions have a predilection for specific skeletal locations. Examples include the tendency for some fibromatoses to involve the hands and feet and for elastofibromas and desmoid tumors to appear about the shoulder. Second, the compartmental localization (juxta-articular, subcutaneous, intermuscular, or intramuscular) may be helpful. Deep masses are more typically malignant.

Certain masses are often multiple, including neurofibromas and other neurogenic tumors, Kaposi's sarcoma, lipomas, and even metastases. Further, multiple soft tissue masses appearing near a primary soft tissue neoplasm may indicate lymph node metastases, an obvious sign of tumor aggressiveness. Most soft tissue sarcomas disseminate hematogenously, although metastasis to regional lymph nodes is not uncommon.

### IMAGING METHODS

#### Radiography

The evaluation of a suspected soft tissue mass begins with a radiograph. Although frequently unrewarding, radiographs may be diagnostic of a palpable lesion caused by an underlying skeletal deformity (such as exuberant callus formation related to prior trauma) or exostosis that may be masquerading as a soft tissue mass. Radiographs may also reveal soft tissue calcifications, which can be suggestive, and at times characteristic, of a specific diagnosis. For example, they may reveal the phleboliths within a hemangioma, the juxta-articular osteocartilaginous masses of synovial chondromatosis, the peripherally more mature ossification of myositis ossificans, or the characteristic bone changes of other processes with associated soft tissue involvement (Fig. 71–1). Even when it is not characteristic of a specific process, soft tissue calcification can suggest certain diagnoses. For example, nonspecific dystrophic calcifications in a slowly growing lower extremity mass in a young adult should suggest synovial sarcoma as the diagnosis of exclusion.

In addition, radiographs are the best initial method of assessing coexistent osseous involvement, such as remodeling, periosteal reaction, or overt osseous invasion and destruction. However, unlike bone tumors, the biologic activity of a soft tissue mass cannot be reliably assessed by its growth rate.

#### Ultrasonography

Ultrasonography has been used successfully to define the nature of certain soft tissue masses, particularly superficial ones, in both the axial and appendicular skeletons. Most notably, synovial cysts, tenosynovitis, and aneurysms are well delineated with ultrasonography, and this technique can be applied to other masses as well (see Chapter 6). Ultrasonography can be used to delineate local recurrence of soft tissue sarcomas and also to guide percutaneous needle aspiration of most lesions. Color Doppler sonography is a useful method for assessing the vascularity of tumors, as well as inflammatory processes.

#### Angiography

In general, the extent of vascularity of a soft tissue tumor correlates positively with the degree of malignancy. Exceptions to this rule are encountered in cases of

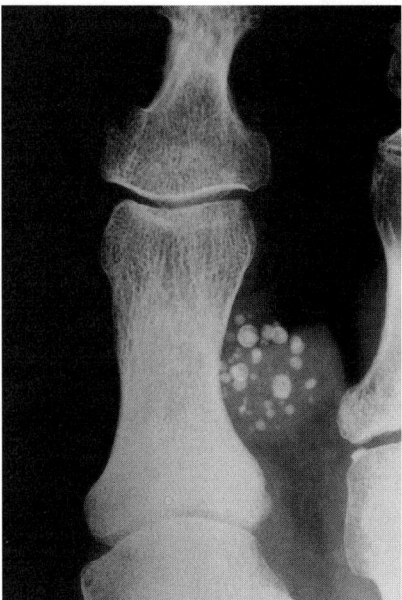

**Figure 71–1.** Soft tissue mass: hemangioma. The circular calcifications, some of which contain lucent centers, within the mass of this great toe represent pleboliths.

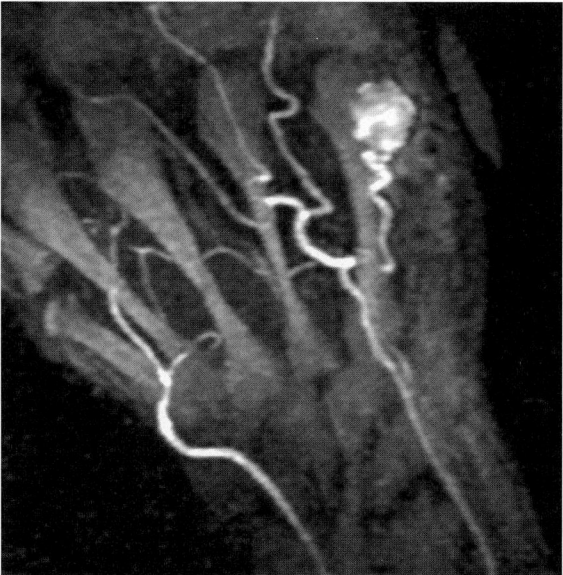

**Figure 71–2.** Soft tissue mass: spindle cell hemangioma. MR angiography accurately reflects the nature and architecture of the vascular mass.

hemangioma, hemangiopericytoma, and hibernoma, and benign and malignant lesions cannot be distinguished based on vascularity. MR angiography is increasingly used as a replacement for standard angiography in providing a "road map" of the regional vascular anatomy about soft tissue tumors (Fig. 71–2).

## Scintigraphy

The vast majority of malignant soft tissue neoplasms accumulate a radiotracer; however, as many as 50% of benign tumors do the same. Because of the diverse nature of the processes that may produce the accumulation of technetium (and other agents), the diagnostic capabilities of this technique are limited. Positive scans can accompany soft tissue neoplasm, infection, and diseases associated with local or widespread calcification. Scintigraphy using bone-seeking radiotracers is capable of predicting osseous involvement with a high degree of accuracy in cases of soft tissue sarcoma and may be more useful than computed tomography (CT) in this respect.

Positron emission tomography (PET) is increasingly being used in the assessment of musculoskeletal neoplasms. The uptake of glucose by tumors (when compared with non-neoplastic processes) can be documented through the use of PET and fludeoxyglucose F 18 (FDG). In vivo, FDG behaves like glucose and provides a means of quantifying glucose metabolism. Unlike glucose, the metabolite of FDG is not a substrate for glycolytic enzymes. Therefore, the radioactive tracer is trapped in the cell, allowing subsequent imaging. The amount of tracer accumulation reflects the tissue's glucose metabolism. Many types of tumors have higher rates of glycolysis than does uninvolved normal tissue. High-grade malignancies tend to have higher rates of glycolysis and FDG uptake than do low-grade malignancies and benign lesions (Fig. 71–3).

## Computed Tomography

With the exception of a few types of masses, such as lipomas, CT attenuation values do not allow a specific histologic diagnosis. The attenuation values of fluid-filled lesions are generally less than those of muscle and greater than those of fat, and the attenuation value of abscesses is usually greater than that of fluid. Most soft tissue tumors have attenuation values that are slightly less than those of normal muscle. CT can be used to monitor percutaneous needle biopsy of soft tissue masses (see Chapter 9).

## Magnetic Resonance Imaging

Despite the superiority of MR imaging in delineating soft tissue tumors, it has a limited ability to precisely characterize them, with most lesions demonstrating prolonged T1 and T2 relaxation times. Findings in the majority of lesions are nonspecific. Wide variations are reported in the ability to establish a correct histologic diagnosis on the basis of imaging studies alone. This ability is greatly influenced by the composition of the population studied, but estimates of approximately 25% to 35% are reasonable. In these cases, a specific diagnosis may be made or strongly suspected on the basis of lesion signal intensity, pattern of growth, location, and associated "signs" and findings. The MR imaging appearance of these lesions (listed in Table 71–1) has been well described.

More commonly, MR imaging reveals a nonspecific appearance, making it impossible to establish a meaningful differential diagnosis or reliably determine whether a lesion is benign or malignant. In such situations, it is useful to formulate a suitably ordered differential diagnosis on the basis of knowledge of tumor prevalence, patient age, and anatomic location of the lesion. This can be

**TABLE 71–1**

### Tumors and Tumor-Like Lesions That Can Be Diagnosed with MR Imaging

Lipomatous lesions
  Lipoma
  Lipoma arborescens
  Lipoblastoma
  Parosteal lipoma
  Fat necrosis
  Fibrolipomatous hamartoma
  Macrodystrophia lipomatosa
  Liposarcoma

Fibrous lesions
  Elastofibroma
  Fibrous hamartoma of infancy
  Generalized fibromatosis
  Musculoaponeurotic fibromatosis
  Recurring digital fibroma
  Palmar/plantar fibromatosis
  Fibromatosis colli
  Retroperitoneal fibromatosis

Lesions of muscle
  Muscle hernia
  Accessory muscle
  Hematoma
  Calcific myonecrosis
  Compartment syndrome
  Myositis ossificans

Myxomatoses
  Ganglion
  Myxoma in fibrous dysplasia

Fibrohistiocytic lesions
  Dermatofibrosarcoma protuberans
  Xanthomatoses

Vascular and lymphatic lesions
  Hemangioma
  Arteriovenous malformation
  Aneurysm/pseudoaneurysm
  Lymphangioma
  Hemangiomatosis/lymphangiomatosis
  Synovial hemangioma
  Glomus tumor

Cartilaginous and osseous lesions
  Chondroma of soft parts
  Tenosynovial osteochondromatosis
  Idiopathic synovial (osteo)chondromatosis

Neurogenic lesions
  Neurilemoma/neurofibroma
  Morton's neuroma
  Traumatic neuroma
  Plexiform neurofibromatosis
  Malignant peripheral nerve sheath tumor

Other lesions
  Synovial sarcoma
  Pigmented villonodular synovitis
  Localized nodular synovitis
  Giant cell tumor of a tendon sheath
  Synovial cyst
  Bursitis/tenosynovitis

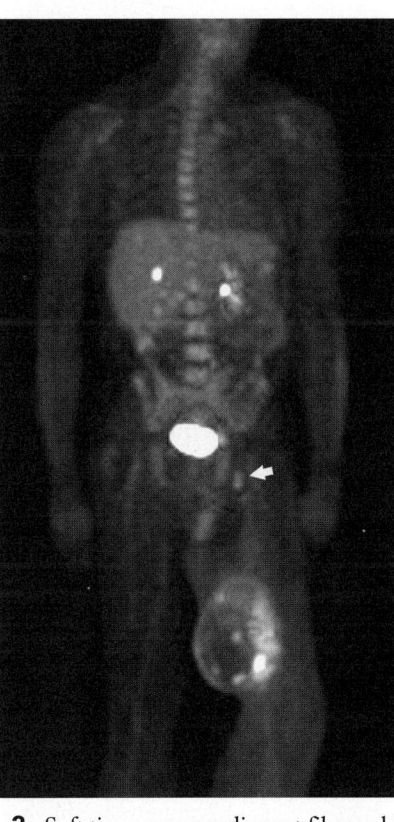

**Figure 71–3.** Soft tissue mass: malignant fibrous histiocytoma. PET reveals hypermetabolic activity at the periphery of this left thigh mass with decreased activity centrally, corresponding to residual foci of high-grade tumor surrounding a large central area of necrosis and hemorrhage. Note the hypermetabolic lymph node in the left groin *(arrow)*.

further refined by considering clinical history and radiographic features, such as pattern of growth, signal intensity, and localization (e.g., subcutaneous, intramuscular, intermuscular). The most common malignant and benign lesions, by tumor location and patient age, are summarized in Tables 71–2 and 71–3.

## PATTERNS OF TUMOR GROWTH

As sarcomas grow, they flatten or compress the surrounding normal soft tissue and produce a pseudocapsule, which on gross pathologic inspection, as well as by various imaging techniques, is easily misinterpreted as encapsulation and can result in an underestimation of tumor aggressiveness.

Distant metastases arising from soft tissue sarcomas are related principally to hematogenous dissemination, although spread to regional lymph nodes may also occur. Osseous involvement in such tumors reflects either local invasion or distant hematogenous dissemination, and the resulting lesions are generally osteolytic in nature.

## STAGING

The purpose of a staging system is to provide a standard manner by which to communicate the state of a malignancy based on local and distant tumor extent. Local staging is best accomplished with MR imaging, which can accurately depict the anatomic spaces (compartments) involved by tumor. Accurate staging is critical for optimal patient care and for planning percutaneous biopsy. It must be emphasized that coordination with the orthopedic surgeon

TABLE 71–2

## Distribution of Common Malignant Soft Tissue Tumors by Anatomic Location and Age

| Age (yr) | Hand and Wrist | No. | Upper Extremity | No. | Axilla and Shoulder | No. | Foot and Ankle | No. | Lower Extremity | No. |
|---|---|---|---|---|---|---|---|---|---|---|
| 0–5 | Fibrosarcoma | 5 (45)* | Fibrosarcoma | 9 (29) | Fibrosarcoma | 9 (56) | Fibrosarcoma | 5 (45) | Fibrosarcoma | 24 (45) |
| | Angiosarcoma | 1 (9) | Rhabdomyosarcoma | 7 (23) | Rhabdomyosarcoma | 4 (25) | DFSP | 2 (18) | Rhabdomyosarcoma | 8 (15) |
| | Epithelioid sarcoma | 1 (9) | Angiomatoid MFH | 3 (10) | Angiomatoid MFH | 1 (6) | MPNST | 2 (18) | Giant cell fibroblastoma | 5 (9) |
| | Malignant GCT of tendon sheath | 1 (9) | DFSP | 2 (6) | Chondrosarcoma | 1 (6) | Rhabdomyosarcoma | 2 (18) | MPNST | 5 (9) |
| | DFSP | 1 (9) | Giant cell fibroblastoma | 2 (6) | MPNST | 1 (6) | | | Angiomatoid MFH | 3 (6) |
| | MPNST | 1 (9) | MPNST | 2 (6) | | | | | DFSP | 3 (6) |
| | Rhabdomyosarcoma | 1 (9) | MFH | 2 (6) | | | | | Angiosarcoma | 2 (4) |
| | | | Other | 4 (13) | | | | | Other | 3 (6) |
| 6–15 | Epithelioid sarcoma | 9 (21) | Angiomatoid MFH | 30 (33) | Angiomatoid MFH | 8 (21) | Synovial sarcoma | 11 (21) | Synovial sarcoma | 28 (22) |
| | Angiomatoid MFH | 7 (16) | Synovial sarcoma | 14 (15) | MFH | 5 (13) | DFSP | 9 (17) | Angiomatoid MFH | 22 (17) |
| | Synovial sarcoma | 5 (12) | Fibrosarcoma | 8 (9) | Ewing's sarcoma | 4 (10) | Rhabdomyosarcoma | 5 (9) | MFH | 13 (10) |
| | MFH | 4 (9) | MPNST | 7 (8) | MPNST | 4 (10) | Angiosarcoma | 4 (8) | Liposarcoma | 11 (9) |
| | Angiosarcoma | 3 (7) | MFH | 7 (8) | Rhabdomyosarcoma | 4 (10) | Clear cell sarcoma | 4 (8) | MPNST | 9 (7) |
| | Rhabdomyosarcoma | 3 (7) | Rhabdomyosarcoma | 7 (8) | Fibrosarcoma | 3 (8) | Fibrosarcoma | 4 (8) | DFSP | 8 (6) |
| | Clear cell sarcoma | 2 (5) | Epithelioid sarcoma | 4 (4) | Synovial sarcoma | 3 (8) | Chondrosarcoma | 3 (6) | Rhabdomyosarcoma | 6 (5) |
| | Other | 10 (23) | Other | 15 (16) | Other | 8 (21) | Other | 13 (25) | Other | 31 (24) |
| 16–25 | Epithelioid sarcoma | 25 (29) | Synovial sarcoma | 32 (23) | Synovial sarcoma | 13 (18) | Synovial sarcoma | 27 (30) | Synovial sarcoma | 76 (22) |
| | MFH | 11 (13) | MFH | 19 (14) | DFSP | 12 (16) | Clear cell sarcoma | 10 (11) | Liposarcoma | 45 (13) |
| | DFSP | 7 (8) | DFSP | 16 (12) | MPNST | 11 (15) | Fibrosarcoma | 7 (8) | MPNST | 44 (13) |
| | Synovial sarcoma | 7 (8) | Synovial sarcoma | 12 (9) | Fibrosarcoma | 8 (11) | DFSP | 7 (8) | MFH | 36 (11) |
| | Rhabdomyosarcoma | 7 (8) | Angiomatoid MFH | 10 (7) | MFH | 8 (11) | MFH | 6 (7) | Fibrosarcoma | 24 (7) |
| | Angiomatoid MFH | 5 (6) | Epithelioid sarcoma | 9 (7) | Rhabdomyosarcoma | 4 (5) | Hemangioendothelioma | 6 (7) | DFSP | 18 (5) |
| | Hemangioendothelioma | 5 (6) | Hemangioendothelioma | 6 (4) | Angiomatoid MFH | 3 (4) | MPNST | 5 (6) | Angiomatoid MFH | 15 (4) |
| | Other | 19 (22) | Other | 34 (25) | Other | 15 (20) | Other | 22 (24) | Other | 80 (24) |
| 26–45 | MFH | 26 (18) | MFH | 65 (28) | DFSP | 55 (33) | Synovial sarcoma | 50 (26) | Liposarcoma | 196 (28) |
| | Epithelioid sarcoma | 24 (16) | MPNST | 29 (12) | MFH | 30 (18) | Clear cell sarcoma | 25 (13) | MFH | 151 (21) |
| | Synovial sarcoma | 21 (14) | Fibrosarcoma | 25 (11) | Liposarcoma | 22 (13) | MFH | 25 (13) | Synovial sarcoma | 78 (11) |
| | Fibrosarcoma | 17 (12) | Synovial sarcoma | 23 (10) | MPNST | 21 (12) | Hemangioendothelioma | 14 (7) | MPNST | 70 (10) |
| | Clear cell sarcoma | 9 (6) | Liposarcoma | 20 (8) | Fibrosarcoma | 10 (6) | DFSP | 13 (7) | DFSP | 47 (7) |
| | Liposarcoma | 9 (6) | DFSP | 18 (8) | Synovial sarcoma | 7 (4) | Liposarcoma | 13 (7) | Leiomyosarcoma | 35 (5) |
| | MPNST | 7 (5) | Epithelioid sarcoma | 13 (6) | Chondrosarcoma | 6 (4) | MPNST | 11 (6) | Fibrosarcoma | 33 (5) |
| | Other | 33 (23) | Other | 43 (18) | Other | 18 (11) | Other | 38 (20) | Other | 98 (14) |
| 46–65 | MFH | 16 (19) | MFH | 133 (46) | MFH | 66 (35) | MFH | 39 (25) | MFH | 399 (43) |
| | Synovial sarcoma | 12 (14) | Liposarcoma | 34 (12) | Liposarcoma | 39 (21) | Synovial sarcoma | 27 (17) | Liposarcoma | 232 (25) |
| | Fibrosarcoma | 8 (10) | Leiomyosarcoma | 22 (8) | DFSP | 22 (12) | Leiomyosarcoma | 19 (12) | Leiomyosarcoma | 63 (7) |
| | Epithelioid sarcoma | 7 (8) | Fibrosarcoma | 18 (6) | MPNST | 20 (11) | Kaposi's sarcoma | 14 (9) | Synovial sarcoma | 40 (4) |
| | Liposarcoma | 7 (8) | MPNST | 17 (6) | Leiomyosarcoma | 14 (7) | Liposarcoma | 9 (6) | MPNST | 38 (4) |
| | Chondrosarcoma | 5 (6) | Synovial sarcoma | 16 (5) | Fibrosarcoma | 8 (4) | Fibrosarcoma | 8 (5) | Chondrosarcoma | 37 (4) |
| | Clear cell sarcoma | 5 (6) | Hemangioendothelioma | 9 (3) | Synovial sarcoma | 4 (2) | Clear cell sarcoma | 7 (5) | Fibrosarcoma | 24 (3) |
| | Other | 22 (26) | Other | 43 (15) | Other | 15 (8) | Other | 32 (21) | Other | 87 (9) |
| 66 | MFH | 28 (35) | MFH | 183 (60) | MFH | 67 (50) | Kaposi's sarcoma | 49 (37) | MFH | 455 (55) |
| | Leiomyosarcoma | 8 (10) | Liposarcoma | 25 (8) | Liposarcoma | 30 (23) | MFH | 26 (19) | Liposarcoma | 178 (22) |
| | Synovial sarcoma | 6 (8) | Leiomyosarcoma | 23 (8) | MPNST | 12 (9) | Leiomyosarcoma | 20 (15) | Leiomyosarcoma | 86 (10) |
| | Kaposi's sarcoma | 5 (6) | MPNST | 20 (7) | DFSP | 6 (5) | Fibrosarcoma | 9 (7) | Fibrosarcoma | 22 (3) |
| | DFSP | 4 (5) | Kaposi's sarcoma | 10 (3) | Fibrosarcoma | 4 (3) | Chondrosarcoma | 6 (4) | Chondrosarcoma | 16 (2) |
| | MPNST | 3 (4) | Fibrosarcoma | 8 (3) | Leiomyosarcoma | 3 (2) | MPNST | 5 (4) | MPNST | 15 (2) |
| | Clear cell sarcoma | 3 (4) | Angiosarcoma | 6 (2) | Chondrosarcoma | 2 (2) | Liposarcoma | 3 (2) | Synovial sarcoma | 11 (1) |
| | Other | 21 (27) | Other | 29 (10) | Other | 9 (7) | Other | 16 (12) | Other | 43 (5) |

**TABLE 71-2**

## Distribution of Common Malignant Soft Tissue Tumors by Anatomic Location and Age *Continued*

| Age (yr) | Hip, Groin, and Buttocks | No. | Head and Neck | No. | Trunk | No. | Retroperitoneum | No. |
|---|---|---|---|---|---|---|---|---|
| 0–5 | Fibrosarcoma | 7 (32) | Fibrosarcoma | 22 (37) | Fibrosarcoma | 13 (26) | Fibrosarcoma | 4 (20) |
| | Giant cell fibroblastoma | 3 (14) | Rhabdomyosarcoma | 20 (33) | Giant cell fibroblastoma | 8 (16) | Neuroblastoma | 4 (20) |
| | Rhabdomyosarcoma | 3 (14) | Malignant hemangiopericytoma | 3 (5) | Rhabdomyosarcoma | 8 (16) | Rhabdomyosarcoma | 4 (20) |
| | DFSP | 2 (9) | Alveolar soft part sarcoma | 2 (3) | Angiomatoid MFH | 6 (12) | Ganglioneuroblastoma | 3 (15) |
| | MFH | 2 (9) | DFSP | 2 (3) | DFSP | 4 (8) | Angiosarcoma | 2 (10) |
| | Leiomyosarcoma | 1 (5) | MPNST | 2 (3) | Ewing's sarcoma | 3 (6) | Leiomyosarcoma | 2 (10) |
| | Synovial sarcoma | 1 (5) | Giant cell fibroblastoma | 2 (3) | Neuroblastoma | 3 (6) | Alveolar soft part sarcoma | 1 (5) |
| | Other | 3 (14) | Other | 7 (12) | Other | 5 (10) | | |
| 6–15 | Angiomatoid MFH | 8 (21) | Rhabdomyosarcoma | 17 (26) | Angiomatoid MFH | 14 (15) | Rhabdomyosarcoma | 9 (31) |
| | Synovial sarcoma | 7 (19) | Fibrosarcoma | 13 (20) | Fibrosarcoma | 13 (14) | MPNST | 5 (17) |
| | Rhabdomyosarcoma | 6 (16) | Synovial sarcoma | 7 (11) | Ewing's sarcoma | 12 (13) | Neuroblastoma | 4 (14) |
| | MFH | 4 (11) | MPNST | 6 (9) | DFSP | 9 (10) | Ewing's sarcoma | 2 (7) |
| | Epithelioid sarcoma | 2 (5) | MFH | 4 (6) | MPNST | 8 (9) | Fibrosarcoma | 2 (7) |
| | Fibrosarcoma | 2 (5) | Angiomatoid MFH | 2 (3) | Rhabdomyosarcoma | 7 (8) | MFH | 2 (7) |
| | MPNST | 2 (5) | DFSP | 2 (3) | MFH | 6 (7) | Malignant hemangiopericytoma | 2 (7) |
| | Other | 7 (18) | Other | 10 (15) | Other | 23 (24) | Other | 3 (10) |
| 16–25 | Synovial sarcoma | 15 (18) | Fibrosarcoma | 15 (17) | DFSP | 37 (23) | MPNST | 9 (20) |
| | MPNST | 13 (16) | DFSP | 14 (16) | MFH | 21 (13) | Ewing's sarcoma | 8 (18) |
| | Liposarcoma | 8 (10) | MPNST | 8 (9) | MPNST | 19 (12) | Leiomyosarcoma | 6 (14) |
| | DFSP | 6 (7) | Synovial sarcoma | 8 (9) | Fibrosarcoma | 15 (9) | Ganglioneuroblastoma | 4 (9) |
| | MFH | 6 (7) | Rhabdomyosarcoma | 8 (9) | Synovial sarcoma | 13 (8) | Neuroblastoma | 4 (9) |
| | Rhabdomyosarcoma | 5 (6) | MFH | 7 (8) | Ewing's sarcoma | 12 (7) | Rhabdomyosarcoma | 3 (7) |
| | Leiomyosarcoma | 4 (5) | Angiomatoid MFH | 6 (7) | Angiomatoid MFH | 6 (4) | Malignant hemangiopericytoma | 2 (5) |
| | Other | 26 (31) | Other | 23 (26) | Other | 38 (24) | Other | 8 (18) |
| 26–45 | Liposarcoma | 45 (18) | DFSP | 59 (30) | DFSP | 129 (30) | Leiomyosarcoma | 57 (32) |
| | DFSP | 42 (17) | MPNST | 27 (14) | MFH | 77 (18) | Liposarcoma | 52 (29) |
| | MFH | 38 (16) | Liposarcoma | 18 (9) | MPNST | 45 (10) | MFH | 22 (12) |
| | Leiomyosarcoma | 26 (11) | MFH | 15 (8) | Liposarcoma | 41 (9) | MPNST | 11 (6) |
| | MPNST | 15 (6) | Fibrosarcoma | 14 (7) | Fibrosarcoma | 36 (8) | Fibrosarcoma | 7 (4) |
| | Synovial sarcoma | 13 (5) | Synovial sarcoma | 10 (5) | Synovial sarcoma | 20 (5) | Malignant hemangiopericytoma | 7 (4) |
| | Fibrosarcoma | 12 (5) | Angiosarcoma | 9 (4) | Angiosarcoma | 15 (3) | Ewing's sarcoma | 3 (2) |
| | Other | 53 (22) | Other | 42 (22) | Other | 70 (16) | Other | 20 (11) |
| 46–65 | Liposarcoma | 67 (24) | MFH | 54 (28) | MFH | 131 (31) | Liposarcoma | 170 (33) |
| | MFH | 66 (23) | DFSP | 28 (15) | Liposarcoma | 80 (19) | Leiomyosarcoma | 154 (30) |
| | Leiomyosarcoma | 40 (14) | MPNST | 23 (12) | DFSP | 60 (14) | MFH | 111 (22) |
| | DFSP | 20 (7) | Liposarcoma | 22 (12) | MPNST | 35 (8) | MPNST | 23 (5) |
| | Fibrosarcoma | 16 (6) | Angiosarcoma | 16 (8) | Leiomyosarcoma | 27 (6) | Malignant mesenchymoma | 10 (2) |
| | Synovial sarcoma | 14 (5) | Atypical fibroxanthoma | 12 (6) | Fibrosarcoma | 24 (6) | Fibrosarcoma | 9 (2) |
| | Chondrosarcoma | 14 (5) | Leiomyosarcoma | 11 (6) | Angiosarcoma | 15 (4) | Malignant hemangiopericytoma | 7 (1) |
| | Other | 46 (16) | Other | 24 (13) | Other | 50 (12) | Other | 27 (5) |
| 66 | MFH | 111 (46) | MFH | 82 (34) | MFH | 137 (44) | Liposarcoma | 164 (39) |
| | Liposarcoma | 49 (20) | Atypical fibroxanthoma | 41 (17) | Liposarcoma | 56 (18) | Leiomyosarcoma | 118 (28) |
| | Leiomyosarcoma | 24 (10) | Angiosarcoma | 27 (11) | Leiomyosarcoma | 23 (7) | MFH | 93 (22) |
| | Angiosarcoma | 11 (5) | Liposarcoma | 20 (8) | MPNST | 20 (6) | MPNST | 13 (3) |
| | MPNST | 11 (5) | MPNST | 16 (7) | DFSP | 17 (5) | Fibrosarcoma | 8 (2) |
| | Fibrosarcoma | 10 (4) | Leiomyosarcoma | 13 (5) | Fibrosarcoma | 12 (4) | Osteosarcoma | 6 (1) |
| | Chondrosarcoma | 7 (3) | Fibrosarcoma | 10 (4) | Chondrosarcoma | 11 (4) | Malignant mesenchymoma | 5 (1) |
| | Other | 20 (8) | Other | 31 (13) | Other | 35 (11) | Other | 9 (2) |

Based on an analysis of 12,370 cases seen in consultation by the Department of Soft Tissue Pathology, Armed Forces Institute of Pathology, over a 10-year period.

*Numbers in parentheses are percentages; for example, 5 (45) indicates that there were five fibrosarcomas in the hands and wrists of patients 0 to 5 years old, and this number represents 45% of all malignant tumors in this location and age group.

DFSP, dermatofibrosarcoma protuberans; GCT, giant cell tumor; MFH, malignant fibrous histiocytoma; MPNST, malignant peripheral nerve sheath tumor.

Adapted from Kransdorf MJ: Malignant soft-tissue tumors in a large referral population: Distribution of diagnoses by age, sex, and location. AJR Am J Roentgenol 164:129, 1995.

## TABLE 71-3

**Distribution of Common Benign Soft Tissue Tumors by Anatomic Location and Age**

| Age (yr) | Hand and Wrist | No. | Upper Extremity | No. | Axilla and Shoulder | No. | Foot and Ankle | No. | Lower Extremity | No. |
|---|---|---|---|---|---|---|---|---|---|---|
| 0–5 | Hemangioma | 15 (15)* | Fibrous hamartoma of infancy | 15 (16) | Fibrous hamartoma of infancy | 23 (29) | Granuloma annulare | 23 (30) | Granuloma annulare | 42 (23) |
| | Granuloma annulare | 14 (14) | Granuloma annulare | 15 (16) | Hemangioma | 12 (15) | Infantile fibromatosis | 11 (14) | Hemangioma | 26 (14) |
| | Infantile fibromatosis | 13 (13) | Hemangioma | 14 (15) | Lipoblastoma | 11 (14) | Hemangioma | 8 (11) | Myofibromatosis | 16 (9) |
| | Infantile digital fibroma | 8 (8) | Infantile fibromatosis | 12 (13) | Fibrous hamartoma | 7 (9) | Fibromatosis | 8 (11) | Fibrous histiocytoma | 15 (8) |
| | Fibromatosis | 8 (8) | Fibrous histiocytoma | 6 (6) | Myofibromatosis | 6 (8) | Infantile digital fibroma | 7 (9) | Lipoblastoma | 13 (7) |
| | Aponeurotic fibroma | 7 (7) | Juvenile xanthogranuloma | 6 (6) | Lymphangioma | 5 (6) | Lipoblastoma | 6 (8) | Lymphangioma | 10 (6) |
| | Fibrous histiocytoma | 5 (5) | Myofibromatosis | 6 (5) | Nodular fasciitis | 4 (5) | Lipoma | 4 (5) | Juvenile xanthogranuloma | 10 (6) |
| | Other | 27 (28) | Other | 20 (21) | Other | 12 (15) | Other | 12 (15) | Other | 48 (27) |
| 6–15 | Fibrous histiocytoma | 32 (14) | Fibrous histiocytoma | 41 (23) | Fibrous histiocytoma | 25 (34) | Fibromatosis | 35 (22) | Hemangioma | 47 (22) |
| | Hemangioma | 31 (13) | Nodular fasciitis | 39 (21) | Nodular fasciitis | 18 (25) | Granuloma annulare | 21 (13) | Fibrous histiocytoma | 34 (16) |
| | Aponeurotic fibroma | 25 (11) | Hemangioma | 24 (13) | Hemangioma | 7 (10) | Hemangioma | 21 (13) | Nodular fasciitis | 22 (10) |
| | Fibroma of tendon sheath | 22 (9) | Granuloma annulare | 12 (7) | Granular cell tumor | 4 (5) | Fibrous histiocytoma | 14 (9) | Granuloma annulare | 20 (9) |
| | GCT of tendon sheath | 17 (7) | Fibromatosis | 11 (6) | Neurofibroma | 3 (4) | GCT of tendon sheath | 13 (8) | Fibromatosis | 14 (6) |
| | Fibromatosis | 13 (6) | Neurofibroma | 7 (4) | Lymphangioma | 2 (3) | Chondroma | 11 (7) | Lipoma | 13 (6) |
| | Lipoma | 9 (4) | Neurothekeoma | 6 (3) | Myofibromatosis | 2 (3) | Lipoma | 9 (6) | Neurofibroma | 8 (4) |
| | Other | 86 (37) | Other | 42 (23) | Other | 12 (16) | Other | 37 (23) | Other | 58 (27) |
| 16–25 | GCT of tendon sheath | 84 (20) | Nodular fasciitis | 130 (35) | Fibrous histiocytoma | 62 (36) | Fibromatosis | 46 (22) | Fibrous histiocytoma | 118 (24) |
| | Fibrous histiocytoma | 57 (14) | Fibrous histiocytoma | 87 (23) | Nodular fasciitis | 35 (20) | GCT of tendon sheath | 29 (14) | Nodular fasciitis | 61 (13) |
| | Hemangioma | 40 (10) | Hemangioma | 36 (10) | Fibromatosis | 16 (9) | Granuloma annulare | 25 (12) | Hemangioma | 55 (11) |
| | Fibroma of tendon sheath | 40 (10) | Neurofibroma | 24 (6) | Lipoma | 14 (8) | Fibrous histiocytoma | 24 (12) | Neurofibroma | 48 (10) |
| | Nodular fasciitis | 26 (6) | Granuloma annulare | 20 (5) | Neurofibroma | 12 (7) | Hemangioma | 13 (6) | Fibromatosis | 38 (8) |
| | Granuloma annulare | 21 (5) | Granular cell tumor | 17 (5) | Hemangioma | 4 (2) | PVNS | 12 (6) | Lipoma | 22 (5) |
| | Ganglion | 20 (5) | Schwannoma | 11 (3) | Schwannoma | 4 (2) | Neurofibroma | 11 (5) | Schwannoma | 20 (4) |
| | Other | 132 (31) | Other | 51 (14) | Other | 25 (15) | Other | 45 (22) | Other | 122 (25) |
| 26–45 | Fibrous histiocytoma | 167 (18) | Nodular fasciitis | 309 (38) | Lipoma | 105 (28) | Fibromatosis | 99 (21) | Fibrous histiocytoma | 245 (25) |
| | GCT of tendon sheath | 148 (16) | Fibrous histiocytoma | 145 (18) | Fibrous histiocytoma | 92 (24) | Fibrous histiocytoma | 74 (16) | Nodular fasciitis | 229 (23) |
| | Fibroma of tendon sheath | 106 (11) | Angiolipoma | 48 (6) | Nodular fasciitis | 55 (14) | GCT of tendon sheath | 41 (9) | Lipoma | 101 (10) |
| | Hemangioma | 86 (10) | Hemangioma | 43 (5) | Fibromatosis | 29 (8) | Hemangioma | 36 (8) | Neurofibroma | 71 (7) |
| | Nodular fasciitis | 79 (8) | Schwannoma | 43 (5) | Hemangioma | 17 (4) | Schwannoma | 30 (6) | Schwannoma | 59 (6) |
| | Fibromatosis | 46 (5) | Neurofibroma | 37 (5) | Neurofibroma | 13 (3) | Neurofibroma | 24 (5) | Myxoma | 53 (5) |
| | Chondroma | 42 (4) | Lipoma | 32 (4) | Schwannoma | 12 (3) | Chondroma | 23 (5) | Hemangioma | 52 (5) |
| | Other | 269 (29) | Other | 153 (19) | Other | 57 (15) | Other | 135 (29) | Other | 185 (19) |
| 46–65 | GCT of tendon sheath | 143 (23) | Nodular fasciitis | 86 (20) | Lipoma | 189 (58) | Fibromatosis | 83 (25) | Lipoma | 157 (23) |
| | Fibrous histiocytoma | 63 (10) | Lipoma | 80 (19) | Fibrous histiocytoma | 28 (9) | Fibrous histiocytoma | 43 (13) | Myxoma | 109 (16) |
| | Hemangioma | 61 (10) | Fibrous histiocytoma | 44 (10) | Myxoma | 16 (5) | Lipoma | 35 (11) | Fibrous histiocytoma | 93 (14) |
| | Lipoma | 59 (9) | Schwannoma | 30 (7) | Fibromatosis | 14 (4) | Schwannoma | 25 (8) | Nodular fasciitis | 40 (6) |
| | Chondroma | 52 (8) | Neurofibroma | 24 (6) | Nodular fasciitis | 13 (4) | GCT of tendon sheath | 21 (6) | Schwannoma | 39 (6) |
| | Fibromatosis | 43 (7) | Myxoma | 24 (6) | Schwannoma | 12 (4) | Chondroma | 21 (6) | Neurofibroma | 31 (5) |
| | Fibroma of tendon sheath | 37 (6) | Hemangioma | 19 (4) | Granular cell tumor | 12 (4) | Hemangioma | 16 (5) | Proliferative fasciitis | 28 (4) |
| | Other | 172 (27) | Other | 125 (29) | Other | 44 (13) | Other | 89 (27) | Other | 186 (27) |
| 66 | GCT of tendon sheath | 51 (21) | Lipoma | 39 (22) | Lipoma | 83 (58) | Fibromatosis | 16 (14) | Lipoma | 68 (26) |
| | Hemangioma | 24 (10) | Myxoma | 19 (11) | Myxoma | 14 (10) | Schwannoma | 15 (13) | Myxoma | 44 (17) |
| | Schwannoma | 24 (10) | Nodular fasciitis | 18 (10) | Schwannoma | 6 (4) | Fibrous histiocytoma | 13 (11) | Fibrous histiocytoma | 33 (13) |
| | Chondroma | 24 (10) | Schwannoma | 17 (9) | Fibromatosis | 5 (3) | Chondroma | 11 (9) | Schwannoma | 31 (12) |
| | Neurofibroma | 21 (9) | Glomus tumor | 12 (7) | Fibrous histiocytoma | 5 (3) | Lipoma | 10 (8) | Hemangiopericytoma | 10 (4) |
| | Fibromatosis | 14 (6) | Neurofibroma | 10 (6) | Proliferative fasciitis | 5 (3) | Granuloma annulare | 8 (7) | Neurofibroma | 9 (4) |
| | Lipoma | 13 (5) | Angiolipoma | 10 (6) | Hemangioma | 4 (3) | GCT of tendon sheath | 6 (5) | Hemangioma | 8 (3) |
| | Other | 71 (29) | Other | 55 (31) | Other | 22 (15) | Other | 39 (33) | Other | 56 (22) |

**TABLE 71-3**

## Distribution of Common Benign Soft Tissue Tumors by Anatomic Location and Age *Continued*

| Age (yr) | Hip, Groin, and Buttocks | No. | Head and Neck | No. | Trunk | No. | Retroperitoneum | No. |
|---|---|---|---|---|---|---|---|---|
| 0–5 | Fibrous hamartoma of infancy | 14 (20) | Nodular fasciitis | 47 (20) | Hemangioma | 36 (18) | Lipoblastoma | 7 (37) |
| | Lipoblastoma | 14 (20) | Hemangioma | 43 (18) | Juvenile xanthogranuloma | 24 (12) | Lymphangioma | 5 (26) |
| | Myofibromatosis | 8 (11) | Myofibromatosis | 27 (11) | Myofibromatosis | 24 (12) | Hemangioma | 4 (21) |
| | Lymphangioma | 7 (10) | Fibromatosis | 17 (7) | Nodular fasciitis | 17 (8) | Ganglioneuroma | 2 (11) |
| | Fibrous histiocytoma | 5 (7) | Granuloma annulare | 14 (6) | Lipoblastoma | 15 (7) | Fibrous hamartoma of infancy | 1 (5) |
| | Nodular fasciitis | 4 (6) | Fibrous histiocytoma | 13 (5) | Infantile fibromatosis | 15 (7) | | |
| | Infantile fibromatosis | 4 (6) | Infantile fibromatosis | 13 (5) | Fibrous hamartoma of infancy | 15 (7) | | |
| | Other | 14 (20) | Other | 63 (27) | Other | 55 (27) | | |
| 6–15 | Nodular fasciitis | 15 (27) | Nodular fasciitis | 75 (33) | Nodular fasciitis | 54 (28) | Lymphangioma | 7 (37) |
| | Fibroma | 7 (13) | Fibrous histiocytoma | 34 (15) | Fibrous histiocytoma | 43 (22) | Ganglioneuroma | 4 (21) |
| | Fibrous histiocytoma | 6 (11) | Neurofibroma | 23 (10) | Hemangioma | 25 (13) | Schwannoma | 2 (11) |
| | Fibromatosis | 5 (9) | Hemangioma | 21 (9) | Lipoma | 9 (5) | Fibromatosis | 2 (11) |
| | Lipoma | 5 (9) | Myofibromatosis | 14 (6) | Neurofibroma | 7 (4) | Paraganglioma | 1 (5) |
| | Lipoblastoma | 3 (5) | Fibromatosis | 12 (5) | Fibromatosis | 6 (3) | Hemangioma | 1 (5) |
| | Neurofibroma | 3 (5) | Lipoma | 6 (3) | Granular cell tumor | 6 (3) | Inflammatory pseudotumor | 1 (5) |
| | Other | 11 (20) | Other | 43 (19) | Other | 45 (23) | Other | 1 (5) |
| 16–25 | Neurofibroma | 20 (16) | Nodular fasciitis | 61 (21) | Nodular fasciitis | 112 (24) | Fibromatosis | 14 (20) |
| | Fibromatosis | 18 (15) | Hemangioma | 48 (17) | Fibromatosis | 72 (16) | Schwannoma | 10 (14) |
| | Fibrous histiocytoma | 18 (15) | Fibrous histiocytoma | 45 (16) | Fibrous histiocytoma | 71 (15) | Neurofibroma | 9 (13) |
| | Nodular fasciitis | 12 (10) | Neurofibroma | 37 (13) | Hemangioma | 52 (11) | Hemangiopericytoma | 8 (11) |
| | Hemangioma | 9 (7) | Schwannoma | 19 (7) | Neurofibroma | 38 (8) | Lymphangioma | 8 (11) |
| | Lipoma | 8 (7) | Fibromatosis | 11 (4) | Lipoma | 21 (5) | Ganglioneuroma | 6 (8) |
| | Hemangiopericytoma | 8 (7) | Lipoma | 10 (4) | Schwannoma | 17 (4) | Hemangioma | 4 (6) |
| | Other | 29 (24) | Other | 56 (19) | Other | 79 (17) | Other | 12 (17) |
| 26–45 | Lipoma | 57 (17) | Lipoma | 168 (22) | Lipoma | 178 (19) | Schwannoma | 38 (23) |
| | Neurofibroma | 38 (12) | Nodular fasciitis | 145 (19) | Nodular fasciitis | 150 (16) | Fibromatosis | 30 (18) |
| | Fibrous histiocytoma | 37 (11) | Fibrous histiocytoma | 137 (18) | Fibromatosis | 148 (16) | Hemangiopericytoma | 25 (15) |
| | Fibromatosis | 36 (11) | Hemangioma | 97 (13) | Fibrous histiocytoma | 98 (10) | Neurofibroma | 13 (8) |
| | Nodular fasciitis | 31 (9) | Neurofibroma | 57 (8) | Hemangioma | 78 (8) | Angiomyolipoma | 10 (6) |
| | Hemangiopericytoma | 24 (7) | Hemangiopericytoma | 37 (5) | Neurofibroma | 65 (7) | Hemangioma | 9 (5) |
| | Myxoma | 22 (7) | Schwannoma | 27 (4) | Schwannoma | 51 (5) | Sclerosing retroperitonitis | 7 (4) |
| | Other | 83 (25) | Other | 91 (12) | Other | 180 (19) | Other | 34 (20) |
| 46–65 | Lipoma | 76 (35) | Lipoma | 306 (46) | Lipoma | 290 (44) | Schwannoma | 33 (19) |
| | Myxoma | 36 (17) | Nodular fasciitis | 66 (10) | Fibromatosis | 63 (9) | Fibromatosis | 25 (14) |
| | Fibrous histiocytoma | 17 (8) | Hemangioma | 55 (8) | Nodular fasciitis | 44 (7) | Sclerosing retroperitonitis | 25 (14) |
| | Schwannoma | 17 (8) | Fibrous histiocytoma | 42 (6) | Hemangioma | 31 (5) | Hemangiopericytoma | 21 (12) |
| | Nodular fasciitis | 11 (5) | Neurofibroma | 30 (4) | Fibrous histiocytoma | 29 (4) | Angiomyolipoma | 12 (7) |
| | Hemangiopericytoma | 11 (5) | Schwannoma | 25 (3) | Neurofibroma | 28 (4) | Lipoma | 10 (6) |
| | Hemangioma | 9 (4) | Myxoma | 23 (3) | Schwannoma | 28 (4) | Paraganglioma | 9 (5) |
| | Other | 40 (18) | Other | 120 (18) | Other | 151 (23) | Other | 40 (23) |
| 66 | Lipoma | 22 (21) | Lipoma | 158 (50) | Lipoma | 124 (42) | Schwannoma | 19 (26) |
| | Myxoma | 16 (15) | Hemangioma | 22 (7) | Fibromatosis | 26 (9) | Hemangiopericytoma | 14 (19) |
| | Neurofibroma | 13 (12) | Schwannoma | 18 (6) | Neurofibroma | 20 (7) | Lipoma | 6 (8) |
| | Schwannoma | 10 (9) | Fibrous histiocytoma | 17 (5) | Schwannoma | 18 (6) | Mesothelioma | 6 (8) |
| | Hemangiopericytoma | 10 (9) | Neurofibroma | 16 (5) | Elastofibroma | 17 (6) | Sclerosing retroperitonitis | 5 (7) |
| | Hemangioma | 8 (8) | Nodular fasciitis | 13 (4) | Myxoma | 16 (5) | Fibromatosis | 4 (6) |
| | Nodular fasciitis | 4 (4) | Myxoma | 12 (4) | Hemangioma | 14 (5) | Paraganglioma | 4 (6) |
| | Other | 23 (22) | Other | 58 (18) | Other | 61 (21) | Other | 14 (19) |

Based on an analysis of 18,677 cases seen in consultation by the Department of Soft Tissue Pathology, Armed Forces Institute of Pathology, over a 10-year period.

*Numbers in parentheses are percentages; for example, 15 (15) indicates that there were 15 hemangiomas in the hands and wrists of patients 0 to 5 years old, and this number represents 15% of all benign tumors in this location and age group.

GCT, giant cell tumor; PVNS, pigmented villonodular synovitis.

Adapted from Kransdorf MJ: Benign soft-tissue tumors in a large referral population: Distribution of specific diagnoses by age, sex, and location. AJR Am J Roentgenol 164:395, 1995.

who will perform the definitive surgery is essential before biopsy. Staging systems for soft tissue sarcomas have been developed to provide information regarding the choice of appropriate therapy and the likelihood of local recurrence or systemic metastasis. Although there are several different systems, the most commonly used are those of Enneking (and the Musculoskeletal Tumor Society) and the American Joint Committee on Cancer (Tables 71–4 and 71–5).

## TYPES OF TUMORS

In general, benign tumors or tumor-like processes are far more frequent than malignant processes are. In many classification systems, benign and malignant subdivisions are entered under each histogenetic group, although transformation of a benign tumor to a malignant one is extremely rare (with the exception of a malignant peripheral nerve sheath tumor originating from a neurofibroma). This chapter takes a histogenetic approach, emphasizing the use of MR imaging and highlighting those diagnoses that may be suggested by imaging.

### Tumors of Fat

**Liposarcoma.** Liposarcoma is the second most frequent malignant neoplasm of soft tissue in adults (after malignant fibrous histiocytoma) and represents approximately 20% of all soft tissue sarcomas. It is usually encountered in middle-aged and elderly patients and is rare in children (most lipomatous tumors in infants and children are lipoblastomas). It is common in the thigh, gluteal region, retroperitoneum, and leg.

Four histologic types of liposarcoma are generally recognized: well differentiated, myxoid, pleomorphic, and dedifferentiated. Well-differentiated and dedifferentiated liposarcomas are encountered most commonly in the retroperitoneum. Myxoid liposarcomas are most common in the extremities.

On radiographs, an ill-defined mass of both water density and fat density may be observed. In general, more malignant lesions have greater radiodensity, whereas less

### TABLE 71–4

**Staging of Soft Tissue Sarcomas: Enneking System**

| Stage | Grade (G) | Site (T) | Metastasis (M) |
| --- | --- | --- | --- |
| IA | 1 | 0 or 1 | 0 |
| IB | 1 | 2 | 0 |
| IIA | 2 | 0 or 1 | 0 |
| IIB | 2 | 2 | 0 |
| IIIA | 1 or 2 | 0 or 1 | 1 |
| IIIB | 1 or 2 | 2 | 1 |

Grade (G) is divided into G0, benign; G1, low-grade malignant; and G2, high-grade malignant. Site (T) is divided into T0, intracompartmental/intracapsular; T1, intracompartmental/extracapsular; and T2, extracompartmental. Metastasis (M) is divided into M0, no evidence of regional or distant metastases; and M1, regional or distant metastases.

From Enneking WF, Spanier SS, Goodman MA: Clin Orthop 153:106, 1980.

### TABLE 71–5

**Staging of Soft Tissue Sarcomas: System of the American Joint Committee on Cancer**

| Stage | Grade (G) | Tumor (T) | Node (N) | Metastasis (M) |
| --- | --- | --- | --- | --- |
| IA | 1 | 1 | 0 | 0 |
| IB | 1 | 2 | 0 | 0 |
| IIA | 2 | 1 | 0 | 0 |
| IIB | 2 | 2 | 0 | 0 |
| IIIA | 3 | 1 | 0 | 0 |
| IIIB | 3 | 2 | 0 | 0 |
| IIIC | 1, 2, or 3 | 1 or 2 | 1 | 0 |
| IVA | 1, 2, or 3 | 3 | 0 or 1 | 0 |
| IVB | 1, 2, or 3 | 1, 2, or 3 | 0 or 1 | 1 |

Grade (G) is divided into G1, well differentiated; G2, moderately differentiated; and G3, poorly differentiated. Tumor (T) is divided into T1, diameter less than 5 cm; T2, diameter 5 cm or greater; and T3, bone or neurovascular invasion. Node (N) is divided into N0, no regional lymph node involvement, and N1, regional lymph node involvement. The category metastasis (M) is divided into M0, no evidence of metastasis, and M1, metastasis.

From Russell WO, Cohen J, Edmonson JH, et al: Semin Oncol 8:156, 1981.

aggressive tumors have a greater fat content and increased radiolucency. Though uncommon, calcification or ossification may be seen (Fig. 71–4). CT may reveal areas of low attenuation in the mass (Fig. 71–5). It must be emphasized that the CT appearance of liposarcomas, with the possible exception of well-differentiated liposarcomas, may not include areas of fat.

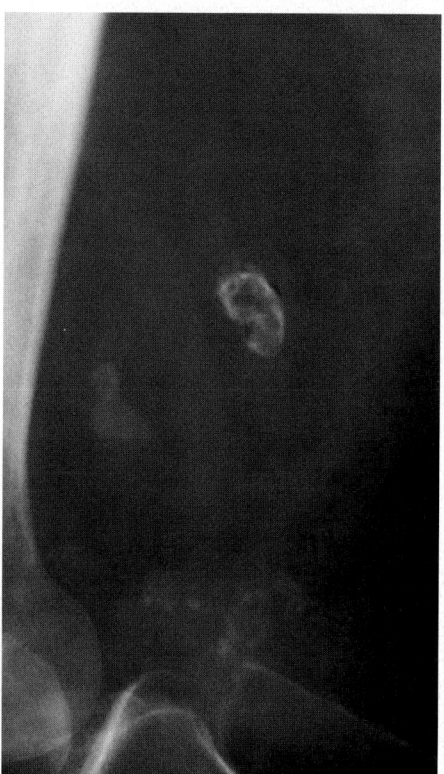

**Figure 71–4.** Liposarcoma. A large mass behind the femur is inhomogeneous in appearance, with some areas of radiolucency and foci of ossification.

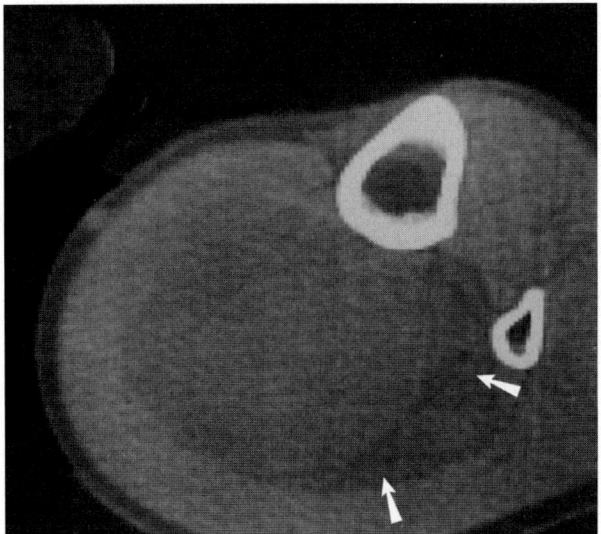

**Figure 71–5.** Liposarcoma. This 37-year-old man had a 1-month history of calf pain and a mass with edema in the ipsilateral ankle. Transaxial CT scan shows an inhomogeneous lesion containing areas with low attenuation *(arrows)*. It extends to the region of the interosseous membrane. Biopsy and subsequent amputation of the leg confirmed a myxoid and pleomorphic liposarcoma. (Courtesy of G. Greenway, MD, Dallas, Tex.)

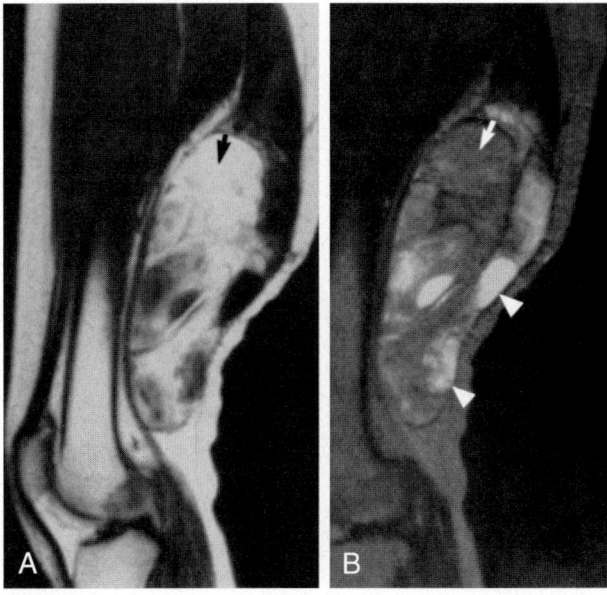

**Figure 71–6.** Liposarcoma. Sagittal T1-weighted (TR/TE, 500/16) *(A)* and T2-weighted (TR/TE, 2500/80) *(B)* spin echo MR images of a myxoid liposarcoma located behind the femur show inhomogeneity of signal intensity. Observe the regions of signal intensity identical to that of fat *(arrows)* and others with high signal intensity *(arrowheads)* in *(B)*. (Courtesy of P. Ellenbogen, MD, Dallas, Tex.)

The MR imaging features of liposarcomas are variable and depend on tumor composition. Fat is seen in approximately 50% to 80% of cases (Fig. 71–6); it is most prominent in well-differentiated liposarcomas. Such well-differentiated tumors are also characterized by septa, which have increased signal intensity on T2-weighted spin echo MR images, a feature that is not typical of most ordinary lipomas. Occasionally, septa are identified in benign lipomatous tumors; the septa of liposarcomas are generally thicker and more irregular than those of benign tumors, however, and they show greater enhancement after intravenous gadolinium administration. Myxoid liposarcomas may be well defined and homogeneous in signal intensity and appear as cystlike lesions on MR (and CT) examinations in about 20% of cases. Inhomogeneous signal intensity is frequently encountered in cases of pleomorphic and round cell liposarcomas. Dedifferentiated liposarcomas, which are best defined as bimorphic neoplasms in which a low-grade liposarcoma is juxtaposed with a high-grade, histologically different sarcoma, are characterized on MR imaging by the presence of a well-defined nonlipomatous mass juxtaposed with a predominantly fatty tumor (Fig. 71–7).

**Lipoma.** Lipomas are common lesions typically encountered in patients 30 to 50 years of age. Women are affected more frequently than men, and solitary lesions predominate. Approximately 5% of all patients with lipomas have multiple tumors, an occurrence that is more frequent in men. Lipomas show a predilection for the subcutaneous tissue of the back, extremities, and thorax. Lipomas arising in subcutaneous tissue are designated superficial lipomas and represent the far more common

type; those arising elsewhere are designated deep lipomas. Superficial lipomas tend to be small, whereas deep lipomas may reach considerable size and are less well defined than their superficial counterparts. Deep lipomas may arise in subfascial tissue or within muscle.

Radiographically, lipomas often appear as radiolucent masses. Ossification in the tumor is occasionally observed (Fig. 71–8), and lipomas located close to a bone may induce cortical thickening or hyperostosis. CT and MR imaging reliably indicate the fatty nature of the tumor (Fig. 71–9). Fibrous connective tissue may be contained within a lipoma, resulting in linear areas or septations with increased attenuation on CT scans and decreased signal intensity on MR imaging.

**Variants of Lipoma.** A number of specific fat-containing lesions differ from ordinary lipomas in their clinical features, multiplicity, specific location, histologic features, or various combinations of these characteristics. Several specific types of infiltrating lipoma have been described. Infiltrating congenital lipomatosis of the face and diffuse lipomatosis are two types that are generally encountered in infants and children. Diffuse lipomatosis typically affects the limbs and may be associated with osseous overgrowth. Shoulder girdle lipomatosis is associated with gradual unilateral enlargement and deformity of the shoulder and proximal portion of the arm, with an accompanying somatic and autonomic neuropathy. Fatty tissue accumulates within and between the muscles connecting the upper portion of the limb to the thoracic wall.

Multiple symmetrical lipomatosis typically affects the neck and shoulders of adult men, often those with alco-

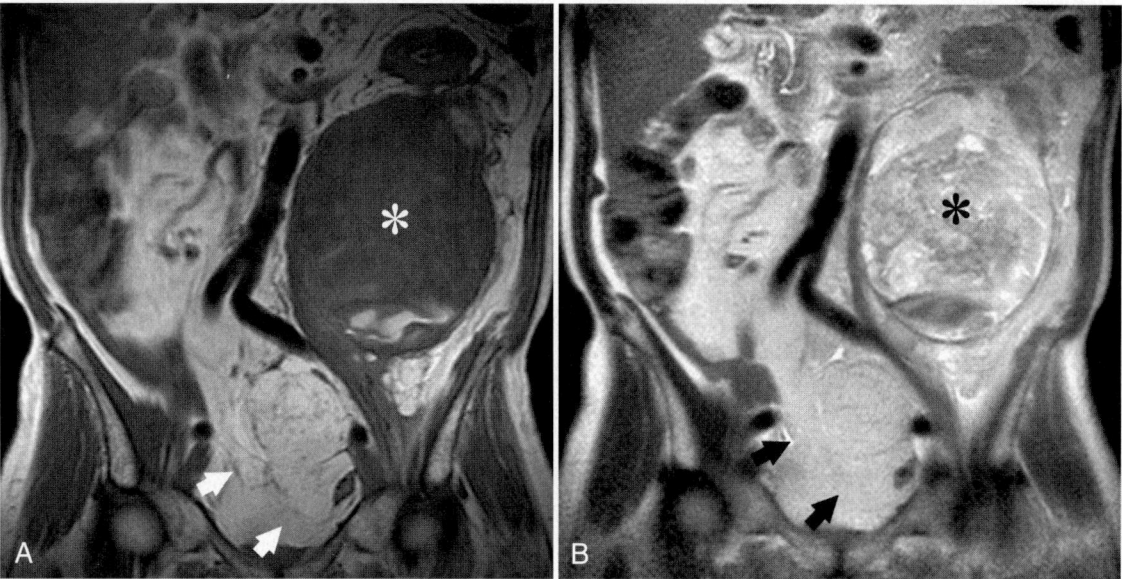

**Figure 71–7.** Dedifferentiated liposarcoma. Coronal T1-weighted (TR/TE, 549/12) spin echo *(A)* and half-Fourier acquisition single shot turbo-spin-echo (TR/TE, 1361/60) *(B)* MR images show a large, well-differentiated retroperitoneal mass with a focal nonadipose component *(asterisk),* representing the dedifferentiated portion of the tumor. Note subacute hemorrhage in the inferior aspect of the high-grade component, as well as superior displacement of the left kidney. The well-differentiated component extends into the pelvis *(arrows)* and is difficult to distinguish from adjacent fat.

holism and liver disease, with or without a family history (Fig. 71–10). This condition is also known as Madelung's disease or syndrome (diffuse and symmetrical distribution of lipomas, with or without calcification or severe peripheral and autonomic neuropathy).

Hibernomas are benign tumors of brown fat in patients who are in the third or fourth decade of life (Fig. 71–11). Although predominating in the interscapular and periscapular regions, hibernomas may be observed elsewhere, such as the thigh, axilla, neck, or chest wall. These lesions

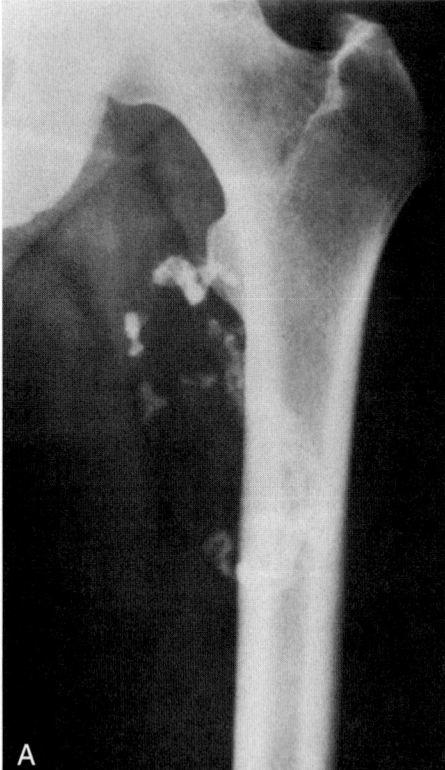

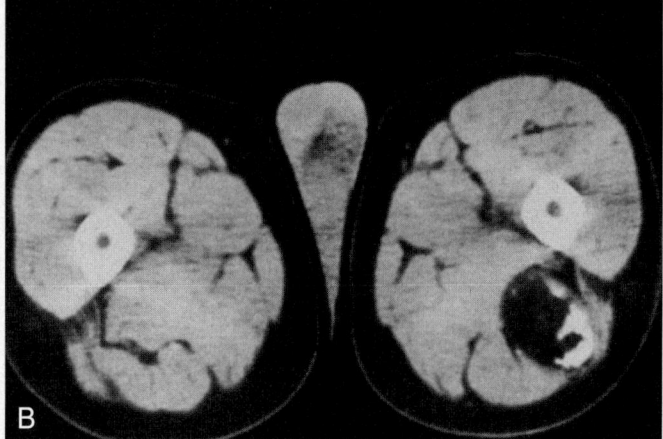

**Figure 71–8.** Lipoma: soft tissue ossification. This 62-year-old man had a mass in his thigh measuring 3 by 3 cm. Conventional radiography *(A)* and CT *(B)* show irregular ossification in a radiolucent mass, which at surgery was found to be well encapsulated and on histologic examination contained areas of necrosis. (Courtesy of G. Greenway, MD, Dallas, Tex.)

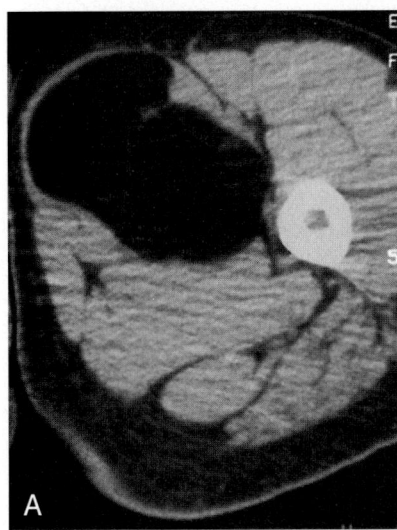 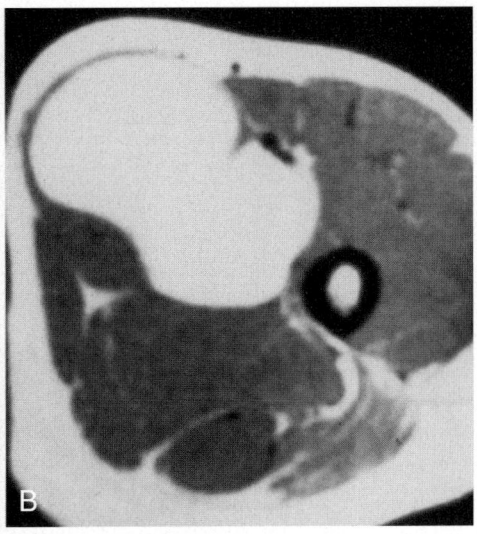

**Figure 71–9.** Lipoma. In this 19-year-old man, a well-encapsulated intramuscular lipoma has a homogeneous appearance, with features of fat, on a transaxial CT scan (A) and transaxial T1-weighted (TR/TE, 600/15) spin echo MR image (B).

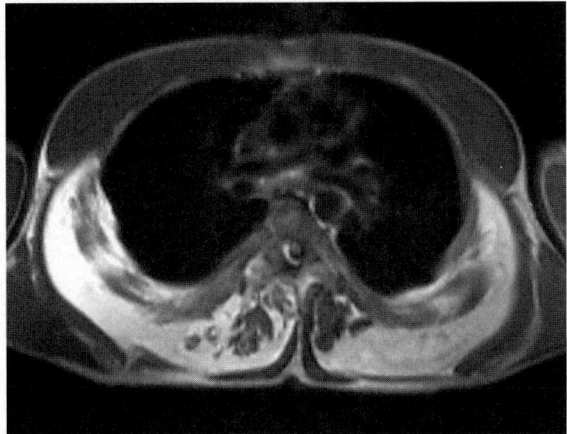

**Figure 71–10.** Multiple symmetrical lipomatosis (Madelung's disease). Axial T1-weighted (TR/TE, 775/20) spin echo MR image shows extensive symmetrical involvement of the chest wall.

often include an admixture of hibernoma and lipoma, and imaging shows variable nonadipose areas.

Lipoblastomas (Fig. 71–12) are tumors of immature and cellular fatty tissue seen in infancy and childhood, generally occurring in the extremities and uncommonly elsewhere. With maturation, lipoblastomas may convert to lipomas. The tumors may be well defined or infiltrative, and on CT or MR imaging, fatty tissue is often present in a portion of the lesion.

Lipoma arborescens (Fig. 71–13) is accompanied by diffuse fatty infiltration of the synovium in a joint (especially the knee), bursa, or tendon sheath, usually occurring idiopathically but sometimes associated with an underlying process such as rheumatoid arthritis or osteo-

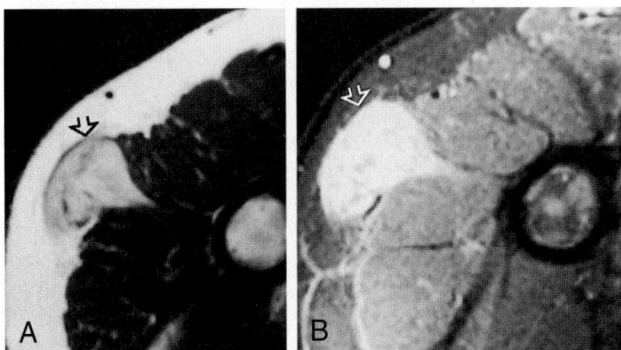

**Figure 71–11.** Hibernoma. In this 50-year-old man, a mass extends from the deltoid muscle into the adjacent subcutaneous tissues. It is of intermediate to high signal intensity on a transaxial T1-weighted (TR/TE, 400/15) spin echo MR image (*arrow* in *A*) and of high signal intensity on a transaxial STIR (TR/TE, 2000/30; inversion time, 140 msec) MR image (*arrow* in *B*). (Courtesy of S. Eilenberg, MD, San Diego, Calif.)

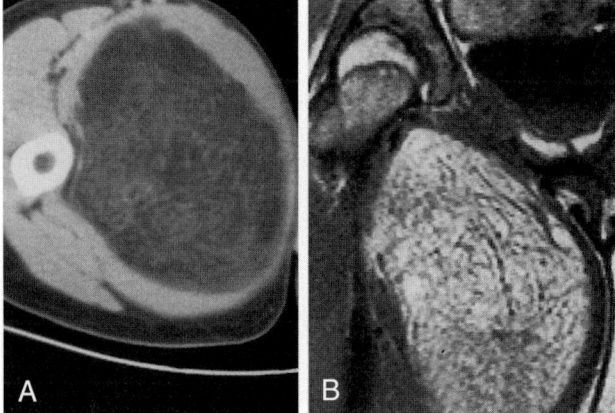

**Figure 71–12.** Lipoblastoma. This 12-year-old girl had a mass in the medial aspect of her right thigh that had developed over several years. It had increased significantly in size over the past few months and was painless. *A*, Transaxial contrast-enhanced CT image shows a rather well-defined radiolucent mass in the adductor muscles. It contains linear regions of increased attenuation. *B*, Coronal T1-weighted (TR/TE, 528/25) spin echo MR image shows that the mass has areas of signal intensity identical to that of fat, as well as linear regions of signal intensity close to that of muscle. (Courtesy of G. Greenway, MD, Dallas, Tex.)

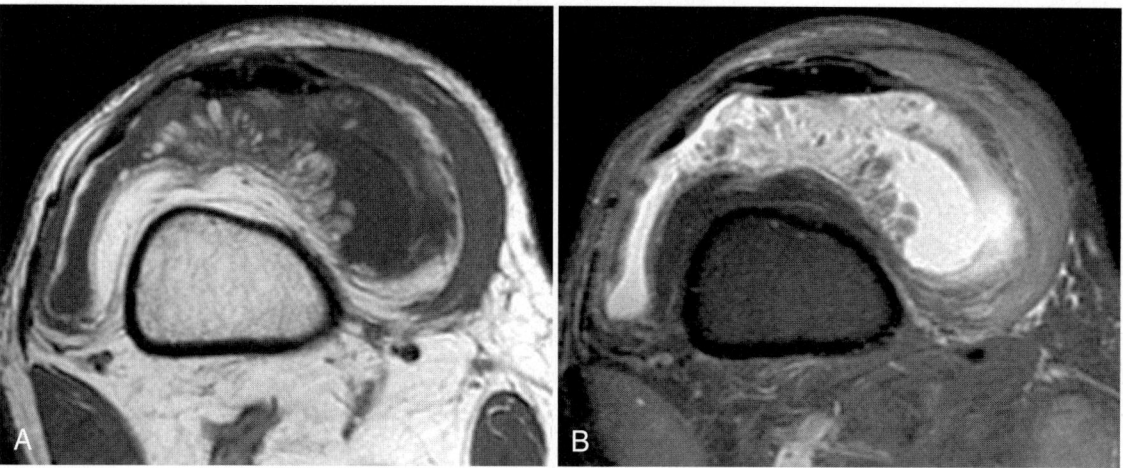

**Figure 71–13.** Lipoma arborescens. Axial T1-weighted (TR/TE, 3500/16) *(A)* and fat-suppressed transverse gradient echo (TR/TE, 610/18; flip angle, 25 degrees) *(B)* spin echo MR images show a moderate joint effusion with multiple synovial-based frondlike areas of fat signal.

arthritis. A frondlike or villous process containing fat with an associated effusion is characteristic on MR imaging.

## Tumors of Fibrous Tissue

**Fibrosarcoma.** Fibrosarcomas occur in both adults and children, and they predominate in the external soft tissues rather than the retroperitoneum, mediastinum, mesentery, or viscera; they are common in the thigh and knee. The frequency of these soft tissue sarcomas has decreased dramatically in recent years in that many lesions previously classified as fibrosarcoma are now designated as malignant fibrous histiocytomas. The neoplasms lack any specific radiographic or MR imaging characteristics. Calcification is seen but is much more frequent in synovial sarcomas.

Infantile fibrosarcoma is a rare but important tumor of infants and children that, although histologically identical to fibrosarcoma in adults, carries a much better prognosis. The peripheral soft tissues are typically affected, and local recurrence after excision is common. With MR imaging and CT, nonspecific findings are evident. The tumors are vascular, and the diagnosis is suggested in an infant or young child with a large soft tissue tumor in an extremity.

**Fibroma and Fibromatoses.** The classification of benign fibrous tumors is complicated (Table 71–6). Certain benign fibrous proliferations are termed fibromatoses. Within this group is the desmoid tumor, which may arise in abdominal or extra-abdominal sites. The designation musculoaponeurotic fibromatosis is sometimes applied to desmoid-like lesions of muscles, fascia, or the aponeurosis, which are observed in the limbs in persons of all ages. As in other forms of fibromatosis, signal heterogeneity characterizes the MR imaging appearance of musculoaponeurotic fibromatosis. Solitary lesions predominate but are not invariable. Recurrences are frequent. The shoulder area is a common site of extra-abdominal desmoid tumors. Other sites of involvement are the upper arm, thigh, neck, pelvis, forearm, and popliteal fossa,

in descending order of frequency. With MR imaging (Fig. 71–14), desmoid tumors show inhomogeneous signal intensity, variable margination, and possible neurovascular and bone involvement, findings not unlike those of malignant tumors. Persistent areas of low signal intensity on T2-weighted MR images, which represent fibrous tissue or regions of increased collagen deposition, allow a more specific diagnosis, especially with involution of the lesion. Inhomogeneous enhancement of signal intensity within a desmoid tumor may follow the intravenous administration of a gadolinium compound.

Palmar and plantar fibromatoses are fibrous proliferations occurring in the palmar fascia (Fig. 71–15) (in association with Dupuytren's contracture) and plantar fascia. These lesions vary in size and commonly recur after local excision. The lesions of plantar fibromatosis occur in patients of variable age but predominate in young adults. Bilateral involvement is evident in 20% to 60% of cases, and multiple sites of abnormality in a single foot are common. A predilection for the medial aspect of the foot has been observed. With MR imaging (Fig. 71–16), persistent low signal intensity in a well-defined or infiltrative mass is often observed, but increased signal intensity on T2-weighted images may be apparent, especially with more aggressive lesions. Similar increased signal intensity may be observed when fat suppression is used, on short tau inversion recovery (STIR) images, and after intravenous gadolinium administration.

Another type of fibrous proliferation is fibromatosis colli (Fig. 71–17), which usually develops in the sternocleidomastoid muscle of infants. Classically, a mass develops in the first few weeks of life, usually in the sternal, clavicular, or both heads of the lower portion of the sternocleidomastoid muscle. After a period of growth, more than half of lesions regress over a period of many months to several years.

Elastofibroma is characterized by unilateral or bilateral reactive lesions containing elastinophilic fibers; they are especially common between the scapula and chest wall (Fig. 71–18) and elsewhere about the shoulders. These

**TABLE 71–6**

**Benign Fibrous Proliferations and Fibromatoses**

| Diagnosis | Typical Age of Onset | Typical Location | Miscellaneous Data |
|---|---|---|---|
| **Fibrous Proliferations of Infancy and Childhood** | | | |
| Fibrous hamartoma | Infancy | Axillary, inguinal regions | Solitary, rarely recurs |
| Congenital generalized fibromatosis (infantile myofibromatosis) | Infancy | Soft tissue, viscera, bone | Solitary or multiple, may regress, rarely recurs |
| Infantile digital fibromatosis | Infancy | Fingers and toes | Solitary or multiple, may regress, commonly recurs |
| Fibromatosis colli | Infancy | Sternocleidomastoid muscle | Solitary, rarely bilateral, may regress, rarely recurs, associated torticollis |
| Juvenile aponeurotic fibroma | Infancy, childhood, or adolescence | Hands and feet | Solitary, may regress, commonly recurs, may calcify |
| Juvenile hyaline fibromatosis | Childhood | Dermis and subcutis | Multiple, does not regress or recur |
| Infantile desmoid-type fibromatosis | Infancy and childhood | Musculature | Solitary, commonly recurs, no regression |
| **Fibrous Proliferations of Adulthood** | | | |
| Nodular fasciitis (pseudosarcomatous fasciitis) | Adulthood | Extremities | Solitary, may regress, rarely recurs |
| Proliferative fasciitis | Adulthood | Extremities | Solitary |
| Proliferative myositis | Late adulthood | Trunk, shoulder girdle | Solitary |
| Elastofibroma | Late adulthood | Chest wall, scapula | Unilateral > bilateral |
| Keloid | Adolescence or adulthood | Face, shoulders, forearms, hands | Solitary or multiple, does not regress, common in blacks |
| **Fibromatoses** | | | |
| Palmar fibromatosis | Late adulthood | Hands | Unilateral or bilateral, associated Dupuytren's contracture |
| Plantar fibromatosis | Childhood or adulthood | Feet | Unilateral or bilateral, associated palmar fibromatosis |
| Peyronie's disease | Adulthood | Penis | May regress, associated palmar and plantar fibromatosis |
| Extra-abdominal fibromatosis (desmoid tumors) | Adulthood | Musculature | Rarely regresses, commonly recurs |
| Abdominal fibromatosis (desmoid tumors) | Early adulthood | Musculature | Commonly recurs, occurs during or after pregnancy |
| Intra-abdominal fibromatosis (pelvic fibromatosis, mesenteric fibromatosis, Gardner's syndrome) | Adulthood | Musculature, mesentery | May recur |

Taken in part from Enzinger FM, Weiss SW: Soft Tissue Tumors. St Louis, CV Mosby, 1983, p 71.

lesions develop in middle-aged and elderly persons, particularly those who are manual laborers or weightlifters. Women are affected more often than men. Based on its location and association with physical activity, mechanical friction appears to be important in the development of elastofibroma. MR imaging reveals a lesion containing both fat and fibrous tissue, which, if located in a periscapular region, is highly characteristic.

Congenital generalized fibromatosis (infantile myofibromatosis) affects mainly infants. In this condition, fibrous proliferation occurs not only in the superficial soft tissues but also in the viscera and bones (Fig. 71–19). Infantile myofibromatosis may be familial in some cases, and the tumors may disappear spontaneously. The osseous lesions can arise at any site; they are typically metaphyseal in location in the tubular bones and are variable in size. The bone lesions may be solitary or, more commonly, multiple; solitary lesions predominate in the craniofacial bones and are accompanied by a benign clinical course, whereas multiple lesions may or may not be associated with visceral involvement, which carries a poor prognosis.

## Tumors of Muscle

**Leiomyosarcoma.** Leiomyosarcomas are uncommon malignant neoplasms of soft tissues that affect primarily

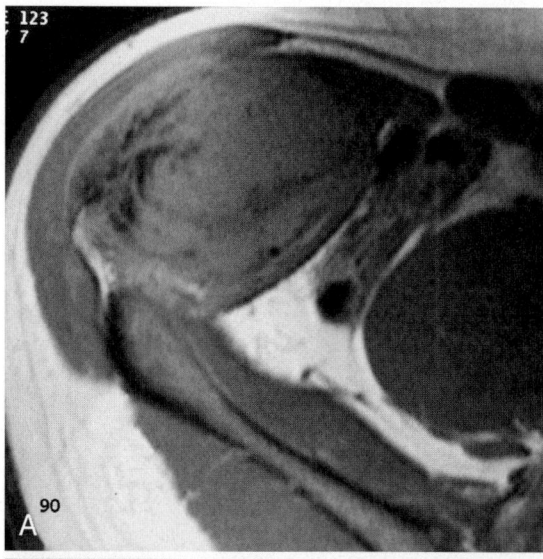

**Figure 71–14.** Extra-abdominal desmoid tumor. Transverse T1-weighted (TR/TE, 874/20) spin echo *(A)*, fat-suppressed fast spin echo (TR/TE, 3204/98) *(B)*, and fat-suppressed T1-weighted (TR/TE, 800/20) spin echo *(C)* MR images are shown, the last image obtained after intravenous gadolinium administration. Note the foci of persistent low signal intensity in this lesion (located just anterior to the ilium), which represent dense collagen tissue. (Courtesy of J. Edwards, MD, Savannah, Ga.)

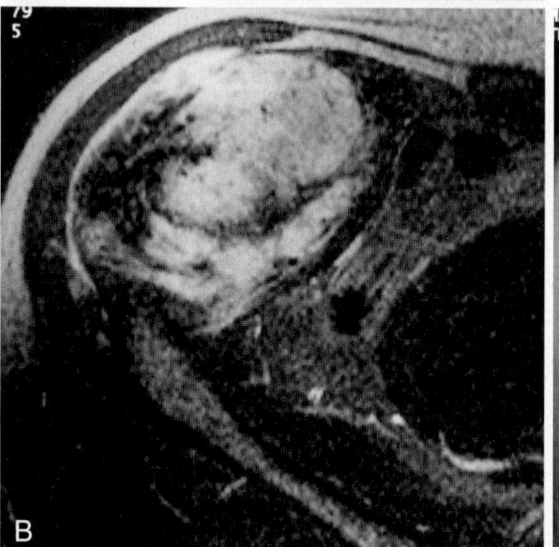

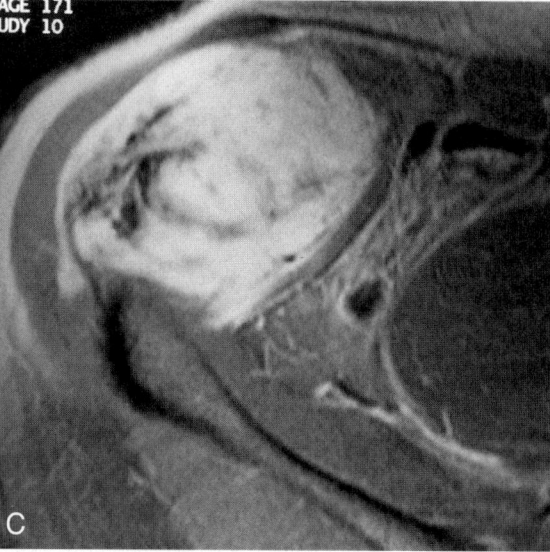

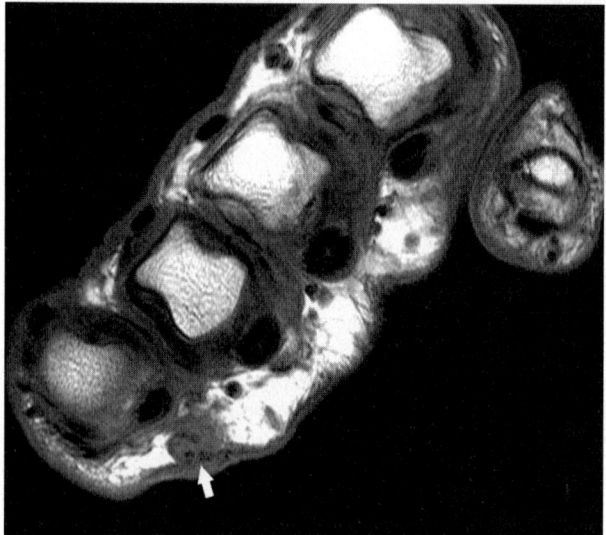

**Figure 71–15.** Palmar fibromatosis. Axial T1-weighted (TR/TE, 656/17) spin echo MR image shows a subcutaneous nodule representing the termination of a cordlike thickening of the palmar aponeurosis.

adults. The tumors predominate in the fifth and sixth decades of life, although they are rarely seen in children. They may arise in the retroperitoneum, peripheral soft tissues (especially in the thigh), or major blood vessels. Those occurring in the retroperitoneal region are the most common. Soft tissue masses of variable size, hypervascularity, and bone invasion are encountered in cases of leiomyosarcoma. Tumors associated with major blood vessels generally arise from veins, not arteries. Typical sites of origin are the inferior vena cava and great saphenous vein; less common sites of origin are the iliac, femoral, and jugular veins and the pulmonary and femoral arteries. Intraluminal or extraluminal growth may occur, and associated thromboses are common. Although findings on CT and MR imaging are nonspecific, large areas of tumor necrosis are typical (Fig. 71–20).

**Leiomyoma.** Leiomyomas, the benign counterparts of leiomyosarcomas, can be found in the skin and subcutaneous or deep soft tissue. They arise at various sites, frequently from the smooth muscle or small blood vessels; are single or multiple; and may ossify or calcify,

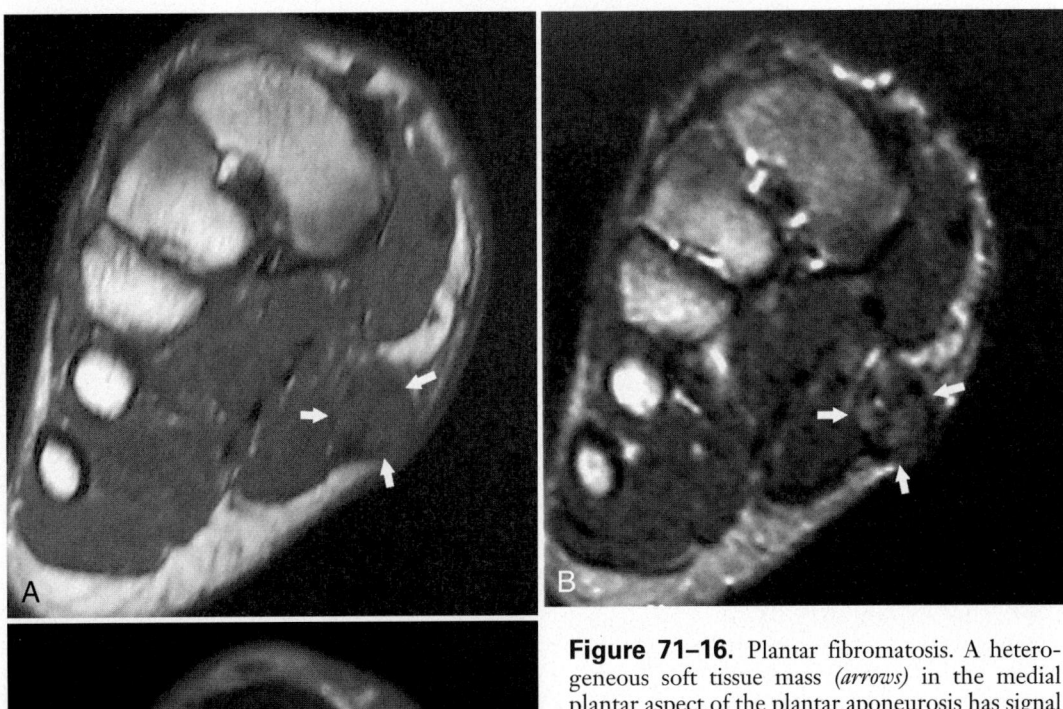

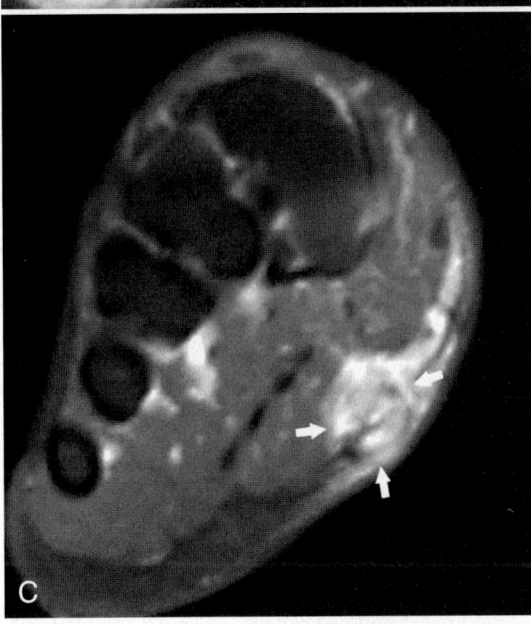

**Figure 71–16.** Plantar fibromatosis. A heterogeneous soft tissue mass *(arrows)* in the medial plantar aspect of the plantar aponeurosis has signal intensity similar to that of muscle on an axial T1-weighted (TR/TE, 500/15) spin echo MR image *(A)* and signal intensity similar to and slightly higher than that of muscle on a conventional T2-weighted (TR/TE, 2500/90) fast spin echo MR image *(B).* Axial fat-suppressed T1-weighted (TR/TE, 600/15) image following contrast *(C)* shows intense enhancement. Apparent enhancement beyond the medial aspect of the lesion is due to inhomogeneous fat suppression.

usually in association with necrosis of part of the tumor. With CT or MR imaging, the lesions may be either well defined or poorly delineated and inhomogeneous; associated vascularity is documented with intravenous contrast administration. With MR imaging, the signal intensity of the tumor is variable and often not homogeneous, although it sometimes follows the signal intensity of muscle (Fig. 71–21).

**Rhabdomyosarcoma.** Rhabdomyosarcoma predominates in children between the ages of 2 and 6 years and in adolescents between the ages of 14 and 18 years. It is rare after age 45 or 50 years. In the pediatric age group, tumors predominate in the head, neck, and urogenital tract and affect both boys and girls. Indeed, rhabdomyosarcoma is the most common malignant tumor of soft tissue in children. Embryonal, alveolar, and pleomorphic histologic types are recognized, with the first type being

most common and the last type predominating in adults. Radiographic examination reveals soft tissue masses that rarely calcify or invade neighboring bone. Skeletal metastasis can resemble neuroblastoma. In adult rhabdomyosarcoma, many of the lesions are located in the deeper tissues of the extremities and torso. The imaging features of rhabdomyosarcoma lack specificity. With MR imaging, the tumor is usually isointense to skeletal muscle on T1-weighted images and has high signal intensity on T2-weighted images (Fig. 71–22). Persistent regions of low signal intensity, prominent vessels, enhancement of signal intensity after intravenous gadolinium administration, and hemorrhage are additional MR imaging features.

**Rhabdomyoma.** Rhabdomyoma is an extremely rare benign tumor composed of striated muscle cells that occurs in both children and adults. Rhabdomyoma in

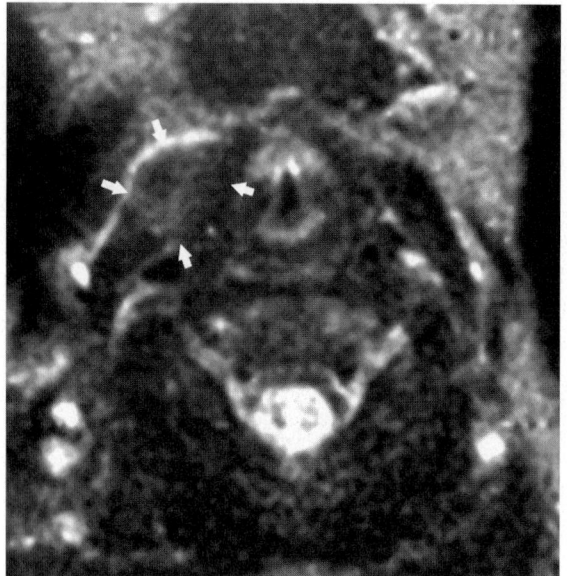

**Figure 71–17.** Fibromatosis colli. Axial T2-weighted (TR/TE, 2000/90) spin echo MR image of a 10-week-old child being evaluated for a palpable neck mass noted at age 2 weeks. The right sternocleidomastoid muscle is enlarged, with slightly increased signal *(arrows)*, but there is no discrete mass.

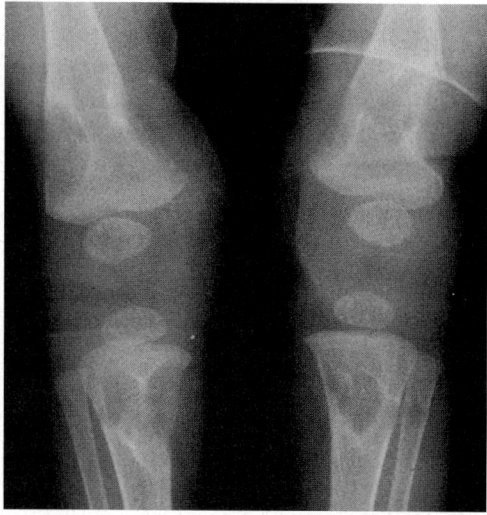

**Figure 71–19.** Infantile myofibromatosis. Radiograph of a 5-month-old girl shows multiple symmetrically distributed radiolucent foci, predominantly in the metaphyses of the tubular bones, representing sites of fibrous proliferation. (Courtesy of D. Weissberg, MD, Orange, Calif.)

infants and children (fetal rhabdomyoma) usually affects boys younger than 2 years and most commonly appears as a subcutaneous nodule in the posterior auricular region. When observed in the cervix, vagina, or vulva in middle-aged women, the tumor is designated genital rhabdomyoma and simulates the appearance of sarcoma botryoides. A special variety of rhabdomyoma occurs in the heart.

## Myxomatoses

Many types of myxoid tumors and tumor-like lesions have been described, and inconstant nomenclature has led to problems in classification. Myxomatous lesions include ganglia, juxta-articular myxomas (also known as cystic myxomas, meniscal cysts, and ganglion cysts with a myxoid lesion), and intramuscular myxomas.

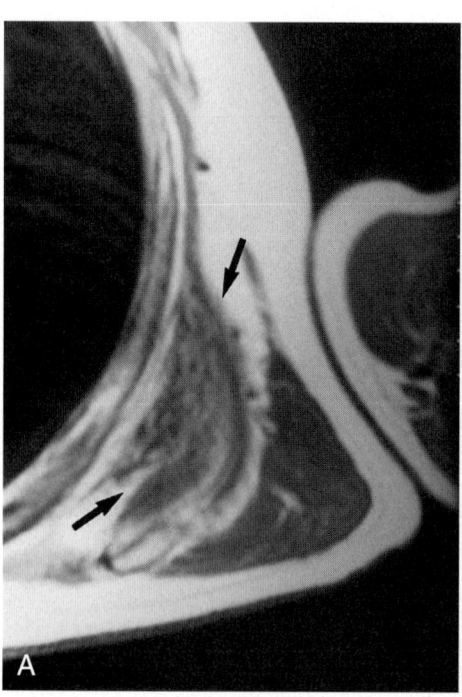
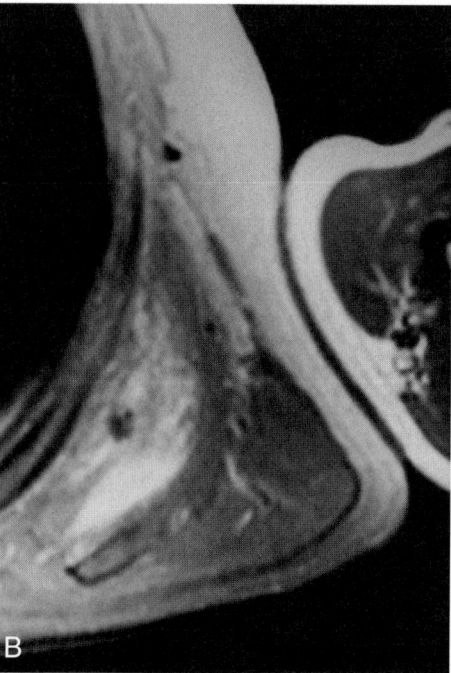

**Figure 71–18.** Elastofibroma. *A,* Transverse T1-weighted (TR/TE, 650/14) spin echo MR image reveals a mass *(arrows)* located between the scapula and chest wall with predominant signal intensity similar to that of muscle. Regions of higher signal intensity within the lesion represent foci of fat. *B,* On a transverse fat-suppressed T1-weighted (TR/TE, 650/14) spin echo MR image, this mass shows irregular enhancement after intravenous gadolinium administration. (Courtesy of J. Jacobson, MD, Ann Arbor, Mich.)

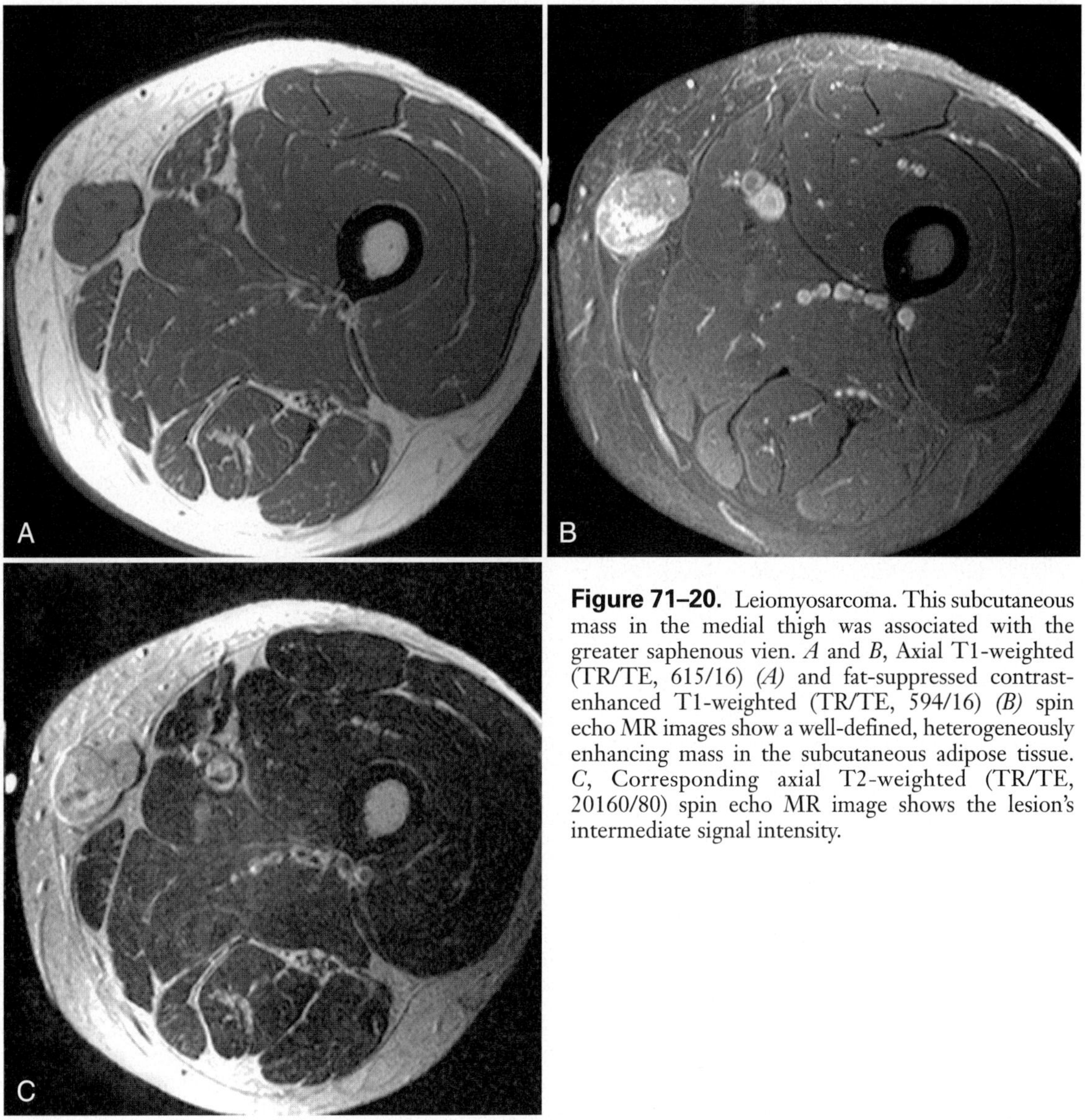

**Figure 71–20.**  Leiomyosarcoma. This subcutaneous mass in the medial thigh was associated with the greater saphenous vien. *A* and *B*, Axial T1-weighted (TR/TE, 615/16) *(A)* and fat-suppressed contrast-enhanced T1-weighted (TR/TE, 594/16) *(B)* spin echo MR images show a well-defined, heterogeneously enhancing mass in the subcutaneous adipose tissue. *C*, Corresponding axial T2-weighted (TR/TE, 20160/80) spin echo MR image shows the lesion's intermediate signal intensity.

**Ganglion.**  As classically described, a ganglion is a cystic tumor-like lesion that is usually attached to a tendon sheath, particularly in the hands, wrists, and feet (Fig. 71–23). It also arises from tendons, muscles, and semi-lunar cartilage. Unilocular or multilocular cystic swellings are observed, although their exact pathogenesis is not clear. Radiographic evaluation may reveal a soft tissue mass, surface bone resorption, and periosteal new bone

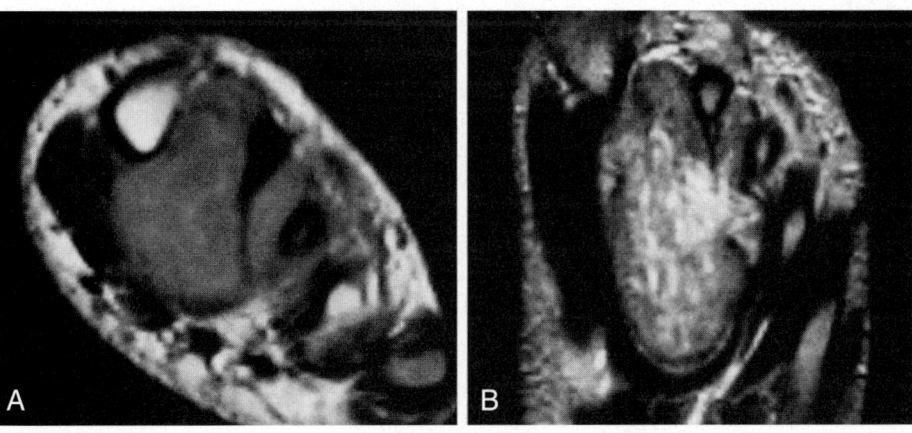

**Figure 71–21.**  Leiomyoma. A vascular leiomyoma (angioleiomyoma) of the foot is seen as a tumor of low signal intensity on a coronal T1-weighted (TR/TE, 750/40) spin echo MR image *(A)* and of inhomogeneous signal intensity on a transverse T2-weighted (TR/TE, 2000/80) spin echo MR image *(B)*. (Courtesy of A. Newberg, MD, Boston, Mass.)

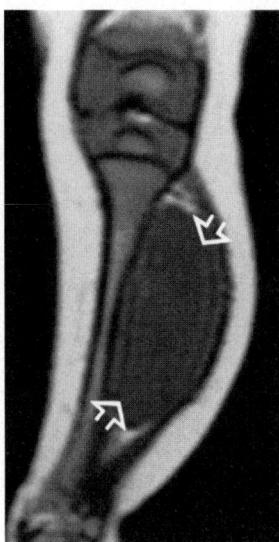

**Figure 71–22.** Rhabdomyosarcoma. Coronal T1-weighted (TR/TE, 500/20) spin echo MR image shows a mass *(arrows)* of low signal intensity producing pressure erosion of the tibia in a 6-month-old girl. (Courtesy of T. Broderick, MD, Orange, Calif.)

formation. Arthrography or tenography may outline communication between the mass and the underlying articular or tendinous structure, especially if delayed images are obtained. Ultrasonography can also be used for diagnosis.

Ganglia arising about the proximal tibiofibular joint are associated with compression of the common peroneal nerve (Fig. 71–24). Those near the hip (and elsewhere) are associated with chronic developmental dysplasia and may communicate with subchondral cystic lesions, which are frequently interpreted as intraosseous ganglia.

**Myxoma.** A myxoma is an uncommon connective tissue tumor characterized by an abundant myxoid matrix and a paucity of spindle-shaped stromal cells. It can appear at any age. These lesions are categorized as intramuscular myxomas, subcutaneous and aponeurotic myxomas, and juxta-articular myxomas.

Intramuscular myxomas are most frequent in the fifth through seventh decades of life, predominate in women, and are most common in the thigh, shoulder, and, to a lesser extent, buttock and upper arm. Solitary lesions are more common than multiple lesions, and multiple myxomas are often associated with fibrous dysplasia, a combination of findings referred to as Mazabraud's syndrome. Intramuscular myxomas are of variable size and usually well circumscribed. Excision is generally curative. MR imaging shows a mass of low signal intensity on T1-weighted images and high signal intensity on T2-weighted images, with a variable pattern of enhancement after intravenous gadolinium administration (Fig. 71–25).

Subcutaneous and aponeurotic myxomas represent about 20% of all soft tissue myxomas. They are often well circumscribed and superficial in location. Juxta-articular, or periarticular, myxomas are usually observed about large joints such as the knee. Histologically, cystic

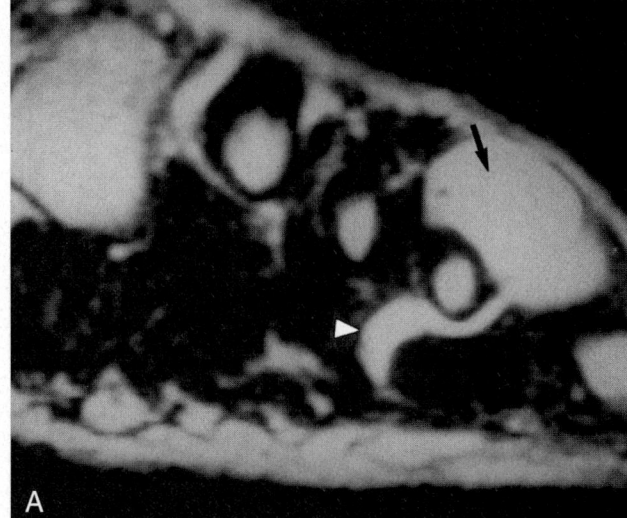

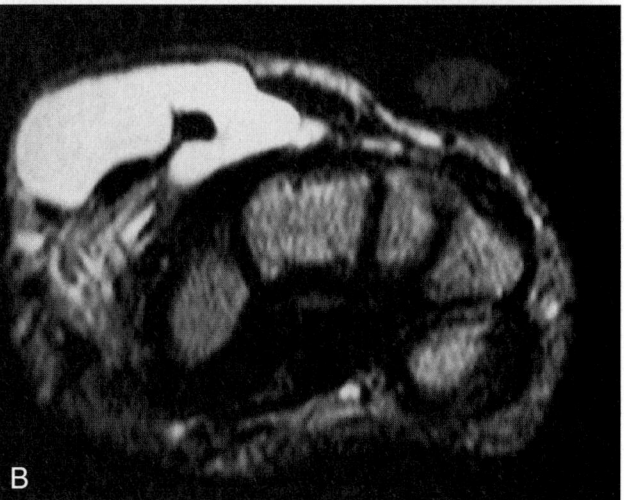

**Figure 71–23.** Ganglion. *A,* Foot. Coronal fast spin echo (TR/TE, 3200/120) MR image shows a ganglion *(arrow)* on the dorsal surface that is communicating via a tract *(arrowhead)* with the plantar tendons. *B,* Wrist. Coronal T2-weighted (TR/TE, 2000/90) spin echo MR image reveals a large dorsal ganglion communicating with a tendon sheath.

changes are often observed, a characteristic that gives these lesions and ganglia overlapping features.

## Tumors of Fibrohistiocytic Composition

Attention has recently been directed toward soft tissue tumors dominated by histiocytes and, specifically, toward a group of tumors composed of cells that resemble fibroblasts and histiocytes. The diversity of opinion regarding the derivation of cells that compose fibrohistiocytic neoplasms has led to shifting nomenclature and complex classification systems and has cast doubt on the validity of data provided by older scientific publications dealing with these or similar tumors. Amid the chaos is the certainty that a number of both benign and malignant neoplasms of soft tissues (as well as neoplasms of bone and supporting structures of various organs) are characterized by a histologic pattern frequently dominated by

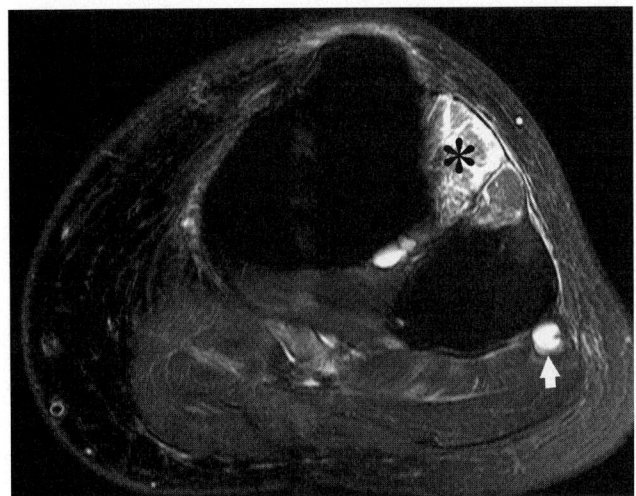

**Figure 71–24.** Ganglion. In a patient with documented peroneal nerve palsy, transaxial fat-suppressed turbo-T2-weighted (TR/TE, 4390/80) spin echo MR image reveals changes of denervation, best seen in the tibialis anterior muscle *(asterisk)*. The lower aspect of the ganglion is just seen along the lateral margin of the fibula *(arrow)*.

spindle cells that exhibit either a storiform pattern (resembling a woven mat) or a fascicular pattern and that may be admixed with myxoid, foam, giant, and inflammatory cells.

**Malignant Fibrous Histiocytoma.** This tumor generally occurs in adults, more frequently in men than in women.

The lower extremity is the most common site of involvement, followed by the upper extremity and retroperitoneum. It typically involves deep fascia or skeletal muscle and only rarely is confined to the subcutis without fascial involvement. It produces a mass of variable size with nonspecific radiographic features. Infrequently, metaplastic bone and cartilage formation in the lesion is visible on conventional radiographs or CT; the resulting radiodense areas predominate at the periphery of the tumor, similar to the characteristics of myositis ossificans. MR imaging features are not specific. The signal intensity characteristics of the tumor vary with but are not specific for histologic variations. Fibrous tissue, calcification, hemorrhage, necrosis, or combinations of these findings influence the single intensity characteristics (Figs. 71–26 and 71–27).

**Benign Fibrous Histiocytoma.** This lesion is also referred to as sclerosing hemangioma, dermatofibroma, and nodular subepidermal fibrosis. It affects both children and adults and is generally seen in the skin or subcutaneous tissue or viscera. Small nodular masses that may be painful are characteristic of superficial tumors. Tumors are multiple in about 30% of cases and may be located in any part of the extremities, even in the fingers and toes. Although the MR imaging features are nonspecific, the tumor may have persistent low signal intensity on T2-weighted images (Fig. 71–28).

**Dermatofibrosarcoma Protuberans.** This tumor, which is composed of fibroblasts with a prominent storiform pattern, represents about 6% of all soft tissue sarcomas.

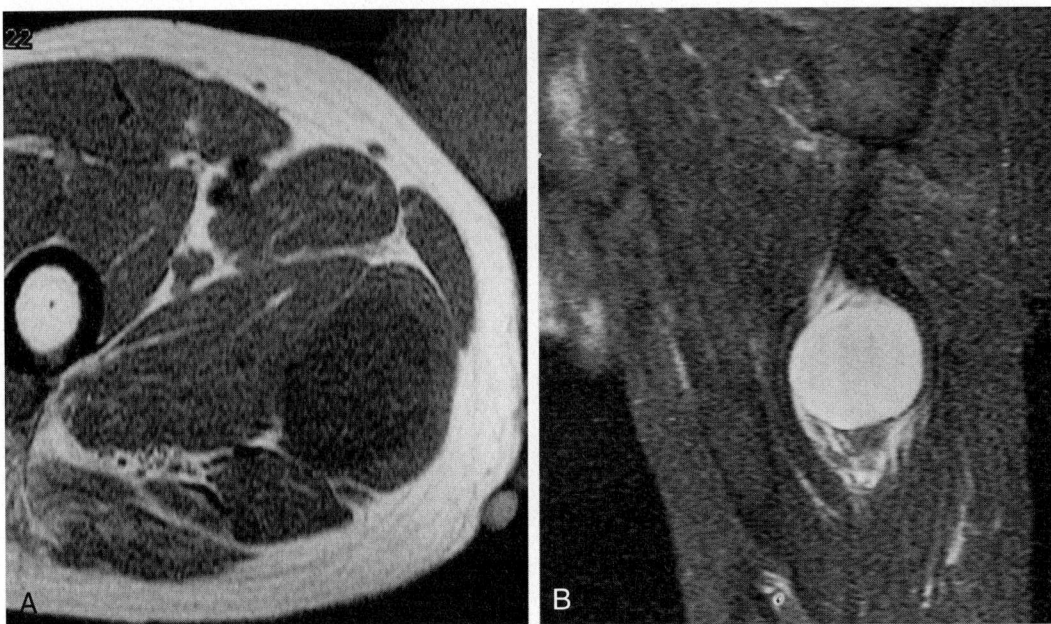

**Figure 71–25.** Myxoma. This intramuscular myxoma of the thigh has signal intensity lower than that of muscle on a transverse T1-weighted (TR/TE, 450/16) spin echo MR image *(A)* and much higher than that of muscle on a sagittal STIR (TR/TE, 5000/34; inversion time, 120 msec) MR image *(B)*. Although generally well defined, adjacent strands of high signal intensity can be seen in *(B)*. (Courtesy of D. Goodwin, MD, Hanover, NH.)

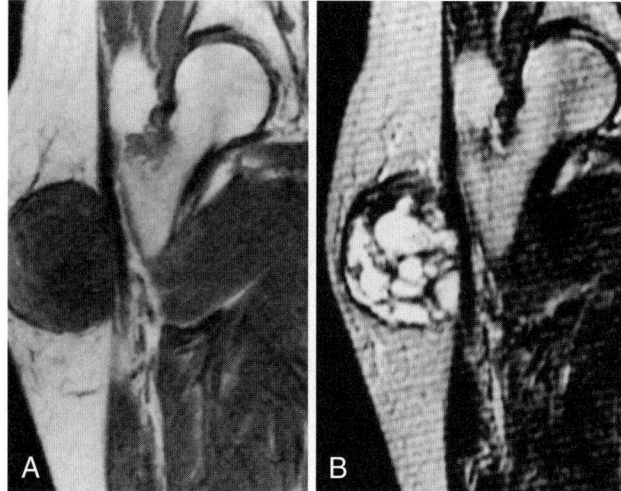

**Figure 71–26.** Malignant fibrous histiocytoma. In this 66-year-old woman, a mass lateral to the proximal portion of the femur is located mainly in subcutaneous tissue but also involves the fascia. It is well circumscribed and of low signal intensity on a coronal T1-weighted (TR/TE, 600/17) spin echo MR image *(A)* and of mixed signal intensity on a coronal T2-weighted (TR/TE, 2000/80) spin echo MR image *(B)*. In *(B)*, note the linear foci of low signal intensity. (Courtesy of M. Schweitzer, MD, Philadelphia, Pa.)

A superficial location in the skin and subcutaneous tissue; involvement of the trunk and, less commonly, the extremities and the head and neck; single or multiple nodules; and discoloration of the overlying skin are other characteristics of this tumor. Most affected patients are in the third to fifth decades of life. The rate of tumor

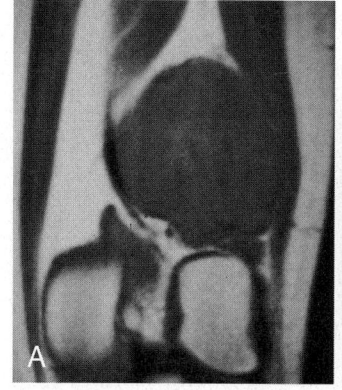
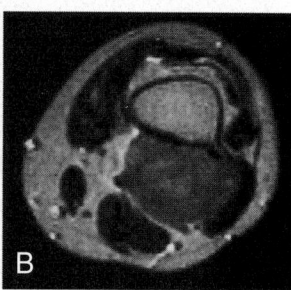

**Figure 71–28.** Fibrous histiocytoma. This 26-year-old woman had a painful mass behind her knee. It is smooth and well marginated and shows predominantly low signal intensity on coronal T1-weighted (TR/TE, 680/21) *(A)* and transaxial T2-weighted (TR/TE, 2000/85) *(B)* spin echo MR images.

growth is slow, but larger lesions may involve deeper soft tissue structures. Dermatofibrosarcoma protuberans appears as a nonmineralized, superficial soft tissue mass. The patterns of tissue attenuation with CT scanning and signal intensity with MR imaging are not specific. This hypervascular tumor enhances after intravenous contrast administration (Fig. 71–29).

**Xanthomatoses.** Xanthomatoses are a group of tumor-like proliferations characterized by the presence of a variable number of foam cells. Some tumors are associated with metabolic and endocrine disorders, such as hypercholesterolemia and diabetes mellitus. Many varieties are

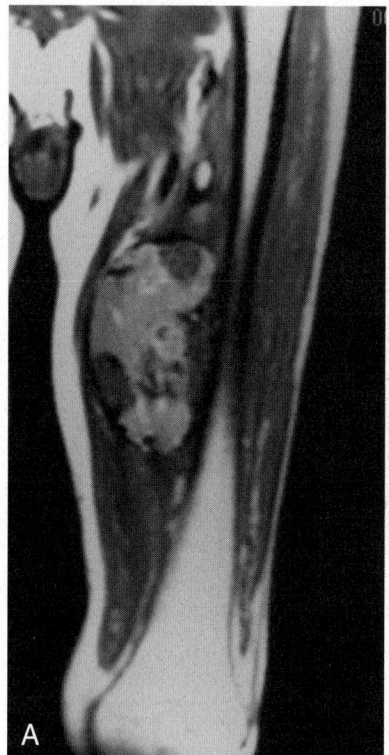
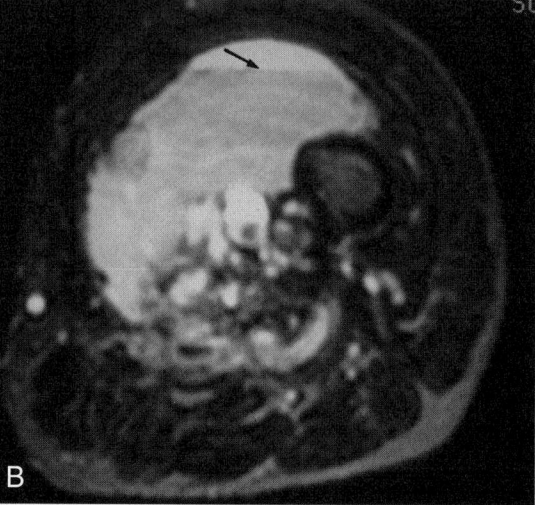

**Figure 71–27.** Malignant fibrous histiocytoma. This hemorrhagic tumor in the thigh of an 80-year-old man is intramuscular, elongated, and irregular in outline, with inhomogeneous signal intensity on a coronal T1-weighted (TR/TE, 500/16) spin echo MR image *(A)* and a transaxial fat-suppressed fast spin echo (TR/TE, 5000/102) MR image *(B)*. Note the fluid level *(arrow in B)*.

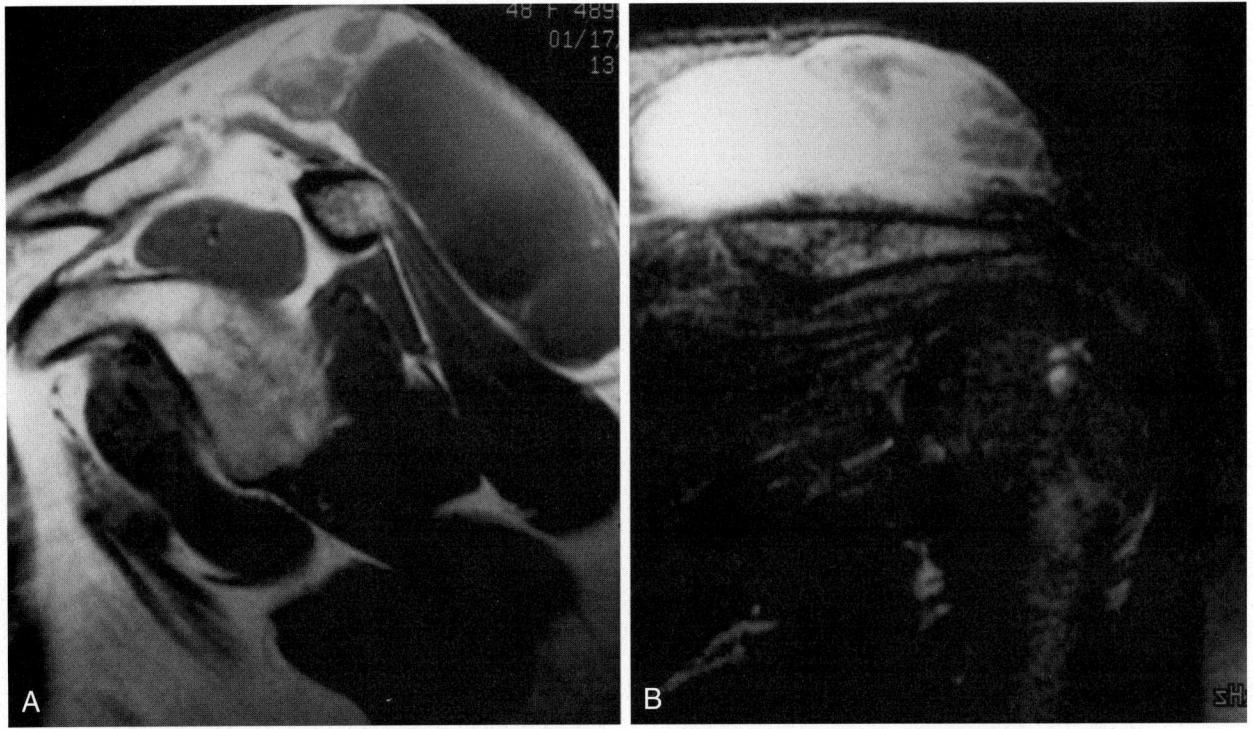

**Figure 71–29.** Dermatofibrosarcoma protuberans. In this 48-year-old woman, note the large superficial tumor in the posterior aspect of the shoulder, as shown on an oblique sagittal T1-weighted (TR/TE, 500/17) spin echo MR image *(A)* and an oblique coronal fat-suppressed fast spin echo (TR/TE, 4000/98) MR image *(B)*. In *(A)*, the signal intensity is similar to that of muscle, whereas inhomogeneous but mainly high signal intensity is seen in *(B)*.

recognized. Tendinous xanthomas are common about the finger, heel, elbow, and knee, where they may erode subjacent bone. Calcification appears in 20% to 25% of cases. MR imaging typically shows thickened tendons with heterogeneous signal intensity, including regions of low signal intensity on T2-weighted spin echo MR images (Fig. 71–30).

## Vascular and Lymphatic Tumors

**Hemangioma.** Hemangioma is the most frequent tumor in the soft tissues and the most common tumor of infancy and childhood. Classification of hemangiomas is based on the type of vascular channel that dominates the histologic appearance. A capillary hemangioma is composed solely of capillaries. This tumor is common and usually appears early in life in the skin or subcutaneous tissue. If histologic analysis shows widely dilated capillaries, the tumor is called a cavernous hemangioma. Cavernous hemangiomas predominate in the deep soft tissues, are less frequent than capillary hemangiomas, and, unlike capillary hemangiomas, do not involute; they commonly calcify (i.e., form phleboliths). If a vascular tumor has thick walls and contains smooth muscle cells, it is called a venous hemangioma. This tumor is less frequent than capillary hemangiomas, and it predominates in children in the upper portion of the body. Slow blood flow typifies venous hemangiomas, and phleboliths may be seen. When histologic analysis shows abnormal communication of

arteries and veins, the tumor is called an arteriovenous hemangioma or arteriovenous malformation. This type of lesion may be associated with arteriovenous shunting of blood and resultant high blood flow.

Radiographs of hemangiomas and related lesions may reveal evidence of soft tissue masses containing circular calcified collections (phleboliths) or, rarely, ossification (see Fig. 71–1); in addition, osseous involvement, overgrowth, and articular abnormalities (especially in the knee, as a result of accompanying synovial lesions) may be encountered. Intramuscular hemangiomas are typically poorly marginated and isointense relative to skeletal muscle on T1-weighted MR images; delicate or coarse strands or bands that contain areas with signal intensity identical to that of fat are seen within the lesion on such images. On T2-weighted MR images, intramuscular hemangiomas are well marginated and hyperintense in comparison with subcutaneous fat and may contain segments that are isointense relative to fat or muscle (Figs. 71–31 and 71–32). On either type of image, foci of low signal intensity representing phleboliths may be evident. Some types of intramuscular hemangiomas, particularly cavernous hemangiomas, contain large amounts of fatty tissue, similar to a lipoma. Serpentine areas within hemangiomas can be a diagnostic aid. Masses of large tortuous vessels accompanied by rapidly flowing blood, which may be found in arteriovenous hemangiomas (Fig. 71–33), are characterized by regions of signal void. Deep and superficial extramuscular hemangiomas, as well

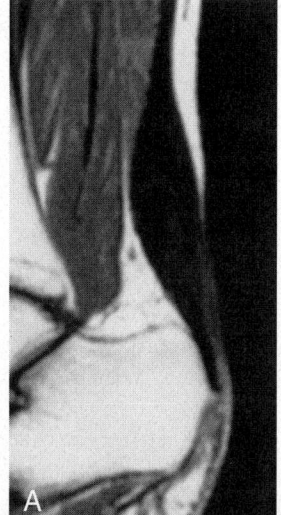

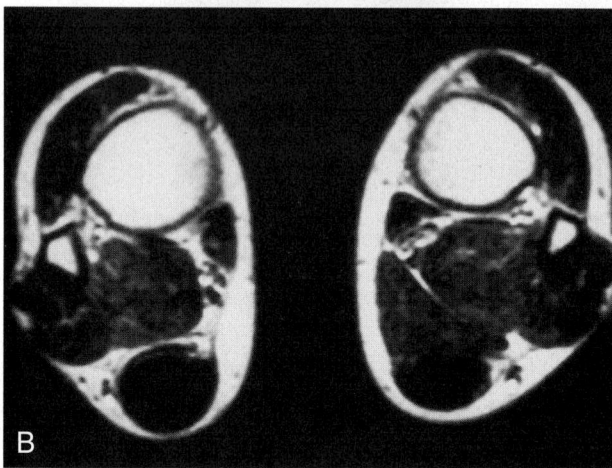

**Figure 71–30.** Xanthoma: tendinous involvement. *A*, Sagittal T1-weighted (TR/TE, 600/12) spin echo MR image shows fusiform enlargement of the Achilles tendon, which is of low signal intensity. *B*, Transaxial T2-weighted (TR/TE, 3600/102) fast spin echo MR image reveals bilateral involvement of the Achilles tendons. The signal intensity of the involved tendons is low and homogeneous. (Courtesy of M. Weisman, MD, Los Angeles, Calif.)

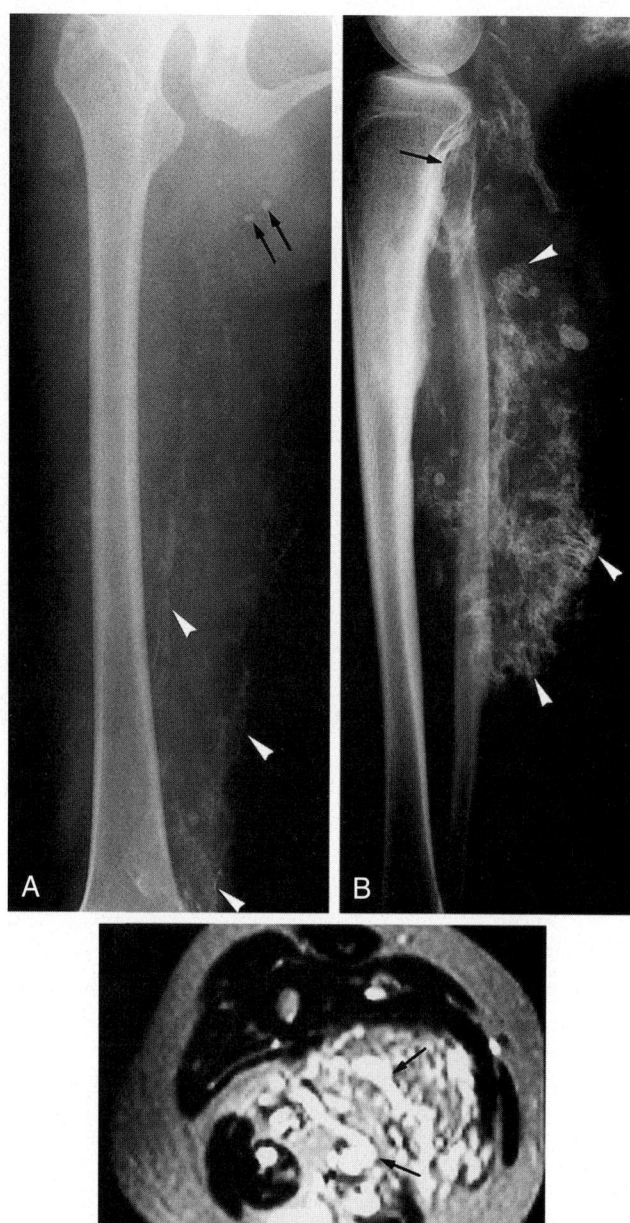

**Figure 71–31.** Hemangioma. *A*, This massive, cavernous hemangioma of the right lower extremity is associated with sheetlike and irregular ossification *(arrowheads)* and phleboliths *(arrows)* in the soft tissues of the thigh and upper portion of the leg. *B*, In the lower portion of the leg, extensive soft tissue ossification *(arrowheads)* and bone erosion *(arrow)* and hyperostosis are evident. *C*, Transaxial T2-weighted (TR/TE, 1000/110) spin echo MR image shows the serpentine areas of high signal intensity *(arrows)* that are typical of hemangioma. (Courtesy of Y.C. Wang, MD, Taipei, Taiwan.)

as synovial hemangiomas, have similar MR imaging features (Fig. 71–34). Some variations in these features reflect modifications in the amount of nonvascular tissue, which includes fat, fibrous tissue, myxoid stroma, smooth muscle, hemosiderin, bone, and thrombus. In some cases, fluid levels reflecting the presence of blood-filled cavities are seen, although this finding is not specific. Synovial hemangiomas predominate in the knee.

**Lymphangioma.** Lymphangiomas are composed of sequestered, noncommunicating lymphoid tissue lined by lymphatic endothelium. These tumors are categorized as capillary lymphangiomas (small subcutaneous lesions), cavernous lymphangiomas (subcutaneous lesions about the mouth, tongue, salivary glands, and intramuscular septa), and cystic lymphangiomas or cystic hygromas (hugely dilated lymphatic spaces typically occurring in

the neck, with possible extension into the mediastinum, pleural spaces, and axilla, in which osteolysis or bone hypertrophy may be present). All types of lymphangioma are typically seen at birth or very early in life (Fig. 71–35), although they are occasionally encountered in older children or even adults, especially when located in the

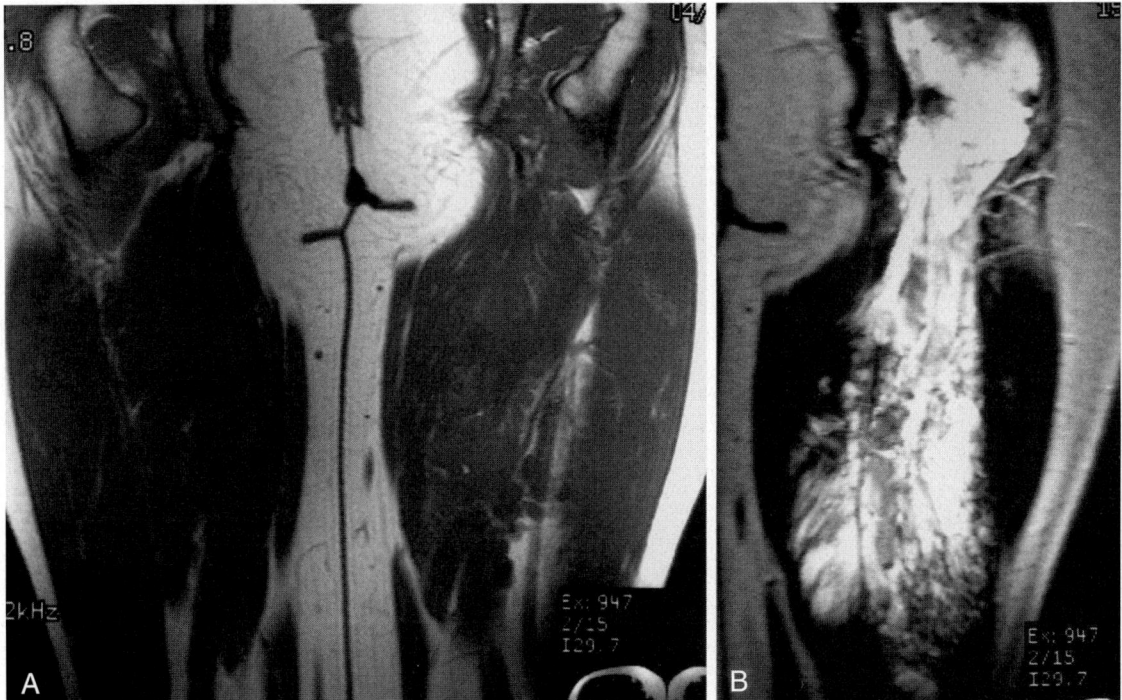

**Figure 71–32.** Hemangioma: intramuscular type. *A*, In this 15-year-old girl with a medial thigh mass, a coronal T1-weighted (TR/TE, 600/10) spin echo MR image shows muscle enlargement but little else. *B*, Coronal T2-weighted (TR/TE, 4000/100) spin echo MR image reveals a large intramuscular hemangioma manifesting as irregular and channel-like regions of high signal intensity. (Courtesy of A. D'Abreu, MD, Porto Alegre, Brazil.)

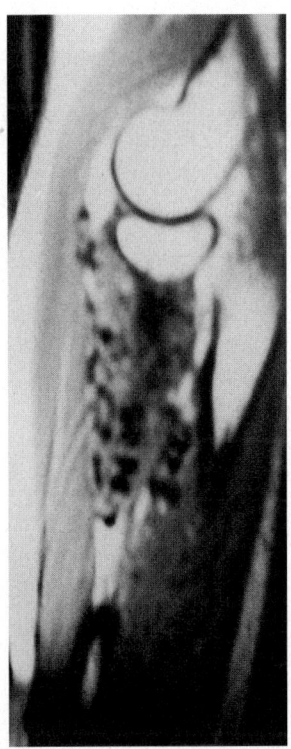

**Figure 71–33.** Arteriovenous hemangioma (arteriovenous malformation). Sagittal T1-weighted (TR/TE, 600/20) spin echo MR image shows tortuous vessels of low signal intensity.

retroperitoneum. With ultrasonography, cystic masses containing septa of variable thickness are observed.

**Glomus Tumor.** A glomus tumor is a benign lesion arising from the neuromyoarterial glomus. This tumor is uncommon, occurs with equal frequency in men and women, and is usually detected in adults. It is typically located beneath the fingernail (subungual glomus tumor) and leads to prominent symptoms that are out of proportion to the size of the lesion (usually <1 cm); radiographs may reveal an eccentric intraosseous lucent lesion or cortical erosion in the terminal phalanx. MR images reveal nodules of low signal intensity on T1-weighted spin echo images and high signal intensity on T2-weighted images (Fig. 71–36). Solitary tumors predominate, but multiple lesions are occasionally encountered, especially in children.

**Angiosarcoma.** Angiosarcoma is a malignant angiomatous tumor that shares features with lymphangiosarcoma, and the two terms are sometimes used interchangeably. Skin or deep soft tissues are involved, and most affected patients are elderly. Lymphangiosarcoma (or angiosarcoma) may be associated with chronic lymphedema, especially in women who have undergone radical mastectomies for carcinoma of the breast, a situation designated the Stewart-Treves syndrome. Lymphangiosarcoma (or angiosarcoma) less commonly complicates congenital, traumatic, or idiopathic lymphedema and is rare in cases of filarial lymphedema.

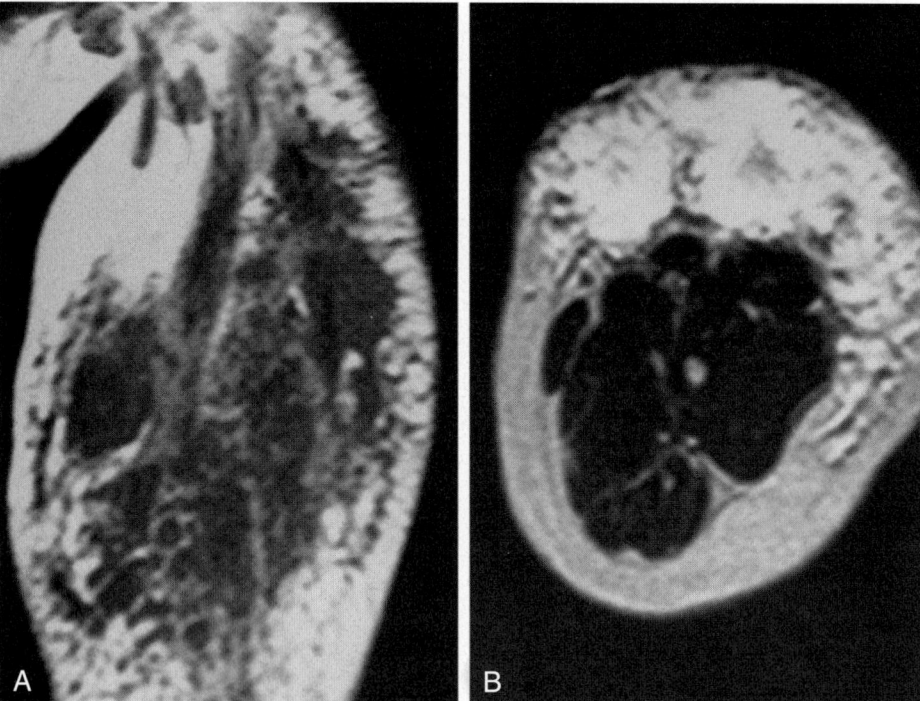

**Figure 71–34.** Hemangioma: superficial type. In this child, a superficial hemangioma in the thigh appears septated, with nodular and linear regions. It is of low signal intensity on a coronal T1-weighted (TR/TE, 700/30) spin echo MR image *(A)* and of high signal intensity on a transaxial T2-weighted (TR/TE, 1800/100) spin echo MR image *(B)*. (Courtesy of T. Mattsson, MD, Riyadh, Saudi Arabia.)

**Kaposi's Sarcoma.** This tumor is a complex vascular growth consisting of both capillaries and fibrosarcoma-like cells. The lesion predominates in adult men and in persons with acquired immunodeficiency syndrome and is especially common in blacks in certain parts of Africa. Cutaneous eruptions or nodules, frequently in the lower extremity, may lead to invasion of underlying bone. Some patients also have evidence of malignant lymphoma, lymphatic leukemia, diabetes mellitus, and varicosities.

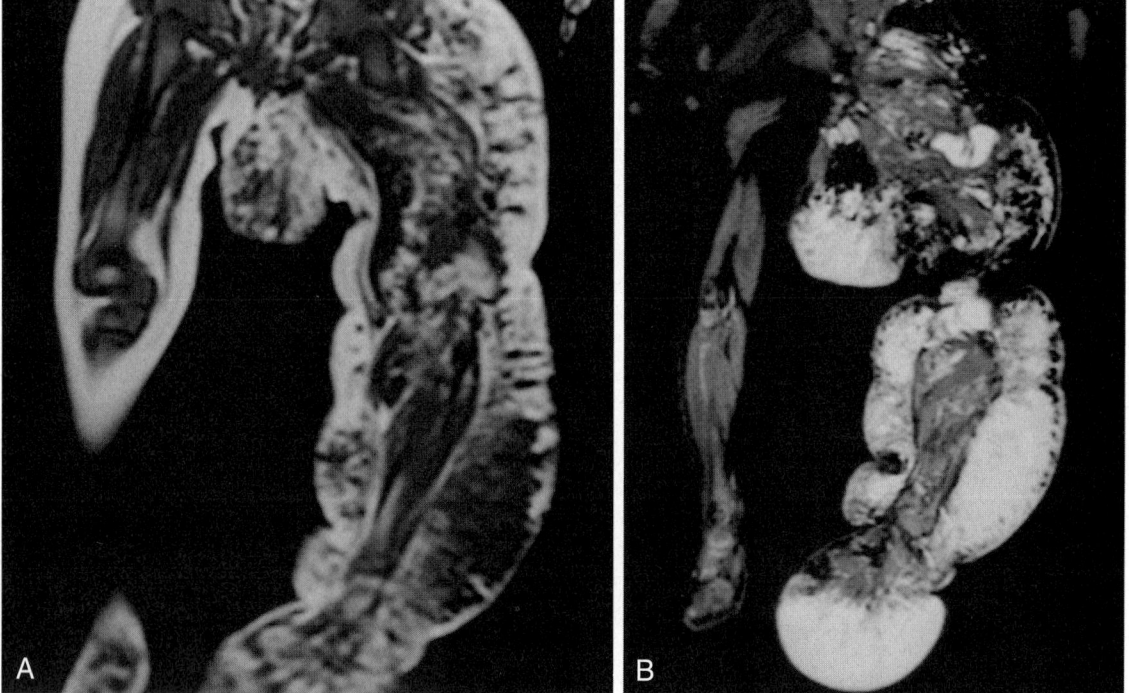

**Figure 71–35.** Lymphangioma. In this 10-month-old patient, coronal T1-weighted (TR/TE, 400/8) spin echo *(A)* and STIR (TR/TE, 6206/33; inversion time, 165 msec) *(B)* MR images show diffuse soft tissue involvement and hypertrophy of the entire leg. (Courtesy of E. Bosch, MD, Santiago, Chile.)

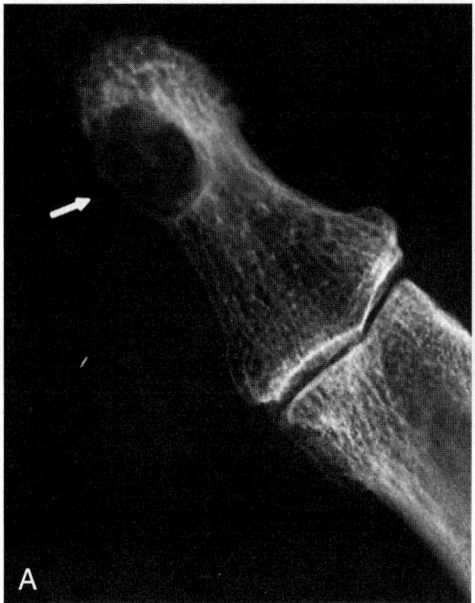

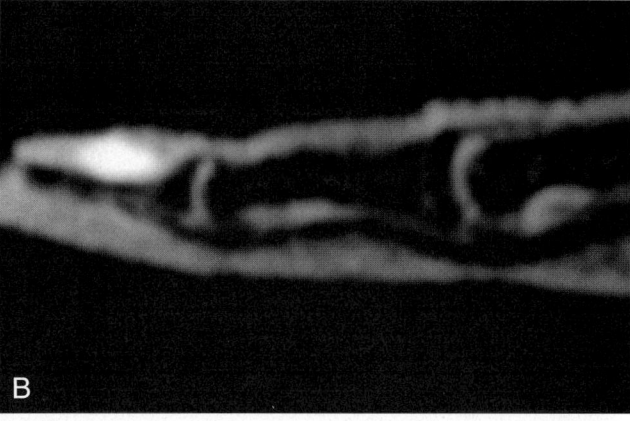

**Figure 71–36.** Glomus tumor. *A*, A well-defined lytic lesion of a terminal tuft is seen *(arrow)*. *B*, In a different patient, the tumor beneath the nail bed is of high signal intensity in a sagittal gradient echo (TR/TE, 77/9; flip angle, 12 degrees) MR image. (Courtesy of J. Campos, MD, Campinos, Brazil.)

## Cartilaginous and Osseous Tumors

**Chondroma.** Soft tissue chondromas (extraskeletal chondromas, chondromas of soft parts) are rare. These tumors occur predominantly in the third and fourth decades of life, especially in the hands and feet. The tumors may be adherent to the periosteum, joint capsule, or synovial membrane (including that in a tendon sheath). They enlarge slowly and are well demarcated and lobulated. Radiographs reveal soft tissue masses frequently containing curvilinear, ringlike, or nodular calcification (Fig. 71–37). Subjacent cortical erosion and sclerosis may simulate the findings in a juxtacortical (periosteal) chondroma. High signal intensity on T2-weighted images is the characteristic MR imaging feature, and a well-defined and lobulated mass of such signal intensity is suggestive of the diagnosis. Intracapsular chondroma is a rare form that most often arises in the knee, typically inferior to the patella (Fig. 71–38). In this location, the lesion may attach to the meniscus, be located in the infrapatellar fat pad, and produce pain and locking of the joint.

**Extra-articular (Tenosynovial) Chondromatosis.** Because extraskeletal chondromas commonly arise in close association with a tendon, tendon sheath, or joint capsule, the designation extra-articular synovial (or tenosynovial) chondromatosis has been used to describe these lesions (Fig. 71–39). Such chondromas should be differentiated from idiopathic (primary) synovial (osteo)chondromatosis, in which metaplasia of the synovial lining in an articulation leads to numerous cartilaginous and osseous bodies; from idiopathic (primary) bursal (osteo)chondromatosis, in which similar metaplasia occurs within a bursal sac that communicates with the joint; and from secondary synovial (osteo)chondromatosis, in which an unrelated articular process is accompanied by disintegration of the joint surface and production of one or more cartilaginous and osseous fragments.

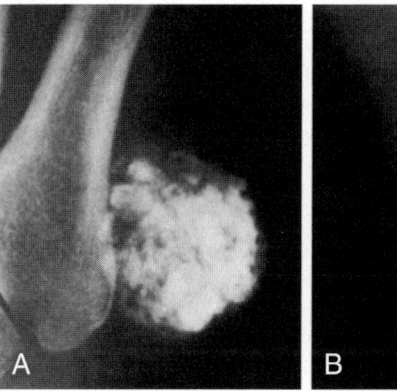
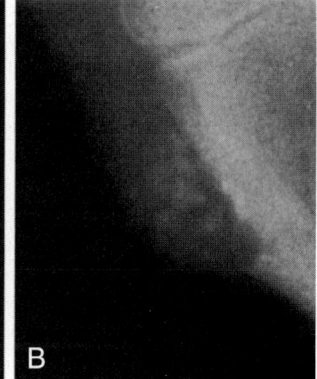

**Figure 71–37.** Chondroma. *A*, Soft tissue chondroma. Observe the calcified soft tissue mass adjacent to the base of the fifth metatarsal bone. *B*, Juxtacortical (periosteal) chondroma. This 8-year-old boy had a lump below the knee. A radiograph reveals a partially calcified and ossified soft tissue mass in the region of the anterior tibial tubercle. Minimal erosion of the cortex is seen. (From Kirchner SJ, et al: Periosteal chondroma of the anterior tibial tubercle: Two cases. AJR Am J Roentgenol 131:1088, 1978.)

**Idiopathic Synovial (Osteo)chondromatosis.** This unusual condition generally involves joints, with or without extension into nearby bursae. It results from metaplasia of subsynovial connective tissue into cartilage nodules that may subsequently calcify or ossify. Enlargement of the resulting intra-articular bodies occurs by proliferation of chondrocytes. The metaplastic or active stage of the disease may be self-limited and followed by an inactive stage in which the synovial membrane is quiescent. The clinical onset of idiopathic synovial (osteo)chondromatosis varies from childhood to the seventh or eighth decade of life, although most affected patients are young and middle-aged adults. The two most frequent sites of involvement

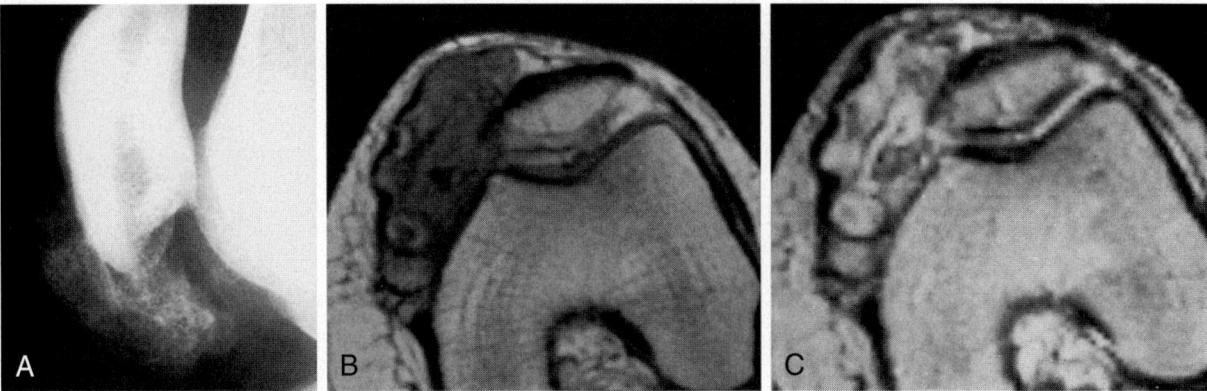

**Figure 71–38.** Intracapsular chondroma. A mass developed below the patella in this 40-year-old woman. With routine radiography *(A)*, the mass is seen to be ossified. Transaxial T1-weighted (TR/TE, 750/24) *(B)* and T2-weighted (TR/TE, 2000/80) *(C)* spin echo MR images show a lobulated soft tissue mass medial to the patella, with distortion of the retinaculum. The mass is of inhomogeneous signal intensity, although its signal intensity is increased in *(C)*. Some of the signal intensity characteristics are those of fat, indicative of ossification with the presence of marrow. (Courtesy of A. Newberg, MD, Boston, Mass.)

are the knee and the hip; however, any articulation may be involved. Monoarticular disease is the rule.

The radiographic features of this condition are variable and classically show multiple calcified or ossified bodies of approximately equal size scattered throughout the involved joint (Fig. 71–40). Unfortunately, this appearance is not often encountered, and in some instances of synovial chondromatosis, the degree of calcification and ossification is limited and is not seen with routine radiography. Osseous erosion is typically encountered in "tight" joints such as the hip (Fig. 71–41). Typically, pressure defects at the articular margins are apparent; these can lead to pathologic fracture and are identical to those produced by pigmented villonodular synovitis. Common sites for such erosion are the femoral neck,

acetabular fossa, humeral head, and proximal metaphysis.

The MR imaging abnormalities are dependent on the stage of the disease. In cases of synovial chondromatosis, in which intrasynovial cartilage nodules are uncalcified, the signal intensity of the process resembles that of fluid—low on T1-weighted spin echo MR images, and high on T2-weighted spin echo MR images (see Fig. 71–41)—and the condition may be misdiagnosed as a joint effusion. In some cases, the cartilage nodules have signal intensity characteristics that differ from those of fluid. In cases of synovial (osteo)chondromatosis, foci of calcification appear as regions of low signal intensity on both T1- and T2-weighted images (Fig. 71–42). With extensive calcification and ossification, ringlike structures with peripheral rims of low signal intensity and central regions of higher signal intensity identical to that of fat or cartilage are seen (Fig. 71–43).

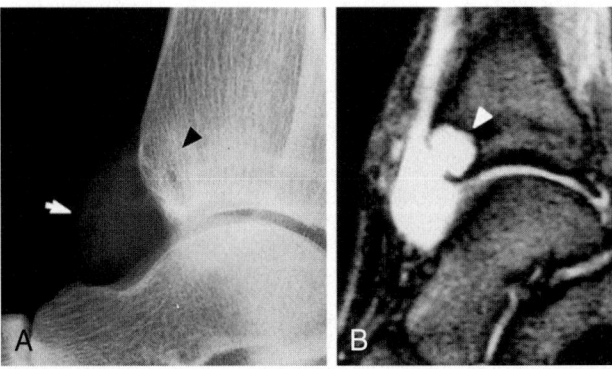

**Figure 71–39.** Tenosynovial chondromatosis. In this 30-year-old man, a mass in the anterior portion of the ankle limited dorsiflexion of the joint. *A*, Routine radiograph shows a soft tissue mass *(arrow)* with bone erosion *(arrowhead)* and spiculated bone reaction. *B*, Sagittal multiplanar gradient recalled (TR/TE, 1000/30; flip angle, 28 degrees) MR image reveals high signal intensity in the mass and along the anterior surface of the tibia, as well as bone erosion *(arrowhead)*. Surgery confirmed that the lesion, which was composed of gelatinous material, was attached to the tibia and the anterior capsule of the ankle joint. (Courtesy of G. Greenway, MD, Dallas, Tex.)

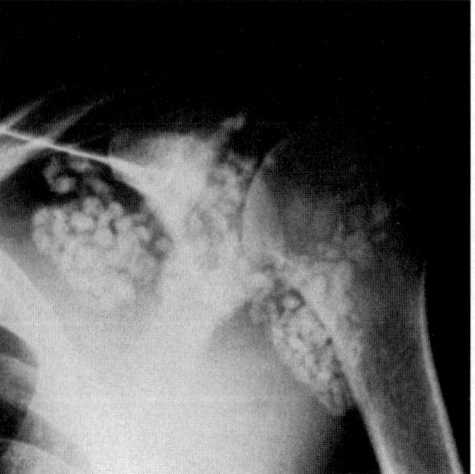

**Figure 71–40.** Idiopathic synovial (osteo)chondromatosis. Observe the uniform size of the radiodense collections, their confinement to the joint cavity, and the relative absence of additional articular abnormalities. (Courtesy of J. Slivka, MD, San Diego, Calif.)

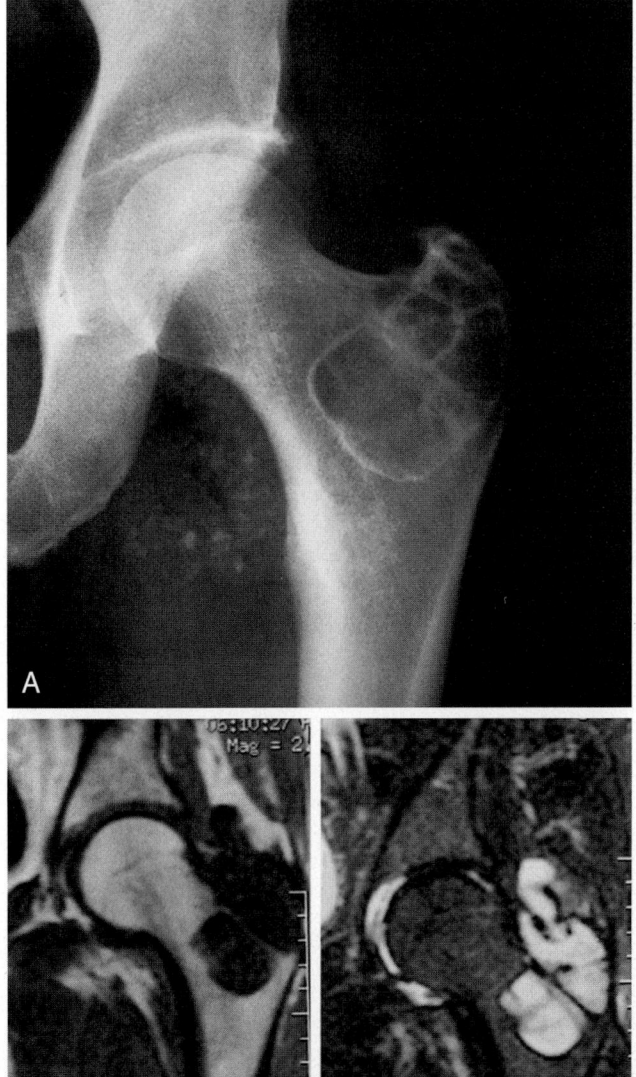

**Figure 71–41.** Idiopathic synovial (osteo)chondromatosis. In this 60-year-old patient, speckled calcification and prominent bone erosion in the femur are evident on a standard radiograph *(A)*. Although the femoral erosions appear cystlike on this radiograph, a lateral radiograph (not shown) confirmed disruption of the cortical surface. The joint space is preserved. Coronal T1-weighted (TR/TE, 666/14) spin echo *(B)* and STIR (TR/TE, 4450/75; inversion time, 120 msec) *(C)* MR images reveal extension of the articular process into the femur. Although the imaging characteristics simulate those of joint fluid, the lobulated appearance of the joint process and its slightly inhomogeneous nature are consistent with cartilage nodules, most of which are not calcified or ossified. (Courtesy of D. Witte, MD, Memphis, Tenn.)

**Synovial Chondrosarcoma.** Chondrosarcoma arising in a joint is extremely rare. The lesion may occur as a primary process or, more commonly, secondary to idiopathic synovial (osteo)chondromatosis. When synovial chondrosarcoma is superimposed on idiopathic synovial (osteo)chondromatosis, the latter disorder has generally been present for many years. An intra-articular mass, often heavily calcified, is evident, and the pattern of calcification may be more irregular than that associated with idiopathic synovial (osteo)chondromatosis; a poorly marginated mass with inhomogeneous signal intensity may be evident on MR images. Distant metastases, including pulmonary foci, may develop.

**Chondrosarcoma.** Extraskeletal soft tissue chondrosarcomas are uncommon. These lesions are distinguished from those arising in bone or in the periosteum and perichondrium. Histologic subtypes include myxoid, mesenchymal, and well-differentiated extraskeletal chondrosarcoma.

Extraskeletal myxoid chondrosarcoma, also designated chordoid sarcoma, is the most common type and is usually observed in middle-aged and elderly patients, especially in the thigh and popliteal fossa. Although the tumors may be located superficially or even in joints, deep lesions predominate. These myxoid tumors are generally of low grade, but both tumor recurrence and distant metastases are encountered. Mesenchymal chondrosarcomas are relatively rare and generally aggressive and have a poor prognosis. Extraskeletal well-differentiated chondrosarcoma is very rare and may be densely calcified.

In any type of chondrosarcoma, a soft tissue mass with calcification and underlying osseous involvement can be detected radiographically. Calcification is more typical of a mesenchymal than a myxoid tumor. In such cases, MR imaging reveals a soft tissue lesion of low signal intensity on T1-weighted spin echo MR images and high signal intensity on T2-weighted spin echo MR images, as well as regions of accentuated signal intensity after intravenous gadolinium administration (Fig. 71–44). A similar MR imaging appearance is evident in cases of myxoid chondrosarcoma, although the signal intensity characteristics of this lesion appear to be more variable on T1-weighted images.

**Osteoma.** Osteoma of soft parts is extremely uncommon. These tumors generally occur in the head, usually in the posterior portion of the tongue, but they have also been described in the thigh (Fig. 71–45).

**Osteosarcoma.** Extraskeletal osteosarcomas are rarely encountered. These lesions are distinguished from osteosarcomas of bone, as well as juxtacortical osteosarcomas. They are usually evident in middle-aged and elderly patients in the deeper tissues of the extremities, thighs, shoulder region, and retroperitoneum. Radiographically, a soft tissue mass with calcification or ossification can be seen in approximately 50% of patients (Fig. 71–46). The malignant potential of these tumors appears to be high. Indeed, widespread metastasis may be seen, including metastasis to bone. MR imaging findings in cases of extraskeletal osteosarcoma lack specificity (see Fig. 71–46). Cystic, solid, and hemorrhagic components account for the variable patterns of signal intensity. Fluid levels have been encountered.

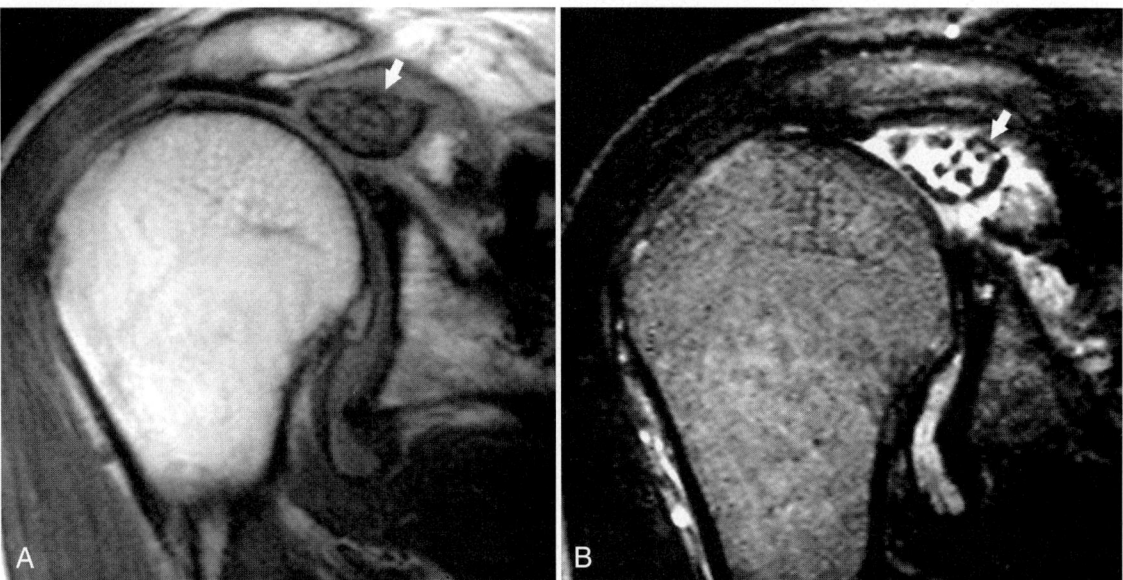

**Figure 71–42.** Idiopathic synovial (osteo)chondromatosis. Coronal oblique T1-weighted (TR/TE, 650/20) *(A)* and T2-weighted (TR/TE, 2500/80) *(B)* spin echo MR images show a distended glenohumeral joint containing fluid of high signal intensity and loose bodies with calcified and ossified areas of low signal intensity *(arrows)*.

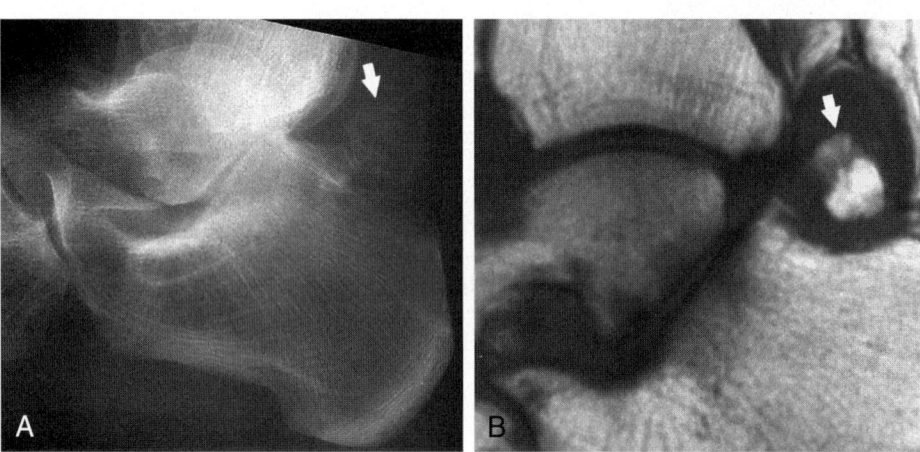

**Figure 71–43.** Idiopathic synovial (osteo)chondromatosis. *A,* Lateral radiograph shows an ossified loose body posterior to the ankle joint *(arrow)*. *B,* Sagittal T1-weighted (TR/TE, 600/20) spin echo MR image demonstrates the loose body to have a fatlike signal intensity centrally *(arrow)*.

**Synovial Sarcoma.** Synovial sarcomas are relatively common malignant neoplasms with a distinct predilection for involvement of the thigh and lower extremity. The single most common site is the region of the knee. Rare sites of involvement are the neck, pharynx, larynx, thoracic and abdominal walls, and heart. Patients of all ages can be affected, including children, although most are in the third and fourth decades of life. On radiographs, a deep or, less commonly, superficial soft tissue mass is seen; there may be evidence of calcification in 20% to 30% of cases and osseous erosion or invasion in 5% to 20% of cases (Fig. 71–47). Extensive bone destruction is rare, and reactive sclerosis is unusual. With MR imaging, synovial sarcomas usually reveal an inhomogeneous septated mass with low signal intensity on T1-weighted spin echo images and high signal intensity on

T2-weighted spin echo images. Because of the common occurrence of cystic and solid areas and hemorrhage within the lesion, T2-weighted MR images may show areas that are hyperintense, isointense, and hypointense to fat (Fig. 71–48). This finding, though not specific, is suggestive of the diagnosis. Fluid levels within the mass may also be evident. Early enhancement of the tumor after intravenous gadolinium administration has been observed.

**Neurogenic Tumors**

Neurogenic tumors, both benign and malignant, are relatively common and represent about 10% of neoplasms in each of these two categories. As opposed to many other soft tissue tumors, certain imaging charac-

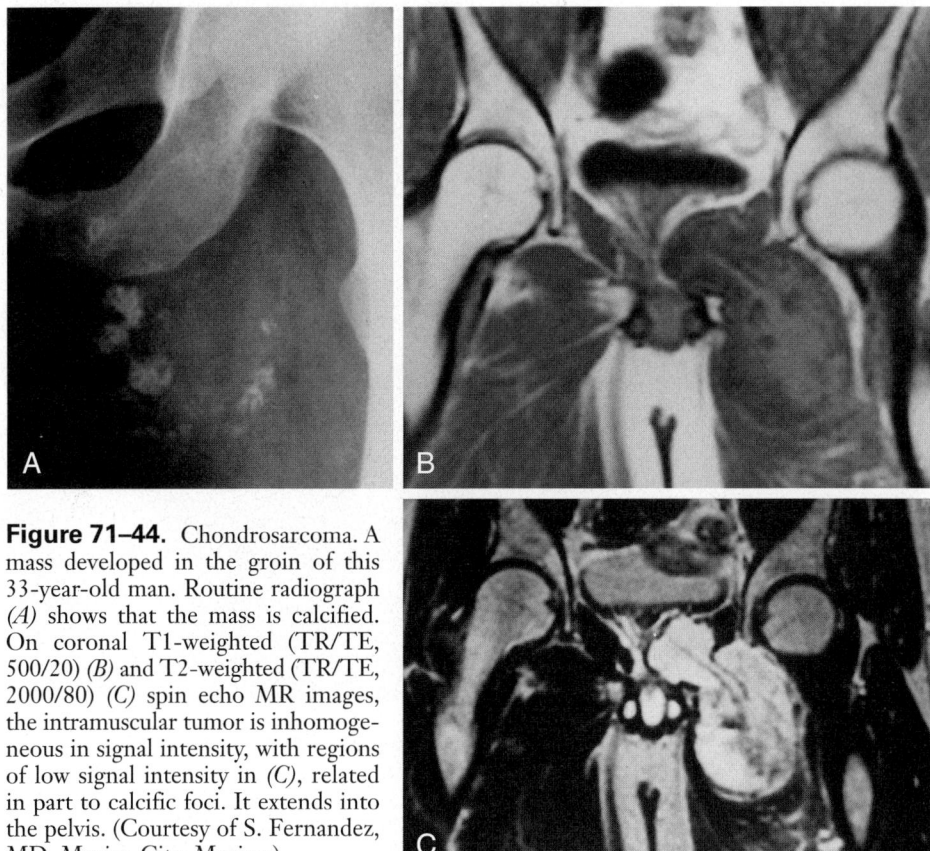

**Figure 71–44.** Chondrosarcoma. A mass developed in the groin of this 33-year-old man. Routine radiograph *(A)* shows that the mass is calcified. On coronal T1-weighted (TR/TE, 500/20) *(B)* and T2-weighted (TR/TE, 2000/80) *(C)* spin echo MR images, the intramuscular tumor is inhomogeneous in signal intensity, with regions of low signal intensity in *(C)*, related in part to calcific foci. It extends into the pelvis. (Courtesy of S. Fernandez, MD, Mexico City, Mexico.)

teristics allow an accurate diagnosis in some cases (Fig. 71–49). These characteristics include a specific clinical situation or anatomic location, relationship to a major or minor nerve, and certain shape and signal intensity patterns.

**Neurilemoma (Schwannoma) and Neurofibroma.** The most important benign tumors of peripheral nerves are neurilemomas (schwannomas) and neurofibromas. Neurilemoma is observed most commonly in adult men and women in the third to fifth decades of life. This

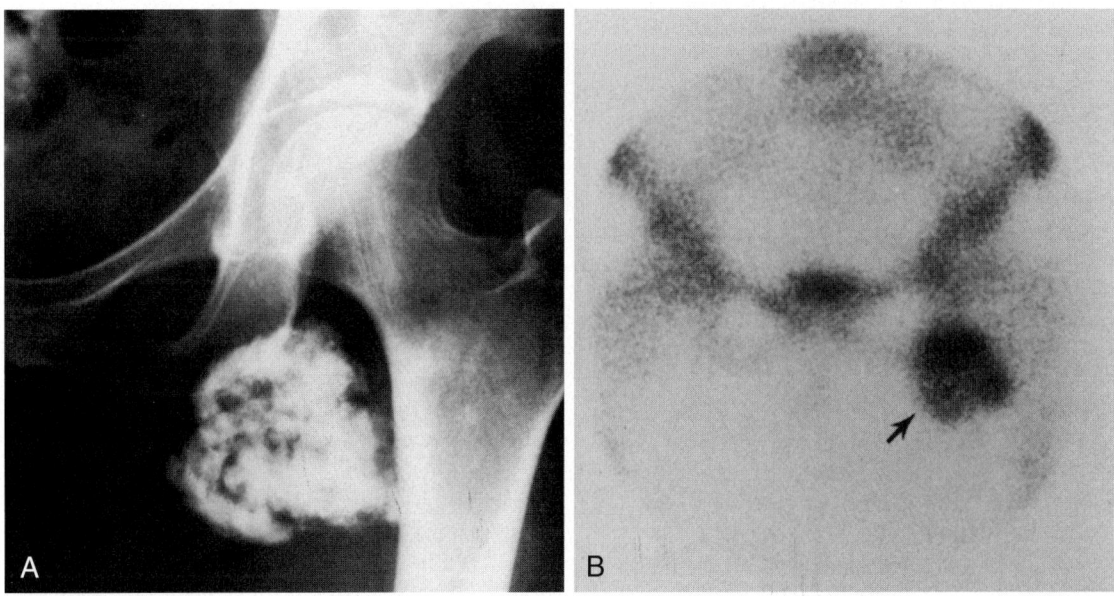

**Figure 71–45.** Osteoma. This 56-year-old woman had a large mass in the thigh. Radiograph *(A)* and bone scan *(B)* document the lesion *(arrow)*, which was interpreted histologically as an osteoma of soft parts. (Courtesy of G. Greenway, MD, Dallas, Tex.)

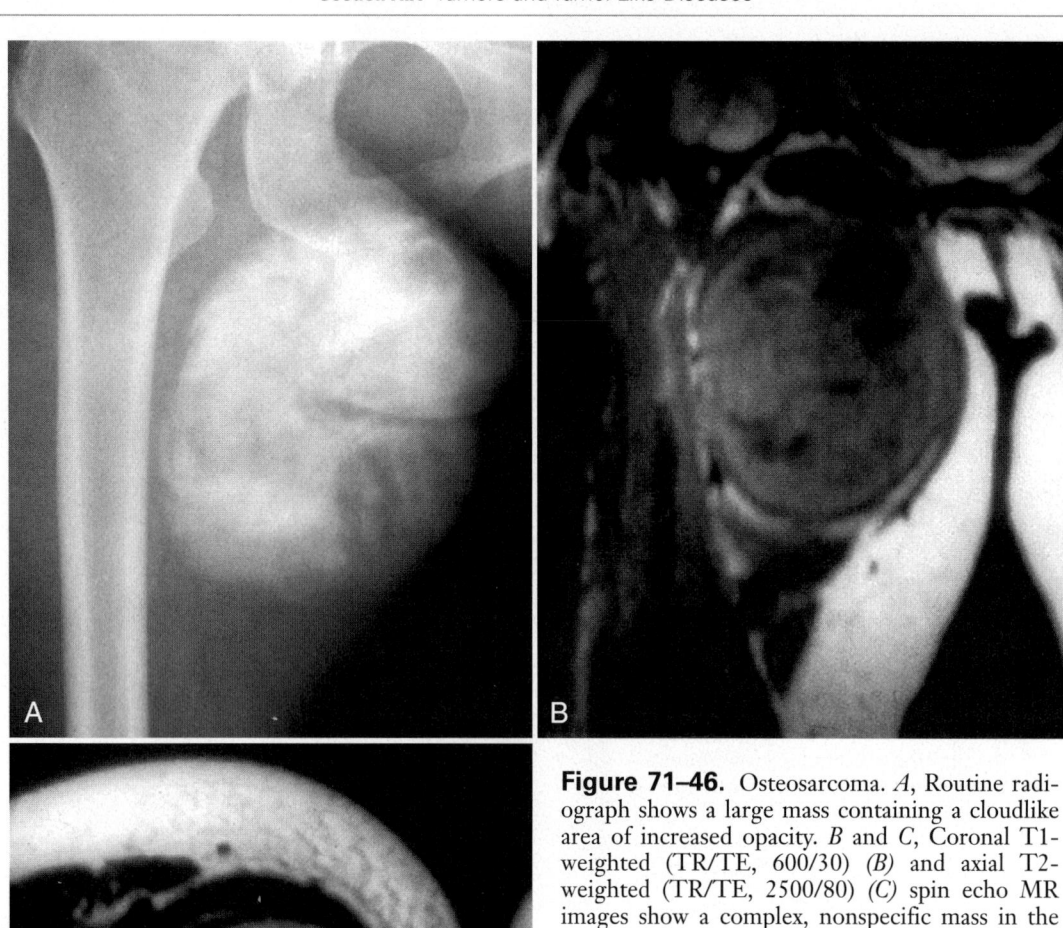

**Figure 71–46.** Osteosarcoma. *A,* Routine radiograph shows a large mass containing a cloudlike area of increased opacity. *B* and *C,* Coronal T1-weighted (TR/TE, 600/30) *(B)* and axial T2-weighted (TR/TE, 2500/80) *(C)* spin echo MR images show a complex, nonspecific mass in the medial aspect of the thigh.

tumor typically arises from the spinal nerve roots and the cervical, sympathetic, vagus, peroneal, and ulnar nerves and appears in the head, neck, and flexor surfaces of the upper and lower extremities. However, virtually any central or peripheral nerve may be affected.

Neurilemoma is predominantly a solitary, slow-growing lesion that, when large, leads to clinical manifestations that include pain, soft tissue prominence, and neurologic findings. Multiple neurilemomas may be encountered, however, with involvement of peripheral, spinal, and intracranial nerves. An association with neurofibromatosis

(von Recklinghausen's disease) is recognized but uncommon. Neurilemomas are benign in their behavior; tumor recurrence is unusual, and malignant transformation is exceedingly rare. As they age, neurilemomas reveal a variety of histologic changes, including cyst formation, calcification, hemorrhage, and hyalinization.

There are three types of neurofibroma: plexiform, localized, and diffuse. Neurofibroma may occur as a solitary lesion unassociated with neurofibromatosis, although plexiform or multiple neurofibromas are characteristic of the latter disease. Localized neurofibroma is

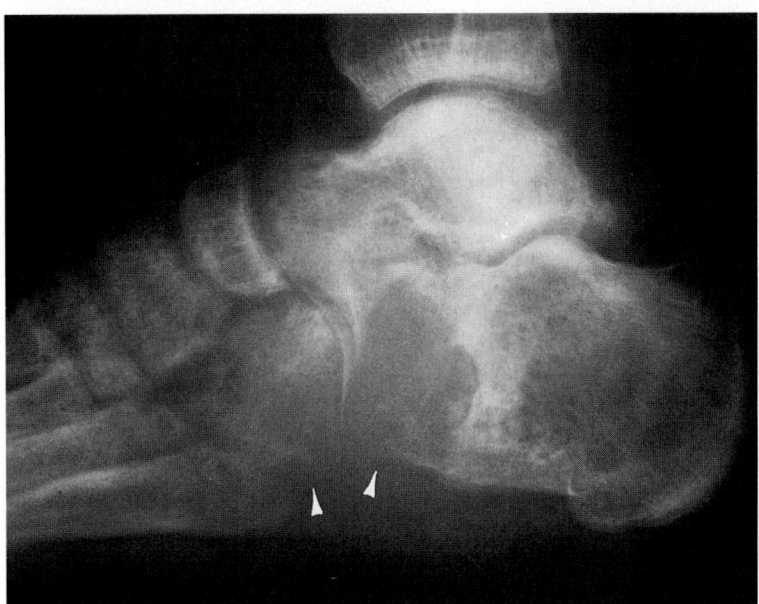

**Figure 71–47.** Synovial sarcoma. Destruction of the calcaneus and cuboid bones is seen *(arrowheads)*. Surrounding sclerosis is apparent, but the patient had previously received cobalt therapy. Osteoporosis is also evident.

the most common type; it is generally solitary and is not associated with neurofibromatosis. The diffuse type of neurofibroma affects primarily children and young adults and typically involves the subcutaneous tissues of the head and neck. Solitary neurofibromas predominate in young adult men and women. They affect all areas of the body and appear in the subcutis or dermis. They grow slowly, erode adjacent bone (such as the pedicle and lamina, where they lead to a widened neural foramen), and rarely undergo malignant degeneration.

Detection of localized neurofibromas or neurilemomas by conventional radiography is difficult unless they are large, are calcified (Fig. 71–50), or affect adja-

cent structures, including the bones, where they lead to scalloped osseous erosions. In this regard, the occurrence of a widened intervertebral foramen is a well-recognized manifestation of dumbbell-shaped lesions extending between the spinal canal and posterior mediastinum (Fig. 71–51). CT and MR imaging are the most effective means of delineating these lesions, particularly those that are deep and nonpalpable, because they can define the tumor's position along the course of a nerve and its relationship to surrounding structures. A characteristic and often diagnostic CT and MR imaging feature of benign (and even malignant) tumors of the peripheral nerve sheath is a fusiform mass with a tubular nerve

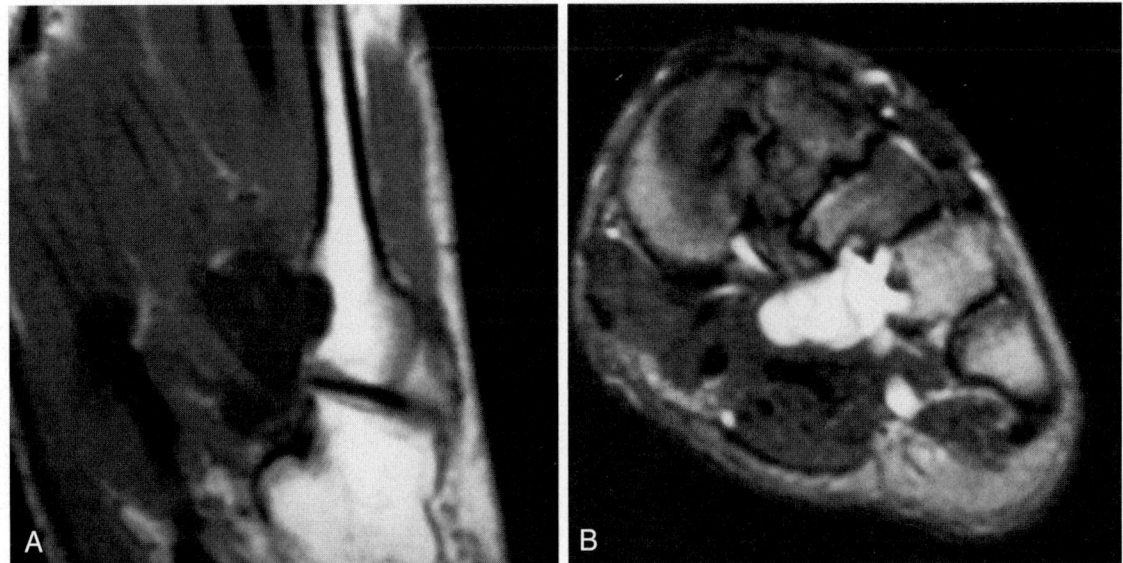

**Figure 71–48.** Synovial sarcoma. *A* and *B*, A synovial sarcoma is evident in the plantar aspect of the foot. Its extent and associated erosion of adjacent bones are seen on transverse T1-weighted (TR/TE, 550/16) *(A)* and coronal T2-weighted (TR/TE, 2700/80) *(B)* spin echo MR images. The lesion has a slightly inhomogeneous appearance in *(A)* and a septated appearance in *(B)*.

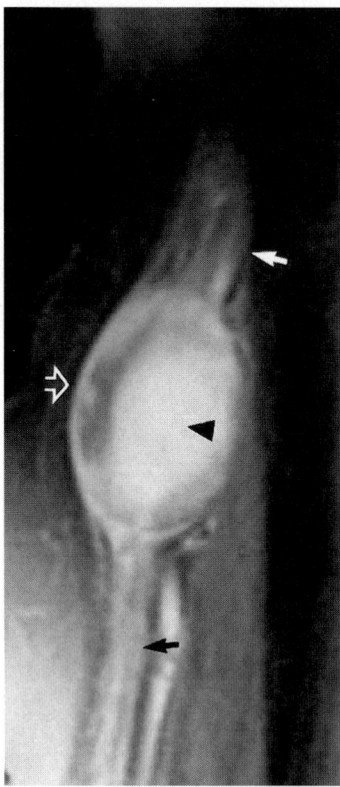

**Figure 71–49.** Neurogenic tumors: general MR imaging characteristics. Coronal fat-suppressed T1-weighted (TR/TE, 450/15) spin echo MR image obtained after intravenous gadolinium administration shows the typical fusiform shape *(open arrow)*, adjacent parent nerves *(closed arrows)*, and central high signal intensity *(arrowhead)*. (Courtesy of D. Goodwin, MD, Hanover, NH.)

entering and exiting the tumor (Fig. 71–52)—an appearance that is more easily recognized when large nerves are involved.

Classically, a neurilemoma is eccentrically located with respect to the parent nerve and easily separated from it, whereas a neurofibroma is more centrally located and intimately related to and inseparable from the parent nerve (Fig. 71–53). In practice, however, such a distinction is not always possible. Further, plexiform neurofibromas produce diffuse thickening and nodularity of the nerve, with a "bag of worms" appearance, and diffuse neurofibromas have a reticulated, linear, or honeycomb appearance. Most lesions have relatively low signal intensity on T1-weighted spin echo MR images and high signal intensity on T2-weighted images. On T1-weighted images, a rim of fat about the tumors, the split fat sign, has been noted (Fig. 71–54). On T2-weighted images, a fascicular sign has been described that consists of small ringlike structures with peripheral high signal intensity. With neurofibromas, however, especially the diffuse variety, low signal intensity may be seen on T2-weighted images. On such images, a target pattern may be identified that consists of increased signal intensity at the periphery of the lesion and low signal intensity in the center (see Fig. 71–54). This pattern corresponds to peripheral myxomatous tissue and central fibrous tissue,

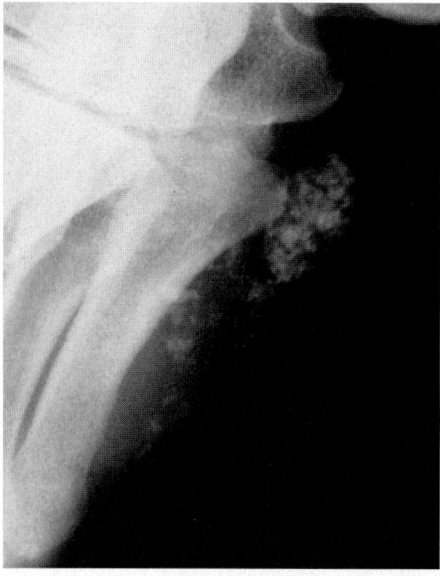

**Figure 71–50.** Neurilemoma. This tumor of the foot is calcified on routine radiograph. (Courtesy of M. Mitchell, MD, Halifax, Nova Scotia, Canada.)

and it is absent in cystic, hemorrhagic, or necrotic lesions. Of interest, a reverse target sign may be seen after intravenous gadolinium administration, with high signal intensity noted centrally.

**Morton's Neuroma.** Morton's neuroma is a perineural fibrosis of a plantar digital nerve. Such neuromas are most commonly seen in the interspace between the third and fourth metatarsal bones. The space between the second and third metatarsal bones is involved less frequently. Multiple neuromas in one or both feet may be encountered. Morton's neuromas predominate in women. Clinical findings include radiating pain and tenderness, although these neuromas may be asymptomatic.

Fat-suppressed T2-weighted and STIR MR images and those obtained after intravenous gadolinium administration are useful because Morton's neuromas, which are generally of low signal intensity, are often of high signal intensity on these images (Fig. 71–55). An associated intermetatarsal bursitis may also be evident.

**Fibrolipomatous Hamartoma.** These hamartomas (also called lipomatosis of the nerve or lipofibromatous hamartomas) are rare lesions related to the gradual infiltration of major nerves and their branches by fibrofatty tissue. The hand is usually involved, and most lesions affect the median nerve (Fig. 71–56). These lesions usually appear in children, adolescents, or young adults and can lead to an enlarging mass, macrodactyly, and a compression neuropathy. A relationship may exist between these hamartomas and macrodystrophia lipomatosa (Fig. 71–57). MR imaging reveals features of both fibrous and fatty tissue, and a serpentine appearance of the enlarged nerves is distinctive.

**Traumatic Neuroma.** Traumatic neuromas develop as a result of non-neoplastic proliferation of the proximal end

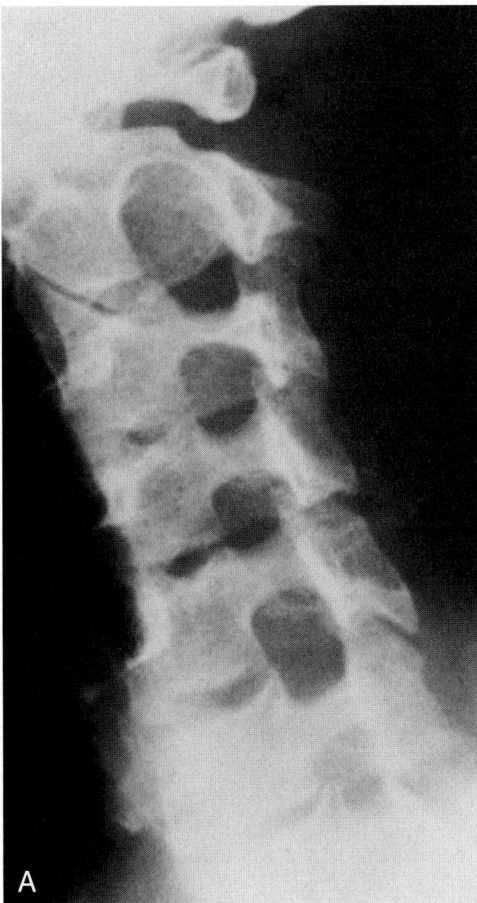

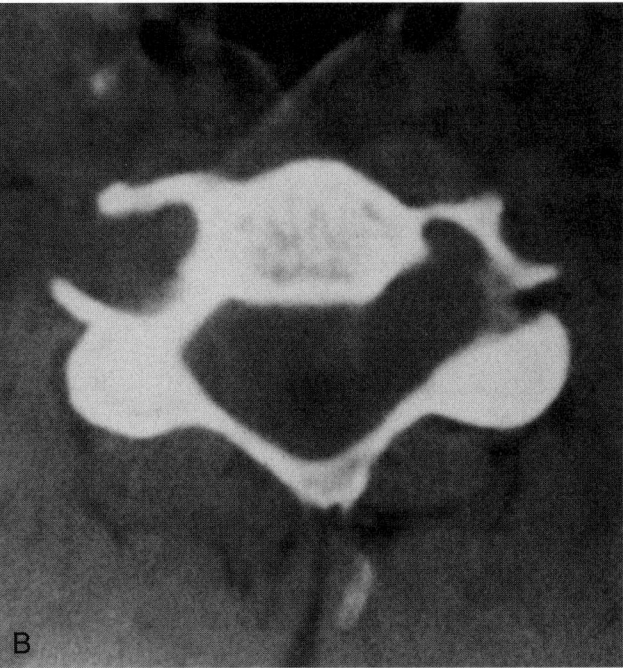

**Figure 71–51.** Neurofibromatosis. Enlargement of the neural foramina in the cervical spine is well shown by both conventional radiography *(A)* and transaxial CT *(B)*. (Courtesy of V. Vint, MD, San Diego, Calif.)

of an injured or severed nerve. Traumatic neuromas may be the consequence of either the nerve injury itself or the abortive attempt at natural repair. Postamputation neuromas become evident approximately 1 to 12 months after transection, are of variable size, have no malignant

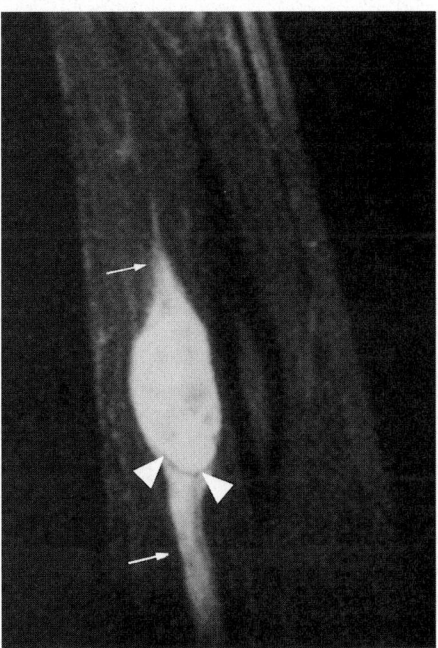

**Figure 71–53.** Neurilemoma. Sagittal STIR (TR/TE, 4890/60; inversion time, 150 msec) MR image of the forearm shows a tumor arising from the median nerve. It has a fusiform shape, with the parent nerve *(arrows)* seen on either side. The meniscus-like contour *(arrowheads)* suggests that the lesion is eccentrically located with respect to the nerve, but this finding is not definite. The tumor is not of homogeneous signal intensity. (Courtesy of R. Boutin, MD, San Francisco, Calif.)

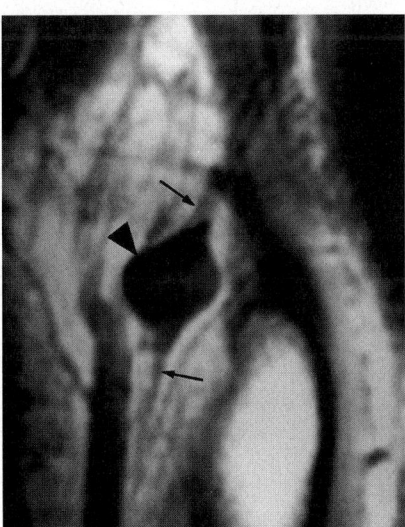

**Figure 71–52.** Neurilemoma (schwannoma). Sagittal T1-weighted (TR/TE, 500/19) spin echo MR image reveals a fusiform mass *(arrowhead)* with an adjacent nerve *(arrows)*, in this case representing a dorsal cutaneous branch of the ulnar nerve at the wrist.

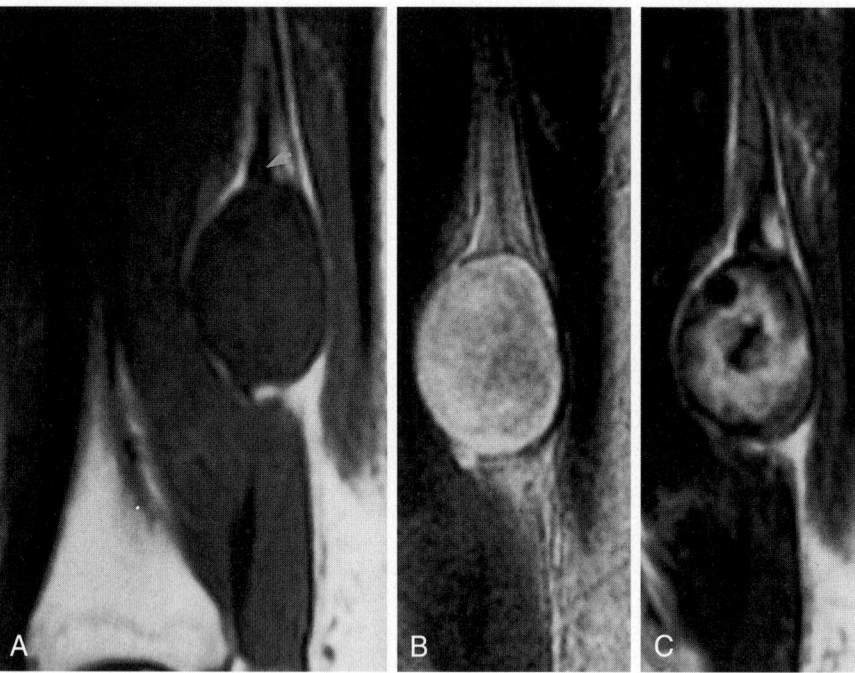

**Figure 71–54.** Neurilemoma. *A* to *C*, Tibial nerve. Sagittal T1-weighted (TR/TE, 540/16) *(A)* and T2-weighted (TR/TE, 1800/80) *(B)* spin echo MR images and sagittal T1-weighted (TR/TE, 540/18) spin echo MR image obtained after the intravenous administration of gadolinium *(C)* show a well-defined mass posterior to the distal portion of the tibia. In *(C)*, the mass is of low signal intensity, and the adjacent nerve *(arrow)* can be seen. Note that the fat is split about the tumor. Regions of high signal intensity in the mass are apparent in *(B)* and *(C)*. In *(B)*, there is a peripheral rim of high signal intensity—the target sign—and in *(C)*, a reverse phenomenon is seen. (Courtesy of P. Kindynis, MD, Geneva, Switzerland.)

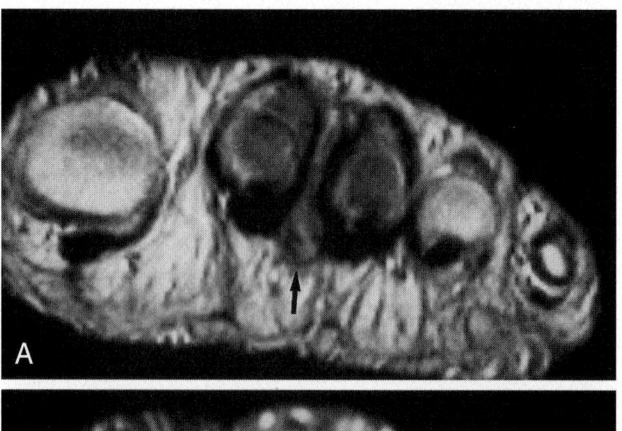

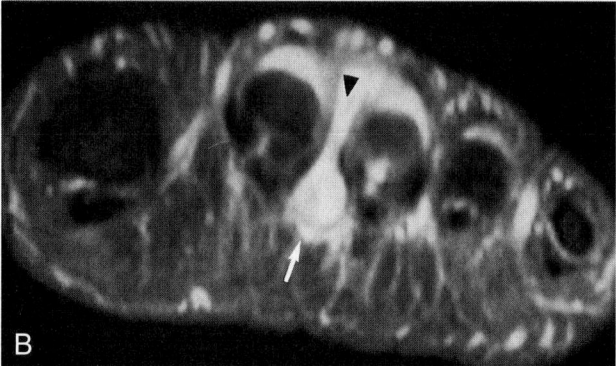

**Figure 71–55.** Morton's neuroma. *A*, Coronal fast spin echo (TR/TE, 3800/96) MR image demonstrates a neuroma *(arrow)* of intermediate to low signal intensity. On a T1-weighted spin echo MR image (not shown), very low signal intensity was evident. *B*, On a coronal fat-suppressed fast spin echo (TR/TE, 4000/15) MR image, the neuroma *(arrow)* has high signal intensity. Note the evidence of intermetatarsal bursitis *(arrowhead)* and nearby marrow edema. Vessels are seen in the lateral interspaces, and a joint effusion is apparent.

potential, and may be asymptomatic. Pain and a mass may be evident, however. When assessing the cause of pain at the stump, other conditions such as soft tissue ulceration, heterotopic bone formation, bursitis and other inflammatory changes, retained foreign bodies, altered musculature, and scar formation must also be considered.

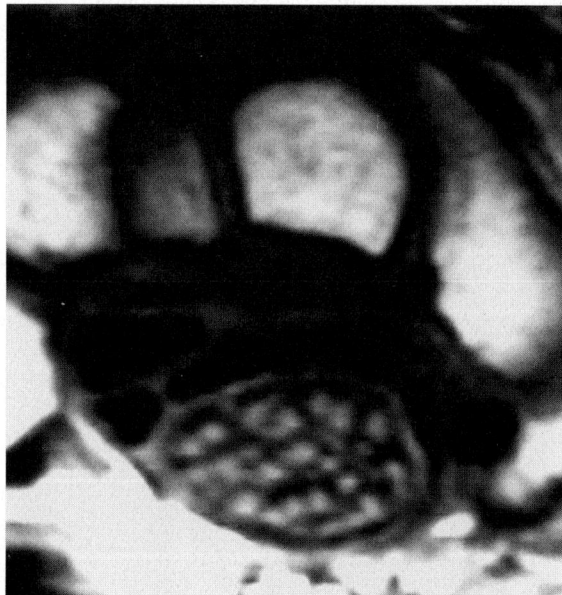

**Figure 71–56.** Fibrolipomatous hamartoma: median nerve. In this 22-year-old man with an enlarging mass in the palm, a T1-weighted (TR/TE, 550/15) transaxial spin echo MR image reveals tubular structures in the lesion of the median nerve. Some regions of the mass demonstrate signal intensity identical to that of fat, and others have low signal intensity.

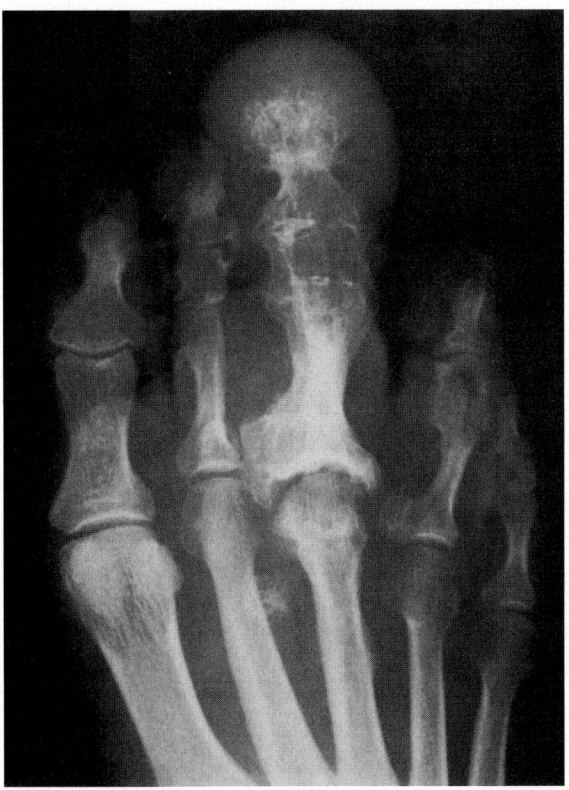

**Figure 71–57.** Macrodystrophia lipomatosa. Massive enlargement of soft tissue and osseous tissue can accompany lipomatosis of the nerve. Observe the degree of joint space narrowing, bony ankylosis, and proliferative alterations. (Courtesy of L. Ginsburg, MD, Long Beach, Calif.)

In addition, paradoxical hypertrophy of nerves after amputation has been described. MR imaging findings include a fusiform mass with inhomogeneous signal intensity. Although most stump neuromas show regions of high signal intensity on T2-weighted images, strand-like regions of low signal intensity may be seen on such images (Fig. 71–58).

**Intraneural Ganglion Cyst.** Intraneural ganglion cysts, also termed peripheral nerve ganglia or mucoid degeneration and intraneural mucoid cysts, are of unknown pathogenesis, are benign in nature, and are encountered most commonly in large nerves, especially those about the knee near the fibular head (e.g., popliteal, peroneal, tibial nerves). Pain and varying degrees of motor and sensory dysfunction in the distribution of the involved nerve, with or without a mass, are the clinical manifestations of these cysts. Although MR imaging findings may resemble those of a neuroma, the pattern of enhancement (which includes increased signal intensity in the rim or septa of a well-defined intraneural mass) after intravenous gadolinium administration provides diagnostic specificity.

**Malignant Peripheral Nerve Sheath Tumor.** The term malignant peripheral nerve sheath tumor (MPNST) is currently accepted as the proper designation for a spindle cell sarcoma arising from a nerve or neurofibroma or demonstrating nerve tissue differentiation. MPNSTs are relatively common soft tissue sarcomas (approximately 10% of all such tumors); they are generally encountered in young adult and middle-aged patients of both sexes.

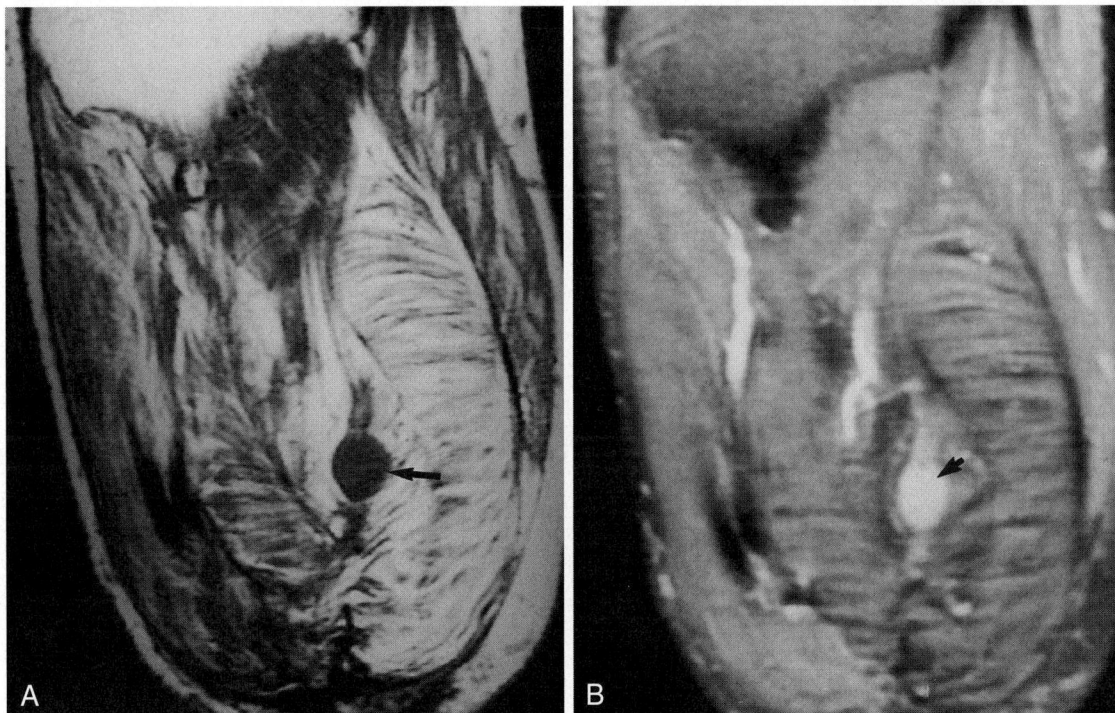

**Figure 71–58.** Stump neuroma. In this 47-year-old man with a previous amputation of the leg below the knee, a neuroma *(arrows)* is shown on coronal T1-weighted (TR/TE, 500/10) spin echo *(A)* and fat-suppressed fast spin echo (TR/TE, 4240/23) *(B)* MR images. Adjacent fatty atrophy of muscle is evident. (Courtesy of A. Pinto Leite, MD, Porto, Portugal.)

When associated with neurofibromas, MPNSTs occur more commonly in a younger age group and in men. MPNSTs dominate in the trunk and proximal portions of the extremities and typically arise from major nerve trunks such as the brachial plexus, sacral plexus, and sciatic nerve. Pain and neurologic manifestations are variable in frequency and intensity, and a mass may be detected. In fact, enlargement of a previously stable neurofibroma may be the first indication of an MPNST. In common with benign neurogenic tumors, MPNSTs are fusiform in shape, intimate with the parent nerve, and accompanied by thickening and irregularity of that nerve.

Thickening of the nerve in either a proximal or distal direction, or both, is compatible with neoplastic spread along the epineurium and perineurium. MR imaging of MPNSTs shows an inhomogeneous mass that is generally of low signal intensity on T1-weighted images and high signal intensity on T2-weighted images (Fig. 71–59). A target pattern, seen in some benign nerve sheath tumors, is absent (Fig. 71–60), although differentiation of benign and malignant lesions may not be possible without histologic analysis. MPNSTs, particularly those occurring in neurofibromatosis, carry a poor prognosis.

## Other Tumors

**Malignant Mesenchymoma.** Malignant mesenchymoma is a sarcoma composed of two or more differentiated mesodermal phenotypes. Foci of osteosarcoma, chondrosarcoma, liposarcoma, leiomyosarcoma, rhabdomyosarcoma, neurogenic sarcoma, angiosarcoma, fibrosarcoma, and malignant fibrous histiocytoma may be included in the tumor. This rare neoplasm accounts for less than 1% of all sarcomas and is usually, but not invariably, seen in older patients; it predominates in the retroperitoneum and thigh.

**Clear Cell Sarcoma.** Clear cell sarcomas, also known as aponeurotic clear cell sarcomas and malignant melanomas of soft parts, are rare malignant neoplasms that arise in the vicinity of tendons and aponeuroses of the upper and lower extremities, especially in the region of the foot and ankle. Although the age range of affected persons is large, most patients are young adults, and many are women. A deep, slowly enlarging mass is typical. Radiographs reveal

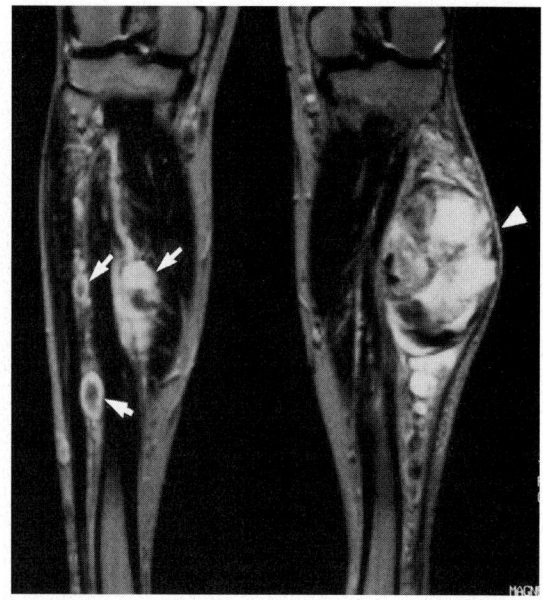

**Figure 71–60.** Neurofibromatosis with malignant peripheral nerve sheath tumor (MPNST). Coronal T2-weighted (TR/TE, 4318/103) fast spin echo MR image of the lower legs reveals multiple neurofibromas (*arrows*) with a typical target pattern and a large MPNST (*arrowhead*) with no such pattern. (Courtesy of D. Levey, MD, Corpus Christi, Tex.)

the mass, the usual absence of calcification, and, rarely, the presence of bone erosion. MR imaging is helpful in making an accurate diagnosis. High signal intensity on T1-weighted spin echo MR images, when compared with the signal intensity of muscle, is related to melanocytic differentiation in the tumor and aids in its correct identification. Low signal intensity on T2-weighted spin echo MR images appears to be related to the effects of melanin, but this feature is not consistently seen. Involvement of subcutaneous tissue and dermis with ulceration is not unusual in cases of clear cell sarcoma (Fig. 71–61). Frequent tumor recurrence and distant metastasis underscore the poor prognosis of this tumor.

**Alveolar Soft Part Sarcoma.** This tumor, also called malignant granular cell myoblastoma, occurs most

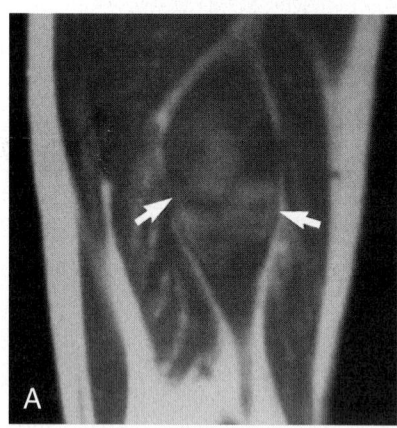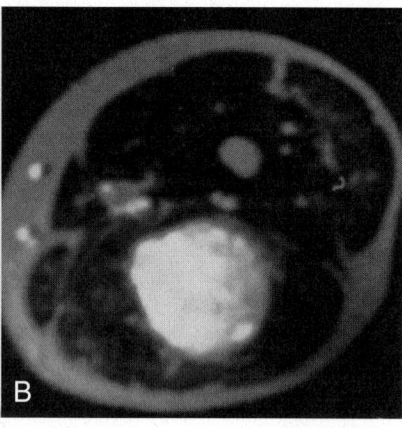

**Figure 71–59.** Malignant peripheral nerve sheath tumor. This 43-year-old man complained of pain in the posterior aspect of the thigh and tingling in the bottom of the foot. A firm posterior mass above the knee was palpated. *A*, Coronal T1-weighted (TR/TE, 500/17) spin echo MR image shows a mass (*arrows*) with slightly inhomogeneous but mainly low signal intensity; it is fusiform in shape and situated in the vicinity of the sciatic nerve. *B*, Transaxial T2-weighted (TR/TE, 2500/90) spin echo MR image reveals inhomogeneous high signal intensity in the mass. Radical excision of the tumor was performed.

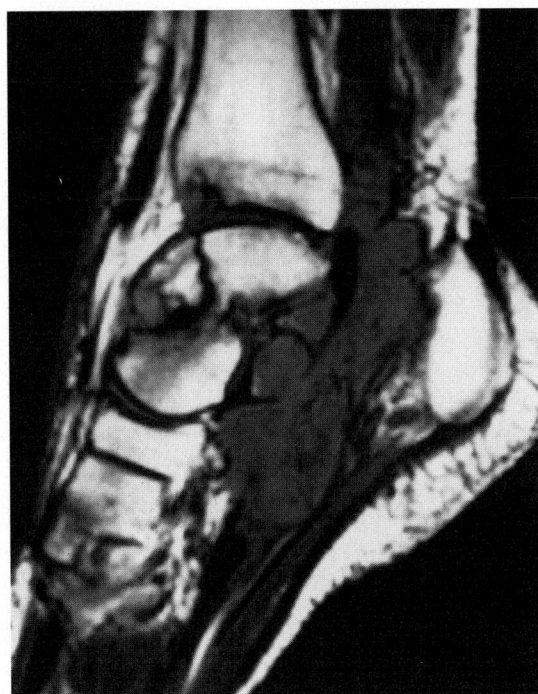

**Figure 71–61.** Clear cell sarcoma. Sagittal T1-weighted (TR/TE, 700/20) spin echo MR image in a 57-year-old woman shows a large tumor involving the plantar aspect of the foot. The tumor extends superiorly along the medial margin of the calcaneus and, posteriorly, behind the tibia in the region of the flexor digitorum longus and flexor hallucis longus tendons. It is of low signal intensity. (Courtesy of C. Gundry, MD, Minneapolis, Minn.)

frequently in young adults, more often in women. It is usually found in muscles but may also appear in the orbit and retroperitoneum; the thigh is a common site of involvement. The tumor grows slowly, may calcify or invade the underlying bone, and may eventually metastasize widely through the bloodstream. Imaging is typically nonspecific; however, in some cases, MR imaging reveals high signal intensity on both T1- and T2-weighted spin echo images (Fig. 71–62), which, when combined with flow voids, suggests the diagnosis.

**Epithelioid Sarcoma.** This sarcoma is a rare neoplasm arising principally in the fingers, hands, and forearms of young adults. Epithelioid sarcomas affect mainly the subcutaneous tissue, fascia, or tendon sheaths. Solitary or multiple firm nodules in the subcutis and deeper tissues are evident. On radiographs, a soft tissue mass may be observed. Calcification, ossification, hyperostosis, and cortical erosion have been described. MR imaging abnormalities, which may include fluid levels and (with intravenous gadolinium administration) rim enhancement, are not specific (Fig. 71–63).

**Granuloma Annulare.** Granuloma annulare, also known as rheumatoid nodule or pseudorheumatoid nodule, is an uncommon benign inflammatory dermatosis that has been divided into localized, generalized, perforating, and subcutaneous types. Granuloma annulare predominates in children, typically presenting as one or more painless, nonmobile subcutaneous masses that may grow rapidly; the lower extremity is involved more often than the upper extremity, and a pretibial localization may be characteristic. Radiographic findings are not specific, and calcification or ossification within the mass is not evident. With CT or MR imaging, an irregular, somewhat poorly defined soft tissue mass is generally evident. Decreased signal intensity on T1-weighted MR images and decreased to intermediate signal intensity on T2-weighted MR images are typical but not invariable features. These imaging characteristics in a subcutaneous soft tissue mass in an otherwise healthy child should suggest the diagnosis (Fig. 71–64).

## Synovial Disorders

A variety of synovial disorders can lead to intra-articular or periarticular masses. Such disorders include inflammatory joint diseases, crystal deposition disorders, idiopathic synovial (osteo)chondromatosis, and septic arthritis, which are discussed elsewhere in this text. Other processes discussed here are pigmented villonodular synovitis and synovial cysts.

**Pigmented Villonodular Synovitis.** This synovial proliferative disorder typically occurs in adults in the third or

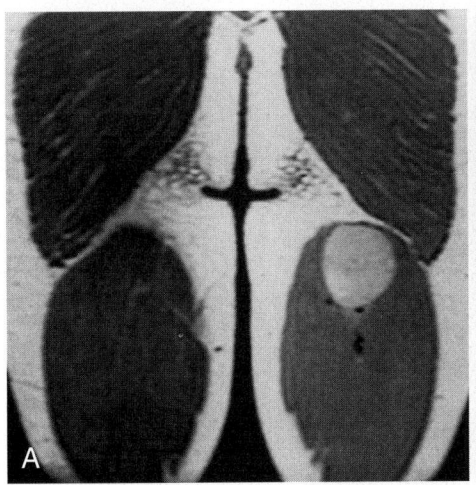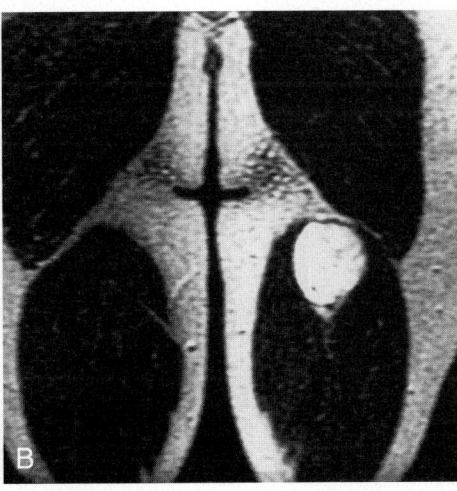

**Figure 71–62.** Alveolar soft part sarcoma. Coronal intermediate-weighted (TR/TE, 2000/20) (A) and T2-weighted (TR/TE, 2000/80) (B) spin echo MR images in an 18-year-old woman show a well-circumscribed mass in the semitendinosus muscle. The high signal intensity in (B) is nonspecific. (Courtesy of G. Greenway, MD, Dallas, Tex.)

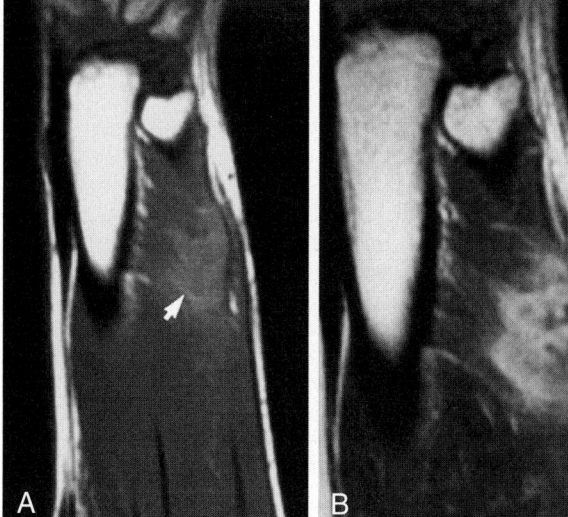

**Figure 71–63.** Epithelioid sarcoma. A forearm mass in this 22-year-old man is well demonstrated with MR imaging. *A,* On a coronal T1-weighted (TR/TE, 650/20) spin echo image, the lesion *(arrow)* is located dorsal to the distal portion of the ulna. Its signal intensity is slightly higher than that of muscle. *B,* Coronal T1-weighted (TR/TE, 650/20) spin echo MR image after the intravenous administration of gadolinium shows enhanced signal intensity of the tumor. The lesion is irregular in outline and not entirely homogeneous in appearance.

fourth decade of life, but it also appears less frequently in older adults, adolescents, and even children. The knee is the most common site of involvement; other frequently involved sites are the hip, elbow, and ankle, but any articulation can be affected. Monoarticular disease is the rule. Clinical manifestations vary according to the type of disease and its specific location. With diffuse involvement of a joint, slowly progressive pain and swelling, sometimes accompanied by warmth, tenderness, and stiffness, may be apparent, and a significant delay in diagnosis is common. With focal or localized involvement of a joint, symptoms and signs of an internal derangement may be apparent. Aspiration of joint contents classically

reveals brown fluid consistent with previous hemorrhage.

The classic radiographic features of diffuse intra-articular pigmented villonodular synovitis include soft tissue swelling or a joint effusion, preservation of joint space, absence of osteoporosis, and presence or absence of bone erosions and cysts. In some cases, radiographs are entirely normal or may show minimal and nonspecific findings such as a joint effusion. Bone erosions, when present, may be prominent, particularly about "tight" joints such as the hip, ankle, elbow, and wrist; less often, they may be observed in joints with large capacities, such as the knee (Fig. 71–65).

Many of the radiographic features of diffuse intra-articular pigmented villonodular synovitis are identical to those seen in idiopathic synovial chondromatosis, in which calcification and ossification are absent. The presence of calcification is quite unusual and generally makes the diagnosis of pigmented villonodular synovitis unlikely and, in the proper setting, favors the diagnosis of idiopathic synovial (osteo)chondromatosis. The radiographic features of diffuse pigmented villonodular synovitis are also modified in cases of bursal or tendon sheath involvement, including the nodular variety of tendon sheath disease known as giant cell tumor. In these instances, a diffuse or localized soft tissue mass (which calcifies only rarely) is observed. Subjacent erosion of bone may be encountered.

Bursal or tenosynovial villonodular synovitis is encountered in a variety of sites, although the subacromial-subdeltoid bursa and the peritenons and tendon sheaths about the wrist and ankle are favored locations (Fig. 71–66). A localized form of pigmented villonodular synovitis, termed nodular synovitis, is encountered in intra-articular locations, particularly the fat pad of Hoffa (infrapatellar fat body) and the suprapatellar recess, or bursae (Fig. 71–67). The tendon sheaths about the ankle are commonly affected by a similar process.

Giant cell tumors of tendon sheaths are one of the most common causes of soft tissue masses in the fingers (Figs. 71–68 and 71–69). Similar lesions have been encountered in other locations, such as about the patellar and quadriceps tendons. A slowly growing and often painless mass is seen. Bone involvement is uncommon,

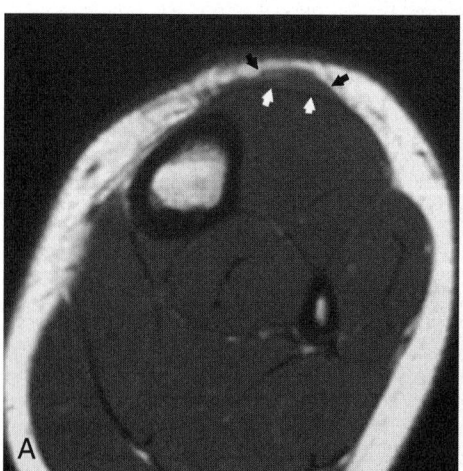
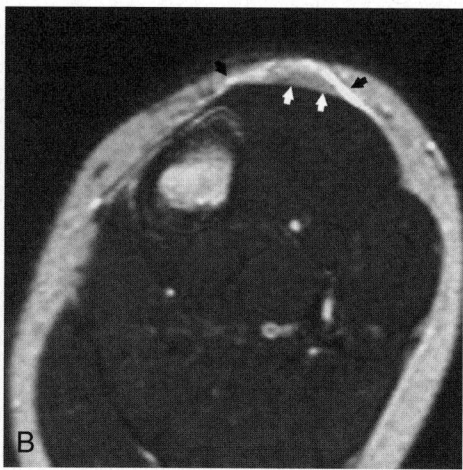

**Figure 71–64.** Granuloma annulare. A crescent-shaped subcutaneous mass *(arrows)* abuts the anterior aspect of the left lower leg. *A,* Coronal T1-weighted (TR/TE, 500/20) spin echo MR image shows a signal intensity similar to that of adjacent skeletal muscle. *B,* On a T2-weighted (TR/TE, 2000/80) spin echo MR image, the lesion has an intermediate signal intensity with a surrounding rind of high signal.

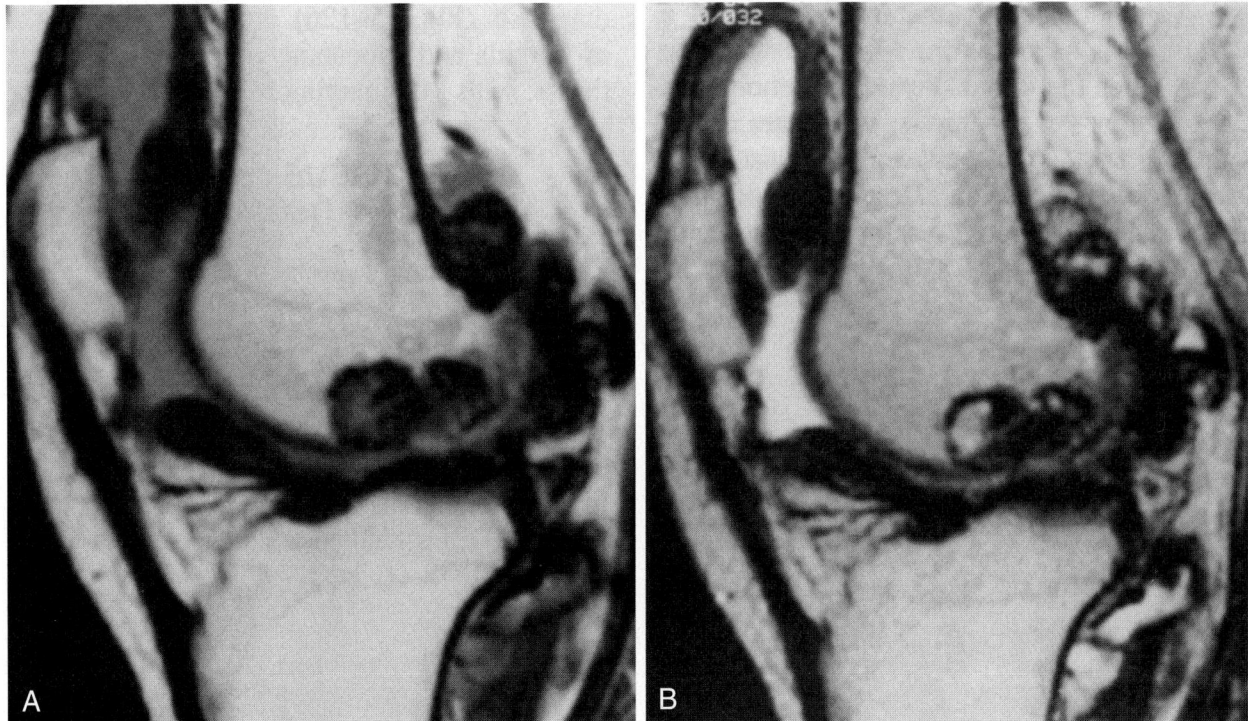

**Figure 71–65.** Diffuse (intra-articular) pigmented villonodular synovitis: knee. Sagittal intermediate-weighted (TR/TE, 2000/20) *(A)* and T2-weighted (TR/TE, 2000/80) *(B)* spin echo MR images show the classic features of this disease. A joint effusion is of intermediate signal intensity in *(A)* and high signal intensity in *(B)*. Hemosiderin deposition accounts for the low signal intensity in the synovial nodules in both images. Note the erosions of the distal end of the femur. (Courtesy of T. Broderick, MD, Orange, Calif.)

and calcification is rarely encountered. A diffuse form of giant cell tumor of tendon sheaths is described and likely represents extra-articular pigmented villonodular synovitis.

The deposition of hemosiderin in some cases of pigmented villonodular synovitis leads to dramatic MR imaging abnormalities characterized by regions of low signal intensity on both T1- and T2-weighted spin echo images (Fig. 71–70) and especially on gradient echo images. High signal intensity on T2-weighted spin echo MR images is also observed and is indicative of joint fluid.

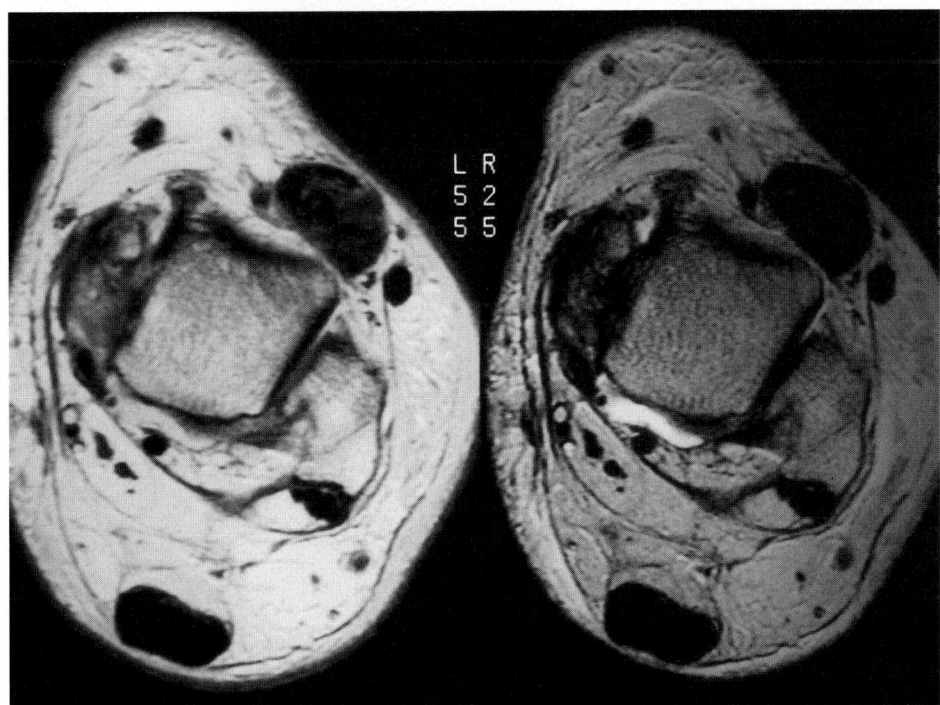

**Figure 71–66.** Tenosynovial villonodular synovitis. Transverse intermediate-weighted *(left)* and T2-weighted *(right)* spin echo MR images of the ankle. Note the enlargement of multiple tendons, including the peroneal and Achilles tendons, as well as the anterior tendons. Hemosiderin deposition accounts for their low signal intensity. (Courtesy of G. Applegate, MD, Van Nuys, Calif.)

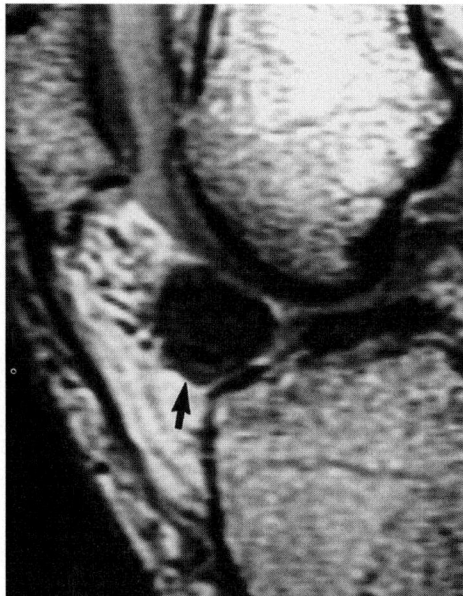

**Figure 71–67.** Localized nodular synovitis. Sagittal three-dimensional gradient echo (TR/TE, 18/4.6; flip angle, 30 degrees) MR image reveals the mass (*arrow*) of low signal intensity. Histologic analysis of the resected lesion revealed findings compatible with the diagnosis of localized nodular synovitis or giant cell tumor of a tendon sheath. (Courtesy of G. Greenway, MD, Dallas, Tex.)

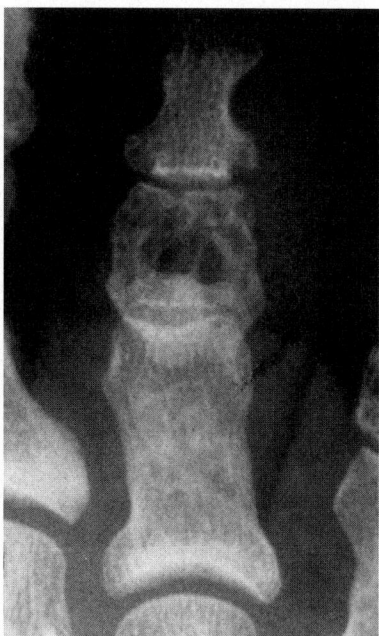

**Figure 71–68.** Giant cell tumor of a tendon sheath. Radiograph reveals a soft tissue mass with involvement of the middle phalanx of the fourth toe.

Although the presence of hemosiderin deposition on MR images is consistent with the diagnosis of pigmented villonodular synovitis, it is also evident in some cases of hemophilia and other bleeding disorders, synovial hemangioma, vascular malformations, neuropathic osteoarthropathy, and other processes associated with chronic hemarthrosis. Enhancement of signal intensity after intravenous gadolinium administration is an inconsistent finding. In some cases, however, such enhancement is profound, and a similar high signal intensity may be evident on STIR images. Although giant cell tumors of tendon sheaths are often characterized by persistent

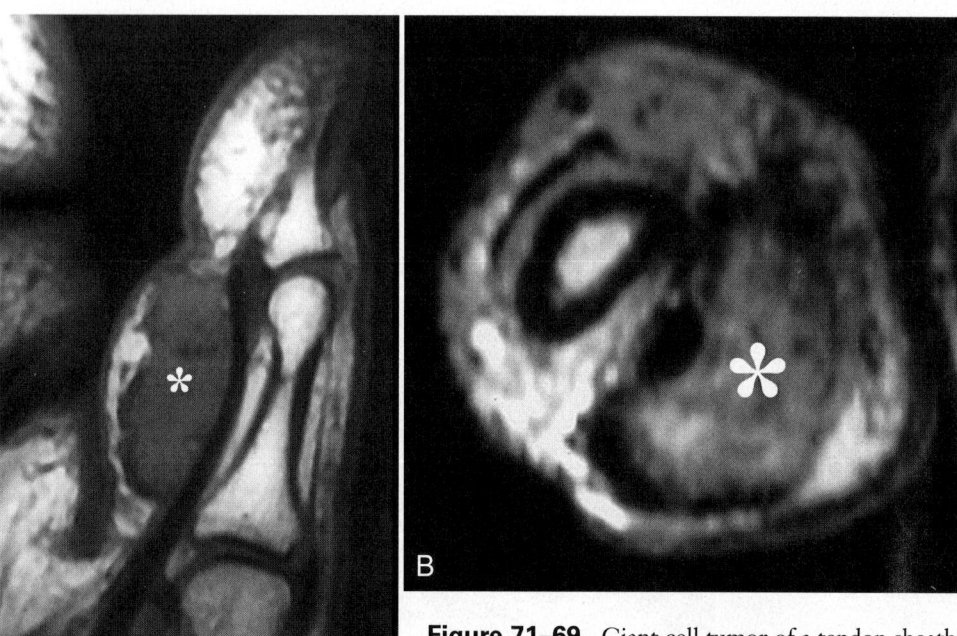

**Figure 71–69.** Giant cell tumor of a tendon sheath. Sagittal T1-weighted (TR/TE, 300/25) (*A*) and transverse T2-weighted (TR/TE, 2000/80) (*B*) spin echo MR images show a lobulated mass of intermediate signal intensity (*asterisks*), intimately associated with the flexor tendon of the thumb.

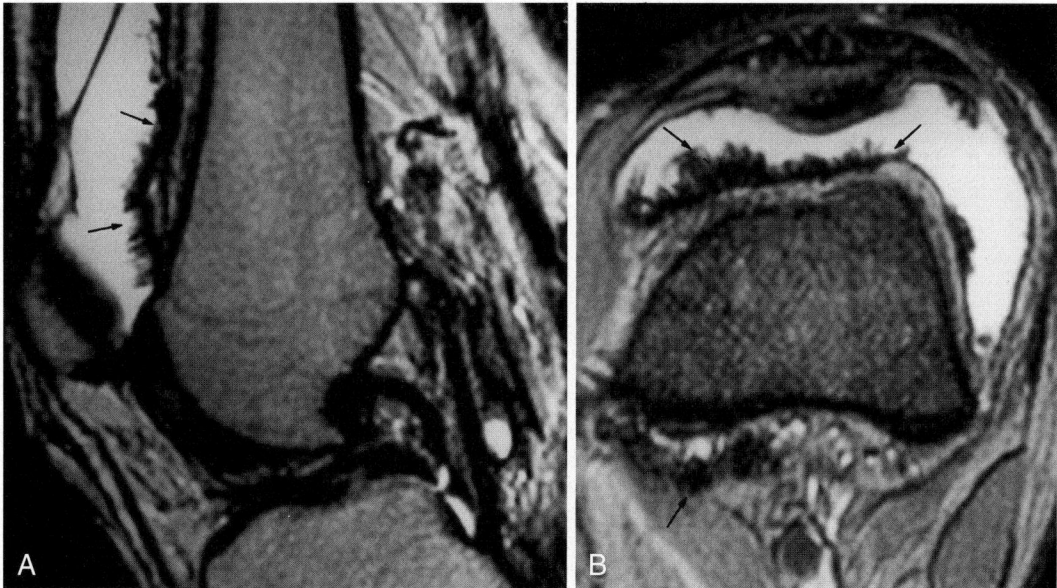

**Figure 71–70.** Diffuse (intra-articular) pigmented villonodular synovitis. *A,* In this 29-year-old man, a sagittal T2-weighted (TR/TE, 2000/75) spin echo MR image reveals a joint effusion and a feathery pattern of hemosiderin deposition of low signal intensity *(arrows),* mainly in the suprapatellar recess of the knee. *B,* Transverse multiplanar gradient recalled (TR/TE, 740/18; flip angle, 18 degrees) MR image confirms hemosiderin deposition *(arrows)* both anteriorly and posteriorly. (Courtesy of E. Bosch, MD, Santiago, Chile.)

regions of low signal intensity, they too may show enhancement when gadolinium-containing contrast agents are used (Fig. 71–71).

**Synovial Cyst.** Synovial cysts are fluid-filled para-articular masses lined by a synovial membrane that may or may not communicate with the neighboring joint. Those that demonstrate such communication commonly distend

with fluid when an effusion, a synovial response, or both appear in the adjacent joint, thereby leading to elevated intra-articular pressure. Synovial cysts can arise at many different periarticular locations, including in the spine, but they are encountered most commonly about the knee and hip. Large synovial cysts are most typical in cases of inflammatory arthritis, whereas small synovial cysts may indicate the presence of an internal derangement of the

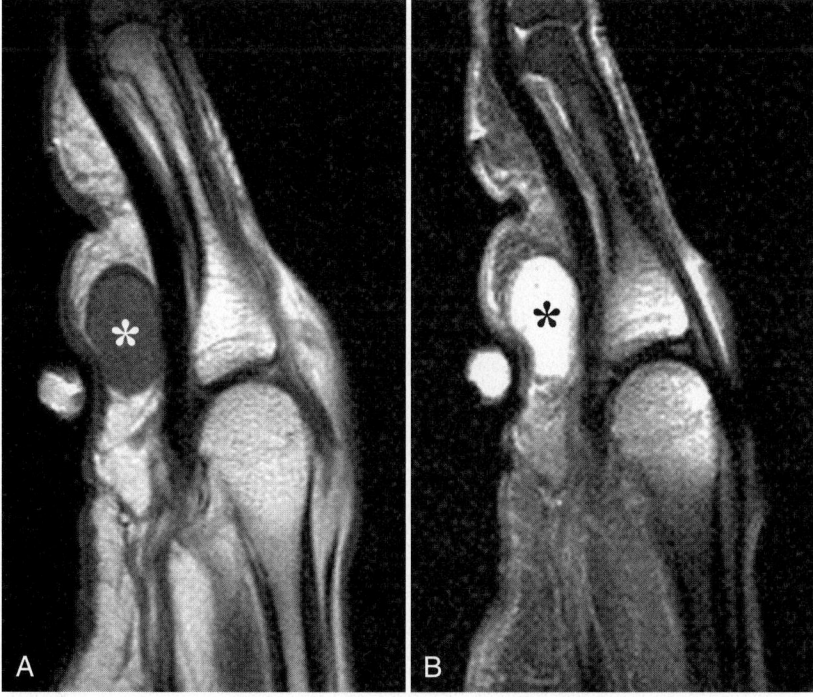

**Figure 71–71.** Giant cell tumor of a tendon sheath. A mass arises from the flexor tendon of the index finger. *A,* The mass *(asterisk)* has a signal intensity similar to that of skeletal muscle on a sagittal T1-weighted (TR/TE, 585/28) spin echo MR image. *B,* Note intense enhancement after intravenous gadolinium administration on a sagittal fat-suppressed T1-weighted (TR/TE, 628/28) spin echo MR image.

joint, such as a torn meniscus of the knee. In some locations, such as the semimembranosus-gastrocnemius region of the knee, a valvelike mechanism allows communication of the joint and cyst as a response to elevations in intra-articular pressure, thus serving as a mechanism for decompression of the joint. In other locations, the cyst and joint communicate freely without such a valve, and some synovial cysts show no communication with the articulation.

The most characteristic location of a synovial cyst is the posterior aspect of the knee, related to distention of the gastrocnemius-semimembranosus bursa in response to a knee effusion. These cysts, which are designated Baker's cysts, may dissect between the muscles of the leg (Fig. 71–72) or rupture and cause extravasation of fluid, which leads to clinical manifestations resembling those of thrombophlebitis. The diagnosis of Baker's cyst can be accomplished with ultrasonography, radionuclide arthrography, standard arthrography, CT, computed arthrotomography, or MR imaging. In addition to dissection or rupture, popliteal cysts may contain chondral or osteochondral bodies or may rarely calcify. About the hip, fluid collections representing synovial cysts, distended iliopsoas bursae, or para-acetabular ganglia may be encountered. The iliopsoas bursa may normally communicate with the hip, so its distention in cases of hip effusion is not unexpected. Chronic developmental dysplasia of the hip may be associated with tears of the acetabular labrum and with intraosseous and para-acetabular ganglion cysts.

**Bursitis.** Accumulation of fluid in bursal cavities may lead to soft tissue masses. Typical examples include subacromial-subdeltoid bursitis, olecranon bursitis, iliopsoas bursitis, anserine bursitis, trochanteric bursitis, cubital bursitis at the elbow, prepatellar and deep infrapatellar bursitis, and bursitis about the Achilles tendon (Haglund's syndrome) (Fig. 71–73). Bursal fluid may result from local irritation or trauma or as a response to systemic rheumatologic conditions or infection. Ultrasonography, CT, or MR imaging can be used for diagnosis.

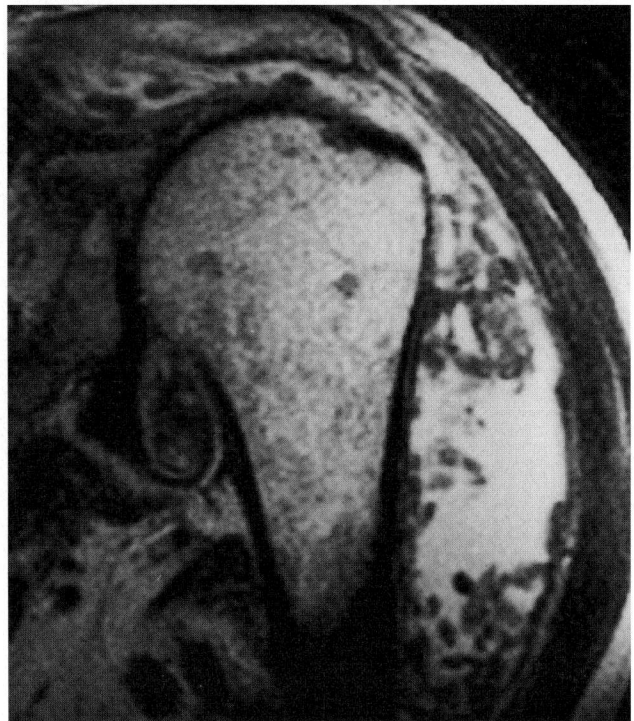

**Figure 71–73.** Subacromial-subdeltoid bursitis. Oblique coronal fast spin echo (TR/TE, 300/99) MR image shows massive distention of this bursa, with fluid of high signal intensity and synovial proliferative tissue and rice bodies of low signal intensity in a patient with probable rheumatoid arthritis. The rotator cuff is torn and retracted, and the glenohumeral joint is also involved. (Courtesy of A. Pinto Leite, MD, Porto, Portugal.)

**Tenosynovitis.** Inflammation of a tendon sheath is a common problem with many causes. Overuse syndromes, rheumatoid arthritis and other articular diseases, and infection are but a few of the processes that can lead to tenosynovitis. Diagnostic methods include CT, ultra-

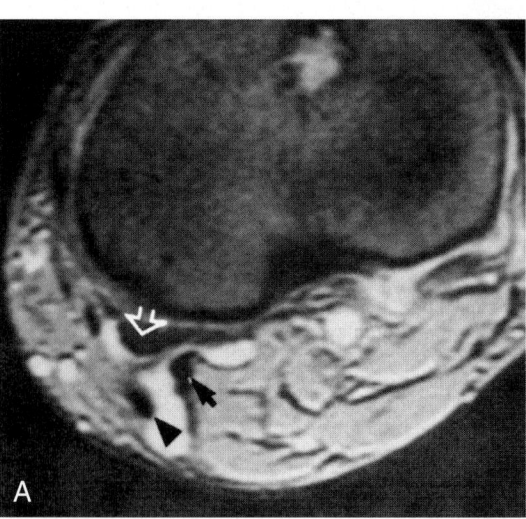
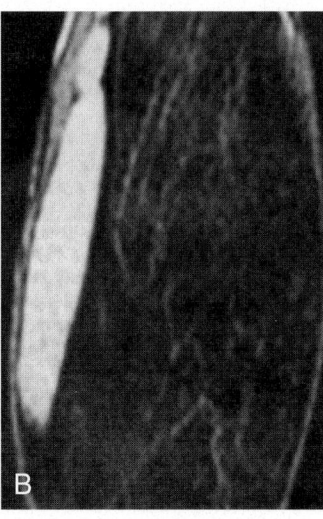

**Figure 71–72.** Synovial cyst: knee. *A,* Transaxial multiplanar gradient recalled (TR/TE, 500/15; flip angle, 20 degrees) MR image shows the site of origin of the synovial cyst. Note the fluid of high signal intensity passing posterior to the semimembranosus tendon *(open arrow),* medial to the tendon of the medial head of the gastrocnemius muscle *(solid arrow),* and lateral to the semitendinosus tendon *(arrowhead). B,* Coronal T2-weighted (TR/TE, 2000/80) spin echo MR image in the same patient shows the more distal extent of the synovial cyst, which is superficial to the medial head of the gastrocnemius muscle.

sonography, and MR imaging. The intravenous administration of a gadolinium-containing contrast agent is a useful ancillary method (Fig. 71–74).

## Hematoma

Hematomas occurring in the extremities or trunk can lead to soft tissue masses that must be distinguished from tumors. Complicating this differentiation is the occurrence of hemorrhage into preexisting neoplasms, leading to the imaging features of both blood products and tumorous tissue. Many previous descriptions of the MR imaging features of hematomas focused on brain involvement, but these concepts can be expanded to explain, in part, the appearance of extracranial hematomas as well.

The presence of hemoglobin and its degradation products, which are the major constituents of hemorrhagic collections, influences the MR imaging appearance of hematomas through alterations in T1 and T2 relaxation times. Because the status of hemoglobin within

a hematoma is dependent on the acute or chronic nature of the hemorrhagic collection, the resulting MR imaging features are not constant but evolve in a somewhat predictable fashion over time. Although the age of a hematoma has the greatest influence on its MR imaging appearance, the application of such terms as acute, subacute, and chronic to the status of the hemorrhagic collection has not been consistent (Table 71–7). As a general guideline, acute hematomas are less than a few days old, subacute hematomas are measured in weeks, and chronic hematomas are measured in months.

In the hyperacute stage of a hematoma (i.e., within the first hours after a bleeding episode), oxyhemoglobin can lead to high signal intensity on both T1- and T2-weighted spin echo MR images (Fig. 71–75), but in clinical practice, because of the rapid conversion of oxyhemoglobin to deoxyhemoglobin, the latter substance influences the MR imaging characteristics of a hematoma, even in its very early stages. Although deoxyhemoglobin is paramagnetic, it does not have a significant ability to shorten T1 relaxation time. On T2-weighted images, however, deoxyhemoglobin can lead to low signal intensity, especially in the center of a hematoma.

In the subacute stage of an evolving hematoma, conversion of deoxyhemoglobin to methemoglobin takes place. With increasing accumulation of methemoglobin, increased signal intensity is observed, particularly at the periphery of a subacute hematoma, designated the concentric ring sign (Fig. 71–76). In the later stages of an evolving hematoma, hemosiderin deposition results in regions of decreased signal intensity, sometimes in a rindlike distribution. Hemosiderin deposition often appears as an outer layer of hypointense signal intensity (relative to that of muscle) in chronic hematomas.

It should be recognized that hematomas can simulate malignant tumors both clinically and on imaging studies. Malignant fibrous histiocytomas and synovial sarcomas are often associated with bleeding, although such bleeding can theoretically be encountered with any type of sarcoma and with benign processes as well (e.g., hemangioma). Contrast-enhanced imaging may be especially useful in distinguishing a hematoma from a hemorrhagic sarcoma (Fig. 71–77).

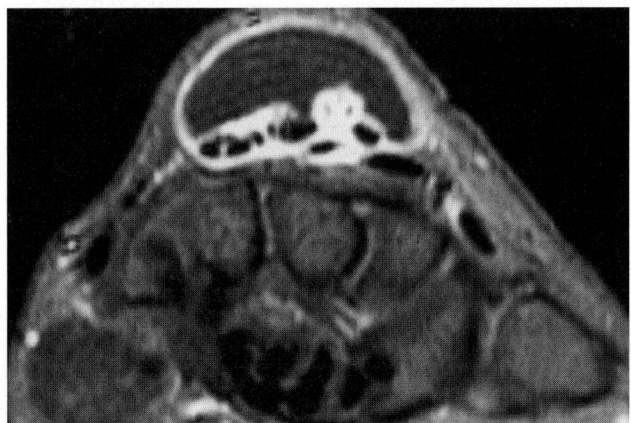

**Figure 71–74.** Tenosynovitis. Transverse fat-suppressed T1-weighted (TR/TE, 600/20) spin echo MR image after intravenous gadolinium administration shows marked distention of the extensor tendon sheath, with enhancement of signal intensity within the synovial membrane of the tendon sheath.

**TABLE 71–7**

**Soft Tissue Hemorrhage (Hematoma)**

|  | Days | RBCs | Hemoglobin | T1 Signal | T2 Signal |
|---|---|---|---|---|---|
| Hyperacute | 0–1 | Intact | OxyHgb | High | Very high |
| Acute | 1–4 | Intact | DeoxyHgb | Low | Very low |
| Early subacute | 2–7 | Intact | MetHgb | Very high | Low |
| Late subacute | 5–21 | Lysed | MetHgb | Very high | High |
| Chronic | >21 | Lysed | Ferritin | Low | Low |

Hgb, hemoglobin; RBC, red blood cell.

From Swenson SJ, Keller PL, Berquist TH, et al: Magnetic resonance imaging of hemorrhage. AJR 145:921, 1985.

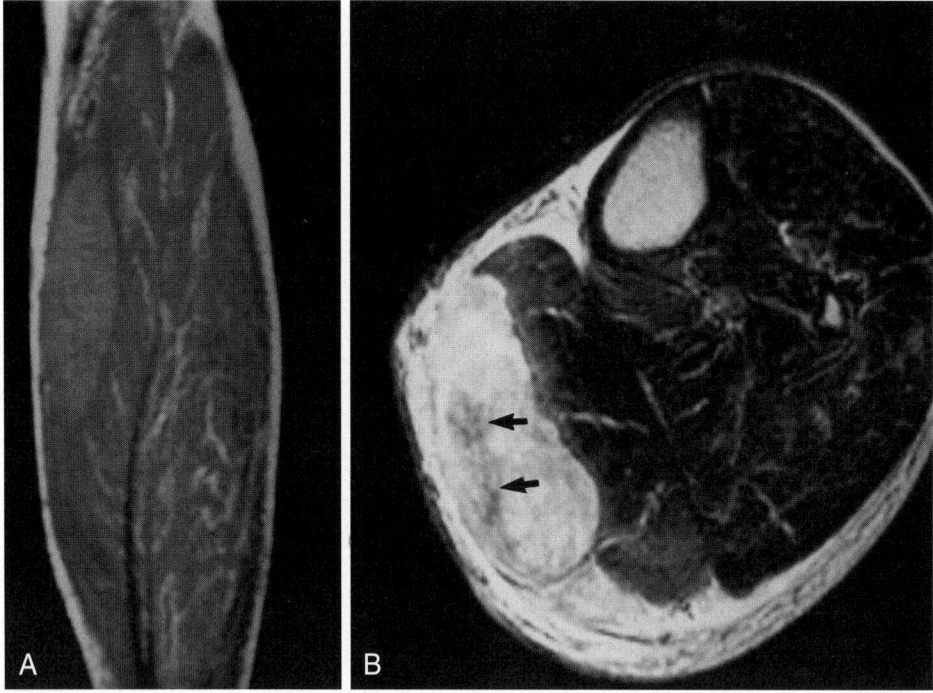

**Figure 71–75.** Hematoma: acute to early subacute stage. A mass developed in the calf of this 55-year-old man after an injury. Imaging was accomplished 3 days later. *A,* Coronal T1-weighted (TR/TE, 500/10) spin echo MR image shows a fusiform mass in the medial head of the gastrocnemius muscle. Its signal intensity is slightly higher than that of muscle. The shape of the mass is characteristic of a hematoma. *B,* Transverse fast spin echo (TR/TE, 3000/102) MR image demonstrates signal inhomogeneity. Regions of low signal intensity are consistent with clots containing intracellular deoxyhemoglobin, methemoglobin, or both *(arrows).*

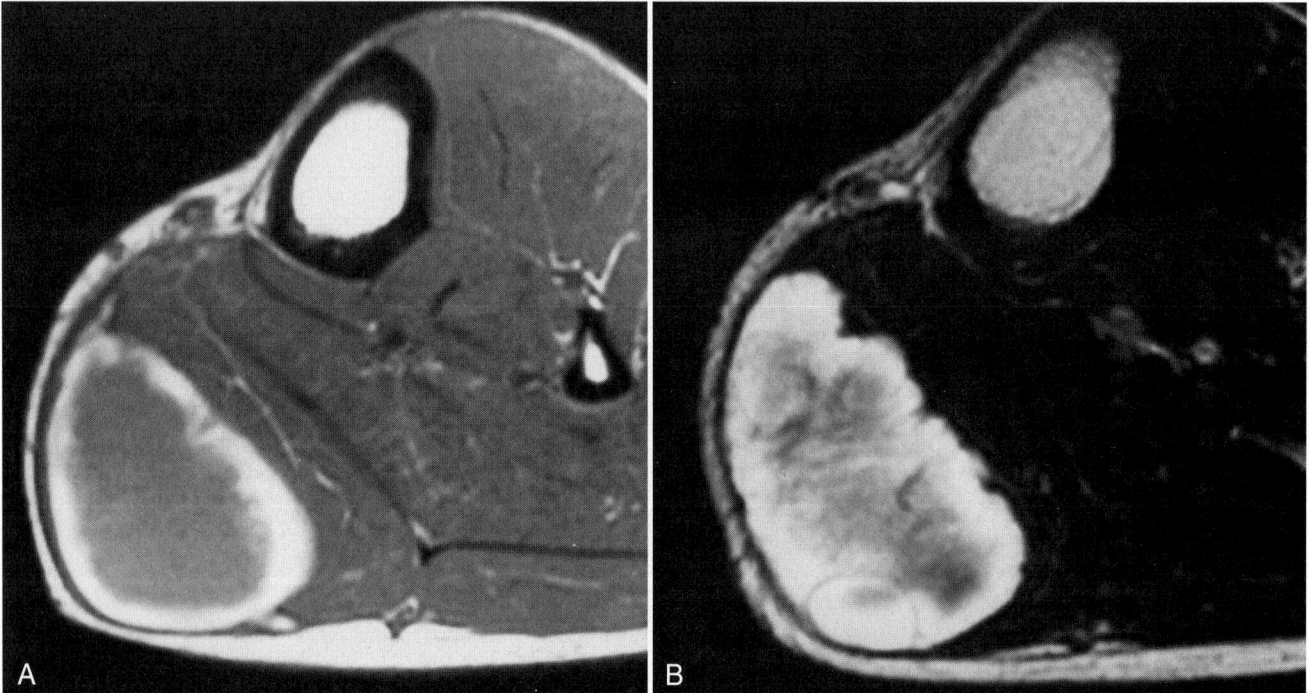

**Figure 71–76.** Hematoma: subacute stage. Transverse T1-weighted (TR/TE, 450/15) *(A)* and fast spin echo (TR/TE, 3616/128) *(B)* MR images show a large hematoma within the gastrocnemius muscle, with an irregular concentric ring of high signal intensity.

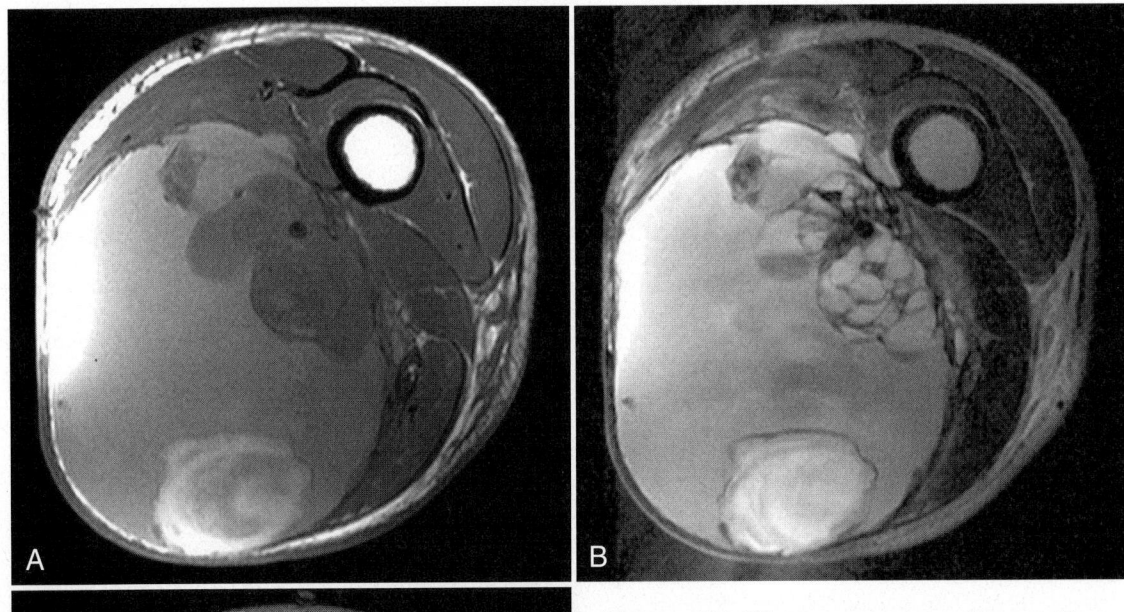

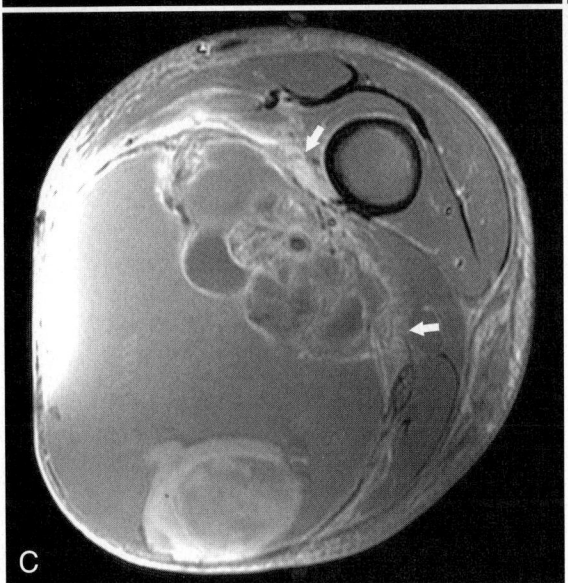

**Figure 71–77.** Hemorrhagic malignant fibrous histiocytoma. *A* and *B*, Axial T1-weighted (TR/TE, 608/16) *(A)* and T2-weighted (TR/TE, 2150/80) *(B)* spin echo MR images show a large hemorrhagic mass in the thigh, with signal characteristics of a hematoma. *C*, Axial fat-suppressed T1-weighted (TR/TE, 653/16) spin echo MR image after the intravenous administration of gadolinium shows the intensely enhancing tumor along the margin of the lesion *(arrows)* and encasing the superficial femoral artery.

## FURTHER READING

Allen PW: The fibromatoses: A clinicopathologic classification based on 140 cases. Am J Surg Pathol 1:255, 1977.

Bliznak J, Staple TW: Radiology of angiodysplasias of the limb. Radiology 110:35, 1974.

Bouhoutsos J, Martin P: Popliteal aneurysm: A review of 116 cases. Br J Surg 61:469, 1974.

Breimer CW, Freiberger RH: Bone lesions associated with villonodular synovitis. AJR Am J Roentgenol 79:618, 1958.

Burleson J, Bickel WH, Dahlin DC: Popliteal cyst: A clinico-pathological survey. J Bone Joint Surg Am 38:1265, 1956.

Cavanagh RC: Tumors of the soft tissues of the extremities. Semin Roentgenol 8:73, 1973.

Cavanagh RC, Schwamm HA: Localized nodular synovitis: RPC of the month from the AFIP. Radiology 100:409, 1971.

Chung EB, Enzinger FM: Benign lipoblastomatosis: An analysis of 35 cases. Cancer 32:482, 1973.

Chung EB, Enzinger FM: Chondroma of soft parts. Cancer 41:1414, 1978.

Chung EB, Enzinger FM: Infantile fibrosarcoma. Cancer 38:729, 1976.

Chung SMK, Janes JM: Diffuse pigmented villonodular synovitis of the hip joint: Review of the literature and report of four cases. J Bone Joint Surg Am 47:293, 1965.

Cohen EK, Kressel HY, Perosio T, et al: MR imaging of soft-tissue hemangiomas: Correlation with pathologic findings. AJR Am J Roentgenol 150:1079, 1988.

Condon VR, Allen RP: Congenital generalized fibromatosis: Case report with roentgen manifestations. Radiology 76:444, 1961.

Craig RM, Pugh DG, Soule EH: Roentgenologic manifestations of synovial sarcoma. Radiology 65:837, 1955.

Dahlin DC, Salvador AH: Cartilaginous tumor of the soft tissues of the hands and feet. Mayo Clin Proc 49:721, 1974.

De Schepper AM, De Beuckeleer L, Vandevenne J, et al: Magnetic resonance imaging of soft tissue tumors. Eur Radiol 10:213, 2000.

Dionne GP, Seemayer TA: Infiltrating lipomas and angiolipomas revisited. Cancer 33:732, 1974.

Donnal JF, Blinder RA, Coblentz CL, et al: MR imaging of stump neuroma. J Comput Assist Tomogr 14:656, 1990.

Dooms GC, Hricak H, Sollitto RA, et al: Lipomatous tumors and tumors with fatty component: MR imaging potential and comparison of MR and CT results. Radiology 157:479, 1985.

Enneking WF, Spanier SS, Malawar MM: The effect of the anatomic setting on the results of surgical procedures for soft part sarcoma of the thigh. Cancer 47:1005, 1981.

Enzi G, Biondetti PR, Fiore D, et al: Computed tomography of deep fat masses in multiple symmetrical lipomatosis. Radiology 144:121, 1982.

Enzinger FM, Weiss SW: Soft Tissue Tumors, 2nd ed. St Louis, CV Mosby, 1988.

Finberg HJ, Levin DC: Angiolipoma: A rare benign soft tissue tumor with a malignant arteriographic appearance. AJR Am J Roentgenol 128:697, 1077.

Fischer HJ, Lois JF, Gomes AS, et al: Radiology and pathology of malignant fibrous histiocytomas of the soft tissues: A report of ten cases. Skeletal Radiol 13:202, 1985.

Fletcher AG Jr, Horn RC Jr: Giant cell tumors of tendon sheath origin: A consideration of bone involvement and report of two cases with extensive bone destruction. Ann Surg 133:374, 1951.

Goergen IG, Resnick D, Niwayama G: Localized nodular synovitis of the knee: A report of two cases with abnormal arthrograms. AJR Am J Roentgenol 126:647, 1976.

Greenfield MM, Wallace KM: Pigmented villonodular synovitis. Radiology 54:350, 1950.

Greenspan A, McGahan JP, Vogelsang P, et al: Imaging strategies in the evaluation of soft-tissue hemangiomas of the extremities: Correlation of the findings on plain films, angiography, CT, MRI, and ultrasonography in 12 histologically proven cases. Skeletal Radiol 21:11, 1992.

Hale DE: Synovioma with special reference to the clinical and roentgenologic aspects. AJR Am J Roentgenol 65:769, 1951.

Heitzman ER, Jones JB: Roentgen characteristics of cavernous hemangioma of striated muscle. Radiology 74:420, 1960.

Horowitz AL, Resnick D, Watson RC: The roentgen features of synovial sarcoma. Clin Radiol 24:481, 1973.

Jacobs P: Parosteal lipoma with hyperostosis. Clin Radiol 23:196, 1972.

Jeffreys TE: Synovial chondromatosis. J Bone Joint Surg Br 49:530, 1967.

Kindblom LG, Angervall L, Stener B, et al: Intermuscular and intramuscular lipomas and hibernomas: A clinical, roentgenologic, histologic, and prognostic study of 46 cases. Cancer 33:754, 1974.

Kindblom LG, Gunterberg B: Pigmented villonodular synovitis involving bone. J Bone Joint Surg Am 60:830, 1978.

Kransdorf MJ: Benign soft-tissue tumors in a large referral population: Distribution of specific diagnoses by age, sex, and location. AJR Am J Roentgenol 164:395, 1995.

Kransdorf MJ: Malignant soft-tissue tumors in a large referral population: Distribution of diagnoses by age, sex, and location. AJR Am J Roentgenol 164:129, 1995.

Kransdorf MJ, Murphey MD: Imaging of Soft Tissue Tumors. Philadelphia, WB Saunders, 1997.

Kransdorf MJ, Murphey MD: Radiologic evaluation of soft-tissue masses: A current perspective. AJR Am J Roentgenol 175:575, 2000.

Levine E, Lee KR, Neff JR, et al: Comparison of computed tomography and other imaging modalities in the evaluation of musculoskeletal tumors. Radiology 131:431, 1979.

Lewis RW: Roentgen recognition of synovioma. AJR Am J Roentgenol 44:170, 1940.

Lichtenstein L: Tumors of synovial joints, bursae and tendon sheaths. Cancer 8:816, 1955.

Lin J, Jacobson JA, Jamadar DA, et al: Pigmented villonodular synovitis and related lesions: The spectrum of imaging findings. AJR Am J Roentgenol 172:191, 1999.

MacKenzie DH: The Differential Diagnosis of Fibroblastic Disorders. Oxford, Blackwell Scientific Publications, 1970.

McMaster MJ, Soule EH, Ivins JC: Hemangiopericytoma: A clinico-pathologic study and long term follow-up of 60 patients. Cancer 36:2232, 1975.

Milgram JW: The classification of loose bodies in human joints. Clin Orthop 124:282, 1977.

Milgram JW: Synovial osteochondromatosis: A histopathological study of thirty cases. J Bone Joint Surg Am 59:792, 1977.

Milgram JW, Dunn EJ: Para-articular chondromas and osteochondromas. Clin Orthop 148:147, 1980.

Moore O, Grossi C: Embryonal rhabdomyosarcoma of the head and neck. Cancer 12:69, 1959.

Murphey MD, Smith WS, Smith SE, et al: Imaging of musculoskeletal neurogenic tumors: Radiologic-pathologic correlation. Radiographics 19:1253, 1999.

Pack GT, Pierson JC: Liposarcoma: A study of 105 cases. Surgery 36:687, 1954.

Piyachon C: Radiology of peripheral arteriovenous malformations. Australas Radiol 21:246, 1977.

Resnick D, Oliphant M: Hemophilia-like arthropathy of the knee associated with cutaneous and synovial hemangiomas: Report of 3 cases and review of the literature. Radiology 114:323, 1975.

Robbin MR, Murphey MD, Temple HT, et al: Imaging of musculoskeletal fibromatosis. Radiographics 21:585, 2001.

Rosenthal DL: Computed tomography in bone and soft tissue neoplasm: Application and pathologic correlation. CRC Crit Rev Diagn Imaging 18:243, 1982.

Sartoris DJ, Danzig L, Gilula L, et al: Synovial cysts of the hip joint and iliopsoas bursitis: A spectrum of imaging abnormalities. Skeletal Radiol 14:85, 1985.

Shnitka TK, Asp DM, Horner RH: Congenital generalized fibromatosis. Cancer 11:627, 1958.

Spjut HJ, Dorfman HD, Fechner RE, et al: Tumors of bone and cartilage. In Atlas of Tumor Pathology, 2nd ser, fascicle 5. Washington, DC, Armed Forces Institute of Pathology, 1971, p 391.

Steinbach L, Hellman D, Petri M, et al: Magnetic resonance imaging: A review of rheumatologic applications. Semin Arthritis Rheum 16:79, 1986.

Stout AP: Pathology and classification of tumors of the soft tissues. AJR Am J Roentgenol 66:903, 1951.

Stout AP, Lattes R: Tumors of the soft tissues. In Atlas of Tumor Pathology, 2nd ser, fascicle 1. Washington, DC, Armed Forces Institute of Pathology, 1967, p 11.

Sundaram M, McGuire MH, Herbold DR: Magnetic resonance imaging of soft tissue masses: An evaluation of fifty-three histologically proven tumors. Magn Reson Imaging 6:237, 1988.

Sundaram M, McGuire MH, Herbold DR, et al: High signal intensity soft tissue masses on T1 weighted pulsing sequences. Skeletal Radiol 16:30, 1987.

Trias A, Quintana O: Synovial chondrometaplasia: Review of world literature and a study of 18 Canadian cases. Can J Surg 19:151, 1976.

Weiss SW, Enzinger FM: Malignant fibrous histiocytoma: An analysis of 200 cases. Cancer 41:2250, 1978.

Weiss SW, Enzinger FM: Myxoid variant of malignant fibrous histiocytoma. Cancer 39:1672, 1977.

Weiss SW, Goldblum JR: Enzinger and Weiss's Soft Tissue Tumors, 4th ed. St Louis, CV Mosby, 2001.

Zimmerman C, Sayegh V: Roentgen manifestations of synovial osteochondromatosis. AJR Am J Roentgenol 83:680, 1960.

Zlatkin MB, Lander PH, Begin LR, et al: Soft-tissue chondromas. AJR Am J Roentgenol 144:1263, 1985.

# CHAPTER 72

## Skeletal Metastases

### SUMMARY OF KEY FEATURES

Metastatic disease of the skeleton can arise from direct extension, lymphatic or hematogenous dissemination, or intraspinal spread of tumor. The osseous response to the neoplasm consists of bone resorption, bone formation, or both. Such metastases predominate in the bones of the axial skeleton, although atypical patterns of distribution are encountered. A variety of diagnostic techniques, including scintigraphy, computed tomography, magnetic resonance imaging, and positron emission tomography, can be used in addition to routine radiography in the initial detection and subsequent monitoring of metastatic foci.

### INTRODUCTION

Metastasis is defined as "the transfer of disease from one organ or part to another not directly connected with it," a process that "may be due either to the transfer of pathogenetic microorganisms . . . or to the transfer of cells, as in malignant tumors." Any malignant neoplasm possesses the capacity to metastasize to the musculoskeletal system, although some do so more frequently than others. Further, nonmalignant tumors can occasionally metastasize if neoplastic cells enter the vascular system through eroded blood vessel walls. Of the potential pathways available for the dissemination of tumor, vascular channels are more important than lymphatic channels; extension of neoplastic cells through lymph vessels to regional lymph nodes is generally followed by entrance into the vascular system. Venous invasion is more common than arterial invasion, because the arterial wall exhibits striking immunity to tumor penetration in the absence of infection.

### GENERAL MECHANISMS OF SKELETAL METASTASIS

The skeleton is one of the most frequent sites of tumor metastasis. As in other locations, successful metastatic implantation requires both the transport of viable tumor cells to the bone and the interaction of these cells with the osseous tissue.

#### Routes of Tumor Spread to Bone

**Direct Extension.** Malignant neoplasms located in the soft tissues adjacent to a bone may penetrate that bone by direct extension. Examples include a carcinoma at the apex of the lung (Pancoast's tumor) that invades the ribs or cervical vertebrae (Fig. 72–1) or a carcinoma of the bladder or rectum that involves the bones of the pelvis. In other instances, contiguous spread of tumor into bone originates from a site that is distant from the primary tumor. Examples of this situation include a carcinoma of the lung that extends into the mediastinum, with subsequent involvement of the spine (Fig. 72–2), or a soft tissue or muscle metastatic deposit resulting from hematogenous or lymphatic dissemination that subsequently invades the adjacent osseous tissue. In all these situations, there is typically a soft tissue mass (of variable size) and osseous destruction (of variable degree).

**Lymphatic Spread.** Tumors generally lack a lymphatic network, such that extension of neoplastic cells into lymphatic channels occurs only at the margin of the tumor. Metastatic deposits in regional draining lymph nodes can secondarily involve the adjacent osseous structures. An important example of this phenomenon is the occurrence of vertebral destruction in cases of pelvic carcinoma arising in such sites as the prostate, bladder, cervix, and uterus. Imaging studies demonstrate characteristic abnormalities, including a paravertebral soft tissue mass and scalloped erosions of one or more vertebral bodies. Predominant involvement of the left side of the lumbar spine is consistent with the fact that the lymph nodes on this side are closer to the spine than are those on the right side. Similar abnormalities are observed in some patients with lymphomas and plasma cell myeloma.

**Hematogenous Dissemination.** The bloodstream is the major pathway allowing dissemination of malignant neoplasms to the skeleton. Two potential vascular routes exist—the arterial system and the venous system, particularly the vertebral plexus of veins described by Batson. The predilection for metastases to occur in the axial skeleton, especially the spine, and the presence of vertebral metastasis in the absence of pulmonary (or other organ) involvement are findings that support the significance of Batson's vertebral plexus in tumor spread.

**Intraspinal Spread.** The cerebrospinal fluid represents an additional pathway for tumor dissemination, allowing secondary deposits in the spinal canal to develop in patients with intracranial neoplasms. Subarachnoid seeding is related to several specific mechanisms, including fragmentation of a tumor bathed with cerebrospinal fluid, ependymal breaching by the primary intracranial tumor or fissuring secondary to hydrocephalus, or shedding of portions of the tumor at the time of craniotomy. Children and adults are affected, and the types of tumors leading to subarachnoid spread (in children) are, in order of decreasing frequency, medulloblastoma, ependymoma, pineal neoplasms, astrocytoma, lymphoma, choroid plexus papilloma, and retinoblastoma. Accurate diagnosis requires the use of methods such as myelography, computed tomography (CT), and magnetic resonance (MR) imaging.

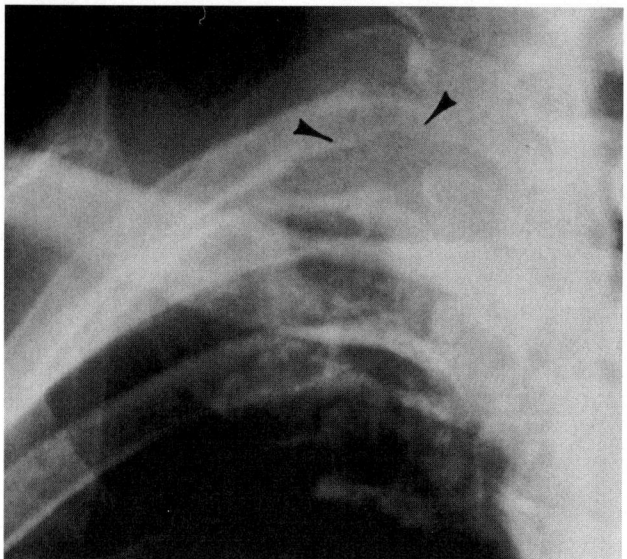

**Figure 72–1.** Routes of tumor spread to bone: direct extension. A carcinoma in the apex of the lung (Pancoast's tumor) has led to destruction of the posterior portion of the second rib (*arrowheads*).

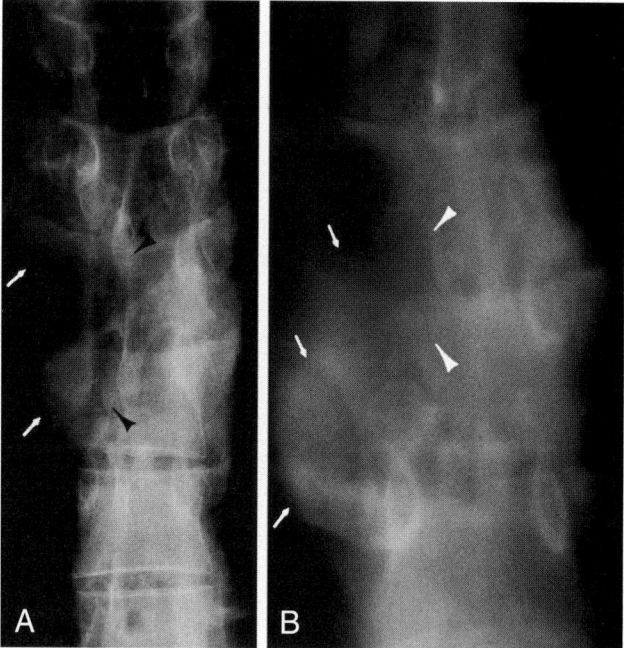

**Figure 72–2.** Routes of tumor spread to bone: lymphatic spread with direct extension. Radiograph (*A*) and tomogram (*B*) in a patient with carcinoma of the lung show evidence of spread to paravertebral lymph nodes (*arrows*), with subsequent extension into several thoracic vertebrae (*arrowheads*). Note the pediculate destruction.

## Osseous Response to Metastatic Tumor

The response of bone to secondary deposits of tumor can be classified broadly into two types: bone resorption and bone formation.

**Bone Resorption.** There is no single unifying mechanism that accounts for the increased bone resorption occurring in patients with malignant disease. Osteoclast-mediated osteolysis is suggested as an early and quantitatively important mechanism of bone loss accompanying skeletal metastasis. A similar pattern of osteolysis is observed in patients with hematologic malignancies, including plasma cell myeloma and lymphoma, in which leukocytes produce an osteoclast-activating factor. In carcinomas, the humoral substance promoting local bone loss may be a prostaglandin, osteoclast-activating factor, alpha transforming growth factor, parathyroid hormone–like substance, tumor necrosis factor, or other unidentified agents. The malignant cells themselves may secrete lytic enzymes responsible for the continued destruction of bone.

**Bone Formation.** Two main mechanisms account for new bone formation associated with skeletal metastasis: stromal bone formation and reactive bone formation. Stromal new bone formation occurs only in those skeletal metastases that are associated with the development of fibrous stroma, particularly those arising from carcinoma of the prostate. Reactive new bone occurs as a response to bone destruction and is similar to the callus that develops in fracture healing. This process is seen to a variable extent in virtually all malignant neoplasms, but it may be a minor or insignificant feature in highly anaplastic, rapidly growing tumors and in plasma cell myeloma, lymphomas, or leukemias.

## GENERAL CLINICAL MANIFESTATIONS

Although the clinical findings accompanying skeletal metastasis are influenced by the age of the patient, the type of tumor, and the site or sites of bone involvement, certain general characteristics deserve emphasis. Bone pain is a common, although not invariable. Pain may be localized to the site of skeletal involvement or referred to a distant site, particularly when the lesion involves the spine. Bone tenderness, a soft tissue mass, and deformity are other possible manifestations.

Laboratory parameters include elevation of the serum calcium level. This hypercalcemia has a complex pathogenesis and is dependent on such factors as the degree of immobilization or bone resorption and destruction; it may be related to the secretion of a humoral substance such as parathyroid hormone, prostaglandins, or osteolytic sterols secreted by the tumor itself. Elevation of the serum alkaline phosphatase level in patients with skeletal metastasis reflects the magnitude of osteoblastic activity in the absence of liver disease. An increase in hydroxyproline excretion in the urine and a myelophthisic anemia are other laboratory abnormalities that may be evident.

## FREQUENCY AND DISTRIBUTION OF SKELETAL METASTASIS

It is well recognized that metastasis to the skeleton represents the most common type of malignant bone tumor. The estimated frequency of skeletal metastasis determined on the basis of radiographic examination is low, owing to the relatively insensitive nature of this diagnostic technique. Scintigraphy using bone-seeking radiopharmaceutical agents is a more sensitive method of analysis, although it, too, is beset with problems, including the known occurrence of false-negative results in some types of malignant tumors. MR imaging is a sensitive diagnostic method, but a survey of the entire skeleton using this technique is impractical.

Previous reports dealing with skeletal metastases generally confirmed the following observations:

1. The skeleton is a common site of metastasis in many types of primary malignant tumor.

2. In accordance with the relative frequency of various types of primary malignant tumors, carcinomas of the breast, prostate, and lung, in decreasing order, are the most common sources of skeletal metastases in a general population.

3. Based on an equal number of various types of primary malignant tumors, carcinomas of the prostate, breast, kidney, lung, and thyroid gland, in order of decreasing frequency, metastasize to the skeleton.

4. The vast majority of metastatic lesions in the skeleton are encountered in middle-aged and elderly patients.

5. Typical causes of skeletal metastasis in children are neuroblastoma, Ewing's sarcoma, osteosarcoma, and malignant tumors of soft tissues.

6. In adults, carcinomas of the prostate, breast, kidney, and lung account for more than 75% of cases of skeletal metastasis. Carcinoma of the prostate is responsible for approximately 60% of such metastases in men, and carcinoma of the breast accounts for approximately 70% of skeletal metastases in women.

Skeletal metastases have a predilection for the axial skeleton, a region rich in red marrow. The vertebral column (thoracolumbar spine and sacrum), bones of the pelvis, ribs, sternum, femoral and humeral shafts, and skull, in decreasing order, are the usual locations for skeletal metastasis. Spinal involvement in the metastatic process should be emphasized, with the frequency of metastasis being greatest in the lumbar region, followed by the thoracic and cervical segments. Metastatic foci are more common in the vertebral bodies than in the posterior osseous elements, although pediculate destruction is more frequent in cases of skeletal metastasis than in those of plasma cell myeloma.

Infrequent sites of skeletal metastasis are the mandible (a site more typically involved in plasma cell myeloma), patella, and bones of the extremities that are distal to the elbow and knee. One exception to this is bronchogenic carcinoma. Such metastases usually, although not invariably, are accompanied by widespread skeletal lesions and are associated with heat, pain, and soft tissue swelling, simulating the findings of osteomyelitis or arthritis. The terminal phalanges and the metacarpal bones are most commonly affected in the hand (Fig. 72–3). In unusual circumstances, metastasis develops at an osseous site that is already altered by disease (osteomyelitis, osteonecrosis, trauma, Paget's disease) or surgical manipulation (metallic implants).

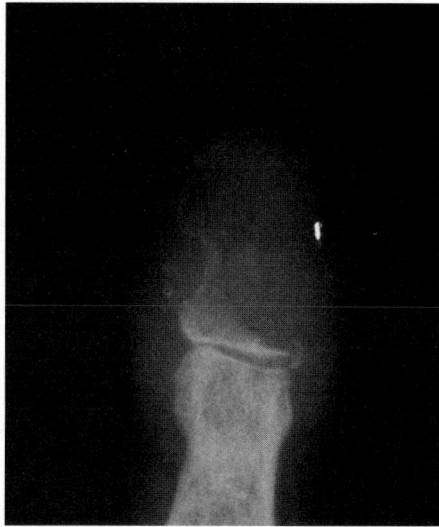

**Figure 72–3.** Skeletal metastasis in the hand: bronchogenic carcinoma. Extensive lysis of the terminal phalanx of the finger is associated with considerable soft tissue swelling. The articular space appears uninvolved.

## RADIOGRAPHIC-PATHOLOGIC CORRELATION

The radiographic characteristics of skeletal metastases are highly variable and are influenced by a number of factors, including the nature of the primary tumor, the age of the patient, the location of the metastatic lesion or lesions, and the timing of the radiographic examination.

### Number of Lesions

Multiplicity is the general rule regarding sites of skeletal metastasis; however, solitary lesions are certainly encountered, especially in patients with carcinoma of the kidney or thyroid. In some instances, only one metastatic lesion is detected on routine radiographs, whereas scintigraphy or MR imaging indicates the presence of many such lesions. In cases of an apparently solitary focus of bone involvement, the radiographic differentiation of an osseous metastasis from a primary bone tumor can be difficult. When multiple lesions are detected on radiographs, they are commonly of variable size, in contrast to the uniform size that is frequently apparent in plasma cell myeloma.

### Patterns of Bone Response

The radiographic appearance of skeletal metastases can be broadly classified as purely osteolytic, purely osteosclerotic, and mixed osteolytic-osteosclerotic, although histologically, a combination of both bone resorption and bone formation is present in the vast majority of lesions. Purely osteolytic lesions typically arise from carcinoma of the thyroid, kidney, adrenal gland, uterus, and gastrointestinal tract, as well as from Wilms' tumor, Ewing's tumor, pheochromocytoma, melanoma, hepatoma, squamous cell carcinoma of the skin, and certain tumors of the head, neck, and vascular and soft tissues; mixed osteolytic-osteosclerotic lesions generally occur in carcinomas of the lung, breast, and cervix and in ovarian and testicular tumors; purely osteosclerotic lesions are encountered in carcinoma of the prostate and, less constantly, in bronchial carcinoid tumor, bladder carcinoma involving the prostate, carcinomas of the nasopharynx and stomach, medulloblastoma, and neuroblastoma (Table 72–1).

None of these patterns is without exception. Osteolytic lesions (Fig. 72–4) may be well circumscribed (geographic bone destruction) or poorly defined (moth-eaten or permeative bone destruction). These patterns reflect varying degrees of aggressiveness of the metastatic deposits. Sclerotic margins about sites of skeletal metastasis are rare unless therapy has been instituted. Osteosclerotic lesions (Fig. 72–5) may be nodular or diffuse in distribution. Typically, nodular osteosclerotic lesions lack the spiculated appearance of a bone island.

## Periosteal Reaction

As a general rule, periosteal new bone is either absent or of limited extent in metastatic lesions, in contrast to the extensive degree of periostitis that commonly accompanies primary malignant tumors of the skeleton. Exuberant periosteal reaction leading to bone spiculation and a sunburst appearance is evident in some cases of skeletal metastasis, however, especially those arising from prostate carcinoma (Fig. 72–6), gastrointestinal malignancies, retinoblastoma, and neuroblastoma.

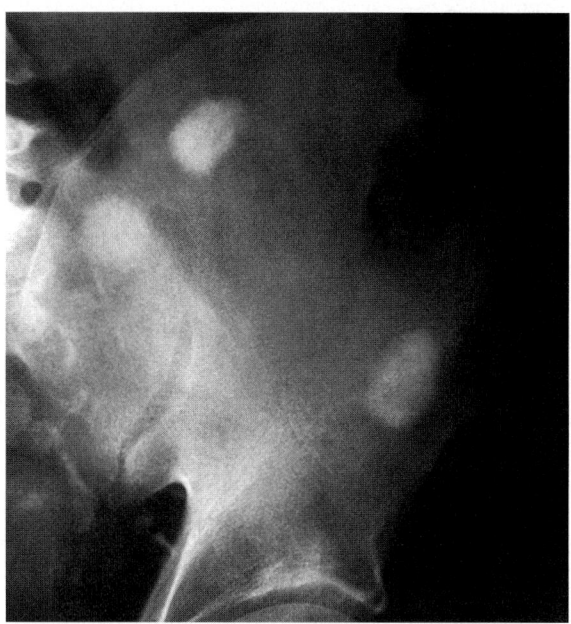

**Figure 72–5.** Skeletal metastasis: purely osteosclerotic pattern. Carcinoma of the prostate resulted in multiple well-defined radiodense lesions of the ilium.

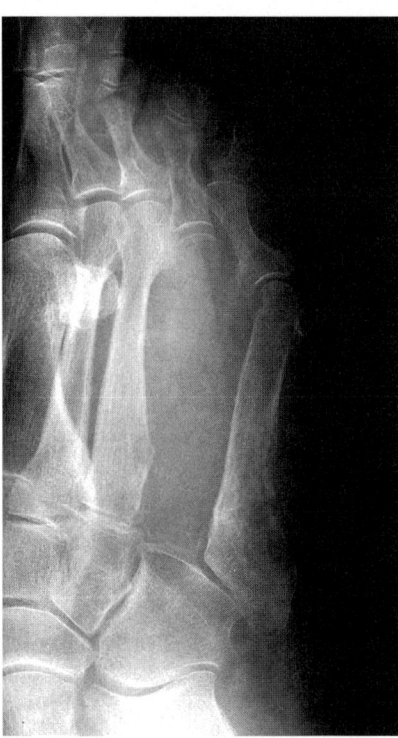

**Figure 72–4.** Skeletal metastasis: purely osteolytic pattern. The entire fourth metatarsal bone reveals lytic destruction, and a similar lesion is present at the base of the fifth metatarsal bone. A poorly differentiated adenocarcinoma of unknown origin was responsible for the defects.

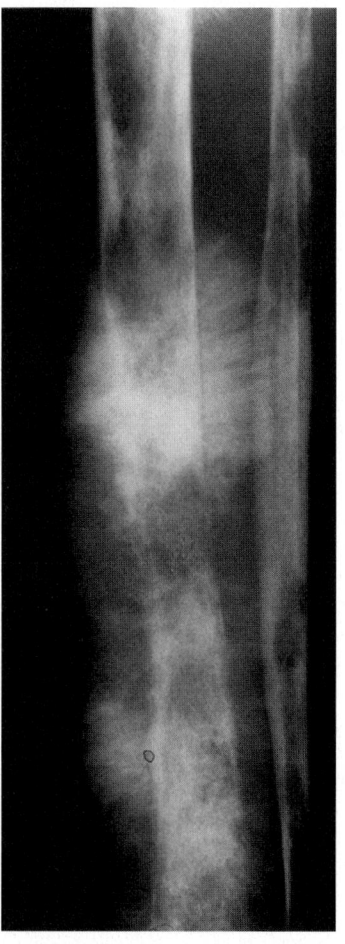

**Figure 72–6.** Skeletal metastasis: periosteal reaction. Metastatic carcinoma of the prostate produced an unusual pattern of exuberant periostitis of the tibia. Osteolytic lesions are seen in the tibia and fibula. (Courtesy of A. Brower, MD, Norfolk, Va.)

## TABLE 72–1

**Sites of Skeletal Metastases**

| Primary Focus | Type of Skeletal Lesion | Relative Frequency of Skeletal Lesion, % Radiograph | Bone Scan | Autopsy |
|---|---|---|---|---|
| **Common primary cancer** | | | | |
| Breast | Lytic; also mixed; frequently blastic | 30–50 | 52–67 | 57–73 |
| Lung | Lytic; also mixed; occasionally blastic | 14–25 | 54–64 | 19–32 |
| Kidney | Invariably lytic | 20–32 | 33–60 | 23–45 |
| Thyroid | Invariably lytic | 8 | 43 | 19–50 |
| Prostate | Usually blastic; occasionally lytic | 33–35 | 62–92 | 57–84 |
| **Head and neck** | | | | |
| Upper respiratory and digestive tract | | | | |
| Nasal fossa and nasopharynx | Lytic; occasionally blastic | 4 | | |
| Oral cavity and oropharynx | Lytic | 14–21 | | |
| Endolarynx and hypopharynx | Lytic | 1–2 | | |
| Maxillary sinuses | Lytic | 12 | | |
| Salivary glands | Lytic | 5 | | 28 |
| Other carcinomas of neck | | | | |
| Parathyroid | Lytic | <1 | | |
| Central nervous system | | | | |
| Brain tumors | Lytic; infrequently blastic | <1 | | |
| Paraganglioma | Lytic | <1 | | |
| Chordoma | Lytic | 15 | | |
| Neuroblastoma | Lytic or mixed; occasionally blastic | 35–75 | | |
| **Chest** | | | | |
| Pleura and pericardium | | | | |
| Mesothelioma | Lytic | <1 | | |
| Mediastinum | | | | |
| Thymoma | Lytic; frequently blastic | <1 | | |
| Teratoma, etc. | Lytic | <1 | | |
| **Gastrointestinal tract** | | | 41 | |
| Esophagus | Lytic or mixed | 3–5 | | 1–2 |
| Stomach | Lytic or mixed; occasionally blastic | 0–2.6 | | 2–17.5 |
| Colon | Lytic or mixed; infrequently blastic | 0.5–1 | 57 | 9–11 |
| Rectum | Lytic or mixed; infrequently blastic | 6–10 | 61 | |
| Pancreas | Lytic or mixed; occasionally blastic | 1.3–3.5 | | |
| Liver | Lytic or mixed | <1 | | |
| Gallbladder and bile ducts | Lytic or mixed | <1 | | |
| **Genitourinary tract** | | | 37 | |
| Urinary bladder | Lytic; infrequently blastic | 5–11 | 43 | 13–26 |
| Adrenal | Lytic | | | 44 |
| **Reproductive system** | | | 29 | |
| Uterine cervix | Lytic or mixed; occasionally blastic | 3–4 | 56 | 8–15 |
| Uterine corpus | Lytic | 6 | | 22 |
| Ovary | Lytic; rarely blastic | 2–7 | | 6 |
| Testis | Lytic; occasionally blastic | 6 | 8 | 10–20 |
| **Skin** | | | | |
| Squamous and basal cell carcinoma | Lytic | <1 | | |
| Malignant melanoma | Lytic | 2–7 | 57 | 44–57 |
| **Primary bone tumors** | | | | |
| Osteosarcoma | Lytic; or mixed, frequently blastic | 4–14 | | |
| Chondrosarcoma | Lytic or mixed; occasionally blastic | 2–18 | | |
| Fibrosarcoma | Lytic | 2–23 | | |
| Malignant fibrous histiocytoma | Lytic | 17 | | |
| Hemangioendothelial sarcoma | Lytic (frequently multifocal) | 1–2 | | |
| Ewing's sarcoma | Lytic (permeative) | 40–50 | | |
| Histiocytic lymphoma | Lytic (permeative) | 49 | | |
| **Primary soft tissue tumors** | | | | |
| Fibrous histiocytoma, angiosarcoma, rhabdomyosarcoma, etc. | Lytic or mixed | 10 | 56 | |
| **Carcinoid tumors** | | | | |
| Bronchial and abdominal carcinoids (other than appendix) | Blastic, frequently mixed, occasionally lytic | 1 | | |

From Wilner D: Radiology of Bone Tumors and Allied Disorders. Philadelphia, WB Saunders, 1982, p 3646.

## Expansile Remodeling

Carcinomas of the kidney or thyroid and hepatomas are among the primary malignant tumors that result in expansile remodeling and an expanded osseous contour. In some of these lesions, such as those arising from renal carcinoma, a distinctive septated appearance accompanies the osseous expansion. Large, expansile osteoblastic lesions are evident in some patients with metastatic prostate carcinoma (Fig. 72–7). On radiographic examination, such lesions may resemble Paget's disease or, when solitary, osteosarcoma.

## Soft Tissue Mass

As a general rule, prominent soft tissue masses are observed infrequently in association with skeletal metastasis, and the detection of such a mass favors the diagnosis of a primary malignant lesion of bone rather than a secondary deposit. Exceptions to this rule are encountered in certain locations. In the ribs, extrapleural extension of metastatic lesions leads to soft tissue masses of variable size, resembling those seen in plasma cell myeloma. Carcinoma of the colon may metastasize to the bones of the pelvis, producing soft tissue masses that occasionally contain calcification.

## Soft Tissue Ossification

Ossification in sites of soft tissue metastases occurring with or without adjacent bone involvement has been identified, particularly with carcinoma of the colon, gastric carcinoma, other gastrointestinal malignancies, transitional cell carcinoma of the bladder, carcinoma of the breast, and bronchogenic carcinoma. Ossification in the soft tissues adjacent to an area of bone destruction simulates the appearance of an osteosarcoma of osseous origin, whereas isolated soft tissue ossific collections in metastases resemble findings in post-traumatic heterotopic ossification, pseudomalignant osseous tumor of soft tissue, osteosarcoma of soft tissue origin, and ossification following burns and neurologic injuries.

## Pathologic Fracture

Metastatic lesions in the skeleton lead to osseous weakening and, frequently, to pathologic fracture (Fig. 72–8). This complication is well recognized in the spine, where compression or collapse of a tumor-containing vertebral body is seen. Pathologic fractures accompanying metastases in tubular bones are evident most commonly in the proximal portion of the femur, although other portions of this bone and other bones may be involved as well. The likelihood of pathologic fracture in a tubular bone becomes more pronounced with increasing degrees of cortical destruction. The majority of pathologic fractures in long tubular bones occur when more than 50% of the cortical surface has been destroyed.

## SPECIFIC SITES OF OSSEOUS INVOLVEMENT
### Skull

Single or multiple osteolytic lesions of variable size are evident in the skull. Perforation of the external surface of the bone may be associated with a soft tissue mass that requires tangential radiographic projections for detec-

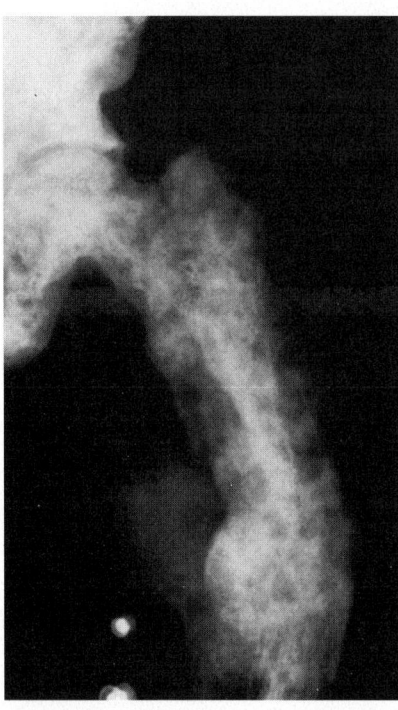

**Figure 72–7.** Skeletal metastasis: bone expansion. Exuberant new and abnormal bone cloaks the original femoral diaphysis in this patient with widespread osseous metastases from carcinoma of the prostate. A previous pathologic fracture of the femoral shaft is apparent. The radiographic findings resemble those of Paget's disease.

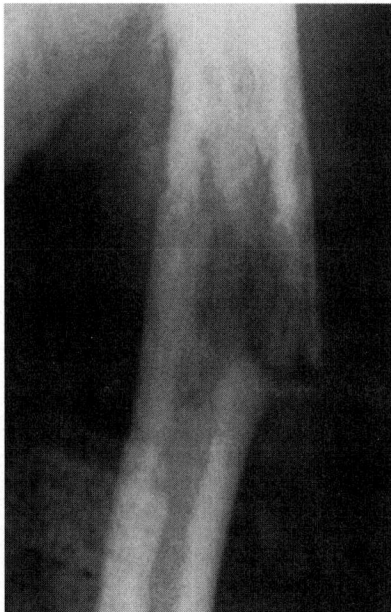

**Figure 72–8.** Skeletal metastasis: pathologic fracture. In this patient with carcinoma of the lung, an oblique fracture has occurred through a "moth-eaten" region of bone destruction in the diaphysis of the humerus.

tion. Rarely, a radiodense focus, the button sequestrum, exists in the center of the lesion, although this finding is more typical of eosinophilic granuloma and is also observed in radiation necrosis, tuberculosis and other infections, fibrous dysplasia, multiple myeloma, Paget's disease, and dermoid and epidermoid tumors.

Other conditions that enter into the differential diagnosis of a solitary osteolytic metastatic lesion of the skull include an epidermoid or dermoid tumor (which appears as a small, well-defined, round or oval radiolucent diploic focus with a sclerotic margin), hemangioma (which possesses a spiculated or reticular pattern), eosinophilic granuloma (which is an oval or lobulated lesion of the diploic portion of the cranium, with differential involvement of the inner and outer tables that produces a beveled margin), fibrous dysplasia (which commonly has a ground-glass or sclerotic appearance, affecting the outer table to a greater degree than the inner table), doughnut lesion (of unknown cause, which produces one or more radiolucent areas, each surrounded by a sclerotic margin of variable thickness; Fig. 72–9), various infections, lymphomas, and sarcoidosis. Other disorders that produce multiple osteolytic areas in the skull are multiple myeloma (in which uniform size and mandibular involvement are characteristic), hyperparathyroidism (which produces the "salt and pepper" appearance), histiocytosis, radiation necrosis, prominent venous lakes, and arachnoid granulations.

Osteosclerotic metastatic lesions of the skull usually arise from carcinoma of the prostate. Osteosclerosis of the base of the skull is a well-recognized manifestation of nasopharyngeal carcinoma and may be accentuated following radiotherapy of this tumor. Additional causes of basal osteosclerosis include meningioma, other tumors, fibrous dysplasia, and adjacent inflammatory processes.

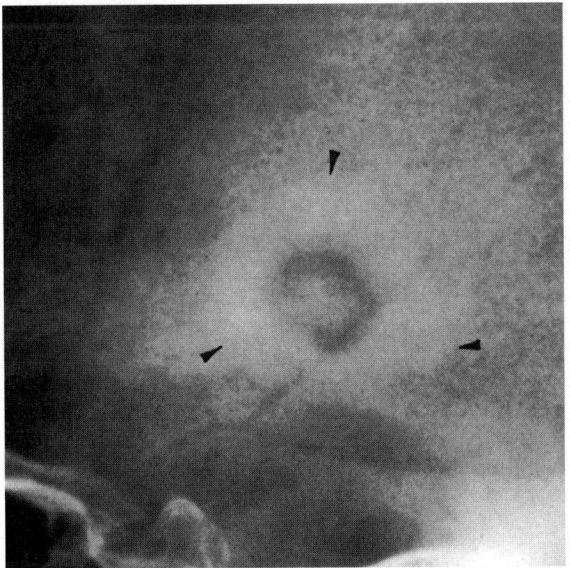

**Figure 72–9.** Doughnut lesion: skull. A radiolucent lesion containing bone is surrounded by a rim of bony sclerosis (*arrowheads*). The radiographic findings are distinctive.

## Spine

The spine represents the most frequent site of skeletal metastasis. Involvement of the thoracic and lumbar levels predominates. Metastases more commonly occur in the vertebral bodies than in the posterior osseous elements. Of the malignant tumors that secondarily involve the spine, carcinomas of the lung, breast, and prostate (as well as lymphomas and plasma cell myeloma) are encountered most often. The radiographic findings of spinal involvement in cases of metastatic disease are variable, although some characteristic patterns emerge.

**Destruction and Collapse of Vertebral Body.** Osteolysis of a vertebral body is difficult to detect with routine radiography until a large portion of the bone is destroyed. Preservation of disc height is remarkable in many cases of skeletal metastasis, serving as a useful diagnostic aid in differentiating tumor from infection, although exceptions to this rule are encountered.

Collapse of a vertebral body (or bodies) is an abnormality that occurs in skeletal metastasis and may be its presenting manifestation. It is also evident in various other disorders, particularly osteoporosis, osteomalacia, and plasma cell myeloma. Carcinomas of the breast, lung, and prostate, in order of decreasing frequency, are the most common causes of such collapse. Findings suggestive of a collapsed vertebral body resulting from metastatic disease (or other malignant tumors) include involvement of the upper thoracic spine (a level of collapse infrequently observed in osteoporosis or osteomalacia), the presence of a soft tissue mass or pediculate destruction, and angular or irregular deformity of the vertebral endplates. Because there is often no specific routine radiographic pattern indicating tumorous vertebral collapse, CT and MR imaging are used as additional diagnostic methods. A biopsy, however, is ultimately required in many patients for an accurate diagnosis.

**Sclerosis of Vertebral Body.** The detection of inhomogeneous or homogeneous sclerotic areas in one or more vertebral bodies in an elderly man is most compatible with a diagnosis of metastatic disease arising from carcinoma of the prostate, although other metastatic tumors, as well as lymphomas and, rarely, chordoma or plasma cell myeloma, must be considered. An entirely radiodense vertebral body (the ivory vertebral body) should be differentiated from the corduroy vertebral body (characterized by accentuated vertical striations) of hemangioma, the rugger-jersey vertebral body (characterized by radiodense stripes at the top and bottom) of renal osteodystrophy (Fig. 72–10), the picture-frame vertebral body (associated with condensation of bone along the margins) of Paget's disease, and the sandwich vertebral body (accompanied by an extreme and uniform increase in radiodensity in the superior and inferior margins) of osteopetrosis.

**Pedicle Involvement.** Destruction of one or both pedicles of a vertebra is a well-known radiographic finding of skeletal metastasis (Fig. 72–11) that is rarely evident in plasma cell myeloma. It is best observed on anteroposterior radiographs as an absence of one or both "eyes"

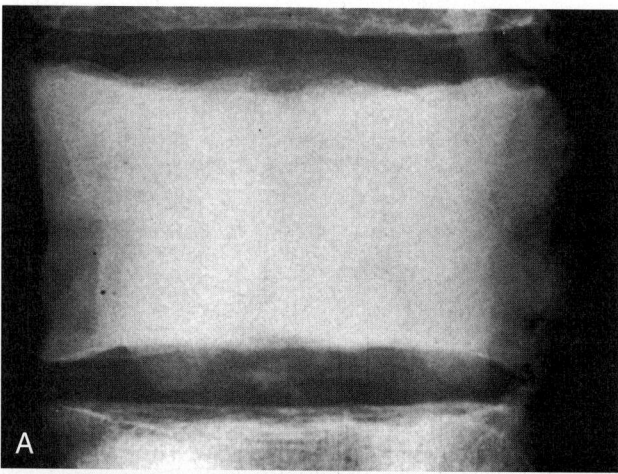

**Figure 72–10.** Skeletal metastasis and mimicking conditions in the spine. *A*, Ivory vertebral body—carcinoma of the prostate. Observe the uniformly increased radiodensity of the entire vertebral body in this radiograph of a spinal specimen. *B*, Corduroy vertebral body—hemangioma. Note the spongy appearance and accentuation of the vertical trabeculae. *C*, Rugger-jersey spine—renal osteodystrophy. The rugger-jersey appearance is accompanied by condensation of bone in the form of stripes at the top and bottom of each vertebral body.

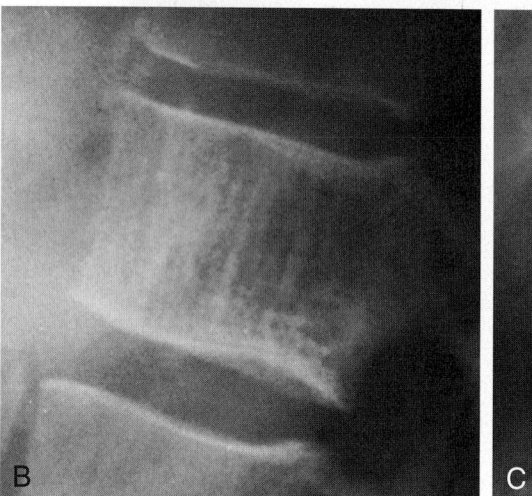

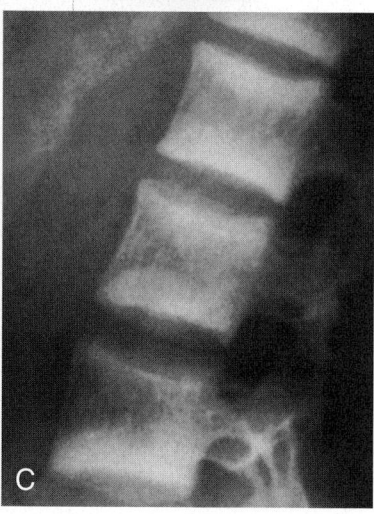

of the vertebral body. The diagnostic importance of pediculate destruction as a sign of skeletal metastasis has led to a misconception that pediculate localization is more frequent than localization in the vertebral body in cases of metastatic disease. Such is not the case, and involvement of the pedicle usually occurs as a result of further extension of a tumorous deposit within the posterior portion of the vertebral body.

### Pelvis

The bones of the pelvis are frequently involved in skeletal metastasis. Typical routes of tumor spread to this region are hematogenous dissemination and direct extension from the primary neoplastic site or from tumorous lymph nodes. Osteolytic, osteosclerotic, or mixed osteolytic-osteosclerotic lesions are seen. Diffuse osteosclerotic metastases, especially from carcinoma of the prostate, should be differentiated from other disorders leading to sclerosis in the pelvic bones (and spine), such as Paget's disease, sickle cell anemia, lymphomas, myelofibrosis, mastocytosis, tuberous sclerosis, fluorosis, and a number of congenital diseases.

### Long Tubular Bones

Of the long tubular bones, the femur and humerus are involved most commonly in cases of skeletal metastasis. Metaphyseal localization predominates, although diaphyseal (Fig. 72–12) or epiphyseal lesions are not infrequent. Typically, spongy bone in the medullary cavity is affected

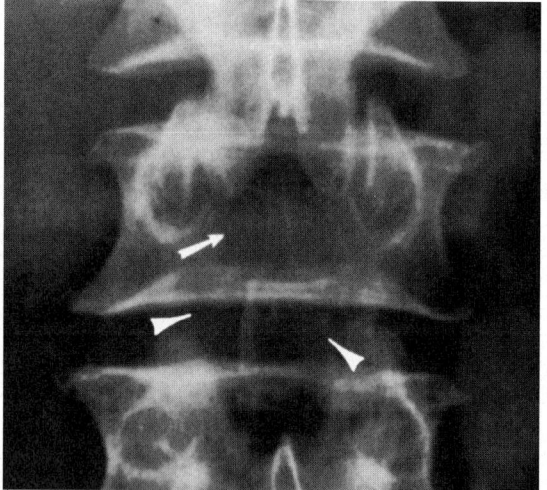

**Figure 72–11.** Skeletal metastasis: pedicle of the spine. Osseous destruction of a portion of the pedicles, the entire lamina, the inferior articulating process *(arrowheads)* and the spinous process is seen. The appearance is that of an empty vertebral body *(arrow)*.

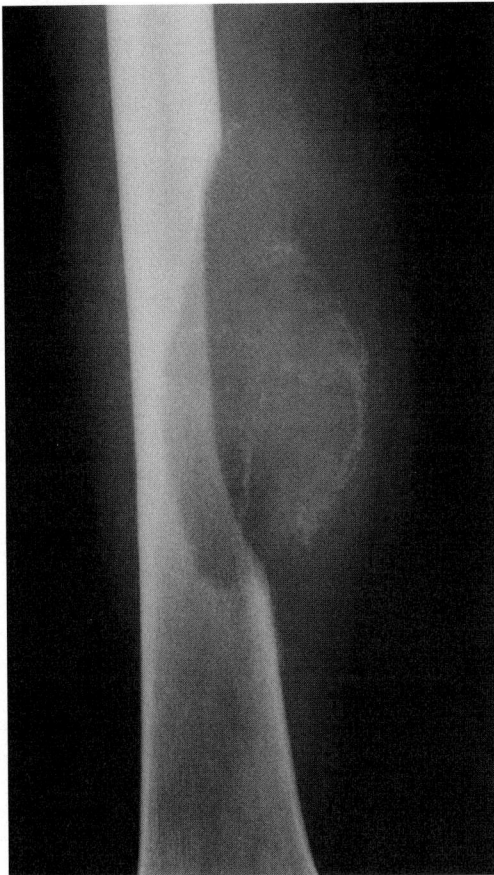

**Figure 72–12.** Skeletal metastasis: long tubular bones. Radiograph shows an osteolytic lesion arising in the shaft of the femur, with extensive cortical disruption. Ossification or calcification is present in the adjacent soft tissue mass. The findings resemble those of a primary malignant tumor of bone.

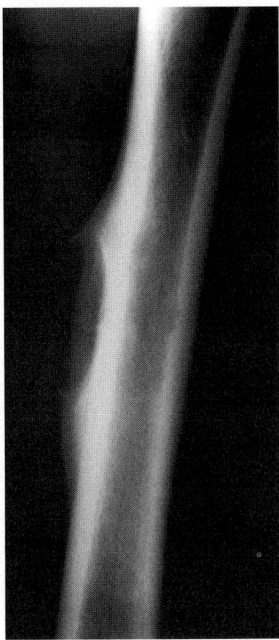

**Figure 72–13.** Skeletal metastasis: long tubular bones. A well-circumscribed erosion of the external surface of the diaphysis of the femur—the cookie-bite sign—is associated with periosteal reaction in this patient with bronchogenic carcinoma. (Courtesy of W. Murphy, MD, St. Louis, Mo.)

first, with secondary involvement of the cortex in instances of hematogenous spread of tumor, although, as indicated previously, cortical destruction is more readily apparent on radiographs. Unusual but characteristic osseous patterns of destruction include small cortical radiolucent foci near the entrance of the nutrient arteries and eccentrically located, scalloped erosions of the external surface of the cortex (cookie-bite sign; Fig. 72–13), particularly in (but not limited to) cases of bronchogenic carcinoma.

A solitary metastatic focus in a long tubular bone may possess radiographic characteristics that simulate those of a primary locally aggressive or malignant osseous tumor. The absence of both extensive periostitis and a prominent soft tissue mass in most metastatic lesions is helpful diagnostically.

### Short Tubular and Irregular Bones

Metastatic lesions in the bones of the hands, wrists, and feet are infrequent, but they have received a great deal of attention. Bronchogenic, renal, and colon carcinomas are the leading causes of such metastases (see Fig. 72–3).

### Sternum and Sacrum

These two bones are relatively common sites of metastasis. In both locations, routine radiographs are often suboptimal, and CT or MR imaging is required for adequate tumor detection (Fig. 72–14). Although primary tumors of the sternum are uncommon, most are malignant, so the differential diagnosis of an aggressive lesion in this bone encompasses lymphomas, chondrosarcoma, and plasma cell myeloma, in addition to skeletal metastasis.

### Chest Wall

Hematogenously derived rib metastases typically produce osteolytic or osteosclerotic lesions without an accompanying soft tissue mass, although the latter finding is occasionally evident, simulating the appearance of plasma cell myeloma. Pathologic fractures are commonly seen with such rib lesions. With regard to contiguous spread of tumor, invasion of the chest wall occurs in approximately 10% of patients with adjacent pulmonary malignancies.

### SPECIFIC TYPES OF TUMOR

### Carcinoma of the Breast

A common cause of hematogenous skeletal metastasis, this tumor usually produces osteolytic or mixed osteolytic-osteosclerotic lesions or, rarely, osteoblastic lesions predominating in the axial skeleton and ribs. Pathologic fractures are frequent. Metastatic breast carcinoma may remain confined to the skeleton, without involvement of other organ systems, for prolonged periods.

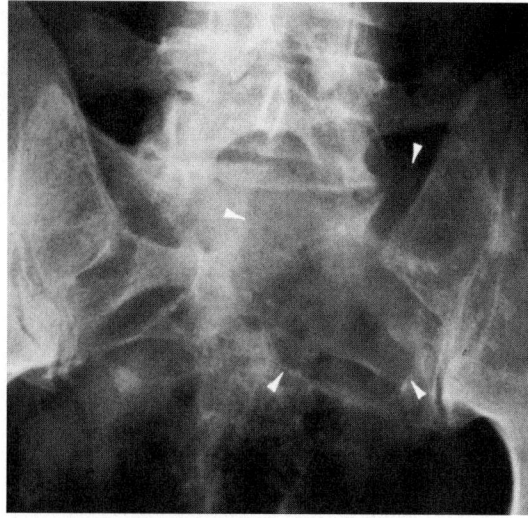

**Figure 72–14.** Skeletal metastasis: carcinoma of the prostate. A large lesion of the sacrum *(arrowheads)* might be missed if comparison with the opposite side were not accomplished.

## Carcinoma of the Lung

Carcinoma of the lung, a common tumor, involves the skeleton as a result of lymphatic spread to regional (mediastinal) lymph nodes, with direct extension to bone; lymphatic spread through the diaphragm to regional (para-aortic) lymph nodes, with direct osseous extension; and invasion of the pulmonary veins, with dissemination via the arterial circulation. In squamous cell and anaplastic large cell carcinomas, osteolytic or mixed osteolytic-osteosclerotic lesions predominate; in small cell carcinoma and adenocarcinoma, osteoblastic lesions may be visible. The latter finding is apparent in less than 15% of patients.

Characteristic patterns of skeletal involvement include rib erosion related to a peripheral tumor of the lung, destruction of vertebrae in association with tumor-containing mediastinal lymph nodes (see Fig. 72–2), destruction of ribs and cervical vertebrae in response to Pancoast's tumor (see Fig. 72–1), and eccentric cookie-bite excavation of the external surface of the cortex (see Fig. 72–13).

## Carcinoma of the Prostate

Carcinoma of the prostate is a common cause of osseous metastasis; potential routes of spread to the skeleton include Batson's venous plexus and extension from tumorous nodes in the pelvic and para-aortic regions. Osteoblastic metastases are characteristic (see Fig. 72–10), though not invariable (see Fig. 72–14), and predominate in the axial skeleton.

## Carcinoma of the Kidney

Renal cell carcinoma spreads principally in three ways: by direct extension; by involvement of lymphatic channels that ultimately drain into the para-aortic, hilar, paratracheal, and mediastinal regions; and by invasion of the renal veins with subsequent extension to the inferior vena

cava, right atrium, and pulmonary vessels. Metastasis to the skeleton is common; infrequently, this occurs in the absence of metastases in other organ systems. Typical sites of involvement are the thoracolumbar spine, pelvic bones, ribs, and femora. Solitary osseous lesions are relatively frequent. Osteolysis is the predominant radiographic finding (Fig. 72–15). Solitary or multiple, small or large areas of bone destruction are seen, and in some cases, massive and expansile lesions are identified.

## Wilms' Tumor

Skeletal metastasis in Wilms' tumor is regarded as uncommon, with a reported frequency of less than 5% in most series. Bone metastases are usually osteolytic and have a widespread distribution in both the axial and appendicular skeletons (Fig. 72–16). A honeycomb pattern of destruction is sometimes seen.

## Carcinoma of the Thyroid

Hematogenous dissemination of thyroid carcinoma to the skeleton results in solitary or multiple osteolytic lesions predominating in the axial skeleton. An expansile nature, small calcific collections, a pathologic fracture, and a tendency to extend across articulations are features of thyroid metastases. Medullary carcinoma of the thyroid accounts for less than 10% of malignancies of the thyroid gland; metastases, though infrequent, are variable in appearance and may be entirely osteosclerotic.

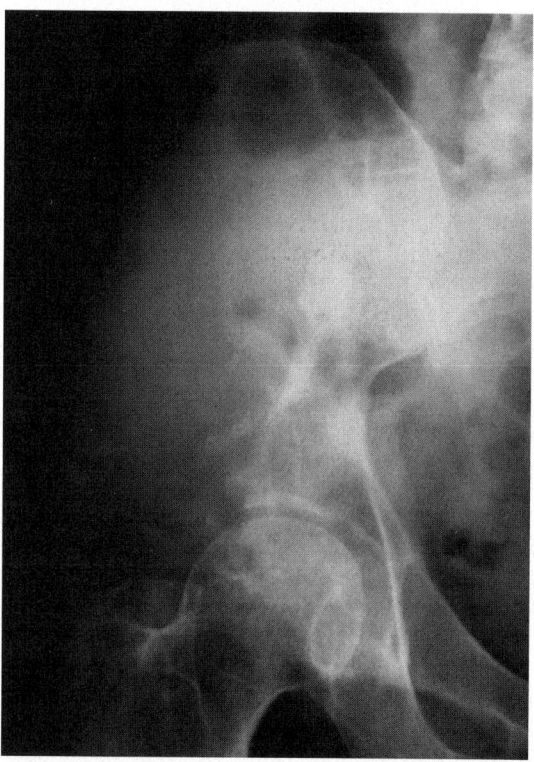

**Figure 72–15.** Skeletal metastasis: carcinoma of the kidney. Radiograph reveals an expansile, osteolytic lesion of the right ilium extending to the subchondral acetabular bone.

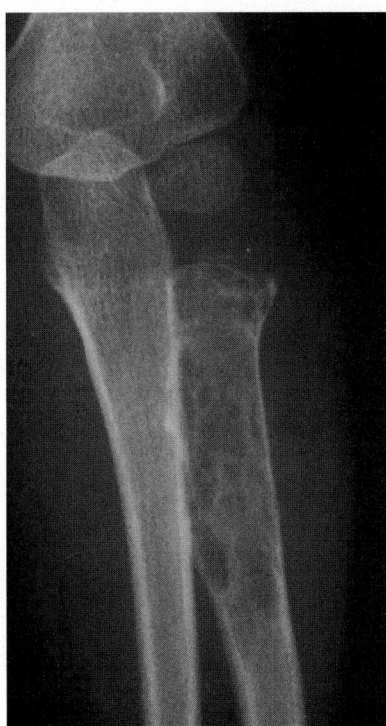

**Figure 72–16.** Skeletal metastasis: Wilms' tumor. Osteolytic lesions are observed in the radius, tibia, and fibula. In the latter two sites, pathologic fractures are evident. In the radius, a honeycomb pattern is apparent.

### Carcinoma of the Bladder

Osseous lesions in carcinoma of the bladder arise from either direct extension from the primary neoplasm and tumorous lymph nodes or hematogenous dissemination. They are relatively infrequent and typically affect the thoracolumbar spine and bones of the pelvis.

### Malignant Melanoma

Skeletal metastasis from melanoma, arising as a result of hematogenous dissemination, is uncommon but not rare. Osteolytic lesions, with or without adjacent soft tissue masses, are observed, principally in the spine, ribs, and bones of the pelvis.

### Carcinoma of the Uterine Cervix

Carcinoma of the uterine cervix may extend to regional lymph nodes and from there to paravertebral and mediastinal lymph nodes; it may also disseminate via the portal and caval venous systems. Osseous involvement results from direct extension into the bones of the pelvis, from tumorous lymph nodes that erode the vertebrae (especially in the lumbar spine) and pelvic bones, or from venous and arterial tumor emboli to any portion of the skeleton. Purely osteolytic lesions are more typical than either mixed osteolytic-osteosclerotic or purely osteosclerotic foci.

## Tumors of the Gastrointestinal System

Metastatic lesions arising from carcinoma of the esophagus are rare and of the osteolytic type. A similar pattern of bone destruction is evident in cases of gastric carcinoma, although diffuse osseous sclerosis may be an initial feature of this tumor. Skeletal metastases from carcinoma of the colon or rectum are generally osteolytic or mixed osteolytic-osteosclerotic; adjacent soft tissue masses containing calcification are occasionally evident.

Pancreatic carcinoma involves the skeleton as a result of posterior extension of the primary tumor into the lower thoracic and upper lumbar vertebral bodies or through hematogenous dissemination to the spine, pelvis, and ribs. Osteolytic lesions predominate.

### Intracranial Tumors

Osseous metastasis is a known manifestation of several types of brain tumor. The typical pathway of spread is along the leptomeninges and, occasionally, via the cerebrospinal fluid into the spinal canal. In some instances, ventricular shunts provide a pathway for extraneural dissemination of tumor; in other circumstances, usually but not invariably following a craniotomy, dural disruption allows more widespread intravascular and perineural lymphatic dissemination.

Medulloblastoma appears to be the intracranial tumor that is most likely to spread outside the central nervous system, and systemic metastases from this tumor are more frequent in children and adolescents than in adults. Skeletal involvement is characterized by osteosclerotic, osteolytic, or mixed osteolytic-osteosclerotic lesions (Fig. 72–17). Widespread involvement may be apparent.

### Neuroblastoma

Characteristics of skeletal metastasis include symmetrical involvement, osteolysis with permeative bone destruc-

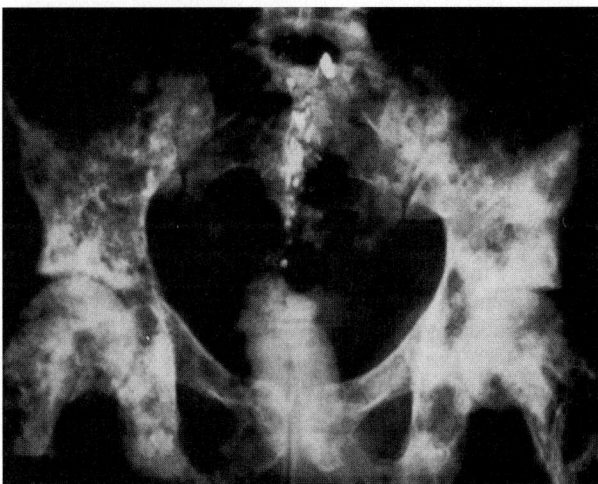

**Figure 72–17.** Skeletal metastasis: medulloblastoma. Following the removal of a medulloblastoma in this 20-year-old man, extensive osteoblastic metastases developed in the spine and, as shown here, throughout the pelvic bones and proximal portions of the femora.

tion, sutural widening, and collapse of vertebral bodies with adjacent soft tissue masses. Spinal cord compression is frequent.

### Retinoblastoma

Retinoblastoma is a common primary tumor of childhood. Patterns of tumor spread include direct extension beyond the orbit, with destruction of the facial bones and sinuses; subdural and subarachnoid invasion, with extension to the spinal canal; and hematogenous dissemination throughout the body, with involvement of the skeleton. Osteolysis with a permeative pattern of bone destruction and periostitis are seen at one or more sites, commonly in a symmetrical distribution. These radiographic features resemble those of neuroblastoma and medulloblastoma.

## ARTICULAR INVOLVEMENT

### Synovial Joints

**Skeletal Metastasis to Periarticular Bone.** Metastases to periarticular foci about synovial joints are not infrequent and are typically encountered in the hip, shoulder, and knee. Radiographs reveal a lytic or sclerotic epiphyseal focus that may extend down to the subchondral bone (Fig. 72–18). Its appearance may be reminiscent of that of a subchondral "cyst."

**Skeletal Metastasis to Periarticular Bone with Intra-articular Extension.** A metastatic focus in subchondral bone may extend into the nearby articulation. Extension of tumor is promoted at sites of tight articulations (e.g., sacroiliac joint) and cartilaginous joints (e.g., discovertebral junction), but such extension is also encountered in the large

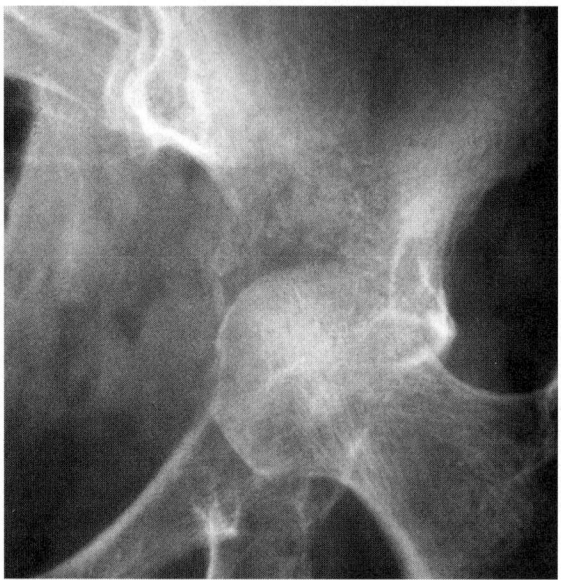

**Figure 72–18.** Skeletal metastasis to periarticular bone: hip. This 65-year-old woman developed a destructive lesion of the left hemipelvis, which was related to metastasis (or direct invasion) from a clear cell carcinoma of the uterus. The loss of acetabular support has allowed inward protrusion of the femoral head. (Courtesy of R. Taketa, MD, Long Beach, Calif.)

synovial articulations of the extremities, especially the knee and hip.

**Metastasis to Synovial Membrane.** Hematogenous spread of tumor to the synovial membrane, with or without adjacent osseous involvement, is occasionally encountered. In these instances, monoarthritis may be unaccompanied by any osseous disruption, with the radiographs revealing a joint effusion or mass. Of tumors metastasizing to the synovium, those of the breast and lung do so most frequently.

### Cartilaginous Joints

**Intervertebral Disc Degeneration (Intervertebral [Osteo]Chondrosis).** Intervertebral chondrosis and (osteo)chondrosis are terms applied to the various stages of disc degeneration that frequently occur in older persons. The presence of intervertebral (osteo)chondrosis adjacent to sites of vertebral body metastasis may represent the coincidental occurrence of two different conditions. Intervertebral (osteo)chondrosis should be particularly prominent when metastatic deposits within the vertebral body are intimate with the subchondral bone plate.

**Cartilaginous Node Formation.** Cartilaginous (Schmorl's) nodes represent protrusions of disc material into the adjacent vertebral body, which occur when defects exist in the cartilaginous endplate. Tumor metastasis to the vertebral body can lead to cartilaginous node formation (Fig. 72–19). If extensive, disc displacement can produce radiographically and pathologically evident disc space loss.

**Disc Invasion by Tumor.** Neoplasms can occur within the intervertebral disc by tumor implantation related to direct hematogenous spread and by invasion of the intervertebral disc from a contiguous source of tumor within the vertebral body. Extensive involvement of the intervertebral disc by tumor may be observed; however, rarely is there evidence of metastatic foci in the disc without contiguous neoplasm in the vertebral body. Instances of bony metastasis adjacent to the subchondral bone plate, with little or no alteration of the bony or cartilaginous endplate, may be identified. Although abnormalities of the intervertebral disc are usually related to metastases arising from carcinoma of the prostate, similar abnormalities may be associated with vertebral metastasis of tumors from other primary sites.

### Differential Diagnosis

The abnormalities occurring at synovial and cartilaginous articulations in patients with skeletal metastasis must be differentiated from other joint manifestations that are indirectly associated with neoplastic disease.

**Secondary Hypertrophic Osteoarthropathy.** Periosteal proliferation is associated with many neoplastic processes, principally those of the lungs and pleurae. The findings are commonly bilateral and symmetrical, affecting predominantly the tibia, fibula, radius, ulna, metacarpals, metatarsals, phalanges, femur, and humerus.

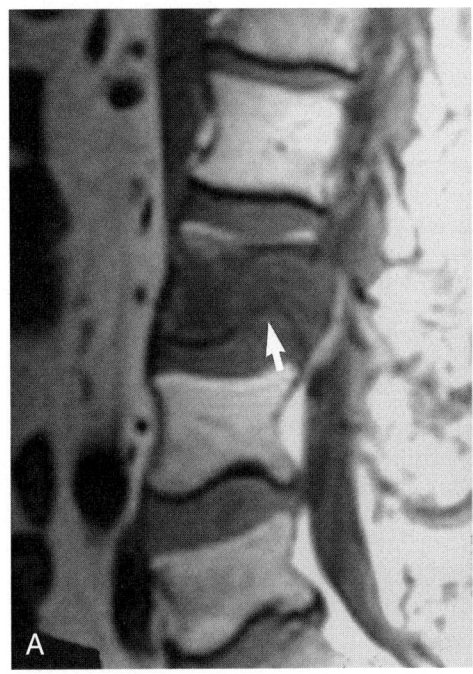 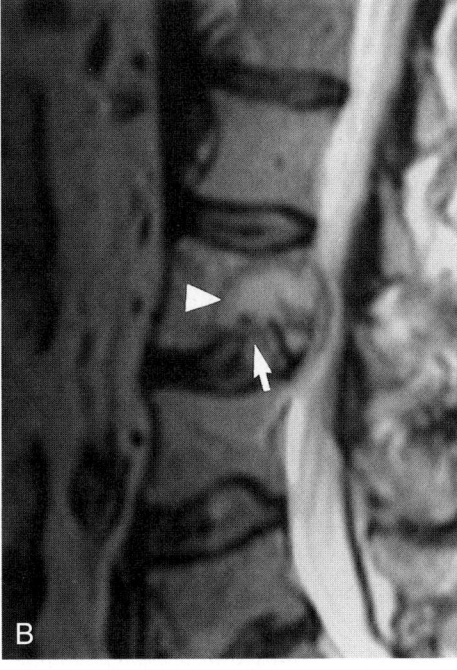

**Figure 72–19.** Vertebral metastasis with cartilaginous node formation. *A,* Sagittal T1-weighted (TR/TE, 500/10) spin echo MR image shows a metastatic deposit related to renal carcinoma within the third lumbar vertebral body. Note deformity of the inferior endplate related to a cartilaginous (Schmorl's) node *(arrow)*. *B,* Sagittal fast spin echo (TR/TE, 3000/102) MR image shows both the tumor *(arrowhead)* and the cartilaginous node *(arrow)*. (Courtesy of D. Goodwin, MD, Hanover, N.H.)

**Secondary Gout.** Secondary hyperuricemia and gout may be encountered in patients with disseminated carcinoma and sarcoma. In these cases, radiographic abnormalities may be mild or absent.

**Carcinomatous Polyarthritis.** A polyarthritis resembling rheumatoid arthritis can be an initial manifestation of malignancy. Articular findings may precede the occurrence of malignant neoplasm by a period of months to years. The cause and pathogenesis of carcinomatous polyarthritis and its relationship to rheumatoid arthritis and tumor are not clear. The radiographic findings, which may consist of soft tissue swelling and osteoporosis, are not related to hypertrophic osteoarthropathy, gout, or joint and bone metastasis.

**Pyogenic Arthritis.** Pyogenic arthritis, due to intestinal flora, has been reported as a complication of advanced neoplastic disease. In fact, the presence of bacteremia due to *Streptococcus bovis* or other enteric organisms causing endocarditis or arthritis may be the first sign of an occult colonic neoplasm. In this situation, neoplastic mucosal ulceration may provide the portal of entry for the organisms.

**Irradiation.** Irradiation of sites of skeletal metastasis can lead to local osseous complications, including osteoporosis, insufficiency fractures, osteonecrosis, and radiation-induced sarcoma. Knowledge of these complications is important, so that the appearance of bony destruction following such treatment is not misinterpreted as evidence of progressive metastasis. This is especially pertinent in neoplasms about the pelvis; acetabular fracture, fragmentation, and protrusion can represent an osseous response to irradiation (Fig. 72–20).

## MUSCLE INVOLVEMENT

Hematogenous metastatic foci in the skeletal muscles are rare. Primary tumors leading to skeletal muscle metastasis arise most frequently in the lung, colon, stomach, and

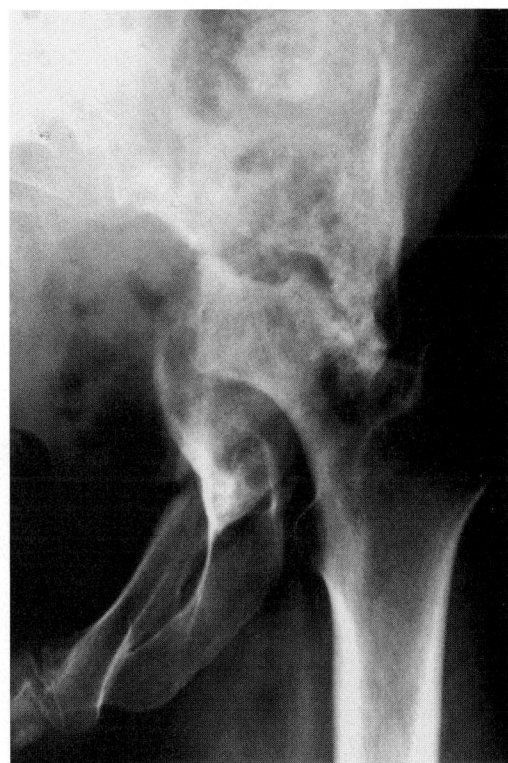

**Figure 72–20.** Irradiation effect. Radiograph obtained 2 years after radiotherapy shows considerable destruction of the acetabulum and femoral head with acetabular protrusion, consistent with irradiation effect.

pancreas. Although other foci of metastasis are usually apparent, skeletal muscle involvement may be the initial manifestation of a distant tumor. Large muscles are involved more commonly than small muscles, and those in either the axial (e.g., erector spinae, psoas, gluteal, abdominal muscles) or the appendicular (e.g., thigh, shoulder, calf muscles) skeleton may be affected. Pain, tenderness, contracture, and a nodular mass may be evident; however, such involvement may be asymptomatic.

Routine radiography generally does not contribute to the diagnosis of such metastasis, unless it is ossified. Scintigraphy, CT, ultrasonography, and MR imaging are more effective diagnostic tools (Fig. 72–21). With contrast-enhanced CT scanning, a mass of variable size with an enhancing rim and central hypoattenuation is most typical. With MR imaging, lobulation, tumor necrosis, and peritumoral edema often are prominent.

## RADIOGRAPHIC MONITORING OF TUMOR RESPONSE TO TREATMENT

The initial manifestation of the healing response of a purely osteolytic lesion to chemotherapy or radiation therapy is the development of a faint sclerotic rim in its periphery. Continued healing is manifested as progressive bone sclerosis proceeding from the outside of the lesion toward its center, the conversion of the osteolytic focus to one that is uniformly or predominantly osteosclerotic (Fig. 72–22), and the eventual shrinkage and disappearance of the osteosclerotic area. In some instances, a successful response to therapy is manifested as sclerotic zones in regions of the bone that initially were radiographically normal. Signs of disease progression are an increase in the size of the osteolytic area, the development of new zones of osteolysis, or progressive osteolytic destruction in an osseous lesion that was responding to therapy in a normal fashion.

With regard to a mixed osteolytic-osteosclerotic lesion, a successful response to chemotherapy or radiation therapy is its gradual conversion to a uniformly sclerotic area. Subsequent stages of the healing process are identical to those of purely osteolytic lesions. Radiographic signs of tumor progression include increasing osteolysis in

sclerotic portions of the lesion and an increase in the overall size of the metastatic focus.

In general, a decrease in size or complete disappearance of an osteoblastic focus is a favorable prognostic sign (Fig. 72–23), whereas increasing size of the osteosclerotic lesion and the development of osseous destruction within an osteosclerotic area are signs of tumor progression. An increase in the number of osteoblastic foci usually indicates progression of the disease; however, it may also signal a healing response of a preexisting lesion that was not identified on the radiographs.

Radiation therapy itself is associated with a number of osseous alterations. Such changes, which include osteopenia, coarsening of the trabecular pattern, insufficiency fractures, ischemic necrosis of bone, and secondary neoplasia, complicate the accurate radiographic appraisal of the metastatic process.

## OTHER DIAGNOSTIC AND THERAPEUTIC TECHNIQUES

### Conventional Radiographic Survey

This survey was originally designed to detect, with a limited number of projections, the majority of metastatic foci in the skeleton, given the propensity of such lesions to be located in the axial skeleton. There is a general consensus that if the radiographic survey examination is used, it should be performed in conjunction with bone scintigraphy; in fact, the latter examination is more appropriately obtained first, so that its results can guide the specific radiographic projections obtained.

### Scintigraphy

Bone scans are highly sensitive in detecting skeletal metastases. The classic (but not invariable) finding of skeletal metastasis is a focus (or foci) of increased accumulation of the radionuclide, called a hot spot (Fig. 72–24). Other abnormalities of a positive bone scan include an area of diminished uptake of the radiotracer (cold spot), a phenomenon related primarily to the absence of blood perfusion to a localized region of bone,

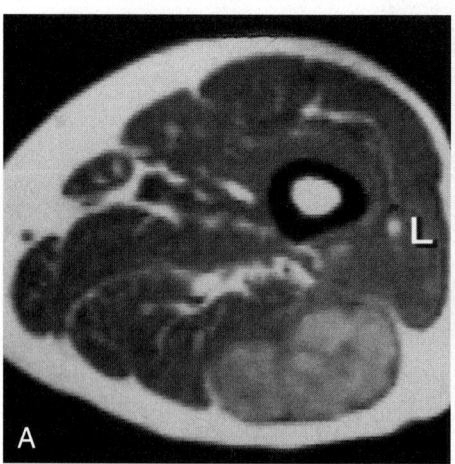
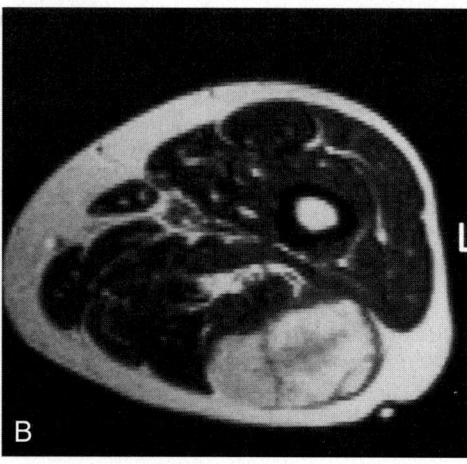

**Figure 72–21.** Muscle metastasis: renal cell carcinoma. Transverse T1-weighted (TR/TE, 500/15) *(A)* and T2-weighted (TR/TE, 2000/60) *(B)* spin echo MR images reveal a metastatic focus infiltrating the biceps femoris muscle. The signal intensity of the tumor is slightly higher than muscle in *(A)* and increases in *(B)*. (Courtesy of J. Robbins, MD, San Diego, Calif.)

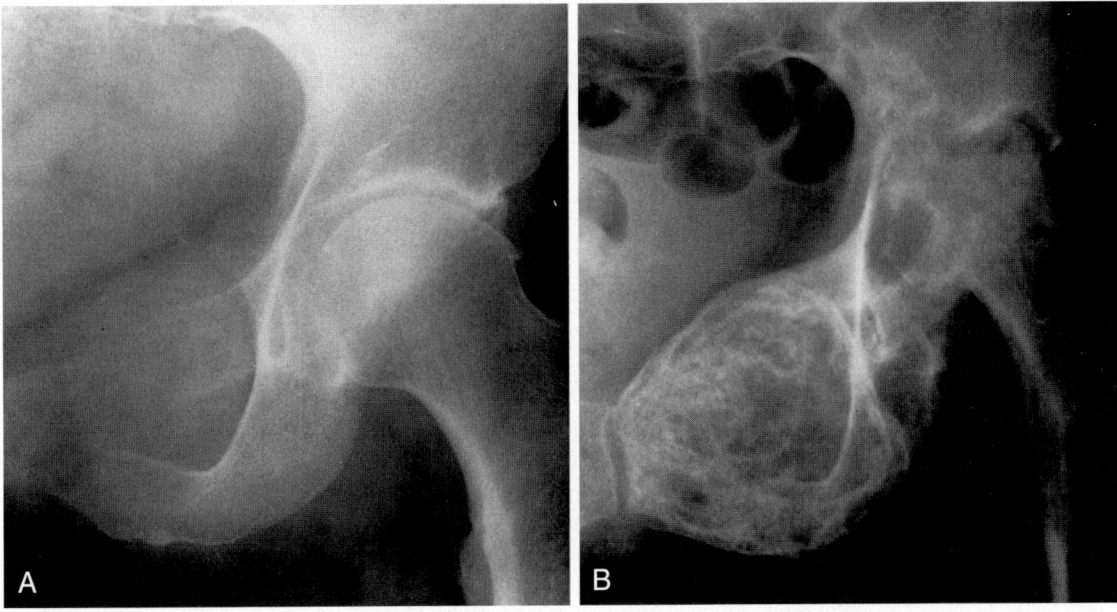

**Figure 72–22.** Osteolytic metastasis: healing with irradiation effect. This 55-year-old woman received radiation therapy for an endometrial carcinoma. *A*, Before therapy, osteolytic destruction of the pubic rami and a soft tissue mass are apparent. Minor changes of osteoarthritis are present in the left hip. *B*, Thirty months after the completion of therapy, mature ossification is indicative of lesion healing. Note the irradiation effects about the left hip. (Courtesy of H. Kroon, MD, Leiden, Netherlands.)

as well as to complete destruction of bone; and an increased accumulation of the radiopharmaceutical agent diffusely throughout the skeleton (superscan; see Fig. 72–24), a phenomenon most frequent in cases of carcinoma of the prostate, in which the scintigraphic pattern is easily misinterpreted as normal unless the absence of renal uptake, the presence of diminished activity in the bones of the appendicular skeleton, and a high ratio of bone to soft tissue activity are recognized.

False-negative bone scans are encountered, especially in certain situations. Any neoplasm that is unaccompanied by ongoing new bone formation may lead to a "cold" region on the bone scan or to an apparently normal examination; this situation is encountered most commonly in plasma cell myeloma, leukemia, and highly aggressive anaplastic carcinomas.

Limitations in the specificity of the bone scan must be recognized by all physicians who interpret its results. A

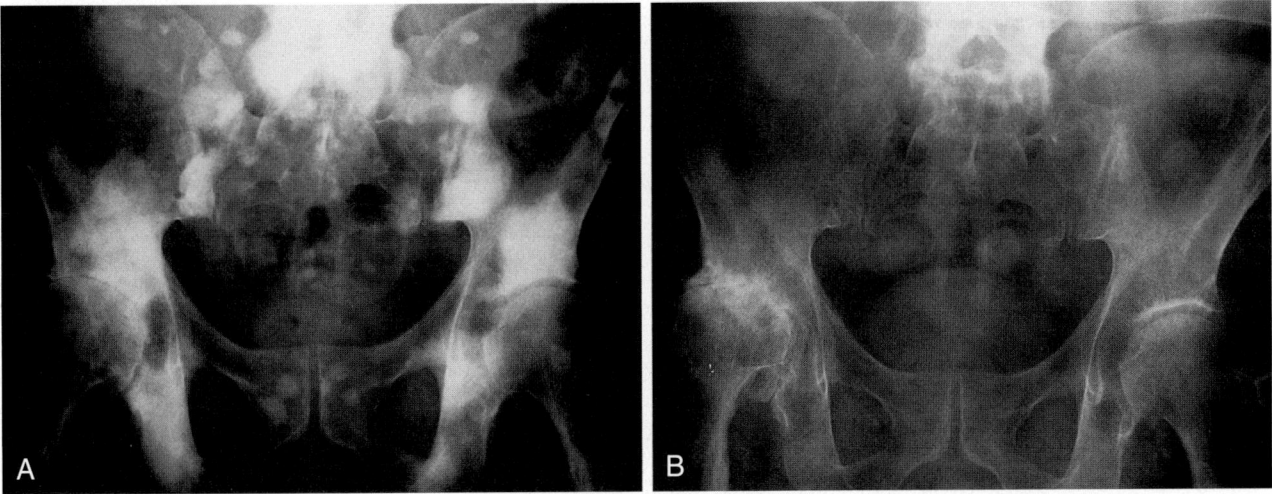

**Figure 72–23.** Osteosclerotic metastasis: healing with chemotherapy. In this 67-year-old patient with metastatic disease related to carcinoma of the prostate, an initial radiograph *(A)* obtained before chemotherapy and orchiectomy shows osteoblastic metastases. Thirty-two months after chemotherapy and orchiectomy *(B)*, dramatic improvement is apparent. Note the progression of osteoarthritis in the right hip.

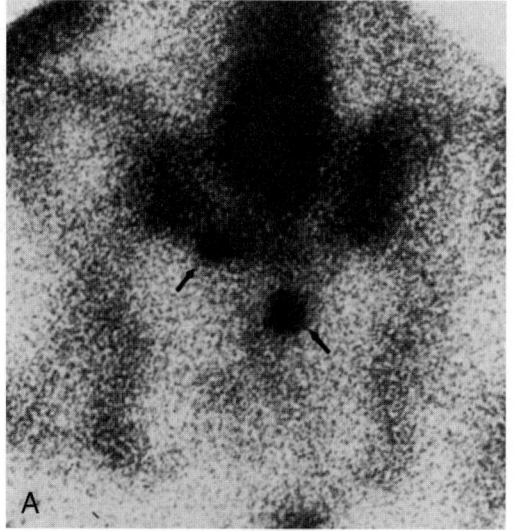

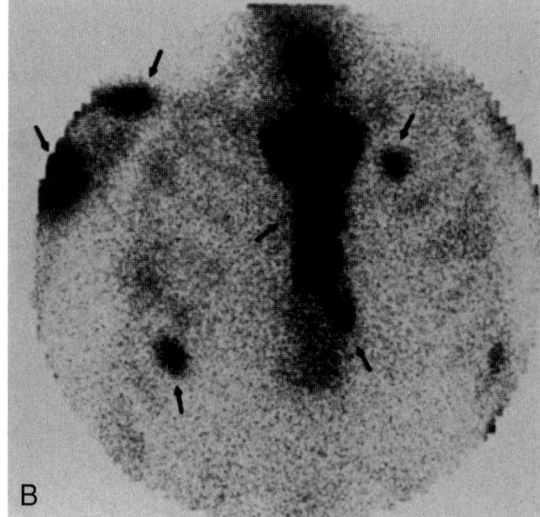

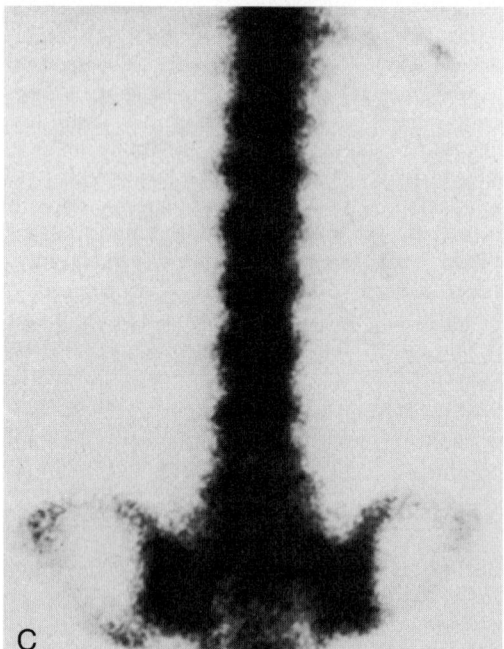

**Figure 72–24.** Skeletal metastasis: abnormal scintigraphic patterns. *A* and *B*, "Hot" spots. Foci of increased accumulation of radionuclide *(arrows)* are shown in the pelvis *(A)* and thorax *(B)*. *C*, Superscan. Diffuse exaggerated uptake of the radiotracer can easily be misinterpreted as normal unless the diminished activity in the soft tissues and kidneys is appreciated.

reliance on the radionuclide study itself, in the belief that a particular scintigraphic pattern is diagnostic of skeletal metastasis and does not require radiographic correlation, will result in diagnostic errors in many patients. The presence of multiple and widespread focal areas of increased accumulation of the radionuclide on the bone scan in a patient with a known primary malignant tumor is the pattern most suggestive of metastases, but it is occasionally simulated by other conditions. As a general rule, solitary lesions of the ribs detected scintigraphically in patients with known primary malignant tumors are most frequently benign and do not represent sites of skeletal metastases. Indeed, even two areas of increased radionuclide uptake in the ribs or any other skeletal site, with the exception of the sternum, commonly denote a nonmalignant process in patients with cancer; however, most sternal lesions are metastases in such patients, particularly those with carcinoma of the breast.

The sequential evaluation of patients with skeletal metastases who are receiving chemotherapy or radiation therapy can be accomplished with bone scintigraphy, although, as with conventional radiography, difficulties in interpretation may arise. The belief that decreasing accumulation of a bone-seeking radionuclide implies tumor healing and that increasing accumulation of this radiotracer suggests tumor progression is inaccurate. As an extreme example of this paradox between tumor behavior and scintigraphic abnormality, a rapidly enlarging osteolytic lesion that completely destroys the adjacent osseous tissue and, with it, the ability to produce new bone is manifested on serial bone scans as conversion of a "hot" lesion to one that may be entirely "cold." Conversely, an increase in the amount of accumulated radionuclide in a lesion, particularly during the early stages of therapy, may indicate tumor healing due to the presence of the flare phenomenon. It has been suggested that the discovery of new lesions on serial bone scintigraphy is a more reliable sign of tumor progression than is an increase in radionuclide uptake at the site of old lesions, although this rule, too, is not without exception. A "flare" response may result in the appearance of apparently new foci of skeletal metastasis during the first months of therapy when, in fact, this is actually an osteoblastic reaction at involved sites not detected on the initial scans. Although quantitative analysis of serial bone scans may increase the accuracy of interpretation, the results should always be correlated with clinical and laboratory parameters, as well as with changing radiographic patterns of disease.

## Computed Tomography

CT can be used to further delineate the nature of a scintigraphically positive osseous region, especially if radiographs fail to document the existence of a metastatic focus. In the spine, CT appears to be more sensitive than conventional radiography in detecting metastatic lesions, and it may also be more specific. In the tubular bones of the appendicular skeleton, CT can detect subtle changes in the attenuation coefficient of the marrow, which may indicate tumor infiltration. CT is an excellent means of defining the extent of any metastatic lesion, especially those in sites that are difficult to evaluate with conventional imaging techniques, such as the vertebral column and pelvis. Paravertebral and intraspinal extension, transarticular spread, and soft tissue involvement with violation of neurovascular structures are examples of information that can be derived from the CT display.

## Magnetic Resonance Imaging

MR imaging has been used most extensively in the evaluation of metastasis in the vertebral column. Its advantages include superior demonstration of paravertebral tumor extension, identification of additional sites of osseous metastasis, and visualization of areas of spinal cord compression between regions of myelographic blocks. On T1-weighted images, intravertebral lesions

are of low signal intensity, and these images are useful in demonstrating spinal cord compression. The signal characteristics of intravertebral lesions are more variable on T2-weighted spin echo MR images, although an increase in signal intensity is most characteristic (Fig. 72–25). In some reports, T2-weighted images have been judged superior to T1-weighted images in showing tumor extension into the subarachnoid space in the absence of cord compression.

Tumorous foci, with their high water content, are generally most conspicuous on T1-weighted images. In elderly patients, whose marrow may appear heterogeneous in composition, and in patients with chronic anemia, in whom increased iron storage in the marrow results in decreased marrow signal intensity on all spin echo sequences, variations in lesion conspicuity are evident. Further, the richly hematopoietic bone marrow of a child's spine reveals low signal intensity on T1-weighted images; metastatic foci may be difficult to detect when such images are used alone. With T2-weighted images, however, hyperintensity of the abnormal marrow becomes evident—a finding designated the flip-flop sign—allowing an accurate diagnosis (Fig. 72–26). Diagnostic difficulty may arise when T1-weighted gadolinium-enhanced MR images are used alone; metastatic lesions in the vertebral bone marrow may enhance so that their signal intensity is similar or identical to that of the marrow itself, significantly decreasing their conspicuity. Because of this possibility, it is important to obtain precontrast spin echo MR images. Short tau inversion recovery (STIR) sequences and fat-suppressed images can be used as an adjunct to unenhanced and gadolinium-enhanced spin echo MR images. When fat suppression is combined with gadolinium administration, accentuated signal intensity in the metastatic focus is more obvious, owing to the suppression of signal intensity in the surrounding marrow.

MR imaging can be useful in the differentiation between nontumorous and tumorous compression fractures of vertebral bodies. Routine spin echo sequences generally allow discrimination between compression fractures related to skeletal metastasis (or other tumors) and those that are

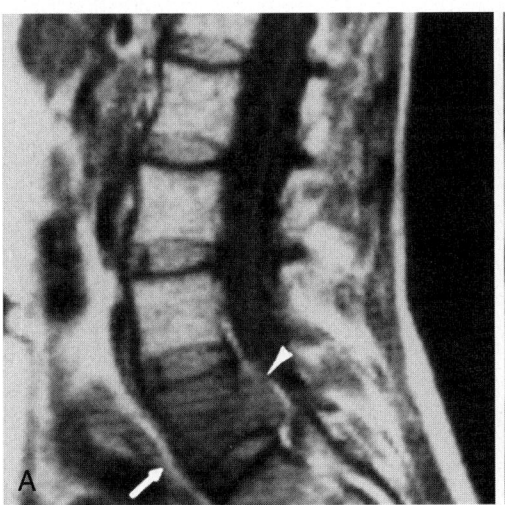
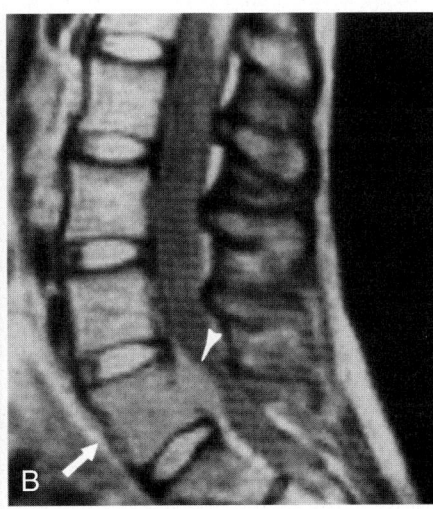

**Figure 72–25.** Skeletal metastasis: standard spin echo MR imaging technique. Sagittal T1-weighted (TR/TE, 600/20) *(A)* and T2-weighted (TR/TE, 2000/80) *(B)* spin echo MR images reveal tumorous replacement of the fifth lumbar vertebral body *(arrows)*, related to metastasis from adenocarcinoma of the breast. A prominent epidural mass is also evident *(arrowheads)*. (Courtesy of M. Solomon, MD, San Jose, Calif.)

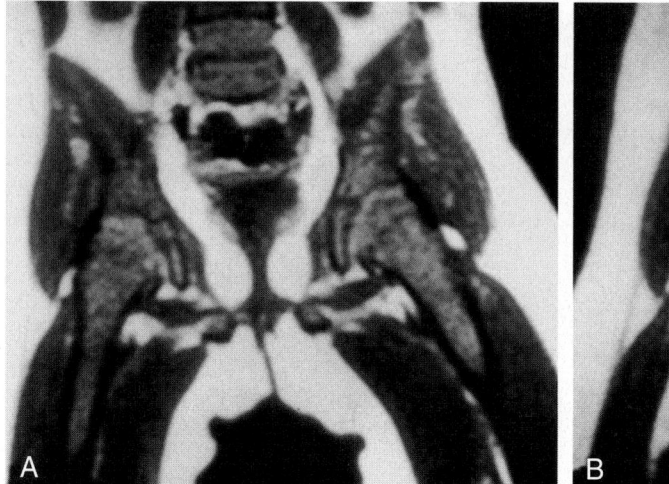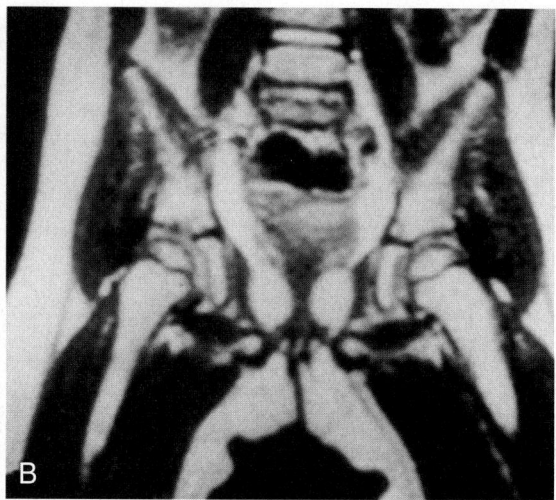

**Figure 72–26.** Skeletal metastasis: flip-flop sign in a 3-year-old child with neuroblastoma. *A,* On this coronal T1-weighted (TR/TE, 500/30) spin echo MR image, diffusely hypointense marrow is seen in the innominate bones and femora. Routine radiographs (not shown) were normal. *B,* On a T2-weighted (TR/TE, 2000/60) spin echo MR image, hyperintensity of the marrow in these sites is evident.

(From Ruzal-Shapiro C, et al: MR imaging of diffuse bone marrow replacement in pediatric patients with cancer. Radiology 181:587, 1991.)

chronic in nature and are related to benign causes such as osteoporosis. The typical appearance of chronic non-tumorous, or benign, fractures of the vertebral body on spin echo sequences relates to the presence of marrow signal intensity in the affected vertebral body that is identical to that of normal vertebrae (Fig. 72–27). Pathologic vertebral fractures caused by metastasis (and other tumors) reveal low signal intensity on T1-weighted images and high signal intensity on T2-weighted images; similar but less pronounced changes in signal intensity accompany acute (<30 days old) benign compression fractures. Morphologic features suggestive of tumorous vertebral collapse include a convex contour of the posterior aspect of the vertebral body, pediculate involvement, and an epidural soft tissue mass. Similar features are used for accurate CT diagnosis.

Although less attention has been given to the MR imaging findings in cases of extraspinal metastatic disease of bone, the general concepts remain the same. The need for gadolinium-enhanced and fat-suppressed techniques is influenced by the signal intensity characteristics of the marrow in the specific skeletal site being evaluated. Fat suppression, when combined with the intravenous administration of gadolinium, is more advantageous when portions of the skeleton that contain abundant fatty marrow, such as the appendicular regions, are being assessed. It should be emphasized that many of the MR imaging abnormalities associated with skeletal metastasis lack specificity and can be simulated by the findings in cases of primary tumors and infections of bone.

With regard to the differentiation between skeletal metastasis and sites of normal hematopoietic marrow, careful attention to the pattern of signal intensity in and about focal lesions may prove diagnostic. On T1-weighted spin echo MR images, one or more areas of high signal intensity (equivalent to that of fat) within a lesion of low signal intensity—a pattern designated the bull's-eye

sign—may be a specific indicator of hematopoietic marrow. Conversely, the presence of a halo sign, defined as a rim of high signal intensity about the lesion on T2-weighted spin echo images, appears to be a reliable indicator of skeletal metastasis, particularly when multiple such lesions are present in a patient with a known malignant tumor.

## METABOLIC CONSEQUENCES OF SKELETAL METASTASIS

### Hypercalcemia

Hypercalcemia is a well-recognized manifestation of cancer, occurring in as many as 10% to 20% of patients. Although generally associated with detectable osseous metastasis, hypercalcemia can appear in patients with malignant tumors in the absence of metastatic involvement of the skeleton, a condition termed pseudohyperparathyroidism. A decrease in serum calcium levels has been observed during the successful treatment of such tumors. Morphologic alterations in the bones of such patients include osteoclastic resorption and fibroblastic proliferation in the marrow, similar or identical to findings in hyperparathyroidism.

### Hypocalcemia

Hypocalcemia is also a well-recognized manifestation in cancer patients who have osteoblastic metastases. In some cases, the laboratory aberration relates to uremia or hypoalbuminemia; in others, the cause is not clear.

### Oncogenic Osteomalacia

In addition to hypocalcemia, hypophosphatemia and elevated serum alkaline phosphatase levels are identified in

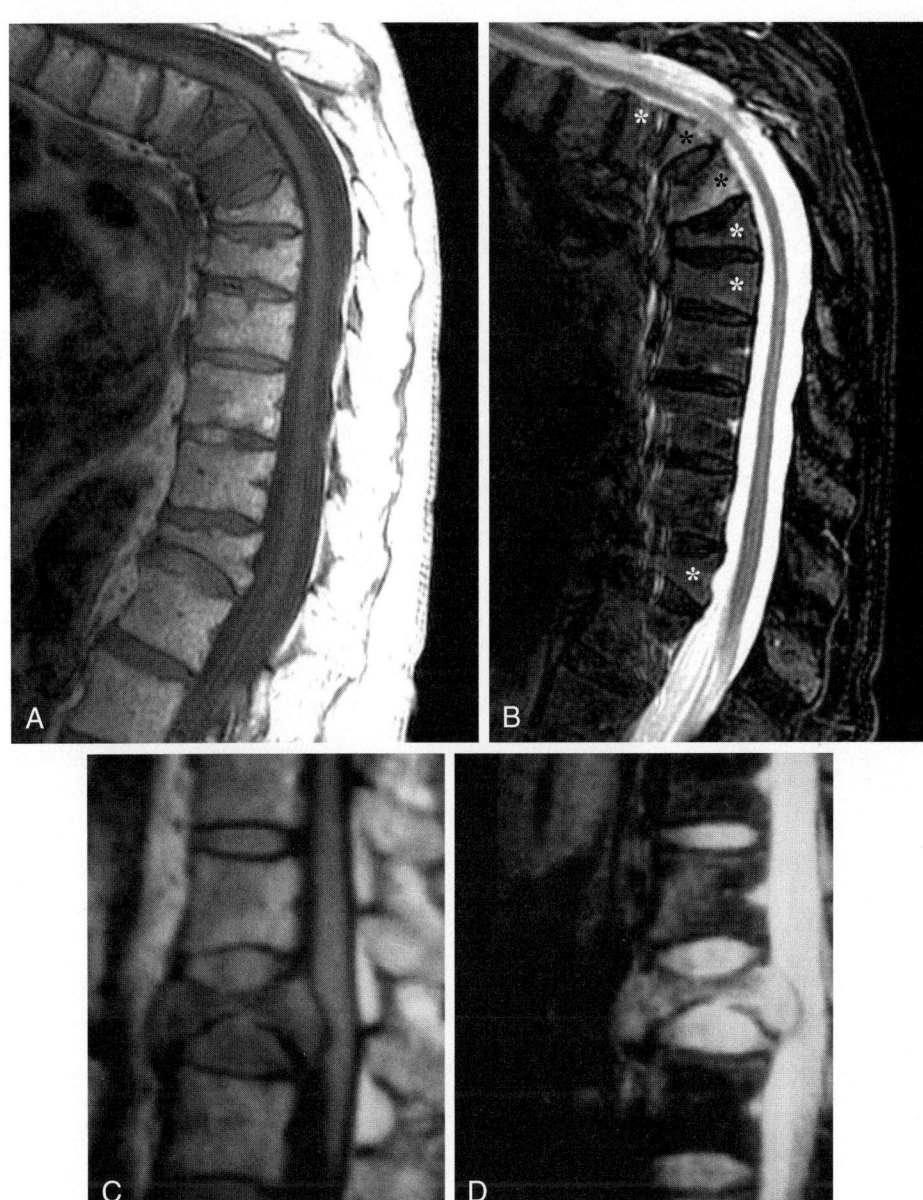

**Figure 72–27.** Nontumorous versus tumorous compression fractures of vertebral bodies: spin echo and gradient echo MR imaging techniques. *A* and *B*, Acute and chronic nontumorous compression fractures. Sagittal T1-weighted (TR/TE, 600/16) *(A)* and fat-suppressed turbo-T2-weighted (TR/TE, 4000/105) *(B)* spin echo MR images show multiple compression fractures. In the chronic compression fractures *(white asterisks)*, the signal intensity in the marrow of the collapsed vertebral body is identical to that in the uninvolved vertebral bodies. Acute nontumorous compression fractures *(black asterisks)* show low signal intensity in the collapsed vertebral body in *(A)* and high signal intensity in this vertebral body on the fluid-sensitive sequence *(B)*. *C* and *D*, Tumorous compression fracture (carcinoma of the breast). In identical T1-weighted spin echo *(C)* and multiplanar gradient recalled *(D)* MR images, note the abnormally low signal intensity in the involved vertebral body in *(C)* and the abnormally high signal intensity in this vertebral body in *(D)*. Compression of the spinal cord is evident.

some patients with extensive osteoblastic metastasis, particularly those arising from carcinoma of the prostate. The diagnosis of osteomalacia has been substantiated in these persons on the basis of histologic findings, as well as depressed serum levels of 1,25-hydroxyvitamin D and normalization of clinical and laboratory abnormalities following the administration of vitamin D derivatives. Oncogenic osteomalacia is typically associated with a number of primary bone and soft tissue neoplasms.

## FURTHER READING

Abrams HL: Skeletal metastases in carcinoma. Radiology 55:534, 1950.

Algra PR, Heimans JJ, Valk J, et al: Do metastases in vertebrae begin in the body or the pedicles? Imaging study in 45 patients. AJR Am J Roentgenol 158:1275, 1992.

Amorosa JK, Weintraub S, Amorosa LF, et al: Sacral destruction: Foraminal lines revisited. AJR Am J Roentgenol 145:773, 1985.

Baker LL, Goodman SB, Perkash I, et al: Benign versus pathologic compression fractures of vertebral bodies: Assessment with conventional spin-echo, chemical-shift, and STIR MR imaging. Radiology 174:495, 1990.

Batson OV: The function of the vertebral veins and their role in the spread of metastases. Ann Surg 112:138, 1940.

Braunstein EM, Kuhns LR: Computed tomographic demonstration of spinal metastases. Spine 8:912, 1983.

Chinn D, Genant HK, Quivey JM, et al: Heterotopic-bone formation in metastatic tumor from transitional-cell carcinoma of the urinary bladder: A case report. J Bone Joint Surg Am 58:881, 1976.

Cuenod CA, Laredo J-D, Chevret S, et al: Acute vertebral collapse due to osteoporosis or malignancy: Appearance on unenhanced and gadolinium-enhanced MR images. Radiology 199:541, 1996.

Debnam JW, Staple TW: Osseous metastases from cerebellar medulloblastoma. Radiology 107:363, 1973.

Deutsch A, Resnick D: Eccentric cortical metastases to the skeleton from bronchogenic carcinoma. Radiology 137:49, 1980.

Eklof O, Mortensson W, Sandstedt B, et al: Bone metastases in Wilms' tumor: Occurrence and radiological appearance. Ann Radiol 27:97, 1984.

Fisher MS: Lumbar spine metastasis in cervical carcinoma: A characteristic pattern. Radiology 134:631, 1980.

Forbes GS, McLeod RA, Hattery RR: Radiographic manifestations of bone metastases from renal carcinoma. AJR Am J Roentgenol 129:61, 1977.

Fornasier VL, Czitrom AA: Collapsed vertebrae: A review of 659 autopsies. Clin Orthop 131:261, 1978.

Fornasier VL, Horne JG: Metastases to the vertebral column. Cancer 36:590, 1975.

Frank JA, Ling A, Patronas NJ, et al: Detection of malignant bone tumors: MR imaging vs scintigraphy. AJR Am J Roentgenol 155:1043, 1990.

Galasko CSB: The anatomy and pathways of skeletal metasasis. In Weiss L, Gilbert HA (eds): Bone Metastasis. Boston, GK Hall, 1981, p 49.

Galasko CSB: Mechanisms of lytic and blastic metastatic disease of bone. Clin Orthop 169:20, 1982.

Goergen TG, Alazraki NP, Halpern SE, et al: "Cold" bone lesions: A newly recognized phenomenon of bone imaging. J Nucl Med 15:1120, 1973.

Harbert JC, George FH, Kerner ML: Differentiation of rib fractures from metastases by bone scanning. Clin Nucl Med 6:359, 1981.

Kerin R: Metastatic tumors of the hand: A review of the literature. J Bone Joint Surg Am 65:1331, 1983.

Lehrer HZ, Maxfield WS, Nice CM: The periosteal "sunburst" pattern in metastatic bone tumors. AJR Am J Roentgenol 108:154, 1970.

McNeil BJ: Value of bone scanning in neoplastic disease. Semin Nucl Med 14:277, 1984.

Mirowitz SA, Apicella P, Reinus WR, et al: MR imaging of bone marrow lesions: Relative conspicuousness on T1-weighted, fat-suppressed T2-weighted, and STIR images. AJR Am J Roentgenol 162:215, 1994.

Mundy GR, Raisz LG, Cooper RA, et al: Evidence for the secretion of an osteoclast activating factor in myeloma. N Engl J Med 291:1041, 1974.

Pagani JJ, Libshitz HI: Imaging bone metastases. Radiol Clin North Am 20:545, 1982.

Pollen JJ, Reznek RH, Talner LB: Lysis of osteoblastic lesions in prostatic cancer: A sign of progression. AJR Am J Roentgenol 142:1175, 1984.

Potter GD: Sclerosis of base of skull as a manifestation of nasopharyngeal carcinoma. Radiology 94:35, 1970.

Punt J, Pritchard J, Pincott JR, et al: Neuroblastoma: A review of 21 cases presenting with spinal cord compression. Cancer 45:3095, 1980.

Ramsey RG, Zacharias CE: MR imaging of the spine after radiation therapy: Easily recognizable effects. AJR Am J Roentgenol 144:1131, 1985.

Reed MH, Culham JAG: Skeletal metastases from retinoblastoma. J Can Assoc Radiol 26:249, 1975.

Resnik CS, Garver P, Resnick D: Bony expansion in skeletal metastasis from carcinoma of the prostate as seen by bone scintigraphy. South Med J 77:1331, 1984.

Rosen IW, Nadel HI: Button sequestrum of the skull. Radiology 92:969, 1969.

Sartoris DJ, Clopton P, Nemcek A, et al: Vertebral-body collapse in focal and diffuse disease: Patterns of pathologic processes. Radiology 160:479, 1986.

Shih TT-F, Huang K-M, Li Y-W: Solitary vertebral collapse: Distinction between benign and malignant causes using MR patterns. J Magn Reson Imaging 9:635, 1999.

Sim FH: Diagnosis and Management of Metastatic Bone Disease: A Multidisciplinary Approach. New York, Raven Press, 1988.

Springfield DS: Mechanisms of metastasis. Clin Orthop 169:15, 1982.

Spuentrup E, Buecker A, Adam G, et al: Diffusion-weighted MR imaging for differentiation of benign fracture edema and tumor infiltration of the vertebral body. AJR Am J Roentgenol 176:351, 2001.

Stanley P, Senac MO Jr, Segali HD: Intraspinal seeding from intracranial tumors in children. AJR Am J Roentgenol 144:157, 1985.

Steckel RJ, Kagan AR: Diagnostic persistence in working up metastatic cancer with an unknown primary site. Radiology 134:367, 1980.

Tofe AJ, Francis MD, Harvey WJ: Correlation of neoplasms with incidence and localization of skeletal metastases: An analysis of 1355 diphosphonate bone scans. J Nucl Med 16:987, 1976.

Weiss L, Gilbert HA: Bone Metastasis. Boston, GK Hall, 1981.

Wilner D: Radiology of Bone Tumors and Allied Disorders. Philadelphia, WB Saunders, 1982, p 3641.

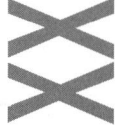

# Congenital Diseases

# CHAPTER 73

## Developmental Dysplasia of the Hip

### Jerry R. Dwek, Christine B. Chung, and David J. Sartoris

## SUMMARY OF KEY FEATURES

Developmental deformity of both sides of the hip joint (dysplasia) may be present at birth or become apparent months to years later. Early diagnosis and treatment are crucial for preventing severe long-term structural abnormalities. Diagnostic methods include the Ortolani and Barlow maneuvers in newborn infants and analysis of radiographic lines drawn on anteroposterior views of the hip and pelvis. Ultrasonography has the lead role in early diagnosis, with conventional radiography becoming more effective after ossification of the femoral head has begun. Conventional tomography, contrast arthrography, computed tomography, and magnetic resonance imaging are valuable both preoperatively and postoperatively in patients with developmental dysplasia of the hip.

## INTRODUCTION

Developmental dysplasia of the hip (DDH) is a disease with extremely variable morphologic patterns. Although early detection through a combination of clinical and imaging evaluation is desirable, the diagnosis is overlooked in many children, who subsequently come to medical attention for evaluation and treatment at several months to years of age. The term DDH replaces the former term congenital dislocation of the hip.

Subluxation and dislocation of the developing hip represent arbitrary designations of static stages in a continuum of disease. The disease is progressive, often insidious in onset, and subtle in its initial clinical and radiographic presentation. A detailed understanding of the pathogenesis of this disorder, as well as of the diagnostic imaging workup and the differential considerations, is essential to an accurate diagnosis and the institution of appropriate therapy.

## CAUSE AND NATURAL HISTORY

Dislocation at 12 to 18 weeks' gestation is termed teratologic, to denote the malformative early development. During this period, congenital neuromuscular abnormalities, including arthrogryposis and myelodysplasia, may cause early dislocation. After this point, mechanical factors are the leading causes of DDH. During the last 4 weeks of gestation, intrauterine positioning puts the hip at risk of dislocation. DDH occurs in approximately 30% of infants with a breech presentation. After delivery, ligamentous laxity caused by the effects of maternal hormones acts to potentiate the risk factors already in place. During the first several days after birth, normal newborn infants may exhibit posterior femoral displacement on stress sonograms. More than 60% of these hips, however, have become stable when reexamined by the Ortolani or Barlow maneuvers within 1 week after birth, and almost 90% are stable by age 2 months.

The acetabulum depends on the correct seating of the femoral head for its proper development. Lateral subluxation causes abnormal modeling of the acetabulum, which becomes shallow and, over time, does not provide a deep cup to properly seat the femoral head. The true acetabulum becomes shallower and fills with fibrofatty material, termed pulvinar. Subsequently, the hip capsule constricts and the hip musculature, especially the adductor group, tightens, making closed reduction difficult. Ossification of the femoral head is delayed (Fig. 73–1). Coxa valga and femoral anteversion are present. Acetabular anteversion is increased on the dislocated side as well.

In many children with DDH, the hip dislocation spontaneously reduces. However, untreated DDH is likely to progress to early osteoarthritis. This includes subluxed forms and reduced forms with acetabular dysplasia.

## EPIDEMIOLOGY

The true incidence of DDH is not known, but the prevalence varies from 1 per 100 births in clinically screened populations to 80 per 1000 births in sonographically screened populations. Female infants are affected approximately eight times more frequently than male infants are. Almost two thirds of infants with DDH are firstborn, suggesting that the maternal uterus and abdominal wall in a primigravida are more confining and perpetuate abnormal stresses on the developing hip joint. In addition, there is an increased incidence of DDH in certain musculoskeletal conditions. For example, the prevalence of DDH in children with infantile idiopathic scoliosis is 6.4%, approximately 10 times its frequency in the general population.

## CLINICAL DETECTION

The Barlow and Ortolani maneuvers represent the mainstay of clinical diagnosis. The Barlow maneuver is performed by progressively adducting the hips. A "clunk" sensation is felt as the femoral head dislocates posterolaterally. The Ortolani test is the reverse: a clunk is palpated as the femoral head reduces into the acetabulum with progressive abduction of the hip. After the initial postnatal

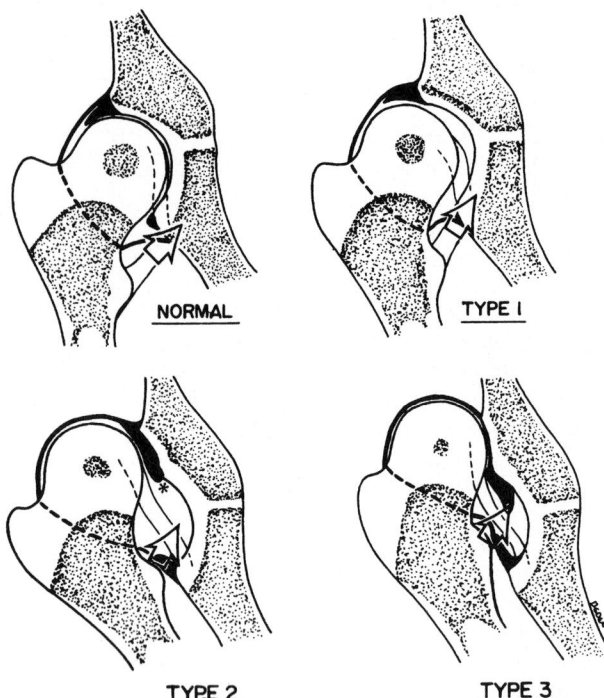

**Figure 73-1.** Schematic diagram of hip dysplasia patterns (*arrows*, course of iliopsoas tendon). *A*, Normal. The acetabular labrum is in an everted position. *B*, Positionally unstable or subluxable hip. The pliable labrum may be deformed slightly. *C*, Subluxed hip, with eversion of the fibrocartilaginous labrum, which may exhibit some inversion (*asterisk*). This type of hip subluxation can be reduced relatively easily in flexion. *D*, Dislocated hip, with inversion and hypertrophy of the labrum, which presents an impediment to reduction. (Courtesy of J. Ogden, MD, Tampa, Fla.)

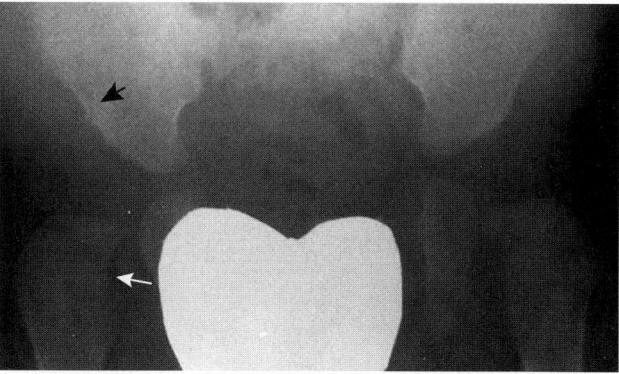

**Figure 73-2.** Subluxed hip. The right femur is slightly lateralized *(white arrow)*, in association with subtle flattening of the lateral acetabular margin *(black arrow)*. The extrapolated femoral head is laterally displaced.

Assessment of the relationship of the femoral head to the acetabulum in a neonate is complicated by the fact that the ossification center is not yet visible; hence, its position must be inferred from the orientation of the femoral metaphysis (Fig. 73–2). Several radiographic lines have been described to distinguish between normal and dislocated hips (Fig. 73–3). The lines are drawn on an anteroposterior view of the pelvis that includes the hips. Accurate positioning is critical; the hips must be extended, with the lower extremities aligned normally and in neutral rotation.

The radiographic lines that are most reliable and helpful in the diagnosis of DDH are as follows:

1. The horizontal line of Hilgenreiner is drawn through the tops of the two triradiate cartilages. Perkins' line is

period, the clinical diagnosis of DDH can be difficult. Owing to muscle contraction and hip capsule constriction, reduction of the femoral head becomes progressively more difficult, and results of the Ortolani and Barlow tests become negative.

## DIAGNOSTIC IMAGING

Before significant femoral head ossification occurs, ultrasonography is the primary imaging technique used for the evaluation of DDH. After ossification, conventional radiography is faster, easier, and as effective as sonography for diagnosis.

### Conventional Radiography

**Neonatal Period.** If the hip is unstable or has dislocated postnatally, conventional radiography in neutral and frog-leg projections will be unrevealing. Both these positions may reduce a dislocatable hip and result in a false-negative study. The pelvis will also be normal. At the earliest, the radiographic changes of a typical dislocated hip can be recognized reliably on a single radiograph at approximately 6 weeks of age.

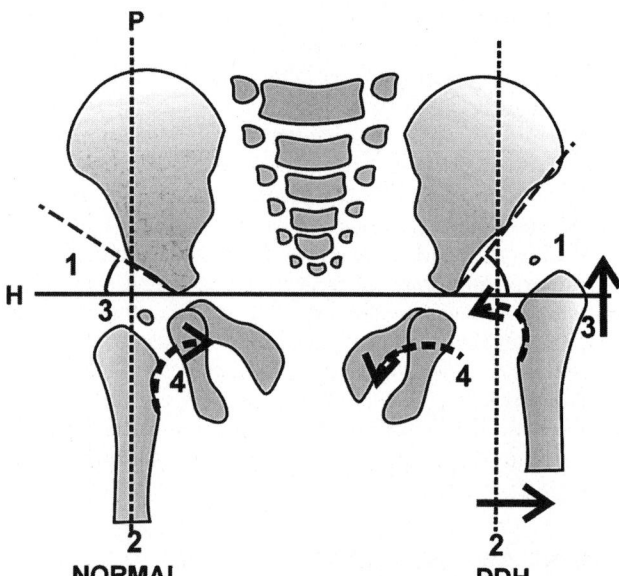

**Figure 73-3.** Radiographic indications of developmental dysplasia of the hip (DDH); the left side is abnormal. 1, acetabular index; 2, lateral migration; H, Hilgenreiner's line; P, Perkins' line; 3, superior migration; 4, Shenton's line. (Courtesy of N. Lektakul, MD, Bangkok, Thailand.)

drawn perpendicular to Hilgenreiner's line, extending inferiorly from the lateral rim of the acetabulum. The intersection of these two lines divides the hip joint into quadrants. The femoral ossific nucleus, if present, or the medial beak of the femoral metaphysis is within the inner lower quadrant if the hip is normal, but it is in the upper outer quadrant if the hip is dislocated.

2. The acetabular index, or angle, is a measurement of the apparent slope of the acetabular roof. It is the angle formed by the intersection of Hilgenreiner's line and a line drawn along the superolateral ossified edge of the acetabulum and the superolateral edge of the triradiate cartilage. At birth it measures 26 ± 5 degrees in males and 30 ± 4 degrees in females. The angle gradually decreases to about 18 ± 4 degrees in boys and 20 ± 3 degrees in girls by 1 year of age. Measurements greater than this strongly suggest acetabular dysplasia.

3. Proximal migration of the femur is measured by observing the shortening of the vertical distance from the femoral ossific nucleus or the femoral metaphysis to Hilgenreiner's line.

4. Shenton's line is drawn along the medial border of the neck of the femur and the superior border of the obturator foramen. The lateral line extends along the lateral border of the ilium and the lateral border of the femoral neck. In the normal hip, these lines form an even, continuous arc, whereas in a dislocated hip with proximal displacement of the femoral head, they are broken and interrupted.

**Childhood Period.** As the child grows, the adaptive changes of the hip joint and femur become more evident on routine radiographs. The characteristic findings include (1) superior and lateral migration of the femur; (2) a shallow, incompletely developed acetabulum (acetabular dysplasia); (3) development of a false acetabulum; and (4) a relatively small femoral ossific nucleus (Fig. 73–4). The normal acetabulum has a slight central concavity and a distinct lateral edge. Absence of either of these findings indicates an abnormal femoral-acetabular relationship.

Several additional measurements have been described in older children, when the femoral head has ossified. The center-edge (CE) angle of Wiberg is constructed by first drawing a horizontal line linking the centers of the two femoral heads. A perpendicular line is then drawn vertically through the center of the femoral head. A third line connects the center of the femoral head to the most lateral point of the acetabulum. The angle is defined by the intersection of these last two lines. Angles greater than 25 degrees are normal, angles of 20 to 25 degrees are borderline, and angles less than 20 degrees are abnormal. Using a false profile view, a similar angle can be constructed by linking the centers of the femoral heads with a horizontal line. A line perpendicular to the center-center line is then constructed. The vertical CE angle is measured between the perpendicular and an oblique line drawn from the center of the femoral head to the most anterior point of the acetabulum. Again, values greater than 25 degrees are normal and those less than 20 degrees are abnormal. Other measurements include the relative lateral displace-

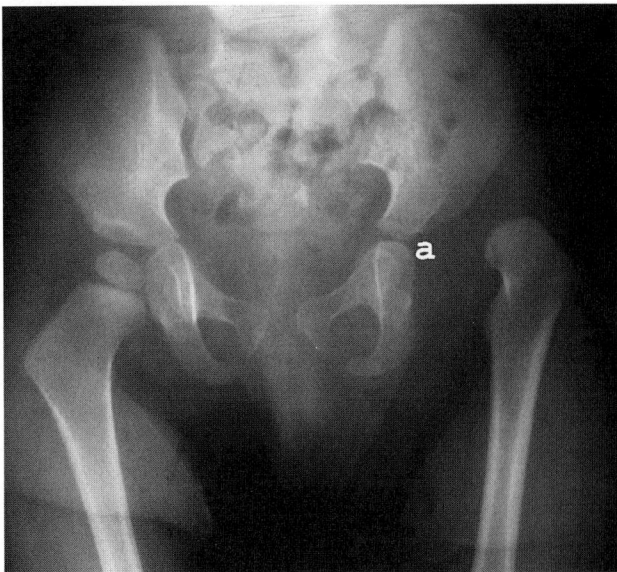

**Figure 73–4.** Left hip dislocation. Delayed development of the left femoral head ossification center is evident by comparison with the normal right side. Note the false acetabulum formation superiorly, with the shallow true acetabulum (a) inferiorly.

ment of the femoral head from the midline, the C/B ratio, the slope of the lateral edge of the acetabulum, and the ratio of acetabular depth to acetabular width (Fig. 73–5).

## Contrast Arthrography

Positive contrast arthrography is helpful when dislocation is discovered late or when sequential radiographic examinations do not document a satisfactory therapeutic response. Arthrography is a useful adjunct to closed or open reduction of an infant hip and is beneficial for preoperative planning of acetabular reconstruction. The method can be combined with computed tomography (CT) or magnetic resonance (MR) imaging, an approach that is particularly valuable for depicting posterior acetabular anatomy.

Arthrographically, the subluxable femoral head lies lateral to and below the margin of the labrum. The labrum may be displaced superiorly or flattened against the pelvis by the femoral head during stress maneuvers, but the femoral head always remains below or lateral to the labral undersurface. Usually the joint capsule is redundant, and the articular cavity is more capacious than normal (Fig. 73–6). The femoral head often lies in a normal position and displaces only with lateral stress. Pooling of contrast material is then observed medial to the lateralized femoral epiphysis. In complete dislocation, the femoral head lies superior and lateral to the margin of the acetabular labrum (Fig. 73–7).

## Ultrasonography

Real-time ultrasonography of an infant's hip provides an accurate image of anatomic relationships, as well as valuable

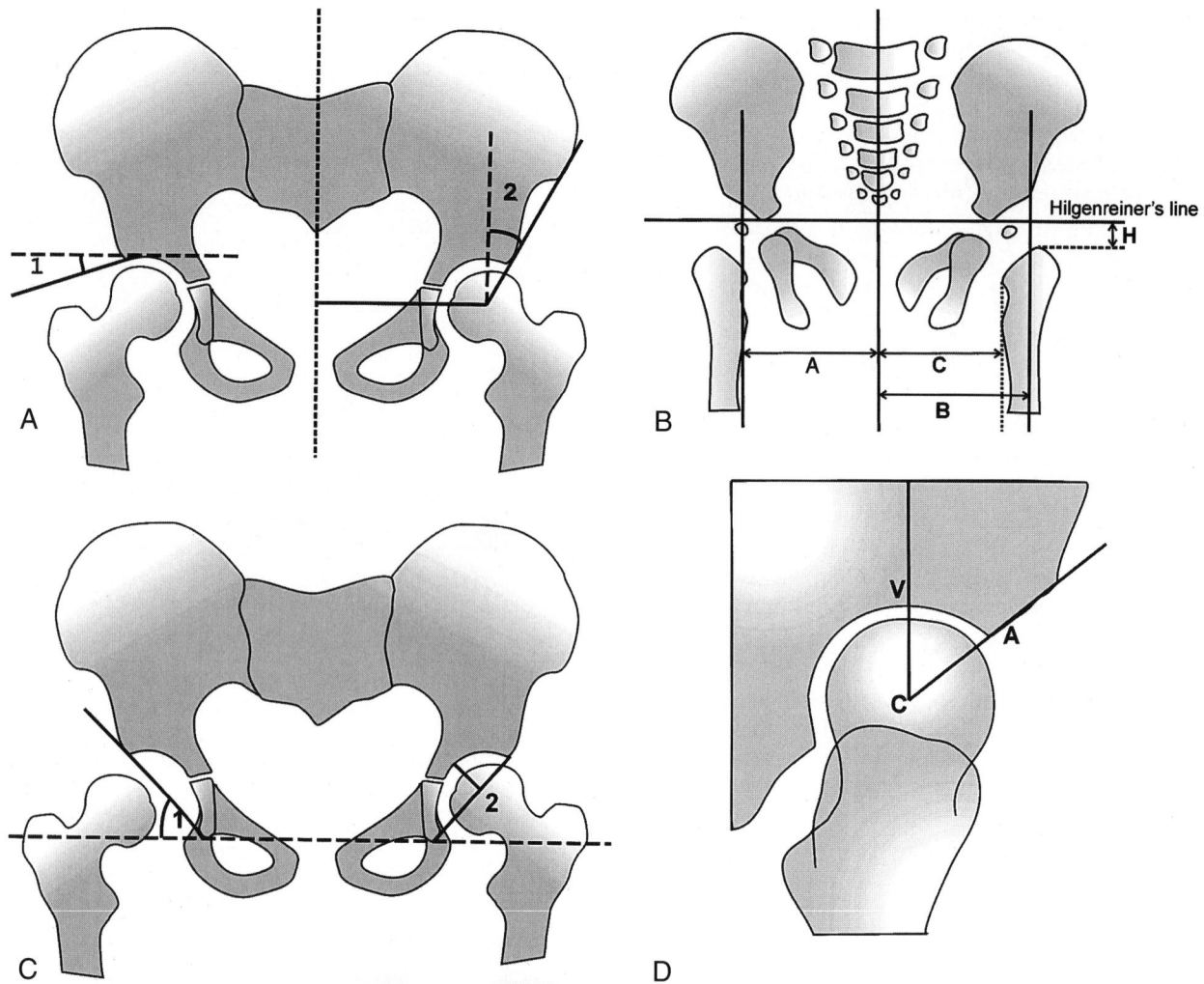

**Figure 73–5.** Additional measurements performed on conventional radiographs in patients with developmental dysplasia of the hip. *A*, 1: Slope of the lateral edge of the acetabulum. The angle formed between a line that is parallel to Hilgenreiner's line and tangent to the roof of the acetabulum and a line that is parallel to the lateral edge of the acetabulum is termed the slope. The normal acetabulum has a slope of the lateral edge that is defined as positive. 2: Center-edge (CE) angle. This angle lies between a line drawn from the center of the femoral head, perpendicular to the line connecting the centers of each femoral head, and a line drawn from the center of the head to the superolateral ossified edge of the acetabulum. In a dislocated hip, in which the center of the femoral head lies lateral to the superolateral ossified edge of the acetabulum, the CE angle has a negative value. *B*, Right hip: The pelvic midline is drawn vertically through the centers of the sacrum and the symphysis pubis. The lateral displacement of each femoral head is indicated by the length of a line (A) drawn horizontally from the pelvic midline to the center of the femoral head. Left hip: The C/B ratio compares C, the distance from the pelvic midline to the medial beak of the femoral metaphysis, and B, the distance from the pelvic midline to the lateral acetabular edge. *C*, 1: The angle that lies between a line connecting the teardrops on the inferior margin of the acetabula and a line drawn from the most superolateral ossified edge of the acetabulum to the teardrop constitutes the adult acetabular index or angle. 2: The greatest perpendicular distance between the medial articular surface of the acetabulum and a line drawn from the teardrop to the superolateral ossified edge of the acetabulum is the acetabular depth. *D*, Vertical center-edge angle, drawn on a false profile view. It is defined as the angle subtended by a line (V–C) drawn from the center of the femoral head extending vertically upward and a line (C–A) drawn from the center of the femoral head obliquely to the anterior edge of the acetabulum. The angle lies between the two lines. (Courtesy of N. Lektakul, MD, Bangkok, Thailand.)

information concerning function. The dynamic relationship of the cartilaginous head to the acetabulum is defined clearly, and instability, subluxation, and dislocation can be demonstrated quantitatively.

The infant is placed supine or on the side. The patient is best scanned via a lateral approach. A linear array high-frequency transducer is used to provide the highest resolution. Static scans include the coronal and transverse planes. The dynamic stress portion of the examination is performed by applying a posteriorly dislocating force to the femur, similar to the Barlow maneuver, while the ultrasonographer watches the femoral head in real time.

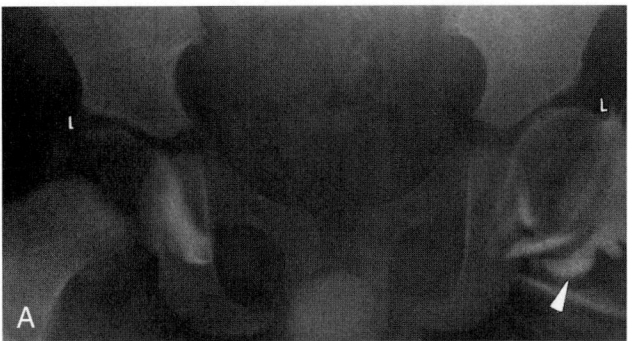

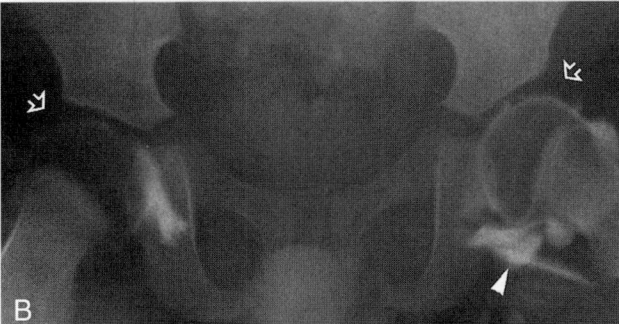

**Figure 73–6.** Arthrography in subluxable developmental dysplasia of the hip. In both the neutral *(A)* and the abducted *(B)* positions, the left acetabular labrum (L, *arrow*) remains in a completely everted configuration, similar to that of the contralateral normal hip. The joint capsule is more redundant on the left *(arrowheads)*.

## Normal Anatomy

The unossified femoral head, composed of hyaline cartilage, is readily identified within the cup of the bony and cartilaginous acetabulum.

**Coronal Image.** The coronal scan of a normal infant hip reveals the femoral head as a discrete, homogeneous sphere of low echogenicity centered over the triradiate cartilage

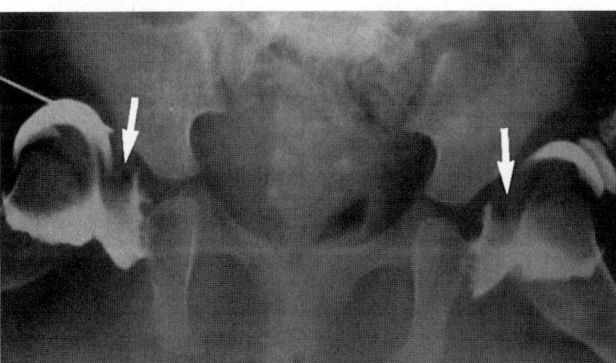

**Figure 73–7.** Arthrography in bilateral dislocations. The acetabular labra *(arrows)* are totally inverted, effectively blocking reduction of the superolaterally displaced femoral heads. The ossified acetabula are shallow, and the joint capsules are capacious.

(Fig. 73–8). The iliac wing is noted as a vertical bony structure, located superiorly, that deviates medially to form the acetabular roof. The point at which the ilium deviates medially is termed the promontory. In the normal mature hip, the promontory has a definite angulated configuration. Rounding of the promontory of various degrees indicates immaturity and that an appropriate seating for the femoral head has not developed. In a frankly dislocated hip, the promontory may have a distinctly flattened contour (Fig. 73–9). The thickness of the cartilage of the acetabular roof that is located inferior to the ossified promontory is increased (>3.4 mm) in infants with DDH.

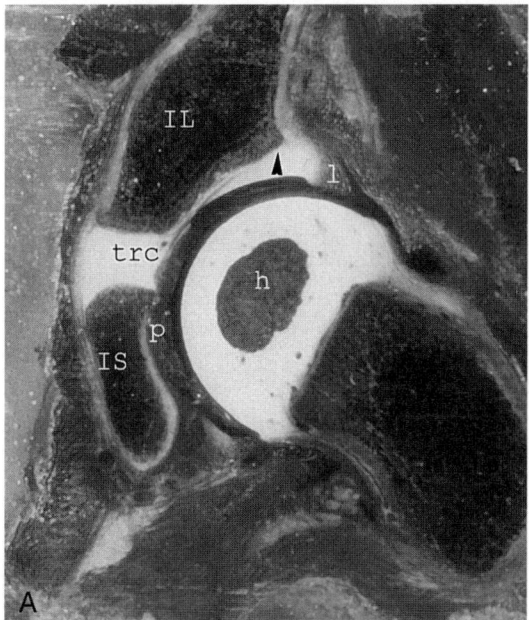

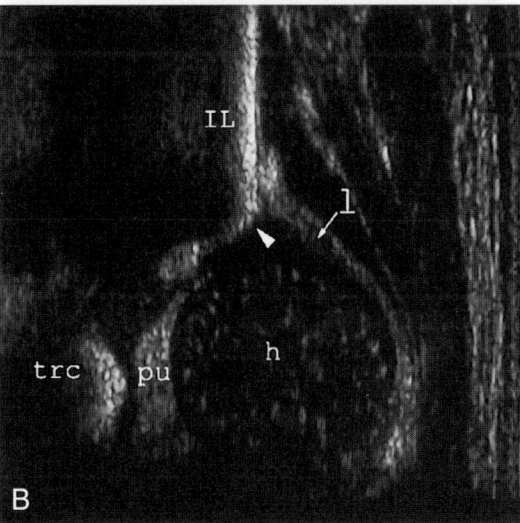

**Figure 73–8.** Normal coronal ultrasound image. *A,* Anatomic section. *B,* Sonographic section rotated 90 degrees to agree with anatomic section. h, femoral head; IL, ilium; IS, ischium; l, labrum; pu, pulvinar; trc, triradiate cartilage; arrowhead, promontory. (*A,* From Johnson ND, Wood BP, Noh KS, et al: MR imaging of the infant hip. AJR Am J Roentgenol 153:127, 1989.)

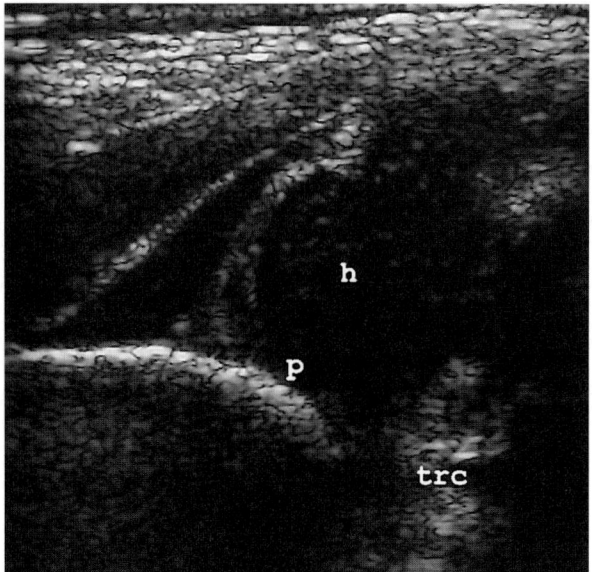

**Figure 73–9.** Coronal sonographic view of a dislocated hip. The femoral head (h) is laterally displaced. The promontory (p) is flattened. trc, triradiate cartilage.

Two important angles are constructed from the coronal scan (Fig. 73–10). The alpha angle is formed by a line running along the iliac wing (termed the baseline) and its intersection with a line drawn along the medially oriented osseous acetabular roof. In normal infants, the alpha angle should be 60 degrees or more. The smaller the angle, the

shallower the acetabular cup, which is indicative of increasing degrees of dysplasia. The beta angle, which is less important, is formed by the intersection of the iliac line and the fibrocartilaginous line of the labrum. This line, termed the labral line, assesses the extent of cartilaginous coverage of the femoral head. A value less than 55 degrees is normal.

**Transverse Image.** The transverse plane provides images of the hip that are analogous to axial CT images (Fig. 73–11). Once again, the femoral head appears as a moderately hypoechogenic, spherical mass cupped within the acetabulum. With the hip flexed, the femoral metaphysis takes the place of the pubis anteriorly. In either position, the hypoechoic zone of the triradiate cartilage is seen at the base of the acetabular cup.

Graf classified hips based on morphologic sonographic information (Table 73–1). This classification system depends not on the position of the femoral head but on the morphology of the acetabulum. Alpha angles greater than 60 degrees are normal. Angles between 50 and 60 degrees indicate immaturity in infants younger than 3 months, whereas the same angle is abnormal in infants older than 3 months. Angles of less than 50 degrees are always abnormal.

## Dynamic Technique

The dynamic portion of the ultrasound examination is based on a sonographic Barlow maneuver; the ultrasonographer watches the hip in real time as it subluxes posteriorly. There are two general methods. In the first

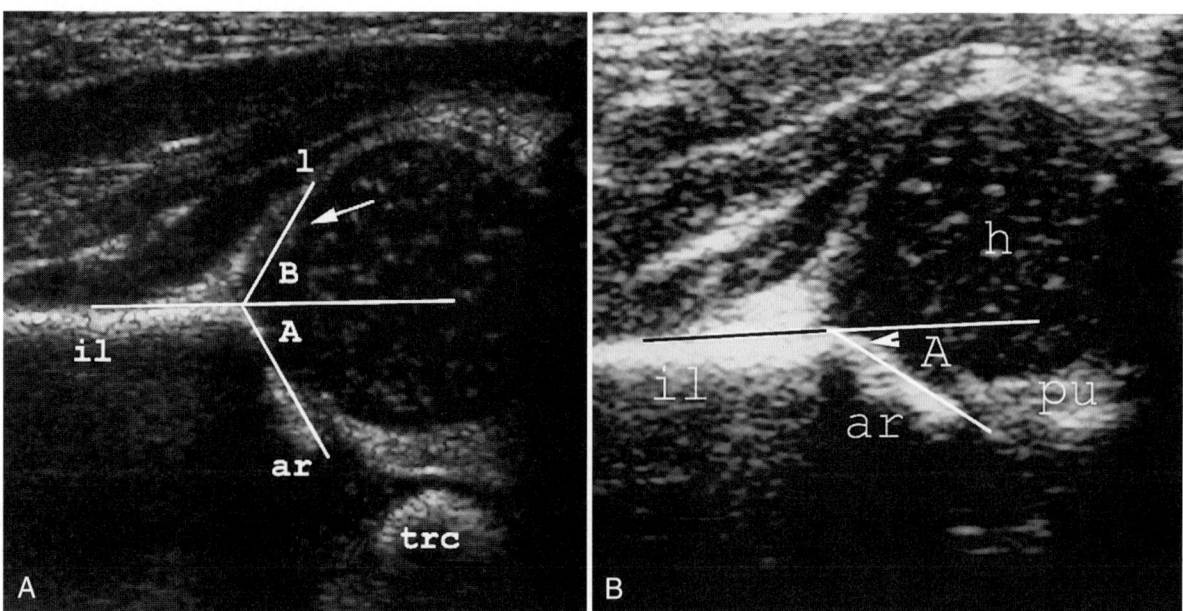

**Figure 73–10.** Normal and abnormal coronal sonographic views. *A*, Normal. The alpha angle (A) and beta angle (B) are shown. The iliac line (il) roughly bisects the femoral head, indicating good acetabular coverage. The *arrow* indicates the labrum. *B*, Abnormal. In this subluxed infant hip, the promontory *(arrowhead)* is flattened. The femoral head (h) is laterally displaced, and there is less than 50% coverage of the femoral head, as indicated by continuation of the iliac line (il) over the femoral head. The alpha angle (A) is low. ar, acetabular roof line; l, labral line; pu, prominent pulvinar; trc, triradiate cartilage.

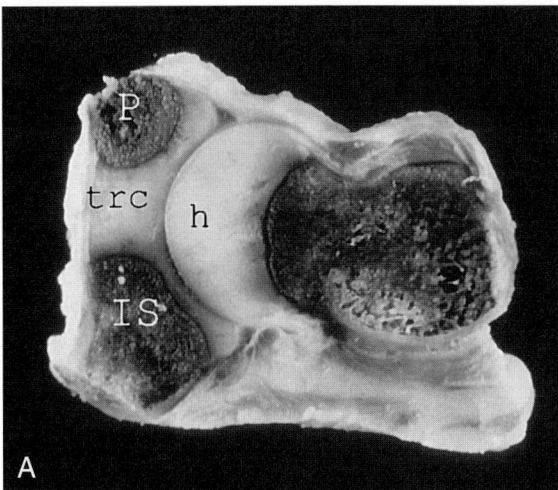

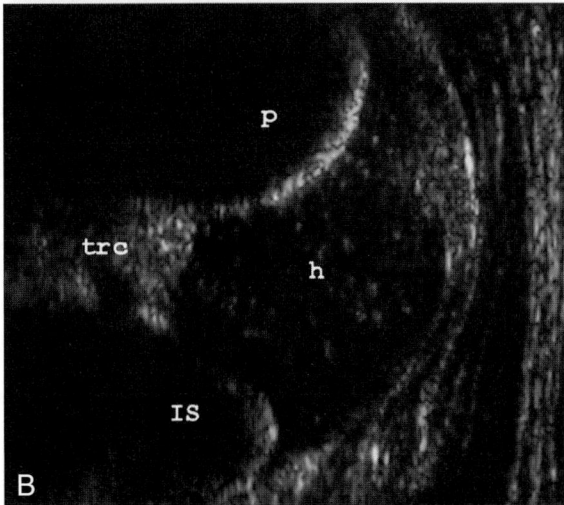

**Figure 73–11.** Transverse section. *A,* Anatomic section. *B,* Sonographic section (rotated 90 degrees clockwise to agree with anatomic orientation). h, femoral head; IS, ischium; P, pubis; trc, triradiate cartilage.

method, the infant is scanned in the transverse plane. As the ultrasonographer focuses on the femoral head in the standard transverse view, the femur is gently positioned posteriorly. A positive examination occurs if the femoral head subluxes posteriorly over the ischium (Fig. 73–12). In the second method, the hip is held in extension. The sonographer establishes a scan plane slightly posterior to the standard coronal view. As a posterior force is applied to the femur, subluxation is identified when a greater diameter of the femoral head is visualized as it subluxes posteriorly. The force exerted need not be great. Because infants up to 2 weeks old may have normal instability, it is preferable to delay the first ultrasound examination until after this time.

### Dislocated Hip

In long-standing, nonreducible dislocation, additional abnormalities may be identified on ultrasonography. The cartilaginous head is situated posterior, lateral, and, fre-

quently, superior to the acetabulum. Consequently, visualization of the acetabulum may be partially obscured by the metaphysis of the dislocated femur. The normally thin joint capsule becomes thickened and echogenic (Fig. 73–13). Fibrofatty tissue, or pulvinar, is identified as echogenic material within the cup of the acetabulum.

### Computed Tomography

CT offers a quick and efficient method of documenting concentric reduction in the postoperative hip without interference from a plaster of Paris cast (Fig. 73–14). CT, particularly with three-dimensional analysis, is extremely useful in characterizing the abnormal acetabular morphology of untreated and postoperative DDH (Fig. 73–15).

### Magnetic Resonance Imaging

MR imaging is capable of accurately depicting the most important determinants of stability in the neonatal hip. These include femoral head shape, acetabular shape, position of the labrum, invagination of the joint capsule by the iliopsoas tendon, degree of femoral and acetabular anteversion, and position of the transverse acetabular ligament (Fig. 73–16).

Scan sequences are tailored to the clinical problem. To document concentric reduction of the femoral head, impediments to such reduction, or osteonecrosis in the acute setting, transverse T1-weighted spin echo MR images are effective. Impediments to concentric reduction include pulvinar hypertrophy, a thickened ligamentum teres, and a labrum or capsule interposed between the femoral head and the acetabulum. The addition of coronal and sagittal sequences improves visualization of acetabular anatomy in cases in which preoperative planning is needed (Figs. 73–17 and 73–18). Assessment of femoral anteversion requires an additional transverse sequence through the femoral condyles, in the same manner as with CT scanning. The abducted position of the hips in a spica cast after reduction of DDH may cause osteonecrosis of the femoral head. A bolus of intravenous contrast material followed by repeated T1-weighted spin echo or three-dimensional spoiled gradient recalled (SPGR) sequences allows the evaluation of femoral head perfusion with scan times of less than 15 seconds per sequence.

### TREATMENT

Treatment of DDH is age dependent. This is true because the modeling capacity of the acetabulum and femoral head is finite and decreases with advancing age.

Before 6 months of age, maintenance of concentric reduction is the key to a favorable outcome. To that end, patients are placed in a splint device that stabilizes the hip in an abducted and flexed position. From 6 months to about 2 years of age, abduction devices lose their utility. Infants are able to crawl, and it is difficult to maintain appropriate harness placement. In addition, there already are secondary changes in the acetabulum and soft tissue that limit reducibility and appropriate development. When treatment with a harness, splint, or pillow fails, closed

**TABLE 73–1**

**Graf Classification of Hip Dysplasia**

| Sonographic Type | Osseous Acetabular Roof | Bony Promontory | Cartilaginous Acetabular Roof | Alpha Angle (°) | Beta Angle (°) |
|---|---|---|---|---|---|
| Mature hip (no age limits) | | | | | |
| Ia | Good | Angular | Narrow, extending far over femoral head | >60 | <55 |
| Ib | Good | Slightly rounded | Stubby, extending short distance over femoral head | >60 | >55 |
| Immature hip (<3 mo of age) | | | | | |
| IIa (+) (physiologic, appropriate for age) | Satisfactory | Rounded | Broad, covering femoral head | 50–59 | >55 |
| IIa (–) (maturational deficit) | Deficient | Rounded | Broad, covering femoral head | 50–59 | >55 |
| IIb Delayed osseous development (>3 mo of age) | Deficient | Rounded | Broad, covering femoral head | 50–59 | >55 |
| IIc Critical zone hip | Deficient to highly deficient | Rounded to flattened | Broad, covering femoral head | 43–49 (critical range) | <77 |
| D (IId) Decentering hip (no age limits) | Highly deficient | Rounded to flattened | Displaced | 43–49 (critical range) | >77 |
| Eccentric hip | | | | | |
| IIIa | Poor | Flattened | Displaced; devoid of echoes, indicating no structural alteration | <43 | >77 |
| IIIb | Poor | Flattened | Displaced; echogenic, indicating structural alteration | <43 | >77 |
| IV | Poor | Flattened | Inverted | <43 | >77 |

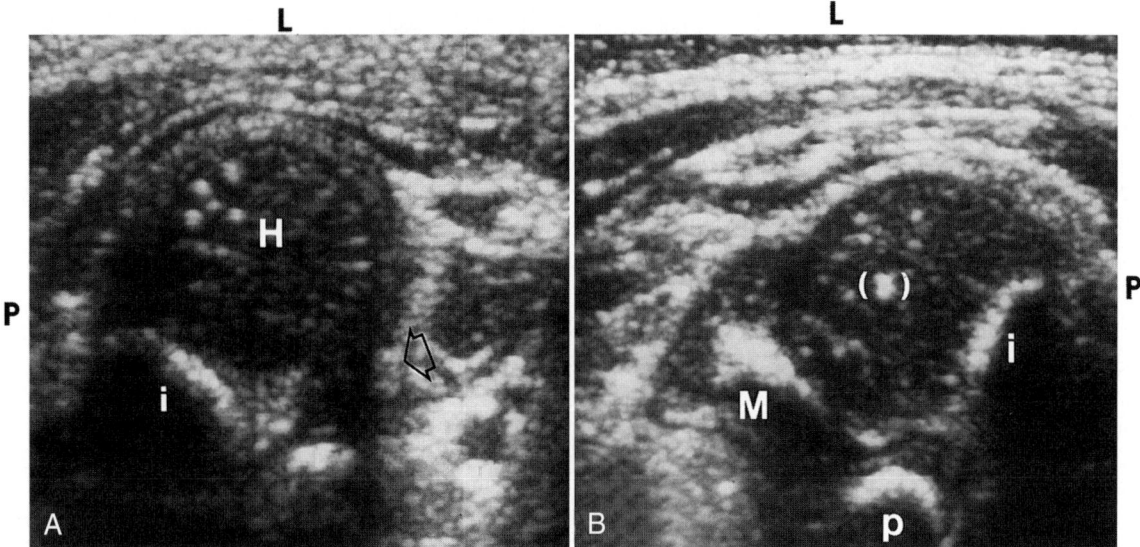

**Figure 73–12.** Transverse dynamic imaging. *A*, Transverse image of a right subluxable hip under stress. The femoral head (H) has subluxed posteriorly and laterally with respect to the acetabulum. *B*, Contralateral normal left hip for comparison. More advanced maturation of the femoral head ossific nucleus *(parentheses)* is evident. i, ischium; L, lateral; M, femoral metaphysis; p, pubis; P, posterior; *arrow*, echogenicity within acetabular fossa.

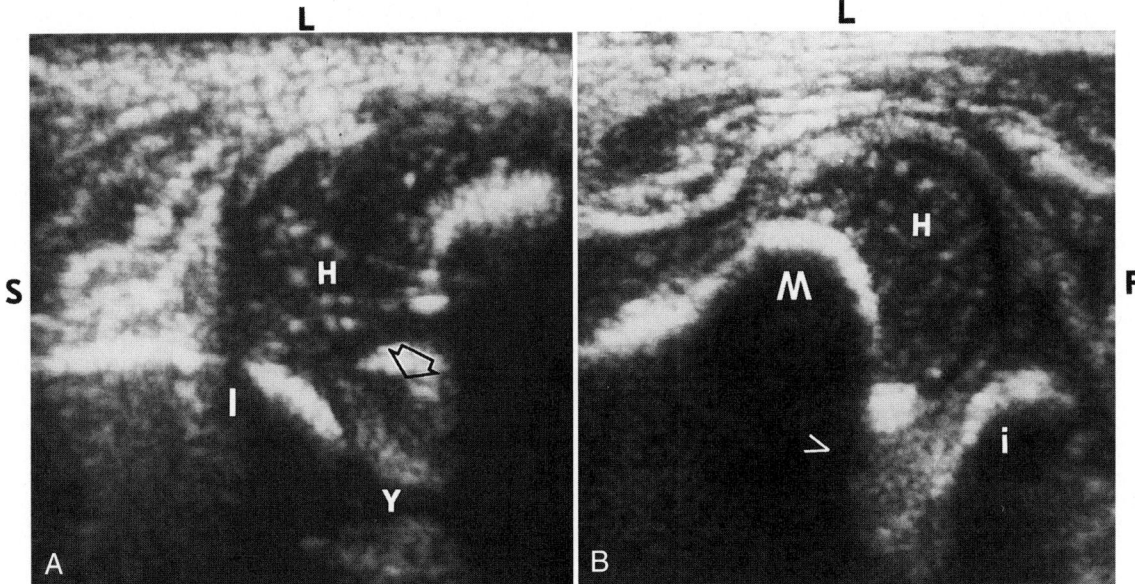

**Figure 73–13.** Long-standing dislocation. *A,* Coronal image of a long-standing dislocation. The femoral head (H) is situated posteriorly, superiorly, and laterally to the acetabulum. The gluteal muscles are displaced laterally, and the joint capsule is echogenic and thick. The poorly defined, echogenic labrum is infolded *(arrow),* preventing reduction. *B,* Transaxial image of the same dislocated hip. The posterior acetabulum (represented by the ischium [i]), the femoral head (H), and the femoral metaphysis (M) are evident. The dislocated femoral head is held laterally by echogenic fibrofatty pulvinar *(arrowhead).* I, ilium; L, lateral; P, posterior; S, superior; Y, triradiate cartilage.

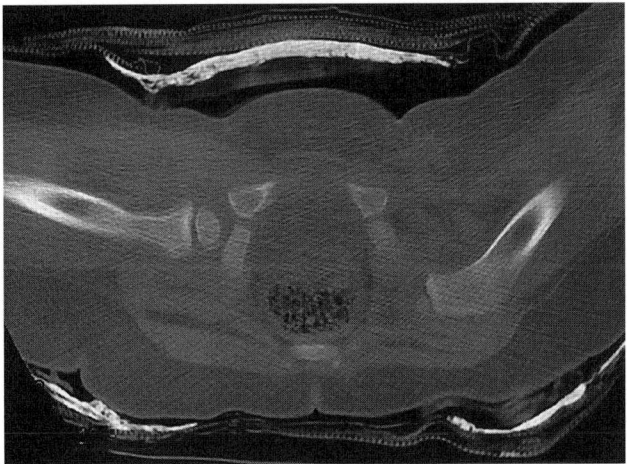

**Figure 73–14.** Failed reduction of unilateral developmental dysplasia of the hip. With the patient in a plaster cast, delayed ossification and posterior displacement of the left femoral head are evident on a CT scan (compared with the normal right side). The left acetabulum is underdeveloped compared with the normal right side.

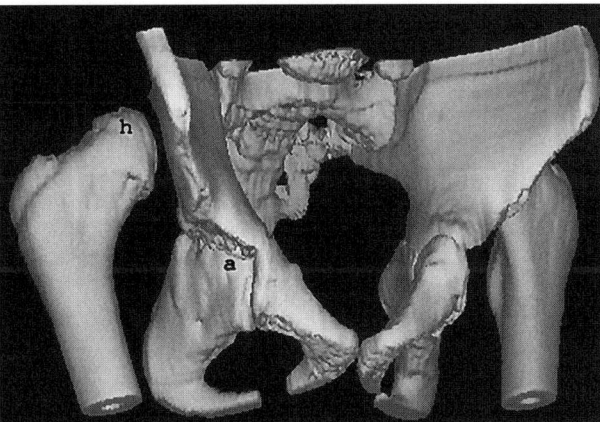

**Figure 73–15.** Three-dimensional reformatted CT scan of untreated developmental dysplasia of the hip. Right anterior oblique images reveal an aspherical, superiorly dislocated femoral head (h), as well as the shallow, featureless acetabulum (a).

reduction may be attempted. Traction applied to the hip is helpful because it stretches the contracted soft tissues and decreases the risk of postoperative osteonecrosis of the femoral head.

After age 2 years, open reduction is usually needed. Operative procedures that provide femoral shortening

and release of soft tissues are helpful in alleviating pressure on the femoral epiphysis after reduction, decreasing the incidence of osteonecrosis of the femoral head. Postoperatively, patients are placed in a spica cast with the hip flexed and abducted. Congruent reductions of the hip accomplished before age 4 years lead to normal hip relationships in more than 95% of patients. There is good evidence that continuous pressure of the femoral head against soft tissue interposed between it and the acetabulum may

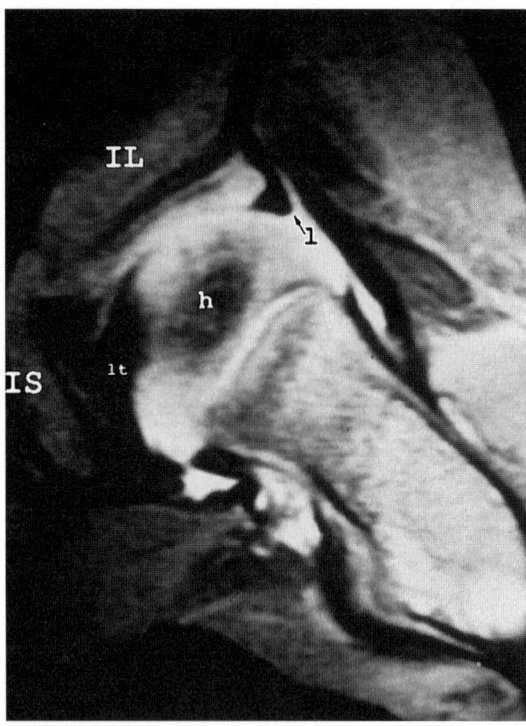

**Figure 73–16.** Coronal T2-weighted (TR/TE, 2000/50) spin echo MR image demonstrates important hip anatomy. h, femoral head; IL, ilium; IS, ischium; l, labrum (arrow); lt, ligamentum teres. (From Johnson ND, Wood BP, Noh KS, et al: MR imaging of the infant hip. AJR Am J Roentgenol 153:127, 1989.)

induce displacement or atrophy of these obstructing structures and lead to normal seating of the femoral head.

Long-standing acetabular dysplasia or dislocation may require a redirective or salvage procedure. Radiographs may be obtained and graded according to the Severin classification system (Table 73–2). A femoral osteotomy is used if the femur needs to be significantly redirected (owing to femoral anteversion or valgus deformity) to achieve reduction. In patients with significant acetabular dysplasia, iliac osteotomies are necessary. The common goals of such intervention are the provision of improved acetabular coverage, enhanced femoral head–acetabular congruence, decreased pressure loading of the femoral head, and increased efficiency of the hip musculature (Fig. 73–19).

In many untreated or unsuccessfully treated cases, pain and disability secondary to residual deformity (Fig. 73–20) or osteoarthritis may necessitate reconstructive surgery or hip replacement, although often not until the fifth or sixth decade of life.

## COMPLICATIONS

Ischemic necrosis of the femoral head occurs in DDH only after treatment and can therefore be considered an iatrogenic complication; it may lead to severe radiographic changes and a painful, dysfunctional hip in early adult life. The reported frequency of ischemic necrosis in early-treated DDH ranges from less than 1% to as high as 12%. Of patients with DDH-associated ischemic necrosis, long-term follow-up assessment reveals a very high prevalence of secondary osteoarthritis, and total hip arthroplasty may ultimately be required in some patients.

Failure of appearance or growth of the femoral ossification center during an interval of approximately 1 year after reduction is good evidence of necrosis. Characteristic manifestations of the process, such as broadening of the femoral neck, may also occur during this time or become evident later. Additional radiographic abnormalities may include irregular physeal margins, metaphyseal cysts, and the "sagging rope" sign—a U-shaped line projecting over the femoral neck that represents either the edge of the malpositioned femoral head or a reactive osseous ridge.

MR imaging allows the diagnosis of an ischemic femoral head immediately after surgery. Ischemia is diagnosed as lack of enhancement after intravenous gadolinium administration on T1-weighted spin echo MR images. Premature fusion of the lateral growth plate with secondary external rotation of the femoral head may result from occlusion of the posterosuperior epiphyseal artery or immobilization-induced physeal compression. Associated findings include shortening of the femoral neck and leg-length discrepancy. Premature closure of the medial physis may induce coxa magna, with mild shortening of the femoral neck. Generalized growth plate injury occurs with compromise of the medial circumflex artery, resulting in severe femoral neck shortening, leg-length discrepancy, and deformity of the femoral head.

Relative trochanteric overgrowth is also a secondary phenomenon resulting from the unbalanced growth rates of the physes of the femoral neck and greater trochanter. This may result in alteration or reversal of the normal relationship between the superior margins of the femoral head and greater trochanter, manifested quantitatively as a decreased or negative articular-trochanteric distance. Inefficient abduction and functional coxa vara despite a normal neck-shaft angle are important biomechanical consequences. Management of this situation includes early trochanteric epiphysiodesis or inferior trochanteric displacement at an older age.

In an older child with initial late reduction of DDH, the radiographic appearance is similar to that of Legg-Calvé-Perthes disease. The sequelae, however, are generally more severe; femoral neck shortening and epiphyseal deformity occur with much higher frequency. Incomplete epiphyseal necrosis is more difficult to recognize radiographically and can occur despite preliminary traction, gentle reduction, and avoidance of extreme immobilization positions. In a review of older children with DDH treated by limbus excision and derotation osteotomy, premature onset of degenerative arthritis was found to be the most important sign of poor long-term prognosis.

## DIFFERENTIAL DIAGNOSIS

### Incomplete Femoral Head Coverage

Inadequate acetabular coverage of the ossified femoral head epiphysis can be observed in a variety of conditions

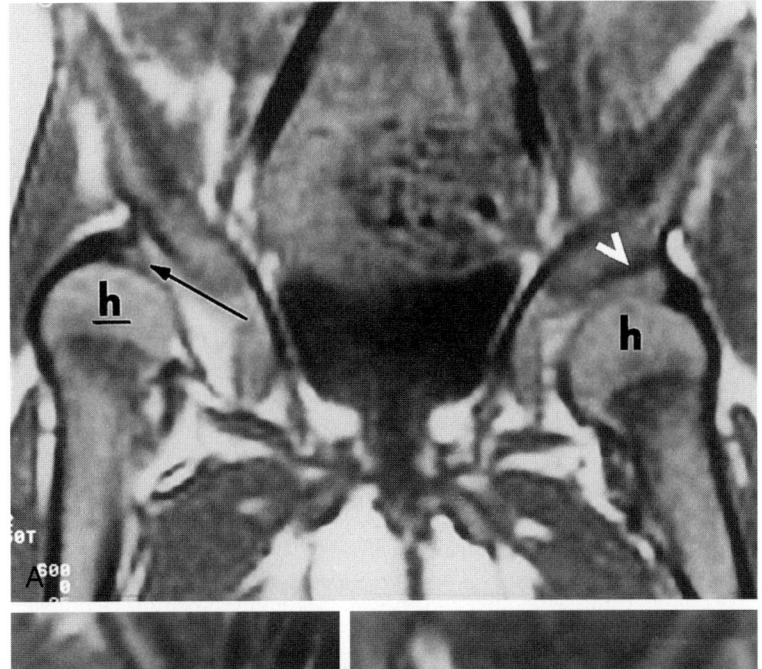

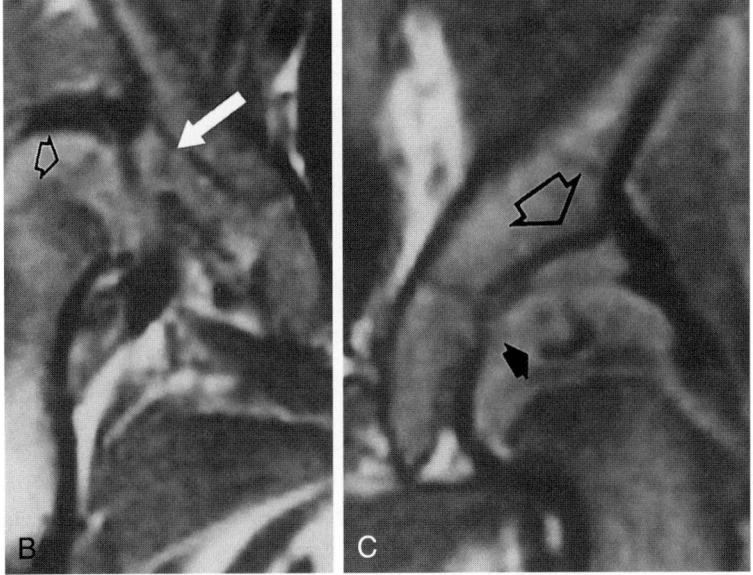

**Figure 73–17.** MR imaging in developmental dysplasia of the hip. *A,* Coronal T1-weighted (TR/TE, 600/25) spin echo MR image reveals superolateral subluxation of the right femoral head (h) when compared with the normal left side. Deformity of the right acetabular labrum *(arrow)* is evident when compared with the normal left side *(arrowhead). B,* At a slightly different level, a similar coronal MR image (TR/TE, 600/25) shows an underdeveloped secondary ossification center for the femoral head *(open arrow).* The acetabular labrum is both flattened and partially inverted *(white arrow). C,* In a coronal T1-weighted (TR/TE, 600/25) spin echo MR image, the normal left hip is shown for comparison *(solid arrow,* femoral head ossification center; *open arrow,* acetabular labrum).

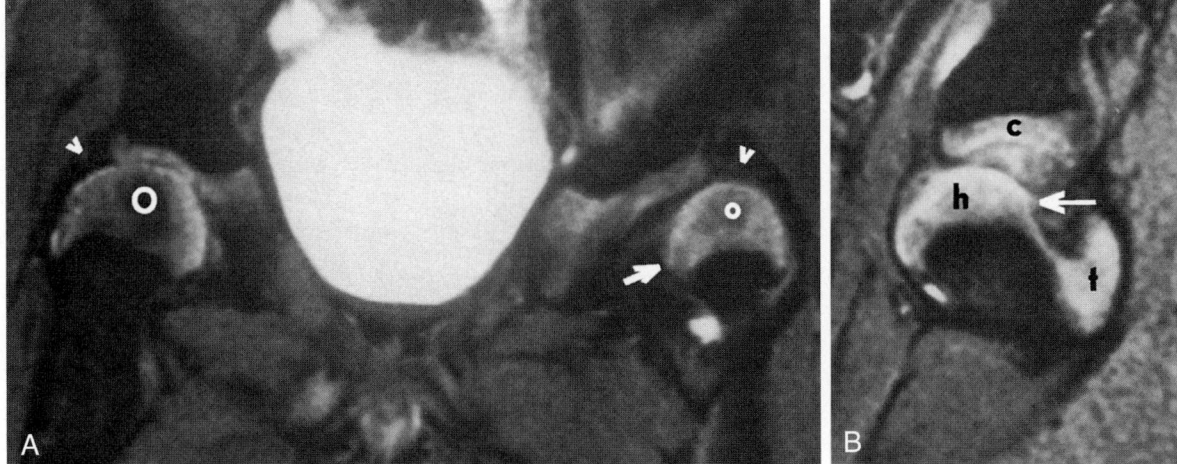

**Figure 73–18.** MR imaging in developmental dysplasia of the hip. *A,* Coronal gradient echo (TR/TE, 100/25) image reveals lateral subluxation of the left femur *(arrow);* its secondary ossification center is delayed in development (O > o). Both acetabular labra are in the normal everted position *(arrowheads). B,* Sagittal gradient echo (TR/TE, 100/25) image demonstrates mild anterior subluxation of the femoral head *(arrow).* Note the continuity between the cartilaginous femoral head (h) and the greater trochanter (t). c, triradiate cartilage.

**TABLE 73-2**

**Severin Classification System**

| Type | Description |
|------|-------------|
| I | Normal |
| Ia | CE angle >19°, age 6 to 13 yr, or CE angle >25°, age 14 yr |
| Ib | CE angle 15° to 19°, age 6 to 13 yr, or CE angle 20° to 25°, age 14 yr |
| II | Moderate deformity of the femoral head or neck or acetabulum, but otherwise as in group Ia or Ib |
| III | Dysplastic but without subluxation—CE angle <15°, age 6 to 13 yr, or CE angle <20°, age 14 yr |
| IV | Subluxation |
| IVa | Moderate, CE angle 0° |
| IVb | Severe, CE angle <0° |
| V | Femoral head articulates with secondary acetabulum in upper part of original acetabulum |
| VI | Redislocation |

CE, center-edge.

From Severin E: Contribution to knowledge of congenital dislocation of the hip joint: Late results of closed reduction and arthrographic studies of recent cases. Acta Chir Scand Suppl 84(Suppl 63):1, 1941.

other than DDH. Lateral uncovering occurs in situations in which the acetabulum is developmentally small or the femoral head is enlarged (e.g., ischemic necrosis). A valgus position and anteversion of the femoral neck tend to rotate the femoral head outward and contribute to poor coverage.

## Inflammatory Disease

Hip subluxation, manifested as lateralization of the femoral metaphysis, occurs in pyogenic arthritis of infancy. Soft tissue swelling in and flexion of the thigh increase the density about the hip region and provide an important clue to the correct radiographic diagnosis.

## Neuromuscular Disease

Superior and lateral displacement of the femoral head is common in patients with meningomyelocele and may occur during infancy. The acetabulum may be shallow owing to the prenatal onset of the disease, and evidence of spinal dysraphism should be present on pelvic radiographs (Fig. 73–21). The hip subluxation of cerebral palsy and other spastic conditions rarely develops during infancy and is associated with severe femoral anteversion and coxa valga.

## Traumatic Epiphyseal Slip

Traumatic epiphyseal slip in the proximal portion of the femur may occur in the setting of infant abuse or birth trauma. If the epiphyseal ossification center is not yet mineralized, lateral shift of the femoral shaft can be misinterpreted as DDH rather than a shearing fracture.

## Congenital Coxa Vara

Congenital coxa vara without femoral shortening is extremely rare and can be distinguished from DDH by clinical examination and arthrography during the neonatal period.

## Abnormal Joint Laxity

Familial joint laxity is probably inherited as an autosomal dominant trait, and most affected persons do not have significant orthopedic problems. Hypotonia and joint laxity occur in Down's syndrome, and recurrent hip dislocation can be observed. Cutaneous and articular hyperlaxity, with inconstant spherical subcutaneous calcifications, is part of the generalized connective tissue derangement

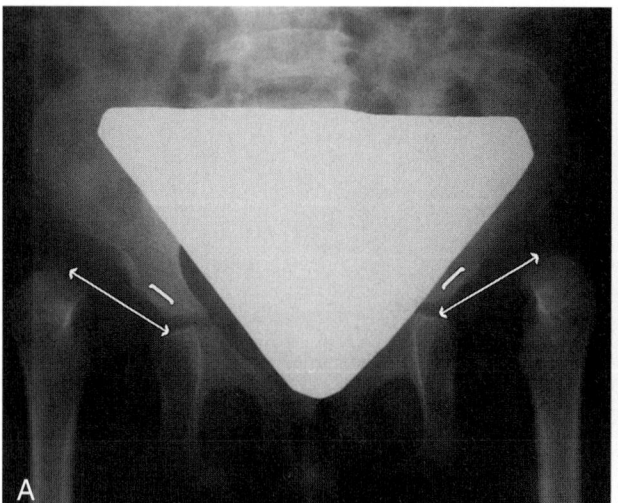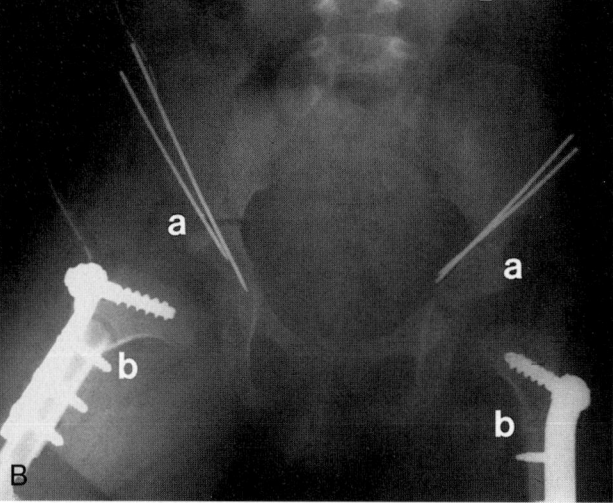

**Figure 73–19.** Bilateral pelvic and proximal femoral osteotomies in the management of developmental dysplasia of the hip. *A,* Preoperative frontal radiograph reveals bilateral and symmetrical dislocation of the femoral heads *(double-headed arrows),* with shallow and underdeveloped acetabula *(brackets). B,* Frontal radiograph in the immediate postoperative period demonstrates supra-acetabular (a) and subtrochanteric (b) varus osteotomy sites with internal fixation hardware and improved femoral-acetabular congruence.

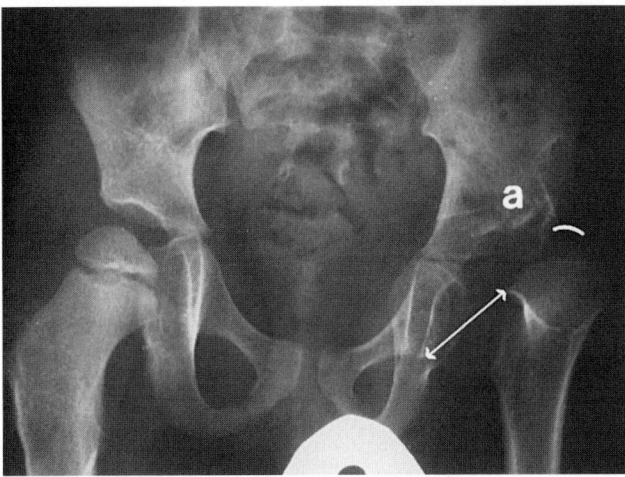

**Figure 73–20.** Recurrent unilateral developmental dysplasia of the hip after pelvic osteotomy. Frontal radiograph demonstrates lateral subluxation *(double-headed arrow)* and rotation of the left femur, which articulates with the lateral edge of the deformed acetabulum (a). Severely delayed ossification of the left femoral head *(bracket)* is evident.

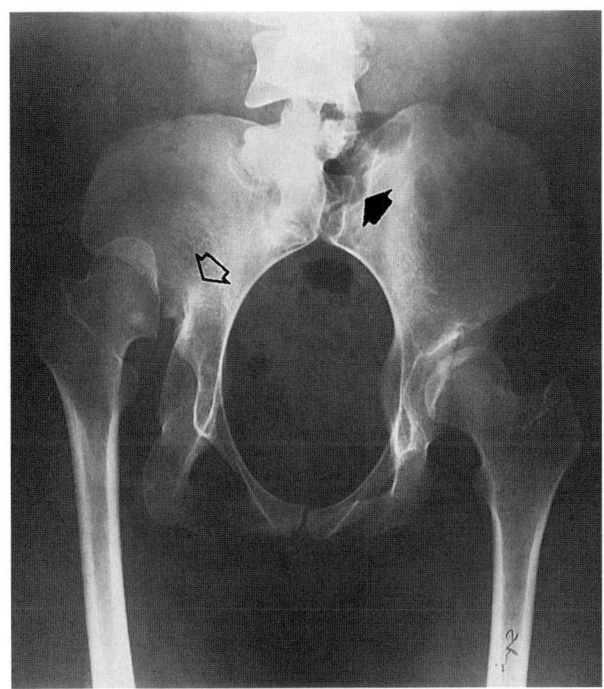

**Figure 73–21.** Developmental dysplasia of the hip associated with caudal regression syndrome. Frontal radiograph of the pelvis reveals sacral agenesis with hypoplasia of L5 *(solid arrow)* and dislocation of the right hip *(open arrow)*.

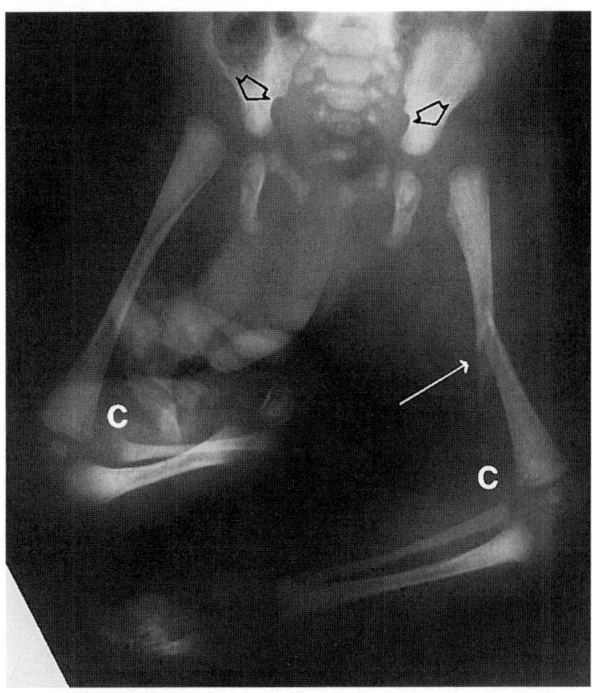

**Figure 73–22.** Developmental dysplasia of the hip associated with arthrogryposis multiplex congenita. Frontal radiograph reveals subluxation of both hips *(open arrows)*, bilateral lower extremity flexion contractures (C), and a fracture of the left femoral shaft *(white arrow)*.

## FURTHER READING

Azuma H, Taneda H, Igarashi H, et al: Preoperative and postoperative assessment of rotational acetabular osteotomy for dysplastic hips in children by three-dimensional surface reconstruction computed tomography imaging. J Pediatr Orthop 10:33, 1990.

Boal DKB, Schwentker EP: Assessment of congenital hip dislocation with real-time ultrasound: A pictorial essay. Clin Imaging 5:77, 1991.

Boal DKB, Schwenkter EP: The infant hip: Assessment with real-time US. Radiology 157:667, 1985.

Delaunay S, Dussault RG, Kaplan PA, et al: Radiographic measurements of dysplastic adult hips. Skeletal Radiol 26:75, 1997.

Eggli KD, King SH, Boal DK, et al: Low-dose CT of developmental dysplasia of the hip after reduction: Diagnostic accuracy and dosimetry. AJR Am J Roentgenol 163:1441, 1994.

Fisher R, OBrien TS, Davis KM: Magnetic resonance imaging in congenital dysplasia of the hip. J Pediatr Orthop 11:617, 1991.

Graf R: Classification of hip joint dysplasia by means of sonography. Arch Orthop Trauma Surg 102:248, 1984.

Graf R: The diagnosis of congenital hip-joint dislocation by the ultrasonic Combound treatment. Arch Orthop Trauma Surg 97:117, 1980.

Hansson G, Jacobsen S: Ultrasonography screening for developmental dysplasia of the hip joint. Acta Paediatr 86:913, 1997.

seen in Ehlers-Danlos syndrome. Among children with arthrogryposis multiplex congenita, recurrent dislocation of many joints or only mild hyperextensibility of the metacarpophalangeal, elbow, or knee joints may be observed. Conventional radiography reveals marked lateral femoral subluxation with relatively normal acetabula (Fig. 73–22).

Harcke HT, Lee MS, Sinning L, et al: Ossification center of the infant hip: Sonographic and radiographic correlation. AJR Am J Roentgenol 147:317, 1986.

Kawaguchi AT, Otsuka NY, Delgado ED, et al: Magnetic resonance arthrography in children with developmental hip dysplasia. Clin Orthop 374:235, 2000.

Lafferty CM, Sartoris DJ, Tyson R, et al: Acetabular alterations in untreated congenital dysplasia of the hip: Computed tomography with multiplanar reformation and three-dimensional analysis. J Comput Assist Tomogr 10:84, 1986.

Ozonoff MB: Pediatric Orthopedic Radiology, 2nd ed. Philadelphia, WB Saunders, 1992, p 164.

Severin E: Contribution to knowledge of congenital dislocation of the hip joint: Late results of closed reduction and arthrographic studies of recent cases. Acta Chir Scand Suppl 84(Suppl 63):1, 1941.

Suzuki S: Deformity of the pelvis in developmental dysplasia of the hip: Three-dimensional evaluation by means of magnetic resonance image. J Pediatr Orthop 15:812, 1995.

# CHAPTER 74

## Heritable Diseases of Connective Tissue, Epiphyseal Dysplasias, and Related Conditions

### Amy Beth Goldman

## SUMMARY OF KEY FEATURES

Included in this chapter are diseases of connective tissue synthesis and disorders of epiphyses. The radiographic changes are diverse, ranging from joint incongruity with secondary degeneration to soft tissue calcification or ossification with or without osseous overgrowth. Although there are clinical and laboratory features in some of these diseases that provide important clues to the correct diagnosis, an awareness of the radiographic alterations allows early and appropriate assessment in cases in which the diagnosis is more obscure.

## INTRODUCTION

Marfan's syndrome, homocystinuria, Ehlers-Danlos syndrome, and osteogenesis imperfecta are all inherited disorders of connective tissue. In varying degrees they involve the skin, ligaments, tendons, eyes, cardiovascular system, and skeleton. The joints of the extremities are not primarily affected by the connective tissue abnormalities. Incongruity resulting from skeletal abnormalities and repetitive subclinical trauma resulting from ligamentous laxity, however, combine to produce precocious osteoarthritis. Fibrodysplasia (myositis) ossificans progressiva is also a primary disorder of connective tissue. It affects the joints of the extremities by causing peripheral ossification, the reverse of the other disorders in this category. Fibrogenesis imperfecta ossium and pseudoxanthoma elasticum do not result in joint changes but are included in this category because of possible similarities in pathogenesis.

The epiphyseal dysplasias are a heterogeneous group of inherited diseases, all of which result in abnormalities of the epiphyseal ends of the bones. Alterations in the contours of the articular surfaces result in incongruity and eventually in premature degeneration of the hyaline cartilage. Degenerative joint disease or degenerative disc disease is often the clinical complaint that brings these patients to medical attention.

Macrodystrophia lipomatosa and the Klippel-Trénaunay-Weber syndrome are two of the causes of congenital macrodactyly. The digital enlargement may be accompanied by articular changes. In macrodystrophia lipomatosa, secondary degenerative changes are dramatic and render the involved digit useless. In Klippel-Trénaunay-Weber

syndrome, the articular changes result from an associated bleeding diathesis.

## MARFAN'S SYNDROME

Marfan's syndrome is a familial disorder of connective tissue that affects primarily the eye, the skeleton, and the cardiovascular system. It usually is an autosomal dominant condition, with a 20% to 30% incidence of spontaneous mutations.

### Pathology and Pathophysiology

The extreme phenotypic heterogeneity of Marfan's syndrome complicates a clinical diagnosis based exclusively on the major physical findings (ectopia lentis, aortic root dilatation or dissection, dural ectasia, and dolichostenomelia). Genetic linkage analysis studies have documented that one or more mutations in a locus (15q15-15q21) of the long arm of chromosome 15 (designated MFS1) result in Marfan's syndrome in both familial and sporadic cases.

Pathologic changes in the tunica media of the aorta are part of the characteristic findings of Marfan's syndrome. Accumulation of collagenous and mucoid material and fragmentation of elastic fibers predispose these patients to aortic dissection and rupture. The changes are most prominent in the ascending aorta, and early dilatation of the proximal portion frequently results in incompetence of the aortic valve and dilatation of the coronary sinuses. In addition to the abnormalities of the great vessels, fibromyxomatous changes may occur in the anulus, leaflets, and chordae tendineae of the aortic and mitral valves, resulting in left-sided cardiac insufficiency related to the "floppy valve" syndrome.

The bilateral ectopia lentis that occurs in a majority of patients with Marfan's syndrome is related to changes in the suspensory ligaments of the lens. The precise cause and pathologic features of the skeletal changes have yet to be elucidated.

### Clinical Findings

No sexual or racial predisposition is seen in Marfan's syndrome. Patients characteristically are tall and thin (>95th percentile by age and sex). The limbs are disproportionately elongated in relation to the trunk, and arm span can exceed height. The increased length of the extremities is most exaggerated distally, particularly in the hands and feet. This gives the patient the typical appearance of arachnodactyly. Chest deformities (pectus carinatum or excavatum) and scoliosis accentuate the limb-trunk discrepancy. Manifestations of ligamentous laxity, including angular deformities of the joints, pes planus, and scoliosis, frequently are evident. Blue sclerae and poor dentition are sometimes present. Intelligence is normal.

The most common ocular abnormalities are bilateral ectopia lentis and myopia, but strabismus and retinal detachments may also be present. The cardiac abnormalities are responsible for the shortened life expectancy of patients with Marfan's syndrome. Cystic medial necrosis of the aorta or pulmonary artery occurs in a majority of patients and predisposes to dissection and rupture. Aortic and mitral valve insufficiency may result from aortic dilatation, floppy valve syndrome, or both.

Certain clinical and radiographic tests are useful to identify the marfanoid phenotype. First, the "thumb sign," with protrusion of the thumb beyond the confines of a clenched fist, is used to reflect the narrow palm and long thumb that characterize arachnodactyly. Second is the segmental measurement, in which the distance from the pubic symphysis to the floor and the distance from the top of the head to the floor are measured and a ratio is calculated. In normal adults, this ratio is less than 0.85; in patients with Marfan's syndrome and dolichostenomelia, the ratio is increased. The third test is the metacarpal index, which is based on the lengths of the second through fifth metacarpal bones as measured on radiographs of the hand. The lengths of the metacarpal bones are then divided by the respective width of each diaphysis, and ratios are obtained. The four ratios are then averaged; this final ratio is increased in patients with Marfan's syndrome (normal is <8.8 in men and <9.4 in women).

## Radiographic Findings

In older children or adults with Marfan's syndrome, radiographs of the hands and feet demonstrate arachnodactyly, with elongation of both the metacarpal bones and the phalanges (Fig. 74–1). Frequently a 90-degree flexion deformity is present in one or both fifth digits of the hands, and a disproportionate elongation of the first digit of the foot may be seen. Other deformities in the hands and feet include hallux valgus, hammer toes, clubfeet, and calcaneal enthesophytes. Pes planus deformities and, rarely, carpal instability result from ligamentous laxity.

The extremities of patients with Marfan's syndrome demonstrate a marked diminution of soft tissue related to both muscular atrophy and sparse subcutaneous fat. The long bones are slender and gracile. Osteoporosis is not present. Joints are hypermobile, predisposing to deformities, dislocations, and joint instability. The hyperlaxity is also responsible for abnormal joint mechanics, repetitive subclinical trauma, and premature degenerative joint disease. Scoliosis occurs in 40% to 60% of patients with Marfan's syndrome, consisting of a major thoracic curve convex to the right (Fig. 74–2). Dural ectasia is observed on computed tomography (CT) or magnetic resonance (MR) imaging studies in two thirds of patients, with scalloping of the posterior aspects of one or more vertebral bodies. A rare but serious complication is atlantoaxial subluxation.

Protrusio acetabuli deformities, associated with a decreased range of motion, have been described. The cause of this finding is unclear, but it may relate to weakened acetabular bone. Chest deformities include asymmetry with pectus excavatum or carinatum resulting from elongation of the ribs.

The radiographic differential diagnosis includes other syndromes associated with marfanoid skeletal changes.

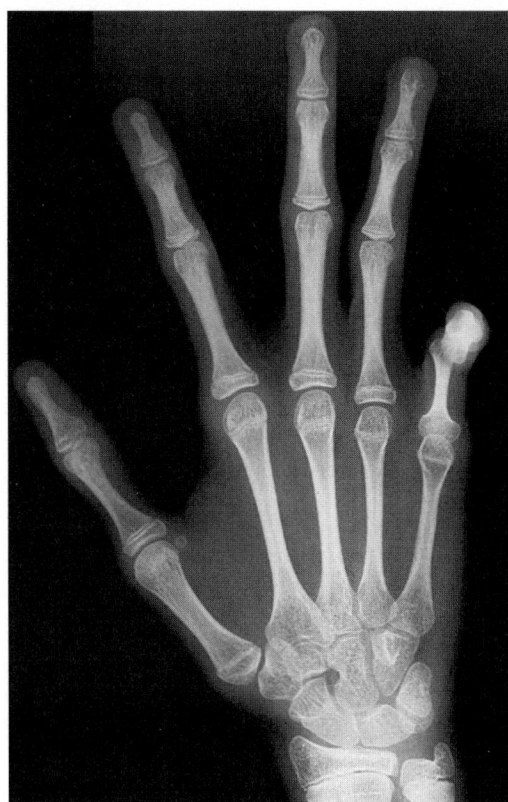

**Figure 74–1.** Marfan's syndrome. Frontal view of hand reveals a 90-degree flexion contracture of the fifth digit and arachnodactyly.

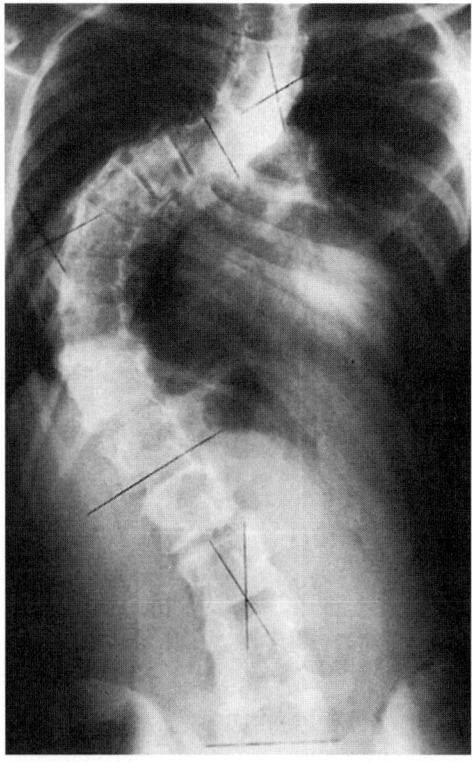

**Figure 74–2.** Marfan's syndrome: scoliosis. The radiographic appearance is indistinguishable from that of idiopathic scoliosis.

Homocystinuria, a congenital disorder of methionine metabolism, is characterized by arachnodactyly, scoliosis, sternal deformities, and ligamentous laxity. Patients are mentally retarded, however, and the skeleton is osteoporotic. Congenital contractural arachnodactyly, another inherited disorder of connective tissue, is also characterized by long, thin limbs; scoliosis; and dolichostenomelia. The absence of eye and cardiac changes and the presence of joint contractures and deformed ears can distinguish the two entities. Slowly progressive myopathies, particularly nemaline myopathy, constitute another possibility. Muscle biopsies and electromyographic studies in these patients are positive for primary abnormalities of the muscle fibers. Multiple endocrine neoplasia syndromes are also associated with marfanoid features, as is Ehlers-Danlos syndrome.

## HOMOCYSTINURIA

Homocystinuria encompasses a group of disorders characterized by inborn errors in methionine metabolism and excessive homocysteine in body fluids. Three different autosomal recessive genetic enzymatic defects that lead to disturbances in homocysteine homeostasis have been described, all of which result in neurologic, ocular, and skeletal abnormalities, as well as premature occlusive vascular disease.

### Pathology and Pathophysiology

Homocystinuria is associated with a defect in collagen synthesis. Arterial and venous thromboses complicate the course of homocystinuria. This phenomenon is likely the result of an increase in platelet "stickiness." The abnormal aggregation of platelets is reported to result from changes in the vessel walls and from the presence of unstable collagen. As in Marfan's syndrome, cystic medial necrosis and fragmentation of elastic fibers are found in the aortas of patients with homocystinuria. In contrast to Marfan's syndrome, however, aortic dissections are not a characteristic feature of homocystinuria. Thromboembolic phenomena are the most common cause of death in patients with homocystinuria.

Mental retardation, seizures, and even schizophrenia may be seen; however, the exact cause of the central nervous system abnormalities is not yet known. The most characteristic ocular abnormality of homocystinuria is bilateral dislocation of the lens.

### Clinical Findings

Homocystinuria occurs most commonly in northern Europeans from Sweden, Germany, the Netherlands, England, Ireland, and Scotland. Patients appear normal at birth and during infancy, with the sole clinical finding being irritability. Even in infants, however, the urine contains increased levels of homocystine and, as in adults, the cyanide nitroprusside test produces a red-purple color.

In early childhood, motor development slows or even regresses. Patients with homocystinuria tend to have thin skin with large pores and prominent venous markings. Striae occur over the buttocks and shoulders. A malar flush is frequently present, and "cigarette paper" scars occur with minor trauma. Hair is thin and sparse, and hair color is abnormal, possibly related to decreased activity of tyrosine (a copper-containing enzyme). A high, arched palate ("gothic" palate) and poor dentition are characteristic. The most frequent physical finding is bilateral lens dislocations, which may be present at birth. Ectopia lentis is present in 90% of untreated patients at 10 years of age and is most often bilateral. The degree of mental retardation varies and may be modified by therapy.

Spontaneous venous and arterial thromboses complicate the clinical course of homocystinuria and are often life threatening. Although it is the main cause of morbidity, vascular thrombosis is rarely the presenting abnormality. Common sites of arterial clotting are the intermediate-sized vessels, including the coronary, renal, and carotid arteries and the other major branches of the aorta. Venous thromboses frequently involve the mesenteric vessels, the vena cava, the iliac vessels, and the pulmonary veins. Surgery may precipitate a major vascular accident.

Between 25% and 60% of patients with homocystinuria have skeletal abnormalities that resemble those of Marfan's syndrome. Patients are tall, with disproportionately long extremities, scoliosis, pectus excavatum, and joint laxity. Several clinical findings differentiate these two entities, however. First, mental retardation, malar flush, and vascular thromboses are not found in Marfan's syndrome. Second, although both entities are characterized by bilateral lens dislocations, this sign can be detected in infancy in patients with homocystinuria. Third, the lens tends to dislocate downward in cases of homocystinuria and upward in Marfan's syndrome. Fourth, in Marfan's syndrome, contractures occur only in the fifth digits of the hands, whereas in homocystinuria, contractures occur in multiple digits as well as in the elbows and knees. Fifth, the primary life-endangering vascular changes in Marfan's syndrome are related to the aorta and its origin, whereas in homocystinuria, sudden death is more commonly the result of thromboembolic phenomena or rupture of medium-sized vessels. Last, unlike in Marfan's syndrome, positive and specific laboratory findings are present in homocystinuria. The plasma levels of homocysteine, homocystine, and methionine are all elevated, and the urine contains abnormal amounts of homocysteine.

### Radiographic Findings

Skeletal changes occur gradually during childhood. The skull can show a variety of changes, including enlargement of the sinuses, widening of the diploic space, extensive dural calcification, or prognathism. Examination of the spine early in childhood can reveal generalized osteoporosis and scoliosis (Fig. 74–3). The vertebral bodies have an increased anteroposterior diameter and may be biconcave in shape. Compression fractures are frequent. Posterior scalloping of the vertebral bodies and premature degenerative disc disease have also been described.

Changes in the extremities include dolichostenomelia, osteoporosis, and multiple growth recovery lines (Fig.

74–4). Frequently seen deformities include flattening of the epiphyses (especially about the knees and hips) and broad metaphyses. A characteristic stippled appearance can occur in the growth plates of the distal radii and ulnae, which contain punctate areas of ossification. Characteristic changes in the hands include arachnodactyly.

The major radiographic differential diagnosis of homocystinuria is Marfan's syndrome. The presence of osteoporosis, metaphyseal flaring, and multiple contractures should distinguish the radiographic appearance of dolichostenomelia in a patient with homocystinuria from that in a patient with Marfan's syndrome.

## EHLERS-DANLOS SYNDROME

Ehlers-Danlos syndrome is a hereditary disorder of connective tissue characterized by three major clinical abnormalities: joint hypermobility, skin bruising and elasticity, and potentially life-threatening vascular abnormalities. The eye, gastrointestinal tract, bronchopulmonary tree, genitourinary system, and cardiovascular system may also be affected by this primary defect in mesenchyme.

Ehlers-Danlos syndrome is not a single entity but is currently classified as a group of 10 syndromes associated with abnormal genes, all concerning the formation of collagen. Collagen synthesis involves genetic heterogenicity, amino acid chain heterogeneity, and multiple genes. The disorders encompassed by Ehlers-Danlos syndrome are almost as protean as the 15 genetic sites so far found in the existent subgroups.

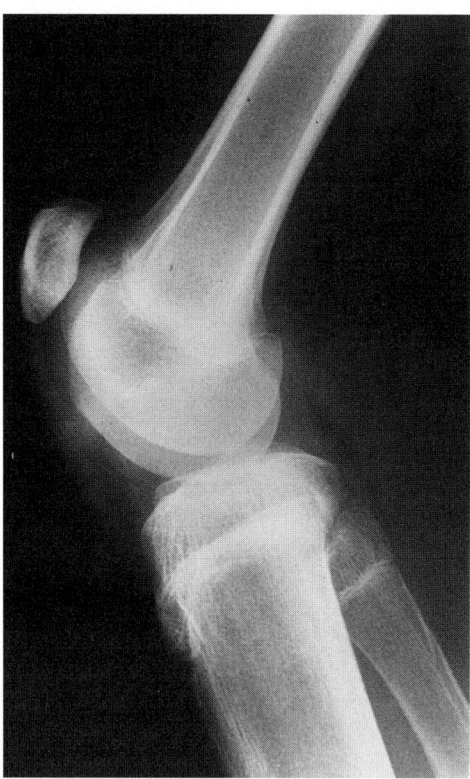

**Figure 74–4.** Homocystinuria. Lateral view of the knee demonstrates an elongated limb and patella alta. The bones are osteoporotic, and the metaphyses are flared. Multiple growth recovery lines are present, although they are not well shown here.

### Pathology and Pathophysiology

Ehlers-Danlos syndrome is primarily a disorder of collagen synthesis. Microscopic and ultrastructural studies have reported abnormal organization and interweaving of collagen bundles and abnormal shortening of the collagen chains. At least 12 different types of collagen, coded by a minimum of 20 genes, have now been identified.

The mesenchymal defect in the various types of Ehlers-Danlos syndrome involves the joint capsules, the ligaments, and the paravertebral supporting tissues. No primary osseous abnormality has been reported in clinical studies of this syndrome. However, immunofluorescent investigations have shown a defect in tetracycline uptake, substantiating the theory of a primary abnormality in collagen production.

### Clinical Findings

The diagnosis of Ehlers-Danlos syndrome continues to rest on the clinical triad of skin fragility, hyperelasticity of joints, and vascular fragility. Molluscoid tumors on pressure points and subcutaneous nodules that form at sites of fatty degeneration are also considered diagnostic criteria. Clinical expression is extremely variable, however; Ehlers-Danlos syndrome can represent a life-threatening disease or a mild disorder of mesenchymal tissues.

Ehlers-Danlos syndrome occurs most frequently in white people of European origin. A male predominance

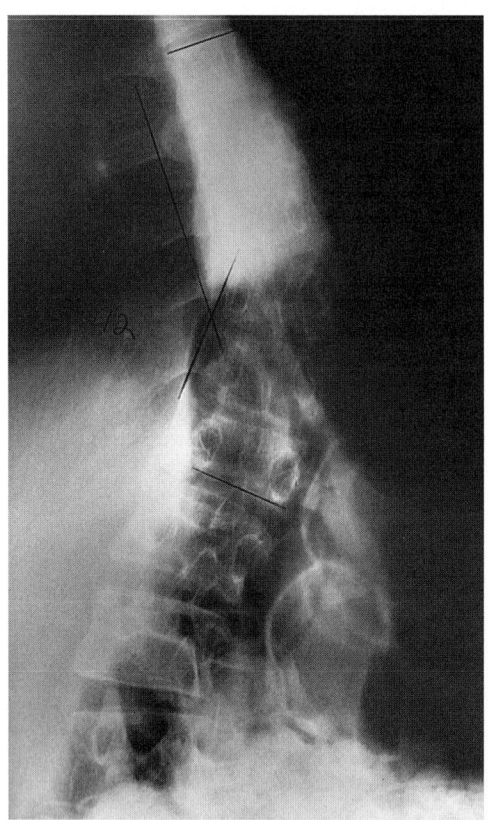

**Figure 74–3.** Homocystinuria. Scoliosis and osteoporosis are seen in the spine of a patient with homocystinuria.

is seen, and many patients are tall. Patients affected with Ehlers-Danlos syndrome walk with a characteristic gait that results from hyperextension of the hips to compensate for genu recurvatum deformities. The skin is velvety, thin, and hyperelastic. It can be raised in high folds and, unlike in cases of cutis laxa, it retracts spontaneously. The skin also is easily bruised and tends to split with minor trauma. Scars are large and are covered by thin skin. The appearance of these scars has been compared to "cigarette paper." Repeated hemorrhage results in a purple discoloration of the pretibial areas.

The passive and active hypermobility of joints in Ehlers-Danlos syndrome has provided many a circus with an "India rubber man." Patients are able to touch their thumbs to their forearms or their little fingers to the dorsum of the hand, passively dorsiflex their fifth fingers beyond 90 degrees, hyperextend their elbows beyond 10 degrees, and hyperextend their knees beyond 10 degrees (recurvatum). Some patients also can touch the tip of the nose with the tongue. Dislocations are frequent, and they correlate with the degree of laxity.

The fragility of the vessel walls and lack of tamponade can result in bleeding from the gastrointestinal tract, the bronchopulmonary tree, or the gums. Dissecting aneurysms of the aorta and spontaneous ruptures of the large vessels may occur and frequently result in death. Raynaud's phenomenon has also been reported. Ocular abnormalities involve the cornea, sclera, fundus, and suspensory mechanism of the lens. Reported changes include strabismus, ectopia lentis, and retinal detachment. Muscle weakness and easy fatigability are also features of Ehlers-Danlos syndrome.

### Radiographic Findings

Calcification of fatty spherules produces multiple dense subcutaneous lesions that are visible on radiographs. They occur primarily in the forearms, shins, and extensor surfaces of the extremities and measure 2 to 8 mm in diameter. These calcifications usually have a dense rim and resemble phleboliths. An increased frequency of heterotopic ossification is seen in patients with Ehlers-Danlos syndrome. Such ossification occurs primarily adjacent to the hips, extending from the inferior iliac spines to the greater trochanters.

Joint findings occur in 20% of patients with Ehlers-Danlos syndrome and include persistent effusions or hemarthroses (Fig. 74–5). The most common sites of joint involvement are the knee and ankle. The fluid is thought to result from ligamentous and capsular laxity, which produces repetitive subclinical trauma. Joint findings are variable but are dominated by ligamentous laxity resulting in varus or valgus deformities or dislocations and subluxations (Fig. 74–6), which complicate the clinical course. The most frequent sites of dislocation are the digits, glenohumeral joints, patellofemoral joints, temporomandibular joints, radial heads, and sternoclavicular and acromioclavicular joints. The prevalence of degenerative changes correlates with the severity of the laxity. Eventually contractures can occur.

The thorax can be asymmetrical, with pectus carinatum. A kyphoscoliosis is often present at the thoracolum-

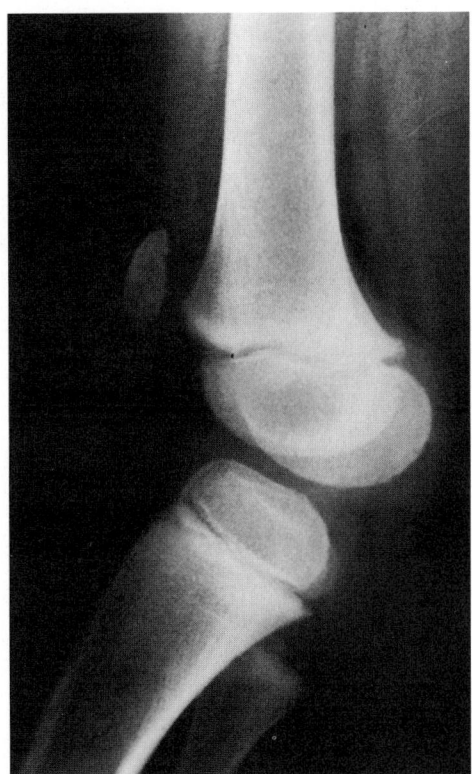

**Figure 74–5.** Ehlers-Danlos syndrome. Lateral view of the knee shows fibular head dislocation and genu recurvatum deformity.

bar junction and is accompanied by decreased bone density. Examination of the spine in early childhood can reveal generalized decreased bone density and scoliosis. The scoliosis is a marfanoid type, with scalloping of the posterior walls of the vertebral bodies caused by dural ectasia and bone with the abnormal "structure" of collagen. Severe spondylolysis and spondylolisthesis have also been reported in association with the scoliosis of Ehlers-Danlos syndrome (Fig. 74–7).

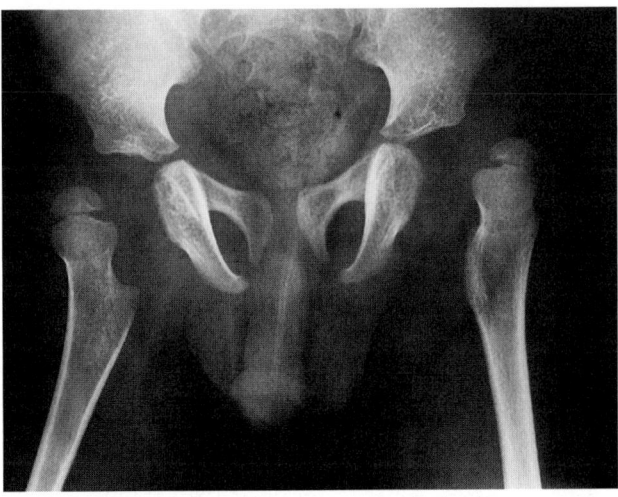

**Figure 74–6.** Ehlers-Danlos syndrome. Bilateral hip dislocations are seen.

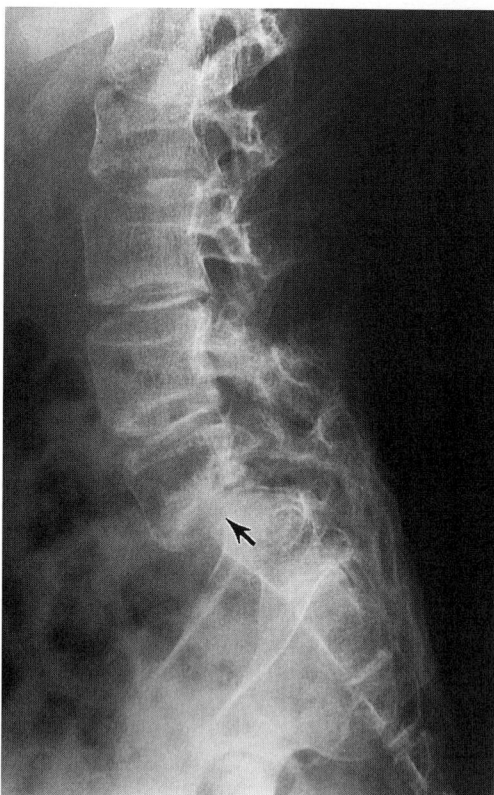

**Figure 74–7.** Ehlers-Danlos syndrome. Lateral view of the lumbar spine shows spondylolysis and spondylolisthesis *(arrow)*. Posterior scalloping of the vertebral bodies is evident.

The radiographic differential diagnosis of joint laxity includes Marfan's syndrome, Larsen's syndrome, cachexia, Down's syndrome, and neuromuscular disorders. The soft tissue calcifications of Ehlers-Danlos syndrome may be mistaken for cysticercosis, vascular tumors, phleboliths, or collagen diseases.

Type IX Ehlers-Danlos syndrome, unlike the other clinical categories, is associated with unique skeletal abnormalities, including horn-shaped excrescences on the occipital bone of the skull and deformed clavicles. The shafts of the long bones are osteopenic and bowed and have wavy, thin cortices.

## OSTEOGENESIS IMPERFECTA

Osteogenesis imperfecta is an inherited disorder of connective tissue that affects the skeleton, ligaments, skin, sclerae, and dentin. In the majority of patients, mutations in one of the two genetic loci that encode type I collagen have been proved. The resultant genetic disorder can be expressed by either abnormal synthesis (quantity) or abnormal structure (quality) of procollagen I. Eighty-five percent of genotypes are heterozygous for an autosomal dominant mutation.

The four major clinical criteria are (1) osteoporosis with abnormal fragility of the skeleton, (2) blue sclerae, (3) dentinogenesis imperfecta, and (4) premature otosclerosis. The presence of two of these abnormalities con-

firms the diagnosis. Other features are ligamentous laxity, episodic diaphoresis with abnormal temperature regulation, easy bruising, constipation, hyperplastic scars, premature vascular calcifications, and inappropriate euphoria.

Classically, osteogenesis imperfecta was subclassified into two syndromes, on the basis of the severity of the skeletal findings: the congenita form, which has a high infant mortality rate, and the tarda form, which is associated with a normal life expectancy. More recent classification schemes divide osteogenesis imperfecta into four types. Type I is both the most common and the mildest phenotype of the disease. Osseous fragility results in an increased number of fractures but not dwarfing or bowing deformities. Type II is the lethal form of osteogenesis imperfecta. Severe osseous fragility results in dwarfing and fractures that occur in utero. Type III is a rare phenotype of osteogenesis imperfecta, and in more than two thirds of cases, fractures are present at birth. Osseous fragility is severe, and patients with type III who survive exhibit the most dramatic dwarfing. Type IV osteogenesis imperfecta has the most variable osseous findings, and patients can range in height from normal to severely dwarfed. Even among these four types, considerable genetic, biochemical, and clinical variability is seen.

## Pathology and Pathophysiology

Osteogenesis imperfecta is an inherited connective tissue syndrome associated clinically with bone fragility and ligamentous laxity and genetically and biochemically with defects (quantitative, qualitative, or both) in fibrillar type I collagen synthesis. Type I collagen composes 90% of the organic matrix of bone. The clinical defects in osteogenesis imperfecta involve tissues with high type I collagen content (bones, ligaments, tendons, fasciae, sclerae, and teeth).

The sclerae are thin and, like the other connective tissues, contain abnormal collagen. The blue translucency results from the brown choroid shining through the abnormal outer layer. The exact reason for premature otosclerosis in osteogenesis imperfecta is unknown.

## Clinical Findings

Osteogenesis imperfecta occurs in all races with an equal sex distribution. The severe forms (10% of cases) have high intrauterine and infant mortality rates caused by respiratory complications resulting from thoracic deformities or intracerebral hemorrhage. In most cases the diagnosis is made at birth or, with the use of ultrasonography, in utero.

Facial characteristics include temporal bulging, flattening of the features, micrognathia, and hypertelorism. Blue sclerae occur in more than 90% of cases. A small ring of sclera surrounding the cornea can retain a normal white color and is called a Saturn's ring or arcus senilis. Abnormal dentition with opalescent blue-gray or brown teeth is termed dentinogenesis imperfecta. It is not as common as blue sclerae, but it is highly specific for osteogenesis imperfecta.

Growth retardation occurs in most cases, and severely affected persons are dwarfed, with short, bowed long bones. The limbs are more involved than the trunk, and the lower extremities are more shortened than the upper extremities. Skeletal deformities include kyphoscoliosis and bowing of the long bones, which exacerbates the limb-trunk discrepancy. The spinal deformities can result in pain, paresthesias, difficulty ambulating, and, in severe congenita-type cases, respiratory failure or paraplegia.

Multiple fractures, resulting from normal daily activities or minor trauma, are the predominant clinical finding in osteogenesis imperfecta. In the severe congenita-type, fractures occur even in the protected environment of the uterus. The frequency of pathologic fractures appears to decrease after puberty.

Otosclerosis can occur before age 40 years. Nerve conduction deafness occurs in 10% of cases, with associated vertigo and tinnitus. As in other hereditary disorders of collagen synthesis, the clinical abnormalities of osteogenesis imperfecta include thin skin, a tendency to form hyperplastic scars, premature vascular calcifications, joint laxity, a high frequency of hernias, and platelet abnormalities. Ligamentous laxity can also result in hypermobile joints, but no increase in the prevalence of dislocations has been reported. Bleeding likewise results from capillary fragility, as it does in Ehlers-Danlos syndrome, but it tends to be less severe in osteogenesis imperfecta. In osteogenesis imperfecta, basilar impression is associated with platybasia or the "tam-o'-shanter" skull.

## Radiographic Findings

The most characteristic radiographic finding of osteogenesis imperfecta is a diffuse decrease in osseous density (Fig. 74–8) that involves the axial and appendicular portions of the skeleton equally. The degree of osteopenia is highly variable, however, and at the mildest end of the spectrum patients can appear to have normal bone density on radiographs.

On the basis of the radiographic appearance of the extremities, patients with osteogenesis imperfecta can be divided into three groups. The first group encompasses those with thin, gracile bones (see Fig. 74–8). This is the most common expression of the disease and includes most patients with type I disease and mildly affected patients with type IV disease. The second group includes those patients with short, thick limbs (Fig. 74–9). This type of radiographic appearance occurs in patients with type II or III disease. As with congenital bowing of the extremities, it is usually associated with severe micromelia and a poor prognosis. Third, and least common, is a group of patients with cystic changes in the extremities (Fig. 74–10). These changes occur in severely affected persons, and the radiographic findings are characterized by flared metaphyses that are hyperlucent and traversed by a honeycomb of coarse trabeculae.

The fractures that complicate the course of osteogenesis imperfecta occur most frequently in the lower extremities and are usually transverse. Avulsion injuries are also common and result from normal muscle pull. Micromelia and bowing deformities are the sequelae of multiple telescoping fractures, which begin to occur during gestation. Fracture healing is usually normal, but tumoral callus and pseudarthroses may occur (Fig. 74–11).

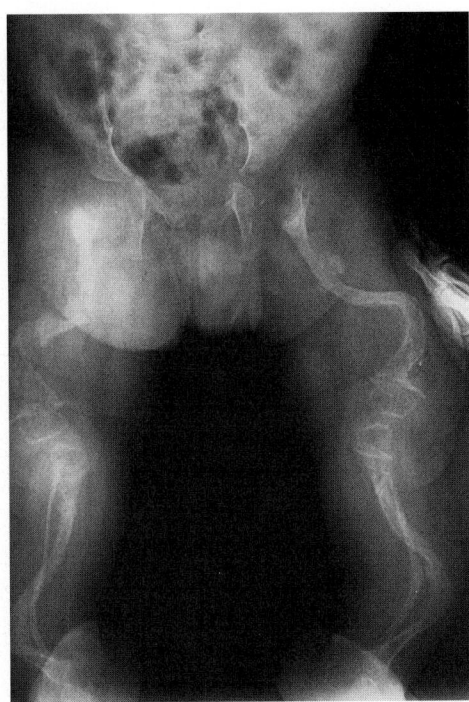

**Figure 74–8.** Osteogenesis imperfecta. Anteroposterior view of pelvis and lower extremities reveals a decrease in osseous density associated with thin, gracile long bones. Multiple fractures in various stages of healing are present. The long bones are bowed.

In children with severe osteogenesis imperfecta, the metaphyses or epiphyses of the long bones may contain multiple scalloped, radiolucent areas with sclerotic margins, referred to as popcorn calcifications (Fig. 74–12).

Radiographs of the skull demonstrate enlargement of the frontal and mastoid sinuses and wormian bones (Fig. 74–13). Platybasia, with or without basilar impression, is a frequent deformity. Spinal studies show flattening of the vertebral bodies, which are either biconcave or wedge shaped anteriorly (see Fig. 74–13). Severe kyphoscoliosis occurs in approximately 40% of patients with osteogenesis imperfecta. The spinal changes are painful and interfere with sitting and ambulation. The pelvis is narrowed and often triradiate in shape, and compression fractures may be present. Protrusion deformities of the acetabula and shepherd's crook deformities of the femora may be present (Fig. 74–14).

The differential diagnosis of osteogenesis imperfecta in infancy includes other entities associated with multiple fractures, such as child abuse syndrome, congenital indifference to pain, scurvy, and Menkes' kinky-hair syndrome. Hypophosphatasia is associated with lucent bones and bowing deformities of the extremities, but the metaphyseal changes of rickets are also present, distinguishing it from osteogenesis imperfecta. The radiographic findings of idiopathic juvenile osteoporosis and Cushing's disease may be indistinguishable from those of osteogenesis imperfecta, and in these instances, clinical correlation is necessary.

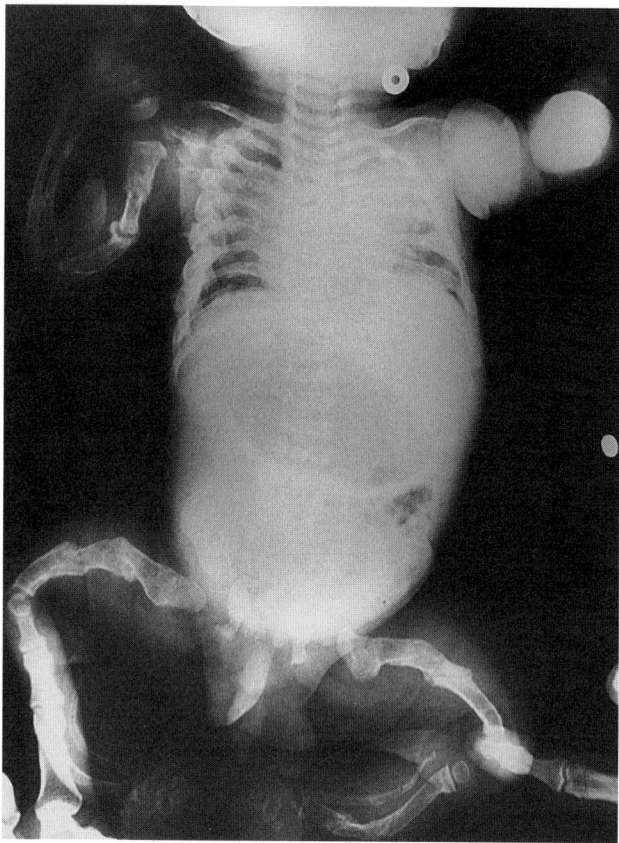

**Figure 74–9.** Osteogenesis imperfecta. Anteroposterior view of the skeleton shows a decrease in osseous density associated with short, thick bones and telescoping fractures. Both the upper and the lower extremities are bowed. Fractures are seen in all the long bones and ribs.

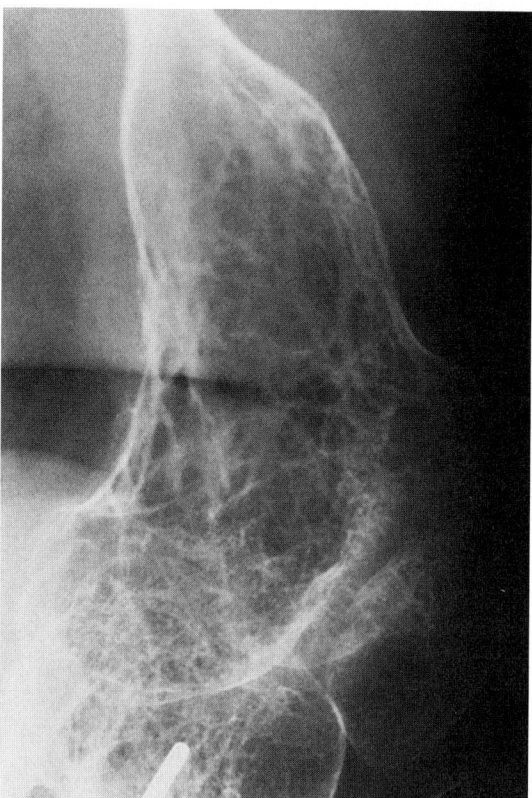

**Figure 74–10.** Osteogenesis imperfecta. Lateral view of the knee demonstrates the rare cystic type of disease. The metaphyses are flared and honeycombed by thick, coarse trabeculae.

## FIBRODYSPLASIA (MYOSITIS) OSSIFICANS PROGRESSIVA

Fibrodysplasia ossificans progressiva is a hereditary disorder characterized by symmetrical congenital anomalies of the great toes and thumbs and progressive chondrogenesis and heterotopic ossification of striated muscles, tendons, ligaments, fasciae, aponeuroses, and occasionally skin. The pattern of transmission is autosomal dominant; however, many cases are the result of spontaneous mutation. The formation of bone is postnatal; the digital anomalies are present at birth.

### Pathology and Pathophysiology

The pathologic abnormalities that characterize the individual lesions are similar but not identical to those of myositis ossificans circumscripta. Mesenchymal proliferation results in the formation of multifocal interconnecting nodules capable of accepting the deposition of calcium salts. Gradually, the nodules coalesce to form large masses, and the abnormal tissue is transformed into membranous bone. Various stages of bone formation are present simultaneously, and in some areas, cartilage formation precedes ossification.

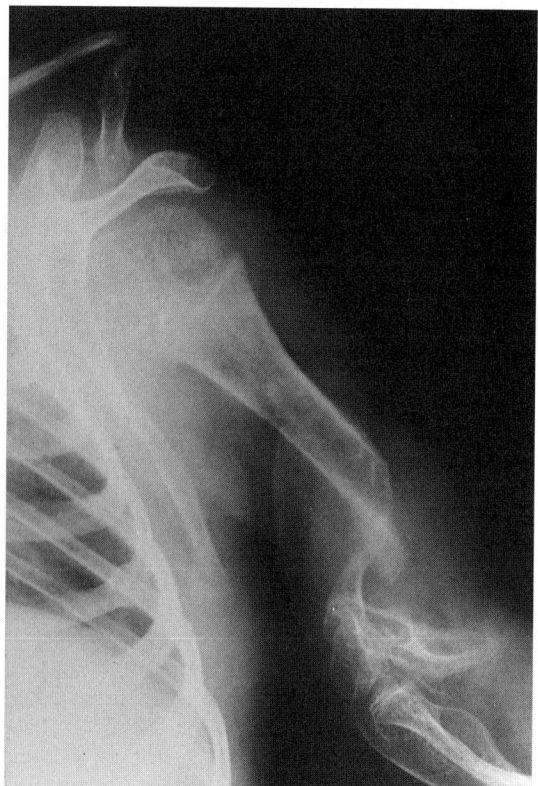

**Figure 74–11.** Osteogenesis imperfecta. Pseudarthroses of the humerus and clavicle complicate fractures.

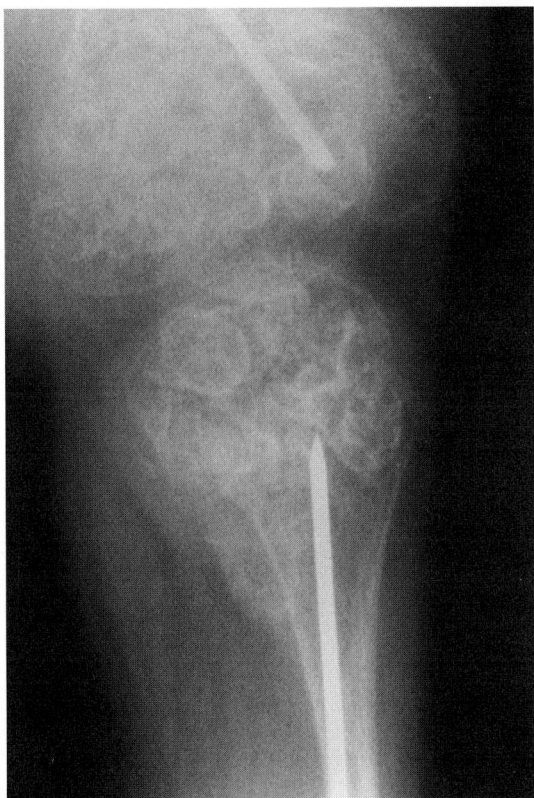

**Figure 74–12.** Osteogenesis imperfecta. Oblique view of the knee shows popcorn calcifications. These lucent areas with sclerotic margins are associated with the absence of a normal horizontal growth plate and severe growth retardation. Previous intramedullary rods have been placed.

In fibrodysplasia ossificans progressiva, the first spicules of bone can appear in the center of the nodules, which is the opposite of the peripheral pattern of ossification (zonal phenomenon) that characterizes myositis

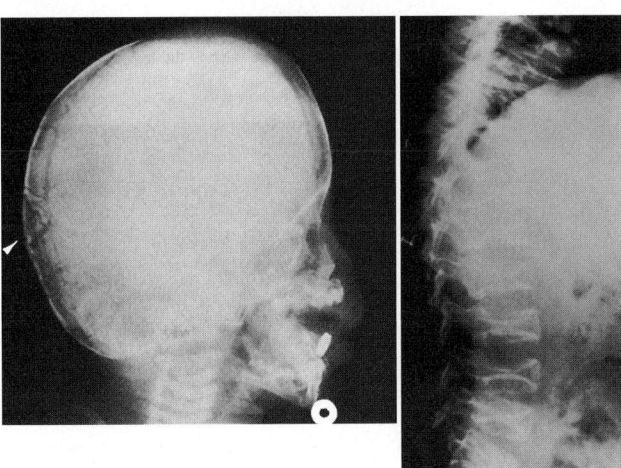

**Figure 74–13.** Osteogenesis imperfecta. *A,* Lateral view of the skull shows decreased osseous density, thinning of both tables, and multiple wormian bones *(arrowhead)*. *B,* In a different patient, lateral view of the spine shows both biconcave and wedged vertebral bodies.

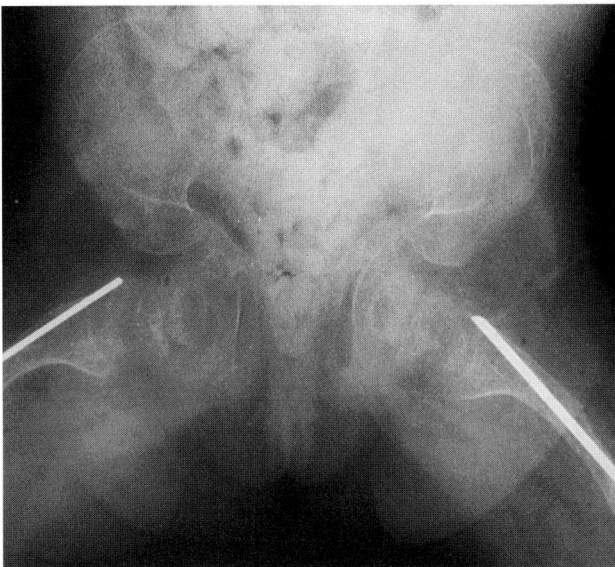

**Figure 74–14.** Osteogenesis imperfecta. Anteroposterior view of the pelvis shows a triradiate shape and protrusion acetabuli deformities. Previous intramedullary rods have been placed.

ossificans circumscripta. Eventually, the entire muscle or muscle group is replaced by columns or plates of lamellar bone, which, like normal bone, contains hematopoietic elements and adipose tissue.

## Clinical Findings

Fibrodysplasia ossificans progressiva is a rare disease. Although the onset of symptoms is usually in the first decade of life (mean age, 3 years), ossification may rarely be present at birth. The most frequent presenting symptom is torticollis resulting from a painful, doughy mass in the sternocleidomastoid muscle. The disease usually progresses from the shoulder girdle to the upper arms, spine, and pelvis. The distal portions of the extremities are involved late in the course of the disease.

Ossification proceeds in a cranial to a caudal direction, from dorsal to ventral, and from axial to appendicular sites. The heart, diaphragm, larynx, tongue, and sphincters are spared, as are all smooth muscle structures. The natural history of fibrodysplasia ossificans progressiva is one of erratic remissions and exacerbations. Quiescent periods may last for years, or the course may be relentless. Joint ankylosis occurs as a result of ossification of the surrounding soft tissues, not due to primary synovial or cartilaginous abnormalities. Fusion of the hips is usually present by the third decade of life, leaving the patient wheelchair bound.

Simple surgical removal of the ectopic bone does little to restore motion. Indeed, the initial lesion recurs, with additional ossification in the scar tissue. Operative intervention or even biopsy has been blamed for accelerating the disease process. Early death is inevitable. It may occur secondary to respiratory failure from constriction of the chest wall and, in many cases, pneumonia.

## Radiographic Findings

Digital abnormalities are present at birth, are symmetrical, and, in the vast majority of cases, precede the soft tissue ossification. The most common type of abnormality is a hallux valgus deformity associated with microdactyly of the first toes, with hypoplasia or synostosis of the phalanges, or with both (Fig. 74–15). The proximal phalanges of the great toes have an abnormal contour (broad and square) and are often fused to the distal phalanges. The first metatarsals are also abnormal, and changes range from rounding of the distal articular surface to a hypoplastic cylindrical ossification center with no epiphysis. In addition to anomalies of the great toes, in almost half of cases the middle phalanx of the fifth digit is small and, in childhood, has an accessory epiphysis. Similar abnormalities are seen in the hand. If the thumbs are involved, the anomalies are less severe than in the toes, and the most common findings are short first metacarpal bones. Other congenital anomalies are hallux valgus deformities, broad femoral necks, bilateral thickening of the medial cortices of the tibias, an abnormal carrying angle at the elbow, and an increased frequency of spina bifida.

The radiographic findings in the individual locations are similar to those seen in the traumatic form of myositis ossificans. The first radiographic finding is a soft tissue mass. The lesion gradually shrinks in size and ossifies. Mineralization often is evident in 3 to 4 weeks. The final appearance of the lesion may be that of a cylindrical column of solid new bone replacing the entire muscle of the neck or extremities (Fig. 74–16). Pseudarthroses can occur within these masses of bone. These lucent areas are attributed to minor trauma. The zonal phenomenon, a characteristic feature of myositis ossificans circumscripta, is not present in progressiva cases. Involvement of the insertions of fasciae, ligaments, and tendons produces pseudoexostoses (not true osteochondromas), which arise from the metaphyses of the long bones, the occiput, and the calcaneus (Fig. 74–17).

Abnormalities in the spine typically consist of ossification of the soft tissues, followed by fusion of the posterior elements and, finally, in adult patients, fusion of the vertebral bodies (Fig. 74–18). Secondary to soft tissue ossification and loss of motion of the posterior elements, the intervertebral discs become hypoplastic and calcified, and the anterior aspects of the vertebral bodies flatten. The findings can mimic the appearance of ankylosing spondylitis (Fig. 74–19). In the cervical spine, the canal appears wide and the pedicles are elongated. These findings result from the small size of the vertebral bodies (particularly their anteroposterior diameters), which stopped growing when motion ceased.

The radiographic differential diagnosis includes the causes of metastatic calcifications (e.g., idiopathic calcinosis universalis, dermatomyositis, idiopathic tumoral calcinosis, disorders of calcium metabolism). In all these conditions, the dense lesions remain calcific and do not mature into trabecular bone. Systemic diseases related to

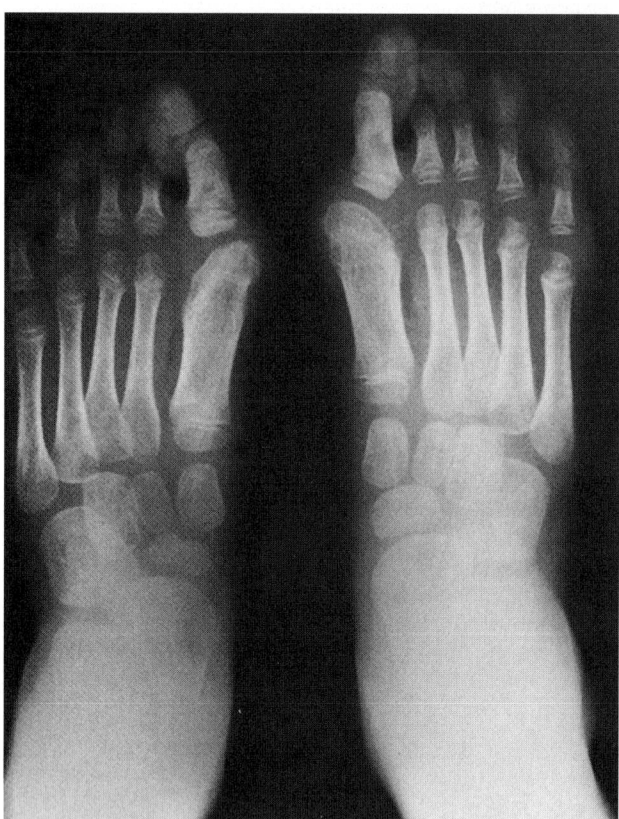

**Figure 74–15.** Fibrodysplasia ossificans progressiva. Anteroposterior view of both feet shows the characteristic congenital anomalies of the first digits.

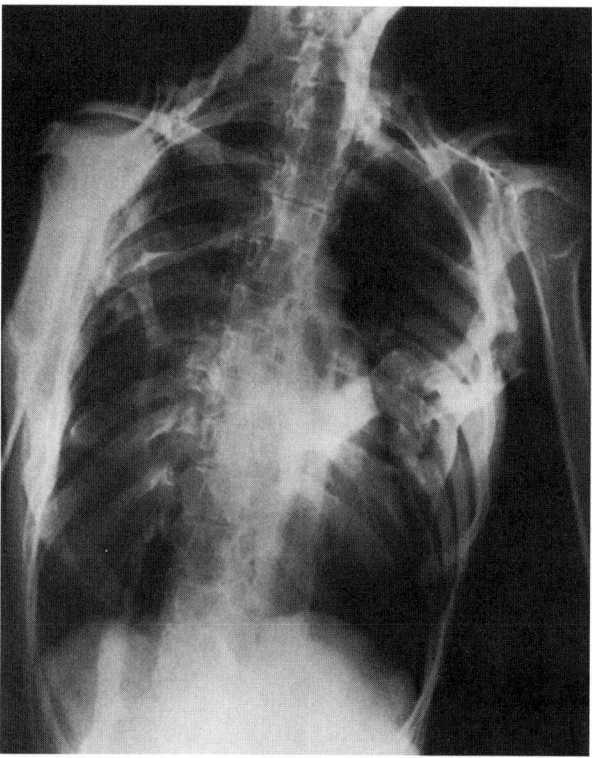

**Figure 74–16.** Fibrodysplasia ossificans progressiva. Anteroposterior view of the thorax shows the early distribution of soft tissue ossification: shoulders, neck, and cervical spine.

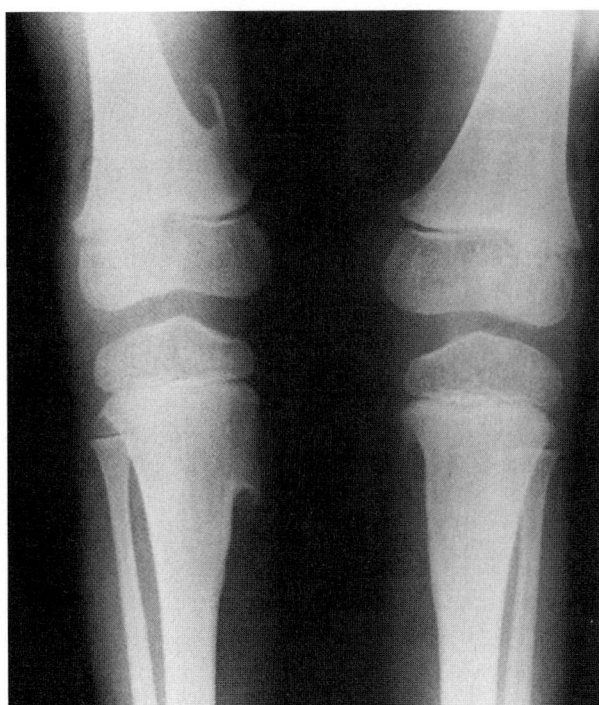

**Figure 74–17.** Fibrodysplasia ossificans progressiva. Ossification of ligamentous insertions has resulted in metaphyseal "exostoses."

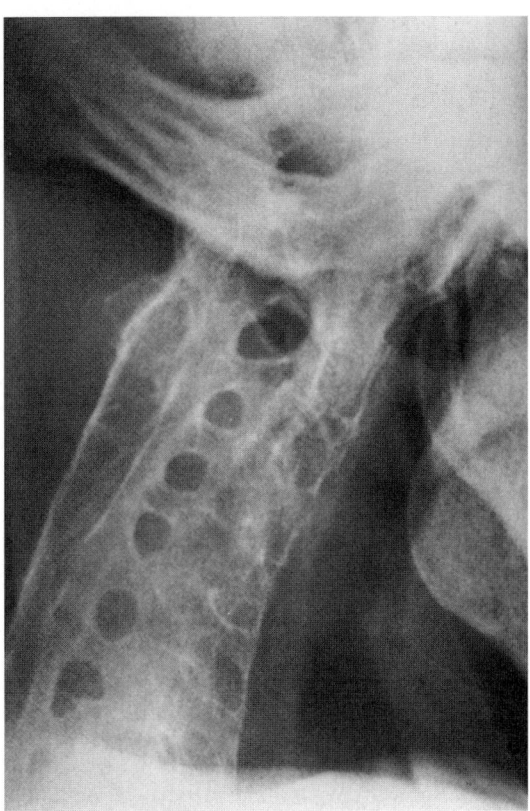

**Figure 74–19.** Fibrodysplasia ossificans progressiva. Lateral view of the cervical spine shows the late changes of the disease, with fusion of the soft tissues, apophyseal joints, and vertebral bodies.

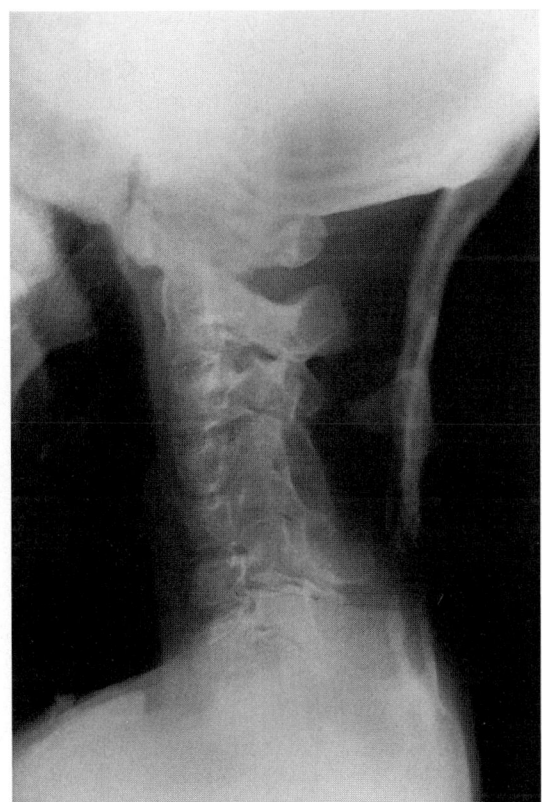

**Figure 74–18.** Fibrodysplasia ossificans progressiva. Lateral view of the cervical spine reveals ossification of the soft tissues and secondary fusion of the apophyseal joints.

multicentric areas of myositis ossificans circumscripta, including tetany, paraplegia, and burns, can mimic fibrodysplasia ossificans progressiva on radiographs; however, the distribution of the ossified lesions is different. For example, in tetanus, the lesions occur on extensor surfaces; in paraplegia, ossification occurs adjacent to pressure points; and in burns, ankylosis is found symmetrically about the elbows. In addition, the clinical history clearly establishes the correct diagnosis. In the cervical spine, other causes of fusion of the posterior elements (Klippel-Feil syndrome, Still's disease, ankylosing spondylitis) can resemble fibrodysplasia ossificans progressiva.

## PSEUDOXANTHOMA ELASTICUM

Pseudoxanthoma elasticum is an inherited disorder characterized by a defect in elastic fibers that involves the skin, eyes, and cardiovascular system. The exact nature of the abnormality is unknown, but the elastic fibers have a tendency to calcify. Because of genetic heterogeneity, the clinical expressions of pseudoxanthoma elasticum are protean.

### Pathology and Pathophysiology

The skin lesions of pseudoxanthoma elasticum are secondary to progressive mineralization of the elastin component of individual fibers. Adjacent to areas of calcified elastin are abnormally thickened, flower-like collagen fibers and a marked increase in ground substance (similar to collagen changes in Ehlers-Danlos syndrome and osteogenesis imperfecta). The abnormal mineralization of the elastic fibers has variously been attributed to an increase in acid mucopolysaccharides that have been sulfated to polyionic deposits (possibly glycoproteins) and to a copper deficiency that results in the production of abnormal elastin.

The ocular changes are characterized by angioid streaks, which represent fissuring and scarring of the membrane beneath the retina. Narrowing and occlusion of the large muscular arteries of the extremities, viscera, and central nervous system are also findings of pseudoxanthoma elasticum. The vascular calcifications of pseudoxanthoma elasticum occur most frequently in the femoral arteries, involve the media of the vessel wall, and are uniform in distribution. In atherosclerosis, the calcifications are more commonly intimal and are distributed in plaques.

## Clinical Findings

Pseudoxanthoma elasticum occurs in all races, and there is a slight female predominance. Skin abnormalities usually become apparent in the second decade of life. Changes in the skin involve primarily those areas that are subjected to mechanical wear and tear (flexion folds), such as the neck, face, axillary and inguinal folds, cubital areas, and periumbilical region. Also affected are the heart and soft palate and the mucosae of the mouth, gastrointestinal tract, and vagina. The earliest clinical findings are accentuation of the normal skin lines; particularly prominent are the nasolabial folds. Later, the skin becomes thickened, redundant, deeply grooved, and hyperextensible. The most characteristic clinical feature is the yellow papules that occur between the thickened folds.

The angioid streaks that characterize the ocular findings of pseudoxanthoma elasticum also begin in the second decade of life. Chorioretinitis, a more severe threat to vision, is another ocular abnormality that may occur in patients with pseudoxanthoma elasticum.

Involvement of the muscular arteries usually occurs in the third decade of life but in some instances may begin in childhood. Physical examination reveals weakening or even absence of the peripheral pulses. Resultant symptoms include intermittent claudication, coronary insufficiency, abdominal angina, hypertension, and bleeding from almost every organ. The gastrointestinal tract is the most frequent location of hemorrhage, and severe gastrointestinal bleeding in a child should suggest the possibility of pseudoxanthoma elasticum.

## Radiographic Findings

Radiographs of the skull frequently demonstrate premature calcification of the falx, tentorium, choroid plexus, and petroclinoid ligaments. Thickening of the calvaria and of the base of the skull has also been reported. Radiographs of the extremities may demonstrate a variety of calcifications. Typically, abnormal lesions with fibrillar linear calcifications are observed in the middle

and deep layers of the dermis, the site of pathologic abnormalities. Calcifications also occur within tendons and ligaments; around the metacarpophalangeal, hip, or elbow joints; and within large peripheral veins and arteries. Angiography of the extremities demonstrates localized occlusion and narrowing of large arteries (resembling fibromuscular dysplasia), as well as the formation of localized aneurysms and arteriovenous malformations. Osseous abnormalities include osteoporosis, bowing, metaphyseal ectasia, and abnormal lucent areas (Fig. 74–20).

The radiographic differential diagnosis includes other entities associated with both soft tissue and vascular calcification, such as renal disease and collagen vascular disease. Ehlers-Danlos syndrome and parasitic disorders can also produce soft tissue calcifications, but their distribution differs from that of pseudoxanthoma elasticum.

## MULTIPLE EPIPHYSEAL DYSPLASIAS

Traditionally, the epiphyseal dysplasias were divided into two broad categories: spondyloepiphyseal dysplasia (with marked spinal changes, including universal platyspondylia and beaking) and multiple epiphyseal dysplasia (with minimal spinal changes or irregular ring apophyses and mild scoliosis). The modern classification of the epiphyseal dysplasias is based on genetic linkage studies. They are defined as hereditary genetic mutations resulting in clinical disorders associated with severe dwarfing to short stature. They are genetically transmitted as autosomal dominant disorders that affect three known loci involved in cartilage formation (not collagen I or III, the main substrates of bone). The phenotypes share the characteristics of relatively short limbs, irregular growth plates before skeletal maturity, delayed ossification, irregular endplates, and premature osteoarthritis.

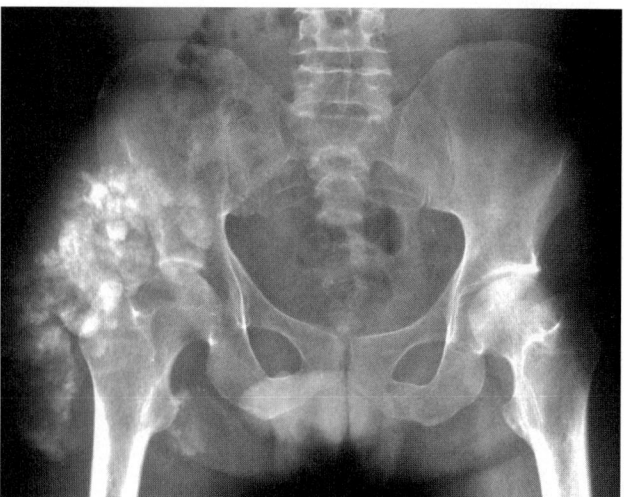

**Figure 74–20.** Pseudoxanthoma elasticum. Radiograph of the pelvis demonstrates large amorphous calcific deposits in the soft tissues around the hip. (From Harle TS, Carroll CL, Leeds NE, et al: Radiographics 15:211, 1995.)

## Pathology and Pathophysiology

The primary defect in dysplasia epiphysealis multiplex appears to involve the epiphyseal chondrocyte. On gross specimens, the growth plate is found to be widened and to have an irregular metaphyseal margin. Tongues of cartilage extend into the osseous metaphysis, and the peripheral trabeculae are irregular. The collagen within the growth plate is normal but with a decreased mucopolysaccharide content, a finding thought to be related to delayed and disorderly ossification of the epiphyseal ends of the bones. The midportions of the secondary ossification centers contain woven bone, and the peripheries are irregular in contour. However, the morphologic abnormalities of the growth plate are not pathognomonic. Joint incongruity inevitably leads to angular deformities (varus or valgus) and to secondary degenerative joint disease.

## Clinical Findings

Dysplasia epiphysealis multiplex affects both sexes equally. Patients have normal intelligence, and osseous involvement is bilateral and symmetrical. This group of conditions is characterized by the disturbance of two or more paired epiphyses; irregular epiphyseal growth; minimal irregularity of the vertebral endplates, particularly at the thoracolumbar junction; and absence of features suggesting other diseases. The most frequent sites of involvement are the hips, knees, shoulders, ankles, and wrists. In the absence of dwarfism, patients usually first manifest the disease early in childhood, and common presenting complaints include articular pain, gait disturbances, and difficulty in running and climbing stairs. In milder cases, symptoms may not occur until adulthood.

The growth disturbance may lead to symmetrical shortening of the skeleton, if the spine is involved, or to micromelia, if only the limbs are affected. In adolescent and young adult patients, precocious degenerative joint disease leads to stiffness and decreased range of motion. The diagnosis of multiple epiphyseal dysplasia is established on the basis of positive radiographic findings in the absence of biochemical abnormalities. The identification of families with autosomal dominant spondyloepiphyseal dysplasia is based on a combination of phenotypic features and appropriate laboratory findings.

## Radiographic Findings

Radiographic abnormalities appear in the second or third year of life and are most marked in the hips, knees, wrists, and ankles. Osseous involvement is always bilaterally symmetrical. In young children, the epiphyseal centers of the long bones are late in appearing and slow in mineralizing, and when they begin to ossify, they are irregularly fragmented (Fig. 74–21). The epiphyses frequently ossify from multiple centers and have a mulberry-like appearance (Fig. 74–22). The secondary centers may be either small (Fig. 74–23) or flattened.

In older children, slipped epiphyses complicate the coxa vara deformities. Incongruity and angular deformities, particularly of the knee and hip joints, result in premature osteoarthritis. In adolescents, apparent improvement in the radiographic appearance is a result of the completion of skeletal growth and fusion of the multiple centers of ossification. Affected articular surfaces of the long bones remain irregular and abnormal in shape. The femoral heads and femoral condyles are flattened. In most cases of multiple epiphyseal dysplasia,

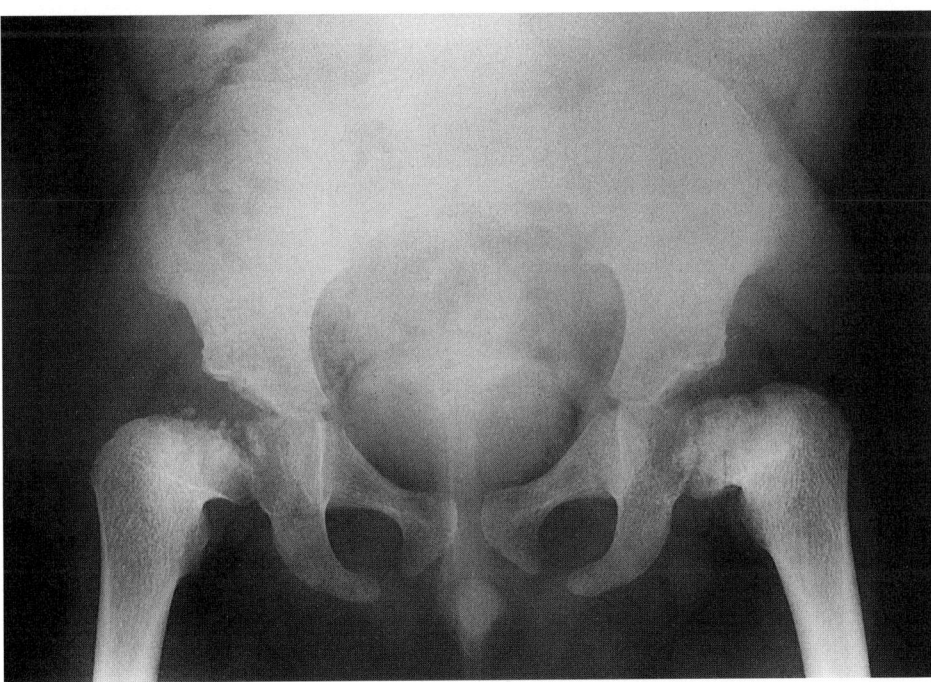

**Figure 74–21.** Multiple epiphyseal dysplasia. Anteroposterior view of the pelvis shows irregular femoral epiphyses and multiple epiphyseal ossification centers. Bilateral coxa vara deformities are present. Mild irregularity of the metaphyses is also noted, and the acetabula show minimal irregularities.

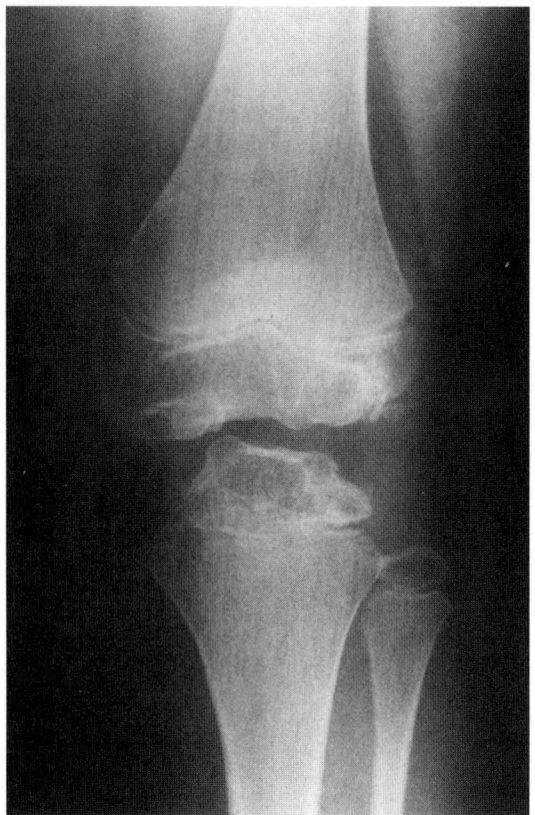

**Figure 74–22.** Multiple epiphyseal dysplasia. Anteroposterior view of a knee demonstrates flattening of the condyles and irregularity of the contours of the epiphyses.

changes of secondary degenerative joint disease are present before the third or fourth decade of life (Fig. 74–24).

The hands and feet of patients with dysplasia epiphysealis multiplex demonstrate small, broad phalanges,

sometimes with irregularity of both epiphyseal and non-epiphyseal ends of the bones (Fig. 74–25). Fusion anomalies or hypoplasia of the carpal bones also occurs in association with this disorder. Bone age is delayed. The spine is affected in two thirds of patients, and the radiographic changes are similar to those of Scheuermann's disease. These changes are usually localized to the midthoracic spine.

The radiographic differential diagnosis includes other causes of irregular articular surfaces, such as juvenile inflammatory arthritis, osteonecrosis, cretinism, the mucopolysaccharidoses, and other dysplasias. Symmetrical changes in the hips in multiple epiphyseal dysplasia differ from the typical appearance of Legg-Calvé-Perthes disease, which is bilateral in 10% of cases.

## Chondrodysplasia Punctata

Chondrodysplasia punctata is a form of multiple epiphyseal dysplasia characterized by calcification of unossified cartilaginous epiphyseal centers during the first year of life (Fig. 74–26). The classic finding is present in the perinatal period and can be diagnosed in utero during the second and third trimesters by ultrasonography and in the first few months of life by radiography.

**Pathophysiology.** To date, six forms (four generalized and two localized) of chondrodysplasia punctata have been defined. The generalized forms can be lethal or nonlethal, and the disease can be autosomal dominant or sporadic. The two localized forms are seen in the tibia and the metacarpals.

**Radiographic Findings.** Four significant shared radiographic abnormalities are seen. First and best known is calcification of the cartilage anlagen at the ends of the bones (see Fig. 74–26). The distribution of the transient

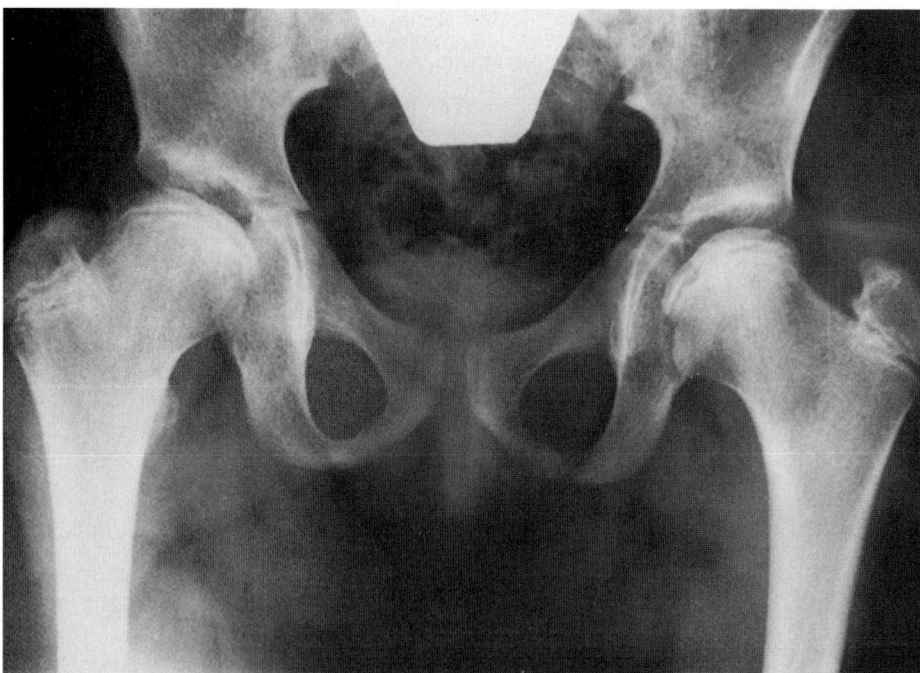

**Figure 74–23.** Multiple epiphyseal dysplasia. Anteroposterior view of both hips shows flattening of the femoral heads and irregularity of the acetabular margins.

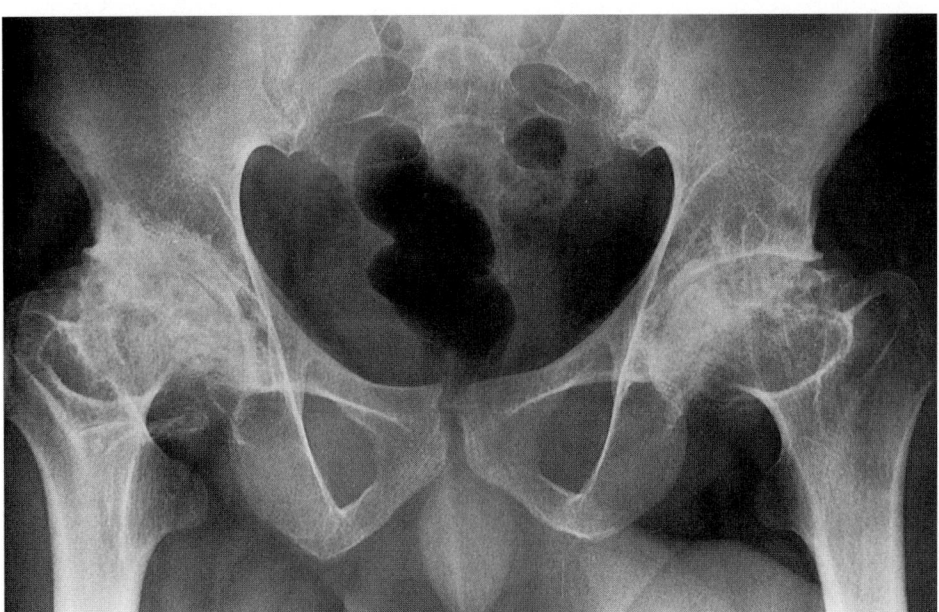

**Figure 74–24.** Multiple epiphyseal dysplasia. Anteroposterior view of the hips shows secondary degenerative changes complicating the epiphyseal dysplasia.

calcification varies with the syndrome. Patients with these syndromes also have hypoplasia of the bones of the midface and nasal flattening. Defective vertebral ossification is associated with transient lucent vertebral clefts that may be replaced by flattening of the vertebral column (especially in Conradi-Hünermann syndrome) or abnormalities of segmentation associated with a cervical and thoracic kyphosis and scoliosis.

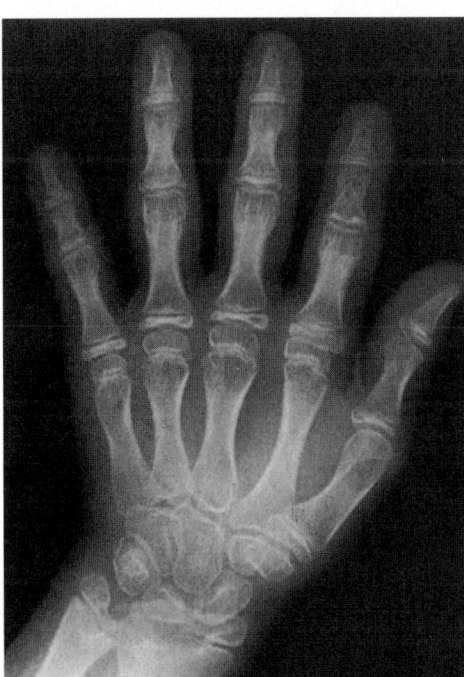

**Figure 74–25.** Multiple epiphyseal dysplasia. Frontal view of the hand shows the characteristic stubby phalanges and a V-shaped deformity of the wrist. The epiphyses of the radius and ulna have an abnormal wedge shape.

The radiographic differential diagnosis of chondrodysplasia punctata includes other causes of "stippled epiphyses." Information regarding the family history and past medical history is necessary to allow differentiation between primary and secondary causes of epiphyseal stippling. The most likely differential diagnosis is Zellweger's cerebrohepatorenal syndrome (a peroxisome disorder). However, in this syndrome, stippling is limited to the patellae, and ultrasonography can reveal abdominal cysts in utero.

## Meyer's Dysplasia

Meyer's dysplasia, also referred to as dysplasia epiphysealis capitis, is thought to be a mild localized dysplasia of the femoral heads. Most cases are discovered incidentally on hip or pelvic radiographs obtained for other reasons. This disorder is more common in boys than in girls, and 50% of cases are bilateral. Occasionally patients complain of mild pain and a limp.

Radiographic studies reveal delayed ossification of the femoral heads, which appear at approximately 2 years of age instead of at 6 months. In unilateral cases, the diagnosis can be suspected before ossification, because the cartilaginous femoral head is smaller on the affected side. As the femoral capital epiphyses begin to ossify, granular foci or multiple irregular centers develop, with an abnormal, flattened appearance (Fig. 74–27). As growth continues, serial radiographic studies reveal consolidation of the granular ossific nuclei and a return to the normal hemispheric shape of the femoral heads.

## MACRODYSTROPHIA LIPOMATOSA

Macrodystrophia lipomatosa is a rare form of localized gigantism characterized by congenital and progressive overgrowth of all the mesenchymal elements of a digit, with a disproportionate increase in the fibroadipose tissue.

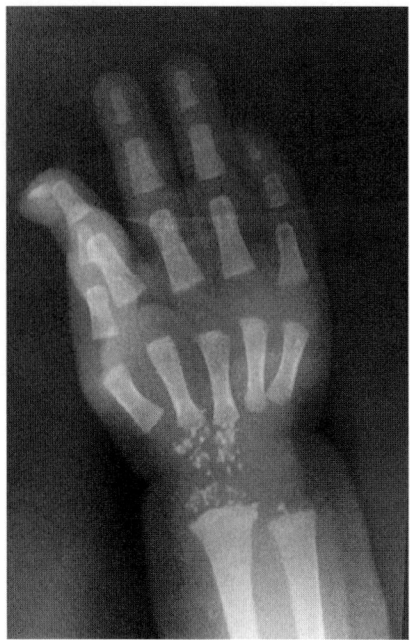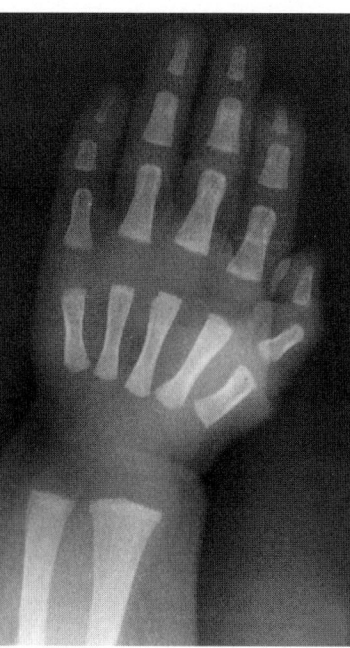

**Figure 74–26.** Chondrodysplasia punctata. Posteroanterior view of the hands obtained at birth demonstrates asymmetrical stippling of cartilage epiphyses.

It is classified as a developmental anomaly and is not hereditary.

True macrodactyly is defined as "a rare congenital malformation characterized by an increase in the size of all elements or structures of a digit or digits." Dramatic proliferation of fatty tissue associated with localized gigantism has been described in the literature under many names, including partial acromegaly, macrosomia, elephantiasis, megalodactyly, dactylomegaly, macrodactyly macrocheiria, and club finger. Recent investigators have classified it as the macrodactyly associated with fibro-lipomatous hamartomas.

## Pathology and Pathophysiology

The most dramatic pathologic finding is the increase in adipose tissue, interspersed in a fine mesh of fibrous tissue. Neural enlargement and irregularity may be prominent, most frequently involving the median nerve in the hand and the plantar nerve in the foot. The phalanges are enlarged by both endosteal and periosteal deposition of bone.

Recent studies of patients with digital macrodactyly have emphasized the coexistence of fibrolipomatous hamartoma of nerve. The cause-and-effect relationship between the hamartomatous changes of nerve sheath origin and macrodystrophia lipomatosa remains unclear. The predilection for involvement of the median nerve is also unexplained. On the basis of this association, macrodystrophia lipomatosa is now referred to as nerve territory–oriented macrodactyly.

## Clinical Findings

The localized gigantism associated with macrodystrophia lipomatosa is recognizable at birth. There is no known sex predilection. Involvement is almost always unilateral, although one or more adjacent digits in the same extremity may be enlarged (Fig. 74–28). The second and third digits are the favored sites in both the upper extremi-

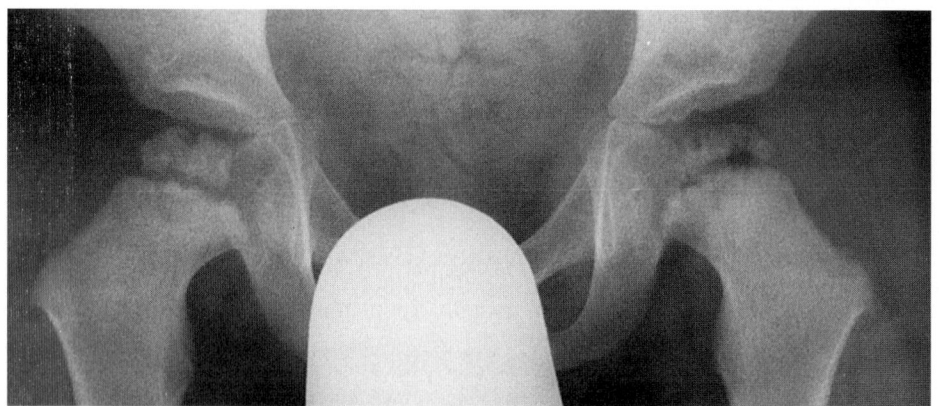

**Figure 74–27.** Meyer's dysplasia in a 2-year-old boy. Anteroposterior view of the pelvis demonstrates irregular ossification of both femoral heads. The irregularity involves the entire epiphysis, and the changes are symmetrical. The femoral heads are of normal density.

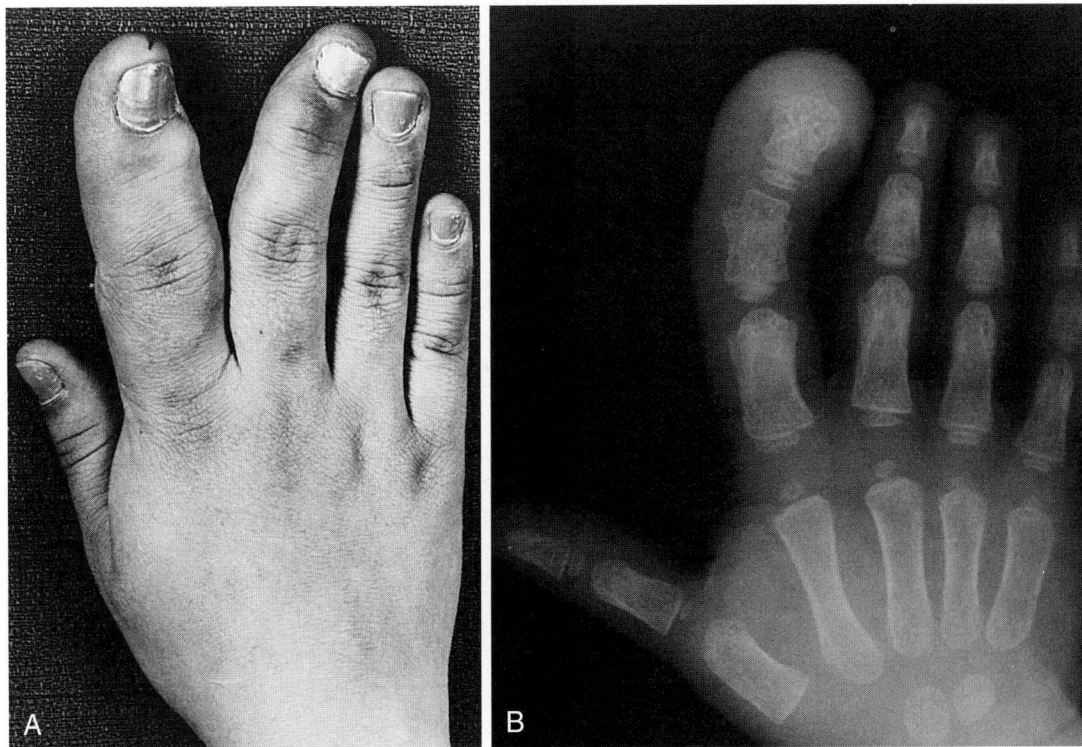

**Figure 74–28.** Macrodystrophia lipomatosa. *A*, Clinical appearance of involvement of the second and third digits of the hand. *B*, Posteroanterior radiograph shows osseous and soft tissue enlargement, affecting predominantly the distal end of the second digit, and splaying of the ends of the phalanges. (From Goldman AB, Kaye JJ: Macrodystrophia lipomatosa: Radiographic diagnosis. AJR Am J Roentgenol 128:101, 1977.)

ties and the lower extremities. Secondary degenerative joint disease reduces function, and large osteophytes result in compression of the neurovascular structures. The affected part is increased in both length and girth. Growth of the digit ceases at puberty.

### Radiographic Findings

Radiographs of patients with macrodystrophia lipomatosa demonstrate abnormalities in both soft tissues and osseous structures (see Fig. 74–28). The soft tissue overgrowth is most marked at the distal end of the digit and along its volar aspect in the distribution of the median and plantar nerves. The phalanges are long, broad, and often splayed at their distal ends. The trabeculae are normal. The distal phalanx or phalanges have a mushroom shape. If more than one digit is involved, the digits are always adjacent to one another. Rare bilateral cases have been observed. A high frequency of associated local anomalies is seen, including syndactyly and polydactyly.

The differential diagnosis of congenital localized gigantism includes angiomatous lesions; however, the tumorous overgrowth of hemangiomatous and lymphangiomatous lesions produces soft tissue hypertrophy and symmetrical overgrowth of the bones. Klippel-Trénaunay-Weber syndrome has obvious cutaneous abnormalities. The absence of enchondromas eliminates the possibility of Ollier's disease. The most difficult differential diagnosis based on radiographs is neurofibromatosis (Fig. 74–29). Macrodactyly in patients with von Recklinghausen's

disease is the result of plexiform neurofibromas (with hemangiomatous and lymphangiomatous elements) combined with a mesodermal dysplasia. The distribution of localized gigantism in neurofibromatosis is not identical to that in macrodystrophia lipomatosa. In neurofibromatosis, the enlarged digits may be bilateral, involvement in one extremity does not necessarily occur in contiguous digits, and the distal phalanges are not the most severely affected. In addition, the hemangiomatous elements of the plexiform neurofibroma can produce premature fusion of the growth plates, whereas the growth in a digit involved by macrodystrophia lipomatosa ceases with puberty.

## KLIPPEL-TRÉNAUNAY-WEBER SYNDROME

Klippel-Trénaunay-Weber syndrome is characterized by the clinical triad of cutaneous capillary hemangiomas (port-wine stains), varicose veins, and local gigantism with both soft tissue and osseous overgrowth, usually in a monomelic distribution. Although not included in the major clinical criteria of this disease, arteriovenous malformations are often present and are responsible for major complications. The cause of this syndrome is unknown, and the majority of cases are sporadic. Some investigators prefer to split Klippel-Trénaunay-Weber syndrome into two forms—those without arteriovenous malformations (Klippel-Trénaunay syndrome) and those with arteriovenous malformations (Parke-Weber syndrome)—but most authors consider them to be a single entity.

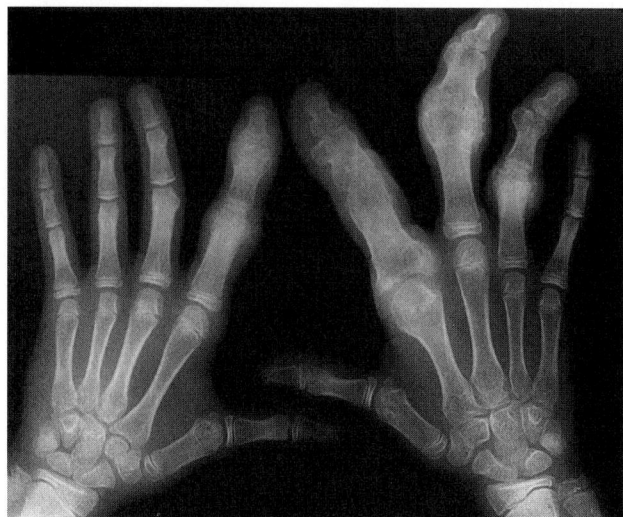

**Figure 74–29.** Neurofibromatosis. Bilateral macrodactyly may be evident in this disease. In addition, digital overgrowth is not most severe in the distal phalanges, premature fusion of the growth plates has occurred, and the cortices of the affected phalanges are dense and wavy. (From Goldman AB, Kaye JJ: Macrodystrophia lipomatosa: Radiographic diagnosis. AJR Am J Roentgenol 128:101, 1977.)

## Pathology and Pathophysiology

Klippel-Trénaunay-Weber syndrome is associated with a variety of vascular abnormalities, including superficial blue and pigmented hemangiomas, varicose veins, arteriovenous fistulas, lymphangiomas, and absence of the deep venous system. Skin biopsies of affected limbs reveal scattered groups of thin-walled vessels and increased collagen proliferation. The arteriovenous malformations, if present, provide a low-resistance pathway for cardiac output. Superficial varicose veins and edema result from agenesis, atresia, or compression of the deep venous system. Lymphatic malformations are also related to the deficient deep veins.

The osseous and soft tissue overgrowth that characterizes Klippel-Trénaunay-Weber syndrome occurs in the same area as the vascular malformations. No specific primary osseous abnormalities seem to occur, and local gigantism is attributed to the abnormal vascular supply.

## Clinical Findings

Klippel-Trénaunay-Weber syndrome is usually monomelic. The lower extremities are more commonly affected than are the upper extremities and trunk. The vascular anomalies may occur in the upper extremity, in two ipsilateral extremities, in the face, or in the trunk.

The most frequent chief complaint is related to the varicosities. Disease progression usually ceases during the second or third decade of life. The port-wine cutaneous hemangiomas (nevus flammeus) represent the earliest clinical finding. They may be present at birth or appear in the first months of life. Extension of the hemangiomatous lesions into the pelvis is common, as is involvement of the viscera, with resultant organomegaly. Varicose veins become obvious when the child begins to

walk. Ulcerations, thrombophlebitis, and edema further complicate the venous changes. Pulmonary varices can also occur in association with this syndrome.

Localized gigantism develops early in childhood and may involve all or only a part of an extremity (Fig. 74–30). The hypertrophy affects both the length and girth of the extremity. Periods of rapid growth alternate with periods of no change. The prepubertal growth spurt and pregnancy are periods of greatest risk for a sudden exacerbation. Arteriovenous malformations, often associated with aneurysmal dilatation of vessels, create both local and systemic complications. To a great extent, their presence and size determine the overall prognosis. In the extremities, vascular fistulas may produce intermittent claudication or high-output congestive heart failure. Physical examination may reveal thrills, bruits, or pulsatile masses. Central nervous system involvement may lead to seizures, mental retardation, migraine headaches, macroencephaly or microcephaly, hemangiomas, fistulas, bifrontal varices, ischemic infarcts, and vascular anomalies.

## Radiographic Findings

The phalanges, metatarsals, and metacarpals are all increased in size (see Fig. 74–30) and may demonstrate cortical thickening. The coarse "sunburst" trabeculae, characteristic of an intraosseous hemangioma, may be observed in isolated bones (skull, hand). Congenital osseous abnormalities are frequent and include syndactyly, polydactyly, and congenital hip dislocations. Calcified phleboliths can be observed in the soft tissues.

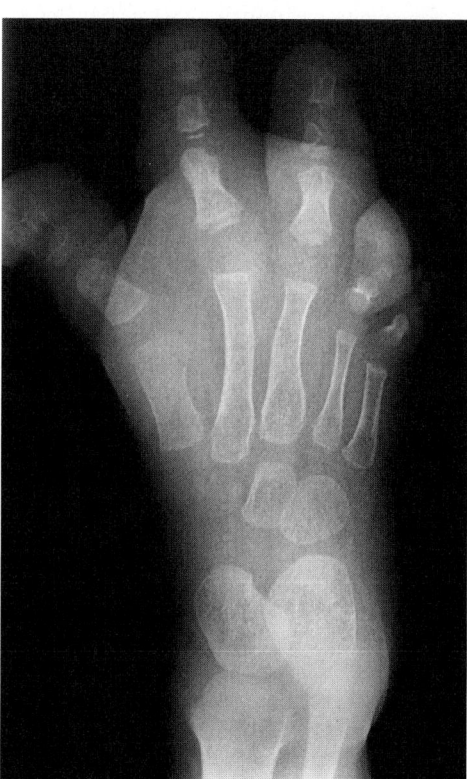

**Figure 74–30.** Klippel-Trénaunay-Weber syndrome. Anteroposterior view of the foot reveals both osseous and soft tissue overgrowth.

Venograms may demonstrate a variety of abnormalities. The deep venous system can be totally absent or demonstrate areas of agenesis, atresia, or extreme obstruction owing to fibrous bands or arteries. Perforators may be incompetent and superficial veins dilated and valveless. The femoral and popliteal veins are involved more frequently than are the deep calf veins. Phleboliths within the varicosities produce multiple soft tissue calcifications. If present, arteriovenous malformations are usually small and numerous. Arteriographic findings are variable; in some cases, the arterial phase is normal, whereas in others, it may demonstrate the presence of arteriovenous malformations.

Arteriovenous malformations also produce skeletal changes, including multiple lytic lesions. Those involving the viscera may be detected on plain films by the presence of a fixed collection of phleboliths. Unlike phleboliths that occur in normal adults, these dense structures are found in children and are located in atypical sites. Barium studies performed on patients with colonic hemangiomas have revealed thickened folds secondary to varices, extrinsic compression by a soft tissue mass, infiltration of the bowel wall, and secondary mucosal ulcerations.

MR imaging studies reveal a variety of findings, including, on T2-weighted sequences, heterogeneous mixed signal and large signal voids at the sites of arteriovenous malformations. Visualization of a persistent sciatic vein, a rare finding in normal persons, is common.

The major radiographic differential diagnoses involve Maffucci's syndrome, macrodystrophia lipomatosa, and neurofibromatosis. Maffucci's syndrome, like Klippel-Trénaunay-Weber syndrome, exhibits both soft tissue and osseous enlargement, soft tissue phleboliths, and brachydactyly; however, unlike Klippel-Trénaunay-Weber syndrome, osseous enchondromas are present. Macrodystrophia lipomatosa is distinguishable from Klippel-Trénaunay-Weber syndrome because overgrowth is limited to the digits. In neurofibromatosis, either the patient or family members have the two classic stigmata of this hereditary disease: café au lait spots and subcutaneous neurofibromas. In addition, unlike in Klippel-Trénaunay-Weber syndrome, the limb overgrowth in neurofibromatosis is associated with an osseous dysplasia, and the bones are grossly deformed, often with sinuous, irregular cortices.

# FURTHER READING

Beals RK, Mason L: The Marfan skull. Radiology 140:723, 1981.

Berg PK: Dysplasia epiphysealis multiplex. AJR Am J Roentgenol 97:31, 1966.

Bjerkreim I, Skogland LB, Trygstad O: Congenital contractural arachnodactyly. Acta Orthop Scand 47:250, 1976.

Blacksin M, Barnes FJ, Lyons MM: MR diagnosis of macrodystrophia lipomatosa. AJR Am J Roentgenol 158:1295, 1992.

Brenton DP, Dow CJ: Homocystinuria and Marfan's syndrome: A comparison. J Bone Joint Surg Br 54:277, 1972.

Briggs MD, Mortier GR, Cole WG, et al: Diverse mutations in the gene for cartilage oligomeric matrix protein in the pseudoachondroplasia multiple epiphyseal dysplasia spectrum. Am J Hum Genet 62:311, 1998.

Brill PW, Mitty JA, Gaull GE: Homocystinuria due to cystathionine synthetase deficiency: Clinical-roentgenologic correlations. AJR Am J Roentgenol 121:45, 1974.

Byers PH, Steiner RD: Osteogenesis imperfecta. Annu Rev Med 43:269, 1992.

Cremin B, Connor M, Beighton P: The radiological spectrum of fibrodysplasia ossificans progressiva. Clin Radiol 33:499, 1982.

Cremin B, Goodman H, Spranger J, et al: Wormian bones in osteogenesis imperfecta and other diseases. Skeletal Radiol 8:35, 1982.

Golding FC: Fibrogenesis imperfecta. J Bone Joint Surg Br 50:619, 1968.

Goldman AB, Davidson D, Pavlov H, et al: "Popcorn calcifications": A prognostic sign of osteogenesis imperfecta. Radiology 136:351, 1980.

Goldman AB, Kaye JJ: Macrodystrophia lipomatosa: Radiographic diagnosis. AJR Am J Roentgenol 128:101, 1977.

Holt JF: The Ehlers-Danlos syndrome. AJR Am J Roentgenol 55:420, 1946.

Hulvey JT, Keats T: Multiple epiphyseal dysplasia: A contribution to the problem of spinal involvement. AJR Am J Roentgenol 106:170, 1969.

Mason RC, Kozlowski K: Chondrodysplasia punctata: A report of 10 cases. Radiology 109:145, 1973.

McCall RE, Bax JA: Hyperplastic callus formation in osteogenesis imperfecta. Pediatr Orthop 4:361, 1984.

McKusick VA: The classification of heritable disorders of connective tissue. Birth Defects 11:1, 1975.

McKusick VA: Heritable Disorders of Connective Tissue, 4th ed. St Louis, CV Mosby, 1972, p 61.

Mitchell GE, Lourie H, Berne AS: The various causes of scalloped vertebrae with notes on their pathogenesis. Radiology 89:67, 1967.

Nuytinck L, Freund M, Lagae L, et al: Classical Ehlers-Danlos syndrome caused by a mutation in type I collagen. Am J Hum Genet 66:1398, 2000.

Paassita P, Lohiniva J, Annumen S, et al: COL9A3: A third locus for multiple epiphyseal dysplasia. Am J Hum Genet 64:1036, 1999.

Prick JJG, Thijssen HDM: Radiodiagnostic signs in pseudoxanthoma elasticum generalisatum (dysgenesis elastofibrillaris mineralisans). Clin Radiol 28:549, 1977.

Rogers JG, Geho WB: Fibrodysplasia ossificans progressiva: A survey of forty-two cases. J Bone Joint Surg Am 61:709, 1979.

Rubin P: Dynamic Classification of Bone Dysplasias. Chicago, Year Book Medical Publishers, 1964.

Sartoris DJ, Luzzatti L, Weaver DD, et al: Type IX Ehlers-Danlos syndrome: A new variant with pathognomonic radiologic features. Radiology 152:665, 1984.

Silengo MC, Luzzatti L, Silverman FN: Clinical and genetic aspects of Conradi-Hünermann disease: A report of three familial cases and review of the literature. J Pediatr 97:911, 1980.

Sillence D: Osteogenesis imperfecta: An expanding panorama of variants. Clin Orthop 159:11, 1981.

Sillence DO, Senn A, Danks DM: Genetic heterogeneity in osteogenesis imperfecta. J Med Genet 16:101, 1979.

Smith SW: Roentgen findings in homocystinuria. AJR Am J Roentgenol 100:147, 1967.

Sofield HA, Millar EA: Fragmentation realignment and intramedullary rod fixation of deformities of the long bones in children: A ten year appraisal. J Bone Joint Surg Am 41:1371, 1959.

Stoddart PGP, Wickremaratchi T, Watt I: Fibrogenesis imperfecta ossium. Br J Radiol 57:744, 1984.

Thickman D, Bonakdar-pour A, Clancy M, et al: Fibrodysplasia ossificans progressiva. AJR Am J Roentgenol 139:935, 1982.

# CHAPTER 75

## Osteochondrodysplasias, Dysostoses, Chromosomal Aberrations, Mucopolysaccharidoses, and Mucolipidoses

William H. McAlister and Thomas E. Herman

## SUMMARY OF KEY FEATURES

The number of skeletal dysplasias is large and continues to increase. Nomenclature is complex and not agreed on. Only the more important dysplasias are covered in this chapter; certain other conditions, such as fibrous dysplasia, osteogenesis imperfecta, and melorheostosis, are discussed elsewhere in this book.

## INTRODUCTION

Until recently, the classification of skeletal dysplasias depended on descriptive features of radiographic and clinical phenotype. Owing to a rapidly expanding knowledge of the human genome, a chromosomal map classification of skeletal dysplasias is increasingly valuable. However, because some osteochondrodysplasias do not yet have a confirmed genetic locus, a workable chromosomal classification of these conditions does not exist.

The approach to the skeletal dysplasias taken here is based primarily on radiographic findings, with the addition of pertinent clinical data, including inheritance patterns.

## OSTEOCHONDRODYSPLASIAS

### Achondroplasias

**Thanatophoric Dysplasia.** Affected children are usually stillborn or die shortly after birth owing to hypoplastic lungs; however, survival into infancy occasionally occurs. The fetus or infant has marked short-limbed dwarfism, a large head with frontal bossing, and a depressed nasal bridge. Numerous skin folds are present. The anteroposterior diameter of the chest is narrow, and the child has a relatively long trunk.

Radiographic findings include marked shortening of the long tubular bones in a rhizomelic pattern of distribution, with metaphyseal flaring and osseous bowing and widening (Fig. 75–1). The bowed femora resemble telephone receivers. Pronounced flattening of the vertebral bodies, with more constriction of their midportions and wide intervertebral disc spaces, is evident.

The appearance of each vertebra on frontal radiographs resembles an inverted U or an H. The thorax is slender, owing to short ribs with flared anterior ends. Small, rectangular iliac bones; small sacroiliac notches; and short, wide pubic and ischial bones are seen. The phalanges are short, relatively broad, and cupped. The base of the skull is short, and the foramen magnum is small. A variety of extraskeletal malformations have been described, including a dysplastic temporal cortex and basal ganglia, megalocephaly, polymicrogyria, heart defects, and some degree of hydronephrosis.

**Classic (Heterozygous) Achondroplasia.** Classic achondroplasia, a relatively common type of dwarfism of autosomal dominant inheritance, is evident at birth and is compatible with a long life span. Clinical manifestations include short limbs, especially of the proximal portions (rhizomelic micromelia); a large head, with a prominent forehead and a depressed nasal bridge; thoracolumbar kyphosis in infancy; and exaggerated lumbar lordosis, with prominent buttocks in children and adults. The hands are stubby and trident. Because of the constricted basicranium, foramen magnum, and spinal canal, persons with achondroplasia may develop compression of the spinal cord, lower brain stem, cauda equina, and nerve roots at any age.

Radiographic findings include a large cranium and a small foramen magnum. The interpediculate distances of the lower lumbar vertebrae, which normally increase proceeding distally, remain the same at all levels or decrease in the lower lumbar region (Fig. 75–2). In the lateral projection of the spine, the pedicles are short, the backs of the vertebral bodies are often concave, and the spinal canal is small (Fig. 75–3). Growth failure occurs at the neurocentral synchondrosis. The vertebral bodies are flattened and appear bullet shaped in infancy and early childhood. The iliac bones are squared, with small sacrosciatic notches and flat acetabular angles (Fig. 75–4). Shortening of the tubular bones, especially the proximal ones, and metaphyseal flaring are seen (Fig. 75–5). A V-shaped configuration of the distal femoral growth plate may be seen. Shortening of the tubular bones in the hands and feet is evident. The ribs are also shortened.

**Homozygous Achondroplasia.** Homozygous achondroplasia is an extremely rare type of congenital short-limbed dwarfism that is lethal; affected infants die within the first days or weeks of life. The condition results when both parents have achondroplasia. Radiographs outline changes that are more severe than those in classic (heterozygous) achondroplasia; indeed, they may be indistinguishable from those of thanatophoric dysplasia.

**Hypochondroplasia.** Hypochondroplasia, an autosomal dominant disorder, first manifests in childhood with clinical and radiographic findings that are similar to but

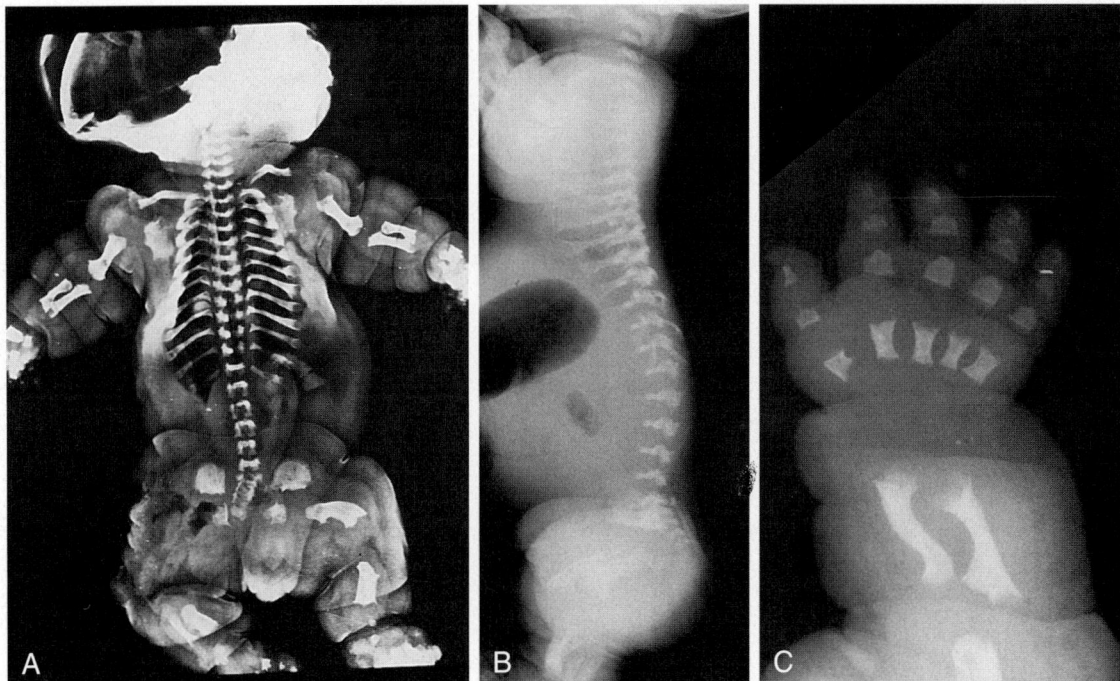

**Figure 75–1.** Thanatophoric dysplasia. Radiographs from three patients are shown. *A*, Findings include short tubular bones with flared metaphyses, squared iliac bones, and short ribs. *B*, The vertebral bodies are markedly flattened, with wide disc spaces. *C*, The tubular bones of the hands are markedly shortened but relatively broad. Bowing and metaphyseal flaring are evident in the bones of the forearm.

less severe than those of achondroplasia. Small stature, increased lumbar lordosis, bowlegs, and limited elbow extension may be noted on clinical evaluation. Radiographic findings include narrowing of the interpediculate distances distally and exaggerated posterior concavity of vertebral bodies in the lumbar region (Fig. 75–6), mild

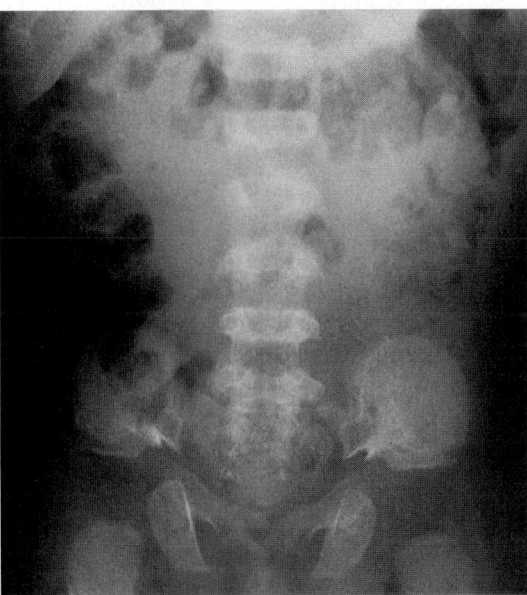

**Figure 75–2.** Heterozygous achondroplasia: spine. The interpediculate distances in the lumbar vertebrae narrow distally. The iliac bones are squared, the sacrosciatic notches are small, and the ischial bones are shortened.

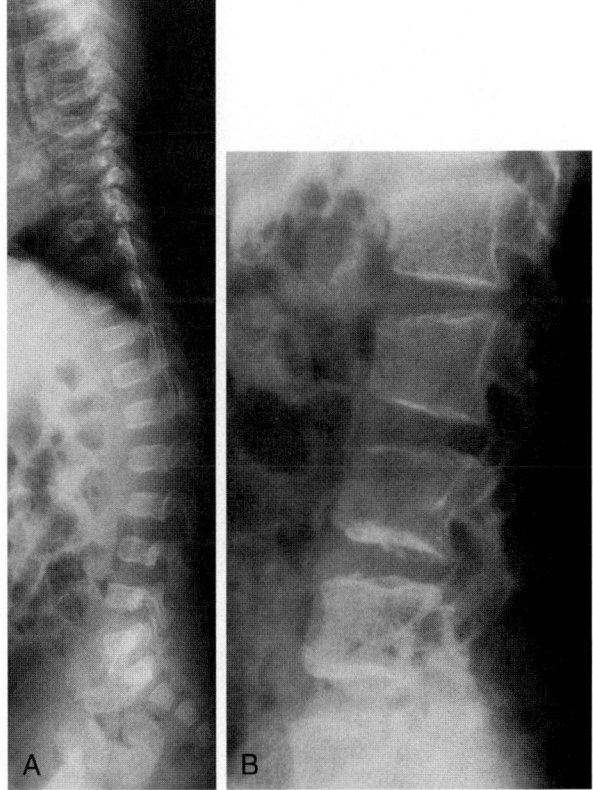

**Figure 75–3.** Heterozygous achondroplasia: lateral spine. *A*, In this 4-month-old child, bullet-shaped vertebral bodies with diminished heights and wide disc spaces are seen. *B*, In an older child, the vertebral bodies have a posterior concavity, diminished height, anterior wedging, and short pedicles, and the spinal canal is small.

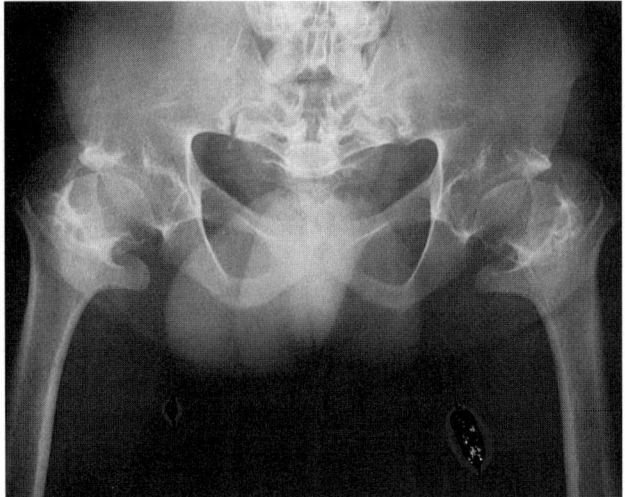

**Figure 75–4.** Heterozygous achondroplasia: pelvis. In this adult patient, findings include spinal stenosis, lack of flaring of the iliac wings (which have rounded corners), and short femoral necks.

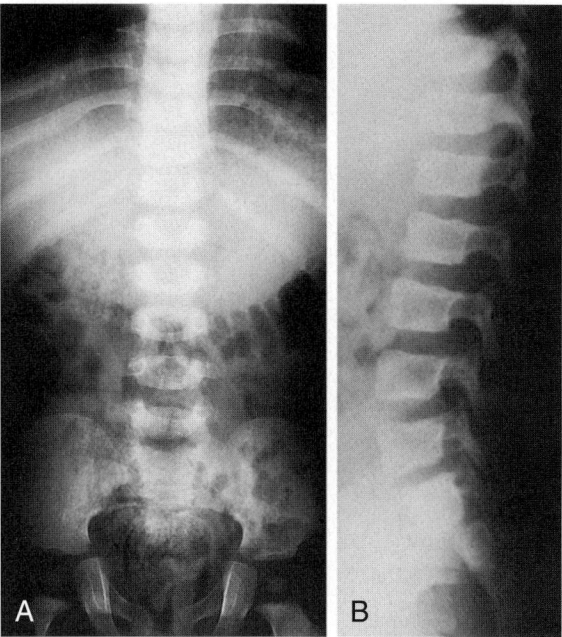

**Figure 75–6.** Hypochondroplasia: spine. *A,* In the lumbar spine of this 7-month-old child, the normal increase in inter-pediculate distances in the lower lumbar spine is not present. Shortening of the iliac bones and small sacrosciatic notches are evident. *B,* In this 8-year-old patient, posterior concavity of the vertebral bodies and slight narrowing of the spinal canal are observed.

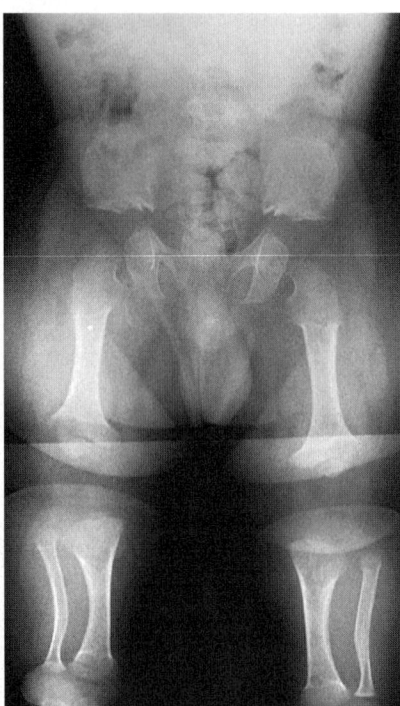

**Figure 75–5.** Heterozygous achondroplasia: lower extremities. In this newborn, rhizomelic shortening of the tubular bones, with metaphyseal flaring and medial slanting of distal femoral metaphyses, is seen.

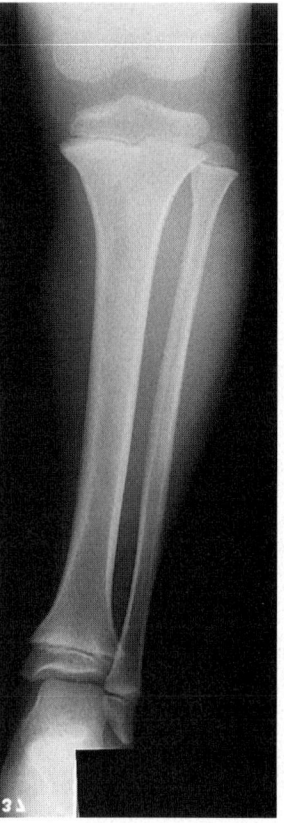

platyspondyly, small spinal canals, shortening of the tubular bones, and a short, broad femoral neck. Mild metaphyseal flaring occurs. The iliac bones are shortened, with flattened acetabular roofs and small sciatic notches. The fibulae may be slightly long (Fig. 75–7), and the distal ends of the ulnae are short, with prominent ulnar styloid processes.

**Figure 75–7.** Hypochondroplasia: long tubular bones. Although both bones are decreased in length, the fibula is long with respect to the tibia.

## Achondrogenesis

Achondrogenesis, a type of dwarfism of neonates, is characterized by a disproportionately large head, short trunk, protuberant abdomen, severe micromelia, and hydrops. It has been divided into types I and II. Type I is subdivided into IA (Houston-Harris) with rib fractures and IB (Fraccaro) without rib fractures. Type II (Langer-Saldino), or hypochondrogenesis, represents the severe end of the spondyloepiphyseal dysplasia congenita spectrum.

Radiographic findings common to both types include severe lack of ossification of the vertebral bodies (especially caudally); small, deformed iliac bones; absent or poor ossification of the pubic and ischial bones, calcaneus, and talus; tubular bones that are strikingly short and malformed, with wide, cupped ends; and short ribs with cupped and flared ends (Fig. 75–8).

## Spondyloepiphyseal Dysplasia Congenita

This short-trunk dwarfism is distinguished by mild shortening of the limbs, flat face, cleft palate, short neck, increased anteroposterior chest diameter, and joint restriction. During growth, progressive kyphoscoliosis, dorsal kyphosis, or lumbar lordosis occurs. The hands and feet are often normal except for the presence of equinovarus deformity. Important additional features include myopia and retinal detachment, which can lead to blindness, and atlantoaxial instability. The pattern of inheritance is usually autosomal dominant.

Radiographic findings include a decreased height of the vertebral bodies and, in infancy, pear-shaped vertebrae (Fig. 75–9). In childhood, anterior wedging, irregularity, and generalized flattening of the vertebral bodies occur. The interpediculate distances in the lower lumbar vertebrae may be narrowed. Hypoplasia of the odontoid process may be associated with atlantoaxial dislocation (see Fig. 75–9). Typical radiographic findings in the pelvis include a marked delay in the ossification of the pubic bones and proximal portion of the femora (Fig. 75–10). The femoral heads often ossify from multiple centers, and a progressive coxa vara develops, with premature osteoarthritis. Prominent shortening of the femoral necks may be evident, with small femoral heads that appear well below

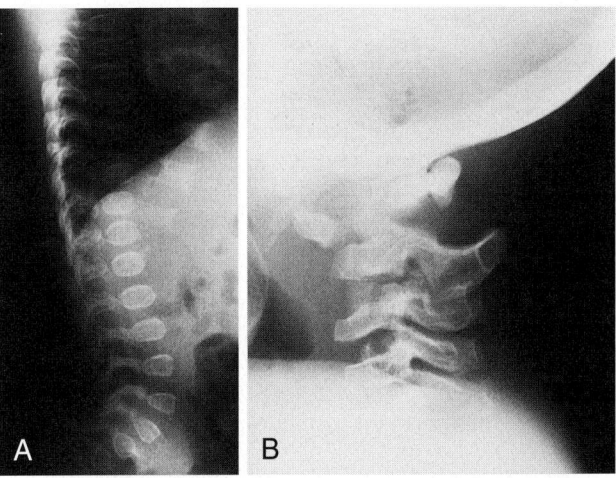

**Figure 75–9.** Spondyloepiphyseal dysplasia congenita. *A,* Decreased height of the vertebral bodies is evident, with pear-shaped vertebrae noted in the thoracic and lower lumbar regions. *B,* Hypoplasia of the odontoid process has resulted in atlantoaxial instability. The vertebral bodies are flat.

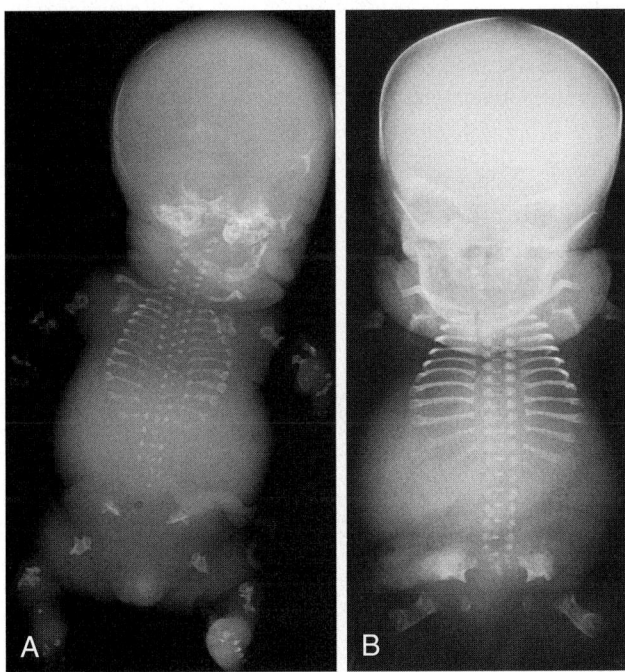

**Figure 75–8.** Achondrogenesis. *A,* Type 1A (Houston-Harris). The vertebrae are poorly ossified. The tubular bones are short, bowed, and deformed; they have wide, cupped ends and metaphyseal osteophytes. Small, deformed iliac bones and short ribs with fractures and cupped ends are also seen. *B,* Type II (Langer-Saldino). The ribs are short; the vertebral bodies are poorly ossified; the tubular bones are short, with mushroom-stem femora; and the iliac bones have a crescent-shaped inner border.

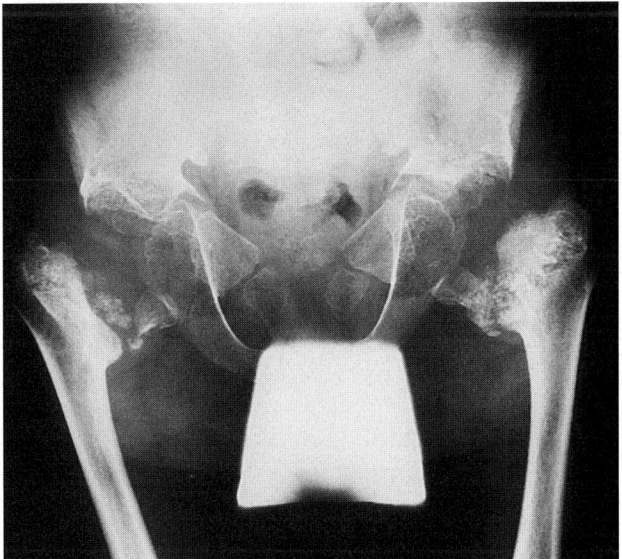

**Figure 75–10.** Spondyloepiphyseal dysplasia congenita. The femoral heads are small and inferiorly placed, and the femoral necks and pubic bones are poorly developed.

the level of the greater trochanters. The long tubular bones have delayed epiphyseal ossification. The epiphyses are irregular, and metaphyses show variable irregularity and flaring.

## Metatropic Dysplasia

Metatropic dysplasia is characterized by short extremities and a normal or elongated trunk at birth and by a short trunk with kyphoscoliosis later in life. At birth, the ends of the long tubular bones are prominent, and joint movement is limited. In infancy, the thorax appears to be long and narrow; a small, soft tissue fold resembling a tail may be present over the sacrum. The hands and feet are initially long and slender but become relatively shortened later in life. Progressive kyphoscoliosis is seen.

The radiographic findings are dramatic. The tubular bones of the extremities are short and have marked metaphyseal widening, resembling a trumpet or dumbbell (Fig. 75–11). The trochanters are particularly large, typically the lesser trochanter, and the appearance simulates that of a battle-ax, especially in infancy. The appearance of the epiphyses is delayed, and they are small, flat, and deformed. The vertebral bodies are rectangular or diamond-shaped in infancy and markedly reduced in height, and the intervertebral disc spaces appear large. The pelvis is characterized by shortened ilia with curved lateral margins, flat acetabular roofs, and small sacro-sciatic and lateral iliac notches. In infancy, the thorax is elongated and has a decreased anteroposterior diameter as a consequence of the short ribs. The tubular bones of the hands and feet have metaphyseal expansion and delayed and irregular epiphyseal ossification. The carpal and tarsal bones are also irregular, with delayed ossification.

## Asphyxiating Thoracic Dystrophy (Jeune's Syndrome)

Initial reports of this autosomal recessive condition described infants with constricted chests and mild shortening of the extremities who died from pulmonary hypoplasia. Later reports included patients with less severe respiratory symptoms, although those who survive to childhood generally succumb to progressive renal disease.

The striking radiographic features are a narrow thorax and short, horizontally oriented ribs with wide, irregular costochondral junctions (Fig. 75–12). The clavicles may have a high, handlebar appearance. The neonatal pelvic findings, similar to those in chondroectodermal dysplasia, are short iliac, pubic, and ischial bones, with the lateral borders of the ilia being rounded. The acetabular roofs are flat, with downward spikelike projections at the medial, lateral, and, sometimes, central aspects of the acetabular roofs, the so-called triradiate or trident acetabulum (Fig. 75–13). The pelvis normalizes with age, but the proximal femoral metaphyses may become progressively irregular. Infants have mild digital shortening, especially in the distal phalanges, and inconstant polydactyly. Later, the epiphyses become cone shaped and fuse prematurely (Fig. 75–14).

Asphyxiating thoracic dystrophy has many radiographic and histopathologic features that are similar to those of chondroectodermal dysplasia, but in contrast to the latter disorder, it is characterized by shorter ribs, a higher prevalence of progressive renal disease, hepatic fibrosis, less prominent nail changes, and less frequent polydactyly.

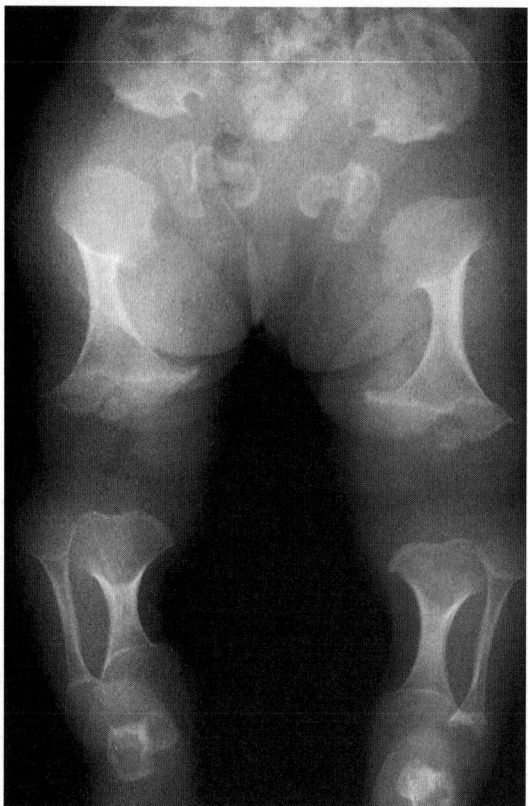

**Figure 75–11.** Metatropic dysplasia. In this newborn infant, the bones are shortened, with marked metaphyseal flaring and large femoral trochanters. The iliac bones are short, with curved lateral margins and small sacrosciatic notches.

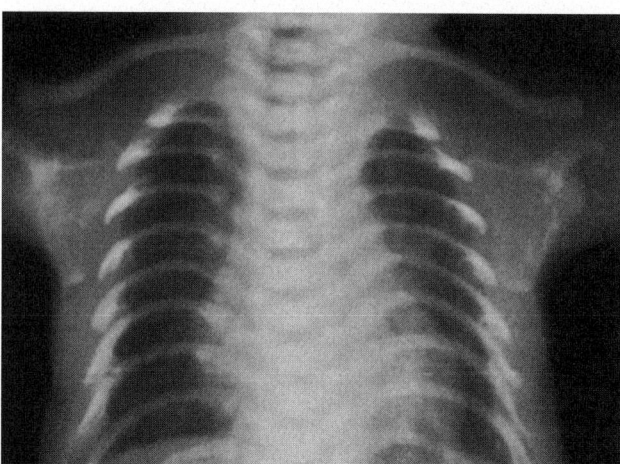

**Figure 75–12.** Asphyxiating thoracic dystrophy: chest. Note the short ribs and handlebar appearance of the clavicles.

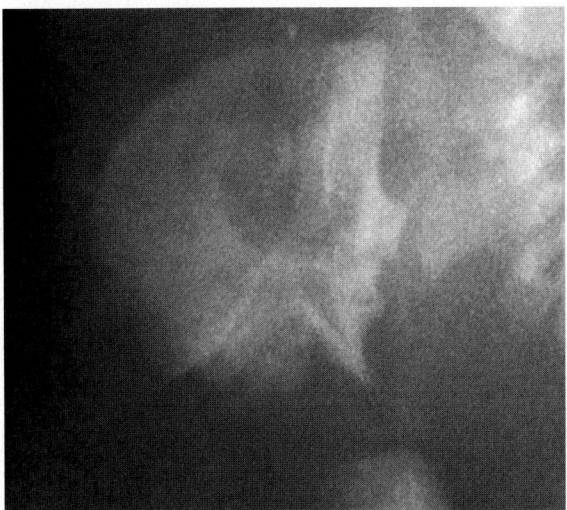

**Figure 75–13.** Asphyxiating thoracic dystrophy: pelvis. Observe the three downward-projecting acetabular spikes.

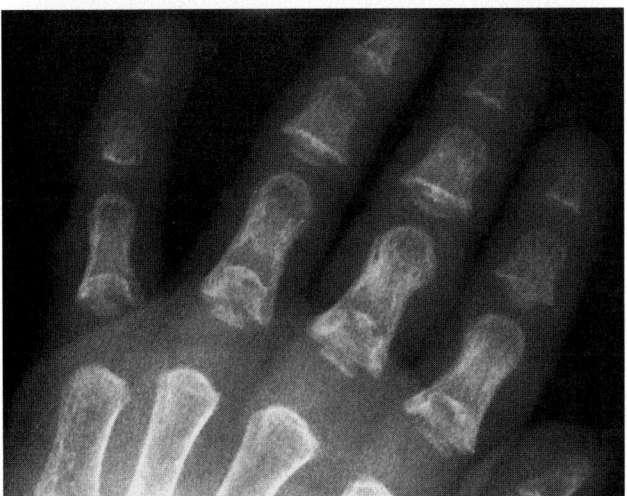

**Figure 75–14.** Asphyxiating thoracic dystrophy: hand. Cone-shaped epiphyses and short phalanges are present.

## Chondroectodermal Dysplasia (Ellis-van Creveld Dysplasia)

Ellis-van Creveld dysplasia, a short-limbed dwarfism, is characterized by ectodermal dysplasia, polydactyly, and congenital heart disease. The condition is inherited as an autosomal recessive trait and is evident at birth. Short stature, distal shortening of limbs, polydactyly (especially in the hands), absent or hypoplastic fingernails or toenails, dysplastic teeth, and upper lip abnormalities are common findings. Cardiac defects, renal abnormalities, and hydrocephalus may be seen. Some radiographic features resemble those of familial asphyxiating thoracic dystrophy. In addition, some patients have shortening of the tubular bones (especially the phalanges), carpal fusion, an extra carpal bone, cone-shaped epiphyses, enlargement of the proximal end of the ulna and distal end of the radius (drumstick appearance), and anterior dislocation

of the radial heads. A wider but hypoplastic lateral aspect of the proximal end of the tibia, medial tibial diaphyseal exostoses, genu valgum, and fibular shortening are typical (Figs. 75–15 and 75–16). The skull and spine are usually normal. Death in childhood is common owing to cardiac and pulmonary complications.

## Spondyloepimetaphyseal Dysplasias

**X-Linked Spondyloepiphyseal Dysplasia Tarda.** The X-linked recessive condition of spondyloepiphyseal dysplasia tarda occurs only in male subjects and generally becomes evident between age 5 and 10 years because of impaired spinal growth. In addition, autosomal dominant and autosomal recessive forms occur. Radiographic findings in the spine predominate in the lumbar area and are quite characteristic, consisting of vertebral bodies that have a hump-shaped area of dense bone on the central and posterior portions of the endplates (Fig. 75–17). The disc spaces appear narrow posteriorly and wide anteriorly. The odontoid process may be deformed. Degenerative spinal changes develop in early adulthood. The bones in the pelvis and the femoral necks may appear slightly small. Coxa vara may be present. The chest has a relative increase in its anteroposterior diameter. Mild flattening of the epiphyses occurs about the major joints, especially the hips and shoulders. Osteoarthritis, particularly in the hips, may eventually become disabling.

**Spondyloepimetaphyseal Dysplasia.** Spondyloepimetaphyseal dysplasia encompasses a heterogeneous group of conditions characterized by involvement of the spine, epiphyses, and metaphyses, resulting in osseous shortening and deformities. These conditions must be distinguished from others that may affect similar portions of

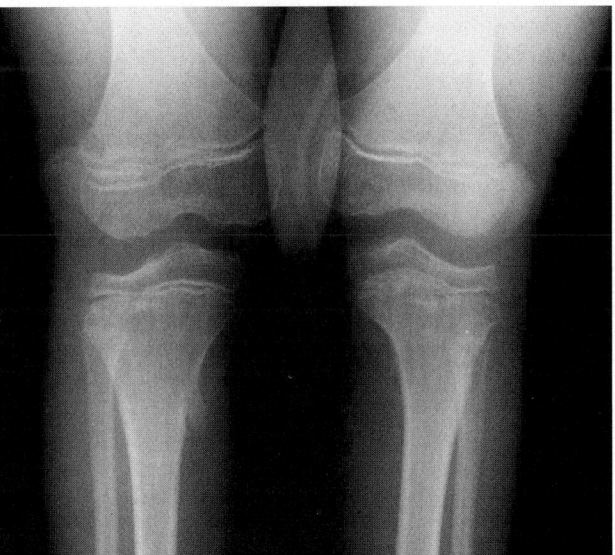

**Figure 75–15.** Chondroectodermal dysplasia. The tubular bones are shortened, with metaphyseal flaring. The lateral portion of the proximal tibial epiphysis is poorly developed. A medial diaphyseal excrescence is present on the tibia, and the patellae are dislocated.

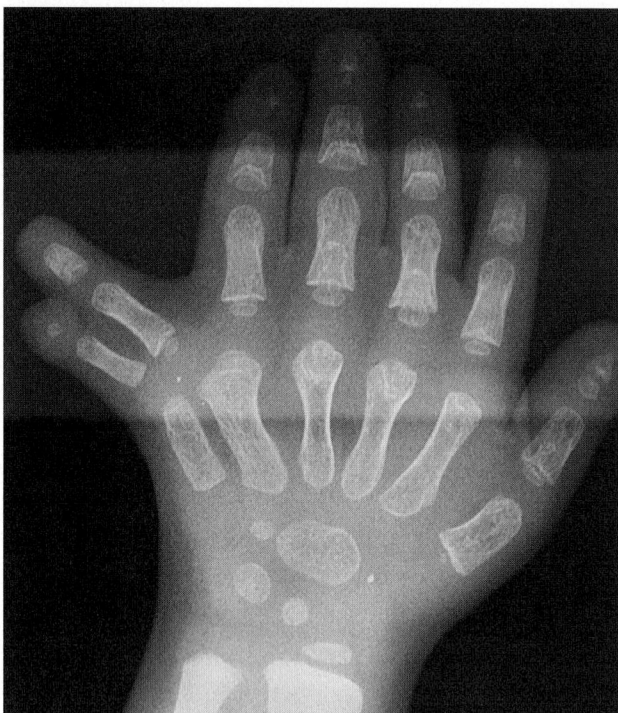

**Figure 75–16.** Chondroectodermal dysplasia. Postaxial polydactyly and shortening of the tubular bones (especially the distal phalanges, which appear as linear streaks) are apparent. Cone-shaped epiphyses are best seen in the middle phalanges. The capitate and hamate are fused, and an extra carpal ossicle appears lateral to the hamate.

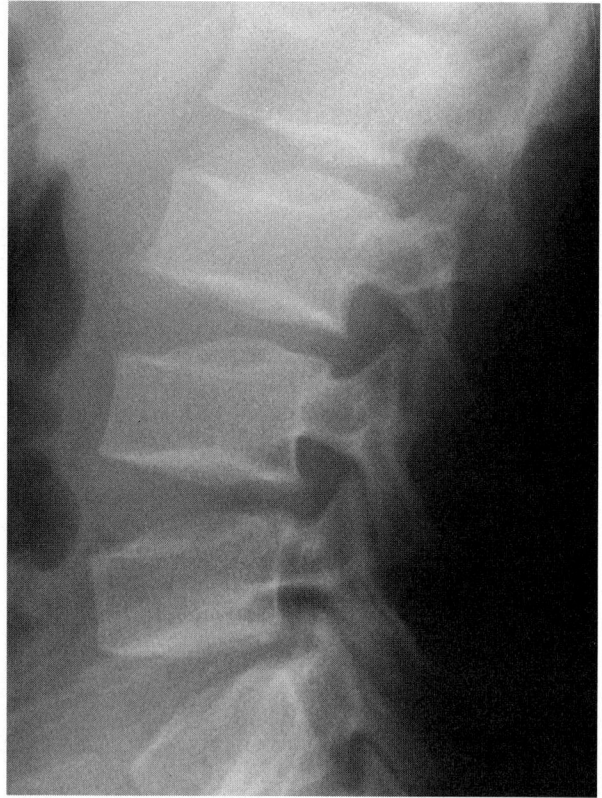

**Figure 75–17.** Spondyloepiphyseal dysplasia tarda: X-linked recessive. The characteristic osseous "humps" are evident in the central and posterior portions of the vertebral endplates. The disc spaces are narrow posteriorly and wide anteriorly.

the skeleton, such as metatropic dysplasia and pseudoachondroplasia. The micromelic type of spondyloepimetaphyseal dysplasia is presumed to be of autosomal recessive inheritance; patients have greatest shortening in the proximal portion of the limbs, relatively long hands and feet, genu valgum, scoliosis, increased lordosis, facial flattening, and hypertelorism. Another variety, the Irapa, is characterized by shortening of the tubular bones, epimetaphyseal dysplasia, platyspondyly, osteopenia, abnormal carpal bones, decreased size of the pelvic bones, coxa vara, and premature degenerative joint disease.

### Spondylometaphyseal Dysplasias

The poorly defined and complex group of diseases known as the spondylometaphyseal dysplasias is characterized by abnormalities in the vertebrae and metaphyses of tubular bones. Considerable heterogeneity can be found in the clinical and radiographic appearances. The most common type of spondylometaphyseal dysplasia (Kozlowski's type) is accompanied by short stature, kyphosis and scoliosis, diminutive hands and feet, bowing of the bones, and, in the lower extremities, joint limitation and gait disturbance. It is an autosomal dominant disorder. Radiographically, the vertebral bodies are flattened appreciably and can be deformed further with spinal curvatures. Irregular metaphyses are most marked in the proximal portion of the femora, where coxa vara is also evident (Fig. 75–18).

Flattening and irregularity in the epiphyses are usually mild, although premature degenerative changes are noted in the joints.

### Multiple Epiphyseal Dysplasias

Multiple epiphyseal dysplasias are discussed in Chapter 74.

### Pseudoachondroplasia

In pseudoachondroplasia, a type of short-stature dwarfism that resembles achondroplasia, the head is normal and the hands and feet are shorter than those seen in true achondroplasia. The legs may be bowed, and the gait is waddling.

Radiographic findings become apparent in late infancy and are modified throughout childhood. Initially, the epiphyses are small and flattened, and the metaphyses are wide. In adults, the tubular bones are short and expanded at their ends. The epiphyses remain abnormal, and premature degenerative arthritis develops as the metaphyseal irregularity resolves. The vertebral bodies are initially oval or biconvex, with central tonguelike anterior projections (Fig. 75–19); later they become wedged or flattened, but the vertebral bodies can have a more normal appearance in adulthood. About half of patients have some vertebral endplate irregularity in childhood. The inferior border of the ilium has a sloping acetabular angle

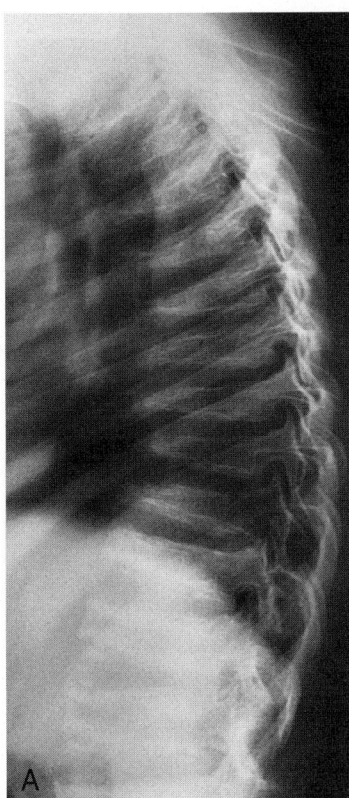

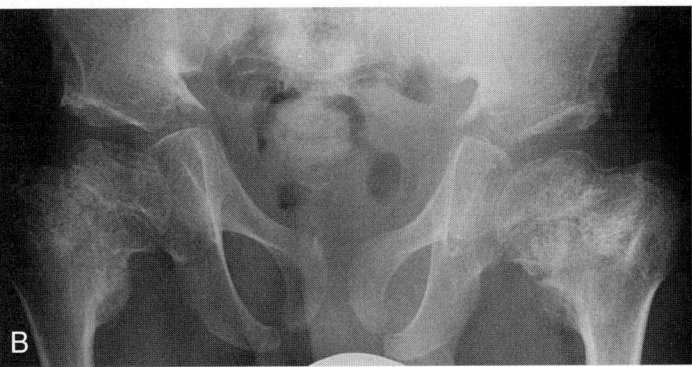

**Figure 75–18.** Spondylometaphyseal dysplasia: Kozlowski's type. *A,* Marked flattening of the vertebral bodies, with anterior wedging in the thoracic spine, is seen. *B,* In the pelvis, shortened femoral necks; metaphyseal and epiphyseal irregularities; flat, broad acetabula; and narrow sacrosciatic notches are evident.

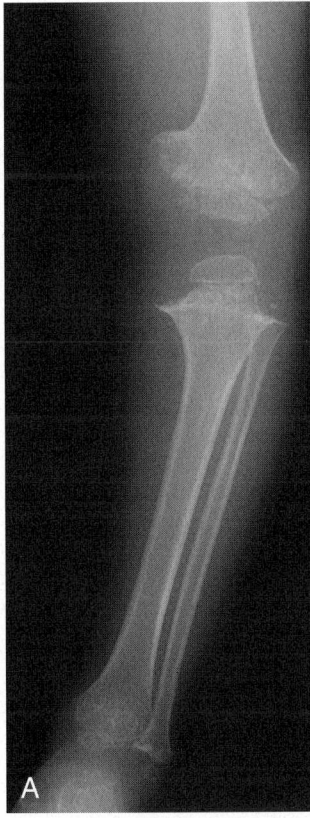

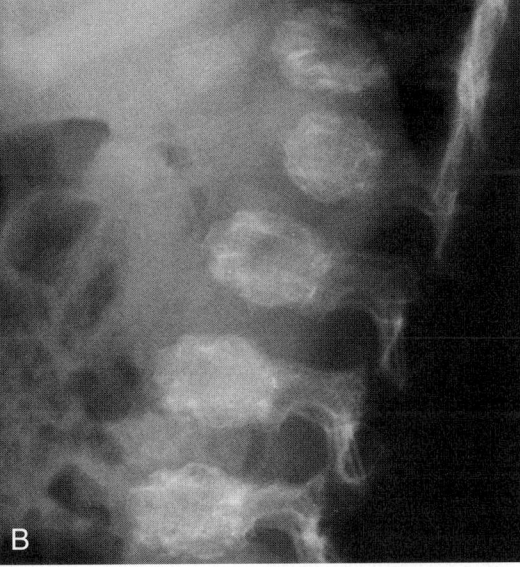

**Figure 75–19.** Pseudoachondroplasia. *A,* Note the small epiphyses and metaphyseal flaring in this 5-year-old child. *B,* The vertebral bodies are rounded, with anterior tongues. Note hypoplasia of the first lumbar vertebra.

and a spiked appearance. The iliac wings may be slightly underdeveloped. As the patient grows, the pelvis becomes more normal in appearance, although coxa vara and deformity of the femoral heads persist.

## Chondrodysplasia Punctata (Stippled Epiphyses)

This dysplasia is reviewed in Chapter 74.

## Metaphyseal Dysplasias

The term metaphyseal dysplasia applies to a number of conditions in which the greatest involvement occurs in the metaphyses, which are flared and irregular; the epiphyses and diaphyses may also be abnormal, however. The spine is normal or involved minimally. There are several types, the most common of which are discussed here.

**Jansen's Type.** The Jansen type of metaphyseal dysplasia is a rare but severe disorder characterized by marked dwarfism, swelling of the joints, and bowed forearms and legs. The face has typical features: frontonasal hyperplasia, hypertelorism, and a receding chin. The inheritance pattern is autosomal dominant. In infancy, radiographs reveal marked irregularity of the metaphyses, widening of the growth plates, diffuse osteopenia, and mild bowing of the long tubular bones. The metaphyseal changes are also apparent in the short tubular bones. In childhood, the metaphyses become cupped, with wide zones of irregular calcification that eventually disappear as the growth plate closes in adulthood. The resultant bones are shortened and bowed and have metaphyseal flaring (Fig. 75–20). The skull is osteopenic. The spine shows minimal platyspondyly, and the anterior ends of the ribs are flared.

**Schmid's Type.** Inheritance of the Schmid type is autosomal dominant. Patients have short stature of variable severity and bowed legs; the disorder usually manifests after infancy. Radiographically, metaphyseal irregularity, flaring, and growth plate widening are present, most obviously about the knees and hips (Fig. 75–21). Proximal femoral metaphyseal involvement with resultant coxa vara is common. The abnormalities in this condition may be confused with the skeletal changes of child abuse, and the widened growth plate may suggest rickets.

**McKusick's Type.** This metaphyseal dysplasia of autosomal recessive inheritance is often termed cartilage-hair hypoplasia. Patients are of normal intelligence and are very short; they have fine, light-colored hair, small hands, bowed legs, and joint laxity. Complex immune deficiencies are seen, with a resultant increase in the frequency of infections and malignant tumors. Radiographic findings include minimal epiphyseal flattening with metaphyseal cupping and flaring (Fig. 75–22). Metaphyseal abnormalities are most prominent in the lower extremities and, when severe, are associated with a short stature. The bones in the hands and feet are small, and the carpal bones appear irregular. The vertebral bodies are small. Additional vertebral abnormalities include atlantoaxial subluxation with odontoid hypoplasia.

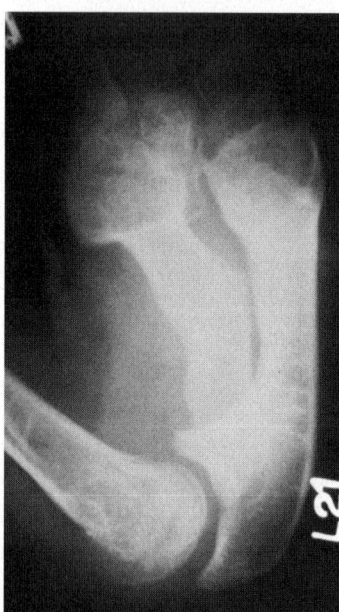

**Figure 75–20.** Metaphyseal dysplasia: Jansen's type. Marked shortening, bowing, and metaphyseal expansion of the bones in the forearm are seen in this 11-year-old patient.

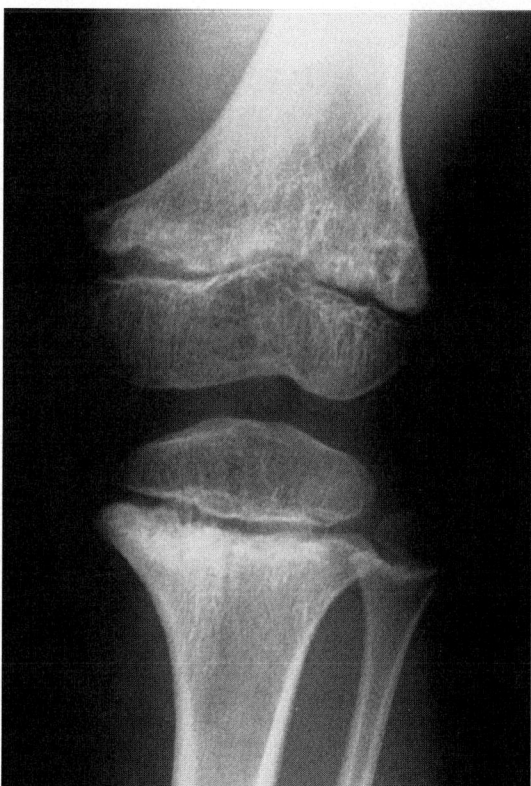

**Figure 75–21.** Metaphyseal dysplasia: Schmid's type. In this 5-year-old child, the tubular bones are short, and V-shaped metaphyseal irregularities are present, best observed in the femur.

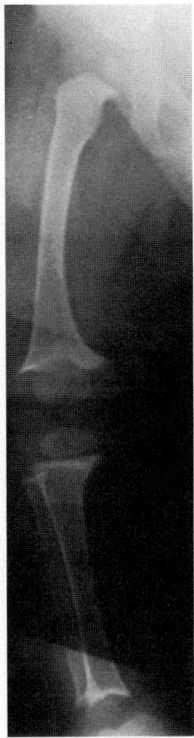

**Figure 75–22.** Metaphyseal dysplasia: McKusick's type. In this 9-month-old child, the tubular bones are short, and V-shaped metaphyseal irregularities are present, best observed in the femur.

## Dyschondrosteosis

Dyschondrosteosis, also called Léri-Weill syndrome, is a common condition characterized by a mild mesomelic type of limb shortening with Madelung's deformity of the forearm. The term mesomelic indicates that limb shortening results primarily from changes in the forearms and lower legs. The inheritance pattern is autosomal dominant, and the disease expresses itself more frequently and more severely in female patients. Radiographic findings include a shortened radius that is bowed dorsally and laterally and a distal segment of the ulna that is often subluxed or dislocated dorsally (Fig. 75–23). Lack of development of the distal radial epiphysis, with premature fusion of the medial side of the physis, is the most characteristic finding in dyschondrosteosis. The carpal bones fit into the resulting V-shaped deformity of the radius and ulna. The distance between the radius and ulna is increased. When accompanied by tibia varum, a relatively long fibula can distort the shape of the ankle mortise. Coxa valga can also occur, and the tubular bones in the hands and feet may be shortened.

## Dysplasias with Prominent Membranous Bone Involvement

**Cleidocranial Dysplasia.** Cleidocranial dysplasia, an autosomal dominant disorder with high penetrance, has a wide range of clinical manifestations. Mild shortening of stature may be seen. The head is large and brachycephalic, with a small face and bossing of the frontal and parietal bones.

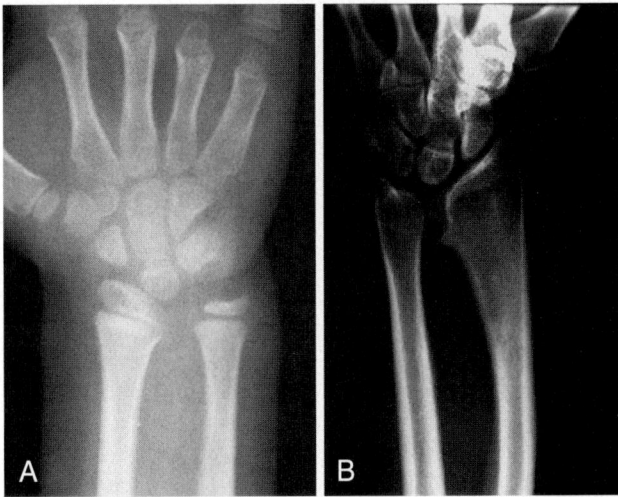

**Figure 75–23.** Dyschondrosteosis. *A,* In this 5-year-old girl, a radiograph shows separation of the radius and ulna and underdevelopment of the medial aspect of the radius. The carpal bones fit into the V-shaped deformity of the wrist. *B,* In the mother of the child in *(A),* a classic V-shaped deformity of the radiocarpal joint is present.

The sutures are wide, and their closure is delayed. Genu valgum and short fingers may be seen.

Radiographic findings include poor ossification of the skull, with wide sutures and multiple wormian bones (Fig. 75–24). Parietal bone ossification may be absent at birth. The mandible may be broad, with persistence of its synchondrosis. Although total clavicular absence is uncommon, any portion of the clavicle may be absent; the middle or outer portion is affected most commonly (Fig. 75–25). The scapula is hypoplastic, with a small glenoid cavity, and the thorax may be bell shaped, especially in patients with more severe clavicular abnormalities. Pelvic alterations occur frequently and consist of a delay in ossification of the pubic bones, a wide symphysis

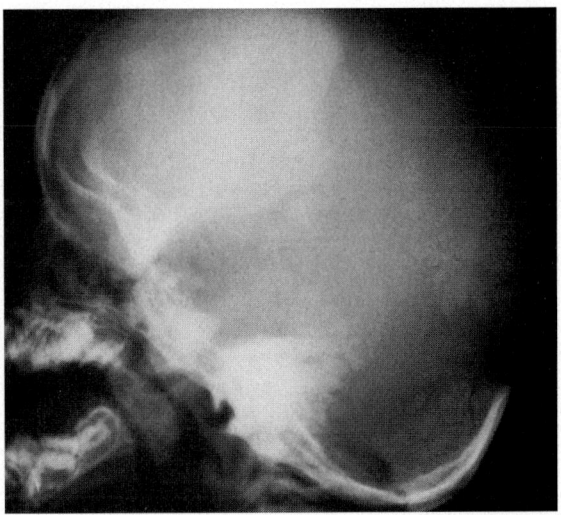

**Figure 75–24.** Cleidocranial dysplasia. Skull radiograph in a 15-month-old patient demonstrates wide sutures, poor ossification of the parietal bone, and multiple wormian bones.

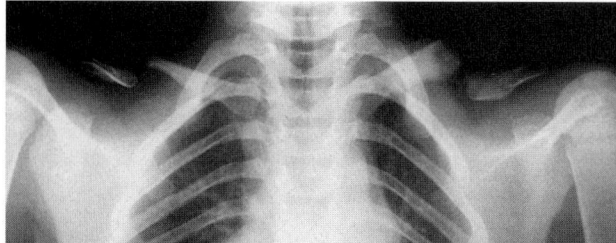

**Figure 75–25.** Cleidocranial dysplasia. In this 8-year-old patient, note clavicular defects at the junction of the outer and middle thirds of the bone.

pubis, and narrow iliac wings (Fig. 75–26). Although coxa valga deformity is more frequent, unilateral or bilateral coxa vara deformity may develop. The spinal changes consist primarily of spina bifida occulta. The findings in the hand include small, tapered distal phalanges; slightly small middle phalanges; pseudoepiphyses in the metacarpal bones; cone-shaped epiphyses; and retarded ossification of the carpal bones.

**Osteodysplasty (Melnick-Needles Syndrome).** The clinical appearance of affected patients is more or less characteristic. Typically, the face is small, with large ears, protruding eyes, micrognathia, and malaligned teeth; the upper portions of the arms are short, and the thorax is narrow. The inheritance pattern of the disorder is X-linked autosomal dominant, and it is lethal in most but not all male subjects.

Radiographically, the cortex of the tubular bones is irregular, with an undulating contour and multiple constrictions of the medullary cavities (Fig. 75–27). Lateral bowing of the tibia is typical. The ribs have a ribbon-like appearance and cortical irregularity. The normal curvature of the clavicle is accentuated, and it may have cortical irregularity and wide medial ends. Sclerosis appears at

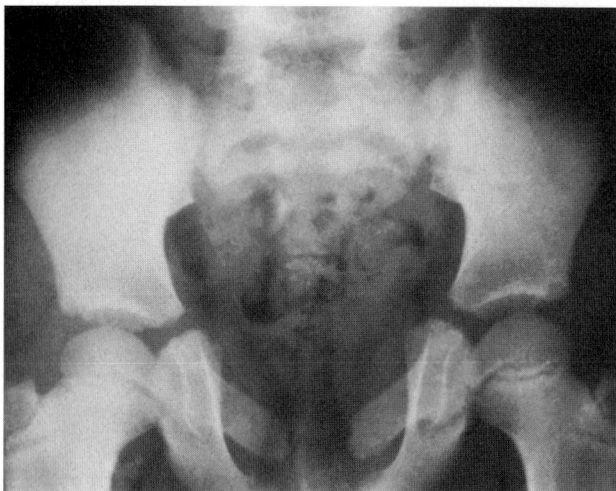

**Figure 75–26.** Cleidocranial dysplasia: pelvis. In this 8-year-old child, incomplete ossification of the pubic bones and narrow iliac wings are evident.

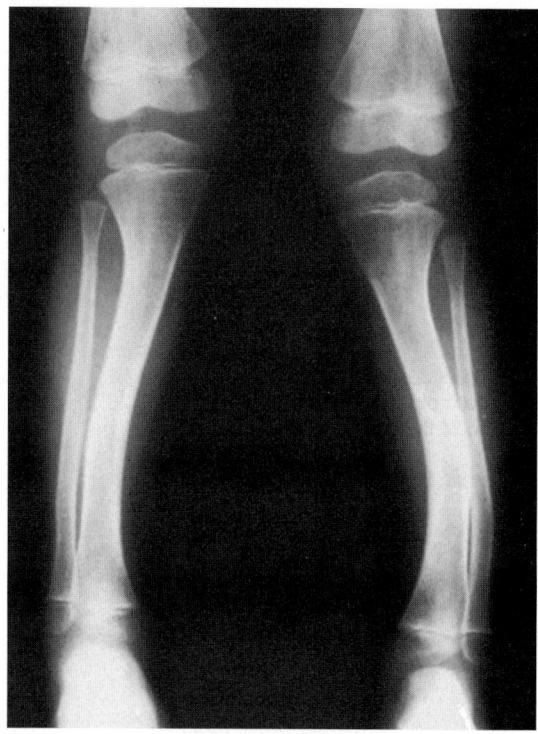

**Figure 75–27.** Osteodysplasty (Melnick-Needles syndrome). Note the characteristic lateral bowing of the tibias.

the base of the skull and mastoid bones, and the anterior portion of the cranial fossa is small. The mandible is thin and small, with an obtuse angle and hypoplastic coronoid processes. In the spine, the vertebral bodies show an increased height and anterior concavity; in the lumbar region, the spinal canal may be enlarged, and the laminae appear thinned. Scoliosis or kyphoscoliosis can occur.

## Dysplasias with Decreased Bone Density

Osteogenesis imperfecta, homocystinuria, and idiopathic juvenile osteoporosis are discussed in chapters 41 and 74.

## Dysplasias with Defective Mineralization

Hypophosphatasia, rickets, and neonatal hyperparathyroidism are discussed in Chapters 42 and 46.

## Dysplasias with Increased Bone Density

### Osteopetrosis

Osteopetrosis is a complex disease with at least four different types that have distinct features.

**Precocious Type.** The precocious type of osteopetrosis is an autosomal recessive form, also called the lethal form; this designation is misleading, however, because some patients survive for a number of years. Clinical abnormalities include failure to thrive, hepatosplenomegaly, and cranial nerve dysfunction, especially blindness and deafness. The head may be large, owing to hydrocephalus.

Obliteration of the marrow cavity by abnormal bone leads to anemia and thrombocytopenia and predisposes to recurrent infections, with early death occurring in most patients.

The radiographic findings are characterized by generalized osteosclerosis. Tubular bones show a failure of differentiation between the cortex and the medullary cavity (Fig. 75–28). Modeling in these bones is defective and, in some instances, leads to a clublike appearance. Longitudinal striations, observed occasionally, are believed to correspond to sites of blood vessels that are surrounded by connective tissue. A "bone within bone" (or "endobone") appearance is an unusual but characteristic finding. Periostitis may be seen, particularly in infants, and fractures, which generally heal, are common. The entire skull is involved, but the cartilaginous portion at its base is affected most frequently and severely (Fig. 75–29). The teeth may be malformed, and the mastoid regions and paranasal sinuses are poorly developed. In the spine, the vertebral bodies tend to be uniformly radiodense, with a prominent anterior vascular notch (see Fig. 75–29B).

**Delayed Type.** The delayed type, an autosomal dominant variety of osteopetrosis, is also called Albers-Schönberg disease. Affected persons may be relatively asymptomatic. The disease may be detected because of a pathologic fracture, problems after tooth extraction, mild anemia, or cranial nerve palsies. The radiographic findings are similar to but less severe than those in the autosomal recessive form of the disease. The bones are diffusely osteosclerotic, with defective tubulation and a thickened cortex. The vertebral endplates become accentuated, especially with advancing age (Fig. 75–30). A "bone within bone" appear-

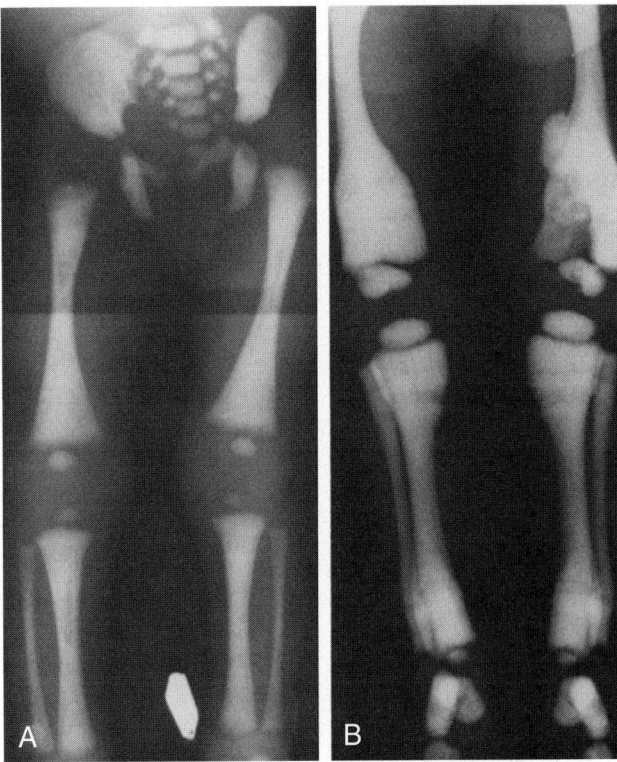

**Figure 75–28.** Osteopetrosis: precocious or autosomal recessive lethal type. *A,* In a newborn infant, diffuse osteosclerosis and slight metaphyseal expansion of the tubular bones are evident. *B,* In a different patient, aged 16 months, marked osteosclerosis and bone expansion are seen. Note the transverse and horizontal radiolucent lines in the metaphyses and a pathologic fracture in the left femur.

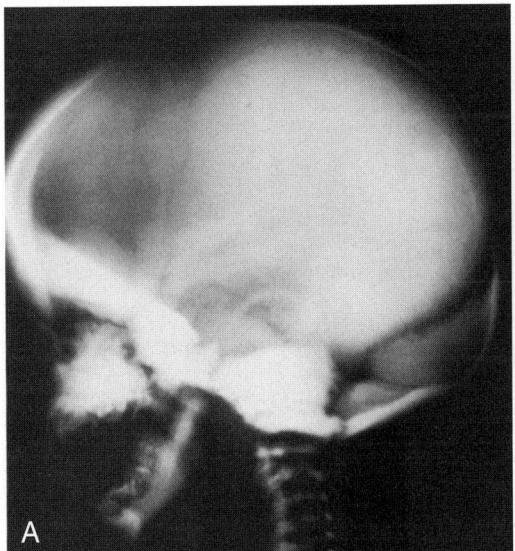

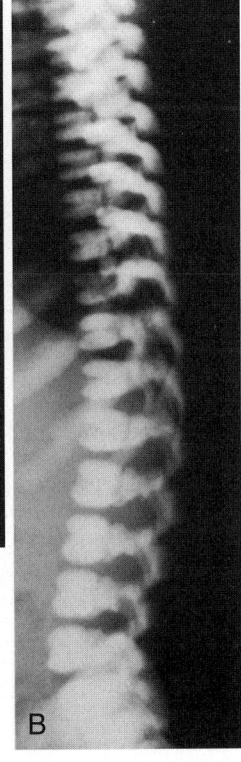

**Figure 75–29.** Osteopetrosis: precocious or autosomal recessive lethal type. *A,* Diffuse osteosclerosis of the skull, most marked at the base, is present. *B,* Diffuse vertebral sclerosis and accentuation of the anterior vascular notches are evident.

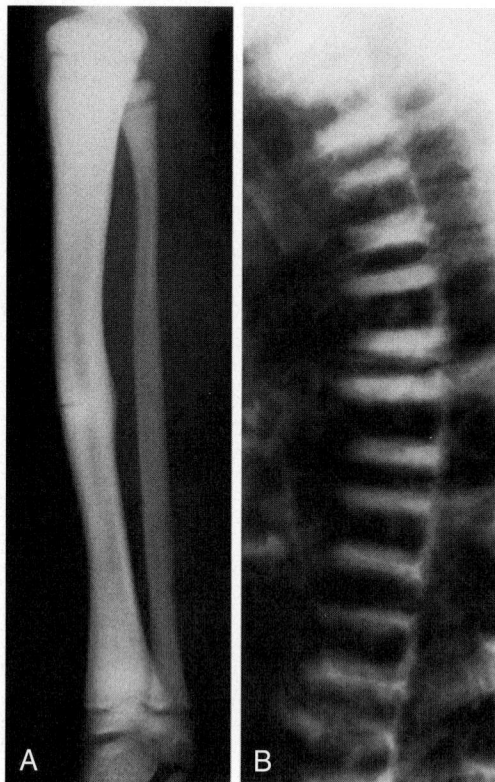

**Figure 75–30.** Osteopetrosis: delayed or autosomal dominant type. *A*, Osteosclerosis, cortical thickening, and an incomplete fracture are evident. *B*, Osteosclerosis in the superior and inferior portions of the vertebral bodies has produced a "sandwich" appearance.

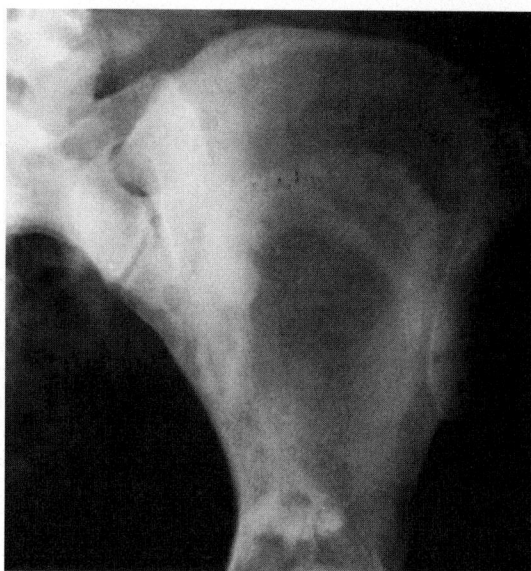

**Figure 75–31.** Osteopetrosis: delayed or autosomal dominant type. The "bone within bone" appearance is seen in the ilium of an adult patient.

ance or radiolucent bands in the ends of the diaphyses are sometimes seen (Fig. 75–31). The autosomal dominant form of osteopetrosis is subdivided into two types. In type I, there is pronounced sclerosis of the cranial vault, and the spine is almost unaffected. In type II, the skull sclerosis is most pronounced at the base; the vertebrae always have endplate thickening; and in the pelvis, the iliac wings contain convex arcs of sclerotic bone.

**Intermediate Recessive Type.** A milder, recessive form of osteopetrosis is distinct from both the more severe recessive form seen in infants and the less severe autosomal dominant form. Affected patients are often of short stature, with pathologic fractures, anemia, and hepatomegaly. The radiographic findings are characterized by diffuse bone sclerosis, interference with normal bone modeling, a "bone within bone" appearance, and retained primary and impacted permanent teeth.

**Tubular Acidosis Type.** This variety, also called "marble brain" disease or Sly's disease, consists of osteopetrosis, renal tubular acidosis, and cerebral calcifications. The inheritance pattern is autosomal recessive, and the clinical course is compatible with long survival; however, many patients are mentally retarded. Typical clinical findings include a failure to thrive, symptoms related to renal tubular acidosis, muscle weakness, and hypotonia. Radiographic findings are detected throughout the skeleton

and include osteosclerosis, obliteration of the medullary cavity, and pathologic fractures. An unusual aspect of this disease is the occurrence of progressive improvement in the radiographic abnormalities. Intracranial calcification can be located anywhere in the brain, but generally it is found in the basal ganglia and periventricular areas (Fig. 75–32).

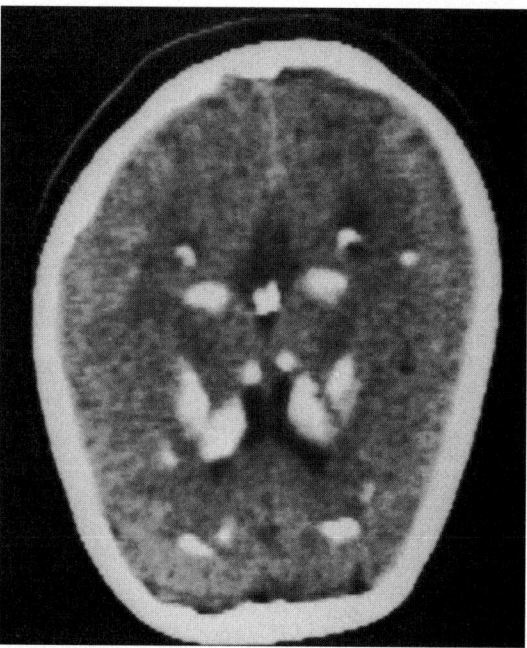

**Figure 75–32.** Osteopetrosis: recessive type with tubular acidosis. In a patient with carbonic anhydrase II deficiency, diffuse intracranial calcifications, particularly in the basal ganglia and periventricular areas, are seen.

## Pyknodysostosis

The syndrome of pyknodysostosis consists of osteosclerosis; short stature; frontal and occipital bossing; a small face with a receding chin; short, broad hands; and hypoplasia of the nails. This disorder is of autosomal recessive inheritance and is often accompanied by multiple fractures. The painter Toulouse-Lautrec is believed to have had this syndrome. Radiographic findings include generalized and uniform osteosclerosis (Fig. 75–33). Metaphyseal modeling is only mildly abnormal, and the medullary cavities may be narrowed. The bones of the hands and feet are short, with hypoplasia or osteolysis of the distal phalanges. In the skull, a marked delay in closure of the sutures is evident, and the anterior fontanelle may remain open, even in adults. Wormian bones are common, especially in the lambdoid sutures. The mandible is hypoplastic, without normal angulation. The vertebral bodies are sclerotic, and errors in vertebral segmentation may be present in the upper portion of the cervical spine. The acromial ends of the clavicles may be resorbed.

## Increased Bone Density with Diaphyseal Involvement

### Diaphyseal Dysplasia (Camurati-Engelmann Disease)

Camurati-Engelmann disease is a generalized, bilaterally symmetrical dysplasia of bone that is characterized by cortical thickening, narrowing of the medullary cavity, and a sclerotic and expanded diaphyseal segment that results from periosteal and endosteal bone formation. The epiphyses are spared. Diaphyseal dysplasia is an autosomal dominant disorder with considerable variability of expression. In some patients, the presenting symptoms appear in the first decade of life, whereas in others, the disease is not discovered until the second, third, or fourth decade of life. Characteristic radiographic features include cortical thickening and sclerosis of the diaphyses of the tubular bones (Fig. 75–34). The osteosclerosis is irregular and inhomogeneous, and endosteal involvement is greater than periosteal involvement. In order of decreasing frequency, the tibia, femur, humerus, ulna, radius, and bones

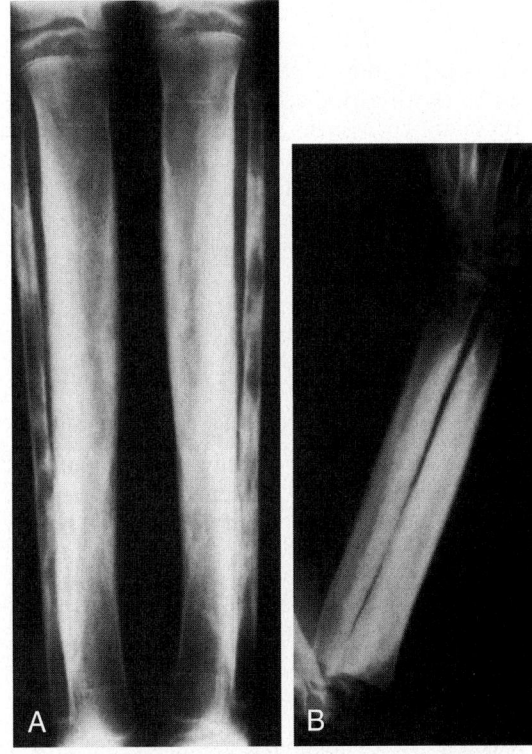

**Figure 75–34.** Diaphyseal dysplasia (Camurati-Engelmann disease). Radiographs of the lower legs *(A)* and forearm *(B)* show widening of the tubular bones with thickened cortices and narrowed medullary canals. Mottled areas of rarefaction are present, best observed in the fibula.

of the hands and feet are affected. A symmetrical distribution is typical but is not present uniformly. Sclerosis of the base of the skull is common.

The course of this disease is variable. Progressive findings are common, but spontaneous improvement in adolescence has also been recognized. Increased intracranial pressure and encroachment on cranial nerves can lead to significant complications in some patients.

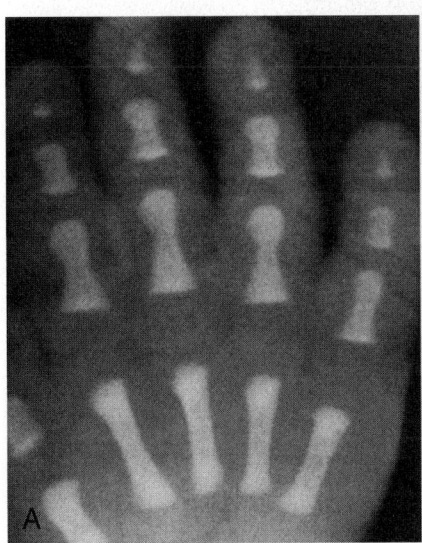
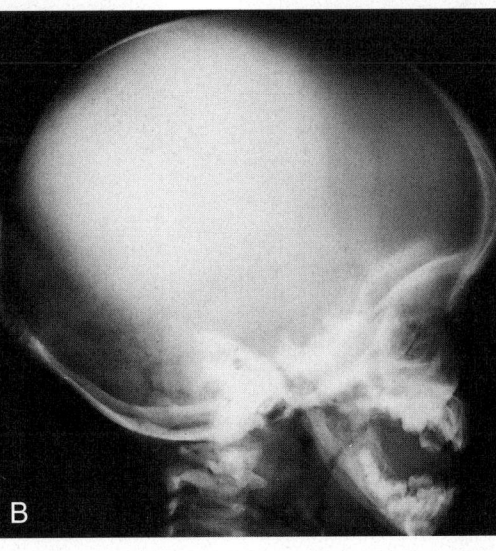

**Figure 75–33.** Pyknodysostosis. *A,* In a newborn infant, diffuse osteosclerosis, with hypoplasia of the distal phalanges, is present. *B,* In a 4-month-old child, wide sutures and basal sclerosis are the significant cranial abnormalities. The mandible is hypoplastic.

## Endosteal Hyperostosis

Although the terminology used to describe the group of diseases termed endosteal hyperostosis is inconstant, and a definitive classification system has yet to be proposed, three types of hyperostosis are considered here: an autosomal recessive type that occurs in childhood (Van Buchem's type), a more severe autosomal recessive syndrome (sclerosteosis), and an autosomal dominant type appearing in late childhood (Worth's type).

**Van Buchem's Type.** Symptoms and signs occur at an earlier age in Van Buchem's syndrome than in the autosomal dominant form of the disease and consist of more severe enlargement of the mandible and more frequent cranial nerve involvement, including facial nerve palsy and deafness. Affected patients also have a prominent forehead and widened nasal bridge, and serum levels of alkaline phosphatase may be elevated. Unlike with sclerosteosis, stature is normal. Radiographic findings are similar to but more severe than those in the dominant form of the disease (Fig. 75–35). Specific abnormalities include periosteal excrescences in the tubular bones, osteosclerotic and enlarged ribs and clavicles, and increased radiodensity of the spine.

**Sclerosteosis.** This autosomal recessive form usually becomes evident in infancy or early childhood. Clinical findings are excessive height and weight; peculiar facies, with a broad, flat nasal bridge; ocular hypertelorism; mandibular prominence; deafness; facial palsy; cutaneous or bony syndactyly of the second and third fingers; absent or dysplastic nails; and radial deviation of the terminal phalanges. Radiographs show a progressive, marked hyperostosis of the skull and mandible. The vertebral endplates and pedicles and the bones of the pelvis are sclerotic. The long bones are enlarged, with cortical hyperostosis.

**Worth's Type.** Worth's syndrome, an autosomal dominant form of endosteal hyperostosis, may be detected incidentally; however, asymmetrical enlargement of portions of the face, particularly the jaw, and the presence of a palatal mass (torus palatinus) are important clinical signs. Radiographic findings include endosteal thickening in the cortex of the tubular bones, with encroachment on the medullary cavity. The bones are not expanded, and abnormal modeling is absent. In the skull, osteosclerosis begins in the base and subsequently involves the facial bones, especially the mandible. The latter bone lacks the normal antegonial notch, and the mandibular canal may be prominent (Fig. 75–36). In the spine, the sclerosis is most evident in the spinous processes. The ribs and osseous pelvis are affected only mildly.

## Pachydermoperiostosis

The clinical and radiographic features of pachydermoperiostosis, which resemble, in part, those of secondary hypertrophic osteoarthropathy, are discussed in Chapter 82.

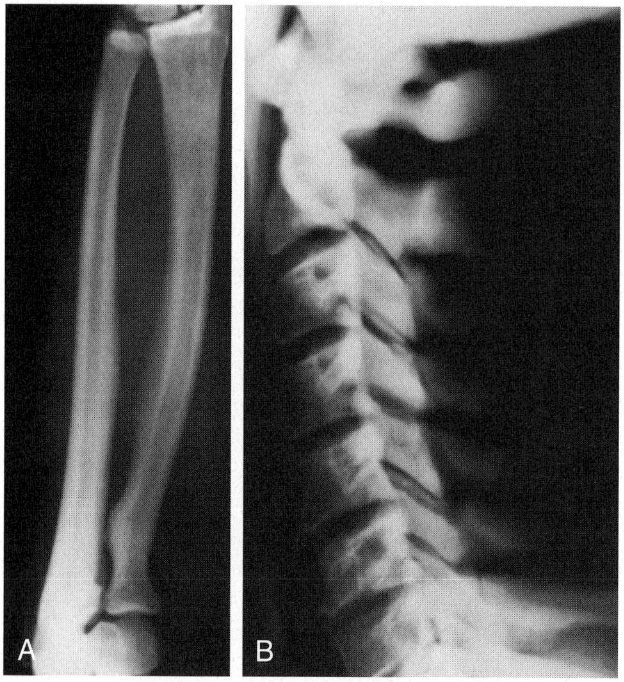

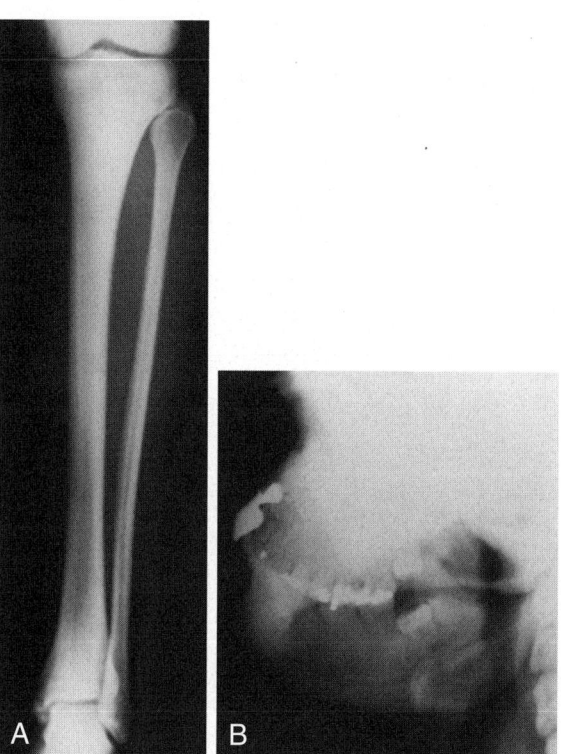

**Figure 75–36.** Endosteal hyperostosis: autosomal dominant (Worth's) syndrome. *A,* In an adult, endosteal thickening of the cortices has led to encroachment of the medullary canals. *B,* Mandibular findings include osteosclerosis, loss of the normal antegonial notch, coarse trabeculation, and a prominent mandibular canal.

**Figure 75–35.** Endosteal hyperostosis: autosomal recessive (Van Buchem's) syndrome. *A,* Note diffuse osteosclerosis and cortical thickening. *B,* Osteosclerosis is especially marked in the neural arches and spinous processes.

## Increased Bone Density with Metaphyseal Involvement

**Frontometaphyseal Dysplasia.** Frontometaphyseal dysplasia encompasses cranial hyperostosis, abnormal tubulation of cylindrical bone, and additional skeletal and extraskeletal abnormalities. Clinical manifestations include childhood onset, prominent hornlike supraorbital ridges, micrognathia, defective dentition, wide nasal bridge, high-arched palate, hearing loss, visual disturbances, short trunk with long extremities, elongated fingers with ulnar deviation of the hands, genu valgum, decreased joint mobility, and contractures. An X-linked recessive inheritance is likely.

Radiographic features consist of a prominent supraorbital ridge, calvarial hyperostosis, absent frontal sinuses, antegonial notching of the mandibular body, hypoplasia of the angle and condylar process of the mandible, dental malformations, accentuated flaring of the iliac wings, metaphyseal splaying in the tubular bones, tibial and fibular waviness and bowing, genu valgum, tibia recurvatum, and elongation and widening of the metacarpal bones and phalanges (Fig. 75–37). In older patients, progressive erosion and fusion of the carpal and tarsal bones have been noted. The presence of prominent cranial abnormalities allows its differentiation from Pyle's dysplasia.

**Craniometaphyseal Dysplasia.** The basic features of both the autosomal dominant and recessive forms of craniometaphyseal dysplasia are facial deformity, cranial hyperostosis, and failure of normal modeling of tubular bones. The recessive forms of the disease are accompanied by more severe facial involvement, which in some cases leads to striking abnormalities consisting of a broad mass at the base of the nose and hypertelorism. Dental mal-occlusion and facial paralysis often occur. Deafness results, in part, from foraminal constriction, with encroachment on the auditory nerve, and from direct involvement of the ossicles in the inner ear.

Radiographically, progressive sclerosis of the base of the skull and about the cranial sutures, obliteration of the paranasal sinuses, and loss of the lamina dura about the teeth are seen. In infancy, osteosclerosis in the diaphysis of the tubular bones, similar to that observed in diaphyseal dysplasia, is evident; it subsequently disappears and is replaced by a severe modeling defect manifesting as metaphyseal expansion, cortical thinning, and club-shaped epiphyses (Fig. 75–38). The spine is rarely affected.

**Pyle's Dysplasia.** Pyle's (or metaphyseal) dysplasia is a rare disorder that demonstrates either recessive or dominant transmission; it manifests at a variable age with mild clinical symptoms and signs, including joint pain, muscular weakness, scoliosis, genu valgum, dental malocclusion, and bone fragility. The radiographic abnormalities include marked expansion of the metaphyseal segments of tubular bones with an Erlenmeyer flask appearance, especially in the distal portion of the femur and proximal portions of the tibia and fibula (Fig. 75–39). The spine may show platyspondyly or biconcave vertebrae. The bones of the pelvis, medial portions of the clavicles, and sternal ends of the ribs are expanded.

## DYSOSTOSES

### Craniosynostosis

The term craniosynostosis implies premature fusion of one or more of the calvarial sutures. Premature closure of

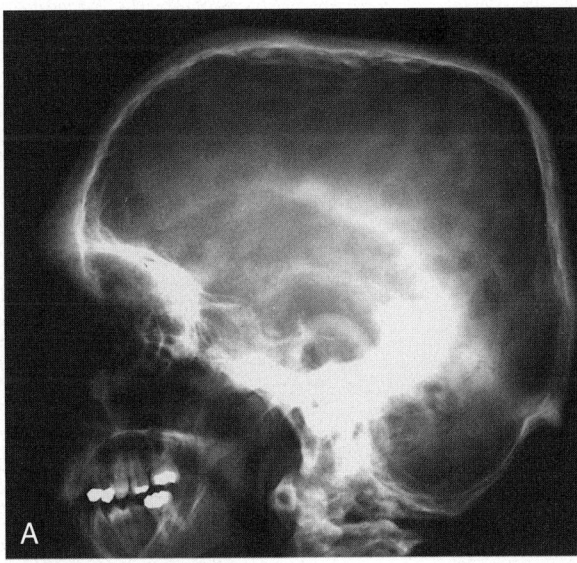
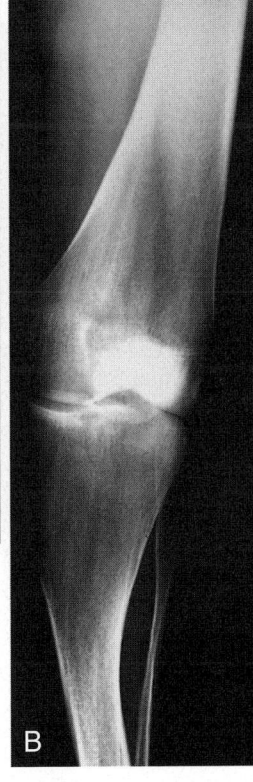

**Figure 75–37.** Frontometaphyseal dysplasia. *A,* Marked thickening of the supraorbital ridges is evident. *B,* The long tubular bones reveal metaphyseal splaying. (Courtesy of L. Langer, MD, Minneapolis, Minn.)

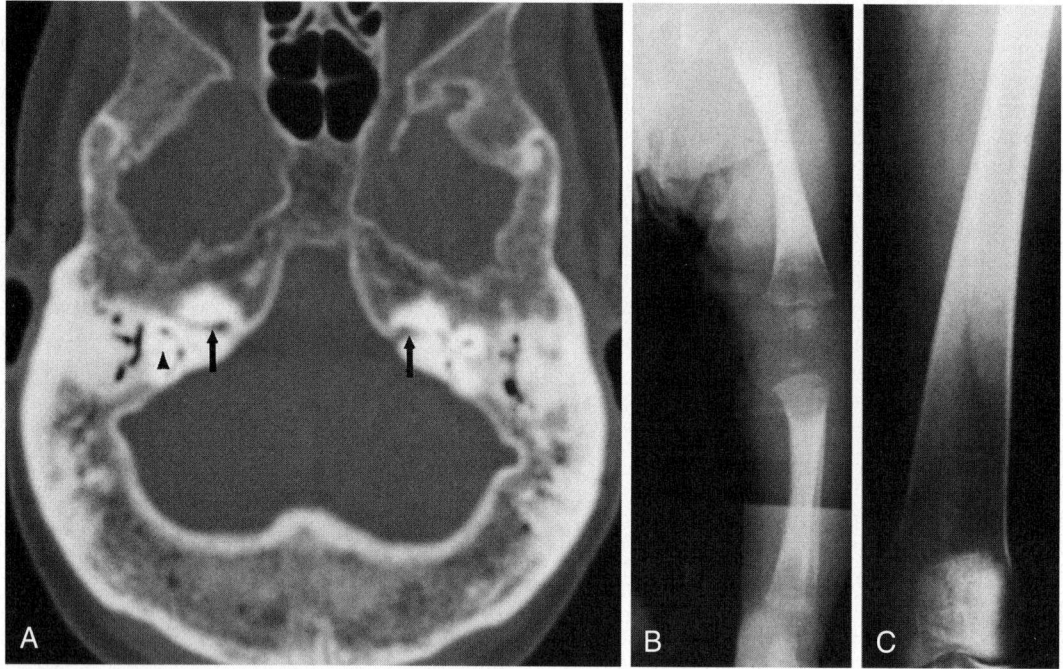

**Figure 75–38.** Craniometaphyseal dysplasia. *A,* CT scan of the temporal bones shows a thick diploic space, narrow internal auditory canals *(arrows),* and sclerotic otic capsules *(arrowhead). B* and *C,* Radiographs of the leg in a 2-month-old child *(B)* and her mother *(C)* show the changing appearance of the abnormalities. The dominant finding in the child is diaphyseal osteosclerosis, and that in the mother is metaphyseal expansion.

a suture results in local cessation of growth and distortion of the calvarial configuration. Accurate radiographic interpretation should be directed toward identifying the affected sutures rather than applying the specific but sometimes confusing terminology that describes the abnormal shape of the skull. The affected suture can be identified by a straight rather than a serrated radiolucent line, osseous proliferation at the suture line, or frank osseous fusion. As a supplement to conventional radiography, CT can be used to delineate any associated abnormalities of the face and central nervous system.

Isolated closure of the sagittal suture is the most common pattern of craniosynostosis, accounting for more than 50% of cases. Closure of the sagittal suture results in an increased anteroposterior diameter of the skull and a decreased biparietal diameter (Fig. 75–40*A* and *B*). Synostosis of both coronal sutures produces a skull that is short in its anteroposterior diameter, often with a decrease in the depth of the orbits and maxillary hypoplasia (see Fig. 75–40*C*). Unilateral closure of a coronal suture produces flattening of the orbit on the involved side, which is best seen on the submentovertical projection of the skull; on the frontal projection, a classic harlequin-shaped orbit is identified (see Fig. 75–40*D*). Unilateral closure of the lambdoid suture leads to flattening of one side of the back of the head, or plagiocephaly. The emphasis on having babies sleep on their backs to prevent sudden infant death syndrome has led to an "epidemic" of flattening of the back of the head without sutural closure. An isolated metopic synostosis creates a triangular forehead with hypotelorism (see Fig. 75–40*E*). In cases of closure of multiple sutures, the skull is variable in shape, although generally it is brachycephalic, and digital

markings in the cranium are quite prominent (see Fig. 75–40*F*). The kleeblattschädel, or cloverleaf skull, is also associated with premature synostosis of multiple sutures

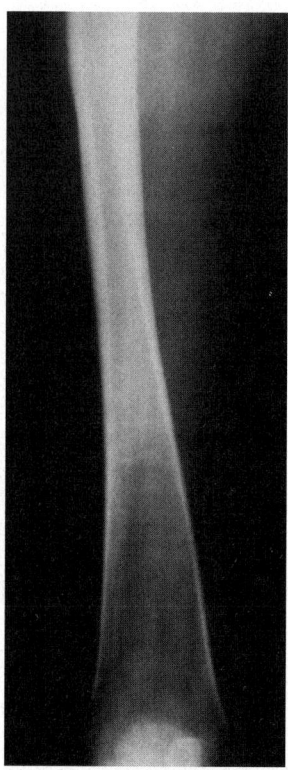

**Figure 75–39.** Metaphyseal dysplasia (Pyle's dysplasia). The femur has an Erlenmeyer flask appearance.

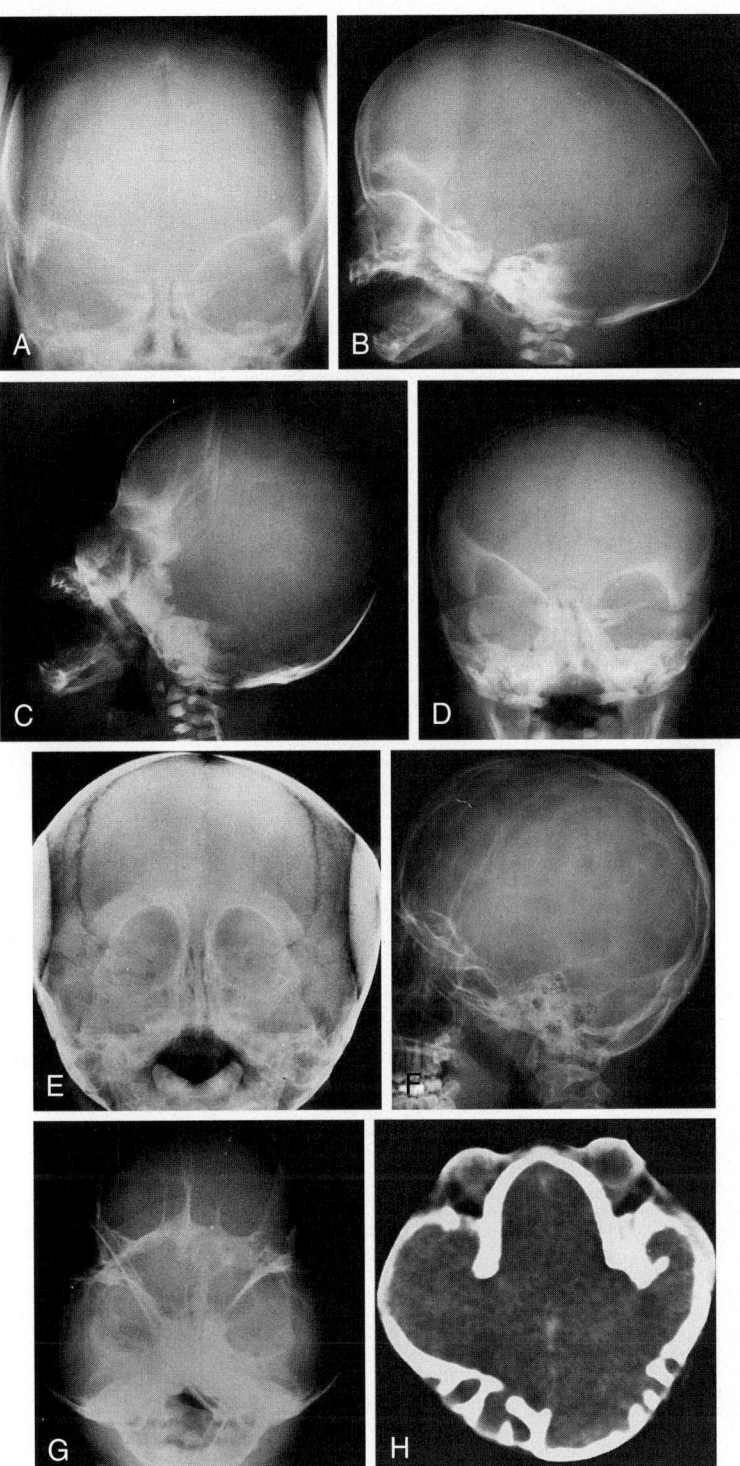

**Figure 75–40.** Craniosynostosis. *A* and *B*, Closure of the sagittal suture. Dolichocephaly has occurred. *C*, Closure of both coronal sutures. The skull is brachycephalic, with a small anterior fossa and a hypoplastic maxilla. *D*, Closure of one coronal suture. Note the harlequin-shaped right orbit. *E*, Closure of the metopic suture. Hypotelorism and a triangular forehead are observed. *F*, Closure of all sutures. The skull is brachycephalic, with prominent digital markings. *G* and *H*, Kleeblattschädel skull. Note osseous scalloping and a trilobed appearance of the cranial vault. The brain projects into the multiple bone channels.

(see Fig. 75–40*G* and *H*). It is frequently accompanied by hypoplasia of the midportion of the face, hydrocephalus, and mental retardation. CT examinations, especially with three-dimensional reconstructions, are useful in surgical planning (Fig. 75–41). Thanatophoric dwarfism, Pfeiffer's syndrome, limb anomalies, and unclassified bone dysplasias can be found in association with kleeblattschädel.

Craniosynostoses can be further classified as primary and secondary types. Primary closure sometimes occurs as an isolated phenomenon or in conjunction with other malformation syndromes. Secondary synostoses are evident in rickets, hypophosphatasia, thyroid disorders, and hypercalcemia, and they may follow surgical decompression of the intracranial contents.

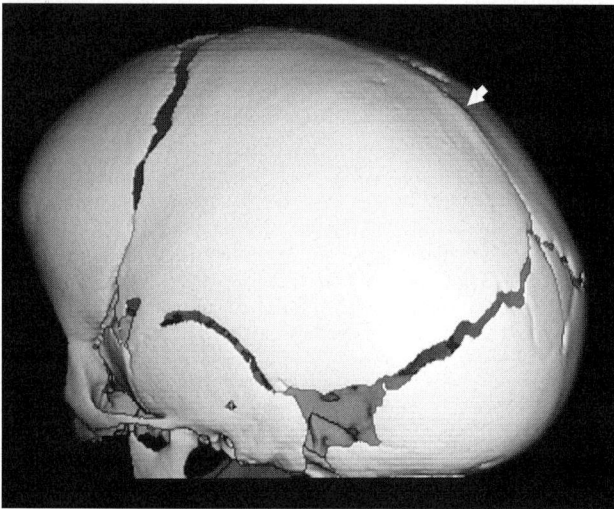

**Figure 75–41.** Craniosynostosis. Three-dimensional reconstruction of CT data in a 3-month-old infant shows isolated closure of the sagittal suture. Note the increased anteroposterior diameter of the skull, with fusion of the sagittal suture and osseous proliferation at the suture line (*arrow*).

## Craniofacial Dysostosis (Crouzon's Syndrome)

Crouzon's syndrome is characterized by craniosynostosis, exophthalmos, and midface retrusion. It has an autosomal dominant mode of transmission. The skull is usually brachycephalic, with fusion of the coronal and sagittal sutures (Fig. 75–42). In addition, fusion of the lambdoid suture has been reported in 80% of patients. Other findings include prominent digital markings in the skull in more than 90% of cases, calcification in the stylohyoid liga-

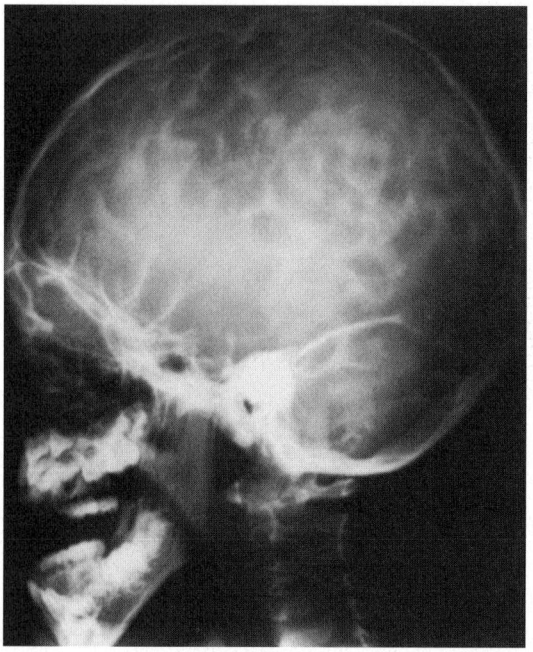

**Figure 75–42.** Craniofacial dysostosis (Crouzon's syndrome). The skull is brachycephalic, and slight maxillary hypoplasia is evident. Abnormal osseous fusion in the cervical spine was also present.

ment, and deviation of the nasal septum. The maxilla is hypoplastic, which is largely responsible for the prognathic appearance of the mandible. Spinal anomalies are seen in approximately one third of patients and usually consist of fusion between the second and third cervical vertebrae.

## Apert's Syndrome

Apert's syndrome is an autosomal dominant acrocephalosyndactyly condition consisting of suture closure, midfacial hypoplasia, and symmetrical syndactyly of the hands and feet involving, at a minimum, the second, third, and fourth digits. The characteristic skull findings at birth are a closed coronal suture area and an extensive midline calvarial defect from the glabella to the posterior fontanelle, often producing a wide metopic suture area (see Fig. 75–40C and D). The calvaria is thin and undermineralized. During the first 4 years of life, islands of ossification occur in the midline defect, coalesce, and, ultimately, close the sagittal suture area. Associated abnormalities include brachycephaly, hypoplastic anterior fossa, and ruminent sella turcica. Hand abnormalities include a short deviated thumb; complex osteocartilaginous syndactyly of the distal phalanges in the second, third, and fourth digits; and simple syndactyly of the fourth and fifth digits. Foot anomalies include complete simple syndactyly, a triangular first proximal phalanx, and progressive osseous fusion of tarsal and metatarsal bones (Fig. 75–43).

Cerebral abnormalities are common and include hydrocephalus, agenesis of the corpus callosum, septal agenesis, septo-optic dysplasia, megencephaly, gyral abnormalities, encephalocele, hypoplasia of white matter, and heterotopic gray matter. Cervical spine fusion is common and almost always involves C5–C6, in contrast to the C2–C3 fusion usually seen in Crouzon's syndrome.

## Mandibulofacial Dysostosis (Treacher Collins Syndrome)

Patients with Treacher Collins syndrome, an autosomal dominant disorder, have characteristic clinical features consisting of an antimongoloid slant to the eyes, flat cheekbones, small mandible, dysplastic ears, deafness, coloboma, and deficient lashes in the lower eyelids. Radiographic findings include marked hypoplasia of the zygomatic arches, maxilla, and paranasal sinuses. The orbits are egg shaped, and the mandible is hypoplastic, with a broad concave curve on the lower border of the body (Fig. 75–44). It appears that this basic shape of the mandible is established in utero and is maintained throughout postnatal development. The coronoid process may be broad, and the condylar process is small. The external auditory canal is sometimes absent, and a poorly formed middle portion of the ear contains abnormal ossicles.

## CHROMOSOMAL ABERRATIONS

Chromosomal abnormalities tend to result from genetic imbalances and involve either autosomal or sex chromosomes. Many are lethal, owing to the severe defects in

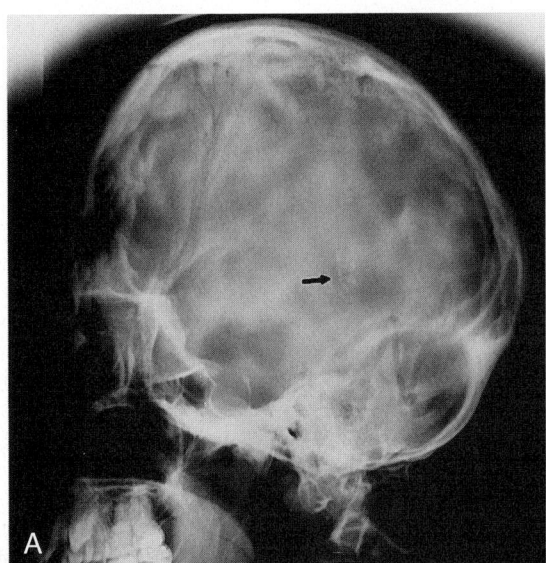

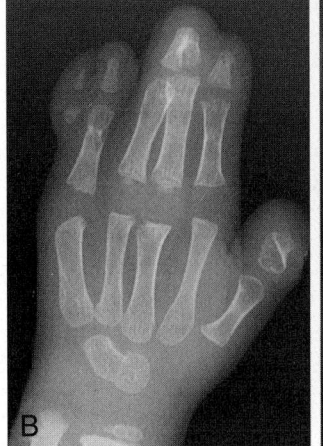

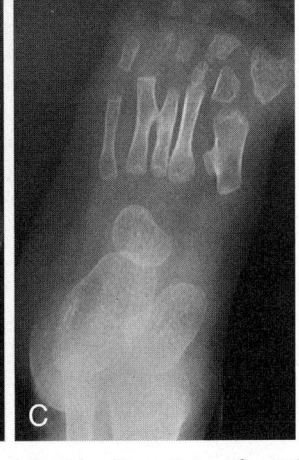

**Figure 75–43.** Acrocephalosyndactyly (Apert's syndrome). *A*, Findings in the skull include brachycephaly, a hypoplastic anterior fossa, a prominent sella turcica, and choroid calcifications *(arrow)*. Cervical spine abnormalities are also present in this adult. *B*, In the hand of a child, symphalangism, osseous and soft tissue syndactyly, phalangeal deformity in the thumb, polydactyly, and carpal fusion are seen. *C*, Similar abnormalities are observed in the foot.

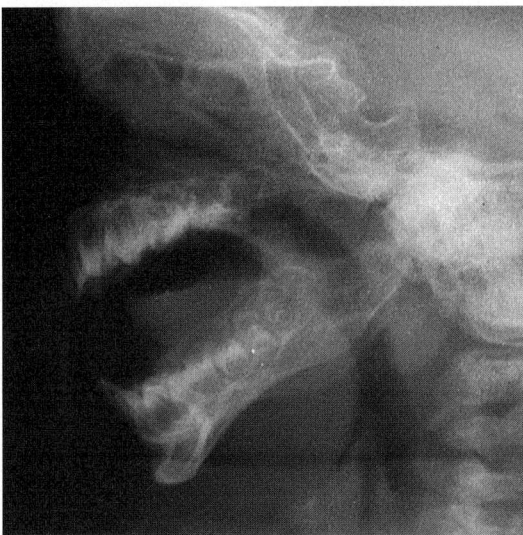

**Figure 75–44.** Mandibulofacial dysostosis (Treacher Collins syndrome). Note the hypoplastic mandible with a broad, concave curve in its lower aspect.

shaped kidneys) are frequent features of this syndrome. Radiographs of the hand reveal adduction of the thumb, superimposition of the second and third fingers, and hypoplasia of the first metacarpal bone. Rocker-bottom feet; metatarsus varus; shortened first toe; hypoplastic terminal phalanges of the toes; hypoplasia of the ribs, clavicles, and sternum; and pelvic deformities complete the radiographic picture (Fig. 75–45). Cerebral anomalies include cerebellar hypoplasia and large choroid plexus cysts.

## Trisomy 21 Syndrome (Down's Syndrome)

Patients with Down's syndrome are identified at birth by ocular abnormalities, hypotonia, brachycephaly, and a

normal morphogenesis they cause. They can be classified as trisomies (in which three rather than the normal pair of chromosomes are present), translocations (in which part of a chromosome is transposed to another chromosome), and deletions (in which a portion of a chromosome is absent). Only a few of the more common chromosomal abnormalities are summarized here.

## Trisomy 18 Syndrome

As with Down's syndrome, trisomy 18 syndrome tends to occur in infants born to older mothers. Affected infants are of low birth weight and possess a narrow head, prominent occiput, malformed ears, micrognathia, high-arched palate, finger deformities, hypertonicity, and hernias. Cardiac abnormalities, omphalocele (10% to 20% of patients), and renal anomalies (especially horseshoe-

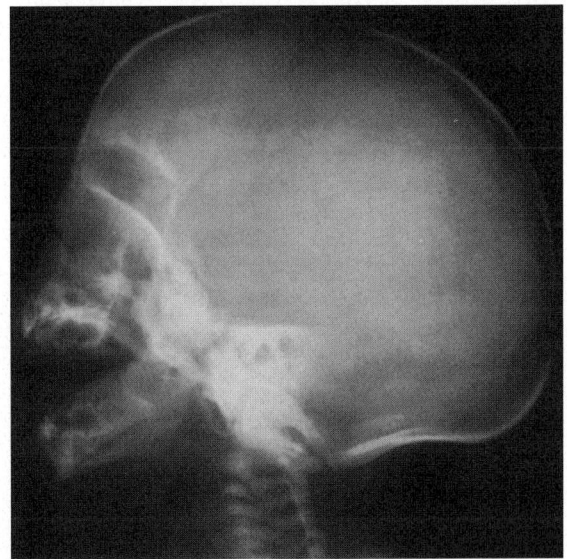

**Figure 75–45.** Trisomy 18 syndrome. The skull is elongated, with a prominent occiput and hypoplastic mandible.

large tongue. Developmental hip dysplasia is evident in approximately 40% of infants. Gastrointestinal abnormalities, including duodenal atresia, Hirschsprung's disease, and tracheoesophageal and anorectal anomalies, are well recognized.

Radiographs of the pelvis reveal flared iliac wings and flattened acetabular roofs. Hypoplasia of the middle phalanx of the fifth finger with clinodactyly, short and irregular metacarpal bones, accessory epiphyses, an extra manubrial ossification center, cuboid vertebral bodies, 11 pairs of ribs, microcephaly, a high-arched and short palate, delayed suture closure, sinus hypoplasia, and absence of widening of the interpediculate distance in the lumbar spine may be identified (Fig. 75–46). Atlanto-occipital and atlantoaxial instability may be associated with neurologic deficits. This instability is generally not symptomatic, however, and may decrease as the patient ages.

### Turner's Syndrome

Turner's syndrome occurs in persons with a female phenotype and a 45,XO chromosome complement. As many as 99.9% of fetuses with this chromosomal complement are aborted spontaneously in the first trimester of pregnancy. Mosaicism is more frequent in live-born infants with Turner's syndrome. In newborn infants, edema of the hands and feet may be evident, and large edematous masses about the neck occur. Secondary sex characteristics do not appear, primary amenorrhea is frequent, and the ovaries are small and streaklike. Clinical manifestations include lymphedema of the lower extremities; loose skin about the neck; congenital anomalies of the heart, great vessels, and kidneys; short stature; and laterally displaced nipples on a shieldlike chest.

Radiographs reveal osteoporosis, except in the very young, likely related to an estrogen deficiency occurring early in life. The decreased bone density is most pronounced in the spine, carpus, and tarsus. Epiphyseal fusion is delayed and may not occur until the third decade of life. Shortening of the metacarpal bones, especially the fourth, and of the metatarsal bones may be evident. Drumstick phalanges have been observed. Deformities of the knees, with flattening of the medial tibial plateau, beaking or exostoses of the medial and proximal portions of the tibia, and enlargement of the medial femoral condyle, are observed. Cubitus valgus, thin clavicles and ribs, vertebral

body irregularities, and abnormalities of the odontoid process and atlas have also been described (Fig. 75–47).

### Klinefelter's Syndrome

Klinefelter's syndrome usually results from the presence of two or more X chromosomes and a Y chromosome, although a number of variant chromosomal patterns are recognized, such as XXYY. Muscle weakness, mental retardation, delayed puberty, azoospermia, and infertility are frequent. A number of nonspecific radiographic changes have been outlined, including metacarpal shortening, clinodactyly, accessory epiphyses, flattened ulnar styloid process, pointed phalangeal tufts, radioulnar synostosis, and retarded bone age (Fig. 75–48).

## DYSOSTOSIS MULTIPLEX

The term mucopolysaccharidosis (MPS) was first used to describe the histologic findings in patients with gargoylism. Currently, various types of MPS are recognized, and additional diseases, such as the mucolipidoses, demonstrate similar clinical and radiographic findings (Table 75–1).

The radiographic abnormalities of these disorders are designated dysostosis multiplex. The skull is usually large and dolichocephalic, with premature closure of the sagittal suture (Fig. 75–49). The mastoids and paranasal sinuses are poorly developed. An elongated J-shaped sella turcica, prominent adenoids, malformed teeth, flattened mandibular condyles, large tongue, and thick diploic space are common. In the spine, there is defective development of the anterosuperior portion of the vertebral bodies at the thoracolumbar junction, with gibbus formation owing to the presence of hook-shaped vertebrae (Fig. 75–50). The vertebral bodies are oval, slightly diminished in height, or flattened (Fig. 75–51). In the pelvis, the superior acetabular region is underdeveloped, resulting in a widened acetabular roof and wide acetabular angle (Fig. 75–52). Coxa valga is frequent, and development of the femoral heads is delayed, causing them to become dysplastic. In the chest, the ribs are widened but taper near their vertebral margins. The clavicles are thick, short, and widened. The changes in the long tubular bones are greater in the upper extremities than in the lower extremities. Constriction of the humeral and

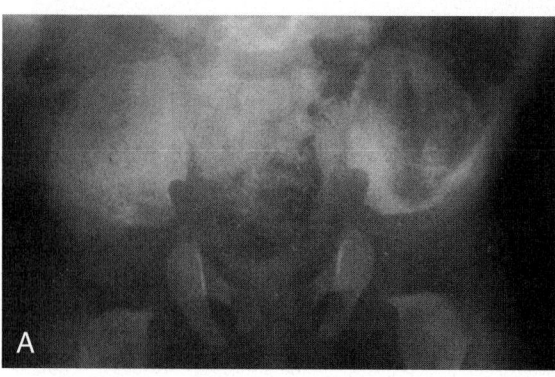
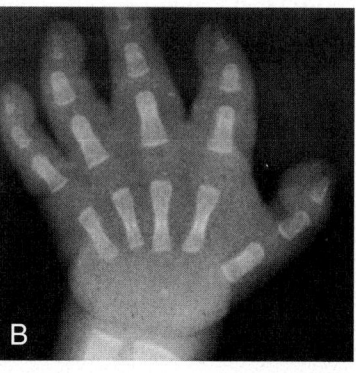

**Figure 75–46.** Trisomy 21 (Down's syndrome). *A,* In a newborn infant, observe flared iliac wings, with resultant decreased acetabular and iliac angles. *B,* Hypoplasia of the middle phalanx of the fifth digit and clinodactyly are present.

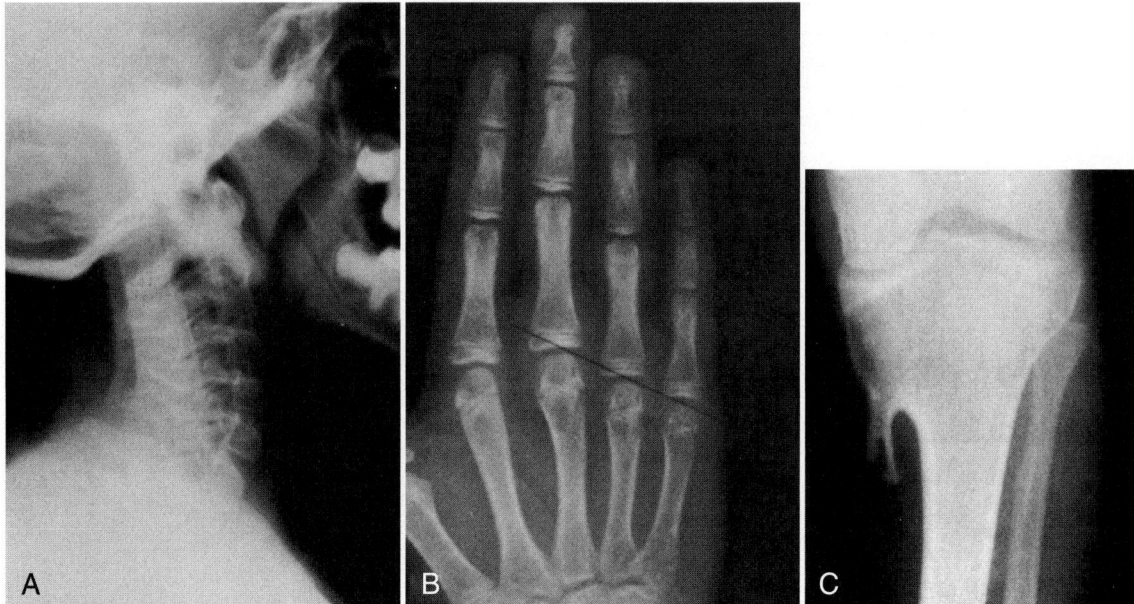

**Figure 75–47.** Turner's syndrome. *A*, In this 8-year-old patient, a soft tissue abnormality, related to webbing of the neck, projects over the posterior portion of the vertebrae. Osteopenia is evident. *B*, The fourth metacarpal bone is relatively short, and the phalanges are relatively long, with a drumstick configuration. *C*, Findings include an exostosis projecting from the medial aspect of the tibia and prominence of the medial femoral condyle.

femoral necks, with resultant varus deformities, may occur. In the hand, diffuse osteopenia, cortical thinning, and proximal tapering of the second to fifth metacarpal bones are observed (Fig. 75–53). The proximal and middle phalanges are short and wide, and the terminal phalanges are hypoplastic. The carpal bones are small

and deformed. Similar but less dramatic changes occur in the foot.

A precise diagnosis also requires clinical information, including the pattern of genetic transmission, and biochemical data, including the pattern of increased urinary excretion of acid mucopolysaccharides. Three clinical-

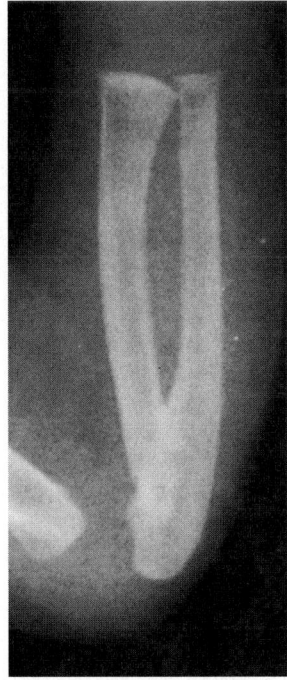

**Figure 75–48.** Klinefelter's syndrome. In a child with an XXY chromosomal pattern, radioulnar synostosis is observed.

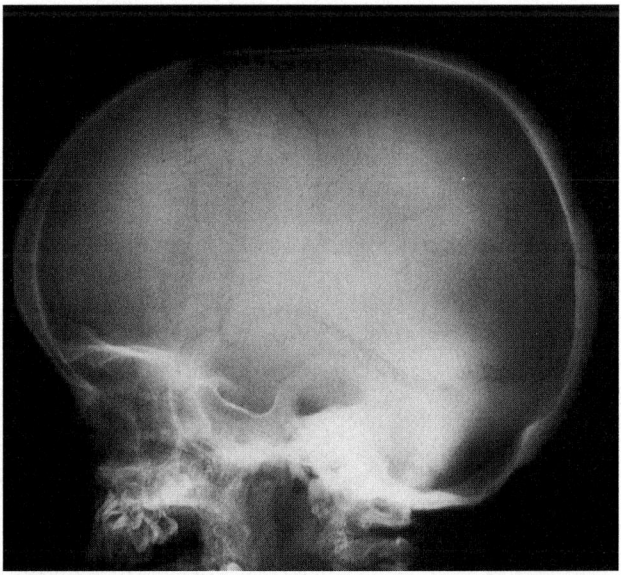

**Figure 75–49.** Dysostosis multiplex: Hurler's syndrome (MPS I). The skull is large, the mastoids are poorly developed, and the sella turcica is J-shaped.

**TABLE 75–1**

**Mucopolysaccharidoses, Mucolipidoses, and Other Conditions with Dysostosis Multiplex**

| Designation | Eponym or Synonym | Enzyme Deficient | Clinical Features |
|---|---|---|---|
| **Mucopolysaccharidoses (MPS)** | | | |
| MPS I-H | Hurler's syndrome | Alpha-L-iduronidase | Early clouding of cornea, mental retardation, heart disease, coarse facial features |
| MPS I-S | Scheie's syndrome | Alpha-L-iduronidase | Late onset, stiff joints, cloudy cornea, aortic valve disease, intelligence unaffected, mild facial dysmorphism |
| MPS I-H-S | Hurler-Scheie syndrome | Alpha-L-iduronidase | Intermediate between Hurler's and Scheie's syndromes |
| MPS II | Hunter's syndrome | Iduronate-2-sulfatase | Severe: diagnosed early, mental retardation, death in second decade |
| | | | Mild: survival into adulthood with little intellectual impairment |
| MPS III | Sanfilippo's syndrome (types A, B, C, D) | IIIA: Heparan N-sulfatase | Severe mental retardation, very mild skeletal and somatic features |
| | | IIIB: Alpha-N-acetyl glucosaminidase | |
| | | IIIC: Acetyl CoA: a-Glucosaminide-N-acetyl transferase | |
| | | IIID: N-acetyl glucosamine-6-sulfate sulfatase | |
| MPS IV | Morquio's syndrome (types A and B) | IVA: Galactosamine-6-sulfate sulfatase | Severe dwarfism, short trunk and neck, knock-knees, corneal changes (seen with slit lamp), intelligence unaffected |
| MPS VI | Maroteaux-Lamy syndome | N-acetylgalactosamine-4-sulfatase | Dwarfism, coarse facial features, corneal clouding, normal intelligence |
| MPS VII | Sly's syndrome | Beta-glucuronidase | Hepatosplenomegaly, variable mental retardation |
| **Other Conditions** | | | |
| Aspartyl-glucosaminuria | | Aspartyl glucosaminidase | Intellectual deterioration, coarse features |
| Alpha-beta-mannosidosis | | Alpha-beta-mannosidase | Variable, mental retardation |
| Fucosidosis | | Alpha-fucosidase | Upper respiratory infections, developmental delay |
| GM$_1$ gangliosidosis (several forms) | | Beta-galactosidase | Severe to mild somatic features, onset in infancy |
| **Mucolipidoses (ML)** | | | |
| ML I (sialidosis) | Lipomucopolysaccharidosis | N-acetyl-neuraminidase | Mild somatic features, progressive neuromuscular symptoms |
| ML II | I-cell disease | UDP-N-acetyl-glucosaminyl-phosphotransferase | Exaggerated somatic features, marked gingival hyperplasia |
| ML III | Pseudo-Hurler's polydystrophy | UDP-N-acetyl-glucosaminyl-phosphotransferase | Variable somatic features, stiff joints, corneal clouding, short stature |

From P Blighton (ed): Heritable Disorders of Connective Tissue, 5th ed. St Louis, CV Mosby, 1993.

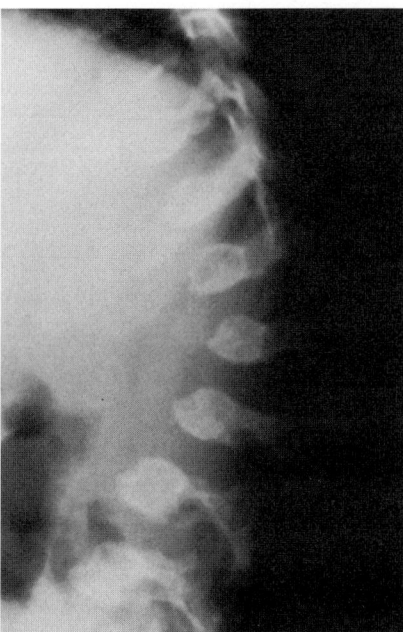

**Figure 75–50.** Dysostosis multiplex: Hurler's syndrome (MPS I). Note the hook-shaped vertebrae and a gibbus deformity at the thoracolumbar junction.

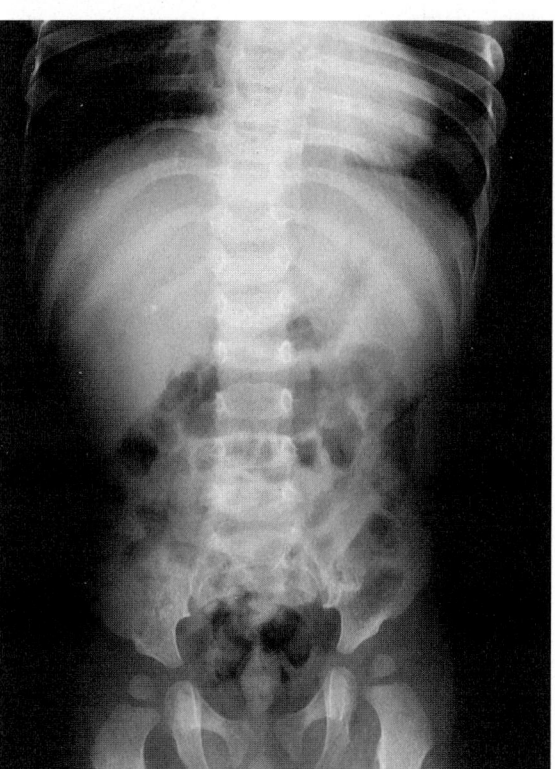

**Figure 75–52.** Dysostosis multiplex: Hunter's syndrome (MPS II). Underdevelopment of the superior acetabular region, wide femoral necks, coxa valga deformity, and wide ribs with posterior tapering are seen.

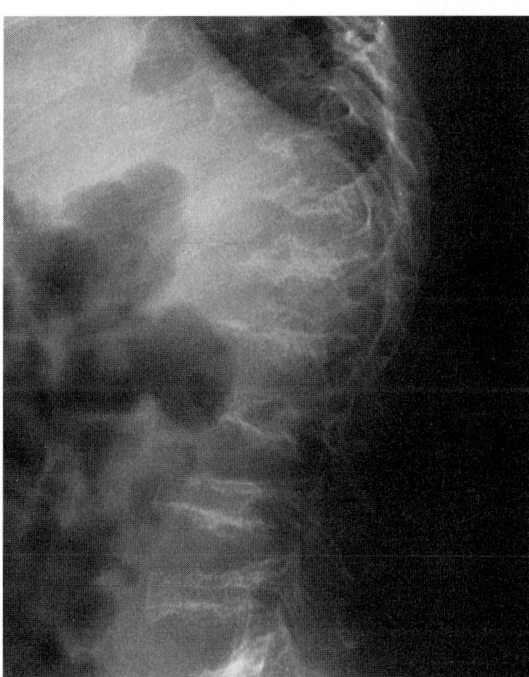

**Figure 75–51.** Dysostosis multiplex: Morquio's syndrome (MPS IV). The vertebral bodies are flattened and possess anterior tongues of bone.

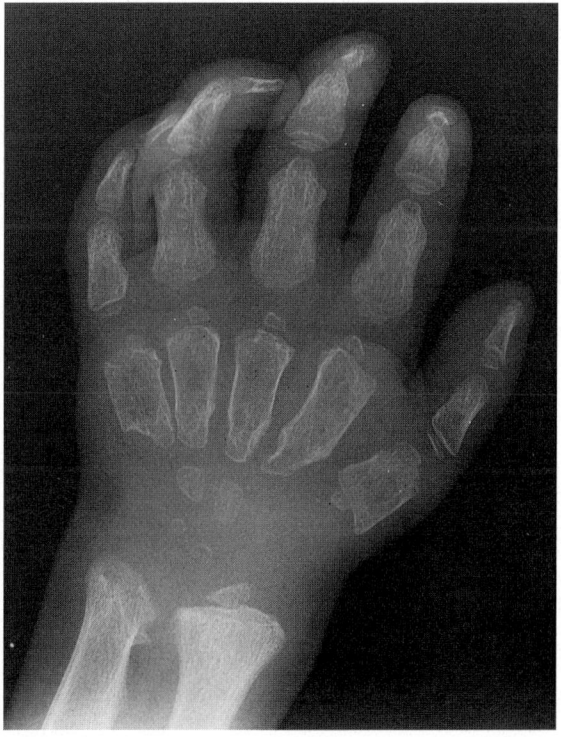

**Figure 75–53.** Dysostosis multiplex: Hurler's syndrome (MPS I). Osteopenia, pointing of the proximal portion of the metacarpal bones, widening of the proximal and middle phalanges, small carpal bones, and a V-shaped deformity of the distal portion of the radius and ulna are evident.

genetic syndromes due to alpha-L-iduronidase deficiency are now recognized: Hurler's syndrome (MPS I-H; the most severe), Scheie's syndrome (MPS I-S), and Hurler-Scheie syndrome (MPS I-H-S), a distinct intermediate syndrome. Additional syndromes are Hunter's (MPS II), Sanfilippo's (MPS III), Morquio's (MPS IV), Maroteaux-Lamy (MPS VI), and Sly's (MPS VII) syndromes.

## Hurler's Syndrome

Hurler's syndrome, an autosomal recessive disorder, manifests in the first few years of life. Patients have distinctive facies, mental retardation, deafness, dwarfism, corneal opacities, hepatosplenomegaly, cardiomegaly, and cardiac murmurs. Radiographs reveal macrocephaly, craniostenosis, J-shaped sella turcica, widening of the anterior portion of the ribs, ovoid vertebral bodies, hypoplasia of vertebrae about the thoracolumbar junction resulting in kyphosis, atlantoaxial subluxation, hypoplasia and stenosis of the bases of the ilia with pseudoenlargement of the acetabulum and coxa valga, shortening and widening of the shafts of the long tubular bones, pointing of the proximal portions of the metacarpal bones, and osteoporosis (see Figs. 75–49, 75–50, and 75–53). Death usually occurs in the first decade of life from heart failure or respiratory complications. Severe involvement of the thoracic and abdominal aorta in Hurler's syndrome, leading to coarctations and occlusions of costal and lumbar arteries, may be common, manifesting clinically as hypertension.

## Scheie's Syndrome

An autosomal recessive disorder, Scheie's syndrome is characterized by a deficiency of alpha-L-iduronidase and manifests primarily as peripheral clouding of the cornea, normal mentality, normal or slightly reduced stature, stiff joints, hirsutism, flexion of the hands, and aortic regurgitation. Airway obstruction may lead to apnea during sleep and require operative intervention. Radiographs demonstrate proximal tapering of the metacarpal bones, widening of the ribs, and mild alterations of the spine and skull. An arthropathy in adult patients with Scheie's syndrome has been described. Periarticular cysts have been seen in the hands, wrists, and hips.

## Hurler-Scheie Syndrome

This syndrome is intermediate between MPS I-H and MPS I-S in its clinical and radiographic severity as a result of the presence of different allelic mutations at the alpha-L-iduronidase locus. Myelography may reveal spinal cord compression, especially in the cervical region, related to thickening of the dura.

## Hunter's Syndrome

Hunter's syndrome, an X-linked recessive disorder, arises from iduronate sulfatase deficiency and is differentiated from MPS I by its occurrence only in male subjects, mild mental retardation, absence of corneal clouding, less significant hearing impairment, and relatively benign clinical course. A severe form of the disease does exist, however, which is often fatal in the second decade of life. The milder form is associated with normal intelligence and less dramatic radiographic abnormalities (Fig. 75–54), although osteoarthritis of the hip may occur.

## Sanfilippo's Syndrome

Sanfilippo's syndrome encompasses a group of diseases that result from deficiencies of lysosomal enzymes involved

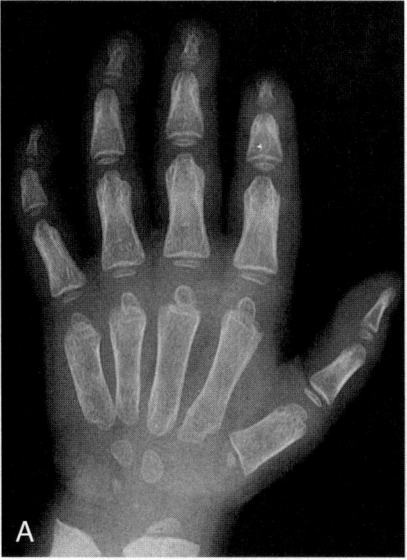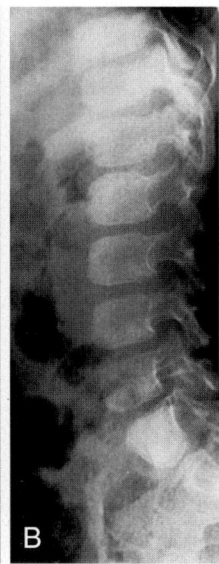

**Figure 75–54.**  Hunter's syndrome (MPS II). *A*, The changes of dysostosis multiplex are mild, with phalangeal widening, metacarpal pointing, and a delay in carpal ossification. *B*, The vertebral bodies are slightly rounded and have an accentuated posterior concavity.

in the degradation of heparan sulfate. The different types are similar clinically but of varying severity. Abnormal facial features, limitation of joint mobility, hepatosplenomegaly, and mental retardation usually become evident after age 2 or 3 years. Radiographic findings of dysostosis multiplex are relatively mild.

## Morquio's and Related Syndromes

MPS IV includes type A, or Morquio's, syndrome, which is related to a deficiency of galactosamine-6-sulfate sulfatase, and type B, which is related to a deficiency of beta-galactosidase. Clinical findings in these syndromes are highly variable but typically include severe dwarfism, spinal shortening and kyphoscoliosis, anterior bulging of the sternum, joint laxity, prominence of the lower face, hypoplasia of the enamel in the deciduous and secondary teeth, short neck, exaggerated lumbar lordosis, and flat feet. Corneal clouding and deafness also occur. Normal intelligence and a variable life span are additional features.

Spinal radiographs are most helpful in the accurate diagnosis of MPS IV. In early infancy, the vertebral bodies are slightly rounded, with a small anterior beak. With subsequent growth, a central tongue or projection appears, protruding from the anterior surface of the vertebral bodies. In adulthood, the vertebrae are flat and rectangular, with irregular margins (see Fig. 75–51). Hypoplasia of the odontoid process, leading to atlantoaxial instability, may result in upper spinal cord damage during anesthesia (Fig. 75–55). In the pelvis, increased obliquity in the lateral aspect of the acetabular roofs and considerable flaring of the iliac wings are observed. Coxa valga deformity and progressive dysplasia of the capital femoral epiphysis are also seen.

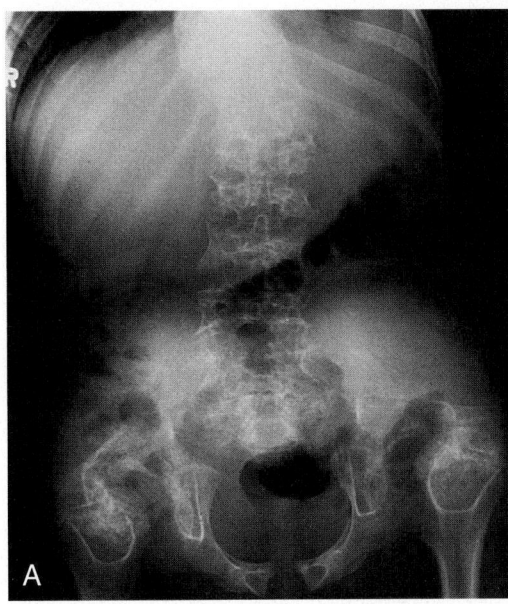 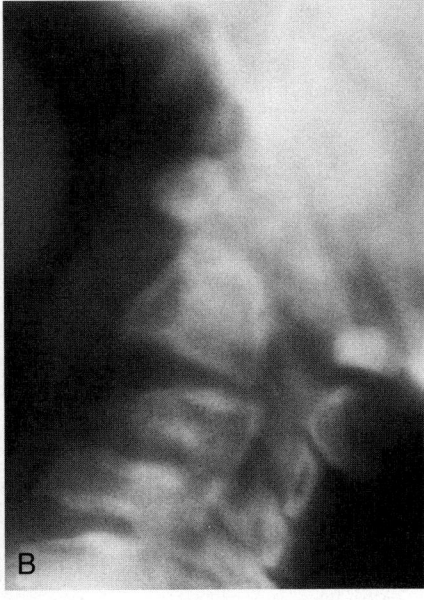

**Figure 75–55.** Morquio's syndrome (MPS IV). *A*, In this 10-year-old patient, marked platyspondyly, flared iliac wings, and severe changes about the hips are evident. *B*, Lateral conventional tomogram of the cervical spine shows odontoid hypoplasia and narrowing of the spinal canal.

## Maroteaux-Lamy Syndrome

Maroteaux-Lamy syndrome, which is an autosomal recessive disorder, is characterized by short stature that usually becomes evident at about 2 years of age in association with lumbar kyphosis, sternal protrusion, knock-knees, abnormal facies, hepatosplenomegaly, and joint contractures. A spectrum of abnormalities ranging from mild to severe is seen. Corneal opacification and normal intelligence are additional clinical findings. Radiographs reveal macrocephaly, enlarged sella turcica, ilial hypoplasia, flared iliac crests, dysplasia of capital femoral epiphyses, constriction of proximal femoral and humeral necks, coxa valga, biconvexity of vertebral endplates, hypoplasia of anterior aspects of the upper lumbar vertebrae and odontoid process, deformities of long tubular bones, narrowing of ribs near their vertebral ends, widening of medial aspects of the clavicles, and shortening, widening, and proximal tapering of metacarpal bones (Fig. 75–56). Cardiac disease develops in adolescence and adulthood and may progress to a severe cardiomyopathy.

## Sly's Syndrome

Sly's syndrome has three recognized forms: a fatal neonatal form, an infantile form with an early onset and with features and a clinical course similar to those of Hurler's syndrome, and a much milder juvenile form with a later clinical onset. Ischemic necrosis of the proximal femoral epiphysis and spinal abnormalities are the dominant radiographic changes (Fig. 75–57). The changes of dysostosis multiplex are most pronounced and progressive in the infantile form.

**Figure 75–56.** Maroteaux-Lamy syndrome (MPS VI). In this 13-year-old patient, note minimal flexion contractures of the fingers and deformity of the distal portion of the radius and ulna.

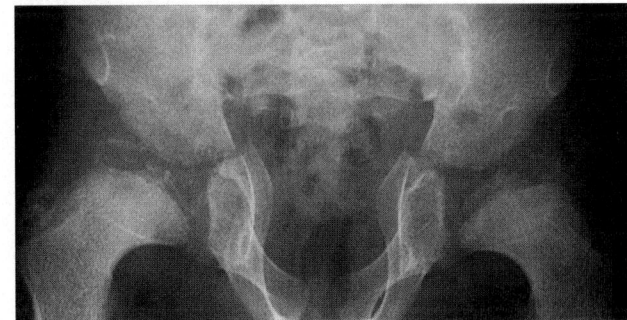

**Figure 75–57.** Sly's syndrome (MPS VII). In this 8-year-old patient, obvious flattening and fragmentation of the capital femoral epiphyses are seen.

## FURTHER READING

Azour EM, Slomic AM, Marton D, et al: The variable manifestations of dysplasia epiphysealis hemimelica. Pediatr Radiol 15:44, 1985.

Baker DH, Berdon WE, Morishima A, et al: Turner's syndrome and pseudo-Turner's syndrome. AJR Am J Roentgenol 100:40, 1967.

Beighton P, Cremin BJ: Sclerosing Bone Dysplasias. New York, Springer-Verlag, 1980.

Beighton P, Emery AEH: Inherited Disorders of the Skeleton. New York, Churchill Livingstone, 1978.

Beligere N, Harris V, Pruzansky S: Progressive bone dysplasia in Apert syndrome. Radiology 139:593, 1981.

Caffey J: Congenital stenosis of the medullary spaces and tubular bones and calvaria in two proportionate dwarfs—mother and son; coupled with transient hypercalcemic tetany. AJR Am J Roentgenol 100:1, 1967.

Carlson DH, Wilkinson RH: Variability of unliateral epiphyseal dysplasia (dysplasia epiphysealis hemimelica). Radiology 133:369, 1969.

Carmel PW, Luken MG, Ascheri GF: Craniosynostosis: Computed tomographic evaluation of skull base and calvarial deformities and associated intracranial changes. Neurosurgery 9:366, 1981.

Cremin BJ: Sclerosteosis in children. Pediatr Radiol 8:173, 1979.

Currarino G, Birch JG, Herring JA: Developmental coxa vara associated with spondylometaphyseal dysplasia (DCV/SMD): "SMD-Corner fracture type" (DCV/SMD-CF) demonstrated in most reported cases. Pediatr Radiol 30:14, 2000.

Elmore SM: Pyknodysostosis: A review. J Bone Joint Surg Am 49:153, 1967.

Engfeld B, Fajers CM, Lodin H, et al: Studies of osteopetrosis: Roentgenological and pathologic-anatomical investigations on some of the bone changes. Acta Pediatr 49:391, 1960.

Gelman MI: Autosomal dominant osteosclerosis. Radiology 125:289, 1977.

Giedion A, Kesztler R, Muggiasca F: The widened spectrum multicartilaginous exostosis (MCE). Pediatr Radiol 3:93, 1975.

Gorlin RJ, Koszalk MS, Spranger J: Pyle's disease (familial metaphyseal dysplasia): A presentation of 2 cases and argument for its separation from craniometaphyseal dysplasia. J Bone Joint Surg Am 52:347, 1970.

Hall BD, Spranger JW: Camptomelic dysplasia. Am J Dis Child 134:285, 1980.

Heselson NG, Raad MS, Hamersma H, et al: Radiologic manifestations of metaphyseal dysplasia (Pyle's disease). Br J Radiol 52:431, 1979.

Holzgrave W, Grobe H, von Figura K, et al: Morquio syndrome: Clinical findings of 11 patients with MPS IV-A and 2 patients with MPS IV-B. Hum Genet 57:360, 1981.

Hungerford GD, Akkaraju V, Rawe SE, et al: Atlanto-occipital and atlanto-axial dislocations with spine cord compression in Down's syndrome: A case report and review of the literature. Br J Radiol 54:758, 1981.

James AE, Adkins L, Feingold M, et al: The cri-du-chat syndrome. Radiology 92:50, 1969.

James AE, Belcourt CL, Atkins L, et al: Trisomy 18. Radiology 92:37, 1969.

Jarvis JL, Keats TE: Cleidocranial dysostosis: The review of 40 cases. AJR Am J Roentgenol 121:5, 1974.

Kaufmann HJ (ed): Intrinsic Diseases of Bones and Joints: Progress in Pediatric Radiology, vol 4. Basel, S Karger, 1973.

Kosowicz J: The roentgen appearance of the hand and wrist in gonadal dysgenesis. AJR Am J Roentgenol 93:354, 1965.

Kozlowski K, Beighton P: Gamut Index of Skeletal Dysplasias. New York, Springer Verlag, 1984.

Kozlowski K, Butzler HO, Galatius-Jensen F, et al: Syndromes of congenital bowing of the long bones. Pediatr Radiol 7:40, 1978.

Kozlowski K, McCrossin R: Early osseous abnormalities in Menkes' kinky hair syndrome. Pediatr Radiol 8:191, 1980.

Lachman RS: International nomenclature and classification of the osteochondrodysplasias (1997). Pediatr Radiol 28:737, 1998.

Lachman RS, Rimoin DL, Hollister DW, et al: The Kniest syndrome. AJR Am J Roentgenol 123:805, 1975.

Langer LO: Diastrophic dwarfism in early infancy. AJR Am J Roentgenol 93:399, 1965.

Langer LO: Dyschondrosteosis of the inheritable bone dysplasia with characteristic roentgenographic features. AJR Am J Roentgenol 95:178, 1965.

Langer LO: Spondyloepiphyseal dysplasia tarda: Hereditary chondrodysplasia with characteristic vertebral configuration in the adult. Radiology 82:833, 1964.

Langer LO Jr: Thoracic-pelvic-phalangeal dystrophy: Asphyxiating thoracic dystrophy of the newborn, infantile thoracic dystrophy. Radiology 91:447, 1968.

Langer LO, Baumann PA, Gorlin RJ: Achondroplasia. AJR Am J Roentgenol 100:12, 1967.

Larsen LJ, Schottstaedt ER, Boist FC: Multiple congenital dislocations associated with a characteristic facial deformity. J Pediatr 37:574, 1950.

Mainzer F, Minagi H, Steinbach HL: The variable manifestation of multiple enchondromatosis. Radiology 99:377, 1971.

McAlister WH: Enchondromatosis with hemangioma. Semin Roentgenol 8:230, 1973.

McAlister WH: Larsen's syndrome. Semin Roentgenol 8:246, 1973.

McAlister WH: Metatropic dwarfism. Semin Roentgenol 8:154, 1973.

McAlister WH: Thanatophoric dwarfism. Semin Roentgenol 8:158, 1973.

McClennan TW, Steinbach HL: Schwachman's syndrome—a broad spectrum of bony abnormality. Radiology 112:167, 1974.

Milgram JW, Jasty M: Osteopetrosis: A morphological study of twenty-one cases. J Bone Joint Surg Am 64:912, 1982.

Naveh Y, Kaftori JK, Alan V, et al: Progressive diaphyseal dysplasia: Genetics and clinical and radiographic manifestations. Pediatrics 74:399, 1984.

Nazara Z, Hernandez A, Corona-Rivera E, et al: Further clinical and radiological features in metaphyseal chondrodysplasia Jansen type. Radiology 140:697, 1981.

Ohsawa T, Furuse M, Kikuchi Y, et al: Roentgenographic manifestation of Kleinfelter syndrome. AJR Am J Roentgenol 112:78, 1971.

Pavone L, Mollica F, Giovanni S, et al: Metaphyseal chondrodysplasia Schmid type. Am J Dis Child 134:699, 1980.

Remes V, Tervahartiala P, Poussa M, Peltonen J: Cervical spine in diastrophic dysplasia: An MRI analysis. J Pediatr Orthop 20:48, 2000.

Rimoin DL, Lachman RS: Genetic disorders of the osseous skeleton. In Beighton P (ed): McKusick's Heritable Disorders of Connective Tissue, 5th ed. St Louis, CV Mosby, 1993, p 557.

Roberts GM, Starey N, Harper P, et al: Radiology of the pelvis and hips in adults with Down's syndrome. Clin Radiol 31:475, 1980.

Robinson LK, Jameds HE, Mubarak SJ, et al: Carpenter syndrome: Natural history and clinical spectrum. Am J Med Genet 20:461, 1985.

Sarafoglou K, Funai EF, Fefferman N, et al: Short rib–polydactyly syndrome: More evidence of a continuous spectrum. Clin Genet 56:145, 1999.

Silverman FN: Caffey's Pediatric X-Ray Diagnosis: An Integrated Imaging Approach. Chicago, Year Book Medical Publishers, 1985.

Spranger JW: International classification of osteochondrodysplasias. Eur J Pediatr 151:407, 1992.

Spranger JW, Langer LO: Spondyloepiphyseal dysplasia congenita. Radiology 94:313, 1970.

Spranger JW, Langer LO, Wiedemann HR: Bone Dysplasias: An Atlas of Constitutional Disorders of Skeletal Development. Philadelphia, WB Saunders, 1974.

Taybi H, Lachman R: Radiology of Syndromes, Metabolic Disorders and Skeletal Dysplasias, 3rd ed. Chicago, Year Book Medical Publishers, 1990.

Taylor GA, Jordan CE, Dorst SK, et al: Polycarpaly and other abnormalities of the wrist in chondroectodermal dysplasia: The Ellis-van Creveld syndrome. Radiology 151:393, 1984.

Thomas SL, Childress MH, Quinton B: Hypoplasia of the odontoid with atlanto-axial subluxation in Hurler's syndrome. Pediatr Radiol 15:353, 1985.

Tishler JM, Martel W: Dislocation of the atlas in mongolism: A preliminary report. Radiology 84:904, 1965.

Whalen JP, Horwith M, Krook L, et al: Calcitonin treatment in hereditary bone dysplasia with hyperphosphatasemia: A radiographic and histologic study of bone. AJR Am J Roentgenol 129:29, 1977.

Wiedemann HR, Kunze J, Grosse FR, et al: Atlas of Clinical Syndromes, 3rd ed. St Louis, Mosby–Year Book, 1992.

Willich E, Fuhr U, Kroll W: Skeletal manifestations in Down's syndrome: Correlation between roentgenologic and cytogenetic findings. Ann Radiol 18:355, 1975.

Wynne-Davies R, Fairbank TJ: Fairbank's Atlas of General Affections of the Skeleton. New York, Churchill Livingstone, 1976.

Wynne-Davies R, Walsh WK, Gormley J: Achondroplasia and hypochondroplasia: Clinical variation and spinal stenosis. J Bone Joint Surg Br 63:508, 1981.

# CHAPTER 76

## Spinal Anomalies and Curvatures

### M. B. Ozonoff

## SUMMARY OF KEY FEATURES

A variety of congenital and developmental anomalies may become evident in the spine. The causes and patterns of abnormal spinal curvature are also varied. Accurate diagnosis of these alterations relies on careful clinical evaluation supplemented by imaging examinations that include routine radiography, computed tomography, sonography, and magnetic resonance imaging.

## INTRODUCTION

Anomalies of the spine are frequent and varied. The emphasis here is on the more important structural abnormalities of the spine.

## CONGENITAL ANOMALIES OF THE SPINE

### Structural Abnormalities

Some anomalies are restricted to skeletal structures, either isolated at one or two levels or part of larger complexes. Other abnormalities are associated with neural tube defects (myelomeningocele, diastematomyelia, congenital intraspinal tumors). Additionally, the skeletal and neural anomalies may be part of a multisystem abnormality, such as the VATER (vertebral, anorectal, tracheal, esophageal, renal/rectal) complex, and numerous dysplasias and syndromes.

Structural spinal abnormalities can generally be classified into those resulting from nondevelopment, from nonfusion, or from nonsegmentation of embryologic structures.

**Anomalies of the Vertebral Body.** The vertebral body originally develops from paired chondral centers and, at a later stage, from a single ossification focus that is transiently separated by the notochord remnant into anterior and posterior centers. Total aplasia can be explained by failure of development of the mesoderm in the involved segment. Lack of development of one of the paired chondral centers produces a lateral hemivertebra, whereas if failure occurs at the ossification stage, anterior agenesis results in a posterior hemivertebra.

Hemivertebrae may vary in size, and the contralateral segment at the same level may be completely absent or hypoplastic (Fig. 76–1). The pedicle on the side of the hemivertebra may be normal or enlarged. A hemivertebra may exist in place of a normal vertebra, or it may

be a supernumerary structure. In many cases, the anomaly in the vertebral body is associated with fusion or segmentation defects in the neural arch.

The vertebral body is occasionally constricted centrally, probably after incomplete fusion of the two chondral centers, with hypoplasia where they join (butterfly vertebra). Two or more vertebral somites may also be subject to nonsegmentation, in which case a block vertebra is formed. The intervertebral discs may be completely absent or may be represented by rudimentary, irregularly calcified structures. Often, a waistlike constriction of the fused structure is found at the level of the intervertebral disc (causing an hourglass appearance), and the total height of the block vertebra is usually less than that expected from the number of segments involved. In the cervical spine, this congenital anomaly may be difficult to differentiate from abnormalities caused by juvenile chronic arthritis.

**Anomalies of the Vertebral Arch.** The same anomalies of formation, segmentation, and maturation may affect the neural arches. Each neural arch develops from a separate chondrification (and subsequently an ossification) center. These paired arches normally unite in the midline by age 2 years, but they frequently remain open at the L5 or S1 spinal level, or both. The frequency of such nonfusion is so high that it must be considered a normal variant. Use of the term spina bifida should be restricted to instances of severe dysraphism with neurologic consequences.

Abnormalities of the neural arch include total absence, underdevelopment with wide osseous separation, and failure of segmentation. When pediculate aplasia occurs, it is most common in the cervical and lumbar regions. The outline of the pedicle on the involved side is absent, and the opposite pedicle at the same level is frequently hyperplastic, although this finding is less common in children than in adults. Hypoplasia of the ipsilateral superior articular facet may be present. Failure of segmentation leads to linkage and fusion of adjacent laminae or pedicles, an abnormality termed congenital vertebral bars. Although such vertebral bars can occur bilaterally, they are usually unilateral and are clinically important because of their restrictive effect on growth on that side.

**Klippel-Feil Syndrome.** Klippel-Feil syndrome is discussed in Chapter 77.

**Craniovertebral Junction Abnormalities.** The craniovertebral junction, like the thoracolumbar and lumbosacral junctions, is a developmentally unstable transitional region where congenital anomalies are common. These anomalies include agenesis of the odontoid process and its base or of the odontoid process alone, incomplete formation of the apex of the dens, os odontoideum, and nonfusion of the apical apophysis of the dens (ossiculum terminale).

In odontoid aplasia, there is no extension of the dens above the body of the axis. The os odontoideum is a well-

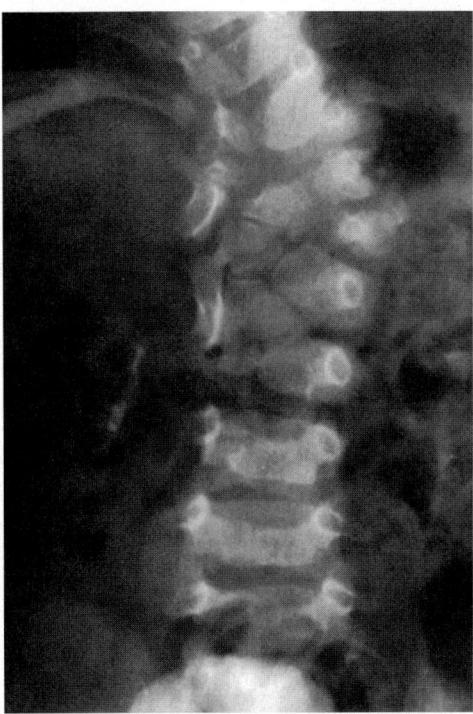

**Figure 76–1.** Congenital scoliosis. Left thoracolumbar scoliosis is associated with right upper lumbar pediculate bars and multiple supernumerary hemivertebrae on the left.

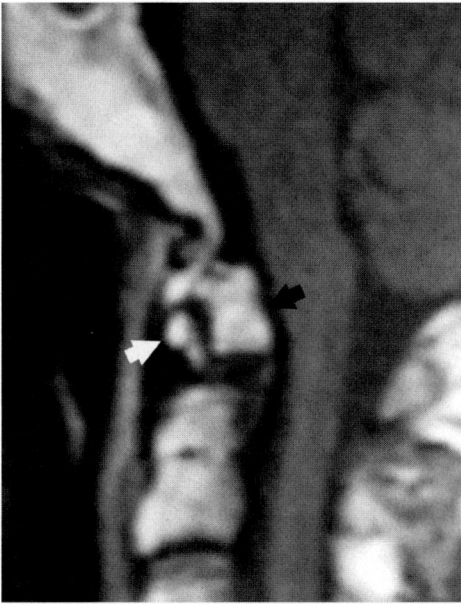

**Figure 76–2.** Os odontoideum. Sagittal T1-weighted (TR/TE, 550/15) spin echo MR image of the skull base demonstrates a well-defined ossicle *(black arrow)* that is about half the size of a normal dens. An irregularly former anterior arch of C1 is seen *(white arrow)*.

defined ossicle that lies above the odontoid process and is about half the size of a normal dens (Fig. 76–2). Strong evidence indicates that this ossicle is an acquired rather than a congenital lesion, as it has been shown to be present after trauma in patients with a previously normal odontoid process. Hypertrophy of the anterior arch of C1, indicative of a long-standing process, may help distinguish os odontoideum from an acute fracture.

Occipitalization (assimilation) of the atlas is a normal variant that is asymptomatic in most cases. Typically, the anterior arch of the atlas is fused to the skull base, and other portions of the ring of the atlas reveal similar fusion in many cases. As many as half of patients with occipitalization of the atlas also have vertebral fusion at the C2–C3 spinal level.

**Sacral Agenesis.** Sacral agenesis is discussed in Chapter 77.

## Spinal Dysraphism Complexes

Dysraphism represents a failure of midline fusion that encompasses not only structural vertebral defects but also associated abnormalities of embryonic tissue in organ systems developing at the same time as the neural tube, including the neurologic, gastrointestinal, and genitourinary systems. Dysraphic abnormalities are described as open (uncovered) or closed (covered or occult) lesions. Open defects, such as myelomeningocele, are usually clinically obvious at birth or may be detected with prenatal sonography. Closed or occult lesions may have a cutaneous marker, such as a nevus, hairy patch, hemangioma, or lipoma, that signals the possible presence of an underlying abnormality.

**Myelomeningocele.** Myelomeningocele, an example of open spinal dysraphism, is clinically evident at birth. The point at which widening of the interpediculate distance and vertebral body occurs is usually considered the superior limit of the anomaly, but the upper extent of the lesion predicted radiographically may not correlate with the functional neurologic level. The expanding neural and meningeal mass causes reorientation of the laminae from an oblique to a sagittal or even coronal plane (Fig. 76–3). Computed tomography (CT), with or without the administration of contrast agents, or magnetic resonance (MR) imaging is necessary to show the vertebral and neural abnormalities.

Vertebral hypoplasia, hemivertebra, laminar and pediculate fusion, diastematomyelia, and lipoma may all be associated with a myelomeningocele. Scoliosis is present at an early age in 50% of patients and in 80% of those older than 10 years; kyphosis is present in about 20% of patients. The status of the urinary tract should be evaluated at standard intervals with cystography, urography, and sonography.

**Occult Spinal Dysraphism.** Dysraphic changes in systems derived from the primitive germ layers but covered with skin are termed occult, closed, or covered spinal dysraphism. The basic pathogenic processes are identical to those causing open lesions: failure of midline fusion, duplication (diplomyelia, diastematomyelia), overgrowth of normal tissue (lipoma, dermoid), herniation of one germ layer through another (neurenteric cyst), and abnormalities caused by differences in the growth patterns of neural and skeletal structures or abnormal fixation (tethered cord). Among the numerous solitary or combined lesions that may occur are abnormal or supernumerary nerve

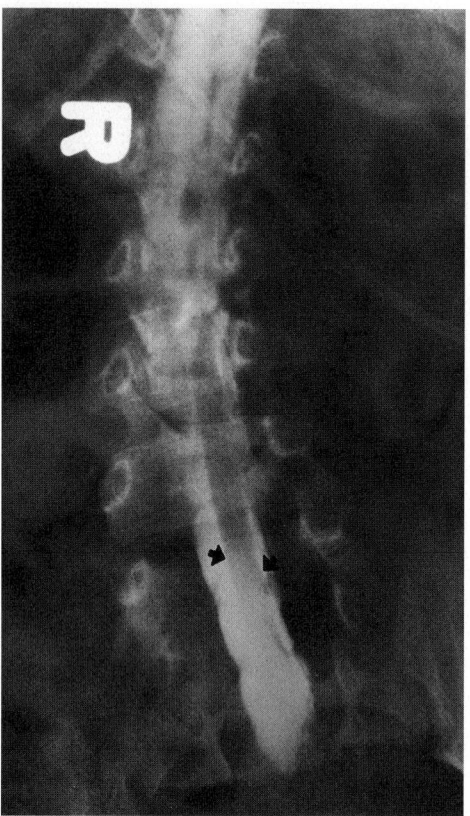

**Figure 76–3.** Myelomeningocele. Dysraphic abnormalities include a widened interpediculate distance at the L3 spinal level and distally. This myelogram demonstrates tethering of the spinal cord *(arrows)* in the sacral area.

osseous structure visible in about 75% of cases (Fig. 76–4). Only 50% of spurs are easily recognized on radiographs, but many can be seen in retrospect once their levels have been identified with CT scanning or MR imaging. The most common radiographic finding in diastematomyelia is an intersegmental laminar fusion associated with a defect in the neural arch at the same or an adjacent level. An increased interpediculate distance and scoliosis are present in about two thirds of patients. Myelography, alone or combined with CT scanning with contrast enhancement or MR imaging, shows the perimedullary space surrounding the normal and divided portions of the spinal cord (Fig. 76–5). Transaxial CT and MR images demonstrate that the two portions of the spinal cord are unequal in size (Fig. 76–6).

The low conus (tethered conus, tight filum terminale, cord traction) syndrome is believed by many investigators to represent another manifestation of occult spinal dysraphism. Intraspinal dermoids, lipomas, congenital bands, and myelomeningoceles (see Fig. 76–3) may all cause tethering of the conus, but in many cases of such tethering, no associated lesions are found. The conus medullaris is considered abnormally low when it lies below the L2–L3 spinal level at the age of 2 months. The

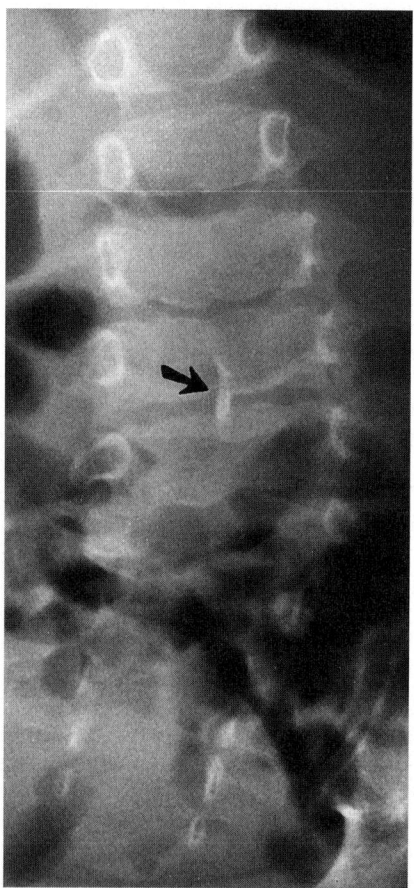

**Figure 76–4.** Diastematomyelia. This 2-year-old girl with myelomeningocele has a well-defined bony spicule projecting over the third lumbar vertebra *(arrow)*. Associated dysraphic changes include widened interpediculate distances, asymmetrical development of the lower vertebral bodies, and undeveloped sacral neural arches.

roots, dural and arachnoid adhesions, spinal cord angiomas and hamartomas, and failure of differentiation of the conus.

Occult dysraphism is twice as common in girls as in boys, whereas open lesions are seen with equal frequency in the two sexes. Approximately half of these abnormalities have cutaneous markers; additional clinical manifestations include leg length and motor power discrepancy, pes cavus and other foot deformities, gait abnormality, and neuropathic bladder. Radiographic evaluation generally reveals structural vertebral defects. Interpediculate widening and enlargement of the spinal canal are often present, and the vertebral bodies may be deformed or scalloped. The most common occult spinal dysraphic lesions are diastematomyelia, low conus (tethered filum), and congenital intraspinal tumors (lipomas and dermoids).

Diastematomyelia, also known as split spinal cord malformation, refers to a congenital longitudinal diastasis in the spinal cord, leading to two parts that are usually of unequal size. Although an osseous spur may be present between the two parts of the spinal cord, approximately half of patients with this anomaly have no true septum. Diastematomyelia occurs in 15% of all patients with congenital scoliosis. Skin changes are noted in about 80% of patients and do not correspond in distribution to the level of any septum or spur. The latter is most common within the L1 to L4 spinal segment, with an abnormal

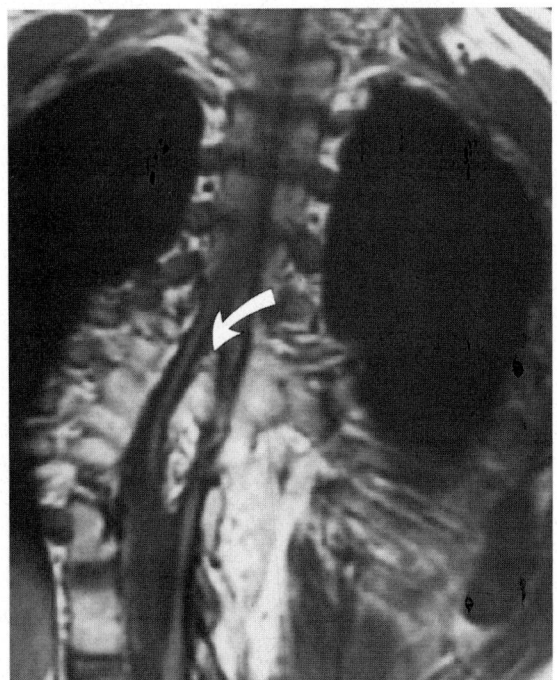

**Figure 76–5.** Diastematomyelia. Coronal T1-weighted (TR/TE, 450/16) spin echo MR image shows a large osseous mound (*arrow*) with an adjacent split spinal cord.
(From Ozonoff MB: Pediatric Orthopedic Radiology. Philadelphia, WB Saunders, 1979.)

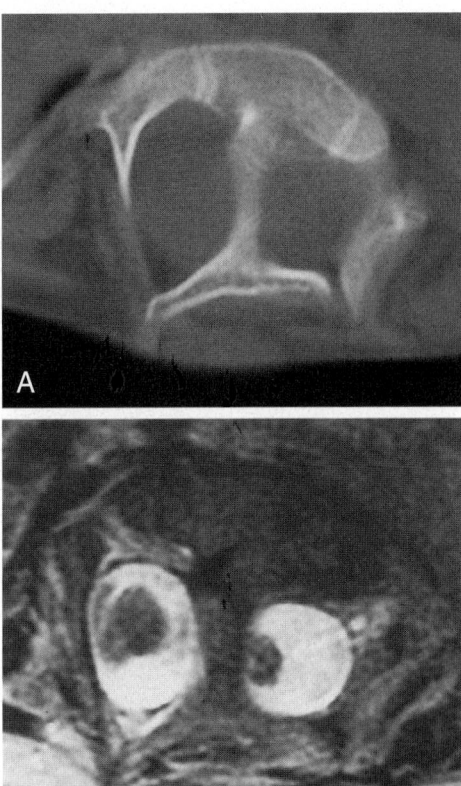

**Figure 76–6.** Diastematomyelia. *A*, Transverse CT scan shows a complete bone septum extending from the vertebral body to a malformed neural arch. *B*, Transverse fast spin echo MR image shows that the two parts of the split cord are of unequal size.

filum terminale may be thickened, often as a result of fatty infiltration; a diameter exceeding 2 mm is considered abnormal.

Congenital intraspinal tumors are associated with vertebral changes, cutaneous manifestations, and clinical symptoms identical to those found in other forms of occult spinal dysraphism. Of these congenital tumors, dermoids and lipomas constitute a large proportion. Vertebral scalloping at the level of an intraspinal tumor is frequent.

## SPINAL CURVATURES

Scoliosis refers to lateral spinal curvature in the coronal plane. Scoliosis may be caused by congenital architectural imbalance or growth asymmetry; neoplastic, traumatic, or infectious damage; radiation injury; reflexive splinting from nerve irritation; bone dysplasias; or asymmetrical neuromuscular control. The great majority of cases, however, are of unknown cause (idiopathic scoliosis) and have an onset during childhood rather than being present at birth.

### Imaging Techniques

The initial radiographic examination should be limited. The entire spine is examined in the erect position with the patient standing without shoes. If a lateral film is needed to evaluate accompanying kyphosis, it should be obtained with the patient standing with his or her forearms resting on a stand so that they are completely hori-zontal. Gonadal shielding is used in all patients. Postero-anterior rather than anteroposterior views are routinely recommended, with the main advantage being reduction of radiation to the breast. Lateral bending films may be helpful to determine whether the curve is structural and to what degree it is correctable.

Rapid progression of scoliosis may occur during the adolescent growth spurt, and examinations during this period may need to be more frequent. Specialized imaging techniques are helpful in certain situations. For example, bone scintigraphy is valuable in confirming the presence of osteoid osteomas, osteoblastomas, or other irritative foci. Sonography can evaluate the contents of the spinal canal in normal infants younger than 6 months and in older children who have an open neural arch or have previously undergone laminectomy. Although MR imaging is certainly of value in the evaluation of congenital scoliosis, its use in the workup of adolescent idiopathic scoliosis is debatable, because only a few unsuspected lesions will be found.

### Radiographic Analysis

On a frontal radiograph, a normal child's spine is straight, without curvature in the coronal plane. On a lateral radiograph, a newborn infant has a relatively straight spine, but thoracic kyphosis and lumbar lordosis develop as the child adopts an upright position. The median T5 to T12 thoracic kyphosis in normal older children is 27 degrees (90th percentile, 40 degrees). The median L1 to L5 lumbar lordosis is normally 40 degrees (90th percentile, 54 degrees). Lumbar lordosis is measured between L1 and L5, not to the superior surface of the sacrum.

The scoliotic curvature should be identified as nonstructural (flexible, with correction to linear alignment by lateral bending) or structural (curvature not completely corrected by lateral bending); associated architectural asymmetry is common in structural curves. Although attempts to label spinal curvatures as primary or secondary are usually speculative, the curvature above or below the level of the major structural curve is usually considered compensatory; it is generally nonstructural and can be corrected by lateral bending.

The first task in the radiographic analysis of scoliosis is identification of the vertebrae at either end of the curvature (the end vertebrae). The most laterally displaced and rotated vertebra is designated the apical vertebra and is located between these two end vertebrae. The degree of rotation and displacement from the midline of the vertebrae above and below the apical vertebra diminishes progressively until the end vertebrae are reached, at which point the spine straightens or a second curve in the opposite direction is detected.

The curvature is conventionally measured by constructing lines along the superior endplate of the highest end vertebra and along the inferior endplate of the lowest end vertebra (Fig. 76–7). If these landmarks are indistinct, the tops or bottoms of the pedicles can be used. (In the case of mild or moderate curvature, drawing lines perpendicular to these endplate lines makes the task of measuring the angle of scoliosis easier.) This technique (Cobb's method) is the standard means of measurement. Rotation of the spine is greatest at the level of the apical vertebra but is quite variable from one patient to another. Scoliotic curves of the same magnitude in two patients may have significantly different degrees of vertebral rotation. Normally, pedicles are placed symmetrically with respect to the vertebral edges, but when spinal rotation occurs, the pedicle moves inward from the edge of the body.

Kyphosis and lordosis are measured in the same manner by constructing lines along the vertebral endplates on the lateral radiograph. In severe scoliosis, the normal patterns of kyphosis and lordosis are diminished, and the lateral profile of the spine is straightened. Evaluation of skeletal maturity is a helpful clinical tool, because most mild or moderate spinal curvatures do not progress after the cessation of growth. Exceptions to this rule occur, however. Skeletal maturity can be estimated by analyzing the ossification of the apophysis of the iliac crest; however, if an exact determination of skeletal maturity is required, it is best to obtain a bone age by standard methods.

## Congenital Scoliosis

Scoliosis initiated and perpetuated by a congenital anomaly of the spine is termed congenital scoliosis. It may be caused by failure of formation (wedge vertebra or hemivertebra), partial duplication (supernumerary hemivertebra), failure of segmentation (unilateral block vertebra,

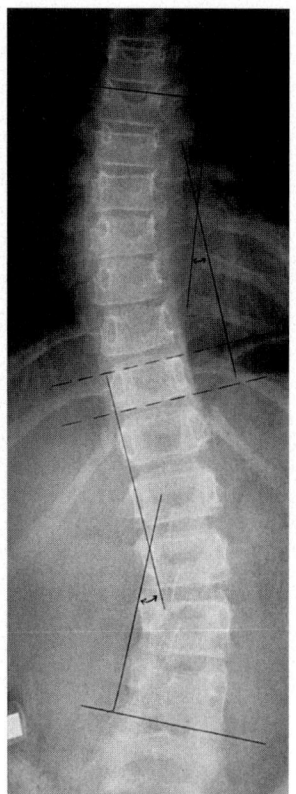

**Figure 76–7.** Measurement of idiopathic scoliosis (Cobb's method). This 10-year-old girl has a T4–T11 right spinal curvature of 20 degrees and a T11–L4 left spinal curvature of 27 degrees. Note that T11 is included in both curve measurements. Minimal rotation occurs in the thoracic region, and essentially none in the lumbar segment.

(From Ozonoff MB: Pediatric Orthopedic Radiology, 2nd ed. Philadelphia, WB Saunders, 1992.)

pediculate bar, neural arch fusion), or a combination of these lesions. The thoracolumbar region is most commonly affected. Progression of congenital scoliosis occurs in about 75% of patients; those with a unilateral bar associated with a contralateral hemivertebra have the poorest prognosis. Associated rib abnormalities are common.

Radiographic evaluation of congenital scoliosis should include erect radiographs of the entire spine and detailed supine spot and oblique radiographs of any area of abnormality. CT (especially with three-dimensional reconstruction) is especially helpful in detecting laminar fusion and defining abnormalities when anomalies of both the centrum and the neural arch are present (Fig. 76–8). MR imaging is an excellent means of determining the status of the neural contents of the spine and is indicated if surgery is contemplated. Examination of the genitourinary tract is indicated in all patients with congenital anomalies of the spine.

## Congenital Lordosis and Kyphosis

Congenital lordosis is uncommon and is usually limited to the thoracic region. The lordosis is caused by fusion of the posterior neural elements and continued anterior vertebral growth.

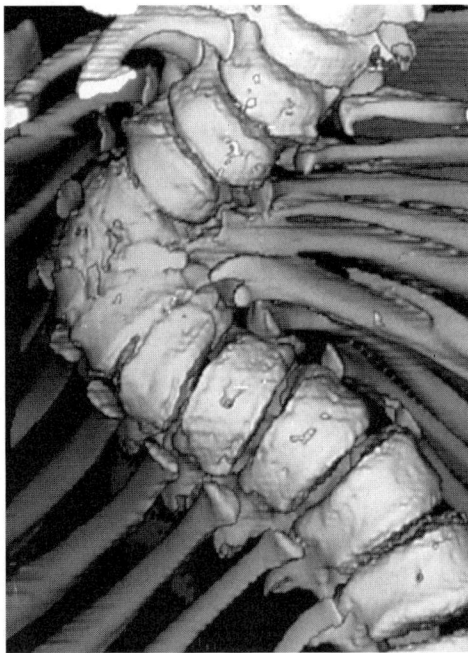

**Figure 76–8.** Congenital scoliosis. CT with three-dimensional reconstruction is especially helpful in defining complex spinal and rib anomalies.

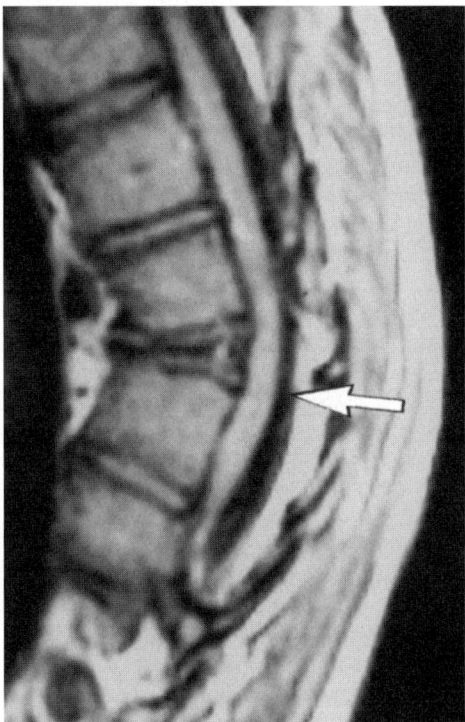

**Figure 76–9.** Congenital kyphosis associated with a posterior hemivertebra in a 15-year-old girl. Sagittal T1-weighted (TR/TE, 550/20) spin echo MR image demonstrates that the spinal cord (*arrow*) is displaced anteriorly and curves around the point of kyphosis.

(From Ozonoff MB: Pediatric Orthopedic Radiology, 2nd ed. Philadelphia, WB Saunders, 1992.)

Congenital kyphosis is much more frequent and is related to agenesis or underdevelopment of the anterior portion of the vertebral centrum and, as a result, a posterior hemivertebra (Fig. 76–9); less commonly, it is related to failure of segmentation anteriorly, with a congenital bar formed between the vertebral bodies. This congenital situation must be distinguished from a developmental anterior fusion occurring in childhood, termed progressive noninfectious anterior vertebral body fusion. Some patients with congenital kyphosis also have Klippel-Feil fusional anomalies in the cervical spine. Congenital kyphosis is common in myelomeningocele, diastrophic dwarfism, and certain other dysplasias.

### Idiopathic Scoliosis

The frequency of idiopathic scoliosis in the normal population depends on the magnitude of the curvature being described. The frequency of scoliosis of more than 25 degrees is 1.5 per 1000 persons in the United States. Adolescent scoliosis is four to eight times more common in girls than in boys, but some evidence indicates that its frequency in the two sexes is nearly equal at younger ages; for unknown reasons, the spinal curvature is more progressive and clinically significant in girls. The ability to predict which curves will progress and which will regress or remain stable is obviously of great clinical importance. The reported frequency of spinal curvature progression varies from 5% to 79%. Curvatures less than 30 degrees generally do not progress after the child is mature, but severe curvatures continue to increase at a rate of about 1 degree per year in adults. Marked tilting and lateral subluxation of vertebral bodies occur in older patients with severe idiopathic scoliosis (Fig. 76–10).

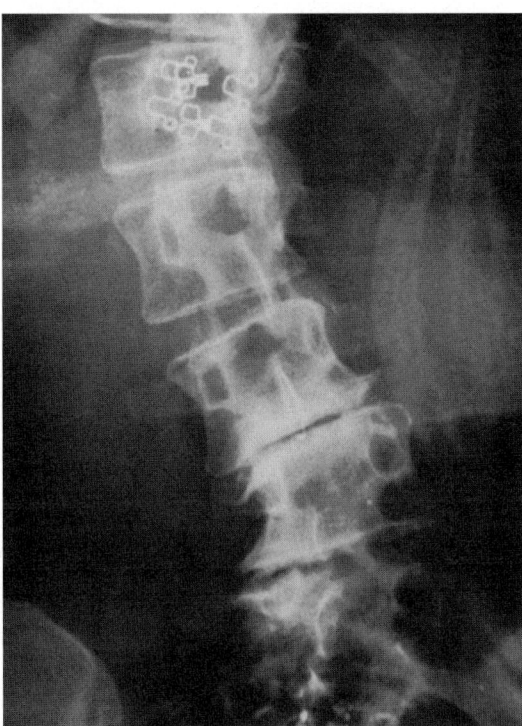

**Figure 76–10.** Idiopathic adolescent scoliosis. The residual effects of this condition are shown in a 43-year-old woman. Disc space narrowing, osteophyte formation, vertebral sclerosis, and lateral vertebral subluxation are present.

One third of first-degree relatives of patients with idiopathic scoliosis have spinal curvatures of 10 degrees or greater. If both parents have idiopathic scoliosis, the possibility of its occurrence in their children is increased by a factor of 50.

**Clinical Patterns.** Idiopathic scoliosis has been divided into three groups—infantile, juvenile, and adolescent—based on the patient's age at the time the condition is recognized.

Infantile scoliosis is detected before age 4 years. Resolution of the spinal curvature occurs in 74% of cases of infantile scoliosis, but scoliotic curves greater than 50 degrees usually progress. Associated plagiocephaly has been noted in 86% of affected infants, with the skull depression invariably located on the convex side of the curve.

Juvenile scoliosis is recognized between age 4 and 10 years. In contrast to adolescent scoliosis, boys are affected predominantly when the diagnosis is established before age 6 years; between the ages of 7 and 10 years, girls are principally affected. Juvenile scoliosis almost invariably progresses with growth.

Adolescent scoliosis is detected between age 10 years and the time of skeletal maturity; it is by far the most common type of idiopathic scoliosis in the United States. The ratio of affected girls to boys ranges from 4:1 to 8:1.

**Radiographic Analysis.** The radiograph remains the mainstay of diagnosis and follow-up, supplemented with specialized projections, CT, and MR imaging, as discussed previously.

**Evolution and Treatment.** As a general rule, spinal curvatures less than 25 degrees are not actively treated unless they occur in preadolescent children and show evidence of rapid progression. With more severe curvature, thoracolumbar orthotic braces are used, with pressure pads placed over the ribs leading to the apical vertebrae. High thoracic curves occasionally require the use of a brace with supports extending into the cervical area. The purpose of bracing is to restrict the ultimate degree of spinal curvature to that encountered when treatment was instituted. The braces are removed when spinal growth is complete.

Surgical treatment is based on the induction of osseous spinal fusion, achieved with an implanted bone graft after excisional decortication and facet fusion. Hardware implants are used to stabilize the fusion length until mature, continuous fusion has occurred. Complications of spinal fusion include breakage of wires or rods, loosening and migration of hooks, spondylolysis, and pseudarthrosis.

### Neuromuscular Scoliosis

Asymmetrical innervation or unbalanced muscular function may lead to scoliosis. The typical neuromuscular curvature is long and C-shaped, extending from the upper thoracic region to the pelvis. Pelvic obliquity is characteristic. In some instances, however, neuromuscular scoliosis may be indistinguishable from idiopathic scoliosis.

Cerebral palsy is the most common cause of neuromuscular scoliosis (Fig. 76–11). Scoliosis is also common in diseases of the spinal cord. It is seen in as many as 70% of patients with syringomyelia and may occur before neurologic symptoms develop. MR imaging assists in differentiating syringomyelia and spinal cord tumors, which may also lead to scoliosis. Abnormal curvatures that develop after traumatic paraplegia or quadriplegia are common as well. In spinal muscular atrophy, scoliosis occurs in more than 60% of patients and usually develops between the ages of 3 and 6 years. Spinal curvature is also common in many other neurologic conditions.

### Scoliosis Associated with or Secondary to Other Conditions

Although most cases of scoliosis are idiopathic, others occur as part of many different syndromes or are associated with systemic disease, regional irritative foci, or fibromuscular changes adjacent to or remote from the spine.

The scoliosis of neurofibromatosis has classically been described as one with sharp angulation and associated kyphosis, but in reality, many abnormal spinal curvatures in this disease resemble those of idiopathic scoliosis. When abrupt angulation of the spine, kyphosis, and adjacent rib dysplasia are evident, however, the radiographic diagnosis of neurofibromatosis is ensured. Associated findings may include a paravertebral soft tissue mass, deformed trans-

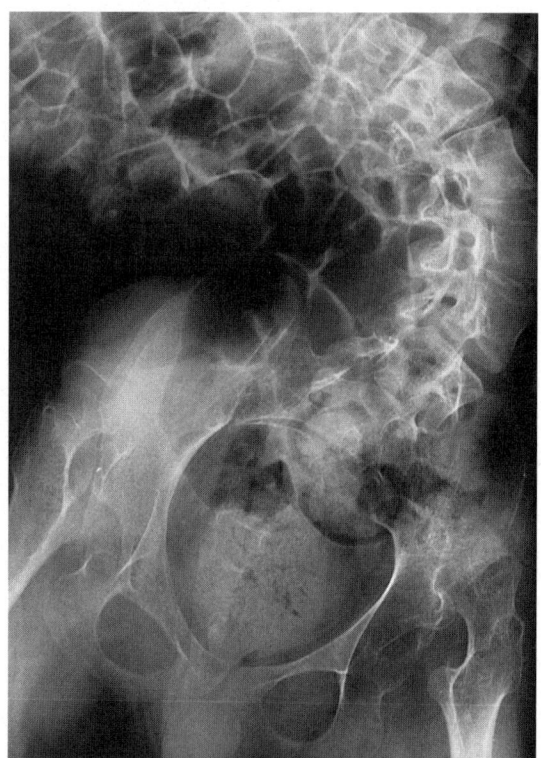

**Figure 76–11.** Neuromuscular scoliosis in cerebral palsy. Severe left lumbar scoliosis with marked rotation is present. The pelvis is oblique, with bilateral hip dislocations.

(From Ozonoff MB: Scoliosis. In Theros EG, Harris JH Jr [eds]: American College of Radiology Bone Syllabus IV. Chicago, American College of Radiology, 1989.)

verse and spinous processes and pedicles, enlarged vertebral foramina, marked rotation of the spinal curvature, and a coarsened and sclerotic trabecular pattern (Fig. 76–12).

Tumors in the vertebrae or adjacent ribs may be associated with scoliosis, presumably on an irritative basis. In this situation, osteoid osteomas or osteoblastomas are generally located on the concave side of the spinal curvature at its apex (Fig. 76–13). Scoliosis is more common in osteoid osteoma than in osteoblastoma.

Radiation therapy for the treatment of malignant tumors of the kidney, thorax, or retroperitoneum can cause both clinical and radiographic spinal deformity. Scoliosis has been reported in 70% of pediatric patients receiving radiation therapy for Wilms' tumor and in 76% of 5-year survivors after treatment of neuroblastoma. Unilateral vertebral body wedging caused by asymmetrical growth on the two sides of the spine is common, as are vertebral contour irregularities and anterior vertebral wedging (Fig. 76–14).

## Scoliosis in Bone Dysplasias and Generalized Syndromes

Scoliosis (or kyphosis) is a common feature of many bone dysplasias and syndromes. A specific diagnosis may not be possible on the basis of spinal deformity alone, although structural features in the individual vertebrae are occasionally distinctive. Bone dysplasias are discussed in Chapter 75.

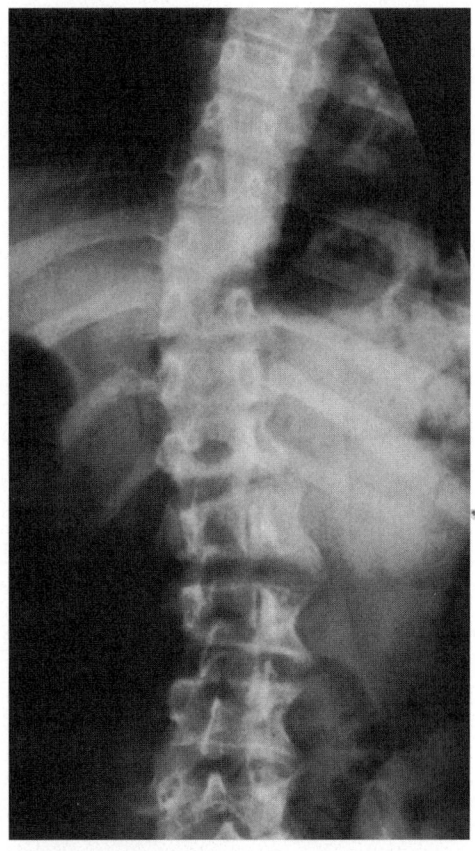

**Figure 76–12.** Neurofibromatosis. Scoliosis is associated with asymmetrical development of the lumbar vertebral bodies, lateral vertebral scalloping, and coarse trabeculae.

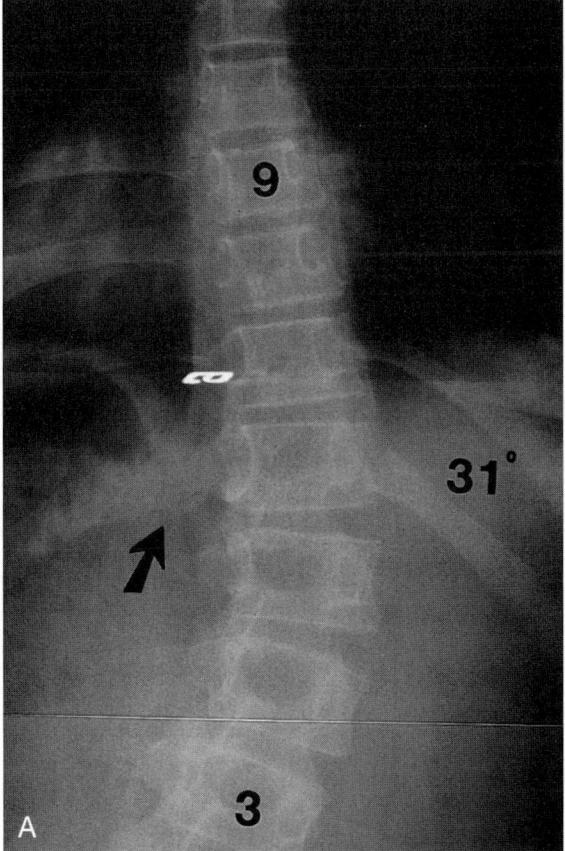

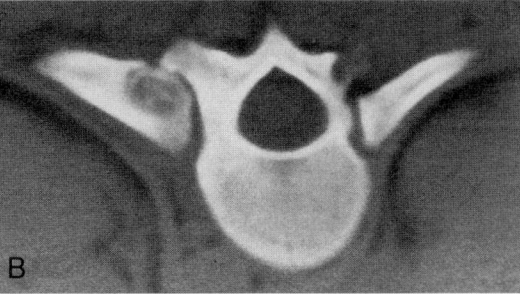

**Figure 76–13.** Scoliosis secondary to osteoid osteoma. *A,* In a posteroanterior projection, expansion of the head of the left 12th rib is present at the concavity of the apex of the thoracolumbar scoliosis *(arrow). B,* CT scanning demonstrates expansion and sclerosis of the proximal portion of the left 12th rib. A central calcific nidus is present. (The orientation of the CT scan was reversed to correspond to that of the other image.)

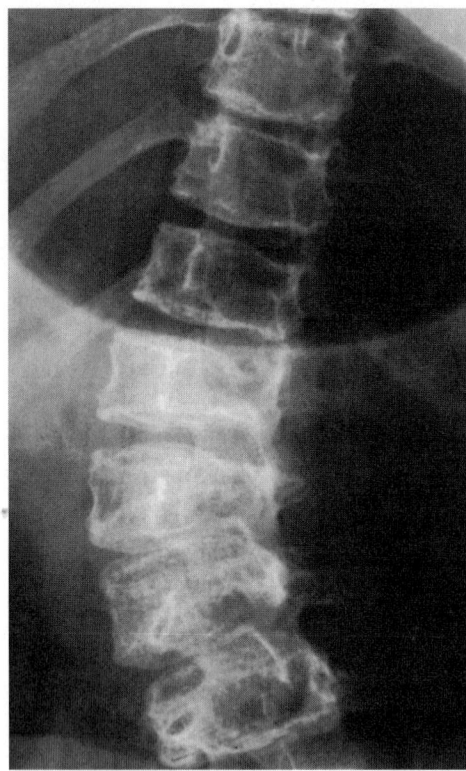

**Figure 76–14.** Kyphoscoliosis after radiation therapy. This 13-year-old boy was treated for Wilms' tumor at 17 months of age. Abnormal bone formation and asymmetrical growth have produced vertebral body wedging and a coarsened trabecular pattern.

(From Ozonoff MB: Scoliosis. In Theros EG, Harris JH Jr [eds]: American College of Radiology Bone Syllabus IV. Chicago, American College of Radiology, 1989.)

## FURTHER READING

Arredondo F, Haughton VM, Hemmy DC, et al: The computed tomographic appearance of the spinal cord in diastematomyelia. Radiology 13:685, 1980.

Bethem D, Winter RB, Lutter L, et al: Spinal disorders of dwarfism: Review of the literature and report of eighty cases. J Bone Joint Surg Am 63:1412, 1981.

Burrows FG: Some aspects of occult spinal dysraphism: A study of 90 cases. Br J Radiol 41:496, 1968.

Bush CH, Kalen V: Three-dimensional computed tomography in the assessment of congenital scoliosis. Skeletal Radiol 28:632, 1999.

Chaglassian JH, Riseborough EJ, Hall JE: Neurofibromatous scoliosis: Natural history and results of treatment in thirty-seven cases. J Bone Joint Surg Am 58:695, 1976.

Dawson EG, Smith L: Atlanto-axial subluxation in children due to vertebral anomalies. J Bone Joint Surg Am 61:582, 1979.

De Smet AA: Radiology of Spinal Curvature. St Louis, CV Mosby, 1985.

DeSousa AL, Kalsbeck JE, Mealey J Jr, et al: Intraspinal tumors in children: A review of 81 cases. J Neurosurg 51:437, 1979.

Fitz CR, Harwood-Nash DC: The tethered conus. AJR Am J Roentgenol 125:515, 1975.

Jaskwhich D, Ali RM, Patel TC, et al: Congenital scoliosis. Curr Opin Pediatr 12:61, 2000.

Jeffries BF, Tarlton M, De Smet AA, et al: Computerized measurement and analysis of scoliosis: A more accurate representation of the shape of the curve. Radiology 134:381, 1980.

Kaplan JO, Quencer RM: The occult tethered conus syndrome in the adult. Radiology 137:387, 1980.

Killian JT, Mayberry S, Wilkinson L: Current concepts in idiopathic scoliosis. Pediatr Ann 28:755, 1999.

Luque ER: Current concepts review: The anatomic basis and development of segmental spinal instrumentation. Spine 7:256, 1982.

MacEwen GD, Conway JJ, Millet WT: Congenital scoliosis with a unilateral bar. Radiology 90:711, 1968.

McAlister WH, Shackelford GD: Classification of spinal curvatures. Radiol Clin North Am 13:93, 1975.

McAlister WH, Shackelford GD: Measurement of spinal curvatures. Radiol Clin North Am 13:113, 1975.

McMaster MJ, Ohtsuka K: The natural history of congenital scoliosis: A study of two hundred and fifty-one patients. J Bone Joint Surg Am 64:1128, 1982.

McRae DL: Bony abnormalities in the region of the foramen magnum: Correlation of the anatomic and neurologic findings. Acta Radiol 40:335, 1953.

Naidich TP, McLone DG, Mutluer S: A new understanding of dorsal dysraphism with lipoma (lipomyeloschisis): Radiologic evaluation and surgical correction. AJNR Am J Neuroradiol 4:103, 1983.

Oestreich AE, Young LW, Young Poussaint T: Scoliosis circa 2000: Radiologic imaging perspective. I. Diagnosis and pretreatment evaluation. Skeletal Radiol 27:591, 1998.

Propst-Proctor SL, Bleck EE: Radiographic determination of lordosis and kyphosis in normal and scoliotic children. J Pediatr Orthop 3:344, 1983.

Schwartz AM, Wechsler RJ, Landy MD, et al: Posterior arch defects of the cervical spine. Skeletal Radiol 8:135, 1982.

Taybi H: Radiology of Syndromes and Metabolic Disorders, 2nd ed. Chicago, Year Book Medical Publishers, 1983.

Tomsick TA, Lebowitz ME, Campbell C: The congenital absence of pedicles in the thoracic spine: Report of two cases. Radiology 111:587, 1974.

Winter RB, Lonstein JE, Leonard AS, et al: Congenital Deformities of the Spine. New York, Thieme-Stratton, 1983.

Winter RB, Moe JH, Bradford DS, et al: Spine deformity in neurofibromatosis: A review of one hundred and two patients. J Bone Joint Surg Am 61:677, 1979.

Winter RB, Moe JH, Wang JF: Congenital kyphosis: Its natural history and treatment as observed in a study of one hundred and thirty patients. J Bone Joint Surg Am 55:223, 1973.

Wright N: Imaging in scoliosis. Arch Dis Child 82:38, 2000.

Yawn BP, Yaw RA, Hodge D, et al: A population-based study of school scoliosis screening. JAMA 282:1427, 1999.

# CHAPTER 77

## Additional Congenital or Heritable Anomalies and Syndromes

### SUMMARY OF KEY FEATURES

There are many congenital and inherited disorders of the skeleton, and these disorders have varied clinical and radiographic manifestations. In some instances, the radiographic features are entirely specific, whereas in others, they must be interpreted with knowledge of the clinical abnormalities to arrive at a correct diagnosis.

### INTRODUCTION

Distinguishing between skeletal anomalies and skeletal variations is not always accomplished with ease. An anomaly represents a marked deviation from normal standards, especially as a result of a congenital or hereditary defect, whereas a variation is a modification of some characteristic that is considered normal (variant of normal) or that is considered typical of a disease (variant of a disease). In some ways, then, the designation of a particular finding as a skeletal anomaly or a skeletal variation is arbitrary and is based on the presence and severity of accompanying clinical manifestations.

### AREAS OF NORMAL AND ANOMALOUS TRABECULAR DIMINUTION OR PROMINENCE

The trabecular architecture of bone coincides with routes of stress. Trabeculae are not uniformly distributed in the human skeleton; rather, they are more prominent and numerous in certain regions and sparse or absent in others. For example, normal areas of rarefaction include the femoral neck (Ward's triangle), the body of the calcaneus, and the proximal portion of the humerus adjacent to the greater tuberosity (Fig. 77–1). Prominent trabeculae are normally encountered at many different sites, particularly in the distal portion of the humerus.

The external surface of bone is not uniformly smooth but possesses normal sites of elevation, depression, and irregularity. Important examples of such sites include the linea aspera on the posterior surface of the middle third of the femur, the soleal line on the posterior surface of the proximal third of the tibia, and the deltoid tuberosity on the lateral surface of the midportion of the humerus.

Cystic areas and cortical irregularities in the posterior aspect of the distal part of the femur at the site of attachment of tendinous fibers of the adductor magnus muscle have been termed fibrous cortical defects; subperiosteal, periosteal, and cortical defects; periosteal and cortical desmoids; and avulsive cortical irregularities. The typical femoral proliferative lesion is consistent with a traumatic pathogenesis (Fig. 77–2).

### SKELETAL CANALS, APERTURES, AND FORAMINA

A channel that extends through a bone is termed a foramen or, when large, an aperture. When the channel is oriented obliquely and is of considerable length, it is referred to as a canal. Nutrient canals, through which pass the nutrient arteries, extend in an oblique fashion from one or more foramina on the osseous surface. In the long tubular bones of the extremities, the nutrient canals typically point away from the dominant growing end of the bone. The resulting radiolucent channels rarely cause diagnostic difficulty, although on occasion, they may resemble a fracture line.

Sites of osseous thinning or true foramina are common in bones containing thin plates, or laminae, such as the parietal and occipital bones of the skull, the sternum, and the scapula. Another commonly encountered aperture, designated a herniation pit, is seen on the anterior surface of the femoral neck. Ingrowth of fibrous and cartilaginous elements occurs through a perforation in the cortex in a roughened reactive area of sclerotic bone and results in unilateral or bilateral small, rounded radiolucent areas in the anterolateral aspect of the femoral neck (Fig. 77–3). Although the lucent regions are generally stable, they may enlarge in persons of all ages. Bone scintigraphy, though typically negative in persons with herniation pits, is occasionally positive, with increased accumulation of the radiopharmaceutical agent.

### ACCESSORY OSSIFICATION CENTERS AND FRAGMENTED SESAMOID BONES

Accessory epiphyseal and apophyseal centers of ossification are frequently encountered in asymptomatic children and adolescents and are generally regarded as a variation of normal. In the past, emphasis was given to differentiating accessory ossicles or ossification centers from fractures; however, the possibility that some of these ossific foci are acquired after injury and may be associated with significant clinical manifestations has led to renewed interest in these "normal" variations.

The os trigonum, near the posterior surface of the talus; os vesalianum, adjacent to the cuboid and base of the fifth metatarsal; os intermetatarseum, between the bases of the first and second metatarsals; os sustentaculi, in the middle facet of the calcaneus; ossicles related to the coracoid process of the scapula; os hamuli proprium, related to the hook of the hamate bone; and os supratrochleare dorsale, in the olecranon fossa, are examples of accessory ossicles that have reportedly been accompanied by pain. Although many ossicles may have clinical significance, several deserve emphasis.

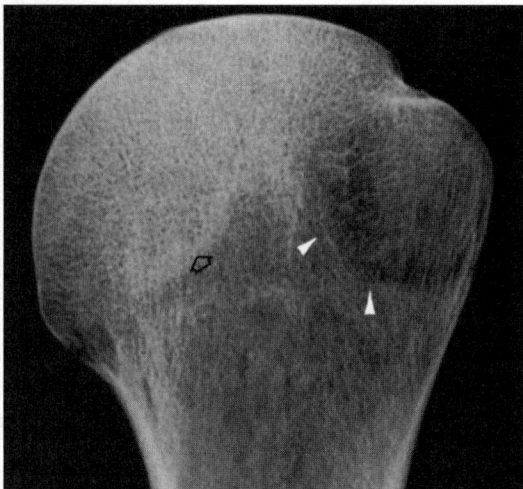

**Figure 77-1.** Normal sites of trabecular diminution: proximal portion of the humerus. The area of rarefaction adjacent to the greater tuberosity is termed a humeral pseudocyst and is a normal finding. The curvilinear inferior margin *(arrowheads)* represents a distinct band of trabeculae that separate the relatively porous region laterally and the more compact spongiosa medially. A fusion line marking the site of closure of a portion of the physis is faintly visible *(arrow)*.

(From Resnick D, Cone RO III: The nature of humeral pseudocysts. Radiology 150:27, 1984.)

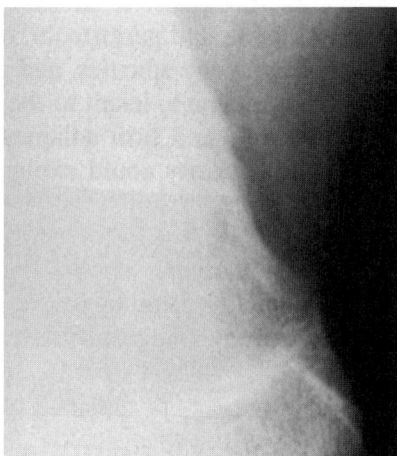

**Figure 77-2.** Normal sites of osseous irregularity: avulsive (proliferative) cortical irregularity in the femur. Observe the normal cortical thickening and small periosteal excrescences extending into soft tissue. The spongiosa is entirely normal, and no soft tissue mass is apparent.

(From Resnick D, Greenway G: Distal femoral cortical defects, irregularities, and excavations: A critical review of the literature with the addition of histologic and paleopathologic data. Radiology 143:345, 1982.)

**Accessory Navicular Bone.** An accessory region of ossification adjacent to the navicular bone is noted in approximately 5% to 10% of feet. Two distinct types of accessory navicular bone have been described: a separate ossicle may occur as a sesamoid bone in the posterior tibial tendon

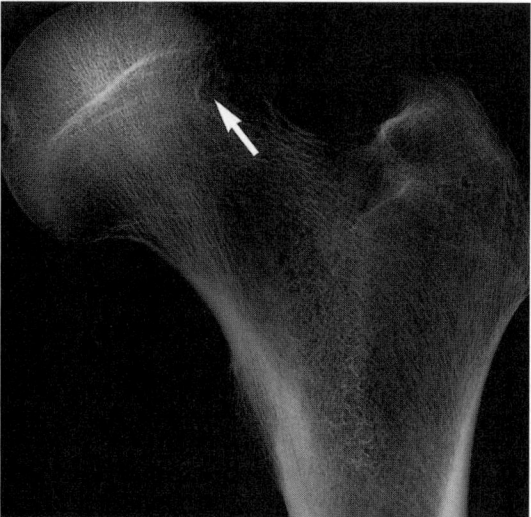

**Figure 77-3.** Herniation pit of the femoral neck. Radiograph of a specimen shows a well-defined radiolucent area *(arrow)*. This corresponds to a roughened area in the femoral neck containing a depression, or pit.

(type I), or an accessory ossification center may appear in the tubercle of the navicular bone (type II) (Fig. 77-4). Another anomaly termed a cornuate navicular involves the medial aspect of the navicular bone and is related to the presence of an osseous bridge connecting the accessory bone with the medial aspect of the navicular. Of these three patterns, the type II ossification center and the cornuate navicular have been associated with clinical manifestations.

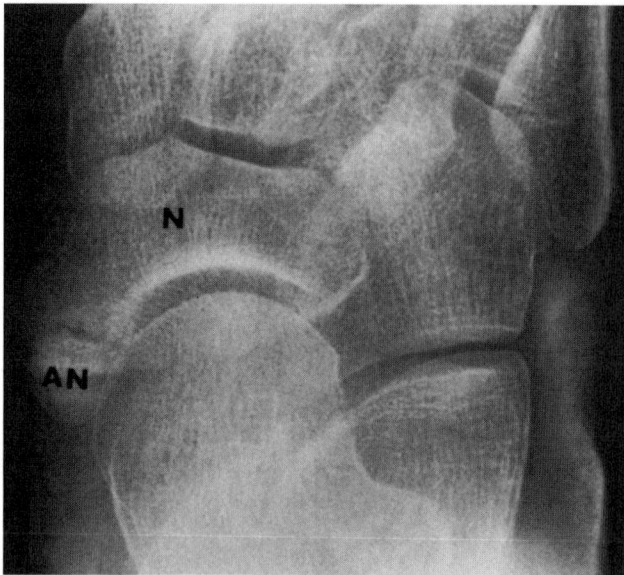

**Figure 77-4.** Accessory navicular bone, type II (accessory ossification center in the tubercle of the navicular bone). Anteroposterior radiograph demonstrates the triangular accessory navicular bone (AN) adjacent to the medial and posterior margin of the navicular (N).

(From Lawson JP, Ogden JA, Sella E, et al: The painful accessory navicular. Skeletal Radiol 12:250, 1984.)

**Carpal Boss (Os Styloideum).** A commonly occurring bony protuberance on the dorsum of the wrist at the base of the second and third metacarpals, adjacent to the capitate and trapezoid bones, is termed a carpal boss, or carpe bossu. It relates to either an osteophyte or an accessory ossification center, the os styloideum. Though generally asymptomatic or associated with only a lump or bump, a carpal boss can occasionally lead to pain.

**Bipartite Patella and Dorsal Defect of the Patella.** A bipartite patella occurs in about 2% of persons. A predilection for the superolateral aspect of the bone (Fig. 77–5) is the radiographic hallmark of this variation and usually allows its differentiation from acute fractures and anomalies of the patella. Dorsal defects of the patella may be related to bipartite patella and are observed in 0.3% to 1% of persons. Recently, a traumatic pathogenesis related to traction in the insertion site of the vastus lateralis muscle has been emphasized. The radiographic characteristics of a dorsal defect of the patella include a well-circumscribed lesion in the superolateral portion of the bone, adjacent to the articular cartilage (Fig. 77–6).

**Os Trigonum.** A separate ossification center in the posterior border of the talar body is designated an os trigonum. A specific syndrome, the os trigonum or talar compression syndrome, has been associated with a persistent and often large os trigonum.

**Os Acromiale.** A persistent ossification center at the free end of the acromion occurs in as many as 15% of persons and is designated an os acromiale (Fig. 77–7). The os

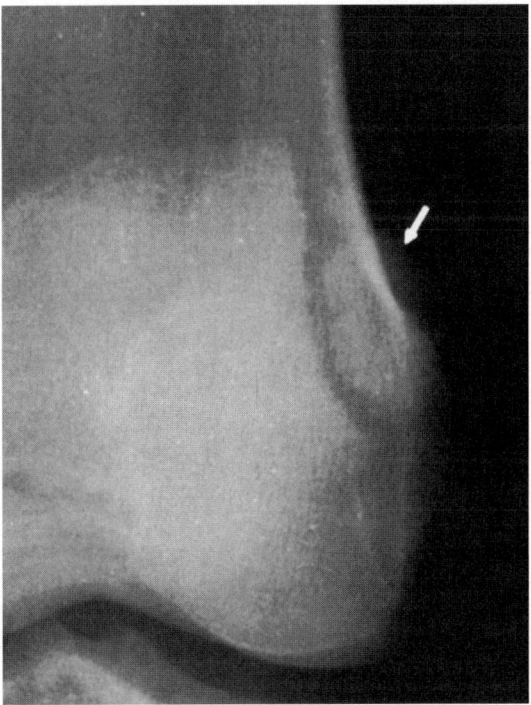

**Figure 77–5.** Bipartite patella. Localization to the superolateral aspect of the patella *(arrow)* is the most characteristic radiographic finding. (Courtesy of A. Pinto Leite, MD, Porto, Portugal.)

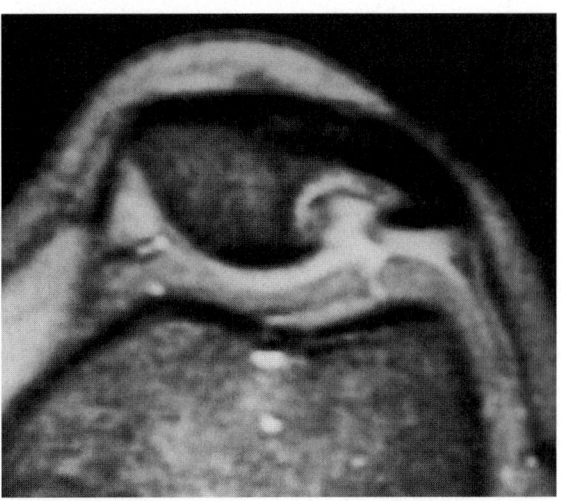

**Figure 77–6.** Dorsal defect of the patella. Note the large patellar defect affecting the superolateral aspect of the bone on an axial gradient (TR/TE, 567/13; flip angle, 25 degrees) MR image. The articular cartilage was slightly depressed but grossly normal.

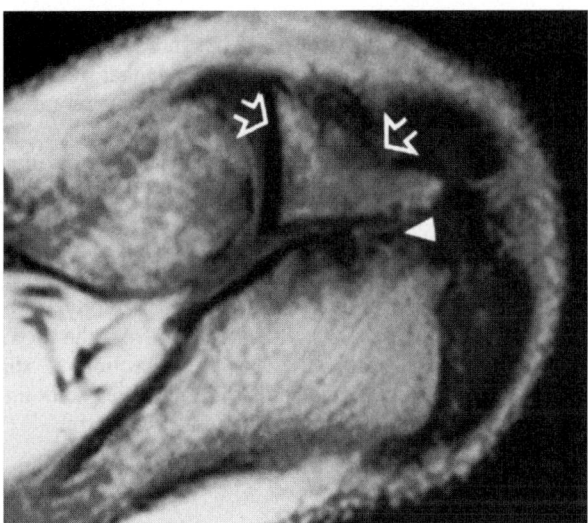

**Figure 77–7.** Os acromiale. Transaxial intermediate-weighted (TR/TE, 1000/20) spin echo MR image shows a triangular os acromiale *(arrows)* articulating with the clavicle and, in an irregular fashion, with the acomion *(arrowhead)*. (Courtesy of S. Eilenberg, MD, San Diego, Calif.)

acromiale is variable in size and is most commonly triangular in shape. Pain and a higher prevalence of the external subacromial shoulder impingement syndrome and tears of the rotator cuff have been associated with an os acromiale.

## SKELETAL APLASIA AND HYPOPLASIA

An entire bone or a portion thereof may fail to form in the normal fashion. Of the major tubular bones, aplasia or hypoplasia typically affects the fibula, radius, femur, ulna, and humerus, in descending order of frequency.

## Fibular Aplasia and Hypoplasia

Congenital absence or severe hypoplasia of the fibula can be combined with ventral and medial bowing of the companion tibia, a skin dimple at the apex of the bow, an equinovalgus foot, absence of one or two of the lateral rays of the foot, tarsal aplasia or fusion, and retarded development or shortening of the ipsilateral femur (Fig. 77–8).

## Radial and Ulnar Aplasia and Hypoplasia

Radial anomalies may include total or partial aplasia or hypoplasia. Bilateral abnormalities are common and may be combined with hypoplasia or absence of the thumb or radial carpal bones. Such radial lesions may be associated with systemic disorders in some cases, including the VATER (vertebral, anal, tracheal, esophageal, radial/renal) syndrome (Fig. 77–9); cardiac abnormalities, including ventricular septal defect, atrial septal defect, pulmonary artery atresia, and patent ductus arteriosus; and thrombocytopenia with absent radius (TAR syndrome).

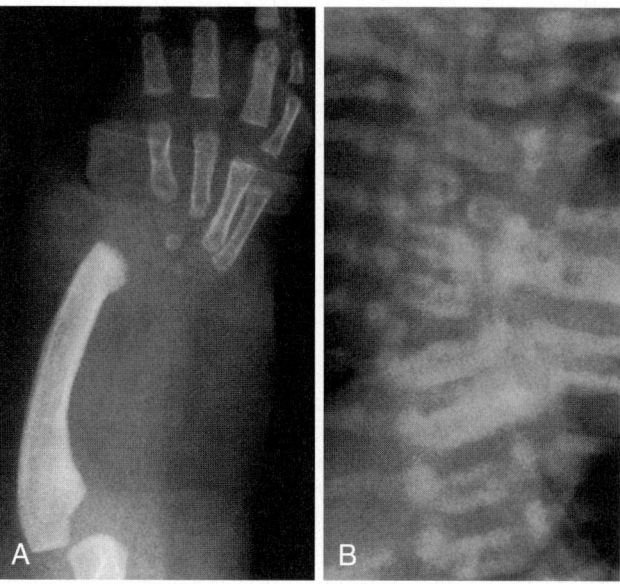

**Figure 77–9.** VATER syndrome. *A,* Anteroposterior radiograph of the forearm in a 2½-year-old child shows radial aplasia and absence of the thumb. *B,* Anteroposterior radiograph of the spine shows severe spinal anomalies. Additional abnormalities included a tracheoesophageal fistula and renal and anal anomalies.

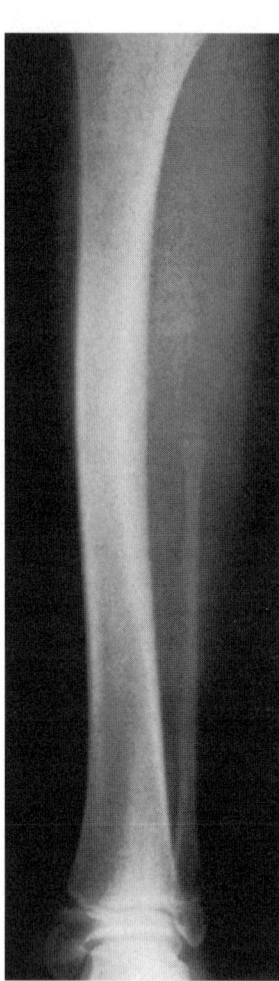

**Figure 77–8.** Hypoplasia and aplasia: fibula. Note the severe hypoplasia of the fibula, with medial bowing of the midshaft of the tibia.

## Proximal Femoral Focal Deficiency

Proximal femoral focal deficiency is the term applied to a spectrum of conditions characterized by partial absence and shortening of the proximal portion of the femur. This disorder is usually an isolated occurrence and appears in a unilateral fashion in 90% of patients. A variety of classification systems have been suggested, based on the presence and location of the femoral head and neck (Table 77–1; Fig. 77–10).

Radiographs of a newborn infant demonstrate a short femur that is displaced superiorly, posteriorly, and laterally to the iliac crest. The distal end of the femur is usually normal. Ossification of the femoral capital epiphysis is invariably delayed. After the second year of life, affected children reveal either dysgenesis or absence of subtrochanteric ossification. At skeletal maturity, changes include subtrochanteric varus deformity or pseudarthrosis, a large unossified gap between the femoral capital epiphysis and dysplastic shaft, or ossification of only the distal femoral epiphysis. Secondary abnormalities of the pelvis and acetabulum are common.

The major differential diagnosis of the radiographic findings is developmental coxa vara, in which familial and bilateral characteristics may be seen. In addition, the abnormalities of coxa vara are less severe, delayed in appearance, progressive, and related to a true decrease in the neck-shaft angle, as opposed to the subtrochanteric varus that appears in proximal femoral focal deficiency.

## Hypoplasia (Dysplasia) of the Glenoid Neck of the Scapula

This entity is also termed glenoid hypoplasia and dentated glenoid anomaly. Men and women are affected with

**TABLE 77–1**

**Classification of Proximal Femoral Focal Deficiency**

| Class | Head of Femur | Acetabulum | Femoral Segment | Relationship among Components of Femur and Acetabulum at Skeletal Maturity |
|-------|---------------|------------|-----------------|---------------------------------------------------------------------------|
| A | Present | Adequate | Short | Bony connection between components of femur; head in acetabulum; subtrochanteric varus, often with pseudarthrosis |
| B | Present | Adequate or moderately dysplastic | Short; usually proximal bony tuft | No osseous connection between head and shaft; head in acetabulum |
| C | Absent or represented by ossicle | Severely dysplastic | Short; usually proximally tapered | May be osseous connection between shaft and proximal ossicle; no osseous connection between femur and acetabulum |
| D | Absent | Absent; obturator foramen enlarged; pelvis squared in bilateral cases | Short, deformed | |

From Levinson ED, Ozonoff MB, Royen PM: Proximal femoral focal deficiency (PFFD). Radiology 125:197, 1977.

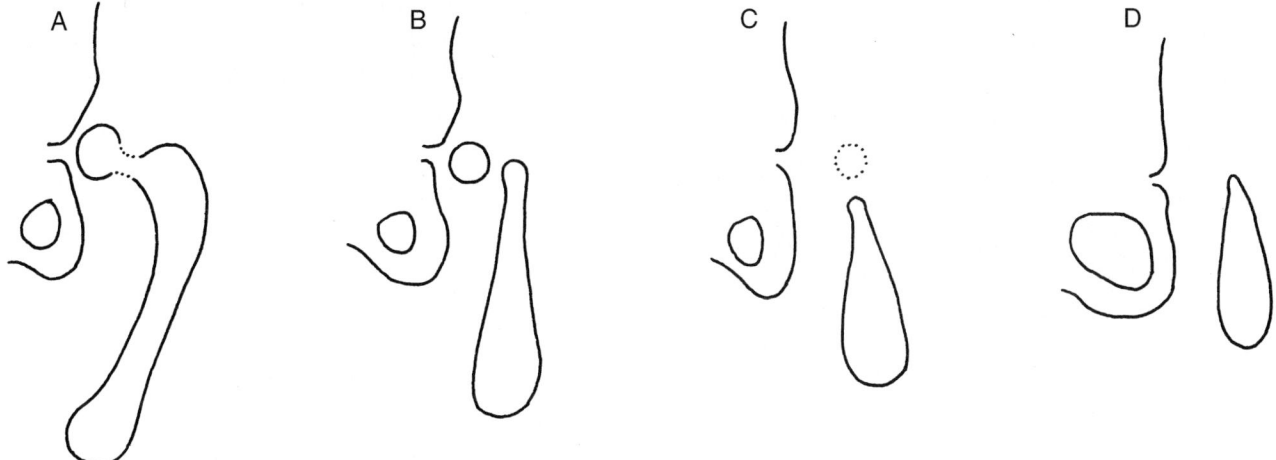

**Figure 77–10.** Proximal femoral focal deficiency: classification system. Classes A to D are shown. In all classes, the femoral shaft is very short. Dashed lines indicate structures that will (class A) or may (class C) ossify at a later date. (After Levinson ED, Ozonoff MB, Royen PM: Proximal femoral focal deficiency (PFFD). Radiology 125:197, 1977.)

about equal frequency. Shoulder pain and limitation of motion are often evident; less commonly, the condition is discovered incidentally. Radiography reveals abnormalities that are usually confined to the shoulder. Bilateral and relatively symmetrical changes predominate and consist of dysplasia of the scapular neck and irregularity of the glenoid surface. A dentate or notched articular surface becomes apparent (Fig. 77–11). Additional findings may include hypoplasia of the humeral head and neck, varus deformity of the proximal portion of the humerus, and enlargement and bowing of the acromion and clavicle. The radiographic abnormalities associated with dysplasia of the neck of the scapula are virtually diagnostic.

## Sacrococcygeal Agenesis (Caudal Regression Syndrome)

This well-known anomaly leads to absence of one or more segments of the sacrum, possibly combined with aplasia of the lower thoracic and upper lumbar spine. Approximately 20% of persons with this syndrome are children of diabetic mothers. Associated abnormalities include neurogenic bladder and serious urologic problems, hip dislocation, flexion contractures of the knees and hips, and foot deformities. Radiographic findings vary with the severity of the anomaly. Complete sacral agenesis is associated with deformed ilia that may articulate with each other or with the lowest vertebral body or that fuse in the

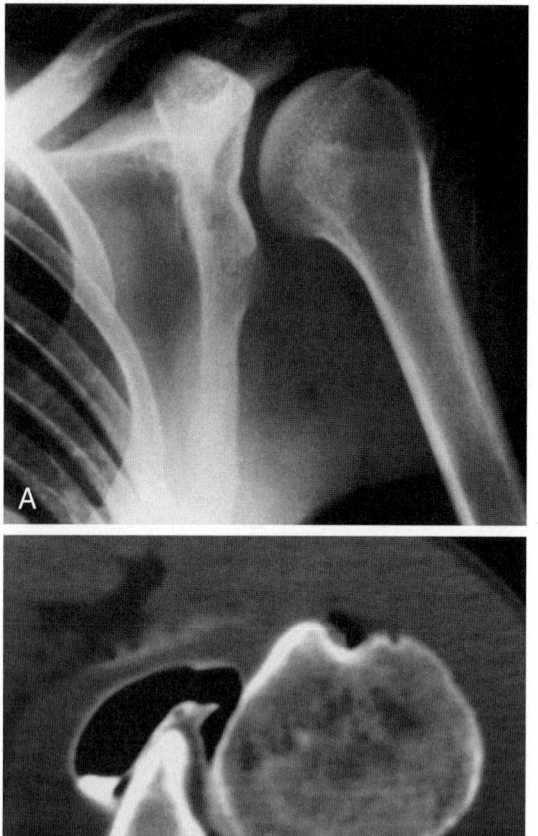

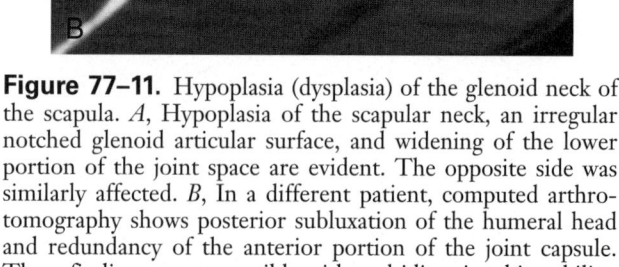

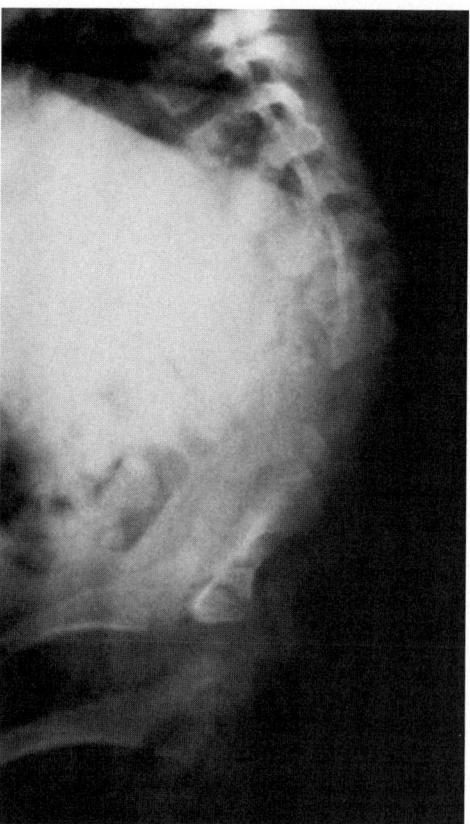

**Figure 77–12.** Sacrococcygeal agenesis (caudal regression syndrome). In this child of a diabetic mother, observe the absence of much of the lumbar spine and all of the sacrum. Deformity of the ilia is evident.

**Figure 77–11.** Hypoplasia (dysplasia) of the glenoid neck of the scapula. *A,* Hypoplasia of the scapular neck, an irregular notched glenoid articular surface, and widening of the lower portion of the joint space are evident. The opposite side was similarly affected. *B,* In a different patient, computed arthrotomography shows posterior subluxation of the humeral head and redundancy of the anterior portion of the joint capsule. These findings are compatible with multidirectional instability.

   (*A,* From Resnick D, Walter RD, Crudale AS: Bilateral dysplasia of the scapular neck. AJR Am J Roentgenol 139:387, 1982. *B,* Courtesy of G. Greenway, MD, Dallas, Tex.)

midline. When combined with complete fusion of the lower extremities, this anomaly has been referred to as the mermaid syndrome (Fig. 77–12). Partial agenesis may lead to a deformed and sickle-shaped sacrum through which an anterior meningocele may protrude.

## MALSEGMENTATION AND FUSION

Errors in segmentation are frequently inherited and result in osseous fusion of neighboring bones, such as the radius and ulna. Bony ankylosis can also occur between longitudinally arranged bones, as in the digits of the hand and foot. On the opposite end of the spectrum, hypersegmentation and duplication anomalies exist.

## Hyperphalangism and Polydactyly

Extra phalanges in humans are virtually confined to the thumb. Although the anomaly can occur as an isolated finding, it may be associated with other anomalies, including polydactyly, duplications, and absent bones, and with certain syndromes, including Holt-Oram syndrome, trisomy 13-15, and Blackfan-Diamond anemia. Accessory phalanges should be differentiated from the pseudoepiphyses of the digits that may accompany certain syndromes, such as cleidocranial dysostosis and hypothyroidism.

   Polydactyly, or an increased number of digits, can occur in the hand or foot. In the foot, the fifth digit is usually involved. Polydactyly on the radial side of the hand (including the thumb) is termed preaxial polydactyly; on the ulnar side of the hand, it is known as postaxial polydactyly. Preaxial polydactyly may be associated with acrocephalosyndactyly, brachydactyly B, acropectorovertebral dysplasia, Fanconi's syndrome, Holt-Oram syndrome, and other conditions; postaxial polydactyly can appear in chondroectodermal dysplasia (Ellis-van Creveld syndrome), Laurence-Moon-Biedl syndrome, trisomy 13, asphyxiating thoracic dystrophy, Goltz's focal dermal hypoplasia, and other diseases.

## Syndactyly

Syndactyly, a common anomaly, refers to a lack of differentiation between two or more digits. It may be divided into cases with either soft tissue or osseous involvement and classified as either partial (involving the proximal segments of a digit) or complete (involving the entire digit). Other classification systems are also used. Most cases are inherited, although some appear in a sporadic fashion. A large number of syndromes have been associated with syndactyly, including Poland's syndrome, in which the pectoral muscles are absent. It has been suggested that Poland's syndrome is present in approximately 10% of patients with syndactyly (Fig. 77–13).

## Carpal Fusion (Coalition)

Carpal fusion, or coalition, is a relatively common abnormality that may occur as an isolated phenomenon or as part of a generalized congenital malformation syndrome. As a rule, isolated fusion involves bones in the same carpal row (proximal or distal), whereas syndrome-related fusion may affect bones in different rows (proximal and distal).

The most common site of an isolated fusion is between the triquetrum and the lunate bones (0.1% to 1.6% of the general population), with little or no clinical significance (Fig. 77–14). The fusion is bilateral in approximately 60% of cases. Widening of the scapholunate interosseous space is a frequent finding in cases of lunotriquetral fusion, although the scapholunate interosseous ligament is generally intact. Other fusions are less common. In most cases, symptoms and signs are entirely lacking, although pain has been observed in some cases.

Massive carpal fusion is usually associated with other anomalies. Similarly, fusion between bones of the proximal and distal carpal rows or between the carpal bones and radius or ulna is generally associated with additional malformations.

## Radioulnar Synostosis

A common site of osseous fusion in the tubular bones of the extremities is between the proximal portions of the radius and ulna (Fig. 77–15). Two distinct types have been recognized: proximal, or true, radioulnar synostosis, in which the radius and ulna are fused smoothly at their proximal borders for a distance of about 2 to 6 cm; and a second variety in which fusion just distal to the proximal radial epiphysis is associated with congenital dislocation of the radial head. In both types, interference with normal forearm supination is seen. The condition is bilateral in approximately 60% of patients.

Additional anomalies that may accompany radioulnar synostosis are clubbed feet, developmental dysplasia of the hip, knee anomalies, hypoplasia of the thumb, carpal fusion, symphalangism, and Madelung's deformity. Radioulnar synostosis may also appear as part of arthrogryposis, multiple hereditary exostoses, acrocephalopolysyndactyly, acrocephalosyndactyly, Holt-Oram syndrome, mandibulofacial dysostosis, Nievergelt-Pearlman syndrome, Klinefelter's syndrome, and other chromosomal aberrations.

## Tarsal Fusion (Coalition)

Tarsal coalition represents abnormal fusion of one or more of the tarsalia. The union may be fibrous, cartilaginous, or osseous and can be congenital (developmental) or acquired in response to infection, trauma, articular disorders, or surgery.

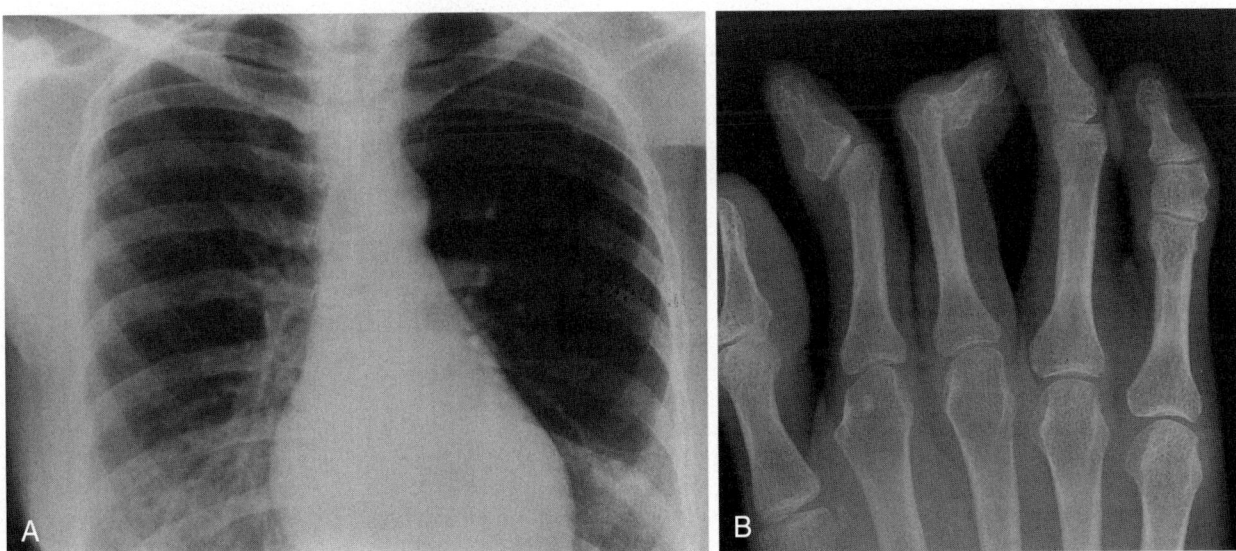

**Figure 77–13.** Poland's syndrome. *A*, Absence of the left pectoral muscles has created increased radiolucency of the left hemithorax. Elevation of the scapula and deformity of the ribs are also seen. *B*, The involved hand reveals aplasia (second, third, and fourth digits) and hypoplasia (fifth digit) of the middle phalanges, partial soft tissue syndactyly between the fourth and fifth fingers and between the second and third fingers, and osseous deformities.

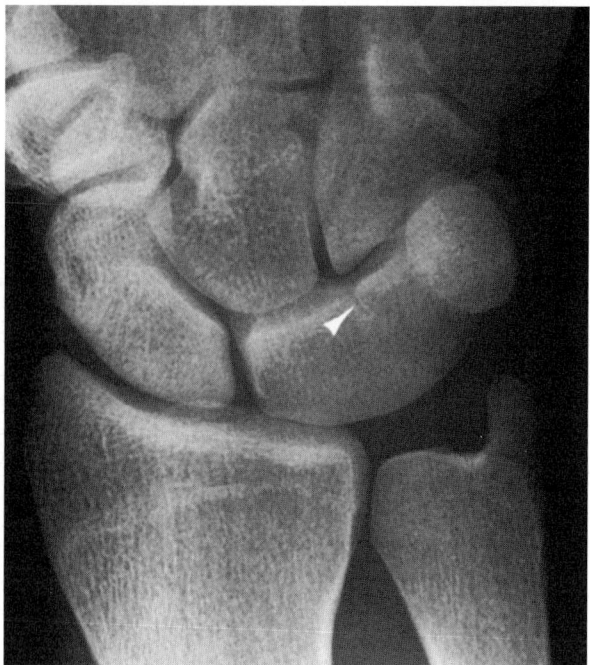

**Figure 77–14.** Carpal fusion (coalition). Note the bony fusion between the lunate and triquetrum, with a small cleft (*arrowhead*) at the site of ankylosis.

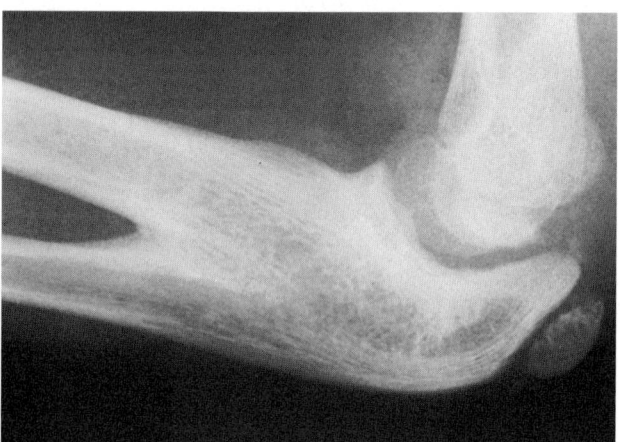

**Figure 77–15.** Radioulnar synostosis. In this patient, note the smooth osseous fusion of the proximal segments of the radius and ulna.

The overall prevalence of tarsal coalition in the general population is about 1%, and bilateral coalitions are apparent in 50% to 60% of cases. Typically, symptoms and signs of tarsal coalition appear in the second or third decade of life. Limited subtalar motion, pes planus, and shortening with persistent or intermittent spasm of the peroneal muscles are seen on physical examination. Coalition can also manifest as a cavus foot or may be an incidental finding in an asymptomatic person.

Isolated partial coalitions can be classified according to the bones affected; calcaneonavicular, talocalcaneal,

talonavicular, and calcaneocuboid fusions, in decreasing order of frequency, may be detected. With the advent of advanced tomographic methods (such as computed tomography [CT] and magnetic resonance [MR] imaging), however, it appears that talocalcaneal coalitions are at least as frequent as, and may be more frequent than, calcaneonavicular coalitions. The most common coalitions are discussed here.

**Calcaneonavicular Coalition.** This type of coalition is one of the most common, is sometimes bilateral, and can be asymptomatic or associated with a rigid flatfoot. Optimally, coalition is identified on a 45-degree medial oblique view of the foot (Fig. 77–16). The diagnosis is simplified by the presence of a solid bony bar extending between the calcaneus and the navicular bone, but it is more difficult in cases of cartilaginous or fibrous coalition. Normally, a joint does not exist between the two bones; a close approximation of their bony contours, especially if adjacent eburnation or sclerosis is evident, should raise the possibility of a nonosseous coalition. Elongation of the anterosuperior portion of the calcaneus also suggests the diagnosis; such elongation, when viewed on a lateral radiograph, has been designated the "anteater nose" sign. Talar "beaking" is uncommon and, when present, may be the result of an associated talocalcaneal fusion. CT and MR imaging may be useful in confirming this diagnosis (Fig. 77–17).

**Talocalcaneal Coalition.** Talocalcaneal fusion is another common type of tarsal coalition. Almost all such fusions occur at the middle facet, between the talus and sustentaculum tali (Fig. 77–18). The condition is bilateral in

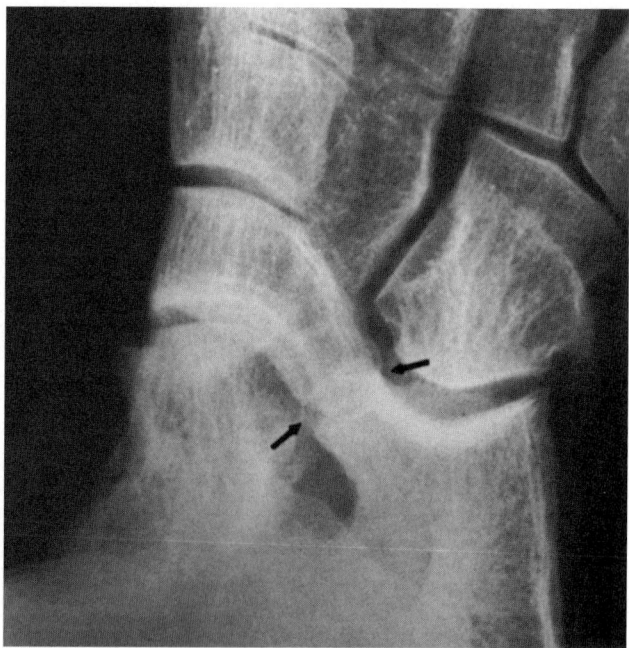

**Figure 77–16.** Calcaneonavicular tarsal coalition. Observe the approximation of the osseous surfaces of the calcaneus and navicular bone (*arrows*) on a medial oblique view. Mild abnormalities are apparent at the calcaneocuboid joint.

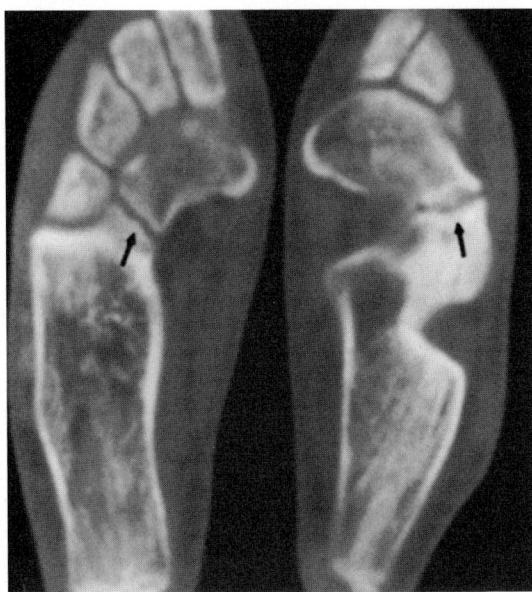

**Figure 77–17.** Calcaneonavicular tarsal coalition. Transverse CT scan confirms the presence of bilateral calcaneonavicular coalitions *(arrows)*. (Courtesy of G. Greenway, MD, Dallas, Tex.)

20% to 25% of patients. Cartilaginous, fibrous, or bony bridges may be identified, although radiographic evaluation often requires special views in addition to standard anteroposterior and lateral projections. In both fibrous and cartilaginous coalitions, CT or MR imaging may be helpful.

Fortunately, a number of secondary radiographic signs have been described in association with talocalcaneal coalition. These signs include the following:

1. *Talar beaking.* Dorsal subluxation of the navicular bone leads to elevation of the periosteum below the talonavicular ligament, along with subperiosteal proliferation and the production of a beak, or excrescence, at the dorsal surface of the talar head adjacent to the talonavicular space (see Fig. 77–18). This "beak" is not pathognomonic of talocalcaneal coalition; it may be identified in other conditions associated with abnormal motion at the talonavicular space. A similar beak may be identified in diffuse idiopathic skeletal hyperostosis.

2. *Broadening of the lateral process of the talus.* Broadening or rounding of this process (see Fig. 77–18) is easily identified by comparing views of the opposite (uninvolved) foot. It is present in 40% to 60% of patients.

3. *Narrowing of the posterior subtalar joint.* This finding may be evident in as many as 50% to 60% of patients.

4. *Continuous C-sign.* A C-shaped line visible on lateral radiographs of the ankle is a sensitive and specific sign of talocalcaneal coalition (Fig. 77–19). This line is formed by the medial outline of the dome of the talus above and the posteroinferior outline of the sustentaculum tali below.

5. *Ball-and-socket ankle joint.* A rounded, convex appearance of the proximal talar articular surface and a concomitant concave appearance of the distal end of the tibia may accompany talocalcaneal coalition (Fig. 77–20).

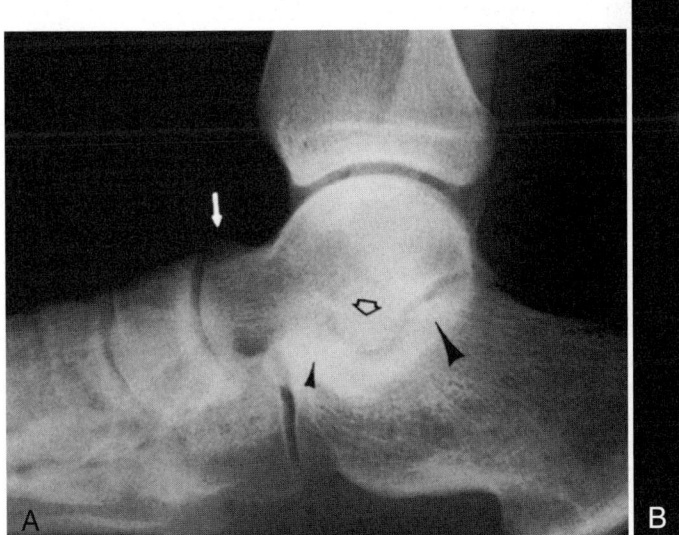
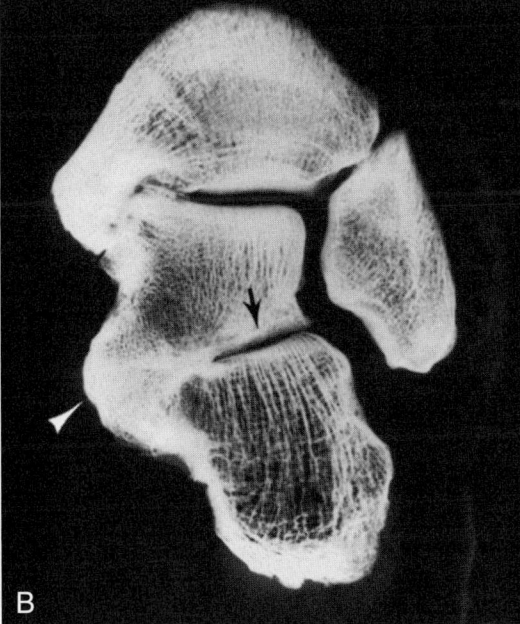

**Figure 77–18.** Talocalcaneal tarsal coalition: middle facets. *A,* Lateral radiograph reveals talar beaking *(solid arrow)*, broadening of the lateral process of the talus *(open arrow)*, narrowing of the posterior subtalar joint *(large arrowhead)*, and nonvisualization of the space between the sustentaculum tali and talus (middle subtalar joint) *(small arrowhead)*. *B,* In a different patient, coronal section of the hindfoot reveals a complete osseous bridge *(arrowhead)* involving the middle facets of the talus and calcaneus. Note the obliquely oriented posterior subtalar joint *(arrow)* and ankle.

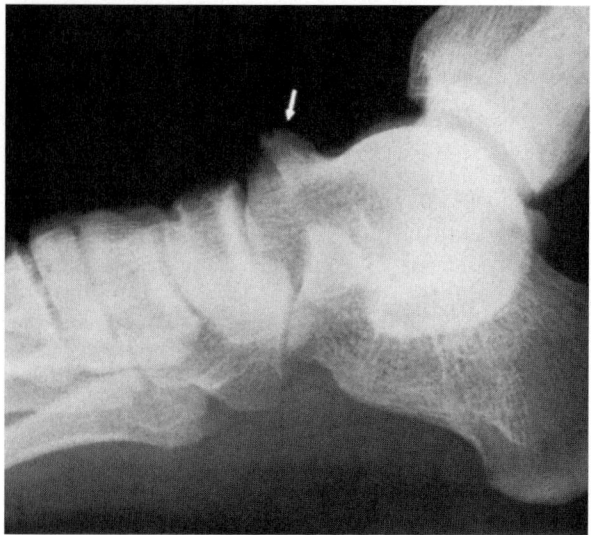

**Figure 77–19.** Talocalcaneal tarsal coalition: talar beak and C-sign. In a patient with a talocalcaneal coalition involving the middle facets, observe a large osseous excrescence *(arrow)* on the dorsal surface of the talus. A continuous C-sign is evident.

(From Sartoris DJ, Resnick D: Tarsal coalition. Arthritis Rheum 28:331, 1985.)

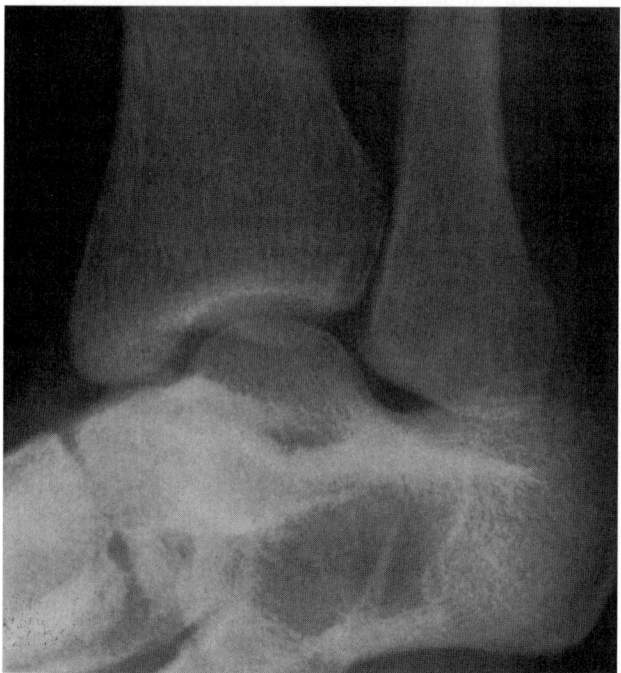

**Figure 77–20.** Tarsal coalition with a ball-and-socket ankle joint (congenital coalition). Oblique radiograph outlines bony coalition among most of the tarsal bones, including the talocalcaneal joints. Note the ball-and-socket appearance of the ankle, with associated deformity of the distal end of the fibula.

CT and MR imaging are especially useful when radiographs are inconclusive, and they can determine the extent of articular involvement. These techniques can also be applied to the assessment of fibrous and cartilaginous coalitions. On MR imaging, marrow edema may be encountered at the sites of coalition.

## Klippel-Feil Syndrome

The term Klippel-Feil deformity is loosely applied to many types of congenital fusion of the cervical vertebrae, but the original syndrome consisted of a triad of signs: short neck, low posterior hairline, and limitation of neck movement. Currently, the designation Klippel-Feil syndrome indicates a congenital fusion of two or more cervical vertebrae; in more than 50% of patients, the classic triad is not apparent.

In most cases, fusion begins at the occiput and first cervical vertebra, at the first and second cervical vertebrae, or at the second and third cervical vertebrae (Fig. 77–21). With involvement of the upper cervical region, the segment of the second and third vertebrae is a typical distal location of the fusion; with involvement of the lower cervical region, the segment between the sixth and seventh vertebrae generally denotes the distal extent of the abnormality. The joints of the second and third and the fifth and sixth cervical vertebrae are altered most frequently.

Patients with Klippel-Feil syndrome or related deformities usually do not have a family history of the disease; exceptions to this rule occur, as documented in several reports. On clinical examination, the patient has a short neck, with restriction of motion. Torticollis may be present in some cases. Neurologic abnormalities are variable.

Many associated malformations have been described:

1. *Sprengel's deformity.* Unilateral or bilateral elevation of the scapula is present in approximately 20% to 25% of cases, especially in those with high and extensive cervical fusions (Fig. 77–22). Sprengel's deformity may be associated with an omovertebral bone connecting the scapula and vertebrae. This bone, which is present in approximately 30% to 40% of cases of fixed elevated scapulae, is not always ossified.

2. *Cervical ribs.* Anomalous ribs are evident in approximately 10% to 15% of cases.

3. *Webbed neck (pterygium colli).*

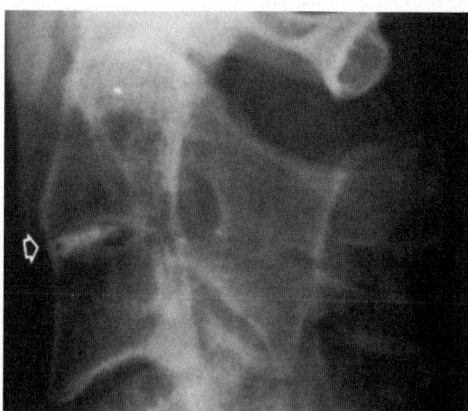

**Figure 77–21.** Klippel-Feil syndrome. Fusion of the second and third cervical vertebrae is seen. Note the ankylosis of the posterior elements and the atrophic intervertebral disc containing calcification *(open arrow).*

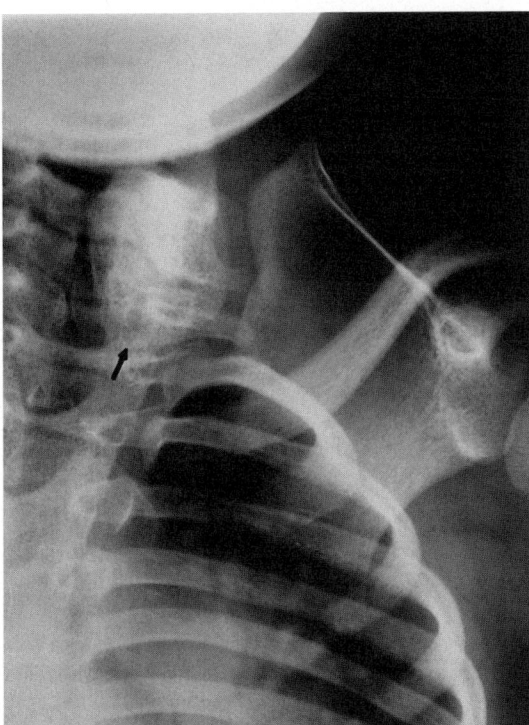

**Figure 77–22.** Klippel-Feil syndrome with Sprengel's deformity. Note the elevated position of the scapula, an omovertebral bone *(arrow)*, and cervical spine abnormalities.

4. *Hemivertebrae.* Hemivertebrae are present in approximately 15% to 20% of cases.

5. *Spina bifida.* Anterior or posterior spina bifida is frequent in patients with cervical fusions.

6. *Other anomalies.* Kyphosis; scoliosis; spinal stenosis; fused, absent, or deformed ribs; basilar impression; cranial asymmetry; congenital defects of the brain or spinal cord; deformed dens; cleft palate; supernumerary lobes of the lung; patent foramen ovale; interventricular septal defect; renal anomalies; and enteric cysts or duplications represent some of the additional malformations that may be apparent.

On radiographs, the fusion may be partial or complete; it may affect the vertebral bodies, pedicles, laminae, or spinous processes. With fusion of the vertebral bodies, small atrophic intervertebral discs may be apparent and can contain calcification. The anteroposterior diameter of the vertebral bodies at the level of an affected discovertebral junction may be smaller than that at the superior and inferior limits of the vertebrae adjacent to uninvolved discs; in such cases, this forms the basis for the "wasp-waist" sign (Fig. 77–23).

The major differential consideration is juvenile chronic arthritis. Although the clinical history is most helpful in differentiating between these two conditions, the radiographic findings of juvenile chronic arthritis do not include ankylosis of adjacent spinous processes. Further, in this articular disease, abnormalities are apparent at other

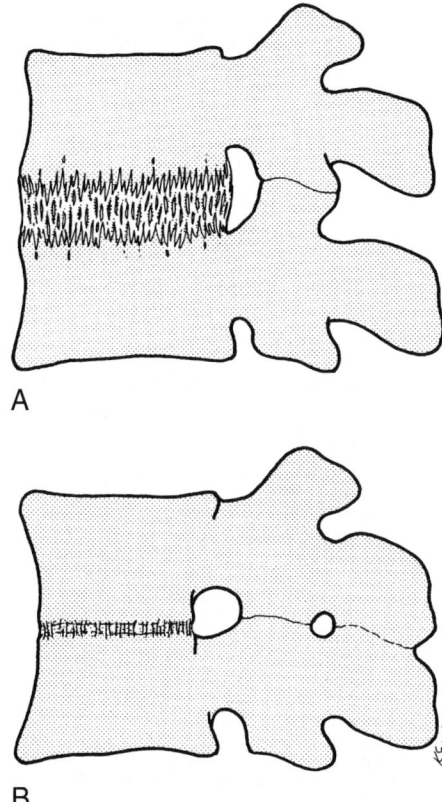

**Figure 77–23.** Acquired versus congenital vertebral fusion. *A,* Acquired ankylosis. Note the absence of constriction at the level of the intervertebral disc and the absence of posterior element fusion. *B,* Congenital ankylosis. A constricted appearance at the level of the intervertebral disc has produced a trapezoidal shape of the bony mass. The posterior elements are also ankylosed, and the intervertebral disc is atrophic.

skeletal sites, and an elevated position of the scapula is not seen.

## Congenital Block Vertebrae

Congenital synostosis of vertebrae in the thoracic and lumbar spine may be encountered, related to a derangement in embryologic development. The anomaly is usually limited in extent and affects two adjacent vertebrae. It is commonly asymptomatic.

## ARTICULAR ABNORMALITIES
### Madelung's Deformity

Madelung's deformity refers to a bowing of the distal end of the radius. Typically, the radial bowing occurs in a volar direction while the ulna continues to grow in a straight fashion. The curvature and growth disturbance of the radius result in its being shorter than the ulna. The carpal angle, formed by the intersection of two lines (one tangent to the proximal surfaces of the scaphoid and lunate bones; the second tangent to the proximal margins of the triquetrum and lunate bones), is normally 130 to 137 degrees; in Madelung's deformity, it is decreased (Table 77–2). Radiographic alterations include the following (Fig. 77–24):

1. *Radial abnormalities.* These include dorsal and ulnar curvature; decreased length; triangular shape of the distal radial epiphysis, with unequal growth of the epiphysis; premature fusion of the medial half of the radial epiphysis; localized area of radiolucency along the ulnar border of the radius; osteophytosis along the inferior ulnar portion of the radius; and ulnar and volar angulation of the distal radial articular surface.

2. *Ulnar abnormalities.* Dorsal subluxation, enlargement and distortion of the ulnar head, and changes in length have been observed.

3. *Carpal abnormalities.* Included are wedging of the carpus between the deformed radius and protruding ulna, a triangular configuration with the lunate at the apex, and an arched curvature in the lateral projection.

A mesomelic variety of dwarfism known as dyschondrosteosis is associated with Madelung's deformity, and there has been considerable debate regarding the relationship between the two disorders.

The isolated variety of Madelung's deformity is more commonly bilateral than unilateral, is asymmetrical, and is at least three to five times more common in female patients. Clinical manifestations usually become evident in adolescents or young adults. Visible deformity, pain, fatigue, and limited range of motion, especially dorsal extension, ulnar deviation, and supination, are noted.

## Infantile Coxa Vara

Normally, the angle of intersection of the axis of the femoral neck with the axis of the femoral shaft varies with age but is approximately 150 degrees at birth and 120 to 130 degrees in adults. The relative valgus position in an infant's femur is due to increased growth of the medial portion of the cartilage plate in the prenatal period. In children, with acceleration of growth in the lateral portion of the plate, a more varus position becomes apparent.

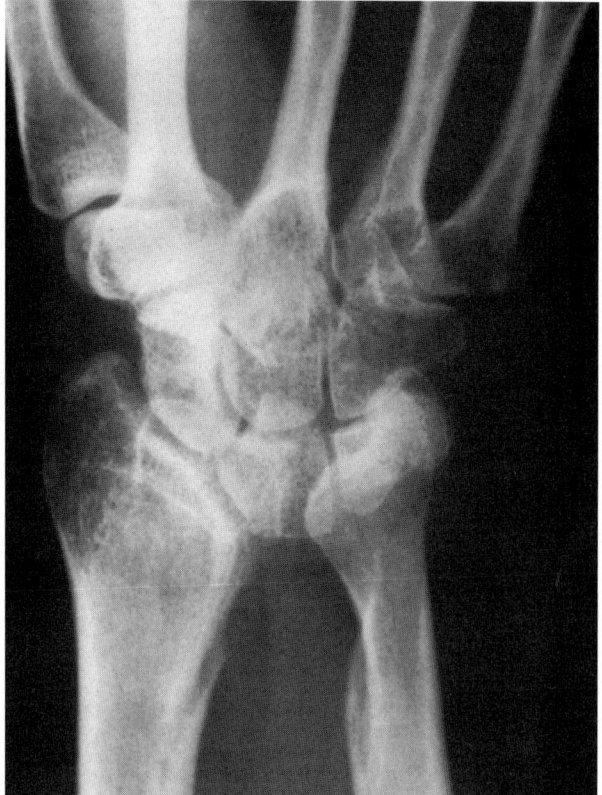

**Figure 77–24.** Madelung's deformity. Abnormalities include increased width between the distal portions of the radius and ulna, an ulna that is relatively long in comparison to the length of the radius, a decreased carpal angle, triangularization of the distal radial epiphysis, osseous excrescences on apposing metaphyseal regions of the radius and ulna, distortion of the ulnar head, and wedging of the carpus between the deformed radius and protruding ulna, with the lunate at the apex of the wedge.

The term coxa vara indicates a neck-shaft angle that is less than 120 degrees, despite the variation in normal values among different age groups. Coxa vara may accompany a number of processes, including proximal femoral focal deficiency, osteogenesis imperfecta, renal osteodystrophy, rickets, and fibrous dysplasia. Infantile, or developmental, coxa vara is the designation given to a proximal femoral deformity that becomes apparent in the first few years of life, especially when the child first walks. Boys and girls are affected with approximately equal frequency, and the condition is unilateral in 60% to 75% of cases. Clinically, affected children have a painless lurching gait or, in the case of bilateral involvement, a "duck-waddle" gait.

Radiographs reveal a decrease in the femoral shaft-neck angle and a medially located triangular piece of bone in the neck adjacent to the head that is bounded by two radiolucent bands traversing the neck and forming an inverted V. The growth plate itself is widened, and its alignment is more vertical than normal. With further growth, the varus deformity frequently progresses, probably related to the forces of weight bearing (Fig. 77–25).

---

**TABLE 77–2**

### Syndromes Associated with Abnormality of the Carpal Angle

| Decreased | Increased |
| --- | --- |
| Madelung's deformity | Arthrogryposis |
| Dyschondrosteosis | Diastrophic dwarfism |
| Turner's syndrome | Epiphyseal dysplasias |
| Morquio's syndrome | Frontometaphyseal dysplasia |
| Hurler's syndrome | Otopalatodigital syndrome |
| | Pfeiffer's syndrome |
| | Spondyloepiphyseal dysplasia |
| | Trisomy 21 |

From Poznanski AK: The Hand in Radiologic Diagnosis. Philadelphia, WB Saunders, 1974, p 140.

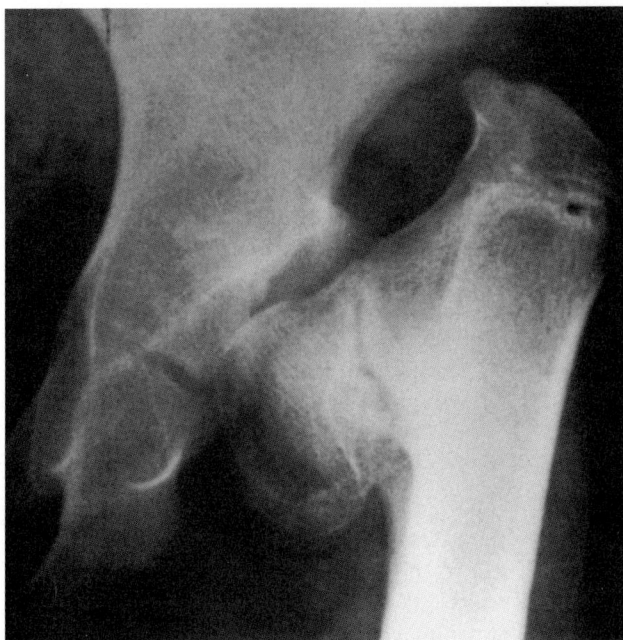

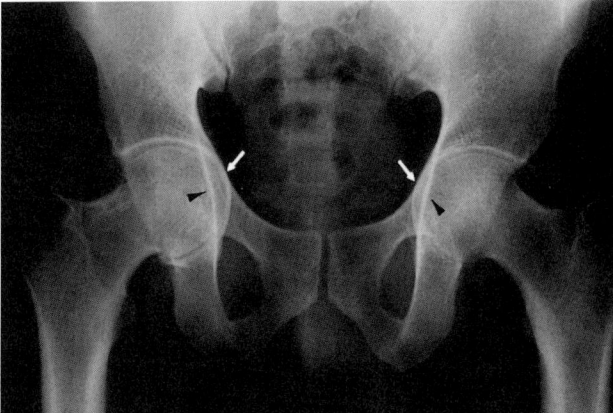

**Figure 77–26.** Primary protrusion of the acetabulum. This 30-year-old man has bilateral acetabular protrusion with concentric loss of joint space. Note that the acetabular line *(arrows)* is located medial to the ilioischial line *(arrowheads)* by a considerable distance.

**Figure 77–25.** Infantile coxa vara. Note the severe varus deformity of the proximal portion of the femur, the vertically located and irregular growth plate, thickening of the medial cortex of the femoral neck, a prominent greater trochanter, and acetabular flattening.

The triangular piece of bone may merge with the shaft, remodeling thickens the medial cortex of the femoral neck, the greater trochanter enlarges, and secondary degenerative joint disease can appear.

## Primary Protrusion of the Acetabulum

Acetabular protrusion refers to intrapelvic displacement of the medial wall of the acetabulum. It may be evident in many articular and nonarticular disorders, including rheumatoid arthritis, ankylosing spondylitis, septic arthritis, degenerative joint disease, osteomalacia, Paget's disease, sickle cell anemia, and neoplasm; after trauma; and as an effect of irradiation. Protrusio acetabuli can also appear in the absence of any recognizable cause, and in such cases, it is termed primary acetabular protrusion, or Otto pelvis.

The cause of primary acetabular protrusion is unknown. It usually affects both hips and is much more frequent in women than in men; a familial nature is noted. With progressive protrusion deformity, the femoral head assumes an intrapelvic location, and the joint space may be normal, narrowed, or obliterated.

A radiographic diagnosis of acetabular protrusion can be made in an adult pelvis when the distance between the medially located acetabular line and the laterally located ilioischial line is 6 mm or more in women and 3 mm or more in men (Fig. 77–26).

## Joint Hypermobility Syndrome

Joint hypermobility syndrome, which is also called congenital laxity of ligaments, refers to hypermobility that is independent of inflammatory conditions, neurologic disorders, diseases of connective tissue (including Ehlers-Danlos syndrome), and other congenital disorders. Although the condition may be entirely asymptomatic, clinical manifestations have been reported and range from minor articular discomfort, acute pain, or joint effusions to recurrent subluxations or dislocations of the patella, hip, elbow, or glenohumeral joint; idiopathic scoliosis; carpal tunnel syndrome and other neuropathies; temporomandibular joint dysfunction; or prolapse of the mitral valve. Foot abnormalities, including equinovarus and calcaneovalgus deformities, are also associated with this syndrome, as are osteoarthritis and chondrocalcinosis.

## Foot Deformities

A detailed discussion of the complexities of the deformed foot is beyond the scope of this chapter, and only a brief summary of the major foot deformities is presented. Proper radiographic analysis requires both anteroposterior and lateral projections during weight bearing. The following terms are applied to foot deformities:

*Talipes:* A long-established term for congenital deformities of the foot (e.g., talipes equinovarus).

*Pes:* A term that should be restricted to acquired deformities of the foot (e.g., pes equinovarus).

*Valgus:* Situation in which the bones distal to a specified joint are oriented in a plane away from the midline of the body.

*Varus:* The opposite of valgus, in which the bones distal to a specified joint are oriented in a plane toward the midline of the body.

*Equinus:* Fixed plantar flexion of the hindfoot.

*Calcaneus:* Fixed dorsiflexion of the hindfoot.

*Cavus:* A raised longitudinal arch of the foot.

*Planus:* A flattened longitudinal arch of the foot.

*Adduction:* Displacement in a transverse plane toward the axis of the body.

*Abduction:* Displacement in a transverse plane away from the axis of the body.

The normal alignment of the foot is inferred from information derived, in large part, from the relationship of the talus and the calcaneus on anteroposterior and lateral radiographs (Figs. 77–27 and 77–28).

In hindfoot (heel) valgus (see Fig. 77–27*C*), an anteroposterior projection reveals an increase in the talocalcaneal angle. A line extended through the longitudinal axis of the talus falls medial to the first metatarsal, and the navicular and other tarsal bones are displaced laterally to the talus. On a lateral projection, the talus is tilted more vertically than normal because of abduction of the calcaneus, which decreases plantar support on the anterior portion of the talus. The long axis of the talus and that of the first metatarsal angulate in a plantar direction. In hindfoot (heel) varus (see Fig. 77–27*B*), on anteroposterior views, the long axis of the talus falls lateral to the base of the first metatarsal because of adduction of the anterior end of the calcaneus. The talocalcaneal angle is decreased, and the talus and calcaneus are more parallel

to each other than in a normal foot. The navicular bone is displaced medially. On a lateral view, the calcaneus and talus are both more horizontal and parallel with each other.

Hindfoot or heel valgus is present in flatfoot, metatarsus varus, congenital vertical talus, and certain congenital and neurologic deformities of the foot. Hindfoot or heel varus is commonly visible in talipes equinovarus and some paralytic deformities.

In hindfoot equinus, on a lateral projection, the calcaneus is flexed in a plantar direction so that the angle between the axes of the calcaneus and the tibia is greater than 90 degrees. This deformity accompanies talipes equinovarus and congenital vertical talus. In calcaneal hindfoot deformity, on a lateral projection, the calcaneus is dorsiflexed abnormally so that its anterior end has a more superior position, and the bone has a boxlike appearance. Calcaneal positions of the calcaneus appear in association with cavus deformities of the foot.

Clubfoot is a condition associated with equinovarus foot deformity and hindfoot varus (Fig. 77–29). The clubfoot deformity is relatively common, occurs more frequently in male children, and can be unilateral or bilateral. Its exact cause is not clear.

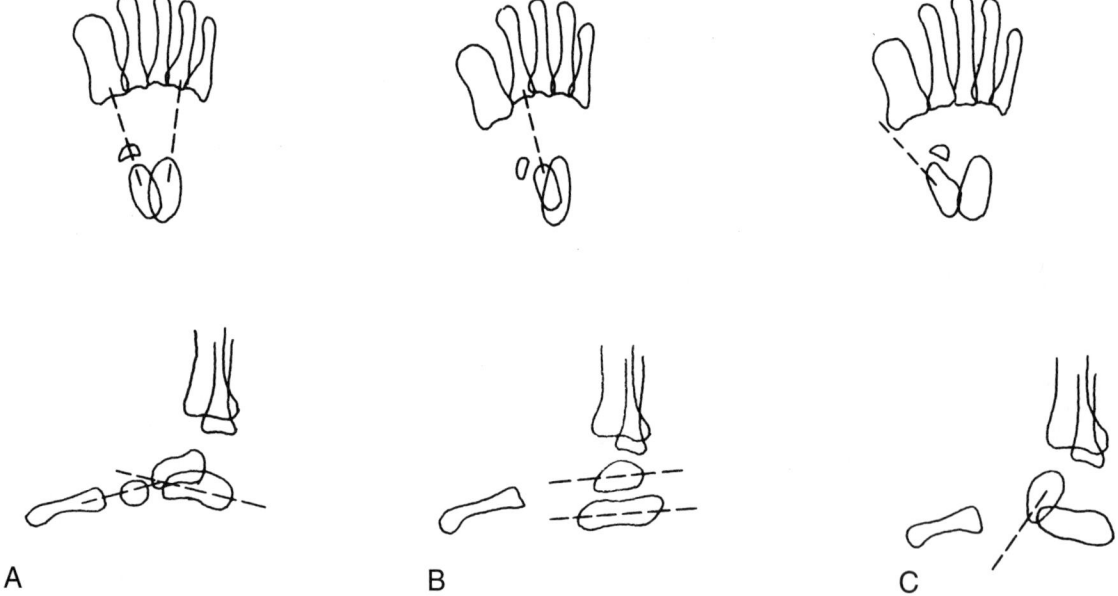

A                              B                              C

**Figure 77–27.** Normal and abnormal hindfoot and forefoot relationship. *A,* Normal. On an anteroposterior radiograph, the talar axis intersects or points slightly medial to the first metatarsal bone, and the navicular bone is situated directly opposite the head of the talus. The calcaneus points toward the fourth metatarsal bone, such that a talocalcaneal angle of approximately 35 degrees is created in an adult (somewhat greater in an infant). On a lateral radiograph, the anterior portion of the talus is mildly flexed in a plantar direction, and the calcaneus is slightly dorsiflexed. A line extended through the longitudinal axis of the talus is directed along the axis of the first metatarsal bone. The talocalcaneal angle is approximately 35 degrees. *B,* Hindfoot varus deformity. Anteroposterior radiograph reveals a decrease in the talocalcaneal angle caused by the two bones lying close together and more parallel to each other. The navicular bone is displaced medially, and the talar axis points lateral to the first metatarsal base. On a lateral projection, the talus and calcaneus are both more horizontal and parallel with each other. *C,* Hindfoot valgus deformity. On an anteroposterior radiograph, the talocalcaneal angle is increased, with the navicular bone and remaining tarsal bones located lateral to the talus. The talar axial line passes medial to the first metatarsal bone. On a lateral radiograph, the talus is oriented more vertically, and the long axis of the talus and that of the first metatarsal bone angulate in a plantar direction. (Adapted from Ozonoff MB: Pediatric Orthopedic Radiology. Philadelphia, WB Saunders, 1979.)

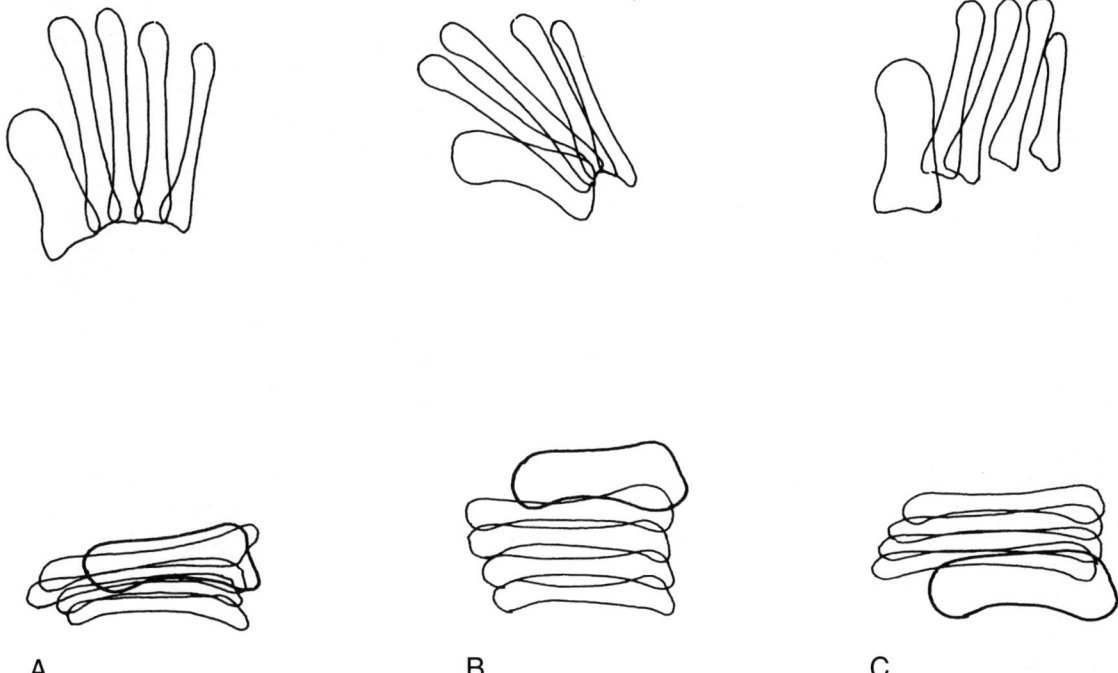

**Figure 77–28.** Normal and abnormal forefoot alignment. *A*, Normal. On an anteroposterior radiograph, the metatarsal bones converge proximally, with overlapping at their bases. On a lateral projection, the fifth metatarsal bone is in the most plantar position, with the other metatarsals superimposed. *B*, Forefoot varus deformity. On a frontal radiograph, the forefoot is narrowed, and increased convergence at the metatarsal bases has resulted in more overlap than normal. On a lateral radiograph, a ladder-like arrangement is seen, with the first metatarsal bone most dorsal. *C*, Forefoot valgus deformity. The forefoot is broadened, with the metatarsal bones more prominent than normal, and with decreased overlap at the metatarsal bases. On a lateral projection, a ladder-like arrangement can be noted in some cases, with the first metatarsal bone in the most plantar position. (Adapted from Ozonoff MB: Pediatric Orthopedic Radiology. Philadelphia, WB Saunders, 1979.)

After inadequate or improper treatment of clubfoot, certain deformities may remain, including the rocker-bottom deformity, which is due to correction of foot dorsiflexion before equinus, and the flattop talus, which is due to flattening of the superior surface of a plantar-flexed talus that is articulating with the tibia.

A congenital vertical talus (congenital flatfoot with talonavicular dislocation) can occur as an isolated condition or as part of a generalized malformation syndrome or disorder. The condition occurs with approximately equal frequency in boys and girls and in a unilateral or bilateral distribution. It is often associated with arthrogryposis or myelomeningocele. On an anteroposterior radiograph, severe heel valgus and forefoot abduction result in an increased talocalcaneal angle, with the talar axis lying medial to the first metatarsal bone. On a lateral radiograph, an equinus heel with plantar flexion of both the calcaneus and the talus is evident (Fig. 77–30). Dorsiflexion of the forefoot at the midtarsal level results in a convex plantar surface of the foot, the rocker-bottom deformity. The navicular bone is dislocated dorsally, thereby locking the talus into its plantar-flexed position.

The cavus foot deformity is a frequent accompaniment of neurologic or muscular disorders, such as peroneal muscular atrophy, poliomyelitis, and meningomyelocele.

An abnormally high longitudinal arch of the foot is seen as a result of dorsiflexion of the calcaneus (calcaneus position) and plantar flexion of the metatarsals (Fig. 77–31).

On an anteroposterior view, the flexible flatfoot deformity is associated with an increase in the talocalcaneal angle, heel valgus, and forefoot abduction. The midtarsal transverse arch is flattened, and the metatarsals are approximately parallel in their orientation. On a lateral projection, hindfoot valgus is noted, with the talus in a more vertical attitude than normal. The calcaneus and metatarsals are aligned horizontally, and the plantar arch is flattened. Although the resulting radiographic picture may superficially resemble that seen in congenital vertical talus, the flexible flatfoot deformity is not associated with equinus, and the navicular bone retains its normal position with regard to the distal surface of the talus.

Metatarsus adductus in association with metatarsus varus is a common deformity of unknown cause (Fig. 77–32). The forefoot is adducted and in varus alignment, with a concave medial border, convex lateral border, and high arch. The hindfoot is normal in mild cases and is in valgus alignment in severe cases. Dorsiflexion of the foot is normal or exaggerated.

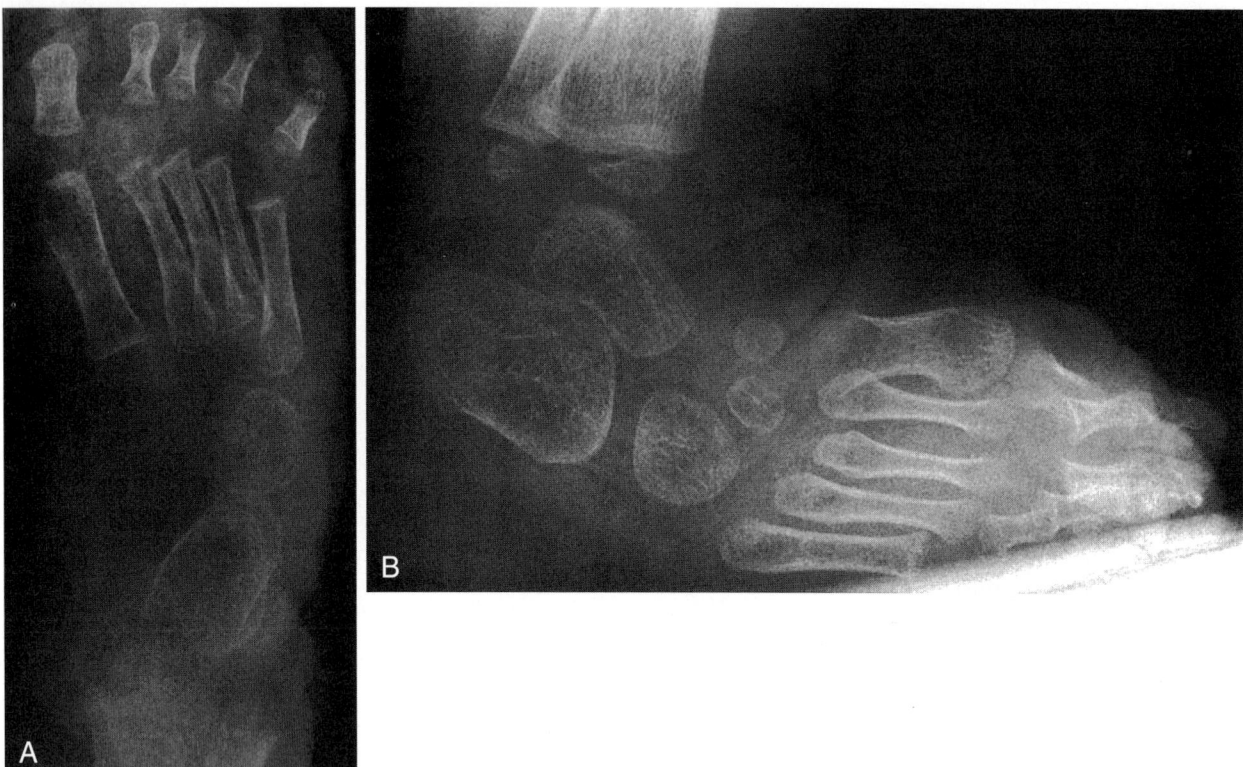

**Figure 77–29.** Clubfoot (equinovarus) deformity. *A*, Anteroposterior projection. The hindfoot is in a marked varus position, with superimposition of the talar and calcaneal centers. A line drawn through the talus would pass far laterally to the first metatarsal bone. The navicular is not ossified, but its abnormal position can be inferred from the location of the first metatarsal base and the first cuneiform center. The forefoot is narrowed, with increased overlap of the metatarsal bases. *B*, Lateral projection. The talus and calcaneus are more parallel than normal. The calcaneus is in an equinus position and abnormally flexed in a plantar direction. Forefoot inversion with a ladder-like arrangement of the metatarsal bones is apparent.
(From Ozonoff MB: Pediatric Orthopedic Radiology. Philadelphia, WB Saunders, 1979.)

## TORSION OF THE FEMUR AND TIBIA

Twisting of a tubular bone on its longitudinal axis is termed torsion. In femoral torsion, the lower or condylar portion of the bone is the segment on which the proximal portion rotates on its longitudinal axis. In anteversion or antetorsion, the axis of the femoral neck is twisted in a forward or anterior direction with respect to the frontal or coronal plane of the femoral condyles; in retroversion or retrotorsion, this axis is rotated posteriorly or directed backward with reference to the coronal condylar plane. In tibial torsion, the distal segment of the tibia is rotated toward either the medial malleolus (internal, or medial, tibial torsion) or the lateral malleolus (external, or lateral, tibial torsion). The precise cause of these torsional deformities is not clear. Accurate diagnosis of tibial torsional malalignment requires knowledge of the changing patterns of tibial torsion in normal infants and children.

## MISCELLANEOUS SYNDROMES AND CONDITIONS

### Osteo-onychodysostosis

Osteo-onychodysostosis, an autosomal dominant disorder, is also referred to as nail-patella syndrome, hereditary osteo-onychodysplasia, and Fong's syndrome. It is characterized by dysplastic fingernails; hypoplastic or absent patellae; additional bony deformities, particularly about the pelvis and elbows; iliac horns; widespread soft tissue changes; and renal dysplasia. Renal osteodystrophy and death can result from the kidney disease. Clinical manifestations are most frequently seen in the second and third decades of life. Hypoplasia or splitting of fingernails, palpable absence of the patellae, presence of iliac protuberances, increased carrying angle of the elbow, abnormal pigmentation of the iris, and proteinuria may be recognized.

In infancy, the demonstration of posterior iliac horns identifies this dysplasia. In the knee, absence or hypoplasia

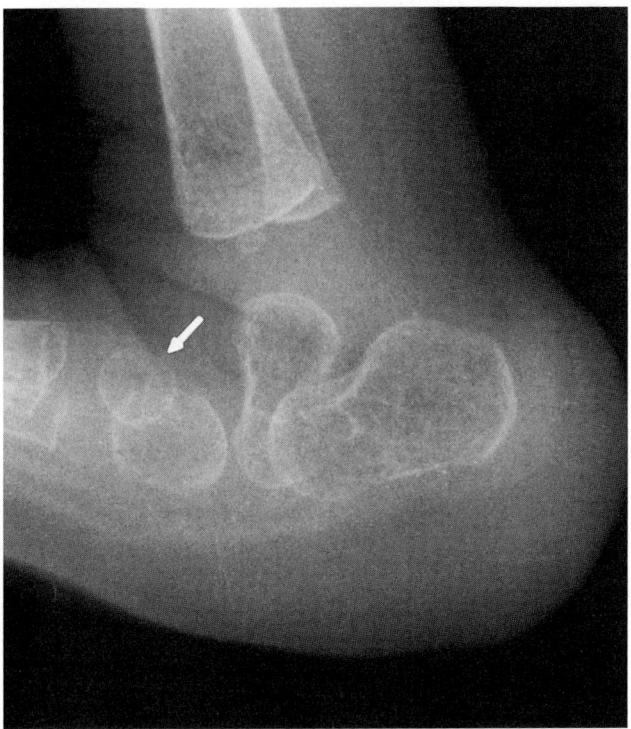

**Figure 77–30.** Congenital vertical talus. The markedly vertical orientation of the talar axis and the equinus position of the calcaneus have produced an inferior convexity of the plantar surface of the foot. The navicular is unossified, but because of the position of the ossified third cuneiform *(arrow)*, it should be displaced dorsally and occupy the space between the cuneiform and the talus.

of the fibula and patella; asymmetrical development of the femoral condyles, with hypoplasia of the lateral condyle and an apparent or true enlargement of the medial condyle; and a sloping tibial plateau with a prominent tibial tubercle are identified (Fig. 77–33). In the elbow, asymmetrical development of the humeral condyles, hypoplasia of the capitulum, and subluxation or dislocation of the radial head are the major changes. Abnormalities of the pelvis consist of dysplasia of the iliac wings and the presence of iliac horns (Fig. 77–34). Bilateral outgrowths from the posterior aspect of the ilium, occasionally capped by an epiphysis, are virtually pathognomonic. Additional bony changes may be evident in the shoulder, wrist, ankle, and subtalar joints.

## Progeria

Progeria is a rare syndrome that was described by Hutchinson in 1886. Infants appear normal at birth, but typical clinical manifestations become evident within the first few years of life. Dwarfism, alopecia, brown pigmentation of the trunk, atrophic skin, loss of subcutaneous fat, impaired extension at the hips and knees, receding chin, beaked nose, and exophthalmos are seen. Radiographic findings include hypoplastic facial bones and mandible, delay in closure of cranial sutures, and coxa valga. Acro-osteolysis of the terminal phalanges of the hands and feet and the clavicles is a distinctive finding. Progressive dissolution of these bones and others, including the ribs and humerus, can lead to pathologic fractures that heal slowly and often progress to nonunion. The pattern and degree of osteolysis may be reminiscent of

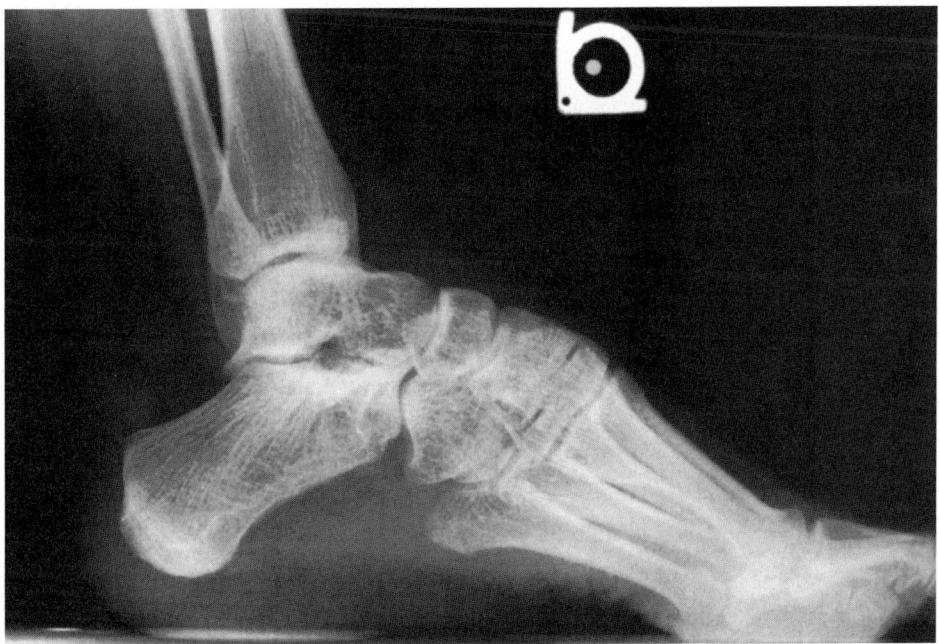

**Figure 77–31.** Cavus foot. After poliomyelitis, this 18-year-old woman has an increased plantar arch, with a calcaneus position of the os calcis and increased plantar flexion of the forefoot.

(From Ozonoff MB: Pediatric Orthopedic Radiology. Philadelphia, WB Saunders, 1979.)

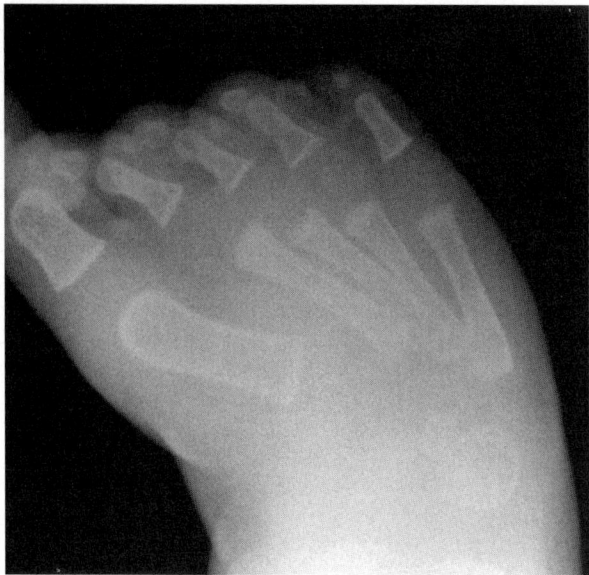

**Figure 77–32.** Metatarsus adductus and metatarsus varus. Note the adducted varus position of the forefoot, with a concave medial border and convex lateral border.

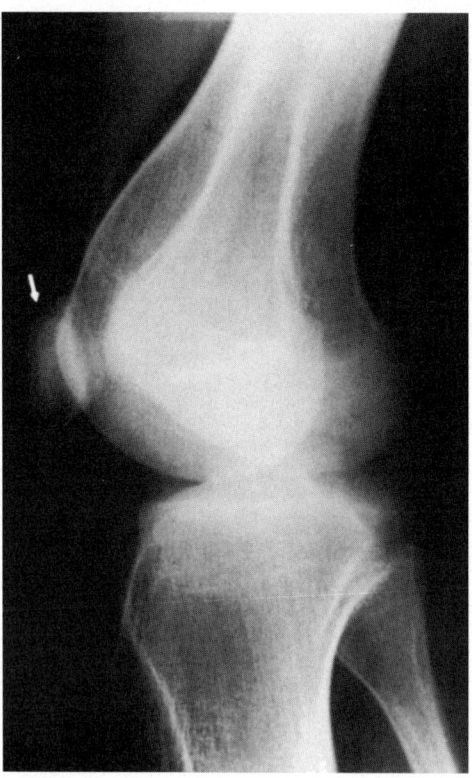

**Figure 77–33.** Osteo-onychodysostosis: knee abnormalities. Observe the hypoplastic patella *(arrow)*. (Courtesy of A. Goldman, MD, New York, N.Y.)

that in hyperparathyroidism or massive Gorham's osteolysis in some cases. Another rare syndrome, acrogeria, resembles progeria and leads to premature aging of the skin. Additional features of acrogeria include a female preponderance, short stature, micrognathia, superficial venous distention, acro-osteolysis of the terminal phalanges, delayed closure of cranial sutures, wormian bones, antegonial notching of the mandible, and linear metaphyseal radiolucent regions.

### Arthrogryposis Multiplex Congenita

The term arthrogryposis is derived from two Greek words meaning curved joints. At birth, affected infants display multiple and frequently symmetrical joint contractures involving many of the peripheral joints, with limitation of both active and passive motion. A "diamond" deformity of the lower extremities is typical, with the hips abducted, flexed, and rotated externally and the knees flexed. Sensation is intact.

Radiographic features include decreased muscle mass and contractures. Equinovarus deformity of the foot, talocalcaneal coalition, clubhand in ulnar deviation, carpal fusion, and dislocation of the hips are frequent (Fig. 77–35).

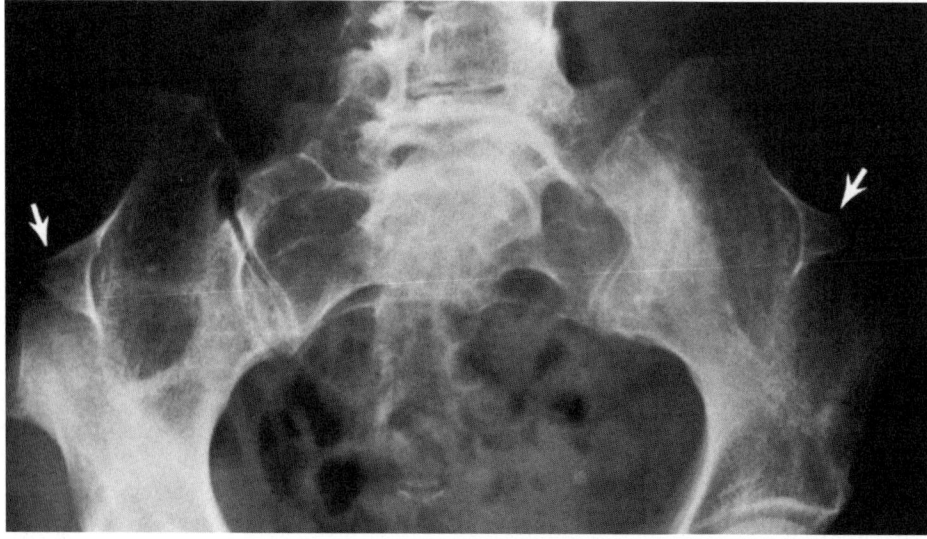

**Figure 77–34.** Osteo-onychodysostosis: pelvic abnormalities. Bilateral posterior iliac outgrowths, or horns, can be identified *(arrows)*.

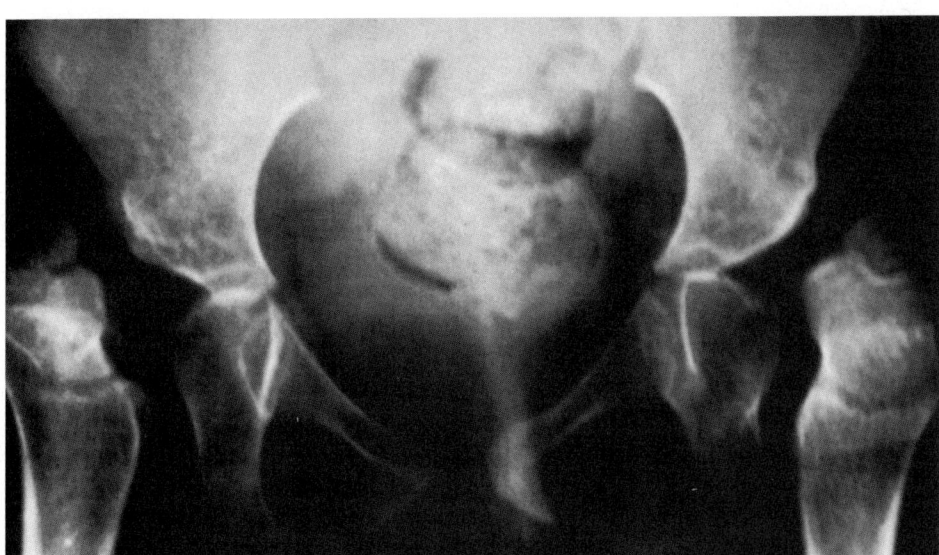

**Figure 77–35.** Arthrogryposis multiplex congenita. Note the bilateral dislocations of the hip.

Additional abnormalities include patellar elongation and malposition, hemophilia-like changes of the distal portion of the femur and proximal end of the tibia, and fibular hypoplasia. Fractures are not unusual, and scoliosis can be detected in many persons.

## Werner's Syndrome

Werner's syndrome is similar to, but distinct from, progeria. Its principal clinical manifestations include symmetrical retardation of growth, with absence of the adolescent growth spurt; graying and loss of hair; voice alterations; cataracts; skin ulcerations; and, in some cases, mild diabetes mellitus. Additional changes are vascular and soft tissue calcification, generalized osteoporosis, atrophy of muscle and fat, and hypogonadism. Neoplasms, especially sarcomas and meningiomas, may complicate the clinical picture in as many as 10% of patients. The exact nature of the disorder remains elusive.

Radiographic evaluation reveals patchy or generalized osteoporosis. Extensive arterial calcification may be evident, particularly in the vessels of the extremities, coronary arteries, and aorta. Soft tissue calcification is observed in approximately one third of cases and predominates about bony protuberances, including the distal ends of the tibia and fibula, and areas about the knees, feet, and hands. Destructive osseous lesions related to osteomyelitis and septic arthritis and neurotrophic changes may be seen.

## Congenital Pseudarthrosis

Congenital pseudarthrosis is an unusual condition associated with fracture followed by nonunion. It is typically identified in the tibia, although pseudarthroses can also occur in the fibula, femur, clavicle, humerus, ulna, radius, rib, and, rarely, other bones. In some patients, pseudarthroses are present at birth (true congenital pseudarthrosis), whereas in other patients, they develop in the first few years of life (infantile pseudarthrosis). Rarely, pseudarthroses first develop in late childhood or adolescence. Some affected persons may have stigmata of neurofibromatosis or fibrous dysplasia, although others do not.

The more common infantile variety usually develops in the first or second year of life. Unilateral changes predominate. Associated abnormalities of the ipsilateral foot include curly and overlapping toes. Initially, anterior bowing of the lower half of the tibia is recognized, with or without abnormality of the adjacent fibula. At the apex of the tibial curve, sclerosis, narrowing of the medullary canal, and cystic abnormality may indicate impending fracture and pseudarthrosis. Once the fracture appears, the margins of the adjacent bone ends taper further (Fig. 77–36). The prognosis for ultimate union at the fracture site varies with the age of the patient (fractures developing before 2 years of age carry a poor prognosis), the pattern of radiographic abnormality (a cystic appearance may be associated with a better prognosis), and the type of therapy instituted.

Congenital pseudarthrosis of the bones of the forearm is rare. The radius and ulna are affected with nearly equal frequency. Pseudarthrosis of the radius or ulna is generally associated with neurofibromatosis. Congenital pseudarthrosis of the clavicle occurs almost exclusively on the right side of the body, although it may be bilateral in 10% of cases. Its occurrence on the left side may be associated with dextrocardia, which suggests that the position of adjacent vascular structures, such as the subclavian artery, may be important in the pathogenesis of this osseous defect. The lesion is usually discovered within the first few months of life because of the presence of a painless lump over the middle third of the clavicle. On radiographs, the medial end of the clavicle is seen to be superior to the lateral end, osseous discontinuity is evident, and callus formation is absent (Fig. 77–37). The absence of pain and visible callus usually allows differentiation from post-traumatic pseudarthrosis.

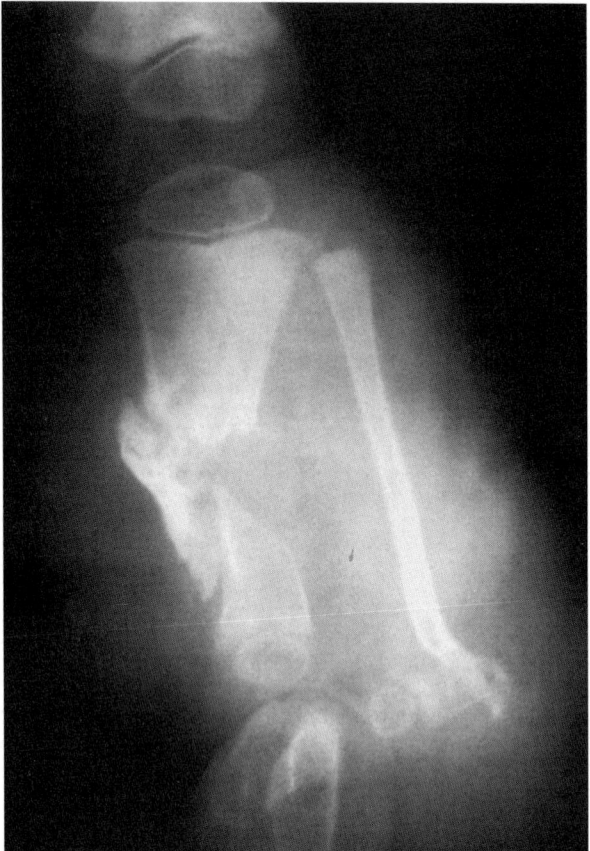

**Figure 77–36.** Congenital pseudarthrosis: tibia and fibula. Fractures with pseudarthroses are observed in the middle third of the tibia and lower third of the fibula. Some of the ends of the fractured bones are tapered. Considerable soft tissue swelling and hypertrophy are evident, although this child had no clinical evidence of neurofibromatosis.

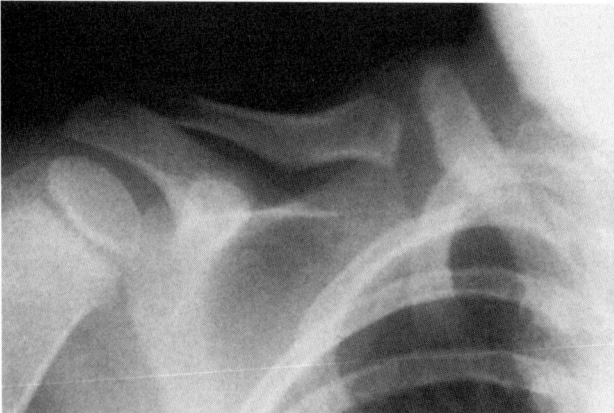

**Figure 77–37.** Congenital pseudarthrosis: clavicle. This girl had a prominent symptomatic mass over the right clavicle. Note the superior position of the medial end of the clavicle and the absence of visible callus.

(From Schnall SB, King JD, Marrero G: Congenital pseudarthrosis of the clavicle: a review of the literature and surgical results of six cases. J Pediatr Orthop 8:316, 1988.)

## FURTHER READING

Alexander C: The aetiology of primary protrusio acetabuli. Br J Radiol 38:567, 1965.

Barnes JC, Smith WL: The VATER association. Radiology 126:445, 1978.

Beckly DE, Anderson PW, Pedegana LR: The radiology of the subtalar joint with special reference to talo-calcaneal coalition. Clin Radiol 26:333, 1975.

Boyd HB: Pathology and natural history of congenital pseudarthrosis of the tibia. Clin Orthop 166:5, 1982.

Brower AC, Culver JE Jr, Keats TE: Histologic nature of the cortical irregularity of the medial posterior distal femoral metaphysis in children. Radiology 99:389, 1971.

Brown GA, Osebold WR, Ponseti IV: Congenital pseudarthrosis of long bones: A clinical, radiographic, histologic, and ultrastructural study. Clin Orthop 128:228, 1977.

Caffey JP: Pediatric X-ray Diagnosis, 7th ed. Chicago, Year Book Medical Publishers, 1978.

Calhoun JD, Pierret G: Infantile coxa vara. AJR Am J Roentgenol 115:561, 1972.

Carlson DH, O'Connor J: Congenital dislocation of the knee. AJR Am J Roentgenol 127:465, 1976.

Conway JJ, Cowell HR: Tarsal coalition: Clinical significance and roentgenographic demonstration. Radiology 92:799, 1969.

Conway WF, Destouet JM, Gilula LA, et al: The carpal boss: An overview of radiographic evaluation. Radiology 156:29, 1985.

Cope JR: Carpal coalition. Clin Radiol 25:261, 1974.

Deutsch AL, Resnick D, Campbell G: Computed tomography and bone scintigraphy in the evaluation of tarsal coalition. Radiology 144:137, 1982.

Felman AH, Kirkpatrick JA Jr: Madelung's deformity: Observations in 17 patients. Radiology 93:1037, 1969.

Freiberger RH, Hersh A, Harrison MO: Roentgen examination of the deformed foot. Semin Roentgenol 5:341, 1970.

Goldman AB, Schneider R, Wilson PD Jr: Proximal focal femoral deficiency. J Can Assoc Radiol 29:101, 1978.

Greenspan A, Norman A: The pelvic digit. Bull Hosp Jt Dis 44:72, 1984.

Greenspan A, Norman A: The "pelvic digit": An unusual developmental anomaly. Skeletal Radiol 9:118, 1982.

Hall JG, Levin J, Kuhn JP, et al: Thrombocytopenia with absent radius (TAR). Medicine 48:411, 1969.

Hensinger RN, Lang JE, MacEwen GD: Klippel-Feil syndrome: A constellation of associated anomalies. J Bone Joint Surg Am 56:1246, 1974.

Hotston S, Carty H: Lumbosacral agenesis: A report of three new cases and review of the literature. Br J Radiol 55:629, 1982.

Jacobsen ST, Crawford AH: Congenital vertical talus. J Pediatr Orthop 3:306, 1983.

Jacobson HG, Rifkin H, Zucker-Franklin D: Werner's syndrome: A clinical-roentgen entity. Radiology. 74:373, 1960.

Kelleher J, O'Connell DJ, MacMahon H: Intrathoracic rib: Radiographic features of two cases. Br J Radiol 52:181, 1979.

Lawson JP: Symptomatic radiographic variants in extremities. Radiology 157:625, 1985.

Lawson JP, Ogden JA, Sella E, et al: The painful accessory navicular. Skeletal Radiol 12:250, 1984.

Manashil G, Laufer S: Congenital pseudarthrosis of the clavicle: Report of three cases. AJR Am J Roentgenol 132:678, 1979.

Margolin FR, Steinbach HL: Progeria: Hutchinson-Gilford syndrome. AJR Am J Roentgenol 103:173, 1968.

McKusick VA: Heritable Disorders of Connective Tissue. St Louis, CV Mosby, 1972.

McNally EG: Posteromedial subtalar coalition: Imaging appearances in three cases. Skeletal Radiol 28:691, 1999.

Miller JH, Bernstein SM: The roentgenographic appearance of the "corrected clubfoot." Foot Ankle 6:177, 1986.

Mital MA: Limb deficiencies: Classification and treatment. Orthop Clin North Am 7:457, 1976.

Newman JS, Newberg AH: Congenital tarsal coalition: Multimodality evaluation with emphasis on CT and MR imaging. Radiographics 20:321, 2000.

Nguyen VD, Tyrrel R: Klippel-Feil syndrome: Patterns of bony fusion and wasp-waist sign. Skeletal Radiol 22:519, 1993.

O'Connor JF, Cranley WR, McCarten KM, et al: Radiographic manifestations of congenital anomalies of the spine. Radiol Clin North Am 29:407, 1991.

Ogden JA, Conlogue GJ, Phillips SB, et al: Sprengel's deformity: Radiology of the pathologic deformation. Skeletal Radiol 4:204, 1979.

Ogden JA, McCarthy SM, Jokl P: The painful bipartite patella. J Pediatr Orthop 2:263, 1982.

Ozonoff MB: Pediatric Orthopedic Radiology. Philadelphia, WB Saunders, 1979.

Ozonoff MB, Clemett AR: Progressive osteolysis in progeria. AJR Am J Roentgenol 100:75, 1967.

Pate D, Kursunoglu S, Resnick D, et al: Scapular foramina. Skeletal Radiol 14:270, 1985.

Pavlov H, Goldman AB, Freiberger RH: Infantile coxa vara. Radiology 135:631, 1980.

Percy EC, Mann DL: Tarsal coalition: A review of the literature and presentation of 13 cases. Foot Ankle 9:40, 1988.

Poznanski AK: The Hand in Radiologic Diagnosis. Philadelphia, WB Saunders, 1974.

Poznanski AK, LaRowe PC: Radiographic manifestations of the arthrogryposis syndrome. Radiology 95:353, 1970.

Preger L, Miller EH, Winfield JS, et al: Hereditary onycho-osteo-arthrodysplasia. AJR Am J Roentgenol 100:546, 1967.

Renshaw TS: Sacral agenesis: A classification and review of twenty-three cases. J Bone Joint Surg Am 60:373, 1978.

Resnick D, Cone RO III: The nature of humeral pseudocysts. Radiology 150:27, 1984.

Resnick D, Greenway G: Distal femoral cortical defects, irregularities, and excavations: A critical review of the literature with the addition of histologic and paleopathologic data. Radiology 143:345, 1982.

Resnick D, Walter RD, Crudale AS: Bilateral dysplasia of the scapular neck. AJR Am J Roentgenol 139:387, 1982.

Resnik CS, Grizzard JD, Simmons BP, et al: Incomplete carpal coalition. AJR Am J Roentgenol 147:301, 1986.

Ritchie GW, Keim HA: A radiographic analysis of major foot deformities. Can Med Assoc J 91:840, 1964.

Rubin P: Dynamic Classification of Bone Dysplasias. Chicago, Year Book Medical Publishers, 1964.

Spranger JW, Langer LO Jr, Wiedemann HR: Bone Dysplasias: An Atlas of Constitutional Disorders of Skeletal Development. Philadelphia, WB Saunders, 1974.

Wechsler RJ, Schweitzer ME, Deely DM, et al: Tarsal coalition: Depiction and characterization with CT and MR imaging. Radiology 193:447, 1994.

Williams HJ, Hoyer JR: Radiographic diagnosis of osteo-onychodysostosis in infancy. Radiology 109:151, 1973.

Wirth MA, Lyons FR, Rockwood CA Jr: Hypoplasia of the glenoid: A review of sixteen patients. J Bone Joint Surg Am 75:1175, 1993.

# Diseases of Soft Tissue and Muscle

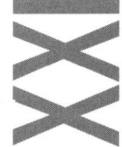

# CHAPTER 78

## Soft Tissue Disorders

## *SUMMARY OF KEY FEATURES*

In many instances, the findings in soft tissue disorders lack specificity, although careful analysis sometimes allows a precise diagnosis. Especially important is the differentiation of myositis ossificans traumatica from various malignant tumors and the recognition that widespread skeletal abnormalities may accompany certain cutaneous syndromes. Other diagnostic techniques, including ultrasonography, computed tomography, magnetic resonance imaging, angiography, and scintigraphy, may be required to supplement the radiographic evaluation and provide more accurate information about the extent of the soft tissue process and its relationship to adjacent structures.

## INTRODUCTION

Soft tissue is broadly defined as being composed of fibrous tissue, fat, and voluntary muscle, as well as the vessels and nerves that supply these structures. Routine radiographic manifestations of soft tissue disorders may include mass formation, alteration in radiodensity, calcification and ossification, and resorption and contracture. In some instances, the constellation of findings is adequate for an accurate diagnosis; more often, supplementary methods such as computed tomography (CT) and magnetic resonance (MR) imaging are needed to further delineate the nature and extent of the process.

## SOFT TISSUE CALCIFICATION AND OSSIFICATION

Although it is helpful to distinguish between calcific and ossific radiodense lesions, this is not always possible, particularly if the collections are small. Documentation of ossification depends on recognition of a trabecular pattern within the dense areas. Calcification appears as irregular punctate, circular, linear, or plaquelike radiodense areas that do not possess a trabecular or cortical structure. It is difficult to differentiate between calcification and ossification with radiographic methods, however, because calcification of ectopic bone does not initially reveal trabeculation, and ossifying neoplasms may produce poorly organized bone that does not possess a trabecular pattern.

## Calcification

Conditions that lead to deposition of calcium within soft tissues can be classified into three types:

1. *Metastatic calcification.* This type of calcification is related to a disturbance in calcium or phosphorus metabolism.
2. *Calcinosis.* Calcinosis results from the deposition of calcium in skin and subcutaneous tissue in the presence of normal calcium metabolism.
3. *Dystrophic calcification.* Dystrophic calcification is related to calcium deposits in damaged or devitalized tissue in the absence of a generalized metabolic derangement.

In most cases of soft tissue calcification, the radiographic appearance does not allow a specific diagnosis. The terms calcinosis universalis and calcinosis circumscripta should be regarded as descriptive designations for widespread and localized calcific deposits, respectively. Many of the disorders leading to calcific deposits in soft tissue are described in other chapters of this book. Two additional entities are noted here.

**Idiopathic Calcinosis Universalis.** This rare disorder of unknown cause affects infants and children. The deposits (calcium phosphate and calcium carbonate) initially appear in the subcutaneous fat of the extremities but subsequently involve other connective tissues, such as muscles, ligaments, and tendons. Calcareous nodules coalesce, become large masses that may violate the skin, and produce sinus tracts. Internal organs are not affected. Serum calcium and phosphorus levels are normal.

Radiographs reveal discrete conglomerations of calcium arranged in longitudinal bands (Fig. 78–1). In infants, the deposits are usually limited to subcutaneous fat, whereas in children, both fat and connective tissue are affected. The major differential diagnosis is dermatomyositis. Other processes such as calcified subcutaneous fat necrosis, extravasation of injected calcium gluconate solutions, and hyperparathyroidism must also be considered.

**Idiopathic Tumoral Calcinosis.** The term tumoral calcinosis is used to describe the appearance of prominent periarticular calcified masses, especially about large joints such as the hip, shoulder, and elbow. Tumoral calcinosis usually manifests in the second and third decades of life. Men are more commonly affected than women, and blacks are especially susceptible. A family history is apparent in 30% to 40% of cases, and an autosomal dominant or recessive pattern of inheritance has been suggested. On clinical evaluation, firm, painless tumor-like swellings are evident, especially about the hips and shoulders, as well as the elbows, knees, and ankles; these swellings may interfere with joint motion. Solitary or, less commonly, multiple foci may be evident. The exact nature of idiopathic

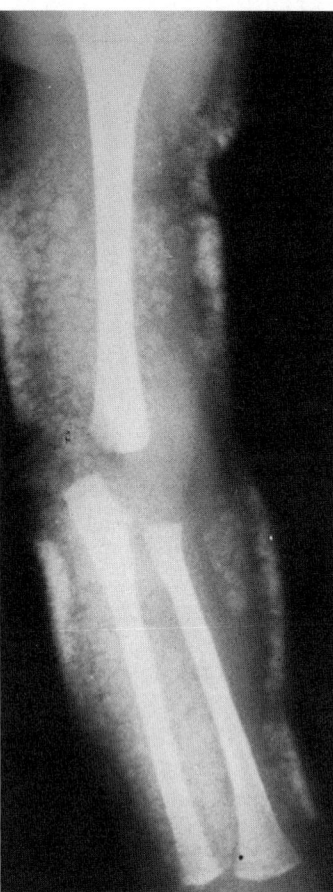

**Figure 78–1.** Calcinosis universalis (idiopathic). Longitudinal bands of calcification in the subcutaneous fat can be identified in this 3-month-old male infant.

tumoral calcinosis is a mystery. The elevated serum phosphorus levels noted in some patients may support the existence of an inborn error of metabolism.

Radiographs reveal circular or oval, well-demarcated masses of calcium about articulations (Fig. 78–2). A lobulated inhomogeneous appearance is characteristic, and subjacent bone erosion may be evident. Radiolucent linear bands separate the calcific foci; the resulting appearance has been likened to chicken wire. The individual lesions vary from 1 to 20 cm in diameter and may reveal fluid levels. This finding can also be demonstrated with CT and MR imaging.

The diagnosis of idiopathic tumoral calcinosis is one of exclusion. Other processes, such as collagen vascular disorders, hyperparathyroidism, hypervitaminosis D, milk-alkali syndrome, and chronic renal disease, must be eliminated by clinical, laboratory, and radiographic examinations. The periarticular localization of the calcifications in idiopathic tumoral calcinosis differs from the intra-articular radiodense deposits of idiopathic synovial (osteo)chondromatosis and calcium pyrophosphate dihydrate crystal deposition disease, although these two disorders occasionally affect extra-articular structures as well.

## Ossification

Disorders leading to soft tissue ossification are fewer in number than those producing soft tissue calcification (Table 78–1). Ossification in soft tissue may occur as a result of intraosseous tumors that extend into the adjacent soft tissue, such as osteosarcoma. Foci of osteoid or new bone may appear in association with melorheostosis (Fig. 78–3), as well as proliferative myositis and ossifying fasciitis. Metastases to soft tissue, including muscle, may subsequently ossify. In most of the situations mentioned previously, as well as those noted later in this chapter, radiographs may outline a definite trabecular structure within the ossific collections, thereby allowing the differentiation of ossification from calcification.

**Ossification of Tendons and Ligaments.** Although calcific tendinitis is common and well recognized, ossification within tendinous structures is relatively rare. Post-traumatic calcification and ossification of tendons or ligaments may be encountered at certain sites, such as the medial collateral ligament of the knee; there, it is termed the Pellegrini-Stieda syndrome and appears as arcuate or curvilinear radiodense collections adjacent to the medial femoral condyle (Fig. 78–4). In some persons with this syndrome, the ossification extends to or involves primarily the adductor magnus tendon. Ossification of the Achilles tendon and patellar tendon has also been recognized. Calcification or ossification in the stylohyoid ligament is a frequent, incidental radiographic finding, although when such ossification is excessive or the styloid process itself is enlarged, or both, a specific syndrome (termed the Eagle syndrome) may occur. Radiographs reveal an elongated and ossified styloid process and ligament with either a smooth or an irregular outline; these findings must be differentiated from normal variations in the length of this process and in the degree of ossification in the ligament.

**Myositis Ossificans Traumatica.** Sixty percent to 75% of patients with localized soft tissue ossification (myositis ossificans circumscripta) have a clear history of trauma. Spontaneous cases may be termed myositis ossificans nontraumatica.

Myositis ossificans traumatica usually appears in adolescents or young adults. The sites of localization are areas susceptible to injury, such as the elbow, thigh, buttocks, and, less often, shoulder and calf. When a history of injury can be elicited, specific radiographic features can be correlated with the time elapsed since the trauma, although in some persons, the initiating injury may be so minor that it is unrecognized or soon forgotten. Shortly after injury, a soft tissue mass or swelling becomes apparent and may be associated with periosteal reaction in 7 to 10 days (Fig. 78–5). Flocculent dense lesions arise in the mass from 11 days to 6 weeks after the injury. The calcific dense areas gradually enlarge, and at 6 to 8 weeks, a lacy pattern of new bone is sharply circumscribed around the periphery of the mass. The soft tissue central core occasionally becomes encysted, and the enlarging central cavity combined with peripheral calcification and ossification resembles an eggshell. Maturity is reached in 5 to 6 months (Fig. 78–6), and the mass then shrinks.

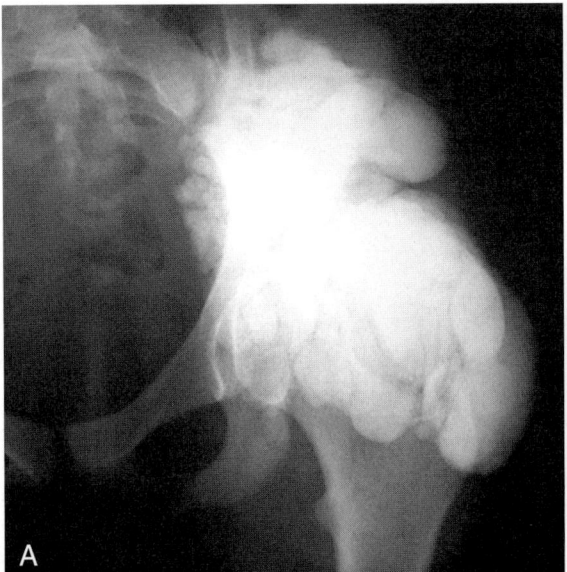
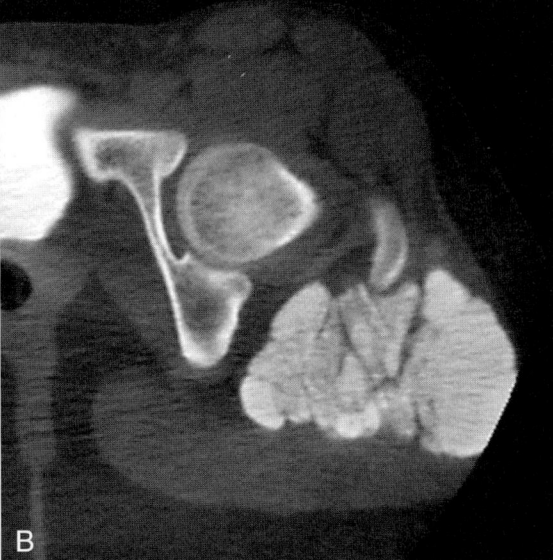
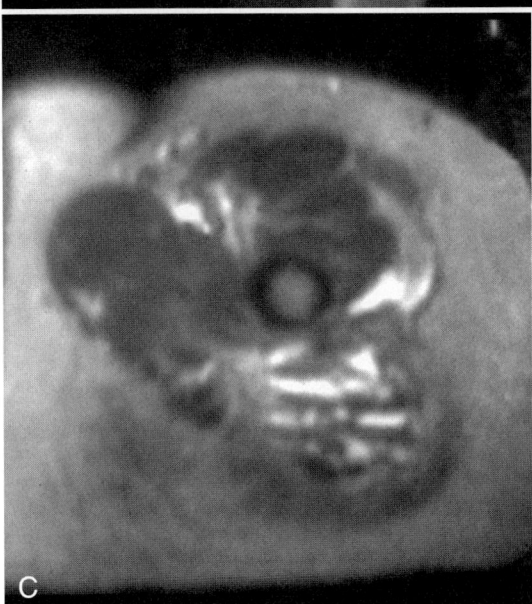

**Figure 78–2.** Tumoral calcinosis (idiopathic). *A*, Radiograph of the hip reveals dense nodular calcific deposits about the hip joint. *B*, CT scan shows the densely mineralized juxta-articular mass. *C*, Axial T2-weighted (TR/TE, 200/80) MR image shows multiple fluid levels.

---

**TABLE 78–1**

**Causes of Soft Tissue Ossification**

Neurologic diseases

Physical and thermal injuries

Venous insufficiency

Neoplasms (e.g., parosteal osteosarcoma, extraskeletal osteosarcoma)

Pseudomalignant osseous tumor of soft tissue

Fibrodysplasia (myositis) ossificans progressiva

Melorheostosis

Surgical scars

Postoperative period

---

Complete or partial resorption of the ossified mass is reportedly more frequent in young persons.

Recognition of a peripheral rim of calcification and ossification around a more lucent center is the most important radiographic manifestation of myositis ossificans traumatica (Figs. 78–7 and 78–8). A radiolucent band or zone between the lesion and the subjacent cortex is also an important finding that reflects a lack of intimacy between the ossified mass and neighboring bone, thus allowing the differentiation of myositis ossificans traumatica from parosteal osteosarcoma. Direct damage to the cambium layer of the periosteum from the traumatic insult can lead to an ossifying subperiosteal hematoma.

Identification of myositis ossificans traumatica is usually possible from the clinical and radiographic findings

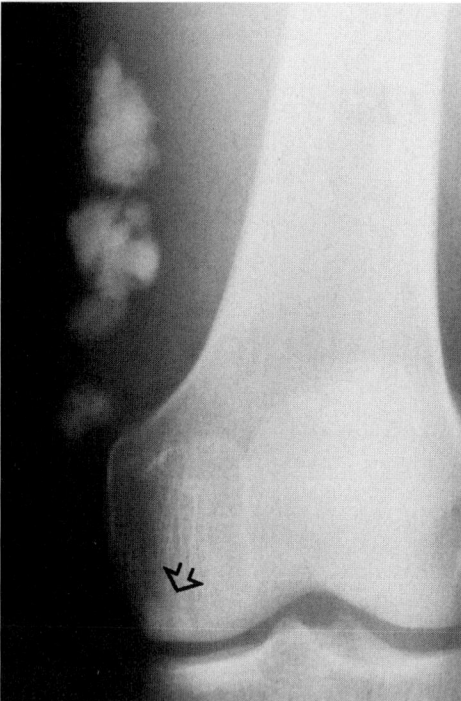

**Figure 78–3.** Melorheostosis. A beaded pattern of soft tissue ossification is characteristic of this disorder. Note the radiodense focus *(arrow)* in the distal end of the femur.

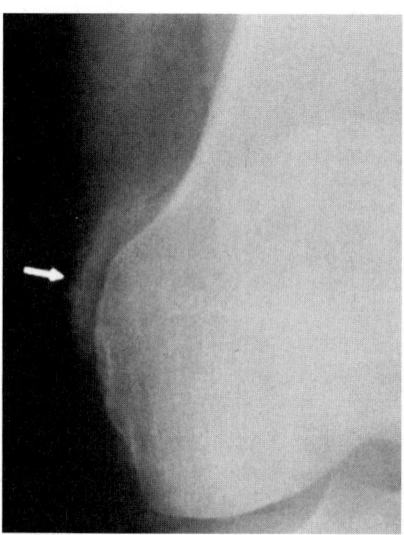

**Figure 78–4.** Pellegrini-Stieda syndrome. Post-traumatic ossification about the medial collateral ligament of the knee *(arrow)* is shown.

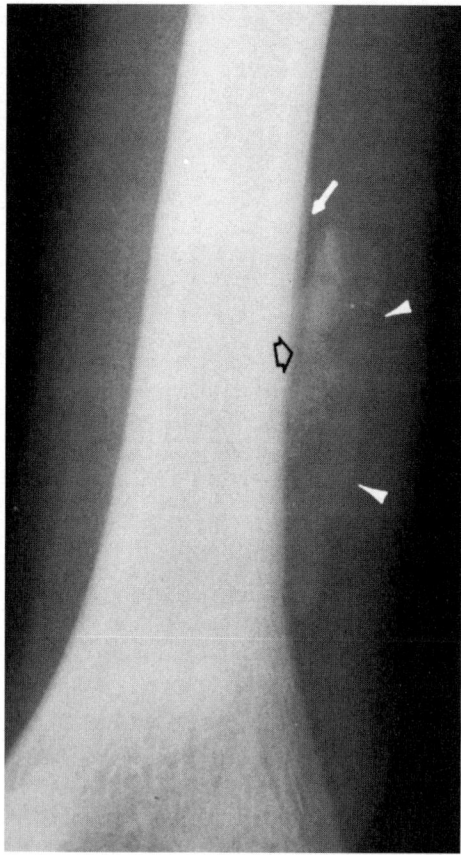

**Figure 78–5.** Myositis ossificans traumatica: radiographic abnormalities. Shortly after injury, a soft tissue swelling appears and may be associated with periostitis *(solid arrow)*. Ill-defined osseous dense areas *(arrowheads)* appear within 2 to 6 weeks after the traumatic insult. Note the lucent area *(open arrow)* between the ossifications and the underlying bone.

(Fig. 78–9). The MR imaging appearance of ossifying lesions varies according to the stage of development. Less diagnostic difficulty is encountered in chronic lesions (see Fig. 78–7), which tend to be well defined, possess a border of low signal intensity, and contain fat (with its characteristic signal intensity), although occasional chronic lesions reveal regions of high signal intensity on T2-weighted images. In the acute or subacute stages of myositis ossificans traumatica, inhomogeneity in signal intensity may be evident; high signal intensity on T2-weighted images may be seen (Fig. 78–10). When a gadolinium-containing contrast agent is administered intravenously, nonspecific diffuse enhancement is observed. When the process begins to calcify and ossify, a thin rim of low signal intensity surrounded by high signal intensity in fluid-sensitive sequences may be observed, a combination of findings that may allow an accurate diagnosis.

Myositis ossificans traumatica must be differentiated from several similar entities. Parosteal osteosarcoma arises in the metaphyses of tubular bones, especially along the posterior aspect of the distal end of the femur. Parosteal osteosarcoma is more heavily calcified in its central portion and base of attachment, the periphery is less dense and is poorly circumscribed, and the tumor enlarges over time. Periosteal osteosarcoma arises in the cortex of the diaphyses of tubular bones and leads to cortical thickening and spiculated osteoid matrix that is progressively denser from the periphery to the cortical base. Extraskeletal osteosarcoma is a rare neoplasm and does not show the zonal pattern seen in myositis ossificans. This tumor

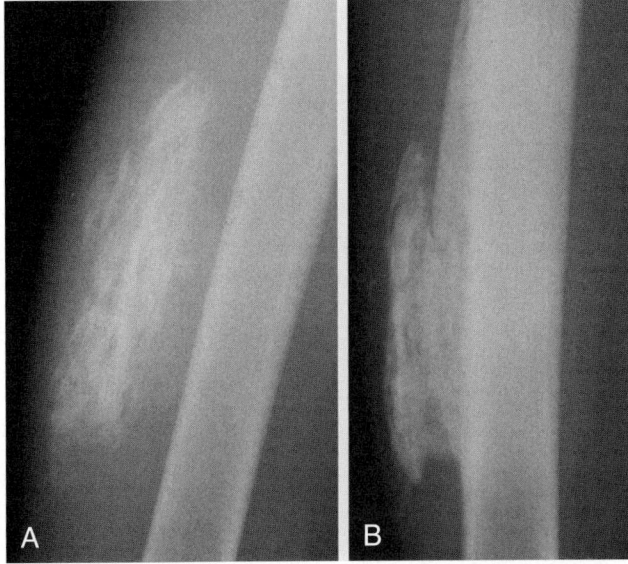

**Figure 78–6.** Myositis ossificans traumatica: maturing ossification. In this 11-year-old boy who fell from the steps of a swimming pool, lateral radiographs of the femur 1 month *(A)* and 5 months *(B)* after the injury show maturation of the ossifying process. Initially separated from the bone, the process subsequently merged with the anterior femoral surface. (Courtesy of G. Greenway, MD, Dallas, Tex.)

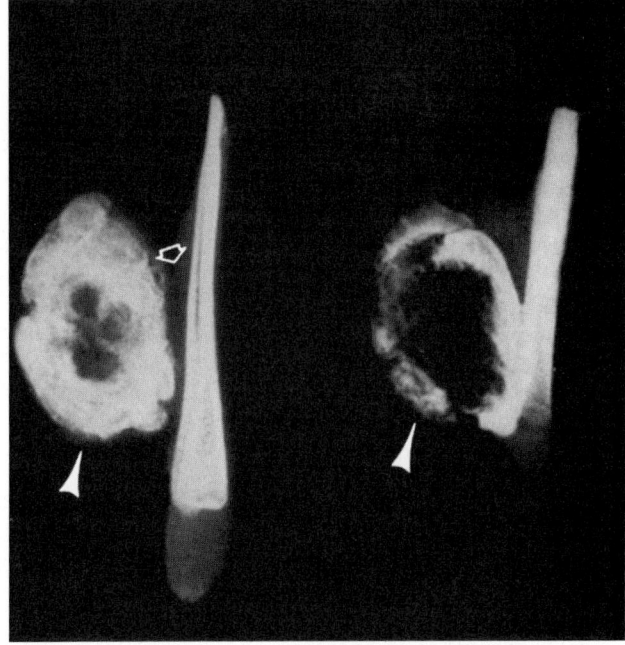

**Figure 78–8.** Myositis ossificans traumatica: radiographic-pathologic correlation. Serial sections through a focus of myositis ossificans delineate a well-encapsulated lesion possessing a peripheral zone of ossification and a lucent center *(arrowheads)*. Note the separation, or clear zone *(arrow)*, between the lesion and the underlying bone. (Courtesy of A. Norman, MD, Valhalla, N.Y.)

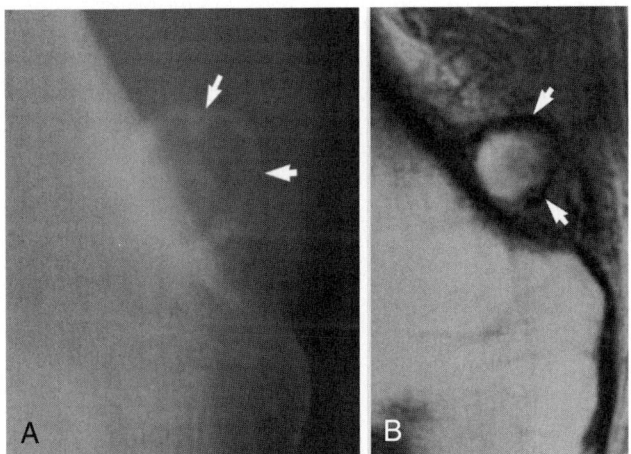

**Figure 78–7.** Myositis ossificans traumatica. *A,* Frontal radiograph shows a lesion on the medial cortex of the distal end of the femur. There is a peripheral rim of calcification and ossification *(arrows)*. Adjacent mature periosteal reaction is seen. *B,* Coronal T1-weighted (TR/TE, 600/20) spin echo MR image shows low signal intensity at the margin of the lesion *(arrows)* and higher signal intensity, identical to that of fat, in the center.

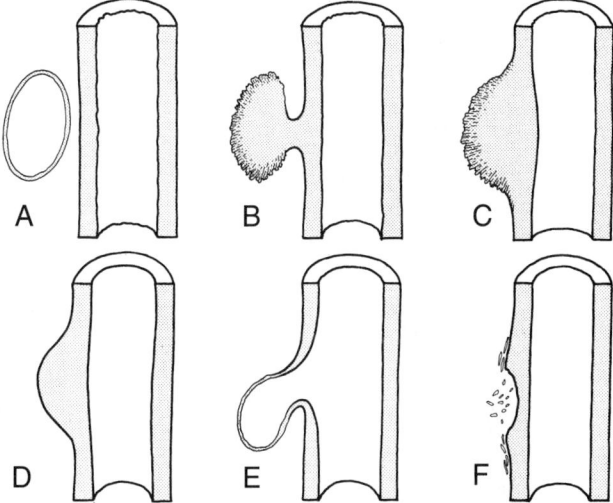

**Figure 78–9.** Myositis ossificans traumatica: differential diagnosis. *A,* Myositis ossificans traumatica. The shell-like configuration of the ossification, with a clear zone between it and the underlying bone, is typical of this condition. *B,* Parosteal osteosarcoma. These lesions appear as central ossifying foci with irregular outlines and may be connected to the underlying bone by a stalk. *C,* Periosteal osteosarcoma. These tumors arise in the cortex of the diaphysis of a tubular bone and produce cortical thickening and spiculated osteoid matrix. *D,* Osteoma. Characteristic of this lesion is a localized excrescence that produces bulging of the cortical contour. *E,* Osteochondroma. An exostosis protrudes from the cortical surface. Its medullary and cortical bone is continuous with that of the underlying osseous structure. *F,* Juxtacortical (periosteal) chondroma. These periosteal lesions produce localized excavation of the cortex, with periostitis. They may contain calcification.

grows slowly and affects older patients. An osteochondroma arises from and is connected to the subjacent bone; both the cortex and the spongiosa of the lesion and parent bone are continuous. An osteoma is an osseous excrescence extending from the outer surface of the cortex and is readily differentiated from myositis ossificans

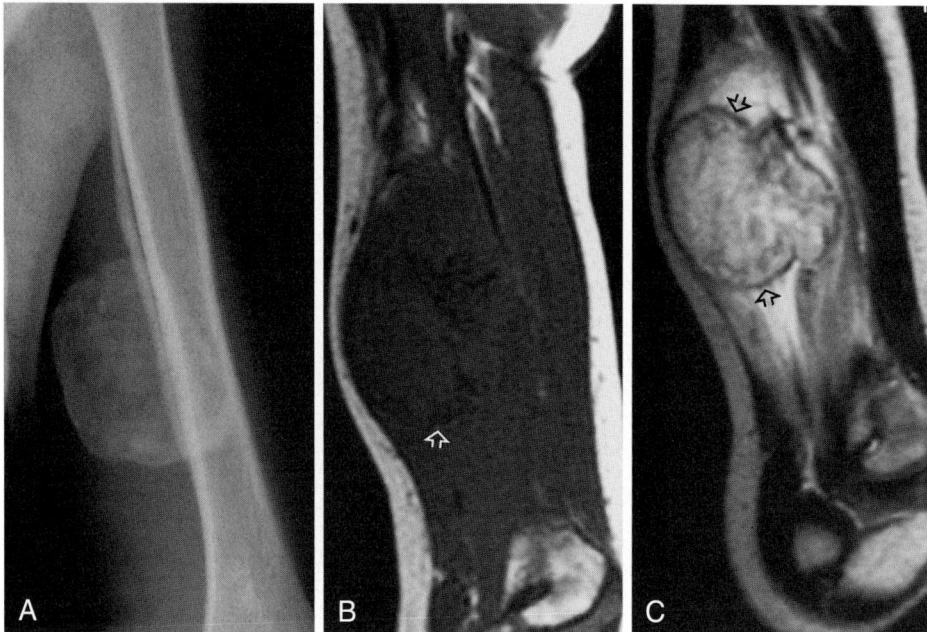

**Figure 78–10.** Myositis ossificans traumatica: radiographic and MR imaging abnormalities. This 4-year-old boy fell on his arm. *A,* Radiograph obtained 4 weeks later shows classic features of myositis ossificans. Note the well-defined ossific mass and mature periosteal new bone formation in the humeral diaphysis. *B,* Sagittal oblique T1-weighted (TR/TE, 600/14) spin echo MR image shows a poorly defined intramuscular mass with signal intensity similar to that of muscle. Some foci of very low signal intensity are seen *(arrow).* *C,* Sagittal oblique T2-weighted (TR/TE, 3000/95) fast spin echo MR image reveals high signal intensity in the mass and surrounding tissues. Note the peripheral rim of low signal intensity *(arrows),* indicative of ossification. This combination of findings is highly suggestive of the diagnosis. (Courtesy of D. Witte, MD, Memphis, Tenn.)

traumatica, whereas a juxtacortical (periosteal) chondroma produces soft tissue calcification, excavation of the cortex, and adjacent periosteal proliferation.

**Pseudomalignant Osseous Tumor of Soft Tissue.** This designation has been used by some as a synonym for myositis ossificans in cases in which there is no known history of antecedent trauma. As with myositis ossificans traumatica, these lesions are well circumscribed, and most tumors are located in the extremities or the gluteal regions. Soft tissue swelling, with or without pain, precedes the appearance of calcification and ossification by approximately 2 to 3 weeks. Radiographs reveal a well-circumscribed ossifying mass with a dense periphery and lucent center. Periostitis may be identified and, in some instances, precedes soft tissue ossification. MR imaging reveals findings typical of those of myositis ossificans traumatica, with extensive surrounding inflammatory changes occurring in some cases (Fig. 78–11). The course is typically benign, and in some cases, the lesions become smaller or disappear.

Pseudomalignant osseous tumor of soft tissue must be distinguished from osteosarcoma of soft tissue. The presence of the zone phenomenon, the peripheral location of the ossification, and the limitation in size are helpful in this regard. The designation of this process as one distinct from myositis ossificans traumatica is based solely on the absence of a history of injury; consequently, it may represent cases in which trauma is occult.

**Florid Reactive Periostitis and Bizarre Parosteal Osteochondromatous Proliferation.** Florid reactive periostitis is best considered a variant of myositis ossificans. It is most

common in the hands and, less commonly, the feet. Involvement of one of the proximal or middle phalanges predominates. A soft tissue mass containing calcification or ossification dominates the radiographic findings and may occur before the development of osseous abnormality. Radiographs typically reveal soft tissue prominence or mass formation, periostitis, or hyperostosis alone or in combination; rarely, cortical erosion or destruction is evident (Fig. 78–12). Over time, the periosteal new bone merges with the underlying bone (Fig. 78–13). Local excision is generally adequate, and the likelihood of lesion recurrence is small.

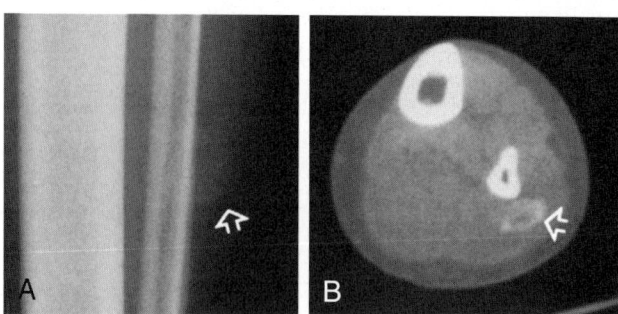

**Figure 78–11.** Pseudomalignant osseous tumor of soft tissue. This 40-year-old woman noted a firm, tender, movable mass in the calf of 3 weeks' duration. She had no history of injury. *A,* Routine radiograph shows a partially ossified soft tissue mass *(arrow)* adjacent to the fibula. The bone appears normal. *B,* Transaxial CT scan demonstrates a peripheral zone of ossification *(arrow).* (Courtesy of G. Greenway, MD, Dallas, Tex.)

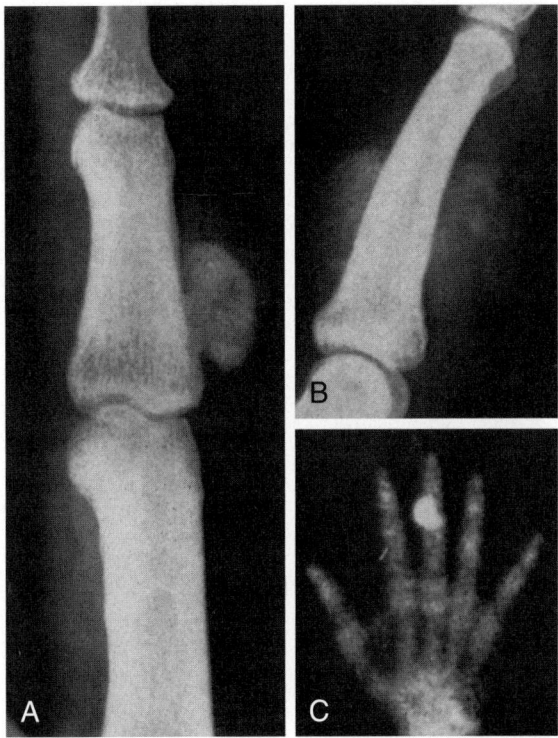

**Figure 78–12.** Florid reactive periostitis. Over a 4-month-period, an enlarging, nontender, slightly hyperemic, firm, fixed mass developed in the dorsolateral aspect of the middle phalanx of the third finger of this 28-year-old man. He had no history of local trauma. *A* and *B*, Posteroanterior *(A)* and oblique *(B)* radiographs reveal a soft tissue mass containing considerable ossification. It appears to be attached to the phalanx by a stalk. *C*, On a bone scan, intense uptake of bone-seeking radionuclide is seen.

(From Porter AR, Tristan TA, Rudy FR, et al: Florid reactive periostitis of the phalanges. AJR Am J Roentgenol 144:617, 1985.)

Common to all descriptions of this lesion is an initial, typically traumatic stimulus, with subsequent hemorrhagic subperiosteal proliferation. If the reaction remains contained within the periosteum, a localized fusiform periostitis develops that, with maturity, becomes incorporated into the cortex, typical of florid reactive periostitis. If the periosteum is breached, the reactive process can extend into the loose areolar tissue around the fingers and produce a lobular lesion attached to the intact cortex. A more limited blood supply to the area of the disruption may lead to incomplete endochondral ossification. Cartilage foci remain, and the lesion is termed bizarre parosteal osteochondromatous proliferation (Fig. 78–14).

**Fibrodysplasia (Myositis) Ossificans Progressiva.** Fibrodysplasia ossificans progressiva is a rare disorder of mesodermal tissue in which inflammatory foci initially appear and proliferate in fibrous tissue. It is discussed in Chapter 74.

## SOFT TISSUE BANDS AND CONTRACTURES

Amniotic (or Streeter's) constriction bands are soft tissue grooves or depressions that can affect any portion of a limb but most frequently involve the fingers. They are the most common cause of a terminal malformation of the limb. The reported frequency of these bands varies widely, from 1 in 5000 to 1 in 45,000 births. Common associated anomalies are clubfoot and cleft lip and palate. Other associated anomalies are craniosynostosis, otic deformations, and dislocated hips. A compression neuropathy of the peroneal nerve caused by a constriction band below the knee is a recognized factor in the genesis of the clubfoot deformity.

On clinical examination, scarred rings are found to encircle a digit or limb. Multiple and symmetrically distributed lesions are typical. Upper extremity abnormalities are more frequent than those in the lower extremities. In the hand, the central digits are affected most often, and the thumb is commonly spared. Radiographs delineate soft tissue constrictions that extend for a variable depth and may contact the subjacent bone. Visualization of the soft tissue deficit allows the differentiation of this condition from congenital defects. The underlying bones may be poorly developed or absent, and distal to the lesions, calcification, lymphedema, or fatty accumulation may be encountered. Syndactyly or amputation may be evident as well (Fig. 78–15).

Soft tissue contractures can accompany many congenital disorders, including arthrogryposis multiplex congenita, Léri's pleonosteosis, and contractural arachnodactyly; acquired conditions such as Volkmann's ischemic contracture, thermal burns, and neurologic injury; and various rheumatologic diseases. The best-known example is Dupuytren's contracture of the palmar fascia, typically seen in middle-aged and elderly adults, more commonly men. Dupuytren's contracture involves the fingers in one or both hands, especially the third through fifth digits. This anatomic distribution may be influenced by the presence of an associated disease, such as diabetes mellitus, in which the third, fourth, and first digits are principally affected. In this disease, well-oriented collagenous matrix increases in amount and is transformed into nodules, cords, and laminated bands. Gross contracture results from an active cellular process in which the digits are drawn closer together as the original tissue is replaced.

MR imaging has been used to define palmar involvement in Dupuytren's contracture. The signal intensity of the subcutaneous nodules and cords shows some variation that appears to be dependent on their cellularity. The cords typically show low signal intensity, similar to that of tendon, on both T1- and T2-weighted spin echo MR images. The nodules usually reveal intermediate signal intensity, similar to that of muscle, on these spin echo MR images, consistent with more cellular tissue (Fig. 78–16). Because highly cellular lesions tend to have higher rates of recurrence after surgery than do hypocellular lesions, MR imaging may have some value in determining the prognosis of this condition.

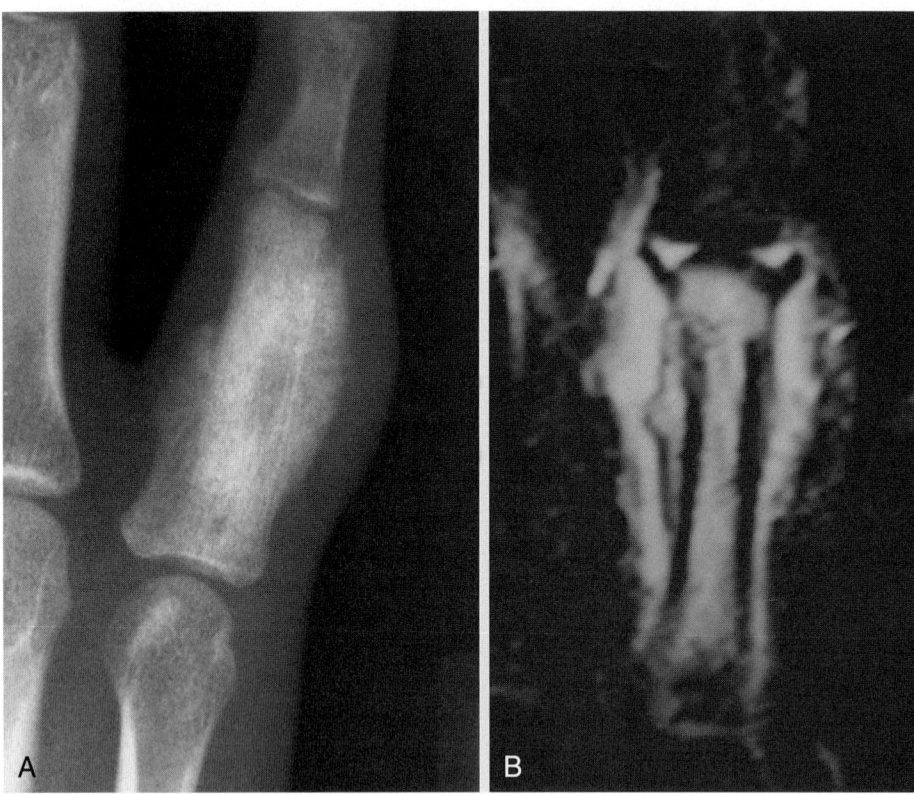

**Figure 78–13.** Florid reactive periostitis. *A,* Periosteal new bone is merging with the adjacent phalanx. *B,* In a different patient, a coronal short tau inversion recovery (TR/TE, 2000/25; inversion time, 80 msec) MR image shows marrow edema and periostitis involving the proximal phalanx of the third finger and surrounding soft tissue edema. (*A,* Courtesy of J. Jacobson, MD, Ann Arbor, Mich.)

## SOFT TISSUE EDEMA

Traumatic or inflammatory processes can lead to localized soft tissue edema. In addition, venous or lymphatic obstruction from many diverse causes can produce edema that is recognized radiographically as enlargement of the soft tissue contour, obliteration of the fascial planes, and a fine or coarsened reticular pattern (Fig. 78–17). Soft tissue calcification or ossification may accompany the process. Lymphedema itself can result from various processes, including primary or congenital disorders, trauma, infection, irradiation, tumor, and surgery. The occurrence of lymphangiosarcomas in areas of long-term lymphedema, termed the Stewart-Treves syndrome, is well documented.

Common causes of diffuse swelling of an extremity include lymphedema, venous obstruction (phlebedema), and lipedema. CT and MR imaging may be effective in differentiating among these conditions. In lymphedema, CT reveals fluid collections in the interstitial spaces of the soft tissue, which, with chronicity, are associated with fibrosis and a honeycomb pattern; in venous obstruction, CT shows an increase in the cross-sectional area of the muscle compartment, with a normal homogeneous layer of subcutaneous fat; and in lipedema, typically seen in overweight women older than 20 years, CT demonstrates fat accumulation, leading to an increase in size but a homogeneous appearance of subcutaneous fat. With regard to MR imaging, lipedema is associated with a homogeneously enlarged subcutaneous layer of fat (Fig. 78–18); phlebedema is accompanied by increased amounts of fluid within muscle and subcutaneous fat, with a moderate increase in signal intensity in muscle and a slight increase in signal intensity in subcutaneous tissue after gadolinium administration; and lymphedema (see Fig. 78–18) is associated with a honeycomb pattern above the fascia between muscle and subcutaneous tissue, with a marked increase in signal intensity on T2-weighted images and a slight increase in signal intensity in subcutaneous tissue after gadolinium administration.

## SOFT TISSUE EMPHYSEMA

Air can be introduced iatrogenically into the soft tissues or joints during puncture for diagnostic or therapeutic purposes. Air can also penetrate the soft tissues in cases of communicating wounds or sinus tracts. Gas formation by bacteria such as *Clostridium* may lead to radiolucent streaks or bubbles in subcutaneous or muscular tissue, a finding not infrequent in diabetic patients. Additional causes of gas or air in soft tissues include irrigation with hydrogen peroxide and accidental injection of compressed air.

## SOFT TISSUE FOREIGN BODIES

A variety of foreign bodies may become embedded or localize in the body's soft tissues. Metallic fragments resulting from various missiles are easily detected on routine radiographs. Identification of particles or fragments of glass, wood, or thorns, substances commonly associated with accidental injury, is more difficult and deserves special emphasis.

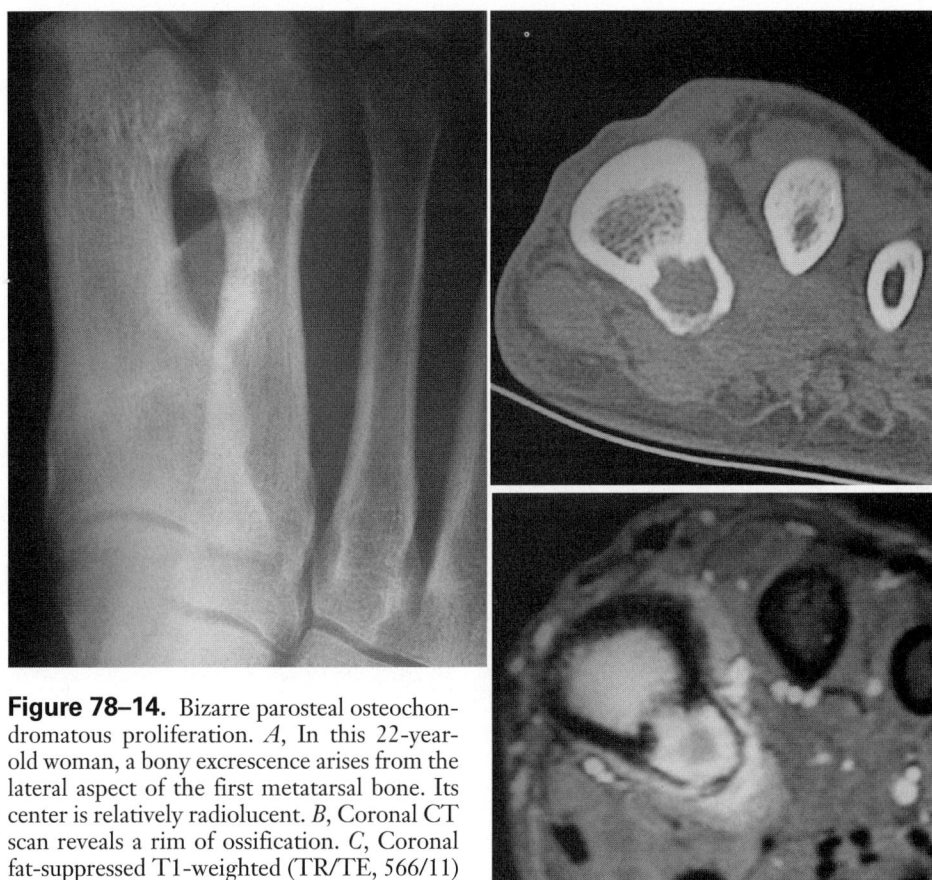

**Figure 78–14.** Bizarre parosteal osteochondromatous proliferation. *A,* In this 22-year-old woman, a bony excrescence arises from the lateral aspect of the first metatarsal bone. Its center is relatively radiolucent. *B,* Coronal CT scan reveals a rim of ossification. *C,* Coronal fat-suppressed T1-weighted (TR/TE, 566/11) spin echo MR image obtained after intravenous gadolinium administration shows the lesion. A rim of low signal intensity is seen; there is peripheral enhancement of signal intensity, as well as adjacent soft tissue enhancement.

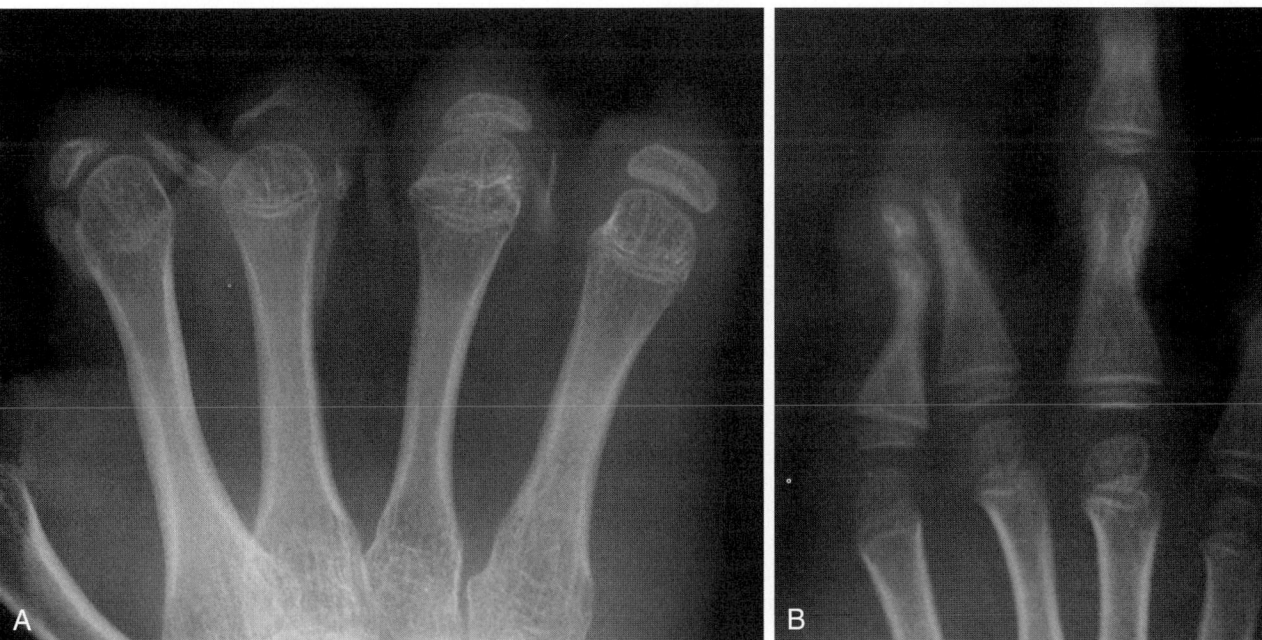

**Figure 78–15.** Amniotic (Streeter's) constriction bands. *A,* Autoamputation of the fingers is presumably the result of amniotic bands, although the presence of small ossific foci about the metacarpal heads may indicate malformed phalanges and congenital defects of the hand. *B,* In this patient, soft tissue and osseous abnormalities involve the second, third, and fourth fingers, with autoamputation of portions of two fingers. (Courtesy of A. D'Abreu, MD, Porto Alegre, Brazil.)

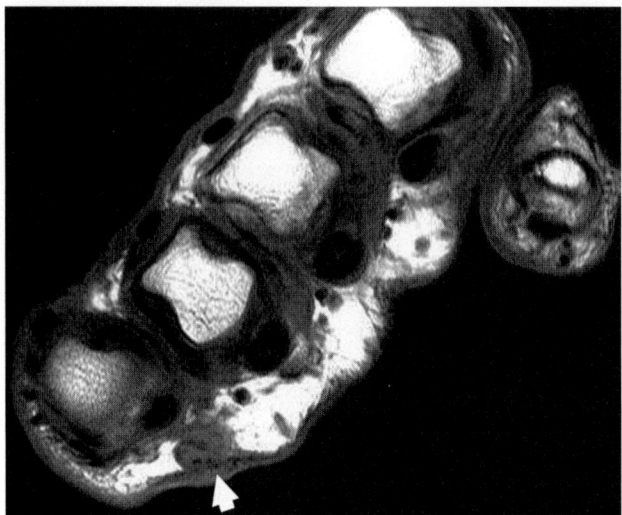

**Figure 78–16.** Dupuytren's contracture. Axial T1-weighted (TR/TE, 656/17) spin echo MR image shows a heterogeneous fibrotic nodule of intermediate signal intensity associated with a contracture of the little finger. The nodule was contiguous with a subcutaneous cord.

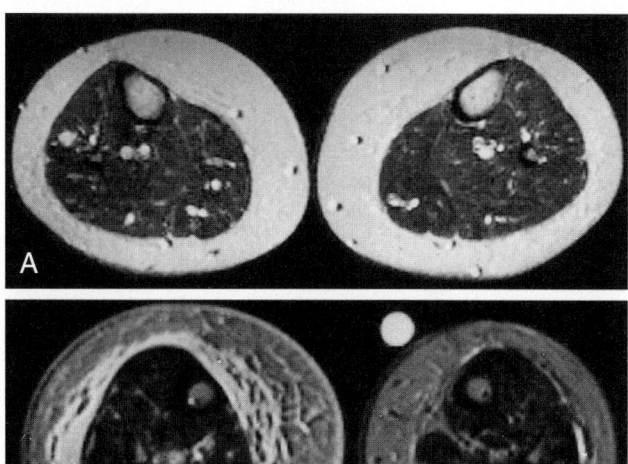

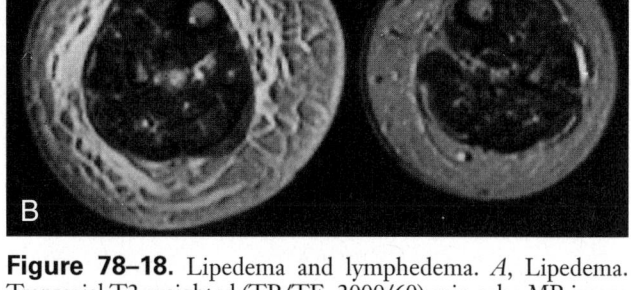

**Figure 78–18.** Lipedema and lymphedema. *A,* Lipedema. Transaxial T2-weighted (TR/TE, 2000/60) spin echo MR image shows homogeneous enlargement of the subcutaneous layer of fat in both legs. *B,* Lymphedema. Transaxial T2-weighted (TR/TE, 2000/60) spin echo MR image shows involvement of the right leg. A honeycomb pattern of increased signal intensity in the subcutaneous fat is evident.
  (From Duewell S, Hagspiel KD, Zuber J, et al: Radiology 184:227, 1992.)

## Glass and Wood

Delineation of glass particles by conventional radiography depends on their size and orientation, their precise anatomic location (thick versus thin body parts), the nature of the surrounding tissue, and the specific radiographic technique used (Fig. 78–19). The radiopacity of some types of glass (e.g., beer and wine bottles) is greater than that of others (e.g., light bulbs). With MR imaging, glass appears as a region of signal void that may be surrounded by a zone of inflammation.

The difficulty of delineating foreign bodies composed of wood with standard radiography is well recognized. Of the other diagnostic techniques available, CT and ultrasonography (Fig. 78–20) have been most successful in detecting wood fragments. Wood appears as a region of signal void on MR images. MR imaging is effective in demonstrating the reactive soft tissue masses that may occur in response to foreign bodies composed of wood (or other substances). These masses, which are sometimes large, simulate the appearance of soft tissue tumors or abscesses, however.

## Plant Thorns

A granulomatous response in the soft tissue, joint, or bone may be seen after the entry of certain types of plant thorns. Although the clinical features vary somewhat according to the specific offending agent and its depth of penetration, the type of human tissue involved, and the presence or absence of associated bacterial infection, certain

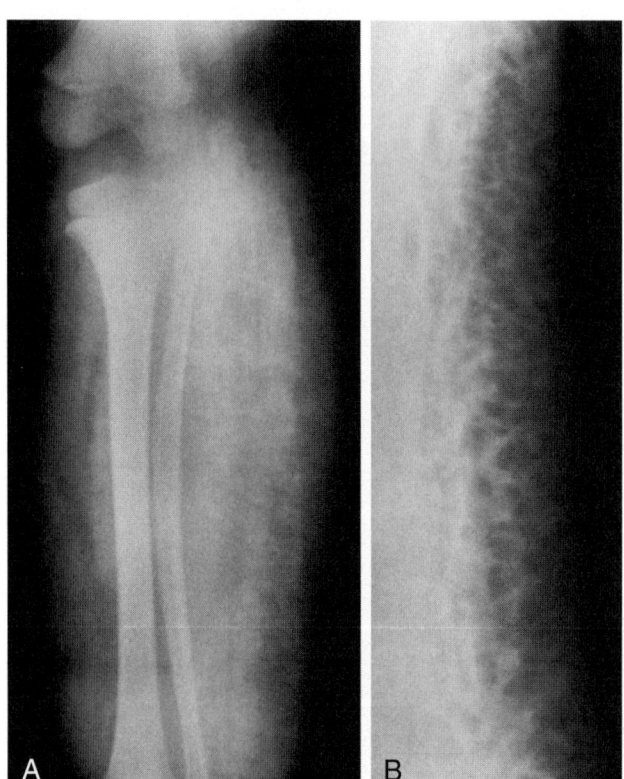

**Figure 78–17.** Lymphedema. *A,* This 5-year-old boy with congenital lymphedema has the typical striated pattern in the enlarged soft tissues. *B,* A coned-down view in another patient delineates the reticular soft tissue pattern.

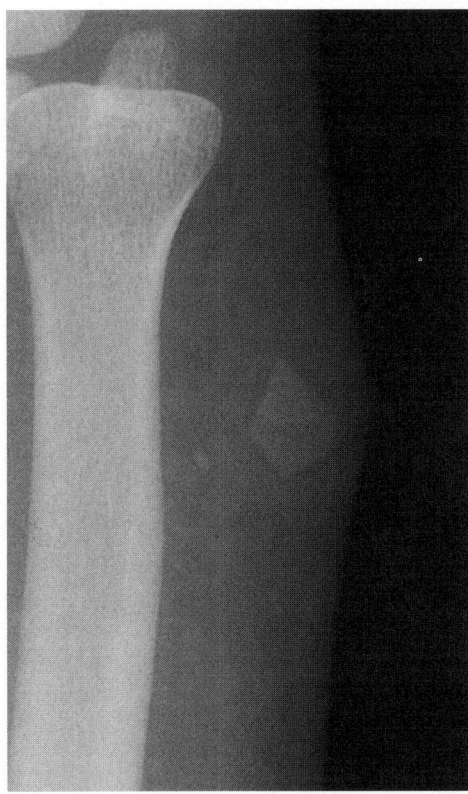

**Figure 78–19.** Foreign bodies: glass shards. Several radiopaque areas in the distal portion of the forearm represent pieces of glass. Note the soft tissue swelling.

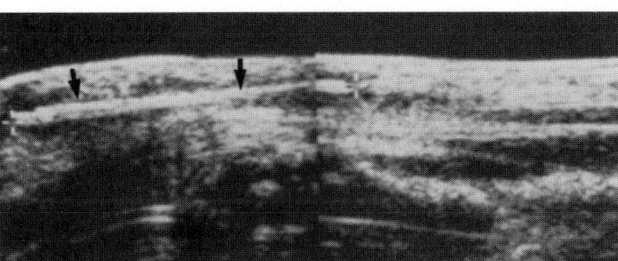

**Figure 78–20.** Foreign bodies: wood splinter. This splinter *(arrows)* lodged in the volar surface of the wrist was not evident on routine radiography but is well shown on a sagittal scan with ultrasonography.

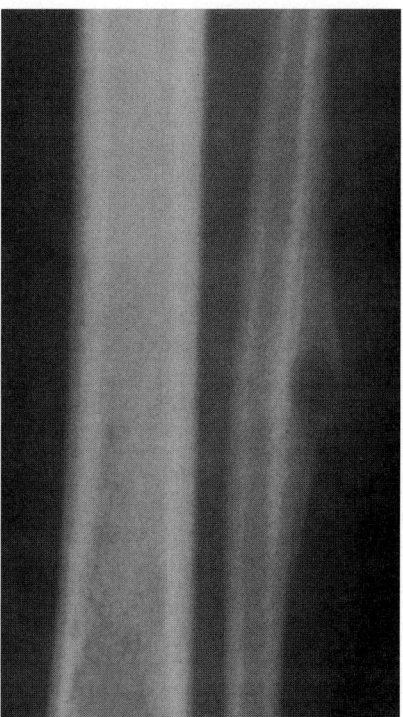

**Figure 78–21.** Foreign bodies: plant thorn. Note the osteolytic lesion related to an embedded plant thorn, with associated periostitis.

typical manifestations can be identified. Children are affected more frequently than adults. The extremities are usually affected, especially the hands and feet. Pain and soft tissue swelling are evident soon after the injury, and a puncture wound may be evident. Subsequently, a period of improvement is common, followed by the reappearance of symptoms and signs.

The radiographic features vary according to the site of granuloma formation. Most often, an articulation, tendon sheath, or bursa is affected; rarely, the bone is the primary site of involvement. In the latter case, a well-circumscribed osteolytic lesion, termed a pseudotumor, with periostitis and soft tissue swelling is typical (Fig. 78–21).

Tenosynovitis or bursitis leads to soft tissue swelling and periosteal reaction and arthritis.

## SOFT TISSUE ATROPHY

Diffuse atrophy of soft tissue, including fat and muscle, is an accompaniment of chronic debilitating illnesses, lipoatrophic diabetes, and malnutrition. Localized atrophy of soft tissue is evident in many different types of disorders, including collagen vascular diseases such as scleroderma, paralysis or prolonged disuse or immobilization of an extremity, thermal injury, and inflammatory or occlusive vascular processes. Muscle atrophy (or, rarely, hypertrophy) occurs in certain neuromuscular disorders and inflammatory conditions. CT and MR imaging are the techniques of choice in evaluating this atrophy.

## SOFT TISSUE HYPERTROPHY

Overgrowth of soft tissue, alone or in combination with osseous enlargement, may occur in a generalized or localized distribution. Generalized hypertrophy is a fundamental part of pituitary gigantism and acromegaly, but it is also encountered in many other conditions, including cerebral gigantism.

Hemihypertrophy refers to overgrowth of one half or one side of the body. It is related to an increase in the size of cells (hypertrophy), an increase in the number of cells (hyperplasia), or both. Hemihypertrophy usually involves the muscular, vascular, skeletal, and nervous systems and may occur on an idiopathic basis or in association with neurocutaneous syndromes (neurofibromatosis, tuberous sclerosis, Sturge-Weber disease, Lindau-von Hippel disease), Beckwith-Wiedemann syndrome, or skin and vascular abnormalities. Additional alterations associated with idiopathic congenital hemihypertrophy include a variety of tumors.

Macrodactyly represents an increase in the size of all the structures (bones, tendons, nerves, vessels, subcutaneous fat, skin) in one or more digits of the hands and feet. It occurs on an idiopathic basis and in association with hemangiomas, lymphangiomas, and arteriovenous malformations. Similar enlargement is seen in neurofibromatosis, epidermal nevus syndrome, fibrolipomatous hamartomas, and macrodystrophia lipomatosa.

The Proteus syndrome (named for the Greek god who could change shape to avoid capture) describes the altered pattern of growth seen in a congenital hamartomatous syndrome associated with partial gigantism of the hands and feet, hemihypertrophy, subcutaneous tumors, pigmented nevi, macrocephaly, and bone exostoses. Clinical findings typically become apparent in the first few years of life. Regional gigantism and lymphangiomatous hamartomas are regarded as the two most essential features of the syndrome (Fig. 78–22). Hyperplasia of subcutaneous tissue is also noted. In the palmar and plantar regions, this hyperplasia manifests as cerebriform or gyriform lesions or, in the lower extremity, as moccasin feet. Macrodactyly is generally present, with enlargement of some of the short tubular bones, and osteochondroma-like lesions arising from the short and long tubular bones are evident. The skull is affected in approximately 50% of cases.

The radiographic abnormalities stemming from musculoskeletal involvement in this syndrome, which consist mainly of bone and soft tissue overgrowth and deformity, resemble those of neurofibromatosis, Ollier's disease, Maffucci's syndrome, macrodystrophia lipomatosa, Klippel-Trénaunay-Weber syndrome, and Bannayan-Zonana syndrome. Indeed, confusion among these syndromes is exemplified by the debate over the cause of the deformities in Joseph Merrick, the "elephant man," who may have had Proteus syndrome rather than neurofibromatosis.

## SPECIAL SYNDROMES OF SKIN AND SOFT TISSUE

Certain afflictions of cutaneous and subcutaneous tissue can be associated with radiographic abnormalities involving not only the soft tissues but also the bones and joints. Some of the important afflictions are described here.

### Epidermolysis Bullosa

This rare, chronic skin disorder results from poor adherence of the epidermis to the dermis. The disorder is inherited in either a dominant or a recessive manner, and the latter form is more severe.

Radiographic findings are characteristic but not specific and vary with the type of disease present. Flexion

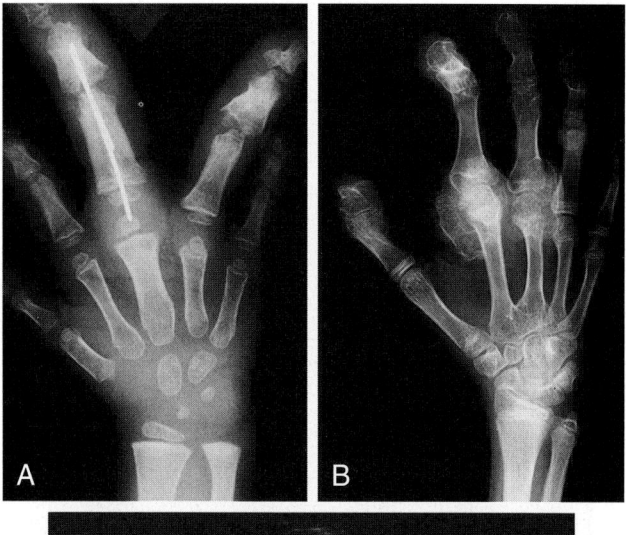

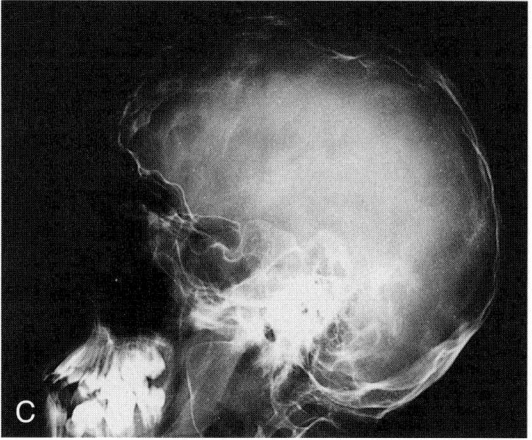

**Figure 78–22.** Proteus syndrome. The radiographic abnormalities of this syndrome are varied. As shown in three affected patients, they include macrodactyly with bone and soft tissue hypertrophy (A), osteochondroma-like lesions of tubular bones (B), and frontal bossing and a "copper-beaten" appearance of the cranial vault (C).

contractures of the metacarpophalangeal and interphalangeal articulations, webbing between the fingers, and distal trophic changes may be encountered (Fig. 78–23). The terminal phalanges of the hands (and, less frequently, the feet) are distorted; they become pointed or wedge shaped and resemble the findings in scleroderma. The combination of flexion deformities of the fingers and toes and webbing is important in the diagnosis of this rare skin disease. Osteoporosis, slender diaphyses of the tubular bones (perhaps caused by chronic muscle atrophy), dental caries, periapical abscesses, loss of teeth, and esophageal strictures may be seen.

### Nevoid Basal Cell Carcinoma Syndrome (Gorlin's Syndrome)

Nevoid basal cell carcinoma syndrome is an inherited disorder characterized by multiple basal cell carcinomas, palmar pits, odontogenic keratocysts, rib and spine anomalies, brachydactyly, and various neurologic and ophthalmic abnormalities. The disorder is inherited in an

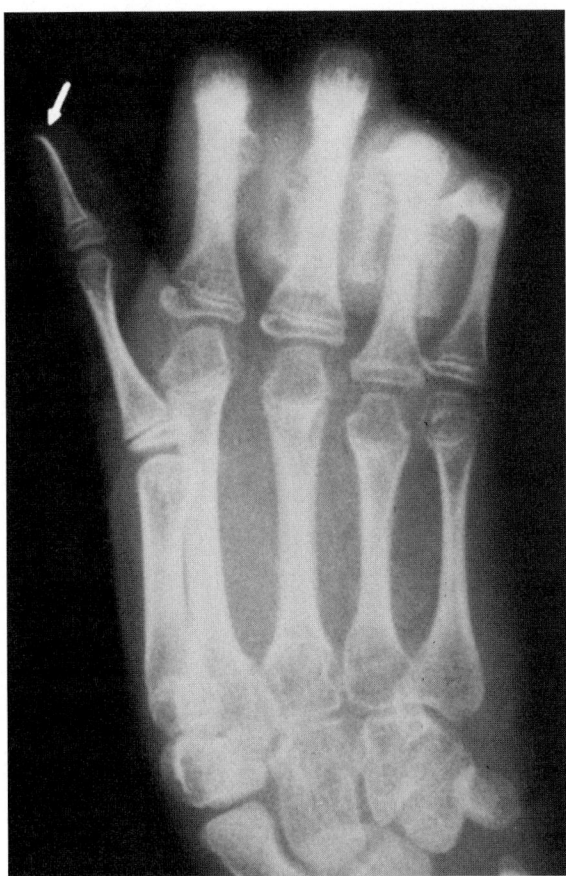

**Figure 78–23.** Epidermolysis bullosa. Observe the contractures of the interphalangeal articulations, webbing between the digits, skin and bone atrophy, osteoporosis, epiphyseal deformity, and pointing of the terminal tufts of the phalanges, most evident in the thumb *(arrow)*.

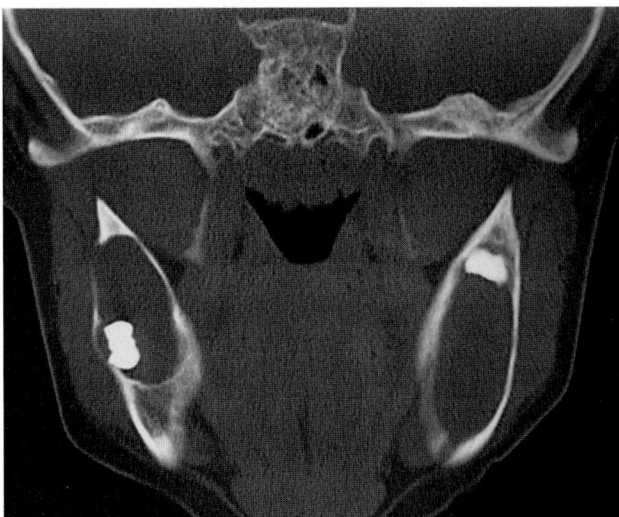

**Figure 78–24.** Nevoid basal cell carcinoma syndrome (Gorlin's syndrome): mandibular abnormalities. Coronal CT scan reveals dentigerous cysts in the ascending ramus on each side of the mandible. Each cyst arises about the crown of a tooth. (Courtesy of D. Wilcox, MD, Kansas City, Mo.)

autosomal dominant pattern with variable expressivity and appears with equal frequency in both sexes.

Basal cell epitheliomas are usually seen near puberty. Typically affected sites are the face and trunk, although other regions may be involved. Dentigerous cysts of the mandible are common in this disorder but rarely produce clinical findings before age 6 to 7 years (Fig. 78–24); they may antedate the appearance of skin lesions. Common rib anomalies are splaying, synostosis, and bifid and cervical ribs (Fig. 78–25A). Unilateral or bilateral alterations

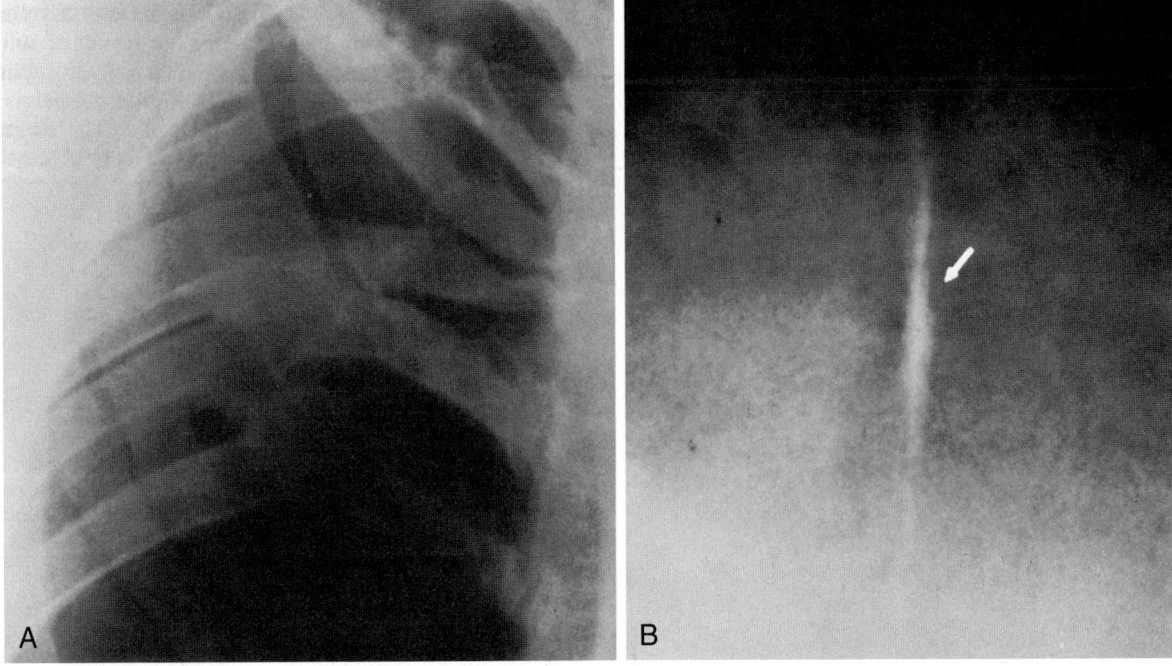

**Figure 78–25.** Nevoid basal cell carcinoma syndrome (Gorlin's syndrome): other abnormalities. *A,* Typical rib anomalies are demonstrated. *B,* Calcification of the falx cerebri *(arrow)* is not unusual in this syndrome.

in the first to fourth ribs are typical. Shortening of the metacarpals, especially the fourth and fifth, is also a relatively common finding. In the spine, kyphoscoliosis, spina bifida occulta, block vertebrae, spondylolysis, spondylolisthesis, and hemivertebrae can be seen. Skull involvement may include calcification of the falx cerebri (see Fig. 78–25B), dura, tentorium, and choroid; partial agenesis of the corpus callosum; hypertelorism; and anosmia. Mental retardation, congenital hydrocephalus, and changes in the eyes (dysgenesis oculi neuroblastica gliomatosa) have been noted.

## Panniculitis and Related Syndromes

Panniculitides are inflammatory disorders of subcutaneous fat. Although several distinct forms of panniculitis have been recognized, clinical manifestations common to most forms include the presence of moderately tender nodules in the soft tissues (Table 78–2), especially in the lower extremities and forearms, that may lead to discharge of liquefied fat and scarring. Factitious panniculitis relates to inflammation and necrosis of fat produced by thermal, mechanical, or chemical trauma.

Inflammation and necrosis of deep and subcutaneous fat (Fig. 78–26) may accompany certain forms of panniculitis, including those related to pancreatic disease, although these changes are more common after an injury. In such cases, routine radiographs may reveal distinctive soft tissue calcifications. MR imaging findings may resemble those accompanying a variety of soft tissue disorders, although a characteristic stellate or nodular lesion containing foci of fat may be evident (Fig. 78–27).

---

**TABLE 78–2**

**Characteristics of Panniculitides in Adults**

| Condition | Clinical Features | Associated Conditions | Histopathologic Characteristics |
|---|---|---|---|
| Erythema nodosum | Tender erythematous nodules on lower extremities<br>Fever<br>Arthritis | Poststreptococcal sarcoidosis<br>Inflammatory bowel disease | Septal panniculitis (no vasculitis) |
| Subacute nodular migratory panniculitis | Painless nodules on lower leg<br>Yellow centers<br>Sclerodermoid changes | None | Septal panniculitis |
| Weber-Christian disease | Chronic, recurrent, tender, erythematous nodules<br>Systemic symptoms of foot necrosis | Pancreatic disease<br>Infections<br>Autoimmune disorders | Lobular panniculitis<br>Foam cells<br>Fibrosis in late stages (no vasculitis) |
| Nodular vasculitis | Tender nodules or plaques on posterior aspect of lower legs | None | Lobular panniculitis with vasculitis |
| Erythema induratum | Nodules on posterior aspects of legs | Tuberculosis | Lobular panniculitis with vasculitis and caseation necrosis |
| Lupus panniculitis | Nodules on face, buttocks, arms<br>Overlying scars | Discoid lupus erythematosus<br>Systemic lupus erythematous | Septal and lobular panniculitis |
| Connective tissue panniculitis | Erythematous, tender plaques and nodules<br>Resolution with atrophy | Unclassified connective tissue disease | Lymphohistiocytic invasion of fat lobules with caseation (no vasculitis) |
| Cytophagic panniculitis | Erythematous, tender nodules<br>Fever<br>Oral ulcers<br>Serositis | Lymphadenopathy<br>Organomegaly<br>Pancytopenia | Lobular panniculitis with fat necrosis and hemorrhage |
| Pancreatic panniculitis | Erythematous nodules | Pancreatitis<br>Pancreatic malignancy | Lobular panniculitis with necrosis of lipocytes and ghost cells |

From Thiers BH: Dermatol Clin North Am 1:537, 1983.

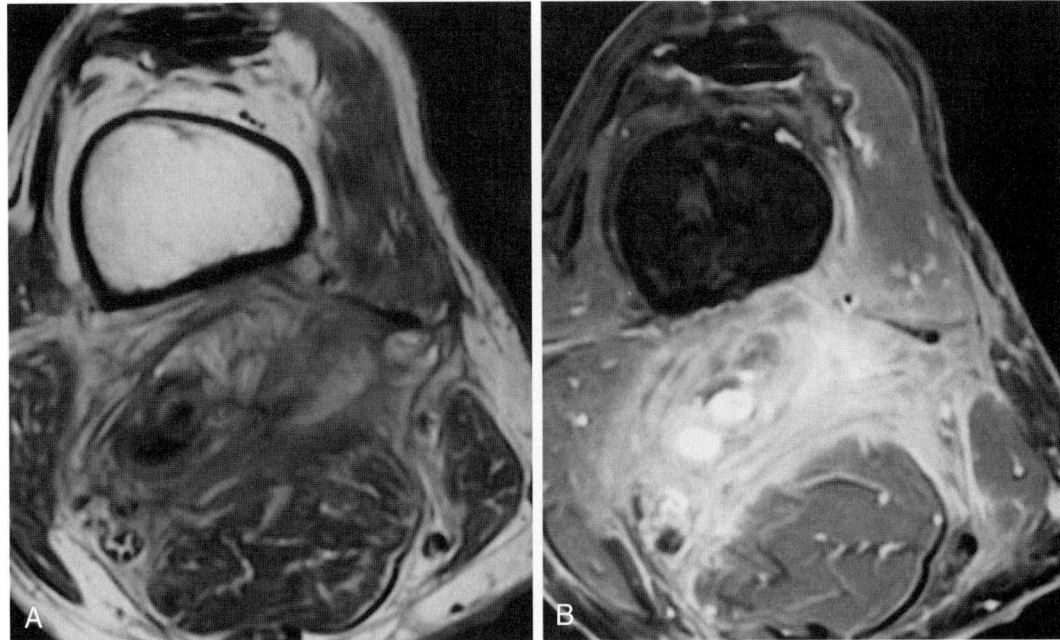

**Figure 78–26.** Panniculitis: MR imaging. This 86-year-old man complained of pain and swelling behind the knee, in the absence of any injury or systemic illness. Biopsy of the lesion confirmed the presence of inflammation and necrosis of fat. *A,* Transverse T1-weighted (TR/TE, 500/15) spin echo MR image reveals regions of low signal intensity posterior to the distal portion of the femur. *B,* After intravenous gadolinium administration, transverse fat-suppressed T1-weighted (TR/TE, 500/21) spin echo MR image shows high signal intensity in these same regions. (Courtesy of Y. Kakitsubata, MD, Miyazaki, Japan.)

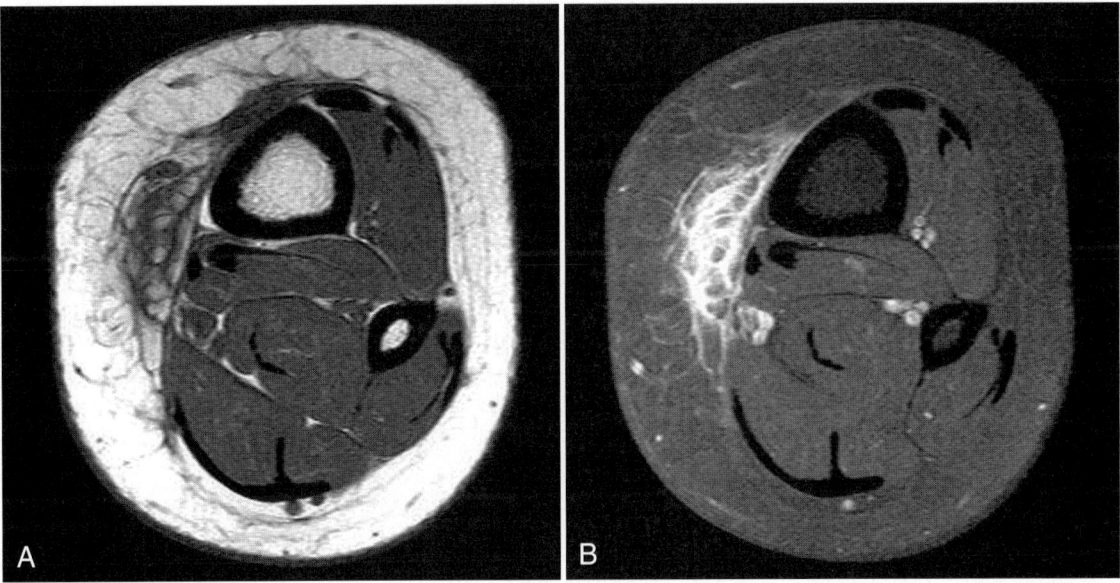

**Figure 78–27.** Fat necrosis: MR imaging. Axial T1-weighted (TR/TE, 552/16) *(A)* and fat-suppressed enhanced T1-weighted (TR/TE, 594/16) *(B)* spin echo MR images reveal a lobular masslike lesion, with preserved central lobules of fat and surrounding enhancing inflammation and edema.

## FURTHER READING

Abel MF, McFarland R III: Hair and thread constriction of the digits in infants: A case report. J Bone Joint Surg Am 75:915, 1993.

Ackerman L, Ramamurthy S, Jablokow V, et al: Case report 488: Post-traumatic myositis ossificans mimicking a soft tissue neoplasm. Skeletal Radiol 17:310, 1988.

Alpert M: Roentgen manifestations of epidermolysis bullosa. AJR Am J Roentgenol 78:66, 1957.

Angervall L, Stener B, Stener I, et al: Pseudomalignant osseous tumour of soft tissue: A clinical, radiological, and pathological study of five cases. J Bone Joint Surg Br 51:654, 1969.

Azouz EM, Costa T, Fitch N: Radiologic findings in the Proteus syndrome. Pediatr Radiol 17:481, 1987.

Ballock RT, Wiesner GL, Myers MT, et al: Hemihypertrophy: Concepts and controversies. J Bone Joint Surg Am 79:1731, 1997.

Bandiera S, Bachini P, Bertoni F: Bizarre parosteal osteochondromatous proliferation of bone. Skeletal Radiol 27:154, 1998.

Bauer W, Marble A, Bennett G: Further studies in a case of calcification of the subcutaneous tissue ("calcinosis universalis") in a child. Am J Med Sci 182:237, 1931.

Becker MH, Kopf AW, Lande A: Basal cell nevus syndrome: Its roentgenographic significance. Review of the literature and report of four cases. AJR Am J Roentgenol 99:817, 1967.

Blackfield HM, Hause DP: Congenital constricting bands of the extremities. Plast Reconstr Surg 8:101, 1951.

Bodne D, Quinn SF, Cochran CF: Imaging foreign glass and wooden bodies of the extremities with CT and MR. J Comput Assist Tomogr 12:608, 1988.

Brickley-Parsons D, Glimcher MJ, Smith RJ, et al: Biochemical changes in the collagen of the palmar fascia in patients with Dupuytren's disease. J Bone Joint Surg Am 63:787, 1981.

Burgio GR, Wiedemann HR: Further and new details on the Proteus syndrome. Eur J Pediatr 143:71, 1984.

Burnstein MI, Kottamasu SR, Weiss L, Katz ME: Case report 509: Proteus syndrome. Skeletal Radiol 17:536, 1988.

Byrne J, Blanc WA, Baker D: Amniotic band syndrome in early fetal life. Birth Defects 18:43, 1982.

Caffey J: Pediatric X-ray Diagnosis, 7th ed. Chicago, Year Book, 1978, p 984.

Canteli B, Saez F, de los Rios A, et al: Fat necrosis. Skeletal Radiol 25:305, 1996.

Chew FS, Crenshaw WB: Idiopathic tumoral calcinosis. AJR Am J Roentgenol 158:330, 1992.

Choi JH, Gu MJ, Kim MJ, et al: Fibrosarcoma in bizarre parosteal osteochondromatous proliferation. Skeletal Radiol 30:44, 2001.

Cracchiolo A: Wooden foreign bodies in the foot. Am J Surg 140:585, 1980.

Crawford SC, Boyer RS, Harnsberger HR, et al: Disorders of histogenesis: The neurocutaneous syndromes. Semin Ultrasound CT MR 9:247, 1988.

Crowley B, Tonkin MA: The proximal interphalangeal joint in Dupuytren's disease. Hand Clin 15:137, 1999.

Cvitanic O, Sedlak J: Acute myositis ossificans. Skeletal Radiol 24:139, 1995.

De Smet AA, Norris MA, Fisher DR: Magnetic resonance imaging of myositis ossificans: Analysis of seven cases. Skeletal Radiol 21:503, 1992.

De Smet L, Vercauteren M: Fast-growing pseudomalignant osseous tumour (myositis ossificans) of the finger: A case report. J Hand Surg [Br] 9:93, 1984.

Dupuytren G: Permanent retraction of the fingers, produced by an affection of the palmar fascia. Lancet 2:222, 1834.

Ehara S, Nakasato T, Tamakawa Y, et al: MRI of myositis ossificans circumscripta. Clin Imaging 15:130, 1991.

Fine G, Stout AP: Osteogenic sarcoma of the extraskeletal soft tissues. Cancer 9:1027, 1956.

Goldman AB: Myositis ossificans circumscripta: A benign lesion with a malignant differential diagnosis. AJR Am J Roentgenol 126:32, 1976.

Greenfield GB: Radiology of Bone Diseases, 2nd ed. Philadelphia, JB Lippincott, 1975, p 491.

Gunn DR, Young WB: Myositis ossificans as a complication of tetanus. J Bone Joint Surg Br 41:535, 1959.

Hermann G, Som P: Case report 135: Multiple basal cell nevus syndrome (Gorlin syndrome). Skeletal Radiol 6:62, 1981.

Holmes WS, Pope TL Jr, de Lange E, et al: Case report 413: Florid reactive periostosis of the proximal phalanx of the fourth finger (parosteal fasciitis, pseudosarcomatous fibromatosis, fasciitis ossificans). Skeletal Radiol 16:163, 1987.

Inclan A, Leon P, Camejo MG: Tumoral calcinosis. JAMA 121:490, 1943.

Johnson MK, Lawrence JF: Metaplastic bone formation (myositis ossificans) in the soft tissue of the hand: Case report. J Bone Joint Surg Am 57:999, 1975.

Kinmonth JB, Taylor GW, Tracy GD, et al: Primary lymphedema: Clinical and lymphangiographic studies of a series of 107 patients in which the lower limbs were affected. Br J Surg 45:1, 1957.

Kirk TS, Simon MA: Tumoral calcinosis. Report of a case with successful medical management. J Bone Joint Surg Am 63:1167, 1981.

Kirks DR, Shackelford GD: Idiopathic congenital hemihypertrophy with associated ipsilateral benign nephromegaly. Radiology 115:145, 1975.

Kolawole TM, Bohrer SP: Tumoral calcinosis with "fluid levels" in the tumoral masses. AJR Am J Roentgenol 120:461, 1974.

Kozlowski K, Baker P, Glasson M: Multiple nevoid basal cell carcinoma syndrome (report of five cases in a family). Pediatr Radiol 2:185, 1974.

Kransdorf MJ, Meis JM, Jelinek JS: Myositis ossificans: MR appearance with radiologic-pathologic correlation. AJR Am J Roentgenol 157:1243, 1991.

Kuhns LR, Borlaza GS, Seigel RS, et al: In vitro comparison of computed tomography and radiography in the detection of soft tissue foreign bodies. Radiology 132:218, 1979.

Lile HA, Rogers JF, Gerald B: The basal cell nevus syndrome. AJR Am J Roentgenol 103:214, 1968.

Ling RS: The genetic factor in Dupuytren's disease. J Bone Joint Surg Br 45:709, 1963.

Lopez JA, Saez F, Larena JA, et al: MRI diagnosis and follow-up of subcutaneous fat necrosis. J Magn Reson Imaging 7:929, 1997.

Martinez S, Vogler JB III, Harrelson JM, et al: Imaging of tumoral calcinosis: New observations. Radiology 174:215, 1990.

Monu JU, McManus CM, Ward WG, et al: Soft-tissue masses caused by long-standing foreign bodies in the extremities: MR imaging findings. AJR Am J Roentgenol 165:395, 1995.

Moses JM, Flatt AE, Cooper RR: Annular constricting bands. J Bone Joint Surg Am 61:562, 1979.

Naschitz JE, Boss JH, Misselevich I, et al: The fasciitis-panniculitis syndromes: Clinical and pathologic features. Medicine (Baltimore) 75:6, 1996.

Ozonoff MB, Flynn FJ Jr: Roentgenologic features of dermatomyositis of childhood. AJR Am J Roentgenol 118:206, 1973.

Paterson DC: Myositis ossificans circumscripta: Report of four cases without history of injury. J Bone Joint Surg Br 52:296, 1970.

Plotkin D: Congenital cicatrizing fibrous bands: Report of 2 cases. Arch Pediatr 68:120, 1951.

Porter AR, Tristan TA, Rudy FR, et al: Florid reactive periostitis of the phalanges. AJR Am J Roentgenol 144:617, 1985.

Poznanski AK: The Hand in Radiologic Diagnosis, 2nd ed. Philadelphia, WB Saunders, 1984.

Resnik CS: Tumoral calcinosis. Arthritis Rheum 32:1484, 1989.

Spjut HJ, Dorfman HD: Florid reactive periostitis of the tubular bones of the hands and feet: A benign lesion which may simulate osteosarcoma. Am J Surg Pathol 5:423, 1981.

Steinbach LS, Johnston JO, Tepper EF, et al: Tumoral calcinosis: Radiologic-pathologic correlation. Skeletal Radiol 24:573, 1995.

Stewart VL, Herling P, Dalinka MK: Calcification in soft tissues. JAMA 250:78, 1983.

Thomson JG: Calcifying collagenolysis (tumoral calcinosis). Br J Radiol 39:526, 1966.

Tibbles JA, Cohen MM Jr: The Proteus syndrome: The Elephant Man diagnosed. BMJ 293:683, 1986.

Totten JR: The multiple nevoid basal cell carcinoma syndrome: Report of its occurrence in four generations of a family. Cancer 46:1456, 1980.

Tsai TS, Evans HA, Donnelly LF, et al: Fat necrosis after trauma: A benign cause of palpable lumps in children. AJR Am J Roentgenol 169:1623, 1997.

Wiedemann HR, Burgio GR, Aldenhoff P, et al: The Proteus syndrome. Eur J Pediatr 140:5, 1983.

Yacoe ME, Bergman AG, Ladd AL, et al: Dupuytren's contracture: MR imaging findings and correlation between MR signal intensity and cellularity of lesions. AJR Am J Roentgenol 160:813, 1993.

Zeanah WR, Hudson TM: Myositis ossificans: Radiologic evaluation of two cases with diagnostic computed tomograms. Clin Orthop 168:187, 1982.

# CHAPTER 79

## Muscle Disorders

### Robert Downey Boutin

## SUMMARY OF KEY FEATURES

This chapter reviews the fundamental elements in interpreting imaging examinations of the neuromuscular system: normal anatomy, imaging techniques, and pathologic conditions. Knowledge of anatomy and of the capabilities of the various techniques is a prerequisite for correctly interpreting the pathologic changes displayed. Imaging examinations also have an impact on patient care by providing meaningful information about the location, extent, severity, and activity of muscular disorders. Further, the muscular abnormalities detected on imaging examinations—some specific and some nonspecific—can be used to plan treatment, predict prognosis, guide invasive procedures, and assess therapeutic response.

## NORMAL ANATOMY
### Muscle Structure

The basic structural element of skeletal muscle is the muscle fiber. Each fiber is a multinucleated cell that may be a few millimeters to a few centimeters long. These fibers are grouped into fascicles, and the fascicles are grouped into muscles. Muscles, in turn, are arranged in compartments that are typically bounded by tough connective tissue termed fascia. Fascia plays a fundamental role in the pathogenesis of certain muscle disorders (e.g., compartment syndrome, fascial herniation) and influences the extent of others (e.g., spread of tumor and infection).

### Muscle Contraction

All muscle fibers in a single motor unit have the same contractile and metabolic properties. At least two general motor unit profiles are recognized widely (Table 79–1). Type I (red, slow-twitch) fibers are relatively slow to contract and relax but are also relatively fatigue resistant. Type II (white, fast-twitch) fibers have the fastest contraction time but are the least resistant to fatigue.

### Muscle Compartments

Compartments are distinct anatomic spaces that are usually bordered by tissues (e.g., fascia, cortical bone) that act as natural barriers to inhibit the spread of pathologic processes. In contradistinction, tissues within or between compartments (e.g., muscle, fat, medullary bone) are relatively poor barriers. Knowledge of compartmental anatomy is of supreme practical significance to radiologists and is especially important in the staging and biopsy of musculoskeletal tumors.

**Arm Compartments.** In the upper arm, muscles are divided into three compartments: anterior, posterior, and deltoid (Fig. 79–1). The deltoid muscle is considered distinct from the two main compartments in the arm. If a biopsy in the proximal portion of the arm requires traversing the deltoid muscle, an approach through the anterior third of the deltoid is favored.

**Forearm Compartments.** The forearm is classically divided into three compartments: radial, dorsal, and volar (Fig. 79–2). The radial compartment is also known as the "mobile wad."

**Thigh Compartments.** There are three compartments in the thigh: anterior, posterior, and medial (Fig. 79–3).

**Leg Compartments.** The four compartments in the leg are the anterior, lateral, superficial posterior, and deep posterior (Fig. 79–4).

**Foot Compartments.** The three compartments in the plantar aspect of the foot are divided by two intermuscular septa that arise from the plantar aponeurosis (Fig. 79–5).

### Anomalous Muscles

Many anatomic variations are of no clinical significance. However, hypertrophied and accessory muscles can be mistaken for neoplasms or for torn muscles that have retracted. Computed tomography (CT), sonography, and magnetic resonance (MR) imaging permit the diagnosis of an anomalous muscle by demonstrating its characteristic morphology, origin, insertion, and course in relation to neighboring anatomic structures. When unperturbed by trauma or other insults, an anomalous muscle has the same appearance (i.e., density, echo texture, and signal intensity) as adjacent skeletal muscles.

Axial T1-weighted or intermediate-weighted images are most reliable in depicting accessory muscles. Additional fat-suppressed T2-weighted or inversion recovery fast spin echo MR images are essential in assessing for superimposed pathologic changes, such as those that accompany an entrapment neuropathy (Fig. 79–6). In this setting, characteristic imaging findings include nerve compression or enlargement, hyperintense T2 signal in a nerve affected by acute or subacute neuritis, hyperintense T2 signal in a muscle affected by subacute denervation, and diminished bulk and fatty infiltration in a muscle affected by chronic denervation. However, anomalous muscles and consequent compressive neuropathy may be underdiagnosed with MR imaging.

**TABLE 79–1**

**Muscle Fiber Types: Common Characteristics**

| Characteristic | Type 1 | Type II |
|---|---|---|
| Strength | Low | High |
| Speed | Slow | Fast |
| Fatigability | Fatigue-resistant | Fatigue-prone |
| Aerobic capacity | High | Low |
| Motor unit size | Small | Large |

## IMAGING TECHNIQUES

### Overview

Radiography is a relatively inexpensive means of screening for abnormal radiodensity in muscle. Specific examples of abnormal radiodensities that help establish the correct diagnosis include the discovery of heterotopic ossification, a phlebolith that may herald the presence of an intramuscular hemangioma, and an avulsion fracture that may result in musculotendinous insufficiency. CT allows cross-sectional assessment of abnormalities detected by radiography and may improve diagnostic confidence in some cases.

Sonography allows the assessment of myotendinous disorders during dynamic maneuvers that may elicit symptoms and clarify the diagnosis (e.g., musculotendinous rupture, muscle herniation through a fascial defect). Power Doppler sonography can be used to measure alterations in muscle blood volume after exercise.

MR imaging is usually the test of choice for evaluating muscle derangements. Provisional indications for MR imaging of muscle are listed in Table 79–2. MR imaging facilitates the diagnostic process by detecting alterations in muscle size, shape, or signal intensity.

## Magnetic Resonance Imaging—Technical Considerations

The MR imaging protocols used for evaluating the musculoskeletal system vary greatly. The field of view should be large enough to allow evaluation of the entire area of interest, but scanning of an asymptomatic contralateral extremity usually is not necessary. Regardless of the technical parameters chosen, a marker should be placed on the skin surface over any palpable mass or focal area of tenderness.

**Imaging Planes.** "Longitudinal" imaging planes are useful for depicting the superior-to-inferior extent of myotendinous abnormalities in relation to bony landmarks. Such longitudinal imaging planes may also display to best advantage the relation between a musculotendinous structure and an avulsion fracture. Transaxial images in the extremities facilitate a cross-sectional evaluation of muscles, compartments, and neurovascular structures.

**Pulse Sequences.** T1-weighted (short TR/short TE) spin echo MR images have a favorable signal-to-noise ratio and can aid in characterizing substances in muscle, such as fat or blood. T1-weighted images are optimal for showing the fatty infiltration and diminished bulk that accompanies muscle atrophy. T1-weighted images also demonstrate characteristic high signal intensity with other muscle derangements, including well-differentiated fat-containing tumors, methemoglobin in subacute hemorrhagic lesions, melanin in well-differentiated metastatic melanomas, proteinaceous debris in necrotic neoplasms, paramagnetic effects of gadolinium-based contrast materials, and various MR artifacts (Table 79–3; Fig. 79–7).

T2-weighted (long TR/long TE) MR images are commonly acquired with a fast spin echo technique. Common causes of high and low signal intensity in muscle on T2-weighted images are listed in Tables 79–4 and 79–5, respectively. Causes of focal mass–like areas of

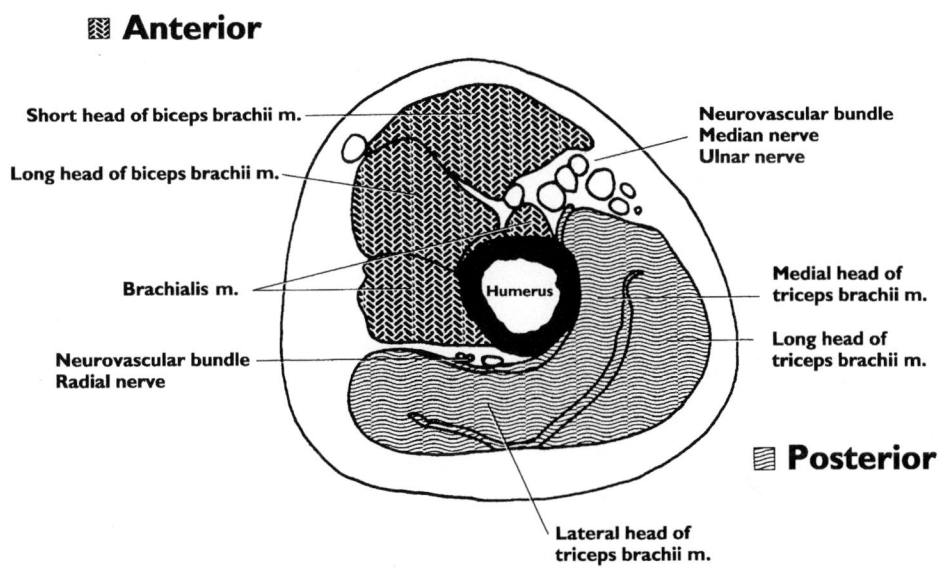

**Anterior**

Short head of biceps brachii m.

Long head of biceps brachii m.

Brachialis m.

Neurovascular bundle
Radial nerve

Humerus

Neurovascular bundle
Median nerve
Ulnar nerve

Medial head of
triceps brachii m.

Long head of
triceps brachii m.

**Posterior**

Lateral head of
triceps brachii m.

**Figure 79–1.** Arm compartments. Section at the level of the midhumerus shows the contents of the anterior and posterior compartments. (The deltoid compartment is not shown at this level.)

(From Anderson MW, Temple HT, Dussault RG, Kaplan PA: Compartmental anatomy: Relevance to staging and biopsy of musculoskeletal tumors. AJR Am J Roentgenol 173:1663, 1999.)

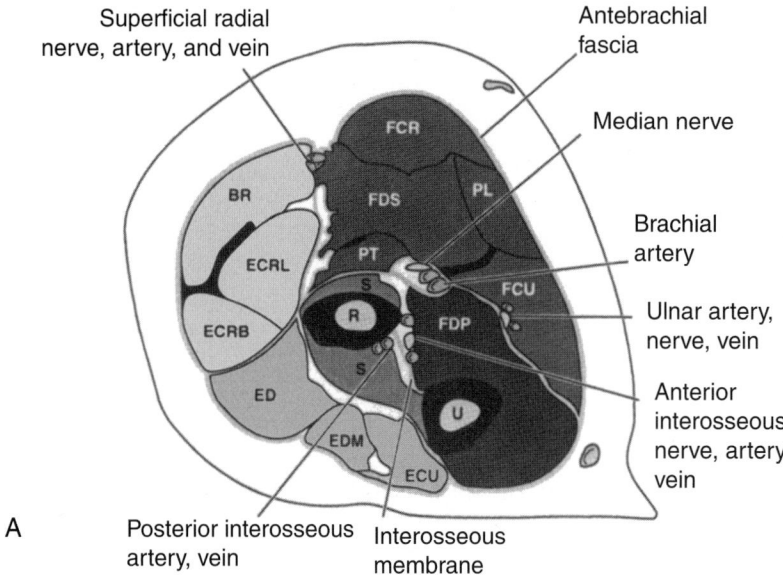

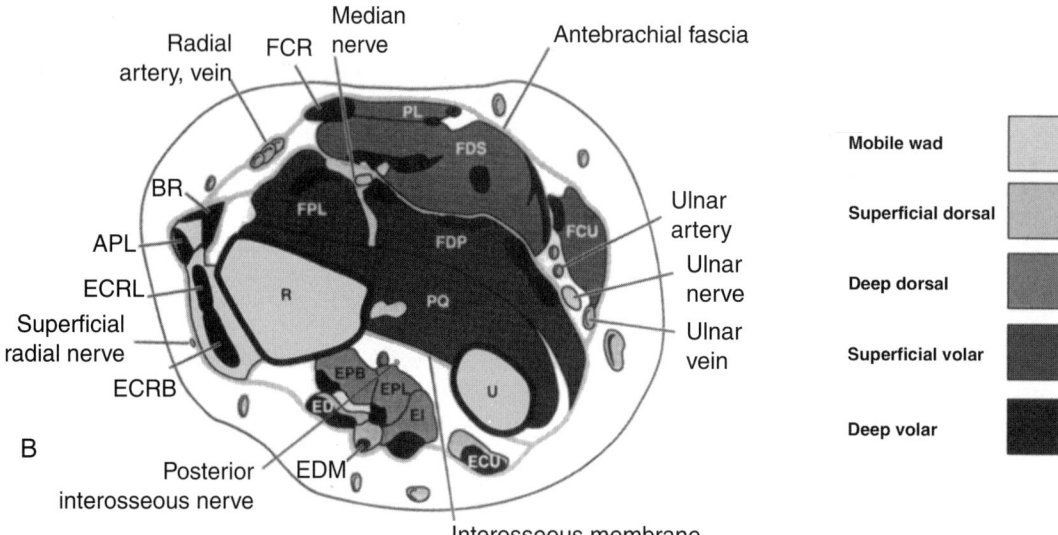

**Figure 79–2.** Forearm compartments. Sections at the level of the proximal forearm *(A)* and the distal forearm at the junction of the radial diaphysis and metaphysis *(B)* are shown. APL, abductor pollicis longus; BR, brachioradialis; ECRB, extensor carpi radialis brevis; ECRL, extensor carpi radialis longus; ECU, extensor carpi ulnaris; ED, extensor digitorum; EDM, extensor digiti minimi; EI, extensor indices; EPB, extensor pollicis brevis; EPL, extensor pollicis longus; FCR, flexor carpi radialis; FCU, flexor carpi ulnaris; FDP, flexor digitorum profundus; FDS, flexor digitorum superficialis; FPL, flexor pollicis longus; PL, palmaris longus; PQ, pronator quadratus; PT, pronator teres; R, radius; S, supinator; U, ulna.

(From Boles CA, Kannam S, Cardwell AB: The forearm: Anatomy of muscle compartments and nerves. AJR Am J Roentgenol 174:151, 2000.)

abnormal signal intensity are listed in Table 79–6. When the suppression of signal from fat is achieved with a frequency-selective technique, intermediate- and T2-weighted fast spin echo MR images become exquisitely sensitive to the presence of edema, fluid collections, most stages of hemorrhage, and most neoplasms. The other technique commonly used for fat suppression, fast spin echo inversion recovery imaging, also tends to have a propitious effect on lesion conspicuity. This imaging technique allows for relatively reliable and uniform fat suppression, even in anatomic areas with complex air-tissue interfaces (e.g., neck, ankle) or that do not fit into a dedicated extremity coil. However, the suppression of signal in fatty tissues is not entirely specific.

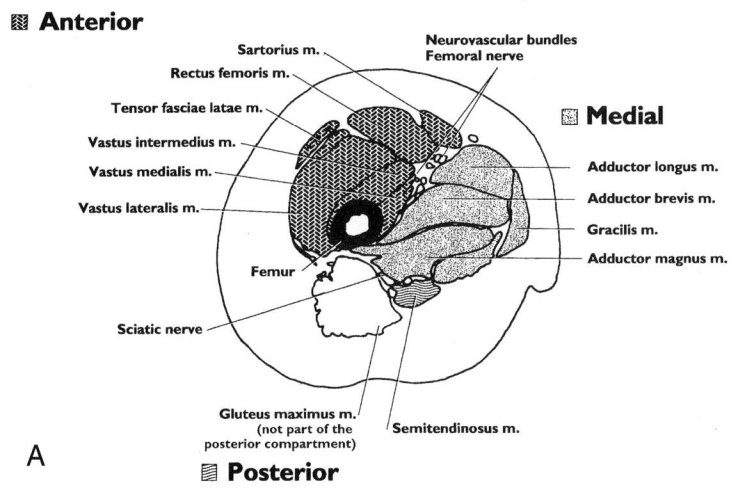

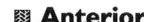

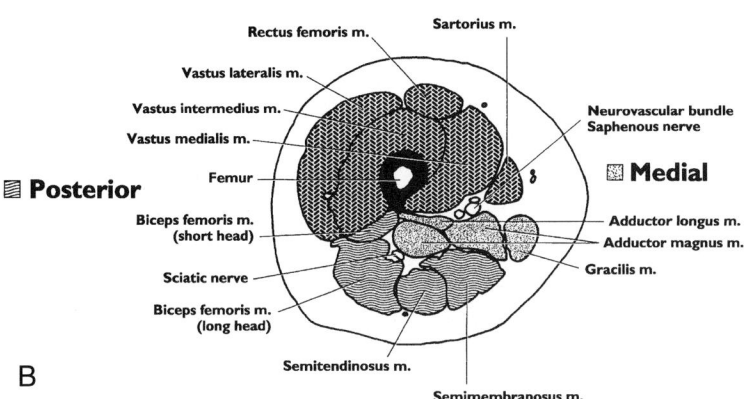

**Figure 79–3.** Thigh compartments. Sections at the level of the proximal *(A)* and mid *(B)* thigh show the contents of the anterior, medial, and posterior compartments.

(From Anderson MW, Temple HT, Dussault RG, Kaplan PA: Compartmental anatomy: Relevance to staging and biopsy of musculoskeletal tumors. AJR Am J Roentgenol 173:1663, 1999.)

**Supplemental Techniques.** T2-weighted gradient echo sequences accentuate certain paramagnetic effects. This "blooming" effect may indicate the presence of hemosiderin, metallic foreign bodies, or gas, helping to hone a differential diagnosis. Fast gradient echo images have been used for high temporal resolution to study anatomic and pathologic changes in muscle. For example, muscle contraction during the MR examination may demonstrate retraction of a torn muscle or herniation of a muscle through a fascial defect. Cine MR imaging may facilitate the diagnosis of an entrapment neuropathy.

The intravenous administration of gadolinium-based contrast material usually is not necessary for the assessment of muscle disorders. Muscle affected by recent trauma, inflammation, or neoplasm is generally displayed conspicuously with fat-suppressed T2-weighted or fast spin echo inversion recovery images. Gadolinium-based contrast material delivered intravenously may be particularly helpful for differentiating between lesions that are solid and those that are cystic, however. In addition, nonenhancing areas help identify a necrotic lesion that has outgrown its own blood supply (pretreatment), guide the selection of an appropriate biopsy site that has viable tissue for histopathologic analysis, and document an appropriate therapeutic response after treatment. Further, the presence of an enhancing nodule in an intramuscular mass often suggests the diagnosis of a neoplasm rather than a hematoma. Detection of torn muscle fibers may be more conspicuous after gadolinium administration, particularly when there is extensive hemorrhage and edema. In addition, contrast material can facilitate the detection of abnormal signal intensity along the periosteum or in the deep posterior compartment muscles of the leg that may occur because of impaired venous outflow.

## IMAGING OF PATHOLOGIC CONDITIONS

A wide array of focal and systemic pathologic conditions can affect muscle. Common categories of derangement include traumatic muscle injuries and their sequelae, ischemia and necrosis, inflammation and infection, congenital and inherited conditions, and neoplasms. Although some of these conditions have similar imaging characteristics, imaging examinations may help hone the clinical differential diagnosis while excluding the possibility of other derangements.

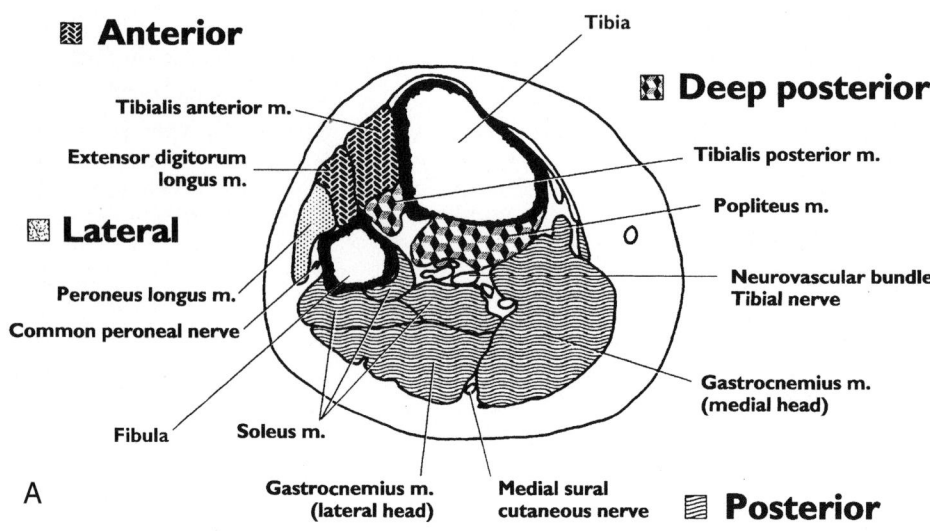

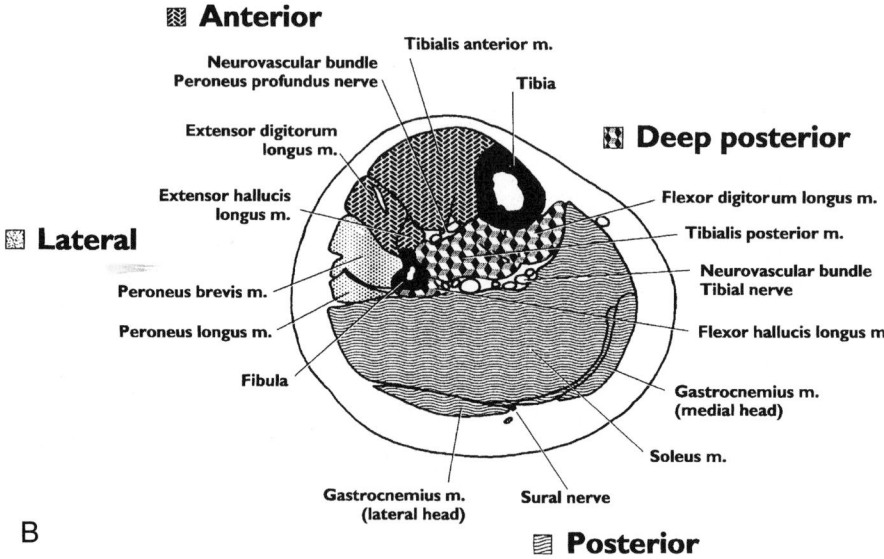

**Figure 79–4.** Leg compartments. Sections at the level of the proximal *(A)* and mid *(B)* calf show contents of the anterior, lateral, superficial posterior, and deep posterior compartments.

(From Anderson MW, Temple HT, Dussault RG, Kaplan PA: Compartmental anatomy: Relevance to staging and biopsy of musculoskeletal tumors. AJR Am J Roentgenol 173:1663, 1999.)

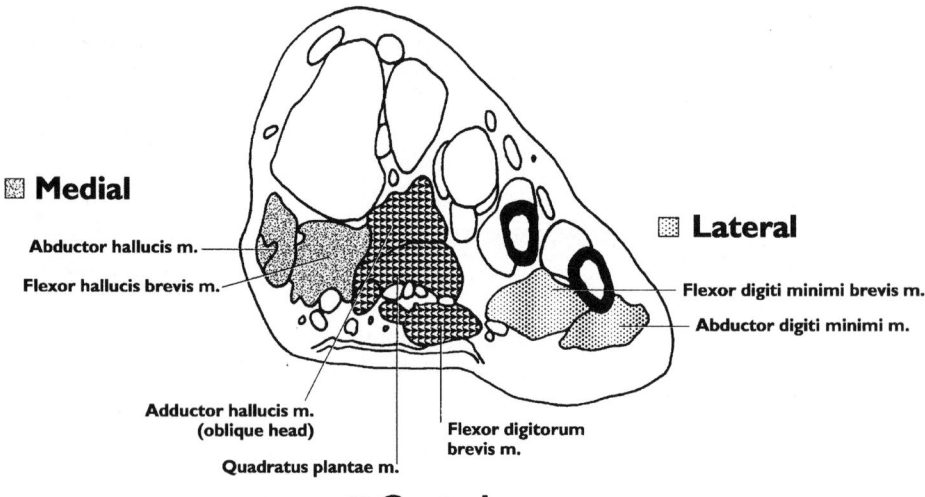

**Figure 79–5.** Foot compartments. Section of the foot shows the medial, central, and lateral compartments.

(From Anderson MW, Temple HT, Dussault RG, Kaplan PA: Compartmental anatomy: Relevance to staging and biopsy of musculoskeletal tumors. AJR Am J Roentgenol 173:1663, 1999.)

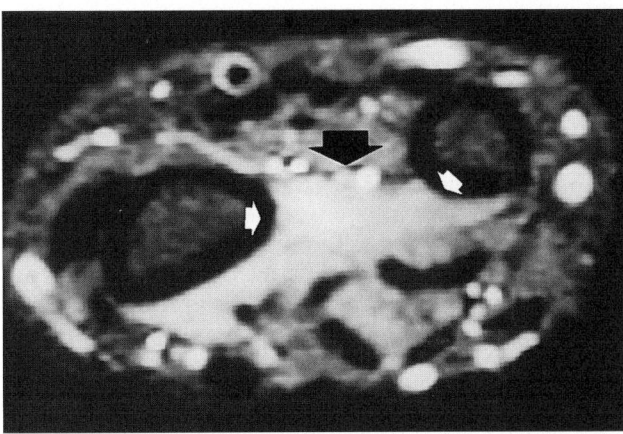

**Figure 79–6.** Subacute denervation. Transverse fat-suppressed T2-weighted fast spin echo MR image demonstrates high signal intensity diffusely in the pronator quadratus muscle (*arrows*), owing to subacute denervation affecting the anterior interosseous nerve.

---

**TABLE 79–3**

**Causes of T1 Hyperintensity in Muscle**

Common causes
  Fat deposition
    Muscular atrophy (e.g., disuse, chronic tendon rupture, chronic denervation, nonacute muscle injury or iatrogenic insult)
    Lipomatous tumor (e.g., intramuscular lipoma)
    Heterotopic ossification (cancellous bone portion)
  Hematoma—subacute (owing to methemoglobin)
  Gadolinium-based contrast material
  Magnetic resonance artifacts (e.g., flow phenomena, coil artifacts)
Uncommon causes
  Proteinaceous material (e.g., in area of necrosis)
  Melanin (e.g., in metastatic melanoma)

---

**TABLE 79–2**

**Indications for Magnetic Resonance Imaging of Muscle**

To provide prompt and accurate diagnosis when crucial for initiating proper treatment

To evaluate a soft tissue mass in a patient without a clear history of trauma

To assess for uncommon sources of muscle pain (e.g., intermittent muscle herniation)

To investigate for an underlying structural cause of neuropathy

To assess the extent and type of infection

To evaluate the location and extent of myopathy, especially before biopsy

---

## Injuries to Muscle

### Avulsion Injury

The age of a patient influences the location of injuries in the bone-tendon-muscle complex. In children and adolescents, the weakest link in this chain is the apophyseal growth plate. The pelvis, with its many apophyses, is a common location of avulsion injuries. Avulsion injuries are multiple at the time of presentation in as many as one third of patients. The single most common site of avulsion is the ischial apophysis. A displaced avulsion fracture fragment can usually be recognized with ease on radiographs. However, in children, radiographs may be interpreted as negative when an apophyseal avulsion is essentially nondisplaced or when the apophysis is unossified. In the subacute or chronic setting, an avulsion injury may resemble a neoplastic or infectious process, especially when no history of trauma is provided.

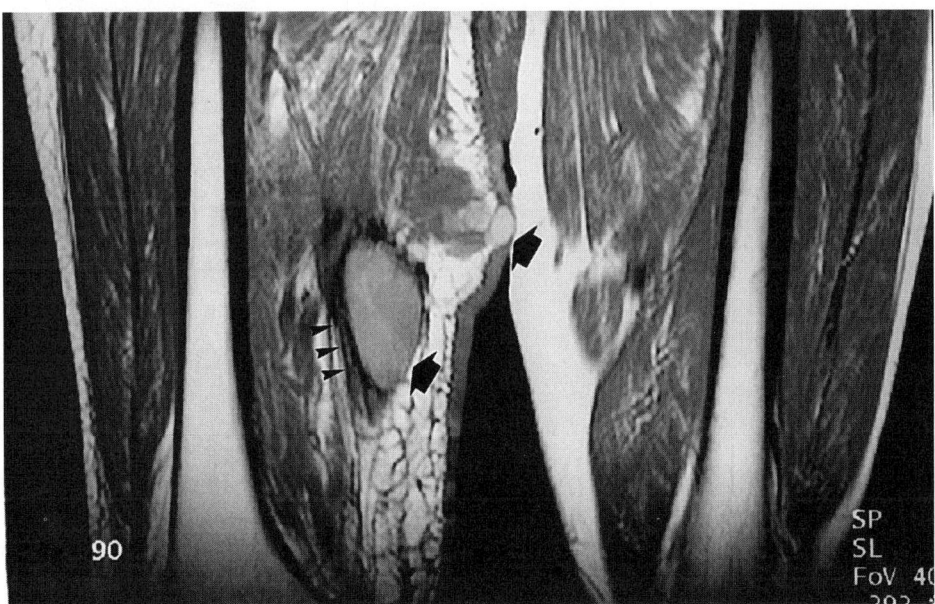

**Figure 79–7.** Hyperintense T1 signal. Coronal T1-weighted spin echo MR image of the thighs shows exophytic, rounded areas of high signal intensity (*arrows*) in a patient with metastatic melanoma and soft tissue hemorrhage. Note the peripheral area of low signal intensity, indicative of hemosiderin (*arrowheads*).

**TABLE 79–4**

**Common Causes of T2 Hyperintensity in Muscle**

| Category of Insult | Examples |
|---|---|
| Muscular exertion | Exercise (a transient physiologic finding) |
| Trauma—direct or indirect | Muscle strain, DOMS, contusion, early myositis ossificans, hemorrhage |
| Vascular insufficiency | Compartment syndrome, deep venous thrombosis, sickle cell crisis |
| Inflammation—infection | Bacterial myositis, inclusion body (viral) myositis |
| Inflammation—autoimmune | Polymyositis, dermatomyositis, sarcoidosis |
| Subacute denervation | Entrapment neuropathy |
| Iatrogenic | Postoperative seroma, radiation therapy, percutaneous injection |
| Infiltrative neoplasm | Lymphoma |
| Muscle cell death | Rhabdomyolysis |

DOMS, delayed-onset muscle soreness.

**TABLE 79–5**

**Common Causes of Focal or Multifocal T2 Hypointensity in Muscle**

Calcification (e.g., metabolic or neoplastic disorders)
Foreign bodies (e.g, surgical clips or micrometallic artifact after surgery)
Gas (e.g., post-traumatic or infectious disorders)
Hemosiderin (e.g., old hemorrhage)
Magnetic resonance artifact (e.g., flowing blood in vessel)

**TABLE 79–6**

**Common Causes of Focal Mass–Like Lesions Involving Muscle***

| Category of Insult | Comments and Examples |
|---|---|
| Neoplasm | Primary or metastatic tumor |
| Inflammation—infection | Abscess, parasitic infection |
| Inflammation—autoimmune | Sarcoidosis (nodular subtype) |
| Trauma—direct or indirect | Retracted muscle tear, nonacute myositis ossificans |
| Muscle cell death | Myonecrosis |

*Many of these disorders are also associated with diffuse areas of abnormal signal intensity in the muscle adjacent to the focal mass–like lesion.

## Strain Injury

Myotendinous strain or tear results from excessive stretch, especially while the muscle is being activated. Strains tend to occur in muscles that cross two joints, have a high proportion of fast-twitch fibers, and undergo eccentric contraction (i.e., stretch during contraction). Accordingly, the most commonly strained muscles are the hamstrings, rectus femoris, and gastrocnemius muscles. Eccentric contraction of certain muscles that do not cross two joints may also result in strain injury; this occurs most commonly in the adductor longus (Fig. 79–8).

In any normal myotendinous unit in adults, the weakest point is the junction between the muscle and tendon. In many aging adults, the myotendinous unit is not normal but is weakened by a process such as tendinosis. In such cases, overload of the myotendinous unit tends to result in biomechanical failure through the abnormal tendon.

The degree of strain can be graded from mild (first-degree) to moderate (second-degree) to severe (third-degree).

**First-Degree Strain.** Mild strains are characterized by microscopic injury to the muscle or tendon (typically with <5% fiber disruption). In the acute setting, edema and hemorrhage at the myotendinous junction create high

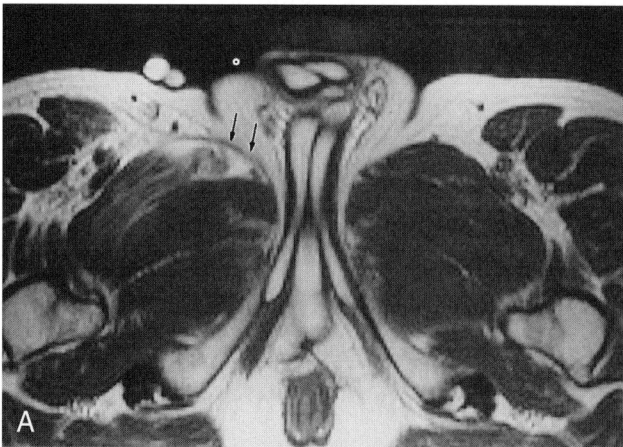
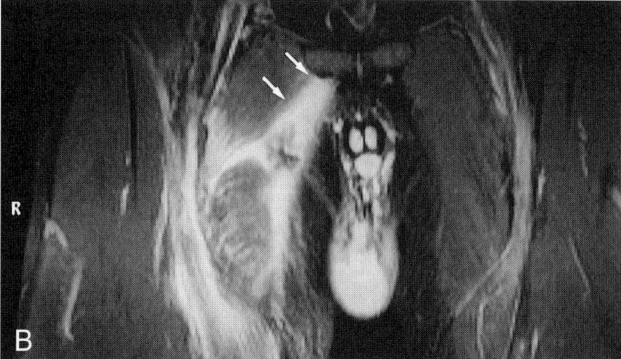

**Figure 79–8.** Adductor muscle strain. Transverse T2-weighted *(A)* and coronal fat-suppressed T2-weighted *(B)* fast spin echo MR images show a retracted, grade III tear of the adductor longus muscle *(arrows)*.

signal intensity focally or diffusely on T2-weighted or fast spin echo inversion recovery MR images (Fig. 79–9). This edema and hemorrhage may track along muscle fascicles, creating a feathery margin. No architectural distortion of the muscle or tendon is present with first-degree strains.

**Second-Degree Strain.** Moderate strains are defined as partial-thickness (macroscopic) tears, with continuity of some fibers near the site of injury. Partial tears are classified as low-grade injuries if less than one third of the fibers are torn, moderate if one third to two thirds are torn, and high-grade if more than two thirds are torn. In the acute setting, high signal intensity on T2-weighted or fast spin echo inversion recovery images reflects the extent of edema and hemorrhage. Hematoma at the myotendinous junction is highly characteristic of second-degree strain injuries (Fig. 79–10). Perifascial fluid is also common in this situation. In the setting of an old second-degree strain, the presence of hemosiderin or fibrosis commonly causes low signal intensity on T2-weighted images. Diminished caliber of the myotendinous unit at the site of injury may also be observed if healing is incomplete. In patients with clinically suspected strain injury in lower extremity muscles, sonography may demonstrate hyperechoic infiltration (in 54% of patients), a soft tissue mass (16%), a compound lesion with characteristics of both infiltration and a mass (14%), or normal findings (16%). Acute and subacute second-degree

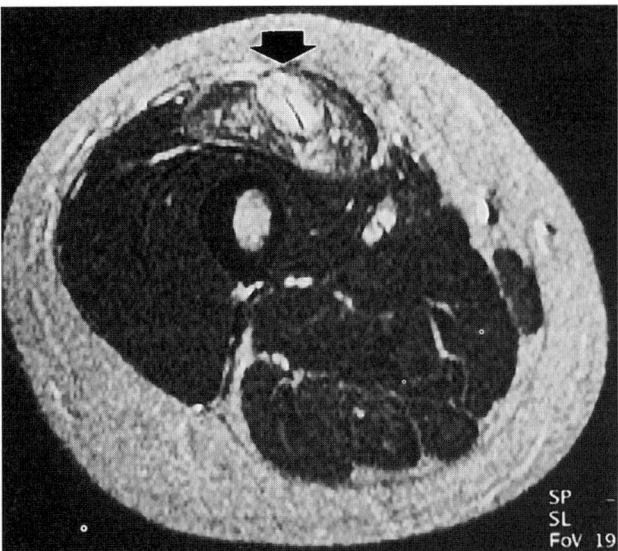

**Figure 79–10.** Second-degree myotendinous strain. Transverse T2-weighted fast spin echo MR image demonstrates high signal intensity in the rectus femoris muscle (*arrow*), especially surrounding the central tendon slip, owing to a second-degree strain.

strains that are diagnosed clinically have a spectrum of sonographic appearances, from small infiltrative lesions to large compound lesions. In the chronic setting, although fibrous tissue may alter muscle echogenicity, fat replacement probably constitutes the main cause of increased muscle echogenicity.

**Third-Degree Strain.** Severe strains are characterized by complete musculotendinous disruption, with or without retraction. Retraction of fibers may result in a palpable defect or a focal soft tissue mass. MR imaging demonstrates complete discontinuity of fibers, commonly with fiber laxity (Fig. 79–11). A focal fluid collection may be seen in the gap created by the tear. Muscular atrophy begins to develop within 10 days after immobilization and may be irreversible by 4 months.

Hematomas may be predominantly intramuscular or intermuscular in location. Intramuscular hematomas often resorb spontaneously over 6 to 8 weeks. Most of the intramuscular hematomas evaluated with MR imaging between 2 days and 5 months after injury display characteristics of methemoglobin, with increased signal intensity on both T1- and T2-weighted images. Pseudo-tumors occurring after a muscle strain most commonly involve the rectus femoris muscle but may be observed at other sites, such as the semimembranosus or semitendinosus muscle (Fig. 79–12). MR imaging may show a ruptured tendon with retraction or an ill-defined signal intensity abnormality at the myotendinous junction that may be interpreted as a soft tissue neoplasm, such as a fibrous tumor or sarcoma.

**Strain Injury of Specific Muscles.** The pectoralis major muscle is the largest, most superficial muscle in the ante-

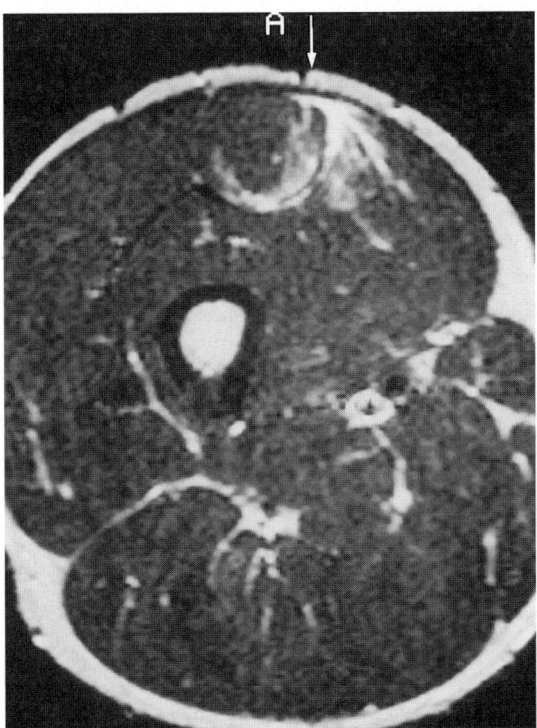

**Figure 79–9.** First-degree muscle strain. Transverse T2-weighted fast spin echo MR image demonstrates high signal intensity in the rectus femoris muscle (*arrow*), with feathery margins but no architectural distortion.

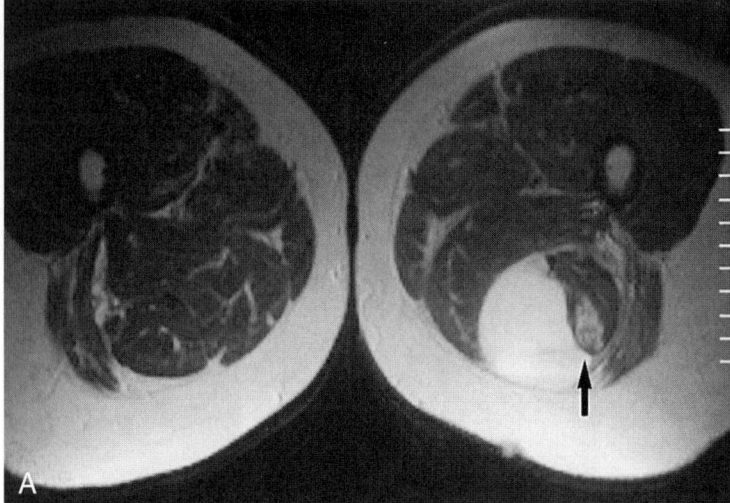

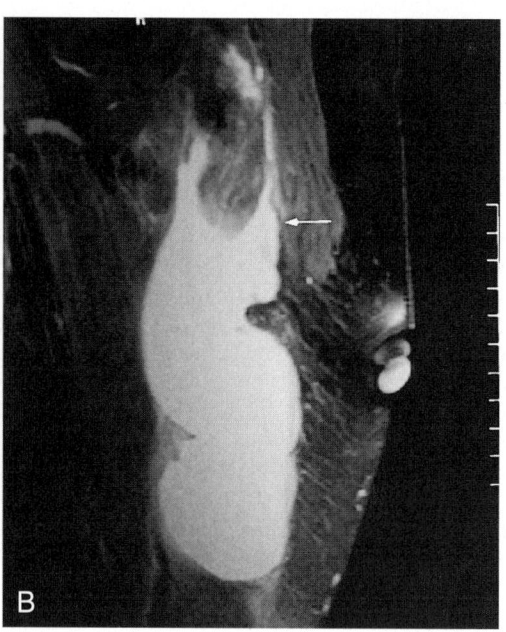

**Figure 79–11.** Third-degree muscle strain. Transverse T2-weighted fast spin echo *(A)* and sagittal fast spin echo inversion recovery *(B)* MR images show a retracted rupture of the semitendinosus muscle with a large hematoma *(arrow)*.

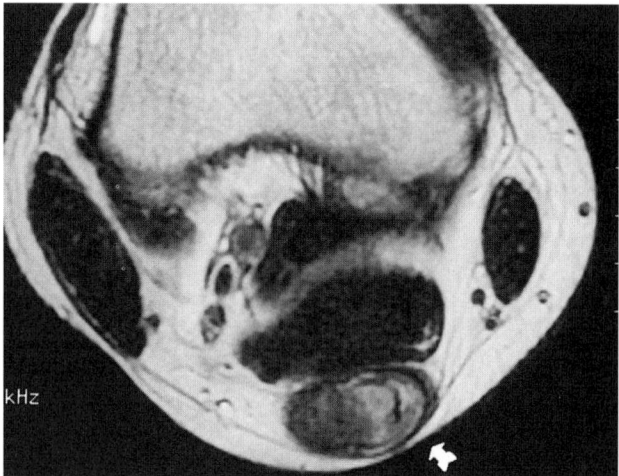

**Figure 79–12.** Pseudotumor after a muscle strain. Transverse T2-weighted fast spin echo MR images show a nonacute midsubstance rupture of the semitendinosus muscle that retracted distally and balled up posterior to the semimembranosus muscle *(arrow)*, resulting in a soft tissue mass that was palpated clinically. (Courtesy of R. C. Fritz, MD, San Francisco, Calif.)

seen superficial to the adjacent cortex as a result of periosteal stripping.

The hamstring muscles (biceps femoris, semitendinosus, and semimembranosus muscles) originate proximally from a conjoined tendon on the posterolateral ischial tuberosity and insert distally into the tibia or fibula. The hamstrings function primarily to flex the knee and extend the hip. In young adults, the majority of hamstring injuries are partial tears; complete hamstring tears or avulsions are relatively uncommon. Of the three hamstring components, the biceps femoris muscle is the most commonly

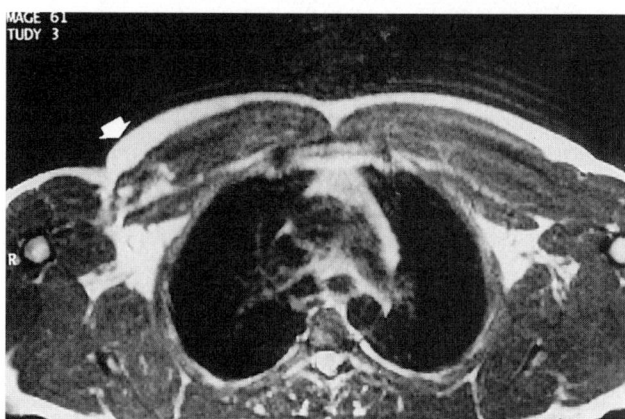

**Figure 79–13.** Pectoralis major muscle strain. Transaxial intermediate-weighted fast spin echo MR image shows a complete tear, indicated by fiber laxity and discontinuity *(arrow)*. The high-signal-intensity edema at the site of this subacute strain is inconspicuous against the background of high-signal-intensity adipose tissue. This tear was repaired surgically, with a good outcome.

rior chest wall. Pectoralis major tears most commonly occur while the arm is abducted during eccentric contraction (e.g., in weightlifters or other athletes) or during a direct blow (e.g., in a motor vehicle accident) (Fig. 79–13). Partial tears of the pectoralis major muscle are more common than complete tears. Partial tears tend to occur at the myotendinous junction and are usually managed nonoperatively. Complete tears usually occur more distally at the enthesis. With avulsion of the tendon from its insertion site, high T2 signal intensity may be injured. Injury to more than one component of the hamstrings is not uncommon (25% to 33% of cases). The myotendinous junction is normally the weakest link in the muscle-tendon-bone "chain" in adults. In the hamstrings, this zone of transition between the muscles and tendons is particularly long. Consequently, when strain injuries occur at the myotendinous junction, these injuries can be located at the ends of the muscle belly or in the muscle belly itself; the proximal myotendinous junction is affected in 33% of cases, the intramuscular myotendinous junction in 53%, and the distal myotendinous junction in 13%.

## Delayed-Onset Muscle Soreness

Delayed-onset muscle soreness (DOMS) refers to the muscular pain, soreness, and swelling that follow unaccustomed exertion. Activities that require eccentric muscle contractions are common culprits, such as downhill hiking or certain types of manual labor. DOMS is thought to occur as a result of reversible structural damage at the cellular level. Symptoms tend to begin within 1 to 2 days after exercise. Soreness crescendos until it peaks 2 to 3 days after the inciting exercise and then generally subsides within 1 week. This soreness may be associated with temporarily diminished strength of up to 50%.

With MR imaging, high signal intensity indicative of interstitial edema is observed on T2-weighted images. Perifascial fluid–like collections occasionally may be seen in the early phase. The MR imaging appearance of DOMS is similar to that of a first-degree strain. The clinical history allows easy differentiation between these two entities in most instances.

## Muscle Contusion

Contusion of muscle is produced by direct trauma, usually by a blunt object. Interstitial edema and hemorrhage result in varying degrees of pain, swelling, ecchymosis, and spasm. In addition, a recognized complication of muscle contusion is myositis ossificans.

Fat-suppressed fast spin echo T2-weighted and fast spin echo inversion recovery MR images provide a conspicuous display of high signal intensity that may have a diffuse or geographic appearance, often with feathery margins (Fig. 79–14). Although the girth of the muscle is typically increased, no fiber discontinuity or laxity is observed. These findings are also observed with CT. With sonography, injuries that appear diffusely hyperechoic reportedly resolve more quickly and have a shorter convalescent period than do injuries displaying a more circumscribed appearance with absent, low, or mixed echogenicity.

## Muscle Laceration

Lacerations are produced by a penetrating injury, such as that caused by a knife. In the acute setting, this type of injury is rarely evaluated with MR imaging, which shows focal, sharply marginated discontinuity of fibers and high T2 signal intensity caused by hemorrhage and edema. In the chronic setting, MR imaging of affected muscle charac-

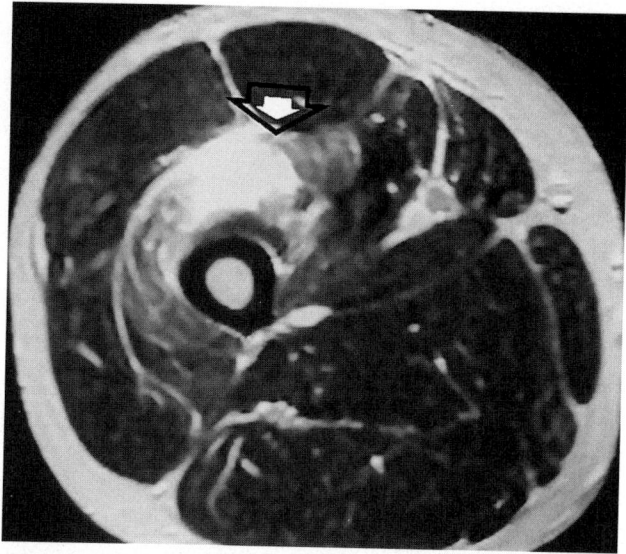

**Figure 79–14.** Muscle contusion. Transverse T2-weighted fast spin echo MR image demonstrates a high-signal-intensity contusion *(arrow)* in the vastus intermedius muscle in a professional football player injured by an opponent's helmet. (Courtesy of R. C. Fritz, MD, San Francisco, Calif.)

teristically demonstrates scarring as low T2 signal intensity and fatty infiltration associated with atrophy as high T1 signal intensity. Sonography may also show the development of a hematoma and fibrous scar.

## Muscle Denervation

MR imaging may be a useful adjunct to electromyography in detecting muscle denervation and its causes (Fig. 79–15). With denervation, the signal intensity and morphology of muscle undergo characteristic changes on MR imaging. Although these denervation changes have been reported as early as 4 days after a nerve insult, hyperintense signal on T2-weighted or fast spin echo inversion recovery MR images is usually not detectable for 2 to 3 weeks. The hyperintense T2 signal in denervated muscle differs from that seen in strained muscle, in that it is not associated with perifascial edema and tends to involve a specific nerve territory.

With chronic denervation, diminished bulk and fatty infiltration occur. These atrophic changes are best displayed on T1-weighted MR images. Whereas the signal intensity changes of acute muscle denervation are reversible, profound atrophic changes seen late in the course of denervation may be irreversible. Pseudohypertrophy refers to prominent accumulation of fat and connective tissue that causes paradoxical enlargement of the affected muscle.

## Sequelae of Muscle Injury

### Hemorrhage and Hematoma

Hematomas may result in pain, anemia, a soft tissue mass, or a compressive neuropathy. Patients with idiopathic intramuscular hemorrhage who are treated conservatively should be monitored until the hemorrhage resolves to

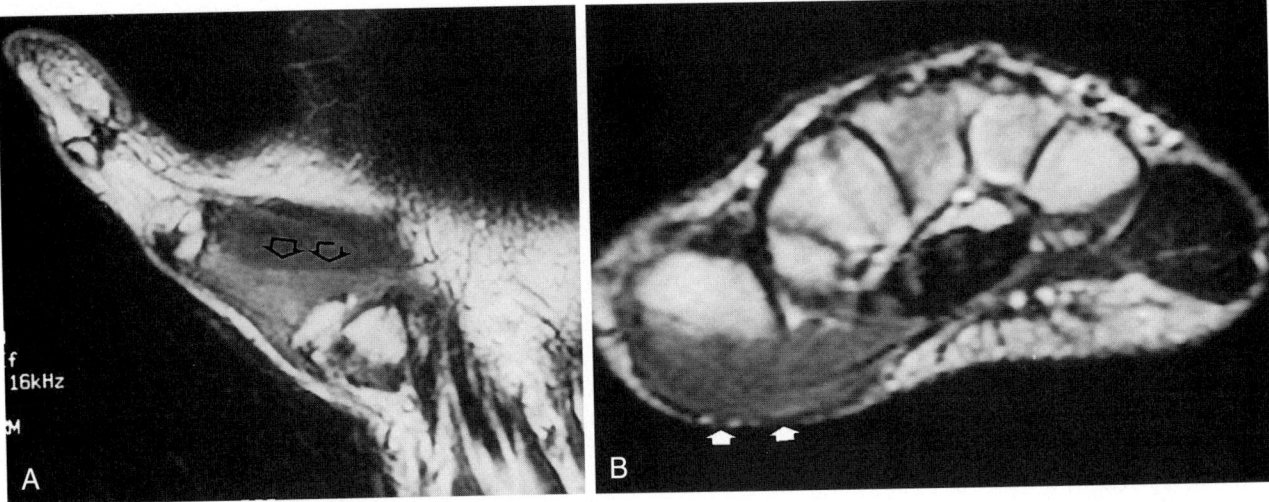

**Figure 79–15.** Subacute denervation. Coronal *(A)* and transverse *(B)* T2-weighted fast spin echo MR images show mildly increased signal intensity in the flexor pollicis brevis and abductor pollicis brevis muscles *(arrows)*, owing to subacute neuropathy affecting the recurrent branch of the median nerve.

exclude an underlying neoplasm as the source of the bleeding.

With sonography, the evolution and resolution of intramuscular hematomas are similar throughout the body. Initially, an intramuscular hematoma tends to appear as a homogeneous, hypoechoic fluid collection. Over the course of several hours, fluid-fluid levels tend to form, and the hematoma takes on a more complex appearance. Over several days, hematomas commonly become uniformly anechoic. With CT, hematomas are seen as space-occupying lesions that evolve through a predictable spectrum of appearances (Fig. 79–16). Initially, hematomas are hyperdense, measuring more than 50 Hounsfield units. Over the course of hours to days, hematomas take

on a more complex appearance, and the density of the hematoma decreases over time.

### Stages of Hematoma

The four principal iron compounds that influence the MR imaging appearance in the various stages of a hematoma are oxyhemoglobin, deoxyhemoglobin, methemoglobin, and hemosiderin (Table 79–7). The circulating erythrocyte contains hemoglobin that binds oxygen (oxyhemoglobin) and releases oxygen (deoxyhemoglobin). When hemorrhage occurs, the resultant hematoma progresses through a number of arbitrarily defined chronologic stages. The actual appearance of any

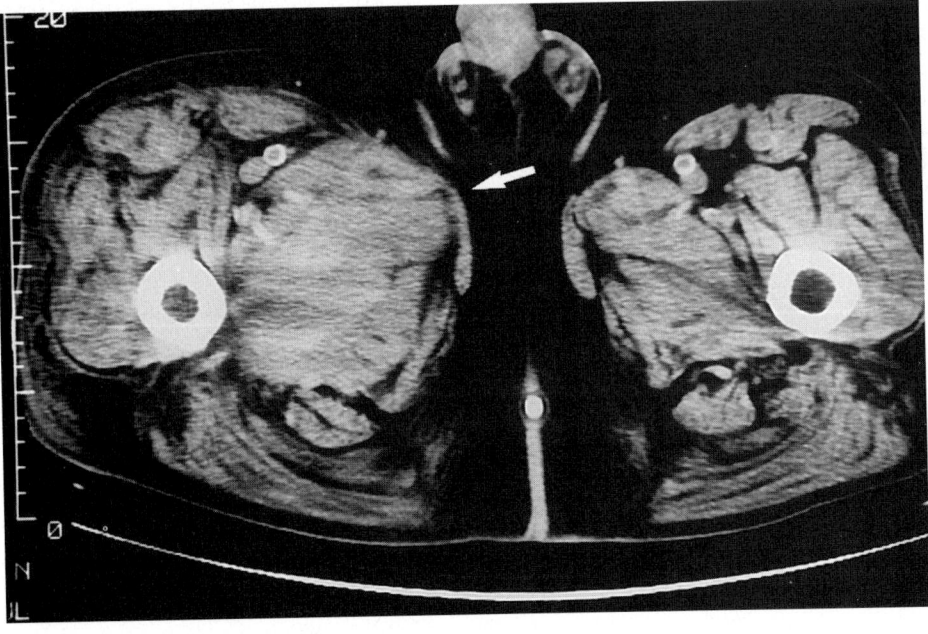

**Figure 79–16.** Hemorrhage. Transverse CT scan shows areas of enlargement and slightly increased attenuation in the adductor musculature *(arrow)*, owing to spontaneous hemorrhage in a patient on warfarin (Coumadin).

**TABLE 79-7**

**Magnetic Resonance Imaging Appearance of Hematomas**

| Stage | Hemoglobin-Related Compound | T1 | Signal Intensity T2 |
|---|---|---|---|
| Hyperacute | Oxyhemoglobin (intracellular) | Intermediate | Intermediate |
| Acute | Deoxyhemoglobin (intracellular) | Intermediate | Hypointenase areas |
| Early subacute | Methemoglobin (intracellular) | Hyperintense | Hypointense areas |
| Late subacute | Methemoglobin (extracellular) | Hyperintense | Heterogeneous, often hyperintense |
| Chronic | Hemosiderin | Hypointense | Hypointense |

given hematoma may differ according to other variables, such as the strength of the MR unit and the location and size of the hematoma (Fig. 79–17).

**Active Hyperacute Hemorrhage—Oxyhemoglobin.** Active hemorrhage is observed with MR imaging only on rare occasions and is characterized by the presence of oxyhemoglobin. Oxyhemoglobin is the only hemoglobin compound occurring in a hematoma that is diamagnetic (not paramagnetic) and therefore does not produce any substantial T1 or T2 shortening.

**Acute Hematoma—Intracellular Deoxyhemoglobin.** In the hypoxic environment of a hematoma, oxyhemoglobin is converted very rapidly to deoxyhemoglobin. Intracellular deoxyhemoglobin does not substantially influence T1 signal intensity, but it can cause hypointensity in the center of acute hematomas on T2-weighted images acquired at 1.5 tesla.

**Early Subacute Hematoma—Intracellular Methemoglobin.** Deoxyhemoglobin is oxidized to methemoglobin, in which the iron in hemoglobin is converted from its reduced (+2) ferrous state to the (+3) ferric state. This change results in increased signal intensity on T1-weighted images. Methemoglobin is often recognized first at the periphery of a subacute hematoma, producing a "concentric ring" sign. On T2-weighted images, intracellular methemoglobin tends to cause T2 shortening, similar to that observed with intracellular deoxyhemoglobin.

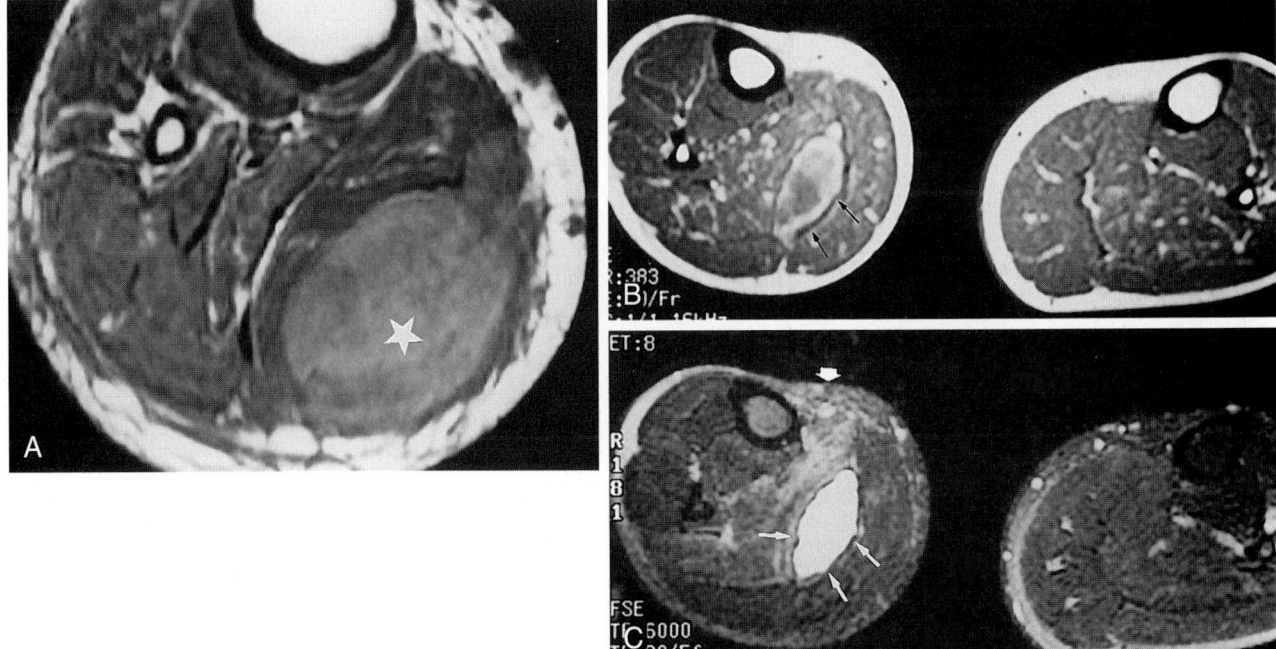

**Figure 79–17.** Hemorrhage. *A,* Transaxial T1-weighted spin echo MR image demonstrates a large sub-acute hematoma *(asterisk)* in the medial head of the gastrocnemius muscle that is hyperintense to muscle, owing to the presence of methemoglobin. *B* and *C,* Transverse T1-weighted spin echo *(B)* and fat-suppressed T2-weighted fast spin echo *(C)* MR images show a subacute hematoma of predominantly high signal intensity, with a faint, thin rim of low signal intensity *(long arrows).* More diffuse high T2 signal in the soleus muscle *(short arrow)* is related to a moderate strain injury.

**Late Subacute Hematoma—Extracellular Methemoglobin.** Later in the subacute stage of a hematoma, lysis of erythrocytes containing methemoglobin occurs. The signal intensity of a hematoma remains hyperintense on T1-weighted images. On T2-weighted images, it tends to be heterogeneous and often predominantly hyperintense in signal.

**Chronic Hematoma—Hemosiderin.** The final iron-containing product of hemoglobin degradation is hemosiderin. On T1- and T2-weighted images, both hemosiderin and the fibrous tissue contribute to the very low signal intensity that may be most conspicuous peripherally in chronic hematomas.

As alluded to earlier, one potential pitfall is the misdiagnosis of a hemorrhagic neoplasm as a simple hematoma. Hemorrhage into soft tissue neoplasms can occur de novo or after treatment with irradiation or chemotherapy. Administration of contrast material aids in excluding a neoplasm when the lesion in question shows no enhancement. If the diagnosis of a probably benign hematoma is in doubt, a follow-up MR imaging examination may be required.

**Chronic Expanding Hematoma.** Although the vast majority of hematomas resolve uneventfully, chronic expanding hematomas mimic aggressive neoplasms by virtue of their slow progressive enlargement, large size, deep location, and bone destruction. The self-perpetuating, expanding nature of these lesions may be secondary to the irritant effects of blood and its breakdown products, which in turn cause repeated exudation or bleeding from capillaries in the granulation tissue that has formed. Radiography and CT show a large soft tissue mass that may be associated with eccentric destruction of adjacent bone, sometimes with small dystrophic calcifications that resemble phleboliths. The mass is of predominantly low attenuation on CT. With MR imaging, a peripheral rim of low T2 signal corresponds to the presence of a fibrous pseudocapsule. Centrally, a heterogeneous area of mixed low and high signal intensity on T2-weighted images corresponds to a combination of hemosiderin deposition, fibrous tissue, granulation tissue, and cavities filled with necrotic debris, fibrin, and clots. On T1-weighted images, high signal intensity may be seen. After intravenous gadolinium administration, T1-weighted images show enhancement caused by the presence of capillaries associated with the granulation tissue.

### Common Sites of Intramuscular Hemorrhage

Although most intramuscular hematomas occur in the extremities, two of the most extensively studied sites of hemorrhage are the rectus abdominis and iliopsoas muscles.

**Rectus Sheath Hematoma.** The onset of an intramuscular hematoma at this site may occur without provocation, particularly in patients with abnormalities in coagulation. The majority of rectus sheath hematomas develop below the umbilicus in the lower third of the abdominal wall. With sonography, a rectus sheath hematoma is described most commonly as a hypoechoic lesion enlarging the rectus abdominis muscle that appears spindle-shaped in the longitudinal plane and ovoid in the transverse plane. These hematomas may appear heterogeneous, with blood-fluid levels or internal echogenicity resulting from blood clots. Color Doppler sonography can be useful in excluding the presence of a vascularized neoplasm. With CT, the acute hematoma appears as an ovoid hyperdense area in an enlarged rectus abdominis muscle. CT may also reveal fluid-fluid levels. Chronic hematomas may be isodense or hypodense to surrounding muscle. MR imaging typically demonstrates changes as described earlier.

Symptoms usually resolve within weeks with supportive treatment. Surgery is reserved for cases complicated by uncontrolled hemodynamic instability or infection. Selective angiographic transcatheter embolization has been described in the post-traumatic setting.

**Iliopsoas Hematoma.** The iliopsoas compartment is composed of the psoas and iliacus muscles. The psoas muscle merges with the iliacus muscle at the L5 through S2 levels to form the iliopsoas muscle, which inserts into the lesser trochanter. Because of its craniocaudal extent, the iliopsoas muscle acts as a potential conduit for the communication of pathologic processes from the mediastinum to the upper thigh.

The most common categories of pathologic processes affecting the iliopsoas are hemorrhagic, neoplastic, inflammatory, and traumatic. Differentiation among these processes may be challenging with current imaging techniques. Given their overlapping imaging characteristics, hematoma, neoplasm, and abscess may be impossible to distinguish on the basis of CT alone. Although follow-up imaging examinations and other techniques, particularly MR imaging, may prove helpful, the correct diagnosis is most often facilitated by the relevant clinical history.

### Heterotopic Calcification and Ossification

When analyzing areas of mineralization in muscle or other soft tissues, an astute examiner attempts to differentiate between calcification and ossification. Calcification refers to the precipitation or deposition of substances such as calcium and phosphate. Soft tissue calcifications consistently appear as amorphous, radiodense foci on radiography and CT, although the size and shape of these foci vary.

Heterotopic ossification refers to the formation of non-neoplastic bonelike tissue in any soft tissue location, including skeletal muscle, tendon, fascia, ligament, or other connective tissue. The most common type of heterotopic ossification occurs in muscle and is commonly referred to as myositis ossificans or myositis ossificans traumatica (see Chapter 78). In contrast to calcification, which has an amorphous appearance, the sine qua non of mature myositis ossificans is its recognizable architecture, which approximates that of native bone: an area of centrally located immature trabecular bone surrounded by compact bone peripherally.

### Proliferative Myositis

Proliferative myositis is an uncommon, self-limited intramuscular lesion that has similarities with myositis ossificans. Although it may mimic a sarcoma or infection, proliferative myositis is considered a reactive (rather than a neoplastic) process, and the pathogenesis most likely involves some type of muscle injury or vascular impairment. Recent trauma is recognized in one third of cases. Resection is not indicated, because these lesions heal spontaneously.

Like proliferative fasciitis, its counterpart arising in the fascia and subcutaneous fat, proliferative myositis is a rapidly growing lesion of fibroblastic tissue that is more common in adults than in children. The thigh and chest wall are affected most often by this process, which diffusely infiltrates muscle tissue. Focal ossification may occur, but it is always less prominent than that seen with myositis ossificans. Radiography and CT may demonstrate a small amount of amorphous calcification or ossification associated with an area of soft tissue swelling. CT may also show nonspecific enlargement, poor definition, and slightly diminished attenuation of the affected muscle. MR imaging displays an ill-defined enlargement of muscle that is slightly hypointense on T1-weighted images and hyperintense on T2-weighted images. Perilesional edema and enhancement of the lesion after intravenous contrast administration have also been reported.

### Muscle Herniation

Muscle herniation refers to protrusion of muscle tissue through a focal fascial defect. These fascial defects most commonly occur secondary to muscle hypertrophy and increased intracompartmental pressure, with subsequent herniation of muscle through relatively weak areas in the fascia. Muscle hernias characteristically occur in the middle to lower portions of the leg. The tibialis anterior muscle is most commonly involved.

Clinically, patients typically present with a small, superficial soft tissue bulge that becomes more prominent and firm with muscle contraction. Although most muscle herniations are asymptomatic, they can cause substantial pain, cramping, and tenderness. Fascial defects may also enlarge over time, resulting in cosmetic complaints. Imaging examinations characteristically demonstrate outward bulging of muscle, sometimes with mild irregularity in contour peripherally (Fig. 79–18). Sonography may demonstrate reduction of the herniated muscle when pressure is applied with the transducer. MR imaging may document muscle herniation, as well as discontinuity in the overlying fascia. Both sonography and MR imaging can be performed dynamically during muscle contraction and relaxation, which may increase the conspicuity of fascial tears or herniated muscle tissue.

### Muscle Ischemia and Necrosis

#### Compartment Syndrome

The term compartment syndrome refers to elevated pressure in a relatively noncompliant anatomic space that may result in ischemia and neuromuscular injury. Volkmann's ischemic contracture refers to the sequelae of compartment syndrome, in which fibrous tissue replaces necrotic muscle and nerve tissue. The fundamental

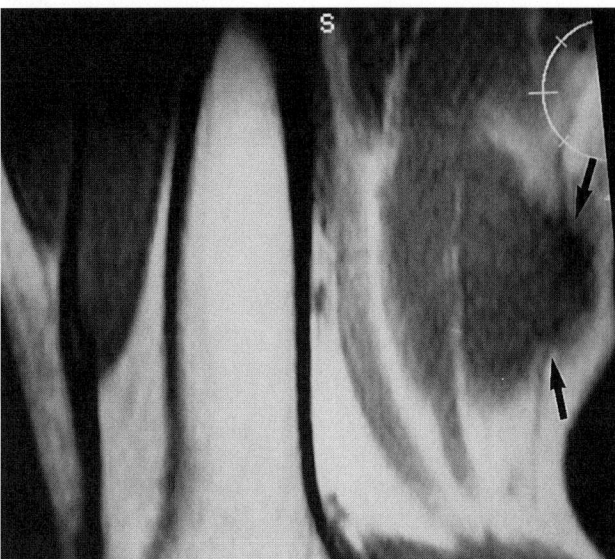

**Figure 79–18.** Muscle herniation. Sagittal T1-weighted spin echo MR image of the distal thigh shows a herniation of the semimembranosus muscle and semitendinosus tendon posteriorly through a defect in the overlying fascia *(arrows)*. This patient was treated with a fascial release. (Courtesy of R. C. Fritz, MD, San Francisco, Calif.)

derangement in patients with compartment syndrome is elevated intracompartmental pressure. A vicious circle can occur in which muscle ischemia results in increased capillary permeability, increased interstitial edema, and increased intramuscular pressure that exceeds the intravascular pressure of small vessels. Regardless of the type of insult, the final result of compartment syndrome is ischemia and, ultimately, tissue necrosis.

Acute compartment syndrome occurs most commonly in male patients younger than 35 years after an acute physical insult, with most cases associated with fractures. Approximately half of these fractures involve the tibia. The second most common cause of compartment syndrome is injury to soft tissues without fracture. Compartment syndrome may affect virtually any noncompliant anatomic compartment. Among the most common sites are the volar compartment of the forearm and the anterior and deep posterior compartments of the leg. Chronic compartment syndrome may occur from exertional causes (e.g., exercise, occupational overuse) or nonexertional causes (e.g., mass lesion, infection). In runners, the most common site of chronic compartment syndrome is the leg. The thigh, forearm, and foot are the next most common sites in athletes.

Patients initially complain of pain. This pain is often described as a sensation of throbbing, aching, cramping, swelling, tightness, or pressure that worsens with palpation and passive stretching of the affected muscles. With acute compartment syndrome, the most important early symptom is pain out of proportion to that expected from the given injury. With chronic exertional compartment syndrome, symptoms typically begin during or immediately after exercise. Direct pressure measurement is usually the procedure of choice to confirm the diagnosis of compartment syndrome. Cross-sectional imaging may complement direct pressure measurements by providing noninvasive data on the compartment or compartments involved. Imaging also helps in the evaluation for an underlying lesion.

CT can show abnormalities such as muscle enlargement and decreased density resulting from edema in patients with acute compartment syndrome. In the chronic setting, major findings include muscle atrophy and fatty infiltration. Both radiography and CT may display sheetlike calcification or ossification in the muscles of patients with a history of compartment syndrome and subsequent myonecrosis (see later discussion).

MR imaging can be used to clarify the location and extent of ischemic damage to muscle. MR imaging findings observed in the setting of acute and chronic compartment syndrome include the following (Fig. 79–19):

1. Increased signal intensity on fat-suppressed T2-weighted images resulting from increased interstitial water or edema (acute or chronic compartment syndrome)

2. Increased signal intensity on T1-weighted images, indicating foci of hemorrhage (acute compartment syndrome) or fatty infiltration (sequela of established compartment syndrome)

3. Decreased signal intensity on T1-weighted images caused by fibrosis (sequela of established compartment syndrome)

4. Increased muscle volume caused by muscle hypertrophy, swelling, or both (acute or chronic compartment syndrome)

5. Decreased muscle volume related to atrophy, fibrosis, or both (sequela of established compartment syndrome)

6. Fascial thickening (sequela of established compartment syndrome)

7. Herniation of muscle through a tear in the surrounding fascia (acute or chronic compartment syndrome)

In patients with impending compartment syndrome, fat-suppressed T1-weighted images after intravenous gadolinium administration show avid contrast enhancement in the affected muscles. This enhancement can be useful in distinguishing between perfused and devitalized muscle.

Although MR imaging may be sensitive in the evaluation of compartment syndrome, it is not specific. Depending on the clinical context, the differential diagnosis may include other causes of painful, swollen extremities such as DOMS, muscle strain, deep venous thrombosis, cellulitis, and lymphedema. Like compartment syndrome, deep venous thrombosis may result in muscle edema, particularly in the deep posterior compartment of the calf. However, unlike compartment syndrome, deep venous thrombosis causes venous occlusion and commonly results in subcutaneous edema and skin thickening, which can all be displayed by sonography and MR imaging. Cellulitis and lymphedema show prominent subcutaneous edema and skin thickening on MR images, but swelling and abnormal signal intensity centered in muscle are often absent.

## Myonecrosis and Rhabdomyolysis

Rhabdomyolysis is defined as the dissolution of skeletal muscle cells caused by insults such as compartment syndrome, blunt trauma, thermal or electrical injury, excessive muscle activity, ischemia, drugs, toxins, infection, inflammation, and congenital enzymatic and metabolic derangements (diabetic muscle infarction is discussed later). Rhabdomyolysis causes the release of myoglobin and toxic intracellular metabolites into the circulation, which results in acute renal failure in 15% to 30% of patients.

Clinically, rhabdomyolysis is characterized by the triad of muscle pain, weakness, and dark brown urine. However, this classic presentation does not occur in the majority of patients, especially early in the disease course, when the patient may complain only of myalgia or weakness. The diagnosis of rhabdomyolysis can be confirmed by detecting myoglobin in the urine or elevated levels of myoglobin in serum. Creatine kinase is thought to be the most sensitive enzyme marker for muscle necrosis, but its concentration can be variable and inconsistent with the degree of muscle damage.

With CT, acute myonecrosis is displayed as diffuse muscle enlargement (attributed to muscle edema), with more sharply marginated intrinsic areas of decreased density at sites of established myonecrosis. Although intravenous contrast material may improve the delineation of avascular areas, it should be avoided in patients who are in danger of renal failure from rhabdomyolysis. Additional CT findings may include hyperdense areas in muscle caused by an acute hematoma or, in the nonacute setting, by dystrophic calcification. MR imaging is the most sensitive method for detecting infarcted musculature. The decreased T1 and increased T2 signal intensity in necrotic muscle reflects the presence of increased water content and increased mobility of water molecules (Fig. 79–20). Repeat MR images often show that these high-intensity areas resolve in parallel with improvement in the clinical course. This reversibility of MR imaging findings suggests that the high-intensity lesions do not reflect permanent myopathic changes but probably represent transient edema in the acute phase of rhabdomyolysis. MR images

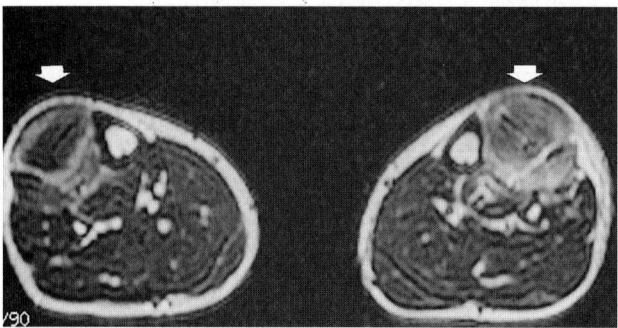

**Figure 79–19.** Compartment syndrome. Transaxial T2-weighted fast spin echo MR image of the legs demonstrates enlarged anterior compartment musculature, with heterogeneous signal intensity and disorganized architecture *(arrows)*.

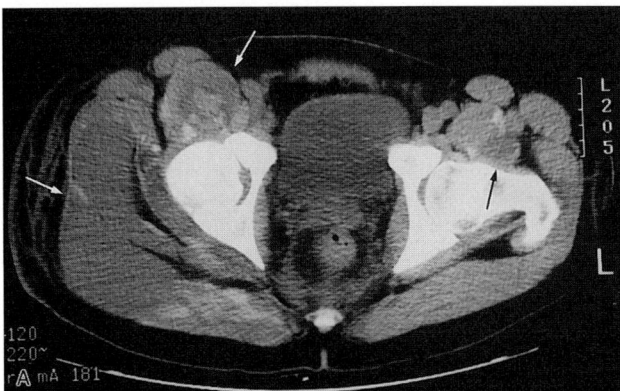

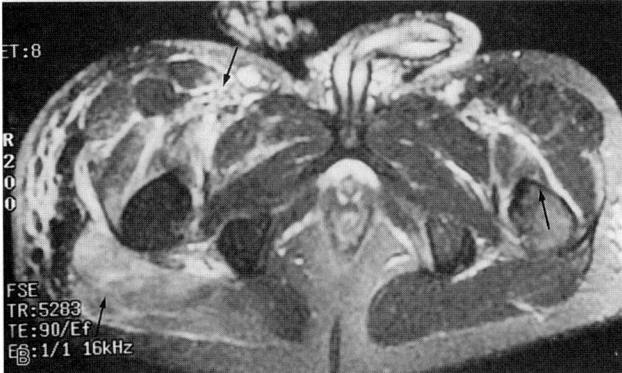

**Figure 79–20.** Rhabdomyolysis. *A*, CT scan performed without contrast material in a patient with acute renal failure shows multiple enlarged muscles of predominantly low attenuation *(arrows)*. *B*, More inferiorly, a transverse fat-suppressed T2-weighted fast spin echo MR image displays ill-defined areas of high signal intensity *(arrows)* in affected muscles and adjacent soft tissues.

acquired without contrast material are not specific, and they may appear identical to the signal intensity changes seen with transient muscle injuries, such as DOMS.

## Calcific Myonecrosis

Calcific myonecrosis is an uncommon late sequela of compartment syndrome that is characterized by cystic degeneration of muscle with plaquelike calcification. Patients present decades after trauma, typically with pain, nerve palsy, or a soft tissue mass in the calf.

Radiographs show a soft tissue mass with dystrophic calcifications involving muscles in the leg. CT and MR imaging demonstrate a fusiform cystic mass with plaque-like peripheral calcifications, most commonly in the anterior compartment of the leg. Calcific tenosynovitis has also been reported in association with calcific myonecrosis. Features mimicking a soft tissue neoplasm include the large size, heterogeneous appearance, and peripheral enhancement of the soft tissue lesion and the smooth, eccentric erosion of bone (Fig. 79–21).

## Diabetic Muscle Infarction

Diabetic muscle infarction is probably caused by extensive thrombosis of small and medium-sized arterioles due to hypercoagulability and associated vascular endothelial damage. The typical patient is middle-aged with poorly controlled or long-standing diabetes. Patients usually present with an abrupt onset of substantial pain that occurs at rest and is exacerbated by movement. The most commonly affected muscles are in the thigh (>80% of patients) and the calf (approximately 15% of patients).

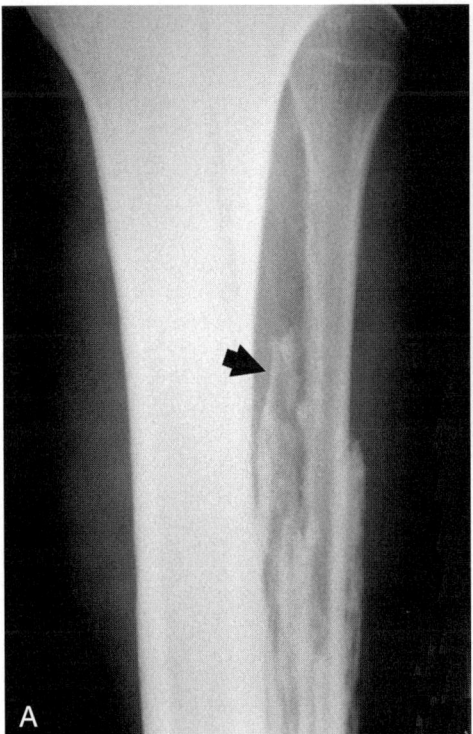

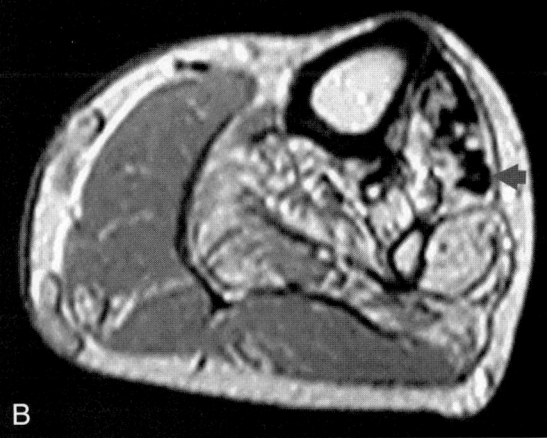

**Figure 79–21.** Calcific myonecrosis. This 44-year-old man had a remote history of post-traumatic compartment syndrome. *A*, Anteroposterior radiograph of the proximal lower leg shows the typical fusiform mass with linear plaquelike calcification *(arrow)*. *B*, Axial proton density (TR/TE, 2350/20) spin echo MR image shows marked muscle atrophy with fatty overgrowth. Note the calcification *(arrow)*.

Muscle infarction in diabetic patients commonly involves multiple muscles and is often bilateral.

CT without intravenous contrast administration typically reveals nonfocal edema in the subcutaneous fat, obscuration of the intermuscular fat planes by inflammation, and enlargement of edematous muscles that may exhibit decreased attenuation. Contrast-enhanced CT may demonstrate a low-attenuation lesion with peripheral enhancement.

MR imaging is generally the test of choice for evaluating diabetic patients with suspected muscle infarction. The acute edema and inflammatory changes caused by muscle infarction are displayed as intermediate signal intensity on T1-weighted images and high signal intensity on T2-weighted, fast spin echo inversion recovery, and gadolinium-enhanced MR images (Fig. 79–22). The pattern of contrast enhancement seen with MR imaging can be diffuse, often with focal areas of low signal intensity that display peripheral enhancement. The common appearance of diffuse enhancement suggests to

some investigators that this entity may be more correctly described as diabetic muscle ischemia, whereas the inconsistently seen areas of low signal intensity with rim enhancement on fat-suppressed T1-weighted images actually correspond to macroscopic areas of muscle infarction. MR imaging is considered essentially 100% sensitive and allows the diagnosis of diabetes-related muscle infarction in the appropriate clinical setting.

## Infectious, Inflammatory, and Idiopathic Acquired Myopathies

The term myositis refers to inflammation of muscle, regardless of its infectious or noninfectious cause. This section reviews the infectious entities known as pyomyositis, necrotizing fasciitis, and human immunodeficiency virus (HIV) infection. Inflammation in muscle may also occur by nonsuppurative autoimmune or idiopathic mechanisms, as is seen with sarcoid myopathy, polymyositis, dermatomyositis, and inclusion body myositis.

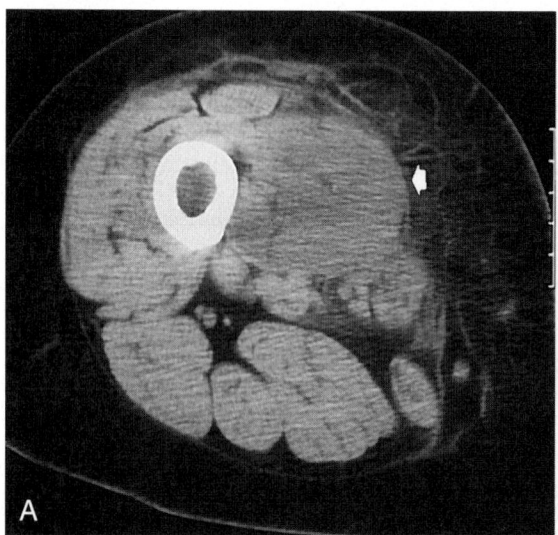

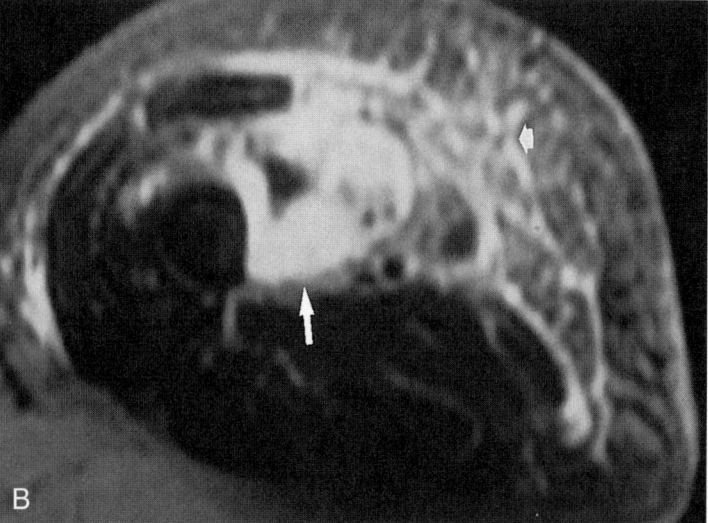

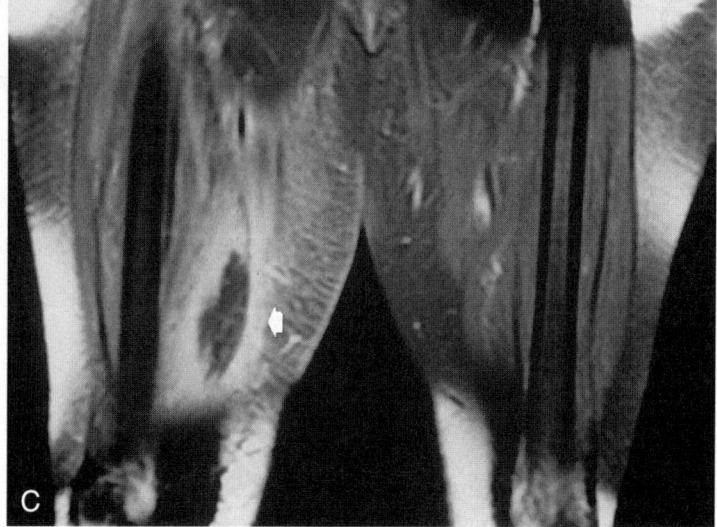

**Figure 79–22.** Diabetic muscle infarction. *A*, CT scan shows enlargement and decreased attenuation in the vastus medialis muscle *(arrow)*, with minimal stranding in the overlying subcutaneous fat, owing to diabetic muscle infarction. *B*, Transverse fat-suppressed T2-weighted fast spin echo MR image demonstrates enlargement and high signal intensity in the vastus medialis muscle *(long arrow)* with increased signal intensity more superficially, indicative of perifascial fluid and subcutaneous edema *(short arrow)*. *C*, Coronal fat-suppressed T1-weighted spin echo MR image after intravenous gadolinium administration reveals a peripheral area of enhancement *(arrow)*. (Courtesy of J. Newman, MD, Boston, Mass.)

## Pyomyositis

Pyomyositis is a primary bacterial (pyogenic) infection of skeletal muscle that rapidly leads to abscess formation. Pyomyositis can be classified as tropical (more common) or temperate (less common). Tropical pyomyositis is endemic to tropical and subtropical areas, where the typical patient is a boy or young man. In temperate climates, such as those in North America and Europe, pyomyositis is less common but afflicts a broader age range of patients.

Although skeletal muscle is generally highly resistant to metastatic infection, specific risk factors for infection have been reported; most commonly, they include some form of immunosuppression or trauma. In the tropics, primary risk factors are HIV and other infections, minor trauma, and malnutrition. In temperate locations, chronic concurrent conditions, including HIV infection, diabetes, and corticosteroid usage, are common risk factors. *Staphylococcus aureus* is the most common pathogen. The typical symptoms and signs of pyomyositis are progressive muscle aches, pain, swelling, erythema, tenderness, and fever. The most frequent presentation is involvement of a single muscle in the thigh, calf, or buttock.

Imaging techniques help delineate the location and extent of pyomyositis and are key to a prompt and accurate diagnosis (Fig. 79–23). Findings observed with cross-sectional imaging techniques generally include muscle enlargement, effacement of intramuscular and intermuscular fat planes, enhancement in the inflamed region after intravenous contrast administration, and a focal fluid collection that may contain septations. Although a purulent fluid collection is usually detected, this is not always the case. With MR imaging, some muscle abscesses show a rim of increased T1 and decreased T2 signal intensity at the margin between the drainable pus and the edematous muscle. Associated findings related to the presence of cellulitis are often observed, including skin thickening, stranding in the subcutaneous fat, and distention of the subcutaneous veins. The presence of cellulitis is a prominent and consistent feature of infectious processes and may militate against the diagnosis of neoplasm (assuming that no surgery or radiation therapy has been performed). MR images may show abnormal signal in the adjacent bone marrow because of the presence of reactive inflammatory changes or coexisting osteomyelitis.

### Necrotizing Fasciitis

Fasciitis refers to inflammation of fascia, the sheets of fibrous tissue that surround muscle compartments and separate different layers of soft tissue. Necrotizing fasciitis is a relatively rare, rapidly progressive, life-threatening bacterial infection involving the fascia. The single most commonly isolated pathogen is group A streptococcus, although polymicrobial infection may occur.

Necrotizing fasciitis is characterized by necrosis predominantly in the superficial fascia and subcutaneous fat; initially, it is not centered inside the muscle, although secondary involvement of muscle is not uncommon. The most common predisposing factors are trauma and an immunocompromised state. Seemingly innocuous events may also be implicated, such as a simple contusion. Clinically, the distinction among early necrotizing fasciitis, uncomplicated infectious fasciitis, and even common soft tissue infection may be challenging. Patients with necrotizing fasciitis typically experience considerable pain, redness, swelling, and fever, which may be followed by fulminant systemic deterioration. Invasive streptococcal infections are associated with a toxic shock syndrome in 10% of patients. Although dusky skin or purplish patches have been reported as typical, the infection can spread unrecognized along fascial planes beneath seemingly normal skin.

Radiographs commonly reveal soft tissue swelling and gas. Although the presence of soft tissue gas is a hallmark finding, it is not universal. Gas is produced most commonly from a mixed infection of aerobic and anaerobic bacteria, rather than from a classic gas-forming organism. Sonographic findings include thickened, distorted fascia and adjacent fluid accumulation. Compared with sonography, contrast-enhanced CT provides better definition of the extent of disease and complications, particularly in areas that are difficult to evaluate by sonography. CT features include fascial thickening, edematous changes in muscle and adipose tissue, soft tissue gas, and focal fluid collections.

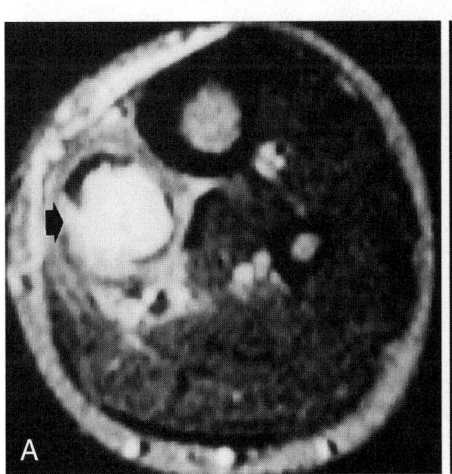
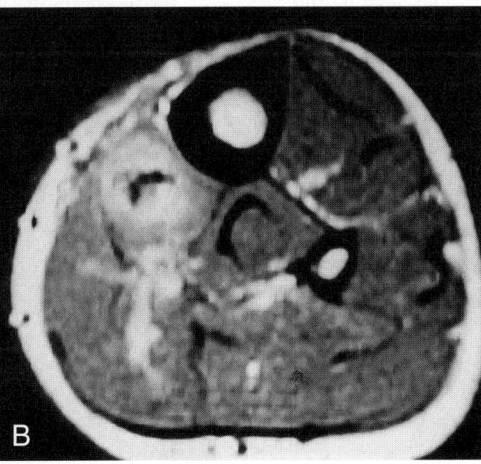

**Figure 79–23.** Pyomyositis. *A*, Transverse T2-weighted fast spin echo MR image in an HIV-positive patient demonstrates high signal intensity involving the tibialis posterior and flexor digitorum longus muscles *(arrow)*, owing to pyomyositis. The surrounding, more ill-defined hyperintensity is indicative of soft tissue edema. *B*, Transverse T1-weighted spin echo MR image (proximal to *A*) after intravenous contrast administration shows enhancement in an adjacent area of myositis. The central portion of the abscess did not enhance.

Diagnostic criteria for necrotizing fasciitis on T2-weighted MR images include thickening, edematous changes, and contrast enhancement in the deep fascia, subcutaneous fat, and often muscle. Superimposed areas of necrosis or abscess formation are identified as areas of hyperintense T2 signal that do not enhance centrally after the intravenous administration of contrast material. Although contrast material may improve diagnostic confidence by delineating abscesses and areas of necrosis more clearly, additional lesions usually are not detected on contrast-enhanced examinations. In contrast to necrotizing fasciitis, cellulitis is diagnosed when soft tissue stranding, thickening, edematous changes, and abnormal contrast enhancement are confined to the subcutis and superficial fascia (Fig. 79–24). Although several investigators have concluded that MR imaging facilitates the differentiation between necrotizing and non-necrotizing soft tissue infections, other investigators have emphasized the nonspecific nature of signal intensity changes on T2-weighted and gadolinium-enhanced MR images.

## Human Immunodeficiency Virus Infection

Skeletal muscle involvement can occur at any stage of HIV infection, and it may be the first manifestation of the disease in some patients. In addition to soft tissue neoplasia, muscle involvement in HIV-infected patients can be divided into several categories, including infectious myositis, HIV-associated myopathy, zidovudine (AZT)-associated myopathy, HIV wasting syndrome, and HIV-associated rhabdomyolysis.

**Infectious Myositis.** Patients may present with mild constitutional symptoms or with exquisite pain. Physical examination may reveal modest muscle swelling or "wooden" stiffness of the tissues in one or more areas. MR imaging is helpful in the detection and characterization of various infections in HIV-infected patients, including the presence or absence of a drainable abscess (Fig. 79–25). The most common pathogen is *S. aureus*.

**HIV-Associated Myopathy.** HIV-associated myopathy is characterized by symptoms similar to those of idiopathic inflammatory myopathies seen in HIV-negative patients. Like patients with polymyositis, those with HIV-associated myopathy typically present with bilateral, symmetrical proximal muscle weakness and an elevated serum creatine kinase concentration. Although HIV does not directly infect myocytes, the virus is found in inflammatory cells surrounding myocytes. As with other myopathies, MR imaging demonstrates high signal intensity particularly well on fat-suppressed T2-weighted and fast spin echo inversion recovery images.

**AZT-Associated Myopathy.** AZT inhibits HIV replication. A potential side effect of this treatment is AZT-associated myopathy, which is a progressive, usually painful condition that causes pronounced muscle wasting, especially in the proximal appendicular skeleton. MR imaging may show nonspecific, abnormally increased T2 signal intensity in affected muscle. Symptoms typically resolve within 4 to 6 weeks after administration of AZT is halted.

**HIV-Associated Rhabdomyolysis.** Acute renal failure syndromes are encountered relatively frequently in patients with HIV infection. Rhabdomyolysis is a common cause of acute renal failure and may be related to a variety of predisposing factors. Although no single cause of rhabdomyolysis has been identified in patients with HIV infection, antiviral medications have been implicated in

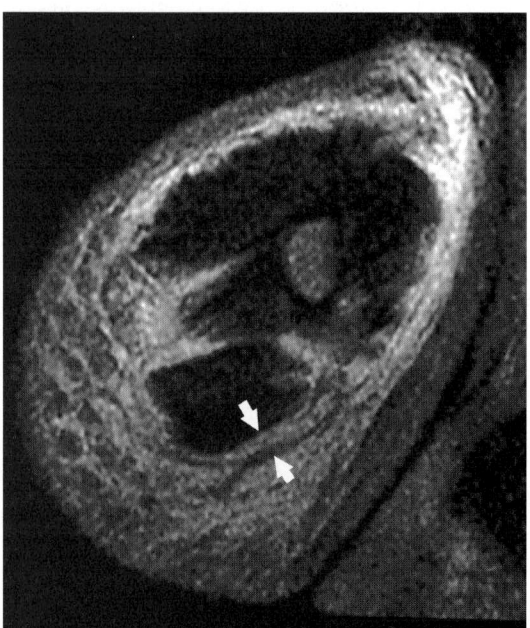

**Figure 79–24.** Necrotizing fasciitis in a 27-year-old woman with systemic lupus erythematosus. Axial T2-weighted (TR/TE, 2250/88) spin echo MR image shows marked fascial thickening (*arrows*), with associated cellulitis. Muscle is relatively spared.

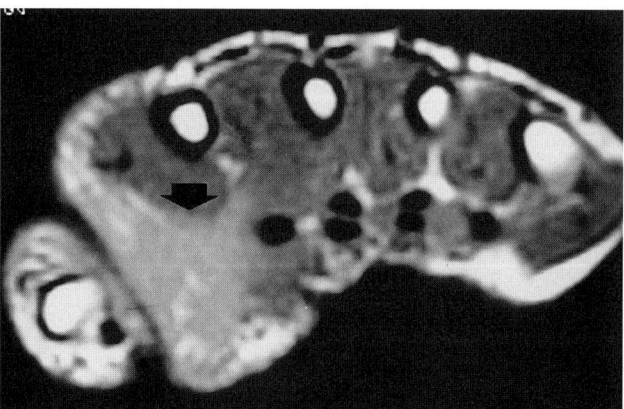

**Figure 79–25.** HIV-associated granulomatous infectious myositis. Transverse intermediate-weighted fast spin echo MR image demonstrates high signal intensity in the abductor pollicis brevis muscle (*arrow*), owing to myositis. No abscess was present.

many cases. MR imaging may be used to document the distribution of rhabdomyolysis and to guide biopsy. With prompt supportive care, the prognosis of acute rhabdomyolysis in this population is reasonably good.

## Sarcoid Myopathy

Sarcoidosis is an idiopathic multisystem disease with truly protean manifestations that is characterized by the presence of noncaseating granulomas. This disease is discussed in Chapter 80.

## Idiopathic Inflammatory Myopathies

The idiopathic inflammatory myopathies (IIMs) are a heterogeneous group of diseases characterized by non-suppurative inflammation in muscle. Although the causes of IIMs are unknown, the favored hypothesis is that they result from immune-mediated damage occurring in the muscles of genetically susceptible persons. For most IIMs, women are affected at least twice as often as men. The most common types of IIMs in adults are polymyositis, dermatomyositis, and inclusion body myositis; other less common types include focal myositis, idiopathic eosinophilic fasciitis, and macrophagic myofasciitis.

Currently, the diagnosis of IIMs is often difficult and can be accomplished only after excluding other causes of myopathy, including infectious, toxic, metabolic, endocrinologic, and dystrophic entities. The subsequent diagnosis of an IIM relies on the detection of clinical, laboratory, electromyographic, histopathologic, and MR imaging abnormalities (Table 79–8). The cardinal symptom of IIMs is the insidious onset of progressive bilateral weakness affecting the proximal musculature, most often in the hip and shoulder girdle regions. Other nonspecific findings include fatigue, myalgias, and muscle atrophy.

MR imaging may be the most sensitive and specific examination for the evaluation of myositis. Abnormal signal intensity is observed in the skeletal muscles of almost all patients. With acute myopathies, signal intensity abnormalities indicative of edema are visible (Fig. 79–26). With chronic myopathies, fatty replacement is commonly observed (Fig. 79–27). Assessment for muscle edema and adiposity can be facilitated by the use of T1-weighted images in combination with corresponding fat-suppressed fast spin echo T2-weighted or fast spin echo inversion recovery images.

In patients with a suspected IIM, biopsy directed by MR imaging is a useful, cost-effective alternative to blind biopsy. MR imaging facilitates the selection of an appropriate biopsy site by displaying areas with the most edema and the least atrophy. These areas usually have active disease and produce the best diagnostic yield on histopathologic examination. Specific myopathies are discussed in Chapter 25.

## Heritable Disorders Affecting Muscle

### Muscular Dystrophies

The term muscular dystrophy refers to a heterogeneous group of heritable disorders characterized by progressive

---

| **TABLE 79–8** |
| --- |
| **Diagnosis of Idiopathic Inflammatory Myopathies\*** |

Clinical
  Bilateral muscle weakness with a predilection for proximal muscles†
  Typical skin rash of dermatomyositis (e.g., Gottron's papule, Gottron's sign, heliotrope rash)
Laboratory
  Serum enzyme elevation (e.g., creatine kinase, aldolase, transaminases)†
  Myositis-specific autoantibodies (e.g., anti-Jo-1, anti-Mi-2)‡
Electromyography
  Abnormal electrical activity in muscle (e.g., myopathic motor unit potentials, positive sharp waves, fibrillations)
Pathology
  Muscle biopsy (e.g., inflammatory infiltration, perifascicular atrophy, fiber degeneration)

---

\*After excluding other causes of myopathy (e.g., infectious, toxic, metabolic, endocrinologic, dystrophic), the following criteria may be used as diagnostic guidelines. The diagnosis of idiopathic inflammatory myopathy is "possible" if two criteria are satisfied, "probable" if three criteria are satisfied, and "definite" if four criteria are satisfied.

†MR imaging demonstration of edema in muscles may be substituted for the diagnostic criterion of proximal muscle weakness or serum enzyme elevation.

‡Myositis-specific autoantibodies are detected in approximately 20% to 85% of patients with idiopathic inflammatory myopathies. These autoantibodies help define specific subtypes of disease that have different prognoses and responses to medication.

Adapted from Targoff IN, Miller FW, Medsger TA Jr, Oddis CV: Classification criteria for the idiopathic inflammatory myopathies. Curr Opin Rheum 9:527, 1997.

---

muscle weakness and loss of muscle tissue. By convention, these disorders are distinguished empirically on the basis of several factors, the most common of which are the age at which symptoms appear, the types of symptoms that develop, the muscles affected, the expected prognosis, and the type of inheritance (e.g., via autosomal dominant genes).

Recent discoveries of new genes and their protein products have led to renewed interest in the microscopic structure of muscle and called into question the traditional clinical classification of the muscular dystrophies. Despite the promise of more precise nosology based on genetics and the dysfunction of muscle cell proteins, this section focuses primarily on three prototypes of muscular dystrophy known by the traditional names Duchenne's muscular dystrophy, Becker's muscular dystrophy, and facioscapulohumeral muscular dystrophy. Numerous other muscular dystrophies have also been described.

**Duchenne's Muscular Dystrophy.** The most common type of muscular dystrophy is Duchenne's muscular dystrophy, an X-linked recessive disorder that affects 20 to 30 males per 100,000 individuals. Females may carry the gene for this disorder, but they rarely develop any symptoms. Although it is an inherited disorder, spontaneous mutations account for one third of cases. Symptoms usually arise before the age of 6 years and include muscle weakness, wasting, and contractures. These abnormalities

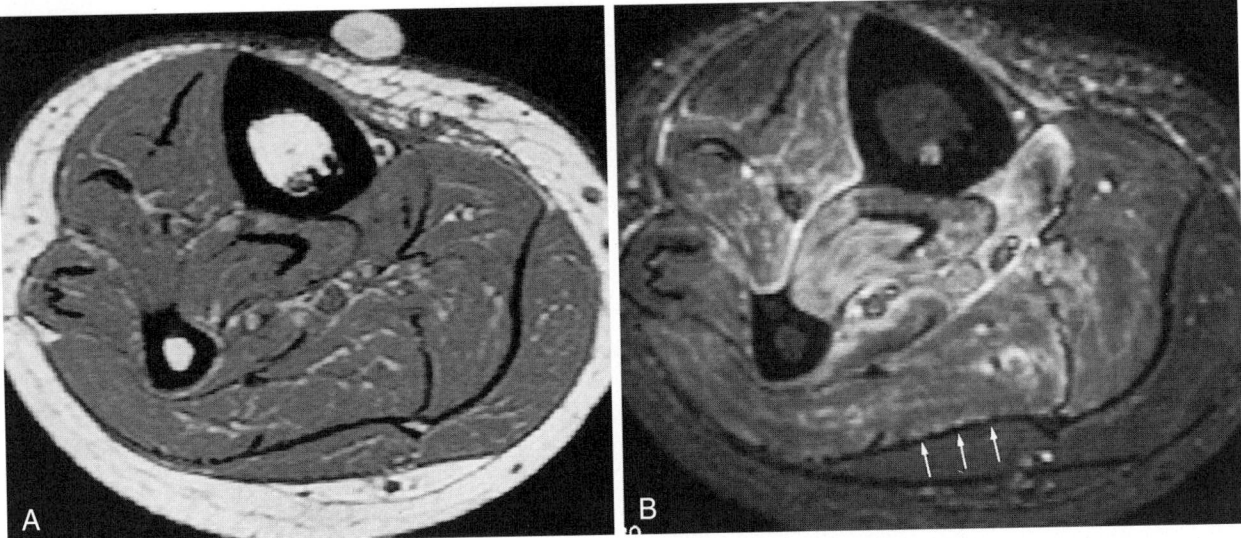

**Figure 79–26.** Acute polymyositis. *A,* Transverse T1-weighted spin echo MR image appears essentially normal. *B,* Transverse fast spin echo inversion recovery MR image shows extensive high signal intensity in the muscles of the leg *(arrows),* which guided the selection of an appropriate biopsy site.

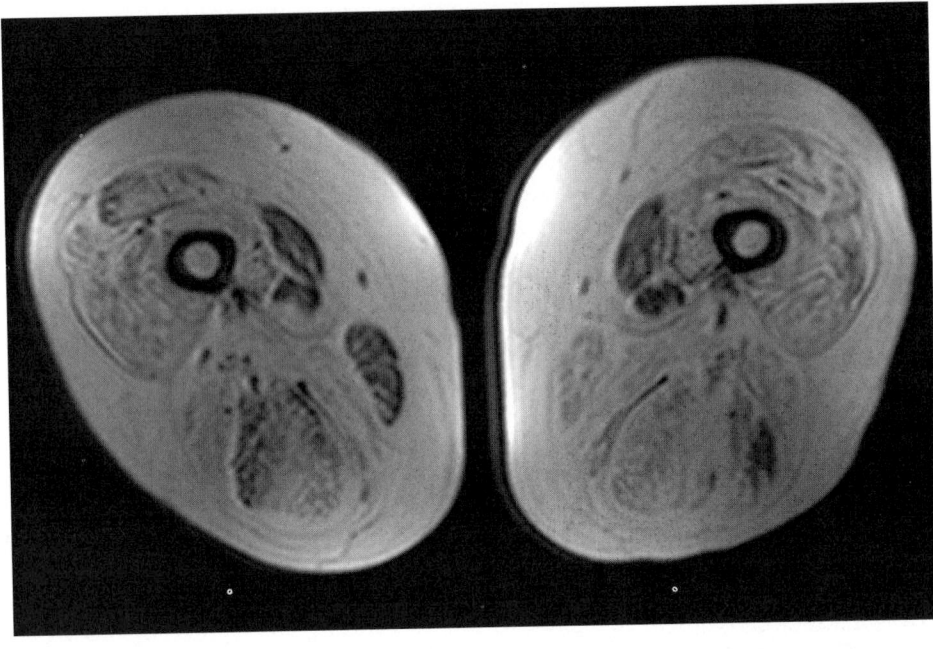

**Figure 79–27.** Chronic myositis. Axial T1-weighted (TR/TE, 748/17) spin echo MR image shows extensive fatty replacement of muscle, which is relatively symmetrical bilaterally.

preferentially affect muscles in the pelvis and lower extremities, especially the hip and knee extensors. In the calf muscles, characteristic replacement of muscle tissue by fat and connective tissue results in pseudohypertrophy. Disability progresses relatively rapidly, so that by age 12 years, most patients with Duchenne's muscular dystrophy are confined to a wheelchair. Common complications of the disease are intellectual retardation, cardiomyopathy, and pneumonitis. This rapidly progressive form of muscular dystrophy usually results in death from respiratory complications by age 15 years.

**Becker's Muscular Dystrophy.** Becker's muscular dystrophy is regarded as less common and less severe than Duchenne's muscular dystrophy. Although the symptoms and signs of Becker's muscular dystrophy are very similar to those of Duchenne's, they begin later and progress more slowly. For example, most patients can ambulate until at least age 16 years. Death typically does not occur until the fourth decade of life, when patients often succumb to cardiopulmonary complications.

**Facioscapulohumeral Muscular Dystrophy.** This disorder is characterized by the insidious onset of progressive muscle weakness and wasting. Because it is an autosomal dominant disorder, men and women are affected equally (prevalence, 5 per 100,000 people). Unlike Duchenne's and Becker's muscular dystrophy, facioscapulohumeral muscular dystrophy targets the upper body, primarily affecting the face, shoulder, and upper arm muscles. The age at onset and the extent and severity of symptoms are extremely variable. Winging deformity of the scapula is characteristic. Intellectual, cardiac, and pulmonary functions are typically normal.

**Imaging Techniques.** Imaging has been used to monitor the presence, location, extent, and progression of muscular dystrophy. With Duchenne's and Becker's muscular dystrophy, early involvement tends to target the gastrocnemius, quadriceps, biceps femoris, gluteus maximus, and gluteus medius muscles. Lower extremity muscles tend to be spared. By comparison, with limb-girdle muscular dystrophy, the highest degree of fat replacement is in the soleus, tibialis anterior, and peroneal muscles; the gastrocnemius and tibialis posterior muscles tend to be less affected. The reason for this particular distribution of muscle involvement, which may be asymmetrical, is not understood. MR imaging is considered the premier method for determining the volume and location of muscle and fat in patients with muscular dystrophy. Early in the course of muscular dystrophy, increased signal intensity on fat-suppressed T2-weighted and fast spin echo inversion recovery images is displayed in affected muscles, presumably because of interstitial edema. Later in the course of the disease, increased T1 signal intensity is indicative of fatty infiltration in diseased muscle and is often accompanied by decreased muscle bulk.

## Chronic Neuromuscular Diseases

Chronic neuromuscular diseases are commonly classified according to the pathologic mechanism or distribution of affected nerves. They include motor neuron diseases, heritable motor and sensory neuropathies, inflammatory neuropathies, and toxic neuropathies. This section focuses on postpolio syndrome and heritable motor and sensory neuropathies, which are two of the most common types of chronic neuromuscular disorders seen in patients undergoing imaging examinations.

**Postpolio Syndrome.** The term postpolio syndrome refers to the neuromuscular symptoms developed by some patients many years after experiencing acute poliomyelitis. New muscle weakness and premature fatigue are two cardinal symptoms. Both CT and MR imaging have been applied to the study of patients with postpolio syndrome (Fig. 79–28). Imaging findings include regions of muscle atrophy that are often large and may involve all extremities. The innervation of muscles in patients with postpolio syndrome may differ from limb to limb or even within the same limb, owing to the segmental nature of the initial involvement.

**Heritable Motor and Sensory Neuropathies.** The heritable motor and sensory neuropathies, also termed Charcot-Marie-Tooth disease, are a diverse group of disorders that are classified based on clinical abnormalities, electromyographic findings, histopathologic results, and genetic features. Accurate classification is becoming more complicated, however, as the number of different mutations implicated in these conditions increases at a rapid rate. A common mutation involves a gene coding for myelin and results in the delayed ability to walk. Lower extremity muscle weakness is common, but patients often remain ambulatory and experience a normal life span. CT or MR imaging techniques demonstrate muscle atrophy targeting the lower extremities (Fig. 79–29). This atrophy is bilateral but may be asymmetrical. The pattern of atrophy is variable and may be patchy or diffuse. Classically, the most profound atrophy is located in the lateral compartment of the midcalf and more diffusely in the distal calf.

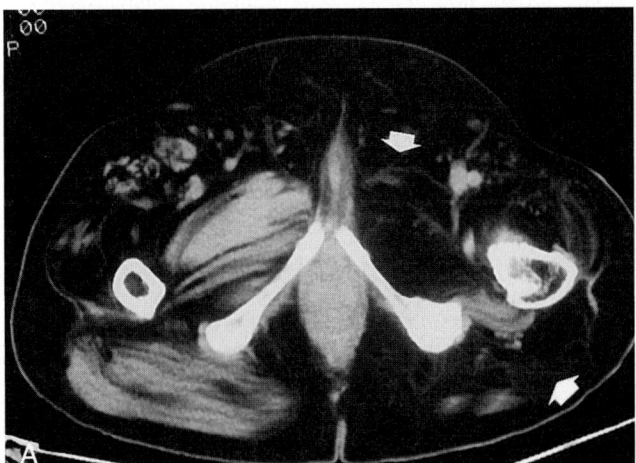
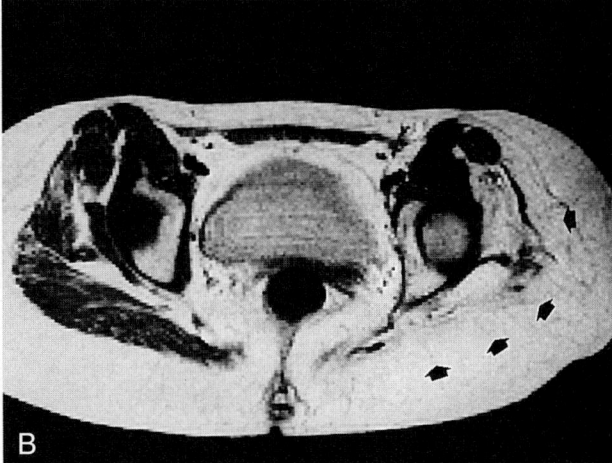

**Figure 79–28.** Postpolio syndrome. *A*, CT scan demonstrates extensive atrophy of the gluteal and adductor musculature *(arrows)* in the left hemipelvis, owing to prior poliomyelitis infection. *B*, Transverse intermediate-weighted fast spin echo MR image in a different patient shows dramatic atrophy of the gluteal musculature *(arrows)* in the left hemipelvis.

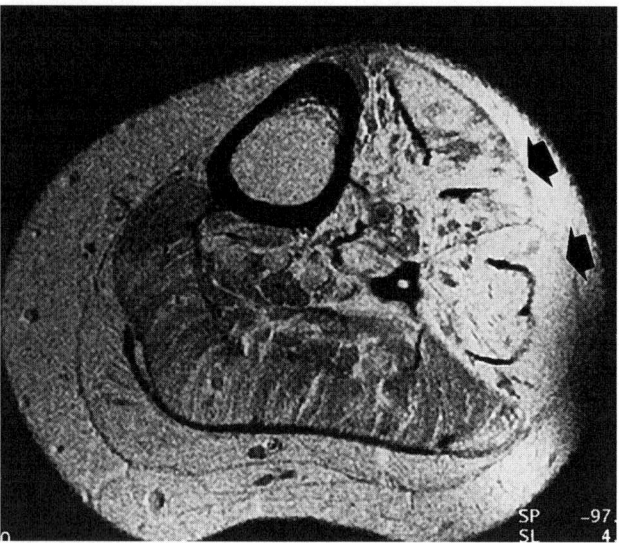

**Figure 79–29.** Heritable motor and sensory neuropathy. Transverse intermediate-weighted fast spin echo MR image of the leg shows dramatic atrophy, particularly affecting the musculature of the anterior and lateral compartments *(arrows)*, owing to Charcot-Marie-Tooth disease.

## FURTHER READING

Adams EM, Chow CK, Premkumar A, Plotz PH: The idiopathic inflammatory myopathies: Spectrum of MR imaging findings. Radiographics 15:563, 1995.

Akman I, Ostrov B, Varma BK, Keenan G: Pyomyositis: Report of three patients and review of the literature. Clin Pediatr (Phila) 35:397, 1996.

Almdahl SM, Due J Jr, Samdal FA: Compartment syndrome with muscle necrosis following repair of hernia of tibialis anterior: Case report. Acta Chir Scand 153:695, 1987.

Anderson MW, Temple HT, Dussault RG, Kaplan PA: Compartmental anatomy: Relevance to staging and biopsy of musculoskeletal tumors. AJR Am J Roentgenol 173:1663, 1999.

Aoki T, Nakata H, Watanabe H, et al: The radiological findings in chronic expanding hematoma. Skeletal Radiol 28:396, 1999.

Bartlett ML, Ginn L, Beitz L, et al: Quantitative assessment of myositis in thigh muscles using magnetic resonance imaging. Magn Reson Imaging 17:183, 1999.

Berna JD, Zuazu I, Madrigal M, et al: Conservative treatment of large rectus sheath hematoma in patients undergoing anticoagulant therapy. Abdom Imaging 25:230, 2000.

Bird TD, Kraft GH, Lipe HP, et al: Clinical and pathological phenotype of the original family with Charcot-Marie-Tooth type 1B: A 20-year study. Ann Neurol 41:463, 1997.

Boles CA, Kannam S, Cardwell AB: The forearm: Anatomy of muscle compartments and nerves. AJR Am J Roentgenol 174:151, 2000.

Braunstein JT, Crues JV 3rd: Magnetic resonance imaging of hereditary hernias of the peroneus longus muscle. Skeletal Radiol 24:601, 1995.

Bush CH: The magnetic resonance imaging of musculoskeletal hemorrhage. Skeletal Radiol 29:1, 2000.

Campellone JV, Lacomis D, Giuliani MJ, Oddis CV: Percutaneous needle muscle biopsy in the evaluation of patients with suspected inflammatory myopathy. Arthritis Rheum 40:1886, 1997.

Chason DP, Fleckenstein JL, Burns DK, et al: Diabetic muscle infarction: Radiologic evaluation. Skeletal Radiol 25:127, 1996.

Chiedozi LC: Pyomyositis: Review of 205 cases in 112 patients. Am J Surg 137:255, 1979.

Connell DA, Potter HG, Sherman NT, Wickiewicz TL: Injuries of the pectoralis major muscle: Evaluation with MR imaging. Radiology 210:785, 1999.

Delfaut EM, Beltran J, Johnson G, et al: Fat suppression in MR imaging: Techniques and pitfalls. Radiographics 19:373, 1999.

De Smet AA: Magnetic resonance findings in skeletal muscle tears. Skeletal Radiol 22:479, 1993.

De Smet AA, Best TM: MR imaging of the distribution and location of acute hamstring injuries in athletes. AJR Am J Roentgenol 174:393, 2000.

De Smet AA, Fisher DR, Heiner JP, Keene JS: Magnetic resonance imaging of muscle tears. Skeletal Radiol 19:283, 1990.

Doyle JR: Anatomy of the upper extremity muscle compartments. Hand Clin 14:343, 1998.

El-Khoury GY, Brandser EA, Kathol MH, et al: Imaging of muscle injuries. Skeletal Radiol 25:3, 1996.

Enzinger FM, Weiss SW: Benign fibrous tissue tumors. In Enzinger FM, Weiss SW (eds): Soft Tissue Tumors, 3rd ed. St Louis, Mosby, 1995, p 165.

Finkelstein JA, Hunter GA, Hu RW: Lower limb compartment syndrome: Course after delayed fasciotomy. J Trauma 40:342, 1996.

Fontes RA Jr, Ogilvie CM, Miclau T: Necrotizing soft-tissue infections. J Am Acad Orthop Surg 8:151, 2000.

Garrett WE, Best TM: Anatomy, physiology, and mechanics of skeletal muscle. In Simon SR (ed): Orthopaedic Basic Science. Rosemont, Ill, American Academy of Orthopaedic Surgeons, 1994, p 89.

Goldberg JS, London WL, Nagel DM: Tropical pyomyositis: A case report and review. Pediatrics 63:298, 1979.

Hansmann Y, Christmann D: Group A streptococcus pyomyositis. Presse Med 27:110, 1998.

Hinton A, Heinrich SD, Craver R: Idiopathic diabetic muscular infarction: The role of ultrasound, CT, NM, and biopsy. Orthopedics 16:623, 1993.

Holscher RS, Leyten FS, Oudenhoven LF, Puylaert JB: Percutaneous decompression of an iliopsoas hematoma. Abdom Imaging 22:114, 1997.

Hutchinson MR, Ireland ML: Common compartment syndromes in athletes: Treatment and rehabilitation. Sports Med 17:200, 1994.

Janzen DL, Connell DG, Vaisler BJ: Calcific myonecrosis of the calf manifesting as an enlarging soft-tissue mass: Imaging features. AJR Am J Roentgenol 160:1072, 1993.

Jelinek JS, Murphey MD, Aboulafia AJ, et al: Muscle infarction in patients with diabetes mellitus: MR imaging findings. Radiology 211:241, 1999.

Joshi MK, Liu HH: Acute rhabdomyolysis and renal failure in HIV-infected patients: Risk factors, presentation, and pathophysiology. AIDS Patient Care STDs 14:541, 2000.

Lefere P, Gryspeerdt S, Van Holsbeeck B, Baekelandt M: Diagnosis and treatment of expanding haematoma of the lateral abdominal wall after blunt abdominal trauma. Eur Radiol 9:1553, 1999.

Liu GC, Jong YJ, Chiang CH, Jaw TS: Duchenne muscular dystrophy: MR grading system with functional correlation. Radiology 186:475, 1993.

Masanes F, Pedrol E, Grau JM, et al: Symptomatic myopathies in HIV-1 infected patients untreated with antiretroviral agents: A clinico-pathological study of 30 consecutive patients. Clin Neuropathol 15:221, 1996.

McQueen MM, Gaston P, Court-Brown CM: Acute compartment syndrome: Who is at risk? J Bone Joint Surg Br 82:200, 2000.

Mellado JM, Perez del Palomar L: Muscle hernias of the lower leg: MRI findings. Skeletal Radiol 28:465, 1999.

Mohler LR, Styf JR, Pedowitz RA, et al: Intramuscular deoxygenation during exercise in patients who have chronic anterior compartment syndrome of the leg. J Bone Joint Surg Am 79:844, 1997.

Mulier S, Stas M, Delabie J, et al: Proliferative myositis in a child. Skeletal Radiol 28:703, 1999.

Nonaka I: Distal myopathies. Curr Opin Neurol 12:493, 1999.

Nordgren B, Falck B, Stalberg E, et al: Postpolio muscular dysfunction: Relationships between muscle energy metabolism, subjective symptoms, magnetic resonance imaging, electromyography, and muscle strength. Muscle Nerve 20:1341, 1997.

Olsen NJ, Park JH: Inflammatory myopathies: Issues in diagnosis and management. Arthritis Care Res 10:200, 1997.

Owens S, Edwards P, Miles K, et al: Chronic compartment syndrome affecting the lower limb: MIBI perfusion imaging as an alternative to pressure monitoring. Two case reports. Br J Sports Med 33:49, 1999.

Palmer WE, Kuong SJ, Elmadbouh HM: MR imaging of myotendinous strain. AJR Am J Roentgenol 173:703, 1999.

Petersilge CA, Pathria MN, Gentili A, et al: Denervation hypertrophy of muscle: MR features. J Comput Assist Tomogr 19:596, 1995.

Reimers CD, Fischer P, Pongratz DE: Histopathological basis of muscle imaging. In Fleckenstein JL, Crues JV, Reimers CD (eds): Muscle Imaging in Health and Disease. New York, Springer, 1996, p 183.

Renwick SE, Naraghi FF, Worrell RV, Spaeth J: Cystic degeneration and calcification of muscle: Late sequelae of compartment syndrome. J Orthop Trauma 8:440, 1994.

Rocca PV, Alloway JA, Hashel DJ: Diabetic muscle infarction. Semin Arthritis Rheum 22:280, 1993.

Rubin DA, Kneeland JB: MR imaging of the musculoskeletal system: Technical considerations for enhancing image quality and diagnostic yield. AJR Am J Roentgenol 163:1155, 1994.

Rubin JI, Gomori JM, Grossman RI, et al: High-field MR imaging of extracranial hematomas. AJR Am J Roentgenol 148:813, 1987.

Ryu KN, Bae DK, Park YK, Lee JH: Calcific tenosynovitis associated with calcific myonecrosis of the leg: Imaging features. Skeletal Radiol 25:273, 1996.

Siliprandi L, Martini G, Chiarelli A, Mazzoleni F: Surgical repair of an anterior tibialis muscle hernia with Mersilene mesh. Plast Reconstr Surg 91:1547, 1993.

Stevens MA, El-Khoury GY, Kathol MH, et al: Imaging features of avulsion injuries. Radiographics 19:655, 1999.

Tuite DJ, Finegan PJ, Saliaris AP, et al: Anatomy of the proximal musculotendinous junction of the adductor longus muscle. Knee Surg Sports Traumatol Arthrosc 6:134, 1998.

Vande Berg B, Malghem J, Puttemans T, et al: Idiopathic muscular infarction in a diabetic patient. Skeletal Radiol 25:183, 1996.

Vogel H: Inclusion body myositis: A review. Adv Anat Pathol 5:164, 1998.

Voit T: Congenital muscular dystrophies: 1997 update. Brain Dev 20:65, 1998.

Wulff EA, Simpson DM: Neuromuscular complications of HIV-1 infection. Curr Infect Dis Rep 1:192, 1999.

Wysoki MG, Santora TA, Shah RM, Friedman AC: Necrotizing fasciitis: CT characteristics. Radiology 203:859, 1997.

Zittergruen M, Grose C: Magnetic resonance imaging for early diagnosis of necrotizing fasciitis. Pediatr Emerg Care 9:26, 1993.

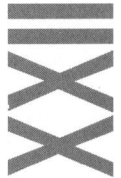

# Miscellaneous Diseases

# CHAPTER 80

## Sarcoidosis

### SUMMARY OF KEY FEATURES

Skeletal abnormalities in sarcoidosis are encountered most frequently in the hand; in this location, a coarsened trabecular pattern, cystic and marginal bone defects, and sclerosis are virtually diagnostic. Although findings can be encountered in other skeletal sites, such as the skull, facial bones, spine, and long tubular bones, as well as in various joints, these alterations are usually not specific.

## INTRODUCTION

Sarcoidosis is a granulomatous disorder of unknown cause that affects multiple organ systems, especially in young adults, and leads principally to bilateral hilar adenopathy, pulmonary infiltrates, and skin or eye lesions. Diagnosis of the disease is substantiated by a combination of clinical, radiographic, and histologic features, the last consisting predominantly of widespread, noncaseating epithelioid cell granulomas. The course of the disease is variable, and it may be associated with significant musculoskeletal abnormalities.

## CLINICAL ABNORMALITIES

Sarcoidosis has a worldwide distribution and is by no means rare in the United States, where the highest concentration of cases occurs in the Southeast. The disease affects men and women equally, although it is particularly common in women of childbearing age. It usually becomes apparent between 20 and 40 years of age. Blacks are more frequently affected than whites; in the United States, the disease is 10 times more common in black patients. Black women are affected about twice as often as black men, and, in general, the disease is more severe in blacks than in whites. Sarcoidosis appears to be rare in Chinese persons.

The clinical manifestations are highly variable. In some patients, radiographic evidence of hilar adenopathy may appear in the absence of any symptoms or signs. In others, an acute or chronic form of the disease becomes evident. One form of acute disease that is accompanied by erythema nodosum, polyarthritis, iritis, and fever is designated Löfgren's syndrome. As many as 90% of patients eventually have pulmonary abnormalities, which include cough, chest pain, and dyspnea. Ocular abnormalities, which occur in about 25% of patients with the disease, include granulomatous uveitis, iritis, and iridocyclitis. Circulating levels of angiotensin-converting enzyme (ACE) are elevated in approximately 80% of patients with acute pulmonary sarcoidosis. ACE levels often correlate with disease activity in patients with sarcoidosis.

## GENERAL PATHOLOGIC ABNORMALITIES

The diagnosis of sarcoidosis is based on compatible clinical and radiographic findings; the presence of supporting laboratory data, such as elevated levels of serum ACE and gamma globulins; and the demonstration of typical noncaseating granulomas in the absence of other identifiable causes for such lesions. As they resolve, the granulomas are frequently replaced with fibrous elements. It is this fibrosis, in addition to mechanical compression of adjacent tissue by the granuloma itself, that accounts for the clinically apparent multisystem organ dysfunction that is characteristic of sarcoidosis.

## MUSCULOSKELETAL ABNORMALITIES

Sarcoidosis can involve muscles, subcutaneous tissues, bones, and joints and results in prominent clinical, radiographic, and pathologic findings.

### Muscle Involvement

Granulomatous involvement of muscular tissue in sarcoidosis can be symptomatic or, more commonly, asymptomatic. Pain, tenderness, and nodular swelling are typical clinical findings. Chronic myopathy, the most common type, is usually accompanied by other manifestations of chronic sarcoidosis; it is characterized by symmetrical involvement, typically of proximal muscle groups. Nodular myopathy is accompanied by small tender nodules in various musculotendinous junctions. Acute myositis, which is rare, leads to muscle tenderness, weakness, and myalgias, usually accompanied by acute polyarthritis or erythema nodosum.

### Subcutaneous Involvement

In addition to a variety of cutaneous manifestations, as well as erythema nodosum, subcutaneous nodules may be identified in approximately 5% of patients with sarcoidosis. These subcutaneous nodules have an insidious onset; are painless, round, and mobile; and are distributed in the extremities, with fewer nodules in the trunk and face (Fig. 80–1).

### Osseous Involvement

#### Frequency

The frequency of radiographic evidence of osseous involvement varies from 1% to 13%, with an average of 5%. Because many of the skeletal lesions of sarcoidosis

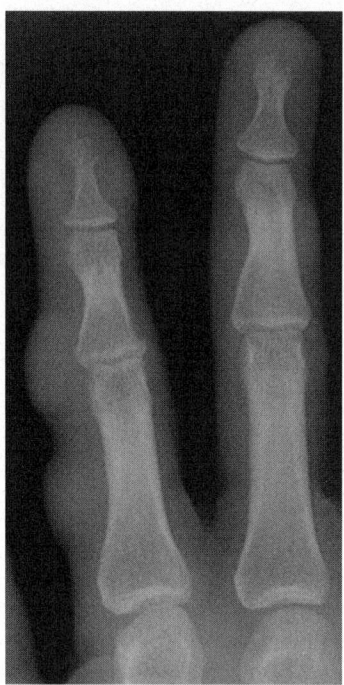

**Figure 80–1.** Sarcoidosis: subcutaneous nodules. Observe the prominent soft tissue nodules in the second and third digits, with acro-osteolysis of the terminal tufts.

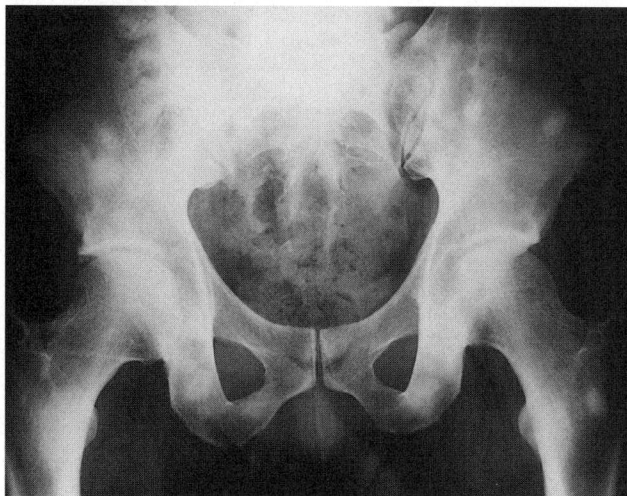

**Figure 80–3.** Sarcoidosis: osteosclerosis. Radiograph of the pelvis shows multiple osteosclerotic lesions of the innominate bones and left femur. (Courtesy of J. Jacobson, MD, Ann Arbor, Mich.)

are asymptomatic, accurate appraisal of the frequency of osseous involvement in this disease is difficult. Osseous sarcoidosis is rarely detected in the absence of skin lesions. In the absence of additional clinical or radiographic manifestations, bone changes are distinctly unusual in this disease.

## Clinical Manifestations

Although bone changes are often entirely asymptomatic, clinical manifestations may be prominent in some cases.

Soft tissue swelling and cutaneous lesions of the hands and, less typically, the feet may accompany osseous disease. Tenderness, stiffness, and restricted motion may be seen.

## Radiographic Manifestations

Osteoporosis producing generalized osteopenia, a decrease in cortical thickness, and striations of the cortex may be observed. A coarsened, reticulated, or lacework trabecular pattern becomes evident (Fig. 80–2). Localized rarefactions or cystic lesions may lead to a "punched-out" appearance that can simulate the findings in a variety of

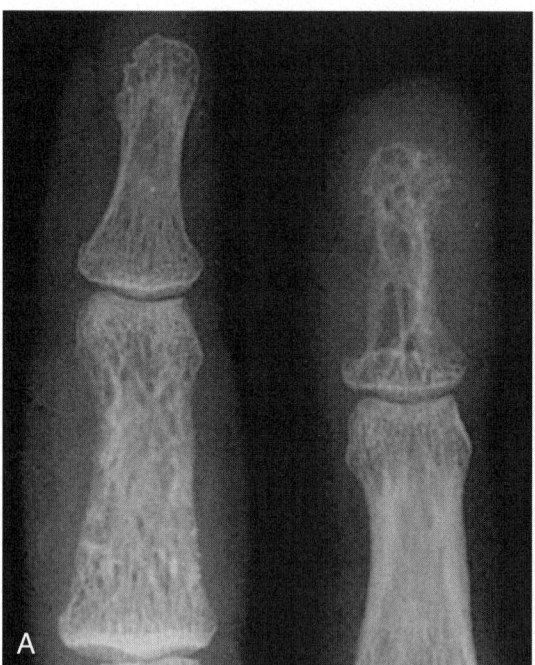

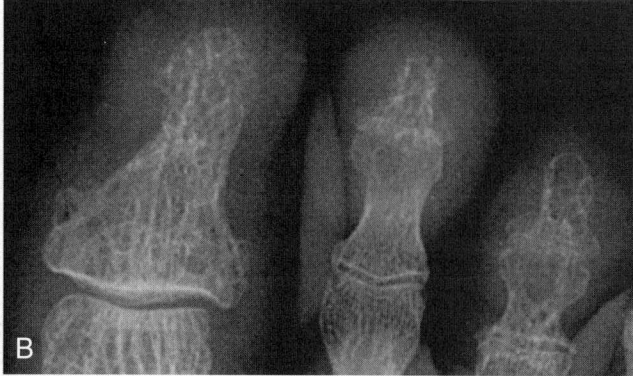

**Figure 80–2.** Sarcoidosis: abnormal trabecular pattern. Observe the coarsened, reticulated, or lacework appearance of the trabeculae in the phalanges of the hand *(A)* and foot *(B)*. Soft tissue swelling is evident. (Courtesy of P. Stern, MD, Covina, Calif.)

benign or malignant processes. These cysts can be located centrally or eccentrically, and they may be sharply marginated. Periostitis is distinctly unusual. Osteosclerosis about these rarefactions is absent or mild. Less typically, localized or generalized osteosclerosis is evident (Fig. 80–3).

**Hands and Feet.** The hand is the predominant site of skeletal sarcoidosis. Unilateral or bilateral asymmetrical changes may be encountered. In the hand, abnormalities are found in the middle and distal phalanges and, less often, the proximal phalanges and metacarpals (Fig. 80–4). Diffuse trabecular alterations are especially characteristic and lead to a honeycomb or latticework configuration. More localized lytic lesions produce cystlike defects that, as they heal, may become surrounded by a thin rim of sclerosis. These lesions can appear centrally or eccentrically. Periostitis is uncommon.

Acro-osteosclerosis has been reported to be a sign of sarcoidosis of the hands (Fig. 80–5). The appearance is characterized by focal opaque areas, frequently in the terminal phalanges, and by endosteal thickening. The finding is not specific and has also been noted in scleroderma, rheumatoid arthritis, systemic lupus erythematosus, Hodgkin's disease, and hematologic disorders.

**Long Tubular Bones.** Destructive lesions of the long tubular bones of the extremities are rare. Single or multiple lytic foci (Fig. 80–6) can lead to cortical erosion and violation, with pathologic fracture.

**Skull and Face.** Calvarial destruction is unusual in sarcoidosis. When present, such destruction may be

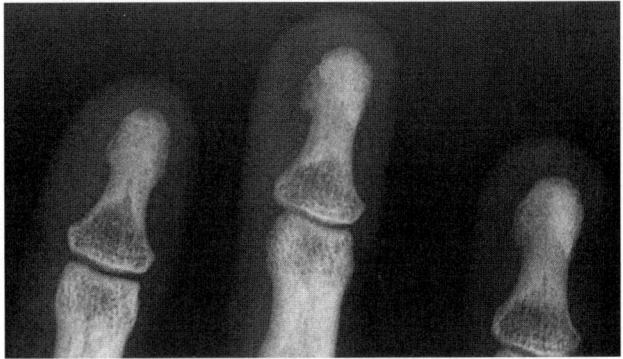

**Figure 80–5.** Sarcoidosis: acro-osteosclerosis. Observe the widespread sclerosis of the terminal aspects of the phalanges. This appearance is not specific.

asymptomatic and is characterized by single or multiple lytic lesions of varying size, usually without adjacent eburnation. Nasal bone destruction is especially characteristic.

**Spine and Spinal Cord.** Although vertebral sarcoidosis is uncommon, postmortem and antemortem studies have verified the localization of granulomas within vertebral marrow. Clinical findings include pain, tenderness, deformity, and neurologic dysfunction. On radiographs, bone lysis with marginal sclerosis can involve one or more contiguous or noncontiguous vertebral bodies, generally with preservation of the intervening intervertebral disc spaces. A predilection for the lower

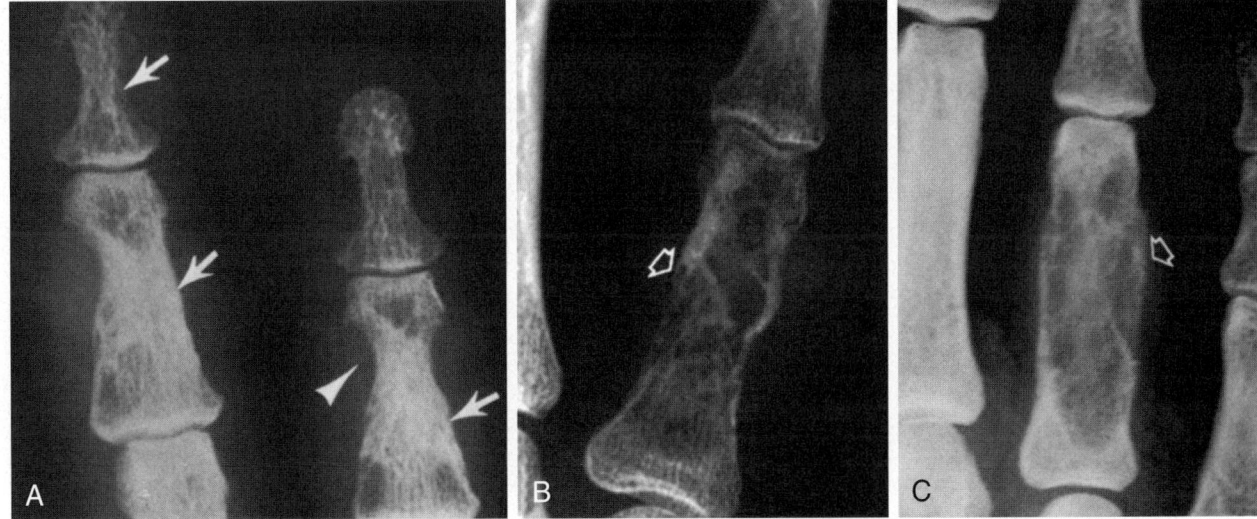

**Figure 80–4.** Sarcoidosis: hand. *A* to *C*, A variety of radiographic changes can be seen. Trabecular alterations can produce a honeycomb or latticework configuration *(solid arrows)*; more localized defects *(open arrows)*; and marginal scalloping of bone *(arrowhead)*. (*A*, Courtesy of A. Brower, MD, Norfolk, Va. *B*, Courtesy of M. Dalinka, MD, Philadelphia, Pa.)

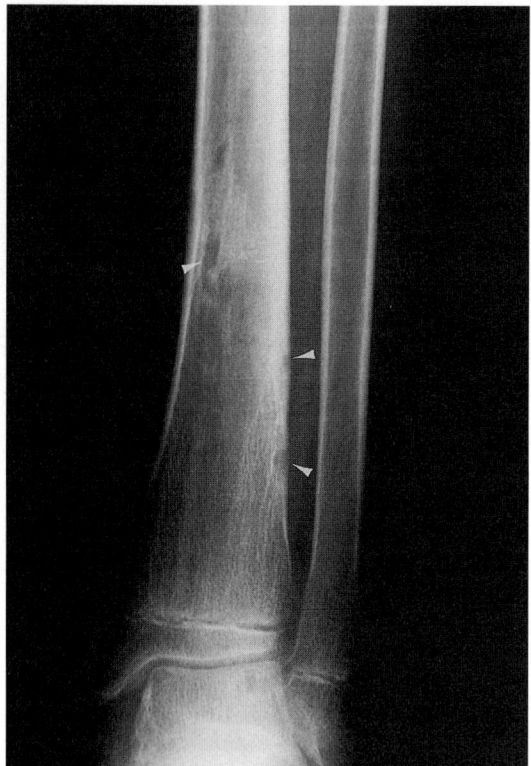

**Figure 80–6.** Sarcoidosis: long tubular bones. Small, eccentric osteolytic lesions *(arrowheads)* in the tibia of a child are observed. They are sharply circumscribed, with minimal marginal sclerosis and no periostitis. (Courtesy of L. Cooperstein, MD, Pittsburgh, Pa.)

thoracic and upper lumbar vertebrae is noted. Magnetic resonance (MR) imaging may reveal an intramedullary or intradural mass or evidence of arachnoiditis and meningeal thickening.

### Articular Involvement

Joint symptoms and signs appear in 10% to 35% of patients with sarcoidosis, more frequently in women than in men. Two fundamental patterns of articular disease occur: acute polyarthritis and chronic polyarthritis (Fig. 80–7).

**Acute Polyarthritis.** Peripheral symmetrical polyarthritis affects small and medium-sized joints, especially the ankles, knees, elbows, wrists, and joints of the hands, in association with erythema nodosum, hilar lymph node enlargement, fever, uveitis, and typical skin lesions. Radiographs generally reveal soft tissue swelling and, perhaps, osteoporosis.

**Chronic Polyarthritis.** In cases of sarcoidosis that have persisted for months to years, a chronic polyarthritis may occur. It generally subsides and recurs and may eventually lead to permanent disability and irreversible joint damage. The joints most typically affected are the ankles, knees, shoulders, wrists, and small joints of the hands. On radiographs, osseous sarcoidosis may or may not be present. In cases in which adjacent bone involvement is evident, articular destruction and collapse may occur secondary to extension of the osseous disease

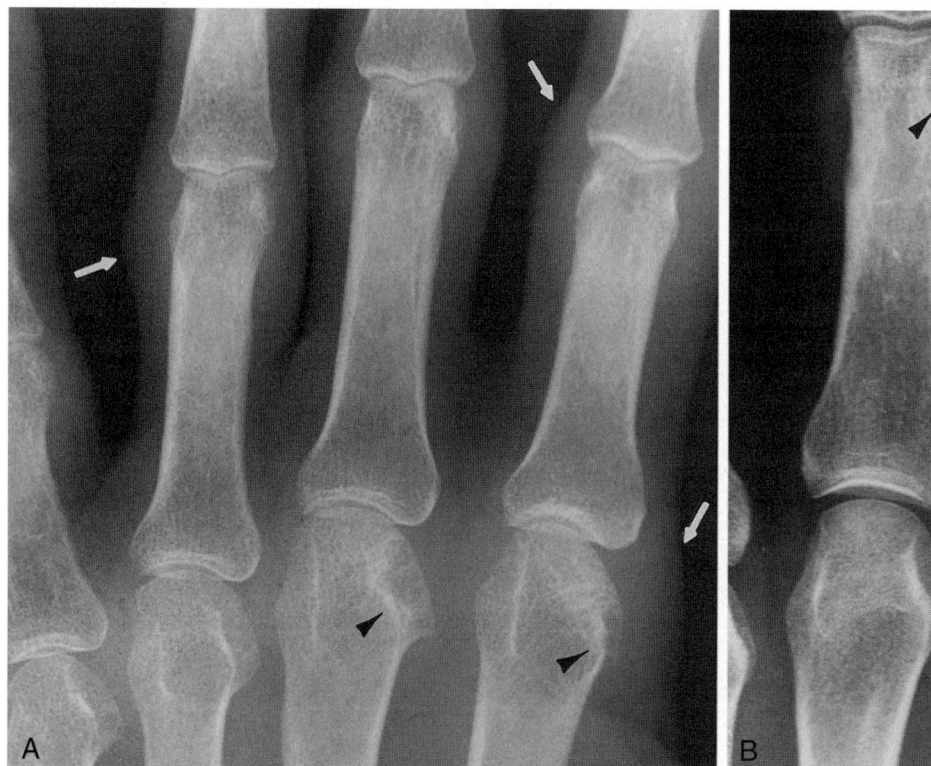
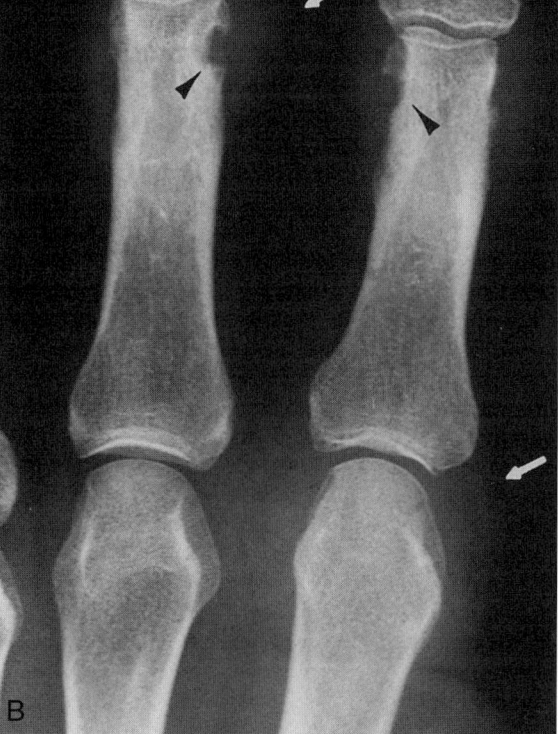

**Figure 80–7.** Sarcoidosis: articular involvement. *A,* Observe the soft tissue swelling of multiple proximal interphalangeal and metacarpophalangeal joints *(arrows),* with articular space narrowing and small osseous defects *(arrowheads).* The absence of obvious osseous sarcoid is unusual in patients with such joint alterations. *B,* In another patient, prominent soft tissue swelling is evident about the proximal interphalangeal and metacarpophalangeal joints *(arrows),* and osseous defects *(arrowheads)* are again seen.

into subchondral bone. Mild, diffuse joint space loss and eccentric and well-defined erosive alterations may also be noted.

**Other Patterns.** Sarcoid arthritis occurring in children may simulate the aberrations seen in some forms of juvenile chronic arthritis. Prominent but painless articular effusions and swelling of tendon sheaths are associated with boggy and thickened synovial membranes. Soft tissue enlargement and osteopenia are the characteristic radiographic abnormalities; rarely, cartilaginous and osseous destruction is apparent.

## DIAGNOSTIC TECHNIQUES

Scintigraphy has been used to delineate the extent of skeletal involvement in sarcoidosis, and scintigraphic abnormalities are more extensive than those depicted on corresponding radiographic studies (Fig. 80–8). MR imaging may document marrow involvement at a time when routine radiographs are normal and bone scan results are equivocal. The signal intensity characteristics of intraosseous lesions in this disease are not unique. Typically, low to intermediate signal intensity is observed on T1-weighted spin echo images, and intermediate to high signal intensity is seen on T2-weighted spin echo images and most fluid-sensitive sequences (Fig. 80–9). Occasionally, a target-like appearance is seen, characterized by a rim of high signal intensity and a central portion of lower signal intensity. A punctate or serpentine appearance, with areas of preserved marrow, is seen in some cases. With involvement of the spine, MR imaging findings resemble those of infective spondylitis or metastatic disease (Fig. 80–10).

The MR imaging appearance of muscular sarcoidosis appears to depend on the type of involvement. Nodular myopathy is characterized by the presence of nodules consisting of a star-shaped area of low signal intensity surrounded by an area of high signal intensity on both T1- and T2-weighted spin echo images (Fig. 80–11).

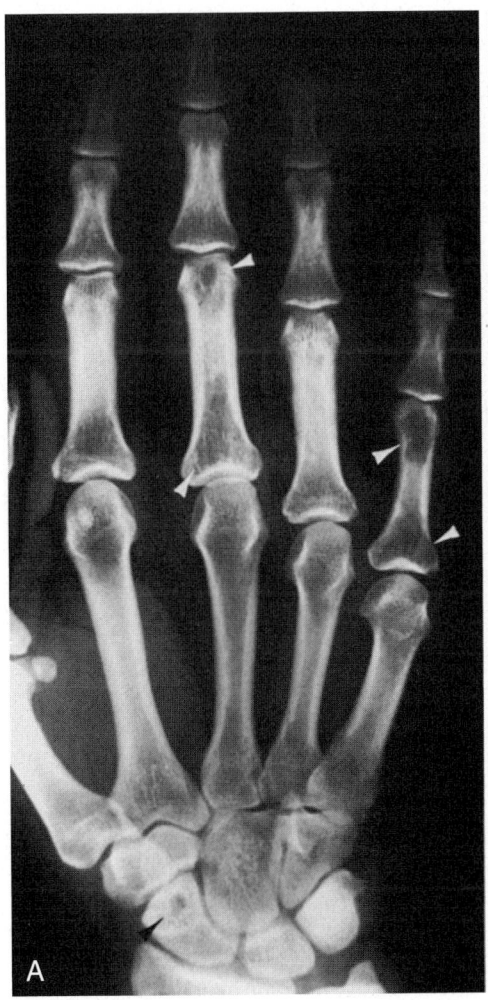
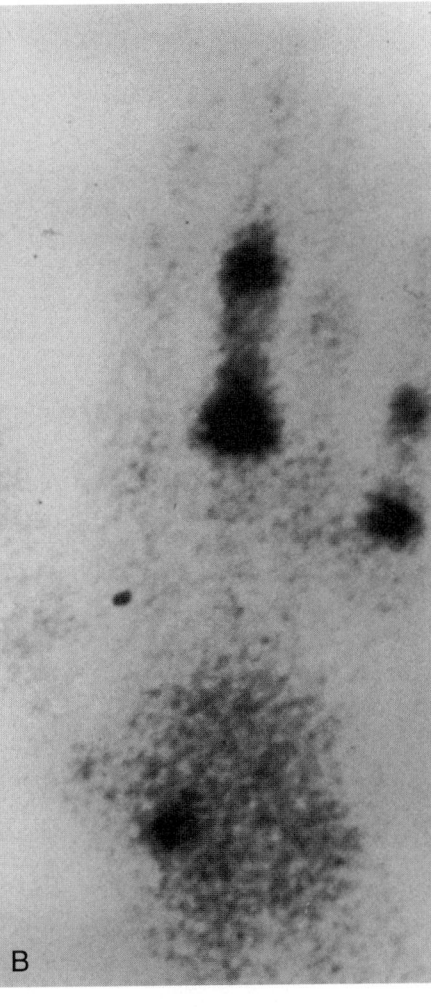

**Figure 80–8.** Sarcoidosis: scintigraphic abnormalities. *A,* Observe the areas of subtle bone destruction in the scaphoid and phalanges *(arrowheads).* These areas are characterized by poorly defined and well-defined osteolytic lesions. *B,* Bone scan shows abnormal accumulation of radiotracer at these sites. (Courtesy of V. Vint, MD, San Diego, Calif.)

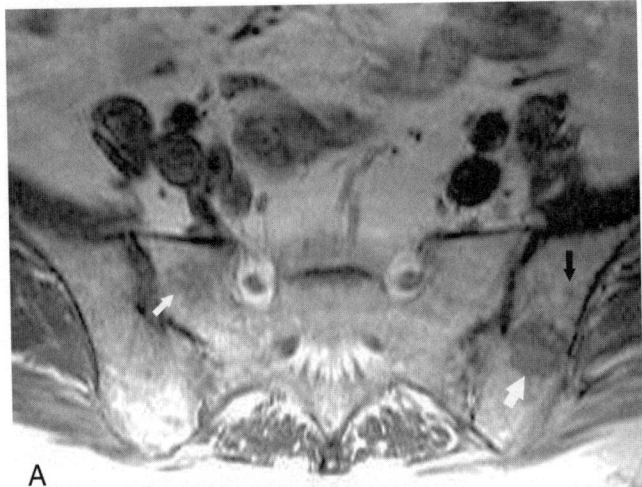

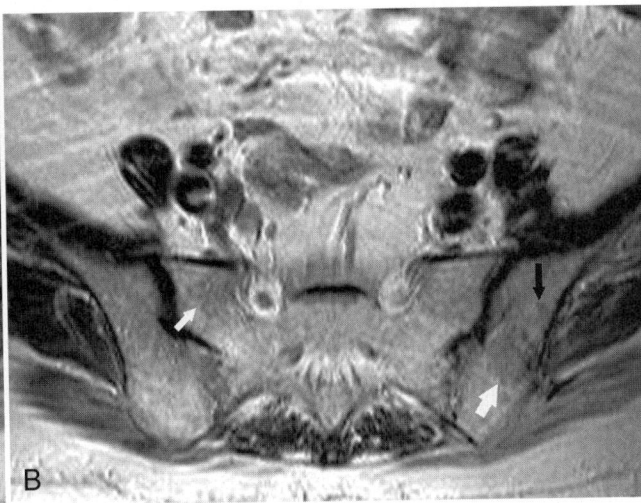

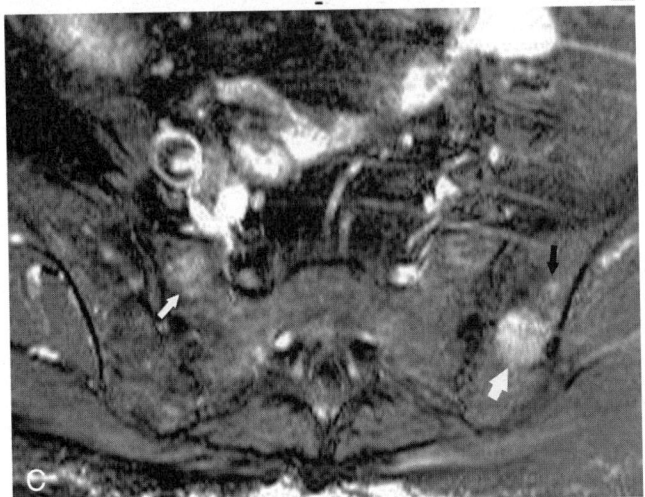

**Figure 80–9.** Sarcoidosis: bone involvement. Corresponding axial T1-weighted (TR/TE, 591/16) spin echo *(A)*, T2-weighted (TR/TE, 4000/71) fast spin echo *(B)*, and fat-suppressed T2-weighted (TR/TE, 4230/73) fast spin echo *(C)* MR images show multiple intramedullary lesions *(arrows)*. The lesions are most conspicuous on T1-weighted and fat-suppressed images. Small central areas of marrow signal are best seen on the T1-weighted image *(A)*.

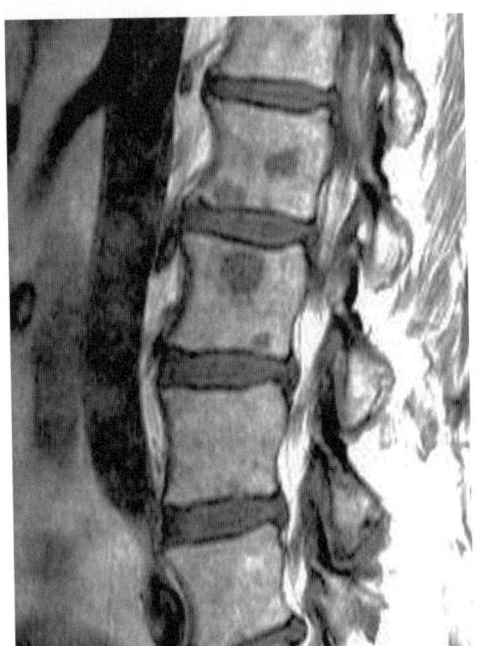

**Figure 80–10.** Sarcoidosis: bone involvement. Sagittal T1-weighted (TR/TE, 619/12) spin echo MR image shows multiple focal intraosseous lesions initially interpreted as metastatic disease.

The foci of inflammatory tissue may show high signal intensity on fat-suppressed MR images (Fig. 80–12) and enhancement of signal intensity after the intravenous administration of a gadolinium compound.

## DIFFERENTIAL DIAGNOSIS

The skeletal alterations in sarcoidosis are sufficiently characteristic in most cases to allow an accurate radiographic diagnosis. Occasionally, the trabecular and cystic changes in the hand may be confused with abnormalities in other disorders (Table 80–1). In tuberous sclerosis, cystlike foci in the phalanges and metacarpals are usually associated with a distinctive variety of periosteal proliferation that leads to nodular excrescences and eburnation. Fibrous dysplasia can produce monostotic or polyostotic abnormalities. A widened medullary space of the phalanges and metacarpals, with a diffuse "ground-glass" appearance, is typical and is commonly combined with more widespread skeletal abnormalities. Enchondromas commonly produce a central rarefied area with or without calcification, as well as scalloping of the endosteal margin of the cortex. Enchondromatosis, a syndrome of multiple enchondromas, produces multiple lucent and calcified lesions, but a more diffuse and bizarre appearance can

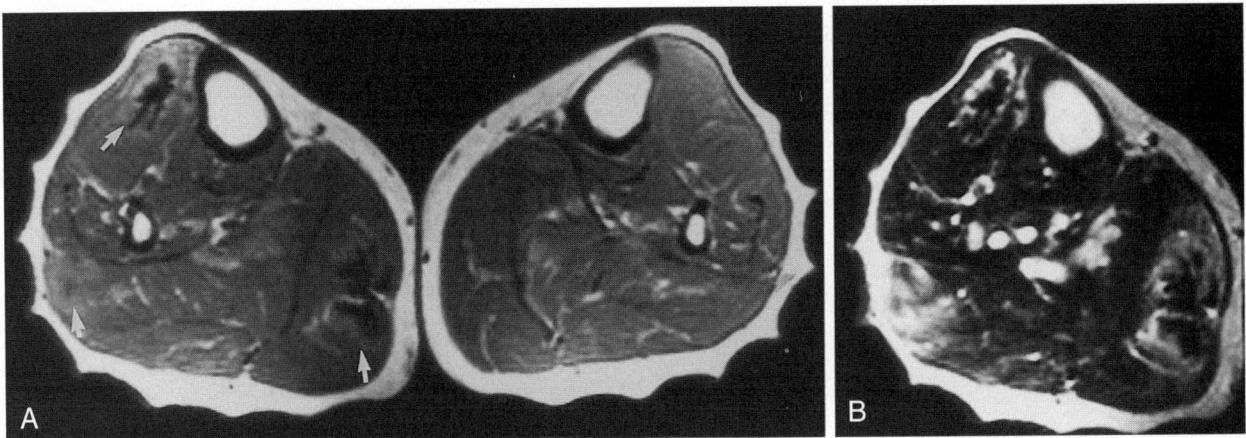

**Figure 80–11.** Sarcoidosis: muscle involvement. This 64-year-old woman had nodular myopathy involving the right lower extremity. *A,* Transaxial T1-weighted (TR/TE, 550/30) spin echo MR image shows three oval nodules—two in the gastrocnemius muscle, and one in the tibialis anterior muscle *(arrows).* In each lesion, a star-shaped area of low signal intensity is surrounded by a region of slightly higher signal intensity. *B,* Transaxial T2-weighted (TR/TE, 1800/100) spin echo MR image reveals high signal intensity in the peripheral portion of each lesion.
(From Otake S, Banno T, Ohba S, et al: Muscular findings at MR imaging. Radiology 176:145, 1990.)

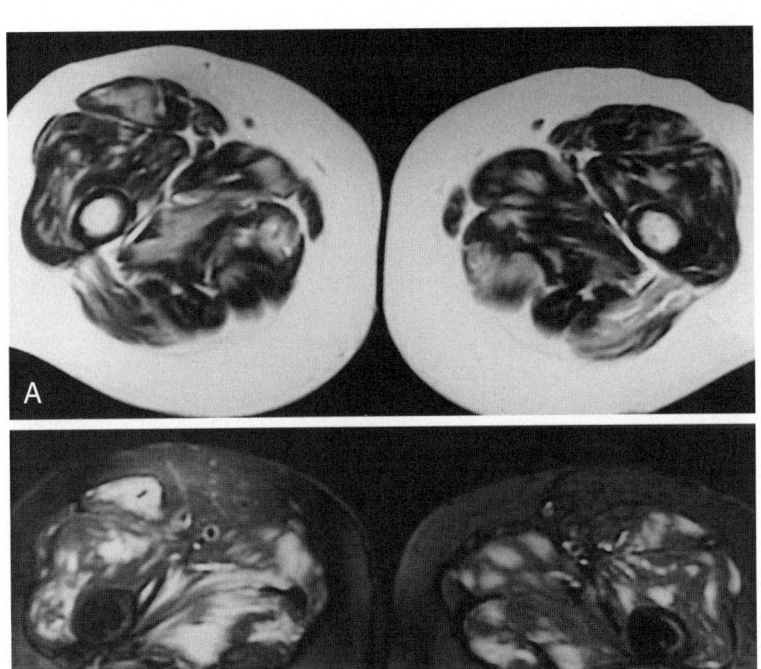

**Figure 80–12.** Sarcoidosis: muscle abnormalities. *A,* In a transverse fast spin echo (TR/TE, 4500/102) MR image, irregular regions of intermediate signal intensity are seen in multiple muscles in both thighs. *B,* These same regions show high signal intensity on a transverse fat-suppressed fast spin echo (TR/TE, 4500/102) MR image. (Courtesy of Y. Kakitsubata, MD, Miyazati, Japan.)

also be seen. When enchondromatosis is combined with cavernous hemangiomas, Maffucci's syndrome is diagnosed.

Multiple lucent lesions of the phalanges, metacarpals, and metatarsals can also accompany tuberculosis and other granulomatous infections, hemangiomatosis, xanthomatosis, fat necrosis, hyperparathyroidism, Gorlin's basal cell nevus syndrome, lipomatosis, plasma cell myeloma, and skeletal metastasis.

**TABLE 80–1**

**Diseases Producing Multiple Cystlike Lesions of the Metacarpal Bones and Phalanges**

Sarcoidosis
Gout
Rheumatoid arthritis
Xanthomatosis
Tuberous sclerosis
Fibrous dysplasia
Enchondromatosis (Ollier's disease)
Tuberculosis
Fungal disease
Metastasis (r)
Plasma cell myeloma (r)
Hyperparathyroidism (r)
Basal cell nevus syndrome (r)
Hemangioma (r)

r, rare manifestation of the disease.

## FURTHER READING

Berk RN, Brower TD: Vertebral sarcoidosis. Radiology 82:660, 1964.

Bonakdarpour A, Levy W, Aergerter EE: Osteosclerotic changes in sarcoidosis. AJR Am J Roentgenol 113:646, 1971.

Boyd RE, Andrews BS: Sarcoidosis presenting as cutaneous ulceration, subcutaneous nodules and chronic arthritis. J Rheumatol 8:311, 1981.

Fisher AJ, Gilula LA, Kyriakos M, et al: MR imaging changes of lumbar vertebral sarcoidosis. AJR Am J Roentgenol 173:354, 1999.

Holt JF, Owens WI: The osseous lesions of sarcoidosis. Radiology 53:11, 1949.

James DG, Neville E, Carstairs LS: Bone and joint sarcoidosis. Semin Arthritis Rheum 6:53, 1976.

Jelinek JS, Mark AS, Barth WF: Sclerotic lesions of the cervical spine in sarcoidosis. Skeletal Radiol 27:702, 1998.

Kaplan H: Sarcoid arthritis: A review. Arch Intern Med 112:924, 1963.

Mayock RL, Bertrand P, Morrison CE, et al: Manifestations of sarcoidosis: Analysis of 145 patients with a review of 9 series selected from the literature. Am J Med 35:67, 1963.

McBrine CS, Fisher MS: Acrosclerosis in sarcoidosis. Radiology 115:279, 1975.

Otake S: Sarcoidosis involving skeletal muscle: Imaging findings and relative value of imaging procedures. AJR Am J Roentgenol 162:369, 1994.

Redman DS, McCarthy RE, Jimenez JF: Sarcoidosis in the long bones of a child: A case report and review of the literature. J Bone Joint Surg Am 65:1010, 1983.

Rosenberg AM, Yee EH, MacKenzie JW: Arthritis in childhood sarcoidosis. J Rheumatol 10:987, 1983.

Sartoris DJ, Resnick D, Resnik C, et al: Musculoskeletal manifestations of sarcoidosis. Semin Roentgenol 20:376, 1985.

Shinozaki T, Watanabe H, Aoki J, et al: Imaging features of subcutaneous sarcoidosis. Skeletal Radiol 27:359, 1998.

Stein GN, Israel HL, Sones M: A roentgenographic study of skeletal lesions in sarcoidosis. Arch Intern Med 97:532, 1956.

Sundaram M, Place H, Shaffer WO, et al: Progressive destructive vertebral sarcoid leading to surgical fusion. Skeletal Radiol 28:717, 1999.

Toomey F, Bautista A: Rare manifestations of sarcoidosis in children. Radiology 94:569, 1970.

Yaghmai I: Radiographic, angiographic and radionuclide manifestations of osseous sarcoidosis. Radiographics 3:375, 1983.

Zimmerman R, Leeds NE: Calvarial and vertebral sarcoidosis: Case report and review of the literature. Radiology 119:384, 1976.

# CHAPTER 81

## Tuberous Sclerosis, Neurofibromatosis, and Fibrous Dysplasia

### Frieda Feldman

## SUMMARY OF KEY FEATURES

Tuberous sclerosis is a widespread aberration that begins during embryonic life and may involve all germ layers. Its classic clinical triad consists of epileptic seizures, mental retardation, and skin lesions. Neurofibromatosis, previously characterized by the classic clinical triad of cutaneous lesions, mental deficiency, and skeletal deformities, has now been reclassified into several subtypes. Fibrous dysplasia is a disorder of unknown cause in which the skeleton is a prominent target tissue. A variety of endocrine abnormalities, including McCune-Albright syndrome, may accompany the osseous abnormalities.

## INTRODUCTION

Tuberous sclerosis, neurofibromatosis, and polyostotic fibrous dysplasia involve multiple systems in multiple ways and are therefore associated with a variety of seemingly unrelated radiographic stigmata. Before discussing dissimilarities, it is important to note that tuberous sclerosis, neurofibromatosis, and fibrous dysplasia share certain characteristics. Although they are grouped with the neuroectodermal and mesodermal dysplasias, all three germ layers may be involved in each of these entities. Moreover, all have been associated with certain classic clinical triads, which are considered aids in their identification. Although mutations do occur, in most cases the three disorders are hereditary or familial diseases.

## TUBEROUS SCLEROSIS

Tuberous sclerosis is a disease of autosomal dominant inheritance. New mutations have been reported in 25% to 90% of cases. It has no known geographic, ethnic, or gender predilection. Tuberous sclerosis was classically characterized by the clinical triad of epileptic seizures, mental retardation, and skin lesions regarded as hamartomas. Hamartomas can occur in many organs, with a variety of clinical manifestations. These traditional criteria have since been modified, and diagnoses are now based on more stringent combinations of clinical, radiographic, and histopathologic signs (Table 81–1).

### Cutaneous, Central Nervous System, and Ocular Abnormalities

Almost all patients have cutaneous stigmata, four of which—adenoma sebaceum, shagreen patches, periungual fibromas, and hypopigmented macules—are believed to be diagnostic. Lesions of the central nervous system are responsible for the epilepsy and mental retardation that constitute the other two components of the classic diagnostic triad.

Routine skull films may also show patchy areas of calvarial sclerosis caused by hyperostosis of the inner table and prominent trabeculae in the diploic spaces (Fig. 81–1). Generalized thickening and increased density of both tables of the vault may also be noted. Evidence of raised intracranial pressure (i.e., sutural diastasis, sellar changes, increased convolutional markings) and thinning adjacent to cortical tubers have been reported. Intracerebral calcifications occur in 50% to 80% of cases (see Fig. 81–1). Calcifications may be multiple, nodular, discrete, and several millimeters in diameter.

Brain lesions in tuberous sclerosis occur predominantly in three main loci: the ventricles, the white matter, and the cortex. Hamartomatous foci, which may or may not calcify, vary in size and number; they typically lie adjacent to cerebrospinal fluid pathways and are either subependymal nodules or cortical tubers located about the ventricles and arising within the basal ganglia (Fig. 81–2). Computed tomography (CT) can demonstrate lesions in the brain at an early stage, particularly if they are calcified; these lesions are detectable on CT scans in 50% of patients by age 10 years.

Ocular abnormalities are seen at birth in more than half of cases. Although many lesions have been described, only retinal hamartomas (phakomas) are clearly part of the syndrome. Hypopigmented spots in the iris analogous to the skin lesions may also occur.

### Extracranial Skeletal Abnormalities

In addition to the skull, the remainder of the skeleton may be focally or diffusely involved with medullary or cortical cystlike radiolucent areas or dense sclerotic deposits. Cortical lesions, as well as irregular, subperiosteal new bone deposition that results in a thickened, undulating cortical contour, most often involve the short tubular bones of the hands and feet (Fig. 81–3) and, occasionally, the long tubular bones. Rounded radiolucent lesions predominate in the distal phalanges of the hand, which rarely may also be eroded by subungual fibromas.

The spine and pelvis are additional sites of medullary osteoblastic deposits ranging from a few millimeters to centimeters in diameter (Fig. 81–4). The usually homogeneously dense intraosseous lesions occasionally have a mottled appearance. Unusual before puberty, these lesions occur as later, asymptomatic manifestations.

## TABLE 81-1

### Revised Diagnostic Criteria for Tuberous Sclerosis Complex

*Major Features*
1. Facial angiofibromas or forehead plaque
2. Nontraumatic ungual or periungual fibroma
3. Hypomelanotic macules (three or more)
4. Shagreen patch (connective tissue nevus)
5. Multiple retinal nodular hamartomas
6. Cortical tuber*
7. Subependymal nodule
8. Subependymal giant cell astrocytoma
9. Cardiac rhabdomyoma, single or multiple
10. Lymphangiomyomatosis†
11. Renal angiomyolipoma†

*Minor Features*
1. Multiple, randomly distributed pits in dental enamel
2. Hamartomatous rectal polyps‡
3. Bone cysts§
4. Cerebral white matter radial migration lines*§‖
5. Gingival fibromas
6. Nonrenal hamartoma‡
7. Retinal achromic patch
8. "Confetti" skin lesions
9. Multiple renal cysts‡

*Definite Tuberous Sclerosis Complex:*
Either 2 major features or 1 major feature plus 2 minor features

*Probable Tuberous Sclerosis Complex:*
One major plus 1 minor feature

*Possible Tuberous Sclerosis Complex:*
Either 1 major feature or 2 or more minor features

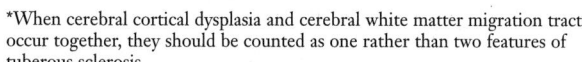

*When cerebral cortical dysplasia and cerebral white matter migration tracts occur together, they should be counted as one rather than two features of tuberous sclerosis.

†When both lymphangiomyomatosis and renal angiomyolipomas are present, other features of tuberous sclerosis should be present before a definite diagnosis is assigned.

‡Histologic confirmation is suggested.

§Radiographic confirmation is sufficient.

‖One panel member believed strongly that three or more radial migration lines should constitute a major sign.

Adapted from Roach ES, Gomez MR, Northrup H: J Child Neurol 13:624, 1998.

## Visceral Abnormalities

The viscera and the skin, eyes, brain, and bones serve as silent sites of tumor-like formations. Approximately 50% of patients with tuberous sclerosis have associated renal lesions, including cysts, angiomyolipomas, and aneurysms. Conversely, 50% of all renal angiomyolipomas occur in patients with tuberous sclerosis. In a patient with epilepsy and "cystic" renal enlargement, tuberous sclerosis is a serious diagnostic consideration, whereas a combination of renal cysts and angiomyolipomas is now thought to be pathognomonic of this disease.

The coincident occurrence of tuberous sclerosis of the brain and rhabdomyoma of the heart is reported in 30% to 50% of patients with tuberous sclerosis. Pulmonary lesions occur in approximately 1% of patients with tuberous sclerosis, almost all of them female.

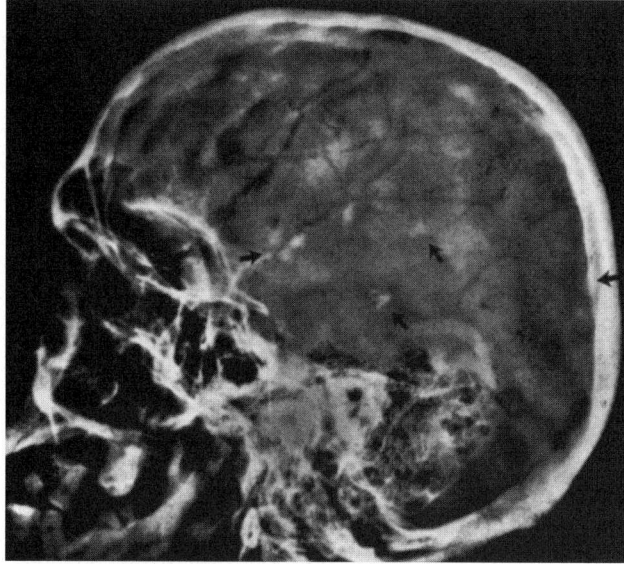

**Figure 81–1.** Tuberous sclerosis: intracerebral calcifications. In a lateral view of the skull, multiple intracerebral calcific deposits are noted, together with several scattered areas of calvarial sclerosis *(arrows)*.

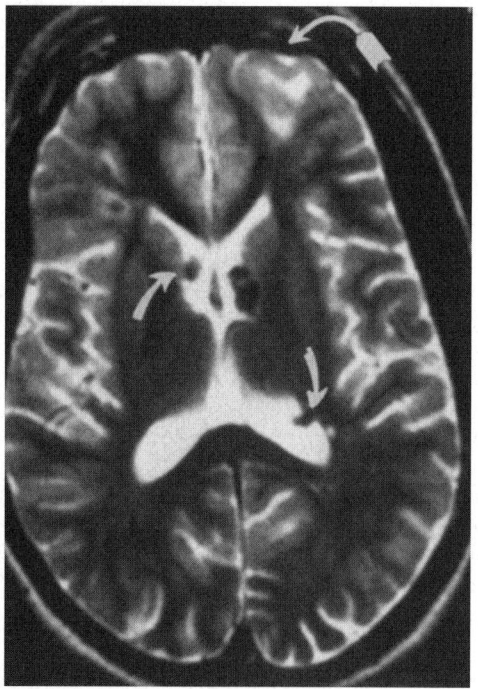

**Figure 81–2.** Tuberous sclerosis: brain. Transaxial fast spin echo (TR/TE, 3000/102) MR image in a 22-year-old man with seizures shows numerous calcified subependymal nodules of low signal intensity *(small arrows)* and a left frontal cortical tuber *(large arrow)*. (Courtesy of R. Mosesson, MD, New York, N.Y.)

## Endocrine Abnormalities

Hepatic, splenic, thyroid, and pancreatic adenomas and lipomyomas have been noted, as have pituitary, adrenal, and thyroid dysfunction and diabetes mellitus. Pancreatic islet cell tumors, though mainly associated with multiple

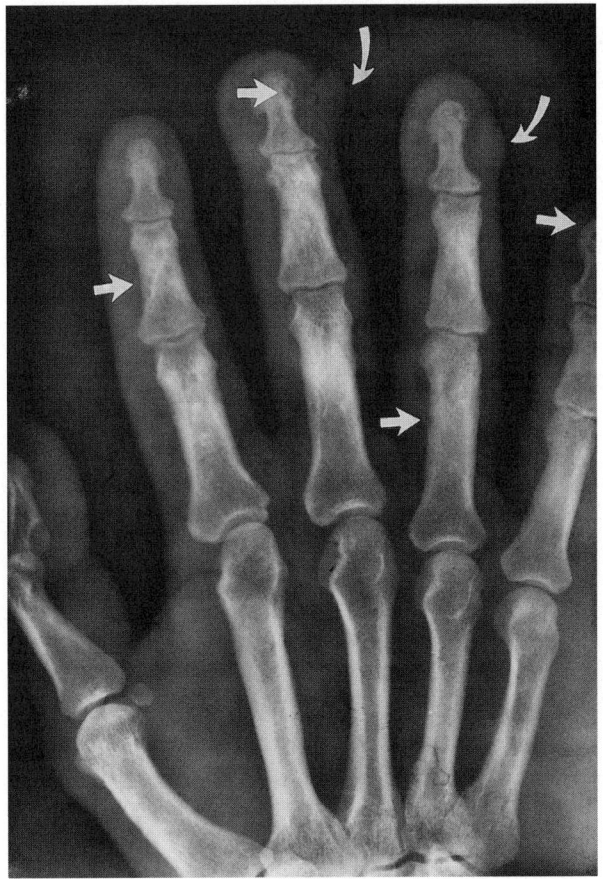

**Figure 81–3.** Tuberous sclerosis: hand. Numerous rounded, intramedullary radiolucent lesions are seen in several phalanges of various digits, together with cortical pitting *(straight arrows)*. Note the neighboring periungual fibromas in the third and fourth digits *(curved arrows)*.

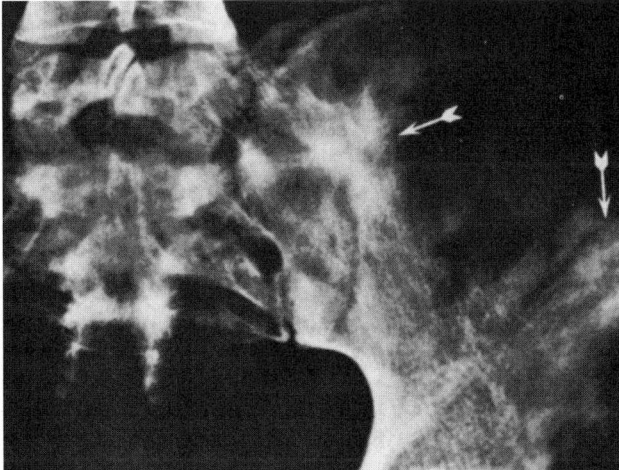

**Figure 81–4.** Tuberous sclerosis: ilium. Irregular intramedullary osteosclerotic deposits are noted in both the ilium and the sacrum. Several are flame-shaped *(arrows)*.

endocrine neoplasia syndrome type 1, have also been noted in association with pancreatic and liver cysts.

## NEUROFIBROMATOSIS

### General Features

Neurofibromatosis 1, previously known as von Recklinghausen's disease, accounts for 97% of cases of neurofibromatosis, and neurofibromatosis 2 (central neurofibromatosis) accounts for 3%. Both subtypes are caused by genetic mutations: neurofibromatosis 1 on chromosome 17, and neurofibromatosis 2 on chromosome 22.

Neurofibromatosis is one of humanity's most common genetic disorders. It is inherited as an autosomal dominant trait with no sex predilection. At least 50% of all index cases are thought to have resulted from mutations. On the basis of genetic and epidemiologic data, eight subtypes have been identified. Diagnostic criteria for neurofibromatosis are summarized in Tables 81–2 and 81–3.

### Cutaneous Abnormalities

Classically, neurofibromatosis consisted of the clinical triad of cutaneous lesions, mental deficiency, and skeletal deformities. In addition to its characteristic tumors, café au lait spots are common. Although café au lait spots are not pathognomonic of neurofibromatosis, differences in their distribution, configuration, and number in comparison with those in tuberous sclerosis and fibrous dysplasia make them useful indicators of neurofibromatosis.

### Osseous Abnormalities

**Cranium.** The orbit frequently displays a characteristic unilateral defect of the greater and lesser wings of the sphenoid bone (Fig. 81–5). The deficient posterosuperior orbital wall may give rise to pulsating exophthalmos.

---

**TABLE 81–2**

**National Institutes of Health Diagnostic Criteria for Neurofibromatosis 1***

6 or more café au lait macules >5 mm in greatest diameter in prepubertal individuals and >15 mm in greatest diameter in postpubertal individuals

2 or more neurofibromas of any type or 1 plexiform neurofibroma

Freckling in the axillary or inguinal regions

Optic glioma

2 or more Lisch nodules (iris hamartomas)

A distinctive osseous lesion such as sphenoid dysplasia or thinning of the long bone cortex with or without pseudarthrosis

A first-degree relative (parent, sibling, or offspring) with neurofibromatosis 1 by the above criteria

*Cardinal clinical features (any two or more are required for diagnosis).
Adapted from Gutmann DH, Aylsworth A, Carey JC, et al: JAMA 278:51, 1997.

## TABLE 81-3

### Diagnostic Criteria for Neurofibromatosis 2 (NF2)

*Individuals with the following clinical features have confirmed (definite) NF2:*
Bilateral vestibular schwannomas (VS)

*or*

Family history of NF2 (first-degree family relative)

*plus*

1. Unilateral VS in individuals <30 yr *or*
2. Any 2 of the following: meningioma, glioma, schwannoma, juvenile posterior subcapsular lenticular opacities/juvenile cortical cataract

*Individuals with the following clinical features should be evaluated for NF2 (presumptive or probable NF2):*
Unilateral VS in individuals <30 yr *plus* at least 1 of the following: meningioma, glioma, schwannoma, juvenile posterior subcapsular lenticular opacities/juvenile cortical cataract
Multiple meningiomas (2 or more) *plus* unilateral VS in individuals <30 yr *or* 1 of the following: glioma, schwannoma, juvenile posterior subcapsular lenticular opacities/juvenile cortical cataract

Adapted from Gutmann DH, Aylsworth A, Carey JC, et al: JAMA 278:51, 1997.

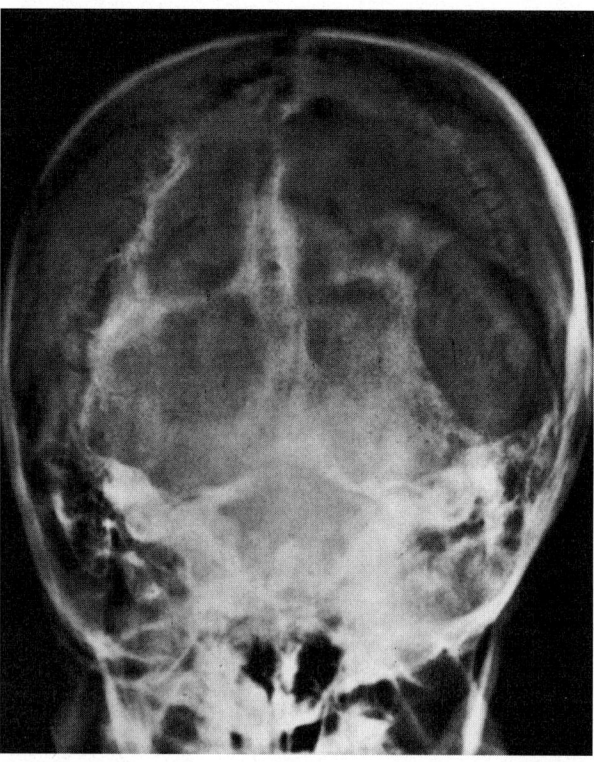

**Figure 81–6.** Neurofibromatosis: sutural defect. In this posteroanterior (Towne's) view of the skull, an oval calvarial defect involves the left lambdoid suture and extends toward the midline. This type of defect usually occurs on the left side.

Another bony defect tends to occur on the left side of the skull in the lambdoid suture just posterior to the junction of the parietomastoid and occipitomastoid sutures (Fig. 81–6). Enlarged ipsilateral middle cranial fossae or orbital fissures, thickened orbital muscles, underdeveloped ipsilateral mastoid, and hypoplastic maxillary and ethmoid sinuses are also common.

**Spine.** Sixty percent of patients with neurofibromatosis have some abnormality of the spine. Scoliosis (with or without kyphosis) is the most common spinal manifestation. The scoliosis has two initial patterns: one resembles an ordinary idiopathic spinal curve; the other is a dysplastic, sharply angulated, short-segment kyphoscoliosis that commonly involves fewer than six middle or lower thoracic vertebrae, may be rapidly progressive, and is considered virtually diagnostic of neurofibromatosis (Fig. 81–7). The spinal deformity in neurofibromatosis is distinguished by the predominance of kyphosis over scoliosis. Severe kyphoscoliosis and many of the other spinal abnormalities, such as vertebral body wedging and scalloping, pedicle erosion, foraminal enlargement, and penciling and spindling of transverse processes and ribs (Figs. 81–8 and 81–9), have been attributed to a primary mesodermal dysplasia.

**Other Sites.** The ribs, pelvis, and long bones are sites of abnormal or deficient bone formation that reflect the basic mesodermal dysplasia (Figs. 81–10 and 81–11). Bowing, pathologic fracture, and pseudarthrosis of long bones occur, and callus formation and fracture healing may be defective. Anterolateral bowing of the tibia, usually evident in the first years of life, is particularly characteristic and may be accompanied by a gracile, abnormally

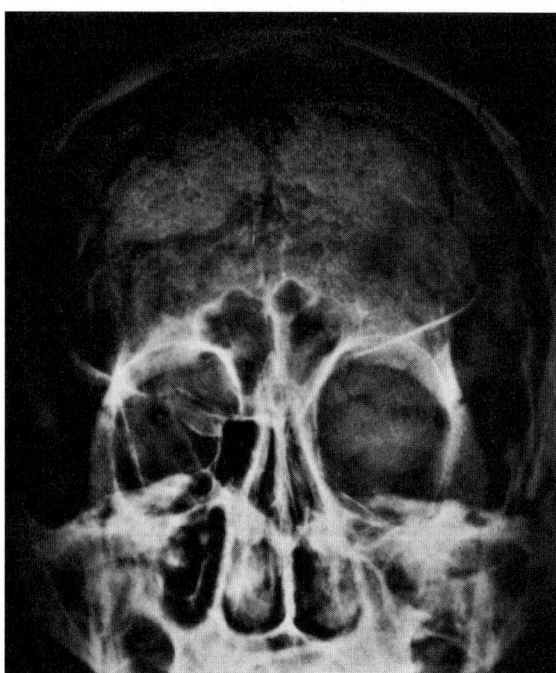

**Figure 81–5.** Neurofibromatosis: pulsating exophthalmos. In this posteroanterior view of the skull, the left orbit is enlarged and appears "empty" because of loss of the normal osseous landmarks, which are present on the right. Note the absence of both sphenoid wings and the small ethmoid sinuses.

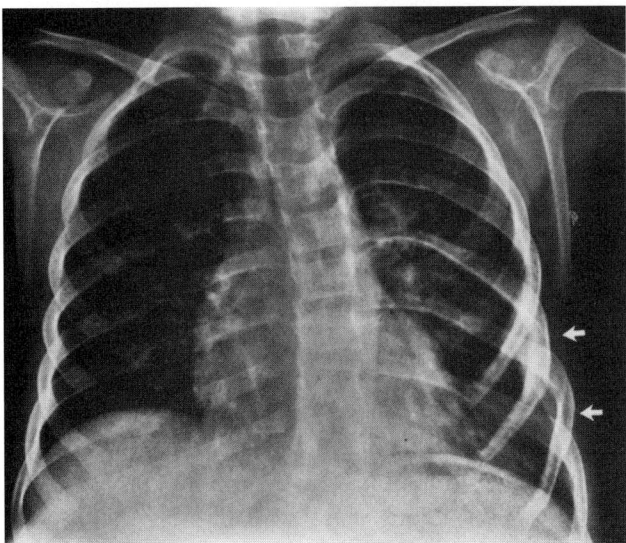

**Figure 81–7.** Neurofibromatosis: scoliosis and rib abnormalities. A moderate degree of thoracic spine scoliosis is associated with widened interpediculate distances of the thoracic vertebrae and deformed, widely spaced, overconstricted, and irregularly contoured ribs on the left side *(arrows)*.

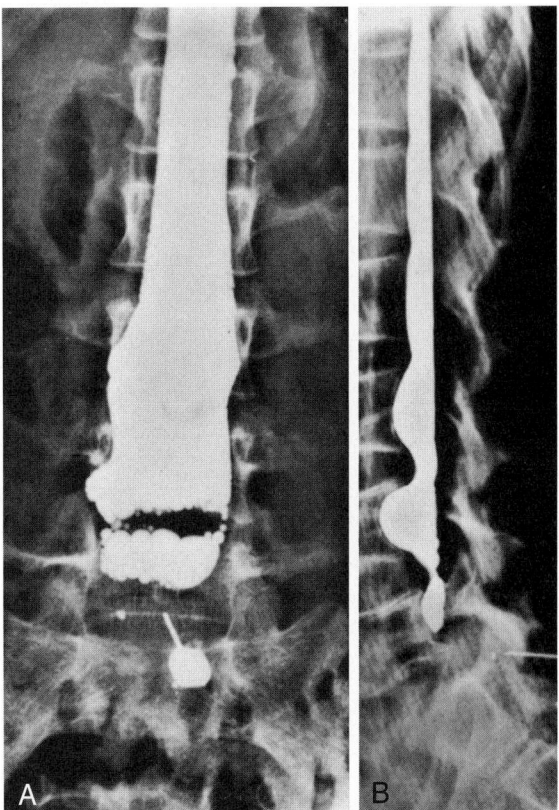

**Figure 81–9.** Neurofibromatosis: dural ectasia—lumbar myelogram. *A,* On a posteroanterior view, the grossly enlarged subarachnoid space has uniform lateral boundaries outlined by the iophendylate column. Note the widened interpediculate distances. *B,* Prone lateral view reveals evidence of localized pooling of the contrast medium at the L3, L4, and L5 levels as a result of dural ectasia. Scalloping usually occurs earlier than interpediculate widening, because the trabecular bone of vertebral bodies offers less resistance to local pressure than does the compact bone of the pedicles.

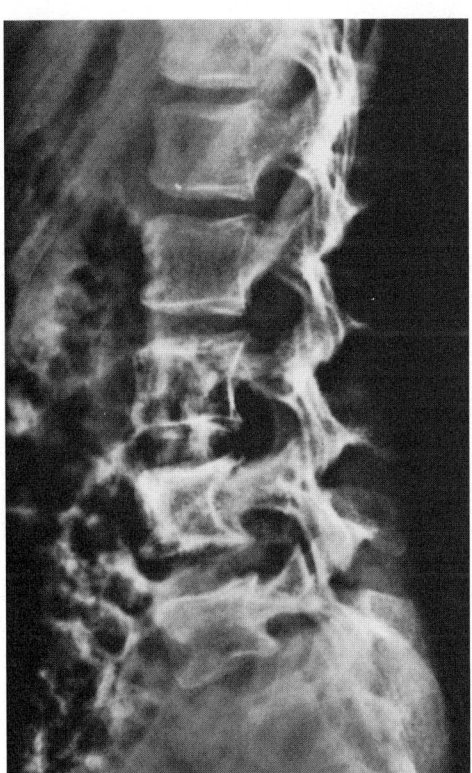

**Figure 81–8.** Neurofibromatosis: marked vertebral scalloping. Posterior vertebral body scalloping is localized to the L3, L4, and L5 levels. No associated scoliosis and no change in the intervertebral disc spaces can be seen. Scalloping may result from the intrinsic dysplastic change within bone, as well as from neighboring dural ectasia (see Fig. 81–9B), rather than from mechanical pressure exerted by a local neurofibroma.

formed, or hypoplastic fibula. When deformed or attenuated bones fracture in this disease, they frequently fail to reunite, and pseudarthroses may ultimately result. The precise cause of defective fracture healing and pseudarthroses in neurofibromatosis is not clear.

## Neural Tumors and Tumor-Like Lesions

**Spinal Nerves.** Two important manifestations of neurofibromatosis are neurofibromas and, far more frequently, meningoceles. In fact, 70% to 80% of all meningoceles occur in patients with neurofibromatosis, in whom they are commonly multiple and often (60% of cases) asymptomatic. Radiographic differentiation of meningoceles and neurofibromas is difficult because both lesions may produce focal, posterior, paravertebral masses protruding laterally from enlarged neural foramina. The presence of eccentric, unilateral spinal column scalloping is thought to favor the diagnosis of an adjacent nerve tumor, whereas central scalloping is believed to be more frequent with

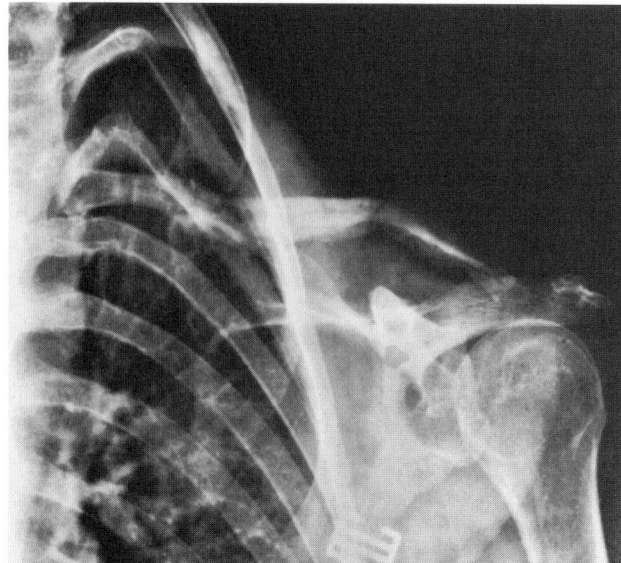

**Figure 81–10.** Neurofibromatosis: rib abnormalities—left upper hemithorax. Typical-appearing ribs are angulated and over-constricted. Some have wavy, undulating, ribbon-like configurations. The upper ribs are widely separated. A pseudarthrosis of the left clavicle is another associated abnormality.

dural ectasia. A paraspinal neuroma may eventually grow centripetally through intervertebral foramina into the spinal canal and assume a dumbbell or hourglass shape identical to that of a meningocele (Figs. 81–12 and 81–13). Focal, paravertebral nerve tumors, with or without intraspinal dumbbell segments, are less frequent. The presence of scoliosis with the convex region directed toward the mass is a feature that favors the diagnosis of meningocele. Calcification within a paraspinal mass, best seen on CT scans, rules against the presence of a meningocele. Conversely, a posterior mediastinal lesion, particularly one that is cystic, in a patient with neurofibromatosis is most likely a meningocele.

The defining lesion of neurofibromatosis is the neurofibroma (Fig. 81–14). Malignant degeneration of neurofibromas is more frequent in association with neurofibromatosis 1 (Fig. 81–15). Many of these lesions are asymptomatic, despite being present at birth or at an early age; however, neurologic sequelae, including paraparesis and paraplegia, may complicate severe kyphoscoliosis, bony dysplasia, or coexistent central nervous system lesions.

**Cranial Nerves.** Tumors of cranial nerves are a recognized manifestation of neurofibromatosis. In neurofibro-

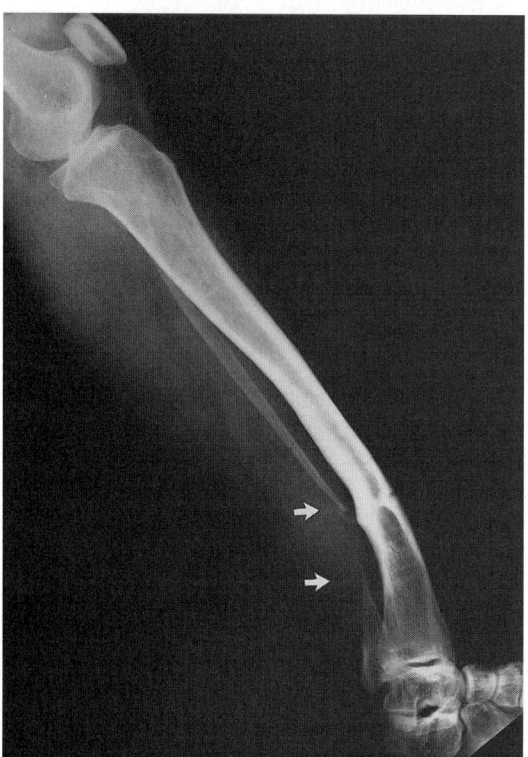

**Figure 81–11.** Neurofibromatosis: pseudarthrosis. On a lateral view of the tibia and fibula, note the pseudarthrosis at the most common site—the junction of the middle and lower thirds of the tibia or fibula, or both, with attenuation and "penciling" of the neighboring fibular segments (*arrows*)—disuse osteoporosis distal to the pseudarthrosis, and secondary deformities of the talus and calcaneus. Anterior bowing of the leg is characteristic and is usually evident in the first years of life. Pseudarthrosis may develop spontaneously, after fracture, or after an osteotomy to correct bowing.

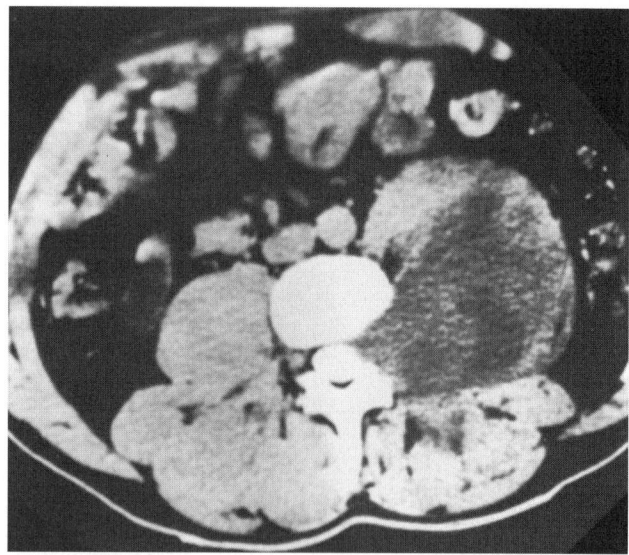

**Figure 81–12.** Neurofibromatosis: neurofibroma. The patient is a 25-year-old black man with known maternal neurofibromatosis, café au lait spots noted at age 13 years, back discomfort since age 18 years, and 6 weeks of progressive left flank pain radiating to the left thigh and knee. Routine films (not shown) revealed a poorly defined mass causing eccentric scalloping of the posterior portion of the vertebral body and superior portion of the L4 transverse process and lateral deviation of the left kidney. Transaxial CT scan at the L3 vertebral level defines a large intradural mass with extradural extension engulfing the nerve root, eroding the posterolateral aspect of the L3 vertebral body and foramen, and involving the psoas and spinothalamic muscles down to the level of the pelvis. The mass, whose rim enhanced irregularly after the injection of contrast material, represents a moderately cellular, focally necrotic, benign neurofibroma.

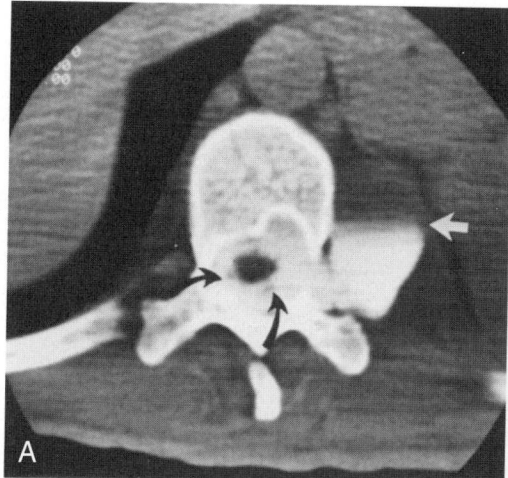

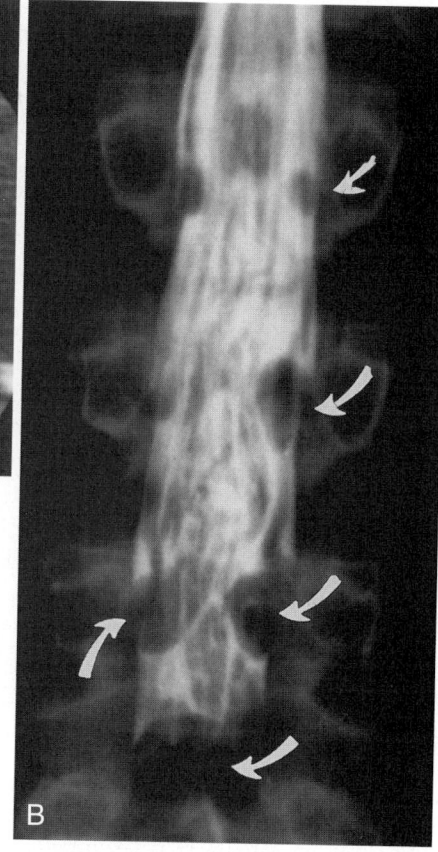

**Figure 81–13.** Neurofibromatosis: meningocele and neurofibroma. *A*, CT scan of the T10 level after a metrizamide myelogram shows a dumbbell-shaped paravertebral mass on the left side arising within the spinal canal. It is causing eccentric erosion of the left pedicle and posterior hemivertebra. Pooled contrast agent with a fluid level within the confines of the mass *(white arrow)* is indicative of a meningocele. Rounded radiolucent shadows represent intradural neurofibromas *(black arrows)*. *B*, Metrizamide myelogram of a 24-year-old man with lower extremity paresthesias shows multiple intrathecal neurofibromas *(arrows)*.

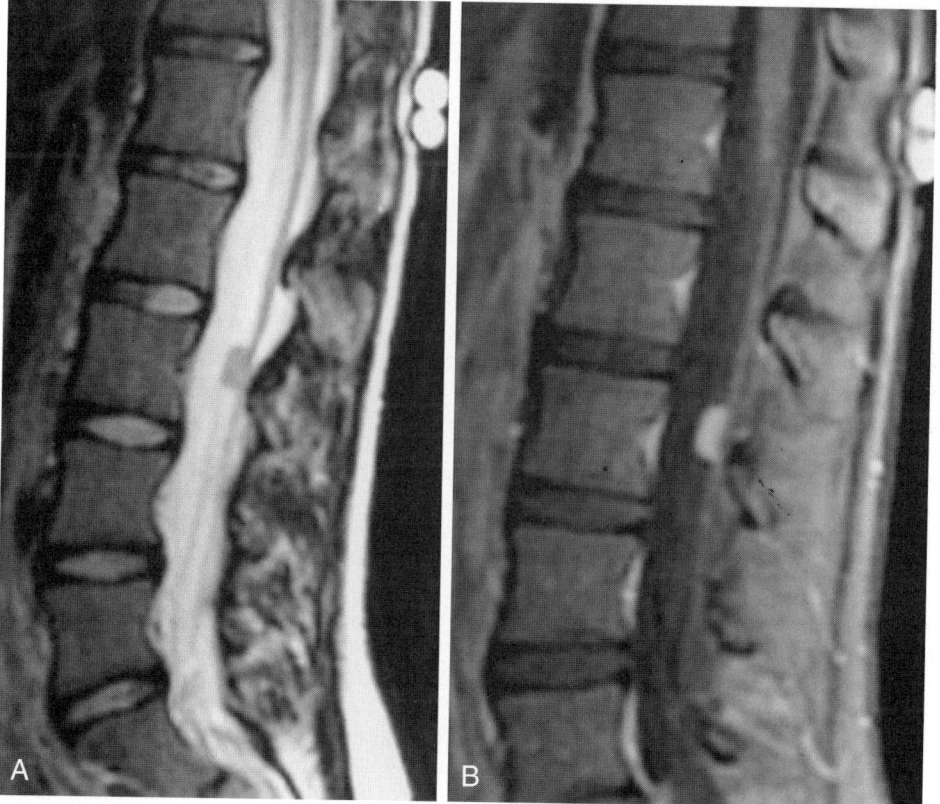

**Figure 81–14.** Neurofibromatosis: neurofibroma. *A*, Sagittal T2-weighted (TR/TE, 3000/112) fat-suppressed spin echo MR image of the lumbar spine in a 19-year-old woman shows an ovoid intraspinal mass with homogeneously decreased signal arising from the filum terminale that represents a neurofibroma. *B*, On a sagittal T1-weighted (TR/TE, 416/21) fat-suppressed spin echo image, the lesion enhances homogeneously after the intravenous administration of a gadolinium-containing contrast agent.

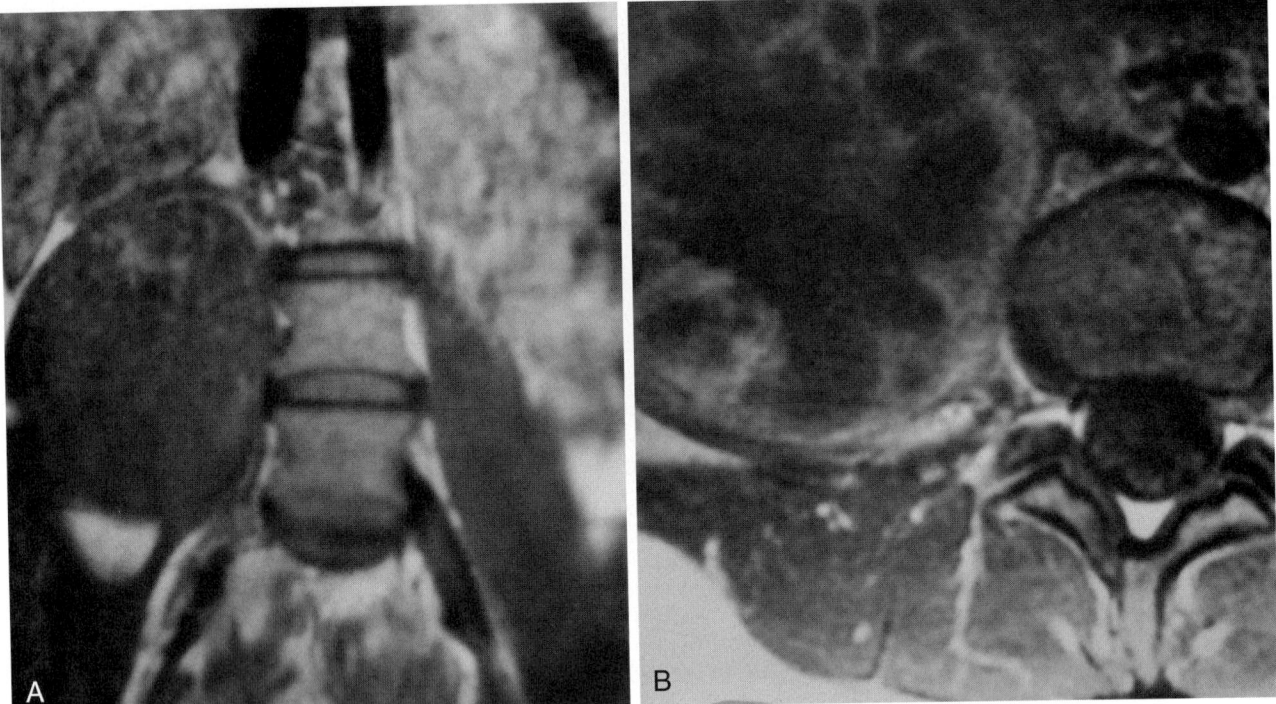

**Figure 81–15.** Neurofibromatosis: retroperitoneal neurofibrosarcoma in a 19-year-old woman. *A,* Coronal T1-weighted (TR/TE, 466/20) spin echo MR image shows a large, apparently well circumscribed, spherical paraspinal mass with homogeneous low signal intensity. *B,* Transverse T1-weighted (TR/TE, 650/19) spin echo MR image after intravenous contrast administration shows peripheral pooling of the contrast agent, with linear extensions into the central substance of the lesion, which subsequently became homogeneously hyperintense.

matosis 1, glial tumors predominate. Optic nerve gliomas are the most common lesions of the central nervous system, with a reported prevalence of 5% to 70%. Conversely, the reported prevalence of neurofibromatosis in patients with optic gliomas varies from 6% to 58%. In neurofibromatosis 2, schwannomas of the cranial (usually the eighth) and spinal nerves are the most common tumors, followed by meningiomas. Bilateral schwannomas usually manifest in the third or fourth decade of life, but they may appear earlier in patients with unilateral lesions.

**Peripheral Nerves.** Peripheral nerve tumors in neurofibromatosis most frequently involve neural supporting tissue. The two most common benign forms are solitary or multiple neurofibromas (Fig. 81–16) and schwannomas (neurilemomas) (Fig. 81–17). The latter are encapsulated lesions that lie on the surface of the nerve. They are more common than neurofibromas, which infiltrate involved nerves diffusely and incorporate all nerve elements. Benign plexiform or cirsoid neurofibromas, observed only in neurofibromatosis, appear as bizarre soft tissue networks that imperceptibly interdigitate with adjacent fat and muscle, recur after resection, and have a potential for malignant degeneration. They are recognized most easily in massively enlarged extremities (e.g., elephantiasis neuromatosa), although the face, head, and trunk may also be involved.

**Malignant Degeneration.** Malignant peripheral nerve sheath tumor (MPNST) has also been referred to as neurofibrosarcoma, malignant neurilemoma, malignant neurofibroma, malignant neurinoma, and malignant schwannoma. MPNSTs can occur at any site but usually arise in the soft tissues of the extremities de novo in a nerve (solitary), in preexisting neurofibromas, or in plexiform neurofibromas of neurofibromatosis 1.

In patients with neurofibromas, approximately half have neurofibromatosis 1. Malignant degeneration occurs in 2% to 29% of patients. MPNST usually manifests as a painless, enlarging, soft tissue mass, most commonly originating from the sciatic nerve or sacral or brachial plexus. Cystic and hemorrhagic degeneration, heterotopic mesenchymal elements such as cartilage, and bone and striated muscle are noted frequently.

With magnetic resonance (MR) imaging, peripheral nerve sheath tumors generally show homogeneous low signal on T1-weighted images and variably increased signal on T2-weighted images. A benign neurogenic tumor is suggested, however, by the presence of a focal homogeneous mass that is isointense or mildly hyperintense to muscle on T1-weighted images, and a central zone of decreased intensity surrounded by a hyperintense rim—the target sign—on T2-weighted images (Fig. 81–18). This sign may correspond to histologic findings in which peripheral myxoid tissue encircles a central collagenous or highly cellular matrix containing Schwann cells, fibroblasts,

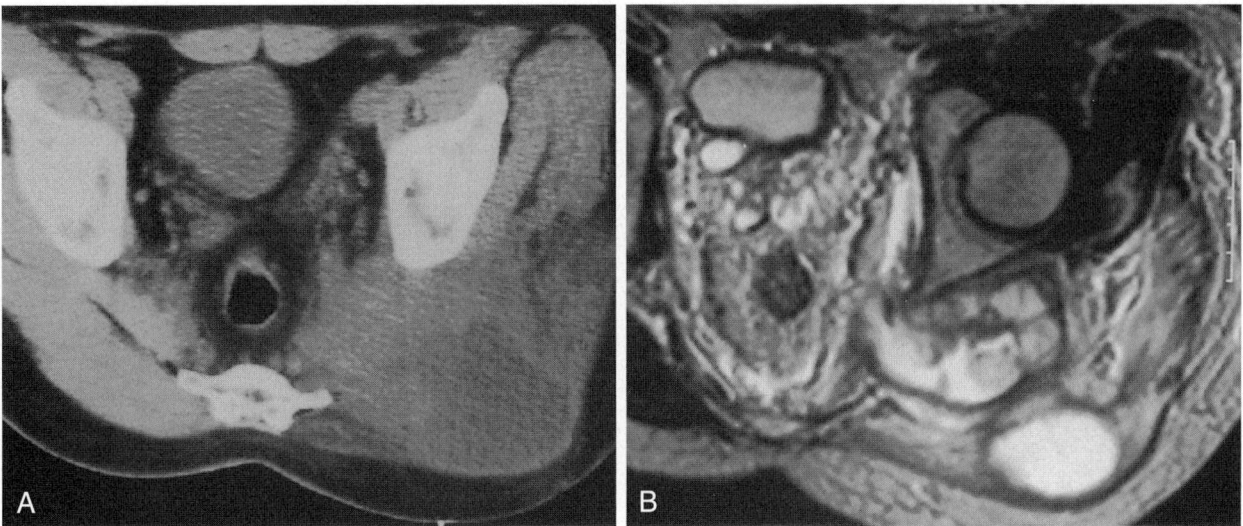

**Figure 81–16.** Neurofibromatosis: plexiform neurofibroma in a 29-year-old man with a painful buttock mass. *A,* Transaxial CT scan at the level of the acetabulum shows a large, poorly circumscribed, inhomogeneous, left-sided buttock mass involving the sacrosciatic notch. *B,* Transaxial T2-weighted (TR/TE, 3000/102) spin echo MR image shows increased signal intensity within rounded masses in the vicinity of the sciatic nerve and in adjacent muscles. Another large, well-defined, more homogeneously hyperintense mass is situated more posteriorly.

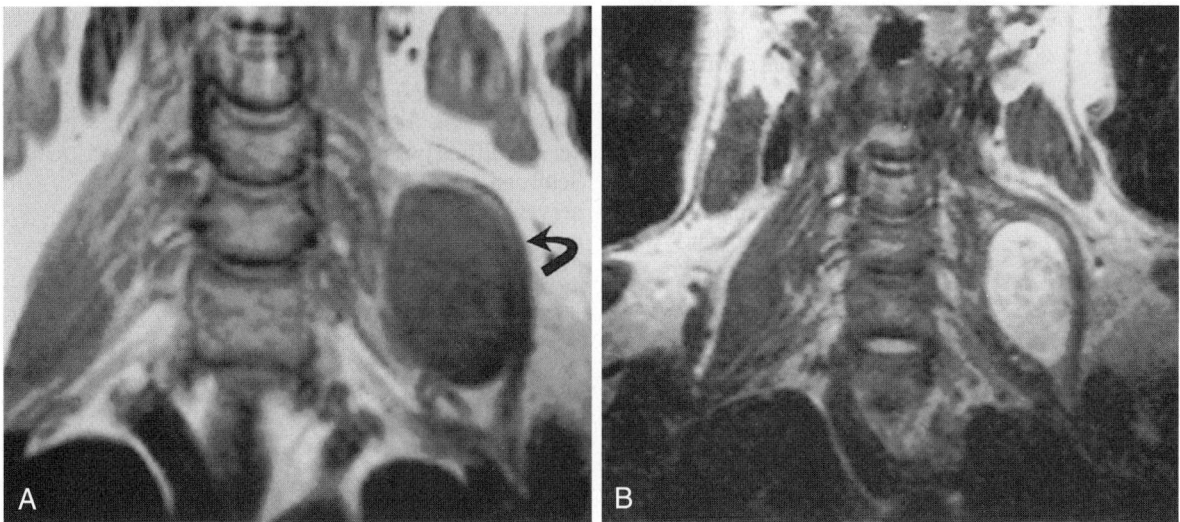

**Figure 81–17.** Neurofibromatosis: schwannoma. In this 38-year-old man with pain and paresthesias in the left arm, coronal T1-weighted (TR/TE, 633/20) *(A)* and T2-weighted (TR/TE, 1800/70) *(B)* spin echo MR images show a well-circumscribed mass in the brachial plexus. It has low signal intensity *(arrow)* in *(A)* and high signal intensity in *(B)*.

and perineurial cells. Benign neurofibromas display either solitary or multiple target signs on MR images, whereas this sign is not seen in MPNSTs. Confounding situations include MPNSTs adjacent to benign neurofibromas or those with gradual regional histologic transition from a benign lesion.

## Miscellaneous Abnormalities

**Other Associated Neoplasms.** Tumors other than those of neural supporting tissue occur much more frequently in patients with neurofibromatosis than in the general population. These tumors include both lesions of neural crest origin (e.g., carcinoid, neuroblastoma, pheochromocy-

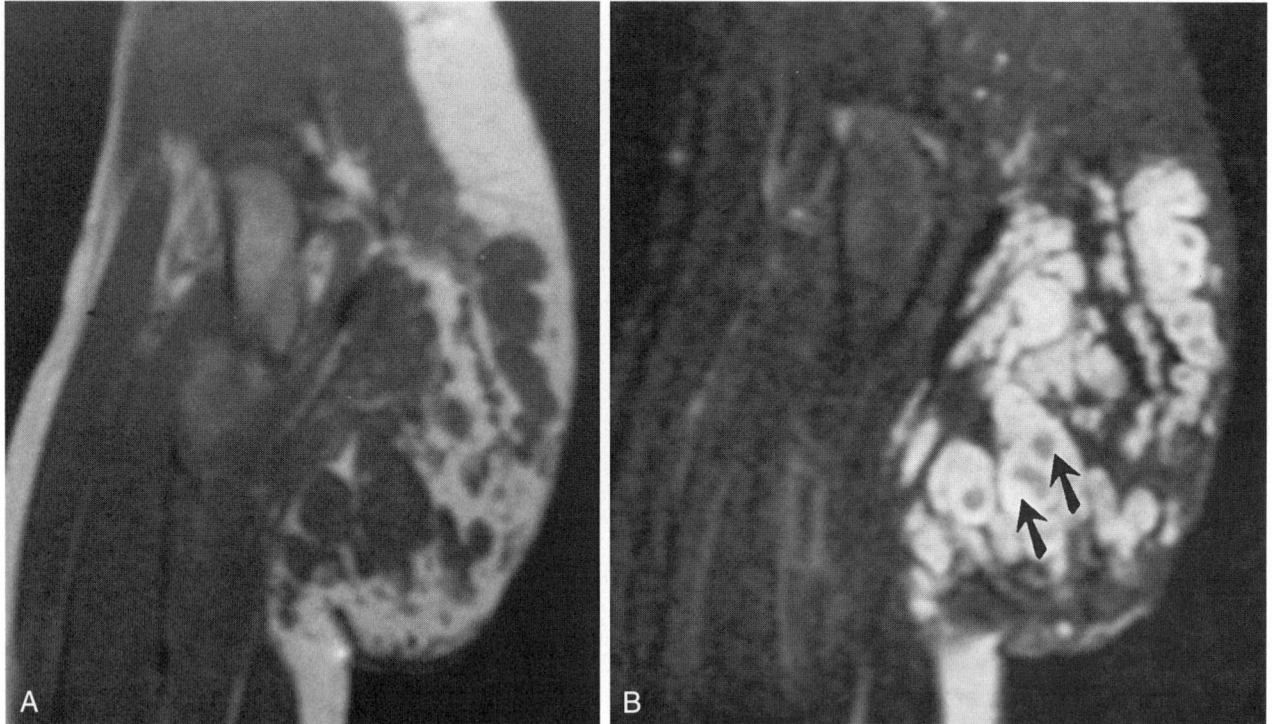

**Figure 81–18.** Neurofibromatosis: plexiform neurofibroma in the right buttock of a 4-year-old girl. *A,* Sagittal T1-weighted (TR/TE, 600/14) spin echo MR image shows lobular and serpentine low-signal masses in the buttock that extend to the superficial subcutaneous tissues, an appearance mimicking that of angiomatosis. *B,* Sagittal fat-suppressed T2-weighted (TR/TE, 6500/80) spin echo image shows that the mass now contains multiple central signal voids—target signs—rimmed by the hyperintense myxoid tissue of the plexiform neurofibroma *(arrows).* (Courtesy of Walter Berdon, MD, New York, N.Y.)

toma, medullary thyroid carcinoma, melanoma) and lesions not clearly derived from the neural crest (e.g., Wilms' tumor, rhabdomyosarcoma, leukemia). In patients with neurofibromatosis, the risk of juvenile chronic myelogenous leukemia and acute myelomonocytic leukemia is 200 to 5000 times normal.

**Aberrations in Growth of Limbs.** The skeletal aberrations frequently associated with neurofibromatosis may be due to deficient or premature cessation of growth, as well as overgrowth of bones and soft tissue. Elephantoid soft tissue hypertrophy of an entire limb or part of a limb, such as gigantism of a finger, may exist with normal-appearing bony structures or with hypertrophied or underdeveloped osseous elements. The cause of these abnormalities is not clear, although hypervascularity, hemorrhage, or both may be important.

**Hemorrhage.** Hemorrhage in neurofibromatosis, which may be massive, recurrent, and fatal, is a commonly unappreciated finding. Subperiosteal and soft tissue hemorrhage has been noted after comparatively minor insults.

**Cystic Lesions in Bone.** Reports of so-called cystic bone lesions in neurofibromatosis have been a source of con-

troversy, particularly when no biopsy has been performed on these lesions. Two types of cysts have been noted: subperiosteal and intraosseous. The subperiosteal form, described as caves, pits, or notches on cortical surfaces, has been attributed to mechanical pressure from adjacent neurogenic tissue and to focal hemorrhage from poorly adherent, dysplastic periosteum, which then proliferates over the lesion. Intraosseous cystic lesions have been attributed to direct invasion of the periosteum, cortex, and haversian canals by neurofibromatous tissue. Most authorities believe that bona fide intraosseous cystic lesions are nonexistent or, at best, are rare expressions of neurofibromatosis.

Jaffe believed that multiple nonossifying fibromas coexisting with brown skin patches might represent a forme fruste of neurofibromatosis. Other investigators thought that nonossifying fibromas were present with increased frequency in neurofibromatosis. Most authors consider nonossifying fibromas to be a coincidental finding in this disorder, however. In one report, patients with neurofibromatosis were noted to have multiple radiolucent bone lesions about the knee. The lesions were variously diagnosed as nonossifying fibromas, fibrous cortical defects, and intraosseous neurofibromas solely on the basis of their radiographic appearance. None was subjected to biopsy.

**Vascular Lesions.** Vascular lesions are common in neurofibromatosis. Arterial abnormalities, including a thickened wall, stenosis, and aneurysms, may involve the genitourinary and gastrointestinal systems, spleen, endocrine glands, brain, heart, and great vessels. Abdominal and thoracic aortic coarctations have been described. Renal artery stenosis is a common underlying cause of hypertension in neurofibromatosis. Approximately 1% of patients with neurofibromatosis have pheochromocytomas, but 5% to 25% of patients with pheochromocytomas have neurofibromatosis.

**Endocrine Abnormalities.** Associated endocrine abnormalities include hyperparathyroidism, osteomalacia, small bowel carcinoid tumors, multiple endocrine adenomatosis, and Sipple's syndrome. Sipple's syndrome is a hereditary disorder consisting of medullary thyroid carcinoma, pheochromocytoma, and multiple mucosal neuromas involving the lips, tongue, eyes, or gastrointestinal tract. It has overlapping features with neurofibromatosis (e.g., multiple neuromas, café au lait spots, and scoliosis), but cutaneous neurofibromas are not present. Precocious sexual development, which is more frequently linked with fibrous dysplasia, has also been reported.

## FIBROUS DYSPLASIA

Fibrous dysplasia is a noninherited, developmental anomaly of bone-forming mesenchyme in which osteoblasts fail to undergo normal morphologic differentiation and maturation. Normal marrow and cancellous bone are replaced by immature woven bone and dense fibrotic stroma. Fibrous dysplasia may affect one bone, a few bones, or many bones. When the polyostotic variety (and, rarely, the monostotic type) is associated with endocrine dysfunction, the disease typically manifests as sexual precocity and cutaneous pigmentation and is known as McCune-Albright syndrome.

## Cutaneous and Mucosal Abnormalities

Abnormal cutaneous pigmentation is the most common extraskeletal manifestation of fibrous dysplasia. Although it is occasionally associated with monostotic involvement, abnormal pigmentation is evident in more than half of persons with polyostotic disease. Abnormal pigmentation may date from birth, but an initial appearance or enlargement of pigmented areas in childhood or even after puberty is not unusual. Pigmentation occasionally precedes the development of skeletal or endocrine abnormalities. The café au lait spots of fibrous dysplasia are usually fewer in number, contoured more irregularly, and darker in color than those of neurofibromatosis.

## Skeletal Abnormalities

Fibrous dysplasia may be associated with either solitary or multiple lesions in one or more bones. Approximately 70% to 80% of cases are monostotic, and 20% to 30% are polyostotic. Monostotic fibrous dysplasia is encountered most frequently in a rib, femur, tibia, gnathic bone, calvaria, and humerus, in decreasing order of frequency.

Polyostotic fibrous dysplasia more frequently involves the skull and facial bones, pelvis, spine, and shoulder girdle.

Polyostotic fibrous dysplasia may be unilateral or bilateral and may affect several bones of a single limb or both limbs, with or without axial skeletal involvement. Despite the designation, however, polyostotic fibrous dysplasia is often limited to just a few osseous sites. The severity and degree of osseous involvement, including gross deformities caused by bowing, angular and curvilinear distortion, fusiform expansion, and linear growth discrepancies, are greater in polyostotic than in monostotic disease. Polyostotic involvement is also correlated with a higher frequency of clinical symptoms, including pain, deformity, limp, and fracture.

Monostotic lesions are recognized most frequently in the second and third decades of life. The age distribution is considerably younger in polyostotic fibrous dysplasia because its more severe manifestations lead to earlier clinical and radiographic recognition. Two thirds of patients are symptomatic before age 10 years. Such differences in degree, distribution, and manifestation of skeletal abnormalities, as well as the absence of well-documented conversion from monostotic to polyostotic involvement, have led some authors to postulate that two independent forms of fibrous dysplasia exist.

**Skull and Facial Bones.** Involvement of the skull and lesions of the facial bones occur with nearly equal frequency and are noted in approximately 10% to 25% of patients with monostotic fibrous dysplasia and in 50% of those with polyostotic involvement (Fig. 81–19). Hypertelorism, displacement of the globe, exophthalmos, diplopia, and visual impairment are related to alterations in the orbital and periorbital bones (Fig. 81–20). Distortion of the sphenoid wing and temporal bone may similarly lead to compromise of the internal auditory canal.

Radiographs commonly reveal radiolucent or sclerotic lesions in the skull, facial bones, or both. Concomitant involvement of the facial bones and prominence of the external occipital protuberance are less frequent in Paget's disease, neurofibromatosis, and meningioma than in fibrous dysplasia. Hazy radiolucent lesions, which are generally the most common manifestations of fibrous dysplasia at all sites, are often associated with widened diploic spaces and expansion of the skull and facial bones. The osseous expansion, which may be focal or widespread, is almost always in an outward direction. Therefore, the outer table of the vault in fibrous dysplasia is invariably convex, whereas both tables, though occasionally thinned, remain essentially intact rather than transgressed or destroyed.

**Spine.** Involvement of the spine is infrequent in polyostotic fibrous dysplasia and rare in monostotic disease. Radiographic characteristics, similar to those noted at sites affected more frequently, include well-defined, expansile radiolucent lesions with multiple internal septations or striations that involve the vertebral body and, occasionally, the pedicles and vertebral arch. Rarely, associated sequelae include paraspinal soft tissue extension and vertebral collapse, which may in turn lead to angular deformity and spinal cord compression (Fig. 81–21).

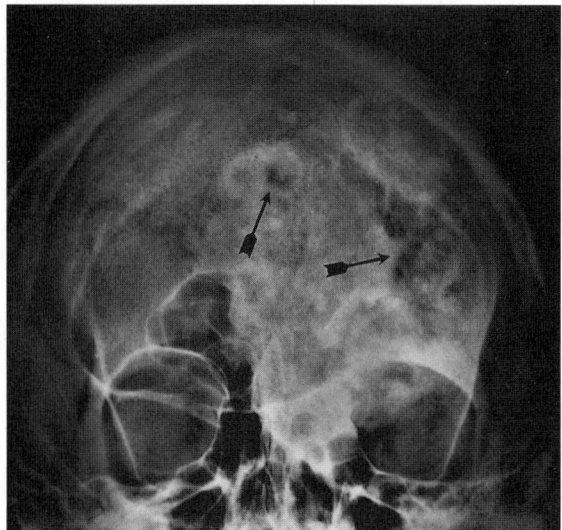

**Figure 81–19.** Fibrous dysplasia: skull abnormalities. In this 22-year-old man, the frontal bone and anterior fossa are predominantly affected. The sphenoid and orbital portions of the frontal bone are markedly involved by the hyperostotic, sharply defined productive process, which is also partially obliterating the left frontal and ethmoid sinuses. Several patchy, well-marginated radiolucent lesions *(arrows)* are evident within the area of sclerosis.

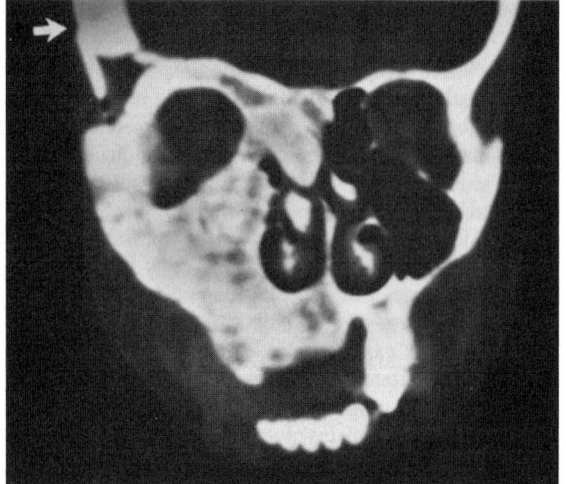

**Figure 81–20.** Fibrous dysplasia: facial bone abnormalities. Coronal CT scan defines the predominantly outward calvarial expansion *(arrow)* with an undisturbed inner table. The dappled, smoky appearance of the expanded bones rimming the right orbit and deforming the right maxilla and maxillary sinus results from their high fibrous and unmineralized osteoid content.

**Tubular Bones.** Lesions in the long bones of the extremities are usually intramedullary and predominantly diaphyseal in location, with only occasional epiphyseal involvement. They may be eccentric or centrally placed and are most often radiolucent, with a hazy quality classically described as a "ground-glass" appearance. The lesions are usually well defined and often bordered by a reactive zone

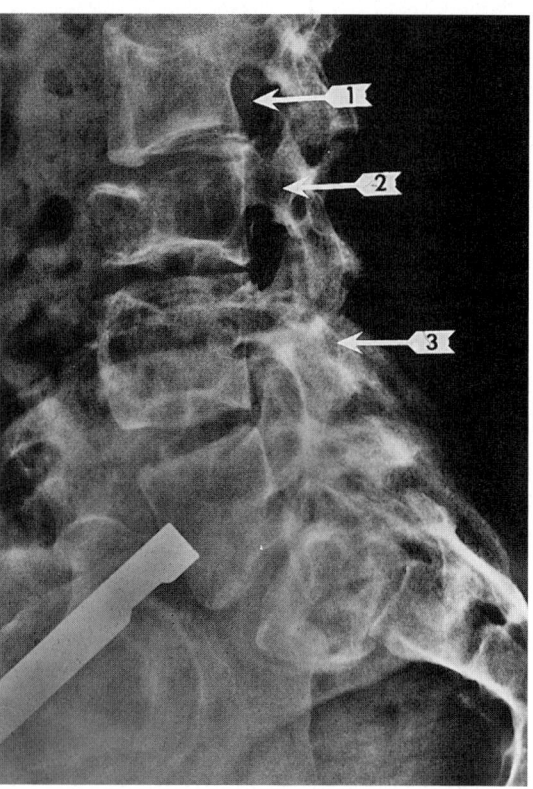

**Figure 81–21.** Fibrous dysplasia: spinal abnormalities. As shown on this lateral view of the lumbar spine, vertebral involvement may take the form of deformed vertebral bodies or posterior elements that have a "ground-glass" appearance *(arrow 1)* or clearer, purely radiolucent lesions having a cystic appearance. The latter most frequently contain a rubbery, fibrous tissue that does not weaken bone *(arrow 3)* as much as the actual cystic, fluid-filled cavities do. Such cysts are presumed to be related to hemorrhage or ischemia and are more prone to compression and collapse *(arrow 2).*

(Figs. 81–22 and 81–23). Occasional endosteal scalloping or erosion may be accompanied by focal cortical thinning. Expansile remodeling contributes the regionally bulging or undulating contours that are a characteristic radiographic feature. An internally loculated or trabeculated configuration and a focally calcified or ossified matrix contribute to the intralesional opaque shadows appreciated on radiographs.

Fibrous dysplasia weakens the structural integrity of involved bone. Weight-bearing bones, in particular, become bowed, with varying degrees of resultant deformity. Pronounced curvature of the femoral neck and proximal portion of the femoral shaft is referred to as a "shepherd's crook" deformity, which is a characteristic stigma of the disease (Fig. 81–24). Fractures frequently follow minor injuries. Stress (insufficiency) fractures are also encountered. The radiographic features of fibrous dysplasia in the metacarpal and metatarsal bones and phalanges are similar to those in the long tubular bones (Fig. 81–25).

**Other Skeletal Sites.** The ribs and innominate bones are affected most commonly, whereas the clavicle, scapula, sacrum, and carpal and tarsal bones are involved only

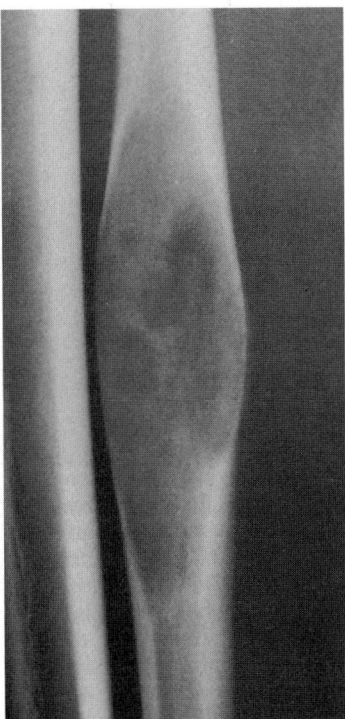

**Figure 81–22.** Fibrous dysplasia: abnormalities of the tubular bones. In this 14-year-old boy, a monostotic lesion in the diaphysis of the fibula is centrally located, hazy in appearance, and well marginated; it shows slight expansile remodeling.

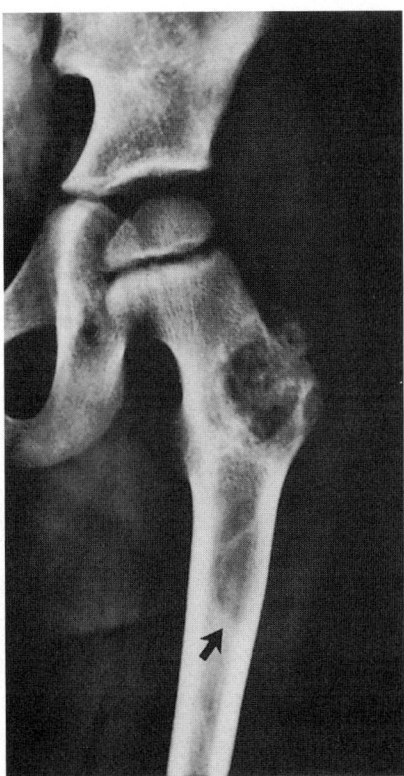

**Figure 81–23.** Fibrous dysplasia: abnormalities of the tubular bones. Anteroposterior view of the femur shows a hazy, irregularly contoured, but well-defined lesion situated in the diametaphysis. Note the partially calcified osseous matrix and the sclerotic rim of the proximal portion of the lesion. Its lowermost extension has an entirely lucent, bladelike configuration that is not as well demarcated *(arrow)*.

occasionally. Of diagnostic importance, fibrous dysplasia is the most frequently occurring benign lesion of the rib cage and represents 30% of primary benign chest wall lesions (Fig. 81–26). Rib involvement, though usually innocuous, may be associated with considerable osseous expansile remodeling and deformity. Unilateral or asymmetrical bilateral involvement of the innominate bones is a frequent eventuality in polyostotic fibrous dysplasia, but it is usually associated with concomitant disease in the proximal portion of the femur (Fig. 81–27). Acetabular deformity, including protrusion, and a markedly distorted triradiate pelvis are often evident.

### Mazabraud's Syndrome

Nonfamilial and noninherited benign myxomatous tumors have also been associated with fibrous dysplasia. Known as Mazabraud's syndrome, this combination is typically seen in polyostotic disease and is more common in women.

Fibrous dysplasia usually precedes the development of myxomas, which occur most often in the thigh, buttock, and pelvic muscles. The most common single site is the thigh, accounting for 75% of cases (Fig. 81–28). On CT, the myxomas appear as soft tissue masses, usually with attenuation between fat and water. MR imaging reveals a mass with the signal intensity of fluid. Often a perilesional fat rind and increased signal in the adjacent muscle are seen on T2-weighted, fluid-sensitive sequences. Although myxomas may appear well defined on imaging

studies, they have no capsule, and the fluid-like perilesional signal results from infiltration of the myxoma into the adjacent atrophic muscle. Contrast enhancement is variable but is most often intense and heterogeneous.

Osteosarcoma of bone has occasionally been reported with Mazabraud's syndrome. Males and patients with polyostotic disease are at greater risk for such malignancy.

### Endocrine Abnormalities

Fibrous dysplasia has no sex predilection. The greater the number of polyostotic cases included in any review of the disease, the greater the likelihood of a female bias. Its characteristically associated endocrinopathy is McCune-Albright syndrome; this syndrome predominates in girls and classically consists of polyostotic fibrous dysplasia, cutaneous pigmentation, and precocious sexual development. Not all patients with fibrous dysplasia characterized by polyostotic disease and cutaneous pigmentation, however, exhibit sexual precocity or endocrine disturbance. Further, incomplete forms of the syndrome include sexual precocity and osseous lesions in the absence of cutaneous pigmentation.

Sexual precocity, rare in boys, occurs in 30% to 50% of affected girls and is characterized by the early appearance

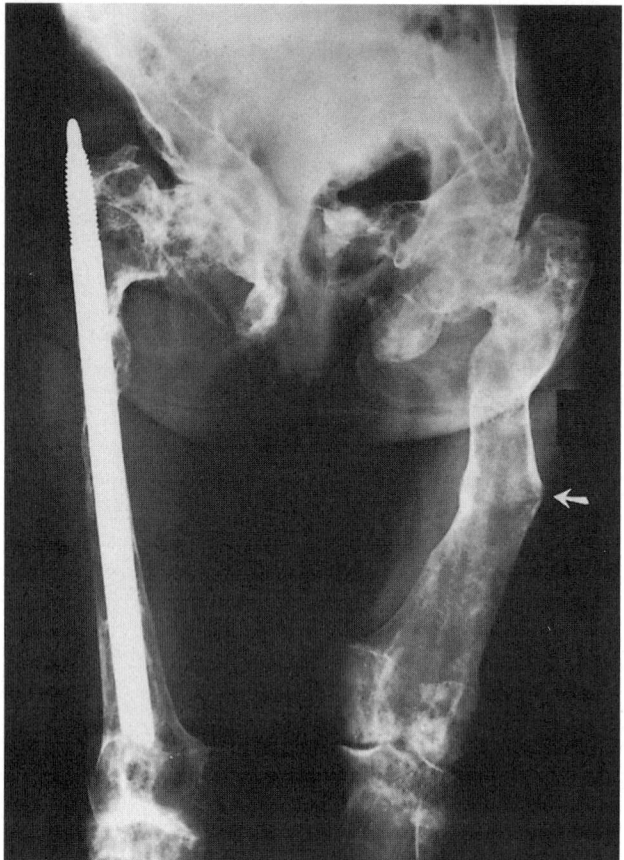

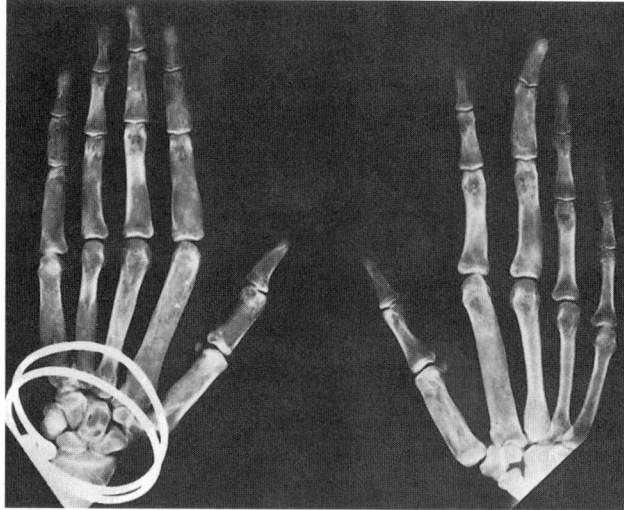

**Figure 81–25.** Fibrous dysplasia: abnormalities of the tubular bones. Posteroanterior view of the hands shows expansion of the spongiosa, cortical thinning, and altered bone texture—common radiographic findings in affected tubular bones. This 16-year-old girl had widespread failure of modeling, with abnormal angulation and localized overgrowth of bones and soft tissues. Several metacarpal bones and phalanges have rectangular or fusiform shapes, with loss of definition between medullary and cortical bone. The hazy or "ground-glass" appearance is particularly uniform in the second metacarpal bones. Localized radiolucent lesions with endosteal scalloping and areas of medullary sclerosis are also seen in several phalanges.

**Figure 81–24.** Fibrous dysplasia: abnormalities of the tubular bones. Anteroposterior view of the pelvis and femora reveals polyostotic involvement in a 20-year-old woman with McCune-Albright syndrome and a history of multiple fractures and surgical interventions. Note the severe pelvic distortion and bilateral proximal femoral varus deformities—the so-called shepherd's crook deformities. The femoral shafts are poorly modeled, with an intrinsic hazy, lucent appearance and little sclerosis or lesional calcification. The entire shafts, including the bone ends, are affected. An acute angulation is seen at the site of a previously healed fracture *(arrow)*.

of vaginal bleeding, breast development, and axillary and pubic hair. The term sexual precocity or precocious pseudopuberty is preferred over precocious puberty, because puberty implies mature gonadal function.

It is noteworthy that even in the absence of overt sexual precocity, apparent hormonal disturbances are reflected in advanced skeletal maturation and accelerated linear growth, with or without subsequent premature closure of the physes.

## Other Abnormalities

Hypophosphatemic rickets and osteomalacia have been noted in patients with either monostotic or polyostotic fibrous dysplasia, both with and without McCune-Albright syndrome. Clinical signs and symptoms, which include skeletal pain, tenderness, and osseous deformity, have been documented in association with pertinent biochemical abnormalities. The findings are analogous to

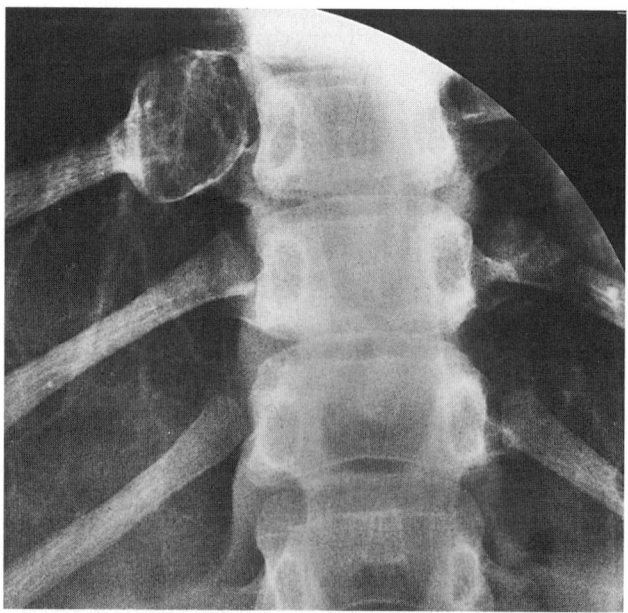

**Figure 81–26.** Fibrous dysplasia: rib abnormalities. This solitary, expansile, multilocular-appearing lesion with an intact cortex was an incidental finding on a chest film of a teenage boy. The most probable cause of such a focal rib lesion is fibrous dysplasia. Rib lesions are more commonly associated with prominent fibrous replacement of bone and are therefore commonly radiolucent.

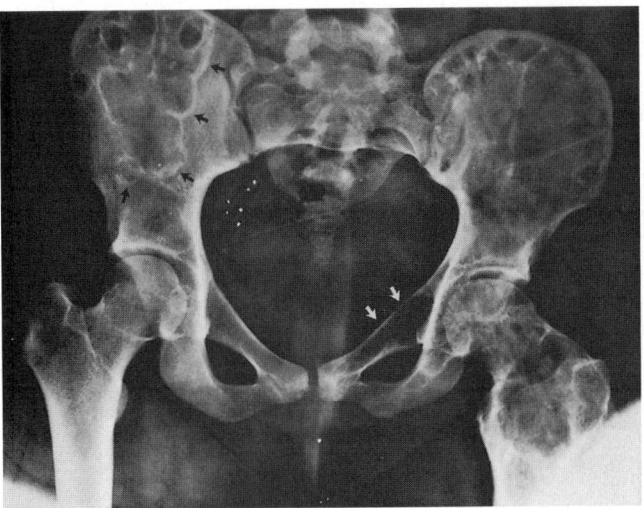

**Figure 81–27.** Fibrous dysplasia: pelvic abnormalities. Anteroposterior view of the pelvis in a 16-year-old girl with polyostotic fibrous dysplasia and McCune-Albright syndrome. The dysplasia has resulted in a thickened, foreshortened femoral neck and shaft held in varus position (shepherd's crook deformity). Note the hazy, "ground-glass" appearance of the involved left femur, with relative sparing of the femoral head. The left pubis and both ilia are also involved by radiographically typical lesions of fibrous dysplasia. The purely radiolucent pubic lesion is expansile and nonmineralized *(white arrows).* The central segments of the right iliac locus appear hazy and smoky because of a high proportion of osteoid and are well demarcated by an almost continuous curvilinear sclerotic rim *(black arrows).*

those seen when rickets and osteomalacia accompany neoplastic disorders of bone or soft tissue. In these instances, as well as in fibrous dysplasia, resection of the lesion may be followed by disappearance of the findings of rickets or osteomalacia. Synthesis of a phosphaturic hormone by a concomitant bone or soft tissue tumor or by benign fibrous lesions, such as fibrous dysplasia, is one hypothesis developed to explain the associated metabolic disorder.

## Imaging Techniques

CT scanning is extremely useful in accurately defining the full extent and nature of the skeletal involvement in fibrous dysplasia, particularly in such complex anatomic areas as the spine, pelvis, and skull. MR imaging can also be applied to the assessment of fibrous dysplasia, but the signal intensity characteristics are variable. Although areas of involvement are typically of low signal intensity on T1-weighted spin echo MR images, low, intermediate, or high signal intensity may be evident on T2-weighted spin echo MR images. The degree of enhancement of signal intensity after the intravenous administration of gadolinium-based contrast agents is also variable (Fig. 81–29).

## Natural History

The prognosis of patients with fibrous dysplasia generally depends on the extent and degree of initial skeletal involvement, as well as the extraskeletal features. Monostotic involvement usually does not convert to polyostotic disease,

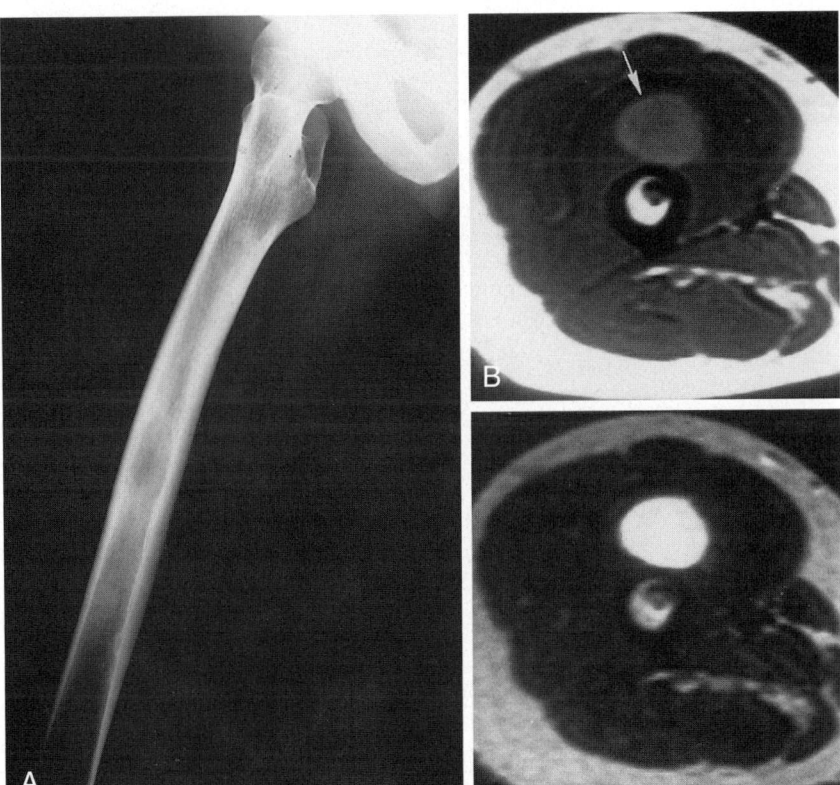

**Figure 81–28.** Fibrous dysplasia: Mazabraud's syndrome. *A,* The long diaphyseal lesion in the right femur has a hazy "ground-glass" appearance, with focal areas of sclerosis and radiolucency. *B,* Transverse intermediate-weighted (TR/TE, 2500/20) spin echo MR image shows a smoothly marginated mass in the vastus intermedius muscle, with its posterior border abutting the anterior femoral cortex. The low-signal intramedullary fibrous component blends imperceptibly with the intact cortex *(arrow).* *C,* Transverse T2-weighted (TR/TE, 2500/160) spin echo MR image shows homogeneously increased signal within a morphologically unchanged mass, an appearance reflecting its myxoid contents. The femoral intramedullary signal remains unchanged. (Courtesy of M. Sundaram, MD, St. Louis, Mo.)

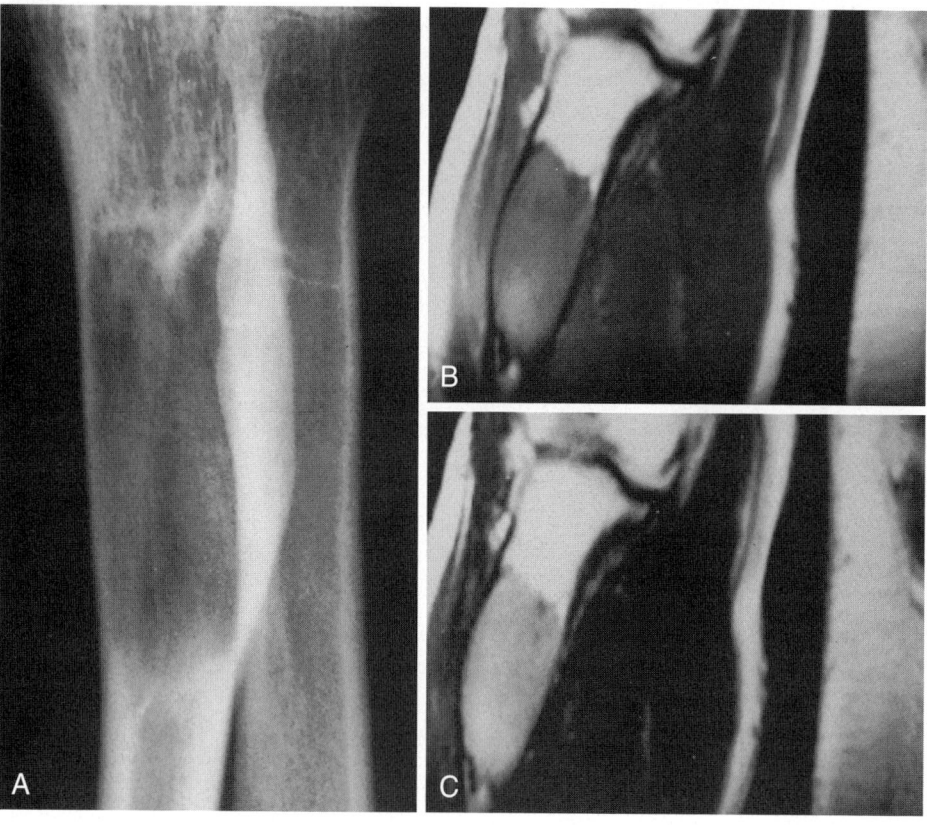

**Figure 81–29.** Fibrous dysplasia. *A*, Routine radiograph shows a slightly expansile osteolytic lesion in the proximal portion of the ulna. *B* and *C*, Coronal intermediate-weighted (TR/TE, 1200/20) *(B)* and T2-weighted (TR/TE, 1200/70) *(C)* spin echo MR images reveal the expansile lesion. It is of low signal intensity in *(B)* and intermediate signal intensity in *(C)*. (Courtesy of C. Sebrechts, MD, San Diego, Calif.)

and in most instances, the size and number of skeletal lesions do not increase after the initial radiographic evaluation. Exceptions to these rules have been documented, however. Although both polyostotic and monostotic fibrous dysplasia generally become quiescent at puberty, activation of skeletal lesions has also been noted during the course of pregnancy and estrogen therapy.

## Malignant Degeneration

Malignant transformation of skeletal lesions is a rare complication of fibrous dysplasia, with an estimated frequency of 0.4% to 1%. In many presumed examples of spontaneous malignant degeneration in fibrous dysplasia, previous irradiation of the involved bones has complicated the picture. Osteosarcoma, fibrosarcoma, and malignant fibrous histiocytoma are the types of tumors encountered most often. Although chondrosarcoma occurs less frequently, its recognition is particularly difficult in view of the intrinsic cartilaginous islands or nodules that frequently coexist with fibrous dysplasia.

## FURTHER READING

Albright F, Butler AM, Hampton AO, et al: Syndrome characterized by osteitis fibrosa disseminata, areas of pigmentation and endocrine dysfunction with precocious puberty in females. N Engl J Med 216:727, 1937.

Brown B: The radiologic features of bone changes in tuberous sclerosis with a case report. J Can Assoc Radiol 12:1, 1961.

Burrows EH: Bone changes in orbital neurofibromatosis. Br J Radiol 36:549, 1963.

Crawford AH Jr, Bogamery N: Osseous manifestations of neurofibromatosis in childhood. J Pediatr Orthop 6:72, 1986.

Drolshagen LF, Reynolds WA, Marcus NW: Fibrocartilaginous dysplasia of bone. Radiology 156:32, 1985.

Ducatman BS, Scheithauer BW, Dahlin DC: Malignant bone tumors associated with neurofibromatosis. Mayo Clin Proc 58:578, 1983.

Dunnick NR: Image interpretation session: 1999. Intraosseous malignant peripheral nerve sheath tumor (malignant schwannoma) in a patient with neurofibromatosis. Radiographics 20:271, 2000.

Gibson MJ, Middlemiss JH: Fibrous dysplasia of bone. Br J Radiol 44:1, 1971.

Green GJ: The radiology of tuberose sclerosis. Clin Radiol 19:135, 1968.

Holt JF, Kuhns LR: Macrocranium and macrencephaly in neurofibromatosis. Skeletal Radiol 1:25, 1976.

Hunt JC, Pugh DG: Skeletal lesions in neurofibromatosis. Radiology 76:1, 1961.

Klatte EC, Franken EA, Smith JA: The radiographic spectrum in neurofibromatosis. Semin Roentgenol 11:17, 1976.

Komar NN, Gabrielsen TO, Holt JF: Roentgenographic appearance of lumbosacral spine and pelvis in tuberous sclerosis. Radiology 89:701, 1967.

Leeds NE, Jacobson HG: Spinal neurofibromatosis. AJR Am J Roentgenol 126:617, 1976.

Leeds N, Seaman WB: Fibrous dysplasia of the skull and its differential diagnosis: A clinical and roentgenographic study of 46 cases. Radiology 78:570, 1962.

Lichtenstein L, Jaffe HL: Fibrous dysplasia of bone: A condition affecting one, several or many bones, the graver cases of which may present abnormal pigmentation of skin, premature sexual development, hyperthyroidism or still other extraskeletal abnormalities. Arch Pathol 33:777, 1942.

Mandell GA, Dalinka MK, Coleman BG: Fibrous lesions in the lower extremities in neurofibromatosis. AJR Am J Roentgenol 133:1135, 1979.

Medley BE, McLeod RA, Houser OW: Tuberous sclerosis. Semin Roentgenol 11:35, 1976.

Murphey MD, McRae GA, Fanburg-Smith JC, et al: Imaging of soft-tissue myxoma with emphasis on CT and MR and comparison of radiologic and pathologic findings. Radiology 225:215, 2002.

Pitt MJ, Mosher JF, Edeiken J: Abnormal periosteum and bone in neurofibromatosis. Radiology 103:143, 1972.

Riddell DH: Malignant change in fibrous dysplasia. J Bone Joint Surg Br 46:251, 1964.

Sack GH Jr: Malignant complications of neurofibromatosis. Clin Oncol 9:17, 1983.

Sundaram M, McDonald DJ, Merenda G: Intramuscular myxoma: A rare but important association. AJR Am J Roentgenol 153:107, 1989.

Warrick CK: Polyostotic fibrous dysplasia—Albright's syndrome: A review of the literature and report of four male cases, two of which were associated with precocious puberty. J Bone Joint Surg Br 31:175, 1949.

Wood B, Lieberman E, Landing B, et al: Tuberous sclerosis. AJR Am J Roentgenol 158:750, 1992.

# CHAPTER 82

## Enostosis, Hyperostosis, and Periostitis

## SUMMARY OF KEY FEATURES

Certain disorders are associated with localized or generalized cortical hyperostosis or periostitis. These include enostoses (bone islands), osteomas with or without associated Gardner's syndrome, osteopoikilosis, osteopathia striata, melorheostosis, pachydermoperiostosis, secondary hypertrophic osteoarthropathy, vascular insufficiency, infantile cortical hyperostosis, hyperostosis frontalis interna, diffuse idiopathic skeletal hyperostosis, sternocostoclavicular hyperostosis, fluorosis, plasma cell dyscrasias, neurofibromatosis, and several rare or poorly defined syndromes. The changes must be distinguished from the periostitis that occurs as a response to an adjacent osseous process (neoplasm, infection, trauma) and from hyperostosis accompanying other congenital disorders.

## INTRODUCTION

Single or multiple areas of increased radiodensity are commonly detected on skeletal radiographs. These may appear as discrete foci within the spongiosa (enostosis) or on the surface of the cortex (osteoma), or there may be more diffuse, widespread areas of cortical hyperostosis or periostitis.

## ENOSTOSIS (BONE ISLAND)

Although the true frequency of these lesions is not known, the prevalence of bone islands of the pelvic bone is about 1%. In the spine, enostoses may be apparent in 1% to 14% of persons. Bone islands are seen in both men and women and in all age groups, with perhaps a lower frequency in pediatric patients. Any osseous site can be affected, but the lesions have a predilection for the pelvis, proximal femur, and ribs.

Enostoses appear radiographically as single or multiple intraosseous sclerotic areas with discrete margins in asymptomatic persons. They may be ovoid, round, or oblong in shape, and they are usually aligned with the long axis of the trabecular architecture. Thorny, radiating bony spicules extend from the center of the lesion, intermingling with the surrounding trabeculae, and lesions do not protrude from the cortical surface of the involved bone (Fig. 82–1). The classic radiographic features of an enostosis include a uniformly radiodense lesion of variable size.

Computed tomography (CT) and magnetic resonance (MR) imaging can be used effectively to further define the morphology and position of enostoses (Fig. 82–2). Typically, with MR imaging, the lesions are of low signal intensity on all pulse sequences. They are located within the medullary cavity of the bone or abut the endosteal surface of the cortex. In the latter situation, the term endosteoma may be applied to the lesion. Rare central resorption of bone within an enostosis has been described, resulting in a central radiolucent area. Bone islands may increase or decrease in size or disappear completely. Bone scintigraphy usually yields normal results, although positive bone scans have been described in patients with large bone islands.

In addition to skeletal metastases, the differential diagnosis of enostoses includes osteomas, osteoid osteomas, enchondromas, bone infarcts, fibrous dysplasia, and osteopoikilosis (Table 82–1).

## OSTEOMA

An osteoma is a protruding mass composed of abnormally dense but otherwise normal bone that is formed in the periosteum. The lesion is confined to areas of the bone that are normally produced by the periosteal membrane. Osteomas predominate in the skull and facial bones, although they may occasionally arise at other sites, including the pelvis and the tubular bones of the extremities. In the latter locations, osteochondromas containing cartilaginous caps are much more frequent and represent different lesions.

Osteomas are very frequent in the sinuses, especially in the frontal and ethmoid sinuses. Their frequency has been estimated to be 0.42% in patients who have had sinus radiographs, and they are usually small. Osteomas also arise from the inner and outer tables of the cranial vault, the mandible, and the maxilla. Osteomas predominate in the fourth and fifth decades of life and are generally asymptomatic unless they protrude significantly into the sinus cavity, encroach on the orbital contents, extend into the cranial cavity, or prohibit normal dental formation or tongue movement.

On radiographs, the lesions appear as a single focus or as multiple radiodense foci that protrude into a sinus or extend from the surface of a parent bone (Figs. 82–3 and 82–4). Their outline is smooth or lobular, and they are frequently homogeneous. Once discovered, osteomas usually remain unchanged on serial studies.

Osteomas arising from the cortical surface of the clavicle, scapula, innominate bone, or tubular bones are sometimes termed parosteal osteomas. The radiographic appearance of parosteal osteoma (Fig. 82–5) simulates that of parosteal osteosarcoma, ossifying parosteal lipoma, or post-traumatic heterotopic bone formation (myositis ossificans). Typically, however, the surface of a parosteal osteoma is smooth, with or without lobulations. CT and MR imaging verify the absence of an adjacent soft tissue mass. Although the signal intensity characteristics of the lesion may vary, low signal intensity is usually dominant. Rarely, intraosseous extension of a parosteal osteoma is seen.

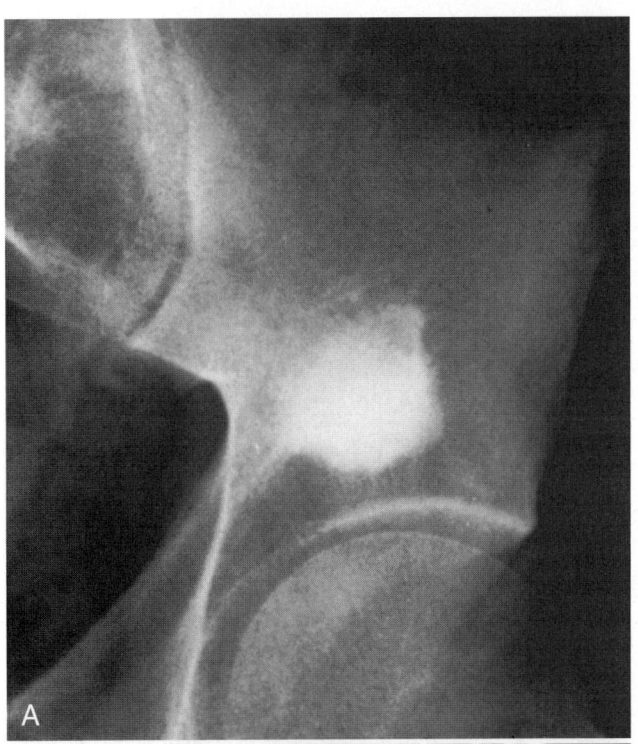

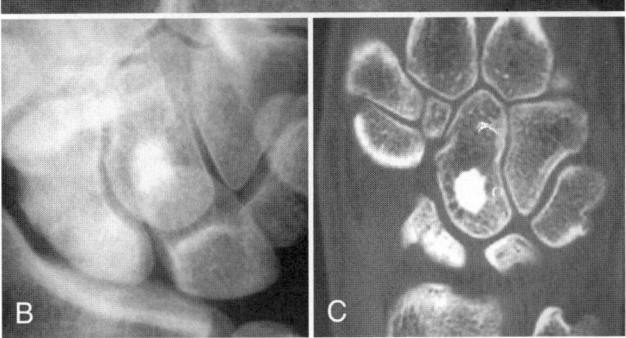

**Figure 82–1.** Enostosis: pelvis and wrist. *A*, Large enostoses of the pelvis. In this location, such lesions are commonly this size. Note the homogeneous nature of the dense area and the radiating spicules extending into the adjacent bone. *B*, In a different patient, a radiograph obtained for a scaphoid fracture reveals incidental enostosis of the capitate. *C*, CT scan demonstrates radiating bony spicules extending from the center of the lesion, intermingling with the surrounding trabeculae.

Multiple osteomas of the mandible, calvaria, or tubular bones can accompany Gardner's syndrome (Table 82–2), a familial autosomal dominant disease consisting of colonic polyposis, osteomatosis, and soft tissue tumors. The soft tissue tumors consist of epidermal or sebaceous cysts, subcutaneous fibromas and lipomas, and desmoid tumors. Desmoid tumors occur in 3% to 29% of patients with Gardner's syndrome. The osseous lesions frequently precede any clinical or radiographic evidence of intestinal polyposis, and as many as half of patients with Gardner's syndrome may have osteomas. The lesions may also be detected in the ribs and long bones; in the latter sites, however, the outgrowths may not be well defined, appearing instead as localized, wavy cortical thickening, especially in the femur, tibia, and ulna (Fig. 82–6).

## OSTEOPOIKILOSIS

Osteopoikilosis (osteopathia condensans disseminata, or "spotted bones") is an asymptomatic osteosclerotic dysplasia. The disorder is seen in both male and female patients, and its appearance before age 3 years is distinctly uncommon. Both inherited and sporadic cases have been reported. Clinical manifestations are usually absent or mild. Cutaneous lesions may be evident in approximately 25% of cases and consist of fibrocollagenous infiltrations, a predisposition to keloid formation, and scleroderma-like lesions.

Radiographic findings are diagnostic. Numerous small, well-defined, homogeneous circular or ovoid foci of increased radiodensity are clustered in periarticular osseous regions. A symmetrical distribution is observed, with a predilection for the epiphyses and metaphyses of the long tubular bones (Fig. 82–7), carpus, tarsus, pelvis, and scapula; involvement of the ribs, clavicle, spine, or skull is rare and, when present, is less marked. Radionuclide examination with bone-seeking radiopharmaceutical agents usually reveals no evidence of increased activity about the skeletal lesions.

Some evidence suggests that a relationship exists between this condition and other osteosclerotic skeletal disorders, especially osteopathia striata and melorheostosis (Table 82–3). The resulting combination of abnormalities is referred to as mixed sclerosing bone dystrophy (see later discussion).

The major differential diagnostic considerations in cases of widespread, focal, round or oval radiodense lesions are osteopoikilosis, osteoblastic metastases, mastocytosis, and tuberous sclerosis. The symmetrical distribution, the propensity for epiphyseal and metaphyseal involvement, and the uniform size of the foci are features that suggest osteopoikilosis, a diagnosis that is supported by a normal-appearing bone scan.

## OSTEOPATHIA STRIATA

Osteopathia striata (Voorhoeve's disease) is a rare disease of unknown cause. Men and women of any age can be affected, and a genetic transmission, probably an autosomal dominant one, has been suggested but is not definite. Clinical manifestations are usually absent.

Radiography reveals linear, regular bands of increased radiodensity that extend from the metaphyses of tubular bones for variable distances into the diaphyses and are interspersed with areas of rarefaction (Fig. 82–8). The length of the striations may be related to the growth rate of the involved bone; the longest lesions are often found in the femur. In the flat bones, especially the ilium, a fanlike arrangement of radiodense striations radiates toward the iliac crests. Involvement of the small bones of the hands and feet, the skull and facial bones, or the spine is unusual. Scintigraphy with bone-seeking radiopharmaceutical agents fails to reveal significant abnormalities. Osteopathia striata may coexist with osteopoikilosis, melorheostosis, or osteopetrosis (see Table 82–3).

The differential diagnosis includes prominent vertical trabecular formation, which may be a normal variant; the adult form of osteopetrosis, in which linear striations of the long bones and pelvis may be encountered; enchon-

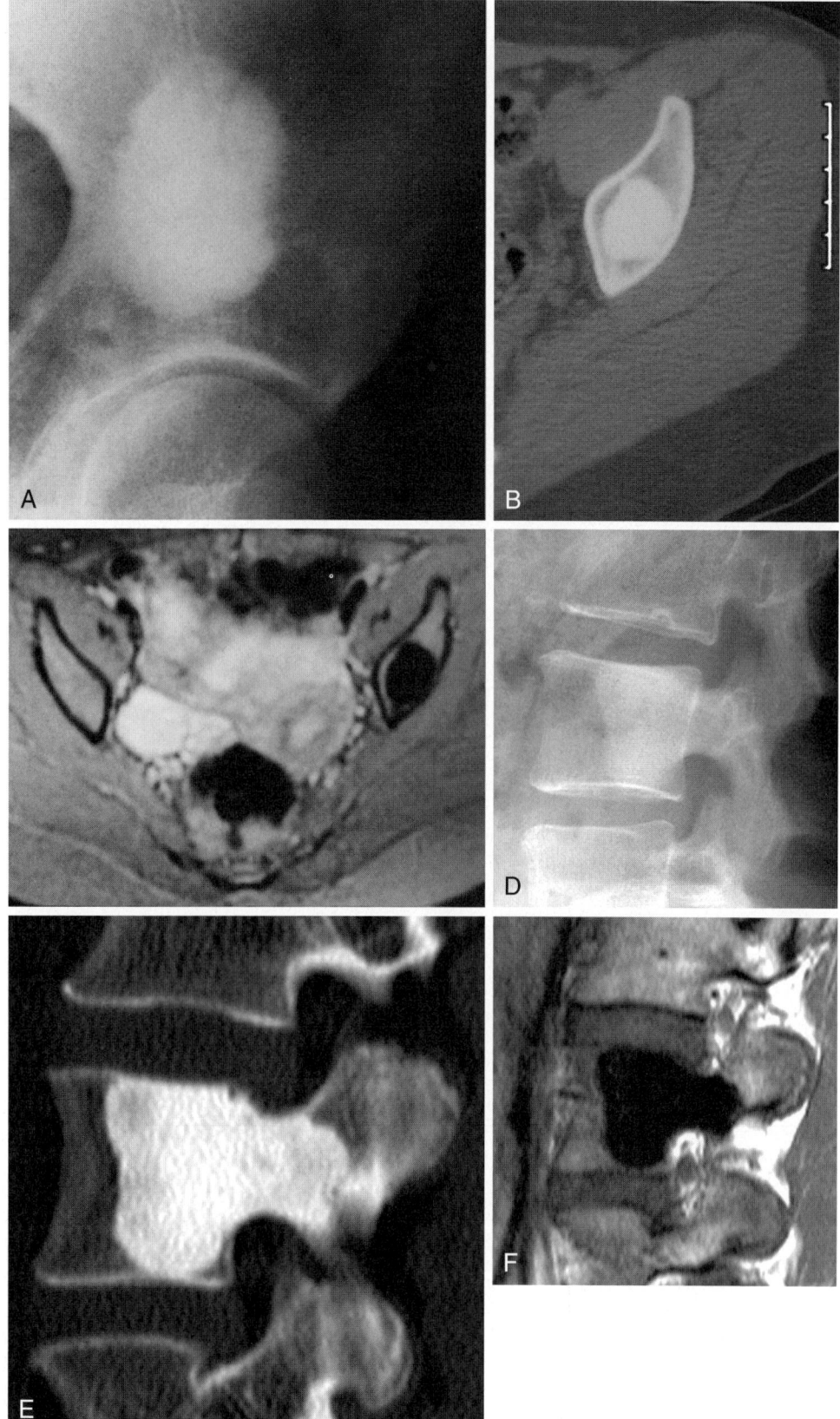

**Figure 82–2.** Enostosis. *A,* On a conventional radiograph, the large radiodense lesion has the typical features of an enostosis. *B,* Transverse CT scan confirms that the lesion is homogeneous in nature. *C,* Transverse intermediate-weighted (TR/TE, 4800/13) spin echo MR image shows a lesion of homogeneously low signal intensity. Similar findings were seen on T1- and T2-weighed pulse sequences. *D,* In a different patient, a large endosteoma of the vertebral body is presented. *E,* CT scan shows the lesion to be relatively homogeneous and well defined, with no expansion of osseous contour. *F,* Sagittal T1-weighted (TR/TE, 658/12) spin echo MR image shows the typical appearance and low signal intensity. Similar findings were seen on T2-weighed pulse images.

**TABLE 82–1**

**Localized Radiodense Lesions**

| Lesion | Location | Appearance |
| --- | --- | --- |
| Enostosis (bone island) | Medullary | Round or oblong, thorny radiating spicules |
| Osteoma | Cortical protrusion | Homogeneous, smooth or lobular, extend from osseous surface |
| Osteochondroma | Cortical and medullary protrusion | Cortical bone and spongiosa are continuous with parent bone, calcified cap |
| Enchondroma | Medullary | Lucent, well-circumscribed, central calcifications |
| Bone infarct | Medullary | Lucent, well or poorly circumscribed, peripheral shell of calcification |
| Osteoid osteoma | Cortical, medullary, or subperiosteal | Cortical: lucent with or without calcification surrounded by sclerotic bone<br>Medullary: lucent or calcified, with little sclerosis<br>Superiosteal: scalloped excavation with or without calcification and sclerosis |

dromatosis (Ollier's disease), in which oval-shaped lesions may produce metaphyseal bands of diminished density; and osteopoikilosis, in which oval or circular radiodense foci are seen.

## MELORHEOSTOSIS

Melorheostosis is a rare bone disorder that usually manifests after early childhood; in approximately 40% to 50% of cases, it is evident by age 20 years. Occasionally, patients in the fourth and fifth decades of life may reveal evidence of melorheostosis. Men and women are affected equally, and no hereditary features have been established.

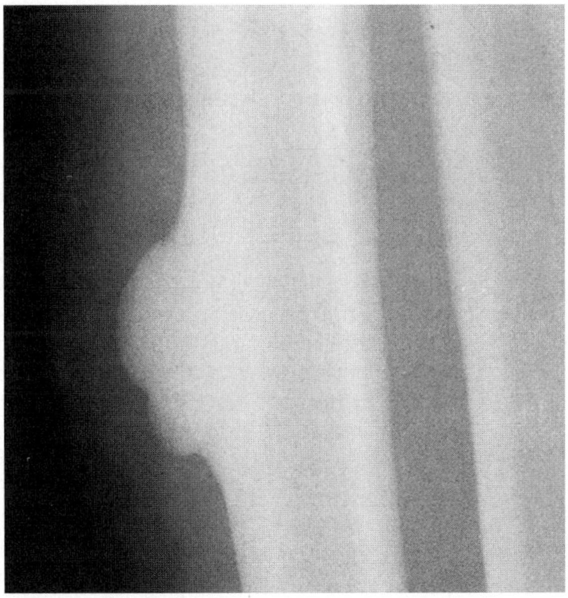

Initial manifestations are variable. Intermittent swelling of joints may be evident. Pain and limitation of motion are more common in adults than in children; with increasing muscle contractures, tendon and ligament shortening, and soft tissue involvement, these findings may become profound. Growth disturbances include increased circumference and angulation of affected limbs and unequal limb length. Soft tissue changes include tense, erythematous, and shiny skin; anomalous pigmentation; induration and edema of subcutaneous tissues; fibrosis; weakness and atrophy of muscles; and linear scleroderma. Soft tissue changes may precede the osseous abnormalities and may be evident at birth. Although life expectancy is not shortened, the disease can result in considerable deformity and disability.

Radiographic alterations are commonly limited to a single limb, in which one or more bones may be affected. The lower extremity is involved more frequently than the upper extremity. Abnormalities may also be encountered in the skull and facial bones, ribs, and vertebrae. Changes

**Figure 82–3.** Osteoma: tubular bones. A protruding, homogeneously dense mass of the ulna is evident. It is of the same radiodensity and appearance as the underlying cortex. Note that there is no connection between the medullary bone of the ulna and the lesion.

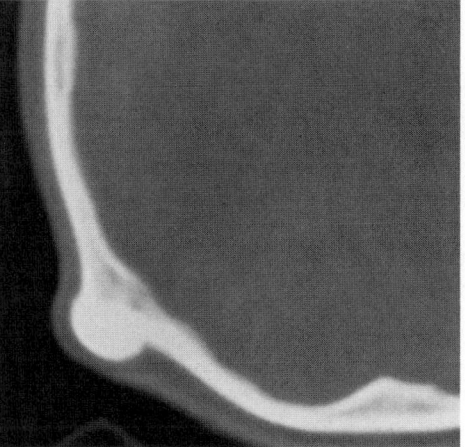

**Figure 82–4.** Osteoma: cranial vault. CT scan reveals an osteoma arising from the external surface of the skull. (Courtesy of M. Taljanovic, MD, Phoenix, Ariz.)

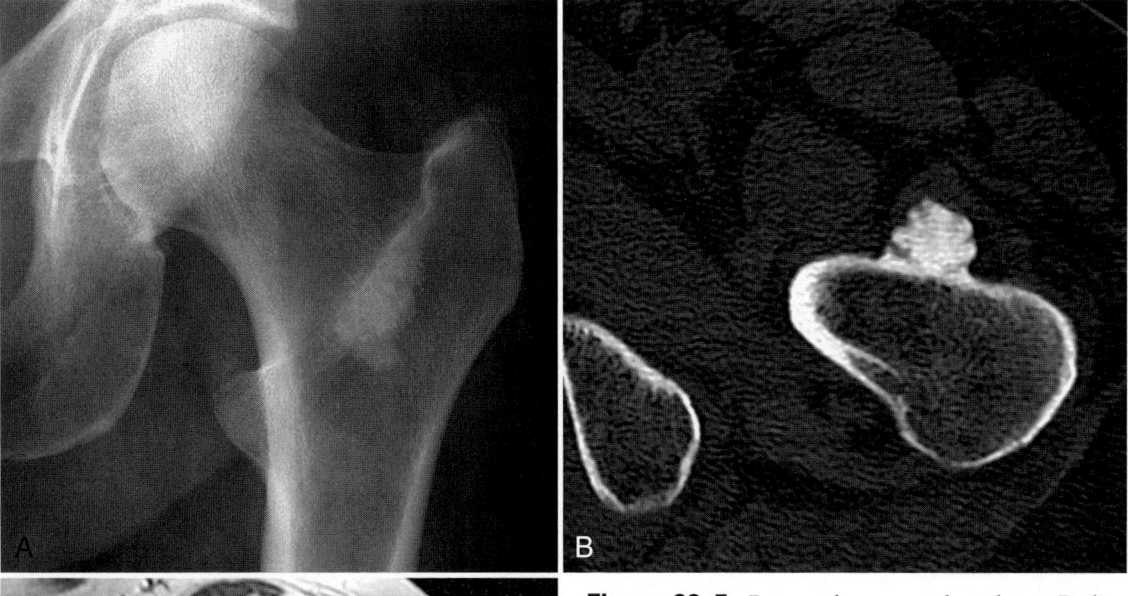

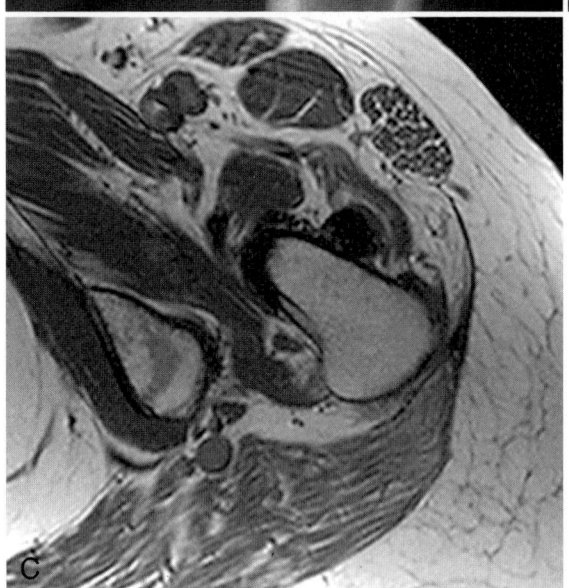

**Figure 82–5.** Parosteal osteoma: long bone. Radiograph *(A)* and transaxial CT scan *(B)* reveal a homogeneous, radiodense lesion arising from the neck of the proximal femur. Axial T1-weighted (TR/TE, 650/20) spin echo MR image *(C)* shows a signal intensity similar to that of cortex and verifies the absence of an adjacent soft tissue mass.

in the scapula, clavicle, and pelvis are frequently combined with alterations in the corresponding limb.

Peripherally located (cortical) hyperostosis is evident in one bone or a series of bones (Figs. 82–9 and 82–10). The appearance of the osseous excrescences extending for the length of the bone simulates that of candle wax flowing down the side of a lit candle. A wavy and sclerotic

---

**TABLE 82–2**

**Major Radiographic Abnormalities in Gardner's Syndrome**

Colonic polyposis
Osteomas
Soft tissue tumors
Dental lesions

---

bony contour is produced that may involve one side of the tubular bones of the upper or lower extremity, reaching the carpus and tarsus as well as the metacarpals, metatarsals, or phalanges. Endosteal hyperostosis is an associated feature that may partially or completely obliterate the medullary cavity. In the carpal and tarsal areas, more discrete round foci may resemble the findings of osteopoikilosis, whereas in the flat bones, such as those in the pelvis or scapula, radiating or localized sclerotic patches are seen (Fig. 82–11). In contrast to the situation in osteopoikilosis and osteopathia striata, scintigraphy can reveal areas of increased skeletal accumulation of radionuclide in cases of melorheostosis, and the resulting scintigraphic image may simulate Paget's disease (see Fig. 82–11). Associated soft tissue calcification and ossification are seen in about 25% of cases and may lead to complete anklyosis of the joint (Fig. 82–12). With MR imaging, bone and soft tissue lesions are usually of low signal intensity on all pulse sequences, although a wider spectrum of imaging findings may be encountered with contrast enhancement.

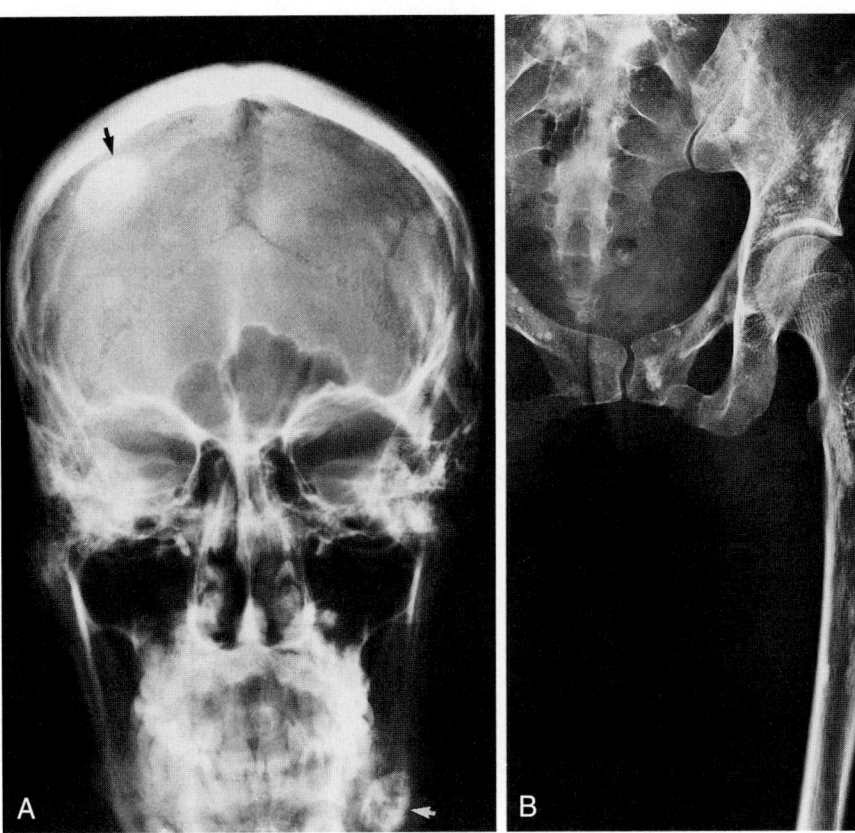

**Figure 82–6.** Gardner's syndrome: bone abnormalities. *A*, Osteomas *(arrows)* of the outer table of the skull and mandible are evident. *B*, Observe wavy cortical thickening of the femur and lesions of the innominate bones that resemble enostoses.

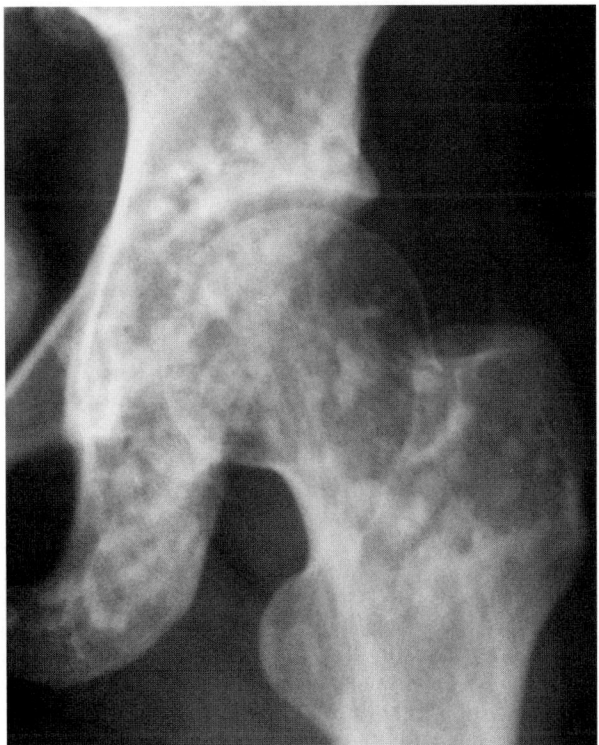

**Figure 82–7.** Osteopoikilosis: hip. Note the circular or ovoid radiodense foci in the femur and pelvis, with no abnormality of the intervening joint space.

Melorheostosis has been reported in association with other disorders (see Table 82–3). The role of sclerotomes in the distribution of hyperostosis in melorheostosis has been emphasized. Sclerotomes represent zones of the skeleton supplied by individual spinal sensory nerves. In many cases of melorheostosis, skeletal alterations correspond to a single sclerotome or to a part thereof.

**TABLE 82–3**

**Diseases Associated with Various Hyperostotic Lesions**

| Lesion | Possible Associated Diseases |
| --- | --- |
| Osteoma | Gardner's syndrome |
| Osteopoikilosis | Osteopathia striata |
| | Melorheostosis |
| | Hyperostosis frontalis interna |
| Osteopathia striata | Osteopoikilosis |
| | Melorheostosis |
| | Osteopetrosis |
| | Cranial sclerosis |
| | Focal dermal hypoplasia |
| Melorheostosis | Linear scleroderma |
| | Osteopoikilosis |
| | Osteopathia striata |
| | Neurofibromatosis |
| | Tuberous sclerosis |
| | Hemangiomas |

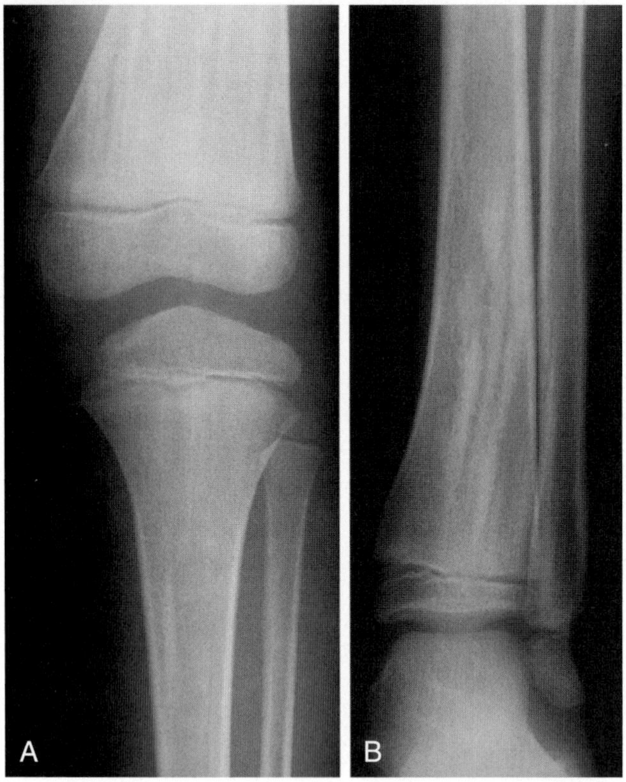

## MIXED SCLEROSING BONE DYSTROPHY

Although osteopoikilosis, osteopathia striata, and melorheostosis each possess characteristic radiographic abnormalities, some patients demonstrate findings of more than one of these disorders (Fig. 82–13). This phenomenon has been termed mixed sclerosing bone dystrophy. Four types of mixed sclerosing bone dystrophy have been described: (1) osteopathia striata, melorheostosis, osteopoikilosis, and focal osteosclerosis; (2) osteopathia striata and cranial sclerosis, with or without osteopoikilosis; (3) osteopathia striata, generalized cortical hyperostosis, and metadiaphyseal widening, with or without cranial sclerosis and osteopoikilosis of the ribs; and (4) osteopoikilosis with diaphyseal periosteal proliferation. These mixed sclerosing bone dystrophies can be associated with a variety of vascular anomalies, including unilateral lymphangiectasia, capillary hemangiomas, and arteriovenous malformations, and with Trevor's disease.

## OTHER SCLEROSING BONE DYSTROPHIES AND DYSPLASIAS

Certain dysplasias of intramembranous ossification lead to dramatic abnormalities of the tubular bones of the extremities, affecting the periosteal or endosteal surfaces (or both) of the diaphyseal cortex.

**Figure 82–8.** Osteopathia striata. *A* and *B*, Note linear radiodense areas principally in the metaphyses of the tibia and femur. (Courtesy of R. Tobin, MD, San Diego, Calif.)

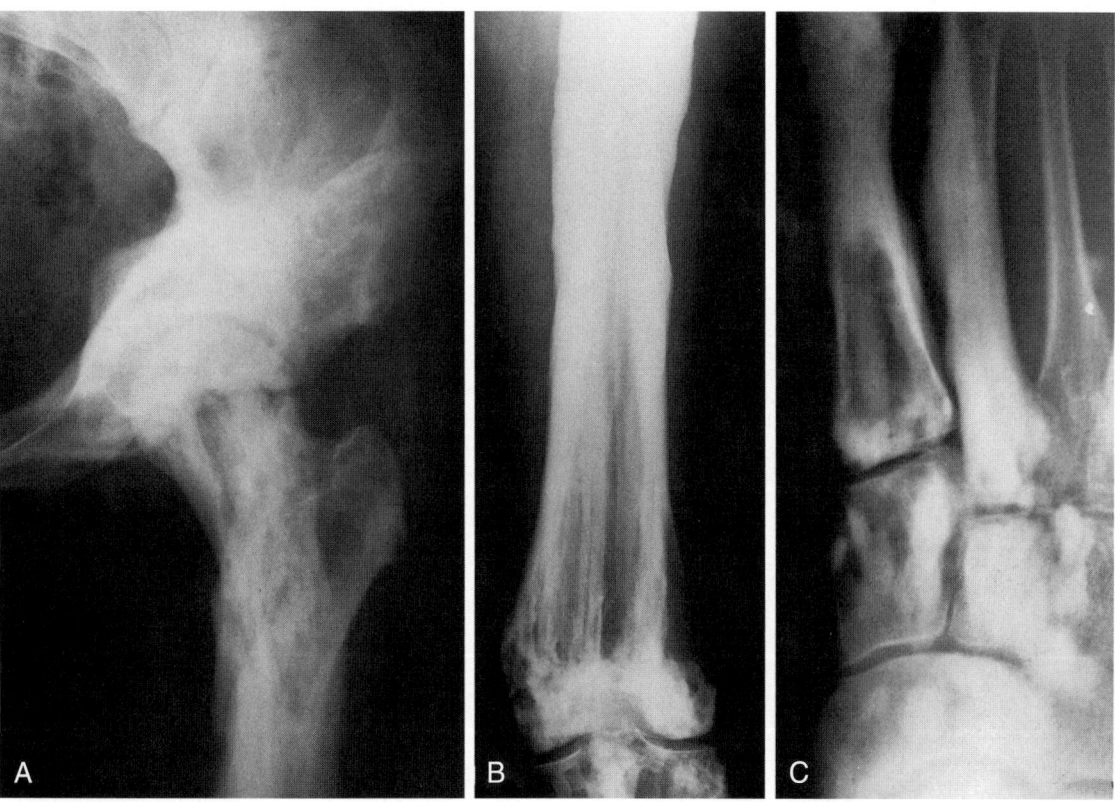

**Figure 82–9.** Melorheostosis. In this patient, characteristic radiographic abnormalities are evident throughout a single extremity. *A*, In the pelvis, note the hyperostosis of the left hemipelvis, para-acetabular region, and medial aspect of the proximal femur. *B*, In the distal femur, a peculiar linear radiodense pattern extends across the knee joint. *C*, Involvement of the medial rays of the foot is also seen. (Courtesy of R. Freiberger, MD, New York, N.Y.)

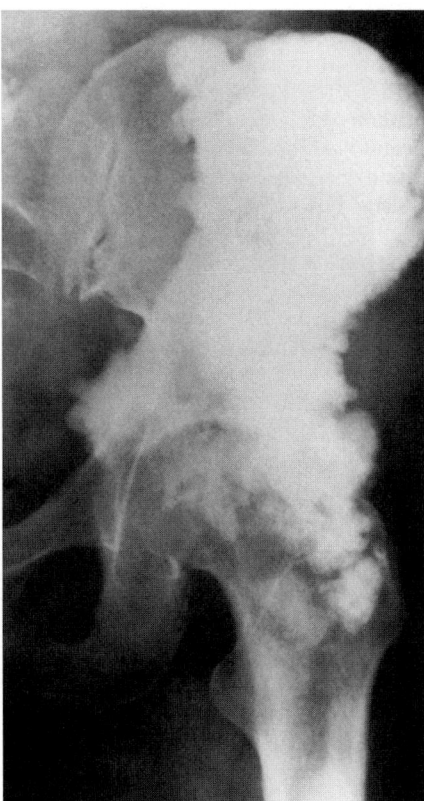

**Figure 82–10.** Melorheostosis. In this 71-year-old woman, osseous excrescences are observed in the lateral portion of the ilium, acetabular region, and anterior surface of the femur, in combination with soft tissue ossification about the hip. (Courtesy of H. R. Fischer, MD, Victoria, British Columbia, Canada.)

## Progressive Diaphyseal Dysplasia

Progressive diaphyseal dysplasia, also known as Camurati-Engelmann disease, usually manifests in the first decade of life. Presenting clinical manifestations include muscle pain, weakness, and atrophy; a waddling and broad-based gait; bone pain; increased fatigability; and delayed puberty. The lower extremities are involved more frequently than the upper extremities. Laboratory parameters are generally normal. Although somewhat variable in its clinical expression and course, the disorder is usually self-limited, resolving by age 30 to 35 years.

Radiographic findings include, foremost, fusiform thickening of the cortex in the diaphyseal portions of the tubular bones, involving (in order of decreasing frequency) the tibia, femur, fibula, humerus, ulna, and radius (Fig. 82–14). Symmetrical in distribution, the thickened cortex occurs as a result of both endosteal and periosteal bone formation. Affected bone is sharply demarcated from normal bone, and the external contour of the bone is usually smooth. Sparing of the metaphyses and epiphyses is characteristic but not invariable. The cause of this disorder is unknown, although reports of families with the disease are most consistent with an autosomal dominant mode of transmission, with variable penetrance.

## Hereditary Multiple Diaphyseal Sclerosis (Ribbing's Disease)

Somewhat similar and perhaps related to progressive diaphyseal dysplasia is hereditary multiple diaphyseal sclerosis. Sometimes referred to as Ribbing's disease, this process gives rise to less extensive clinical and radiographic features; in fact, it is often entirely asymptomatic

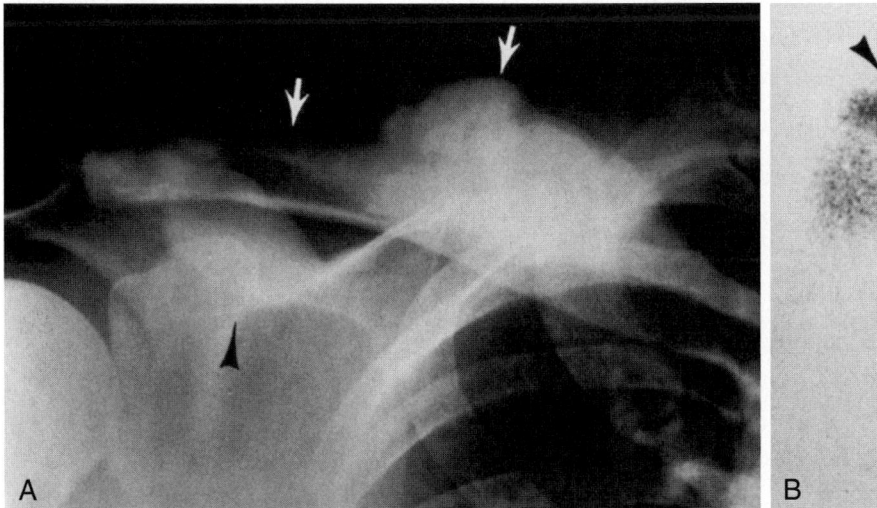

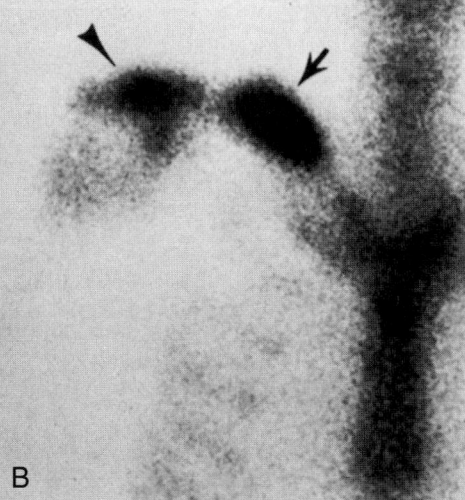

**Figure 82–11.** Melorheostosis. This 29-year-old man had painful swelling of the right clavicle, and a biopsy revealed findings of melorheostosis. *A,* Observe localized hyperostosis of the middle and distal portions of the clavicle *(arrows)* and the scapula *(arrowhead).* The process extends down the proximal aspect of the humerus. *B,* Technetium bone scan delineates increased activity in the clavicle *(arrow)* and scapula *(arrowhead).* (Courtesy of W. Pogue, MD, San Diego, Calif.)

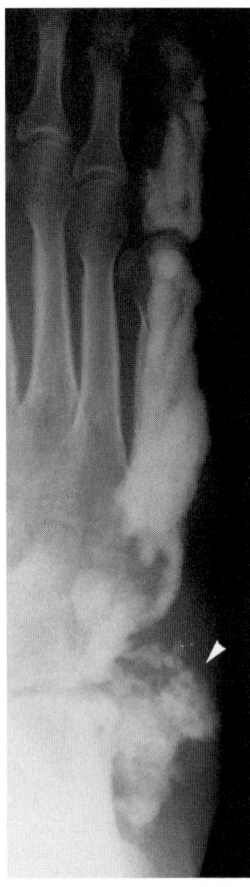

**Figure 82–12.** Melorheostosis. In addition to the typical osseous changes in the tarsus, metatarsal bone, and phalanges, observe prominent soft tissue ossification *(arrowhead)*. (Courtesy of G. Greenway, MD, Dallas, Tex.)

or causes only minor pain and tenderness in the affected extremity or extremities. Like progressive diaphyseal dysplasia, hereditary multiple diaphyseal sclerosis leads to osteosclerosis and hyperostosis of the diaphyses of tubular bones, especially the femur and tibia, but also the fibula and radius (Fig. 82–15). The cortex is thickened, the medullary cavity is narrowed, and slight expansion of the bone may be evident. However, skeletal involvement in Ribbing's disease is much less widespread than in progressive diaphyseal dysplasia, and asymmetry is the rule. Some regard the two disorders as related entities that differ only in severity.

### Idiopathic Intramedullary Osteosclerosis

Idiopathic intramedullary osteosclerosis is a recently described entity involving the midportion of the tibia, the distal portion of the tibia, the distal portion of the fibula, or the entire lower extremity. Patients show a wide age distribution and present with pain referred to the lower extremity. The pain is mild to moderate and increases with physical activity. In this disease, sclerosis is limited to an intramedullary location, with an absence of significant periosteal reaction. Bone scintigraphy is positive in areas of involvement.

Despite minor differences, the radiographic features of idiopathic intramedullary osteosclerosis resemble those of Ribbing's disease (Fig. 82–16) and also bear some resemblance to stress-induced changes in the tubular bones of the lower extremities. Features that should suggest the presence of idiopathic intramedullary osteosclerosis include the following: a female patient in the third through sixth decades of life, absence of a family history of a similar disorder, and presence of endosteal hyperostosis involving

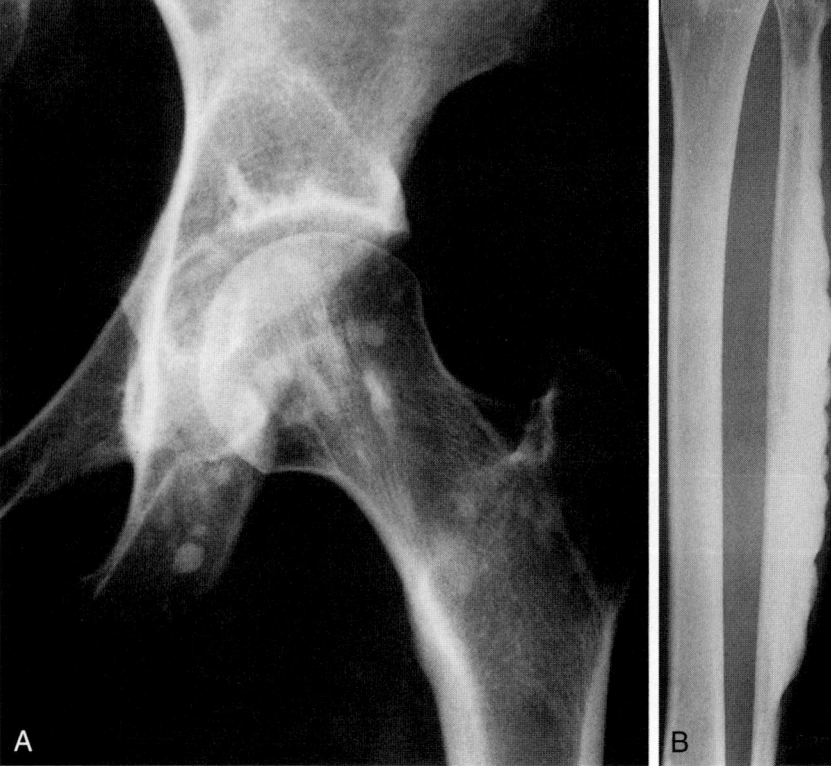

**Figure 82–13.** Mixed sclerosing bone dystrophy. *A*, The changes in the hip are diagnostic of osteopoikilosis, although some of the foci are elongated or linear in shape. *B*, Involvement of the fibula in the same patient consists of flowing, eccentrically located ossification, an appearance typical of melorheostosis. (Courtesy of A. Brower, MD, Norfolk, Va.)

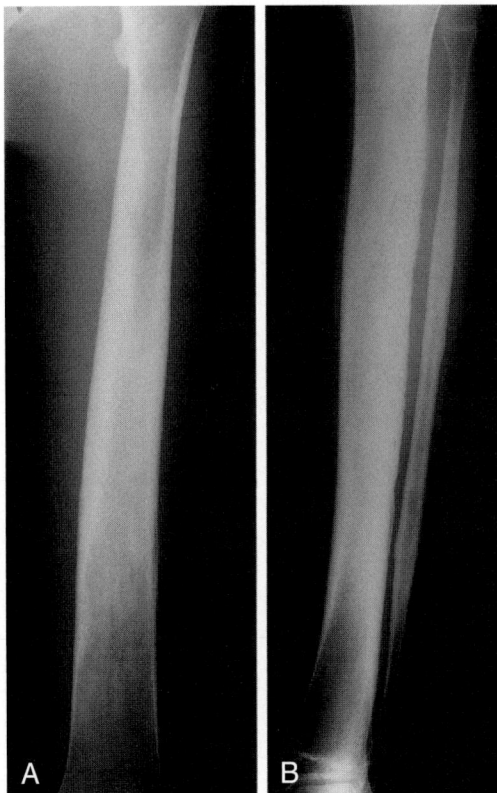

**Figure 82–14.** Progressive diaphyseal dysplasia (Camurati-Engelmann disease). Periosteal and endosteal bone formation has led to cortical thickening in the diaphyses of the femur *(A)* and tibia and fibula *(B)*. (Courtesy of M. de Maeseneer, MD, Brussels, Belgium.)

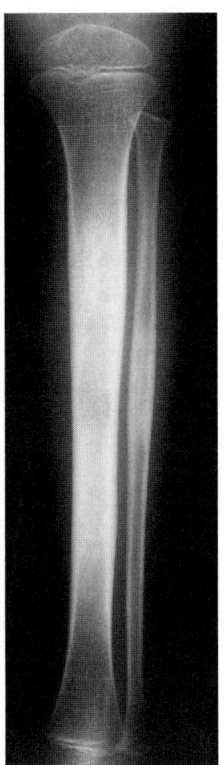

**Figure 82–15.** Hereditary multiple diaphyseal sclerosis (Ribbing's disease). Note the sclerotic regions in the diaphyses of the tibia and fibula. Radiolucent foci are also evident.

the diaphyseal segment of one or more tubular bones in the lower extremities, especially the tibia but also the fibula and femur.

## PRIMARY HYPERTROPHIC OSTEOARTHROPATHY (PACHYDERMOPERIOSTOSIS)

Hypertrophic osteoarthropathy is a clinical syndrome consisting of clubbing of the digits of the hands and feet, enlargement of the extremities secondary to periarticular and osseous proliferation, and painful and swollen joints. The syndrome can be divided into two categories: primary (hereditary or idiopathic) and secondary. The primary form accounts for approximately 3% to 5% of all cases. In either variety, the syndrome may be incomplete; alternatively, additional features, such as thickening of skin on the face and scalp (pachyderma), may be prominent. Primary hypertrophic osteoarthropathy is also called pachydermoperiostosis.

### Clinical Abnormalities

Pachydermoperiostosis is a rare disease that demonstrates an autosomal dominant genetic transmission, with marked variability of expression. More than one third of

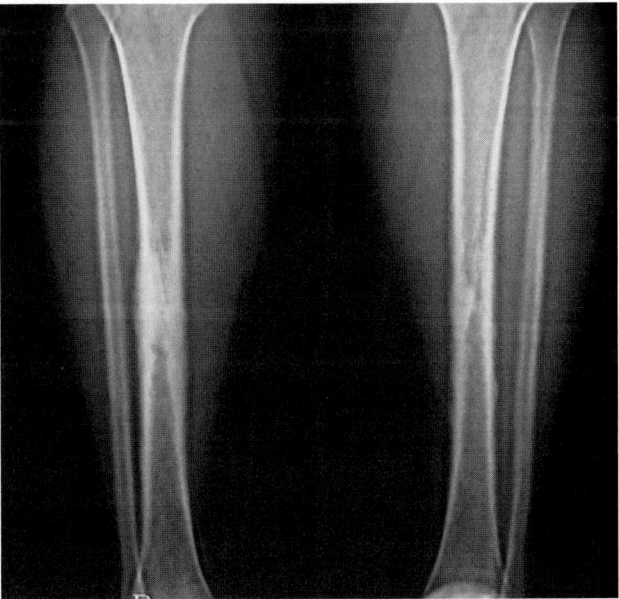

**Figure 82–16.** Idiopathic intramedullary osteosclerosis. Note the bilateral involvement of the tibial shafts in this 39-year-old woman. The right side is involved more severely. The process is dominated by endosteal hyperostosis, although mature periosteal new bone is also evident in the right tibia. (Courtesy of B. Sosnow, MD, Phoenix, Ariz.)

the reported patients have an affected relative. It predominates and is more severe in blacks. There is an insidious onset of enlargement of the hands and feet that produces a pawlike appearance, clubbing of the distal ends of the fingers and toes, and convexity of the nails. Coarsening of the skin of the face and scalp, ptosis, furrowing of the cutaneous tissue, enlargement and disruption of the normal contour of the extremities, and vague pains in the bones and joints are also encountered. Pachydermoperiostosis usually progresses for approximately 10 years before arresting spontaneously.

### Radiographic Abnormalities

The predominant radiographic feature of pachydermoperiostosis is periostitis (Fig. 82–17). Widespread and symmetrical findings occur, although osseous thickening is most pronounced in the tubular bones of the extremities, especially the tibia, fibula, radius, and ulna. Involvement of the carpus, tarsus, metacarpals, metatarsals, phalanges, and pelvis is also frequent. Thickening of the calvaria and base of the skull may be detected; however, changes in the spine are unusual.

Superficially, the periosteal proliferation of the tubular bones resembles that typically seen in secondary hypertrophic osteoarthropathy (Table 82–4). Although the diaphyses and metaphyses can be affected in both conditions, periostitis commonly extends into the epiphyseal region in pachydermoperiostosis, producing shaggy, ill-defined, bony excrescences about various articulations that are especially characteristic of this disease (differing from the linear deposits that typically accompany secondary hypertrophic osteoarthropathy).

In more advanced cases of pachydermoperiostosis, expansion of the diaphyses of the tubular bones and sclerosis of the spongiosa in both appendicular and axial skeletal sites are evident. Soft tissue prominence of the distal digits may be associated with tuftal osteolysis. Osteolysis may occur after phalangeal hypertrophy, perhaps indicating that an orderly sequence of bone formation followed by bone destruction is typical of the tuftal abnormalities.

### Differential Diagnosis

The irregular periosteal deposits that appear about the metaphyses and epiphyses of tubular bones and at axial skeletal sites are distinctive and are usually not encountered in secondary hypertrophic osteoarthropathy. This characteristic may indicate only that more irregular and extensive periostitis is seen in cases of hypertrophic osteoarthropathy with an earlier onset or longer duration (as is typical of pachydermoperiostosis). Early age at onset,

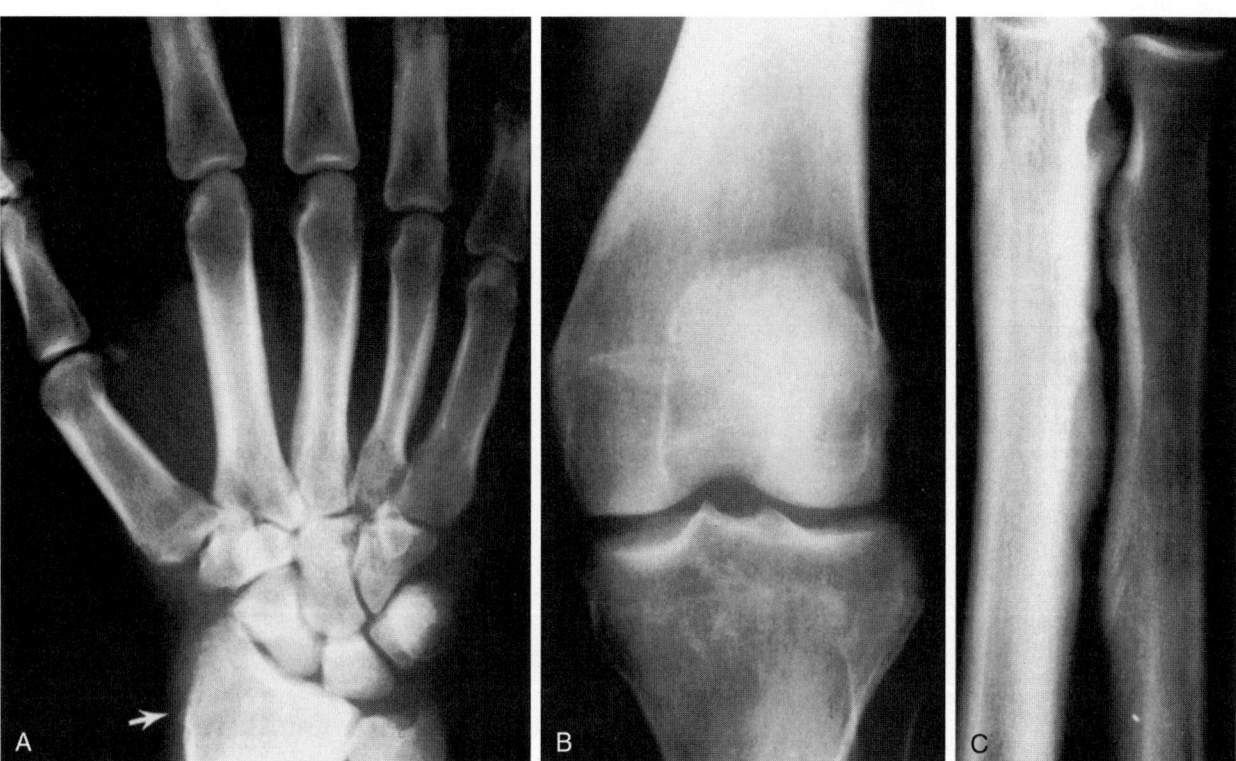

**Figure 82–17.** Primary hypertrophic osteoarthropathy (pachydermoperiostosis). This 26-year-old man developed acromegalic features and cutaneous abnormalities. *A,* In addition to periosteal proliferation of the distal radius *(arrow),* note the widened metacarpals and phalanges. *B,* An expanded contour of the distal femur is associated with cortical thickening. *C,* Exuberant osseous proliferation is evident along apposing surfaces of the radius and ulna.

**TABLE 82-4**

**Causes of Diffuse Periostitis**

| Disease | Location | Characteristics |
|---------|----------|-----------------|
| Primary hypertrophic osteoarthropathy (pachydermoperiostosis) | Tibia, fibula, radius, ulna (less commonly, carpus, tarsus, metacarpals, metatarsals, phalanges, pelvis, ribs, clavicle) | Diaphyseal, metaphyseal, and epiphyseal involvement<br>Shaggy, irregular excrescences<br>Diaphyseal expansion<br>Clubbing<br>Ligamentous ossification<br>Cranial and facial changes |
| Secondary hypertrophic osteoarthropathy | Tibia, fibula, radius, ulna (less commonly, femur, humerus, metacarpals, metatarsals, phalanges) | Diaphyseal and metaphyseal involvement<br>Single or laminated, regular or irregular proliferation<br>Clubbing<br>Periarticular osteoporosis, soft tissue swelling<br>Underlying primary lesion |
| Thyroid acropachy | Metacarpals, metatarsals, phalanges (less commonly, other tubular bones) | Diaphyseal involvement<br>Radial side predilection in the hands<br>Dense, solid, and spiculated proliferation<br>Clubbing<br>Soft tissue swelling<br>Thyroid gland abnormalities |
| Venous stasis | Tibia, fibula, femur, metatarsals, phalanges | Diaphyseal and metaphyseal involvement<br>Undulating osseous contour<br>Cortical thickening<br>Soft tissue swelling, ulceration, ossification<br>Phleboliths |
| Hypervitaminosis A | Ulna, metatarsals, clavicle, tibia, fibula | Diaphyseal involvement<br>Undulating contour<br>Epiphyseal deformities<br>Soft tissue nodules<br>Intracranial hypertension |
| Infantile cortical hyperostosis (Caffey's disease) | Mandible, clavicle, scapula, ribs, tubular bones | Periostitis and cortical hyperostosis<br>May become extreme<br>Cranial destruction<br>Soft tissue nodules<br>Deformities |

family history of the disease, and absence of significant joint pain are clinical characteristics of pachydermoperiostosis that differ from those of secondary hypertrophic osteoarthropathy. In thyroid acropachy, fluffy, spiculated periosteal bone is encountered in the hands and feet but is rarely observed elsewhere. In endosteal hyperostosis (van Buchem's disease), thickening of the cranial vault and cortices of the tubular bones is not combined with digital clubbing, skin changes, enlargement of paranasal sinuses, or irregular para-articular osseous excrescences. Similarly, in diaphyseal dysplasia (Camurati-Engelmann disease), endosteal and periosteal proliferation of the diaphyses of the tubular bones is characteristic.

## SECONDARY HYPERTROPHIC OSTEOARTHROPATHY

Secondary hypertrophic osteoarthropathy is sometimes called hypertrophic pulmonary osteoarthropathy, emphasizing the fact that pulmonary problems are a major cause of the periostitis. Although reports vary widely, a 5% incidence appears to be a good estimate of the frequency of this complication in cases of bronchogenic carcinoma. Some other causes are listed in Table 82–5. Of all the

**TABLE 82-5**

**Causes of Secondary Hypertrophic Osteoarthropathy**

| | |
|---|---|
| Pulmonary | Bronchogenic carcinoma<br>Abscess<br>Bronchiectasis<br>Emphysema<br>Hodgkin's disease<br>Metastasis<br>Cystic fibrosis |
| Pleural, diaphragmatic | Mesothelioma |
| Cardiac | Cyanotic congenital heart disease |
| Abdominal | Portal or biliary cirrhosis<br>Ulcerative colitis<br>Crohn's disease<br>Dysentery<br>Gastrointestinal polyposis<br>Neoplasms<br>Biliary atresia |
| Miscellaneous | Nasopharyngeal carcinoma<br>Esophageal carcinoma<br>Infected aortic or axillary artery grafts |

potential intrathoracic causes, however, bronchogenic carcinoma is by far the most common underlying lesion.

## Clinical Abnormalities

Digital clubbing is a frequent but not invariable feature of hypertrophic osteoarthropathy. Articular symptoms and signs are apparent in approximately 30% to 40% of patients and may be the presenting manifestation. Hypertrophic osteoarthropathy due to pulmonary neoplasm is commonly associated with an acute onset of digital clubbing, warmth and burning of the fingertips, and, occasionally, skin thickening and hyperhidrosis. Joint findings appear in approximately 30% to 35% of cases and may precede pulmonary symptoms and signs.

In cases of hypertrophic osteoarthropathy secondary to intrathoracic causes, thoracotomy frequently leads to prominent remission of the joint symptoms and signs within 24 hours, although radiographic findings may recede more slowly. Even patients with nonresectable tumors may benefit from thoracotomy. Regrowth of the neoplasm is commonly associated with exacerbation of the clinical and radiographic findings.

## Radiographic Abnormalities

Periostitis is the radiographic hallmark of hypertrophic osteoarthropathy. Periosteal bone deposition initially appears in the proximal and distal diaphyses of the tibia, fibula, radius, and ulna and, less frequently, the femur, humerus, metacarpals, metatarsals, and phalanges (Fig. 82–18). With progression, periostitis becomes prominent in the metaphyseal regions as well as at musculotendinous insertions, but it usually does not extend into the epiphyses. Epiphyseal extension of periostitis may be observed in patients with hypertrophic osteoarthropathy secondary to congenital cyanotic heart disease, however.

Various types of periostitis are seen: simple elevation of the periosteum, with a radiolucent area between the periosteal bone and subjacent cortex; laminated or "onion-skin" appearance, with smooth layers of new bone formation; irregular areas of periosteal elevation; irregular, solid areas of periosteal cloaking with a wavy contour; and cortical thickening, with application of the periosteal bone to the outer surface of the cortex. Digital clubbing leading to radiographically detectable soft tissue swelling is also evident.

## Articular Abnormalities

Pain and swelling about the knees, ankles, wrists, and even the fingers may be the presenting manifestation of hypertrophic osteoarthropathy. The joint manifestations are not specific, however, nor are they inflammatory in nature. Articular space narrowing, marginal and central erosions (as noted in patients with rheumatoid arthritis), and osseous excrescences and bony ankylosis (seen in patients with primary hypertrophic osteoarthropathy) are not found in persons with secondary hypertrophic osteoarthropathy.

## Radionuclide Abnormalities

Radionuclide bone imaging is a highly sensitive method for detecting abnormalities of primary or secondary hypertrophic osteoarthropathy. A diffuse, symmetrical, increased uptake in the diaphyses and metaphyses of tubular bones along their cortical margins creates a distinctive "double stripe" or "parallel track" sign (Fig. 82–19). Associated synovitis can lead to increased radionuclide uptake in periarticular regions as well. The scintigraphic abnormalities frequently appear before the radiographic findings, correspond well with clinical manifestations, and decrease after appropriate therapeutic regimens (e.g., surgery, radiation therapy). Tumor recurrence is followed by the return of abnormal radionuclide patterns.

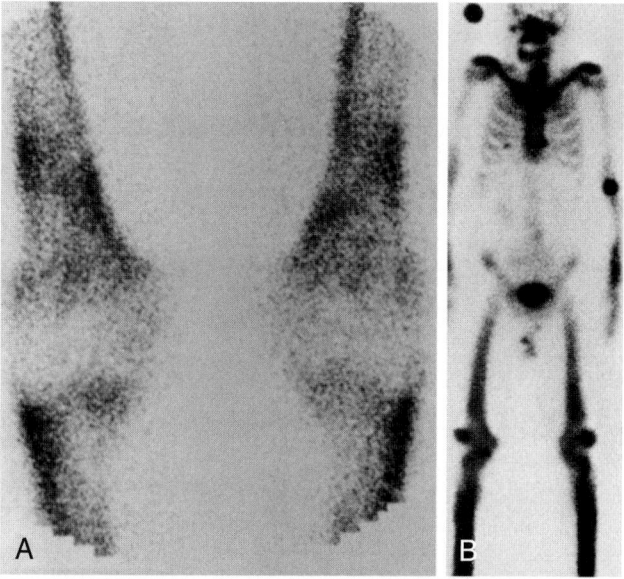

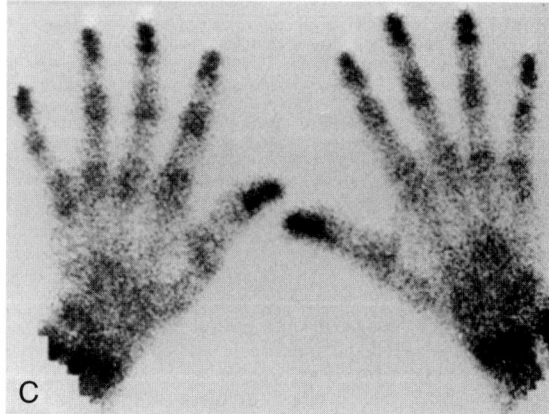

**Figure 82–19.** Secondary hypertrophic osteoarthropathy: radionuclide abnormalities. *A*, The "double stripe" or "parallel track" sign is present in the femur and tibia. *B*, Diffuse uptake is observed in both the appendicular skeleton and the axial skeleton. *C*, Digital accumulation of radionuclide is evident. (*B*, Courtesy of V. Vint, MD, San Diego, Calif.)

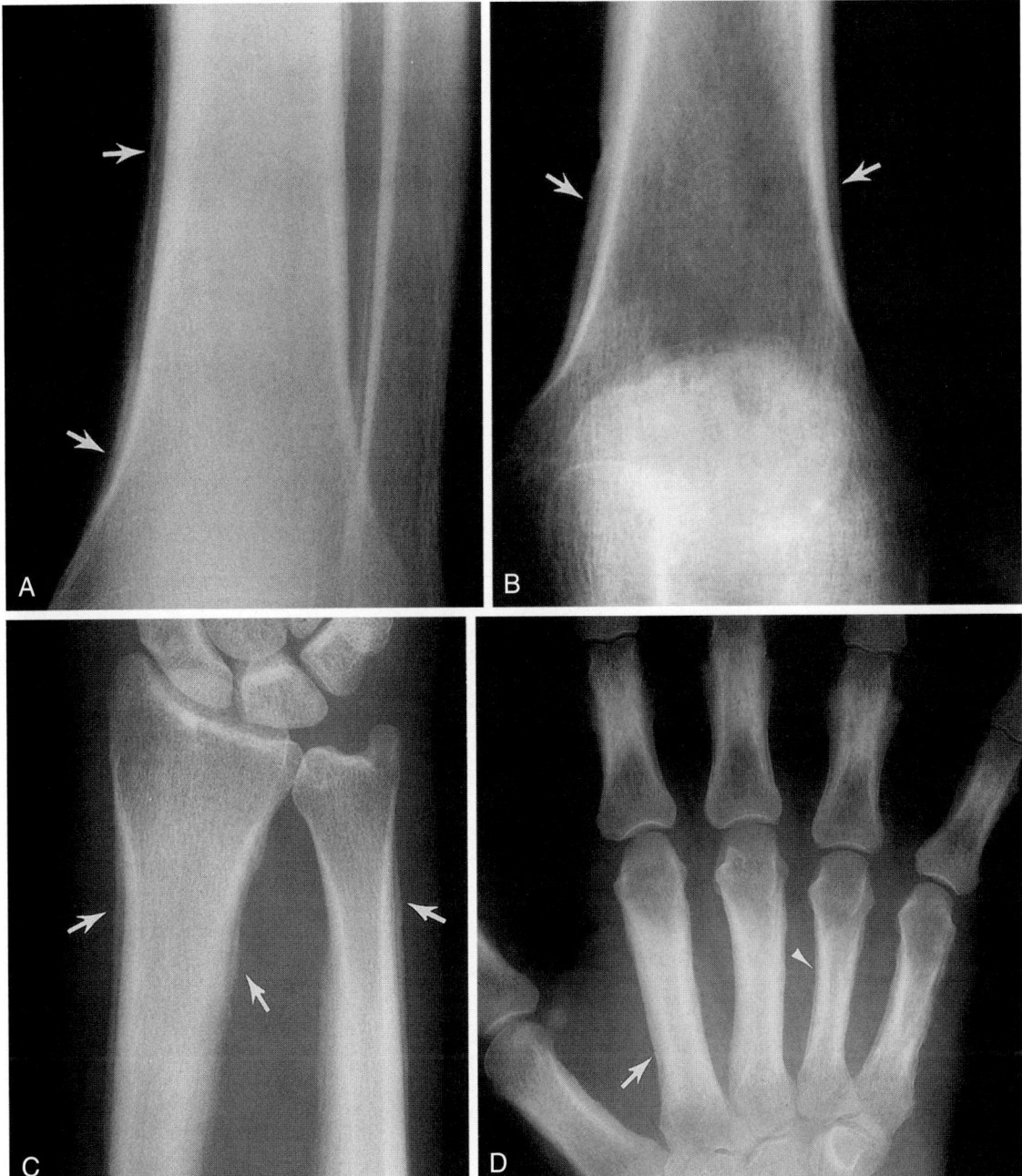

**Figure 82–18.** Secondary hypertrophic osteoarthropathy: periostitis. *A*, Distal tibia and fibula. Elevation of the periosteal membrane in the diaphyses of these bones has resulted in linear deposition of new bone *(arrows)*. Involvement ends at the metaphyses. *B*, Femur. Observe thick linear periosteal bone formation on the medial and lateral aspects of the femur *(arrows)*. The endosteal surface of the cortex is not affected. *C*, Distal radius and ulna. In another classic location, observe linear periostitis of the diaphyses extending to the metaphyses of both bones *(arrows)*. *D*, Metacarpal bones and phalanges. Linear periostitis of the metacarpal bones has produced bone that is either separated from *(arrowhead)* or firmly merged with *(arrow)* the underlying osseous tissue. Bony proliferation at muscular insertions of the phalanges is also seen. Note some degree of periarticular osteoporosis.

## Differential Diagnosis

Periostitis (and clubbing) can also be observed in primary hypertrophic osteoarthropathy (pachydermoperiostosis) and in thyroid acropachy (see Table 82–4; Fig. 82–20). In the former condition, the osseous excrescences are more irregular and extend into the epiphyses of the tubular bones, and a family history of the disease is evident. In thyroid acropachy, periosteal proliferation has a predilection for the small bones of the hands and feet; significant or isolated abnormalities of the major tubular bones are

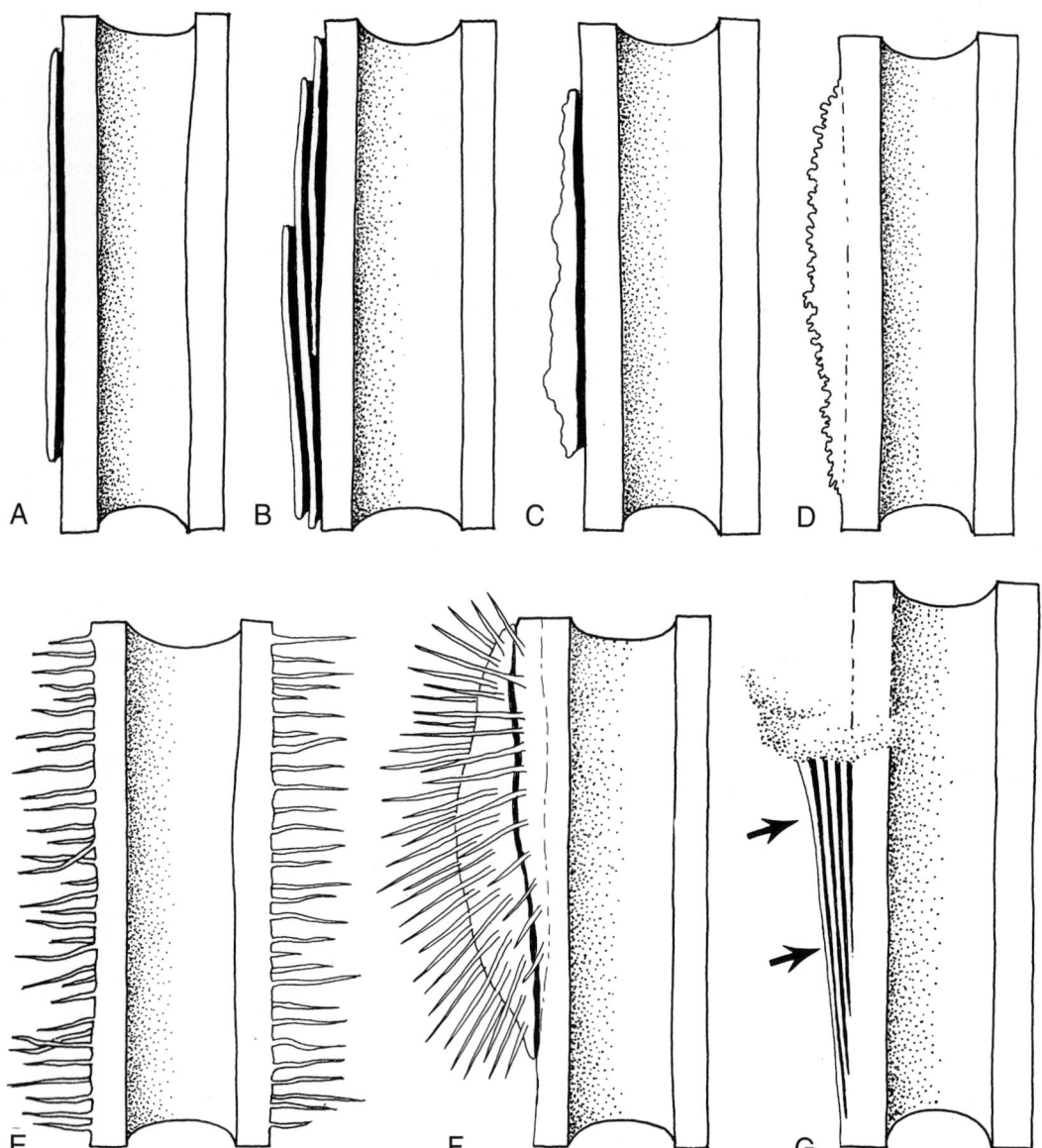

**Figure 82–20.** Differential diagnosis of periosteal new bone formation: various types of periostitis. *A,* A single layer of new bone may be observed in benign or malignant tumors, infection, and secondary hypertrophic osteoarthropathy. *B,* Multiple layers of new bone, or "onion-skinning," may be evident in infection, malignant tumors such as Ewing's sarcoma, hypertrophic osteoarthropathy, and other conditions. *C,* A thick, linear osseous deposit may be separate from (as indicated here) or merged with the underlying bone. This pattern is common in hypertrophic osteoarthropathy and venous stasis. *D,* An irregular osseous excrescence with a spiculated contour merges with the underlying cortex. This pattern may be observed in thyroid acropachy or primary hypertrophic osteoarthropathy (pachydermoperiostosis). *E,* Thin, linear osseous deposits extend in a direction perpendicular to the underlying cortex, a pattern that is highly characteristic of Ewing's sarcoma. *F,* A sunburst pattern, in which linear deposits fan out from a single focus, may be evident in osteosarcoma. *G,* Codman's triangle, consisting of triangular elevation of the periosteum with one or more layers of new bone *(arrows),* is a pattern suggestive but not diagnostic of malignancy.

distinctly unusual. Chronic venous stasis can produce periostitis, usually confined to the lower extremities. Additional causes of diffuse periostitis or bone proliferation, such as hypervitaminosis A, infantile cortical hyperostosis, diffuse idiopathic skeletal hyperostosis, and fluorosis, are usually not confused with hypertrophic osteoarthropathy.

## VASCULAR INSUFFICIENCY

Periosteal bone formation has been noted in association with chronic venous insufficiency. The lower extremities are affected almost exclusively, with involvement of the tibia, fibula, femur, metatarsals, and phalanges (see Table 82–4). The diaphyseal and metaphyseal segments are predominantly altered, and an undulating osseous contour is produced, with considerable new bone appearing on the outer aspect of the cortex (Fig. 82–21). Although initially separated from the underlying bone, the periosteal deposits soon merge with the cortex.

The frequency of periostitis increases with the severity and duration of the venous insufficiency, and the disorder may be detected in 10% to 60% of patients with chronic disabling venous stasis. The pathogenesis of the periostitis may be related to the hypoxia created by vascular stasis or hypertension, but a single mechanism has yet to be substantiated. Soft tissue edema and ossification represent radiographic findings that are commonly associated with venous insufficiency and periostitis (Fig. 82–22). Single or multiple phleboliths may be apparent, and in some cases, a diffuse reticular ossific pattern is evident. Arterial insufficiency has also been associated with periosteal bone proliferation.

## INFANTILE CORTICAL HYPEROSTOSIS

Infantile cortical hyperostosis (Caffey's disease) is an uncommon disease that usually commences in infancy and affects predominantly the skeleton and adjacent fascial, muscular, and connective tissues. Infantile cortical hyperostosis has a worldwide distribution, is evident in all racial strains, and affects boys and girls with approximately equal frequency.

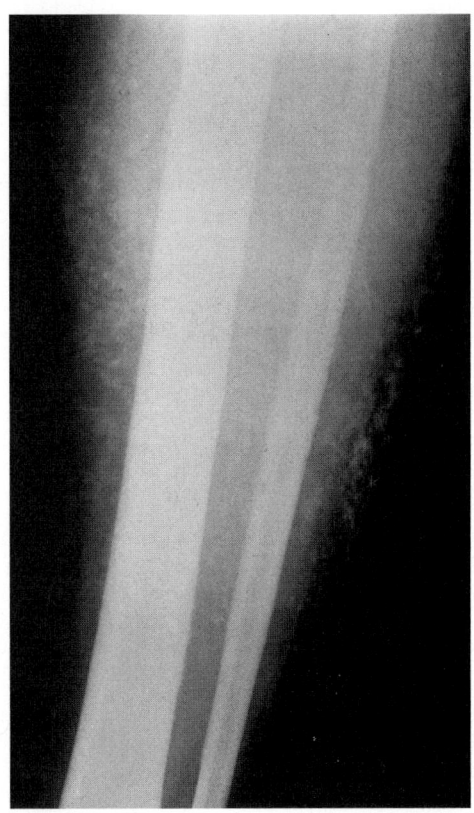

**Figure 82–22.** Chronic venous stasis. An example of reticular ossification is seen.

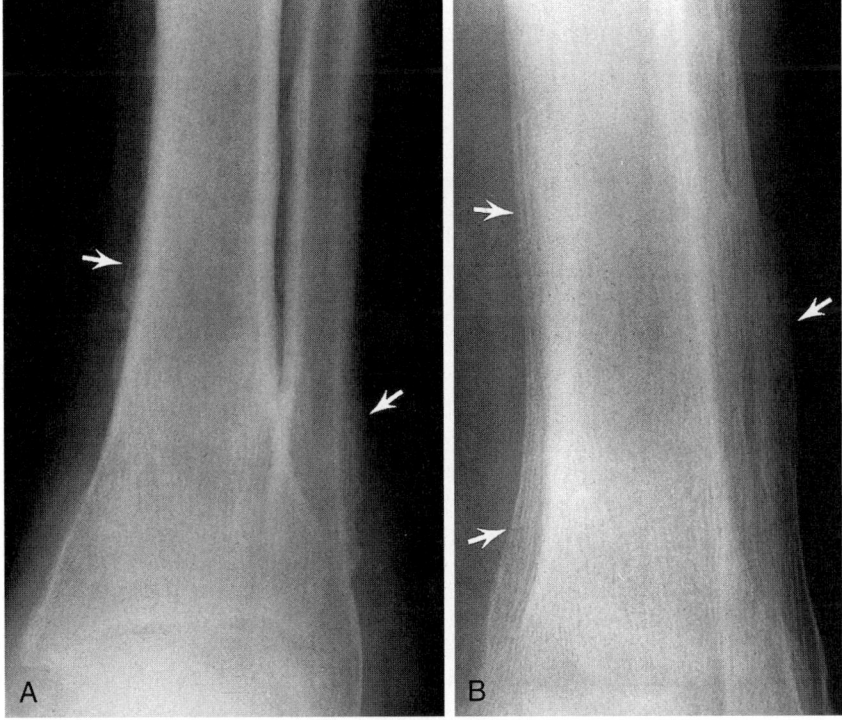

**Figure 82–21.** Chronic venous stasis: periostitis. *A,* Observe undulating periosteal new bone in the diaphyses and metaphyses of the distal tibia and fibula *(arrows).* Soft tissue edema is present. *B,* In this patient, a laminated or solid coat of periosteal bone surrounds the distal tibia and fibula *(arrows).*

## Clinical Abnormalities

Almost without exception, the disease becomes evident in infants younger than 5 months old; it may be apparent in the first days or weeks of life. The average age at onset is 9 to 10 weeks. Familial cases are recognized. Fever of abrupt onset, hyperirritability, and soft tissue swelling are typical. The swelling is especially prominent over the mandible but can also appear at other sites. On palpation, indurated, hard, and tender soft tissue masses are noted, and these may be attached to the underlying bones. The clinical course is extremely variable, and in many instances, the clinical and radiographic features subside slowly over a few months to a few years, but this self-limited quality is not uniform.

## Radiographic Abnormalities

In any patient, a single bone or many bones may be involved (see Table 82–4). Sequential involvement is typical, with one area being affected initially, followed later by changes at other sites. The mandible, clavicle, and ribs are involved most often, and changes in these bones may be symmetrical (Fig. 82–23). Thoracic cage abnormalities may be combined with pleural effusions. In the tubular bones, asymmetry predominates, and the ulna is involved most frequently, although changes in the tibia, fibula, humerus, femur, radius, metacarpals, and metatarsals may be seen (Fig. 82–24).

Cortical hyperostosis is the hallmark of this disease. New bone formation begins in the soft tissue swelling

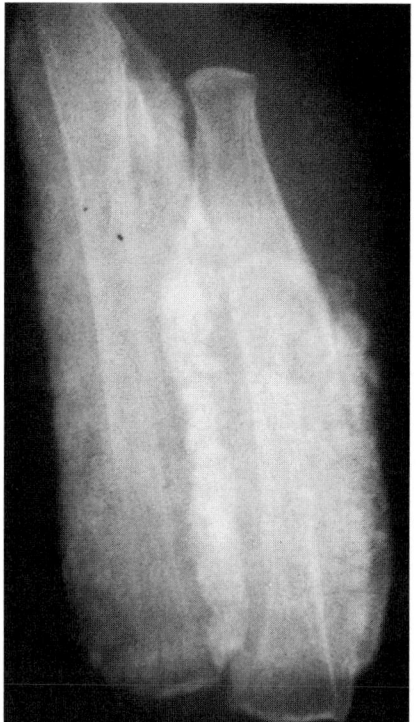

**Figure 82–24.** Infantile cortical hyperostosis: tubular bones. Note involvement of the radius and ulna. The extent of new bone formation is remarkable. These deposits are initially evident in the soft tissues and later merge with the underlying bone.

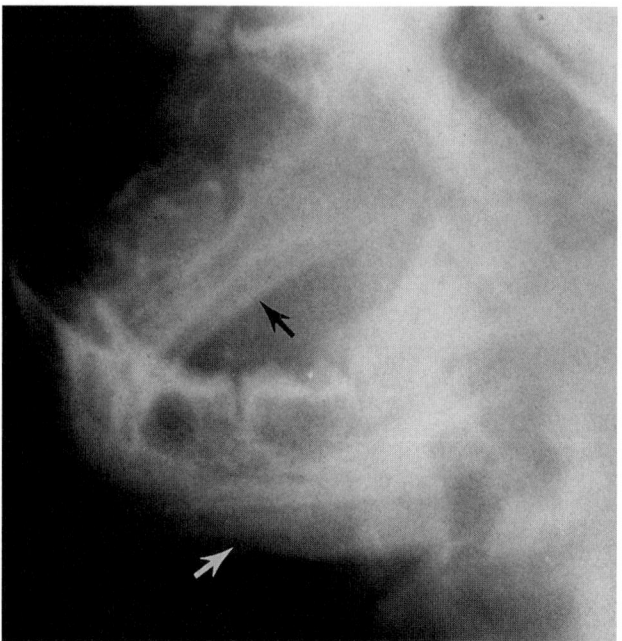

**Figure 82–23.** Infantile cortical hyperostosis: mandible. Observe diffuse periosteal proliferation of the mandible *(arrows)*.

directly contiguous to the original cortex; it becomes progressively more dense and may reach profound proportions. The deposits of bone merge with the underlying osseous tissue, doubling or tripling the normal width of the parent bone. A predilection for the lateral arches of the ribs and for the diaphyses and metaphyses of the tubular bones is evident. The epiphyseal ossification centers are generally spared. Destructive lesions have been identified rarely. Radiographic improvement can occur in a period of weeks to months (Fig. 82–25).

## Cause and Pathogenesis

There are many clinical and pathologic features suggesting that an infectious agent is responsible for infantile cortical hyperostosis; however, the cause remains unknown. The appearance of the disease in many members of a single family over one or more generations underscores the importance of genetic factors in its pathogenesis. An autosomal dominant pattern of inheritance, with incomplete penetrance and variable expressivity, is seen. With a decrease in the number of sporadic cases encountered, familial infantile cortical hyperostosis may represent the major pattern of disease evident today.

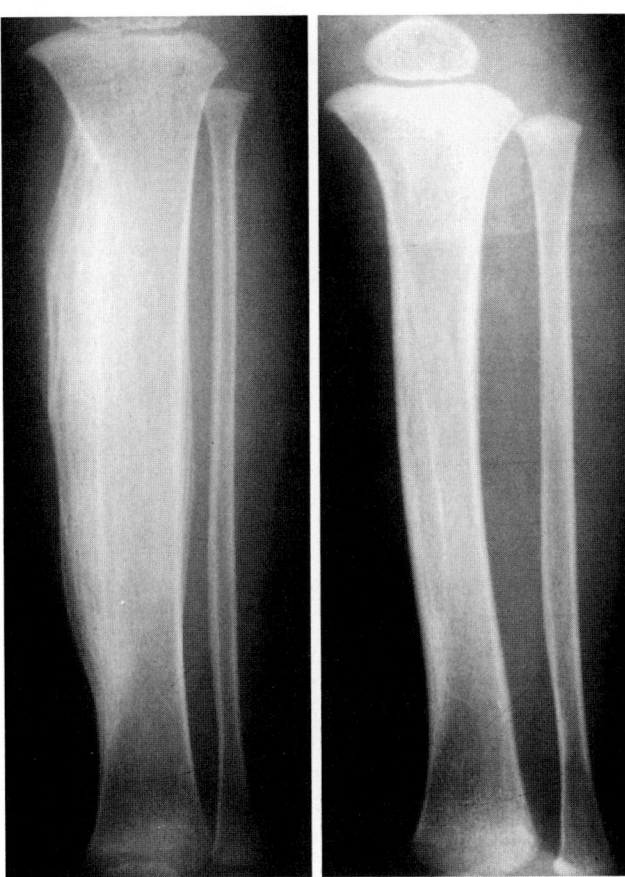

**Figure 82–25.** Infantile cortical hyperostosis: improvement of skeletal lesions. Radiographs of this child at age 6 months *(A)* and 10 months *(B)* show marked improvement of the skeletal abnormalities. (Courtesy of H. S. Kang, MD, Seoul, Korea.)

Radiographically, the disorder leads to mild to moderate thickening of the inner table that is sessile or nodular in outline (Fig. 82–26). The outer cranial contour generally is not altered, although in some cases, CT indicates mild thickening of the outer table of the cranium. Scintigraphically, increased uptake of bone-seeking radionuclide is evident at an early stage of the process, and such uptake may be prominent when radiographic abnormalities are mild. The radiographic findings are virtually diagnostic, although in some cases they may be misinterpreted as evidence of meningioma, Paget's disease, skeletal metastasis, or acromegaly.

## OTHER DISORDERS

Numerous other congenital disorders can lead to hyperostosis and increased skeletal density. These include osteopetrosis, pyknodysostosis, sclerosteosis, endosteal hyperostosis (van Buchem's disease, hyperostosis corticalis generalisata), hereditary hyperphosphatasia (juvenile Paget's disease), and idiopathic hypercalcemia (Williams' syndrome), some of which are discussed elsewhere in this book.

### Plasma Cell Dyscrasia with Polyneuropathy, Organomegaly, Endocrinopathy, M Protein, and Skin Changes

The acronym POEMS (polyneuropathy, organomegaly, endocrinopathy, M protein, and skin changes) refers to a unique syndrome characterized by severe progressive sensorimotor polyneuropathy that might be associated with a plasma cell dyscrasia, osteosclerotic bone lesions, production of M protein, hepatosplenomegaly, lym-

## Differential Diagnosis

Although periostitis and hyperostosis in an infant can also be observed in rickets and scurvy, the absence of epiphyseal or metaphyseal alterations and the resolution of clinical and radiographic features over a period of months allow infantile cortical hyperostosis to be differentiated from these other disorders. Similarly, trauma, including that in an abused child, can lead to calcifying subperiosteal hematomas, but additional findings such as microfractures and metaphyseal irregularity are evident. In hypervitaminosis A, clinical and radiographic manifestations initially appear toward the end of the first year of life, a metatarsal predilection is apparent, facial swelling and mandibular involvement are rare, and serologic testing indicates increased vitamin A levels.

## HYPEROSTOSIS FRONTALIS INTERNA AND RELATED CONDITIONS

Hyperostosis frontalis interna is a descriptive term applied to hyperostosis involving predominantly the inner table of the frontal squama. Hyperostosis frontalis interna is usually observed in patients who are older than 40 years. The disease affects women more often than men, and many of them are postmenopausal.

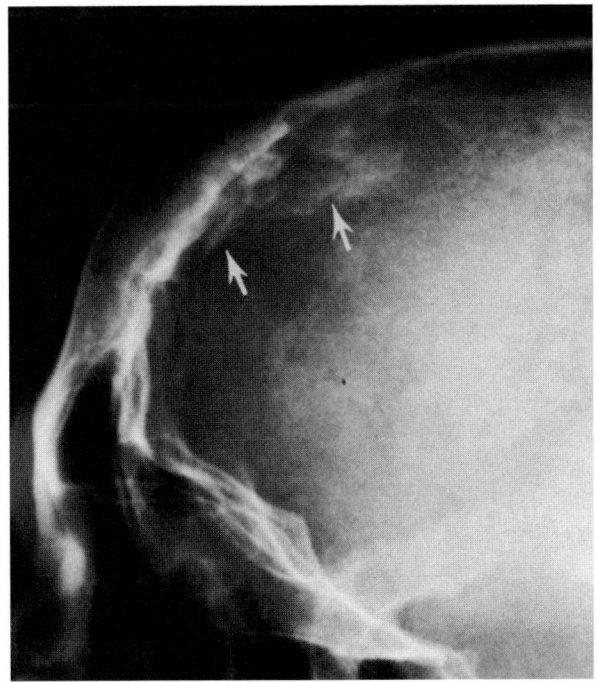

**Figure 82–26.** Hyperostosis frontalis interna. Note nodular hyperostosis of the inner table of the frontal bone *(arrows).*

**TABLE 82–6**

**SAPHO Syndrome**

| Disorder | Typical Age at Onset | Pustulosis Palmaris et Plantaris | Anterior Chest Wall Involvement | Other Skeletal Sites of Involvement |
|---|---|---|---|---|
| Chronic recurrent multifocal osteomyelitis | First 2 decades of life | Evident in <40% of patients | ± | ± |
| Sternocostoclavicular hyperostosis | Fourth to sixth decades of life | Evident in 30% to 50% of patients | +* | ± |
| Pustulotic arthro-osteitis | Adult | +* | − | +* |

*Must be present to establish the diagnosis.

+, present; ±, may be present; −, not present.

SAPHO, synovitis, acne, pustulosis, hyperostosis, osteitis.

phadenopathy, endocrine dysfunction (diabetes mellitus, amenorrhea, gynecomastia, impotence, hypothyroidism), skin thickening and hyperpigmentation, papilledema, and episodes of anasarca. Although some of its radiographic features, including single or multiple solid or "bull's-eye" osteosclerotic lesions, resemble findings in skeletal metastasis, plasma cell myeloma, cystic angiomatosis, or tuberous sclerosis, a peculiar pattern of bone proliferation appears to be unique to this condition. It consists of fluffy, spiculated, hyperostotic areas that show a predilection for the sites of ligamentous attachment in the spine (apophyseal joints, transverse processes, laminae), as well as other axial and extra-axial locations (see Chapter 49). The genesis of the osteosclerotic lesions and bone proliferation is obscure.

## Neurofibromatosis

Massive subperiosteal proliferation is seen in patients with neurofibromatosis. Involvement of the tubular bones of the lower extremity is characterized by bizarre, undulating periosteal deposits of varying size (see Chapter 81).

## Diffuse Idiopathic Skeletal Hyperostosis

Hyperostosis is a common manifestation of this disorder, which is discussed in Chapter 31. Such hyperostosis affects spinal and extraspinal sites, leading to a diagnostic picture of flowing ossification of the spine, bony excrescences at sites of tendinous and ligamentous attachment, para-articular osteophytes, and ligamentous calcification and ossification.

## Syndromes of Hyperostosis, Osteitis, and Skin Lesions (SAPHO Syndrome)

During the last 2 or 3 decades, extraordinary attention has been given to musculoskeletal problems associated with a variety of cutaneous lesions, including acne conglobata, pustulosis palmaris et plantaris, and psoriasis. The acronym SAPHO (representing the major findings of synovitis, acne, pustulosis, hyperostosis, and osteitis) has been used to designate this group of disorders, whose most common manifestation is osteitis of the anterior chest wall (Table 82–6). Although the term is gaining support, it has not yet been fully accepted.

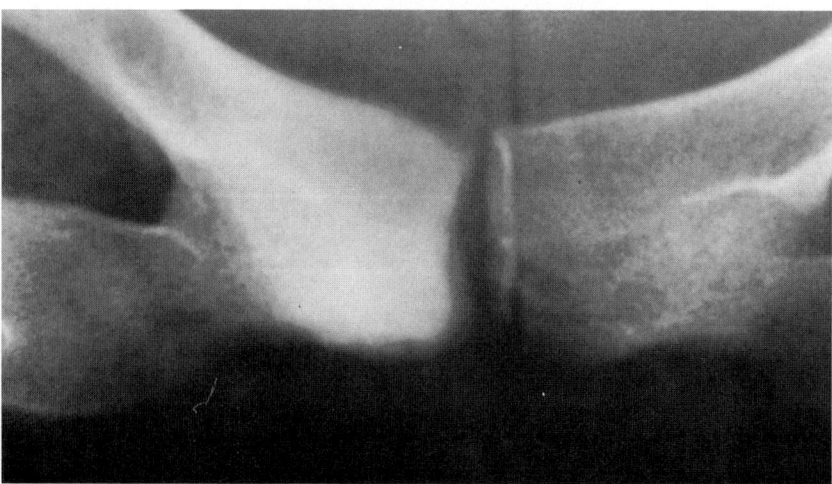

**Figure 82–27.** SAPHO syndrome: involvement of the symphysis pubis. Unilateral osteosclerosis is evident. (Courtesy of J. Schils, MD, Cleveland, Ohio.)

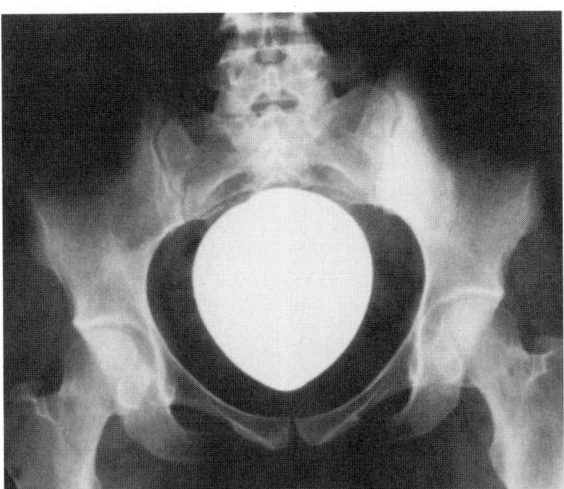

**Figure 82–28.** SAPHO syndrome: involvement of synovial joints. Note ilial sclerosis adjacent to the left sacroiliac joint. The right side is normal.

(From Wetzel R, Wetzel R, Gondolph-Zink B, Puhl W: Pustular osteoarthropathy and its differential diagnosis. Intern Orthop [SICOT] 15:101, 1991.)

SAPHO syndrome encompasses the disorders previously designated sternocostoclavicular hyperostosis, arthro-osteitis associated with pustulosis palmaris et plantaris, and arthro-osteitis associated with severe acne. These disorders share the following findings: (1) pustulosis and severe acne that share the same basic histologic process (i.e., neutrophilic pseudoabscesses); (2) bone involvement that is radiographically and anatomically identical in patients with pustulosis, with acne, or without skin lesions; (3) preferential localization to the anterior chest wall; (4) acute arthritis simulating infection observed with pustulosis, acne, and even psoriasis; and (5) sacroiliac joint involvement.

Involvement of the sternum, clavicles, and anterior portions of the ribs is fundamental to the identification of adult patients with sternocostoclavicular hyperostosis, but it also occurs in children with chronic recurrent multifocal osteomyelitis; in both situations, such involvement may be seen with or without pustulosis palmaris et plantaris. Similar localization is encountered in some patients with cutaneous evidence of psoriasis or acne conglobata. Elsewhere, subchondral lesions may be evident in many of these syndromes, particularly about cartilaginous joints such as the discovertebral junction and symphysis pubis (Fig. 82–27), but also about synovial articulations such as the sacroiliac joints (Fig. 82–28). The distribution of lesions in tubular bones is more variable, although metaphyseal localization in chronic recurrent multifocal osteomyelitis is well known. Bone sclerosis is a dominant radiographic abnormality. Depending on its localization, such sclerosis may simulate that of osteitis condensans ilii, osteitis pubis, spondylitis, or condensing osteitis of the clavicle.

Is SAPHO an appropriate designation for these syndromes of bone and skin? At this time, it is appropriate to consider SAPHO syndrome as comprising several disorders that share some clinical, radiographic, and pathologic characteristics. At one end of the spectrum of such disorders is chronic recurrent multifocal osteomyelitis, and at the other end is sternocostoclavicular hyperostosis. Between these extremes are a number of less well defined

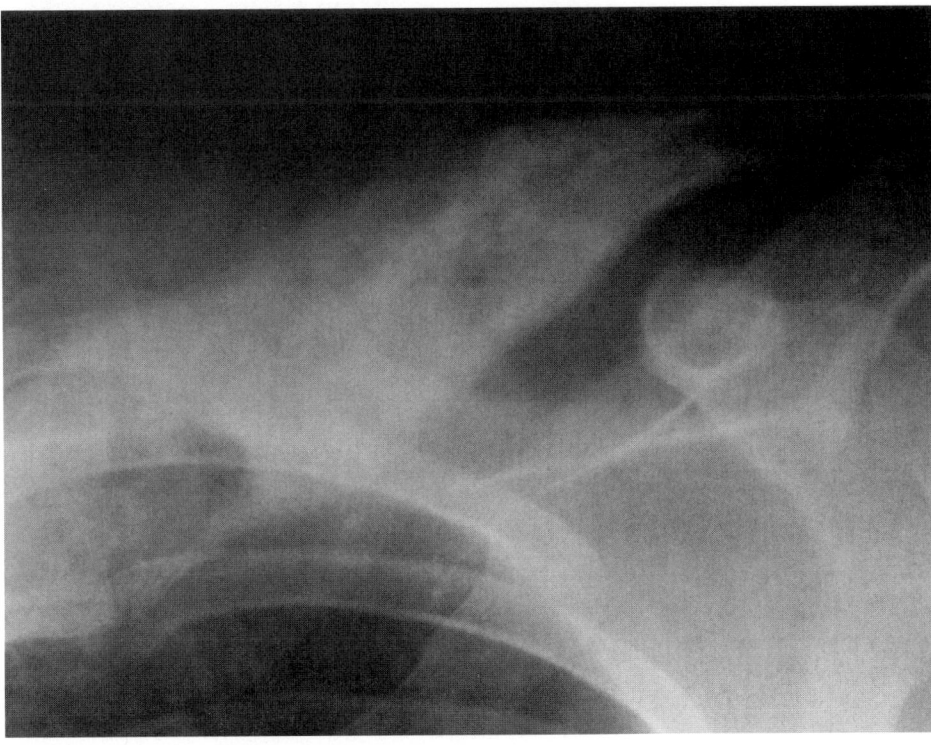

**Figure 82–29.** Chronic recurrent multifocal osteomyelitis. Observe bizarre bone proliferation and osteolytic foci in the clavicle of a 19-year-old man.

musculoskeletal manifestations associated with pustulosis palmaris et plantaris that are perhaps best described as pustulotic arthro-osteitis.

**Chronic Recurrent Multifocal Osteomyelitis.** This disorder, which is discussed more fully in Chapter 53, has also been called plasma cell osteomyelitis, cleidometaphyseal osteomyelitis, and chronic symmetrical osteomyelitis. As classically described, chronic recurrent multifocal osteomyelitis is a disease of unknown causation that affects primarily children and adolescents and is accompanied by local pain and swelling and, less commonly, by systemic manifestations such as fever and weight loss. A significant relationship between this disorder and pustulosis palmaris et plantaris has been emphasized repeatedly in the literature, although less than 40% of patients with chronic recurrent multifocal osteomyelitis have this skin lesion. Also, as classically described, chronic recurrent multifocal osteomyelitis affects a variety of tubular bones, especially the tibia and femur, with or without clavicular involvement (Fig. 82–29). In the tubular bones, a metaphyseal localization is frequent, and involvement of the diaphysis of the femur may be characteristic (Fig. 82–30). The radiographic abnormalities include, eventually, sclerosis and periostitis, with expansion and enlargement of the bone.

The diagnosis of chronic recurrent multifocal osteomyelitis can be applied most confidently to an illness of children and adolescents that demonstrates remissions and exacerbations, affects metaphyseal and subphyseal portions of tubular bones, produces clavicular sclerosis and enlargement, is accompanied histologically by findings of bone inflammation, is unassociated with recoverable microorganisms, and occurs in the clinical setting of pustular lesions of the hands and feet.

**Sternocostoclavicular Hyperostosis.** In its classic form, sternocostoclavicular hyperostosis is characterized by distinctive bone overgrowth and soft tissue ossification of the clavicle, anterior portion of the upper ribs, and sternum. Patients are usually in the fourth to sixth decades of life; men are affected more frequently than women. Bilateral alterations predominate. Clinical findings include pain, swelling, tenderness, and local heat in the anterior upper chest. Osseous overgrowth may lead to occlusion of the subclavian veins. Approximately 30% to 50% of patients with sternocostoclavicular hyperostosis have evidence of pustulosis palmaris et plantaris.

The major radiographic abnormalities of sternocostoclavicular hyperostosis are seen in the anterior and upper portion of the chest wall (Fig. 82–31). Hyperostosis occurs in the sternum, clavicle, upper ribs, and, in some cases, manubriosternal junction. Sternocostoclavicular hyperostosis follows a protracted course, with periods of exacerbation and remission.

The diagnosis of sternocostoclavicular hyperostosis can be applied most confidently to an illness of adults in which bone hypertrophy and ligamentous ossification involve the structures of the anterior chest wall and in which other features, including pustular skin lesions, spinal

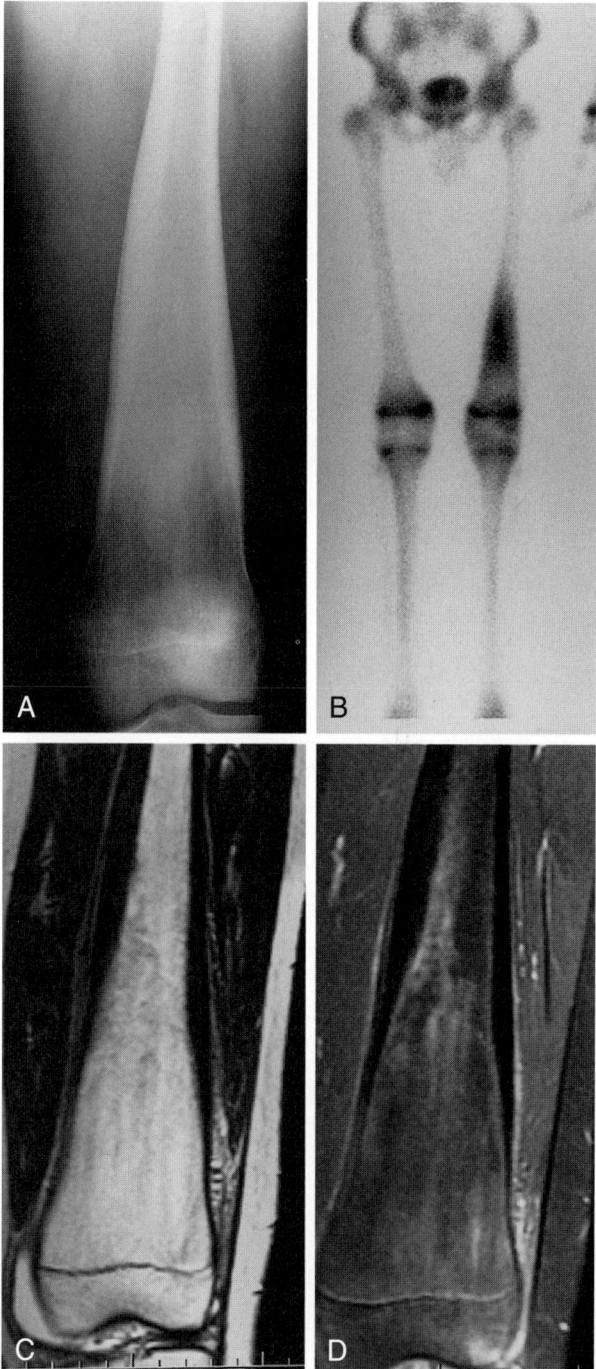

**Figure 82–30.** Chronic recurrent multifocal osteomyelitis. *A,* In this 18-year-old male patient, a conventional radiograph shows fusiform enlargement and cortical thickening of the femoral shaft. *B,* Bone scan confirms accumulation of the radionuclide in the left femoral diaphysis. *C,* On a coronal fast spin echo (TR/TE, 4300/77) MR image, the cortex of the femur is thickened, and patchy increased signal intensity is evident in the medullary bone. *D,* Coronal fat-suppressed T1-weighted (TR/TE, 667/9) spin echo MR image obtained after the intravenous administration of a gadolinium-containing contrast agent shows enhancement of signal intensity in portions of the medullary bone and cortical thickening. (Courtesy of D. Goodwin, MD, Hanover, N.H.)

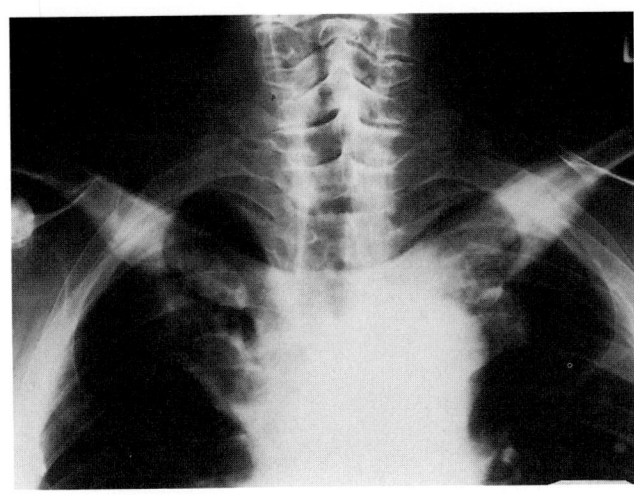

**Figure 82–31.** Sternocostoclavicular hyperostosis. Radiograph shows hyperostosis of the sternum, clavicles, and anterior portions of the first ribs.

(From Wetzel R, Gondolph-Zink B, Puhl W: Pustular osteoarthropathy and its differential diagnosis. Intern Orthop [SICOT] 15:101, 1991.)

and tubular bone involvement, and subclavian venous obstruction, may or may not be present.

**Pustulotic Arthro-osteitis.** Currently, this designation is best applied to adult patients with pustulosis palmaris et plantaris who have inflammatory changes of peripheral joints or sclerotic bone lesions (or both) in sites other than the anterior chest wall. In a child or adolescent with similar findings, the diagnosis of chronic recurrent multifocal osteomyelitis is more appropriate. There are few documented cases of adult patients who meet these diagnostic criteria for pustulotic arthro-osteitis.

Almost all reported cases of the SAPHO syndrome, when analyzed according to these criteria, can be categorized as examples of chronic recurrent multifocal osteomyelitis, sternocostoclavicular hyperostosis, or pustulotic arthro-osteitis.

## FURTHER READING

Ali A, Tetalman MR, Fordham EW, et al: Distribution of hypertrophic pulmonary osteoarthropathy. AJR Am J Roentgenol 134:771, 1980.

Beauvais P, Faur C, Montagne JP, et al: Leri's melorheostosis: Three pediatric cases and a review of the literature. Pediatr Radiol 6:153, 1977.

Caffey J: On some late skeletal changes in chronic infantile cortical hyperostosis. Radiology 59:651, 1952.

Caffey J, Silverman WA: Infantile cortical hyperostoses. Preliminary report on a new syndrome. AJR Am J Roentgenol 54:1, 1945.

Camp JD, Scanlan R: Chronic idiopathic hypertrophic osteoarthropathy. Radiology 50:581, 1948.

Chang CH, Piatt ED, Thomas KE, et al: Bone abnormalities in Gardner's syndrome. AJR Am J Roentgenol 103:645, 1968.

Clarke E, Swischuk LE, Hayden CK Jr: Tumoral calcinosis, diaphysitis, and hyperphosphatemia. Radiology 151:643, 1984.

DeKeyser J, Bruyland M, DeGreve J, et al: Osteopathia striata with cranial sclerosis: Report of a case and review of the literature. Clin Neurol Neurosurg 85:41, 1983.

Dolan KD, Seibert J, Seibert RW: Gardner's syndrome: A model for correlative radiology. AJR Am J Roentgenol 119:359, 1973.

Fairbank HAT: Osteopathia striata. J Bone Joint Surg Br 32:117, 1950.

Garver P, Resnick D, Haghighi P, Guerra J: Melorheostosis of the axial skeleton with associated fibrolipomatous lesions. Skeletal Radiol 9:41, 1982.

Gehweiler JA, Bland WR, Carden TS Jr, et al: Osteopathia striata—Voorhoeve's disease: Review of the roentgen manifestations. AJR Am J Roentgenol 118:450, 1973.

Gershon-Cohen J, Schraer H, Blumberg N: Hyperostosis frontalis interna among the aged. AJR Am J Roentgenol 73:396, 1955.

Goldbloom RB, Stein PB, Eisen A, et al: Idiopathic periosteal hyperostosis with dysproteinemia: A new clinical entity. N Engl J Med 274:873, 1966.

Greenfield GB, Schorsch HA, Shkolnik A: The various roentgen appearances of pulmonary hypertrophic osteoarthropathy. AJR Am J Roentgenol 101:927, 1967.

Greenspan A: Sclerosing bone dysplasias: A target-site approach. Skeletal Radiol 20:561, 1991.

Guyot-Drouot M-H, Solau-Gervais E, Cortet B, et al: Rheumatologic manifestations of pachydermoperiostosis and preliminary experience with biphosphonates. J Rheumatol 27:2418, 2000.

Hall FM, Goldberg RP, Davies JA, Fainsinger MH: Scintigraphic assessment of bone islands. Radiology 135:737, 1980.

Harbison JB, Nice CM Jr: Familial pachydermoperiostosis presenting as an acromegaly-like syndrome. AJR Am J Roentgenol 112:532, 1971.

Joseph B, Chacko V: Acro-osteolysis associated with hypertrophic pulmonary osteoarthropathy and pachydermoperiostosis. Radiology 154:343, 1985.

Kahn MF, Chamot AM: SAPHO syndrome. Rheum Dis Clin North Am 18:225, 1992.

Kasperczyk A, Freyschmidt J: Pustulotic arthroosteitis: Spectrum of bone lesions with palmoplantar pustulosis. Radiology 191:207, 1994.

Kay CJ, Rosenberg MA, Burd R: Hypertrophic osteoarthropathy and childhood Hodgkin's disease. Radiology 112:177, 1974.

Kim SK, Barry WF Jr: Bone island. AJR Am J Roentgenol 92:1301, 1964.

Lagier R, Mbakop A, Bigler A: Osteopoikilosis: A radiological and pathological study. Skeletal Radiol 11:161, 1984.

Lippmann HI, Goldin RR: Subcutaneous ossification of the legs in chronic venous insufficiency. Radiology 74:279, 1960.

Martinez-Lavin M, Pineda C, Valdez T, et al: Primary hypertrophic osteoarthropathy. Semin Arthritis Rheum 17:156, 1988.

Melhem RE, Najjar SS, Knachadurian AK: Cortical hyperostosis with hyperphosphatemia: A new syndrome? J Pediatr 77:986, 1970.

Melnick JC: Osteopathia condensans disseminata (osteopoikilosis): Study of a family of 4 generations. AJR Am J Roentgenol 82:229, 1959.

Murray RO, McCredie J: Melorheostosis and the sclerotomes: A radiological correlation. Skeletal Radiol 4:57, 1979.

Nathanson I, Riddlesberger MM Jr: Pulmonary hypertrophic osteoarthropathy in cystic fibrosis. Radiology 135:649, 1980.

Neiman HL, Gompels BM, Martel W: Pachydermoperiostosis with bone marrow failure and gross extramedullary hematopoiesis: Report of a case. Radiology 110:553, 1974.

Onitsuka H: Roentgenologic aspects of bone islands. Radiology 123:607, 1977.

Pitt MJ, Mosher JF, Edeiken J: Abnormal periosteum and bone in neurofibromatosis. Radiology 103:143, 1972.

Resnick D: Sternocostoclavicular hyperostosis. AJR Am J Roentgenol 135:1278, 1980.

Resnick D, Vint V, Poteshman NL: Sternocostoclavicular hyperostosis: A report of three new cases. J Bone Joint Surg Am 63:1329, 1981.

Rosenthal L, Kirsh J: Observations on the radionuclide imaging in hypertrophic pulmonary osteoarthropathy. Radiology 120:359, 1976.

Sartoris DJ, Schreiman JS, Kerr R, et al: Sternocostoclavicular hyperostosis: A review and report of 11 cases. Radiology 158:125, 1986.

Saul RA, Lee WH, Stevenson RE: Caffey's disease revisited: Further evidence for autosomal dominant inheritance with incomplete penetrance. Am J Dis Child 136:56, 1982.

Silverman FN: Virus diseases of bone: Do they exist? AJR Am J Roentgenol 126:677, 1976.

Smith J: Giant bone islands. Radiology 107:35, 1973.

Sonozaki H, Azuma A, Okai K, et al: Clinical features of 22 cases with "inter-sterno-costo-clavicular ossification." Arch Orthop Trauma Surg 95:13, 1979.

Sonozaki H, Kawashima M, Hongo O, et al: Incidence of arthro-osteitis in patients with pustulosis palmaris. Ann Rheum Dis 40:554, 1981.

Sonozaki H, Mitsui H, Miyanaga Y, et al: Clinical features of 53 cases with pustulosis arthro-osteitis. Ann Rheum Dis 40:547, 1981.

Sundaram M, Falbo S, McDonald D, Janney C: Surface osteomas of the appendicular skeleton. AJR Am J Roentgenol 167:1529, 1996.

Swerdloff BA, Ozonoff MB, Gyepes MT: Late recurrence of infantile cortical hyperostosis (Caffey's disease). AJR Am J Roentgenol 108:461, 1970.

Temple HL, Jaspin G: Hypertrophic osteoarthropathy. AJR Am J Roentgenol 60:232, 1948.

Van Buskirk FW, Tampas JP, Peterson OS Jr: Infantile cortical hyperostosis: Inquiry into its familial aspects. AJR Am J Roentgenol 85:613, 1961.

Vogl A, Goldfischer S: Pachydermoperiostosis: Primary or idiopathic hypertrophic osteoarthropathy. Am J Med 33:166, 1962.

Walter RD, Resnick D: Hypertrophic osteoarthropathy of a lower extremity in association with arterial graft sepsis. AJR Am J Roentgenol 137:1059, 1981.

Whyte MP, Murphy WA, Fallon MD, et al: Mixed-sclerosing-bone-dystrophy: Report of a case and review of the literature. Skeletal Radiol 6:95, 1981.

Wilcox LF: Osteopoikilosis. AJR Am J Roentgenol 30:615, 1933.

Yaghmai I, Tafazoli M: Massive subperiosteal hemorrhage in neurofibromatosis. Radiology 122:439, 1977.

# CHAPTER 83

## Osteolysis and Chondrolysis

### SUMMARY OF KEY FEATURES

A variety of disorders can lead to osteolysis and chondrolysis. In some, bone resorption is especially prominent in the phalanges of the hand and foot and may be related to occupational or inherited factors. Post-traumatic osteolysis can occur at many sites, particularly the distal end of the clavicle, pubic and ischial rami, and femoral neck. Massive osteolysis of Gorham can lead to regional destruction and disappearance of bone. Idiopathic multicentric osteolysis shows a predilection for the carpal and tarsal areas and must be differentiated from juvenile chronic arthritis, Winchester's syndrome, and Farber's disease. Additional osteolysis syndromes include neurogenic acro-osteolysis, acro-osteolysis of Joseph or of Shinz, osteolysis with detritic synovitis, and familial expansile osteolysis. Chondrolysis of the hip can accompany a slipped capital femoral epiphysis, or it can appear on an idiopathic basis. It must be differentiated from juvenile chronic arthritis, infection, and regional osteoporosis.

### INTRODUCTION

Destruction of bone (osteolysis) or cartilage (chondrolysis) can occur in numerous neoplastic, infectious, metabolic, traumatic, vascular, congenital, and articular disorders that are discussed elsewhere in this book. A group of heterogeneous conditions remains in which significant and severe osteolysis and chondrolysis may manifest; these disorders are described in this chapter.

### OSTEOLYSIS

#### Occupational Acro-osteolysis

During the 1960s, several investigators implicated exposure to vinyl chloride monomer in the pathogenesis of acro-osteolysis. Routine radiographic surveys of employees in certain industrial plants revealed that as many as 1% to 2% of workers involved in the polymerization of vinyl chloride develop acro-osteolysis. Occasionally, exposure to vapors of other synthetic materials used in the manufacture of plastic products can produce similar abnormalities. Initial clinical manifestations include fatigue, asthenia, nervousness, and insomnia. Additional clinical findings can include scleroderma-like plaques on the hands, wrists, and forearms; soft tissue nodules; hyperhidrosis and discoloration; and medial nerve compression in the carpal tunnel.

The radiographic hallmark of the disorder is osteolysis that predominates in the terminal phalanges of the hands, although it may also affect other phalanges, the sacroiliac joint, and the foot. Bandlike radiolucent areas across the waist of one or more terminal phalanges may be combined with tuftal resorption and beveling and osseous fragmentation (Fig. 83–1). The thumb is affected more commonly than the other digits. Similar changes may appear in the foot, and bone erosion and sclerosis about one or both sacroiliac joints resemble the changes of sacroiliitis. If the exposure to polyvinyl chloride is halted, slow improvement of the radiographic abnormalities may occur.

#### Post-Traumatic Osteolysis

Some degree of bone loss is common after a traumatic insult, particularly when complicated by a fracture; in certain situations and sites, however, the degree of post-traumatic osteolysis may be excessive (Table 83–1). Knowledge of the existence and appearance of such osteolysis is important so that the resorption of bone that accompanies a traumatic insult is not mistaken for an inflammatory or neoplastic process.

Post-traumatic osteolysis can lead to progressive resorption of the outer end of the clavicle. The process becomes apparent after single or repeated episodes of local trauma. Frequently, the traumatic insult is minor and is unassociated with obvious fracture or dislocation. The osteolytic process may begin as early as 2 to 3 weeks and as late as several years after the injury. When untreated, it leads to lysis of 0.5 to 3 cm of bony substance from the distal end of the clavicle over 12 to 18 months, which may be associated with erosion and cupping of the acromion, soft tissue swelling, and dystrophic calcification (Fig. 83–2). After the lytic phase stabilizes, reparative changes occur over 4 to 6 months, emphasizing the self-limited nature of the process. Eventually, the subchondral bone becomes reconstituted, although the acromioclavicular joint can remain permanently widened.

Post-traumatic osteolysis of one or both clavicles is also observed in athletes, particularly weightlifters, owing to chronic stress rather than acute injury. A similar process can evolve in persons who lift heavy weights as part of their occupational activities. Clinical and radiographic abnormalities are virtually identical to those that occur after acute injury.

The magnetic resonance (MR) imaging features of clavicular osteolysis caused by acute trauma or chronic stress are similar. Marrow edema in the distal portion of the clavicle and, less commonly, the acromion is typical (Fig. 83–3). Additional abnormalities, in decreasing order of frequency, include prominence of the capsule of the acromioclavicular joint, irregularity of subchondral bone, joint fluid, and bone fragmentation (Fig. 83–4).

The differential diagnosis of osteolysis about the acromioclavicular joint includes, in addition to trauma, hyperparathyroidism, collagen vascular disorders, infection, rheumatoid arthritis, and other articular processes. Osteolysis of the distal clavicle has also been noted after spinal cord injury and on an idiopathic basis.

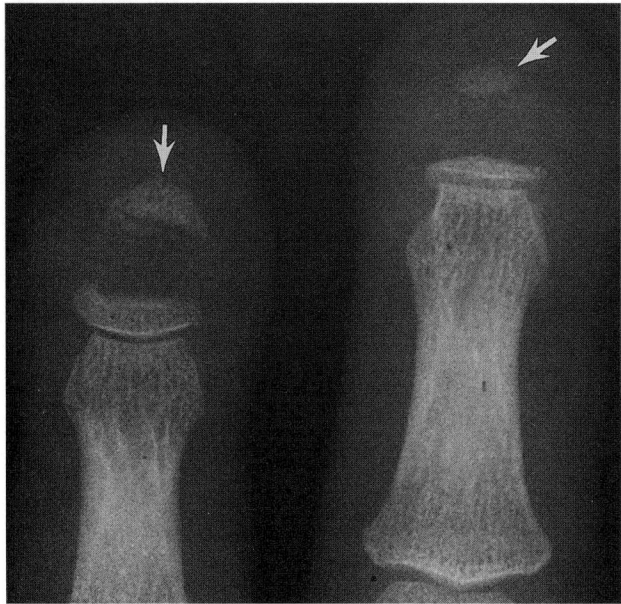

**Figure 83–1.** Occupational acro-osteolysis. Note bandlike resorption of the terminal phalanges of two digits, isolating small osseous fragments in the terminal tufts *(arrows)*. Observe that the distal interphalangeal joints are intact.

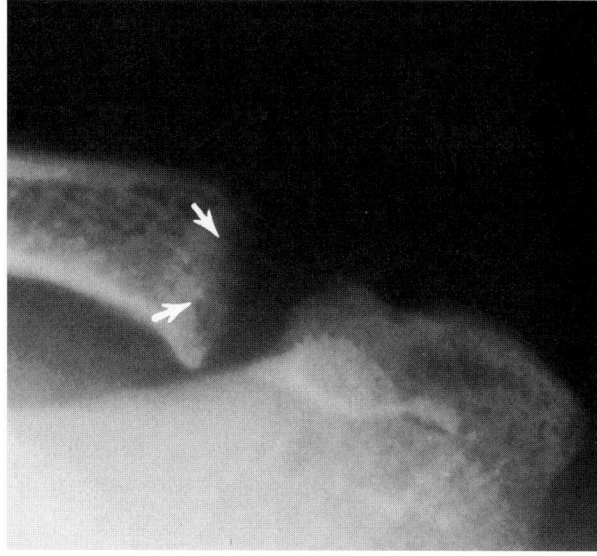

**Figure 83–2.** Post-traumatic osteolysis: clavicle. In this 23-year-old weightlifter, irregular erosion of the distal portion of the clavicle *(arrows)* and, to a lesser extent, the acromion, with widening of the acromioclavicular joint, is seen. (Courtesy of P. Kaplan, MD, Boston, Mass.)

---

**TABLE 83–1**

**Common Sites of Post-Traumatic Osteolysis**

Distal portion of clavicle
Pubic and ischial rami
Distal portion of ulna
Distal portion of radius
Carpus
Femoral neck

---

Post-traumatic osteolysis can also be seen in the pubic or ischial rami, where exaggerated resorption of bone about a fracture, with or without associated sclerosis, can simulate the appearance of a malignant process (Fig. 83–5). Such fractures occur after direct trauma or often as a result of chronic stress in an osteopenic skeleton (insufficiency fractures), sometimes in combination with similar fractures of the sacrum.

### Primary Osteolysis Syndromes

A diverse group of idiopathic disorders can lead to significant skeletal lysis. They differ in the presence or absence of genetic transmission, the associated clinical manifestations, and the major locations of osteolysis (Table 83–2).

### Acro-osteolysis Syndrome of Hajdu and Cheney

This unusual syndrome may be familial, with a dominant mode of inheritance, or it may be sporadic. It is manifested by short stature, low-set ears, recessed mandible, malocclusion and early loss of teeth, coarse hairs, pseudoclubbing of the digits, joint laxity, conductive hearing loss, and speech impairment. Radiographic features include osteolysis of distal phalanges of the hands and feet; a bizarre-shaped dolichocephalic skull, with basilar impression, delayed closure of cranial sutures, multiple wormian bones, hypoplastic or absent frontal sinuses, prominent occipital ridge, and enlarged sella turcica; diminutive mandible and maxilla, with poor dentition; generalized osteoporosis, with vertebral compressions and deformities and fractures of tubular bones; kyphosis or kyphoscoliosis; valgus deformities of the knees; and hypoplasia and subluxation of the proximal portion of the radius. Laboratory analysis is usually unremarkable, and renal function, which is altered in other osteolysis syndromes, is normal in this condition.

Osteolysis of the distal phalanges is especially characteristic (Fig. 83–6). Changes in the phalanges, which consist of resorption of tufts and bandlike areas of lucency, simulate the abnormalities in occupational (polyvinyl chloride) acro-osteolysis, renal osteodystrophy, pyknodysostosis, Rothmund's syndrome, and collagen vascular disorders. Osteolysis may also be apparent in the tubular bones, mandibular rami, tarsal and metatarsal bones, and acromioclavicular joints. The radionuclide examination is characterized by abnormal accumulation of bone-seeking radiopharmaceutical agents at sites of osteolysis. MR imaging can be used to study the degree of involvement

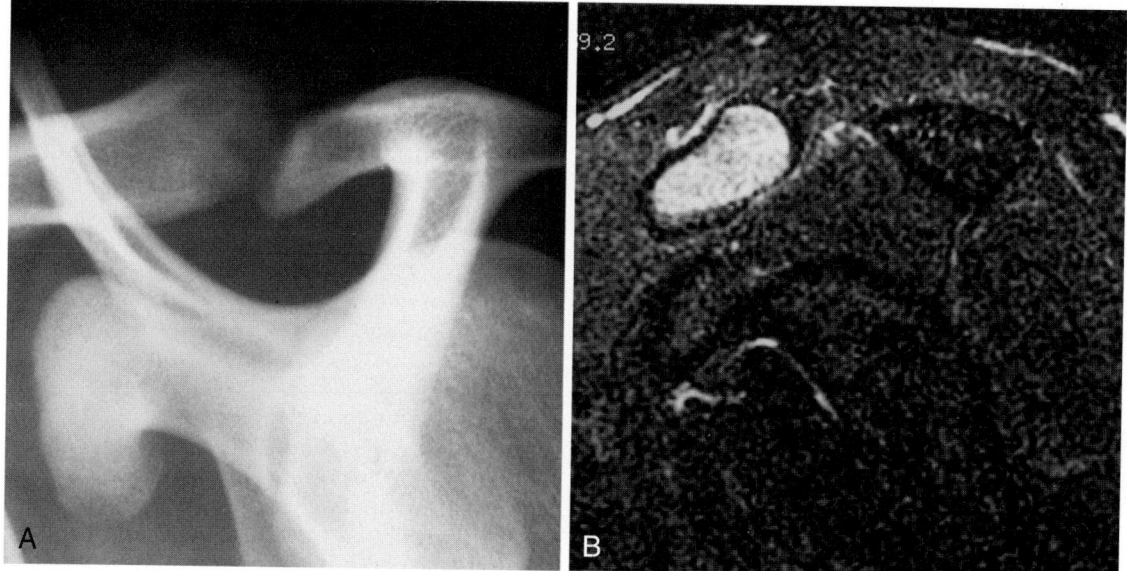

**Figure 83–3.** Post-traumatic osteolysis: clavicle. This 35-year-old man, who was a recreational body-builder, developed progressive shoulder pain. *A,* Lateral scapular view shows osteolysis and ill-defined bone proliferation in the distal portion of the clavicle. *B,* Oblique sagittal fat-suppressed fast spin echo (TR/TE, 3000/98) MR image reveals increased signal intensity in this portion of the clavicle.

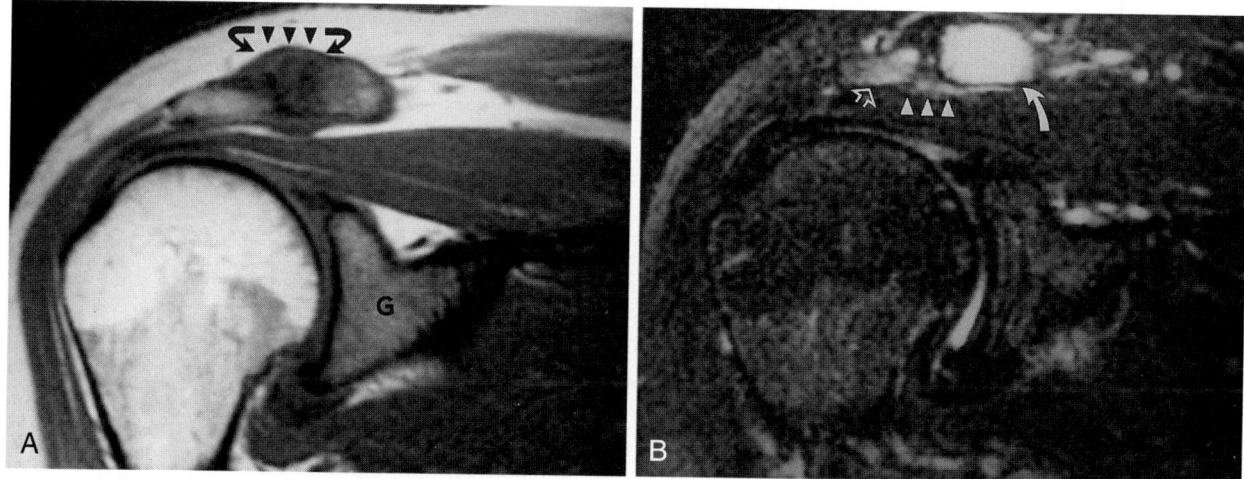

**Figure 83–4.** Post-traumatic osteolysis: clavicle. This 46-year-old woman developed chronic shoulder pain after a jet-ski accident. *A,* Oblique coronal T1-weighted (TR/TE, 433/17) spin echo MR image shows prominence of the capsule *(arrows, arrowheads)* about the acromioclavicular joint. *B,* Corresponding oblique coronal fat-suppressed fast spin echo (TR/TE, 3416/96) MR image shows edema of high signal intensity in the distal portion of the clavicle *(curved arrow)* and, to a lesser extent, the acromion *(open arrow),* with capsular distention of the acromioclavicular joint without an effusion *(arrowheads).*

(From de la Puente R, Boutin RD, Theodorou DJ, et al: Post-traumatic and stress-induced osteolysis of the distal clavicle: MR imaging findings in 17 patients. Skeletal Radiol 28:202, 1999.)

of the spinal cord in patients who have basilar impression and in those rare patients who develop instability of the cervical spine.

## Massive Osteolysis of Gorham

Also termed hemangiomatosis, massive osteolysis, disappearing bone disease, vanishing bone disease, and Gorham's disease, this rare disease can be seen in patients of any age, although most cases are discovered before age 40 years. The disease affects both men and women, and a family history is not apparent. Clinical manifestations vary. Some patients have a relatively abrupt onset of pain and swelling; others describe an insidious onset of soft tissue atrophy and limitation of motion that is painless unless an associated pathologic fracture develops; still others note

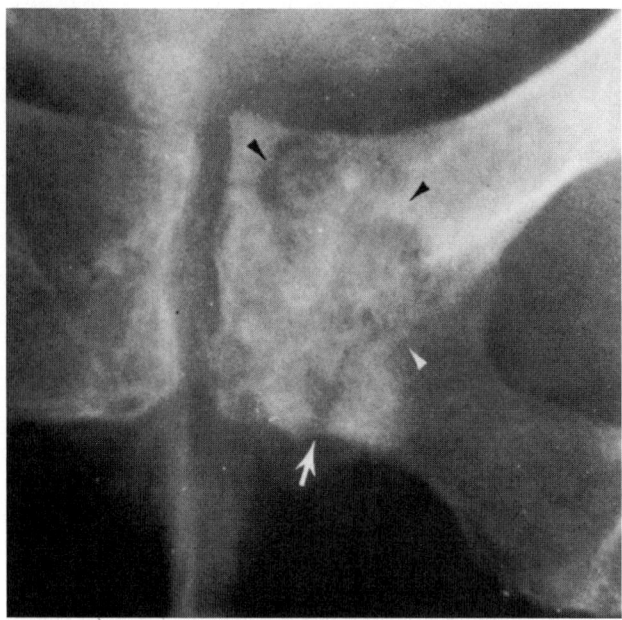

**Figure 83–5.** Post-traumatic osteolysis: pubis. This 54-year-old alcoholic woman complained of a dull left groin ache of 4 months' duration. The patient later developed fractures of the sternum and ribs, although she continued to deny any significant trauma. Preoperative radiograph reveals a mixed lytic and sclerotic lesion of the left pubis *(arrowheads)* with a fracture *(arrow)*.

the onset of the disorder after significant trauma. The process may affect either the axial or the appendicular skeleton; numerous cases document the frequency of changes in the pelvic or shoulder region. Laboratory analysis may show unremarkable results, with slight elevation of the serum alkaline phosphatase level.

The most dramatic aspect of massive osteolysis is its radiographic appearance (Fig. 83–7). Initially, radiolucent foci appear in the intramedullary or subcortical regions, resembling the findings in patchy osteoporosis. Slowly progressive atrophy, dissolution, fracture, fragmentation, and disappearance of a portion of the bone then occur, with tapering or "pointing" of the remaining osseous tissue and atrophy of soft tissue. The process subsequently extends to contiguous bones, with the intervening joints affording no protection. Thus, osteolysis of the ilium may be associated with resorption of the proximal portion of the femur, resembling the findings of idiopathic, rapidly destructive hip disease; changes in the scapula may later be combined with osteolysis of the proximal end of the humerus, clavicle, and ribs. This pattern of regional destruction is dramatic and should suggest the correct diagnosis. The degree of osseous destruction generally increases relentlessly over a period of years, although eventually it may stabilize. Rarely, two or more anatomic regions are affected, separated by normal osseous structures. Apparently, any bone can be involved, including the small tubular bones of the hands and feet, the spine, the skull, and the mandible.

**TABLE 83–2**

**Osteolysis Syndromes**

| Syndrome | Age at Onset | Major Site of Osteolysis | Patterns of Inheritance | Associated Features |
|---|---|---|---|---|
| Acro-osteolysis of Hajdu and Cheney | Second decade | Distal phalanges; rarely tubular bones, mandible, acromioclavicular joints | Dominant or sporadic | Generalized bone dysplasia, fractures, osteoporosis |
| Massive osteolysis of Gorham | Young adult | Variable; pelvic or shoulder girdles | Sporadic | Slowly progressive, extreme dissolution |
| Carpal-tarsal osteolysis | | | | |
|   Multicentric osteolysis with nephropathy | Infant, child | Carpal and tarsal areas, elbows | Sporadic; occasionally dominant | Osteoporosis, deformity, hypertension, renal failure, death |
|   Hereditary multicentric osteolysis | 1–5 yr | Carpal and tarsal areas, elbows, digits | Dominant; occasionally recessive or sporadic | Progressive deformity |
| Neurogenic osteolysis | Childhood | Phalanges | Dominant or recessive | Sensory neuropathy, skin ulcerations |
| Acro-osteolysis of Joseph | Childhood | Distal phalanges | Recessive | Otherwise healthy |
| Acro-osteolysis of Shinz | Second decade | Phalanges | Dominant | Skin ulcerations, no neurologic defect |
| Farber's disease | Infancy | Elbows, wrists, knees, ankles | Sporadic | Subcutaneous nodules |
| Winchester's syndrome | Infancy | Carpal and tarsal areas, elbows | Recessive | Osteoporosis, joint contractures, thick skin, corneal opacities |
| Osteolysis with detritic synovitis | Adulthood | Widespread | Sporadic | Progressive |

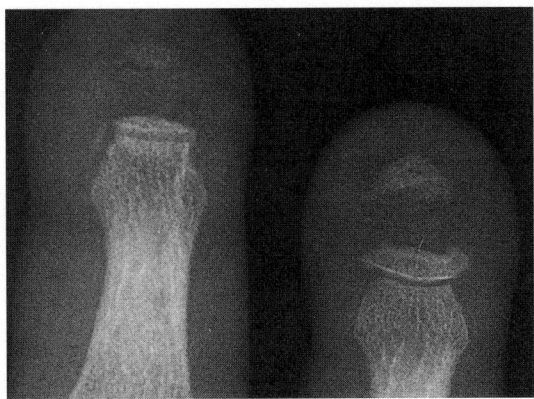

**Figure 83–6.** Acro-osteolysis of Hajdu and Cheney. The typical pattern of osteolysis of the digits is demonstrated. Note that resorption occurs in a bandlike fashion across the waist of the terminal phalanges, isolating one or more phalangeal fragments. Soft tissue swelling is also evident. The appearance is identical to that in occupational acro-osteolysis. (Courtesy of M. Dalinka, MD, Philadelphia, Pa.)

Scintigraphy using bone-seeking radiopharmaceutical agents may demonstrate increased vascularity on initial images, followed by an area of decreased uptake corresponding to the site of diminished or absent bone tissue. These results are variable, however. The reported MR imaging features of this form of osteolysis are also variable.

T1-weighted spin echo MR images reveal the bone lesions to be either of uniformly low signal intensity or characterized by regions of high signal intensity. Increased signal intensity is generally observed on T2-weighted spin echo images, and enhancement of the lesions is usually evident after intravenous gadolinium administration.

### Idiopathic Multicentric Osteolysis (Carpal-Tarsal Osteolysis)

Idiopathic multicentric osteolysis is a rare disorder associated with extensive osteolysis, usually in the carpal or tarsal areas. It was previously called by a variety of names, including idiopathic osteolysis, essential osteolysis, progressive essential osteolysis, essential acro-osteolysis, familial osteolysis, hereditary osteolysis, carpal and tarsal agenesis, familial dysostosis carpi, and bilateral carpal necrosis. Idiopathic multicentric osteolysis can be classified into two basic types: multicentric osteolysis with nephropathy, and hereditary multicentric osteolysis. Not all cases fit neatly into one of these categories, however, so a third designation—miscellaneous patterns—is required.

**Multicentric Osteolysis with Nephropathy.** This entity, which has been recognized in only a handful of cases, is characterized by early-onset (within the first few years of life) osteolysis associated with progressive renal failure that is commonly fatal by the third decade of life. No family history of either osteolysis or renal disease is present. Presenting clinical manifestations include swollen, painful

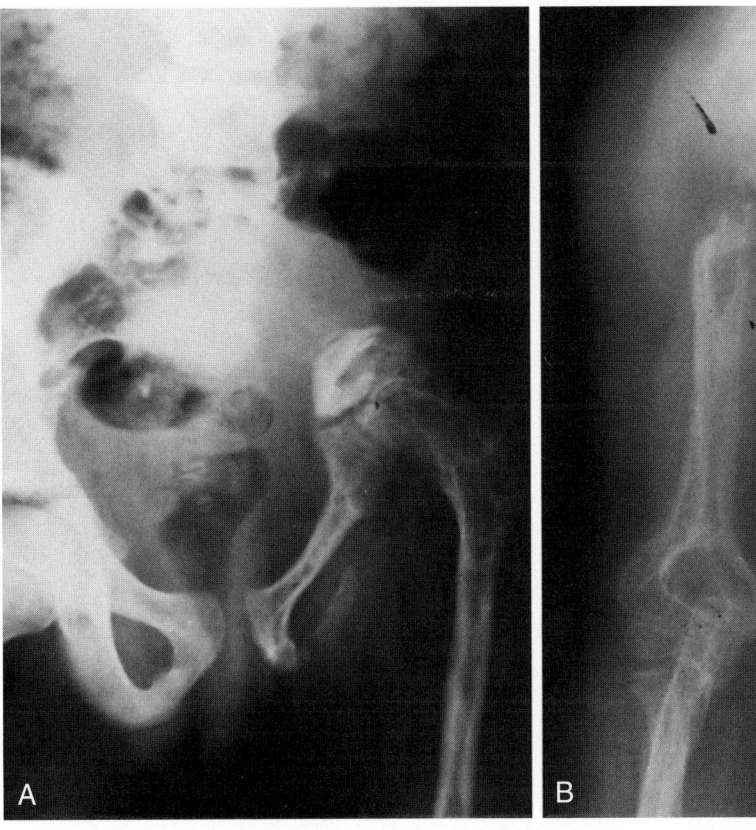

**Figure 83–7.** Massive osteolysis of Gorham. *A,* In this 14-year-old boy, observe the dissolution of most of the left hemipelvis and the narrowed and tapered left femur. Radiolucent foci and a coarsened trabecular pattern are seen in the femur and pubic bone. *B,* In this 6-year-old girl, resorption of the proximal half of the humerus is evident. The remaining bone is osteoporotic, with lucent lesions.

wrists, with or without foot deformities. Radiographs reveal progressive disappearance of the carpus and, less strikingly, the tarsus, with tapering of the adjacent tubular bones. Osteolysis and subluxation about the elbow and congenital foot deformities may also be apparent. Rarely, other sites are affected. Renal alterations accompany the onset of osteolysis. Chronic glomerulonephritis results in hypertension, azotemia, and death in early adulthood.

**Hereditary Multicentric Osteolysis.** This condition has a familial distribution, with most cases exhibiting a dominant mode of transmission, although the trait is occasionally recessive. In the dominant variety, disease onset usually occurs at age 3 to 4 years, with articular complaints involving the wrists and ankles. Subsequently, an asymptomatic period arises in adolescence in which a varying amount of carpal and tarsal osteolysis is associated with progressive deformity. In the recessive variety, the clinical course is basically similar.

Radiographs in both dominant and recessive forms of the disease outline dissolution of the carpus and tarsus that, in most cases, is not associated with tapering of the adjacent tubular bones (Fig. 83–8). This latter characteristic differs from the "penciling" of tubular bones evident in multicentric osteolysis with nephropathy; this feature is not constant, however, and patients with hereditary multicentric osteolysis can have tapering of the metacarpals, distal end of the radius, and ulna. Rarely, osteolysis is encountered at additional sites, including the elbows, shoulders, clavicles, hips, knees, ankles, feet, and ribs.

**Miscellaneous Patterns.** Some cases of idiopathic multicentric osteolysis do not fall precisely into one of the two groups just described. Nonfamilial cases of carpal and tarsal osteolysis may be discovered that do not involve renal disease. Similar sporadic cases with a late onset or involvement of osseous sites other than the carpal and tarsal areas have been described. Conversely, examples of carpal-tarsal osteolysis with evidence of renal involvement may demonstrate familial patterns (dominant mode of inheritance), although the nephropathy may differ in type and degree from that in sporadic (nonfamilial) cases.

## Other Osteolysis Syndromes

**Neurogenic Acro-osteolysis.** Both recessive and dominant forms of progressive peripheral bone destruction associated with sensory neuropathy have been described. The disease becomes clinically apparent in childhood and is associated with skin ulcerations and progressive resorption of phalanges of the hands and feet. A somewhat similar pattern of osteolysis, with more widespread bone destruction, has been noted in Vietnamese patients with severe scarring of the skin, no neurologic alterations, and positive serologic tests for syphilis.

**Acro-osteolysis of Joseph or of Shinz.** Joseph and associates described a single sibship with recessive inheritance of osteolysis of the distal phalanges in otherwise normal boys. Shinz observed a form of peripheral osteolysis charac-

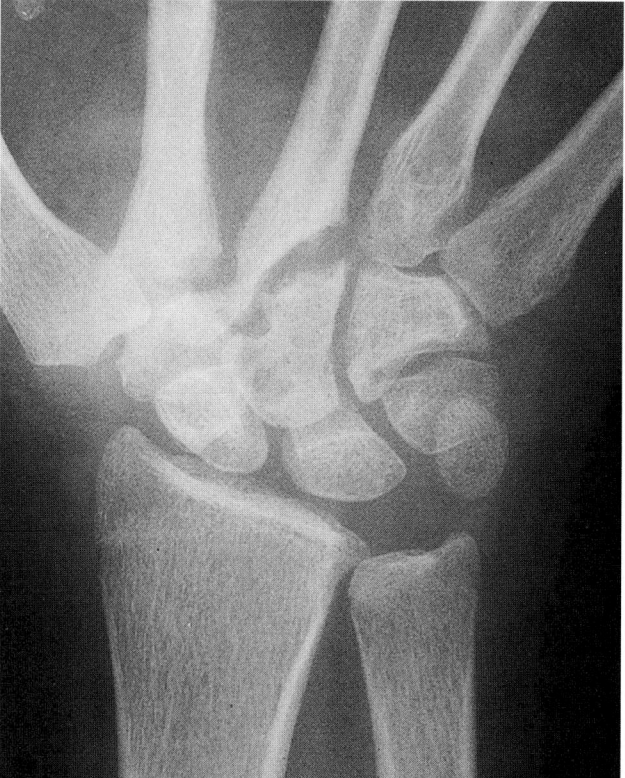

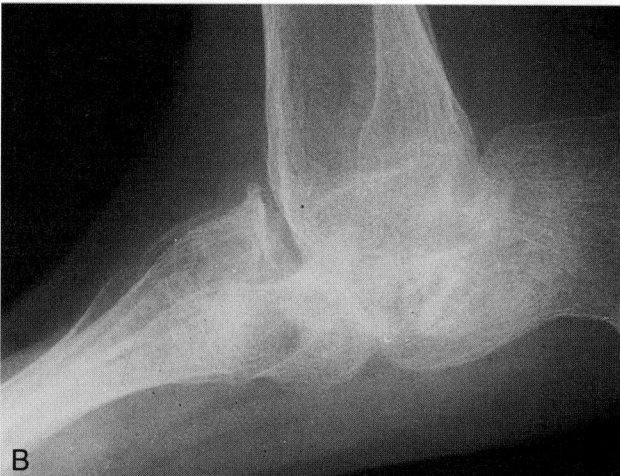

**Figure 83–8.** Hereditary multicentric osteolysis. This child developed progressive osteolysis at multiple skeletal sites, without evidence of renal disease. *A,* Radiograph of the wrist obtained at age 16 years reveals progressive resorption of the carpus and metacarpal bases, with soft tissue swelling. The tapered appearance of the proximal metacarpal bones and the osseous erosions at several metacarpophalangeal joints are readily apparent. *B,* Radiograph of the foot at age 16 years demonstrates the great degree of lysis of most of the tarsal bones. The tibia is articulating with the calcaneus. (Courtesy of A. Brower, MD, Norfolk, Va.)

terized by a dominant inheritance, onset in the second decade of life, destruction of phalanges of the hands and feet, and ulcerating skin lesions, without neurologic abnormalities. Acro-osteolysis syndromes similar to those of Joseph and of Shinz have been identified in adult patients without a family history of disease.

**Farber's Disease.** Farber's disease is characterized by the onset in infancy of progressive, painful periarticular swelling, joint rigidity and contracture, osteolysis, and subcutaneous nodules. It may represent a disorder of mucopolysaccharide metabolism.

**Winchester's Syndrome.** Winchester and associates described a disorder with recessive inheritance that manifests as extensive and progressive destruction of the carpus, tarsus, and elbows beginning in infancy. Additional findings include dwarfism, coarsened facial features, peripheral corneal opacities, arthralgias and joint stiffening, progressive deformities of the trunk and limbs, and generalized and profound osteoporosis. Although originally classified as a form of mucopolysaccharidosis, Winchester's syndrome is more accurately regarded as a nonlysosomal connective tissue disease.

**Osteolysis with Detritic Synovitis.** In 1978, a new pattern of osteolysis in both the appendicular and the axial skeleton was described in a 71-year-old woman with no family history of similar abnormalities. A severely destructive and mutilating arthropathy of the hands was associated with bone resorption of the phalanges, metacarpals, metatarsals, clavicles, tubular bones, and spine (Fig. 83–9). The radiographic characteristics resembled, in part, the findings of hyperparathyroidism; however, the absence of the classic features of subperiosteal and subchondral resorption, the presence of severe digital deformities, and normal values for serum calcium, phosphorus, and parathyroid hormone concentrations made this latter diagnosis untenable.

**Familial Expansile Osteolysis.** A rare autosomal dominant bone disorder beginning in childhood, adolescence, or early adulthood, familial expansile osteolysis shares some clinical, radiographic, and histologic features with Paget's disease. Hearing loss is an early clinical manifestation, sometimes becoming apparent before 5 years of age. Bone pain and dental manifestations, consisting of tooth mobility and fracture, are also observed. Radiographic abnormalities may be both generalized and focal. In the former category, disordered modeling and a coarsened trabecular pattern are evident, especially in the humerus, radius, ulna, and tibia. Trabecular changes include small radiolucent foci that have been characterized as having a "fishnet" appearance. Three grades of focal changes, all of which predominate in the appendicular skeleton, have also been

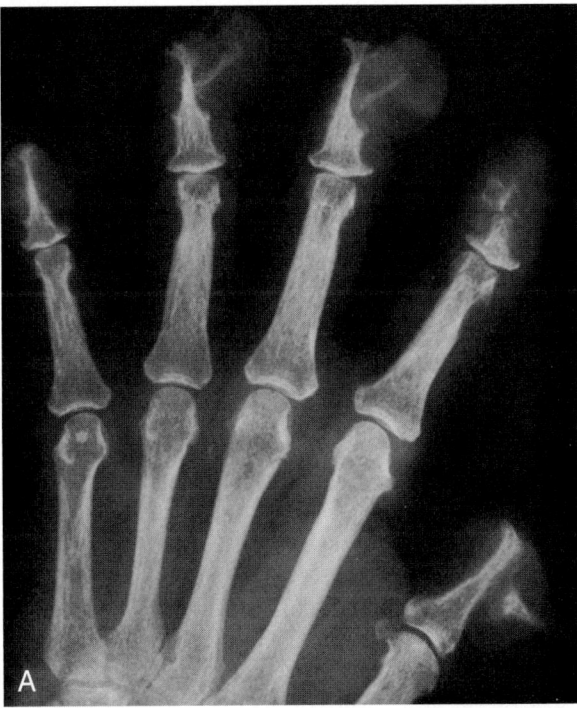
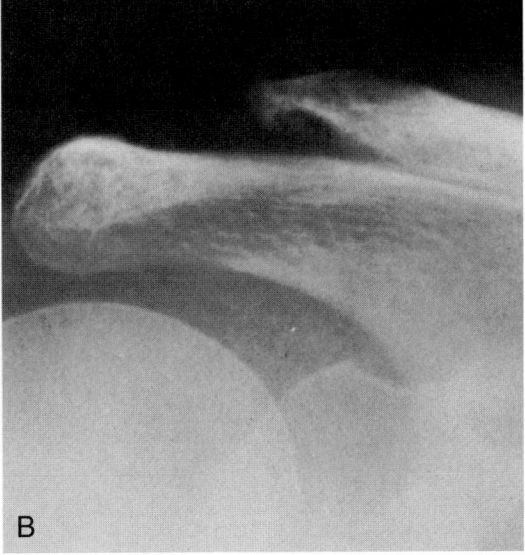

**Figure 83–9.** Osteolysis with detritic synovitis. This 71-year-old woman developed a severely destructive and mutilating arthropathy of the hands. She had no pertinent family, occupational, or traumatic history. *A,* Note almost complete resorption of all terminal phalanges, with proximal subluxation of the remaining bone, resorption along both radial and ulnar aspects of the phalanges and metacarpal bones, and articular spaces that appear unremarkable. *B,* Lysis of the distal end of the clavicle has produced a shortened and tapered osseous contour.

(From Resnick D, Weisman M, Goergen TG, Feldman PS: Osteolysis with detritic synovitis. A new syndrome. Arch Intern Med 138:1003, 1978.)

identified: osteolytic lesions leading to cortical thinning and involving increasing portions of the bone, advancing with a flame-shaped osteolytic front; multiloculated and trabeculated osteolytic lesions producing bone expansion; and marked deformity and expansion of the bone, with or without pathologic fractures (Fig. 83–10).

## Differential Diagnosis

The major radiographic characteristic of the various forms of idiopathic multicentric osteolysis is the striking resorption of bone that predominates in the carpal and tarsal areas (and occasionally in the elbows). This distribution differs from that typically associated with other varieties of osteolysis, such as occupational acro-osteolysis (phalanges), post-traumatic osteolysis (distal end of the clavicle, pubic and ischial rami, femoral neck, ulna, radius), acro-osteolysis syndrome of Hajdu and Cheney (phalanges), massive osteolysis of Gorham (variable distribution, with a predilection for pelvic and shoulder girdles), multicentric reticulohistiocytosis

(hands, feet, wrists, ankles), acro-osteolysis syndrome of Joseph or of Shinz (phalanges), and neurogenic acro-osteolysis (phalanges).

## CHONDROLYSIS

Cartilage loss or destruction is an important complication of many articular disorders, including rheumatoid arthritis, seronegative spondyloarthropathies, septic arthritis, degenerative joint disease, and relapsing polychondritis. In addition, cartilage atrophy can appear after disuse, immobilization, or paralysis, perhaps related to interruption of the normal patterns of chondral nutrition. Finally, chondrolysis may appear as a complication of a slipped capital femoral epiphysis or on an idiopathic basis.

### Chondrolysis Occurring after Slipped Capital Femoral Epiphysis

Chondrolysis is a well-recognized and important complication of slippage of the capital femoral epiphysis, with a reported frequency that varies from approximately 1% to 40%. A high rate of occurrence is recorded among black, Hawaiian, and Hispanic patients. Both men and women are affected, but the frequency of chondrolysis in women is relatively high in view of the male predominance in cases of uncomplicated slipped epiphysis. Chondrolysis may be more common among patients treated with long-term immobilization or by surgical procedures other than in situ fixations. A greater frequency of chondrolysis has also been recorded among patients whose symptoms were of longer duration at the time of treatment of the slipped capital femoral epiphysis, as well as among those in whom the pins used to treat the slipped epiphysis penetrated the femoral head.

Clinical manifestations of chondrolysis usually appear within 1 year after the epiphyseal separation and occasionally occur simultaneously with the slippage. Pain, tenderness, limitation of motion, and flexion contracture are noted. These findings may not allow a precise or early diagnosis, because similar manifestations can accompany the slippage itself. In addition, the severity of the clinical abnormalities is extremely variable, and other complications of epiphyseal slippage can produce almost identical clinical alterations, underscoring the importance of correct interpretation of the radiographic findings.

There are three main radiographic features of chondrolysis (Fig. 83–11). Initially, periarticular osteoporosis appears and may persist for a variable period, probably reflecting the increased vascularity of the subchondral osseous tissue. The second finding is rapid narrowing of the joint space, which typically affects the entire articulation or is isolated to the superior aspect of the joint. Superior joint space diminution is especially common when osteonecrosis is also present (7% to 25% of cases) or when osteotomies have been used to treat the epiphyseal slippage. Third, thinning and disappearance of the subchondral bone plate, osseous erosion, and osseous flattening can be seen, particularly at sites of chondral

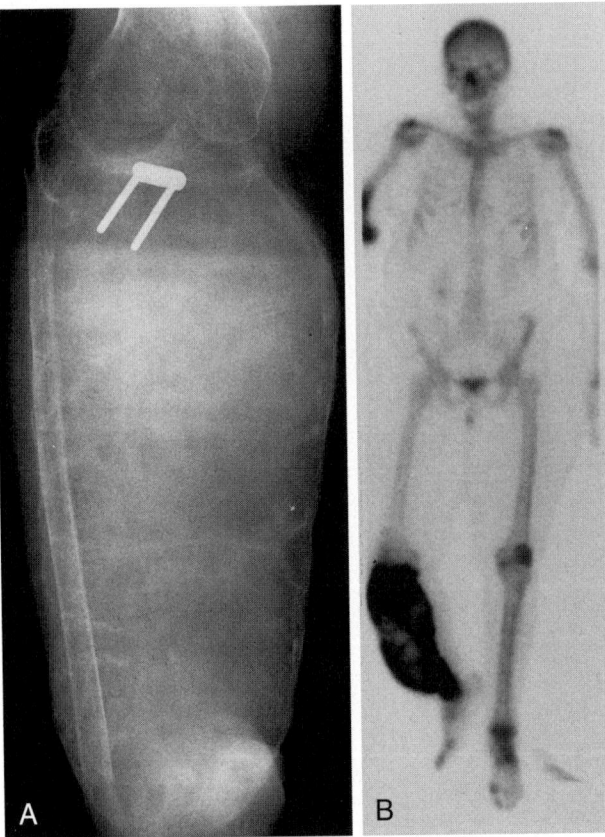

**Figure 83–10.** Familial expansile osteolysis in a 45-year-old woman with "familial Paget's disease." *A*, Frontal radiograph of the lower leg shows bizarre expansion of the tibia. The bone appears to have disappeared. *B*, Bone scan reveals extensive accumulation of radionuclide in the expanded tibia. The right humerus is also affected. (Courtesy of J. Jacobson, MD, Ann Arbor, Mich.)

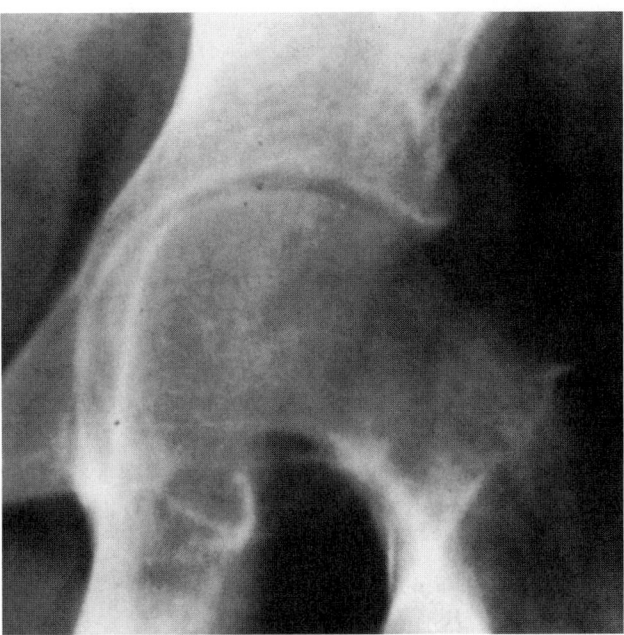

**Figure 83–11.** Chondrolysis after slipped capital femoral epiphysis. Note osteoporosis, concentric joint space narrowing, protrusio acetabuli deformity, and abnormal alignment of the femoral head and femoral neck.

destruction, about the fovea, and on both femoral and acetabular surfaces. Acetabular protrusion (which is usually mild), subchondral cysts (which are usually small or medium-size), and premature fusion of adjacent growth plates may be apparent.

The radiographic findings appear in a relatively short time and can stabilize, followed by changes of cartilaginous and osseous repair characterized by partial or complete "recovery" of the articular space, bony eburnation or sclerosis, and osteophytosis. In other cases, especially in the presence of osteonecrosis, progressive deterioration of the joint is seen. Intra-articular bone fusion may be noted.

The differential diagnosis of the radiographic features of chondrolysis accompanying slipped capital femoral epiphysis varies with the stage of the process. Initially, the osteoporosis observed in chondrolysis mimics that seen in various inflammatory synovial disorders and in regional forms of osteoporosis. In the later stages of chondrolysis, loss of the articular space and subchondral osseous thinning and erosion simulate the changes seen in infection, rheumatoid arthritis, and other inflammatory disorders, but they differ from the typical findings of reflex sympathetic dystrophy, regional migratory osteoporosis, and transient osteoporosis of the hip. In advanced stages of chondrolysis, the differential diagnosis includes other disorders such as pigmented villonodular synovitis and

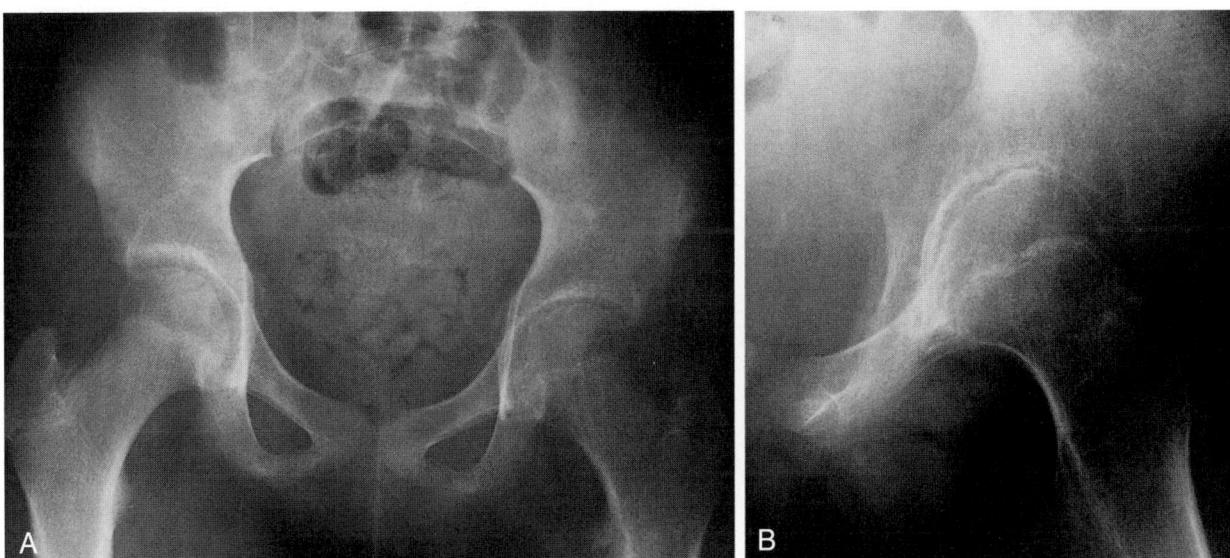

**Figure 83–12.** Idiopathic chondrolysis of the hip. This 10-year-old black girl presented with a 4-month history of pain in the left hip, which appeared suddenly while she was running. *A*, Radiograph demonstrates osteoporosis and diffuse joint space narrowing in the left hip. Conventional tomography confirmed the presence of these findings and revealed focal irregularity within the subchondral cortex of the capital femoral epiphysis. Aspiration arthrography demonstrated decreased thickness of the cartilage of both the acetabulum and the femoral head. Cultures of the joint fluid were sterile. The diagnosis at the time of this initial admission was synovitis of unknown cause. The patient was treated with restriction of weight bearing and aspirin. *B*, Three months later, the patient was readmitted for evaluation of progressive loss of motion of the left hip. Radiograph at this time demonstrates a joint contracture with the hip held in external rotation. Progressive cartilage loss has occurred, and diffuse osteoporosis persists. The findings are those of idiopathic chondrolysis of the hip. (Courtesy of G. Greenway, MD, Dallas, Tex.)

idiopathic synovial (osteo)chondromatosis. At all stages, the history and the clinical and radiographic manifestations of a slipped capital femoral epiphysis should serve as important indicators of the possible presence of chondrolysis.

## Idiopathic Chondrolysis of the Hip

Chondrolysis is also known to occur in the hip joint in adolescent girls, particularly blacks, who do not have a slipped capital femoral epiphysis. It is also occasionally seen in men, Hispanics, other whites, and Native Americans and in persons older than 20 years. Idiopathic chondrolysis of the hip is a monoarticular disease. Typical clinical findings include pain, stiffness, restriction of motion, and absence of a history of trauma. Radiographs outline periarticular osteoporosis, joint space narrowing that is usually diffuse or maximal on the weight-bearing surface, and irregularity and erosion of the subchondral bone (Fig. 83–12). In addition, slight enlargement and alteration in shape of the femoral head, increased width and periosteal bone formation of the femoral neck, narrowing of the growth plate, and mild protrusio acetabuli may be evident. The last-mentioned feature is reminiscent of that seen in primary protrusio acetabuli (Otto pelvis); differentiating between the two conditions may be difficult, and some regard them as manifestations of a single disorder. Joint aspiration usually confirms the absence of an effusion or of organisms, and arthrography may demonstrate the irregularity and narrowing of the chondral surface (Fig. 83–13). Later stages of the process may be associated with obliteration of the articular space, cysts, osteophytes, and deformity.

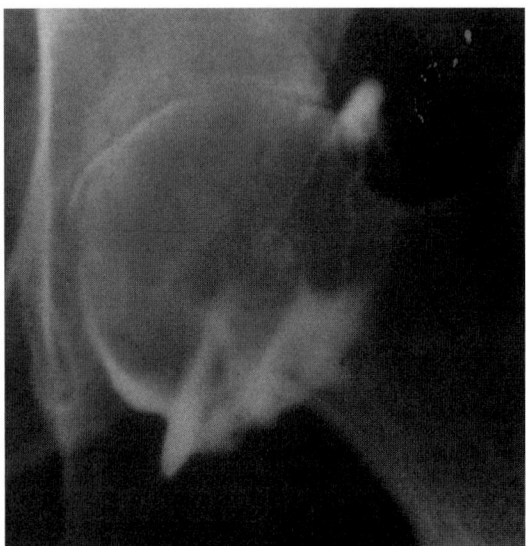

**Figure 83–13.** Idiopathic chondrolysis of the hip. In this teenage girl with clinical and radiographic manifestations of idiopathic chondrolysis, hip arthrography reveals diffuse loss of acetabular and femoral cartilage.

## FURTHER READING

Boles CA, El-Khoury GY: Slipped capital femoral epiphysis. Radiographics 17:809, 1997.

Branch HE: Acute spontaneous absorption of bone: Report of a case involving a clavicle and a scapula. J Bone Joint Surg 27:706, 1945.

Chung C, Yu J, Resnick D, et al: Gorham syndrome of the thorax and cervical spine: CT and MRI findings. Skeletal Radiol 26:55, 1997.

de la Puente R, Boutin RD, Theodorou DJ, et al: Post-traumatic and stress-induced osteolysis of the distal clavicle: MR imaging findings in 17 patients. Skeletal Radiol 28:202, 1999.

Dodson VN, Dinman BD, Whitehouse WM, et al: Occupational acroosteolysis. III. A clinical study. Arch Environ Health 22:83, 1971.

Downing ND, Garnavos C, Lunn PG: Idiopathic multicentric osteolysis principally affecting the phalanges of the hands and feet. J Hand Surg [Br] 21:656, 1996.

Gama C, Meira JB: Occupational acro-osteolysis. J Bone Joint Surg Am 60:86, 1975.

Garcia ADC, Fernandez PL, Gonzalez MP, et al: Idiopathic chondrolysis of the hip: Long-term evolution. J Pediatr Orthop 19:449, 1999.

Gilula LA, Bliznak J, Staple TW: Idiopathic nonfamilial acro-osteolysis with cortical defects and mandibular ramus osteolysis. Radiology 121:63, 1976.

Goergen TG, Resnick D, Riley RR: Post-traumatic abnormalities of the pubic bone simulating malignancy. Radiology 126:85, 1978.

Hall FM: Post-traumatic pubic osteolysis simulating malignancy. J Bone Joint Surg Am 66:975, 1984.

Hardegger F, Simpson LA, Segmueller G: The syndrome of idiopathic osteolysis: Classification, review, and case report. J Bone Joint Surg Br 67:89, 1985.

Harris DK, Adams WG: Acro-osteolysis occurring in men engaged in the polymerization of vinyl chloride. BMJ 3:712, 1967.

Hawkins BJ, Covey DC, Thiel BG: Distal clavicle osteolysis unrelated to trauma, overuse, or metabolic disease. Clin Orthop 370:208, 2000.

Kaplan PA, Resnick D: Stress-induced osteolysis of the clavicle. Radiology 158:139, 1986.

Levine AH, Pais MJ, Schwartz EE: Posttraumatic osteolysis of the distal clavicle with emphasis on early radiologic changes. AJR Am J Roentgenol 127:781, 1976.

Moller G, Priemel M, Amling M, et al: The Gorham-Stout syndrome (Gorham's massive osteolysis). J Bone Joint Surg Br 81:501, 1999.

Murphy OB, Bellamy R, Wheeler W, et al: Post-traumatic osteolysis of the distal clavicle. Clin Orthop 109:108, 1975.

Schulze R, Gulbin O: Beitrag zum Problem der Akroosteolyse (gleichzeitig ein Beitrag zur Kenntner der Patella profunda). Rofo 109:209, 1968.

Shaw DG: Acro-osteolysis and bone fragility. Br J Radiol 42:934, 1969.

Simpson BS: An unusual case of post-traumatic decalcification of the bones of the foot. J Bone Joint Surg 19:223, 1937.

Spieth ME, Greenspan A, Forrester D, et al: Gorham's disease of the radius: Radiographic, scintigraphic, and MRI findings with pathologic correlation. A case report and review of the literature. Skeletal Radiol 26:659, 1997.

# Index